OTHER PMIC TITLES OF INTEREST

CODING AND REIMBURSEMENT TITLES
Collections Made Easy!
CPT Coders Choice®, Thumb Indexed
CPT & HCPCS Coding Made Easy!
CPT Easy Links
CPT Plus!
DRG Plus!
E/M Coding Made Easy!
Getting Paid for What You Do
HCPCS Coders Choice®, Color Coded, Thumb Indexed
Health Insurance Carrier Directory
HIPAA Compliance Manual
ICD-9-CM, Coders Choice®, Thumb Indexed
ICD-9-CM Coding for Physicians' Offices
ICD-9-CM Coding Made Easy!
ICD-9-CM, Home Health Edition
Medical Fees in the United States
Medicare Compliance Manual
Medicare Rules & Regulations
Physicians Fee Guide
Reimbursement Manual for the Medical Office

PRACTICE MANAGEMENT TITLES
Accounts Receivable Management for the Medical Practice
Achieving Profitability With a Medical Office System
Encyclopedia of Practice and Financial Management
Managed Care Organizations
Managing Medical Office Personnel
Marketing Strategies for Physicians
Medical Marketing Handbook
Medical Office Policy Manual
Medical Practice Forms
Medical Practice Handbook
Medical Staff Privileges
Negotiating Managed Care Contracts
Patient Satisfaction
Performance Standards for the Laboratory
Professional and Practice Development
Promoting Your Medical Practice
Starting in Medical Practice
Working With Insurance and Managed Care Plans

**AVAILABLE FROM YOUR LOCAL MEDICAL
BOOK STORE OR CALL 1-800-MED-SHOP**

OTHER PMIC TITLES OF INTEREST

RISK MANAGEMENT TITLES
Malpractice Depositions
Medical Risk Management
Preparing for Your Deposition
Preventing Emergency Malpractice
Testifying in Court

FINANCIAL MANAGEMENT TITLES
A Physician's Guide to Financial Independence
Business Ventures for Physicians
Financial Valuation of Your Practice
Personal Money Management for Physicians
Personal Pension Plan Strategies for Physicians
Securing Your Assets

DICTIONARIES AND OTHER REFERENCE TITLES
Drugs of Abuse
Health and Medicine on the Internet
Medical Acronyms and Abbreviations
Medical Phrase Index
Medical Word Building
Medico Mnemonica
Medico-Legal Glossary
Spanish/English Handbook for Medical Professionals

MEDICAL REFERENCE AND CLINICAL TITLES
Advance Medical Directives
Clinical Research Opportunities
Gastroenterology: Problems in Primary Care
Manual of IV Therapy
Medical Care of the Adolescent Athlete
Medical Procedures for Referral
Neurology: Problems in Primary Care
Orthopaedics: Problems in Primary Care
Patient Care Emergency Handbook
Patient Care Flowchart Manual
Patient Care Procedures for Your Practice
Physician's Office Laboratory
Pulmonary Medicine: Problems in Primary Care
Questions and Answers on AIDS

ICD·9·CM

International Classification of Diseases
9th Revision

Clinical Modification
Sixth Edition

Color Coded

2012

Volumes 1 & 2 : Office Edition

ISBN 978-1-936977-04-8   (Coder's Choice® Soft cover)
ISBN 978-1-936977-05-5   (Spiral)
ISBN 978-1-57066-697-1   (e-book)

Volumes 1, 2, & 3 : Hospital Edition

ISBN 978-1-936977-01-7   (Coder's Choice® Soft cover)
ISBN 978-1-936977-02-4   (Spiral)
ISBN 978-1-57066-698-8   (e-book)

Volumes 1, 2, & 3 : Home Health Edition

ISBN 978-1-936977-00-0   (Coder's Choice® Soft cover)
ISBN 978-1-57066-699-5   (e-book)

Practice Management Information Corporation [PMIC]
4727 Wilshire Boulevard, Suite 300
Los Angeles, California 90010
1-800-MED-SHOP
http://www.pmiconline.com

Printed in China

Preface

Health care professionals have long used coding systems to describe procedures, services, and supplies. However, most described the reason for the procedure, service or supply with a diagnostic statement. Of those health care professionals who do code the diagnosis, either due to a requirement for a computer billing system and/or electronic claims filing, many do not code completely or accurately. With the passage of the Medicare Catastrophic Coverage Act of 1988, diagnostic coding using *ICD-9-CM* became mandatory for Medicare claims. In the area of health care reimbursement rules and regulations, the typical progression is that changes required for Medicare are followed shortly by similar changes for Medicaid and private insurance carriers.

To some professionals, the requirement to use diagnostic coding may have seemed like a burden or simply another excuse for Medicare intermediaries to delay or deny payment. However, it is important to understand that the proper use of coding systems for both procedures and diagnoses gives the professional absolute control over his or her billing and reimbursement. Accurate diagnosis coding is not easy. It requires a good working knowledge of medical terminology and a fundamental understanding of *ICD-9-CM*. In addition, the coder must know the rules and regulations required to comply with Medicare requirements for coding.

This edition of the *International Classification of Diseases, 9th Revision, Clinical Modification (ICD-9-CM)* is published by Practice Management Information Corporation in recognition of its responsibility to promulgate this classification throughout the United States for morbidity coding and billing purposes. *The International Classification of Diseases, 9th Revision*, originally published by the World Health Organization (WHO) is the foundation of the *ICD-9-CM* and continues to be the classification employed in cause-of-death coding in the United States.

The *ICD-9-CM* is recommended for use in all clinical settings, but is required for reporting diagnoses and diseases to all U.S. Public Health Service and Department of Health and Human Services programs, such as Medicare and Medicaid. This version faithfully follows and contains the same information found in the official U.S. government version of the *ICD-9-CM*.

All official authorized addenda effective October 1, 2011, have been included in this edition. A new revision will be available approximately September 15th of each year. Revised editions may be purchased from:

Practice Management Information Corporation
4727 Wilshire Boulevard, Suite 300
Los Angeles, California 90010
1-800-MED-SHOP

Or by contacting our web site at http://www.pmionline.com.

Disclaimer

This publication includes all official ICD-9-CM codes, descriptions, annotations and guidelines as maintained by the U.S. Department of Health and Human Services with the exception that this publication includes special symbols to indicate additions and revisions from the previous edition and special symbols to facilitate identification of diagnostic codes that require 4th or 5th digit specificity, the use of color coding to alert the user to special coding considerations, and thumb indexing to make locating codes easier. This publication is revised annually so that we may present the most current information possible. Though all of the information is carefully researched and checked for accuracy and completeness, the publisher accepts no responsibility with regard to errors, omissions, misuse or misinterpretation.

Table of Contents

PREFACE iii
DISCLAIMER iv
INTRODUCTION 1
  Historical Perspective 1
    ICD-9-CM Background 2
    Use of ICD-9-CM Codes for Professional Billing 2
  Terminology 3
  Format of ICD-9-CM 5
    The Tabular List (Volume 1) 5
      Classification of Diseases and Injuries 5
      Supplementary Classifications 6
      Appendices 6
      Specifications for the Tabular List 6
    The Alphabetic Index (Volume 2) 7
      Supplementary Sections 8
      Special Tables 8
      Specifications for the Alphabetic Index 8
    Procedures: Tabular List and Alphabetic Index (Volume 3) 8
      Tabular List of Procedures 8
      Alphabetic Index to Procedures 9
      Specifications for the Procedure Classification 9
  Conventions Used in the Tabular List 9
    Abbreviations 9
    Punctuation 10
    Symbols 10
    Other Conventions 10
    Instructional Notations 11
    Related Terms 11
  Color Coding 12
    Volume 1 12
    Volume 3 12
ICD-9-CM OFFICIAL GUIDELINES FOR CODING & REPORTING . . . 13
  Conventions, General Coding Guidelines and Chapter Specific Guidelines . . 14
    Conventions for ICD-9-CM 14
    General Coding Guidelines 16
    Chapter Specific Coding Guidelines 20
  Selection of Principal Diagnosis 83
  Reporting Additional Diagnoses 85
  Diagnostic Coding and Reporting Guidelines for Outpatient Services 86
  Present on Admission (POA) Reporting Guidelines 90
  ICD-10 99
  Where to Get Answers About ICD-9-CM 100

TABLE OF CONTENTS

ANATOMICAL ILLUSTRATIONS 101

DISEASES: TABULAR LIST VOLUME 1 151

   1. Infectious and Parasitic Diseases 153
   2. Neoplasms 207
   3. Endocrine, Nutritional, and Metabolic Diseases,
      and Immunity Disorders 255
   4. Diseases of the Blood and Blood-Forming Organs 281
   5. Mental, Behavioral and Neurodevelopmental Disorders 297
   6. Diseases of the Nervous System and Sense Organs 325
   7. Diseases of the Circulatory System 391
   8. Diseases of the Respiratory System 427
   9. Diseases of the Digestive System 451
  10. Diseases of the Genitourinary System 487
  11. Complications of Pregnancy, Childbirth, and the Puerperium 517
  12. Diseases of the Skin and Subcutaneous Tissue 545
  13. Diseases of the Musculoskeletal System and Connective Tissue 563
  14. Congenital Anomalies 591
  15. Certain Conditions Originating in the Perinatal Period 619
  16. Symptoms, Signs, and Ill-Defined Conditions 637
  17. Injury and Poisoning 663

SUPPLEMENTARY CLASSIFICATIONS

   V CODES: Classification of Factors Influencing Health Status and
      Contact With Health Services 751
   E CODES: Classification of External Causes of Injury and Poisoning 801

APPENDICES

   A. Morphology of Neoplasms 871
   B. Glossary of Mental Disorders (Removed from FY2005 ICD-9-CM) . . 885
   C. Classification of Drugs by American Hospital Formulary Service List
      Number and Their ICD-9-CM Equivalents 887
   D. Classification of Industrial Accidents According to Agency 893
   E. List of Three-Digit Categories 897

DISEASES: ALPHABETIC INDEX VOLUME 2 921

   Hypertension Chart 1254
   Neoplasm Chart 1358
   Table of Drugs and Chemicals 1599
   Index to External Causes 1681

SUMMARY OF ADDITIONS, DELETIONS, REVISIONS, VOL. 1 1727

PROCEDURES: TABULAR LIST VOLUME 3 [1] 1735

   1. Operations on the Nervous System (01-05) 1737
   2. Operations on the Endocrine System (06-07) 1755
   3. Operations on the Eye (08-16) 1759
  3A. Other Miscellaneous Diagnostic and Therapeutic Procedures (17) . . . 1769
   4. Operations on the Ear (18-20) 1773
   5. Operations on the Nose, Mouth and Pharynx (21-29) 1777
   6. Operations on the Respiratory System (30-34) 1787
   7. Operations on the Cardiovascular System (35-39) 1795
   8. Operations on the Hemic and Lymphatic Systems (40-41) 1821

TABLE OF CONTENTS

9. Operations on the Digestive System (42-54) 1825

10. Operations on the Urinary System (55-59) 1851

11. Operations on the Male Genital Organs (60-64) 1861

12. Operations on the Female Genital Organs (65-71) 1867

13. Obstetrical Procedures (72-75) 1879

14. Operations on the Musculoskeletal System (76-84) 1883

15. Operations on the Integumentary System (85-86) 1905

16. Miscellaneous Diagnostic and Therapeutic Procedures (87-99) 1912

PROCEDURES: ALPHABETIC INDEX VOLUME 3 [1] 1943

SUMMARY OF ADDITIONS, DELETIONS, REVISIONS, VOL. 3 [1]. . 2117

[1] These listings appear only in the three volume edition

TABLE OF CONTENTS

Introduction to ICD-9-CM

ICD-9-CM is an acronym for *International Classification of Diseases, 9th Revision, Clinical Modification*, published under different names since 1900. *ICD-9-CM* is a statistical classification system that arranges diseases and injuries into groups according to established criteria. Most *ICD-9-CM* codes are numeric and consist of three, four or five numbers and a description. The codes are revised approximately every 10 years by the World Health Organization and annual updates are published by Center for Medicare and Medicaid Services (CMS).

HISTORICAL PERSPECTIVE

The *International Classification of Diseases, 9th Revision, Clinical Modification (ICD-9-CM)* is based on the official version of the *World Health Organization's (WHO) 9th Revision, International Classification of Diseases (ICD-9)*. *ICD-9* is designed for the classification of morbidity and mortality information for statistical purposes, and for the indexing of medical records by disease and operations, and for data storage and retrieval. *ICD-9-CM* replaced the Eighth Revision International Classification of Diseases, Adapted for Use in the United States commonly referred to as *ICDA*.

The concept of extending the International Classification of Diseases for use in hospital indexing was originally developed in response to a need for a more efficient basis for storage and retrieval of diagnostic data. In 1950, the U.S. Public Health Service and the Veterans Administration began independent tests of the International Classification of Diseases for hospital indexing purposes. In the following year, the Columbia Presbyterian Medical Center in New York City adopted the International Classification of Diseases, 6th Revision for use in its medical record department. A few years later, the Commission on Professional and Hospital Activities adopted the International Classification of Diseases for use in hospitals participating in the Professional Activity Study (PAS).

In view of the growing interest in the use of the International Classification of Diseases for hospital indexing, a study was undertaken in 1956 by the American Medical Association and the American Medical Record Association of the relative efficiencies of coding systems for diagnostic indexing. Following this study, the major uses of the International Classification of Diseases for hospital indexing purposes consolidated their experiences and an adaptation was published in December 1959. A revision containing the first "Classification of Operations and Treatments" was published in 1962.

In 1968, following a study by the American Hospital Association, the United States Public Health Service published the Eighth Revision International Classification of Diseases, Adapted for Use in the United States. This publication became commonly known as ICDA, and served as the basis for coding diagnostic data for official morbidity and mortality statistics in the United States.

ICD-9-CM Background

In February 1977, a committee was convened by the National Center for Health Statistics to provide advice and counsel for the development of clinical modification of the ICD-9. The organizations represented on the committee included:

American Association of Health Data Systems
American Hospital Association
American Medical Record Association
Association for Health Records
Commission on Professional and Hospital Activities
Council on Clinical Classifications, sponsored by:

American Academy of Pediatrics
American College of Obstetricians and Gynecologists
American College of Physicians
American College of Surgeons
American Psychiatric Association

Health Care Financing Administration
WHO Center for Classification of Diseases

The resulting *ICD-9-CM* is a clinical modification of the *World Health Organization's International Classification of Diseases, 9th Revision (ICD-9)*. The term "clinical" is used to emphasize the modifications intent; namely, to serve as a useful tool in the area of classification of morbidity data for indexing of medical records, medical care review, ambulatory and other medical care programs, as well as for basic health statistics.

In use since January 1979, *ICD-9-CM* provides a diagnostic coding system that is more precise than those needed only for statistical groupings and trend analysis. Official addenda (updates) to *ICD-9-CM* are issued in October each year by the National Center for Health Statistics (NCHS), part of the Centers for Disease Control (CDC).

Use of ICD-9-CM Codes for Professional Billing

Until passage of the Medicare Catastrophic Coverage Act of 1988, health care professionals were not required to report *ICD-9-CM* codes when billing government or private insurance carriers for reimbursement. The exception to this requirement was for those health care professionals who filed insurance claims electronically and those who used "code driven" computer billing services or computer systems.

Most health care professionals simply included the text or description of the injury, illness, sign or symptom that was the reason for the encounter. Insurance carriers who used *ICD-9-CM* coding had to code the diagnostic statements prior to input into their computer systems for reimbursement processing.

A specific requirement of the Medicare Catastrophic Coverage Act of 1988 required health care professionals to include *ICD-9-CM* codes on their Medicare claim forms effective April 1, 1989. After a two-month grace period, the requirement was officially implemented on June 1, 1989. The Medicare Catastrophic Coverage Act was repealed in November, 1989; however the ICD-9-CM coding requirement was continued.

TERMINOLOGY

There are terms used throughout this publication that are important for a proper understanding of *ICD-9-CM*. The following terms are defined specifically as they are used for *ICD-9-CM* with the knowledge that some terms may have other definitions and meanings.

acute
refers to the condition that is the primary reason for the current encounter.

addenda
official updates to ICD-9-CM published continuously since 1986, that become effective on October 1st of each year.

adverse
any response to a drug that is noxious and unintended and occurs with proper dosage.

aftercare
an encounter for something planned in advance, for example, cast removal.

AHFS
American Hospital Formulary Service.

alphabetic index
the portion of ICD-9-CM that lists definitions and codes in alphabetic order. Also called Volume 2.

category
refers to diagnoses codes listed within a specific three-digit category, for example category 250, Diabetes Mellitus.

cause
that which brings about any condition or produces any effect.

chronic
continuing over a long period of time or recurring frequently.

coding
the process of transferring written or verbal descriptions of diseases, injuries and procedures into numerical designations.

combination
a code that combines a diagnosis with an associated secondary process or complication.

complication
the occurrence of two or more diseases in the same patient at the same time.

concurrent
when a patient is being treated by more than one provider for different care conditions at the same time.

conventions
refers to the use of certain abbreviations, punctuation, symbols, type faces, and other instructions that must be clearly understood in order to use ICD-9-CM.

CPT
Current Procedural Terminology. Listing of codes and descriptions for procedures, services and supplies published by the American Medical Association. Used to bill insurance carriers.

diagnosis
a written description of the reason(s) for the procedure, service, supply or encounter.

down coding
the process where insurance carriers reduce the value of a procedure, and the resulting reimbursement, due to either 1) a mismatch of CPT code and description or 2) ICD-9-CM code does not justify the procedure or level of service.

E codes
specific ICD-9-CM codes used to identify the cause of injury, poisoning and other adverse effects.

eponyms
medical procedures or conditions named after a person or a place.

etiology
the cause(s) or origin of a disease.

HCFA1500	Uniform health insurance claim form used for billing services to Medicare and other insurance carriers.
hierarchy	a system that ranks items one above another.
ICD-9-CM	International Classification of Diseases, 9th Revision, Clinical Modification.
ICD-10	International Classification of Diseases, 10th Revision
late effect	a residual effect (condition produced) after the acute phase of an illness or injury has ended.
main term	refers to listings in the Alphabetic Index appearing **BOLDFACE** type.
manifestation	characteristic signs or symptoms of an illness.
multiple	refers to the need to use more than one ICD-9-CM code to fully identify coding a condition.
primary code	the ICD-9-CM code that defines the main reason for the current encounter.
residual	the long-term condition(s) resulting from a previous acute illness or injury.
rule out	refers to a method used to indicate that a condition is probable, suspected, or questionable but unconfirmed. ICD-9-CM has no provisions for the use of this term.
secondary	code(s) listed after the primary code that further indicate the cause(s) code for the current encounter or define the need for higher levels of care.
sections	refers to portions of the Tabular List that are organized in groups of three-digit code numbers. For example, Malignant Neoplasm of Lip, Oral Cavity and Pharynx (140-149).
sequencing	the process of listing ICD-9-CM codes in the proper order.
specificity	refers to the requirement to code to the highest number of digits possible, 3, 4 or 5, when choosing an ICD-9-CM code.
sub term	refers to listings appearing in the Alphabetic Index under MAIN TERMS and always indented two spaces to the right.
subcategories	refers to groupings of four-digit codes listed under three-digit categories.
Tabular List	the portion of ICD-9-CM that lists codes and definitions in numeric order. Also referred to as Volume 1.
V codes	specific ICD-9-CM codes used to identify encounters for reasons other than illness or injury, for example, immunization.
Volume 1	see TABULAR LIST
Volume 2	see ALPHABETIC INDEX
Volume 3	procedure codes used only for hospital coding. Volume 3 contains both a numeric listing and an alphabetic index.

FORMAT OF ICD-9-CM

The *International Classification of Diseases, 9th Revision, Clinical Modification* was originally published as a three volume set (2nd edition). Newer versions of *ICD-9-CM* are available as two separate books containing Volume 1 and Volume 2 in one book and Volumes 1, 2 and 3 in the other. It is also now available on CD-ROM from the U.S. Government.

This edition of *ICD-9-CM* includes all official addenda from October 1986 through October 2010.

The Tabular List (Volume 1)

The Tabular List (Volume 1) is a *numeric* listing of diagnosis codes and descriptions consisting of 17 chapters that classify diseases and injuries, two sections containing supplementary codes (V codes and E codes) and four appendices.

Classification of Diseases and Injuries

The Classification of Diseases and Injuries includes the following 17 chapters:

Chapter 1   Infectious and Parasitic Diseases (001-139)

Chapter 2   Neoplasms (140-239)

Chapter 3   Endocrine, Nutritional and Metabolic Diseases, and Immunity Disorders (240-279)

Chapter 4   Diseases of the Blood and Blood-Forming Organs (280-289)

Chapter 5   Mental, Behavioral and Neurodevelopmental Disorders (290-319)

Chapter 6   Diseases of the Nervous System and Sense Organs (320-389)

Chapter 7   Diseases of the Circulatory System (390-459)

Chapter 8   Diseases of the Respiratory System (460-519)

Chapter 9   Diseases of the Digestive System (520-579)

Chapter 10   Diseases of the Genitourinary System (580-629)

Chapter 11   Complications of Pregnancy, Childbirth, and the Puerperium (630-677)

Chapter 12   Diseases of the Skin and Subcutaneous Tissue (680-709)

Chapter 13   Diseases of the Musculoskeletal System and Connective Tissue (710-739)

Chapter 14   Congenital Anomalies (740-759)

Chapter 15   Certain Conditions Originating in the Perinatal Period (760-779)

Chapter 16   Symptoms, Signs and Ill-defined Conditions (780-799)

Chapter 17   Injury and Poisoning (800-999)

Each chapter of the Tabular List (Volume 1) is structured into four components, namely:

Sections: groups of three-digit code numbers

Categories: three-digit code numbers

Subcategories: four-digit code numbers

Fifth-Digit Subclassifications: five-digit code numbers

Supplementary Classifications

There are two supplementary classifications included in the Tabular List (Volume 1). These are:

V Codes   Supplementary Classification of Factors Influencing Health Status and Contact with Health Services (V01-V91)

E Codes   Supplementary Classification of External Causes of Injury and Poisoning (E000-E999)

Appendices

The Tabular List (Volume 1) includes four appendices. These are:

Appendix A   Morphology of Neoplasms

Appendix C   Classification of Drugs by American Hospital Formulary Service List Number and Their ICD-9-CM Equivalents

Appendix D   Classification of Industrial Accidents According to Agency

Appendix E   List of Three-Digit Categories

Specifications for the Tabular List

1. Three-digit rubrics and their contents are unchanged from *ICD-9*.

2. The sequence of three-digit rubrics is unchanged from *ICD-9*.

3. Three-digit rubrics are not added to the main body of the classification.

4.   Unsubdivided three-digit rubrics are subdivided where necessary to:

    a) Add clinical detail

    b) Isolate terms for clinical accuracy

5.   The modification in *ICD-9-CM* is accomplished by the addition of a fifth digit to existing *ICD-9* rubrics, except as noted under number 7 below.

6.   Four-digit rubrics are added to subdivided three-digit codes only when there is no other means of achieving desired detail. These codes, unique to *ICD-9-CM* (28 three-digit categories) are marked with the symbol in the Tabular List.

7.   The optional dual classification in *ICD-9* is modified.

    a) Duplicate rubrics are deleted:

        1) Four-digit manifestation categories duplicating etiology entries.

        2) Manifestation inclusion terms duplicating etiology entries.

    b) Manifestations of diseases are identified, to the extent possible, by creating five digit codes in the etiology rubrics.

    c) When the manifestation of a disease cannot be included in the etiology rubrics, provision for its identification is made by retaining the *ICD-9* rubrics used for classifying manifestations of disease.

8.   The format of *ICD-9-CM* is revised from that used in *ICD-9*.

    a) American spelling of medical terms is used.

    b) Inclusion terms are indented beneath the titles of codes.

    c) Codes not to be used for primary tabulation of disease are printed in italics with the notation, "code also underlying disease."

The Alphabetic Index (Volume 2)

The Alphabetic Index (Volume 2) of *ICD-9-CM* consists of an alphabetic list of terms and codes, two supplementary Sections following the alphabetic listing, plus two special tables found within the alphabetic listing. The Alphabetic Index (Volume 2) is structured as follows:

MAIN TERMS: appear in **BOLDFACE** type

SUBTERMS: are always indented two spaces to the right under main terms

CARRY-OVER   are always indented more than two spaces from the level of
LINES: the preceding line

Supplementary Sections

The supplementary sections following the Alphabetic Index are:

TABLE OF DRUGS AND CHEMICALS

This table contains a classification of drugs and other chemical substances to identify poisoning states and external causes of adverse effects.

INDEX TO EXTERNAL CAUSES OF INJURIES & POISONINGS (E-CODES)

This section contains the index to the codes that classify environmental events, circumstances, and other conditions as the cause of injury and other adverse effects.

Special Tables

The two special tables, located within the Alphabetic Index, and found under the main terms as underlined below, are:

HYPERTENSION TABLE

NEOPLASM TABLE

Specifications for the Alphabetic Index

1. Format of the Alphabetic Index follows the format of the ICD-9.

2. Main terms in the Alphabetic Index are printed in bold face type.

3. When two codes are required to indicate etiology and manifestation, the manifestation code appears in brackets, e.g., diabetic cataract 250.5 [366.41].

Procedures: Tabular List and Alphabetic Index (Volume 3)

Volume 3 consists of two sections, a Tabular List of codes and an alphabetic index. These codes define procedures instead of diagnoses. Frequently used incorrectly by health care professionals, codes from Volume 3 are intended only for use by hospitals.

The ICD-9-CM Procedure Classification is a modification of WHO's *Fascicle V, Surgical Procedures*, and is published as Volume 3 of ICD-9-CM. It contains both a Tabular List and an Alphabetic Index. Greater detail has been added to the ICD-9-CM Procedure Classification necessitating expansion of the codes from three to four digits. Approximately 90% of the rubrics refer to surgical procedures with the remaining 10% accounting for other investigative and therapeutic procedures.

Tabular List of Procedures

The Tabular List includes 16 chapters containing codes and descriptions for surgical procedures and miscellaneous diagnostic and therapeutic procedures.

Alphabetic Index to Procedures

The Alphabetic Index provides an alphabetic index to the Tabular List of Volume 3

Specifications for the Procedure Classification

1. The ICD-9-CM Procedure Classification is published in its own volume containing both a Tabular List and an Alphabetic Index.

2. The classification is a modification of *Fascicle V Surgical Procedures* of the ICD-9 Classification of Procedures in Medicine, working from the draft dated Geneva, 30 September-6 October 1975, and labeled WHO/ICD-9/Rev. Conf. 75.4.

3. All three-digit rubrics in the range 01-86 are maintained as they appear in *Fascicle V*, whenever feasible.

4. Nonsurgical procedures are segregated from the surgical procedures and confined to the rubrics 87-99, whenever feasible.

5. Selected detail contained in the remaining fascicles of the *ICD-9 Classification of Procedures in Medicine* is accommodated where possible.

6. The structure of the classification is based on anatomy rather than surgical specialty.

7. The *ICD-9-CM* Procedure Classification is numeric only, i.e., no alphabetic characters are used.

8. The classification is based on a two-digit structure with two decimal digits where necessary.

9. Compatibility with the *ICD-9 Classification of Procedures in Medicine* was not maintained when a different axis was deemed more clinically appropriate.

CONVENTIONS USED IN THE TABULAR LIST

The *ICD-9-CM* Tabular List (Volume 1) makes use of certain abbreviations, punctuation, symbols, and other conventions that must be clearly understood. The purpose of these conventions is to first, provide special coding instructions, and second, to conserve space.

Abbreviations

NOS   Not Otherwise Specified. Equivalent to Unspecified. This abbreviation refers to a lack of sufficient detail in the statement of diagnosis to be able to assign it to a more specific sub division within the classification.

NEC   Not Elsewhere Classified. Used with ill-defined terms to alert the coder that a specified form of the condition is classified differently. The category number for the term including NEC is to be used only when the coder lacks the information necessary to code the term to a more specific category.

Punctuation

( )   PARENTHESES are used to enclose supplementary words that may be present or absent in a statement of disease without affecting the code assignment.

[ ]   SQUARE BRACKETS are used to enclose synonyms, alternate wordings or explanatory phrases.

:   COLONS are used after an incomplete phrase or term that requires one or more of the modifiers indented under it to make it assignable to a given category. EXCEPTION to this rule pertains to the abbreviation NOS.

Symbols

●   A filled BLACK CIRCLE preceding a code indicates that the code is new to this revision of ICD-9-CM. A symbol key appears on all left-hand pages of the Tabular List, Volume 1 and Volume 3.

▲   A filled BLACK TRIANGLE preceding a code indicates that there is a revision to the text of an existing code. A symbol key appears on all left-hand pages of the Tabular List, Volume 1 and Volume 3.

④ ⑤   A circle containing the number 4 or the number 5 preceding a code indicates that a fourth or fifth digit is required for coding to the highest level of specificity. Valid digits are in [brackets] under each code if the fourth- and fifth-digit codes themselves are not listed. Definitions of valid fifth digits are found under the major category.

Other conventions

Type Face:

BOLD: Bold type face is used for all codes and titles in the Tabular List.

Italics: Italicized type face is used for all exclusion notes and to identify those rubrics that are not to be used for primary tabulations of disease.

Format: ICD-9-CM uses an indented format for ease in reference.

ALERT!   References alternate codes for personal history/late effects or other coding alerts.

DEFINITION   Definition of a common word or phrase.

Instructional Notations

Instructional terms define what is, or what is not, included in a given subdivision. This is accomplished by using both inclusion and exclusion terms.

INCLUDES: Indicates separate terms, such as, modifying adjectives, sites and conditions, entered under a subdivision, such as a category, to further define or give examples of, the content of the category.

Excludes: Exclusion terms are enclosed in a box and are printed in italics to draw attention to their presence. The importance of this instructional term is its use as a guideline to direct the coder to the proper code assignment. In other words, all terms following the word EXCLUDES: are to be coded elsewhere as indicated in each instance.

NOTES These are used to define terms and give coding instructions. Often used to list the fifth-digit subclassifications for certain categories.

SEE The "see" instruction following a main term in the index indicates that another term should be referenced. It is necessary to go to the main term referenced with the "see" note to locate the correct code.

SEE CATEGORY A variation of the instructional term SEE. This refers the coder to a specific category. You must *always* follow this instructional term.

SEE ALSO A "see also" instruction following a main term in the index instructs that there is another main term that may also be referenced that may provide additional index entries that may be useful. It is not necessary to follow the "see also" note when the original main term provides the necessary code.

CODE FIRST This instructional note is used for those codes not intended to be used as a principal diagnosis, or not to be sequenced before the underlying disease. The note requires that the underlying disease (etiology) be coded first with the code the note is applied to being coded second. This note appears only in the Tabular List (Vol. 1).

USE ADDITIONAL CODE This instruction is placed in the Tabular List in those categories where the coder may wish to add further information, by using an additional code, to give a more complete picture of the diagnosis or procedure.

Related terms

AND The word "and" should be interpreted to mean either "and" or "or" when it appears in a title.

WITH The word "with" in the alphabetic index is sequenced immediately following the main term, not in alphabetical order.

COLOR CODING

A PMIC versions of ICD-9-CM include color-coding to alert the user to special coding situations or conditions that require additional attention. The use of color-coding is found in the Tabular List of Volume 1 and the Tabular List of Volume 3. The color is applied as solid rectangular bars over the codes only so that the descriptions remain clear and legible. The color codes and definitions are printed at the bottom of all right-sided pages of Volume 1 and Volume 3.

Volume 1

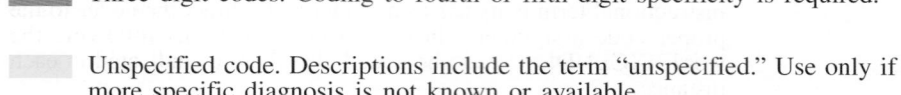 Three digit codes. Coding to fourth or fifth digit specificity is required.

Unspecified code. Descriptions include the term "unspecified." Use only if a more specific diagnosis is not known or available.

 Nonspecific code. Descriptions include the term "nonspecific, unspecified, other specified or other." A report *may* be required by insurance carriers.

Manifestation codes. Used only to code the manifestation of an underlying disease. Code the underlying disease first.

Medicare secondary payer (MSP) alert. Diagnoses that may trigger a post-payment review by Medicare. Medicare is usually the secondary payer for these diagnoses.

Secondary diagnosis only. V codes that may only be used as additional codes, not as first-listed codes.

Primary diagnosis only. V codes which are only acceptable as first listed codes.

Volume 3[*]

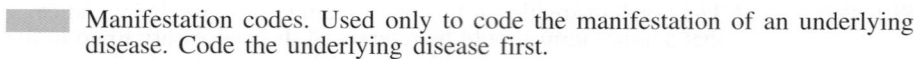 Noncovered operating room procedure. An operating room procedure that is not covered by Medicare.

Non-operating room procedure. A procedure that is not performed in the operating room that affects DRG assignment.

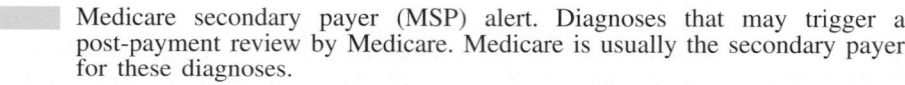 Bilateral procedure.

Valid operating room procedure. Prompts a change in DRG assignment.

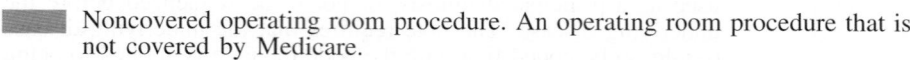 Nonspecific operating room procedure. Choose a more precise code if possible.

---

*These colors appear only in the three-volume edition

ICD-9-CM OFFICIAL GUIDELINES FOR CODING AND REPORTING

Guidelines effective as of publication date. For updates, visit http://pmiconline.com
The guidelines include the updated V Code Table

The Centers for Medicare and Medicaid Services (CMS) and the National Center for Health Statistics (NCHS), two departments within the U.S. Federal Government's Department of Health and Human Services (DHHS) provide the following guidelines for coding and reporting using the International Classification of Diseases, 9th Revision, Clinical Modification (ICD-9-CM). These guidelines should be used as a companion document to the official version of the ICD-9-CM as published on CD-ROM by the U.S. Government Printing Office (GPO).

These guidelines have been approved by the four organizations that make up the Cooperating Parties for the ICD-9-CM: the American Hospital Association (AHA), the American Health Information Management Association (AHIMA), CMS, and NCHS. These guidelines are included on the official government version of the ICD-9-CM, and also appear in "Coding Clinic for ICD-9-CM" published by the AHA.

These guidelines are a set of rules that have been developed to accompany and complement the official conventions and instructions provided within the ICD-9-CM itself. The instructions and conventions of the classification take precedence over guidelines. These guidelines are based on the coding and sequencing instructions in Volumes I, II and III of ICD-9-CM, but provide additional instruction. Adherence to these guidelines when assigning ICD-9-CM diagnosis and procedure codes is required under the Health Insurance Portability and Accountability Act (HIPAA). The diagnosis codes (Volumes 1-2) have been adopted under HIPAA for all healthcare settings. Volume 3 procedure codes have been adopted for inpatient procedures reported by hospitals. A joint effort between the healthcare provider and the coder is essential to achieve complete and accurate documentation, code assignment, and reporting of diagnoses and procedures. These guidelines have been developed to assist both the healthcare provider and the coder in identifying those diagnoses and procedures that are to be reported. The importance of consistent, complete documentation in the medical record cannot be overemphasized. Without such documentation accurate coding cannot be achieved. The entire record should be reviewed to determine the specific reason for the encounter and the conditions treated.

The term encounter is used for all settings, including hospital admissions. In the context of these guidelines, the term provider is used throughout the guidelines to mean physician or any qualified health care practitioner who is legally accountable for establishing the patient's diagnosis. Only this set of guidelines, approved by the Cooperating Parties, is official.

The guidelines are organized into sections. Section I includes the structure and conventions of the classification and general guidelines that apply to the entire classification, and chapter-specific guidelines that correspond to the chapters as they are arranged in the classification.

Section II includes guidelines for selection of principal diagnosis for non-outpatient settings. Section III includes guidelines for reporting additional diagnoses in non-outpatient settings. Section IV is for outpatient coding and reporting.

SECTION I. CONVENTIONS, GENERAL CODING GUIDELINES AND CHAPTER SPECIFIC GUIDELINES

The conventions, general guidelines and chapter-specific guidelines are applicable to all health care settings unless otherwise indicated. The conventions and instructions of the classification take precedence over guidelines.

A. Conventions for the ICD-9-CM

The conventions for the ICD-9-CM are the general rules for use of the classification independent of the guidelines. These conventions are incorporated within the index and tabular of the ICD-9-CM as instructional notes. The conventions are as follows:

1. Format:

The ICD-9-CM uses an indented format for ease in reference

2. Abbreviations

a. Index abbreviations
NEC   "Not elsewhere classifiable"
This abbreviation in the index represents "other specified" when a specific code is not available for a condition the index directs the coder to the "other specified" code in the tabular.

b. Tabular abbreviations
NEC   "Not elsewhere classifiable"
This abbreviation in the tabular represents "other specified". When a specific code is not available for a condition the tabular includes an NEC entry under a code to identify the code as the "other specified" code.
(See Section I.A.5.a. "Other" codes").
NOS   "Not otherwise specified"
This abbreviation is the equivalent of unspecified.
(See Section I.A.5.b., "Unspecified" codes)

3. Punctuation

[ ]   Brackets are used in the tabular list to enclose synonyms, alternative wording or explanatory phrases. Brackets are used in the index to identify manifestation codes.
(See Section I.A.6. "Etiology/manifestations")

( )   Parentheses are used in both the index and tabular to enclose supplementary words that may be present or absent in the statement of a disease or procedure without affecting the code number to which it is assigned. The terms within the parentheses are referred to as nonessential modifiers.

:   Colons are used in the Tabular list after an incomplete term which needs one or more of the modifiers following the colon to make it assignable to a given category.

4. Includes and Excludes Notes and Inclusion terms

Includes: This note appears immediately under a three-digit code title to further define, or give examples of, the content of the category.

Excludes: An excludes note under a code indicates that the terms excluded from the code are to be coded elsewhere. In some cases the codes for the excluded terms should not be used in conjunction with the code from which it is excluded. An example of this is a congenital condition excluded from an acquired form of the same condition. The congenital and acquired codes should not be used together. In other cases, the excluded terms may be used together with an excluded code. An example of this is when fractures of different bones are coded to different codes. Both codes may be used together if both types of fractures are present.

Inclusion terms: List of terms is included under certain four and five digit codes. These terms are the conditions for which that code number is to be used. The terms may be synonyms of the code title, or, in the case of "other specified" codes, the terms are a list of the various conditions assigned to that code. The inclusion terms are not necessarily exhaustive. Additional terms found only in the index may also be assigned to a code.

5. Other and Unspecified codes

a. "Other" codes

Codes titled "other" or "other specified" (usually a code with a 4th digit 8 or fifth-digit 9 for diagnosis codes) are for use when the information in the medical record provides detail for which a specific code does not exist. Index entries with NEC in the line designate "other" codes in the tabular. These index entries represent specific disease entities for which no specific code exists so the term is included within an "other" code.

b. "Unspecified" codes

Codes (usually a code with a 4th digit 9 or 5th digit 0 for diagnosis codes) titled "unspecified" are for use when the information in the medical record is insufficient to assign a more specific code.

6. Etiology/manifestation convention ("code first", "use additional code" and "in diseases classified elsewhere" notes)

Certain conditions have both an underlying etiology and multiple body system manifestations due to the underlying etiology. For such conditions, the ICD-9-CM has a coding convention that requires the underlying condition be sequenced first followed by the manifestation. Wherever such a combination exists, there is a "use additional code" note at the etiology code, and a "code first" note at the manifestation code. These instructional notes indicate the proper sequencing order of the codes, etiology followed by manifestation. In most cases the manifestation codes will have in the code title, "in diseases classified elsewhere." Codes with this title are a component of the etiology/manifestation convention. The code title indicates that it is a manifestation code. "In diseases classified elsewhere" codes are never permitted to be used as first listed or principal diagnosis codes. They must be used in conjunction with an underlying condition code and they must be listed following the underlying condition.

There are manifestation codes that do not have "in diseases classified elsewhere" in the title. For such codes a "use additional code" note will still be present and the rules for sequencing apply.

In addition to the notes in the tabular, these conditions also have a specific index entry structure. In the index both conditions are listed together with the etiology code first followed by the manifestation codes in brackets. The code in brackets is always to be sequenced second.

The most commonly used etiology/manifestation combinations are the codes for Diabetes mellitus, category 250. For each code under category 250 there is a use additional code note for the manifestation that is specific for that particular diabetic manifestation. Should a patient have more than one manifestation of diabetes, more than one code from category 250 may be used with as many manifestation codes as are needed to fully describe the patient's complete diabetic condition. The category 250 diabetes codes should be sequenced first, followed by the manifestation codes.

"Code first" and "Use additional code" notes are also used as sequencing rules in the classification for certain codes that are not part of an etiology/manifestation combination.

See - Section I.B.9. "Multiple coding for a single condition".

7. "And"

The word "and" should be interpreted to mean either "and" or "or" when it appears in a title.

8. "With"

The word "with" should be interpreted to mean "associated with" or "due to" when it appears in a code title, the Alphabetic Index, or an instructional note in the Tabular List. The word "with" in the alphabetic index is sequenced immediately following the main term, not in alphabetical order.

9. "See" and "See Also"

The "see" instruction following a main term in the index indicates that another term should be referenced. It is necessary to go to the main term referenced with the "see" note to locate the correct code.

A "see also" instruction following a main term in the index instructs that there is another main term that may also be referenced that may provide additional index entries that may be useful. It is not necessary to follow the "see also" note when the original main term provides the necessary code.

B. General Coding Guidelines

1. Use of Both Alphabetic Index and Tabular List

Use both the Alphabetic Index and the Tabular List when locating and assigning a code. Reliance on only the Alphabetic Index or the Tabular List leads to errors in code assignments and less specificity in code selection.

2. Locate each term in the Alphabetic Index

Locate each term in the Alphabetic Index and verify the code selected in the Tabular List. Read and be guided by instructional notations that appear in both the Alphabetic Index and the Tabular List.

3. Level of Detail in Coding

Diagnosis and procedure codes are to be used at their highest number of digits available. ICD-9-CM diagnosis codes are composed of codes with 3, 4, or 5 digits. Codes with three digits are included in ICD-9-CM as the heading of a category of codes that may be further subdivided by the use of fourth and/or fifth digits, which provide greater detail.

A three-digit code is to be used only if it is not further subdivided. Where fourth-digit subcategories and/or fifth-digit subclassifications are provided, they must be assigned. A code is invalid if it has not been coded to the full number of digits required for that code. For example, Acute myocardial infarction, code 410, has fourth digits that describe the location of the infarction (e.g., 410.2, Of inferolateral wall), and fifth digits that identify the episode of care. It would be incorrect to report a code in category 410 without a fourth and fifth digit.

ICD-9-CM Volume 3 procedure codes are composed of codes with either 3 or 4 digits. Codes with two digits are included in ICD-9-CM as the heading of a category of codes that may be further subdivided by the use of third and/or fourth digits, which provide greater detail.

4. Code or codes from 001.0 through V91.99

The appropriate code or codes from 001.0 through V91.99 must be used to identify diagnoses, symptoms, conditions, problems, complaints or other reason(s) for the encounter/visit.

5. Selection of codes 001.0 through 999.9

The selection of codes 001.0 through 999.9 will frequently be used to describe the reason for the admission/encounter. These codes are from the section of ICD-9-CM for the classification of diseases and injuries (e.g., infectious and parasitic diseases; neoplasms; symptoms, signs, and ill-defined conditions, etc.).

6. Signs and symptoms

Codes that describe symptoms and signs, as opposed to diagnoses, are acceptable for reporting purposes when a related definitive diagnosis has not been established (confirmed) by the provider. Chapter 16 of ICD-9-CM, Symptoms, Signs, and Ill-defined conditions (codes 780.0 - 799.9) contain many, but not all codes for symptoms.

7. Conditions that are an integral part of a disease process

Signs and symptoms that are associated routinely with a disease process should not be assigned as additional codes, unless otherwise instructed by the classification.

8. Conditions that are not an integral part of a disease process

Additional signs and symptoms that may not be associated routinely with a disease process should be coded when present.

9. Multiple coding for a single condition

In addition to the etiology/manifestation convention that requires two codes to fully describe a single condition that affects multiple body systems, there are other single conditions that also require more than one code. "Use additional code" notes are found in the tabular at codes that are not part of an etiology/manifestation pair where a secondary code is useful to fully describe a condition. The sequencing rule is the same as the etiology/manifestation pair - , "use additional code" indicates that a secondary code should be added.

For example, for infections that are not included in chapter 1, a secondary code from category 041, Bacterial infection in conditions classified elsewhere and of unspecified site, may be required to identify the bacterial organism causing the infection. A "use additional code" note will normally be found at the infectious disease code, indicating a need for the organism code to be added as a secondary code.

"Code first" notes are also under certain codes that are not specifically manifestation codes but may be due to an underlying cause. When a "code first" note is present and an underlying condition is present the underlying condition should be sequenced first.

"Code, if applicable, any causal condition first", notes indicate that this code may be assigned as a principal diagnosis when the causal condition is unknown or not applicable. If a causal condition is known, then the code for that condition should be sequenced as the principal or first-listed diagnosis.

Multiple codes may be needed for late effects, complication codes and obstetric codes to more fully describe a condition. See the specific guidelines for these conditions for further instruction.

10. Acute and Chronic Conditions

If the same condition is described as both acute (subacute) and chronic, and separate subentries exist in the Alphabetic Index at the same indentation level, code both and sequence the acute (subacute) code first.

11. Combination Code

A combination code is a single code used to classify:

— Two diagnoses, or
— A diagnosis with an associated secondary process (manifestation), or
— A diagnosis with an associated complication

Combination codes are identified by referring to subterm entries in the Alphabetic Index and by reading the inclusion and exclusion notes in the Tabular List.

Assign only the combination code when that code fully identifies the diagnostic conditions involved or when the Alphabetic Index so directs. Multiple coding should not be used when the classification provides a combination code that clearly identifies all of the elements documented in the diagnosis. When the combination code lacks necessary specificity in describing the manifestation or complication, an additional code should be used as a secondary code.

12. Late Effects

A late effect is the residual effect (condition produced) after the acute phase of an illness or injury has terminated. There is no time limit on when a late effect code can be used. The residual may be apparent early, such as in cerebrovascular accident cases, or it may occur months or years later, such as that due to a previous injury. Coding of late effects generally requires two codes sequenced in the following order: The condition or nature of the late effect is sequenced first. The late effect code is sequenced second.

An exception to the above guidelines are those instances where the code for late effect is followed by a manifestation code identified in the Tabular List and title, or the late effect code has been expanded (at the fourth and fifth-digit levels) to include the manifestation(s). The code for the acute phase of an illness or injury that led to the late effect is never used with a code for the late effect.

13. Impending or Threatened Condition

Code any condition described at the time of discharge as "impending" or "threatened" as follows:

If it did occur, code as confirmed diagnosis.

If it did not occur, reference the Alphabetic Index to determine if the condition has a subentry term for "impending" or "threatened" and also reference main term entries for "Impending" and for "Threatened."

If the subterms are listed, assign the given code.

If the subterms are not listed, code the existing underlying condition(s) and not the condition described as impending or threatened.

14. Reporting Same Diagnosis Code More Than Once

Each unique ICD-9-CM diagnosis code may be reported only once for an encounter. This applies to bilateral conditions or two different conditions classified to the same ICD-9-CM diagnosis code.

15. Admissions/Encounters for Rehabilitation

When the purpose for the admission/encounter is rehabilitation, sequence the appropriate V code from category V57, Care involving use of rehabilitation procedures, as the principal/first-listed diagnosis. The code for the condition for which the service is being performed should be reported as an additional diagnosis.
Only one code from category V57 is required. Code V57.89, Other specified rehabilitation procedures, should be assigned if more than one type of rehabilitation is performed during a single encounter. A procedure code should be reported to identify each type of rehabilitation therapy actually performed.

16. Documentation of BMI and Pressure Ulcer Stages

For the Body Mass Index (BMI) and pressure ulcer stage codes, code assignment may be based on medical record documentation from clinicians who are not the patient's provider (i.e., physician or other qualified healthcare practitioner legally accountable for establishing the patient's diagnosis), since this information is typically documented by other clinicians involved in the care of the patient (e.g., a dietitian often documents the BMI and nurses often documents the pressure ulcer stages). However, the associated diagnosis (such as overweight, obesity, or pressure ulcer) must be documented by the patient's provider. If there is conflicting medical record documentation, either from the same clinician or different clinicians, the patient's attending provider should be queried for clarification.

The BMI and pressure ulcer stage codes should only be reported as secondary diagnoses. As with all other secondary diagnosis codes, the BMI and pressure ulcer stage codes should only be assigned when they meet the definition of a reportable additional diagnosis (see Section III, Reporting Additional Diagnoses).

17. Syndromes

Follow the Alphabetic Index guidance when coding syndromes. In the absence of index guidance, assign codes for the documented manifestations of the syndrome.

C. Chapter-Specific Coding Guidelines

In addition to general coding guidelines, there are guidelines for specific diagnoses and/or conditions in the classification. Unless otherwise indicated, these guidelines apply to all health care settings. Please refer to Section II for guidelines on the selection of principal diagnosis.

1. Chapter 1: Infectious and Parasitic Diseases (001-139)

a. Human Immunodeficiency Virus (HIV) Infections

1) Code only confirmed cases

Code only confirmed cases of HIV infection/illness. This is an exception to the hospital inpatient guideline Section II, H. In this context, "confirmation" does not require documentation of positive serology or culture for HIV; the provider's diagnostic statement that the patient is HIV positive, or has an HIV-related illness is sufficient.

2) Selection and sequencing of HIV codes

(a) Patient admitted for HIV-related condition

If a patient is admitted for an HIV-related condition, the principal diagnosis should be 042, followed by additional diagnosis codes for all reported HIV-related conditions.

(b) Patient with HIV disease admitted for unrelated condition

If a patient with HIV disease is admitted for an unrelated condition (such as a traumatic injury), the code for the unrelated condition (e.g., the nature of injury code) should be the principal diagnosis. Other diagnoses would be 042 followed by additional diagnosis codes for all reported HIV-related conditions.

(c) Whether the patient is newly diagnosed

Whether the patient is newly diagnosed or has had previous admissions/encounters for HIV conditions is irrelevant to the sequencing decision.

(d) Asymptomatic human immunodeficiency virus V08

V08 Asymptomatic human immunodeficiency virus [HIV] infection, is to be applied when the patient without any documentation of symptoms is listed as being "HIV positive," "known HIV," "HIV test positive," or similar terminology. Do not use this code if the term "AIDS" is used or if the patient is treated for any HIV-related illness or is described as having any condition(s) resulting from his/her HIV positive status; use 042 in these cases.

(e) Patients with inconclusive HIV serology

Patients with inconclusive HIV serology, but no definitive diagnosis or manifestations of the illness, may be assigned code 795.71, Inconclusive serologic test for Human Immuno deficiency Virus [HIV].

(f) Previously diagnosed HIV-related illness

Patients with any known prior diagnosis of an HIV-related illness should be coded to 042. Once a patient has developed an HIV-related illness, the patient should always be assigned code 042 on every subsequent admission/encounter.

Patients previously diagnosed with any HIV illness (042) should never be assigned to 795.71 or V08.

(g) HIV Infection in Pregnancy, Childbirth and the Puerperium

During pregnancy, childbirth or the puerperium, a patient admitted (or presenting for a health care encounter) because of an HIV-related illness should receive a principal diagnosis code of 647.6X, Other specified infectious and parasitic diseases in the mother classifiable elsewhere, but complicating the pregnancy, childbirth or the puerperium, followed by 042 and the code(s) for the HIV-related illness(es). Codes from Chapter 15 always take sequencing priority.

Patients with asymptomatic HIV infection status admitted (or presenting for a health care encounter) during pregnancy, childbirth, or the puerperium should receive codes of 647.6X and V08.

(h) Encounters for testing for HIV

If a patient is being seen to determine his/her HIV status, use code V73.89, Screening for other specified viral disease. Use code V69.8, Other problems related to lifestyle, as a secondary code if an asymptomatic patient is in a known high risk group for HIV. Should a patient with signs or symptoms or illness, or a confirmed HIV related diagnosis be tested for HIV, code the signs and symptoms or the diagnosis. An additional counseling code V65.44 may be used if counseling is provided during the encounter for the test.

When a patient returns to be informed of his/her HIV test results use code V65.44, HIV counseling, if the results of the test are negative.

If the results are positive but the patient is asymptomatic use code V08, Asymptomatic HIV infection. If the results are positive and the patient is symptomatic use code 042, HIV infection, with codes for the HIV related symptoms or diagnosis. The HIV counseling code may also be used if counseling is provided for patients with positive test results.

b. Septicemia, Systemic Inflammatory Response Syndrome (SIRS), Sepsis, Severe Sepsis, and Septic Shock

1) SIRS, Septicemia, and Sepsis

(a) The terms septicemia and sepsis are often used interchangeably by providers, however they are not considered synonymous terms. The following descriptions are provided for reference but do not preclude querying the provider for clarification about terms used in the documentation:

(i) Septicemia generally refers to a systemic disease associated with the presence of pathological microorganisms or toxins in the blood, which can include bacteria, viruses, fungi or other organisms.

(ii) Systemic inflammatory response syndrome (SIRS) generally refers to the systemic response to infection, trauma/burns, or other insult (such as cancer) with symptoms including fever, tachycardia, tachypnea, and leukocytosis.

(iii) Sepsis generally refers to SIRS due to infection.

(iv) Severe sepsis generally refers to sepsis with associated acute organ dysfunction.

(b) The coding of SIRS, sepsis and severe sepsis requires a minimum of 2 codes: a code for the underlying cause (such as infection or trauma) and a code from subcategory 995.9 Systemic inflammatory response syndrome (SIRS)..

(i)   The code for the underlying cause (such as infection or trauma) must be sequenced before the code from subcategory 995.9 Systemic inflammatory response syndrome (SIRS).

(ii) Sepsis and severe sepsis require a code for the systemic infection (038.xx, 112.5, etc.) and either code 995.91, Sepsis, or 995.92, Severe sepsis. If the causal organism is not documented, assign code 038.9, Unspecified septicemia.

(iii) Severe sepsis requires additional code(s) for the associated acute organ dysfunction(s).

(iv) If a patient has sepsis with multiple organ dysfunctions, follow the instructions for coding severe sepsis.

(v)   Either the term sepsis or SIRS must be documented to assign a code from subcategory 995.9.

(vi) See Section I.C.17.g), Injury and poisoning, for information regarding systemic inflammatory response syndrome (SIRS) due to trauma/burns and other non-infectious processes.

(c) Due to the complex nature of sepsis and severe sepsis, some cases may require querying the provider prior to assignment of the codes.

2) Sequencing sepsis and severe sepsis

(a) Sepsis and severe sepsis as principal diagnosis

If sepsis or severe sepsis is present on admission, and meets the definition of principal diagnosis, the systemic infection code (e.g., 038.xx, 112.5, etc) should be assigned as the principal diagnosis, followed by code 995.91, Sepsis, or 995.92, Severe sepsis, as required by the sequencing rules in the Tabular List. Codes from subcategory 995.9 can never be assigned as a principal diagnosis. A code should also be assigned for any localized infection, if present.

If the sepsis or severe sepsis is due to a postprocedural infection, see Section I.C.10 for guidelines related to sepsis due to postprocedural infection.

(b) Sepsis and severe sepsis as secondary diagnoses

When sepsis or severe sepsis develops during the encounter (it was not present on admission), the systemic infection code and code 995.91 or 995.92 should be assigned as secondary diagnoses.

(c) Documentation unclear as to whether sepsis or severe sepsis is present on admission

Sepsis or severe sepsis may be present on admission but the diagnosis may not be confirmed until sometime after admission. If the documentation is not clear whether the sepsis or severe sepsis was present on admission, the provider should be queried.

3) **Sepsis/SIRS with Localized Infection**

If the reason for admission is both sepsis, severe sepsis, or SIRS and a localized infection, such as pneumonia or cellulitis, a code for the systemic infection (038.xx, 112.5, etc) should be assigned first, then code 995.91 or 995.92, followed by the code for the localized infection. If the patient is admitted with a localized infection, such as pneumonia, and sepsis/SIRS doesn't develop until after admission, see guideline I.C.1.b.2.b).

If the localized infection is postprocedural, see Section I.C.10 for guidelines related to sepsis due to postprocedural infection.

Note: The term urosepsis is a nonspecific term. If that is the only term documented then only code 599.0 should be assigned based on the default for the term in the ICD-9-CM index, in addition to the code for the causal organism if known.

4) **Bacterial Sepsis and Septicemia**

In most cases, it will be a code from category 038, Septicemia, that will be used in conjunction with a code from subcategory 995.9 such as the following:

(a) Streptococcal sepsis

If the documentation in the record states streptococcal sepsis, codes 038.0, Streptococcal septicemia, and code 995.91 should be used, in that sequence.

(b) Streptococcal septicemia

If the documentation states streptococcal septicemia, only code 038.0 should be assigned, however, the provider should be queried whether the patient has sepsis, an infection with SIRS.

5) **Acute organ dysfunction that is not clearly associated with the sepsis**

If a patient has sepsis and an acute organ dysfunction, but the medical record documentation indicates that the acute organ dysfunction is related to a medical condition other than the sepsis, do not assign code 995.92, Severe sepsis. An acute organ dysfunction must be associated with the sepsis in order to assign the severe sepsis code. If the documentation is not clear as to whether an acute organ dysfunction is related to the sepsis or another medical condition, query the provider.

6) Septic shock

(a) Sequencing of septic shock

Septic shock generally refers to circulatory failure associated with severe sepsis, and, therefore, it represents a type of acute organ dysfunction.

For all cases of septic shock, the code for the systemic infection should be sequenced first, followed by codes 995.92 and 785.52. Any additional codes for other acute organ dysfunctions should also be assigned. As noted in the sequencing instructions in the Tabular List, the code for septic shock cannot be assigned as a principal diagnosis.

(b) Septic Shock without documentation of severe sepsis

Septic shock indicates the presence of severe sepsis. Code 995.92, Severe sepsis, must be assigned with code 785.52, Septic shock, even if the term severe sepsis is not documented in the record. The "use additional code" note and the "code first" note in the tabular support this guideline.

7) Sepsis and septic shock complicating abortion and pregnancy

Sepsis and septic shock complicating abortion, ectopic pregnancy, and molar pregnancy are classified to category codes in Chapter 11 (630-639). *See section I.C.11.*

8) Negative or inconclusive blood cultures

Negative or inconclusive blood cultures do not preclude a diagnosis of septicemia or sepsis in patients with clinical evidence of the condition, however, the provider should be queried.

9) Newborn sepsis

See Section I.C.15.j for information on the coding of newborn sepsis.

10) Sepsis due to a Postprocedural Infection

(a) Documentation of causal relationship

As with all postprocedural complications, code assign-ment is based on the provider's documentation of the relationship between the infection and the procedure.

(b) Sepsis due to postprocedural infection

In cases of postprocedural sepsis, the complication code, such as code 998.59, Other postoperative infection, or 674.3x, Other complications of obstetrical surgical wounds should be coded first followed by the appropriate sepsis codes (systemic infection code and either code 995.91or 995.92). An additional code(s) for any acute organ dysfunction should also be assigned for cases of severe sepsis.

11) External cause of injury codes with SIRS

Refer to Section I.C.19.a.7 for instruction on the use of external cause of injury codes with codes for SIRS resulting from trauma.

12) Sepsis and Severe Sepsis Associated with Noninfectious Process

In some cases, a non-infectious process, such as trauma, may lead to an infection which can result in sepsis or severe sepsis. If sepsis or severe sepsis is documented as associated with a non-infectious condition, such as a burn or serious injury, and this condition meets the definition for principal diagnosis, the code for the noninfectious condition should be sequenced first, followed by the code for the systemic infection and either code 995.91, Sepsis, or 995.92, Severe sepsis. Additional codes for any associated acute organ dysfunction(s) should also be assigned for cases of severe sepsis. If the sepsis or severe sepsis meets the definition of principal diagnosis, the systemic infection and sepsis codes should be sequenced before the non-infectious condition. When both the associated non-infectious condition and the sepsis or severe sepsis meet the definition of principal diagnosis, either may be assigned as principal diagnosis.

See Section I.C.1.b.2)(a) for guidelines pertaining to sepsis or severe sepsis as the principal diagnosis.

Only one code from subcategory 995.9 should be assigned. Therefore, when a non-infectious condition leads to an infection resulting in sepsis or severe sepsis, assign either code 995.91 or 995.92. Do not additionally assign code 995.93, Systemic inflammatory response syndrome due to non-infectious process without acute organ dysfunction, or 995.94, Systemic inflammatory response syndrome with acute organ dysfunction.

See Section I.C.17.g for information on the coding of SIRS due to trauma/burns or other non-infectious disease processes.

c. Methicillin Resistant Staphylococcus aureus (MRSA) Conditions

1) Selection and sequencing of MRSA codes

(a) Combination codes for MRSA infection

When a patient is diagnosed with an infection that is due to methicillin resistant Staphylococcus aureus (MRSA), and that infection has a combination code that includes the causal organism (e.g., septicemia, pneumonia) assign the appropriate code for the condition (e.g., code 038.12, Methicillin resistant Staphylococcus aureus septicemia or code 482.42, Methicillin resistant pneumonia due to Staphylococcus aureus). Do not assign code 041.12, Methicillin resistant Staphylococcus aureus, as an additional code because the code includes the type of infection and the MRSA organism. Do not assign a code from subcategory V09.0, Infection with microorganisms resistant to penicillins, as an additional diagnosis.

See Section C.1.b.1 for instructions on coding and sequencing of septicemia.

(b) Other codes for MRSA infection

When there is documentation of a current infection (e.g., wound infection, stitch abscess, urinary tract infection) due to MRSA, and that infection does not have a combination code that includes the causal organism, select the appropriate code to identify the condition along with code 041.12, Methicillin resistant Staphylococcus aureus, for the MRSA infection. Do not assign a code from subcategory V09.0, Infection with microorganisms resistant to penicillins.

(c) Methicillin susceptible Staphylococcus aureus (MSSA) and MRSA colonization

The condition or state of being colonized or carrying MSSA or MRSA is called colonization or carriage, while an individual person is described as being colonized or being a carrier. Colonization means that MSSA or MSRA is present on or in the body without necessarily causing illness. A positive MRSA colonization test might be documented by the provider as "MRSA screen positive" or "MRSA nasal swab positive".

Assign code V02.54, Carrier or suspected carrier, Methicillin resistant Staphylococcus aureus, for patients documented as having MRSA colonization. Assign code V02.53, Carrier or suspected carrier, Methicillin susceptible Staphylococcus aureus, for patient documented as having MSSA colonization. Colonization is not necessarily indicative of a disease process or as the cause of a specific condition the patient may have unless documented as such by the provider.

Code V02.59, Other specified bacterial diseases, should be assigned for other types of staphylococcal colonization (e.g., S. epidermidis, S. saprophyticus). Code V02.59 should not be assigned for colonization with any type of Staphylococcus aureus (MRSA, MSSA).

(d) MRSA colonization and infection

If a patient is documented as having both MRSA colonization and infection during a hospital admission, code V02.54, Carrier or suspected carrier, Methicillin resistant Staphylococcus aureus, and a code for the MRSA infection may both be assigned.

2. **Chapter 2: Neoplasms (140-239)**

General guidelines

Chapter 2 of the ICD-9-CM contains the codes for most benign and all malignant neoplasms. Certain benign neoplasms, such as prostatic adenomas, may be found in the specific body system chapters. To properly code a neoplasm it is necessary to determine from the record if the neoplasm is benign, in-situ, malignant, or of uncertain histologic behavior. If malignant, any secondary (metastatic) sites should also be determined.

The neoplasm table in the Alphabetic Index should be referenced first. However, if the histological term is documented, that term should be referenced first, rather than going immediately to the Neoplasm Table, in order to determine which column in the Neoplasm Table is appropriate. For example, if the documentation indicates "adenoma," refer to the term in the Alphabetic Index to review the entries under this term and the instructional note to "see also neoplasm, by site, benign." The table provides the proper code based on the type of neoplasm and the site. It is important to select the proper column in the table that corresponds to the type of neoplasm. The tabular should then be referenced to verify that the correct code has been selected from the table and that a more specific site code does not exist. *See Section I. C. 18.d.4. for information regarding V codes for genetic susceptibility to cancer.*

a. Treatment directed at the malignancy

If the treatment is directed at the malignancy, designate the malignancy as the principal diagnosis. The only exception to this guideline is if a patient admission/encounter is solely for the administration of chemotherapy, immunotherapy or radiation therapy, assign the appropriate V58.x code as the first-listed or principal diagnosis, and the diagnosis or problem for which the service is being performed as a secondary diagnosis.

b. Treatment of secondary site

When a patient is admitted because of a primary neoplasm with metastasis and treatment is directed toward the secondary site only, the secondary neoplasm is designated as the principal diagnosis even though the primary malignancy is still present.

c. Coding and sequencing of complications

Coding and sequencing of complications associated with the malignancies or with the therapy thereof are subject to the following guidelines:

1) Anemia associated with malignancy

When admission/encounter is for management of an anemia associated with the malignancy, and the treatment is only for anemia, the appropriate anemia code (such as code 285.22, Anemia in neoplastic disease) is designated as the principal diagnosis and is followed by the appropriate code(s) for the malignancy. Code 285.22 may also be used as a secondary code if the patient suffers from anemia and is being treated for the malignancy.

Code 285.22, Anemia in neoplastic disease, and code 285.3, Antineoplastic chemotherapy induced anemia, may both be assigned if anemia in neoplastic disease and anemia due to antineoplastic chemotherapy are both documented.

2) Anemia associated with chemotherapy, immunotherapy and radiation therapy

When the admission/encounter is for management of an anemia associated with chemotherapy, immunotherapy or radiotherapy and the only treatment is for the anemia, the anemia is sequenced first. The appropriate neoplasm code should be assigned as an additional code.

3) Management of dehydration due to the malignancy

When the admission/encounter is for management of dehydration due to the malignancy or the therapy, or a combination of both, and only the dehydration is being treated (intravenous rehydration), the dehydration is sequenced first, followed by the code(s) for the malignancy.

4) Treatment of a complication resulting from a surgical procedure

When the admission/encounter is for treatment of a complication resulting from a surgical procedure, designate the complication as the principal or first-listed diagnosis if treatment is directed at resolving the complication.

d. Primary malignancy previously excised

When a primary malignancy has been previously excised or eradicated from its site and there is no further treatment directed to that site and there is no evidence of any existing primary malignancy, a code from category V10, Personal history of malignant neoplasm, should be used to indicate the former site of the malignancy. Any mention of extension, invasion, or metastasis to another site is coded as a secondary malignant neoplasm to that site. The secondary site may be the principal or first-listed with the V10 code used as a secondary code.

e. Admissions/Encounters involving chemotherapy, immunotherapy and radiation therapy

1) Episode of care involves surgical removal of neoplasm

When an episode of care involves the surgical removal of a neoplasm, primary or secondary site, followed by adjunct chemotherapy or radiation treatment during the same episode of care, the neoplasm code should be assigned as principal or first-listed diagnosis, using codes in the 140-198 series or where appropriate in the 200-203 series.

2) Patient admission/encounter solely for administration of chemotherapy, immunotherapy and radiation therapy

If a patient admission/encounter is solely for the administration of chemotherapy, immunotherapy or radiation therapy assign code V58.0, Encounter for radiation therapy, or V58.11, Encounter for antineoplastic chemotherapy, or V58.12, Encounter for antineoplastic immunotherapy as the first-listed or principal diagnosis. If a patient receives more than one of these therapies during the same admission more than one of these codes may be assigned, in any sequence.

The malignancy for which the therapy is being administered should be assigned as a secondary diagnosis.

3) Patient admitted for radiotherapy/chemotherapy and immunotherapy and develops complications

When a patient is admitted for the purpose of radiotherapy, immunotherapy or chemotherapy and develops complications such as uncontrolled nausea and vomiting or dehydration, the principal or first-listed diagnosis is V58.0, Encounter for radiotherapy, or V58.11, Encounter for antineoplastic chemotherapy, or V58.12, Encounter for antineoplastic immunotherapy followed by any codes for the complications.

f. Admission/encounter to determine extent of malignancy

When the reason for admission/encounter is to determine the extent of the malignancy, or for a procedure such as paracentesis or thoracentesis, the primary malignancy or appropriate metastatic site is designated as the principal or first-listed diagnosis, even though chemotherapy or radiotherapy is administered.

g. Symptoms, signs, and ill-defined conditions listed in Chapter 16 associated with neoplasms

Symptoms, signs, and ill-defined conditions listed in Chapter 16 characteristic of, or associated with, an existing primary or secondary site malignancy cannot be used to replace the malignancy as principal or first-listed diagnosis, regardless of the number of admissions or encounters for treatment and care of the neoplasm.

h. Admission/encounter for pain control/management

See Section I.C.6.a.5 for information on coding admission / encounter for pain control/management.

i. Malignant neoplasm associated with transplanted organ

A malignant neoplasm of a transplanted organ should be coded as a transplant complication. Assign first the appropriate code from subcategory 996.8, Complications of transplanted organ, followed by code 199.2, Malignant neoplasm associated with transplanted organ. Use an additional code for the specific malignancy.

3. Chapter 3: Endocrine, Nutritional, and Metabolic Diseases and Immunity Disorders (240-279)

a. Diabetes mellitus
Codes under category 250, Diabetes mellitus, identify complications/ manifestations associated with diabetes mellitus. A fifth-digit is required for all category 250 codes to identify the type of diabetes mellitus and whether the diabetes is controlled or uncontrolled.
See I.C.3.a.7 for secondary diabetes

1) **Fifth-digits for category 250:**

The following are the fifth-digits for the codes under category 250:

0 type II or unspecified type, not stated as uncontrolled
1 type I, [juvenile type], not stated as uncontrolled
2 type II or unspecified type, uncontrolled
3 type I, [juvenile type], uncontrolled

The age of a patient is not the sole determining factor, though most type I diabetics develop the condition before reaching puberty. For this reason type I diabetes mellitus is also referred to as juvenile diabetes.

2) **Type of diabetes mellitus not documented**

If the type of diabetes mellitus is not documented in the medical record the default is type II.

3) **Diabetes mellitus and the use of insulin**

All type I diabetics must use insulin to replace what their bodies do not produce. However, the use of insulin does not mean that a patient is a type I diabetic. Some patients with type II diabetes mellitus are unable to control their blood sugar through diet and oral medication alone and do require insulin. If the documentation in a medical record does not indicate the type of diabetes but does indicate that the patient uses insulin, the appropriate fifth-digit for type II must be used.

For type II patients who routinely use insulin, code V58.67, Long-term (current) use of insulin, should also be assigned to indicate that the patient uses insulin. Code V58.67 should not be assigned if insulin is given temporarily to bring a type II patient's blood sugar under control during an encounter.

4) **Assigning and sequencing diabetes codes and associated conditions**

When assigning codes for diabetes and its associated conditions, the code(s) from category 250 must be sequenced before the codes for the associated conditions. The diabetes codes and the secondary codes that correspond to them are paired codes that follow the etiology/manifestation convention of the classification (See SectionI.A.6., Etiology/manifestation convention).

Assign as many codes from category 250 as needed to identify all of the associated conditions that the patient has. The corresponding secondary codes are listed under each of the diabetes codes.

(a) Diabetic retinopathy/diabetic macular edema

Diabetic macular edema, code 362.07, is only present with diabetic retinopathy. Another code from subcategory 362.0, Diabetic retinopathy, must be used with code 362.07. Codes under subcategory 362.0 are diabetes manifestation codes, so they must be used following the appropriate diabetes code.

5) Diabetes mellitus in pregnancy and gestational diabetes

(a) For diabetes mellitus complicating pregnancy, see Section I.C.11.f., Diabetes mellitus in pregnancy.

(b) For gestational diabetes, see Section I.C.11, g., Gestational diabetes.

6) Insulin pump malfunction

(a) Underdose of insulin due insulin pump failure

An underdose of insulin due to an insulin pump failure should be assigned 996.57, Mechanical complication due to insulin pump, as the principal or first listed code, followed by the appropriate diabetes mellitus code based on documentation.

(b) Overdose of insulin due to insulin pump failure

The principal or first listed code for an encounter due to an insulin pump malfunction resulting in an overdose of insulin, should also be 996.57, Mechanical complication due to insulin pump, followed by code 962.3, Poisoning by insulins and antidiabetic agents, and the appropriate diabetes mellitus code based on documentation.

7) Secondary Diabetes Mellitus

Codes under category 249, Secondary diabetes mellitus, identify complications/manifestations associated with secondary diabetes mellitus. Secondary diabetes is always caused by another condition or event (e.g., cystic fibrosis, malignant neoplasm of pancreas, pancreatectomy, adverse effect of drug, or poisoning).

(a) Fifth-digits for category 249:

A fifth-digit is required for all category 249 codes to identify whether the diabetes is controlled or uncontrolled.

(b) Secondary diabetes mellitus and the use of insulin

For patients who routinely use insulin, code V58.67, Long-term (current) use of insulin, should also be assigned. Code V58.67 should not be assigned if insulin is given temporarily to bring a patient's blood sugar under control during an encounter.

(c) Assigning and sequencing secondary diabetes codes and associated conditions

When assigning codes for secondary diabetes and its associated conditions (e.g. renal manifestations), the code(s) from category 249 must be sequenced before the codes for the associated conditions. The secondary diabetes codes and the diabetic manifestation codes that correspond to them are paired codes that follow the etiology/manifestation convention of the classification.

Assign as many codes from category 249 as needed to identify all of the associated conditions that the patient has. The corresponding codes for the associated conditions are listed under each of the secondary diabetes codes. For example, secondary diabetes with diabetic nephrosis is assigned to code 249.40, followed by 581.81.

(d)　Assigning and sequencing secondary diabetes codes and its causes

The sequencing of the secondary diabetes codes in relationship to codes for the cause of the diabetes is based on the reason for the encounter, applicable ICD-9-CM sequencing conventions, and chapter-specific guidelines.

If a patient is seen for treatment of the secondary diabetes or one of its associated conditions, a code from category 249 is sequenced as the principal or first-listed diagnosis, with the cause of the secondary diabetes (e.g. cystic fibrosis) sequenced as an additional diagnosis.

If, however, the patient is seen for the treatment of the condition causing the secondary diabetes (e.g., malignant neoplasm of pancreas), the code for the cause of the secondary diabetes should be sequenced as the principal or first-listed diagnosis followed by a code from category 249.

(i)　Secondary diabetes mellitus due to pancreatectomy

For postpancreatectomy diabetes mellitus (lack of insulin due to the surgical removal of all or part of the pancreas), assign code 251.3, Postsurgical hypoinsulinemia. Assign a code from subcategory 249, Secondary diabetes mellitus and a code from subcategory V88.1, Acquired absence of pancreas as additional codes. Code also any diabetic manifestations (e.g. diabetic nephrosis 581.81).

(ii)　Secondary diabetes due to drugs

Secondary diabetes may be caused by an adverse effect of correctly administered medications, poisoning or late effect of poisoning.

See section I.C.17.e for coding of adverse effects and poisoning, and section I.C.19 for E code reporting.

4.　Chapter 4: Diseases of Blood and Blood Forming Organs (280-289)

a. Anemia of chronic disease

Subcategory 285.2, Anemia in chronic illness, has codes for anemia in chronic kidney disease, code 285.21; anemia in neoplastic disease, code 285.22; and anemia in other chronic illness, code 285.29. These codes can be used as the principal/first listed code if the reason for the encounter is to treat the anemia. They may also be used as secondary codes if treatment of the anemia is a component of an encounter, but not the primary reason for the encounter. When using a code from subcategory 285 it is also necessary to use the code for the chronic condition causing the anemia.

1) Anemia in chronic kidney disease

When assigning code 285.21, Anemia in chronic kidney disease, it is also necessary to assign a code from category 585, Chronic kidney disease, to indicate the stage of chronic kidney disease.
See I.C.10.a. Chronic kidney disease (CKD).

2) Anemia in neoplastic disease

When assigning code 285.22, Anemia in neoplastic disease, it is also necessary to assign the neoplasm code that is responsible for the anemia. Code 285.22 is for use for anemia that is due to the malignancy, not for anemia due to antineoplastic chemotherapy drugs. Assign code 285.3 for anemia due to antineoplastic chemotherapy.

See I.C.2.c.I Anemia associated with malignancy. See I.C.2.c.2 Anemia associated with chemotherapy ,immunotherapy and radiation therapy.

5. Chapter 5: Mental Disorders (290-319)

Reserved for future guideline expansion

6. Chapter 6: Diseases of Nervous System and Sense Organs (320-389)

a. Pain - Category 338

1) General coding information

Codes in category 338 may be used in conjunction with codes from other categories and chapters to provide more detail about acute or chronic pain and neoplasm-related pain, unless otherwise indicated below.

If the pain is not specified as acute or chronic, do not assign codes from category 338, except for post-thoracotomy pain, postoperative pain, neoplasm related pain, or central pain syndrome. A code from subcategories 338.1 and 338.2 should not be assigned if the underlying (definitive) diagnosis is known, unless the reason for the encounter is pain control/management and not management of the underlying condition.

(a) Category 338 Codes as Principal or First-Listed Diagnosis

Category 338 codes are acceptable as principal diagnosis or the first-listed code:

- When pain control or pain management is the reason for the admission/encounter (e.g., a patient with displaced intervertebral disc, nerve impingement and severe back pain presents for injection of steroid into the spinal canal). The underlying cause of the pain should be reported as an additional diagnosis, if known.

- When an admission or encounter is for a procedure aimed at treating the underlying condition (e.g., spinal fusion, kyphoplasty), a code for the underlying condition (e.g., vertebral fracture, spinal stenosis) should be assigned as the principal diagnosis. No code from category 338 should be assigned.

- When a patient is admitted for the insertion of a neurostimulator for pain control, assign the appropriate pain code as the principal or first listed diagnosis. When an admission or encounter is for a procedure aimed at treating the underlying condition and a neurostimulator is inserted for pain control during the same admission/encounter, a code for the underlying condition should be assigned as the principal diagnosis and the appropriate pain code should be assigned as a secondary diagnosis.

(b) Use of Category 338 Codes in Conjunction with Site-Specific Pain Codes

(i) Assigning Category 338 Codes and Site Specific Pain Codes

Codes from category 338 may be used in conjunction with codes that identify the site of pain (including codes from chapter 16) if the category 338 code provides additional information. For example, if the code describes the site of the pain, but does not fully describe whether the pain is acute or chronic, then both codes should be assigned.

(ii) Sequencing of Category 338 Codes with Site Specific Pain Codes

The sequencing of category 338 codes with site-specific pain codes (including chapter 16 codes), is dependent on the circumstances of the encounter/ admission as follows:

- If the encounter is for pain control or pain management, assign the code from category 338 followed by the code identifying the specific site of pain (e.g., encounter for pain management for acute neck pain from trauma is assigned code 338.11, Acute pain due to trauma, followed by code 723.1, Cervicalgia, to identify the site of pain).

- If the encounter is for any other reason except pain control or pain management, and a related definitive diagnosis has not been established (confirmed) by the provider, assign the code for the specific site of pain first, followed by the appropriate code from category 338.

2) **Pain due to devices, implants and grafts**

Pain associated with devices, implants or grafts left in a surgical site (for example painful hip prosthesis) is assigned to the appropriate code(s) found in Chapter 17, Injury and Poisoning. Use additional code(s) from category 338 to identify acute or chronic pain due to presence of the device, implant or graft (338.18-338.19 or 338.28-338.29).

3) **Postoperative Pain**

Post-thoracotomy pain and other postoperative pain are classified to subcategories 338.1 and 338.2, depending on whether the pain is acute or chronic. The default for post-thoracotomy and other postoperative pain not specified as acute or chronic is the code for the acute form.

Routine or expected postoperative pain immediately after surgery should not be coded.

(a) Postoperative pain not associated with specific postoperative complication

Postoperative pain not associated with a specific postoperative complication is assigned to the appropriate postoperative pain code in category 338.

(b) Postoperative pain associated with specific postoperative complication

Postoperative pain associated with a specific postoperative complication (such as painful wire sutures) is assigned to the appropriate code(s) found in Chapter 17, Injury and Poisoning. If appropriate, use additional code(s) from category 338 to identify acute or chronic pain (338.18 or 338.28). If pain control/management is the reason for the encounter, a code from category 338 should be assigned as the principal or first-listed diagnosis in accordance with Section I.C.6.a.I.a above.

(c) Postoperative pain as principal or first-listed diagnosis

Postoperative pain may be reported as the principal or first-listed diagnosis when the stated reason for the admission/encounter is documented as postoperative pain control/management.

(d) Postoperative pain as secondary diagnosis

Postoperative pain may be reported as a secondary diagnosis code when a patient presents for outpatient surgery and develops an unusual or inordinate amount of postoperative pain.

The provider's documentation should be used to guide the coding of postoperative pain, as well as *Section III. Reporting Additional Diagnoses* and *Section IV. Diagnostic Coding and Reporting in the Outpatient Setting.*

See Section II.I.2 for information on sequencing of diagnoses for patients admitted to hospital inpatient care following post-operative observation.

See Section II.J for information on sequencing of diagnoses for patients admitted to hospital inpatient care from outpatient surgery.

See Section IV.A.2 for information on sequencing of diagnoses for patients admitted for observation.

4) **Chronic pain**

Chronic pain is classified to subcategory 338.2. There is no time frame defining when pain becomes chronic pain. The provider's documentation should be used to guide use of these codes.

5) **Neoplasm Related Pain**

Code 338.3 is assigned to pain documented as being related, associated or due to cancer, primary or secondary malignancy, or tumor. This code is assigned regardless of whether the pain is acute or chronic.

This code may be assigned as the principal or first-listed code when the stated reason for the admission/encounter is documented as pain control/pain management. The underlying neoplasm should be reported as an additional diagnosis.

When the reason for the admission/encounter is management of the neoplasm and the pain associated with the neoplasm is also documented, code 338.3 may be assigned as an additional diagnosis.

See Section I.C.2 for instructions on the sequencing of neoplasms for all other stated reasons for the admission/encounter (except for pain control/pain management).

6) **Chronic pain syndrome**

This condition is different than the term "chronic pain," and therefore this code should only be used when the provider has specifically documented this condition.

7. **Chapter 7: Diseases of Circulatory System (390-459)**

a. **Hypertension**

Hypertension Table

The Hypertension Table, found under the main term, "Hypertension", in the Alphabetic Index, contains a complete listing of all conditions due to or associated with hypertension and classifies them according to malignant, benign, and unspecified.

1) Hypertension, Essential, or NOS

Assign hypertension (arterial) (essential) (primary) (systemic) (NOS) to category code 401 with the appropriate fourth digit to indicate malignant (.0), benign (.1), or unspecified (.9). Do not use either .0 malignant or .1 benign unless medical record documentation supports such a designation.

2) Hypertension with Heart Disease

Heart conditions (425.8, 429.0-429.3, 429.8, and 429.9) are assigned to a code from category 402 when a causal relationship is stated (due to hypertension) or implied (hypertensive). Use an additional code from category 428 to identify the type of heart failure in those patients with heart failure. More than one code from category 428 may be assigned if the patient has systolic or diastolic failure and congestive heart failure.

The same heart conditions (425.8, 429.0-429.3, 429.8, and 429.9) with hypertension, but without a stated causal relationship, are coded separately. Sequence according to the circumstances of the admission/encounter.

3) Hypertensive Chronic Kidney Disease

Assign codes from category 403, Hypertensive chronic kidney disease, when conditions classified to category 585 or code 587 are present with hypertension. Unlike hypertension with heart disease, ICD-9-CM presumes a cause-and-effect relationship and classifies chronic kidney disease (CKD) with hypertension as hypertensive chronic kidney disease.

Fifth digits for category 403 should be assigned as follows:

0 with CKD stage I through stage IV, or unspecified.

1 with CKD stage V or end stage renal disease.

The appropriate code from category 585, Chronic kidney disease, should be used as a secondary code with a code from category 403 to identify the stage of chronic kidney disease.

See Section I.C.10.a for information on the coding of chronic kidney disease.

4) Hypertensive Heart and Chronic Kidney Disease

Assign codes from combination category 404, Hypertensive heart and chronic kidney disease, when both hypertensive kidney disease and hypertensive heart disease are stated in the diagnosis. Assume a relationship between the hypertension and the chronic kidney disease, whether or not the condition is so designated. Assign an additional code from category 428, to identify the type of heart failure. More than one code from category 428 may be assigned if the patient has systolic or diastolic failure and congestive heart failure.

Fifth digits for category 404 should be assigned as follows:

0 without heart failure and with chronic kidney disease (CKD) stage I through stage IV, or unspecified

1 with heart failure and with CKD stage I through stage IV, or unspecified

2 without heart failure and with CKD stage V or end stage renal disease

3 with heart failure and with CKD stage V or end stage renal disease

The appropriate code from category 585, Chronic kidney disease, should be used as a secondary code with a code from category 404 to identify the stage of kidney disease. *See Section I.C.10.a for information on the coding of chronic kidney disease.*

5) Hypertensive Cerebrovascular Disease

First assign codes from 430-438, Cerebrovascular disease, then the appropriate hypertension code from categories 401-405.

6) Hypertensive Retinopathy

Two codes are necessary to identify the condition. First assign the code from subcategory 362.11, Hypertensive retinopathy, then the appropriate code from categories 401-405 to indicate the type of hypertension.

7) Hypertension, Secondary

Two codes are required: one to identify the underlying etiology and one from category 405 to identify the hypertension.Sequencing of codes is determined by the reason for admission/encounter.

8) Hypertension, Transient

Assign code 796.2, Elevated blood pressure reading without diagnosis of hypertension, unless patient has an established diagnosis of hypertension. Assign code 642.3x for transient hypertension of pregnancy.

9) Hypertension, Controlled

Assign appropriate code from categories 401-405. This diagnostic statement usually refers to an existing state of hypertension under control by therapy.

10) Hypertension, Uncontrolled

Uncontrolled hypertension may refer to untreated hypertension or hypertension not responding to current therapeutic regimen. In either case, assign the appropriate code from categories 401-405 to designate the stage and type of hypertension. Code to the type of hypertension.

11) Elevated Blood Pressure

For a statement of elevated blood pressure without further specificity, assign code 796.2, Elevated blood pressure reading without diagnosis of hypertension, rather than a code from category 401.

b. Cerebral infarction/stroke/cerebrovascular accident (CVA)

The terms stroke and CVA are often used interchangeably to refer to a cerebral infarction. The terms stroke, CVA, and cerebral infarction NOS are all indexed to the default code 434.91, Cerebral artery occlusion, unspecified, with infarction.

Additional code(s) should be assigned for any neurologic deficits associated with the acute CVA, regardless of whether or not the neurologic deficit resolves prior to discharge.

See Section I.C.18.d.3 for information on coding status post administration of tPA in a different facility within the last 24 hours.

c. Postoperative cerebrovascular accident

A cerebrovascular hemorrhage or infarction that occurs as a result of medical intervention is coded to 997.02, Iatrogenic cerebrovascular infarction or hemorrhage. Medical record documentation should clearly specify the cause- and-effect relationship between the medical intervention and the cerebrovascular accident in order to assign this code. A secondary code from the code range 430-432 or from a code from subcategories 433 or 434 with a fifth digit of "1" should also be used to identify the type of hemorrhage or infarct.

This guideline conforms to the use additional code note instruction at category 997. Code 436, Acute, but ill-defined, cerebrovascular disease, should not be used as a secondary code with code 997.02.

d. Late Effects of Cerebrovascular Disease

1) Category 438, Late Effects of Cerebrovascular disease

Category 438 is used to indicate conditions classifiable to categories 430-437 as the causes of late effects (neurologic deficits), themselves classified elsewhere. These "late effects" include neurologic deficits that persist after initial onset of conditions classifiable to 430-437. The neurologic deficits caused by cerebrovascular disease may be present from the onset or may arise at any time after the onset of the condition classifiable to 430-437.

Codes in category 438 are only for use for late effects of cerebrovascular disease, not for neurologic deficits associated with an acute CVA.

2) Codes from category 438 with codes from 430-437

Codes from category 438 may be assigned on a health care record with codes from 430-437, if the patient has a current cerebrovascular accident (CVA) and deficits from an old CVA.

3) Code V12.54

Assign code V12.54, Transient ischemic attack (TIA), and cerebral infarction without residual deficits (and not a code from category 438) as an additional code for history of cerebrovascular disease when no neurologic deficits are present.

e. Acute myocardial infarction (AMI)

1) ST elevation myocardial infarction (STEMI) and non ST elevation myocardial infarction (NSTEMI)

The ICD-9-CM codes for acute myocardial infarction (AMI) identify the site, such as anterolateral wall or true posterior wall. Subcategories 410.0-410.6 and 410.8 are used for ST elevation myocardial infarction (STEMI). Subcategory 410.7, Subendocardial infarction, is used for non ST elevation myocardial infarction (NSTEMI) and nontransmural MIs.

2) Acute myocardial infarction, unspecified

Subcategory 410.9 is the default for the unspecified term acute myocardial infarction. If only STEMI or transmural MI without the site is documented, query the provider as to the site, or assign a code from subcategory 410.9.

3) AMI documented as nontransmural or subendocardial but site provided

If an AMI is documented as nontransmural or subendocardial, but the site is provided, it is still coded as a subendocardial AMI. If NSTEMI evolves to STEMI, assign the STEMI code. If STEMI converts to NSTEMI due to thrombolytic therapy, it is still coded as STEMI.

See Section I.C.18.d.3 for information on coding status post administration of tPA in a different facility within the last 24 hours.

8. Chapter 8: Diseases of Respiratory System (460-519)

See I.C.17.f. for ventilator-associated pneumonia.

a. Chronic Obstructive Pulmonary Disease [COPD] and Asthma

1) Conditions that comprise COPD and Asthma
The conditions that comprise COPD are obstructive chronic bronchitis, subcategory 491.2, and emphysema, category 492. All asthma codes are under category 493, Asthma. Code 496, Chronic airway obstruction, not elsewhere classified, is a nonspecific code that should only be used when the documentation in a medical record does not specify the type of COPD being treated.

2) Acute exacerbation of chronic obstructive bronchitis and asthma

The codes for chronic obstructive bronchitis and asthma distinguish between uncomplicated cases and those in acute exacerbation. An acute exacerbation is a worsening or a decompensation of a chronic condition. An acute exacerbation is not equivalent to an infection superimposed on a chronic condition, though an exacerbation may be triggered by an infection.

3) Overlapping nature of the conditions that comprise COPD and asthma

Due to the overlapping nature of the conditions that make up COPD and asthma, there are many variations in the way these conditions are documented. Code selection must be based on the terms as documented. When selecting the correct code for the documented type of COPD and asthma, it is essential to first review the index, and then verify the code in the tabular list. There are many instructional notes under the different COPD subcategories and codes. It is important that all such notes be reviewed to assure correct code assignment.

4) Acute exacerbation of asthma and status asthmaticus

An acute exacerbation of asthma is an increased severity of the asthma symptoms, such as wheezing and shortness of breath. Status asthmaticus refers to a patient's failure to respond to therapy administered during an asthmatic episode and is a life threatening complication that requires emergency care. If status asthmaticus is documented by the provider with any type of COPD or with acute bronchitis, the status asthmaticus should be sequenced first. It supersedes any type of COPD including that with acute exacerbation or acute bronchitis.

It is inappropriate to assign an asthma code with 5th digit 2, with acute exacerbation, together with an asthma code with 5th digit 1, with status asthmatics. Only the 5th digit 1 should be assigned.

b. Chronic Obstructive Pulmonary Disease [COPD] and Bronchitis

1) Acute bronchitis with COPD

Acute bronchitis, code 466.0, is due to an infectious organism. When acute bronchitis is documented with COPD, code 491.22, Obstructive chronic bronchitis with acute bronchitis, should be assigned. It is not necessary to also assign code 466.0. If a medical record documents acute bronchitis with COPD with acute exacerbation, only code 491.22 should be assigned. The acute bronchitis included in code 491.22 supersedes the acute exacerbation. If a medical record documents COPD with acute exacerbation without mention of acute bronchitis, only code 491.21 should be assigned.

c. **Acute Respiratory Failure**

1) **Acute respiratory failure as principal diagnosis**

Code 518.81, Acute respiratory failure, may be assigned as a principal diagnosis when it is the condition established after study to be chiefly responsible for occasioning the admission to the hospital, and the selection is supported by the Alphabetic Index and Tabular List. However, chapter-specific coding guidelines (such as obstetrics, poisoning, HIV, newborn) that provide sequencing direction take precedence.

2) **Acute respiratory failure as secondary diagnosis**

Respiratory failure may be listed as a secondary diagnosis if it occurs after admission, or if it is present on admission, but does not meet the definition of principal diagnosis.

3) **Sequencing of acute respiratory failure and another acute condition**

When a patient is admitted with respiratory failure and another acute condition, (e.g., myocardial infarction, cerebrovascular accident, aspiration pneumonia), the principal diagnosis will not be the same in every situation. This applies whether the other acute condition is a respiratory or nonrespiratory condition. Selection of the principal diagnosis will be dependent on the circumstances of admission. If both the respiratory failure and the other acute condition are equally responsible for occasioning the admission to the hospital, and there are no chapter-specific sequencing rules, the guideline regarding two or more diagnoses that equally meet the definition for principal diagnosis (Section II, C.) may be applied in these situations.

If the documentation is not clear as to whether acute respiratory failure and another condition are equally responsible for occasioning the admission, query the provider for clarification.

d. **Influenza due to certain identified viruses**

Code only confirmed cases of avian influenza (codes 488.01-488.02, 488.09, Influenza due to identified avian influenza virus) or novel H1N1 influenza virus (H1N1 or swine flu, code 488.11-488.12, 488.19). This is an exception to the hospital inpatient guideline Section II, H. (Uncertain Diagnosis). In this context, "confirmation" does not require documentation of positive laboratory testing specific for avian or novel H1N1 influenza. However, coding should be based on the provider's diagnostic statement that the patient has avian or novel H1N1 (H1N1 or swine flu) influenza.

If the provider records "suspected or possible or probable avian or novel H1N1 influenza (H1N1 or swine flu)," the appropriate influenza code from category 487 should be assigned. A code from category 488, Influenza due to certain identified influenza viruses, should not be assigned.

9. **Chapter 9: Diseases of Digestive System (520-579)**

Reserved for future guideline expansion

10. Chapter 10: Diseases of Genitourinary System (580-629)

a. Chronic kidney disease

1) Stages of chronic kidney disease (CKD)

The ICD-9-CM classifies CKD based on severity. The severity of CKD is designated by stages I-V. Stage II, code 585.2, equates to mild CKD; stage III, code 585.3, equates to moderate CKD; and stage IV, code 585.4, equates to severe CKD. Code 585.6, End stage renal disease (ESRD), is assigned when the provider has documented end-stage-renal disease (ESRD).

If both a stage of CKD and ESRD are documented, assign code 585.6 only.

2) Chronic kidney disease and kidney transplant status

Patients who have undergone kidney transplant may still have some form of CKD, because the kidney transplant may not fully restore kidney function. Therefore, the presence of CKD alone does not constitute a transplant complication. Assign the appropriate 585 code for the patient's stage of CKD and code V42.0. If a transplant complication such as failure or rejection is documented, see section I.C.17.f.2.b for information on coding complications of a kidney transplant. If the documentation is unclear as to whether the patient has a complication of the transplant, query the provider.

3) Chronic kidney disease with other conditions

Patients with CKD may also suffer from other serious conditions, most commonly diabetes mellitus and hypertension. The sequencing of the CKD code in relationship to codes for other contributing conditions is based on the conventions in the tabular list.

See I.C.3.a.4 for sequencing instructions for diabetes. See I.C.4.a.1 for anemia in CKD. See I.C.7.a.3 for hypertensive chronic kidney disease. See I.C.I7.f.2.b, Kidney transplant complications, for instructions on coding of documented rejection or failure.

11. Chapter 11: Complications of Pregnancy, Childbirth, and the Puerperium (630-679)

a. General Rules for Obstetric Cases

1) Codes from chapter 11 and sequencing priority

Obstetric cases require codes from chapter 11, codes in the range 630-679, Complications of Pregnancy, Childbirth, and the Puerperium. Chapter 11 codes have sequencing priority over codes from other chapters. Additional codes from other chapters may be used in conjunction with chapter 11 codes to further specify conditions. Should the provider document that the pregnancy is incidental to the encounter, then code V22.2 should be used in place of any chapter 11 codes. It is the provider's responsibility to state that the condition being treated is not affecting the pregnancy.

2) Chapter 11 codes used only on the maternal record

Chapter 11 codes are to be used only on the maternal record, never on the record of the newborn.

3) Chapter 11 fifth-digits

Categories 640-648, 651-676 have required fifth-digits, which indicate whether the encounter is antepartum, postpartum and whether a delivery has also occurred.

4) Fifth-digits, appropriate for each code

The fifth-digits, which are appropriate for each code number, are listed in brackets under each code. The fifth-digits on each code should all be consistent with each other. That is, should a delivery occur all of the fifth-digits should indicate the delivery.

b. Selection of OB Principal or First-listed Diagnosis

1) Routine outpatient prenatal visits

For routine outpatient prenatal visits when no complications are present codes V22.0, Supervision of normal first pregnancy, and V22.1, Supervision of other normal pregnancy, should be used as the first-listed diagnoses. These codes should not be used in conjunction with chapter 11 codes.

2) Prenatal outpatient visits for high-risk patients

For routine prenatal outpatient visits for patients with high-risk pregnancies, a code from category V23, Supervision of high-risk pregnancy, should be used as the first-listed diagnosis. Secondary chapter 11 codes may be used in conjunction with these codes if appropriate.

3) Episodes when no delivery occurs

In episodes when no delivery occurs, the principal diagnosis should correspond to the principal complication of the pregnancy, which necessitated the encounter. Should more than one complication exist, all of which are treated or monitored, any of the complications codes may be sequenced first.

4) When a delivery occurs

When a delivery occurs, the principal diagnosis should correspond to the main circumstances or complication of the delivery. In cases of cesarean delivery, the selection of the principal diagnosis should be the condition established after study that was responsible for the patient's admission. If the patient was admitted with a condition that resulted in the performance of a cesarean procedure, that condition should be selected as the principal diagnosis. If the reason for the admission/encounter was unrelated to the condition resulting in the cesarean delivery, the condition related to the reason for the admission/encounter should be selected as the principal diagnosis, even if a cesarean was performed.

5) Outcome of delivery

An outcome of delivery code, V27.0-V27.9, should be included on every maternal record when a delivery has occurred. These codes are not to be used on subsequent records or on the newborn record.

c. Fetal Conditions Affecting the Management of the Mother

1) Codes from category 655 and 656

Codes from categories 655, Known or suspected fetal abnormality affecting management of the mother, and 656, Other known or suspected fetal and placental problems affecting the management of the mother, are assigned only when the fetal condition is actually responsible for modifying the management of the mother, i.e., by requiring diagnostic studies, additional observation, special care, or termination of pregnancy. The fact that the fetal condition exists does not justify assigning a code from this series to the mother's record..

See I.C.I8.d. for suspected maternal and fetal conditions not found

2) In utero surgery

In cases when surgery is performed on the fetus, a diagnosis code from category 655, Known or suspected fetal abnormalities affecting management of the mother, should be assigned identifying the fetal condition. Procedure code 75.36, Correction of fetal defect, should be assigned on the hospital inpatient record.

No code from Chapter 15, the perinatal codes, should be used on the mother's record to identify fetal conditions. Surgery performed in utero on a fetus is still to be coded as an obstetric encounter.

d. HIV Infection in Pregnancy, Childbirth and the Puerperium

During pregnancy, childbirth or the puerperium, a patient admitted because of an HIV-related illness should receive a principal diagnosis of 647.6X, Other specified infectious and parasitic diseases in the mother classifiable elsewhere, but complicating the pregnancy, childbirth or the puerperium, followed by 042 and the code(s) for the HIV-related illness(es).

Patients with asymptomatic HIV infection status admitted during pregnancy, childbirth, or the puerperium should receive codes of 647.6X and V08.

e. Current Conditions Complicating Pregnancy

Assign a code from subcategory 648.x for patients that have current conditions when the condition affects the management of the pregnancy, childbirth, or the puerperium. Use additional secondary codes from other chapters to identify the conditions, as appropriate.

f.   Diabetes mellitus in pregnancy

Diabetes mellitus is a significant complicating factor in pregnancy. Pregnant women who are diabetic should be assigned code 648.0x, Diabetes mellitus complicating pregnancy, and a secondary code from category 250, Diabetes mellitus, or category 249, Secondary diabetes to identify the type of diabetes.

Code V58.67, Long-term (current) use of insulin, should also be assigned if the diabetes mellitus is being treated with insulin.

g.   Gestational diabetes

Gestational diabetes can occur during the second and third trimester of pregnancy in women who were not diabetic prior to pregnancy. Gestational diabetes can cause complications in the pregnancy similar to those of pre-existing diabetes mellitus. It also puts the woman at greater risk of developing diabetes after the pregnancy. Gestational diabetes is coded to 648.8x, Abnormal glucose tolerance. Codes 648.0x and 648.8x should never be used together on the same record. Code V58.67, Long-term (current) use of insulin, should also be assigned if the gestational diabetes is being treated with insulin.

h.   Normal Delivery, Code 650

1) Normal delivery

Code 650 is for use in cases when a woman is admitted for a full-term normal delivery and delivers a single, healthy infant without any complications antepartum, during the delivery, or postpartum during the delivery episode. Code 650 is always a principal diagnosis. It is not to be used if any other code from chapter 11 is needed to describe a current complication of the antenatal, delivery, or perinatal period. Additional codes from other chapters may be used with code 650 if they are not related to or are in any way complicating the pregnancy.

2) Normal delivery with resolved antepartum complication

Code 650 may be used if the patient had a complication at some point during her pregnancy, but the complication is not present at the time of the admission for delivery.

3) V27.0, Single liveborn, outcome of delivery

V27.0, Single liveborn, is the only outcome of delivery code appropriate for use with 650.

i.   The Postpartum and Peripartum Periods

1) Postpartum and peripartum periods

The postpartum period begins immediately after delivery and continues for six weeks following delivery. The peripartum period is defined as the last month of pregnancy to five months postpartum.

2) **Postpartum complication**

A postpartum complication is any complication occurring within the six-week period.

3) **Pregnancy-related complications after 6 week period**

Chapter 11 codes may also be used to describe pregnancy-related complications after the six-week period should the provider document that a condition is pregnancy related.

4) **Postpartum complications occurring during the same admission as delivery**

Postpartum complications that occur during the same admission as the delivery are identified with a fifth digit of "2." Subsequent admissions/encounters for postpartum complications should be identified with a fifth digit of "4."

5) **Admission for routine postpartum care following delivery outside hospital**

When the mother delivers outside the hospital prior to admission and is admitted for routine postpartum care and no complications are noted, code V24.0, Postpartum care and examination immediately after delivery, should be assigned as the principal diagnosis.

6) **Admission following delivery outside hospital with postpartum conditions**

A delivery diagnosis code should not be used for a woman who has delivered prior to admission to the hospital. Any postpartum conditions and/or postpartum procedures should be coded.

7) **Puerperal sepsis**

Code 670.2x, Puerperal sepsis, should be assigned with a secondary code to identify the causal organism (e.g., for a bacterial infection, assign a code from category 041, Bacterial infections in conditions classified elsewhere and of unspecified site). A code from category 038, Septicemia, should not be used for puerperal sepsis. Do not assign code 995.91, Sepsis, as code 670.2x describes the sepsis. If applicable, use additional codes to identify severe sepsis (995.92) and any associated acute organ dysfunction.

j. **Code 677, Late effect of complication of pregnancy**

1) **Code 677**

Code 677, Late effect of complication of pregnancy, childbirth, and the puerperium is for use in those cases when an initial complication of a pregnancy develops a sequelae requiring care or treatment at a future date.

2) **After the initial postpartum period**

This code may be used at any time after the initial postpartum period.

3) Sequencing of Code 677

This code, like all late effect codes, is to be sequenced following the code describing the sequelae of the complication.

k. Abortions

1) Fifth-digits required for abortion categories

Fifth-digits are required for abortion categories 634-637. Fifth digit assignment is based on the status of the patient at the beginning (or start) of the encounter. Fifth-digit 1, incomplete, indicates that all of the products of conception have not been expelled from the uterus. Fifth-digit 2, complete, indicates that all products of conception have been expelled from the uterus.

2) Code from categories 640-648 and 651-659

A code from categories 640-648 and 651-659 may be used as additional codes with an abortion code to indicate the complication leading to the abortion.

Fifth digit 3 is assigned with codes from these categories when used with an abortion code because the other fifth digits will not apply. Codes from the 660-669 series are not to be used for complications of abortion.

3) Code 639 for complications

Code 639 is to be used for all complications following abortion. Code 639 cannot be assigned with codes from categories 634-638.

4) Abortion with Liveborn Fetus

When an attempted termination of pregnancy results in a liveborn fetus assign code 644.21, Early onset of delivery, with an appropriate code from category V27, Outcome of Delivery. The procedure code for the attempted termination of pregnancy should also be assigned.

5) Retained Products of Conception following an abortion

Subsequent admissions for retained products of conception following a spontaneous or legally induced abortion are assigned the appropriate code from category 634, Spontaneous abortion, or 635 Legally induced abortion, with a fifth digit of "1" (incomplete). This advice is appropriate even when the patient was discharged previously with a discharge diagnosis of complete abortion.

12. Chapter 12: Diseases Skin and Subcutaneous Tissue (680-709)

a. Pressure ulcer stage codes

1) Pressure ulcer stages

Two codes are needed to completely describe a pressure ulcer: A code from subcategory 707.0, Pressure ulcer, to identify the site of the pressure ulcer and a code from subcategory 707.2, Pressure ulcer stages.

The codes in subcategory 707.2, Pressure ulcer stages, are to be used as an additional diagnosis with a code(s) from subcategory 707.0, Pressure Ulcer. Codes from 707.2, Pressure ulcer stages, may not be assigned as a principal or first-listed diagnosis. The pressure ulcer stage codes should only be used with pressure ulcers and not with other types of ulcers (e.g., stasis ulcer).

The ICD-9-CM classifies pressure ulcer stages based on severity, which is designated by stages I-IV and unstageable.

2) **Unstageable pressure ulcers**

Assignment of code 707.25, Pressure ulcer, unstageable, should be based on the clinical documentation. Code 707.25 is used for pressure ulcers whose stage cannot be clinically determined (e.g., the ulcer is covered by eschar or has been treated with a skin or muscle graft) and pressure ulcers that are documented as deep tissue injury but not documented as due to trauma.

This code should not be confused with code 707.20, Pressure ulcer, stage unspecified. Code 707.20 should be assigned when there is no documentation regarding the stage of the pressure ulcer.

3) **Documented pressure ulcer stage**

Assignment of the pressure ulcer stage code should be guided by clinical documentation of the stage or documentation of the terms found in the index. For clinical terms describing the stage that are not found in the index, and there is no documentation of the stage, the provider should be queried.

4) **Bilateral pressure ulcers with same stage**

When a patient has bilateral pressure ulcers (e.g., both buttocks) and both pressure ulcers are documented as being the same stage, only the code for the site and one code for the stage should be reported.

5) **Bilateral pressure ulcers with different stages**

When a patient has bilateral pressure ulcers at the same site (e.g., both buttocks) and each pressure ulcer is documented as being at a different stage, assign one code for the site and the appropriate codes for the pressure ulcer stage.

6) **Multiple pressure ulcers of different sites and stages**

When a patient has multiple pressure ulcers at different sites (e.g., buttock, heel, shoulder) and each pressure ulcer is documented as being at different stages (e.g., stage 3 and stage 4), assign the appropriate codes for each different site and a code for each different pressure ulcer stage.

7) **Patients admitted with pressure ulcers documented as healed**

No code is assigned if the documentation states that the pressure ulcer is completely healed.

8) **Patients admitted with pressure ulcers documented as healing**

Pressure ulcers described as healing should be assigned the appropriate pressure ulcer stage code based on the documentation in the medical record. If the documentation does not provide information about the stage of the healing pressure ulcer, assign code 707.20, Pressure ulcer stage, unspecified.

If the documentation is unclear as to whether the patient has a current (new) pressure ulcer or if the patient is being treated for a healing pressure ulcer, query the provider.

9) **Patient admitted with pressure ulcer evolving into another stage during the admission**

If a patient is admitted with a pressure ulcer at one stage and it progresses to a higher stage, assign the code for highest stage reported for that site.

13. Chapter 13: Diseases of Musculoskeletal and Connective Tissue (710-739)

a. **Coding of Pathologic Fractures**

1) **Acute Fractures vs. Aftercare**

Pathologic fractures are reported using subcategory 733.1, when the fracture is newly diagnosed. Subcategory 733.1 may be used while the patient is receiving active treatment for the fracture. Examples of active treatment are: surgical treatment, emergency department encounter, evaluation and treatment by a new physician.

Fractures are coded using the aftercare codes (subcategories V54.0, V54.2, V54.8 or V54.9) for encounters after the patient has completed active treatment of the fracture and is receiving routine care for the fracture during the healing or recovery phase. Examples of fracture aftercare are: cast change or removal, removal of external or internal fixation device, medication adjustment, and follow up visits following fracture treatment.

Care for complications of surgical treatment for fracture repairs during the healing or recovery phase should be coded with the appropriate complication codes.

Care of complications of fractures, such as malunion and nonunion, should be reported with the appropriate codes. *See Section I. C. 17.b for information on the coding of traumatic fractures.*

14. Chapter 14: Congenital Anomalies (740-759)

a. **Codes in categories 740-759, Congenital Anomalies**

Assign an appropriate code(s) from categories 740-759, Congenital Anomalies, when an anomaly is documented. A congenital anomaly may be the principal/first listed diagnosis on a record or a secondary diagnosis.

When a congenital anomaly does not have a unique code assignment, assign additional code(s) for any manifestations that may be present.

When the code assignment specifically identifies the congenital anomaly, manifestations that are an inherent component of the anomaly should not be coded separately. Additional codes should be assigned for manifestations that are not an inherent component.

Codes from Chapter 14 may be used throughout the life of the patient. If a congenital anomaly has been corrected, a personal history code should be used to identify the history of the anomaly. Although present at birth, a congenital anomaly may not be identified until later in life. Whenever the condition is diagnosed by the physician, it is appropriate to assign a code from codes 740-759.

For the birth admission, the appropriate code from category V30, Liveborn infants, according to type of birth should be sequenced as the principal diagnosis, followed by any congenital anomaly codes, 740-759.

15. Chapter 15: Newborn (Perinatal) Guidelines (760-779)

For coding and reporting purposes the perinatal period is defined as before birth through the 28th day following birth. The following guidelines are provided for reporting purposes. Hospitals may record other diagnoses as needed for internal data use.

a. General Perinatal Rules

1) Chapter 15 Codes

They are never for use on the maternal record. Codes from Chapter 11, the obstetric chapter, are never permitted on the newborn record. Chapter 15 code may be used throughout the life of the patient if the condition is still present.

2) Sequencing of perinatal codes

Generally, codes from Chapter 15 should be sequenced as the principal/first-listed diagnosis on the newborn record, with the exception of the appropriate V30 code for the birth episode, followed by codes from any other chapter that provide additional detail.

The "use additional code" note at the beginning of the chapter supports this guideline. If the index does not provide a specific code for a perinatal condition, assign code 779.89, Other specified conditions originating in the perinatal period, followed by the code from another chapter that specifies the condition. Codes for signs and symptoms may be assigned when a definitive diagnosis has not been established.

3) Birth process or community acquired conditions

If a newborn has a condition that may be either due to the birth process or community acquired and the documentation does not indicate which it is, the default is due to the birth process and the code from Chapter 15 should be used. If the condition is community-acquired, a code from Chapter 15 should not be assigned.

4) Code all clinically significant conditions

All clinically significant conditions noted on routine newborn examination should be coded. A condition is clinically significant if it requires:

- clinical evaluation; or
- therapeutic treatment; or
- diagnostic procedures; or
- extended length of hospital stay; or
- increased nursing care and/or monitoring; or
- has implications for future health care needs

Note: The perinatal guidelines listed above are the same as the general coding guidelines for "additional diagnoses", except for the final point regarding implications for future health care needs. Codes should be assigned for conditions that have been specified by the provider as having implications for future health care needs. Codes from the perinatal chapter should not be assigned unless the provider has established a definitive diagnosis.

b. Use of codes V30-V39

When coding the birth of an infant, assign a code from categories V30-V39, according to the type of birth. A code from this series is assigned as a principal diagnosis, and assigned only once to a newborn at the time of birth.

c. Newborn transfers

If the newborn is transferred to another institution, the V30 series is not used at the receiving hospital.

d. Use of category V29

1) Assigning a code from category V29

Assign a code from category V29, Observation and evaluation of newborns and infants for suspected conditions not found, to identify those instances when a healthy newborn is evaluated for a suspected condition that is determined after study not to be present. Do not use a code from category V29 when the patient has identified signs or symptoms of a suspected problem; in such cases, code the sign or symptom.

A code from category V29 may also be assigned as a principal code for readmissions or encounters when the V30 code no longer applies. Codes from category V29 are for use only for healthy newborns and infants for which no condition after study is found to be present.

2) V29 code on a birth record

A V29 code is to be used as a secondary code after the V30, Outcome of delivery, code.

e. Use of other V codes on perinatal records

V codes other than V30 and V29 may be assigned on a perinatal or newborn record code. The codes may be used as a principal or first-listed diagnosis for specific types of encounters or for readmissions or encounters when the V30 code no longer applies.

See Section I.C.18 for information regarding the assignment of V codes.

f. Maternal Causes of Perinatal Morbidity

Codes from categories 760-763, Maternal causes of perinatal morbidity and mortality, are assigned only when the maternal condition has actually affected the fetus or newborn. The fact that the mother has an associated medical condition or experiences some complication of pregnancy, labor or delivery does not justify the routine assignment of codes from these categories to the newborn record.

g. Congenital Anomalies in Newborns

For the birth admission, the appropriate code from category V30, Liveborn infants according to type of birth, should be used, followed by any congenital anomaly codes, categories 740-759. Use additional secondary codes from other chapters to specify conditions associated with the anomaly, if applicable.

Also, see Section I.C.14 for information on the coding of congenital anomalies.

h. Coding Additional Perinatal Diagnoses

1) Assigning codes for conditions that require treatment

Assign codes for conditions that require treatment or further investigation, prolong the length of stay, or require resource utilization.

2) Codes for conditions specified as having implications for future health care needs

Assign codes for conditions that have been specified by the provider as having implications for future health care needs.

Note: This guideline should not be used for adult patients.

3) Codes for newborn conditions originating in the perinatal period

Assign a code for newborn conditions originating in the perinatal period (categories 760-779), as well as complications arising during the current episode of care classified in other chapters, only if the diagnoses have been documented by the responsible provider at the time of transfer or discharge as having affected the fetus or newborn.

i. Prematurity and Fetal Growth Retardation

Providers utilize different criteria in determining prematurity. A code for prematurity should not be assigned unless it is documented. The 5th digit assignment for codes from category 764 and subcategories 765.0 and 765.1 should be based on the recorded birth weight and estimated gestational age.

A code from subcategory 765.2, Weeks of gestation, should be assigned as an additional code with category 764 and codes from 765.0 and 765.1 to specify weeks of gestation as documented by the provider in the record.

j. Newborn sepsis

Code 771.81, Septicemia [sepsis] of newborn, should be assigned with a secondary code from category 041, Bacterial infections in conditions classified elsewhere and of unspecified site, to identify the organism. A code from category 038, Septicemia, should not be used on a newborn record. Do not assign code 995.91, Sepsis, as code 771.81 describes the sepsis. If applicable, use additional codes to identify severe sepsis (995.92) and any associated acute organ dysfunction.

16. Chapter 16: Signs, Symptoms and Ill-Defined Conditions (780-799)

Reserved for future guideline expansion

17. Chapter 17: Injury and Poisoning (800-999)

a. Coding of Injuries

When coding injuries, assign separate codes for each injury unless a combination code is provided, in which case the combination code is assigned. Multiple injury codes are provided in ICD-9-CM, but should not be assigned unless information for a more specific code is not available. These traumatic injury codes are not to be used for normal, healing surgical wounds or to identify complications of surgical wounds.

The code for the most serious injury, as determined by the provider and the focus of treatment, is sequenced first.

1) Superficial injuries

Superficial injuries such as abrasions or contusions are not coded when associated with more severe injuries of the same site.

2) Primary injury with damage to nerves/blood vessels

When a primary injury results in minor damage to peripheral nerves or blood vessels, the primary injury is sequenced first with additional code(s) from categories 950-957, Injury to nerves and spinal cord, and/or 900-904, Injury to blood vessels. When the primary injury is to the blood vessels or nerves, that injury should be sequenced first.

b. **Coding of Traumatic Fractures**

The principles of multiple coding of injuries should be followed in coding fractures. Fractures of specified sites are coded individually by site in accordance with both the provisions within categories 800-829 and the level of detail furnished by medical record content.

Combination categories for multiple fractures are provided for use when there is insufficient detail in the medical record (such as trauma cases transferred to another hospital), when the reporting form limits the number of codes that can be used in reporting pertinent clinical data, or when there is insufficient specificity at the fourth-digit or fifth-digit level. More specific guidelines are as follows:

1) **Acute Fractures vs. Aftercare**

Traumatic fractures are coded using the acute fracture codes (800-829) while the patient is receiving active treatment for the fracture. Examples of active treatment are: surgical treatment, emergency department encounter, and evaluation and treatment by a new physician.

Fractures are coded using the aftercare codes (subcategories V54.0, V54.1, V54.8, or V54.9) for encounters after the patient has completed active treatment of the fracture and is receiving routine care for the fracture during the healing or recovery phase. Examples of fracture aftercare are: cast change or removal, removal of external or internal fixation device, medication adjustment, and follow up visits following fracture treatment.

Care for complications of surgical treatment for fracture repairs during the healing or recovery phase should be coded with the appropriate complication codes.

Care of complications of fractures, such as malunion and nonunion, should be reported with the appropriate codes.

Pathologic fractures are not coded in the 800-829 range, but instead are assigned to subcategory 733.1. *See Section I.C.13.a for additional information.*

2) **Multiple fractures of same limb**

Multiple fractures of same limb classifiable to the same three-digit or four-digit category are coded to that category.

3) **Multiple unilateral or bilateral fractures of same bone**

Multiple unilateral or bilateral fractures of same bone(s) but classified to different fourth-digit subdivisions (bone part) within the same three-digit category are coded individually by site.

4) **Multiple fracture categories 819 and 828**

Multiple fracture categories 819 and 828 classify bilateral fractures of both upper limbs (819) and both lower limbs (828), but without any detail at the fourth-digit level other than open and closed type of fractures.

5) Multiple fractures sequencing

Multiple fractures are sequenced in accordance with the severity of the fracture. The provider should be asked to list the fracture diagnoses in the order of severity.

c. Coding of Burns

Current burns (940-948) are classified by depth, extent and by agent (E code). Burns are classified by depth as first degree (erythema), second degree (blistering), and third degree (full-thickness involvement).

1) Sequencing of burn and related condition codes

Sequence first the code that reflects the highest degree of burn when more than one burn is present.

(a.) When the reason for the admission or encounter is for treatment of external multiple burns, sequence first the code that reflects the burn of the highest degree.

(b.) When a patient has both internal and external burns, the circumstances of admission govern the selection of the principal diagnosis or first-listed diagnosis.

(c.) When a patient is admitted for burn injuries and other related conditions such as smoke inhalation and/or respiratory failure, the circumstances of admission govern the selection of the principal or first-listed diagnosis.

2) Burns of the same local site

Classify burns of the same local site (three-digit category level, 940-947) but of different degrees to the subcategory identifying the highest degree recorded in the diagnosis.

3) Non-healing burns

Non-healing burns are coded as acute burns. Necrosis of burned skin should be coded as a non-healed burn.

4) Code 958.3, Posttraumatic wound infection

Assign code 958.3, Posttraumatic wound infection, not elsewhere classified, as an additional code for any documented infected burn site.

5) Assign separate codes for each burn site

When coding burns, assign separate codes for each burn site. Category 946 Burns of Multiple specified sites, should only be used if the location of the burns are not documented. Category 949, Burn, unspecified, is extremely vague and should rarely be used.

6) Assign codes from category 948, Burns

Burns classified according to extent of body surface involved, when the site of the burn is not specified or when there is a need for additional data. It is advisable to use category 948 as additional coding when needed to provide data for evaluating burn mortality, such as that needed by burn units. It is also advisable to use category 948 as an additional code for reporting purposes when there is mention of a third-degree burn involving 20 percent or more of the body surface.

In assigning a code from category 948:

- Fourth-digit codes are used to identify the percentage of total body surface involved in a burn (all degree).

- Fifth-digits are assigned to identify the percentage of body surface involved in third-degree burn.

- Fifth-digit zero (0) is assigned when less than 10 percent or when no body surface is involved in a third-degree burn.

Category 948 is based on the classic "rule of nines" in estimating body surface involved: head and neck are assigned nine percent, each arm nine percent, each leg 18 percent, the anterior trunk 18 percent, posterior trunk 18 percent, and genitalia one percent. Providers may change these percentage assignments where necessary to accommodate infants and children who have proportionally larger heads than adults and patients who have large buttocks, thighs, or abdomen that involve burns.

7) **Encounters for treatment of late effects of burns**

Encounters for the treatment of the late effects of burns (i.e., scars or joint contractures) should be coded to the residual condition (sequelae) followed by the appropriate late effect code (906.5-906.9). A late effect E code may also be used, if desired.

8) **Sequelae with a late effect code and current burn**

When appropriate, both a sequelae with a late effect code, and a current burn code may be assigned on the same record (when both a current burn and sequelae of an old burn exist).

d. **Coding of Debridement of Wound, Infection, or Burn**

Excisional debridement involves surgical removal or cutting away, as opposed to a mechanical (brushing, scrubbing, washing) debridement. For coding purposes, excisional debridement is assigned to code 86.22. Nonexcisional debridement is assigned to code 86.28

e. **Adverse Effects, Poisoning and Toxic Effects**

The properties of certain drugs, medicinal and biological substances or combinations of such substances, may cause toxic reactions. The occurrence of drug toxicity is classified in ICD-9-CM as follows:

1) **Adverse Effect**

When the drug was correctly prescribed and properly administered, code the reaction plus the appropriate code from the E930-E949 series. Codes from the E930-E949 series must be used to identify the causative substance for an adverse effect of drug, medicinal and biological substances, correctly prescribed and properly administered. The effect, such as tachycardia, delirium, gastrointestinal hemorrhaging, vomiting, hypokalemia, hepatitis, renal failure, or respiratory failure, is coded and followed by the appropriate code from the E930-E949 series.

Adverse effects of therapeutic substances correctly prescribed and properly administered (toxicity, synergistic reaction, side effect, and idiosyncratic reaction) may be due to (1) differences among patients, such as age, sex, disease, and genetic factors, and (2) drug-related factors, such as type of drug, route of administration, duration of therapy, dosage, and bioavailability.

2) Poisoning

(a) Error was made in drug prescription

Errors made in drug prescription or in the administration of the drug by provider, nurse, patient, or other person, use the appropriate poisoning code from the 960-979 series.

(b) Overdose of a drug intentionally taken

If an overdose of a drug was intentionally taken or administered and resulted in drug toxicity, it would be coded as a poisoning (960-979 series).

(c) Nonprescribed drug taken with correctly prescribed and properly administered drug

If a nonprescribed drug or medicinal agent was taken in combination with a correctly prescribed and properly administered drug, any drug toxicity or other reaction resulting from the interaction of the two drugs would be classified as a poisoning.

(d) Interaction of drug(s) and alcohol

When a reaction results from the interaction of a drug(s) and alcohol, this would be classified as poisoning.

(e) Sequencing of poisoning

When coding a poisoning or reaction to the improper use of a medication (e.g., wrong dose, wrong substance, wrong route of administration) the poisoning code is sequenced first, followed by a code for the manifestation. If there is also a diagnosis of drug abuse or dependence to the substance, the abuse or dependence is coded as an additional code. *See Section I.C.3.a.6.b. if poisoning is the result of insulin pump malfunctions and Section I.C.19 for general use of E-codes.*

3) Toxic Effects

(a) Toxic effect codes

When a harmful substance is ingested or comes in contact with a person, this is classified as a toxic effect. The toxic effect codes are in categories 980-989.

(b) Sequencing toxic effect codes

A toxic effect code should be sequenced first, followed by the code(s) that identify the result of the toxic effect.

(c) External cause codes for toxic effects

An external cause code from categories E860-E869 for accidental exposure, codes E950.6 or E950.7 for intentional self-harm, category E962 for assault, or categories E980-E982, for undetermined, should also be assigned to indicate intent.

f. Complications of care

1) Complications of care

(a) Documentation of complications of care

As with all procedural or postprocedural complications, code assignment is based on the provider's documentation of the relationship between the condition and the procedure.

2) Transplant complications

(a) Transplant complications other than kidney

Codes under subcategory 996.8, Complications of transplanted organ, are for use for both complications and rejection of transplanted organs. A transplant complication code is only assigned if the complication affects the function of the transplanted organ. Two codes are required to fully describe a transplant complication, the appropriate code from subcategory 996.8 and a secondary code that identifies the complication.

Pre-existing conditions or conditions that develop after the transplant are not coded as complications unless they affect the function of the transplanted organs.

See I.C.18.d.3) for transplant organ removal status. See I.C.2.i for malignant neoplasm associated with transplanted organ.

(b) Chronic kidney disease and kidney transplant complications

Patients who have undergone kidney transplant may still have some form of chronic kidney disease (CKD) because the kidney transplant may not fully restore kidney function. Code 996.81 should be assigned for documented complications of a kidney transplant, such as transplant failure or rejection or other transplant complication. Code 996.81 should not be assigned for post kidney transplant patients who have chronic kidney (CKD) unless a transplant complication such as transplant failure or rejection is documented. If the documentation is unclear as to whether the patient has a complication of the transplant, query the provider.

For patients with CKD following a kidney transplant, but who do not have a complication such as failure or rejection, *see section I.C.10.a.2, Chronic kidney disease and kidney transplant status*

3) Ventilator associated pneumonia

(a) Documentation of Ventilator associated pneumonia

As with all procedural or postprocedural complications, code assignment is based on the provider's documentation of the relationship between the condition and the procedure.

Code 997.31, Ventilator associated pneumonia, should be assigned only when the provider has documented ventilator associated pneumonia (VAP). An additional code to identify the organism (e.g., Pseudomonas aeruginosa, code 041.7) should also be assigned. Do not assign an additional code from categories 480-484 to identify the type of pneumonia.

Code 997.31 should not be assigned for cases where the patient has pneumonia and is on a mechanical ventilator but the provider has not specifically stated that the pneumonia is ventilator-associated pneumonia.

If the documentation is unclear as to whether the patient has a pneumonia that is a complication attributable to the mechanical ventilator, query the provider.

(b) Patient admitted with pneumonia and develops VAP

A patient may be admitted with one type of pneumonia (e.g., code 481, Pneumococcal pneumonia) and subsequently develop VAP. In this instance, the principal diagnosis would be the appropriate code from categories 480-484 for the pneumonia diagnosed at the time of admission. Code 997.31, Ventilator associated neumonia, would be assigned as an additional diagnosis when the provider has also documented the presence of ventilator associated pneumonia.

g. SIRS due to Non-infectious Process

The systemic inflammatory response syndrome (SIRS) can develop as a result of certain non-infectious disease processes, such as trauma, malignant neoplasm, or pancreatitis. When SIRS is documented with a noninfectious condition, and no subsequent infection is documented, the code for the underlying condition, such as an injury, should be assigned, followed by code 995.93, Systemic inflammatory response syndrome due to noninfectious process without acute organ dysfunction, or 995.94, Systemic inflammatory response syndrome due to non-infectious process with acute organ dysfunction.

If an acute organ dysfunction is documented, the appropriate code(s) for the associated acute organ dysfunction(s) should be assigned in addition to code 995.94. If acute organ dysfunction is documented, but it cannot be determined if the acute organ dysfunction is associated with SIRS or due to another condition (e.g., directly due to the trauma), the provider should be queried.

When the non-infectious condition has led to an infection that results in SIRS, *see Section I.C.Lb.12 for the guideline for sepsis and severe sepsis associated with a non-infectious process.*

18. Classification of Factors Influencing Health Status and Contact with Health Service (Supplemental V01-V91)

Note: The chapter specific guidelines provide additional information about the use of V codes for specified encounters.

a. Introduction

ICD-9-CM provides codes to deal with encounters for circumstances other than a disease or injury. The Supplementary Classification of Factors Influencing Health Status and Contact with Health Services (V01.0 - V91.99) is provided to deal with occasions when circumstances other than a disease or injury (codes 001-999) are recorded as a diagnosis or problem.

There are four primary circumstances for the use of V codes:

1) A person who is not currently sick encounters the health services for some specific reason, such as to act as an organ donor, to receive prophylactic care, such as inoculations or health screenings, or to receive counseling on health related issues.

2) A person with a resolving disease or injury, or a chronic, long term condition requiring continuous care, encounters the health care system for specific aftercare of that disease or injury (e.g., dialysis for renal disease; chemotherapy for malignancy; cast change). A diagnosis/symptom code should be used whenever a current, acute, diagnosis is being treated or a sign or symptom is being studied.

3) Circumstances or problems influence a person's health status but are not in themselves a current illness or injury.

4) Newborns, to indicate birth status

b. V codes use in any healthcare setting

V codes are for use in any healthcare setting. V codes may be used as either a first listed (principal diagnosis code in the inpatient setting) or secondary code, depending on the circumstances of the encounter. Certain V codes may only be used as first listed, others only as secondary codes.

See Section I.C.18.e, V Codes That May Only be Principal/ First-Listed Diagnosis.

c. **V Codes indicate a reason for an encounter**

They are not procedure codes. A corresponding procedure code must accompany a V code to describe the procedure performed.

d. **Categories of V Codes**

1) **Contact/Exposure**

Category V01 indicates contact with or exposure to communicable diseases. These codes are for patients who do not show any sign or symptom of a disease but have been exposed to it by close personal contact with an infected individual or are in an area where a disease is epidemic. These codes may be used as a first listed code to explain an encounter for testing, or, more commonly, as a secondary code to identify a potential risk.

2) **Inoculations and vaccinations**

Categories V03-V06 are for encounters for inoculations and vaccinations. They indicate that a patient is being seen to receive a prophylactic inoculation against a disease. The injection itself must be represented by the appropriate procedure code. A code from V03-V06 may be used as a secondary code if the inoculation is given as a routine part of preventive health care, such as a well-baby visit.

3) **Status**

Status codes indicate that a patient is a carrier of a disease, has the sequelae or residual of a past disease or condition, or has another factor influencing a person's health status. This includes such things as the presence of prosthetic or mechanical devices resulting from past treatment. A status code is informative, because the status may affect the course of treatment and its outcome. A status code is distinct from a history code. The history code indicates that the patient no longer has the condition.

A status code should not be used with a diagnosis code from one of the body system chapters, if the diagnosis code includes the information provided by the status code. For example, code V42.1, Heart transplant status, should not be used with code 996.83, Complications of transplanted heart. The status code does not provide additional information. The complication code indicates that the patient is a heart transplant patient.

The status V codes/categories are:

V02   Carrier or suspected carrier of infectious diseases

Carrier status indicates that a person harbors the specific organisms of a disease without manifest symptoms and is capable of transmitting the infection

V07.5x Use of agents affecting estrogen receptors and estrogen level

This code indicates when a patient is receiving a drug that affects estrogen receptors and estrogen levels for prevention of cancer.

V08   Asymptomatic HIV infection status

This code indicates that a patient has tested positive for HIV but has manifested no signs or symptoms of the disease.

V09   Infection with drug-resistant microorganisms

This category indicates that a patient has an infection that is resistant to drug treatment. Sequence the infection code first.

V21   Constitutional states in development

V22.2   Pregnant state, incidental

This code is a secondary code only for use when the pregnancy is in no way complicating the reason for visit. Otherwise, a code from the obstetric chapter is required.

V26.5x   Sterilization status

V42   Organ or tissue replaced by transplant

V43   Organ or tissue replaced by other means

V44   Artificial opening status

V45   Other postsurgical states

Assign code V45.87, Transplant organ removal status, to indicate that a transplanted organ has been previously removed. This code should not be assigned for the encounter in which the transplanted organ is removed. The complication necessitating removal of the transplant organ should be assigned for that encounter.

See section I.C17.f.2. for information on the coding of organ transplant complications.

Assign code V45.88, Status post administration of tPA (rtPA) in a different facility within the last 24 hours prior to admission to the current facility, as a secondary diagnosis when a patient is received by transfer into a facility and documentation indicates they were administered tissue plasminogen activator (tPA) within the last 24 hours prior to admission to the current facility.

This guideline applies even if the patient is still receiving the tPA at the time they are received into the current facility.

The appropriate code for the condition for which the tPA was administered (such as cerebrovascular disease or myocardial infarction) should be assigned first.

Code V45.88 is only applicable to the receiving facility record and not to the transferring facility record..

V46   Other dependence on machines

V49.6   Upper limb amputation status

V49.7   Lower limb amputation status

Note: Categories V42-V46, and subcategories V49.6, V49.7 are for use only if there are no complications or malfunctions of the organ or tissue replaced, the amputation site or the equipment on which the patient is dependent.

V49.81   Asymptomatic postmenopausal status (age-related) (natural)

V49.82   Dental sealant status

V49.83   Awaiting organ transplant status

V49.86   Do not resuscitate status

This code may be used when it is documented by the provider that a patient is on do not resuscitate status at any time during the stay.

V49.87   Physical restraint status

This code may be used when it is documented by the provider that a patient has been put in restraints during the current encounter. Please note that this code should not be reported when it is documented by the provider that a patient is temporarily restrained during a procedure.

V58.6x   Long-term (current) drug use

Codes from this subcategory indicate a patient's continuous use of a prescribed drug (including such things as aspirin therapy) for the long-term treatment of a condition or for prophylactic use. It is not for use for patients who have addictions to drugs. This subcategory is not for use of medications for detoxification or maintenance programs to prevent withdrawal symptoms in patients with drug dependence (e.g., methadone maintenance for opiate dependence). Assign the appropriate code for the drug dependence instead.

Assign a code from subcategory V58.6, Long-term (current) drug use, if the patient is receiving a medication for an extended period as a prophylactic measure (such as for the prevention of deep vein thrombosis) or as treatment of a chronic condition (such as arthritis) or a disease requiring a lengthy course of treatment (such as cancer). Do not assign a code from subcategory V58.6 for medication being administered for a brief period of time to treat an acute illness or injury (such as a course of antibiotics to treat acute bronchitis).

V83   Genetic carrier status

Genetic carrier status indicates that a person carries a gene, associated with a particular disease, which may be passed to offspring who may develop that disease. The person does not have the disease and is not at risk of developing the disease.

V84   Genetic susceptibility status

Genetic susceptibility indicates that a person has a gene that increases the risk of that person developing the disease.

Codes from category V84, Genetic susceptibility to disease, should not be used as principal or first-listed codes. If the patient has the condition to which he/she is susceptible, and that condition is the reason for the encounter, the code for the current condition should be sequenced first. If the patient is being seen for follow-up after completed treatment for this condition, and the condition no longer exists, a follow-up code should be sequenced first, followed by the appropriate personal history and genetic susceptibility codes. If the purpose of the encounter is genetic counseling associated with procreative management, a code from subcategory V26.3, Genetic counseling and testing, should be assigned as the first-listed code, followed by a code from category V84. Additional codes should be assigned for any applicable family or personal history.

See Section I.C. 18.d.14 for information on prophylactic organ removal due to a genetic susceptibility.

V85   Body Mass Index (BMI)

V86   Estrogen receptor status

V88   Acquired absence of other organs and tissue

V90   Retained foreign body

4) History (of)

There are two types of history V codes, personal and family. Personal history codes explain a patient's past medical condition that no longer exists and is not receiving any treatment, but that has the potential for recurrence, and therefore may require continued monitoring. The exceptions to this general rule are category V14, Personal history of allergy to medicinal agents, and subcategory V15.0, Allergy, other than to medicinal agents. A person who has had an allergic episode to a substance or food in the past should always be considered allergic to the substance.

Family history codes are for use when a patient has a family member(s) who has had a particular disease that causes the patient to be at higher risk of also contracting the disease.

Personal history codes may be used in conjunction with follow-up codes and family history codes may be used in conjunction with screening codes to explain the need for a test or procedure. History codes are also acceptable on any medical record regardless of the reason for visit. A history of an illness, even if no longer present, is important information that may alter the type of treatment ordered.

The history V code categories are:

V10   Personal history of malignant neoplasm

V12   Personal history of certain other diseases

V13   Personal history of other diseases

Except: V13.4, Personal history of arthritis, and subcategory V13.6, Personal history of congenital (corrected) malformations. These conditions are life-long so are not true history codes.

V14   Personal history of allergy to medicinal agents

V15   Other personal history presenting hazards to health
Except: V15.7, Personal history of contraception.

V16   Family history of malignant neoplasm

V17   Family history of certain chronic disabling diseases

V18   Family history of certain other specific diseases

V19   Family history of other conditions

V87   Other specified personal exposures and history presenting hazards to health

5) Screening

Screening is the testing for disease or disease precursors in seemingly well individuals so that early detection and treatment can be provided for those who test positive for the disease. Screenings that are recommended for many subgroups in a population include: routine mammograms for women over 40, a fecal occult blood test for everyone over 50, an amniocentesis to rule out a fetal anomaly for pregnant women over 35, because the incidence of breast cancer and colon cancer in these subgroups is higher than in the general population, as is the incidence of Down's syndrome in older mothers.

The testing of a person to rule out or confirm a suspected diagnosis because the patient has some sign or symptom is a diagnostic examination, not a screening. In these cases, the sign or symptom is used to explain the reason for the test. A screening code may be a first listed code if the reason for the visit is specifically the screening exam. It may also be used as an additional code if the screening is done during an office visit for other health problems. A screening code is not necessary if the screening is inherent to a routine examination, such as a pap smear done during a routine pelvic examination.

Should a condition be discovered during the screening then the code for the condition may be assigned as an additional diagnosis.

The V code indicates that a screening exam is planned. A procedure code is required to confirm that the screening was performed.

The screening V code categories:

V28   Antenatal screening

V73-V82 Special screening examinations

6)   Observation

There are three observation V code categories. They are for use in very limited circumstances when a person is being observed for a suspected condition that is ruled out. The observation codes are not for use if an injury or illness or any signs or symptoms related to the suspected condition are present. In such cases the diagnosis/symptom code is used with the corresponding E code to identify any external cause.

The observation codes are to be used as principal diagnosis only. The only exception to this is when the principal diagnosis is required to be a code from the V30, Live born infant, category. Then the V29 observation code is sequenced after the V30 code. Additional codes may be used in addition to the observation code but only if they are unrelated to the suspected condition being observed.

Codes from subcategory V89.0, Suspected maternal and fetal conditions not found, may either be used as a first listed or as an additional code assignment depending on the case. They are for use in very limited circumstances on a maternal record when an encounter is for a suspected maternal or fetal condition that is ruled out during that encounter (for example, a maternal or fetal condition may be suspected due to an abnormal test result). These codes should not be used when the condition is confirmed. In those cases, the confirmed condition should be coded. In addition, these codes are not for use if an illness or any signs or symptoms related to the suspected condition or problem are present. In such cases the diagnosis/symptom code is used.
Additional codes may be used in addition to the code from subcategory V89.0, but only if they are unrelated to the suspected condition being evaluated.

Codes from subcategory V89.0 may not be used for encounters for antenatal screening of mother. See Section I.C.18.d., Screening).

For encounters for suspected fetal condition that are inconclusive following testing and evaluation, assign the appropriate code from category 655, 656, 657 or 658.

The observation V code categories:

V29   Observation and evaluation of newborns for suspected condition not found

For the birth encounter, a code from category V30 should be sequenced before the V29 code.

V71   Observation and evaluation for suspected condition not found

V89   Suspected maternal and fetal conditions not found

7) Aftercare

Aftercare visit codes cover situations when the initial treatment of a disease or injury has been performed and the patient requires continued care during the healing or recovery phase, or for the long-term consequences of the disease. The aftercare V code should not be used if treatment is directed at a current, acute disease or injury. The diagnosis code is to be used in these cases. Exceptions to this rule are codes V58.0, Radiotherapy, and codes from subcategory V58.1, Encounter for chemotherapy and immunotherapy for neoplastic conditions. These codes are to be first listed, followed by the diagnosis code when a patient's encounter is solely to receive radiation therapy or chemotherapy for the treatment of a neoplasm. Should a patient receive both chemotherapy and radiation therapy during the same encounter code V58.0 and V58.1 may be used together on a record with either one being sequenced first.

The aftercare codes are generally first listed to explain the specific reason for the encounter. An aftercare code may be used as an additional code when some type of aftercare is provided in addition to the reason for admission and no diagnosis code is applicable. An example of this would be the closure of a colostomy during an encounter for treatment of another condition.

Aftercare codes should be used in conjunction with any other aftercare codes or other diagnosis codes to provide better detail on the specifics of an aftercare encounter visit, unless otherwise directed by the classification. The sequencing of multiple aftercare codes is discretionary.

Certain aftercare V code categories need a secondary diagnosis code to describe the resolving condition or sequelae, for others, the condition is inherent in the code title.

Additional V code aftercare category terms include fitting and adjustment, and attention to artificial openings.

Status V codes may be used with aftercare V codes to indicate the nature of the aftercare. For example code V45.81, Aortocoronary bypass status, may be used with code V58.73, Aftercare following surgery of the circulatory system, NEC, to indicate the surgery for which the aftercare is being performed. Also, a transplant status code may be used following code V58.44, Aftercare following organ transplant, to identify the organ transplanted. A status code should not be used when the aftercare code indicates the type of status, such as using V55.0, Attention to tracheostomy with V44.0, Tracheostomy status.*See Section I. B.16 Admissions/Encounter for Rehabilitation*

The aftercare V category/codes:

V51.0   Encounter for breast reconstruction following mastectomy

V52   Fitting and adjustment of prosthetic device and implant

V53   Fitting and adjustment of other device

V54   Other orthopedic aftercare

V55   Attention to artificial openings

V56   Encounter for dialysis and dialysis catheter care

V57   Care involving the use of rehabilitation procedures

V58.0   Radiotherapy

V58.11   Encounter for antineoplastic chemotherapy

V58.12   Encounter for antineoplastic immunotherapy

V58.3x   Attention to dressings and sutures

V58.41   Encounter for planned post-operative wound closure

V58.42   Aftercare, surgery, neoplasm

V58.43   Aftercare, surgery, trauma

V58.44   Aftercare involving organ transplant

V58.49   Other specified aftercare following surgery

V58.7x   Aftercare following surgery

V58.81   Fitting and adjustment of vascular catheter

V58.82   Fitting and adjustment of non-vascular catheter

V58.83   Monitoring therapeutic drug

V58.89   Other specified aftercare

8) Follow-up

The follow-up codes are used to explain continuing surveillance following completed treatment of a disease, condition, or injury. They imply that the condition has been fully treated and no longer exists. They should not be confused with aftercare codes that explain current treatment for a healing condition or its sequelae. Follow-up codes may be used in conjunction with history codes to provide the full picture of the healed condition and its treatment. The follow-up code is sequenced first, followed by the history code.

A follow-up code may be used to explain repeated visits. Should a condition be found to have recurred on the follow-up visit, then the diagnosis code should be used in place of the follow-up code.

The follow-up V code categories:

V24   Postpartum care and evaluation

V67   Follow-up examination

9) Donor

Category V59 is the donor codes. They are used for living individuals who are donating blood or other body tissue. These codes are only for individuals donating for others, not for self donations. They are not for use to identify cadaveric donations.

10) Counseling

Counseling V codes are used when a patient or family member receives assistance in the aftermath of an illness or injury, or when support is required in coping with family or social problems. They are not necessary for use in conjunction with a diagnosis code when the counseling component of care is considered integral to standard treatment.

The counseling V categories/codes:

V25.0   General counseling and advice for contraceptive management

V26.3   Genetic counseling

V26.4   General counseling and advice for procreative management

V61.x   Other family circumstances

V65.1   Person consulted on behalf of another person

V65.3   Dietary surveillance and counseling

V65.4   Other counseling, not elsewhere classified

11) Obstetrics and related conditions

See Section I.C.11., the Obstetrics guidelines for further instruction on the use of these codes.
V codes for pregnancy are for use in those circumstances when none of the problems or complications included in the codes from the Obstetrics chapter exist (a routine prenatal visit or postpartum care). Codes V22.0, Supervision of normal first pregnancy, and V22.1, Supervision of other normal pregnancy, are always first listed and are not to be used with any other code from the OB chapter.

The outcome of delivery, category V27, should be included on all maternal delivery records. It is always a secondary code. V codes for family planning (contraceptive) or procreative management and counseling should be included on an obstetric record either during the pregnancy or the postpartum stage, if applicable.
Obstetrics and related conditions V code categories:

V22   Normal pregnancy

V23   Supervision of high-risk pregnancy

Except: V23.2, Pregnancy with history of abortion. Code 646.3, Recurrent pregnancy loss, from the OB chapter is required to indicate a history of abortion during a pregnancy.

V24   Postpartum care and evaluation

V25   Encounter for contraceptive management

Except V25.0x
(See Section I.C.18.d.11, Counseling)

V26   Procreative management

Except V26.5x, Sterilization status, V26.3 and V26.4
(See Section I.C.18.d.11., Counseling)

V27   Outcome of delivery

V28   Antenatal screening

V91   Multiple gestation placenta status

(See Section I.C.18.d.6., Screening)

12) Newborn, infant and child

See Section I.C.15, the Newborn guidelines for further instruction on the use of these codes.

Newborn V code categories:

V20   Health supervision of infant or child

V29   Observation and evaluation of newborns for suspected condition not found

(See Section I.C.18.d.7, Observation)

V30-V39 Liveborn infant according to type of birth

13) Routine and administrative examinations

The V codes allow for the description of encounters for routine examinations, such as, a general check-up, or examinations for administrative purposes, such as a pre-employment physical. The codes are not to be used if the examination is for diagnosis of a suspected condition or for treatment purposes. In such cases the diagnosis code is used. During a routine exam, should a diagnosis or condition be discovered, it should be coded as an additional code. Pre-existing and chronic conditions and history codes may also be included as additional codes as long as the examination is for administrative purposes and not focused on any particular condition.

Pre-operative examination and pre-procedural laboratory examination V codes are for use only in those situations when a patient is being cleared for a procedure or surgery and no treatment is given.

The V codes categories/code for routine and administrative examinations:

V20.2 Routine infant or child health check

Any injections given should have a corresponding procedure code.

V70 General medical examination

V72 Special investigations and examinations

Codes V72.5 and V72.62 may be used if the reason for the patient encounter is for routine laboratory/radiology testing in the absence of any signs, symptoms, or associated diagnosis. If routine testing is performed during the same encounter as a test to evaluate a sign, symptom, or diagnosis, it is appropriate to assign both the V code and the code describing the reason for the non-routine test.

14) Miscellaneous V codes

The miscellaneous V codes capture a number of other health care encounters that do not fall into one of the other categories. Certain of these codes identify the reason for the encounter, others are for use as additional codes that provide useful information on circumstances that may affect a patient's care and treatment.

Prophylactic Organ Removal

For encounters specifically for prophylactic removal of breasts, ovaries, or another organ due to a genetic susceptibility to cancer or a family history of cancer, the principal or first listed code should be a code from subcategory V50.4, Prophylactic organ removal, followed by the appropriate genetic susceptibility code and the appropriate family history code. If the patient has a malignancy of one site and is having prophylactic removal at another site to prevent either a new primary malignancy or metastatic disease, a code for the malignancy should also be assigned in addition to a code from subcategory V50.4. A V50.4 code should not be assigned if the patient is having organ removal for treatment of a malignancy, such as the removal of the testes for the treatment of prostate cancer.

Miscellaneous V code categories/codes:

V07 Need for isolation and other prophylactic or treatment measures

Except V07.5X, Use of agents affecting estrogen receptors and estrogen levels

V50 Elective surgery for purposes other than remedying health states

V58.5   Orthodontics

V60   Housing, household, and economic circumstances

V62   Other psychosocial circumstances

V63   Unavailability of other medical facilities for care

V64   Persons encountering health services for specific procedures, not carried out

V66   Convalescence and Palliative Care

V68   Encounters for administrative purposes

V69   Problems related to lifestyle

15) Nonspecific V codes

Certain V codes are so non-specific, or potentially redundant with other codes in the classification, that there can be little justification for their use in the inpatient setting. Their use in the outpatient setting should be limited to those instances when there is no further documentation to permit more precise coding. Otherwise, any sign or symptom or any other reason for visit that is captured in another code should be used.

Nonspecific V code categories/codes:

V11   Personal history of mental disorder

         A code from the mental disorders chapter, with an in remission fifth-digit, should be used.

V13.4   Personal history of arthritis

V13.6   Personal history of congenital malformations

V15.7   Personal history of contraception

V23.2   Pregnancy with history of abortion

V40   Mental and behavioral problems

V41   Problems with special senses and other special functions

V47   Other problems with internal organs

V48   Problems with head, neck, and trunk

V49   Problems with limbs and other problems
         Exceptions:

         V49.6   Upper limb amputation status

         V49.7   Lower limb amputation status

          V49.81 Asymptomatic postmenopausal status (age-related) (natural)

          V49.82 Dental sealant status

          V49.83 Awaiting organ transplant status

          V49.86 Do not resuscitate status

          V49.87 Physical restraints status

V51.8   Other aftercare involving the use of plastic surgery

V58.2   Blood transfusion, without reported diagnosis

V58.9   Unspecified aftercare

See Section IV.K. and Section IV.L. of the Outpatient guidelines.

e. V Codes That May Only be Principal/First-Listed Diagnosis

The list of V codes/categories below may only be reported as the principal/first-listed diagnosis, except when there are multiple encounters on the same day and the medical records for the encounters are combined or when there is more than one V code that meets the definition of principal diagnosis (e.g., a patient is admitted to home healthcare for both aftercare and rehabilitation and they equally meet the definition of principal diagnosis). These codes should not be reported if they do not meet the definition of principal or first-listed diagnosis.

See Section II and Section IV. A for information on selection of principal and first-listed diagnosis.

See Section II. C for information on two or more diagnoses that equally meet the definition for principal diagnosis.

V20.X   Health supervision of infant or child

V22.0   Supervision of normal first pregnancy

V22.1   Supervision of other normal pregnancy

V24.X   Postpartum care and examination

V26.81 Encounter for assisted reproductive fertility procedure cycle

V26.82 Encounter for fertility preservation procedure

V30.X   Single liveborn

V31.X   Twin, mate liveborn

V32.X   Twin, mate stillborn

V33.X   Twin, unspecified

V34.X   Other multiple, mates all liveborn

V35.X   Other multiple, mates all stillborn

V36.X   Other multiple, mates live- and stillborn

V37.X   Other multiple, unspecified
V39.X   Unspecified

V46.12 Encounter for respirator dependence during power failure

V46.13 Encounter for weaning from respirator [ventilator]

V51.0   Encounter for breast reconstruction following mastectomy

V56.0   Extracorporeal dialysis

V57.X   Care involving use of rehabilitation procedures

V58.0   Radiotherapy

V58.11 Encounter for antineoplastic chemotherapy

V58.12 Encounter for antineoplastic immunotherapy

V59.X   Donors

V66.0   Convalescence and palliative care following surgery

V66.1   Convalescence and palliative care following radiotherapy

V66.2   Convalescence and palliative care following chemotherapy

V66.3   Convalescence and palliative care following psychotherapy and other treatment for mental disorder

V66.4   Convalescence and palliative care following treatment of fracture

V66.5   Convalescence and palliative care following other treatment

V66.6   Convalescence and palliative care following combined treatment

V66.9   Unspecified convalescence

V68.X   Encounters for administrative purposes

V70.0   Routine general medical examination at a health care facility

V70.1   General psychiatric examination, requested by the authority

V70.2   General psychiatric examination, other and unspecified

V70.3   Other medical examination for administrative purposes

V70.4   Examination for medicolegal reasons

V70.5   Health examination of defined subpopulations

V70.6   Health examination in population surveys

V70.8　Other specified general medical examinations

V70.9　Unspecified general medical examination

V71.X　Observation and evaluation for suspected conditions not found

19. Supplemental Classification of External Causes of Injury and Poisoning (E-codes, E800-E999)

Introduction

These guidelines are provided for those who are currently collecting E codes in order that there will be standardization in the process. If your institution plans to begin collecting E codes, these guidelines are to be applied. The use of E codes is supplemental to the application of ICD-9-CM diagnosis codes.

External causes of injury and poisoning codes (categories E000 and E800-E999) are intended to provide data for injury research and evaluation of injury prevention strategies. Activity codes (categories E001-E030) are intended to be used to describe the activity of a person seeking care for injuries as well as other health conditions, when the injury or other health condition resulted from an activity or the activity contributed to a condition. E codes capture how the injury, poisoning, or adverse effect happened (cause), the intent (unintentional or accidental; or intentional, such as suicide or assault), the person's status (e.g. civilian, military), the associated activity and the place where the event occurred.

Some major categories of E codes include:

> transport accidents
> poisoning and adverse effects of drugs, medicinal substances and biologicals
> accidental falls
> accidents caused by fire and flames
> accidents due to natural and environmental factors
> late effects of accidents, assaults or self injury
> assaults or purposely inflicted injury
> suicide or self inflicted injury

These guidelines apply for the coding and collection of E codes from records in hospitals, outpatient clinics, emergency departments, other ambulatory care settings and provider offices, and nonacute care settings, except when other specific guidelines apply.

a.　General E Code Coding Guidelines

1)　Used with any code in the range of 001-V91

An E code from categories E800-E999 may be used with any code in the range of 001-V91, which indicates an injury, poisoning, or adverse effect due to an external cause.

An activity E code (categories E001-E030) may be used with any code in the range of 001-V91 that indicates an injury, or other health condition that resulted from an activity, or the activity contributed to a condition.

2) **Assign the appropriate E code for all initial treatment**

Assign the appropriate E code for the initial encounter of an injury, poisoning, or adverse effect of drugs, not for subsequent treatment.

External cause of injury codes (E-codes) may be assigned while the acute fracture codes are still applicable.

See Section I.C.17.b.1 for coding of acute fractures.

3) **Use the full range of E codes**

Use the full range of E codes (E800 - E999) to completely describe the cause, the intent and the place of occurrence, if applicable, for all injuries, poisonings, and adverse effects of drugs.

See a.1.), j.), and k.) in this section for information on the use of status and activity E codes.

4) **Assign as many E codes as necessary**

Assign as many E codes as necessary to fully explain each cause.

5) **The selection of the appropriate E code**

The selection of the appropriate E code is guided by the Index to External Causes, which is located after the alphabetical index to diseases and by Inclusion and Exclusion notes in the Tabular List.

6) **E code can never be a principal diagnosis**

An E code can never be a principal (first listed) diagnosis.

7) **External cause code(s) with systemic inflammatory response syndrome (SIRS)**

An external cause code is not appropriate with a code from subcategory 995.9, unless the patient also has another condition for which an E code would be appropriate (such as an injury, poisoning, or adverse effect of drugs.

8) **Multiple Cause E Code Coding Guidelines**

More than one E-code is required to fully describe the external cause of an illness, injury or poisoning. The assignment of E-codes should be sequenced in the following priority:

If two or more events cause separate injuries, an E code should be assigned for each cause. The first listed E code will be selected in the following order:

E codes for child and adult abuse take priority over all other E codes.

See Section I.C.19.e., Child and Adult abuse guidelines.

E codes for terrorism events take priority over all other E codes except child and adult abuse.

E codes for cataclysmic events take priority over all other E codes except child and adult abuse and terrorism.

E codes for transport accidents take priority over all other E codes except cataclysmic events, child and adult abuse and terrorism. Activity and external cause status codes are assigned following all causal (intent) E codes.

The first-listed E code should correspond to the cause of the most serious diagnosis due to an assault, accident, or self-harm, following the order of hierarchy listed above.

9) If the reporting format limits the number of E codes

If the reporting format limits the number of E codes that can be used in reporting clinical data, report the code for the cause/intent most related to the principal diagnosis. If the format permits capture of additional E codes, the cause/intent, including medical misadventures, of the additional events should be reported rather than the codes for place, activity or external status.

b. Place of Occurrence Guideline

Use an additional code from category E849 to indicate the Place of Occurrence. The Place of Occurrence describes the place where the event occurred and not the patient's activity at the time of the event.

Do not use E849.9 if the place of occurrence is not stated.

c. Adverse Effects of Drugs, Medicinal and Biological Substances Guidelines

1) Do not code directly from the Table of Drugs

Do not code directly from the Table of Drugs and Chemicals. Always refer back to the Tabular List.

2) Use as many codes as necessary to describe

Use as many codes as necessary to describe completely all drugs, medicinal or biological substances.

If the reporting format limits the number of E codes, and there are different fourth digit codes in the same three digit category, use the code for "Other specified" of that category of drugs, medicinal or biological substances. If there is no "Other specified" code in that category, use the appropriate "Unspecified" code in that category.

If the reporting format limits the number of E codes, and the codes are in different three digit categories, assign the appropriate E code for other multiple drugs and medicinal substances.

3) If the same E code would describe the causative agent

If the same E code would describe the causative agent for more than one adverse reaction, assign the code only once.

4) If two or more drugs, medicinal or biological substances

If two or more drugs, medicinal or biological substances are reported, code each individually unless the combination code is listed in the Table of Drugs and Chemicals. In that case, assign the E code for the combination.

5) When a reaction results from the interaction of a drug(s)

When a reaction results from the interaction of a drug(s) and alcohol, use poisoning codes and E codes for both.

6) Codes from the E930-E949 series

Codes from the E930-E949 series must be used to identify the causative substance for an adverse effect of drug, medicinal and biological substances, correctly prescribed and properly administered. The effect, such as tachycardia, delirium, gastrointestinal hemorrhaging, vomiting, hypokalemia, hepatitis, renal failure, or respiratory failure, is coded and followed by the appropriate code from the E930-E949 series.

d. Child and Adult Abuse Guideline

1) Intentional injury

When the cause of an injury or neglect is intentional child or adult abuse, the first listed E code should be assigned from categories E960-E968, Homicide and injury purposely inflicted by other persons, (except category E967). An E code from category E967, Child and adult battering and other maltreatment, should be added as an additional code to identify the perpetrator, if known.

2) Accidental intent

In cases of neglect when the intent is determined to be accidental E code E904.0, Abandonment or neglect of infant and helpless person, should be the first listed E code.

e. Unknown or Suspected Intent Guideline

1) If the intent (accident, self-harm, assault) of the cause of an injury or poisoning is unknown

If the intent (accident, self-harm, assault) of the cause of an injury or poisoning is unknown or unspecified, code the intent as undetermined E980-E989.

2) If the intent (accident, self-harm, assault) of the cause of an injury or poisoning is questionable

If the intent (accident, self-harm, assault) of the cause of an injury or poisoning is questionable, probable or suspected, code the intent as undetermined E980-E989.

f. Undetermined Cause

When the intent of an injury or poisoning is known, but the cause is unknown, use codes: E928.9, Unspecified accident, E958.9, Suicide and self-inflicted injury by unspecified means, and E968.9, Assault by unspecified means.

These E codes should rarely be used, as the documentation in the medical record, in both the inpatient outpatient and other settings, should normally provide sufficient detail to determine the cause of the injury.

g. Late Effects of External Cause Guidelines

1) Late effect E codes

Late effect E codes exist for injuries and poisonings but not for adverse effects of drugs, misadventures and surgical complications.

2) Late effect E codes (E929, E959, E969, E977, E989, or E999.1)

A late effect E code (E929, E959, E969, E977, E989, or E999.1) should be used with any report of a late effect or sequela resulting from a previous injury or poisoning (905-909).

3) Late effect E code with a related current injury

A late effect E code should never be used with a related current nature of injury code.

4) Use of late effect E codes for subsequent visits

Use a late effect E code for subsequent visits when a late effect of the initial injury or poisoning is being treated. There is no late effect E code for adverse effects of drugs.

Do not use a late effect E code for subsequent visits for follow-up care (e.g., to assess healing, to receive rehabilitative therapy) of the injury or poisoning when no late effect of the injury has been documented.

h. Misadventures and Complications of Care Guidelines

1) Code range E870-E876

Assign a code in the range of E870-E876 if misadventures are stated by the provider. When applying the E code guidelines pertaining to sequencing, these E codes are considered causal codes.

2) Code range E878-E879

Assign a code in the range of E878-E879 if the provider attributes an abnormal reaction or later complication to a surgical or medical procedure, but does not mention misadventure at the time of the procedure as the cause of the reaction.

i. Terrorism Guidelines

1) Cause of injury identified by the Federal Government (FBI) as terrorism

When the cause of an injury is identified by the Federal Government (FBI) as terrorism, the first-listed E-code should be a code from category E979, Terrorism. The definition of terrorism employed by the FBI is found at the inclusion note at E979. The terrorism E-code is the only E-code that should be assigned. Additional E codes from the assault categories should not be assigned.

2) Cause of an injury is suspected to be the result of terrorism

When the cause of an injury is suspected to be the result of terrorism a code from category E979 should not be assigned. Assign a code in the range of E codes based circumstances on the documentation of intent and mechanism.

3) Code E979.9, Terrorism, secondary effects

Assign code E979.9, Terrorism, secondary effects, for conditions occurring subsequent to the terrorist event. This code should not be assigned for conditions that are due to the initial terrorist act.

4) Statistical tabulation of terrorism codes

For statistical purposes these codes will be tabulated within the category for assault, expanding the current category from E960-E969 to include E979 and E999.1.

j. Activity Code Guidelines

Assign a code from category E001-E030 to describe the activity that caused or contributed to the injury or other health condition.

Unlike other E codes, activity E codes may be assigned to indicate a health condition (not just injuries) resulted from an activity, or the activity contributed to the condition. The activity codes are not applicable to poisonings, adverse effects, misadventures or late effects.

Do not assign E030, Unspecified activity, if the activity is not stated.

k. External cause status

A code from category E000, External cause status, should be assigned whenever any other E code is assigned for an encounter, including an Activity E code, except for the events noted below. Assign a code from category E000, External cause status, to indicate the work status of the person at the time the event occurred. The status code indicates whether the event occurred during military activity, whether a non-military person was at work, whether an individual including a student or volunteer was involved in a non-work activity at the time of the causal event.

A code from E000, External cause status, should be assigned, when applicable, with other external cause codes, such as transport accidents and falls. The external cause status codes are not applicable to poisonings, adverse effects, misadventures or late effects.

Do not assign a code from category E000 if no other E codes (cause, activity) are applicable for the encounter.

Do not assign code E000.9, Unspecified external cause status, if the status is not stated.

SECTION II. SELECTION OF PRINCIPAL DIAGNOSIS

The circumstances of inpatient admission always govern the selection of principal diagnosis. The principal diagnosis is defined in the Uniform Hospital Discharge Data Set (UHDDS) as "that condition established after study to be chiefly responsible for occasioning the admission of the patient to the hospital for care."

The UHDDS definitions are used by hospitals to report inpatient data elements in a standardized manner. These data elements and their definitions can be found in the July 31, 1985, Federal Register (Vol. 50, No, 147), pp. 31038-40.

Since that time the application of the UHDDS definitions has been expanded to include all non-outpatient settings (acute care, short term, long term care and psychiatric hospitals; home health agencies; rehab facilities; nursing homes, etc).

In determining principal diagnosis the coding conventions in the ICD-9-CM, Volumes I and II take precedence over these official coding guidelines.

(See Section I. A., Conventions for the ICD-9-CM)

The importance of consistent, complete documentation in the medical record cannot be overemphasized. Without such documentation the application of all coding guidelines is a difficult, if not impossible, task.

A. Codes for symptoms, signs, and ill-defined conditions

Codes for symptoms, signs, and ill-defined conditions from Chapter 16 are not to be used as principal diagnosis when a related definitive diagnosis has been established.

B. Two or more interrelated conditions, each potentially meeting the definition for principal diagnosis.

When there are two or more interrelated conditions (such as diseases in the same ICD-9-CM chapter or manifestations characteristically associated with a certain disease) potentially meeting the definition of principal diagnosis, either condition may be sequenced first, unless the circumstances of the admission, the therapy provided, the Tabular List, or the Alphabetic Index indicate otherwise.

C. Two or more diagnoses that equally meet the definition for principal diagnosis

In the unusual instance when two or more diagnoses equally meet the criteria for principal diagnosis as determined by the circumstances of admission, diagnostic workup and/or therapy provided, and the Alphabetic Index, Tabular List, or another coding guidelines does not provide sequencing direction, any one of the diagnoses may be sequenced first.

D. Two or more comparative or contrasting conditions.

In those rare instances when two or more contrasting or comparative diagnoses are documented as "either/or" (or similar terminology), they are coded as if the diagnoses were confirmed and the diagnoses are sequenced according to the circumstances of the admission. If no further determination can be made as to which diagnosis should be principal, either diagnosis may be sequenced first.

E. A symptom(s) followed by contrasting/comparative diagnoses

When a symptom(s) is followed by contrasting/comparative diagnoses, the symptom code is sequenced first. All the contrasting/comparative diagnoses should be coded as additional diagnoses.

F. Original treatment plan not carried out

Sequence as the principal diagnosis the condition, which after study occasioned the admission to the hospital, even though treatment may not have been carried out due to unforeseen circumstances.

G. Complications of surgery and other medical care

When the admission is for treatment of a complication resulting from surgery or other medical care, the complication code is sequenced as the principal diagnosis. If the complication is classified to the 996-999 series and the code lacks the necessary specificity in describing the complication, an additional code for the specific complication should be assigned.

H. Uncertain Diagnosis

If the diagnosis documented at the time of discharge is qualified as "probable", "suspected", "likely", "questionable", "possible", or "still to be ruled out", or other similar terms indicating uncertainty, code the condition as if it existed or was established. The bases for these guidelines are the diagnostic workup, arrangements for further workup or observation, and initial therapeutic approach that correspond most closely with the established diagnosis.

Note: This guideline is applicable only to inpatient admissions to short-term, acute, long-term care and psychiatric hospitals.

I. Admission from Observation Unit

1. Admission Following Medical Observation

When a patient is admitted to an observation unit for a medical condition, which either worsens or does not improve, and is subsequently admitted as an inpatient of the same hospital for this same medical condition, the principal diagnosis would be the medical condition which led to the hospital admission.

2. Admission Following Post-Operative Observation

When a patient is admitted to an observation unit to monitor a condition (or complication) that develops following outpatient surgery, and then is subsequently admitted as an inpatient of the same hospital, hospitals should apply the Uniform Hospital Discharge Data Set (UHDDS) definition of principal diagnosis as "that condition established after study to be chiefly responsible for occasioning the admission of the patient to the hospital for care."

J. Admission from Outpatient Surgery

When a patient receives surgery in the hospital's outpatient surgery department and is subsequently admitted for continuing inpatient care at the same hospital, the following guidelines should be followed in selecting the principal diagnosis for the inpatient admission:

■ If the reason for the inpatient admission is a complication, assign the complication as the principal diagnosis.

■ If no complication, or other condition, is documented as the reason for the inpatient admission, assign the reason for the outpatient surgery as the principal diagnosis.

■ If the reason for the inpatient admission is another condition unrelated to the surgery, assign the unrelated condition as the principal diagnosis.

SECTION III. REPORTING ADDITIONAL DIAGNOSES

General Rules For Other (Additional) Diagnoses

For reporting purposes the definition for "other diagnoses" is interpreted as additional conditions that affect patient care in terms of requiring:

clinical evaluation; or
therapeutic treatment; or
diagnostic procedures; or
extended length of hospital stay; or
increased nursing care and/or monitoring.

The UHDDS item #11-b defines Other Diagnoses as "all conditions that coexist at the time of admission, that develop subsequently, or that affect the treatment received and/or the length of stay. Diagnoses that relate to an earlier episode which have no bearing on the current hospital stay are to be excluded." UHDDS definitions apply to inpatients in acute care, short-term, long term care and psychiatric hospital setting. The UHDDS definitions are used by acute care short- term hospitals to report inpatient data elements in a standardized manner. These data elements and their definitions can be found in the July 31, 1985, Federal Register (Vol. 50, No, 147), pp. 31038-40.

Since that time the application of the UHDDS definitions has been expanded to include all non-outpatient settings (acute care, short term, long term care and psychiatric hospitals; home health agencies; rehab facilities; nursing homes, etc).

The following guidelines are to be applied in designating "other diagnoses" when neither the Alphabetic Index nor the Tabular List in ICD-9-CM provide direction. The listing of the diagnoses in the patient record is the responsibility of the attending provider.

A. Previous conditions

If the provider has included a diagnosis in the final diagnostic statement, such as the discharge summary or the face sheet, it should ordinarily be coded. Some providers include in the diagnostic statement resolved conditions or diagnoses and status-post procedures from previous admission that have no bearing on the current stay. Such conditions are not to be reported and are coded only if required by hospital policy.

However, history codes (V10-V19) may be used as secondary codes if the historical condition or family history has an impact on current care or influences treatment.

B. Abnormal findings

Abnormal findings (laboratory, x-ray, pathologic, and other diagnostic results) are not coded and reported unless the provider indicates their clinical significance. If the findings are outside the normal range and the attending provider has ordered other tests to evaluate the condition or prescribed treatment, it is appropriate to ask the provider whether the abnormal finding should be added.

Please note: This differs from the coding practices in the outpatient setting for coding encounters for diagnostic tests that have been interpreted by a provider.

C. Uncertain Diagnosis

If the diagnosis documented at the time of discharge is qualified as "probable", "suspected", "likely", "questionable", "possible", or "still to be ruled out" or other similar terms indicating uncertainty, code the condition as if it existed or was established. The bases for these guidelines are the diagnostic workup, arrangements for further workup or observation, and initial therapeutic approach that correspond most closely with the established diagnosis.

Note: This guideline is applicable only to inpatient admissions to short-term, acute, long-term care and psychiatric hospitals.

SECTION IV. DIAGNOSTIC CODING AND REPORTING GUIDELINES FOR OUTPATIENT SERVICES

These coding guidelines for outpatient diagnoses have been approved for use by hospitals/providers in coding and reporting hospital-based outpatient services and provider-based office visits.

Information about the use of certain abbreviations, punctuation, symbols, and other conventions used in the ICD-9-CM Tabular List (code numbers and titles), can be found in Section IA of these guidelines, under "Conventions Used in the Tabular List." Information about the correct sequence to use in finding a code is also described in Section I.

The terms encounter and visit are often used interchangeably in describing outpatient service contacts and, therefore, appear together in these guidelines without distinguishing one from the other.

Though the conventions and general guidelines apply to all settings, coding guidelines for outpatient and provider reporting of diagnoses will vary in a number of instances from those for inpatient diagnoses, recognizing that:

The Uniform Hospital Discharge Data Set (UHDDS) definition of principal diagnosis applies only to inpatients in acute, short-term, long-term care and psychiatric hospitals.

Coding guidelines for inconclusive diagnoses (probable, suspected, rule out, etc.) were developed for inpatient reporting and do not apply to outpatients.

A. Selection of first-listed condition

In the outpatient setting, the term first-listed diagnosis is used in lieu of principal diagnosis.

In determining the first-listed diagnosis the coding conventions of ICD-9-CM, as well as the general and disease specific guidelines take precedence over the outpatient guidelines.

Diagnoses often are not established at the time of the initial encounter/visit. It may take two or more visits before the diagnosis is confirmed.

The most critical rule involves beginning the search for the correct code assignment through the Alphabetic Index. Never begin searching initially in the Tabular List as this will lead to coding errors.

1. Outpatient Surgery

When a patient presents for outpatient surgery, code the reason for the surgery as the first-listed diagnosis (reason for the encounter), even if the surgery is not performed due to a contraindication.

2. Observation Stay

When a patient is admitted for observation for a medical condition, assign a code for the medical condition as the first-listed diagnosis.

When a patient presents for outpatient surgery and develops complications requiring admission to observation, code the reason for the surgery as the first reported diagnosis (reason for the encounter), followed by codes for the complications as secondary diagnoses.

B. Codes from 001.0 through V91

The appropriate code or codes from 001.0 through V91.99 must be used to identify diagnoses, symptoms, conditions, problems, complaints, or other reason(s) for the encounter/visit.

C. Accurate reporting of ICD-9-CM diagnosis codes

For accurate reporting of ICD-9-CM diagnosis codes, the documentation should describe the patient's condition, using terminology which includes specific diagnoses as well as symptoms, problems, or reasons for the encounter. There are ICD-9-CM codes to describe all of these.

D. Selection of codes 001.0 through 999.9

The selection of codes 001.0 through 999.9 will frequently be used to describe the reason for the encounter. These codes are from the section of ICD-9-CM for the classification of diseases and injuries (e.g. infectious and parasitic diseases; neoplasms; symptoms, signs, and ill-defined conditions, etc.).

E. Codes that describe symptoms and signs

Codes that describe symptoms and signs, as opposed to diagnoses, are acceptable for reporting purposes when a diagnosis has not been established (confirmed) by the provider. Chapter 16 of ICD-9-CM, Symptoms, Signs, and Ill-defined conditions (codes 780.0-799.9) contain many, but not all codes for symptoms.

F. Encounters for circumstances other than a disease or injury

ICD-9-CM provides codes to deal with encounters for circumstances other than a disease or injury. The Supplementary Classification of factors Influencing Health Status and Contact with Health Services (V01.0-V89) is provided to deal with occasions when circumstances other than a disease or injury are recorded as diagnosis or problems. See Section I.C. 18for information on V-codes.

G. Level of Detail in Coding

1. ICD-9-CM codes with 3, 4, or 5 digits

ICD-9-CM is composed of codes with either 3, 4, or 5 digits. Codes with three digits are included in ICD-9-CM as the heading of a category of codes that may be further subdivided by the use of fourth and/or fifth digits, which provide greater specificity.

2. Use of full number of digits required for a code

A three-digit code is to be used only if it is not further subdivided. Where fourth-digit subcategories and/or fifth-digit subclassifications are provided, they must be assigned. A code is invalid if it has not been coded to the full number of digits required for that code.

See also discussion under Section I.b.3., General Coding Guidelines, Level of Detail in Coding.

H. ICD-9-CM code for the diagnosis, condition, problem, or other reason for encounter/visit

List first the ICD-9-CM code for the diagnosis, condition, problem, or other reason for encounter/visit shown in the medical record to be chiefly responsible for the services provided. List additional codes that describe any coexisting conditions. In some cases the first-listed diagnosis may be a symptom when a diagnosis has not been established (confirmed) by the physician.

I. Uncertain diagnosis

Do not code diagnoses documented as "probable", "suspected," "questionable," "rule out," or "working diagnosis" or other similar terms indicating uncertainty. Rather, code the condition(s) to the highest degree of certainty for that encounter/visit, such as symptoms, signs, abnormal test results, or other reason for the visit.

Please note: This differs from the coding practices used by short-term, acute care, long-term care and psychiatric hospitals.

J. Chronic diseases

Chronic diseases treated on an ongoing basis may be coded and reported as many times as the patient receives treatment and care for the condition(s)

K. Code all documented conditions that coexist

Code all documented conditions that coexist at the time of the encounter/visit, and require or affect patient care treatment or management. Do not code conditions that were previously treated and no longer exist. However, history codes (V10-V19) may be used as secondary codes if the historical condition or family history has an impact on current care or influences treatment.

L. Patients receiving diagnostic services only

For patients receiving diagnostic services only during an encounter/visit, sequence first the diagnosis, condition, problem, or other reason for encounter/visit shown in the medical record to be chiefly responsible for the outpatient services provided during the encounter/visit. Codes for other diagnoses (e.g., chronic conditions) may be sequenced as additional diagnoses.

For encounters for routine laboratory/radiology testing in the absence of any signs, symptoms, or associated diagnosis, assign V72.5 and a code from subcategory V72.6. If routine testing is performed during the same encounter as a test to evaluate a sign, symptom, or diagnosis, it is appropriate to assign both the V code and the code describing the reason for the non-routine test.

For outpatient encounters for diagnostic tests that have been interpreted by a physician, and the final report is available at the time of coding, code any confirmed or definitive diagnosis(es) documented in the interpretation. Do not code related signs and symptoms as additional diagnoses.

Please note: This differs from the coding practice in the hospital inpatient setting regarding abnormal findings on test results.

M. Patients receiving therapeutic services only

For patients receiving therapeutic services only during an encounter/visit, sequence first the diagnosis, condition, problem, or other reason for encounter/visit shown in the medical record to be chiefly responsible for the outpatient services provided during the encounter/visit. Codes for other diagnoses (e.g., chronic conditions) may be sequenced as additional diagnoses.

The only exception to this rule is that when the primary reason for the admission/encounter is chemotherapy, radiation therapy, or rehabilitation, the appropriate V code for the service is listed first, and the diagnosis or problem for which the service is being performed listed second.

N. Patients receiving preoperative evaluations only

For patients receiving preoperative evaluations only, sequence first a code from category V72.8, Other specified examinations, to describe the pre-op consultations. Assign a code for the condition to describe the reason for the surgery as an additional diagnosis. Code also any findings related to the pre-op evaluation.

O. Ambulatory surgery

For ambulatory surgery, code the diagnosis for which the surgery was performed. If the postoperative diagnosis is known to be different from the preoperative diagnosis at the time the diagnosis is confirmed, select the postoperative diagnosis for coding, since it is the most definitive.

P. Routine outpatient prenatal visits

For routine outpatient prenatal visits when no complications are present, codes V22.0, Supervision of normal first pregnancy, or V22.1, Supervision of other normal pregnancy, should be used as the principal diagnosis. These codes should not be used in conjunction with chapter 11 codes.

APPENDIX I

Present On Admission (POA) Reporting Guidelines

Introduction

These guidelines are to be used as a supplement to the ICD-9-CM Official Guidelines for Coding and Reporting to facilitate the assignment of the Present on Admission (POA) indicator for each diagnosis and external cause of injury code reported on claim forms (UB-04 and 837 Institutional).

These guidelines are not intended to replace any guidelines in the main body of the ICD-9-CM Official Guidelines for Coding and Reporting. The POA guidelines are not intended to provide guidance on when a condition should be coded, but rather, how to apply the POA indicator to the final set of diagnosis codes that have been assigned in accordance with Sections I, II, and III of the official coding guidelines. Subsequent to the assignment of the ICD-9-CM codes, the POA indicator should then be assigned to those conditions that have been coded.

As stated in the Introduction to the ICD-9-CM Official Guidelines for Coding and Reporting, a joint effort between the healthcare provider and the coder is essential to achieve complete and accurate documentation, code assignment, and reporting of diagnoses and procedures. The importance of consistent, complete documentation in the medical record cannot be overemphasized. Medical record documentation from any provider involved in the care and treatment of the patient may be used to support the determination of whether a condition was present on admission or not. In the context of the official coding guidelines, the term "provider" means a physician or any qualified healthcare practitioner who is legally accountable for establishing the patient's diagnosis.

These guidelines are not a substitute for the provider's clinical judgment as to the determination of whether a condition was/was not present on admission. The provider should be queried regarding issues related to the linking of signs/symptoms, timing of test results, and the timing of findings.

General Reporting Requirements

All claims involving inpatient admissions to general acute care hospitals or other facilities that are subject to a law or regulation mandating collection of present on admission information.

Present on admission is defined as present at the time the order for inpatient admission occurs -- conditions that develop during an outpatient encounter, including emergency department, observation, or outpatient surgery, are considered as present on admission.

POA indicator is assigned to principal and secondary diagnoses (as defined in Section II of the Official Guidelines for Coding and Reporting) and the external cause of injury codes.

Issues related to inconsistent, missing, conflicting or unclear documentation must still be resolved by the provider.

If a condition would not be coded and reported based on UHDDS definitions and current official coding guidelines, then the POA indicator would not be reported.

Reporting Options

Y -   Yes
N -   No
U -   Unknown
W -   Clinically undetermined
Unreported/Not used (or "1" for Medicare usage) - (Exempt from POA reporting)

Reporting Definitions

Y =   present at the time of inpatient admission

N =   not present at the time of inpatient admission

U =   documentation is insufficient to determine if condition is present on admission

W = provider is unable to clinically determine whether condition was present on admission or not

Timeframe for POA Identification and Documentation

There is no required timeframe as to when a provider (per the definition of "provider" used in these guidelines) must identify or document a condition to be present on admission. In some clinical situations, it may not be possible for a provider to make a definitive diagnosis (or a condition may not be recognized or reported by the patient) for a period of time after admission. In some cases it may be several days before the provider arrives at a definitive diagnosis. This does not mean that the condition was not present on admission. Determination of whether the condition was present on admission or not will be based on the applicable POA guideline as identified in this document, or on the provider's best clinical judgment.

If at the time of code assignment the documentation is unclear as to whether a condition was present on admission or not, it is appropriate to query the provider for clarification.

Assigning The POA Indicator

Condition is on the "Exempt from Reporting" list

Leave the "present on admission" field blank if the condition is on the list of ICD-9-CM codes for which this field is not applicable. This is the only circumstance in which the field may be left blank.

POA Explicitly Documented

Assign Y for any condition the provider explicitly documents as being present on admission.

Assign N for any condition the provider explicitly documents as not present at the time of admission.

Conditions diagnosed prior to inpatient admission

Assign "Y" for conditions that were diagnosed prior to admission (example: hypertension, diabetes mellitus, asthma)

Conditions diagnosed during the admission but clearly present before admission

Assign "Y" for conditions diagnosed during the admission that were clearly present but not diagnosed until after admission occurred.

Diagnoses subsequently confirmed after admission are considered present on admission if at the time of admission they are documented as suspected, possible, rule out, differential diagnosis, or constitute an underlying cause of a symptom that is present at the time of admission.

Condition develops during outpatient encounter prior to inpatient admission

Assign Y for any condition that develops during an outpatient encounter prior to a written order for inpatient admission.

Documentation does not indicate whether condition was present on admission

Assign "U" when the medical record documentation is unclear as to whether the condition was present on admission. "U" should not be routinely assigned and used only in very limited circumstances. Coders are encouraged to query the providers when the documentation is unclear.

Documentation states that it cannot be determined whether the condition was or was not present on admission

Assign "W" when the medical record documentation indicates that it cannot be clinically determined whether or not the condition was present on admission.

Chronic condition with acute exacerbation during the admission

If the code is a combination code that identifies both the chronic condition and the acute exacerbation, see POA guidelines pertaining to combination codes.

If the combination code only identifies the chronic condition and not the acute exacerbation (e.g., acute exacerbation of CHF), assign "Y."

Conditions documented as possible, probable, suspected, or rule out at the time of discharge

If the final diagnosis contains a possible, probable, suspected, or rule out diagnosis, and this diagnosis was based on signs, symptoms or clinical findings suspected at the time of inpatient admission, assign "Y."

If the final diagnosis contains a possible, probable, suspected, or rule out diagnosis, and this diagnosis was based on signs, symptoms or clinical findings that were not present on admission, assign "N".

Conditions documented as impending or threatened at the time of discharge

If the final diagnosis contains an impending or threatened diagnosis, and this diagnosis is based on symptoms or clinical findings that were present on admission, assign "Y".

If the final diagnosis contains an impending or threatened diagnosis, and this diagnosis is based on symptoms or clinical findings that were not present on admission, assign "N".

Acute and Chronic Conditions

Assign "Y" for acute conditions that are present at time of admission and N for acute conditions that are not present at time of admission.

Assign "Y" for chronic conditions, even though the condition may not be diagnosed until after admission.

If a single code identifies both an acute and chronic condition, see the POA guidelines for combination codes.

Combination Codes

Assign "N" if any part of the combination code was not present on admission (e.g., obstructive chronic bronchitis with acute exacerbation and the exacerbation was not present on admission; gastric ulcer that does not start bleeding until after admission; asthma patient develops status asthmaticus after admission)

Assign "Y" if all parts of the combination code were present on admission (e.g., patient with diabetic nephropathy is admitted with uncontrolled diabetes)

If the final diagnosis includes comparative or contrasting diagnoses, and both were present, or suspected, at the time of admission, assign "Y".

For infection codes that include the causal organism, assign "Y" if the infection (or signs of the infection) was present on admission, even though the culture results may not be known until after admission (e.g., patient is admitted with pneumonia and the provider documents pseudomonas as the causal organism a few days later).

Same Diagnosis Code for Two or More Conditions

When the same ICD-9-CM diagnosis code applies to two or more conditions during the same encounter (e.g. bilateral condition, or two separate conditions classified to the same ICD-9-CM diagnosis code):

Assign "Y" if all conditions represented by the single ICD-9-CM code were present on admission (e.g. bilateral fracture of the same bone, same site, and both fractures were present on admission)

Assign "N" if any of the conditions represented by the single ICD-9-CM code was not present on admission (e.g. dehydration with hyponatremia is assigned to code 276.1, but only one of these conditions was present on admission).

Obstetrical conditions

Whether or not the patient delivers during the current hospitalization does not affect assignment of the POA indicator. The determining factor for POA assignment is whether the pregnancy complication or obstetrical condition described by the code was present at the time of admission or not.

If the pregnancy complication or obstetrical condition was present on admission (e.g., patient admitted in preterm labor), assign "Y".

If the pregnancy complication or obstetrical condition was not present on admission (e.g., 2nd degree laceration during delivery, postpartum hemorrhage that occurred during current hospitalization, fetal distress develops after admission), assign "N".

If the obstetrical code includes more than one diagnosis and any of the diagnoses identified by the code were not present on admission assign "N". (e.g., Code 642.7, Pre-eclampsia or eclampsia superimposed on pre-existing hypertension).

If the obstetrical code includes information that is not a diagnosis, do not consider that information in the POA determination. (e.g. Code 652.1x, Breech or other malpresentation successfully converted to cephalic presentation should be reported as present on admission if the fetus was breech on admission but was converted to cephalic presentation after admission (since the conversion to cephalic presentation does not represent a diagnosis, the fact that the conversion occurred after admission has no bearing on the POA determination).

Perinatal conditions

Newborns are not considered to be admitted until after birth. Therefore, any condition present at birth or that developed in utero is considered present at admission and should be assigned "Y". This includes conditions that occur during delivery (e.g., injury during delivery, meconium aspiration, exposure to streptococcus B in the vaginal canal).

Congenital conditions and anomalies

Assign "Y" for congenital conditions and anomalies. Congenital conditions are always considered present on admission.

External cause of injury codes

Assign "Y" for any E code representing an external cause of injury or poisoning that occurred prior to inpatient admission (e.g., patient fell out of bed at home, patient fell out of bed in emergency room prior to admission)

Assign "N" for any E code representing an external cause of injury or poisoning that occurred during inpatient hospitalization (e.g., patient fell out of hospital bed during hospital stay, patient experienced an adverse reaction to a medication administered after inpatient admission)

Categories and Codes Exempt from Diagnosis Present on Admission Requirement (Effective Oct. 1, 2008)

Note: "Diagnosis present on admission" for these code categories are exempt because they represent circumstances regarding the healthcare encounter or factors influencing health status that do not represent a current disease or injury or are always present on admission

Categories or subcategories listed are inclusive of all codes within those categories or subcategories, unless otherwise indicated. In order to streamline the POA exempt list and make it easier to read, where all of the codes in a code range are POA exempt, only the code range is shown, rather than listing each of the individual codes in the range.

137-139	Late effects of infectious and parasitic diseases
268.1	Rickets, late effect
326	Late effects of intracranial abscess or pyogenic infection
412	Old myocardial infarction
438	Late effects of cerebrovascular disease
650	Normal delivery
660.7	Failed forceps or vacuum extractor, unspecified
677	Late effect of complication of pregnancy, childbirth, and the puerperium
740-759	Congenital anomalies
905-909	Late effects of injuries, poisonings, toxic effects, and other external causes

V02	Carrier or suspected carrier of infectious diseases
V03	Need for prophylactic vaccination and inoculation against bacterial diseases
V04	Need for prophylactic vaccination and inoculation against certain viral diseases
V05	Need for other prophylactic vaccination and inoculation against single diseases
V06	Need for prophylactic vaccination and inoculation against combinations of diseases
V07	Need for isolation and other prophylactic or treatment measures
V10	Personal history of malignant neoplasm
V11	Personal history of mental disorder
V12	Personal history of certain other diseases
V13	Personal history of other diseases
V14	Personal history of allergy to medicinal agents
V15	Other personal history presenting hazards to health
V16	Family history of malignant neoplasm
V17	Family history of certain chronic disabling diseases
V18	Family history of certain other specific conditions
V19	Family history of other conditions
V20	Health supervision of infant or child
V21	Constitutional states in development
V22	Normal pregnancy
V23	Supervision of high-risk pregnancy
V24	Postpartum care and examination
V25	Encounter for contraceptive management
V26	Procreative management
V27	Outcome of delivery
V28	Antenatal screening
V29	Observation and evaluation of newborns for suspected condition not found
V30-V39	Liveborn infants according to type of birth
V42	Organ or tissue replaced by transplant
V43	Organ or tissue replaced by other means
V44	Artificial opening status
V45	Other postprocedural states
V46	Other dependence on machines and devices
V49.60-V49.77	Upper and lower limb amputation status
V49.81-V49.85	Other specified conditions influencing health status
V50	Elective surgery for purposes other than remedying health states
V51	Aftercare involving the use of plastic surgery
V52	Fitting and adjustment of prosthetic device and implant
V53	Fitting and adjustment of other device
V54	Other orthopedic aftercare
V55	Attention to artificial openings
V56	Encounter for dialysis and dialysis catheter care
V57	Care involving use of rehabilitation procedures
V58	Encounter for other and unspecified procedures and aftercare
V59	Donors
V60	Housing, household, and economic circumstances
V61	Other family circumstances

V62	Other psychosocial circumstances
V64	Persons encountering health services for specific procedures, not carried out
V65	Other persons seeking consultation
V66	Convalescence and palliative care
V67	Follow-up examination
V68	Encounters for administrative purposes
V69	Problems related to lifestyle
V70	General medical examination
V71	Observation and evaluation for suspected condition not found
V72	Special investigations and examinations
V73	Special screening examination for viral and chlamydial diseases
V74	Special screening examination for bacterial and spirochetal diseases
V75	Special screening examination for other infectious diseases
V76	Special screening for malignant neoplasms
V77	Special screening for endocrine, nutritional, metabolic, and immunity disorders
V78	Special screening for disorders of blood and blood-forming organs
V79	Special screening for mental disorders and developmental handicaps
V80	Special screening for neurological, eye, and ear diseases
V81	Special screening for cardiovascular, respiratory, and genitourinary diseases
V82	Special screening for other conditions
V83	Genetic carrier status
V84	Genetic susceptibility to disease
V85	Body Mass Index
V86	Estrogen receptor status
V87.32	Contact with and (suspected) exposure to algae bloom
V87.4	Personal history of drug therapy
V88	Acquired absence of other organs and tissue
V89	Suspected maternal and fetal conditions not found
V90	Retained foreign body
V91	Multiple gestation placenta status
E000	External cause status
E001-E030	Activity
E800-E807	Railway accidents
E810-E819	Motor vehicle traffic accidents
E820-E825	Motor vehicle nontraffic accidents
E826-E829	Other road vehicle accidents
E830-E838	Water transport accidents
E840-E845	Air and space transport accidents
E846-E848	Vehicle accidents not elsewhere classifiable
E849	Place of occurrence (except E849.7)
E883.1	Accidental fall into well
E883.2	Accidental fall into storm drain or manhole
E884.0	Fall from playground equipment
E884.1	Fall from cliff
E885.0	Fall from (nonmotorized) scooter
E885.1	Fall from roller skates

E885.2	Fall from skateboard
E885.3	Fall from skis
E885.4	Fall from snowboard
E886.0	Fall on same level from collision, pushing, or shoving, by or with other person, In sports
E890.0-E890.9	Conflagration in private dwelling
E893.0	Accident caused by ignition of clothing, from controlled fire in private dwelling
E893.2	Accident caused by ignition of clothing, from controlled fire not in building or structure
E894	Ignition of highly inflammable material
E895	Accident caused by controlled fire in private dwelling
E897	Accident caused by controlled fire not in building or structure
E917.0	Striking against or struck accidentally by objects or persons, in sports without subsequent fall
E917.1	Striking against or struck accidentally by objects or persons, caused by a crowd, by collective fear or panic without subsequent fall
E917.2	Striking against or struck accidentally by objects or persons, in running water without subsequent fall
E917.5	Striking against or struck accidentally by objects or persons, object in sports with subsequent fall
E917.6	Striking against or struck accidentally by objects or persons, caused by a crowd, by collective fear or panic with subsequent fall
E919	Accidents caused by machinery (except E919.2)
E921	Accident caused by explosion of pressure vessel
E922	Accident caused by firearm and air gun missile
E926.2	Visible and ultraviolet light sources
E928.0-E928.8	Other and unspecified environmental and accidental causes
E929.0-E929.9	Late effects of accidental injury
E959	Late effects of self-inflicted injury
E970-E978	Legal intervention
E979	Terrorism
E981	Poisoning by gases in domestic use, undetermined whether accidentally or purposely inflicted
E982	Poisoning by other gases, undetermined whether accidentally or purposely inflicted
E985	Injury by firearms, air guns and explosives, undetermined whether accidentally or purposely inflicted
E987.0	Falling from high place, undetermined whether accidentally or purposely inflicted, residential premises
E987.2	Falling from high place, undetermined whether accidentally or purposely inflicted, natural sites
E989	Late effects of injury, undetermined whether accidentally or purposely inflicted
E990-E999	Injury resulting from operations of war

POA Examples

The POA examples have been removed from the guidelines.

ICD-10

Subject to possible legislative delays, ICD-10-CM codes must be used on all HIPAA transactions, including outpatient claims with dates of service, and inpatient claims with dates of discharge on and after <u>October 1, 2013</u>. In addition, ICD-10-PCS will replace the current ICD-9-CM Volume 3 procedures list. This change does not affect CPT coding for outpatient procedures and there will continue to be ICD-9-CM updates until ICD-10-CM is implemented.

Differences Between ICD-10-CM and ICD-9-CM

ICD-10-CM uses 3-7 alpha and numeric digits and full code titles, but the format is very much the same as ICD-9-CM. Primarily, changes in ICD-10-CM are in its organization and structure, code composition, and level of detail.

Format of ICD-10-CM

- 3-7 digits
- Digit 1 is alpha; Digit 2 is numeric
- Digits 3-7 are alpha or numeric (alpha characters are not case sensitive)
- Decimal is used after third character.

Examples of ICD-10-CM Codes

A78 Q fever

A69.21 Meningitis due to Lyme disease

S52.131A Displaced fracture of neck of right radius, initial encounter for closed fracture.

Due to the additional digits, there will be over 85,000 potential codes in ICD-10-CM versus about 16,000 codes in ICD-9-CM.

WHERE TO GET ANSWERS TO QUESTIONS ABOUT ICD-9-CM

Questions regarding the use and interpretation of the *International Classification of Diseases, 9th Revision, Clinical Modification* should be directed in writing to any of the organizations listed below.

Coding Advice/Central Office on ICD-9-CM
American Hospital Association
One North Franklin
Chicago, Illinois 60606
Vols. 1 and 2: kayala@aha.org

World Health Organization Collaborating Center
    for Classification of Diseases in North America
National Center for Health Statistics
Department of Health and Human Services
6525 Belcrest Road
Hyattsville, Maryland 20782

Morbidity Classification Branch
National Center for Health Statistics
Department of Health and Human Services
6525 Belcrest Road, Room 1100
Hyattsville, Maryland 20782

Center for Medicare and Medicaid Services (CMS)
Division of Prospective Payment
Mail Stop C5-06-27
7500 Security Blvd.
Baltimore, MD   21244-1850
Vol. 3: pbrooks@cms.hhs.gov

Comments, questions or suggestions regarding the PMIC version of ICD-9-CM should be directed in writing to:

Managing Editor
Practice Management Information Corporation
4727 Wilshire Boulevard, Suite 300
Los Angeles, California 90010
http://www.pmiconline.com

Anatomical Illustrations

A fundamental knowledge and understanding of basic human anatomy and physiology is a prerequisite for accurate diagnosis coding. While a comprehensive treatment of anatomy and physiology is beyond the scope of this text, the large scale, full color anatomical illustrations on the following pages are designed to facilitate the diagnosis coding process for both beginning and experienced coders.

The illustrations provide an anatomical perspective of diagnosis coding by providing a side-by-side view of the major systems of the human body and a corresponding list of the most common diagnoses categories used to support medical, surgical and diagnostic services performed on the illustrated system.

The diagnostic categories listed on the left facing page of each anatomical illustration are three-digit categories and may not be used for coding. These categories are provided as "pointers" to the appropriate section of the ICD-9-CM Volume 1 where the complete listings, including 4th and 5th digits if appropriate, may be found.

Plate	System	Page
Plate 1	Skin and subcutaneous tissue — male	103
Plate 2	Skin and subcutaneous tissue — female	105
Plate 3	Skin and subcutaneous tissue — female breast	107
Plate 4	Muscular system and connective tissue — anterior view	109
Plate 5	Muscular system and connective tissue — posterior view	111
Plate 6	Shoulder and elbow	113
Plate 7	Hand and wrist	115
Plate 8	Hip and knee	117
Plate 9	Foot and ankle	119
Plate 10	Skeletal system — anterior view	121
Plate 11	Skeletal system — posterior view	123
Plate 12	Vertebral column	125
Plate 13	Respiratory system	127
Plate 14	Heart and pericardium	129
Plate 15	Circulatory system	131
Plate 16	Digestive system	133
Plate 17	Genitourinary system	135
Plate 18	Male reproductive system	137
Plate 19	Female reproductive system	139
Plate 20	Female reproductive system — pregnancy, lateral view	141
Plate 21	Brain	143
Plate 22	Nervous system	145
Plate 23	Right eye — horizontal section	147
Plate 24	The Ear	149

PLATE 1. SKIN AND SUBCUTANEOUS TISSUE — MALE

Viral diseases accompanied by exanthem   050-057

Neoplasms
Malignant melanoma of skin	172
Other malignant neoplasm of skin	173
Malignant neoplasm of male breast	175
Kaposi's sarcoma	176
Benign neoplasm of skin	216
Carcinoma in situ of skin	232

Infections of skin and subcutaneous tissue
Carbuncle and furuncle	680
Cellulitis and abscess of finger and toe	681
Other cellulitis and abscess	682
Acute lymphadenitis	683
Impetigo	684
Pilonidal cyst	685
Other local infections of skin and subcutaneous tissue	686

Other inflammatory conditions of skin and subcutaneous tissue
Erythematosquamous dermatosis	690
Atopic dermatitis and related conditions	691
Contact dermatitis and other eczema	692
Dermatitis due to substances taken internally	693
Bullous dermatoses	694
Erythematous conditions	695
Psoriasis and similar disorders	696
Lichen	697
Pruritus and related conditions	698

Other diseases of skin and subcutaneous tissue
Corns and callosities	700
Other hypertrophic and atrophic conditions of skin	701
Diseases of nail	703
Diseases of hair and hair follicles	704
Disorders of sweat glands	705
Diseases of sebaceous glands	706
Chronic ulcer of skin	707
Urticaria	708
Other disorders of skin and subcutaneous tissue	709
Symptoms involving skin and other integumentary tissue	782

Symptoms, signs and ill-defined conditions   780-799

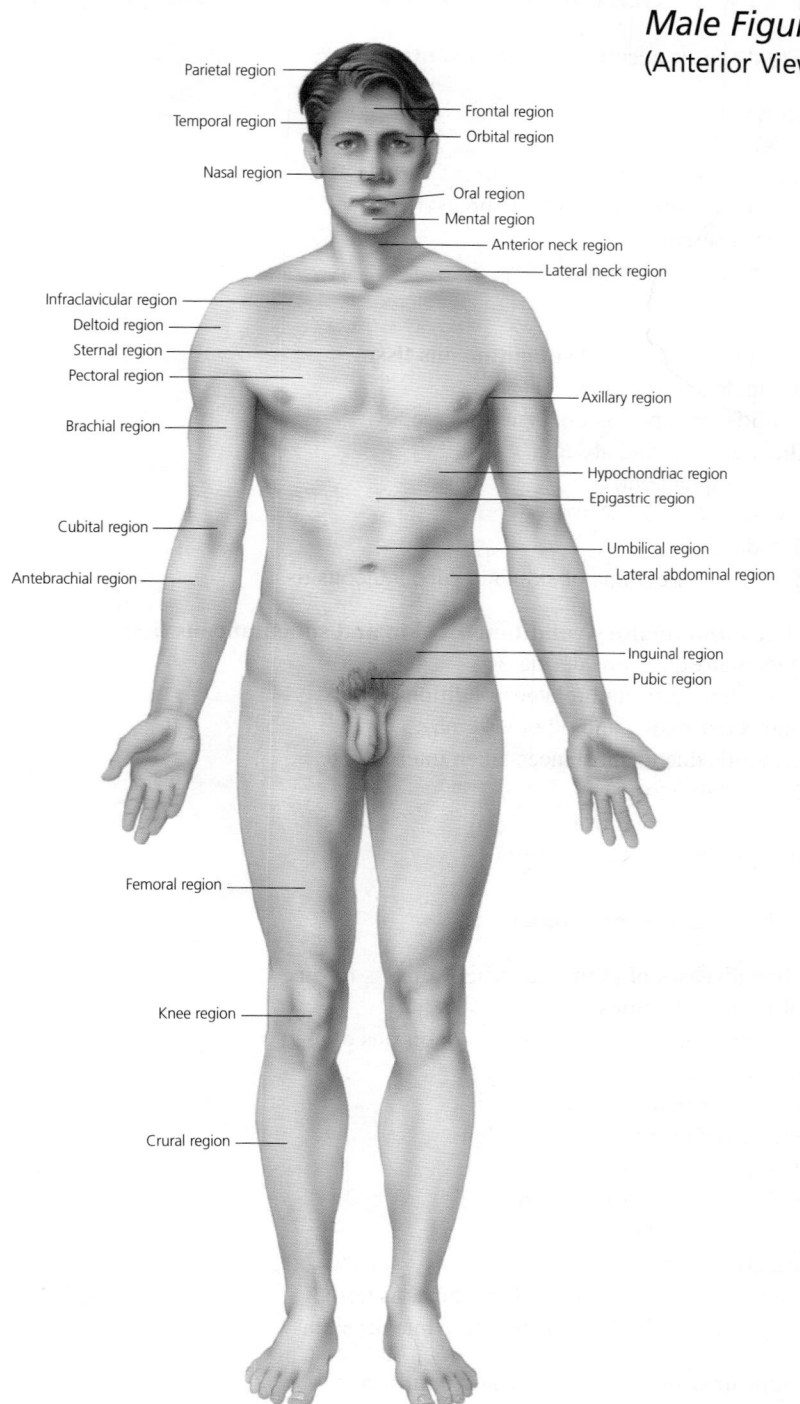

Male Figure
(Anterior View)

Parietal region

Temporal region

Frontal region

Orbital region

Nasal region

Oral region

Mental region

Anterior neck region

Lateral neck region

Infraclavicular region

Deltoid region

Sternal region

Pectoral region

Axillary region

Brachial region

Hypochondriac region

Epigastric region

Cubital region

Umbilical region

Antebrachial region

Lateral abdominal region

Inguinal region

Pubic region

Femoral region

Knee region

Crural region

©Practice Management Information Corp., Los Angeles, CA

PLATE 2. SKIN AND SUBCUTANEOUS TISSUE — FEMALE

Viral diseases accompanied by exanthem	050-057

Neoplasms

Malignant melanoma of skin	172
Other malignant neoplasm of skin	173
Malignant neoplasm of female breast	174
Kaposi's sarcoma	176
Benign neoplasm of skin	216
Carcinoma in situ of skin	232

Infections of skin and subcutaneous tissue

Carbuncle and furuncle	680
Cellulitis and abscess of finger and toe	681
Other cellulitis and abscess	682
Acute lymphadenitis	683
Impetigo	684
Pilonidal cyst	685
Other local infections of skin and subcutaneous tissue	686

Other inflammatory conditions of skin and subcutaneous tissue

Erythematosquamous dermatosis	690
Atopic dermatitis and related conditions	691
Contact dermatitis and other eczema	692
Dermatitis due to substances taken internally	693
Bullous dermatoses	694
Erythematous conditions	695
Psoriasis and similar disorders	696
Lichen	697
Pruritus and related conditions	698

Other diseases of skin and subcutaneous tissue

Corns and callosities	700
Other hypertrophic and atrophic conditions of skin	701
Other dermatoses	702
Diseases of nail	703
Diseases of hair and hair follicles	704
Disorders of sweat glands	705
Diseases of sebaceous glands	706
Chronic ulcer of skin	707
Urticaria	708
Other disorders of skin and subcutaneous tissue	709
Symptoms involving skin and other integumentary tissue	782

Symptoms, signs and ill-defined conditions	780-799

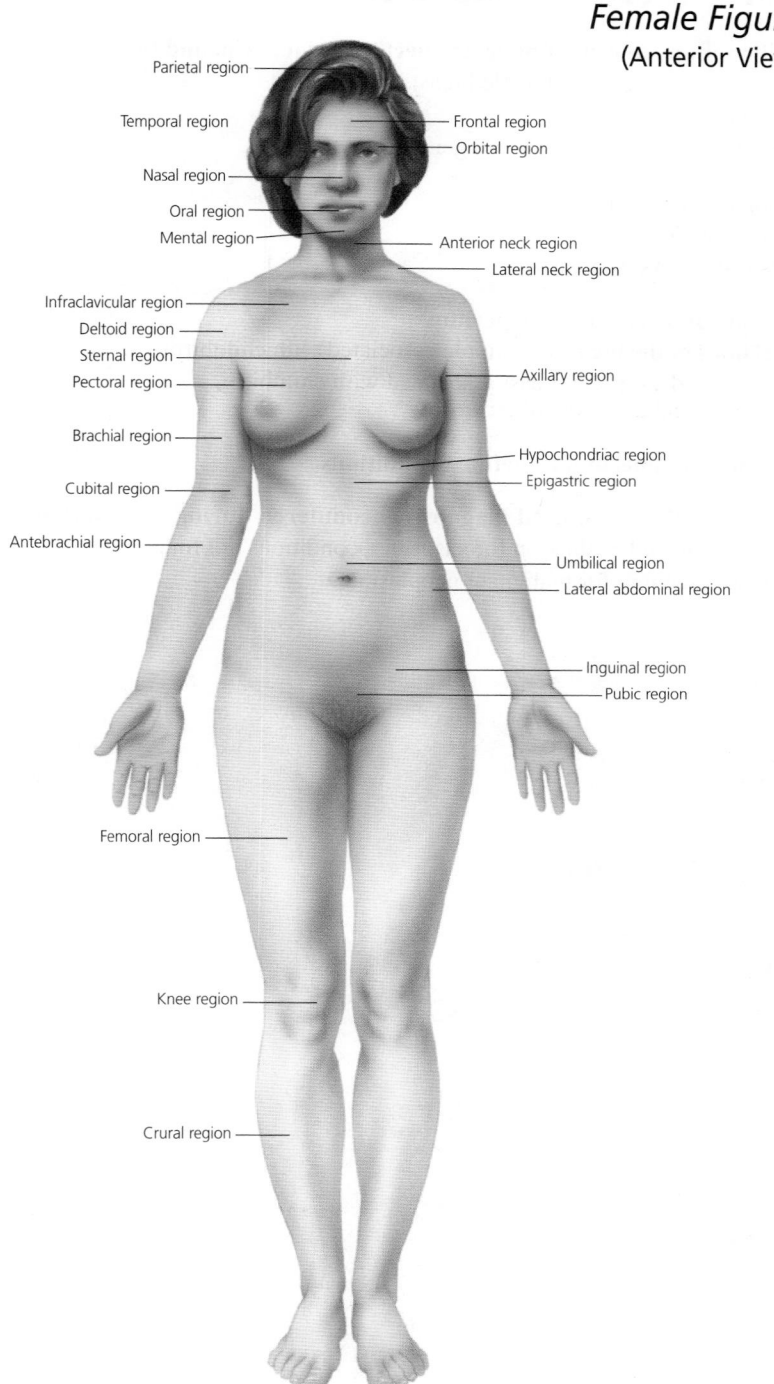

Female Figure
(Anterior View)

Parietal region

Temporal region

Frontal region

Orbital region

Nasal region

Oral region

Mental region

Anterior neck region

Lateral neck region

Infraclavicular region

Deltoid region

Sternal region

Pectoral region

Axillary region

Brachial region

Hypochondriac region

Epigastric region

Cubital region

Antebrachial region

Umbilical region

Lateral abdominal region

Inguinal region

Pubic region

Femoral region

Knee region

Crural region

PLATE 3. FEMALE BREAST

Malignant neoplasm of bone, connective tissue, skin, and breast
Malignant neoplasm of female breast   174
Benign neoplasm of breast   217
Carcinoma in situ of breast and genitourinary system   233

Disorders of breast
Benign mammary dysplasias   610
Other disorders of breast   611

Complications of the puerperium
Infections of the breast and nipple associated with childbirth   675
Other disorders of the breast associated with childbirth,
      and disorders of lactation   676

Symptoms, signs and ill-defined conditions   780-799

Persons without reported diagnosis encountered during examination
Observation and evaluation for suspected conditions not found   V71
Special screening for malignant neoplasms   V76

Female Breast

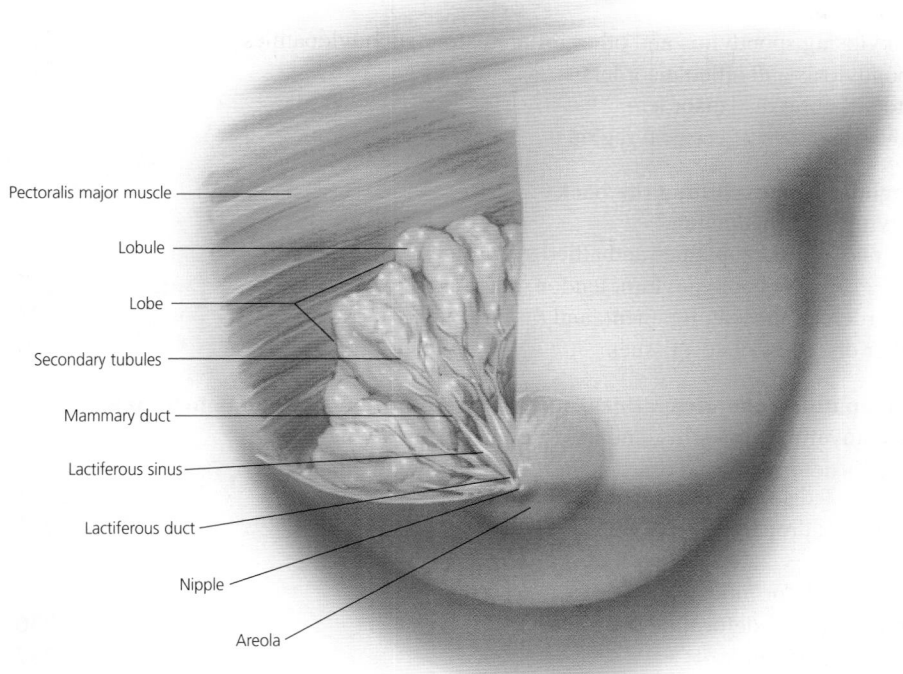

Pectoralis major muscle

Lobule

Lobe

Secondary tubules

Mammary duct

Lactiferous sinus

Lactiferous duct

Nipple

Areola

PLATE 4. MUSCULAR SYSTEM AND CONNECTIVE TISSUE — ANTERIOR VIEW

Arthropathies and related disorders
Diffuse diseases of connective tissue 710
Arthropathy associated with infections 711
Crystal arthropathies 712
Arthropathy associated with other disorders classified elsewhere 713
Rheumatoid arthritis and other inflammatory polyarthropathies 714
Osteoarthrosis and allied disorders 715
Internal derangement of knee 717
Other derangement of joint 718

Dorsopathies
Ankylosing spondylitis and other inflammatory spondylopathies 720
Spondylosis and allied disorders 721
Intervertebral disc disorders 722
Other disorders of cervical region 723

Rheumatism, excluding the back
Polymyalgia rheumatica 725
Peripheral enthesopathies and allied syndromes 726
Other disorders of synovium, tendon, and bursa 727
Disorders of muscle, ligament, and fascia 728
Other disorders of soft tissues 729

Osteopathies, chondropathies, and acquired musculoskeletal deformities
Osteomyelitis, periostitis, and other infections involving bone 730
Osteitis deformans and osteopathies associated with other
    disorders classified elsewhere 731
Osteochondropathies 732
Flat foot 734
Acquired deformities of toe 735
Other acquired deformities of limbs 736
Curvature of spine 737
Other acquired deformity 738
Nonallopathic lesions, not elsewhere classified 739

Symptoms, signs and ill-defined conditions 780-799

Muscular System
(Anterior View)

Temporalis m.
Orbicularis oculi m.
Masseter m.
Sternocleidomastoid m.
Trapezius m.
Levator scapulae m.

Frontalis m.
Buccinator
Orbicularis oris m.
Depressor anguli oris m.

Deltoid m.
Pectoralis major m.

Serratus anterior m.
Biceps m.
External abdominal oblique m.
Brachialis m.
Brachioradialis m.
Extensor carpi radialis longus m.
Palmaris longus m.
Flexor carpi radialis m.
Superficial inguinal ring

Tensor fasciae latae m.
Sartorius m.
Rectus femoris m.
Adductor longus m.
Vastus lateralis m.

Pectoralis minor m.
Internal intercostal m.
Coracobrachialis m.
Brachialis m.
Rectus sheath
Rectus abdominis m.
Linea alba
Internal abdominal oblique m.
Transversus abdominis m.
Flexor digitorum superficialis m.
Flexor pollicis longus m.
Abductor digiti minimi m.
Abductor pollicis brevis m.
Flexor pollicis brevis m.
Iliopsoas m.
Pectineus m.
Adductor brevis m.

Gracilis m.
Adductor magnus m.
Vastus medialis m.
Vastus lateralis m.

Iliotibial tract
Vastus medialis m.

Sartorius m.

Lateral patellar retinaculum

Tibialis anterior m.
Gastrocnemius m.
Extensor digitorum longus m.
Peroneus longus m.
Soleus m.
Peroneus brevis m.
Extensor hallucis longus m.
Extensor hallucis brevis m.
Extensor digitorum brevis m.

Patella
Patellar ligament
Medial patellar retinaculum

Gastrocnemius m.
Soleus m.
Tibia

Flexor digitorum longus m.
Extensor hallucis brevis m.
Abductor hallucis m.

PLATE 5. MUSCULAR SYSTEM AND CONNECTIVE TISSUE — POSTERIOR VIEW

Arthropathies and related disorders
Diffuse diseases of connective tissue   710
Arthropathy associated with infections   711
Crystal arthropathies   712
Arthropathy associated with other disorders classified elsewhere   713
Rheumatoid arthritis and other inflammatory polyarthropathies   714
Osteoarthrosis and allied disorders   715
Other and unspecified arthropathies   716
Internal derangement of knee   717
Other derangement of joint   718
Other and unspecified disorders of joint   719

Dorsopathies
Ankylosing spondylitis and other inflammatory spondylopathies   720
Spondylosis and allied disorders   721
Intervertebral disc disorders   722
Other disorders of cervical region   723
Other and unspecified disorders of back   724

Rheumatism, excluding the back
Polymyalgia rheumatica   725
Peripheral enthesopathies and allied syndromes   726
Other disorders of synovium, tendon, and bursa   727
Disorders of muscle, ligament, and fascia   728
Other disorders of soft tissues   729

Osteopathies, chondropathies, and acquired musculoskeletal deformities
Osteomyelitis, periostitis, and other infections involving bone   730
Osteitis deformans and osteopathies associated with other
                    disorders classified elsewhere   731
Osteochondropathies   732
Other disorders of bone and cartilage   733
Flat foot   734
Acquired deformities of toe   735
Other acquired deformities of limbs   736
Curvature of spine   737
Other acquired deformity   738
Nonallopathic lesions, not elsewhere classified   739

Symptoms, signs and ill-defined conditions   780-799

Muscular System
(Posterior View)

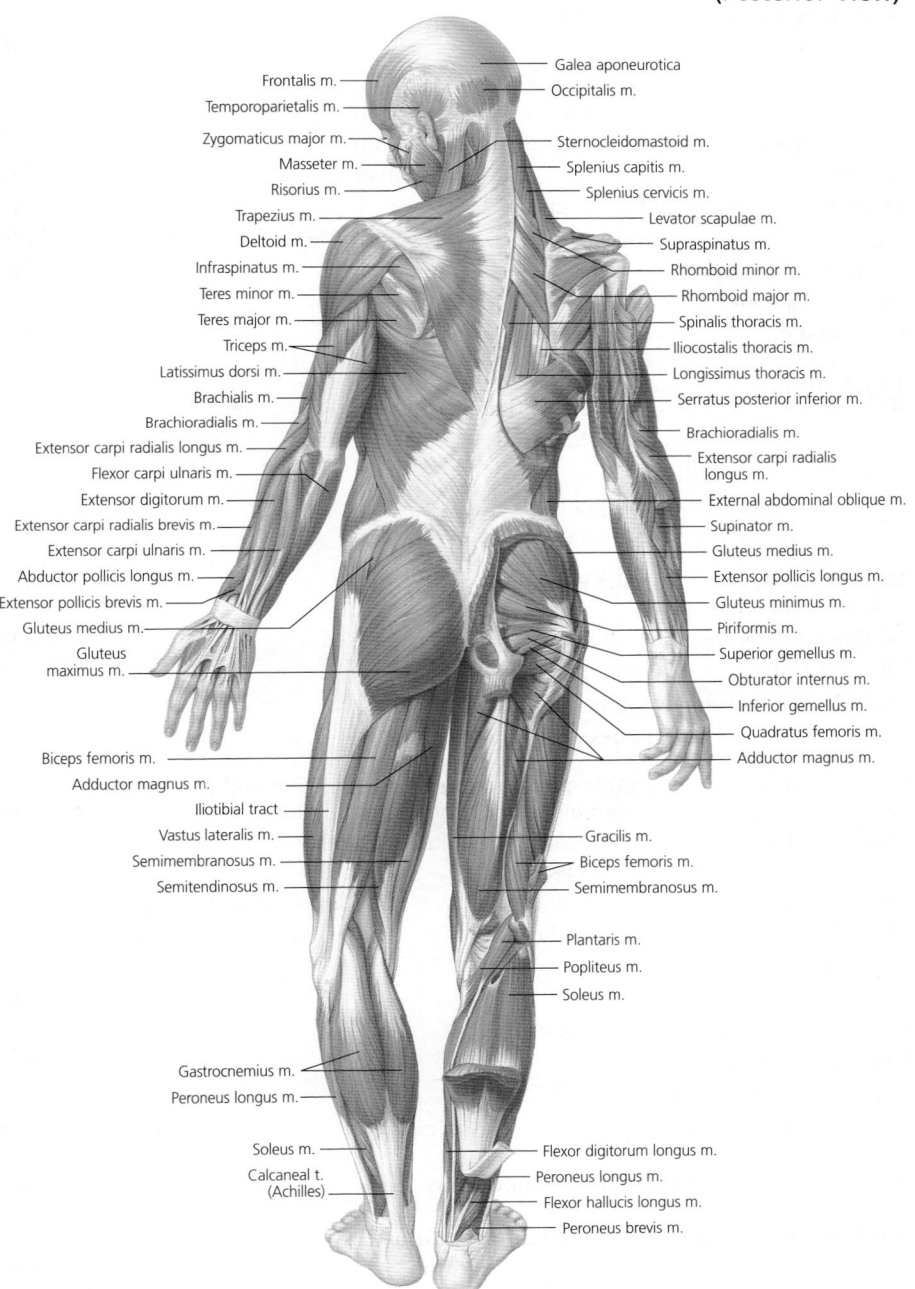

Galea aponeurotica
Occipitalis m.
Frontalis m.
Temporoparietalis m.
Zygomaticus major m.
Masseter m.
Risorius m.
Sternocleidomastoid m.
Splenius capitis m.
Splenius cervicis m.
Trapezius m.
Deltoid m.
Infraspinatus m.
Teres minor m.
Teres major m.
Triceps m.
Latissimus dorsi m.
Brachialis m.
Brachioradialis m.
Extensor carpi radialis longus m.
Flexor carpi ulnaris m.
Extensor digitorum m.
Extensor carpi radialis brevis m.
Extensor carpi ulnaris m.
Abductor pollicis longus m.
Extensor pollicis brevis m.
Gluteus medius m.
Gluteus maximus m.
Levator scapulae m.
Supraspinatus m.
Rhomboid minor m.
Rhomboid major m.
Spinalis thoracis m.
Iliocostalis thoracis m.
Longissimus thoracis m.
Serratus posterior inferior m.
Brachioradialis m.
Extensor carpi radialis longus m.
External abdominal oblique m.
Supinator m.
Gluteus medius m.
Extensor pollicis longus m.
Gluteus minimus m.
Piriformis m.
Superior gemellus m.
Obturator internus m.
Inferior gemellus m.
Quadratus femoris m.
Adductor magnus m.
Biceps femoris m.
Adductor magnus m.
Iliotibial tract
Vastus lateralis m.
Semimembranosus m.
Semitendinosus m.
Gracilis m.
Biceps femoris m.
Semimembranosus m.
Plantaris m.
Popliteus m.
Soleus m.
Gastrocnemius m.
Peroneus longus m.
Soleus m.
Calcaneal t. (Achilles)
Flexor digitorum longus m.
Peroneus longus m.
Flexor hallucis longus m.
Peroneus brevis m.

PLATE 6. MUSCULAR SYSTEM — SHOULDER AND ELBOW

Arthropathies and related disorders

Diffuse diseases of connective tissue	710
Arthropathy associated with infections	711
Crystal arthropathies	712
Arthropathy associated with other disorders classified elsewhere	713
Rheumatoid arthritis and other inflammatory polyarthropathies	714
Osteoarthrosis and allied disorders	715
Other and unspecified arthropathies	716
Internal derangement of knee	717
Other derangement of joint	718
Other and unspecified disorders of joint	719

Dorsopathies

Ankylosing spondylitis and other inflammatory spondylopathies	720
Spondylosis and allied disorders	721
Intervertebral disc disorders	722
Other disorders of cervical region	723
Other and unspecified disorders of back	724

Rheumatism, excluding the back

Polymyalgia rheumatica	725
Peripheral enthesopathies and allied syndromes	726
Other disorders of synovium, tendon, and bursa	727
Disorders of muscle, ligament, and fascia	728
Other disorders of soft tissues	729

Osteopathies, chondropathies, and acquired musculoskeletal deformities

Osteomyelitis, periostitis, and other infections involving bone	730
Osteitis deformans and osteopathies associated with other disorders classified elsewhere	731
Osteochondropathies	732
Other disorders of bone and cartilage	733
Flat foot	734
Acquired deformities of toe	735
Other acquired deformities of limbs	736
Curvature of spine	737
Other acquired deformity	738
Nonallopathic lesions, not elsewhere classified	739

Symptoms, signs and ill-defined conditions

	780-799

Sprains and strains of joints and adjacent muscles

Sprains and strains of shoulder and upper arm	840
Sprains and strains of elbow and forearm	841
Other and ill-defined sprains and strains	848

Shoulder and Elbow
(Anterior View)

Coracoclavicular ligament
Acromioclavicular ligament
Coracoacromial ligament
Supraspinatus tendon
Coracohumeral ligament
Transverse humeral ligament
Tendon of long head of biceps muscle
Subscapularis tendon
Articular capsule

Acromion
Clavicle

Coracoid process
Scapular notch
Subscapular fossa
Head of humerus
Lesser tubercle
Greater tubercle
Scapula
Nutrient foramen
Humerus
Deltoid tuberosity

Articular capsule
Radial collateral ligament
Annular ligament
Ulnar collateral ligament

Interosseous membrane
Radius
Ulna

Lateral epicondyle
Capitulum
Coronoid fossa
Medial epicondyle
Trochlea
Coronoid process
Head of radius
Ulnar tuberosity
Radial tuberosity

PLATE 7. MUSCULAR SYSTEM — HAND AND WRIST

Arthropathies and related disorders

Diffuse diseases of connective tissue 710
Arthropathy associated with infections 711
Crystal arthropathies 712
Arthropathy associated with other disorders classified elsewhere 713
Rheumatoid arthritis and other inflammatory polyarthropathies 714
Osteoarthrosis and allied disorders 715
Other and unspecified arthropathies 716
Other derangement of joint 718
Other and unspecified disorders of joint 719

Rheumatism, excluding the back

Polymyalgia rheumatica 725
Peripheral enthesopathies and allied syndromes 726
Other disorders of synovium, tendon, and bursa 727
Disorders of muscle, ligament, and fascia 728
Other disorders of soft tissues 729

Osteopathies, chondropathies, and acquired musculoskeletal deformities

Osteomyelitis, periostitis, and other infections involving bone 730
Osteitis deformans and osteopathies associated with other
disorders classified elsewhere 731
Osteochondropathies 732
Other disorders of bone and cartilage 733
Other acquired deformities of limbs 736
Other acquired deformity 738
Nonallopathic lesions, not elsewhere classified 739

Symptoms, signs and ill-defined conditions 780-799

Sprains and strains of joints and adjacent muscles

Sprains and strains of wrist and hand 842
Other and ill-defined sprains and strains 848

Hand and Wrist

Abductor pollicis longus muscle

Extensor pollicis brevis muscle

Extensor digitorum tendons

Extensor pollicis brevis tendon

Extensor pollicis longus tendon

Extensor carpi radialis brevis tendon

Extensor carpi radialis longus tendon

1st dorsal interosseous muscle

Extensor digiti minimi muscle

Extensor carpi ulnaris muscle

Extensor retinaculum

Extensor digiti minimi tendons

Extensor digitorum tendons

2nd, 3rd, 4th dorsal interosseous muscles

Brachioradialis tendon

Flexor carpi radialis tendon

Flexor pollicis longus muscle

Abductor pollicis longus tendon

Opponens pollicis muscle

Abductor pollicis brevis muscle

Flexor digitorum superficialis muscle & tendons

Flexor carpi ulnaris tendon

Palmaris longus tendon

Opponens digiti minimi muscle

Flexor digiti minimi brevis muscle

Abductor digiti minimi muscle

Flexor digitorum superficialis tendons

Palmar interosseous muscles

Fibrous digital sheath: anular part cruciform part

Flexor pollicis brevis muscle

Adductor pollicis muscle

Lumbrical muscles

Flexor digitorum profundus tendon

PLATE 8. MUSCULOSKELETAL SYSTEM — HIP AND KNEE

Arthropathies and related disorders
Diffuse diseases of connective tissue 710
Arthropathy associated with infections 711
Crystal arthropathies 712
Arthropathy associated with other disorders classified elsewhere 713
Rheumatoid arthritis and other inflammatory polyarthropathies 714
Osteoarthrosis and allied disorders 715
Other and unspecified arthropathies 716
Internal derangement of knee 717
Other derangement of joint 718
Other and unspecified disorders of joint 719

Rheumatism, excluding the back
Polymyalgia rheumatica 725
Peripheral enthesopathies and allied syndromes 726
Other disorders of synovium, tendon, and bursa 727
Disorders of muscle, ligament, and fascia 728
Other disorders of soft tissues 729

Osteopathies, chondropathies, and acquired musculoskeletal deformities
Osteomyelitis, periostitis, and other infections involving bone 730
Osteitis deformans and osteopathies associated with other
disorders classified elsewhere 731
Osteochondropathies 732
Other disorders of bone and cartilage 733
Other acquired deformities of limbs 736
Curvature of spine 737
Other acquired deformity 738
Nonallopathic lesions, not elsewhere classified 739

Symptoms, signs and ill-defined conditions 780-799

Sprains and strains of joints and adjacent muscles
Sprains and strains of hip and thigh 843
Sprains and strains of knee and leg 844
Other and ill-defined sprains and strains 848

Hip and Knee
(Anterior View)

Sacral promontory
Sacrum
Iliac crest
Ilium
Anterior superior iliac spine
Spine of ischium
Anterior inferior iliac spine
Head of femur
Greater trochanter
Obturator foramen
Pubis
Lesser trochanter

Anterior longitudinal ligament
Iliolumbar ligament
Anterior sacroiliac ligament
Coccyx
Sacrotuberous ligament
Sacrospinous ligament
Inguinal ligament
Iliofemoral ligament
Pubofemoral ligament
Obturator membrane
Pubic symphysis
Femur

Medial epicondyle
Lateral epicondyle
Patella
Lateral condyles
Head of fibula
Tibial tuberosity
Medial condyles

Tibia

Fibula

Quadriceps femoris tendon
Medial patellar retinaculum
Fibular collateral ligament
Tibial collateral ligament
Lateral patellar retinaculum
Patellar ligament

Interosseous
membrane

PLATE 9. MUSCULOSKELETAL SYSTEM — FOOT AND ANKLE

Arthropathies and related disorders

Diffuse diseases of connective tissue	710
Arthropathy associated with infections	711
Crystal arthropathies	712
Arthropathy associated with other disorders classified elsewhere	713
Rheumatoid arthritis and other inflammatory polyarthropathies	714
Osteoarthrosis and allied disorders	715
Other and unspecified arthropathies	716
Other derangement of joint	718
Other and unspecified disorders of joint	719

Rheumatism, excluding the back

Polymyalgia rheumatica	725
Peripheral enthesopathies and allied syndromes	726
Other disorders of synovium, tendon, and bursa	727
Disorders of muscle, ligament, and fascia	728
Other disorders of soft tissues	729

Osteopathies, chondropathies, and acquired musculoskeletal deformities

Osteomyelitis, periostitis, and other infections involving bone	730
Osteitis deformans and osteopathies associated with other disorders classified elsewhere	731
Osteochondropathies	732
Other disorders of bone and cartilage	733
Flat foot	734
Acquired deformities of toe	735
Other acquired deformities of limbs	736
Other acquired deformity	738
Nonallopathic lesions, not elsewhere classified	739

Symptoms, signs and ill-defined conditions — 780-799

Sprains and strains of joints and adjacent muscles

Sprains and strains of ankle and foot	845
Other and ill-defined sprains and strains	848

Foot and Ankle

Soleus muscle

Tibia

Tibialis anterior muscle

Peroneus brevis muscle

Peroneus longus tendon

Extensor digitorum longus muscle

Flexor digitorum longus muscle

Flexor hallucis tendon

Achilles tendon

Medial malleolus

Tibialis posterior tendon

Retinaculum

Tibia

Fibula

Extensor hallucis longus muscle

Tibialis posterior tendon

Tibialis anterior tendon

Extensor hallucis brevis muscle

Abductor hallucis muscle

Lateral malleous

Retinaculum

Peroneus longus tendon

Extensor digitorum brevis muscle

Calcaneus

Peroneus brevis tendon

Peroneus tertius tendon

Opponens digiti minimi muscle

Dorsal interosseous muscles

Extensor hallucis longus tendon

Extensor hallucis brevis muscle

Extensor digitorum longus tendons

PLATE 10. SKELETAL SYSTEM — ANTERIOR VIEW

Symptoms, signs and ill-defined conditions   780-799

Fracture of skull

Fracture of vault of skull   800
Fracture of base of skull   801
Fracture of face bones   802
Multiple fractures involving skull or face with other bones   804

Fracture of neck and trunk

Fracture of vertebral column without mention of spinal cord injury   805
Fracture of vertebral column with spinal cord injury   806
Fracture of rib(s), sternum, larynx and trachea   807
Fracture of pelvis   808

Fracture of upper limb

Fracture of clavicle   810
Fracture of scapula   811
Fracture of humerus   812
Fracture of radius and ulna   813
Fracture of carpal bone(s)   814
Fracture of metacarpal bone(s)   815
Fracture of one or more phalanges of hand   816
Multiple fractures of hand bones   817

Fracture of lower limb

Fracture of neck of femur   820
Fracture of other and unspecified parts of femur   821
Fracture of patella   822
Fracture of tibia and fibula   823
Fracture of ankle   824
Fracture of one or more tarsal and metatarsal bones   825
Fracture of one or more phalanges of foot   826

Dislocation

Dislocation of jaw   830
Dislocation of shoulder   831
Dislocation of elbow   832
Dislocation of wrist   833
Dislocation of finger   834
Dislocation of hip   835
Dislocation of knee   836
Dislocation of ankle   837
Dislocation of foot   838

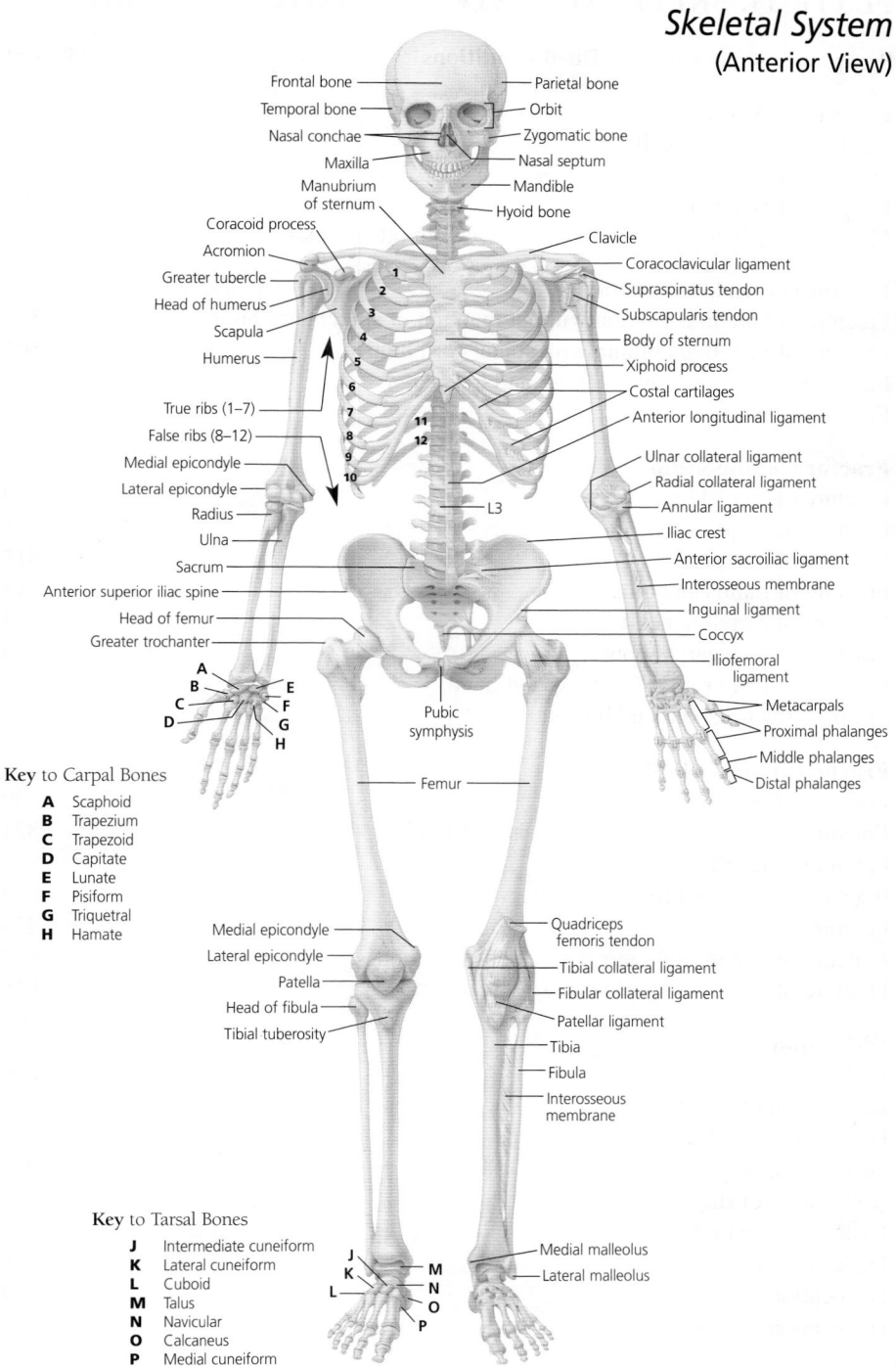

Skeletal System
(Anterior View)

Frontal bone
Parietal bone
Temporal bone
Orbit
Nasal conchae
Zygomatic bone
Maxilla
Nasal septum
Manubrium of sternum
Mandible
Coracoid process
Hyoid bone
Acromion
Clavicle
Greater tubercle
Coracoclavicular ligament
Head of humerus
Suprasupinatus tendon
Scapula
Subscapularis tendon
Humerus
Body of sternum
Xiphoid process
Costal cartilages
True ribs (1–7)
Anterior longitudinal ligament
False ribs (8–12)
Medial epicondyle
Ulnar collateral ligament
Lateral epicondyle
Radial collateral ligament
Radius
Annular ligament
Ulna
Iliac crest
Sacrum
Anterior sacroiliac ligament
Anterior superior iliac spine
Interosseous membrane
Head of femur
Inguinal ligament
Greater trochanter
Coccyx
Iliofemoral ligament
Metacarpals
Proximal phalanges
Pubic symphysis
Middle phalanges
Distal phalanges

1
2
3
4
5
6
7
8
9
10
11
12
L3

A
B
C
D
E
F
G
H

Key to Carpal Bones
A Scaphoid
B Trapezium
C Trapezoid
D Capitate
E Lunate
F Pisiform
G Triquetral
H Hamate

Femur

Medial epicondyle
Lateral epicondyle
Patella
Head of fibula
Tibial tuberosity
Quadriceps femoris tendon
Tibial collateral ligament
Fibular collateral ligament
Patellar ligament
Tibia
Fibula
Interosseous membrane

Key to Tarsal Bones
J Intermediate cuneiform
K Lateral cuneiform
L Cuboid
M Talus
N Navicular
O Calcaneus
P Medial cuneiform

J
K
M
L
N
O
P

Medial malleolus
Lateral malleolus

PLATE 11. SKELETAL SYSTEM — POSTERIOR VIEW

Symptoms, signs and ill-defined conditions   780-799

Fracture of skull
Fracture of vault of skull   800
Fracture of base of skull   801
Fracture of face bones   802
Multiple fractures involving skull or face with other bones   804

Fracture of neck and trunk
Fracture of vertebral column without mention of spinal cord injury   805
Fracture of vertebral column with spinal cord injury   806
Fracture of rib(s), sternum, larynx and trachea   807
Fracture of pelvis   808

Fracture of upper limb
Fracture of clavicle   810
Fracture of scapula   811
Fracture of humerus   812
Fracture of radius and ulna   813
Fracture of carpal bone(s)   814
Fracture of metacarpal bone(s)   815
Fracture of one or more phalanges of hand   816
Multiple fractures of hand bones   817

Fracture of lower limb
Fracture of neck of femur   820
Fracture of other and unspecified parts of femur   821
Fracture of patella   822
Fracture of tibia and fibula   823
Fracture of ankle   824
Fracture of one or more tarsal and metatarsal bones   825
Fracture of one or more phalanges of foot   826

Dislocation
Dislocation of jaw   830
Dislocation of shoulder   831
Dislocation of elbow   832
Dislocation of wrist   833
Dislocation of finger   834
Dislocation of hip   835
Dislocation of knee   836
Dislocation of ankle   837
Dislocation of foot   838

Skeletal System
(Posterior View)

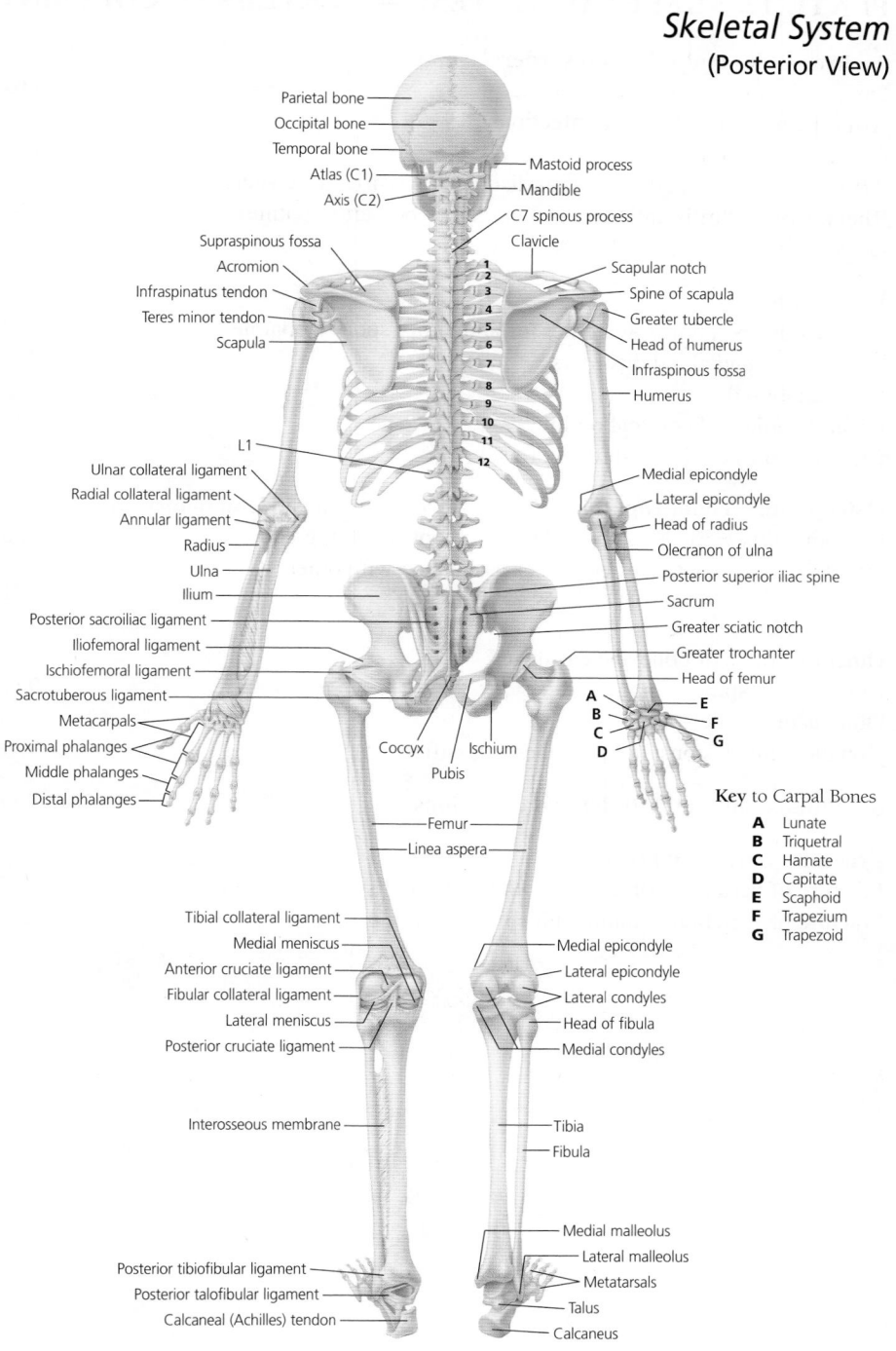

Parietal bone
Occipital bone
Temporal bone
Atlas (C1)
Axis (C2)
Mastoid process
Mandible
C7 spinous process
Supraspinous fossa
Acromion
Clavicle
Scapular notch
Infraspinatus tendon
Spine of scapula
Teres minor tendon
Greater tubercle
Scapula
Head of humerus
Infraspinous fossa
Humerus
1
2
3
4
5
6
7
8
9
10
11
12
L1
Ulnar collateral ligament
Radial collateral ligament
Annular ligament
Radius
Ulna
Ilium
Medial epicondyle
Lateral epicondyle
Head of radius
Olecranon of ulna
Posterior superior iliac spine
Sacrum
Posterior sacroiliac ligament
Greater sciatic notch
Iliofemoral ligament
Greater trochanter
Ischiofemoral ligament
Head of femur
Sacrotuberous ligament
Metacarpals
Proximal phalanges
Middle phalanges
Distal phalanges
Coccyx
Ischium
Pubis
A
B
C
D
E
F
G
Femur
Linea aspera

Key to Carpal Bones
A Lunate
B Triquetral
C Hamate
D Capitate
E Scaphoid
F Trapezium
G Trapezoid

Tibial collateral ligament
Medial meniscus
Anterior cruciate ligament
Fibular collateral ligament
Lateral meniscus
Posterior cruciate ligament
Medial epicondyle
Lateral epicondyle
Lateral condyles
Head of fibula
Medial condyles

Interosseous membrane
Tibia
Fibula

Medial malleolus
Lateral malleolus
Metatarsals
Posterior tibiofibular ligament
Posterior talofibular ligament
Calcaneal (Achilles) tendon
Talus
Calcaneus

PLATE 12. SKELETAL SYSTEM — VERTEBRAL COLUMN

Arthropathies and related disorders
Diffuse diseases of connective tissue 710
Arthropathy associated with infections 711
Crystal arthropathies 712
Arthropathy associated with other disorders classified elsewhere 713
Rheumatoid arthritis and other inflammatory polyarthropathies 714
Osteoarthrosis and allied disorders 715

Dorsopathies
Ankylosing spondylitis and other inflammatory spondylopathies 720
Spondylosis and allied disorders 721
Intervertebral disc disorders 722
Other disorders of cervical region 723
Other and unspecified disorders of back 724

Osteopathies, chondropathies, and acquired musculoskeletal deformities
Osteomyelitis, periostitis, and other infections involving bone 730
Osteitis deformans and osteopathies associated with other
 disorders classified elsewhere 731
Osteochondropathies 732
Other disorders of bone and cartilage 733
Curvature of spine 737
Other acquired deformity 738
Nonallopathic lesions, not elsewhere classified 739

Symptoms, signs and ill-defined conditions 780-799

Fracture of neck and trunk
Fracture of vertebral column without mention of spinal cord injury 805
Fracture of vertebral column with spinal cord injury 806

Vertebral Column
(Lateral View)

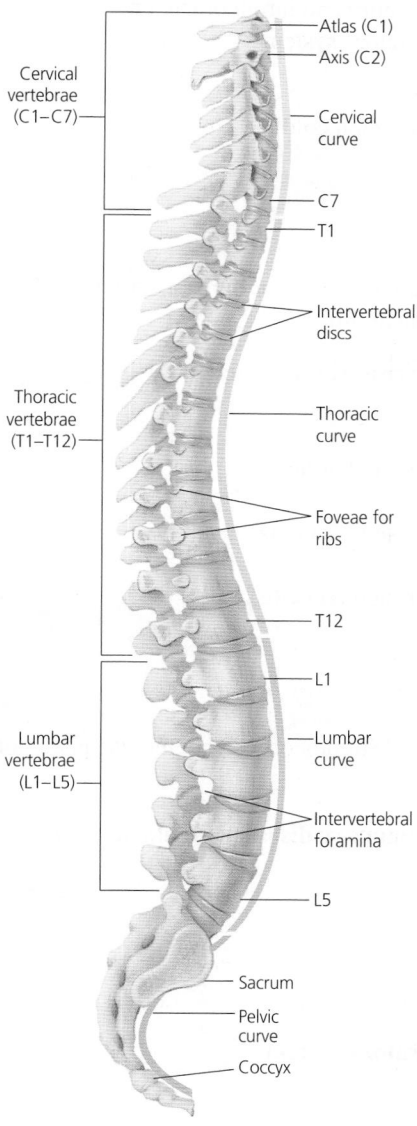

Cervical vertebrae (C1–C7)

Thoracic vertebrae (T1–T12)

Lumbar vertebrae (L1–L5)

Atlas (C1)

Axis (C2)

Cervical curve

C7

T1

Intervertebral discs

Thoracic curve

Foveae for ribs

T12

L1

Lumbar curve

Intervertebral foramina

L5

Sacrum

Pelvic curve

Coccyx

PLATE 13. RESPIRATORY SYSTEM

Malignant neoplasm of respiratory and intrathoracic organs   160-165
Malignant neoplasm of larynx   161
Malignant neoplasm of trachea, bronchus, and lung   162
Benign neoplasm of respiratory and intrathoracic organs   212
Carcinoma in situ of respiratory system   231

Acute respiratory infections
Acute nasopharyngitis [common cold]   460
Acute sinusitis   461
Acute pharyngitis   462
Acute tonsillitis   463
Acute laryngitis and tracheitis   464
Acute upper respiratory infections of multiple or unspecified sites   465
Acute bronchitis and bronchiolitis   466

Other diseases of upper respiratory tract
Deviated nasal septum   470
Nasal polyps   471
Chronic pharyngitis and nasopharyngitis   472
Chronic sinusitis   473
Chronic disease of tonsils and adenoids   474
Peritonsillar abscess   475
Chronic laryngitis and laryngotracheitis   476
Allergic rhinitis   477

Pneumonia and influenza
Viral pneumonia   480
Pneumococcal pneumonia [Streptococcus pneumoniae pneumonia]   481
Influenza   487

Chronic obstructive pulmonary disease and allied conditions
Chronic bronchitis   491
Emphysema   492
Asthma   493
Bronchiectasis   494
Extrinsic allergic alveolitis   495

Other diseases of respiratory system
Empyema   510
Pleurisy   511
Pneumothorax   512
Abscess of lung and mediastinum   513
Pulmonary congestion and hypostasis   514
Postinflammatory pulmonary fibrosis   515

Respiratory System

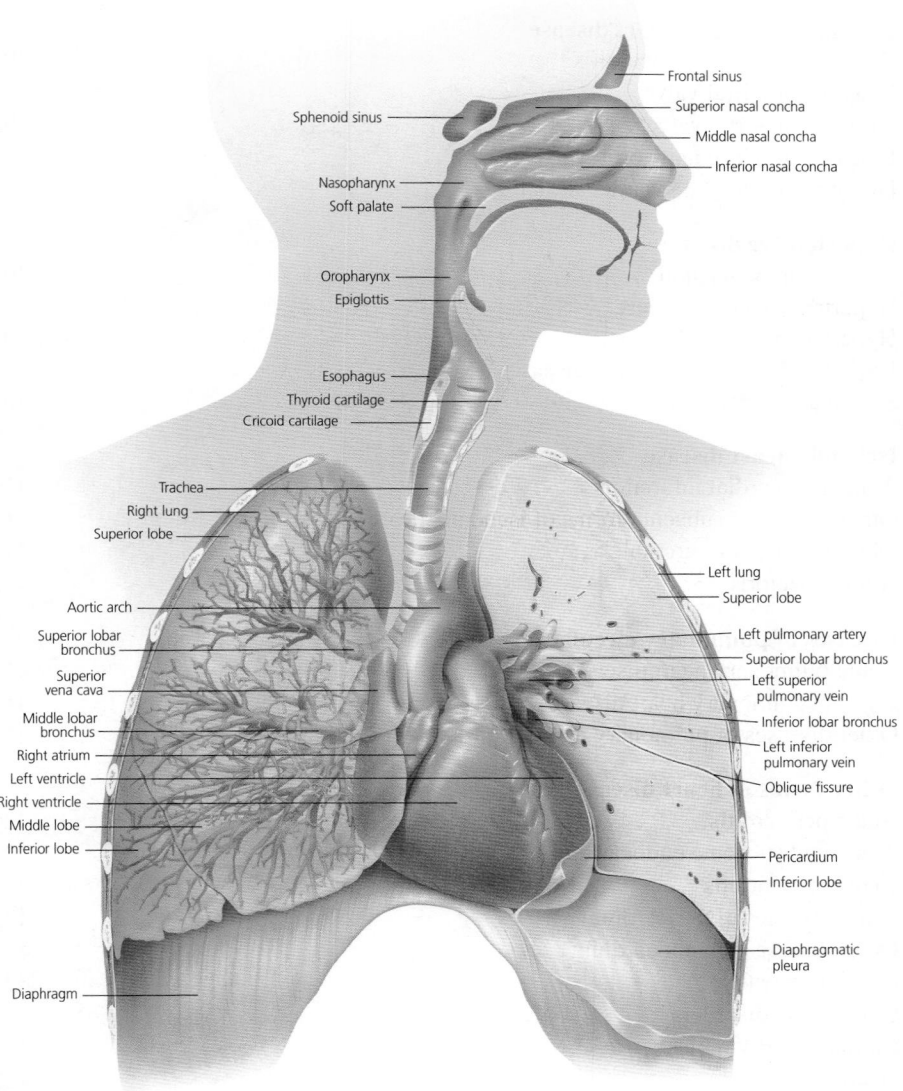

Frontal sinus

Superior nasal concha

Sphenoid sinus

Middle nasal concha

Inferior nasal concha

Nasopharynx

Soft palate

Oropharynx

Epiglottis

Esophagus

Thyroid cartilage

Cricoid cartilage

Trachea

Right lung

Superior lobe

Left lung

Superior lobe

Aortic arch

Left pulmonary artery

Superior lobar bronchus

Superior lobar bronchus

Superior vena cava

Left superior pulmonary vein

Middle lobar bronchus

Inferior lobar bronchus

Right atrium

Left inferior pulmonary vein

Left ventricle

Oblique fissure

Right ventricle

Middle lobe

Inferior lobe

Pericardium

Inferior lobe

Diaphragmatic pleura

Diaphragm

PLATE 14. HEART AND PERICARDIUM

Acute rheumatic fever
Rheumatic fever without mention of heart involvement   390
Rheumatic fever with heart involvement   391
Rheumatic chorea   392

Chronic rheumatic heart disease
Chronic rheumatic pericarditis   393
Diseases of mitral valve   394
Diseases of aortic valve   395
Diseases of mitral and aortic valves   396
Diseases of other endocardial structures   397

Hypertensive disease
Essential hypertension   401
Hypertensive heart disease   402
Hypertensive renal disease   403
Hypertensive heart and renal disease   404
Secondary hypertension   405

Ischemic heart disease
Acute myocardial infarction   410
Other acute and subacute forms of ischemic heart disease   411
Old myocardial infarction   412
Angina pectoris   413

Diseases of pulmonary circulation
Acute pulmonary heart disease   415
Chronic pulmonary heart disease   416
Other diseases of pulmonary circulation   417

Other forms of heart disease
Acute pericarditis   420
Acute and subacute endocarditis   421
Acute myocarditis   422
Other diseases of pericardium   423
Other diseases of endocardium   424
Cardiomyopathy   425
Conduction disorders   426
Cardiac dysrhythmias   427
Heart failure   428

Symptoms, signs and ill-defined conditions   780-799

Heart
(External View)

Left common carotid artery
Brachiocephalic artery
Left subclavian artery
Aortic arch
Ligamentum arteriosum
Superior vena cava
Left pulmonary artery
Ascending aorta
Pulmonary trunk
Left auricle
Right coronary artery
Circumflex artery
Right atrium
Great cardiac vein
Right ventricle
Anterior descending (interventricular) artery
Anterior cardiac vein
Left ventricle
Right marginal artery
Small cardiac vein
Apex

Heart
(Internal View)

Superior vena cava
Right pulmonary artery branches
Left pulmonary artery
Aorta
Pulmonary trunk
Left pulmonary veins
Right pulmonary veins
Left atrium
Pulmonary semilunar valve
Aortic semilunar valve
Right atrium
Bicuspid (left AV) valve
Left ventricle
Tricuspid (right AV) valve
Papillary muscle
Interventricular septum
Chordae tendineae
Inferior vena cava
Myocardium
Right ventricle
Trabeculae carneae

PLATE 15. CIRCULATORY SYSTEM

Diseases of arteries, arterioles, and capillaries
Atherosclerosis   440
Aortic aneurysm and dissection   441
Arterial embolism and thrombosis   444
Polyarteritis nodosa and allied conditions   446
Other disorders of arteries and arterioles   447
Diseases of capillaries   448

Diseases of veins and lymphatics, and other circulatory system
Phlebitis and thrombophlebitis   451
Portal vein thrombosis   452
Varicose veins of lower extremities   454
Hemorrhoids   455
Varicose veins of other sites   456
Noninfectious disorders of lymphatic channels   457
Hypotension   458

Symptoms, signs and ill-defined conditions   780-799

Injury to blood vessels
Injury to blood vessels of head and neck   900
Injury to blood vessels of thorax   901
Injury to blood vessels of abdomen and pelvis   902
Injury to blood vessels of upper extremity   903
Injury to blood vessels of lower extremity and unspecified sites   904

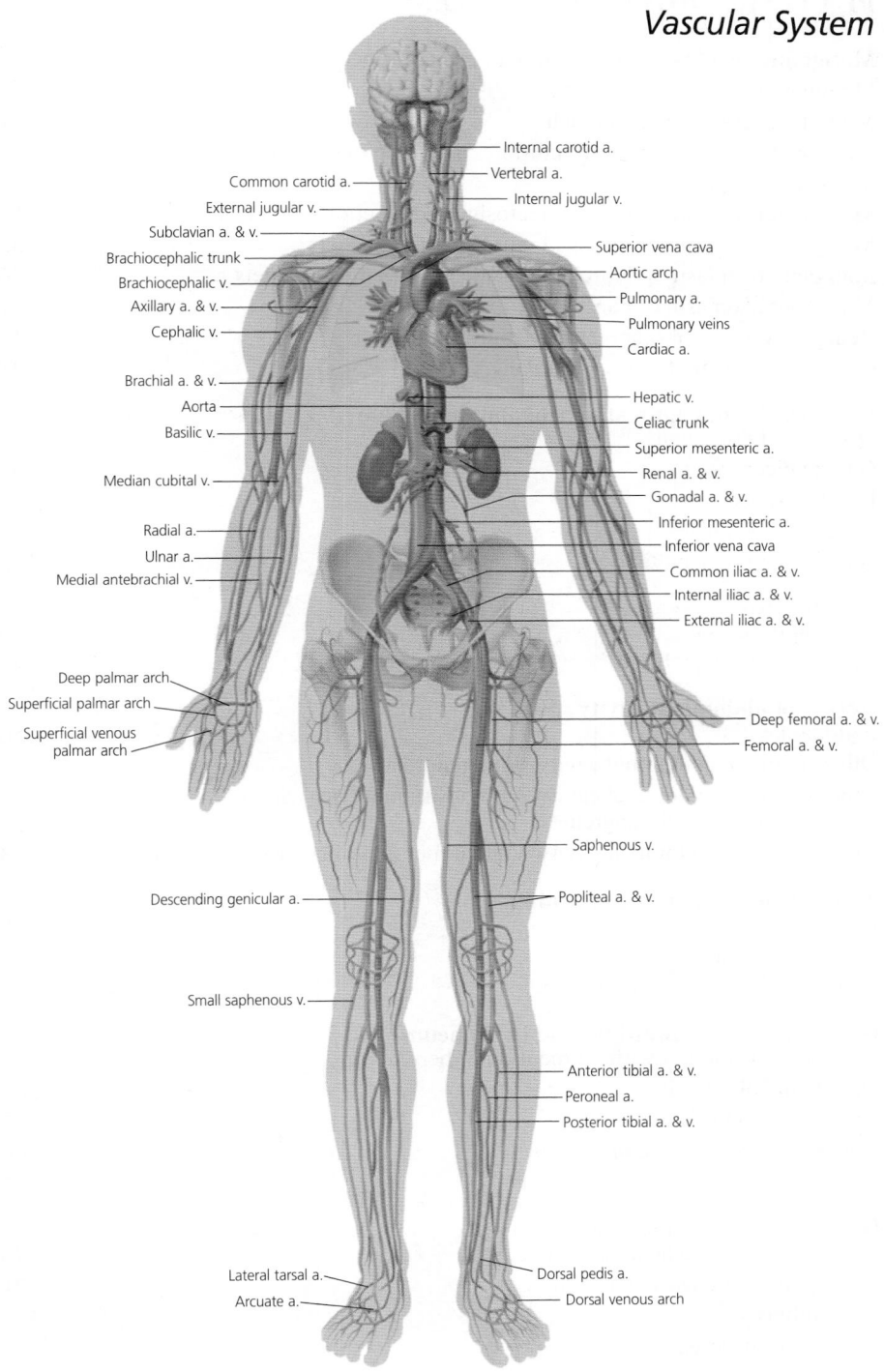

Vascular System

Internal carotid a.
Common carotid a.
Vertebral a.
External jugular v.
Internal jugular v.
Subclavian a. & v.
Brachiocephalic trunk
Superior vena cava
Brachiocephalic v.
Aortic arch
Axillary a. & v.
Pulmonary a.
Cephalic v.
Pulmonary veins
Cardiac a.
Brachial a. & v.
Hepatic v.
Aorta
Celiac trunk
Basilic v.
Superior mesenteric a.
Median cubital v.
Renal a. & v.
Gonadal a. & v.
Radial a.
Inferior mesenteric a.
Ulnar a.
Inferior vena cava
Medial antebrachial v.
Common iliac a. & v.
Internal iliac a. & v.
External iliac a. & v.
Deep palmar arch
Superficial palmar arch
Superficial venous palmar arch
Deep femoral a. & v.
Femoral a. & v.
Saphenous v.
Descending genicular a.
Popliteal a. & v.
Small saphenous v.
Anterior tibial a. & v.
Peroneal a.
Posterior tibial a. & v.
Lateral tarsal a.
Dorsal pedis a.
Arcuate a.
Dorsal venous arch

PLATE 16. DIGESTIVE SYSTEM

Malignant neoplasms of digestive organs and peritoneum
Malignant neoplasm of esophagus 150
Malignant neoplasm of stomach 151
Malignant neoplasm of small intestine, including duodenum 152
Malignant neoplasm of colon 153
Malignant neoplasm of rectum, rectosigmoid junction, and anus 154
Malignant neoplasm of liver and intrahepatic bile ducts 155
Malignant neoplasm of gallbladder and extrahepatic bile ducts 156
Malignant neoplasm of pancreas 157
Benign neoplasm of other parts of digestive system 211
Carcinoma in situ of digestive organs 230

Diseases of esophagus, stomach, and duodenum
Diseases of esophagus 530
Gastric ulcer 531
Duodenal ulcer 532
Gastrojejunal ulcer 534
Gastritis and duodenitis 535

Appendicitis
Acute appendicitis 540
Appendicitis, unqualified 541

Hernia of abdominal cavity
Inguinal hernia 550
Other hernia of abdominal cavity, with gangrene 551
Other hernia of abdominal cavity, with obstruction, but without
    mention of gangrene 552
Other hernia of abdominal cavity without mention of obstruction or gangrene 553

Noninfectious enteritis and colitis
Regional enteritis 555
Ulcerative colitis 556
Vascular insufficiency of intestine 557

Other diseases of intestines and peritoneum
Intestinal obstruction without mention of hernia 560
Diverticula of intestine 562
Anal fissure and fistula 565
Abscess of anal and rectal regions 566
Peritonitis 567

Other diseases of digestive system
Acute and subacute necrosis of liver 570
Chronic liver disease and cirrhosis 571
Cholelithiasis 574
Diseases of pancreas 577
Gastrointestinal hemorrhage 578

Digestive System

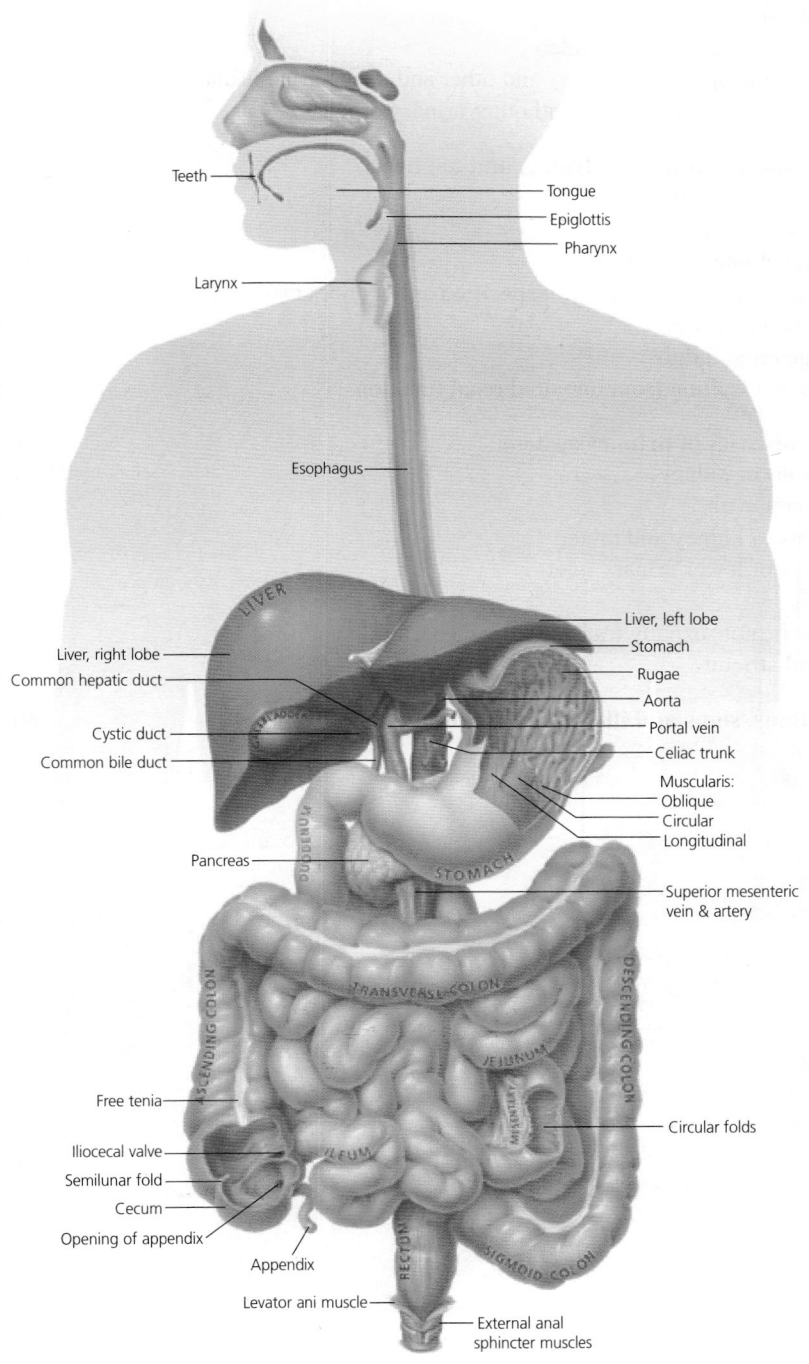

Teeth

Tongue

Epiglottis

Pharynx

Larynx

Esophagus

Liver, left lobe

Stomach

Liver, right lobe

Common hepatic duct

Rugae

Aorta

Portal vein

Cystic duct

Celiac trunk

Common bile duct

Muscularis:
Oblique
Circular
Longitudinal

Pancreas

Superior mesenteric
vein & artery

Free tenia

Circular folds

Iliocecal valve

Semilunar fold

Cecum

Opening of appendix

Appendix

Levator ani muscle

External anal
sphincter muscles

PLATE 17. GENITOURINARY SYSTEM

Neoplasms

Malignant neoplasm of bladder   188
Malignant neoplasm of kidney and other and unspecified urinary organs   189
Benign neoplasm of kidney and other urinary organs   223

Nephritis, nephrotic syndrome, and nephrosis

Acute glomerulonephritis   580
Nephrotic syndrome   581
Chronic glomerulonephritis   582
Nephritis and nephropathy, not specified as acute or chronic   583
Acute renal failure   584
Chronic renal failure   585
Disorders resulting from impaired renal function   588

Other diseases of urinary system

Infections of kidney   590
Hydronephrosis   591
Calculus of kidney and ureter   592
Calculus of lower urinary tract   594
Cystitis   595
Urethritis, not sexually transmitted, and urethral syndrome   597
Urethral stricture   598

Symptoms, signs and ill-defined conditions   780-799

Urinary System

PLATE 18. MALE REPRODUCTIVE SYSTEM

Neoplasms

Malignant neoplasm of prostate   185
Malignant neoplasm of testis   186
Malignant neoplasm of penis and other male genital organs   187
Benign neoplasm of male genital organs   222

Diseases of male genital organs

Hyperplasia of prostate   600
Inflammatory diseases of prostate   601
Hydrocele   603
Orchitis and epididymitis   604
Redundant prepuce and phimosis   605
Infertility, male   606
Disorders of penis   607

Symptoms, signs and ill-defined conditions   780-799

Male Reproductive System

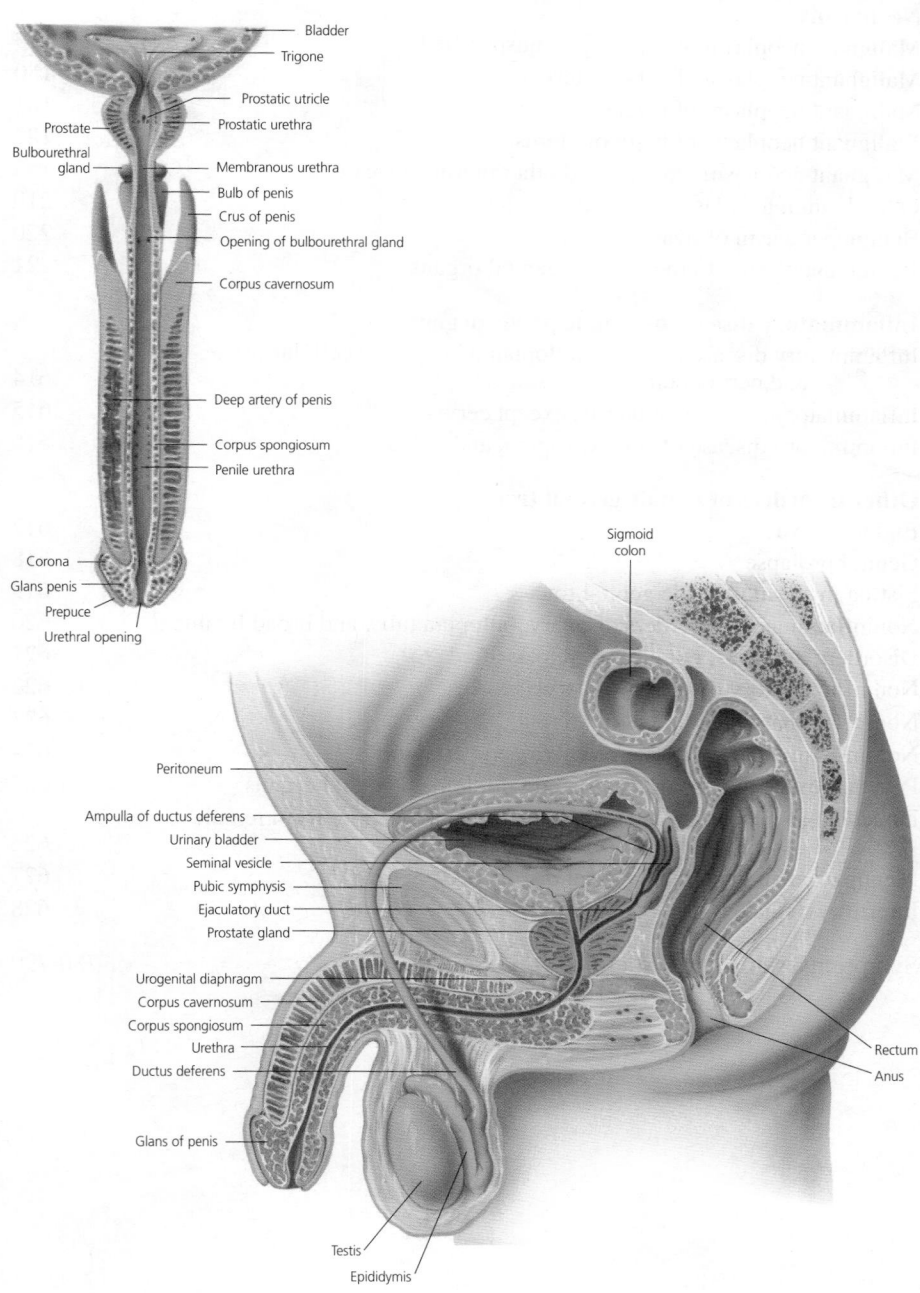

PLATE 19. FEMALE REPRODUCTIVE SYSTEM

Neoplasms

Malignant neoplasm of uterus, part unspecified	179
Malignant neoplasm of cervix uteri	180
Malignant neoplasm of placenta	181
Malignant neoplasm of body of uterus	182
Malignant neoplasm of ovary and other uterine adnexa	183
Other benign neoplasm of uterus	219
Benign neoplasm of ovary	220
Benign neoplasm of other female genital organs	221

Inflammatory disease of female pelvic organs

Inflammatory disease of ovary, fallopian tube, pelvic cellular tissue, and peritoneum	614
Inflammatory diseases of uterus, except cervix	615
Inflammatory disease of cervix, vagina, and vulva	616

Other disorders of female genital tract

Endometriosis	617
Genital prolapse	618
Fistula involving female genital tract	619
Noninflammatory disorders of ovary, fallopian tube, and broad ligament	620
Disorders of uterus, not elsewhere classified	621
Noninflammatory disorders of cervix	622
Noninflammatory disorders of vagina	623
Noninflammatory disorders of vulva and perineum	624
Pain and other symptoms associated with female genital organs	625
Disorders of menstruation and other abnormal bleeding from female genital tract	626
Menopausal and postmenopausal disorders	627
Infertility, female	628

Symptoms, signs and ill-defined conditions 780-799

Female Reproductive System

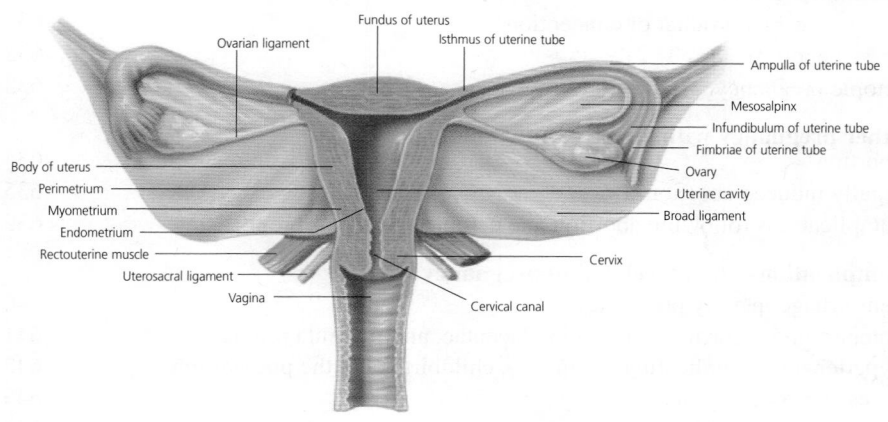

Fundus of uterus
Ovarian ligament
Isthmus of uterine tube
Ampulla of uterine tube
Mesosalpinx
Infundibulum of uterine tube
Fimbriae of uterine tube
Ovary
Body of uterus
Perimetrium
Uterine cavity
Myometrium
Broad ligament
Endometrium
Rectouterine muscle
Uterosacral ligament
Cervix
Vagina
Cervical canal

Sacrum
Suspensory ligament of ovary
Sigmoid colon
Uterine tube
Rectouterine pouch
Ovary
Round ligament of uterus
Uterus
Cervix
Urinary bladder
Pubic symphysis
Urethra
Rectum
Vagina
Clitoris
Anus
Labium minus
Labium majus
Vaginal opening

PLATE 20. PREGNANCY, CHILDBIRTH AND THE PUERPERIUM

Ectopic and molar pregnancy
Hydatidiform mole   630
Other abnormal product of conception   631
Missed abortion   632
Ectopic pregnancy   633

Other pregnancy with abortive outcome
Abortion   634
Legally induced abortion   635
Complications following abortion and ectopic and molar pregnancies   639

Complications mainly related to pregnancy
Hemorrhage in early pregnancy   640
Antepartum hemorrhage, abruptio placentae, and placenta previa   641
Hypertension complicating pregnancy, childbirth, and the puerperium   642
Excessive vomiting in pregnancy   643
Early or threatened labor   644
Late pregnancy   645

Normal delivery, other indications for care in pregnancy and delivery
Normal delivery   650
Multiple gestation   651
Malposition and malpresentation of fetus   652
Disproportion   653
Polyhydramnios   657

Complications occurring mainly in the course of labor and delivery
Obstructed labor   660
Abnormality of forces of labor   661
Long labor   662
Umbilical cord complications   663
Trauma to perineum and vulva during delivery   664
Postpartum hemorrhage   666
Retained placenta or membranes, without hemorrhage   667

Complications of the puerperium
Major puerperal infection   670
Venous complications in pregnancy and the puerperium   671
Pyrexia of unknown origin during the puerperium   672
Obstetrical pulmonary embolism   673

Persons encountering health services in circumstances related to reproduction
Normal pregnancy   V22
Supervision of high-risk pregnancy   V23
Postpartum care and examination   V24
Encounter for contraceptive management   V25
Procreative management   V26

Female Reproductive System: Pregnancy
(Lateral View)

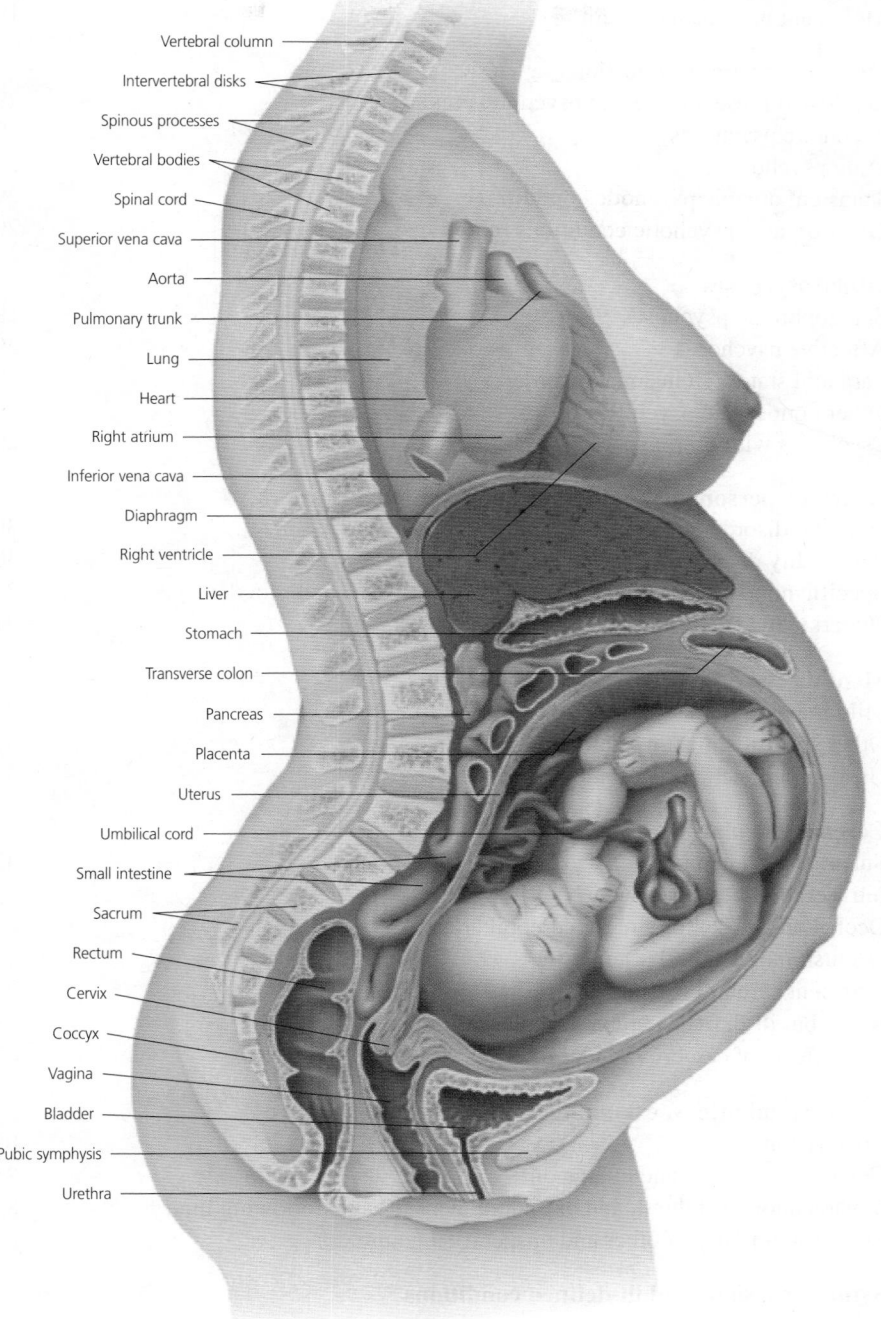

Vertebral column
Intervertebral disks
Spinous processes
Vertebral bodies
Spinal cord
Superior vena cava
Aorta
Pulmonary trunk
Lung
Heart
Right atrium
Inferior vena cava
Diaphragm
Right ventricle
Liver
Stomach
Transverse colon
Pancreas
Placenta
Uterus
Umbilical cord
Small intestine
Sacrum
Rectum
Cervix
Coccyx
Vagina
Bladder
Pubic symphysis
Urethra

PLATE 21. NERVOUS SYSTEM — BRAIN

Neoplasms
Malignant neoplasm of brain   191

Organic psychotic conditions
Senile and presenile organic psychotic conditions   290
Alcoholic psychoses   291
Drug psychoses   292
Transient organic psychotic conditions   293
Other organic psychotic conditions (chronic)   294

Other psychoses
Schizophrenic psychoses   295
Affective psychoses   296
Paranoid states (Delusional disorders)   297
Other nonorganic psychoses   298
Psychoses with origin specific to childhood   299

Neurotic, personality, and other nonpsychotic disorders
Neurotic disorders   300
Personality disorders   301
Specific nonpsychotic mental disorders due to organic brain damage   310
Hyperkinetic syndrome of childhood   314

Mental retardation
Mild mental retardation   317
Other specified mental retardation   318
Unspecified mental retardation   319

Cerebrovascular disease
Subarachnoid hemorrhage   430
Intracerebral hemorrhage   431
Occlusion and stenosis of precerebral arteries   433
Occlusion of cerebral arteries   434
Transient cerebral ischemia   435
Acute but ill-defined cerebrovascular disease   436
Late effects of cerebrovascular disease   438

Intracranial injury, excluding those with skull fracture
Concussion   850
Cerebral laceration and contusion   851
Subarachnoid, subdural, and extradural hemorrhage, following injury   852
Intracranial injury of other and unspecified nature   854

Symptoms, signs and ill-defined conditions   780-799

Brain
(Base View)

Olfactory bulb

Cerebrum

Olfactory tract (I)

Anterior communicating artery

Anterior cerebral artery

Optic nerve (II)

Optic chiasm

Middle cerebral artery

Internal carotid artery

Posterior communicating artery

Pituitary gland

Posterior cerebral artery

Oculomotor nerve (III)

Superior cerebellar artery

Troclear nerve (IV)

Basilar artery

Trigeminal nerve (V)

Abducens nerve

Pons

Abducens nerve (VI)

Facial nerve (VII)

Vestibulocochlear nerve (VIII)

Glossopharyngeal nerve (IX)

Hypoglossal nerve (XII)

Vagus nerve (X)

Accessory nerve (XI)

Anterior inferior cerebellar artery

Vertebral artery

Medulla oblongata

Anterior spinal artery

Cerebellum

Spinal cord

Posterior inferior cerebellar artery

PLATE 22. NERVOUS SYSTEM

Inflammatory diseases of the central nervous system
Bacterial meningitis 320
Meningitis due to other organisms 321
Encephalitis, myelitis, and encephalomyelitis 323
Intracranial and intraspinal abscess 324
Phlebitis and thrombophlebitis of intracranial venous sinuses 325

Hereditary and degenerative diseases of the central nervous system
Cerebral degenerations usually manifest in childhood 330
Other cerebral degenerations 331
Parkinson's disease 332
Spinocerebellar disease 334
Anterior horn cell disease 335
Other diseases of spinal cord 336
Disorders of the autonomic nervous system 337

Other disorders of the central nervous system
Multiple sclerosis 340
Other demyelinating diseases of central nervous system 341
Hemiplegia and hemiparesis 342
Infantile cerebral palsy 343
Other paralytic syndromes 344
Epilepsy 345
Migraine 346
Cataplexy and narcolepsy 347

Disorders of the peripheral nervous system
Trigeminal nerve disorders 350
Facial nerve disorders 351
Disorders of other cranial nerves 352
Nerve root and plexus disorders 353
Mononeuritis of upper limb and mononeuritis multiplex 354
Mononeuritis of lower limb and unspecified site 355
Hereditary and idiopathic peripheral neuropathy 356
Inflammatory and toxic neuropathy 357
Myoneural disorders 358
Muscular dystrophies and other myopathies 359

Injury to nerves and spinal cord
Injury to optic nerve and pathways 950
Injury to other cranial nerve(s) 951
Spinal cord injury without evidence of spinal bone injury 952
Injury to nerve roots and spinal plexus 953
Injury to other nerve(s) of trunk, excluding shoulder and pelvic girdles 954
Injury to peripheral nerve(s) of shoulder girdle and upper limb 955
Injury to peripheral nerve(s) of pelvic girdle and lower limb 956

Nervous System

Brain
Cerebrum
Brain stem
Cerebellum
Cervical plexus
Lateral cord
Spinal cord
Medial cord
Brachial plexus
Posterior cord
Phrenic nerve
Musculocutaneous nerve
Intercostal nerves
Ulnar nerve
Median nerve
Subcostal nerve
Radial nerve
Iliohypogastric nerve
Lumbar plexus
Ilioinguinal nerve
Genitofemoral nerve
Deep branch of radial nerve
Sacral plexus
Lateral femoral cutaneous nerve
Coccygeal plexus
Superficial branch of radial nerve
Femoral nerve
Obturator nerve
Pudendal nerve
Sciatic nerve
Muscular branches of femoral nerve
Saphenous nerve
Common peroneal nerve
Deep peroneal nerve
Superficial peroneal nerve
Tibial nerve

PLATE 23. EYE AND OCULAR ADNEXA

Disorders of the eye and adnexa
Disorders of the globe 360
Retinal detachments and defects 361
Other retinal disorders 362
Chorioretinal inflammations, scars, and other disorders of choroid 363
Disorders of iris and ciliary body 364
Glaucoma 365
Cataract 366
Disorders of refraction and accommodation 367
Visual disturbances 368
Blindness and low vision 369
Keratitis 370
Corneal opacity and other disorders of cornea 371
Disorders of conjunctiva 372
Inflammation of eyelids 373
Other disorders of eyelids 374
Disorders of lacrimal system 375
Disorders of the orbit 376
Disorders of optic nerve and visual pathways 377
Strabismus and other disorders of binocular eye movements 378

Symptoms, signs and ill-defined conditions 780-799

Right Eye
(Horizontal Section)

Lateral rectus muscle

Conjunctiva

Canal of Schlemm

Zonular fibers

Iris

Lens

Cornea

Pupil

Aqueous humor

Anterior chamber

Posterior chamber

Ciliary body

Sclera

Ora serrata

Choroid

Medial rectus muscle

Vitreous body

Hyaloid canal

Macula lutea

Optic disc

Retinal vessels

Optic nerve

Nerve sheath

Retina

PLATE 24. AUDITORY SYSTEM

Diseases of the ear and mastoid process
Disorders of external ear   380
Nonsuppurative otitis media and Eustachian tube disorders   381
Suppurative and unspecified otitis media   382
Mastoiditis and related conditions   383
Other disorders of tympanic membrane   384
Other disorders of middle ear and mastoid   385
Vertiginous syndromes and other disorders of vestibular system   386
Otosclerosis   387
Hearing loss   389

Symptoms, signs and ill-defined conditions   780-799

The Ear

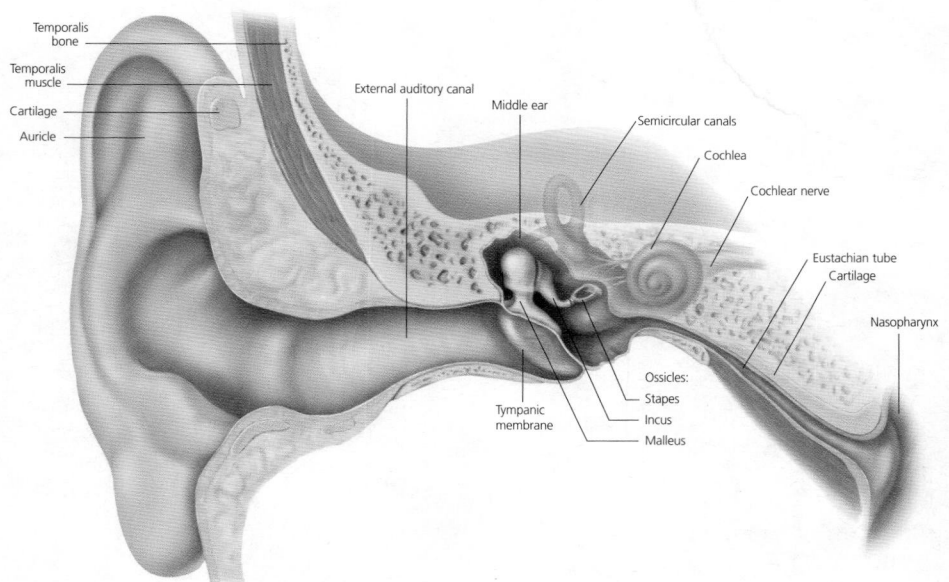

Temporalis bone

Temporalis muscle

Cartilage

Auricle

External auditory canal

Middle ear

Semicircular canals

Cochlea

Cochlear nerve

Eustachian tube
Cartilage

Nasopharynx

Ossicles:
Stapes
Incus
Malleus

Tympanic membrane

This page intentionally left blank.

DISEASES: TABULAR LIST

VOLUME 1

This page intentionally left blank.

Chapter 1: Infectious and Parasitic Diseases (001-139)

DEFINITIONS AND CODING ALERTS

This chapter includes definitions of selected key words, terms and phrases and coding alerts for adding points to the clinical domain, references to coding late effects where appropriate, and references to personal history V-codes in situations where the acute or chronic condition is no longer active. An example from this chapter is as follows:

049 **Other non-arthropod borne viral diseases of central nervous system**

> **DEFINITION** Non-arthropod-borne viral diseases refers to diseases caused by a virus that is not carried by insects, spiders, crustaceans, centipedes or millipedes
> **ALERT!** For coding late effects of viral encephalitis see 139.0.
> **ALERT!** For personal history of other specified infectious and parasitic disease see V12.09.

MULTIPLE CODING FOR A SINGLE CONDITION

In addition to the etiology or manifestation convention that requires two codes to fully describe a single condition that affects multiple body systems, there are other single conditions that also require more than one code. "Use additional code" notes are found in the tabular at codes that are not part of an etiology or manifestation pair where a secondary code is useful to fully describe a condition. The sequencing rule is the same as the etiology or manifestation pair - , "use additional code" indicates that a secondary code should be added. For example, for infections that are not included in chapter 1, a secondary code from category 041, Bacterial infection in conditions classified elsewhere and of unspecified site, may be required to identify the bacterial organism causing the infection. A "use additional code" note will normally be found at the infectious disease code, indicating a need for the organism code to be added as a secondary code.

"Code first" notes are also under certain codes that are not specifically manifestation codes but may be due to an underlying cause. When a "code first" note is present and an underlying condition is present the underlying condition should be sequenced first.

"Code, if applicable, any causal condition first", notes indicate that this code may be assigned as a principal diagnosis when the causal condition is unknown or not applicable. If a causal condition is known, then the code for that condition should be sequenced as the principal or first-listed diagnosis. Multiple codes may be needed for late effects, complication codes and obstetric codes to more fully describe a condition. See the specific guidelines for these conditions for further instruction.

COMBINATION CODE

A combination code is a single code used to classify: two diagnoses, or a diagnosis with an associated secondary process (manifestation) A diagnosis with an associated complication Combination codes are identified by referring to subterm entries in the Alphabetic Index and by reading the inclusion and exclusion notes in the Tabular List.

Assign only the combination code when that code fully identifies the diagnostic conditions involved or when the Alphabetic Index so directs. Multiple coding should not be used when the classification provides a combination code that clearly identifies all of the elements documented in the diagnosis. When the combination code lacks necessary specificity in describing the manifestation or complication, an additional code should be used as a secondary code.

CODING LATE EFFECTS

A late effect is the residual effect (condition produced) after the acute phase of an illness or injury has terminated. There is no time limit on when a late effect code can be used. The residual may be apparent early, such as in cerebrovascular accident cases, or it may occur months or years later, such as that due to a previous injury. Coding of late effects generally requires two codes sequenced in the following order: The condition or nature of the late effect is sequenced first. The late effect code is sequenced second.

An exception to the above guidelines are those instances where the code for late effect is followed by a manifestation code identified in the Tabular List and title, or the late effect code has been expanded (at the fourth and fifth-digit levels) to include the manifestation(s). The code for the acute phase of an illness or injury that led to the late effect is never used with a code for the late effect.

	Add 4th or 5th digit		Nonspecific code		Unspecified code		Manifestation code

HUMAN IMMUNODEFICIENCY VIRUS (HIV) INFECTIONS

Code only confirmed cases

Code only confirmed cases of HIV infection or illness. This is an exception to the hospital inpatient guideline Official Guidelines, Section II, H. In this context, "confirmation" does not require documentation of positive serology or culture for HIV; the provider's diagnostic statement that the patient is HIV positive, or has an HIV-related illness is sufficient.

Selection and sequencing of HIV codes

A. Patient admitted for HIV-related condition

   If a patient is admitted for an HIV-related condition, the principal diagnosis should be 042, followed by additional diagnosis codes for all reported HIV-related conditions.

B. Patient with HIV disease admitted for unrelated condition

   If a patient with HIV disease is admitted for an unrelated condition (such as a traumatic injury), the code for the unrelated condition (e.g., the nature of injury code) should be the principal diagnosis. Other diagnoses would be 042 followed by additional diagnosis codes for all reported HIV-related conditions.

C. Whether the patient is newly diagnosed

   Whether the patient is newly diagnosed or has had previous admissions or encounters for HIV conditions is irrelevant to the sequencing decision.

D. Asymptomatic human immunodeficiency virus V08

   Asymptomatic human immunodeficiency virus [HIV] infection, is to be applied when the patient without any documentation of symptoms is listed as being "HIV positive," "known HIV," "HIV test positive," or similar terminology. Do not use this code if the term "AIDS" is used or if the patient is treated for any HIV-related illness or is described as having any condition(s) resulting from his or her HIV positive status; use 042 in these cases.

E. Patients with inconclusive HIV serology

   Patients with inconclusive HIV serology, but no definitive diagnosis or manifestations of the illness, may be assigned code 795.71, Inconclusive serologic test for Human Immunodeficiency Virus [HIV].

F. Previously diagnosed HIV-related illness

   Patients with any known prior diagnosis of an HIV-related illness should be coded to 042. Once a patient has developed an HIV-related illness, the patient should always be assigned code 042 on every subsequent admission or encounter. Patients previously diagnosed with any HIV illness 042 should never be assigned to 795.71 or V08.

G. HIV Infection in Pregnancy, Childbirth and the Puerperium

   During pregnancy, childbirth or the puerperium, a patient admitted (or presenting for a health care encounter) because of an HIV-related illness should receive a principal diagnosis code of 647.6X, Other specified infectious and parasitic diseases in the mother classifiable elsewhere, but complicating the pregnancy, childbirth or the puerperium, followed by 042 and the code(s) for the HIV-related illness(es). Codes from Chapter 15 always take sequencing priority.

   Patients with asymptomatic HIV infection status admitted (or presenting for a health care encounter) during pregnancy, childbirth, or the puerperium should receive codes of 647.6X and V08.

H. Encounters for testing for HIV

   If a patient is being seen to determine his or her HIV status, use code V73.89, Screening for other specified viral disease. Use code V69.8, Other problems related to lifestyle, as a secondary code if an asymptomatic patient is in a known high risk group for HIV. Should a patient with signs or symptoms or illness, or a confirmed HIV related diagnosis be tested for HIV, code the signs and symptoms or the diagnosis. An additional counseling code V65.44 may be used if counseling is provided during the encounter for the test.

   When a patient returns to be informed of his or her HIV test results use code V65.44, HIV counseling, if the results of the test are negative.

● Code new
   to this edition

▲ Revision of
   existing code

④ ⑤ Fourth or fifth
   digit required

If the results are positive but the patient is asymptomatic use code V08, Asymptomatic HIV infection. If the results are positive and the patient is symptomatic use code 042, HIV infection, with codes for the HIV related symptoms or diagnosis. The HIV counseling code may also be used if counseling is provided for patients with positive test results.

SEPTICEMIA, SYSTEMIC INFLAMMATORY RESPONSE SYNDROME (SIRS), SEPSIS, SEVERE SEPSIS, AND SEPTIC SHOCK

SIRS, Septicemia, and Sepsis

A.   The terms septicemia and sepsis are often used interchangeably by providers, however they are not considered synonymous terms. The following descriptions are provided for reference but do not preclude querying the provider for clarification about terms used in the documentation:

   1)   Septicemia generally refers to a systemic disease associated with the presence of pathological microorganisms or toxins in the blood, which can include bacteria, viruses, fungi or other organisms.

   2)   Systemic inflammatory response syndrome (SIRS) generally refers to the systemic response to infection, trauma or burns, or other insult (such as cancer) with symptoms including fever, tachycardia, tachypnea, and leukocytosis.

   3)   Sepsis generally refers to SIRS due to infection.

   4)   Severe sepsis generally refers to sepsis with associated acute organ dysfunction.

B.   The Coding of SIRS, sepsis and severe sepsis requires a minimum of 2 codes: a code for the underlying cause (such as infection or trauma) and a code from subcategory 995.9 Systemic inflammatory response syndrome (SIRS).

   1)   The code for the underlying cause (such as infection or trauma) must be sequenced before the code from subcategory 995.9 Systemic inflammatory response syndrome (SIRS).

   2)   Sepsis and severe sepsis require a code for the systemic infection (038.xx, 112.5, etc.) and either code 995.91, Sepsis, or 995.92, Severe sepsis. If the causal organism is not documented, assign code 038.9, Unspecified septicemia.

   3)   Severe sepsis requires additional code(s) for the associated acute organ dysfunction(s).

   4)   If a patient has sepsis with multiple organ dysfunctions, follow the instructions for coding severe sepsis.

   5)   Either the term sepsis or SIRS must be documented to assign a code from subcategory 995.9.

   6)   See Official Guidelines, Section I.C.17 g, Injury And Poisoning, Due To Non-Infectious Process, for information regarding systemic inflammatory response syndrome (SIRS) due to trauma or burns and other non-infectious processes.

C.   Due to the complex nature of sepsis and severe sepsis, some cases may require querying the provider prior to assignment of the codes.

Sequencing sepsis and severe sepsis

A.   Sepsis and severe sepsis as principal diagnosis

   If sepsis or severe sepsis is present on admission, and meets the definition of principal diagnosis, the systemic infection code (e.g., 038.xx, 112.5, etc) should be assigned as the principal diagnosis, followed by code 995.91, Sepsis, or 995.92, Severe sepsis, as required by the sequencing rules in the Tabular List. Codes from subcategory 995.9 can never be assigned as a principal diagnosis. A code should also be assigned for any localized infection, if present.

   If the sepsis or severe sepsis is due to a postprocedural infection, see Official Guidelines, Section I.C.10 for guidelines related to sepsis due to postprocedural infection.

B.   Sepsis and severe sepsis as secondary diagnoses

   When sepsis or severe sepsis develops during the encounter (it was not present on admission), the systemic infection code and code 995.91 or 995.92 should be assigned as secondary diagnoses.

	Add 4th or 5th digit		Nonspecific code		Unspecified code		Manifestation code

C.   Documentation unclear as to whether sepsis or severe sepsis is present on admission

Sepsis or severe sepsis may be present on admission but the diagnosis may not be confirmed until sometime after admission. If the documentation is not clear whether the sepsis or severe sepsis was present on admission, the provider should be queried.

Sepsis or SIRS with Localized Infection

If the reason for admission is both sepsis, severe sepsis, or SIRS and a localized infection, such as pneumonia or cellulitis, a code for the systemic infection (038.xx, 112.5, etc) should be assigned first, then code 995.91 or 995.92, followed by the code for the localized infection. If the patient is admitted with a localized infection, such as pneumonia, and sepsis or SIRS doesn't develop until after admission, see Official Guidelines, Section I.c.1.b.2.b).

If the localized infection is postprocedural, see Official Guidelines, Section I.c.10 for guidelines related to sepsis due to postprocedural infection.

Note: The term urosepsis is a nonspecific term. If that is the only term documented then only code 599.0 should be assigned based on the default for the term in the ICD-9-CM index, in addition to the code for the causal organism if known.

Bacterial Sepsis and Septicemia

In most cases, it will be a code from category 038, Septicemia, that will be used in conjunction with a code from subcategory 995.9 such as the following:

A.   Streptococcal sepsis

If the documentation in the record states streptococcal sepsis, codes 038.0, Streptococcal septicemia, and code 995.91 should be used, in that sequence.

B.   Streptococcal septicemia

If the documentation states streptococcal septicemia, only code 038.0 should be assigned, however, the provider should be queried whether the patient has sepsis, an infection with SIRS.

Acute organ dysfunction that is not clearly associated with the sepsis

If a patient has sepsis and an acute organ dysfunction, but the medical record documentation indicates that the acute organ dysfunction is related to a medical condition other than the sepsis, do not assign code 995.92, Severe sepsis. An acute organ dysfunction must be associated with the sepsis in order to assign the severe sepsis code. If the documentation is not clear as to whether an acute organ dysfunction is related to the sepsis or another medical condition, query the provider.

Septic shock

A.   Sequencing of septic shock

Septic shock generally refers to circulatory failure associated with severe sepsis, and, therefore, it represents a type of acute organ dysfunction.

For all cases of septic shock, the code for the systemic infection should be sequenced first, followed by codes 995.92 and 785.52. Any additional codes for other acute organ dysfunctions should also be assigned. As noted in the sequencing instructions in the Tabular List, the code for septic shock cannot be assigned as a principal diagnosis.

B.   Septic Shock without documentation of severe sepsis

Septic shock indicates the presence of severe sepsis.

Code 995.92, Severe sepsis, must be assigned with code 785.52, Septic shock, even if the term severe sepsis is not documented in the record. The "use additional code" note and the "code first" note in the tabular support this guideline.

● Code new to this edition   ▲ Revision of existing code   ④ ⑤ Fourth or fifth digit required

Sepsis and septic shock complicating abortion and pregnancy

Sepsis and septic shock complicating abortion, ectopic pregnancy, and molar pregnancy are classified to category codes in Chapter 11 (630-639).

Negative or inconclusive blood cultures

Negative or inconclusive blood cultures do not preclude a diagnosis of septicemia or sepsis in patients with clinical evidence of the condition, however, the provider should be queried.

Newborn sepsis

Code 771.81, Septicemia [sepsis] of newborn, should be assigned with a secondary code from category 041, Bacterial infections in conditions classified elsewhere and of unspecified site, to identify the organism.

Sepsis due to a Postprocedural Infection

A. Documentation of causal relationship

As with all postprocedural complications, code assignment is based on the provider's documentation of the relationship between the infection and the procedure.

B. Sepsis due to postprocedural infection

In cases of postprocedural sepsis, the complication code, such as code 998.59, Other postoperative infection, or 674.3x, Other complications of obstetrical surgical wounds should be coded first followed by the appropriate sepsis codes (systemic infection code and either code 995.91or 995.92. An additional code(s) for any acute organ dysfunction should also be assigned for cases of severe sepsis.

External cause of injury codes with SIRS

An external cause code with systemic inflammatory response syndrome (SIRS) is not appropriate with a code from subcategory 995.9, unless the patient also has an injury, poisoning, or adverse effect of drugs.

Sepsis and Severe Sepsis Associated with Noninfectious Process

In some cases, a non-infectious process, such as trauma, may lead to an infection which can result in sepsis or severe sepsis. If sepsis or severe sepsis is documented as associated with a non-infectious condition, such as a burn or serious injury, and this condition meets the definition for principal diagnosis, the code for the noninfectious condition should be sequenced first, followed by the code for the systemic infection and either code 995.91, Sepsis, or 995.92, Severe sepsis. Additional codes for any associated acute organ dysfunction(s) should also be assigned for cases of severe sepsis. If the sepsis or severe sepsis meets the definition of principal diagnosis, the systemic infection and sepsis codes should be sequenced before the non-infectious condition. When both the associated non-infectious condition and the sepsis or severe sepsis meet the definition of principal diagnosis, either may be assigned as principal diagnosis.

See Official Guidelines, Section I.C.1.b.2.a for guidelines pertaining to sepsis or severe sepsis as the principal diagnosis.

Only one code from subcategory 995.9 should be assigned. Therefore, when a non-infectious condition leads to an infection resulting in sepsis or severe sepsis, assign either code 995.91 or 995.92. Do not additionally assign code 995.93, Systemic inflammatory response syndrome due to non-infectious process without acute organ dysfunction, or 995.94, Systemic inflammatory response syndrome with acute organ dysfunction.

SIRS Due To Trauma Or Burns Or Other Non-Infectious Disease Processes

The systemic inflammatory response syndrome (SIRS) can develop as a result of certain non-infectious disease processes, such as trauma, malignant neoplasm, or pancreatitis. When SIRS is documented with a noninfectious condition, and no subsequent infection is documented, the code for the underlying condition, such as an injury, should be assigned, followed by code 995.93, Systemic inflammatory response syndrome due to noninfectious process without acute organ dysfunction, or 995.94, Systemic inflammatory response syndrome due to non-infectious process with acute organ dysfunction. If an acute organ dysfunction is documented, the appropriate code(s) for the associated acute organ dysfunction(s) should be assigned in addition to code 995.94. If acute organ dysfunction is documented, but it cannot be determined if the acute organ dysfunction is associated with SIRS or due to another condition (e.g., directly due to the trauma), the provider should be queried.

Add 4th or 5th digit   Nonspecific code   Unspecified code   Manifestation code

METHICILLIN RESISTANT STAPHYLOCOCCUS AUREUS (MRSA) CONDITIONS

Selection and sequencing of MRSA codes

A.   Combination codes for MRSA infection

When a patient is diagnosed with an infection that is due to methicillin resistant Staphylococcus aureus (MRSA), and that infection has a combination code that includes the causal organism (e.g., septicemia, pneumonia) assign the appropriate code for the condition (e.g., code 038.12, Methicillin resistant Staphylococcus aureus septicemia or code 482.42, Methicillin resistant pneumonia due to Staphylococcus aureus). Do not assign code 041.12, Methicillin resistant Staphylococcus aureus, as an additional code because the code includes the type of infection and the MRSA organism. Do not assign a code from subcategory V09.0, Infection with microorganisms resistant to penicillins, as an additional diagnosis.

See Section C.1.b.1 for instructions on coding and sequencing of septicemia.

B.   Other codes for MRSA infection

When there is documentation of a current infection (e.g., wound infection, stitch abscess, urinary tract infection) due to MRSA, and that infection does not have a combination code that includes the causal organism, select the appropriate code to identify the condition along with code 041.12, Methicillin resistant Staphylococcus aureus, for the MRSA infection. Do not assign a code from subcategory V09.0, Infection with microorganisms resistant to penicillins.

C.   Methicillin susceptible Staphylococcus aureus (MSSA) and MRSA colonization

The condition or state of being colonized or carrying MSSA or MRSA is called colonization or carriage, while an individual person is described as being colonized or being a carrier. Colonization means that MSSA or MSRA is present on or in the body without necessarily causing illness. A positive MRSA colonization test might be documented by the provider as "MRSA screen positive" or "MRSA nasal swab positive".

Assign code V02.54, Carrier or suspected carrier, Methicillin resistant Staphylococcus aureus, for patients documented as having MRSA colonization. Assign code V02.53, Carrier or suspected carrier, Methicillin susceptible Staphylococcus aureus, for patient documented as having MSSA colonization. Colonization is not necessarily indicative of a disease process or as the cause of a specific condition the patient may have unless documented as such by the provider.

Code V02.59, Other specified bacterial diseases, should be assigned for other types of staphylococcal colonization (e.g., S. epidermidis, S. saprophyticus).

Code V02.59 should not be assigned for colonization with any type of Staphylococcus aureus (MRSA, MSSA).

D.   MRSA colonization and infection

If a patient is documented as having both MRSA colonization and infection during a hospital admission, code V02.54, Carrier or suspected carrier, Methicillin resistant Staphylococcus aureus, and a code for the MRSA infection may both be assigned.

● Code new to this edition   ▲ Revision of existing code   ④ ⑤ Fourth or fifth digit required

1. INFECTIOUS AND PARASITIC DISEASES (001-139)

ALERT! For personal history of infectious and parasitic disease see V12.0

Note: Categories for "late effects" of infectious and parasitic diseases are to be found at 137-139.

Includes: diseases generally recognized as communicable or transmissible as well as a few diseases of unknown but possibly infectious origin

Excludes: *acute respiratory infections (460-466)*
carrier or suspected carrier of infectious organism (V02.0-V02.9)
certain localized infections
influenza (487.0-487.8, 488.01-488.19)

INTESTINAL INFECTIOUS DISEASES (001-009)

Excludes: *helminthiases (120.0-129)*

001 Cholera

DEFINITION Cholera, aka asiatic or epidemic cholera, is an infectious gastroenteritis caused by enterotoxin-producing strains of the bacterium vibrio cholerae.

001.0 Due to Vibrio cholerae

001.1 Due to Vibrio cholerae el tor

001.9 Cholera, unspecified

002 Typhoid and paratyphoid fevers

DEFINITION Typhoid fever, aka enteric fever, salmonella typhi is an illness caused by the bacterium salmonella enterica serovar typhi.

002.0 Typhoid fever
Typhoid (fever) (infection) [any site]

002.1 Paratyphoid fever A

002.2 Paratyphoid fever B

002.3 Paratyphoid fever C

002.9 Paratyphoid fever, unspecified

003 Other salmonella infections
Includes: infection or food poisoning by Salmonella [any serotype]

DEFINITION Salmonellosis is an infection with salmonella bacteria. Most persons infected with salmonella develop diarrhea, fever, vomiting, and abdominal cramps.

003.0 Salmonella gastroenteritis
Salmonellosis

003.1 Salmonella septicemia

⑤ **003.2** Localized salmonella infections

003.20 Localized salmonella infection, unspecified

003.21 Salmonella meningitis

003.22 Salmonella pneumonia

003.23 Salmonella arthritis

003.24 Salmonella osteomyelitis

003.29 Other

003.8 Other specified salmonella infections

003.9 Salmonella infection, unspecified

004 Shigellosis
Includes: bacillary dysentery

DEFINITION Shigellosis, aka bacillary dysentery, is a food borne illness caused by infection by bacteria of the genus shigella.

004.0 Shigella dysenteriae
Infection by group A Shigella (Schmitz) (Shiga)

004.1 Shigella flexneri
Infection by group B Shigella

004.2 Shigella boydii
Infection by group C Shigella

004.3 Shigella sonnei
Infection by group D Shigella

004.8 Other specified shigella infections

004.9 Shigellosis, unspecified

| | Add 4th or 5th digit | | Nonspecific code | | Unspecified code | | Manifestation code |

005 **Other food poisoning (bacterial)**

> Excludes: *salmonella infections (003.0-003.9)*
>> *toxic effect of:*
>>> *food contaminants (989.7)*
>>> *noxious foodstuffs (988.0-988.9)*

DEFINITION Food poisoning (bacterial) is any illness resulting from the consumption of contaminated food.

005.0 **Staphylococcal food poisoning**
> Staphylococcal toxemia specified as due to food

005.1 **Botulism food poisoning**
> Botulism NOS
> Food poisoning due to Clostridium botulinum

> Excludes: *infant botulism (040.41)*
>> *wound botulism (040.42)*

DEFINITION Botulism is food poisoning resulting from the toxin produced by botulinus bacteria, sometimes found in foods improperly canned or preserved; often fatal.

005.2 **Food poisoning due to Clostridium perfringens [C. welchii]**
> Enteritis necroticans

005.3 **Food poisoning due to other Clostridia**

005.4 **Food poisoning due to Vibrio parahaemolyticus**

⑤ **005.8** **Other bacterial food poisoning**

> Excludes: *salmonella food poisoning (003.0-003.9)*

> **005.81** **Food poisoning due to Vibrio vulnificus**

> **005.89** **Other bacterial food poisoning**
>> Food poisoning due to Bacillus cereus

005.9 **Food poisoning, unspecified**

006 **Amebiasis**
> Includes: infection due to Entamoeba histolytica

> Excludes: *amebiasis due to organisms other than Entamoeba histolytica (007.8)*

DEFINITION Amebiasis is an inflammation of the intestines caused by infection with entamoeba histolytica characterized by frequent, loose stools flecked with blood and mucus.
DEFINITION Amebic dysentery is an inflammation of the intestines caused by endamoeba histolytica; usually acquired by ingesting food or water contaminated with feces; characterized by severe diarrhea.

006.0 **Acute amebic dysentery without mention of abscess**
> Acute amebiasis

006.1 **Chronic intestinal amebiasis without mention of abscess**
> Chronic:
>> amebiasis
>> amebic dysentery

006.2 **Amebic nondysenteric colitis**

006.3 **Amebic liver abscess**
> Hepatic amebiasis

006.4 **Amebic lung abscess**
> Amebic abscess of lung (and liver)

006.5 **Amebic brain abscess**
> Amebic abscess of brain (and liver) (and lung)

006.6 **Amebic skin ulceration**
> Cutaneous amebiasis

006.8 **Amebic infection of other sites**
> Amebic: Ameboma
>> appendicitis
>> balanitis

> Excludes: *specific infections by free-living amebae (136.21-136.29)*

006.9 **Amebiasis, unspecified**
> Amebiasis NOS

● Code new
  to this edition
▲ Revision of
  existing code
④ ⑤ Fourth or fifth
  digit required

007 **Other protozoal intestinal diseases**

Includes: protozoal:
colitis
diarrhea
dysentery

DEFINITION Protozoal intestinal diseases refers to diseases of the intestinal system caused by protozoa, which are single-cell organisms that can only divide within a host organism. Malaria ,giardia and toxoplasmosis are examples of diseases caused by protozoa.

ALERT! For personal history of other specified infectious and parasitic disease see V12.09.

007.0 **Balantidiasis**
Infection by Balantidium coli

007.1 **Giardiasis**
Infection by Giardia lamblia
Lambliasis

007.2 **Coccidiosis**
Infection by Isospora belli and Isospora hominis
Isosporiasis

007.3 **Intestinal trichomoniasis**

007.4 **Cryptosporidiosis**

007.5 **Cyclosporiasis**

007.8 **Other specified protozoal intestinal diseases**
Amebiasis due to organisms other than Entamoeba histolytica

007.9 **Unspecified protozoal intestinal disease**
Flagellate diarrhea   Protozoal dysentery NOS

008 **Intestinal infections due to other organisms**

Includes: any condition classifiable to 009.0-009.3 with mention of the responsible organisms

Excludes: food poisoning by these organisms (005.0-005.9)

⑤ **008.0** **Escherichia coli [E. coli]**

008.00 **E. coli, unspecified**
E. coli enteritis NOS

008.01 **Enteropathogenic E. coli**

008.02 **Enterotoxigenic E. coli**

008.03 **Enteroinvasive E. coli**

008.04 **Enterohemorrhagic E. coli**

008.09 **Other intestinal E. coli infections**

008.1 **Arizona group of paracolon bacilli**

008.2 **Aerobacter aerogenes**
Enterobacter aerogenes

008.3 **Proteus (mirabilis) (morganii)**

⑤ **008.4** **Other specified bacteria**

008.41 **Staphylococcus**
Staphylococcal enterocolitis

008.42 **Pseudomonas**

008.43 **Campylobacter**

008.44 **Yersinia enterocolitica**

008.45 **Clostridium difficile**
Pseudomembranous colitis

008.46 **Other anaerobes**
Anaerobic enteritis NOS
Bacteroides (fragilis)
Gram-negative anaerobes

008.47 **Other Gram-negative bacteria**
Gram-negative enteritis NOS

Excludes: Gram-negative anaerobes (008.46)

008.49 **Other**

008.5 **Bacterial enteritis, unspecified**

⑤ **008.6** **Enteritis due to specified virus**

008.61 **Rotavirus**

161

| | Add 4th or 5th digit | | Nonspecific code | | Unspecified code | | Manifestation code |

008.62 **Adenovirus**

008.63 **Norwalk virus**
Norovirus
Norwalk-like agent

008.64 **Other small round viruses [SRV's]**
Small round virus NOS

008.65 **Calicivirus**

008.66 **Astrovirus**

008.67 **Enterovirus NEC**
Coxsackie virus
Echovirus

Excludes: *poliovirus (045.0-045.9)*

008.69 **Other viral enteritis**
Torovirus

008.8 **Other organism, not elsewhere classified**
Viral:
enteritis NOS
gastroenteritis

Excludes: *influenza with involvement of gastrointestinal tract (487.8, 488.09, 488.19)*

009 **Ill-defined intestinal infections**

Excludes: *diarrheal disease or intestinal infection due to specified organism (001.0-008.8)*
diarrhea following gastrointestinal surgery (564.4)
intestinal malabsorption (579.0-579.9)
ischemic enteritis (557.0-557.9)
other noninfectious gastroenteritis and colitis (558.1-558.9)
regional enteritis (555.0-555.9)
ulcerative colitis (556)

009.0 **Infectious colitis, enteritis, and gastroenteritis**
Colitis, septic
Enteritis, septic
Gastroenteritis, septic
Dysentery:
NOS
catarrhal
hemorrhagic

009.1 **Colitis, enteritis, and gastroenteritis of presumed infectious origin**
Excludes: *colitis NOS (558.9)*
enteritis NOS (558.9)
gastroenteritis NOS (558.9)

009.2 **Infectious diarrhea**
Diarrhea:
dysenteric
epidemic
Infectious diarrheal disease NOS

009.3 **Diarrhea of presumed infectious origin**
Excludes: *diarrhea NOS (787.91)*

TUBERCULOSIS (010-018)

Includes: infection by Mycobacterium tuberculosis (human) (bovine)

Excludes: *congenital tuberculosis (771.2)*
late effects of tuberculosis (137.0-137.4)

DEFINITION Tuberculosis is a common and often deadly infectious disease caused by mycobacteria, in humans mainly mycobacterium tuberculosis. Tuberculosis usually attacks the lungs but can also affect the central nervous system, the lymphatic system, the circulatory system, the genitourinary system, the gastrointestinal system, bones, joints, and even the skin.

ALERT! For personal history of tuberculosis see V12.01

The following fifth-digit subclassification is for use with categories 010-018:

0 unspecified

1 bacteriological or histological examination not done

2 bacteriological or histological examination unknown (at present)

3 tubercle bacilli found (in sputum) by microscopy

4 tubercle bacilli not found (in sputum) by microscopy, but found by bacterial culture

5 tubercle bacilli not found by bacteriological examination, but tuberculosis confirmed histologically

6 tubercle bacilli not found by bacteriological or histological examination but tuberculosis confirmed by other methods [inoculation of animals]

⑤ **010** **Primary tuberculous infection**

> *Excludes:* *nonspecific reaction to test for tuberculosis without active tuberculosis (795.51-795.52)*
> *positive PPD (795.51)*
> *positive tuberculin skin test without active tuberculosis (795.51)*

> **ALERT!** For coding late effects of tuberculosis see 137

⑤ **010.0** **Primary tuberculous complex**
[0-6]

⑤ **010.1** **Tuberculous pleurisy in primary progressive tuberculosis**
[0-6]

⑤ **010.8** **Other primary progressive tuberculosis**
[0-6]

> *Excludes:* *tuberculous erythema nodosum (017.1)*

⑤ **010.9** **Primary tuberculous infection, unspecified**
[0-6]

⑤ **011** **Pulmonary tuberculosis**

Use additional code, if desired, to identify any associated silicosis (502)

> **ALERT!** For coding late effects of respiratory or unspecified tuberculosis see 137.0

⑤ **011.0** **Tuberculosis of lung, infiltrative**
[0-6]

⑤ **011.1** **Tuberculosis of lung, nodular**
[0-6]

⑤ **011.2** **Tuberculosis of lung with cavitation**
[0-6]

⑤ **011.3** **Tuberculosis of bronchus**
[0-6]

> *Excludes:* *isolated bronchial tuberculosis (012.2)*

⑤ **011.4** **Tuberculous fibrosis of lung**
[0-6]

⑤ **011.5** **Tuberculous bronchiectasis**
[0-6]

⑤ **011.6** **Tuberculous pneumonia [any form]**
[0-6]

⑤ **011.7** **Tuberculous pneumothorax**
[0-6]

⑤ **011.8** **Other specified pulmonary tuberculosis**
[0-6]

⑤ **011.9** **Pulmonary tuberculosis, unspecified**
[0-6] Respiratory tuberculosis NOS
Tuberculosis of lung NOS

⑤ **012** **Other respiratory tuberculosis**

> *Excludes:* *respiratory tuberculosis, unspecified (011.9)*

> **ALERT!** For coding late effects of respiratory or unspecified tuberculosis see 137.0
> **ALERT!** For personal history of other specified infectious and parasitic disease see V12.09

	Add 4th or 5th digit		Nonspecific code		Unspecified code		Manifestation code

⑤ **012.0 Tuberculous pleurisy**
[0-6]   Tuberculosis of pleura
            Tuberculous empyema
            Tuberculous hydrothorax

Excludes: *pleurisy with effusion without mention of cause (511.9)*
          tuberculous pleurisy in primary progressive tuberculosis (010.1)

⑤ **012.1 Tuberculosis of intrathoracic lymph nodes**
[0-6]   Tuberculosis of lymph nodes:
              hilar
              mediastinal
              tracheobronchial
            Tuberculous tracheobronchial adenopathy

Excludes: *that specified as primary (010.0-010.9)*

⑤ **012.2 Isolated tracheal or bronchial tuberculosis**
[0-6]

⑤ **012.3 Tuberculous laryngitis**
[0-6]   Tuberculosis of glottis

⑤ **012.8 Other specified respiratory tuberculosis**
[0-6]   Tuberculosis of: Tuberculosis of:
              mediastinum   nose (septum)
              nasopharynx   sinus [any nasal]

⑤ **013 Tuberculosis of meninges and central nervous system**
     ALERT! For coding late effects of central nervous system tuberculosis see 137.1

⑤ **013.0 Tuberculous meningitis**
[0-6]   Tuberculosis of meninges   Tuberculous:
              (cerebral) (spinal)   leptomeningitis
                                            meningoencephalitis

Excludes: *tuberculoma of meninges (013.1)*

⑤ **013.1 Tuberculoma of meninges**
[0-6]

⑤ **013.2   Tuberculoma of brain**
[0-6]   Tuberculosis of brain (current disease)

⑤ **013.3 Tuberculous abscess of brain**
[0-6]

⑤ **013.4 Tuberculoma of spinal cord**
[0-6]

⑤ **013.5 Tuberculous abscess of spinal cord**
[0-6]

⑤ **013.6 Tuberculous encephalitis or myelitis**
[0-6]

⑤ **013.8 Other specified tuberculosis of central nervous system**
[0-6]

⑤ **013.9 Unspecified tuberculosis of central nervous system**
[0-6]   Tuberculosis of central nervous system NOS

⑤ **014 Tuberculosis of intestines, peritoneum, and mesenteric glands**

⑤ **014.0 Tuberculous peritonitis**
[0-6]   Tuberculous ascites

⑤ **014.8 Other**
[0-6]   Tuberculosis (of):   Tuberculous enteritis
              anus
              intestine (large) (small)
              mesenteric glands
              rectum
              retroperitoneal (lymph nodes)

● Code new   ▲ Revision of   ④ ⑤ Fourth or fifth
     to this edition   existing code   digit required

⑤ **015** **Tuberculosis of bones and joints**
Use additional code, if desired, to identify manifestation, as:
tuberculous:
    arthropathy (711.4)
    necrosis of bone (730.8)
    osteitis (730.8)
    osteomyelitis (730.8)
    synovitis (727.01)
    tenosynovitis (727.01)
    ALERT! For coding late effects of tuberculosis of bones and joints see 137.3

⑤ **015.0** **Vertebral column**
[0-6]   Pott's disease
Use additional code, if desired, to identify manifestation, as:
    curvature of spine [Pott's] (737.4)
    kyphosis (737.4)
    spondylitis (720.81)

⑤ **015.1** **Hip**
[0-6]

⑤ **015.2** **Knee**
[0-6]

⑤ **015.5** **Limb bones**
[0-6]   Tuberculous dactylitis

⑤ **015.6** **Mastoid**
[0-6]   Tuberculous mastoiditis

⑤ **015.7** **Other specified bone**
[0-6]

⑤ **015.8** **Other specified joint**
[0-6]

⑤ **015.9** **Tuberculosis of unspecified bones and joints**
[0-6]

⑤ **016** **Tuberculosis of genitourinary system**
    ALERT! For coding late effects of genitourinary tuberculosis see 137.2

⑤ **016.0** **Kidney**
[0-6]   Renal tuberculosis
Use additional code, if desired, to identify manifestation, as:
    tuberculous:
      nephropathy (583.81)
      pyelitis (590.81)
      pyelonephritis (590.81)

⑤ **016.1** **Bladder**
[0-6]

⑤ **016.2** **Ureter**
[0-6]

⑤ **016.3** **Other urinary organs**
[0-6]

⑤ **016.4** **Epididymis**
[0-6]

⑤ **016.5** **Other male genital organs**
[0-6]
Use additional code, if desired, to identify manifestation, as:
    tuberculosis of:
      prostate (601.4)
      seminal vesicle (608.81)
      testis (608.81)

⑤ **016.6** **Tuberculous oophoritis and salpingitis**
[0-6]

⑤ **016.7** **Other female genital organs**
[0-6]   Tuberculous:
      cervicitis
      endometritis

⑤ **016.9** **Genitourinary tuberculosis, unspecified**
[0-6]

| | Add 4th or 5th digit | | Nonspecific code | | Unspecified code | | Manifestation code |

⑤ **017** **Tuberculosis of other organs**

  ALERT! For coding late effects of tuberculosis of other specified organs see 137.4

⑤ **017.0** **Skin and subcutaneous cellular tissue**
[0-6]

Lupus:
  exedens
  vulgaris
Scrofuloderma

Tuberculosis:
  colliquativa
  cutis
  lichenoides
  papulonecrotica
  verrucosa cutis

Excludes: lupus erythematosus (695.4)
  disseminated (710.0)
  lupus NOS (710.0)
  nonspecific reaction to test for tuberculosis without active tuberculosis
    (795.51-795.52)
  positive PPD (795.51)
  positive tuberculin skin test without active tuberculosis (795.51)

⑤ **017.1** **Erythema nodosum with hypersensitivity reaction in tuberculosis**
[0-6]

Bazin's disease
Erythema:
  induratum
  nodosum, tuberculous

Tuberculosis indurativa

Excludes: erythema nodosum NOS (695.2)

⑤ **017.2** **Peripheral lymph nodes**
[0-6]

Scrofula
Scrofulous abscess

Tuberculous adenitis

Excludes: tuberculosis of lymph nodes:
  bronchial and mediastinal (012.1)
  mesenteric and retroperitoneal (014.8)
  tuberculous tracheobronchial adenopathy (012.1)

⑤ **017.3** **Eye**
[0-6]

Use additional code, if desired, to identify manifestation, as:
  tuberculous:
    chorioretinitis, disseminated (363.13)
    episcleritis (379.09)
    interstitial keratitis (370.59)
    iridocyclitis, chronic (364.11)
    keratoconjunctivitis (phlyctenular) (370.31)

⑤ **017.4** **Ear**
[0-6]

Tuberculosis of ear
Tuberculous otitis media

Excludes: tuberculous mastoiditis (015.6)

⑤ **017.5** **Thyroid gland**
[0-6]

⑤ **017.6** **Adrenal glands**
[0-6]

Addison's disease, tuberculous

⑤ **017.7** **Spleen**
[0-6]

⑤ **017.8** **Esophagus**
[0-6]

⑤ **017.9** **Other specified organs**
[0-6]

Use additional code, if desired, to identify manifestation, as:
  tuberculosis of:
    endocardium [any valve] (424.91)
    myocardium (422.0)
    pericardium (420.0)

● Code new
  to this edition

▲ Revision of
  existing code

④ ⑤ Fourth or fifth
  digit required

⑤ **018** **Miliary tuberculosis**
Includes: tuberculosis:
     disseminated
     generalized
     miliary, whether of a single specified site, multiple sites, or unspecified site
     polyserositis
DEFINITION Miliary tuberculosis acute tuberculosis characterized by the appearance of tiny tubercles on one or more organs of the body.

⑤ **018.0**   **Acute miliary tuberculosis**
[0-6]

⑤ **018.8**   **Other specified miliary tuberculosis**
[0-6]

⑤ **018.9**   **Miliary tuberculosis, unspecified**
[0-6]

ZOONOTIC BACTERIAL DISEASES (020-027)

020 **Plague**
Includes: infection by Yersinia [Pasteurella] pestis
DEFINITION Plague is a deadly infectious disease caused by the enterobacteria yersinia pestis (pasteurella pestis).

020.0   **Bubonic**

020.1   **Cellulocutaneous**

020.2   **Septicemic**

020.3   **Primary pneumonic**

020.4   **Secondary pneumonic**

020.5   **Pneumonic, unspecified**

020.8   **Other specified types of plague**
Abortive plague   Pestis minor
Ambulatory plague

020.9   **Plague, unspecified**

021 **Tularemia**
Includes: deerfly fever
     infection by Francisella [Pasteurella] tularensis
     rabbit fever
DEFINITION Tularemia, aka rabbit fever, deer fly fever, O'Hara's fever is a serious infectious disease caused by the bacterium francisella tularensis.

021.0   **Ulceroglandular tularemia**

021.1   **Enteric tularemia**
Tularemia:
     cryptogenic
     intestinal
     typhoidal

021.2   **Pulmonary tularemia**
Bronchopneumonic tularemia

021.3   **Oculoglandular tularemia**

021.8   **Other specified tularemia**
Tularemia:
     generalized or disseminated
     glandular

021.9   **Unspecified tularemia**

022 **Anthrax**
DEFINITION Anthrax is an acute disease in humans and animals caused by the bacterium bacillus anthracis which is highly lethal in some forms.

022.0   **Cutaneous anthrax**
Malignant pustule

022.1   **Pulmonary anthrax**
Respiratory anthrax
Wool-sorters' disease

022.2   **Gastrointestinal anthrax**

022.3   **Anthrax septicemia**

022.8   **Other specified manifestations of anthrax**

022.9   **Anthrax, unspecified**

	Add 4th or 5th digit		Nonspecific code		Unspecified code		Manifestation code

023 **Brucellosis**

Includes: fever:
        Malta
        Mediterranean
        undulant

`DEFINITION` Brucellosis, aka undulant fever, or malta fever is a highly contagious zoonosis caused by ingestion of unsterilized milk or meat from infected animals, or close contact with their secretions.

023.0 **Brucella melitensis**

023.1 **Brucella abortus**

023.2 **Brucella suis**

023.3 **Brucella canis**

023.8 **Other brucellosis**
Infection by more than one organism

023.9 **Brucellosis, unspecified**

024 **Glanders**

Infection by: Farcy
  Actinobacillus mallei   Malleus
  Malleomyces mallei
  Pseudomonas mallei

`DEFINITION` Glanders is an infectious disease that occurs primarily in horses, mules, and donkeys and other animals such as dogs, cats and goats that can be transmitted to humans. It is caused by infection with the bacterium burkholderia mallei.

025 **Melioidosis**

Infection by:
  Malleomyces pseudomallei
  Pseudomonas pseudomallei
  Whitmore's bacillus
Pseudoglanders

`DEFINITION` Melioidosis aka Whitmore disease or Nightcliff Gardener's disease, is an infectious disease caused by a gram-negative bacterium, burkholderia pseudomallei, found in soil and water.

026 **Rat-bite fever**

`DEFINITION` Rat-bite fever is an acute, febrile human illness caused by bacteria transmitted by rodents, rats in most cases, which is passed from rodent to human via the rodent's urine or mucous secretions. Two types of gram-negative facultative anaerobic bacteria can cause the infection.

026.0 **Spirillary fever**
Rat-bite fever due to Spirillum minor [S. minus]
Sodoku

026.1 **Streptobacillary fever**
Epidemic arthritic erythema
Haverhill fever
Rat-bite fever due to Streptobacillus moniliformis

026.9 **Unspecified rat-bite fever**

027 **Other zoonotic bacterial diseases**

`DEFINITION` Zoonotic refers to other diseases that can be passed from animals, whether wild or domesticated, to humans.

`ALERT!` For personal history of other specified infectious and parasitic disease see V12.09

027.0 **Listeriosis**
Infection by Listeria monocytogenes
Septicemia by Listeria monocytogenes

Use additional code to identify manifestations, as meningitis (320.7)

Excludes: congenital listeriosis (771.2)

027.1 **Erysipelothrix infection**
Erysipeloid (of Rosenbach)
Infection by Erysipelothrix insidiosa [E. rhusiopathiae]
Septicemia by Erysipelothrix insidiosa [E. rhusiopathiae]

● Code new
  to this edition
    ▲ Revision of
      existing code
        ④ ⑤ Fourth or fifth
           digit required

027.2 Pasteurellosis
Pasteurella pseudotuberculosis infection
Mesenteric adenitis by Pasteurella multocida [P. septica]
Septic infection (cat bite) (dog bite) by Pasteurella multocida [P. septica]

Excludes: *infection by:*
Francisella [Pasteurella] tularensis (021.0-021.9)
Yersinia [Pasteurella] pestis (020.0-020.9)

027.8 Other specified zoonotic bacterial diseases

027.9 Unspecified zoonotic bacterial disease

OTHER BACTERIAL DISEASES (030-041)

Excludes: *bacterial venereal diseases (098.0-099.9)*
bartonellosis (088.0)

030 Leprosy
Includes: Hansen's disease
infection by Mycobacterium leprae

DEFINITION Leprosy is an infectious disease characterized by disfiguring skin sores, nerve damage, and progressive debilitation. Leprosy is caused by the organism mycobacterium leprae.

030.0 Lepromatous [type L]
Lepromatous leprosy (macular) (diffuse) (infiltrated) (nodular) (neuritic)

030.1 Tuberculoid [type T]
Tuberculoid leprosy (macular) (maculoanesthetic) (major) (minor) (neuritic)

030.2 Indeterminate [group I]
Indeterminate [uncharacteristic] leprosy (macular) (neuritic)

030.3 Borderline [group B]
Borderline or dimorphous leprosy (infiltrated) (neuritic)

030.8 Other specified leprosy

030.9 Leprosy, unspecified

031 Diseases due to other mycobacteria

031.0 Pulmonary
Infection by Mycobacterium:
avium
intracellulare [Battey bacillus]
kansasii
Battey disease

031.1 Cutaneous
Buruli ulcer
Infection by Mycobacterium:
marinum [M. balnei]
ulcerans

031.2 Disseminated
Disseminated mycobacterium avium-intracellulare complex (DMAC)
Mycobacterium avium-intracellulare complex (MAC) bacteremia

031.8 Other specified mycobacterial diseases

031.9 Unspecified diseases due to mycobacteria
Atypical mycobacterium infection NOS

032 Diphtheria
Includes: infection by Corynebacterium diphtheriae

DEFINITION Diphtheria is a highly infectious disease of the upper respiratory tract characterised by a sore throat, fever and causing difficulty in breathing.

032.0 Faucial diphtheria
Membranous angina, diphtheritic

032.1 Nasopharyngeal diphtheria

032.2 Anterior nasal diphtheria

032.3 Laryngeal diphtheria
Laryngotracheitis, diphtheritic

⑤ **032.8 Other specified diphtheria**

032.81 Conjunctival diphtheria
Pseudomembranous diphtheritic conjunctivitis

032.82 Diphtheritic myocarditis

032.83 Diphtheritic peritonitis

169

| | Add 4th or 5th digit | | Nonspecific code | | Unspecified code | | Manifestation code |

032.84 **Diphtheritic cystitis**

032.85 **Cutaneous diphtheria**

032.89 **Other**

032.9 **Diphtheria, unspecified**

033 **Whooping cough**

Includes: pertussis

Use additional code, if desired, to identify any associated pneumonia (484.3)

DEFINITION Whooping cough, aka pertussis, is a highly contagious disease caused by bacteria. The most prominent symptom of whooping cough is a distinctive, uncontrollable cough, followed by a sharp, high-pitched intake of air.

033.0 **Bordetella pertussis [B. pertussis]**

033.1 **Bordetella parapertussis [B. parapertussis]**

033.8 **Whooping cough due to other specified organism**

Bordetella bronchiseptica [B. bronchiseptica]

033.9 **Whooping cough, unspecified organism**

034 **Streptococcal sore throat and scarlet fever**

DEFINITION Streptococcal sore throat is an infection of the oral pharynx and tonsils by streptococcus. Scarlet fever is an infection caused by a bacterium called streptococcus.

034.0 **Streptococcal sore throat**

Septic:
  angina
  sore throat
Streptococcal:
  angina
  laryngitis
  pharyngitis
  tonsillitis

034.1 **Scarlet fever**

Scarlatina

Excludes: *parascarlatina (057.8)*

035 **Erysipelas**

Excludes: *postpartum or puerperal erysipelas (670.8)*

DEFINITION Erysipelas is an acute febrile disease that is associated with intense often vesicular and edematous local inflammation of the skin and subcutaneous tissues and that is caused by a hemolytic streptococcus.

036 **Meningococcal infection**

DEFINITION Meningococcal infection is an infection with the bacterium neisseria meningitidis. Neisseria was formerly called meningococcus but the term meningococcal is still common.

036.0 **Meningococcal meningitis**

Cerebrospinal fever
  (meningococcal)
Meningitis:
  cerebrospinal
  epidemic

036.1 **Meningococcal encephalitis**

036.2 **Meningococcemia**

Meningococcal septicemia

036.3 **Waterhouse-Friderichsen syndrome, meningococcal**

Meningococcal hemorrhagic adrenalitis
Meningococcic adrenal syndrome
Waterhouse-Friderichsen syndrome NOS

⑤ 036.4 **Meningococcal carditis**

036.40 **Meningococcal carditis, unspecified**

036.41 **Meningococcal pericarditis**

036.42 **Meningococcal endocarditis**

036.43 **Meningococcal myocarditis**

⑤ 036.8 **Other specified meningococcal infections**

036.81 **Meningococcal optic neuritis**

036.82 **Meningococcal arthropathy**

036.89 **Other**

● Code new
to this edition

▲ Revision of
existing code

④ ⑤ Fourth or fifth
digit required

036.9 Meningococcal infection, unspecified
Meningococcal infection NOS

037 Tetanus

Excludes: *tetanus:*
   complicating:
      abortion (634-638 with .0, 639.0)
      ectopic or molar pregnancy (639.0)
   neonatorum (771.3)
   puerperal (670.8)

DEFINITION Tetanus is an often fatal infectious disease caused by the bacteria clostridium tetani (c. Tetani) which usually enters the body through a puncture, cut, or open wound.

038 Septicemia

Excludes: *bacteremia (790.7)*
   during labor (659.3)
   following ectopic or molar pregnancy (639.0)
   following infusion, injection, transfusion, or vaccination (999.3)
   postpartum, puerperal (670)
   septicemia (sepsis) of newborn (771.81)
   that complicating abortion (634-638 with .0, 639.0)

Use additional code for systemic inflammatory response syndrome (SIRS) (995.91-995.92)

DEFINITION Septicemia, aka blood poisoning, is a systemic illness with toxicity due to invasion of the bloodstream by virulent bacteria coming from a local seat of infection. The symptoms of chills, fever and exhaustion are caused by the bacteria and substances they produce.

038.0 Streptococcal septicemia

⑤ **038.1 Staphylococcal septicemia**

   038.10 Staphylococcal septicemia, unspecified

   038.11 Methicillin susceptible Staphylococcus aureus septicemia
      MSSA septicemia
      Staphylococcus aureus septicemia NOS

   038.12 Methicillin resistant Staphylococcus aureus septicemia

   038.19 Other staphylococcal septicemia

038.2 Pneumococcal septicemia

038.3 Septicemia due to anaerobes
Septicemia due to bacteroides

Excludes: *gas gangrene (040.0)*
   that due to anaerobic streptococci (038.0)

⑤ **038.4 Septicemia due to other gram-negative organisms**

   038.40 Gram-negative organism, unspecified
      Gram-negative septicemia NOS

   038.41 Hemophilus influenzae [H. influenzae]

   038.42 Escherichia coli [E. coli]

   038.43 Pseudomonas

   038.44 Serratia

   038.49 Other

038.8 Other specified septicemias

Excludes: *septicemia (due to):*
   anthrax (022.3)
   gonococcal (098.89)
   herpetic (054.5)
   meningococcal (036.2)
septicemic plague (020.2)

038.9 Unspecified septicemia
Septicemia NOS

Excludes: *bacteremia NOS (790.7)*

039 Actinomycotic infections
Includes: actinomycotic mycetoma
      infection by Actinomycetales, such as species of Actinomyces, Actinomadura,
        Nocardia, Streptomyces
      maduromycosis (actinomycotic)
      schizomycetoma (actinomycotic)

| | Add 4th or 5th digit | | Nonspecific code | | Unspecified code | | Manifestation code |

DEFINITION Actinomycosis is an infection primarily caused by the bacterium actinomyces israelii. Infection most often occurs in the face and neck region and is characterized by the presence of a slowly enlarging, hard, red lump.

039.0 Cutaneous
Erythrasma   Trichomycosis axillaris

039.1 Pulmonary
Thoracic actinomycosis

039.2 Abdominal

039.3 Cervicofacial

039.4 Madura foot
Excludes: *madura foot due to mycotic infection (117.4)*

039.8 Of other specified sites

039.9 Of unspecified site
Actinomycosis NOS   Nocardiosis NOS
Maduromycosis NOS

040 Other bacterial diseases
Excludes: *bacteremia NOS (790.7)*
bacterial infection NOS (041.9)

ALERT! For personal history of other specified infectious and parasitic disease see V12.09

040.0 Gas gangrene
Gas bacillus infection   Malignant edema
or gangrene   Myonecrosis, clostridial
Infection by Clostridium: Myositis, clostridial
histolyticum
oedematiens
perfringens [welchii]
septicum
sordellii

040.1 Rhinoscleroma

040.2 Whipple's disease
Intestinal lipodystrophy

040.3 Necrobacillosis

⑤ **040.4 Other specified botulism**
Non-foodborne intoxication due to toxins of Clostridium botulinum [*C. botulinum*]
Excludes: *botulism NOS (005.1)*
food poisoning due to toxins of Clostridium botulinum (005.1)

040.41 Infant botulism

040.42 Wound botulism
Non-foodborne botulism NOS
Use additional code to identify complicated open wound

⑤ **040.8 Other specified bacterial diseases**

040.81 Tropical pyomyositis

040.82 Toxic shock syndrome
Use additional code to identify the organism

040.89 Other

041 Bacterial infection in conditions classified elsewhere and of unspecified site
Note: This category is provided to be used as an additional code where it is desired to identify the bacterial agent in diseases classified elsewhere. This category will also be used to classify bacterial infections of unspecified nature or site.
Excludes: *septicemia (038.0-038.9)*

⑤ **041.0 Streptococcus**

041.00 Streptococcus, unspecified

041.01 Group A

041.02 Group B

041.03 Group C

041.04 Group D [Enterococcus]

041.05 Group G

041.09 Other Streptococcus

● Code new   ▲ Revision of   ④ ⑤ Fourth or fifth
to this edition   existing code   digit required

⑤ **041.1 Staphylococcus**

> **ALERT!** For personal history of methicillin resistant staphylococcus aureus see V12.04

> **041.10 Staphylococcus, unspecified**

> **041.11 Methicillin susceptible Staphylococcus aureus**
> MSSA
> Staphylococcus aureus NOS

> **041.12 Methicillin resistant Staphylococcus aureus**
> Methicillin-resistant Staphylococcus aureus (MRSA)

> **041.19 Other Staphylococcus**

041.2 Pneumococcus

041.3 Klebsiella pneumoniae

⑤ **041.4 Escherichia coli [E. coli]**

● **041.41 Shiga toxin-producing Escherichia coli [E. coli] (STEC) O157**
E. coli O157:H- (nonmotile) with confirmation of Shiga toxin
E. coli O157 with confirmation of Shiga toxin when H antigen is unknown, or is not H7
O157:H7 Escherichia coli [E.coli] with or without confirmation of Shiga toxin-production
Shiga toxin-producing Escherichia coli [E.coli] O157:H7 with or without confirmation of Shiga toxin-production
STEC O157:H7 with or without confirmation of Shiga toxin-production

● **041.42 Other specified Shiga toxin-producing Escherichia coli [E. coli] (STEC)**
Non-O157 Shiga toxin-producing Escherichia coli [E.coli]
Non-O157 Shiga toxin-producing Escherichia coli [E.coli] with known O group

● **041.43 Shiga toxin-producing Escherichia coli [E. coli] (STEC), unspecified**
Shiga toxin-producing Escherichia coli [E. coli] with unspecified O group
STEC NOS

● **041.49 Other and unspecified Escherichia coli [E. coli]**
Escherichia coli [E. coli] NOS
Non-Shiga toxin-producing E. coli

041.5 Hemophilus influenzae [H. influenzae]

041.6 Proteus (mirabilis) (morganii)

041.7 Pseudomonas

⑤ **041.8 Other specified bacterial infections**

> **041.81 Mycoplasma**
> Eaton's agent
> Pleuropneumonia-like organisms [PPLO]

> **041.82 Bacteroides fragilis**

> **041.83 Clostridium perfringens**

> **041.84 Other anaerobes**
> Gram-negative anaerobes

> *Excludes:* *Helicobacter pylori (041.86)*

> **041.85 Other Gram-negative organisms**
> Aerobacter aerogenes
> Gram-negative bacteria NOS
> Mima polymorpha
> Serratia

> *Excludes:* *Gram-negative anaerobes (041.84)*

> **041.86 Helicobacter pylori [H. pylori]**

> **041.89 Other specified bacteria**

041.9 Bacterial infection, unspecified

HUMAN IMMUNODEFICIENCY VIRUS (HIV) INFECTION (042)

042 Human immunodeficiency virus [HIV] disease
Acquired immune deficiency syndrome
Acquired immunodeficiency syndrome
AIDS
AIDS-like syndrome
AIDS-related complex
ARC
HIV infection, symptomatic

Use additional code(s) to identify all manifestations of HIV

| | Add 4th or 5th digit | | Nonspecific code | | Unspecified code | | Manifestation code |

Use additional code, if desired, to identify HIV-2 infection (079.53)

Excludes: *asymptomatic HIV infection status (V08)*
exposure to HIV virus (V01.79)
nonspecific serologic evidence of HIV (795.71)

DEFINITION Human immunodeficiency virus (HIV) disease is a virus that can lead to acquired immunodeficiency syndrome (AIDS), a condition in humans in which the immune system begins to fail, leading to life-threatening opportunistic infections.

POLIOMYELITIS AND OTHER NON-ARTHROPOD-BORNE VIRAL DISEASES AND PRION DISEASES OF CENTRAL NERVOUS SYSTEM (045-049)

⑤ **045 Acute poliomyelitis**

Excludes: *late effects of acute poliomyelitis (138)*

DEFINITION Poliomyelitis, aka polio or infantile paralysis, is a highly infectious viral disease that may attack the central nervous system and is characterized by symptoms that range from a mild nonparalytic infection to total paralysis in a matter of hours.

ALERT! For coding late effects of acute poliomyelitis see 138

ALERT! For personal history of poliomyelitis see V12.02

The following fifth-digit subclassification is for use with category 045:

  0 poliovirus, unspecified type

  1 poliovirus type I

  2 poliovirus type II

  3 poliovirus type III

⑤ **045.0 Acute paralytic poliomyelitis specified as bulbar**
[0-3]   Infantile paralysis (acute) specified as bulbar
Poliomyelitis (acute) (anterior) specified as bulbar
Polioencephalitis (acute) (bulbar)
Polioencephalomyelitis (acute) (anterior) (bulbar)

⑤ **045.1 Acute poliomyelitis with other paralysis**
[0-3]   Paralysis:
    acute atrophic, spinal
    infantile, paralytic
Poliomyelitis (acute):
    anterior, with paralysis except bulbar
    epidemic, with paralysis except bulbar

⑤ **045.2 Acute nonparalytic poliomyelitis**
[0-3]   Poliomyelitis (acute):
    anterior, specified as nonparalytic
    epidemic, specified as nonparalytic

⑤ **045.9 Acute poliomyelitis, unspecified**
[0-3]   Infantile paralysis, unspecified whether paralytic or nonparalytic
Poliomyelitis (acute):
    anterior, unspecified whether paralytic or nonparalytic
    epidemic, unspecified whether paralytic or nonparalytic

046 Slow virus infections and prion diseases of central nervous system

046.0 Kuru

⑤ **046.1 Jakob-Creutzfeldt disease**
Use additional code to identify dementia:
    with behavioral disturbance (294.11)
    without behavioral disturbance (294.10)

    046.11 Variant Creutzfeldt-Jakob disease
      vCJD

    046.19 Other and unspecified Creutzfeldt-Jakob disease
      CJD
      Familial Creutzfeldt-Jakob disease
      Iatrogenic Creutzfeldt-Jakob disease
      Jakob-Creutzfeldt disease, unspecified
      Sporadic Creutzfeldt-Jakob disease
      Subacute spongiform encephalopathy

Excludes: *variant Creutzfeldt-Jakob disease (vCJD) (046.11)*

046.2 Subacute sclerosing panencephalitis
Dawson's inclusion body encephalitis
Van Bogaert's sclerosing leukoencephalitis

  ● Code new to this edition   ▲ Revision of existing code   ④ ⑤ Fourth or fifth digit required

046.3 Progressive multifocal leukoencephalopathy
Multifocal leukoencephalopathy NOS

⑤ **046.7 Other specified prion diseases of central nervous system**

Excludes: Creutzfeldt-Jakob disease (046.11-046.19)
Jakob-Creutzfeldt disease (046.11-046.19)
kuru (046.0)
variant Creutzfeldt-Jakob disease (vCJD) (046.11)

046.71 Gerstmann-Straussler-Scheinker syndrome
GSS syndrome

046.72 Fatal familial insomnia
FFI

046.79 Other and unspecified prion disease of central nervous system

046.8 Other specified slow virus infection of central nervous system

046.9 Unspecified slow virus infection of central nervous system

047 Meningitis due to enterovirus
Includes: meningitis:
abacterial
aseptic
viral

Excludes: meningitis due to:
adenovirus (049.1)
arthropod-borne virus (060.0-066.9)
leptospira (100.81)
virus of:
herpes simplex (054.72)
herpes zoster (053.0)
lymphocytic choriomeningitis (049.0)
mumps (072.1)
poliomyelitis (045.0-045.9)
any other infection specifically classified elsewhere

DEFINITION Meningitis due to enterovirus refers to any of a subgroup of picornaviruses, including polioviruses, coxsackie viruses, and echoviruses, that infect the gastrointestinal tract and often spread to other areas of the body, especially the nervous system.

047.0 Coxsackie virus

047.1 ECHO virus
Meningo-eruptive syndrome

047.8 Other specified viral meningitis

047.9 Unspecified viral meningitis
Viral meningitis NOS

048 Other enterovirus diseases of central nervous system
Boston exanthem

ALERT! For personal history of other specified infectious and parasitic disease see V12.09

049 Other non-arthropod-borne viral diseases of central nervous system

Excludes: late effects of viral encephalitis (139.0)

DEFINITION Non-arthropod-borne viral diseases refers to diseases caused by a virus that is not carried by insects, spiders, crustaceans, centipedes or millipedes.

ALERT! For coding late effects of viral encephalitis see 139.0

ALERT! For personal history of other specified infectious and parasitic disease see V12.09

049.0 Lymphocytic choriomeningitis
Lymphocytic:
meningitis (serous) (benign)
meningoencephalitis (serous) (benign)

049.1 Meningitis due to adenovirus

049.8 Other specified non-arthropod-borne viral diseases of central nervous system

Encephalitis:	Encephalitis:
acute:	lethargica
inclusion body	Rio Bravo
necrotizing	von Economo's disease
epidemic	

Excludes: human herpesvirus 6 encephalitis (058.21)
other human herpesvirus encephalitis (058.29)

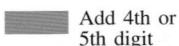

| | Add 4th or 5th digit | | Nonspecific code | | Unspecified code | | Manifestation code |

049.9 **Unspecified non-arthropod-borne viral diseases of central nervous system**
Viral encephalitis NOS

VIRAL DISEASES GENERALLY ACCOMPANIED BY EXANTHEM (050-059)

Excludes: *arthropod-borne viral diseases (060.0-066.9)*
Boston exanthem (048)

050 **Smallpox**
DEFINITION Smallpox, aka variola, a highly contagious and frequently fatal viral disease characterized by a biphasic fever and a distinctive skin rash that left pock marks in its wake. The disease is caused by the variola virus.

050.0 **Variola major**
Hemorrhagic (pustular)   Malignant smallpox
smallpox   Purpura variolosa

050.1 **Alastrim**
Variola minor

050.2 **Modified smallpox**
Varioloid

050.9 **Smallpox, unspecified**

051 **Cowpox and paravaccinia**
DEFINITION Cowpox and paravaccinia is a mild contagious skin disease of cattle, usually affecting the udder that is caused by a virus and characterized by the eruption of a pustular rash. When the virus is transmitted to humans, as by vaccination, it can confer immunity to smallpox.

⑤ **051.0** **Cowpox and vaccinia not from vaccination**

051.01 **Cowpox**

051.02 **Vaccinia not from vaccination**

Excludes: *vaccinia (generalized) (from vaccination) (999.0)*

051.1 **Pseudocowpox**
Milkers' node

051.2 **Contagious pustular dermatitis**
Ecthyma contagiosum   Orf

051.9 **Paravaccinia, unspecified**

052 **Chickenpox**
DEFINITION Chickenpox is an acute contagious disease caused by herpes varicella zoster virus; causes a rash of vesicles on the face and body.

052.0 **Postvaricella encephalitis**
Postchickenpox encephalitis

052.1 **Varicella (hemorrhagic) pneumonitis**

052.2 **Postvaricella myelitis**
Postchickenpox myelitis

052.7 **With other specified complications**

052.8 **With unspecified complication**

052.9 **Varicella without mention of complication**
Chickenpox NOS
Varicella NOS

053 **Herpes zoster**
Includes: shingles
zona
DEFINITION Herpes zoster is a viral disease characterized by a painful skin rash with blisters in a limited area on one side of the body, often in a stripe.

053.0 **With meningitis**

⑤ **053.1** **With other nervous system complications**

053.10 **With unspecified nervous system complication**

053.11 **Geniculate herpes zoster**
Herpetic geniculate ganglionitis

053.12 **Postherpetic trigeminal neuralgia**

053.13 **Postherpetic polyneuropathy**

053.14 **Herpes zoster myelitis**

053.19 **Other**

● Code new   ▲ Revision of   ④ ⑤ Fourth or fifth
to this edition   existing code   digit required

⑤ **053.2 With ophthalmic complications**

    053.20 Herpes zoster dermatitis of eyelid
        Herpes zoster ophthalmicus

    053.21 Herpes zoster keratoconjunctivitis

    053.22 Herpes zoster iridocyclitis

    053.29 Other

⑤ **053.7 With other specified complications**

    053.71 Otitis externa due to herpes zoster

    053.79 Other

053.8 With unspecified complication

053.9 Herpes zoster without mention of complication
    Herpes zoster NOS

054 Herpes simplex

    Excludes: *congenital herpes simplex (771.2)*

    DEFINITION Herpes simplex is an infection caused by the herpes simplex virus; affects the skin and nervous system; produces small temporary blisters on the skin and mucous membranes.

054.0 Eczema herpeticum
    Kaposi's varicelliform eruption

⑤ **054.1 Genital herpes**

    054.10 Genital herpes, unspecified
        Herpes progenitalis

    054.11 Herpetic vulvovaginitis

    054.12 Herpetic ulceration of vulva

    054.13 Herpetic infection of penis

    054.19 Other

054.2 Herpetic gingivostomatitis

054.3 Herpetic meningoencephalitis
    Herpes encephalitis
    Simian B disease

    Excludes: *human herpesvirus 6 encephalitis (058.21)*
             other human herpesvirus encephalitis (058.29)

⑤ **054.4 With ophthalmic complications**

    054.40 With unspecified ophthalmic complication

    054.41 Herpes simplex dermatitis of eyelid

    054.42 Dendritic keratitis

    054.43 Herpes simplex disciform keratitis

    054.44 Herpes simplex iridocyclitis

    054.49 Other

054.5 Herpetic septicemia

054.6 Herpetic whitlow
    Herpetic felon

⑤ **054.7 With other specified complications**

    054.71 Visceral herpes simplex

    054.72 Herpes simplex meningitis

    054.73 Herpes simplex otitis externa

    054.74 Herpes simplex myelitis

    054.79 Other

054.8 With unspecified complication

054.9 Herpes simplex without mention of complication

055 Measles
    Includes: morbilli
            rubeola

    DEFINITION Measles is a viral infection which causes an illness displaying a characteristic skin rash. Measles is also sometimes called rubeola, 5-day measles, or hard measles.

	Add 4th or 5th digit		Nonspecific code		Unspecified code		Manifestation code

055.0 Postmeasles encephalitis

055.1 Postmeasles pneumonia

055.2 Postmeasles otitis media

⑤ **055.7 With other specified complications**

055.71 Measles keratoconjunctivitis
Measles keratitis

055.79 Other

055.8 With unspecified complication

055.9 Measles without mention of complication

056 Rubella
Includes: German measles

Excludes: *congenital rubella (771.0)*

DEFINITION Rubella is a highly contagious viral disease, aka german measles. The symptoms include swollen glands, joint pain, low fever, and a fine red rash.

⑤ **056.0 With neurological complications**

056.00 With unspecified neurological complication

056.01 Encephalomyelitis due to rubella
Encephalitis due to rubella
Meningoencephalitis due to rubella

056.09 Other

⑤ **056.7 With other specified complications**

056.71 Arthritis due to rubella

056.79 Other

056.8 With unspecified complications

056.9 Rubella without mention of complication

057 Other viral exanthemata

DEFINITION Viral exanthemata refers to other skin eruptions occurring as a symptom of an acute viral or coccal disease.

ALERT! For personal history of other specified infectious and parasitic disease see V12.09

057.0 Erythema infectiosum [fifth disease]

057.8 Other specified viral exanthemata
Dukes (-Filatow) disease   Parascarlatina
Fourth disease   Pseudoscarlatina

Excludes: *exanthema subitum [sixth disease] (058.10-058.12)*
roseola infantum (058.10-058.12)

057.9 Viral exanthem, unspecified

⑤ **058 Other human herpesvirus**

Excludes: *congenital herpes (771.2)*
cytomegalovirus (078.5)
Epstein-Barr virus (075)
herpes NOS (054.0-054.9)
herpes simplex (054.0-054.9)
herpes zoster (053.0-053.9)
human herpesvirus NOS (054.0-054.9)
human herpesvirus 1 (054.0-054.9)
human herpesvirus 2 (054.0-054.9)
human herpesvirus 3 (052.0-053.9)
human herpesvirus 4 (075)
human herpesvirus 5 (078.5)
varicella (052.0-052.9)
varicella-zoster virus (052.0-053.9)

DEFINITION Human herpes viruses, refers to a family of viruses including herpes simplex, varicella zoster, and Epstein-Barr.

ALERT! For personal history of other specified infectious and parasitic disease see V12.09

⑤ **058.1 Roseola infantum**
Exanthema subitum [sixth disease]

058.10 Roseola infantum, unspecified
Exanthema subitum [sixth disease], unspecified

058.11 Roseola infantum due to human herpesvirus 6
Exanthema subitum [sixth disease] due to human herpesvirus 6

058.12 **Roseola infantum due to human herpesvirus 7**
Exanthema subitum [sixth disease] due to human herpesvirus 7

⑤ **058.2** **Other human herpesvirus encephalitis**

Excludes: *herpes encephalitis NOS (054.3)*
herpes simplex encephalitis (054.3)
human herpesvirus encephalitis NOS (054.3)
simian B herpes virus encephalitis (054.3)

058.21 **Human herpesvirus 6 encephalitis**

058.29 **Other human herpesvirus encephalitis**
Human herpesvirus 7 encephalitis

⑤ **058.8** **Other human herpesvirus infections**

058.81 **Human herpesvirus 6 infection**

058.82 **Human herpesvirus 7 infection**

058.89 **Other human herpesvirus infection**
Human herpesvirus 8 infection
Kaposi's sarcoma-associated herpesvirus infection

059 **Other poxvirus infections**

Excludes: *contagious pustular dermatitis (051.2)*
cowpox (051.01)
ecthyma contagiosum (051.2)
milker's nodule (051.1)
orf (051.2)
paravaccinia NOS (051.9)
pseudocowpox (051.1)
smallpox (050.0-050.9)
vaccinia (generalized) (from vaccination) (999.0)
vaccinia not from vaccination (051.02)

DEFINITION Poxvirus infections refers to a group of viruses that produce spreading vesicular lesions, including smallpox, vaccinia, and molluscum contagiosum.

ALERT! For personal history of other specified infectious and parasitic disease see V12.09

⑤ **059.0** **Other orthopoxvirus infections**

059.00 **Orthopoxvirus infection, unspecified**

059.01 **Monkeypox**

059.09 **Other orthopoxvirus infection**

⑤ **059.1** **Other parapoxvirus infections**

059.10 **Parapoxvirus infection, unspecified**

059.11 **Bovine stomatitis**

059.12 **Sealpox**

059.19 **Other parapoxvirus infections**

⑤ **059.2** **Yatapoxvirus infections**

059.20 **Yatapoxvirus infection, unspecified**

059.21 **Tanapox**

059.22 **Yaba monkey tumor virus**

059.8 **Other poxvirus infections**

059.9 **Poxvirus infections, unspecified**

ARTHROPOD-BORNE VIRAL DISEASES (060-066)

Use additional code, if desired, to identify any associated meningitis (321.2)

Excludes: *late effects of viral encephalitis (139.0)*

060 **Yellow fever**
DEFINITION Yellow fever is an acute systemic (body wide) illness caused by a virus called a flavivirus. In severe cases, the viral infection causes a high fever, bleeding into the skin, and necrosis (death) of cells in the kidney and liver.

ALERT! For coding late effects of viral encephalitis see 139.0

060.0 **Sylvatic**
Yellow fever:
jungle
sylvan

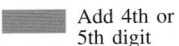 Add 4th or
5th digit

 Nonspecific
code

Unspecified
code

 Manifestation
code

060.1 Urban

060.9 Yellow fever, unspecified

061 Dengue
Breakbone fever

Excludes: *hemorrhagic fever caused by dengue virus (065.4)*

DEFINITION Dengue is an acute febrile and sometimes hemorrhagic disease endemic to the tropics, caused by any of four species of the virus genus flavivirus, and primarily transmitted to humans from mosquitoes, though human-to-human transmission is also well documented.

062 Mosquito-borne viral encephalitis
DEFINITION Mosquito-borne viral encephalitis is an inflammation of the brain, caused by a mosquito-bourne virus.

ALERT! For coding late effects of viral encephalitis see 139.0

062.0 Japanese encephalitis
Japanese B encephalitis

062.1 Western equine encephalitis

062.2 Eastern equine encephalitis

Excludes: *Venezuelan equine encephalitis (066.2)*

062.3 St. Louis encephalitis

062.4 Australian encephalitis
Australian arboencephalitis
Australian X disease
Murray Valley encephalitis

062.5 California virus encephalitis
Encephalitis: Tahyna fever
    California
    La Crosse

062.8 Other specified mosquito-borne viral encephalitis
Encephalitis by Ilheus virus

Excludes: *West Nile virus (066.40-066.49)*

062.9 Mosquito-borne viral encephalitis, unspecified

063 Tick-borne viral encephalitis
Includes: diphasic meningoencephalitis
DEFINITION Tick-borne viral encephalitis is an inflammation of the brain, caused by a tick-bourne virus.

ALERT! For coding late effects of viral encephalitis see 139.0

063.0 Russian spring-summer [taiga] encephalitis

063.1 Louping ill

063.2 Central European encephalitis

063.8 Other specified tick-borne viral encephalitis
Langat encephalitis
Powassan encephalitis

063.9 Tick-borne viral encephalitis, unspecified

064 Viral encephalitis transmitted by other and unspecified arthropods
Arthropod-borne viral encephalitis, vector unknown
Negishi virus encephalitis

Excludes: *viral encephalitis NOS (049.9)*

DEFINITION Viral encephalitis is an inflammation of the brain.

ALERT! For coding late effects of viral encephalitis see 139.0

065 Arthropod-borne hemorrhagic fever
DEFINITION Hemorrhagic fever is a group of viral infections characterized by fever, chills, headache, malaise, and respiratory or gastrointestinal symptoms, followed by capillary hemorrhages and, in severe infection, by oliguria, kidney failure, hypotension, and possibly death.

ALERT! For coding late effects of viral encephalitis see 139.0

065.0 Crimean hemorrhagic fever [CHF Congo virus]
Central Asian hemorrhagic fever

065.1 Omsk hemorrhagic fever

065.2 Kyasanur Forest disease

065.3 Other tick-borne hemorrhagic fever

● Code new
   to this edition

▲ Revision of
   existing code

④ ⑤ Fourth or fifth
   digit required

065.4 Mosquito-borne hemorrhagic fever
　　Chikungunya hemorrhagic fever
　　Dengue hemorrhagic fever

　Excludes: *Chikungunya fever (066.3)*
　　　　　dengue (061)
　　　　　yellow fever (060.0-060.9)

065.8 Other specified arthropod-borne hemorrhagic fever
　　Mite-borne hemorrhagic fever

065.9 Arthropod-borne hemorrhagic fever, unspecified
　　Arbovirus hemorrhagic fever NOS

066 Other arthropod-borne viral diseases
　　DEFINITION Arthropod-borne viral diseases, refers to other viral diseases caused by insects.
　　ALERT! For coding late effects of viral encephalitis see 139.0
　　ALERT! For personal history of other specified infectious and parasitic disease see V12.09

066.0 Phlebotomus fever
　　Changuinola fever
　　Sandfly fever

066.1 Tick-borne fever
　　Nairobi sheep disease　　　Tick fever:
　　Tick fever:　　　　　　　　Kemerovo
　　　American mountain　　　　Quaranfil
　　　Colorado

066.2 Venezuelan equine fever
　　Venezuelan equine encephalitis

066.3 Other mosquito-borne fever
　　Fever (viral):　　　　　　Fever (viral):
　　　Bunyamwera　　　　　　Oropouche
　　　Bwamba　　　　　　　　Pixuna
　　　Chikungunya　　　　　　Rift valley
　　　GuamaR Mayaro　　　　　Ross river
　　　Mucambo　　　　　　　　Wesselsbron
　　　O'nyong-nyong　　　　　Zika

　Excludes: *dengue (061)*
　　　　　yellow fever (060.0-060.9)

⑤ **066.4 West Nile fever**

　　066.40 West Nile fever, unspecified
　　　　West Nile fever NOS
　　　　West Nile fever without complications
　　　　West Nile virus NOS

　　066.41 West Nile fever with encephalitis
　　　　West Nile encephalitis
　　　　West Nile encephalomyelitis

　　066.42 West Nile fever with other neurologic manifestation
　　Use additional code to specify the neurologic manifestation

　　066.49 West Nile fever with other complications
　　Use additional code to specify the other conditions

066.8 Other specified arthropod-borne viral diseases
　　Chandipura fever
　　Piry fever

066.9 Arthropod-borne viral disease, unspecified
　　Arbovirus infection NOS

OTHER DISEASES DUE TO VIRUSES AND CHLAMYDIAE (070-079)

070 Viral hepatitis
　　Includes: viral hepatitis (acute) (chronic)

　Excludes: *cytomegalic inclusion virus hepatitis (078.5)*

The following fifth-digit subclassification is for use with categories 070.2 and 070.3:

　　0 acute or unspecified, without mention of hepatitis delta

　　1 acute or unspecified, with hepatitis delta

　　2 chronic, without mention of hepatitis delta

　　3 chronic, with hepatitis delta

Add 4th or 5th digit　　Nonspecific code　　Unspecified code　　Manifestation code

DEFINITION Viral hepatitis is a liver inflammation due to a viral infection. It may present in acute or chronic forms. The most common causes of viral hepatitis are the five unrelated hepatotropic viruses hepatitis A, hepatitis B, hepatitis C, hepatitis D, and hepatitis E.

070.0 Viral hepatitis A with hepatic coma

070.1 Viral hepatitis A without mention of hepatic coma
Infectious hepatitis

⑤ **070.2 Viral hepatitis B with hepatic coma**
[0-3]

⑤ **070.3 Viral hepatitis B without mention of hepatic coma**
[0-3]   Serum hepatitis

⑤ **070.4 Other specified viral hepatitis with hepatic coma**

070.41 Acute hepatitis C with hepatic coma

070.42 Hepatitis delta without mention of active hepatitis B disease with hepatic coma
Hepatitis delta with hepatitis B carrier state

070.43 Hepatitis E with hepatic coma

070.44 Chronic hepatitis C with hepatic coma

070.49 Other specified viral hepatitis with hepatic coma

⑤ **070.5 Other specified viral hepatitis without mention of hepatic coma**

070.51 Acute hepatitis C without mention of hepatic coma

070.52 Hepatitis delta without mention of active hepatitis B disease or hepatic coma

070.53 Hepatitis E without mention of hepatic coma

070.54 Chronic hepatitis C without mention of hepatic coma

070.59 Other specified viral hepatitis without mention of hepatic coma

070.6 Unspecified viral hepatitis with hepatic coma
Excludes: unspecified viral hepatitis C with hepatic coma (070.71)

⑤ **070.7 Unspecified viral hepatitis C**

070.70 Unspecified viral hepatitis C without hepatic coma
Unspecified viral hepatitis C NOS

070.71 Unspecified viral hepatitis C with hepatic coma

070.9 Unspecified viral hepatitis without mention of hepatic coma
Viral hepatitis NOS
Excludes: unspecified viral hepatitis C without hepatic coma (070.70)

071 Rabies
Hydrophobia
Lyssa
DEFINITION Rabies is a viral disease that causes acute encephalitis in warm-blooded animals and people, characterised by abnormal behaviour such as excitement, aggressiveness, and dementia, followed by paralysis and death.

072 Mumps
DEFINITION Mumps, aka parotitis, is a viral disease of the human species, caused by the mumps virus. It is an acute contagious viral disease characterized by fever and by swelling of the parotid glands

072.0 Mumps orchitis

072.1 Mumps meningitis

072.2 Mumps encephalitis
Mumps meningoencephalitis

072.3 Mumps pancreatitis

⑤ **072.7 Mumps with other specified complications**

072.71 Mumps hepatitis

072.72 Mumps polyneuropathy

072.79 Other

072.8 Mumps with unspecified complication

072.9 Mumps without mention of complication
Epidemic parotitis
Infectious parotitis

● Code new   ▲ Revision of   ④ ⑤ Fourth or fifth
   to this edition   existing code   digit required

073 **Ornithosis**
Includes: parrot fever
psittacosis
DEFINITION Ornithosis is an atypical pneumonia caused by a rickettsia microorganism and transmitted to humans from infected birds.

073.0 **With pneumonia**
Lobular pneumonitis due to ornithosis

073.7 **With other specified complications**

073.8 **With unspecified complication**

073.9 **Ornithosis, unspecified**

074 **Specific diseases due to Coxsackie virus**
Excludes: Coxsackie virus:
infection NOS (079.2)
meningitis (047.0)
DEFINITION Coxsackie virus is any of a group of enteroviruses that are associated with a variety of diseases, including meningitis myocarditis and pericarditis and primarily affect children during the summer months.

074.0 **Herpangina**
Vesicular pharyngitis

074.1 **Epidemic pleurodynia**
Bornholm disease   Epidemic:
Devil's grip   myalgia
                          myositis

⑤ **074.2** **Coxsackie carditis**

074.20 **Coxsackie carditis, unspecified**

074.21 **Coxsackie pericarditis**

074.22 **Coxsackie endocarditis**

074.23 **Coxsackie myocarditis**
Aseptic myocarditis of newborn

074.3 **Hand, foot, and mouth disease**
Vesicular stomatitis and exanthem

074.8 **Other specified diseases due to Coxsackie virus**
Acute lymphonodular pharyngitis

075 **Infectious mononucleosis**
Glandular fever   Pfeiffer's disease
Monocytic angina
DEFINITION Infectious mononucleosis, aka mono, glandular fever, kissing disease is an acute disease characterized by fever and swollen lymph nodes and an abnormal increase of mononuclear leucocytes or monocytes in the bloodstream.

076 **Trachoma**
Excludes: late effect of trachoma (139.1)
DEFINITION Trachoma is a severe, chronic and contagious conjunctival eyelid and corneal infection caused by a virus that leads to corneal blood vessel formation, corneal clouding, conjunctival and eyelid scarring, and dry eyes.
ALERT! For coding late effects of trachoma see 139.1

076.0 **Initial stage**
Trachoma dubium

076.1 **Active stage**
Granular conjunctivitis (trachomatous)
Trachomatous:
follicular conjunctivitis
pannus

076.9 **Trachoma, unspecified**
Trachoma NOS

077 **Other diseases of conjunctiva due to viruses and Chlamydiae**
Excludes: ophthalmic complications of viral diseases classified elsewhere
ALERT! For personal history of other specified infectious and parasitic disease see V12.09

	Add 4th or 5th digit		Nonspecific code		Unspecified code		Manifestation code

077.0 Inclusion conjunctivitis
    Paratrachoma
    Swimming pool conjunctivitis
    Excludes: *inclusion blennorrhea (neonatal) (771.6)*

077.1 Epidemic keratoconjunctivitis
    Shipyard eye

077.2 Pharyngoconjunctival fever
    Viral pharyngoconjunctivitis

077.3 Other adenoviral conjunctivitis
    Acute adenoviral follicular conjunctivitis

077.4 Epidemic hemorrhagic conjunctivitis
    Apollo:
       conjunctivitis
       disease
    Conjunctivitis due to enterovirus type 70
    Hemorrhagic conjunctivitis (acute) (epidemic)

077.8 Other viral conjunctivitis
    Newcastle conjunctivitis

⑤ **077.9 Unspecified diseases of conjunctiva due to viruses and Chlamydiae**

    077.98 Due to Chlamydiae

    077.99 Due to viruses
       Viral conjunctivitis NOS

078 Other diseases due to viruses and Chlamydiae
    Excludes: *viral infection NOS (079.0-079.9)*
           viremia NOS (790.8)
    ALERT! For personal history of other specified infectious and parasitic disease see V12.09

078.0 Molluscum contagiosum

⑤ **078.1 Viral warts**
    Viral warts due to Human papillomavirus

    078.10 Viral warts, unspecified
       Verruca vulgaris
       Warts (infectious)

    078.11 Condyloma acuminatum
       Condyloma NOS
       Genital warts NOS

    078.12 Plantar wart
       Verruca plantaris

    078.19 Other specified viral warts
       Common wart
       Flat wart
       Verruca plana

078.2 Sweating fever
    Miliary fever
    Sweating disease

078.3 Cat-scratch disease
    Benign lymphoreticulosis (of inoculation)
    Cat-scratch fever

078.4 Foot and mouth disease
    Aphthous fever
    Epizootic:
       aphthae
       stomatitis

078.5 Cytomegaloviral disease
    Cytomegalic inclusion disease
    Salivary gland virus disease
    Use additional code, if desired, to identify manifestation, as:
       cytomegalic inclusion virus:
          hepatitis (573.1)
          pneumonia (484.1)
    Excludes: *congenital cytomegalovirus infection (771.1)*

    ● Code new
       to this edition
    ▲ Revision of
       existing code
    ④ ⑤ Fourth or fifth
       digit required

078.6 Hemorrhagic nephrosonephritis

Hemorrhagic fever:
    epidemic
    Korean

Hemorrhagic fever:
    Russian
    with renal syndrome

078.7 Arenaviral hemorrhagic fever

Hemorrhagic fever:
    Argentine
    Bolivian

Hemorrhagic fever:
    Junin virus
    Machupo virus

⑤ **078.8 Other specified diseases due to viruses and Chlamydiae**

Excludes: *epidemic diarrhea (009.2)*
lymphogranuloma venereum (099.1)

078.81 Epidemic vertigo

078.82 Epidemic vomiting syndrome
Winter vomiting disease

078.88 Other specified diseases due to Chlamydiae

078.89 Other specified diseases due to viruses
Epidemic cervical myalgia
Marburg disease

079 Viral and Chlamydial infection in conditions classified elsewhere and of unspecified site

Note: This category is provided to be used as an additional code where it is desired to identify the viral agent in diseases classifiable elsewhere. This category will also be used to classify virus infection of unspecified nature or site.

ALERT! For personal history of other specified infectious and parasitic disease see V12.09

079.0 Adenovirus

079.1 ECHO virus

079.2 Coxsackievirus

079.3 Rhinovirus

079.4 Human papillomavirus

⑤ **079.5 Retrovirus**

Excludes: *human immunodeficiency virus, type 1 [HIV-1] (042)*
human T-cell lymphotrophic virus, type III [HTLV-III] (042)
lymphadenopathy-associated virus [LAV] (042)

079.50 Retrovirus, unspecified

079.51 Human T-cell lymphotrophic virus, type I [HTLV-I]

079.52 Human T-cell lymphotrophic virus, type II [HTLV-II]

079.53 Human immunodeficiency virus, type 2 [HIV-2]

079.59 Other specified retrovirus

079.6 Respiratory syncytial virus (RSV)

⑤ **079.8 Other specified viral and chlamydial infections**

079.81 Hantavirus

079.82 SARS-associated coronavirus

079.83 Parvovirus B19
Human parvovirus
Parvovirus NOS

Excludes: *erythema infectiosum [fifth disease] (057.0)*

079.88 Other specified chlamydial infection

079.89 Other specified viral infection

⑤ **079.9 Unspecified viral and chlamydial infections**

Excludes: *viremia NOS (790.8)*

079.98 Unspecified chlamydial infection
Chlamydial infection NOS

079.99 Unspecified viral infection
Viral infection NOS

| | Add 4th or 5th digit | | Nonspecific code | | Unspecified code | | Manifestation code |

RICKETTSIOSES AND OTHER ARTHROPOD-BORNE DISEASES (080-088)

Excludes: arthropod-borne viral diseases (060.0-066.9)

080 Louse-borne [epidemic] typhus

Typhus (fever):
  classical
  epidemic

Typhus (fever):
  exanthematic NOS
  louse-borne

DEFINITION Louse-borne typhus is any of several forms of infectious disease caused by rickettsia, especially those transmitted by fleas, lice, or mites, and characterized generally by severe headache, sustained high fever, depression, delirium, and the eruption of red rashes on the skin. Also called prison fever, ship fever, typhus fever.

081 Other typhus

ALERT! For personal history of other specified infectious and parasitic disease see V12.09

081.0 Murine [endemic] typhus
Typhus (fever):
  endemic
  flea-borne

081.1 Brill's disease
Brill-Zinsser disease
Recrudescent typhus (fever)

081.2 Scrub typhus
Japanese river fever   Mite-borne typhus
Kedani fever   Tsutsugamushi

081.9 Typhus, unspecified
Typhus (fever) NOS

082 Tick-borne rickettsioses

082.0 Spotted fevers
Rocky mountain spotted fever
São Paulo fever

082.1 Boutonneuse fever
African tick typhus   Marseilles fever
India tick typhus   Mediterranean tick fever
Kenya tick typhus

082.2 North Asian tick fever
Siberian tick typhus

082.3 Queensland tick typhus

⑤ **082.4 Ehrlichiosis**

082.40 Ehrlichiosis, unspecified

082.41 Ehrlichiosis chafeensis (E. chafeensis)

082.49 Other ehrlichiosis

082.8 Other specified tick-borne rickettsioses
Lone star fever

082.9 Tick-borne rickettsiosis, unspecified
Tick-borne typhus NOS

083 Other rickettsioses

DEFINITION Rickettsioses is a disease caused by intracellular bacteria. Examples of rickettsioses include typhus, Rocky Mountain spotted fever, and Rickettsialpox.

ALERT! For personal history of other specified infectious and parasitic disease see V12.09

083.0 Q fever

083.1 Trench fever
Quintan fever
Wolhynian fever

083.2 Rickettsialpox
Vesicular rickettsiosis

083.8 Other specified rickettsioses

083.9 Rickettsiosis, unspecified

084 Malaria

Note: Subcategories 084.0-084.6 exclude the listed conditions with mention of pernicious complications (084.8-084.9).

Excludes: congenital malaria (771.2)

● Code new
to this edition

▲ Revision of
existing code

④ ⑤ Fourth or fifth
digit required

DEFINITION Malaria is an infective disease caused by sporozoan parasites that are transmitted through the bite of an infected anopheles mosquito; marked by paroxysms of chills and fever.

ALERT! For personal history of malaria see V12.03

084.0 Falciparum malaria [malignant tertian]
Malaria (fever):
by Plasmodium falciparum
subtertian

084.1 Vivax malaria [benign tertian]
Malaria (fever) by Plasmodium vivax

084.2 Quartan malaria
Malaria (fever) by Plasmodium malariae
Malariae malaria

084.3 Ovale malaria
Malaria (fever) by Plasmodium ovale

084.4 Other malaria
Monkey malaria

084.5 Mixed malaria
Malaria (fever) by more than one parasite

084.6 Malaria, unspecified
Malaria (fever) NOS

084.7 Induced malaria
Therapeutically induced malaria

Excludes: accidental infection from syringe, blood transfusion, etc. (084.0-084.6, above, according to parasite species)
transmission from mother to child during delivery (771.2)

084.8 Blackwater fever
Hemoglobinuric: Malarial hemoglobinuria
fever (bilious)
malaria

084.9 Other pernicious complications of malaria
Algid malaria
Cerebral malaria
Use additional code, if desired, to identify complication, as:
malarial:
hepatitis (573.2)
nephrosis (581.81)

085 Leishmaniasis

DEFINITION Leishmaniasis is a disease caused by protozoan parasites that belong to the genus leishmania and is transmitted by the bite of certain species of sand fly.

085.0 Visceral [kala-azar]
Dumdum fever   Leishmaniasis:
Infection by Leishmania: dermal, post-kala-azar
donovani   Mediterranean
infantum   visceral (Indian)

085.1 Cutaneous, urban
Aleppo boil   Leishmaniasis, cutaneous:
Baghdad boil   dry form
Delhi boil   late
Infection by Leishmania   recurrent
tropica (minor)   ulcerating
Oriental sore

085.2 Cutaneous, Asian desert
Infection by Leishmania tropica major
Leishmaniasis, cutaneous:
acute necrotizing
rural
wet form
zoonotic form

085.3 Cutaneous, Ethiopian
Infection by Leishmania ethiopica
Leishmaniasis, cutaneous:
diffuse
lepromatous

Add 4th or 5th digit | Nonspecific code | Unspecified code | Manifestation code

085.4 Cutaneous, American
Chiclero ulcer
Infection by Leishmania mexicana
Leishmaniasis tegumentaria diffusa

085.5 Mucocutaneous (American)
Espundia
Infection by Leishmania braziliensis
Uta

085.9 Leishmaniasis, unspecified

086 Trypanosomiasis
Use additional code, if desired, to identify manifestations, as:
trypanosomiasis:
encephalitis (323.2)
meningitis (321.3)
DEFINITION Trypanosomiasis is an infection caused by a type of protozoan parasite of the genus trypanosoma that causes sleeping sickness and other diseases in man and animals (usually transmitted by insects).

086.0 Chagas' disease with heart involvement
American trypanosomiasis with heart involvement
Infection by Trypanosoma cruzi with heart involvement
Any condition classifiable to 086.2 with heart involvement

086.1 Chagas' disease with other organ involvement
American trypanosomiasis with involvement of organ other than heart
Infection by Trypanosoma cruzi with involvement of organ other than heart
Any condition classifiable to 086.2 with involvement of organ other than heart

086.2 Chagas' disease without mention of organ involvement
American trypanosomiasis
Infection by Trypanosoma cruzi

086.3 Gambian trypanosomiasis
Gambian sleeping sickness
Infection by Trypanosoma gambiense

086.4 Rhodesian trypanosomiasis
Infection by Trypanosoma rhodesiense
Rhodesian sleeping sickness

086.5 African trypanosomiasis, unspecified
Sleeping sickness NOS

086.9 Trypanosomiasis, unspecified

087 Relapsing fever
Includes: recurrent fever
DEFINITION Relapsing fever is an infection caused by certain bacteria in the genus borrelia. It is a vector-borne disease that is transmitted through louse or soft-bodied tick bites.

087.0 Louse-borne

087.1 Tick-borne

087.9 Relapsing fever, unspecified

088 Other arthropod-borne diseases
DEFINITION Arthropod-borne diseases are transmitted by insects, spiders and crustaceans.
ALERT! For personal history of other specified infectious and parasitic disease see V12.09

088.0 Bartonellosis
Carrión's disease   Verruga peruana
Oroya fever

⑤ **088.8 Other specified arthropod-borne diseases**

088.81   Lyme Disease
Erythema chronicum migrans

088.82   Babesiosis
Babesiasis

088.89   Other

088.9 Arthropod-borne disease, unspecified

● Code new to this edition   ▲ Revision of existing code   ④ ⑤ Fourth or fifth digit required

SYPHILIS AND OTHER VENEREAL DISEASES (090-099)

> Excludes: nonvenereal endemic syphilis (104.0)
> urogenital trichomoniasis (131.0)

090 **Congenital syphilis**

DEFINITION Congenital syphilis is syphilis present in utero and at birth, and occurs when a child is born to a mother with secondary or tertiary syphilis.

090.0 Early congenital syphilis, symptomatic

Congenital syphilitic:
  choroiditis
  coryza (chronic)
  hepatomegaly
  mucous patches
  periostitis
  splenomegaly

Syphilitic (congenital):
  epiphysitis
  osteochondritis
  pemphigus
Any congenital syphilitic condition specified as early or manifest less than two years after birth

090.1 Early congenital syphilis, latent

Congenital syphilis without clinical manifestations, with positive serological reaction and negative spinal fluid test, less than two years after birth

090.2 Early congenital syphilis, unspecified

Congenital syphilis NOS, less than two years after birth

090.3 Syphilitic interstitial keratitis

Syphilitic keratitis:
  parenchymatous
  punctata profunda

> Excludes: interstitial keratitis NOS (370.50)

⑤ **090.4 Juvenile neurosyphilis**

Use additional code, if desired, to identify any associated mental disorder

090.40 Juvenile neurosyphilis, unspecified

Congenital neurosyphilis
Dementia paralytica juvenilis
Juvenile:
  general paresis
  tabes
  taboparesis

090.41 Congenital syphilitic encephalitis

090.42 Congenital syphilitic meningitis

090.49 Other

090.5 Other late congenital syphilis, symptomatic

Gumma due to congenital syphilis
Hutchinson's teeth
Syphilitic saddle nose
Any congenital syphilitic condition specified as late or manifest two years or more after birth

090.6 Late congenital syphilis, latent

Congenital syphilis without clinical manifestations, with positive serological reaction and negative spinal fluid test, two years or more after birth

090.7 Late congenital syphilis, unspecified

Congenital syphilis NOS, two years or more after birth

090.9 Congenital syphilis, unspecified

091 **Early syphilis, symptomatic**

> Excludes: early cardiovascular syphilis (093.0-093.9)
> early neurosyphilis (094.0-094.9)

DEFINITION Early syphilis is defined as the stages of syphilis (primary, secondary, and early latent syphilis) that typically occur within the first year after acquisition of the infection.

091.0 Genital syphilis (primary)

Genital chancre

091.1 Primary anal syphilis

091.2 Other primary syphilis

Primary syphilis of:
  breast
  fingers

Primary syphilis of:
  lip
  tonsils

Add 4th or 5th digit   Nonspecific code   Unspecified code   Manifestation code

091.3 Secondary syphilis of skin or mucous membranes
    Condyloma latum
    Secondary syphilis of:
      anus
      mouth
      pharynx
    Secondary syphilis of:
      skin
      tonsils
      vulva

091.4 Adenopathy due to secondary syphilis
    Syphilitic adenopathy (secondary)
    Syphilitic lymphadenitis (secondary)

⑤ **091.5 Uveitis due to secondary syphilis**

    091.50 Syphilitic uveitis, unspecified

    091.51 Syphilitic chorioretinitis (secondary)

    091.52 Syphilitic iridocyclitis (secondary)

⑤ **091.6 Secondary syphilis of viscera and bone**

    091.61 Secondary syphilitic periostitis

    091.62 Secondary syphilitic hepatitis
        Secondary syphilis of liver

    091.69 Other viscera

091.7 Secondary syphilis, relapse
    Secondary syphilis, relapse (treated) (untreated)

⑤ **091.8 Other forms of secondary syphilis**

    091.81 Acute syphilitic meningitis (secondary)

    091.82 Syphilitic alopecia

    091.89 Other

091.9 Unspecified secondary syphilis

092 Early syphilis, latent
    Includes: syphilis (acquired) without clinical manifestations, with positive serological
             reaction and negative spinal fluid test, less than two years after infection

092.0 Early syphilis, latent, serological relapse after treatment

092.9 Early syphilis, latent, unspecified

093 Cardiovascular syphilis
    DEFINITION Cardiovascular syphilis refers to the involvement of the cardiovascular system in
    late syphilis usually resulting in aortitis aneurysm formation, and aortic valvular insufficiency.

093.0 Aneurysm of aorta, specified as syphilitic
    Dilatation of aorta, specified as syphilitic

093.1 Syphilitic aortitis

⑤ **093.2 Syphilitic endocarditis**

    093.20 Valve, unspecified
        Syphilitic ostial coronary disease

    093.21 Mitral valve

    093.22 Aortic valve
        Syphilitic aortic incompetence or stenosis

    093.23 Tricuspid valve

    093.24 Pulmonary valve

⑤ **093.8 Other specified cardiovascular syphilis**

    093.81 Syphilitic pericarditis

    093.82 Syphilitic myocarditis

    093.89 Other

093.9 Cardiovascular syphilis, unspecified

094 Neurosyphilis
    Use additional code, if desired, to identify any associated mental disorder
    DEFINITION Neurosyphilis, aka tabes dorsalis, is the slowly progressive degeneration of the
    spinal cord that occurs in the late (tertiary) phase of syphilis a decade or more after
    contracting the infection.

● Code new
  to this edition
▲ Revision of
  existing code
④ ⑤ Fourth or fifth
    digit required

094.0 Tabes dorsalis
Locomotor ataxia (progressive)
Posterior spinal sclerosis (syphilitic)
Tabetic neurosyphilis
Use additional code, if desired, to identify manifestation, as:
  neurogenic arthropathy [Charcot's joint disease] (713.5)

094.1 General paresis
Dementia paralytica   Paretic neurosyphilis
General paralysis (of the   Taboparesis
  insane) (progressive)

094.2 Syphilitic meningitis
Meningovascular syphilis

Excludes: acute syphilitic meningitis (secondary) (091.81)

094.3 Asymptomatic neurosyphilis

⑤ **094.8 Other specified neurosyphilis**

094.81 Syphilitic encephalitis

094.82 Syphilitic Parkinsonism

094.83 Syphilitic disseminated retinochoroiditis

094.84 Syphilitic optic atrophy

094.85 Syphilitic retrobulbar neuritis

094.86 Syphilitic acoustic neuritis

094.87 Syphilitic ruptured cerebral aneurysm

094.89 Other

094.9 Neurosyphilis, unspecified
Gumma (syphilitic) of central nervous system NOS
Syphilis (early) (late) of central nervous system NOS
Syphiloma of central nervous system NOS

095 Other forms of late syphilis, with symptoms
Includes: gumma (syphilitic)
           syphilis, late, tertiary, or unspecified stage
ALERT! For personal history of other specified infectious and parasitic disease see V12.09

095.0 Syphilitic episcleritis

095.1 Syphilis of lung

095.2 Syphilitic peritonitis

095.3 Syphilis of liver

095.4 Syphilis of kidney

095.5 Syphilis of bone

095.6 Syphilis of muscle
Syphilitic myositis

095.7 Syphilis of synovium, tendon, and bursa
Syphilitic:
  bursitis
  synovitis

095.8 Other specified forms of late symptomatic syphilis

Excludes: cardiovascular syphilis (093.0-093.9)
            neurosyphilis (094.0-094.9)

095.9 Late symptomatic syphilis, unspecified

096 Late syphilis, latent
Syphilis (acquired) without clinical manifestations, with positive serological reaction and
  negative spinal fluid test, two years or more after infection

097 Other and unspecified syphilis
ALERT! For personal history of other specified infectious and parasitic disease see V12.09

097.0 Late syphilis, unspecified

097.1 Latent syphilis, unspecified
Positive serological reaction for syphilis

097.9 Syphilis, unspecified
Syphilis (acquired) NOS

Excludes: syphilis NOS causing death under two years of age (090.9)

| | Add 4th or 5th digit | | Nonspecific code | | Unspecified code | | Manifestation code |

098 **Gonococcal infections**

DEFINITION Gonococcal infection is a sexually transmitted disease caused by gonococcal bacteria that affects the mucous membrane chiefly of the genital and urinary tracts and is characterized by an acute purulent discharge and painful or difficult urination, though women often have no symptoms.

098.0 Acute, of lower genitourinary tract

Gonococcal:	Gonorrhea (acute):
Bartholinitis (acute)	NOS
urethritis (acute)	genitourinary (tract) NOS
vulvovaginitis (acute)	

⑤ **098.1 Acute, of upper genitourinary tract**

098.10 Gonococcal infection (acute) of upper genitourinary tract, site unspecified

098.11 Gonococcal cystitis (acute)
Gonorrhea (acute) of bladder

098.12 Gonococcal prostatitis (acute)

098.13 Gonococcal epididymo-orchitis (acute)
Gonococcal orchitis (acute)

098.14 Gonococcal seminal vesiculitis (acute)
Gonorrhea (acute) of seminal vesicle

098.15 Gonococcal cervicitis (acute)
Gonorrhea (acute) of cervix

098.16 Gonococcal endometritis (acute)
Gonorrhea (acute) of uterus

098.17 Gonococcal salpingitis, specified as acute

098.19 Other

098.2 Chronic, of lower genitourinary tract
Gonococcal:
Bartholinitis specified as chronic or with duration of two months or more
urethritis specified as chronic or with duration of two months or more
vulvovaginitis specified as chronic or with duration of two months or more
Gonorrhea:
NOS specified as chronic or with duration of two months or more
genitourinary (tract) specified as chronic or with duration of two months or more
Any condition classifiable to 098.0 specified as chronic or with duration of two months or more

⑤ **098.3 Chronic, of upper genitourinary tract**
Includes: any condition classifiable to 098.1 stated as chronic or with a duration of two months or more

098.30 Chronic gonococcal infection of upper genitourinary tract, site unspecified

098.31 Gonococcal cystitis, chronic
Any condition classifiable to 098.11, specified as chronic
Gonorrhea of bladder, chronic

098.32 Gonococcal prostatitis, chronic
Any condition classifiable to 098.12, specified as chronic

098.33 Gonococcal epididymo-orchitis, chronic
Any condition classifiable to 098.13, specified as chronic
Chronic gonococcal orchitis

098.34 Gonococcal seminal vesiculitis, chronic
Any condition classifiable to 098.14, specified as chronic
Gonorrhea of seminal vesicle, chronic

098.35 Gonococcal cervicitis, chronic
Any condition classifiable to 098.15, specified as chronic
Gonorrhea of cervix, chronic

098.36 Gonococcal endometritis, chronic
Any condition classifiable to 098.16, specified as chronic

098.37 Gonococcal salpingitis (chronic)

098.39 Other

⑤ **098.4 Gonococcal infection of eye**

098.40 Gonococcal conjunctivitis (neonatorum)
Gonococcal ophthalmia (neonatorum)

098.41 Gonococcal iridocyclitis

098.42 Gonococcal endophthalmia

● Code new to this edition   ▲ Revision of existing code   ④ ⑤ Fourth or fifth digit required

098.43   **Gonococcal keratitis**

`098.49`   **Other**

⑤ **098.5**   **Gonococcal infection of joint**

098.50   **Gonococcal arthritis**
Gonococcal infection of joint NOS

098.51   **Gonococcal synovitis and tenosynovitis**

098.52   **Gonococcal bursitis**

098.53   **Gonococcal spondylitis**

`098.59`   **Other**
Gonococcal rheumatism

098.6   Gonococcal infection of pharynx

098.7   Gonococcal infection of anus and rectum
Gonococcal proctitis

⑤ **098.8**   **Gonococcal infection of other specified sites**

098.81   **Gonococcal keratosis (blennorrhagica)**

098.82   **Gonococcal meningitis**

098.83   **Gonococcal pericarditis**

098.84   **Gonococcal endocarditis**

`098.85`   **Other gonococcal heart disease**

098.86   **Gonococcal peritonitis**

`098.89`   **Other**
Gonococcemia

`099`   **Other venereal diseases**

DEFINITION Venereal disease is a disease that is contracted and transmitted by sexual contact, caused by microorganisms that survive on the skin or mucus membranes.

ALERT! For personal history of other specified infectious and parasitic disease see V12.09

099.0   Chancroid

Bubo (inguinal):	Chancre:
chancroidal	Ducrey's
due to Hemophilus ducreyi	simple
	soft
	Ulcus molle (cutis) (skin)

099.1   Lymphogranuloma venereum

Climatic or tropical bubo	Esthiomene
(Durand-) Nicolas- Favre	Lymphogranuloma inguinale
disease	

099.2   Granuloma inguinale

Donovanosis	Granuloma venereum
Granuloma pudendi	Pudendal ulcer
(ulcerating)	

099.3   Reiter's disease
Reactive arthritis
Reiter's syndrome
Use additional code for associated:
arthropathy (711.1)
conjunctivitis (372.33)

⑤ **099.4   Other nongonococcal urethritis [NGU]**

`099.40`   **Unspecified**
Nonspecific urethritis

099.41   **Chlamydia trachomatis**

`099.49`   **Other specified organism**

⑤ **099.5   Other venereal diseases due to Chlamydia trachomatis**

Excludes: *Chlamydia trachomatis infection of conjunctiva (076.0-076.9, 077.0, 077.9)*
Lymphogranuloma venereum (099.1)

`099.50`   **Unspecified site**

099.51   **Pharynx**

099.52   **Anus and rectum**

Add 4th or 5th digit	Nonspecific code	Unspecified code	Manifestation code

099.53 Lower genitourinary sites

Excludes: urethra (099.41)

Use additional code, if desired, to specify site of infection, such as:
    bladder (595.4)
    cervix (616.0)
    vagina and vulva (616.11)

099.54 Other genitourinary sites

Use additional code, if desired, to specify site of infection, such as:
    pelvic inflammatory disease NOS (614.9)
    testis and epididymis (604.91)

099.55 Unspecified genitourinary site

099.56 Peritoneum
    Perihepatitis

099.59 Other specified site

099.8 Other specified venereal diseases

099.9 Venereal disease, unspecified

OTHER SPIROCHETAL DISEASES (100-104)

100 Leptospirosis

DEFINITION Leptospirosis, aka swamp fever, is an acute, infectious, febrile disease of both humans and animals, caused by spirochetes of the genus leptospira.

100.0 Leptospirosis icterohemorrhagica
    Leptospiral or spirochetal jaundice (hemorrhagic)
    Weil's disease

⑤ **100.8 Other specified leptospiral infections**

    100.81 Leptospiral meningitis (aseptic)

    100.89 Other
        Fever: Infection by Leptospira:
          Fort Bragg   australis
          pretibial   bataviae
          swamp   pyrogenes

100.9 Leptospirosis, unspecified

101 Vincent's angina
    Acute necrotizing ulcerative: Spirochetal stomatitis
      gingivitis   Trench mouth
      stomatitis   Vincent's:
    Fusospirochetal pharyngitis   gingivitis
                        infection [any site]

DEFINITION Vincent's angina, aka trench mouth, is an acute communicable infection of the respiratory tract and mouth marked by ulceration of the mucous membrane.

102 Yaws
    Includes: frambesia
             pian

DEFINITION Yaws is a contagious tropical disease caused by the spirochete treponema pertenue, characterized by yellowish or reddish tumors, which often resemble currants, strawberries, or raspberries.

102.0 Initial lesions
    Chancre of yaws   Initial frambesial ulcer
    Frambesia, initial or primary Mother yaw

102.1 Multiple papillomata and wet crab yaws
    Butter yaws   Planter or palmer papilloma of yaws
    Frambesioma
    Pianoma

102.2 Other early skin lesions
    Early yaws (cutaneous) (macular) (papular) (maculopapular) (micropapular)
    Frambeside of early yaws
    Cutaneous yaws, less than five years after infection

102.3 Hyperkeratosis
    Ghoul hand
    Hyperkeratosis, palmer or plantar (early) (late) due to yaws
    Worm-eaten soles

102.4 Gummata and ulcers
    Nodular late yaws (ulcerated)
    Gummatous frambeside

● Code new to this edition   ▲ Revision of existing code   ④ ⑤ Fourth or fifth digit required

102.5 Gangosa
>Rhinopharyngitis mutilans

102.6 Bone and joint lesions
>Goundou, of yaws (late)
>Gumma, bone, of yaws (late)
>Gummatous osteitis or periostitis, of yaws (late)
>Hydrarthrosis, of yaws (early) (late)
>Osteitis, of yaws (early) (late)
>Periostitis (hypertrophic), of yaws (early) (late)

102.7 Other manifestations
>Juxta-articular nodules of yaws
>Mucosal yaws

102.8 Latent yaws
>Yaws without clinical manifestations, with positive serology

102.9 Yaws, unspecified

103 Pinta
>**DEFINITION** Pinta is a human skin disease endemic to Mexico, Central America, and South America caused by infection with a spirochete, treponema pallidum carateum, which is morphologically and serologically indistinguishable from the organism that causes syphilis.

103.0 Primary lesions
>Chancre (primary) of pinta [carate]
>Papule (primary) of pinta [carate]
>Pintid of pinta [carate]

103.1 Intermediate lesions
>Erythematous plaques of pinta [carate]
>Hyperchromic lesions of pinta [carate]
>Hyperkeratosis of pinta [carate]

103.2 Late lesions
>Cardiovascular lesions, of pinta [carate]
>Skin lesions:
> achromic of pinta [carate]
> cicatricial of pinta [carate]
> dyschromic of pinta [carate]
>Vitiligo of pinta [carate]

103.3 Mixed lesions
>Achromic and hyperchromic skin lesions of pinta [carate]

103.9 Pinta, unspecified

104 Other spirochetal infection
>**ALERT!** For personal history of other specified infectious and parasitic disease see V12.09

104.0 Nonvenereal endemic syphilis
>Bejel   Njovera

104.8 Other specified spirochetal infections
>*Excludes:* *relapsing fever (087.0-087.9)*
>   *syphilis (090.0-097.9)*

104.9 Spirochetal infection, unspecified

MYCOSES (110-118)

Use additional code, if desired, to identify manifestation, as:
arthropathy (711.6)
meningitis (321.0-321.1)
otitis externa (380.15)

>*Excludes:* *infection by Actinomycetales, such as species of Actinomyces, Actinomadura,*
>   *Nocardia, Streptomyces (039.0-039.9)*

110 Dermatophytosis
>Includes: infection by species of Epidermophyton, Microsporum, and Trichophyton
>   tinea, any type except those in 111
>**DEFINITION** Dermatophytosis, aka tinea or ringworm, is a disease that can affect the scalp (tinea capitis), body (tinea corporis), nails (tinea unguium), feet (tinea pedis), groin (tinea cruris), and bearded skin (tinea harbae).

110.0 Of scalp and beard
>Kerion
>Sycosis, mycotic
>Trichophytic tinea [black dot tinea], scalp

Add 4th or 5th digit	Nonspecific code	Unspecified code	Manifestation code

110.1 Of nail
Dermatophytic onychia   Tinea unguium
Onychomycosis

110.2 Of hand
Tinea manuum

110.3 Of groin and perianal area
Dhobie itch   Tinea cruris
Eczema marginatum

110.4 Of foot
Athlete's foot   Tinea pedis

110.5 Of the body
Herpes circinatus
Tinea imbricata [Tokelau]

110.6 Deep seated dermatophytosis
Granuloma trichophyticum
Majocchi's granuloma

110.8 Of other specified sites

110.9 Of unspecified site
Favus NOS   Ringworm NOS
Microsporic tinea NOS

111 Dermatomycosis, other and unspecified

   DEFINITION Dermatomycosis is a superficial fungal infection of the skin or its appendages.

111.0 Pityriasis versicolor
Infection by Malassezia [Pityrosporum] furfur
Tinea flava
Tinea versicolor

111.1 Tinea nigra
Infection by   Microsporosis nigra
   Cladosporium species   Pityriasis nigra
Keratomycosis nigricans   Tinea palmaris nigra

111.2 Tinea blanca
Infection by Trichosporon (beigelii) cutaneum
White piedra

111.3 Black piedra
Infection by Piedraia hortai

111.8 Other specified dermatomycoses

111.9 Dermatomycosis, unspecified

112 Candidiasis
Includes: infection by Candida species
         moniliasis

   Excludes: neonatal monilial infection (771.7)

   DEFINITION Candidiasis is an infection caused by a species of the yeast candida, usually candida albicans. Candidiasis is a common cause of vaginal infections in women.

112.0 Of mouth
Thrush (oral)

112.1 Of vulva and vagina
Candidal vulvovaginitis   Monilial vulvovaginitis

112.2 Of other urogenital sites
Candidal balanitis

112.3 Of skin and nails
Candidal intertrigo   Candidal perionyxis [paronychia]
Candidal onychia

112.4 Of lung
Candidal pneumonia

112.5 Disseminated
Systemic candidiasis

⑤ **112.8 Of other specified sites**

     112.81 Candidal endocarditis

     112.82 Candidal otitis externa
        Otomycosis in moniliasis

● Code new   ▲ Revision of   ④ ⑤ Fourth or fifth
    to this edition   existing code   digit required

112.83   **Candidal meningitis**

112.84   **Candidal esophagitis**

112.85   **Candidal enteritis**

112.89   **Other**

112.9 **Of unspecified site**

114 **Coccidioidomycosis**

    Includes: infection by Coccidioides (immitis)
                  Posada-Wernicke disease

    DEFINITION Coccidioidomycosis is an infection caused by inhaling the microscopic spores of the fungus coccidioides immitis. The chronic form can develop as many as 20 years after initial infection and, in the lungs, can produce inflamed, injured areas that can fill with pus.

114.0 **Primary coccidioidomycosis (pulmonary)**
      Acute pulmonary coccidioidomycosis
      Coccidioidomycotic pneumonitis
      Desert rheumatism
      Pulmonary coccidioidomycosis
      San Joaquin Valley fever

114.1 **Primary extrapulmonary coccidioidomycosis**
      Chancriform syndrome
      Primary cutaneous coccidioidomycosis

114.2 **Coccidioidal meningitis**

114.3 **Other forms of progressive coccidioidomycosis**
      Coccidioidal granuloma
      Disseminated coccidioidomycosis

114.4 **Chronic pulmonary coccidioidomycosis**

114.5 **Pulmonary coccidioidomycosis, unspecified**

114.9 **Coccidioidomycosis, unspecified**

⑤ **115** **Histoplasmosis**

    The following fifth-digit subclassification is for use with category 115:

    0   **without mention of manifestation**

    1   **meningitis**

    2   **retinitis**

    3   **pericarditis**

    4   **endocarditis**

    5   **pneumonia**

    9   **other**

    DEFINITION Histoplasmosis, aka Darling's disease, is a disease caused by the fungus histoplasma capsulatum. Symptoms vary greatly, but the disease primarily affects the lungs. Histoplasmosis is common among aids patients because of their lowered immune system.

⑤ **115.0** **Infection by Histoplasma capsulatum**
  [0-5, 9]   American histoplasmosis
             Darling's disease
             Reticuloendothelial cytomycosis
             Small form histoplasmosis

⑤ **115.1** **Infection by Histoplasma duboisii**
  [0-5, 9]   African histoplasmosis   Large form histoplasmosis

⑤ **115.9** **Histoplasmosis, unspecified**
  [0-5, 9]   Histoplasmosis NOS

116 **Blastomycotic infection**
    DEFINITION Blastomycotic infection, aka North American blastomycosis, blastomycetic dermatitis, and gilchrist's disease, is a fungal infection caused by the organism blastomyces dermatitidis. Endemic to portions of north america, blastomycosis causes clinical symptoms similar to histoplasmosis.

116.0 **Blastomycosis**
      Blastomycotic dermatitis
      Chicago disease
      Cutaneous blastomycosis
      Disseminated blastomycosis
      Gilchrist's disease
      Infection by Blastomyces [Ajellomyces] dermatitidis
      North American blastomycosis
      Primary pulmonary blastomycosis

	Add 4th or 5th digit		Nonspecific code		Unspecified code		Manifestation code

116.1 Paracoccidioidomycosis
Brazilian blastomycosis
Infection by Paracoccidioides [Blastomyces] brasiliensis
Lutz-Splendore-Almeida disease
Mucocutaneous-lymphangitic paracoccidioidomycosis
Pulmonary paracoccidioidomycosis
South American blastomycosis
Visceral paracoccidioidomycosis

116.2 Lobomycosis
Infections by Loboa [Blastomyces] loboi
Keloidal blastomycosis
Lobo's disease

117 Other mycoses
DEFINITION Mycoses is a fungal infection in or on a part of the body.

ALERT! For personal history of other specified infectious and parasitic disease see V12.09

117.0 Rhinosporidiosis
Infection by Rhinosporidium seeberi

117.1 Sporotrichosis
Cutaneous sporotrichosis
Disseminated sporotrichosis
Infection by Sporothrix [Sporotrichum] schenckii
Lymphocutaneous sporotrichosis
Pulmonary sporotrichosis
Sporotrichosis of the bones

117.2 Chromoblastomycosis
Chromomycosis
Infection by Cladosporidium carrionii, Fonsecaea compactum, Fonsecaea pedrosoi, Phialophora verrucosa

117.3 Aspergillosis
Infection by Aspergillus species, mainly A. fumigatus, A. flavus group, A. terreus group

117.4 Mycotic mycetomas
Infection by various genera and species of Ascomycetes and Deuteromycetes, such as Acremonium [Cephalosporium] falciforme, Neotestudina rosatii, Madurella grisea, Madurella mycetomii, Pyrenochaeta romeroi, Zopfia [Leptosphaeria] senegalensis
Madura foot, mycotic
Maduromycosis, mycotic

Excludes: actinomycotic mycetomas (039.0-039.9)

117.5 Cryptococcosis
Busse-Buschke's disease
European cryptococcosis
Infection by Cryptococcus neoformans
Pulmonary cryptococcosis
Systemic cryptococcosis
Torula

117.6 Allescheriosis [Petriellidosis]
Infections by Allescheria [Petriellidium] boydii [Monosporium apiospermum]

Excludes: mycotic mycetoma (117.4)

117.7 Zygomycosis [Phycomycosis or Mucormycosis]
Infection by species of Absidia, Basidiobolus, Conidiobolus, Cunninghamella, Entomophthora, Mucor, Rhizopus, Saksenaea

117.8 Infection by dematiacious fungi, [Phaehyphomycosis]
Infection by dematiacious fungi, such as Cladosporium trichoides [bantianum], Dreschlera hawaiiensis, Phialophora gougerotii, Phialophora jeanselmi

117.9 Other and unspecified mycoses

118 Opportunistic mycoses
Infection of skin, subcutaneous tissues, and/or organs by a wide variety of fungi generally considered to be pathogenic to compromised hosts only (e.g., infection by species of Alternaria, Dreschlera, Fusarium)

Use additional code to identify manifestation, such as:
keratitis (370.8)

● Code new to this edition   ▲ Revision of existing code   ④ ⑤ Fourth or fifth digit required

HELMINTHIASES (120-129)

120 **Schistosomiasis [bilharziasis]**

DEFINITION Schistosomiasis [bilharziasis], aka bilharzia, bilharziosis or snail fever, is a parasitic disease caused by several species of fluke of the genus schistosoma. Schistosomiasis often is a chronic illness that can damage internal organs and, in children, impair growth and cognitive development.

120.0 Schistosoma haematobium
Vesical schistosomiasis NOS

120.1 Schistosoma mansoni
Intestinal schistosomiasis NOS

120.2 Schistosoma japonicum
Asiatic schistosomiasis NOS
Katayama disease or fever

120.3 Cutaneous
Cercarial dermatitis   Schistosome dermatitis
Infection by cercariae   Swimmers' itch
  of Schistosoma

120.8 Other specified schistosomiasis
Infection by Schistosoma: Infection by Schistosoma spindale
  bovis   Schistosomiasis chestermani
  intercalatum
  mattheii

120.9 Schistosomiasis, unspecified
Blood flukes NOS   Hemic distomiasis

121 **Other trematode infections**

DEFINITION A trematode infection is the infection of the digestive tract by adult parasitic flatworms called cestodes or tapeworms.

ALERT! For personal history of other specified infectious and parasitic disease see V12.09

121.0 Opisthorchiasis
Infection by:
  cat liver fluke
  Opisthorchis (felineus) (tenuicollis) (viverrini)

121.1 Clonorchiasis
Biliary cirrhosis due to clonorchiasis
Chinese liver fluke disease
Hepatic distomiasis due to Clonorchis sinensis
Oriental liver fluke disease

121.2 Paragonimiasis
Infection by Paragonimus   Pulmonary distomiasis
Lung fluke disease (oriental)

121.3 Fascioliasis
Infection by Fasciola: Liver flukes NOS
  gigantica   Sheep liver fluke infection
  hepatica

121.4 Fasciolopsiasis
Infection by Fasciolopsis [buski]
Intestinal distomiasis

121.5 Metagonimiasis
Infection by Metagonimus yokogawai

121.6 Heterophyiasis
Infection by:
  Heterophyes heterophyes
  Stellantchasmus falcatus

121.8 Other specified trematode infections
Infection by:
  Dicrocoelium dendriticum
  Echinostoma ilocanum
  Gastrodiscoides hominis

121.9 Trematode infection, unspecified
Distomiasis NOS
Fluke disease NOS

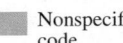 Add 4th or 5th digit

 Nonspecific code

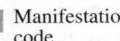 Unspecified code

Manifestation code

122 Echinococcosis

Includes: echinococciasis
hydatid disease
hydatidosis

DEFINITION Echinococcosis, aka hydatid disease, hydatid cyst, unilocular hydatid disease or cystic echinococcosis is a potentially fatal parasitic disease that can affect many animals, including wildlife, commercial livestock and humans. The disease results from infection by tapeworm larvae of the genus echinococcus.

122.0 Echinococcus granulosus infection of liver

122.1 Echinococcus granulosus infection of lung

122.2 Echinococcus granulosus infection of thyroid

122.3 Echinococcus granulosus infection, other

122.4 Echinococcus granulosus infection, unspecified

122.5 Echinococcus multilocularis infection of liver

122.6 Echinococcus multilocularis infection, other

122.7 Echinococcus multilocularis infection, unspecified

122.8 Echinococcosis, unspecified, of liver

122.9 Echinococcosis, other and unspecified

123 Other cestode infection

DEFINITION Cestode infection refers to infestation by any of various parasitic flatworms of the class cestoda, including the tapeworms.

ALERT! For personal history of other specified infectious and parasitic disease see V12.09

123.0 Taenia solium infection, intestinal form
Pork tapeworm (adult) (infection)

123.1 Cysticercosis
Cysticerciasis
Infection by Cysticercus cellulosae [larval form of Taenia solium]

123.2 Taenia saginata infection
Beef tapeworm (infection)
Infection by Taeniarhynchus saginatus

123.3 Taeniasis, unspecified

123.4 Diphyllobothriasis, intestinal
Diphyllobothrium (adult) (latum) (pacificum) infection
Fish tapeworm (infection)

123.5 Sparganosis [larval diphyllobothriasis]
Infection by:
Diphyllobothrium larvae
Sparganum (mansoni) (proliferum)
Spirometra larvae

123.6 Hymenolepiasis
Dwarf tapeworm (infection)
Hymenolepis (diminuta) (nana) infection
Rat tapeworm (infection)

123.8 Other specified cestode infection
Diplogonoporus (grandis) infection
Dipylidium (caninum) infection
Dog tapeworm (infection) infection

123.9 Cestode infection, unspecified
Tapeworm (infection) NOS

124 Trichinosis

Trichinella spiralis infection
Trichinellosis
Trichiniasis

DEFINITION Trichinosis, aka trichinellosis or trichiniasis, is a parasitic disease caused by eating raw or undercooked pork and wild game infected with the larvae of a species of roundworm trichinella spiralis commonly called the trichina worm.

● Code new
to this edition

▲ Revision of
existing code

④ ⑤ Fourth or fifth
digit required

125 **Filarial infection and dracontiasis**

> **DEFINITION** Filarial infection and dracontiasis is a group of tropical diseases caused by various thread-like parasitic round worms (nematodes) and their larvae transmitted to humans through a mosquito bite. Filariasis is characterized by fever, chills, headache, and skin lesions in the early stages and, if untreated, can progress to include gross enlargement of the limbs and genitalia in a condition called elephantiasis. Dracunculiasis more commonly known as guinea worm disease (GWD), dracontiasis or medina worm is a parasitic infection caused by the nematode dracunculus medinensis.

125.0 **Bancroftian filariasis**
Chyluria due to Wuchereria bancrofti
Elephantiasis due to Wuchereria bancrofti
Infection due to Wuchereria bancrofti
Lymphadenitis due to Wuchereria bancrofti
Lymphangitis due to Wuchereria bancrofti
Wuchereriasis

125.1 **Malayan filariasis**
Brugia filariasis due to Brugia [Wuchereria] malayi
Chyluria due to Brugia [Wuchereria] malayi
Elephantiasis due to Brugia [Wuchereria] malayi
Infection due to Brugia [Wuchereria] malayi
Lymphadenitis due to Brugia [Wuchereria] malayi
Lymphangitis due to Brugia [Wuchereria] malayi

125.2 **Loiasis**
Eyeworm disease of Africa
Loa loa infection

125.3 **Onchocerciasis**
Onchocerca volvulus infection
Onchocercosis

125.4 **Dipetalonemiasis**
Infection by:
Acanthocheilonema perstans
Dipetalonema perstans

125.5 **Mansonella ozzardi infection**
Filariasis ozzardi

125.6 **Other specified filariasis**
Dirofilaria infection
Infection by:
Acanthocheilonema streptocerca
Dipetalonema streptocerca

125.7 **Dracontiasis**
Guinea-worm infection
Infection by Dracunculus medinensis

125.9 **Unspecified filariasis**

126 **Ancylostomiasis and necatoriasis**
Includes: cutaneous larva migrans due to Ancylostoma
hookworm (disease) (infection)
uncinariasis

> **DEFINITION** Ancylostomiasis and necatoriasis ancylostomiasis, aka hookworm disease or tunnel disease, is a disease caused by hookworm infestation and marked by progressive anemia. Necatoriasis is a hookworm disease caused by necator, the resulting anemia being usually less severe than that from ancylostomiasis.

126.0 **Ancylostoma duodenale**

126.1 **Necator americanus**

126.2 **Ancylostoma braziliense**

126.3 **Ancylostoma ceylanicum**

126.8 **Other specified Ancylostoma**

126.9 **Ancylostomiasis and necatoriasis, unspecified**
Creeping eruption NOS
Cutaneous larva migrans NOS

127 **Other intestinal helminthiases**

> **DEFINITION** Helminthiases is a disease in which a part of the body is infested with worms such as pinworm, roundworm or tapeworm.

> **ALERT!** For personal history of other specified infectious and parasitic disease see V12.09

| | Add 4th or 5th digit | | Nonspecific code | | Unspecified code | | Manifestation code |

127.0 Ascariasis
    Ascaridiasis
    Infection by Ascaris lumbricoides
    Roundworm infection

127.1 Anisakiasis
    Infection by Anisakis larva

127.2 Strongyloidiasis
    Infection by Strongyloides stercoralis
    Excludes: trichostrongyliasis (127.6)

127.3 Trichuriasis
    Infection by Trichuris trichiuria
    Trichocephaliasis
    Whipworm (disease) (infection)

127.4 Enterobiasis
    Infection by Enterobius vermicularis
    Oxyuriasis
    Oxyuris vermicularis infection
    Pinworn (disease) (infection)
    Threadworm infection

127.5 Capillariasis
    Infection by Capillaria philippinensis
    Excludes: infection by Capillaria hepatica (128.8)

127.6 Trichostrongyliasis
    Infection by Trichostrongylus species

127.7 Other specified intestinal helminthiasis
    Infection by:
        Oesophagostomum apiostomum and related species
        Ternidens diminutus
        other specified intestinal helminth
    Physalopteriasis

127.8 Mixed intestinal helminthiasis
    Infection by intestinal helminths classified to more than one of the categories
        120.0-127.7
    Mixed helminthiasis NOS

127.9 Intestinal helminthiasis, unspecified

128 Other and unspecified helminthiases
    ALERT! For personal history of other specified infectious and parasitic disease see V12.09

128.0 Toxocariasis
    Larva migrans visceralis
    Toxocara (canis) (cati) infection
    Visceral larva migrans syndrome

128.1 Gnathostomiasis
    Infection by Gnathostoma spinigerum and related species

128.8 Other specified helminthiasis
    Infection by:
        Angiostrongylus cantonensis
        Capillaria hepatica
        other specified helminth

128.9 Helminth infection, unspecified
    Helminthiasis NOS
    Worms NOS

129 Intestinal parasitism, unspecified

● Code new   ▲ Revision of   ④ ⑤ Fourth or fifth
      to this edition   existing code   digit required

OTHER INFECTIOUS AND PARASITIC DISEASES (130-136)

ALERT! For coding late effects of other infectious and parasitic diseases see 139

130 Toxoplasmosis

Includes: infection by toxoplasma gondii
toxoplasmosis (acquired)

Excludes: congenital toxoplasmosis (771.2)

DEFINITION Toxoplasmosis is an infection caused by the parasite named toxoplasma gondii that can invade tissues and damage the brain, especially in a fetus and in a newborn baby. Symptoms include fever, fatigue, headache, swollen lymph glands, and muscle aches and pains.

130.0 Meningoencephalitis due to toxoplasmosis
Encephalitis due to acquired toxoplasmosis

130.1 Conjunctivitis due to toxoplasmosis

130.2 Chorioretinitis due to toxoplasmosis
Focal retinochoroiditis due to acquired toxoplasmosis

130.3 Myocarditis due to toxoplasmosis

130.4 Pneumonitis due to toxoplasmosis

130.5 Hepatitis due to toxoplasmosis

130.7 Toxoplasmosis of other specified sites

130.8 Multisystemic disseminated toxoplasmosis
Toxoplasmosis of multiple sites

130.9 Toxoplasmosis, unspecified

131 Trichomoniasis

Includes: infection due to Trichomonas (vaginalis)

DEFINITION Trichomoniasis is a common sexually transmitted disease caused by the parasite trichomonas vaginalis and infecting the urinary tract or vagina.

ALERT! For coding late effects of other infectious and parasitic diseases see 139

⑤ **131.0 Urogenital trichomoniasis**

131.00 Urogenital trichomoniasis, unspecified
Fluor (vaginalis) trichomonal or due to Trichomonas (vaginalis)
Leukorrhea (vaginalis) trichomonal or due to Trichomonas (vaginalis)

131.01 Trichomonal vulvovaginitis
Vaginitis, trichomonal or due to Trichomonas (vaginalis)

131.02 Trichomonal urethritis

131.03 Trichomonal prostatitis

131.09 Other

131.8 Other specified sites

Excludes: intestinal (007.3)

131.9 Trichomoniasis, unspecified

132 Pediculosis and phthirus infestation

DEFINITION Pediculosis and phthirus infestation is an infestation with lice (pediculus humanus) or true lice or crab lice (phthirius) resulting in severe itching.

ALERT! For coding late effects of other infectious and parasitic diseases see 139

132.0 Pediculus capitis [head louse]

132.1 Pediculus corporis [body louse]

132.2 Phthirus pubis [pubic louse]
Pediculus pubis

132.3 Mixed infestation
Infestation classifiable to more than one of the categories 132.0-132.2

132.9 Pediculosis, unspecified

133 Acariasis

DEFINITION Acariasis is an infestation with arthropod parasites of the order acarina including the ticks and mites.

ALERT! For coding late effects of other infectious and parasitic diseases see 139

133.0 Scabies
Infestation by Sarcoptes scabiei
Norwegian scabies
Sarcoptic itch

| | Add 4th or 5th digit | | Nonspecific code | | Unspecified code | | Manifestation code |

133.8 Other acariasis
Chiggers
Infestation by:
Demodex folliculorum
Trombicula

133.9 Acariasis, unspecified
Infestation by mites NOS

134 Other infestation
ALERT! For coding late effects of other infectious and parasitic diseases see 139

134.0 Myiasis
Infestation by:
Dermatobia (hominis)
fly larvae
Gasterophilus (intestinalis)
Infestation by:
maggots
Oestrus ovis

134.1 Other arthropod infestation
Infestation by:
chigoe
sand flea
Tunga penetrans
Jigger disease
Scarabiasis
Tungiasis

134.2 Hirudiniasis
Hirudiniasis (external) (internal)
Leeches (aquatic) (land)

134.8 Other specified infestations

134.9 Infestation, unspecified
Infestation (skin) NOS
Skin parasites NOS

135 Sarcoidosis
Besnier-Boeck- Schaumann disease
Lupoid (miliary) of Boeck
Lupus pernio (Besnier)
Lymphogranulomatosis, benign
(Schaumann's)
Sarcoid (any site):
NOS
Boeck
Darier-Roussy
Uveoparotid fever
DEFINITION Sarcoidosis is a disease of unknown origin that causes small lumps (granulomas) due to chronic inflammation to develop in a great range of body tissues. Sarcoidosis can appear in almost any body organ, but most often starts in the lungs or lymph nodes.
ALERT! For coding late effects of other infectious and parasitic diseases see 139

136 Other and unspecified infectious and parasitic diseases
ALERT! For coding late effects of other and unspecified infectious and parasitic diseases see 139.8
ALERT! For personal history of unspecified infectious and parasitic disease see V12.00

136.0 Ainhum
Dactylolysis spontanea

136.1 Behçet's syndrome

⑤ **136.2 Specific infections by free-living amebae**

136.21 Specific infection due to acanthamoeba
Use additional code to identify manifestation, such as:
keratitis (370.8)

136.29 Other specific infections by free-living amebae
Meningoencephalitis due to Naegleria

136.3 Pneumocystosis
Pneumonia due to Pneumocystis carinii
Pneumonia due to Pneumocystis jiroveci

136.4 Psorospermiasis

136.5 Sarcosporidiosis
Infection by Sarcocystis lindemanni

136.8 Other specified infectious and parasitic diseases
Candiru infestation

136.9 Unspecified infectious and parasitic diseases
Infectious disease NOS
Parasitic disease NOS

● Code new to this edition   ▲ Revision of existing code   ④ ⑤ Fourth or fifth digit required

LATE EFFECTS OF INFECTIOUS AND PARASITIC DISEASES (137-139)

137 **Late effects of tuberculosis**

Note: This category is to be used to indicate conditions classifiable to 010-018 as the cause of late effects, which are themselves classified elsewhere. The "late effects" include those specified as such, as sequelae, or as due to old or inactive tuberculosis, without evidence of active disease.

DEFINITION Late effects of tuberculosis refers to condition that appears after the acute phase of tuberculosis has run its course.

137.0 **Late effects of respiratory or unspecified tuberculosis**

137.1 **Late effects of central nervous system tuberculosis**

137.2 **Late effects of genitourinary tuberculosis**

137.3 **Late effects of tuberculosis of bones and joints**

137.4 **Late effects of tuberculosis of other specified organs**

138 **Late effects of acute poliomyelitis**

Note: This category is to be used to indicate conditions classifiable to 045 as the cause of late effects, which are themselves classified elsewhere. The "late effects" include conditions specified as such, or as sequelae, or as due to old or inactive poliomyelitis, without evidence of active disease.

DEFINITION Late effects of acute poliomyelitis refers to condition that appears after the acute phase of poliomyelitis has run its course.

139 **Late effects of other infectious and parasitic diseases**

Note: This category is to be used to indicate conditions classifiable to categories 001-009, 020-041, 046-136 as the cause of late effects, which are themselves classified elsewhere. The "late effects" include conditions specified as such; they also include sequela of diseases classifiable to the above categories if there is evidence that the disease itself is no longer present.

DEFINITION Late effects of other infectious and parasitic diseases refers to condition that appears after the acute phase of other infectious and/or parasitic diseases has run its course.

139.0 **Late effects of viral encephalitis**
Late effects of conditions classifiable to 049.8-049.9, 062-064

139.1 **Late effects of trachoma**
Late effects of conditions classifiable to 076

139.8 **Late effects of other and unspecified infectious and parasitic diseases**

Add 4th or 5th digit   Nonspecific code   Unspecified code   Manifestation code

This page intentionally left blank.

Chapter 2: Neoplasms (140-239)

GENERAL GUIDELINES

Chapter 2 of the ICD-9-CM contains the codes for most benign and all malignant neoplasms. Certain benign neoplasms, such as prostatic adenomas, may be found in the specific body system chapters. To properly code a neoplasm it is necessary to determine from the record if the neoplasm is benign, in-situ, malignant, or of uncertain histologic behavior. If malignant, any secondary (metastatic) sites should also be determined.

The neoplasm table in the Alphabetic Index should be referenced first. However, if the histological term is documented, that term should be referenced first, rather than going immediately to the Neoplasm Table, in order to determine which column in the Neoplasm Table is appropriate. For example, if the documentation indicates "adenoma," refer to the term in the Alphabetic Index to review the entries under this term and the instructional note to "see also neoplasm, by site, benign." The table provides the proper code based on the type of neoplasm and the site. It is important to select the proper column in the table that corresponds to the type of neoplasm. The tabular should then be referenced to verify that the correct code has been selected from the table and that a more specific site code does not exist.

See Chapter 18 "History (of)" for information regarding V codes for genetic susceptibility to cancer.

DEFINITIONS AND CODING ALERTS

This chapter includes definitions of selected key words, terms and phrases and coding alerts for adding points to the clinical domain, references to coding late effects where appropriate, and references to personal history V-codes in situations where the acute or chronic condition is no longer active. An example from this chapter is as follows:

⑤ **200** **Lymphosarcoma and reticulosarcoma and other specified malignant tumors of lymphatic tissue**
> **DEFINITION** Lymphosarcoma is a type of cancer that originates in lymphocytes of the immune system. The diseases often originates in lymph nodes, presenting as an enlargement of the node (a tumor). A reticulosarcoma is a malignant lymphoma, histiocytic or undifferentiated.
> **ALERT!** For personal history of other lymphatic and hematopoietic neoplasms see V10.7

MULTIPLE CODING FOR A SINGLE CONDITION

In addition to the etiology or manifestation convention that requires two codes to fully describe a single condition that affects multiple body systems, there are other single conditions that also require more than one code. "Use additional code" notes are found in the tabular at codes that are not part of an etiology or manifestation pair where a secondary code is useful to fully describe a condition. The sequencing rule is the same as the etiology or manifestation pair - , "use additional code" indicates that a secondary code should be added.

"Code first" notes are also under certain codes that are not specifically manifestation codes but may be due to an underlying cause. When a "code first" note is present and an underlying condition is present the underlying condition should be sequenced first.

"Code, if applicable, any causal condition first", notes indicate that this code may be assigned as a principal diagnosis when the causal condition is unknown or not applicable. If a causal condition is known, then the code for that condition should be sequenced as the principal or first-listed diagnosis. Multiple codes may be needed for late effects, complication codes and obstetric codes to more fully describe a condition. See the specific guidelines for these conditions for further instruction.

COMBINATION CODE

A combination code is a single code used to classify: two diagnoses, or a diagnosis with an associated secondary process (manifestation) A diagnosis with an associated complication Combination codes are identified by referring to subterm entries in the Alphabetic Index and by reading the inclusion and exclusion notes in the Tabular List.

Assign only the combination code when that code fully identifies the diagnostic conditions involved or when the Alphabetic Index so directs. Multiple coding should not be used when the classification provides a combination code that clearly identifies all of the elements documented in the diagnosis. When the combination code lacks necessary specificity in describing the manifestation or complication, an additional code should be used as a secondary code.

▓	Add 4th or 5th digit	▓	Nonspecific code	▓	Unspecified code	▓	Manifestation code

CODING LATE EFFECTS

A late effect is the residual effect (condition produced) after the acute phase of an illness or injury has terminated. There is no time limit on when a late effect code can be used. The residual may be apparent early, such as in cerebrovascular accident cases, or it may occur months or years later, such as that due to a previous injury. Coding of late effects generally requires two codes sequenced in the following order: The condition or nature of the late effect is sequenced first. The late effect code is sequenced second.

An exception to the above guidelines are those instances where the code for late effect is followed by a manifestation code identified in the Tabular List and title, or the late effect code has been expanded (at the fourth and fifth-digit levels) to include the manifestation(s). The code for the acute phase of an illness or injury that led to the late effect is never used with a code for the late effect.

TREATMENT DIRECTED AT THE MALIGNANCY

If the treatment is directed at the malignancy, designate the malignancy as the principal diagnosis.

The only exception to this guideline is if a patient admission or encounter is solely for the administration of chemotherapy, immunotherapy or radiation therapy, assign the appropriate V58.x code as the first-listed or principal diagnosis, and the diagnosis or problem for which the service is being performed as a secondary diagnosis.

TREATMENT OF SECONDARY SITE

When a patient is admitted because of a primary neoplasm with metastasis and treatment is directed toward the secondary site only, the secondary neoplasm is designated as the principal diagnosis even though the primary malignancy is still present.

CODING AND SEQUENCING OF COMPLICATIONS

Coding and sequencing of complications associated with the malignancies or with the therapy thereof are subject to the following guidelines:

Anemia associated with malignancy

When admission or encounter is for management of an anemia associated with the malignancy, and the treatment is only for anemia, the appropriate anemia code (such as code 285.22, Anemia in neoplastic disease) is designated as the principal diagnosis and is followed by the appropriate code(s) for the malignancy.

Code 285.22 may also be used as a secondary code if the patient suffers from anemia and is being treated for the malignancy.

Anemia associated with chemotherapy, immunotherapy and radiation therapy

When the admission or encounter is for management of an anemia associated with chemotherapy, immunotherapy or radiotherapy and the only treatment is for the anemia, the anemia is sequenced first followed by code E933.1. The appropriate neoplasm code should be assigned as an additional code.

Management of dehydration due to the malignancy

When the admission or encounter is for management of dehydration due to the malignancy or the therapy, or a combination of both, and only the dehydration is being treated (intravenous rehydration), the dehydration is sequenced first, followed by the code(s) for the malignancy.

Treatment of a complication resulting from a surgical procedure

When the admission or encounter is for treatment of a complication resulting from a surgical procedure, designate the complication as the principal or first-listed diagnosis if treatment is directed at resolving the complication.

Primary malignancy previously excised

When a primary malignancy has been previously excised or eradicated from its site and there is no further treatment directed to that site and there is no evidence of any existing primary malignancy, a code from category V10, Personal history of malignant neoplasm, should be used to indicate the former site of the malignancy. Any mention of extension, invasion, or metastasis to another site is coded as a secondary malignant neoplasm to that site. The secondary site may be the principal or first-listed with the V10 code used as a secondary code.

ADMISSIONS OR ENCOUNTERS INVOLVING CHEMOTHERAPY, IMMUNOTHERAPY AND RADIATION THERAPY

A. Episode of care involves surgical removal of neoplasm

When an episode of care involves the surgical removal of a neoplasm, primary or secondary site, followed by adjunct chemotherapy or radiation treatment during the same episode of care, the neoplasm code should be assigned as principal or first-listed diagnosis, using codes in the 140-198 series or where appropriate in the 200-203 series.

B. Patient admission or encounter solely for administration of chemotherapy, immunotherapy and radiation therapy

If a patient admission or encounter is solely for the administration of chemotherapy, immunotherapy or radiation therapy assign code V58.0, Encounter for radiation therapy, or V58.11, Encounter for antineoplastic chemotherapy, or V58.12, Encounter for antineoplastic immunotherapy as the first-listed or principal diagnosis. If a patient receives more than one of these therapies during the same admission more than one of these codes may be assigned, in any sequence.

The malignancy for which the therapy is being administered should be assigned as a secondary diagnosis.

C. Patient admitted for radiotherapy or chemotherapy and immunotherapy and develops complications

When a patient is admitted for the purpose of radiotherapy, immunotherapy or chemotherapy and develops complications such as uncontrolled nausea and vomiting or dehydration, the principal or first-listed diagnosis is V58.0, Encounter for radiotherapy, or V58.11, Encounter for antineoplastic chemotherapy, or V58.12, Encounter for antineoplastic immunotherapy followed by any codes for the complications.

ADMISSION OR ENCOUNTER TO DETERMINE EXTENT OF MALIGNANCY

When the reason for admission or encounter is to determine the extent of the malignancy, or for a procedure such as paracentesis or thoracentesis, the primary malignancy or appropriate metastatic site is designated as the principal or first-listed diagnosis, even though chemotherapy or radiotherapy is administered.

SYMPTOMS, SIGNS, AND ILL-DEFINED CONDITIONS LISTED IN CHAPTER 16 ASSOCIATED WITH NEOPLASMS

Symptoms, signs, and ill-defined conditions listed in Chapter 16 characteristic of, or associated with, an existing primary or secondary site malignancy cannot be used to replace the malignancy as principal or first-listed diagnosis, regardless of the number of admissions or encounters for treatment and care of the neoplasm.

See Chapter 18, "Prophylactic organ removal" for information regarding prophylactic organ removal..

ADMISSION OR ENCOUNTER FOR PAIN CONTROL OR MANAGEMENT

A malignant neoplasm of a transplanted organ should be coded as a transplant complication. Assign first the appropriate code from subcategory 996.8, Complications of transplanted organ, followed by code 199.2, Malignant neoplasm associated with transplanted organ. Use an additional code for the specific malignancy.

| | Add 4th or 5th digit | | Nonspecific code | | Unspecified code | | Manifestation code |

This page intentionally left blank.

● Code new
to this edition

▲ Revision of
existing code

④ ⑤ Fourth or fifth
digit required

2. NEOPLASMS (140-239)

Notes:

1. Content
This chapter contains the following broad groups:

140-195	**Malignant neoplasms, stated or presumed to be primary, of specified sites, except of lymphatic and hematopoietic tissue**
196-198	**Malignant neoplasms, stated or presumed to be secondary, of specified sites**
199	**Malignant neoplasms, without specification of site**
200-208	**Malignant neoplasms, stated or presumed to be primary, of lymphatic and hematopoietic tissue**
209	**Neuroendocrine tumors**
210-229	**Benign neoplasms**
230-234	**Carcinoma in situ**
235-238	**Neoplasms of uncertain behavior**
239	**Neoplasms of unspecified nature**

2. Functional activity
All neoplasms are classified in this chapter, whether or not functionally active. An additional code from Chapter 3 may be used, if desired, to identify such functional activity associated with any neoplasm, e.g.:
   catecholamine-producing malignant pheochromocytoma of adrenal:
      code 194.0, additional code 255.6
   basophil adenoma of pituitary with Cushing's syndrome:
      code 227.3, additional code 255.0

3. Morphology [Histology]
For those wishing to identify the histological type of neoplasms, a comprehensive coded nomenclature, which comprises the morphology rubrics of the ICD-Oncology, is given in Appendix A.

4. Malignant neoplasms overlapping site boundaries
Categories 140-195 are for the classification of primary malignant neoplasms according to their point of origin. A malignant neoplasm that overlaps two or more subcategories within a three-digit rubric and whose point of origin cannot be determined should be classified to the subcategory .8 "Other." For example, "carcinoma involving tip and ventral surface of tongue" should be assigned to 141.8. On the other hand, "carcinoma of tip of tongue, extending to involve the ventral surface" should be coded to 141.2, as the point of origin, the tip, is known. Three subcategories (149.8, 159.8, 165.8) have been provided for malignant neoplasms that overlap the boundaries of three-digit rubrics within certain systems. Overlapping malignant neoplasms that cannot be classified as indicated above should be assigned to the appropriate subdivision of category 195 (Malignant neoplasm of other and ill-defined sites).

MALIGNANT NEOPLASM OF LIP, ORAL CAVITY, AND PHARYNX (140-149)

   Excludes: *carcinoma in situ (230.0)*

140 Malignant neoplasm of lip

   Excludes: *malignant melanoma of skin of lip (172.0)*
   malignant neoplasm of skin of lip (173.00-173.09)

   DEFINITION Malignant neoplasm refers to a tumor that tends to grow, invade, and metastasize. The tumor usually has an irregular shape and is composed of poorly differentiated cells. If untreated, it may result in death.

   ALERT! For personal history of malignant neoplasm see V10

   140.0 Upper lip, vermilion border
      Upper lip:
         NOS
         external
         lipstick area

   140.1 Lower lip, vermilion border
      Lower lip:
         NOS
         external
         lipstick area

   140.3 Upper lip, inner aspect
      Upper lip   Upper lip:
         buccal aspect   mucosa
         frenulum   oral aspect

   140.4 Lower lip, inner aspect
      Lower lip: Lower lip:
         buccal aspect   mucosa
         frenulum   oral aspect

▬ Add 4th or 5th digit	▬ Nonspecific code	▬ Unspecified code	▬ Manifestation code

140.5 Lip, unspecified, inner aspect
Lip, not specified whether upper or lower:
buccal aspect	frenulum
mucosa	oral aspect

140.6 Commissure of lip
Labial commissure

140.8 Other sites of lip
Malignant neoplasm of contiguous or overlapping sites of lip whose point of origin cannot be determined

140.9 Lip, unspecified, vermilion border
Lip, not specified as upper or lower:
NOS
external
lipstick area

141 Malignant neoplasm of tongue
ALERT! For personal history of malignant neoplasm of tongue see V10.01

141.0 Base of tongue
Dorsal surface of base of tongue
Fixed part of tongue NOS

141.1 Dorsal surface of tongue
Anterior two-thirds of tongue, dorsal surface
Dorsal tongue NOS
Midline of tongue
Excludes: dorsal surface of base of tongue (141.0)

141.2 Tip and lateral border of tongue

141.3 Ventral surface of tongue
Anterior two-thirds of tongue, ventral surface
Frenulum linguae

141.4 Anterior two-thirds of tongue, part unspecified
Mobile part of tongue NOS

141.5 Junctional zone
Border of tongue at junction of fixed and mobile parts at insertion of anterior tonsillar pillar

141.6 Lingual tonsil

141.8 Other sites of tongue
Malignant neoplasm of contiguous or overlapping sites of tongue whose point of origin cannot be determined

141.9 Tongue, unspecified
Tongue NOS

142 Malignant neoplasm of major salivary glands
Includes: salivary ducts
Excludes: malignant neoplasm of minor salivary glands:
NOS (145.9)
buccal mucosa (145.0)
soft palate (145.3)
tongue (141.0-141.9)
tonsil, palatine (146.0)

142.0 Parotid gland

142.1 Submandibular gland
Submaxillary gland

142.2 Sublingual gland

142.8 Other major salivary glands
Malignant neoplasm of contiguous or overlapping sites of salivary glands and ducts whose point of origin cannot be determined

142.9 Salivary gland, unspecified
Salivary gland (major) NOS

143 Malignant neoplasm of gum
Includes: alveolar (ridge) mucosa
gingiva (alveolar) (marginal)
interdental papillae
Excludes: malignant odontogenic neoplasms (170.0-170.1)

● Code new
   to this edition
▲ Revision of
   existing code
④ ⑤ Fourth or fifth
   digit required

143.0 Upper gum

143.1 Lower gum

143.8 Other sites of gum
Malignant neoplasm of contiguous or overlapping sites of gum whose point of origin cannot be determined

143.9 Gum, unspecified

144 Malignant neoplasm of floor of mouth

144.0 Anterior portion
Anterior to the premolar-canine junction

144.1 Lateral portion

144.8 Other sites of floor of mouth
Malignant neoplasm of contiguous or overlapping sites of floor of mouth whose point of origin cannot be determined

144.9 Floor of mouth, part unspecified

145 Malignant neoplasm of other and unspecified parts of mouth
Excludes: mucosa of lips (140.0-140.9)

145.0 Cheek mucosa
Buccal mucosa   Cheek, inner aspect

145.1 Vestibule of mouth
Buccal sulcus (upper) (lower)
Labial sulcus (upper) (lower)

145.2 Hard palate

145.3 Soft palate
Excludes: nasopharyngeal [posterior] [superior] surface of soft palate (147.3)

145.4 Uvula

145.5 Palate, unspecified
Junction of hard and soft palate
Roof of mouth

145.6 Retromolar area

145.8 Other specified parts of mouth
Malignant neoplasm of contiguous or overlapping sites of mouth whose point of origin cannot be determined

145.9 Mouth, unspecified
Buccal cavity NOS
Minor salivary gland, unspecified site
Oral cavity NOS

146 Malignant neoplasm of oropharynx

146.0 Tonsil
Tonsil:
  NOS
  faucial
  palatine
Excludes: lingual tonsil (141.6)
          pharyngeal tonsil (147.1)

146.1 Tonsillar fossa

146.2 Tonsillar pillars (anterior) (posterior)
Faucial pillar   Palatoglossal arch
Glossopalatine fold   Palatopharyngeal arch

146.3 Vallecula
Anterior and medial surface of the pharyngoepiglottic fold

146.4 Anterior aspect of epiglottis
Epiglottis, free border [margin]
Glossoepiglottic fold(s)
Excludes: epiglottis:
            NOS (161.1)
            suprahyoid portion (161.1)

146.5 Junctional region
Junction of the free margin of the epiglottis, the aryepiglottic fold, and the pharyngoepiglottic fold

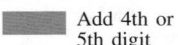
Add 4th or   Nonspecific   Unspecified   Manifestation
5th digit   code   code   code

146.6 Lateral wall of oropharynx

146.7 Posterior wall of oropharynx

146.8 Other specified sites of oropharynx
Branchial cleft
Malignant neoplasm of contiguous or overlapping sites of oropharynx whose point of origin cannot be determined

146.9 Oropharynx, unspecified

147 Malignant neoplasm of nasopharynx

147.0 Superior wall
Roof of nasopharynx

147.1 Posterior wall
Adenoid   Pharyngeal tonsil

147.2 Lateral wall
Fossa of Rosenmüller   Pharyngeal recess
Opening of auditory tube

147.3 Anterior wall
Floor of nasopharynx
Nasopharyngeal [posterior] [superior] surface of soft palate
Posterior margin of nasal septum and choanae

147.8 Other specified sites of nasopharynx
Malignant neoplasm of contiguous or overlapping sites of nasopharynx whose point of origin cannot be determined

147.9 Nasopharynx, unspecified
Nasopharyngeal wall NOS

148 Malignant neoplasm of hypopharynx

148.0 Postcricoid region

148.1 Pyriform sinus
Pyriform fossa

148.2 Aryepiglottic fold, hypopharyngeal aspect
Aryepiglottic fold or interarytenoid fold:
NOS
marginal zone

Excludes: *aryepiglottic fold or interarytenoid fold, laryngeal aspect (161.1)*

148.3 Posterior hypopharyngeal wall

148.8 Other specified sites of hypopharynx
Malignant neoplasm of contiguous or overlapping sites of hypopharynx whose point of origin cannot be determined

148.9 Hypopharynx, unspecified
Hypopharyngeal wall NOS   Hypopharynx NOS

149 Malignant neoplasm of other and ill-defined sites within the lip, oral cavity, and pharynx
ALERT! For personal history of malignant neoplasm of other sites see V10.8

149.0 Pharynx, unspecified

149.1 Waldeyer's ring

149.8 Other
Malignant neoplasms of lip, oral cavity, and pharynx whose point of origin cannot be assigned to any one of the categories 140-148

Excludes: *"book leaf" neoplasm [ventral surface of tongue and floor of mouth] (145.8)*

149.9 Ill-defined

MALIGNANT NEOPLASM OF DIGESTIVE ORGANS AND PERITONEUM (150-159)

Excludes: *carcinoma in situ (230.1-230.9)*

ALERT! For personal history of malignant neoplasm of gastrointestinal tract see V10.0

150 Malignant neoplasm of esophagus
ALERT! For personal history of malignant neoplasm of esophagus see V10.03

150.0 Cervical esophagus

150.1 Thoracic esophagus

150.2 Abdominal esophagus

Excludes: *adenocarcinoma (151.0)*
cardio-esophageal junction (151.0)

● Code new
to this edition

▲ Revision of
existing code

④ ⑤ Fourth or fifth
digit required

150.3 Upper third of esophagus
Proximal third of esophagus

150.4 Middle third of esophagus

150.5 Lower third of esophagus
Distal third of esophagus

Excludes: *adenocarcinoma (151.0)*
cardio-esophageal junction (151.0)

150.8 Other specified part
Malignant neoplasm of contiguous or overlapping sites of esophagus whose point of origin cannot be determined

150.9 Esophagus, unspecified

151 Malignant neoplasm of stomach

Excludes: *benign carcinoid tumor of stomach (209.63)*
malignant carcinoid tumor of stomach (209.23)

ALERT! For personal history of malignant neoplasm of stomach see V10.04

151.0 Cardia
Cardiac orifice   Cardio-esophageal junction

Excludes: *squamous cell carcinoma (150.2, 150.5)*

151.1 Pylorus
Prepylorus   Pyloric canal

151.2 Pyloric antrum
Antrum of stomach NOS

151.3 Fundus of stomach

151.4 Body of stomach

151.5 Lesser curvature, unspecified
Lesser curvature, not classifiable to 151.1-151.4

151.6 Greater curvature, unspecified
Greater curvature, not classifiable to 151.0-151.4

151.8 Other specified sites of stomach
Anterior wall, not classifiable to 151.0-151.4
Posterior wall, not classifiable to 151.0-151.4
Malignant neoplasm of contiguous or overlapping sites of stomach whose point of origin cannot be determined

151.9 Stomach, unspecified
Carcinoma ventriculi   Gastric cancer

152 Malignant neoplasm of small intestine, including duodenum

Excludes: *benign carcinoid tumor of small intestine and duodenum (209.40-209.43)*
malignant carcinoid tumor of small intestine and duodenum (209.00-209.03)

152.0 Duodenum

152.1 Jejunum

152.2 Ileum

Excludes: *ileocecal valve (153.4)*

152.3 Meckel's diverticulum

152.8 Other specified sites of small intestine
Duodenojejunal junction
Malignant neoplasm of contiguous or overlapping sites of small intestine whose point of origin cannot be determined

152.9 Small intestine, unspecified

153 Malignant neoplasm of colon

Excludes: *benign carcinoid tumor of colon (209.50-209.56)*
malignant carcinoid tumor of colon (209.10-209.16)

ALERT! For personal history of colonic polyps see V12.72

153.0 Hepatic flexure

153.1 Transverse colon

153.2 Descending colon
Left colon

	Add 4th or 5th digit		Nonspecific code		Unspecified code		Manifestation code

153.3 Sigmoid colon
Sigmoid (flexure)

Excludes: rectosigmoid junction (154.0)

153.4 Cecum
Ileocecal valve

153.5 Appendix

153.6 Ascending colon
Right colon

153.7 Splenic flexure

153.8 Other specified sites of large intestine
Malignant neoplasm of contiguous or overlapping sites of colon whose point of origin cannot be determined

Excludes: ileocecal valve (153.4)
rectosigmoid junction (154.0)

153.9 Colon, unspecified
Large intestine NOS

154 Malignant neoplasm of rectum, rectosigmoid junction, and anus

Excludes: benign carcinoid tumor of rectum (209.57)
malignant carcinoid tumor of rectum (209.17)

ALERT! For personal history of malignant neoplasm of rectum rectosigmoid junction and anus see V10.06

154.0 Rectosigmoid junction
Colon with rectum   Rectosigmoid (colon)

154.1 Rectum
Rectal ampulla

154.2 Anal canal
Anal sphincter

Excludes: malignant melanoma of skin of anus (172.5)
malignant neoplasm of skin of anus (173.50-173.59)

154.3 Anus, unspecified

Excludes: malignant melanoma of
anus:
margin (172.5)
skin (172.5)
perianal skin (172.5)
malignant neoplasm of
anus:
margin (173.50-173.59)
skin (173.50-173.59)
perianal skin (173.50-173.59)

154.8 Other
Anorectum
Cloacogenic zone
Malignant neoplasm of contiguous or overlapping sites of rectum, rectosigmoid junction, and anus whose point of origin cannot be determined

155 Malignant neoplasm of liver and intrahepatic bile ducts
ALERT! For personal history of malignant neoplasm of liver see V10.07

155.0 Liver, primary
Carcinoma:
liver, specified as primary
hepatocellular
liver cell
Hepatoblastoma

155.1 Intrahepatic bile ducts
Canaliculi biliferi   Intrahepatic:
Interlobular: biliary passages
bile ducts   canaliculi
biliary canals   gall duct

Excludes: hepatic duct (156.1)

155.2 Liver, not specified as primary or secondary

● Code new to this edition   ▲ Revision of existing code   ④ ⑤ Fourth or fifth digit required

156 **Malignant neoplasm of gallbladder and extrahepatic bile ducts**

156.0 **Gallbladder**

156.1 **Extrahepatic bile ducts**
Biliary duct or passage NOS   Cystic duct
Common bile duct   Hepatic duct
          Sphincter of Oddi

156.2 **Ampulla of Vater**

156.8 **Other specified sites of gallbladder and extrahepatic bile ducts**
Malignant neoplasm of contiguous or overlapping sites of gallbladder and extrahepatic bile ducts whose point of origin cannot be determined

156.9 **Biliary tract, part unspecified**
Malignant neoplasm involving both intrahepatic and extrahepatic bile ducts

157 **Malignant neoplasm of pancreas**

157.0 **Head of pancreas**

157.1 **Body of pancreas**

157.2 **Tail of pancreas**

157.3 **Pancreatic duct**
Duct of:
    Santorini
    Wirsung

157.4 **Islets of Langerhans**
Islets of Langerhans, any part of pancreas
Use additional code, if desired, to identify any functional activity

157.8 **Other specified sites of pancreas**
Ectopic pancreatic tissue
Malignant neoplasm of contiguous or overlapping sites of pancreas whose point of origin cannot be determined

157.9 **Pancreas, part unspecified**

158 **Malignant neoplasm of retroperitoneum and peritoneum**

158.0 **Retroperitoneum**
Periadrenal tissue   Perirenal tissue
Perinephric tissue   Retrocecal tissue

158.8 **Specified parts of peritoneum**
Cul-de-sac (of Douglas)
Mesentery
Mesocolon
Omentum
Peritoneum:
    parietal
    pelvic
Rectouterine pouch
Malignant neoplasm of contiguous or overlapping sites of retroperitoneum and peritoneum whose point of origin cannot be determined

158.9 **Peritoneum, unspecified**

159 **Malignant neoplasm of other and ill-defined sites within the digestive organs and peritoneum**

ALERT! For personal history of malignant neoplasm of other sites in gastrointestinal tract see V10.09

ALERT! For personal history of malignant neoplasm of other sites see V10.8

ALERT! For personal history of malignant neoplasm of unspecified site in gastrointestinal tract see V10.00

159.0 **Intestinal tract, part unspecified**
Intestine NOS

159.1 **Spleen, not elsewhere classified**
Angiosarcoma of spleen
Fibrosarcoma of spleen

Excludes: Hodgkin's disease (201.0-201.9)
          lymphosarcoma (200.1)
          reticulosarcoma (200.0)

Add 4th or 5th digit   Nonspecific code   Unspecified code   Manifestation code

159.8 **Other sites of digestive system and intra-abdominal organs**
Malignant neoplasm of digestive organs and peritoneum whose point of origin cannot be assigned to any one of the categories 150-158

Excludes: *anus and rectum (154.8)*
cardio-esophageal junction (151.0)
colon and rectum ORANGE (154.0)

159.9 **Ill-defined**
Alimentary canal or tract NOS
Gastrointestinal tract NOS

Excludes: *abdominal NOS (195.2)*
intra-abdominal NOS (195.2)

MALIGNANT NEOPLASM OF RESPIRATORY AND INTRATHORACIC ORGANS (160-165)

Excludes: *carcinoma in situ (231.0-231.9)*

160 **Malignant neoplasm of nasal cavities, middle ear, and accessory sinuses**
ALERT! For personal history of malignant neoplasm of nasal cavities middle ear and accessory sinuses see V10.22

160.0 **Nasal cavities**
Cartilage of nose   Septum of nose
Conchae, nasal   Vestibule of nose
Internal nose

Excludes: *nasal bone (170.0)*
nose NOS (195.0)
olfactory bulb (192.0)
posterior margin of septum and choanae (147.3)
malignant melanoma of skin of nose (172.3)
malignant neoplasm of skin of nose (173.30-173.39)
turbinates (170.0)

160.1 **Auditory tube, middle ear, and mastoid air cells**
Antrum tympanicum   Tympanic cavity
Eustachian tube

Excludes: *bone of ear (meatus) (170.0)*
cartilage of ear (171.0)
malignant melanoma of:
auditory canal (external) (172.2)
ear (external) (skin) (172.2)
malignant neoplasm of:
auditory canal (external) (173.20-173.29)
ear (external) (skin) (173.20-173.29)

160.2 **Maxillary sinus**
Antrum (Highmore) (maxillary)

160.3 **Ethmoidal sinus**

160.4 **Frontal sinus**

160.5 **Sphenoidal sinus**

160.8 **Other**
Malignant neoplasm of contiguous or overlapping sites of nasal cavities, middle ear, and accessory sinuses whose point of origin cannot be determined

160.9 **Accessory sinus, unspecified**

161 **Malignant neoplasm of larynx**
ALERT! For personal history of malignant neoplasm of larynx see V10.21

161.0 **Glottis**
Intrinsic larynx   True vocal cord
Laryngeal commissure   Vocal cord NOS
(anterior) (posterior)

● Code new   ▲ Revision of   ④ ⑤ Fourth or fifth
to this edition   existing code   digit required

161.1 Supraglottis
Aryepiglottic fold or interarytenoid fold, laryngeal aspect
Epiglottis (suprahyoid portion) NOS
Extrinsic larynx
False vocal cords
Posterior (laryngeal) surface of epiglottis
Ventricular bands

Excludes: anterior aspect of epiglottis (146.4)
aryepiglottic fold or interarytenoid fold:
NOS (148.2)
hypopharyngeal aspect (148.2)
marginal zone (148.2)

161.2 Subglottis

161.3 Laryngeal cartilages
Cartilage: Cartilage:
arytenoid   cuneiform
cricoid   thyroid

161.8 Other specified sites of larynx
Malignant neoplasm of contiguous or overlapping sites of larynx whose point of origin cannot be determined

161.9 Larynx, unspecified

162 Malignant neoplasm of trachea, bronchus, and lung

Excludes: benign carcinoid tumor of bronchus (209.61)
malignant carcinoid tumor of bronchus (209.21)

ALERT! For personal history of malignant neoplasm of bronchus and lung see V10.11
ALERT! For personal history of malignant neoplasm of trachea see V10.12

162.0 Trachea
Cartilage of trachea
Mucosa of trachea

162.2 Main bronchus
Carina   Hilus of lung

162.3 Upper lobe, bronchus or lung

162.4 Middle lobe, bronchus or lung

162.5 Lower lobe, bronchus or lung

162.8 Other parts of bronchus or lung
Malignant neoplasm of contiguous or overlapping sites of bronchus or lung whose point of origin cannot be determined

162.9 Bronchus and lung, unspecified

163 Malignant neoplasm of pleura

163.0 Parietal pleura

163.1 Visceral pleura

163.8 Other specified sites of pleura
Malignant neoplasm of contiguous or overlapping sites of pleura whose point of origin cannot be determined

163.9 Pleura, unspecified

164 Malignant neoplasm of thymus, heart, and mediastinum

164.0 Thymus

Excludes: benign carcinoid tumor of thymus (209.62)
malignant carcinoid tumor of thymus (209.22)

164.1 Heart
Endocardium   Myocardium
Epicardium   Pericardium

Excludes: great vessels (171.4)

164.2 Anterior mediastinum

164.3 Posterior mediastinum

164.8 Other
Malignant neoplasm of contiguous or overlapping sites of thymus, heart, and mediastinum whose point of origin cannot be determined

164.9 Mediastinum, part unspecified

Add 4th or 5th digit | Nonspecific code | Unspecified code | Manifestation code

165 **Malignant neoplasm of other and ill-defined sites within the respiratory system and intrathoracic organs**

> ALERT! For personal history of malignant neoplasm of other respiratory and intrathoracic organs see V10.29
>
> ALERT! For personal history of malignant neoplasm of other sites see V10.8
>
> ALERT! For personal history of malignant neoplasm of unspecified respiratory organ see V10.20

165.0 **Upper respiratory trace, part unspecified**

165.8 **Other**

> Malignant neoplasm of respiratory and intrathoracic organs whose point of origin cannot be assigned to any one of the categories 160-164
>
> ALERT! For personal history of malignant neoplasm of other respiratory and intrathoracic organs see V10.2

165.9 **Ill-defined sites within the respiratory system**

> Respiratory tract NOS

> Excludes: *intrathoracic NOS (195.1)*
> *thoracic NOS (195.1)*

MALIGNANT NEOPLASM OF BONE, CONNECTIVE TISSUE, SKIN, AND BREAST (170-176)

> Excludes: *carcinoma in situ:*
> *breast (233.0)*
> *skin (232.0-232.9)*

170 **Malignant neoplasm of bone and articular cartilage**

> Includes: cartilage (articular) (joint)
> periosteum

> Excludes: *bone marrow NOS (202.9)*
> *cartilage:*
> *ear (171.0)*
> *eyelid (171.0)*
> *larynx (161.3)*
> *nose (160.0)*
> *synovia (171.0-171.9)*

> ALERT! For personal history of malignant neoplasm of bone see V10.81

170.0 **Bones of skull and face, except mandible**

Bone:	Bone:
ethmoid	sphenoid
frontal	temporal
malar	zygomatic
nasal	Maxilla (superior)
occipital	Turbinate
orbital	Upper jaw bone
parietal	Vomer

> Excludes: *carcinoma, any type except intraosseous or odontogenic:*
> *maxilla, maxillary (sinus) (160.2)*
> *upper jaw bone (143.0)*
> *jaw bone (lower) (170.1)*

170.1 **Mandible**

> Inferior maxilla   Lower jaw bone
> Jaw bone NOS

> Excludes: *carcinoma, any type except intraosseous or odontogenic:*
> *jaw bone NOS (143.9)*
> *lower (143.1)*
> *upper jaw bone (170.0)*

170.2 **Vertebral column, excluding sacrum and coccyx**

> Spinal column   Vertebra
> Spine

> Excludes: *sacrum and coccyx (170.6)*

170.3 **Ribs, sternum, and clavicle**

> Costal cartilage   Xiphoid process
> Costovertebral joint

● Code new to this edition   ▲ Revision of existing code   ④ ⑤ Fourth or fifth digit required

170.4 Scapula and long bones of upper limb

Acromion	Radius
Bones NOS of upper limb	Ulna
Humerus	

170.5 Short bones of upper limb

Carpal	Scaphoid (of hand)
Cuneiform, wrist	Semilunar or lunate
Metacarpal	Trapezium
Navicular, of hand	Trapezoid
Phalanges of hand	Unciform
Pisiform	

170.6 Pelvic bones, sacrum, and coccyx

Coccygeal vertebra	Pubic bone
Ilium	Sacral vertebra
Ischium	

170.7 Long bones of lower limb

Bones NOS of lower limb	Fibula
Femur	Tibia

170.8 Short bones of lower limb

Astragalus [talus]	Navicular (of ankle)
Calcaneus	Patella
Cuboid	Phalanges of foot
Cuneiform, ankle	Tarsal
Metatarsal	

170.9 Bone and articular cartilage, site unspecified

171 Malignant neoplasm of connective and other soft tissue

Includes: blood vessel
bursa
fascia
fat
ligament, except uterine
muscle
peripheral, sympathetic, and parasympathetic nerves and ganglia
synovia
tendon (sheath)

Excludes: *cartilage (of):*
articular (170.0-170.9)
larynx (161.3)
nose (160.0)
connective tissue:
breast (174.0-175.9)
internal organs—code to malignant neoplasm of the site [e.g., leiomyosarcoma of stomach, 151.9]
heart (164.1)
uterine ligament (183.4)

171.0 Head, face, and neck

Cartilage of:
ear
eyelid

171.2 Upper limb, including shoulder

Arm	Forearm
Finger	Hand

171.3 Lower limb, including hip

Foot	Thigh
Leg	Toe
Popliteal space	

171.4 Thorax

Axilla	Great vessels
Diaphragm	

Excludes: *heart (164.1)*
mediastinum (164.2-164.9)
thymus (164.0)

Add 4th or 5th digit	Nonspecific code	Unspecified code	Manifestation code

171.5 Abdomen
    Abdominal wall
    Hypochondrium

Excludes: *peritoneum (158.8)*
      retroperitoneum (158.0)

171.6 Pelvis
    Buttock   Inguinal region
    Groin   Perineum

Excludes: *pelvic peritoneum (158.8)*
      retroperitoneum (158.0)
      uterine ligament, any (183.3-183.5)

171.7 Trunk, unspecified
    Back NOS
    Flank NOS

171.8 Other specified sites of connective and other soft tissue
    Malignant neoplasm of contiguous or overlapping sites of connective tissue whose point
      of origin cannot be determined

171.9 Connective and other soft tissue, site unspecified

172 Malignant melanoma of skin
    Includes: melanocarcinoma
          melanoma in situ of skin
          melanoma (skin) NOS

Excludes: *skin of genital organs (184.0-184.9, 187.1-187.9)*
      sites other than skin—code to malignant neoplasm of the site

ALERT! For personal history of malignant melanoma of skin see V10.82

172.0 Lip

Excludes: *vermilion border of lip (140.0-140.1, 140.9)*

172.1 Eyelid, including canthus

172.2 Ear and external auditory canal
    Auricle (ear)
    Auricular canal, external
    External [acoustic] meatus
    Pinna

172.3 Other and unspecified parts of face
    Cheek (external)   Forehead
    Chin   Nose, external
    Eyebrow   Temple

172.4 Scalp and neck

172.5 Trunk, except scrotum
    Axilla   Perianal skin
    Breast   Perineum
    Buttock   Umbilicus
    Groin

Excludes: *anal canal (154.2)*
      anus NOS (154.3)
      scrotum (187.7)

172.6 Upper limb, including shoulder
    Arm   Forearm
    Finger   Hand

172.7 Lower limb, including hip
    Ankle   Leg
    Foot   Popliteal area
    Heel   Thigh
    Knee   Toe

172.8 Other specified sites of skin
    Malignant melanoma of contiguous or overlapping sites of skin whose point of origin
      cannot be determined

172.9 Melanoma of skin, site unspecified

● Code new
   to this edition
▲ Revision of
   existing code
④ ⑤ Fourth or fifth
     digit required

▲ **173** **Other and unspecified malignant neoplasm of skin**
Includes: malignant neoplasm of:
sebaceous glands
sudoriferous, sudoriparous glands
sweat glands

Excludes: *Kaposi's sarcoma (176.0-176.9)*
malignant melanoma of skin (172.0-172.9)
Merkel cell carcinoma of skin (209.31-209.36)
skin of genital organs (184.0-184.9, 187.1-187.9)

ALERT! For personal history of other malignant neoplasm of skin see V10.83

▲ **173.0** **Other and unspecified malignant neoplasm of skin of lip**
Excludes: *vermilion border of lip (140.0-140.1, 140.9)*

● **173.00** Unspecified malignant neoplasm of skin of lip

● **173.01** Basal cell carcinoma of skin of lip

● **173.02** Squamous cell carcinoma of skin of lip

● **173.09** Other specified malignant neoplasm of skin of lip

▲ **173.1** **Other and unspecified malignant neoplasm of eyelid, including canthus**
Excludes: *cartilage of eyelid (171.0)*

● **173.10** Unspecified malignant neoplasm of eyelid, including canthus

● **173.11** Basal cell carcinoma of eyelid, including canthus

● **173.12** Squamous cell carcinoma of eyelid, including canthus

● **173.19** Other specified malignant neoplasm of eyelid, including canthus

▲ **173.2** **Other and unspecified malignant neoplasm of skin of ear and external auditory canal**
Auricle (ear)   External meatus
Auricular canal, external   Pinna
Excludes: *cartilage of ear (171.0)*

● **173.20** Unspecified malignant neoplasm of skin of ear and external auditory canal

● **173.21** Basal cell carcinoma of skin of ear and external auditory canal

● **173.22** Squamous cell carcinoma of skin of ear and external auditory canal

● **173.29** Other specified malignant neoplasm of skin of ear and external auditory canal

▲ **173.3** **Other and unspecified malignant neoplasm of skin of other and unspecified parts of face**
Cheek, external   Forehead
Chin   Nose, external
Eyebrow   Temple

● **173.30** Unspecified malignant neoplasm of skin of other and unspecified parts of face

● **173.31** Basal cell carcinoma of skin of other and unspecified parts of face

● **173.32** Squamous cell carcinoma of skin of other and unspecified parts of face

● **173.39** Other specified malignant neoplasm of skin of other and unspecified parts of face

▲ **173.4** **Other and unspecified malignant neoplasm of scalp and skin of neck**

● **173.40** Unspecified malignant neoplasm of scalp and skin of neck

● **173.41** Basal cell carcinoma of scalp and skin of neck

● **173.42** Squamous cell carcinoma of scalp and skin of neck

● **173.49** Other specified malignant neoplasm of scalp and skin of neck

Add 4th or   Nonspecific   Unspecified   Manifestation
5th digit   code   code   code

▲ **173.5** **Other and unspecified malignant neoplasm of skin of trunk, except scrotum**
Axillary fold
Perianal skin
Skin of:
abdominal wall
anus
back
breast

Skin of:
buttock
chest wall
groin
perineum
Umbilicus

Excludes: anal canal (154.2)
anus NOS (154.3)
skin of scrotum (187.7)

● **173.50** Unspecified malignant neoplasm of skin of trunk, except scrotum
● **173.51** Basal cell carcinoma of skin of trunk, except scrotum
● **173.52** Squamous cell carcinoma of skin of trunk, except scrotum
● **173.59** Other specified malignant neoplasm of skin of trunk, except scrotum

▲ **173.6** **Other and unspecified malignant neoplasm of skin of upper limb, including shoulder**
Arm
Finger
Forearm
Hand

● **173.60** Unspecified malignant neoplasm of skin of upper limb, including shoulder
● **173.61** Basal cell carcinoma of skin of upper limb, including shoulder
● **173.62** Squamous cell carcinoma of skin of upper limb, including shoulder
● **173.69** Other specified malignant neoplasm of skin of upper limb, including shoulder

▲ **173.7** **Other and unspecified malignant neoplasm of skin of lower limb, including hip**
Ankle
Foot
Heel
Knee

Leg
Popliteal area
Thigh
Toe

● **173.70** Unspecified malignant neoplasm of skin of lower limb, including hip
● **173.71** Basal cell carcinoma of skin of lower limb, including hip
● **173.72** Squamous cell carcinoma of skin of lower limb, including hip
● **173.79** Other specified malignant neoplasm of skin of lower limb, including hip

▲ **173.8** **Other and unspecified malignant neoplasm of other specified sites of skin**
Malignant neoplasm of contiguous or overlapping sites of skin whose point of origin cannot be determined

● **173.80** Unspecified malignant neoplasm of other specified sites of skin
● **173.81** Basal cell carcinoma of other specified sites of skin
● **173.82** Squamous cell carcinoma of other specified sites of skin
● **173.89** Other specified malignant neoplasm of other specified sites of skin

▲ **173.9** **Other and unspecified malignant neoplasm of skin, site unspecified**
● **173.90** Unspecified malignant neoplasm of skin, site unspecified
Malignant neoplasm of skin, NOS
● **173.91** Basal cell carcinoma of skin, site unspecified
● **173.92** Squamous cell carcinoma of skin, site unspecified
● **173.99** Other specified malignant neoplasm of skin, site unspecified

174 **Malignant neoplasm of female breast**
Use additional code to identify estrogen receptor status (V86.0,V86.1)
Includes: breast (female)
connective tissue
soft parts
Paget's disease of:
breast
nipple

Excludes: malignant melanoma of skin of breast (172.5)
malignant neoplasm of skin of breast (173.50-173.59)

ALERT! For personal history of malignant neoplasm of breast see V10.3

174.0 **Nipple and areola**
174.1 **Central portion**
174.2 **Upper-inner quadrant**

● Code new to this edition　　▲ Revision of existing code　　④ ⑤ Fourth or fifth digit required

174.3 **Lower-inner quadrant**

174.4 **Upper-outer quadrant**

174.5 **Lower-outer quadrant**

174.6 **Axillary tail**

174.8 **Other specified sites of female breast**
    Ectopic sites
    Inner breast
    Lower breast
    Midline of breast
    Outer breast
    Upper breast
    Malignant neoplasm of contiguous or overlapping sites of breast whose point of origin
      cannot be determined

174.9 **Breast (female), unspecified**

175 **Malignant neoplasm of male breast**
Use additional code to identify estrogen receptor status (V86.0,V86.1)

    Excludes: *malignant melanoma of skin of breast (172.5)*
                malignant neoplasm of skin of breast (173.50-173.59)

175.0 **Nipple and areola**

175.9 **Other and unspecified sites of male breast**
    Ectopic breast tissue, male

176 **Kaposi's sarcoma**
    DEFINITION Kaposi's sarcoma is a form of skin cancer that can involve internal organs. It is most often found in patients with acquired immunodeficiency syndrome (AIDS), and can be fatal.

176.0 **Skin**

176.1 **Soft tissue**
    Includes: Blood vessel
               Connective tissue
               Fascia
               Ligament
               Lymphatic(s) NEC
               Muscle

    Excludes: *lymph glands and nodes (176.5)*

176.2 **Palate**

176.3 **Gastrointestinal sites**

176.4 **Lung**

176.5 **Lymph nodes**

176.8 **Other specified sites**
    Includes: Oral cavity NEC

176.9 **Unspecified**
    Viscera NOS

MALIGNANT NEOPLASM OF GENITOURINARY ORGANS (179-189)

    Excludes: *carcinoma in situ (233.1-233.9)*

    ALERT! For personal history of malignant neoplasm of genital organs see V10.4

179 **Malignant neoplasm of uterus, part unspecified**

180 **Malignant neoplasm of cervix uteri**
    Includes: invasive malignancy [carcinoma]

    Excludes: *carcinoma in situ (233.1)*

    ALERT! For personal history of malignant neoplasm of cervix uteri see V10.41

180.0 **Endocervix**
    Cervical canal NOS   Endocervical gland
    Endocervical canal

180.1 **Exocervix**

180.8 **Other specified sites of cervix**
    Cervical stump
    Squamocolumnar junction of cervix
    Malignant neoplasm of contiguous or overlapping sites of cervix uteri whose point of
      origin cannot be determined

225

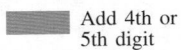 Add 4th or 5th digit   Nonspecific code   Unspecified code   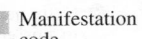 Manifestation code

180.9 Cervix uteri, unspecified

181 Malignant neoplasm of placenta
Choriocarcinoma NOS
Chorioepithelioma NOS

> *Excludes:* *chorioadenoma (destruens) (236.1)*
> *hydatidiform mole (630)*
> *malignant (236.1)*
> *invasive mole (236.1)*
> *male choriocarcinoma NOS (186.0-186.9)*

182 Malignant neoplasm of body of uterus

> *Excludes:* *carcinoma in situ (233.2)*

182.0 Corpus uteri, except isthmus
Cornu   Fundus
Endometrium   Myometrium

182.1 Isthmus
Lower uterine segment

182.8 Other specified sites of body of uterus
Malignant neoplasm of contiguous or overlapping sites of body of uterus whose point
of origin cannot be determined

> *Excludes:* *uterus NOS (179)*

ALERT! For personal history of malignant neoplasm of other parts of uterus see V10.42

183 Malignant neoplasm of ovary and other uterine adnexa

> *Excludes:* *Douglas' cul-de-sac (158.8)*

ALERT! For personal history of malignant neoplasm of ovary see V10.43

183.0 Ovary
Use additional code, if desired, to identify any functional activity

183.2 Fallopian tube
Oviduct
Uterine tube

183.3 Broad ligament
Mesovarium
Parovarian region

183.4 Parametrium
Uterine ligament NOS
Uterosacral ligament

183.5 Round ligament

183.8 Other specified sites of uterine adnexa
Tubo-ovarian
Utero-ovarian
Malignant neoplasm of contiguous or overlapping sites of ovary and other uterine
adnexa whose point of origin cannot be determined

183.9 Uterine adnexa, unspecified

184 Malignant neoplasm of other and unspecified female genital organs

> *Excludes:* *carcinoma in situ (233.30-233.39)*

ALERT! For personal history of malignant neoplasm of other female genital organs see V10.44
ALERT! For personal history of malignant neoplasm of unspecified female genital organ see
V10.40

184.0 Vagina
Gartner's duct
Vaginal vault

184.1 Labia majora
Greater vestibular [Bartholin's] gland

184.2 Labia minora

184.3 Clitoris

184.4 Vulva, unspecified
External female genitalia NOS
Pudendum

184.8 Other specified sites of female genital organs
Malignant neoplasm of contiguous or overlapping sites of female genital organs whose
point of origin cannot be determined

● Code new   ▲ Revision of   ④ ⑤ Fourth or fifth
to this edition   existing code   digit required

184.9 Female genital organ, site unspecified
Female genitourinary tract NOS

185 Malignant neoplasm of prostate
Excludes: seminal vesicles (187.8)
ALERT! For personal history of malignant neoplasm of prostate see V10.46

186 Malignant neoplasm of testis
Use additional code, if desired, to identify any functional activity
ALERT! For personal history of malignant neoplasm of testis see V10.47

186.0 Undescended testis
Ectopic testis
Retained testis

186.9 Other and unspecified testis
Testis:
NOS
descended
scrotal

187 Malignant neoplasm of penis and other male genital organs

187.1 Prepuce
Foreskin

187.2 Glans penis

187.3 Body of penis
Corpus cavernosum

187.4 Penis, part unspecified
Skin of penis NOS

187.5 Epididymis
ALERT! For personal history of malignant neoplasm of epididymis see V10.48

187.6 Spermatic cord
Vas deferens

187.7 Scrotum
Skin of scrotum

187.8 Other specified sites of male genital organs
Seminal vesicle
Tunica vaginalis
Malignant neoplasm of contiguous or overlapping sites of penis and other male genital organs whose point of origin cannot be determined
ALERT! For personal history of malignant neoplasm of other male genital organs see V10.49

187.9 Male genital organ, site unspecified
Male genital organ or tract NOS
ALERT! For personal history of malignant neoplasm of other male genital organs see V10.49
ALERT! For personal history of malignant neoplasm of unspecified male genital organ see V10.45

188 Malignant neoplasm of bladder
Excludes: carcinoma in situ (233.7)
ALERT! For personal history of malignant neoplasm of bladder see V10.51
ALERT! For personal history of malignant neoplasm of urinary organs see V10.5

188.0 Trigone of urinary bladder

188.1 Dome of urinary bladder

188.2 Lateral wall of urinary bladder

188.3 Anterior wall of urinary bladder

188.4 Posterior wall of urinary bladder

188.5 Bladder neck
Internal urethral orifice

188.6 Ureteric orifice

188.7 Urachus

188.8 Other specified sites of bladder
Malignant neoplasm of contiguous or overlapping sites of bladder whose point of origin cannot be determined

188.9 Bladder, part unspecified
Bladder wall NOS

Add 4th or 5th digit   Nonspecific code   Unspecified code   Manifestation code

189 **Malignant neoplasm of kidney and other and unspecified urinary organs**

> *Excludes:* benign carcinoid tumor of kidney (209.64)
>   malignant carcinoid tumor of kidney (209.24)

ALERT! For personal history of malignant neoplasm of kidney see V10.52

ALERT! For personal history of malignant neoplasm of unspecified urinary organ see V10.50

189.0 **Kidney, except pelvis**
Kidney NOS
Kidney parenchyma

189.1 **Renal pelvis**
Renal calyces
Ureteropelvic junction

ALERT! For personal history of malignant neoplasm of renal pelvis see V10.53

189.2 **Ureter**

> *Excludes:* ureteric orifice of bladder (188.6)

189.3 **Urethra**

> *Excludes:* urethral orifice of bladder (188.5)

189.4 **Paraurethral glands**

189.8 **Other specified sites of urinary organs**
Malignant neoplasm of contiguous or overlapping sites of kidney and other urinary organs whose point of origin cannot be determined

ALERT! For personal history of malignant neoplasm of other urinary organs see V10.59

189.9 **Urinary organ, site unspecified**
Urinary system NOS

MALIGNANT NEOPLASM OF OTHER AND UNSPECIFIED SITES (190-199)

> *Excludes:* carcinoma in situ (234.0-234.9)

190 **Malignant neoplasm of eye**

> *Excludes:* carcinoma in situ (234.0)
>   dark area on retina and choroid (239.81)
>   malignant melanoma of eyelid (skin) (172.1)
>   cartilage (171.0)
>   malignant neoplasm of eyelid (skin) (173.10-173.19)
>   optic nerve (192.0)
>   orbital bone (170.0)
>   retinal freckle (239.81)

ALERT! For personal history of malignant neoplasm of eye see V10.84

190.0 **Eyeball, except conjunctiva, cornea, retina, and choroid**
Ciliary body   Sclera
Crystalline lens   Uveal tract
Iris

190.1 **Orbit**
Connective tissue of orbit
Extraocular muscle
Retrobulbar

> *Excludes:* bone of orbit (170.0)

190.2 **Lacrimal gland**

190.3 **Conjunctiva**

190.4 **Cornea**

190.5 **Retina**

190.6 **Choroid**

190.7 **Lacrimal duct**
Lacrimal sac
Nasolacrimal duct

190.8 **Other specified sites of eye**
Malignant neoplasm of contiguous or overlapping sites of eye whose point of origin cannot be determined

190.9 **Eye, part unspecified**

● Code new to this edition ▲ Revision of existing code ④ ⑤ Fourth or fifth digit required

191 **Malignant neoplasm of brain**

> *Excludes:* cranial nerves (192.0)
> retrobulbar area (190.1)

> **ALERT!** For personal history of malignant neoplasm of brain see V10.85

191.0 **Cerebrum, except lobes and ventricles**

Basal ganglia	Globus pallidus
Cerebral cortex	Hypothalamus
Corpus striatum	Thalamus

191.1 **Frontal lobe**

191.2 **Temporal lobe**
Hippocampus
Uncus

191.3 **Parietal lobe**

191.4 **Occipital lobe**

191.5 **Ventricles**
Choroid plexus
Floor of ventricle

191.6 **Cerebellum NOS**
Cerebellopontine angle

191.7 **Brain stem**

Cerebral peduncle	Midbrain
Medulla oblongata	Pons

191.8 **Other parts of brain**
Corpus callosum
Tapetum
Malignant neoplasm of contiguous or overlapping sites of brain whose point of origin cannot be determined

191.9 **Brain, unspecified**
Cranial fossa NOS

192 **Malignant neoplasm of other and unspecified parts of nervous system**

> *Excludes:* peripheral, sympathetic, and parasympathetic nerves and ganglia (171.0-171.9)

> **ALERT!** For personal history of malignant neoplasm of other parts of nervous system see V10.86

192.0 **Cranial nerves**
Olfactory bulb

192.1 **Cerebral meninges**

Dura (mater)	Meninges NOS
Falx (cerebelli) (cerebri)	Tentorium

192.2 **Spinal cord**
Cauda equina

192.3 **Spinal meninges**

192.8 **Other specified sites of nervous system**
Malignant neoplasm of contiguous or overlapping sites of other parts of nervous system whose point of origin cannot be determined

192.9 **Nervous system, part unspecified**
Nervous system (central) NOS

> *Excludes:* meninges NOS (192.1)

193 **Malignant neoplasm of thyroid gland**
Thyroglossal duct

Use additional code, if desired, to identify any functional activity

> **ALERT!** For personal history of malignant neoplasm of thyroid see V10.87

194 **Malignant neoplasm of other endocrine glands and related structures**

> *Excludes:* islets of Langerhans (157.4)
> neuroendocrine tumors (209.00-209.69)
> ovary (183.0)
> testis (186.0-186.9)
> thymus (164.0)

> **ALERT!** For personal history of malignant neoplasm of other endocrine glands and related structures see V10.88

	Add 4th or 5th digit		Nonspecific code		Unspecified code		Manifestation code

194.0 Adrenal gland
Adrenal cortex   Suprarenal gland
Adrenal medulla

194.1 Parathyroid gland

194.3 Pituitary gland and craniopharyngeal duct
Craniobuccal pouch   Rathke's pouch
Hypophysis   Sella turcica

194.4 Pineal gland

194.5 Carotid body

194.6 Aortic body and other paraganglia
Coccygeal body   Para-aortic body
Glomus jugulare

194.8 Other
Pluriglandular involvement NOS

Note: If the sites of multiple involvements are known, they should be coded separately.

194.9 Endocrine gland, site unspecified

195 Malignant neoplasm of other and ill-defined sites
Includes: malignant neoplasms of contiguous sites, not elsewhere classified, whose point of origin cannot be determined

Excludes: *malignant neoplasm:*
lymphatic and hematopoietic tissue (200.0-208.9)
secondary sites (196.0-198.8)
unspecified site (199.0-199.1)

ALERT! For personal history of malignant neoplasm of other sites see V10.89

195.0 Head, face, and neck
Cheek NOS   Nose NOS
Jaw NOS   Supraclavicular region NOS

195.1 Thorax
Axilla   Intrathoracic NOS
Chest (wall) NOS

195.2 Abdomen
Intra-abdominal NOS

195.3 Pelvis
Groin
Inguinal region NOS
Presacral region
Sacrococcygeal region
Sites overlapping systems within pelvis, as:
    rectovaginal (septum)
    rectovesical (septum)

195.4 Upper limb

195.5 Lower limb

195.8 Other specified sites
Back NOS   Trunk NOS
Flank NOS

196 Secondary and unspecified malignant neoplasm of lymph nodes
Excludes: *any malignant neoplasm of lymph nodes, specified as primary (200.0-202.9)*
Hodgkin's disease (201.0-201.9)
lymphosarcoma (200.1)
reticulosarcoma (200.0)
other forms of lymphoma (202.0-202.9)
secondary neuroendocrine tumor of (distant) lymph nodes (209.71)

ALERT! For personal history of unspecified type of malignant neoplasm see V10.90

196.0 Lymph nodes of head, face, and neck
Cervical   Scalene
Cervicofacial   Supraclavicular

196.1 Intrathoracic lymph nodes
Bronchopulmonary   Mediastinal
Intercostal   Tracheobronchial

196.2 Intra-abdominal lymph nodes
Intestinal   Retroperitoneal
Mesenteric

● Code new   ▲ Revision of   ④ ⑤ Fourth or fifth
   to this edition   existing code   digit required

196.3 Lymph nodes of axilla and upper limb
    Brachial   Infraclavicular
    Epitrochlear   Pectoral

196.5 Lymph nodes of inguinal region and lower limb
    Femoral   Popliteal
    Groin   Tibial

196.6 Intrapelvic lymph nodes
    Hypogastric   Obturator
    Iliac   Parametrial

196.8 Lymph nodes of multiple sites

196.9 Site unspecified
    Lymph nodes NOS

197 Secondary malignant neoplasm of respiratory and digestive systems

Excludes: lymph node metastasis (196.0-196.9)
      secondary neuroendocrine tumor of liver (209.72)
      secondary neuroendocrine tumor of respiratory organs (209.79)

ALERT! For personal history of unspecified type of malignant neoplasm see V10.90

197.0 Lung
    Bronchus

197.1 Mediastinum

197.2 Pleura

197.3 Other respiratory organs
    Trachea

ALERT! For personal history of malignant neoplasm of other respiratory and intrathoracic organs see V10.2

197.4 Small intestine, including duodenum

197.5 Large intestine and rectum

197.6 Retroperitoneum and peritoneum

197.7 Liver, specified as secondary

197.8 Other digestive organs and spleen

198 Secondary malignant neoplasm of other specified sites

Excludes: lymph node metastasis (196.0-196.9)
      secondary neuroendocrine tumor of other specified sites (209.79)

ALERT! For personal history of malignant neoplasm of other sites see V10.8

ALERT! For personal history of unspecified type of malignant neoplasm see V10.90

198.0 Kidney

198.1 Other urinary organs

198.2 Skin
    Skin of breast

198.3 Brain and spinal cord

198.4 Other parts of nervous system
    Meninges (cerebral) (spinal)

198.5 Bone and bone marrow

198.6 Ovary

198.7 Adrenal gland
    Suprarenal gland

⑤ **198.8 Other specified sites**

    198.81 Breast

Excludes: skin of breast (198.2)

    198.82 Genital organs

    198.89 Other

Excludes: retroperitoneal lymph nodes (196.2)

199 Malignant neoplasm without specification of site

Excludes: malignant carcinoid tumor of unknown primary site (209.20)
      malignant (poorly differentiated) neuroendocrine carcinoma, any site (209.30)
      malignant (poorly differentiated) neuroendocrine tumor, any site (209.30)
      neuroendocrine carcinoma (high grade), any site (209.30)

Add 4th or 5th digit   Nonspecific code   Unspecified code   Manifestation code

ALERT! For personal history of unspecified type of malignant neoplasm see V10.90

199.0 Disseminated
  Carcinomatosis unspecified site (primary) (secondary)
  Generalized:
    cancer unspecified site (primary) (secondary)
    malignancy unspecified site (primary) (secondary)
  Multiple cancer unspecified site (primary) (secondary)

199.1 Other
  Cancer unspecified site (primary) (secondary)
  Carcinoma unspecified site (primary) (secondary)
  Malignancy unspecified site (primary) (secondary)

199.2 Malignant neoplasm associated with transplanted organ
Code first complication of transplanted organ (996.80-996.89)
  Use additional code for specific malignancy

MALIGNANT NEOPLASM OF LYMPHATIC AND HEMATOPOIETIC TISSUE (200-208)

Excludes: *autoimmune lymphoproliferative syndrome (279.41)*
      secondary neoplasm of:
        bone marrow (198.5)
        spleen (197.8)
      secondary and unspecified neoplasm of lymph nodes (196.0-196.9)

The following fifth-digit subclassification is for use with categories 200-202:

  0 unspecified site, extranodal and solid organ sites

  1 lymph nodes of head, face, and neck

  2 intrathoracic lymph nodes

  3 intra-abdominal lymph nodes

  4 lymph nodes of axilla and upper limb

  5 lymph nodes of inguinal region and lower limb

  6 intrapelvic lymph nodes

  7 spleen

  8 lymph nodes of multiple sites

⑤ **200 Lymphosarcoma and reticulosarcoma and other specified malignant tumors of lymphatic tissue**
  DEFINITION Lymphosarcoma is a type of cancer that originates in lymphocytes of the immune system. The diseases often originates in lymph nodes, presenting as an enlargement of the node (a tumor). A reticulosarcoma is a malignant lymphoma, histiocytic or undifferentiated.
  ALERT! For personal history of other lymphatic and hematopoietic neoplasms see V10.7

⑤ **200.0 Reticulosarcoma**
[0-8]   Lymphoma (malignant):
      histiocytic (diffuse):
        nodular
        pleomorphic cell type
      reticulum cell type
    Reticulum cell sarcoma:
      NOS
      pleomorphic cell type

⑤ **200.1 Lymphosarcoma**
[0-8]   Lymphoblastoma (diffuse)
    Lymphoma (malignant):   Lymphosarcoma:
      lymphoblastic (diffuse)   NOS
      lymphocytic (cell type)   diffuse NOS
        (diffuse)   lymphoblastic (diffuse)
      lymphosarcoma type   lymphocytic (diffuse)
                                     prolymphocytic

    Excludes: *lymphosarcoma:*
          follicular or nodular (202.0)
          mixed cell type (200.8)
          lymphosarcoma cell leukemia (207.8)

⑤ **200.2 Burkitt's tumor or lymphoma**
[0-8]   Malignant lymphoma, Burkitt's type

● Code new   ▲ Revision of   ④ ⑤ Fourth or fifth
      to this edition   existing code   digit required

⑤ **200.3 Marginal zone lymphoma**
[0-8]   Extranodal marginal zone B-cell lymphoma
         Mucosa associated lymphoid tissue [MALT]
         Nodal marginal zone B-cell lymphoma
         Splenic marginal zone B-cell lymphoma

⑤ **200.4 Mantle cell lymphoma**
[0-8]

⑤ **200.5 Primary central nervous system lymphoma**
[0-8]

⑤ **200.6 Anaplastic large cell lymphoma**
[0-8]

⑤ **200.7 Large cell lymphoma**
[0-8]

⑤ **200.8 Other named variants**
[0-8]   Lymphoma (malignant):
            lymphoplasmacytoid type
            mixed lymphocytic-histiocytic (diffuse)
         Lymphosarcoma, mixed cell type (diffuse)
         Reticulolymphosarcoma (diffuse)

⑤ **201 Hodgkin's disease**
         DEFINITION Hodgkin's disease is a malignant disease of the lymphatic system is characterized
         by painless enlargement of lymph nodes, the spleen, or other lymphatic tissue. It is
         sometimes accompanied by symptoms such as fever, weight loss, fatigue and night sweats.
         ALERT! For personal history of hodgkin's disease see V10.72

⑤ **201.0 Hodgkin's paragranuloma**
[0-8]

⑤ **201.1 Hodgkin's granuloma**
[0-8]

⑤ **201.2 Hodgkin's sarcoma**
[0-8]

⑤ **201.4 Lymphocytic-histiocytic predominance**
[0-8]

⑤ **201.5 Nodular sclerosis**
[0-8]   Hodgkin's disease, nodular sclerosis:
            NOS
            cellular phase

⑤ **201.6 Mixed cellularity**
[0-8]

⑤ **201.7 Lymphocytic depletion**
[0-8]   Hodgkin's disease, lymphocytic depletion:
            NOS
            diffuse fibrosis
            reticular type

⑤ **201.9 Hodgkin's disease, unspecified**
[0-8]   Hodgkin's: Malignant:
            disease NOS   lymphogranuloma
            lymphoma NOS   lymphogranulomatosis

⑤ **202 Other malignant neoplasms of lymphoid and histiocytic tissue**
         ALERT! For personal history of other lymphatic and hematopoietic neoplasms see V10.79

⑤ **202.0 Nodular lymphoma**
[0-8]   Brill-Symmers disease
         Lymphoma: Lymphosarcoma:
            follicular (giant) (large cell)   follicular (giant)
            lymphocytic, nodular   nodular

⑤ **202.1 Mycosis fungoides**
[0-8]
         Excludes: peripheral T-cell lymphoma (202.7)

⑤ **202.2 Sézary's disease**
[0-8]

 Add 4th or
5th digit

 Nonspecific
code

 Unspecified
code

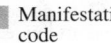 Manifestation
code

⑤ **202.3 Malignant histiocytosis**
[0-8]   Histiocytic medullary reticulosis
          Malignant:
              reticuloendotheliosis
              reticulosis

⑤ **202.4 Leukemic reticuloendotheliosis**
[0-8]   Hairy-cell leukemia

⑤ **202.5 Letterer-Siwe disease**
[0-8]   Acute:
              differentiated progressive histiocytosis
              histiocytosis X (progressive)
              infantile reticuloendotheliosis
              reticulosis of infancy

  Excludes: *adult pulmonary Langerhans cell histiocytic tissue (516.5)*
            Hand-Schüller-Christian disease (277.89)
            histiocytosis (acute) (chronic) (277.89)
            histiocytosis X (chronic) (277.89)

⑤ **202.6 Malignant mast cell tumors**
[0-8]   Malignant: Mast cell sarcoma
              mastocytoma   Systemic tissue mast cell disease
              mastocytosis

  Excludes: *mast cell leukemia (207.8)*

⑤ **202.7 Peripheral T-cell lymphoma**
[0-8]

⑤ **202.8 Other lymphomas**
[0-8]   Lymphoma (malignant):
              NOS
              diffuse

  Excludes: *benign lymphoma (229.0)*

⑤ **202.9 Other and unspecified malignant neoplasms of lymphoid and histiocytic tissue**
[0-8]   Follicular dendritic cell sarcoma
          Interdigitating dendritic cell sarcoma
          Langerhans cell sarcoma
          Malignant neoplasm of bone marrow NOS

⑤ **203 Multiple myeloma and immunoproliferative neoplasms**
  The following fifth-digit subclassification is for use with category 203

     **0   without mention of having achieved remission
          failed remission**

     1   in remission

     2   in relapse

  DEFINITION Multiple myeloma and immunoproliferative neoplasms is a cancer in which there
  is a uncontrolled proliferation and disordered function of cells called plasma cells in the bone
  marrow., aka a plasma cell neoplasm.

⑤ **203.0 Multiple myeloma**
[0-2]   Kahler's disease
          Myelomatosis

  Excludes: *solitary myeloma (238.6)*

⑤ **203.1 Plasma cell leukemia**
[0-2]   Plasmacytic leukemia

⑤ **203.8 Other immunoproliferative neoplasms**
[0-2]

● Code new   ▲ Revision of   ④ ⑤ Fourth or fifth
      to this edition   existing code   digit required

⑤ **204 Lymphoid leukemia**
  Includes: leukemia:
              lymphatic
              lymphoblastic
              lymphocytic
              lymphogenous

The following fifth-digit subclassification is for use with category 204

> **0   without mention of having achieved remission**
>   **failed remission**
>
> **1   in remission**
>
> **2   in relapse**

DEFINITION Lymphoid leukemia is a form of leukemia associated with hyperplasia and overactivity of the lymphoid tissue, with increased levels of circulating malignant lymphocytes or lymphoblasts.

ALERT! For personal history of leukemia see V10.6

⑤ **204.0 Acute**
  [0-2]

> Excludes: acute exacerbation of chronic lymphoid leukemia (204.1)

⑤ **204.1 Chronic**
  [0-2]

⑤ **204.2 Subacute**
  [0-2]

⑤ **204.8 Other lymphoid leukemia**
  [0-2]   Aleukemic leukemia:
              lymphatic
              lymphocytic
              lymphoid

⑤ **204.9 Unspecified lymphoid leukemia**
  [0-2]

⑤ **205 Myeloid leukemia**
  Includes: leukemia:
              granulocytic   myelomonocytic
              myeloblastic   myelosclerotic
              myelocytic   myelosis
              myelogenous

The following fifth-digit subclassification is for use with category 205

> **0   without mention of having achieved remission**
>   **failed remission**
>
> **1   in remission**
>
> **2   in relapse**

DEFINITION Myeloid leukemia is a type of leukemia affecting myeloid tissue (bone marrow).

ALERT! For personal history of myeloid leukemia see V10.62

⑤ **205.0 Acute**
  [0-2]   Acute promyelocytic leukemia

> Excludes: acute exacerbation of chronic myeloid leukemia (205.1)

⑤ **205.1 Chronic**
  [0-2]   Eosinophilic leukemia   Neutrophilic leukemia

⑤ **205.2 Subacute**
  [0-2]

⑤ **205.3 Myeloid sarcoma**
  [0-2]   Chloroma
            Granulocytic sarcoma

⑤ **205.8 Other myeloid leukemia**
  [0-2]   Aleukemic leukemia:
              granulocytic
              myelogenous
              myeloid
            Aleukemic myelosis

⑤ **205.9 Unspecified myeloid leukemia**
  [0-2]

  ALERT! For personal history of unspecified leukemia see V10.60

235

| Add 4th or 5th digit | Nonspecific code | Unspecified code | Manifestation code |

⑤ **206** **Monocytic leukemia**
       Includes: leukemia:
               histiocytic
               monoblastic
               monocytoid

The following fifth-digit subclassification is for use with category 206

    0 **without mention of having achieved remission**
        failed remission

    1 **in remission**

    2 **in relapse**

DEFINITION Monocytic leukemia is a type of leukemia characterized by the proliferation of monocytes and monoblasts in the blood .

ALERT! ICD-9-CM codes in the Category 206 add points to the clinical domain as a Cancer & benign neoplasms diagnosis.

ALERT! For personal history of monocytic leukemia see V10.63

⑤ **206.0** **Acute**
[0-2]
> Excludes: acute exacerbation of chronic monocytic leukemia (206.1)

⑤ **206.1** **Chronic**
[0-2]

⑤ **206.2** **Subacute**
[0-2]

⑤ **206.8** **Other monocytic leukemia**
[0-2]   Aleukemic:
      monocytic leukemia
      monocytoid leukemia

⑤ **206.9** **Unspecified monocytic leukemia**
[0-2]
ALERT! For personal history of unspecified leukemia see V10.60

⑤ **207** **Other specified leukemia**
> Excludes: leukemic reticuloendotheliosis (202.4)
>   plasma cell leukemia (203.1)

The following fifth-digit subclassification is for use with category 207

    0 **without mention of having achieved remission**
        failed remission

    1 **in remission**

    2 **in relapse**

ALERT! For personal history of other leukemia see V10.69

⑤ **207.0** **Acute erythremia and erythroleukemia**
[0-2]   Acute erythremic myelosis
      Di Guglielmo's disease
      Erythremic myelosis

⑤ **207.1** **Chronic erythremia**
[0-2]   Heilmeyer-Schöner disease

⑤ **207.2** **Megakaryocytic leukemia**
[0-2]   Megakaryocytic myelosis   Thrombocytic leukemia

⑤ **207.8** **Other specified leukemia**
[0-2]   Lymphosarcoma cell leukemia

⑤ **208** **Leukemia of unspecified cell type**
The following fifth-digit subclassification is for use with category 208

    0 **without mention of having achieved remission**
        failed remission

    1 **in remission**

    2 **in relapse**

ALERT! For personal history of unspecified leukemia see V10.60

● Code new to this edition   ▲ Revision of existing code   ④ ⑤ Fourth or fifth digit required

⑤ **208.0** **Acute**
[0-2]   Acute leukemia NOS
         Blast cell leukemia
         Stem cell leukemia

> *Excludes:* acute exacerbation of chronic unspecified leukemia (208.1)

⑤ **208.1** **Chronic**
[0-2]   Chronic leukemia NOS

⑤ **208.2** **Subacute**
[0-2]   Subacute leukemia NOS

⑤ **208.8** **Other leukemia of unspecified cell type**
[0-2]

⑤ **208.9** **Unspecified leukemia**
[0-2]   Leukemia NOS

NEUROENDOCRINE TUMORS (209)

⑤ **209** **Neuroendocrine tumors**
Code first any associated multiple endocrine neoplasia syndrome (258.01-258.03)
Use additional code to identify associated endocrine syndrome, such as: carcinoid syndrome (259.2)

> *Excludes:* benign pancreatic islet cell tumors (211.7)
>   malignant pancreatic islet cell tumors (157.4)

DEFINITION Neuroendocrine tumor is a tumor derived from cells that release a hormone in response to a signal from the nervous system. Examples of neuroendocrine tumors include carcinoid tumors islet cell tumors, medullary thyroid carcinoma, and pheochromocytoma.

ALERT! For personal history of malignant neuroendocrine tumor see V10.91

⑤ **209.0** **Malignant carcinoid tumors of the small intestine**

   209.00 **Malignant carcinoid tumor of the small intestine, unspecified portion**

   209.01 **Malignant carcinoid tumor of the duodenum**

   209.02 **Malignant carcinoid tumor of the jejunum**

   209.03 **Malignant carcinoid tumor of the ileum**

⑤ **209.1** **Malignant carcinoid tumors of the appendix, large intestine, and rectum**

   209.10 **Malignant carcinoid tumor of the large intestine, unspecified portion**
             Malignant carcinoid tumor of the colon NOS

   209.11 **Malignant carcinoid tumor of the appendix**

   209.12 **Malignant carcinoid tumor of the cecum**

   209.13 **Malignant carcinoid tumor of the ascending colon**

   209.14 **Malignant carcinoid tumor of the transverse colon**

   209.15 **Malignant carcinoid tumor of the descending colon**

   209.16 **Malignant carcinoid tumor of the sigmoid colon**

   209.17 **Malignant carcinoid tumor of the rectum**

⑤ **209.2** **Malignant carcinoid tumors of other and unspecified sites**

   209.20 **Malignant carcinoid tumor of unknown primary site**

   209.21 **Malignant carcinoid tumor of the bronchus and lung**

   209.22 **Malignant carcinoid tumor of the thymus**

   209.23 **Malignant carcinoid tumor of the stomach**

   209.24 **Malignant carcinoid tumor of the kidney**

   209.25 **Malignant carcinoid tumor of the foregut NOS**

   209.26 **Malignant carcinoid tumor of the midgut NOS**

   209.27 **Malignant carcinoid tumor of the hindgut NOS**

   209.29 **Malignant carcinoid tumors of other sites**

⑤ **209.3** **Malignant poorly differentiated neuroendocrine tumors**

   209.30 **Malignant poorly differentiated neuroendocrine carcinoma, any site**
             High grade neuroendocrine carcinoma, any site
             Malignant poorly differentiated neuroendocrine tumor NOS

> *Excludes:* Merkel cell carcinoma (209.31-209.36)

Add 4th or 5th digit   Nonspecific code   Unspecified code   Manifestation code

209.31 Merkel cell carcinoma of the face
Merkel cell carcinoma of the ear
Merkel cell carcinoma of the eyelid, including canthus
Merkel cell carcinoma of the lip

209.32 Merkel cell carcinoma of the scalp and neck

209.33 Merkel cell carcinoma of the upper limb

209.34 Merkel cell carcinoma of the lower limb

209.35 Merkel cell carcinoma of the trunk

209.36 Merkel cell carcinoma of other sites
Merkel cell carcinoma of the buttock
Merkel cell carcinoma of the genitals
Merkel cell carcinoma NOS

⑤ **209.4 Benign carcinoid tumors of the small intestine**

209.40 Benign carcinoid tumor of the small intestine, unspecified portion

209.41 Benign carcinoid tumor of the duodenum

209.42 Benign carcinoid tumor of the jejunum

209.43 Benign carcinoid tumor of the ileum

⑤ **209.5 Benign carcinoid tumors of the appendix, large intestine, and rectum**

209.50 Benign carcinoid tumor of the large intestine, unspecified portion
Benign carcinoid tumor of the colon NOS

209.51 Benign carcinoid tumor of the appendix

209.52 Benign carcinoid tumor of the cecum

209.53 Benign carcinoid tumor of the ascending colon

209.54 Benign carcinoid tumor of the transverse colon

209.55 Benign carcinoid tumor of the descending colon

209.56 Benign carcinoid tumor of the sigmoid colon

209.57 Benign carcinoid tumor of the rectum

⑤ **209.6 Benign carcinoid tumors of other and unspecified sites**

209.60 Benign carcinoid tumor of unknown primary site
Carcinoid tumor NOS
Neuroendocrine tumor NOS

209.61 Benign carcinoid tumor of the bronchus and lung

209.62 Benign carcinoid tumor of the thymus

209.63 Benign carcinoid tumor of the stomach

209.64 Benign carcinoid tumor of the kidney

209.65 Benign carcinoid tumor of the foregut NOS

209.66 Benign carcinoid tumor of the midgut NOS

209.67 Benign carcinoid tumor of the hindgut NOS

209.69 Benign carcinoid tumors of other sites

⑤ **209.7 Secondary neuroendocrine tumors**
Secondary carcinoid tumors

209.70 Secondary neuroendocrine tumor, unspecified site

209.71 Secondary neuroendocrine tumor of distant lymph nodes

209.72 Secondary neuroendocrine tumor of liver

209.73 Secondary neuroendocrine tumor of bone

209.74 Secondary neuroendocrine tumor of peritoneum
Mesentary metastasis of neuroendocrine tumor

209.75 Secondary Merkel cell carcinoma
Merkel cell carcinoma nodal presentation
Merkel cell carcinoma visceral metastatic presentation
Secondary Merkel cell carcinoma, any site

209.79 Secondary neuroendocrine tumor of other sites

● Code new
  to this edition

▲ Revision of
  existing code

④ ⑤ Fourth or fifth
  digit required

BENIGN NEOPLASMS (210-229)

210 Benign neoplasm of lip, oral cavity, and pharynx

> Excludes: cyst (of):
>> jaw (526.0-526.2, 526.89)
>> oral soft tissue (528.4)
>> radicular (522.8)

DEFINITION A benign neoplasm is a localized tumor that has a fibrous capsule, limited potential for growth, a regular shape, and cells that are well differentiated. A benign neoplasm does not invade surrounding tissue or metastasize to distant sites. Some kinds of benign neoplasms are adenoma, fibroma, hemangioma, and lipoma.

210.0 Lip
Frenulum labii
Lip (inner aspect) (mucosa) (vermilion border)

> Excludes: labial commissure (210.4)
>> skin of lip (216.0)

210.1 Tongue
Lingual tonsil

210.2 Major salivary glands
Gland:
parotid
sublingual
submandibular

> Excludes: benign neoplasms of minor salivary glands:
>> NOS (210.4)
>> buccal mucosa (210.4)
>> lips (210.0)
>> palate (hard) (soft) (210.4)
>> tongue (210.1)
>> tonsil, palatine (210.5)

210.3 Floor of mouth

210.4 Other and unspecified parts of mouth
Gingiva   Oral mucosa
Gum (upper) (lower)   Palate (hard) (soft)
Labial commissure   Uvula
Oral cavity NOS

> Excludes: benign odontogenic neoplasms of bone (213.0-213.1)
>> developmental odontogenic cysts (526.0)
>> mucosa of lips (210.0)
>> nasopharyngeal [posterior] [superior] surface of soft palate (210.7)

210.5 Tonsil
Tonsil (faucial) (palatine)

> Excludes: lingual tonsil (210.1)
>> pharyngeal tonsil (210.7)
>> tonsillar:
>>> fossa (210.6)
>>> pillars (210.6)

210.6 Other parts of oropharynx
Branchial cleft or vestiges
Epiglottis, anterior aspect
Fauces NOS
Mesopharynx NOS
Tonsillar:
fossa
pillars
Vallecula

> Excludes: epiglottis:
>> NOS (212.1)
>> suprahyoid portion (212.1)

210.7 Nasopharynx
Adenoid tissue   Pharyngeal tonsil
Lymphadenoid tissue   Posterior nasal septum

210.8 Hypopharynx
Arytenoid fold   Postcricoid region
Laryngopharynx   Pyriform fossa

	Add 4th or 5th digit		Nonspecific code		Unspecified code		Manifestation code

210.9 Pharynx, unspecified
  Throat NOS

211 Benign neoplasm of other parts of digestive system

Excludes: benign stromal tumors of digestive system (215.5)

211.0 Esophagus

211.1 Stomach
  Body of stomach   Cardiac orifice
  Cardia of stomach   Pylorus
  Fundus of stomach

Excludes: benign carcinoid tumors of the stomach (209.63)

211.2 Duodenum, jejunum, and ileum
  Small intestine NOS

Excludes: ampulla of Vater (211.5)

  benign carcinoid tumors of the small intestine (209.40-209.43)
  ileocecal valve (211.3)

211.3 Colon
  Appendix   Ileocecal valve
  Cecum   Large intestine NOS

Excludes: benign carcinoid tumors of the large intestine (209.50-209.56)
  rectosigmoid junction (211.4)

ALERT! For personal history of colonic polyps see V12.72

211.4 Rectum and anal canal
  Anal canal or sphincter   Rectosigmoid junction
  Anus NOS

Excludes: anus:
    margin (216.5)
    skin (216.5)
  benign carcinoid tumors of the rectum (209.57)
  perianal skin (216.5)

211.5 Liver and biliary passages
  Ampulla of Vater   Gallbladder
  Common bile duct   Hepatic duct
  Cystic duct   Sphincter of Oddi

211.6 Pancreas, except islets of Langerhans

211.7 Islets of Langerhans
  Islet cell tumor

Use additional code, if desired, to identify any functional activity

211.8 Retroperitoneum and peritoneum
  Mesentery   Omentum
  Mesocolon   Retroperitoneal tissue

211.9 Other and unspecified site
  Alimentary tract NOS   Intestinal tract NOS
  Digestive system NOS   Intestine NOS
  Gastrointestinal tract NOS   Spleen, not elsewhere classified

● Code new
  to this edition

▲ Revision of
  existing code

④ ⑤ Fourth or fifth
  digit required

212 **Benign neoplasm of respiratory and intrathoracic organs**

212.0 Nasal cavities, middle ear, and accessory sinuses

Cartilage of nose
Eustachian tube
Nares
Septum of nose

Sinus:
 ethmoidal
 frontal
 maxillary
 sphenoidal

Excludes: *auditory canal (external) (216.2)*
bone of:
 ear (213.0)
 nose [turbinates] (213.0)
cartilage of ear (215.0)
ear (external) (skin) (216.2)
nose NOS (229.8)
 skin (216.3)
olfactory bulb (225.1)
polyp of:
 accessory sinus (471.8)
 ear (385.30-385.35)
 nasal cavity (471.0)
posterior margin of septum and choanae (210.7)

212.1 Larynx

Cartilage:
 arytenoid
 cricoid
 cuneiform
 thyroid

Epiglottis (suprahyoid portion) NOS
Glottis
Vocal cords (false) (true)

Excludes: *epiglottis, anterior aspect (210.6)*
polyp of vocal cord or larynx (478.4)

212.2 Trachea

212.3 Bronchus and lung
Carina
Hilus of lung

Excludes: *benign carcinoid tumors of bronchus and lung (209.61)*

212.4 Pleura

212.5 Mediastinum

212.6 Thymus

Excludes: *benign carcinoid tumors of thymus (209.62)*

212.7 Heart

Excludes: *great vessels (215.4)*

212.8 Other specified sites

212.9 Site unspecified
Respiratory organ NOS
Upper respiratory tract NOS

Excludes: *intrathoracic NOS (229.8)*
thoracic NOS (229.8)

213 **Benign neoplasm of bone and articular cartilage**
Includes: cartilage (articular) (joint)
 periosteum

Excludes: *cartilage of:*
 ear (215.0)
 eyelid (215.0)
 larynx (212.1)
 nose (212.0)
exostosis NOS (726.91)
synovia (215.0-215.9)

213.0 Bones of skull and face
Excludes: *lower jaw bone (213.1)*

213.1 Lower jaw bone

213.2 Vertebral column, excluding sacrum and coccyx

213.3 Ribs, sternum, and clavicle

Add 4th or 5th digit   Nonspecific code   Unspecified code   Manifestation code

213.4 **Scapula and long bones of upper limb**

213.5 **Short bones of upper limb**

213.6 **Pelvic bones, sacrum, and coccyx**

213.7 **Long bones of lower limb**

213.8 **Short bones of lower limb**

213.9 **Bone and articular cartilage, site unspecified**

214 **Lipoma**

Includes: angiolipoma
fibrolipoma
hibernoma
lipoma (fetal) (infiltrating) (intramuscular)
myelolipoma
myxolipoma

DEFINITION Lipoma is a benign tumor composed chiefly of fat cells.

214.0 **Skin and subcutaneous tissue of face**

214.1 **Other skin and subcutaneous tissue**

214.2 **Intrathoracic organs**

214.3 **Intra-abdominal organs**

214.4 **Spermatic cord**

214.8 **Other specified sites**

214.9 **Lipoma, unspecified site**

215 **Other benign neoplasm of connective and other soft tissue**

Includes: blood vessel
bursa
fascia
ligament
muscle
peripheral, sympathetic, and parasympathetic nerves and ganglia
synovia
tendon (sheath)

Excludes: *cartilage:*
articular (213.0-213.9)
larynx (212.1)
nose (212.0)
connective tissue of:
breast (217)
internal organ, except lipoma and hemangioma — code to benign neoplasm of the site
lipoma (214.0-214.9)

215.0 **Head, face, and neck**

215.2 **Upper limb, including shoulder**

215.3 **Lower limb, including hip**

215.4 **Thorax**

Excludes: *heart (212.7)*
mediastinum (212.5)
thymus (212.6)

215.5 **Abdomen**
Abdominal wall
Benign stromal tumors of abdomen
Hypochondrium

215.6 **Pelvis**
Buttock   Inguinal region
Groin   Perineum

Excludes: *uterine:*
leiomyoma (218.0-218.9)
ligament, any (221.0)

215.7 **Trunk, unspecified**
Back NOS
Flank NOS

215.8 **Other specified sites**

215.9 **Site unspecified**

● Code new   ▲ Revision of   ④ ⑤ Fourth or fifth
to this edition   existing code   digit required

216 Benign neoplasm of skin
Includes: blue nevus
dermatofibroma
hydrocystoma
pigmented nevus
syringoadenoma
syringoma

Excludes: *skin of genital organs (221.0-222.9)*

216.0 Skin of lip
Excludes: *vermilion border of lip (210.0)*

216.1 Eyelid, including canthus
Excludes: *cartilage of eyelid (215.0)*

216.2 Ear and external auditory canal
Auricle (ear)   External meatus
Auricular canal, external   Pinna
Excludes: *cartilage of ear (215.0)*

216.3 Skin of other and unspecified parts of face
Cheek, external   Nose, external
Eyebrow   Temple

216.4 Scalp and skin of neck

216.5 Skin of trunk, except scrotum
Axillary fold   Skin of:
Perianal skin   buttock
Skin of: chest wall
  abdominal wall   groin
  anus   perineum
  back   Umbilicus
  breast

Excludes: *anal canal (211.4)*
anus NOS (211.4)
skin of scrotum (222.4)

216.6 Skin of upper limb, including shoulder

216.7 Skin of lower limb, including hip

216.8 Other specified sites of skin

216.9 Skin, site unspecified

217 Benign neoplasm of breast
Breast (male) (female)
connective tissue
glandular tissue
soft parts

Excludes: *adenofibrosis (610.2)*
benign cyst of breast (610.0)
fibrocystic disease (610.1)
skin of breast (216.5)

218 Uterine leiomyoma
Includes: fibroid (bleeding) (uterine)
uterine:
  fibromyoma
  myoma

DEFINITION Uterine leiomyoma refers to one or more smooth, firm, painful, often waxy nodules arising from cutaneous or subcutaneous of the uterus.

218.0 Submucous leiomyoma of uterus

218.1 Intramural leiomyoma of uterus
Interstitial leiomyoma of uterus

218.2 Subserous leiomyoma of uterus
Subperitoneal leiomyoma of uterus

218.9 Leiomyoma of uterus, unspecified

219 Other benign neoplasm of uterus

219.0 Cervix uteri

Add 4th or   Nonspecific   Unspecified   Manifestation
5th digit   code   code   code

219.1 Corpus uteri
Endometrium   Myometrium
Fundus

219.8 Other specified parts of uterus

219.9 Uterus, part unspecified

220 Benign neoplasm of ovary
Use additional code, if desired, to identify any functional activity (256.0-256.1)

Excludes: cyst:
corpus albicans (620.2)
corpus luteum (620.1)
endometrial (617.1)
follicular (atretic) (620.0)
graafian follicle (620.0)
ovarian NOS (620.2)
retention (620.2)

221 Benign neoplasm of other female genital organs
Includes: adenomatous polyp
benign teratoma

Excludes: cyst:
epoophoron (752.11)
fimbrial (752.11)
Gartner's duct (752.11)
parovarian (752.11)

221.0 Fallopian tube and uterine ligaments
Oviduct   Uterine ligament (broad) (round) (uterosacral)
Parametrium   Uterine tube

221.1 Vagina

221.2 Vulva
Clitoris
External female genitalia NOS
Greater vestibular [Bartholin's] gland
Labia (majora) (minora)
Pudendum

Excludes: Bartholin's (duct) (gland) cyst (616.2)

221.8 Other specified sites of female genital organs

221.9 Female genital organ, site unspecified
Female genitourinary tract NOS

222 Benign neoplasm of male genital organs

222.0 Testis
Use additional code, if desired, to identify any functional activity

222.1 Penis
Corpus cavernosum   Prepuce
Glans penis

222.2 Prostate
Excludes: adenomatous hyperplasia of prostate (600.20-600.21)
prostatic:
adenoma (600.20-600.21)
enlargement (600.00-600.01)
hypertrophy (600.00-600.01)

222.3 Epididymis

222.4 Scrotum
Skin of scrotum

222.8 Other specified sites of male genital organs
Seminal vesicle
Spermatic cord

222.9 Male genital organ, site unspecified
Male genitourinary tract NOS

223 Benign neoplasm of kidney and other urinary organs

● Code new to this edition   ▲ Revision of existing code   ④ ⑤ Fourth or fifth digit required

223.0 Kidney, except pelvis
   Kidney NOS

   Excludes: *benign carcinoid tumors of kidney (209.64)*
         renal:
            calyces (223.1)
            pelvis (223.1)

223.1 Renal pelvis

223.2 Ureter

   Excludes: *ureteric orifice of bladder (223.3)*

223.3 Bladder

⑤ **223.8 Other specified sites of urinary organs**

      223.81 Urethra

      Excludes: *urethral orifice of bladder (223.3)*

         223.89 Other
            Paraurethral glands

223.9 Urinary organ, site unspecified
   Urinary system NOS

224 Benign neoplasm of eye

   Excludes: *cartilage of eyelid (215.0)*
         eyelid (skin) (216.1)
         optic nerve (225.1)
         orbital bone (213.0)

224.0 Eyeball, except conjunctiva, cornea, retina, and choroid
   Ciliary body   Sclera
   Iris   Uveal tract

224.1 Orbit

   Excludes: *bone of orbit (213.0)*

224.2 Lacrimal gland

224.3 Conjunctiva

224.4 Cornea

224.5 Retina

   Excludes: *hemangioma of retina (228.03)*

224.6 Choroid

224.7 Lacrimal duct
   Lacrimal sac
   Nasolacrimal duct

224.8 Other specified parts of eye

224.9 Eye, part unspecified

225 Benign neoplasm of brain and other parts of nervous system

   Excludes: *hemangioma (228.02)*
         neurofibromatosis (237.70-237.79)
         peripheral, sympathetic, and parasympathetic nerves and ganglia (215.0-215.9)
         retrobulbar (224.1)

   ALERT! For personal history of benign neoplasm of the brain see V12.41

225.0 Brain

225.1 Cranial nerves

225.2 Cerebral meninges
   Meninges NOS
   Meningioma (cerebral)

225.3 Spinal cord
   Cauda equina

225.4 Spinal meninges
   Spinal meningioma

225.8 Other specified sites of nervous system

225.9 Nervous system, part unspecified
   Nervous system (central) NOS

   Excludes: *meninges NOS (225.2)*

| ▨ | Add 4th or 5th digit | ▨ | Nonspecific code | ▨ | Unspecified code | ▨ | Manifestation code |

226 Benign neoplasm of thyroid glands
Use additional code, if desired, to identify any functional activity

227 Benign neoplasm of other endocrine glands and related structures
Use additional code, if desired, to identify any functional activity

> Excludes: *ovary (220)*
> *pancreas (211.6)*
> *testis (222.0)*

227.0 Adrenal gland
Suprarenal gland

227.1 Parathyroid gland

227.3 Pituitary gland and craniopharyngeal duct (pouch)
Craniobuccal pouch   Rathke's pouch
Hypophysis   Sella turcica

227.4 Pineal gland
Pineal body

227.5 Carotid body

227.6 Aortic body and other paraganglia
Coccygeal body   Para-aortic body
Glomus jugulare

227.8 Other

227.9 Endocrine gland, site unspecified

228 Hemangioma and lymphangioma, any site
Includes: angioma (benign) (cavernous) (congenital) NOS
cavernous nevus
glomus tumor
hemangioma (benign) (congenital)

> Excludes: *benign neoplasm of spleen, except hemangioma and lymphangioma (211.9)*
> *glomus jugulare (227.6)*
> *nevus:*
> *NOS (216.0-216.9)*
> *blue or pigmented (216.0-216.9)*
> *vascular (757.32)*

DEFINITION Hemangioma is a benign skin lesion consisting of dense, usually elevated masses of dilated blood vessels. Lymphangioma is a benign neoplasm characterized by lymph vessel proliferation.

⑤ **228.0 Hemangioma, any site**

228.00 Of unspecified site

228.01 Of skin and subcutaneous tissue

228.02 Of intracranial structures

228.03 Of retina

228.04 Of intra-abdominal structures
Peritoneum
Retroperitoneal tissue

228.09 Of other sites
Systemic angiomatosis

228.1 Lymphangioma, any site
Congenital lymphangioma
Lymphatic nevus

229 Benign neoplasm of other and unspecified sites

229.0 Lymph nodes

> Excludes: *lymphangioma (228.1)*

229.8 Other specified sites
Intrathoracic NOS
Thoracic NOS

229.9 Site unspecified

● Code new   ▲ Revision of   ④ ⑤ Fourth or fifth
to this edition   existing code   digit required

CARCINOMA IN SITU (230-234)

Includes: Bowen's disease
erythroplasia
Queyrat's erythroplasia

Excludes: *leukoplakia—see Alphabetic Index*

230 **Carcinoma in situ of digestive organs**

> **DEFINITION** Carcinoma in situ is a cluster of malignant cells that has not yet invaded the deeper epithelial tissue or spread to other parts of the body.

230.0 **Lip, oral cavity, and pharynx**

Gingiva	Oropharynx
Hypopharynx	Salivary gland or duct
Mouth [any part]	Tongue
Nasopharynx	

Excludes: *aryepiglottic fold or interarytenoid fold, laryngeal aspect (231.0)*
     epiglottis:
      NOS (231.0)
      suprahyoid portion (231.0)
     skin of lip (232.0)

230.1 **Esophagus**

230.2 **Stomach**

Body of stomach	Cardiac orifice
Cardia of stomach	Pylorus
Fundus of stomach	

230.3 **Colon**

Appendix	
Cecum	Ileocecal valve
	Large intestine NOS

Excludes: *rectosigmoid junction (230.4)*

230.4 **Rectum**

Rectosigmoid junction

230.5 **Anal canal**

Anal sphincter

230.6 **Anus, unspecified**

Excludes: *anus:*
     margin (232.5)
     skin (232.5)
     perianal skin (232.5)

230.7 **Other and unspecified parts of intestine**

Duodenum	Jejunum
Ileum	Small intestine NOS

Excludes: *ampulla of Vater (230.8)*

230.8 **Liver and biliary system**

Ampulla of Vater	Gallbladder
Common bile duct	Hepatic duct
Cystic duct	Sphincter of Oddi

230.9 **Other and unspecified digestive organs**

Digestive organ NOS	Pancreas
Gastrointestinal tract NOS	Spleen

231 **Carcinoma in situ of respiratory system**

231.0 **Larynx**

Cartilage:	Epiglottis:
arytenoid	NOS
cricoid	posterior surface
cuneiform	suprahyoid portion
thyroid	Vocal cords (false) (true)

Excludes: *aryepiglottic fold or interarytenoid fold:*
     NOS (230.0)
     hypopharyngeal aspect (230.0)
     marginal zone (230.0)

231.1 **Trachea**

231.2 **Bronchus and lung**

Carina
Hilus of lung

Add 4th or 5th digit	Nonspecific code	Unspecified code	Manifestation code

231.8 Other specified parts of respiratory system
Accessory sinuses   Nasal cavities
Middle ear   Pleura

Excludes: *ear (external) (skin) (232.2)*
       nose NOS (234.8)
       skin (232.3)

231.9 Respiratory system, part unspecified
Respiratory organ NOS

232 Carcinoma in situ of skin
Includes: pigment cells

Excludes: *melanoma in situ of skin (172.0-172.9)*

232.0 Skin of lip

Excludes: *vermilion border of lip (230.0)*

232.1 Eyelid, including canthus

232.2 Ear and external auditory canal

232.3 Skin of other and unspecified parts of face

232.4 Scalp and skin of neck

232.5 Skin of trunk, except scrotum
Anus, margin   Skin of:
Axillary fold   breast
Perianal skin   buttock
Skin of: chest wall
   abdominal wall   groin
   anus   perineum
   back   Umbilicus

Excludes: *anal canal (230.5)*
       anus NOS (230.6)
       skin of genital organs (233.30-233.39, 233.5-233.6)

232.6 Skin of upper limb, including shoulder

232.7 Skin of lower limb, including hip

232.8 Other specified sites of skin

232.9 Skin, site unspecified

233 Carcinoma in situ of breast and genitourinary system

233.0 Breast

Excludes: *Paget's disease (174.0-174.9)*
       skin of breast (232.5)

233.1 Cervix uteri
Adenocarcinoma in situ of cervix
Cervical intraepithelial glandular neoplasia, grade III
Cervical intraepithelial neoplasia III [CIN III]
Severe dysplasia of cervix

Excludes: *cervical intraepithelial neoplasia II [CIN II] (622.12)*
       cytologic evidence of malignancy without histologic confirmation (795.06)
       high grade squamous intraepithelial lesion (HGSIL) (795.04)
       moderate dysplasia of cervix (622.12)

233.2 Other and unspecified parts of uterus

⑤ **233.3 Other and unspecified female genital organs**

233.30 Unspecified female genital organ

233.31 Vagina
Severe dysplasia of vagina
Vaginal intraepithelial neoplasia III [VAIN III]

233.32 Vulva
Severe dysplasia of vulva
Vulvar intraepithelial neoplasia III [VIN III]

233.39 Other female genital organ

233.4 Prostate

233.5 Penis

233.6 Other and unspecified male genital organs

233.7 Bladder

● Code new   ▲ Revision of   ④ ⑤ Fourth or fifth
   to this edition   existing code   digit required

233.9 Other and unspecified urinary organs

234 Carcinoma in situ of other and unspecified sites

234.0 Eye

> *Excludes:* cartilage of eyelid (234.8)
> eyelid (skin) (232.1)
> optic nerve (234.8)
> orbital bone (234.8)

234.8 Other specified sites
Endocrine gland [any]

234.9 Site unspecified
Carcinoma in situ NOS

NEOPLASMS OF UNCERTAIN BEHAVIOR (235-238)

Note: Categories 235-238 classify by site certain histo-morphologically well-defined neoplasms, the subsequent behavior of which cannot be predicted from the present appearance.

235 Neoplasm of uncertain behavior of digestive and respiratory systems

> *Excludes:* stromal tumors of uncertain behavior of digestive system (238.1)

235.0 Major salivary glands
Gland:
parotid
sublingual
submandibular

> *Excludes:* minor salivary glands (235.1)

235.1 Lip, oral cavity, and pharynx

Gingiva	Nasopharynx
Hypopharynx	Oropharynx
Minor salivary glands	Tongue
Mouth	

> *Excludes:* aryepiglottic fold or interarytenoid fold, laryngeal aspect (235.6)
> epiglottis:
> NOS (235.6)
> suprahyoid portion (235.6)
> skin of lip (238.2)

235.2 Stomach, intestines, and rectum
ALERT! For personal history of colonic polyps see V12.72

235.3 Liver and biliary passages

Ampulla of Vater	Gallbladder
Bile ducts [any]	Liver

235.4 Retroperitoneum and peritoneum

235.5 Other and unspecified digestive organs

Anal:	Esophagus
canal	Pancreas
sphincter	Spleen
Anus NOS	

> *Excludes:* anus:
> margin (238.2)
> skin (238.2)
> perianal skin (238.2)

235.6 Larynx

> *Excludes:* aryepiglottic fold or interarytenoid fold:
> NOS (235.1)
> hypopharyngeal aspect (235.1)
> marginal zone (235.1)

235.7 Trachea, bronchus, and lung

235.8 Pleura, thymus, and mediastinum

Add 4th or
5th digit

Nonspecific
code

Unspecified
code

Manifestation
code

235.9 **Other and unspecified respiratory organs**
    Accessory sinuses   Nasal cavities
    Middle ear   Respiratory organ NOS

    Excludes: ear (external) (skin) (238.2)
             nose (238.8)
             skin (238.2)

236 **Neoplasm of uncertain behavior of genitourinary organs**

236.0 **Uterus**

236.1 **Placenta**
    Chorioadenoma (destruens)
    Invasive mole
    Malignant hydatid mole
    Malignant hydatidiform mole

236.2 **Ovary**
Use additional code, if desired, to identify any functional activity

236.3 **Other and unspecified female genital organs**

236.4 **Testis**
Use additional code, if desired, to identify any functional activity

236.5 **Prostate**

236.6 **Other and unspecified male genital organs**

236.7 **Bladder**

⑤ **236.9** **Other and unspecified urinary organs**

    236.90 **Urinary organ, unspecified**

    236.91 **Kidney and ureter**

    236.99 **Other**

237 **Neoplasm of uncertain behavior of endocrine glands and nervous system**

237.0 **Pituitary gland and craniopharyngeal duct**
Use additional code, if desired, to identify any functional activity

237.1 **Pineal gland**

237.2 **Adrenal gland**
    Suprarenal gland
Use additional code, if desired, to identify any functional activity

237.3 **Paraganglia**
    Aortic body
    Carotid body
    Coccygeal body
    Glomus jugulare

237.4 **Other and unspecified endocrine glands**
    Parathyroid gland
    Thyroid gland

237.5 **Brain and spinal cord**

237.6 **Meninges**
    Meninges:
      NOS
      cerebral
      spinal

⑤ **237.7** **Neurofibromatosis**

    237.70 **Neurofibromatosis, unspecified**

    237.71 **Neurofibromatosis, Type I [von Recklinghausen's disease]**

    237.72 **Neurofibromatosis, Type II [acoustic neurofibromatosis]**

    237.73 **Schwannomatosis**

    237.79 **Other neurofibromatosis**

237.9 **Other and unspecified parts of nervous system**
    Cranial nerves

    Excludes: peripheral, sympathetic, and parasympathetic nerves and ganglia (238.1)

● Code new   ▲ Revision of   ④ ⑤ Fourth or fifth
  to this edition   existing code   digit required

238 **Neoplasm of uncertain behavior of other and unspecified sites and tissues**

238.0 Bone and articular cartilage

Excludes: *cartilage:*
ear (238.1)
eyelid (238.1)
larynx (235.6)
nose (235.9)
synovia (238.1)

238.1 Connective and other soft tissue
Peripheral, sympathetic, and parasympathetic nerves and ganglia
Stromal tumors of digestive system

Excludes: *cartilage (of):*
articular (238.0)
larynx (235.6)
nose (235.9)
connective tissue of breast (238.3)

238.2 Skin

Excludes: *anus NOS (235.5)*
skin of genital organs (236.3, 236.6)
vermilion border of lip (235.1)

238.3 Breast

Excludes: *skin of breast (238.2)*

238.4 Polycythemia vera

238.5 Histiocytic and mast cells
Mast cell tumor NOS
Mastocytoma NOS

238.6 Plasma cells
Plasmacytoma NOS
Solitary myeloma

⑤ **238.7 Other lymphatic and hematopoietic tissues**

Excludes: *acute myelogenous leukemia (205.0)*
chronic myelomonocytic leukemia (205.1)
myelosclerosis NOS (289.89)
myelosis:
NOS (205.9)
megakaryocytic (207.2)

238.71 Essential thrombocythemia
Essential hemorrhagic thrombocythemia
Essential thrombocytosis
Idiopathic (hemorrhagic) thrombocythemia
Primary thrombocytosis

238.72 Low grade myelodysplastic syndrome lesions
Refractory anemia (RA)
Refractory anemia (RA) with excess blasts-1 (RAEB-1)
Refractory anemia with ringed sideroblasts (RARS)
Refractory cytopenia with multilineage dysplasia (RCMD)
Refractory cytopenia with multilineage dysplasia and ringed sideroblasts
(RCMD-RS)

238.73 High grade myelodysplastic syndrome lesions
Refractory anemia with excess blasts-2 (RAEB-2)

238.74 Myelodysplastic syndrome with 5q deletion
5q minus syndrome NOS

Excludes: *constitutional 5q deletion (758.39)*
high grade myelodysplastic syndrome with 5q deletion (238.73)

238.75 Myelodysplastic syndrome, unspecified

| | Add 4th or 5th digit | | Nonspecific code | | Unspecified code | | Manifestation code |

238.76 Myelofibrosis with myeloid metaplasia
Agnogenic myeloid metaplasia
Idiopathic myelofibrosis (chronic)
Myelosclerosis with myeloid metaplasia
Primary myelofibrosis

Excludes: *myelofibrosis NOS (289.83)*
myelophthisic anemia (284.2)
myelophthisis (284.2)
secondary myelofibrosis (289.83)

238.77 Post-transplant lymphoproliferative disorder (PTLD)
Code first complications of transplant (996.80-996.89)

238.79 Other lymphatic and hematopoietic tissues
Lymphoproliferative disease (chronic) NOS
Megakaryocytic myelosclerosis
Myeloproliferative disease (chronic) NOS
Panmyelosis (acute)

238.8 Other specified sites
Eye
Heart

Excludes: *eyelid (skin) (238.2)*
cartilage (238.1)

238.9 Site unspecified

NEOPLASMS OF UNSPECIFIED NATURE (239)

239 Neoplasms of unspecified nature
Note: Category 239 classifies by site neoplasms of unspecified morphology and behavior. The term "mass," unless otherwise stated, is not to be regarded as a neoplastic growth.
Includes: "growth" NOS
neoplasm NOS
new growth NOS
tumor NOS

239.0 Digestive system
Excludes: *anus:*
margin (239.2)
skin (239.2)
perianal skin (239.2)

239.1 Respiratory system

239.2 Bone, soft tissue, and skin
Excludes: *anal canal (239.0)*
anus NOS (239.0)
bone marrow (202.9)
cartilage:
larynx (239.1)
nose (239.1)
connective tissue of breast (239.3)
skin of genital organs (239.5)
vermilion border of lip (239.0)

239.3 Breast
Excludes: *skin of breast (239.2)*

239.4 Bladder

239.5 Other genitourinary organs

239.6 Brain
Excludes: *cerebral meninges (239.7)*
cranial nerves (239.7)

239.7 Endocrine glands and other parts of nervous system
Excludes: *peripheral, sympathetic, and parasympathetic nerves and ganglia (239.2)*

⑤ **239.8 Other specified sites**
Excludes: *eyelids (skin) (239.2)*
cartilage (239.2)
great vessels (239.2)
optic nerve (239.7)

● Code new
to this edition

▲ Revision of
existing code

④ ⑤ Fourth or fifth
digit required

239.81 **Retina and choroid**
Dark area on retina
Retinal freckle

239.89 **Other specified sites**

239.9 **Site unspecified**

Add 4th or 5th digit   Nonspecific code   Unspecified code   Manifestation code

This page intentionally left blank.

● Code new
to this edition

▲ Revision of
existing code

④ ⑤ Fourth or fifth
digit required

Chapter 3: Endocrine, Nutritional, and Metabolic Diseases and Immunity Disorders (240-279)

DEFINITIONS AND CODING ALERTS

This chapter includes definitions of selected key words, terms and phrases and coding alerts for adding points to the clinical domain, references to coding late effects where appropriate, and references to personal history V-codes in situations where the acute or chronic condition is no longer active. An example from this chapter is as follows:

240 **Simple and unspecified goiter**

DEFINITION Simple and unspecified goiter is a simple enlargement of the thyroid gland, causing a swelling in the front part of the neck.

ALERT! For personal history of endocrine metabolic and immunity disorders see V12.2

MULTIPLE CODING FOR A SINGLE CONDITION

In addition to the etiology or manifestation convention that requires two codes to fully describe a single condition that affects multiple body systems, there are other single conditions that also require more than one code. "Use additional code" notes are found in the tabular at codes that are not part of an etiology or manifestation pair where a secondary code is useful to fully describe a condition. The sequencing rule is the same as the etiology or manifestation pair - , "use additional code" indicates that a secondary code should be added.

"Code first" notes are also under certain codes that are not specifically manifestation codes but may be due to an underlying cause. When a "code first" note is present and an underlying condition is present the underlying condition should be sequenced first.

"Code, if applicable, any causal condition first", notes indicate that this code may be assigned as a principal diagnosis when the causal condition is unknown or not applicable. If a causal condition is known, then the code for that condition should be sequenced as the principal or first-listed diagnosis. Multiple codes may be needed for late effects, complication codes and obstetric codes to more fully describe a condition. See the specific guidelines for these conditions for further instruction.

COMBINATION CODE

A combination code is a single code used to classify: two diagnoses, or a diagnosis with an associated secondary process (manifestation) A diagnosis with an associated complication Combination codes are identified by referring to subterm entries in the Alphabetic Index and by reading the inclusion and exclusion notes in the Tabular List.

Assign only the combination code when that code fully identifies the diagnostic conditions involved or when the Alphabetic Index so directs. Multiple coding should not be used when the classification provides a combination code that clearly identifies all of the elements documented in the diagnosis. When the combination code lacks necessary specificity in describing the manifestation or complication, an additional code should be used as a secondary code.

CODING LATE EFFECTS

A late effect is the residual effect (condition produced) after the acute phase of an illness or injury has terminated. There is no time limit on when a late effect code can be used. The residual may be apparent early, such as in cerebrovascular accident cases, or it may occur months or years later, such as that due to a previous injury. Coding of late effects generally requires two codes sequenced in the following order: The condition or nature of the late effect is sequenced first. The late effect code is sequenced second.

An exception to the above guidelines are those instances where the code for late effect is followed by a manifestation code identified in the Tabular List and title, or the late effect code has been expanded (at the fourth and fifth-digit levels) to include the manifestation(s). The code for the acute phase of an illness or injury that led to the late effect is never used with a code for the late effect.

DIABETES MELLITUS

Codes under category 250, Diabetes mellitus, identify complications or manifestations associated with diabetes mellitus. A fifth-digit is required for all category 250 codes to identify the type of diabetes mellitus and whether the diabetes is controlled or uncontrolled.

| | Add 4th or 5th digit | | Nonspecific code | | Unspecified code | | Manifestation code |

Fifth-digits for category 250:

The following are the fifth-digits for the codes under category 250:

0   type II or unspecified type, not stated as uncontrolled
1   type I, [juvenile type], not stated as uncontrolled
2   type II or unspecified type, uncontrolled
3   type I, [juvenile type], uncontrolled

The age of a patient is not the sole determining factor, though most type I diabetics develop the condition before reaching puberty. For this reason type I diabetes mellitus is also referred to as juvenile diabetes.

Type of diabetes mellitus not documented

If the type of diabetes mellitus is not documented in the medical record the default is type II.

Diabetes mellitus and the use of insulin

All type I diabetics must use insulin to replace what their bodies do not produce. However, the use of insulin does not mean that a patient is a type I diabetic. Some patients with type II diabetes mellitus are unable to control their blood sugar through diet and oral medication alone and do require insulin. If the documentation in a medical record does not indicate the type of diabetes but does indicate that the patient uses insulin, the appropriate fifth-digit for type II must be used. For type II patients who routinely use insulin, code V58.67, Long-term (current) use of insulin, should also be assigned to indicate that the patient uses insulin. Code V58.67 should not be assigned if insulin is given temporarily to bring a type II patient's blood sugar under control during an encounter.

Assigning and sequencing diabetes codes and associated conditions

When assigning codes for diabetes and its associated conditions, the code(s) from category 250 must be sequenced before the codes for the associated conditions. The diabetes codes and the secondary codes that correspond to them are paired codes that follow the etiology or manifestation convention of the classification (See Official Guidelines, Section I.A.6., Etiology or manifestation convention). Assign as many codes from category 250 as needed to identify all of the associated conditions that the patient has. The corresponding secondary codes are listed under each of the diabetes codes.

A.   Diabetic retinopathy or diabetic macular edema

Diabetic macular edema, code 362.07, is only present with diabetic retinopathy. Another code from subcategory 362.0, Diabetic retinopathy, must be used with code 362.07. Codes under subcategory 362.0 are diabetes manifestation codes, so they must be used following the appropriate diabetes code.

Diabetes mellitus in pregnancy and gestational diabetes

A.   Diabetes mellitus in pregnancy

Diabetes mellitus is a significant complicating factor in pregnancy. Pregnant women who are diabetic should be assigned code 648.0x, Diabetes mellitus complicating pregnancy, and a secondary code from category 250, Diabetes mellitus, or category 249, Secondary diabetes to identify the type of diabetes.

Code V58.67, Long-term (current) use of insulin, should also be assigned if the diabetes mellitus is being treated with insulin.

B.   Gestational diabetes

Gestational diabetes can occur during the second and third trimester of pregnancy in women who were not diabetic prior to pregnancy. Gestational diabetes can cause complications in the pregnancy similar to those of pre-existing diabetes mellitus. It also puts the woman at greater risk of developing diabetes after the pregnancy. Gestational diabetes is coded to 648.8x, Abnormal glucose tolerance. Codes 648.0x and 648.8x should never be used together on the same record.

Code V58.67, Long-term (current) use of insulin, should also be assigned if the gestational diabetes is being treated with insulin.

256   ● Code new
      to this edition   ▲ Revision of
                               existing code   ④ ⑤ Fourth or fifth
                                                          digit required

Insulin pump malfunction

A. Underdose of insulin due insulin pump failure

An underdose of insulin due to an insulin pump failure should be assigned 996.57, Mechanical complication due to insulin pump, as the principal or first listed code, followed by the appropriate diabetes mellitus code based on documentation.

B. Overdose of insulin due to insulin pump failure

The principal or first listed code for an encounter due to an insulin pump malfunction resulting in an overdose of insulin, should also be 996.57, Mechanical complication due to insulin pump, followed by code 962.3, Poisoning by insulins and antidiabetic agents, and the appropriate diabetes mellitus code based on documentation.

Secondary Diabetes Mellitus

Codes under category 249, Secondary diabetes mellitus, identify complications or manifestations associated with secondary diabetes mellitus. Secondary diabetes is always caused by another condition or event (e.g., cystic fibrosis, malignant neoplasm of pancreas, pancreatectomy, adverse effect of drug, or poisoning).

A. Fifth-digits for category 249:

A fifth-digit is required for all category 249 codes to identify whether the diabetes is controlled or uncontrolled.

B. Secondary diabetes mellitus and the use of insulin

For patients who routinely use insulin, code V58.67, Long-term (current) use of insulin, should also be assigned. Code V58.67 should not be assigned if insulin is given temporarily to bring a patient's blood sugar under control during an encounter.

C. Assigning and sequencing secondary diabetes codes and associated conditions

When assigning codes for secondary diabetes and its associated conditions (e.g. renal manifestations), the code(s) from category 249 must be sequenced before the codes for the associated conditions. The secondary diabetes codes and the diabetic manifestation codes that correspond to them are paired codes that follow the etiology or manifestation convention of the classification. Assign as many codes from category 249 as needed to identify all of the associated conditions that the patient has. The corresponding codes for the associated conditions are listed under each of the secondary diabetes codes. For example, secondary diabetes with diabetic nephrosis is assigned to code 249.40, followed by 581.81.

D. Assigning and sequencing secondary diabetes codes and its causes

The sequencing of the secondary diabetes codes in relationship to codes for the cause of the diabetes is based on the reason for the encounter, applicable ICD-9-CM sequencing conventions, and chapter-specific guidelines.

If a patient is seen for treatment of the secondary diabetes or one of its associated conditions, a code from category 249 is sequenced as the principal or first-listed diagnosis, with the cause of the secondary diabetes (e.g. cystic fibrosis) sequenced as an additional diagnosis.

If, however, the patient is seen for the treatment of the condition causing the secondary diabetes (e.g., malignant neoplasm of pancreas), the code for the cause of the secondary diabetes should be sequenced as the principal or first-listed diagnosis followed by a code from category 249.

1) Secondary diabetes mellitus due to pancreatectomy

For postpancreatectomy diabetes mellitus (lack of insulin due to the surgical removal of all or part of the pancreas), assign code 251.3, Postsurgical hypoinsulinemia. A code from subcategory 249 should not be assigned for secondary diabetes mellitus due to pancreatectomy. Code also any diabetic manifestations (e.g. diabetic nephrosis 581.81).

2) Secondary diabetes due to drugs

Secondary diabetes may be caused by an adverse effect of correctly administered medications, poisoning or late effect of poisoning.

| Add 4th or 5th digit | Nonspecific code | Unspecified code | Manifestation code |

See Chapter 17 for coding of adverse effects and poisoning.

See Chapter 19 for reporting of E codes.

● Code new
to this edition

▲ Revision of
existing code

④ ⑤ Fourth or fifth
digit required

3. ENDOCRINE, NUTRITIONAL AND METABOLIC DISEASES, AND IMMUNITY DISORDERS (240-279)

> **Excludes:** *endocrine and metabolic disturbances specific to the fetus and newborn (775.0-775.9)*

Note: All neoplasms, whether functionally active or not, are classified in Chapter 2. Codes in Chapter 3 (i.e., 242.8, 246.0, 251-253, 255-259) may be used, if desired, to identify such functional activity associated with any neoplasm, or by ectopic endocrine tissue.

DISORDERS OF THYROID GLAND (240-246)

240 **Simple and unspecified goiter**

> **DEFINITION** Simple and unspecified goiter is a simple enlargement of the thyroid gland, causing a swelling in the front part of the neck.
>
> **ALERT!** For personal history of endocrine metabolic and immunity disorders see V12.2

240.0 Goiter, specified as simple
Any condition classifiable to 240.9, specified as simple

240.9 Goiter, unspecified
Enlargement of thyroid
Goiter or struma:
  NOS
  diffuse colloid
  endemic
Goiter or struma:
  hyperplastic
  nontoxic (diffuse)
  parenchymatous
  sporadic

> **Excludes:** *congenital (dyshormonogenic) goiter (246.1)*

241 **Nontoxic nodular goiter**

> **Excludes:** *adenoma of thyroid (226)*
> *cystadenoma of thyroid (226)*
>
> **DEFINITION** Nontoxic nodular goiter is a type of simple goiter with enlargement caused by nodules, or lumps, on the thyroid.

241.0 Nontoxic uninodular goiter
Thyroid nodule
Uninodular goiter (nontoxic)

241.1 Nontoxic multinodular goiter
Multinodular goiter (nontoxic)

241.9 Unspecified nontoxic nodular goiter
Adenomatous goiter
Nodular goiter (nontoxic) NOS
Struma nodosa (simplex)

⑤ **242** **Thyrotoxicosis with or without goiter**

> **Excludes:** *neonatal thyrotoxicosis (775.3)*

The following fifth-digit subclassification is for use with category 242:

  0 **without mention of thyrotoxic crisis or storm**

  1 **with mention of thyrotoxic crisis or storm**

> **DEFINITION** Thyrotoxicosis with or without goiter is a condition resulting from excessive concentrations of thyroid hormones in the body, as in hyperthyroidism.

⑤ **242.0 Toxic diffuse goiter**
[0-1]
  Basedow's disease
  Exophthalmic or toxic goiter NOS
  Graves' disease
  Primary thyroid hyperplasia

⑤ **242.1 Toxic uninodular goiter**
[0-1]
  Thyroid nodule, toxic or with hyperthyroidism
  Uninodular goiter, toxic or with hyperthyroidism

⑤ **242.2 Toxic multinodular goiter**
[0-1]
  Secondary thyroid hyperplasia

⑤ **242.3 Toxic nodular goiter, unspecified**
[0-1]
  Adenomatous goiter, toxic or with hyperthyroidism
  Nodular goiter, toxic or with hyperthyroidism
  Struma nodosa, toxic or with hyperthyroidism
  Any condition classifiable to 241.9 specified as toxic or with hyperthyroidism

⑤ **242.4 Thyrotoxicosis from ectopic thyroid nodule**
[0-1]

| | Add 4th or 5th digit | | Nonspecific code | | Unspecified code | | Manifestation code |

⑤ **242.8 Thyrotoxicosis of other specified origin**
[0-1]   Overproduction of thyroid-stimulating hormone [TSH]
Thyrotoxicosis:
  factitia
  from ingestion of excessive thyroid material
Use additional E code to identify cause, if drug-induced

⑤ **242.9 Thyrotoxicosis without mention of goiter or other cause**
[0-1]   Hyperthyroidism NOS
Thyrotoxicosis NOS

243 Congenital hypothyroidism
Congenital thyroid insufficiency
Cretinism (athyrotic) (endemic)
Use additional code to identify associated intellectual disabilities

Excludes: congenital (dyshormonogenic) goiter (246.1)

DEFINITION Congenital hypothyroidism is a congenital glandular disorder resulting from insufficient production of thyroid hormones .

244 Acquired hypothyroidism
Includes: athyroidism (acquired)
  hypothyroidism (acquired)
  myxedema (adult) (juvenile)
  thyroid (gland) insufficiency (acquired)

DEFINITION Acquired hypothyroidism is an acquired glandular disorder resulting from insufficient production of thyroid hormones .

244.0 Postsurgical hypothyroidism

244.1 Other postablative hypothyroidism
Hypothyroidism following therapy, such as irradiation

244.2 Iodine hypothyroidism
Hypothyroidism resulting from administration or ingestion of iodide

Excludes: hypothyroidism resulting from administration of radioactive iodine (244.1)
Use additional E code to identify drug

244.3 Other iatrogenic hypothyroidism
Hypothyroidism resulting from:
  P-aminosalicylic acid [PAS]
  Phenylbutazone
  Resorcinol
Iatrogenic hypothyroidism NOS
Use additional E code to identify drug

244.8 Other specified acquired hypothyroidism
Secondary hypothyroidism NEC

244.9 Unspecified hypothyroidism
Hypothyroidism, primary or NOS
Myxedema, primary or NOS

245 Thyroiditis
DEFINITION Thyroiditis is an inflammation of the thyroid gland.

245.0 Acute thyroiditis
Abscess of thyroid
Thyroiditis:
  nonsuppurative, acute
  pyogenic
  suppurative
Use additional code to identify organism

245.1 Subacute thyroiditis
Thyroiditis: Thyroiditis:
  de Quervain's   granulomatous
  giant cell   viral

245.2 Chronic lymphocytic thyroiditis
Hashimoto's disease   Thyroiditis:
Struma lymphomatosa   autoimmune
                                  lymphocytic (chronic)

● Code new
  to this edition
▲ Revision of
  existing code
④ ⑤ Fourth or fifth
  digit required

245.3 Chronic fibrous thyroiditis
Struma fibrosa
Thyroiditis:
invasive (fibrous)
ligneous
Riedel's

245.4 Iatrogenic thyroiditis
Use additional code to identify cause

245.8 Other and unspecified chronic thyroiditis
Chronic thyroiditis:
NOS
nonspecific

245.9 Thyroiditis, unspecified
Thyroiditis NOS

246 Other disorders of thyroid

246.0 Disorders of thyrocalcitonin secretion
Hypersecretion of calcitonin or thyrocalcitonin

246.1 Dyshormonogenic goiter
Congenital (dyshormonogenic) goiter
Goiter due to enzyme defect in synthesis of thyroid hormone
Goitrous cretinism (sporadic)

246.2 Cyst of thyroid
Excludes: cystadenoma of thyroid (226)

246.3 Hemorrhage and infarction of thyroid

246.8 Other specified disorders of thyroid

Abnormality of	Hyper-TBG-nemia
thyroid-binding globulin	Hypo-TBG-nemia
Atrophy of thyroid	

246.9 Unspecified disorder of thyroid

DISEASES OF OTHER ENDOCRINE GLANDS (249-259)

⑤ 249 Secondary diabetes mellitus
Includes: diabetes mellitus (due to) (in) (secondary) (with):
drug-induced or chemical induced
infection

Excludes: gestational diabetes (648.8)
hyperglycemia NOS (790.29)
neonatal diabetes mellitus (775.1)
nonclinical diabetes (790.29)
Type I diabetes - see category 250
Type II diabetes - see category 250

The following fifth-digit subclassification is for use with category 249:

0 not stated as uncontrolled, or unspecified

1 uncontrolled

Use additional code to identify any associated insulin use (V58.67)

DEFINITION Secondary diabetes is always caused by another condition or event, such as cystic fibrosis, malignant neoplasm of the pancreas, pancreatectomy, adverse effect or drug or poisoning

ALERT! Codes under this category identify complications or manifestations associated with secondary diabetes

ALERT! When assigning codes for secondary diabetes and its associated conditions (e.g., renal manifestations), the code(s) from category 249 must be sequenced before the codes for the associated conditions

⑤ 249.0 Secondary diabetes mellitus without mention of complication
[0-1]   Secondary diabetes mellitus without mention of complication or manifestation
classifiable to 249.1-249.9
Secondary diabetes mellitus NOS

⑤ 249.1 Secondary diabetes mellitus with ketoacidosis
[0-1]   Secondary diabetes mellitus with diabetic acidosis without mention of coma
Secondary diabetes mellitus with diabetic ketosis without mention of coma

⑤ 249.2 Secondary diabetes mellitus with hyperosmolarity
[0-1]   Secondary diabetes mellitus with hyperosmolar (nonketotic) coma

Add 4th or 5th digit   Nonspecific code   Unspecified code   Manifestation code

⑤ **249.3 Secondary diabetes mellitus with other coma**
[0-1]   Secondary diabetes mellitus with diabetic coma (with ketoacidosis)
          Secondary diabetes mellitus with diabetic hypoglycemic coma
          Secondary diabetes mellitus with insulin coma NOS

> Excludes: *secondary diabetes mellitus with hyperosmolar coma (249.2)*

⑤ **249.4 Secondary diabetes mellitus with renal manifestations**
[0-1]

Use additional code to identify manifestation, as:
  chronic kidney disease (585.1-585.9)
  diabetic nephropathy NOS (583.81)
  diabetic nephrosis (581.81)
  intercapillary glomerulosclerosis (581.81)
  Kimmelstiel-Wilson syndrome (581.81)

⑤ **249.5 Secondary diabetes mellitus with ophthalmic manifestations**
[0-1]

Use additional code to identify manifestation, as:
  diabetic blindness (369.00-369.9)
  diabetic cataract (366.41)
  diabetic glaucoma (365.44)
  diabetic macular edema (362.07)
  diabetic retinal edema (362.07)
  diabetic retinopathy (362.01-362.07)

⑤ **249.6 Secondary diabetes mellitus with neurological manifestations**
[0-1]

Use additional code to identify manifestation, as:
  diabetic amyotrophy (353.5)
  diabetic gastroparalysis (536.3)
  diabetic gastroparesis (536.3)
  diabetic mononeuropathy (354.0-355.9)
  diabetic neurogenic arthropathy (713.5)
  diabetic peripheral autonomic neuropathy (337.1)
  diabetic polyneuropathy (357.2)

⑤ **249.7 Secondary diabetes mellitus with peripheral circulatory disorders**
[0-1]

Use additional code to identify manifestation, as:
  diabetic gangrene (785.4)
  diabetic peripheral angiopathy (443.81)

⑤ **249.8 Secondary diabetes mellitus with other specified manifestations**
[0-1]   Secondary diabetic hypoglycemia in diabetes mellitus
          Secondary hypoglycemic shock in diabetes mellitus

Use additional code to identify manifestation, as:
  any associated ulceration (707.10-707.19, 707.8, 707.9)
  diabetic bone changes (731.8)

⑤ **249.9 Secondary diabetes mellitus with unspecified complication**
[0-1]

⑤ **250 Diabetes mellitus**

> Excludes: *gestational diabetes (648.8)*
>   *hyperglycemia NOS (790.29)*
>   *neonatal diabetes mellitus (775.1)*
>   *nonclinical diabetes (790.29)*
>   *secondary diabetes (249.0-249.9)*

The following fifth-digit subclassification is for use with category 250:

  0 type II or unspecified type, not stated as uncontrolled

    Fifth-digit 0 is for use with type II patients, even if the patient requires insulin
    Use additional code, if applicable, for associated long-term (current) insulin use V58.67

  1 type I [juvenile type], not stated as uncontrolled

  2 type II or unspecified type, uncontrolled

    Fifth-digit 2 is for use with type II patients, even if the patient requires insulin
    Use additional code, if applicable, for associated long-term (current) insulin use V58.67

  3 type I [juvenile type], uncontrolled

● Code new
  to this edition
▲ Revision of
  existing code
④ ⑤ Fourth or fifth
  digit required

DEFINITION Diabetes mellitus is a condition in which the pancreas no longer produces enough insulin or cells stop responding to the insulin that is produced, so that glucose in the blood cannot be absorbed into the cells of the body. Symptoms include frequent urination, lethargy, excessive thirst, and hunger.

ALERT! A fifth-digit is required for all category 250 codes to identify the type of diabetes mellitus and whether the diabetes is controlled or uncontrolled

⑤ **250.0 Diabetes mellitus without mention of complication**
[0-3]   Diabetes mellitus without mention of complication or manifestation classifiable to
             250.1-250.9
         Diabetes (mellitus) NOS

⑤ **250.1 Diabetes with ketoacidosis**
[0-3]   Diabetic:
             acidosis without mention of coma
             ketosis without mention of coma

⑤ **250.2 Diabetes with hyperosmolarity**
[0-3]   Hyperosmolar (nonketotic) coma

⑤ **250.3 Diabetes with other coma**
[0-3]   Diabetic coma (with ketoacidosis)
         Diabetic hypoglycemic coma
         Insulin coma NOS

   Excludes: _diabetes with hyperosmolar coma (250.2)_

⑤ **250.4 Diabetes with renal manifestations**
[0-3]
Use additional code to identify manifestation, as:
         chronic kidney disease (585.1-585.9)
         diabetic:
             nephropathy NOS (583.81)
             nephrosis (581.81)
         intercapillary glomerulosclerosis (581.81)
         Kimmelstiel-Wilson syndrome (581.81)

⑤ **250.5 Diabetes with ophthalmic manifestations**
[0-3]
Use additional code to identify manifestation, as:
         diabetic:
             blindness (369.00-369.9)
             cataract (366.41)
             glaucoma (365.44)
             macular edema (362.07)
             retinal edema (362.07)
             retinopathy (362.01-362.07)   ·

⑤ **250.6 Diabetes with neurological manifestations**
[0-3]
Use additional code to identify manifestation, as:
         diabetic:
             amyotrophy (353.5)
             gastroparalysis (536.3)
             gastroparesis (536.3)
             mononeuropathy (354.0-355.9)
             neurogenic arthropathy (713.5)
             peripheral autonomic neuropathy (337.1)
             polyneuropathy (357.2)

⑤ **250.7 Diabetes with peripheral circulatory disorders**
[0-3]
Use additional code to identify manifestation, as:
         diabetic:
             gangrene (785.4)
             peripheral angiopathy (443.81)

⑤ **250.8 Diabetes with other specified manifestations**
[0-3]   Diabetic hypoglycemia NOS
         Hypoglycemic shock NOS
Use additional code to identify manifestation, as:
         any associated ulceration (707.10-707.19, 707.8, 707.9)
         diabetic bone changes (731.8)

⑤ **250.9 Diabetes with unspecified complication**
[0-3]

Add 4th or   Nonspecific   Unspecified   Manifestation
5th digit   code   code   code

251 **Other disorders of pancreatic internal secretion**

251.0 **Hypoglycemic coma**
Iatrogenic hyperinsulinism
Non-diabetic insulin coma

Use additional E code to identify cause, if drug-induced

Excludes: *hypoglycemic coma in diabetes mellitus (249.3, 250.3)*

251.1 **Other specified hypoglycemia**
Hyperinsulinism:
NOS
ectopic
functional
Hyperplasia of pancreatic islet beta cells NOS

Excludes: *hypoglycemia in diabetes mellitus (249.8, 250.8)*
hypoglycemia in infant of diabetic mother (775.0)
hypoglycemic coma (251.0)
neonatal hypoglycemia (775.6)

Use additional E code to identify cause, if drug-induced

251.2 **Hypoglycemia, unspecified**
Hypoglycemia:
NOS
reactive
spontaneous

Excludes: *hypoglycemia:*
with coma (251.0)
in diabetes mellitus (249.8, 250.8)
leucine-induced (270.3)

DEFINITION Hypoglycemia is the medical term for abnormally low blood sugar usually resulting from excessive insulin or a poor diet.

251.3 **Postsurgical hypoinsulinemia**
Hypoinsulinemia following complete or partial pancreatectomy
Postpancreatectomy hyperglycemia

Use additional code to identify (any associated):
acquired absence of pancreas (V88.11-V88.12)
insulin use (V58.67)
secondary diabetes mellitus (249.00-249.91)

Excludes: *transient hyperglycemia post procedure (790.29)*
transient hypoglycemia post procedure (251.2)

251.4 **Abnormality of secretion of glucagon**
Hyperplasia of pancreatic islet alpha cells with glucagon excess

251.5 **Abnormality of secretion of gastrin**
Hyperplasia of pancreatic alpha cells with gastrin excess
Zollinger-Ellison syndrome

251.8 **Other specified disorders of pancreatic internal secretion**

251.9 **Unspecified disorder of pancreatic internal secretion**
Islet cell hyperplasia NOS

252 **Disorders of parathyroid gland**

Excludes: *hungry bone syndrome (275.5)*

⑤ **252.0** **Hyperparathyroidism**

Excludes: *ectopic hyperparathyroidism (259.3)*

252.00 **Hyperparathyroidism, unspecified**

252.01 **Primary hyperparathyroidism**
Hyperplasia of parathyroid

252.02 **Secondary hyperparathyroidism, non-renal**

Excludes: *secondary hyperparathyroidism (of renal origin) (588.81)*

252.08 **Other hyperparathyroidism**
Tertiary hyperparathyroidism

● Code new
to this edition
▲ Revision of
existing code
④ ⑤ Fourth or fifth
digit required

252.1 Hypoparathyroidism
Parathyroiditis (autoimmune)
Tetany:
parathyroid
parathyroprival

Excludes: *pseudohypoparathyroidism (275.4)*
pseudo-pseudohypoparathyroidism (275.4)
tetany NOS (781.7)
transitory neonatal hypoparathyroidism (775.4)

252.8 Other specified disorders of parathyroid gland
Cyst of parathyroid gland
Hemorrhage of parathyroid gland

252.9 Unspecified disorder of parathyroid gland

253 Disorders of the pituitary gland and its hypothalamic control
Includes: the listed conditions whether the disorder is in the pituitary or the hypothalamus

Excludes: *Cushing's syndrome (255.0)*

DEFINITION Disorders of the pituitary gland and its hypothalamic control refers to congenital or acquired abnormalities in the structure or function of the pituitary gland.

253.0 Acromegaly and gigantism
Overproduction of growth hormone

253.1 Other and unspecified anterior pituitary hyperfunction
Forbes-Albright syndrome

Excludes: *overproduction of:*
ACTH (255.3)
thyroid-stimulating hormone [TSH] (242.8)

253.2 Panhypopituitarism
Cachexia, pituitary   Sheehan's syndrome
Necrosis of pituitary   Simmonds' disease
(postpartum)
Pituitary insufficiency NOS

Excludes: *iatrogenic hypopituitarism (253.7)*

253.3 Pituitary dwarfism
Isolated deficiency of (human) growth hormone [HGH]
Lorain-Levi dwarfism

253.4 Other anterior pituitary disorders
Isolated or partial deficiency of an anterior pituitary hormone, other than growth hormone
Prolactin deficiency

253.5 Diabetes insipidus
Vasopressin deficiency

Excludes: *nephrogenic diabetes insipidus (588.1)*

253.6 Other disorders of neurohypophysis
Syndrome of inappropriate secretion of antidiuretic hormone [ADH]

Excludes: *ectopic antidiuretic hormone secretion (259.3)*

253.7 Iatrogenic pituitary disorders
Hypopituitarism:
hormone-induced
hypophysectomy-induced
postablative
radiotherapy-induced

Use additional E code to identify cause

253.8 Other disorders of the pituitary and other syndromes of diencephalohypophyseal origin
Abscess of pituitary   Cyst of Rathke's pouch
Adiposogenital dystrophy   Fröhlich's syndrome

Excludes: *craniopharyngioma (237.0)*

253.9 Unspecified
Dyspituitarism

	Add 4th or 5th digit		Nonspecific code		Unspecified code		Manifestation code

254 **Diseases of thymus gland**

Excludes: *aplasia or dysplasia with immunodeficiency (279.2)*
hypoplasia with immunodeficiency (279.2)
myasthenia gravis (358.00-358.01)

DEFINITION The thymus is a gland located behind the breastbone that functions in the development of the immune system. The thymus is large in infancy and early childhood but begins to atrophy between ages eight and ten.

254.0 Persistent hyperplasia of thymus
Hypertrophy of thymus

254.1 Abscess of thymus

254.8 Other specified diseases of thymus gland
Atrophy of thymus
Cyst of thymus

Excludes *thymoma (212.6)*

254.9 Unspecified disease of thymus gland

255 **Disorders of adrenal glands**
Includes: the listed conditions whether the basic disorder is in the adrenals or is pituitary-induced

DEFINITION The adrenal glands are located on each kidney and secrete hormones regulating metabolism, sexual function, water balance, and stress.

255.0 Cushing's syndrome
Adrenal hyperplasia due to Ectopic ACTH syndrome
excess ACTH Iatrogenic syndrome of excess cortisol
Cushing's syndrome: Overproduction of cortisol
NOS
iatrogenic
idiopathic
pituitary-dependent

Excludes: *congenital adrenal hyperplasia (255.2)*
Use additional E code to identify cause, if drug-induced

⑤ **255.1 Hyperaldosteronism**

255.10 Hyperaldosteronism, unspecified
Aldosteronism NOS
Primary aldosteronism, unspecified

Excludes: *Conn's syndrome (255.12)*

255.11 Glucocorticoid-remediable aldosteronism
Familial aldosteronism type I

Excludes: *Conn's syndrome (255.12)*

255.12 Conn's syndrome

255.13 Bartter's syndrome

255.14 Other secondary aldosteronism

255.2 Adrenogenital disorders
Adrenogenital syndromes, virilizing or feminizing, whether acquired or associated with congenital adrenal hyperplasia consequent on inborn enzyme defects in hormone synthesis
Achard-Thiers syndrome
Congenital adrenal hyperplasia
Female adrenal pseudohermaphroditism
Male:
macrogenitosomia praecox
sexual precocity with adrenal hyperplasia
Virilization (female) (suprarenal)

Excludes: *adrenal hyperplasia due to excess ACTH (255.0)*
isosexual virilization (256.4)

255.3 Other corticoadrenal overactivity
Acquired benign adrenal androgenic overactivity
Overproduction of ACTH

⑤ **255.4 Corticoadrenal insufficiency**

Excludes: *tuberculous Addison's disease (017.6)*

● Code new ▲ Revision of ④ ⑤ Fourth or fifth
to this edition existing code digit required

255.41 Glucocorticoid deficiency
Addisonian crisis
Addison's disease NOS
Adrenal atrophy (autoimmune)
Adrenal calcification
Adrenal crisis
Adrenal hemorrhage
Adrenal infarction
Adrenal insufficiency NOS
Combined glucocorticoid and mineralocorticoid deficiency
Corticoadrenal insufficiency NOS

255.42 Mineralocorticoid deficiency
Hypoaldosteronism

Excludes: *combined glucocorticoid and mineralocorticoid deficiency (255.41)*

255.5 Other adrenal hypofunction
Adrenal medullary insufficiency

Excludes: *Waterhouse-Friderichsen syndrome (meningococcal) (036.3)*

255.6 Medulloadrenal hyperfunction
Catecholamine secretion by pheochromocytoma

255.8 Other specified disorders of adrenal glands
Abnormality of cortisol-binding globulin

255.9 Unspecified disorder of adrenal glands

256 Ovarian dysfunction
DEFINITION Ovarian dysfunction refers to improper functioning of the ovaries.

256.0 Hyperestrogenism

256.1 Other ovarian hyperfunction
Hypersecretion of ovarian androgens

256.2 Postablative ovarian failure
Use additional code for states associated with artifical menopause (627.4)
Ovarian failure:
iatrogenic
postirradiation
postsurgical

Excludes: *asymptomatic age-related (natural) postmenopausal status (V49.81)*
acquired absence of ovary (V45.77)

⑤ **256.3 Other ovarian failure**
Use additional code for states associated with natural menopause (627.2)

Excludes: *asymptomatic age-related (natural) postmenopausal status (V49.81)*

256.31 Premature menopause

256.39 Other ovarian failure
Delayed menarche
Ovarian hypofunction
Primary ovarian failure NOS

256.4 Polycystic ovaries
Isosexual virilization
Stein-Leventhal syndrome

256.8 Other ovarian dysfunction

256.9 Unspecified ovarian dysfunction

257 Testicular dysfunction
DEFINITION Testicular dysfunction refers to improper functioning of the testicles.

257.0 Testicular hyperfunction
Hypersecretion of testicular hormones

257.1 Postablative testicular hypofunction
Testicular hypofunction:
iatrogenic
postirradiation
postsurgical

Add 4th or
5th digit

Nonspecific
code

Unspecified
code

Manifestation
code

257.2 **Other testicular hypofunction**
Defective biosynthesis of testicular androgen
Eunuchoidism:
  NOS
  hypogonadotropic
Failure:
  Leydig's cell, adult
  seminiferous tubule, adult
Testicular hypogonadism

Excludes: *azoospermia (606.0)*

257.8 **Other testicular dysfunction**
Excludes: *androgen insensitivity syndromes (259.50-259.52)*

257.9 **Unspecified testicular dysfunction**

258 **Polyglandular dysfunction and related disorders**
DEFINITION Polyglandular dysfunction and related disorders refers to dysfunctional disorders involving multiple glands.

⑤ **258.0** **Polyglandular activity in multiple endocrine adenomatosis**
Multiple endocrine neoplasia [MEN] syndromes

Use additional codes to identify any malignancies and other conditions associated with the syndromes

    258.01 **Multiple endocrine neoplasia [MEN] type I**
    Wermer's syndrome

    258.02 **Multiple endocrine neoplasia [MEN] type IIA**
    Sipple's syndrome

    258.03 **Multiple endocrine neoplasia [MEN] type IIB**

258.1 **Other combinations of endocrine dysfunction**
Lloyd's syndrome   Schmidt's syndrome

258.8 **Other specified polyglandular dysfunction**

258.9 **Polyglandular dysfunction, unspecified**

259 **Other endocrine disorders**
DEFINITION Endocrine disorders refers to disorders which involve the over-production or under-production of hormone substances from an endocrine gland. Examples include diabetes, hypothyroidism, hyperthyroidism, hyperparathyroidism, cushing's disease, cushing's syndrome and acromegaly.

259.0 **Delay in sexual development and puberty, not elsewhere classified**
Delayed puberty

259.1 **Precocious sexual development and puberty, not elsewhere classified**
Sexual precocity:
  NOS
  constitutional
  cryptogenic
  idiopathic

259.2 **Carcinoid syndrome**
Hormone secretion by carcinoid tumors

259.3 **Ectopic hormone secretion, not elsewhere classified**
Ectopic:
  antidiuretic hormone secretion [ADH]
  hyperparathyroidism

Excludes: *ectopic ACTH syndrome (255.0)*

259.4 **Dwarfism, not elsewhere classified**
Dwarfism:
  NOS
  constitutional

Excludes: *dwarfism:*
    achondroplastic (756.4)
    intrauterine (759.7)
    nutritional (263.2)
    pituitary (253.3)
    renal (588.0)
  progeria (259.8)

● Code new
  to this edition
▲ Revision of
  existing code
④ ⑤ Fourth or fifth
    digit required

⑤ **259.5 Androgen insensitivity syndrome**

    259.50 Androgen insensitivity, unspecified

    259.51 Androgen insensitivity syndrome
        Complete androgen insensitivity
        de Quervain's syndrome
        Goldberg-Maxwell Syndrome

    259.52 Partial androgen insensitivity
        Partial androgen insensitivity syndrome
        Reifenstein syndrome

259.8 Other specified endocrine disorders
    Pineal gland dysfunction
    Progeria

259.9 Unspecified endocrine disorder
    Disturbance: Infantilism NOS
      endocrine NOS
      hormone NOS

NUTRITIONAL DEFICIENCIES (260-269)

    Excludes: deficiency anemias (280.0-281.9)

    ALERT! For personal history of nutritional deficiency see V12.1

260 Kwashiorkor
    Nutritional edema with dyspigmentation of skin and hair
    DEFINITION Kwashiorkor is a virulent form of childhood malnutrition characterized by edema, irritability, anorexia, ulcerating dermatoses, and an enlarged liver with fatty infiltrates.

261 Nutritional marasmus
    Nutritional atrophy   Severe malnutrition NOS
    Severe calorie deficiency
    DEFINITION Nutritional marasmus is extreme malnutrition and emaciation, especially in children; resulting from inadequate intake of food.

262 Other severe protein-calorie malnutrition
    Nutritional edema without mention of dyspigmentation of skin and hair

263 Other and unspecified protein-calorie malnutrition

    263.0 Malnutrition of moderate degree

    263.1 Malnutrition of mild degree

    263.2 Arrested development following protein-calorie malnutrition
        Nutritional dwarfism   Physical retardation due to malnutrition

    263.8 Other protein-calorie malnutrition

    263.9 Unspecified protein-calorie malnutrition
        Dystrophy due to malnutrition
        Malnutrition (calorie) NOS

    Excludes: nutritional deficiency NOS (269.9)

264 Vitamin A deficiency
    DEFINITION Vitamin A deficiency may result in abnormal visual adaptation to darkness (night blindness), dry skin, dry hair, broken fingernails, and decreased resistance to infections .

    264.0 With conjunctival xerosis

    264.1 With conjunctival xerosis and Bitot's spot
        Bitot's spot in the young child

    264.2 With corneal xerosis

    264.3 With corneal ulceration and xerosis

    264.4 With keratomalacia

    264.5 With night blindness

    264.6 With xerophthalmic scars of cornea

    264.7 Other ocular manifestations of vitamin A deficiency
        Xerophthalmia due to vitamin A deficiency

    264.8 Other manifestations of vitamin A deficiency
        Follicular keratosis due to vitamin A deficiency
        Xeroderma due to vitamin A deficiency

    264.9 Unspecified vitamin A deficiency
        Hypovitaminosis A NOS

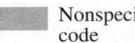

| Add 4th or 5th digit | Nonspecific code | Unspecified code | Manifestation code |

265 **Thiamine and niacin deficiency states**

> **DEFINITION** Thiamine, aka vitamin B1, is a vitamin of the B complex, found in meat, yeast, and the bran coat of grains, necessary for carbohydrate metabolism and normal neural activity. Niacin, aka nicotinic acid, is a component of the vitamin b complex found in meat, wheat germ, dairy products, and yeast. .

265.0 Beriberi

265.1 Other and unspecified manifestations of thiamine deficiency
Other vitamin B_1 deficiency states

265.2 Pellagra
Deficiency:
niacin (-tryptophan)
nicotinamide
nicotinic acid
vitamin PP
Pellagra (alcoholic)

266 Deficiency of B-complex components

266.0 Ariboflavinosis
Riboflavin [vitamin B_2] deficiency

266.1 Vitamin B_6 deficiency
Deficiency: Vitamin B_6 deficiency syndrome
pyridoxal
pyridoxamine
pyridoxine

> Excludes: vitamin B_6-responsive sideroblastic anemia (285.0)

266.2 Other B-complex deficiencies
Deficiency:
cyanocobalamin
folic acid
vitamin B_{12}

> Excludes: combined system disease with anemia (281.0-281.1)
> deficiency anemias (281.0-281.9)
> subacute degeneration of spinal cord with anemia (281.0-281.1)

266.9 Unspecified vitamin B deficiency

267 Ascorbic acid deficiency
Deficiency of vitamin C
Scurvy

> Excludes: scorbutic anemia (281.8)

> **DEFINITION** Ascorbic acid deficiency, refers to a deficiency of ascorbic acid, aka vitamin c is found in citrus fruits, tomatoes, potatoes, and leafy green vegetables and used to prevent scurvy.

268 Vitamin D deficiency

> Excludes: vitamin D-resistant:
> osteomalacia (275.3)
> rickets (275.3)

> **DEFINITION** Vitamin D deficiency, refers to a deficiency of vitamin D2 or D3, required for normal growth of teeth and bones, and produced in general by ultraviolet irradiation of sterols found in milk, fish, and eggs.

268.0 Rickets, active

> Excludes: celiac rickets (579.0)
> renal rickets (588.0)

268.1 Rickets, late effect
Any condition specified as due to rickets and stated to be a late effect or sequela of rickets

Code first the nature of late effect

268.2 Osteomalacia, unspecified

268.9 Unspecified vitamin D deficiency
Avitaminosis D

269 Other nutritional deficiencies

> **DEFINITION** Nutritional deficiencies refers to a disease caused by a deficiency of a particular nutrient such as minerals, vitamins, carbohydrates, fats and proteins.

● Code new
    to this edition

▲ Revision of
    existing code

④ ⑤ Fourth or fifth
    digit required

269.0 Deficiency of vitamin K

Excludes: *deficiency of coagulation factor due to vitamin K deficiency (286.7)*
vitamin K deficiency of newborn (776.0)

269.1 Deficiency of other vitamins
Deficiency:
vitamin E
vitamin P

269.2 Unspecified vitamin deficiency
Multiple vitamin deficiency NOS

269.3 Mineral deficiency, not elsewhere classified
Deficiency:
calcium, dietary
iodine

Excludes: *deficiency:*
calcium NOS (275.4)
potassium (276.8)
sodium (276.1)

269.8 Other nutritional deficiency

Excludes: *adult failure to thrive (783.7)*
failure to thrive in childhood (783.41)
feeding problems (783.3)
newborn (779.31-779.34)

269.9 Unspecified nutritional deficiency

OTHER METABOLIC AND IMMUNITY DISORDERS (270-279)

Use additional code to identify any associated intellectual disabilities

270 Disorders of amino-acid transport and metabolism

Excludes: *abnormal findings without manifest disease (790.0-796.9)*
disorders of purine and pyrimidine metabolism (277.1-277.2)
gout (274.00-274.9)

270.0 Disturbances of amino-acid transport
Cystinosis
Cystinuria
Fanconi (-de Toni) (-Debré) syndrome
Glycinuria (renal)
Hartnup disease

270.1 Phenylketonuria [PKU]
Hyperphenylalaninemia

270.2 Other disturbances of aromatic amino-acid metabolism

Albinism	Hypertyrosinemia
Alkaptonuria	Indicanuria
Alkaptonuric ochronosis	Kynureninase defects
Disturbances of metabolism	Oasthouse urine disease
of tyrosine and	Ochronosis
tryptophan	Tyrosinosis
Homogentisic acid defects	Tyrosinuria
Hydroxykynureninuria	Waardenburg syndrome

Excludes: *vitamin B$_6$-deficiency syndrome (266.1)*

270.3 Disturbances of branched-chain amino-acid metabolism
Disturbances of metabolism of leucine, isoleucine, and valine
Hypervalinemia
Intermittent branched-chain ketonuria
Leucine-induced hypoglycemia
Leucinosis
Maple syrup urine disease

270.4 Disturbances of sulphur-bearing amino-acid metabolism
Cystathioninemia
Cystathioninuria
Disturbances of metabolism of methionine, homocystine, and cystathionine
Homocystinuria
Hypermethioninemia
Methioninemia

Add 4th or   Nonspecific   Unspecified   Manifestation
5th digit   code   code   code

270.5 Disturbances of histidine metabolism
Carnosinemia
Histidinemia
Hyperhistidinemia
Imidazole aminoaciduria

270.6 Disorders of urea cycle metabolism
Argininosuccinic aciduria
Citrullinemia
Disorders of metabolism of ornithine, citrulline, argininosuccinic acid, arginine, and ammonia
Hyperammonemia
Hyperornithinemia

270.7 Other disturbances of straight-chain amino-acid metabolism
Glucoglycinuria
Glycinemia (with methyl-malonic acidemia)
Hyperglycinemia
Hyperlysinemia
Pipecolic acidemia
Saccharopinuria
Other disturbances of metabolism of glycine, threonine, serine, glutamine, and lysine

270.8 Other specified disorders of amino-acid metabolism
Alaninemia
Ethanolaminuria
Glycoprolinuria
Hydroxyprolinemia
Hyperprolinemia
Iminoacidopathy
Prolinemia
Prolinuria
Sarcosinemia

270.9 Unspecified disorder of amino-acid metabolism

271 Disorders of carbohydrate transport and metabolism

Excludes: abnormality of secretion of glucagon (251.4)
diabetes mellitus (249.0-249.9, 250.0-250.9)
hypoglycemia NOS (251.2)
mucopolysaccharidosis (277.5)

271.0 Glycogenosis
Amylopectinosis
Glucose-6-phosphatase deficiency
Glycogen storage disease
McArdle's disease
Pompe's disease
von Gierke's disease

271.1 Galactosemia
Galactose-1-phosphate uridyl transferase deficiency
Galactosuria

271.2 Hereditary fructose intolerance
Essential benign fructosuria
Fructosemia

271.3 Intestinal disaccharidase deficiencies and disaccharide malabsorption
Intolerance or malabsorption (congenital) (of):
glucose-galactose
lactose
sucrose-isomaltose

271.4 Renal glycosuria
Renal diabetes

271.8 Other specified disorders of carbohydrate transport and metabolism
Essential benign pentosuria
Fucosidosis
Glycolic aciduria
Hyperoxaluria (primary)
Mannosidosis
Oxalosis
Xylosuria
Xylulosuria

271.9 Unspecified disorder of carbohydrate transport and metabolism

272 Disorders of lipoid metabolism

Excludes: localized cerebral lipidoses (330.1)

272.0 Pure hypercholesterolemia
Familial hypercholesterolemia
Fredrickson Type IIa hyperlipoproteinemia
Hyperbetalipoproteinemia
Hyperlipidemia, Group A
Low-density-lipoid-type [LDL] hyperlipoproteinemia

● Code new to this edition   ▲ Revision of existing code   ④ ⑤ Fourth or fifth digit required

272.1 Pure hyperglyceridemia
  Endogenous hyperglyceridemia
  Frederickson Type IV hyperlipoproteinemia
  Hyperlipidemia, Group B
  Hyperprebetalipoproteinemia
  Hypertriglyceridemia, essential
  Very-low-density-lipoid-type [VLDL] hyperlipoproteinemia

272.2 Mixed hyperlipidemia
  Broad- or floating-betalipoproteinemia
  Combined hyperlipidemia
  Elevated cholesterol with elevated triglycerides NEC
  Fredrickson Type IIb or III hyperlipoproteinemia
  Hypercholesterolemia with endogenous hyperglyceridemia
  Hyperbetalipoproteinemia with prebetalipoproteinemia
  Tubo-eruptive xanthoma
  Xanthoma tuberosum

272.3 Hyperchylomicronemia
  Bürger-Grütz syndrome
  Fredrickson type I or V hyperlipoproteinemia
  Hyperlipidemia, Group D
  Mixed hyperglyceridemia

272.4 Other and unspecified hyperlipidemia
  Alpha-lipoproteinemia
  Hyperlipidemia NOS
  Hyperlipoproteinemia NOS

272.5 Lipoprotein deficiencies
  Abetalipoproteinemia
  Bassen-Kornzweig syndrome
  High-density lipoid deficiency
  Hypoalphalipoproteinemia
  Hypobetalipoproteinemia (familial)

272.6 Lipodystrophy
  Barraquer-Simons disease
  Progressive lipodystrophy

Use additional E code to identify cause, if iatrogenic

  Excludes: intestinal lipodystrophy (040.2)

272.7 Lipidoses

Chemically-induced lipidosis	Disease:
Disease:	triglyceride storage, Type I or II
Anderson's	Wolman's or triglyceride storage, Type III
Fabry's	Mucolipidosis II
Gaucher's	Primary familial xanthomatosis
I cell [mucolipidosis I]	
lipoid storage NOS	
Neimann-Pick	
pseudo-Hurler's or	
mucolipidosis III	

  Excludes: cerebral lipidoses (330.1)
        Tay-Sachs disease (330.1)

272.8 Other disorders of lipoid metabolism
  Hoffa's disease or liposynovitis prepatellaris
  Launois-Bensaude's lipomatosis
  Lipoid dermatoarthritis

272.9 Unspecified disorder of lipoid metabolism

273 Disorders of plasma protein metabolism

  Excludes: agammaglobulinemia and hypogammaglobulinemia (279.0 -279.2)
        coagulation defects (286.0-286.9)
        hereditary hemolytic anemias (282.0-282.9)

273.0 Polyclonal hypergammaglobulinemia
  Hypergammaglobulinemic purpura:
  benign primary
  Waldenström's

273.1 Monoclonal paraproteinemia
Benign monoclonal hypergammaglobulinemia [BMH]
Monoclonal gammopathy:
  NOS
  associated with lymphoplasmacytic dyscrasias
  benign
Paraproteinemia:
  benign (familial)
  secondary to malignant or inflammatory disease

273.2 Other paraproteinemias
Cryoglobulinemic: Mixed cryoglobulinemia
  purpura
  vasculitis

273.3 Macroglobulinemia
Macroglobulinemia (idiopathic) (primary)
Waldenström's macroglobulinemia

273.4 Alpha-1-antitrypsin deficiency
AAT deficiency

273.8 Other disorders of plasma protein metabolism
Abnormality of transport protein
Bisalbuminemia

273.9 Unspecified disorder of plasma protein metabolism

274 Gout

Excludes: lead gout (984.0-984.9)

DEFINITION Gout is a painful inflammation of the big toe and foot caused by defects in uric acid metabolism resulting in deposits of the acid and its salts in the blood and joints.

⑤ **274.0 Gouty arthropathy**

274.00 Gout arthropathy, unspecified

274.01 Acute gouty arthropathy
Acute gout
Gout attack
Gout flare
Podagra

274.02 Chronic gouty arthropathy without mention of tophus (tophi)
Chronic gout

274.03 Chronic gouty arthropathy with tophus (tophi)
Chronic tophaceous gout
Gout with tophi NOS

⑤ **274.1 Gouty nephropathy**

274.10 Gouty nephropathy, unspecified

274.11 Uric acid nephrolithiasis

274.19 Other

⑤ **274.8 Gout with other specified manifestations**

274.81 Gouty tophi of ear

274.82 Gouty tophi of other sites
Gouty tophi of heart

Excludes: gout with tophi NOS (274.03)
        gouty arthropathy with tophi (274.03)

274.89 Other
Use additional code to identify manifestations, as:
        gouty:
          iritis (364.11)
          neuritis (357.4)

274.9 Gout, unspecified

275 Disorders of mineral metabolism

Excludes: abnormal findings without manifest disease (790.0-796.9)

⑤ **275.0 Disorders of iron metabolism**

Excludes: anemia:
        iron deficiency (280.0-280.9)
        sideroblastic (285.0)

● Code new   ▲ Revision of   ④ ⑤ Fourth or fifth
         to this edition   existing code   digit required

275.01 Hereditary hemochromatosis
Bronzed diabetes
Pigmentary cirrhosis (of liver)
Primary (hereditary) hemochromatosis

275.02 Hemochromatosis due to repeated red blood cell transfusions
Iron overload due to repeated red blood cell transfusions
Transfusion (red blood cell) associated hemochromatosis

275.03 Other hemochromatosis
Hemochromatosis NOS

275.09 Other disorders of iron metabolism

275.1 Disorders of copper metabolism
Hepatolenticular degeneration
Wilson's disease

275.2 Disorders of magnesium metabolism
Hypermagnesemia
Hypomagnesemia

275.3 Disorders of phosphorus metabolism
Familial hypophosphatemia
Hypophosphatasia
Vitamin D-resistant:
  osteomalacia
  rickets

⑤ **275.4 Disorders of calcium metabolism**

Excludes: *hungry bone syndrome (275.5)*
parathyroid disorders (252.00-252.9)
vitamin D deficiency (268.0-268.9)

275.40 Unspecified disorder of calcium metabolism

275.41 Hypocalcemia

275.42 Hypercalcemia

275.49 Other disorders of calcium metabolism
Nephrocalcinosis
Pseudohypoparathyroidism
Pseudopseudohypoparathyroidism

275.5 Hungry bone syndrome

275.8 Other specified disorders of mineral metabolism

275.9 Unspecified disorder of mineral metabolism

276 Disorders of fluid, electrolyte, and acid-base balance

Excludes: *diabetes insipidus (253.5)*
familial periodic paralysis (359.3)

276.0 Hyperosmolality and/or hypernatremia
Sodium [Na] excess
Sodium [Na] overload

276.1 Hyposmolality and/or hyponatremia
Sodium [Na] deficiency

276.2 Acidosis
Acidosis:
  NOS
  lactic
  metabolic
  respiratory

Excludes: *diabetic acidosis (249.1, 250.1)*

276.3 Alkalosis
Alkalosis:
  NOS
  metabolic
  respiratory

276.4 Mixed acid-base balance disorder
Hypercapnia with mixed acid-base disorder

| | Add 4th or 5th digit | | Nonspecific code | | Unspecified code | | Manifestation code |

⑤ **276.5 Volume depletion**

Excludes: *hypovolemic shock:*
postoperative (998.09)

> **276.50 Volume depletion, unspecified**
> **276.51 Dehydration**
> **276.52 Hypovolemia**
> Depletion of volume of plasma

⑤ **276.6 Fluid overload**

Excludes: *ascites (789.51-789.59)*
localized edema (782.3)

> **276.61 Transfusion associated circulatory overload**
> Fluid overload due to transfusion (blood) (blood components)
> TACO

> **276.69 Other fluid overload**
> Fluid retention

276.7 Hyperpotassemia
Hyperkalemia
Potassium [K]:
  excess
  intoxication
  overload

276.8 Hypopotassemia
Hypokalemia
Potassium [K] deficiency

276.9 Electrolyte and fluid disorders not elsewhere classified
Electrolyte imbalance
Hyperchloremia
Hypochloremia

Excludes: *electrolyte imbalance:*
associated with hyperemesis gravidarum (643.1)
complicating labor and delivery (669.0)
following abortion and ectopic or molar pregnancy (634-638 with .4, 639.4)

277 Other and unspecified disorders of metabolism

⑤ **277.0 Cystic fibrosis**
Fibrocystic disease of the pancreas
Mucoviscidosis

> **277.00 Without mention of meconium ileus**
> Cystic fibrosis NOS

> **277.01 With meconium ileus**
> Meconium:
>   ileus (of newborn)
>   obstruction of intestine in mucoviscidosis

> **277.02 With pulmonary manifestations**
> Cystic fibrosis with pulmonary exacerbation

Use additional code to identify any infectious organism present, such as:
  pseudomonas (041.7)

> **277.03 With gastrointestinal manifestations**

Excludes: *with meconium ileus (277.01)*

> **277.09 With other manifestations**

277.1 Disorders of porphyrin metabolism

Hematoporphyria   Porphyrinuria
Hematoporphyrinuria   Protocoproporphyria
Hereditary coproporphyria Protoporphyria
Porphyria   Pyrroloporphyria

277.2 Other disorders of purine and pyrimidine metabolism
Hypoxanthine-guanine-phosphoribosyltransferase deficiency [HG-PRT deficiency]
Lesch-Nyhan syndrome
Xanthinuria

Excludes: *gout (274.00-274.9)*
orotic aciduric anemia (281.4)

⑤ **277.3 Amyloidosis**

● Code new
to this edition

▲ Revision of
existing code

④ ⑤ Fourth or fifth
digit required

277.30 **Amyloidosis, unspecified**
Amyloidosis NOS

277.31 **Familial Mediterranean fever**
Benign paroxysmal peritonitis
Hereditary amyloid nephropathy
Periodic familial polyserositis
Recurrent polyserositis

277.39 **Other amyloidosis**
Hereditary cardiac amyloidosis
Inherited systemic amyloidosis
Neuropathic (Portuguese) (Swiss) amyloidosis
Secondary amyloidosis

277.4 **Disorders of bilirubin excretion**
Hyperbilirubinemia:
congenital
constitutional
Syndrome:
Crigler-Najjar
Dubin-Johnson
Gilbert's
Rotor's

Excludes: *hyperbilirubinemias specific to the perinatal period (774.0-774.7)*

277.5 **Mucopolysaccharidosis**
Gargoylism   Morquio-Brailsford disease
Hunter's syndrome   Osteochondrodystrophy
Hurler's syndrome   Sanfilippo's syndrome
Lipochondrodystrophy   Scheie's syndrome
Maroteaux-Lamy syndrome

277.6 **Other deficiencies of circulating enzymes**
Hereditary angioedema

277.7 **Dysmetabolic syndrome X**
Use additional code for associated manifestation, such as:
cardiovascular disease (414.00-414.07)
obesity (278.00-278.03)

⑤ **277.8** **Other specified disorders of metabolism**

277.81 **Primary carnitine deficiency**

277.82 **Carnitine deficiency due to inborn errors of metabolism**

277.83 **Iatrogenic carnitine deficiency**
Carnitine deficiency due to:
hemodialysis
valproic acid therapy

277.84 **Other secondary carnitine deficiency**

277.85 **Disorders of fatty acid oxidation**
Carnitine palmitoyltransferase deficiencies (CPT1, CPT2)
Glutaric aciduria type II (type IIA, IIB, IIC)
Long chain 3-hydroxyacyl CoA dehydrogenase deficiency (LCHAD)
Long chain/very long chain acyl CoA dehydrogenase deficiency (LCAD, VLCAD)
Medium chain acyl CoA dehydrogenase deficiency (MCAD)
Short chain acyl CoA dehydrogenase deficiency (SCAD)

Excludes: *primary carnitine deficiency (277.81)*

277.86 **Peroxisomal disorders**
Adrenomyeloneuropathy
Neonatal adrenoleukodystrophy
Rhizomelic chrondrodysplasia punctata
X-linked adrenoleukodystrophy
Zellweger syndrome

Excludes: *infantile Refsum disease (356.3)*

Add 4th or   Nonspecific   Unspecified   Manifestation
5th digit   code   code   code

277.87 Disorders of mitochondrial metabolism
Kearns-Sayre syndrome
Mitochondrial Encephalopathy, Lactic Acidosis and Stroke-like episodes (MELAS syndrome)
Mitochondrial Neurogastrointestinal Encephalopathy syndrome (MNGIE)
Myoclonus with Epilepsy and with Ragged Red Fibers (MERRF syndrome)
Neuropathy, Ataxia and Retinitis Pigmentosa (NARP syndrome)
Use additional code for associated conditions

Excludes: *disorders of pyruvate metabolism (271.8)*
Leber's optic atrophy (377.16)
Leigh's subacute necrotizing encephalopathy (330.8)
Reye's syndrome (331.81)

277.88 Tumor lysis syndrome
Spontaneous tumor lysis syndrome
Tumor lysis syndrome following antineoplastic drug therapy
Use additional E code to identify cause, if drug-induced

277.89 Other specified disorders of metabolism
Hand-Schuller-Christian disease
Histiocytosis (acute) (chronic)
Histiocytosis X (chronic)

Excludes: *histiocytosis:*
acute differentiatied progressive (202.5)
adult pulmonary Langerhans cell (516.5)
X, acute (progressive) (202.5)

277.9 Unspecified disorder of metabolism
Enzymopathy NOS

278 Overweight, obesity and other hyperalimentation

Excludes: *hyperalimentation NOS (783.6)*
poisoning by vitamins NOS (963.5)
polyphagia (783.6)
Use additional code to identify Body Mass Index (BMI), if known (V85.21-V85.25, V85.30-V85.39, V85.4, V85.53, V85.54)

⑤ **278.0 Overweight and obesity**
Use additional code to identify Body Mass Index (BMI), if known (V85.0-V85.54)

Excludes: *adiposogenital dystrophy (253.8)*
obesity of endocrine origin NOS (259.9)

278.00 Obesity, unspecified
Obesity NOS

278.01 Morbid obesity
Severe obesity

278.02 Overweight

278.03 Obesity hypoventilation syndrome
Pickwickian syndrome

278.1 Localized adiposity
Fat pad

278.2 Hypervitaminosis A

278.3 Hypercarotinemia

278.4 Hypervitaminosis D

278.8 Other hyperalimentation

279 Disorders involving the immune mechanism
Use additional code for associated manifestations

⑤ **279.0 Deficiency of humoral immunity**

279.00 Hypogammaglobulinemia, unspecified
Agammaglobulinemia NOS

279.01 Selective IgA immunodeficiency

279.02 Selective IgM immunodeficiency

279.03 Other selective immunoglobulin deficiencies
Selective deficiency of IgG

● Code new
to this edition
▲ Revision of
existing code
④ ⑤ Fourth or fifth
digit required

279.04 **Congenital hypogammaglobulinemia**
Agammaglobulinemia:
Bruton's type
X-linked

279.05 **Immunodeficiency with increased IgM**
Immunodeficiency with hyper-IgM:
autosomal recessive
X-linked

279.06 **Common variable immunodeficiency**
Dysgammaglobulinemia (acquired) (congenital) (primary)
Hypogammaglobulinemia:
acquired primary
congenital non-sex-linked
sporadic

279.09 **Other**
Transient hypogammaglobulinemia of infancy

⑤ **279.1** **Deficiency of cell-mediated immunity**

279.10 **Immunodeficiency with predominant T-cell defect, unspecified**

279.11 **DiGeorge's syndrome**
Pharyngeal pouch syndrome
Thymic hypoplasia

279.12 **Wiskott-Aldrich syndrome**

279.13 **Nezelof's syndrome**
Cellular immunodeficiency with abnormal immunoglobulin deficiency

279.19 **Other**

Excludes: *ataxia-telangiectasia (334.8)*

279.2 **Combined immunity deficiency**
Agammaglobulinemia:
autosomal recessive
Swiss-type
x-linked recessive
Severe combined immunodeficiency [SCID]
Thymic:
alymphoplasia
aplasia or dysplasia with immunodeficiency

Excludes: *thymic hypoplasia (279.11)*

279.3 **Unspecified immunity deficiency**

⑤ **279.4** **Autoimmune disease, not elsewhere classified**

Excludes: *transplant failure or rejection (996.80-996.89)*

279.41 **Autoimmune lymphoproliferative syndrome**
ALPS

279.49 **Autoimmune disease, not elsewhere classified**
Autoimmune disease NOS

⑤ **279.5** **Graft-versus-host disease**

Code first underlying cause, such as:
complication of blood transfusion (999.89)
complication of transplanted organ (996.80-996.89)

Use additional code to identify associated manifestations, such as:
desquamative dermatitis (695.89)
diarrhea (787.91)
elevated bilirubin (782.4)
hair loss (704.09)

279.50 **Graft-versus-host disease, unspecified**

279.51 **Acute graft-versus-host disease**

279.52 **Chronic graft-versus-host disease**

279.53 **Acute on chronic graft-versus-host disease**

279.8 **Other specified disorders involving the immune mechanism**
Single complement [C_1-C_9] deficiency or dysfunction

279.9 **Unspecified disorder of immune mechanism**

279

	Add 4th or 5th digit		Nonspecific code		Unspecified code		Manifestation code

This page intentionally left blank.

Chapter 4: Diseases of Blood and Blood Forming Organs (280-289)

DEFINITIONS AND CODING ALERTS

This chapter includes definitions of selected key words, terms and phrases and coding alerts for adding points to the clinical domain, references to coding late effects where appropriate, and references to personal history V-codes in situations where the acute or chronic condition is no longer active. An example from this chapter is as follows:

282 Hereditary hemolytic anemias
> **DEFINITION** Hereditary hemolytic anemias are caused by the destruction of red blood cells by a disease process. Occurs in newborns as a result of blood- group incompatibility between mother and baby. It is also caused by abnormal red cell membranes or abnormal hemoglobin, ie, sickle cell anemia and thallassemia.

MULTIPLE CODING FOR A SINGLE CONDITION

In addition to the etiology or manifestation convention that requires two codes to fully describe a single condition that affects multiple body systems, there are other single conditions that also require more than one code. "Use additional code" notes are found in the tabular at codes that are not part of an etiology or manifestation pair where a secondary code is useful to fully describe a condition. The sequencing rule is the same as the etiology or manifestation pair - , "use additional code" indicates that a secondary code should be added.

"Code first" notes are also under certain codes that are not specifically manifestation codes but may be due to an underlying cause. When a "code first" note is present and an underlying condition is present the underlying condition should be sequenced first.

"Code, if applicable, any causal condition first", notes indicate that this code may be assigned as a principal diagnosis when the causal condition is unknown or not applicable. If a causal condition is known, then the code for that condition should be sequenced as the principal or first-listed diagnosis. Multiple codes may be needed for late effects, complication codes and obstetric codes to more fully describe a condition. See the specific guidelines for these conditions for further instruction.

COMBINATION CODE

A combination code is a single code used to classify: two diagnoses, or a diagnosis with an associated secondary process (manifestation) A diagnosis with an associated complication Combination codes are identified by referring to subterm entries in the Alphabetic Index and by reading the inclusion and exclusion notes in the Tabular List.

Assign only the combination code when that code fully identifies the diagnostic conditions involved or when the Alphabetic Index so directs. Multiple coding should not be used when the classification provides a combination code that clearly identifies all of the elements documented in the diagnosis. When the combination code lacks necessary specificity in describing the manifestation or complication, an additional code should be used as a secondary code.

CODING LATE EFFECTS

A late effect is the residual effect (condition produced) after the acute phase of an illness or injury has terminated. There is no time limit on when a late effect code can be used. The residual may be apparent early, such as in cerebrovascular accident cases, or it may occur months or years later, such as that due to a previous injury. Coding of late effects generally requires two codes sequenced in the following order: The condition or nature of the late effect is sequenced first. The late effect code is sequenced second.

An exception to the above guidelines are those instances where the code for late effect is followed by a manifestation code identified in the Tabular List and title, or the late effect code has been expanded (at the fourth and fifth-digit levels) to include the manifestation(s). The code for the acute phase of an illness or injury that led to the late effect is never used with a code for the late effect.

ANEMIA OF CHRONIC DISEASE

Subcategory 285.2, Anemia in chronic illness, has codes for anemia in chronic kidney disease, code 285.21; anemia in neoplastic disease, code 285.22; and anemia in other chronic illness, code 285.29. These codes can be used as the principal or first listed code if the reason for the encounter is to treat the anemia. They may also be used as secondary codes if treatment of the anemia is a component of an encounter, but not the primary reason for the encounter. When using a code from subcategory 285 it is also necessary to use the code for the chronic condition causing the anemia.

Add 4th or 5th digit | Nonspecific code | Unspecified code | Manifestation code

Anemia in chronic kidney disease

When assigning code 285.21, Anemia in chronic kidney disease, it is also necessary to assign a code from category 585, Chronic kidney disease, to indicate the stage of chronic kidney disease.

See Chapter 10 for information regarding. Chronic kidney disease (CKD).

Anemia in neoplastic disease

When assigning code 285.22, Anemia in neoplastic disease, it is also necessary to assign the neoplasm code that is responsible for the anemia. Code 285.22 is for use for anemia that is due to the malignancy, not for anemia due to antineoplastic chemotherapy drugs, which is an adverse effect.

See Chapter 2 for information regarding anemia associated with malignancy, chemotherapy, immunotherapy and radiation therapy.

See Chapter 17 for information regarding adverse effects.

● Code new
to this edition

▲ Revision of
existing code

④ ⑤ Fourth or fifth
digit required

4. DISEASES OF THE BLOOD AND BLOOD-FORMING ORGANS (280-289)

Excludes: anemia complicating pregnancy or the puerperium (648.2)

ALERT! For personal history of diseases of blood and blood-forming organs see V12.3

280 Iron deficiency anemias
Includes: anemia:
    asiderotic
    hypochromic-microcytic
    sideropenic

Excludes: familial microcytic anemia (282.49)

DEFINITION Iron deficiency anemia is a form of anemia due to lack of iron in the diet or to iron loss as a result of chronic bleeding.

280.0 Secondary to blood loss (chronic)
Normocytic anemia due to blood loss

Excludes: acute posthemorrhagic anemia (285.1)

280.1 Secondary to inadequate dietary iron intake

280.8 Other specified iron deficiency anemias
Paterson-Kelly syndrome
Plummer-Vinson syndrome
Sideropenic dysphagia

280.9 Iron deficiency anemia, unspecified
Anemia:
    achlorhydric
    chlorotic
    idiopathic hypochromic
    iron [Fe] deficiency NOS

281 Other deficiency anemias

281.0 Pernicious anemia
Anemia: Congenital intrinsic factor [Castle's] deficiency
    Addison's
    Biermer's
    congenital pernicious

Excludes: combined system disease without mention of anemia (266.2)
    subacute degeneration of spinal cord without mention of anemia (266.2)

281.1 Other vitamin B_{12} deficiency anemia
Anemia:
    vegan's
    vitamin B_{12} deficiency (dietary)
    due to selective vitamin B_{12} malabsorption with proteinuria
Syndrome:
    Imerslund's
    Imerslund-Gräsbeck

Excludes: combined system disease without mention of anemia (266.2)
    subacute degeneration of spinal cord without mention of anemia (266.2)

281.2 Folate-deficiency anemia
Congenital folate malabsorption
Folate or folic acid deficiency anemia:
    NOS
    dietary
    drug-induced
Goat's milk anemia
Nutritional megaloblastic anemia (of infancy)

Use additional E code, if desired, to identify drug

281.3 Other specified megaloblastic anemias not elsewhere classified
Combined B_{12} and folate-deficiency anemia
Refractory megaloblastic anemia

281.4 Protein-deficiency anemia
Amino-acid-deficiency anemia

281.8 Anemia associated with other specified nutritional deficiency
Scorbutic anemia

Add 4th or 5th digit   Nonspecific code   Unspecified code   Manifestation code

281.9 Unspecified deficiency anemia
Anemia:
dimorphic
macrocytic
megaloblastic NOS

Anemia:
nutritional NOS
simple chronic

282 Hereditary hemolytic anemias
DEFINITION Hereditary hemolytic anemias are caused by the destruction of red blood cells by a disease process. Occurs in newborns as a result of blood- group incompatibility between mother and baby. It is also caused by abnormal red cell membranes or abnormal hemoglobin, ie, sickle cell anemia and thalassemia.

282.0 Hereditary spherocytosis
Acholuric (familial) jaundice
Congenital hemolytic anemia (spherocytic)
Congenital spherocytosis
Minkowski-Chauffard syndrome
Spherocytosis (familial)

Excludes: hemolytic anemia of newborn (773.0-773.5)

282.1 Hereditary elliptocytosis
Elliptocytosis (congenital)
Ovalocytosis (congenital) (hereditary)

282.2 Anemias due to disorders of glutathione metabolism
Anemia:
6-phosphogluconic dehydrogenase deficiency
enzyme deficiency, drug-induced
erythrocytic glutathione deficiency
glucose-6-phosphate dehydrogenase [G-6-PD] deficiency
glutathione-reductase deficiency
hemolytic nonspherocytic (hereditary), type I
Disorder of pentose phosphate pathway
Favism

282.3 Other hemolytic anemias due to enzyme deficiency
Anemia:
hemolytic nonspherocytic (hereditary), type II
hexokinase deficiency
pyruvate kinase [PK] deficiency
triosephosphate isomerase deficiency

⑤ **282.4 Thalassemias**
Excludes: sickle-cell:
disease (282.60-282.69)
trait (282.5)

● **282.40 Thalassemia, unspecified**
Thalassemia NOS

282.41 Sickle-cell thalassemia without crisis
Sickle-cell thalassemia NOS
Microdrepanocytosis
Thalassemia Hb-S disease without crisis

282.42 Sickle-cell thalassemia with crisis
Sickle-cell thalassemia with vaso-occlusive pain
Thalassemia Hb-S disease with crisis
Use additional code for types of crisis, such as:
acute chest syndrome (517.3)
splenic sequestration (289.52)

● **282.43 Alpha thalassemia**
Alpha thalassemia major
Hemoglobin H Constant Spring
Hemoglobin H disease
Hydrops fetalis due to alpha thalassemia
Severe alpha thalassemia
Triple gene defect alpha thalassemia

Excludes: alpha thalassemia trait or minor (282.46)
hydrops fetalis due to isoimmunization (773.3)
hydrops fetalis not due to immune hemolysis (778.0)

● Code new
to this edition
▲ Revision of
existing code
④ ⑤ Fourth or fifth
digit required

● **282.44 Beta thalassemia**
  Beta thalassemia major
  Cooley's anemia
  Homozygous beta thalassemia
  Severe beta thalassemia
  Thalassemia intermedia
  Thalassemia major

Excludes: beta thalassemia minor (282.46)
  beta thalassemia trait (282.46)
  delta-beta thalassemia (282.45)
  hemoglobin E beta thalassemia (282.47)
  sickle-cell beta thalassemia (282.41, 282.42)

● **282.45 Delta-beta thalassemia**
  Homozygous delta-beta thalassemia

Excludes: delta-beta thalassemia trait (282.46)

● **282.46 Thalassemia minor**
  Alpha thalassemia minor
  Alpha thalassemia silent carrier
  Alpha thalassemia trait
  Beta thalassemia minor
  Beta thalassemia trait
  Delta-beta thalassemia trait
  Thalassemia trait NOS

Excludes: alpha thalassemia (282.43)
  beta thalassemia (282.44)
  delta-beta thalassemia (282.45)
  hemoglobin E-beta thalassemia (282.47)
  sickle-cell trait (282.5)

● **282.47 Hemoglobin E-beta thalassemia**

Excludes: beta thalassemia (282.44)
  beta thalassemia minor (282.46)
  beta thalassemia trait (282.46)
  delta-beta thalassemia (282.45)
  delta-beta thalassemia trait (282.46)
  hemoglobin E disease (282.7)
  other hemoglobinopathies (282.7)
  sickle-cell beta thalassemia (282.41, 282.42)

282.49 Other thalassemia
  Dominant thalassemia
  Hemoglobin C thalassemia
  Hereditary leptocytosis
  Mediterranean anemia (with other hemoglobinopathy)
  Mixed thalassemia
  Thalassemia with other hemoglobinopathy

Excludes: hemoglobin C disease (282.7)
  hemoglobin E disease (282.7)
  other hemoglobinopathies (282.7)
  sickle-cell anemias (282.60-282.69)
  sickle-cell beta thalassemia (282.41-282.42)

282.5 Sickle-cell trait
  Hb-AS genotype   Heterozygous:
  Hemoglobin S [Hb-S] trait   hemoglobin S
                              Hb-S

Excludes: that with other hemoglobinopathy (282.60-282.69)
  that with thalassemia (282.41-282.42)

⑤ **282.6 Sickle-cell disease**
  Sickle-cell anemia

Excludes: sickle-cell thalassemia (282.41-282.42)
  sickle-cell trait (282.5)

282.60 Sickle-cell disease, unspecified
  Sickle-cell anemia NOS

282.61 Hb-SS disease without crisis

Add 4th or 5th digit | Nonspecific code | Unspecified code | Manifestation code

282.62 Hb-SS disease with crisis
Hb-SS disease with vaso-occlusive pain
Sickle-cell crisis NOS

Use additional code for type of crisis, such as:
acute chest syndrome (517.3)
splenic sequestration (289.52)

282.63 Sickle-cell/Hb-C disease without crisis
Hb-S/Hb-C disease without crisis

282.64 Sickle-cell/Hb-C disease with crisis
Hb-S/Hb-C disease with crisis
Sickle-cell/Hb-C disease with vaso-occlusive pain

Use additional code for type of crisis, such as:
acute chest syndrome (517.3)
splenic sequestration (289.52)

282.68 Other sickle-cell disease without crisis
Hb-S/Hb-D disease without crisis
Hb-S/Hb-E disease without crisis
Sickle-cell/Hb-D disease without crisis
Sickle-cell/Hb-E disease without crisis

282.69 Other sickle-cell disease with crisis
Hb-S/Hb-D disease with crisis
Hb-S/Hb-E disease with crisis
Other sickle-cell disease with vaso-occlusive pain
Sickle-cell/Hb-D disease with crisis
Sickle-cell/Hb-E disease with crisis

Use additional code for type of crisis, such as:
acute chest syndrome (517.3)
splenic sequestration (289.52)

282.7 Other hemoglobinopathies
Abnormal hemoglobin NOS
Congenital Heinz-body anemia
Disease:
hemoglobin C [Hb-C]
hemoglobin D [Hb-D]
hemoglobin E [Hb-E]
hemoglobin Zurich [Hb-Zurich]
Hemoglobinopathy NOS
Hereditary persistence of fetal hemoglobin [HPFH]
Unstable hemoglobin hemolytic disease

Excludes: *familial polycythemia (289.6)*
hemoglobin E-beta thalassemia (282.47)
hemoglobin M [Hb-M] disease (289.7)
high-oxygen-affinity hemoglobin (289.0)
other hemoglobinopathies with thalassemia (282.49)

282.8 Other specified hereditary hemolytic anemias
Stomatocytosis

282.9 Hereditary hemolytic anemia, unspecified
Hereditary hemolytic anemia NOS

283 Acquired hemolytic anemias

283.0 Autoimmune hemolytic anemias
Autoimmune hemolytic anemias (cold type) (warm type)
Chronic cold hemagglutinin disease
Cold agglutinin disease or hemoglobinuria
Hemolytic anemia:
cold type (secondary) (symptomatic)
drug-induced
warm type (secondary) (symptomatic)

Use additional E code, if desired, to identify cause, if drug-induced

Excludes: *Evans' syndrome (287.32)*
hemolytic disease of newborn (773.0-773.5)

⑤ **283.1 Non-autoimmune hemolytic anemias**

283.10 Non-autoimmune hemolytic anemia, unspecified

● Code new
to this edition

▲ Revision of
existing code

④ ⑤ Fourth or fifth
digit required

283.11   Hemolytic-uremic syndrome
Use additional code to identify associated:
  E. coli infection (041.41-041.49)
  Pneumococcal pnemonia (481)
  Shigella dysenteriae (004.0)

283.19   Other non-autoimmune hemolytic anemias
  Hemolytic anemia:
    mechanical
    microangiopathic
    toxic
Use additional E code, if desired, to identify cause

283.2   Hemoglobinuria due to hemolysis from external causes
  Acute intravascular hemolysis
  Hemoglobinuria:
    from exertion
    march
    paroxysmal (cold) (nocturnal)
    due to other hemolysis
  Marchiafava-Micheli syndrome
Use additional E code, if desired, to identify cause

283.9   Acquired hemolytic anemia, unspecified
  Acquired hemolytic anemia NOS
  Chronic idiopathic hemolytic anemia

284   Aplastic anemia and other bone marrow failure syndromes
  DEFINITION Anemia is a condition where bone marrow does not produce sufficient new cells to replenish blood cells.

⑤ **284.0   Constitutional aplastic anemia**

  284.01   Constitutional red blood cell aplasia
    Aplasia, (pure) red cell:
      congenital
      of infants
      primary
    Blackfan-Diamond syndrome
    Familial hypoplastic anemia

  284.09   Other constitutional aplastic anemia
    Fanconi's anemia
    Pancytopenia with malformations

⑤ **284.1   Pancytopenia**
  Excludes: *pancytopenia (due to) (with):*
    aplastic anemia NOS (284.9)
    bone marrow infiltration (284.2)
    constitutional red blood cell aplasia (284.01)
    hairy cell leukemia (202.4)
    human immunodeficiency virus disease (042)
    leukoerythroblastic anemia (284.2)
    malformations (284.09)
    myelodysplastic syndromes (238.72-238.75)
    myeloproliferative disease (238.79)
    other constitutional aplastic anemia (284.09)

  ● **284.11   Antineoplastic chemotherapy induced pancytopenia**
  Excludes: *aplastic anemia due to antineoplastic chemotherapy (284.89)*

  ● **284.12   Other drug-induced pancytopenia**
  Excludes: *aplastic anemia due to drugs (284.89)*

  ● **284.19   Other pancytopenia**

	Add 4th or 5th digit		Nonspecific code		Unspecified code		Manifestation code

284.2 Myelophthisis
Leukoerythroblastic anemia
Myelophthisic anemia

Code first the underlying disorder, such as:
malignant neoplasm of breast (174.0-174.9, 175.0-175.9)
tuberculosis (015.0-015.9)

Excludes: *idiopathic myelofibrosis (238.76)*
myelofibrosis NOS (289.83)
myelofibrosis with myeloid metaplasia (238.76)
primary myelofibrosis (238.76)
secondary myelofibrosis (289.83)

⑤ **284.8 Other specified aplastic anemias**

284.81 Red cell aplasia (acquired) (adult) (with thymoma)
Red cell aplasia NOS

284.89 Other specified aplastic anemias
Aplastic anemia (due to):
chronic systemic disease
drugs
infection
radiation
toxic (paralytic)

Use additional E code to identify cause

284.9 Aplastic anemia, unspecified
Anemia: Anemia:
aplastic (idiopathic) NOS   nonregenerative
aregenerative   Medullary hypoplasia
hypoplastic NOS

Excludes: *refractory anemia (238.72)*

285 Other and unspecified anemias
ALERT! When using a code from this category it is also necessary to use the code for the chronic condition causing the anemia

285.0 Sideroblastic anemia
Anemia:
hypochromic with iron loading
sideroachrestic
sideroblastic:
acquired
congenital
hereditary
primary
secondary (drug-induced) (due to disease)
sex-linked hypochromic
vitamin B_6-responsive
Pyridoxine-responsive (hypochromic) anemia

Use additional E code, if desired, to identify cause, if drug induced

Excludes: *refractory sideroblastic anemia (238.72)*

285.1 Acute posthemorrhagic anemia
Anemia due to acute blood loss

Excludes: *anemia due to chronic blood loss (280.0)*
blood loss anemia NOS (280.0)

⑤ **285.2 Anemia of chronic disease**
Anemia in (due to) (with) chronic illness

285.21 Anemia in chronic kidney disease
Anemia in end stage renal disease
Erythropoietin-resistant anemia (EPO resistant anemia)

ALERT! When assigning this code it is also necessary to assign a code from Category 585 to indicate the stage of chronic kidney disease.

● Code new to this edition   ▲ Revision of existing code   ④ ⑤ Fourth or fifth digit required

285.22 Anemia in neoplastic disease

Excludes: *anemia due to antineoplastic chemotherapy (285.3)*

aplastic anemia due to antineoplastic chemotherapy (284.89)

ALERT! Code 285.22 is for use for anemia that is due to the malignancy, not for anemia due to antineoplastic chemotherapy drugs, which is an adverse effect. May be used as a secondary code if the patient suffers from anemia and is being treated for the malignancy. When assigning code 285.22, it is also necessary to assign the neoplasm code that is responsible for the anemia.

285.29 Anemia of other chronic disease
Anemia in other chronic illness

285.3 Antineoplastic chemotherapy induced anemia
Anemia due to antineoplastic chemotherapy

Excludes: *anemia due to drug NEC – code to type of anemia*

anemia in neoplastic disease (285.22)

aplastic anemia due to antineoplastic chemotherapy (284.89)

285.8 Other specified anemias
Anemia:
dyserythropoietic (congenital)
dyshematopoietic (congenital)
von Jaksch's
Infantile pseudoleukemia

285.9 Anemia, unspecified
Anemia:
NOS
essential
normocytic, not due to blood loss

Anemia:
profound
progressive
secondary
Oligocythemia

Excludes: *anemia (due to):*

blood loss:
acute (285.1)
chronic or unspecified (280.0)
iron deficiency (280.0-280.9)

286 Coagulation defects

DEFINITION Coagulation defects, aka coagulopathy, clotting disorder, and bleeding disorder, refers to defect in the body's mechanism for blood clotting

286.0 Congenital factor VIII disorder
Antihemophilic globulin [AHG] deficiency
Factor VIII (functional) deficiency
Hemophilia:
NOS
A
classical
familial
hereditary
Subhemophilia

Excludes: *factor VIII deficiency with vascular defect (286.4)*

286.1 Congenital factor IX disorder
Christmas disease
Deficiency:
factor IX (functional)
plasma thromboplastin component [PTC]
Hemophilia B

286.2 Congenital factor XI deficiency
Hemophilia C
Plasma thromboplastin antecedent [PTA] deficiency
Rosenthal's disease

| Add 4th or 5th digit | Nonspecific code | Unspecified code | Manifestation code |

286.3 Congenital deficiency of other clotting factors

Congenital afibrinogenemia
Deficiency:
  AC globulin factor:
    I [fibrinogen]
    II [prothrombin]
    V [labile]
    VII [stable]
    X [Stuart-Prower]
    XII [Hageman]
    XIII [fibrin stabilizing]

Deficiency:
  Laki-Lorand factor
  proaccelerin
Disease:
  Owren's
  Stuart-Prower
Dysfibrinogenemia (congenital)
Dysprothrombinemia (constitutional)
Hypoproconvertinemia
Hypoprothrombinemia (hereditary)
Parahemophilia

286.4 von Willebrand's disease

Angiohemophilia (A) (B)
Constitutional thrombopathy
Factor VIII deficiency with vascular defect
Pseudohemophilia type B
Vascular hemophilia
von Willebrand's (-Jürgens') disease

Excludes: factor VIII deficiency:
  NOS (286.0)
  with functional defect (286.0)
  hereditary capillary fragility (287.8)

▲ **286.5 Hemorrhagic disorder due to intrinsic circulating anticoagulants, antibodies or inhibitors**

● **286.52 Acquired hemophilia**
Autoimmune hemophilia
Autoimmune inhibitors to clotting factors
Secondary hemophilia

● **286.53 Antiphospholipid antibody with hemorrhagic disorder**
Lupus anticoagulant (LAC) with hemorrhagic disorder
Systemic lupus erythematosus [SLE] inhibitor with hemorrhagic disorder

Excludes: antiphospholipid antibody, finding without diagnosis (795.79)
  antiphospholipid antibody syndrome (289.81)
  antiphospholipid antibody with hypercoagulable state (289.81)
  lupus anticoagulant (LAC) finding without diagnosis (795.79)
  lupus anticoagulant (LAC) with hypercoagulable state (289.81)
  systemic lupus erythematosus [SLE] inhibitor finding without diagnosis (795.79)
  systemic lupus erythematosus [SLE] inhibitor with hypercoagulable state (289.81)

● **286.59 Other hemorrhagic disorder due to intrinsic circulating anticoagulants, antibodies, or inhibitors**
Antithrombinemia
Antithromboplastinemia
Antithromboplastinogenemia
Increase in:
  anti-II (prothrombin)
  anti-VIIIa
  anti-IXa
  anti-XIa

286.6 Defibrination syndrome

Afibrinogenemia, acquired
Consumption coagulopathy
Diffuse or disseminated intravascular coagulation [DIC syndrome]
Fibrinolytic hemorrhage, acquired
Hemorrhagic fibrinogenolysis
Pathologic fibrinolysis
Purpura:
  fibrinolytic
  fulminans

Excludes: that complicating:
  abortion (634-638 with .1, 639.1)
  pregnancy or the puerperium (641.3, 666.3)
  disseminated intravascular coagulation in newborn (776.2)

● Code new to this edition   ▲ Revision of existing code   ④ ⑤ Fourth or fifth digit required

286.7 Acquired coagulation factor deficiency
Deficiency of coagulation factor due to:
liver disease
vitamin K deficiency
Hypoprothrombinemia, acquired

Excludes: *vitamin K deficiency of newborn (776.0)*

Use additional E-code, if desired, to identify cause, if drug induced

286.9 Other and unspecified coagulation defects
Defective coagulation NOS
Deficiency, coagulation factor NOS
Delay, coagulation
Disorder:
coagulation
hemostasis

Excludes: *abnormal coagulation profile (790.92)*
hemorrhagic disease of newborn (776.0)
that complicating:
abortion (634-638 with .1, 639.1)
pregnancy or the puerperium (641.3, 666.3)

287 Purpura and other hemorrhagic conditions

Excludes: *hemorrhagic thrombocythemia (238.79)*
purpura fulminans (286.6)

DEFINITION Purpura are purple-colored spots and patches that occur on the skin, organs, and in mucus membranes, including the lining of the mouth.

287.0 Allergic purpura
Peliosis rheumatica
Purpura:
anaphylactoid
autoimmune
Henoch's

Purpura:
nonthrombocytopenic:
hemorrhagic
idiopathic
rheumatica
Schönlein-Henoch
vascular
Vasculitis, allergic

Excludes: *hemorrhagic purpura (287.39)*
purpura annularis telangiectodes (709.1)

287.1 Qualitative platelet defects
Thrombasthenia (hemorrhagic) (hereditary)
Thrombocytasthenia
Thrombocytopathy (dystrophic)
Thrombopathy (Bernard-Soulier)

Excludes: *von Willebrand's disease (286.4)*

287.2 Other nonthrombocytopenic purpuras
Purpura:
NOS
senile
simplex

⑤ **287.3 Primary thrombocytopenia**

287.30 Primary thrombocytopenia, unspecified
Megakaryocytic hypoplasia

287.31 Immune thrombocytopenic purpura
Idiopathic thrombocytopenic purpura
Tidal platelet dysgenesis

287.32 Evans' syndrome

287.33 Congenital and hereditary thrombocytopenic purpura
Congenital and hereditary thrombocytopenia
Thrombocytopenia with absent radii (TAR) syndrome

Excludes: *Wiskott-Aldrich syndrome (279.12)*

287.39 Other primary thrombocytopenia

⑤ **287.4 Secondary thrombocytopenia**
Use additional E code, if desired, to identify cause

Excludes: *heparin-induced thrombocytopenia (HIT) (289.84)*
transient thrombocytopenia of newborn (776.1)

| | Add 4th or 5th digit | | Nonspecific code | | Unspecified code | | Manifestation code |

287.41 Posttransfusion purpura
Posttransfusion purpura from whole blood (fresh) or blood products
PTP

287.49 Other secondary thrombocytopenia
Thrombocytopenia (due to):
dilutional
drugs
extracorporeal circulation of blood
massive blood transfusion
platelet alloimmunization
secondary NOS

287.5 Thrombocytopenia, unspecified

287.8 Other specified hemorrhagic conditions
Capillary fragility (hereditary)
Vascular pseudohemophilia

287.9 Unspecified hemorrhagic conditions
Hemorrhagic diathesis (familial)

288 Diseases of white blood cells

Excludes: leukemia (204.0-208.9)

DEFINITION White blood cells, aka leukocyte, refers to Any of various blood cells that help protect the body from infection and disease. White blood cells include neutrophils, eosinophils, basophils, lymphocytes, and monocytes.

⑤ **288.0 Neutropenia**
Decreased Absolute Neutrophil Count (ANC)
Use additional code for any associated:
fever (780.61)
mucositis (478.11, 528.00-528.09, 538, 616.81)

Excludes: neutropenic splenomegaly (289.53)
transitory neonatal neutropenia (776.7)

288.00 Neutropenia, unspecified

288.01 Congenital neutropenia
Congenital agranulocytosis
Infantile genetic agranulocytosis
Kostmann's syndrome

288.02 Cyclic neutropenia
Cyclic hematopoiesis
Periodic neutropenia

288.03 Drug induced neutropenia
Use additional E code to identify drug

288.04 Neutropenia due to infection

288.09 Other neutropenia
Agranulocytosis
Neutropenia:
immune
toxic

288.1 Functional disorders of polymorphonuclear neutrophils
Chronic (childhood) granulomatous disease
Congenital dysphagocytosis
Job's syndrome
Lipochrome histiocytosis (familial)
Progressive septic granulomatosis

288.2 Genetic anomalies of leukocytes
Anomaly (granulation) (granulocyte) or syndrome:
Alder's (-Reilly)
Chédiak-Steinbrinck (-Higashi)
Jordan's
May-Hegglin
Pelger-Huet
Hereditary:
hypersegmentation
hyposegmentation
leukomelanopathy

● Code new
to this edition

▲ Revision of
existing code

④ ⑤ Fourth or fifth
digit required

288.3 Eosinophilia
Eosinophilia
allergic
hereditary
idiopathic
secondary
Eosinophilic leukocytosis

Excludes: *Löffler's syndrome (518.3)*
pulmonary eosinophilia (518.3)

288.4 Hemophagocytic syndromes
Familial hemophagocytic lymphohistiocytosis
Familial hemophagocytic reticulosis
Hemophagocytic syndrome, infection-associated
Histiocytic syndromes
Macrophage activation syndrome

⑤ **288.5 Decreased white blood cell count**

Excludes: *neutropenia (288.01-288.09)*

288.50 Leukocytopenia, unspecified
Decreased leukocytes, unspecified
Decreased white blood cell count, unspecified
Leukopenia NOS

288.51 Lymphocytopenia
Decreased lymphocytes

288.59 Other decreased white blood cell count
Basophilic leukopenia
Eosinophilic leukopenia
Monocytopenia
Plasmacytopenia

⑤ **288.6 Elevated white blood cell count**

Excludes: *eosinophilia (288.3)*

288.60 Leukocytosis, unspecified
Elevated leukocytes, unspecified
Elevated white blood cell count, unspecified

288.61 Lymphocytosis (symptomatic)
Elevated lymphocytes

288.62 Leukemoid reaction
Basophilic leukemoid reaction
Lymphocytic leukemoid reaction
Monocytic leukemoid reaction
Myelocytic leukemoid reaction
Neutrophilic leukemoid reaction

288.63 Monocytosis (symptomatic)

Excludes: *infectious mononucleosis (075)*

288.64 Plasmacytosis

288.65 Basophilia

288.66 Bandemia
Bandemia without diagnosis of specific infection

Excludes: *confirmed infection – code to infection leukemia (204.00-208.9)*

288.69 Other elevated white blood cell count

288.8 Other specified disease of white blood cells

Excludes: *decreased white blood cell counts (288.50-288.59)*
elevated white blood cell counts (288.60-288.69)
immunity disorders (279.0-279.9)

288.9 Unspecified disease of white blood cells

	Add 4th or 5th digit		Nonspecific code		Unspecified code		Manifestation code

289 **Other diseases of blood and blood-forming organs**

289.0 **Polycythemia, secondary**

High-oxygen-affinity
  hemoglobin
Polycythemia:
  acquired
  benign
  due to:
    fall in plasma volume
    high altitude

Polycythemia:
  emotional
  erythropoietin
  hypoxemic
  nephrogenous
  relative
  spurious
  stress

Excludes: *polycythemia:*
    neonatal (776.4)
    primary (238.4)
    vera (238.4)

289.1 **Chronic lymphadenitis**

Chronic:
  adenitis, any lymph node except mesenteric
  lymphadenitis, any lymph node except mesenteric

Excludes: *acute lymphadenitis (683)*
    mesenteric (289.2)
    enlarged glands NOS (785.6)

289.2 **Nonspecific mesenteric lymphadenitis**

Mesenteric lymphadenitis (acute) (chronic)

289.3 **Lymphadenitis, unspecified, except mesenteric**

289.4 **Hypersplenism**

"Big spleen" syndrome   Hypersplenia
Dyssplenism

Excludes: *primary splenic neutropenia (289.53)*

⑤ **289.5** **Other diseases of spleen**

289.50 **Disease of spleen, unspecified**

289.51 **Chronic congestive splenomegaly**

289.52 **Splenic sequestration**

Code first sickle-cell disease in crisis (282.42, 282.62, 282.64, 282.69)

289.53 **Neutropenic splenomegaly**

289.59 **Other**

Lien migrans
Perisplenitis
Splenic:
  abscess
  atrophy
  cyst

Splenic:
  fibrosis
  infarction
  rupture, nontraumatic
Splenitis
Wandering spleen

Excludes: *bilharzial splenic fibrosis (120.0-120.9)*
    hepatolienal fibrosis (571.5)
    splenomegaly NOS (789.2)

289.6 **Familial polycythemia**

Familial benign polycythemia
Familial erythrocytosis

289.7 **Methemoglobinemia**

Congenital NADH [DPNH]-methemoglobin-reductase deficiency
Hemoglobin M [Hb-M] disease
Methemoglobinemia:
  NOS
  acquired (with sulfhemoglobinemia)
  hereditary
  toxic
Stokvis' disease
Sulfhemoglobinemia

Use additional E code, if desired, to identify cause

● Code new
  to this edition

▲ Revision of
  existing code

④ ⑤ Fourth or fifth
  digit required

⑤ **289.8   Other specified diseases of blood and blood-forming organs**

289.81   Primary hypercoagulable state
Activated protein C resistance
Antiphospholipid antibody syndrome
Antithrombin III deficiency
Factor V Leiden mutation
Lupus anticoagulant with hypercoagulable state
Protein C deficiency
Protein S deficiency
Prothrombin gene mutation
Systemic lupus erythematosus [SLE] inhibitor with hypercoagulable state

Excludes: *anti-phospholipid antibody, finding without diagnosis (795.79)*
anti-phospholipid antibody with hemorrhagic disorder (286.53)
lupus anticoagulant (LAC) finding without diagnosis (795.79)
lupus anticoagulant (LAC) with hemorrhagic disorder (286.53)
secondary activated protein C resistance (289.82)
secondary antiphospholipid antibody syndrome (289.82)
secondary lupus anticoagulant with hypercoagulable state (289.82)
secondary systemic lupus erythematosus [SLE] inhibitor with hypercoagulable state (289.82)
systemic lupus erythematosus [SLE] inhibitor finding without diagnosis (795.79)
systemic lupus erythematosus [SLE] inhibitor with hemorrhagic disorder (286.53)

289.82   Secondary hypercoagulable state

Excludes: *heparin-induced thrombocytopenia (HIT) (289.84)*

289.83   Myelofibrosis
Myelofibrosis NOS
Secondary myelofibrosis

Code first the underlying disorder, such as:
malignant neoplasm of breast (174.0-174.9, 175.0-175.9)

Use additional code for associated therapy-related
myelodysplastic syndrome, if applicable (238.72, 238.73)

Use additional external cause code if due to anti-neoplastic chemotherapy (E933.1)

Excludes: *idiopathic myelofibrosis (238.76)*
leukoerythroblastic anemia (284.2)
myelofibrosis with myeloid metaplasia (238.76)
myelophthisic anemia (284.2)
myelophthisis (284.2)
primary myelofibrosis (238.76)

289.84   Heparin-induced thrombocytopenia (HIT)

289.89   Other specified diseases of blood and blood-forming organs
Hypergammaglobulinemia
Pseudocholinesterase deficiency

289.9   Unspecified diseases of blood and blood-forming organs
Blood dyscrasia NOS
Erythroid hyperplasia

| | Add 4th or 5th digit | | Nonspecific code | | Unspecified code | | Manifestation code |

This page intentionally left blank.

● Code new
to this edition

▲ Revision of
existing code

④ ⑤ Fourth or fifth
digit required

Chapter 5: Mental, Behavioral and Neurodevelopmental Disorders (290-319)

DEFINITIONS AND CODING ALERTS

This chapter includes definitions of selected key words, terms and phrases and coding alerts for adding points to the clinical domain, references to coding late effects where appropriate, and references to personal history V-codes in situations where the acute or chronic condition is no longer active. An example from this chapter is as follows:

⑤ **295** **Schizophrenic disorders**

> **DEFINITION** Schizophrenia is a psychotic disorder marked by severely impaired thinking, emotions, and behaviors. Schizophrenic patients are typically unable to filter sensory stimuli and may have enhanced perceptions of sounds, colors, and other features of their environment.
> **ALERT!** For personal history of schizophrenia see V11.0

MULTIPLE CODING FOR A SINGLE CONDITION

In addition to the etiology or manifestation convention that requires two codes to fully describe a single condition that affects multiple body systems, there are other single conditions that also require more than one code. "Use additional code" notes are found in the tabular at codes that are not part of an etiology or manifestation pair where a secondary code is useful to fully describe a condition. The sequencing rule is the same as the etiology or manifestation pair - , "use additional code" indicates that a secondary code should be added.

"Code first" notes are also under certain codes that are not specifically manifestation codes but may be due to an underlying cause. When a "code first" note is present and an underlying condition is present the underlying condition should be sequenced first.

"Code, if applicable, any causal condition first", notes indicate that this code may be assigned as a principal diagnosis when the causal condition is unknown or not applicable. If a causal condition is known, then the code for that condition should be sequenced as the principal or first-listed diagnosis. Multiple codes may be needed for late effects, complication codes and obstetric codes to more fully describe a condition. See the specific guidelines for these conditions for further instruction.

COMBINATION CODE

A combination code is a single code used to classify: two diagnoses, or a diagnosis with an associated secondary process (manifestation) A diagnosis with an associated complication Combination codes are identified by referring to subterm entries in the Alphabetic Index and by reading the inclusion and exclusion notes in the Tabular List.

Assign only the combination code when that code fully identifies the diagnostic conditions involved or when the Alphabetic Index so directs. Multiple coding should not be used when the classification provides a combination code that clearly identifies all of the elements documented in the diagnosis. When the combination code lacks necessary specificity in describing the manifestation or complication, an additional code should be used as a secondary code.

CODING LATE EFFECTS

A late effect is the residual effect (condition produced) after the acute phase of an illness or injury has terminated. There is no time limit on when a late effect code can be used. The residual may be apparent early, such as in cerebrovascular accident cases, or it may occur months or years later, such as that due to a previous injury. Coding of late effects generally requires two codes sequenced in the following order: The condition or nature of the late effect is sequenced first. The late effect code is sequenced second.

An exception to the above guidelines are those instances where the code for late effect is followed by a manifestation code identified in the Tabular List and title, or the late effect code has been expanded (at the fourth and fifth-digit levels) to include the manifestation(s). The code for the acute phase of an illness or injury that led to the late effect is never used with a code for the late effect.

	Add 4th or 5th digit		Nonspecific code		Unspecified code		Manifestation code

This page intentionally left blank.

● Code new
  to this edition

▲ Revision of
  existing code

④ ⑤ Fourth or fifth
   digit required

5. MENTAL, BEHAVIORAL AND NEURODEVELOPMENTAL DISORDERS (290-319)

PSYCHOSES (290-299)

> Excludes: intellectual disabilities (317-319)

ORGANIC PSYCHOTIC CONDITIONS (290-294)

> Includes: psychotic organic brain syndrome
>
> Excludes: nonpsychotic syndromes of organic etiology (310.0-310.9)
>
> psychoses classifiable to 295-298 and without impairment of orientation, comprehension, calculation, learning capacity, and judgement, but associated with physical disease, injury, or condition affecting the brain [e.g., following childbirth] (295.0-298.8)

ALERT! For personal history of mental disorder see V11.

290 Dementias

Code first the associated neurological condition

> Excludes: dementia due to alcohol (291.0-291.2)
>
> dementia due to drugs (292.82)
> dementia not classified as senile, presenile, or arteriosclerotic (294.10-294.11)
> psychoses classifiable to 295-298 occurring in the senium without dementia or delirium (295.0-298.8)
> senility with mental changes of nonpsychotic severity (310.1)
> transient organic psychotic conditions (293.0-293.9)

DEFINITION Dementia refers to a group of symptoms caused by disorders that affect the brain. It is not a specific disease.

290.0 Senile dementia, uncomplicated

Senile dementia:
NOS
simple type

> Excludes: mild memory disturbances, not amounting to dementia, associated with senile brain disease (310.89)
>
> senile dementia with:
> delirium or confusion (290.3)
> delusional [paranoid] features (290.20)
> depressive features (290.21)

⑤ **290.1 Presenile dementia**

Brain syndrome with presenile brain disease

> Excludes: arteriosclerotic dementia (290.40-290.43)
>
> dementia associated with other cerebral conditions (294.10-294.11)

290.10 Presenile dementia, uncomplicated

Presenile dementia:
NOS
simple type

290.11 Presenile dementia with delirium

Presenile dementia with acute confusional state

290.12 Presenile dementia with delusional features

Presenile dementia, paranoid type

290.13 Presenile dementia with depressive features

Presenile dementia, depressed type

⑤ **290.2 Senile dementia with delusional or depressive features**

> Excludes: senile dementia:
>
> NOS (290.0)
> with delirium and/or confusion (290.3)

290.20 Senile dementia with delusional features

Senile dementia, paranoid type
Senile psychosis NOS

290.21 Senile dementia with depressive features

290.3 Senile dementia with delirium

Senile dementia with acute confusional state

> Excludes: senile:
>
> dementia NOS (290.0)
> psychosis NOS (290.20)

⑤ **290.4 Vascular dementia**
　　　Multi-infarct dementia or psychosis

Use additional code to identify cerebral atherosclerosis (437.0)

> *Excludes:* suspected cases with no clear evidence of arteriosclerosis (290.9)

290.40 Vascular dementia, uncomplicated
　　　Arteriosclerotic dementia:
　　　　NOS
　　　　simple type

290.41 Vascular dementia with delirium
　　　Arteriosclerotic dementia with acute confusional state

290.42 Vascular dementia with delusions
　　　Arteriosclerotic dementia, paranoid type

290.43 Vascular dementia with depressed mood
　　　Arteriosclerotic dementia, depressed type

290.8 Other specified senile psychotic conditions
　　　Presbyophrenic psychosis

290.9 Unspecified senile psychotic condition

291 Alcohol-induced mental disorders

> *Excludes:* alcoholism without psychosis (303.0-303.9)

DEFINITION Alcohol-induced mental disorders is an alcohol-induced psychological or behavioral pattern that occurs in an individual and is thought to cause distress or disability that is not expected as part of normal development or culture.

291.0 Alcohol withdrawal delirium
　　　Alcoholic delirium
　　　Delirium tremens

> *Excludes:* alcohol withdrawal (291.81)

291.1 Alcohol-induced persisting amnestic disorder
　　　Alcoholic polyneuritic psychosis
　　　Korsakoff's psychosis, alcoholic
　　　Wernicke-Korsakoff syndrome (alcoholic)

291.2 Alcohol-induced persisting dementia
　　　Alcoholic dementia NOS
　　　Alcoholism associated with dementia NOS
　　　Chronic alcoholic brain syndrome

291.3 Alcohol-induced psychotic disorder with hallucinations
　　　Alcoholic:
　　　　hallucinosis (acute)
　　　　psychosis with hallucinosis

> *Excludes:* alcohol withdrawal with delirium (291.0)
>　　　schizophrenia (295.0-295.9) and paranoid states (297.0-297.9) taking the form of chronic hallucinosis with clear consciousness in an alcoholic

291.4 Idiosyncratic alcohol intoxication
　　　Pathologic:
　　　　alcohol intoxication
　　　　drunkenness

> *Excludes:* acute alcohol intoxication (305.0)
>　　　in alcoholism (303.0)
>　　　simple drunkenness (305.0)

291.5 Alcohol-induced psychotic disorder with delusions
　　　Alcoholic:
　　　　paranoia
　　　　psychosis, paranoid type

> *Excludes:* nonalcoholic paranoid states (297.0-297.9)
>　　　schizophrenia, paranoid type (295.3)

⑤ **291.8 Other specified alcohol induced mental disorders**
　　ALERT! For personal history of other mental disorders see V11.8

● Code new to this edition　　▲ Revision of existing code　　④ ⑤ Fourth or fifth digit required

291.81 Alcohol withdrawal
Alcohol:
withdrawal syndrome or symptoms
abstinence syndrome or symptoms

Excludes: *alcohol withdrawal:*
delirium (291.0)
hallucinosis (291.3)
delirium tremens (291.0)

291.82 Alcohol induced sleep disorders
Alcohol induced circadian rhythm sleep disorders
Alcohol induced hypersomnia
Alcohol induced insomnia
Alcohol induced parasomnia

291.89 Other
Alcohol induced anxiety disorder
Alcohol induced mood disorder
Alcohol induced sexual dysfunction

291.9 Unspecified alcohol-induced mental disorders
Alcohol-related disorder NOS
Alcoholic:
mania NOS
psychosis NOS
Alcoholism (chronic) with psychosis

292 Drug induced mental disorders
Includes: organic brain syndrome associated with consumption of drugs

Use additional code for any associated drug dependence (304.0-304.9)

Use additional E code, if desired, to identify drug

DEFINITION Drug-induced mental disorders is a drug-induced psychological or behavioral pattern that occurs in an individual and is thought to cause distress or disability that is not expected as part of normal development or culture.

292.0 Drug withdrawal
Drug:
abstinence syndrome or symptoms
withdrawal syndrome or symptoms

⑤ **292.1 Drug-induced psychotic disorders**

292.11 Drug-induced psychotic disorder with delusions
Paranoid state induced by drugs

292.12 Drug-induced psychotic disorder with hallucinations
Hallucinatory state induced by drugs

Excludes: *states following LSD or other hallucinogens, lasting only a few days or less ["bad trips"] (305.3)*

292.2 Pathological drug intoxication
Drug reaction:
NOS resulting in brief psychotic states
idiosyncratic resulting in brief psychotic states
pathologic resulting in brief psychotic states

Excludes: *expected brief psychotic reactions to hallucinogens ["bad trips"] (305.3)*
physiological side-effects of drugs (e.g., dystonias)

⑤ **292.8 Other specified drug induced mental disorders**
ALERT! For personal history of other mental disorders see V11.8

292.81 Drug induced delirium

292.82 Drug induced persisting dementia

292.83 Drug induced persisting amnestic disorder

292.84 Drug induced mood disorder
Depressive state induced by drugs

292.85 Drug induced sleep disorders
Drug induced circadian rhythm sleep disorder
Drug induced hypersomnia
Drug induced insomnia
Drug induced parasomnia

292.89 Other
Drug induced anxiety disorder
Drug induced organic personality syndrome
Drug induced sexual dysfunction
Drug intoxication

292.9 Unspecified drug-induced mental disorder
Drug-related disorder NOS
Organic psychosis NOS due to or associated with drugs

293 Transient mental disorders due to conditions classified elsewhere
Includes: transient organic mental disorders not associated with alcohol or drugs
Code first the associated physical or neurological condition

Excludes: *confusional state or delirium superimposed on senile dementia (290.3)*
dementia due to:
alcohol (291.0-291.9)
arteriosclerosis (290.40-290.43)
drugs (292.82)
senility (290.0)

293.0 Delirium due to conditions classified elsewhere
Acute:
confusional state
infective psychosis
organic reaction
posttraumatic organic psychosis
psycho-organic syndrome
Acute psychosis associated with endocrine, metabolic, or cerebrovascular disorder
Epileptic:
confusional state
twilight state

293.1 Subacute delirium
Subacute:
confusional state
infective psychosis
organic reaction
posttraumatic organic psychosis
psycho-organic syndrome
psychosis associated with endocrine or metabolic disorder

⑤ **293.8 Other specified transient mental disorders due to conditions classified elsewhere**
ALERT! For personal history of other mental disorders see V11.8

293.81 Psychotic disorder with delusions in conditions classified elsewhere
Transient organic psychotic condition, paranoid type

293.82 Psychotic disorder with hallucinations in conditions classified elsewhere
Transient organic psychotic condition, hallucinatory type

293.83 Mood disorder in conditions classified elsewhere
Transient organic psychotic condition, depressive type

293.84 Anxiety disorder in conditions classified elsewhere

293.89 Other
Catatonic disorder in conditions classified elsewhere

293.9 Unspecified transient mental disorder in conditions classified elsewhere
Organic psychosis:
infective NOS
posttraumatic NOS
transient NOS
Psycho-organic syndrome

294 Persistent mental disorders due to conditions classified elsewhere
Includes: organic psychotic brain syndromes (chronic), not elsewhere classified

294.0 Amnestic disorder in conditions classified elsewhere
Korsakoff's psychosis or syndrome (nonalcoholic)
Code first underlying condition
Excludes: *alcoholic:*
amnestic syndrome (291.1)
Korsakoff's psychosis (291.1)

● Code new to this edition   ▲ Revision of existing code   ④ ⑤ Fourth or fifth digit required

⑤ *294.1 Dementia in conditions classified elsewhere*
Dementia of the Alzheimer's type

Code first any underlying physical condition, as:
Alzheimer's disease (331.0)
cerebral lipidoses (330.1)
dementia with Lewy bodies (331.82)
dementia with Parkinsonism (331.82)
epilepsy (345.0-345.9)
frontal dementia (331.19)
frontotemporal dementia (331.19)
general paresis [syphilis] (094.1)
hepatolenticular degeneration (275.1)
Huntington's chorea (333.4)
Jakob-Creutzfeldt disease (046.11-046.19)
multiple sclerosis (340)
Parkinson's disease (332.0)
Pick's disease of the brain (331.11)
polyarteritis nodosa (446.0)
syphilis (094.1)

Excludes: *dementia:*
arteriosclerotic (290.40-290.43)
presenile (290.10-290.13)
senile (290.0)
epileptic psychosis NOS (294.8)

294.10 Dementia in conditions classified elsewhere without behavioral disturbance
Dementia in conditions classified elsewhere NOS

294.11 Dementia in conditions classified elsewhere with behavioral disturbance
Aggressive behavior
Combative behavior
Violent behavior

Use additional code, where applicable, to identify:
wandering in conditions classified elsewhere (V40.31)

● **294.2 Dementia, unspecified**

Excludes: *mild memory disturbances, not amounting to dementia (310.89)*

● **294.20 Dementia, unspecified, without behavioral disturbance**
Dementia NOS

● **294.21 Dementia, unspecified, with behavioral disturbance**
Aggressive behavior
Combative behavior
Violent behavior

Use additional code, where applicable, to identify:
wandering in conditions classified elsewhere (V40.31)

294.8 Other persistent mental disorders due to conditions classified elsewhere
Amnestic disorder NOS
Epileptic psychosis NOS
Mixed paranoid and affective organic psychotic states

Use additional code for associated epilepsy (345.0-345.9)

Excludes: *mild memory disturbances, not amounting to dementia (310.89)*

ALERT! For personal history of other mental disorders see V11.8

294.9 Unspecified persistent mental disorders due to conditions classified elsewhere
Cognitive disorder NOS
Organic psychosis (chronic)

Add 4th or
5th digit
Nonspecific
code
Unspecified
code
Manifestation
code

OTHER PSYCHOSES (295-299)

Use additional code to identify any associated physical disease, injury, or condition affecting the brain with psychoses classifiable to 295-298

⑤ **295** **Schizophrenic disorders**

Includes: schizophrenia of the types described in 295.0-295.9 occurring in children

Excludes: *childhood type schizophrenia (299.9)*

infantile autism (299.0)

The following fifth-digit subclassification is for use with category 295:

0 **unspecified**

1 **subchronic**

2 **chronic**

3 **subchronic with acute exacerbation**

4 **chronic with acute exacerbation**

5 **in remission**

DEFINITION Schizophrenia is a psychotic disorder marked by severely impaired thinking, emotions, and behaviors. Schizophrenic patients are typically unable to filter sensory stimuli and may have enhanced perceptions of sounds, colors, and other features of their environment.

ALERT! For personal history of schizophrenia see V11.0

⑤ **295.0** **Simple type**
[0-5]   Schizophrenia simplex

Excludes: *latent schizophrenia (295.5)*

⑤ **295.1** **Disorganized type**
[0-5]   Hebephrenia
Hebephrenic type schizophrenia

⑤ **295.2** **Catatonic type**
[0-5]   Catatonic (schizophrenia):   Schizophrenic:
agitation   catalepsy
excitation   catatonia
excited type   flexibilitas cerea
stupor
withdrawn type

⑤ **295.3** **Paranoid type**
[0-5]   Paraphrenic schizophrenia

Excludes: *involutional paranoid state (297.2)*

paranoia (297.1)

paraphrenia (297.2)

⑤ **295.4** **Schizophreniform disorder**
[0-5]   Oneirophrenia
Schizophreniform:
attack
psychosis, confusional type

Excludes: *acute forms of schizophrenia of:*

catatonic type (295.2)
hebephrenic type (295.1)
paranoid type (295.3)
simple type (295.0)
undifferentiated type (295.8)

⑤ **295.5** **Latent schizophrenia**
[0-5]   Latent schizophrenic reaction
Schizophrenia:
borderline
incipient
Schizophrenia:
prepsychotic
prodromal
pseudoneurotic
pseudopsychopathic

Excludes: *schizoid personality (301.20-301.22)*

● Code new
to this edition   ▲ Revision of
existing code   ④ ⑤ Fourth or fifth
digit required

⑤ **295.6 Residual type**
[0-5]   Chronic undifferentiated schizophrenia
         Restzustand (schizophrenic)
         Schizophrenic residual state

⑤ **295.7 Schizoaffective disorder**
[0-5]   Cyclic schizophrenia
         Mixed schizophrenic and affective psychosis
         Schizoaffective psychosis
         Schizophreniform psychosis, affective type

⑤ **295.8 Other specified types of schizophrenia**
[0-5]   Acute (undifferentiated) schizophrenia
         Atypical schizophrenia
         Cenesthopathic schizophrenia

    Excludes: infantile autism (299.0)

⑤ **295.9 Unspecified schizophrenia**
[0-5]   Schizophrenia: Schizophrenic reaction NOS
           NOS   Schizophreniform psychosis NOS
           mixed NOS
           undifferentiated NOS
           undifferentiated type

296 Episodic mood disorders
         Includes: episodic affective disorders

    Excludes: neurotic depression (300.4)
                reactive depressive psychosis (298.0)
                reactive excitation (298.1)

The following fifth-digit subclassification is for use with categories 296.0-296.6:

   0   unspecified
   1   mild
   2   moderate
   3   severe, without mention of psychotic behavior
   4   severe, specified as with psychotic behavior
   5   in partial or unspecified remission
   6   in full remission

DEFINITION Episodic mood disorders are psychological disorders that may include depression, bipolar disorder (manic-depression), major depression, dysthymia, and cyclothymia.

ALERT! For personal history of affective disorders see V11.1

⑤ **296.0 Bipolar I disorder, single manic episode**
[0-6]   Hypomania (mild) NOS, single episode or unspecified
         Hypomanic psychosis, single episode or unspecified
         Mania (monopolar) NOS, single episode or unspecified
         Manic-depressive psychosis or reaction:
           hypomanic, single episode or unspecified
           manic, single episode or unspecified

    Excludes: circular type, if there was a previous attack of depression (296.4)

⑤ **296.1 Manic disorder, recurrent episode**
[0-6]   Any condition classifiable to 296.0, stated to be recurrent

    Excludes: circular type, if there was a previous attack of depression (296.4)

⑤ **296.2 Major depressive disorder, single episode**
[0-6]   Depressive psychosis, single episode or unspecified
         Endogenous depression, single episode or unspecified
         Involutional melancholia, single episode or unspecified
         Manic-depressive psychosis or reaction, depressed type, single episode or unspecified
         Monopolar depression, single episode or unspecified
         Psychotic depression, single episode or unspecified

    Excludes: circular type, if previous attack was of manic type (296.5)
                depression NOS (311)
                reactive depression (neurotic) (300.4)
                  psychotic (298.0)

⑤ **296.3 Major depressive disorder, recurrent episode**
[0-6]   Any condition classifiable to 296.2, stated to be recurrent

   Excludes: *circular type, if previous attack was of manic type (296.5)*
                 depression NOS (311)
                 reactive depression (neurotic) (300.4)
                 psychotic (298.0)

⑤ **296.4 Bipolar I disorder, most recent episode (or current) manic**
[0-6]   Bipolar disorder, now manic
            Manic-depressive psychosis, circular type but currently manic

   Excludes: *brief compensatory or rebound mood swings (296.99)*

⑤ **296.5 Bipolar I disorder, most recent episode (or current) depressed**
[0-6]   Bipolar disorder, now depressed
            Manic-depressive psychosis, circular type but currently depressed

   Excludes: *brief compensatory or rebound mood swings (296.99)*

⑤ **296.6 Bipolar I disorder, most recent episode (or current) mixed**
[0-6]   Manic-depressive psychosis, circular type, mixed

   296.7 Bipolar I disorder, most recent episode (or current) unspecified
            Atypical bipolar affective disorder NOS
            Manic-depressive psychosis, circular type, current condition not specified as either
               manic or depressive

⑤ **296.8 Other and unspecified bipolar disorders**

   296.80 Bipolar disorder, unspecified
            Bipolar disorder NOS
            Manic-depressive:
               reaction NOS
               syndrome NOS

   296.81 Atypical manic disorder

   296.82 Atypical depressive disorder

   296.89 Other
            Bipolar II disorder
            Manic-depressive psychosis, mixed type

⑤ **296.9 Other and unspecified episodic mood disorder**

   Excludes: *psychogenic affective psychoses (298.0-298.8)*

   296.90 Unspecified episodic mood disorder
            Affective psychosis NOS
            Melancholia NOS
            Mood disorder NOS

   296.99 Other specified episodic mood disorder
            Mood swings:
               brief compensatory
               rebound

297 Delusional disorders
      Includes: paranoid disorders

   Excludes: *acute paranoid reaction (298.3)*
                 alcoholic jealousy or paranoid state (291.5)
                 paranoid schizophrenia (295.3)

   DEFINITION Delusional disorders refers to any mental disorder in which delusions play a
   significant role.

297.0 Paranoid state, simple

297.1 Delusional disorder
         Chronic paranoid psychosis
         Sander's disease
         Systematized delusions

   Excludes: *paranoid personality disorder (301.0)*

297.2 Paraphrenia
         Involutional paranoid state
         Late paraphrenia
         Paraphrenia (involutional)

297.3 Shared psychotic disorder
         Folie à deux
         Induced psychosis or paranoid disorder

● Code new   ▲ Revision of   ④ ⑤ Fourth or fifth
          to this edition   existing code   digit required

297.8 **Other specified paranoid states**
Paranoia querulans
Sensitiver Beziehungswahn

Excludes: *acute paranoid reaction or state (298.3)*
senile paranoid state (290.20)

297.9 **Unspecified paranoid state**
Paranoid: Paranoid:
  disorder NOS   reaction NOS
  psychosis   state NOS

298 **Other nonorganic psychoses**
Includes: psychotic conditions due to or provoked by:
emotional stress
environmental factors as major part of etiology

298.0 **Depressive type psychosis**
Psychogenic depressive psychosis
Psychotic reactive depression
Reactive depressive psychosis

Excludes: *manic-depressive psychosis, depressed type (296.2-296.3)*
neurotic depression (300.4)
reactive depression NOS (300.4)

298.1 **Excitative type psychosis**
Acute hysterical psychosis   Reactive excitation
Psychogenic excitation

Excludes: *manic-depressive psychosis, manic type (296.0-296.1)*

298.2 **Reactive confusion**
Psychogenic confusion
Psychogenic twilight state

Excludes: *acute confusional state (293.0)*

298.3 **Acute paranoid reaction**
Acute psychogenic paranoid psychosis
Bouffée délirante

Excludes: *paranoid states (297.0-297.9)*

298.4 **Psychogenic paranoid psychosis**
Protracted reactive paranoid psychosis

298.8 **Other and unspecified reactive psychosis**
Brief psychotic disorder
Brief reactive psychosis NOS
Hysterical psychosis
Psychogenic psychosis NOS
Psychogenic stupor

Excludes: *acute hysterical psychosis (298.1)*

298.9 **Unspecified psychosis**
Atypical psychosis
Psychosis NOS
Psychotic disorder NOS

⑤ **299** **Pervasive developmental disorders**

Excludes: *adult type psychoses occurring in childhood, as:*
affective disorders (296.0-296.9)
manic-depressive disorders (296.0-296.9)
schizophrenia (295.0-295.9)

The following fifth-digit subclassification is for use with category 299:

0 **current or active state**

1 **residual state**

⑤ **299.0** **Autistic disorder**
[0-1]   Childhood autism
Infantile psychosis
Kanner's syndrome

Excludes: *disintegrative psychosis (299.1)*
Heller's syndrome (299.1)
schizophrenic syndrome of childhood (299.9)

Add 4th or   Nonspecific   Unspecified   Manifestation
5th digit   code   code   code

⑤ **299.1 Childhood disintegrative disorder**
[0-1]   Heller's syndrome
Use additional code to identify any associated neurological disorder

Excludes: *infantile autism (299.0)*

  schizophrenic syndrome of childhood (299.9)

⑤ **299.8 Other specified pervasive developmental disorders**
[0-1]   Asperger's disorder
          Atypical childhood psychosis
          Borderline psychosis of childhood

Excludes: *simple stereotypies without psychotic disturbance (307.3)*

⑤ **299.9 Unspecified pervasive developmental disorder**
[0-1]   Child psychosis NOS
          Pervasive developmental disorder NOS
          Schizophrenia, childhood type NOS
          Schizophrenic syndrome of childhood NOS

Excludes: *schizophrenia of adult type occurring in childhood (295.0-295.9)*

NEUROTIC DISORDERS, PERSONALITY DISORDERS, AND OTHER NONPSYCHOTIC MENTAL DISORDERS (300-316)

ALERT! For personal history of neurosis see V11.2

300 **Anxiety, dissociative and somatoform disorders**

⑤ **300.0 Anxiety states**

Excludes: *anxiety in:*

  acute stress reaction (308.0)
  transient adjustment reaction (309.24)
neurasthenia (300.5)
psychophysiological disorders (306.0-306.9)
separation anxiety (309.21)

300.00   Anxiety state, unspecified
          Anxiety:
            neurosis
            reaction
            state (neurotic)
          Atypical anxiety disorder

300.01   Panic disorder without agoraphobia
          Panic:
            attack
            state

Excludes: *panic disorder with agoraphobia (300.21)*

300.02   Generalized anxiety disorder

300.09   Other

⑤ **300.1 Dissociative, conversion and factitious disorders**

Excludes: *adjustment reaction (309.0-309.9)*

  anorexia nervosa (307.1)
  gross stress reaction (308.0-308.9)
  hysterical personality (301.50-301.59)
  psychophysiologic disorders (306.0-306.9)

300.10   Hysteria, unspecified

300.11   Conversion disorder
          Astasia-abasia, hysterical
          Conversion hysteria or reaction
          Hysterical:
            blindness
            deafness
            paralysis

300.12   Dissociative amnesia
          Hysterical amnesia

300.13   Dissociative fugue
          Hysterical fugue

300.14   Dissociative identity disorder

300.15   Dissociative disorder or reaction, unspecified

● Code new   ▲ Revision of   ④ ⑤ Fourth or fifth
       to this edition   existing code   digit required

300.16 Factitious disorder with predominantly psychological signs and symptoms
Compensation neurosis
Ganser's syndrome, hysterical

300.19 Other and unspecified factitious illness
Factitious disorder (with combined psychological and physical signs and symptoms) (with predominantly physical signs and symptoms) NOS

Excludes: *multiple operations or hospital addiction syndrome (301.51)*

⑤ **300.2 Phobic disorders**

Excludes: *anxiety state not associated with a specific situation or object (300.0-300.09)*
obsessional phobias (300.3)

300.20 Phobia, unspecified
Anxiety-hysteria NOS
Phobia NOS

300.21 Agoraphobia with panic disorder
Fear of:
open spaces with panic attacks
streets with panic attacks
travel with panic attacks
Panic disorder with agoraphobia

Excludes: *agoraphobia without panic disorder (300.22)*
panic disorder without agoraphobia (300.01)

300.22 Agoraphobia without mention of panic attacks
Any condition classifiable to 300.21 without mention of panic attacks

300.23 Social phobia
Fear of:
eating in public
public speaking
washing in public

300.29 Other isolated or specific phobias
Acrophobia   Claustrophobia
Animal phobias   Fear of crowds

300.3 Obsessive-compulsive disorders
Anancastic neurosis   Obsessional phobia [any]
Compulsive neurosis

Excludes: *obsessive-compulsive symptoms occurring in:*
endogenous depression (296.2-296.3)
organic states (e.g., encephalitis)
schizophrenia (295.0-295.9)

300.4 Dysthymic disorder
Anxiety depression   Neurotic depressive state
Depression with anxiety   Reactive depression
Depressive reaction

Excludes: *adjustment reaction with depressive symptoms (309.0-309.1)*
depression NOS (311)
manic-depressive psychosis, depressed type (296.2-296.3)
reactive depressive psychosis (298.0)

300.5 Neurasthenia
Fatigue neurosis
Nervous debility
Psychogenic:
asthenia
general fatigue

Use additional code to identify any associated physical disorder

Excludes: *anxiety state (300.00-300.09)*
neurotic depression (300.4)
psychophysiological disorders (306.0-306.9)
specific nonpsychotic mental disorders following organic brain damage (310.0-310.9)

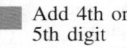 Add 4th or 5th digit
 Nonspecific code
 Unspecified code
 Manifestation code

300.6 Depersonalization disorder
Derealization (neurotic)
Neurotic state with depersonalization episode

Excludes: *depersonalization associated with:*
anxiety (300.00-300.09)
depression (300.4)
manic-depressive disorder or psychosis (296.0-296.9)
schizophrenia (295.0-295.9)

300.7 Hypochondriasis
Body dysmorphic disorder

Excludes: *hypochondriasis in:*
hysteria (300.10-300.19)
manic-depressive psychosis, depressed type (296.2-296.3)
neurasthenia (300.5)
obsessional disorder (300.3)
schizophrenia (295.0-295.9)

⑤ **300.8 Somatoform disorders**

300.81 Somatization disorder
Briquet's disorder
Severe somatoform disorder

300.82 Undifferentiated somatoform disorder
Atypical somatoform disorder
Somatoform disorder NOS

300.89 Other somatoform disorders
Occupational neurosis, including writers' cramp
Psychasthenia
Psychasthenic neurosis

300.9 Unspecified nonpsychotic mental disorder
Psychoneurosis NOS

301 Personality disorders
Includes: character neurosis

Use additional code to identify any associated neurosis or psychosis, or physical condition

Excludes: *nonpsychotic personality disorder associated with organic brain syndromes*
(310.0-310.9)

DEFINITION Personality disorders, formerly referred to as character disorders, are a class of personality types which deviate from the contemporary expectations of a society. Common types of personality disorders include paranoia, schizoid tendencies, antisocial behavior, narcissism, and obsessive-compulsive disorders.

301.0 Paranoid personality disorder
Fanatic personality
Paranoid personality (disorder)
Paranoid traits

Excludes: *acute paranoid reaction (298.3)*
alcoholic paranoia (291.5)
paranoid schizophrenia (295.3)
paranoid states (297.0-297.9)

⑤ **301.1 Affective personality disorder**

Excludes: *affective psychotic disorders (296.0-296.9)*
neurasthenia (300.5)
neurotic depression (300.4)

301.10 Affective personality disorder, unspecified

301.11 Chronic hypomanic personality disorder
Chronic hypomanic disorder
Hypomanic personality

301.12 Chronic depressive personality disorder
Chronic depressive disorder
Depressive character or personality

301.13 Cyclothymic disorder
Cycloid personality
Cyclothymia
Cyclothymic personality

● Code new
to this edition
▲ Revision of
existing code
④ ⑤ Fourth or fifth
digit required

⑤ **301.2 Schizoid personality disorder**

Excludes: schizophrenia (295.0-295.9)

　　301.20 Schizoid personality disorder, unspecified
　　301.21 Introverted personality
　　301.22 Schizotypal personality disorder

301.3 Explosive personality disorder

Aggressive:　　　　　　　　　Emotional instability (excessive)
　personality　　　　　　　　Pathological emotionality
　reaction　　　　　　　　　Quarrelsomeness
Aggressiveness

Excludes: dyssocial personality (301.7)
　　　　　hysterical neurosis (300.10-300.19)

301.4 Obsessive-compulsive personality disorder

Anancastic personality
Obsessional personality

Excludes: obsessive-compulsive disorder (300.3)
　　　　　phobic state (300.20-300.29)

⑤ **301.5 Histrionic personality disorder**

Excludes: hysterical neurosis (300.10-300.19)

　　301.50 Histrionic personality disorder, unspecified
　　　　Hysterical personality NOS

　　301.51 Chronic factitious illness with physical symptoms
　　　　Hospital addiction syndrome
　　　　Multiple operations syndrome
　　　　Munchausen syndrome

　　301.59 Other histrionic personality disorder
　　　　Personality:
　　　　　emotionally unstable
　　　　　labile
　　　　　psychoinfantile

301.6 Dependent personality disorder

Asthenic personality　　　Passive personality
Inadequate personality

Excludes: neurasthenia (300.5)
　　　　　passive-aggressive personality (301.84)

301.7 Antisocial personality disorder

Amoral personality
Asocial personality
Dyssocial personality
Personality disorder with predominantly sociopathic or asocial manifestation

Excludes: disturbance of conduct without specifiable personality disorder (312.0-312.9)
　　　　　explosive personality (301.3)

⑤ **301.8 Other personality disorders**

　　301.81 Narcissistic personality disorder
　　301.82 Avoidant personality disorder
　　301.83 Borderline personality disorder
　　301.84 Passive-aggressive personality
　　301.89 Other
　　　　Personality:　　　　　Personality:
　　　　　eccentric　　　　　　masochistic
　　　　　"haltlose" type　　　　psychoneurotic
　　　　　immature

Excludes: psychoinfantile personality (301.59)

301.9 Unspecified personality disorder

Pathological personality　　Psychopathic:
NOS　　　　　　　　　　constitutional state
Personality disorder NOS　　personality (disorder)

302 **Sexual and gender identity disorders**
Excludes: sexual disorder manifest in:
   organic brain syndrome (290.0-294.9, 310.0-310.9)
   psychosis (295.0-298.9)

302.0 Ego-dystonic sexual orientation
Ego-dystonic lesbianism
Sexual orientation conflict disorder
Excludes: homosexual pedophilia (302.2)

302.1 Zoophilia
Bestiality

302.2 Pedophilia

302.3 Transvestic fetishism
Excludes: trans-sexualism (302.5)

302.4 Exhibitionism

⑤ **302.5 Trans-sexualism**
Sex reassignment surgery status
Excludes: transvestism (302.3)

302.50 With unspecified sexual history

302.51 With asexual history

302.52 With homosexual history

302.53 With heterosexual history

302.6 Gender identity disorder in children
Feminism in boys
Gender identity disorder NOS
Excludes: gender identity disorder in adult (302.85)
   trans-sexualism (302.50-302.53)
   transvestism (302.3)

⑤ **302.7 Psychosexual dysfunction**
Excludes: impotence of organic origin (607.84)
   normal transient symptoms from ruptured hymen
   transient or occasional failures of erection due to fatigue, anxiety, alcohol, or
   drugs

302.70 Psychosexual dysfunction, unspecified
Sexual dysfunction NOS

302.71 Hypoactive sexual desire disorder
Excludes: decreased sexual desire NOS (799.81)

302.72 With inhibited sexual excitement
Female sexual arousal disorder
Frigidity
Impotence
Male erectile disorder

302.73 Female orgasmic disorder

302.74 Male orgasmic disorder

302.75 Premature ejaculation

302.76 Dyspareunia, psychogenic

302.79 With other specified psychosexual dysfunctions
Sexual aversion disorder

⑤ **302.8 Other specified psychosexual disorders**

302.81 Fetishism

302.82 Voyeurism

302.83 Sexual masochism

302.84 Sexual sadism

302.85 Gender identity disorder in adolescents or adults
Use additional code to identify sex reassignment surgery status (302.5)
Excludes: gender identity disorder NOS (302.6)
   gender identity disorder in children (302.6)

● Code new to this edition   ▲ Revision of existing code   ④ ⑤ Fourth or fifth digit required

302.89 **Other**
Frotteurism
Nymphomania
Satyriasis

302.9 **Unspecified psychosexual disorder**
Paraphilia NOS
Pathologic sexuality NOS
Sexual deviation NOS
Sexual disorder NOS

⑤ **303 Alcohol dependence syndrome**
Use additional code to identify any associated condition, as:
alcoholic psychoses (291.0-291.9)
drug dependence (304.0-304.9)
physical complications of alcohol, such as:
cerebral degeneration (331.7)
cirrhosis of liver (571.2)
epilepsy (345.0-345.9)
gastritis (535.3)
hepatitis (571.1)
liver damage NOS (571.3)

Excludes: drunkenness NOS (305.0)

The following fifth-digit subclassification is for use with category 303:

0 **unspecified**

1 **continuous**

2 **episodic**

3 **in remission**

DEFINITION Alcohol dependence syndrome, aka, alcoholism, is the most severe stage of a group of drinking problems which begins with binge drinking and alcohol abuse.
ALERT! For personal history of alcoholism see V11.3

⑤ **303.0 Acute alcoholic intoxication**
[0-3] Acute drunkenness in alcoholism

⑤ **303.9 Other and unspecified alcohol dependence**
[0-3] Chronic alcoholism
Dipsomania

⑤ **304 Drug dependence**
Excludes: nondependent abuse of drugs (305.1-305.9)

The following fifth-digit subclassification is for use with category 304:

0 **unspecified**

1 **continuous**

2 **episodic**

3 **in remission**

⑤ **304.0 Opioid type dependence**
[0-3] Heroin
Meperidine
Methadone
Morphine
Opium
Opium alkaloids and their derivatives
Synthetics with morphine-like effects

⑤ **304.1 Sedative, hypnotic or anxiolytic dependence**
[0-3] Barbiturates
Nonbarbiturate sedatives and tranquilizers with a similar effect:
chlordiazepoxide
diazepam
glutethimide
meprobamate
methaqualone

⑤ **304.2 Cocaine dependence**
[0-3] Coca leaves and derivatives

	Add 4th or 5th digit		Nonspecific code		Unspecified code		Manifestation code

⑤ **304.3 Cannabis dependence**
[0-3]   Hashish
         Hemp
         Marijuana

⑤ **304.4 Amphetamine and other psychostimulant dependence**
[0-3]   Methylphenidate
         Phenmetrazine

⑤ **304.5 Hallucinogen dependence**
[0-3]   Dimethyltryptamine [DMT]
         Lysergic acid diethylamide [LSD] and derivatives
         Mescaline
         Psilocybin

⑤ **304.6 Other specified drug dependence**
[0-3]   Absinthe addiction
         Glue sniffing
         Inhalant dependence
         Phencyclidine dependence

   Excludes: *tobacco dependence (305.1)*

⑤ **304.7 Combinations of opioid type drug with any other**
[0-3]

⑤ **304.8 Combinations of drug dependence excluding opioid type drug**
[0-3]

⑤ **304.9 Unspecified drug dependence**
[0-3]   Drug addiction NOS
         Drug dependence NOS

305 Nondependent abuse of drugs
   Note: Includes cases where a person, for whom no other diagnosis is possible, has come under medical care because of the maladaptive effect of a drug on which he is not dependent and that he has taken on his own initiative to the detriment of his health or social functioning.

   Excludes: *alcohol dependence syndrome (303.0-303.9)*
              drug dependence (304.0-304.9)
              drug withdrawal syndrome (292.0)
              poisoning by drugs or medicinal substances (960.0-979.9)

   The following fifth-digit subclassification is for use with codes 305.0, 305.2-305.9:

      0 unspecified
      1 continuous
      2 episodic
      3 in remission

⑤ **305.0 Alcohol abuse**
[0-3]   Drunkenness NOS
         Excessive drinking of alcohol NOS
         "Hangover" (alcohol)
         Inebriety NOS

   Excludes: *acute alcohol intoxication in alcoholism (303.0)*
              alcoholic psychoses (291.0-291.9)

305.1 Tobacco use disorder
   Tobacco dependence

   Excludes: *history of tobacco use (V15.82)*
              smoking complicating pregnancy (649.0)
              tobacco use disorder complicating pregnancy (649.0)

   ALERT! For personal history of tobacco use see V15.82

⑤ **305.2 Cannabis abuse**
[0-3]

⑤ **305.3 Hallucinogen abuse**
[0-3]   Acute intoxication from hallucinogens ["bad trips"]
         LSD reaction

⑤ **305.4 Sedative, hypnotic or anxiolytic abuse**
[0-3]

⑤ **305.5 Opioid abuse**
[0-3]

⑤ **305.6 Cocaine abuse**
[0-3]

⑤ **305.7 Amphetamine or related acting sympathomimetic abuse**
[0-3]

⑤ **305.8 Antidepressant type abuse**
[0-3]

⑤ **305.9 Other, mixed, or unspecified drug abuse**
[0-3]   Caffeine intoxication
Inhalant abuse
"Laxative habit"
Misuse of drugs NOS
Nonprescribed use of drugs or patent medicinals
Phencyclidine abuse

306 Physiological malfunction arising from mental factors
Includes: psychogenic:
physical symptoms not involving tissue damage
physiological manifestation not involving tissue damage

Excludes: *hysteria (300.11-300.19)*

physical symptoms secondary to a psychiatric disorder classified elsewhere
psychic factors associated with physical conditions involving tissue damage
classified elsewhere (316)
specific nonpsychotic mental disorders following organic brain damage
(310.0-310.9)

306.0 Musculoskeletal
Psychogenic paralysis
Psychogenic torticollis

Excludes: *Gilles de la Tourette's syndrome (307.23)*

paralysis as hysterical or conversion reaction (300.11)
tics (307.20-307.22)

306.1 Respiratory
Psychogenic: Psychogenic:
air hunger   hyperventilation
cough   yawning
hiccough

Excludes: *psychogenic asthma (316 and 493.9)*

306.2 Cardiovascular
Cardiac neurosis
Cardiovascular neurosis
Neurocirculatory asthenia
Psychogenic cardiovascular disorder

Excludes: *psychogenic paroxysmal tachycardia (316 and 427.2)*

306.3 Skin
Psychogenic pruritus

Excludes: *psychogenic:*

alopecia (316 and 704.00)
dermatitis (316 and 692.9)
eczema (316 and 691.8 or 692.9)
urticaria (316 and 708.0-708.9)

306.4 Gastrointestinal
Aerophagy   Diarrhea, psychogenic
Cyclical vomiting,   Nervous gastritis
psychogenic   Psychogenic dyspepsia

Excludes: *cyclical vomiting NOS (536.2)*

associated with migraine (346.2)
globus hystericus (300.11)
mucous colitis (316 and 564.9)
psychogenic:
cardiospasm (316 and 530.0)
duodenal ulcer (316 and 532.0-532.9)
gastric ulcer (316 and 531.0-531.9)
peptic ulcer NOS (316 and 533.0-533.9)
vomiting NOS (307.54)

| | Add 4th or 5th digit | | Nonspecific code | | Unspecified code | | Manifestation code |

⑤ **306.5 Genitourinary**

Excludes: *enuresis, psychogenic (307.6)*
frigidity (302.72)
impotence (302.72)
psychogenic dyspareunia (302.76)

306.50 Psychogenic genitourinary malfunction, unspecified

306.51 Psychogenic vaginismus
Functional vaginismus

306.52 Psychogenic dysmenorrhea

306.53 Psychogenic dysuria

306.59 Other

306.6 Endocrine

306.7 Organs of special sense

Excludes: *hysterical blindness or deafness (300.11)*
psychophysical visual disturbances (368.16)

306.8 Other specified psychophysiological malfunction
Bruxism
Teeth grinding

306.9 Unspecified psychophysiological malfunction
Psychophysiologic disorder NOS
Psychosomatic disorder NOS

307 Special symptoms or syndromes, not elsewhere classified

Note: This category is intended for use if the psychopathology is manifested by a single specific symptom or group of symptoms which is not part of an organic illness or other mental disorder classifiable elsewhere.

Excludes: *those due to mental disorders classified elsewhere*
those of organic origin

307.0 Adult onset fluency disorder

Excludes: *childhood onset fluency disorder (315.35)*
dysphasia (784.59)
lisping or lalling (307.9)
retarded development of speech (315.31-315.39)
fluency disorder due to late effect of cerebrovascular accident (438.14)
fluency disorder in conditions classified elsewhere (784.52)

307.1 Anorexia nervosa

Excludes: *eating disturbance NOS (307.50)*
feeding problem (783.3)
of nonorganic origin (307.59)
loss of appetite (783.0)
of nonorganic origin (307.59)

⑤ **307.2 Tics**

Excludes: *nail-biting or thumb-sucking (307.9)*
stereotypies occurring in isolation (307.3)
tics of organic origin (333.3)

307.20 Tic disorder, unspecified
Tic disorder NOS

307.21 Transient tic disorder

307.22 Chronic motor or vocal tic disorder

307.23 Tourette's disorder
Motor-verbal tic disorder

307.3 Stereotypic movement disorder
Body-rocking   Spasmus nutans
Head banging   Stereotypies NOS

Excludes: *tics (307.20-307.23)*
of organic origin (333.3)

● Code new
to this edition   ▲ Revision of
existing code   ④ ⑤ Fourth or fifth
digit required

⑤ **307.4 Specific disorders of sleep of nonorganic origin**

Excludes: narcolepsy (347.00-347.11)
organic hypersomnia (327.10-327.19)
organic insomnia (327.00-327.09)
those of unspecified cause (780.50-780.59)

307.40 Nonorganic sleep disorder, unspecified

307.41 Transient disorder of initiating or maintaining sleep
Adjustment insomnia
Hyposomnia associated with acute or intermittent emotional reactions or conflicts
Insomnia associated with acute or intermittent emotional reactions or conflicts
Sleeplessness associated with acute or intermittent emotional reactions or conflicts

307.42 Persistent disorder of initiating or maintaining sleep
Hyposomnia, insomnia, or sleeplessness associated with:
anxiety
conditioned arousal
depression (major) (minor)
psychosis
Idiopathic insomnia
Paradoxical insomnia
Primary insomnia
Psychophysiological insomnia

307.43 Transient disorder of initiating or maintaining wakefulness
Hypersomnia associated with acute or intermittent emotional reactions or conflicts

307.44 Persistent disorder of initiating or maintaining wakefulness
Hypersomnia associated with depression (major) (minor)
Insufficient sleep syndrome
Primary hypersomnia

Excludes: sleep deprivation (V69.4)

307.45 Circadian rhythm sleep disorder of nonorganic origin

307.46 Sleep arousal disorder
Night terror disorder
Night terrors
Sleep terror disorder
Sleepwalking
Somnambulism

307.47 Other dysfunctions of sleep stages or arousal from sleep
Dyssomnia NOS
Nightmare disorder
Nightmares:
NOS
REM-sleep type
Parasomnia NOS
Sleep drunkenness

307.48 Repetitive intrusions of sleep
Repetitive intrusion of sleep with:
atypical polysomnographic features
environmental disturbances
repeated REM-sleep interruptions

307.49 Other
"Short-sleeper"
Subjective insomnia complaint

⑤ **307.5 Other and unspecified disorders of eating**

Excludes: anorexia:
nervosa (307.1)
of unspecified cause (783.0)
overeating, of unspecified cause (783.6)
vomiting:
NOS (787.03)
cyclical (536.2)
associated with migraine (346.2)
psychogenic (306.4)

Add 4th or 5th digit   Nonspecific code   Unspecified code   Manifestation code

307.50 Eating disorder, unspecified
Eating disorder NOS

307.51 Bulimia nervosa
Overeating of nonorganic origin

307.52 Pica
Perverted appetite of nonorganic origin

307.53 Rumination disorder
Regurgitation, of nonorganic origin, of food with reswallowing

Excludes: obsessional rumination (300.3)

307.54 Psychogenic vomiting

307.59 Other
Feeding disorder of infancy or early childhood of nonorganic origin
Infantile feeding disturbances of nonorganic origin
Loss of appetite of nonorganic origin

307.6 Enuresis
Enuresis (primary) (secondary) of nonorganic origin

Excludes: enuresis of unspecified cause (788.3)

307.7 Encopresis
Encopresis (continuous) (discontinuous) of nonorganic origin

Excludes: encopresis of unspecified cause (787.60-787.63)

⑤ **307.8 Pain disorders related to psychological factors**

307.80 Psychogenic pain, site unspecified

307.81 Tension headache

Excludes: headache:
NOS (784.0)
migraine (346.0-346.9)
syndromes (339.00-339.89)
tension type (339.10-339.12)

307.89 Other

Code first to type or site of pain

Excludes: pain disorder exclusively attributed to psychological factors (307.80)
psychogenic pain (307.80)

307.9 Other and unspecified special symptoms or syndromes, not elsewhere classified
Communication disorder NOS
Hair plucking
Lalling
Lisping
Masturbation
Nail-biting
Thumb-sucking

308 Acute reaction to stress
Includes: catastrophic stress
combat and operational stress reaction
combat fatigue
gross stress reaction (acute)
transient disorders in response to exceptional physical or mental stress which
usually subside within hours or days

Excludes: adjustment reaction or disorder (309.0-309.9)
chronic stress reaction (309.1-309.9)

308.0 Predominant disturbance of emotions
Anxiety as acute reaction to exceptional [gross] stress
Emotional crisis as acute reaction to exceptional [gross] stress
Panic state as acute reaction to exceptional [gross] stress

308.1 Predominant disturbance of consciousness
Fugues as acute reaction to exceptional [gross] stress

308.2 Predominant psychomotor disturbance
Agitation states as acute reaction to exceptional [gross] stress
Stupor as acute reaction to exceptional [gross] stress

● Code new
to this edition

▲ Revision of
existing code

④ ⑤ Fourth or fifth
digit required

308.3 Other acute reactions to stress
Acute situational disturbance
Acute stress disorder

Excludes: *prolonged posttraumatic emotional disturbance (309.81)*

308.4 Mixed disorders as reaction to stress

308.9 Unspecified acute reaction to stress

309 Adjustment reaction
Includes: adjustment disorders
reaction (adjustment) to chronic stress

Excludes: *acute reaction to major stress (308.0-308.9)*
neurotic disorders (300.0-300.9)

ALERT! For personal history of psychological trauma presenting hazards to health see V15.4

309.0 Adjustment disorder with depressed mood
Grief reaction

Excludes: *affective psychoses (296.0-296.9)*
neurotic depression (300.4)
prolonged depressive reaction (309.1)
psychogenic depressive psychosis (298.0)

309.1 Prolonged depressive reaction

Excludes: *affective psychoses (296.0-296.9)*
brief depressive reaction (309.0)
neurotic depression (300.4)
psychogenic depressive psychosis (298.0)

⑤ **309.2 With predominant disturbance of other emotions**

309.21 Separation anxiety disorder

309.22 Emancipation disorder of adolescence and early adult life

309.23 Specific academic or work inhibition

309.24 Adjustment disorder with anxiety

309.28 Adjustment disorder with mixed anxiety and depressed mood
Adjustment reaction with anxiety and depression

309.29 Other
Culture shock

309.3 Adjustment disorder with disturbance of conduct
Conduct disturbance as adjustment reaction
Destructiveness as adjustment reaction

Excludes: *destructiveness in child (312.9)*
disturbance of conduct NOS (312.9)
dyssocial behavior without manifest psychiatric disorder (V71.01-V71.02)
personality disorder with predominantly sociopathic or asocial manifestations (301.7)

309.4 Adjustment disorder with mixed disturbance of emotions and conduct

⑤ **309.8 Other specified adjustment reactions**

309.81 Posttraumatic stress disorder
Chronic posttraumatic stress disorder
Concentration camp syndrome
Posttraumatic stress disorder NOS
Post-Traumatic Stress Disorder (PTSD)

Excludes: *acute stress disorder (308.3)*
posttraumatic brain syndrome:
nonpsychotic (310.2)
psychotic (293.0-293.9)

309.82 Adjustment reaction with physical symptoms

309.83 Adjustment reaction with withdrawal
Elective mutism as adjustment reaction
Hospitalism (in children) NOS

309.89 Other

309.9 Unspecified adjustment reaction
Adaptation reaction NOS
Adjustment reaction NOS

| | Add 4th or 5th digit | | Nonspecific code | | Unspecified code | | Manifestation code |

310 **Specific nonpsychotic mental disorders due to brain damage**

> Excludes: *neuroses, personality disorders, or other nonpsychotic conditions occurring in a form similar to that seen with functional disorders but in association with a physical condition (300.0-300.9, 301.0-301.9)*

> **ALERT!** For personal history of unspecified mental disorder see V11.9

310.0 **Frontal lobe syndrome**
Lobotomy syndrome
Postleucotomy syndrome [state]

> Excludes: *postcontusion syndrome (310.2)*

310.1 **Personality change due to conditions classified elsewhere**
Cognitive or personality change of other type, of nonpsychotic severity
Organic psychosyndrome of nonpsychotic severity
Presbyophrenia NOS
Senility with mental changes of nonpsychotic severity

> Excludes: *mild cognitive impairment (331.83)*
> *postconcussion syndrome (310.2)*
> *signs and symptoms involving emotional state (799.21-799.29)*

310.2 **Postconcussion syndrome**
Postcontusion syndrome or encephalopathy
Posttraumatic brain syndrome, nonpsychotic
Status postcommotio cerebri

Use additional code to identify associated post-traumatic headache, if applicable (339.20-339.22)

> Excludes: *frontal lobe syndrome (310.0)*
> *postencephalitic syndrome (310.89)*
> *any organic psychotic conditions following head injury (293.0—294.0)*

⑤ **310.8** **Other specified nonpsychotic mental disorders following organic brain damage**

● **310.81** **Pseudobulbar affect**
Involuntary emotional expression disorder

Code first underlying cause, if known, such as:
amyotrophic lateral sclerosis (335.20)
late effect of cerebrovascular accident (438.89)
late effect of traumatic brain injury (907.0)
multiple sclerosis (340)

● **310.89** **Other specified nonpsychotic mental disorders following organic brain damage**
Mild memory disturbance
Other focal (partial) organic psychosyndromes
Postencephalitic syndrome

> Excludes: *memory loss of unknown cause (780.93)*

310.9 **Unspecified nonpsychotic mental disorder following organic brain damage**

311 **Depressive disorder, not elsewhere classified**
Depressive disorder NOS
Depressive state NOS
Depression NOS

> Excludes: *acute reaction to major stress with depressive symptoms (308.0)*
> *affective personality disorder (301.10-301.13)*
> *affective psychoses (296.0-296.9)*
> *brief depressive reaction (309.0)*
> *depressive states associated with stressful events (309.0-309.1)*
> *disturbance of emotions specific to childhood and adolescence, with misery and unhappiness (313.1)*
> *mixed adjustment reaction with depressive symptoms (309.4)*
> *neurotic depression (300.4)*
> *prolonged depressive adjustment reaction (309.1)*
> *psychogenic depressive psychosis (298.0)*

> **ALERT!** For personal history of unspecified mental disorder see V11.9

312 **Disturbance of conduct, not elsewhere classified**

> Excludes: *adjustment reaction with disturbance of conduct (309.3)*
> *drug dependence (304.0-304.9)*
> *dyssocial behavior without manifest psychiatric disorder (V71.01-V71.02)*
> *personality disorder with predominantly sociopathic or asocial manifestations (301.7)*
> *sexual deviations (302.0-302.9)*

● Code new to this edition   ▲ Revision of existing code   ④ ⑤ Fourth or fifth digit required

The following fifth-digit subclassification is for use with categories 312.0-312.2:

0   unspecified

1   mild

2   moderate

3   severe

ALERT! For personal history of unspecified mental disorder see V11.9

⑤ **312.0   Undersocialized conduct disorder, aggressive type**
[0-3] Aggressive outburst
Anger reaction
Unsocialized aggressive disorder

⑤ **312.1   Undersocialized conduct disorder, unaggressive type**
[0-3] Childhood truancy,   Solitary stealing
unsocialized   Tantrums

⑤ **312.2   Socialized conduct disorder**
[0-3] Childhood truancy, socialized
Group delinquency

Excludes: gang activity without manifest psychiatric disorder (V71.01)

⑤ **312.3   Disorders of impulse control, not elsewhere classified**

312.30   Impulse control disorder, unspecified

312.31   Pathological gambling

312.32   Kleptomania

312.33   Pyromania

312.34   Intermittent explosive disorder

312.35   Isolated explosive disorder

312.39   Other
Trichotillomania

312.4   Mixed disturbance of conduct and emotions
Neurotic delinquency

Excludes: compulsive conduct disorder (312.3)

⑤ **312.8   Other specified disturbances of conduct, not elsewhere classified**

312.81   Conduct disorder, childhood onset type

312.82   Conduct disorder, adolescent onset type

312.89   Other conduct disorder
Conduct disorder of unspecified onset

312.9   Unspecified disturbance of conduct
Delinquency (juvenile)
Disruptive behavior disorder NOS

313   Disturbance of emotions specific to childhood and adolescence

Excludes: adjustment reaction (309.0-309.9)

emotional disorder of neurotic type (300.0-300.9)
masturbation, nail-biting, thumb-sucking, and other isolated symptoms (307.0-307.9)

313.0   Overanxious disorder
Anxiety and fearfulness of childhood and adolescence
Overanxious disorder of childhood and adolescence

Excludes: abnormal separation anxiety (309.21)

anxiety states (300.00-300.09)
hospitalism in children (309.83)
phobic state (300.20-300.29)

313.1   Misery and unhappiness disorder

Excludes: depressive neurosis (300.4)

⑤ **313.2   Sensitivity, shyness, and social withdrawal disorder**

Excludes: infantile autism (299.0)

schizoid personality (301.20-301.22)
schizophrenia (295.0-295.9)

313.21   Shyness disorder of childhood
Sensitivity reaction of childhood or adolescence

| Add 4th or 5th digit | Nonspecific code | Unspecified code | Manifestation code |

313.22 Introverted disorder of childhood
Social withdrawal of childhood and adolescence
Withdrawal reaction of childhood and adolescence

313.23 Selective mutism

Excludes: *elective mutism as adjustment reaction (309.83)*

313.3 Relationship problems
Sibling jealousy

Excludes: *relationship problems associated with aggression, destruction, or other forms of conduct disturbance (312.0-312.9)*

⑤ **313.8 Other or mixed emotional disturbances of childhood or adolescence**

313.81 Oppositional defiant disorder

313.82 Identity disorder
Identity problem

313.83 Academic underachievement disorder

313.89 Other
Reactive attachment disorder of infancy or early childhood

313.9 Unspecified emotional disturbance of childhood or adolescence
Mental disorder of infancy, childhood or adolescence NOS

314 Hyperkinetic syndrome of childhood

Excludes: *hyperkinesis as symptom of underlying disorder—code the underlying disorder*

DEFINITION Hyperkinetic syndrome of childhood is a childhood or adolescent disorder characterized by excessive activity, emotional instability, significantly reduced attention span, and an absence of shyness and fear, and that occasionally develops in individuals with brain injury, mental defect, or epilepsy.

⑤ **314.0 Attention deficit disorder**
Adult
Child

314.00 Without mention of hyperactivity
Predominantly inattentive type

314.01 With hyperactivity
Combined type
Overactivity NOS
Predominantly hyperactive/impulsive type
Simple disturbance of attention with overactivity

314.1 Hyperkinesis with developmental delay
Developmental disorder of hyperkinesis
Use additional code to identify any associated neurological disorder

314.2 Hyperkinetic conduct disorder
Hyperkinetic conduct disorder without developmental delay

Excludes: *hyperkinesis with significant delays in specific skills (314.1)*

314.8 Other specified manifestations of hyperkinetic syndrome

314.9 Unspecified hyperkinetic syndrome
Hyperkinetic reaction of childhood or adolescence NOS
Hyperkinetic syndrome NOS

315 Specific delays in development

Excludes: *that due to a neurological disorder (320.0-389.9)*

⑤ **315.0 Specific reading disorder**

315.00 Reading disorder, unspecified

315.01 Alexia

315.02 Developmental dyslexia

315.09 Other
Specific spelling difficulty

315.1 Mathematics disorder
Dyscalculia

315.2 Other specific learning difficulties
Disorder of written expression

Excludes: *specific arithmetical disorder (315.1)*
specific reading disorder (315.00-315.09)

● Code new
to this edition   ▲ Revision of
existing code   ④ ⑤ Fourth or fifth
digit required

⑤ **315.3 Developmental speech or language disorder**

315.31 Expressive language disorder
Developmental aphasia
Word deafness

Excludes: *acquired aphasia (784.3)*
elective mutism (309.83, 313.0, 313.23)

315.32 Mixed receptive-expressive language disorder
Central auditory processing disorder

Excludes: *acquired auditory processing disorder (388.45)*

315.34 Speech and language developmental delay due to hearing loss

315.35 Childhood onset fluency disorder
Cluttering NOS
Stuttering NOS

Excludes: *adult onset fluency disorder (307.0)*
fluency disorder due to late effect of cerebrovascular accident (438.14)
fluency disorder in conditions classified elsewhere (784.52)

315.39 Other
Developmental articulation disorder
Dyslalia
Phonological disorder

Excludes: *lisping and lalling (307.9)*

315.4 Developmental coordination disorder
Clumsiness syndrome
Dyspraxia syndrome
Specific motor development disorder

315.5 Mixed development disorder

315.8 Other specified delays in development

315.9 Unspecified delay in development
Developmental disorder NOS
Learning disorder NOS

316 Psychic factors associated with diseases classified elsewhere
Psychologic factors in physical conditions classified elsewhere

Use additional code to identify the associated physical condition, as:
psychogenic:
asthma (493.9)
dermatitis (692.9)
duodenal ulcer (532.0-532.9)
eczema (691.8, 692.9)
gastric ulcer (531.0-531.9)
mucous colitis (564.9)
paroxysmal tachycardia (427.2)
ulcerative colitis (556)
urticaria (708.0-708.9)
psychosocial dwarfism (259.4)

Excludes: *physical symptoms and physiological malfunctions, not involving tissue damage, of mental origin (306.0-306.9)*

INTELLECTUAL DISABILITIES (317-319)

Use additional code(s) to identify any associated psychiatric or physical condition(s)

▲ **317 Mild intellectual disabilities**
High-grade defect   Mild mental subnormality
IQ 50-70

DEFINITION Intellectual disabilities is a generalized disorder, characterized by sub average cognitive functioning and deficits in two or more adaptive behaviors with onset before the age of 18.

▲ **318 Other specified intellectual disabilities**

▲ **318.0 Moderate intellectual disabilities**
IQ 35-49
Moderate mental subnormality

▲ **318.1 Severe intellectual disabilities**
IQ 20-34
Severe mental subnormality

Add 4th or   Nonspecific   Unspecified   Manifestation
5th digit   code   code   code

▲ **318.2 Profound intellectual disabilities**
　　　IQ under 20
　　　Profound mental subnormality

▲ **319 Unspecified intellectual disabilities**
　　　Mental deficiency NOS
　　　Mental subnormality NOS

● Code new
　to this edition
▲ Revision of
　existing code
④ ⑤ Fourth or fifth
　　digit required

Chapter 6: Diseases of Nervous System and Sense Organs (320-389)

DEFINITIONS AND CODING ALERTS

This chapter includes definitions of selected key words, terms and phrases and coding alerts for adding points to the clinical domain, references to coding late effects where appropriate, and references to personal history V-codes in situations where the acute or chronic condition is no longer active. An example from this chapter is as follows:

> **324** **Intracranial and intraspinal abscess**
> **DEFINITION** Intracranial and intraspinal abscess refers to an abcess occuring inside the cranium or the spinal column
> **ALERT!** For coding late effects of intracranial abscess or pyogenic infection see 326

MULTIPLE CODING FOR A SINGLE CONDITION

In addition to the etiology or manifestation convention that requires two codes to fully describe a single condition that affects multiple body systems, there are other single conditions that also require more than one code. "Use additional code" notes are found in the tabular at codes that are not part of an etiology or manifestation pair where a secondary code is useful to fully describe a condition. The sequencing rule is the same as the etiology or manifestation pair - , "use additional code" indicates that a secondary code should be added.

"Code first" notes are also under certain codes that are not specifically manifestation codes but may be due to an underlying cause. When a "code first" note is present and an underlying condition is present the underlying condition should be sequenced first.

"Code, if applicable, any causal condition first", notes indicate that this code may be assigned as a principal diagnosis when the causal condition is unknown or not applicable. If a causal condition is known, then the code for that condition should be sequenced as the principal or first-listed diagnosis. Multiple codes may be needed for late effects, complication codes and obstetric codes to more fully describe a condition. See the specific guidelines for these conditions for further instruction.

COMBINATION CODE

A combination code is a single code used to classify: two diagnoses, or a diagnosis with an associated secondary process (manifestation) A diagnosis with an associated complication Combination codes are identified by referring to subterm entries in the Alphabetic Index and by reading the inclusion and exclusion notes in the Tabular List.

Assign only the combination code when that code fully identifies the diagnostic conditions involved or when the Alphabetic Index so directs. Multiple coding should not be used when the classification provides a combination code that clearly identifies all of the elements documented in the diagnosis. When the combination code lacks necessary specificity in describing the manifestation or complication, an additional code should be used as a secondary code.

CODING LATE EFFECTS

A late effect is the residual effect (condition produced) after the acute phase of an illness or injury has terminated. There is no time limit on when a late effect code can be used. The residual may be apparent early, such as in cerebrovascular accident cases, or it may occur months or years later, such as that due to a previous injury. Coding of late effects generally requires two codes sequenced in the following order: The condition or nature of the late effect is sequenced first. The late effect code is sequenced second.

An exception to the above guidelines are those instances where the code for late effect is followed by a manifestation code identified in the Tabular List and title, or the late effect code has been expanded (at the fourth and fifth-digit levels) to include the manifestation(s). The code for the acute phase of an illness or injury that led to the late effect is never used with a code for the late effect.

PAIN - CATEGORY 338

General coding information

Codes in category 338 may be used in conjunction with codes from other categories and chapters to provide more detail about acute or chronic pain and neoplasm-related pain, unless otherwise indicated below.

	Add 4th or 5th digit		Nonspecific code		Unspecified code		Manifestation code

If the pain is not specified as acute or chronic, do not assign codes from category 338, except for post-thoracotomy pain, postoperative pain, neoplasm related pain, or central pain syndrome.

A code from subcategories 338.1 and 338.2 should not be assigned if the underlying (definitive) diagnosis is known, unless the reason for the encounter is pain control or management and not management of the underlying condition.

A.   Category 338 Codes as Principal or First-Listed Diagnosis

Category 338 codes are acceptable as principal diagnosis or the first-listed code:

1)   When pain control or pain management is the reason for the admission or encounter (e.g., a patient with displaced intervertebral disc, nerve impingement and severe back pain presents for injection of steroid into the spinal canal). The underlying cause of the pain should be reported as an additional diagnosis, if known.

2)   When an admission or encounter is for a procedure aimed at treating the underlying condition (e.g., spinal fusion, kyphoplasty), a code for the underlying condition (e.g., vertebral fracture, spinal stenosis) should be assigned as the principal diagnosis. No code from category 338 should be assigned.

3)   When a patient is admitted for the insertion of a neurostimulator for pain control, assign the appropriate pain code as the principal or first listed diagnosis. When an admission or encounter is for a procedure aimed at treating the underlying condition and a neurostimulator is inserted for pain control during the same admission or encounter, a code for the underlying condition should be assigned as the principal diagnosis and the appropriate pain code should be assigned as a secondary diagnosis.

B.   Use of Category 338 Codes in Conjunction with Site-Specific Pain Codes

1)   Assigning Category 338 Codes and Site Specific Pain Codes

Codes from category 338 may be used in conjunction with codes that identify the site of pain including codes from chapter 16. If the category 338 code provides additional information. For example, if the code describes the site of the pain, but does not fully describe whether the pain is acute or chronic, then both codes should be assigned.

2)   Sequencing of Category 338 Codes with Site Specific Pain Codes

The sequencing of category 338 codes with site specific pain codes (including chapter 16 codes), is dependent on the circumstances of the encounter or admission as follows:

a)   If the encounter is for pain control or pain management, assign the code from category 338 followed by the code identifying the specific site of pain (e.g., encounter for pain management for acute neck pain from trauma is assigned code 338.11, Acute pain due to trauma, followed by code 723.1, Cervicalgia, to identify the site of pain).

b)   If the encounter is for any other reason except pain control or pain management, and a related definitive diagnosis has not been established (confirmed) by the provider, assign the code for the specific site of pain first, followed by the appropriate code from category 338.

Pain due to devices, implants and grafts

Pain associated with devices, implants or grafts left in a surgical site (for example painful hip prosthesis) is assigned to the appropriate code(s) found in Chapter 17, Injury and Poisoning. Use additional code(s) from category 338 to identify acute or chronic pain due to presence of the device, implant or graft (338.18-338.19 or 338.28-338.29).

Postoperative Pain

Post-thoracotomy pain and other postoperative pain are classified to subcategories 338.1 and 338.2, depending on whether the pain is acute or chronic. The default for post-thoracotomy and other postoperative pain not specified as acute or chronic is the code for the acute form.

Routine or expected postoperative pain immediately after surgery should not be coded.

A.   Postoperative pain not associated with specific postoperative complication

Postoperative pain not associated with a specific postoperative complication is assigned to the appropriate postoperative pain code in category 338.

● Code new
     to this edition
     ▲ Revision of
       existing code
     ④ ⑤ Fourth or fifth
         digit required

B. Postoperative pain associated with specific postoperative complication

Postoperative pain associated with a specific postoperative complication (such as painful wire sutures) is assigned to the appropriate code(s) found in Chapter 17, Injury and Poisoning. If appropriate, use additional code(s) from category 338 to identify acute or chronic pain (338.18 or 338.28). If pain control or management is the reason for the encounter, a code from category 338 should be assigned as the principal or first-listed diagnosis in accordance with Official Guidelines, Section I.C.6.a.1.a above.

C. Postoperative pain as principal or first-listed diagnosis

Postoperative pain may be reported as the principal or first-listed diagnosis when the stated reason for the admission or encounter is documented as postoperative pain control or management.

D. Postoperative pain as secondary diagnosis

Postoperative pain may be reported as a secondary diagnosis code when a patient presents for outpatient surgery and develops an unusual or inordinate amount of postoperative pain.

The provider's documentation should be used to guide the coding of postoperative pain, as well as Official Guidelines, Section III. Reporting Additional Diagnoses and Official Guidelines, Section IV. Diagnostic Coding and Reporting in the Outpatient Setting.

See Official Guidelines, Section II.I.2 for information on sequencing of diagnoses for patients admitted to hospital inpatient care following post-operative observation.

See Official Guidelines, Section II.J for information on sequencing of diagnoses for patients admitted to hospital inpatient care from outpatient surgery.

See Official Guidelines, Section IV.A.2 for information on sequencing of diagnoses for patients admitted for observation.

CHRONIC PAIN

Chronic pain is classified to subcategory 338.2. There is no time frame defining when pain becomes chronic pain. The provider's documentation should be used to guide use of these codes.

NEOPLASM RELATED PAIN

Code 338.3 is assigned to pain documented as being related, associated or due to cancer, primary or secondary malignancy, or tumor. This code is assigned regardless of whether the pain is acute or chronic.

This code may be assigned as the principal or first listed code when the stated reason for the admission or encounter is documented as pain control or pain management. The underlying neoplasm should be reported as an additional diagnosis.

When the reason for the admission or encounter is management of the neoplasm and the pain associated with the neoplasm is also documented, code 338.3 may be assigned as an additional diagnosis.

See Chapter 2 for instructions on the sequencing of neoplasms for all other stated reasons for the admission or encounter (except for pain control or pain management).

CHRONIC PAIN SYNDROME

This condition is different than the term "chronic pain," and therefore this code should only be used when the provider has specifically documented this condition.

Add 4th or 5th digit   Nonspecific code   Unspecified code   Manifestation code

This page intentionally left blank.

● Code new
  to this edition

▲ Revision of
  existing code

④ ⑤ Fourth or fifth
  digit required

6. DISEASES OF THE NERVOUS SYSTEM AND SENSE ORGANS (320-389)

ALERT! For personal history of disorders of nervous system and sense organs see V12.4

INFLAMMATORY DISEASES OF THE CENTRAL NERVOUS SYSTEM (320-326)

ALERT! For personal history of infections of the central nervous system see V12.42

320 Bacterial meningitis

Includes: arachnoiditis, bacterial
leptomeningitis, bacterial
meningitis, bacterial
meningoencephalitis, bacterial
meningomyelitis, bacterial
pachymeningitis, bacterial

DEFINITION Meningitis is an infectious disease characterized by inflammation of the meninges (the tissues that surround the brain or spinal cord) usually caused by a bacterial infection; symptoms include headache and stiff neck and fever and nausea.

320.0 Hemophilus meningitis
Meningitis due to Hemophilus influenzae [H. influenzae]

320.1 Pneumococcal meningitis

320.2 Streptococcal meningitis

320.3 Staphylococcal meningitis

320.7 *Meningitis in other bacterial diseases classified elsewhere*
Code first underlying disease, as:
actinomycosis (039.8)
listeriosis (027.0)
typhoid fever (002.0)
whooping cough (033.0-033.9)

Excludes: *meningitis (in):*
epidemic (036.0)
gonococcal (098.82)
meningococcal (036.0)
salmonellosis (003.21)
syphilis:
NOS (094.2)
congenital (090.42)
meningovascular (094.2)
secondary (091.81)
tuberculous (013.0)

⑤ **320.8 Meningitis due to other specified bacteria**

320.81 Anaerobic meningitis
Bacteroides (fragilis)
Gram-negative anaerobes

320.82 Meningitis due to Gram-negative bacteria, not elsewhere classified
Aerobacter aerogenes
Escherichia coli [E. coli]
Friedlander bacillus
Klebsiella pneumoniae
Proteus morganii
Pseudomonas

Excludes: *Gram-negative anaerobes (320.81)*

320.89 Meningitis due to other specified bacteria
Bacillus pyocyaneus

320.9 Meningitis due to unspecified bacterium

Meningitis:	Meningitis:
bacterial NOS	pyogenic NOS
purulent NOS	suppurative NOS

321 Meningitis due to other organisms

Includes: arachnoiditis due to organisms other than bacteria
leptomeningitis due to organisms other than bacteria
meningitis due to organisms other than bacteria
pachymeningitis due to organisms other than bacteria

321.0 *Cryptococcal meningitis*
Code first underlying disease (117.5)

	Add 4th or 5th digit		Nonspecific code		Unspecified code		Manifestation code

321.1 Meningitis in other fungal diseases
  Code first underlying disease (110.0-118)

  Excludes: meningitis in:
  candidiasis (112.83)
  coccidioidomycosis (114.2)
  histoplasmosis (115.01, 115.11, 115.91)

321.2 Meningitis due to viruses not elsewhere classified
  Code first underlying disease, as:
  meningitis due to arbovirus (060.0-066.9)

  Excludes: meningitis (due to):
  abacterial (047.0-047.9)
  adenovirus (049.1)
  aseptic NOS (047.9)
  Coxsackie (virus) (047.0)
  ECHO virus (047.1)
  enterovirus (047.0-047.9)
  herpes simplex virus (054.72)
  herpes zoster virus (053.0)
  lymphocytic choriomeningitis virus (049.0)
  mumps (072.1)
  viral NOS (047.9)
  meningo-eruptive syndrome (047.1)

321.3 Meningitis due to trypanosomiasis
  Code first underlying disease (086.0-086.9)

321.4 Meningitis in sarcoidosis
  Code first underlying disease (135)

321.8 Meningitis due to other nonbacterial organisms classified elsewhere
  Code first underlying disease

  Excludes: leptospiral meningitis (100.81)

322 Meningitis of unspecified cause
  Includes: arachnoiditis with no organism specified as cause
  leptomeningitis with no organism specified as cause
  meningitis with no organism specified as cause
  pachymeningitis with no organism specified as cause

322.0 Nonpyogenic meningitis
  Meningitis with clear cerebrospinal fluid

322.1 Eosinophilic meningitis

322.2 Chronic meningitis

322.9 Meningitis, unspecified

323 Encephalitis, myelitis, and encephalomyelitis
  Includes: acute disseminated encephalomyelitis
  meningoencephalitis, except bacterial
  meningomyelitis, except bacterial
  myelitis:
  ascending
  transverse

  Excludes: acute transverse myelitis NOS (341.20)
  acute transverse myelitis in conditions classified elsewhere (341.21)
  bacterial:
  meningoencephalitis (320.0-320.9)
  meningomyelitis (320.0-320.9)
  idiopathic transverse myelitis (341.22)
  idiopathic transverse myelitis (341.22)

  DEFINITION Encephalitis is an inflammation of the brain, usually caused by a direct viral infection or a hypersensitivity reaction to a virus or foreign protein. Myelitis is an inflammation of the spinal column. Encephalomyelitis is an inflammation of the brain and spinal cord.

⑤ 323.0 Encephalitis, myelitis, and encephalomyelitis in viral diseases classified elsewhere
  Code first underlying disease, as:
  cat-scratch disease (078.3)
  infectious mononucleosis (075)
  human immunodeficiency virus [HIV] disease (042)
  ornithosis (073.7)

● Code new
  to this edition

▲ Revision of
  existing code

④ ⑤ Fourth or fifth
  digit required

323.01 *Encephalitis and encephalomyelitis in viral diseases classified elsewhere*

Excludes: *encephalitis (in):*

> *arthropod-borne viral (062.0-064)*
> *herpes simplex (054.3)*
> *mumps (072.2)*
> *other viral diseases of central nervous system (049.8-049.9)*
> *poliomyelitis (045.0-045.9)*
> *rubella (056.01)*
> *slow virus infections of central nervous system (046.0-046.9)*
> *viral NOS (049.9)*
> *West Nile (066.41)*

323.02 *Myelitis in viral diseases classified elsewhere*

Excludes: *myelitis (in):*

> *herpes simplex (054.74)*
> *herpes zoster (053.14)*
> *poliomyelitis (045.0-045.9)*
> *rubella (056.01)*
> *other viral diseases of central nervous system (049.8-049.9)*

323.1 *Encephalitis, myelitis, and encephalomyelitis in rickettsial diseases classified elsewhere*
Code first underlying disease (080-083.9)

323.2 *Encephalitis, myelitis, and encephalomyelitis in protozoal diseases classified elsewhere*
Code first underlying disease, as:
malaria (084.0-084.9)
trypanosomiasis (086.0-086.9)

▲ **323.4** *Other encephalitis, myelitis, and encephalomyelitis due to other infections classified elsewhere*
Code first underlying disease

▲ **323.41** *Other encephalitis and encephalomyelitis due to other infections classified elsewhere*

Excludes: *encephalitis (in):*

> *meningococcal (036.1)*
> *syphilis:*
>> *NOS (094.81)*
>> *congenital (090.41)*
> *toxoplasmosis (130.0)*
> *tuberculosis (013.6)*
> *meningoencephalitis due to free-living ameba [Naegleria] (136.29)*

▲ **323.42** *Other myelitis due to other infections classified elsewhere*

Excludes: *myelitis (in):*

> *syphilis (094.89)*
> *tuberculosis (013.6)*

⑤ **323.5 Encephalitis, myelitis, and encephalomyelitis following immunization procedures**
Use additional E code, if desired, to identify vaccine

323.51 Encephalitis and encephalomyelitis following immunization procedures
Encephalitis postimmunization or postvaccinal
Encephalomyelitis postimmunization or postvaccinal

323.52 Myelitis following immunization procedures
Myelitis postimmunization or postvaccinal

⑤ **323.6** *Postinfectious encephalitis, myelitis, and encephalomyelitis*
Code first underlying disease

323.61 *Infectious acute disseminated encephalomyelitis (ADEM)*
Acute necrotizing hemorrhagic encephalopathy

Excludes: *noninfectious acute disseminated encephalomyelitis (ADEM) (323.81)*

323.62 *Other postinfectious encephalitis and encephalomyelitis*

Excludes: *encephalitis:*

> *postchickenpox (052.0)*
> *postmeasles (055.0)*

323.63 *Postinfectious myelitis*

Excludes: *postchickenpox myelitis (052.2)*

> *herpes simplex myelitis (054.74)*
> *herpes zoster myelitis (053.14)*

| ▮ Add 4th or 5th digit | ▮ Nonspecific code | ▮ Unspecified code | ▮ Manifestation code |

⑤ **323.7** *Toxic encephalitis, myelitis, and encephalomyelitis*
> *Code first underlying cause, as:*
>> carbon tetrachloride (982.1)
>> hydroxyquinoline derivatives (961.3)
>> lead (984.0-984.9)
>> mercury (985.0)
>> thallium (985.8)

> **323.71** *Toxic encephalitis and encephalomyelitis*

> **323.72** *Toxic myelitis*

⑤ **323.8 Other causes of encephalitis, myelitis, and encephalomyelitis**

> **323.81 Other causes of encephalitis and encephalomyelitis**
>> Noninfectious acute disseminated encephalomyelitis (ADEM)

> **323.82 Other causes of myelitis**
>> Transverse myelitis NOS

323.9 Unspecified causes of encephalitis, myelitis, and encephalomyelitis

324 Intracranial and intraspinal abscess
> **DEFINITION** Intracranial and intraspinal abscess refers to an abcess occuring inside the cranium or the spinal column.
> **ALERT!** For coding late effects of intracranial abscess or pyogenic infection see 326

324.0 Intracranial abscess

Abscess (embolic):	Abscess (embolic) of brain [any part]:
cerebellar	epidural
cerebral	extradural
	otogenic
	subdural

> *Excludes:* *tuberculous (013.3)*

324.1 Intraspinal abscess
> Abscess (embolic) of spinal cord [any part]:
>> epidural
>> extradural
>> subdural

> *Excludes:* *tuberculous (013.5)*

324.9 Of unspecified site
> Extradural or subdural abscess NOS

325 Phlebitis and thrombophlebitis of intracranial venous sinuses
> Embolism, of cavernous, lateral, or other intracranial or unspecified intracranial venous sinus
> Endophlebitis, of cavernous, lateral, or other intracranial or unspecified intracranial venous sinus
> Phlebitis, septic or suppurative, of cavernous, lateral, or other intracranial or unspecified intracranial venous sinus
> Thrombophlebitis of cavernous, lateral, or other intracranial or unspecified intracranial venous sinus
> Thrombosis of cavernous, lateral, or other intracranial or unspecified intracranial venous sinus

> *Excludes:* *that specified as:*
>> *complicating pregnancy, childbirth, or the puerperium (671.5)*
>> *of nonpyogenic origin (437.6)*

> **DEFINITION** Phlebitis and thrombophlebitis of intracranial venous sinuses refers to the inflammation of a vein or phlebitis related to a blood clot of the intracranial venous sinuses.
> **ALERT!** For personal history of venous thrombosis and embolism see V12.51

326 Late effects of intracranial abscess or pyogenic infection
> Note: This category is to be used to indicate conditions whose primary classification is to 320-325 [excluding 320.7, 321.0-321.8, 323.01-323.42, 323.61-323.72] as the cause of late effects, themselves classifiable elsewhere. The "late effects" include conditions specified as such, or as sequelae, which may occur at any time after the resolution of the causal condition.

> Use additional code, if desired, to identify condition, as:
> hydrocephalus (331.4)
> paralysis (342.0-342.9, 344.0-344.9)

> **DEFINITION** Late effects of intracranial abscess or pyogenic infection refers to a condition that appears after the acute phase of an intracranial abscess or pyogenic infection ha run its course.

● Code new
   to this edition

▲ Revision of
   existing code

④ ⑤ Fourth or fifth
   digit required

ORGANIC SLEEP DISORDERS (327)

327 Organic sleep disorders

> **DEFINITION** Organic sleep disorders are sleep disorders that are the result of an anatomic or physiologic abnormality or disease process.

⑤ **327.0** **Organic disorders of initiating and maintaining sleep [Organic insomnia]**

> Excludes: insomnia NOS (780.52)
>
> insomnia not due to a substance or known physiological condition (307.41-307.42)
> insomnia with sleep apnea NOS (780.51)

327.00 **Organic insomnia, unspecified**

327.01 **Insomnia due to medical condition classified elsewhere**
Code first underlying condition

> Excludes: insomnia due to mental disorder (327.02)

327.02 **Insomnia due to mental disorder**
Code first mental disorder

> Excludes: alcohol induced insomnia (291.82)
>
> drug induced insomnia (292.85)

327.09 **Other organic insomnia**

⑤ **327.1** **Organic disorder of excessive somnolence [Organic hypersomnia]**

> Excludes: hypersomnia NOS (780.54)
>
> hypersomnia not due to a substance or known physiological condition (307.43-307.44)
> hypersomnia with sleep apnea NOS (780.53)

327.10 **Organic hypersomnia, unspecified**

327.11 **Idiopathic hypersomnia with long sleep time**

327.12 **Idiopathic hypersomnia without long sleep time**

327.13 **Recurrent hypersomnia**
Kleine-Levin syndrome
Menstrual related hypersomnia

327.14 **Hypersomnia due to medical condition classified elsewhere**
Code first underlying condition

> Excludes: hypersomnia due to mental disorder (327.15)

327.15 **Hypersomnia due to mental disorder**
Code first mental disorder

> Excludes: alcohol induced hypersomnia (291.82)
>
> drug induced hypersomnia (292.85)

327.19 **Other organic hypersomnia**

⑤ **327.2** **Organic sleep apnea**

> Excludes: Cheyne-Stokes breathing (786.04)
>
> hypersomnia with sleep apnea NOS (780.53)
> insomnia with sleep apnea NOS (780.51)
> sleep apnea in newborn (770.81-770.82)
> sleep apnea NOS (780.57)

327.20 **Organic sleep apnea, unspecified**

327.21 **Primary central sleep apnea**

327.22 **High altitude periodic breathing**

327.23 **Obstructive sleep apnea (adult) (pediatric)**

327.24 **Idiopathic sleep related nonobstructive alveolar hypoventilation**
Sleep related hypoxia

327.25 **Congenital central alveolar hypoventilation syndrome**

327.26 **Sleep related hypoventilation/hypoxemia in conditions classifiable elsewhere**
Code first underlying condition

327.27 **Central sleep apnea in conditions classified elsewhere**
Code first underlying condition

327.29 **Other organic sleep apnea**

| | Add 4th or 5th digit | | Nonspecific code | | Unspecified code | | Manifestation code |

⑤ **327.3 Circadian rhythm sleep disorder**
   Organic disorder of sleep wake cycle
   Organic disorder of sleep wake schedule

   Excludes: *alcohol induced circadian rhythm sleep disorder (291.82)*
   circadian rhythm sleep disorder of nonorganic origin (307.45)
   disruption of 24 hour sleep wake cycle NOS (780.55)
   drug induced circadian rhythm sleep disorder (292.85)

   327.30 Circadian rhythm sleep disorder, unspecified

   327.31 Circadian rhythm sleep disorder, delayed sleep phase type

   327.32 Circadian rhythm sleep disorder, advanced sleep phase type

   327.33 Circadian rhythm sleep disorder, irregular sleep-wake type

   327.34 Circadian rhythm sleep disorder, free-running type

   327.35 Circadian rhythm sleep disorder, jet lag type

   327.36 Circadian rhythm sleep disorder, shift work type

   327.37 Circadian rhythm sleep disorder in conditions classified elsewhere
   Code first underlying condition

   327.39 Other circadian rhythm sleep disorder

⑤ **327.4 Organic parasomnia**

   Excludes: *alcohol induced parasomnia (291.82)*
   drug induced parasomnia (292.85)
   parasomnia not due to a known physiological condition (307.47)

   327.40 Organic parasomnia, unspecified

   327.41 Confusional arousals

   327.42 REM sleep behavior disorder

   327.43 Recurrent isolated sleep paralysis

   327.44 Parasomnia in conditions classified elsewhere
   Code first underlying condition

   327.49 Other organic parasomnia

⑤ **327.5 Organic sleep related movement disorders**

   Excludes: *restless legs syndrome (333.94)*
   sleep related movement disorder NOS (780.58)

   327.51 Periodic limb movement disorder
   Periodic limb movement sleep disorder

   327.52 Sleep related leg cramps

   327.53 Sleep related bruxism

   327.59 Other organic sleep related movement disorders

327.8 Other organic sleep disorders

HEREDITARY AND DEGENERATIVE DISEASES OF THE CENTRAL NERVOUS SYSTEM (330-337)

   Excludes: *hepatolenticular degeneration (275.1)*
   multiple sclerosis (340)
   other demyelinating diseases of central nervous system (341.0-341.9)

330 Cerebral degenerations usually manifest in childhood
   Use additional code, if desired, to identify associated intellectual disabilities

   330.0 Leukodystrophy

Krabbe's disease	Leukodystrophy:
Leukodystrophy:	metachromatic
NOS	sudanophilic
globoid cell	Pelizaeus-Merzbacher disease
	Sulfatide lipidosis

   330.1 Cerebral lipidoses

Amaurotic (familial) idiocy	Disease:
Disease:	Kufs'
Batten	Spielmeyer-Vogt
Jansky-Bielschowsky	Tay-Sachs
	Gangliosidosis

● Code new
   to this edition

▲ Revision of
   existing code

④ ⑤ Fourth or fifth
   digit required

330.2 Cerebral degeneration in generalized lipidoses
Code first underlying disease, as:
Fabry's disease (272.7)
Gaucher's disease (272.7)
Neimann-Pick disease (272.7)
sphingolipidosis (272.7)

330.3 Cerebral degeneration of childhood in other diseases classified elsewhere
Code first underlying disease, as:
Hunter's disease (277.5)
mucopolysaccharidosis (277.5)

330.8 Other specified cerebral degenerations in childhood
Alpers' disease or gray-matter degeneration
Infantile necrotizing encephalomyelopathy
Leigh's disease
Subacute necrotizing encephalopathy or encephalomyelopathy

330.9 Unspecified cerebral degeneration in childhood

331 Other cerebral degenerations
Use additional code, where applicable, to identify dementia:
with behavioral disturbance (294.11)
without behavioral disturbance (294.10)
ALERT! For personal history of other disorders of nervous system and sense organs see V12.49

331.0 Alzheimer's disease

⑤ **331.1 Frontotemporal dementia**

331.11 Pick's disease

331.19 Other frontotemporal dementia
Frontal dementia

331.2 Senile degeneration of brain
Excludes: senility NOS (797)

331.3 Communicating hydrocephalus
Secondary normal pressure hydrocephalus
Excludes: congenital hydrocephalus (742.3)
idiopathic normal pressure hydrocephalus (331.5)
normal pressure hydrocephalus (331.5)
spina bifida with hydrocephalus (741.0)

331.4 Obstructive hydrocephalus
Acquired hydrocephalus NOS
Excludes: congenital hydrocephalus (742.3)
idiopathic normal pressure hydrocephalus (331.5)
normal pressure hydrocephalus (331.5)
spina bifida with hydrocephalus (741.0)

331.5 Idiopathic normal pressure hydrocephalus (INPH)
Normal pressure hydrocephalus NOS
Excludes: congenital hydrocephalus (742.3)
secondary normal pressure hydrocephalus (331.3)
spina bifida with hydrocephalus (741.0)

● **331.6 Corticobasal degeneration**

331.7 Cerebral degeneration in diseases classified elsewhere
Code first underlying disease, as:
alcoholism (303.0-303.9)
beriberi (265.0)
cerebrovascular disease (430-438)
congenital hydrocephalus (741.0, 742.3)
neoplastic disease (140.0-239.9)
myxedema (244.0-244.9)
vitamin B_{12} deficiency (266.2)
Excludes: cerebral degeneration in:
Jakob-Creutzfeldt disease (046.11-046.19)
progressive multifocal leukoencephalopathy (046.3)
subacute spongiform encephalopathy (046.1)

⑤ **331.8 Other cerebral degeneration**

331.81 Reye's syndrome

Add 4th or 5th digit	Nonspecific code	Unspecified code	Manifestation code

331.82 Dementia with Lewy bodies
Dementia with Parkinsonism
Lewy body dementia
Lewy body disease

331.83 Mild cognitive impairment, so stated

Excludes: altered mental status (780.97)
cerebral degeneration (331.0-331.9)
change in mental status (780.97)
cognitive deficits following (late effects of) cerebral hemorrhage or infarction
  (438.0)
cognitive impairment due to intracranial or head injury (850-854, 959.01)
cognitive impairment due to late effect of intracranial injury (907.0)
cognitive impairment due to skull fracture (800-801, 803-804)
dementia (290.0-290.43, 294.20-294.21)
mild memory disturbance (310.89)
neurologic neglect syndrome (781.8)
personality change, nonpsychotic (310.1)

331.89 Other
Cerebral ataxia

331.9 Cerebral degeneration, unspecified

332 Parkinson's disease

Excludes: dementia with Parkinsonism (331.82)

DEFINITION Parkinson's disease is a degenerative disease of the brain (central nervous system) that often impairs motor skills, speech, and other functions.

332.0 Paralysis agitans
Parkinsonism or Parkinson's disease:
  NOS
  idiopathic
  primary

332.1 Secondary Parkinsonism
Neuroleptic-induced Parkinsonism
Parkinsonism due to drugs

Use additional E code, if desired, to identify drug, if drug-induced

Excludes: Parkinsonism (in):
  Huntington's disease (333.4)
  progressive supranuclear palsy (333.0)
  Shy-Drager syndrome (333.0)
  syphilitic (094.82)

333 Other extrapyramidal disease and abnormal movement disorders
Includes: other forms of extrapyramidal, basal ganglia, or striatopallidal disease

Excludes: abnormal movements of head NOS (781.0)
  sleep related movement disorders (327.51-327.59)

DEFINITION Extrapyramidal disease is a general term for a number of disorders caused by abnormalities of the basal ganglia or certain brain stem or thalamic nuclei; characterised by motor deficits, loss of postural reflexes, bradykinesia, tremor, rigidity, and various involuntary movements.

ALERT! For personal history of other disorders of nervous system and sense organs see V12.49

333.0 Other degenerative diseases of the basal ganglia
Atrophy or degeneration:
  olivopontocerebellar [Déjérine-Thomas syndrome]
  pigmentary pallidal [Hallervorden-Spatz disease]
  striatonigral
Parkinsonian syndrome associated with:
  idiopathic orthostatic hypotension
  symptomatic orthostatic hypotension
Progressive supranuclear ophthalmoplegia
Shy-Drager syndrome

333.1 Essential and other specified forms of tremor
Benign essential tremor
Familial tremor
Medication-induced postural tremor

Use additional E code, if desired, to identify drug, if drug-induced

Excludes: tremor NOS (781.0)

● Code new
to this edition

▲ Revision of
existing code

④ ⑤ Fourth or fifth
digit required

333.2 Myoclonus
 Familial essential myoclonus
 Palatal myoclonus

Excludes:	*progressive myoclonic epilepsy (345.1)*
	Unverricht-Lundborg disease (345.1)

Use additional E code, if desired, to identify drug, if drug-induced

333.3 Tics of organic origin

Excludes:	*Gilles de la Tourette's syndrome (307.23)*
	habit spasm (307.22)
	tic NOS (307.20)

Use additional E code, if desired, to identify drug, if drug-induced

333.4 Huntington's chorea

333.5 Other choreas
 Hemiballism(us)
 Paroxysmal choreo-athetosis

Excludes:	*Sydenham's or rheumatic chorea (392.0-392.9)*

Use additional E code, if desired, to identify drug, if drug-induced

333.6 Genetic torsion dystonia
 Dystonia:
  deformans progressiva
  musculorum deformans
  (Schwalbe-) Ziehen-Oppenheim disease

⑤ **333.7 Acquired torsion dystonia**

 333.71 Athetoid cerebral palsy
  Double athetosis (syndrome)
  Vogt's disease

Excludes:	*infantile cerebral palsy (343.0-343.9)*

 333.72 Acute dystonia due to drugs
  Acute dystonic reaction due to drugs
  Neuroleptic induced acute dystonia

Use additional E code to identify drug

Excludes:	*blepharospasm due to drugs (333.85)*
	orofacial dyskinesia due to drugs (333.85)
	secondary Parkinsonism (332.1)
	subacute dyskinesia due to drugs (333.85)
	tardive dyskinesia (333.85)

 333.79 Other acquired torsion dystonia

⑤ **333.8 Fragments of torsion dystonia**
 Use additional E code, if desired, to identify drug, if drug-induced

 333.81 Blepharospasm

Excludes:	*blepharospasm due to drugs (333.85)*

 333.82 Orofacial dyskinesia

Excludes:	*orofacial dyskinesia due to drugs (333.85)*

 333.83 Spasmodic torticollis

Excludes:	*torticollis:*
	NOS (723.5)
	hysterical (300.11)
	psychogenic (306.0)

 333.84 Organic writers' cramp

Excludes:	*psychogenic (300.89)*

 333.85 Subacute dyskinesia due to drugs
  Blepharospasm due to drugs
  Orofacial dyskinesia due to drugs
  Tardive dyskinesia

Use additional E code to identify drug

Excludes:	*acute dystonia due to drugs (333.72)*
	acute dystonic reaction due to drugs (333.72)
	secondary Parkinsonism (332.1)

 333.89 Other

	Add 4th or 5th digit		Nonspecific code		Unspecified code		Manifestation code

⑤ **333.9 Other and unspecified extrapyramidal diseases and abnormal movement disorders**

333.90 Unspecified extrapyramidal disease and abnormal movement disorder
Medication-induced movement disorders NOS
Use additional E code to identify drug, if drug-induced

333.91 Stiff-man syndrome

333.92 Neuroleptic malignant syndrome
Use additional E code to identify drug

Excludes: neuroleptic induced Parkinsonism (332.1)

333.93 Benign shuddering attacks

333.94 Restless legs syndrome (RLS)

333.99 Other
Neuroleptic-induced acute akathisia
Use additional E code to identify drug, if drug-induced

334 Spinocerebellar disease

Excludes: olivopontocerebellar degeneration (333.0)
peroneal muscular atrophy (356.1)

DEFINITION Spinocerebellar disease refers to a disease involving both the spinal cord and the cerebellum.

334.0 Friedreich's ataxia

334.1 Hereditary spastic paraplegia

334.2 Primary cerebellar degeneration
Cerebellar ataxia:
Marie's
Sanger-Brown
Dyssynergia cerebellaris myoclonica
Primary cerebellar degeneration:
NOS
hereditary
sporadic

334.3 Other cerebellar ataxia
Cerebellar ataxia NOS
Use additional E code, if desired, to identify drug, if drug-induced

334.4 Cerebellar ataxia in diseases classified elsewhere
Code first underlying disease, as:
alcoholism (303.0-303.9)
myxedema (244.0-244.9)
neoplastic disease (140.0-239.9)

334.8 Other spinocerebellar diseases
Ataxia-telangiectasia [Louis-Bar syndrome]
Corticostriatal-spinal degeneration

334.9 Spinocerebellar disease, unspecified

335 Anterior horn cell disease
DEFINITION Anterior horn cell disease refers to diseases characterized by a selective degeneration of the motor neurons of the spinal cord, brainstem, or motor cortex. Clinical subtypes are distinguished by the major site of degeneration

335.0 Werdnig-Hoffmann disease
Infantile spinal muscular atrophy
Progressive muscular atrophy of infancy

⑤ **335.1 Spinal muscular atrophy**

335.10 Spinal muscular atrophy, unspecified

335.11 Kugelberg-Welander disease
Spinal muscular atrophy:
familial
juvenile

335.19 Other
Adult spinal muscular atrophy

⑤ **335.2 Motor neuron disease**

335.20 Amyotrophic lateral sclerosis
Motor neuron disease (bulbar) (mixed type)

335.21 Progressive muscular atrophy
Duchenne-Aran muscular atrophy
Progressive muscular atrophy (pure)

● Code new to this edition ▲ Revision of existing code ④ ⑤ Fourth or fifth digit required

335.22   **Progressive bulbar palsy**

335.23   **Pseudobulbar palsy**

335.24   **Primary lateral sclerosis**

335.29   Other

335.8 **Other anterior horn cell diseases**

335.9 **Anterior horn cell disease, unspecified**

336 **Other diseases of spinal cord**

> **ALERT!** For personal history of other disorders of nervous system and sense organs see V12.49

336.0   **Syringomyelia and syringobulbia**

336.1   **Vascular myelopathies**
Acute infarction of spinal cord (embolic) (nonembolic)
Arterial thrombosis of spinal cord
Edema of spinal cord
Hematomyelia
Subacute necrotic myelopathy

336.2   *Subacute combined degeneration of spinal cord in diseases classified elsewhere*
Code first underlying disease, as:
pernicious anemia (281.0)
other vitamin B_{12} deficiency anemia (281.1)
vitamin B_{12} deficiency (266.2)

336.3   *Myelopathy in other diseases classified elsewhere*
Code first underlying disease, as:
myelopathy in neoplastic disease (140.0-239.9)

> *Excludes:* *myelopathy in:*
> *intervertebral disc disorder (722.70-722.73)*
> *spondylosis (721.1, 721.41-721.42, 721.91)*

336.8 **Other myelopathy**
Myelopathy:
drug-induced
radiation-induced

Use additional E code, if desired, to identify cause

336.9   **Unspecified disease of spinal cord**
Cord compression NOS   Myelopathy NOS

> *Excludes:* *myelitis (323.02, 323.1, 323.2, 323.42, 323.52, 323.63, 323.72, 323.82, 323.9)*
> *spinal (canal) stenosis (723.0, 724.00-724.09)*

337 **Disorders of the autonomic nervous system**
Includes: disorders of peripheral autonomic, sympathetic, parasympathetic, or vegetative system

> *Excludes:* *familial dysautonomia [Riley-Day syndrome] (742.8)*

> **DEFINITION** Disorders of the autonomic nervous system refers to disorders of the part of the nervous system that regulates involuntary action, as of the intestines, heart, and glands.

⑤ 337.0   **Idiopathic peripheral autonomic neuropathy**

337.00   **Idiopathic peripheral autonomic neuropathy, unspecified**

337.01   **Carotid sinus syndrome**
Carotid sinus syncope

337.09   **Other idiopathic peripheral autonomic neuropathy**
Cervical sympathetic dystrophy or paralysis

337.1   *Peripheral autonomic neuropathy in disorders classified elsewhere*
Code first underlying disease, as:
amyloidosis (277.30-277.39)
diabetes (249.6, 250.6)

⑤ 337.2   **Reflex sympathetic dystrophy**

337.20   **Reflex sympathetic dystrophy, unspecified**
Complex regional pain syndrome type I, unspecified

337.21   **Reflex sympathetic dystrophy of the upper limb**
Complex regional pain syndrome type I of the upper limb

337.22   **Reflex sympathetic dystrophy of the lower limb**
Complex regional pain syndrome type I of the lower limb

337.29   **Reflex sympathetic dystrophy of other specified site**
Complex regional pain syndrome type I of other specified site

| | Add 4th or 5th digit | | Nonspecific code | | Unspecified code | | Manifestation code |

TABULAR LIST

337.3 Autonomic dysreflexia
Use additional code to identify the cause, such as:
  fecal impaction (560.32)
  pressure ulcer (707.00-707.09)
  urinary tract infection (599.0)

337.9 Unspecified disorder of autonomic nervous system

PAIN (338)

338 Pain, not elsewhere classified
Use additional code to identify:
  pain associated with psychological factors (307.89)

Excludes: *generalized pain (780.96)*
  headache syndromes (339.00-339.89)
  localized pain, unspecified type – code to pain by site
  migraines (346.0-346.9)
  pain disorder exclusively attributed to psychological factors (307.80)
  vulvar vestibulitis (625.71)
  vulvodynia (625.70-625.79)

ALERT! Codes in category 338 may be used in conjunction with codes from other categories and chapters to provide more detail about acute or chronic pain and neoplasm-related pain, unless otherwise indicated.

338.0 Central pain syndrome
  Déjérine-Roussy syndrome
  Myelopathic pain syndrome
  Thalamic pain syndrome (hyperesthetic)

⑤ 338.1 Acute pain

  338.11 Acute pain due to trauma

  338.12 Acute post-thoracotomy pain
    Post-thoracotomy pain NOS

  338.18 Other acute postoperative pain
    Postoperative pain NOS

  338.19 Other acute pain

Excludes: *neoplasm related acute pain (338.3)*

⑤ 338.2 Chronic pain

Excludes: *causalgia (355.9)*
  lower limb (355.71)
  upper limb (354.4)
  chronic pain syndrome (338.4)
  myofascial pain syndrome (729.1)
  neoplasm related chronic pain (338.3)
  reflex sympathetic dystrophy (337.20-337.29)

ALERT! Chronic pain is classified to this subcategory. There is no time frame defining when pain becomes chronic pain. The provider's documentation should be used to guide use of these codes

  338.21 Chronic pain due to trauma

  338.22 Chronic post-thoracotomy pain

  338.28 Other chronic postoperative pain

  338.29 Other chronic pain

338.3 Neoplasm related pain (acute) (chronic)
  Cancer associated pain
  Pain due to malignancy (primary) (secondary)
  Tumor associated pain

338.4 Chronic pain syndrome
  Chronic pain associated with significant psychosocial dysfunction

OTHER HEADACHE SYNDROMES (339)

339 Other headache syndromes
Excludes: *headache:*
  NOS (784.0)
  due to lumbar puncture (349.0)
  migraine (346.0-346.9)

● Code new to this edition ▲ Revision of existing code ④ ⑤ Fourth or fifth digit required

⑤ **339.0 Cluster headaches and other trigeminal autonomic cephalgias**
TACS

339.00 Cluster headache syndrome, unspecified
Ciliary neuralgia
Cluster headache NOS
Histamine cephalgia
Lower half migraine
Migrainous neuralgia

339.01 Episodic cluster headache

339.02 Chronic cluster headache

339.03 Episodic paroxysmal hemicrania
Paroxysmal hemicrania NOS

339.04 Chronic paroxysmal hemicrania

339.05 Short lasting unilateral neuralgiform headache with conjunctival injection and tearing
SUNCT

339.09 Other trigeminal autonomic cephalgias

⑤ **339.1 Tension type headache**

Excludes: *tension headache NOS (307.81)*
tension headache related to psychological factors (307.81)

339.10 Tension type headache, unspecified

339.11 Episodic tension type headache

339.12 Chronic tension type headache

⑤ **339.2 Post-traumatic headache**

339.20 Post-traumatic headache, unspecified

339.21 Acute post-traumatic headache

339.22 Chronic post-traumatic headache

339.3 Drug induced headache not elsewhere classified
Medication overuse headache
Rebound headache

⑤ **339.4 Complicated headache syndromes**

339.41 Hemicrania continua

339.42 New daily persistent headache
NDPH

339.43 Primary thunderclap headache

339.44 Other complicated headache syndrome

⑤ **339.8 Other specified headache syndromes**

339.81 Hypnic headache

339.82 Headache associated with sexual activity
Orgasmic headache
Preorgasmic headache

339.83 Primary cough headache

339.84 Primary exertional headache

339.85 Primary stabbing headache

339.89 Other specified headache syndromes

OTHER DISORDERS OF THE CENTRAL NERVOUS SYSTEM (340-349)

340 Multiple sclerosis
Disseminated or multiple sclerosis:
NOS
brain stem
cord
generalized
DEFINITION Multiple sclerosis is a chronic autoimmune disorder affecting movement, sensation, and bodily functions. It is caused by destruction of the myelin insulation covering nerve fibers in the central nervous system.

| | Add 4th or 5th digit | | Nonspecific code | | Unspecified code | | Manifestation code |

341 **Other demyelinating diseases of central nervous system**

DEFINITION Demyelinating diseases of the central nervous system is any disease of the nervous system in which the myelin sheath of neurons is damaged.

ALERT! For personal history of other disorders of nervous system and sense organs see V12.49

341.0 **Neuromyelitis optica**

341.1 **Schilder's disease**
Baló's concentric sclerosis
Encephalitis periaxialis:
concentrica [Baló's]
diffusa [Schilder's]

⑤ **341.2** **Acute (transverse) myelitis**
Excludes: acute (transverse)myelitis (in) (due to):
following immunization procedures (323.52)
infection classified elsewhere (323.42)
postinfectious (323.63)
protozoal diseases classified elsewhere (323.2)
rickettsial diseases classified elsewhere (323.1)
toxic (323.72)
viral diseases classified elsewhere (323.02)
transverse myelitis NOS (323.82)

341.20 **Acute (transverse) myelitis NOS**

341.21 **Acute (transverse) myelitis in conditions classified elsewhere**
Code first underlying condition

341.22 **Idiopathic transverse myelitis**

341.8 **Other demyelinating diseases of central nervous system**
Central demyelination of corpus callosum
Central pontine myelinosis
Marchiafava (-Bignami) disease

341.9 **Demyelinating disease of central nervous system, unspecified**

342 **Hemiplegia and hemiparesis**
Excludes: congenital (343.1)
hemiplegia due to late effect of cerebrovascular accident (438.20-438.22)
infantile NOS (343.4)

Note: This category is to be used when hemiplegia (complete) (incomplete) is reported without further specification, or is stated to be old or long-standing but of unspecified cause. The category is also for use in multiple coding to identify these types of hemiplegia resulting from any cause.

The following fifth-digits are for use with codes 342.0-342.9

0 **affecting unspecified side**

1 **affecting dominant side**

2 **affecting nondominant side**

DEFINITION Hemiplegia is defined as paralysis or loss of voluntary motion, on one side of the body; may include head and neck, trunk and/or limbs. Hemiparesis is weakness on one side of the body.

⑤ **342.0** **Flaccid hemiplegia**
[0-2]

⑤ **342.1** **Spastic hemiplegia**
[0-2]

⑤ **342.8** **Other specified hemiplegia**
[0-2]

⑤ **342.9** **Hemiplegia, unspecified**
[0-2]

● Code new to this edition   ▲ Revision of existing code   ④ ⑤ Fourth or fifth digit required

343 **Infantile cerebral palsy**
Includes: cerebral:
palsy NOS
spastic infantile paralysis
congenital spastic paralysis (cerebral)
Little's disease
paralysis (spastic) due to birth injury:
intracranial
spinal

Excludes: *athetoid cerebral palsy (333.71)*
hereditary cerebral paralysis, such as:
hereditary spastic paraplegia (334.1)
Vogt's disease (333.71)
spastic paralysis specified as noncongenital or noninfantile (344.0-344.9)

DEFINITION Infantile cerebral palsy is the term used for a group of nonprogressive disorders of movement and posture caused by abnormal development of, or damage to, motor control centers of the brain. Cerebral palsy is caused by events before, during, or after birth. The abnormalities of muscle control that define cp are often accompanied by other neurological and physical abnormalities.

343.0 Diplegic
Congenital diplegia   Congenital paraplegia

343.1 Hemiplegic
Congenital hemiplegia

Excludes: *infantile hemiplegia NOS (343.4)*

343.2 Quadriplegic
Tetraplegic

343.3 Monoplegic

343.4 Infantile hemiplegia
Infantile hemiplegia (postnatal) NOS

343.8 Other specified infantile cerebral palsy

343.9 Infantile cerebral palsy, unspecified
Cerebral palsy NOS

344 **Other paralytic syndromes**
Note: This category is to be used when the listed conditions are reported without further specification or are stated to be old or long-standing but of unspecified cause. The category is also for use in multiple coding to identify these conditions resulting from any cause.

Includes: paralysis (complete) (incomplete), except as classifiable to 342 and 343

Excludes: *congenital or infantile cerebral palsy (343.0-343.9)*
hemiplegia (342.0-342.9)
congenital or infantile (343.1, 343.4)

DEFINITION Paralytic syndromes refers to other forms of paralysis resulting in the complete loss of muscle function for one or more muscle groups.

ALERT! For personal history of other disorders of nervous system and sense organs see V12.49

⑤ **344.0 Quadriplegia and quadriparesis**

344.00 Quadriplegia, unspecified

344.01 C1-C4, complete

344.02 C1-C4, incomplete

344.03 C5-C7, complete

344.04 C5-C7, incomplete

344.09 Other

344.1 Paraplegia
Paralysis of both lower limbs
Paraplegia (lower)

344.2 Diplegia of upper limbs
Diplegia (upper)
Paralysis of both upper limbs

⑤ **344.3 Monoplegia of lower limb**
Paralysis of lower limb

Excludes: *monoplegia of lower limb due to late effect of cerebrovascular accident (438.40-438.42)*

Add 4th or 5th digit	Nonspecific code	Unspecified code	Manifestation code

344.30   affecting **unspecified** side

344.31   affecting **dominant** side

344.32   affecting **nondominant** side

⑤ **344.4 Monoplegia of upper limb**
Paralysis of upper limb

Excludes: *monoplegia of upper limb due to late effect of cerebrovascular accident (438.30-438.32)*

344.40   affecting **unspecified** side

344.41   affecting **dominant** side

344.42   affecting **nondominant** side

344.5 Unspecified monoplegia

⑤ **344.6 Cauda equina syndrome**

344.60   **Without mention of neurogenic bladder**

344.61   **With neurogenic bladder**
Acontractile bladder
Autonomic hyperreflexia of bladder
Cord bladder
Detrusor hyperreflexia

⑤ **344.8 Other specified paralytic syndromes**

344.81   **Locked-in state**

344.89   **Other specified paralytic syndrome**

344.9 Paralysis, unspecified

345 Epilepsy and recurrent seizures
The following fifth-digit subclassification is for use with categories 345.0, 345.1, 345.4-345.9:

0   **without mention of intractable epilepsy**

1   **with intractable epilepsy**
pharmacoresistant (pharmacologically resistant)
poorly controlled
refractory (medically)
treatment resistant

Excludes: *hippocampal sclerosis (348.81)*
mesial temporal sclerosis (348.81)
temporal sclerosis (348.81)

DEFINITION Epilepsy and recurrent seizures is a common chronic neurological disorder characterized by recurrent unprovoked seizures. These seizures are transient signs and/or symptoms of abnormal, excessive or synchronous neuronal activity in the brain.

⑤ **345.0 Generalized nonconvulsive epilepsy**
[0-1]   Absences:
atonic
typical
Minor epilepsy
Petit mal
Pykno-epilepsy
Seizures:
akinetic
atonic

⑤ **345.1 Generalized convulsive epilepsy**
[0-1]   Epileptic seizures:
clonic
myoclonic
tonic
tonic-clonic
Grand mal
Major epilepsy
Progressive myoclonic epilepsy
Unverricht-Lundborg disease

Excludes: *convulsions:*
NOS (780.39)
infantile (780.39)
newborn (779.0)
infantile spasms (345.6)

● Code new
to this edition   ▲ Revision of
existing code   ④ ⑤ Fourth or fifth
digit required

345.2 Petit mal status
Epileptic absence status

345.3 Grand mal status
Status epilepticus NOS

Excludes: *epilepsia partialis continua (345.7)*
status:
psychomotor (345.7)
temporal lobe (345.7)

⑤ **345.4 Localization-related (focal) (partial) epilepsy and epileptic syndromes with complex partial seizures**
[0-1]   Epilepsy:
limbic system
partial:
secondarily generalized
with impairment of consciousness
with memory and ideational disturbances
psychomotor
psychosensory
temporal lobe
Epileptic automatism

⑤ **345.5 Localization-related (focal) (partial) epilepsy and epileptic syndromes with simple partial seizures**
[0-1]
Epilepsy: Epilepsy:
Bravais-Jacksonian NOS   sensory-induced
focal (motor) NOS   somatomotor
Jacksonian NOS   somatosensory
motor partial   visceral
partial NOS: visual
without impairment of consciousness

⑤ **345.6 Infantile spasms**
[0-1]   Hypsarrhythmia
Lightning spasms
Salaam attacks

Excludes: *salaam tic (781.0)*

⑤ **345.7 Epilepsia partialis continua**
[0-1]   Kojevnikov's epilepsy

⑤ **345.8 Other forms of epilepsy and recurrent seizures**
[0-1]   Epilepsy:
cursive [running]
gelastic

⑤ **345.9 Epilepsy, unspecified**
[0-1]   Epileptic convulsions, fits, or seizures NOS

Excludes: *convulsion (convulsive) disorder (780.39)*
convulsive seizure or fit NOS (780.39)
recurrent convulsions (780.39)

⑤ **346 Migraine**

Excludes: *headache:*
NOS (784.0)
syndromes (339.00-339.89)

The following fifth-digit subclassification is for use with category 346:

0   without mention of intractable migraine without mention of status migrainosus
without mention of refractory migraine without mention of status migrainosus

1   with intractable migraine, so stated, without mention of status migrainosus
with refractory migraine, so stated, without mention of status migrainosus

2   without mention of intractable migraine with status migrainosus
without mention of refractory migraine with status migrainosus

3   with intractable migraine, so stated, with status migrainosus
with refractory migraine, so stated, with status migrainosus

DEFINITION Migraine is a severe, disabling headache, usually affecting only one side of the head, and often accompanied by nausea, vomiting, photophobia and visual disturbances.

Add 4th or   Nonspecific   Unspecified   Manifestation
5th digit   code   code   code

⑤ **346.0 Migraine with aura**
[0-3]   Basilar migraine
Classic migraine
Migraine preceded or accompanied by transient focal neurological phenomena
Migraine triggered seizures
Migraine with acute-onset aura
Migraine with aura without headache (migraine equivalents)
Migraine with prolonged aura
Migraine with typical aura
Retinal migraine

Excludes: *persistent migraine aura (346.5, 346.6)*

⑤ **346.1 Migraine without aura**
[0-3]   Common migraine

⑤ **346.2 Variants of migraine, not elsewhere classified**
[0-3]   Abdominal migraine
Cyclical vomiting associated with migraine
Ophthalmoplegic migraine
Periodic headache syndromes in child or adolescent

Excludes: *cyclical vomiting NOS (536.2)*
psychogenic cyclical vomiting (306.4)

⑤ **346.3 Hemiplegic migraine**
[0-3]   Familial migraine
Sporadic migraine

⑤ **346.4 Menstrual migraine**
[0-3]   Menstrual headache
Menstrually related migraine
Premenstrual headache
Premenstrual migraine
Pure menstrual migraine

⑤ **346.5 Persistent migraine aura without cerebral infarction**
[0-3]   Persistent migraine aura NOS

⑤ **346.6 Persistent migraine aura with cerebral infarction**
[0-3]

⑤ **346.7 Chronic migraine without aura**
[0-3]   Transformed migraine without aura

⑤ **346.8 Other forms of migraine**
[0-3]

⑤ **346.9 Migraine, unspecified**
[0-3]

347 Cataplexy and narcolepsy
DEFINITION Cataplexy is a sudden loss of muscle tone and reflexes that leads to muscle weakness, paralysis or postural collapse. Usually caused by an outburst of emotion such as laughter. Cataplexy is one of the first symptoms of narcolepsy, a chronic sleep disorder (a dyssomnia) which often causes sufferers to feel extreme tiredness, or spontaneously fall asleep.

⑤ **347.0 Narcolepsy**

347.00 Without cataplexy
Narcolepsy NOS

347.01 With cataplexy

⑤ **347.1 Narcolepsy in conditions classified elsewhere**
Code first underlying condition

347.10 Without cataplexy

347.11 With cataplexy

348 Other conditions of brain
ALERT! For personal history of other disorders of nervous system and sense organs see V12.49

348.0 Cerebral cysts
Arachnoid cyst   Porencephaly, acquired
Porencephalic cyst   Pseudoporencephaly

Excludes: *porencephaly (congenital) (742.4)*

● Code new to this edition   ▲ Revision of existing code   ④ ⑤ Fourth or fifth digit required

348.1 Anoxic brain damage
Excludes: *that occurring in:*
　　　abortion (634-638 with .7, 639.8)
　　　ectopic or molar pregnancy (639.8)
　　　labor or delivery (668.2, 669.4)
　　　that of newborn (767.0, 768.0-768.9, 772.1-772.2)
Use additional E code, if desired, to identify cause

348.2 Benign intracranial hypertension
　　Pseudotumor cerebri
Excludes: *hypertensive encephalopathy (437.2)*

⑤ **348.3 Encephalopathy, not elsewhere classified**

　　348.30 Encephalopathy, unspecified

　　348.31 Metabolic encephalopathy
　　　Septic encephalopathy
Excludes: *toxic metabolic encephalopathy (349.82)*

　　348.39 Other encephalopathy
Excludes: *encephalopathy:*
　　　alcoholic (291.2)
　　　hepatic (572.2)
　　　hypertensive (437.2)
　　　toxic (349.82)

348.4 Compression of brain
　　Compression, brain (stem)
　　Herniation, brain (stem)
　　Posterior fossa compression syndrome

348.5 Cerebral edema

⑤ **348.8 Other conditions of brain**

　　348.81 Temporal sclerosis
　　　Hippocampal sclerosis
　　　Mesial temporal sclerosis

● **348.82 Brain death**

　　348.89 Other conditions of brain
　　　Cerebral:
　　　　calcification
　　　　fungus
Excludes: *brain death (348.82)*

348.9 Unspecified condition of brain

349 Other and unspecified disorders of the nervous system
　　ALERT! For personal history of other disorders of nervous system and sense organs see V12.49
　　ALERT! For personal history of unspecified disorder of nervous system and sense organs see V12.40

349.0 Reaction to spinal or lumbar puncture
　　Headache following lumbar puncture

349.1 Nervous system complications from surgically implanted device

349.2 Disorders of meninges, not elsewhere classified
Excludes: *immediate postoperative complications (997.00-997.09)*
　　　mechanical complications of nervous system device (996.2)
　　Adhesions, meningeal (cerebral) (spinal)
　　Cyst, spinal meninges
　　Meningocele, acquired
　　Pseudomeningocele, acquired

⑤ **349.3 Dural tear**

　　349.31 Accidental puncture or laceration of dura during a procedure
　　　Incidental (inadvertent) durotomy

　　349.39 Other dural tear

⑤ **349.8 Other specified disorders of nervous system**

　　349.81 Cerebrospinal fluid rhinorrhea
Excludes: *cerebrospinal fluid otorrhea (388.61)*

	Add 4th or 5th digit		Nonspecific code		Unspecified code		Manifestation code

349.82 Toxic encephalopathy
Toxic metabolic encephalopathy

Use additional E code, if desired, to identify cause

349.89 Other

349.9 Unspecified disorders of nervous system
Disorder of nervous system (central) NOS

DISORDERS OF THE PERIPHERAL NERVOUS SYSTEM (350-359)

Excludes: diseases of:
> acoustic [8th] nerve (388.5)
> oculomotor [3rd, 4th, 6th] nerves (378.0-378.9)
> optic [2nd] nerve (377.0-377.9)
> peripheral autonomic nerves (337.0-337.9)
> neuralgia NOS or "rheumatic" (729.2)
> neuritis NOS or "rheumatic" (729.2)
> radiculitis NOS or "rheumatic" (729.2)
> peripheral neuritis in pregnancy (646.4)

350 Trigeminal nerve disorders
Includes: disorders of 5th cranial nerve

DEFINITION The trigeminal nerve is the main sensory nerve of the face and motor nerve for the muscles of chewing.

350.1 Trigeminal neuralgia
Tic douloureux
Trifacial neuralgia
Trigeminal neuralgia NOS

Excludes: postherpetic (053.12)

350.2 Atypical face pain

350.8 Other specified trigeminal nerve disorders

350.9 Trigeminal nerve disorder, unspecified

351 Facial nerve disorders
Includes: disorders of 7th cranial nerve

Excludes: that in newborn (767.5)

DEFINITION Facial nerve disorders refers to a disorder resulting from a weakness of the facial nerve. Bell's palsy is an example of a facial nerve disorder.

351.0 Bell's palsy
Facial palsy

351.1 Geniculate ganglionitis
Geniculate ganglionitis NOS

Excludes: herpetic (053.11)

351.8 Other facial nerve disorders
Facial myokymia
Melkersson's syndrome

351.9 Facial nerve disorder, unspecified

352 Disorders of other cranial nerves
DEFINITION Cranial nerves arise from the base of the brain or the brainstem that provide sensory and motor function to the eyes, nose, ears, tongue, and face.

352.0 Disorders of olfactory [1st] nerve

352.1 Glossopharyngeal neuralgia

352.2 Other disorders of glossopharyngeal [9th] nerve

352.3 Disorders of pneumogastric [10th] nerve
Disorders of vagal nerve

Excludes: paralysis of vocal cords or larynx (478.30-478.34)

352.4 Disorders of accessory [11th] nerve

352.5 Disorders of hypoglossal [12th] nerve

352.6 Multiple cranial nerve palsies
Collet-Sicard syndrome
Polyneuritis cranialis

352.9 Unspecified disorder of cranial nerves

● Code new to this edition   ▲ Revision of existing code   ④ ⑤ Fourth or fifth digit required

353 **Nerve root and plexus disorders**

> *Excludes:* conditions due to:
>> intervertebral disc disorders (722.0-722.9)
>> spondylosis (720.0-721.9)
>> vertebrogenic disorders (723.0-724.9)

> **DEFINITION** A nerve root is the initial segment of a nerve leaving the central nervous system. Plexus refers to a network of intersecting nerves and blood vessels or of lymphatic vessels. The body contains many plexuses, such as the brachial plexus, the cardiac plexus, the cervical plexus, and the lumbar plexus.

353.0 Brachial plexus lesions

Cervical rib syndrome
Costoclavicular syndrome

Scalenus anticus syndrome
Thoracic outlet syndrome

> *Excludes:* brachial neuritis or radiculitis NOS (723.4)
>> that in newborn (767.6)

353.1 Lumbosacral plexus lesions

353.2 Cervical root lesions, not elsewhere classified

353.3 Thoracic root lesions, not elsewhere classified

353.4 Lumbosacral root lesions, not elsewhere classified

353.5 Neuralgic amyotrophy

Parsonage-Aldren-Turner syndrome

> *Code first any associated underlying disease, such as:*
>> diabetes mellitus (249.6, 250.6)

353.6 Phantom limb (syndrome)

353.8 Other nerve root and plexus disorders

353.9 Unspecified nerve root and plexus disorder

354 **Mononeuritis of upper limb and mononeuritis multiplex**

> **DEFINITION** Mononeuritis is the inflammation of a single nerve of a upper limb. There are many causes of mononeuritis including diabetes mellitus, carpal tunnel syndrome, rheumatoid arthritis and lyme disease.

354.0 Carpal tunnel syndrome

Median nerve entrapment
Partial thenar atrophy

354.1 Other lesion of median nerve

Median nerve neuritis

354.2 Lesion of ulnar nerve

Cubital tunnel syndrome
Tardy ulnar nerve palsy

354.3 Lesion of radial nerve

Acute radial nerve palsy

354.4 Causalgia of upper limb

Complex regional pain syndrome type II of the upper limb

> *Excludes:* causalgia:
>> NOS (355.9)
>> lower limb (355.71)
>> complex regional pain syndrome type II of the lower limb (355.71)

354.5 Mononeuritis multiplex

Combinations of single conditions classifiable to 354 or 355

354.8 Other mononeuritis of upper limb

354.9 Mononeuritis of upper limb, unspecified

355 **Mononeuritis of lower limb and unspecified site**

355.0 Lesion of sciatic nerve

> *Excludes:* sciatica NOS (724.3)

355.1 Meralgia paresthetica

Lateral cutaneous femoral nerve of thigh compression or syndrome

355.2 Other lesion of femoral nerve

355.3 Lesion of lateral popliteal nerve

Lesion of common peroneal nerve

355.4 Lesion of medial popliteal nerve

355.5 Tarsal tunnel syndrome

| | Add 4th or 5th digit | | Nonspecific code | | Unspecified code | | Manifestation code |

355.6 Lesion of plantar nerve
Morton's metatarsalgia, neuralgia, or neuroma

⑤ **355.7 Other mononeuritis of lower limb**

355.71 Causalgia of lower limb

Excludes: *causalgia:*
NOS (355.9)
upper limb (354.4)
complex regional pain syndrome type II of upper limb (354.4)

355.79 Other mononeuritis of lower limb

355.8 Mononeuritis of lower limb, unspecified

355.9 Mononeuritis of unspecified site
Causalgia NOS
Complex regional pain syndrome NOS

Excludes: *causalgia:*
lower limb (355.71)
upper limb (354.4)
complex regional pain syndrome:
lower limb (355.71)
upper limb (354.4)

356 Hereditary and idiopathic peripheral neuropathy
DEFINITION Peripheral neuropathy refers to damage to nerves of the peripheral nervous system which may be caused either by diseases of the nerve or from the side-effects of systemic illness.

356.0 Hereditary peripheral neuropathy
Déjérine-Sottas disease

356.1 Peroneal muscular atrophy
Charcot-Marie-Tooth disease
Neuropathic muscular atrophy

356.2 Hereditary sensory neuropathy

356.3 Refsum's disease
Heredopathia atactica polyneuritiformis

356.4 Idiopathic progressive polyneuropathy

356.8 Other specified idiopathic peripheral neuropathy
Supranuclear paralysis

356.9 Unspecified

357 Inflammatory and toxic neuropathy
DEFINITION Inflammatory and toxic neuropathy refers to pathology of the peripheral nerves caused by inflammation or toxins

357.0 Acute infective polyneuritis
Guillain-Barré syndrome
Postinfectious polyneuritis

357.1 Polyneuropathy in collagen vascular disease
Code first underlying disease, as:
disseminated lupus erythematosus (710.0)
polyarteritis nodosa (446.0)
rheumatoid arthritis (714.0)

357.2 Polyneuropathy in diabetes
Code first underlying disease (249.6, 250.6)

357.3 Polyneuropathy in malignant disease
Code first underlying disease (140.0-208.9)

● Code new to this edition   ▲ Revision of existing code   ④ ⑤ Fourth or fifth digit required

357.4 Polyneuropathy in other diseases classified elsewhere
Code first underlying disease, as:
amyloidosis (277.30-277.39)
beriberi (265.0)
chronic uremia (585.9)
deficiency of B vitamins (266.0-266.9)
diphtheria (032.0-032.9)
hypoglycemia (251.2)
pellagra (265.2)
porphyria (277.1)
sarcoidosis (135)
uremia NOS (586)

Excludes: polyneuropathy in:
herpes zoster (053.13)
mumps (072.72)

357.5 Alcoholic polyneuropathy

357.6 Polyneuropathy due to drugs
Use additional E code, if desired, to identify drug

357.7 Polyneuropathy due to other toxic agents
Use additional E code, if desired, to identify toxic agent

⑤ **357.8 Other**

357.81 Chronic inflammatory demyelinating polyneuritis

357.82 Critical illness polyneuropathy
Acute motor neuropathy

357.89 Other inflammatory and toxic neuropathy

357.9 Unspecified

358 Myoneural disorders
DEFINITION Myoneural disorders refers to disorders affecting both muscles and nerves, especially to nerve endings in muscle tissue

⑤ **358.0 Myasthenia gravis**

358.00 Myasthenia gravis without (acute) exacerbation
Myasthenia gravis NOS

358.01 Myasthenia gravis with (acute) exacerbation
Myasthenia gravis in crisis

358.1 Myasthenic syndromes in diseases classified elsewhere
Code first underlying disease, as:
botulism (005.1, 040.41-040.42)
hypothyroidism (244.0-244.9)
malignant neoplasm (140.0-208.9)
pernicious anemia (281.0)
thyrotoxicosis (242.0-242.9)

358.2 Toxic myoneural disorders
Use additional E code, if desired, to identify toxic agent

● **358.3 Lambert-Eaton syndrome**
Eaton-Lambert syndrome

● **358.30 Lambert-Eaton syndrome, unspecified**
Lambert-Eaton syndrome NOS

● **358.31 Lambert-Eaton syndrome in neoplastic disease**
Code first the underlying neoplastic disease

● **358.39 Lambert-Eaton syndrome in other diseases classified elsewhere**
Code first the underlying condition

358.8 Other specified myoneural disorders

358.9 Myoneural disorders, unspecified

359 Muscular dystrophies and other myopathies
Excludes: idiopathic polymyositis (710.4)

DEFINITION Muscular dystrophy refers to a group of genetic, hereditary muscle diseases that weaken the muscles that move the human body. Muscular dystrophies are characterized by progressive skeletal muscle weakness, defects in muscle proteins, and the death of muscle cells and tissue.

Add 4th or 5th digit | Nonspecific code | Unspecified code | Manifestation code

359.0 Congenital hereditary muscular dystrophy
Benign congenital myopathy
Central core disease
Centronuclear myopathy
Myotubular myopathy
Nemaline body disease

Excludes: *arthrogryposis multiplex congenita (754.89)*

359.1 Hereditary progressive muscular dystrophy

Muscular dystrophy:
 NOS
 distal
 Duchenne
 Erb's
 fascioscapulohumeral

Muscular dystrophy:
 Gower's
 Landouzy-Déjérine
 limb-girdle
 ocular
 oculopharyngeal

⑤ **359.2 Myotonic disorders**

Excludes: *periodic paralysis (359.3)*

359.21 Myotonic muscular dystrophy
Dystrophia myotonica
Myotonia atrophica
Myotonic dystrophy
Proximal myotonic myopathy (PROMM)
Steinert's disease

359.22 Myotonia congenita
Acetazolamide responsive myotonia congenita
Dominant form (Thomsen's disease)
Myotonia levior
Recessive form (Becker's disease)

359.23 Myotonic chondrodystrophy
Congenital myotonic chondrodystrophy
Schwartz-Jampel disease

359.24 Drug-induced myotonia
Use additional E code to identify drug

359.29 Other specified myotonic disorder
Myotonia fluctuans
Myotonia permanens
Paramyotonia congenita (of von Eulenburg)

359.3 Periodic paralysis
Familial periodic paralysis
Hyperkalemic periodic paralysis
Hypokalemic familial periodic paralysis
Hypokalemic periodic paralysis
Potassium sensitive periodic paralysis

Excludes: *paramyotonia congenita (of von Eulenburg) (359.29)*

359.4 Toxic myopathy
Use additional E code, if desired, to identify toxic agent

359.5 Myopathy in endocrine diseases classified elsewhere
Code first underlying disease, as:
Addison's disease (255.41)
Cushing's syndrome (255.0)
hypopituitarism (253.2)
myxedema (244.0-244.9)
thyrotoxicosis (242.0-242.9)

359.6 Symptomatic inflammatory myopathy in diseases classified elsewhere
Code first underlying disease, as:
amyloidosis (277.30-277.39)
disseminated lupus erythematosus (710.0)
malignant neoplasm (140.0-208.9)
polyarteritis nodosa (446.0)
rheumatoid arthritis (714.0)
sarcoidosis (135)
scleroderma (710.1)
Sjögren's disease (710.2)

⑤ **359.7 Inflammatory and immune myopathies, NEC**

● Code new
to this edition   ▲ Revision of
existing code   ④ ⑤ Fourth or fifth
digit required

359.71 Inclusion body myositis
IBM

359.79 Other inflammatory and immune myopathies, NEC
Inflammatory myopathy NOS

⑤ **359.8 Other myopathies**

359.81 Critical illness myopathy
Acute necrotizing myopathy
Acute quadriplegic myopathy
Intensive care (ICU) myopathy
Myopathy of critical illness

359.89 Other myopathies

359.9 Myopathy, unspecified

DISORDERS OF THE EYE AND ADNEXA (360-379)

Use additional external cause code, if applicable, to identify the cause of the eye condition

360 Disorders of the globe
Includes: disorders affecting multiple structures of eye
DEFINITION Disorders of the globe refers to disorders affecting the outer membranes of the eye.

⑤ **360.0 Purulent endophthalmitis**
Excludes: *bleb associated endophthalmitis (379.63)*

360.00 Purulent endophthalmitis, unspecified

360.01 Acute endophthalmitis

360.02 Panophthalmitis

360.03 Chronic endophthalmitis

360.04 Vitreous abscess

⑤ **360.1 Other endophthalmitis**
Excludes: *bleb associated endophthalmitis (379.63)*

360.11 Sympathetic uveitis

360.12 Panuveitis

360.13 Parasitic endophthalmitis NOS

360.14 Ophthalmia nodosa

360.19 Other
Phacoanaphylactic endophthalmitis

⑤ **360.2 Degenerative disorders of globe**

360.20 Degenerative disorder of globe, unspecified

360.21 Progressive high (degenerative) myopia
Malignant myopia

360.23 Siderosis

360.24 Other metallosis
Chalcosis

360.29 Other
Excludes: *xerophthalmia (264.7)*

⑤ **360.3 Hypotony of eye**

360.30 Hypotony, unspecified

360.31 Primary hypotony

360.32 Ocular fistula causing hypotony

360.33 Hypotony associated with other ocular disorders

360.34 Flat anterior chamber

⑤ **360.4 Degenerated conditions of globe**

360.40 Degenerated globe or eye, unspecified

360.41 Blind hypotensive eye
Atrophy of globe
Phthisis bulbi

360.42 Blind hypertensive eye
Absolute glaucoma

Add 4th or 5th digit	Nonspecific code	Unspecified code	Manifestation code

360.43 Hemophthalmos, except current injury

Excludes: *traumatic (871.0-871.9, 921.0-921.9)*

360.44 Leucocoria

⑤ **360.5 Retained (old) intraocular foreign body, magnetic**
Use additional code to identify foreign body (V90.11)

Excludes: *current penetrating injury with magnetic foreign body (871.5)*
retained (old) foreign body of orbit (376.6)

360.50 Foreign body, magnetic, intraocular, unspecified

360.51 Foreign body, magnetic, in anterior chamber

360.52 Foreign body, magnetic, in iris or ciliary body

360.53 Foreign body, magnetic, in lens

360.54 Foreign body, magnetic, in vitreous

360.55 Foreign body, magnetic, in posterior wall

360.59 Foreign body, magnetic, in other or multiple sites

⑤ **360.6 Retained (old) intraocular foreign body, nonmagnetic**
Retained (old) foreign body:
   NOS
   nonmagnetic
Use additional code to identify foreign body (V90.01-V90.10, V90.12, V90.2-V90.9)

Excludes: *current penetrating injury with (nonmagnetic) foreign body (871.6)*
retained (old) foreign body in orbit (376.6)

360.60 Foreign body, intraocular, unspecified

360.61 Foreign body in anterior chamber

360.62 Foreign body in iris or ciliary body

360.63 Foreign body in lens

360.64 Foreign body in vitreous

360.65 Foreign body in posterior wall

360.69 Foreign body in other or multiple sites

⑤ **360.8 Other disorders of globe**

360.81 Luxation of globe

360.89 Other

360.9 Unspecified disorder of globe

361 Retinal detachments and defects
DEFINITION Retinal detachment is a disorder of the eye in which the retina peels away from its underlying layer of support tissue

⑤ **361.0 Retinal detachment with retinal defect**
Rhegmatogenous retinal detachment

Excludes: *detachment of retinal pigment epithelium (362.42-362.43)*
retinal detachment (serous) (without defect) (361.2)

361.00 Retinal detachment with retinal defect, unspecified

361.01 Recent detachment, partial, with single defect

361.02 Recent detachment, partial, with multiple defects

361.03 Recent detachment, partial, with giant tear

361.04 Recent detachment, partial, with retinal dialysis
Dialysis (juvenile) of retina (with detachment)

361.05 Recent detachment, total or subtotal

361.06 Old detachment, partial
Delimited old retinal detachment

361.07 Old detachment, total or subtotal

⑤ **361.1 Retinoschisis and retinal cysts**

Excludes: *juvenile retinoschisis (362.73)*
microcystoid degeneration of retina (362.62)
parasitic cyst of retina (360.13)

361.10 Retinoschisis, unspecified

361.11 Flat retinoschisis

361.12 Bullous retinoschisis

● Code new
to this edition
▲ Revision of
existing code
④ ⑤ Fourth or fifth
digit required

361.13 **Primary retinal cysts**

361.14 **Secondary retinal cysts**

361.19 **Other**
Pseudocyst of retina

361.2 **Serous retinal detachment**
Retinal detachment without retinal defect

Excludes: *central serous retinopathy (362.41)*
retinal pigment epithelium detachment (362.42-362.43)

⑤ 361.3 **Retinal defects without detachment**

Excludes: *chorioretinal scars after surgery for detachment (363.30-363.35)*
peripheral retinal degeneration without defect (362.60-362.66)

361.30 **Retinal defect, unspecified**
Retinal break(s) NOS

361.31 **Round hole of retina without detachment**

361.32 **Horseshoe tear of retina without detachment**
Operculum of retina without mention of detachment

361.33 **Multiple defects of retina without detachment**

⑤ 361.8 **Other forms of retinal detachment**

361.81 **Traction detachment of retina**
Traction detachment with vitreoretinal organization

361.89 **Other**

361.9 **Unspecified retinal detachment**

362 **Other retinal disorders**

Excludes: *chorioretinal scars (363.30-363.35)*
chorioretinitis (363.0-363.2)

ALERT! For personal history of other disorders of nervous system and sense organs see V12.49

⑤ *362.0 Diabetic retinopathy*
Code first diabetes (249.5, 250.5)

362.01 *Background diabetic retinopathy*
Diabetic retinal microaneurysms
Diabetic retinopathy NOS

362.02 *Proliferative diabetic retinopathy*

362.03 **Nonproliferative diabetic retinopathy NOS**

362.04 **Mild nonproliferative diabetic retinopathy**

362.05 **Moderate nonproliferative diabetic retinopathy**

362.06 **Severe nonproliferative diabetic retinopathy**

362.07 **Diabetic macular edema**
Diabetic retinal edema
Note: Code 362.07 must be used with a code for diabetic retinopathy (362.01-362.06)

⑤ 362.1 **Other background retinopathy and retinal vascular changes**

362.10 **Background retinopathy, unspecified**

362.11 **Hypertensive retinopathy**

362.12 **Exudative retinopathy**
Coats' syndrome

362.13 **Changes in vascular appearance**
Vascular sheathing of retina
Use additional code for any associated atherosclerosis (440.8)

362.14 **Retinal microaneurysms NOS**

362.15 **Retinal telangiectasia**

362.16 **Retinal neovascularization NOS**
Neovascularization:
choroidal
subretinal

362.17 **Other intraretinal microvascular abnormalities**
Retinal varices

362.18 Retinal vasculitis
    Eales' disease
    Retinal:
      arteritis
      endarteritis
    Retinal:
      perivasculitis
      phlebitis

⑤ **362.2 Other proliferative retinopathy**

362.20 Retinopathy of prematurity, unspecified
    Retinopathy of prematurity NOS

362.21 Retrolental fibroplasia
    Cicatricial retinopathy of prematurity

362.22 Retinopathy of prematurity, stage 0

362.23 Retinopathy of prematurity, stage 1

362.24 Retinopathy of prematurity, stage 2

362.25 Retinopathy of prematurity, stage 3

362.26 Retinopathy of prematurity, stage 4

362.27 Retinopathy of prematurity, stage 5

362.29 Other nondiabetic proliferative retinopathy

⑤ **362.3 Retinal vascular occlusion**

362.30 Retinal vascular occlusion, unspecified

362.31 Central retinal artery occlusion

362.32 Arterial branch occlusion

362.33 Partial arterial occlusion
    Hollenhorst plaque
    Retinal microembolism

362.34 Transient arterial occlusion
    Amaurosis fugax

362.35 Central retinal vein occlusion

362.36 Venous tributary (branch) occlusion

362.37 Venous engorgement
    Occlusion:
      incipient of retinal vein
      partial of retinal vein

⑤ **362.4 Separation of retinal layers**

Excludes: *retinal detachment (serous) (361.2)*
           rhegmatogenous (361.00-361.07)

362.40 Retinal layer separation, unspecified

362.41 Central serous retinopathy

362.42 Serous detachment of retinal pigment epithelium
    Exudative detachment of retinal pigment epithelium

362.43 Hemorrhagic detachment of retinal pigment epithelium

⑤ **362.5 Degeneration of macula and posterior pole**

Excludes: *degeneration of optic disc (377.21-377.24)*
           hereditary retinal degeneration [dystrophy] (362.70-362.77)

362.50 Macular degeneration (senile), unspecified

362.51 Nonexudative senile macular degeneration
    Senile macular degeneration:
      atrophic
      dry

362.52 Exudative senile macular degeneration
    Kuhnt-Junius degeneration
    Senile macular degeneration:
      disciform
      wet

362.53 Cystoid macular degeneration
    Cystoid macular edema

362.54 Macular cyst, hole, or pseudohole

362.55 Toxic maculopathy
Use additional E code, if desired, to identify drug, if drug induced

● Code new   ▲ Revision of   ④ ⑤ Fourth or fifth
      to this edition   existing code   digit required

362.56　**Macular puckering**
Preretinal fibrosis

362.57　**Drusen (degenerative)**

⑤ **362.6　Peripheral retinal degenerations**

Excludes: *hereditary retinal degeneration [dystrophy] (362.70-362.77)*
retinal degeneration with retinal defect (361.00-361.07)

362.60　**Peripheral retinal degeneration, unspecified**

362.61　**Paving stone degeneration**

362.62　**Microcystoid degeneration**
Blessig's cysts　　　　Iwanoff's cysts

362.63　**Lattice degeneration**
Palisade degeneration of retina

362.64　**Senile reticular degeneration**

362.65　**Secondary pigmentary degeneration**
Pseudoretinitis pigmentosa

362.66　**Secondary vitreoretinal degenerations**

⑤ **362.7　Hereditary retinal dystrophies**

362.70　**Hereditary retinal dystrophy, unspecified**

362.71　***Retinal dystrophy in systemic or cerebroretinal lipidoses***
Code first underlying disease, as:
cerebroretinal lipidoses (330.1)
systemic lipidoses (272.7)

362.72　***Retinal dystrophy in other systemic disorders and syndromes***
Code first underlying disease, as:
Bassen-Kornzweig syndrome (272.5)
Refsum's disease (356.3)

362.73　**Vitreoretinal dystrophies**
Juvenile retinoschisis

362.74　**Pigmentary retinal dystrophy**
Retinal dystrophy, albipunctate
Retinitis pigmentosa

362.75　**Other dystrophies primarily involving the sensory retina**
Progressive cone (-rod) dystrophy
Stargardt's disease

362.76　**Dystrophies primarily involving the retinal pigment epithelium**
Fundus flavimaculatus
Vitelliform dystrophy

362.77　**Dystrophies primarily involving Bruch's membrane**
Dystrophy:
hyaline
pseudoinflammatory foveal
Hereditary drusen

⑤ **362.8　Other retinal disorders**

Excludes: *chorioretinal inflammations (363.0-363.2)*
chorioretinal scars (363.30-363.35)

362.81　**Retinal hemorrhage**
Hemorrhage:
preretinal
retinal (deep) (superficial)
subretinal

362.82　**Retinal exudates and deposits**

362.83　**Retinal edema**
Retinal:
cotton wool spots
edema (localized) (macular) (peripheral)

362.84　**Retinal ischemia**

362.85　**Retinal nerve fiber bundle defects**

362.89　**Other retinal disorders**

362.9　Unspecified retinal disorder

Add 4th or 5th digit	Nonspecific code	Unspecified code	Manifestation code

363 **Chorioretinal inflammations, scars, and other disorders of choroid**

DEFINITION Chorioretinal inflammations, scars and other disorders of choroid is an inflammation affecting the choroid and the retina of the eye.

⑤ **363.0 Focal chorioretinitis and focal retinochoroiditis**

Excludes: *focal chorioretinitis or retinochoroiditis in:*
  histoplasmosis (115.02, 115.12, 115.92)
  toxoplasmosis (130.2)
    congenital infection (771.2)

  363.00 Focal chorioretinitis, unspecified
    Focal:
      choroiditis or chorioretinitis NOS
      retinitis or retinochoroiditis NOS

  363.01 Focal choroiditis and chorioretinitis, juxtapapillary

  363.03 Focal choroiditis and chorioretinitis of other posterior pole

  363.04 Focal choroiditis and chorioretinitis, peripheral

  363.05 Focal retinitis and retinochoroiditis, juxtapapillary
    Neuroretinitis

  363.06 Focal retinitis and retinochoroiditis, macular or paramacular

  363.07 Focal retinitis and retinochoroiditis of other posterior pole

  363.08 Focal retinitis and retinochoroiditis, peripheral

⑤ **363.1 Disseminated chorioretinitis and disseminated retinochoroiditis**

Excludes: *disseminated choroiditis or chorioretinitis in secondary syphilis (091.51)*
  neurosyphilitic disseminated retinitis or retinochoroiditis (094.83)
  retinal (peri)vasculitis (362.18)

  363.10 Disseminated chorioretinitis, unspecified
    Disseminated:
      choroiditis or chorioretinitis NOS
      retinitis or retinochoroiditis NOS

  363.11 Disseminated choroiditis and chorioretinitis, posterior pole

  363.12 Disseminated choroiditis and chorioretinitis, peripheral

  363.13 Disseminated choroiditis and chorioretinitis, generalized
  Code first any underlying disease, as:
    tuberculosis (017.3)

  363.14 Disseminated retinitis and retinochoroiditis, metastatic

  363.15 Disseminated retinitis and retinochoroiditis, pigment epitheliopathy
    Acute posterior multifocal placoid pigment epitheliopathy

⑤ **363.2 Other and unspecified forms of chorioretinitis and retinochoroiditis**

Excludes: *panophthalmitis (360.02)*
  sympathetic uveitis (360.11)
  uveitis NOS (364.3)

  363.20 Chorioretinitis, unspecified
    Choroiditis NOS
    Retinitis NOS
    Uveitis, posterior NOS

  363.21 Pars planitis
    Posterior cyclitis

  363.22 Harada's disease

⑤ **363.3 Chorioretinal scars**
    Scar (postinflammatory) (postsurgical) (posttraumatic):
      choroid
      retina

  363.30 Chorioretinal scar, unspecified

  363.31 Solar retinopathy

  363.32 Other macular scars

  363.33 Other scars of posterior pole

  363.34 Peripheral scars

  363.35 Disseminated scars

⑤ **363.4 Choroidal degenerations**

● Code new   ▲ Revision of   ④ ⑤ Fourth or fifth
  to this edition   existing code   digit required

363.40 **Choroidal degeneration, unspecified**
Choroidal sclerosis NOS

363.41 **Senile atrophy of choroid**

363.42 **Diffuse secondary atrophy of choroid**

363.43 **Angioid streaks of choroid**

⑤ **363.5** **Hereditary choroidal dystrophies**
Hereditary choroidal atrophy:
partial [choriocapillaris]
total [all vessels]

363.50 **Hereditary choroidal dystrophy or atrophy, unspecified**

363.51 **Circumpapillary dystrophy of choroid, partial**

363.52 **Circumpapillary dystrophy of choroid, total**
Helicoid dystrophy of choroid

363.53 **Central dystrophy of choroid, partial**
Dystrophy, choroidal:
central areolar
circinate

363.54 **Central choroidal atrophy, total**
Dystrophy, choroidal:
central gyrate
serpiginous

363.55 **Choroideremia**

363.56 **Other diffuse or generalized dystrophy, partial**
Diffuse choroidal sclerosis

363.57 **Other diffuse or generalized dystrophy, total**
Generalized gyrate atrophy, choroid

⑤ **363.6** **Choroidal hemorrhage and rupture**

363.61 **Choroidal hemorrhage, unspecified**

363.62 **Expulsive choroidal hemorrhage**

363.63 **Choroidal rupture**

⑤ **363.7** **Choroidal detachment**

363.70 **Choroidal detachment, unspecified**

363.71 **Serous choroidal detachment**

363.72 **Hemorrhagic choroidal detachment**

363.8 **Other disorders of choroid**

363.9 **Unspecified disorder of choroid**

364 **Disorders of iris and ciliary body**
DEFINITION The iris is a muscular diaphragm that controls the size of the pupil which in turn controls the amount of light that enters the eye. The ciliary body is part of the middle layer of the wall of the eye that includes the ring-shaped muscle that changes the size of the pupil and the shape of the lens when the eye focuses and also produces the fluid that fills the eye.

⑤ **364.0** **Acute and subacute iridocyclitis**
Anterior uveitis, acute, subacute
Cyclitis, acute, subacute
Iridocyclitis, acute, subacute
Iritis, acute, subacute

Excludes: gonococcal (098.41)
herpes simplex (054.44)
herpes zoster (053.22)

364.00 **Acute and subacute iridocyclitis, unspecified**

364.01 **Primary iridocyclitis**

364.02 **Recurrent iridocyclitis**

364.03 **Secondary iridocyclitis, infectious**

364.04 **Secondary iridocyclitis, noninfectious**
Aqueous:
cells
fibrin
flare

364.05 **Hypopyon**

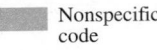 Add 4th or 5th digit

 Nonspecific code

Unspecified code

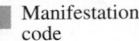 Manifestation code

⑤ **364.1** **Chronic iridocyclitis**
> *Excludes:* posterior cyclitis (363.21)

364.10 **Chronic iridocyclitis, unspecified**

364.11 *Chronic iridocyclitis in diseases classified elsewhere*
Code first underlying disease, as:
  sarcoidosis (135)
  tuberculosis (017.3)
> *Excludes:* syphilitic iridocyclitis (091.52)

⑤ **364.2** **Certain types of iridocyclitis**
> *Excludes:* posterior cyclitis (363.21)
> sympathetic uveitis (360.11)

364.21 **Fuchs' heterochromic cyclitis**

364.22 **Glaucomatocyclitic crises**

364.23 **Lens-induced iridocyclitis**

364.24 **Vogt-Koyanagi syndrome**

364.3 **Unspecified iridocyclitis**
  Uveitis NOS

⑤ **364.4** **Vascular disorders of iris and ciliary body**

364.41 **Hyphema**
  Hemorrhage of iris or ciliary body

364.42 **Rubeosis iridis**
  Neovascularization of iris or ciliary body

⑤ **364.5** **Degenerations of iris and ciliary body**

364.51 **Essential or progressive iris atrophy**

364.52 **Iridoschisis**

364.53 **Pigmentary iris degeneration**
  Acquired heterochromia of iris
  Pigment dispersion syndrome of iris
  Translucency of iris

364.54 **Degeneration of pupillary margin**
  Atrophy of sphincter of iris
  Ectropion of pigment epithelium of iris

364.55 **Miotic cysts of pupillary margin**

364.56 **Degenerative changes of chamber angle**

364.57 **Degenerative changes of ciliary body**

364.59 **Other iris atrophy**
  Iris atrophy (generalized) (sector shaped)

⑤ **364.6** **Cysts of iris, ciliary body, and anterior chamber**
> *Excludes:* miotic pupillary cyst (364.55)
> parasitic cyst (360.13)

364.60 **Idiopathic cysts**

364.61 **Implantation cysts**
  Epithelial down-growth, anterior chamber
  Implantation cysts (surgical) (traumatic)

364.62 **Exudative cysts of iris or anterior chamber**

364.63 **Primary cyst of pars plana**

364.64 **Exudative cyst of pars plana**

⑤ **364.7** **Adhesions and disruptions of iris and ciliary body**
> *Excludes:* flat anterior chamber (360.34)

364.70 **Adhesions of iris, unspecified**
  Synechiae (iris) NOS

364.71 **Posterior synechiae**

364.72 **Anterior synechiae**

364.73 **Goniosynechiae**
  Peripheral anterior synechiae

● Code new
  to this edition

▲ Revision of
  existing code

④ ⑤ Fourth or fifth
  digit required

364.74 Pupillary membranes
Iris bombé
Pupillary:
 occlusion
 seclusion

364.75 Pupillary abnormalities
Deformed pupil   Rupture of sphincter, pupil
Ectopic pupil

364.76 Iridodialysis

364.77 Recession of chamber angle

⑤ **364.8 Other disorders of iris and ciliary body**

364.81 Floppy iris syndrome
Intraoperative floppy iris syndrome (IFIS)

Use additional E code to identify cause, such as:
sympatholytics [antiadrenergics] causing adverse effect in therapeutic use (E941.3)

364.82 Plateau iris syndrome

364.89 Other disorders of iris and ciliary body
Prolapse of iris NOS

Excludes: *prolapse of iris in recent wound (871.1)*

364.9 Unspecified disorder of iris and ciliary body

365 Glaucoma

Excludes: *blind hypertensive eye [absolute glaucoma] (360.42)*
congenital glaucoma (743.20-743.22)

DEFINITION Glaucoma is a group of eye diseases characterized by damage to the optic nerve usually due to excessively high intraocular pressure.

⑤ **365.0 Borderline glaucoma [glaucoma suspect]**

365.00 Preglaucoma, unspecified

▲ 365.01 **Open angle with borderline findings, low risk**
Open angle, low risk

365.02 Anatomical narrow angle
Primary angle closure suspect

365.03 Steroid responders

365.04 Ocular hypertension

● 365.05 **Open angle with borderline findings, high risk**
Open angle, high risk

● 365.06 **Primary angle closure without glaucoma damage**

⑤ **365.1 Open-angle glaucoma**

365.10 Open-angle glaucoma, unspecified
Wide-angle glaucoma NOS

Use additional code to identify glaucoma stage (365.70-365.74)

365.11 Primary open angle glaucoma
Chronic simple glaucoma

Use additional code to identify glaucoma stage (365.70-365.74)

365.12 Low tension glaucoma

Use additional code to identify glaucoma stage (365.70-365.74)

365.13 Pigmentary glaucoma

Use additional code to identify glaucoma stage (365.70-365.74)

365.14 Glaucoma of childhood
Infantile or juvenile glaucoma

365.15 Residual stage of open angle glaucoma

⑤ **365.2 Primary angle-closure glaucoma**

365.20 Primary angle-closure glaucoma, unspecified
Use additional code to identify glaucoma stage (365.70-365.74)

365.21 Intermittent angle-closure glaucoma
Angle-closure glaucoma:
 interval
 subacute

	Add 4th or 5th digit		Nonspecific code		Unspecified code		Manifestation code

365.22 Acute angle-closure glaucoma
Acute angle-closure glaucoma attack
Acute angle-closure glaucoma crisis

365.23 Chronic angle-closure glaucoma
Chronic primary angle closure glaucoma
Use additional code to identify glaucoma stage (365.70-365.74)

365.24 Residual stage of angle-closure glaucoma

⑤ 365.3 **Corticosteroid-induced glaucoma**

365.31 Glaucomatous stage
Use additional code to identify glaucoma stage (365.70-365.74)

365.32 Residual stage

⑤ 365.4 **Glaucoma associated with congenital anomalies, dystrophies, and systemic syndromes**

365.41 *Glaucoma associated with chamber angle anomalies*

365.42 *Glaucoma associated with anomalies of iris*

365.43 *Glaucoma associated with other anterior segment anomalies*

365.44 *Glaucoma associated with systemic syndromes*

Code first associated disease, as:
neurofibromatosis (237.70-237.79)
Sturge-Weber (-Dimitri) syndrome (759.6)

⑤ 365.5 **Glaucoma associated with disorders of the lens**

365.51 Phacolytic glaucoma

365.52 Pseudoexfoliation glaucoma
Use additional code to identify glaucoma stage (365.70-365.74)

365.59 **Glaucoma associated with other lens disorders**

⑤ 365.6 **Glaucoma associated with other ocular disorders**

365.60 **Glaucoma associated with unspecified ocular disorder**

365.61 Glaucoma associated with pupillary block

365.62 Glaucoma associated with ocular inflammations
Use additional code to identify glaucoma stage (365.70-365.74)

365.63 Glaucoma associated with vascular disorders
Use additional code to identify glaucoma stage (365.70-365.74)

365.64 Glaucoma associated with tumors or cysts

365.65 Glaucoma associated with ocular trauma
Use additional code to identify glaucoma stage (365.70-365.74)

● **365.7** **Glaucoma stage**
Code first associated type of glaucoma (365.10-365.13, 365.20, 365.23, 365.31, 365.52, 365.62-365.63, 365.65)

● **365.70** **Glaucoma stage, unspecified**
Glaucoma stage NOS

● **365.71** **Mild stage glaucoma**
Early stage glaucoma

● **365.72** **Moderate stage glaucoma**

● **365.73** **Severe stage glaucoma**
Advanced stage glaucoma
End-stage glaucoma

● **365.74** **Indeterminate stage glaucoma**

⑤ 365.8 **Other specified forms of glaucoma**

365.81 Hypersecretion glaucoma

365.82 Glaucoma with increased episcleral venous pressure

365.83 Aqueous misdirection
Malignant glaucoma

365.89 **Other specified glaucoma**

365.9 **Unspecified glaucoma**

● Code new to this edition   ▲ Revision of existing code   ④ ⑤ Fourth or fifth digit required

366 Cataract

Excludes: congenital cataract (743.30-743.34)

DEFINITION A cataract is a clouding that develops in the crystalline lens of the eye or in its envelope, varying in degree from slight to complete opacity and obstructing the passage of light.

⑤ **366.0 Infantile, juvenile, and presenile cataract**

366.00 Nonsenile cataract, unspecified

366.01 Anterior subcapsular polar cataract

366.02 Posterior subcapsular polar cataract

366.03 Cortical, lamellar, or zonular cataract

366.04 Nuclear cataract

366.09 Other and combined forms of nonsenile cataract

⑤ **366.1 Senile cataract**

366.10 Senile cataract, unspecified

366.11 Pseudoexfoliation of lens capsule

366.12 Incipient cataract
Cataract: Water clefts
  coronary
  immature NOS
  punctate

366.13 Anterior subcapsular polar senile cataract

366.14 Posterior subcapsular polar senile cataract

366.15 Cortical senile cataract

366.16 Nuclear sclerosis
Cataracta brunescens
Nuclear cataract

366.17 Total or mature cataract

366.18 Hypermature cataract
Morgagni cataract

366.19 Other and combined forms of senile cataract

⑤ **366.2 Traumatic cataract**

366.20 Traumatic cataract, unspecified

366.21 Localized traumatic opacities
Vossius' ring

366.22 Total traumatic cataract

366.23 Partially resolved traumatic cataract

⑤ **366.3 Cataract secondary to ocular disorders**

366.30 Cataracts complicata, unspecified

366.31 *Glaucomatous flecks (subcapsular)*
Code first underlying glaucoma (365.0-365.9)

366.32 *Cataract in inflammatory disorders*
Code first underlying condition, as:
chronic choroiditis (363.0-363.2)

366.33 *Cataract with neovascularization*
Code first underlying condition, as:
chronic iridocyclitis (364.10)

366.34 *Cataract in degenerative disorders*
Sunflower cataract
Code first underlying condition, as:
chalcosis (360.24)
degenerative myopia (360.21)
pigmentary retinal dystrophy (362.74)

⑤ **366.4 Cataract associated with other disorders**

366.41 *Diabetic cataract*
Code first diabetes (249.5, 250.5)

Add 4th or 5th digit   Nonspecific code   Unspecified code   Manifestation code

366.42 Tetanic cataract
Code first underlying disease, as:
    calcinosis (275.4)
    hypoparathyroidism (252.1)

366.43 Myotonic cataract
Code first underlying disorder (359.21, 359.23)

366.44 Cataract associated with other syndromes
Code first underlying condition, as:
    craniofacial dysostosis (756.0)
    galactosemia (271.1)

366.45 Toxic cataract
    Drug-induced cataract

Use additional E code, if desired, to identify drug or other toxic substance

366.46 Cataract associated with radiation and other physical influences
Use additional E code, if desired, to identify cause

⑤ **366.5 After-cataract**

366.50 After-cataract, unspecified
    Secondary cataract NOS

366.51 Soemmering's ring

366.52 Other after-cataract, not obscuring vision

366.53 After-cataract, obscuring vision

366.8 Other cataract
    Calcification of lens

366.9 Unspecified cataract

367 Disorders of refraction and accommodation

    DEFINITION Refraction is the ability of the eye to bend light so that an image is focused on the retina. Accommodation is the automatic adjustment in focal length of the natural lens of the eye.

367.0 Hypermetropia
    Far-sightedness
    Hyperopia

367.1 Myopia
    Near-sightedness

⑤ **367.2 Astigmatism**

367.20 Astigmatism, unspecified

367.21 Regular astigmatism

367.22 Irregular astigmatism

⑤ **367.3 Anisometropia and aniseikonia**

367.31 Anisometropia

367.32 Aniseikonia

367.4 Presbyopia

⑤ **367.5 Disorders of accommodation**

367.51 Paresis of accommodation
    Cycloplegia

367.52 Total or complete internal ophthalmoplegia

367.53 Spasm of accommodation

⑤ **367.8 Other disorders of refraction and accommodation**

367.81 Transient refractive change

367.89 Other
    Drug-induced disorders of refraction and accommodation
    Toxic disorders of refraction and accommodation

367.9 Unspecified disorder of refraction and accommodation

368 Visual disturbances

    Excludes: *electrophysiological disturbances (794.11-794.14)*

⑤ **368.0 Amblyopia ex anopsia**

368.00 Amblyopia, unspecified

● Code new
    to this edition
▲ Revision of
    existing code
④ ⑤ Fourth or fifth
    digit required

368.01 **Strabismic amblyopia**
Suppression amblyopia

368.02 **Deprivation amblyopia**

368.03 **Refractive amblyopia**

⑤ **368.1** **Subjective visual disturbances**

368.10 **Subjective visual disturbance, unspecified**

368.11 **Sudden visual loss**

368.12 **Transient visual loss**
Concentric fading
Scintillating scotoma

368.13 **Visual discomfort**
Asthenopia   Photophobia
Eye strain

368.14 **Visual distortions of shape and size**
Macropsia   Micropsia
Metamorphopsia

368.15 **Other visual distortions and entoptic phenomena**
Photopsia   Visual halos
Refractive:
diplopia
polyopia

368.16 **Psychophysical visual disturbances**
Prosopagnosia
Visual:
agnosia
disorientation syndrome
hallucinations
object agnosia

368.2 **Diplopia**
Double vision

⑤ **368.3** **Other disorders of binocular vision**

368.30 **Binocular vision disorder, unspecified**

368.31 **Suppression of binocular vision**

368.32 **Simultaneous visual perception without fusion**

368.33 **Fusion with defective stereopsis**

368.34 **Abnormal retinal correspondence**

⑤ **368.4** **Visual field defects**

368.40 **Visual field defect, unspecified**

368.41 **Scotoma involving central area**
Scotoma:
central
centrocecal
paracentral

368.42 **Scotoma of blind spot area**
Enlarged: Paracecal scotoma
angioscotoma
blind spot

368.43 **Sector or arcuate defects**
Scotoma:
arcuate
Bjerrum
Seidel

368.44 **Other localized visual field defect**
Scotoma: Visual field defect:
NOS   nasal step
ring   peripheral

368.45 **Generalized contraction or constriction**

368.46 **Homonymous bilateral field defects**
Hemianopsia (altitudinal) (homonymous)
Quadrant anopia

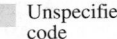 Add 4th or
5th digit

Nonspecific
code

Unspecified
code

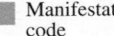 Manifestation
code

368.47 Heteronymous bilateral field defects
Hemianopsia:
binasal
bitemporal

⑤ **368.5 Color vision deficiencies**
Color blindness

368.51 Protan defect
Protanomaly
Protanopia

368.52 Deutan defect
Deuteranomaly
Deuteranopia

368.53 Tritan defect
Tritanomaly
Tritanopia

368.54 Achromatopsia
Monochromatism (cone) (rod)

368.55 Acquired color vision deficiencies

368.59 Other color vision deficiencies

⑤ **368.6 Night blindness**
Nyctalopia

368.60 Night blindness, unspecified

368.61 Congenital night blindness
Hereditary night blindness
Oguchi's disease

368.62 Acquired night blindness

Excludes: that due to vitamin A deficiency (264.5)

368.63 Abnormal dark adaptation curve
Abnormal threshold of cones or rods
Delayed adaptation of cones or rods

368.69 Other night blindness

368.8 Other specified visual disturbances
Blurred vision NOS

368.9 Unspecified visual disturbance

● Code new to this edition   ▲ Revision of existing code   ④ ⑤ Fourth or fifth digit required

369 **Blindness and low vision**

Note: Visual impairment refers to a functional limitation of the eye (e.g., limited visual acuity or visual field). It should be distinguished from visual disability, indicating a limitation of the abilities of the individual (e.g., limited reading skills, vocational skills), and from visual handicap, indicating a limitation of personal and socioeconomic independence (e.g., limited mobility, limited employability.)

The levels of impairment defined in the table in this section are based on the recommendations of the WHO Study Group on Prevention of Blindness (Geneva, November 6-10, 1972; WHO Technical Report Series 518), and of the International Council of Ophthalmology (1976).

Note that definitions of blindness vary in different settings.

For international reporting WHO defines blindness as profound impairment. This definition can be applied to blindness of one eye (369.1, 369.6) and to blindness of the individual (369.0).

For determination of benefits in the U.S.A., the definition of legal blindness as severe impairment is often used. This definition applies to blindness of the individual only.

Excludes: correctable impaired vision due to refractive errors (367.0-367.9)

Classification		LEVELS OF VISUAL IMPAIRMENT					Additional Descriptors
"legal"	WHO	Visual Acuity and/or Visual Field Limitation (whichever is worse)					which may be encountered
LEGAL BLINDNESS	(NEAR-) NORMAL VISION	**RANGE OF NORMAL VISION**					
		20/10 0.7	20/13 0.6	20/16 0.5	20/20 0.4	20/25 0.8	
		NEAR-NORMAL VISION					
		0.7	20/30 0.6	20/40 0.5	20/50 0.4	20/60 0.4	
	LOW VISION	**MODERATE VISUAL IMPAIRMENT**					Moderate low vision
		20/70	20/80 0.25	20/100 0.20	20/125 0.16	20/160 0.12	
		SEVERE VISUAL IMPAIRMENT					Severe low vision, "legal blindness"
			20/200 0.10	20/250 0.08	20/320 0.06	20/400 0.05	
		Visual Field:	20 degrees or less				
	BLINDNESS	**PROFOUND VISUAL IMPAIRMENT**					Profound low vision, moderate blindness
			20/500 0.04	20/630 0.03	20/800 0.025	20/1000 0.02	
		Count Fingers at:	less than 3 m (10ft)				
		Visual Field:	10 degrees or less				
		NEAR-TOTAL VISUAL IMPAIRMENT					Severe blindness
		Visual Acuity:	less than 0.02 (20/1000)				
		Count Fingers at:	1 m (3 ft) or less				
		Hand Movements:	5m (15ft) or less				Near-Total blindness
(USA) both eyes	(WHO) one or both eyes	Light projection, light perception					
		Visual Field:	5 degrees or less				
		TOTAL VISUAL IMPAIRMENT					Total blindness
		No light perception (NLP)					

Visual acuity refers to best achievable acuity with correction

Non-listed Snellen fractions may be classified by converting to the nearest decimal equivalent, e.g., 10/200=0.05, 6/30=0.20

CF (count fingers) without designation of distance, may be classified to profound impairment

HM (hand motion) without designation of distance, may be classified to near-total impairment.

Visual field measurements refer to the largest field diameter for a 1/100 white test object.

⑤ **369.0 Profound impairment, both eyes**

  369.00 **Impairment level not further specified**
      Blindness:
         NOS according to WHO definition
         both eyes

	Add 4th or 5th digit		Nonspecific code		Unspecified code		Manifestation code

369.01 Better eye: total impairment;
lesser eye: total impairment

369.02 Better eye: near-total impairment;
lesser eye: not further specified

369.03 Better eye: near-total impairment;
lesser eye: total impairment

369.04 Better eye: near-total impairment;
lesser eye: near-total impairment

369.05 Better eye: profound impairment;
lesser eye: not further specified

369.06 Better eye: profound impairment;
lesser eye: total impairment

369.07 Better eye: profound impairment;
lesser eye: near-total impairment

369.08 Better eye: profound impairment;
lesser eye: profound impairment

⑤ 369.1 Moderate or severe impairment, better eye, profound impairment lesser eye

369.10 Impairment level not further specified
Blindness, one eye, low vision other eye

369.11 Better eye: severe impairment;
lesser eye: blind, not further specified

369.12 Better eye: severe impairment;
lesser eye: total impairment

369.13 Better eye: severe impairment;
lesser eye: near-total impairment

369.14 Better eye: severe impairment;
lesser eye: profound impairment

369.15 Better eye: moderate impairment;
lesser eye: blind, not further specified

369.16 Better eye: moderate impairment;
lesser eye: total impairment

369.17 Better eye: moderate impairment;
lesser eye: near-total impairment

369.18 Better eye: moderate impairment;
lesser eye: profound impairment

⑤ 369.2 Moderate or severe impairment, both eyes

369.20 Impairment level not further specified
Low vision, both eyes NOS

369.21 Better eye: severe impairment;
lesser eye: not further specified

369.22 Better eye: severe impairment;
lesser eye: severe impairment

369.23 Better eye: moderate impairment;
lesser eye: not further specified

369.24 Better eye: moderate impairment;
lesser eye: severe impairment

369.25 Better eye: moderate impairment;
lesser eye: moderate impairment

369.3 Unqualified visual loss, both eyes
Excludes: blindness NOS:
legal [U.S.A. definition] (369.4)
WHO definition (369.00)

369.4 Legal blindness, as defined in U.S.A.
Blindness NOS according to U.S.A. definition
Excludes: legal blindness with specification of impairment level (369.01-369.08,
369.11-369.14, 369.21-369.22)

⑤ 369.6 Profound impairment, one eye

369.60 Impairment level not further specified
Blindness, one eye

369.61 One eye: total impairment; other eye: not specified

● Code new to this edition ▲ Revision of existing code ④ ⑤ Fourth or fifth digit required

369.62　One eye: total impairment; other eye: near-normal vision

369.63　One eye: total impairment; other eye: normal vision

369.64　One eye: near-total impairment; other eye: not specified

369.65　One eye: near-total impairment; other eye: near-normal vision

369.66　One eye: near-total impairment; other eye: normal vision

369.67　One eye: profound impairment; other eye: not specified

369.68　One eye: profound impairment; other eye: near-normal vision

369.69　One eye: profound impairment; other eye: normal vision

⑤ 369.7　Moderate or severe impairment, one eye

369.70　Impairment level not further specified
Low vision, one eye

369.71　One eye: severe impairment; other eye: not specified

369.72　One eye: severe impairment; other eye: near-normal vision

369.73　One eye: severe impairment; other eye: normal vision

369.74　One eye: moderate impairment; other eye: not specified

369.75　One eye: moderate impairment; other eye: near-normal vision

369.76　One eye: moderate impairment; other eye: normal vision

369.8　Unqualified visual loss, one eye

369.9　Unspecified visual loss

370　Keratitis

DEFINITION Keratitis is an infection or inflammation of the cornea which can be caused by a variety of conditions, including infections, dry eyes, foreign objects, contact lenses, intense light, vitamin a deficiency or allergies.

⑤ 370.0　Corneal ulcer

Excludes: that due to vitamin A deficiency (264.3)

370.00　Corneal ulcer, unspecified

370.01　Marginal corneal ulcer

370.02　Ring corneal ulcer

370.03　Central corneal ulcer

370.04　Hypopyon ulcer
Serpiginous ulcer

370.05　Mycotic corneal ulcer

370.06　Perforated corneal ulcer

370.07　Mooren's ulcer

⑤ 370.2　Superficial keratitis without conjunctivitis

Excludes: dendritic [herpes simplex] keratitis (054.42)

370.20　Superficial keratitis, unspecified

370.21　Punctate keratitis
Thygeson's superficial punctate keratitis

370.22　Macular keratitis
Keratitis:	Keratitis:
areolar	stellate
nummular	striate

370.23　Filamentary keratitis

370.24　Photokeratitis
Snow blindness
Welders' keratitis

⑤ 370.3　Certain types of keratoconjunctivitis

370.31　Phlyctenular keratoconjunctivitis
Phlyctenulosis
Use additional code for any associated tuberculosis (017.3)

370.32　Limbar and corneal involvement in vernal conjunctivitis
Use additional code for vernal conjunctivitis (372.13)

370.33　Keratoconjunctivitis sicca, not specified as Sjögren's

Excludes: Sjögren's syndrome (710.2)

370.34　Exposure keratoconjunctivitis

369

	Add 4th or 5th digit		Nonspecific code		Unspecified code		Manifestation code

370.35 **Neurotrophic keratoconjunctivitis**

⑤ **370.4 Other and unspecified keratoconjunctivitis**

370.40 **Keratoconjunctivitis, unspecified**
Superficial keratitis with conjunctivitis NOS

370.44 ***Keratitis or keratoconjunctivitis in exanthema***
Code first underlying condition (050.0-052.9)

Excludes: *herpes simplex (054.43)*
herpes zoster (053.21)
measles (055.71)

370.49 **Other**

Excludes: *epidemic keratoconjunctivitis (077.1)*

⑤ **370.5 Interstitial and deep keratitis**

370.50 **Interstitial keratitis, unspecified**

370.52 **Diffuse interstitial keratitis**
Cogan's syndrome

370.54 **Sclerosing keratitis**

370.55 **Corneal abscess**

370.59 **Other**

Excludes: *disciform herpes simplex keratitis (054.43)*
syphilitic keratitis (090.3)

⑤ **370.6 Corneal neovascularization**

370.60 **Corneal neovascularization, unspecified**

370.61 **Localized vascularization of cornea**

370.62 **Pannus (corneal)**

370.63 **Deep vascularization of cornea**

370.64 **Ghost vessels (corneal)**

370.8 Other forms of keratitis
Code first underlying condition, such as:
Acanthamoeba (136.21)
Fusarium (118)

370.9 Unspecified keratitis

371 Corneal opacity and other disorders of cornea
DEFINITION Corneal opacity is a cloudy spot in the cornea, which is normally transparent. Causes include corneal scar tissue and infection.

⑤ **371.0 Corneal scars and opacities**

Excludes: *that due to vitamin A deficiency (264.6)*

371.00 **Corneal opacity, unspecified**
Corneal scar NOS

371.01 **Minor opacity of cornea**
Corneal nebula

371.02 **Peripheral opacity of cornea**
Corneal macula not interfering with central vision

371.03 **Central opacity of cornea**
Corneal:
leucoma interfering with central vision
macula interfering with central vision

371.04 **Adherent leucoma**

371.05 ***Phthisical cornea***
Code first underlying tuberculosis (017.3)

⑤ **371.1 Corneal pigmentations and deposits**

371.10 **Corneal deposit, unspecified**

371.11 **Anterior pigmentations**
Stähli's lines

371.12 **Stromal pigmentations**
Hematocornea

● Code new to this edition   ▲ Revision of existing code   ④ ⑤ Fourth or fifth digit required

371.13 **Posterior pigmentations**
Krukenberg spindle

371.14 **Kayser-Fleischer ring**

371.15 **Other deposits associated with metabolic disorders**

371.16 **Argentous deposits**

⑤ 371.2 **Corneal edema**

371.20 **Corneal edema, unspecified**

371.21 **Idiopathic corneal edema**

371.22 **Secondary corneal edema**

371.23 **Bullous keratopathy**

371.24 **Corneal edema due to wearing of contact lenses**

⑤ 371.3 **Changes of corneal membranes**

371.30 **Corneal membrane change, unspecified**

371.31 **Folds and rupture of Bowman's membrane**

371.32 **Folds in Descemet's membrane**

371.33 **Rupture in Descemet's membrane**

⑤ 371.4 **Corneal degenerations**

371.40 **Corneal degeneration, unspecified**

371.41 **Senile corneal changes**
Arcus senilis
Hassall-Henle bodies

371.42 **Recurrent erosion of cornea**

Excludes: *Mooren's ulcer (370.07)*

371.43 **Band-shaped keratopathy**

371.44 **Other calcerous degenerations of cornea**

371.45 **Keratomalacia NOS**

Excludes: *that due to vitamin A deficiency (264.4)*

371.46 **Nodular degeneration of cornea**
Salzmann's nodular dystrophy

371.48 **Peripheral degenerations of cornea**
Marginal degeneration of cornea [Terrien's]

371.49 **Other**
Discrete colliquative keratopathy

⑤ 371.5 **Hereditary corneal dystrophies**

371.50 **Corneal dystrophy, unspecified**

371.51 **Juvenile epithelial corneal dystrophy**

371.52 **Other anterior corneal dystrophies**
Corneal dystrophy:
microscopic cystic
ring-like

371.53 **Granular corneal dystrophy**

371.54 **Lattice corneal dystrophy**

371.55 **Macular corneal dystrophy**

371.56 **Other stromal corneal dystrophies**
Crystalline corneal dystrophy

371.57 **Endothelial corneal dystrophy**
Combined corneal dystrophy
Cornea guttata
Fuchs' endothelial dystrophy

371.58 **Other posterior corneal dystrophies**
Polymorphous corneal dystrophy

⑤ 371.6 **Keratoconus**

371.60 **Keratoconus, unspecified**

371.61 **Keratoconus, stable condition**

371.62 **Keratoconus, acute hydrops**

 Add 4th or
5th digit

 Nonspecific
code

 Unspecified
code

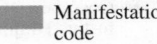 Manifestation
code

⑤ **371.7 Other corneal deformities**

    371.70   Corneal deformity, unspecified

    371.71   Corneal ectasia

    371.72   Descemetocele

    371.73   Corneal staphyloma

⑤ **371.8 Other corneal disorders**

    371.81   Corneal anesthesia and hypoesthesia

    371.82   Corneal disorder due to contact lens

    Excludes: *corneal edema due to contact lens (371.24)*

    371.89   **Other**

  371.9 Unspecified corneal disorder

372 **Disorders of conjunctiva**

    Excludes: *keratoconjunctivitis (370.3-370.4)*

    DEFINITION Disorders of conjunctiva are disorders of the mucous membrane that lines the inner surface of the eyelid and the exposed surface of the eyeball.

⑤ **372.0 Acute conjunctivitis**

    372.00   **Acute conjunctivitis, unspecified**

    372.01   **Serous conjunctivitis, except viral**

    Excludes: *viral conjunctivitis NOS (077.9)*

    372.02   **Acute follicular conjunctivitis**
        Conjunctival folliculosis NOS

    Excludes: *conjunctivitis:*

        adenoviral (acute follicular) (077.3)
        epidemic hemorrhagic (077.4)
        inclusion (077.0)
        Newcastle (077.8)
      epidemic keratoconjunctivitis (077.1)
      pharyngoconjunctival fever (077.2)

    372.03   **Other mucopurulent conjunctivitis**
        Catarrhal conjunctivitis

    Excludes: *blennorrhea neonatorum (gonococcal) (098.40)*
      neonatal conjunctivitis (771.6)
      ophthalmia neonatorum NOS (771.6)

    372.04   **Pseudomembranous conjunctivitis**
        Membranous conjunctivitis

    Excludes: *diphtheritic conjunctivitis (032.81)*

    372.05   **Acute atopic conjunctivitis**

    372.06   **Acute chemical conjunctivitis**
        Acute toxic conjunctivitis

    Use addtional E code to identify the chemical or toxic agent

    Excludes: *burn of eye and adnexa (940.0-940.9)*
      chemical corrosion injury of eye (940.2-940.3)

⑤ **372.1 Chronic conjunctivitis**

    372.10   **Chronic conjunctivitis, unspecified**

    372.11   **Simple chronic conjunctivitis**

    372.12   **Chronic follicular conjunctivitis**

    372.13   **Vernal conjunctivitis**

    372.14   **Other chronic allergic conjunctivitis**

    372.15   *Parasitic conjunctivitis*
    Code first underlying disease, as:
      filariasis (125.0-125.9)
      mucocutaneous leishmaniasis (085.5)

⑤ **372.2 Blepharoconjunctivitis**

    372.20   **Blepharoconjunctivitis, unspecified**

    372.21   **Angular blepharoconjunctivitis**

    372.22   **Contact blepharoconjunctivitis**

● Code new to this edition   ▲ Revision of existing code   ④ ⑤ Fourth or fifth digit required

⑤ **372.3 Other and unspecified conjunctivitis**

    372.30 Conjunctivitis, unspecified

    372.31 *Rosacea conjunctivitis*
    Code first underlying rosacea dermatitis (695.3)

    372.33 *Conjunctivitis in mucocutaneous disease*
    Code first underlying disease, as:
        erythema multiforme (695.10-695.19)
        Reiter's disease (099.3)
    Excludes: *ocular pemphigoid (694.61)*

    372.34 Pingueculitis
    Excludes: *pinguecula (372.51)*

    372.39 Other

⑤ **372.4 Pterygium**
    Excludes: *pseudopterygium (372.52)*

    372.40 Pterygium, unspecified

    372.41 Peripheral pterygium, stationary

    372.42 Peripheral pterygium, progressive

    372.43 Central pterygium

    372.44 Double pterygium

    372.45 Recurrent pterygium

⑤ **372.5 Conjunctival degenerations and deposits**

    372.50 Conjunctival degeneration, unspecified

    372.51 Pinguecula
    Excludes: *pingueculitis (372.34)*

    372.52 Pseudopterygium

    372.53 Conjunctival xerosis
    Excludes: *conjunctival xerosis due to vitamin A deficiency (264.0, 264.1, 264.7)*

    372.54 Conjunctival concretions

    372.55 Conjunctival pigmentations
        Conjunctival argyrosis

    372.56 Conjunctival deposits

⑤ **372.6 Conjunctival scars**

    372.61 Granuloma of conjunctiva

    372.62 Localized adhesions and strands of conjunctiva

    372.63 Symblepharon
        Extensive adhesions of conjunctiva

    372.64 Scarring of conjunctiva
        Contraction of eye socket (after enucleation)

⑤ **372.7 Conjunctival vascular disorders and cysts**

    372.71 Hyperemia of conjunctiva

    372.72 Conjunctival hemorrhage
        Hyposphagma
        Subconjunctival hemorrhage

    372.73 Conjunctival edema
        Chemosis of conjunctiva
        Subconjunctival edema

    372.74 Vascular abnormalities of conjunctiva
        Aneurysm(ata) of conjunctiva

    372.75 Conjunctival cysts

⑤ **372.8 Other disorders of conjunctiva**

    372.81 Conjunctivochalasis

    372.89 Other disorders of conjunctiva

372.9 Unspecified disorder of conjunctiva

	Add 4th or 5th digit		Nonspecific code		Unspecified code		Manifestation code

373 Inflammation of eyelids

DEFINITION Inflammation of eyelids refers to swelling or redness of the eyelids caused by infection or injury.

⑤ **373.0 Blepharitis**

Excludes: *blepharoconjunctivitis (372.20-372.22)*

373.00 Blepharitis, unspecified
373.01 Ulcerative blepharitis
373.02 Squamous blepharitis

⑤ **373.1 Hordeolum and other deep inflammation of eyelid**

373.11 Hordeolum externum
Hordeolum NOS
Stye

373.12 Hordeolum internum
Infection of meibomian gland

373.13 Abscess of eyelid
Furuncle of eyelid

373.2 Chalazion
Meibomian (gland) cyst

Excludes: *infected meibomian gland (373.12)*

⑤ **373.3 Noninfectious dermatoses of eyelid**

373.31 Eczematous dermatitis of eyelid
373.32 Contact and allergic dermatitis of eyelid
373.33 Xeroderma of eyelid
373.34 Discoid lupus erythematosus of eyelid

373.4 Infective dermatitis of eyelid of types resulting in deformity
Code first underlying disease, as:
leprosy (030.0-030.9)
lupus vulgaris (tuberculous) (017.0)
yaws (102.0-102.9)

373.5 Other infective dermatitis of eyelid
Code first underlying disease, as:
actinomycosis (039.3)
impetigo (684)
mycotic dermatitis (110.0-111.9)
vaccinia (051.0)
postvaccination (999.0)

Excludes: *herpes:*
simplex (054.41)
zoster (053.20)

373.6 Parasitic infestation of eyelid
Code first underlying disease, as:
leishmaniasis (085.0-085.9)
loiasis (125.2)
onchocerciasis (125.3)
pediculosis (132.0)

373.8 Other inflammations of eyelids

373.9 Unspecified inflammation of eyelid

374 Other disorders of eyelids

ALERT! For personal history of other disorders of nervous system and sense organs see V12.49

⑤ **374.0 Entropion and trichiasis of eyelid**

374.00 Entropion, unspecified
374.01 Senile entropion
374.02 Mechanical entropion
374.03 Spastic entropion
374.04 Cicatricial entropion
374.05 Trichiasis without entropion

⑤ **374.1 Ectropion**

● Code new to this edition   ▲ Revision of existing code   ④ ⑤ Fourth or fifth digit required

> **374.10** Ectropion, unspecified
374.11 Senile ectropion
374.12 Mechanical ectropion
374.13 Spastic ectropion
374.14 Cicatricial ectropion

⑤ **374.2** Lagophthalmos
> **374.20** Lagophthalmos, unspecified
374.21 Paralytic lagophthalmos
374.22 Mechanical lagophthalmos
374.23 Cicatricial lagophthalmos

⑤ **374.3** Ptosis of eyelid
> **374.30** Ptosis of eyelid, unspecified
374.31 Paralytic ptosis
374.32 Myogenic ptosis
374.33 Mechanical ptosis
374.34 Blepharochalasis
Pseudoptosis

⑤ **374.4** Other disorders affecting eyelid function
> Excludes: blepharoclonus (333.81)
blepharospasm (333.81)
facial nerve palsy (351.0)
third nerve palsy or paralysis (378.51-378.52)
tic (psychogenic) (307.20-307.23)
organic (333.3)

> **374.41** Lid retraction or lag
374.43 Abnormal innervation syndrome
Jaw-blinking
Paradoxical facial movements
374.44 Sensory disorders
374.45 Other sensorimotor disorders
Deficient blink reflex
374.46 Blepharophimosis
Ankyloblepharon

⑤ **374.5** Degenerative disorders of eyelid and periocular area
> **374.50** Degenerative disorder of eyelid, unspecified
374.51 *Xanthelasma*
Xanthoma (planum) (tuberosum) of eyelid
Code first underlying condition (272.0-272.9)
374.52 Hyperpigmentation of eyelid
Chloasma
Dyspigmentation
374.53 Hypopigmentation of eyelid
Vitiligo of eyelid
374.54 Hypertrichosis of eyelid
374.55 Hypotrichosis of eyelid
Madarosis of eyelid
374.56 Other degenerative disorders of skin affecting eyelid

⑤ **374.8** Other disorders of eyelid
> **374.81** Hemorrhage of eyelid
> Excludes: black eye (921.0)

> **374.82** Edema of eyelid
Hyperemia of eyelid
374.83 Elephantiasis of eyelid
374.84 Cysts of eyelids
Sebaceous cyst of eyelid
374.85 Vascular anomalies of eyelid
374.86 Retained foreign body of eyelid
Use additional code to identify foreign body (V90.01-V90.9)

Add 4th or 5th digit · Nonspecific code · Unspecified code · Manifestation code

374.87 Dermatochalasis

374.89 Other disorders of eyelid

374.9 Unspecified disorder of eyelid

375 Disorders of lacrimal system

> **DEFINITION** Disorders of lacrimal system refers to disorders of the lacrimal gland, lake, puncta, canaliculi, sac, and nasolacrimal duct.

⑤ 375.0 Dacryoadenitis

375.00 Dacryoadenitis, unspecified

375.01 Acute dacryoadenitis

375.02 Chronic dacryoadenitis

375.03 Chronic enlargement of lacrimal gland

⑤ 375.1 Other disorders of lacrimal gland

375.11 Dacryops

375.12 Other lacrimal cysts and cystic degeneration

375.13 Primary lacrimal atrophy

375.14 Secondary lacrimal atrophy

375.15 Tear film insufficiency, unspecified
Dry eye syndrome

375.16 Dislocation of lacrimal gland

⑤ 375.2 Epiphora

375.20 Epiphora, unspecified as to cause

375.21 Epiphora due to excess lacrimation

375.22 Epiphora due to insufficient drainage

⑤ 375.3 Acute and unspecified inflammation of lacrimal passages

Excludes: neonatal dacryocystitis (771.6)

375.30 Dacryocystitis, unspecified

375.31 Acute canaliculitis, lacrimal

375.32 Acute dacryocystitis
Acute peridacryocystitis

375.33 Phlegmonous dacryocystitis

⑤ 375.4 Chronic inflammation of lacrimal passages

375.41 Chronic canaliculitis

375.42 Chronic dacryocystitis

375.43 Lacrimal mucocele

⑤ 375.5 Stenosis and insufficiency of lacrimal passages

375.51 Eversion of lacrimal punctum

375.52 Stenosis of lacrimal punctum

375.53 Stenosis of lacrimal canaliculi

375.54 Stenosis of lacrimal sac

375.55 Obstruction of nasolacrimal duct, neonatal

Excludes: congenital anomaly of nasolacrimal duct (743.65)

375.56 Stenosis of nasolacrimal duct, acquired

375.57 Dacryolith

⑤ 375.6 Other changes of lacrimal passages

375.61 Lacrimal fistula

375.69 Other

⑤ 375.8 Other disorders of lacrimal system

375.81 Granuloma of lacrimal passages

375.89 Other

375.9 Unspecified disorder of lacrimal system

376 Disorders of the orbit

> **DEFINITION** Disorders of the orbit refers to disorders of the eye socket.

● Code new
to this edition

▲ Revision of
existing code

④ ⑤ Fourth or fifth
digit required

⑤ **376.0 Acute inflammation of orbit**

　　376.00 Acute inflammation of orbit, unspecified

　　376.01 Orbital cellulitis
　　　　Abscess of orbit

　　376.02 Orbital periostitis

　　376.03 Orbital osteomyelitis

　　376.04 Tenonitis

⑤ **376.1 Chronic inflammatory disorders of orbit**

　　376.10 Chronic inflammation of orbit, unspecified

　　376.11 Orbital granuloma
　　　　Pseudotumor (inflammatory) of orbit

　　376.12 Orbital myositis

　　376.13 Parasitic infestation of orbit
　　Code first underlying disease, as:
　　　　hydatid infestation of orbit (122.3, 122.6, 122.9)
　　　　myiasis of orbit (134.0)

⑤ *376.2 Endocrine exophthalmos*
　　Code first underlying thyroid disorder (242.0-242.9)

　　376.21 Thyrotoxic exophthalmos

　　376.22 Exophthalmic ophthalmoplegia

⑤ **376.3 Other exophthalmic conditions**

　　376.30 Exophthalmos, unspecified

　　376.31 Constant exophthalmos

　　376.32 Orbital hemorrhage

　　376.33 Orbital edema or congestion

　　376.34 Intermittent exophthalmos

　　376.35 Pulsating exophthalmos

　　376.36 Lateral displacement of globe

⑤ **376.4 Deformity of orbit**

　　376.40 Deformity of orbit, unspecified

　　376.41 Hypertelorism of orbit

　　376.42 Exostosis of orbit

　　376.43 Local deformities due to bone disease

　　376.44 Orbital deformities associated with craniofacial deformities

　　376.45 Atrophy of orbit

　　376.46 Enlargement of orbit

　　376.47 Deformity due to trauma or surgery

⑤ **376.5 Enophthalmos**

　　376.50 Enophthalmos, unspecified as to cause

　　376.51 Enophthalmos due to atrophy of orbital tissue

　　376.52 Enophthalmos due to trauma or surgery

　　376.6 Retained (old) foreign body following penetrating wound of orbit
　　　　Retrobulbar foreign body
　　Use additional code to identify foreign body (V90.01-V90.9)

⑤ **376.8 Other orbital disorders**

　　376.81 Orbital cysts
　　　　Encephalocele of orbit

　　376.82 Myopathy of extraocular muscles

　　376.89 Other

　　376.9 Unspecified disorder of orbit

377 Disorders of optic nerve and visual pathways
　　DEFINITION The optic nerve transmits visual information from the retina to the brain.

⑤ **377.0 Papilledema**

　　377.00 Papilledema, unspecified

　　377.01 Papilledema associated with increased intracranial pressure

Add 4th or 5th digit	Nonspecific code	Unspecified code	Manifestation code

377.02   **Papilledema associated with decreased ocular pressure**

377.03   **Papilledema associated with retinal disorder**

377.04   **Foster-Kennedy syndrome**

⑤ **377.1   Optic atrophy**

   377.10   **Optic atrophy, unspecified**

   377.11   **Primary optic atrophy**

   Excludes: *neurosyphilitic optic atrophy (094.84)*

   377.12   **Postinflammatory optic atrophy**

   377.13   **Optic atrophy associated with retinal dystrophies**

   377.14   **Glaucomatous atrophy [cupping] of optic disc**

   377.15   **Partial optic atrophy**
       Temporal pallor of optic disc

   377.16   **Hereditary optic atrophy**
       Optic atrophy:
         dominant hereditary
         Leber's

⑤ **377.2   Other disorders of optic disc**

   377.21   **Drusen of optic disc**

   377.22   **Crater-like holes of optic disc**

   377.23   **Coloboma of optic disc**

   377.24   **Pseudopapilledema**

⑤ **377.3   Optic neuritis**

   Excludes: *meningococcal optic neuritis (036.81)*

   377.30   **Optic neuritis, unspecified**

   377.31   **Optic papillitis**

   377.32   **Retrobulbar neuritis (acute)**

   Excludes: *syphilitic retrobulbar neuritis (094.85)*

   377.33   **Nutritional optic neuropathy**

   377.34   **Toxic optic neuropathy**
       Toxic amblyopia

   377.39   **Other**

   Excludes: *ischemic optic neuropathy (377.41)*

⑤ **377.4   Other disorders of optic nerve**

   377.41   **Ischemic optic neuropathy**

   377.42   **Hemorrhage in optic nerve sheaths**

   377.43   **Optic nerve hypoplasia**

   377.49   **Other**
       Compression of optic nerve

⑤ **377.5   Disorders of optic chiasm**

   377.51   **Associated with pituitary neoplasms and disorders**

   377.52   **Associated with other neoplasms**

   377.53   **Associated with vascular disorders**

   377.54   **Associated with inflammatory disorders**

⑤ **377.6   Disorders of other visual pathways**

   377.61   **Associated with neoplasms**

   377.62   **Associated with vascular disorders**

   377.63   **Associated with inflammatory disorders**

⑤ **377.7   Disorders of visual cortex**

   Excludes: *visual:*
       agnosia (368.16)
       hallucinations (368.16)
       halos (368.15)

   377.71   **Associated with neoplasms**

   377.72   **Associated with vascular disorders**

   ● Code new   ▲ Revision of   ④ ⑤ Fourth or fifth
         to this edition   existing code   digit required

377.73 Associated with inflammatory disorders

377.75 Cortical blindness

377.9 Unspecified disorder of optic nerve and visual pathways

378 Strabismus and other disorders of binocular eye movements

Excludes: nystagmus and other irregular eye movements (379.50-379.59)

DEFINITION Strabismus, aka crossed eyes, is a visual defect in which the eyes are misaligned and point in different directions. Strabismus usually occurs in childhood but can occur later in life.

⑤ **378.0 Esotropia**
Convergent concomitant strabismus

Excludes: intermittent esotropia (378.20-378.22)

378.00 Esotropia, unspecified

378.01 Monocular esotropia

378.02 Monocular esotropia with A pattern

378.03 Monocular esotropia with V pattern

378.04 Monocular esotropia with other noncomitancies
Monocular esotropia with X or Y pattern

378.05 Alternating esotropia

378.06 Alternating esotropia with A pattern

378.07 Alternating esotropia with V pattern

378.08 Alternating esotropia with other noncomitancies
Alternating esotropia with X or Y pattern

⑤ **378.1 Exotropia**
Divergent concomitant strabismus

Excludes: intermittent exotropia (378.20, 378.23-378.24)

378.10 Exotropia, unspecified

378.11 Monocular exotropia

378.12 Monocular exotropia with A pattern

378.13 Monocular exotropia with V pattern

378.14 Monocular exotropia with other noncomitancies
Monocular exotropia with X or Y pattern

378.15 Alternating exotropia

378.16 Alternating exotropia with A pattern

378.17 Alternating exotropia with V pattern

378.18 Alternating exotropia with other noncomitancies
Alternating exotropia with X or Y pattern

⑤ **378.2 Intermittent heterotropia**

Excludes: vertical heterotropia (intermittent) (378.31)

378.20 Intermittent heterotropia, unspecified
Intermittent:
esotropia NOS
exotropia NOS

378.21 Intermittent esotropia, monocular

378.22 Intermittent esotropia, alternating

378.23 Intermittent exotropia, monocular

378.24 Intermittent exotropia, alternating

⑤ **378.3 Other and unspecified heterotropia**

378.30 Heterotropia, unspecified

378.31 Hypertropia
Vertical heterotropia (constant) (intermittent)

378.32 Hypotropia

378.33 Cyclotropia

378.34 Monofixation syndrome
Microtropia

378.35 Accommodative component in esotropia

	Add 4th or 5th digit		Nonspecific code		Unspecified code		Manifestation code

⑤ **378.4 Heterophoria**

> **378.40** Heterophoria, unspecified
>
> **378.41** Esophoria
>
> **378.42** Exophoria
>
> **378.43** Vertical heterophoria
>
> **378.44** Cyclophoria
>
> **378.45** Alternating hyperphoria

⑤ **378.5 Paralytic strabismus**

> **378.50** Paralytic strabismus, unspecified
>
> **378.51** Third or oculomotor nerve palsy, partial
>
> **378.52** Third or oculomotor nerve palsy, total
>
> **378.53** Fourth or trochlear nerve palsy
>
> **378.54** Sixth or abducens nerve palsy
>
> **378.55** External ophthalmoplegia
>
> **378.56** Total ophthalmoplegia

⑤ **378.6 Mechanical strabismus**

> **378.60** Mechanical strabismus, unspecified
>
> **378.61** Brown's (tendon) sheath syndrome
>
> **378.62** Mechanical strabismus from other musculofascial disorders
>
> **378.63** Limited duction associated with other conditions

⑤ **378.7 Other specified strabismus**

> **378.71** Duane's syndrome
>
> **378.72** Progressive external ophthalmoplegia
>
> **378.73** Strabismus in other neuromuscular disorders

⑤ **378.8 Other disorders of binocular eye movements**

> Excludes: nystagmus (379.50-379.56)
>
> **378.81** Palsy of conjugate gaze
>
> **378.82** Spasm of conjugate gaze
>
> **378.83** Convergence insufficiency or palsy
>
> **378.84** Convergence excess or spasm
>
> **378.85** Anomalies of divergence
>
> **378.86** Internuclear ophthalmoplegia
>
> **378.87** Other dissociated deviation of eye movements
>   Skew deviation

378.9 Unspecified disorder of eye movements
  Ophthalmoplegia NOS
  Strabismus NOS

379 **Other disorders of eye**

> **ALERT!** For personal history of other disorders of nervous system and sense organs see V12.49

⑤ **379.0 Scleritis and episcleritis**

> Excludes: syphilitic episcleritis (095.0)
>
> **379.00** Scleritis, unspecified
>   Episcleritis NOS
>
> **379.01** Episcleritis periodica fugax
>
> **379.02** Nodular episcleritis
>
> **379.03** Anterior scleritis
>
> **379.04** Scleromalacia perforans
>
> **379.05** Scleritis with corneal involvement
>   Scleroperikeratitis
>
> **379.06** Brawny scleritis
>
> **379.07** Posterior scleritis
>   Sclerotenonitis

● Code new   ▲ Revision of   ④ ⑤ Fourth or fifth
     to this edition   existing code   digit required

379.09 **Other**
Scleral abscess

⑤ **379.1 Other disorders of sclera**
Excludes: blue sclera (743.47)

379.11 **Scleral ectasia**
Scleral staphyloma NOS

379.12 **Staphyloma posticum**

379.13 **Equatorial staphyloma**

379.14 **Anterior staphyloma, localized**

379.15 **Ring staphyloma**

379.16 **Other degenerative disorders of sclera**

379.19 **Other**

⑤ **379.2 Disorders of vitreous body**

379.21 **Vitreous degeneration**
Vitreous:
cavitation
detachment
liquefaction

379.22 **Crystalline deposits in vitreous**
Asteroid hyalitis
Synchysis scintillans

379.23 **Vitreous hemorrhage**

379.24 **Other vitreous opacities**
Vitreous floaters

379.25 **Vitreous membranes and strands**

379.26 **Vitreous prolapse**

● 379.27 **Vitreomacular adhesion**
Vitreomacular traction

Excludes: traction detachment with vitreoretinal organization (361.81)

379.29 **Other disorders of vitreous**

Excludes: vitreous abscess (360.04)

⑤ **379.3 Aphakia and other disorders of lens**
Excludes: after-cataract (366.50-366.53)

379.31 **Aphakia**

Excludes: cataract extraction status (V45.61)

379.32 **Subluxation of lens**

379.33 **Anterior dislocation of lens**

379.34 **Posterior dislocation of lens**

379.39 **Other disorders of lens**

⑤ **379.4 Anomalies of pupillary function**

379.40 **Abnormal pupillary function, unspecified**

379.41 **Anisocoria**

379.42 **Miosis (persistent), not due to miotics**

379.43 **Mydriasis (persistent) not due to mydriatics**

379.45 **Argyll Robertson pupil, atypical**
Argyll Robertson phenomenon or pupil, nonsyphilitic

Excludes: Argyll Robertson pupil (syphilitic) (094.89)

379.46 **Tonic pupillary reaction**
Adie's pupil or syndrome

379.49 **Other**
Hippus
Pupillary paralysis

⑤ **379.5 Nystagmus and other irregular eye movements**

379.50 **Nystagmus, unspecified**

379.51 **Congenital nystagmus**

379.52 **Latent nystagmus**

Add 4th or 5th digit | Nonspecific code | Unspecified code | Manifestation code

379.53 **Visual deprivation nystagmus**

379.54 **Nystagmus associated with disorders of the vestibular system**

379.55 **Dissociated nystagmus**

379.56 **Other forms of nystagmus**

379.57 **Deficiencies of saccadic eye movements**
Abnormal optokinetic response

379.58 **Deficiencies of smooth pursuit movements**

379.59 **Other irregularities of eye movements**
Opsoclonus

⑤ 379.6 **Inflammation (infection) of postprocedural bleb**
Postprocedural blebitis

379.60 **Inflammation (infection) of postprocedural bleb, unspecified**

379.61 **Inflammation (infection) of postprocedural bleb, stage 1**

379.62 **Inflammation (infection) of postprocedural bleb, stage 2**

379.63 **Inflammation (infection) of postprocedural bleb, stage 3**
Bleb associated endophthalmitis

379.8 **Other specified disorders of eye and adnexa**

⑤ 379.9 **Unspecified disorder of eye and adnexa**

379.90 **Disorder of eye, unspecified**

379.91 **Pain in or around eye**

379.92 **Swelling or mass of eye**

379.93 **Redness or discharge of eye**

379.99 **Other ill-defined disorders of eye**

Excludes: blurred vision NOS (368.8)

DISEASES OF THE EAR AND MASTOID PROCESS (380-389)

Use additional external cause code, if applicable, to identify the cause of the ear condition

380 **Disorders of external ear**

⑤ 380.0 **Perichondritis and chondritis of pinna**
Chondritis of auricle
Perichondritis of auricle

380.00 **Perichondritis of pinna, unspecified**

380.01 **Acute perichondritis of pinna**

380.02 **Chronic perichondritis of pinna**

380.03 **Chondritis of pinna**

⑤ 380.1 **Infective otitis externa**

380.10 **Infective otitis externa, unspecified**
Otitis externa (acute):
NOS
circumscribed
diffuse
hemorrhagica
infective NOS

380.11 **Acute infection of pinna**

Excludes: furuncular otitis externa (680.0)

380.12 **Acute swimmers' ear**
Beach ear
Tank ear

380.13 *Other acute infections of external ear*
Code first underlying disease, as:
erysipelas (035)
impetigo (684)
seborrheic dermatitis (690.10-690.18)

Excludes: herpes simplex (054.73)
herpes zoster (053.71)

380.14 **Malignant otitis externa**

● Code new to this edition ▲ Revision of existing code ④ ⑤ Fourth or fifth digit required

380.15 *Chronic mycotic otitis externa*
Code first underlying disease, as:
    aspergillosis (117.3)
    otomycosis NOS (111.9)
Excludes: *candidal otitis externa (112.82)*

380.16 **Other chronic infective otitis externa**
    Chronic infective otitis externa NOS

⑤ **380.2 Other otitis externa**

380.21 **Cholesteatoma of external ear**
    Keratosis obturans of external ear (canal)

Excludes: *cholesteatoma NOS (385.30-385.35)*
    postmastoidectomy (383.32)

380.22 **Other acute otitis externa**
    Acute otitis externa:
      actinic
      chemical
      contact
      eczematoid
      reactive

380.23 **Other chronic otitis externa**
    Chronic otitis externa NOS

⑤ **380.3 Noninfectious disorders of pinna**

380.30 **Disorder of pinna, unspecified**

380.31 **Hematoma of auricle or pinna**

380.32 **Acquired deformities of auricle or pinna**

Excludes: *cauliflower ear (738.7)*

380.39 **Other**

Excludes: *gouty tophi of ear (274.81)*

380.4 Impacted cerumen
    Wax in ear

⑤ **380.5 Acquired stenosis of external ear canal**
    Collapse of external ear canal

380.50 **Acquired stenosis of external ear canal, unspecified as to cause**

380.51 **Secondary to trauma**

380.52 **Secondary to surgery**

380.53 **Secondary to inflammation**

⑤ **380.8 Other disorders of external ear**

380.81 **Exostosis of external ear canal**

380.89 **Other**

380.9 Unspecified disorder of external ear

381 **Nonsuppurative otitis media and Eustachian tube disorders**
    DEFINITION Nonsuppurative otitis media and eustachian tube disorders, otitis media is an inflammation of the middle ear without the formation or discharge of pus.

⑤ **381.0 Acute nonsuppurative otitis media**
    Acute tubotympanic catarrh
    Otitis media, acute or subacute:
      catarrhal
      exudative
      transudative
      with effusion

Excludes: *otitic barotrauma (993.0)*

381.00 **Acute nonsuppurative otitis media, unspecified**

381.01 **Acute serous otitis media**
    Acute or subacute secretory otitis media

381.02 **Acute mucoid otitis media**
    Acute or subacute seromucinous otitis media
    Blue drum syndrome

381.03 **Acute sanguinous otitis media**

381.04 **Acute allergic serous otitis media**

	Add 4th or 5th digit		Nonspecific code		Unspecified code		Manifestation code

381.05   Acute allergic mucoid otitis media

381.06   Acute allergic sanguinous otitis media

⑤ **381.1   Chronic serous otitis media**
Chronic tubotympanic catarrh

381.10   Chronic serous otitis media, simple or unspecified

381.19   **Other**
Serosanguinous chronic otitis media

⑤ **381.2   Chronic mucoid otitis media**
Glue ear

Excludes: *adhesive middle ear disease (385.10-385.19)*

381.20   Chronic mucoid otitis media, simple or unspecified

381.29   **Other**
Mucosanguinous chronic otitis media

381.3   Other and unspecified chronic nonsuppurative otitis media
Otitis media, chronic: Otitis media, chronic:
 allergic   seromucinous
 exudative   transudative
 secretory   with effusion

381.4   Nonsuppurative otitis media, not specified as acute or chronic
Otitis media: Otitis media:
 allergic   secretory
 catarrhal   seromucinous
 exudative   serous
 mucoid   transudative
                                                         with effusion

⑤ **381.5   Eustachian salpingitis**

381.50   Eustachian salpingitis, unspecified

381.51   Acute Eustachian salpingitis

381.52   Chronic Eustachian salpingitis

⑤ **381.6   Obstruction of Eustachian tube**
Stenosis of Eustachian tube
Stricture of Eustachian tube

381.60   **Obstruction of Eustachian tube, unspecified**

381.61   **Osseous obstruction of Eustachian tube**
Obstruction of Eustachian tube from cholesteatoma, polyp, or other osseous lesion

381.62   **Intrinsic cartilagenous obstruction of Eustachian tube**

381.63   **Extrinsic cartilagenous obstruction of Eustachian tube**
Compression of Eustachian tube

381.7   Patulous Eustachian tube

⑤ **381.8   Other disorders of Eustachian tube**

381.81   **Dysfunction of Eustachian tube**

381.89   **Other**

381.9   Unspecified Eustachian tube disorder

382   Suppurative and unspecified otitis media
DEFINITION Suppurative and unspecified otitis media is an inflammation of the middle ear including the formation or discharge of pus.

⑤ **382.0   Acute suppurative otitis media**
Otitis media, acute:
 necrotizing NOS
 purulent

382.00   **Acute suppurative otitis media without spontaneous rupture of ear drum**

382.01   **Acute suppurative otitis media with spontaneous rupture of ear drum**

382.02   *Acute suppurative otitis media in diseases classified elsewhere*
Code first underlying disease, as:
 influenza (487.8, 488.09, 488.19)
 scarlet fever (034.1)

Excludes: *postmeasles otitis (055.2)*

● Code new   ▲ Revision of   ④ ⑤ Fourth or fifth
      to this edition   existing code   digit required

382.1 Chronic tubotympanic suppurative otitis media
Benign chronic suppurative otitis media (with anterior perforation of ear drum)
Chronic tubotympanic disease (with anterior perforation of ear drum)

382.2 Chronic atticoantral suppurative otitis media
Chronic atticoantral disease (with posterior or superior marginal perforation of ear drum)
Persistent mucosal disease (with posterior or superior marginal perforation of ear drum)

382.3 Unspecified chronic suppurative otitis media
Chronic purulent otitis media

Excludes: *tuberculous otitis media (017.4)*

382.4 Unspecified suppurative otitis media
Purulent otitis media NOS

382.9 Unspecified otitis media
Otitis media:
  NOS
  acute NOS
  chronic NOS

383 Mastoiditis and related conditions
DEFINITION Mastoiditis is an infection of the spaces within the mastoid bone. It is almost always associated with otitis media, an infection of the middle ear. In the most serious cases, the bone itself becomes infected.

⑤ **383.0 Acute mastoiditis**
Abscess of mastoid
Empyema of mastoid

383.00 Acute mastoiditis without complications

383.01 Subperiosteal abscess of mastoid

383.02 Acute mastoiditis with other complications
Gradenigo's syndrome

383.1 Chronic mastoiditis
Caries of mastoid
Fistula of mastoid

Excludes: *tuberculous mastoiditis (015.6)*

⑤ **383.2 Petrositis**
Coalescing osteitis of petrous bone
Inflammation of petrous bone
Osteomyelitis of petrous bone

383.20 Petrositis, unspecified

383.21 Acute petrositis

383.22 Chronic petrositis

⑤ **383.3 Complications following mastoidectomy**

383.30 Postmastoidectomy complication, unspecified

383.31 Mucosal cyst of postmastoidectomy cavity

383.32 Recurrent cholesteatoma of postmastoidectomy cavity

383.33 Granulations of postmastoidectomy cavity
Chronic inflammation of postmastoidectomy cavity

⑤ **383.8 Other disorders of mastoid**

383.81 Postauricular fistula

383.89 Other

383.9 Unspecified mastoiditis

384 Other disorders of tympanic membrane
DEFINITION The tympanic membrane is a thin membrane that separates the external ear from the middle ear.

ALERT! For personal history of other disorders of nervous system and sense organs see V12.49

⑤ **384.0 Acute myringitis without mention of otitis media**

384.00 Acute myringitis, unspecified
Acute tympanitis NOS

384.01 Bullous myringitis
Myringitis bullosa hemorrhagica

	Add 4th or 5th digit		Nonspecific code		Unspecified code		Manifestation code

385

384.09 Other

384.1 Chronic myringitis without mention of otitis media
Chronic tympanitis

⑤ **384.2 Perforation of tympanic membrane**
Perforation of ear drum:
NOS
persistent posttraumatic
postinflammatory

Excludes: otitis media with perforation of tympanic membrane (382.00-382.9)
traumatic perforation [current injury] (872.61)

384.20 Perforation of tympanic membrane, unspecified

384.21 Central perforation of tympanic membrane

384.22 Attic perforation of tympanic membrane
Pars flaccida

384.23 Other marginal perforation of tympanic membrane

384.24 Multiple perforations of tympanic membrane

384.25 Total perforation of tympanic membrane

⑤ **384.8 Other specified disorders of tympanic membrane**

384.81 Atrophic flaccid tympanic membrane
Healed perforation of ear drum

384.82 Atrophic nonflaccid tympanic membrane

384.9 Unspecified disorder of tympanic membrane

385 Other disorders of middle ear and mastoid

Excludes: mastoiditis (383.0-383.9)

DEFINITION The middle ear is the space between the eardrum and the inner ear that contains the three auditory ossicles, which convey vibrations through the oval window to the cochlea. The mastoid is the bone located directly behind the external ear.

ALERT! For personal history of other disorders of nervous system and sense organs see V12.49

⑤ **385.0 Tympanosclerosis**

385.00 Tympanosclerosis, unspecified as to involvement

385.01 Tympanosclerosis involving tympanic membrane only

385.02 Tympanosclerosis involving tympanic membrane and ear ossicles

385.03 Tympanosclerosis involving tympanic membrane, ear ossicles, and middle ear

385.09 Tympanosclerosis involving other combination of structures

⑤ **385.1 Adhesive middle ear disease**
Adhesive otitis
Otitis media:
chronic adhesive
fibrotic

Excludes: glue ear (381.20-381.29)

385.10 Adhesive middle ear disease, unspecified as to involvement

385.11 Adhesions of drum head to incus

385.12 Adhesions of drum head to stapes

385.13 Adhesions of drum head to promontorium

385.19 Other adhesions and combinations

⑤ **385.2 Other acquired abnormality of ear ossicles**

385.21 Impaired mobility of malleus
Ankylosis of malleus

385.22 Impaired mobility of other ear ossicles
Ankylosis of ear ossicles, except malleus

385.23 Discontinuity or dislocation of ear ossicles

385.24 Partial loss or necrosis of ear ossicles

● Code new
to this edition
▲ Revision of
existing code
④ ⑤ Fourth or fifth
digit required

⑤ **385.3 Cholesteatoma of middle ear and mastoid**
    Cholesterosis of (middle) ear
    Epidermosis of (middle) ear
    Keratosis of (middle) ear
    Polyp of (middle) ear

> *Excludes:* *cholesteatoma:*
> *external ear canal (380.21)*
> *recurrent of postmastoidectomy cavity (383.32)*

    385.30 Cholesteatoma, unspecified

    385.31 Cholesteatoma of attic

    385.32 Cholesteatoma of middle ear

    385.33 Cholesteatoma of middle ear and mastoid

    385.35 Diffuse cholesteatosis

⑤ **385.8 Other disorders of middle ear and mastoid**

    385.82 Cholesterin granuloma

    385.83 Retained foreign body of middle ear
    Use additional code to identify foreign body (V90.01-V90.9)

    385.89 Other

385.9 Unspecified disorder of middle ear and mastoid

386 Vertiginous syndromes and other disorders of vestibular system

> *Excludes:* *vertigo NOS (780.4)*

DEFINITION Vertiginous syndromes are disorders that cause vertigo (dizziness).

⑤ **386.0 Ménière's disease**
    Endolymphatic hydrops   Ménière's syndrome or vertigo
    Lermoyez's syndrome

    386.00 Ménière's disease, unspecified
    Ménière's disease (active)

    386.01 Active Ménière's disease, cochleovestibular

    386.02 Active Ménière's disease, cochlear

    386.03 Active Ménière's disease, vestibular

    386.04 Inactive Ménière's disease
    Ménière's disease in remission

⑤ **386.1 Other and unspecified peripheral vertigo**

> *Excludes:* *epidemic vertigo (078.81)*

    386.10 Peripheral vertigo, unspecified

    386.11 Benign paroxysmal positional vertigo
    Benign paroxysmal positional nystagmus

    386.12 Vestibular neuronitis
    Acute (and recurrent) peripheral vestibulopathy

    386.19 Other
    Aural vertigo
    Otogenic vertigo

386.2 Vertigo of central origin
    Central positional nystagmus
    Malignant positional vertigo

⑤ **386.3 Labyrinthitis**

    386.30 Labyrinthitis, unspecified

    386.31 Serous labyrinthitis
    Diffuse labyrinthitis

    386.32 Circumscribed labyrinthitis
    Focal labyrinthitis

    386.33 Suppurative labyrinthitis
    Purulent labyrinthitis

    386.34 Toxic labyrinthitis

    386.35 Viral labyrinthitis

⑤ **386.4 Labyrinthine fistula**

    386.40 Labyrinthine fistula, unspecified

    386.41 Round window fistula

| ▓ Add 4th or 5th digit | ▓ Nonspecific code | ░ Unspecified code | ▓ Manifestation code |

386.42   Oval window fistula

386.43   Semicircular canal fistula

386.48   Labyrinthine fistula of combined sites

⑤ 386.5 Labyrinthine dysfunction

386.50   Labyrinthine dysfunction, unspecified

386.51   Hyperactive labyrinth, unilateral

386.52   Hyperactive labyrinth, bilateral

386.53   Hypoactive labyrinth, unilateral

386.54   Hypoactive labyrinth, bilateral

386.55   Loss of labyrinthine reactivity, unilateral

386.56   Loss of labyrinthine reactivity, bilateral

386.58   Other forms and combinations

386.8   Other disorders of labyrinth

386.9   Unspecified vertiginous syndromes and labyrinthine disorders

387   Otosclerosis
Includes: otospongiosis
DEFINITION   Otosclerosis is a hereditary disorder in which ossification of the labyrinth of the inner ear causes tinnitus and eventual deafness .

387.0   Otosclerosis involving oval window, nonobliterative

387.1   Otosclerosis involving oval window, obliterative

387.2   Cochlear otosclerosis
Otosclerosis involving:
   otic capsule
   round window

387.8   Other otosclerosis

387.9   Otosclerosis, unspecified

388   Other disorders of ear
ALERT!   For personal history of other disorders of nervous system and sense organs see V12.49

⑤ 388.0 Degenerative and vascular disorders of ear

388.00   Degenerative and vascular disorders, unspecified

388.01   Presbyacusis

388.02   Transient ischemic deafness

⑤ 388.1 Noise effects on inner ear

388.10   Noise effects on inner ear, unspecified

388.11   Acoustic trauma (explosive) to ear
Otitic blast injury

388.12   Noise-induced hearing loss

388.2   Sudden hearing loss, unspecified

⑤ 388.3 Tinnitus

388.30   Tinnitus, unspecified

388.31   Subjective tinnitus

388.32   Objective tinnitus

⑤ 388.4 Other abnormal auditory perception

388.40   Abnormal auditory perception, unspecified

388.41   Diplacusis

388.42   Hyperacusis

388.43   Impairment of auditory discrimination

388.44   Recruitment

388.45   Acquired auditory processing disorder
Auditory processing disorder NOS

Excludes: central auditory processing disorder (315.32)

● Code new
   to this edition
▲ Revision of
   existing code
④ ⑤ Fourth or fifth
   digit required

388.5 Disorders of acoustic nerve
Acoustic neuritis
Degeneration of acoustic or eighth nerve
Disorder of acoustic or eighth nerve
Excludes: *acoustic neuroma (225.1)*
syphilitic acoustic neuritis (094.86)

⑤ **388.6 Otorrhea**

388.60 Otorrhea, unspecified
Discharging ear NOS

388.61 Cerebrospinal fluid otorrhea
Excludes: *cerebrospinal fluid rhinorrhea (349.81)*

388.69 Other
Otorrhagia

⑤ **388.7 Otalgia**

388.70 Otalgia, unspecified
Earache NOS

388.71 Otogenic pain

388.72 Referred pain

388.8 Other disorders of ear

388.9 Unspecified disorder of ear

389 Hearing loss
DEFINITION Hearing loss refers to the partial or complete loss of hearing

⑤ **389.0 Conductive hearing loss**
Conductive deafness
Excludes: *mixed conductive and sensorineural hearing loss (389.20-389.22)*

389.00 Conductive hearing loss, unspecified

389.01 Conductive hearing loss, external ear

389.02 Conductive hearing loss, tympanic membrane

389.03 Conductive hearing loss, middle ear

389.04 Conductive hearing loss, inner ear

389.05 Conductive hearing loss, unilateral

389.06 Conductive hearing loss, bilateral

389.08 Conductive hearing loss of combined types

⑤ **389.1 Sensorineural hearing loss**
Perceptive hearing loss or deafness
Excludes: *abnormal auditory perception (388.40-388.44)*
mixed conductive and sensorineural hearing loss (389.20-389.22)
psychogenic deafness (306.7)

389.10 Sensorineural hearing loss, unspecified

389.11 Sensory hearing loss, bilateral

389.12 Neural hearing loss, bilateral

389.13 Neural hearing loss, unilateral

389.14 Central hearing loss

389.15 Sensorineural hearing loss, unilateral

389.16 Sensorineural hearing loss, asymmetrical

389.17 Sensory hearing loss, unilateral

389.18 Sensorineural hearing loss, bilateral

⑤ **389.2 Mixed conductive and sensorineural hearing loss**
Deafness or hearing loss of type classifiable to 389.00-389.08 with type classifiable to 389.10-389.18

389.20 Mixed hearing loss, unspecified

389.21 Mixed hearing loss, unilateral

389.22 Mixed hearing loss, bilateral

389.7 Deaf nonspeaking, not elsewhere classifiable

389.8 Other specified forms of hearing loss

Add 4th or 5th digit | Nonspecific code | Unspecified code | Manifestation code

389.9 Unspecified hearing loss
Deafness NOS

● Code new
   to this edition

▲ Revision of
   existing code

④ ⑤ Fourth or fifth
     digit required

Chapter 7: Diseases of Circulatory System (390-459)

DEFINITIONS AND CODING ALERTS

This chapter includes definitions of selected key words, terms and phrases and coding alerts for adding points to the clinical domain, references to coding late effects where appropriate, and references to personal history V-codes in situations where the acute or chronic condition is no longer active. An example from this chapter is as follows:

435 **Transient cerebral ischemia**

> **DEFINITION** Transition cerebral ischemia is the reduction or loss of oxygen to the cerebrum; prolonged ischemia may lead to cerebral infarction.
> **ALERT** For personal history of transient ischemic attack (tia), and cerebral infarction without residual deficits see v12.54.

MULTIPLE CODING FOR A SINGLE CONDITION

In addition to the etiology or manifestation convention that requires two codes to fully describe a single condition that affects multiple body systems, there are other single conditions that also require more than one code. "Use additional code" notes are found in the tabular at codes that are not part of an etiology or manifestation pair where a secondary code is useful to fully describe a condition. The sequencing rule is the same as the etiology or manifestation pair - , "use additional code" indicates that a secondary code should be added.

"Code first" notes are also under certain codes that are not specifically manifestation codes but may be due to an underlying cause. When a "code first" note is present and an underlying condition is present the underlying condition should be sequenced first.

"Code, if applicable, any causal condition first", notes indicate that this code may be assigned as a principal diagnosis when the causal condition is unknown or not applicable. If a causal condition is known, then the code for that condition should be sequenced as the principal or first-listed diagnosis. Multiple codes may be needed for late effects, complication codes and obstetric codes to more fully describe a condition. See the specific guidelines for these conditions for further instruction.

COMBINATION CODE

A combination code is a single code used to classify: two diagnoses, or a diagnosis with an associated secondary process (manifestation) A diagnosis with an associated complication Combination codes are identified by referring to subterm entries in the Alphabetic Index and by reading the inclusion and exclusion notes in the Tabular List.

Assign only the combination code when that code fully identifies the diagnostic conditions involved or when the Alphabetic Index so directs. Multiple coding should not be used when the classification provides a combination code that clearly identifies all of the elements documented in the diagnosis. When the combination code lacks necessary specificity in describing the manifestation or complication, an additional code should be used as a secondary code.

CODING LATE EFFECTS

A late effect is the residual effect (condition produced) after the acute phase of an illness or injury has terminated. There is no time limit on when a late effect code can be used. The residual may be apparent early, such as in cerebrovascular accident cases, or it may occur months or years later, such as that due to a previous injury. Coding of late effects generally requires two codes sequenced in the following order: The condition or nature of the late effect is sequenced first. The late effect code is sequenced second.

An exception to the above guidelines are those instances where the code for late effect is followed by a manifestation code identified in the Tabular List and title, or the late effect code has been expanded (at the fourth and fifth-digit levels) to include the manifestation(s). The code for the acute phase of an illness or injury that led to the late effect is never used with a code for the late effect.

HYPERTENSION

Hypertension Table

The Hypertension Table, found under the main term, "Hypertension", in the Alphabetic Index, contains a complete listing of all conditions due to or associated with hypertension and classifies them according to malignant, benign, and unspecified.

	Add 4th or 5th digit		Nonspecific code		Unspecified code		Manifestation code

Hypertension, Essential, or NOS

Assign hypertension (arterial) (essential) (primary) (systemic) (NOS) to category code 401 with the appropriate fourth digit to indicate malignant (.0), benign (.1), or unspecified (.9). Do not use either .0 malignant or .1 benign unless medical record documentation supports such a designation.

Hypertension with Heart Disease

Heart conditions (425.8, 429.0-429.3, 429.8, 429.9) are assigned to a code from category 402 when a causal relationship is stated (due to hypertension) or implied (hypertensive). Use an additional code from category 428 to identify the type of heart failure in those patients with heart failure. More than one code from category 428 may be assigned if the patient has systolic or diastolic failure and congestive heart failure.

The same heart conditions (425.8, 429.0-429.3, 429.8, 429.9) with hypertension, but without a stated causal relationship, are coded separately. Sequence according to the circumstances of the admission or encounter.

Hypertensive Chronic Kidney Disease

Assign codes from category 403, Hypertensive chronic kidney disease, when conditions classified to categories 585-587 are present. Unlike hypertension with heart disease, ICD-9-CM presumes a cause-and-effect relationship and classifies chronic kidney disease (CKD) with hypertension as hypertensive chronic kidney disease.

Fifth digits for category 403 should be assigned as follows:

0 with CKD stage I through stage IV, or unspecified.
1 with CKD stage V or end stage renal disease.

The appropriate code from category 585, Chronic kidney disease, should be used as a secondary code with a code from category 403 to identify the stage of chronic kidney disease.

See Chapter 10 for information on the coding of chronic kidney disease.

Hypertensive Heart And Chronic Kidney Disease

Assign codes from combination category 404, Hypertensive heart and chronic kidney disease, when both hypertensive kidney disease and hypertensive heart disease are stated in the diagnosis. Assume a relationship between the hypertension and the chronic kidney disease, whether or not the condition is so designated. Assign an additional code from category 428, to identify the type of heart failure. More than one code from category 428 may be assigned if the patient has systolic or diastolic failure and congestive heart failure.

Fifth digits for category 404 should be assigned as follows:

0 without heart failure and with chronic kidney disease (CKD) stage I through stage IV, or unspecified
1 with heart failure and with CKD stage I through stage IV, or unspecified
2 without heart failure and with CKD stage V or end stage renal disease
3 with heart failure and with CKD stage V or end stage renal disease

The appropriate code from category 585, Chronic kidney disease, should be used as a secondary code with a code from category 404 to identify the stage of kidney disease.

See Chapter 10 for information on the coding of chronic kidney disease.

Hypertensive Cerebrovascular Disease

First assign codes from 430-438, Cerebrovascular disease, then the appropriate hypertension code from categories 401-405.

Hypertensive Retinopathy

Two codes are necessary to identify the condition. First assign the code from subcategory 362.11, Hypertensive retinopathy, then the appropriate code from categories 401-405 to indicate the type of hypertension.

● Code new
to this edition

▲ Revision of
existing code

④ ⑤ Fourth or fifth
digit required

Hypertension, Secondary

Two codes are required: one to identify the underlying etiology and one from category 405 to identify the hypertension. Sequencing of codes is determined by the reason for admission or encounter.

Hypertension, Transient

Assign code 796.2, Elevated blood pressure reading without diagnosis of hypertension, unless patient has an established diagnosis of hypertension. Assign code 642.3x for transient hypertension of pregnancy.

Hypertension, Controlled

Assign appropriate code from categories 401-405. This diagnostic statement usually refers to an existing state of hypertension under control by therapy.

Hypertension, Uncontrolled

Uncontrolled hypertension may refer to untreated hypertension or hypertension not responding to current therapeutic regimen. In either case, assign the appropriate code from categories 401-405 to designate the stage and type of hypertension. Code to the type of hypertension.

Elevated Blood Pressure

For a statement of elevated blood pressure without further specificity, assign code 796.2, Elevated blood pressure reading without diagnosis of hypertension, rather than a code from category 401.

CEREBRAL INFARCTION OR STROKE OR CEREBROVASCULAR ACCIDENT (CVA)

The terms stroke and CVA are often used interchangeably to refer to a cerebral infarction. The terms stroke, CVA, and cerebral infarction NOS are all indexed to the default code 434.91, Cerebral artery occlusion, unspecified, with infarction. Code 436, Acute, but ill-defined, cerebrovascular disease, should not be used when the documentation states stroke or CVA.

See Chapter 18 for information on coding status post administration of tPA in a different facility within the last 24 hours.

POSTOPERATIVE CEREBROVASCULAR ACCIDENT

A cerebrovascular hemorrhage or infarction that occurs as a result of medical intervention is coded to 997.02, Iatrogenic cerebrovascular infarction or hemorrhage. Medical record documentation should clearly specify the cause- and-effect relationship between the medical intervention and the cerebrovascular accident in order to assign this code. A secondary code from the code range 430-432 or from a code from subcategories 433 or 434 with a fifth digit of "1" should also be used to identify the type of hemorrhage or infarct.

This guideline conforms to the use additional code note instruction at category 997. Code 436, Acute, but ill-defined, cerebrovascular disease, should not be used as a secondary code with code 997.02.

LATE EFFECTS OF CEREBROVASCULAR DISEASE

Category 438, Late Effects of Cerebrovascular disease

Category 438 is used to indicate conditions classifiable to categories 430-437 as the causes of late effects (neurologic deficits), themselves classified elsewhere. These "late effects" include neurologic deficits that persist after initial onset of conditions classifiable to 430-437. The neurologic deficits caused by cerebrovascular disease may be present from the onset or may arise at any time after the onset of the condition classifiable to 430-437.

Codes from category 438 with codes from 430-437

Codes from category 438 may be assigned on a health care record with codes from 430-437, if the patient has a current cerebrovascular accident (CVA) and deficits from an old CVA.

Code V12.54

Assign code V12.54, Transient ischemic attack (TIA), and cerebral infarction without residual deficits (and not a code from category 438 as an additional code for history of cerebrovascular disease when no neurologic deficits are present.

Add 4th or 5th digit | Nonspecific code | Unspecified code | Manifestation code

ACUTE MYOCARDIAL INFARCTION (AMI)

ST elevation myocardial infarction (STEMI) and non ST elevation myocardial infarction (NSTEMI)

The ICD-9-CM codes for acute myocardial infarction (AMI) identify the site, such as anterolateral wall or true posterior wall. Subcategories 410.0-410.6 and 410.8 are used for ST elevation myocardial infarction (STEMI). Subcategory 410.7, Subendocardial infarction, is used for non ST elevation myocardial infarction (NSTEMI) and nontransmural myocardial infarctions.

Acute myocardial infarction, unspecified

Subcategory 410.9 is the default for the unspecified term acute myocardial infarction. If only STEMI or transmural myocardial infarction without the site is documented, query the provider as to the site, or assign a code from subcategory 410.9.

AMI documented as nontransmural or subendocardial but site provided

If an AMI is documented as nontransmural or subendocardial, but the site is provided, it is still coded as a subendocardial AMI. If NSTEMI evolves to STEMI, assign the STEMI code. If STEMI converts to NSTEMI due to thrombolytic therapy, it is still coded as STEMI.

See Chapter 18 for information on coding status post administration of tPA in a different facility within the last 24 hours.

● Code new to this edition ▲ Revision of existing code ④ ⑤ Fourth or fifth digit required

7. DISEASES OF THE CIRCULATORY SYSTEM (390-459)

ALERT! For personal history of diseases of circulatory system see V12.5

ACUTE RHEUMATIC FEVER (390-392)

390 Rheumatic fever without mention of heart involvement
Arthritis, rheumatic, acute or subacute
Rheumatic fever (active) (acute)
Rheumatism, articular, acute or subacute

Excludes: that with heart involvement (391.0-391.9)

DEFINITION Rheumatic fever is an illness which arises as a complication of untreated or inadequately treated strep throat infection. Rheumatic fever can seriously damage the valves of the heart.

391 Rheumatic fever with heart involvement

Excludes: chronic heart diseases of rheumatic origin (393-398.99) unless rheumatic fever is also present or there is evidence of recrudescence or activity of the rheumatic process

391.0 Acute rheumatic pericarditis
Rheumatic:
fever (active) (acute) with pericarditis
pericarditis (acute)
Any condition classifiable to 390 with pericarditis

Excludes: that not specified as rheumatic (420.0-420.9)

391.1 Acute rheumatic endocarditis
Rheumatic:
endocarditis, acute
fever (active) (acute) with endocarditis or valvulitis
valvulitis acute
Any condition classifiable to 390 with endocarditis or valvulitis

391.2 Acute rheumatic myocarditis
Rheumatic fever (active) (acute) with myocarditis
Any condition classifiable to 390 with myocarditis

391.8 Other acute rheumatic heart disease
Rheumatic:
fever (active) (acute) with other or multiple types of heart involvement
pancarditis, acute
Any condition classifiable to 390 with other or multiple types of heart involvement

391.9 Acute rheumatic heart disease, unspecified
Rheumatic:
carditis, acute
fever (active) (acute) with unspecified type of heart involvement
heart disease, active or acute
Any condition classifiable to 390 with unspecified type of heart involvement

392 Rheumatic chorea
Includes: Sydenham's chorea

Excludes: chorea:
NOS (333.5)
Huntington's (333.4)

DEFINITION Rheumatic chorea, aka Sydenham's chorea or Saint Vitus' Dance, is a disease characterized by rapid, uncoordinated jerking movements affecting primarily the face, feet and hands.

392.0 With heart involvement
Rheumatic chorea with heart involvement of any type classifiable to 391

392.9 Without mention of heart involvement

CHRONIC RHEUMATIC HEART DISEASE (393-398)

393 Chronic rheumatic pericarditis
Adherent pericardium, rheumatic
Chronic rheumatic:
mediastinopericarditis
myopericarditis

Excludes: pericarditis NOS or not specified as rheumatic (423.0-423.9)

DEFINITION Chronic rheumatic pericarditis is an inflammation of the pericardium resulting from rheumatic heart disease.

| | Add 4th or 5th digit | | Nonspecific code | | Unspecified code | | Manifestation code |

394 Diseases of mitral valve

Excludes: that with aortic valve involvement (396.0-396.9)

DEFINITION The mitral valve is the valve that separates the two chambers on the left side of the heart. The mitral valve prevents blood from regurgitating backwards into the upper heart chambers during cardiac contractions.

394.0 Mitral stenosis
Mitral (valve):
　obstruction (rheumatic)
　stenosis NOS

394.1 Rheumatic mitral insufficiency
Rheumatic mitral:
　incompetence
　regurgitation

Excludes: that not specified as rheumatic (424.0)

394.2 Mitral stenosis with insufficiency
Mitral stenosis with incompetence or regurgitation

394.9 Other and unspecified mitral valve diseases
Mitral (valve):
　disease (chronic)
　failure

395 Diseases of aortic valve

Excludes: that not specified as rheumatic (424.1)
　　　　that with mitral valve involvement (396.0-396.9)

DEFINITION The aortic valve is a semilunar valve between the left ventricle and the aorta; prevents blood from flowing from the aorta back into the heart.

395.0 Rheumatic aortic stenosis
Rheumatic aortic (valve) obstruction

395.1 Rheumatic aortic insufficiency
Rheumatic aortic:
　incompetence
　regurgitation

395.2 Rheumatic aortic stenosis with insufficiency
Rheumatic aortic stenosis with incompetence or regurgitation

395.9 Other and unspecified rheumatic aortic diseases
Rheumatic aortic (valve) disease

396 Diseases of mitral and aortic valves

Includes: involvement of both mitral and aortic valves, whether specified as rheumatic or not

DEFINITION The mitral valve is the valve that separates the two chambers on the left side of the heart. The aortic vale is a valve between the left ventricle and the aorta; prevents blood from flowing from the aorta back into the heart.

396.0 Mitral valve stenosis and aortic valve stenosis
Atypical aortic (valve) stenosis
Mitral and aortic (valve) obstruction (rheumatic)

396.1 Mitral valve stenosis and aortic valve insufficiency

396.2 Mitral valve insufficiency and aortic valve stenosis

396.3 Mitral valve insufficiency and aortic valve insufficiency
Mitral and aortic (valve):
　incompetence
　regurgitation

396.8 Multiple involvement of mitral and aortic valves
Stenosis and insufficiency of mitral or aortic valve with stenosis or insufficiency, or both, of the other valve

396.9 Mitral and aortic valve diseases, unspecified

397 Diseases of other endocardial structures

397.0 Diseases of tricuspid valve
Tricuspid (valve) (rheumatic):
　disease
　insufficiency
　obstruction
　regurgitation
　stenosis

● Code new　　　　▲ Revision of　　　④ ⑤ Fourth or fifth
　to this edition　　　existing code　　　　digit required

397.1 Rheumatic diseases of pulmonary valve

Excludes: | *that not specified as rheumatic (424.3)*

397.9 Rheumatic diseases of endocarditis, valve unspecified
Rheumatic:
    endocarditis (chronic)
    valvulitis (chronic)

Excludes: | *that not specified as rheumatic (424.90-424.99)*

398 Other rheumatic heart disease

DEFINITION Rheumatic heart disease refers to a thickening and stenosis of one or more of the heart valves and often requires surgery to repair or replace the involved valve(s).

398.0 Rheumatic myocarditis
Rheumatic degeneration of myocardium

Excludes: | *myocarditis not specified as rheumatic (429.0)*

⑤ **398.9 Other and unspecified rheumatic heart diseases**

398.90 Rheumatic heart disease, unspecified
Rheumatic:
    carditis
    heart disease NOS

Excludes: | *carditis not specified as rheumatic (429.89)*
heart disease NOS not specified as rheumatic (429.9)

398.91 Rheumatic heart failure (congestive)
Rheumatic left ventricular failure

398.99 Other

HYPERTENSIVE DISEASE (401-405)

Excludes: | *that complicating pregnancy, childbirth, or the puerperium (642.0-642.9)*
that involving coronary vessels (410.00-414.9)

401 Essential hypertension
Includes: high blood pressure
    hyperpiesia
    hyperpiesis
    hypertension (arterial) (essential) (primary) (systemic)
    hypertensive vascular:
      degeneration
      disease

Excludes: | *elevated blood pressure without diagnosis of hypertension (796.2)*
pulmonary hypertension (416.0-416.9)
that involving vessels of:
  brain (430-438)
  eye (362.11)

DEFINITION Essential hypertension is defined as hypertension without known cause.

401.0 Malignant

401.1 Benign

401.9 Unspecified

402 Hypertensive heart disease
Use additional code to specify type of heart failure (428.0-428.43), if known
Includes: hypertensive:
      cardiomegaly
      cardiopathy
      cardiovascular disease
      heart (disease) (failure)
    any condition classifiable to 429.0-429.3, 429.8, 429.9 due to hypertension
    any condition classifiable to 429.0-429.3, 429.8, 429.9 due to hypertension

DEFINITION Hypertensive heart disease refers to heart disease caused by high blood pressure, especially localised high blood pressure.

ALERT! Heart conditions (425.8, 429.0-429.3, 429.8, 429.9) are assigned to a code from category 402 when a causal relationship is stated (due to hypertension) or implied (hypertensive)

⑤ **402.0 Malignant**

402.00 Without heart failure

402.01 With heart failure

| | Add 4th or 5th digit | | Nonspecific code | | Unspecified code | | Manifestation code |

⑤ **402.1 Benign**

      402.10 Without heart failure

      402.11 With heart failure

⑤ **402.9 Unspecified**

      402.90 Without heart failure

      402.91 With heart failure

⑤ **403 Hypertensive chronic kidney disease**

The following fifth-digit subclassification is for use with category 403:

    0 with chronic kidney disease stage I through stage IV, or unspecified

      Use additional code to identify the stage of chronic kidney disease (585.1-585.4, 585.9)

    1 with chronic kidney disease stage V or end stage renal disease

      Use additional code to identify the stage of chronic kidney disease (585.5, 585.6)

    Includes: arteriolar nephritis
             arteriosclerosis of:
               kidney
               renal arterioles
             arteriosclerotic nephritis (chronic) (interstitial)
             hypertensive:
               nephropathy
               renal failure
               uremia (chronic)
             nephrosclerosis
             renal sclerosis with hypertension
             any condition classifiable to 585 and 587 with any condition classifiable to 401

    Excludes: *acute kidney failure (584.5-584.9)*
           renal disease stated as not due to hypertension
           renovascular hypertension (405.0-405.9 with fifth-digit 1)

    DEFINITION Hypertensive chronic kidney disease, refers to diseases of the kidney caused by high blood pressure.

    ALERT! The appropriate code from category 585, Chronic kidney disease, should be used as a secondary code with a code from category 403 to identify the stage of chronic kidney disease

⑤ **403.0 Malignant**
[0-1]

⑤ **403.1 Benign**
[0-1]

⑤ **403.9 Unspecified**
[0-1]

⑤ **404 Hypertensive heart and chronic kidney disease**

Use additional code to specify type of heart failure (428.0-428.43), if known

The following fifth-digit subclassification is for use with category 404:

    0 without heart failure and with chronic kidney disease stage I through stage IV, or unspecified

      Use additional code to identify the stage of chronic kidney disease (585.1-585.4, 585.9)

    1 with heart failure and with chronic kidney disease stage I through stage IV, or unspecified

      Use additional code to identify the stage of chronic kidney disease (585.1-585.4, 585.9)

    2 without heart failure and with chronic kidney disease stage V or end stage renal disease

      Use additional code to identify the stage of chronic kidney disease (585.5, 585.6)

    3 with heart failure and chronic kidney disease stage V or end stage renal disease

      Use additional code to identify the stage of chronic kidney disease (585.5-585.6)

    Includes: disease:
           cardiornal
           cardiovascular renal
          any condition classifiable to 402 with any condition classifiable to 403

    DEFINITION Hypertensive heart and chronic kidney disease, refers to diseases of the heart and kidneys cause by high blood pressure.

    ALERT! The appropriate code from category 585, Chronic kidney disease, should be used as a secondary code with a code from category 404 to identify the stage of kidney disease

● Code new to this edition   ▲ Revision of existing code   ④ ⑤ Fourth or fifth digit required

⑤ **404.0 Malignant**
[0-3]

⑤ **404.1 Benign**
[0-3]

⑤ **404.9 Unspecified**
[0-3]

405 Secondary hypertension
> DEFINITION Secondary hypertension is a type of hypertension caused by an identifiable underlying secondary cause

⑤ **405.0 Malignant**

    405.01 Renovascular
    405.09 Other

⑤ **405.1 Benign**

    405.11 Renovascular
    405.19 Other

⑤ **405.9 Unspecified**

    405.91 Renovascular
    405.99 Other

ISCHEMIC HEART DISEASE (410-414)

> Includes: that with mention of hypertension
> Use additional code, if desired, to identify presence of hypertension (401.0-405.9)

⑤ **410 Acute myocardial infarction**
> ST elevation (STEMI) and non-ST elevation (NSTEMI) myocardial infarction
> Includes: cardiac infarction
> coronary (artery):
>   embolism
>   occlusion
>   rupture
>   thrombosis
> infarction of heart, myocardium, or ventricle
> rupture of heart, myocardium, or ventricle
> any condition classifiable to 414.1-414.9 specified as acute or with a stated duration of 8 weeks or less

The following fifth-digit subclassification is for use with category 410:

0 episode of care unspecified
> Use when the source document does not contain sufficient information for the assignment of fifth digit 1 or 2.

1 initial episode of care
> Use fifth digit 1 to designate the first episode of care (regardless of facility site) for a newly diagnosed myocardial infarction. The fifth digit 1 is assigned regardless of the number of times a patient may be transferred during the initial episode of care

2 subsequent episode of care
> Use fifth digit 2 to designate an episode of care following the initial episode when the patient is admitted for further observation, evaluation, or treatment for a myocardial infarction that has received initial treatment, but is still less than 8 weeks old.

> DEFINITION Myocardial infarction, commonly known as a heart attack, occurs when the blood supply to part of the heart is interrupted causing some heart cells to die.

⑤ **410.0 Of anterolateral wall**
[0-2]   ST elevation myocardial infarction (STEMI) of anterolateral wall

⑤ **410.1 Of other anterior wall**
[0-2]   ST elevation myocardial infarction (STEMI) of other anterior wall
    Infarction:
      anterior (wall) NOS (with contiguous portion of intraventricular septum)
      anteroapical (with contiguous portion of intraventricular septum)
      anteroseptal (with contiguous portion of intraventricular septum)

⑤ **410.2 Of inferolateral wall**
[0-2]   ST elevation myocardial infarction (STEMI) of inferolateral wall

⑤ **410.3 Of inferoposterior wall**
[0-2]   ST elevation myocardial infarction (STEMI) of inferoposterior wall

	Add 4th or 5th digit		Nonspecific code		Unspecified code		Manifestation code

⑤ **410.4** **Of other inferior wall**
[0-2] ST elevation myocardial infarction (STEMI) of other inferior wall
Infarction:
   diaphragmatic wall NOS (with contiguous portion of intraventricular septum)
   inferior (wall) NOS (with contiguous portion of intraventricular septum)

⑤ **410.5** **Of other lateral wall**
[0-2] ST elevation myocardial infarction (STEMI) of other lateral wall
Infarction: Infarction:
   apical-lateral   high lateral
   basal-lateral   posterolateral

⑤ **410.6** **True posterior wall infarction**
[0-2] ST elevation myocardial infarction (STEMI) of true posterior wall
Infarction:
   posterobasal
   strictly posterior

⑤ **410.7** **Subendocardial infarction**
[0-2] Non-ST elevation myocardial infarction (NSTEMI)
Nontransmural infarction

⑤ **410.8** **Other specified sites**
[0-2] ST elevation myocardial infarction (STEMI) of other specified sites
Infarction of:
   atrium
   papillary muscle
   septum alone

⑤ **410.9** **Unspecified site**
[0-2] Acute myocardial infarction NOS
Coronary occlusion NOS
Myocardial infarction NOS
ALERT! Subcategory 410.9 is the default for the unspecified term acute myocardial infarction. If only STEMI or transmural MI without the site is documented, query the provider as to the site, or assign a code from subcategory 410.9.

411 **Other acute and subacute forms of ischemic heart disease**
DEFINITION Ischemic heart disease is caused by deposits of fat or plaque that occur in the walls of the coronary arteries.

411.0 **Postmyocardial infarction syndrome**
Dressler's syndrome

411.1 **Intermediate coronary syndrome**
Impending infarction   Preinfarction syndrome
Preinfarction angina   Unstable angina
Excludes: angina (pectoris) (413.9)
             decubitus (413.0)

⑤ **411.8** **Other**

411.81 **Acute coronary occlusion without myocardial infarction**
Acute coronary (artery):
   embolism without or not resulting in myocardial infarction
   obstruction without or not resulting in myocardial infarction
   occlusion without or not resulting in myocardial infarction
   thrombosis without or not resulting in myocardial infarction
Excludes: obstruction without infarction due to atherosclerosis (414.00-414.07)
             occlusion without infarction due to atherosclerosis (414.00-414.07)

411.89 **Other**
Coronary insufficiency (acute)
Subendocardial ischemia

412 **Old myocardial infarction**
Healed myocardial infarction
Past myocardial infarction diagnosed on ECG [EKG] or other special investigation, but currently presenting no symptoms
DEFINITION Old myocardial infarction refers to an old occlusion or blockage of arteries supplying the muscles of the heart, resulting in injury or necrosis of the heart muscle.

413 **Angina pectoris**
DEFINITION Angina pectoris, commonly known as angina, is severe chest pain due to ischemia (a lack of blood and hence oxygen supply) of the heart muscle

413.0 **Angina decubitus**
Nocturnal angina

● Code new to this edition   ▲ Revision of existing code   ④ ⑤ Fourth or fifth digit required

413.1 Prinzmetal angina
Variant angina pectoris

413.9 Other and unspecified angina pectoris

Angina:
  equivalent
  NOS
  cardiac
  of effort

Anginal syndrome
Status anginosus
Stenocardia
Syncope anginosa

Use additional code(s) for symptoms associated with angina equivalent

Excludes: *preinfarction angina (411.1)*

414 Other forms of chronic ischemic heart disease

Excludes: *arteriosclerotic cardiovascular disease [ASCVD] (429.2)*
cardiovascular:
arteriosclerosis or sclerosis (429.2)
degeneration or disease (429.2)

DEFINITION Ischemic heart disease is a disease characterized by reduced blood supply to the heart muscle, usually due to coronary artery disease (atherosclerosis of the coronary arteries).

⑤ **414.0 Coronary atherosclerosis**
Arteriosclerotic heart disease [ASHD]
Atherosclerotic heart disease
Coronary (artery):
  arteriosclerosis
  arteritis or endarteritis
  atheroma
  sclerosis
  stricture

Use additional code, if applicable, to identify chronic total occlusion of coronary artery (414.2)

Excludes: *embolism of graft (996.72)*
occlusion NOS of graft (996.72)
thrombus of graft (996.72)

414.00 Of unspecified type of vessel, native or graft

414.01 Of native coronary artery

414.02 Of autologous vein bypass graft

414.03 Of nonautologous biological bypass graft

414.04 Of artery bypass graft
Internal mammary artery

414.05 Of unspecified type of bypass graft
Bypass graft NOS

414.06 Of native coronary artery of transplanted heart

414.07 Of bypass graft (artery) (vein) of transplanted heart

⑤ **414.1 Aneurysm and dissection of heart**

414.10 Aneurysm of heart (wall)
Aneurysm (arteriovenous):
  mural
  ventricular

414.11 Aneurysm of coronary vessels
Aneurysm (arteriovenous) of coronary vessels

414.12 Dissection of coronary artery

414.19 Other aneurysm of heart
Arteriovenous fistula, acquired, of heart

414.2 Chronic total occlusion of coronary artery
Complete occlusion of coronary artery
Total occlusion of coronary artery

Code first coronary atherosclerosis (414.00-414.07)

Excludes: *acute coronary occlusion with myocardial infarction (410.00-410.92)*
acute coronary occlusion without myocardial infarction (411.81)

414.3 Coronary atherosclerosis due to lipid rich plaque
Code first coronary atherosclerosis (414.00-414.07)

	Add 4th or 5th digit		Nonspecific code		Unspecified code		Manifestation code

● **414.4 Coronary atherosclerosis due to calcified coronary lesion**
Coronary atherosclerosis due to severely calcified coronary lesion

Code first coronary atherosclerosis (414.00-414.07)

414.8 Other specified forms of chronic ischemic heart disease
Chronic coronary insufficiency
Ischemia, myocardial (chronic)
Any condition classifiable to 410 specified as chronic, or presenting with symptoms
after 8 weeks from date of infarction

Excludes: *coronary insufficiency (acute) (411.89)*

414.9 Chronic ischemic heart disease, unspecified
Ischemic heart disease NOS

DISEASES OF PULMONARY CIRCULATION (415-417)

415 Acute pulmonary heart disease
DEFINITION Pulmonary heart disease is the enlargement and eventual failure of the right
ventricle of the heart due to disorders of the lungs or their blood vessels or chest wall
abnormalities.

415.0 Acute cor pulmonale

Excludes: *cor pulmonale NOS (416.9)*

⑤ **415.1 Pulmonary embolism and infarction**
Pulmonary (artery) (vein):
apoplexy
embolism
infarction (hemorrhagic)
thrombosis

Excludes: *chronic pulmonary embolism (416.2)*
personal history of pulmonary embolism (V12.55)
that complicating:
abortion (634-638 with .6, 639.6)
ectopic or molar pregnancy (639.6)
pregnancy, childbirth, or the puerperium (673.0-673.8)

415.11 Iatrogenic pulmonary embolism and infarction
Use additional code for associated septic pulmonary embolism, if applicable, 415.12

415.12 Septic pulmonary embolism
Septic embolism NOS

Code first underlying infection, such as:
septicemia (038.0-038.9)

Excludes: *septic arterial embolism (449)*

● **415.13 Saddle embolus of pulmonary artery**

415.19 Other

416 Chronic pulmonary heart disease

416.0 Primary pulmonary hypertension
Idiopathic pulmonary arteriosclerosis
Pulmonary hypertension (essential) (idiopathic) (primary)

Excludes: *pulmonary hypertension NOS (416.8)*
secondary pulmonary hypertension (416.8)

416.1 Kyphoscoliotic heart disease

416.2 Chronic pulmonary embolism
Use additional code, if applicable, for associated long-term (current) use of anticoagulants
(V58.61)

Excludes: *personal history of pulmonary embolism (V12.55)*

416.8 Other chronic pulmonary heart diseases
Pulmonary hypertension NOS
Pulmonary hypertension, secondary

416.9 Chronic pulmonary heart disease, unspecified
Chronic cardiopulmonary disease
Cor pulmonale (chronic) NOS

417 Other diseases of pulmonary circulation
DEFINITION Pulmonary circulation is the circulation of blood through the lungs for the
purpose of oxygenation and the release of carbon dioxide. Also known as lesser circulation.

● Code new
to this edition
▲ Revision of
existing code
④ ⑤ Fourth or fifth
digit required

417.0 Arteriovenous fistula of pulmonary vessels
> *Excludes:* *congenital arteriovenous fistula (747.32)*

417.1 Aneurysm of pulmonary artery
> *Excludes:* *congenital aneurysm (747.39)*
> *congenital arteriovenous aneurysm (747.32)*

417.8 Other specified diseases of pulmonary circulation
Pulmonary:
  arteritis
  endarteritis
Rupture of pulmonary vessel
Stricture of pulmonary vessel

417.9 Unspecified disease of pulmonary circulation

OTHER FORMS OF HEART DISEASE (420-429)

420 Acute pericarditis
Includes: acute:
         mediastinopericarditis
         myopericarditis
         pericardial effusion
         pleuropericarditis
         pneumopericarditis

> *Excludes:* *acute rheumatic pericarditis (391.0)*
> *postmyocardial infarction syndrome [Dressler's] (411.0)*

DEFINITION Pericarditis is an inflammation of the two layers of the thin, sac-like membrane that surrounds the heart.

420.0 *Acute pericarditis in diseases classified elsewhere*
Code first underlying disease, as:
    actinomycosis (039.8)
    amebiasis (006.8)
    chronic uremia (585.9)
    nocardiosis (039.8)
    tuberculosis (017.9)
    uremia NOS (586)

> *Excludes:* *pericarditis (acute) (in):*
> *Coxsackie (virus) (074.21)*
> *gonococcal (098.83)*
> *histoplasmosis (115.0-115.9 with fifth-digit 3)*
> *meningococcal infection (036.41)*
> *syphilitic (093.81)*

⑤ **420.9 Other and unspecified acute pericarditis**

420.90 Acute pericarditis, unspecified
Pericarditis (acute):
  NOS
  infective NOS
  sicca

420.91 Acute idiopathic pericarditis
Pericarditis, acute:
  benign
  nonspecific
  viral

420.99 Other
Pericarditis (acute):	Pericarditis (acute):
pneumococcal	streptococcal
purulent	suppurative
staphylococcal	Pneumopyopericardium
	Pyopericardium

> *Excludes:* *pericarditis in diseases classified elsewhere (420.0)*

421 Acute and subacute endocarditis
DEFINITION Endocarditis is an infection of the lining of the heart chambers and heart valves that is caused by bacteria, fungi, or other infectious substances.

Add 4th or   Nonspecific   Unspecified   Manifestation
5th digit   code   code   code

421.0 Acute and subacute bacterial endocarditis

Endocarditis (acute) (chronic) (subacute):
bacterial
infective NOS
lenta
malignant
purulent

Endocarditis (acute) (chronic) (subacute):
septic
ulcerative
vegetative
Infective aneurysm
Subacute bacterial endocarditis [SBE]

Use additional code, if desired, to identify infectious organism [e.g., Streptococcus 041.0, Staphylococcus 041.1]

421.1 *Acute and subacute infective endocarditis in diseases classified elsewhere*

Code first underlying disease, as:
blastomycosis (116.0)
Q fever (083.0)
typhoid (fever) (002.0)

Excludes: *endocarditis (in):*
Coxsackie (virus) (074.22)
gonococcal (098.84)
histoplasmosis (115.0-115.9 with fifth-digit 4)
meningococcal infection (036.42)
monilial (112.81)

421.9 Acute endocarditis, unspecified

Endocarditis, acute or subacute
Myoendocarditis, acute or subacute
Periendocarditis, acute or subacute

Excludes: *acute rheumatic endocarditis (391.1)*

422 Acute myocarditis

Excludes: *acute rheumatic myocarditis (391.2)*

DEFINITION Myocarditis is inflammation of the myocardium, the muscular tissue of the heart.

422.0 *Acute myocarditis in diseases classified elsewhere*

Code first underlying disease, as:
myocarditis (acute):
influenzal (487.8, 488.09, 488.19)
tuberculous (017.9)

Excludes: *myocarditis (acute) (due to):*
aseptic, of newborn (074.23)
Coxsackie (virus) (074.23)
diphtheritic (032.82)
meningococcal infection (036.43)
syphilitic (093.82)
toxoplasmosis (130.3)

⑤ **422.9 Other and unspecified acute myocarditis**

422.90 Acute myocarditis, unspecified
Acute or subacute (interstitial) myocarditis

422.91 Idiopathic myocarditis
Myocarditis (acute or subacute):
Fiedler's
giant cell
isolated (diffuse) (granulomatous)
nonspecific granulomatous

422.92 Septic myocarditis
Myocarditis, acute or subacute:
pneumococcal
staphylococcal

Use additional code, if desired, to identify infectious organism [e.g., Staphylococcus 041.1]

Excludes: *myocarditis, acute or subacute:*
in bacterial diseases classified elsewhere (422.0)
streptococcal (391.2)

422.93 Toxic myocarditis

422.99 Other

● Code new to this edition   ▲ Revision of existing code   ④ ⑤ Fourth or fifth digit required

423 Other diseases of pericardium

> *Excludes:* *that specified as rheumatic (393)*

> **DEFINITION** The pericardium is a double-walled sac that contains the heart and the roots of the great vessels

423.0 Hemopericardium

423.1 Adhesive pericarditis

Adherent pericardium
Fibrosis of pericardium
Milk spots

Pericarditis:
  adhesive
  obliterative
Soldiers' patches

423.2 Constrictive pericarditis

Concato's disease
Pick's disease of heart (and liver)

423.3 Cardiac tamponade

Code first the underlying cause

423.8 Other specified diseases of pericardium

Calcification of pericardium
Fistula of pericardium

423.9 Unspecified disease of pericardium

424 Other diseases of endocardium

> *Excludes:* *bacterial endocarditis (421.0-421.9)*
> *rheumatic endocarditis (391.1, 394.0-397.9)*
> *syphilitic endocarditis (093.20-093.24)*

> **DEFINITION** The endocardium is the membrane that lines the cavities of the heart and forms part of the heart valves .

424.0 Mitral valve disorders

Mitral (valve):
  incompetence NOS of specified cause, except rheumatic
  insufficiency NOS of specified cause, except rheumatic
  regurgitation NOS of specified cause, except rheumatic

> *Excludes:* *mitral (valve):*
> *disease (394.9)*
> *failure (394.9)*
> *stenosis (394.0)*
> *the listed conditions:*
> *specified as rheumatic (394.1)*
> *unspecified as to cause but with mention of:*
> *diseases of aortic valve (396.0-396.9)*
> *mitral stenosis or obstruction (394.2)*

424.1 Aortic valve disorders

Aortic (valve):
  incompetence NOS of specified cause, except rheumatic
  insufficiency NOS of specified cause, except rheumatic
  regurgitation NOS of specified cause, except rheumatic
  stenosis NOS of specified cause, except rheumatic

> *Excludes:* *hypertrophic subaortic stenosis (425.11)*
> *that specified as rheumatic (395.0-395.9)*
> *that of unspecified cause but with mention of diseases of mitral valve*
> *(396.0-396.9)*

424.2 Tricuspid valve disorders, specified as nonrheumatic

Tricuspid valve:
  incompetence of specified cause, except rheumatic
  insufficiency of specified cause, except rheumatic
  regurgitation of specified cause, except rheumatic
  stenosis of specified cause, except rheumatic

> *Excludes:* *rheumatic or of unspecified cause (397.0)*

424.3 Pulmonary valve disorders

Pulmonic:
  incompetence NOS
  insufficiency NOS

Pulmonic:
  regurgitation NOS
  stenosis NOS

> *Excludes:* *that specified as rheumatic (397.1)*

⑤ **424.9 Endocarditis, valve unspecified**

	Add 4th or 5th digit		Nonspecific code		Unspecified code		Manifestation code

424.90 Endocarditis, valve unspecified, unspecified cause
Endocarditis (chronic):
  NOS
  nonbacterial thrombotic
Valvular:
  incompetence of unspecified valve, unspecified cause
  insufficiency of unspecified valve, unspecified cause
  regurgitation of unspecified valve, unspecified cause
  stenosis of unspecified valve, unspecified cause
Valvulitis (chronic)

424.91 *Endocarditis in diseases classified elsewhere*
Code first underlying disease, as:
  atypical verrucous endocarditis [Libman-Sacks] (710.0)
  disseminated lupus erythematosus (710.0)
  tuberculosis (017.9)

Excludes: *syphilitic (093.20-093.24)*

424.99 Other
Any condition classifiable to 424.90 with specified cause, except rheumatic

Excludes: *endocardial fibroelastosis (425.3)*
  that specified as rheumatic (397.9)

425 Cardiomyopathy
Includes: myocardiopathy
DEFINITION Cardiomyopathy is a weakening of the heart muscle or a change in heart muscle structure. It is often associated with inadequate heart pumping or other heart function problems.

425.0 Endomyocardial fibrosis

▲ **425.1 Hypertrophic cardiomyopathy**

Excludes: *ventricular hypertrophy (429.3)*

● **425.11 Hypertrophic obstructive cardiomyopathy**
Hypertrophic subaortic stenosis (idiopathic)

● **425.18 Other hypertrophic cardiomyopathy**
Nonobstructive hypertrophic cardiomyopathy

425.2 Obscure cardiomyopathy of Africa
Becker's disease
Idiopathic mural endomyocardial disease

425.3 Endocardial fibroelastosis
Elastomyofibrosis

425.4 Other primary cardiomyopathies
Cardiomyopathy: Cardiomyopathy:
  NOS   idiopathic
  congestive   obstructive
  constrictive   restrictive
  familial   Cardiovascular collagenosis

425.5 Alcoholic cardiomyopathy

425.7 *Nutritional and metabolic cardiomyopathy*
Code first underlying disease, as:
  amyloidosis (277.30-277.39)
  beriberi (265.0)
  cardiac glycogenosis (271.0)
  mucopolysaccharidosis (277.5)
  thyrotoxicosis (242.0-242.9)

Excludes: *gouty tophi of heart (274.82)*

425.8 *Cardiomyopathy in other diseases classified elsewhere*
Code first underlying disease, as:
  Friedreich's ataxia (334.0)
  myotonia atrophica (359.21)
  progressive muscular dystrophy (359.1)
  sarcoidosis (135)

Excludes: *cardiomyopathy in Chagas' disease (086.0)*

425.9 Secondary cardiomyopathy, unspecified

● Code new   ▲ Revision of   ④ ⑤ Fourth or fifth
   to this edition   existing code   digit required

426 Conduction disorders

DEFINITION Conduction disorders refers to interference with the normal electrical conduction in the heart

426.0 Atrioventricular block, complete
Third degree atrioventricular block

⑤ **426.1 Atrioventricular block, other and unspecified**

426.10 Atrioventricular block, unspecified
Atrioventricular [AV] block (incomplete) (partial)

426.11 First degree atrioventricular block
Incomplete atrioventricular block, first degree
Prolonged P-R interval NOS

426.12 Mobitz (type) II atrioventricular block
Incomplete atrioventricular block:
Mobitz (type) II
second degree, Mobitz (type) II

426.13 Other second degree atrioventricular block
Incomplete atrioventricular block:
Mobitz (type) I [Wenckebach's]
second degree:
NOS
Mobitz (type) I
with 2:1 atrioventricular response [block]
Wenckebach's phenomenon

426.2 Left bundle branch hemiblock
Block:
left anterior fascicular
left posterior fascicular

426.3 Other left bundle branch block
Left bundle branch block:
NOS
anterior fascicular with posterior fascicular
complete
main stem

426.4 Right bundle branch block

⑤ **426.5 Bundle branch block, other and unspecified**

426.50 Bundle branch block, unspecified

426.51 Right bundle branch block and left posterior fascicular block

426.52 Right bundle branch block and left anterior fascicular block

426.53 Other bilateral bundle branch block
Bifascicular block NOS
Bilateral bundle branch block NOS
Right bundle branch with left bundle branch block (incomplete) (main stem)

426.54 Trifascicular block

426.6 Other heart block
Intraventricular block: Sinoatrial block
NOS   Sinoauricular block
diffuse
myofibrillar

426.7 Anomalous atrioventricular excitation
Atrioventricular conduction:
accelerated
accessory
pre-excitation
Ventricular pre-excitation
Wolff-Parkinson-White syndrome

⑤ **426.8 Other specified conduction disorders**

426.81 Lown-Ganong-Levine syndrome
Syndrome of short P-R interval, normal QRS complexes, and supraventricular tachycardias

426.82 Long QT syndrome

	Add 4th or 5th digit		Nonspecific code		Unspecified code		Manifestation code

426.89 Other
  Dissociation:
    atrioventricular [AV]
    interference
    isorhythmic
  Nonparoxysmal AV nodal tachycardia

426.9 Conduction disorder, unspecified
  Heart block NOS
  Stokes-Adams syndrome

427 Cardiac dysrhythmias

  Excludes: *that complicating:*
    abortion (634-638 with .7, 639.8)
    ectopic or molar pregnancy (639.8)
    labor or delivery (668.1, 669.4)

  DEFINITION Cardiac dysrhythmias is a term for any of a large and heterogeneous group of conditions in which there is abnormal electrical activity in the heart. The heart beat may be too fast or too slow, and may be regular or irregular.

427.0 Paroxysmal supraventricular tachycardia
  Paroxysmal tachycardia:
    atrial [PAT]
    atrioventricular [AV]
    junctional
    nodal

427.1 Paroxysmal ventricular tachycardia
  Ventricular tachycardia (paroxysmal)

427.2 Paroxysmal tachycardia, unspecified
  Bouveret-Hoffmann syndrome
  Paroxysmal tachycardia:
    NOS
    essential

⑤ **427.3 Atrial fibrillation and flutter**

  427.31 Atrial fibrillation

  427.32 Atrial flutter

⑤ **427.4 Ventricular fibrillation and flutter**

  427.41 Ventricular fibrillation

  427.42 Ventricular flutter

427.5 Cardiac arrest
  Cardiorespiratory arrest

  ALERT! For personal history of sudden cardiac arrest see V12.53

⑤ **427.6 Premature beats**

  427.60 Premature beats, unspecified
    Ectopic beats
    Extrasystoles
    Extrasystolic arrhythmia
    Premature contractions or systoles NOS

  427.61 Supraventricular premature beats
    Atrial premature beats, contractions, or systoles

  427.69 Other
    Ventricular premature beats, contractions, or systoles

⑤ **427.8 Other specified cardiac dysrhythmias**

  427.81 Sinoatrial node dysfunction

Sinus bradycardia:	Syndrome:
persistent	sick sinus
severe	tachycardia-bradycardia

  Excludes: *sinus bradycardia NOS (427.89)*

● Code new
 to this edition

▲ Revision of
 existing code

④ ⑤ Fourth or fifth
 digit required

CIRCULATORY SYSTEM

427.89 Other

Rhythm disorder:
  coronary sinus
  ectopic

Rhythm disorder:
  nodal
Wandering (atrial) pacemaker

Excludes: *carotid sinus syncope (337.0)*
neonatal bradycardia (779.81)
neonatal tachycardia (779.82)
reflex bradycardia (337.0)
tachycardia (785.0)

427.9 Cardiac dysrhythmia, unspecified

Arrhythmia (cardiac) NOS

428 Heart failure

Code, if applicable, heart failure due to hypertension first (402.0-402.9, with fifth-digit 1 or 404.0-404.9 with fifth digit 1 or 3)

Excludes: *following cardiac surgery (429.4)*
rheumatic (398.91)
that complicating:
  abortion (634-638 with .7, 639.8)
  ectopic or molar pregnancy (639.8)
  labor or delivery (668.1, 669.4)

DEFINITION Heart failure is a condition where there is ineffective pumping of the heart leading to an accumulation of fluid in the lungs. Typical symptoms include shortness of breath with exertion, difficulty breathing when lying flat and leg or ankle swelling

428.0 Congestive heart failure, unspecified

Congestive heart disease
Right heart failure (secondary to left heart failure)

Excludes: *fluid overload NOS (276.69)*

428.1 Left heart failure

Acute edema of lung with heart disease NOS or heart failure
Acute pulmonary edema with heart disease NOS or heart failure
Cardiac asthma
Left ventricular failure

⑤ **428.2 Systolic heart failure**

Excludes: *combined systolic and diastolic heart failure (428.40-428.43)*

  428.20 Unspecified
  428.21 Acute
  428.22 Chronic
  428.23 Acute on chronic

⑤ **428.3 Diastolic heart failure**

Excludes: *combined systolic and diastolic heart failure (428.40-428.43)*

  428.30 Unspecified
  428.31 Acute
  428.32 Chronic
  428.33 Acute on chronic

⑤ **428.4 Combined systolic and diastolic heart failure**

  428.40 Unspecified
  428.41 Acute
  428.42 Chronic
  428.43 Acute on chronic

428.9 Heart failure, unspecified

Cardiac failure NOS
Heart failure NOS

Myocardial failure NOS
Weak heart

Add 4th or 5th digit · Nonspecific code · Unspecified code · Manifestation code

429 Ill-defined descriptions and complications of heart disease

429.0 Myocarditis, unspecified
> Myocarditis:
>> NOS (with mention of arteriosclerosis)
>> chronic (interstitial) (with mention of arteriosclerosis)
>> fibroid (with mention of arteriosclerosis)
>> senile (with mention of arteriosclerosis)

Use additional code, if desired, to identify presence of arteriosclerosis

> Excludes: *acute or subacute (422.0-422.9)*
>> *rheumatic (398.0)*
>>> *acute (391.2)*
>> *that due to hypertension (402.0-402.9)*

429.1 Myocardial degeneration
> Degeneration of heart or myocardium:
>> fatty (with mention of arteriosclerosis)
>> mural (with mention of arteriosclerosis)
>> muscular (with mention of arteriosclerosis)
> Myocardial:
>> degeneration (with mention of arteriosclerosis)
>> disease (with mention of arteriosclerosis)

Use additional code, if desired, to identify presence of arteriosclerosis

> Excludes: *that due to hypertension (402.0-402.9)*

429.2 Cardiovascular disease, unspecified
> Arteriosclerotic cardiovascular disease [ASCVD]
> Cardiovascular arteriosclerosis
> Cardiovascular:
>> degeneration (with mention of arteriosclerosis)
>> disease (with mention of arteriosclerosis)
>> sclerosis (with mention of arteriosclerosis)

Use additional code, if desired, to identify presence of arteriosclerosis

> Excludes: *that due to hypertension (402.0-402.9)*

429.3 Cardiomegaly
> Cardiac: Ventricular dilatation
>> dilatation
>> hypertrophy

> Excludes: *that due to hypertension (402.0-402.9)*

429.4 Functional disturbances following cardiac surgery
> Cardiac insufficiency following cardiac surgery or due to prosthesis
> Heart failure following cardiac surgery or due to prosthesis
> Postcardiotomy syndrome
> Postvalvulotomy syndrome

> Excludes: *cardiac failure in the immediate postoperative period (997.1)*

429.5 Rupture of chordae tendineae

429.6 Rupture of papillary muscle

⑤ **429.7 Certain sequelae of myocardial infarction, not elsewhere classified**
Use additional code to identify the associated myocardial infarction:
> with onset of 8 weeks or less (410.00-410.92)
> with onset of more than 8 weeks (414.8)

> Excludes: *congenital defects of heart (745, 746)*
>> *coronary aneurysm (414.11)*
>> *disorders of papillary muscle (429.6, 429.81)*
>> *postmyocardial infarction syndrome (411.0)*
>> *rupture of chordae tendineae (429.5)*

> **429.71 Acquired cardiac septal defect**

> Excludes: *acute septal infarction (410.00-410.92)*

>> **429.79 Other**
>>> Mural thrombus (atrial) (ventricular), acquired, following myocardial infarction

⑤ **429.8 Other ill-defined heart diseases**

 ● Code new   ▲ Revision of   ④ ⑤ Fourth or fifth
   to this edition   existing code   digit required

429.81 **Other disorders of papillary muscle**

Papillary muscle:
  atrophy
  degeneration
  dysfunction

Papillary muscle:
  incompetence
  incoordination
  scarring

429.82 **Hyperkinetic heart disease**

429.83 **Takotsubo syndrome**
Broken heart syndrome
Reversible left ventricular dysfunction following sudden emotional stress
Stress induced cardiomyopathy
Transient left ventricular apical ballooning syndrome

429.89 **Other**
Carditis

Excludes: *that due to hypertension (402.0-402.9)*

429.9 **Heart disease, unspecified**
Heart disease (organic) NOS
Morbus cordis NOS

Excludes: *that due to hypertension (402.0-402.9)*

CEREBROVASCULAR DISEASE (430-438)

Includes: with mention of hypertension (conditions classifiable to 401-405)

Use additional code, if desired, to identify presence of hypertension

Excludes: *any condition classifiable to 430-434, 436, 437 occurring during pregnancy,*
childbirth, or the puerperium, or specified as puerperal (674.0)
iatrogenic cerebrovascular infarction or hemorrhage (997.02)

430 **Subarachnoid hemorrhage**
Meningeal hemorrhage
Ruptured:
  berry aneurysm
  (congenital) cerebral aneurysm NOS

Excludes: *berry aneurysm, nonruptured (437.3)*
syphilitic ruptured cerebral aneurysm (094.87)

DEFINITION Subarachnoid hemorrhage refers to bleeding within the head into the space between two membranes that surround the brain.

ALERT! For coding late effects of cerebrovascular disease see 438

ALERT! For coding late effects of cerebrovascular disease, dysarthria see 438.13

ALERT! For coding late effects of cerebrovascular disease, fluency disorder see 438.14

431 **Intracerebral hemorrhage**
Hemorrhage (of):
  basilar
  bulbar
  cerebellar
  cerebral
  cerebromeningeal
  cortical
  internal capsule

Hemorrhage (of):
  intrapontine
  pontine
  subcortical
  ventricular
Rupture of blood vessel in brain

DEFINITION Intracerebral hemorrhage is a medical condition indicated by the rupturing of a blood vessel in the brain and the subsequent bleeding into the tissues of the brain.

432 **Other and unspecified intracranial hemorrhage**
DEFINITION Intracranial hemorrhage is bleeding in the brain caused by the breaking (rupture) of a blood vessel in the head.

432.0 **Nontraumatic extradural hemorrhage**
Nontraumatic epidural hemorrhage

432.1 **Subdural hemorrhage**
Subdural hematoma, nontraumatic

432.9 **Unspecified intracranial hemorrhage**
Intracranial hemorrhage NOS

| | Add 4th or 5th digit | | Nonspecific code | | Unspecified code | | Manifestation code |

⑤ **433** **Occlusion and stenosis of precerebral arteries**

Use additional code, if applicable, to identify status post administration of tPA (rtPA) in a different facility within the last 24 hours prior to admission to current facility (V45.88)

The following fifth-digit subclassification is for use with category 433:

0 **without mention of cerebral infarction**

1 **with cerebral infarction**

Includes: embolism of basilar, carotid, and vertebral arteries
narrowing of basilar, carotid, and vertebral arteries
obstruction of basilar, carotid, and vertebral arteries
thrombosis of basilar, carotid, and vertebral arteries

Excludes: insufficiency NOS of precerebral arteries (435.0-435.9)

⑤ **433.0** **Basilar artery**
[0-1]

⑤ **433.1** **Carotid artery**
[0-1]

⑤ **433.2** **Vertebral artery**
[0-1]

⑤ **433.3** **Multiple and bilateral**
[0-1]

⑤ **433.8** **Other specified precerebral artery**
[0-1]

⑤ **433.9** **Unspecified precerebral artery**
[0-1] Precerebral artery NOS

⑤ **434** **Occlusion of cerebral arteries**

Use additional code, if applicable, to identify status post administration of tPA (rtPA) in a different facility within the last 24 hours prior to admission to current facility (V45.88)

The following fifth-digit subclassification is for use with category 434:

0 **without mention of cerebral infarction**

1 **with cerebral infarction**

DEFINITION Occlusion of cerebral arteries, refers to any of the arteries supplying blood to the cerebral cortex.

⑤ **434.0** **Cerebral thrombosis**
[0-1] Thrombosis of cerebral arteries

⑤ **434.1** **Cerebral embolism**
[0-1]

⑤ **434.9** **Cerebral artery occlusion, unspecified**
[0-1]

ALERT! The terms stroke and CVA are often used interchangeably to refer to a cerebral infarction. The terms stroke, CVA, and cerebral infarction NOS are all indexed to the default code 434.91

435 **Transient cerebral ischemia**

Includes: cerebrovascular insufficiency (acute) with transient focal neurological signs and symptoms
insufficiency of basilar, carotid, and vertebral arteries
spasm of cerebral arteries

Excludes: acute cerebrovascular insufficiency NOS (437.1)
that due to any condition classifiable to 433 (433.0-433.9)

DEFINITION Transient cerebral ischemia is the reduction or loss of oxygen to the cerebrum; prolonged ischemia may lead to cerebral infarction

ALERT! For personal history of transient ischemic attack (tia), and cerebral infarction without residual deficits see V12.54

435.0 **Basilar artery syndrome**

435.1 **Vertebral artery syndrome**

435.2 **Subclavian steal syndrome**

435.3 **Vertebrobasilar artery syndrome**

435.8 **Other specified transient cerebral ischemias**

435.9 **Unspecified transient cerebral ischemia**
Impending cerebrovascular accident
Intermittent cerebral ischemia
Transient ischemic attack [TIA]

● Code new
to this edition
▲ Revision of
existing code
④ ⑤ Fourth or fifth
digit required

436 Acute, but ill-defined, cerebrovascular disease

Apoplexy, apoplectic:
NOS
attack
cerebral
seizure
Cerebral seizure

Excludes: *any condition classifiable to categories 430-435*
cerebrovascular accident (434.91)
CVA (ischemic) (434.91)
embolic (434.11)
hemorrhagic (430, 431, 432.0-432.9)
thrombotic (434.01)
postoperative cerebrovascular accident (997.02)
stroke (ischemic) (434.91)
embolic (434.11)
hemorrhagic (430, 431, 432.0-432.9)
thrombotic (434.01)

DEFINITION Cerebrovascular disease is a disease of the blood vessels, especially, the arteries that supply the brain. Cerebrovascular disease is usually caused by atherosclerosis and can lead to a stroke.

ALERT! Code 436 should not be used when the documentation states stroke or CVA

ALERT! Code 436 should not be used as a secondary code with code 997.02.

437 Other and ill-defined cerebrovascular disease

437.0 Cerebral atherosclerosis
Atheroma of cerebral arteries
Cerebral arteriosclerosis

437.1 Other generalized ischemic cerebrovascular disease
Acute cerebrovascular insufficiency NOS
Cerebral ischemia (chronic)

437.2 Hypertensive encephalopathy

437.3 Cerebral aneurysm, nonruptured
Internal carotid artery, intracranial portion
Internal carotid artery NOS

Excludes: *congenital cerebral aneurysm, nonruptured (747.81)*
internal carotid artery, extracranial portion (442.81)

437.4 Cerebral arteritis

437.5 Moyamoya disease

437.6 Nonpyogenic thrombosis of intracranial venous sinus

Excludes: *pyogenic (325)*

437.7 Transient global amnesia

437.8 Other

437.9 Unspecified
Cerebrovascular disease or lesion NOS

438 Late effects of cerebrovascular disease

Note: This category is to be used to indicate conditions in 430-437 as the cause of late effects. The "late effects" include conditions specified as such, as sequelae, which may occur at any time after the onset of the causal condition.

Excludes: *personal history of:*
cerebral infarction without residual deficits (V12.54)
PRIND (Prolonged reversible ischemic neurologic deficit) (V12.54)
RIND (Reversible ischemic neurological deficit) (V12.54)
transient ischemic attack (TIA) (V12.54)

DEFINITION Late effects of cerebrovascular disease refers to a condition that appears after the acute phase of cerebral vascular disease has run its course

ALERT! Category 438 is used to indicate conditions classifiable to categories 430-437 as the causes of late effects (neurologic deficits), themselves classified elsewhere. These "late effects" include neurologic deficits that persist after initial onset of conditions classifiable to 430-437.

438.0 Cognitive deficits

⑤ **438.1 Speech and language deficits**

438.10 Speech and language deficit, unspecified

| | Add 4th or 5th digit | | Nonspecific code | | Unspecified code | | Manifestation code |

	438.11	**Aphasia**
	438.12	**Dysphasia**
	438.13	**Dysarthria**
	438.14	**Fluency disorder**

Stuttering due to late effect of cerebrovascular accident

438.19 **Other speech and language deficits**

⑤ **438.2 Hemiplegia/hemiparesis**

438.20 **Hemiplegia affecting unspecified side**

438.21 **Hemiplegia affecting dominant side**

438.22 **Hemiplegia affecting nondominant side**

⑤ **438.3 Monoplegia of upper limb**

438.30 **Monoplegia of upper limb affecting unspecified side**

438.31 **Monoplegia of upper limb affecting dominant side**

438.32 **Monoplegia of upper limb affecting nondominant side**

⑤ **438.4 Monoplegia of lower limb**

438.40 **Monoplegia of lower limb affecting unspecified side**

438.41 **Monoplegia of lower limb affecting dominant side**

438.42 **Monoplegia of lower limb affecting nondominant side**

⑤ **438.5 Other paralytic syndrome**

Use additional code to identify type of paralytic syndrome, such as:
    locked-in state (344.81)
    quadriplegia (344.00-344.09)

[Excludes:] *late effects of cerebrovascular accident with:*
    hemiplegia/hemiparesis (438.20-438.22)
    monoplegia of lower limb (438.40-438.42)
    monoplegia of upper limb (438.30-438.32)

438.50 **Other paralytic syndrome affecting unspecified side**

438.51 **Other paralytic syndrome affecting dominant side**

438.52 **Other paralytic syndrome affecting nondominant side**

438.53 **Other paralytic syndrome, bilateral**

438.6 Alterations of sensations

Use additional code to identify the altered sensation

438.7 Disturbances of vision

Use additional code to identify the visual disturbance

⑤ **438.8 Other late effects of cerebrovascular disease**

438.81 **Apraxia**

438.82 **Dysphagia**

Use additional code to identify the type of dysphagia, if known (787.20-787.29)

438.83 **Facial weakness**
        Facial droop

438.84 **Ataxia**

438.85 **Vertigo**

438.89 **Other late effects of cerebrovascular disease**
Use additional code to identify the late effect

438.9 Unspecified late effects of cerebrovascular disease

● Code new
to this edition

▲ Revision of
existing code

④ ⑤ Fourth or fifth
digit required

DISEASES OF ARTERIES, ARTERIOLES, AND CAPILLARIES (440-449)

440   Atherosclerosis

Includes: arteriolosclerosis
arteriosclerosis (obliterans) (senile)
arteriosclerotic vascular disease
atheroma
degeneration:
arterial
arteriovascular
vascular
endarteritis deformans or obliterans
senile arteritis
senile endarteritis

Excludes: *atheroembolism (445.01-445.89)*
atherosclerosis of bypass graft of the extremities (440.30-440.32)

DEFINITION Atherosclerosis is a condition in which an artery wall thickens as the result of a build up of fatty materials such as cholesterol. It is a syndrome affecting arterial blood vessels.

440.0   Of aorta

440.1   Of renal artery

Excludes: *atherosclerosis of renal arterioles (403.00-403.91)*

⑤ **440.2   Of native arteries of the extremities**

Use additional code, if applicable, to identify chronic total occlusion of artery of the extremities (440.4)

Excludes: *atherosclerosis of bypass graft of the extremities (440.30-440.32)*

440.20   Atherosclerosis of the extremities, unspecified

440.21   Atherosclerosis of the extremities with intermittent claudication

440.22   Atherosclerosis of the extremities with rest pain
Any condition classifiable to 440.21

440.23   Atherosclerosis of the extremities with ulceration
Any condition classifiable to 440.21 and 440.22

Use additional code for any associated ulceration (707.10-707.19, 707.8, 707.9)

440.24   Atherosclerosis of the extremities with gangrene
Any condition classifiable to 440.21, 440.22, and 440.23 with ischemic gangrene 785.4

Use additional code for any associated ulceration (707.10-707.19, 707.8, 707.9)

Excludes: *gas gangrene 040.0*

440.29   Other

⑤ **440.3   Of bypass graft of the extremities**

Excludes: *atherosclerosis of native artery of the extremity (440.21-440.24)*
embolism [occlusion NOS] [thrombus]
of graft (996.74)

440.30   Of unspecified graft

440.31   Of autologous vein bypass graft

440.32   Of nonautologous biological bypass graft

440.4   Chronic total occlusion of artery of the extremities
Complete occlusion of artery of the extremities
Total occlusion of artery of the extremities

Code first atherosclerosis of arteries of the extremities (440.20-440.29, 440.30-440.32)

Excludes: *acute occlusion of artery of extremity (444.21- 444.22)*

440.8   Of other specified arteries

Excludes: *basilar (433.0)*
carotid (433.1)
cerebral (437.0)
coronary (414.00-414.07)
mesenteric (557.1)
precerebral (433.0-433.9)
pulmonary (416.0)
vertebral (433.2)

█ Add 4th or   █ Nonspecific   █ Unspecified   █ Manifestation
  5th digit   code   code   code

440.9 Generalized and unspecified atherosclerosis
Arteriosclerotic vascular disease NOS

Excludes: arteriosclerotic cardiovascular disease [ASCVD] (429.2)

441 Aortic aneurysm and dissection

Excludes: aortic ectasia (447.70-447.73)
syphilitic aortic aneurysm (093.0)
traumatic aortic aneurysm (901.0, 902.0)

DEFINITION Aortic aneurysm and dissection is a localized, abnormal and persistent dilation of a section of the aorta. This usually results from a weakness in the vessel wall. If severe enough, rupture of the aorta with severe hemorrhage is a potential hazard.

⑤ **441.0 Dissection of aorta**

441.00 Unspecified site

441.01 Thoracic

441.02 Abdominal

441.03 Thoracoabdominal

441.1 Thoracic aneurysm, ruptured

441.2 Thoracic aneurysm without mention of rupture

441.3 Abdominal aneurysm, ruptured

441.4 Abdominal aneurysm without mention of rupture

441.5 Aortic aneurysm of unspecified site, ruptured
Rupture of aorta NOS

441.6 Thoracoabdominal aneurysm, ruptured

441.7 Thoracoabdominal aneurysm, without mention of rupture

441.9 Aortic aneurysm of unspecified site without mention of rupture
Aneurysm
Dilatation of aorta
Hyaline necrosis of aorta

442 Other aneurysm
Includes: aneurysm (ruptured) (cirsoid) (false) (varicose)
aneurysmal varix

Excludes: arteriovenous aneurysm or fistula:
acquired (447.0)
congenital (747.60-747.69)
traumatic (900.0-904.9)

DEFINITION Aneurysm is a cardiovascular disease characterized by a saclike widening of an artery resulting from weakening of the artery wall.

442.0 Of artery of upper extremity

442.1 Of renal artery

442.2 Of iliac artery

442.3 Of artery of lower extremity
Aneurysm:
femoral artery
popliteal artery

⑤ **442.8 Of other specified artery**

442.81 Artery of neck
Aneurysm of carotid artery (common) (external) (internal, extracranial portion)

Excludes: internal carotid artery, intracranial portion (437.3)

442.82 Subclavian artery

442.83 Splenic artery

442.84 Other visceral artery
Aneurysm:
celiac artery
gastroduodenal artery
gastroepiploic artery
hepatic artery
pancreaticoduodenal artery
superior mesenteric artery

● Code new to this edition   ▲ Revision of existing code   ④ ⑤ Fourth or fifth digit required

442.89 Other
Aneurysm:
mediastinal artery
spinal artery

Excludes: *cerebral (nonruptured) (437.3)*
congenital (747.81)
ruptured (430)
coronary (414.11)
heart (414.10)
pulmonary (417.1)

442.9 Of unspecified site

443 Other peripheral vascular disease
DEFINITION Peripheral vascular disease (PVD), aka peripheral artery disease (PAD) or peripheral artery occlusive disease (PAOD), includes all diseases caused by the obstruction of large arteries in the arms and legs

443.0 Raynaud's syndrome
Raynaud's:
disease
phenomenon (secondary)
Use additional code, if desired, to identify gangrene (785.4)

443.1 Thromboangiitis obliterans [Buerger's disease]
Presenile gangrene

⑤ **443.2 Other arterial dissection**

Excludes: *dissection of aorta (441.00-441.03)*
dissection of coronary arteries (414.12)

443.21 Dissection of carotid artery

443.22 Dissection of iliac artery

443.23 Dissection of renal artery

443.24 Dissection of vertebral artery

443.29 Dissection of other artery

⑤ **443.8 Other specified peripheral vascular diseases**

443.81 *Peripheral angiopathy in diseases classified elsewhere*
Code first underlying disease, as:
diabetes mellitus (249.7, 250.7)

443.82 Erythromelalgia

443.89 Other
Acrocyanosis
Acroparesthesia:
simple [Schultze's type]
vasomotor [Nothnagel's type]
Erythrocyanosis

Excludes: *chilblains (991.5)*
frostbite (991.0-991.3)
immersion foot (991.4)

443.9 Peripheral vascular disease, unspecified
Intermittent claudication NOS
Peripheral:
angiopathy NOS
vascular disease NOS
Spasm of artery

Excludes: *atherosclerosis of the arteries of the extremities (440.20-440.22)*
spasm of cerebral artery (435.0-435.9)

Add 4th or 5th digit   Nonspecific code   Unspecified code   Manifestation code

444 Arterial embolism and thrombosis

Includes: infarction:
  embolic
  thrombotic
  occlusion

Excludes: *atheroembolism (445.01-445.89)*

  septic arterial embolism (449)
  that complicating:
    abortion (634-638 with .6, 639.6)
    ectopic or molar pregnancy (639.6)
    pregnancy, childbirth, or the puerperium (673.0-673.8)

DEFINITION An embolism is a sudden interruption in arterial blood flow to an organ or body extremity. The blockage is caused by a blood clot or foreign object. A Thrombosis is the formation or presence of a thrombus (a clot of coagulated blood) in a blood vessel.

⑤ **444.0 Of abdominal aorta**

● **444.01 Saddle embolus of abdominal aorta**

● **444.09 Other arterial embolism and thrombosis of abdominal aorta**
  Aortic bifurcation syndrome
  Aortoiliac obstruction
  Leriche's syndrome

444.1 Of thoracic aorta
  Embolism or thrombosis of aorta (thoracic)

⑤ **444.2 Of arteries of the extremities**

444.21 Upper extremity

444.22 Lower extremity
  Arterial embolism or thrombosis:
    femoral
    peripheral NOS
    popliteal

Excludes: *iliofemoral (444.81)*

⑤ **444.8 Of other specified artery**

444.81 Iliac artery

444.89 Other

Excludes: *basilar (433.0)*
  carotid (433.1)
  cerebral (434.0-434.9)
  coronary (410.00-410.92)
  mesenteric (557.0)
  ophthalmic (362.30-362.34)
  precerebral (433.0-433.9)
  pulmonary (415.11-415.19)
  renal (593.81)
  retinal (362.30-362.34)
  vertebral (433.2)

444.9 Of unspecified artery

445 Atheroembolism

Includes: Atherothrombotic microembolism
  Cholesterol embolism

DEFINITION Atheroembolism is the obstruction of a blood vessel by an atherosclerotic embolism originating from an atheroma in a major artery

⑤ **445.0 Of extremities**

445.01 Upper extremity

445.02 Lower extremity

⑤ **445.8 Of other sites**

445.81 Kidney
  Use additional code for any associated acute kidney failure or chronic kidney disease (584, 585)

445.89 Other site

● Code new
  to this edition

▲ Revision of
  existing code

④ ⑤ Fourth or fifth
  digit required

446 **Polyarteritis nodosa and allied conditions**

> **DEFINITION** Polyarteritis nodosa is a progressive disease of connective tissue that is characterized by nodules along arteries; nodules may block the artery and result in inadequate circulation to the particular area

446.0 **Polyarteritis nodosa**
Disseminated necrotizing periarteritis
Necrotizing angiitis
Panarteritis (nodosa)
Periarteritis (nodosa)

446.1 **Acute febrile mucocutaneous lymph node syndrome [MLNS]**
Kawasaki disease

⑤ **446.2** **Hypersensitivity angiitis**

> *Excludes:* *antiglomerular basement membrane disease without pulmonary hemorrhage (583.89)*

  446.20 **Hypersensitivity angiitis, unspecified**

  446.21 **Goodpasture's syndrome**
  Antiglomerular basement membrane antibody-mediated nephritis with pulmonary hemorrhage

  Use additional code, if desired, to identify renal disease (583.81)

  446.29 **Other specified hypersensitivity angiitis**

446.3 **Lethal midline granuloma**
Malignant granuloma of face

446.4 **Wegener's granulomatosis**
Necrotizing respiratory granulomatosis
Wegener's syndrome

446.5 **Giant cell arteritis**
Cranial arteritis   Temporal arteritis
Horton's disease

446.6 **Thrombotic microangiopathy**
Moschcowitz's syndrome
Thrombotic thrombocytopenic purpura

446.7 **Takayasu's disease**
Aortic arch arteritis
Pulseless disease

447 **Other disorders of arteries and arterioles**

> **DEFINITION** Arteries are blood vessels that carry blood away from the heart. An arteriole is a small diameter blood vessel that extends and branches out from an artery and leads to capillaries.

447.0 **Arteriovenous fistula, acquired**
Arteriovenous aneurysm, acquired

> *Excludes:* *cerebrovascular (437.3)*
> *coronary (414.19)*
> *pulmonary (417.0)*
> *surgically created arteriovenous shunt or fistula:*
> *complication (996.1, 996.61-996.62)*
> *status or presence (V45.11)*
> *traumatic (900.0-904.9)*

447.1 **Stricture of artery**

447.2 **Rupture of artery**
Erosion of artery
Fistula, except arteriovenous of artery
Ulcer of artery

> *Excludes:* *traumatic rupture of artery (900.0-904.9)*

447.3 **Hyperplasia of renal artery**
Fibromuscular hyperplasia of renal artery

447.4 **Celiac artery compression syndrome**
Celiac axis syndrome
Marable's syndrome

447.5 **Necrosis of artery**

Add 4th or   Nonspecific   Unspecified   Manifestation
5th digit   code   code   code

447.6 Arteritis, unspecified
Aortitis NOS
Endarteritis NOS

Excludes: *arteritis, endarteritis:*
aortic arch (446.7)
cerebral (437.4)
coronary (414.00-414.07)
deformans (440.0-440.9)
obliterans (440.0-440.9)
pulmonary (417.8)
senile (440.0-440.9)
polyarteritis NOS (446.0)
syphilitic aortitis (093.1)

⑤ **447.7 Aortic ectasia**
Ectasis aorta

Excludes: *aortic aneurysm and dissection (441.00-441.9)*

447.70 Aortic ectasia, unspecified site
447.71 Thoracic aortic ectasia
447.72 Abdominal aortic ectasia
447.73 Thoracoabdominal aortic ectasia

447.8 Other specified disorders of arteries and arterioles
Fibromuscular hyperplasia of arteries, except renal

447.9 Unspecified disorders of arteries and arterioles

448 Disease of capillaries

DEFINITION Capillaries are the smallest of blood vessels. They serve to distribute oxygenated blood from arteries to the tissues of the body and to feed deoxygenated blood from the tissues back into the veins.

448.0 Hereditary hemorrhagic telangiectasia
Rendu-Osler-Weber disease

448.1 Nevus, non-neoplastic

Nevus:
araneus
senile

Nevus:
spider
stellar

Excludes: *neoplastic (216.0-216.9)*
port wine (757.32)
strawberry (757.32)

448.9 Other and unspecified capillary diseases
Capillary:
hemorrhage
hyperpermeability
thrombosis

Excludes: *capillary fragility (hereditary) (287.8)*

449 Septic arterial embolism
Code first underlying infection, such as:
infective endocarditis (421.0)
lung abscess (513.0)

Use additional code to identify the site of the embolism (433.0-433.9, 444.01-444.9)

Excludes: *septic pulmonary embolism (415.12)*

DEFINITION Septic arterial embolism is a sudden interruption in arterial blood flow to an organ or body extremity. The blockage is caused by a bacterial infection in the bloodstream.

● Code new
to this edition

▲ Revision of
existing code

④ ⑤ Fourth or fifth
digit required

DISEASES OF VEINS AND LYMPHATICS, AND OTHER DISEASES OF CIRCULATORY SYSTEM (451-459)

451 **Phlebitis and thrombophlebitis**

Includes: endophlebitis
inflammation, vein
periphlebitis
suppurative phlebitis

Use additional E Code, if desired, to identify drug, if drug-induced

Excludes: *that complicating:*
abortion (634-638 with .7, 639.8)
ectopic or molar pregnancy (639.8)
pregnancy, childbirth, or the puerperium (671.0-671.9)
that due to or following:
implant or catheter device (996.61-996.62)
infusion, perfusion, or transfusion (999.2)

DEFINITION Phlebitis is the inflammation of a vein. Thrombophlebitis is a phlebitis related to a blood clot or thrombus.

ALERT! For personal history of thrombophlebitis see V12.52

451.0 **Of superficial vessels of lower extremities**
Saphenous vein (greater) (lesser)

⑤ **451.1** **Of deep vessels of lower extremities**

451.11 **Femoral vein (deep) (superficial)**

451.19 **Other**
Femoropopliteal vein
Popliteal vein
Tibial vein

451.2 **Of lower extremities, unspecified**

⑤ **451.8** **Of other sites**

Excludes: *intracranial venous sinus (325)*
nonpyogenic (437.6)
portal (vein) (572.1)

451.81 **Iliac vein**

451.82 **Of superficial veins of upper extremities**
Antecubital vein
Basilic vein
Cephalic vein

451.83 **Of deep veins of upper extremities**
Brachial vein
Radial vein
Ulnar vein

451.84 **Of upper extremities, unspecified**

451.89 **Other**
Axillary vein
Jugular vein
Subclavian vein
Thrombophlebitis of breast (Mondor's disease)

451.9 **Of unspecified site**

452 **Portal vein thrombosis**
Portal (vein) obstruction

Excludes: *hepatic vein thrombosis (453.0)*
phlebitis of portal vein (572.1)

DEFINITION Portal vein thrombosis is a form of venous thrombosis affecting the hepatic portal vein, which can lead to portal hypertension and reduction in the blood supply to the liver.

453 **Other venous embolism and thrombosis**

Excludes: *that complicating:*
abortion (634-638 with .7, 639.8)
ectopic or molar pregnancy (639.8)
pregnancy, childbirth, or the puerperium (671.0-671.9)

DEFINITION Venous embolism and thrombosis is a mass of clotted blood or other material moved by the blood from one vein and forced into a smaller one

ALERT! For personal history of venous thrombosis and embolism see V12.51

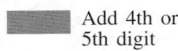 Add 4th or 5th digit   Nonspecific code   Unspecified code   Manifestation code

453.0 Budd-Chiari syndrome
Hepatic vein thrombosis

453.1 Thrombophlebitis migrans

453.2 Of inferior vena cava

453.3 Of renal vein

⑤ **453.4 Acute venous embolism and thrombosis of deep vessels of lower extremity**

> **453.40 Acute venous embolism and thrombosis of unspecified deep vessels of lower extremity**
> Deep vein thrombosis NOS
> DVT NOS

> **453.41 Acute venous embolism and thrombosis of deep vessels of proximal lower extremity**
> Femoral
> Iliac
> Popliteal
> Thigh
> Upper leg NOS

> **453.42 Acute venous embolism and thrombosis of deep vessels of distal lower extremity**
> Calf
> Lower leg NOS
> Peroneal
> Tibial

⑤ **453.5 Chronic venous embolism and thrombosis of deep vessels of lower extremity**
Use additional code, if applicable, for associated long-term (current) use of anticoagulants (V58.61)

> Excludes: *personal history of venous thrombosis and embolism (V12.51)*

> **453.50 Chronic venous embolism and thrombosis of unspecified deep vessels of lower extremity**

> **453.51 Chronic venous embolism and thrombosis of deep vessels of proximal lower extremity**
> Femoral
> Iliac
> Popliteal
> Thigh
> Upper leg NOS

> **453.52 Chronic venous embolism and thrombosis of deep vessels of distal lower extremity**
> Calf
> Lower leg NOS
> Peroneal
> Tibial

453.6 Venous embolism and thrombosis of superficial vessels of lower extremity
Saphenous vein (greater) (lesser)
Use additional code, if applicable, for associated long-term (current) use of anticoagulants (V58.61)

⑤ **453.7 Chronic venous embolism and thrombosis of other specified vessels**
Use additional code, if applicable, for associated long-term (current) use of anticoagulants (V58.61)

> Excludes: *personal history of venous thrombosis and embolism (V12.51)*

> **453.71 Chronic venous embolism and thrombosis of superficial veins of upper extremity**
> Antecubital vein
> Basilic vein
> Cephalic vein

> **453.72 Chronic venous embolism and thrombosis of deep veins of upper extremity**
> Brachial vein
> Radial vein
> Ulnar vein

> **453.73 Chronic venous embolism and thrombosis of upper extremity, unspecified**

> **453.74 Chronic venous embolism and thrombosis of axillary veins**

> **453.75 Chronic venous embolism and thrombosis of subclavian veins**

> **453.76 Chronic venous embolism and thrombosis of internal jugular veins**

● Code new
to this edition
▲ Revision of
existing code
④ ⑤ Fourth or fifth
digit required

453.77 **Chronic venous embolism and thrombosis of other thoracic veins**
Brachiocephalic (innominate)
Superior vena cava

453.79 **Chronic venous embolism and thrombosis of other specified veins**

⑤ **453.8** **Acute venous embolism and thrombosis of other specified veins**

Excludes: *cerebral (434.0-434.9)*
coronary (410.00-410.92)
intracranial venous sinus (325)
nonpyogenic (437.6)
mesenteric (557.0)
portal (452)
precerebral (433.0-433.9)
pulmonary (415.19)

453.81 **Acute venous embolism and thrombosis of superficial veins of upper extremity**
Antecubital vein
Basilic vein
Cephalic vein

453.82 **Acute venous embolism and thrombosis of deep veins of upper extremity**
Brachial vein
Radial vein
Ulnar vein

453.83 **Acute venous embolism and thrombosis of upper extremity, unspecified**

453.84 **Acute venous embolism and thrombosis of axillary veins**

453.85 **Acute venous embolism and thrombosis of subclavian veins**

453.86 **Acute venous embolism and thrombosis of internal jugular veins**

453.87 **Acute venous embolism and thrombosis of other thoracic veins**
Brachiocephalic (innominate)
Superior vena cava

453.89 **Acute venous embolism and thrombosis of other specified veins**

453.9 **Of unspecified site**
Embolism of vein
Thrombosis (vein)

454 **Varicose veins of lower extremities**

Excludes: *that complicating pregnancy, childbirth, or the puerperium (671.0)*

DEFINITION Varicose veins are dilated (widened) tortuous (twisting) veins, usually involving a superficial vein in the leg, often associated with incompetency of the valves in the vein.

454.0 **With ulcer**
Varicose ulcer (lower extremity, any part)
Varicose veins with ulcer of lower extremity [any part] or of unspecified site
Any condition classifiable to 454.9 with ulcer or specified as ulcerated

454.1 **With inflammation**
Stasis dermatitis
Varicose veins with inflammation of lower extremity [any part] or of unspecified site
Any condition classifiable to 454.9 with inflammation or specified as inflamed

454.2 **With ulcer and inflammation**
Varicose veins with ulcer and inflammation of lower extremity [any part] or of unspecified site
Any condition classifiable to 454.9 with ulcer and inflammation

454.8 **With other complications**
Edema
Pain
Swelling

454.9 **Asymptomatic varicose veins**
Phlebectasia of lower extremity [any part] or of unspecified site
Varicose veins NOS
Varicose veins of lower extremity [any part] or of unspecified site
Varix of lower extremity [any part] or of unspecified site

| | Add 4th or 5th digit | | Nonspecific code | | Unspecified code | | Manifestation code |

455 **Hemorrhoids**

Includes: hemorrhoids (anus) (rectum)
piles
varicose veins, anus or rectum

Excludes: *that complicating pregnancy, childbirth or the puerperium (671.8)*

DEFINITION Hemorrhoids are swollen blood vessels in and around the anus that cause itching, pain, and sometimes bleeding

455.0 **Internal hemorrhoids without mention of complication**

455.1 **Internal thrombosed hemorrhoids**

455.2 **Internal hemorrhoids with other complication**

Internal hemorrhoids: Internal hemorrhoids:
bleeding   strangulated
prolapsed   ulcerated

455.3 **External hemorrhoids without mention of complication**

455.4 **External thrombosed hemorrhoids**

455.5 **External hemorrhoids with other complication**

External hemorrhoids: External hemorrhoids:
bleeding   strangulated
prolapsed   ulcerated

455.6 **Unspecified hemorrhoids without mention of complication**
Hemorrhoids NOS

455.7 **Unspecified thrombosed hemorrhoids**
Thrombosed hemorrhoids, unspecified whether internal or external

455.8 **Unspecified hemorrhoids with other complication**
Hemorrhoids, unspecified whether internal or external:
bleeding
prolapsed
strangulated
ulcerated

455.9 **Residual hemorrhoidal skin tags**
Skin tags, anus or rectum

456 **Varicose veins of other sites**

DEFINITION Varicose veins are dilated (widened) tortuous (twisting) veins, often associated with incompetency of the valves in the vein.

456.0 **Esophageal varices with bleeding**

456.1 **Esophageal varices without mention of bleeding**

⑤ **456.2** *Esophageal varices in diseases classified elsewhere*
Code first underlying cause, as:
cirrhosis of liver (571.0-571.9)
portal hypertension (572.3)

456.20 *With bleeding*

456.21 *Without mention of bleeding*

456.3 **Sublingual varices**

456.4 **Scrotal varices**
Varicocele

456.5 **Pelvic varices**
Varices of broad ligament

456.6 **Vulval varices**
Varices of perineum

Excludes: *that complicating pregnancy, childbirth, or the puerperium (671.1)*

456.8 **Varices of other sites**
Varicose veins of nasal septum (with ulcer)

Excludes: *placental varices (656.7)*
retinal varices (362.17)
varicose ulcer of unspecified site (454.0)
varicose veins of unspecified site (454.9)

457 **Noninfectious disorders of lymphatic channels**

457.0 **Postmastectomy lymphedema syndrome**
Elephantiasis due to mastectomy
Obliteration of lymphatic vessel due to mastectomy

● Code new
to this edition

▲ Revision of
existing code

④ ⑤ Fourth or fifth
digit required

457.1 Other lymphedema
    Elephantiasis (nonfilarial) NOS
    Lymphangiectasis
    Lymphedema:
      acquired (chronic)
      praecox
      secondary
    Obliteration, lymphatic vessel

Excludes: *elephantiasis (nonfilarial):*
        congenital (757.0)
        eyelid (374.83)
        vulva (624.8)

457.2 Lymphangitis
    Lymphangitis:
      NOS
      chronic
      subacute

Excludes: *acute lymphangitis (682.0-682.9)*

457.8 Other noninfectious disorders of lymphatic channels
    Chylocele (nonfilarial)   Lymph node or vessel:
    Chylous: fistula
      ascites   infarction
      cyst   rupture

Excludes: *chylocele:*
        filarial (125.0-125.9)
        tunica vaginalis (nonfilarial) (608.84)

457.9 Unspecified noninfectious disorder of lymphatic channels

458 Hypotension
    Includes: hypopiesis

Excludes: *cardiovascular collapse (785.50)*
        maternal hypotension syndrome (669.2)
        shock (785.50-785.59)
        Shy-Drager syndrome (333.0)

DEFINITION Hypotension is the medical term for abnormally low blood pressure.

458.0 Orthostatic hypotension
    Hypotension:
      orthostatic (chronic)
      postural

458.1 Chronic hypotension
    Permanent idiopathic hypotension

⑤ **458.2 Iatrogenic hypotension**

    458.21 Hypotension of hemodialysis
        Intra-dialytic hypotension

    458.29 Other iatrogenic hypotension
        Postoperative hypotension

458.8 Other specified hypotension

458.9 Hypotension, unspecified
    Hypotension (arterial) NOS

459 Other disorders of circulatory system
    ALERT! For personal history of other diseases of circulatory system not elsewhere classified see V12.59

459.0 Hemorrhage, unspecified
    Rupture of blood vessel NOS
    Spontaneous hemorrhage NEC

Excludes: *hemorrhage:*
        gastrointestinal NOS (578.9)
        in newborn NOS (772.9)
        secondary or recurrent following trauma (958.2)
        nontraumatic hematoma of soft tissue (729.92)
        traumatic rupture of blood vessel (900.0-904.9)

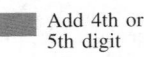
Add 4th or 5th digit   Nonspecific code   Unspecified code   Manifestation code

⑤ **459.1 Postphlebitic syndrome**
Chronic venous hypertension due to deep vein thrombosis

Excludes: *chronic venous hyptertension without deep vein thrombosis (459.30-459.39)*

459.10 Postphlebetic syndrome without complications
Asymptomatic postphlebetic syndrome
Postphlebetic syndrome NOS

459.11 Postphlebetic syndrome with ulcer

459.12 Postphlebetic syndrome with inflammation

459.13 Postphlebetic syndrome with ulcer and inflammation

459.19 Postphlebetic syndrome with other complication

459.2 Compression of vein
Stricture of vein
Vena cava syndrome (inferior) (superior)

⑤ **459.3 Chronic venous hypertension (idiopathic)**
Statis edema

Excludes: *chronic venous hypertension due to deep vein thrombosis (459.10-459.19)*
varicose veins (454.0-454.9)

459.30 Chronic venous hypertension without complications
Asymptomatic chronic venous hypertension
Chronic venous hypertension NOS

459.31 Chronic venous hypertension with ulcer

459.32 Chronic venous hypertension with inflammation

459.33 Chronic venous hypertension with ulcer and inflammation

459.39 Chronic venous hypertension with other complication

⑤ **459.8 Other specified disorders of circulatory system**

459.81 Venous (peripheral) insufficiency, unspecified
Chronic venous insufficiency NOS

Use additional code for any associated ulceration (707.10-707.19, 707.8, 707.9)

459.89 Other
Collateral circulation (venous), any site
Phlebosclerosis
Venofibrosis

459.9 Unspecified circulatory system disorder

● Code new
to this edition
▲ Revision of
existing code
④ ⑤ Fourth or fifth
digit required

Chapter 8: Diseases of Respiratory System (460-519)

DEFINITIONS AND CODING ALERTS

This chapter includes definitions of selected key words, terms and phrases and coding alerts for adding points to the clinical domain, references to coding late effects where appropriate, and references to personal history V-codes in situations where the acute or chronic condition is no longer active. An example from this chapter is as follows:

501 Asbestosis

DEFINITION Asbestosis is a condition featuring scarring of the lungs caused by inhaled asbestos fibers.

ALERT! For personal history of contact with and (suspected) exposure to asbestos see V15.84

MULTIPLE CODING FOR A SINGLE CONDITION

In addition to the etiology or manifestation convention that requires two codes to fully describe a single condition that affects multiple body systems, there are other single conditions that also require more than one code. "Use additional code" notes are found in the tabular at codes that are not part of an etiology or manifestation pair where a secondary code is useful to fully describe a condition. The sequencing rule is the same as the etiology or manifestation pair - , "use additional code" indicates that a secondary code should be added.

"Code first" notes are also under certain codes that are not specifically manifestation codes but may be due to an underlying cause. When a "code first" note is present and an underlying condition is present the underlying condition should be sequenced first.

"Code, if applicable, any causal condition first", notes indicate that this code may be assigned as a principal diagnosis when the causal condition is unknown or not applicable. If a causal condition is known, then the code for that condition should be sequenced as the principal or first-listed diagnosis. Multiple codes may be needed for late effects, complication codes and obstetric codes to more fully describe a condition. See the specific guidelines for these conditions for further instruction.

COMBINATION CODE

A combination code is a single code used to classify: two diagnoses, or a diagnosis with an associated secondary process (manifestation) A diagnosis with an associated complication Combination codes are identified by referring to subterm entries in the Alphabetic Index and by reading the inclusion and exclusion notes in the Tabular List.

Assign only the combination code when that code fully identifies the diagnostic conditions involved or when the Alphabetic Index so directs. Multiple coding should not be used when the classification provides a combination code that clearly identifies all of the elements documented in the diagnosis. When the combination code lacks necessary specificity in describing the manifestation or complication, an additional code should be used as a secondary code.

CODING LATE EFFECTS

A late effect is the residual effect (condition produced) after the acute phase of an illness or injury has terminated. There is no time limit on when a late effect code can be used. The residual may be apparent early, such as in cerebrovascular accident cases, or it may occur months or years later, such as that due to a previous injury. Coding of late effects generally requires two codes sequenced in the following order: The condition or nature of the late effect is sequenced first. The late effect code is sequenced second.

An exception to the above guidelines are those instances where the code for late effect is followed by a manifestation code identified in the Tabular List and title, or the late effect code has been expanded (at the fourth and fifth-digit levels) to include the manifestation(s). The code for the acute phase of an illness or injury that led to the late effect is never used with a code for the late effect.

CHRONIC OBSTRUCTIVE PULMONARY DISEASE [COPD] AND ASTHMA

Conditions that comprise COPD and Asthma

The conditions that comprise COPD are obstructive chronic bronchitis, subcategory 491.2, and emphysema, category 492. All asthma codes are under category 493, Asthma. Code 496, Chronic airway obstruction, not elsewhere classified, is a nonspecific code that should only be used when the documentation in a medical record does not specify the type of COPD being treated.

| | Add 4th or 5th digit | | Nonspecific code | | Unspecified code | | Manifestation code |

Acute exacerbation of chronic obstructive bronchitis and asthma

The codes for chronic obstructive bronchitis and asthma distinguish between uncomplicated cases and those in acute exacerbation. An acute exacerbation is a worsening or a decompensation of a chronic condition. An acute exacerbation is not equivalent to an infection superimposed on a chronic condition, though an exacerbation may be triggered by an infection.

Overlapping nature of the conditions that comprise COPD and asthma

Due to the overlapping nature of the conditions that make up COPD and asthma, there are many variations in the way these conditions are documented. Code selection must be based on the terms as documented. When selecting the correct code for the documented type of COPD and asthma, it is essential to first review the index, and then verify the code in the tabular list. There are many instructional notes under the different COPD subcategories and codes. It is important that all such notes be reviewed to assure correct code assignment.

Acute exacerbation of asthma and status asthmaticus

An acute exacerbation of asthma is an increased severity of the asthma symptoms, such as wheezing and shortness of breath. Status asthmaticus refers to a patient's failure to respond to therapy administered during an asthmatic episode and is a life threatening complication that requires emergency care. If status asthmaticus is documented by the provider with any type of COPD or with acute bronchitis, the status asthmaticus should be sequenced first. It supersedes any type of COPD including that with acute exacerbation or acute bronchitis. It is inappropriate to assign an asthma code with 5th digit 2, with acute exacerbation, together with an asthma code with 5th digit 1, with status asthmatics. Only the 5th digit 1 should be assigned.

CHRONIC OBSTRUCTIVE PULMONARY DISEASE [COPD] AND BRONCHITIS

Acute bronchitis with COPD

Acute bronchitis, code 466.0, is due to an infectious organism. When acute bronchitis is documented with COPD, code 491.22, Obstructive chronic bronchitis with acute bronchitis, should be assigned. It is not necessary to also assign code 466.0. If a medical record documents acute bronchitis with COPD with acute exacerbation, only code 491.22 should be assigned. The acute bronchitis included in code 491.22 supersedes the acute exacerbation. If a medical record documents COPD with acute exacerbation without mention of acute bronchitis, only code 491.21 should be assigned.

ACUTE RESPIRATORY FAILURE

Acute respiratory failure as principal diagnosis

Code 518.81, Acute respiratory failure, may be assigned as a principal diagnosis when it is the condition established after study to be chiefly responsible for occasioning the admission to the hospital, and the selection is supported by the Alphabetic Index and Tabular List. However, chapter-specific coding guidelines (such as obstetrics, poisoning, HIV, newborn) that provide sequencing direction take precedence.

Acute respiratory failure as secondary diagnosis

Respiratory failure may be listed as a secondary diagnosis if it occurs after admission, or if it is present on admission, but does not meet the definition of principal diagnosis.

Sequencing of acute respiratory failure and another acute condition

When a patient is admitted with respiratory failure and another acute condition, (e.g., myocardial infarction, cerebrovascular accident, aspiration pneumonia), the principal diagnosis will not be the same in every situation. This applies whether the other acute condition is a respiratory or nonrespiratory condition. Selection of the principal diagnosis will be dependent on the circumstances of admission. If both the respiratory failure and the other acute condition are equally responsible for occasioning the admission to the hospital, and there are no chapter-specific sequencing rules, the guideline regarding two or more diagnoses that equally meet the definition for principal diagnosis (Official Guidelines, Section II) may be applied in these situations.

If the documentation is not clear as to whether acute respiratory failure and another condition are equally responsible for occasioning the admission, query the provider for clarification.

● Code new
to this edition   ▲ Revision of
existing code   ④ ⑤ Fourth or fifth
digit required

INFLUENZA DUE TO IDENTIFIED AVIAN INFLUENZA VIRUS (AVIAN INFLUENZA)

Code only confirmed cases of avian influenza. This is an exception to the hospital inpatient guideline Official Guidelines, Section II, H. (Uncertain Diagnosis).

In this context, "confirmation" does not require documentation of positive laboratory testing specific for avian influenza. However, coding should be based on the provider's diagnostic statement that the patient has avian influenza.

If the provider records "suspected or possible or probable avian influenza," the appropriate influenza code from category 487 should be assigned. Code 488, Influenza due to identified avian influenza virus, should not be assigned.

| | Add 4th or 5th digit | | Nonspecific code | | Unspecified code | | Manifestation code |

This page intentionally left blank.

● Code new
to this edition

▲ Revision of
existing code

④ ⑤ Fourth or fifth
digit required

8. DISEASES OF THE RESPIRATORY SYSTEM (460-519)

Use additional code, if desired, to identify infectious organism

ALERT! For personal history of diseases of respiratory system see V12.6

ACUTE RESPIRATORY INFECTIONS (460-466)

Excludes: pneumonia and influenza (480.0-488.19)

460 Acute nasopharyngitis [common cold]
Coryza (acute)
Nasal catarrh, acute
Nasopharyngitis:
NOS
acute
infective NOS
Rhinitis:
acute
infective

Excludes: nasopharyngitis, chronic (472.2)
pharyngitis:
acute or unspecified (462)
chronic (472.1)
rhinitis:
allergic (477.0-477.9)
chronic or unspecified (472.0)
sore throat:
acute or unspecified (462)
chronic (472.1)

DEFINITION Nasopharyngitis, usually known as the common cold, is a viral infectious disease of the upper respiratory system.

461 Acute sinusitis
Includes: abscess acute, of sinus (accessory) (nasal)
empyema acute, of sinus (accessory) (nasal)
infection acute, of sinus (accessory) (nasal)
inflammation acute, of sinus (accessory) (nasal)
suppuration acute, of sinus (accessory) (nasal)

Excludes: chronic or unspecified sinusitis (473.0-473.9)

DEFINITION Sinusitis is an infection of the small, air-filled cavities inside the cheekbones and forehead.

461.0 Maxillary
Acute antritis

461.1 Frontal

461.2 Ethmoidal

461.3 Sphenoidal

461.8 Other acute sinusitis
Acute pansinusitis

461.9 Acute sinusitis, unspecified
Acute sinusitis NOS

Add 4th or
5th digit

Nonspecific
code

Unspecified
code

Manifestation
code

462 Acute pharyngitis

Acute sore throat NOS
Pharyngitis (acute):
NOS
gangrenous
infective
phlegmonous
pneumococcal
staphylococcal
suppurative
ulcerative
Sore throat (viral) NOS
Viral pharyngitis

Excludes: *abscess:*
peritonsillar [quinsy] (475)
pharyngeal NOS (478.29)
retropharyngeal (478.24)
chronic pharyngitis (472.1)
infectious mononucleosis (075)
that specified as (due to):
Coxsackie (virus) (074.0)
gonococcus (098.6)
herpes simplex (054.79)
influenza (487.1, 488.02, 488.12)
septic (034.0)
streptococcal (034.0)

DEFINITION Pharyngitis, aka sore throat, is an inflammation of the pharynx. Most sore throats are viral and will not respond to antibiotics. Bacterial causes include group a streptococcus.

463 Acute tonsillitis

Tonsillitis (acute):
NOS
follicular
gangrenous
infective
pneumococcal

Tonsillitis (acute):
septic
staphylococcal
suppurative
ulcerative
viral

Excludes: *chronic tonsillitis (474.0)*
hypertrophy of tonsils (474.1)
peritonsillar abscess [quinsy] (475)
sore throat:
acute or NOS (462)
septic (034.0)
streptococcal tonsillitis (034.0)

DEFINITION Tonsillitis is an infection and swelling of the tonsils.

464 Acute laryngitis and tracheitis

Excludes: *that associated with influenza (487.1, 488.02, 488.12)*
that due to Streptococcus (034.0)

DEFINITION Laryngitis and tracheitis is an inflammation of the mucous membrane of the larynx and trachea; characterized by hoarseness or loss of voice and coughing .

⑤ **464.0 Acute laryngitis**

Laryngitis (acute):
NOS
edematous
Hemophilus influenza
[H. influenzae]

Laryngitis (acute):
pneumococcal
septic
suppurative
ulcerative

Excludes: *chronic laryngitis (476.0-476.1)*
influenzal laryngitis (487.1, 488.02, 488.12)

464.00 Without mention of obstruction

464.01 With obstruction

⑤ **464.1 Acute tracheitis**

Tracheitis (acute):
NOS
catarrhal
viral

Excludes: *chronic tracheitis (491.8)*

464.10 Without mention of obstruction

● Code new to this edition   ▲ Revision of existing code   ④ ⑤ Fourth or fifth digit required

464.11 **With obstruction**

⑤ **464.2** **Acute laryngotracheitis**
Laryngotracheitis (acute)
Tracheitis (acute) with laryngitis (acute)

Excludes: chronic laryngotracheitis (476.1)

464.20 **Without mention of obstruction**

464.21 **With obstruction**

⑤ **464.3** **Acute epiglottitis**
Viral epiglottitis

Excludes: epiglottitis, chronic (476.1)

464.30 **Without mention of obstruction**

464.31 **With obstruction**

464.4 **Croup**
Croup syndrome

⑤ **464.5** **Supraglottitis, unspecified**

464.50 **Without mention of obstruction**

464.51 **With obstruction**

465 **Acute upper respiratory infections of multiple or unspecified sites**

Excludes: upper respiratory infection due to:
influenza (487.1, 488.02, 488.12)
Streptococcus (034.0)

DEFINITION Upper respiratory infection is an inflammation of the nose, sinuses, ears or throat, caused by a viral infection.

465.0 **Acute laryngopharyngitis**

465.8 **Other multiple sites**
Multiple URI

465.9 **Unspecified site**
Acute URI NOS
Upper respiratory infection (acute)

466 **Acute bronchitis and bronchiolitis**
Includes: that with:
bronchospasm
obstruction

DEFINITION Bronchitis and bronchiolitis is an inflammation of the membranes lining the bronchial tubes

466.0 **Acute bronchitis**
Bronchitis, acute or subacute:
fibrinous
membranous
pneumococcal
purulent
septic
viral
with tracheitis
Croupous bronchitis
Tracheobronchitis, acute

Excludes: acute bronchitis with chronic obstructive pulmonary disease (491.22)

⑤ **466.1** **Acute bronchiolitis**
Bronchiolitis (acute)
Capillary pneumonia

Excludes: respiratory bronchiolitis interstitial lung disease (516.34)

466.11 **Acute bronchiolitis due to respiratory syncytial virus (RSV)**

466.19 **Acute bronchiolitis due to other infectious organisms**
Use additional code to identify organism

| | Add 4th or 5th digit | | Nonspecific code | | Unspecified code | | Manifestation code |

OTHER DISEASES OF THE UPPER RESPIRATORY TRACT (470-478)

470 Deviated nasal septum
>   Deflected septum (nasal) (acquired)

> *Excludes:* *congenital (754.0)*

> **DEFINITION** A Deviated nasal septum is an abnormal shift in location of the nasal septum; a common condition causing obstruction of the nasal passages and difficulty in breathing and recurrent nosebleeds.

471 Nasal polyps

> *Excludes:* *adenomatous polyps (212.0)*

> **DEFINITION** Nasal polyps are small, sac-like growths made up of inflamed tissue lining the nose (nasal mucosa).

471.0 Polyp of nasal cavity
>   Polyp:
>   choanal
>   nasopharyngeal

471.1 Polypoid sinus degeneration
>   Woakes' syndrome or ethmoiditis

471.8 Other polyp of sinus
>   Polyp of sinus: Polyp of sinus:
>   accessory   maxillary
>   ethmoidal   sphenoidal

471.9 Unspecified nasal polyp
>   Nasal polyp NOS

472 Chronic pharyngitis and nasopharyngitis

> **DEFINITION** Pharyngitis and nasopharyngitis, aka sore throat, is an inflammation of the pharynx. Most sore throats are viral and will not respond to antibiotics. Bacterial causes include group a streptococcus.

472.0 Chronic rhinitis
>   Ozena   Rhinitis:
>   Rhinitis: hypertrophic
>   NOS   obstructive
>   atrophic   purulent
>   granulomatous   ulcerative

> *Excludes:* *allergic rhinitis (477.0-477.9)*

472.1 Chronic pharyngitis
>   Chronic sore throat
>   Pharyngitis:
>   atrophic
>   granular (chronic)
>   hypertrophic

472.2 Chronic nasopharyngitis

> *Excludes:* *acute or unspecified nasopharyngitis (460)*

473 Chronic sinusitis
>   Includes: abscess (chronic) of sinus (accessory) (nasal)
>   empyema (chronic) of sinus (accessory) (nasal)
>   infection (chronic) of sinus (accessory) (nasal)
>   suppuration (chronic) of sinus (accessory) (nasal)

> *Excludes:* *acute sinusitis (461.0-461.9)*

> **DEFINITION** Sinusitis is an infection of the small, air-filled cavities inside the cheekbones and forehead.

473.0 Maxillary
>   Antritis (chronic)

473.1 Frontal

473.2 Ethmoidal

> *Excludes:* *Woakes' ethmoiditis (471.1)*

473.3 Sphenoidal

473.8 Other chronic sinusitis
>   Pansinusitis (chronic)

473.9 Unspecified sinusitis (chronic)
>   Sinusitis (chronic) NOS

474 Chronic disease of tonsils and adenoids

● Code new to this edition   ▲ Revision of existing code   ④ ⑤ Fourth or fifth digit required

⑤ **474.0 Chronic tonsillitis and adenoiditis**
Excludes: acute or unspecified tonsillitis (463)

474.00 Chronic tonsillitis

474.01 Chronic adenoiditis

474.02 Chronic tonsillitis and adenoiditis

⑤ **474.1 Hypertrophy of tonsils and adenoids**
Enlargement of tonsils or adenoids
Hyperplasia of tonsils or adenoids
Hypertrophy of tonsils or adenoids

Excludes: that with adenoiditis (474.01)
that with adenoiditis and tonsillitis (474.02)
that with tonsillitis (474.00)

474.10 Tonsils with adenoids

474.11 Tonsils alone

474.12 Adenoids alone

474.2 Adenoid vegetations

474.8 Other chronic disease of tonsils and adenoids
Amygdalolith
Calculus, tonsil
Cicatrix of tonsil (and adenoid)
Tonsillar tag
Ulcer, tonsil

474.9 Unspecified chronic disease of tonsils and adenoids
Disease (chronic) of tonsils (and adenoids)

475 Peritonsillar abscess
Abscess of tonsil
Peritonsillar cellulitis
Quinsy

Excludes: tonsillitis:
acute or NOS (463)
chronic (474.0)

DEFINITION A Peritonsillar abscess is an abscess forming in acute tonsillitis around one or both tonsils.

476 Chronic laryngitis and laryngotracheitis
DEFINITION Chronic laryngitis and laryngotracheitis refer to an inflammation of the mucous membrane of the larynx and trachea; characterized by hoarseness or loss of voice and coughing .

476.0 Chronic laryngitis
Laryngitis:
catarrhal
hypertrophic
Sicca

476.1 Chronic laryngotracheitis
Laryngitis, chronic, with tracheitis (chronic)
Tracheitis, chronic, with laryngitis

Excludes: chronic tracheitis (491.8)
laryngitis and tracheitis, acute or unspecified (464.00-464.51)

477 Allergic rhinitis
Includes: allergic rhinitis (nonseasonal) (seasonal)
hay fever
spasmodic rhinorrhea

Excludes: allergic rhinitis with asthma (bronchial) (493.0)

DEFINITION Allergic rhinitis refers to a group of symptoms similar to those of a cold such as runny nose and sore throat, caused by an allergic reaction to an allergen such as dust, plant pollens or animal dander.

477.0 Due to pollen
Pollinosis

477.1 Due to food

477.2 Due to animal (cat) (dog) hair and dander

477.8 Due to other allergen

477.9 Cause unspecified

| | Add 4th or 5th digit | | Nonspecific code | | Unspecified code | | Manifestation code |

478 **Other diseases of upper respiratory tract**

> **DEFINITION** Diseases of upper respiratory tract refers to the part of the respiratory system including the nose, nasal passages, and nasopharynx.

478.0 **Hypertrophy of nasal turbinates**

⑤ **478.1** **Other diseases of nasal cavity and sinuses**

> *Excludes:* *varicose ulcer of nasal septum (456.8)*

    478.11 **Nasal mucositis (ulcerative)**

Use additional E code to identify adverse effects of therapy, such as:
    antineoplastic and immunosuppressive drugs (E930.7, E933.1)
    radiation therapy (E879.2)

    478.19 **Other disease of nasal cavity and sinuses**
        Abscess of nose (septum)
        Necrosis of nose (septum)
        Ulcer of nose (septum)
        Cyst or mucocele of sinus (nasal)
        Rhinolith

⑤ **478.2** **Other diseases of pharynx, not elsewhere classified**

    478.20 **Unspecified disease of pharynx**

    478.21 **Cellulitis of pharynx or nasopharynx**

    478.22 **Parapharyngeal abscess**

    478.24 **Retropharyngeal abscess**

    478.25 **Edema of pharynx or nasopharynx**

    478.26 **Cyst of pharynx or nasopharynx**

    478.29 **Other**
        Abscess of pharynx or nasopharynx

> *Excludes:* *ulcerative pharyngitis (462)*

⑤ **478.3** **Paralysis of vocal cords or larynx**

    478.30 **Paralysis, unspecified**
        Laryngoplegia
        Paralysis of glottis

    478.31 **Unilateral, partial**

    478.32 **Unilateral, complete**

    478.33 **Bilateral, partial**

    478.34 **Bilateral, complete**

478.4 **Polyp of vocal cord or larynx**

> *Excludes:* *adenomatous polyps (212.1)*

478.5 **Other diseases of vocal cords**
    Abscess of vocal cords
    Cellulitis of vocal cords
    Granuloma of vocal cords
    Leukoplakia of vocal cords
    Chorditis (fibrinous) (nodosa) (tuberosa)
    Singers' nodes

478.6 **Edema of larynx**
    Edema (of):
        glottis
        subglottic
        supraglottic

⑤ **478.7** **Other diseases of larynx, not elsewhere classified**

    478.70 **Unspecified disease of larynx**

    478.71 **Cellulitis and perichondritis of larynx**

    478.74 **Stenosis of larynx**

    478.75 **Laryngeal spasm**
        Laryngismus (stridulus)

    478.79 **Other**
        Abscess of larynx
        Necrosis of larynx
        Obstruction of larynx
        Pachyderma of larynx
        Ulcer of larynx

● Code new
  to this edition

▲ Revision of
  existing code

④ ⑤ Fourth or fifth
    digit required

> *Excludes:* ulcerative laryngitis (464.00-464.01)

478.8 Upper respiratory tract hypersensitivity reaction, site unspecified

> *Excludes:* hypersensitivity reaction of lower respiratory tract, as:
>> extrinsic allergic alveolitis (495.0-495.9)
>> pneumoconiosis (500-505)

478.9 Other and unspecified diseases of upper respiratory tract
   Abscess of trachea
   Cicatrix of trachea

PNEUMONIA AND INFLUENZA (480-488)

> *Excludes:* pneumonia:
>> allergic or eosinophilic (518.3)
>> aspiration:
>>> NOS (507.0)
>>> newborn (770.18)
>>> solids and liquids (507.0-507.8)
>> congenital (770.0)
>> lipoid (507.1)
>> passive (514)
>> rheumatic (390)
>> ventilator-associated (997.31)

ALERT! For personal history of pneumonia (recurrent) see V12.61

480 Viral pneumonia
   DEFINITION Viral pneumonia is an inflammation of the lungs caused by infection with a virus.

480.0 Pneumonia due to adenovirus

480.1 Pneumonia due to respiratory syncytial virus

480.2 Pneumonia due to parainfluenza virus

480.3 Pneumonia due to SARS-associated coronavirus

480.8 Pneumonia due to other virus not elsewhere classified

> *Excludes:* congenital rubella pneumonitis (771.0)
>> pneumonia complicating viral diseases classified elsewhere (484.1-484.8)

480.9 Viral pneumonia, unspecified

481 Pneumococcal pneumonia [*Streptococcus pneumoniae* pneumonia]
   Lobar pneumonia, organism unspecified

482 Other bacterial pneumonia

482.0 Pneumonia due to Klebsiella pneumoniae

482.1 Pneumonia due to Pseudomonas

482.2 Pneumonia due to Hemophilus influenzae [H. influenzae]

⑤ **482.3 Pneumonia due to Streptococcus**

> *Excludes:* Streptococcus pneumoniae pneumonia (481)

   482.30 Streptococcus, unspecified

   482.31 Group A

   482.32 Group B

   482.39 Other Streptococcus

⑤ **482.4 Pneumonia due to Staphylococcus**

   482.40 Pneumonia due to Staphylococcus, unspecified

   482.41 Methicillin susceptible pneumonia due to Staphylococcus aureus
      MSSA pneumonia
      Pneumonia due to Staphylococcus aureus NOS

   482.42 Methicillin resistant pneumonia due to Staphylococcus aureus

   482.49 Other Staphylococcus pneumonia

⑤ **482.8 Pneumonia due to other specified bacteria**

> *Excludes:* pneumonia complicating infectious disease classified elsewhere (484.1-484.8)

   482.81 Anaerobes
      Bacteroides (melaninogenicus)
      Gram-negative anaerobes

   482.82 Escherichia coli [E. coli]

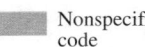 Add 4th or 5th digit

 Nonspecific code

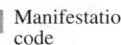 Unspecified code

Manifestation code

482.83 Other gram-negative bacteria
Gram-negative pneumonia NOS
Proteus
Serratia marcescens

Excludes: Gram-negative anaerobes (482.81)
Legionnaires' disease (482.84)

482.84 Legionnaires' disease

482.89 Other specified bacteria

482.9 Bacterial pneumonia unspecified

483 Pneumonia due to other specified organism

483.0 Mycoplasma pneumoniae
Eaton's agent
Pleuropneumonia-like organism [PPLO]

483.1 Chlamydia

483.8 Other specified organism

484 Pneumonia in infectious diseases classified elsewhere

484.1 Pneumonia in cytomegalic inclusion disease
Code first underlying disease (078.5)

484.3 Pneumonia in whooping cough
Code first underlying disease (033.0-033.9)

484.5 Pneumonia in anthrax
Code first underlying disease (022.1)

484.6 Pneumonia in aspergillosis
Code first underlying disease (117.3)

484.7 Pneumonia in other systemic mycoses
Code first underlying disease

Excludes: pneumonia in:
candidiasis (112.4)
coccidioidomycosis (114.0)
histoplasmosis (115.0-115.9 with fifth-digit 5)

484.8 Pneumonia in other infectious diseases classified elsewhere
Code first underlying disease, as:
Q fever (083.0)
typhoid fever (002.0)

Excludes: pneumonia in:
actinomycosis (039.1)
measles (055.1)
nocardiosis (039.1)
ornithosis (073.0)
Pneumocystis carinii (136.3)
salmonellosis (003.22)
toxoplasmosis (130.4)
tuberculosis (011.6)
tularemia (021.2)
varicella (052.1)

485 Bronchopneumonia, organism unspecified
Bronchopneumonia: Pneumonia:
hemorrhagic   lobular
terminal   segmental
Pleurobronchopneumonia

Excludes: bronchiolitis (acute) (466.11-466.19)
chronic (491.8)
lipoid pneumonia (507.1)

DEFINITION Bronchopneumonia is a pneumonia characterized by acute inflammation of the walls of the bronchioles

486 Pneumonia, organism unspecified

Excludes: hypostatic or passive pneumonia (514)
inhalation or aspiration pneumonia due to foreign materials (507.0-507.8)
pneumonitis due to fumes and vapors (506.0)

● Code new to this edition   ▲ Revision of existing code   ④ ⑤ Fourth or fifth digit required

487 **Influenza**

Influenza caused by unspecified influenza virus

Excludes: *Hemophilus influenzae [H. influenzae]:*
  infection NOS (041.5)
  laryngitis (464.00-464.01)
  meningitis (320.0)
  influenza due to 2009 H1N1 [swine] influenza virus (488.11-488.19)
  influenza due to identified avian influenza virus (488.01-488.09)
  influenza due to identified (novel) 2009 H1N1 influenza virus (488.11-488.19)

DEFINITION Influenza, usually referred to as the flu, is a highly infectious respiratory disease. The disease is caused by certain strains of the influenza virus.

487.0 **With pneumonia**

Influenza with pneumonia, any form
Influenzal:
  bronchopneumonia
  pneumonia
Use additional code to identify the type of pneumonia (480.0-480.9, 481, 482.0-482.9, 483.0-483.8, 485)

487.1 **With other respiratory manifestations**

Influenza NEC
Influenza NOS
Influenzal:
  laryngitis
  pharyngitis
  respiratory infection (upper) (acute)

487.8 **With other manifestations**

Encephalopathy due to influenza
Influenza with involvement of gastrointestinal tract

Excludes: *"intestinal flu" [viral gastroenteritis] (008.8)*

488 **Influenza due to certain identified influenza viruses**

Excludes: *influenza caused by unspecified or seasonal influenza viruses (487.0-487.8)*

⑤ **488.0** **Influenza due to identified avian influenza virus**

Avian influenza
Bird flu
Influenza A/H5N1

488.01 **Influenza due to identified avian influenza virus with pneumonia**

Avian influenzal:
  bronchopneumonia
  pneumonia
Influenza due to identified avian influenza virus with pneumonia, any form

Use additional code to identify the type of pneumonia (480.0-480.9, 481, 482.0-482.9, 483.0-483.8, 485)

488.02 **Influenza due to identified avian influenza virus with other respiratory manifestations**

Avian influenzal:
  laryngitis
  pharyngitis
  respiratory infection (acute) (upper)
Identified avian influenza NOS

488.09 **Influenza due to identified avian influenza virus with other manifestations**

Avian influenza with involvement of gastrointestinal tract
Encephalopathy due to identified avian influenza

Excludes: *"intestinal flu" [viral gastroenteritis] (008.8)*

▲ **488.1** **Influenza due to identified 2009 H1N1 influenza virus**

2009 H1N1 swine influenza virus
(Novel) 2009 influenza H1N1
Novel H1N1 influenza
Novel influenza A/H1N1

Excludes: *bird influenza virus infection (488.01-488.09)*
  influenza A/H5N1 (488.01-488.09)
  other human infection with influenza virus of animal origin (488.81-488.89)
  swine influenza virus infection (488.81-488.89)

Add 4th or 5th digit | Nonspecific code | Unspecified code | Manifestation code

▲ **488.11 Influenza due to identified 2009 H1N1 influenza virus with pneumonia**
Influenza due to identified (novel) 2009 H1N1 with pneumonia, any form
(Novel) 2009 H1N1 influenzal:
  bronchopneumonia
  pneumonia

Use additional code to identify the type of pneumonia (480.0-480.9, 481, 482.0-482.9, 483.0-483.8, 485)

▲ **488.12 Influenza due to identified 2009 H1N1 influenza virus with other respiratory manifestations**
(Novel) 2009 H1N1 influenza NOS
(Novel) 2009 H1N1 influenzal:
  laryngitis
  pharyngitis
  respiratory infection (acute) (upper)

▲ **488.19 Influenza due to identified 2009 H1N1 influenza virus with other manifestations**
Encephalopathy due to identified (novel) 2009 H1N1 influenza
(Novel) 2009 H1N1 influenza with involvement of gastrointestinal tract

Excludes: *"intestinal flu" [viral gastroenteritis] (008.8)*

● **488.8 Influenza due to novel influenza A**
Influenza due to animal origin influenza virus
Infection with influenza viruses occurring in pigs or other animals
Other novel influenza A viruses not previously found in humans

Excludes: *bird influenza virus infection (488.01-488.09)*
  influenza A/H5N1 (488.01-488.09)
  influenza due to identified 2009 H1N1 influenza virus (488.11- 488.19)

● **488.81 Influenza due to identified novel influenza A virus with pneumonia**
Influenza due to animal origin influenza virus with pneumonia, any form
Novel influenza A:
  bronchopneumonia
  pneumonia

Use additional code to identify the type of pneumonia (480.0-480.9, 481, 482.0-482.9, 483.0-483.8, 485)

● **488.82 Influenza due to identified novel influenza A virus with other respiratory manifestations**
Influenza due to animal origin influenza A virus with other respiratory manifestations
Novel influenza A:
  laryngitis
  pharyngitis
  respiratory infection (acute) (upper)

● **488.89 Influenza due to identified novel influenza A virus with other manifestations**
Encephalopathy due to novel influenza A
Influenza due to animal origin influenza virus with encephalopathy
Influenza due to animal origin influenza virus with involvement of gastrointestinal tract
Novel influenza A with involvement of gastrointestinal tract

Excludes: *"intestinal flu" [viral gastroenteritis] (008.8)*

CHRONIC OBSTRUCTIVE PULMONARY DISEASE AND ALLIED CONDITIONS (490-496)

490 Bronchitis, not specified as acute or chronic
Bro nchitis NOS: Tracheobronchitis NOS
  catarrhal
  with tracheitis NOS

Excludes: *bronchitis:*
  allergic NOS (493.9)
  asthmatic NOS (493.9)
  due to fumes and vapors (506.0)

DEFINITION Bronchitis is an inflammation of the membranes lining the bronchial tubes.

491 Chronic bronchitis

Excludes: *chronic obstructive asthma (493.2)*

DEFINITION Chronic bronchitis is an inflammation of the membranes lining the bronchial tubes.

● Code new   ▲ Revision of   ④ ⑤ Fourth or fifth
  to this edition   existing code   digit required

491.0 Simple chronic bronchitis
   Catarrhal bronchitis, chronic
   Smokers' cough

491.1 Mucopurulent chronic bronchitis
   Bronchitis (chronic) (recurrent):
      fetid
      mucopurulent
      purulent

⑤ **491.2 Obstructive chronic bronchitis**

Bronchitis:	Bronchitis with:
emphysematous	chronic airway obstruction
obstructive (chronic) (diffuse)	emphysema

Excludes: *asthmatic bronchitis (acute) NOS (493.9)*
   chronic obstructive asthma (493.2)

   491.20 Without exacerbation
      Emphysema with chronic bronchitis

   491.21 With (acute) exacerbation
      Acute exacerbation of chronic obstructive pulmonary disease [COPD]
      Decompensated chronic obstructive pulmonary disease [COPD]
      Decompensated chronic obstructive pulmonary disease [COPD] with
         exacerbation

   Excludes: *chronic obstructive asthma with acute exacerbation (493.22)*

   491.22 With acute bronchitis

491.8 Other chronic bronchitis
   Chronic:
      traeheitis
      tracheobronchitis

491.9 Unspecified chronic bronchitis

492 Emphysema
   DEFINITION Emphysema is a chronic respiratory disease where there is over-inflation of the
   air sacs (alveoli) in the lungs, causing a decrease in lung function, and often, breathlessness.

492.0 Emphysematous bleb
   Giant bullous emphysema
   Ruptured emphysematous bleb
   Tension pneumatocele
   Vanishing lung

492.8 Other emphysema

Emphysema (lung or pulmonary):	Emphysema (lung or pulmonary):
NOS	panlobular
centriacinar	unilateral
centrilobular	vesicular
obstructive	MacLeod's syndrome
panacinar	Swyer-James syndrome
	Unilateral hyperlucent lung

   Excludes: *emphysema:*
      compensatory (518.2)
      due to fumes and vapors (506.4)
      interstitial (518.1)
         newborn (770.2)
      mediastinal (518.1)
      surgical (subcutaneous) (998.81)
      traumatic (958.7)
      with chronic bronchitis (491.20-491.22)

493 Asthma
   Excludes: *wheezing NOS (786.07)*

The following fifth-digit subclassification is for use with codes 493.0-493.2, 493.9:

   0 unspecified

   1 with status asthmaticus

   2 with (acute) exacerbation
   DEFINITION Asthma is a condition often of allergic origin that is marked by labored breathing
   accompanied by wheezing and a sense of constriction in the chest, and often by attacks of
   coughing or gasping

Add 4th or 5th digit	Nonspecific code	Unspecified code	Manifestation code

⑤ **493.0 extrinsic asthma**
[0-2]   Asthma:
          allergic with stated cause
          atopic
          childhood
          hay
          platinum
       Hay fever with asthma

   Excludes: *asthma:*
              allergic NOS (493.9)
              detergent (507.8)
              miners' (500)
              wood (495.8)

⑤ **493.1 Intrinsic asthma**
[0-2]   Late-onset asthma

⑤ **493.2 Chronic obstructive asthma**
[0-2]   Asthma with chronic obstructive pulmonary disease [COPD]
          Chronic asthmatic bronchitis

   Excludes: *chronic obstructive bronchitis (491.20-491.22)*
              acute bronchitis (466.0)

⑤ **493.8 Other forms of asthma**

       493.81 Exercise induced bronchospasm

       493.82 Cough variant asthma

⑤ **493.9 Asthma, unspecified**
[0-2]   Asthma (bronchial) (allergic NOS)
          Bronchitis:
            allergic
            asthmatic

494 Bronchiectasis
       Bronchiectasis (fusiform) (postinfectious) (recurrent)
       Bronchiolectasis

   Excludes: *congenital (748.61)*
              tuberculous bronchiectasis (current disease) (011.5)

   DEFINITION Bronchiectasis is a condition characterized by abnormal dilatation of the bronchi
   (airways) and excessive mucus production. The mucus accumulation may obstruct the
   bronchi. Is often associated with repeated bronchial infections.

   494.0 Bronchiectasis without acute exacerbation

   494.1 Bronchiectasis with acute exacerbation

495 Extrinsic allergic alveolitis
       Includes: allergic alveolitis and pneumonitis due to inhaled organic dust particles of fungal,
                  thermophilic actinomycete, or other origin

   DEFINITION Extrinsic allergic alveolitis is an inflammation of the alveoli in the lungs caused
   by inhaling dust.

   495.0 Farmers' lung

   495.1 Bagassosis

   495.2 Bird-fanciers' lung
          Budgerigar-fanciers' disease or lung
          Pigeon-fanciers' disease or lung

   495.3 Suberosis
          Cork-handlers' disease or lung

   495.4 Malt workers' lung
          Alveolitis due to Aspergillus clavatus

   495.5 Mushroom workers' lung

   495.6 Maple bark-strippers' lung
          Alveolitis due to Cryptostroma corticale

   495.7 "Ventilation" pneumonitis
          Allergic alveolitis due to fungal, thermophilic actinomycete, and other organisms
          growing in ventilation [air conditioning] systems

● Code new   ▲ Revision of   ④ ⑤ Fourth or fifth
     to this edition   existing code   digit required

495.8 **Other specified allergic alveolitis and pneumonitis**

Cheese-washers' lung
Coffee workers' lung
Fish-meal workers' lung
Furriers' lung
Grain-handlers' disease or lung

Pituitary snuff-takers' disease
Sequoiosis or red-cedar asthma
Wood asthma

495.9 **Unspecified allergic alveolitis and pneumonitis**

Alveolitis, allergic (extrinsic)
Hypersensitivity pneumonitis

496 **Chronic airway obstruction, not elsewhere classified**

Note: This code is not to be used with any code from categories 491-493

Chronic:
nonspecific lung disease
obstructive lung disease
obstructive pulmonary disease [COPD] NOS

Excludes: *chronic obstructive lung disease [COPD] specified (as) (with):*
allergic alveolitis (495.0-495.9)
asthma (493.2)
bronchiectasis (494.0-494.1)
bronchitis (491.20-491.22)
with emphysema (491.20-491.22)
decompensated (491.21)
emphysema (492.0-492.8)

DEFINITION Chronic airway obstruction is a pulmonary disorder, such as emphysema or chronic bronchitis, in which the upper or lower airway is chronically obstructed.

ALERT! Code 496 is a nonspecific code that should only be used when the documentation in a medical record does not specify the type of COPD being treated.

PNEUMOCONIOSES AND OTHER LUNG DISEASES DUE TO EXTERNAL AGENTS (500-508)

500 **Coal workers' pneumoconiosis**

Anthracosilicosis
Anthracosis
Black lung disease

Coal workers' lung
Miner's asthma

DEFINITION Coal workers' pneumoconiosis is a diseases characterized by fibrosis and scarring of the lungs caused by repeated inhalation of occupationally associated dust, such as silica, asbestos, and coal dust.

501 **Asbestosis**

DEFINITION Asbestosis is a condition featuring scarring of the lungs caused by inhaled asbestos fibers.

ALERT! For personal history of contact with and (suspected) exposure to asbestos see V15.84

502 **Pneumoconiosis due to other silica or silicates**

Pneumoconiosis due to talc
Silicotic fibrosis (massive) of lung
Silicosis (simple) (complicated)

DEFINITION Pneumoconiosis is a fibrosis and scarring of the lungs caused by repeated inhalation of occupationally associated dust, such as silica, asbestos, and coal dust.

503 **Pneumoconiosis due to other inorganic dust**

Aluminosis (of lung)
Bauxite fibrosis (of lung)
Berylliosis

Graphite fibrosis (of lung)
Siderosis
Stannosis

504 **Pneumonopathy due to inhalation of other dust**

Byssinosis
Cannabinosis

Flax-dressers' disease

Excludes: *allergic alveolitis (495.0-495.9)*
asbestosis (501)
bagassosis (495.1)
farmers' lung (495.0)

DEFINITION Pneumopathy due to inhalation of other dust is any disease of the lungs caused by dust inhalation

505 **Pneumoconiosis, unspecified**

DEFINITION Pneumoconiosis is fibrosis and scarring of the lungs as a result of repeated inhalation of occupationally associated dust, such as silica, asbestos, and coal dust.

500

	Add 4th or 5th digit		Nonspecific code		Unspecified code		Manifestation code

506 **Respiratory conditions due to chemical fumes and vapors**
Use additional E code, if desired, to identify cause
Use additional code to identify associated respiratory conditions, such as:
acute respiratory failure (518.81)

506.0 **Bronchitis and pneumonitis due to fumes and vapors**
Chemical bronchitis (acute)

506.1 **Acute pulmonary edema due to fumes and vapors**
Chemical pulmonary edema (acute)

Excludes: *acute pulmonary edema NOS (518.4)*
chronic or unspecified pulmonary edema (514)

506.2 **Upper respiratory inflammation due to fumes and vapors**

506.3 **Other acute and subacute respiratory conditions due to fumes and vapors**

506.4 **Chronic respiratory conditions due to fumes and vapors**
Emphysema (diffuse) (chronic) due to inhalation of chemical fumes and vapors
Obliterative bronchiolitis (chronic) (subacute) due to inhalation of chemical fumes and vapors
Pulmonary fibrosis (chronic) due to inhalation of chemical fumes and vapors

506.9 **Unspecified respiratory conditions due to fumes and vapors**
Silo-fillers' disease

507 **Pneumonitis due to solids and liquids**

Excludes: *fetal aspiration pneumonitis (770.18)*
postprocedural pneumonitis (997.32)

507.0 **Due to inhalation of food or vomitus**
Aspiration pneumonia (due to):
NOS
food (regurgitated)
gastric secretions
milk
saliva
vomitus

507.1 **Due to inhalation of oils and essences**
Lipoid pneumonia (exogenous)

Excludes: *endogenous lipoid pneumonia (516.8)*

507.8 **Due to other solids and liquids**
Detergent asthma

508 **Respiratory conditions due to other and unspecified external agents**
Use additional E code, if desired, to identify cause
Use additional code to identify associated respiratory conditions, such as:
acute respiratory failure (518.81)

508.0 **Acute pulmonary manifestations due to radiation**
Radiation pneumonitis

508.1 **Chronic and other pulmonary manifestations due to radiation**
Fibrosis of lung following radiation

● **508.2** **Respiratory conditions due to smoke inhalation**
Smoke inhalation NOS

Excludes: *smoke inhalation due to chemical fumes and vapors (506.9)*

508.8 **Respiratory conditions due to other specified external agents**

508.9 **Respiratory conditions due to unspecified external agent**

OTHER DISEASES OF RESPIRATORY SYSTEM (510-519)

510 **Empyema**
Use additional code, if desired, to identify infectious organism (041.0-041.9)

Excludes: *abscess of lung (513.0)*

DEFINITION Empyema is a collection of pus within a naturally existing anatomical cavity

510.0 **With fistula**

Fistula:	Fistula:
bronchocutaneous	mediastinal
bronchopleural	pleural
hepatopleural	thoracic

Any condition classifiable to 510.9 with fistula

● Code new
to this edition
▲ Revision of
existing code
④ ⑤ Fourth or fifth
digit required

510.9 Without mention of fistula

Abscess:
   pleura
   thorax
Empyema (chest) (lung)
   (pleura)
Fibrinopurulent pleurisy

Pleurisy:
   purulent
   septic
   seropurulent
   suppurative
Pyopneumothorax
Pyothorax

511 Pleurisy

Excludes: *pleurisy with mention of tuberculosis, current disease (012.0)*

DEFINITION Pleurisy is an inflammation of the membrane that surrounds and protects the lungs (the pleura). Inflammation occurs when an infection or damaging agent irritates the pleural surface.

511.0 Without mention of effusion or current tuberculosis

Adhesion, lung or pleura
Calcification of pleura
Pleurisy (acute) (sterile):
   diaphragmatic
   fibrinous
   interlobar

Pleurisy:
   NOS
   pneumococcal
   staphylococcal
   streptococcal
Thickening of pleura

511.1 With effusion, with mention of a bacterial cause other than tuberculosis

Pleurisy with effusion (exudative) (serous):
   pneumococcal
   staphylococcal
   streptococcal
   other specified nontuberculous bacterial cause

⑤ 511.8 Other specified forms of effusion, except tuberculous

Excludes: *traumatic (860.2-860.5, 862.29, 862.39)*

511.81 Malignant pleural effusion

Code first malignant neoplasm, if known

511.89 Other specified forms of effusion, except tuberculous

Encysted pleurisy
Hemopneumothorax
Hemothorax
Hydropneumothorax
Hydrothorax

511.9 Unspecified pleural effusion

Pleural effusion NOS
Pleurisy:
   exudative
   serofibrinous

Pleurisy:
   serous
   with effusion NOS

▲ 512 Pneumothorax and air leak

DEFINITION Pneumothorax is a collection of air or gas in the chest or pleural space that causes part or all of a lung to collapse

512.0 Spontaneous tension pneumothorax

512.1 Iatrogenic pneumothorax

Postoperative pneumothorax

● 512.2 Postoperative air leak

▲ 512.8 Other pneumothorax and air leak

Excludes: *pneumothorax:*
   congenital (770.2)
   traumatic (860.0-860.1, 860.4-860.5)
   tuberculous, current disease (011.7)

● 512.81 Primary spontaneous pneumothorax

Add 4th or 5th digit	Nonspecific code	Unspecified code	Manifestation code

- ● 512.82 *Secondary spontaneous pneumothorax*
  Code first underlying condition, such as:
  cancer metastatic to lung (197.0)
  catamenial pneumothorax due to endometriosis (617.8)
  cystic fibrosis (277.02)
  eosinophilic pneumonia (518.3)
  lymphangioleiomyomatosis (516.4)
  Marfan syndrome (759.82)
  pneumocystis carinii pneumonia (136.3)
  primary lung cancer (162.3-162.9)
  spontaneous rupture of the esophagus (530.4)

  - ● 512.83 **Chronic pneumothorax**

  - ● 512.84 **Other air leak**
    Persistent air leak

  - ● 512.89 **Other pneumothorax**
    Acute pneumothorax
    Pneumothorax NOS
    Spontaneous pneumothorax NOS

513 **Abscess of lung and mediastinum**
  DEFINITION The mediastinum refers to the area in the middle of the chest containing the heart, great vessels, esophagus and other structures.

  513.0 **Abscess of lung**
    Abscess (multiple) of lung
    Gangrenous or necrotic pneumonia
    Pulmonary gangrene or necrosis

  513.1 **Abscess of mediastinum**

514 **Pulmonary congestion and hypostasis**
    Hypostatic:
    bronchopneumonia
    pneumonia
    Passive pneumonia
    Pulmonary congestion (chronic) (passive)
    Pulmonary edema:
    NOS
    chronic

    Excludes: *acute pulmonary edema:*
        NOS (518.4)
        with mention of heart disease or failure (428.1)
        hypostatic pneumonia due to or specified as a specific type of pneumonia – code to the type of pneumonia (480.0-480.9, 481, 482.0-482.9, 483.0-483.8, 487.0, 488.01, 488.11)

    DEFINITION Pulmonary congestion and hypostasis refers to excess fluid or blood in the lungs

515 **Postinflammatory pulmonary fibrosis**
    Cirrhosis of lung, chronic or unspecified
    Fibrosis of lung (atrophic) (confluent) (massive) (perialveolar) (peribronchial), chronic or unspecified
    Induration of lung, chronic or unspecified

    DEFINITION Pulmonary fibrosis is a condition characterized by deposition of fibrous tissue in the lung. It decreases lung compliance and results in a restrictive ventilatory defect as seen on pulmonary function testing.

516 **Other alveolar and parietoalveolar pneumonopathy**

  516.0 **Pulmonary alveolar proteinosis**

  516.1 *Idiopathic pulmonary hemosiderosis*
    Essential brown induration of lung

    Code first underlying disease (275.01-275.09)

    Excludes: *acute idiopathic pulmonary hemorrhage in infants [AIPHI] (786.31)*

  516.2 **Pulmonary alveolar microlithiasis**

▲ 516.3 **Idiopathic interstitial pneumonia**

  - ● 516.30 **Idiopathic interstitial pneumonia, not otherwise specified**
    Idiopathic fibrosing alveolitis

  - ● 516.31 **Idiopathic pulmonary fibrosis**
    Cryptogenic fibrosing alveolitis

● Code new
to this edition   ▲ Revision of
existing code   ④ ⑤ Fourth or fifth
digit required

● **516.32 Idiopathic non-specific interstitial pneumonitis**
Excludes: *non-specific interstitial pneumonia NOS, or due to known underlying cause (516.8)*

● **516.33 Acute interstitial pneumonitis**
Hamman-Rich syndrome
Excludes: *pneumocystis pneumonia (136.3)*

● **516.34 Respiratory bronchiolitis interstitial lung disease**

● **516.35 Idiopathic lymphoid interstitial pneumonia**
Idiopathic lymphocytic interstitial pneumonitis
Excludes: *lymphoid interstitial pneumonia NOS, or due to known underlying cause (516.8)*
pneumocystis pneumonia (136.3)

● **516.36 Cryptogenic organizing pneumonia**
Excludes: *organizing pneumonia NOS, or due to known underlying cause (516.8)*

● **516.37 Desquamative interstitial pneumonia**

● **516.4 Lymphangioleiomyomatosis**
Lymphangiomyomatosis

● **516.5 Adult pulmonary Langerhans cell histiocytosis**
Adult PLCH

● **516.6 Interstitial lung diseases of childhood**

● **516.61 Neuroendocrine cell hyperplasia of infancy**

● **516.62 Pulmonary interstitial glycogenosis**

● **516.63 Surfactant mutations of the lung**

● **516.64 Alveolar capillary dysplasia with vein misalignment**

● **516.69 Other interstitial lung diseases of childhood**

516.8 Other specified alveolar and parietoalveolar pneumonopathies
Endogenous lipoid pneumonia
Interstitial pneumonia
Lymphoid interstitial pneumonia due to known underlying cause
Lymphoid interstitial pneumonia NOS
Non-specific interstitial pneumonia due to known underlying cause
Non-specific interstitial pneumonia NOS
Organizing pneumonia due to known underlying cause
Organizing pneumonia NOS
Code first, if applicable, underlying cause of pneumonopathy, if known
Use additional E code, if applicable, for drug-induced or toxic pneumonopathy
Excludes: *cryptogenic organizing pneumonia (516.36)*
idiopathic lymphoid interstitial pneumonia (516.35)
idiopathic non-specific interstitial pneumonitis (516.32)
lipoid pneumonia, exogenous or unspecified (507.1)

516.9 Unspecified alveolar and parietoalveolar pneumonopathy

517 Lung involvement in conditions classified elsewhere
Excludes: *rheumatoid lung (714.81)*

517.1 Rheumatic pneumonia
Code first underlying disease (390)

517.2 Lung involvement in systemic sclerosis
Code first underlying disease (710.1)

517.3 Acute chest syndrome
Code first sickle-cell disease in crisis (282.42, 282.62, 282.64, 282.69)

517.8 Lung involvement in other diseases classified elsewhere
Code first underlying disease, as:
amyloidosis (277.30-277.39)
polymyositis (710.4)
sarcoidosis (135)
Sjögren's disease (710.2)
systemic lupus erythematosus (710.0)
Excludes: *syphilis (095.1)*

518 Other diseases of lung

Add 4th or 5th digit   Nonspecific code   Unspecified code   Manifestation code

518.0 Pulmonary collapse
Atelectasis
Collapse of lung
Middle lobe syndrome

Excludes: atelectasis:
congenital (partial) (770.5)
primary (770.4)
tuberculous, current disease (011.8)

518.1 Interstitial emphysema
Mediastinal emphysema

Excludes: surgical (subcutaneous) emphysema (998.81)
that in fetus or newborn (770.2)
traumatic emphysema (958.7)

518.2 Compensatory emphysema

518.3 Pulmonary eosinophilia
Eosinophilic asthma   Tropical eosinophilia
Löffler's syndrome
Pneumonia:
allergic
eosinophilic

Excludes: pulmonary infiltrate NOS (793.19)

518.4 Acute edema of lung, unspecified
Acute pulmonary edema NOS
Pulmonary edema, postoperative

Excludes: pulmonary edema:
acute, with mention of heart disease or failure (428.1)
chronic or unspecified (514)
due to external agents (506.0-508.9)

⑤ **518.5 Pulmonary insufficiency following trauma and surgery**

Excludes: adult respiratory distress syndrome associated with other conditions (518.82)
pneumonia:
aspiration (507.0)
hypostatic (514)
respiratory failure in other conditions (518.81, 518.83-518.84)

● **518.51 Acute respiratory failure following trauma and surgery**
Respiratory failure, not otherwise specified, following trauma and surgery

Excludes: acute respiratory failure in other conditions (518.81)

● **518.52 Other pulmonary insufficiency, not elsewhere classified, following trauma and surgery**
Adult respiratory distress syndrome
Pulmonary insufficiency following surgery
Pulmonary insufficiency following trauma
Shock lung related to trauma and surgery

Excludes: adult respiratory distress syndrome associated with other conditions (518.82)
aspiration pneumonia (507.0)
hypostatic pneumonia (514)
shock lung, not related to trauma or surgery (518.82)

● **518.53 Acute and chronic respiratory failure following trauma and surgery**

Excludes: acute and chronic respiratory failure in other conditions (518.84)

518.6 Allergic bronchopulmonary aspergillosis

518.7 Transfusion related acute lung injury (TRALI)

⑤ **518.8 Other diseases of lung**

518.81   Acute respiratory failure
Respiratory failure NOS

Excludes: *acute and chronic respiratory failure (518.84)*
acute respiratory distress (518.82)
acute respiratory failure following trauma and surgery (518.51)
chronic respiratory failure (518.83)
respiratory arrest (799.1)
respiratory failure, newborn (770.84)

ALERT! Code 518.81 may be assigned as a principal diagnosis when it is the condition established after study to be chiefly responsible for occasioning the admission to the hospital, and the selection is supported by the Alphabetic Index and Tabular List

518.82   Other pulmonary insufficiency, not elsewhere classified
Acute respiratory distress
Acute respiratory insufficiency
Adult respiratory distress syndrome NEC

Excludes: *acute interstitial pneumonitis (516.33)*
adult respiratory distress syndrome associated with trauma or surgery (518.52)
pulmonary insufficiency following trauma or surgery (518.52)
respiratory distress:
 NOS (786.09)
 newborn (770.89)
 syndrome, newborn (769)

518.83   Chronic respiratory failure

518.84   Acute and chronic respiratory failure
Acute or chronic respiratory failure

Excludes: *acute and chronic respiratory failure following trauma or surgery (518.53)*

518.89   Other diseases of lung, not elsewhere classified
Broncholithiasis   Lung disease NOS
Calcification of lung   Pulmolithiasis

519 **Other diseases of respiratory system**

ALERT! For personal history of other diseases of respiratory system see V12.69

⑤ **519.0   Tracheostomy complications**

519.00   Tracheostomy complication, unspecified

519.01   Infection of tracheostomy
Use additional code to identify type of infection, such as:
 abscess or cellulitis of neck (682.1)
 septicemia (038.0-038.9)
Use additional code to identify organism (041.00-041.9)

519.02   Mechanical complication of tracheostomy
Tracheal stenosis due to tracheostomy

519.09   Other tracheostomy complications
Hemorrhage due to tracheostomy
Tracheoesophageal fistula due to tracheostomy

⑤ **519.1   Other diseases of trachea and bronchus, not elsewhere classified**

519.11   Acute bronchospasm
Bronchospasm NOS

Excludes: *acute bronchitis with bronchospasm (466.0)*
asthma (493.00-493.92)
exercise induced bronchospasm (493.81)

519.19   Other diseases of trachea and bronchus
Calcification of bronchus or trachea
Stenosis of bronchus or trachea
Ulcer of bronchus or trachea

519.2   Mediastinitis

519.3   Other diseases of mediastinum, not elsewhere classified
Fibrosis of mediastinum
Hernia of mediastinum
Retraction of mediastinum

Add 4th or 5th digit   Nonspecific code   Unspecified code   Manifestation code

519.4 Disorders of diaphragm
    Diaphragmitis
    Paralysis of diaphragm
    Relaxation of diaphragm

    Excludes: *congenital defect of diaphragm (756.6)*
             diaphragmatic hernia (551-553 with .3)
                congenital (756.6)

519.8 Other diseases of respiratory system, not elsewhere classified

519.9 Unspecified disease of respiratory system
    Respiratory disease (chronic) NOS

    ALERT! For personal history of unspecified disease of respiratory system see V12.60

● Code new
   to this edition
▲ Revision of
   existing code
④ ⑤ Fourth or fifth
     digit required

Chapter 9: Diseases of Digestive System (520-579)

DEFINITIONS AND CODING ALERTS

This chapter includes definitions of selected key words, terms and phrases and coding alerts for adding points to the clinical domain, references to coding late effects where appropriate, and references to personal history V-codes in situations where the acute or chronic condition is no longer active. An example from this chapter is as follows:

⑤ **533** **Peptic ulcer, site unspecified**

> **DEFINITION** A Peptic ulcer is an ulcer of the mucous membrane lining of the alimentary tract.
>
> **ALERT!** For personal history of peptic ulcer disease see V12.71

MULTIPLE CODING FOR A SINGLE CONDITION

In addition to the etiology or manifestation convention that requires two codes to fully describe a single condition that affects multiple body systems, there are other single conditions that also require more than one code. "Use additional code" notes are found in the tabular at codes that are not part of an etiology or manifestation pair where a secondary code is useful to fully describe a condition. The sequencing rule is the same as the etiology or manifestation pair - , "use additional code" indicates that a secondary code should be added.

"Code first" notes are also under certain codes that are not specifically manifestation codes but may be due to an underlying cause. When a "code first" note is present and an underlying condition is present the underlying condition should be sequenced first.

"Code, if applicable, any causal condition first", notes indicate that this code may be assigned as a principal diagnosis when the causal condition is unknown or not applicable. If a causal condition is known, then the code for that condition should be sequenced as the principal or first-listed diagnosis. Multiple codes may be needed for late effects, complication codes and obstetric codes to more fully describe a condition. See the specific guidelines for these conditions for further instruction.

COMBINATION CODE

A combination code is a single code used to classify: two diagnoses, or a diagnosis with an associated secondary process (manifestation) A diagnosis with an associated complication Combination codes are identified by referring to subterm entries in the Alphabetic Index and by reading the inclusion and exclusion notes in the Tabular List.

Assign only the combination code when that code fully identifies the diagnostic conditions involved or when the Alphabetic Index so directs. Multiple coding should not be used when the classification provides a combination code that clearly identifies all of the elements documented in the diagnosis. When the combination code lacks necessary specificity in describing the manifestation or complication, an additional code should be used as a secondary code.

CODING LATE EFFECTS

A late effect is the residual effect (condition produced) after the acute phase of an illness or injury has terminated. There is no time limit on when a late effect code can be used. The residual may be apparent early, such as in cerebrovascular accident cases, or it may occur months or years later, such as that due to a previous injury. Coding of late effects generally requires two codes sequenced in the following order: The condition or nature of the late effect is sequenced first. The late effect code is sequenced second.

An exception to the above guidelines are those instances where the code for late effect is followed by a manifestation code identified in the Tabular List and title, or the late effect code has been expanded (at the fourth and fifth-digit levels) to include the manifestation(s). The code for the acute phase of an illness or injury that led to the late effect is never used with a code for the late effect.

| Add 4th or 5th digit | Nonspecific code | Unspecified code | Manifestation code |

This page intentionally left blank.

● Code new
   to this edition
▲ Revision of
   existing code
④ ⑤ Fourth or fifth
   digit required

9. DISEASES OF THE DIGESTIVE SYSTEM (520-579)

ALERT! For personal history of digestive disease see V12.7

DISEASES OF ORAL CAVITY, SALIVARY GLANDS, AND JAWS (520-529)

520 Disorders of tooth development and eruption

520.0 Anodontia
Absence of teeth (complete) (congenital) (partial)
Hypodontia
Oligodontia

Excludes: acquired absence of teeth (525.10-525.19)

520.1 Supernumerary teeth
Distomolar   Paramolar
Fourth molar   Supplemental teeth
Mesiodens

Excludes: supernumerary roots (520.2)

520.2 Abnormalities of size and form
Concrescence of teeth   Macrodontia
Fusion of teeth   Microdontia
Gemination of teeth   Peg-shaped [conical] teeth
Dens evaginatus   Supernumerary roots
Dens in dente   Taurodontism
Dens invaginatus   Tuberculum paramolare
Enamel pearls

Excludes: that due to congenital syphilis (090.5)
tuberculum Carabelli, which is regarded as a normal variation

520.3 Mottled teeth
Dental fluorosis
Mottling of enamel
Nonfluoride enamel opacities

520.4 Disturbances of tooth formation
Aplasia and hypoplasia of cementum   Horner's teeth
Dilaceration of tooth   Hypocalcification of teeth
Enamel hypoplasia (neonatal) (postnatal) Regional odontodysplasia
(prenatal)   Turner's tooth

Excludes: Hutchinson's teeth and mulberry molars in congenital syphilis (090.5)
mottled teeth (520.3)

520.5 Hereditary disturbances in tooth structure, not elsewhere classified
Amelogenesis imperfecta
Dentinogenesis imperfecta
Odontogenesis imperfecta
Dentinal dysplasia
Shell teeth

520.6 Disturbances of tooth eruption
Teeth: Tooth eruption:
embedded   late
impacted   obstructed
natal   premature
neonatal
prenatal
primary [deciduous]:
persistent
shedding, premature

Excludes: exfoliation of teeth (attributable to disease of surrounding tissues) (525.0-525.19)

520.7 Teething syndrome

520.8 Other specified disorders of tooth development and eruption
Color changes during tooth formation
Pre-eruptive color changes

Excludes: posteruptive color changes (521.7)

520.9 Unspecified disorder of tooth development and eruption

521 Diseases of hard tissue of teeth

⑤ **521.0 Dental caries**

521.00 Dental caries, unspecified

| | Add 4th or 5th digit | | Nonspecific code | | Unspecified code | | Manifestation code |

521.01 Dental caries limited to enamel
Initial caries
White spot lesion

521.02 Dental caries extending into dentine

521.03 Dental caries extending into pulp

521.04 Arrested dental caries

521.05 Odontoclasia
Infantile melanodontia
Melanodontoclasia

Excludes: *internal and external resorption of teeth (521.40-521.49)*

521.06 Dental caries pit and fissure
Primary dental caries, pit and fissure origin

521.07 Dental caries of smooth surface
Primary dental caries, smooth surface origin

521.08 Dental caries of root surface
Primary dental caries, root surface

521.09 Other dental caries

⑤ **521.1 Excessive attrition (approximal wear) (occlusal wear)**

521.10 Excessive attrition, unspecified

521.11 Excessive attrition, limited to enamel

521.12 Excessive attrition, extending into dentine

521.13 Excessive attrition, extending into pulp

521.14 Excessive attrition, localized

521.15 Excessive attrition, generalized

⑤ **521.2 Abrasion**
Abrasion of teeth:
dentifrice
habitual
occupational
ritual
traditional
Wedge defect NOS of teeth

521.20 Abrasion, unspecified

521.21 Abrasion, limited to enamel

521.22 Abrasion, extending into dentine

521.23 Abrasion, extending into pulp

521.24 Abrasion, localized

521.25 Abrasion, generalized

⑤ **521.3 Erosion**
Erosion of teeth: Erosion of teeth:
NOS   idiopathic
due to: occupational
medicine
persistent vomiting

521.30 Erosion, unspecified

521.31 Erosion, limited to enamel

521.32 Erosion, extending into dentine

521.33 Erosion, extending into pulp

521.34 Erosion, localized

521.35 Erosion, generalized

⑤ **521.4 Pathological resorption**

521.40 Pathological resorption, unspecified

521.41 Pathological resorption, internal

521.42 Pathological resorption, external

521.49 Other pathological resorption
Internal granuloma of pulp

521.5 Hypercementosis
Cementation hyperplasia

● Code new
to this edition

▲ Revision of
existing code

④ ⑤ Fourth or fifth
digit required

521.6   Ankylosis of teeth

521.7   Intrinsic posteruptive color changes
  Staining [discoloration] of teeth:
    NOS
    due to:
      drugs
      metals
      pulpal bleeding

  Excludes: *accretions [deposits] on teeth (523.6)*
         extrinsic color changes (523.6)
         pre-eruptive color changes (520.8)

⑤ **521.8   Other specific diseases of hard tissues of teeth**

   521.81   Cracked tooth

   Excludes: *asymptomatic craze lines in enamel – omit code*
          broken tooth due to trauma (873.63, 873.73)
          fractured tooth due to trauma (873.63, 873.73)

   521.89   Other specific diseases of hard tissues of teeth
         Irradiated enamel
         Sensitive dentin

521.9   Unspecified disease of hard tissues of teeth

522   Diseases of pulp and periapical tissues
   DEFINITION Pulp is the part in the center of a tooth made up of living soft tissue and cells called odontoblasts.

522.0   Pulpitis
  Pulpal: Pulpitis:
    abscess   acute
    polyp   chronic (hyperplastic) (ulcerative)
                              suppurative

522.1   Necrosis of the pulp
  Pulp gangrene

522.2   Pulp degeneration
  Denticles
  Pulp calcifications
  Pulp stones

522.3   Abnormal hard tissue formation in pulp
  Secondary or irregular dentin

522.4   Acute apical periodontitis of pulpal origin

522.5   Periapical abscess without sinus
  Abscess:
    dental
    dentoalveolar

  Excludes: *periapical abscess with sinus (522.7)*

522.6   Chronic apical periodontitis
  Apical or periapical granuloma
  Apical periodontitis NOS

522.7   Periapical abscess with sinus
  Fistula:
    alveolar process
    dental

522.8   Radicular cyst
  Cyst:
    apical (periodontal)
    periapical
    radiculodental
    residual radicular

  Excludes: *lateral developmental or lateral periodontal cyst (526.0)*

522.9   Other and unspecified diseases of pulp and periapical tissues

523   Gingival and periodontal diseases
   DEFINITION Gingival and periodontal diseases are diseases of the gums and/or tissue and bones that support the teeth

| | Add 4th or 5th digit | | Nonspecific code | | Unspecified code | | Manifestation code |

⑤ **523.0 Acute gingivitis**

> Excludes: *acute necrotizing ulcerative gingivitis (101)*
> *herpetic gingivostomatitis (054.2)*

523.00 Acute gingivitis, plaque induced
Acute gingivitis NOS

523.01 Acute gingivitis, non-plaque induced

⑤ **523.1 Chronic gingivitis**

Gingivitis (chronic):   Gingivitis (chronic):
desquamative   simple marginal
hyperplastic   ulcerative

> Excludes: *herpetic gingivostomatitis (054.2)*

523.10 Chronic gingivitis, plaque induced
Chronic gingivitis NOS
Gingivitis NOS

523.11 Chronic gingivitis, non-plaque induced

⑤ **523.2 Gingival recession**
Gingival recession (postinfective) (postoperative)

523.20 Gingival recession, unspecified

523.21 Gingival recession, minimal

523.22 Gingival recession, moderate

523.23 Gingival recession, severe

523.24 Gingival recession, localized

523.25 Gingival recession, generalized

⑤ **523.3 Aggressive and acute periodontitis**
Acute:
pericementitis
pericoronitis

> Excludes: *acute apical periodontitis (522.4)*
> *periapical abscess (522.5, 522.7)*

523.30 Aggressive periodontitis, unspecified

523.31 Aggressive periodontitis, localized
Periodontal abscess

523.32 Aggressive periodontitis, generalized

523.33 Aggressive periodontitis

⑤ **523.4 Chronic periodontitis**
Chronic pericoronitis
Pericementitis (chronic)
Periodontitis:
NOS
complex
simplex

> Excludes: *chronic apical periodontitis (522.6)*

523.40 Chronic periodontitis, unspecified

523.41 Chronic periodontitis, localized

523.42 Chronic periodontitis, generalized

523.5 Periodontosis

523.6 Accretions on teeth
Dental calculus:
subgingival
supragingival
Deposits on teeth:
betel
materia alba
soft
tartar
tobacco
Extrinsic discoloration of teeth

> Excludes: *intrinsic discoloration of teeth (521.7)*

523.8 Other specified periodontal diseases

Giant cell:
　epulis
　peripheral granuloma
Gingival:
　cysts
　enlargement NOS
　fibromatosis

Gingival polyp
Periodontal lesions due to traumatic occlusion
Peripheral giant cell granuloma

Excludes: *leukoplakia of gingiva (528.6)*

523.9 Unspecified gingival and periodontal disease

524 Dentofacial anomalies, including malocclusion

DEFINITION Dentofacial anomalies, including malocclusion, malocclusion is a misalignment of teeth and/or incorrect relation between the teeth of the two dental arches.

⑤ **524.0 Major anomalies of jaw size**

Excludes: *hemifacial atrophy or hypertrophy (754.0)*
　　　unilateral condylar hyperplasia or hypoplasia of mandible (526.89)

　524.00 Unspecified anomaly

　524.01 Maxillary hyperplasia

　524.02 Mandibular hyperplasia

　524.03 Maxillary hypoplasia

　524.04 Mandibular hypoplasia

　524.05 Macrogenia

　524.06 Microgenia

　524.07 Excessive tuberosity of jaw
　　Entire maxillary tuberosity

　524.09 Other specified anomaly

⑤ **524.1 Anomalies of relationship of jaw to cranial base**

　524.10 Unspecified anomaly
　　prognathism
　　retrognathism

　524.11 Maxillary asymmetry

　524.12 Other jaw asymmetry

　524.19 Other specified anomaly

⑤ **524.2 Anomalies of dental arch relationship**
　Anomaly of dental arch

Excludes: *hemifacial atrophy or hypertrophy (754.0)*
　　　soft tissue impingement (524.81-524.82)
　　　unilateral condylar hyperplasia or hypoplasia of mandible (526.89)

　524.20 Unspecified anomaly of dental arch relationship

　524.21 Malocclusion, Angle's class I
　　Neutro-occlusion

　524.22 Malocclusion, Angle's class II
　　Disto-occlusion Division I
　　Disto-occlusion Division II

　524.23 Malocclusion, Angle's class III
　　Mesio-occlusion

　524.24 Open anterior occlusal relationship
　　Anterior open bite

　524.25 Open posterior occlusal relationship
　　Posterior open bite

　524.26 Excessive horizontal overlap
　　Excessive horizontal overjet

　524.27 Reverse articulation
　　Anterior articulation
　　Crossbite
　　Posterior articulation

　524.28 Anomalies of interarch distance
　　Excessive interarch distance
　　Inadequate interarch distance

| | Add 4th or 5th digit | | Nonspecific code | | Unspecified code | | Manifestation code |

524.29 Other anomalies of dental arch relationship
  Other anomalies of dental arch

⑤ **524.3** Anomalies of tooth position of fully erupted teeth

Excludes: *impacted or embedded teeth with abnormal position of such teeth or adjacent teeth (520.6)*

524.30 Unspecified anomaly of tooth position
  Diastema of teeth NOS
  Displacement of teeth NOS
  Transposition of teeth NOS

524.31 Crowding of teeth

524.32 Excessive spacing of teeth

524.33 Horizontal displacement of teeth
  Tipped teeth
  Tipping of teeth

524.34 Vertical displacement of teeth
  Extruded tooth
  Infraeruption of teeth
  Intruded tooth
  Supraeruption of teeth

524.35 Rotation of tooth/teeth

524.36 Insufficient interocclusal distance of teeth (ridge)
  Lack of adequate intermaxillary vertical dimension

524.37 Excessive interocclusal distance of teeth
  Excessive intermaxillary vertical dimension
  Loss of occlusal vertical dimension

524.39 Other anomalies of tooth position

524.4 Malocclusion, unspecified

⑤ **524.5** Dentofacial functional abnormalities

524.50 Dentofacial functional abnormality, unspecified

524.51 Abnormal jaw closure

524.52 Limited mandibular range of motion

524.53 Deviation in opening and closing of the mandible

524.54 Insufficient anterior guidance
  Insufficient anterior occlusal guidance

524.55 Centric occlusion maximum intercuspation discrepancy
  Centric occlusion of teeth discrepancy

524.56 Non-working side interference
  Balancing side interference

524.57 Lack of posterior occlusal support

524.59 Other dentofacial functional abnormalities
  Abnormal swallowing
  Mouth breathing
  Sleep postures
  Tongue, lip, or finger habits

⑤ **524.6** Temporomandibular joint disorders

Excludes: *current temporomandibular joint:*
  dislocation (830.0-830.1)
  strain (848.1)

524.60 Temporomandibular joint disorders, unspecified
  Temporomandibular joint-pain-dysfunction syndrome [TMJ]

524.61 Adhesions and ankylosis (bony or fibrous)

524.62 Arthralgia of temporomandibular joint

524.63 Articular disc disorder (reducing or non-reducing)

524.64 Temporomandibular joint sounds on opening and/or closing the jaw

524.69 Other specified temporomandibular joint disorders

⑤ **524.7** Dental alveolar anomalies

524.70 Unspecified alveolar anomaly

524.71 Alveolar maxillary hyperplasia

524.72 Alveolar mandibular hyperplasia

● Code new
to this edition
▲ Revision of
existing code
④ ⑤ Fourth or fifth
digit required

524.73　Alveolar maxillary hypoplasia

524.74　Alveolar mandibular hypoplasia

524.75　Vertical displacement of alveolus and teeth
　　　　Extrusion of alveolus and teeth

524.76　Occlusal plane deviation

524.79　Other specified alveolar anomaly

⑤ 524.8　Other specified dentofacial anomalies

524.81　Anterior soft tissue impingement

524.82　Posterior soft tissue impingement

524.89　Other specified dentofacial anomalies

524.9　Unspecified dentofacial anomalies

525　Other diseases and conditions of the teeth and supporting structures
　　　ALERT! For personal history of other specified digestive system diseases see V12.79

525.0　Exfoliation of teeth due to systemic causes

⑤ 525.1　Loss of teeth due to trauma, extraction, or periodontal disease
Code first class of edentulism (525.40-525.44, 525.50-525.54)

525.10　Acquired absence of teeth, unspecified
　　　　Tooth extraction status, NOS

525.11　Loss of teeth due to trauma

525.12　Loss of teeth due to periodontal disease

525.13　Loss of teeth due to caries

525.19　Other loss of teeth

⑤ 525.2　Atrophy of edentulous alveolar ridge

525.20　Unspecified atrophy of edentulous alveolar ridge
　　　　Atrophy of the mandible NOS
　　　　Atrophy of the maxilla NOS

525.21　Minimal atrophy of the mandible

525.22　Moderate atrophy of the mandible

525.23　Severe atrophy of the mandible

525.24　Minimal atrophy of the maxilla

525.25　Moderate atrophy of the maxilla

525.26　Severe atrophy of the maxilla

525.3　Retained dental root

⑤ 525.4　Complete edentulism
Use additional code to identify cause of edentulism (525.10-525.19)

525.40　Complete edentulism, unspecified
　　　　Edentulism NOS

525.41　Complete edentulism, class I

525.42　Complete edentulism, class II

525.43　Complete edentulism, class III

525.44　Complete edentulism, class IV

⑤ 525.5　Partial edentulism
Use additional code to identify cause of edentulism (525.10-525.19)

525.50　Partial edentulism, unspecified

525.51　Partial edentulism, class I

525.52　Partial edentulism, class II

525.53　Partial edentulism, class III

525.54　Partial edentulism, class IV

⑤ 525.6　Unsatisfactory restoration of tooth
　　　　Defective bridge, crown, fillings
　　　　Defective dental restoration

Excludes: *dental restoration status (V45.84)*
　　　　　unsatisfactory endodontic treatment (526.61-526.69)

525.60　Unspecified unsatisfactory restoration of tooth
　　　　Unspecified defective dental restoration

459

	Add 4th or 5th digit		Nonspecific code		Unspecified code		Manifestation code

525.61 **Open restoration margins**
Dental restoration failure of marginal integrity
Open margin on tooth restoration

525.62 **Unrepairable overhanging of dental restorative materials**
Overhanging of tooth restoration

525.63 **Fractured dental restorative material without loss of material**
Excludes: *cracked tooth (521.81)*
fractured tooth (873.63, 873.73)

525.64 **Fractured dental restorative material with loss of material**
Excludes: *cracked tooth (521.81)*
fractured tooth (873.63, 873.73)

525.65 **Contour of existing restoration of tooth biologically incompatible with oral health**
Dental restoration failure of periodontal anatomical integrity
Unacceptable contours of existing restoration
Unacceptable morphology of existing restoration

525.66 **Allergy to existing dental restorative material**
Use additional code to identify the specific type of allergy

525.67 **Poor aesthetics of existing restoration**
Dental restoration aesthetically inadequate or displeasing

525.69 **Other unsatisfactory restoration of existing tooth**

⑤ **525.7 Endosseous dental implant failure**

525.71 **Osseointegration failure of dental implant**
Failure of dental implant due to infection
Failure of dental implant due to unintentional loading
Failure of dental implant osseointegration due to premature loading
Failure of dental implant to osseointegrate prior to intentional prosthetic loading
Hemorrhagic complications of dental implant placement
Iatrogenic osseointegration failure of dental implant
Osseointegration failure of dental implant due to complications of systemic disease
Osseointegration failure of dental implant due to poor bone quality
Pre-integration failure of dental implant NOS
Pre-osseointegration failure of dental implant

525.72 **Post-osseointegration biological failure of dental implant**
Failure of dental implant due to lack of attached gingiva
Failure of dental implant due to occlusal trauma (caused by poor prosthetic design)
Failure of dental implant to osseointegrate following intentional prosthetic loading
Failure of dental implant due to parafunctional habits
Failure of dental implant due to periodontal infection (peri-implantitis)
Failure of dental implant due to poor oral hygiene
Iatrogenic post-osseointegration failure of dental implant
Post-osseointegration failure of dental implant due to complications of systemic disease

525.73 **Post-osseointegration mechanical failure of dental implant**
Failure of dental prosthesis causing loss of dental implant
Fracture of dental implant
Mechanical failure of dental implant NOS

Excludes: *cracked tooth (521.81)*
fractured dental restorative material with loss of material (525.64)
fractured dental restorative material without loss of material (525.63)
fractured tooth (873.63, 873.73)

525.79 **Other endosseous dental implant failure**
Dental implant failure NOS

525.8 Other specified disorders of the teeth and supporting structures
Enlargement of alveolar ridge NOS
Irregular alveolar process

525.9 Unspecified disorder of the teeth and supporting structures

● Code new
to this edition
▲ Revision of
existing code
④ ⑤ Fourth or fifth
digit required

526 Diseases of the jaws

526.0 Developmental odontogenic cysts

Cyst:
  dentigerous
  eruption
  follicular
  lateral developmental

Cyst:
  lateral periodontal
  primordial
  Keratocyst

Excludes: radicular cyst (522.8)

526.1 Fissural cysts of jaw

Cyst:
  globulomaxillary
  incisor canal
  median anterior maxillary
  median palatal
  nasopalatine
  palatine of papilla

Excludes: cysts of oral soft tissues (528.4)

526.2 Other cysts of jaws

Cyst of jaw:
  NOS
  aneurysmal

Cyst of jaw:
  hemorrhagic
  traumatic

526.3 Central giant cell (reparative) granuloma

Excludes: peripheral giant cell granuloma (523.8)

526.4 Inflammatory conditions

Abscess of jaw (acute) (chronic) (suppurative)
Osteitis of jaw (acute) (chronic) (suppurative)
Osteomyelitis (neonatal) of jaw (acute) (chronic) (suppurative)
Periostitis of jaw (acute) (chronic) (suppurative)
Sequestrum of jaw bone

Excludes: alveolar osteitis (526.5)
         osteonecrosis of jaw (733.45)

526.5 Alveolitis of jaw

Alveolar osteitis
Dry socket

⑤ **526.6 Periradicular pathology associated with previous endodontic treatment**

526.61 Perforation of root canal space

526.62 Endodontic overfill

526.63 Endodontic underfill

526.69 Other periradicular pathology associated with previous endodontic treatment

⑤ **526.8 Other specified diseases of the jaws**

526.81 Exostosis of jaw
Torus mandibularis
Torus palatinus

526.89 Other
Cherubism of jaw(s)
Fibrous dysplasia of jaw(s)
Latent bone cyst of jaw(s)
Osteoradionecrosis of jaw(s)
Unilateral condylar hyperplasia or hypoplasia of mandible

526.9 Unspecified disease of the jaws

527 Diseases of the salivary glands

DEFINITION The salivary gland is a gland that secretes saliva, especially any of three pairs of large glands, the parotid, submaxillary, and sublingual, whose secretions enter the mouth and mingle in saliva

527.0 Atrophy

527.1 Hypertrophy

■■■ Add 4th or 5th digit   ■■■ Nonspecific code   ▢ Unspecified code   ■■■ Manifestation code

527.2 Sialoadenitis
Parotitis:
NOS
allergic
toxic
Sialoangitis
Sialodochitis

> Excludes: epidemic or infectious parotitis (072.0-072.9)
> uveoparotid fever (135)

527.3 Abscess

527.4 Fistula

> Excludes: congenital fistula of salivary glands (750.24)

527.5 Sialolithiasis
Calculus of salivary gland or duct
Stone of salivary gland or duct
Sialodocholithiasis

527.6 Mucocele
Mucous:
extravasation cyst of salivary gland
retention cyst of salivary gland
Ranula

527.7 Disturbance of salivary secretion
Hyposecretion
Ptyalism
Sialorrhea
Xerostomia

527.8 Other specified diseases of the salivary glands
Benign lymphoepithelial lesion of salivary gland
Sialectasia
Sialosis
Stenosis of salivary duct
Stricture of salivary duct

527.9 Unspecified disease of the salivary glands

528 Diseases of the oral soft tissues, excluding lesions specific for gingiva and tongue

⑤ **528.0 Stomatitis and mucositis (ulcerative)**

> Excludes: cellulitis and abscess of mouth (528.3)
> diphtheritic stomatitis (032.0)
> epizootic stomatitis (078.4)
> gingivitis (523.0-523.1)
> oral thrush (112.0)
> Stevens-Johnson syndrome (695.13)
> stomatitis:
> acute necrotizing ulcerative (101)
> aphthous (528.2)
> gangrenous (528.1)
> herpetic (054.2)
> Vincent's (101)

528.00 Stomatitis and mucositis, unspecified
Mucositis NOS
Ulcerative mucositis NOS
Ulcerative stomatitis NOS
Vesicular stomatitis NOS

528.01 Mucositis (ulcerative) due to antineoplastic therapy
Use additional E code to identify adverse effects of therapy, such as:
antineoplastic and immunosuppressive drugs (E930.7, E933.1)
radiation therapy (E879.2)

ALERT! For personal history of antineoplastic chemotherapy see V87.41

528.02 Mucositis (ulcerative) due to other drugs
Use additional E code to identify drug

528.09 Other stomatitis and mucositis (ulcerative)

528.1 Cancrum oris
Gangrenous stomatitis
Noma

462
● Code new
to this edition
▲ Revision of
existing code
④ ⑤ Fourth or fifth
digit required

528.2 Oral aphthae
Aphthous stomatitis
Canker sore
Periadenitis mucosa necrotica recurrens
Recurrent aphthous ulcer
Stomatitis herpetiformis

Excludes: herpetic stomatitis (054.2)

528.3 Cellulitis and abscess
Cellulitis of mouth (floor)
Ludwig's angina
Oral fistula

Excludes: abscess of tongue (529.0)
cellulitis or abscess of lip (528.5)
fistula (of):
  dental (522.7)
  lip (528.5)
gingivitis (523.00-523.11)

528.4 Cysts
Dermoid cyst of mouth
Epidermoid cyst of mouth
Epstein's pearl of mouth
Lymphoepithelial cyst of mouth
Nasoalveolar cyst of mouth
Nasolabial cyst of mouth

Excludes: cyst:
  gingiva (523.8)
  tongue (529.8)

528.5 Diseases of lips
Abscess of lip(s)
Cellulitis of lip(s)
Fistula of lip(s)
Hypertrophy of lip(s)
Cheilitis:
  NOS
  angular
Cheilodynia
Cheilosis

Excludes: actinic cheilitis (692.79)
congenital fistula of lip (750.25)
leukoplakia of lips (528.6)

528.6 Leukoplakia of oral mucosa, including tongue
Leukokeratosis of oral mucosa
Leukoplakia of:
  gingiva
  lips
  tongue

Excludes: carcinoma in situ (230.0, 232.0)
leukokeratosis nicotina palati (528.79)

⑤ 528.7 Other disturbances of oral epithelium, including tongue

Excludes: carcinoma in situ (230.0, 232.0)
leukokeratosis NOS (702.8)

528.71 Minimal keratinized residual ridge mucosa
Minimal keratinization of alveolar ridge mucosa

528.72 Excessive keratinized residual ridge mucosa
Excessive keratinization of alveolar ridge mucosa

528.79 Other disturbances of oral epithelium, including tongue
Erythroplakia of mouth or tongue
Focal epithelial hyperplasia of mouth or tongue
Leukoedema of mouth or tongue
Leukokeratosis nicotina palate
Other oral epithelium disturbances

528.8 Oral submucosal fibrosis, including of tongue

Add 4th or 5th digit   Nonspecific code   Unspecified code   Manifestation code

528.9 **Other and unspecified diseases of the oral soft tissues**
Cheek and lip biting
Denture sore mouth
Denture stomatitis
Melanoplakia
Papillary hyperplasia of palate
Eosinophilic granuloma of oral mucosa
Irritative hyperplasia of oral mucosa
Pyogenic granuloma of oral mucosa
Ulcer (traumatic) of oral mucosa

529 **Diseases and other conditions of the tongue**

529.0 **Glossitis**
Abscess of tongue
Ulceration (traumatic) of tongue

Excludes: glossitis:
benign migratory (529.1)
Hunter's (529.4)
median rhomboid (529.2)
Moeller's (529.4)

529.1 **Geographic tongue**
Benign migratory glossitis
Glossitis areata exfoliativa

529.2 **Median rhomboid glossitis**

529.3 **Hypertrophy of tongue papillae**
Black hairy tongue
Coated tongue
Hypertrophy of foliate papillae
Lingua villosa nigra

529.4 **Atrophy of tongue papillae**
Bald tongue   Glossodynia exfoliativa
Glazed tongue   Smooth atrophic tongue
Glossitis:
   Hunter's
   Moeller's

529.5 **Plicated tongue**
Fissured tongue
Furrowed tongue
Scrotal tongue

Excludes: *fissure of tongue, congenital (750.13)*

529.6 **Glossodynia**
Glossopyrosis
Painful tongue

Excludes: *glossodynia exfoliativa (529.4)*

529.8 **Other specified conditions of the tongue**
Atrophy (of) tongue
Crenated (of) tongue
Enlargement (of) tongue
Hypertrophy (of) tongue
Glossocele
Glossoptosis

Excludes: *erythroplasia of tongue (528.79)*
leukoplakia of tongue (528.6)
macroglossia (congenital) (750.15)
microglossia (congenital) (750.16)
oral submucosal fibrosis (528.8)

529.9 **Unspecified condition of the tongue**

DISEASES OF ESOPHAGUS, STOMACH, AND DUODENUM (530-539)

530 **Diseases of esophagus**

Excludes: *esophageal varices (456.0-456.2)*

DEFINITION The esophagus, the muscular membranous tube for the passage of food from the pharynx to the stomach; the gullet.

● Code new   ▲ Revision of   ④ ⑤ Fourth or fifth
   to this edition   existing code   digit required

530.0   Achalasia and cardiospasm
Achalasia (of cardia)
Aperistalsis of esophagus
Megaesophagus

Excludes: *congenital cardiospasm (750.7)*

⑤ **530.1   Esophagitis**
Esophagitis:
   chemical
   peptic
   postoperative
   regurgitant

Use additional E code, if desired, to identify cause, if induced by chemical

Excludes: *tuberculous esophagitis (017.8)*

   530.10   Esophagitis, unspecified
   Esophagitis NOS

   530.11   Reflux esophagitis

   530.12   Acute esophagitis

   530.13   Eosinophilic esophagitis

   530.19   Other esophagitis
   Abscess of esophagus

⑤ **530.2   Ulcer of esophagus**
Ulcer of esophagus
   fungal
   peptic
Ulcer of esophagus due to ingestion of:
   aspirin
   chemicals
   medicines

Use additional E code, if desired, to identify cause, if induced by chemical or drug

   530.20   Ulcer of esophagus without bleeding
   Ulcer of esophagus NOS

   530.21   Ulcer of esophagus with bleeding

Excludes: *bleeding esophageal varices (456.0, 456.20)*

530.3   Stricture and stenosis of esophagus
Compression of esophagus
Obstruction of esophagus

Excludes: *congenital stricture of esophagus (750.3)*

530.4   Perforation of esophagus
Rupture of esophagus

Excludes: *traumatic perforation of esophagus (862.22, 862.32, 874.4-874.5)*

530.5   Dyskinesia of esophagus
Corkscrew esophagus   Esophagospasm
Curling esophagus   Spasm of esophagus

Excludes: *cardiospasm (530.0)*

530.6   Diverticulum of esophagus, acquired
Diverticulum, acquired:
   epiphrenic
   pharyngoesophageal
   pulsion
   subdiaphragmatic
   traction
   Zenker's (hypopharyngeal)
Esophageal pouch, acquired
Esophagocele, acquired

Excludes: *congenital diverticulum of esophagus (750.4)*

530.7   Gastroesophageal laceration-hemorrhage syndrome
Mallory-Weiss syndrome

⑤ **530.8   Other specified disorders of esophagus**

   530.81   Esophageal reflux
   Gastroesophageal reflux

Excludes: *reflux esophagitis (530.11)*

 Add 4th or 5th digit   Nonspecific code   Unspecified code   Manifestation code

530.82 Esophageal hemorrhage

Excludes: *hemorrhage due to esophageal varices (456.0-456.2)*

530.83 Esophageal leukoplakia

530.84 Tracheoesophageal fistula

Excludes: *congenital tracheoesophageal fistula (750.3)*

530.85 Barrett's esophagus

530.86 Infection of esophagostomy

Use additional code to specify infection

530.87 Mechanical complication of esophagostomy

Malfunction of esophagostomy

530.89 Other

Excludes: *Paterson-Kelly syndrome (280.8)*

530.9 Unspecified disorder of esophagus

ALERT! For personal history of unspecified digestive disease see V12.70

⑤ **531 Gastric ulcer**

Includes: ulcer (peptic):
            prepyloric
            pylorus
            stomach

Use additional E code, if desired, to identify drug, if drug-induced

Excludes: *peptic ulcer NOS (533.0-533.9)*

The following fifth-digit subclassification is for use with category 531:

   0   without mention of obstruction

   1   with obstruction

   DEFINITION A Gastric ulcer is a hole in the lining of the stomach corroded by the acidic digestive juices which are secreted by the stomach cells.

⑤ **531.0 Acute with hemorrhage**
[0-1]

⑤ **531.1 Acute with perforation**
[0-1]

⑤ **531.2 Acute with hemorrhage and perforation**
[0-1]

⑤ **531.3 Acute without mention of hemorrhage or perforation**
[0-1]

⑤ **531.4 Chronic or unspecified with hemorrhage**
[0-1]

⑤ **531.5 Chronic or unspecified with perforation**
[0-1]

⑤ **531.6 Chronic or unspecified with hemorrhage and perforation**
[0-1]

⑤ **531.7 Chronic without mention of hemorrhage or perforation**
[0-1]

⑤ **531.9 Unspecified as acute or chronic, without mention of hemorrhage or perforation**
[0-1]

⑤ **532 Duodenal ulcer**

Includes: erosion (acute) of duodenum
            ulcer (peptic):
              duodenum
              postpyloric

Use additional E code, if desired, to identify drug, if drug-induced

Excludes: *peptic ulcer NOS (533.0-533.9)*

The following fifth-digit subclassification is for use with category 532:

   0   without mention of obstruction

   1   with obstruction

   DEFINITION A Duodenal ulcer is a ulcer in the lining of the first part of the small intestine (duodenum)

● Code new   ▲ Revision of   ④ ⑤ Fourth or fifth
         to this edition   existing code   digit required

⑤ **532.0** **Acute with hemorrhage**
[0-1]

⑤ **532.1** **Acute with perforation**
[0-1]

⑤ **532.2** **Acute with hemorrhage and perforation**
[0-1]

⑤ **532.3** **Acute without mention of hemorrhage or perforation**
[0-1]

⑤ **532.4** **Chronic or unspecified with hemorrhage**
[0-1]

⑤ **532.5** **Chronic or unspecified with perforation**
[0-1]

⑤ **532.6** **Chronic or unspecified with hemorrhage and perforation**
[0-1]

⑤ **532.7** **Chronic without mention of hemorrhage or perforation**
[0-1]

⑤ **532.9** **Unspecified as acute or chronic, without mention of hemorrhage or perforation**
[0-1]

⑤ **533** **Peptic ulcer, site unspecified**
    Includes: gastroduodenal ulcer NOS
              peptic ulcer NOS
              stress ulcer NOS

Use additional E code, if desired, to identify drug, if drug-induced

Excludes: *peptic ulcer:*
            duodenal (532.0-532.9)
            gastric (531.0-531.9)

The following fifth-digit subclassification is for use with category 533:

0 **without mention of obstruction**

1 **with obstruction**

DEFINITION A Peptic ulcer is an ulcer of the mucous membrane lining of the alimentary tract.

ALERT! For personal history of peptic ulcer disease see V12.71

⑤ **533.0** **Acute with hemorrhage**
[0-1]

⑤ **533.1** **Acute with perforation**
[0-1]

⑤ **533.2** **Acute with hemorrhage and perforation**
[0-1]

⑤ **533.3** **Acute without mention of hemorrhage and perforation**
[0-1]

⑤ **533.4** **Chronic or unspecified with hemorrhage**
[0-1]

⑤ **533.5** **Chronic or unspecified with perforation**
[0-1]

⑤ **533.6** **Chronic or unspecified with hemorrhage and perforation**
[0-1]

⑤ **533.7** **Chronic without mention of hemorrhage or perforation**
[0-1]

⑤ **533.9** **Unspecified as acute or chronic, without mention of hemorrhage or perforation**
[0-1]

ALERT! For personal history of unspecified digestive disease see V12.70

| | Add 4th or 5th digit | | Nonspecific code | | Unspecified code | | Manifestation code |

⑤ 534 **Gastrojejunal ulcer**
    Includes: ulcer (peptic) or erosion:
                anastomotic
                gastrocolic
                gastrointestinal
                gastrojejunal
                jejunal
                marginal
                stomal

   Excludes: *primary ulcer of small intestine (569.82)*
   The following fifth-digit subclassification is for use with category 534:

      0   without mention of obstruction

      1   with obstruction

⑤ **534.0 Acute with hemorrhage**
   [0-1]

⑤ **534.1 Acute with perforation**
   [0-1]

⑤ **534.2 Acute with hemorrhage and perforation**
   [0-1]

⑤ **534.3 Acute without mention of hemorrhage or perforation**
   [0-1]

⑤ **534.4 Chronic or unspecified with hemorrhage**
   [0-1]

⑤ **534.5 Chronic or unspecified with perforation**
   [0-1]

⑤ **534.6 Chronic or unspecified with hemorrhage and perforation**
   [0-1]

⑤ **534.7 Chronic without mention of hemorrhage or perforation**
   [0-1]

⑤ **534.9 Unspecified as acute or chronic, without mention of hemorrhage or perforation**
   [0-1]
      ALERT! For personal history of unspecified digestive disease see V12.70

⑤ 535 **Gastritis and duodenitis**
   The following fifth-digit subclassification is for use with category 535

      0   without mention of hemorrhage

      1   with hemorrhage
      DEFINITION Gastritis is an inflammation of the lining of the stomach; nausea and loss of appetite and discomfort after eating. Duodenitis is an inflammation of the duodenum. It may persist acutely or chronically

⑤ **535.0 Acute gastritis**
   [0-1]

⑤ **535.1 Atrophic gastritis**
   [0-1]   Gastritis:
                atrophic-hyperplastic
                chronic (atrophic)

⑤ **535.2 Gastric mucosal hypertrophy**
   [0-1]   Hypertrophic gastritis

⑤ **535.3 Alcoholic gastritis**
   [0-1]

⑤ **535.4 Other specified gastritis**
   [0-1]   Gastritis:
                allergic
                bile induced
                irritant
                superficial
                toxic

   Excludes: *eosinophilic gastritis (535.7)*

⑤ **535.5 Unspecified gastritis and gastroduodenitis**
   [0-1]

      ALERT! For personal history of unspecified digestive disease see V12.70

● Code new   ▲ Revision of   ④ ⑤ Fourth or fifth
              to this edition   existing code   digit required

⑤ **535.6 Duodenitis**
[0-1]

⑤ **535.7 Eosinophilic gastritis**
[0-1]

536 **Disorders of function of stomach**

Excludes: functional disorders of stomach specified as psychogenic (306.4)

536.0 Achlorhydria

536.1 Acute dilatation of stomach
Acute distention of stomach

536.2 Persistent vomiting
Cyclical vominting
Habit vomiting
Persistent vomiting [not of pregnancy]
Uncontrollable vomiting

Excludes: bilious emesis (vomiting) (787.04)
excessive vomiting in pregnancy (643.0-643.9)
vomiting NOS (787.03)
cyclical, associated with migraine (346.2)
vomiting of fecal matter (569.87)

536.3 Gastroparesis
Gastroparalysis
Code first underlying disease, if known, such as:
diabetes mellitus (249.6, 250.6)

⑤ **536.4 Gastrostomy complications**

536.40 Gastrostomy complications, unspecified

536.41 Infection of gastrostomy
Use additional code to specify type of infection, such as:
abscess or cellulitis of abdomen (682.2)
septicemia (038.0-038.9)
Use additional code to identify organism (041.00-041.9)

536.42 Mechanical complication of gastrostomy

536.49 Other gastrostomy complications

536.8 Dyspepsia and other specified disorders of function of stomach
Achylia gastrica   Hyperchlorhydria
Hourglass contraction of   Hypochlorhydria
  stomach   Indigestion
Hyperacidity   Tachygastria

Excludes: achlorhydria (536.0)
heartburn (787.1)

536.9 Unspecified functional disorder of stomach
Functional gastrointestinal:
disorder
disturbance
irritation

ALERT! For personal history of unspecified digestive disease see V12.70

537 **Other disorders of stomach and duodenum**
DEFINITION The duodenum is the beginning portion of the small intestine, starting at the lower end of the stomach and extending to the jejunum
ALERT! For personal history of other specified digestive system diseases see V12.79

537.0 Acquired hypertrophic pyloric stenosis
Constriction of pylorus, acquired or adult
Obstruction of pylorus, acquired or adult
Stricture of pylorus, acquired or adult

Excludes: congenital or infantile pyloric stenosis (750.5)

537.1 Gastric diverticulum

Excludes: congenital diverticulum of stomach (750.7)

537.2 Chronic duodenal ileus

| | Add 4th or 5th digit | | Nonspecific code | | Unspecified code | | Manifestation code |

537.3 Other obstruction of duodenum
Cicatrix of duodenum
Stenosis of duodenum
Stricture of duodenum
Volvulus of duodenum

Excludes: congenital obstruction of duodenum (751.1)

537.4 Fistula of stomach or duodenum
Gastrocolic fistula
Gastrojejunocolic fistula

537.5 Gastroptosis

537.6 Hourglass stricture or stenosis of stomach
Cascade stomach

Excludes: congenital hourglass stomach (750.7)
hourglass contraction of stomach (536.8)

⑤ **537.8 Other specified disorders of stomach and duodenum**

537.81 Pylorospasm

Excludes: congenital pylorospasm (750.5)

537.82 Angiodysplasia of stomach and duodenum without mention of hemorrhage

537.83 Angiodysplasia of stomach and duodenum with hemorrhage

537.84 Dieulafoy lesion (hemorrhagic) of stomach and duodenum

537.89 Other
Gastric or duodenal:
  prolapse
  rupture
Intestinal metaplasia of gastric mucosa
Passive congestion of stomach

Excludes: diverticula of duodenum (562.00-562.01)
gastrointestinal hemorrhage (578.0-578.9)

537.9 Unspecified disorder of stomach and duodenum
ALERT! For personal history of unspecified digestive disease see V12.70

538 Gastrointestinal mucositis (ulcerative)
Use additional E code to identify adverse effects of therapy, such as:
  antineoplastic and immunosuppressive drugs (E930.7, E933.1)
  radiation therapy (E879.2)

Excludes: mucositis (ulcerative) of mouth and oral soft tissue (528.00-528.09)

DEFINITION Gastrointestinal mucositis (ulcerative) is the inflammation of a mucous membrane of the gastrointestinal system

● **539 Complications of bariatric procedures**
  ● **539.0 Complications of gastric band procedure**
    ● **539.01 Infection due to gastric band procedure**
    Use additional code to specify type of infection, such as:
      abscess or cellulitis of abdomen (682.2)
      septicemia (038.0-038.9)
    Use additional code to identify organism (041.00-041.9)

    ● **539.09 Other complications of gastric band procedure**
    Use additional code(s) to further specify complication

  ● **539.8 Complications of other bariatric procedure**
    Excludes: complications of gastric band surgery (539.01-539.09)

    ● **539.81 Infection due to other bariatric procedure**
    Use additional code to specify type of infection, such as:
      abscess or cellulitis of abdomen (682.2)
      septicemia (038.0-038.9)
    Use additional code to identify organism (041.00-041.9)

    ● **539.89 Other complications of other bariatric procedure**
    Use additional code(s) to further specify complication

● Code new
to this edition
▲ Revision of
existing code
④ ⑤ Fourth or fifth
digit required

APPENDICITIS (540-543)

540 **Acute appendicitis**

> **DEFINITION** Appendicitis is an inflammation of the appendix, which is the worm-shaped pouch attached to the cecum, the beginning of the large intestine

540.0 With generalized peritonitis
Appendicitis (acute):
  fulminating with: perforation, peritonitis (generalized), rupture
  gangrenous with: perforation, peritonitis (generalized), rupture
  obstructive with: perforation, peritonitis (generalized), rupture
Cecitis (acute) with: perforation peritonitis (generalized) rupture
Rupture of appendix

> Excludes: acute appendicitis with peritoneal abscess (540.1)

540.1 With peritoneal abscess
Abscess of appendix
With generalized peritonitis

540.9 Without mention of peritonitis
Acute:
  appendicitis:
    fulminating without mention of perforation, peritonitis, or rupture
    gangrenous without mention of perforation, peritonitis, or rupture
    inflamed without mention of perforation, peritonitis, or rupture
    obstructive without mention of perforation, peritonitis, or rupture
    cecitis without mention of perforation, peritonitis, or rupture

541 **Appendicitis, unqualified**

542 **Other appendicitis**

Appendicitis: Appendicitis:
  chronic   relapsing
  recurrent   subacute

> Excludes: hyperplasia (lymphoid) of appendix (543.0)

> **ALERT!** For personal history of other specified digestive system diseases see V12.79

543 **Other diseases of appendix**

> **ALERT!** For personal history of other specified digestive system diseases see V12.79

543.0 Hyperplasia of appendix (lymphoid)

543.9 Other and unspecified diseases of appendix
Appendicular or appendiceal:
  colic
  concretion
  fistula
Diverticulum of appendix
Fecalith of appendix
Intussusception of appendix
Mucocele of appendix
Stercolith of appendix

HERNIA OF ABDOMINAL CAVITY (550-553)

Includes: hernia:
             acquired
             congenital, except diaphragmatic or hiatal

⑤ **550** **Inguinal hernia**
Includes: bubonocele
             inguinal hernia (direct) (double) (indirect) (oblique) (sliding)
             scrotal hernia

The following fifth-digit subclassification is for use with category 550:

0 **unilateral or unspecified (not specified as recurrent)**
       Unilateral NOS

1 **unilateral or unspecified, recurrent**

2 **bilateral (not specified as recurrent)**
       Bilateral NOS

3 **bilateral, recurrent**

> **DEFINITION** Inguinal hernia, protrusion of the abdominal viscera through the inguinal canal.

⑤ **550.0 Inguinal hernia, with gangrene**
[0-3]   Inguinal hernia with gangrene (and obstruction)

	Add 4th or 5th digit		Nonspecific code		Unspecified code		Manifestation code

⑤ **550.1 Inguinal hernia, with obstruction, without mention of gangrene**
[0-3] Inguinal hernia with mention of incarceration, irreducibility, or strangulation

⑤ **550.9 Inguinal hernia, without mention of obstruction or gangrene**
[0-3] Inguinal hernia NOS

551 Other hernia of abdominal cavity, with gangrene
Includes: that with gangrene (and obstruction)

DEFINITION Gangrene is the decay or death of an organ or tissue caused by a lack of blood supply. It is a complication resulting from infectious or inflammatory processes, injury, or degenerative changes associated with chronic diseases, such as diabetes mellitus.

ALERT! For personal history of other specified digestive system diseases see V12.79

⑤ **551.0 Femoral hernia with gangrene**

 551.00 Unilateral or unspecified (not specified as recurrent)
Femoral hernia NOS with gangrene

 551.01 Unilateral or unspecified, recurrent

 551.02 Bilateral (not specified as recurrent)

 551.03 Bilateral, recurrent

551.1 Umbilical hernia with gangrene
Parumbilical hernia specified as gangrenous

⑤ **551.2 Ventral hernia with gangrene**

 551.20 Ventral, unspecified, with gangrene

 551.21 Incisional, with gangrene
Hernia:
  postoperative specified as gangrenous
  recurrent, ventral specified as gangrenous

 551.29 Other
Epigastric hernia specified as gangrenous

551.3 Diaphragmatic hernia with gangrene
Hernia:
  hiatal (esophageal) (sliding) specified as gangrenous
  paraesophageal specified as gangrenous
Thoracic stomach specified as gangrenous

Excludes: congenital diaphragmatic hernia (756.6)

551.8 Hernia of other specified sites, with gangrene
Any condition classifiable to 553.8 if specified as gangrenous

551.9 Hernia of unspecified site, with gangrene
Any condition classifiable to 553.9 if specified as gangrenous

552 Other hernia of abdominal cavity, with obstruction, but without mention of gangrene

Excludes: that with mention of gangrene (551.0-551.9)

ALERT! For personal history of other specified digestive system diseases see V12.79

⑤ **552.0 Femoral hernia with obstruction**
Femoral hernia specified as incarcerated, irreducible, strangulated, or causing obstruction

 552.00 Unilateral or unspecified (not specified as recurrent)

 552.01 Unilateral or unspecified, recurrent

 552.02 Bilateral (not specified as recurrent)

 552.03 Bilateral, recurrent

552.1 Umbilical hernia with obstruction
Parumbilical hernia specified as incarcerated, irreducible, strangulated, or causing obstruction

⑤ **552.2 Ventral hernia with obstruction**
Ventral hernia specified as incarcerated, irreducible, strangulated, or causing obstruction

 552.20 Ventral, unspecified, with obstruction

 552.21 Incisional, with obstruction
Hernia:
  postoperative specified as incarcerated, irreducible, strangulated, or causing obstruction
  recurrent, ventral specified as incarcerated, irreducible, strangulated, or causing obstruction

 552.29 Other
Epigastric hernia specified as incarcerated, irreducible, strangulated, or causing obstruction

● Code new to this edition   ▲ Revision of existing code   ④ ⑤ Fourth or fifth digit required

552.3 Diaphragmatic hernia with obstruction
Hernia:
hiatal (esophageal) (sliding), specified as incarcerated, irreducible, strangulated, or causing obstruction
paraesophageal, specified as incarcerated, irreducible, strangulated, or causing obstruction
Thoracic stomach, specified as incarcerated, irreducible, strangulated, or causing obstruction

Excludes: congenital diaphragmatic hernia (756.6)

552.8 Hernia of other specified sites, with obstruction
Any condition classifiable to 553.8 if specified as incarcerated, irreducible, strangulated, or causing obstruction

552.9 Hernia of unspecified site, with obstruction
Any condition classifiable to 553.9 if specified as incarcerated, irreducible, strangulated, or causing obstruction

553 Other hernia of abdominal cavity without mention of obstruction or gangrene

Excludes: the listed conditions with mention of:
gangrene (and obstruction) (551.0-551.9)
obstruction (552.0-552.9)

ALERT! For personal history of other specified digestive system diseases see V12.79

⑤ **553.0 Femoral hernia**

553.00 Unilateral or unspecified (not specified as recurrent)
Femoral hernia NOS

553.01 Unilateral or unspecified, recurrent

553.02 Bilateral (not specified as recurrent)

553.03 Bilateral, recurrent

553.1 Umbilical hernia
Parumbilical hernia

⑤ **553.2 Ventral hernia**

553.20 Ventral, unspecified

553.21 Incisional
Hernia:
postoperative
recurrent, ventral

553.29 Other
Hernia:
epigastric
spigelian

553.3 Diaphragmatic hernia
Hernia:
hiatal (esophageal) (sliding)
paraesophageal
Thoracic stomach

Excludes: congenital:
diaphragmatic hernia (756.6)
hiatal hernia (750.6)
esophagocele (530.6)

553.8 Hernia of other specified sites
Hernia:
ischiatic
ischiorectal
lumbar
obturator
pudendal

Hernia:
retroperitoneal
sciatic
Other abdominal hernia of specified site

Excludes: vaginal enterocele (618.6)

553.9 Hernia of unspecified site
Enterocele
Epiplocele
Hernia:
NOS
interstitial

Hernia:
intestinal
intra-abdominal
Rupture (nontraumatic)
Sarcoepiplocele

Add 4th or 5th digit | Nonspecific code | Unspecified code | Manifestation code

NONINFECTIOUS ENTERITIS AND COLITIS (555-558)

555 Regional enteritis
Includes: Crohn's disease
Granulomatous enteritis

Excludes: ulcerative colitis (556)

DEFINITION Regional enteritis refers to inflammation of the intestinal tract, especially of the small intestine

555.0 Small intestine
Ileitis:
regional
segmental
terminal

Regional enteritis or Crohn's disease of:
duodenum
ileum
jejunum

555.1 Large intestine
Colitis:
granulomatous
regional
transmural

Regional enteritis or Crohn's disease of:
colon
large bowel
rectum

555.2 Small intestine with large intestine
Regional ileocolitis

555.9 Unspecified site
Crohn's disease NOS
Regional enteritis NOS

556 Ulcerative colitis
DEFINITION Ulcerative colitis ulcerative colitis is a form of inflammatory bowel disease (ibd). It causes swelling, ulcerations, and loss of function of the large intestine

556.0 Ulcerative (chronic) enterocolitis

556.1 Ulcerative (chronic) ileocolitis

556.2 Ulcerative (chronic) proctitis

556.3 Ulcerative (chronic) proctosigmoiditis

556.4 Pseudopolyposis of colon

556.5 Left-sided ulcerative (chronic) colitis

556.6 Universal ulcerative (chronic) colitis
Pancolitis

556.8 Other ulcerative colitis

556.9 Ulcerative colitis, unspecified
Ulcerative enteritis NOS
ALERT! For personal history of unspecified digestive disease see V12.70

557 Vascular insufficiency of intestine
Excludes: necrotizing enterocolitis of the newborn (777.50-777.53)

DEFINITION Vascular insufficiency of intestine, refers to inadequate peripheral blood flow to the intestines

557.0 Acute vascular insufficiency of intestine
Acute:
hemorrhagic enterocolitis
ischemic colitis, enteritis, or enterocolitis
massive necrosis of intestine
Bowel infarction
Embolism of mesenteric artery
Fulminant enterocolitis
Hemorrhagic necrosis of intestine
Infarction of appendices epiploicae
Intestinal gangrene
Intestinal infarction (acute) (agnogenic) (hemorrhagic) (nonocclusive)
Mesenteric infarction (embolic) (thrombotic)
Necrosis of intestine
Terminal hemorrhagic enteropathy
Thrombosis of mesenteric artery

● Code new to this edition   ▲ Revision of existing code   ④ ⑤ Fourth or fifth digit required

557.1 Chronic vascular insufficiency of intestine
Angina, abdominal
Chronic ischemic colitis, enteritis, or enterocolitis
Ischemic stricture of intestine
Mesenteric:
angina
artery syndrome (superior)
vascular insufficiency

557.9 Unspecified vascular insufficiency of intestine
Alimentary pain due to vascular insufficiency
Ischemic colitis, enteritis, or enterocolitis NOS
ALERT! For personal history of unspecified digestive disease see V12.70

558 Other and unspecified noninfectious gastroenteritis and colitis
Excludes: infectious:
colitis, enteritis, or gastroenteritis (009.0-009.1)
diarrhea (009.2-009.3)
ALERT! For personal history of other specified digestive system diseases see V12.79

558.1 Gastroenteritis and colitis due to radiation
Radiation enterocolitis

558.2 Toxic gastroenteritis and colitis
Use additional E code, if desired, to identify cause

558.3 Allergic gastroenteritis and colitis
Use additional code to identify type of food allergy (V15.01-V15.05)

⑤ **558.4 Eosinophilic gastroenteritis and colitis**

   558.41 Eosinophilic gastroenteritis
   Eosinophilic enteritis

   558.42 Eosinophilic colitis

558.9 Other and unspecified noninfectious gastroenteritis and colitis
Colitis NOS, dietetic, or noninfectious
Enteritis NOS, dietetic, or noninfectious
Gastroenteritis NOS, dietetic, or noninfectious
Ileitis NOS, dietetic, or noninfectious
Jejunitis NOS, dietetic, or noninfectious
Sigmoiditis NOS, dietetic, or noninfectious

OTHER DISEASES OF INTESTINES AND PERITONEUM (560-569)

560 Intestinal obstruction without mention of hernia
Excludes: duodenum (537.2-537.3)
inguinal hernia with obstruction (550.1)
intestinal obstruction complicating hernia (552.0-552.9)
mesenteric:
embolism (557.0)
infarction (557.0)
thrombosis (557.0)
neonatal intestinal obstruction (277.01, 777.1-777.2, 777.4)
DEFINITION Intestinal obstruction without mention of hernia, a blockage in the intestine which prevents the normal flow of waste down the length of the intestine

560.0 Intussusception
Intussusception (colon) (intestine) (rectum)
Invagination of intestine or colon
Excludes: intussusception of appendix (543.9)

560.1 Paralytic ileus
Adynamic ileus
Ileus (of intestine) (of bowel) (of colon)
Paralysis of intestine or colon
Excludes: gallstone ileus (560.31)

560.2 Volvulus
Knotting of intestine, bowel, or colon
Strangulation of intestine, bowel, or colon
Torsion of intestine, bowel, or colon
Twist of intestine, bowel, or colon

| | Add 4th or 5th digit | | Nonspecific code | | Unspecified code | | Manifestation code |

⑤ **560.3 Impaction of intestine**

> **560.30** **Impaction of intestine, unspecified**
> Impaction of colon

> **560.31** **Gallstone ileus**
> Obstruction of intestine by gallstone

> **560.32** **Fecal impaction**

> *Excludes:* *constipation (564.00-564.09)*
> *incomplete defecation (787.61)*

> **560.39** **Other**
> Concretion of intestine
> Enterolith

⑤ **560.8 Other specified intestinal obstruction**

> **560.81** **Intestinal or peritoneal adhesions with obstruction (postoperative)**
> **(postinfection)**

> *Excludes:* *adhesions without obstruction (568.0)*

> **560.89** **Other**
> Acute pseudo-obstruction of intestine
> Mural thickening causing obstruction

> *Excludes:* *ischemic stricture of intestine (557.1)*

560.9 Unspecified intestinal obstruction
> Enterostenosis
> Obstruction of intestine or colon
> Occlusion of intestine or colon
> Stenosis of intestine or colon
> Stricture of intestine or colon

> *Excludes:* *congenital stricture or stenosis of intestine (751.1-751.2)*

> **ALERT!** For personal history of unspecified digestive disease see V12.70

562 **Diverticula of intestine**
Use additional code, if desired, to identify any associated:
> peritonitis (567.0-567.9)

> *Excludes:* *congenital diverticulum of colon (751.5)*
> *diverticulum of appendix (543.9)*
> *Meckel's diverticulum (751.0)*

> **DEFINITION** A diverticulum of the colon is a sac or pouch in the colon walls which is usually asymptomatic (without symptoms) but may cause difficulty if it becomes inflamed

⑤ **562.0 Small intestine**

> **562.00** **Diverticulosis of small intestine (without mention of hemorrhage)**
> Diverticulosis:
> duodenum without mention of diverticulitis
> ileum without mention of diverticulitis
> jejunum without mention of diverticulitis

> **562.01** **Diverticulitis of small intestine (without mention of hemorrhage)**
> Diverticulitis (with diverticulosis):
> duodenum
> ileum
> jejunum
> small intestine

> **562.02** **Diverticulosis of small intestine with hemorrhage**

> **562.03** **Diverticulitis of small intestine with hemorrhage**

⑤ **562.1 Colon**

> **562.10** **Diverticulosis of colon (without mention of hemorrhage)**
> Diverticulosis:
> NOS without mention of diverticulitis
> intestine (large) without mention of diverticulitis
> Diverticular disease (colon) without mention of diverticulitis

> **562.11** **Diverticulitis of colon (without mention of hemorrhage)**
> Diverticulitis (with diverticulosis):
> NOS
> colon
> intestine (large)

> **562.12** **Diverticulosis of colon with hemorrhage**

> **562.13** **Diverticulitis of colon with hemorrhage**

● Code new
to this edition

▲ Revision of
existing code

④ ⑤ Fourth or fifth
digit required

564 **Functional digestive disorders, not elsewhere classified**

> *Excludes:* *functional disorders of stomach (536.0-536.9)*
> *those specified as psychogenic (306.4)*

DEFINITION Functional digestive disorders are a group of disorders, which include irritable bowel syndrome or ibs, dyspepsia, gerd, and chronic constipation or diarrhea

⑤ **564.0** **Constipation**

> *Excludes:* *fecal impaction (560.32)*
> *incomplete defecation (787.61)*

     564.00 **Constipation, unspecified**

     564.01 **Slow transit constipation**

     564.02 **Outlet dysfunction constipation**

     564.09 **Other constipation**

564.1 **Irritable bowel syndrome**
Irritable colon   Spastic colon

564.2 **Postgastric surgery syndromes**
Dumping syndrome   Postgastrectomy syndrome
Jejunal syndrome   Postvagotomy syndrome

> *Excludes:* *malnutrition following gastrointestinal surgery (579.3)*
> *postgastrojejunostomy ulcer (534.0-534.9)*

564.3 **Vomiting following gastrointestinal surgery**
Vomiting (bilious) following gastrointestinal surgery

564.4 **Other postoperative functional disorders**
Diarrhea following gastrointestinal surgery

> *Excludes:* *colostomy and enterostomy complications (569.60-569.69)*

564.5 **Functional diarrhea**

> *Excludes:* *diarrhea:*
> *NOS (787.91)*
> *psychogenic (306.4)*

564.6 **Anal spasm**
Proctalgia fugax

564.7 **Megacolon, other than Hirschsprung's**
Dilatation of colon

> *Excludes:* *megacolon:*
> *congenital [Hirschsprung's] (751.3)*
> *toxic (556)*

⑤ **564.8** **Other specified functional disorders of intestine**

> *Excludes:* *malabsorption (579.0-579.9)*

     564.81 **Neurogenic bowel**

     564.89 **Other functional disorders of intestine**
             Atony of colon

564.9 **Unspecified functional disorder of intestine**

ALERT! For personal history of unspecified digestive disease see V12.70

565 **Anal fissure and fistula**

DEFINITION An anal fissure is a crack-like sore in the anal region. It is the commonest reason for pain in this area. An anal fistula is a channel that develops between the anus and the skin. Most fistulas are the result of an abscess that spreads to the skin

565.0 **Anal fissure**

> *Excludes:* *anal sphincter tear (healed) (non-traumatic) (old) (569.43)*
> *traumatic (863.89, 863.99)*

565.1 **Anal fistula**
Fistula:
     anorectal
     rectal
     rectum to skin

> *Excludes:* *fistula of rectum to internal organs—see Alphabetic Index*
> *ischiorectal fistula (566)*
> *rectovaginal fistula (619.1)*

| | Add 4th or 5th digit | | Nonspecific code | | Unspecified code | | Manifestation code |

566   Abscess of anal and rectal regions
  Abscess:
    ischiorectal
    perianal
    perirectal
  Cellulitis:
    anal
    perirectal
    rectal
  Ischiorectal fistula
  ALERT! ICD-9-CM codes in the Category 566 add points to the clinical domain as a Skin 2 diagnosis

567   Peritonitis and retroperitoneal infections
  Excludes: peritonitis:
      benign paroxysmal (277.31)
      pelvic, female (614.5, 614.7)
      periodic familial (277.31)
      puerperal (670.8)
      with or following:
        abortion (634-638 with .0, 639.0)
        appendicitis (540.0-540.1)
        ectopic or molar pregnancy (639.0)
  DEFINITION Peritonitis is an inflammation of the membrane which lines the inside of the abdomen and all of the internal organs.

  567.0   Peritonitis in infectious diseases classified elsewhere
    Code first underlying disease
    Excludes: peritonitis:
        gonococcal (098.86)
        syphilitic (095.2)
        tuberculous (014.0)

  567.1   Pneumococcal peritonitis
  ⑤ **567.2   Other suppurative peritonitis**
      567.21   Peritonitis (acute) generalized
        Pelvic peritonitis, male

      567.22   Peritoneal abscess
        Abscess (of):   Abscess (of):
          abdominopelvic   retrocecal
          mesenteric   subdiaphragmatic
          omentum   subhepatic
          peritoneum   subphrenic

      567.23   Spontaneous bacterial peritonitis
      Excludes: bacterial peritonitis NOS (567.29)

        567.29   Other suppurative peritonitis
          Subphrenic peritonitis

  ⑤ **567.3   Retroperitoneal infections**
      567.31   Psoas muscle abscess
      567.38   Other retroperitoneal abscess
      567.39   Other retroperitoneal infections
  ⑤ **567.8   Other specified peritonitis**
      567.81   Choleperitonitis
        Peritonitis due to bile

      567.82   Sclerosing mesenteritis
        Fat necrosis of peritoneum
        (Idiopathic) sclerosing mesenteric fibrosis
        Mesenteric lipodystrophy
        Mesenteric panniculitis
        Retractile mesenteritis

      567.89   Other specified peritonitis
        Chronic proliferative peritonitis
        Mesenteric saponification
        Peritonitis due to urine

● Code new to this edition   ▲ Revision of existing code   ④ ⑤ Fourth or fifth digit required

567.9 Unspecified peritonitis
Peritonitis:
NOS
of unspecified cause *

ALERT! For personal history of unspecified digestive disease see V12.70

568 Other disorders of peritoneum

DEFINITION The peritoneum is the membrane that lines the abdominal cavity and covers most of the abdominal organs

ALERT! For personal history of other specified digestive system diseases see V12.79

568.0 Peritoneal adhesions (postoperative) (postinfection)

Adhesions (of):	Adhesions (of):
abdominal (wall)	mesenteric
diaphragm	omentum
intestine	stomach
male pelvis	Adhesive bands

Excludes: adhesions:
pelvic, female (614.6)
with obstruction:
duodenum (537.3)
intestine (560.81)

⑤ **568.8 Other specified disorders of peritoneum**

568.81 Hemoperitoneum (nontraumatic)

568.82 Peritoneal effusion (chronic)

Excludes: ascites NOS (789.51-789.59)

568.89 Other
Peritoneal:
cyst
granuloma

568.9 Unspecified disorder of peritoneum

ALERT! For personal history of unspecified digestive disease see V12.70

569 Other disorders of intestine

ALERT! For personal history of other specified digestive system diseases see V12.79

569.0 Anal and rectal polyp
Anal and rectal polyp NOS

Excludes: adenomatous anal and rectal polyp (211.4)

569.1 Rectal prolapse

Procidentia:	Prolapse:
anus (sphincter)	anal canal
rectum (sphincter)	rectal mucosa
Proctoptosis	

Excludes: prolapsed hemorrhoids (455.2, 455.5)

569.2 Stenosis of rectum and anus
Stricture of anus (sphincter)

569.3 Hemorrhage of rectum and anus

Excludes: gastrointestinal bleeding NOS (578.9)
melena (578.1)

⑤ **569.4 Other specified disorders of rectum and anus**

569.41 Ulcer of anus and rectum
Solitary ulcer of anus (sphincter) or rectum (sphincter)
Stercoral ulcer of anus (sphincter) or rectum (sphincter)

569.42 Anal or rectal pain

569.43 Anal sphincter tear (healed) (old)
Tear of anus, nontraumatic

Use additional code for any associated fecal incontinence (787.60-787.63)

Excludes: anal fissure (565.0)
anal sphincter tear (healed) (old) complicating delivery (654.8)

Add 4th or 5th digit	Nonspecific code	Unspecified code	Manifestation code

569.44 Dysplasia of anus
Anal intraepithelial neoplasia I and II (AIN I and II) (histologically confirmed)
Dysplasia of anus NOS
Mild and moderate dysplasia of anus (histologically confirmed)

Excludes: *abnormal results from anal cytologic examination without histologic confirmation*
(796.70-796.79)
anal intraepithelial neoplasia III (230.5, 230.6)
carcinoma in situ of anus (230.5, 230.6)
HGSIL of anus (796.74)
severe dysplasia of anus (230.5, 230.6)

569.49 Other
Granuloma of rectum (sphincter)
Rupture of rectum (sphincter)
Hypertrophy of anal papillae
Proctitis NOS

Use additional code for any associated fecal incontinence (787.60-787.63)

Excludes: *fistula of rectum to:*
internal organs—see Alphabetic Index
skin (565.1)
hemorrhoids (455.0-455.9)

569.5 Abscess of intestine
Excludes: *appendiceal abscess (540.1)*

⑤ **569.6 Colostomy and enterostomy complications**

569.60 Colostomy and enterostomy complication, unspecified

569.61 Infection of colostomy or enterostomy
Use additional code to specify type of infection, such as:
abscess or cellulitis of abdomen (682.2)
septicemia (038.0-038.9)
Use additional code to identify organism (041.00-041.9)

569.62 Mechanical complication of colostomy and enterostomy
Malfunction of colostomy and enterostomy

569.69 Other complication
Fistula
Hernia
Prolapse

⑤ **569.7 Complications of intestinal pouch**

569.71 Pouchitis
Inflammation of internal ileoanal pouch

569.79 Other complications of intestinal pouch

⑤ **569.8 Other specified disorders of intestine**

569.81 Fistula of intestine, excluding rectum and anus
Fistula: Fistula:
abdominal wall   enteroenteric
enterocolic   ileorectal

Excludes: *fistula of intestine to internal organs —see Alphabetic Index*
persistent postoperative fistula (998.6)

569.82 Ulceration of intestine
Primary ulcer of intestine
Ulceration of colon

Excludes: *that with perforation (569.83)*

569.83 Perforation of intestine

569.84 Angiodysplasia of intestine (without mention of hemorrhage)

569.85 Angiodysplasia of intestine with hemorrhage

569.86 Dieulafoy lesion (hemorrhagic) of intestine

569.87 Vomiting of fecal matter

● Code new   ▲ Revision of   ④ ⑤ Fourth or fifth
to this edition   existing code   digit required

569.89 **Other**
Enteroptosis
Granuloma of intestine
Prolapse of intestine
Pericolitis
Perisigmoiditis
Visceroptosis

Excludes: *gangrene of intestine, mesentery, or omentum (557.0)*
hemorrhage of intestine NOS (578.9)
obstruction of intestine (560.0-560.9)

569.9 **Unspecified disorder of intestine**
ALERT! For personal history of unspecified digestive disease see V12.70

OTHER DISEASES OF DIGESTIVE SYSTEM (570-579)

570 **Acute and subacute necrosis of liver**
Acute hepatic failure
Acute or subacute hepatitis, not specified as infective
Necrosis of liver (acute) (diffuse) (massive) (subacute)
Parenchymatous degeneration of liver
Yellow atrophy (liver) (acute) (subacute)

Excludes: *icterus gravis of newborn (773.0-773.2)*
serum hepatitis (070.2-070.3)
that with:
abortion (634-638 with .7, 639.8)
ectopic or molar pregnancy (639.8)
pregnancy, childbirth, or the puerperium (646.7)
viral hepatitis (070.0-070.9)

571 **Chronic liver disease and cirrhosis**
DEFINITION Cirrhosis is the chronic scarring of the liver, leading to loss of normal liver function.

571.0 **Alcoholic fatty liver**

571.1 **Acute alcoholic hepatitis**
Acute alcoholic liver disease

571.2 **Alcoholic cirrhosis of liver**
Florid cirrhosis
Laennec's cirrhosis (alcoholic)

571.3 **Alcoholic liver damage, unspecified**

⑤ **571.4** **Chronic hepatitis**

Excludes: *viral hepatitis (acute) (chronic) (070.0-070.9)*

571.40 **Chronic hepatitis, unspecified**

571.41 **Chronic persistent hepatitis**

571.42 **Autoimmune hepatitis**

571.49 **Other**
Chronic hepatitis:
active
aggressive
Recurrent hepatitis

571.5 **Cirrhosis of liver without mention of alcohol**
Cirrhosis of liver: Cirrhosis of liver:
NOS   posthepatitic
cryptogenic   postnecrotic
macronodular   Healed yellow atrophy (liver)
micronodular   Portal cirrhosis
Code first, if applicable, viral hepatitis (acute) (chronic) (070.0-070.9)

571.6 **Biliary cirrhosis**
Chronic nonsuppurative destructive cholangitis
Cirrhosis:
cholangitic
cholestatic

571.8 **Other chronic nonalcoholic liver disease**
Chronic yellow atrophy (liver)
Fatty liver, without mention of alcohol

Add 4th or 5th digit   Nonspecific code   Unspecified code   Manifestation code

571.9 Unspecified chronic liver disease without mention of alcohol

ALERT! For personal history of unspecified digestive disease see V12.70

572 Liver abscess and sequelae of chronic liver disease

572.0 Abscess of liver

Excludes: amebic liver abscess (006.3)

572.1 Portal pyemia
Phlebitis of portal vein
Portal thrombophlebitis
Pylephlebitis
Pylethrombophlebitis

572.2 Hepatic encephalopathy
Hepatic coma
Hepatocerebral intoxication
Portal-systemic encephalopathy

Excludes: hepatic coma associated with viral hepatitis – see category 070

572.3 Portal hypertension
Use additional code for any associated complications, such as:
portal hypertensive gastropathy (537.89)

572.4 Hepatorenal syndrome

Excludes: that following delivery (674.8)

572.8 Other sequelae of chronic liver disease

Excludes: hepatopulmonary syndrome (573.5)

573 Other disorders of liver

Excludes: amyloid or lardaceous degeneration of liver (277.39)
congenital cystic disease of liver (751.62)
glycogen infiltration of liver (271.0)
hepatomegaly NOS (789.1)
portal vein obstruction (452)

ALERT! For personal history of other specified digestive system diseases see V12.79

573.0 Chronic passive congestion of liver

573.1 Hepatitis in viral diseases classified elsewhere
Code first underlying disease as:
Coxsackie virus disease (074.8)
cytomegalic inclusion virus disease (078.5)
infectious mononucleosis (075)

Excludes: hepatitis (in):
mumps (072.71)
viral (070.0-070.9)
yellow fever (060.0-060.9)

573.2 Hepatitis in other infectious diseases classified elsewhere
Code first underlying disease, as:
malaria (084.9)

Excludes: hepatitis in:
late syphilis (095.3)
secondary syphilis (091.62)
toxoplasmosis (130.5)

573.3 Hepatitis, unspecified
Toxic (noninfectious) hepatitis
Use additional E code, if desired, to identify cause

573.4 Hepatic infarction

● **573.5 Hepatopulmonary syndrome**
Code first underlying liver disease, such as:
alcoholic cirrhosis of liver (571.2)
cirrhosis of liver without mention of alcohol (571.5)

573.8 Other specified disorders of liver
Hepatoptosis

573.9 Unspecified disorder of liver

● Code new to this edition   ▲ Revision of existing code   ④ ⑤ Fourth or fifth digit required

⑤ **574** **Cholelithiasis**

The following fifth-digit subclassification is for use with category 574:

    0   **without mention of obstruction**

    1   **with obstruction**

DEFINITION Cholelithiasis the presence or formation of gallstones in the gallbladder or bile ducts

Excludes: *retained cholelithiasis following cholecystecomy (997.41)*

⑤ **574.0** **Calculus of gallbladder with acute cholecystitis**
[0-1]   Biliary calculus with acute cholecystitis
        Calculus of cystic duct with acute cholecystitis
        Cholelithiasis with acute cholecystitis
        Any condition classifiable to 574.2 with acute cholecystitis

⑤ **574.1** **Calculus of gallbladder with other cholecystitis**
[0-1]   Biliary calculus with cholecystitis
        Calculus of cystic duct with cholecystitis
        Cholelithiasis with cholecystitis
        Cholecystitis with cholelithiasis NOS
        Any condition classifiable to 574.2 with cholecystitis (chronic)

⑤ **574.2** **Calculus of gallbladder without mention of cholecystitis**
[0-1]   Biliary:
        calculus NOS
        colic NOS
        Calculus of cystic duct
        Cholelithiasis NOS
        Colic (recurrent) of
        gallbladder
        Gallstone (impacted)

⑤ **574.3** **Calculus of bile duct with acute cholecystitis**
[0-1]   Calculus of bile duct [any] with acute cholecystitis
        Choledocholithiasis with acute cholecystitis
        Any condition classifiable to 574.5 with acute cholecystitis

⑤ **574.4** **Calculus of bile duct with other cholecystitis**
[0-1]   Calculus of bile duct [any] with cholecystitis (chronic)
        Choledocholithiasis with cholecystitis (chronic)
        Any condition classifiable to 574.5 with cholecystitis (chronic)

⑤ **574.5** **Calculus of bile duct without mention of cholecystitis**
[0-1]   Calculus of:
        bile duct [any]
        common duct
        hepatic duct
        Choledocholithiasis
        Hepatic:
        colic (recurrent)
        lithiasis

⑤ **574.6** **Calculus of gallbladder and bile duct with acute cholecystitis**
[0-1]   Any condition classifiable to 574.0 and 574.3

⑤ **574.7** **Calculus of gallbladder and bile duct with other cholecystitis**
[0-1]   Any condition classifiable to 574.1 and 574.4

⑤ **574.8** **Calculus of gallbladder and bile duct with acute and chronic cholecystitis**
[0-1]   Any condition classifiable to 574.6 and 574.7

⑤ **574.9** **Calculus of gallbladder and bile duct without cholecystitis**
[0-1]   Any condition classifiable to 574.2 and 574.5

575 **Other disorders of gallbladder**

DEFINITION The gallbladder is a small, pear-shaped muscular sac, located under the right lobe of the liver, in which bile secreted by the liver is stored until needed by the body for digestion.

ALERT! For personal history of other specified digestive system diseases see V12.79

	Add 4th or 5th digit		Nonspecific code		Unspecified code		Manifestation code

575.0 Acute cholecystitis
Abscess of gallbladder without mention of calculus
Angiocholecystitis without mention of calculus
Cholecystitis without mention of calculus:
 emphysematous (acute)
 gangrenous
 suppurative
Empyema of gallbladder without mention of calculus
Gangrene of gallbladder without mention of calculus

Excludes: *that with:*
> *acute and chronic cholecystitis (575.12)*
> *choledocholithiasis (574.3)*
> *choledocholithiasis and cholelithiasis (574.6)*
> *cholelithiasis (574.0)*

⑤ **575.1 Other cholecystitis**
Cholecystitis:
 NOS without mention of calculus
 chronic without mention of calculus

Excludes: *that with:*
> *choledocholithiasis (574.4)*
> *choledocholithiasis and cholelithiasis (574.8)*
> *cholelithiasis (574.1)*

575.10 Cholecystitis, unspecified
 Cholecystitis NOS

575.11 Chronic cholecystitis

575.12 Acute and chronic cholecystits

575.2 Obstruction of gallbladder
Occlusion of cystic duct or gallbladder without mention of calculus
Stenosis of cystic duct or gallbladder without mention of calculus
Stricture of cystic duct or gallbladder without mention of calculus

Excludes: *that with calculus (574.0-574.2 with fifth-digit 1)*

575.3 Hydrops of gallbladder
Mucocele of gallbladder

575.4 Perforation of gallbladder
Rupture of cystic duct or gallbladder

575.5 Fistula of gallbladder
Fistula:
 cholecystoduodenal
 cholecystoenteric

575.6 Cholesterolosis of gallbladder
Strawberry gallbladder

575.8 Other specified disorders of gallbladder
Adhesions (of) cystic duct or gallbladder
Atrophy (of) cystic duct or gallbladder
Cyst (of) cystic duct or gallbladder
Hypertrophy (of) cystic duct or gallbladder
Nonfunctioning (of) cystic duct or gallbladder
Ulcer (of) cystic duct or gallbladder
Biliary dyskinesia

Excludes: *nonvisualization of gallbladder (793.3)*
> *Hartmann's pouch of intestine (V44.3)*

575.9 Unspecified disorder of gallbladder

576 Other disorders of biliary tract

Excludes: *that involving the:*
> *cystic duct (575.0-575.9)*
> *gallbladder (575.0-575.9)*

DEFINITION The biliary tract is the system of organs and ducts through which bile is made and transported from the liver. Bile is a liquid produced in the liver whose function is to remove waste from the liver and break down fats as food is digested

ALERT! For personal history of other specified digestive system diseases see V12.79

576.0 Postcholecystectomy syndrome

● Code new to this edition   ▲ Revision of existing code   ④ ⑤ Fourth or fifth digit required

576.1 Cholangitis

Cholangitis:
  NOS
  acute
  ascending
  chronic
  primary

Cholangitis:
  recurrent
  sclerosing
  secondary
  stenosing
  suppurative

576.2 Obstruction of bile duct
Occlusion of bile duct, except cystic duct, without mention of calculus
Stenosis of bile duct, except cystic duct, without mention of calculus
Stricture of bile duct, except cystic duct, without mention of calculus

Excludes: *congenital (751.61)*
  that with calculus (574.3-574.5 with fifth-digit 1)

576.3 Perforation of bile duct
Rupture of bile duct, except cystic duct

576.4 Fistula of bile duct
Choledochoduodenal fistula

576.5 Spasm of sphincter of Oddi

576.8 Other specified disorders of biliary tract
Adhesions of bile duct [any]
Atrophy of bile duct [any]
Cyst of bile duct [any]
Hypertrophy of bile duct [any]
Stasis of bile duct [any]
Ulcer of bile duct [any]

Excludes: *congenital choledochal cyst (751.69)*

576.9 Unspecified disorder of biliary tract
ALERT! For personal history of unspecified digestive disease see V12.70

577 Diseases of pancreas

DEFINITION The pancreas is gland that lies in the abdomen behind the stomach. It produces enzymes that are released into the small intestine to help with digestion. It also contains clusters of cells called islets that produce hormones such as insulin and glucagon, which help control the level of glucose in the blood.

577.0 Acute pancreatitis

Abscess of pancreas
Necrosis of pancreas:
  acute
  infective

Pancreatitis:
  NOS
  acute (recurrent)
  apoplectic
  hemorrhagic
  subacute
  suppurative

Excludes: *mumps pancreatitis (072.3)*

577.1 Chronic pancreatitis

Chronic pancreatitis:
  NOS
  infectious
  interstitial

Pancreatitis:
  painless
  recurrent
  relapsing

577.2 Cyst and pseudocyst of pancreas

577.8 Other specified diseases of pancreas

Atrophy of pancreas
Calculus of pancreas
Cirrhosis of pancreas
Fibrosis of pancreas

Pancreatic:
  infantilism
  necrosis:
    NOS
    aseptic
    fat
Pancreatolithiasis

Excludes: *fibrocystic disease of pancreas (277.00-277.09)*
  islet cell tumor of pancreas (211.7)
  pancreatic steatorrhea (579.4)

577.9 Unspecified disease of pancreas
ALERT! For personal history of unspecified digestive disease see V12.70

Add 4th or 5th digit   Nonspecific code   Unspecified code   Manifestation code

578 Gastrointestinal hemorrhage

Excludes: *that with mention of:*
    angiodysplasia of stomach and duodenum (537.83)
    angiodysplasia of intestine (569.85)
    diverticulitis, intestine:
      large (562.13)
      small (562.03)
    diverticulosis, intestine:
      large (562.12)
      small (562.02)
    gastritis and duodenitis (535.0-535.6)
    ulcer:
      duodenal (532.0-532.9)
      gastric (531.0-531.9)
      gastrojejunal (534.0-534.9)
      peptic (533.0-533.9)

DEFINITION Gastrointestinal hemorrhage refers to bleeding in any segment of the gastrointestinal tract from esophagus to rectum

578.0 Hematemesis
    Vomiting of blood

578.1 Blood in stool
    Melena

Excludes: *occult blood (792.1)*

578.9 Hemorrhage of gastrointestinal tract, unspecified
    Gastric hemorrhage
    Intestinal hemorrhage

ALERT! For personal history of unspecified digestive disease see V12.70

579 Intestinal malabsorption

DEFINITION Intestinal malabsorption is a state arising from abnormality in digestion or absorption of food nutrients across the gastrointestinal(GI) tract.

579.0 Celiac disease
Celiac:	Gee (-Herter) disease
crisis	Gluten enteropathy
infantilism	Idiopathic steatorrhea
rickets	Nontropical sprue

579.1 Tropical sprue
Sprue:	Tropical steatorrhea
NOS	
tropical	

579.2 Blind loop syndrome
    Postoperative blind loop syndrome

579.3 Other and unspecified postsurgical nonabsorption
    Hypoglycemia following gastrointestinal surgery
    Malnutrition following gastrointestinal surgery

579.4 Pancreatic steatorrhea

579.8 Other specified intestinal malabsorption
Enteropathy:	Steatorrhea (chronic)
exudative	
protein-losing	

579.9 Unspecified intestinal malabsorption
    Malabsorption syndrome NOS

ALERT! For personal history of unspecified digestive disease see V12.70

  ● Code new
     to this edition
    ▲ Revision of
      existing code
    ④ ⑤ Fourth or fifth
       digit required

Chapter 10: Diseases of Genitourinary System (580-629)

DEFINITIONS AND CODING ALERTS

This chapter includes definitions of selected key words, terms and phrases and coding alerts for adding points to the clinical domain, references to coding late effects where appropriate, and references to personal history V-codes in situations where the acute or chronic condition is no longer active. An example from this chapter is as follows:

581 **Nephrotic syndrome**

> **DEFINITION** Nephrotic syndrome is a collection of symptoms which occur because the glomeruli (tiny blood vessels) in the kidney become leaky. This allows protein, normally never passed out in the urine, to leave the body in large amounts.
> **ALERT!** For personal history of nephrotic syndrome see V13.03

MULTIPLE CODING FOR A SINGLE CONDITION

In addition to the etiology or manifestation convention that requires two codes to fully describe a single condition that affects multiple body systems, there are other single conditions that also require more than one code. "Use additional code" notes are found in the tabular at codes that are not part of an etiology or manifestation pair where a secondary code is useful to fully describe a condition. The sequencing rule is the same as the etiology or manifestation pair - , "use additional code" indicates that a secondary code should be added.

"Code first" notes are also under certain codes that are not specifically manifestation codes but may be due to an underlying cause. When a "code first" note is present and an underlying condition is present the underlying condition should be sequenced first.

"Code, if applicable, any causal condition first", notes indicate that this code may be assigned as a principal diagnosis when the causal condition is unknown or not applicable. If a causal condition is known, then the code for that condition should be sequenced as the principal or first-listed diagnosis. Multiple codes may be needed for late effects, complication codes and obstetric codes to more fully describe a condition. See the specific guidelines for these conditions for further instruction.

COMBINATION CODE

A combination code is a single code used to classify: two diagnoses, or a diagnosis with an associated secondary process (manifestation) A diagnosis with an associated complication Combination codes are identified by referring to subterm entries in the Alphabetic Index and by reading the inclusion and exclusion notes in the Tabular List.

Assign only the combination code when that code fully identifies the diagnostic conditions involved or when the Alphabetic Index so directs. Multiple coding should not be used when the classification provides a combination code that clearly identifies all of the elements documented in the diagnosis. When the combination code lacks necessary specificity in describing the manifestation or complication, an additional code should be
used as a secondary code.

CODING LATE EFFECTS

A late effect is the residual effect (condition produced) after the acute phase of an illness or injury has terminated. There is no time limit on when a late effect code can be used. The residual may be apparent early, such as in cerebrovascular accident cases, or it may occur months or years later, such as that due to a previous injury. Coding of late effects generally requires two codes sequenced in the following order: The condition or nature of the late effect is sequenced first. The late effect code is sequenced second.

An exception to the above guidelines are those instances where the code for late effect is followed by a manifestation code identified in the Tabular List and title, or the late effect code has been expanded (at the fourth and fifth-digit levels) to include the manifestation(s). The code for the acute phase of an illness or injury that led to the late effect is never used with a code for the late effect.

CHRONIC KIDNEY DISEASE

Stages of chronic kidney disease (CKD)

The ICD-9-CM classifies CKD based on severity. The severity of CKD is designated by stages I-V. Stage II, code 585.2, equates to mild CKD; stage III, code 585.3, equates to moderate CKD; and stage IV, code

| | Add 4th or 5th digit | | Nonspecific code | | Unspecified code | | Manifestation code |

585.4, equates to severe CKD. Code 585.6, End stage renal disease (ESRD), is assigned when the provider has documented end-stage-renal disease (ESRD).

If both a stage of CKD and ESRD are documented, assign code 585.6 only.

Chronic kidney disease and kidney transplant status

Patients who have undergone kidney transplant may still have some form of CKD, because the kidney transplant may not fully restore kidney function. Therefore, the presence of CKD alone does not constitute a transplant complication. Assign the appropriate 585 code for the patient's stage of CKD and code V42.0. If a transplant complication such as failure or rejection is documented, see Official Guidelines, Section I.C.17.f.1.b for information on coding complications of a kidney transplant. If the documentation is unclear as to whether the patient has a complication of the transplant, query the provider.

Chronic kidney disease with other conditions

Patients with CKD may also suffer from other serious conditions, most commonly diabetes mellitus and hypertension. The sequencing of the CKD code in relationship to codes for other contributing conditions is based on the conventions in the tabular list.

See Chapter 3 for sequencing instructions for diabetes.
See Chapter 4 for anemia in CKD.
See Chapter 7 for hypertensive chronic kidney disease.
See Chapter 17 for instructions on coding of documented rejection or failure of kidney transplant.

● Code new
  to this edition

▲ Revision of
  existing code

④ ⑤ Fourth or fifth
  digit required

10. DISEASES OF THE GENITOURINARY SYSTEM (580-629)

NEPHRITIS, NEPHROTIC SYNDROME, AND NEPHROSIS (580-589)

> Excludes: *hypertensive chronic kidney disease (403.00-403.91, 404.00-404.93)*
>
> **ALERT!** For personal history of disorders of the urinary system see V13.0

580 Acute glomerulonephritis

Includes: acute nephritis

DEFINITION Glomerulonephritis is a form of nephritis with inflammation of the capillary loops in the renal glomeruli. The acute form is characterized by proteinuria, edema, hematuria, renal failure, and hypertension, sometimes preceded by tonsillitis or febrile pharyngitis

580.0 With lesion of proliferative glomerulonephritis

Acute (diffuse) proliferative glomerulonephritis
Acute poststreptococcal glomerulonephritis

580.4 With lesion of rapidly progressive glomerulonephritis

Acute nephritis with lesion of necrotizing glomerulitis

⑤ **580.8 With other specified pathological lesion in kidney**

> **580.81 Acute glomerulonephritis in diseases classified elsewhere**
>
> *Code first underlying disease, as:*
> infectious hepatitis (070.0-070.9)
> mumps (072.79)
> subacute bacterial endocarditis (421.0)
> typhoid fever (002.0)

580.89 Other

Glomerulonephritis, acute, with lesion of:
exudative nephritis
interstitial (diffuse) (focal) nephritis

580.9 Acute glomerulonephritis with unspecified pathological lesion in kidney

Glomerulonephritis:
NOS specified as acute
hemorrhagic specified as acute
Nephritis specified as acute
Nephropathy specified as acute

581 Nephrotic syndrome

DEFINITION Nephrotic syndrome is a collection of symptoms which occur because the glomeruli (tiny blood vessels) in the kidney become leaky. This allows protein, normally never passed out in the urine, to leave the body in large amounts

ALERT! For personal history of nephrotic syndrome see V13.03

581.0 With lesion of proliferative glomerulonephritis

581.1 With lesion of membranous glomerulonephritis

Epimembranous nephritis
Idiopathic membranous glomerular disease
Nephrotic syndrome with lesion of:
focal glomerulosclerosis
sclerosing membranous glomerulonephritis
segmental hyalinosis

581.2 With lesion of membranoproliferative glomerulonephritis

Nephrotic syndrome with lesion (of):
endothelial glomerulonephritis
hypocomplementemic persistent glomerulonephritis
lobular glomerulonephritis
mesangiocapillary glomerulonephritis
mixed membranous and proliferative glomerulonephritis

581.3 With lesion of minimal change glomerulonephritis

Foot process disease	Minimal change:
Lipoid nephrosis	glomerular disease
	glomerulitis
	nephrotic syndrome

⑤ **581.8 With other specified pathological lesion in kidney**

> **581.81 Nephrotic syndrome in diseases classified elsewhere**
>
> *Code first underlying disease, as:*
> amyloidosis (277.30-277.39)
> diabetes mellitus (249.4, 250.4)
> malaria (084.9)
> polyarteritis (446.0)
> systemic lupus erythematosus (710.0)

Add 4th or 5th digit	Nonspecific code	Unspecified code	Manifestation code

> Excludes: *nephrosis in epidemic hemorrhagic fever (078.6)*

581.89 Other
Glomerulonephritis with edema and lesion of:
  exudative nephritis
  interstitial (diffuse) (focal) nephritis

581.9 Nephrotic syndrome with unspecified pathological lesion in kidney
Glomerulonephritis with edema NOS
Nephritis:
  nephrotic NOS
  with edema NOS
Nephrosis NOS
Renal disease with edema NOS

582 Chronic glomerulonephritis
Includes: chronic nephritis

582.0 With lesion of proliferative glomerulonephritis
Chronic (diffuse) proliferative glomerulonephritis

582.1 With lesion of membranous glomerulonephritis
Chronic glomerulonephritis:
  membranous
  sclerosing
Focal glomerulosclerosis
Segmental hyalinosis

582.2 With lesion of membranoproliferative glomerulonephritis
Chronic glomerulonephritis:
  endothelial
  hypocomplementemic persistent
  lobular
  membranoproliferative
  mesangiocapillary
  mixed membranous and proliferative

582.4 With lesion of rapidly progressive glomerulonephritis
Chronic nephritis with lesion of necrotizing glomerulitis

⑤ **582.8 With other specified pathological lesion in kidney**

582.81 *Chronic glomerulonephritis in diseases classified elsewhere*
Code first underlying disease, as:
  amyloidosis (277.30-277.39)
  systemic lupus erythematosus (710.0)

582.89 Other
Chronic glomerulonephritis with lesion of:
  exudative nephritis
  interstitial (diffuse) (focal) nephritis

582.9 Chronic glomerulonephritis with unspecified pathological lesion in kidney
Glomerulonephritis:
  NOS specified as chronic
  hemorrhagic specified as chronic
Nephritis specified as chronic
Nephropathy specified as chronic

583 Nephritis and nephropathy, not specified as acute or chronic
Includes: "renal disease" so stated, not specified as acute or chronic but with stated
      pathology or cause
DEFINITION Nephritis and nephropathy refers to inflammation or other damage to the kidney

583.0 With lesion of proliferative glomerulonephritis
Proliferative:
  glomerulonephritis (diffuse) NOS
  nephritis NOS
  nephropathy NOS

583.1 With lesion of membranous glomerulonephritis
Membranous: Membranous nephropathy NOS
  glomerulonephritis NOS
  nephritis NOS

● Code new to this edition   ▲ Revision of existing code   ④ ⑤ Fourth or fifth digit required

583.2 With lesion of membranoproliferative glomerulonephritis
Membranoproliferative:
glomerulonephritis NOS
nephritis NOS
nephropathy NOS
Nephritis NOS, with lesion of:
hypocomplementemic persistent glomerulonephritis
lobular glomerulonephritis
mesangiocapillary glomerulonephritis
mixed membranous and proliferative glomerulonephritis

583.4 With lesion of rapidly progressive glomerulonephritis
Necrotizing or rapidly progressive:
glomerulitis NOS
glomerulonephritis NOS
nephritis NOS
nephropathy NOS
Nephritis, unspecified, with lesion of necrotizing glomerulitis

583.6 With lesion of renal cortical necrosis
Nephritis NOS with (renal) cortical necrosis
Nephropathy NOS with (renal) cortical necrosis
Renal cortical necrosis NOS

583.7 With lesion of renal medullary necrosis
Nephritis NOS with (renal) medullary [papillary] necrosis
Nephropathy NOS with (renal) medullary [papillary] necrosis

⑤ **583.8 With other specified pathological lesion in kidney**

> **583.81 *Nephritis and nephropathy, not specified as acute or chronic, in diseases classified elsewhere***

Code first underlying disease, as:
amyloidosis (277.30-277.39)
diabetes mellitus (249.4, 250.4)
gonococcal infection (098.19)
Goodpasture's syndrome (446.21)
systemic lupus erythematosus (710.0)
tuberculosis (016.0)

Excludes: *gouty nephropathy (274.10)*
syphilitic nephritis (095.4)

583.89 Other
Glomerulitis with lesion of:
exudative nephritis
interstitial nephritis
Glomerulonephritis with lesion of:
exudative nephritis
interstitial nephritis
Nephritis with lesion of:
exudative nephritis
interstitial nephritis
Nephropathy with lesion of:
exudative nephritis
interstitial nephritis
Renal disease with lesion of:
exudative nephritis
interstitial nephritis

583.9 With unspecified pathological lesion in kidney
Glomerulitis NOS
Glomerulonephritis NOS
Nephritis NOS
Nephropathy NOS

Excludes: *nephropathy complicating pregnancy, labor, or the puerperium (642.0-642.9, 646.2)*
renal disease NOS with no stated cause (593.9)

584 Acute kidney failure
Includes: Acute renal failure

Excludes: *following labor and delivery (669.3)*
posttraumatic (958.5)
that complicating:
abortion (634-638 with .3, 639.3)
ectopic or molar pregnancy (639.3)

DEFINITION Kidney failure is the sudden loss of the kidneys' ability to eliminate excess fluid and electrolytes as well as waste material from the blood

584.5 Acute kidney failure with lesion of tubular necrosis
Lower nephron nephrosis
Renal failure with (acute) tubular necrosis
Tubular necrosis:
  NOS
  acute

584.6 Acute kidney failure with lesion of renal cortical necrosis

584.7 Acute kidney failure with lesion of renal medullary [papillary] necrosis
Necrotizing renal papillitis

584.8 Acute kidney failure with other specified pathological lesion in kidney

584.9 Acute kidney failure, unspecified
Acute kidney injury (nontraumatic)

Excludes: *traumatic kidney injury (866.00-866.13)*

585 Chronic kidney disease (CKD)
Code first hypertensive chronic kidney disease, if applicable, (403.00-403.91, 404.00-404.93)
Use additional code to identify kidney transplant status, if applicable (V42.0)

DEFINITION Chronic kidney disease (CKD), aka chronic renal disease, is a progressive loss of renal function over a period of months or years

585.1 Chronic kidney disease, Stage I

585.2 Chronic kidney disease, Stage II (mild)

585.3 Chronic kidney disease, Stage III (moderate)

585.4 Chronic kidney disease, Stage IV (severe)

585.5 Chronic kidney disease, Stage V

Excludes: *chronic kidney disease, stage V requiring chronic dialysis (585.6)*

585.6 End stage renal disease
Chronic kidney disease requiring chronic dialysis

585.9 Chronic kidney disease, unspecified
Chronic renal disease
Chronic renal failure NOS
Chronic renal insufficiency

586 Renal failure, unspecified
Uremia NOS

Excludes: *following labor and delivery (669.3)*
posttraumatic renal failure (958.5)
that complicating:
abortion (634-638 with .3, 639.3)
ectopic or molar pregnancy (639.3)
uremia:
extrarenal (788.9)
prerenal (788.9)

DEFINITION Renal failure refers to severe malfunction of the kidneys, producing uremia and the resulting constitutional symptoms

587 Renal sclerosis, unspecified
Includes: Atrophy of kidney
Contracted kidney
Renal:
  cirrhosis
  fibrosis

DEFINITION Renal sclerosis is a sclerosis or hardening of the kidney due to renovascular disease

● Code new
  to this edition
▲ Revision of
  existing code
④ ⑤ Fourth or fifth
  digit required

588 **Disorders resulting from impaired renal function**

588.0 Renal osteodystrophy
Azotemic osteodystrophy
Phosphate-losing tubular
disorders

Renal:
dwarfism
infantilism
rickets

588.1 Nephrogenic diabetes insipidus
Excludes: *diabetes insipidus NOS (253.5)*

⑤ **588.8 Other specified disorders resulting from impaired renal function**
Excludes: *secondary hypertension (405.0-405.9)*

588.81 Secondary hyperparathyroidism (of renal origin)
Secondary hyperparathyroidism NOS

588.89 Other specified disorders resulting from impaired renal function
Hypokalemic nephropathy

588.9 Unspecified disorder resulting from impaired renal function

589 **Small kidney of unknown cause**

589.0 Unilateral small kidney

589.1 Bilateral small kidneys

589.9 Small kidney, unspecified

OTHER DISEASES OF URINARY SYSTEM (590-599)

590 **Infections of kidney**
Use additional code to identify organism, such as Escherichia coli [E. coli] (041.41-041.49)

⑤ **590.0 Chronic pyelonephritis**
Chronic pyelitis
Chronic pyonephrosis

Code, if applicable, any causal condition first

590.00 Without lesion of renal medullary necrosis

590.01 With lesion of renal medullary necrosis

⑤ **590.1 Acute pyelonephritis**
Acute pyelitis
Acute pyonephrosis

590.10 Without lesion of renal medullary necrosis

590.11 With lesion of renal medullary necrosis

590.2 Renal and perinephric abscess
Abscess:
kidney
nephritic
perirenal

Carbuncle of kidney

590.3 Pyeloureteritis cystica
Infection of renal pelvis and ureter
Ureteritis cystica

⑤ **590.8 Other pyelonephritis or pyonephrosis, not specified as acute or chronic**

590.80 Pyelonephritis, unspecified
Pyelitis NOS
Pyelonephritis NOS

590.81 *Pyelitis or pyelonephritis in diseases classified elsewhere*
Code first underlying disease, as:
tuberculosis (016.0)

590.9 Infection of kidney, unspecified
Excludes: *urinary tract infection NOS (599.0)*

591 Hydronephrosis
Hydrocalycosis
Hydronephrosis

Hydroureteronephrosis

Excludes: *congenital hydronephrosis (753.29)*
hydroureter (593.5)

DEFINITION Hydronephrosis is a condition that occurs as a result of urine accumulation in the upper urinary tract. This usually occurs from a blockage somewhere along the urinary tract.

Add 4th or
5th digit

Nonspecific
code

Unspecified
code

Manifestation
code

592 Calculus of kidney and ureter

> *Excludes:* nephrocalcinosis (275.4)

ALERT! For personal history of urinary calculi see V13.01

592.0 Calculus of kidney
Nephrolithiasis NOS Staghorn calculus
Renal calculus or stone Stone in kidney

> *Excludes:* uric acid nephrolithiasis (274.11)

592.1 Calculus of ureter
Ureteric stone
Ureterolithiasis

592.9 Urinary calculus, unspecified

593 Other disorders of kidney and ureter

ALERT! For personal history of other specified urinary system disorders see V13.09

593.0 Nephroptosis
Floating kidney
Mobile kidney

593.1 Hypertrophy of kidney

593.2 Cyst of kidney, acquired
Cyst (multiple) (solitary) of kidney, not congenital
Peripelvic (lymphatic) cyst

> *Excludes:* calyceal or pyelogenic cyst of kidney (591)
> congenital cyst of kidney (753.1)
> polycystic (disease of) kidney (753.1)

593.3 Stricture or kinking of ureter
Angulation of ureter (postoperative)
Constriction of ureter (postoperative)
Stricture of pelviureteric junction

593.4 Other ureteric obstruction
Idiopathic retroperitoneal fibrosis
Occlusion NOS of ureter

> *Excludes:* that due to calculus (592.1)

593.5 Hydroureter

> *Excludes:* congenital hydroureter (753.22)
> hydroureteronephrosis (591)

593.6 Postural proteinuria
Benign postural proteinuria
Orthostatic proteinuria

> *Excludes:* proteinuria NOS (791.0)

⑤ **593.7 Vesicoureteral reflux**

593.70 Unspecified or without reflux nephropathy

593.71 With reflux nephropathy, unilateral

593.72 With reflux nephropathy, bilateral

593.73 With reflux nephropathy NOS

⑤ **593.8 Other specified disorders of kidney and ureter**

593.81 Vascular disorders of kidney
Renal (artery): Renal infarction
embolism
hemorrhage
thrombosis

593.82 Ureteral fistula
Intestinoureteral fistula

> *Excludes:* fistula between ureter and female genital tract (619.0)

● Code new ▲ Revision of ④ ⑤ Fourth or fifth
to this edition existing code digit required

593.89 Other
Adhesions, kidney or ureter
Periureteritis
Polyp of ureter
Pyelectasia
Ureterocele

Excludes: *tuberculosis of ureter (016.2)*
ureteritis cystica (590.3)

593.9 Unspecified disorder of kidney and ureter
Acute renal disease
Acute renal insufficiency
Renal disease NOS
Salt-losing nephritis or syndrome

Excludes: *chronic renal insufficiency (585.9)*
cystic kidney disease (753.1)
nephropathy, so stated (583.0-583.9)
renal disease:
arising in pregnancy or the puerperium (642.1-642.2, 642.4-642.7, 646.2)
not specified as acute or chronic, but with stated pathology or cause (583.0-583.9)

594 Calculus of lower urinary tract
DEFINITION A Calculus of lower urinary tract is a stone (calculus) located in the lower urinary tract.

594.0 Calculus in diverticulum of bladder

594.1 Other calculus in bladder
Urinary bladder stone

Excludes: *staghorn calculus (592.0)*

594.2 Calculus in urethra

594.8 Other lower urinary tract calculus

594.9 Calculus of lower urinary tract, unspecified

Excludes: *calculus of urinary tract NOS (592.9)*

595 Cystitis

Excludes: *prostatocystitis (601.3)*

Use additional code to identify organism, such as Escherichia coli [E. coli] (041.41-041.49)
DEFINITION Cystitis is an inflammation of the urinary bladder and ureters

595.0 Acute cystitis

Excludes: *trigonitis (595.3)*

595.1 Chronic interstitial cystitis
Hunner's ulcer   Submucous cystitis
Panmural fibrosis of bladder

595.2 Other chronic cystitis
Chronic cystitis NOS
Subacute cystitis

Excludes: *trigonitis (595.3)*

595.3 Trigonitis
Follicular cystitis
Trigonitis (acute) (chronic)
Urethrotrigonitis

595.4 *Cystitis in diseases classified elsewhere*
Code first underlying disease, as:
actinomycosis (039.8)
amebiasis (006.8)
bilharziasis (120.0-120.9)
Echinococcus infestation (122.3, 122.6)

Excludes: *cystitis:*
diphtheritic (032.84)
gonococcal (098.11, 098.31)
monilial (112.2)
trichomonal (131.09)
tuberculous (016.1)

Add 4th or 5th digit   Nonspecific code   Unspecified code   Manifestation code

⑤ **595.8 Other specified types of cystitis**

    595.81 Cystitis cystica

    595.82 Irradiation cystitis
    Use additional E code, if desired, to identify cause

    595.89 Other
        Abscess of bladder
        Cystitis:
            bullous
            emphysematous
            glandularis

595.9 Cystitis, unspecified

596 Other disorders of bladder
Use additional code, if desired, to identify urinary incontinence (625.6, 788.30-788.39)
    ALERT! For personal history of other specified urinary system disorders see V13.09

596.0 Bladder neck obstruction
    Contracture (acquired) of bladder neck or vesicourethral orifice
    Obstruction (acquired) of bladder neck or vesicourethral orifice
    Stenosis (acquired) of bladder neck or vesicourethral orifice
    Excludes: congenital (753.6)

596.1 Intestinovesical fistula
    Fistula: Fistula:
      enterovesical   vesicoenteric
      vesicocolic   vesicorectal

596.2 Vesical fistula, not elsewhere classified
    Fistula: Fistula:
      bladder NOS   vesicocutaneous
      urethrovesical   vesicoperineal
    Excludes: fistula between bladder and female genital tract (619.0)

596.3 Diverticulum of bladder
    Diverticulitis of bladder
    Diverticulum (acquired) (false) of bladder
    Excludes: that with calculus in diverticulum of bladder (594.0)

596.4 Atony of bladder
    High compliance bladder, of bladder
    Hypotonicity of bladder
    Inertia of bladder
    Excludes: neurogenic bladder (596.54)

⑤ **596.5 Other functional disorders of bladder**
    Excludes: cauda equina syndrome
               with neurogenic bladder (344.61)

    596.51 Hypertonicity of bladder
        Hyperactivity
        Overactive bladder

    596.52 Low bladder compliance

    596.53 Paralysis of bladder

    596.54 Neurogenic bladder NOS

    596.55 Detrusor sphincter dyssynergia

    596.59 Other functional disorder of bladder
        Detrusor instability

596.6 Rupture of bladder, nontraumatic

596.7 Hemorrhage into bladder wall
    Hyperemia of bladder
    Excludes: acute hemorrhagic cystitis (595.0)

⑤ **596.8 Other specified disorders of bladder**
    Excludes: cystocele, female (618.01-618.02, 618.09, 618.2-618.4)
           hernia or prolapse of bladder, female (618.01-618.02, 618.09, 618.2-618.4)

● Code new   ▲ Revision of   ④ ⑤ Fourth or fifth
    to this edition   existing code   digit required

● **596.81   Infection of cystostomy**
Use additional code to specify type of infection, such as:
abscess or cellulitis of abdomen (682.2)
septicemia (038.0-038.9)
Use additional code to identify organism (041.00-041.9)

● **596.82   Mechanical complication of cystostomy**
Malfunction of cystostomy

● **596.83   Other complication of cystostomy**
Fistula
Hernia
Prolapse

● **596.89   Other specified disorders of bladder**
Bladder hemorrhage
Bladder hypertrophy
Calcified bladder
Contracted bladder

596.9 Unspecified disorder of bladder

597 Urethritis, not sexually transmitted, and urethral syndrome

Excludes: nonspecific urethritis, so stated (099.4)

DEFINITION Urethritis is inflammation of the urethra; resulting in painful urination. Urethral syndrome is a term used to describe symptoms of urethritis , without any evidence of bacterial or viral infection as a cause.

597.0 Urethral abscess

Abscess of:
bulbourethral gland
Cowper's gland
Littré's gland

Abscess:
periurethral
urethral (gland)
Periurethral cellulitis

Excludes: urethral caruncle (599.3)

⑤ **597.8 Other urethritis**

597.80   Urethritis, unspecified

597.81   Urethral syndrome NOS

597.89   Other
Adenitis, Skene's
glands
Cowperitis

Meatitis, urethral
Ulcer, urethra (meatus)
Verumontanitis

Excludes: trichomonal (131.02)

598 Urethral stricture
Includes: pinhole meatus
stricture of urinary meatus

Excludes: congenital stricture of urethra and urinary meatus (753.6)
Use additional code to identify urinary incontinence (625.6, 788.30-788.39)

DEFINITION Urethral stricture is a narrowing of the urethra caused by injury or disease such as urinary tract infections or other forms of urethritis

⑤ **598.0 Urethral stricture due to infection**

598.00   Due to unspecified infection

598.01   *Due to infective diseases classified elsewhere*
Code first underlying disease, as:
gonococcal infection (098.2)
schistosomiasis (120.0-120.9)
syphilis (095.8)

598.1 Traumatic urethral stricture
Stricture of urethra:
late effect of injury
postobstetric

Excludes: postoperative following surgery on genitourinary tract (598.2)

598.2 Postoperative urethral stricture
Postcatheterization stricture of urethra

598.8 Other specified causes of urethral stricture

598.9 Urethral stricture, unspecified

| | Add 4th or 5th digit | | Nonspecific code | | Unspecified code | | Manifestation code |

599 **Other disorders of urethra and urinary tract**
> **ALERT!** For personal history of other specified urinary system disorders see V13.09
> **ALERT!** For personal history of urinary (tract) infection see V13.02

599.0 **Urinary tract infection, site not specified**
> Pyuria
> **Excludes:** *candidiasis of urinary tract (112.2)*
> *urinary tract infection of newborn (771.82)*

Use additional code to identify organism, such as Escherichia coli [E. coli] (041.41-041.49)

599.1 **Urethral fistula**
> Fistula: Urinary fistula NOS
> urethroperineal
> urethrorectal
> **Excludes:** *fistula:*
> *urethroscrotal (608.89)*
> *urethrovaginal (619.0)*
> *urethrovesicovaginal (619.0)*

599.2 **Urethral diverticulum**

599.3 **Urethral caruncle**
> Polyp of urethra

599.4 **Urethral false passage**

599.5 **Prolapsed urethral mucosa**
> Prolapse of urethra
> Urethrocele
> **Excludes:** *urethrocele, female (618.03, 618.09, 618.2-618.4)*

⑤ **599.6** **Urinary obstruction**

> **599.60** **Urinary obstruction, unspecified**
> Obstructive uropathy NOS
> Urinary (tract) obstruction NOS

> **599.69** **Urinary obstruction, not elsewhere classified**
> Code, if applicable, any causal condition first, such as:
> hyperplasia of prostate (600.0-600.9 with fifth-digit 1)

⑤ **599.7** **Hematuria**
> Hematuria (benign) (essential)
> **Excludes:** *hemoglobinuria (791.2)*

> **599.70** **Hematuria, unspecified**

> **599.71** **Gross hematuria**

> **599.72** **Microscopic hematuria**

⑤ **599.8** **Other specified disorders of urethra and urinary tract**
> **Excludes:** *symptoms and other conditions classifiable to 788.0-788.9, 791.0-791.9*
> Use additional code, if desired, to identify urinary incontinence (625.6, 788.30-788.39)

> **599.81** **Urethral hypermobility**

> **599.82** **Intrinsic (urethral) sphincter deficiency [ISD]**

> **599.83** **Urethral instability**

> **599.84** **Other specified disorders of urethra**
> Rupture of urethra (nontraumatic)
> Urethral:
> cyst
> granuloma

> **599.89** **Other specified disorders of urinary tract**

599.9 **Unspecified disorder of urethra and urinary tract**
> **ALERT!** For personal history of unspecified urinary disorder see V13.00

DISEASES OF MALE GENITAL ORGANS (600-608)

600 **Hyperplasia of prostate**
> Includes: enlarged prostate
> **DEFINITION** Hyperplasia of prostate is a nonmalignant enlargement of the prostate gland commonly occurring in men after the age of 50, and sometimes leading to compression of the urethra and obstruction of the flow of urine

● Code new
to this edition

▲ Revision of
existing code

④ ⑤ Fourth or fifth
digit required

⑤ **600.0 Hypertrophy (benign) of prostate**
Benign prostatic hypertrophy
Enlargement of prostate
Smooth enlarged prostate
Soft enlarged prostate

600.00 Hypertrophy (benign) of prostate without urinary obstruction and other lower urinary tract symptoms (LUTS)
Hypertrophy (benign) of prostate NOS

600.01 Hypertrophy (benign) of prostate with urinary obstruction and other lower urinary tract symptoms (LUTS)
Hypertrophy (benign) of prostate with urinary retention

Use additional code to identify symptoms:
incomplete bladder emptying (788.21)
nocturia (788.43)
straining on urination (788.65)
urinary frequency (788.41)
urinary hesitancy (788.64)
urinary incontinence (788.30-788.39)
urinary obstruction (599.69)
urinary retention (788.20)
urinary urgency (788.63)
weak urinary stream (788.62)

⑤ **600.1 Nodular prostate**
Hard, firm prostate
Multinodular prostate

Excludes: *malignant neoplasm of prostate (185)*

600.10 Nodular prostate without urinary obstruction
Nodular prostate NOS

600.11 Nodular prostate with urinary obstruction
Nodular prostate with urinary retention

⑤ **600.2 Benign localized hyperplasia of prostate**
Adenofibromatous hypertrophy of prostate
Adenoma of prostate
Fibroadenoma of prostate
Fibroma of prostate
Myoma of prostate
Polyp of prostate

Excludes: *benign neoplasms of prostate (222.2)*
hypertrophy of prostate (600.00-600.01)
malignant neoplasm of prostate (185)

600.20 Benign localized hyperplasia of prostate without urinary obstruction and other lower urinary tract symptoms (LUTS)
Benign localized hyperplasia of prostate NOS

600.21 Benign localized hyperplasia of prostate with urinary obstruction and other lower urinary tract symptoms (LUTS)
Benign localized hyperplasia of prostate with urinary retention

Use additional code to identify symptoms:
incomplete bladder emptying (788.21)
nocturia (788.43)
straining on urination (788.65)
urinary frequency (788.41)
urinary hesitancy (788.64)
urinary incontinence (788.30-788.39)
urinary obstruction (599.69)
urinary retention (788.20)
urinary urgency (788.63)
weak urinary stream (788.62)

600.3 Cyst of prostate

⑤ **600.9 Hyperplasia of prostate, unspecified**
Median bar
Prostatic obstruction NOS

600.90 Hyperplasia of prostate, unspecified, without urinary obstruction and other lower urinary symptoms (LUTS)
Hyperplasia of prostate NOS

600

| ■ | Add 4th or 5th digit | ■ | Nonspecific code | ■ | Unspecified code | ■ | Manifestation code |

600.91 Hyperplasia of prostate, unspecified, with urinary obstruction and other lower urinary symptoms (LUTS)
Hyperplasia of prostate, unspecified, with urinary retention

Use additional code to identify symptoms:
incomplete bladder emptying (788.21)
nocturia (788.43)
straining on urination (788.65)
urinary frequency (788.41)
urinary hesitancy (788.64)
urinary incontinence (788.30-788.39)
urinary obstruction (599.69)
urinary retention (788.20)
urinary urgency (788.63)
weak urinary stream (788.62)

601 Inflammatory diseases of prostate
Use additional code, if desired, to identify organism, such as Staphylococcus (041.1), or Streptococcus (041.0)

601.0 Acute prostatitis

601.1 Chronic prostatitis

601.2 Abscess of prostate

601.3 Prostatocystitis

601.4 *Prostatitis in diseases classified elsewhere*
Code first underlying disease, as:
actinomycosis (039.8)
blastomycosis (116.0)
syphilis (095.8)
tuberculosis (016.5)

Excludes: *prostatitis:*
gonococcal (098.12, 098.32)
monilial (112.2)
trichomonal (131.03)

601.8 Other specified inflammatory diseases of prostate
Prostatitis:
cavitary
diverticular
granulomatous

601.9 Prostatitis, unspecified
Prostatitis NOS

602 Other disorders of prostate

602.0 Calculus of prostate
Prostatic stone

602.1 Congestion or hemorrhage of prostate

602.2 Atrophy of prostate

602.3 Dysplasia of prostate
Prostatic intraepithelial neoplasia I (PIN I)
Prostatic intraepithelial neoplasia II (PIN II)

Excludes: *Prostatic intraepithelial neoplasia III (PIN III) (233.4)*

602.8 Other specified disorders of prostate
Fistula of prostate
Infarction of prostate
Stricture of prostate
Periprostatic adhesions

602.9 Unspecified disorder of prostate

603 Hydrocele
Includes: hydrocele of spermatic cord, testis, or tunica vaginalis

Excludes: *congenital (778.6)*

DEFINITION A Hydrocele is a painless swelling of the scrotum, caused by a collection of fluid around the testicle; commonly occurs in middle-aged men

603.0 Encysted hydrocele

603.1 Infected hydrocele
Use additional code, if desired, to identify organism

● Code new
to this edition

▲ Revision of
existing code

④ ⑤ Fourth or fifth
digit required

603.8 Other specified types of hydrocele

603.9 Hydrocele, unspecified

604 Orchitis and epididymitis

Use additional code to identify organism, such as:
  Escherichia coli [E. coli] (041.41-041.49)
  Staphylococcus (041.10-041.19)
  Streptococcus (041.00-041.09)

DEFINITION Orchitis is the inflammation and swelling of the testes as a result of infection or physical injury. Epididymitis is an inflammation of the epididymis which is located along the posterior aspect of the testicle.

604.0 Orchitis, epididymitis, and epididymo-orchitis, with abscess
  Abscess of epididymis or testis

⑤ **604.9** Other orchitis, epididymitis, and epididymo-orchitis, without mention of abscess

604.90 Orchitis and epididymitis, unspecified

604.91 *Orchitis and epididymitis in diseases classified elsewhere*
  Code first underlying disease, as:
    diphtheria (032.89)
    filariasis (125.0-125.9)
    syphilis (095.8)

  Excludes: *orchitis:*
    gonococcal (098.13, 098.33)
    mumps (072.0)
    tuberculous (016.5)
    tuberculous epididymitis (016.4)

604.99 Other

605 Redundant prepuce and phimosis

Adherent prepuce   Phimosis (congenital)
Paraphimosis   Tight foreskin

DEFINITION Redundant prepuce is a condition where the foreskin of the penis more than covers the glans when not erect and does not automatically fully retract upon erection. Phimosis is a constriction of the foreskin of the penis resulting in the inability to retract the prepuce over the glans

606 Infertility, male

DEFINITION Male Infertility refers to the biological inability of the male to contribute to conception

606.0 Azoospermia
  Absolute infertility
  Infertility due to:
    germinal (cell) aplasia
    spermatogenic arrest (complete)

606.1 Oligospermia
  Infertility due to:
    germinal cell desquamation
    hypospermatogenesis
    incomplete spermatogenic arrest

606.8 Infertility due to extratesticular causes
  Infertility due to:
    drug therapy
    infection
    obstruction of efferent ducts
    radiation
    systemic disease

ALERT! For personal history of drug therapy see V87.4

606.9 Male infertility, unspecified

607 Disorders of penis

Excludes: *phimosis (605)*

607.0 Leukoplakia of penis
  Kraurosis of penis

Excludes: *carcinoma in situ of penis (233.5)*
    erythroplasia of Queyrat (233.5)

607.1 Balanoposthitis
  Balanitis

Use additional code, if desired, to identify organism

| | Add 4th or 5th digit | | Nonspecific code | | Unspecified code | | Manifestation code |

607.2 Other inflammatory disorders of penis
Abscess of corpus cavernosum or penis
Boil of corpus cavernosum or penis
Carbuncle of corpus cavernosum or penis
Cellulitis of corpus cavernosum or penis
Cavernitis (penis)
Use additional code, if desired, to identify organism
Excludes: herpetic infection (054.13)

607.3 Priapism
Painful erection

⑤ **607.8 Other specified disorders of penis**

607.81 Balanitis xerotica obliterans
Induratio penis plastica

607.82 Vascular disorders of penis
Embolism of corpus cavernosum or penis
Hematoma (nontraumatic) of corpus cavernosum or penis
Hemorrhage of corpus cavernosum or penis
Thrombosis of corpus cavernosum or penis

607.83 Edema of penis

607.84 Impotence of organic origin
Excludes: nonorganic (302.72)

607.85 Peyronie's disease

607.89 Other
Atrophy of corpus cavernosum or penis
Fibrosis of corpus cavernosum or penis
Hypertrophy of corpus cavernosum or penis
Ulcer (chronic) of corpus cavernosum or penis

607.9 Unspecified disorder of penis

608 Other disorders of male genital organs
ALERT! For personal history of other genital system and obstetric disorders see V13.2

608.0 Seminal vesiculitis
Abscess of seminal vesicle
Cellulitis of seminal vesicle
Vesiculitis (seminal)
Use additional code, if desired, to identify organism
Excludes: gonococcal infection (098.14, 098.34)

608.1 Spermatocele

⑤ **608.2 Torsion of testis**

608.20 Torsion of testis, unspecified

608.21 Extravaginal torsion of spermatic cord

608.22 Intravaginal torsion of spermatic cord
Torsion of spermatic cord NOS

608.23 Torsion of appendix testis

608.24 Torsion of appendix epididymis

608.3 Atrophy of testis

608.4 Other inflammatory disorders of male genital organs
Abscess of scrotum, spermatic cord, testis [except abscess], tunica vaginalis, or vas deferens
Boil of scrotum, spermatic cord, testis [except abscess], tunica vaginalis, or vas deferens
Carbuncle of scrotum, spermatic cord, testis [except abscess], tunica vaginalis, or vas deferens
Cellulitis of scrotum, spermatic cord, testis [except abscess], tunica vaginalis, or vas deferens
Vasitis
Use additional code, if desired, to identify organism
Excludes: abscess of testis (604.0)

⑤ **608.8 Other specified disorders of male genital organs**

608.81 Disorders of male genital organs in diseases classified elsewhere
Code first underlying disease, as:
filariasis (125.0-125.9)
tuberculosis (016.5)

608.82 Hematospermia

● Code new to this edition   ▲ Revision of existing code   ④ ⑤ Fourth or fifth digit required

608.83 Vascular disorders
Hematoma (nontraumatic) of seminal vesicle, spermatic cord, testis, scrotum, tunica vaginalis, or vas deferens
Hemorrhage of seminal vesicle, spermatic cord, testis, scrotum, tunica vaginalis, or vas deferens
Thrombosis of seminal vesicle, spermatic cord, testis, scrotum, tunica vaginalis, or vas deferens
Hematocele NOS, male

608.84 Chylocele of tunica vaginalis

608.85 Stricture
Stricture of:
  spermatic cord
  tunica vaginalis
  vas deferens

608.86 Edema

608.87 Retrograde ejaculation

608.89 Other
Atrophy of seminal vesicle, spermatic cord, testis, scrotum, tunica vaginalis, or vas deferens
Fibrosis of seminal vesicle, spermatic cord, testis, scrotum, tunica vaginalis, or vas deferens
Hypertrophy of seminal vesicle, spermatic cord, testis, scrotum, tunica vaginalis, or vas deferens
Ulcer of seminal vesicle, spermatic cord, testis, scrotum, tunica vaginalis, or vas deferens

Excludes: atrophy of testis (608.3)

608.9 Unspecified disorder of male genital organs

DISORDERS OF BREAST (610-612)

610 Benign mammary dysplasias
DEFINITION Mammary dysplasia is a common condition marked by benign (noncancerous) changes in breast tissue. These changes may include irregular lumps or cysts, breast discomfort, sensitive nipples, and itching.

610.0 Solitary cyst of breast
Cyst (solitary) of breast

610.1 Diffuse cystic mastopathy
Chronic cystic mastitis   Fibrocystic disease of breast
Cystic breast

610.2 Fibroadenosis of breast
Fibroadenosis of breast: Fibroadenosis of breast:
  NOS   diffuse
  chronic   periodic
  cystic   segmental

610.3 Fibrosclerosis of breast

610.4 Mammary duct ectasia
Comedomastitis   Mastitis:
Dust ectasia   periductal
                          plasma cell

610.8 Other specified benign mammary dysplasias
Mazoplasia
Sebaceous cyst of breast

610.9 Benign mammary dysplasia, unspecified

611 Other disorders of breast

Excludes: that associated with lactation or the puerperium (675.0-676.9)

Add 4th or 5th digit   Nonspecific code   Unspecified code   Manifestation code

611.0 Inflammatory disease of breast
    Abscess (acute) (chronic) (nonpuerperal) of:
      areola
      breast
    Mammillary fistula
    Mastitis (acute) (subacute) (nonpuerperal):
      NOS
      infective
      retromammary
      submammary

    | Excludes: | *carbuncle of breast (680.2)*
        chronic cystic mastitis (610.1)
        neonatal infective mastitis (771.5)
        thrombophlebitis of breast [Mondor's disease] (451.89)

611.1 Hypertrophy of breast
    Gynecomastia
    Hypertrophy of breast:
      NOS
      massive pubertal

    | Excludes: | *breast engorgement in newborn (778.7)*
        disproportion of reconstructed breast (612.1)

611.2 Fissure of nipple

611.3 Fat necrosis of breast
    Fat necrosis (segmental) of breast
Code first breast necrosis due to breast graft (996.79)

611.4 Atrophy of breast

611.5 Galactocele

611.6 Galactorrhea not associated with childbirth

⑤ **611.7 Signs and symptoms in breast**

    611.71 Mastodynia
      Pain in breast

    611.72 Lump or mass in breast

    611.79 Other
      Induration of breast   Nipple discharge
      Inversion of nipple   Retraction of nipple

⑤ **611.8 Other specified disorders of breast**

    611.81 Ptosis of breast

    | Excludes: | *ptosis of native breast in relation to reconstructed breast (612.1)*

    611.82 Hypoplasia of breast
      Micromastia

    | Excludes: | *congenital absence of breast (757.6)*
        hypoplasia of native breast in relation to reconstructed breast (612.1)

    611.83 Capsular contracture of breast implant

    611.89 Other specified disorders of breast
      Hematoma (nontraumatic) of breast
      Infarction of breast
      Occlusion of breast duct
      Subinvolution of breast (postlactational) (postpartum)

611.9 Unspecified breast disorder

612 Deformity and disproportion of reconstructed breast

612.0 Deformity of reconstructed breast
    Contour irregularity in reconstructed breast
    Excess tissue in reconstructed breast
    Misshapen reconstructed breast

612.1 Disproportion of reconstructed breast
    Breast asymmetry between native breast and reconstructed breast
    Disproportion between native breast and reconstructed breast

INFLAMMATORY DISEASE OF FEMALE PELVIC ORGANS (614-616)

Use additional code, if desired, to identify organism, such as Staphylococcus (041.1), or Streptococcus (041.0)

> *Excludes:* *that associated with pregnancy, abortion, childbirth, or the puerperium (630-676.9)*

614 **Inflammatory disease of ovary, fallopian tube, pelvic cellular tissue, and peritoneum**

> *Excludes:* *endometritis (615.0-615.9)*
> *major infection following delivery (670.0-670.8)*
> *that complicating:*
> *abortion (634-638 with .0, 639.0)*
> *ectopic or molar pregnancy (639.0)*
> *pregnancy or labor (646.6)*

DEFINITION Inflammatory disease is a general term for infection of the uterus lining, fallopian tubes, or ovaries.

614.0 Acute salpingitis and oophoritis
Any condition classifiable to 614.2, specified as acute or subacute

614.1 Chronic salpingitis and oophoritis
Hydrosalpinx
Salpingitis:
 follicularis
 isthmica nodosa
Any condition classifiable to 614.2, specified as chronic

614.2 Salpingitis and oophoritis not specified as acute, subacute, or chronic

Abscess (of):	Perisalpingitis
fallopian tube	Pyosalpinx
ovary	Salpingitis
tubo-ovarian	Salpingo-oophoritisRTubo-ovarian inflammatory disease
Oophoritis	
Perioophoritis	

> *Excludes:* *gonococcal infection (chronic) (098.37)*
> *acute (098.17)*
> *tuberculous (016.6)*

614.3 Acute parametritis and pelvic cellulitis
Acute inflammatory pelvic disease
Any condition classifiable to 614.4, specified as acute

614.4 Chronic or unspecified parametritis and pelvic cellulitis
Abscess (of):
 broad ligament, chronic or NOS
 parametrium, chronic or NOS
 pelvis, female, chronic or NOS
 pouch of Douglas, chronic or NOS
Chronic inflammatory pelvic disease
Pelvic cellulitis, female

> *Excludes:* *tuberculous (016.7)*

614.5 Acute or unspecified pelvic peritonitis, female

614.6 Pelvic peritoneal adhesions, female (postoperative) (postinfection)
Adhesions:
 peritubal
 tubo-ovarian

Use additional code, if desired, to identify any associated infertility (628.2)

614.7 Other chronic pelvic peritonitis, female

> *Excludes:* *tuberculous (016.7)*

614.8 Other specified inflammatory disease of female pelvic organs and tissues

614.9 Unspecified inflammatory disease of female pelvic organs and tissues
Pelvic infection or inflammation, female NOS
Pelvic inflammatory disease [PID]

615 **Inflammatory diseases of uterus, except cervix**

> *Excludes:* *following delivery (670.0-670.8)*
> *hyperplastic endometritis (621.30-621.35)*
> *that complicating:*
> *abortion (634-638 with .0, 639.0)*
> *ectopic or molar pregnancy (639.0)*
> *pregnancy or labor (646.6)*

	Add 4th or 5th digit		Nonspecific code		Unspecified code		Manifestation code

615.0 Acute
Any condition classifiable to 615.9, specified as acute or subacute

615.1 Chronic
Any condition classifiable to 615.9, specified as chronic

615.9 Unspecified inflammatory disease of uterus

Endometritis	Perimetritis
Endomyometritis	Pyometra
Metritis	Uterine abscess
Myometritis	

616 Inflammatory disease of cervix, vagina, and vulva

Excludes: *that complicating:*
> *abortion (634-638 with .0, 639.0)*
> *ectopic or molar pregnancy (639.0)*
> *pregnancy, childbirth, or the puerperium (646.6)*

616.0 Cervicitis and endocervicitis
Cervicitis with or without mention of erosion or ectropion
Endocervicitis with or without mention of erosion or ectropion
Nabothian (gland) cyst or follicle

Excludes: *erosion or ectropion without mention of cervicitis (622.0)*

⑤ **616.1 Vaginitis and vulvovaginitis**

Excludes: *vulvar vestibulitis (625.71)*

616.10 Vaginitis and vulvovaginitis, unspecified
Vaginitis:
  NOS
  postirradiation
Vulvitis NOS
Vulvovaginitis NOS

Use additional code to identify organism, such as:
  Escherichia coli [E. coli] (041.41-041.49)
  Staphylococcus (041.10-041.19)
  Streptococcus (041.00-041.09)

Excludes: *noninfective leukorrhea (623.5)*
> *postmenopausal or senile vaginitis (627.3)*

616.11 Vaginitis and vulvovaginitis in diseases classified elsewhere
Code first underlying disease, as:
  pinworm vaginitis (127.4)

Excludes: *herpetic vulvovaginitis (054.11)*
> *monilial vulvovaginitis (112.1)*
> *trichomonal vaginitis or vulvovaginitis (131.01)*

616.2 Cyst of Bartholin's gland
Bartholin's duct cyst

616.3 Abscess of Bartholin's gland
Vulvovaginal gland abscess

616.4 Other abscess of vulva
Abscess of vulva
Carbuncle of vulva
Furuncle of vulva

⑤ **616.5 Ulceration of vulva**

616.50 Ulceration of vulva, unspecified
Ulcer NOS of vulva

616.51 Ulceration of vulva in diseases classified elsewhere
Code first underlying disease, as:
  Behçet's syndrome (136.1)
  tuberculosis (016.7)

Excludes: *vulvar ulcer (in):*
> *gonococcal (098.0)*
> *herpes simplex (054.12)*
> *syphilitic (091.0)*

● Code new
to this edition

▲ Revision of
existing code

④ ⑤ Fourth or fifth
digit required

⑤ **616.8 Other specified inflammatory diseases of cervix, vagina, and vulva**

Excludes: *noninflammatory disorders of:*
cervix (622.0-622.9)
vagina (623.0-623.9)
vulva (624.0-624.9)

> **616.81 Mucositis (ulcerative) of cervix, vagina, and vulva**
> Use additional E code to identify adverse effects of therapy, such as:
> antineoplastic and immunosuppressive drugs (E930.7, E933.1)
> radiation therapy (E879.2)

> **616.89 Other inflammatory disease of cervix, vagina and vulva**
> Caruncle, vagina or labium
> Ulcer, vagina

616.9 Unspecified inflammatory disease of cervix, vagina, and vulva

OTHER DISORDERS OF FEMALE GENITAL TRACT (617-629)

617 Endometriosis
> **DEFINITION** Endometriosis is a condition where tissue that normally lines the uterus grows in other areas of the body. This can cause pain, irregular menstrual bleeding, and infertility for some women.

617.0 Endometriosis of uterus
Adenomyosis
Endometriosis:
cervix
internal
myometrium

Excludes: *stromal endometriosis (236.0)*

617.1 Endometriosis of ovary
Chocolate cyst of ovary
Endometrial cystoma of ovary

617.2 Endometriosis of fallopian tube

617.3 Endometriosis of pelvic peritoneum
Endometriosis: Endometriosis:
broad ligament   parametrium
cul-de-sac (Douglas')   round ligament

617.4 Endometriosis of rectovaginal septum and vagina

617.5 Endometriosis of intestine
Endometriosis:
appendix
colon
rectum

617.6 Endometriosis in scar of skin

617.8 Endometriosis of other specified sites
Endometriosis: Endometriosis:
bladder   umbilicus
lung   vulva

617.9 Endometriosis, site unspecified

618 Genital prolapse
Use additional code, if desired, to identify urinary incontinence (625.6, 788.31, 788.33-788.39)
> *Excludes:* *that complicating pregnancy, labor, or delivery (654.4)*
> **DEFINITION** Genital prolapse is a condition in which the vaginal wall or uterus descend below their normal positions; part of the bladder or rectum may protrude from the vagina

⑤ **618.0 Prolapse of vaginal walls without mention of uterine prolapse**
> *Excludes:* *that with uterine prolapse (618.2-618.4)*
> *enterocele (618.6)*
> *vaginal vault prolapse following hysterectomy (618.5)*

> **618.00 Unspecified prolapse of vaginal walls**
> Vaginal prolapse NOS

> **618.01 Cystocele, midline**
> Cystocele NOS

> **618.02 Cystocele, lateral**
> Paravaginal

> **618.03 Urethrocele**

507

Add 4th or 5th digit   Nonspecific code   Unspecified code   Manifestation code

618.04 Rectocele
　　Proctocele
Use additional code for any associated fecal incontinence (787.60-787.63)

618.05 Perineocele

618.09 Other prolapse of vaginal walls without mention of uterine prolapse
　　Cystourethrocele

618.1 Uterine prolapse without mention of vaginal wall prolapse

Descensus uteri	Uterine prolapse:
Uterine prolapse:	first degree
NOS	second degree
complete	third degree

　Excludes: that with mention of cystocele, urethrocele, or rectocele (618.2-618.4)

618.2 Uterovaginal prolapse, incomplete

618.3 Uterovaginal prolapse, complete

618.4 Uterovaginal prolapse, unspecified

618.5 Prolapse of vaginal vault after hysterectomy

618.6 Vaginal enterocele, congenital or acquired
　　Pelvic enterocele, congenital or acquired

618.7 Old laceration of muscles of pelvic floor

⑤ **618.8 Other specified genital prolapse**

　　618.81 Incompetence or weakening of pubocervical tissue

　　618.82 Incompetence or weakening of rectovaginal tissue

　　618.83 Pelvic muscle wasting
　　　　Disuse atrophy of pelvic muscles and anal sphincter

　　618.84 Cervical stump prolapse

　　618.89 Other specified genital prolapse

618.9 Unspecified genital prolapse

619 Fistula involving female genital tract

　Excludes: vesicorectal and intestinovesical fistula (596.1)

　DEFINITION A fistula involving female genital tract is a fistula that has formed in the wall of the vagina. A vaginal fistula may open into the urinary tract, the rectum, the colon, or the small bowel

619.0 Urinary-genital tract fistula, female

Fistula:	Fistula:
cervicovesical	uteroureteric
ureterovaginal	uterovesical
urethrovaginal	vesicocervicovaginal
urethrovesicovaginal	vesicovaginal

619.1 Digestive-genital tract fistula, female

Fistula:	Fistula:
intestinouterine	rectovulval
intestinovaginal	sigmoidovaginal
rectovaginal	uterorectal

619.2 Genital tract-skin fistula, female
　　Fistula:
　　　uterus to abdominal wall
　　　vaginoperinea

619.8 Other specified fistulas involving female genital tract

Fistula:	Fistula:
cervix	uterus
cul-de-sac (Douglas')	vagina

619.9 Unspecified fistula involving female genital tract

620 Noninflammatory disorders of ovary, fallopian tube, and broad ligament

　Excludes: hydrosalpinx (614.1)

　DEFINITION Noninflammatory disorders of ovary, fallopian tube, and broad ligament, noninflammatory refer to degenerative and/or neoplastic disorders of the ovary, fallopian tube, and broad ligament.

620.0 Follicular cyst of ovary
　　Cyst of graafian follicle

● Code new	▲ Revision of	④ ⑤ Fourth or fifth
to this edition	existing code	digit required

620.1 Corpus luteum cyst or hematoma
Corpus luteum hemorrhage or rupture
Lutein cyst

620.2 Other and unspecified ovarian cyst
Cyst of ovary:
NOS
corpus albicans
retention NOS
serous
theca-lutein
Simple cystoma of ovary

Excludes: cystadenoma (benign) (serous) (220)
developmental cysts (752.0)
neoplastic cysts (220)
polycystic ovaries (256.4)
Stein-Leventhal syndrome (256.4)

620.3 Acquired atrophy of ovary and fallopian tube
Senile involution of ovary

620.4 Prolapse or hernia of ovary and fallopian tube
Displacement of ovary and fallopian tube
Salpingocele

620.5 Torsion of ovary, ovarian pedicle, or fallopian tube
Torsion:
accessory tube
hydatid of Morgagni

620.6 Broad ligament laceration syndrome
Masters-Allen syndrome

620.7 Hematoma of broad ligament
Hematocele, broad ligament

620.8 Other noninflammatory disorders of ovary, fallopian tube, and broad ligament
Cyst of broad ligament or fallopian tube
Polyp of broad ligament or fallopian tube
Infarction of ovary or fallopian tube
Rupture of ovary or fallopian tube
Hematosalpinx of ovary or fallopian tube

Excludes: hematosalpinx in ectopic pregnancy (639.2)
peritubal adhesions (614.6)
torsion of ovary, ovarian pedicle, or fallopian tube (620.5)

620.9 Unspecified noninflammatory disorder of ovary, fallopian tube, and broad ligament

621 Disorders of uterus, not elsewhere classified

621.0 Polyp of corpus uteri
Polyp:
endometrium
uterus NOS

Excludes: cervical polyp NOS (622.7)

621.1 Chronic subinvolution of uterus

Excludes: puerperal (674.8)

621.2 Hypertrophy of uterus
Bulky or enlarged uterus

Excludes: puerperal (674.8)

⑤ **621.3 Endometrial hyperplasia**

621.30 Endometrial hyperplasia, unspecified
Endometrial hyperplasia NOS
Hyperplasia (adenomatous) (cystic) (glandular) of endometrium
Hyperplastic endometritis

621.31 Simple endometrial hyperplasia without atypia

Excludes: benign endometrial hyperplasia (621.34)

621.32 Complex endometrial hyperplasia without atypia

Excludes: benign endometrial hyperplasia (621.34)

621.33 Endometrial hyperplasia with atypia

Excludes: endometrial intraepithelial neoplasia [EIN] (621.35)

| | Add 4th or 5th digit | | Nonspecific code | | Unspecified code | | Manifestation code |

621.34 **Benign endometrial hyperplasia**

621.35 **Endometrial intraepithelial neoplasia [EIN]**

Excludes: *malignant neoplasm of endometrium with endometrial intraepithelial neoplasia [EIN] (182.0)*

621.4 Hematometra
Hemometra

Excludes: *that in congenital anomaly (752.2-752.39)*

621.5 Intrauterine synechiae
Adhesions of uterus
Band(s) of uterus

621.6 Malposition of uterus
Anteversion of uterus
Retroflexion of uterus
Retroversion of uterus

Excludes: *malposition complicating pregnancy, labor, or delivery (654.3-654.4)*
prolapse of uterus (618.1-618.4)

621.7 Chronic inversion of uterus

Excludes: *current obstetrical trauma (665.2)*
prolapse of uterus (618.1-618.4)

621.8 Other specified disorders of uterus, not elsewhere classified
Atrophy, acquired of uterus
Cyst of uterus
Fibrosis NOS of uterus
Old laceration (postpartum) of uterus
Ulcer of uterus

Excludes: *bilharzial fibrosis (120.0-120.9)*
endometriosis (617.0)
fistulas (619.0-619.8)
inflammatory diseases (615.0-615.9)

621.9 Unspecified disorder of uterus

622 Noninflammatory disorders of cervix

Excludes: *abnormality of cervix complicating pregnancy, labor, or delivery (654.5-654.6)*
fistula (619.0-619.8)

622.0 Erosion and ectropion of cervix
Eversion of cervix
Ulcer of cervix

Excludes: *that in chronic cervicitis (616.0)*

⑤ **622.1 Dysplasia of cervix (uteri)**

Excludes: *abnormal results from cervical cytologic examination without histologic confirmation (795.00-795.09)*
carcinoma in situ of cervix (233.1)
cervical intraepithelial neoplasia III [CIN III] (233.1)
HGSIL of cervix (795.04)

ALERT! For personal history of cervical dysplasia see V13.22

622.10 **Dysplasia of cervix, unspecified**
Anaplasia of cervix
Cervical atypism
Cervical dysplasia NOS

622.11 **Mild dysplasia of cervix**
Cervical intraepithelial neoplasia I [CIN I]

622.12 **Moderate dysplasia of cervix**
Cervical intraepithelial neoplasia II [CIN II]

Excludes: *carcinoma in situ of cervix (233.1)*
cervical intraepithelial neoplasia III [CIN III] (233.1)
severe dysplasia (233.1)

622.2 Leukoplakia of cervix (uteri)

Excludes: *carcinoma in situ of cervix (233.1)*

● Code new
to this edition

▲ Revision of
existing code

④ ⑤ Fourth or fifth
digit required

622.3 Old laceration of cervix
 Adhesions of cervix
 Band(s) of cervix
 Cicatrix (postpartum) of cervix

Excludes: *current obstetrical trauma (665.3)*

622.4 Stricture and stenosis of cervix
 Atresia (acquired) of cervix
 Contracture of cervix
 Occlusion of cervix
 Pinpoint os uteri

Excludes: *congenital (752.49)*
 that complicating labor (654.6)

622.5 Incompetence of cervix

Excludes: *complicating pregnancy (654.5)*
 that affecting fetus or newborn (761.0)

622.6 Hypertrophic elongation of cervix

622.7 Mucous polyp of cervix
 Polyp NOS of cervix

Excludes: *adenomatous polyp of cervix (219.0)*

622.8 Other specified noninflammatory disorders of cervix
 Atrophy (senile) of cervix
 Cyst of cervix
 Fibrosis of cervix
 Hemorrhage of cervix

Excludes: *endometriosis (617.0)*
 fistula (619.0-619.8)
 inflammatory diseases (616.0)

622.9 Unspecified noninflammatory disorder of cervix

623 Noninflammatory disorders of vagina

Excludes: *abnormality of vagina complicating pregnancy, labor, or delivery (654.7)*
 congenital absence of vagina (752.49)
 congenital diaphragm or bands (752.49)
 fistulas involving vagina (619.0-619.8)

623.0 Dysplasia of vagina
 Mild and moderate dysplasia of vagina
 Vaginal intraepithelial neoplasia I and II [VAIN I and II]

Excludes: *abnormal results from vaginal cytological examination without histologic confirmation (795.10-795.19)*
 carcinoma in situ of vagina (233.31)
 HGSIL of vagina (795.14)
 severe dysplasia of vagina (233.31)
 vaginal intraepithelial neoplasia III [VAIN III] (233.31)

623.1 Leukoplakia of vagina

623.2 Stricture or atresia of vagina
 Adhesions (postoperative) (postradiation) of vagina
 Occlusion of vagina
 Stenosis, vagina

Use additional E code, if desired, to identify any external cause

Excludes: *congenital atresia or stricture (752.49)*

623.3 Tight hymenal ring
 Rigid hymen acquired or congenital
 Tight hymenal ring acquired or congenital
 Tight introitus acquired or congenital

Excludes: *imperforate hymen (752.42)*

623.4 Old vaginal laceration

Excludes: *old laceration involving muscles of pelvic floor (618.7)*

623.5 Leukorrhea, not specified as infective
 Leukorrhea NOS of vagina
 Vaginal discharge NOS

Excludes: *trichomonal (131.00)*

| | Add 4th or 5th digit | | Nonspecific code | | Unspecified code | | Manifestation code |

623.6 Vaginal hematoma

Excludes: *current obstetrical trauma (665.7)*

623.7 Polyp of vagina

623.8 Other specified noninflammatory disorders of vagina
Cyst of vagina
Hemorrhage of vagina

623.9 Unspecified noninflammatory disorder of vagina

624 Noninflammatory disorders of vulva and perineum

Excludes: *abnormality of vulva and perineum complicating pregnancy, labor, or delivery (654.8)*
condyloma acuminatum (078.11)
fistulas involving:
perineum—see Alphabetic Index
vulva (619.0-619.8)
vulval varices (456.6)
vulvar involvement in skin conditions (690-709.9)

⑤ **624.0 Dystrophy of vulva**

Excludes: *carcinoma in situ of vulva (233.32)*
severe dysplasia of vulva (233.32)
vulvar intraepithelial neoplasia III [VIN III] (233.32)

624.01 Vulvar intraepithelial neoplasia I [VIN I]
Mild dysplasia of vulva

624.02 Vulvar intraepithelial neoplasia II [VIN II]
Moderate dysplasia of vulva

624.09 Other dystrophy of vulva
Kraurosis of vulva
Leukoplakia of vulva

624.1 Atrophy of vulva

624.2 Hypertrophy of clitoris

Excludes: *that in endocrine disorders (255.2, 256.1)*

624.3 Hypertrophy of labia
Hypertrophy of vulva NOS

624.4 Old laceration or scarring of vulva

624.5 Hematoma of vulva

Excludes: *that complicating delivery (664.5)*

624.6 Polyp of labia and vulva

624.8 Other specified noninflammatory disorders of vulva and perineum
Cyst of vulva
Edema of vulva
Stricture of vulva

624.9 Unspecified noninflammatory disorder of vulva and perineum

625 Pain and other symptoms associated with female genital organs

625.0 Dyspareunia

Excludes: *psychogenic dyspareunia (302.76)*

625.1 Vaginismus
Colpospasm
Vulvismus

Excludes: *psychogenic vaginismus (306.51)*

625.2 Mittelschmerz
Intermenstrual pain
Ovulation pain

625.3 Dysmenorrhea
Painful menstruation

Excludes: *psychogenic dysmenorrhea (306.52)*

● Code new
to this edition
▲ Revision of
existing code
④ ⑤ Fourth or fifth
digit required

625.4 Premenstrual tension syndromes
Menstrual molimen
Premenstrual dysphoric disorder
Premenstrual syndrome
Premenstrual tension NOS

Excludes: menstrual migraine (346.4)

625.5 Pelvic congestion syndrome
Congestion-fibrosis syndrome
Taylor's syndrome

625.6 Stress incontinence, female

Excludes: mixed incontinence (788.33)
stress incontinence, male (788.32)

⑤ **625.7 Vulvodynia**

625.70 Vulvodynia, unspecified
Vulvodynia NOS

625.71 Vulvar vestibulitis

625.79 Other vulvodynia

625.8 Other specified symptoms associated with female genital organs

625.9 Unspecified symptom associated with female genital organs

626 Disorders of menstruation and other abnormal bleeding from female genital tract

Excludes: menopausal and premenopausal bleeding (627.0)
pain and other symptoms associated with menstrual cycle (625.2-625.4)
postmenopausal bleeding (627.1)
precocious puberty (259.1)

626.0 Absence of menstruation
Amenorrhea (primary) (secondary)

626.1 Scanty or infrequent menstruation
Hypomenorrhea
Oligomenorrhea

626.2 Excessive or frequent menstruation
Heavy periods   Menorrhagia
Menometrorrhagia   Polymenorrhea

Excludes: premenopausal (627.0)
that in puberty (626.3)

626.3 Puberty bleeding
Excessive bleeding associated with onset of menstrual periods
Pubertal menorrhagia

626.4 Irregular menstrual cycle
Irregular:
bleeding NOS
menstruation
periods

626.5 Ovulation bleeding
Regular intermenstrual bleeding

626.6 Metrorrhagia
Bleeding unrelated to menstrual cycle
Irregular intermenstrual bleeding

626.7 Postcoital bleeding

626.8 Other
Dysfunctional or functional uterine hemorrhage NOS
Menstruation:
retained
suppression of

626.9 Unspecified

627 Menopausal and postmenopausal disorders

Excludes: asymptomatic age-related (natural) postmenopausal status (V49.81)

DEFINITION Menopausal and postmenopausal disorders refer to disorders occuring during and after the menopausal period.

Add 4th or
5th digit

Nonspecific
code

Unspecified
code

Manifestation
code

627.0 Premenopausal menorrhagia
Excessive bleeding associated with onset of menopause
Menorrhagia:
    climacteric
    menopausal
    preclimacteric

627.1 Postmenopausal bleeding

627.2 Symptomatic menopausal or female climacteric states
Symptoms, such as flushing, sleeplessness, headache, lack of concentration, associated with the menopause

627.3 Postmenopausal atrophic vaginitis
Senile (atrophic) vaginitis

627.4 Symptomatic states associated with artificial menopause
Postartificial menopause syndromes
Any condition classifiable to 627.1, 627.2, or 627.3 which follows induced menopause

627.8 Other specified menopausal and postmenopausal disorders
Excludes: premature menopause NOS (256.31)

627.9 Unspecified menopausal and postmenopausal disorder

628 Infertility, female
Includes: primary and secondary sterility
DEFINITION Female Infertility refers to the biological inability of the female to contribute to conception.

628.0 Associated with anovulation
Anovulatory cycle
Use additional code for any associated Stein-Leventhal syndrome (256.4)

628.1 *Of pituitary-hypothalamic origin*
Code first underlying cause, as:
    adiposogenital dystrophy (253.8)
    anterior pituitary disorder (253.0-253.4)

628.2 Of tubal origin
Infertility associated with congenital anomaly of tube
Tubal:
    block
    occlusion
    stenosis
Use additional code for any associated peritubal adhesions (614.6)

628.3 Of uterine origin
Infertility associated with congenital anomaly of uterus
Nonimplantation
Use additional code for any associated tuberculous endometritis (016.7)

628.4 Of cervical or vaginal origin
Infertility associated with:
    anomaly of cervical mucus
    congenital structural anomaly
    dysmucorrhea

628.8 Of other specified origin

628.9 Of unspecified origin

629 Other disorders of female genital organs
ALERT! For personal history of other genital system and obstetric disorders see V13.2

629.0 Hematocele, female, not elsewhere classified
Excludes: hematocele or hematoma:
    broad ligament (620.7)
    fallopian tube (620.8)
    that associated with ectopic pregnancy (633.00-633.91)
    uterus (621.4)
    vagina (623.6)
    vulva (624.5)

629.1 Hydrocele, canal of Nuck
Cyst of canal of Nuck (acquired)
Excludes: congenital (752.41)

● Code new   ▲ Revision of   ④ ⑤ Fourth or fifth
     to this edition   existing code   digit required

⑤ **629.2 Female genital mutilation status**
Female circumcision status
Female genital cutting

    629.20 Female genital mutilation status, unspecified
Female genital cutting status, unspecified
Female genital mutilation status NOS
Female genital mutilation status, type 4

    629.21 Female genital mutilation Type I status
Clitorectomy status
Female genital cutting Type I status

    629.22 Female genital mutilation Type II status
Clitorectomy with excision of labia minor status
Female genital cutting Type II status

    629.23 Female genital mutilation Type III status
Female genital cutting Type III status
Infibulation status

    629.29 Other female genital mutilation status
Female genital cutting Type IV status
Female genital mutilation Type IV status
Other female genital cutting status

● **629.3 Complication of implanted vaginal mesh and other prosthetic materials**

  ● **629.31 Erosion of implanted vaginal mesh and other prosthetic materials to surrounding organ or tissue**
Erosion of implanted vaginal mesh and other prosthetic materials into pelvic floor muscles

  ● **629.32 Exposure of implanted vaginal mesh and other prosthetic materials into vagina**
Exposure of vaginal mesh and other prosthetic materials through vaginal wall

⑤ **629.8 Other specified disorders of female genital organs**

    629.81 Recurrent pregnancy loss without current pregnancy

    Excludes: recurrent pregnancy loss with current pregnancy (646.3)

    629.89 Other specified disorders of female genital organs

629.9 Unspecified disorder of female genital organs

	Add 4th or 5th digit		Nonspecific code		Unspecified code		Manifestation code

This page intentionally left blank

● Code new
to this edition

▲ Revision of
existing code

④ ⑤ Fourth or fifth
digit required

Chapter 11: Complications of Pregnancy, Childbirth, and the Puerperium (630-679)

DEFINITIONS AND CODING ALERTS

This chapter includes definitions of selected key words, terms and phrases and coding alerts for adding points to the clinical domain, references to coding late effects where appropriate, and references to personal history V-codes in situations where the acute or chronic condition is no longer active. An example from this chapter is as follows:

⑤ **679** **Complications of in utero procedures**

> **DEFINITION** Complications of in utero procedures, refers to problems caused by procedures performed on the unborn fetus.
>
> **ALERT!** For personal history of undergoing in utero procedure during pregnancy see V15.21
>
> **ALERT!** For personal history of undergoing in utero procedure while a fetus see V15.22

MULTIPLE CODING FOR A SINGLE CONDITION

In addition to the etiology or manifestation convention that requires two codes to fully describe a single condition that affects multiple body systems, there are other single conditions that also require more than one code. "Use additional code" notes are found in the tabular at codes that are not part of an etiology or manifestation pair where a secondary code is useful to fully describe a condition. The sequencing rule is the same as the etiology or manifestation pair - , "use additional code" indicates that a secondary code should be added.

"Code first" notes are also under certain codes that are not specifically manifestation codes but may be due to an underlying cause. When a "code first" note is present and an underlying condition is present the underlying condition should be sequenced first.

"Code, if applicable, any causal condition first", notes indicate that this code may be assigned as a principal diagnosis when the causal condition is unknown or not applicable. If a causal condition is known, then the code for that condition should be sequenced as the principal or first-listed diagnosis. Multiple codes may be needed for late effects, complication codes and obstetric codes to more fully describe a condition. See the specific guidelines for these conditions for further instruction.

COMBINATION CODE

A combination code is a single code used to classify: two diagnoses, or a diagnosis with an associated secondary process (manifestation) A diagnosis with an associated complication Combination codes are identified by referring to subterm entries in the Alphabetic Index and by reading the inclusion and exclusion notes in the Tabular List.

Assign only the combination code when that code fully identifies the diagnostic conditions involved or when the Alphabetic Index so directs. Multiple coding should not be used when the classification provides a combination code that clearly identifies all of the elements documented in the diagnosis. When the combination code lacks necessary specificity in describing the manifestation or complication, an additional code should be used as a secondary code.

CODING LATE EFFECTS

A late effect is the residual effect (condition produced) after the acute phase of an illness or injury has terminated. There is no time limit on when a late effect code can be used. The residual may be apparent early, such as in cerebrovascular accident cases, or it may occur months or years later, such as that due to a previous injury. Coding of late effects generally requires two codes sequenced in the following order: The condition or nature of the late effect is sequenced first. The late effect code is sequenced second.

An exception to the above guidelines are those instances where the code for late effect is followed by a manifestation code identified in the Tabular List and title, or the late effect code has been expanded (at the fourth and fifth-digit levels) to include the manifestation(s). The code for the acute phase of an illness or injury that led to the late effect is never used with a code for the late effect.

GENERAL RULES FOR OBSTETRIC CASES

Codes from chapter 11 and sequencing priority

Obstetric cases require codes from chapter 11, codes in the range 630-677, Complications of Pregnancy, Childbirth, and the Puerperium. Chapter 11 codes have sequencing priority over codes from other chapters. Additional codes from other chapters may be used in conjunction with chapter 11 codes to further specify

| ▨ Add 4th or 5th digit | ▨ Nonspecific code | ▨ Unspecified code | ▨ Manifestation code |

conditions. Should the provider document that the pregnancy is incidental to the encounter, then code V22.2 should be used in place of any chapter 11 codes. It is the provider's responsibility to state that the condition being treated is not affecting the pregnancy.

Chapter 11 codes are to be used only on the maternal record, never on the record of the newborn.

Chapter 11 fifth-digits

Categories 640-648, 651-676 have required fifth-digits, which indicate whether the encounter is antepartum, postpartum and whether a delivery has also occurred.

The fifth-digits, which are appropriate for each code number, are listed in brackets under each code. The fifth-digits on each code should all be consistent with each other. That is, should a delivery occur all of the fifth-digits should indicate the delivery.

SELECTION OF OB PRINCIPAL OR FIRST-LISTED DIAGNOSIS

Routine outpatient prenatal visits

For routine outpatient prenatal visits when no complications are present codes V22.0, Supervision of normal first pregnancy, and V22.1, Supervision of other normal pregnancy, should be used as the first-listed diagnoses. These codes should not be used in conjunction with chapter 11 codes.

Prenatal outpatient visits for high-risk patients

For prenatal outpatient visits for patients with high-risk pregnancies, a code from category V23, Supervision of high-risk pregnancy, should be used as the first-listed diagnosis. Secondary chapter 11 codes may be used in conjunction with these codes if appropriate.

Episodes when no delivery occurs

In episodes when no delivery occurs, the principal diagnosis should correspond to the principal complication of the pregnancy, which necessitated the encounter. Should more than one complication exist, all of which are treated or monitored, any of the complications codes may be sequenced first.

When a delivery occurs

When a delivery occurs, the principal diagnosis should correspond to the main circumstances or complication of the delivery. In cases of cesarean delivery, the selection of the principal diagnosis should correspond to the reason the cesarean delivery was performed unless the reason for admission or encounter was unrelated to the condition resulting in the cesarean delivery.

Outcome of delivery

An outcome of delivery code, V27.0-V27.9, should be included on every maternal record when a delivery has occurred. These codes are not to be used on subsequent records or on the newborn record.

FETAL CONDITIONS AFFECTING THE MANAGEMENT OF THE MOTHER

Codes from category 655

Known or suspected fetal abnormality affecting management of the mother, and category 656, Other fetal and placental problems affecting the management of the mother, are assigned only when the fetal condition is actually responsible for modifying the management of the mother, i.e., by requiring diagnostic studies, additional observation, special care, or termination of pregnancy. The fact that the fetal condition exists does not justify assigning a code from this series to the mother's record.

See Chapter 18 for suspected maternal and fetal conditions not found.

In utero surgery

In cases when surgery is performed on the fetus, a diagnosis code from category 655, Known or suspected fetal abnormalities affecting management of the mother, should be assigned identifying the fetal condition. Procedure code 75.36, Correction of fetal defect, should be assigned on the hospital inpatient record.

No code from Chapter 15, the perinatal codes, should be used on the mother's record to identify fetal conditions. Surgery performed in utero on a fetus is still to be coded as an obstetric encounter.

HIV INFECTION IN PREGNANCY, CHILDBIRTH AND THE PUERPERIUM

During pregnancy, childbirth or the puerperium, a patient admitted because of an HIV-related illness should receive a principal diagnosis of 647.6X, Other specified infectious and parasitic diseases in the mother classifiable elsewhere, but complicating the pregnancy, childbirth or the puerperium, followed by 042 and the code(s) for the HIV-related illness(es).

Patients with asymptomatic HIV infection status admitted during pregnancy, childbirth, or the puerperium should receive codes of 647.6X and V08.

CURRENT CONDITIONS COMPLICATING PREGNANCY

Assign a code from subcategory 648.x for patients that have current conditions when the condition affects the management of the pregnancy, childbirth, or the puerperium. Use additional secondary codes from other chapters to identify the conditions, as appropriate.

DIABETES MELLITUS IN PREGNANCY

Diabetes mellitus is a significant complicating factor in pregnancy. Pregnant women who are diabetic should be assigned code 648.0x, Diabetes mellitus complicating pregnancy, and a secondary code from category 250, Diabetes mellitus, or category 249, Secondary diabetes, to identify the type of diabetes.

Code V58.67, Long-term (current) use of insulin, should also be assigned if the diabetes mellitus is being treated with insulin.

GESTATIONAL DIABETES

Gestational diabetes can occur during the second and third trimester of pregnancy in women who were not diabetic prior to pregnancy. Gestational diabetes can cause complications in the pregnancy similar to those of pre-existing diabetes mellitus. It also puts the woman at greater risk of developing diabetes after the pregnancy. Gestational diabetes is coded to 648.8x, Abnormal glucose tolerance. Codes 648.0x and 648.8x should never be used together on the same record.

Code V58.67, Long-term (current) use of insulin, should also be assigned if the gestational diabetes is being treated with insulin.

NORMAL DELIVERY, CODE 650

Normal delivery

Code 650 is for use in cases when a woman is admitted for a full-term normal delivery and delivers a single, healthy infant without any complications antepartum, during the delivery, or postpartum during the delivery episode. Code 650 is always a principal diagnosis. It is not to be used if any other code from chapter 11 is needed to describe a current complication of the antenatal, delivery, or perinatal period. Additional codes from other chapters may be used with code 650 if they are not related to or are in any way complicating the pregnancy.

Normal delivery with resolved antepartum complication

Code 650 may be used if the patient had a complication at some point during her pregnancy, but the complication is not present at the time of the admission for delivery.

V27.0, Single liveborn, outcome of delivery

V27.0, Single liveborn, is the only outcome of delivery code appropriate for use with 650.

THE POSTPARTUM AND PERIPARTUM PERIODS

Postpartum and peripartum periods

The postpartum period begins immediately after delivery and continues for six weeks following delivery. The peripartum period is defined as the last month of pregnancy to five months postpartum.

Complications

A postpartum complication is any complication occurring within the six-week period.

| | Add 4th or 5th digit | | Nonspecific code | | Unspecified code | | Manifestation code |

Chapter 11 codes may also be used to describe pregnancy-related complications after the six-week period should the provider document that a condition is pregnancy related.

Postpartum complications that occur during the same admission as the delivery are identified with a fifth digit of "2." Subsequent admissions or encounters for postpartum complications should be identified with a fifth digit of "4."

Admission for routine postpartum care following delivery outside hospital

When the mother delivers outside the hospital prior to admission and is admitted for routine postpartum care and no complications are noted, code V24.0, Postpartum care and examination immediately after delivery, should be assigned as the principal diagnosis.

Admission following delivery outside hospital with postpartum conditions

A delivery diagnosis code should not be used for a woman who has delivered prior to admission to the hospital. Any postpartum conditions and/or postpartum procedures should be coded.

CODE 677, LATE EFFECT OF COMPLICATION OF PREGNANCY

Code 677, Late effect of complication of pregnancy, childbirth, and the puerperium is for use in those cases when an initial complication of a pregnancy develops a sequelae requiring care or treatment at a future date.

This code may be used at any time after the initial postpartum period.

This code, like all late effect codes, is to be sequenced following the code describing the sequelae of the complication.

ABORTIONS

Fifth-digits required for abortion categories

Fifth-digits are required for abortion categories 634-637. Fifth-digit 1, incomplete, indicates that all of the products of conception have not been expelled from the uterus. Fifth-digit 2, complete, indicates that all products of conception have been expelled from the uterus prior to the episode of care.

Code from categories 640-648 and 651-659

A code from categories 640-648 and 651-659 may be used as additional codes with an abortion code to indicate the complication leading to the abortion.
Fifth digit 3 is assigned with codes from these categories when used with an abortion code because the other fifth digits will not apply. Codes from the 660-669 series are not to be used for complications of abortion.

Code 639 for complications

Code 639 is to be used for all complications following abortion. Code 639 cannot be assigned with codes from categories 634-638.

Abortion with Liveborn Fetus

When an attempted termination of pregnancy results in a liveborn fetus assign code 644.21, Early onset of delivery, with an appropriate code from category V27, Outcome of Delivery. The procedure code for the attempted termination of pregnancy should also be assigned.

Retained Products of Conception following an abortion

Subsequent admissions for retained products of conception following a spontaneous or legally induced abortion are assigned the appropriate code from category 634, Spontaneous abortion, or 635 Legally induced abortion, with a fifth digit of "1" (incomplete). This advice is appropriate even when the patient was discharged previously with a discharge diagnosis of complete abortion.

11. COMPLICATIONS OF PREGNANCY, CHILDBIRTH, AND THE PUERPERIUM (630-679)

ECTOPIC AND MOLAR PREGNANCY (630-633)

Use additional code from category 639 to identify any complications

630 Hydatidiform mole
Trophoblastic disease NOS
Vesicular mole

Excludes: *chorioadenoma (destruens) (236.1)*
chorionepithelioma (181)
malignant hydatidiform mole (236.1)

DEFINITION A Hydatidiform mole is a rare mass or growth that forms inside the uterus at the beginning of a pregnancy. It is a type of gestational trophoblastic disease (GTD)
ALERT! For personal history of trophoblastic disease see V13.1

631 Other abnormal product of conception

- **631.0 Inappropriate change in quantitative human chorionic gonadotropin (hCG) in early pregnancy**
Biochemical pregnancy
Chemical pregnancy
Inappropriate level of quantitative human chorionic gonadotropin (hCG) for gestational age in early pregnancy

Excludes: *blighted ovum (631.8)*
molar pregnancy (631.8)

- **631.8 Other abnormal products of conception**
Blighted ovum

632 Missed abortion
Early fetal death before completion of 22 weeks' gestation with retention of dead fetus
Retained products of conception, not following spontaneous or induced abortion or delivery

Excludes: *failed induced abortion (638.0-638.9)*
fetal death (intrauterine) (late) (656.4)
missed delivery (656.4)
that with hydatiform mole (630)
that with other abnormal products of conception (631.8)

DEFINITION Missed abortion refers to retention in the uterus of an fetus that has been dead for at least eight weeks.

633 Ectopic pregnancy
Includes: ruptured ectopic pregnancy

DEFINITION Ectopic pregnancy occurs with the implantation and subsequent development of a fertilized ovum outside the uterus, as in a fallopian tube.

⑤ **633.0 Abdominal pregnancy**
Intraperitoneal pregnancy

   633.00 Abdominal pregnancy without intrauterine pregnancy

   633.01 Abdominal pregnancy with intrauterine pregnancy

⑤ **633.1 Tubal pregnancy**
Fallopian pregnancy
Rupture of (fallopian) tube due to pregnancy
Tubal abortion

   633.10 Tubal pregnancy without intrauterine pregnancy

   633.11 Tubal pregnancy with intrauterine pregnancy

⑤ **633.2 Ovarian pregnancy**

   633.20 Ovarian pregnancy without intrauterine pregnancy

   633.21 Ovarian pregnancy with intrauterine pregnancy

⑤ **633.8 Other ectopic pregnancy**
Pregnancy: Pregnancy:
   cervical   intraligamentous
   combined   mesometric
   cornual   mural

   633.80 Other ectopic pregnancy without intrauterine pregnancy

   633.81 Other ectopic pregnancy with intrauterine pregnancy

⑤ **633.9 Unspecified ectopic pregnancy**

   633.90 Unspecified ectopic pregnancy without intrauterine pregnancy

Add 4th or 5th digit	Nonspecific code	Unspecified code	Manifestation code

633.91 Unspecified ectopic pregnancy with intrauterine pregnancy

OTHER PREGNANCY WITH ABORTIVE OUTCOME (634-639)

Note: Use the following fifth-digit subclassification with categories 634-637:

0 **Unspecified**

1 **Incomplete**

2 **Complete**

The following fourth-digit subdivisions are for use with categories 634-638:

.0 **Complicated by genital tract and pelvic infection**
   Endometritis
   Salpingo-oophoritis
   Sepsis NOS
   Septicemia NOS
   Any condition classifiable to 639.0, with condition classifiable to 634-638

   Excludes: urinary tract infection (634-638 with .7)

.1 **Complicated by delayed or excessive hemorrhage**
   Afibrinogenemia
   Defibrination syndrome
   Intravascular hemolysis
   Any condition classifiable to 639.1, with condition classifiable to 634-638

.2 **Complicated by damage to pelvic organs and tissues**
   Laceration, perforation, or tear of:
     bladder
     uterus
   Any condition classifiable to 639.2, with condition classifiable to 634-638

.3 **Complicated by renal failure**
   Oliguria
   Uremia
   Any condition classifiable to 639.3, with condition classifiable to 634-638

.4 **Complicated by metabolic disorder**
   Electrolyte imbalance with conditions classifiable to 634-638

.5 **Complicated by shock**
   Circulatory collapse
   Shock (postoperative) (septic)
   Any condition classifiable to 639.5, with condition classifiable to 634-638

.6 **Complicated by embolism**
   Embolism:
     NOS
     amniotic fluid
     pulmonary
   Any condition classifiable to 639.6, with condition classifiable to 634-638

.7 **With other specified complications**
   Cardiac arrest or failure
   Urinary tract infection
   Any condition classifiable to 639.8, with condition classifiable to 634-638

.8 **With unspecified complication**

.9 **Without mention of complication**

⑤ **634** Spontaneous abortion
   Includes: miscarriage
         spontaneous abortion

   DEFINITION An abortion is the termination of a pregnancy by the removal or expulsion from the uterus of a fetus/embryo, resulting in or caused by its death. An abortion can occur spontaneously due to complications during pregnancy or can be induced.

⑤ **634.0** **Complicated by genital tract and pelvic infection**
   [0-2]

⑤ **634.1** **Complicated by delayed or excessive hemorrhage**
   [0-2]

⑤ **634.2** **Complicated by damage to pelvic organs or tissues**
   [0-2]

⑤ **634.3** **Complicated by renal failure**
   [0-2]

⑤ **634.4** **Complicated by metabolic disorder**
   [0-2]

● Code new
        to this edition
        ▲ Revision of
        existing code
        ④ ⑤ Fourth or fifth
        digit required

⑤ **634.5 Complicated by shock**
[0-2]

⑤ **634.6 Complicated by embolism**
[0-2]

⑤ **634.7 With other specified complications**
[0-2]

⑤ **634.8 With unspecified complication**
[0-2]

⑤ **634.9 Without mention of complication**
[0-2]

⑤ **635 Legally induced abortion**
    Includes: abortion or termination of pregnancy:
                        elective
                        legal
                        therapeutic

    Excludes: *menstrual extraction or regulation (V25.3)*

    DEFINITION Legally induced abortion refers to an abortion performed by medical professionals conforming to the legal guidelines of the state where the abortion is performed.

⑤ **635.0 Complicated by genital tract and pelvic infection**
[0-2]

⑤ **635.1 Complicated by delayed or excessive hemorrhage**
[0-2]

⑤ **635.2 Complicated by damage to pelvic organs or tissues**
[0-2]

⑤ **635.3 Complicated by renal failure**
[0-2]

⑤ **635.4 Complicated by metabolic disorder**
[0-2]

⑤ **635.5 Complicated by shock**
[0-2]

⑤ **635.6 Complicated by embolism**
[0-2]

⑤ **635.7 With other specified complications**
[0-2]

⑤ **635.8 With unspecified complication**
[0-2]

⑤ **635.9 Without mention of complication**
[0-2]

⑤ **636 Illegally induced abortion**
    Includes: abortion:
                        criminal
                        illegal
                        self-induced

    DEFINITION Illegally induced abortion refers to an abortion performed by medical professionals or non-medical persons outside the legal guidelines of the state where the abortion is performed.

⑤ **636.0 Complicated by genital tract and pelvic infection**
[0-2]

⑤ **636.1 Complicated by delayed or excessive hemorrhage**
[0-2]

⑤ **636.2 Complicated by damage to pelvic organs or tissues**
[0-2]

⑤ **636.3 Complicated by renal failure**
[0-2]

⑤ **636.4 Complicated by metabolic disorder**
[0-2]

⑤ **636.5 Complicated by shock**
[0-2]

⑤ **636.6 Complicated by embolism**
[0-2]

⑤ **636.7 With other specified complications**
[0-2]

	Add 4th or 5th digit		Nonspecific code		Unspecified code		Manifestation code

⑤ **636.8 With unspecified complication**
[0-2]

⑤ **636.9 Without mention of complication**
[0-2]

⑤ **637 Unspecified abortion**
Includes: abortion NOS
retained products of conception following abortion, not classifiable elsewhere

⑤ **637.0 Complicated by genital tract and pelvic infection**
[0-2]

⑤ **637.1 Complicated by delayed or excessive hemorrhage**
[0-2]

⑤ **637.2 Complicated by damage to pelvic organs or tissues**
[0-2]

⑤ **637.3 Complicated by renal failure**
[0-2]

⑤ **637.4 Complicated by metabolic disorder**
[0-2]

⑤ **637.5 Complicated by shock**
[0-2]

⑤ **637.6 Complicated by embolism**
[0-2]

⑤ **637.7 With other specified complications**
[0-2]

⑤ **637.8 With unspecified complication**
[0-2]

⑤ **637.9 Without mention of complication**
[0-2]

638 Failed attempted abortion
Includes: failure of attempted induction of (legal) abortion

Excludes: *incomplete abortion (634.0-637.9)*

DEFINITION Failed attempted abortion refers to an attempted abortion that is incomplete.

638.0 Complicated by genital tract and pelvic infection

638.1 Complicated by delayed or excessive hemorrhage

638.2 Complicated by damage to pelvic organs or tissues

638.3 Complicated by renal failure

638.4 Complicated by metabolic disorder

638.5 Complicated by shock

638.6 Complicated by embolism

638.7 With other specified complications

638.8 With unspecified complication

638.9 Without mention of complication

639 Complications following abortion and ectopic and molar pregnancies
Note: This category is provided for use when it is required to classify separately the
complications classifiable to the fourth-digit level in categories 634-638; for example:
  a) when the complication itself was responsible for an episode of medical care, the
abortion, ectopic or molar pregnancy itself having been dealt with at a previous
episode
  b) when these conditions are immediate complications of ectopic or molar pregnancies
classifiable to 630-633 where they cannot be identified at fourth-digit level.

DEFINITION Ectopic pregnancy is the implantation and subsequent development of a fertilized
ovum outside the uterus, as in a fallopian tube. Molar pregnancy is the conversion of the
early embryo into a mole.

ALERT! Code 639 is to be used for all complications following abortion. Code 639 cannot be
assigned with codes from categories 634-638

639.0 Genital tract and pelvic infection
Endometritis following conditions classifiable to 630-638
Parametritis following conditions classifiable to 630-638
Pelvic peritonitis following conditions classifiable to 630-638
Salpingitis following conditions classifiable to 630-638
Salpingo-oophoritis following conditions classifiable to 630-638
Sepsis NOS following conditions classifiable to 630-638

● Code new
to this edition
▲ Revision of
existing code
④ ⑤ Fourth or fifth
digit required

Septicemia NOS following conditions classifiable to 630-638

Excludes: *urinary tract infection (639.8)*

639.1 Delayed or excessive hemorrhage
Afibrinogenemia following conditions classifiable to 630-638
Defibrination syndrome following conditions classifiable to 630-638
Intravascular hemolysis following conditions classifiable to 630-638

639.2 Damage to pelvic organs and tissues
Laceration, perforation, or tear of:
bladder following conditions classifiable to 630-638
bowel following conditions classifiable to 630-638
broad ligament following conditions classifiable to 630-638
cervix following conditions classifiable to 630-638
periurethral tissue following conditions classifiable to 630-638
uterus following conditions classifiable to 630-638
vagina following conditions classifiable to 630-638

639.3 Kidney failure
Oliguria following conditions classifiable to 630-638
Renal (kidney):
failure (acute) following conditions classifiable to 630-638
shutdown following conditions classifiable to 630-638
tubular necrosis following conditions classifiable to 630-638
Uremia following conditions classifiable to 630-638

639.4 Metabolic disorders
Electrolyte imbalance following conditions classifiable to 630-638

639.5 Shock
Circulatory collapse following conditions classifiable to 630-638
Shock (postoperative) (septic) following conditions classifiable to 630-638

639.6 Embolism
Embolism:
NOS following conditions classifiable to 630-638
air following conditions classifiable to 630-638
amniotic fluid following conditions classifiable to 630-638
blood-clot following conditions classifiable to 630-638
fat following conditions classifiable to 630-638
pulmonary following conditions classifiable to 630-638
pyemic following conditions classifiable to 630-638
septic following conditions classifiable to 630-638
soap following conditions classifiable to 630-638

639.8 Other specified complications following abortion or ectopic and molar pregnancy
Acute yellow atrophy or necrosis of liver following conditions classifiable to 630-638
Cardiac arrest or failure following conditions classifiable to 630-638
Cerebral anoxia following conditions classifiable to 630-638
Urinary tract infection following conditions classifiable to 630-638

639.9 Unspecified complication following abortion or ectopic and molar pregnancy
Complication(s) not further specified following conditions classifiable to 630-638

COMPLICATIONS MAINLY RELATED TO PREGNANCY (640-649)

Includes: the listed conditions even if they arose or were present during labor, delivery, or the puerperium

The following fifth-digit subclassification is for use with categories 640-649 to denote the current episode of care:

0 unspecified as to episode of care or not applicable

1 delivered, with or without mention of antepartum condition
Antepartum condition with delivery
Delivery NOS (with mention of antepartum complication during current episode of care)
Intrapartum obstetric condition (with mention of antepartum complication during current episode of care)
Pregnancy, delivered (with mention of antepartum complication during current episode of care)

2 delivered, with mention of postpartum complication
Delivery with mention of puerperal complication during current episode of care

3 antepartum condition or complication
Antepartum obstetric condition, not delivered during the current episode of care

 Add 4th or 5th digit   Nonspecific code   Unspecified code   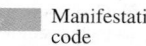 Manifestation code

4   postpartum condition or complication
>   Postpartum or puerperal obstetric condition or complication following delivery that
>   occurred:
>   during previous episode of care
>   outside hospital, with subsequent admission for observation or care

⑤ **640   Hemorrhage in early pregnancy**
>   Includes: hemorrhage before completion of 22 weeks' gestation
>
> Requires fifth digit; valid digits are in [brackets] under each code. See beginning of section
>   640-649 for definitions.
>
> **ALERT!** For coding late effect of complication of pregnancy childbirth the puerperium see 677

⑤ **640.0   Threatened abortion**
[0,1,3]

⑤ **640.8   Other specified hemorrhage in early pregnancy**
[0,1,3]

⑤ **640.9   Unspecified hemorrhage in early pregnancy**
[0,1,3]

⑤ **641   Antepartum hemorrhage, abruptio placentae, and placenta previa**
>   Requires fifth digit; valid digits are in [brackets] under each code. See beginning of section
>   640-649 for definitions.
>
> **DEFINITION** Antepartum hemorrhage refers to bleeding before delivery. Abruptio placentae is
> the premature separation of the placenta from the wall of the uterus. Placenta previa is a
> pregnancy in which the placenta is implanted in the lower uterine segment instead of the
> upper segmen

⑤ **641.0   Placenta previa without hemorrhage**
[0,1,3]   Low implantation of placenta without hemorrhage
>   Placenta previa noted:
>   during pregnancy without hemorrhage
>   before labor (and delivered by cesarean delivery) without hemorrhage

⑤ **641.1   Hemorrhage from placenta previa**
[0,1,3]   Low-lying placenta NOS or with hemorrhage (intrapartum)
>   Placenta previa:
>   incomplete NOS or with hemorrhage (intrapartum)
>   marginal NOS or with hemorrhage (intrapartum)
>   partial NOS or with hemorrhage (intrapartum)
>   total NOS or with hemorrhage (intrapartum)
>
> Excludes: *hemorrhage from vasa previa (663.5)*

⑤ **641.2   Premature separation of placenta**
[0,1,3]   Ablatio placentae
>   Abruptio placentae
>   Accidental antepartum hemorrhage
>   Couvelaire uterus
>   Detachment of placenta (premature)
>   Premature separation of normally implanted placenta

⑤ **641.3   Antepartum hemorrhage associated with coagulation defects**
[0,1,3]   Antepartum or intrapartum hemorrhage associated with:
>   afibrinogenemia
>   hyperfibrinolysis
>   hypofibrinogenemia
>
> Excludes: *coagulation defects not associated with antepartum hemorrhage (649.3)*

⑤ **641.8   Other antepartum hemorrhage**
[0,1,3]   Antepartum or intrapartum hemorrhage associated with:
>   trauma
>   uterine leiomyoma

⑤ **641.9   Unspecified antepartum hemorrhage**
[0,1,3]   Hemorrhage:
>   antepartum NOS
>   intrapartum NOS
>   of pregnancy NOS

⑤ **642   Hypertension complicating pregnancy, childbirth, and the puerperium**
>   Requires fifth digit; valid digits are in [brackets] under each code. See beginning of section
>   640-649 for definitions.

● Code new   ▲ Revision of   ④ ⑤ Fourth or fifth
          to this edition   existing code   digit required

DEFINITION Pregnancy-induced hypertension is a rise in blood pressure, without proteinuria, during the second half of pregnancy. Pre-eclampsia is a multisystem disorder, unique to pregnancy, that is usually associated with raised blood pressure and proteinuria. Eclampsia is one or more convulsions in association with the syndrome of pre-eclampsia.

⑤ **642.0 Benign essential hypertension complicating pregnancy, childbirth, and the puerperium**
[0-4]   Hypertension:
          benign essential specified as complicating, or as a reason for obstetric care during
              pregnancy, childbirth, or the puerperium
          chronic NOS specified as complicating, or as a reason for obstetric care during
              pregnancy, childbirth, or the puerperium
          essential specified as complicating, or as a reason for obstetric care during
              pregnancy, childbirth, or the puerperium
          pre-existing NOS specified as complicating, or as a reason for obstetric care during
              pregnancy, childbirth, or the puerperium

⑤ **642.1 Hypertension secondary to renal disease, complicating pregnancy, childbirth, and the
          puerperium**
[0-4]   Hypertension secondary to renal disease, specified as complicating, or as a reason for
              obstetric care during pregnancy, childbirth, or the puerperium

⑤ **642.2 Other pre-existing hypertension complicating pregnancy, childbirth, and the puerperium**
[0-4]   Hypertensive:
          chronic kidney disease specified as complicating, or as a reason for obstetric care
              during pregnancy, childbirth, or the puerperium
          heart and chronic kidney disease specified as complicating, or as a reason for obstetric
              care during pregnancy, childbirth, or the puerperium
          heart disease specified as complicating, or as a reason for obstetric care during
              pregnancy, childbirth, or the puerperium
          Malignant hypertension specified as complicating, or as a reason for obstetric care
              during pregnancy, childbirth, or the puerperium

⑤ **642.3 Transient hypertension of pregnancy**
[0-4]   Gestational hypertension
          Transient hypertension, so described, in pregnancy, childbirth, or the puerperium

⑤ **642.4 Mild or unspecified pre-eclampsia**
[0-4]   Hypertension in pregnancy, childbirth, or the puerperium, not specified as pre-existing,
              with either albuminuria or edema, or both; mild or unspecified
          Pre-eclampsia: Toxemia (pre-eclamptic):
            NOS   NOS
            mild   mild

          Excludes: albuminuria in pregnancy, without mention of hypertension (646.2)
                    edema in pregnancy, without mention of hypertension (646.1)

⑤ **642.5 Severe pre-eclampsia**
[0-4]   Hypertension in pregnancy, childbirth, or the puerperium, not specified as pre-existing,
              with either albuminuria or edema, or both; specified as severe
          Pre-eclampsia, severe
          Toxemia (pre-eclamptic), severe

⑤ **642.6 Eclampsia**
[0-4]   Toxemia:
            eclamptic
            with convulsions

⑤ **642.7 Pre-eclampsia or eclampsia superimposed on pre-existing hypertension**
[0-4]   Conditions classifiable to 642.4-642.6, with conditions classifiable to 642.0-642.2

⑤ **642.9 Unspecified hypertension complicating pregnancy, childbirth, or the puerperium**
[0-4]   Hypertension NOS, without mention of albuminuria or edema, complicating pregnancy,
              childbirth, or the puerperium

⑤ **643 Excessive vomiting in pregnancy**
      Includes: hyperemesis arising during pregnancy
                 vomiting:
                   persistent arising during pregnancy
                   vicious arising during pregnancy
                 hyperemesis gravidarum

      Requires fifth digit; valid digits are in [brackets] under each code. See beginning of section
          640-649 for definitions.

          DEFINITION Excessive vomiting in pregnancy, aka hyperemesis gravidarum, refers to excessive
      vomiting in early pregnancy.

⑤ **643.0 Mild hyperemesis gravidarum**
[0,1,3]   Hyperemesis gravidarum, mild or unspecified, starting before the end of the 22nd week
              of gestation

▓	Add 4th or	▒	Nonspecific	▒	Unspecified	▓	Manifestation
	5th digit		code		code		code

⑤ **643.1 Hyperemesis gravidarum with metabolic disturbance**
[0,1,3] Hyperemesis gravidarum, starting before the end of the 22nd week of gestation, with metabolic disturbance, such as:
carbohydrate depletion
dehydration
electrolyte imbalance

⑤ **643.2 Late vomiting of pregnancy**
[0,1,3] Excessive vomiting starting after 22 completed weeks of gestation

⑤ **643.8 Other vomiting complicating pregnancy**
[0,1,3] Vomiting due to organic disease or other cause, specified as complicating pregnancy, or as a reason for obstetric care during pregnancy
Use additional code, if desired, to specify cause

⑤ **643.9 Unspecified vomiting of pregnancy**
[0,1,3] Vomiting as a reason for care during pregnancy, length of gestation unspecified

⑤ **644 Early or threatened labor**
Requires fifth digit; valid digits are in [brackets] under each code. See beginning of section 640-649 for definitions.
ALERT! For personal history of pre-term labor see V13.21

⑤ **644.0 Threatened premature labor**
[0,3] Premature labor after 22 weeks, but before 37 completed weeks of gestation without delivery

Excludes: *that occurring before 22 completed weeks of gestation (640.0)*

⑤ **644.1 Other threatened labor**
[0,3] False labor:
NOS without delivery
after 37 completed weeks of gestation without delivery
Threatened labor NOS without delivery

⑤ **644.2 Early onset of delivery**
[0,1] Onset (spontaneous) of delivery before 37 completed weeks of gestation
Premature labor with onset of delivery before 37 completed weeks of gestation
ALERT! Assign code 644.21 with an appropriate code from category V27 when an attempted termination of pregnancy results in a liveborn fetus. The procedure code for the attempted termination of pregnancy should also be assigned

⑤ **645 Late pregnancy**
Requires fifth digit; valid digits are in [brackets] under each code. See beginning of section 640-649 for definitions.

⑤ **645.1 Post term pregnancy**
[0,1,3] Pregnancy over 40 completed weeks to 42 completed weeks gestation

⑤ **645.2 Prolonged pregnancy**
[0,1,3] Pregnancy which has advanced beyond 42 completed weeks gestation

⑤ **646 Other complications of pregnancy, not elsewhere classified**
Requires fifth digit; valid digits are in [brackets] under each code. See beginning of section 640-649 for definitions.
Use additional code(s) to further specify complication
ALERT! For personal history of other genital system and obstetric disorders see V13.2

⑤ **646.0 Papyraceous fetus**
[0,1,3]

⑤ **646.1 Edema or excessive weight gain in pregnancy, without mention of hypertension**
[0-4] Gestational edema
Maternal obesity syndrome

Excludes: *that with mention of hypertension (642.0-642.9)*

⑤ **646.2 Unspecified renal disease in pregnancy, without mention of hypertension**
[0-4] Albuminuria in pregnancy or the puerperium, without mention of hypertension
Nephropathy NOS in pregnancy or the puerperium, without mention of hypertension
Renal disease NOS in pregnancy or the puerperium, without mention of hypertension
Uremia in pregnancy or the puerperium, without mention of hypertension
Gestational proteinuria in pregnancy or the puerperium, without mention of hypertension

Excludes: *that with mention of hypertension (642.0-642.9)*

⑤ **646.3 Recurrent pregnancy loss**
[0,1,3]

Excludes: *with current abortion (634.0-634.9)*
without current pregnancy (629.81)

● Code new to this edition   ▲ Revision of existing code   ④ ⑤ Fourth or fifth digit required

⑤ **646.4 Peripheral neuritis in pregnancy**
[0-4]

⑤ **646.5 Asymptomatic bacteriuria in pregnancy**
[0-4]

⑤ **646.6 Infections of genitourinary tract in pregnancy**
[0-4] Conditions classifiable to 590, 595, 597, 599.0, 616 complicating pregnancy, childbirth, or the puerperium
Conditions classifiable to (614.0-614.5, 617.7-614.9, 615) complicating pregnancy or labor

Excludes: *major puerperal infection (670.0-670.8)*

▲ **646.7 Liver and biliary tract disorders in pregnancy**
[0,1,3] Acute yellow atrophy of liver (obstetric) (true) of pregnancy
Icterus gravis of pregnancy
Necrosis of liver of pregnancy

Excludes: *hepatorenal syndrome following delivery (674.8)*
viral hepatitis (647.6)

⑤ **646.8 Other specified complications of pregnancy**
[0-4] Fatigue during pregnancy
Herpes gestationis
Insufficient weight gain of pregnancy

⑤ **646.9 Unspecified complication of pregnancy**
[0,1,3]

⑤ **647 Infectious and parasitic conditions in the mother classifiable elsewhere, but complicating pregnancy, childbirth, or the puerperium**
Includes: the listed conditions when complicating the pregnant state, aggravated by the pregnancy, or when a main reason for obstetric care

Excludes: *those conditions in the mother known or suspected to have affected the fetus (655.0-655.9)*

Requires fifth digit; valid digits are in [brackets] under each code. See beginning of section 640-649 for definitions.

Use additional code(s) to further specify complication

⑤ **647.0 Syphilis**
[0-4] Conditions classifiable to 090-097

⑤ **647.1 Gonorrhea**
[0-4] Conditions classifiable to 098

⑤ **647.2 Other venereal diseases**
[0-4] Conditions classifiable to 099

⑤ **647.3 Tuberculosis**
[0-4] Conditions classifiable to 010-018

⑤ **647.4 Malaria**
[0-4] Conditions classifiable to 084

⑤ **647.5 Rubella**
[0-4] Conditions classifiable to 056

⑤ **647.6 Other viral diseases**
[0-4] Conditions classifiable to 042, 050-055, 057-079, 795.05, 795.15, 795.75

⑤ **647.8 Other specified infectious and parasitic diseases**
[0-4]

⑤ **647.9 Unspecified infection or infestation**
[0-4]

⑤ **648 Other current conditions in the mother classifiable elsewhere, but complicating pregnancy, childbirth, or the puerperium**
Includes: the listed conditions when complicating the pregnant state, aggravated by the pregnancy, or when a main reason for obstetric care

Excludes: *those conditions in the mother known or suspected to have affected the fetus (655.0-655.9)*

Requires fifth digit; valid digits are in [brackets] under each code. See beginning of section 640-649 for definitions.

Use additional code(s) to identify the condition

⑤ **648.0 Diabetes mellitus**
[0-4] Conditions classifiable to 249, 250

Excludes: *gestational diabetes (648.8)*

| | Add 4th or 5th digit | | Nonspecific code | | Unspecified code | | Manifestation code |

⑤ **648.1 Thyroid dysfunction**
[0-4]   Conditions classifiable to 240-246

⑤ **648.2 Anemia**
[0-4]   Conditions classifiable to 280-285

⑤ **648.3 Drug dependence**
[0-4]   Conditions classifiable to 304

⑤ **648.4 Mental disorders**
[0-4]   Conditions classifiable to 290-303, 305.0, 305.2-305.9, 306-316, 317-319

⑤ **648.5 Congenital cardiovascular disorders**
[0-4]   Conditions classifiable to 745-747

⑤ **648.6 Other cardiovascular diseases**
[0-4]   Conditions classifiable to 390-398, 410-429

> Excludes: *cerebrovascular disorders in the puerperium (674.0)*
> *peripartum cardiomyopathy (674.5)*
> *venous complications (671.0-671.9)*

⑤ **648.7 Bone and joint disorders of back, pelvis, and lower limbs**
[0-4]   Conditions classifiable to 720-724, and those classifiable to 711-719 or 725-738, specified as affecting the lower limbs

⑤ **648.8 Abnormal glucose tolerance**
[0-4]   Conditions classifiable to 790.21-790.29
Gestational diabetes
Use additional code, if applicable, for associated long-term (current) insulin use (V58.67)

⑤ **648.9 Other current conditions classifiable elsewhere**
[0-4]   Conditions classifiable to 440-459, 795.01-795.04, 795.06, 795.10-795.14, 795.16, 796.70-796.74, 796.76
Nutritional deficiencies [conditions classifiable to 260-269]

649 Other conditions or status of the mother complicating pregnancy, childbirth, or the puerperium
The following fifth-digit subclassification is for use with categories 640-649 to denote the current episode of care:

  0 **unspecified as to episode of care or not applicable**

  1 **delivered, with or without mention of antepartum condition**
     Antepartum condition with delivery
     Delivery NOS (with mention of antepartum complication during current episode of care)
     Intrapartum obstetric condition (with mention of antepartum complication during current episode of care)
     Pregnancy, delivered (with mention of antepartum complication during current episode of care)

  2 **delivered, with mention of postpartum complication**
     Delivery with mention of puerperal complication during current episode of care

  3 **antepartum condition or complication**
     Antepartum obstetric condition, not delivered during the current episode of care

  4 **postpartum condition or complication**
     Postpartum or puerperal obstetric condition or complication following delivery that occurred:
     during previous episode of care
     outside hospital, with subsequent admission for observation or care

    ALERT! For personal history of tobacco use see V15.82

⑤ **649.0 Tobacco use disorder complicating pregnancy, childbirth, or the puerperium**
[0-4]   Smoking complicating pregnancy, childbirth, or the puerperium

⑤ **649.1 Obesity complicating pregnancy, childbirth, or the puerperium**
[0-4]
Use additional code to identify the obesity (278.00-278.03)

⑤ **649.2 Bariatric surgery status complicating pregnancy, childbirth, or the puerperium**
[0-4]   Gastric banding status complicating pregnancy, childbirth, or the puerperium
     Gastric bypass status for obesity complicating pregnancy, childbirth, or the puerperium
     Obesity surgery status complicating pregnancy, childbirth, or the puerperium

⑤ **649.3 Coagulation defects complicating pregnancy, childbirth, or the puerperium**
[0-4]   Conditions classifiable to 286, 287, 289
Use additional code to identify the specific coagulation defect (286.0-286.9, 287.0-287.9, 289.0-289.9)

    ● Code new to this edition   ▲ Revision of existing code   ④ ⑤ Fourth or fifth digit required

Excludes: coagulation defects causing antepartum hemorrhage (641.3)
postpartum coagulation defects (666.3)

⑤ **649.4 Epilepsy complicating pregnancy, childbirth, or the puerperium**
[0-4]   Conditions classifiable to 345

Use additional code to identify the specific type of epilepsy (345.00-345.91)

Excludes: eclampsia (642.6)

⑤ **649.5 Spotting complicating pregnancy**
[0,1,3]

Excludes: antepartum hemorrhage (641.0-641.9)
hemorrhage in early pregnancy (640.0-640.9)

⑤ **649.6 Uterine size date discrepancy**
[0-4]

Excludes: suspected problem with fetal growth not found (V89.04)

⑤ **649.7 Cervical shortening**
[0,1,3]

Excludes: suspected cervical shortening not found (V89.05)

● **649.8** **Onset (spontaneous) of labor after 37 completed weeks of gestation but before 39 completed weeks gestation, with delivery by (planned) cesarean section**
[1-2]   Delivery by (planned) cesarean section occurring after 37 completed weeks of gestation but before 39 completed weeks gestation due to (spontaneous) onset of labor

Use additional code to specify reason for planned cesarean section such as:
cephalopelvic disproportion (normally formed fetus) (653.4)
previous cesarean delivery (654.2)

NORMAL DELIVERY, AND OTHER INDICATIONS FOR CARE IN PREGNANCY, LABOR, AND DELIVERY (650-659)

650 Normal delivery
Delivery requiring minimal or no assistance, with or without episiotomy, without fetal manipulation [e.g., rotation version] or instrumentation [forceps] of spontaneous, cephalic, vaginal, full-term, single, live born infant. This code is for use as a single diagnosis code and is not to be used with any other code in the range 630-676.

Excludes: breech delivery (assisted) (spontaneous) NOS (652.2)
delivery by vacuum extractor, forceps, cesarean section, or breech extraction, without specified complication (669.5-669.7)

Use additional code to indicate outcome of delivery (V27.0)

ALERT! Code 650 is for use in cases when a woman is admitted for a full-term normal delivery and delivers a single, healthy infant without any complications antepartum, during the delivery, or postpartum during the delivery episode. Code 650 is always a principal diagnosis

ALERT! V27.0, Single liveborn, is the only outcome of delivery code appropriate for use with 650.

The following fifth-digit subclassification is for use with categories 651-659 to denote the current episode of care:

0   unspecified as to episode of care or not applicable

1   delivered, with or without mention of antepartum condition

2   delivered, with mention of postpartum complication

3   antepartum condition or complication

4   postpartum condition or complication

⑤ **651 Multiple gestation**
Use additional code to specify placenta status (V91.00-V91.99)

DEFINITION Multiple gestation is a multiple birth occurs when more than one fetus is carried to term in a single pregnancy

⑤ **651.0 Twin pregnancy**
[0,1,3]

Excludes: fetal conjoined twins (678.1)

⑤ **651.1 Triplet pregnancy**
[0,1,3]

⑤ **651.2 Quadruplet pregnancy**
[0,1,3]

▩ Add 4th or 5th digit	▩ Nonspecific code	▩ Unspecified code	▩ Manifestation code

⑤ **651.3 Twin pregnancy with fetal loss and retention of one fetus**
[0,1,3]

⑤ **651.4 Triplet pregnancy with fetal loss and retention of one or more fetus(es)**
[0,1,3]

⑤ **651.5 Quadruplet pregnancy with fetal loss and retention of one or more fetus(es)**
[0,1,3]

⑤ **651.6 Other multiple pregnancy with fetal loss and retention of one or more fetus(es)**
[0,1,3]

⑤ **651.7 Multiple gestation following (elective) fetal reduction**
Fetal reduction of multiple fetuses reduced to single fetus

> **651.70 Multiple gestation following (elective) fetal reduction, unspecified as to episode of care or not applicable**

> **651.71 Multiple gestation following (elective) fetal reduction, delivered, with or without mention of antepartum condition**

> **651.73 Multiple gestation following (elective) fetal reduction, antepartum condition or complication**

⑤ **651.8 Other specified multiple gestation**
[0,1,3]

⑤ **651.9 Unspecified multiple gestation**
[0,1,3]

⑤ **652 Malposition and malpresentation of fetus**
Code first any associated obstructed labor (660.0)
DEFINITION Malposition and malpresentation of fetus refers to presentation of the fetal parts in inappropriate positions for the easiest passage through the cervix, e.g. Retention of the head, breech presentation.

⑤ **652.0 Unstable lie**
[0,1,3]

⑤ **652.1 Breech or other malpresentation successfully converted to cephalic presentation**
[0,1,3]   Cephalic version NOS

⑤ **652.2 Breech presentation without mention of version**
[0,1,3]   Breech delivery (assisted) (spontaneous) NOS
Buttocks presentation
Complete breech
Frank breech

> Excludes: *footling presentation (652.8)*
> *incomplete breech (652.8)*

⑤ **652.3 Transverse or oblique presentation**
[0,1,3]   Oblique lie   Transverse lie

> Excludes: *transverse arrest of fetal head (660.3)*

⑤ **652.4 Face or brow presentation**
[0,1,3]   Mentum presentation

⑤ **652.5 High head at term**
[0,1,3]   Failure of head to enter pelvic brim

⑤ **652.6 Multiple gestation with malpresentation of one fetus or more**
[0,1,3]

⑤ **652.7 Prolapsed arm**
[0,1,3]

⑤ **652.8 Other specified malposition or malpresentation**
[0,1,3]   Compound presentation

⑤ **652.9 Unspecified malposition or malpresentation**
[0,1,3]

⑤ **653 Disproportion**
Code first any associated obstructed labor (660.1)

⑤ **653.0 Major abnormality of bony pelvis, not further specified**
[0,1,3]   Pelvic deformity NOS

⑤ **653.1 Generally contracted pelvis**
[0,1,3]   Contracted pelvis NOS

⑤ **653.2 Inlet contraction of pelvis**
[0,1,3]   Inlet contraction (pelvis)

⑤ **653.3 Outlet contraction of pelvis**
[0,1,3]   Outlet contraction (pelvis)

● Code new
  to this edition

▲ Revision of
  existing code

④ ⑤ Fourth or fifth
  digit required

⑤ **653.4 Fetopelvic disproportion**
[0,1,3]   Cephalopelvic disproportion NOS
            Disproportion of mixed maternal and fetal origin, with normally formed fetus

⑤ **653.5 Unusually large fetus causing disproportion**
[0,1,3]   Disproportion of fetal origin with normally formed fetus
            Fetal disproportion NOS

  Excludes: *that when the reason for medical care was concern for the fetus (656.6)*

⑤ **653.6 Hydrocephalic fetus causing disproportion**
[0,1,3]

  Excludes: *that when the reason for medical care was concern for the fetus (655.0)*

⑤ **653.7 Other fetal abnormality causing disproportion**
[0,1,3]   Fetal:
              ascites
              hydrops
              myelomeningocele
              sacral teratoma
              tumor

  Excludes: *conjoined twins causing disproportion (678.1)*

⑤ **653.8 Disproportion of other origin**
[0,1,3]

  Excludes: *shoulder (girdle) dystocia (660.4)*

⑤ **653.9 Unspecified disproportion**
[0,1,3]

⑤ **654 Abnormality of organs and soft tissues of pelvis**
        Includes: the listed conditions during pregnancy, childbirth, or the puerperium
        Code first any associated obstructed labor (660.2)

  Excludes: *trauma to perineum and vulva complicating current delivery (664.0-664.9)*

⑤ **654.0 Congenital abnormalities of uterus**
[0-4]   Double uterus   Uterus bicornis

⑤ **654.1 Tumors of body of uterus**
[0-4]   Uterine fibroids

⑤ **654.2 Previous cesarean delivery NOS**
[0,1,3]   Uterine scar from previous cesarean delivery

⑤ **654.3 Retroverted and incarcerated gravid uterus**
[0-4]

⑤ **654.4 Other abnormalities in shape or position of gravid uterus and of neighboring
        structures**
[0-4]   Cystocele
            Pelvic floor repair
            Pendulous abdomen
            Prolapse of gravid uterus
            Rectocele
            Rigid pelvic floor

⑤ **654.5 Cervical incompetence**
[0-4]   Presence of Shirodkar suture with or without mention of cervical incompetence

⑤ **654.6 Other congenital or acquired abnormality of cervix**
[0-4]   Cicatricial cervix
            Polyp of cervix
            Previous surgery to cervix
            Rigid cervix (uteri)
            Stenosis or stricture of cervix
            Tumor of cervix

⑤ **654.7 Congenital or acquired abnormality of vagina**
[0-4]   Previous surgery to vagina
            Septate vagina
            Stenosis of vagina (acquired) (congenital)
            Stricture of vagina
            Tumor of vagina

| | Add 4th or 5th digit | | Nonspecific code | | Unspecified code | | Manifestation code |

⑤ **654.8 Congenital or acquired abnormality of vulva**
[0-4]   Anal sphincter tear (healed) (old) complicating delivery
Fibrosis of perineum
Persistent hymen
Previous surgery to perineum or vulva
Rigid perineum
Tumor of vulva

Excludes: *anal sphincter tear (healed) (old) not associated with delivery (569.43)*
varicose veins of vulva (671.1)

⑤ **654.9 Other and unspecified**
[0-4]   Uterine scar NEC

⑤ **655 Known or suspected fetal abnormality affecting management of mother**
Includes: the listed conditions in the fetus as a reason for observation or obstetrical care of
the mother, or for termination of pregnancy

ALERT! In cases where surgery is performed on the fetus a diagnosis code from this category
should be assigned to identify the fetal condition

⑤ **655.0 Central nervous system malformation in fetus**
[0,1,3]   Fetal or suspected fetal:
anencephaly
hydrocephalus
spina bifida (with myelomeningocele)

⑤ **655.1 Chromosomal abnormality in fetus**
[0,1,3]

⑤ **655.2 Hereditary disease in family possibly affecting fetus**
[0,1,3]

⑤ **655.3 Suspected damage to fetus from viral disease in the mother**
[0,1,3]   Suspected damage to fetus from maternal rubella

⑤ **655.4 Suspected damage to fetus from other disease in the mother**
[0,1,3]   Suspected damage to fetus from maternal:
alcohol addiction
listeriosis
toxoplasmosis

⑤ **655.5 Suspected damage to fetus from drugs**
[0,1,3]

⑤ **655.6 Suspected damage to fetus from radiation**
[0,1,3]

⑤ **655.7 Decreased fetal movements**
[0,1,3]

⑤ **655.8 Other known or suspected fetal abnormality, not elsewhere classified**
[0,1,3]   Suspected damage to fetus from:
environmental toxins
intrauterine contraceptive device

⑤ **655.9 Unspecified**
[0,1,3]

⑤ **656 Other known or suspected fetal and placental problems affecting management of mother**
Excludes: *fetal hematologic conditions (678.0)*
suspected placental problems not found (V89.02)

⑤ **656.0 Fetal-maternal hemorrhage**
[0,1,3]   Leakage (microscopic) of fetal blood into maternal circulation

⑤ **656.1 Rhesus isoimmunization**
[0,1,3]   Anti-D [Rh] antibodies
Rh incompatibility

⑤ **656.2 Isoimmunization from other and unspecified blood-group incompatibility**
[0,1,3]   ABO isoimmunization

⑤ **656.3 Fetal distress**
[0,1,3]   Fetal metabolic acidemia

Excludes: *abnormal fetal acid-base balance (656.8)*
abnormality in fetal heart rate or rhythm (659.7)
fetal bradycardia (659.7)
fetal tachycardia (659.7)
meconium in liquor (656.8)

⑤ **656.4 Intrauterine death**
[0,1,3]   Fetal death:
                   NOS
                   after completion of 22 weeks' gestation
                   late
             Missed delivery

      Excludes: missed abortion (632)

⑤ **656.5 Poor fetal growth**
[0,1,3]   "Light-for-dates"   "Small-for-dates"
             "Placental insufficiency"

⑤ **656.6 Excessive fetal growth**
[0,1,3]   "Large-for-dates"

⑤ **656.7 Other placental conditions**
[0,1,3]   Abnormal placenta   Placental infarct

      Excludes: placental polyp (674.4)
                   placentitis (658.4)

⑤ **656.8 Other specified fetal and placental problems**
[0,1,3]   Abnormal acid-base balance
             Intrauterine acidosis
             Lithopedian
             Meconium in liquor
             Subchorionic hematoma

⑤ **656.9 Unspecified fetal and placental problem**
[0,1,3]

⑤ **657 Polyhydramnios**
[0,1,3]   Hydramnios

      Excludes: suspected polyhydramnios not found (V89.01)

      DEFINITION Polyhydramnios is a condition that exists when there is too much amniotic fluid
      in the uterus.
      Use 0 as fourth-digit for this category

⑤ **658 Other problems associated with amniotic cavity and membranes**

      Excludes: amniotic fluid embolism (673.1)
                   suspected problems with amniotic cavity and membranes not found (V89.01)

      DEFINITION The amniotic cavity is the fluid-filled cavity that surrounds the developing embryo

⑤ **658.0 Oligohydramnios**
[0,1,3]   Oligohydramnios without mention of rupture of membranes

⑤ **658.1 Premature rupture of membranes**
[0,1,3]   Rupture of amniotic sac less than 24 hours prior to the onset of labor

⑤ **658.2 Delayed delivery after spontaneous or unspecified rupture of membranes**
[0,1,3]   Prolonged rupture of membranes NOS
             Rupture of amniotic sac 24 hours or more prior to the onset of labor

⑤ **658.3 Delayed delivery after artificial rupture of membranes**
[0,1,3]

⑤ **658.4 Infection of amniotic cavity**
[0,1,3]   Amnionitis
             Chorioamnionitis
             Membranitis
             Placentitis

⑤ **658.8 Other**
[0,1,3]   Amnion nodosum
             Amniotic cyst

⑤ **658.9 Unspecified**
[0,1,3]

⑤ **659 Other indications for care or intervention related to labor and delivery, not elsewhere
         classified**

⑤ **659.0 Failed mechanical induction**
[0,1,3]   Failure of induction of labor by surgical or other instrumental methods

⑤ **659.1 Failed medical or unspecified induction**
[0,1,3]   Failed induction NOS
             Failure of induction of labor by medical methods, such as oxytocic drugs

	Add 4th or 5th digit		Nonspecific code		Unspecified code		Manifestation code

⑤ **659.2 Maternal pyrexia during labor, unspecified**
[0,1,3]

⑤ **659.3 Generalized infection during labor**
[0,1,3]   Septicemia during labor

⑤ **659.4 Grand multiparity**
[0,1,3]

  Excludes: *supervision only, in pregnancy (V23.3)*
          without current pregnancy (V61.5)

⑤ **659.5 Elderly primigravida**
[0,1,3]   First pregnancy in a woman who will be 35 years of age or older at expected date of
          delivery

  Excludes: *supervision only, in pregnancy (V23.81)*

⑤ **659.6 Elderly multigravida**
[0,1,3]   Second or more pregnancy in a woman who will be 35 years of age or older at
          expected date of delivery

  Excludes: *elderly primigravida 659.5*
          supervision only, in pregnancy (V23.82)

⑤ **659.7 Abnormality in fetal heart rate or rhythm**
[0,1,3]   Depressed fetal heart tones
          Fetal:
            bradycardia
            tachycardia
          Fetal heart rate decelerations
          Non-reassuring fetal heart rate or rhythm

⑤ **659.8 Other specified indications for care or intervention related to labor and delivery**
[0,1,3]   Pregnancy in female less than 16 years old at expected date of delivery
          Very young maternal age

⑤ **659.9 Unspecified indication for care or intervention related to labor and delivery**
[0,1,3]

COMPLICATIONS OCCURRING MAINLY IN THE COURSE OF LABOR AND DELIVERY (660-669)

The following fifth-digit subclassification is for use with categories 660-669 to denote the current episode of care:

  0   unspecified as to episode of care or not applicable

  1   delivered, with or without mention of antepartum condition

  2   delivered, with mention of postpartum complication

  3   antepartum condition or complication

  4   postpartum condition or complication

⑤ **660 Obstructed labor**
    DEFINITION Obstructed labor is a labor in which delivery is prevented by mechanical factors;
    delivery often requires cesarean section.

⑤ **660.0 Obstruction caused by malposition of fetus at onset of labor**
[0,1,3]   Any condition classifiable to 652, causing obstruction during labor
    Use additional code from 652.0-652.9, if desired, to identify condition

⑤ **660.1 Obstruction by bony pelvis**
[0,1,3]   Any condition classifiable to 653, causing obstruction during labor
    Use additional code from 653.0-653.9, if desired, to identify condition

⑤ **660.2 Obstruction by abnormal pelvic soft tissues**
[0,1,3]   Prolapse of anterior lip of cervix
          Any condition classifiable to 654, causing obstruction during labor
    Use additional code from 654.0-654.9, if desired, to identify condition

⑤ **660.3 Deep transverse arrest and persistent occipitoposterior position**
[0,1,3]

⑤ **660.4 Shoulder (girdle) dystocia**
[0,1,3]   Impacted shoulders

⑤ **660.5 Locked twins**
[0,1,3]

⑤ **660.6 Failed trial of labor, unspecified**
[0,1,3]   Failed trial of labor, without mention of condition or suspected condition

● Code new   ▲ Revision of   ④ ⑤ Fourth or fifth
  to this edition   existing code   digit required

⑤ **660.7 Failed forceps or vacuum extractor, unspecified**
[0,1,3]   Application of ventouse or forceps, without mention of condition

⑤ **660.8 Other causes of obstructed labor**
[0,1,3]   Use additional code to identify condition

⑤ **660.9 Unspecified obstructed labor**
[0,1,3]   Dystocia:
    NOS
    fetal NOS
    maternal NOS

⑤ **661 Abnormality of forces of labor**

⑤ **661.0 Primary uterine inertia**
[0,1,3]   Failure of cervical dilation
    Hypotonic uterine dysfunction, primary
    Prolonged latent phase of labor

⑤ **661.1 Secondary uterine inertia**
[0,1,3]   Arrested active phase of labor
    Hypotonic uterine dysfunction, secondary

⑤ **661.2 Other and unspecified uterine inertia**
[0,1,3]   Atony of uterus without hemorrhage
    Desultory labor   Poor contractions
    Irregular labor   Slow slope active phase of labor

Excludes: atony of uterus with hemorrhage (666.1)
    postpartum atony of uterus without hemorrhage (669.8)

⑤ **661.3 Precipitate labor**
[0,1,3]

⑤ **661.4 Hypertonic, incoordinate, or prolonged uterine contractions**
[0,1,3]   Cervical spasm
    Contraction ring (dystocia)
    Dyscoordinate labor
    Hourglass contraction of uterus
    Hypertonic uterine dysfunction
    Incoordinate uterine action
    Retraction ring (Bandl's) (pathological)
    Tetanic contractions
    Uterine dystocia NOS
    Uterine spasm

⑤ **661.9 Unspecified abnormality of labor**
[0,1,3]

⑤ **662 Long labor**

⑤ **662.0 Prolonged first stage**
[0,1,3]

⑤ **662.1 Prolonged labor, unspecified**
[0,1,3]

⑤ **662.2 Prolonged second stage**
[0,1,3]

⑤ **662.3 Delayed delivery of second twin, triplet, etc.**
[0,1,3]

⑤ **663 Umbilical cord complications**
DEFINITION The Umbilical cord is the cord that transports blood, oxygen and nutrients to the baby from the placenta.

⑤ **663.0 Prolapse of cord**
[0,1,3]   Presentation of cord

⑤ **663.1 Cord around neck, with compression**
[0,1,3]   Cord tightly around neck

⑤ **663.2 Other and unspecified cord entanglement, with compression**
[0,1,3]   Entanglement of cords of twins in mono-amniotic sac
    Knot in cord (with compression)

⑤ **663.3 Other and unspecified cord entanglement, without mention of compression**
[0,1,3]

⑤ **663.4 Short cord**
[0,1,3]

⑤ **663.5 Vasa previa**
[0,1,3]

Add 4th or 5th digit   Nonspecific code   Unspecified code   Manifestation code

537

⑤ **663.6 Vascular lesions of cord**
[0,1,3]   Bruising of cord
               Hematoma of cord
               Thrombosis of vessels of cord

⑤ **663.8 Other umbilical cord complications**
[0,1,3]   Velamentous insertion of umbilical cord

⑤ **663.9 Unspecified umbilical cord complication**
[0,1,3]

⑤ **664 Trauma to perineum and vulva during delivery**
               Includes: damage from instruments
                          that from extension of episiotomy
               DEFINITION The perineum is the area between the vagina and the rectum.

⑤ **664.0 First-degree perineal laceration**
[0,1,4]   Perineal laceration, rupture, or tear involving:
               fourchette
               hymen
               labia
               skin
               vagina
               vulva

⑤ **664.1 Second-degree perineal laceration**
[0,1,4]   Perineal laceration, rupture, or tear (following episiotomy) involving:
               pelvic floor
               perineal muscles
               vaginal muscles

               Excludes: that involving anal sphincter (664.2)

⑤ **664.2 Third-degree perineal laceration**
[0,1,4]   Perineal laceration, rupture, or tear (following episiotomy) involving:
               anal sphincter
               rectovaginal septum
               sphincter NOS

               Excludes: anal sphincter tear during delivery not associated with third-degree perineal
                           laceration (664.6)
                           that with anal or rectal mucosal laceration (664.3)

⑤ **664.3 Fourth-degree perineal laceration**
[0,1,4]   Perineal laceration, rupture, or tear as classifiable to 664.2 and involving also:
               anal mucosa
               rectal mucosa

⑤ **664.4 Unspecified perineal laceration**
[0,1,4]   Central laceration

⑤ **664.6 Anal sphincter tear complicating delivery, not associated with third-degree perineal
           laceration**
[0,1,4]

               Excludes: third-degree perineal laceration (664.2)

⑤ **664.5 Vulval and perineal hematoma**
[0,1,4]

⑤ **664.8 Other specified trauma to perineum and vulva**
[0,1,4]   Periurethral trauma

⑤ **664.9 Unspecified trauma to perineum and vulva**
[0,1,4]

⑤ **665 Other obstetrical trauma**
               Includes: damage from instruments
               ALERT! For personal history of other genital system and obstetric disorders see V13.2

⑤ **665.0 Rupture of uterus before onset of labor**
[0,1,3]

⑤ **665.1 Rupture of uterus during labor**
[0,1]   Rupture of uterus NOS

⑤ **665.2 Inversion of uterus**
[0,2,4]

⑤ **665.3 Laceration of cervix**
[0,1,4]

⑤ **665.4 High vaginal laceration**
[0,1,4]   Laceration of vaginal wall or sulcus without mention of perineal laceration

● Code new   ▲ Revision of   ④ ⑤ Fourth or fifth
          to this edition   existing code   digit required

⑤ **665.5** **Other injury to pelvic organs**
[0,1,4]   Injury to:
                bladder
                urethra

Excludes: periurethral trauma (664.8)

⑤ **665.6** **Damage to pelvic joints and ligaments**
[0,1,4]   Avulsion of inner symphyseal cartilage
                Damage to coccyx
                Separation of symphysis (pubis)

⑤ **665.7** **Pelvic hematoma**
[0,1,2,4]   Hematoma of vagina

⑤ **665.8** **Other specified obstetrical trauma**
[0-4]

⑤ **665.9** **Unspecified obstetrical trauma**
[0-4]

⑤ **666** **Postpartum hemorrhage**
DEFINITION Postpartum hemorrhage refers to abnormal bleeding after delivery.

⑤ **666.0** **Third-stage hemorrhage**
[0,2,4]   Hemorrhage associated with retained, trapped, or adherent placenta
                Retained placenta NOS

⑤ **666.1** **Other immediate postpartum hemorrhage**
[0,2,4]   Atony of uterus with hemorrhage
                Hemorrhage within the first 24 hours following delivery of placenta
                Postpartum atony of uterus with hemorrhage
                Postpartum hemorrhage (atonic) NOS

Excludes: atony of uterus without hemorrhage (661.2)
                postpartum atony of uterus without hemorrhage (669.8)

⑤ **666.2** **Delayed and secondary postpartum hemorrhage**
[0,2,4]   Hemorrhage:
                    after the first 24 hours following delivery
                    associated with retained portions of placenta or membranes
                Postpartum hemorrhage specified as delayed or secondary
                Retained products of conception NOS, following delivery

⑤ **666.3** **Postpartum coagulation defects**
[0,2,4]   Postpartum afibrinogenemia
                Postpartum fibrinolysis

⑤ **667** **Retained placenta or membranes, without hemorrhage**
DEFINITION A Retained placenta is a placenta that remains inside the womb after the birth of the baby.

⑤ **667.0** **Retained placenta without hemorrhage**
[0,2,4]   Placenta accreta without hemorrhage
                Retained placenta: without hemorrhage
                    NOS without hemorrhage
                    total without hemorrhage

⑤ **667.1** **Retained portions of placenta or membranes, without hemorrhage**
[0,2,4]   Retained products of conception following delivery, without hemorrhage

⑤ **668** **Complications of the administration of anesthetic or other sedation in labor and delivery**
Includes: complications arising from the administration of a general or local anesthetic,
                analgesic, or other sedation in labor and delivery

Excludes: reaction to spinal or lumbar puncture (349.0)
                spinal headache (349.0)

Use additional code(s) to further specify complication
ALERT! For personal history of failed moderate sedation see V15.80

⑤ **668.0** **Pulmonary complications**
[0-4]   Inhalation [aspiration] of stomach contents or secretions following anesthesia or other
                sedation in labor or delivery
             Mendelson's syndrome following anesthesia or other sedation in labor or delivery
             Pressure collapse of lung following anesthesia or other sedation in labor or delivery

⑤ **668.1** **Cardiac complications**
[0-4]   Cardiac arrest or failure following anesthesia or other sedation in labor and delivery

⑤ **668.2** **Central nervous system complications**
[0-4]   Cerebral anoxia following anesthesia or other sedation in labor and delivery

---

| | Add 4th or 5th digit | | Nonspecific code | | Unspecified code | | Manifestation code |

⑤ **668.8** Other complications of anesthesia or other sedation in labor and delivery
[0-4]

⑤ **668.9** Unspecified complication of anesthesia and other sedation
[0-4]

⑤ **669** Other complications of labor and delivery, not elsewhere classified
ALERT! For personal history of other genital system and obstetric disorders see V13.2

⑤ **669.0** **Maternal distress**
[0-4]   Metabolic disturbance in labor and delivery

⑤ **669.1** **Shock during or following labor and delivery**
[0-4]   Obstetric shock

⑤ **669.2** **Maternal hypotension syndrome**
[0-4]

⑤ **669.3** **Acute kidney failure following labor and delivery**
[0,2,4]

⑤ **669.4** **Other complications of obstetrical surgery and procedures**
[0-4]   Cardiac:
           arrest following cesarean or other obstetrical surgery or procedure, including delivery NOS
           failure following cesarean or other obstetrical surgery or procedure, including delivery NOS
       Cerebral anoxia following cesarean or other obstetrical surgery or procedure, including
           delivery NOS

> Excludes: complications of obstetrical surgical wounds (674.1-674.3)

⑤ **669.5** **Forceps or vacuum extractor delivery without mention of indication**
[0,1]   Delivery by ventouse, without mention of indication

⑤ **669.6** **Breech extraction, without mention of indication**
[0,1]

> Excludes: breech delivery NOS (652.2)

⑤ **669.7** **Cesarean delivery, without mention of indication**
[0,1]

⑤ **669.8** **Other complications of labor and delivery**
[0-4]

⑤ **669.9** **Unspecified complication of labor and delivery**
[0-4]

COMPLICATIONS OF THE PUERPERIUM (670-677)

Note: Categories 671 and 673-676 include the listed conditions even if they occur during pregnancy or childbirth.

The following fifth-digit subclassification is for use with categories 670-676 to denote the current episode of care:

0 unspecified as to episode of care or not applicable

1 delivered, with or without mention of antepartum condition

2 delivered, with mention of postpartum complication

3 antepartum condition or complication

4 postpartum condition or complication

⑤ **670** **Major puerperal infection**

> Excludes: infection following abortion (639.0)
> minor genital tract infection following delivery (646.6)
> puerperal pyrexia NOS (672)
> puerperal fever NOS (672)
> puerperal pyrexia of unknown origin (672)
> urinary tract infection following delivery (646.6)

DEFINITION Major puerperal infection refers to a bacterial infection following childbirth. The infection may also be referred to as puerperal or postpartum fever.

⑤ **670.0** **Major puerperal infection, unspecified**
[0,2,4]

⑤ **670.1** **Puerperal endometritis**
[0,2,4]

⑤ **670.2** **Puerperal sepsis**
[0,2,4]   Puerperal pyemia
Use additional code to identify severe sepsis (995.92) and any associated acute organ dysfunction, if applicable

● Code new   ▲ Revision of   ④ ⑤ Fourth or fifth
  to this edition   existing code   digit required

⑤ **670.3 Puerperal septic thrombophlebitis**
[0,2,4]

⑤ **670.8 Other major puerperal infection**
[0,2,4]   Puerperal:
              pelvic cellulitis
              peritonitis
              salpingitis

⑤ **671 Venous complications in pregnancy and the puerperium**

> *Excludes:* personal history of venous complications prior to pregnancy, such as:
>   thrombophlebitis (V12.52)
>   thrombosis and embolism (V12.51)

⑤ **671.0 Varicose veins of legs**
[0-4]   Varicose veins NOS

⑤ **671.1 Varicose veins of vulva and perineum**
[0-4]

⑤ **671.2 Superficial thrombophlebitis**
[0-4]   Phlebitis NOS
          Thrombophlebitis (superficial)
          Thrombosis NOS

Use additional code to identify the superficial thrombophlebitis (453.6, 453.71, 453.81)

⑤ **671.3 Deep phlebothrombosis, antepartum**
[0,1,3]   Deep-vein thrombosis, antepartum

Use additional code to identify the deep vein thrombosis (453.40-453.42, 453.50-453.52, 453.72-453.79, 453.82-453.89)

Use additional code for long term (current) use of anticoagulants, if applicable (V58.61)

⑤ **671.4 Deep phlebothrombosis, postpartum**
[0,2,4]   Deep-vein thrombosis, postpartum
          Pelvic thrombophlebitis, postpartum
          Phlegmasia alba dolens (puerperal)

Use additional code to identify the deep vein thrombosis (453.40-453.42, 453.50-453.52, 453.72-453.79, 453.82-453.89)

Use additional code for long term (current) use of anticoagulants, if applicable (V58.61)

⑤ **671.5 Other phlebitis and thrombosis**
[0-4]   Cerebral venous thrombosis
          Thrombosis of intracranial venous sinus
          ALERT! For personal history of venous thrombosis and embolism see V12.51

⑤ **671.8 Other venous complications**
[0-4]   Hemorrhoids

⑤ **671.9 Unspecified venous complication**
[0-4]

⑤ **672 Pyrexia of unknown origin during the puerperium**
[0,2,4]   Puerperal fever NOS
          Postpartum fever NOS

Use 0 as fourth-digit for this category
DEFINITION Pyrexia of unknown origin during the puerperium, refers to a fever or febrile condition during the period following childbirth.

⑤ **673 Obstetrical pulmonary embolism**
        Includes: pulmonary emboli in pregnancy, childbirth, or the puerperium, or specified as puerperal

> *Excludes:* embolism following abortion (639.6)

DEFINITION Obstetrical pulmonary embolism is a blood clot that lodges in the lungs and blocks the lung arteries during pregnancy so the flow of blood to the lungs and heart is reduced

⑤ **673.0 Obstetrical air embolism**
[0-4]

⑤ **673.1 Amniotic fluid embolism**
[0-4]

⑤ **673.2 Obstetrical blood-clot embolism**
[0-4]   Puerperal pulmonary embolism NOS

⑤ **673.3 Obstetrical pyemic and septic embolism**
[0-4]

| ▨ Add 4th or 5th digit | ▨ Nonspecific code | ▨ Unspecified code | ▨ Manifestation code |

⑤ `673.8` **Other pulmonary embolism**
[0-4] Fat embolism

⑤ `674` **Other and unspecified complications of the puerperium, not elsewhere classified**
> **ALERT!** For personal history of other genital system and obstetric disorders see V13.2

⑤ 674.0 **Cerebrovascular disorders in the puerperium**
[0-4] Any condition classifiable to 430-434, 436-437 occurring during pregnancy, childbirth, or the puerperium, or specified as puerperal
> Excludes: *intracranial venous sinus thrombosis (671.5)*

⑤ 674.1 **Disruption of cesarean wound**
[0,2,4] Dehiscence or disruption of uterine wound
> Excludes: *uterine rupture before onset of labor (665.0)*
> *uterine rupture during labor (665.1)*

⑤ 674.2 **Disruption of perineal wound**
[0,2,4] Breakdown of perineum
Disruption of wound of:
episiotomy
perineal laceration
Secondary perineal tear

⑤ `674.3` **Other complications of obstetrical surgical wounds**
[0,2,4] Hematoma of cesarean section or perineal wound
Hemorrhage of cesarean section or perineal wound
Infection of cesarean section or perineal wound
> Excludes: *damage from instruments in delivery (664.0-665.9)*

⑤ 674.4 **Placental polyp**
[0,2,4]

⑤ 674.5 **Peripartum cardiomyopathy**
[0-4] Postpartum cardiomyopathy

⑤ `674.8` **Other**
[0,2,4] Hepatorenal syndrome, following delivery
Postpartum:
subinvolution of uterus
uterine hypertrophy

⑤ 674.9 **Unspecified**
[0,2,4] Sudden death of unknown cause during the puerperium

⑤ `675` **Infections of the breast and nipple associated with childbirth**
Includes: the listed conditions during pregnancy, childbirth, or the puerperium

⑤ 675.0 **Infections of nipple**
[0-4] Abscess of nipple

⑤ 675.1 **Abscess of breast**
[0-4] Abscess:
mammary
subareolar
submammary
Mastitis:
purulent
retromammary
submammary

⑤ 675.2 **Nonpurulent mastitis**
[0-4] Lymphangitis of breast
Mastitis:
NOS
interstitial
parenchymatous

⑤ `675.8` **Other specified infections of the breast and nipple**
[0-4]

⑤ 675.9 **Unspecified infection of the breast and nipple**
[0-4]

⑤ `676` **Other disorders of the breast associated with childbirth and disorders of lactation**
Includes: the listed conditions during pregnancy, the puerperium, or lactation

⑤ 676.0 **Retracted nipple**
[0-4]

⑤ 676.1 **Cracked nipple**
[0-4] Fissure of nipple

● Code new
to this edition

▲ Revision of
existing code

④ ⑤ Fourth or fifth
digit required

⑤ **676.2 Engorgement of breasts**
[0-4]

⑤ **676.3 Other and unspecified disorder of breast**
[0-4]

⑤ **676.4 Failure of lactation**
[0-4]   Agalactia

⑤ **676.5 Suppressed lactation**
[0-4]

⑤ **676.6 Galactorrhea**
[0-4]

> *Excludes:* galactorrhea not associated with childbirth (611.6)

⑤ **676.8 Other disorders of lactation**
[0-4]   Galactocele

⑤ **676.9 Unspecified disorder of lactation**
[0-4]

677 Late effect of complication of pregnancy, childbirth, and the puerperium

Note: This category is to be used to indicate conditions in 632-648.9 and 651-676.9 as the cause of the late effect, themselves classifiable elsewhere. The "late effects" include conditions specified as such, or as sequelae, which may occur at any time after the puerperium.

Code first any sequelae

DEFINITION Late effect of complication of pregnancy, childbirth, and the puerperium is a condition that appears after the acute phase of the pregnancy complication has run its course

ALERT! Code 677 is for use in those cases when an initial complication of a pregnancy develops a sequelae requiring care or treatment at a future date. This code, like all late effect codes, is to be sequenced following the code describing the sequelae of the complication.

OTHER MATERNAL AND FETAL COMPLICATIONS (678-679)

The following fifth-digit subclassification is for use with categories 678-679 to denote the current episode of care:

0   unspecified as to episode of care or not applicable

1   delivered, with or without mention of antepartum condition

2   delivered, with mention of postpartum complication

3   antepartum condition or complication

4   postpartum condition or complication

⑤ **678 Other fetal conditions**

Requires fifth digit; valid digits are in [brackets] under each code. See beginning of section 678-679 for definitions.

⑤ **678.0 Fetal hematologic conditions**
[0,1,3]   Fetal anemia
Fetal thrombocytopenia
Fetal twin to twin transfusion

> *Excludes:* fetal and neonatal hemorrhage (772.0-772.9)
> fetal hematologic disorders affecting newborn (776.0-776.9)
> fetal-maternal hemorrhage (656.00-656.03)
> isoimmunization incompatibility (656.10-656.13, 656.20-656.23)

⑤ **678.1 Fetal conjoined twins**
[0,1,3]

⑤ **679 Complications of in utero procedures**

Requires fifth digit; valid digits are in [brackets] under each code. See beginning of section 678-679 for definitions.

DEFINITION Complications of in utero procedures, refers to problems caused by procedures performed on the unborn fetus.

ALERT! For personal history of undergoing in utero procedure during pregnancy see V15.21

ALERT! For personal history of undergoing in utero procedure while a fetus see V15.22

⑤ **679.0 Maternal complications from in utero procedure**
[0-4]

> *Excludes:* maternal history of in utero procedure during previous pregnancy (V23.86)

⑤ **679.1 Fetal complications from in utero procedure**
[0-4]   Fetal complications from amniocentesis

> *Excludes:* newborn affected by in utero procedure (760.61-760.64)

| | Add 4th or 5th digit | | Nonspecific code | | Unspecified code | | Manifestation code |

This page intentionally left blank.

● Code new
to this edition

▲ Revision of
existing code

④ ⑤ Fourth or fifth
digit required

Chapter 12: Diseases Skin and Subcutaneous Tissue (680-709)

DEFINITIONS AND CODING ALERTS

This chapter includes definitions of selected key words, terms and phrases and coding alerts for adding points to the clinical domain, references to coding late effects where appropriate, and references to personal history V-codes in situations where the acute or chronic condition is no longer active. An example from this chapter is as follows:

706 **Diseases of sebaceous glands**

> **DEFINITION** Sebaceous glands are microscopic glands in the skin which secrete an oily matter (sebum) in the hair follicles to lubricate the skin and hair.

⑤ **707.2 Pressure ulcer stages**

> **ALERT!** Two codes are needed to completely describe a pressure ulcer: a code from subcategory 707.0 to identify the site of the pressure ulcer, and a code from subcategory 707.2

MULTIPLE CODING FOR A SINGLE CONDITION

In addition to the etiology or manifestation convention that requires two codes to fully describe a single condition that affects multiple body systems, there are other single conditions that also require more than one code. "Use additional code" notes are found in the tabular at codes that are not part of an etiology or manifestation pair where a secondary code is useful to fully describe a condition. The sequencing rule is the same as the etiology or manifestation pair - , "use additional code" indicates that a secondary code should be added.

"Code first" notes are also under certain codes that are not specifically manifestation codes but may be due to an underlying cause. When a "code first" note is present and an underlying condition is present the underlying condition should be sequenced first.

"Code, if applicable, any causal condition first", notes indicate that this code may be assigned as a principal diagnosis when the causal condition is unknown or not applicable. If a causal condition is known, then the code for that condition should be sequenced as the principal or first-listed diagnosis. Multiple codes may be needed for late effects, complication codes and obstetric codes to more fully describe a condition. See the specific guidelines for these conditions for further instruction.

COMBINATION CODE

A combination code is a single code used to classify: two diagnoses, or a diagnosis with an associated secondary process (manifestation) A diagnosis with an associated complication Combination codes are identified by referring to subterm entries in the Alphabetic Index and by reading the inclusion and exclusion notes in the Tabular List.

Assign only the combination code when that code fully identifies the diagnostic conditions involved or when the Alphabetic Index so directs. Multiple coding should not be used when the classification provides a combination code that clearly identifies all of the elements documented in the diagnosis. When the combination code lacks necessary specificity in describing the manifestation or complication, an additional code should be used as a secondary code.

CODING LATE EFFECTS

A late effect is the residual effect (condition produced) after the acute phase of an illness or injury has terminated. There is no time limit on when a late effect code can be used. The residual may be apparent early, such as in cerebrovascular accident cases, or it may occur months or years later, such as that due to a previous injury. Coding of late effects generally requires two codes sequenced in the following order: The condition or nature of the late effect is sequenced first. The late effect code is sequenced second.

An exception to the above guidelines are those instances where the code for late effect is followed by a manifestation code identified in the Tabular List and title, or the late effect code has been expanded (at the fourth and fifth-digit levels) to include the manifestation(s). The code for the acute phase of an illness or injury that led to the late effect is never used with a code for the late effect.

	Add 4th or 5th digit		Nonspecific code		Unspecified code		Manifestation code

PRESSURE ULCER STAGE CODES

Pressure ulcer stages

Two codes are needed to completely describe a pressure ulcer: A code from subcategory 707.0, Pressure ulcer, to identify the site of the pressure ulcer and a code from subcategory 707.2, Pressure ulcer stages.

The codes in subcategory 707.2, Pressure ulcer stages, are to be used as an additional diagnosis with a code(s) from subcategory 707.0, Pressure Ulcer. Codes from 707.2, Pressure ulcer stages, may not be assigned as a principal or first-listed diagnosis. The pressure ulcer stage codes should only be used with pressure ulcers and not with other types of ulcers (e.g., stasis ulcer).

The ICD-9-CM classifies pressure ulcer stages based on severity, which is designated by stages I-IV and unstageable.

Unstageable pressure ulcers

Assignment of code 707.25, Pressure ulcer, unstageable, should be based on the clinical documentation. Code 707.25 is used for pressure ulcers whose stage cannot be clinically determined (e.g., the ulcer is covered by eschar or has been treated with a skin or muscle graft) and pressure ulcers that are documented as deep tissue injury but not documented as due to trauma. This code should not be confused with code 707.20, Pressure ulcer, stage unspecified. Code 707.20 should be assigned when there is no documentation regarding the stage of the pressure ulcer.

Documented pressure ulcer stage

Assignment of the pressure ulcer stage code should be guided by clinical documentation of the stage or documentation of the terms found in the index. For clinical terms describing the stage that are not found in the index, and there is no documentation of the stage, the provider should be queried.

Bilateral pressure ulcers with same stage

When a patient has bilateral pressure ulcers (e.g., both buttocks) and both pressure ulcers are documented as being the same stage, only the code for the site and one code for the stage should be reported.

Bilateral pressure ulcers with different stages

When a patient has bilateral pressure ulcers at the same site (e.g., both buttocks) and each pressure ulcer is documented as being at a different stage, assign one code for the site and the appropriate codes for the pressure ulcer stage.

Multiple pressure ulcers of different sites and stages

When a patient has multiple pressure ulcers at different sites (e.g., buttock, heel, shoulder) and each pressure ulcer is documented as being at different stages (e.g., stage 3 and stage 4), assign the appropriate codes for each different site and a code for each different pressure ulcer stage.

No code is assigned if the documentation states that the pressure ulcer is completely healed.

Pressure ulcers described as healing should be assigned the appropriate pressure ulcer stage code based on the documentation in the medical record. If the documentation does not provide information about the stage of the healing pressure ulcer, assign code 707.20, Pressure ulcer stage, unspecified.

If the documentation is unclear as to whether the patient has a current (new) pressure ulcer or if the patient is being treated for a healing pressure ulcer, query the provider.

If a patient is admitted with a pressure ulcer at one stage and it progresses to a higher stage, assign the code for highest stage reported for that site.

● Code new
to this edition

▲ Revision of
existing code

④ ⑤ Fourth or fifth
digit required

12. DISEASES OF THE SKIN AND SUBCUTANEOUS TISSUE (680-709)

INFECTIONS OF SKIN AND SUBCUTANEOUS TISSUE (680-686)

Excludes: *certain infections of skin classified under "Infectious and Parasitic Diseases," such as:*
  erysipelas (035)
  erysipeloid of Rosenbach (027.1)
  herpes:
    simplex (054.0-054.9)
    zoster (053.0-053.9)
  molluscum contagiosum (078.0)
  viral warts (078.10-078.19)

ALERT! For personal history of diseases of skin and subcutaneous tissue see V13.3

680   Carbuncle and furuncle
  Includes: boil
          furunculosis

DEFINITION A carbuncle is an abscess larger than a boil, usually with one or more openings draining pus onto the skin. It is usually caused by bacterial infection, most commonly staphylococcus aureus. A furuncle is a skin disease caused by the infection of hair follicles, resulting in the localized accumulation of pus and dead tissue

680.0   Face
    Ear [any part]
    Face [any part, except eye]
    Nose (septum)
    Temple (region)

  Excludes: *eyelid (373.13)*
        lacrimal apparatus (375.31)
        orbit (376.01)

680.1   Neck

680.2   Trunk
    Abdominal wall   Flank
    Back [any part, except   Groin
        buttocks]   Pectoral region
    Breast   Perineum
    Chest wall   Umbilicus

  Excludes: *buttocks (680.5)*
        external genital organs:
        female (616.4)
        male (607.2, 608.4)

680.3   Upper arm and forearm
    Arm [any part, except hand]
    Axilla
    Shoulder

680.4   Hand
    Finger [any]   Wrist
    Thumb

680.5   Buttock
    Anus
    Gluteal region

680.6   Leg, except foot
    Ankle   Knee
    Hip   Thigh

680.7   Foot
    Heel
    Toe

680.8   Other specified sites
    Head [any part, except face]
    Scalp

  Excludes: *external genital organs:*
        female (616.4)
        male (607.2, 608.4)

680.9   Unspecified site
    Boil NOS   Furuncle NOS
    Carbuncle NOS

| Add 4th or 5th digit | Nonspecific code | Unspecified code | Manifestation code |

681 **Cellulitis and abscess of finger and toe**
Includes: that with lymphangitis

Use additional code, if desired, to identify organism, such as Staphylococcus (041.1)

DEFINITION Cellulitis is an infection of the finger or toe, usually caused by normal skin bacteria that get under the top layer of skin. Signs of infection include red, warm, tender skin, swelling, fever, and/or chills.

⑤ **681.0 Finger**

    681.00 Cellulitis and abscess, unspecified

    681.01 Felon
        Pulp abscess
        Whitlow

    Excludes: *herpetic whitlow (054.6)*

    681.02 Onychia and paronychia of finger
        Panaritium of finger
        Perionychia of finger

⑤ **681.1 Toe**

    681.10 Cellulitis and abscess, unspecified

    681.11 Onychia and paronychia of toe
        Panaritium of toe
        Perionychia of toe

681.9 Cellulitis and abscess of unspecified digit
    Infection of nail NOS

682 **Other cellulitis and abscess**
Includes: abscess (acute) (with lymphangitis) except of finger or toe
        cellulitis (diffuse) (with lymphangitis) except of finger or toe
        lymphangitis, acute (with lymphangitis) except of finger or toe

Use additional code, if desired, to identify organism, such as Staphylococcus (041.1)

    Excludes: *lymphangitis (chronic) (subacute) (457.2)*

682.0 Face
Cheek, external	Nose, external
Chin	Submandibular
Forehead	Temple (region)

    Excludes: *ear [any part] (380.10-380.16)*
        eyelid (373.13)
        lacrimal apparatus (375.31)
        lip (528.5)
        mouth (528.3)
        nose (internal) (478.1)
        orbit (376.01)

682.1 Neck

682.2 Trunk
Abdominal wall	Groin
Back [any part, except buttock]	Pectoral region
Chest wall	Perineum
Flank	Umbilicus, except newborn

    Excludes: *anal and rectal regions (566)*
        breast:
          NOS (611.0)
          puerperal (675.1)
        external genital organs:
          female (616.3-616.4)
          male (604.0, 607.2, 608.4)
        umbilicus, newborn (771.4)

682.3 Upper arm and forearm
    Arm [any part, except hand]
    Axilla
    Shoulder

    Excludes: *hand (682.4)*

682.4 Hand, except fingers and thumb
    Wrist

    Excludes: *finger and thumb (681.00-681.02)*

● Code new to this edition	▲ Revision of existing code	④ ⑤ Fourth or fifth digit required

682.5 Buttock
    Gluteal region

> *Excludes:* *anal and rectal regions (566)*

682.6 Leg, except foot

Ankle	Knee
Hip	Thigh

682.7 Foot, except toes
    Heel

> *Excludes:* *toe (681.10-681.11)*

682.8 Other specified sites
    Head [except face]
    Scalp

> *Excludes:* *face (682.0)*

682.9 Unspecified site

Abscess NOS	Lymphangitis, acute NOS
Cellulitis NOS	

> *Excludes:* *lymphangitis NOS (457.2)*

683 Acute lymphadenitis
    Abscess (acute), lymph gland or node, except mesenteric
    Adenitis, acute, lymph gland or node, except mesenteric
    Lymphadenitis, acute, lymph gland or node, except mesenteric
Use additional code, if desired, to identify organism, such as Staphylococcus (041.1)

> *Excludes:* *enlarged glands NOS (785.6)*
>
>   *lymphadenitis:*
>   *chronic or subacute, except mesenteric (289.1)*
>   *mesenteric (acute) (chronic) (subacute) (289.2)*
>   *unspecified (289.3)*

> **DEFINITION** Lymphadenitis is an inflammation of a lymph node. It is often a complication of a bacterial infection of a wound, although it can also be caused by viruses or other disease agents

684 Impetigo
    Impetiginization of other dermatoses
    Impetigo (contagiosa) [any site] [any organism]:
      bullous
      circinate
      neonatorum
      simplex
    Pemphigus neonatorum

> *Excludes:* *impetigo herpetiformis (694.3)*

> **DEFINITION** Impetigo is a contagious bacterial skin disease forming pustules and yellow crusty sores, chiefly on the face and hands.

685 Pilonidal cyst
    Includes:
      fistula, coccygeal or pilonidal
      sinus, coccygeal or pilonidal

> **DEFINITION** Pilonidal cyst is a special kind of abscess that occurs in the cleft between the buttocks. Forms frequently in adolescence after long trips that involve sitting.

685.0 With abscess

685.1 Without mention of abscess

686 Other local infections of skin and subcutaneous tissue
Use additional code, if desired, to identify any infectious organism (041.0-041.8)

> **DEFINITION** Subcutaneous tissue is the bottom layer of he skin and is composed of fat cells, connective tissue, blood vessels and nerves.

⑤ **686.0 Pyoderma**
    Dermatitis:
      purulent
      septic
      suppurative

    686.00 Pyoderma, unspecified

    686.01 Pyoderma gangrenosum

    686.09 Other pyoderma

Add 4th or 5th digit	Nonspecific code	Unspecified code	Manifestation code

686.1 Pyogenic granuloma
Granuloma:
septic
suppurative
telangiectaticum

Excludes: pyogenic granuloma of oral mucosa (528.9)

686.8 Other specified local infections of skin and subcutaneous tissue
Bacterid (pustular)   Ecthyma
Dermatitis vegetans   Perlèche

Excludes: dermatitis infectiosa eczematoides (690.8)
panniculitis (729.30-729.39)

686.9 Unspecified local infection of skin and subcutaneous tissue
Fistula of skin NOS
Skin infection NOS

Excludes: fistula to skin from internal organs—see Alphabetic Index

OTHER INFLAMMATORY CONDITIONS OF SKIN AND SUBCUTANEOUS TISSUE (690-698)

Excludes: panniculitis (729.30-729.39)

690 Erythematosquamous dermatosis

Excludes: eczematous dermatitis of eyelid (373.31)
parakeratosis variegata (696.2)
psoriasis (696.0-696.1)
seborrheic keratosis (702.11-702.19)

DEFINITION Erythematosquamous dermatosis is a skin disease, especially one that is not accompanied by inflammation.

⑤ **690.1 Seborrheic dermatitis**

690.10 Seborrheic dermatitis, unspecified
Seborrheic dermatitis NOS

690.11 Seborrhea capitis
Cradle cap

690.12 Seborrheic infantile dermatitis

690.18 Other seborrheic dermatitis

690.8 Other erythematosquamous dermatosis

691 Atopic dermatitis and related conditions

DEFINITION Atopic dermatitis and related conditions, aka eczema, is a chronic, recurring inflammatory skin disorder that usually first appears in babies or very young children and may last through adulthood. Eczema causes the skin to itch and develop a red, scaly, patchy rash.

691.0 Diaper or napkin rash
Ammonia dermatitis
Diaper or napkin:
dermatitis
erythema
rash
Psoriasiform napkin eruption

691.8 Other atopic dermatitis and related conditions
Atopic dermatitis   Neurodermatitis:
Besnier's prurigo   atopic
Eczema: diffuse (of Brocq)
atopic
flexural
intrinsic (allergic)

● Code new   ▲ Revision of   ④ ⑤ Fourth or fifth
to this edition   existing code   digit required

692 Contact dermatitis and other eczema
  Includes:

dermatitis:	eczema (acute) (chronic):
NOS	NOS
contact	allergic
occupational	erythematous
venenata	occupational

Excludes: *allergy NOS (995.3)*
  contact dermatitis of eyelids (373.32)
  dermatitis due to substances taken internally (693.0-693.9)
  eczema of external ear (380.22)
  perioral dermatitis (695.3)
  urticarial reactions (708.0-708.9, 995.1)

DEFINITION Contact dermatitis refers to a skin reaction resulting from exposure to allergens (allergic contact dermatitis) or irritants (irritant contact dermatitis). Phototoxic dermatitis occurs when the allergen or irritant is activated by sunlight.

692.0 Due to detergents

692.1 Due to oils and greases

692.2 Due to solvents
  Dermatitis due to solvents of:
    chlorocompound group
    cyclohexane group
    ester group
    glycol group
    hydrocarbon group
    ketone group

692.3 Due to drugs and medicines in contact with skin
  Dermatitis (allergic) (contact) due to:
    arnica
    fungicides
    iodine
    keratolytics
    mercurials
    neomycin
    pediculocides
    phenols
    scabicides
    any drug applied to skin
  Dermatitis medicamentosa due to drug applied to skin
Use additional E code, if desired, to identify drug

Excludes: *allergy NOS due to drugs (995.27)*
  dermatitis due to ingested drugs (693.0)
  dermatitis medicamentosa NOS (693.0)

692.4 Due to other chemical products

Dermatitis due to:	Dermatitis due to:
acids	insecticide
adhesive plaster	nylon
alkalis	plastic
caustics	rubber
dichromate	

692.5 Due to food in contact with skin

Dermatitis, contact, due to:	Dermatitis, contact, due to:
cereals	fruit
fish	meat
flour	milk

Excludes: *dermatitis due to:*
  dyes (692.89)
  ingested foods (693.1)
  preservatives (692.89)

Add 4th or 5th digit Nonspecific code Unspecified code Manifestation code

692.6 Due to plants [except food]
　　　　Dermatitis due to:
　　　　　　lacquer tree [Rhus verniciflua]
　　　　　　poison ivy [Rhus toxicodendron]
　　　　　　poison oak [Rhus diversiloba]
　　　　　　poison sumac [Rhus venenata]
　　　　　　poison vine [Rhus radicans]
　　　　　　primrose [Primula]
　　　　　　ragweed [Senecio jacobae]
　　　　　　other plants in contact with the skin

Excludes: *allergy NOS due to pollen (477.0)*
　　　　　　　nettle rash (708.8)

⑤ **692.7 Due to solar radiation**

Excludes: *sunburn due to other ultraviolet radiation exposure (692.82)*

　　692.70 Unspecified dermatitis due to sun

　　692.71 Sunburn
　　　　　　First degree sunburn
　　　　　　Sunburn NOS

　　692.72 Acute dermatitis due to solar radiation
　　　　　　Berloque dermatitis
　　　　　　Photoallergic response
　　　　　　Phototoxic response
　　　　　　Polymorphus light eruption
　　　　　　Acute solar skin damage NOS

Excludes: *sunburn (692.71, 692.76-692.77)*
　　Use additional E code, if desired, to identify drug, if drug induced

　　692.73 Actinic reticuloid and actinic granuloma

　　692.74 Other chronic dermatitis due to solar radiation
　　　　　　Solar elastosis
　　　　　　Chronic solar skin damage NOS

Excludes: *actinic [solar] keratosis (702.0)*

　　692.75 Disseminated superficial actinic porokeratosis (DSAP)

　　692.76 Sunburn of second degree

　　692.77 Sunburn of third degree

　　692.79 Other dermatitis due to solar radiation
　　　　　　Hydroa aestivale
　　　　　　Photodermatitis due to sun
　　　　　　Photosensitiveness due to sun
　　　　　　Solar skin damage NOS

⑤ **692.8 Due to other specified agents**

　　692.81 Dermatitis due to cosmetics

　　692.82 Dermatitis due to other radiation
　　　　　　Infrared rays
　　　　　　Light, except from sun
　　　　　　Radiation NOS
　　　　　　Ultraviolet rays, except from sun
　　　　　　X-rays
　　　　　　Tanning bed

Excludes: *that due to solar radiation (692.70-692.79)*

　　692.83 Dermatitis due to metals
　　　　　　Jewelry

　　692.84 Due to animal (cat) (dog) dander
　　　　　　Due to animal (cat) (dog) hair

　　692.89 Other
　　　　　　Dermatitis due to:
　　　　　　　cold weather
　　　　　　　dyes
　　　　　　　hot weather
　　　　　　　preservatives

Excludes: *allergy (NOS) (rhinitis) due to animal hair or dander (477.2)*
　　　　　　　allergy to dust (477.8)
　　　　　　　sunburn (692.71, 692.76-692.77)

　● Code new　　　　▲ Revision of　　　④ ⑤ Fourth or fifth
　　　　to this edition　　　existing code　　　digit required

692.9 Unspecified cause
 Dermatitis: Eczema NOS
  NOS
  contact NOS
  venenata NOS

693 Dermatitis due to substances taken internally
 Excludes: *adverse effect NOS of drugs and medicines (995.20)*
   allergy NOS (995.3)
   contact dermatitis (692.0-692.9)
   urticarial reactions (708.0-708.9, 995.1)

693.0 Due to drugs and medicines
 Dermatitis medicamentosa NOS
Use additional E code, if desired, to identify drug
 Excludes: *that due to drugs in contact with skin (692.3)*

693.1 Due to food

693.8 Due to other specified substances taken internally

693.9 Due to unspecified substance taken internally
 Excludes: *dermatitis NOS (692.9)*

694 Bullous dermatoses
 DEFINITION Bullous dermatoses is a skin disease, especially one that is not accompanied by inflammation

694.0 Dermatitis herpetiformis
 Dermatosis herpetiformis
 Duhring's disease
 Hydroa herpetiformis

 Excludes: *herpes gestationis (646.8)*
   dermatitis herpetiformis:
   juvenile (694.2)
   senile (694.5)

694.1 Subcorneal pustular dermatosis
 Sneddon-Wilkinson disease or syndrome

694.2 Juvenile dermatitis herpetiformis
 Juvenile pemphigoid

694.3 Impetigo herpetiformis

694.4 Pemphigus
 Pemphigus: Pemphigus:
  NOS   malignant
  erythematosus   vegetans
  foliaceus   vulgaris

 Excludes: *pemphigus neonatorum (684)*

694.5 Pemphigoid
 Benign pemphigus NOS
 Bullous pemphigoid
 Herpes circinatus bullosus
 Senile dermatitis herpetiformis

⑤ **694.6 Benign mucous membrane pemphigoid**
 Cicatricial pemphigoid
 Mucosynechial atrophic bullous dermatitis

  694.60 Without mention of ocular involvement

  694.61 With ocular involvement
   Ocular pemphigus

694.8 Other specified bullous dermatoses
 Excludes: *herpes gestationis (646.8)*

694.9 Unspecified bullous dermatoses

695 Erythematous conditions
 DEFINITION Erythematous conditions refers to conditions causing diffuse or patchy redness of skin

695.0 Toxic erythema
 Erythema venenatum

	Add 4th or 5th digit		Nonspecific code		Unspecified code		Manifestation code

⑤ **695.1 Erythema multiforme**

Use additional code to identify associated manifestations, such as:
  arthropathy associated with dermatological disorders (713.3)
  conjunctival edema (372.73)
  conjunctivitis (372.04, 372.33)
  corneal scars and opacities (371.00-371.05)
  corneal ulcer (370.00-370.07)
  edema of eyelid (374.82)
  inflammation of eyelid (373.8)
  keratoconjunctivitis sicca (370.33)
  mechanical lagophthalmos (374.22)
  mucositis (478.11, 528.00, 538, 616.81)
  stomatitis (528.00)
  symblepharon (372.63)

Use additional E-code to identify drug, if drug-induced

Use additional code to identify percentage of skin exfoliation (695.50-695.59)

Excludes: *(staphylococcal) scalded skin syndrome (695.81)*

695.10 Erythema multiforme, unspecified
  Erythema iris
  Herpes iris

695.11 Erythema multiforme minor

695.12 Erythema multiforme major

695.13 Stevens-Johnson syndrome

695.14 Stevens-Johnson syndrome-toxic epidermal
  necrolysis overlap syndrome
  SJS-TEN overlap syndrome

695.15 Toxic epidermal necrolysis
  Lyell's syndrome

695.19 Other erythema multiforme

695.2 Erythema nodosum

Excludes: *tuberculous erythema nodosum (017.1)*

695.3 Rosacea

Acne: Perioral dermatitis
  erythematosa   Rhinophyma
  rosacea

695.4 Lupus erythematosus
  Lupus:
    erythematodes (discoid)
    erythematosus (discoid), not disseminated

Excludes: *lupus (vulgaris) NOS (017.0)*
  systemic [disseminated] lupus erythematosus (710.0)

⑤ **695.5 Exfoliation due to erythematous conditions according to extent of body surface involved**

Code first erythematous condition causing exfoliation, such as:
  Ritter's disease (695.81)
  (Staphylococcal) scalded skin syndrome (695.81)
  Stevens-Johnson syndrome (695.13)
  Stevens-Johnson syndrome-toxic epidermal necrolysis overlap syndrome (695.14)
  Toxic epidermal necrolysis (695.15)

695.50 *Exfoliation due to erythematous condition involving less than 10 percent of body surface*
  Exfoliation due to erythematous condition NOS

695.51 *Exfoliation due to erythematous condition involving 10-19 percent of body surface*

695.52 *Exfoliation due to erythematous condition involving 20-29 percent of body surface*

695.53 *Exfoliation due to erythematous condition involving 30-39 percent of body surface*

695.54 *Exfoliation due to erythematous condition involving 40-49 percent of body surface*

695.55 *Exfoliation due to erythematous condition involving 50-59 percent of body surface*

● Code new   ▲ Revision of   ④ ⑤ Fourth or fifth
       to this edition   existing code   digit required

695.56 *Exfoliation due to erythematous condition involving 60-69 percent of body surface*

695.57 *Exfoliation due to erythematous condition involving 70-79 percent of body surface*

695.58 *Exfoliation due to erythematous condition involving 80-89 percent of body surface*

695.59 *Exfoliation due to erythematous condition involving 90 percent or more of body surface*

⑤ **695.8 Other specified erythematous conditions**

    695.81 Ritter's disease
        Dermatitis exfoliativa neonatorum
        (Staphylococcal) Scalded skin syndrome

Use additional code to identify percentage of skin exfoliation (695.50-695.59)

    695.89 Other
        Erythema intertrigo
        Intertrigo
        Pityriasis rubra (Hebra)

Excludes: mycotic intertrigo (111.0-111.9)

695.9 Unspecified erythematous condition
    Erythema NOS
    Erythroderma (secondary)

696 Psoriasis and similar disorders

DEFINITION Psoriasis is a chronic, noncontagious genetic disease of the immune system that prompts skin cells to regenerate too quickly, causing red, scaly lesions that crack and bleed. .

696.0 Psoriatic arthropathy

696.1 Other psoriasis
    Acrodermatitis continua
    Dermatitis repens
    Psoriasis:
      NOS
      any type, except arthropathic

Excludes: psoriatic arthropathy (696.0)

696.2 Parapsoriasis
    Parakeratosis variegata
    Parapsoriasis lichenoides chronica
    Pityriasis lichenoides et varioliformis

696.3 Pityriasis rosea
    Pityriasis circinata (et maculata)

696.4 Pityriasis rubra pilaris
    Devergie's disease
    Lichen ruber acuminatus

Excludes: pityriasis rubra (Hebra) (695.89)

696.5 Other and unspecified pityriasis
    Pityriasis:
      NOS
      alba
      streptogenes

Excludes: pityriasis simplex (690.18)
          pityriasis versicolor (111.0)

696.8 Other

697 Lichen

Excludes: lichen:
        obtusus corneus (698.3)
        pilaris (congenital) (757.39)
        ruber acuminatus (696.4)
        sclerosus et atrophicus (701.0)
        scrofulosus (017.0)
        simplex chronicus (698.3)
        spinulosus (congenital) (757.39)
        urticatus (698.2)

DEFINITION Lichen refers to any of several eruptive skin diseases characterized by hard thick lesions grouped together and resembling lichens growing on rocks.

	Add 4th or 5th digit		Nonspecific code		Unspecified code		Manifestation code

697.0 Lichen planus
Lichen:
planopilaris
ruber planus

697.1 Lichen nitidus
Pinkus' disease

697.8 Other lichen, not elsewhere classified
Lichen:
ruber moniliforme
striata

697.9 Lichen, unspecified

698 Pruritus and related conditions

Excludes: pruritus specified as psychogenic (306.3)

DEFINITION Pruritus is the medical term for itching. Pruritus can result from drug reaction, food allergy, kidney or liver disease, cancers, parasites, aging or dry skin, contact skin reaction, such as poison ivy, and for unknown reasons.

698.0 Pruritus ani
Perianal itch

698.1 Pruritus of genital organs

698.2 Prurigo
Lichen urticatus
Prurigo:
NOS
Hebra's
mitis
simplex
Urticaria papulosa (Hebra)

Excludes: prurigo nodularis (698.3)

698.3 Lichenification and lichen simplex chronicus
Hyde's disease
Neurodermatitis (circumscripta) (local)
Prurigo nodularis

Excludes: neurodermatitis, diffuse (of Brocq) (691.8)

698.4 Dermatitis factitia [artefacta]
Dermatitis ficta
Neurotic excoriation

Use additional code, if desired, to identify any associated mental disorder

698.8 Other specified pruritic conditions
Pruritus:
hiemalis
senilis
Winter itch

698.9 Unspecified pruritic disorder
Itch NOS
Pruritus NOS

OTHER DISEASES OF SKIN AND SUBCUTANEOUS TISSUE (700-709)

Excludes: conditions confined to eyelids (373.0-374.9)
congenital conditions of skin, hair, and nails (757.0-757.9)

700 Corns and callosities
Callus
Clavus

DEFINITION Corns and callosities is an especially toughened area of skin which has become relatively thick and hard in response to repeated friction, pressure or other irritation.

701 Other hypertrophic and atrophic conditions of skin

Excludes: dermatomyositis (710.3)
hereditary edema of legs (757.0)
scleroderma (generalized) (710.1)

DEFINITION Hypertrophic and atrophic conditions of skin, are conditions that cause enlargement or wasting away of the skin.

● Code new
to this edition
▲ Revision of
existing code
④ ⑤ Fourth or fifth
digit required

701.0 Circumscribed scleroderma
Addison's keloid
Dermatosclerosis, localized
Lichen sclerosus et atrophicus
Morphea
Scleroderma, circumscribed or localized

701.1 Keratoderma, acquired
Acquired:
ichthyosis
keratoderma palmaris et plantaris
Elastosis perforans serpiginosa
Hyperkeratosis:
NOS
follicularis in cutem penetrans
palmoplantaris climacterica
Keratoderma:
climactericum
tylodes, progressive
Keratosis (blennorrhagica)

Excludes: *Darier's disease [keratosis follicularis] (congenital) (757.39)*
keratosis:
arsenical (692.4)
gonococcal (098.81)

701.2 Acquired acanthosis nigricans
Keratosis nigricans

701.3 Striae atrophicae
Atrophic spots of skin
Atrophoderma maculatum
Atrophy blanche (of Milian)
Degenerative colloid atrophy
Senile degenerative atrophy
Striae distensae

701.4 Keloid scar
Cheloid
Hypertrophic scar
Keloid

701.5 Other abnormal granulation tissue
Excessive granulation

701.8 Other specified hypertrophic and atrophic conditions of skin
Acrodermatitis atrophicans chronica
Atrophia cutis senilis
Atrophoderma neuriticum
Confluent and reticulate papillomatosis
Cutis laxa senilis
Elastosis senilis
Folliculitis ulerythematosa reticulata
Gougerot-Carteaud syndrome or disease

701.9 Unspecified hypertrophic and atrophic conditions of skin
Atrophoderma

702 Other dermatoses
Excludes: *carcinoma in situ (232.0-232.9)*

DEFINITION Dermatoses are other skin diseases, especially those not accompanied by inflammation.

702.0 Actinic keratosis
⑤ **702.1 Seborrheic keratosis**

702.11 Inflamed seborrheic keratosis

702.19 Other seborrheic keratosis
Seborrheic keratosis NOS

702.8 Other specified dermatoses

703 Diseases of nail
Excludes: *congenital anomalies (757.5)*
onychia and paronychia (681.02, 681.11)

700

Add 4th or 5th digit	Nonspecific code	Unspecified code	Manifestation code

703.0 Ingrowing nail
Ingrowing nail with infection
Unguis incarnatus

Excludes: *infection, nail NOS (681.9)*

703.8 Other specified diseases of nail
Dystrophia unguium   Onychauxis
Hypertrophy of nail   Onychogryposis
Koilonychia   Onycholysis
Leukonychia (punctata) (striata)

703.9 Unspecified disease of nail

704 Diseases of hair and hair follicles

Excludes: *congenital anomalies (757.4)*

DEFINITION A hair follicle is part of the skin that grows hair by packing old cells together. Attached to the follicle is a sebaceous gland,

⑤ **704.0 Alopecia**

Excludes: *madarosis (374.55)*
syphilitic alopecia (091.82)

704.00 Alopecia, unspecified
Baldness
Loss of hair

704.01 Alopecia areata
Ophiasis

704.02 Telogen effluvim

704.09 Other
Folliculitis decalvans
Hypotrichosis:
NOS
postinfectional NOS
Pseudopelade

704.1 Hirsutism
Hypertrichosis:
NOS
lanuginosa, acquired
Polytrichia

Excludes: *hypertrichosis of eyelid (374.54)*

704.2 Abnormalities of the hair
Atrophic hair   Trichiasis:
Clastothrix   NOS
Fragilitas crinium   cicatrical
                       Trichorrhexis (nodosa)

Excludes: *trichiasis of eyelid (374.05)*

704.3 Variations in hair color
Canities (premature)   Poliosis:
Grayness, hair (premature)   NOS
Heterochromia of hair   circumscripta, acquired

● **704.4 Pilar and trichilemmal cysts**

● **704.41 Pilar cyst**

● **704.42 Trichilemmal cyst**
Trichilemmal proliferating cyst

704.8 Other specified diseases of hair and hair follicles
Folliculitis: Sycosis:
NOS   NOS
abscedens et suffodiens   barbae [not parasitic]
pustular   lupoid
Perifolliculitis: vulgaris
NOS
capitis abscedens et suffodiens
scalp

704.9 Unspecified disease of hair and hair follicles

● Code new   ▲ Revision of   ④ ⑤ Fourth or fifth
to this edition   existing code   digit required

705 **Disorders of sweat glands**

> **DEFINITION** Sweat glands are numerous small, tubular glands that are found nearly everywhere in the skin of humans and that secrete perspiration externally through pores to help regulate body temperature.

705.0 **Anhidrosis**
　　Hypohidrosis
　　Oligohidrosis

705.1 **Prickly heat**
　　Heat rash
　　Miliaria rubra (tropicalis)
　　Sudamina

⑤ **705.2** **Focal hyperhidrosis**

> *Excludes:* *generalized (secondary) hyperhidrosis (780.8)*

705.21 **Primary focal hyperhidrosis**
　　Focal hyperhidrosis NOS
　　Hyperhidrosis NOS
　　Hyperhidrosis of:
　　　axilla
　　　face
　　　palms
　　　soles

705.22 **Secondary focal hyperhidrosis**
　　Frey's syndrome

⑤ **705.8** **Other specified disorders of sweat glands**

705.81 **Dyshidrosis**
　　Cheiropompholyx
　　Pompholyx

705.82 **Fox-Fordyce disease**

705.83 **Hidradenitis**
　　Hidradenitis suppurativa

705.89 **Other**
　　Bromhidrosis　　　　Granulosis rubra nasi
　　Chromhidrosis　　　Urhidrosis

> *Excludes:* *generalized hyperhidrosis (780.8)*
> 　　　*hidrocystoma (216.0-216.9)*

705.9 **Unspecified disorder of sweat glands**
　　Disorder of sweat glands NOS

706 **Diseases of sebaceous glands**

> **DEFINITION** Sebaceous glands are microscopic glands in the skin which secrete an oily matter (sebum) in the hair follicles to lubricate the skin and hair.

706.0 **Acne varioliformis**
　　Acne:
　　　frontalis
　　　necrotica

706.1 **Other acne**
　　Acne:　　　　　　　Blackhead
　　　NOS　　　　　　　Comedo
　　　conglobata
　　　cystic
　　　pustular
　　　vulgaris

> *Excludes:* *acne rosacea (695.3)*

706.2 **Sebaceous cyst**
　　Atheroma, skin
　　Keratin cyst
　　Wen

> *Excludes:* *pilar cyst (704.41)*
> 　　　*trichilemmal (proliferating) cyst (704.42)*

	Add 4th or 5th digit		Nonspecific code		Unspecified code		Manifestation code

706.3 Seborrhea
> Excludes: *seborrhea:*
>> *capitis (690.11)*
>> *sicca (690.18)*
>> *seborrheic dermatitis (690.11)*
>> *seborrheic keratosis (702.11-702.19)*

706.8 Other specified diseases of sebaceous glands
> Asteatosis (cutis)
> Xerosis cutis

706.9 Unspecified disease of sebaceous glands

707 Chronic ulcer of skin
> Includes: non-infected sinus of skin
>> non-healing ulcer

> Excludes: *varicose ulcer (454.0, 454.2)*

⑤ **707.0 Pressure ulcer**
> Bed sore
> Decubitus ulcer
> Plaster ulcer

Use additional code to identify pressure ulcer stage (707.20 -707.25)

> **ALERT!** Two codes are needed to completely describe a pressure ulcer: a code from subcategory 707.0 to identify the site of the pressure ulcer, and a code from subcategory 707.2

> **707.00 Unspecified site**

> **707.01 Elbow**

> **707.02 Upper back**
>> Shoulder blades

> **707.03 Lower back**
>> Coccyx
>> Sacrum

> **707.04 Hip**

> **707.05 Buttock**

> **707.06 Ankle**

> **707.07 Heel**

> **707.09 Other site**
>> Head

⑤ **707.1 Ulcer of lower limbs, except pressure ulcer**
> Ulcer, chronic, of lower limb:
>> neurogenic of lower limb
>> trophic of lower limb

> Code, if applicable, any causal condition first:
>> atherosclerosis of the extremities with ulceration (440.23)
>> chronic venous hypertension with ulcer (459.31)
>> chronic venous hypertension with ulcer and inflammation (459.33)
>> diabetes mellitus (249.80-249.81, 250.80-250.83)
>> postphlebetic syndrome with ulcer (459.11)
>> postphlebetic syndrome with ulcer and inflammation (459.13)

> **707.10 Ulcer of lower limb, unspecified**

> **707.11 Ulcer of thigh**

> **707.12 Ulcer of calf**

> **707.13 Ulcer of ankle**

> **707.14 Ulcer of heel and midfoot**
>> Plantar surface of midfoot

> **707.15 Ulcer of other part of foot**
>> Toes

> **707.19 Ulcer of other part of lower limb**

⑤ **707.2 Pressure ulcer stages**
> *Code first site of pressure ulcer (707.00-707.09)*

> **ALERT!** Two codes are needed to completely describe a pressure ulcer: a code from subcategory 707.0 to identify the site of the pressure ulcer, and a code from subcategory 707.2

● Code new
   to this edition

▲ Revision of
   existing code

④ ⑤ Fourth or fifth
     digit required

707.20 **Pressure ulcer, unspecified stage**
Healing pressure ulcer NOS
Healing pressure ulcer, unspecified stage

707.21 **Pressure ulcer stage I**
Healing pressure ulcer, stage I
Pressure pre-ulcer skin changes limited to persistent focal erythema

707.22 **Pressure ulcer stage II**
Healing pressure ulcer, stage II
Pressure ulcer with abrasion, blister, partial thickness skin loss involving
epidermis and/or dermis

707.23 **Pressure ulcer stage III**
Healing pressure ulcer, stage III
Pressure ulcer with full thickness skin loss involving damage or necrosis of
subcutaneous tissue

707.24 **Pressure ulcer stage IV**
Healing pressure ulcer, stage IV
Pressure ulcer with necrosis of soft tissues through to underlying muscle,
tendon, or bone

707.25 **Pressure ulcer, unstageable**
`ALERT!` Code 707.25 is used for pressure ulcers whose stage cannot be clinically determined
(e.g., the ulcer is covered by eschar or has been treated with a skin or muscle graft) and
pressure ulcers that are documented as deep tissue injury but not documented as due to
trauma. This code should not be confused with code 707.20, Pressure ulcer, stage unspecified

707.8 **Chronic ulcer of other specified sites**
Ulcer, chronic, of other specified sites:
neurogenic of other specified sites
trophic of other specified sites

707.9 **Chronic ulcer of unspecified site**

Chronic ulcer NOS	Tropical ulcer NOS
Trophic ulcer NOS	Ulcer of skin NOS

708 **Urticaria**

`Excludes:` edema:

angioneurotic (995.1)
Quincke's (995.1)
hereditary angioedema (277.6)
urticaria:
giant (995.1)
papulosa (Hebra) (698.2)
pigmentosa (juvenile) (congenital) (757.33)

`DEFINITION` Urticaria, aka hives, is the transient appearance of slightly raised patches of skin
which are redder or paler than the surrounding skin and often attended by severe itching.

708.0 **Allergic urticaria**

708.1 **Idiopathic urticaria**

708.2 **Urticaria due to cold and heat**
Thermal urticaria

708.3 **Dermatographic urticaria**
Dermatographia
Factitial urticaria

708.4 **Vibratory urticaria**

708.5 **Cholinergic urticaria**

708.8 **Other specified urticaria**
Nettle rash
Urticaria:
chronic
recurrent periodic

708.9 **Urticaria, unspecified**
Hives NOS

709 **Other disorders of skin and subcutaneous tissue**

⑤ **709.0** **Dyschromia**

`Excludes:` albinism (270.2)

pigmented nevus (216.0-216.9)
that of eyelid (374.52-374.53)

▓ Add 4th or 5th digit	▓ Nonspecific code	▓ Unspecified code	▓ Manifestation code

709.00 Dyschromia, unspecified

709.01 Vitiligo

709.09 Other

709.1 Vascular disorders of skin
Angioma serpiginosum
Purpura (primary) annularis telangiectodes

709.2 Scar conditions and fibrosis of skin
Adherent scar (skin)
Cicatrix
Disfigurement (due to scar)
Fibrosis, skin NOS
Scar NOS

Excludes: keloid scar (701.4)

709.3 Degenerative skin disorders

Calcinosis:	Degeneration, skin
circumscripta	Deposits, skin
cutis	Senile dermatosis NOS
Colloid milium	Subcutaneous calcification

709.4 Foreign body granuloma of skin and subcutaneous tissue

Excludes: residual foreign body without granuloma of skin and subcutaneous tissue (729.6)
that of muscle (728.82)

Use additional code to identify foreign body (V90.01-V90.9)

709.8 Other specified disorders of skin
Epithelial hyperplasia
Menstrual dermatosis
Vesicular eruption

709.9 Unspecified disorder of skin and subcutaneous tissue
Dermatosis NOS

● Code new to this edition　　▲ Revision of existing code　　④ ⑤ Fourth or fifth digit required

Chapter 13: Diseases of Musculoskeletal and Connective Tissue (710-739)

DEFINITIONS AND CODING ALERTS

This chapter includes definitions of selected key words, terms and phrases and coding alerts for adding points to the clinical domain, references to coding late effects where appropriate, and references to personal history V-codes in situations where the acute or chronic condition is no longer active. An example from this chapter is as follows:

710 **Diffuse diseases of connective tissue**
> **DEFINITION** Connective tissue is a type of tissue made up of fibers forming a framework and support structure for body tissues and organs.
> **ALERT!** For personal history of arthritis see V13.4

MULTIPLE CODING FOR A SINGLE CONDITION

In addition to the etiology or manifestation convention that requires two codes to fully describe a single condition that affects multiple body systems, there are other single conditions that also require more than one code. "Use additional code" notes are found in the tabular at codes that are not part of an etiology or manifestation pair where a secondary code is useful to fully describe a condition. The sequencing rule is the same as the etiology or manifestation pair - , "use additional code" indicates that a secondary code should be added.

"Code first" notes are also under certain codes that are not specifically manifestation codes but may be due to an underlying cause. When a "code first" note is present and an underlying condition is present the underlying condition should be sequenced first.

"Code, if applicable, any causal condition first", notes indicate that this code may be assigned as a principal diagnosis when the causal condition is unknown or not applicable. If a causal condition is known, then the code for that condition should be sequenced as the principal or first-listed diagnosis. Multiple codes may be needed for late effects, complication codes and obstetric codes to more fully describe a condition. See the specific guidelines for these conditions for further instruction.

COMBINATION CODE

A combination code is a single code used to classify: two diagnoses, or a diagnosis with an associated secondary process (manifestation) A diagnosis with an associated complication Combination codes are identified by referring to subterm entries in the Alphabetic Index and by reading the inclusion and exclusion notes in the Tabular List.

Assign only the combination code when that code fully identifies the diagnostic conditions involved or when the Alphabetic Index so directs. Multiple coding should not be used when the classification provides a combination code that clearly identifies all of the elements documented in the diagnosis. When the combination code lacks necessary specificity in describing the manifestation or complication, an additional code should be used as a secondary code.

CODING LATE EFFECTS

A late effect is the residual effect (condition produced) after the acute phase of an illness or injury has terminated. There is no time limit on when a late effect code can be used. The residual may be apparent early, such as in cerebrovascular accident cases, or it may occur months or years later, such as that due to a previous injury. Coding of late effects generally requires two codes sequenced in the following order: The condition or nature of the late effect is sequenced first. The late effect code is sequenced second.

An exception to the above guidelines are those instances where the code for late effect is followed by a manifestation code identified in the Tabular List and title, or the late effect code has been expanded (at the fourth and fifth-digit levels) to include the manifestation(s). The code for the acute phase of an illness or injury that led to the late effect is never used with a code for the late effect.

CODING OF PATHOLOGIC FRACTURES

Acute Fractures vs. Aftercare

Pathologic fractures are reported using subcategory 733.1, when the fracture is newly diagnosed. Subcategory 733.1 may be used while the patient is receiving active treatment for the fracture. Examples of active treatment are: surgical treatment, emergency department encounter, evaluation and treatment by a new physician.

	Add 4th or 5th digit		Nonspecific code		Unspecified code		Manifestation code

Fractures are coded using the aftercare codes (subcategories V54.0, V54.2, V54.8 or V54.9) for encounters after the patient has completed active treatment of the fracture and is receiving routine care for the fracture during the healing or recovery phase. Examples of fracture aftercare are: cast change or removal, removal of external or internal fixation device, medication adjustment, and follow up visits following fracture treatment.

Care for complications of surgical treatment for fracture repairs during the healing or recovery phase should be coded with the appropriate complication codes.

Care of complications of fractures, such as malunion and nonunion, should be reported with the appropriate codes. See Official Guidelines, Section I. C. 17.b for information on the coding of traumatic fractures.

● Code new to this edition ▲ Revision of existing code ④ ⑤ Fourth or fifth digit required

13. DISEASES OF THE MUSCULOSKELETAL SYSTEM AND CONNECTIVE TISSUE (710-739)

Use additional external cause code, if applicable, to identify the cause of the musculoskeletal condition

The following fifth-digit subclassification is for use with categories 711-712, 715-716, 718-719, and 730:

0 site unspecified

1 shoulder region
Acromioclavicular joint(s)
Glenohumeral joint(s)
Sternoclavicular joint(s)
Clavicle
Scapula

2 upper arm
Elbow joint   Humerus

3 forearm
Radius   Wrist joint
Ulna

4 hand
Carpus   Phalanges [fingers]
Metacarpus

5 pelvic region and thigh
Buttock   Hip (joint)
Femur

6 lower leg
Fibula   Patella
Knee joint   Tibia

7 ankle and foot
Ankle joint   Phalanges, foot
Digits [toes]   Tarsus
Metatarsus   Other joints in foot

8 other specified sites
Head   Skull
Neck   Trunk
Ribs   Vertebral column

9 multiple sites

ARTHROPATHIES AND RELATED DISORDERS (710-719)

Excludes: *disorders of spine (720.0-724.9)*

710 Diffuse diseases of connective tissue
Includes: all collagen diseases whose effects are not mainly confined to a single system

Excludes: *those affecting mainly the cardiovascular system, i.e., polyarteritis nodosa and allied conditions (446.0-446.7)*

DEFINITION Connective tissue is a type of tissue made up of fibers forming a framework and support structure for body tissues and organs.

ALERT! For personal history of arthritis see V13.4

710.0 Systemic lupus erythematosus
Disseminated lupus erythematosus
Libman-Sacks disease

Use additional code, if desired, to identify manifestation, as:
endocarditis (424.91)
nephritis (583.81)
chronic (582.81)
nephrotic syndrome (581.81)

Excludes: *lupus erythematosus (discoid) NOS (695.4)*

710.1 Systemic sclerosis
Acrosclerosis
CRST syndrome
Progressive systemic sclerosis
Scleroderma

Use additional code, if desired, to identify manifestation, as:
lung involvement (517.2)
myopathy (359.6)

Excludes: *circumscribed scleroderma (701.0)*

	Add 4th or 5th digit		Nonspecific code		Unspecified code		Manifestation code

710.2 Sicca syndrome
Keratoconjunctivitis sicca
Sjögren's disease

710.3 Dermatomyositis
Poikilodermatomyositis
Polymyositis with skin involvement

710.4 Polymyositis

710.5 Eosinophilia myalgia syndrome
Toxic oil syndrome

Use additional E code, if desired, to identify drug, if drug induced

710.8 Other specified diffuse diseases of connective tissue
Multifocal fibrosclerosis (idiopathic) NEC
Systemic fibrosclerosing syndrome

710.9 Unspecified diffuse connective tissue disease
Collagen disease NOS

⑤ **711 Arthropathy associated with infections**
Includes: arthritis associated with conditions classifiable below
arthropathy associated with conditions classifiable below
polyarthritis associated with conditions classifiable below
polyarthropathy associated with conditions classifiable below

Excludes: *rheumatic fever (390)*

The following fifth-digit subclassification is for use with category 711; valid digits are in [brackets] under each code. For definitions, see the beginning of this chapter:

0 **site unspecified**

1 **shoulder region**

2 **upper arm**

3 **forearm**

4 **hand**

5 **pelvic region and thigh**

6 **lower leg**

7 **ankle and foot**

8 **other specified sites**

9 **multiple sites**

DEFINITION Arthropathy is any disease or abnormal condition affecting a joint

⑤ **711.0 Pyogenic arthritis**
[0-9] Arthritis or polyarthritis (due to):
coliform [Escherichia coli]
Hemophilus influenzae [H. influenzae]
pneumococcal
Pseudomonas
staphylococcal
streptococcal
Pyarthrosis

Use additional code, if desired, to identify infectious organism (041.0-041.8)

⑤ **711.1 *Arthropathy associated with Reiter's disease and nonspecific urethritis***
[0-9] *Code first underlying disease, as:*
nonspecific urethritis (099.4)
Reiter's disease (099.3)

⑤ **711.2 *Arthropathy in Behçet's syndrome***
[0-9] *Code first underlying disease (136.1)*

⑤ **711.3 *Postdysenteric arthropathy***
[0-9] *Code first underlying disease, as:*
dysentery (009.0)
enteritis, infectious (008.0-009.3)
paratyphoid fever (002.1-002.9)
typhoid fever (002.0)

Excludes: *salmonella arthritis (003.23)*

⑤ **711.4 *Arthropathy associated with other bacterial diseases***
[0-9] *Code first underlying disease, as:*
diseases classifiable to 010-040, 090-099, except as in 711.1, 711.3, and 713.5
leprosy (030.0-030.9)
tuberculosis (015.0-015.9)

● Code new
to this edition
▲ Revision of
existing code
④ ⑤ Fourth or fifth
digit required

Excludes: *gonococcal arthritis (098.50)*
meningococcal arthritis (036.82)

⑤ **711.5 *Arthropathy associated with other viral diseases***
[0-9]   *Code first underlying disease, as:*
    diseases classifiable to 045-049, 050-079, 480, 487
    O'nyong nyong (066.3)

Excludes: *that due to rubella (056.71)*

⑤ **711.6 *Arthropathy associated with mycoses***
[0-9]   *Code first underlying disease (110.0-118)*

⑤ **711.7 *Arthropathy associated with helminthiasis***
[0-9]   *Code first underlying disease, as:*
    filariasis (125.0-125.9)

⑤ **711.8 *Arthropathy associated with other infectious and parasitic diseases***
[0-9]   *Code first underlying disease, as:*
    diseases classifiable to 080-088, 100-104, 130-136

Excludes: *arthropathy associated with sarcoidosis (713.7)*

⑤ **711.9 Unspecified infective arthritis**
[0-9]   Infective arthritis or polyarthritis (acute) (chronic) (subacute) NOS

⑤ **712 Crystal arthropathies**
    Includes: crystal-induced arthritis and synovitis

Excludes: *gouty arthropathy (274.00-274.03)*

The following fifth-digit subclassification is for use with category 712; valid digits are in
    [brackets] under each code. See beginning of this chapter for definitions:

0 site unspecified

1 shoulder region

2 upper arm

3 forearm

4 hand

5 pelvic region and thigh

6 lower leg

7 ankle and foot

8 other specified sites

9 multiple sites

DEFINITION Crystal arthropathies refers to a type of arthropathy characterized by accumulation of crystals in joints.

⑤ **712.1 *Chondrocalcinosis due to dicalcium phosphate crystals***
[0-9]   Chondrocalcinosis due to dicalcium phosphate crystals (with other crystals)
    Code first underlying disease (275.4)

⑤ **712.2 *Chondrocalcinosis due to pyrophosphate crystals***
[0-9]   *Code first underlying disease (275.4)*

⑤ **712.3 *Chondrocalcinosis, unspecified***
[0-9]   *Code first underlying disease (275.4)*

⑤ **712.8 Other specified crystal arthropathies**
[0-9]

⑤ **712.9 Unspecified crystal arthropathy**
[0-9]

713 Arthropathy associated with other disorders classified elsewhere
    Includes: arthritis associated with conditions classifiable below
        arthropathy associated with conditions classifiable below
        polyarthritis associated with conditions classifiable below
        polyarthropathy associated with conditions classifiable below

    DEFINITION Arthropathy is any disease or abnormal condition affecting a joint

713.0 *Arthropathy associated with other endocrine and metabolic disorders*
> *Code first underlying disease, as:*
> acromegaly (253.0)
> hemochromatosis (275.01-275.09)
> hyperparathyroidism (252.00-252.08)
> hypogammaglobulinemia (279.00-279.09)
> hypothyroidism (243-244.9)
> lipoid metabolism disorder (272.0-272.9)
> ochronosis (270.2)

> | *Excludes:* | *arthropathy associated with:* |
> | --- | --- |
> *amyloidosis (713.7)*
> *crystal deposition disorders, except gout (712.1-712.9)*
> *diabetic neuropathy (713.5)*
> *gout (274.00-274.03)*

713.1 *Arthropathy associated with gastrointestinal conditions other than infections*
> *Code first underlying disease, as:*
> regional enteritis (555.0-555.9)
> ulcerative colitis (556)

713.2 *Arthropathy associated with hematological disorders*
> *Code first underlying disease, as:*
> hemoglobinopathy (282.4-282.7)
> hemophilia (286.0-286.2)
> leukemia (204.0-208.9)
> malignant reticulosis (202.3)
> multiple myelomatosis (203.0)

> | *Excludes:* | *arthropathy associated with Henoch-Schönlein purpura (713.6)* |
> | --- | --- |

713.3 *Arthropathy associated with dermatological disorders*
> *Code first underlying disease, as:*
> erythema multiforme (695.10-695.19)
> erythema nodosum (695.2)

> | *Excludes:* | *psoriatic arthropathy (696.0)* |
> | --- | --- |

713.4 *Arthropathy associated with respiratory disorders*
> *Code first underlying disease, as:*
> diseases classifiable to 490-519

> | *Excludes:* | *arthropathy associated with respiratory infections (711.0, 711.4-711.8)* |
> | --- | --- |

713.5 *Arthropathy associated with neurological disorders*
> Charcot's arthropathy associated with diseases classifiable elsewhere
> Neuropathic arthritis associated with diseases classifiable elsewhere
>
> *Code first underlying disease, as:*
> neuropathic joint disease [Charcot's joints]:
> NOS (094.0)
> diabetic (249.6, 250.6)
> syringomyelic (336.0)
> tabetic [syphilitic] (094.0)

713.6 *Arthropathy associated with hypersensitivity reaction*
> *Code first underlying disease, as:*
> Henoch (-Schönlein) purpura (287.0)
> serum sickness (999.51-999.59)

> | *Excludes:* | *allergic arthritis NOS (716.2)* |
> | --- | --- |

713.7 *Other general diseases with articular involvement*
> *Code first underlying disease, as:*
> amyloidosis (277.30-277.39)
> familial Mediterranean fever (277.31)
> sarcoidosis (135)

713.8 *Arthropathy associated with other conditions classifiable elsewhere*
> *Code first underlying disease, as:*
> conditions classifiable elsewhere except as in 711.1-711.8, 712, and 713.0-713.7

● Code new   ▲ Revision of   ④ ⑤ Fourth or fifth
to this edition   existing code   digit required

714 **Rheumatoid arthritis and other inflammatory polyarthropathies**

Excludes: rheumatic fever (390)

rheumatoid arthritis of spine NOS (720.0)

DEFINITION Rheumatoid arthritis is a chronic, systemic inflammatory disorder that may affect many tissues and organs, but principally attacks the joints producing a inflammatory synovitis that often progresses to destruction of the articular cartilage and ankylosis of the joints.

714.0 Rheumatoid arthritis

Arthritis or polyarthritis:

atrophic

rheumatic (chronic)

Use additional code, if desired, to identify manifestation, as:

myopathy (359.6)

polyneuropathy (357.1)

Excludes: juvenile rheumatoid arthritis NOS (714.30)

714.1 Felty's syndrome

Rheumatoid arthritis with splenoadenomegaly and leukopenia

714.2 Other rheumatoid arthritis with visceral or systemic involvement

Rheumatoid carditis

⑤ **714.3 Juvenile chronic polyarthritis**

714.30 Polyarticular juvenile rheumatoid arthritis, chronic or unspecified

Juvenile rheumatoid arthritis NOS

Still's disease

714.31 Polyarticular juvenile rheumatoid arthritis, acute

714.32 Pauciarticular juvenile rheumatoid arthritis

714.33 Monoarticular juvenile rheumatoid arthritis

714.4 Chronic postrheumatic arthropathy

Chronic rheumatoid nodular fibrositis

Jaccoud's syndrome

⑤ **714.8 Other specified inflammatory polyarthropathies**

714.81 Rheumatoid lung

Caplan's syndrome

Diffuse interstitial rheumatoid disease of lung

Fibrosing alveolitis, rheumatoid

714.89 Other

714.9 Unspecified inflammatory polyarthropathy

Inflammatory polyarthropathy or polyarthritis NOS

Excludes: polyarthropathy NOS (716.5)

⑤ **715 Osteoarthrosis and allied disorders**

Note: Localized, in the subcategories below, includes bilateral involvement of the same site.

Includes: arthritis or polyarthritis:

degenerative

hypertrophic

degenerative joint disease

osteoarthritis

Excludes: Marie-Strümpell spondylitis (720.0)

osteoarthrosis [osteoarthritis] of spine (721.0-721.9)

The following fifth-digit subclassification is for use with category 715; valid digits are in [brackets] under each code. See beginning of this chapter for definitions:

0 **site unspecified**

1 **shoulder region**

2 **upper arm**

3 **forearm**

4 **hand**

5 **pelvic region and thigh**

6 **lower leg**

7 **ankle and foot**

8 **other specified sites**

9 **multiple sites**

Add 4th or 5th digit   Nonspecific code   Unspecified code   Manifestation code

DEFINITION Osteoarthrosis is a chronic degenerative non-inflammatory condition of the joint characterized by structural changes of the joint surfaces

⑤ **715.0 Osteoarthrosis, generalized**
[0,4,9]   Degenerative joint disease, involving multiple joints
Primary generalized hypertrophic osteoarthrosis

⑤ **715.1 Osteoarthrosis, localized, primary**
[0-8]   Localized osteoarthropathy, idiopathic

⑤ **715.2 Osteoarthrosis, localized, secondary**
[0-8]   Coxae malum senilis

⑤ **715.3 Osteoarthrosis, localized, not specified whether primary or secondary**
[0-8]   Otto's pelvis

⑤ **715.8 Osteoarthrosis involving, or with mention of more than one site, but not specified as**
[0,9]   **generalized**

⑤ **715.9 Osteoarthrosis, unspecified whether generalized or localized**
[0-8]

⑤ **716 Other and unspecified arthropathies**

    Excludes: cricoarytenoid arthropathy (478.79)

The following fifth-digit subclassification is for use with category 716; valid digits are in [brackets] under each code. See beginning of this chapter for definitions:

    0 site unspecified

    1 shoulder region

    2 upper arm

    3 forearm

    4 hand

    5 pelvic region and thigh

    6 lower leg

    7 ankle and foot

    8 other specified sites

    9 multiple sites

DEFINITION Arthropathy refers to any disease or abnormal condition affecting a joint.

ALERT! For personal history of other musculoskeletal disorders see V13.5

⑤ **716.0 Kaschin-Beck disease**
[0-9]   Endemic polyarthritis

⑤ **716.1 Traumatic arthropathy**
[0-9]

⑤ **716.2 Allergic arthritis**
[0-9]

    Excludes: arthritis associated with Henoch-Schönlein purpura or serum sickness (713.6)

⑤ **716.3 Climacteric arthritis**
[0-9]   Menopausal arthritis

⑤ **716.4 Transient arthropathy**
[0-9]

    Excludes: palindromic rheumatism (719.3)

⑤ **716.5 Unspecified polyarthropathy or polyarthritis**
[0-9]

⑤ **716.6 Unspecified monoarthritis**
[0-8]   Coxitis

⑤ **716.8 Other specified arthropathy**
[0-9]

⑤ **716.9 Arthropathy, unspecified**
[0-9]   Arthritis (acute) (chronic) (subacute)
Arthropathy (acute) (chronic) (subacute)
Articular rheumatism (chronic)
Inflammation of joint NOS

● Code new to this edition   ▲ Revision of existing code   ④ ⑤ Fourth or fifth digit required

717 **Internal derangement of knee**

Includes: degeneration of articular cartilage or meniscus of knee
rupture, old, of articular cartilage or meniscus of knee
tear, old, of articular cartilage or meniscus of knee

Excludes: *acute derangement of knee (836.0-836.6)*
ankylosis (718.5)
contracture (718.4)
current injury (836.0-836.6)
deformity (736.4-736.6)
recurrent dislocation (718.3)

DEFINITION Internal derangement of knee is a term that describes internal damage to the knee joint, generally caused by trauma. It is a nonspecific term that usually must be further refined by history, physical exam, x-rays, and frequently mri studies.

717.0 **Old bucket handle tear of medial meniscus**
Old bucket handle tear of unspecified cartilage

717.1 **Derangement of anterior horn of medial meniscus**

717.2 **Derangement of posterior horn of medial meniscus**

717.3 **Other and unspecified derangement of medial meniscus**
Degeneration of internal semilunar cartilage

⑤ **717.4** **Derangement of lateral meniscus**

    717.40 **Derangement of lateral meniscus, unspecified**

    717.41 **Bucket handle tear of lateral meniscus**

    717.42 **Derangement of anterior horn of lateral meniscus**

    717.43 **Derangement of posterior horn of lateral meniscus**

    717.49 **Other**

717.5 **Derangement of meniscus, not elsewhere classified**
Congenital discoid meniscus
Cyst of semilunar cartilage
Derangement of semilunar cartilage NOS

717.6 **Loose body in knee**
Joint mice, knee
Rice bodies, knee (joint)

717.7 **Chondromalacia of patella**
Chondromalacia patellae
Degeneration [softening] of articular cartilage of patella

⑤ **717.8** **Other internal derangement of knee**

    717.81 **Old disruption of lateral collateral ligament**

    717.82 **Old disruption of medial collateral ligament**

    717.83 **Old disruption of anterior cruciate ligament**

    717.84 **Old disruption of posterior cruciate ligament**

    717.85 **Old disruption of other ligaments of knee**
Capsular ligament of knee

    717.89 **Other**
Old disruption of ligaments of knee NOS

717.9 **Unspecified internal derangement of knee**
Derangement NOS of knee

⑤ **718** **Other derangement of joint**

Excludes: *current injury (830.0-848.9)*
jaw (524.60-524.69)

The following fifth-digit subclassification is for use with category 718; valid digits are in [brackets] under each code. See beginning of this chapter for definitions:

    0 **site unspecified**

    1 **shoulder region**

    2 **upper arm**

    3 **forearm**

    4 **hand**

    5 **pelvic region and thigh**

    6 **lower leg**

    7 **ankle and foot**

	Add 4th or 5th digit		Nonspecific code		Unspecified code		Manifestation code

8 other specified sites

9 multiple sites

ALERT! For personal history of other musculoskeletal disorders see V13.5

⑤ **718.0 Articular cartilage disorder**
[0-5, 7-9] Meniscus:
    disorder
    rupture, old
    tear, old
    Old rupture of ligament(s) of joint NOS

Excludes: *articular cartilage disorder:*
    in ochronosis (270.2)
    knee (717.0-717.9)
    chondrocalcinosis (275.4)
    metastatic calcification (275.4)

⑤ **718.1 Loose body in joint**
[0-5, 7-9] Joint mice

Excludes: *knee (717.6)*

⑤ **718.2 Pathological dislocation**
[0-9] Dislocation or displacement of joint, not recurrent and not current injury
Spontaneous dislocation (joint)

⑤ **718.3 Recurrent dislocation of joint**
[0-9]

⑤ **718.4 Contracture of joint**
[0-9]

⑤ **718.5 Ankylosis of joint**
[0-9] Ankylosis of joint (fibrous) (osseous)

Excludes: *spine (724.9)*
    stiffness of joint without mention of ankylosis (719.5)

⑤ **718.6 Unspecified intrapelvic protrusion of acetabulum**
[5] Protrusio acetabuli, unspecified

⑤ **718.7 Developmental dislocation of joint**
[0-9]

Excludes: *congenital dislocation of joint (754.0-755.8)*
    traumatic dislocation of joint (830-839)

⑤ **718.8 Other joint derangement, not elsewhere classified**
[0-9] Flail joint (paralytic)   Instability of joint

Excludes: *deformities classifiable to 736 (736.0-736.9)*

⑤ **718.9 Unspecified derangement of joint**
[0-5, 7-9]

Excludes: *knee (717.9)*

719 **Other and unspecified disorders of joint**

Excludes: *jaw (524.60-524.69)*

The following fifth-digit subclassification is for use with codes 719.0-719.6, 719.8-719.9; valid digits are in [brackets] under each code. See list at beginning of chapter for definitions:

0 site unspecified

1 shoulder region

2 upper arm

3 forearm

4 hand

5 pelvic region and thigh

6 lower leg

7 ankle and foot

8 other specified sites

9 multiple sites

ALERT! For personal history of other musculoskeletal disorders see V13.5

● Code new
to this edition
    ▲ Revision of
existing code
    ④ ⑤ Fourth or fifth
digit required

⑤ **719.0 Effusion of joint**
[0-9]   Hydrarthrosis
             Swelling of joint, with or without pain
Excludes: intermittent hydrarthrosis (719.3)

⑤ **719.1 Hemarthrosis**
[0-9]
Excludes: current injury (840.0-848.9)

⑤ **719.2 Villonodular synovitis**
[0-9]

⑤ **719.3 Palindromic rheumatism**
[0-9]   Hench-Rosenberg syndrome
             Intermittent hydrarthrosis

⑤ **719.4 Pain in joint**
[0-9]   Arthralgia

⑤ **719.5 Stiffness of joint, not elsewhere classified**
[0-9]

⑤ **719.6 Other symptoms referable to joint**
[0-9]   Joint crepitus   Snapping hip

719.7 Difficulty in walking
Excludes: abnormality of gait (781.2)

⑤ **719.8 Other specified disorders of joint**
[0-9]   Calcification of joint   Fistula of joint
Excludes: temporomandibular joint-pain-dysfunction syndrome [Costen's syndrome] (524.60)

⑤ **719.9 Unspecified disorder of joint**
[0-9]

DORSOPATHIES (720-724)

Excludes: curvature of spine (737.0-737.9)
            osteochondrosis of spine (juvenile) (732.0)
            adult (732.8)

DEFINITION Dorsopathy is a term used to describe various diseases of the back and or spine.

720 Ankylosing spondylitis and other inflammatory spondylopathies
DEFINITION Ankylosing spondylitis is a long-term disease that causes inflammation of the joints between the spinal bones and the joints between the spine and the pelvis. It eventually causes the affected spinal bones to join together.

720.0 Ankylosing spondylitis
        Rheumatoid arthritis of spine NOS
        Spondylitis:
          Marie-Strümpell
          rheumatoid

720.1 Spinal enthesopathy
        Disorder of peripheral ligamentous or muscular attachments of spine
        Romanus lesion

720.2 Sacroiliitis, not elsewhere classified
        Inflammation of sacroiliac joint NOS

⑤ **720.8 Other inflammatory spondylopathies**

720.81 Inflammatory spondylopathies in diseases classified elsewhere
Code first underlying disease, as:
        tuberculosis (015.0)

720.89 Other

720.9 Unspecified inflammatory spondylopathy
        Spondylitis NOS

721 Spondylosis and allied disorders
DEFINITION Spondylosis is degenerative arthritis (osteoarthritis) of the spinal vertebra and related tissue.

721.0 Cervical spondylosis without myelopathy
        Cervical or cervicodorsal:
          arthritis
          osteoarthritis
          spondylarthritis

| Add 4th or 5th digit | Nonspecific code | Unspecified code | Manifestation code |

721.1 Cervical spondylosis with myelopathy
   Anterior spinal artery compression syndrome
   Spondylogenic compression of cervical spinal cord
   Vertebral artery compression syndrome

721.2 Thoracic spondylosis without myelopathy
   Thoracic:
      arthritis
      osteoarthritis
      spondylarthritis

721.3 Lumbosacral spondylosis without myelopathy
   Lumbar or lumbosacral:
      arthritis
      osteoarthritis
      spondylarthritis

⑤ **721.4 Thoracic or lumbar spondylosis with myelopathy**

   721.41 Thoracic region
      Spondylogenic compression of thoracic spinal cord

   721.42 Lumbar region

721.5 Kissing spine
   Baastrup's syndrome

721.6 Ankylosing vertebral hyperostosis

721.7 Traumatic spondylopathy
   Kümmell's disease or spondylitis

`721.8` **Other allied disorders of spine**

⑤ **721.9 Spondylosis of unspecified site**

   721.90 Without mention of myelopathy
      Spinal:
         arthritis (deformans) (degenerative) (hypertrophic)
         osteoarthritis NOS
      Spondylarthrosis NOS

   721.91 With myelopathy
      Spondylogenic compression of spinal cord NOS

`722` **Intervertebral disc disorders**
   `DEFINITION` Intervertebral disc disorders result from a protrusion or herniation of one of the gel-like cushions (discs) that separate the vertebrae of the spine.

722.0 Displacement of cervical intervertebral disc without myelopathy
   Neuritis (brachial) or radiculitis due to displacement or rupture of cervical intervertebral disc
   Any condition classifiable to 722.2 of the cervical or cervicothoracic intervertebral disc

⑤ **722.1 Displacement of thoracic or lumbar intervertebral disc without myelopathy**

   722.10 Lumbar intervertebral disc without myelopathy
      Lumbago or sciatica due to displacement of intervertebral disc
      Neuritis or radiculitis due to displacement or rupture of lumbar intervertebral disc
      Any condition classifiable to 722.2 of the lumbar or lumbosacral intervertebral disc

   722.11 Thoracic intervertebral disc without myelopathy
      Any condition classifiable to 722.2 of thoracic intervertebral disc

722.2 Displacement of intervertebral disc, site unspecified, without myelopathy
   Discogenic syndrome NOS
   Herniation of nucleus pulposus NOS
   Intervertebral disc NOS:
      extrusion
      prolapse
      protrusion
      rupture
   Neuritis or radiculitis due to displacement or rupture of intervertebral disc

⑤ **722.3 Schmorl's nodes**

   722.30 Unspecified region

   722.31 Thoracic region

   722.32 Lumbar region

   722.39 Other

● Code new
   to this edition
▲ Revision of
   existing code
④ ⑤ Fourth or fifth
   digit required

722.4 Degeneration of cervical intervertebral disc
Degeneration of cervicothoracic intervertebral disc

⑤ **722.5 Degeneration of thoracic or lumbar intervertebral disc**

    722.51 Thoracic or thoracolumbar intervertebral disc

    722.52 Lumbar or lumbosacral intervertebral disc

722.6 Degeneration of intervertebral disc, site unspecified
Degenerative disc disease NOS
Narrowing of intervertebral disc or space NOS

⑤ **722.7 Intervertebral disc disorder with myelopathy**

    722.70 Unspecified region

    722.71 Cervical region

    722.72 Thoracic region

    722.73 Lumbar region

⑤ **722.8 Postlaminectomy syndrome**

    722.80 Unspecified region

    722.81 Cervical region

    722.82 Thoracic region

    722.83 Lumbar region

⑤ **722.9 Other and unspecified disc disorder**
Calcification of intervertebral cartilage or disc
Discitis

    722.90 Unspecified region

    722.91 Cervical region

    722.92 Thoracic region

    722.93 Lumbar region

723 Other disorders of cervical region

    Excludes: *conditions due to:*
        intervertebral disc disorders (722.0-722.9)
        spondylosis (721.0-721.9)

    ALERT! For personal history of other musculoskeletal disorders see V13.5

723.0 Spinal stenosis in cervical region

723.1 Cervicalgia
Pain in neck

723.2 Cervicocranial syndrome
Barré-Liéou syndrome
Posterior cervical sympathetic syndrome

723.3 Cervicobrachial syndrome (diffuse)

723.4 Brachial neuritis or radiculitis NOS
Cervical radiculitis
Radicular syndrome of upper limbs

723.5 Torticollis, unspecified
Contracture of neck

    Excludes: *congenital (754.1)*
        due to birth injury (767.8)
        hysterical (300.11)
        ocular torticollis (781.93)
        psychogenic (306.0)
        spasmodic (333.83)
        traumatic, current (847.0)

723.6 Panniculitis specified as affecting neck

723.7 Ossification of posterior longitudinal ligament in cervical region

723.8 Other syndromes affecting cervical region
Cervical syndrome NEC
Klippel's disease
Occipital neuralgia

723.9 Unspecified musculoskeletal disorders and symptoms referable to neck
Cervical (region) disorder NOS

---

724 **Other and unspecified disorders of back**

> *Excludes:* *collapsed vertebra (code to cause, e.g., osteoporosis, 733.00-733.09)*
> *conditions due to:*
> *intervertebral disc disorders (722.0-722.9)*
> *spondylosis (721.0-721.9)*

ALERT! For personal history of other musculoskeletal disorders see V13.5

⑤ **724.0** **Spinal stenosis, other than cervical**

724.00 **Spinal stenosis, unspecified region**

724.01 **Thoracic region**

724.02 **Lumbar region, without neurogenic claudication**
Lumbar region NOS

724.03 **Lumbar region, with neurogenic claudication**

724.09 **Other**

724.1 **Pain in thoracic spine**

724.2 **Lumbago**
Low back pain
Low back syndrome
Lumbalgia

724.3 **Sciatica**
Neuralgia or neuritis of sciatic nerve

> *Excludes:* *specified lesion of sciatic nerve (355.0)*

724.4 **Thoracic or lumbosacral neuritis or radiculitis, unspecified**
Radicular syndrome of lower limbs

724.5 **Backache, unspecified**
Vertebrogenic (pain) syndrome NOS

724.6 **Disorders of sacrum**
Ankylosis, lumbosacral or sacroiliac (joint)
Instability, lumbosacral or sacroiliac (joint)

⑤ **724.7** **Disorders of coccyx**

724.70 **Unspecified disorder of coccyx**

724.71 **Hypermobility of coccyx**

724.79 **Other**
Coccygodynia

724.8 **Other symptoms referable to back**
Ossification of posterior longitudinal ligament NOS
Panniculitis specified as sacral or affecting back

724.9 **Other unspecified back disorders**
Ankylosis of spine NOS
Compression of spinal nerve root NEC
Spinal disorder NOS

> *Excludes:* *sacroiliitis (720.2)*

RHEUMATISM, EXCLUDING THE BACK (725-729)

> Includes: disorders of muscles and tendons and their attachments, and of other soft tissues

725 **Polymyalgia rheumatica**
DEFINITION Polymyalgia rheumatica is a rheumatic disorder that is associated with moderate to severe muscle pain and stiffness in the neck, shoulder and hip areas.

726 **Peripheral enthesopathies and allied syndromes**
Note: Enthesopathies are disorders of peripheral ligamentous or muscular attachments.

> *Excludes:* *spinal enthesopathy (720.1)*

DEFINITION Peripheral enthesopathies and allied syndromes refers to any pathological condition of the enthesis (teno-osseous junction), for example tennis elbow, and jumper's knee

726.0 **Adhesive capsulitis of shoulder**

⑤ **726.1** **Rotator cuff syndrome of shoulder and allied disorders**

726.10 **Disorders of bursae and tendons in shoulder region, unspecified**
Rotator cuff syndrome NOS
Supraspinatus syndrome NOS

● Code new   ▲ Revision of   ④ ⑤ Fourth or fifth
       to this edition   existing code   digit required

726.11 **Calcifying tendinitis of shoulder**

726.12 **Bicipital tenosynovitis**

● 726.13 **Partial tear of rotator cuff**

Excludes: *complete rupture of rotator cuff, nontraumatic (727.61)*

726.19 **Other specified disorders**

Excludes: *complete rupture of rotator cuff, nontraumatic (727.61)*

726.2 **Other affections of shoulder region, not elsewhere classified**
Periarthritis of shoulder
Scapulohumeral fibrositis

⑤ 726.3 **Enthesopathy of elbow region**

726.30 **Enthesopathy of elbow, unspecified**

726.31 **Medial epicondylitis**

726.32 **Lateral epicondylitis**
Epicondylitis NOS
Golfers' elbow
Tennis elbow

726.33 **Olecranon bursitis**
Bursitis of elbow

726.39 **Other**

726.4 **Enthesopathy of wrist and carpus**
Bursitis of hand or wrist
Periarthritis of wrist

726.5 **Enthesopathy of hip region**
Bursitis of hip   Psoas tendinitis
Gluteal tendinitis   Trochanteric tendinitis
Iliac crest spur

⑤ 726.6 **Enthesopathy of knee**

726.60 **Enthesopathy of knee, unspecified**
Bursitis of knee NOS

726.61 **Pes anserinus tendinitis or bursitis**

726.62 **Tibial collateral ligament bursitis**
Pellegrini-Stieda syndrome

726.63 **Fibular collateral ligament bursitis**

726.64 **Patellar tendinitis**

726.65 **Prepatellar bursitis**

726.69 **Other**
Bursitis:
  infrapatellar
  subpatellar

⑤ 726.7 **Enthesopathy of ankle and tarsus**

726.70 **Enthesopathy of ankle and tarsus, unspecified**
Metatarsalgia NOS

Excludes: *Morton's metatarsalgia (355.6)*

726.71 **Achilles bursitis or tendinitis**

726.72 **Tibialis tendinitis**
Tibialis (anterior) (posterior) tendinitis

726.73 **Calcaneal spur**

726.79 **Other**
Peroneal tendinitis

726.8 **Other peripheral enthesopathies**

⑤ 726.9 **Unspecified enthesopathy**

726.90 **Enthesopathy of unspecified site**
Capsulitis NOS
Periarthritis NOS
Tendinitis NOS

726.91 **Exostosis of unspecified site**
Bone spur NOS

| | Add 4th or 5th digit | | Nonspecific code | | Unspecified code | | Manifestation code |

727 **Other disorders of synovium, tendon, and bursa**
    DEFINITION Synovium is a tissue that surrounds and protects the joints. It produces synovial fluid that nourishes and lubricates the joints
    ALERT! For personal history of other musculoskeletal disorders see V13.5

⑤ **727.0** **Synovitis and tenosynovitis**

    727.00 **Synovitis and tenosynovitis, unspecified**
        Synovitis NOS
        Tenosynovitis NOS

    727.01 *Synovitis and tenosynovitis in diseases classified elsewhere*
    Code first underlying disease, as:
        tuberculosis (015.0-015.9)
    Excludes: *crystal-induced (275.4)*
        gonococcal (098.51)
        gout (274.00-274.03)
        syphilitic (095.7)

    727.02 **Giant cell tumor of tendon sheath**

    727.03 **Trigger finger (acquired)**

    727.04 **Radial styloid tenosynovitis**
        de Quervain's disease

    727.05 **Other tenosynovitis of hand and wrist**

    727.06 **Tenosynovitis of foot and ankle**

    727.09 **Other**

727.1 **Bunion**

727.2 **Specific bursitides often of occupational origin**
    Beat:
        elbow
        hand
        knee
    Chronic crepitant synovitis of wrist
    Miners':
        elbow
        knee

727.3 **Other bursitis**
    Bursitis NOS
    Excludes: *bursitis:*
        gonococcal (098.52)
        subacromial (726.19)
        subcoracoid (726.19)
        subdeltoid (726.19)
        syphilitic (095.7)
        "frozen shoulder" (726.0)

⑤ **727.4** **Ganglion and cyst of synovium, tendon, and bursa**

    727.40 **Synovial cyst, unspecified**
    Excludes: *that of popliteal space (727.51)*

    727.41 **Ganglion of joint**

    727.42 **Ganglion of tendon sheath**

    727.43 **Ganglion, unspecified**

    727.49 **Other**
        Cyst of bursa

⑤ **727.5** **Rupture of synovium**

    727.50 **Rupture of synovium, unspecified**

    727.51 **Synovial cyst of popliteal space**
        Baker's cyst (knee)

    727.59 **Other**

⑤ **727.6** **Rupture of tendon, nontraumatic**

    727.60 **Nontraumatic rupture of unspecified tendon**

    727.61 **Complete rupture of rotator cuff**
    Excludes: *partial tear of rotator cuff (726.13)*

   ● Code new   ▲ Revision of   ④ ⑤ Fourth or fifth
       to this edition   existing code   digit required

727.62   **Tendons of biceps (long head)**

727.63   **Extensor tendons of hand and wrist**

727.64   **Flexor tendons of hand and wrist**

727.65   **Quadriceps tendon**

727.66   **Patellar tendon**

727.67   **Achilles tendon**

727.68   **Other tendons of foot and ankle**

727.69   **Other**

⑤ **727.8   Other disorders of synovium, tendon, and bursa**

727.81   **Contracture of tendon (sheath)**
Short Achilles tendon (acquired)

727.82   **Calcium deposits in tendon and bursa**
Calcification of tendon NOS
Calcific tendinitis NOS

Excludes: peripheral ligamentous or muscular attachments (726.0-726.9)

727.83   **Plica syndrome**
Plica knee

727.89   **Other**
Abscess of bursa or tendon

Excludes: xanthomatosis localized to tendons (272.7)

727.9   Unspecified disorder of synovium, tendon, and bursa

728   Disorders of muscle, ligament, and fascia

Excludes: enthesopathies (726.0-726.9)
muscular dystrophies (359.0-359.1)
myoneural disorders (358.00-358.9)
myopathies (359.2-359.9)
nontraumatic hematoma of muscle (729.92)
old disruption of ligaments of knee (717.81-717.89)

DEFINITION Disorders of muscle, ligament, and fascia, fascia is a flat band of tissue below the skin that covers the underlying tissues and separates different layers of tissue.

728.0   Infective myositis
Myositis:
purulent
suppurative

Excludes: myositis:
epidemic (074.1)
interstitial (728.81)
syphilitic (095.6)
tropical (040.81)

⑤ **728.1   Muscular calcification and ossification**

728.10   **Calcification and ossification, unspecified**
Massive calcification (paraplegic)

728.11   **Progressive myositis ossificans**

728.12   **Traumatic myositis ossificans**
Myositis ossificans (circumscripta)

728.13   **Postoperative heterotopic calcification**

728.19   **Other**
Polymyositis ossificans

728.2   Muscular wasting and disuse atrophy, not elsewhere classified
Amyotrophia NOS
Myofibrosis

Excludes: neuralgic amyotrophy (353.5)
pelvic muscle wasting and disuse atrophy (618.83)
progressive muscular atrophy (335.0-335.9)

728.3   Other specific muscle disorders
Arthrogryposis
Immobility syndrome (paraplegic)

Excludes: arthrogryposis multiplex congenita (754.89)
stiff-man syndrome (333.91)

| | Add 4th or 5th digit | | Nonspecific code | | Unspecified code | | Manifestation code |

728.4 Laxity of ligament

728.5 Hypermobility syndrome

728.6 Contracture of palmar fascia
Dupuytren's contracture

⑤ **728.7 Other fibromatoses**

    728.71 Plantar fascial fibromatosis
        Contracture of plantar fascia
        Plantar fasciitis (traumatic)

    728.79 Other
        Garrod's or knuckle pads
        Nodular fasciitis
        Pseudosarcomatous fibromatosis (proliferative) (subcutaneous)

⑤ **728.8 Other disorders of muscle, ligament, and fascia**

    728.81 Interstitial myositis

    728.82 Foreign body granuloma of muscle
        Talc granuloma of muscle
  Use additional code to identify foreign body (V90.01-V90.9)

    728.83 Rupture of muscle, nontraumatic

    728.84 Diastasis of muscle
        Diastasis recti (abdomen)

  Excludes: *diastasis recti complicating pregnancy, labor, and delivery (665.8)*

    728.85 Spasm of muscle

    728.86 Necrotizing fasciitis
        Use additional code to identify:
          infectious organism (041.00 - 041.89)
          gangrene (785.4), if applicable

    728.87 Muscle weakness (generalized)

  Excludes: *generalized weakness (780.79)*

    728.88 Rhabdomyolysis

    728.89 Other
        Eosinophilic fasciitis
  Use additional E code, if desired, to identify drug, if drug induced

728.9 Unspecified disorder of muscle, ligament, and fascia

729 Other disorders of soft tissues

  Excludes: *acroparesthesia (443.89)*
        carpal tunnel syndrome (354.0)
        disorders of the back (720.0-724.9)
        entrapment syndromes (354.0-355.9)
        palindromic rheumatism (719.3)
        periarthritis (726.0-726.9)
        psychogenic rheumatism (306.0)

  DEFINITION Disorders of soft tissues, refers to tissues that connect, support, or surround other structures and organs of the body.

  ALERT! For personal history of other musculoskeletal disorders see V13.5

729.0 Rheumatism, unspecified and fibrositis

729.1 Myalgia and myositis, unspecified
    Fibromyositis NOS

729.2 Neuralgia, neuritis, and radiculitis, unspecified

  Excludes: *brachial radiculitis (723.4)*
        cervical radiculitis (723.4)
        lumbosacral radiculitis (724.4)
        mononeuritis (354.0-355.9)
        radiculitis due to intervertebral disc involvement (722.0-722.2, 722.7)
        sciatica (724.3)

⑤ **729.3 Panniculitis, unspecified**

    729.30 Panniculitis, unspecified site
        Weber-Christian disease

    729.31 Hypertrophy of fat pad, knee
        Hypertrophy of infrapatellar fat pad

● Code new
to this edition

▲ Revision of
existing code

④ ⑤ Fourth or fifth
digit required

729.39 **Other site**

Excludes: panniculitis specified as (affecting):
    back (724.8)
    neck (723.6)
    sacral (724.8)

729.4 Fasciitis, unspecified

Excludes: necrotizing fasciitis (728.86)
    nodular fasciitis (728.79)

729.5 Pain in limb

729.6 Residual foreign body in soft tissue
Use additional code to identify foreign body (V90.01-V90.9)

Excludes: foreign body granuloma:
    muscle (728.82)
    skin and subcutaneous tissue (709.4)

⑤ **729.7 Nontraumatic compartment syndrome**
    Code first, if applicable, postprocedural complication (998.89)

Excludes: compartment syndrome NOS (958.90)
    traumatic compartment syndrome (958.90-958.99)

729.71 **Nontraumatic compartment syndrome of upper extremity**
    Nontraumatic compartment syndrome of shoulder, arm, forearm, wrist, hand and fingers

729.72 **Nontraumatic compartment syndrome of lower extremity**
    Nontraumatic compartment syndrome of hip, buttock, thigh, leg, foot and toes

729.73 **Nontraumatic compartment syndrome of abdomen**

729.79 **Nontraumatic compartment syndrome of other sites**

⑤ **729.8 Other musculoskeletal symptoms referable to limbs**

729.81 **Swelling of limb**

729.82 **Cramp**

729.89 **Other**

Excludes: abnormality of gait (781.2)
    tetany (781.7)
    transient paralysis of limb (781.4)

⑤ **729.9 Other and unspecified disorders of soft tissue**

729.90 **Disorders of soft tissue, unspecified**

729.91 **Post-traumatic seroma**

Excludes: seroma complicating a procedure (998.13)

729.92 **Nontraumatic hematoma of soft tissue**
    Nontraumatic hematoma of muscle

729.99 **Other disorders of soft tissue**
    Polyalgia

OSTEOPATHIES, CHONDROPATHIES, AND ACQUIRED MUSCULOSKELETAL DEFORMITIES (730-739)

⑤ **730 Osteomyelitis, periostitis, and other infections involving bone**

Excludes: jaw (526.4-526.5)
    petrous bone (383.2)

Use additional code, if desired, to identify organism, such as Staphylococcus (041.1)

The following fifth-digit subclassification is for use with category 730; valid digits are in [brackets] under each code. See beginning of this chapter for definitions:

0 site unspecified

1 shoulder region

2 upper arm

3 forearm

4 hand

5 pelvic region and thigh

6 lower leg

7 ankle and foot

	Add 4th or 5th digit		Nonspecific code		Unspecified code		Manifestation code

8 other specified sites

9 multiple sites

DEFINITION Osteomyelitis is an inflammation of bone and bone marrow (usually caused by bacterial infection). Periostitis is an inflammation of the membrane which covers bones .

⑤ **730.0 Acute osteomyelitis**
[0-9]   Abscess of any bone except accessory sinus, jaw, or mastoid
Acute or subacute osteomyelitis, with or without mention of periostitis
Use additional code to identify major osseous defect, if applicable (731.3)

⑤ **730.1 Chronic osteomyelitis**
[0-9]   Brodie's abscess
Chronic or old osteomyelitis, with or without mention of periostitis
Sequestrum of bone
Sclerosing osteomyelitis of Garré
Use additional code to identify major osseous defect, if applicable (731.3)

   Excludes: aseptic necrosis of bone (733.40-733.49)

⑤ **730.2 Unspecified osteomyelitis**
[0-9]   Osteitis or osteomyelitis NOS, with or without mention of periostitis
Use additional code to identify major osseous defect, if applicable (731.3)

⑤ **730.3 Periostitis without mention of osteomyelitis**
[0-9]   Abscess of periosteum without mention of osteomyelitis
Periostosis without mention of osteomyelitis

   Excludes: that in secondary syphilis (091.61)

⑤ **730.7 Osteopathy resulting from poliomyelitis**
[0-9]   Code first underlying disease (045.0-045.9)

⑤ **730.8 Other infections involving bone in diseases classified elsewhere**
[0-9]   Code first underlying disease, as:
tuberculosis (015.0-015.9)
typhoid fever (002.0)

   Excludes: syphilis of bone NOS (095.5)

⑤ **730.9 Unspecified infection of bone**
[0-9]

731 Osteitis deformans and osteopathies associated with other disorders classified elsewhere
DEFINITION Osteitis deformans, aka paget's disease, is a disease of bone occurring in the middle aged and elderly; excessive bone destruction sometimes leading to bone pain and fractures and skeletal deformities.

731.0 Osteitis deformans without mention of bone tumor
Paget's disease of bone

731.1 Osteitis deformans in diseases classified elsewhere
Code first underlying disease, as:
malignant neoplasm of bone (170.0-170.9)

731.2 Hypertrophic pulmonary osteoarthropathy
Bamberger-Marie disease

731.3 Major osseous defects
Code first underlying disease, if known, such as:
aseptic necrosis (733.40-733.49)
malignant neoplasm of bone (170.0-170.9)
osteomyelitis (730.00-730.29)
osteoporosis (733.00-733.09)
peri-prosthetic osteolysis (996.45)

731.8 Other bone involvement in diseases classified elsewhere
Code first underlying disease, as:
diabetes mellitus (249.8, 250.8)
Use additional code to specify bone condition, such as:
acute osteomyelitis (730.00-730.09)

732 Osteochondropathies
DEFINITION Osteochondropathies refers to diseases involving both bone and cartilage

● Code new to this edition   ▲ Revision of existing code   ④ ⑤ Fourth or fifth digit required

732.0 Juvenile osteochondrosis of spine
　　Juvenile osteochondrosis (of):
　　　marginal or vertebral epiphysis (of Scheuermann)
　　　spine NOS
　　Vertebral epiphysitis

　　Excludes: adolescent postural kyphosis (737.0)

732.1 Juvenile osteochondrosis of hip and pelvis
　　Coxa plana
　　Ischiopubic synchondrosis (of van Neck)
　　Osteochondrosis (juvenile) of:
　　　acetabulum
　　　head of femur (of Legg-Calvé-Perthes)
　　　iliac crest (of Buchanan)
　　　symphysis pubis (of Pierson)
　　Pseudocoxalgia

732.2 Nontraumatic slipped upper femoral epiphysis
　　Slipped upper femoral epiphysis NOS

732.3 Juvenile osteochondrosis of upper extremity
　　Osteochondrosis (juvenile) of:
　　　capitulum of humerus (of Panner)
　　　carpal lunate (of Kienbock)
　　　hand NOS
　　　head of humerus (of Haas)
　　　heads of metacarpals (of Mauclaire)
　　　lower ulna (of Burns)
　　　radial head (of Brailsford)
　　　upper extremity NOS

732.4 Juvenile osteochondrosis of lower extremity, excluding foot
　　Osteochondrosis (juvenile) of:
　　　lower extremity NOS
　　　primary patellar center (of Köhler)
　　　proximal tibia (of Blount)
　　　secondary patellar center (of Sinding-Larsen)
　　　tibial tubercle (of Osgood-Schlatter)
　　Tibia vara

732.5 Juvenile osteochondrosis of foot
　　Calcaneal apophysitis
　　Epiphysitis, os calcis
　　Osteochondrosis (juvenile) of:
　　　astragalus (of Diaz)
　　　calcaneum (of Sever)
　　　foot NOS
　　　metatarsal
　　　　second (of Freiberg)
　　　　fifth (of Iselin)
　　　os tibiale externum (Haglund)
　　　tarsal navicular (of Köhler)

732.6 Other juvenile osteochondrosis
　　Apophysitis specified as juvenile, of other site, or site NOS
　　Epiphysitis specified as juvenile, of other site, or site NOS
　　Osteochondritis specified as juvenile, of other site, or site NOS
　　Osteochondrosis specified as juvenile, of other site, or site NOS

732.7 Osteochondritis dissecans

732.8 Other specified forms of osteochondropathy
　　Adult osteochondrosis of spine

732.9 Unspecified osteochondropathy
　　Apophysitis
　　　NOS
　　　not specified as adult or juvenile, of unspecified site
　　Epiphysitis
　　　NOS
　　　not specified as adult or juvenile, of unspecified site
　　Osteochondritis
　　　NOS
　　　not specified as adult or juvenile, of unspecified site
　　Osteochondrosis
　　　NOS
　　　not specified as adult or juvenile, of unspecified site

	Add 4th or 5th digit		Nonspecific code		Unspecified code		Manifestation code

733 **Other disorders of bone and cartilage**

Excludes: *bone spur (726.91)*
cartilage of, or loose body in, joint (717.0-717.9, 718.0-718.9)
giant cell granuloma of jaw (526.3)
osteitis fibrosa cystica generalisata (252.01)
osteomalacia (268.2)
polyostotic fibrous dysplasia of bone (756.54)
prognathism, retrognathism (524.1)
xanthomatosis localized to bone (272.7)

DEFINITION Bone cartilage is a tough, elastic, fibrous connective tissue found in various parts of the body, such as the joints, outer ear, and larynx

ALERT! For personal history of other musculoskeletal disorders see V13.5

⑤ **733.0** **Osteoporosis**
Use additional code to identify major osseous defect, if applicable (731.3)
Use additional code to identify personal history of pathologic (healed) fracture (V13.51)

    733.00 **Osteoporosis, unspecified**
        Wedging of vertebra NOS

    733.01 **Senile osteoporosis**
        Postmenopausal osteoporosis

    733.02 **Idiopathic osteoporosis**

    733.03 **Disuse osteoporosis**

    733.09 **Other**
        Drug-induced osteoporosis

    Use additional E code, if desired, to identify drug

⑤ **733.1** **Pathologic fracture**
    Chronic fracture
    Spontaneous fracture

Excludes: *traumatic fracture (800-829)*
stress fracture (733.93-733.95)

ALERT! Code 733.1 is used to report pathologic fractures when the fracture is newly diagnosed. Subcategory 733.1 may be used while the patient is receiving active treatment for the fracture

ALERT! For personal history of pathologic fracture see V13.51

    733.10 **Pathologic fracture, unspecified site**

    733.11 **Pathologic fracture of humerus**

    733.12 **Pathologic fracture of distal radius and ulna**
        Wrist NOS

    733.13 **Pathologic fracture of vertebrae**
        Collapse of vertebra NOS

    733.14 **Pathologic fracture of neck of femur**
        Femur NOS
        Hip NOS

    733.15 **Pathologic fracture of other specified part of femur**

    733.16 **Pathologic fracture of tibia or fibula**
        Ankle NOS

    733.19 **Pathologic fracture of other specified site**

⑤ **733.2** **Cyst of bone**

    733.20 **Cyst of bone (localized), unspecified**

    733.21 **Solitary bone cyst**
        Unicameral bone cyst

    733.22 **Aneurysmal bone cyst**

    733.29 **Other**
        Fibrous dysplasia (monostotic)

Excludes: *cyst of jaw (526.0-526.2, 526.89)*
osteitis fibrosa cystica (252.01)
polyostotic fibrous dysplasia of bone (756.54)

733.3 **Hyperostosis of skull**
    Hyperostosis interna frontalis
    Leontiasis ossium

⑤ **733.4** **Aseptic necrosis of bone**
Use additional code to identify major osseous defect, if applicable (731.3)

● Code new to this edition   ▲ Revision of existing code   ④ ⑤ Fourth or fifth digit required

Excludes: *osteochondropathies (732.0-732.9)*

733.40 **Aseptic necrosis of bone, site unspecified**

733.41 **Head of humerus**

733.42 **Head and neck of femur**
Femur NOS

Excludes: *Legg-Calvé-Perthes disease (732.1)*

733.43 **Medial femoral condyle**

733.44 **Talus**

733.45 **Jaw**
Use additional E code to identify drug, if drug-induced

Excludes: *osteoradionecrosis of jaw (526.89)*

733.49 **Other**

733.5 Osteitis condensans
Piriform sclerosis of ilium

733.6 Tietze's disease
Costochondral junction syndrome
Costochondritis

733.7 Algoneurodystrophy
Disuse atrophy of bone
Sudeck's atrophy

⑤ **733.8 Malunion and nonunion of fracture**

733.81 **Malunion of fracture**

733.82 **Nonunion of fracture**
Pseudoarthrosis (bone)

⑤ **733.9 Other and unspecified disorders of bone and cartilage**
ALERT! For personal history of stress fracture see V13.52

733.90 **Disorder of bone and cartilage, unspecified**

733.91 **Arrest of bone development or growth**
Epiphyseal arrest

733.92 **Chondromalacia**
Chondromalacia:
NOS
localized, except patella
systemic
tibial plateau

Excludes: *chondromalacia of patella (717.7)*

733.93 **Stress fracture of tibia or fibula**
Stress reaction of tibia or fibula

Use additional external cause code(s) to identify the cause of the stress fracture

733.94 **Stress fracture of the metatarsals**
Stress reaction of metatarsals

Use additional external cause code(s) to identify the cause of the stress fracture

733.95 **Stress fracture of other bone**
Stress reaction of other bone

Use additional external cause code(s) to identify the cause of the stress fracture

Excludes: *stress fracture of:*
femoral neck (733.96)
fibula (733.93)
metatarsals (733.94)
pelvis (733.98)
shaft of femur (733.97)
tibia (733.93)

733.96 **Stress fracture of femoral neck**
Stress reaction of femoral neck

Use additional external cause code(s) to identify the cause of the stress fracture

733.97 **Stress fracture of shaft of femur**
Stress reaction of shaft of femur

Use additional external cause code(s) to identify the cause of the stress fracture

	Add 4th or 5th digit		Nonspecific code		Unspecified code		Manifestation code

733.98 Stress fracture of pelvis
Stress reaction of pelvis
Use additional external cause code(s) to identify the cause of the stress fracture

733.99 Other
Diaphysitis
Hypertrophy of bone
Relapsing polychondritis

734 Flat foot
Pes planus (acquired)
Talipes planus (acquired)
Excludes: *congenital (754.61)*
rigid flat foot (754.61)
spastic (everted) flat foot (754.61)
DEFINITION Flat foot, aka pes planus or fallen arches, is an informal reference to a medical condition in which the arch of the foot collapses.

735 Acquired deformities of toe
Excludes: *congenital (754.60-754.69, 755.65-755.66)*
DEFINITION Acquired deformities of toe is a deformity of the toe acquired after birth resulting from injury or disease.

735.0 Hallux valgus (acquired)
735.1 Hallux varus (acquired)
735.2 Hallux rigidus
735.3 Hallux malleus
735.4 Other hammer toe (acquired)
735.5 Claw toe (acquired)
735.8 Other acquired deformities of toe
735.9 Unspecified acquired deformity of toe

736 Other acquired deformities of limbs
Excludes: *congenital (754.3-755.9)*
DEFINITION Acquired deformities of limbs, refers to other deformities of the limbs acquired after birth resulting from injury or disease
ALERT! For personal history of other musculoskeletal disorders see V13.5

⑤ **736.0 Acquired deformities of forearm, excluding fingers**
736.00 Unspecified deformity
Deformity of elbow, forearm, hand, or wrist (acquired) NOS
736.01 Cubitus valgus (acquired)
736.02 Cubitus varus (acquired)
736.03 Valgus deformity of wrist (acquired)
736.04 Varus deformity of wrist (acquired)
736.05 Wrist drop (acquired)
736.06 Claw hand (acquired)
736.07 Club hand, acquired
736.09 Other

736.1 Mallet finger
⑤ **736.2 Other acquired deformities of finger**
736.20 Unspecified deformity
Deformity of finger (acquired) NOS
736.21 Boutonniere deformity
736.22 Swan-neck deformity
736.29 Other
Excludes: *trigger finger (727.03)*

⑤ **736.3 Acquired deformities of hip**
736.30 Unspecified deformity
Deformity of hip (acquired) NOS
736.31 Coxa valga (acquired)
736.32 Coxa vara (acquired)

● Code new to this edition   ▲ Revision of existing code   ④ ⑤ Fourth or fifth digit required

`736.39` Other

⑤ **736.4 Genu valgum or varum (acquired)**

736.41 Genu valgum (acquired)

736.42 Genu varum (acquired)

736.5 Genu recurvatum (acquired)

`736.6` **Other acquired deformities of knee**
Deformity of knee (acquired) NOS

⑤ **736.7 Other acquired deformities of ankle and foot**

Excludes: *deformities of toe (acquired) (735.0-735.9)*
pes planus (acquired) (734)

`736.70` Unspecified deformity of ankle and foot, acquired

736.71 Acquired equinovarus deformity
Clubfoot, acquired

Excludes: *clubfoot not specified as acquired (754.5-754.7)*

736.72 Equinus deformity of foot, acquired

736.73 Cavus deformity of foot

Excludes: *that with claw foot (736.74)*

736.74 Claw foot, acquired

736.75 Cavovarus deformity of foot, acquired

`736.76` Other calcaneus deformity

`736.79` Other
Acquired:
pes not elsewhere classified
talipes not elsewhere classified

⑤ **736.8 Acquired deformities of other parts of limbs**

736.81 Unequal leg length (acquired)

`736.89` Other
Deformity (acquired):
arm or leg, not elsewhere classified
shoulder

`736.9` **Acquired deformity of limb, site unspecified**

`737` **Curvature of spine**

Excludes: *congenital (754.2)*

DEFINITION Curvature of spine, aka scoliosis, is an abnormal curving of the spine, especially in a lateral direction.

737.0 Adolescent postural kyphosis

Excludes: *osteochondrosis of spine (juvenile) (732.0)*
adult (732.8)

⑤ **737.1 Kyphosis (acquired)**

737.10 Kyphosis (acquired) (postural)

737.11 Kyphosis due to radiation

737.12 Kyphosis, postlaminectomy

`737.19` Other

Excludes: *that associated with conditions classifiable elsewhere (737.41)*

⑤ **737.2 Lordosis (acquired)**

737.20 Lordosis (acquired) (postural)

737.21 Lordosis, postlaminectomy

`737.22` Other postsurgical lordosis

`737.29` Other

Excludes: *that associated with conditions classifiable elsewhere (737.42)*

⑤ **737.3 Kyphoscoliosis and scoliosis**

737.30 Scoliosis [and kyphoscoliosis], idiopathic

737.31 Resolving infantile idiopathic scoliosis

737.32 Progressive infantile idiopathic scoliosis

	Add 4th or 5th digit		Nonspecific code		Unspecified code		Manifestation code

737.33 Scoliosis due to radiation

737.34 Thoracogenic scoliosis

737.39 Other

Excludes: *that associated with conditions classifiable elsewhere (737.43)*
that in kyphoscoliotic heart disease (416.1)

⑤ **737.4 Curvature of spine associated with other conditions**
Code first associated condition, as:
Charcot-Marie-Tooth disease (356.1)
mucopolysaccharidosis (277.5)
neurofibromatosis (237.70-237.79)
osteitis deformans (731.0)
osteitis fibrosa cystica (252.01)
osteoporosis (733.00-733.09)
poliomyelitis (138)
tuberculosis [Pott's curvature] (015.0)

737.40 *Curvature of spine, unspecified*

737.41 *Kyphosis*

737.42 *Lordosis*

737.43 *Scoliosis*

737.8 **Other curvatures of spine**

737.9 **Unspecified curvature of spine**
Curvature of spine (acquired) (idiopathic) NOS
Hunchback, acquired

Excludes: *deformity of spine NOS (738.5)*

738 **Other acquired deformity**

Excludes: *congenital (754.0-756.9, 758.0-759.9)*
dentofacial anomalies (524.0-524.9)

DEFINITION An Acquired deformity is a deformity acquired after birth from injury or disease.

ALERT! For personal history of other musculoskeletal disorders see V13.5

738.0 **Acquired deformity of nose**
Deformity of nose (acquired)
Overdevelopment of nasal bones

Excludes: *deflected or deviated nasal septum (470)*

⑤ **738.1 Other acquired deformity of head**

738.10 **Unspecified deformity**

738.11 **Zygomatic hyperplasia**

738.12 **Zygomatic hypoplasia**

738.19 **Other specified deformity**

738.2 **Acquired deformity of neck**

738.3 **Acquired deformity of chest and rib**
Deformity: Pectus:
chest (acquired)   carinatum, acquired
rib (acquired)   excavatum, acquired

738.4 **Acquired spondylolisthesis**
Degenerative spondylolisthesis
Spondylolysis, acquired

Excludes: *congenital (756.12)*

738.5 **Other acquired deformity of back or spine**
Deformity of spine NOS

Excludes: *curvature of spine (737.0-737.9)*

738.6 **Acquired deformity of pelvis**
Pelvic obliquity

Excludes: *intrapelvic protrusion of acetabulum (718.6)*
that in relation to labor and delivery (653.0-653.4, 653.8-653.9)

738.7 **Cauliflower ear**

738.8 **Acquired deformity of other specified site**
Deformity of clavicle

738.9 **Acquired deformity of unspecified site**

● Code new
to this edition

▲ Revision of
existing code

④ ⑤ Fourth or fifth
digit required

739 Nonallopathic lesions, not elsewhere classified
    Includes: segmental dysfunction
              somatic dysfunction

739.0 Head region
    Occipitocervical region

739.1 Cervical region
    Cervicothoracic region

739.2 Thoracic region
    Thoracolumbar region

739.3 Lumbar region
    Lumbosacral region

739.4 Sacral region
    Sacrococcygeal region
    Sacroiliac region

739.5 Pelvic region
    Hip region
    Pubic region

739.6 Lower extremities

739.7 Upper extremities
    Acromioclavicular region
    Sternoclavicular region

739.8 Rib cage
    Costochondral region   Sternochondral region
    Costovertebral region

739.9 Abdomen and other

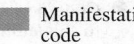

Add 4th or 5th digit   Nonspecific code   Unspecified code   Manifestation code

This page intentionally left blank.

● Code new
to this edition

▲ Revision of
existing code

④ ⑤ Fourth or fifth
digit required

Chapter 14: Congenital Anomalies (740-759)

DEFINITIONS AND CODING ALERTS

This chapter includes definitions of selected key words, terms and phrases and coding alerts for adding points to the clinical domain, references to coding late effects where appropriate, and references to personal history V-codes in situations where the acute or chronic condition is no longer active. An example from this chapter is as follows:

746 **Other congenital anomalies of heart**

> **DEFINITION** Congenital anomalies of heart refers to other defects of the heart that are present at birth.
>
> **ALERT!** For personal history of other congenital malformations see V13.69

MULTIPLE CODING FOR A SINGLE CONDITION

In addition to the etiology or manifestation convention that requires two codes to fully describe a single condition that affects multiple body systems, there are other single conditions that also require more than one code. "Use additional code" notes are found in the tabular at codes that are not part of an etiology or manifestation pair where a secondary code is useful to fully describe a condition. The sequencing rule is the same as the etiology or manifestation pair - , "use additional code" indicates that a secondary code should be added.

"Code first" notes are also under certain codes that are not specifically manifestation codes but may be due to an underlying cause. When a "code first" note is present and an underlying condition is present the underlying condition should be sequenced first.

"Code, if applicable, any causal condition first", notes indicate that this code may be assigned as a principal diagnosis when the causal condition is unknown or not applicable. If a causal condition is known, then the code for that condition should be sequenced as the principal or first-listed diagnosis. Multiple codes may be needed for late effects, complication codes and obstetric codes to more fully describe a condition. See the specific guidelines for these conditions for further instruction.

COMBINATION CODE

A combination code is a single code used to classify: two diagnoses, or a diagnosis with an associated secondary process (manifestation) A diagnosis with an associated complication Combination codes are identified by referring to subterm entries in the Alphabetic Index and by reading the inclusion and exclusion notes in the Tabular List.

Assign only the combination code when that code fully identifies the diagnostic conditions involved or when the Alphabetic Index so directs. Multiple coding should not be used when the classification provides a combination code that clearly identifies all of the elements documented in the diagnosis. When the combination code lacks necessary specificity in describing the manifestation or complication, an additional code should be used as a secondary code.

CODING LATE EFFECTS

A late effect is the residual effect (condition produced) after the acute phase of an illness or injury has terminated. There is no time limit on when a late effect code can be used. The residual may be apparent early, such as in cerebrovascular accident cases, or it may occur months or years later, such as that due to a previous injury. Coding of late effects generally requires two codes sequenced in the following order: The condition or nature of the late effect is sequenced first. The late effect code is sequenced second.

An exception to the above guidelines are those instances where the code for late effect is followed by a manifestation code identified in the Tabular List and title, or the late effect code has been expanded (at the fourth and fifth-digit levels) to include the manifestation(s). The code for the acute phase of an illness or injury that led to the late effect is never used with a code for the late effect.

CODES IN CATEGORIES 740-759, CONGENITAL ANOMALIES

Assign an appropriate code(s) from categories 740-759, Congenital Anomalies, when an anomaly is documented. A congenital anomaly may be the principal or first listed diagnosis on a record or a secondary diagnosis.

When a congenital anomaly does not have a unique code assignment, assign additional code(s) for any manifestations that may be present.

	Add 4th or 5th digit		Nonspecific code		Unspecified code		Manifestation code

When the code assignment specifically identifies the congenital anomaly, manifestations that are an inherent component of the anomaly should not be coded separately. Additional codes should be assigned for manifestations that are not an inherent component.

Codes from Chapter 14 may be used throughout the life of the patient. If a congenital anomaly has been corrected, a personal history code should be used to identify the history of the anomaly. Although present at birth, a congenital anomaly may not be identified until later in life. Whenever the condition is diagnosed by the physician, it is appropriate to assign a code from codes 740-759.

For the birth admission, the appropriate code from category V30, Liveborn infants, according to type of birth should be sequenced as the principal diagnosis, followed by any congenital anomaly codes, 740-759.

14. CONGENITAL ANOMALIES (740-759)

ALERT! For personal history of congenital malformations see V13.6

740 Anencephalus and similar anomalies

DEFINITION Anencephalus and similar anomalies, refers to the congenital absence of most of the brain and spinal cord

740.0 Anencephalus

Acrania	Hemianencephaly
Amyelencephalus	Hemicephaly

740.1 Craniorachischisis

740.2 Iniencephaly

⑤ 741 Spina bifida

Excludes: spina bifida occulta (756.17)

The following fifth-digit subclassification is for use with category 741:

0 unspecified region

1 cervical region

2 dorsal [thoracic] region

3 lumbar region

DEFINITION Spina bifida is a serious birth abnormality in which the spinal cord is malformed and lacks its usual protective skeletal and soft tissue coverings

⑤ 741.0 With hydrocephalus
[0-3]   Arnold-Chiari syndrome, type II
          Any condition classifiable to 741.9 with any condition classifiable to 742.3
          Chiari malformation, type II

⑤ 741.9 Without mention of hydrocephalus
[0-3]   Hydromeningocele (spinal)

Hydromyelocele	Myelocystocele
Meningocele (spinal)	Rachischisis
Meningomyelocele	Spina bifida (aperta)
Myelocele	Syringomyelocele

742 Other congenital anomalies of nervous system

Excludes: congenital central alveolar hypoventilation syndrome (327.25)

DEFINITION Congenital anomalies of nervous system refers to defects of the nervous system that are present at birth.

ALERT! For personal history of other congenital malformations see V13.69

742.0 Encephalocele

Encephalocystocele	Meningocele, cerebral
Encephalomyelocele	Meningoencephalocele
Hydroencephalocele	
Hydromeningocele, cranial	

742.1 Microcephalus
     Hydromicrocephaly
     Micrencephaly

742.2 Reduction deformities of brain
     Absence of part of brain
     Agenesis of part of brain
     Agyria
     Aplasia of part of brain
     Arhinencephaly
     Hypoplasia of part of brain
     Holoprosencephaly
     Microgyria

	Add 4th or 5th digit		Nonspecific code		Unspecified code		Manifestation code

742.3 Congenital hydrocephalus
Aqueduct of Sylvius:
anomaly
obstruction, congenital
stenosis
Atresia of foramina of Magendie and Luschka
Hydrocephalus in newborn

Excludes: hydrocephalus:
acquired (331.3-331.4)
due to congenital toxoplasmosis (771.2)
with any condition classifiable to 741.9 (741.0)

742.4 Other specified anomalies of brain
Congenital cerebral cyst   Multiple anomalies of brain NOS
Macroencephaly   Porencephaly
Macrogyria   Ulegyria
Megalencephaly

⑤ **742.5 Other specified anomalies of spinal cord**

742.51 Diastematomyelia

742.53 Hydromyelia
Hydrorhachis

742.59 Other
Amyelia
Atelomyelia
Congenital anomaly of spinal meninges
Defective development of cauda equina
Hypoplasia of spinal cord
Myelatelia
Myelodysplasia

742.8 Other specified anomalies of nervous system
Agenesis of nerve   Jaw-winking syndrome
Displacement of brachial   Marcus-Gunn syndrome
plexus   Riley-Day syndrome
Familial dysautonomia

Excludes: neurofibromatosis (237.70-237.79)

742.9 Unspecified anomaly of brain, spinal cord, and nervous system
Anomaly of brain, nervous system, and spinal cord
Congenital:
disease of brain, nervous system, and spinal cord
lesion of brain, nervous system, and spinal cord
Deformity of brain, nervous system, and spinal cord

743 Congenital anomalies of eye
DEFINITION Congenital anomalies of eye, refers to defects of the eye and ocular adnexa that
are present at birth.

⑤ **743.0 Anophthalmos**

743.00 Clinical anophthalmos, unspecified
Agenesis of eye
Congenital absence of eye
Anophthalmos NOS

743.03 Cystic eyeball, congenital

743.06 Cryptophthalmos

⑤ **743.1 Microphthalmos**
Dysplasia of eye
Hypoplasia of eye
Rudimentary eye

743.10 Microphthalmos, unspecified

743.11 Simple microphthalmos

743.12 Microphthalmos associated with other anomalies of eye and adnexa

⑤ **743.2 Buphthalmos**
Glaucoma: Hydrophthalmos
congenital
newborn

Excludes: glaucoma of childhood (365.14)
traumatic glaucoma due to birth injury (767.8)

● Code new   ▲ Revision of   ④ ⑤ Fourth or fifth
to this edition   existing code   digit required

743.20 Buphthalmos, unspecified

743.21 **Simple buphthalmos**

743.22 Buphthalmos associated with other ocular anomalies
Keratoglobus, congenital associated with buphthalmos
Megalocornea associated with buphthalmos

⑤ **743.3 Congenital cataract and lens anomalies**
Excludes: *infantile cataract (366.00-366.09)*

743.30 Congenital cataract, unspecified

743.31 **Capsular and subcapsular cataract**

743.32 **Cortical and zonular cataract**

743.33 **Nuclear cataract**

743.34 **Total and subtotal cataract, congenital**

743.35 **Congenital aphakia**
Congenital absence of lens

743.36 **Anomalies of lens shape**
Microphakia
Spherophakia

743.37 **Congenital ectopic lens**

743.39 Other

⑤ **743.4 Coloboma and other anomalies of anterior segment**

743.41 **Anomalies of corneal size and shape**
Microcornea

Excludes: *that associated with buphthalmos (743.22)*

743.42 **Corneal opacities, interfering with vision, congenital**

743.43 Other corneal opacities, congenital

743.44 Specified anomalies of anterior chamber, chamber angle, and related structures
Anomaly:
Axenfeld's
Peters'
Rieger's

743.45 **Aniridia**

743.46 Other specified anomalies of iris and ciliary body
Anisocoria, congenital
Atresia of pupil
Coloboma of iris
Corectopia

743.47 Specified anomalies of sclera

743.48 Multiple and combined anomalies of anterior segment

743.49 Other

⑤ **743.5 Congenital anomalies of posterior segment**

743.51 **Vitreous anomalies**
Congenital vitreous opacity

743.52 **Fundus coloboma**

743.53 **Chorioretinal degeneration, congenital**

743.54 **Congenital folds and cysts of posterior segment**

743.55 **Congenital macular changes**

743.56 Other retinal changes, congenital

743.57 Specified anomalies of optic disc
Coloboma of optic disc (congenital)

743.58 **Vascular anomalies**
Congenital retinal aneurysm

743.59 Other

⑤ **743.6 Congenital anomalies of eyelids, lacrimal system, and orbit**

743.61 **Congenital ptosis**

▓	Add 4th or 5th digit	▓	Nonspecific code	▓	Unspecified code	▓	Manifestation code

743.62 Congenital deformities of eyelids
Ablepharon   Congenital:
Absence of eyelid   ectropion
Accessory eyelid   entropion

743.63 Other specified congenital anomalies of eyelid
Absence, agenesis, of cilia

743.64 Specified congenital anomalies of lacrimal gland

743.65 Specified congenital anomalies of lacrimal passages
Absence, agenesis of:
    lacrimal apparatus
    punctum lacrimale
Accessory lacrimal canal

743.66 Specified congenital anomalies of orbit

743.69 Other
Accessory eye muscles

743.8 Other specified anomalies of eye
Excludes: *congenital nystagmus (379.51)*
      ocular albinism (270.2)
      optic nerve hypoplasia (377.43)
      retinitis pigmentosa (362.74)

743.9 Unspecified anomaly of eye
Congenital:
    anomaly NOS of eye [any part]
    deformity NOS of eye [any part]

744 Congenital anomalies of ear, face, and neck
Excludes: *anomaly of:*
      cervical spine (754.2, 756.10-756.19)
      larynx (748.2-748.3)
      nose (748.0-748.1)
      parathyroid gland (759.2)
      thyroid gland (759.2)
      cleft lip (749.10-749.25)

DEFINITION Congenital anomalies of ear, face, and neck, refers to defects of the ear, face and/or neck that are present at birth.

⑤ **744.0 Anomalies of ear causing impairment of hearing**
Excludes: *congenital deafness without mention of cause (389.0-389.9)*

744.00 Unspecified anomaly of ear with impairment of hearing

744.01 Absence of external ear
Absence of:
    auditory canal (external)
    auricle (ear) (with stenosis or atresia of auditory canal)

744.02 Other anomalies of external ear with impairment of hearing
Atresia or stricture of auditory canal (external)

744.03 Anomaly of middle ear, except ossicles
Atresia or stricture of osseous meatus (ear)

744.04 Anomalies of ear ossicles
Fusion of ear ossicles

744.05 Anomalies of inner ear
Congenital anomaly of:
    membranous labyrinth
    organ of Corti

744.09 Other
Absence of ear, congenital

744.1 Accessory auricle
Accessory tragus   Supernumerary:
Polyotia   ear
Preauricular appendage   lobule

⑤ **744.2 Other specified anomalies of ear**
Excludes: *that with impairment of hearing (744.00-744.09)*

744.21 Absence of ear lobe, congenital

744.22 Macrotia

744.23 Microtia

● Code new
   to this edition   ▲ Revision of
              existing code   ④ ⑤ Fourth or fifth
                                     digit required

744.24 Specified anomalies of Eustachian tube
Absence of Eustachian tube

744.29 Other

Bat ear
Darwin's tubercle
Pointed ear

Prominence of auricle
Ridge ear

Excludes: *preauricular sinus (744.46)*

744.3 Unspecified anomaly of ear
Congenital:
anomaly NOS of ear, not elsewhere classified
deformity NOS of ear, not elsewhere classified

⑤ **744.4 Branchial cleft cyst or fistula; preauricular sinus**

744.41 Branchial cleft sinus or fistula
Branchial:
sinus (external) (internal)
vestige

744.42 Branchial cleft cyst

744.43 Cervical auricle

744.46 Preauricular sinus or fistula

744.47 Preauricular cyst

744.49 Other
Fistula (of):
auricle, congenital
cervicoaural

744.5 Webbing of neck
Pterygium colli

⑤ **744.8 Other specified anomalies of face and neck**

744.81 Macrocheilia
Hypertrophy of lip, congenital

744.82 Microcheilia

744.83 Macrostomia

744.84 Microstomia

744.89 Other

Excludes: *congenital fistula of lip (750.25)*
musculoskeletal anomalies (754.0-754.1, 756.0)

744.9 Unspecified anomalies of face and neck
Congenital:
anomaly NOS of face [any part] or neck [any part]
deformity NOS of face [any part] or neck [any part]

745 Bulbus cordis anomalies and anomalies of cardiac septal closure
DEFINITION Bulbus cordis anomalies and anomalies of cardiac septal closure, bulbus cordis is a transitory dilation in the embryonic heart where the arterial trunk joins the ventral roots of the aortic arches

745.0 Common truncus
Absent septum between aorta and pulmonary artery
Communication (abnormal) between aorta and pulmonary artery
Aortic septal defect
Common aortopulmonary trunk
Persistent truncus arteriosus

⑤ **745.1 Transposition of great vessels**

745.10 Complete transposition of great vessels
Transposition of great vessels:
NOS
classical

745.11 Double outlet right ventricle
Dextratransposition of aorta
Incomplete transposition of great vessels
Origin of both great vessels from right ventricle
Taussig-Bing syndrome or defect

745.12 Corrected transposition of great vessels

745.19 Other

	Add 4th or 5th digit		Nonspecific code		Unspecified code		Manifestation code

745.2 Tetralogy of Fallot
Fallot's pentalogy
Ventricular septal defect with pulmonary stenosis or atresia, dextraposition of aorta, and
hypertrophy of right ventricle

Excludes: *Fallot's triad (746.09)*

745.3 Common ventricle
Cor triloculare biatriatum
Single ventricle

745.4 Ventricular septal defect
Eisenmenger's defect or complex
Gerbode defect
Interventricular septal defect
Left ventricular-right atrial communication
Roger's disease

Excludes: *common atrioventricular canal type (745.69)*
single ventricle (745.3)

745.5 Ostium secundum type atrial septal defect
Defect: Patent or persistent:
   atrium secundum   foramen ovale
   fossa ovalis   ostium secundum
   Lutembacher's syndrome

⑤ **745.6 Endocardial cushion defects**

   745.60 Endocardial cushion defect, unspecified type

   745.61 Ostium primum defect
       Persistent ostium primum

   745.69 Other
       Absence of atrial septum
       Atrioventricular canal type ventricular septal defect
       Common atrioventricular canal
       Common atrium

745.7 Cor biloculare
Absence of atrial and ventricular septa

745.8 Other

745.9 Unspecified defect of septal closure
Septal defect NOS

746 Other congenital anomalies of heart

Excludes: *endocardial fibroelastosis (425.3)*

DEFINITION Congenital anomalies of heart refers to other defects of the heart that are present
at birth.

ALERT! For personal history of other congenital malformations see V13.69

⑤ **746.0 Anomalies of pulmonary valve**

Excludes: *infundibular or subvalvular pulmonic stenosis (746.83)*
tetralogy of Fallot (745.2)

   746.00 Pulmonary valve anomaly, unspecified

   746.01 Atresia, congenital
       Congenital absence of pulmonary valve

   746.02 Stenosis, congenital

   746.09 Other
       Congenital insufficiency of pulmonary valve
       Fallot's triad or trilogy

746.1 Tricuspid atresia and stenosis, congenital
Absence of tricuspid valve

746.2 Ebstein's anomaly

746.3 Congenital stenosis of aortic valve
Congenital aortic stenosis

Excludes: *congenital:*
subaortic stenosis (746.81)
supravalvular aortic stenosis (747.22)

746.4 Congenital insufficiency of aortic valve
Bicuspid aortic valve
Congenital aortic insufficiency

   ● Code new
      to this edition
         ▲ Revision of
              existing code
                 ④ ⑤ Fourth or fifth
                    digit required

746.5 **Congenital mitral stenosis**
Fused commissure of mitral valve
Parachute deformity of mitral valve
Supernumerary cusps of mitral valve

746.6 **Congenital mitral insufficiency**

746.7 **Hypoplastic left heart syndrome**
Atresia, or marked hypoplasia, of aortic orifice or valve, with hypoplasia of ascending aorta and defective development of left ventricle (with mitral valve atresia)

⑤ **746.8** **Other specified anomalies of heart**

746.81 **Subaortic stenosis**

746.82 **Cor triatriatum**

746.83 **Infundibular pulmonic stenosis**
Subvalvular pulmonic stenosis

746.84 **Obstructive anomalies of heart, not elsewhere classified**
Shone's syndrome
Uhl's disease
Use additional code for associated anomalies, such as:
coarctation of aorta (747.10)
congenital mitral stenosis (746.5)
subaortic stenosis (746.81)

746.85 **Coronary artery anomaly**
Anomalous origin or communication of coronary artery
Arteriovenous malformation of coronary artery
Coronary artery:
absence
arising from aorta or pulmonary trunk
single

746.86 **Congenital heart block**
Complete or incomplete atrioventricular [AV] block

746.87 **Malposition of heart and cardiac apex**
Abdominal heart   Levocardia (isolated)
Dextrocardia   Mesocardia
Ectopia cordis

Excludes: *dextrocardia with complete transposition of viscera (759.3)*

746.89 **Other**
Atresia of cardiac vein
Hypoplasia of cardiac vein
Congenital:
cardiomegaly
diverticulum, left ventricle
pericardial defect

746.9 **Unspecified anomaly of heart**
Congenital:
anomaly of heart NOS
heart disease NOS

747 **Other congenital anomalies of circulatory system**
DEFINITION Congenital anomalies of circulatory system refers to other defects of the circulatory system that are present at birth.
ALERT! For personal history of other congenital malformations see V13.69

747.0 **Patent ductus arteriosus**
Patent ductus Botalli
Persistent ductus arteriosus

⑤ **747.1** **Coarctation of aorta**

747.10 **Coarctation of aorta (preductal) (postductal)**
Hypoplasia of aortic arch

747.11 **Interruption of aortic arch**

⑤ **747.2** **Other anomalies of aorta**

747.20 **Anomaly of aorta, unspecified**

| Add 4th or 5th digit | Nonspecific code | Unspecified code | Manifestation code |

747.21 Anomalies of aortic arch
Anomalous origin, right subclavian artery
Dextraposition of aorta
Double aortic arch
Kommerell's diverticulum
Overriding aorta
Persistent:
    convolutions, aortic arch
    right aortic arch
Vascular ring

Excludes: *hypoplasia of aortic arch (747.10)*

747.22 Atresia and stenosis of aorta
Absence of aorta
Aplasia of aorta
Hypoplasia of aorta
Stricture of aorta
Supra (valvular)-aortic stenosis

Excludes: *congenital aortic (valvular) stenosis or stricture, so stated (746.3)*
hypoplasia of aorta in hypoplastic left heart syndrome (746.7)

747.29 Other
Aneurysm of sinus of Valsalva
Congenital:
    aneurysm of aorta
    dilation of aorta

⑤ **747.3 Anomalies of pulmonary artery**

● **747.31 Pulmonary artery coarctation and atresia**
Agenesis of pulmonary artery
Atresia of pulmonary artery
Coarctation of pulmonary artery
Hypoplasia of pulmonary artery
Stenosis of pulmonary artery

● **747.32 Pulmonary arteriovenous malformation**
Pulmonary arteriovenous aneurysm

Excludes: *acquired pulmonary arteriovenous fistula (417.0)*

● **747.39 Other anomalies of pulmonary artery and pulmonary circulation**
Anomaly of pulmonary artery

⑤ **747.4 Anomalies of great veins**

747.40 Anomaly of great veins, unspecified
Anomaly NOS of:
    pulmonary veins
    vena cava

747.41 Total anomalous pulmonary venous connection
Total anomalous pulmonary venous return [TAPVR]:
    subdiaphragmatic
    supradiaphragmatic

747.42 Partial anomalous pulmonary venous connection
Partial anomalous pulmonary venous return

747.49 Other anomalies of great veins
Absence of vena cava (inferior) (superior)
Congenital stenosis of vena cava (inferior) (superior)
Persistent:
    left posterior cardinal vein
    left superior vena cava
Scimitar syndrome
Transposition of pulmonary veins NOS

747.5 Absence or hypoplasia of umbilical artery
Single umbilical artery

● Code new
to this edition

▲ Revision of
existing code

④ ⑤ Fourth or fifth
digit required

⑤ **747.6 Other anomalies of peripheral vascular system**
  Absence of artery or vein, not elsewhere classified
  Anomaly of artery or vein, not elsewhere classified
  Atresia of artery or vein, not elsewhere classified
  Arteriovenous aneurysm (peripheral)
  Arteriovenous malformation of the peripheral vascular system
  Congenital:
    aneurysm (peripheral)
    phlebectasia
    stricture, artery
    varix
  Multiple renal arteries

  Excludes: *anomalies of:*
      cerebral vessels (747.81)
      pulmonary artery (747.39)
      congenital retinal aneurysm (743.58)
      hemangioma (228.00-228.09)
      lymphangioma (228.1)

  747.60 Anomaly of the peripheral vascular system, unspecified site

  747.61 Gastrointestinal vessel anomaly

  747.62 Renal vessel anomaly

  747.63 Upper limb vessel anomaly

  747.64 Lower limb vessel anomaly

  747.69 Anomalies of other specified sites of peripheral vascular system

⑤ **747.8 Other specified anomalies of circulatory system**

  747.81 Anomalies of cerebrovascular system
      Arteriovenous malformation of brain
      Cerebral arteriovenous aneurysm, congenital
      Congenital anomalies of cerebral vessels

  Excludes: *ruptured cerebral (arteriovenous) aneurysm (430)*

  747.82 Spinal vessel anomaly
      Arteriovenous malformation of spinal vessel

  747.83 Persistent fetal circulation
      Persistent pulmonary hypertension
      Primary pulmonary hypertension of newborn

  747.89 Other
      Aneurysm, congenital, specified site not elsewhere classified

  Excludes: *congenital aneurysm:*
      coronary (746.85)
      peripheral (747.6)
      pulmonary (747.39)
        arteriovenous (747.32)
      retinal (743.58)

747.9 Unspecified anomaly of circulatory system

748 Congenital anomalies of respiratory system

  Excludes: *congenital central alveolar hypoventilation syndrome (327.25)*
      congenital defect of diaphragm (756.6)

  DEFINITION Congenital anomalies of respiratory system refers to other defects of the respiratory system that are present at birth.

748.0 Choanal atresia
    Atresia of nares (anterior) (posterior)
    Congenital stenosis of nares (anterior) (posterior)

748.1 Other anomalies of nose

Absent nose	Congenital:
Accessory nose	deformity of nose
Cleft nose	notching of tip of nose
Deformity of wall of nasal	perforation of wall of nasal sinus
sinus	

  Excludes: *congenital deviation of nasal septum (754.0)*

▬ Add 4th or 5th digit	▬ Nonspecific code	▬ Unspecified code	▬ Manifestation code

748.2 Web of larynx
Web of larynx:
NOS
glottic
subglottic

748.3 Other anomalies of larynx, trachea, and bronchus

Absence or agenesis of:
  bronchus
  larynx
  trachea
Anomaly (of):
  cricoid cartilage
  epiglottis
  thyroid cartilage
  tracheal cartilage
Atresia (of):
  epiglottis
  glottis
  larynx
  trachea
Cleft thyroid, cartilage, congenital

Congenital:
  dilation, trachea
  stenosis:
    larynx
    trachea
  tracheocele
Diverticulum:
  bronchus
  trachea
Fissure of epiglottis
Laryngocele
Posterior cleft of cricoid cartilage (congenital)
Rudimentary tracheal bronchus
Stridor, laryngeal, congenital

748.4 Congenital cystic lung
Disease, lung:
  cystic, congenital
  polycystic, congenital
Honeycomb lung, congenital

Excludes: acquired or unspecified cystic lung (518.89)

748.5 Agenesis, hypoplasia, and dysplasia of lung
Absence of lung (fissures) (lobe)
Aplasia of lung
Hypoplasia of lung (lobe)
Sequestration of lung

⑤ **748.6 Other anomalies of lung**
  748.60 Anomaly of lung, unspecified
  748.61 Congenital bronchiectasis
  748.69 Other
    Accessory lung (lobe)
    Azygos lobe (fissure), lung

748.8 Other specified anomalies of respiratory system
Abnormal communication between pericardial and pleural sacs
Anomaly, pleural folds
Atresia of nasopharynx
Congenital cyst of mediastinum

748.9 Unspecified anomaly of respiratory system
Anomaly of respiratory system NOS

749 Cleft palate and cleft lip
DEFINITION Cleft palate is a congenital fissure in the roof of the mouth, resulting from incomplete fusion of the palate during embryonic development. Cleft lip is a congenital deformity characterized by a vertical cleft or pair of clefts in the upper lip, with or without involvement of the palate.

⑤ **749.0 Cleft palate**
  749.00 Cleft palate, unspecified
  749.01 Unilateral, complete
  749.02 Unilateral, incomplete
    Cleft uvula
  749.03 Bilateral, complete
  749.04 Bilateral, incomplete

⑤ **749.1 Cleft lip**
Cheiloschisis
Congenital fissure of lip
Harelip
Labium leporinum
  749.10 Cleft lip, unspecified
  749.11 Unilateral, complete
  749.12 Unilateral, incomplete

● Code new to this edition ▲ Revision of existing code ④ ⑤ Fourth or fifth digit required

749.13 **Bilateral, complete**

749.14 **Bilateral, incomplete**

⑤ 749.2 **Cleft palate with cleft lip**
Cheilopalatoschisis

749.20 **Cleft palate with cleft lip, unspecified**

749.21 **Unilateral, complete**

749.22 **Unilateral, incomplete**

749.23 **Bilateral, complete**

749.24 **Bilateral, incomplete**

749.25 **Other combinations**

750 **Other congenital anomalies of upper alimentary tract**

Excludes: *dentofacial anomalies (524.0-524.9)*

DEFINITION Congenital anomalies of upper alimentary tract refers to other defects of the upper alimentary tract that are present at birth.

ALERT! For personal history of other congenital malformations see V13.69

750.0 **Tongue tie**
Ankyloglossia

⑤ 750.1 **Other anomalies of tongue**

750.10 **Anomaly of tongue, unspecified**

750.11 **Aglossia**

750.12 **Congenital adhesions of tongue**

750.13 **Fissure of tongue**
Bifid tongue
Double tongue

750.15 **Macroglossia**
Congenital hypertrophy of tongue

750.16 **Microglossia**
Hypoplasia of tongue

750.19 **Other**

⑤ 750.2 **Other specified anomalies of mouth and pharynx**

750.21 **Absence of salivary gland**

750.22 **Accessory salivary gland**

750.23 **Atresia, salivary duct**
Imperforate salivary duct

750.24 **Congenital fistula of salivary gland**

750.25 **Congenital fistula of lip**
Congenital (mucus) lip pits

750.26 **Other specified anomalies of mouth**
Absence of uvula

750.27 **Diverticulum of pharynx**
Pharyngeal pouch

750.29 **Other specified anomalies of pharynx**
Imperforate pharynx

750.3 **Tracheoesophageal fistula, esophageal atresia and stenosis**

Absent esophagus	Congenital fistula:
Atresia of esophagus	esophagobronchial
Congenital:	esophagotracheal
esophageal ring	Imperforate esophagus
stenosis of esophagus	Webbed esophagus
stricture of esophagus	

Add 4th or 5th digit	Nonspecific code	Unspecified code	Manifestation code

750.4 Other specified anomalies of esophagus
Dilatation, congenital (of) esophagus
Displacement, congenital (of) esophagus
Diverticulum (of) esophagus
Duplication (of) esophagus
Giant esophagus
Esophageal pouch

Excludes: *congenital hiatus hernia (750.6)*

750.5 Congenital hypertrophic pyloric stenosis
Congenital or infantile:
constriction of pylorus
hypertrophy of pylorus
spasm of pylorus
stenosis of pylorus
stricture of pylorus

750.6 Congenital hiatus hernia
Displacement of cardia through esophageal hiatus

Excludes: *congenital diaphragmatic hernia (756.6)*

750.7 Other specified anomalies of stomach
Congenital:
cardiospasm
hourglass stomach
Displacement of stomach
Diverticulum of stomach,
congenital
Duplication of stomach
Megalogastria
Microgastria
Transposition of stomach

750.8 Other specified anomalies of upper alimentary tract

750.9 Unspecified anomaly of upper alimentary tract
Congenital:
anomaly NOS of upper alimentary tract [any part, except tongue]
deformity NOS of upper alimentary tract [any part, except tongue]

751 Other congenital anomalies of digestive system
DEFINITION Congenital anomalies of digestive system refers to other defects of the digestive system that are present at birth.
ALERT! For personal history of other congenital malformations see V13.69

751.0 Meckel's diverticulum
Meckel's diverticulum (displaced) (hypertrophic)
Persistent:
omphalomesenteric duct
vitelline duct

751.1 Atresia and stenosis of small intestine
Atresia of:
duodenum
ileum
intestine NOS
Congenital:
absence of small intestine or intestine NOS
obstruction of small intestine or intestine NOS
stenosis of small intestine or intestine NOS
stricture of small intestine or intestine NOS
Imperforate jejunum

751.2 Atresia and stenosis of large intestine, rectum, and anal canal
Absence:
anus (congenital)
appendix, congenital
large intestine, congenital
rectum
Atresia of:
anus
colon
rectum
Congenital or infantile:
obstruction of large intestine
occlusion of anus
stricture of anus
Imperforate:
anus
rectum
Stricture of rectum, congenital

751.3 Hirschsprung's disease and other congenital functional disorders of colon
Aganglionosis
Congenital dilation of colon
Congenital megacolon
Macrocolon

● Code new
to this edition   ▲ Revision of
existing code   ④ ⑤ Fourth or fifth
digit required

751.4   Anomalies of intestinal fixation

Congenital adhesions:
  omental, anomalous
  peritoneal
Jackson's membrane
Malrotation of colon

Rotation of cecum or colon:
  failure of
  incomplete
  insufficient
Universal mesentery

751.5   Other anomalies of intestine

Congenital diverticulum,
  colon
Dolichocolon
Duplication of:
  anus
  appendix
  cecum
  intestine
Ectopic anus

Megaloappendix
Megaloduodenum
Microcolon
Persistent cloaca
Transposition of:
  appendix
  colon
  intestine

⑤ **751.6   Anomalies of gallbladder, bile ducts, and liver**

751.60   Unspecified anomaly of gallbladder, bile ducts, and liver

751.61   Biliary atresia

Congenital:
  absence of bile duct (common) or passage
  hypoplasia of bile duct (common) or passage
  obstruction of bile duct (common) or passage
  stricture of bile duct (common) or passage

751.62   Congenital cystic disease of liver

Congenital polycystic disease of liver
Fibrocystic disease of liver

751.69   Other anomalies of gallbladder, bile ducts, and liver

Absence of:
  gallbladder, congenital
  liver (lobe)
Accessory:
  hepatic ducts
  liver
Congenital:
  choledochal cyst
  hepatomegaly

Duplication of:
  biliary duct
  cystic duct
  gallbladder
  liver
Floating:
  gallbladder
  liver
Intrahepatic gallbladder

751.7   Anomalies of pancreas

Absence of pancreas
Accessory pancreas
Agenesis of pancreas
Annular pancreas
Ectopic pancreatic tissue
Hypoplasia of pancreas
Pancreatic heterotopia

Excludes: *diabetes mellitus (249.0-249.9, 250.0-250.9)*
  fibrocystic disease of pancreas (277.00-277.09)
  neonatal diabetes mellitus (775.1)

751.8   Other specified anomalies of digestive system

Absence (complete) (partial) of alimentary tract NOS
Duplication of digestive organs NOS
Malposition, congenital of digestive organs NOS

Excludes: *congenital diaphragmatic hernia (756.6)*
  congenital hiatus hernia (750.6)

751.9   Unspecified anomaly of digestive system

Congenital:
  anomaly NOS of digestive system NOS
  deformity NOS of digestive system NOS

752   Congenital anomalies of genital organs

Excludes: *syndromes associated with anomalies in the number and form of chromosomes (758.0-758.9)*

DEFINITION Congenital anomalies of genital organs refers to defects of the genital organs that are present at birth.

| | Add 4th or 5th digit | | Nonspecific code | | Unspecified code | | Manifestation code |

752.0 Anomalies of ovaries
  Absence, congenital (of) ovary
  Accessory ovary
  Ectopic ovary
  Streak of ovary

⑤ **752.1 Anomalies of fallopian tubes and broad ligaments**

  752.10 Unspecified anomaly of fallopian tubes and broad ligaments

  752.11 Embryonic cyst of fallopian tubes and broad ligaments
    Cyst:
      epoophoron
      fimbrial
      parovarian

  752.19 Other
    Absence of fallopian tube or broad ligament
    Accessory fallopian tube or broad ligament
    Atresia of fallopian tube or broad ligament

752.2 Doubling of uterus
  Didelphic uterus
  Doubling of uterus [any degree] (associated with doubling of cervix and vagina)

⑤ **752.3 Other anomalies of uterus**

  752.31 Agenesis of uterus
    Congenital absence of uterus

  752.32 Hypoplasia of uterus

  752.33 Unicornuate uterus
    Unicornate uterus with or without a separate uterine horn
    Uterus with only one functioning horn

  752.34 Bicornuate uterus
    Bicornuate uterus, complete or partial

  752.35 Septate uterus
    Septate uterus, complete or partial

  752.36 Arcuate uterus

  752.39 Other anomalies of uterus
    Aplasia of uterus NOS
    Müllerian anomaly of the uterus, NEC

  Excludes: *anomaly of uterus due to exposure to diethylstilbestrol [DES] in utero (760.76)*
    didelphic uterus (752.2)
    doubling of uterus (752.2)

⑤ **752.4 Anomalies of cervix, vagina, and external female genitalia**

  752.40 Unspecified anomaly of cervix, vagina, and external female genitalia

  752.41 Embryonic cyst of cervix, vagina, and external female genitalia
    Cyst of: Cyst of:
      canal of Nuck, congenital   vagina, embryonal
      Gartner's duct   vulva, congenital

  752.42 Imperforate hymen

  752.43 Cervical agenesis
    Cervical hypoplasia

  752.44 Cervical duplication

  752.45 Vaginal agenesis
    Agenesis of vagina, total or partial

  752.46 Transverse vaginal septum

  752.47 Longitudinal vaginal septum
    Longitudinal vaginal septum with or without obstruction

  752.49 Other anomalies of cervix, vagina, and external female genitalia
    Absence of clitoris or vulva
    Agenesis of clitoris or vulva
    Anomalies of cervix, NEC
    Anomalies of hymen, NEC
    Congenital stenosis or stricture of:
      cervical canal
      vagina
    Müllerian anomalies of the cervix and vagina, NEC

  Excludes: *double vagina associated with total duplication (752.2)*

● Code new
  to this edition
▲ Revision of
  existing code
④ ⑤ Fourth or fifth
  digit required

⑤ **752.5 Undescended and retractile testicle**

    752.51 Undescended testis
       Cryptorchism
       Ectopic testis

    752.52 Retractile testis

⑤ **752.6 Hypospadias and epispadias and other penile anomalies**

    ALERT! For personal history of hypospadias see V13.61

    752.61 Hypospadias

    752.62 Epispadias
       Anaspadias

    752.63 Congenital chordee

    752.64 Micropenis

    752.65 Hidden penis

    752.69 Other penile anomalies

  752.7 Indeterminate sex and pseudohermaphroditism
    Gynandrism   Pseudohermaphroditism (male) (female)
    Hermaphroditism   Pure gonadal dysgenesis
    Ovotestis

    Excludes: *androgen insensitivity (259.50-259.52)*

          pseudohermaphroditism:
            female, with adrenocortical disorder (255.2)
            male, with gonadal disorder (257.8)
            with specified chromosomal anomaly (758.0-758.9)
          testicular feminization syndrome (259.50-259.72)

⑤ **752.8 Other specified anomalies of genital organs**

    Excludes: *congenital hydrocele (778.6)*

          penile anomalies (752.61-752.69)
          phimosis or paraphimosis (605)

    752.81 Scrotal transposition

    752.89 Other specified anomalies of genital organs
       Absence of:
         prostate
         spermatic cord
         vas deferens
       Anorchism
       Aplasia (congenital) of:
         prostate
         round ligament
         testicle
       Atresia of:
         ejaculatory duct
         vas deferens
       Fusion of testes
       Hypoplasia of testes
       Monorchism
       Polyorchism

  752.9 Unspecified anomaly of genital organs
     Congenital:
       anomaly NOS of genital organ, NEC
       deformity NOS of genital organ, NEC

753 Congenital anomalies of urinary system

    DEFINITION Congenital anomalies of urinary system refers to defects of the urinary system that are present at birth

  753.0 Renal agenesis and dysgenesis
    Atrophy of kidney: Congenital absence of kidney(s)
      congenital   Hypoplasia of kidney(s)
      infantile

⑤ **753.1 Cystic kidney disease**

    Excludes: *acquired cyst of kidney (593.2)*

    753.10 Cystic kidney disease, unspecified

    753.11 Congenital single renal cyst

    753.12 Polycystic kidney, unspecified type

	Add 4th or 5th digit		Nonspecific code		Unspecified code		Manifestation code

753.13   **Polycystic kidney, autosomal dominant**

753.14   **Polycystic kidney, autosomal recessive**

753.15   **Renal dysplasia**

753.16   **Medullary cystic kidney**
    Nephronopthisis

753.17   **Medullary sponge kidney**

753.19   **Other specified cystic kidney disease**
    Multicystic kidney

⑤ **753.2   Obstructive defects of renal pelvis and ureter**

753.20   **Unspecified obstructive defect of renal pelvis and ureter**

753.21   **Congenital obstruction of ureteropelvic junction**

753.22   **Congenital obstruction of ureterovesical junction**
    Adynamic ureter
    Congenital hydroureter

753.23   **Congenital ureterocele**

753.29   **Other**

753.3   Other specified anomalies of kidney

Accessory kidney	Fusion of kidneys
Congenital:	Giant kidney
calculus of kidney	Horseshoe kidney
displaced kidney	Hyperplasia of kidney
Discoid kidney	Lobulation of kidney
Double kidney with double	Malrotation of kidney
pelvis	Trifid kidney (pelvis)
Ectopic kidney	

753.4   Other specified anomalies of ureter

Absent ureter	Double ureter
Accessory ureter	Ectopic ureter
Deviation of ureter	Implantation, anomalous of ureter
Displaced ureteric orifice	

753.5   Exstrophy of urinary bladder

Ectopia vesicae	Extroversion of bladder

753.6   Atresia and stenosis of urethra and bladder neck

Congenital obstruction:	Imperforate urinary meatus
bladder neck	Impervious urethra
urethra	Urethral valve formation
Congenital stricture of:	
urethra (valvular)	
urinary meatus	
vesicourethral orifice	

753.7   Anomalies of urachus

Cyst (of) urachus	Persistent umbilical sinus
Fistula (of) urachus	
Patent (of) urachus	

753.8   Other specified anomalies of bladder and urethra

Absence, congenital of:	Congenital urethrorectal fistula
bladder	Congenital prolapse of:
urethra	bladder (mucosa)
Accessory:	urethra
bladder	Double:
urethra	urethra
Congenital:	urinary meatus
diverticulum of bladder	
hernia of bladder	

753.9   Unspecified anomaly of urinary system
    Congenital:
      anomaly NOS of urinary system [any part, except urachus]
      deformity NOS of urinary system [any part, except urachus]

754   Certain congenital musculoskeletal deformities
    Includes: nonteratogenic deformities which are considered to be due to intrauterine
            malposition and pressure

DEFINITION Certain congenital musculoskeletal deformities refers to defects of the
musculoskeletal system that are present at birth.

● Code new
  to this edition
▲ Revision of
  existing code
④ ⑤ Fourth or fifth
     digit required

754.0 Of skull, face, and jaw

Asymmetry of face
Compression facies
Depressions in skull
Deviation of nasal
  septum, congenital

Dolichocephaly
Plagiocephaly
Potter's facies
Squashed or bent nose, congenital

Excludes: *dentofacial anomalies (524.0-524.9)*
        syphilitic saddle nose (090.5)

754.1 Of sternocleidomastoid muscle

Congenital sternomastoid torticollis
Congenital wryneck
Contracture of sternocleidomastoid (muscle)
Sternomastoid tumor

754.2 Of spine

Congenital postural:
  lordosis
  scoliosis

⑤ **754.3 Congenital dislocation of hip**

  754.30 Congenital dislocation of hip, unilateral
      Congenital dislocation of hip NOS

  754.31 Congenital dislocation of hip, bilateral

  754.32 Congenital subluxation of hip, unilateral
      Congenital flexion deformity, hip or thigh
      Predislocation status of hip at birth
      Preluxation of hip, congenital

  754.33 Congenital subluxation of hip, bilateral

  754.35 Congenital dislocation of one hip with subluxation of other hip

⑤ **754.4 Congenital genu recurvatum and bowing of long bones of leg**

  754.40 Genu recurvatum

  754.41 Congenital dislocation of knee (with genu recurvatum)

  754.42 Congenital bowing of femur

  754.43 Congenital bowing of tibia and fibula

  754.44 Congenital bowing of unspecified long bones of leg

⑤ **754.5 Varus deformities of feet**

Excludes: *acquired (736.71, 736.75, 736.79)*

  754.50 Talipes varus
      Congenital varus deformity of foot, unspecified
      Pes varus

  754.51 Talipes equinovarus
      Equinovarus (congenital)

  754.52 Metatarsus primus varus

  754.53 Metatarsus varus

  754.59 Other
      Talipes calcaneovarus

⑤ **754.6 Valgus deformities of feet**

Excludes: *valgus deformity of foot (acquired) (736.79)*

  754.60 Talipes valgus
      Congenital valgus deformity of foot, unspecified

  754.61 Congenital pes planus
      Congenital rocker bottom flat foot
      Flat foot, congenital

Excludes: *pes planus (acquired) (734)*

  754.62 Talipes calcaneovalgus

  754.69 Other
      Talipes:
        equinovalgus
        planovalgus

⑤ **754.7 Other deformities of feet**

Excludes: *acquired (736.70-736.79)*

| | Add 4th or 5th digit | | Nonspecific code | | Unspecified code | | Manifestation code |

754.70 Talipes, unspecified
Congenital deformity of foot NOS

754.71 Talipes cavus
Cavus foot (congenital)

754.79 Other
Asymmetric talipes
Talipes:
calcaneus
equinus

⑤ **754.8 Other specified nonteratogenic anomalies**

754.81 Pectus excavatum
Congenital funnel chest

754.82 Pectus carinatum
Congenital pigeon chest [breast]

754.89 Other
Club hand (congenital)
Congenital:
deformity of chest wall
dislocation of elbow
Generalized flexion contractures of lower limb joints, congenital
Spade-like hand (congenital)

755 Other congenital anomalies of limbs

Excludes: *those deformities classifiable to 754.0-754.8*

DEFINITION Congenital anomalies of limbs refers to other defects of the limbs that are present at birth

ALERT! For personal history of other congenital malformations see V13.69

⑤ **755.0 Polydactyly**

755.00 Polydactyly, unspecified digits
Supernumerary digits

755.01 Of fingers
Accessory fingers

755.02 Of toes
Accessory toes

⑤ **755.1 Syndactyly**
Symphalangy
Webbing of digits

755.10 Of multiple and unspecified sites

755.11 Of fingers without fusion of bone

755.12 Of fingers with fusion of bone

755.13 Of toes without fusion of bone

755.14 Of toes with fusion of bone

⑤ **755.2 Reduction deformities of upper limb**

DEFINITION A reduction deformity is a congenital deformity in which a body part, especially a limb, is shorter than normal or missing.

755.20 Unspecified reduction deformity of upper limb
Ectromelia NOS of upper limb
Hemimelia NOS of upper limb
Shortening of arm, congenital

755.21 Transverse deficiency of upper limb
Amelia of upper limb
Congenital absence of:
fingers, all (complete or partial)
forearm, including hand and fingers
upper limb, complete
Congenital amputation of upper limb
Transverse hemimelia of upper limb

755.22 Longitudinal deficiency of upper limb, not elsewhere classified
Phocomelia NOS of upper limb
Rudimentary arm

● Code new
to this edition

▲ Revision of
existing code

④ ⑤ Fourth or fifth
digit required

755.23 Longitudinal deficiency, combined, involving humerus, radius, and ulna (complete or incomplete)
Congenital absence of arm and forearm (complete or incomplete) with or without metacarpal deficiency and/or phalangeal deficiency, incomplete
Phocomelia, complete, of upper limb

755.24 Longitudinal deficiency, humeral, complete or partial (with or without distal deficiencies, incomplete)
Congenital absence of humerus (with or without absence of some [but not all] distal elements)
Proximal phocomelia of upper limb

755.25 Longitudinal deficiency, radioulnar, complete or partial (with or without distal deficiencies, incomplete)
Congenital absence of radius and ulna (with or without absence of some [but not all] distal elements)
Distal phocomelia of upper limb

755.26 Longitudinal deficiency, radial, complete or partial (with or without distal deficiencies, incomplete)
Agenesis of radius
Congenital absence of radius (with or without absence of some [but not all] distal elements)

755.27 Longitudinal deficiency, ulnar, complete or partial (with or without distal deficiencies, incomplete)
Agenesis of ulna
Congenital absence of ulna (with or without absence of some [but not all] distal elements)

755.28 Longitudinal deficiency, carpals or metacarpals, complete or partial (with or without incomplete phalangeal deficiency)

755.29 Longitudinal deficiency, phalanges, complete or partial
Absence of finger, congenital
Aphalangia of upper limb, terminal, complete or partial

Excludes: *terminal deficiency of all five digits (755.21)*
transverse deficiency of phalanges (755.21)

⑤ **755.3 Reduction deformities of lower limb**
DEFINITION A reduction deformity is a congenital deformity in which a body part, especially a limb, is shorter than normal or missing.

755.30 Unspecified reduction deformity of lower limb
Ectromelia NOS of lower limb
Hemimelia NOS of lower limb
Shortening of leg, congenital

755.31 Transverse deficiency of lower limb
Amelia of lower limb
Congenital absence of:
   foot
   leg, including foot and toes
   lower limb, complete
   toes, all, complete
Transverse hemimelia of lower limb

755.32 Longitudinal deficiency of lower limb, not elsewhere classified
Phocomelia NOS of lower limb

755.33 Longitudinal deficiency, combined, involving femur, tibia, and fibula (complete or incomplete)
Congenital absence of thigh and (lower) leg (complete or incomplete) with or without metacarpal deficiency and/or phalangeal deficiency, incomplete
Phocomelia, complete, of lower limb

755.34 Longitudinal deficiency, femoral, complete or partial (with or without distal deficiencies, incomplete)
Congenital absence of femur (with or without absence of some [but not all] distal elements)
Proximal phocomelia of lower limb

755.35 Longitudinal deficiency, tibiofibular, complete or partial (with or without distal deficiencies, incomplete)
Congenital absence of tibia and fibula (with or without absence of some [but not all] distal elements)
Distal phocomelia of lower limb

Add 4th or 5th digit	Nonspecific code	Unspecified code	Manifestation code

755.36 Longitudinal deficiency, tibia, complete or partial (with or without distal deficiencies, incomplete)
Agenesis of tibia
Congenital absence of tibia (with or without absence of some [but not all] distal elements)

755.37 Longitudinal deficiency, fibular, complete or partial (with or without distal deficiencies, incomplete)
Agenesis of fibula
Congenital absence of fibula (with or without absence of some [but not all] distal elements)

755.38 Longitudinal deficiency, tarsals or metatarsals, complete or partial (with or without incomplete phalangeal deficiency)

755.39 Longitudinal deficiency, phalanges, complete or partial
Absence of toe, congenital
Aphalangia of lower limb, terminal, complete or partial

Excludes: *terminal deficiency of all five digits (755.31)*
transverse deficiency of phalanges (755.31)

755.4 Reduction deformities, unspecified limb
Absence, congenital (complete or partial) of limb NOS
Amelia of unspecified limb
Ectromelia of unspecified limb
Hemimelia of unspecified limb
Phocomelia of unspecified limb

⑤ **755.5 Other anomalies of upper limb, including shoulder girdle**

755.50 Unspecified anomaly of upper limb

755.51 Congenital deformity of clavicle

755.52 Congenital elevation of scapula
Sprengel's deformity

755.53 Radioulnar synostosis

755.54 Madelung's deformity

755.55 Acrocephalosyndactyly
Apert's syndrome

755.56 Accessory carpal bones

755.57 Macrodactylia (fingers)

755.58 Cleft hand, congenital
Lobster-claw hand

755.59 Other
Cleidocranial dysostosis
Cubitus:
  valgus, congenital
  varus, congenital

Excludes: *club hand (congenital) (754.89)*
congenital dislocation of elbow (754.89)

⑤ **755.6 Other anomalies of lower limb, including pelvic girdle**

755.60 Unspecified anomaly of lower limb

755.61 Coxa valga, congenital

755.62 Coxa vara, congenital

755.63 Other congenital deformity of hip (joint)
Congenital anteversion of femur (neck)

Excludes: *congenital dislocation of hip (754.30-754.35)*

755.64 Congenital deformity of knee (joint)
Congenital:
  absence of patella
  genu valgum [knock-knee]
  genu varum [bowleg]
Rudimentary patella

755.65 Macrodactylia of toes

755.66 Other anomalies of toes
Congenital:
  hallux valgus
  hallux varus
  hammer toe

● Code new
  to this edition

▲ Revision of
  existing code

④ ⑤ Fourth or fifth
  digit required

755.67 Anomalies of foot, not elsewhere classified
Astragaloscaphoid synostosis
Calcaneonavicular bar
Coalition of calcaneus
Talonavicular synostosis
Tarsal coalitions

755.69 Other
Congenital:
 angulation of tibia
 deformity (of):
  ankle (joint)
  sacroiliac (joint)
 fusion of sacroiliac joint

755.8 Other specified anomalies of unspecified limb

755.9 Unspecified anomaly of unspecified limb
Congenital:
 anomaly NOS of unspecified limb
 deformity NOS of unspecified limb

Excludes: *reduction deformity of unspecified limb (755.4)*

756 Other congenital musculoskeletal anomalies

Excludes: *congenital myotonic chondrodystrophy (359.23)*
those deformities classifiable to 754.0-754.8

DEFINITION Congenital musculoskeletal anomalies refers to other defects of the musculoskeletal system that are present at birth.
ALERT! For personal history of other congenital malformations see V13.69

756.0 Anomalies of skull and face bones
Absence of skull bones
Acrocephaly
Congenital deformity of
 forehead
Craniosynostosis
Crouzon's disease
Hypertelorism
Imperfect fusion of skull
Oxycephaly
Platybasia
Premature closure of cranial sutures
Tower skull
Trigonocephaly

Excludes: *acrocephalosyndactyly [Apert's syndrome] (755.55)*
dentofacial anomalies (524.0-524.9)
skull defects associated with brain anomalies, such as:
anencephalus (740.0)
encephalocele (742.0)
hydrocephalus (742.3)
microcephalus (742.1)

⑤ **756.1 Anomalies of spine**

756.10 Anomaly of spine, unspecified

756.11 Spondylolysis, lumbosacral region
Prespondylolisthesis (lumbosacral)

756.12 Spondylolisthesis

756.13 Absence of vertebra, congenital

756.14 Hemivertebra

756.15 Fusion of spine [vertebra], congenital

756.16 Klippel-Feil syndrome

756.17 Spina bifida occulta

Excludes: *spina bifida (aperta) (741.0-741.9)*

756.19 Other
Platyspondylia
Supernumerary vertebra

756.2 Cervical rib
Supernumerary rib in the cervical region

Add 4th or 5th digit   Nonspecific code   Unspecified code   Manifestation code

756.3 Other anomalies of ribs and sternum
Congenital absence of:
  rib
  sternum
Congenital:
  fissure of sternum
  fusion of ribs
Sternum bifidum

Excludes: nonteratogenic deformity of chest wall (754.81-754.89)

756.4 Chondrodystrophy
Achondroplasia
Chondrodystrophia (fetalis)
Dyschondroplasia
Enchondromatosis
Ollier's disease

Excludes: congenital myotonic chondrodystrophy (359.23)
  lipochondrodystrophy [Hurler's syndrome] (277.5)
  Morquio's disease (277.5)

⑤ **756.5 Osteodystrophies**

756.50 Osteodystrophy, unspecified

756.51 Osteogenesis imperfecta
Fragilitas ossium
Osteopsathyrosis

756.52 Osteopetrosis

756.53 Osteopoikilosis

756.54 Polyostotic fibrous dysplasia of bone

756.55 Chondroectodermal dysplasia
Ellis-van Creveld syndrome

756.56 Multiple epiphyseal dysplasia

756.59 Other
Albright (-McCune)-Sternberg syndrome

756.6 Anomalies of diaphragm
Absence of diaphragm
Congenital hernia:
  diaphragmatic
  foramen of Morgagni
Eventration of diaphragm

Excludes: congenital hiatus hernia (750.6)

⑤ **756.7 Anomalies of abdominal wall**

756.70 Anomaly of abdominal wall, unspecified

756.71 Prune belly syndrome
Eagle-Barrett syndrome
Prolapse of bladder mucosa

756.72 Omphalocele
Exomphalos

756.73 Gastroschisis

756.79 Other congenital anomalies of abdominal wall

Excludes: umbilical hernia (551-553 with .1)

⑤ **756.8 Other specified anomalies of muscle, tendon, fascia, and connective tissue**

756.81 Absence of muscle and tendon
Absence of muscle (pectoral)

756.82 Accessory muscle

756.83 Ehlers-Danlos syndrome

756.89 Other
Amyotrophia congenita
Congenital shortening of tendon

756.9 Other and unspecified anomalies of musculoskeletal system
Congenital:
  anomaly NOS of musculoskeletal system, not elsewhere classified
  deformity NOS of musculoskeletal system, not elsewhere classified

● Code new
  to this edition

▲ Revision of
  existing code

④ ⑤ Fourth or fifth
  digit required

757 Congenital anomalies of the integument
Includes: anomalies of skin, subcutaneous tissue, hair, nails, and breast
Excludes: *hemangioma (228.00-228.09)*
pigmented nevus (216.0-216.9)

DEFINITION Congenital anomalies of the integument refers to defects of the integumentary system that are present at birth.

757.0 Hereditary edema of legs
Congenital lymphedema   Milroy's disease
Hereditary trophedema

757.1 Ichthyosis congenita
Congenital ichthyosis
Harlequin fetus
Ichthyosiform erythroderma

757.2 Dermatoglyphic anomalies
Abnormal palmar creases

⑤ **757.3 Other specified anomalies of skin**

757.31 Congenital ectodermal dysplasia

757.32 Vascular hamartomas
Birthmarks
Port-wine stain
Strawberry nevus

757.33 Congenital pigmentary anomalies of skin
Congenital poikiloderma
Urticaria pigmentosa
Xeroderma pigmentosum

Excludes: *albinism (270.2)*

757.39 Other
Accessory skin tags, congenital
Congenital scar
Epidermolysis bullosa
Keratoderma (congenital)

Excludes: *pilonidal cyst (685.0-685.1)*

757.4 Specified anomalies of hair
Congenital: Congenital:
alopecia   hypertrichosis
atrichosis   monilethrix
beaded hair   Persistent lanugo

757.5 Specified anomalies of nails
Anonychia   Congenital:
Congenital: leukonychia
clubnail   onychauxis
koilonychia   pachyonychia

757.6 Specified congenital anomalies of breast
Congenital absent breast or nipple
Accessory breast or nipple
Supernumerary breast or nipple

Excludes: *absence of pectoral muscle (756.81)*
hypoplasia of breast (611.82)
micromastia (611.82)

757.8 Other specified anomalies of the integument

757.9 Unspecified anomaly of the integument
Congenital:
anomaly NOS of integument
deformity NOS of integument

758 Chromosomal anomalies
Includes: syndromes associated with anomalies in the number and form of chromosomes
Use additional codes for conditions associated with the chromosomal anomalies

DEFINITION Chromosomal anomalies refer to changes in the normal structure or number of chromosomes; often resulting in physical or mental abnormalities

758.0 Down's syndrome
Mongolism   Trisomy:
Translocation Down's   21 or 22
syndrome   G

| Add 4th or 5th digit | Nonspecific code | Unspecified code | Manifestation code |

758.1 Patau's syndrome
Trisomy:
13
D$_1$

758.2 Edwards' syndrome
Trisomy:
18
E$_3$

⑤ **758.3 Autosomal deletion syndromes**

    758.31 Cri-du-chat syndrome
    Deletion 5p

    758.32 Velo-cardio-facial syndrome
    Deletion 22q11.2

    758.33 Other microdeletions
    Miller-Dieker syndrome
    Smith-Magenis syndrome

    758.39 Other autosomal deletions

758.4 Balanced autosomal translocation in normal individual

758.5 Other conditions due to autosomal anomalies
Accessory autosomes NEC

758.6 Gonadal dysgenesis
Ovarian dysgenesis
Turner's syndrome
XO syndrome

   Excludes: *pure gonadal dysgenesis (752.7)*

758.7 Klinefelter's syndrome
XXY syndrome

⑤ **758.8 Other conditions due to chromosome anomalies**

    758.81 Other conditions due to sex chromosome anomalies

    758.89 Other

758.9 Conditions due to anomaly of unspecified chromosome

759 Other and unspecified congenital anomalies

759.0 Anomalies of spleen

Aberrant spleen	Congenital splenomegaly
Absent spleen	Ectopic spleen
Accessory spleen	Lobulation of spleen

759.1 Anomalies of adrenal gland
Aberrant adrenal gland
Absent adrenal gland
Accessory adrenal gland

   Excludes: *adrenogenital disorders (255.2)*
        congenital disorders of steroid metabolism (255.2)

759.2 Anomalies of other endocrine glands
Absent parathyroid gland
Accessory thyroid gland
Persistent thyroglossal or thyrolingual duct
Thyroglossal (duct) cyst

   Excludes: *congenital:*
        goiter (246.1)
        hypothyroidism (243)

759.3 Situs inversus
Situs inversus or transversus:
abdominalis
thoracis
Transposition of viscera:
abdominal
thoracic

   Excludes: *dextrocardia without mention of complete transposition (746.87)*

759.4 Conjoined twins

Craniopagus	Thoracopagus
Dicephalus	Xiphopagus
Pygopagus	

● Code new
   to this edition

▲ Revision of
   existing code

④ ⑤ Fourth or fifth
     digit required

759.5 Tuberous sclerosis
Bourneville's disease
Epiloia

759.6 Other hamartoses, not elsewhere classified
Syndrome:
Peutz-Jeghers
Sturge-Weber (-Dimitri)
von Hippel-Lindau

Excludes: *neurofibromatosis (237.70-237.79)*

759.7 Multiple congenital anomalies, so described
Congenital:
anomaly, multiple NOS
deformity, multiple NOS

⑤ **759.8 Other specified anomalies**

759.81 Prader-Willi syndrome

759.82 Marfan syndrome

759.83 Fragile X syndrome

759.89 Other
Congenital malformation syndromes affecting multiple systems, not elsewhere
classified
Laurence-Moon-Biedl syndrome

759.9 Congenital anomaly, unspecified

This page intentionally left blank.

● Code new
  to this edition
▲ Revision of
  existing code
④ ⑤ Fourth or fifth
  digit required

Chapter 15: Newborn (Perinatal) Guidelines (760-779)

DEFINITIONS AND CODING ALERTS

This chapter includes definitions of selected key words, terms and phrases and coding alerts for adding points to the clinical domain, references to coding late effects where appropriate, and references to personal history V-codes in situations where the acute or chronic condition is no longer active. An example from this chapter is as follows:

> **771.81   Septicemia [sepsis] of newborn**
> **ALERT** This code should be assigned with a secondary code from category 041, Bacterial infections in conditions classified elsewhere and of unspecified site, to identify the organism. A code from 038, Septicemia should not be used on a newborn record. Do not assign code 995.91, Sepsis, as code 771.81 describes the sepsis.
> **ALERT** If applicable, use additional codes to identify severe sepsis (995.92) and any associated acute organ dysfunction.

MULTIPLE CODING FOR A SINGLE CONDITION

In addition to the etiology or manifestation convention that requires two codes to fully describe a single condition that affects multiple body systems, there are other single conditions that also require more than one code. "Use additional code" notes are found in the tabular at codes that are not part of an etiology or manifestation pair where a secondary code is useful to fully describe a condition. The sequencing rule is the same as the etiology or manifestation pair - , "use additional code" indicates that a secondary code should be added.

"Code first" notes are also under certain codes that are not specifically manifestation codes but may be due to an underlying cause. When a "code first" note is present and an underlying condition is present the underlying condition should be sequenced first.

"Code, if applicable, any causal condition first", notes indicate that this code may be assigned as a principal diagnosis when the causal condition is unknown or not applicable. If a causal condition is known, then the code for that condition should be sequenced as the principal or first-listed diagnosis. Multiple codes may be needed for late effects, complication codes and obstetric codes to more fully describe a condition. See the specific guidelines for these conditions for further instruction.

COMBINATION CODE

A combination code is a single code used to classify: two diagnoses, or a diagnosis with an associated secondary process (manifestation) A diagnosis with an associated complication Combination codes are identified by referring to subterm entries in the Alphabetic Index and by reading the inclusion and exclusion notes in the Tabular List.

Assign only the combination code when that code fully identifies the diagnostic conditions involved or when the Alphabetic Index so directs. Multiple coding should not be used when the classification provides a combination code that clearly identifies all of the elements documented in the diagnosis. When the combination code lacks necessary specificity in describing the manifestation or complication, an additional code should be used as a secondary code.

CODING LATE EFFECTS

A late effect is the residual effect (condition produced) after the acute phase of an illness or injury has terminated. There is no time limit on when a late effect code can be used. The residual may be apparent early, such as in cerebrovascular accident cases, or it may occur months or years later, such as that due to a previous injury. Coding of late effects generally requires two codes sequenced in the following order: The condition or nature of the late effect is sequenced first. The late effect code is sequenced second.

An exception to the above guidelines are those instances where the code for late effect is followed by a manifestation code identified in the Tabular List and title, or the late effect code has been expanded (at the fourth and fifth-digit levels) to include the manifestation(s). The code for the acute phase of an illness or injury that led to the late effect is never used with a code for the late effect.

For coding and reporting purposes the perinatal period is defined as before birth through the 28th day following birth. The following guidelines are provided for reporting purposes. Hospitals may record other diagnoses as needed for internal data use.

Add 4th or 5th digit	Nonspecific code	Unspecified code	Manifestation code

GENERAL PERINATAL RULES

Chapter 15 Codes

They are never for use on the maternal record. Codes from Chapter 11, the obstetric chapter, are never permitted on the newborn record. Chapter 15 code may be used throughout the life of the patient if the condition is still present.

Sequencing of perinatal codes

Generally, codes from Chapter 15 should be sequenced as the principal or first-listed diagnosis on the newborn record, with the exception of the appropriate V30 code for the birth episode, followed by codes from any other chapter that provide additional detail. The "use additional code" note at the beginning of the chapter supports this guideline. If the index does not provide a specific code for a perinatal condition, assign code 779.89, Other specified conditions originating in the perinatal period, followed by the code from another chapter that specifies the condition. Codes for signs and symptoms may be assigned when a definitive diagnosis has not been established.

Birth process or community acquired conditions

If a newborn has a condition that may be either due to the birth process or community acquired and the documentation does not indicate which it is, the default is due to the birth process and the code from Chapter 15 should be used. If the condition is community-acquired, a code from Chapter 15 should not be assigned.

Code all clinically significant conditions

All clinically significant conditions noted on routine newborn examination should be coded. A condition is clinically significant if it requires:

- clinical evaluation; or
- therapeutic treatment; or
- diagnostic procedures; or
- extended length of hospital stay; or
- increased nursing care and/or monitoring; or
- has implications for future health care needs

Note: The perinatal guidelines listed above are the same as the general coding guidelines for "additional diagnoses", except for the final point regarding implications for future health care needs. Codes should be assigned for conditions that have been specified by the provider as having implications for future health care needs. Codes from the perinatal chapter should not be assigned unless the provider has established a definitive diagnosis.

USE OF CODES V30-V39

When coding the birth of an infant, assign a code from categories V30-V39, according to the type of birth. A code from this series is assigned as a principal diagnosis, and assigned only once to a newborn at the time of birth.

NEWBORN TRANSFERS

If the newborn is transferred to another institution, the V30 series is not used at the receiving hospital.

USE OF CATEGORY V29

Assigning a code from category V29

Assign a code from category V29, Observation and evaluation of newborns and infants for suspected conditions not found, to identify those instances when a healthy newborn is evaluated for a suspected condition that is determined after study not to be present. Do not use a code from category V29 when the patient has identified signs or symptoms of a suspected problem; in such cases, code the sign or symptom.

A code from category V29 may also be assigned as a principal code for readmissions or encounters when the V30 code no longer applies. Codes from category V29 are for use only for healthy newborns and infants for which no condition after study is found to be present.

A V29 code is to be used as a secondary code after the V30, Outcome of delivery, code.

USE OF OTHER V CODES ON PERINATAL RECORDS

V codes other than V30 and V29 may be assigned on a perinatal or newborn record code. The codes may be used as a principal or first listed diagnosis for specific types of encounters or for readmissions or encounters when the V30 code no longer applies.

See Official Guidelines, Section I.C.18 for information regarding the assignment of V codes.

MATERNAL CAUSES OF PERINATAL MORBIDITY

Codes from categories 760-763, Maternal causes of perinatal morbidity and mortality, are assigned only when the maternal condition has actually affected the fetus or newborn. The fact that the mother has an associated medical condition or experiences some complication of pregnancy, labor or delivery does not justify the routine assignment of codes from these categories to the newborn record.

CONGENITAL ANOMALIES IN NEWBORNS

For the birth admission, the appropriate code from category V30, Liveborn infants according to type of birth, should be used, followed by any congenital anomaly codes, categories 740-759. Use additional secondary codes from other chapters to specify conditions associated with the anomaly, if applicable.

Also, see Official Guidelines, Section I.C.14 for information on the coding of congenital anomalies.

CODING ADDITIONAL PERINATAL DIAGNOSES

Assigning codes for conditions that require treatment

Assign codes for conditions that require treatment or further investigation, prolong the length of stay, or require resource utilization.

Codes for conditions specified as having implications for future health care needs

Assign codes for conditions that have been specified by the provider as having implications for future health care needs. This guideline should not be used for adult patients.

Codes for newborn conditions originating in the perinatal period

Assign a code for newborn conditions originating in the perinatal period (categories 760-779, as well as complications arising during the current episode of care classified in other chapters, only if the diagnoses have been documented by the responsible provider at the time of transfer or discharge as having affected the fetus or newborn.

PREMATURITY AND FETAL GROWTH RETARDATION

Providers utilize different criteria in determining prematurity. A code for prematurity should not be assigned unless it is documented. The 5th digit assignment for codes from category 764 and subcategories 765.0 and 765.1 should be based on the recorded birth weight and estimated gestational age.

A code from subcategory 765.2, Weeks of gestation, should be assigned as an additional code with category 764 and codes from 765.0 and 765.1 to specify weeks of gestation as documented by the provider in the record.

NEWBORN SEPSIS

Code 771.81, Septicemia [sepsis] of newborn, should be assigned with a secondary code from category 041, Bacterial infections in conditions classified elsewhere and of unspecified site, to identify the organism.

A code from category 038, Septicemia, should not be used on a newborn record. Do not assign code 995.91, Sepsis, as code 771.81 describes the sepsis. If applicable, use additional codes to identify severe sepsis (995.92) and any associated acute organ dysfunction.

	Add 4th or 5th digit		Nonspecific code		Unspecified code		Manifestation code

This page intentionally left blank.

● Code new
to this edition

▲ Revision of
existing code

④ ⑤ Fourth or fifth
digit required

15. CERTAIN CONDITIONS ORIGINATING IN THE PERINATAL PERIOD (760-779)

Includes: conditions which have their origin in the perinatal period, before birth through the first 28 days after birth, even though death or morbidity occurs later

Use additional code(s) to further specify condition

MATERNAL CAUSES OF PERINATAL MORBIDITY AND MORTALITY (760-763)

ALERT! For personal history of perinatal problems see V13.7

760 Fetus or newborn affected by maternal conditions which may be unrelated to present pregnancy

Includes: the listed maternal conditions only when specified as a cause of mortality or morbidity of the fetus or newborn

Excludes: *maternal endocrine and metabolic disorders affecting fetus or newborn (775.0-775.9)*

760.0 Maternal hypertensive disorders
Fetus or newborn affected by maternal conditions classifiable to 642

760.1 Maternal renal and urinary tract diseases
Fetus or newborn affected by maternal conditions classifiable to 580-599

760.2 Maternal infections
Fetus or newborn affected by maternal infectious disease classifiable to 001-136 and 487, but fetus or newborn not manifesting that disease

Excludes: *congenital infectious diseases (771.0-771.8)*
maternal genital tract and other localized infections (760.8)

760.3 Other chronic maternal circulatory and respiratory diseases
Fetus or newborn affected by chronic maternal conditions classifiable to 390-459, 490-519, 745-748

760.4 Maternal nutritional disorders
Fetus or newborn affected by:
maternal disorders classifiable to 260-269
maternal malnutrition NOS

Excludes: *fetal malnutrition (764.10-764.29)*

760.5 Maternal injury
Fetus or newborn affected by maternal conditions classifiable to 800-995

⑤ **760.6 Surgical operation on mother and fetus**

Excludes: *cesarean section for present delivery (763.4)*
damage to placenta from amniocentesis, cesarean section, or surgical induction (762.1)

    760.61 Newborn affected by amniocentesis

Excludes: *fetal complications from amniocentesis (679.1)*

    760.62 Newborn affected by other in utero procedure

Excludes: *fetal complications of in utero procedure (679.1)*

    760.63 Newborn affected by other surgical operations on mother during pregnancy

Excludes: *newborn affected by previous surgical procedure on mother not associated with pregnancy (760.64)*

    760.64 Newborn affected by previous surgical procedure on mother not associated with pregnancy

⑤ **760.7 Noxious influences affecting fetus or newborn via placenta or breast milk**
Fetus or newborn affected by noxious substance transmitted via placenta or breast milk

Excludes: *anesthetic and analgesic drugs administered during labor and delivery (763.5)*
drug withdrawal syndrome in newborn (779.5)

    760.70 Unspecified noxious substance
Fetus or newborn affected by:
Drug NEC

    760.71 Alcohol
Fetal alcohol syndrome

    760.72 Narcotics

    760.73 Hallucinogenic agents

    760.74 Anti-infectives
Antibiotics
Antifungals

    760.75 Cocaine

	Add 4th or 5th digit		Nonspecific code		Unspecified code		Manifestation code

760.76 Diethylstilbestrol (DES)

760.77 Anticonvulsants
Carbamazepine
Phenobarbital
Phenytoin
Valproic acid

760.78 Antimetabolic agents
Methotrexate
Retinoic acid
Statins

760.79 Other
Fetus or newborn affected by:
immune sera transmitted via placenta or breast milk
medicinal agents NEC transmitted via placenta or breast milk
toxic substance NEC transmitted via placenta or breast milk

760.8 Other specified maternal conditions affecting fetus or newborn
Maternal genital tract and other localized infection affecting fetus or newborn, but fetus or newborn not manifesting that disease

Excludes: maternal urinary tract infection affecting fetus or newborn (760.1)

760.9 Unspecified maternal condition affecting fetus or newborn

761 Fetus or newborn affected by maternal complications of pregnancy
Includes: the listed maternal conditions only when specified as a cause of mortality or morbidity of the fetus or newborn

761.0 Incompetent cervix

761.1 Premature rupture of membranes

761.2 Oligohydramnios

Excludes: that due to premature rupture of membranes (761.1)

761.3 Polyhydramnios
Hydramnios (acute) (chronic)

761.4 Ectopic pregnancy
Pregnancy:
abdominal
intraperitoneal
tubal

761.5 Multiple pregnancy
Triplet (pregnancy)
Twin (pregnancy)

761.6 Maternal death

761.7 Malpresentation before labor
Breech presentation before labor
External version before labor
Oblique lie before labor
Transverse lie before labor
Unstable lie before labor

761.8 Other specified maternal complications of pregnancy affecting fetus or newborn
Spontaneous abortion, fetus

761.9 Unspecified maternal complication of pregnancy affecting fetus or newborn

762 Fetus or newborn affected by complications of placenta, cord, and membranes
Includes: the listed maternal conditions only when specified as a cause of mortality or morbidity in the fetus or newborn

762.0 Placenta previa

762.1 Other forms of placental separation and hemorrhage
Abruptio placentae
Antepartum hemorrhage
Damage to placenta from amniocentesis, cesarean section, or surgical induction
Maternal blood loss
Premature separation of placenta
Rupture of marginal sinus

762.2 Other and unspecified morphological and functional abnormalities of placenta
Placental:
dysfunction
infarction
insufficiency

● Code new
to this edition

▲ Revision of
existing code

④ ⑤ Fourth or fifth
digit required

762.3 Placental transfusion syndromes
> Placental and cord abnormality resulting in twin-to-twin or other transplacental transfusion

Use additional code to indicate resultant condition in newborn:
> fetal blood loss (772.0)
> polycythemia neonatorum (776.4)

762.4 Prolapsed cord
> Cord presentation

762.5 Other compression of umbilical cord
> Cord around neck   Knot in cord
> Entanglement of cord   Torsion of cord

762.6 Other and unspecified conditions of umbilical cord
> Short umbilical cord
> Thrombosis of umbilical cord
> Varices of umbilical cord
> Velamentous insertion of umbilical cord
> Vasa previa

> *Excludes:* *infection of umbilical cord (771.4)*
> *single umbilical artery (747.5)*

762.7 Chorioamnionitis
> Amnionitis
> Membranitis
> Placentitis

762.8 Other specified abnormalities of chorion and amnion

762.9 Unspecified abnormality of chorion and amnion

763 Fetus or newborn affected by other complications of labor and delivery
> Includes: the listed conditions only when specified as a cause of mortality or morbidity in the fetus or newborn

> *Excludes:* *newborn affected by surgical procedures on mother (760.61-760.64)*

763.0 Breech delivery and extraction

763.1 Other malpresentation, malposition, and disproportion during labor and delivery
> Fetus or newborn affected by:
> abnormality of bony pelvis
> contracted pelvis
> persistent occipitoposterior position
> shoulder presentation
> transverse lie
> conditions classifiable to 652, 653, and 660

763.2 Forceps delivery
> Fetus or newborn affected by forceps extraction

763.3 Delivery by vacuum extractor

763.4 Cesarean delivery
> *Excludes:* *placental separation or hemorrhage from cesarean section (762.1)*

763.5 Maternal anesthesia and analgesia
> Reactions and intoxications from maternal opiates and tranquilizers during labor and delivery

> *Excludes:* *drug withdrawal syndrome in newborn (779.5)*

763.6 Precipitate delivery
> Rapid second stage

763.7 Abnormal uterine contractions
> Fetus or newborn affected by:
> contraction ring
> hypertonic labor
> hypotonic uterine dysfunction
> uterine inertia or dysfunction
> conditions classifiable to 661, except 661.3

⑤ **763.8 Other specified complications of labor and delivery affecting fetus or newborn**

> **763.81 Abnormality in fetal heart rate or rhythm before the onset of labor**

> **763.82 Abnormality in fetal heart rate or rhythm during labor**

> **763.83 Abnormality in fetal heart rate or rhythm, unspecified as to time of onset**

	Add 4th or 5th digit		Nonspecific code		Unspecified code		Manifestation code

763.84 Meconium passage during delivery

Excludes: *meconium aspiration (770.11, 770.12)*
meconium staining (779.84)

763.89 Other specified complications of labor and delivery affecting fetus or newborn

Fetus or newborn affected by:
abnormality of maternal soft tissues
destructive operation on live fetus to facilitate delivery
induction of labor (medical)
other conditions classifiable to 650-669
other procedures used in labor and delivery

763.9 Unspecified complication of labor and delivery affecting fetus or newborn

OTHER CONDITIONS ORIGINATING IN THE PERINATAL PERIOD (764-779)

The following fifth-digit subclassification is for use with categories 764 and codes 765.0 and 765.1 to denote birthweight:

0 unspecified [weight]
1 less than 500 grams
2 500-749 grams
3 750-999 grams
4 1,000- 1,249 grams
5 1,250-1,499 grams
6 1,500-1,749 grams
7 1,750-1,999 grams
8 2,000-2,499 grams
9 2,500 grams and over

⑤ **764** Slow fetal growth and fetal malnutrition

⑤ 764.0 "Light-for-dates" without mention of fetal malnutrition
[0-9] Infants underweight for gestational age
"Small-for-dates"

⑤ 764.1 "Light-for-dates" with signs of fetal malnutrition
[0-9] Infants "light-for-dates" classifiable to 764.0, who in addition show signs of fetal malnutrition, such as dry peeling skin and loss of subcutaneous tissue

⑤ 764.2 Fetal malnutrition without mention of "light-for-dates"
[0-9] Infants, not underweight for gestational age, showing signs of fetal malnutrition, such as dry peeling skin and loss of subcutaneous tissue
Intrauterine malnutrition

⑤ 764.9 Fetal growth retardation, unspecified
[0-9] Intrauterine growth retardation

765 Disorders relating to short gestation and low birthweight
Includes: the listed conditions, without further specification, as causes of mortality, morbidity, or additional care, in fetus or newborn

⑤ 765.0 Extreme immaturity
[0-9]
Note: Usually implies a birthweight of less than 1000 grams
Use additional code for weeks of gestation (765.20-765.29)

⑤ 765.1 Other preterm infants
[0-9] Prematurity NOS
Prematurity or small size, not classifiable to 765.0 or as "light-for-dates" in 764
Note: Usually implies a birthweight of 1000-2499 grams
Use additional code for weeks of gestation (765.20-765.29)

⑤ 765.2 Weeks of gestation
765.20 Unspecified weeks of gestation
765.21 Less than 24 completed weeks of gestation
765.22 24 completed weeks of gestation
765.23 25-26 completed weeks of gestation
765.24 27-28 completed weeks of gestation
765.25 29-30 completed weeks of gestation
765.26 31-32 completed weeks of gestation

● Code new to this edition ▲ Revision of existing code ④ ⑤ Fourth or fifth digit required

765.27 33-34 completed weeks of gestation

765.28 35-36 completed weeks of gestation

765.29 37 or more completed weeks of gestation

766 **Disorders relating to long gestation and high birthweight**
Includes: the listed conditions, without further specification, as causes of mortality, morbidity, or additional care, in fetus or newborn

766.0 Exceptionally large baby
Note: Usually implies a birthweight of 4500 grams or more.

766.1 Other "heavy-for-dates" infants
Other fetus or infant "heavy-" or "large-for-dates" regardless of period of gestation

⑤ **766.2 Late infant, not "heavy-for-dates"**

766.21 Post-term infant
Infant with gestation period over 40 completed weeks to 42 completed weeks

766.22 Prolonged gestation of infant
Infant with gestation period over 42 completed weeks
Postmaturity NOS

767 **Birth trauma**

767.0 Subdural and cerebral hemorrhage
Subdural and cerebral hemorrhage, whether described as due to birth trauma or to intrapartum anoxia or hypoxia
Subdural hematoma (localized)
Tentorial tear
Use additional code, if desired, to identify cause

Excludes: *intraventricular hemorrhage (772.10-772.14)*
subarachnoid hemorrhage (772.2)

⑤ **767.1 Injuries to scalp**

767.11 Epicranial subaponeurotic hemorrhage (massive)
Subgaleal hemorrhage

767.19 Other injuries to scalp
Caput succedaneum
Cephalhematoma
Chignon (from vacuum extraction)

767.2 Fracture of clavicle

767.3 Other injuries to skeleton
Fracture of:
long bones
skull

Excludes: *congenital dislocation of hip (754.30-754.35)*
fracture of spine, congenital (767.4)

767.4 Injury to spine and spinal cord
Dislocation of spine or spinal cord due to birth trauma
Fracture of spine or spinal cord due to birth trauma
Laceration of spine or spinal cord due to birth trauma
Rupture of spine or spinal cord due to birth trauma

767.5 Facial nerve injury
Facial palsy

767.6 Injury to brachial plexus
Palsy or paralysis:
brachial
Erb (-Duchenne)
Klumpke (-Déjérine)

767.7 Other cranial and peripheral nerve injuries
Phrenic nerve paralysis

767.8 Other specified birth trauma

Eye damage	Rupture of:
Hematoma of:	liver
liver (subcapsular)	spleen
testes	Scalpel wound
vulva	Traumatic glaucoma

Excludes: *hemorrhage classifiable to 772.0-772.9*

767.9 Birth trauma, unspecified
Birth injury NOS

Add 4th or 5th digit	Nonspecific code	Unspecified code	Manifestation code

768 **Intrauterine hypoxia and birth asphyxia**
Use only when associated with newborn morbidity classifiable elsewhere

> Excludes: *acidemia NOS of newborn (775.81)*
> *acidosis NOS of newborn (775.81)*
> *cerebral ischemia NOS (779.2)*
> *hypoxia NOS of newborn (770.88)*
> *mixed metabolic and respiratory acidosis of newborn (775.81)*
> *respiratory arrest of newborn (770.87)*

768.0 **Fetal death from asphyxia or anoxia before onset of labor or at unspecified time**

768.1 **Fetal death from asphyxia or anoxia during labor**

768.2 **Fetal distress before onset of labor, in liveborn infant**
Fetal metabolic acidemia before onset of labor, in liveborn infant

768.3 **Fetal distress first noted during labor and delivery, in liveborn infant**
Fetal metabolic acidemia first noted during labor and delivery, in liveborn infant

768.4 **Fetal distress, unspecified as to time of onset, in liveborn infant**
Fetal metabolic acidemia unspecified as to time of onset, in liveborn infant

768.5 **Severe birth asphyxia**
Birth asphyxia with neurologic involvement

> Excludes: *hypoxic-ischemic encephalopathy (HIE) (768.70-768.73)*

768.6 **Mild or moderate birth asphyxia**
Other specified birth asphyxia (without mention of neurologic involvement)

> Excludes: *hypoxic-ischemic encephalopathy (HIE) (768.70-768.73)*

⑤ **768.7** **Hypoxic-ischemic encephalopathy (HIE)**

768.70 **Hypoxic-ischemic encephalopathy, unspecified**

768.71 **Mild hypoxic-ischemic encephalopathy**

768.72 **Moderate hypoxic-ischemic encephalopathy**

768.73 **Severe hypoxic-ischemic encephalopathy**

768.9 **Unspecified birth asphyxia in liveborn infant**
Anoxia NOS, in liveborn infant
Asphyxia NOS, in liveborn infant

769 **Respiratory distress syndrome**
Cardiorespiratory distress syndrome of newborn
Hyaline membrane disease (pulmonary)
Idiopathic respiratory distress syndrome [IRDS or RDS] of newborn
Pulmonary hypoperfusion syndrome

> Excludes: *transient tachypnea of newborn (770.6)*

770 **Other respiratory conditions of fetus and newborn**

770.0 **Congenital pneumonia**
Infective pneumonia acquired prenatally

> Excludes: *pneumonia from infection acquired after birth (480.0-486)*

⑤ **770.1** **Fetal and newborn aspiration**

> Excludes: *aspiration of postnatal stomach contents (770.85, 770.86)*
> *meconium passage during delivery (763.84)*
> *meconium staining (779.84)*

770.10 **Fetal and newborn aspiration, unspecified**

770.11 **Meconium aspiration without respiratory symptoms**
Meconium aspiration NOS

770.12 **Meconium aspiration with respiratory symptoms**
Meconium aspiration pneumonia
Meconium aspiration pneumonitis
Meconium aspiration syndrome NOS
Use additional code to identify any secondary pulmonary hypertension (416.8), if applicable

770.13 **Aspiration of clear amniotic fluid without respiratory symptoms**
Aspiration of clear amniotic fluid NOS

770.14 **Aspiration of clear amniotic fluid with respiratory symptoms**
Aspiration of clear amniotic fluid with pneumonia
Aspiration of clear amniotic fluid with pneumonitis
Use additional code to identify any secondary pulmonary hypertension (416.8), if applicable

● Code new to this edition　　▲ Revision of existing code　　④ ⑤ Fourth or fifth digit required

770.15 Aspiration of blood without respiratory symptoms
Aspiration of blood NOS

770.16 Aspiration of blood with respiratory symptoms
Aspiration of blood with pneumonia
Aspiration of blood with pneumonitis
Use additional code to identify any secondary pulmonary hypertension (416.8), if applicable

770.17 Other fetal and newborn aspiration without respiratory symptoms

770.18 Other fetal and newborn aspiration with respiratory symptoms
Other aspiration pneumonia
Other aspiration pneumonitis
Use additional code to identify any secondary pulmonary hypertension (416.8), if applicable

770.2 Interstitial emphysema and related conditions
Pneumomediastinum originating in the perinatal period
Pneumopericardium originating in the perinatal period
Pneumothorax originating in the perinatal period

770.3 Pulmonary hemorrhage
Hemorrhage:
alveolar (lung) originating in the perinatal period
intra-alveolar (lung) originating in the perinatal period
massive pulmonary originating in the perinatal period

770.4 Primary atelectasis
Pulmonary immaturity NOS

770.5 Other and unspecified atelectasis
Atelectasis:
NOS, originating in the perinatal period
partial, originating in the perinatal period
secondary, originating in the perinatal period
Pulmonary collapse, originating in the perinatal period

770.6 Transitory tachypnea of newborn
Idiopathic tachypnea of newborn
Wet lung syndrome

Excludes: respiratory distress syndrome (769)

770.7 Chronic respiratory disease arising in the perinatal period
Bronchopulmonary dysplasia
Interstitial pulmonary fibrosis of prematurity
Wilson-Mikity syndrome

⑤ **770.8 Other respiratory problems after birth**

Excludes: mixed metabolic and respiratory acidosis of newborn (775.81)

770.81 Primary apnea of newborn
Apneic spells of newborn NOS
Essential apnea of newborn
Sleep apnea of newborn

770.82 Other apnea of newborn
Obstructure apnea of newborn

770.83 Cyanotic attacks of newborn

770.84 Respiratory failure of newborn

Excludes: respiratory distress syndrome (769)

770.85 Aspiration of postnatal stomach contents without respiratory symptoms
Aspiration of postnatal stomach contents NOS

770.86 Aspiration of postnatal stomach contents with respiratory symptoms
Aspiration of postnatal stomach contents with pneumonia
Aspiration of postnatal stomach contents with pneumonitis
Use additional code to identify any secondary pulmonary hypertension (416.8), if applicable

770.87 Respiratory arrest of newborn

770.88 Hypoxemia of newborn
Hypoxia NOS of newborn

770.89 Other respiratory problems after birth

770.9 Unspecified respiratory condition of fetus and newborn

| Add 4th or 5th digit | Nonspecific code | Unspecified code | Manifestation code |

771 **Infections specific to the perinatal period**
  Includes: infections acquired before or during birth via the umbilicus or during the first 28 days after birth

  Excludes: congenital pneumonia (770.0)
    congenital syphilis (090.0-090.9)
    infant botulism (040.41)
    maternal infectious disease as a cause of mortality or morbidity in fetus or newborn, but fetus or newborn not manifesting the disease (760.2)
    ophthalmia neonatorum due to gonococcus (098.40)
    other infections not specifically classified to this category

771.0 **Congenital rubella**
  Congenital rubella pneumonitis

771.1 **Congenital cytomegalovirus infection**
  Congenital cytomegalic inclusion disease

771.2 **Other congenital infections**
  Congenital:
    herpes simplex
    listeriosis
    malaria
  Congenital:
    toxoplasmosis
    tuberculosis

771.3 **Tetanus neonatorum**
  Tetanus omphalitis

  Excludes: hypocalcemic tetany (775.4)

771.4 **Omphalitis of the newborn**
  Infection:
    navel cord
    umbilical stump

  Excludes: tetanus omphalitis (771.3)

771.5 **Neonatal infective mastitis**

  Excludes: noninfective neonatal mastitis (778.7)

771.6 **Neonatal conjunctivitis and dacryocystitis**
  Ophthalmia neonatorum NOS

  Excludes: ophthalmia neonatorum due to gonococcus (098.40)

771.7 **Neonatal Candida infection**
  Neonatal moniliasis
  Thrush in newborn

⑤ **771.8** **Other infections specific to the perinatal period**
  Use additional code to identify organism or specific infection

  771.81 **Septicemia [sepsis] of newborn**
    Use additional code(s) to identify severe sepsis (995.92) and any associated acute organ dysfunction, if applicable

    ALERT This code should be assigned with a secondary code from category 041, Bacterial infections in conditions classified elsewhere and of unspecified site, to identify the organism. A code from 038, Septicemia should not be used on a newborn record. Do not assign code 995.91, Sepsis, as code 771.81 describes the sepsis.
    ALERT If applicable, use additional codes to identify severe sepsis (995.92) and any associated acute organ dysfunction.

  771.82 **Urinary tract infection of newborn**

  771.83 **Bacteremia of newborn**

  771.89 **Other infections specific to the perinatal period**
    Intra-amniotic infection of fetus NOS
    Infection of newborn NOS

772 **Fetal and neonatal hemorrhage**

  Excludes: fetal hematologic conditions complicating pregnancy (678.0)
    hematological disorders of fetus and newborn (776.0-776.9)

772.0 **Fetal blood loss affecting newborn**
  Fetal blood loss from:
    cut end of co-twin's cord
    placenta
    ruptured cord
    vasa previa
  Fetal exsanguination
  Fetal hemorrhage into:
    co-twin
    mother's circulation

⑤ **772.1** **Intraventricular hemorrhage**
  Intraventricular hemorrhage from any perinatal cause

● Code new to this edition ▲ Revision of existing code ④ ⑤ Fourth or fifth digit required

772.10 Unspecified grade

772.11 Grade I
Bleeding into germinal matrix

772.12 Grade II
Bleeding into ventricle

772.13 Grade III
Bleeding with enlargement of ventricle

772.14 Grade IV
Bleeding into cerebral cortex

772.2 Subarachnoid hemorrhage
Subarachnoid hemorrhage from any perinatal cause

Excludes: *subdural and cerebral hemorrhage (767.0)*

772.3 Umbilical hemorrhage after birth
Slipped umbilical ligature

772.4 Gastrointestinal hemorrhage

Excludes: *swallowed maternal blood (777.3)*

772.5 Adrenal hemorrhage

772.6 Cutaneous hemorrhage
Bruising in fetus or newborn
Ecchymoses in fetus or newborn
Petechiae in fetus or newborn
Superficial hematoma in fetus or newborn

772.8 Other specified hemorrhage of fetus or newborn

Excludes: *hemorrhagic disease of newborn (776.0)*
pulmonary hemorrhage (770.3)

772.9 Unspecified hemorrhage of newborn

773 Hemolytic disease of fetus or newborn, due to isoimmunization

773.0 Hemolytic disease due to Rh isoimmunization
Anemia due to RH:
  antibodies
  isoimmunization
  maternal/fetal incompatibility
Erythroblastosis (fetalis) due to RH:
  antibodies
  isoimmunization
  maternal/fetal incompatibility
Hemolytic disease (fetus) (newborn) due to RH:
  antibodies
  isoimmunization
  maternal/fetal incompatibility
Jaundice due to RH:
  antibodies
  isoimmunization
  maternal/fetal incompatibility
Rh hemolytic disease
Rh isoimmunization

773.1 Hemolytic disease due to ABO isoimmunization
ABO hemolytic disease
ABO isoimmunization
Anemia due to ABO: antibodies, isoimmunization, or maternal/fetal incompatibility
Erythroblastosis (fetalis) due to ABO:
  antibodies
  isoimmunization
  maternal/fetal incompatibility
Hemolytic disease (fetus) (newborn) due to ABO:
  antibodies
  isoimmunization
  maternal/fetal incompatibility
Jaundice due to ABO:
  antibodies
  isoimmunization
  maternal/fetal incompatibility

773.2 Hemolytic disease due to other and unspecified isoimmunization
Erythroblastosis (fetalis) (neonatorum) NOS
Hemolytic disease (fetus) (newborn) NOS
Jaundice or anemia due to other and unspecified blood-group incompatibility

773.3 Hydrops fetalis due to isoimmunization
Use additional code, if desired, to identify type of isoimmunization (773.0-773.2)

773.4 Kernicterus due to isoimmunization
Use additional code, if desired, to identify type of isoimmunization (773.0-773.2)

773.5 Late anemia due to isoimmunization

774 Other perinatal jaundice
DEFINITION Jaundice is a condition in which a person's skin and the whites of the eyes are discolored yellow due to an increased level of bile pigments in the blood.

774.0 *Perinatal jaundice from hereditary hemolytic anemias*
Code first underlying disease (282.0-282.9)

774.1 Perinatal jaundice from other excessive hemolysis
Fetal or neonatal jaundice from:
bruising
drugs or toxins transmitted from mother
infection
polycythemia
swallowed maternal blood
Use additional code, if desired, to identify cause
Excludes: *jaundice due to isoimmunization (773.0-773.2)*

774.2 Neonatal jaundice associated with preterm delivery
Hyperbilirubinemia of prematurity
Jaundice due to delayed conjugation associated with preterm delivery

⑤ **774.3 Neonatal jaundice due to delayed conjugation from other causes**

774.30 Neonatal jaundice due to delayed conjugation, cause unspecified

774.31 *Neonatal jaundice due to delayed conjugation in diseases classified elsewhere*
Code first underlying diseases, as:
congenital hypothyroidism (243)
Crigler-Najjar syndrome (277.4)
Gilbert's syndrome (277.4)

774.39 Other
Jaundice due to delayed conjugation from causes, such as:
breast milk inhibitors
delayed development of conjugating system

774.4 Perinatal jaundice due to hepatocellular damage
Fetal or neonatal hepatitis
Giant cell hepatitis
Inspissated bile syndrome

774.5 *Perinatal jaundice from other causes*
Code first underlying cause, as:
congenital obstruction of bile duct (751.61)
galactosemia (271.1)
mucoviscidosis (277.00-277.09)

774.6 Unspecified fetal and neonatal jaundice
Icterus neonatorum
Neonatal hyperbilirubinemia (transient)
Physiologic jaundice NOS in newborn
Excludes: *that in preterm infants (774.2)*

774.7 Kernicterus not due to isoimmunization
Bilirubin encephalopathy
Kernicterus of newborn NOS
Excludes: *kernicterus due to isoimmunization (773.4)*

775 Endocrine and metabolic disturbances specific to the fetus and newborn
Includes: transitory endocrine and metabolic disturbances caused by the infant's response to maternal endocrine and metabolic factors, its removal from them, or its adjustment to extrauterine existence
ALERT! For personal history of endocrine metabolic and immunity disorders see V12.2

775.0 Syndrome of "infant of a diabetic mother"
Maternal diabetes mellitus affecting fetus or newborn (with hypoglycemia)

● Code new
to this edition
▲ Revision of
existing code
④ ⑤ Fourth or fifth
digit required

775.1 Neonatal diabetes mellitus
Diabetes mellitus syndrome in newborn infant

775.2 Neonatal myasthenia gravis

775.3 Neonatal thyrotoxicosis
Neonatal hyperthyroidism (transient)

775.4 Hypocalcemia and hypomagnesemia of newborn
Cow's milk hypocalcemia
Hypocalcemic tetany, neonatal
Neonatal hypoparathyroidism
Phosphate-loading hypocalcemia

775.5 Other transitory neonatal electrolyte disturbances
Dehydration, neonatal

775.6 Neonatal hypoglycemia
Excludes: infant of mother with diabetes mellitus (775.0)

775.7 Late metabolic acidosis of newborn

⑤ **775.8 Other neonatal endocrine and metabolic disturbances**

   775.81 Other acidosis of newborn
   Acidemia NOS of newborn
   Acidosis of newborn NOS
   Mixed metabolic and respiratory acidosis of newborn

   775.89 Other neonatal endocrine and metabolic disturbances
   Amino-acid metabolic disorders described as transitory

775.9 Unspecified endocrine and metabolic disturbances specific to the fetus and newborn

776 Hematological disorders of newborn
Includes: disorders specific to the newborn though possibly originating in utero
Excludes: fetal hematologic conditions (678.0)

776.0 Hemorrhagic disease of newborn
Hemorrhagic diathesis of newborn
Vitamin K deficiency of newborn
Excludes: fetal or neonatal hemorrhage (772.0-772.9)

776.1 Transient neonatal thrombocytopenia
Neonatal thrombocytopenia due to:
   exchange transfusion
   idiopathic maternal thrombocytopenia
   isoimmunization

776.2 Disseminated intravascular coagulation in newborn

776.3 Other transient neonatal disorders of coagulation
Transient coagulation defect, newborn

776.4 Polycythemia neonatorum
Plethora of newborn
Polycythemia due to:
   donor twin transfusion
   maternal-fetal transfusion

776.5 Congenital anemia
Anemia following fetal blood loss
Excludes: anemia due to isoimmunization (773.0-773.2, 773.5)
   hereditary hemolytic anemias (282.0-282.9)

776.6 Anemia of prematurity

776.7 Transient neonatal neutropenia
Isoimmune neutropenia
Maternal transfer neutropenia
Excludes: congenital neutropenia (nontransient) (288.01)

776.8 Other specified transient hematological disorders

776.9 Unspecified hematological disorder specific to newborn

777 Perinatal disorders of digestive system
Includes: disorders specific to the fetus and newborn
Excludes: intestinal obstruction classifiable to 560.0-560.9

| | Add 4th or 5th digit | | Nonspecific code | | Unspecified code | | Manifestation code |

777.1 Meconium obstruction
Congenital fecaliths
Delayed passage of meconium
Meconium ileus NOS
Meconium plug syndrome

Excludes: *meconium ileus in cystic fibrosis (277.01)*

777.2 Intestinal obstruction due to inspissated milk

777.3 Hematemesis and melena due to swallowed maternal blood
Swallowed blood syndrome in newborn

Excludes: *that not due to swallowed maternal blood (772.4)*

777.4 Transitory ileus of newborn

Excludes: *Hirschsprung's disease (751.3)*

⑤ **777.5 Necrotizing enterocolitis in newborn**

777.50 Necrotizing enterocolitis in newborn, unspecified
Necrotizing enterocolitis in newborn, NOS

777.51 Stage I necrotizing enterocolitis in newborn
Necrotizing enterocolitis without pneumatosis, without perforation

777.52 Stage II necrotizing enterocolitis in newborn
Necrotizing enterocolitis with pneumatosis, without perforation

777.53 Stage III necrotizing enterocolitis in newborn
Necrotizing enterocolitis with perforation
Necrotizing enterocolitis with pneumatosis and perforation

777.6 Perinatal intestinal perforation
Meconium peritonitis

777.8 Other specified perinatal disorders of digestive system

777.9 Unspecified perinatal disorder of digestive system

778 Conditions involving the integument and temperature regulation of fetus and newborn

778.0 Hydrops fetalis not due to isoimmunization
Idiopathic hydrops

Excludes: *hydrops fetalis due to isoimmunization (773.3)*

778.1 Sclerema neonatorum
Subcutaneous fat necrosis

778.2 Cold injury syndrome of newborn

778.3 Other hypothermia of newborn

778.4 Other disturbances of temperature regulation of newborn
Dehydration fever in newborn
Environmentally-induced pyrexia
Hyperthermia in newborn
Transitory fever of newborn

778.5 Other and unspecified edema of newborn
Edema neonatorum

778.6 Congenital hydrocele
Congenital hydrocele of tunica vaginalis

778.7 Breast engorgement in newborn
Noninfective mastitis of newborn

Excludes: *infective mastitis of newborn (771.5)*

778.8 Other specified conditions involving the integument of fetus and newborn
Urticaria neonatorum

Excludes: *impetigo neonatorum (684)*
pemphigus neonatorum (684)

778.9 Unspecified condition involving the integument and temperature regulation of fetus and newborn

779 Other and ill-defined conditions originating in the perinatal period

779.0 Convulsions in newborn
Fits in newborn
Seizures in newborn

779.1 Other and unspecified cerebral irritability in newborn

● Code new
to this edition   ▲ Revision of
existing code   ④ ⑤ Fourth or fifth
digit required

779.2　Cerebral depression, coma, and other abnormal cerebral signs
　　Cerebral ischemia NOS of newborn
　　CNS dysfunction in newborn NOS

　Excludes:　*cerebral ischemia due to birth trauma (767.0)*
　　　　　　　intrauterine cerebral ischemia (768.2-768.9)
　　　　　　　intraventricular hemorrhage (772.10-772.14)

⑤ **779.3　Disorder of stomach function and feeding problems in newborn**

　　779.31　Feeding problems in newborn
　　　　Slow feeding in newborn

　Excludes:　*feeding problem in child over 28 days old　(783.3)*

　　779.32　Bilious vomiting in newborn

　Excludes:　*bilious vomiting in child over 28 days old (787.04)*

　　779.33　Other vomiting in newborn
　　　　Regurgitation of food in newborn

　Excludes:　*vomiting in child over 28 days old (536.2,787.01-787.03, 787.04)*

　　779.34　Failure to thrive in newborn

　Excludes:　*failure to thrive in child over 28 days old (783.41)*

779.4　Drug reactions and intoxications specific to newborn
　　Gray syndrome from chloramphenicol administration in newborn

　Excludes:　*fetal alcohol syndrome (760.71)*
　　　　　　　reactions and intoxications from maternal opiates and tranquilizers (763.5)

779.5　Drug withdrawal syndrome in newborn
　　Drug withdrawal syndrome in infant of dependent mother

　Excludes:　*fetal alcohol syndrome (760.71)*

779.6　Termination of pregnancy (fetus)
　　Fetus death due to:
　　　induced abortion
　　　termination of pregnancy

　Excludes:　*spontaneous abortion (fetus) (761.8)*

779.7　Periventricular leukomalacia

⑤ **779.8　Other specified conditions originating in the perinatal period**

　　779.81　Neonatal bradycardia

　Excludes:　*abnormality in fetal heart rate or rhythm complicating labor and delivery*
　　　　　　　(763.81-763.83)
　　　　　　　bradycardia due to birth asphyxia (768.5-768.9)

　　779.82　Neonatal tachycardia

　Excludes:　*abnormality in fetal heart rate or rhythm complicating labor and delivery*
　　　　　　　(763.81-763.83)

　　779.83　Delayed separation of umbilical cord

　　779.84　Meconium staining

　Excludes:　*meconium aspiration (770.11, 770.12)*
　　　　　　　meconium passage during delivery (763.84)

　　779.85　Cardiac arrest of newborn

　　779.89　Other specified conditions originating in the perinatal period
　　Use additional code to specify condition

779.9　Unspecified condition originating in the perinatal period
　　Congenital debility NOS
　　Stillbirth NEC

	Add 4th or 5th digit		Nonspecific code		Unspecified code		Manifestation code

This page intentionally left blank.

● Code new
to this edition

▲ Revision of
existing code

④ ⑤ Fourth or fifth
digit required

Chapter 16: Symptoms, Signs and Ill-Defined Conditions (780-799)

DEFINITIONS AND CODING ALERTS

This chapter includes definitions of selected key words, terms and phrases and coding alerts for adding points to the clinical domain, references to coding late effects where appropriate, and references to personal history V-codes in situations where the acute or chronic condition is no longer active. An example from this chapter is as follows:

780.5 Sleep disturbances
DEFINITION A sleep disorder (somnipathy) is a medical disorder of the sleep patterns. Some sleep disorders are serious enough to interfere with normal physical, mental and emotional functioning..

MULTIPLE CODING FOR A SINGLE CONDITION

In addition to the etiology or manifestation convention that requires two codes to fully describe a single condition that affects multiple body systems, there are other single conditions that also require more than one code. "Use additional code" notes are found in the tabular at codes that are not part of an etiology or manifestation pair where a secondary code is useful to fully describe a condition. The sequencing rule is the same as the etiology or manifestation pair - , "use additional code" indicates that a secondary code should be added. For example, for infections that are not included in chapter 1, a secondary code from category 041, Bacterial infection in conditions classified elsewhere and of unspecified site, may be required to identify the bacterial organism causing the infection. A "use additional code" note will normally be found at the infectious disease code, indicating a need for the organism code to be added as a secondary code.

"Code first" notes are also under certain codes that are not specifically manifestation codes but may be due to an underlying cause. When a "code first" note is present and an underlying condition is present the underlying condition should be sequenced first.

"Code, if applicable, any causal condition first", notes indicate that this code may be assigned as a principal diagnosis when the causal condition is unknown or not applicable. If a causal condition is known, then the code for that condition should be sequenced as the principal or first-listed diagnosis. Multiple codes may be needed for late effects, complication codes and obstetric codes to more fully describe a condition. See the specific guidelines for these conditions for further instruction.

COMBINATION CODE

A combination code is a single code used to classify: two diagnoses, or a diagnosis with an associated secondary process (manifestation) A diagnosis with an associated complication Combination codes are identified by referring to subterm entries in the Alphabetic Index and by reading the inclusion and exclusion notes in the Tabular List.

Assign only the combination code when that code fully identifies the diagnostic conditions involved or when the Alphabetic Index so directs. Multiple coding should not be used when the classification provides a combination code that clearly identifies all of the elements documented in the diagnosis. When the combination code lacks necessary specificity in describing the manifestation or complication, an additional code should be used as a secondary code.

CODING LATE EFFECTS

A late effect is the residual effect (condition produced) after the acute phase of an illness or injury has terminated. There is no time limit on when a late effect code can be used. The residual may be apparent early, such as in cerebrovascular accident cases, or it may occur months or years later, such as that due to a previous injury. Coding of late effects generally requires two codes sequenced in the following order: The condition or nature of the late effect is sequenced first. The late effect code is sequenced second.

An exception to the above guidelines are those instances where the code for late effect is followed by a manifestation code identified in the Tabular List and title, or the late effect code has been expanded (at the fourth and fifth-digit levels) to include the manifestation(s). The code for the acute phase of an illness or injury that led to the late effect is never used with a code for the late effect.

Add 4th or 5th digit Nonspecific code Unspecified code Manifestation code

This page intentionally left blank.

● Code new
to this edition

▲ Revision of
existing code

④ ⑤ Fourth or fifth
digit required

16. SYMPTOMS, SIGNS, AND ILL-DEFINED CONDITIONS (780-799)

This section includes symptoms, signs, abnormal results of laboratory or other investigative procedures, and ill-defined conditions regarding which no diagnosis classifiable elsewhere is recorded.

Signs and symptoms that point rather definitely to a given diagnosis are assigned to some category in the preceding part of the classification. In general, categories 780-796 include the more ill-defined conditions and symptoms that point with perhaps equal suspicion to two or more diseases or to two or more systems of the body, and without the necessary study of the case to make a final diagnosis. Practically all categories in this group could be designated as "not otherwise specified," or as "unknown etiology," or as "transient." The Alphabetic Index should be consulted to determine which symptoms and signs are to be allocated here and which to more specific sections of the classification; the residual subcategories numbered .9 are provided for other relevant symptoms which cannot be allocated elsewhere in the classification.

The conditions and signs or symptoms included in categories 780-796 consist of: (a) cases for which no more specific diagnosis can be made even after all facts bearing on the case have been investigated; (b) signs or symptoms existing at the time of initial encounter that proved to be transient and whose causes could not be determined; (c) provisional diagnoses in a patient who failed to return for further investigation or care; (d) cases referred elsewhere for investigation or treatment before the diagnosis was made; (e) cases in which a more precise diagnosis was not available for any other reason; (f) certain symptoms which represent important problems in medical care and which it might be desired to classify in addition to a known cause.

SYMPTOMS (780-789)

780 General symptoms

⑤ **780.0 Alteration of consciousness**

Excludes: *alteration of consciousness due to:*
intracranial injuries (850.0-854.19)
skull fractures (800.00-801.99, 803.00-804.99)
coma:
diabetic (249.2-249.3, 250.2-250.3)
hepatic (572.2)
originating in the perinatal period (779.2)

780.01 Coma

780.02 Transient alteration of awareness

780.03 Persistent vegetative state

780.09 Other
Drowsiness	Somnolence
Semicoma	Stupor
Unconsciousness	

780.1 Hallucinations
Hallucinations:	Hallucinations:
NOS	olfactory
auditory	tactile
gustatory	

Excludes: *those associated with mental disorders, as functional psychoses (295.0-298.9)*
organic brain syndromes (290.0-294.9, 310.0-310.9)
visual hallucinations (368.16)

780.2 Syncope and collapse
Blackout	(Near) (Pre) syncope
Fainting	Vasovagal attack

Excludes: *carotid sinus syncope (337.0)*
heat syncope (992.1)
neurocirculatory asthenia (306.2)
orthostatic hypotension (458.0)
shock NOS (785.50)

⑤ **780.3 Convulsions**

Excludes: *convulsions:*
epileptic (345.10-345.91)
in newborn (779.0)

780.31 Febrile convulsions (simple), unspecified
Febrile seizure NOS

Add 4th or 5th digit	Nonspecific code	Unspecified code	Manifestation code

780.32 Complex febrile convulsions
Febrile seizure:
   atypical
   complex
   complicated

Excludes: *status epilepticus (345.3)*

780.33 Post traumatic seizures

Excludes: *post traumatic epilepsy (345.00-345.91)*

780.39 Other convulsions
Convulsive disorder NOS
Fit NOS
Recurrent convulsions NOS
Seizure NOS

780.4 Dizziness and giddiness
Light-headedness
Vertigo NOS

Excludes: *Ménière's disease and other specified vertiginous syndromes (386.0-386.9)*

⑤ **780.5 Sleep disturbances**

Excludes: *circadian rhythm sleep disorders (327.30-327.39)*
organic hypersomnia (327.10-327.19)
organic insomnia (327.00-327.09)
organic sleep apnea (327.20-327.29)
organic sleep related movement disorders (327.51-327.59)
parasomnias (327.40-327.49)
that of nonorganic origin (307.40-307.49)

DEFINITION A sleep disorder (somnipathy) is a medical disorder of the sleep patterns. Some sleep disorders are serious enough to interfere with normal physical, mental and emotional functioning.

780.50 Sleep disturbance, unspecified

780.51 Insomnia with sleep apnea, unspecified

780.52 Insomnia, unspecified

780.53 Hypersomnia with sleep apnea, unspecified

780.54 Hypersomnia, unspecified

780.55 Disruption of 24 hour sleep wake cycle, unspecified

780.56 Dysfunctions associated with sleep stages or arousal from sleep

780.57 Unspecified sleep apnea

780.58 Sleep related movement disorder, unspecified

Excludes: *restless legs syndrome (333.94)*

780.59 Other

⑤ **780.6 Fever and other physiologic disturbances of temperature regulation**

Excludes: *effects of reduced environmental temperature (991.0-991.9)*
effects of heat and light (992.0-992.9)
fever, chills or hypothermia associated with confirmed infection - code to infection

780.60 Fever, unspecified
Chills with fever
Fever NOS
Fever of unknown origin (FUO)
Hyperpyrexia NOS
Pyrexia NOS
Pyrexia of unknown origin

Excludes: *chills without fever (780.64)*
neonatal fever (778.4)
pyrexia of unknown origin (during):
  in newborn (778.4)
  labor (659.2)
  the puerperium (672)

780.61 Fever presenting with conditions classified elsewhere
Code first underlying condition when associated fever is present, such as with:
leukemia (conditions classifiable to 204-208)
neutropenia (288.00-288.09)
sickle-cell disease (282.60-282.69)

● Code new
to this edition
▲ Revision of
existing code
④ ⑤ Fourth or fifth
digit required

780.62 Postprocedural fever

Excludes: posttransfusion fever (780.66)
postvaccination fever (780.63)

780.63 Postvaccination fever
Postimmunization fever

780.64 Chills (without fever)
Chills NOS

Excludes: chills with fever (780.60)

780.65 Hypothermia not associated with low environmental temperature

Excludes: hypothermia:
associated with low environmental temperature (991.6)
due to anesthesia (995.89)
of newborn (778.2, 778.3)

780.66 Febrile nonhemolytic transfusion reaction
FNHTR
Posttransfusion fever

⑤ **780.7 Malaise and fatigue**

Excludes: debility, unspecified (799.3)
fatigue (during):
combat (308.0-308.9)
heat (992.6)
pregnancy (646.8)
neurasthenia (300.5)
senile asthenia (797.5)

780.71 Chronic fatigue syndrome

780.72 Functional quadriplegia
Complete immobility due to severe physical disability or frailty

Excludes: hysterical paralysis (300.11)
immobility syndrome (728.3)
neurologic quadriplegia (344.00-344.09)
quadriplegia NOS (344.00)

780.79 Other malaise and fatigue
Asthenia NOS
Lethargy
Postviral (asthenic) syndrome
Tiredness

780.8 Generalized hyperhidrosis
Diaphoresis
Excessive sweating
Secondary hyperhidrosis

Excludes: focal (localized) (primary) (secondary) hyperhidrosis (705.21-705.22)
Frey's syndrome (705.22)

⑤ **780.9 Other general symptoms**

Excludes: hypothermia:
NOS (accidental) (991.6)
due to anesthesia (995.89)
of newborn (778.2-778.3)
memory disturbance as part of a pattern of mental disorder

780.91 Fussy infant (baby)

780.92 Excessive crying of infant (baby)

Excludes: excessive crying of child, adolescent or adult (780.95)

780.93 Memory loss
Amnesia (retrograde)
Memory loss NOS

Excludes: memory loss due to:
intracranial injuries (850.0-854.19)
skull fractures (800.00-801.99, 803.00-804.99)
mild memory disturbance due to organic brain damage (310.89)
transient global amnesia (437.7)

780.94 Early satiety

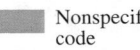 Add 4th or 5th digit   Nonspecific code   Unspecified code   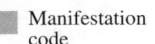 Manifestation code

780.95 Excessive crying of child, adolescent, or adult

Excludes: *excessive crying of infant (baby) (780.92)*

780.96 Generalized pain
Pain NOS

780.97 Altered mental status
Change in mental status

Excludes: *altered level of consciousness (780.01-780.09)*

altered mental status due to known condition — code to condition
delirium NOS (780.09)

780.99 Other general symptoms

781 Symptoms involving nervous and musculoskeletal systems

Excludes: *depression NOS (311)*

disorders specifically relating to:
back (724.0-724.9)
hearing (388.0-389.9)
joint (718.0-719.9)
limb (729.0-729.9)
neck (723.0-723.9)
vision (368.0-369.9)
pain in limb (729.5)

781.0 Abnormal involuntary movements
Abnormal head movements
Fasciculation
Spasms NOS
Tremor NOS

Excludes: *abnormal reflex (796.1)*

chorea NOS (333.5)
infantile spasms (345.60-345.61)
spastic paralysis (342.1, 343.0-344.9)
specified movement disorders classifiable to 333 (333.0-333.9)
that of nonorganic origin (307.2-307.3)

781.1 Disturbances of sensation of smell and taste
Anosmia   Parosmia
Parageusia

781.2 Abnormality of gait
Gait: Gait:
  ataxic   spastic
  paralytic   staggering

Excludes: *ataxia:*

NOS (781.3)
locomotor (progressive) (094.0)
difficulty in walking (719.7)

781.3 Lack of coordination
Ataxia NOS
Muscular incoordination

Excludes: *ataxic gait (781.2)*

cerebellar ataxia (334.0-334.9)
difficulty in walking (719.7)
vertigo NOS (780.4)

781.4 Transient paralysis of limb
Monoplegia, transient NOS

Excludes: *paralysis (342.0-344.9)*

781.5 Clubbing of fingers

781.6 Meningismus
Dupré's syndrome
Meningism

● Code new
to this edition

▲ Revision of
existing code

④ ⑤ Fourth or fifth
digit required

781.7 Tetany
Carpopedal spasm

Excludes: *tetanus neonatorum (771.3)*

tetany:
hysterical (300.11)
newborn (hypocalcemic) (775.4)
parathyroid (252.1)
psychogenic (306.0)

781.8 Neurologic neglect syndrome

Asomatognosia
Hemi-akinesia
Hemi-inattention
Hemispatial neglect

Left-sided neglect
Sensory extinction
Sensory neglect
Visuospatial neglect

Excludes: *visuospatial deficit (799.53)*

⑤ **781.9 Other symptoms involving nervous and musculoskeletal systems**

    781.91 Loss of height

Excludes: *osteoporosis (733.00-733.09)*

    781.92 Abnormal posture

    781.93 Ocular torticollis

    781.94 Facial weakness
        Facial droop

Excludes: *facial weakness due to late effect of cerebrovascular accident (438.83)*

    781.99 Other symptoms involving nervous and musculoskeletal systems

782 Symptoms involving skin and other integumentary tissue

Excludes: *symptoms relating to breast (611.71-611.79)*

782.0 Disturbance of skin sensation

Anesthesia of skin
Burning or prickling
  sensation
Hyperesthesia

Hypoesthesia
Numbness
Paresthesia
Tingling

782.1 Rash and other nonspecific skin eruption
Exanthem

Excludes: *vesicular eruption (709.8)*

782.2 Localized superficial swelling, mass, or lump
Subcutaneous nodules

Excludes: *localized adiposity (278.1)*

782.3 Edema
Anasarca
Dropsy
                       Localized edema NOS

Excludes: *ascites (789.51-789.59)*

edema of:
newborn NOS (778.5)
pregnancy (642.0-642.9, 646.1)
fluid retention (276.69)
hydrops fetalis (773.3, 778.0)
hydrothorax (511.81-511.89)
nutritional edema (260, 262)

782.4 Jaundice, unspecified, not of newborn
Cholemia NOS
Icterus NOS

Excludes: *jaundice in newborn (774.0-774.7)*
due to isoimmunization (773.0-773.2, 773.4)

782.5 Cyanosis

Excludes: *newborn (770.83)*

⑤ **782.6 Pallor and flushing**

    782.61 Pallor

    782.62 Flushing
        Excessive blushing

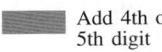 Add 4th or
5th digit

     Nonspecific
code

 Unspecified
code

     Manifestation
code

782.7 Spontaneous ecchymoses
Petechiae

Excludes: *ecchymosis in fetus or newborn (772.6)*
purpura (287.0-287.9)

782.8 Changes in skin texture
Induration of skin
Thickening of skin

782.9 Other symptoms involving skin and integumentary tissues

783 Symptoms concerning nutrition, metabolism, and development

783.0 Anorexia
Loss of appetite

Excludes: *anorexia nervosa (307.1)*
loss of appetite of nonorganic origin (307.59)

783.1 Abnormal weight gain

Excludes: *excessive weight gain in pregnancy (646.1)*
obesity (278.00)
morbid (278.01)

⑤ **783.2 Abnormal loss of weight and underweight**
Use additional code to identify Body Mass Index (BMI), if known (V85.0-V85.54)

783.21 Loss of weight

783.22 Underweight

783.3 Feeding difficulties and mismanagement
Feeding problem (elderly) (infant)

Excludes: *feeding disturbance or problems:*
in newborn (779.31-779.34)
of nonorganic origin (307.50-307.59)

⑤ **783.4 Lack of expected normal physiological development in childhood**

Excludes: *delay in sexual development and puberty (259.0)*
gonadal dysgenesis (758.6)
pituitary dwarfism (253.3)
slow fetal growth and fetal malnutrition (764.00-764.99)
specific delays in mental development (315.0-315.9)

783.40 Lack of normal physiological development, unspecified
Inadequate development
Lack of development

783.41 Failure to thrive
Failure to gain weight

Excludes: *failure to thrive in newborn (779.34)*

783.42 Delayed milestones
Late talker
Late walker

783.43 Short stature
Growth failure
Growth retardation
Lack of growth
Physical retardation

783.5 Polydipsia
Excessive thirst

783.6 Polyphagia
Excessive eating
Hyperalimentation NOS

Excludes: *disorders of eating of nonorganic origin (307.50-307.59)*

783.7 Adult failure to thrive

783.9 Other symptoms concerning nutrition, metabolism, and development
Hypometabolism

Excludes: *abnormal basal metabolic rate (794.7)*
dehydration (276.51)
other disorders of fluid, electrolyte, and acid-base balance (276.0-276.9)

● Code new to this edition   ▲ Revision of existing code   ④ ⑤ Fourth or fifth digit required

784 **Symptoms involving head and neck**

> *Excludes:* encephalopathy NOS (348.30)
> specific symptoms involving neck classifiable to 723 (723.0-723.9)

784.0 **Headache**
Facial pain
Pain in head NOS

> *Excludes:* atypical face pain (350.2)
> migraine (346.0-346.9)
> tension headache (307.81)

784.1 **Throat pain**

> *Excludes:* dysphagia (787.20-787.29)
> neck pain (723.1)
> sore throat (462)
> chronic (472.1)

784.2 **Swelling, mass, or lump in head and neck**
Space-occupying lesion, intracranial NOS

784.3 **Aphasia**

> *Excludes:* aphasia due to late effects of cerebrovascular disease (438.11)
> developmental aphasia (315.31)

⑤ **784.4** **Voice and resonance disorders**

> **784.40** **Voice and resonance disorder, unspecified**
>
> **784.41** **Aphonia**
> Loss of voice
>
> **784.42** **Dysphonia**
> Hoarseness
>
> **784.43** **Hypernasality**
>
> **784.44** **Hyponasality**
>
> **784.49** **Other voice and resonance disorders**
> Change in voice

⑤ **784.5** **Other speech disturbance**

> *Excludes:* speech disorder due to late effect of cerebrovascular accident (438.10 - 438.19)
> stuttering (315.35)

> **784.51** **Dysarthria**

> *Excludes:* dysarthria due to late effect of cerebrovascular accident (438.13)

> **784.52** **Fluency disorder in conditions classified elsewhere**
> Stuttering in conditions classified elsewhere
>
> *Code first underlying disease or condition, such as:*
> Parkinson's disease (332.0)

> *Excludes:* adult onset fluency disorder (307.0)
> childhood onset fluency disorder (315.35)
> fluency disorder due to late effect of cerebrovascular accident (438.14)

> **784.59** **Other speech disturbance**
> Dysphasia
> Slurred speech
> Speech disturbance NOS

⑤ **784.6** **Other symbolic dysfunction**

> *Excludes:* developmental learning delays (315.0-315.9)

> **784.60** **Symbolic dysfunction, unspecified**
>
> **784.61** **Alexia and dyslexia**
> Alexia (with agraphia)
>
> **784.69** **Other**
> Acalculia   Agraphia NOS
> Agnosia   Apraxia

784.7 **Epistaxis**
Hemorrhage from nose
Nosebleed

784.8 **Hemorrhage from throat**

> *Excludes:* hemoptysis (786.30-786.39)

| � Add 4th or 5th digit | ▪ Nonspecific code | ▪ Unspecified code | ▪ Manifestation code |

⑤ **784.9 Other symptoms involving head and neck**

    784.91 Postnasal drip

    784.92 Jaw pain
        Mandibular pain
        Maxilla pain

   Excludes: temporomandibular joint arthralgia (524.62)

    784.99 Other symptoms involving head and neck
        Choking sensation
        Feeling of foreign body in throat
        Halitosis
        Mouth breathing
        Sneezing

   Excludes: foreign body in throat (933.0)

785 Symptoms involving cardiovascular system

   Excludes: heart failure NOS (428.9)

785.0 Tachycardia, unspecified
    Rapid heart beat

   Excludes: neonatal tachycardia (779.82)
             paroxysmal tachycardia (427.0-427.2)

785.1 Palpitations
    Awareness of heart beat

   Excludes: specified dysrhythmias (427.0-427.9)

785.2 Undiagnosed cardiac murmurs
    Heart murmur NOS

785.3 Other abnormal heart sounds
    Cardiac dullness, increased or decreased
    Friction fremitus, cardiac
    Precordial friction

785.4 Gangrene
    Gangrene NOS
    Gangrene spreading cutaneous
    Gangrenous cellulitis
    Phagedena

   Code first any associated underlying condition, as:
    diabetes (250.7)
    Raynaud's syndrome (443.0)

   Excludes: gangrene of certain sites—see Alphabetic Index
             gangrene with atherosclerosis of the extremities (440.24)
             gas gangrene (040.0)

⑤ **785.5 Shock without mention of trauma**

    785.50 Shock, unspecified
        Failure of peripheral circulation

    785.51 Cardiogenic shock

    785.52 *Septic shock*
        endotoxic
        gram-negative

   Code first underlying infection
   Use additional code, if applicable, to identify systemic inflammatory response syndrome
    due to infectious process with organ dysfunction (995.92)

● Code new   ▲ Revision of   ④ ⑤ Fourth or fifth
   to this edition   existing code   digit required

785.59 **Other**
Shock:
hypovolemic

Excludes: *shock (due to):*
anesthetic (995.4)
anaphylactic (995.0)
due to serum (999.41-999.49)
electric (994.8)
following abortion (639.5)
lightning (994.0)
obstetrical (669.1)
postoperative (998.00-998.09)
traumatic (958.4)

785.6 **Enlargement of lymph nodes**
Lymphadenopathy
"Swollen glands"

Excludes: *lymphadenitis (chronic) (289.1-289.3)*
acute (683)

785.9 **Other symptoms involving cardiovascular system**
Bruit (arterial)
Weak pulse

786 **Symptoms involving respiratory system and other chest symptoms**

⑤ **786.0** **Dyspnea and respiratory abnormalities**

786.00 **Respiratory abnormality, unspecified**

786.01 **Hyperventilation**

Excludes: *hyperventilation, psychogenic (306.1)*

786.02 **Orthopnea**

786.03 **Apnea**

Excludes: *apnea of newborn (770.81, 770.82)*
sleep apnea (780.51, 780.53, 780.57)

786.04 **Cheyne-Stokes respiration**

786.05 **Shortness of breath**

786.06 **Tachypnea**

Excludes: *transitory tachypnea of newborn (770.6)*

786.07 **Wheezing**

Excludes: *asthma (493.00-493.92)*

786.09 **Other**
Respiratory:
distress
insufficiency

Excludes: *respiratory distress:*
following trauma and surgery (518.52)
newborn (770.89)
syndrome (newborn) (769)
adult (518.52)
respiratory failure (518.81, 518.83-518.84)
newborn (770.84)

786.1 **Stridor**

Excludes: *congenital laryngeal stridor (748.3)*

786.2 **Cough**

Excludes: *cough:*
psychogenic (306.1)
smokers' (491.0)
with hemorrhage (786.39)

⑤ **786.3** **Hemoptysis**

786.30 **Hemoptysis, unspecified**
Pulmonary hemorrhage NOS

	Add 4th or 5th digit		Nonspecific code		Unspecified code		Manifestation code

786.31 **Acute idiopathic pulmonary hemorrhage in infants [AIPHI]**
Acute idiopathic pulmonary hemorrhage in infant over 28 days old

Excludes: *pulmonary hemorrhage of newborn under 28 days old (770.3)*
von Willebrand's disease (286.4)

786.39 **Other hemoptysis**
Cough with hemorrhage

786.4 **Abnormal sputum**
Abnormal:
amount (of) sputum
color (of) sputum
odor (of) sputum
Excessive sputum

⑤ **786.5** **Chest pain**

786.50 **Chest pain, unspecified**

786.51 **Precordial pain**

786.52 **Painful respiration**
Pain:
anterior chest wall
pleuritic
Pleurodynia

Excludes: *epidemic pleurodynia (074.1)*

786.59 **Other**
Discomfort in chest
Pressure in chest
Tightness in chest

Excludes: *pain in breast (611.71)*

786.6 **Swelling, mass, or lump in chest**

Excludes: *lump in breast (611.72)*

786.7 **Abnormal chest sounds**
Abnormal percussion, chest   Rales
Friction sounds, chest   Tympany, chest

Excludes: *wheezing (786.07)*

786.8 **Hiccough**

Excludes: *psychogenic hiccough (306.1)*

786.9 **Other symptoms involving respiratory system and chest**
Breath-holding spell

787 **Symptoms involving digestive system**

Excludes: *constipation (564.00-564.09)*
pylorospasm (537.81)
congenital (750.5)

⑤ **787.0** **Nausea and vomiting**
Emesis

Excludes: *hematemesis NOS (578.0)*
vomiting:
bilious, following gastrointestinal surgery (564.3)
cyclical (536.2)
associated with migraine (346.2)
psychogenic (306.4)
excessive, in pregnancy (643.0-643.9)
fecal matter (569.87)
habit (536.2)
of newborn (779.32, 779.33)
persistent (536.2)
psychogenic NOS (307.54)

787.01 **Nausea with vomiting**

787.02 **Nausea alone**

787.03 **Vomiting alone**

787.04 **Bilious emesis**
Bilious vomiting

Excludes: *bilious emesis (vomiting) in newborn (779.32)*

787.1 Heartburn
　　Pyrosis
　　Waterbrash

　　Excludes: *dyspepsia or indigestion (536.8)*

⑤ **787.2 Dysphagia**
Code first, if applicable, dysphagia due to late effect of cerebrovascular accident (438.82)

　　787.20 Dysphagia, unspecified
　　　　Difficulty in swallowing NOS

　　787.21 Dysphagia, oral phase

　　787.22 Dysphagia, oropharyngeal phase

　　787.23 Dysphagia, pharyngeal phase

　　787.24 Dysphagia, pharyngoesophageal phase

　　787.29 Other dysphagia
　　　　Cervical dysphagia
　　　　Neurogenic dysphagia

787.3 Flatulence, eructation, and gas pain
　　Abdominal distention (gaseous)
　　Bloating
　　Tympanites (abdominal) (intestinal)

　　Excludes: *aerophagy (306.4)*

787.4 Visible peristalsis
　　Hyperperistalsis

787.5 Abnormal bowel sounds
　　Absent bowel sounds
　　Hyperactive bowel sounds

⑤ **787.6 Incontinence of feces**
　　Encopresis NOS
　　Incontinence of sphincter ani

　　Excludes: *that of nonorganic origin (307.7)*

　　787.60 Full incontinence of feces
　　　　Fecal incontinence NOS

　　787.61 Incomplete defecation

　　Excludes: *constipation (564.00-564.09)*
　　　　　　fecal impaction (560.32)

　　787.62 Fecal smearing
　　　　Fecal soiling

　　787.63 Fecal urgency

787.7 Abnormal feces
　　Bulky stools

　　Excludes: *abnormal stool content (792.1)*
　　　　　　melena:
　　　　　　　NOS (578.1)
　　　　　　　newborn (772.4, 777.3)

⑤ **787.9 Other symptoms involving digestive system**

　　Excludes: *gastrointestinal hemorrhage (578.0-578.9)*
　　　　　　intestinal obstruction (560.0-560.9)
　　　　　　specific functional digestive disorders:
　　　　　　　esophagus (530.0-530.9)
　　　　　　　stomach and duodenum (536.0-536.9)
　　　　　　　those not elsewhere classified (564.00-564.9)

　　787.91 Diarrhea
　　　　Diarrhea NOS

　　787.99 Other
　　　　Change in bowel habitsTenesmus (rectal)

788 Symptoms involving urinary system

　　Excludes: *hematuria (599.70-599.72)*
　　　　　　nonspecific findings on examination of the urine (791.0-791.9)
　　　　　　small kidney of unknown cause (589.0-589.9)
　　　　　　uremia NOS (586)
　　　　　　urinary obstruction (599.60, 599.69)

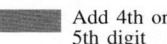 Add 4th or
5th digit
 Nonspecific
code
Unspecified
code
Manifestation
code

788.0 Renal colic
　　Colic (recurrent) of:
　　　kidney
　　　ureter

788.1 Dysuria
　　Painful urination
　　Strangury

⑤ **788.2 Retention of urine**
Code, if applicable, any causal condition first, such as:
　　hyperplasia of prostate (600.0-600.9 with fifth-digit 1)

　　788.20 Retention of urine, unspecified

　　788.21 Incomplete bladder emptying

　　788.29 Other specified retention of urine

⑤ **788.3 Urinary incontinence**

　　Excludes: *functional urinary incontinence (788.91)*
　　　　　　　that of nonorganic origin (307.6)
　　　　　　　urinary incontinence associated with cognitive impairment (788.91)

Code, if applicable, any causal condition first, such as:
　　congenital ureterocele (753.23)
　　genital prolapse (618.00-618.9)
　　hyperplasia of prostate (600.0-600.9 with fifth-digit 1)

　　788.30 Urinary incontinence, unspecified
　　　　Enuresis NOS

　　788.31 Urge incontinence

　　788.32 Stress incontinence, male

　　Excludes: *stress incontinence (female) (625.6)*

　　788.33 Mixed incontinence (male) (female)
　　　　Urge and stress

　　788.34 Incontinence without sensory awareness

　　788.35 Post-void dribbling

　　788.36 Nocturnal enuresis

　　788.37 Continuous leakage

　　788.38 Overflow incontinence

　　788.39 Other urinary incontinence

⑤ **788.4 Frequency of urination and polyuria**
Code, if applicable, any causal condition first, such as:
　　hyperplasia of prostate (600.0-600.9 with fifth-digit 1)

　　788.41 Urinary frequency
　　　　Frequency of micturition

　　788.42 Polyuria

　　788.43 Nocturia

788.5 Oliguria and anuria
　　Deficient secretion of urine
　　Suppression of urinary secretion

　　Excludes: *that complicating:*
　　　　abortion (634-638 with .3, 639.3)
　　　　ectopic or molar pregnancy (639.3)
　　　　pregnancy, childbirth, or the puerperium (642.0-642.9, 646.2)

⑤ **788.6 Other abnormality of urination**
Code, if applicable, any causal condition first, such as:
　　hyperplasia of prostate (600.0-600.9 with fifth-digit 1)

　　788.61 Splitting of urinary stream
　　　　Intermittent urinary stream

　　788.62 Slowing of urinary stream
　　　　Weak stream

　　788.63 Urgency of urination
　　Excludes: *urge incontinence (788.31, 788.33)*

　　788.64 Urinary hesitancy

　　788.65 Straining on urination

　● Code new　　　▲ Revision of　　④ ⑤ Fourth or fifth
　　to this edition　　existing code　　　digit required

788.69 Other

788.7 Urethral discharge
Penile discharge
Urethrorrhea

788.8 Extravasation of urine

⑤ **788.9 Other symptoms involving urinary system**

788.91 Functional urinary incontinence
Urinary incontinence due to cognitive impairment, or severe physical disability or immobility

Excludes: *urinary incontinence due to physiologic condition (788.30-788.39)*

788.99 Other symptoms involving urinary system
Extrarenal uremia
Vesical:
pain
tenesmus

789 Other symptoms involving abdomen and pelvis
The following fifth-digit subclassification is to be used for codes 789.0, 789.3, 789.4, 789.6

0 unspecified site

1 right upper quadrant

2 left upper quadrant

3 right lower quadrant

4 left lower quadrant

5 periumbilic

6 epigastric

7 generalized

9 other specified site
multiple sites

789.1

Excludes: *symptoms referable to genital organs:*
female (625.0-625.9)
male (607.0-608.9)
psychogenic (302.70-302.79)

⑤ **789.0 Abdominal pain**
[0-7,9] Cramps, abdominal

789.1 Hepatomegaly
Enlargement of liver

789.2 Splenomegaly
Enlargement of spleen

⑤ **789.3 Abdominal or pelvic swelling, mass, or lump**
[0-7,9] Diffuse or generalized swelling or mass:
abdominal NOS
umbilical

Excludes: *abdominal distention (gaseous) (787.3)*
ascites (789.51-789.59)

⑤ **789.4 Abdominal rigidity**
[0-7,9]

⑤ **789.5 Ascites**
Fluid in peritoneal cavity

789.51 Malignant ascites
Code first malignancy, such as:
malignant neoplasm of ovary (183.0)
secondary malignant neoplasm of retroperitoneum and peritoneum (197.6)

789.59 Other ascites

⑤ **789.6 Abdominal tenderness**
[0-7,9] Rebound tenderness

789.7 Colic
Colic NOS
Infantile colic

Excludes: *colic in adult and child over 12 months old (789.0)*
renal colic (788.0)

Add 4th or 5th digit   Nonspecific code   Unspecified code   Manifestation code

789.9 **Other symptoms involving abdomen and pelvis**
Umbilical:
bleeding
discharge

NONSPECIFIC ABNORMAL FINDINGS (790-796)

790 **Nonspecific findings on examination of blood**

Excludes: *abnormalities of:*
platelets (287.0-287.9)
thrombocytes (287.0-287.9)
white blood cells (288.00-288.9)

⑤ **790.0** **Abnormality of red blood cells**

Excludes: *anemia:*
congenital (776.5)
newborn, due to isoimmunization (773.0-773.2, 773.5)
of premature infant (776.6)
other specified types (280.0-285.9)
hemoglobin disorders (282.5-282.7)
polycythemia:
familial (289.6)
neonatorum (776.4)
secondary (289.0)
vera (238.4)

790.01 **Precipitous drop in hematocrit**
Drop in hematocrit
Drop in hemoglobin

790.09 **Other abnormality of red blood cells**
Abnormal red cell morphology NOS
Abnormal red cell volume NOS
Anisocytosis
Poikilocytosis

790.1 **Elevated sedimentation rate**

⑤ **790.2** **Abnormal glucose**

Excludes: *diabetes mellitus (249.00-249.91, 250.00-250.93)*
dysmetabolic syndrome X (277.7)
gestational diabetes (648.8)
glycosuria (791.5)
hypoglycemia (251.2)
that complicating pregnancy, childbirth, or the puerperium (648.8)

790.21 **Impaired fasting glucose**
Elevated fasting glucose

790.22 **Impaired glucose tolerance test (oral)**
Elevated glucose tolerance test

790.29 **Other abnormal glucose**
Abnormal glucose NOS
Abnormal non-fasting glucose
Hyperglycemia NOS
Pre-diabetes NOS

790.3 **Excessive blood level of alcohol**
Elevated blood-alcohol

790.4 **Nonspecific elevation of levels of transaminase or lactic acid dehydrogenase [LDH]**

790.5 **Other nonspecific abnormal serum enzyme levels**
Abnormal serum level of: Abnormal serum level of:
acid phosphatase   amylase
alkaline phosphatase   lipase

Excludes: *deficiency of circulating enzymes (277.6)*

● Code new   ▲ Revision of   ④ ⑤ Fourth or fifth
to this edition   existing code   digit required

790.6 Other abnormal blood chemistry

Abnormal blood level of:
  cobalt
  copper
  iron
  lead

Abnormal blood level of:
  lithium
  magnesium
  mineral
  zinc

Excludes: *abnormality of electrolyte or acid-base balance (276.0-276.9)*
hypoglycemia NOS (251.2)
lead poisoning (984.0-984.9)
specific finding indicating abnormality of:
amino-acid transport and metabolism (270.0-270.9)
carbohydrate transport and metabolism (271.0-271.9)
lipid metabolism (272.0-272.9)
uremia NOS (586)

790.7 Bacteremia

Excludes: *bacteremia of newborn (771.83)*
septicemia (038)

Use additional code, if desired, to identify organism (041)

790.8 Viremia, unspecified

⑤ **790.9 Other nonspecific findings on examination of blood**

790.91 Abnormal arterial blood gases

790.92 Abnormal coagulation profile
Abnormal or prolonged:
  bleeding time
  coagulation time
  partial thromboplastin time [PTT]
  prothrombin time [PT]

Excludes: *coagulation (hemorrhagic) disorders (286.0-286.9)*

790.93 Elevated prostate specific antigen (PSA)

790.94 Euthyroid sick syndrome

790.95 Elevated C-reactive protein (CRP)

790.99 Other

791 Nonspecific findings on examination of urine

Excludes: *hematuria NOS (599.70-599.72)*
specific findings indicating abnormality of:
amino-acid transport and metabolism (270.0-270.9)
carbohydrate transport and metabolism (271.0-271.9)

791.0 Proteinuria
Albuminuria
Bence-Jones proteinuria

Excludes: *postural proteinuria (593.6)*
that arising during pregnancy or the puerperium (642.0-642.9, 646.2)

791.1 Chyluria

Excludes: *filarial (125.0-125.9)*

791.2 Hemoglobinuria

791.3 Myoglobinuria

791.4 Biliuria

791.5 Glycosuria

Excludes: *renal glycosuria (271.4)*

791.6 Acetonuria
Ketonuria

791.7 Other cells and casts in urine

| | Add 4th or 5th digit | | Nonspecific code | | Unspecified code | | Manifestation code |

791.9 Other nonspecific findings on examination of urine
Crystalluria
Elevated urine levels of:
17-ketosteroids
catecholamines
indolacetic acid
vanillylmandelic acid [VMA]
Melanuria

792 Nonspecific abnormal findings in other body substances

Excludes: that in chromosomal analysis (795.2)

792.0 Cerebrospinal fluid

792.1 Stool contents
Abnormal stool color
Fat in stool   Occult blood
Mucus in stool   Pus in stool

Excludes: blood in stool [melena] (578.1)
newborn (772.4, 777.3)

792.2 Semen
Abnormal spermatozoa

Excludes: azoospermia (606.0)
oligospermia (606.1)

792.3 Amniotic fluid

792.4 Saliva

Excludes: that in chromosomal analysis (795.2)

792.5 Cloudy (hemodialysis) (peritoneal) dialysis effluent

792.9 Other nonspecific abnormal findings in body substances
Peritoneal fluid   Synovial fluid
Pleural fluid   Vaginal fluids

793 Nonspecific (abnormal) findings on radiological and other examinations of body structure
Includes: nonspecific abnormal findings of:
thermography
ultrasound examination [echogram]
x-ray examination

Excludes: abnormal results of function studies and radioisotope scans (794.0-794.9)

793.0 Skull and head

Excludes: nonspecific abnormal echoencephalogram (794.01)

⑤ **793.1 Lung field**

● **793.11 Solitary pulmonary nodule**
Coin lesion lung
Solitary pulmonary nodule, subsegmental branch of the bronchial tree

● **793.19 Other nonspecific abnormal finding of lung field**
Pulmonary infiltrate NOS
Shadow, lung

793.2 Other intrathoracic organ
Abnormal: Mediastinal shift
echocardiogram
heart shadow
ultrasound cardiogram

793.3 Biliary tract
Nonvisualization of gallbladder

793.4 Gastrointestinal tract

793.5 Genitourinary organs
Filling defect:
bladder
kidney
ureter

793.6 Abdominal area, including retroperitoneum

793.7 Musculoskeletal system

⑤ **793.8 Breast**

793.80 Abnormal mammogram, unspecified

● Code new
to this edition
▲ Revision of
existing code
④ ⑤ Fourth or fifth
digit required

793.81 Mammographic microcalcification

Excludes: *mammographic calcification (793.89)*
mammographic calculus (793.89)

793.82 Inconclusive mammogram
Dense breasts NOS
Inconclusive mammogram NEC
Inconclusive mammography due to dense breasts
Inconclusive mammography NEC

793.89 Other (abnormal) findings on radiological examination of breast
Mammographic calcification
Mammographic calculus

⑤ **793.9 Other**

Excludes: *abnormal finding by radioisotope localization of placenta (794.9)*

793.91 Image test inconclusive due to excess body fat
Use additional code to identify Body Mass Index (BMI), if known (V85.0-V85.54)

793.99 Other nonspecific (abnormal) findings on radiological and other examinations of body structure
Abnormal:
placental finding by x-ray or ultrasound method
radiological findings in skin and subcutaneous tissue

794 Nonspecific abnormal results of function studies
Includes: radioisotope:
scans
uptake studies
scintiphotography

⑤ **794.0 Brain and central nervous system**

794.00 Abnormal function study, unspecified

794.01 Abnormal echoencephalogram

794.02 Abnormal electroencephalogram [EEG]

794.09 Other
Abnormal brain scan

⑤ **794.1 Peripheral nervous system and special senses**

794.10 Abnormal response to nerve stimulation, unspecified

794.11 Abnormal retinal function studies
Abnormal electroretinogram [ERG]

794.12 Abnormal electro-oculogram [EOG]

794.13 Abnormal visually evoked potential

794.14 Abnormal oculomotor studies

794.15 Abnormal auditory function studies

794.16 Abnormal vestibular function studies

794.17 Abnormal electromyogram [EMG]

Excludes: *that of eye (794.14)*

794.19 Other

794.2 Pulmonary
Abnormal lung scan
Reduced:
ventilatory capacity
vital capacity

⑤ **794.3 Cardiovascular**

794.30 Abnormal function study, unspecified

794.31 Abnormal electrocardiogram [ECG] [EKG]

Excludes: *long QT syndrome (426.82)*

794.39 Other
Abnormal:
ballistocardiogram
phonocardiogram
vectorcardiogram

794.4 Kidney
Abnormal renal function test

| | Add 4th or 5th digit | | Nonspecific code | | Unspecified code | | Manifestation code |

794.5 Thyroid
Abnormal thyroid:
scan
uptake

794.6 Other endocrine function study

794.7 Basal metabolism
Abnormal basal metabolic rate [BMR]

794.8 Liver
Abnormal liver scan

794.9 Other
Bladder
Pancreas
Placenta
Spleen

795 Other and nonspecific abnormal cytological, histological, immunological and DNA test findings

Excludes: *abnormal cytologic smear of anus and anal HPV (796.70-796.79)*
nonspecific abnormalities of red blood cells (790.01-790.09)

⑤ **795.0 Abnormal Papanicolaou smear of cervix and cervical HPV**
Abnormal thin preparation smear of cervix
Abnormal cervical cytology

Excludes: *abnormal cytologic smear of vagina and vaginal HPV (795.10-795.19)*
carcinoma in situ of cervix (233.1)
cervical intraepithelial neoplasia I [CIN I] (622.11)
cervical intraepithelial neoplasia II [CIN II] (622.12)
cervical intraepithelial neoplasia III [CIN III] (233.1)
dysplasia (histologically confirmed) of cervix (uteri) NOS (622.10)
mild cervical dysplasia (histologically confirmed) (622.11)
moderate cervical dysplasia (histologically confirmed) (622.12)
severe cervical dysplasia (histologically confirmed) (233.1)

795.00 Abnormal glandular Papanicolaou smear of cervix
Atypical cervical glandular cells NOS
Atypical endocervical cells NOS
Atypical endometrial cells NOS

795.01 Papanicolaou smear of cervix with atypical squamous cells of undetermined significance (ASC-US)

795.02 Papanicolaou smear of cervix with atypical squamous cells cannot exclude high grade squamous intraepithelial lesion (ASC-H)

795.03 Papanicolaou smear of cervix with low grade squamous intraepithelial lesion (LGSIL)

795.04 Papanicolaou smear of cervix with high grade squamous intraepithelial lesion (HGSIL)

795.05 Cervical high risk human papillomavirus (HPV) DNA test positive

795.06 Papanicolaou smear of cervix with cytologic evidence of malignancy

795.07 Satisfactory cervical smear but lacking transformation zone

795.08 Unsatisfactory cervical cytology smear
Inadequate cervical cytology sample

795.09 Other abnormal Papanicolaou smear of cervix and cervical HPV
Cervical low risk human papillomavirus (HPV) DNA test positive
Papanicolaou smear of cervix with low risk human papillomavirus (HPV) DNA test positive
Use additional code for associated human papillomavirus (HPV) (079.4)

Excludes: *encounter for Papanicolaou cervical smear to confirm findings of recent normal smear following initial abnormal smear (V72.32)*

● Code new
to this edition
▲ Revision of
existing code
④ ⑤ Fourth or fifth
digit required

⑤ **795.1 Abnormal Papanicolaou smear of vagina and vaginal HPV**
Abnormal thin preparation smear of vagina NOS
Abnormal vaginal cytology NOS

Use additional code to identify acquired absence of uterus and cervix, if applicable (V88.01-V88.03)

Excludes: *abnormal cytologic smear of cervix and cervical HPV (795.00-795.09)*
carcinoma in situ of vagina (233.31)
carcinoma in situ of vulva (233.32)
dysplasia (histologically confirmed) of vagina NOS (623.0, 233.31)
dysplasia (histologically confirmed) of vulva NOS (624.01, 624.02, 233.32)
mild vaginal dysplasia (histologically confirmed) (623.0)
mild vulvar dysplasia (histologically confirmed) (624.01)
moderate vaginal dysplasia (histologically confirmed) (623.0)
moderate vulvar dysplasia (histologically confirmed) (624.02)
severe vaginal dysplasia (histologically confirmed) (233.31)
severe vulvar dysplasia (histologically confirmed) (233.32)
vaginal intraepithelial neoplasia I (VAIN I) (623.0)
vaginal intraepithelial neoplasia II (VAIN II) (623.0)
vaginal intraepithelial neoplasia III (VAIN III) (233.31)
vulvar intraepithelial neoplasia I (VIN I) (624.01)
vulvar intraepithelial neoplasia II (VIN II) (624.02)
vulvar intraepithelial neoplasia III (VIN III) (233.32)

795.10 Abnormal glandular Papanicolaou smear of vagina
Atypical vaginal glandular cells NOS

795.11 Papanicolaou smear of vagina with atypical squamous cells of undetermined significance (ASC-US)

795.12 Papanicolaou smear of vagina with atypical squamous cells cannot exclude high grade squamous intraepithelial lesion (ASC-H)

795.13 Papanicolaou smear of vagina with low grade squamous intraepithelial lesion (LGSIL)

795.14 Papanicolaou smear of vagina with high grade squamous intraepithelial lesion (HGSIL)

795.15 Vaginal high risk human papillomavirus (HPV) DNA test positive

Excludes: *condyloma acuminatum (078.11)*
genital warts (078.11)

795.16 Papanicolaou smear of vagina with cytologic evidence of malignancy

795.18 Unsatisfactory vaginal cytology smear
Inadequate vaginal cytology sample

795.19 Other abnormal Papanicolaou smear of vagina and vaginal HPV
Vaginal low risk human papillomavirus (HPV) DNA test positive

Use additional code for associated human papillomavirus (079.4)

795.2 Nonspecific abnormal findings on chromosomal analysis
Abnormal karyotype

⑤ **795.3 Nonspecific positive culture findings**
Positive culture findings in:
nose
sputum
throat
wound

Excludes: *that of:*
blood (790.7-790.8)
urine (791.9)

795.31 Nonspecific positive findings for anthrax
Positive findings by nasal swab

795.39 Other nonspecific positive culture findings

Excludes: *colonization status (V02.0-V02.9)*

795.4 Other nonspecific abnormal histological findings

| | Add 4th or 5th digit | | Nonspecific code | | Unspecified code | | Manifestation code |

▲ **795.5** **Nonspecific reaction to test for tuberculosis**

● **795.51** **Nonspecific reaction to tuberculin skin test without active tuberculosis**
Abnormal result of Mantoux test
PPD positive
Tuberculin (skin test) positive
Tuberculin (skin test) reactor

Excludes: *nonspecific reaction to cell mediated immunity measurement of gamma interferon*
antigen response without active tuberculosis (795.52)

● **795.52** **Nonspecific reaction to cell mediated immunity measurement of gamma interferon antigen response without active tuberculosis**
Nonspecific reaction to QuantiFERON-TB test (QFT) without active tuberculosis

Excludes: *nonspecific reaction to tuberculin skin test without active tuberculosis (795.51)*
positive tuberculin skin test (795.51)

795.6 **False positive serological test for syphilis**
False positive Wassermann reaction

⑤ **795.7** **Other nonspecific immunological findings**

Excludes: *abnormal tumor markers (795.81-795.89)*
elevated prostate specific antigen [PSA] (790.93)
elevated tumor associated antigens (795.81-795.89)
isoimmunization, in pregnancy (656.1-656.2)
affecting fetus or newborn (773.0-773.2)

795.71 **Nonspecific serologic evidence of human immunodeficiency virus [HIV]**
Inconclusive human immunodeficiency virus [HIV] test (adult) (infant)

Note: This code is ONLY to be used when a test finding is reported as nonspecific. Asymptomatic positive findings are coded to V08. If any HIV infection symptom or condition is present, see code 042. Negative findings are not coded.

Excludes: *acquired immunodeficiency syndrome [AIDS] (042)*
asymptomatic human immunodeficiency virus, [HIV] infection status (V08)
HIV infection, symptomatic (042)
human immunodeficiency virus [HIV] disease (042)
positive (status) NOS (V08)

795.79 **Other and unspecified nonspecific immunological findings**
Raised antibody titer
Raised level of immunoglobulins

⑤ **795.8** **Abnormal tumor markers**
Elevated tumor associated antigens [TAA]
Elevated tumor specific antigens [TSA]

Excludes: *elevated prostate specific antigen [PSA] (790.93)*

795.81 **Elevated carcinoembryonic antigen (CEA)**

795.82 **Elevated cancer antigen 125 (CA 125)**

795.89 **Other abnormal tumor markers**

796 **Other nonspecific abnormal findings**

796.0 **Nonspecific abnormal toxicological findings**
Abnormal levels of heavy metals or drugs in blood, urine, or other tissue
Use additional code for retained foreign body, if applicable, (V90.01-V90.9)

Excludes: *excessive blood level of alcohol (790.3)*

796.1 **Abnormal reflex**

796.2 **Elevated blood pressure reading without diagnosis of hypertension**
Note: This category is to be used to record an episode of elevated blood pressure in a patient in whom no formal diagnosis of hypertension has been made, or as an incidental finding.

796.3 **Nonspecific low blood pressure reading**

796.4 **Other abnormal clinical findings**

796.5 **Abnormal finding on antenatal screening**

796.6 **Abnormal findings on neonatal screening**

Excludes: *nonspecific serologic evidence of human immunodeficiency virus [HIV] (795.71)*

● Code new
to this edition

▲ Revision of
existing code

④ ⑤ Fourth or fifth
digit required

⑤ **796.7 Abnormal cytologic smear of anus and anal HPV**

> Excludes: *abnormal cytologic smear of cervix and cervical HPV (795.00-795.09)*
> *abnormal cytologic smear of vagina and vaginal HPV (795.10-795.19)*
> *anal intraepithelial neoplasia I (AIN I) (569.44)*
> *anal intraepithelial neoplasia II (AIN II) (569.44)*
> *anal intraepithelial neoplasia III (AIN III) (230.5, 230.6)*
> *carcinoma in situ of anus (230.5, 230.6)*
> *dysplasia (histologically confirmed) of anus NOS (569.44)*
> *mild anal dysplasia (histologically confirmed) (569.44)*
> *moderate anal dysplasia (histologically confirmed) (569.44)*
> *severe anal dysplasia (histologically confirmed) (230.5, 230.6)*

   796.70 Abnormal glandular Papanicolaou smear of anus
   Atypical anal glandular cells NOS

   796.71 Papanicolaou smear of anus with atypical squamous cells of undetermined significance (ASC-US)

   796.72 Papanicolaou smear of anus with atypical squamous cells cannot exclude high grade squamous intraepithelial lesion (ASC-H)

   796.73 Papanicolaou smear of anus with low grade squamous intraepithelial lesion (LGSIL)

   796.74 Papanicolaou smear of anus with high grade squamous intraepithelial lesion (HGSIL)

   796.75 Anal high risk human papillomavirus (HPV) DNA test positive

   796.76 Papanicolaou smear of anus with cytologic evidence of malignancy

   796.77 Satisfactory anal smear but lacking transformation zone

   796.78 Unsatisfactory anal cytology smear
   Inadequate anal cytology sample

   796.79 Other abnormal Papanicolaou smear of anus and anal HPV
   Anal low risk human papillomavirus (HPV)
   DNA test positive

   Use additional code for associated human papillomavirus (079.4)

796.9 Other

ILL-DEFINED AND UNKNOWN CAUSES OF MORBIDITY AND MORTALITY (797-799)

797 Senility without mention of psychosis
   Frailty
   Old age
   Senescence
   Senile asthenia
   Senile debility
   Senile exhaustion

> Excludes: *senile psychoses (290.0-290.9)*

798 Sudden death, cause unknown

   798.0 Sudden infant death syndrome
   Cot death
   Crib death
   Sudden death of nonspecific cause in infancy

   798.1 Instantaneous death

   798.2 Death occurring in less than 24 hours from onset of symptoms, not otherwise explained
   Death known not to be violent or instantaneous, for which no cause could be discovered
   Died without sign of disease

   798.9 Unattended death
   Death in circumstances where the body of the deceased was found and no cause could be discovered
   Found dead

799 Other ill-defined and unknown causes of morbidity and mortality

⑤ **799.0 Asphyxia and hypoxemia**

> Excludes: *asphyxia and hypoxemia (due to)*
> *hypercapnia (786.09)*

   799.01 Asphyxia

   799.02 Hypoxemia

	Add 4th or 5th digit		Nonspecific code		Unspecified code		Manifestation code

799.1 Respiratory arrest
Cardiorespiratory failure

Excludes: cardiac arrest (427.5)
failure of peripheral circulation (785.50)
respiratory distress:
NOS (786.09)
acute (518.82)
following trauma or surgery (518.52)
newborn (770.89)
syndrome (newborn) (769)
adult (following trauma or surgery) (518.52)
other (518.82)
respiratory failure (518.81, 518.83-518.84)
newborn (770.84)
respiratory insufficiency (786.09)
acute (518.82)

⑤ **799.2 Signs and symptoms involving emotional state**

Excludes: anxiety (293.84, 300.00-300.09)
depression (311)

799.21 Nervousness
Nervous

799.22 Irritability
Irritable

799.23 Impulsiveness
Impulsive

Excludes: impulsive neurosis (300.3)

799.24 Emotional lability

799.25 Demoralization and apathy
Apathetic

799.29 Other signs and symptoms involving emotional state

799.3 Debility, unspecified

Excludes: asthenia (780.79)
nervous debility (300.5)
neurasthenia (300.5)
senile asthenia (797)

799.4 Cachexia
Wasting disease

Code first underlying condition, if known

⑤ **799.5 Signs and symptoms involving cognition**

Excludes: amnesia (780.93)
amnestic syndrome (294.0)
attention deficit disorder (314.00-314.01)
late effects of cerebrovascular disease (438)
memory loss (780.93)
mild cognitive impairment, so stated (331.83)
specific problems in developmental delay (315.00-315.9)
transient global amnesia (437.7)
visuospatial neglect (781.8)

799.51 Attention or concentration deficit

799.52 Cognitive communication deficit

799.53 Visuospatial deficit

799.54 Psychomotor deficit

799.55 Frontal lobe and executive function deficit

799.59 Other signs and symptoms involving cognition

⑤ **799.8 Other ill-defined conditions**

799.81 Decreased libido
Decreased sexual desire

Excludes: psychosexual dysfunction with inhibited sexual desire (302.71)

● Code new to this edition   ▲ Revision of existing code   ④ ⑤ Fourth or fifth digit required

799.82 Apparent life threatening event in infant

ALTE

Apparent life threatening event in newborn and infant

Code first confirmed diagnosis, if known

Use additional code(s) for associated signs and symptoms if no confirmed diagnosis established, or if signs and symptoms are not associated routinely with confirmed diagnosis, or provide additional information for cause of ALTE

799.89 Other ill-defined conditions

799.9 Other unknown and unspecified cause

Undiagnosed disease, not specified as to site or system involved

Unknown cause of morbidity or mortality

| | Add 4th or 5th digit | | Nonspecific code | | Unspecified code | | Manifestation code |

This page intentionally left blank.

● Code new
to this edition

▲ Revision of
existing code

④ ⑤ Fourth or fifth
digit required

Chapter 17: Injury and Poisoning (800-999)

DEFINITIONS AND CODING ALERTS

This chapter includes definitions of selected key words, terms and phrases and coding alerts for adding points to the clinical domain, references to coding late effects where appropriate, and references to personal history V-codes in situations where the acute or chronic condition is no longer active. An example from this chapter is as follows:

⑤ `800` **Fracture of vault of skull**

> `DEFINITION` A fracture is a complete or incomplete break in a bone resulting from the application of excessive force
>
> `ALERT!` For coding late effect of fracture of skull and face bones see 905.0

MULTIPLE CODING FOR A SINGLE CONDITION

In addition to the etiology or manifestation convention that requires two codes to fully describe a single condition that affects multiple body systems, there are other single conditions that also require more than one code. "Use additional code" notes are found in the tabular at codes that are not part of an etiology or manifestation pair where a secondary code is useful to fully describe a condition. The sequencing rule is the same as the etiology or manifestation pair - , "use additional code" indicates that a secondary code should be added.

"Code first" notes are also under certain codes that are not specifically manifestation codes but may be due to an underlying cause. When a "code first" note is present and an underlying condition is present the underlying condition should be sequenced first.

"Code, if applicable, any causal condition first", notes indicate that this code may be assigned as a principal diagnosis when the causal condition is unknown or not applicable. If a causal condition is known, then the code for that condition should be sequenced as the principal or first-listed diagnosis. Multiple codes may be needed for late effects, complication codes and obstetric codes to more fully describe a condition. See the specific guidelines for these conditions for further instruction.

COMBINATION CODE

A combination code is a single code used to classify: two diagnoses, or a diagnosis with an associated secondary process (manifestation) A diagnosis with an associated complication Combination codes are identified by referring to subterm entries in the Alphabetic Index and by reading the inclusion and exclusion notes in the Tabular List.

Assign only the combination code when that code fully identifies the diagnostic conditions involved or when the Alphabetic Index so directs. Multiple coding should not be used when the classification provides a combination code that clearly identifies all of the elements documented in the diagnosis. When the combination code lacks necessary specificity in describing the manifestation or complication, an additional code should be used as a secondary code.

CODING LATE EFFECTS

A late effect is the residual effect (condition produced) after the acute phase of an illness or injury has terminated. There is no time limit on when a late effect code can be used. The residual may be apparent early, such as in cerebrovascular accident cases, or it may occur months or years later, such as that due to a previous injury. Coding of late effects generally requires two codes sequenced in the following order: The condition or nature of the late effect is sequenced first. The late effect code is sequenced second.

An exception to the above guidelines are those instances where the code for late effect is followed by a manifestation code identified in the Tabular List and title, or the late effect code has been expanded (at the fourth and fifth-digit levels) to include the manifestation(s). The code for the acute phase of an illness or injury that led to the late effect is never used with a code for the late effect.

CODING OF INJURIES

When coding injuries, assign separate codes for each injury unless a combination code is provided, in which case the combination code is assigned. Multiple injury codes are provided in ICD-9-CM, but should not be assigned unless information for a more specific code is not available. These codes are not to be used for normal, healing surgical wounds or to identify complications of surgical wounds.

The code for the most serious injury, as determined by the provider and the focus of treatment, is sequenced first.

| | Add 4th or 5th digit | | Nonspecific code | | Unspecified code | | Medicare secondary payer (MSP) alert |

Superficial injuries

Superficial injuries such as abrasions or contusions are not coded when associated with more severe injuries of the same site.

Primary injury with damage to nerves or blood vessels

When a primary injury results in minor damage to peripheral nerves or blood vessels, the primary injury is sequenced first with additional code(s) from categories 950-957, Injury to nerves and spinal cord, and/or 900-904, Injury to blood vessels. When the primary injury is to the blood vessels or nerves, that injury should be sequenced first.

CODING OF TRAUMATIC FRACTURES

The principles of multiple coding of injuries should be followed in coding fractures. Fractures of specified sites are coded individually by site in accordance with both the provisions within categories 800-829 and the level of detail furnished by medical record content.

Combination categories for multiple fractures are provided for use when there is insufficient detail in the medical record (such as trauma cases transferred to another hospital), when the reporting form limits the number of codes that can be used in reporting pertinent clinical data, or when there is insufficient specificity at the fourth-digit or fifth-digit level. More specific guidelines are as follows:

Acute Fractures vs. Aftercare

Traumatic fractures are coded using the acute fracture codes (800-829) while the patient is receiving active treatment for the fracture. Examples of active treatment are: surgical treatment, emergency department encounter, and evaluation and treatment by a new physician.

Fractures are coded using the aftercare codes (subcategories V54.0, V54.1, V54.8, or V54.9) for encounters after the patient has completed active treatment of the fracture and is receiving routine care for the fracture during the healing or recovery phase. Examples of fracture aftercare are: cast change or removal, removal of external or internal fixation device, medication adjustment, and follow up visits following fracture treatment.

Care for complications of surgical treatment for fracture repairs during the healing or recovery phase should be coded with the appropriate complication codes.

Care of complications of fractures, such as malunion and nonunion, should be reported with the appropriate codes.

Pathologic fractures are not coded in the 800-829 range, but instead are assigned to subcategory 733.1. See Official Guidelines, Section I.C.13.a for additional information.

Multiple fractures

Multiple fractures of same limb classifiable to the same three-digit or four-digit category are coded to that category.

Multiple unilateral or bilateral fractures of same bone(s) but classified to different fourth-digit subdivisions (bone part) within the same three-digit category are coded individually by site.

Multiple fracture categories 819 and 828 classify bilateral fractures of both upper limbs (819) and both lower limbs (828), but without any detail at the fourth-digit level other than open and closed type of fractures.

Multiple fractures sequencing

Multiple fractures are sequenced in accordance with the severity of the fracture. The provider should be asked to list the fracture diagnoses in the order of severity.

CODING OF BURNS

Current burns (940-948) are classified by depth, extent and by agent (E code). Burns are classified by depth as first degree (erythema), second degree (blistering), and third degree (full-thickness involvement).

Sequencing of burn and related condition codes

Sequence first the code that reflects the highest degree of burn when more than one burn is present.

● Code new
  to this edition
▲ Revision of
  existing code
④ ⑤ Fourth or fifth
  digit required

When the reason for the admission or encounter is for treatment of external multiple burns, sequence first the code that reflects the burn of the highest degree.

When a patient has both internal and external burns, the circumstances of admission govern the selection of the principal diagnosis or first-listed diagnosis.

When a patient is admitted for burn injuries and other related conditions such as smoke inhalation and/or respiratory failure, the circumstances of admission govern the selection of the principal or first-listed diagnosis.

Burns of the same local site

Classify burns of the same local site (three-digit category level, 940-947). but of different degrees to the subcategory identifying the highest degree recorded in the diagnosis.

Non-healing burns

Non-healing burns are coded as acute burns. Necrosis of burned skin should be coded as a non-healed burn.

Code 958.3, Posttraumatic wound infection

Assign code 958.3, Posttraumatic wound infection, not elsewhere classified, as an additional code for any documented infected burn site.

Assign separate codes for each burn site

When coding burns, assign separate codes for each burn site. Category 946 Burns of Multiple specified sites, should only be used if the location of the burns are not documented.

Category 949, Burn, unspecified, is extremely vague and should rarely be used.

Assign codes from category 948, Burns

Burns classified according to extent of body surface involved, when the site of the burn is not specified or when there is a need for additional data. It is advisable to use category 948 as additional coding when needed to provide data for evaluating burn mortality, such as that needed by burn units. It is also advisable to use category 948 as an additional code for reporting purposes when there is mention of a third-degree burn involving 20 percent or more of the body surface.

In assigning a code from category 948:

Fourth-digit codes are used to identify the percentage of total body surface involved in a burn (all degree).

Fifth-digits are assigned to identify the percentage of body surface involved in third-degree burn.

Fifth-digit zero (0) is assigned when less than 10 percent or when no body surface is involved in a third-degree burn.

Category 948 is based on the classic "rule of nines" in estimating body surface involved: head and neck are assigned nine percent, each arm nine percent, each leg 18 percent, the anterior trunk 18 percent, posterior trunk 18 percent, and genitalia one percent. Providers may change these percentage assignments where necessary to accommodate infants and children who have proportionately larger heads than adults and patients who have large buttocks, thighs, or abdomen that involve burns.

Encounters for treatment of late effects of burns

Encounters for the treatment of the late effects of burns (i.e., scars or joint contractures) should be coded to the residual condition (sequelae) followed by the appropriate late effect code (906.5-906.9). A late effect E code may also be used, if desired.

Sequelae with a late effect code and current burn

When appropriate, both a sequelae with a late effect code, and a current burn code may be assigned on the same record (when both a current burn and sequelae of an old burn exist).

█ Add 4th or 5th digit   █ Nonspecific code   █ Unspecified code   █ Medicare secondary payer (MSP) alert

CODING OF DEBRIDEMENT OF WOUND, INFECTION, OR BURN

Excisional debridement involves surgical removal or cutting away, as opposed to a mechanical (brushing, scrubbing, washing) debridement.

For coding purposes, excisional debridement is assigned to code 86.22. Nonexcisional debridement is assigned to code 86.28.

ADVERSE EFFECTS, POISONING AND TOXIC EFFECTS

The properties of certain drugs, medicinal and biological substances or combinations of such substances, may cause toxic reactions. The occurrence of drug toxicity is classified in ICD-9-CM as follows:

Adverse Effect

When the drug was correctly prescribed and properly administered, code the reaction plus the appropriate code from the E930-E949 series. Codes from the E930-E949 series must be used to identify the causative substance for an adverse effect of drug, medicinal and biological substances, correctly prescribed and properly administered. The effect, such as tachycardia, delirium, gastrointestinal hemorrhaging, vomiting, hypokalemia, hepatitis, renal failure, or respiratory failure, is coded and followed by the appropriate code from the E930-E949 series.

Adverse effects of therapeutic substances correctly prescribed and properly administered (toxicity, synergistic reaction, side effect, and idiosyncratic reaction) may be due to (1) differences among patients, such as age, sex, disease, and genetic factors, and (2) drug-related factors, such as type of drug, route of administration, duration of therapy, dosage, and bioavailability.

Poisoning

A. Error was made in drug prescription

Errors made in drug prescription or in the administration of the drug by provider, nurse, patient, or other person, use the appropriate poisoning code from the 960-979 series.

B. Overdose of a drug intentionally taken

If an overdose of a drug was intentionally taken or administered and resulted in drug toxicity, it would be coded as a poisoning (960-979 series).

C. Nonprescribed drug taken with correctly prescribed and properly administered drug

If a nonprescribed drug or medicinal agent was taken in combination with a correctly prescribed and properly administered drug, any drug toxicity or other reaction resulting from the interaction of the two drugs would be classified as a poisoning.

D. Interaction of drug(s) and alcohol

When a reaction results from the interaction of a drug(s) and alcohol, this would be classified as poisoning.

E. Sequencing of poisoning

When coding a poisoning or reaction to the improper use of a medication (e.g., wrong dose, wrong substance, wrong route of administration) the poisoning code is sequenced first, followed by a code for the manifestation. If there is also a diagnosis of drug abuse or dependence to the substance, the abuse or dependence is coded as an additional code.

See Official Guidelines, Section I.C.3.a.6.b. if poisoning is the result of insulin pump malfunctions and Official Guidelines, Section I.C.19 for general use of E-codes.

Toxic Effects

A. Toxic effect codes

When a harmful substance is ingested or comes in contact with a person, this is classified as a toxic effect. The toxic effect codes are in categories 980-989.

B. Sequencing toxic effect codes

A toxic effect code should be sequenced first, followed by the code(s) that identify the result of the toxic effect.

● Code new to this edition   ▲ Revision of existing code   ④ ⑤ Fourth or fifth digit required

C.   External cause codes for toxic effects

An external cause code from categories E860-E869 for accidental exposure, codes E950.6 or E950.7 for intentional self-harm, category E962 for assault, or categories E980-E982, for undetermined, should also be assigned to indicate intent.

COMPLICATIONS OF CARE

Documentation of complications of care

As with all procedural or postprocedural complications, code assignment is based on the provider's documentation of the relationship between the condition and the procedure.

Transplant complications

A.   Transplant complications other than kidney

Codes under subcategory 996.8, Complications of transplanted organ, are for use for both complications and rejection of transplanted organs. A transplant complication code is only assigned if the complication affects the function of the transplanted organ. Two codes are required to fully describe a transplant complication, the appropriate code from subcategory 996.8 and a secondary code that identifies the complication.

Pre-existing conditions or conditions that develop after the transplant are not coded as complications unless they affect the function of the transplanted organs.

See I.C.18.d.3.for transplant organ removal status. See I.C.2.i for malignant neoplasm associated with transplanted organ.

B.   Chronic kidney disease and kidney transplant complications

Patients who have undergone kidney transplant may still have some form of chronic kidney disease (CKD) because the kidney transplant may not fully restore kidney function. Code 996.81 should be assigned for documented complications of a kidney transplant, such as transplant failure or rejection or other transplant complication. Code 996.81 should not be assigned for post kidney transplant patients who have chronic kidney (CKD) unless a transplant complication such as transplant failure or rejection is documented. If the documentation is unclear as to whether the patient has a complication of the transplant, query the provider.

For patients with CKD following a kidney transplant, but who do not have a complication such as failure or rejection, see Chapter 10.

Ventilator associated pneumonia

A.   Documentation of Ventilator associated pneumonia

As with all procedural or postprocedural complications, code assignment is based on the provider's documentation of the relationship between the condition and the procedure.

Code 997.31, Ventilator associated pneumonia, should be assigned only when the provider has documented ventilator associated pneumonia (VAP). An additional code to identify the organism (e.g., Pseudomonas aeruginosa, code 041.7) should also be assigned. Do not assign an additional code from categories 480-484 to identify the type of pneumonia.

Code 997.31 should not be assigned for cases where the patient has pneumonia and is on a mechanical ventilator but the provider has not specifically stated that the pneumonia is ventilator-associated pneumonia.

If the documentation is unclear as to whether the patient has a pneumonia that is a complication attributable to the mechanical ventilator, query the provider.

B.   Patient admitted with pneumonia and develops VAP

A patient may be admitted with one type of pneumonia (e.g., code 481, Pneumococcal pneumonia) and subsequently develop VAP. In this instance, the principal diagnosis would be the appropriate code from categories 480-484 for the pneumonia diagnosed at the time of admission. Code 997.31, Ventilator associated pneumonia, would be assigned as an additional diagnosis when the provider has also documented the presence of ventilator associated pneumonia.

| | Add 4th or 5th digit | | Nonspecific code | | Unspecified code | | Medicare secondary payer (MSP) alert |

SIRS DUE TO NON-INFECTIOUS PROCESS

The systemic inflammatory response syndrome (SIRS) can develop as a result of certain non-infectious disease processes, such as trauma, malignant neoplasm, or pancreatitis. When SIRS is documented with a noninfectious condition, and no subsequent infection is documented, the code for the underlying condition, such as an injury, should be assigned, followed by code 995.93, Systemic inflammatory response syndrome due to noninfectious process without acute organ dysfunction, or 995.94, Systemic inflammatory response syndrome due to non-infectious process with acute organ dysfunction. If an acute organ dysfunction is documented, the appropriate code(s) for the associated acute organ dysfunction(s) should be assigned in addition to code 995.94. If acute organ dysfunction is documented, but it cannot be determined if the acute organ dysfunction is associated with SIRS or due to another condition (e.g., directly due to the trauma), the provider should be queried.

Sepsis and Severe Sepsis Associated with Non-infectious Process

In some cases, a non-infectious process, such as trauma, may lead to an infection which can result in sepsis or severe sepsis. If sepsis or severe sepsis is documented as associated with a non-infectious condition, such as a burn or serious injury, and this condition meets the definition for principal diagnosis, the code for the non-infectious condition should be sequenced first, followed by the code for the systemic infection and either code 995.91, Sepsis, or 995.92, Severe sepsis. Additional codes for any associated acute organ dysfunction(s) should also be assigned for cases of severe sepsis. If the sepsis or severe sepsis meets the definition of principal diagnosis, the systemic infection and sepsis codes should be sequenced before the non-infectious condition. When both the associated non-infectious condition and the sepsis or severe sepsis meet the definition of principal diagnosis, either may be assigned as principal diagnosis.

● Code new
to this edition
▲ Revision of
existing code
④ ⑤ Fourth or fifth
digit required

17. INJURY AND POISONING (800-999)

Use E code(s) to identify the cause and intent of the injury or poisoning (E800-E999)
Use additional code for retained foreign body, if applicable, V90.01- V90.9)
Note:

1. The principle of multiple coding of injuries should be followed wherever possible. Combination categories for multiple injuries are provided for use when there is insufficient detail as to the nature of the individual conditions, or for primary tabulation purposes when it is more convenient to record a single code; otherwise, the component injuries should be coded separately.

    Where multiple sites of injury are specified in the titles, the word "with" indicates involvement of both sites, and the word "and" indicates involvement of either or both sites. The word "finger" includes thumb.

2. Categories for "late effect" of injuries are to be found at 905-909.

FRACTURES (800-829)

Excludes: malunion (733.81)
nonunion (733.82)
pathologic or spontaneous fracture (733.10-733.19)
stress fractures (733.93-733.95)

The terms "condyle," "coronoid process," "ramus," and "symphysis" indicate the portion of the bone fractured, not the name of the bone involved.

The descriptions "closed" and "open" used in the fourth-digit subdivisions include the following terms:

closed (with or without delayed healing):
comminuted   impacted
depressed   linear
elevated   simple
fissured   slipped epiphysis
fracture NOS   spiral
greenstick

open (with or without delayed healing):
compound   puncture
infected   with foreign body
missile

A fracture not indicated as closed or open should be classified as closed.

DEFINITION A fracture is a complete or incomplete break in a bone resulting from the application of excessive force.

ALERT! For coding late effects of musculoskeletal and connective tissue injuries see 905

ALERT! For personal history of traumatic fracture see V15.51

FRACTURE OF SKULL (800-804)

Includes: traumatic brain injury due to fracture of skull

The following fifth-digit subclassification is for use with the appropriate codes in categories 800, 801, 803, and 804:

0 unspecified state of consciousness

1 with no loss of consciousness

2 with brief [less than one hour] loss of consciousness

3 with moderate [1-24 hours] loss of consciousness and return to pre-existing conscious level

4 with prolonged [more than 24 hours] loss of consciousness and return to pre-existing conscious level

5 with prolonged [more than 24 hours] loss of consciousness, without return to pre-existing conscious level
    Use fifth-digit 5 to designate when a patient is unconscious and dies before regaining consciousness, regardless of the duration of the loss of consciousness

6 with loss of consciousness of unspecified duration

9 with concussion, unspecified

⑤ **800** Fracture of vault of skull
Includes: frontal bone
parietal bone
DEFINITION A fracture is a complete or incomplete break in a bone resulting from the application of excessive force
ALERT! For coding late effect of fracture of skull and face bones see 905.0

Add 4th or 5th digit | Nonspecific code | Unspecified code | Medicare secondary payer (MSP) alert

⑤ **800.0** Closed without mention of intracranial injury
[0-6,9]

⑤ **800.1** Closed with cerebral laceration and contusion
[0-6,9]

⑤ **800.2** Closed with subarachnoid, subdural, and extradural hemorrhage
[0-6,9]

⑤ **800.3** Closed with other and unspecified intracranial hemorrhage
[0-6,9]

⑤ **800.4** Closed with intracranial injury of other and unspecified nature
[0-6,9]

⑤ **800.5** Open without mention of intracranial injury
[0-6,9]

⑤ **800.6** Open with cerebral laceration and contusion
[0-6,9]

⑤ **800.7** Open with subarachnoid, subdural, and extradural hemorrhage
[0-6,9]

⑤ **800.8** Open with other and unspecified intracranial hemorrhage
[0-6,9]

⑤ **800.9** Open with intracranial injury of other and unspecified nature
[0-6,9]

⑤ **801** Fracture of base of skull
Includes:

fossa:	sinus:
anterior	ethmoid
middle	frontal
posterior	sphenoid bone
occiput bone	temporal bone
orbital roof	

ALERT! For coding late effect of fracture of skull and face bones see 905.0

⑤ **801.0** Closed without mention of intracranial injury
[0-6,9]

⑤ **801.1** Closed with cerebral laceration and contusion
[0-6,9]

⑤ **801.2** Closed with subarachnoid, subdural, and extradural hemorrhage
[0-6,9]

⑤ **801.3** Closed with other and unspecified intracranial hemorrhage
[0-6,9]

⑤ **801.4** Closed with intracranial injury of other and unspecified nature
[0-6,9]

⑤ **801.5** Open without mention of intracranial injury
[0-6,9]

⑤ **801.6** Open with cerebral laceration and contusion
[0-6,9]

⑤ **801.7** Open with subarachnoid, subdural, and extradural hemorrhage
[0-6,9]

⑤ **801.8** Open with other and unspecified intracranial hemorrhage
[0-6,9]

⑤ **801.9** Open with intracranial injury of other and unspecified nature
[0-6,9]

802 Fracture of face bones
ALERT! For coding late effect of fracture of skull and face bones see 905.0

802.0 Nasal bones, closed

802.1 Nasal bones, open

⑤ **802.2** Mandible, closed
Inferior maxilla
Lower jaw (bone)

802.20 Unspecified site

802.21 Condylar process

802.22 Subcondylar

802.23 Coronoid process

● Code new
to this edition

▲ Revision of
existing code

④ ⑤ Fourth or fifth
digit required

802.24 **Ramus, unspecified**

802.25 **Angle of jaw**

802.26 **Symphysis of body**

802.27 **Alveolar border of body**

802.28 **Body, other and unspecified**

802.29 **Multiple sites**

⑤ 802.3 **Mandible, open**

802.30 **Unspecified site**

802.31 **Condylar process**

802.32 **Subcondylar**

802.33 **Coronoid process**

802.34 **Ramus, unspecified**

802.35 **Angle of jaw**

802.36 **Symphysis of body**

802.37 **Alveolar border of body**

802.38 **Body, other and unspecified**

802.39 **Multiple sites**

802.4 **Malar and maxillary bones, closed**
Superior maxilla   Zygoma
Upper jaw (bone)   Zygomatic arch

802.5 **Malar and maxillary bones, open**

802.6 **Orbital floor (blow-out), closed**

802.7 **Orbital floor (blow-out), open**

802.8 **Other facial bones, closed**
Alveolus
Orbit:
  NOS
  part other than roof or floor
Palate

Excludes: *orbital:*
    floor (802.6)
    roof (801.0-801.9)

802.9 **Other facial bones, open**

⑤ **803** **Other and unqualified skull fractures**
Includes: skull NOS
           skull multiple NOS

ALERT! For coding late effect of fracture of skull and face bones see 905.0

⑤ **803.0** **Closed without mention of intracranial injury**
[0-6,9]

⑤ **803.1** **Closed with cerebral laceration and contusion**
[0-6,9]

⑤ **803.2** **Closed with subarachnoid, subdural, and extradural hemorrhage**
[0-6,9]

⑤ **803.3** **Closed with other and unspecified intracranial hemorrhage**
[0-6,9]

⑤ **803.4** **Closed with intracranial injury of other and unspecified nature**
[0-6,9]

⑤ **803.5** **Open without mention of intracranial injury**
[0-6,9]

⑤ **803.6** **Open with cerebral laceration and contusion**
[0-6,9]

⑤ **803.7** **Open with subarachnoid, subdural, and extradural hemorrhage**
[0-6,9]

⑤ **803.8** **Open with other and unspecified intracranial hemorrhage**
[0-6,9]

⑤ **803.9** **Open with intracranial injury of other and unspecified nature**
[0-6,9]

| | Add 4th or 5th digit | | Nonspecific code | | Unspecified code | | Medicare secondary payer (MSP) alert |

⑤ **804** **Multiple fractures involving skull or face with other bones**
ALERT! For coding late effect of fracture of skull and face bones see 905.0

⑤ **804.0** **Closed without mention of intracranial injury**
[0-6,9]

⑤ **804.1** **Closed with cerebral laceration and contusion**
[0-6,9]

⑤ **804.2** **Closed with subarachnoid, subdural, and extradural hemorrhage**
[0-6,9]

⑤ **804.3** **Closed with other and unspecified intracranial hemorrhage**
[0-6,9]

⑤ **804.4** **Closed with intracranial injury of other and unspecified nature**
[0-6,9]

⑤ **804.5** **Open without mention of intracranial injury**
[0-6,9]

⑤ **804.6** **Open with cerebral laceration and contusion**
[0-6,9]

⑤ **804.7** **Open with subarachnoid, subdural, and extradural hemorrhage**
[0-6,9]

⑤ **804.8** **Open with other and unspecified intracranial hemorrhage**
[0-6,9]

⑤ **804.9** **Open with intracranial injury of other and unspecified nature**
[0-6,9]

FRACTURE OF NECK AND TRUNK (805-809)

805 **Fracture of vertebral column without mention of spinal cord injury**
Includes: neural arch
spine
spinous process
transverse process
vertebra

The following fifth-digit subclassification is for use with codes 805.0-805.1:

0 **cervical vertebra, unspecified level**

1 **first cervical vertebra**

2 **second cervical vertebra**

3 **third cervical vertebra**

4 **fourth cervical vertebra**

5 **fifth cervical vertebra**

6 **sixth cervical vertebra**

7 **seventh cervical vertebra**

8 **multiple cervical vertebrae**

ALERT! For coding late effect of fracture of spine and trunk without spinal cord lesion see 905.1

⑤ **805.0** **Cervical, closed**
[0-8] Atlas
Axis

⑤ **805.1** **Cervical, open**
[0-8]

805.2 **Dorsal [thoracic], closed**

805.3 **Dorsal [thoracic], open**

805.4 **Lumbar, closed**

805.5 **Lumbar, open**

805.6 **Sacrum and coccyx, closed**

805.7 **Sacrum and coccyx, open**

805.8 **Unspecified, closed**

805.9 **Unspecified, open**

● Code new
to this edition

▲ Revision of
existing code

④ ⑤ Fourth or fifth
digit required

806 **Fracture of vertebral column with spinal cord injury**

Includes: any condition classifiable to 805 with:
         complete or incomplete transverse lesion (of cord)
         hematomyelia
      injury to:
         cauda equina
         nerve
      paralysis
      paraplegia
      quadriplegia
      spinal concussion

ALERT! For coding late effect of fracture of spine and trunk without spinal cord lesion see 905.1

⑤ **806.0 Cervical, closed**

  806.00 C_1-C_4 level with unspecified spinal cord injury
        Cervical region NOS with spinal cord injury NOS

  806.01 C_1-C_4 level with complete lesion of cord

  806.02 C_1-C_4 level with anterior cord syndrome

  806.03 C_1-C_4 level with central cord syndrome

  806.04 C_1-C_4 level with other specified spinal cord injury
        C_1-C_4 level with:
          incomplete spinal cord lesion NOS
          posterior cord syndrome

  806.05 C_5-C_7 level with unspecified spinal cord injury

  806.06 C_5-C_7 level with complete lesion of cord

  806.07 C_5-C_7 level with anterior cord syndrome

  806.08 C_5-C_7 level with central cord syndrome

  806.09 C_5-C_7 level with other specified spinal cord injury
        C_5-C_7 level with:
          incomplete spinal cord lesion NOS
          posterior cord syndrome

⑤ **806.1 Cervical, open**

  806.10 C_1-C_4 level with unspecified spinal cord injury

  806.11 C_1-C_4 level with complete lesion of cord

  806.12 C_1-C_4 level with anterior cord syndrome

  806.13 C_1-C_4 level with central cord syndrome

  806.14 C_1-C_4 level with other specified spinal cord injury
        C_1-C_4 level with:
          incomplete spinal cord lesion NOS
          posterior cord syndrome

  806.15 C_5-C_7 level with unspecified spinal cord injury

  806.16 C_5-C_7 level with complete lesion of cord

  806.17 C_5-C_7 level with anterior cord syndrome

  806.18 C_5-C_7 level with central cord syndrome

  806.19 C_5-C_7 level with other specified spinal cord injury
        C_5-C_7 level with:
          incomplete spinal cord lesion NOS
          posterior cord syndrome

⑤ **806.2 Dorsal [thoracic], closed**

  806.20 T_1-T_6 level with unspecified spinal cord injury
        Thoracic region NOS with spinal cord injury NOS

  806.21 T_1-T_6 level with complete lesion of cord

  806.22 T_1-T_6 level with anterior cord syndrome

  806.23 T_1-T_6 level with central cord syndrome

  806.24 T_1-T_6 level with other specified spinal cord injury
        T_1-T_6 level with:
          incomplete spinal cord lesion NOS
          posterior cord syndrome

  806.25 T_7-T_{12} level with unspecified spinal cord injury

  806.26 T_7-T_{12} level with complete lesion of cord

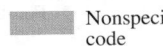 Add 4th or 5th digit   Nonspecific code   Unspecified code   Medicare secondary payer (MSP) alert

806.27	T_7-T_{12} level with anterior cord syndrome
806.28	T_7-T_{12} level with central cord syndrome
806.29	T_7-T_{12} level with other specified spinal cord injury

T_7-T_{12} level with:
   incomplete spinal cord lesion NOS
   posterior cord syndrome

⑤ **806.3 Dorsal [thoracic], open**

806.30	T_1-T_6 level with unspecified spinal cord injury
806.31	T_1-T_6 level with complete lesion of cord
806.32	T_1-T_6 level with anterior cord syndrome
806.33	T_1-T_6 level with central cord syndrome
806.34	T_1-T_6 level with other specified spinal cord injury

T_1-T_6 level with:
   incomplete spinal cord lesion NOS
   posterior cord syndrome

806.35	T_7-T_{12} level with unspecified spinal cord injury
806.36	T_7-T_{12} level with complete lesion of cord
806.37	T_7-T_{12} level with anterior cord syndrome
806.38	T_7-T_{12} level with central cord syndrome
806.39	T_7-T_{12} level with other specified spinal cord injury

T_7-T_{12} level with:
   incomplete spinal cord lesion NOS
   posterior cord syndrome

806.4 Lumbar, closed

806.5 Lumbar, open

⑤ **806.6 Sacrum and coccyx, closed**

806.60	With unspecified spinal cord injury
806.61	With complete cauda equina lesion
806.62	With other cauda equina injury
806.69	With other spinal cord injury

⑤ **806.7 Sacrum and coccyx, open**

806.70	With unspecified spinal cord injury
806.71	With complete cauda equina lesion
806.72	With other cauda equina injury
806.79	With other spinal cord injury

806.8 Unspecified, closed

806.9 Unspecified, open

807 Fracture of rib(s), sternum, larynx, and trachea

The following fifth-digit subclassification is for use with codes 807.0-807.1:

  0 rib(s), unspecified
  1 one rib
  2 two ribs
  3 three ribs
  4 four ribs
  5 five ribs
  6 six ribs
  7 seven ribs
  8 eight or more ribs
  9 multiple ribs, unspecified

ALERT! For coding late effect of fracture of spine and trunk without spinal cord lesion see 905.1

⑤ **807.0 Rib(s), closed**
[0-9]

⑤ **807.1 Rib(s), open**
[0-9]

● Code new
  to this edition

▲ Revision of
  existing code

④ ⑤ Fourth or fifth
  digit required

807.2 Sternum, closed

807.3 Sternum, open

807.4 Flail chest

807.5 Larynx and trachea, closed
    Hyoid bone   Trachea
    Thyroid cartilage

807.6 Larynx and trachea, open

808 Fracture of pelvis

> **ALERT!** For coding late effect of fracture of spine and trunk without spinal cord lesion see 905.1

808.0 Acetabulum, closed

808.1 Acetabulum, open

808.2 Pubis, closed

808.3 Pubis, open

⑤ **808.4 Other specified part, closed**

    808.41 Ilium

    808.42 Ischium

▲ **808.43 Multiple closed pelvic fractures with disruption of pelvic circle**
    Multiple closed pelvic fractures with disruption of pelvic ring

● **808.44 Multiple closed pelvic fractures without disruption of pelvic circle**
    Multiple closed pelvic fractures without disruption of pelvic ring

    808.49 Other
    Innominate bone
    Pelvic rim

⑤ **808.5 Other specified part, open**

    808.51 Ilium

    808.52 Ischium

    808.53 Multiple open pelvic fractures with disruption of pelvic circle
    Multiple open pelvic fractures with disruption of pelvic ring

● **808.54 Multiple open pelvic fractures without disruption of pelvic circle**
    Multiple open pelvic fractures without disruption of pelvic ring

    808.59 Other

808.8 Unspecified, closed

808.9 Unspecified, open

809 Ill-defined fractures of bones of trunk
    Includes: bones of trunk with other bones except those of skull and face
               multiple bones of trunk

> Excludes: *multiple fractures of:*
>   *pelvic bones alone (808.0-808.9)*
>   *ribs alone (807.0-807.1, 807.4)*
>   *ribs or sternum with limb bones (819.0-819.1, 828.0-828.1)*
>   *skull or face with other bones (804.0-804.9)*

> **ALERT!** For coding late effect of fracture of spine and trunk without spinal cord lesion see 905.1

809.0 Fracture of bones of trunk, closed

809.1 Fracture of bones of trunk, open

FRACTURE OF UPPER LIMB (810-819)

⑤ **810 Fracture of clavicle**
    Includes: collar bone
               interligamentous part of clavicle
The following fifth-digit subclassification is for use with category 810:

    0 unspecified part
        Clavicle NOS

    1 sternal end of clavicle

    2 shaft of clavicle

    3 acromial end of clavicle

> **ALERT!** For coding late effect of fracture of upper extremities see 905.2

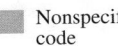

Add 4th or 5th digit	Nonspecific code	Unspecified code	Medicare secondary payer (MSP) alert

⑤ **810.0 Closed**
[0-3]

⑤ **810.1 Open**
[0-3]

⑤ **811 Fracture of scapula**
Includes: shoulder blade
The following fifth-digit subclassification is for use with category 811:

0 unspecified part

1 acromial process
Acromion (process)

2 coracoid process

3 glenoid cavity and neck of scapula

9 other
Scapula body

ALERT! For coding late effect of fracture of upper extremities see 905.2

⑤ **811.0 Closed**
[0-3,9]

⑤ **811.1 Open**
[0-3,9]

812 Fracture of humerus
ALERT! For coding late effect of fracture of upper extremities see 905.2

⑤ **812.0 Upper end, closed**

812.00 Upper end, unspecified part
Proximal end
Shoulder

812.01 Surgical neck
Neck of humerus NOS

812.02 Anatomical neck

812.03 Greater tuberosity

812.09 Other
Head
Upper epiphysis

⑤ **812.1 Upper end, open**

812.10 Upper end, unspecified part

812.11 Surgical neck

812.12 Anatomical neck

812.13 Greater tuberosity

812.19 Other

⑤ **812.2 Shaft or unspecified part, closed**

812.20 Unspecified part of humerus
Humerus NOS
Upper arm NOS

812.21 Shaft of humerus

⑤ **812.3 Shaft or unspecified part, open**

812.30 Unspecified part of humerus

812.31 Shaft of humerus

⑤ **812.4 Lower end, closed**
Distal end of humerus
Elbow

812.40 Lower end, unspecified part

812.41 Supracondylar fracture of humerus

812.42 Lateral condyle
External condyle

812.43 Medial condyle
Internal epicondyle

812.44 Condyle(s), unspecified
Articular process NOS
Lower epiphysis NOS

● Code new
to this edition   ▲ Revision of
existing code   ④ ⑤ Fourth or fifth
digit required

812.49 **Other**
Multiple fractures of lower end
Trochlea

⑤ **812.5** **Lower end, open**

812.50 **Lower end, unspecified part**

812.51 **Supracondylar fracture of humerus**

812.52 **Lateral condyle**

812.53 **Medial condyle**

812.54 **Condyle(s), unspecified**

812.59 **Other**

813 **Fracture of radius and ulna**
ALERT! For coding late effect of fracture of upper extremities see 905.2

⑤ **813.0** **Upper end, closed**
Proximal end

813.00 **Upper end of forearm, unspecified**

813.01 **Olecranon process of ulna**

813.02 **Coronoid process of ulna**

813.03 **Monteggia's fracture**

813.04 **Other and unspecified fractures of proximal end of ulna (alone)**
Multiple fractures of ulna, upper end

813.05 **Head of radius**

813.06 **Neck of radius**

813.07 **Other and unspecified fractures of proximal end of radius (alone)**
Multiple fractures of radius, upper end

813.08 **Radius with ulna, upper end [any part]**

⑤ **813.1** **Upper end, open**

813.10 **Upper end of forearm, unspecified**

813.11 **Olecranon process of ulna**

813.12 **Coronoid process of ulna**

813.13 **Monteggia's fracture**

813.14 **Other and unspecified fractures of proximal end of ulna (alone)**

813.15 **Head of radius**

813.16 **Neck of radius**

813.17 **Other and unspecified fractures of proximal end of radius (alone)**

813.18 **Radius with ulna, upper end [any part]**

⑤ **813.2** **Shaft, closed**

813.20 **Shaft, unspecified**

813.21 **Radius (alone)**

813.22 **Ulna (alone)**

813.23 **Radius with ulna**

⑤ **813.3** **Shaft, open**

813.30 **Shaft, unspecified**

813.31 **Radius (alone)**

813.32 **Ulna (alone)**

813.33 **Radius with ulna**

⑤ **813.4** **Lower end, closed**
Distal end

813.40 **Lower end of forearm, unspecified**

813.41 **Colles' fracture**
Smith's fracture

813.42 **Other fractures of distal end of radius (alone)**
Dupuytren's fracture, radius
Radius, lower end

Add 4th or 5th digit   Nonspecific code   Unspecified code   Medicare secondary payer (MSP) alert

813.43 Distal end of ulna (alone)
Ulna: Ulna:
  head   lower epiphysis
  lower end   styloid process

813.44 Radius with ulna, lower end

813.45 Torus fracture of radius (alone)

Excludes: *Torus fracture of radius and ulna (813.47)*

813.46 Torus fracture of ulna (alone)

Excludes: *Torus fracture of radius and ulna (813.47)*

813.47 Torus fracture of radius and ulna

⑤ **813.5 Lower end, open**

813.50 Lower end of forearm, unspecified

813.51 Colles' fracture

813.52 Other fractures of distal end of radius (alone)

813.53 Distal end of ulna (alone)

813.54 Radius with ulna, lower end

⑤ **813.8 Unspecified part, closed**

813.80 Forearm, unspecified

813.81 Radius (alone)

813.82 Ulna (alone)

813.83 Radius with ulna

⑤ **813.9 Unspecified part, open**

813.90 Forearm, unspecified

813.91 Radius (alone)

813.92 Ulna (alone)

813.93 Radius with ulna

⑤ **814 Fracture of carpal bone(s)**

The following fifth-digit subclassification is for use with category 814:

0 carpal bone, unspecified
Wrist NOS

1 navicular [scaphoid] of wrist

2 lunate [semilunar] bone of wrist

3 triquetral [cuneiform] bone of wrist

4 pisiform

5 trapezium bone [larger multangular]

6 trapezoid bone [smaller multangular]

7 capitate bone [os magnum]

8 hamate [unciform] bone

9 other

ALERT! For coding late effect of fracture of upper extremities see 905.2

⑤ **814.0 Closed**
[0-9]

⑤ **814.1 Open**
[0-9]

⑤ **815 Fracture of metacarpal bone(s)**
Includes: hand [except finger]
          metacarpus

The following fifth-digit subclassification is for use with category 815:

0 metacarpal bone(s), site unspecified

1 base of thumb [first] metacarpal
Bennett's fracture

2 base of other metacarpal bone(s)

3 shaft of metacarpal bone(s)

4 neck of metacarpal bone(s)

9 multiple sites of metacarpus

● Code new
to this edition

▲ Revision of
existing code

④ ⑤ Fourth or fifth
digit required

ALERT! For coding late effect of fracture of upper extremities see 905.2

⑤ **815.0 Closed**
[0-4,9]

⑤ **815.1 Open**
[0-4,9]

⑤ **816 Fracture of one or more phalanges of hand**
Includes: finger(s)
thumb

The following fifth-digit subclassification is for use with category 816:

0 phalanx or phalanges, unspecified

1 middle or proximal phalanx or phalanges

2 distal phalanx or phalanges

3 multiple sites

ALERT! For coding late effect of fracture of upper extremities see 905.2

⑤ **816.0 Closed**
[0-3]

⑤ **816.1 Open**
[0-3]

817 Multiple fractures of hand bones
Includes: metacarpal bone(s) with phalanx or phalanges of same hand
ALERT! For coding late effect of fracture of upper extremities see 905.2

817.0 Closed

817.1 Open

818 Ill-defined fractures of upper limb
Includes: arm NOS
multiple bones of same upper limb

Excludes: *multiple fractures of:*
metacarpal bone(s) with phalanx or phalanges (817.0-817.1)
phalanges of hand alone (816.0-816.1)
radius with ulna (813.0-813.9)

ALERT! For coding late effect of fracture of upper extremities see 905.2

818.0 Closed

818.1 Open

819 Multiple fractures involving both upper limbs, and upper limb with rib(s) and sternum
Includes: arm(s) with rib(s) or sternum
both arms [any bones]
ALERT! For coding late effect of fracture of upper extremities see 905.2

819.0 Closed

819.1 Open

FRACTURE OF LOWER LIMB (820-829)

820 Fracture of neck of femur
ALERT! For coding late effect of fracture of neck of femur see 905.3

⑤ **820.0 Transcervical fracture, closed**

820.00 Intracapsular section, unspecified

820.01 Epiphysis (separation) (upper)
Transepiphyseal

820.02 Midcervical section
Transcervical NOS

820.03 Base of neck
Cervicotrochanteric section

820.09 Other
Head of femur
Subcapital

⑤ **820.1 Transcervical fracture, open**

820.10 Intracapsular section, unspecified

820.11 Epiphysis (separation) (upper)

820.12 Midcervical section

820.13 Base of neck

| Add 4th or 5th digit | Nonspecific code | Unspecified code | Medicare secondary payer (MSP) alert |

820.19 Other

⑤ **820.2 Pertrochanteric fracture, closed**

820.20 **Trochanteric section, unspecified**
Trochanter:
  NOS
  greater
  lesser

820.21 **Intertrochanteric section**

820.22 **Subtrochanteric section**

⑤ **820.3 Pertrochanteric fracture, open**

820.30 **Trochanteric section, unspecified**

820.31 **Intertrochanteric section**

820.32 **Subtrochanteric section**

820.8 Unspecified part of neck of femur, closed
Hip NOS
Neck of femur NOS

820.9 Unspecified part of neck of femur, open

821 **Fracture of other and unspecified parts of femur**
ALERT! For coding late effect of fracture of lower extremities see 905.4

⑤ **821.0 Shaft or unspecified part, closed**

821.00 **Unspecified part of femur**
Thigh
Upper leg

Excludes: hip NOS (820.8)

821.01 **Shaft**

⑤ **821.1 Shaft or unspecified part, open**

821.10 **Unspecified part of femur**

821.11 **Shaft**

⑤ **821.2 Lower end, closed**
Distal end

821.20 **Lower end, unspecified part**

821.21 **Condyle, femoral**

821.22 **Epiphysis, lower (separation)**

821.23 **Supracondylar fracture of femur**

821.29 **Other**
Multiple fractures of lower end

⑤ **821.3 Lower end, open**

821.30 **Lower end, unspecified part**

821.31 **Condyle, femoral**

821.32 **Epiphysis, lower (separation)**

821.33 **Supracondylar fracture of femur**

821.39 **Other**

822 **Fracture of patella**
ALERT! For coding late effect of fracture of lower extremities see 905.4

822.0 Closed

822.1 Open

⑤ **823** **Fracture of tibia and fibula**

Excludes: Dupuytren's fracture (824.4-824.5)
  ankle (824.4-824.5)
  radius (813.42, 813.52)
  Pott's fracture (824.4-824.5)
  that involving ankle (824.0-824.9)

The following fifth-digit subclassification is for use with category 823:

0 **tibia alone**

1 **fibula alone**

2 **fibula with tibia**

● Code new
to this edition
▲ Revision of
existing code
④ ⑤ Fourth or fifth
digit required

ALERT! For coding late effect of fracture of lower extremities see 905.4

⑤ **823.0 Upper end, closed**
[0-2] Head
     Proximal end
     Tibia:
       condyles
       tuberosity

⑤ **823.1 Upper end, open**
[0-2]

⑤ **823.2 Shaft, closed**
[0-2]

⑤ **823.3 Shaft, open**
[0-2]

⑤ **823.4 Torus fracture**
[0-2]

⑤ **823.8 Unspecified part, closed**
[0-2] Lower leg NOS

⑤ **823.9 Unspecified part, open**
[0-2]

824 Fracture of ankle

ALERT! For coding late effect of fracture of lower extremities see 905.4

824.0 Medial malleolus, closed
   Tibia involving:
     ankle
     malleolus

824.1 Medial malleolus, open

824.2 Lateral malleolus, closed
   Fibula involving:
     ankle
     malleolus

824.3 Lateral malleolus, open

824.4 Bimalleolar, closed
   Dupuytren's fracture, fibula
   Pott's fracture

824.5 Bimalleolar, open

824.6 Trimalleolar, closed
   Lateral and medial malleolus with anterior or posterior lip of tibia

824.7 Trimalleolar, open

824.8 Unspecified, closed
   Ankle NOS

824.9 Unspecified, open

825 Fracture of one or more tarsal and metatarsal bones

ALERT! For coding late effect of fracture of lower extremities see 905.4

825.0 Fracture of calcaneus, closed
   Heel bone
   Os calcis

825.1 Fracture of calcaneus, open

⑤ **825.2 Fracture of other tarsal and metatarsal bones, closed**

   825.20 Unspecified bone(s) of foot [except toes]
       Instep

   825.21 Astragalus
       Talus

   825.22 Navicular [scaphoid], foot

   825.23 Cuboid

   825.24 Cuneiform, foot

   825.25 Metatarsal bone(s)

   825.29 Other
       Tarsal with metatarsal bone(s) only

   Excludes: calcaneus (825.0)

⑤ **825.3 Fracture of other tarsal and metatarsal bones, open**

| | Add 4th or 5th digit | | Nonspecific code | | Unspecified code | | Medicare secondary payer (MSP) alert |

825.30 **Unspecified bone(s) of foot [except toes]**

825.31 **Astragalus**

825.32 **Navicular [scaphoid], foot**

825.33 **Cuboid**

825.34 **Cuneiform, foot**

825.35 **Metatarsal bone(s)**

825.39 **Other**

826 Fracture of one or more phalanges of foot
Includes: toe(s)

ALERT! For coding late effect of fracture of lower extremities see 905.4

826.0 **Closed**

826.1 **Open**

827 Other, multiple, and ill-defined fractures of lower limb
Includes: leg NOS
multiple bones of same lower limb

Excludes: *multiple fractures of:*
ankle bones alone (824.4-824.9)
phalanges of foot alone (826.0-826.1)
tarsal with metatarsal bones (825.29, 825.39)
tibia with fibula (823.0-823.9 with fifth-digit 2)

ALERT! For coding late effect of fracture of lower extremities see 905.4

827.0 **Closed**

827.1 **Open**

828 Multiple fractures involving both lower limbs, lower with upper limb, and lower limb(s) with rib(s) and sternum
Includes: arm(s) with leg(s) [any bones]
both legs [any bones]
leg(s) with rib(s) or sternum

ALERT! For coding late effect of fracture of lower extremities see 905.4

828.0 **Closed**

828.1 **Open**

829 Fracture of unspecified bones

ALERT! For coding late effect of fracture of multiple and unspecified bones see 905.5

829.0 **Unspecified bone, closed**

829.1 **Unspecified bone, open**

DISLOCATION (830-839)

Includes: displacement
subluxation

Excludes: *congenital dislocation (754.0-755.8)*
pathological dislocation (718.2)
recurrent dislocation (718.3)

The descriptions "closed" and "open", used in the fourth-digit subdivisions, include the following terms:

closed:
  complete
  dislocation NOS
  partial
  simple
  uncomplicated

open:
  compound
  infected
  with foreign body

A dislocation not indicated as closed or open should be classified as closed.

830 Dislocation of jaw
Includes: jaw (cartilage) (meniscus)
mandible
maxilla (inferior)
temporomandibular (joint)

DEFINITION Dislocation refers to the displacement of bones that form a joint, often resulting from trauma.

ALERT! For coding late effect of dislocation see 905.6

830.0 **Closed dislocation**

830.1 **Open dislocation**

● Code new
  to this edition

▲ Revision of
  existing code

④ ⑤ Fourth or fifth
  digit required

⑤ **831** **Dislocation of shoulder**

> *Excludes:* *sternoclavicular joint (839.61, 839.71)*
> *sternum (839.61, 839.71)*

The following fifth-digit subclassification is for use with category 831:

0 **shoulder, unspecified**
Humerus NOS

1 **anterior dislocation of humerus**

2 **posterior dislocation of humerus**

3 **inferior dislocation of humerus**

4 **acromioclavicular (joint)**
Clavicle

9 **other**
Scapula

ALERT! For coding late effect of dislocation see 905.6

⑤ **831.0** **Closed dislocation**
[0-4,9]

⑤ **831.1** **Open dislocation**
[0-4,9]

832 **Dislocation of elbow**

The following fifth-digit subclassification is for use with subcategories 832.0 and 832.1:

0 **elbow unspecified**

1 **anterior dislocation of elbow**

2 **posterior dislocation of elbow**

3 **medial dislocation of elbow**

4 **lateral dislocation of elbow**

9 **other**

ALERT! For coding late effect of dislocation see 905.6

⑤ **832.0** **Closed dislocation**
[0-4,9]

⑤ **832.1** **Open dislocation**
[0-4,9]

832.2 **Nursemaid's elbow**
Subluxation of radial head

⑤ **833** **Dislocation of wrist**

The following fifth-digit subclassification is for use with category 833:

0 **wrist, unspecified part**
Carpal (bone)   Radius, distal end

1 **radioulnar (joint), distal**

2 **radiocarpal (joint)**

3 **midcarpal (joint)**

4 **carpometacarpal (joint)**

5 **metacarpal (bone), proximal end**

9 **other**
Ulna, distal end

ALERT! For coding late effect of dislocation see 905.6

⑤ **833.0** **Closed dislocation**
[0-5,9]

⑤ **833.1** **Open dislocation**
[0-5,9]

	Add 4th or 5th digit		Nonspecific code		Unspecified code		Medicare secondary payer (MSP) alert

⑤ **834** **Dislocation of finger**
Includes: finger(s)
phalanx of hand
thumb

The following fifth-digit subclassification is for use with category 834:

0 **finger, unspecified part**

1 **metacarpophalangeal (joint)**
Metacarpal (bone), distal end

2 **interphalangeal (joint), hand**
ALERT! For coding late effect of dislocation see 905.6

⑤ **834.0** **Closed dislocation**
[0-2]

⑤ **834.1** **Open dislocation**
[0-2]

⑤ **835** **Dislocation of hip**
The following fifth-digit subclassification is for use with category 835:

0 **dislocation of hip, unspecified**

1 **posterior dislocation**

2 **obturator dislocation**

3 **other anterior dislocation**
ALERT! For coding late effect of dislocation see 905.6

⑤ **835.0** **Closed dislocation**
[0-3]

⑤ **835.1** **Open dislocation**
[0-3]

836 **Dislocation of knee**
Excludes: *dislocation of knee:*
old or pathological (718.2)
recurrent (718.3)
internal derangement of knee joint (717.0-717.5, 717.8-717.9)
old tear of cartilage or meniscus of knee (717.0-717.5, 717.8-717.9)
ALERT! For coding late effect of dislocation see 905.6

836.0 **Tear of medial cartilage or meniscus of knee, current**
Bucket handle tear:
NOS current injury
medial meniscus current injury

836.1 **Tear of lateral cartilage or meniscus of knee, current**

836.2 **Other tear of cartilage or meniscus of knee, current**
Tear of:
cartilage (semilunar) current injury, not specified as medial or lateral
meniscus current injury, not specified as medial or lateral

836.3 **Dislocation of patella, closed**

836.4 **Dislocation of patella, open**

⑤ **836.5** **Other dislocation of knee, closed**

836.50 **Dislocation of knee, unspecified**

836.51 **Anterior dislocation of tibia, proximal end**
Posterior dislocation of femur, distal end, closed

836.52 **Posterior dislocation of tibia, proximal end**
Anterior dislocation of femur, distal end, closed

836.53 **Medial dislocation of tibia, proximal end**

836.54 **Lateral dislocation of tibia, proximal end**

836.59 **Other**

⑤ **836.6** **Other dislocation of knee, open**

836.60 **Dislocation of knee, unspecified**

836.61 **Anterior dislocation of tibia, proximal end**
Posterior dislocation of femur, distal end, open

836.62 **Posterior dislocation of tibia, proximal end**
Anterior dislocation of femur, distal end, open

836.63 **Medial dislocation of tibia, proximal end**

● Code new
to this edition
▲ Revision of
existing code
④ ⑤ Fourth or fifth
digit required

836.64 **Lateral dislocation of tibia, proximal end**

836.69 **Other**

837 **Dislocation of ankle**
Includes: astragalus
fibula, distal end
navicular, foot
scaphoid, foot
tibia, distal end
ALERT! For coding late effect of dislocation see 905.6

837.0 **Closed dislocation**

837.1 **Open dislocation**

838 **Dislocation of foot**
The following fifth-digit subclassification is for use with category 838:

0 **foot, unspecified**

1 **tarsal (bone), joint unspecified**

2 **midtarsal (joint)**

3 **tarsometatarsal (joint)**

4 **metatarsal (bone), joint unspecified**

5 **metatarsophalangeal (joint)**

6 **interphalangeal (joint), foot**

9 **other**
Phalanx of foot
Toe(s)
ALERT! For coding late effect of dislocation see 905.6

838.0 **Closed dislocation**
[0-6,9]

838.1 **Open dislocation**
[0-6,9]

839 **Other, multiple, and ill-defined dislocations**
ALERT! For coding late effect of dislocation see 905.6

839.0 **Cervical vertebra, closed**
Cervical spine
Neck

839.00 **Cervical vertebra, unspecified**

839.01 **First cervical vertebra**

839.02 **Second cervical vertebra**

839.03 **Third cervical vertebra**

839.04 **Fourth cervical vertebra**

839.05 **Fifth cervical vertebra**

839.06 **Sixth cervical vertebra**

839.07 **Seventh cervical vertebra**

839.08 **Multiple cervical vertebrae**

839.1 **Cervical vertebra, open**

839.10 **Cervical vertebra, unspecified**

839.11 **First cervical vertebra**

839.12 **Second cervical vertebra**

839.13 **Third cervical vertebra**

839.14 **Fourth cervical vertebra**

839.15 **Fifth cervical vertebra**

839.16 **Sixth cervical vertebra**

839.17 **Seventh cervical vertebra**

839.18 **Multiple cervical vertebrae**

839.2 **Thoracic and lumbar vertebra, closed**

839.20 **Lumbar vertebra**

839.21 **Thoracic vertebra**
Dorsal [thoracic] vertebra

Add 4th or
5th digit

Nonspecific
code

Unspecified
code

Medicare secondary
payer (MSP) alert

⑤ **839.3** **Thoracic and lumbar vertebra, open**

    839.30 **Lumbar vertebra**

    839.31 **Thoracic vertebra**

⑤ **839.4** **Other vertebra, closed**

    839.40 **Vertebra, unspecified site**
        Spine NOS

    839.41 **Coccyx**

    839.42 **Sacrum**
        Sacroiliac (joint)

    839.49 **Other**

⑤ **839.5** **Other vertebra, open**

    839.50 **Vertebra, unspecified site**

    839.51 **Coccyx**

    839.52 **Sacrum**

    839.59 **Other**

⑤ **839.6** **Other location, closed**

    839.61 **Sternum**
        Sternoclavicular joint

    839.69 **Other**
        Pelvis

⑤ **839.7** **Other location, open**

    839.71 **Sternum**

    839.79 **Other**

839.8 **Multiple and ill-defined, closed**
    Arm
    Back
    Hand
    Multiple locations, except fingers or toes alone
    Other ill-defined locations
    Unspecified location

839.9 **Multiple and ill-defined, open**

SPRAINS AND STRAINS OF JOINTS AND ADJACENT MUSCLES (840-848)

Includes: avulsion of: joint capsule, ligament, muscle, tendon
        hemarthrosis of: joint capsule, ligament, muscle, tendon
        laceration of: joint capsule, ligament, muscle, tendon
        rupture of: joint capsule, ligament, muscle, tendon
        sprain of: joint capsule, ligament, muscle, tendon
        strain of: joint capsule, ligament, muscle, tendon
        tear of: joint capsule, ligament, muscle, tendon

Excludes: *laceration of tendon in open wounds (880-884 and 890-894 with .2)*

840 **Sprains and strains of shoulder and upper arm**
    DEFINITION Sprain refers to damage or tearing of ligaments or a joint capsule
    ALERT! For coding late effect of sprain and strain without tendon injury see 905.7
    ALERT! For coding late effect of tendon injury see 905.8

    840.0 **Acromioclavicular (joint) (ligament)**

    840.1 **Coracoclavicular (ligament)**

    840.2 **Coracohumeral (ligament)**

    840.3 **Infraspinatus (muscle) (tendon)**

    840.4 **Rotator cuff (capsule)**

    Excludes: *complete rupture of rotator cuff, nontraumatic (727.61)*

    840.5 **Subscapularis (muscle)**

    840.6 **Supraspinatus (muscle) (tendon)**

    840.7 **Superior glenoid labrum lesion**
        SLAP lesion

    840.8 **Other specified sites of shoulder and upper arm**

● Code new   ▲ Revision of   ④ ⑤ Fourth or fifth
  to this edition   existing code   digit required

840.9 Unspecified site of shoulder and upper arm
Arm NOS
Shoulder NOS

841 Sprains and strains of elbow and forearm
ALERT! For coding late effect of sprain and strain without tendon injury see 905.7
ALERT! For coding late effect of tendon injury see 905.8

841.0 Radial collateral ligament

841.1 Ulnar collateral ligament

841.2 Radiohumeral (joint)

841.3 Ulnohumeral (joint)

841.8 Other specified sites of elbow and forearm

841.9 Unspecified site of elbow and forearm
Elbow NOS

842 Sprains and strains of wrist and hand
ALERT! For coding late effect of sprain and strain without tendon injury see 905.7
ALERT! For coding late effect of tendon injury see 905.8

⑤ **842.0 Wrist**

842.00 Unspecified site

842.01 Carpal (joint)

842.02 Radiocarpal (joint) (ligament)

842.09 Other
Radioulnar joint, distal

⑤ **842.1 Hand**

842.10 Unspecified site

842.11 Carpometacarpal (joint)

842.12 Metacarpophalangeal (joint)

842.13 Interphalangeal (joint)

842.19 Other
Midcarpal (joint)

843 Sprains and strains of hip and thigh
ALERT! For coding late effect of sprain and strain without tendon injury see 905.7
ALERT! For coding late effect of tendon injury see 905.8

843.0 Iliofemoral (ligament)

843.1 Ischiocapsular (ligament)

843.8 Other specified sites of hip and thigh

843.9 Unspecified site of hip and thigh
Hip NOS
Thigh NOS

844 Sprains and strains of knee and leg
ALERT! For coding late effect of sprain and strain without tendon injury see 905.7
ALERT! For coding late effect of tendon injury see 905.8

844.0 Lateral collateral ligament of knee

844.1 Medial collateral ligament of knee

844.2 Cruciate ligament of knee

844.3 Tibiofibular (joint) (ligament), superior

844.8 Other specified sites of knee and leg

844.9 Unspecified site of knee and leg
Knee NOS
Leg NOS

845 Sprains and strains of ankle and foot
ALERT! For coding late effect of sprain and strain without tendon injury see 905.7
ALERT! For coding late effect of tendon injury see 905.8

⑤ **845.0 Ankle**

845.00 Unspecified site

845.01 Deltoid (ligament), ankle
Internal collateral (ligament), ankle

| | Add 4th or 5th digit | | Nonspecific code | | Unspecified code | | Medicare secondary payer (MSP) alert |

845.02   **Calcaneofibular (ligament)**

845.03   **Tibiofibular (ligament), distal**

`845.09`   **Other**
      Achilles tendon

⑤ **845.1   Foot**

`845.10`   **Unspecified site**

845.11   **Tarsometatarsal (joint) (ligament)**

845.12   **Metatarsophalangeal (joint)**

845.13   **Interphalangeal (joint), toe**

`845.19`   **Other**

`846` **Sprains and strains of sacroiliac region**

    `ALERT!` For coding late effect of sprain and strain without tendon injury see 905.7

    `ALERT!` For coding late effect of tendon injury see 905.8

846.0   Lumbosacral (joint) (ligament)

846.1   Sacroiliac ligament

846.2   Sacrospinatus (ligament)

846.3   Sacrotuberous (ligament)

`846.8`   **Other specified sites of sacroiliac region**

846.9   Unspecified site of sacroiliac region

`847` **Sprains and strains of other and unspecified parts of back**

    Excludes: *lumbosacral (846.0)*

    `ALERT!` For coding late effect of sprain and strain without tendon injury see 905.7

    `ALERT!` For coding late effect of tendon injury see 905.8

`847.0`   **Neck**
      Anterior longitudinal (ligament), cervical
      Atlanto-axial (joints)
      Atlanto-occipital (joints)
      Whiplash injury

    Excludes: *neck injury NOS (959.0)*
          thyroid region (848.2)

847.1   Thoracic

847.2   Lumbar

847.3   Sacrum
      Sacrococcygeal (ligament)

847.4   Coccyx

`847.9`   **Unspecified site of back**
      Back NOS

`848` **Other and ill-defined sprains and strains**

    `ALERT!` For coding late effect of sprain and strain without tendon injury see 905.7

    `ALERT!` For coding late effect of tendon injury see 905.8

848.0   Septal cartilage of nose

848.1   Jaw
      Temporomandibular (joint) (ligament)

848.2   Thyroid region
      Cricoarytenoid (joint) (ligament)
      Cricothyroid (joint) (ligament)
      Thyroid cartilage

848.3   Ribs
      Chondrocostal (joint) without mention of injury to sternum
      Costal cartilage without mention of injury to sternum

⑤ **848.4   Sternum**

`848.40`   **Unspecified site**

848.41   **Sternoclavicular (joint) (ligament)**

848.42   **Chondrosternal (joint)**

`848.49`   **Other**
      Xiphoid cartilage

   ● Code new   ▲ Revision of   ④ ⑤ Fourth or fifth
          to this edition   existing code   digit required

848.5 Pelvis
> Symphysis pubis
> *Excludes:* *that in childbirth (665.6)*

848.8 Other specified sites of sprains and strains

848.9 Unspecified site of sprain and strain

INTRACRANIAL INJURY, EXCLUDING THOSE WITH SKULL FRACTURE (850-854)

> *Excludes:* *intracranial injury with skull fracture (800-801 and 803-804, except .0 and .5)*
> *open wound of head without intracranial injury (870.0-873.9)*
> *skull fracture alone (800-801 and 803-804 with .0, .5)*

Includes: traumatic brain injury without skull fracture

The description "with open intracranial wound," used in the fourth-digit subdivisions, includes those specified as open or with mention of infection or foreign body.

The following fifth-digit subclassification is for use with categories 851-854:

  0 unspecified state of consciousness

  1 with no loss of consciousness

  2 with brief [less than one hour] loss of consciousness

  3 with moderate [1-24 hours] loss of consciousness

  4 with prolonged [more than 24 hours] loss of consciousness and return to pre-existing conscious level

  5 with prolonged [more than 24 hours] loss of consciousness, without return to pre-existing conscious level

  Use fifth-digit 5 to designate when a patient is unconscious and dies before regaining consciousness, regardless of the duration of the loss of consciousness

  6 with loss of consciousness of unspecified duration

  9 with concussion, unspecified

  ALERT! For coding late effect of intracranial injury without skull fracture see 907.0

850 Concussion
> Includes: commotio cerebri
> *Excludes:* *concussion with:*
> *cerebral laceration or contusion (851.0-851.9)*
> *cerebral hemorrhage (852-853)*
> *head injury NOS (959.01)*

DEFINITION Concussion is a trauma-induced change in mental status, with confusion and amnesia, and with or without a brief loss of consciousness

ALERT! For personal history of traumatic brain injury see V15.52

850.0 With no loss of consciousness
> Concussion with mental confusion or disorientation, without loss of consciousness

⑤ **850.1 With brief loss of consciousness**
> Loss of consciousness for less than one hour

  850.11 With loss of consciousness of 30 minutes or less

  850.12 With loss of consciousness from 31 to 59 minutes

850.2 With moderate loss of consciousness
> Loss of consciousness for 1-24 hours

850.3 With prolonged loss of consciousness and return to pre-existing conscious level
> Loss of consciousness for more than 24 hours with complete recovery

850.4 With prolonged loss of consciousness, without return to pre-existing conscious level

850.5 With loss of consciousness of unspecified duration

850.9 Concussion, unspecified

⑤ **851 Cerebral laceration and contusion**
> **DEFINITION** Cerebral laceration and contusion is a type of traumatic brain injury that occurs when the tissue of the brain is mechanically cut or torn.
> **ALERT!** For personal history of traumatic brain injury see V15.52

⑤ **851.0 Cortex (cerebral) contusion without mention of open intracranial wound**
[0-6,9]

⑤ **851.1 Cortex (cerebral) contusion with open intracranial wound**
[0-6,9]

⑤ **851.2 Cortex (cerebral) laceration without mention of open intracranial wound**
[0-6,9]

| ▮ Add 4th or 5th digit | ▮ Nonspecific code | ▮ Unspecified code | ▮ Medicare secondary payer (MSP) alert |

⑤ **851.3** **Cortex (cerebral) laceration with open intracranial wound**
[0-6,9]

⑤ **851.4** **Cerebellar or brain stem contusion without mention of open intracranial wound**
[0-6,9]

⑤ **851.5** **Cerebellar or brain stem contusion with open intracranial wound**
[0-6,9]

⑤ **851.6** **Cerebellar or brain stem laceration without mention of open intracranial wound**
[0-6,9]

⑤ **851.7** **Cerebellar or brain stem laceration with open intracranial wound**
[0-6,9]

⑤ **851.8** **Other and unspecified cerebral laceration and contusion, without mention of open intracranial wound**
[0-6,9]   Brain (membrane) NOS

⑤ **851.9** **Other and unspecified cerebral laceration and contusion, with open intracranial wound**
[0-6,9]

⑤ **852** **Subarachnoid, subdural, and extradural hemorrhage, following injury**

> *Excludes:* *Cerebral contusion or laceration (with hemorrhage) (851.0-851.9)*

> **DEFINITION** Subarachnoid, subdural, and extradural hemorrhage, following injury, refers to an abnormal condition in which blood collects beneath the arachnoid mater or the dura mater or outside the dura mater

> **ALERT!** For personal history of traumatic brain injury see V15.52

⑤ **852.0** **Subarachnoid hemorrhage following injury without mention of open intracranial wound**
[0-6,9]   Middle meningeal hemorrhage following injury

⑤ **852.1** **Subarachnoid hemorrhage following injury with open intracranial wound**
[0-6,9]

⑤ **852.2** **Subdural hemorrhage following injury without mention of open intracranial wound**
[0-6,9]

⑤ **852.3** **Subdural hemorrhage following injury with open intracranial wound**
[0-6,9]

⑤ **852.4** **Extradural hemorrhage following injury without mention of open intracranial wound**
[0-6,9]   Epidural hematoma following injury

⑤ **852.5** **Extradural hemorrhage following injury with open intracranial wound**
[0-6,9]

⑤ **853** **Other and unspecified intracranial hemorrhage following injury**

> **DEFINITION** Intracranial hemorrhage refers to bleeding within the cranium due to the loss of integrity of vascular channels and frequently leading to formation of a hematoma.

> **ALERT!** For personal history of traumatic brain injury see V15.52

⑤ **853.0** **Without mention of open intracranial wound**
[0-6,9]   Cerebral compression due to injury
          Intracranial hematoma following injury
          Traumatic cerebral hemorrhage

⑤ **853.1** **With open intracranial wound**
[0-6,9]

⑤ **854** **Intracranial injury of other and unspecified nature**
Includes: injury
                brain NOS
                intracranial
                traumatic brain NOS
            cavernous sinus

> *Excludes:* *any condition classifiable to 850-853*
>   *head injury NOS (959.01)*

> **ALERT!** For personal history of traumatic brain injury see V15.52

⑤ **854.0** **Without mention of open intracranial wound**
[0-6,9]

⑤ **854.1** **With open intracranial wound**
[0-6,9]

● Code new   ▲ Revision of   ④ ⑤ Fourth or fifth
  to this edition   existing code   digit required

INTERNAL INJURY OF THORAX, ABDOMEN, AND PELVIS (860-869)

Includes:
> blast injuries of internal organs
> blunt trauma of internal organs
> bruise of internal organs
> concussion injuries (except cerebral) of internal organs
> crushing of internal organs
> hematoma of internal organs
> laceration of internal organs
> puncture of internal organs
> tear of internal organs
> traumatic rupture of internal organs

Excludes: *concussion NOS (850.0-850.9)*
> *flail chest (807.4)*
> *foreign body entering through orifice (930.0-939.9)*
> *injury to blood vessels (901.0-902.9)*

The description "with open wound," used in the fourth-digit subdivisions, includes those with mention of infection or foreign body.

860 Traumatic pneumothorax and hemothorax

DEFINITION Pneumothorax is a collection of air or gas in the chest or pleural space that causes part or all of a lung to collapse. Hemothorax is the accumulation of blood in the pleural cavity.

860.0 Pneumothorax without mention of open wound into thorax

860.1 Pneumothorax with open wound into thorax

860.2 Hemothorax without mention of open wound into thorax

860.3 Hemothorax with open wound into thorax

860.4 Pneumohemothorax without mention of open wound into thorax

860.5 Pneumohemothorax with open wound into thorax

861 Injury to heart and lung

Excludes: *injury to blood vessels of thorax (901.0-901.9)*

⑤ **861.0 Heart, without mention of open wound into thorax**

  861.00 Unspecified injury

  861.01 Contusion
  > Cardiac contusion
  > Myocardial contusion

  861.02 Laceration without penetration of heart chambers

  861.03 Laceration with penetration of heart chambers

⑤ **861.1 Heart, with open wound into thorax**

  861.10 Unspecified injury

  861.11 Contusion

  861.12 Laceration without penetration of heart chambers

  861.13 Laceration with penetration of heart chambers

⑤ **861.2 Lung, without mention of open wound into thorax**

  861.20 Unspecified injury

  861.21 Contusion

  861.22 Laceration

⑤ **861.3 Lung, with open wound into thorax**

  861.30 Unspecified injury

  861.31 Contusion

  861.32 Laceration

862 Injury to other and unspecified intrathoracic organs

Excludes: *injury to blood vessels of thorax (901.0-901.9)*

862.0 Diaphragm, without mention of open wound into cavity

862.1 Diaphragm, with open wound into cavity

⑤ **862.2 Other specified intrathoracic organs, without mention of open wound into cavity**

  862.21 Bronchus

  862.22 Esophagus

	Add 4th or 5th digit		Nonspecific code		Unspecified code		Medicare secondary payer (MSP) alert

862.29 **Other**
    Pleura
    Thymus gland

⑤ **862.3 Other specified intrathoracic organs, with open wound into cavity**

862.31 **Bronchus**

862.32 **Esophagus**

862.39 **Other**

862.8 **Multiple and unspecified intrathoracic organs, without mention of open wound into cavity**
    Crushed chest
    Multiple intrathoracic organs

862.9 **Multiple and unspecified intrathoracic organs, with open wound into cavity**

863 **Injury to gastrointestinal tract**

> Excludes: *anal sphincter laceration during delivery (664.2)*
> *bile duct (868.0-868.1 with fifth-digit 2)*
> *gallbladder (868.0-868.1 with fifth-digit 2)*

863.0 **Stomach, without mention of open wound into cavity**

863.1 **Stomach, with open wound into cavity**

⑤ **863.2 Small intestine, without mention of open wound into cavity**

863.20 **Small intestine, unspecified site**

863.21 **Duodenum**

863.29 **Other**

⑤ **863.3 Small intestine, with open wound into cavity**

863.30 **Small intestine, unspecified site**

863.31 **Duodenum**

863.39 **Other**

⑤ **863.4 Colon or rectum, without mention of open wound into cavity**

863.40 **Colon, unspecified site**

863.41 **Ascending [right] colon**

863.42 **Transverse colon**

863.43 **Descending [left] colon**

863.44 **Sigmoid colon**

863.45 **Rectum**

863.46 **Multiple sites in colon and rectum**

863.49 **Other**

⑤ **863.5 Colon or rectum, with open wound into cavity**

863.50 **Colon, unspecified site**

863.51 **Ascending [right] colon**

863.52 **Transverse colon**

863.53 **Descending [left] colon**

863.54 **Sigmoid colon**

863.55 **Rectum**

863.56 **Multiple sites in colon and rectum**

863.59 **Other**

⑤ **863.8 Other and unspecified gastrointestinal sites, without mention of open wound into cavity**

863.80 **Gastrointestinal tract, unspecified site**

863.81 **Pancreas, head**

863.82 **Pancreas, body**

863.83 **Pancreas, tail**

863.84 **Pancreas, multiple and unspecified sites**

863.85 **Appendix**

863.89 **Other**
    Intestine NOS

● Code new
to this edition
▲ Revision of
existing code
④ ⑤ Fourth or fifth
digit required

⑤ **863.9** **Other and unspecified gastrointestinal sites, with open wound into cavity**

- **863.90** **Gastrointestinal tract, unspecified site**
- **863.91** **Pancreas, head**
- **863.92** **Pancreas, body**
- **863.93** **Pancreas, tail**
- **863.94** **Pancreas, multiple and unspecified sites**
- **863.95** **Appendix**
- **863.99** **Other**

⑤ **864** **Injury to liver**

The following fifth-digit subclassification is for use with category 864:

- **0** **unspecified injury**
- **1** **hematoma and contusion**
- **2** **laceration, minor**
  Laceration involving capsule only, or without significant involvement of hepatic parenchyma [i.e., less than 1 cm deep]
- **3** **laceration, moderate**
  Laceration involving parenchyma but without major disruption of parenchyma [i.e., less than 10 cm long and less than 3 cm deep]
- **4** **laceration, major**
  Laceration with significant disruption of hepatic parenchyma [i.e., 10 cm long and 3 cm deep]
  Multiple moderate lacerations, with or without hematoma
  Stellate lacerations of liver
- **5** **laceration, unspecified**
- **9** **other**

⑤ **864.0** **Without mention of open wound into cavity**
  [0-5,9]

⑤ **864.1** **With open wound into cavity**
  [0-5,9]

⑤ **865** **Injury to spleen**

The following fifth-digit subclassification is for use with category 865:

- **0** **unspecified injury**
- **1** **hematoma without rupture of capsule**
- **2** **capsular tears, without major disruption of parenchyma**
- **3** **laceration extending into parenchyma**
- **4** **massive parenchymal disruption**
- **9** **other**

⑤ **865.0** **Without mention of open wound into cavity**
  [0-4,9]

⑤ **865.1** **With open wound into cavity**
  [0-4,9]

⑤ **866** **Injury to kidney**

  Excludes: *acute kidney injury (nontraumatic) (584.9)*

The following fifth-digit subclassification is for use with category 866:

- **0** **unspecified injury**
- **1** **hematoma without rupture of capsule**
- **2** **laceration**
- **3** **complete disruption of kidney parenchyma**

⑤ **866.0** **Without mention of open wound into cavity**
  [0-3]

⑤ **866.1** **With open wound into cavity**
  [0-3]

867 **Injury to pelvic organs**

  Excludes: *injury during delivery (664.0-665.9)*

- **867.0** **Bladder and urethra, without mention of open wound into cavity**
- **867.1** **Bladder and urethra, with open wound into cavity**

Add 4th or 5th digit   Nonspecific code   Unspecified code   Medicare secondary payer (MSP) alert

867.2 Ureter, without mention of open wound into cavity

867.3 Ureter, with open wound into cavity

867.4 Uterus, without mention of open wound into cavity

867.5 Uterus, with open wound into cavity

867.6 Other specified pelvic organs, without mention of open wound into cavity

Fallopian tube   Seminal vesicle
Ovary   Vas deferens
Prostate

867.7 Other specified pelvic organs, with open wound into cavity

867.8 Unspecified pelvic organs, without mention of open wound into cavity

867.9 Unspecified pelvic organ, with open wound into cavity

⑤ **868** Injury to other intra-abdominal organs

The following fifth-digit subclassification is for use with category 868:

  0   unspecified intra-abdominal organ

  1   adrenal gland

  2   bile duct and gallbladder

  3   peritoneum

  4   retroperitoneum

  9   other and multiple intra-abdominal organs

  ⑤ **868.0** Without mention of open wound into cavity
      [0-4,9]

  ⑤ **868.1** With open wound into cavity
      [0-4,9]

869 Internal injury to unspecified or ill-defined organs

Includes: internal injury NOS
          multiple internal injury NOS

869.0 Without mention of open wound into cavity

869.1 With open wound into cavity

OPEN WOUNDS (870-897)

Includes: animal bite
          avulsion
          cut
          laceration
          puncture wound
          traumatic amputation

Excludes: *burn (940.0-949.5)*
        crushing (925-929.9)
        puncture of internal organs (860.0-869.1)
        superficial injury (910.0-919.9)
        that incidental to:
          dislocation (830.0-839.9)
          fracture (800.0-829.1)
          internal injury (860.0-869.1)
          intracranial injury (851.0-854.1)

Note: The description "complicated" used in the fourth-digit subdivisions includes those with mention of delayed healing, delayed treatment, foreign body, or infection.

OPEN WOUND OF HEAD, NECK, AND TRUNK (870-879)

870 Open wound of ocular adnexa

ALERT! For coding late effect of open wound of head neck and trunk see 906.0

870.0 Laceration of skin of eyelid and periocular area

870.1 Laceration of eyelid, full-thickness, not involving lacrimal passages

870.2 Laceration of eyelid involving lacrimal passages

870.3 Penetrating wound of orbit, without mention of foreign body

870.4 Penetrating wound of orbit with foreign body

Excludes: *retained (old) foreign body in orbit (376.6)*

870.8 Other specified open wounds of ocular adnexa

870.9 Unspecified open wound of ocular adnexa

  ● Code new
     to this edition
       ▲ Revision of
          existing code
           ④ ⑤ Fourth or fifth
                 digit required

871 Open wound of eyeball

> *Excludes:* *2nd cranial nerve [optic] injury (950.0-950.9)*
> *3rd cranial nerve [oculomotor] injury (951.0)*

> **ALERT!** For coding late effect of open wound of head neck and trunk see 906.0

871.0 Ocular laceration without prolapse of intraocular tissue

871.1 Ocular laceration with prolapse or exposure of intraocular tissue

871.2 Rupture of eye with partial loss of intraocular tissue

871.3 Avulsion of eye
Traumatic enucleation

871.4 Unspecified laceration of eye

871.5 Penetration of eyeball with magnetic foreign body

> *Excludes:* *retained (old) magnetic foreign body in globe (360.50-360.59)*

871.6 Penetration of eyeball with (nonmagnetic) foreign body

> *Excludes:* *retained (old) (nonmagnetic) foreign body in globe (360.60-360.69)*

871.7 Unspecified ocular penetration

871.9 Unspecified open wound of eyeball

872 Open wound of ear

> **ALERT!** For coding late effect of open wound of head neck and trunk see 906.0

⑤ **872.0 External ear, without mention of complication**

    872.00 External ear, unspecified site

    872.01 Auricle, ear
       Pinna

    872.02 Auditory canal

⑤ **872.1 External ear, complicated**

    872.10 External ear, unspecified site

    872.11 Auricle, ear

    872.12 Auditory canal

⑤ **872.6 Other specified parts of ear, without mention of complication**

    872.61 Ear drum
       Drumhead
       Tympanic membrane

    872.62 Ossicles

    872.63 Eustachian tube

    872.64 Cochlea

    872.69 Other and multiple sites

⑤ **872.7 Other specified parts of ear, complicated**

    872.71 Ear drum

    872.72 Ossicles

    872.73 Eustachian tube

    872.74 Cochlea

    872.79 Other and multiple sites

872.8 Ear, part unspecified, without mention of complication
Ear NOS

872.9 Ear, part unspecified, complicated

873 Other open wound of head

> **ALERT!** For coding late effect of open wound of head neck and trunk see 906.0

873.0 Scalp, without mention of complication

873.1 Scalp, complicated

⑤ **873.2 Nose, without mention of complication**

    873.20 Nose, unspecified site

    873.21 Nasal septum

    873.22 Nasal cavity

    873.23 Nasal sinus

    873.29 Multiple sites

| | Add 4th or 5th digit | | Nonspecific code | | Unspecified code | | Medicare secondary payer (MSP) alert |

⑤ **873.3 Nose, complicated**

    873.30   Nose, unspecified site

    873.31   Nasal septum

    873.32   Nasal cavity

    873.33   Nasal sinus

    873.39   Multiple sites

⑤ **873.4 Face, without mention of complication**

    873.40   Face, unspecified site

    873.41   Cheek

    873.42   Forehead
                    Eyebrow

    873.43   Lip

    873.44   Jaw

    873.49   Other and multiple sites

⑤ **873.5 Face, complicated**

    873.50   Face, unspecified site

    873.51   Cheek

    873.52   Forehead

    873.53   Lip

    873.54   Jaw

    873.59   Other and multiple sites

⑤ **873.6 Internal structures of mouth, without mention of complication**

    873.60   Mouth, unspecified site

    873.61   Buccal mucosa

    873.62   Gum (alveolar process)

    873.63   Tooth (broken) (fractured) (due to trauma)

    Excludes: *cracked tooth (521.81)*

    873.64   Tongue and floor of mouth

    873.65   Palate

    873.69   Other and multiple sites

⑤ **873.7 Internal structures of mouth, complicated**

    873.70   Mouth, unspecified site

    873.71   Buccal mucosa

    873.72   Gum (alveolar process)

    873.73   Tooth (broken) (fractured) (due to trauma)

    Excludes: *cracked tooth (521.81)*

    873.74   Tongue and floor of mouth

    873.75   Palate

    873.79   Other and multiple sites

873.8   **Other and unspecified open wound of head without mention of complication**
    Head NOS

873.9   **Other and unspecified open wound of head, complicated**

874 **Open wound of neck**

    ALERT! For coding late effect of open wound of head neck and trunk see 906.0

⑤ **874.0 Larynx and trachea, without mention of complication**

    874.00   Larynx with trachea

    874.01   Larynx

    874.02   Trachea

⑤ **874.1 Larynx and trachea, complicated**

    874.10   Larynx with trachea

    874.11   Larynx

    874.12   Trachea

● Code new   ▲ Revision of   ④ ⑤ Fourth or fifth
   to this edition   existing code   digit required

874.2 Thyroid gland, without mention of complication

874.3 Thyroid gland, complicated

874.4 Pharynx, without mention of complication
Cervical esophagus

874.5 Pharynx, complicated

874.8 Other and unspecified parts, without mention of complication
Nape of neck   Throat NOS
Supraclavicular region

874.9 Other and unspecified parts, complicated

875 Open wound of chest (wall)
Excludes: *open wound into thoracic cavity (860.0-862.9)*
traumatic pneumothorax and hemothorax (860.1, 860.3, 860.5)
ALERT! For coding late effect of open wound of head neck and trunk see 906.0

875.0 Without mention of complication

875.1 Complicated

876 Open wound of back
Includes: loin
lumbar region
Excludes: *open wound into thoracic cavity (860.0-862.9)*
traumatic pneumothorax and hemothorax (860.1, 860.3, 860.5)
ALERT! For coding late effect of open wound of head neck and trunk see 906.0

876.0 Without mention of complication

876.1 Complicated

877 Open wound of buttock
Includes: sacroiliac region
ALERT! For coding late effect of open wound of head neck and trunk see 906.0

877.0 Without mention of complication

877.1 Complicated

878 Open wound of genital organs (external), including traumatic amputation
Excludes: *injury during delivery (664.0-665.9)*
internal genital organs (867.0-867.9)
ALERT! For coding late effect of open wound of head neck and trunk see 906.0
ALERT! For coding late effect of traumatic amputation see 905.9

878.0 Penis, without mention of complication

878.1 Penis, complicated

878.2 Scrotum and testes, without mention of complication

878.3 Scrotum and testes, complicated

878.4 Vulva, without mention of complication
Labium (majus) (minus)

878.5 Vulva, complicated

878.6 Vagina, without mention of complication

878.7 Vagina, complicated

878.8 Other and unspecified parts, without mention of complication

878.9 Other and unspecified parts, complicated

879 Open wound of other and unspecified sites, except limbs
ALERT! For coding late effect of open wound of head neck and trunk see 906.0

879.0 Breast, without mention of complication

879.1 Breast, complicated

879.2 Abdominal wall, anterior, without mention of complication
Abdominal wall NOS   Pubic region
Epigastric region   Umbilical region
Hypogastric region

879.3 Abdominal wall, anterior, complicated

879.4 Abdominal wall, lateral, without mention of complication
Flank   Iliac (region)
Groin   Inguinal region
Hypochondrium

| Add 4th or 5th digit | Nonspecific code | Unspecified code | Medicare secondary payer (MSP) alert |

879.5 Abdominal wall, lateral, complicated

879.6 Other and unspecified parts of trunk, without mention of complication
Pelvic region   Trunk NOS
Perineum

879.7 Other and unspecified parts of trunk, complicated

879.8 Open wound(s) (multiple) of unspecified site(s) without mention of complication
Multiple open wounds NOS
Open wound NOS

879.9 Open wound(s) (multiple) of unspecified site(s), complicated

OPEN WOUND OF UPPER LIMB (880-887)

⑤ 880 Open wound of shoulder and upper arm
The following fifth-digit subclassification is for use with category 880:

    0   shoulder region

    1   scapular region

    2   axillary region

    3   upper arm

    9   multiple sites

ALERT! For coding late effect of open wound of extremities without tendon injury see 906.1

⑤ 880.0 Without mention of complication

⑤ 880.1 Complicated

⑤ 880.2 With tendon involvement

⑤ 881 Open wound of elbow, forearm, and wrist
The following fifth-digit subclassification is for use with category 881:

    0   forearm

    1   elbow

    2   wrist

ALERT! For coding late effect of open wound of extremities without tendon injury see 906.1

⑤ 881.0 Without mention of complication

⑤ 881.1 Complicated

⑤ 881.2 With tendon involvement

882 Open wound of hand except finger(s) alone
ALERT! For coding late effect of open wound of extremities without tendon injury see 906.1

882.0 Without mention of complication

882.1 Complicated

882.2 With tendon involvement

883 Open wound of finger(s)
Includes: fingernail
           thumb (nail)
ALERT! For coding late effect of open wound of extremities without tendon injury see 906.1

883.0 Without mention of complication

883.1 Complicated

883.2 With tendon involvement

884 Multiple and unspecified open wound of upper limb
Includes: arm NOS
           multiple sites of one upper limb
           upper limb NOS
ALERT! For coding late effect of open wound of extremities without tendon injury see 906.1

884.0 Without mention of complication

884.1 Complicated

884.2 With tendon involvement

885 Traumatic amputation of thumb (complete) (partial)
Includes: thumb(s) (with finger(s) of either hand)
ALERT! For coding late effect of traumatic amputation see 905.9

885.0 Without mention of complication

885.1 Complicated

    ● Code new   ▲ Revision of   ④ ⑤ Fourth or fifth
            to this edition   existing code   digit required

886 **Traumatic amputation of other finger(s) (complete) (partial)**
Includes: finger(s) of one or both hands, without mention of thumb(s)
ALERT! For coding late effect of traumatic amputation see 905.9

886.0 **Without mention of complication**

886.1 **Complicated**

887 **Traumatic amputation of arm and hand (complete) (partial)**
ALERT! For coding late effect of traumatic amputation see 905.9

887.0 **Unilateral, below elbow, without mention of complication**

887.1 **Unilateral, below elbow, complicated**

887.2 **Unilateral, at or above elbow, without mention of complication**

887.3 **Unilateral, at or above elbow, complicated**

887.4 **Unilateral, level not specified, without mention of complication**

887.5 **Unilateral, level not specified, complicated**

887.6 **Bilateral [any level], without mention of complication**
One hand and other arm

887.7 **Bilateral [any level], complicated**

OPEN WOUND OF LOWER LIMB (890-897)

890 **Open wound of hip and thigh**
ALERT! For coding late effect of open wound of extremities without tendon injury see 906.1

890.0 **Without mention of complication**

890.1 **Complicated**

890.2 **With tendon involvement**

891 **Open wound of knee, leg [except thigh], and ankle**
Includes: leg NOS
multiple sites of leg, except thigh

Excludes: that of thigh (890.0-890.2)
with multiple sites of lower limb (894.0-894.2)

ALERT! For coding late effect of open wound of extremities without tendon injury see 906.1

891.0 **Without mention of complication**

891.1 **Complicated**

891.2 **With tendon involvement**

892 **Open wound of foot except toe(s) alone**
Includes: heel
ALERT! For coding late effect of open wound of extremities without tendon injury see 906.1

892.0 **Without mention of complication**

892.1 **Complicated**

892.2 **With tendon involvement**

893 **Open wound of toe(s)**
Includes: toenail
ALERT! For coding late effect of open wound of extremities without tendon injury see 906.1

893.0 **Without mention of complication**

893.1 **Complicated**

893.2 **With tendon involvement**

894 **Multiple and unspecified open wound of lower limb**
Includes: lower limb NOS
multiple sites of one lower limb, with thigh

ALERT! For coding late effect of open wound of extremities without tendon injury see 906.1

894.0 **Without mention of complication**

894.1 **Complicated**

894.2 **With tendon involvement**

895 **Traumatic amputation of toe(s) (complete) (partial)**
Includes: toe(s) of one or both feet
ALERT! For coding late effect of traumatic amputation see 905.9

895.0 **Without mention of complication**

895.1 **Complicated**

Add 4th or 5th digit Nonspecific code Unspecified code Medicare secondary payer (MSP) alert

896 **Traumatic amputation of foot (complete) (partial)**

> **ALERT!** For coding late effect of traumatic amputation see 905.9

896.0 **Unilateral, without mention of complication**

896.1 **Unilateral, complicated**

896.2 **Bilateral, without mention of complication**

> *Excludes:* *one foot and other leg (897.6-897.7)*

896.3 **Bilateral, complicated**

897 **Traumatic amputation of leg(s) (complete) (partial)**

> **ALERT!** For coding late effect of traumatic amputation see 905.9

897.0 **Unilateral, below knee, without mention of complication**

897.1 **Unilateral, below knee, complicated**

897.2 **Unilateral, at or above knee, without mention of complication**

897.3 **Unilateral, at or above knee, complicated**

897.4 **Unilateral, level not specified, without mention of complication**

897.5 **Unilateral, level not specified, complicated**

897.6 **Bilateral [any level], without mention of complication**
One foot and other leg

897.7 **Bilateral [any level], complicated**

INJURY TO BLOOD VESSELS (900-904)

> Includes: arterial hematoma of blood vessel, secondary to other injuries e.g., fracture or open wound
> avulsion of blood vessel, secondary to other injuries e.g., fracture or open wound
> cut of blood vessel, secondary to other injuries e.g., fracture or open wound
> laceration of blood vessel, secondary to other injuries e.g., fracture or open wound
> rupture of blood vessel, secondary to other injuries e.g., fracture or open wound
> traumatic aneurysm or fistula (arteriovenous) of blood vessel, secondary to other injuries e.g., fracture or open wound

> *Excludes:* *accidental puncture or laceration during medical procedure (998.2)*
> *intracranial hemorrhage following injury (851.0-854.1)*

900 **Injury to blood vessels of head and neck**

> **ALERT!** For coding late effect of injury to blood vessel of head neck and extremities see 908.3

⑤ **900.0** **Carotid artery**

900.00 **Carotid artery, unspecified**

900.01 **Common carotid artery**

900.02 **External carotid artery**

900.03 **Internal carotid artery**

900.1 **Internal jugular vein**

⑤ **900.8** **Other specified blood vessels of head and neck**

900.81 **External jugular vein**
Jugular vein NOS

900.82 **Multiple blood vessels of head and neck**

900.89 **Other**

900.9 **Unspecified blood vessel of head and neck**

901 **Injury to blood vessels of thorax**

> *Excludes:* *traumatic hemothorax (860.2-860.5)*

> **ALERT!** For coding late effect of injury to blood vessel of thorax abdomen and pelvis see 908.4

901.0 **Thoracic aorta**

901.1 **Innominate and subclavian arteries**

901.2 **Superior vena cava**

901.3 **Innominate and subclavian veins**

⑤ **901.4** **Pulmonary blood vessels**

901.40 **Pulmonary vessel(s), unspecified**

901.41 **Pulmonary artery**

● Code new to this edition   ▲ Revision of existing code   ④ ⑤ Fourth or fifth digit required

901.42   **Pulmonary vein**

⑤ **901.8**   **Other specified blood vessels of thorax**

901.81   **Intercostal artery or vein**

901.82   **Internal mammary artery or vein**

901.83   **Multiple blood vessels of thorax**

901.89   **Other**
Azygos vein
Hemiazygos vein

901.9   **Unspecified blood vessel of thorax**

902   **Injury to blood vessels of abdomen and pelvis**
ALERT! For coding late effect of injury to blood vessel of thorax abdomen and pelvis see 908.4

902.0   **Abdominal aorta**

⑤ **902.1**   **Inferior vena cava**

902.10   **Inferior vena cava, unspecified**

902.11   **Hepatic veins**

902.19   **Other**

⑤ **902.2**   **Celiac and mesenteric arteries**

902.20   **Celiac and mesenteric arteries, unspecified**

902.21   **Gastric artery**

902.22   **Hepatic artery**

902.23   **Splenic artery**

902.24   **Other specified branches of celiac axis**

902.25   **Superior mesenteric artery (trunk)**

902.26   **Primary branches of superior mesenteric artery**
Ileo-colic artery

902.27   **Inferior mesenteric artery**

902.29   **Other**

⑤ **902.3**   **Portal and splenic veins**

902.31   **Superior mesenteric vein and primary subdivisions**
Ileo-colic vein

902.32   **Inferior mesenteric vein**

902.33   **Portal vein**

902.34   **Splenic vein**

902.39   **Other**
Cystic vein
Gastric vein

⑤ **902.4**   **Renal blood vessels**

902.40   **Renal vessel(s), unspecified**

902.41   **Renal artery**

902.42   **Renal vein**

902.49   **Other**
Suprarenal arteries

⑤ **902.5**   **Iliac blood vessels**

902.50   **Iliac vessel(s), unspecified**

902.51   **Hypogastric artery**

902.52   **Hypogastric vein**

902.53   **Iliac artery**

902.54   **Iliac vein**

902.55   **Uterine artery**

902.56   **Uterine vein**

902.59   **Other**

⑤ **902.8**   **Other specified blood vessels of abdomen and pelvis**

902.81   **Ovarian artery**

902.82   **Ovarian vein**

| | Add 4th or 5th digit | | Nonspecific code | | Unspecified code | | Medicare secondary payer (MSP) alert |

902.87 Multiple blood vessels of abdomen and pelvis

902.89 Other

902.9 Unspecified blood vessel of abdomen and pelvis

903 Injury to blood vessels of upper extremity

ALERT! For coding late effect of injury to blood vessel of head neck and extremities see 908.3

⑤ 903.0 Axillary blood vessels

903.00 Axillary vessel(s), unspecified

903.01 Axillary artery

903.02 Axillary vein

903.1 Brachial blood vessels

903.2 Radial blood vessels

903.3 Ulnar blood vessels

903.4 Palmar artery

903.5 Digital blood vessels

903.8 Other specified blood vessels of upper extremity
Multiple blood vessels of upper extremity

903.9 Unspecified blood vessel of upper extremity

904 Injury to blood vessels of lower extremity and unspecified sites

ALERT! For coding late effect of injury to blood vessel of head neck and extremities see 908.3

904.0 Common femoral artery
Femoral artery above profunda origin

904.1 Superficial femoral artery

904.2 Femoral veins

904.3 Saphenous veins
Saphenous vein (greater) (lesser)

⑤ 904.4 Popliteal blood vessels

904.40 Popliteal vessel(s), unspecified

904.41 Popliteal artery

904.42 Popliteal vein

⑤ 904.5 Tibial blood vessels

904.50 Tibial vessel(s), unspecified

904.51 Anterior tibial artery

904.52 Anterior tibial vein

904.53 Posterior tibial artery

904.54 Posterior tibial vein

904.6 Deep plantar blood vessels

904.7 Other specified blood vessels of lower extremity
Multiple blood vessels of lower extremity

904.8 Unspecified blood vessel of lower extremity

904.9 Unspecified site
Injury to blood vessel NOS

LATE EFFECTS OF INJURIES, POISONINGS, TOXIC EFFECTS, AND OTHER EXTERNAL CAUSES (905-909)

Note: These categories are to be used to indicate conditions classifiable to 800-999 as the cause of late effects, which are themselves classified elsewhere. The "late effects" include those specified as such, or as sequelae, which may occur at any time after the acute injury.

905 Late effects of musculoskeletal and connective tissue injuries

DEFINITION Late effects of musculoskeletal and connective tissue injuries refers to a condition that appears after the acute phase of the musculoskeletal and connective tissue injuries has run its course

905.0 Late effect of fracture of skull and face bones
Late effect of injury classifiable to 800-804

905.1 Late effect of fracture of spine and trunk without mention of spinal cord lesion
Late effect of injury classifiable to 805, 807-809

905.2 Late effect of fracture of upper extremities
Late effect of injury classifiable to 810-819

● Code new
to this edition

▲ Revision of
existing code

④ ⑤ Fourth or fifth
digit required

905.3 Late effect of fracture of neck of femur
Late effect of injury classifiable to 820

905.4 Late effect of fracture of lower extremities
Late effect of injury classifiable to 821-827

905.5 Late effect of fracture of multiple and unspecified bones
Late effect of injury classifiable to 828-829

905.6 Late effect of dislocation
Late effect of injury classifiable to 830-839

905.7 Late effect of sprain and strain without mention of tendon injury
Late effect of injury classifiable to 840-848, except tendon injury

905.8 Late effect of tendon injury
Late effect of tendon injury due to:
open wound [injury classifiable to 880-884 with .2, 890-894 with .2]
sprain and strain [injury classifiable to 840-848]

905.9 Late effect of traumatic amputation
Late effect of injury classifiable to 885-887, 895-897

Excludes: *late amputation stump complication (997.60-997.69)*

906 Late effects of injuries to skin and subcutaneous tissues
DEFINITION Late effects of injuries to skin and subcutaneous tissues refers to a condition that appears after the acute phase of the skin and subcutaneous tissues injuries has run its course

906.0 Late effect of open wound of head, neck, and trunk
Late effect of injury classifiable to 870-879

906.1 Late effect of open wound of extremities without mention of tendon injury
Late effect of injury classifiable to 880-884, 890-894 except .2

906.2 Late effect of superficial injury
Late effect of injury classifiable to 910-919

906.3 Late effect of contusion
Late effect of injury classifiable to 920-924

906.4 Late effect of crushing
Late effect of injury classifiable to 925-929

906.5 Late effect of burn of eye, face, head, and neck
Late effect of injury classifiable to 940-941

906.6 Late effect of burn of wrist and hand
Late effect of injury classifiable to 944

906.7 Late effect of burn of other extremities
Late effect of injury classifiable to 943 or 945

906.8 Late effect of burns of other specified sites
Late effect of injury classifiable to 942, 946-947

906.9 Late effect of burn of unspecified site
Late effect of injury classifiable to 948-949

907 Late effects of injuries to the nervous system
DEFINITION Late effects of injuries to the nervous system refers to a condition that appears after the acute phase of the nervous system has run its course.

907.0 Late effect of intracranial injury without mention of skull fracture
Late effect of injury classifiable to 850-854

907.1 Late effect of injury to cranial nerve
Late effect of injury classifiable to 950-951

907.2 Late effect of spinal cord injury
Late effect of injury classifiable to 806, 952

907.3 Late effect of injury to nerve root(s), spinal plexus(es), and other nerves of trunk
Late effect of injury classifiable to 953-954

907.4 Late effect of injury to peripheral nerve of shoulder girdle and upper limb
Late effect of injury classifiable to 955

907.5 Late effect of injury to peripheral nerve of pelvic girdle and lower limb
Late effect of injury classifiable to 956

907.9 Late effect of injury to other and unspecified nerve
Late effect of injury classifiable to 957

908 Late effects of other and unspecified injuries
908.0 Late effect of internal injury to chest
Late effect of injury classifiable to 860-862

| | Add 4th or 5th digit | | Nonspecific code | | Unspecified code | | Medicare secondary payer (MSP) alert |

908.1 Late effect of internal injury to intra-abdominal organs
Late effect of injury classifiable to 863-866, 868

908.2 Late effect of internal injury to other internal organs
Late effect of injury classifiable to 867 or 869

908.3 Late effect of injury to blood vessel of head, neck, and extremities
Late effect of injury classifiable to 900, 903-904

908.4 Late effect of injury to blood vessel of thorax, abdomen, and pelvis
Late effect of injury classifiable to 901-902

908.5 Late effect of foreign body in orifice
Late effect of injury classifiable to 930-939

908.6 Late effect of certain complications of trauma
Late effect of complications classifiable to 958

908.9 Late effect of unspecified injury
Late effect of injury classifiable to 959

909 Late effects of other and unspecified external causes

909.0 Late effect of poisoning due to drug, medicinal or biological substance
Late effect of conditions classifiable to 960-979

Excludes: *late effect of adverse effect of drug, medicinal or biological substance (909.5)*

909.1 Late effect of toxic effects of nonmedical substances
Late effect of conditions classifiable to 980-989

909.2 Late effect of radiation
Late effect of conditions classifiable to 990

909.3 Late effect of complications of surgical and medical care
Late effect of conditions classifiable to 996-999

909.4 Late effect of certain other external causes
Late effect of conditions classifiable to 991-994

909.5 Late effect of adverse effect of drug, medicinal or biological substance

Excludes: *late effect of poisoning due to drug, medicinal or biological substance (909.0)*

909.9 Late effect of other and unspecified external causes

SUPERFICIAL INJURY (910-919)

Excludes: *burn (blisters) (940.0-949.5)*
contusion (920-924.9)
foreign body:
 granuloma (728.82)
 inadvertently left in operative wound (998.4)
 residual, in soft tissue (729.6)
insect bite, venomous (989.5)
open wound with incidental foreign body (870.0-897.7)

910 Superficial injury of face, neck, and scalp except eye
Includes: cheek
 ear
 gum
 lip
 nose
 throat

Excludes: *eye and adnexa (918.0-918.9)*

ALERT! For coding late effect of superficial injury see 906.2

910.0 Abrasion or friction burn without mention of infection

910.1 Abrasion or friction burn, infected

910.2 Blister without mention of infection

910.3 Blister, infected

910.4 Insect bite, nonvenomous, without mention of infection

910.5 Insect bite, nonvenomous, infected

910.6 Superficial foreign body (splinter) without major open wound and without mention of infection

910.7 Superficial foreign body (splinter) without major open wound, infected

910.8 Other and unspecified superficial injury of face, neck, and scalp without mention of infection

910.9 Other and unspecified superficial injury of face, neck, and scalp, infected

● Code new
to this edition
▲ Revision of
existing code
④ ⑤ Fourth or fifth
digit required

911 **Superficial injury of trunk**
Includes:

abdominal wall	interscapular region
anus	labium (majus) (minus)
back	penis
breast	perineum
buttock	scrotum
chest wall	testis
flank	vagina
groin	vulva

Excludes: hip (916.0-916.9)
scapular region (912.0-912.9)

ALERT! For coding late effect of superficial injury see 906.2

911.0 **Abrasion or friction burn without mention of infection**

911.1 **Abrasion or friction burn, infected**

911.2 **Blister without mention of infection**

911.3 **Blister, infected**

911.4 **Insect bite, nonvenomous, without mention of infection**

911.5 **Insect bite, nonvenomous, infected**

911.6 **Superficial foreign body (splinter) without major open wound and without mention of infection**

911.7 **Superficial foreign body (splinter) without major open wound, infected**

911.8 **Other and unspecified superficial injury of trunk without mention of infection**

911.9 **Other and unspecified superficial injury of trunk, infected**

912 **Superficial injury of shoulder and upper arm**
Includes: axilla   scapular region

ALERT! For coding late effect of superficial injury see 906.2

912.0 **Abrasion or friction burn without mention of infection**

912.1 **Abrasion or friction burn, infected**

912.2 **Blister without mention of infection**

912.3 **Blister, infected**

912.4 **Insect bite, nonvenomous, without mention of infection**

912.5 **Insect bite, nonvenomous, infected**

912.6 **Superficial foreign body (splinter) without major open wound and without mention of infection**

912.7 **Superficial foreign body (splinter) without major open wound, infected**

912.8 **Other and unspecified superficial injury of shoulder and upper arm without mention of infection**

912.9 **Other and unspecified superficial injury of shoulder and upper arm, infected**

913 **Superficial injury of elbow, forearm, and wrist**
ALERT! For coding late effect of superficial injury see 906.2

913.0 **Abrasion or friction burn without mention of infection**

913.1 **Abrasion or friction burn, infected**

913.2 **Blister without mention of infection**

913.3 **Blister, infected**

913.4 **Insect bite, nonvenomous, without mention of infection**

913.5 **Insect bite, nonvenomous, infected**

913.6 **Superficial foreign body (splinter) without major open wound and without mention of infection**

913.7 **Superficial foreign body (splinter) without major open wound, infected**

913.8 **Other and unspecified superficial injury of elbow, forearm, and wrist without mention of infection**

913.9 **Other and unspecified superficial injury of elbow, forearm, and wrist, infected**

914 **Superficial injury of hand(s) except finger(s) alone**
ALERT! For coding late effect of superficial injury see 906.2

914.0 **Abrasion or friction burn without mention of infection**

914.1 **Abrasion or friction burn, infected**

Add 4th or 5th digit	Nonspecific code	Unspecified code	Medicare secondary payer (MSP) alert

914.2 Blister without mention of infection

914.3 Blister, infected

914.4 Insect bite, nonvenomous, without mention of infection

914.5 Insect bite, nonvenomous, infected

914.6 Superficial foreign body (splinter) without major open wound and without mention of infection

914.7 Superficial foreign body (splinter) without major open wound, infected

914.8 Other and unspecified superficial injury of hand without mention of infection

914.9 Other and unspecified superficial injury of hand, infected

915 Superficial injury of finger(s)

Includes: fingernail   thumb (nail)

   ALERT! For coding late effect of superficial injury see 906.2

915.0 Abrasion or friction burn without mention of infection

915.1 Abrasion or friction burn, infected

915.2 Blister without mention of infection

915.3 Blister, infected

915.4 Insect bite, nonvenomous, without mention of infection

915.5 Insect bite, nonvenomous, infected

915.6 Superficial foreign body (splinter) without major open wound and without mention of infection

915.7 Superficial foreign body (splinter) without major open wound, infected

915.8 Other and unspecified superficial injury of fingers without mention of infection

915.9 Other and unspecified superficial injury of fingers, infected

916 Superficial injury of hip, thigh, leg, and ankle

   ALERT! For coding late effect of superficial injury see 906.2

916.0 Abrasion or friction burn without mention of infection

916.1 Abrasion or friction burn, infected

916.2 Blister without mention of infection

916.3 Blister, infected

916.4 Insect bite, nonvenomous, without mention of infection

916.5 Insect bite, nonvenomous, infected

916.6 Superficial foreign body (splinter) without major open wound and without mention of infection

916.7 Superficial foreign body (splinter) without major open wound, infected

916.8 Other and unspecified superficial injury of hip, thigh, leg, and ankle without mention of infection

916.9 Other and unspecified superficial injury of hip, thigh, leg, and ankle, infected

917 Superficial injury of foot and toe(s)

Includes: heel   toenail

   ALERT! For coding late effect of superficial injury see 906.2

917.0 Abrasion or friction burn without mention of infection

917.1 Abrasion or friction burn, infected

917.2 Blister without mention of infection

917.3 Blister, infected

917.4 Insect bite, nonvenomous, without mention of infection

917.5 Insect bite, nonvenomous, infected

917.6 Superficial foreign body (splinter) without major open wound and without mention of infection

917.7 Superficial foreign body (splinter) without major open wound, infected

917.8 Other and unspecified superficial injury of foot and toes without mention of infection

917.9 Other and unspecified superficial injury of foot and toes, infected

● Code new to this edition   ▲ Revision of existing code   ④ ⑤ Fourth or fifth digit required

918 **Superficial injury of eye and adnexa**

> Excludes: *burn (940.0-940.9)*
> *foreign body on external eye (930.0-930.9)*

> **ALERT!** For coding late effect of superficial injury see 906.2

918.0 **Eyelids and periocular area**
Abrasion   Superficial foreign body (splinter)
Insect bite

918.1 **Cornea**
Corneal abrasion
Superficial laceration

> Excludes: *corneal injury due to contact lens (371.82)*

918.2 **Conjunctiva**

918.9 **Other and unspecified superficial injuries of eye**
Eye (ball) NOS

919 **Superficial injury of other, multiple, and unspecified sites**

> Excludes: *multiple sites classifiable to the same three-digit category (910.0-918.9)*

> **ALERT!** For coding late effect of superficial injury see 906.2

919.0 **Abrasion or friction burn without mention of infection**

919.1 **Abrasion or friction burn, infected**

919.2 **Blister without mention of infection**

919.3 **Blister, infected**

919.4 **Insect bite, nonvenomous, without mention of infection**

919.5 **Insect bite, nonvenomous, infected**

919.6 **Superficial foreign body (splinter) without major open wound and without mention of infection**

919.7 **Superficial foreign body (splinter) without major open wound, infected**

919.8 **Other and unspecified superficial injury without mention of infection**

919.9 **Other and unspecified superficial injury, infected**

CONTUSION WITH INTACT SKIN SURFACE (920-924)

Includes: bruise without fracture or open wound
hematoma without fracture or open wound

> Excludes: *concussion (850.0-850.9)*
> *hemarthrosis (840.0-848.9)*
> *internal organs (860.0-869.1)*
> *that incidental to:*
> *crushing injury (925-929.9)*
> *dislocation (830.0-839.9)*
> *fracture (800.0-829.1)*
> *internal injury (860.0-869.1)*
> *intracranial injury (850.0-854.1)*
> *nerve injury (950.0-957.9)*
> *open wound (870.0-897.7)*

920 **Contusion of face, scalp, and neck except eye(s)**
Cheek   Mandibular joint area
Ear (auricle)   Nose
Gum   Throat
Lip

> **DEFINITION** A Contusion, aka bruise, is an injury caused by a blow to the muscle, tendon or ligament; occurs when blood pools around the injury and discolors the skin.

> **ALERT!** For coding late effect of contusion see 906.3

921 **Contusion of eye and adnexa**

> **ALERT!** For coding late effect of contusion see 906.3

921.0 **Black eye, not otherwise specified**

921.1 **Contusion of eyelids and periocular area**

921.2 **Contusion of orbital tissues**

921.3 **Contusion of eyeball**

921.9 **Unspecified contusion of eye**
Injury of eye NOS

| | Add 4th or 5th digit | | Nonspecific code | | Unspecified code | | Medicare secondary payer (MSP) alert |

922 **Contusion of trunk**
> **ALERT!** For coding late effect of contusion see 906.3

922.0 **Breast**

922.1 **Chest wall**

922.2 **Abdominal wall**
Flank
Groin

⑤ **922.3** **Back**
> *Excludes:* scapular region (923.01)

> **922.31** **Back**
> *Excludes:* interscapular region (922.33)

> **922.32** **Buttock**

> **922.33** **Interscapular region**

922.4 **Genital organs**
Labium (majus) (minus)   Testis
Penis   Vagina
Perineum   Vulva
Scrotum

922.8 **Multiple sites of trunk**

922.9 **Unspecified part**
Trunk NOS

923 **Contusion of upper limb**
> **ALERT!** For coding late effect of contusion see 906.3

⑤ **923.0** **Shoulder and upper arm**

> **923.00** **Shoulder region**

> **923.01** **Scapular region**

> **923.02** **Axillary region**

> **923.03** **Upper arm**

> **923.09** **Multiple sites**

⑤ **923.1** **Elbow and forearm**

> **923.10** **Forearm**

> **923.11** **Elbow**

⑤ **923.2** **Wrist and hand(s), except finger(s) alone**

> **923.20** **Hand(s)**

> **923.21** **Wrist**

923.3 **Finger**
Fingernail
Thumb (nail)

923.8 **Multiple sites of upper limb**

923.9 **Unspecified part of upper limb**
Arm NOS

924 **Contusion of lower limb and of other and unspecified sites**
> **ALERT!** For coding late effect of contusion see 906.3

⑤ **924.0** **Hip and thigh**

> **924.00** **Thigh**

> **924.01** **Hip**

⑤ **924.1** **Knee and lower leg**

> **924.10** **Lower leg**

> **924.11** **Knee**

⑤ **924.2** **Ankle and foot, excluding toe(s)**

> **924.20** **Foot**
> Heel

> **924.21** **Ankle**

924.3 **Toe**
Toenail

● Code new   ▲ Revision of   ④ ⑤ Fourth or fifth
 to this edition   existing code   digit required

924.4 **Multiple sites of lower limb**

924.5 **Unspecified part of lower limb**
Leg NOS

924.8 **Multiple sites, not elsewhere classified**

924.9 **Unspecified site**

CRUSHING INJURY (925-929)

Use additional code to identify any associated injuries, such as:
fractures (800-829)
internal injuries (860.0-869.1)
intracranial injury (850.0-854.1)

925 **Crushing injury of face, scalp, and neck**
Cheek   Pharynx
Ear   Throat
Larynx

ALERT! For coding late effect of crushing see 906.4

925.1 **Crushing injury of face and scalp**
Cheek   Ear

925.2 **Crushing injury of neck**
Larynx   Throat
Pharynx

926 **Crushing injury of trunk**
DEFINITION A crushing injury occurs when a body part is subjected to a high degree of force or pressure, usually after being squeezed between two heavy objects
ALERT! For coding late effect of crushing see 906.4

926.0 **External genitalia**
Labium (majus) (minus)   Testis
Penis   Vulva
Scrotum

⑤ **926.1** **Other specified sites**

926.11 **Back**

926.12 **Buttock**

926.19 **Other**
Breast

926.8 **Multiple sites of trunk**

926.9 **Unspecified site**
Trunk NOS

927 **Crushing injury of upper limb**
ALERT! For coding late effect of crushing see 906.4

⑤ **927.0** **Shoulder and upper arm**

927.00 **Shoulder region**

927.01 **Scapular region**

927.02 **Axillary region**

927.03 **Upper arm**

927.09 **Multiple sites**

⑤ **927.1** **Elbow and forearm**

927.10 **Forearm**

927.11 **Elbow**

⑤ **927.2** **Wrist and hand(s), except finger(s) alone**

927.20 **Hand(s)**

927.21 **Wrist**

927.3 **Finger(s)**

927.8 **Multiple sites of upper limb**

927.9 **Unspecified site**
Arm NOS

928 **Crushing injury of lower limb**
ALERT! For coding late effect of crushing see 906.4

⑤ **928.0** **Hip and thigh**

Add 4th or 5th digit | Nonspecific code | Unspecified code | Medicare secondary payer (MSP) alert

928.00 Thigh

928.01 Hip

⑤ 928.1 Knee and lower leg

928.10 Lower leg

928.11 Knee

⑤ 928.2 Ankle and foot, excluding toe(s) alone

928.20 Foot
Heel

928.21 Ankle

928.3 Toe(s)

928.8 Multiple sites of lower limb

928.9 Unspecified site
Leg NOS

929 Crushing injury of multiple and unspecified sites
ALERT! For coding late effect of crushing see 906.4

929.0 Multiple sites, not elsewhere classified

929.9 Unspecified site

EFFECTS OF FOREIGN BODY ENTERING THROUGH ORIFICE (930-939)

Excludes: foreign body:
granuloma (728.82)
inadvertently left in operative wound (998.4, 998.7)
in open wound (800-839, 851-897)
residual, in soft tissues (729.6)
superficial without major open wound (910-919 with .6 or .7)

930 Foreign body on external eye

Excludes: foreign body in penetrating wound of:
eyeball (871.5-871.6)
retained (old) (360.5-360.6)
ocular adnexa (870.4)
retained (old) (376.6)
ALERT! For coding late effect of foreign body in orifice see 908.5

930.0 Corneal foreign body

930.1 Foreign body in conjunctival sac

930.2 Foreign body in lacrimal punctum

930.8 Other and combined sites

930.9 Unspecified site
External eye NOS

931 Foreign body in ear
Auditory canal
Auricle
ALERT! For coding late effect of foreign body in orifice see 908.5

932 Foreign body in nose
Nasal sinus
Nostril
ALERT! For coding late effect of foreign body in orifice see 908.5

933 Foreign body in pharynx and larynx
ALERT! For coding late effect of foreign body in orifice see 908.5

933.0 Pharynx
Nasopharynx
Throat NOS

933.1 Larynx
Asphyxia due to foreign body
Choking due to:
food (regurgitated)
phlegm

934 Foreign body in trachea, bronchus, and lung
ALERT! For coding late effect of foreign body in orifice see 908.5

934.0 Trachea

● Code new to this edition ▲ Revision of existing code ④ ⑤ Fourth or fifth digit required

934.1 Main bronchus

934.8 Other specified parts
Bronchioles
Lung

934.9 Respiratory tree, unspecified
Inhalation of liquid or vomitus, lower respiratory tract NOS

935 Foreign body in mouth, esophagus, and stomach
ALERT! For coding late effect of foreign body in orifice see 908.5

935.0 Mouth

935.1 Esophagus

935.2 Stomach

936 Foreign body in intestine and colon
ALERT! For coding late effect of foreign body in orifice see 908.5

937 Foreign body in anus and rectum
Rectosigmoid (junction)
ALERT! For coding late effect of foreign body in orifice see 908.5

938 Foreign body in digestive system, unspecified
Alimentary tract NOS
Swallowed foreign body
ALERT! For coding late effect of foreign body in orifice see 908.5

939 Foreign body in genitourinary tract
ALERT! For coding late effect of foreign body in orifice see 908.5

939.0 Bladder and urethra

939.1 Uterus, any part
Excludes: intrauterine contraceptive device:
complications from (996.32, 996.65)
presence of (V45.51)

939.2 Vulva and vagina

939.3 Penis

939.9 Unspecified site

BURNS (940-949)

Includes: burns from:
electrical heating appliance
electricity
flame
hot object
lightning
radiation
chemical burns (external) (internal)
scalds
Excludes: friction burns (910-919 with .0, .1)
sunburn (692.71, 692.76-692.77)

940 Burn confined to eye and adnexa
ALERT! For coding late effect of burn of eye face head and neck see 906.5

940.0 Chemical burn of eyelids and periocular area

940.1 Other burns of eyelids and periocular area

940.2 Alkaline chemical burn of cornea and conjunctival sac

940.3 Acid chemical burn of cornea and conjunctival sac

940.4 Other burn of cornea and conjunctival sac

940.5 Burn with resulting rupture and destruction of eyeball

940.9 Unspecified burn of eye and adnexa

⑤ **941 Burn of face, head, and neck**
Excludes: mouth (947.0)
The following fifth-digit subclassification is for use with category 941:

0 face and head, unspecified site

1 ear [any part]

2 eye (with other parts of face, head, and neck)

| | Add 4th or 5th digit | | Nonspecific code | | Unspecified code | | Medicare secondary payer (MSP) alert |

3 lip(s)

4 chin

5 nose (septum)

6 scalp [any part]
    Temple (region)

7 forehead and cheek

8 neck

9 multiple sites [except with eye] of face, head, and neck

ALERT! For coding late effect of burn of eye face head and neck see 906.5

⑤ **941.0** Unspecified degree
[0-9]

⑤ **941.1** Erythema [first degree]
[0-9]

⑤ **941.2** Blisters, epidermal loss [second degree]
[0-9]

⑤ **941.3** Full-thickness skin loss [third degree NOS]
[0-9]

⑤ **941.4** Deep necrosis of underlying tissues [deep third degree] without mention of loss of a body part
[0-9]

⑤ **941.5** Deep necrosis of underlying tissues [deep third degree] with loss of a body part
[0-9]

⑤ **942** Burn of trunk

    Excludes: scapular region (943.0-943.5 with fifth-digit 6)

The following fifth-digit subclassification is for use with category 942:

  0 trunk, unspecified site

  1 breast

  2 chest wall, excluding breast and nipple

  3 abdominal wall
      Flank   Groin

  4 back [any part]
      Buttock   Interscapular region

  5 genitalia
      Labium (majus) (minus)   Scrotum
      Penis   Testis
      Perineum   Vulva

  9 other and multiple sites of trunk

ALERT! For coding late effect of burn of eye face head and neck see 906.5

⑤ **942.0** Unspecified degree
[0-5,9]

⑤ **942.1** Erythema [first degree]
[0-5,9]

⑤ **942.2** Blisters, epidermal loss [second degree]
[0-5,9]

⑤ **942.3** Full-thickness skin loss [third degree NOS]
[0-5,9]

⑤ **942.4** Deep necrosis of underlying tissues [deep third degree] without mention of loss of a body part
[0-5,9]

⑤ **942.5** Deep necrosis of underlying tissues [deep third degree] with loss of a body part
[0-5,9]

⑤ **943** Burn of upper limb, except wrist and hand

The following fifth-digit subclassification is for use with category 943:

  0 upper limb, unspecified site

  1 forearm

  2 elbow

  3 upper arm

  4 axilla

● Code new
to this edition
▲ Revision of
existing code
④ ⑤ Fourth or fifth
digit required

     5 **shoulder**

     6 **scapular region**

     9 **multiple sites of upper limb, except wrist and hand**

⑤ **943.0** **Unspecified degree**
[0-6,9]

⑤ **943.1** **Erythema [first degree]**
[0-6,9]

⑤ **943.2** **Blisters, epidermal loss [second degree]**
[0-6,9]

⑤ **943.3** **Full-thickness skin loss [third degree NOS]**
[0-6,9]

⑤ **943.4** **Deep necrosis of underlying tissues [deep third degree] without mention of loss of a body part**
[0-6,9]

⑤ **943.5** **Deep necrosis of underlying tissues [deep third degree] with loss of a body part**
[0-6,9]

⑤ **944** **Burn of wrist(s) and hand(s)**

The following fifth-digit subclassification is for use with category 944:

     0 **hand, unspecified site**

     1 **single digit [finger (nail)] other than thumb**

     2 **thumb (nail)**

     3 **two or more digits, not including thumb**

     4 **two or more digits including thumb**

     5 **palm**

     6 **back of hand**

     7 **wrist**

     8 **multiple sites of wrist(s) and hand(s)**

ALERT! For coding late effect of burn of wrist and hand see 906.6

⑤ **944.0** **Unspecified degree**
[0-8]

⑤ **944.1** **Erythema [first degree]**
[0-8]

⑤ **944.2** **Blisters, epidermal loss [second degree]**
[0-8]

⑤ **944.3** **Full-thickness skin loss [third degree NOS]**
[0-8]

⑤ **944.4** **Deep necrosis of underlying tissues [deep third degree] without mention of loss of a body part**
[0-8]

⑤ **944.5** **Deep necrosis of underlying tissues [deep third degree] with loss of a body part**
[0-8]

⑤ **945** **Burn of lower limb(s)**

The following fifth-digit subclassification is for use with category 945:

     0 **lower limb [leg], unspecified site**

     1 **toe(s) (nail)**

     2 **foot**

     3 **ankle**

     4 **lower leg**

     5 **knee**

     6 **thigh [any part]**

     9 **multiple sites of lower limb(s)**

ALERT! For coding late effect of burn of other extremities see 906.7

⑤ **945.0** **Unspecified degree**
[0-6,9]

⑤ **945.1** **Erythema [first degree]**
[0-6,9]

⑤ **945.2** **Blisters, epidermal loss [second degree]**
[0-6,9]

| | Add 4th or 5th digit | | Nonspecific code | | Unspecified code | | Medicare secondary payer (MSP) alert |

⑤ **945.3 Full-thickness skin loss [third degree NOS]**
[0-6,9]

⑤ **945.4 Deep necrosis of underlying tissues [deep third degree] without mention of loss of a body part**
[0-6,9]

⑤ **945.5 Deep necrosis of underlying tissues [deep third degree] with loss of a body part**
[0-6,9]

946 Burns of multiple specified sites

Includes: burns of sites classifiable to more than one three-digit category in 940-945

Excludes: *multiple burns NOS (949.0-949.5)*

ALERT! For coding late effect of burns of other specified sites see 906.8

946.0 Unspecified degree

946.1 Erythema [first degree]

946.2 Blisters, epidermal loss [second degree]

946.3 Full-thickness skin loss [third degree NOS]

946.4 Deep necrosis of underlying tissues [deep third degree] without mention of loss of a body part

946.5 Deep necrosis of underlying tissues [deep third degree] with loss of a body part

947 Burn of internal organs

Includes: burns from chemical agents (ingested)

947.0 Mouth and pharynx
Gum
Tongue

947.1 Larynx, trachea, and lung

947.2 Esophagus

947.3 Gastrointestinal tract
Colon   Small intestine
Rectum   Stomach

947.4 Vagina and uterus

947.8 Other specified sites

947.9 Unspecified site

⑤ **948 Burns classified according to extent of body surface involved**

Excludes: *sunburn (692.71, 692.76-692.77)*

Note: This category is to be used when the site of the burn is unspecified, or with categories 940-947 when the site is specified.

The following fifth-digit subclassification is for use with category 948 to indicate the percent of *body surface* with *third degree burn*; valid digits are in [brackets] under each code:

  0 less than 10 percent or unspecified

  1   10-19%

  2   20-29%

  3   30-39%

  4   40-49%

  5   50-59%

  6   60-69%

  7   70-79%

  8   80-89%

  9   90% or more of body surface

ALERT! It is advisable to use category 948 as additional coding when needed to provide data for evaluating burn mortality, such as that needed by burn units. It is also advisable to use category 948 as an additional code for reporting purposes when there is mention of a third-degree burn involving 20 percent or more of the body surface.

⑤ **948.0 Burn [any degree] involving less than 10 percent of body surface**
[0]

⑤ **948.1 10-19 percent of body surface**
[0-1]

⑤ **948.2 20-29 percent of body surface**
[0-2]

● Code new
  to this edition
▲ Revision of
  existing code
④ ⑤ Fourth or fifth
  digit required

⑤ **948.3 30-39 percent of body surface**
[0-3]

⑤ **948.4 40-49 percent of body surface**
[0-4]

⑤ **948.5 50-59 percent of body surface**
[0-5]

⑤ **948.6 60-69 percent of body surface**
[0-6]

⑤ **948.7 70-79 percent of body surface**
[0-7]

⑤ **948.8 80-89 percent of body surface**
[0-8]

⑤ **948.9 90 percent or more of body surface**
[0-9]

949 Burn, unspecified
> Includes: burn NOS
> multiple burns NOS

> Excludes: *burn of unspecified site but with statement of the extent of body surface involved (948.0-948.9)*

> **ALERT!** For coding late effect of burn of unspecified site see 906.9

949.0 Unspecified degree

949.1 Erythema [first degree]

949.2 Blisters, epidermal loss [second degree]

949.3 Full-thickness skin loss [third degree NOS]

949.4 Deep necrosis of underlying tissues [deep third degree] without mention of loss of a body part

949.5 Deep necrosis of underlying tissues [deep third degree] with loss of a body part

INJURY TO NERVES AND SPINAL CORD (950-957)

> Includes:
> division of nerve (with open wound)
> lesion in continuity (with open wound)
> traumatic neuroma (with open wound)
> traumatic transient paralysis (with open wound)

> Excludes: *accidental puncture or laceration during medical procedure (998.2)*

950 Injury to optic nerve and pathways
> **ALERT!** For coding late effects of injuries to the nervous system see 907

950.0 Optic nerve injury
Second cranial nerve

950.1 Injury to optic chiasm

950.2 Injury to optic pathways

950.3 Injury to visual cortex

950.9 Unspecified
Traumatic blindness NOS

951 Injury to other cranial nerve(s)
> **ALERT!** For coding late effect of injury to cranial nerve see 907.1
> **ALERT!** For coding late effects of injuries to the nervous system see 907

951.0 Injury to oculomotor nerve
Third cranial nerve

951.1 Injury to trochlear nerve
Fourth cranial nerve

951.2 Injury to trigeminal nerve
Fifth cranial nerve

951.3 Injury to abducens nerve
Sixth cranial nerve

951.4 Injury to facial nerve
Seventh cranial nerve

951.5 Injury to acoustic nerve
Auditory nerve   Traumatic deafness NOS
Eighth cranial nerve

| | Add 4th or 5th digit | | Nonspecific code | | Unspecified code | | Medicare secondary payer (MSP) alert |

951.6 Injury to accessory nerve
Eleventh cranial nerve

951.7 Injury to hypoglossal nerve
Twelfth cranial nerve

951.8 Injury to other specified cranial nerves
Glossopharyngeal [9th cranial] nerve
Olfactory [1st cranial] nerve
Pneumogastric [10th cranial] nerve
Traumatic anosmia NOS
Vagus [10th cranial] nerve

951.9 Injury to unspecified cranial nerve

952 Spinal cord injury without evidence of spinal bone injury

ALERT! For coding late effect of spinal cord injury see 907.2

ALERT! For coding late effects of injuries to the nervous system see 907

⑤ **952.0 Cervical**

952.00 C_1-C_4 **level with unspecified spinal cord injury**
Spinal cord injury, cervical region NOS

952.01 C_1-C_4 **level with complete lesion of spinal cord**

952.02 C_1-C_4 **level with anterior cord syndrome**

952.03 C_1-C_4 **level with central cord syndrome**

952.04 C_1-C_4 **level with other specified spinal cord injury**
Incomplete spinal cord lesion at C_1-C_4 level:
  NOS
  with posterior cord syndrome

952.05 C_5-C_7 **level with unspecified spinal cord injury**

952.06 C_5-C_7 **level with complete lesion of spinal cord**

952.07 C_5-C_7 **level with anterior cord syndrome**

952.08 C_5-C_7 **level with central cord syndrome**

952.09 C_5-C_7 **level with other specified spinal cord injury**
Incomplete spinal cord lesion at C_5-C_7 level:
  NOS
  with posterior cord syndrome

⑤ **952.1 Dorsal [thoracic]**

952.10 T_1-T_6 **level with unspecified spinal cord injury**
Spinal cord injury, thoracic region NOS

952.11 T_1-T_6 **level with complete lesion of spinal cord**

952.12 T_1-T_6 **level with anterior cord syndrome**

952.13 T_1-T_6 **level with central cord syndrome**

952.14 T_1-T_6 **level with other specified spinal cord injury**
Incomplete spinal cord lesion at T_1-T_6 level:
  NOS
  with posterior cord syndrome

952.15 T_7-T_{12} **level with unspecified spinal cord injury**

952.16 T_7-T_{12} **level with complete lesion of spinal cord**

952.17 T_7-T_{12} **level with anterior cord syndrome**

952.18 T_7-T_{12} **level with central cord syndrome**

952.19 T_7-T_{12} **level with other specified spinal cord injury**
Incomplete spinal cord lesion at T_7-T_{12} level:
  NOS
  with posterior cord syndrome

952.2 Lumbar

952.3 Sacral

952.4 Cauda equina

952.8 Multiple sites of spinal cord

952.9 Unspecified site of spinal cord

953 Injury to nerve roots and spinal plexus

ALERT! For coding late effect of injury to nerve root(s) spinal plexus(es) and other nerves of trunk see 907.3

ALERT! For coding late effects of injuries to the nervous system see 907

● Code new
  to this edition
▲ Revision of
  existing code
④ ⑤ Fourth or fifth
  digit required

953.0 **Cervical root**

953.1 **Dorsal root**

953.2 **Lumbar root**

953.3 **Sacral root**

953.4 **Brachial plexus**

953.5 **Lumbosacral plexus**

953.8 **Multiple sites**

953.9 **Unspecified site**

954 Injury to other nerve(s) of trunk, excluding shoulder and pelvic girdles
> ALERT! For coding late effects of injuries to the nervous system see 907

954.0 **Cervical sympathetic**

954.1 **Other sympathetic**
> Celiac ganglion or plexus   Splanchnic nerve(s)
> Inferior mesenteric plexus   Stellate ganglion

954.8 **Other specified nerve(s) of trunk**

954.9 **Unspecified nerve of trunk**

955 Injury to peripheral nerve(s) of shoulder girdle and upper limb
> ALERT! For coding late effect of injury to peripheral nerve of shoulder girdle and upper limb see 907.4
> ALERT! For coding late effects of injuries to the nervous system see 907

955.0 **Axillary nerve**

955.1 **Median nerve**

955.2 **Ulnar nerve**

955.3 **Radial nerve**

955.4 **Musculocutaneous nerve**

955.5 **Cutaneous sensory nerve, upper limb**

955.6 **Digital nerve**

955.7 **Other specified nerve(s) of shoulder girdle and upper limb**

955.8 **Multiple nerves of shoulder girdle and upper limb**

955.9 **Unspecified nerve of shoulder girdle and upper limb**

956 Injury to peripheral nerve(s) of pelvic girdle and lower limb
> ALERT! For coding late effect of injury to peripheral nerve of pelvic girdle and lower limb see 907.5
> ALERT! For coding late effects of injuries to the nervous system see 907

9956.0 **Sciatic nerve**

956.1 **Femoral nerve**

956.2 **Posterior tibial nerve**

956.3 **Peroneal nerve**

956.4 **Cutaneous sensory nerve, lower limb**

956.5 **Other specified nerve(s) of pelvic girdle and lower limb**

956.8 **Multiple nerves of pelvic girdle and lower limb**

956.9 **Unspecified nerve of pelvic girdle and lower limb**

957 Injury to other and unspecified nerves
> ALERT! For coding late effect of injury to other and unspecified nerve see 907.9
> ALERT! For coding late effects of injuries to the nervous system see 907

957.0 **Superficial nerves of head and neck**

957.1 **Other specified nerve(s)**

957.8 **Multiple nerves in several parts**
> Multiple nerve injury NOS

957.9 **Unspecified site**
> Nerve injury NOS

| | Add 4th or 5th digit | | Nonspecific code | | Unspecified code | | Medicare secondary payer (MSP) alert |

CERTAIN TRAUMATIC COMPLICATIONS AND UNSPECIFIED INJURIES (958-959)

958 **Certain early complications of trauma**

> *Excludes:* *adult respiratory distress syndrome (518.52)*
> *flail chest (807.4)*
> *post-traumatic seroma (729.91)*
> *shock lung related to trauma and surgery (518.52)*
> *that occurring during or following medical procedures (996.0-999.9)*

ALERT! For coding late effect of certain complications of trauma see 908.6

ALERT! For coding late effects of other and unspecified injuries see 908

958.0 Air embolism
    Pneumathemia

> *Excludes:* *that complicating:*
> *abortion (634-638 with .6, 639.6)*
> *ectopic or molar pregnancy (639.6)*
> *pregnancy, childbirth, or the puerperium (673.0)*

958.1 Fat embolism

> *Excludes:* *that complicating:*
> *abortion (634-638 with .6, 639.6)*
> *pregnancy, childbirth, or the puerperium (673.8)*

958.2 Secondary and recurrent hemorrhage

958.3 Posttraumatic wound infection, not elsewhere classified

> *Excludes:* *infected open wounds—code to complicated open wound of site*

ALERT! Assign code 958.3 as an additional code for any documented infected burn site

958.4 **Traumatic shock**
    Shock (immediate) (delayed) following injury

> *Excludes:* *shock:*
> *anaphylactic (995.0)*
>   *due to serum (999.41-999.49)*
> *anesthetic (995.4)*
> *electric (994.8)*
> *following abortion (639.5)*
> *lightning (994.0)*
> *nontraumatic NOS (785.50)*
> *obstetric (669.1)*
> *postoperative (998.00-998.09)*

958.5 **Traumatic anuria**
    Crush syndrome
    Renal failure following crushing

> *Excludes:* *that due to a medical procedure (997.5)*

958.6 Volkmann's ischemic contracture
    Posttraumatic muscle contracture

958.7 Traumatic subcutaneous emphysema

> *Excludes:* *subcutaneous emphysema resulting from a procedure (998.81)*

958.8 **Other early complications of trauma**

⑤ **958.9 Traumatic compartment syndrome**

> *Excludes:* *nontraumatic compartment syndrome (729.71-729.79)*

   958.90 Compartment syndrome, unspecified

   958.91 Traumatic compartment syndrome of upper extremity
       Traumatic compartment syndrome of shoulder, arm, forearm, wrist, hand, and
          fingers

   958.92 Traumatic compartment syndrome of lower extremity
       Traumatic compartment syndrome of hip, buttock, thigh, leg, foot, and toes

   958.93 Traumatic compartment syndrome of abdomen

   958.99 **Traumatic compartment syndrome of other sites**

● Code new
    to this edition   ▲ Revision of
                              existing code   ④ ⑤ Fourth or fifth
                                                      digit required

959 **Injury, other and unspecified**
    Includes: injury NOS

    Excludes: *injury NOS of:*
        blood vessels (900.0-904.9)
        eye (921.0-921.9)
        internal organs (860.0-869.1)
        intracranial sites (854.0-854.1)
        nerves (950.0-951.9, 953.0-957.9)
        spinal cord (952.0-952.9)

    ALERT! For coding late effect of unspecified injury see 908.9
    ALERT! For coding late effects of other and unspecified injuries see 908

⑤ **959.0** **Head, face and neck**
    Cheek   Mouth
    Ear   Nose
    Eyebrow   Throat
    Lip

    959.01 **Head injury, unspecified**
    Excludes: *concussion (850.1-850.9)*
        with head injury NOS (850.1-850.9)
        head injury NOS with loss of consciousness (850.1-850.5)
        specified intracranial injuries (850.0-854.1)

    959.09 **Injury of face and neck**

⑤ **959.1** **Trunk**
    Excludes: *scapular region (959.2)*

    959.11 **Other injury of chest wall**

    959.12 **Other injury of abdomen**

    959.13 **Fracture of corpus cavernosum penis**

    959.14 **Other injury of external genitals**

    959.19 **Other injury of other sites of trunk**
        Injury of trunk NOS

  959.2 **Shoulder and upper arm**
    Axilla
    Scapular region

  959.3 **Elbow, forearm, and wrist**

  959.4 **Hand, except finger**

  959.5 **Finger**
    Fingernail
    Thumb (nail)

  959.6 **Hip and thigh**
    Upper leg

  959.7 **Knee, leg, ankle, and foot**

  959.8 **Other specified sites, including multiple**
    Excludes: *multiple sites classifiable to the same four-digit category (959.0-959.7)*

  959.9 **Unspecified site**

POISONING BY DRUGS, MEDICINAL AND BIOLOGICAL SUBSTANCES (960-979)

Includes: overdose of these substances
wrong substances given or taken in error

Excludes: *adverse effects ["hypersensitivity," "reaction," etc.] of correct substance properly administered. Such cases are to be classified according to the nature of the adverse effect, such as:*
adverse effect NOS (995.20)
allergic lymphadenitis (289.3)
aspirin gastritis (535.4)
blood disorders (280.0-289.9)
dermatitis:
  contact (692.0-692.9)
  due to ingestion (693.0-693.9)
nephropathy (583.9)
[The drug giving rise to the adverse effect may be identified by use of categories E930-E949]
drug dependence (304.0-304.9)
drug reaction and poisoning affecting the newborn (760.0-779.9)
nondependent abuse of drugs (305.0-305.9)
pathological drug intoxication (292.2)

Use additional code to specify the effects of the poisoning

ALERT! For coding late effect of poisoning due to drug medicinal or biological substance see 909.0

ALERT! For personal history of poisoning presenting hazards to health see V15.6

960 Poisoning by antibiotics

Excludes: *antibiotics:*
ear, nose, and throat (976.6)
eye (976.5)
local (976.0)

960.0 Penicillins
Ampicillin   Cloxacillin
Carbenicillin   Penicillin G

960.1 Antifungal antibiotics
Amphotericin B   Nystatin
Griseofulvin   Trichomycin

Excludes: *preparations intended for topical use (976.0-976.9)*

960.2 Chloramphenicol group
Chloramphenicol
Thiamphenicol

960.3 Erythromycin and other macrolides
Oleandomycin
Spiramycin

960.4 Tetracycline group
Doxycycline   Oxytetracycline
Minocycline

960.5 Cephalosporin group
Cephalexin   Cephaloridine
Cephaloglycin   Cephalothin

960.6 Antimycobacterial antibiotics
Cycloserine   Rifampin
Kanamycin   Streptomycin

960.7 Antineoplastic antibiotics
Actinomycin such as: Bleomycin
  Cactinomycin   Daunorubicin
  Dactinomycin   Mitomycin

960.8 Other specified antibiotics

960.9 Unspecified antibiotic

● Code new to this edition   ▲ Revision of existing code   ④ ⑤ Fourth or fifth digit required

961 **Poisoning by other anti-infectives**

> *Excludes:* anti-infectives:
>> ear, nose, and throat (976.6)
>> eye (976.5)
>> local (976.0)

ALERT! For coding late effect of poisoning due to drug medicinal or biological substance see 909.0

961.0 **Sulfonamides**

Sulfadiazine   Sulfamethoxazole
Sulfafurazole

961.1 **Arsenical anti-infectives**

961.2 **Heavy metal anti-infectives**

Compounds of: Compounds of:
  antimony   lead
  bismuth   mercury

> *Excludes:* mercurial diuretics (974.0)

ALERT! For personal history of contact with and (suspected) exposure to lead see V15.86

961.3 **Quinoline and hydroxyquinoline derivatives**

Chiniofon
Diiodohydroxyquin

> *Excludes:* antimalarial drugs (961.4)

961.4 **Antimalarials and drugs acting on other blood protozoa**

Chloroquine   Proguanil [chloroguanide]
Cycloguanil   Pyrimethamine
Primaquine   Quinine

961.5 **Other antiprotozoal drugs**

Emetine

961.6 **Anthelmintics**

Hexylresorcinol   Thiabendazole
Piperazine

961.7 **Antiviral drugs**

Methisazone

> *Excludes:* amantadine (966.4)
>> cytarabine (963.1)
>> idoxuridine (976.5)

961.8 **Other antimycobacterial drugs**

Ethambutol   Para-aminosalicylic acid derivatives
Ethionamide   Sulfones
Isoniazid

961.9 **Other and unspecified anti-infectives**

Flucytosine
Nitrofuran derivatives

962 **Poisoning by hormones and synthetic substitutes**

> *Excludes:* oxytocic hormones (975.0)

ALERT! For coding late effect of poisoning due to drug medicinal or biological substance see 909.0

ALERT! For personal history of inhaled steroid therapy see V87.44

ALERT! For personal history of systemic steroid therapy see V87.45

962.0 **Adrenal cortical steroids**

Cortisone derivatives
Desoxycorticosterone derivatives
Fluorinated corticosteroids

962.1 **Androgens and anabolic congeners**

Methandriol   Oxymetholone
Nandrolone   Testosterone

962.2 **Ovarian hormones and synthetic substitutes**

Contraceptives, oral
Estrogens
Estrogens and progestogens, combined
Progestogens

ALERT! For personal history of estrogen therapy see V87.43

| | Add 4th or 5th digit | | Nonspecific code | | Unspecified code | | Medicare secondary payer (MSP) alert |

962.3 Insulins and antidiabetic agents
Acetohexamide
Biguanide derivatives, oral
Chlorpropamide
Glucagon
Insulin
Phenformin
Sulfonylurea derivatives, oral
Tolbutamide

962.4 Anterior pituitary hormones
Corticotropin
Gonadotropin
Somatotropin [growth hormone]

962.5 Posterior pituitary hormones
Vasopressin

Excludes: oxytocic hormones (975.0)

962.6 Parathyroid and parathyroid derivatives

962.7 Thyroid and thyroid derivatives
Dextrothyroxin
Levothyroxine sodium
Liothyronine
Thyroglobulin

962.8 Antithyroid agents
Iodides
Thiouracil
Thiourea

962.9 Other and unspecified hormones and synthetic substitutes

963 Poisoning by primarily systemic agents

ALERT! For coding late effect of poisoning due to drug medicinal or biological substance see 909.0

963.0 Antiallergic and antiemetic drugs
Antihistamines
Chlorpheniramine
Diphenhydramine
Diphenylpyraline
Thonzylamine
Tripelennamine

Excludes: phenothiazine-based tranquilizers (969.1)

963.1 Antineoplastic and immunosuppressive drugs
Azathioprine
Busulfan
Chlorambucil
Cyclophosphamide
Cytarabine
Fluorouracil
Mercaptopurine
thio-TEPA

Excludes: antineoplastic antibiotics (960.7)

ALERT! For personal history of antineoplastic chemotherapy see V87.41
ALERT! For personal history of immunosuppressive therapy see V87.46

963.2 Acidifying agents

963.3 Alkalizing agents

963.4 Enzymes, not elsewhere classified
Penicillinase

963.5 Vitamins, not elsewhere classified
Vitamin A
Vitamin D

Excludes: nicotinic acid (972.2)
vitamin K (964.3)

963.8 Other specified systemic agents
Heavy metal antagonists

963.9 Unspecified systemic agent

964 Poisoning by agents primarily affecting blood constituents

ALERT! For coding late effect of poisoning due to drug medicinal or biological substance see 909.0

964.0 Iron and its compounds
Ferric salts
Ferrous sulfate and other ferrous salts

964.1 Liver preparations and other antianemic agents
Folic acid

964.2 Anticoagulants
Coumarin
Heparin
Phenindione
Warfarin sodium

964.3 Vitamin K [phytonadione]

● Code new
to this edition
▲ Revision of
existing code
④ ⑤ Fourth or fifth
digit required

964.4 Fibrinolysis-affecting drugs
Aminocaproic acid   Streptokinase
Streptodornase   Urokinase

964.5 Anticoagulant antagonists and other coagulants
Hexadimethrine
Protamine sulfate

964.6 Gamma globulin

964.7 Natural blood and blood products
Blood plasma   Packed red cells
Human fibrinogen   Whole blood

> Excludes: *transfusion reactions (999.41-999.8)*

964.8 Other specified agents affecting blood constituents
Macromolecular blood substitutes
Plasma expanders

964.9 Unspecified agent affecting blood constituents

965 Poisoning by analgesics, antipyretics, and antirheumatics

> Excludes: *drug dependence (304.0-304.9)*
> *nondependent abuse (305.0-305.9)*

ALERT! For coding late effect of poisoning due to drug medicinal or biological substance see 909.0

⑤ **965.0 Opiates and related narcotics**

    965.00 Opium (alkaloids), unspecified

    965.01 Heroin
        Diacetylmorphine

    965.02 Methadone

    965.09 Other
        Codeine [methylmorphine]
        Meperidine [pethidine]
        Morphine

965.1 Salicylates
Acetylsalicylic acid [aspirin]
Salicylic acid salts

965.4 Aromatic analgesics, not elsewhere classified
Acetanilid
Paracetamol [acetaminophen]
Phenacetin [acetophenetidin]

965.5 Pyrazole derivatives
Aminophenazone [aminopyrine]
Phenylbutazone

⑤ **965.6 Antirheumatics [antiphlogistics]**

> Excludes: *salicylates (965.1)*
> *steroids (962.0-962.9)*

    965.61 Propionic acid derivatives
        Fenoprofen   Ketoprofen
        Flurbiprofen   Naproxen
        Ibuprofen   Oxaprozin

    965.69 Other antirheumatics
        Gold salts
        Indomethacin

965.7 Other non-narcotic analgesics
Pyrabital

965.8 Other specified analgesics and antipyretics
Pentazocine

965.9 Unspecified analgesic and antipyretic

966 Poisoning by anticonvulsants and anti-Parkinsonism drugs

ALERT! For coding late effect of poisoning due to drug medicinal or biological substance see 909.0

966.0 Oxazolidine derivatives
Paramethadione
Trimethadione

| ■ Add 4th or 5th digit | ■ Nonspecific code | ■ Unspecified code | ■ Medicare secondary payer (MSP) alert |

966.1 Hydantoin derivatives
Phenytoin

966.2 Succinimides
Ethosuximide
Phensuximide

966.3 Other and unspecified anticonvulsants
Primidone

Excludes: *barbiturates (967.0)*
sulfonamides (961.0)

966.4 Anti-Parkinsonism drugs
Amantadine
Ethopropazine [profenamine]
Levodopa [L-dopa]

967 Poisoning by sedatives and hypnotics

Excludes: *drug dependence (304.0-304.9)*
nondependent abuse (305.0-305.9)

ALERT! For coding late effect of poisoning due to drug medicinal or biological substance see 909.0

967.0 Barbiturates
Amobarbital [amylobarbitone]
Barbital [barbitone]
Butabarbital [butabarbitone]
Pentobarbital [pentobarbitone]
Phenobarbital [phenobarbitone]
Secobarbital [quinalbarbitone]

Excludes: *thiobarbiturate anesthetics (968.3)*

967.1 Chloral hydrate group

967.2 Paraldehyde

967.3 Bromine compounds
Bromide
Carbromal (derivatives)

967.4 Methaqualone compounds

967.5 Glutethimide group

967.6 Mixed sedatives, not elsewhere classified

967.8 Other sedatives and hypnotics

967.9 Unspecified sedative or hypnotic
Sleeping:
drug NOS
pill NOS
tablet NOS

968 Poisoning by other central nervous system depressants and anesthetics

Excludes: *drug dependence (304.0-304.9)*
nondependent abuse (305.0-305.9)

ALERT! For coding late effect of poisoning due to drug medicinal or biological substance see 909.0

968.0 Central nervous system muscle-tone depressants
Chlorphenesin (carbamate)   Methocarbamol
Mephenesin

968.1 Halothane

968.2 Other gaseous anesthetics
Ether
Halogenated hydrocarbon derivatives, except halothane
Nitrous oxide

968.3 Intravenous anesthetics

Excludes: *Methohexital [methohexitone]*
Thiobarbiturates, such as thiopental sodium

968.4 Other and unspecified general anesthetics

● Code new
to this edition

▲ Revision of
existing code

④ ⑤ Fourth or fifth
digit required

▲ **968.5 Surface (topical) and infiltration anesthetics**

    Cocaine (topical)   Procaine

    Lidocaine [lignocaine]   Tetracaine

    Excludes: *poisoning by cocaine used as a central nervous system stimulant (970.81)*

968.6 Peripheral nerve and plexus-blocking anesthetics

968.7 Spinal anesthetics

968.9 Other and unspecified local anesthetics

969 Poisoning by psychotropic agents

    Excludes: *drug dependence (304.0-304.9)*

                nondependent abuse (305.0-305.9)

    ALERT! For coding late effect of poisoning due to drug medicinal or biological substance see 909.0

⑤ **969.0 Antidepressants**

    969.00 Antidepressant, unspecified

    969.01 Monoamine oxidase inhibitors

        MAOI

    969.02 Selective serotonin and norepinephrine reuptake inhibitors

        SSNRI antidepressants

    969.03 Selective serotonin reuptake inhibitors

        SSRI antidepressants

    969.04 Tetracyclic antidepressants

    969.05 Tricyclic antidepressants

    969.09 Other antidepressants

969.1 Phenothiazine-based tranquilizers

    Chlorpromazine   Prochlorperazine

    Fluphenazine   Promazine

969.2 Butyrophenone-based tranquilizers

    Haloperidol   Trifluperidol

    Spiperone

969.3 Other antipsychotics, neuroleptics, and major tranquilizers

969.4 Benzodiazepine-based tranquilizers

    Chlordiazepoxide   Lorazepam

    Diazepam   Medazepam

    Flurazepam   Nitrazepam

969.5 Other tranquilizers

    Hydroxyzine

    Meprobamate

969.6 Psychodysleptics [hallucinogens]

    Cannabis (derivatives)   Mescaline

    Lysergide [LSD]   Psilocin

    Marijuana (derivatives)   Psilocybin

⑤ **969.7 Psychostimulants**

    Excludes: *central appetite depressants (977.0)*

    969.70 Psychostimulant, unspecified

    969.71 Caffeine

    969.72 Amphetamines

        Methamphetamines

    969.73 Methylphenidate

    969.79 Other psychostimulants

969.8 Other specified psychotropic agents

969.9 Unspecified psychotropic agent

970 Poisoning by central nervous system stimulants

    ALERT! For coding late effect of poisoning due to drug medicinal or biological substance see 909.0

970.0 Analeptics

    Lobeline

    Nikethamide

| | Add 4th or 5th digit | | Nonspecific code | | Unspecified code | | Medicare secondary payer (MSP) alert |

970.1 Opiate antagonists
Levallorphan   Naloxone
Nalorphine

⑤ **970.8 Other specified central nervous system stimulants**

    970.81 Cocaine
      Crack

    970.89 Other central nervous system stimulants

970.9 Unspecified central nervous system stimulant

971 Poisoning by drugs primarily affecting the autonomic nervous system
ALERT! For coding late effect of poisoning due to drug medicinal or biological substance see 909.0

971.0 Parasympathomimetics [cholinergics]
Acetylcholine   Pilocarpine
Anticholinesterase:
  organophosphorus
  reversible

971.1 Parasympatholytics [anticholinergics and antimuscarinics] and spasmolytics
Atropine   Hyoscine [scopolamine]
Homatropine   Quaternary ammonium derivatives
Excludes: papaverine (972.5)

971.2 Sympathomimetics [adrenergics]
Epinephrine [adrenalin]
Levarterenol [noradrenalin]

971.3 Sympatholytics [antiadrenergics]
Phenoxybenzamine
Tolazoline hydrochloride

971.9 Unspecified drug primarily affecting autonomic nervous system

972 Poisoning by agents primarily affecting the cardiovascular system
ALERT! For coding late effect of poisoning due to drug medicinal or biological substance see 909.0

972.0 Cardiac rhythm regulators
Practolol   Propranolol
Procainamide   Quinidine
Excludes: lidocaine (968.5)

972.1 Cardiotonic glycosides and drugs of similar action
Digitalis glycosides   Strophanthins
Digoxin

972.2 Antilipemic and antiarteriosclerotic drugs
Clofibrate
Nicotinic acid derivatives

972.3 Ganglion-blocking agents
Pentamethonium bromide

972.4 Coronary vasodilators
Dipyridamole   Nitrites
Nitrates [nitroglycerin]

972.5 Other vasodilators
Cyclandelate   Papaverine
Diazoxide
Excludes: nicotinic acid (972.2)

972.6 Other antihypertensive agents
Clonidine   Rauwolfia alkaloids
Guanethidine   Reserpine

972.7 Antivaricose drugs, including sclerosing agents
Sodium morrhuate
Zinc salts

972.8 Capillary-active drugs
Adrenochrome derivatives
Metaraminol

972.9 Other and unspecified agents primarily affecting the cardiovascular system

● Code new to this edition   ▲ Revision of existing code   ④ ⑤ Fourth or fifth digit required

973 **Poisoning by agents primarily affecting the gastrointestinal system**

> **ALERT!** For coding late effect of poisoning due to drug medicinal or biological substance see 909.0

973.0 Antacids and antigastric secretion drugs
Aluminum hydroxide
Magnesium trisilicate

973.1 Irritant cathartics
Bisacodyl   Phenolphthalein
Castor oil

973.2 Emollient cathartics
Dioctyl sulfosuccinates

973.3 Other cathartics, including intestinal atonia drugs
Magnesium sulfate

973.4 Digestants
Pancreatin   Pepsin
Papain

973.5 Antidiarrheal drugs
Kaolin
Pectin

> *Excludes:* anti-infectives (960.0-961.9)

973.6 Emetics

973.8 Other specified agents primarily affecting the gastrointestinal system

973.9 Unspecified agent primarily affecting the gastrointestinal system

974 **Poisoning by water, mineral, and uric acid metabolism drugs**

> **ALERT!** For coding late effect of poisoning due to drug medicinal or biological substance see 909.0

974.0 Mercurial diuretics
Chlormerodrin
Mercaptomerin
Mersalyl

974.1 Purine derivative diuretics
Theobromine
Theophylline

> *Excludes:* aminophylline [theophylline ethylenediamine] (975.7)
>   caffeine (969.71)

974.2 Carbonic acid anhydrase inhibitors
Acetazolamide

974.3 Saluretics
Benzothiadiazides
Chlorothiazide group

974.4 Other diuretics
Ethacrynic acid
Furosemide

974.5 Electrolytic, caloric, and water-balance agents

974.6 Other mineral salts, not elsewhere classified

974.7 Uric acid metabolism drugs
Allopurinol   Probenecid
Colchicine

975 **Poisoning by agents primarily acting on the smooth and skeletal muscles and respiratory system**

> **ALERT!** For coding late effect of poisoning due to drug medicinal or biological substance see 909.0

975.0 Oxytocic agents
Ergot alkaloids   Prostaglandins
Oxytocin

975.1 Smooth muscle relaxants
Adiphenine
Metaproterenol [orciprenaline]

> *Excludes:* papaverine (972.5)

| | Add 4th or 5th digit | | Nonspecific code | | Unspecified code | | Medicare secondary payer (MSP) alert |

975.2 **Skeletal muscle relaxants**

975.3 **Other and unspecified drugs acting on muscles**

975.4 **Antitussives**
Dextromethorphan
Pipazethate

975.5 **Expectorants**
Acetylcysteine   Terpin hydrate
Guaifenesin

975.6 **Anti-common cold drugs**

975.7 **Antiasthmatics**
Aminophylline [theophylline ethylenediamine]

975.8 **Other and unspecified respiratory drugs**

976 **Poisoning by agents primarily affecting skin and mucous membrane, ophthalmological, otorhinolaryngological, and dental drugs**
ALERT! For coding late effect of poisoning due to drug medicinal or biological substance see 909.0

976.0 **Local anti-infectives and anti-inflammatory drugs**

976.1 **Antipruritics**

976.2 **Local astringents and local detergents**

976.3 **Emollients, demulcents, and protectants**

976.4 **Keratolytics, keratoplastics, other hair treatment drugs and preparations**

976.5 **Eye anti-infectives and other eye drugs**
Idoxuridine

976.6 **Anti-infectives and other drugs and preparations for ear, nose, and throat**

976.7 **Dental drugs topically applied**
Excludes: anti-infectives (976.0)
              local anesthetics (968.5)

976.8 **Other agents primarily affecting skin and mucous membrane**
Spermicides [vaginal contraceptives]

976.9 **Unspecified agent primarily affecting skin and mucous membrane**

977 **Poisoning by other and unspecified drugs and medicinal substances**
ALERT! For coding late effect of poisoning due to drug medicinal or biological substance see 909.0

977.0 **Dietetics**
Central appetite depressants

977.1 **Lipotropic drugs**

977.2 **Antidotes and chelating agents, not elsewhere classified**

977.3 **Alcohol deterrents**

977.4 **Pharmaceutical excipients**
Pharmaceutical adjuncts

977.8 **Other specified drugs and medicinal substances**
Contrast media used for diagnostic x-ray procedures
Diagnostic agents and kits

977.9 **Unspecified drug or medicinal substance**

978 **Poisoning by bacterial vaccines**
ALERT! For coding late effect of poisoning due to drug medicinal or biological substance see 909.0

978.0 **BCG**

978.1 **Typhoid and paratyphoid**

978.2 **Cholera**

978.3 **Plague**

978.4 **Tetanus**

978.5 **Diphtheria**

978.6 **Pertussis vaccine, including combinations with a pertussis component**

978.8 **Other and unspecified bacterial vaccines**

978.9 **Mixed bacterial vaccines, except combinations with a pertussis component**

● Code new
to this edition

▲ Revision of
existing code

④ ⑤ Fourth or fifth
digit required

979 **Poisoning by other vaccines and biological substances**

> *Excludes:* gamma globulin (964.6)

> **ALERT!** For coding late effect of poisoning due to drug medicinal or biological substance see 909.0

979.0 **Smallpox vaccine**

979.1 **Rabies vaccine**

979.2 **Typhus vaccine**

979.3 **Yellow fever vaccine**

979.4 **Measles vaccine**

979.5 **Poliomyelitis vaccine**

979.6 **Other and unspecified viral and rickettsial vaccines**
Mumps vaccine

979.7 **Mixed viral-rickettsial and bacterial vaccines, except combinations with a pertussis component**

> *Excludes:* combinations with a pertussis component (978.6)

979.9 **Other and unspecified vaccines and biological substances**

TOXIC EFFECTS OF SUBSTANCES CHIEFLY NONMEDICINAL AS TO SOURCE (980-989)

> *Excludes:* burns from chemical agents (ingested) (947.0-947.9)
> localized toxic effects indexed elsewhere (001.0-799.9)
> respiratory conditions due to external agents (506.0-508.9)
> respiratory conditions due to smoke inhalation NOS (508.2)

Use additional code to specify the nature of the toxic effect

Use additional code to identify:
personal history of retained foreign body fully removed (V15.53)
retained foreign body status, if applicable (V90.01-V90.9)

980 **Toxic effect of alcohol**

> **ALERT!** For coding late effect of toxic effects of nonmedical substances see 909.1

980.0 **Ethyl alcohol**
Denatured alcohol
Ethanol
Grain alcohol

Use additional code to identify any associated:
acute alcohol intoxication (305.0)
in alcoholism (303.0)
drunkenness (simple) (305.0)
pathological (291.4)

980.1 **Methyl alcohol**
Methanol
Wood alcohol

980.2 **Isopropyl alcohol**
Dimethyl carbinol
Isopropanol
Rubbing alcohol

980.3 **Fusel oil**
Alcohol:
amyl
butyl
propyl

980.8 **Other specified alcohols**

980.9 **Unspecified alcohol**

981 **Toxic effect of petroleum products**
Benzine
Gasoline
Kerosene
Paraffin wax
Petroleum:
ether
naphtha
spirit

> **ALERT!** For coding late effect of toxic effects of nonmedical substances see 909.1

982 **Toxic effect of solvents other than petroleum-based**

> **ALERT!** For coding late effect of toxic effects of nonmedical substances see 909.1

982.0 **Benzene and homologues**

982.1 **Carbon tetrachloride**

Add 4th or 5th digit | Nonspecific code | Unspecified code | Medicare secondary payer (MSP) alert

982.2 Carbon disulfide
Carbon bisulfide

982.3 Other chlorinated hydrocarbon solvents
Tetrachloroethylene
Trichloroethylene

Excludes: chlorinated hydrocarbon preparations other than solvents (989.2)

982.4 Nitroglycol

982.8 Other nonpetroleum-based solvents
Acetone

983 Toxic effect of corrosive aromatics, acids, and caustic alkalis
ALERT! For coding late effect of toxic effects of nonmedical substances see 909.1

983.0 Corrosive aromatics
Carbolic acid or phenol
Cresol

983.1 Acids
Acid:
  hydrochloric
  nitric
  sulfuric

983.2 Caustic alkalis
Lye
Potassium hydroxide
Sodium hydroxide

983.9 Caustic, unspecified

984 Toxic effect of lead and its compounds (including fumes)
Includes: that from all sources except medicinal substances
ALERT! For coding late effect of toxic effects of nonmedical substances see 909.1
ALERT! For personal history of contact with and (suspected) exposure to lead see V15.86

984.0 Inorganic lead compounds
Lead dioxide
Lead salts

984.1 Organic lead compounds
Lead acetate
Tetraethyl lead

984.8 Other lead compounds

984.9 Unspecified lead compound

985 Toxic effect of other metals
Includes: that from all sources except medicinal substances
ALERT! For coding late effect of toxic effects of nonmedical substances see 909.1

985.0 Mercury and its compounds
Minamata disease

985.1 Arsenic and its compounds

985.2 Manganese and its compounds

985.3 Beryllium and its compounds

985.4 Antimony and its compounds

985.5 Cadmium and its compounds

985.6 Chromium

985.8 Other specified metals
Brass fumes   Iron compounds
Copper salts   Nickel compounds

985.9 Unspecified metal

986 Toxic effect of carbon monoxide
Carbon monoxide from any source
ALERT! For coding late effect of toxic effects of nonmedical substances see 909.1

987 Toxic effect of other gases, fumes, or vapors
ALERT! For coding late effect of toxic effects of nonmedical substances see 909.1

987.0 Liquefied petroleum gases
Butane
Propane

● Code new   ▲ Revision of   ④ ⑤ Fourth or fifth
to this edition   existing code   digit required

987.1 **Other hydrocarbon gas**

987.2 **Nitrogen oxides**
Nitrogen dioxide
Nitrous fumes

987.3 **Sulfur dioxide**

987.4 **Freon**
Dichloromonofluoromethane

987.5 **Lacrimogenic gas**
Bromobenzyl cyanide
Chloroacetophenone
Ethyliodoacetate

987.6 **Chlorine gas**

987.7 **Hydrocyanic acid gas**

987.8 **Other specified gases, fumes, or vapors**
Phosgene
Polyester fumes

987.9 **Unspecified gas, fume, or vapor**

988 **Toxic effect of noxious substances eaten as food**

Excludes: *allergic reaction to food, such as:*
gastroenteritis (558.3)
rash (692.5, 693.1)
food poisoning (bacterial) (005.0-005.9)
toxic effects of food contaminants, such as:
aflatoxin and other mycotoxin (989.7)
mercury (985.0)

ALERT! For coding late effect of toxic effects of nonmedical substances see 909.1

988.0 **Fish and shellfish**

988.1 **Mushrooms**

988.2 **Berries and other plants**

988.8 **Other specified noxious substances eaten as food**

988.9 **Unspecified noxious substance eaten as food**

989 **Toxic effect of other substances, chiefly nonmedicinal as to source**

ALERT! For coding late effect of toxic effects of nonmedical substances see 909.1

989.0 **Hydrocyanic acid and cyanides**
Potassium cyanide
Sodium cyanide

Excludes: *gas and fumes (987.7)*

989.1 **Strychnine and salts**

989.2 **Chlorinated hydrocarbons**
Aldrin   DDT
Chlordane   Dieldrin

Excludes: *chlorinated hydrocarbon solvents (982.0-982.3)*

989.3 **Organophosphate and carbamate**
Carbaryl   Parathion
Dichlorvos   Phorate
Malathion   Phosdrin

989.4 **Other pesticides, not elsewhere classified**
Mixtures of insecticides

989.5 **Venom**
Bites of venomous snakes, lizards, and spiders
Tick paralysis

989.6 **Soaps and detergents**

989.7 **Aflatoxin and other mycotoxin [food contaminants]**

⑤ **989.8** **Other substances, chiefly nonmedicinal as to source**

ALERT! For personal history of contact with and (suspected) exposure to asbestos see V15.84

989.81 **Asbestos**

Excludes: *asbestosis (501)*
exposure to asbestos (V15.84)

989.82 **Latex**

Add 4th or 5th digit   Nonspecific code   Unspecified code   Medicare secondary payer (MSP) alert

989.83 Silicone

Excludes: *silicone used in medical devices, implants and grafts (996.00-996.79)*

989.84 Tobacco

989.89 Other

989.9 Unspecified substance, chiefly nonmedicinal as to source

OTHER AND UNSPECIFIED EFFECTS OF EXTERNAL CAUSES (990-995)

990 Effects of radiation, unspecified

Complication of phototherapy   Radiation sickness
Complication of radiation therapy

Excludes: *specified adverse effects of radiation*

> *Such conditions are to be classified according to the nature of the adverse effect, as:*
> *burns (940.0-949.5)*
> *dermatitis (692.7-692.8)*
> *leukemia (204.0-208.9)*
> *pneumonia (508.0)*
> *sunburn (692.71, 692.76-692.77)*
> *[The type of radiation giving rise to the adverse effect may be identified by use of the E codes.]*

ALERT! For coding late effect of radiation see 909.2

ALERT! For personal history of irradiation presenting hazards to health see V15.3

991 Effects of reduced temperature

991.0 Frostbite of face

991.1 Frostbite of hand

991.2 Frostbite of foot

991.3 Frostbite of other and unspecified sites

991.4 Immersion foot
Trench foot

991.5 Chilblains
Erythema pernio
Perniosis

991.6 Hypothermia
Hypothermia (accidental)

Excludes: *hypothermia following anesthesia (995.89)*
hypothermia not associated with low environmental temperature (780.65)

991.8 Other specified effects of reduced temperature

991.9 Unspecified effect of reduced temperature
Effects of freezing or excessive cold NOS

992 Effects of heat and light

Excludes: *burns (940.0-949.5)*
diseases of sweat glands due to heat (705.0-705.9)
malignant hyperpyrexia following anesthesia (995.86)
sunburn (692.71, 692.76-692.77)

992.0 Heat stroke and sunstroke
Heat apoplexy
Heat pyrexia
Ictus solaris
Siriasis
Thermoplegia

Use additional code(s) to identify any associated complications of heat stroke, such as:
alterations of consciousness (780.01-780.09)
systemic inflammatory response syndrome (995.93-995.94)

992.1 Heat syncope
Heat collapse

992.2 Heat cramps

992.3 Heat exhaustion, anhydrotic
Heat prostration due to water depletion

Excludes: *that associated with salt depletion (992.4)*

992.4 Heat exhaustion due to salt depletion
Heat prostration due to salt (and water) depletion

● Code new   ▲ Revision of   ④ ⑤ Fourth or fifth
to this edition   existing code   digit required

992.5 Heat exhaustion, unspecified
    Heat prostration NOS

992.6 Heat fatigue, transient

992.7 Heat edema

992.8 Other specified heat effects

992.9 Unspecified

993 Effects of air pressure

993.0 Barotrauma, otitic
    Aero-otitis media
    Effects of high altitude on ears

993.1 Barotrauma, sinus
    Aerosinusitis
    Effects of high altitude on sinuses

993.2 Other and unspecified effects of high altitude
    Alpine sickness
    Andes disease
    Anoxia due to high altitude
    Hypobaropathy
    Mountain sickness

993.3 Caisson disease
    Bends
    Compressed-air disease
    Decompression sickness
    Divers' palsy or paralysis

993.4 Effects of air pressure caused by explosion

993.8 Other specified effects of air pressure

993.9 Unspecified effect of air pressure

994 Effects of other external causes

Excludes: certain adverse effects not elsewhere classified (995.0-995.8)

994.0 Effects of lightning
    Shock from lightning
    Struck by lightning NOS

Excludes: burns (940.0-949.5)

994.1 Drowning and nonfatal submersion
    Bathing cramp
    Immersion

994.2 Effects of hunger
    Deprivation of food
    Starvation

994.3 Effects of thirst
    Deprivation of water

994.4 Exhaustion due to exposure

994.5 Exhaustion due to excessive exertion
    Exhaustion due to overexertion

994.6 Motion sickness
    Air sickness
    Seasickness
    Travel sickness

994.7 Asphyxiation and strangulation
    Suffocation (by):   Suffocation (by):
      bedclothes   plastic bag
      cave-in   pressure
      constriction   strangulation
      mechanical

Excludes: asphyxia from:
    carbon monoxide (986)
    inhalation of food or foreign body (932-934.9)
    other gases, fumes, and vapors (987.0-987.9)

Add 4th or 5th digit   Nonspecific code   Unspecified code   Medicare secondary payer (MSP) alert

994.8 Electrocution and nonfatal effects of electric current
Shock from electric current
Shock from electroshock gun (taser)

Excludes: electric burns (940.0-949.5)

994.9 Other effects of external causes
Effects of:
abnormal gravitational [G] forces or states
weightlessness

995 Certain adverse effects not elsewhere classified

Excludes: complications of surgical and medical care (996.0-999.9)

ALERT! For personal history of allergy other than to medicinal agents see V15.0

▲ **995.0 Other anaphylactic reaction**
Allergic shock NOS or due to adverse effect of correct medicinal substance properly
administered
Anaphylactic reaction NOS or due to adverse effect of correct medicinal substance
properly administered
Anaphylactic shock NOS or due to adverse effect of correct medicinal substance
properly administered
Anaphylactoid reaction NOS
Anaphylaxis NOS or due to adverse effect of correct medicinal substance properly
administered

Excludes: anaphylactic reaction to serum (999.41-999.49)
anaphylactic shock or reaction due to adverse food reaction (995.60-995.69)

Use additional E code, if desired, to identify external cause, such as:
adverse effects of correct medicinal substance properly administered (E930-E949)

995.1 Angioneurotic edema
Allergic angioedema
Giant urticaria

Excludes: Urticaria:
due to serum (999.51-999.59)
other specified (698.2, 708.0-708.9, 757.33)

⑤ **995.2 Other and unspecified adverse effect of drug, medicinal and biological substance**

Excludes: pathological drug intoxication (292.2)

ALERT! For coding late effect of adverse effect of drug medicinal or biological substance see
909.5

**995.20 Unspecified adverse effect of unspecified drug, medicinal and biological
substance**
Unspecified adverse effect of unspecified medicinal substance properly
administered

995.21 Arthus phenomenon
Arthus reaction

995.22 Unspecified adverse effect of anesthesia

995.23 Unspecified adverse effect of insulin

995.24 Failed moderate sedation during procedure
Failed conscious sedation during procedure

995.27 Other drug allergy
Allergic reaction NEC (due) to correct medical substance properly
administered
Drug allergy NOS
Drug hypersensitivity NOS
Hypersensitivity (due) to correct medical substance properly administered

995.29 Unspecified adverse effect of other drug, medicinal and biological substance
Unspecified adverse effect of medicinal substance NEC properly administered

● Code new
to this edition

▲ Revision of
existing code

④ ⑤ Fourth or fifth
digit required

995.3 Allergy, unspecified
　　Allergic reaction NOS　　　　　Idiosyncrasy NOS
　　Hypersensitivity NOS

　　Excludes: *allergic reaction NOS to correct medicinal substance properly administered*
　　　　　　　(995.27)
　　　　　　allergy to existing dental restorative materials (525.66)
　　　　　　specific types of allergic reaction, such as:
　　　　　　　allergic diarrhea (558.3)
　　　　　　　dermatitis (691.0-693.9)
　　　　　　　hay fever (477.0-477.9)

995.4 Shock due to anesthesia
　　Shock due to anesthesia in which the correct substance was properly administered

　　Excludes: *complications of anesthesia in labor or delivery (668.0-668.9)*
　　　　　　　overdose or wrong substance given (968.0-969.9)
　　　　　　　postoperative shock NOS (998.00)
　　　　　　　specified adverse effects of anesthesia classified elsewhere, such as:
　　　　　　　　anoxic brain damage (348.1)
　　　　　　　　hepatitis (070.0-070.9), etc.
　　　　　　　unspecified adverse effect of anesthesia (995.22)

⑤ **995.5 Child maltreatment syndrome**
Use additional code(s), if applicable, to identify any associated injuries
Use additional E code to identify:
　　　　nature of abuse (E960-E968)
　　　　perpetrator (E967.0-E967.9)

　　995.50　Child abuse, unspecified

　　995.51　Child emotional/psychological abuse
　　ALERT! For personal history of emotional abuse see V15.42

　　995.52　Child neglect (nutritional)

　　995.53　Child sexual abuse

　　995.54　Child physical abuse
　　　　　Battered baby or child syndrome
　　Excludes: *Shaken infant syndrome (995.55)*
　　ALERT! For personal history of physical abuse see V15.41

　　995.55　Shaken infant syndrome
Use additional code(s) to identify any associated injuries

　　995.59　Other child abuse and neglect
　　　　　Multiple forms of abuse

▲ **995.6 Anaphylactic reaction due to food**
　　Anaphylactic reaction due to adverse food reaction
　　Anaphylactic shock or reaction due to nonpoisonous foods
　　Anaphylactoid reaction due to food

　　▲ **995.60　Anaphylactic reaction due to unspecified food**

　　▲ **995.61　Anaphylactic reaction due to peanuts**

　　▲ **995.62　Anaphylactic reaction due to crustaceans**

　　▲ **995.63　Anaphylactic reaction due to fruits and vegetables**

　　▲ **995.64　Anaphylactic reaction due to tree nuts and seeds**

　　▲ **995.65　Anaphylactic reaction due to fish**

　　▲ **995.66　Anaphylactic reaction due to food additives**

　　▲ **995.67　Anaphylactic reaction due to milk products**

　　▲ **995.68　Anaphylactic reaction due to eggs**

　　▲ **995.69　Anaphylactic reaction due to other specified food**

995.7 Other adverse food reactions, not elsewhere classified
Use additional code to identify the type of reaction, such as:
　　　　hives (708.0)
　　　　wheezing (786.07)

　　Excludes: *anaphylactic reaction or shock due to adverse food reaction (995.60-995.69)*
　　　　　　　asthma (493.0, 493.9)
　　　　　　　dermatitis due to food (693.1)
　　　　　　　　in contact with the skin (692.5)
　　　　　　　gastroenteritis and colitis due to food (558.3)
　　　　　　　rhinitis due to food (477.1)

Add 4th or　　　Nonspecific　　　Unspecified　　　Medicare secondary
5th digit　　　　code　　　　　　code　　　　　　payer (MSP) alert

⑤ **995.8 Other specified adverse effects, not elsewhere classified**

995.80 Adult maltreatment, unspecified
Abused person NOS

Use additional code to identify:
any associated injury
perpetrator (E967.0-E967.9)

995.81 Adult physical abuse
Battered:
person syndrome NEC
man
spouse
woman

Use additional code to identify:
any associated injury
nature of abuse (E960-E968)
perpetrator (E967.0-E967.9)

ALERT! For personal history of physical abuse see V15.41

995.82 Adult emotional/psychological abuse
Use additional E code to identify perpetrator (E967.0-E967.9)

ALERT! For personal history of emotional abuse see V15.42

995.83 Adult sexual abuse
Use additional code to identify:
any associated injury
perpetrator (E967.0-E967.9)

995.84 Adult neglect (nutritional)
Use additional code to identify:
intent of neglect (E904.0, E968.4)
perpetrator (E967.0-967.9)

995.85 Other adult abuse and neglect
Multiple forms of abuse and neglect

Use additional code to identify:
any associated injury
intent of neglect (E904.0, E968.4)
nature of abuse (E960-E968)
perpetrator (E967.0-E967.9)

995.86 Malignant hyperthermia
Malignant hyperpyrexia due to anesthesia

995.89 Other
Hypothermia due to anesthesia

⑤ **995.9 Systemic inflammatory response syndrome (SIRS)**

995.90 Systemic inflammatory response syndrome, unspecified
SIRS NOS

995.91 Sepsis
Systemic inflammatory response syndrome due to infectious process without acute organ dysfunction

Code first underlying infection

Excludes: *sepsis with acute organ dysfunction (995.92)*
sepsis with multiple organ dysfunction (995.92)
severe sepsis (995.92)

995.92 Severe sepsis
Sepsis with acute organ dysfunction
Sepsis with multiple organ dysfunction (MOD)
Systemic inflammatory response syndrome due to infectious process with acute organ dysfunction

Code first underlying infection

Use additional code to specify acute organ dysfunction, such as:
acute kidney failure (584.5-584.9)
acute respiratory failure (518.81)
critical illness myopathy (359.81)
critical illness polyneuropathy (357.82)
disseminated intravascular coagulopathy (DIC) syndrome (286.6)
encephalopathy (348.31)
hepatic failure (570)
septic shock (785.52)

● Code new
to this edition

▲ Revision of
existing code

④ ⑤ Fourth or fifth
digit required

995.93 Systemic inflammatory response syndrome due to noninfectious process without acute organ dysfunction

Code first underlying conditions, such as:
    acute pancreatitis (577.0)
    trauma

Excludes: *systemic inflammatory response syndrome due to noninfectious process with acute organ dysfunction (995.94)*

995.94 Systemic inflammatory response syndrome due to non-infectious process with acute organ dysfunction

Code first underlying condition, such as:
    acute pancreatitis (577.0)
    heat stroke (992.0)
    trauma

Use additional code to specify acute organ dysfunction, such as:
    acute kidney failure (584.5-584.9)
    acute respiratory failure (518.81)
    critical illness myopathy (359.81)
    critical illness polyneuropathy (357.82)
    disseminated intravascular coagulopathy (DIC) syndrome (286.6)
    encephalopathy (348.31)
    hepatic failure (570)

Excludes: *severe sepsis (995.92)*

COMPLICATIONS OF SURGICAL AND MEDICAL CARE, NOT ELSEWHERE CLASSIFIED (996-999)

Excludes: *adverse effects of medicinal agents (001.0-799.9, 995.0-995.8)*
    burns from local applications and irradiation (940.0-949.5)
    complications of:
      conditions for which the procedure was performed
      surgical procedures during abortion, labor, and delivery (630-676.9)
    poisoning and toxic effects of drugs and chemicals (960.0-989.9)
    postoperative conditions in which no complications are present, such as:
      artificial opening status (V44.0-V44.9)
      closure of external stoma (V55.0-V55.9)
      fitting of prosthetic device (V52.0-V52.9)
    specified complications classified elsewhere
      anesthetic shock (995.4)
      electrolyte imbalance (276.0-276.9)
      postlaminectomy syndrome (772.80-722.83)
      postmastectomy lymphedema syndrome (457.0)
      postoperative psychosis (293.0-293.9)
      any other condition classified elsewhere in the Alphabetic Index when described as due to a procedure

996 Complications peculiar to certain specified procedures

Includes: complications, not elsewhere classified, in the use of artificial substitutes [e.g., Dacron, metal, Silastic, Teflon] or natural sources [e.g., bone] involving:
    anastomosis (internal)
    graft (bypass) (patch)
    implant
    internal device:
      catheter
      electronic
      fixation
      prosthetic
    reimplant
    transplant

Excludes: *accidental puncture or laceration during procedure (998.2)*
    capsular contracture of breast implant (611.83)
    complications of internal anastomosis of:
      gastrointestinal tract (997.49)
      urinary tract (997.5)
    endosseous dental implant failures (525.71-525.79)
    intraoperative floppy iris syndrome (IFIS) (364.81)
    mechanical complication of respirator (V46.14)
    other specified complications classified elsewhere, such as:

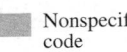 Add 4th or 5th digit   Nonspecific code   Unspecified code   Medicare secondary payer (MSP) alert

> *hemolytic anemia (283.1)*
> *functional cardiac disturbances (429.4)*
> *serum hepatitis (070.2-070.3)*

ALERT! For coding late effect of complications of surgical and medical care see 909.3

ALERT! For personal history of surgery to other organs see V15.29

⑤ **996.0 Mechanical complication of cardiac device, implant, and graft**

Breakdown (mechanical)	Obstruction, mechanical
Displacement	Perforation
Leakage	Protrusion

> **996.00 Unspecified device, implant, and graft**

> **996.01 Due to cardiac pacemaker (electrode)**

> **996.02 Due to heart valve prosthesis**

> **996.03 Due to coronary bypass graft**

Excludes: *atherosclerosis of graft (414.02, 414.03)*
> *embolism [occlusion NOS] [thrombus] of graft (996.72)*

> **996.04 Due to automatic implantable cardiac defibrillator**

> **996.09 Other**

996.1 Mechanical complication of other vascular device, implant, and graft
Mechanical complications involving:
aortic (bifurcation) graft (replacement)
arteriovenous:
dialysis catheter
fistula surgically created
shunt surgicall created
balloon (counterpulsation) device, intra-aortic
carotid artery bypass graft
femoral-popliteal bypass graft
umbrella device, vena cava

Excludes: *atherosclerosis of biological graft (440.30-440.32)*
> *embolism [occlusion NOS] [thrombus] of (biological) (synthetic) graft (996.74)*
> *peritoneal dialysis catheter (996.56)*

996.2 Mechanical complication of nervous system device, implant, and graft
Mechanical complications involving:
dorsal column stimulator
electrodes implanted in brain [brain "pacemaker"]
peripheral nerve graft
ventricular (communicating) shunt

⑤ **996.3 Mechanical complication of genitourinary device, implant, and graft**

> **996.30 Unspecified device, implant, and graft**

> **996.31 Due to urethral [indwelling] catheter**

> **996.32 Due to intrauterine contraceptive device**

> **996.39 Other**
> Prosthetic reconstruction of vas deferens
> Repair (graft) of ureter without mention of resection

Excludes: *complications due to:*
> *external stoma of urinary tract (596.81-596.83)*
> *internal anastomosis of urinary tract (997.5)*

⑤ **996.4 Mechanical complication of internal orthopedic device, implant, and graft**
Use additional code to identify prosthetic joint with mechanical complication (V43.60-V43.69)

> **996.40 Unspecified mechanical complication of internal orthopedic device, implant, and graft**

> **996.41 Mechanical loosening of prosthetic joint**
> Aseptic loosening

> **996.42 Dislocation of prosthetic joint**
> Instability of prosthetic joint
> Subluxation of prosthetic joint

> **996.43 Broken prosthetic joint implant**
> Breakage (fracture) of prosthetic joint

> **996.44 Peri-prosthetic fracture around prosthetic joint**

> **996.45 Peri-prosthetic osteolysis**
Use additional code to identify major osseous defect, if applicable (731.3)

● Code new	▲ Revision of	④ ⑤ Fourth or fifth
to this edition	existing code	digit required

996.46   Articular bearing surface wear of prosthetic joint

996.47   **Other mechanical complication of prosthetic joint implant**
      Mechanical complication of prosthetic joint NOS
      Prosthetic joint implant failure NOS

996.49   **Other mechanical complication of other internal orthopedic device, implant, and graft**
      Breakage of internal fixation device in bone
      Dislocation of internal fixation device in bone

Excludes: *mechanical complication of prosthetic joint implant (996.41-996.47)*

⑤ **996.5**   **Mechanical complication of other specified prosthetic device, implant, and graft**
      Mechanical complications involving:
      prosthetic implant in:
        bile duct
        breast
        chin
        orbit of eye
      nonabsorbable surgical material NOS
      other graft, implant, and internal device, not elsewhere classified

  996.51   **Due to corneal graft**

  996.52   **Due to graft of other tissue, not elsewhere classified**
      Skin graft failure or rejection

Excludes: *failure of artificial skin graft (996.55)*
       failure of decellularized allodermis (996.55)
       sloughing of temporary skin allografts or xenografts (pigskin)—omit code

  996.53   **Due to ocular lens prosthesis**

Excludes: *contact lenses—code to condition*

  996.54   **Due to breast prosthesis**
      Breast capsule (prosthesis)
      Mammary implant

  996.55   **Due to artificial skin graft and decellularized allodermis**
      Dislodgement   Displacement
      Failure   Non-adherence
      Poor incorporation   Shearing

  996.56   **Due to peritoneal dialysis catheter**

Excludes: *mechanical complication of arteriovenous dialysis catheter (996.1)*

  996.57   **Due to insulin pump**

  996.59   **Due to other implant and internal device, not elsewhere classified**
      Nonabsorbable surgical material NOS
      Prosthetic implant in:
        bile duct
        chin
        orbit of eye

⑤ **996.6**   **Infection and inflammatory reaction due to internal prosthetic device, implant, and graft**
      Infection (causing obstruction) due to (presence of) any device, implant and graft classifiable to 996.0-996.5
      Inflammation due to (presence of) any device, implant and graft classifiable to 996.0-996.5
      Use additional code to identify specified infections

  996.60   **Due to unspecified device, implant, and graft**

  996.61   **Due to cardiac device, implant, and graft**
      Cardiac pacemaker or defibrillator:
        electrode(s), lead(s)
        pulse generator
        subcutaneous pocket
      Coronary artery bypass graft
      Heart valve prosthesis

Add 4th or 5th digit	Nonspecific code	Unspecified code	Medicare secondary payer (MSP) alert

996.62 Due to other vascular device, implant, and graft
Arterial graft
Arteriovenous fistula or shunt
Infusion pump
Vascular catheter (arterial) (dialysis) (peripheral venous)

Excludes: *infection due to:*
central venous catheter (999.31-999.32)
Hickman catheter (999.31-999.32)
peripherally inserted central catheter (PICC) (999.31-999.32)
portacath (port-a-cath) (999.31999.32)
triple lumen catheter (999.31-999.32)
umbilical venous catheter (999.31-999.32)

996.63 Due to nervous system device, implant, and graft
Electrodes implanted in brain
Peripheral nerve graft
Spinal canal catheter
Ventricular (communicating) shunt (catheter)

996.64 Due to indwelling urinary catheter
Use additional code to identify specified infections, such as:
Cystitis (595.0-595.9)
Sepsis (038.0-038.9)

Excludes: *complications due to:*
external stoma of urinary tract (596.81-596.83)

996.65 Due to other genitourinary device, implant, and graft
Intrauterine contraceptive device

996.66 Due to internal joint prosthesis
Use additional code to identify infected prosthetic joint (V43.60-V43.69)

996.67 Due to other internal orthopedic device, implant, and graft
Bone growth stimulator (electrode)
Internal fixation device (pin) (rod) (screw)

996.68 Due to peritoneal dialysis catheter
Exit-site infection or inflammation

996.69 Due to other internal prosthetic device, implant, and graft
Breast prosthesis
Ocular lens prosthesis
Prosthetic orbital implant

⑤ **996.7 Other complications of internal (biological) (synthetic) prosthetic device, implant, and graft**
Complication NOS due to (presence of) any device, implant, and graft classifiable to 996.0-996.5
occlusion NOS
Embolism due to (presence of) any device, implant, and graft classifiable to 996.0-996.5
Fibrosis due to (presence of) any device, implant, and graft classifiable to 996.0-996.5
Hemorrhage due to (presence of) any device, implant, and graft classifiable to 996.0-996.5
Pain due to (presence of) any device, implant, and graft classifiable to 996.0-996.5
Stenosis due to (presence of) any device, implant, and graft classifiable to 996.0-996.5
Thrombus due to (presence of) any device, implant, and graft classifiable to 996.0-996.5
Use additional code to identify complication, such as:
pain due to presence of device, implant or graft (338.18-338.19,338.28-338.29)
venous embolism and thrombosis (453.2-453.9)

Excludes: *disruption (dehiscence) of internal suture material (998.31)*
transplant rejection (996.80-996.89)

996.70 Due to unspecified device, implant, and graft

996.71 Due to heart valve prosthesis

996.72 Due to other cardiac device, implant, and graft
Cardiac pacemaker or defibrillator:
electrode(s), lead(s)
subcutaneous pocket
Coronary artery bypass (graft)

Excludes: *occlusion due to atherosclerosis (414.02-414.06)*

996.73 Due to renal dialysis device, implant, and graft

996.74 Due to other vascular device, implant, and graft

Excludes: *occlusion of biological graft due to atherosclerosis (440.30-440.32)*

● Code new
to this edition
▲ Revision of
existing code
④ ⑤ Fourth or fifth
digit required

996.75 Due to nervous system device, implant, and graft

996.76 Due to genitourinary device, implant, and graft

Excludes: *complications of implanted vaginal mesh (629.31-629.32)*

996.77 Due to internal joint prosthesis
Use additional code to identify prosthetic joint (V43.60 - V43.69)

996.78 Due to other internal orthopedic device, implant, and graft

996.79 Due to other internal prosthetic device, implant, and graft

⑤ **996.8 Complications of transplanted organ**
Use additional code, if desired, to identify nature of complication, such as:
  cytomegalovirus (CMV) infection (078.5)
  graft-versus-host disease (279.50-279.53)
  malignancy associated with organ transplant (199.2)
  post-transplant lymphoproliferative disorder (PTLD) (238.77)
  transplant failure or rejection

ALERT! Codes under subcategory 996.8 are for use for both complications and rejection of transplanted organs. A transplant complication code is only assigned if the complication affects the function of the transplanted organ. Two codes are required to fully describe a transplant complication, the appropriate code from subcategory 996.8 and a secondary code that identifies the complication.

996.80 Transplanted organ, unspecified

996.81 Kidney
ALERT! Code 996.81 should be assigned for documented complications of a kidney transplant, such as transplant failure or rejection or other transplant complication
ALERT! Code 996.81 should not be assigned for post kidney transplant patients who have chronic kidney (CKD) unless a transplant complication such as transplant failure or rejection is documented. If the documentation is unclear as to whether the patient has a complication of the transplant, query the provider

996.82 Liver

996.83 Heart

996.84 Lung

996.85 Bone Marrow

996.86 Pancreas

996.87 Intestine

● **996.88 Stem cell**
  Complications from stem cells from:
    peripheral blood
    umbilical cord

996.89 Other specified transplanted organ

⑤ **996.9 Complications of reattached extremity or body part**

996.90 Unspecified extremity

996.91 Forearm

996.92 Hand

996.93 Finger(s)

996.94 Upper extremity, other and unspecified

996.95 Foot and toe(s)

996.96 Lower extremity, other and unspecified

996.99 Other specified body part

| Add 4th or 5th digit | Nonspecific code | Unspecified code | Medicare secondary payer (MSP) alert |

997 **Complications affecting specified body systems, not elsewhere classified**
Use additional code to identify complication
Excludes: *the listed conditions when specified as:*
causing shock (998.00-998.09)
complications of:
anesthesia:
adverse effect (001.0-799.9, 995.0-995.8)
in labor or delivery (668.0-668.9)
poisoning (968.0-969.9)
implanted device or graft (996.0-996.9)
obstetrical procedures (669.0-669.4)
reattached extremity (996.90-996.96)
transplanted organ (996.80-996.89)
ALERT! For coding late effect of complications of surgical and medical care see 909.3

⑤ **997.0** **Nervous system complications**

997.00 **Nervous system complication, unspecified**

997.01 **Central nervous system complication**
Anoxic brain damage
Cerebral hypoxia

Excludes: *cerebrovascular hemorrhage or infarction (997.02)*

997.02 **Iatrogenic cerebrovascular infarction or hemorrhage**
Postoperative stroke

997.09 **Other nervous system complications**

997.1 **Cardiac complications**
Cardiac arrest during or resulting from a procedure
Cardiac insufficiency during or resulting from a procedure
Cardiorespiratory failure during or resulting from a procedure
Heart failure during or resulting from a procedure

Excludes: *the listed conditions as long-term effects of cardiac surgery or due to the presence of cardiac prosthetic device (429.4)*

997.2 **Peripheral vascular complications**
Phlebitis or thrombophlebitis during or resulting from a procedure

Excludes: *the listed conditions due to:*
implant or catheter device (996.62)
infusion, perfusion, or transfusion (999.2)
complications affecting blood vessels (997.71-997.79)

⑤ **997.3** **Respiratory complications**

Excludes: *iatrogenic [postoperative] pneumothorax (512.1)*
iatrogenic pulmonary embolism (415.11)
specified complications classified elsewhere, such as:
adult respiratory distress syndrome (518.52)
pulmonary edema, postoperative (518.4)
respiratory insufficiency, acute, postoperative (518.52)
shock lung related to trauma and surgery (518.52)
tracheostomy complications (519.00-519.09)
transfusion related acute lung injury (TRALI) (518.7)

997.31 **Ventilator associated pneumonia**
Ventilator associated pneumonitis
Use additional code to identify organism
ALERT! Code 997.31 should be assigned only when the provider has documented ventilator associated pneumonia (VAP). An additional code to identify the organism (e.g., Pseudomonas aeruginosa, code 041.7) should also be assigned.
ALERT! Code 997.31 should not be assigned for cases where the patient has pneumonia and is on a mechanical ventilator but the provider has not specifically stated that the pneumonia is ventilator-associated pneumonia

● **997.32** **Postprocedural aspiration pneumonia**
Chemical pneumonitis resulting from a procedure
Mendelson's syndrome resulting from a procedure

Excludes: *aspiration pneumonia during labor and delivery (668.0)*

997.39 **Other respiratory complications**

● Code new
to this edition
▲ Revision of
existing code
④ ⑤ Fourth or fifth
digit required

⑤ **997.4 Digestive system complications**
Complications of intestinal (internal) anastomosis and bypass, not elsewhere classified, except that involving urinary tract
Hepatic failure specified as due to a procedure
Hepatorenal syndrome specified as due to a procedure
Intestinal obstruction NOS specified as due to a procedure

Excludes: *complications of gastric band procedure (539.01-539.09)*
complications of other bariatric procedure (539.81-539.89)
specified gastrointestinal complications classified elsewhere, such as:
blind loop syndrome (579.2)
colostomy or enterostomy complications (569.60-569.69)
complications of intestinal pouch (569.71-569.79)
gastrostomy complications (536.40-536.49)
gastrojejunal ulcer (534.0-534.9)
infection of esophagostomy (530.86)
infection of external stoma (569.61)
mechanical complication of esophagostomy (530.87)
pelvic peritoneal adhesions, female (614.6)
peritoneal adhesions (568.0)
peritoneal adhesions with obstruction (560.81)
postcholecystectomy syndrome (576.0)
postgastric surgery syndromes (564.2)
pouchitis (569.71)
vomiting following gastrointestinal surgery (564.3)

● **997.41 Retained cholelithiasis following cholecystectomy**
● **997.49 Other digestive system complications**

997.5 Urinary complications
Complications of:
internal anastomosis and bypass of urinary tract, including that involving intestinal tract
Oliguria or anuria specified as due to procedure
Renal (kidney):
failure (acute) specified as due to procedure
insufficiency (acute) specified as due to procedure
Tubular necrosis (acute) specified as due to procedure

Excludes: *complications of cystostomy (596.81-596.83)*
complications of external stoma of urinary tract (596.81-596.83)
specified complications classified elsewhere, such as:
postoperative stricture of:
ureter (593.3)
urethra (598.2)

⑤ **997.6 Amputation stump complication**

Excludes: *admission for treatment for a current traumatic amputation; code to complicated traumatic amputation*
phantom limb (syndrome) (353.6)

997.60 Unspecified complication
997.61 Neuroma of amputation stump
997.62 Infection (chronic)
Use additional code to identify the organism
997.69 Other

⑤ **997.7 Vascular complications of other vessels**

Excludes: *peripheral vascular complications (997.2)*

997.71 Vascular complications of mesenteric artery
997.72 Vascular complications of renal artery
997.79 Vascular complications of other vessels

⑤ **997.9 Complications affecting other specified body systems, not elsewhere classified**

Excludes: *specified complications classified elsewhere, such as:*
broad ligament laceration syndrome (620.6)
postartificial menopause syndrome (627.4)
postoperative stricture of vagina (623.2)

997.91 Hypertension
Excludes: *essential hypertension (401.0-401.9)*

Add 4th or 5th digit | Nonspecific code | Unspecified code | Medicare secondary payer (MSP) alert

997.99 **Other**
Vitreous touch syndrome

998 **Other complications of procedures, not elsewhere classified**

Excludes: *fluid overload due to transfusion (blood) (276.61)*
TACO (276.61)
transfusion associated circulatory overload (276.61)

ALERT! For coding late effect of complications of surgical and medical care see 909.3

⑤ **998.0 Postoperative shock**
Shock during or resulting from a surgical procedure

Excludes: *shock:*
anaphylactic due to serum (999.41-999.49)
anesthetic (995.4)
electric (994.8)
following abortion (639.5)
obstetric (669.1)
traumatic (958.4)

● **998.00 Postoperative shock, unspecified**
Collapse, not otherwise specified, during or resulting from a surgical procedure
Failure of peripheral circulation, postoperative

● **998.01 Postoperative shock, cardiogenic**

● **998.02 Postoperative shock, septic**
Postoperative endotoxic shock
Postoperative gram-negative shock

Code first underlying infection

Use additional code, to identify severe sepsis (995.92) and any associated acute organ dysfunction, if applicable

● **998.09 Postoperative shock, other**
Postoperative hypovolemic shock

⑤ **998.1 Hemorrhage or hematoma or seroma complicating a procedure**

Excludes: *hemorrhage due to implanted device or graft (996.70-996.79)*
hemorrhage, hematoma or seroma complicating cesarean section or puerperal perineal wound (674.3)

998.11 Hemorrhage complicating a procedure

998.12 Hematoma complicating a procedure

998.13 Seroma complicating a procedure

998.2 Accidental puncture or laceration during a procedure
Accidental perforation by catheter or other instrument during a procedure on:
blood vessel
nerve
organ

Excludes: *iatrogenic [postoperative] pneumothorax (512.1)*
puncture or laceration caused by implanted device intentionally left in operation wound (996.0-996.5)
specified complications classified elsewhere, such as:
broad ligament laceration syndrome (620.6)
dural tear (349.31)
incidental durotomy (349.31)
trauma from instruments during delivery (664.0-665.9)

⑤ **998.3 Disruption of wound**
Dehiscence of operation wound
Disruption of any suture materials or other closure method
Rupture of operation wound

Excludes: *disruption of:*
cesarean wound (674.1)
perineal wound, puerperal (674.2)

998.30 Disruption of wound, unspecified
Disruption of wound NOS

● Code new
to this edition
▲ Revision of
existing code
④ ⑤ Fourth or fifth
digit required

998.31 **Disruption of internal operation (surgical) wound**
Disruption or dehiscence of closure of:
fascia, superficial or muscular
internal organ
muscle or muscle flap
ribs or rib cage
skull or craniotomy
sternum or sternotomy
tendon or ligament
Deep disruption or dehiscence of operation wound NOS

Excludes: *complications of internal anastomosis of:*
gastrointestinal tract (997.49)
urinary tract (997.5)

998.32 **Disruption of external operation (surgical) wound**
Disruption or dehiscence of closure of:
cornea
mucosa
skin
subcutaneous tissue
Disruption of operation wound NOS
Full-thickness skin disruption or dehiscence
Superficial disruption or dehiscence of operation wound

998.33 **Disruption of traumatic injury wound repair**
Disruption or dehiscence of closure of traumatic laceration (external) (internal)

998.4 Foreign body accidentally left during a procedure
Adhesions due to foreign body accidentally left in operative wound or body cavity
during a procedure
Obstruction due to foreign body accidentally left in operative wound or body cavity
during a procedure
Perforation due to foreign body accidentally left in operative wound or body cavity
during a procedure

Excludes: *obstruction or perforation caused by implanted device intentionally left in body*
(996.0-996.5)

⑤ **998.5 Postoperative infection**

Excludes: *bleb associated endophthalmitis (379.63)*
infection due to:
implanted device (996.60-996.69)
infusion, perfusion, or transfusion (999.31-999.39)
postoperative obstetrical wound infection (674.3)

998.51 **Infected postoperative seroma**
Use additional code to identify organism

998.59 **Other postoperative infection**
Abscess: postoperative
intra-abdominal postoperative
stitch postoperative
subphrenic postoperative
wound postoperative
Septicemia postoperative
Use additional code to identify infection

998.6 Persistent postoperative fistula

998.7 Acute reaction to foreign substance accidentally left during a procedure
Peritonitis:
aseptic
chemical

⑤ **998.8 Other specified complications of procedures, not elsewhere classified**

998.81 **Emphysema (subcutaneous) (surgical) resulting from a procedure**

998.82 **Cataract fragments in eye following cataract surgery**

998.83 **Non-healing surgical wound**

998.89 **Other specified complications**

| | Add 4th or 5th digit | | Nonspecific code | | Unspecified code | | Medicare secondary payer (MSP) alert |

998.9 Unspecified complication of procedure, not elsewhere classified
Postoperative complication NOS

Excludes: *complication NOS of obstetrical surgery or procedure (669.4)*

999 Complications of medical care, not elsewhere classified
Use additional code, where applicable, to identify specific complication

Includes: complications, not elsewhere classified, of:
dialysis (hemodialysis) (peritoneal) (renal)
extracorporeal circulation
hyperalimentation therapy
immunization
infusion
inhalation therapy
injection
inoculation
perfusion
transfusion
vaccination
ventilation therapy

Excludes: *specified complications classified elsewhere such as:*
complications of implanted device (996.0-996.9)
contact dermatitis due to drugs (692.3)
dementia dialysis (294.8)
  transient (293.9)
dialysis disequilibrium syndrome (276.0-276.9)
poisoning and toxic effects of drugs and chemicals (960.0-989.9)
postvaccinal encephalitis (323.51)
water and electrolyte imbalance (276.0-276.9)

ALERT! For coding late effect of complications of surgical and medical care see 909.3

999.0 Generalized vaccinia

Excludes: *vaccinia not from vaccine (051.02)*

999.1 Air embolism
Air embolism to any site following infusion, perfusion, or transfusion

Excludes: *embolism specified as:*
complicating:
abortion (634-638 with .6, 639.6)
ectopic or molar pregnancy (639.6)
pregnancy, childbirth, or the puerperium (673.0)
due to implanted device (996.7)
traumatic (958.0)

999.2 Other vascular complications
Phlebitis following infusion, perfusion, or transfusion
Thromboembolism following infusion, perfusion, or transfusion
Thrombophlebitis following infusion, perfusion, or transfusion

Excludes: *extravasation of vesicant drugs (999.81, 999.82)*
the listed conditions when specified as:
due to implanted device (996.61-996.62, 996.72-996.74)
postoperative NOS (997.2, 997.71-997.79)

⑤ **999.3 Other infection**
Infection following infusion, injection, transfusion, or vaccination
Sepsis following infusion, injection, transfusion, or vaccination
Septicemia following infusion, injection, transfusion, or vaccination
Use additional code to identify the specified infection, such as:
septicemia (038.0-038.9)

Excludes: *the listed conditions when specified as:*
due to implanted device (996.60-996.69)
postoperative NOS (998.51-998.59)

● Code new
   to this edition
▲ Revision of
   existing code
④ ⑤ Fourth or fifth
   digit required

▲ **999.31 Other and unspecified infection due to central venous catheter**
Central line-associated infection
Infection due to:
  central venous catheter NOS
  Hickman catheter
  peripherally inserted central catheter (PICC)
  triple lumen catheter
  umbilical venous catheter

Excludes: *infection due to:*
  arterial catheter (996.62)
  catheter NOS (996.69)
  peripheral venous catheter (996.62)
  urinary catheter (996.64)

● **999.32 Bloodstream infection due to central venous catheter**
Bloodstream infection due to:
  Hickman catheter
  peripherally inserted central catheter (PICC)
  portacath (port-a-cath)
  triple lumen catheter
  umbilical venous catheter
Catheter-related bloodstream infection (CRBSI) NOS
Central line-associated bloodstream infection (CLABSI)

● **999.33 Local infection due to central venous catheter**
Exit or insertion site infection
Local infection due to:
  Hickman catheter
  peripherally inserted central catheter (PICC)
  portacath (port-a-cath)
  triple lumen catheter
  umbilical venous catheter
Port or reservoir infection
Tunnel infection

● **999.34 Acute infection following transfusion, infusion, or injection of blood and blood products**

999.39 Infection following other infusion, injection, transfusion, or vaccination

▲ **999.4 Anaphylactic reaction due to serum**
Allergic shock
Anaphylactic shock due to serum
Anaphylactoid reaction due to serum
Anaphylaxis

Excludes: *ABO incompatibility reaction due to transfusion of blood or blood products*
  (999.60-999.69)
  reaction:
  allergic NOS (995.0)
  anaphylactic:
  NOS (995.0)
  due to drugs and chemicals (995.0)
  other serum (999.51-999.59)
  shock:
  allergic NOS (995.0)
  anaphylactic:
  NOS (995.0)
  due to drugs and chemicals (995.0)

● **999.41 Anaphylactic reaction due to administration of blood and blood products**
● **999.42 Anaphylactic reaction due to vaccination**
● **999.49 Anaphylactic reaction due to other serum**

⑤ **999.5 Other serum reaction**
  Intoxication by serum   Serum sickness
  Protein sickness   Urticaria due to serum
  Serum rash

Excludes: *serum hepatitis (070.2-070.3)*

● **999.51 Other serum reaction due to administration of blood and blood products**
● **999.52 Other serum reaction due to vaccination**
● **999.59 Other serum reaction**

Add 4th or 5th digit | Nonspecific code | Unspecified code | Medicare secondary payer (MSP) alert

⑤ **999.6 ABO incompatibility reaction due to transfusion of blood or blood products**

> Excludes: *minor blood group antigens reactions (Duffy) (E) (K(ell)) (Kidd) (Lewis) (M) (N) (P) (S) (999.75-999.79)*

999.60 ABO incompatibility reaction, unspecified
ABO incompatible blood transfusion NOS
Reaction to ABO incompatibility from transfusion NOS

999.61 ABO incompatibility with hemolytic transfusion reaction not specified as acute or delayed
ABO incompatibility with hemolytic transfusion reaction at unspecified time after transfusion
Hemolytic transfusion reaction (HTR) due to ABO incompatibility

999.62 ABO incompatibility with acute hemolytic transfusion reaction
ABO incompatibility with hemolytic transfusion reaction less than 24 hours after transfusion
Acute hemolytic transfusion reaction (AHTR) due to ABO incompatibility

999.63 ABO incompatibility with delayed hemolytic transfusion reaction
ABO incompatibility with hemolytic transfusion reaction 24 hours or more after transfusion
Delayed hemolytic transfusion reaction (DHTR) due to ABO incompatibility

999.69 Other ABO incompatibility reaction
Delayed serologic transfusion reaction (DSTR) from ABO incompatibility
Other ABO incompatible blood transfusion
Other reaction to ABO incompatibility from transfusion

⑤ **999.7 Rh and other non-ABO incompatibility reaction due to transfusion of blood or blood products**

999.70 Rh incompatibility reaction, unspecified
Reaction due to Rh factor in transfusion NOS
Rh incompatible blood transfusion NOS
Unspecified reaction due to incompatibility related to Rh antigens (C) (c) (D) (E) (e)
Unspecified reaction to Rh incompatibility

999.71 Rh incompatibility with hemolytic transfusion reaction not specified as acute or delayed
Hemolytic transfusion reaction (HTR) due to Rh incompatibility
HTR due to incompatibility related to Rh antigens (C) (c) (D) (E) (e), not specified as acute or delayed
Rh incompatibility with hemolytic transfusion reaction at unspecified time after transfusion

999.72 Rh incompatibility with acute hemolytic transfusion reaction
Acute hemolytic transfusion reaction (AHTR) due to Rh incompatibility
AHTR due to incompatibility related to Rh antigens (C) (c) (D) (E) (e)
Rh incompatibility with hemolytic transfusion reaction less than 24 hours after transfusion

999.73 Rh incompatibility with delayed hemolytic transfusion reaction
Delayed hemolytic transfusion reaction (DHTR) due to Rh incompatibility
DHTR due to incompatibility related to Rh antigens (C) (c) (D) (E) (e)
Rh incompatibility with hemolytic transfusion reaction 24 hours or more after transfusion

999.74 Other Rh incompatibility reaction
Delayed serologic transfusion reaction (DSTR) from Rh incompatibility
Other reaction due to incompatibility related to Rh antigens (C) (c) (D) (E) (e)
Other reaction to Rh incompatible blood transfusion

999.75 Non-ABO incompatibility reaction, unspecified
Non-ABO incompatible blood transfusion NOS
Reaction to non-ABO antigen incompatibility from transfusion NOS
Unspecified reaction due to incompatibility related to minor antigens (Duffy) (Kell) (Kidd) (Lewis) (M) (N) (P) (S)

999.76 Non-ABO incompatibility with hemolytic transfusion reaction not specified as acute or delayed
Hemolytic transfusion reaction (HTR) due to non-ABO incompatibility
HTR from incompatibility related to minor antigens (Duffy) (Kell) (Kidd) (Lewis) (M) (N) (P) (S)
Non-ABO incompatibility with hemolytic transfusion reaction at unspecified time after transfusion

● Code new to this edition   ▲ Revision of existing code   ④ ⑤ Fourth or fifth digit required

999.77 **Non-ABO incompatibility with acute hemolytic transfusion reaction**
Acute hemolytic transfusion reaction (AHTR) due to non-ABO incompatibility
AHTR from incompatibility related to minor antigens (Duffy) (Kell) (Kidd) (Lewis) (M) (N) (P) (S)
Non-ABO incompatibility with hemolytic transfusion reaction less than 24 hours after transfusion

999.78 **Non-ABO incompatibility with delayed hemolytic transfusion reaction**
Delayed hemolytic transfusion reaction (DHTR) due to non-ABO incompatibility
DHTR from incompatibility related to minor antigens (Duffy) (Kell) (Kidd) (Lewis) (M) (N) (P) (S)
Non-ABO incompatibility with hemolytic transfusion reaction 24 hours or more after transfusion

999.79 **Other non-ABO incompatibility reaction**
Delayed serologic transfusion reaction (DSTR) from non-ABO incompatibility
Other non-ABO incompatible blood transfusion
Other reaction due to incompatibility related to minor antigens (Duffy) (Kell) (Kidd) (Lewis) (M) (N) (P) (S)
Other reaction to non-ABO incompatibility from transfusion

⑤ **999.8 Other and unspecified infusion and transfusion reaction**
Excludes: ABO incompatibility reactions (999.60-999.69)
febrile nonhemolytic transfusion reaction (FNHTR) (780.66)
hemochromatosis due to repeated red blood cell transfusions (275.02)
non-ABO incompatibility reactions (999.70-999.79)
postoperative shock (998.00-998.09)
posttransfusion purpura (287.41)
Rh incompatibility reactions (999.70-999.74)
transfusion associated circulatory overload (TACO) (276.61)
transfusion related acute lung injury (TRALI) (518.7)

999.80 **Transfusion reaction, unspecified**
Incompatible blood transfusion NOS
Reaction to blood group incompatibility in infusion or transfusion NOS

999.81 **Extravasation of vesicant chemotherapy**
Infiltration of vesicant chemotherapy

999.82 **Extravasation of other vesicant agent**
Infiltration of other vesicant agent

999.83 **Hemolytic transfusion reaction, incompatibility unspecified**
Hemolytic transfusion reaction (HTR) with antigen incompatibility unspecified, not specified as acute or delayed
HTR with incompatibility unspecified at unspecified time after transfusion

999.84 **Acute hemolytic transfusion reaction, incompatibility unspecified**
Acute hemolytic transfusion reaction (AHTR) with antigen incompatibility unspecified
AHTR, incompatibility unspecified

999.85 **Delayed hemolytic transfusion reaction, incompatibility unspecified**
Delayed hemolytic transfusion reaction (DHTR) with antigen incompatibility unspecified
DHTR, incompatibility unspecified

999.88 **Other infusion reaction**

999.89 **Other transfusion reaction**
Delayed serologic transfusion reaction (DSTR), incompatibility unspecified
Use additional code to identify graft-versus-host reaction (279.5)

999.9 Other and unspecified complications of medical care, not elsewhere classified
Complications, not elsewhere classified, of:
electroshock therapy
inhalation therapy
ultrasound therapy
ventilation therapy
Unspecified misadventure of medical care

Excludes: unspecified complication of:
phototherapy (990)
radiation therapy (990)
ventilator associated pneumonia (997.31)

| | Add 4th or 5th digit | | Nonspecific code | | Unspecified code | | Medicare secondary payer (MSP) alert |

This page intentionally left blank

● Code new
  to this edition

▲ Revision of
  existing code

④ ⑤ Fourth or fifth
  digit required

Chapter 18: Classification of Factors Influencing Health Status and Contact with Health Service (Supplemental V01-V91)

DEFINITIONS AND CODING ALERTS

This chapter includes definitions of selected key words, terms and phrases and coding alerts for adding points to the clinical domain, references to coding late effects where appropriate, and references to personal history V-codes in situations where the acute or chronic condition is no longer active. An example from this chapter is as follows:

V22.0 Supervision of normal first pregnancy
> **ALERT!** Codes V22.0 and V22.1 are always first listed and are not to be used with any other code from the OB chapter.

V23 Supervision of high-risk pregnancy
> **DEFINITION** A high risk pregnancy is one in which some condition puts the mother, the developing fetus, or both at higher-than-normal risk for complications during or after the pregnancy and birth.

MULTIPLE CODING FOR A SINGLE CONDITION

In addition to the etiology or manifestation convention that requires two codes to fully describe a single condition that affects multiple body systems, there are other single conditions that also require more than one code. "Use additional code" notes are found in the tabular at codes that are not part of an etiology or manifestation pair where a secondary code is useful to fully describe a condition. The sequencing rule is the same as the etiology or manifestation pair - , "use additional code" indicates that a secondary code should be added.

"Code first" notes are also under certain codes that are not specifically manifestation codes but may be due to an underlying cause. When a "code first" note is present and an underlying condition is present the underlying condition should be sequenced first.

"Code, if applicable, any causal condition first", notes indicate that this code may be assigned as a principal diagnosis when the causal condition is unknown or not applicable. If a causal condition is known, then the code for that condition should be sequenced as the principal or first-listed diagnosis. Multiple codes may be needed for late effects, complication codes and obstetric codes to more fully describe a condition. See the specific guidelines for these conditions for further instruction.

COMBINATION CODE

A combination code is a single code used to classify: two diagnoses, or a diagnosis with an associated secondary process (manifestation) A diagnosis with an associated complication Combination codes are identified by referring to subterm entries in the Alphabetic Index and by reading the inclusion and exclusion notes in the Tabular List.

Assign only the combination code when that code fully identifies the diagnostic conditions involved or when the Alphabetic Index so directs. Multiple coding should not be used when the classification provides a combination code that clearly identifies all of the elements documented in the diagnosis. When the combination code lacks necessary specificity in describing the manifestation or complication, an additional code should be used as a secondary code.

CODING LATE EFFECTS

A late effect is the residual effect (condition produced) after the acute phase of an illness or injury has terminated. There is no time limit on when a late effect code can be used. The residual may be apparent early, such as in cerebrovascular accident cases, or it may occur months or years later, such as that due to a previous injury. Coding of late effects generally requires two codes sequenced in the following order: The condition or nature of the late effect is sequenced first. The late effect code is sequenced second.

An exception to the above guidelines are those instances where the code for late effect is followed by a manifestation code identified in the Tabular List and title, or the late effect code has been expanded (at the fourth and fifth-digit levels) to include the manifestation(s). The code for the acute phase of an illness or injury that led to the late effect is never used with a code for the late effect.

▨	Add 4th or 5th digit	▨	Nonspecific code	▨	Unspecific code	▨	Secondary Dx Only	▨	Primary Dx Only

INTRODUCTION

ICD-9-CM provides codes to deal with encounters for circumstances other than a disease or injury. The Supplementary Classification of Factors Influencing Health Status and Contact with Health Services (V01.0 - V89.09) is provided to deal with occasions when circumstances other than a disease or injury (codes 001-999) are recorded as a diagnosis or problem.

There are four primary circumstances for the use of V codes:

1. A person who is not currently sick encounters the health services for some specific reason, such as to act as an organ donor, to receive prophylactic care, such as inoculations or health screenings, or to receive counseling on health related issues.

2. A person with a resolving disease or injury, or a chronic, long term condition requiring continuous care, encounters the health care system for specific aftercare of that disease or injury (e.g., dialysis for renal disease; chemotherapy for malignancy; cast change). A diagnosis or symptom code should be used whenever a current, acute, diagnosis is being treated or a sign or symptom is being studied.

3. Circumstances or problems influence a person's health status but are not in themselves a current illness or injury.

4. Newborns, to indicate birth status

V CODES USE IN ANY HEALTH CARE SETTING

V codes are for use in any health care setting. V codes may be used as either a first listed (principal diagnosis code in the inpatient setting) or secondary code, depending on the circumstances of the encounter. Certain V codes may only be used as first listed, others only as secondary codes.

V CODES INDICATE A REASON FOR AN ENCOUNTER

They are not procedure codes. A corresponding procedure code must accompany a V code to describe the procedure performed.

CATEGORIES OF V CODES

Contact or Exposure

Category V01 indicates contact with or exposure to communicable diseases. These codes are for patients who do not show any sign or symptom of a disease but have been exposed to it by close personal contact with an infected individual or are in an area where a disease is epidemic. These codes may be used as a first listed code to explain an encounter for testing, or, more commonly, as a secondary code to identify a potential risk.

Inoculations and vaccinations

Categories V03-V06 are for encounters for inoculations and vaccinations. They indicate that a patient is being seen to receive a prophylactic inoculation against a disease. The injection itself must be represented by the appropriate procedure code. A code from V03-V06 may be used as a secondary code if the inoculation is given as a routine part of preventive health care, such as a well-baby visit.

Status

Status codes indicate that a patient is either a carrier of a disease or has the sequelae or residual of a past disease or condition. This includes such things as the presence of prosthetic or mechanical devices resulting from past treatment. A status code is informative, because the status may affect the course of treatment and its outcome. A status code is distinct from a history code. The history code indicates that the patient no longer has the condition.

A status code should not be used with a diagnosis code from one of the body system chapters, if the diagnosis code includes the information provided by the status code. For example, code V42.1, Heart transplant status, should not be used with code 996.83, Complications of transplanted heart. The status code does not provide additional information. The complication code indicates that the patient is a heart transplant patient.

● Code new to this edition   ▲ Revision of existing code   ④ ⑤ Fourth or fifth digit required

History (of)

There are two types of history V codes, personal and family. Personal history codes explain a patient's past medical condition that no longer exists and is not receiving any treatment, but that has the potential for recurrence, and therefore may require continued monitoring. The exceptions to this general rule are category V14, Personal history of allergy to medicinal agents, and subcategory V15.0, Allergy, other than to medicinal agents. A person who has had an allergic episode to a substance or food in the past should always be considered allergic to the substance.

Family history codes are for use when a patient has a family member(s) who has had a particular disease that causes the patient to be at higher risk of also contracting the disease.

Personal history codes may be used in conjunction with followup codes and family history codes may be used in conjunction with screening codes to explain the need for a test or procedure. History codes are also acceptable on any medical record regardless of the reason for visit. A history of an illness, even if no longer present, is important information that may alter the type of treatment ordered.

Screening

Screening is the testing for disease or disease precursors in seemingly well individuals so that early detection and treatment can be provided for those who test positive for the disease. Screenings that are recommended for many subgroups in a population include: routine mammograms for women over 40, a fecal occult blood test for everyone over 50, an amniocentesis to rule out a fetal anomaly for pregnant women over 35, because the incidence of breast cancer and colon cancer in these subgroups is higher than in the general population, as is the incidence of Down's syndrome in older mothers.

The testing of a person to rule out or confirm a suspected diagnosis because the patient has some sign or symptom is a diagnostic examination, not a screening. In these cases, the sign or symptom is used to explain the reason for the test. A screening code may be a first listed code if the reason for the visit is specifically the screening exam. It may also be used as an additional code if the screening is done during an office visit for other health problems. A screening code is not necessary if the screening is inherent to a routine examination, such as a pap smear done during a routine pelvic examination.

Should a condition be discovered during the screening then the code for the condition may be assigned as an additional diagnosis.

The V code indicates that a screening exam is planned. A procedure code is required to confirm that the screening was performed.

Observation

There are three observation V code categories. They are for use in very limited circumstances when a person is being observed for a suspected condition that is ruled out. The observation codes are not for use if an injury or illness or any signs or symptoms related to the suspected condition are present. In such cases the diagnosis or symptom code is used with the corresponding E code to identify any external cause.

The observation codes are to be used as principal diagnosis only. The only exception to this is when the principal diagnosis is required to be a code from the V30, Live born infant, category. Then the V29 observation code is sequenced after the V30 code. Additional codes may be used in addition to the observation code but only if they are unrelated to the suspected condition being observed.

Codes from subcategory V89.0, Suspected maternal and fetal conditions not found, may either be used as a first listed or as an additional code assignment depending on the case. They are for use in very limited circumstances on a maternal record when an encounter is for a suspected maternal or fetal condition that is ruled out during that encounter (for example, a maternal or fetal condition may be suspected due to an abnormal test result). These codes should not be used when the condition is confirmed. In those cases, the confirmed condition should be coded. In addition, these codes are not for use if an illness or any signs or symptoms related to the suspected condition or problem are present. In such cases the diagnosis or symptom code is used.

Additional codes may be used in addition to the code from subcategory V89.0, but only if they are unrelated to the suspected condition being evaluated.

Codes from subcategory V89.0 may not be used for encounters for antenatal screening of mother. See Official Guidelines, Section I.C.18.d., Screening).

For encounters for suspected fetal condition that are inconclusive following testing and evaluation, assign the appropriate code from category 655, 656, 657 or 658.

Add 4th or 5th digit | Nonspecific code | Unspecific code | Secondary Dx Only | Primary Dx Only

Aftercare

Aftercare visit codes cover situations when the initial treatment of a disease or injury has been performed and the patient requires continued care during the healing or recovery phase, or for the long-term consequences of the disease. The aftercare V code should not be used if treatment is directed at a current, acute disease or injury. The diagnosis code is to be used in these cases. Exceptions to this rule are codes V58.0, Radiotherapy, and codes from subcategory V58.1, Encounter for chemotherapy and immunotherapy for neoplastic conditions. These codes are to be first listed, followed by the diagnosis code when a patient's encounter is solely to receive radiation therapy or chemotherapy for the treatment of a neoplasm. Should a patient receive both chemotherapy and radiation therapy during the same encounter code V58.0 and V58.1 may be used together on a record with either one being sequenced first.

The aftercare codes are generally first listed to explain the specific reason for the encounter. An aftercare code may be used as an additional code when some type of aftercare is provided in addition to the reason for admission and no diagnosis code is applicable. An example of this would be the closure of a colostomy during an encounter for treatment of another condition.

Aftercare codes should be used in conjunction with any other aftercare codes or other diagnosis codes to provide better detail on the specifics of an aftercare encounter visit, unless otherwise directed by the classification. The sequencing of multiple aftercare codes is discretionary.

Certain aftercare V code categories need a secondary diagnosis code to describe the resolving condition or sequelae, for others, the condition is inherent in the code title.

Additional V code aftercare category terms include, fitting and adjustment, and attention to artificial openings. Status V codes may be used with aftercare V codes to indicate the nature of the aftercare. For example code V45.81, Aortocoronary bypass status, may be used with code V58.73, Aftercare following surgery of the circulatory system, NEC, to indicate the surgery for which the aftercare is being performed. Also, a transplant status code may be used following code V58.44, Aftercare following organ transplant, to identify the organ transplanted. A status code should not be used when the aftercare code indicates the type of status, such as using V55.0, Attention to tracheostomy with V44.0, Tracheostomy status.

See Chapter 16 for admissions or encounter for rehabilitation.

Follow-up

The follow-up codes are used to explain continuing surveillance following completed treatment of a disease, condition, or injury. They imply that the condition has been fully treated and no longer exists. They should not be confused with aftercare codes that explain current treatment for a healing condition or its sequelae. Follow-up codes may be used in conjunction with history codes to provide the full picture of the healed condition and its treatment. The follow-up code is sequenced first, followed by the history code.

A follow-up code may be used to explain repeated visits.

Should a condition be found to have recurred on the follow-up visit, then the diagnosis code should be used in place of the follow-up code.

Donor

Category V59 is the donor codes. They are used for living individuals who are donating blood or other body tissue. These codes are only for individuals donating for others, not for self donations. They are not for use to identify cadaveric donations.

Counseling

Counseling V codes are used when a patient or family member receives assistance in the aftermath of an illness or injury, or when support is required in coping with family or social problems. They are not necessary for use in conjunction with a diagnosis code when the counseling component of care is considered integral to standard treatment.

Obstetrics and related conditions

See Chapter 11, obstetrics guidelines for further instruction on the use of these codes.

V codes for pregnancy are for use in those circumstances when none of the problems or complications included in the codes from the Obstetrics chapter exist (a routine prenatal visit or postpartum care). Codes V22.0, Supervision of normal first pregnancy, and V22.1, Supervision of other normal pregnancy, are always first listed and are not to be used with any other code from the OB chapter.

● Code new to this edition   ▲ Revision of existing code   ④ ⑤ Fourth or fifth digit required

The outcome of delivery, category V27, should be included on all maternal delivery records. It is always a secondary code.

V codes for family planning (contraceptive) or procreative management and counseling should be included on an obstetric record either during the pregnancy or the postpartum stage, if applicable.

Routine and administrative examinations

The V codes allow for the description of encounters for routine examinations, such as, a general check-up, or, examinations for administrative purposes, such as, a pre-employment physical. The codes are not to be used if the examination is for diagnosis of a suspected condition or for treatment purposes. In such cases the diagnosis code is used. During a routine exam, should a diagnosis or condition be discovered, it should be coded as an additional code. Pre-existing and chronic conditions and history codes may also be included as additional codes as long as the examination is for administrative purposes and not focused on any particular condition.

Pre-operative examination V codes are for use only in those situations when a patient is being cleared for surgery and no treatment is given.

Miscellaneous V codes

The miscellaneous V codes capture a number of other health care encounters that do not fall into one of the other categories. Certain of these codes identify the reason for the encounter, others are for use as additional codes that provide useful information on circumstances that may affect a patient's care and treatment.

PROPHYLACTIC ORGAN REMOVAL

For encounters specifically for prophylactic removal of breasts, ovaries, or another organ due to a genetic susceptibility to cancer or a family history of cancer, the principal or first listed code should be a code from subcategory V50.4, Prophylactic organ removal, followed by the appropriate genetic susceptibility code and the appropriate family history code.

If the patient has a malignancy of one site and is having prophylactic removal at another site to prevent either a new primary malignancy or metastatic disease, a code for the malignancy should also be assigned in addition to a code from subcategory V50.4. A V50.4 code should not be assigned if the patient is having organ removal for treatment of a malignancy, such as the removal of the testes for the treatment of prostate cancer.

Nonspecific V codes

Certain V codes are so non-specific, or potentially redundant with other codes in the classification, that there can be little justification for their use in the inpatient setting. Their use in the outpatient setting should be limited to those instances when there is no further documentation to permit more precise coding. Otherwise, any sign or symptom or any other reason for visit that is captured in another code should be used.

See Official Guidelines, Section IV, .K. and Official Guidelines, Section IV.L. of the Outpatient guidelines.

V CODE TABLE

The V code table in the Official Coding Guidelines contains columns for 1st listed, 1st or additional, additional only, and non-specific. Each code or category is listed on the left hand column and the allowable sequencing of the code or codes within the category is noted under the appropriate column.

The V codes designated as first-listed only are generally intended to be limited for use as a first-listed only diagnosis, but may be reported as an additional diagnosis in those situations when the patient has more than one encounter on a single day and the codes for the multiple encounters are combined, or when there is more than one V code that meets the definition of principal diagnosis (e.g., a patient is admitted to home healthcare for both aftercare and rehabilitation and they equally meet the definition of principal diagnosis). The V codes designated as first-listed only should not be reported if they do not meet the definition of principal or first-listed diagnosis.

See Official Guidelines, Section II and Official Guidelines, Section IV,.A for information on selection of principal and first-listed diagnosis.

See Official Guidelines, Section II.C for information on two or more diagnoses that equally meet the definition for principal diagnosis.

Add 4th or 5th digit | Nonspecific code | Unspecific code | Secondary Dx Only | Primary Dx Only

This page intentionally left blank.

● Code new
  to this edition

▲ Revision of
  existing code

④ ⑤ Fourth or fifth
     digit required

SUPPLEMENTARY CLASSIFICATION OF FACTORS INFLUENCING HEALTH STATUS AND CONTACT WITH HEALTH SERVICES (V01-V91)

This classification is provided to deal with occasions when circumstances other than a disease or injury classifiable to categories 001-999 (the main part of ICD) are recorded as "diagnoses" or "problems." This can arise mainly in three ways:

a) When a person who is not currently sick encounters the health services for some specific purpose, such as to act as a donor of an organ or tissue, to receive prophylactic vaccination, or to discuss a problem which is in itself not a disease or injury. This will be a fairly rare occurrence among hospital inpatients, but will be relatively more common among hospital outpatients and patients of family practitioners, health clinics, etc.

b) When a person with a known disease or injury, whether it is current or resolving, encounters the health care system for a specific treatment of that disease or injury (e.g., dialysis for renal disease; chemotherapy for malignancy; cast change).

c) When some circumstance or problem is present which influences the person's health status but is not in itself a current illness or injury. Such factors may be elicited during population surveys, when the person may or may not be currently sick, or be recorded as an additional factor to be borne in mind when the person is receiving care for some current illness or injury classifiable to categories 001-999.

In the latter circumstances the V code should be used only as a supplementary code and should not be the one selected for use in primary, single cause tabulations. Examples of these circumstances are a personal history of certain diseases, or a person with an artificial heart valve in situ.

PERSONS WITH POTENTIAL HEALTH HAZARDS RELATED TO COMMUNICABLE DISEASES (V01-V06)

> Excludes: family history of infectious and parasitic diseases (V18.8)
> personal history of infectious and parasitic diseases (V12.0)

V01 **Contact with or exposure to communicable diseases**

ALERT! Category V01 indicates contact with or exposure to communicable diseases. These codes are for patients who do not show any sign or symptom of a disease but have been exposed to it by close personal contact with an infected individual or are in an area where a disease is epidemic. These codes may be used as a first listed code to explain an encounter for testing, or, more commonly, as a secondary code to identify a potential risk

V01.0 Cholera
Conditions classifiable to 001

V01.1 Tuberculosis
Conditions classifiable to 010-018

V01.2 Poliomyelitis
Conditions classifiable to 045

V01.3 Smallpox
Conditions classifiable to 050

V01.4 Rubella
Conditions classifiable to 056

V01.5 Rabies
Conditions classifiable to 071

V01.6 Venereal diseases
Conditions classifiable to 090-099

⑤ **V01.7 Other viral diseases**
Conditions classifiable to 042-078 and V08, except as above

    V01.71 Varicella

    V01.79 Other viral diseases

⑤ **V01.8 Other communicable diseases**
Conditions classifiable to 001-136, except as above

    V01.81 Anthrax

    V01.82 Exposure to SARS-associated coronavirus

    V01.83 Escherichia coli (E. coli)

    V01.84 Meningococcus

    V01.89 Other communicable diseases

  V01.9 Unspecified communicable disease

V02 **Carrier or suspected carrier of infectious diseases**
Includes: Colonization status

  V02.0 Cholera

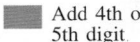

| | Add 4th or 5th digit | | Nonspecific code | | Unspecific code | | Secondary Dx Only | | Primary Dx Only |

V02.1 Typhoid

V02.2 Amebiasis

V02.3 Other gastrointestinal pathogens

V02.4 Diphtheria

⑤ **V02.5 Other specified bacterial diseases**

    V02.51 Group B streptococcus

    V02.52 Other streptococcus

    V02.53 Methicillin susceptible Staphylococcus aureus
        MSSA colonization

   ALERT! Assign this code for patients documented as having MSRA colonization

    V02.54 Methicillin resistant Staphylococcus aureus
        MRSA colonization

   ALERT! Assign this code for patients documented as having MSRA colonization

    V02.59 Other specified bacterial diseases
        Meningococcal
        Staphylococcal

⑤ **V02.6 Viral hepatitis**
    Hepatitis Australian-antigen [HAA] [SH] carrier
    Serum hepatitis carrier

    V02.60 Viral hepatitis carrier, unspecified

    V02.61 Hepatitis B carrier

    V02.62 Hepatitis C carrier

    V02.69 Other viral hepatitis carrier

V02.7 Gonorrhea

V02.8 Other venereal diseases

V02.9 Other specified infectious organism

V03 Need for prophylactic vaccination and inoculation against bacterial diseases

    Excludes: *vaccination not carried out (V64.00-V64.09)*
          vaccines against combinations of diseases (V06.0-V06.9)

    DEFINITION Prophylactic vaccination performed to prevent infectious diseases. Suspension of attenuated or killed viruses or bacteria or parts thereof that is capable of producing a protective immune response to such infectious agents.

V03.0 Cholera alone

V03.1 Typhoid-paratyphoid alone [TAB]

V03.2 Tuberculosis [BCG]

V03.3 Plague

V03.4 Tularemia

V03.5 Diphtheria alone

V03.6 Pertussis alone

V03.7 Tetanus toxoid alone

⑤ **V03.8 Other specified vaccinations against single bacterial diseases**

    V03.81 Hemophilus influenza, type B [Hib]

    V03.82 Streptococcus pneumoniae [pneumococcus]

    V03.89 Other specified vaccination

V03.9 Unspecified single bacterial disease

V04 Need for prophylactic vaccination and inoculation against certain viral diseases

    Excludes: *vaccines against combinations of diseases (V06.0-V06.9)*

V04.0 Poliomyelitis

V04.1 Smallpox

V04.2 Measles alone

V04.3 Rubella alone

V04.4 Yellow fever

V04.5 Rabies

V04.6 Mumps alone

V04.7 Common cold

● Code new
   to this edition

▲ Revision of
   existing code

④ ⑤ Fourth or fifth
     digit required

⑤ **V04.8 Other viral diseases**

    V04.81 Influenza

    V04.82 Respiratory syncytial virus (RSV)

    V04.89 Other viral diseases

V05 Need for other prophylactic vaccination and inoculation against single diseases

    Excludes: vaccines against combinations of diseases (V06.0-V06.9)

    V05.0 Arthropod-borne viral encephalitis

    V05.1 Other arthropod-borne viral diseases

    V05.2 Leishmaniasis

    V05.3 Viral hepatitis

    V05.4 Varicella
        Chickenpox

    V05.8 Other specified disease

    V05.9 Unspecified single disease

V06 Need for prophylactic vaccination and inoculation against combinations of diseases

    Note: Use additional single vaccination codes from categories V03-V05 to identify any vaccinations not included in a combination code.

    V06.0 Cholera with typhoid-paratyphoid [cholera + TAB]

    V06.1 Diphtheria-tetanus-pertussis, combined [DTP] [DTaP]

    V06.2 Diphtheria-tetanus-pertussis with typhoid-paratyphoid [DTP + TAB]

    V06.3 Diphtheria-tetanus-pertussis with poliomyelitis [DTP + polio]

    V06.4 Measles-mumps-rubella [MMR]

    V06.5 Tetanus-diphtheria [Td] [DT]

    V06.6 Streptococcus pneumoniae [pneumococcus] and influenza

    V06.8 Other combinations

    Excludes: multiple single vaccination codes (V03.0-V05.9)

    V06.9 Unspecified combined vaccine

PERSONS WITH NEED FOR ISOLATION, OTHER POTENTIAL HEALTH HAZARDS AND PROPHYLACTIC MEASURES (V07-V09)

V07 Need for isolation and other prophylactic or treatment measures

    Excludes: long-term (current) (prophylactic) use of certain specific drugs (V58.61-V58.69)
               prophylactic organ removal (V50.41-V50.49)

    V07.0 Isolation
        Admission to protect the individual from his surroundings or for isolation of individual after contact with infectious diseases

    V07.1 Desensitization to allergens

    V07.2 Prophylactic immunotherapy
        Administration of:
           antivenin
           immune sera [gamma globulin]
           RhoGAM
           tetanus antitoxin

⑤ **V07.3 Other prophylactic chemotherapy**

    V07.31 Prophylactic fluoride administration

    V07.39 Other prophylactic chemotherapy

    Excludes: maintenance chemotherapy following disease (V58.11)

    V07.4 Hormone replacement therapy (postmenopausal)

 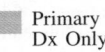

Add 4th or 5th digit   Nonspecific code   Unspecific code   Secondary Dx Only   Primary Dx Only

⑤ **V07.5 Use of agents affecting estrogen receptors and estrogen levels**

Code first, if applicable:
    malignant neoplasm of breast (174.0-174.9, 175.0-175.9)
    malignant neoplasm of prostate (185)

Use additional code, if applicable, to identify:
    estrogen receptor positive status (V86.0)
    family history of breast cancer (V16.3)
    genetic susceptibility to cancer (V84.01-V84.09)
    personal history of breast cancer (V10.3)
    personal history of prostate cancer (V10.46)
    postmenopausal status (V49.81)

Excludes: *hormone replacement therapy (postmenopausal) (V07.4)*

  V07.51 Use of selective estrogen receptor modulators (SERMs)
      Use of:
        raloxifene (Evista)
        tamoxifen (Nolvadex)
        toremifene (Fareston)

  V07.52 Use of aromatase inhibitors
      Use of:
        anastrozole (Arimidex)
        exemestane (Aromasin)
        letrozole (Femara)

  V07.59 Use of other agents affecting estrogen receptors and estrogen levels
      Use of:
        estrogen receptor downregulators
        fulvestrant (Faslodex)
        gonadotropin-releasing hormone (GnRH) agonist
        goserelin acetate (Zoladex)
        leuprolide acetate (leuprorelin) (Lupron)
        megestrol acetate (Megace)

V07.8 Other specified prophylactic or treatment measure

V07.9 Unspecified prophylactic or treatment measure

V08 Asymptomatic human immunodeficiency virus [HIV] infection status
  HIV positive NOS

Note: This code is ONLY to be used when NO HIV infection symptoms or conditions are present. If any HIV infection symptoms or conditions are present, see code 042.

Excludes: *AIDS (042)*
    human immunodeficiency virus [HIV] disease (042)
    exposure to HIV (V01.79)
    nonspecific serologic evidence of HIV (795.71)
    symptomatic human immunodeficiency virus [HIV] infection (042)

V09 Infection with drug-resistant microorganisms

Note: This category is intended for use as an additional code for infectious conditions classified elsewhere to indicate the presence of drug-resistance of the infectious organism.

V09.0 Infection with microorganisms resistant to penicillins

V09.1 Infection with microorganisms resistant to cephalosporins and other B-lactam antibiotics

V09.2 Infection with microorganisms resistant to macrolides

V09.3 Infection with microorganisms resistant to tetracyclines

V09.4 Infection with microorganisms resistant to aminoglycosides

⑤ **V09.5 Infection with microorganisms resistant to quinolones and fluoroquinolones**

  V09.50 Without mention of resistance to multiple quinolones and fluoroquinolones

  V09.51 With resistance to multiple quinolones and fluoroquinolones

V09.6 Infection with microorganisms resistant to sulfonamides

⑤ **V09.7 Infection with microorganisms resistant to other specified antimycobacterial agents**

Excludes: *Amikacin (V09.4)*
    Kanamycin (V09.4)
    Streptomycin [SM] (V09.4)

  V09.70 Without mention of resistance to multiple antimycobacterial agents

  V09.71 With resistance to multiple antimycobacterial agents

● Code new to this edition   ▲ Revision of existing code   ④ ⑤ Fourth or fifth digit required

⑤ **V09.8 Infection with microorganisms resistant to other specified drugs**
Vancomycin (glycopeptide) intermediate staphylococcus aureus (VISA/GISA)
Vancomycin (glycopeptide) resistant enterococcus (VRE)
Vancomycin (glycopeptide) resistant staphylococcus aureus (VRSA/GRSA)

V09.80 Without mention of resistance to multiple drugs

V09.81 With resistance to multiple drugs

⑤ **V09.9 Infection with drug-resistant microorganisms, unspecified**
Drug resistance NOS

V09.90 Without mention of multiple drug resistance

V09.91 With multiple drug resistance
Multiple drug resistance NOS

PERSONS WITH POTENTIAL HEALTH HAZARDS RELATED TO PERSONAL AND FAMILY HISTORY (V10-V19)

Excludes: *obstetric patients where the possibility that the fetus might be affected is the reason for observation or management during pregnancy (655.0-655.9)*

V10 **Personal history of malignant neoplasm**

⑤ **V10.0 Gastrointestinal tract**
History of conditions classifiable to 140-159

Excludes: *personal history of malignant carcinoid tumor (V10.91)*
personal history of malignant neuroendocrine tumor (V10.91)

V10.00 Gastrointestinal tract, unspecified

V10.01 Tongue

V10.02 Other and unspecified oral cavity and pharynx

V10.03 Esophagus

V10.04 Stomach

V10.05 Large intestine

V10.06 Rectum, rectosigmoid junction, and anus

V10.07 Liver

V10.09 Other

⑤ **V10.1 Trachea, bronchus, and lung**
History of conditions classifiable to 162

Excludes: *personal history of malignant carcinoid tumor (V10.91)*
personal history of malignant neuroendocrine tumor (V10.91)

V10.11 Bronchus and lung

V10.12 Trachea

⑤ **V10.2 Other respiratory and intrathoracic organs**
History of conditions classifiable to 160, 161, 163-165

V10.20 Respiratory organ, unspecified

V10.21 Larynx

V10.22 Nasal cavities, middle ear, and accessory sinuses

V10.29 Other

V10.3 Breast
History of conditions classifiable to 174 and 175

⑤ **V10.4 Genital organs**
History of conditions classifiable to 179-187

V10.40 Female genital organ, unspecified

V10.41 Cervix uteri

V10.42 Other parts of uterus

V10.43 Ovary

V10.44 Other female genital organs

V10.45 Male genital organ, unspecified

V10.46 Prostate

V10.47 Testis

V10.48 Epididymis

V10.49 Other male genital organs

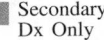 Add 4th or 5th digit   Nonspecific code   Unspecific code   Secondary Dx Only   Primary Dx Only

⑤ **V10.5 Urinary organs**
History of conditions classifiable to 188 and 189

Excludes: *personal history of malignant carcinoid tumor (V10.91)*
personal history of malignant neuroendocrine tumor (V10.91)

V10.50 Urinary organ, unspecified

V10.51 Bladder

V10.52 Kidney

Excludes: *renal pelvis (V10.53)*

V10.53 Renal pelvis

V10.59 Other

⑤ **V10.6 Leukemia**
Conditions classifiable to 204-208

Excludes: *leukemia in remission (204-208)*

V10.60 Leukemia, unspecified

V10.61 Lymphoid leukemia

V10.62 Myeloid leukemia

V10.63 Monocytic leukemia

V10.69 Other

⑤ **V10.7 Other lymphatic and hematopoietic neoplasms**
Conditions classifiable to 200-203

Excludes: *listed conditions in 200-203 in remission*

V10.71 Lymphosarcoma and reticulosarcoma

V10.72 Hodgkin's disease

V10.79 Other

⑤ **V10.8 Personal history of malignant neoplasm of other sites**
History of conditions classifiable to 170-173, 190-195

Excludes: *personal history of malignant carcinoid tumor (V10.91)*
personal history of malignant neuroendocrine tumor (V10.91)

V10.81 Bone

V10.82 Malignant melanoma of skin

V10.83 Other malignant neoplasm of skin

V10.84 Eye

V10.85 Brain

V10.86 Other parts of nervous system

Excludes: *peripheral, sympathetic, and parasympathetic nerves (V10.89)*

V10.87 Thyroid

V10.88 Other endocrine glands and related structures

V10.89 Other

⑤ **V10.9 Other and unspecified personal history of malignant neoplasm**

V10.90 Personal history of unspecified malignant neoplasm
Personal history of malignant neoplasm NOS

Excludes: *personal history of malignant carcinoid tumor (V10.91)*
personal history of malignant neuroendocrine tumor (V10.91)
personal history of Merkel cell carcinoma (V10.91)

V10.91 Personal history of malignant neuroendocrine tumor
Personal history of malignant carcinoid tumor NOS
Personal history of malignant neuroendocrine tumor NOS
Personal history of Merkel cell carcinoma NOS

Code first any continuing functional activity, such as: carcinoid syndrome (259.2)

V11 Personal history of mental disorder

V11.0 Schizophrenia

Excludes: *that in remission (295.0-295.9 with fifth-digit 5)*

● Code new
to this edition

▲ Revision of
existing code

④ ⑤ Fourth or fifth
digit required

V11.1 Affective disorders
Personal history of manic-depressive psychosis
Excludes: that in remission (296.0-296.6 with fifth-digit 5, 6)

V11.2 Neurosis

V11.3 Alcoholism

V11.4 Combat and operational stress reaction

V11.8 Other mental disorders

V11.9 Unspecified mental disorder

V12 Personal history of certain other diseases

⑤ **V12.0 Infectious and parasitic diseases**
Excludes: personal history of infectious diseases specific to a body system

   V12.00 Unspecified infectious and parasitic disease

   V12.01 Tuberculosis

   V12.02 Poliomyelitis

   V12.03 Malaria

   V12.04 Methicillin resistant Staphylococcus aureus
    MRSA

   V12.09 Other

V12.1 Nutritional deficiency

⑤ **V12.2 Endocrine, metabolic, and immunity disorders**
Excludes: history of allergy (V14.0-V14.9, V15.01-V15.09)

   ● **V12.21 Gestational diabetes**

   ● **V12.29 Other endocrine, metabolic, and immunity disorders**

V12.3 Diseases of blood and blood-forming organs

⑤ **V12.4 Disorders of nervous system and sense organs**

   V12.40 Unspecified disorder of nervous system and sense organs

   V12.41 Benign neoplasm of the brain

   V12.42 Infections of the central nervous system
    Encephalitis
    Meningitis

   V12.49 Other disorders of nervous system and sense organs

⑤ **V12.5 Diseases of circulatory system**
Excludes: history of anaphylactic shcok (V13.81)
    old myocardial infarction (412)
    postmyocardial infarction syndrome (411.0)

   V12.50 Unspecified circulatory disease

   V12.51 Venous thrombosis and embolism
Excludes: pulmonary embolism V12.55

   V12.52 Thrombophlebitis

   V12.53 Sudden cardiac arrest
    Sudden cardiac death successfully resuscitated

   V12.54 Transient ischemic attack (TIA), and cerebral infarction without residual deficits
    Prolonged reversible ischemic neurological deficit (PRIND)
    Reversible ischemic neurologic deficit (RIND)
    Stroke NOS without residual deficits
Excludes: history of traumatic brain injury (V15.52)
    late effects of cerebrovascular disease (438.0-438.9)

ALERT! Assign code V12.54, not a code from category 438 as an additional code for history of cerebrovascular disease when no neurologic deficits are present

   ● **V12.55 Pulmonary embolism**

   V12.59 Other
Note: Assign code V12.59 (and not a code from category 438) as an additional code for history of cerebrovascular disease when no neurologic deficits are present.

Add 4th or 5th digit | Nonspecific code | Unspecific code | Secondary Dx Only | Primary Dx Only

⑤ **V12.6 Diseases of respiratory system**
> *Excludes:* tuberculosis (V12.01)

    V12.60   Unspecified disease of respiratory system
    V12.61   Pneumonia (recurrent)
    V12.69   Other diseases of respiratory system

⑤ **V12.7 Diseases of digestive system**

    V12.70   Unspecified digestive disease
    V12.71   Peptic ulcer disease
    V12.72   Colonic polyps
    V12.79   Other

V13 **Personal history of other diseases**

⑤ **V13.0 Disorders of urinary system**

    V13.00   Unspecified urinary disorder
    V13.01   Urinary calculi
    V13.02   Urinary (tract) infection
    V13.03   Nephrotic syndrome
    V13.09   Other

V13.1 Trophoblastic disease
> *Excludes:* supervision during a current pregnancy (V23.1)

⑤ **V13.2 Other genital system and obstetric disorders**
> *Excludes:* supervision during a current pregnancy of a woman with poor obstetric history (V23.0-V23.9)
> recurrent pregnancy loss (646.3)
> without current pregnancy (629.81)

    V13.21   Personal history of pre-term labor
> *Excludes:* current pregnancy with history of pre-term labor (V23.41)

    V13.22   Personal history of cervical dysplasia
        Personal history of conditions classifiable to 622.10-622.12
> *Excludes:* personal history of malignant neoplasm of cervix uteri (V10.41)

    V13.23   Personal history of vaginal dysplasia
        Personal history of conditions classifiable to 623.0
> *Excludes:* personal history of malignant neoplasm of vagina (V10.44)

    V13.24   Personal history of vulvar dysplasia
        Personal history of conditions classifiable to 624.01-624.02
> *Excludes:* personal history of malignant neoplasm of vulva (V10.44)

    V13.29   Other genital system and obstetric disorders

V13.3 Diseases of skin and subcutaneous tissue

V13.4 Arthritis

⑤ **V13.5 Other musculoskeletal disorders**

    V13.51   Pathologic fracture
        Healed pathologic fracture
> *Excludes:* personal history of traumatic fracture (V15.51)

    V13.52   Stress fracture
        Healed stress fracture
> *Excludes:* personal history of traumatic fracture (V15.51)

    V13.59   Other musculoskeletal disorders

⑤ **V13.6 Congenital (corrected) malformations**

    V13.61   Personal history of (corrected) hypospadias
    V13.62   Personal history of other (corrected) congenital malformations of genitourinary system
    V13.63   Personal history of (corrected) congenital malformations of nervous system
    V13.64   Personal history of (corrected) congenital malformations of eye, ear, face and neck
        Corrected cleft lip and palate

● Code new to this edition   ▲ Revision of existing code   ④ ⑤ Fourth or fifth digit required

V13.65 **Personal history of (corrected) congenital malformations of heart and circulatory system**

V13.66 **Personal history of (corrected) congenital malformations of respiratory system**

V13.67 **Personal history of (corrected) congenital malformations of digestive system**

V13.68 **Personal history of (corrected) congenital malformations of integument, limbs, and musculoskeletal systems**

V13.69 **Personal history of other (corrected) congenital malformations**

V13.7 **Perinatal problems**

Excludes: *low birth weight status (V21.30-V21.35)*

⑤ V13.8 **Other specified diseases**

● V13.81 **Anaphylaxis**

● V13.89 **Other specified diseases**

V13.9 **Unspecified disease**

V14 **Personal history of allergy to medicinal agents**

V14.0 **Penicillin**

V14.1 **Other antibiotic agent**

V14.2 **Sulfonamides**

V14.3 **Other anti-infective agent**

V14.4 **Anesthetic agent**

V14.5 **Narcotic agent**

V14.6 **Analgesic agent**

V14.7 **Serum or vaccine**

V14.8 **Other specified medicinal agents**

V14.9 **Unspecified medicinal agent**

V15 **Other personal history presenting hazards to health**

Excludes: *personal history of drug therapy (V87.41-V87.49)*

⑤ V15.0 **Allergy, other than to medicinal agents**

Excludes: *allergy to food substance used as base for medicinal agent (V14.0-V14.9)*

V15.01 **Allergy to peanuts**

V15.02 **Allergy to milk products**

Excludes: *lactose intolerance (271.3)*

V15.03 **Allergy to eggs**

V15.04 **Allergy to seafood**
Seafood (octopus) (squid) ink
Shellfish

V15.05 **Allergy to other foods**
Food additives
Nuts other than peanuts

V15.06 **Allergy to insects and arachnids**
Bugs
Insect bites and stings
Spiders

V15.07 **Allergy to latex**
Latex sensitivity

V15.08 **Allergy to radiographic dye**
Contrast media used for diagnostic x-ray procedures

V15.09 **Other allergy, other than to medicinal agents**

V15.1 **Surgery to heart and great vessels**

Excludes: *replacement by transplant or other means (V42.1-V42.2, V43.2-V43.4)*

⑤ V15.2 **Surgery to other organs**

Excludes: *replacement by transplant or other means (V42.0-V43.8)*

V15.21 **Personal history of undergoing in utero procedure during pregnancy**

V15.22 **Personal history of undergoing in utero procedure while a fetus**

V15.29 **Surgery to other organs**

765

Add 4th or 5th digit   Nonspecific code   Unspecific code   Secondary Dx Only   Primary Dx Only

V15.3 Irradiation
Previous exposure to therapeutic or other ionizing radiation

⑤ **V15.4 Psychological trauma**
Excludes: history of condition classifiable to 290-316 (V11.0-V11.9)

V15.41 History of physical abuse
Rape

V15.42 History of emotional abuse
Neglect

V15.49 Other

⑤ **V15.5 Injury**

V15.51 Traumatic fracture
Healed traumatic fracture
Excludes: personal history of pathologic and stress fracture (V13.51, V13.52)

V15.52 History of traumatic brain injury
Excludes: personal history of cerebrovascular accident (cerebral infarction) without residual deficits (V12.54)

V15.53 Personal history of retained foreign body fully removed
V15.59 Other injury

V15.6 Poisoning
V15.7 Contraception
Excludes: current contraceptive management (V25.0-V25.4)
presence of intrauterine contraceptive device as incidental finding (V45.5)

⑤ **V15.8 Other specified personal history presenting hazards to health**
Excludes: contact with and (suspected) exposure to:
aromatic compounds and dyes (V87.11-V87.19)
arsenic and other metals (V87.01-V87.09)
molds (V87.31)

V15.80 History of failed moderate sedation
History of failed conscious sedation

V15.81 Noncompliance with medical treatment
Excludes: noncompliance with renal dialysis (V45.12)

V15.82 History of tobacco use
Excludes: tobacco dependence (305.1)

V15.83 Underimmunization status
Delinquent immunization status
Lapsed immunization schedule status

V15.84 Contact with and (suspected) exposure to asbestos
V15.85 Contact with and (suspected) exposure to potentially hazardous body fluids
V15.86 Contact with and (suspected) exposure to lead
V15.87 History of extracorporeal membrane oxygenation [ECMO]
V15.88 History of fall
At risk for falling

V15.89 Other
Excludes: contact with and (suspected) exposure to other potentially hazardous chemicals (V87.2)
contact with and (suspected) exposure to other potentially hazardous substances (V87.39)

V15.9 Unspecified personal history presenting hazards to health
V16 Family history of malignant neoplasm

V16.0 Gastrointestinal tract
Family history of condition classifiable to 140-159

V16.1 Trachea, bronchus, and lung
Family history of condition classifiable to 162

V16.2 Other respiratory and intrathoracic organs
Family history of condition classifiable to 160-161, 163-165

V16.3 Breast
Family history of condition classifiable to 174

● Code new to this edition   ▲ Revision of existing code   ④ ⑤ Fourth or fifth digit required

⑤ **V16.4 Genital organs**
Family history of condition classifiable to 179-187

    V16.40 Genital organ, unspecified

    V16.41 Ovary

    V16.42 Prostate

    V16.43 Testis

    V16.49 Other

⑤ **V16.5 Urinary organs**
Family history of condition classifiable to 188-189

    V16.51 Kidney

    V16.52 Bladder

    V16.59 Other

V16.6 Leukemia
Family history of condition classifiable to 204-208

V16.7 Other lymphatic and hematopoietic neoplasms
Family history of condition classifiable to 200-203

V16.8 Other specified malignant neoplasm
Family history of other condition classifiable to 140-199

V16.9 Unspecified malignant neoplasm

V17 Family history of certain chronic disabling diseases

V17.0 Psychiatric condition
Excludes: family history of intellectual disabilities (V18.4)

V17.1 Stroke (cerebrovascular)

V17.2 Other neurological diseases
Epilepsy
Huntington's chorea

V17.3 Ischemic heart disease

⑤ **V17.4 Other cardiovascular diseases**

    V17.41 Family history of sudden cardiac death (SCD)
Excludes: family history of ischemic heart disease (V17.3)
        family history of myocardial infarction (V17.3)

    V17.49 Family history of other cardiovascular diseases
Family history of cardiovascular disease NOS

V17.5 Asthma

V17.6 Other chronic respiratory conditions

V17.7 Arthritis

⑤ **V17.8 Other musculoskeletal diseases**

    V17.81 Osteoporosis

    V17.89 Other musculoskeletal diseases

V18 Family history of certain other specific conditions

V18.0 Diabetes mellitus

⑤ **V18.1 Other endocrine and metabolic diseases**

    V18.11 Multiple endocrine neoplasia [MEN] syndrome

    V18.19 Other endocrine and metabolic diseases

V18.2 Anemia

V18.3 Other blood disorders

▲ **V18.4 Intellectual disabilities**

⑤ **V18.5 Digestive disorders**

    V18.51 Colonic polyps
Excludes: family history of malignant neoplasm of gastrointestinal tract (V16.0)

    V18.59 Other digestive disorders

⑤ **V18.6 Kidney diseases**

    V18.61 Polycystic kidney

    V18.69 Other kidney diseases

Add 4th or 5th digit	Nonspecific code	Unspecific code	Secondary Dx Only	Primary Dx Only

V18.7 Other genitourinary diseases

V18.8 Infectious and parasitic diseases

V18.9 Genetic disease carrier

V19 Family history of other conditions

V19.0 Blindness or visual loss

⑤ **V19.1** Other eye disorders

- ● **V19.11** Glaucoma
- ● **V19.19** Other specified eye disorder

V19.2 Deafness or hearing loss

V19.3 Other ear disorders

V19.4 Skin conditions

V19.5 Congenital anomalies

V19.6 Allergic disorders

V19.7 Consanguinity

V19.8 Other condition

PERSONS ENCOUNTERING HEALTH SERVICES IN CIRCUMSTANCES RELATED TO REPRODUCTION AND DEVELOPMENT (V20-V29)

V20 Health supervision of infant or child

V20.0 Foundling

V20.1 Other healthy infant or child receiving care
Medical or nursing care supervision of healthy infant in cases of:
maternal illness, physical or psychiatric
socioeconomic adverse condition at home
too many children at home preventing or interfering with normal care

V20.2 Routine infant or child health check
Developmental testing of infant or child
Health check for child over 28 days old
Immunizations appropriate for age
Routine vision and hearing testing

Excludes: health check for child under 29 days old (V20.31-V20.32)
newborn health supervision (V20.31-V20.32)
special screening for developmental handicaps (V79.3)

Use additional code(s) to identify:
Special screening examination(s) performed (V73.0-V82.9)

⑤ **V20.3** Newborn health supervision
Health check for child under 29 days old

Excludes: health check for child over 28 days old (V20.2)

V20.31 Health supervision for newborn under 8 days old
Health check for newborn under 8 days old

V20.32 Health supervision for newborn 8 to 28 days old
Health check for newborn 8 to 28 days old
Newborn weight check

V21 Constitutional states in development

V21.0 Period of rapid growth in childhood

V21.1 Puberty

V21.2 Other adolescence

⑤ **V21.3** Low birth weight status

Excludes: history of perinatal problems (V13.7)

V21.30 Low birth weight status, unspecified

V21.31 Low birth weight status, less than 500 grams

V21.32 Low birth weight status, 500-999 grams

V21.33 Low birth weight status, 1000-1499 grams

V21.34 Low birth weight status, 1500-1999 grams

V21.35 Low birth weight status, 2000-2500 grams

V21.8 Other specified constitutional states in development

V21.9 Unspecified constitutional state in development

● Code new to this edition　▲ Revision of existing code　④ ⑤ Fourth or fifth digit required

V22 Normal pregnancy

> *Excludes:* *pregnancy examination or test, pregnancy unconfirmed (V72.40)*

V22.0 Supervision of normal first pregnancy

> **ALERT!** Codes V22.0 and V22.1 are always first listed and are not to be used with any other code from the OB chapter.

V22.1 Supervision of other normal pregnancy

> **ALERT!** Codes V22.0 and V22.1 are always first listed and are not to be used with any other code from the OB chapter.

V22.2 Pregnant state, incidental
Pregnant state NOS

V23 Supervision of high-risk pregnancy

V23.0 Pregnancy with history of infertility

V23.1 Pregnancy with history of trophoblastic disease
Pregnancy with history of:
hydatidiform mole
vesicular mole

> *Excludes:* *that without current pregnancy (V13.1)*

V23.2 Pregnancy with history of abortion
Pregnancy with history of conditions classifiable to 634-638

> *Excludes:* *recurrent pregnancy loss:*
> *care during pregnancy (646.3)*
> *that without current pregnancy (629.81)*

V23.3 Grand multiparity

> *Excludes:* *care in relation to labor and delivery (659.4)*
> *that without current pregnancy (V61.5)*

⑤ **V23.4 Pregnancy with other poor obstetric history**
Pregnancy with history of other conditions classifiable to 630-676

> **V23.41 Pregnancy with history of pre-term labor**

● **V23.42 Pregnancy with history of ectopic pregnancy**

V23.49 Pregnancy with other poor obstetric history

V23.5 Pregnancy with other poor reproductive history
Pregnancy with history of stillbirth or neonatal death

V23.7 Insufficient prenatal care
History of little or no prenatal care

⑤ **V23.8 Other high-risk pregnancy**

> **V23.81 Elderly primigravida**
> First pregnancy in a woman who will be 35 years of age or older at expected date of delivery

> *Excludes:* *elderly primigravida complicating pregnancy (659.5)*

> **V23.82 Elderly multigravida**
> Second or more pregnancy in a woman who will be 35 years of age or older at expected date of delivery

> *Excludes:* *elderly multigravida complicating pregnancy (659.6)*

> **V23.83 Young primigravida**
> First pregnancy in a female less than 16 years old at expected date of delivery

> *Excludes:* *young primigravida complicating pregnancy (659.8)*

> **V23.84 Young multigravida**
> Second or more pregnancy in a female less than 16 years old at expected date of delivery

> *Excludes:* *young multigravida complicating pregnancy (659.8)*

> **V23.85 Pregnancy resulting from assisted reproductive technology**
> Pregnancy resulting from in vitro fertilization

> **V23.86 Pregnancy with history of in utero procedure during previous pregnancy**

> *Excludes:* *management of pregnancy affected by in utero procedure during current pregnancy (679.0-679.1)*

● **V23.87 Pregnancy with inconclusive fetal viability**
Encounter to determine fetal viability of pregnancy

V23.89 Other high-risk pregnancy

	Add 4th or 5th digit		Nonspecific code		Unspecific code		Secondary Dx Only		Primary Dx Only

V23.9 Unspecified high-risk pregnancy

V24 Postpartum care and examination

> **DEFINITION** A high risk pregnancy is one in which some condition puts the mother, the developing fetus, or both at higher-than-normal risk for complications during or after the pregnancy and birth.

V24.0 Immediately after delivery
Care and observation in uncomplicated cases

V24.1 Lactating mother
Supervision of lactation

V24.2 Routine postpartum follow-up

V25 Encounter for contraceptive management

⑤ **V25.0 General counseling and advice**

V25.01 Prescription of oral contraceptives

V25.02 Initiation of other contraceptive measures
Fitting of diaphragm
Prescription of foams, creams, or other agents

V25.03 Encounter for emergency contraceptive counseling and prescription
Encounter for postcoital contraceptive counseling and prescription

V25.04 Counseling and instruction in natural family planning to avoid pregnancy

V25.09 Other
Family planning advice

⑤ **V25.1 Encounter for insertion or removal of intrauterine contraceptive device**

> *Excludes:* *encounter for routine checking of intrauterine contraceptive device (V25.42)*

V25.11 Encounter for insertion of intrauterine contraceptive device

V25.12 Encounter for removal of intrauterine contraceptive device

V25.13 Encounter for removal and reinsertion of intrauterine contraceptive device
Encounter for replacement of intrauterine contraceptive device

V25.2 Sterilization
Admission for interruption of fallopian tubes or vas deferens

V25.3 Menstrual extraction
Menstrual regulation

⑤ **V25.4 Surveillance of previously prescribed contraceptive methods**
Checking, reinsertion, or removal of contraceptive device
Repeat prescription for contraceptive method
Routine examination in connection with contraceptive maintenance

V25.40 Contraceptive surveillance, unspecified

V25.41 Contraceptive pill

V25.42 Intrauterine contraceptive device
Checking of intrauterine device

> *Excludes:* *insertion or removal of intrauterine contraceptive device (V25.11-V25.13)*
> *presence of intrauterine contraceptive device as incidental finding (V45.5)*

V25.43 Implantable subdermal contraceptive

V25.49 Other contraceptive method

V25.5 Insertion of implantable subdermal contraceptive

V25.8 Other specified contraceptive management
Postvasectomy sperm count

> *Excludes:* *sperm count following sterilization reversal (V26.22)*
> *sperm count for fertility testing (V26.21)*

V25.9 Unspecified contraceptive management

V26 Procreative management

V26.0 Tuboplasty or vasoplasty after previous sterilization

V26.1 Artificial insemination

⑤ **V26.2 Investigation and testing**

> *Excludes:* *postvasectomy sperm count (V25.8)*

● Code new
  to this edition

▲ Revision of
  existing code

④ ⑤ Fourth or fifth
      digit required

⑤ **V26.21 Fertility testing**
　　　　Fallopian insufflation
　　　　Sperm count for fertility testing

Excludes: *genetic counseling and testing (V26.31-V26.39)*

　　V26.22 Aftercare following sterilization reversal
　　　　Fallopian insufflation following sterilization reversal
　　　　Sperm count following sterilization reversal

　V26.29 Other investigation and testing

⑤ **V26.3 Genetic counseling and testing**

Excludes: *fertility testing (V26.21)*
　　　　　nonprocreative genetic screening (V82.71, V82.79)

　　V26.31 Testing of female for genetic disease carrier status

　V26.32 Other genetic testing of female
Use additional code to identify recurrent pregnancy loss (629.81, 646.3)

　　V26.33 Genetic counseling

　　V26.34 Testing of male for genetic disease carrier status

　　V26.35 Encounter for testing of male partner of female with recurrent pregnancy loss

　V26.39 Other genetic testing of male

⑤ **V26.4 General counseling and advice**

　　V26.41 Procreative counseling and advice using natural family planning

　　V26.42 Encounter for fertility preservation counseling
　　　　Encounter for fertility preservation counseling prior to cancer therapy
　　　　Encounter for fertility preservation counseling prior to surgical removal of gonads

　V26.49 Other procreative management counseling and advice

⑤ **V26.5 Sterilization status**

　V26.51 Tubal ligation status

Excludes: *infertility not due to previous tubal ligation (628.0-628.9)*

　V26.52 Vasectomy status

⑤ **V26.8 Other specified procreative management**

　V26.81 Encounter for assisted reproductive fertility procedure cycle
　　　　Patient undergoing in vitro fertilization cycle
Use additional code to identify the type of infertility

Excludes: *pre-cycle diagnosis and testing – code to reason for encounter*

　　V26.82 Encounter for fertility preservation procedure
　　　　Encounter for fertility preservation procedure prior to cancer therapy
　　　　Encounter for fertility preservation procedure prior to surgical removal of gonads

　V26.89 Other specified procreative management

V26.9 Unspecified procreative management

V27 **Outcome of delivery**
Note: This category is intended for the coding of the outcome of delivery on the mother's record.
　　ALERT! The outcome of delivery, category V27, should be included on all maternal delivery records. It is always a secondary code.

V27.0 Single liveborn

V27.1 Single stillborn

V27.2 Twins, both liveborn

V27.3 Twins, one liveborn and one stillborn

V27.4 Twins, both stillborn

V27.5 Other multiple birth, all liveborn

V27.6 Other multiple birth, some liveborn

V27.7 Other multiple birth, all stillborn

V27.9 Unspecified outcome of delivery
　　　Single birth, outcome to infant unspecified
　　　Multiple birth, outcome to infant unspecified

| | Add 4th or 5th digit | | Nonspecific code | | Unspecific code | | Secondary Dx Only | | Primary Dx Only |

V28 **Encounter for antenatal screening of mother**

> Excludes: *abnormal findings on screening—code to findings*
> *routine prenatal care (V22.0-V23.9)*
> *suspected fetal conditions affecting management of pregnancy (655.00-655.93,*
> *656.00-656.93, 657.00-657.03, 658.00 -658.93)*
> *suspected fetal conditions not found (V89.01-V89.09)*

V28.0 **Screening for chromosomal anomalies by amniocentesis**

V28.1 **Screening for raised alpha-fetoprotein levels in amniotic fluid**

V28.2 **Other screening based on amniocentesis**

V28.3 **Encounter for routine screening for malformation using ultrasonics**
Encounter for routine fetal ultrasound NOS

> Excludes: *encounter for feal anatomic survey (V28.81)*
> *genetic counseling and testing (V26.31-V26.39)*

V28.4 **Screening for fetal growth retardation using ultrasonics**

V28.5 **Screening for isoimmunization**

V28.6 **Screening for Streptococcus B**

⑤ **V28.8** **Other specified antenatal screening**

> **V28.81** **Encounter for fetal anatomic survey**
>
> **V28.82** **Encounter for screening for risk of pre-term labor**
>
> **V28.89** **Other specified antenatal screening**
> Chorionic villus sampling
> Genomic screening
> Nuchal translucency testing
> Proteomic screening

V28.9 **Unspecified antenatal screening**

V29 **Observation and evaluation of newborns for suspected condition not found**

Note: This category is to be used for newborns, within the neonatal period, (the first 28 days of life) who are suspected of having an abnormal condition resulting from exposure from the mother or the birth process, but without signs or symptoms, and, which after examination and observation, is found not to exist.

> Excludes: *suspected fetal conditions not found (V89.01-V89.09)*

ALERT! Assign a code from category V29 to identify those instances when a healthy newborn is evaluated for a suspected condition that is determined after study not to be present.

ALERT! Do not use a code from category V29 when the patient has identified signs or symptoms of a suspected problem; in such cases, code the sign or symptom.

V29.0 **Observation for suspected infectious condition**

V29.1 **Observation for suspected neurological condition**

V29.2 **Observation for suspected respiratory condition**

V29.3 **Observation for suspected genetic or metabolic condition**

V29.8 **Observation for other specified suspected condition**

V29.9 **Observation for unspecified suspected condition**

LIVEBORN INFANTS ACCORDING TO TYPE OF BIRTH (V30-V39)

Note: These categories are intended for the coding of liveborn infants who are consuming health care [e.g., crib or bassinet occupancy].

The following fourth-digit subdivisions are for use with categories V30-V39:

⑤ **.0** **Born in hospital**

.1 **Born before admission to hospital**

.2 **Born outside hospital and not hospitalized**

The following two fifth-digits are for use with the fourth-digit .0, Born in hospital:

0 **delivered without mention of cesarean delivery**

1 **delivered by cesarean delivery**

④ **V30** **Single liveborn**

④ **V31** **Twin, mate liveborn**

④ **V32** **Twin, mate stillborn**

④ **V33** **Twin, unspecified**

④ **V34** **Other multiple, mates all liveborn**

● Code new
to this edition   ▲ Revision of
existing code   ④ ⑤ Fourth or fifth
digit required

④ **V35** Other multiple, mates all stillborn

④ **V36** Other multiple, mates live- and stillborn

④ **V37** Other multiple, unspecified

④ **V39** Unspecified

PERSONS WITH A CONDITION INFLUENCING THEIR HEALTH STATUS (V40-V49)

> Note: These categories are intended for use when these conditions are recorded as "diagnoses" or "problems."

V40 Mental and behavioral problems

  V40.0 Problems with learning

  V40.1 Problems with communication [including speech]

  V40.2 Other mental problems

⑤ V40.3 Other behavioral problems

    ● V40.31 Wandering in diseases classified elsewhere

      Code first underlying disorder such as:
        Alzheimer's disease (331.0)
        autism or pervasive developmental disorder (299.0-299.9)
        dementia, unspecified, with behavioral disturbance (294.21)
        intellectual disabilities (317-319)

    ● **V40.39** Other specified behavioral problem

  V40.9 Unspecified mental or behavioral problem

V41 Problems with special senses and other special functions

  V41.0 Problems with sight

  V41.1 Other eye problems

  V41.2 Problems with hearing

  V41.3 Other ear problems

  V41.4 Problems with voice production

  V41.5 Problems with smell and taste

  V41.6 Problems with swallowing and mastication

  V41.7 Problems with sexual function

    Excludes: marital problems (V61.10)
            psychosexual disorders (302.0-302.9)

  V41.8 Other problems with special functions

  V41.9 Unspecified problem with special function

V42 Organ or tissue replaced by transplant
    Includes: homologous or heterologous (animal) (human) transplant organ status

  V42.0 Kidney

  V42.1 Heart

  V42.2 Heart valve

  V42.3 Skin

  V42.4 Bone

  V42.5 Cornea

  V42.6 Lung

  V42.7 Liver

⑤ V42.8 Other specified organ or tissue

    V42.81 Bone marrow

    V42.82 Peripheral stem cells

    V42.83 Pancreas

    V42.84 Intestines

    V42.89 Other

  V42.9 Unspecified organ or tissue

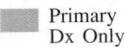

| | Add 4th or 5th digit | | Nonspecific code | | Unspecific code | | Secondary Dx Only | | Primary Dx Only |

V43 **Organ or tissue replaced by other means**
Includes: organ or tissue assisted by other means
replacement of organ by:
artificial device
mechanical device
prosthesis

Excludes: *cardiac pacemaker in situ (V45.01)*
fitting and adjustment of prosthetic device (V52.0-V52.9)
renal dialysis status (V45.11)

V43.0   **Eye globe**

V43.1   **Lens**
Pseudophakos

⑤ **V43.2**   **Heart**

V43.21   **Heart assist device**

V43.22   **Fully implantable artificial heart**

V43.3   **Heart valve**

V43.4   **Blood vessel**

V43.5   **Bladder**

⑤ **V43.6**   **Joint**

V43.60   **Unspecified joint**

V43.61   **Shoulder**

V43.62   **Elbow**

V43.63   **Wrist**

V43.64   **Hip**

V43.65   **Knee**

V43.66   **Ankle**

V43.69   **Other**

V43.7   **Limb**

⑤ **V43.8**   **Other organ or tissue**

V43.81   **Larynx**

V43.82   **Breast**

V43.83   **Artificial skin**

V43.89   **Other**

V44 **Artificial opening status**

Excludes: *artificial openings requiring attention or management (V55.0-V55.9)*

V44.0   **Tracheostomy**

V44.1   **Gastrostomy**

V44.2   **Ileostomy**

V44.3   **Colostomy**

V44.4   **Other artificial opening of gastrointestinal tract**

⑤ **V44.5**   **Cystostomy**

V44.50   **Cystostomy, unspecified**

V44.51   **Cutaneous-vesicostomy**

V44.52   **Appendico-vesicostomy**

V44.59   **Other cystostomy**

V44.6   **Other artificial opening of urinary tract**
Nephrostomy
Ureterostomy
Urethrostomy

V44.7   **Artificial vagina**

V44.8   **Other artificial opening status**

V44.9   **Unspecified artificial opening status**

V45 **Other postprocedural states**

Excludes: *aftercare management (V51-V58.9)*
malfunction or other complication—code to condition

● Code new
to this edition   ▲ Revision of
existing code   ④ ⑤ Fourth or fifth
digit required

⑤ **V45.0 Cardiac device in situ**

Excludes: artificial heart (V43.22)
                heart assist device (V43.21)

V45.00 Unspecified cardiac device

V45.01 Cardiac pacemaker

Excludes: cardiac defibrillator with synchronous cardiac pacemaker (V45.02)

V45.02 Automatic implantable cardiac defibrillator
          With synchronous cardiac pacemaker

V45.09 Other specified cardiac device
          Carotid sinus pacemaker in situ

⑤ **V45.1 Renal dialysis status**

Excludes: admission for dialysis treatment, or session (V56.0)

V45.11 Renal dialysis status
          Hemodialysis status
          Patient requiring intermittent renal dialysis
          Peritoneal dialysis status
          Presence of arterial-venous shunt (for dialysis)

V45.12 Noncompliance with renal dialysis

V45.2 Presence of cerebrospinal fluid drainage device
          Cerebral ventricle (communicating) shunt, valve, or device in situ

Excludes: malfunction (996.2)

V45.3 Intestinal bypass or anastomosis status

Excludes: bariatric surgery status (V45.86)
                gastric bypass status (V45.86)
                obesity surgery status (V45.86)

V45.4 Arthrodesis status

⑤ **V45.5 Presence of contraceptive device**

V45.51 Intrauterine contraceptive device

Excludes: checking of device (V25.42)
                complication from device (996.32)
                insertion and removal of device (V25.11-V25.13)

V45.52 Subdermal contraceptive implant

V45.59 Other

⑤ **V45.6 States following surgery of eye and adnexa**
          Cataract extraction state following eye surgery
          Filtering bleb state following eye surgery
          Surgical eyelid adhesion state following eye surgery

Excludes: aphakia (379.31)
                artificial eye globe (V43.0)

V45.61 Cataract extraction status
          Use additional code for associated artificial lens status (V43.1)

V45.69 Other states following surgery of eye and adnexa

⑤ **V45.7 Acquired absence of organ**

V45.71 Acquired absence of breast and nipple

Excludes: congenital absence of breast and nipple (757.6)

V45.72 Acquired absence of intestine (large) (small)

V45.73 Acquired absence of kidney

V45.74 Other parts of urinary tract
          Bladder

V45.75 Stomach

V45.76 Lung

V45.77 Genital organs

Excludes: acquired absence of cervix and uterus (V88.01-V88.03)
                female genital mutilation status (629.20-629.29)

V45.78 Eye

V45.79 Other acquired absence of organ
Excludes: *acquired absence of pancreas (V88.11-V88.12)*

⑤ **V45.8 Other postprocedural status**

V45.81 Aortocoronary bypass status

V45.82 Percutaneous transluminal coronary angioplasty status

V45.83 Breast implant removal status

V45.84 Dental restoration status
Dental crowns status
Dental fillings status

V45.85 Insulin pump status

V45.86 Bariatric surgery status
Gastric banding status
Gastric bypass status for obesity
Obesity surgery status

Excludes: *bariatric surgery status complicating pregnancy, childbirth or the puerperium*
(649.2)
intestinal bypass or anastomosis status (V45.3)

V45.87 Transplanted organ removal status
Transplanted organ previously removed due to complication, failure, rejection
or infection

Excludes: *encounter for removal of transplanted organ - code to complication of*
transplanted organ (996.80-996.89)

V45.88 Status post administration of tPA (rtPA) in a different facility within the
last 24 hours prior to admission to current facility
Code first condition requiring tPA administration, such as:
acute cerebral infarction (433.0-433.9 with fifth-digit 1, 434.0-434.9 with fifth digit 1)
acute myocardial infarction (410.00-410.92)
ALERT! Assign code V45.88 as a secondary diagnosis when a patient is received by transfer
into a facility and documentation indicates they were administered tissue plasminogen
activator (tPA) within the last 24 hours prior to admission to the current facility.

V45.89 Other
Presence of neuropacemaker or other electronic device

Excludes: *artificial heart valve in situ (V43.3)*
vascular prosthesis in situ (V43.4)

V46 Other dependence on machines and devices

V46.0 Aspirator

⑤ **V46.1 Respirator [Ventilator]**
Iron lung

V46.11 Dependence on respirator, status

V46.12 Encounter for respirator dependence during power failure

V46.13 Encounter for weaning from respirator [ventilator]

V46.14 Mechanical complication of respirator [ventilator]
Mechanical failure of respirator [ventilator]

V46.2 Supplemental oxygen
Long-term oxygen therapy

V46.3 Wheelchair dependence
Wheelchair confinement status

Code first cause of dependence, such as:
muscular dystrophy (359.1)
obesity (278.00-278.03)

V46.8 Other enabling machines
Hyperbaric chamber
Possum [Patient-Operated-Selector-Mechanism]

Excludes: *cardiac pacemaker (V45.0)*
kidney dialysis machine (V45.11)

V46.9 Unspecified machine dependence

V47 Other problems with internal organs

V47.0 Deficiencies of internal organs

V47.1 Mechanical and motor problems with internal organs

● Code new
 to this edition

▲ Revision of
 existing code

④ ⑤ Fourth or fifth
 digit required

V47.2 **Other cardiorespiratory problems**
Cardiovascular exercise intolerance with pain (with):
at rest
less than ordinary activity
ordinary activity

V47.3 **Other digestive problems**

V47.4 **Other urinary problems**

V47.5 **Other genital problems**

V47.9 **Unspecified**

V48 **Problems with head, neck, and trunk**

V48.0 **Deficiencies of head**
Excludes: deficiencies of ears, eyelids, and nose (V48.8)

V48.1 **Deficiencies of neck and trunk**

V48.2 **Mechanical and motor problems with head**

V48.3 **Mechanical and motor problems with neck and trunk**

V48.4 **Sensory problem with head**

V48.5 **Sensory problem with neck and trunk**

V48.6 **Disfigurements of head**

V48.7 **Disfigurements of neck and trunk**

V48.8 **Other problems with head, neck, and trunk**

V48.9 **Unspecified problem with head, neck, or trunk**

V49 **Other conditions influencing health status**

V49.0 **Deficiencies of limbs**

V49.1 **Mechanical problems with limbs**

V49.2 **Motor problems with limbs**

V49.3 **Sensory problems with limbs**

V49.4 **Disfigurements of limbs**

V49.5 **Other problems of limbs**

⑤ **V49.6** **Upper limb amputation status**

V49.60 **Unspecified level**

V49.61 **Thumb**

V49.62 **Other finger(s)**

V49.63 **Hand**

V49.64 **Wrist**
Disarticulation of wrist

V49.65 **Below elbow**

V49.66 **Above elbow**
Disarticulation of elbow

V49.67 **Shoulder**
Disarticulation of shoulder

⑤ **V49.7** **Lower limb amputation status**

V49.70 **Unspecified level**

V49.71 **Great toe**

V49.72 **Other toe(s)**

V49.73 **Foot**

V49.74 **Ankle**
Disarticulation of ankle

V49.75 **Below knee**

V49.76 **Above knee**
Disarticulation of knee

V49.77 **Hip**
Disarticulation of hip

⑤ **V49.8** **Other specified conditions influencing health status**

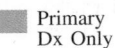

| | Add 4th or 5th digit | | Nonspecific code | | Unspecific code | | Secondary Dx Only | | Primary Dx Only |

V49.81 Asymptomatic postmenopausal status (age-related) (natural)

Excludes: *menopausal and premenopausal disorders (627.0-627.9)*
postsurgical menopause (256.2)
premature menopause (256.31)
symptomatic menopause (627.0-627.9)

V49.82 Dental sealant status

V49.83 Awaiting organ transplant status

V49.84 Bed confinement status

V49.85 Dual sensory impairment
Blindness with deafness
Combined visual hearing impairment

Code first:
hearing impairment (389.00-389.9)
visual impairment (369.00-369.9)

V49.86 Do not resuscitate status

V49.87 Physical restraints status

Excludes: *restraint due to a procedure – omit code*

V49.89 Other specified conditions influencing health status

V49.9 Unspecified

PERSONS ENCOUNTERING HEALTH SERVICES FOR SPECIFIC PROCEDURES AND AFTERCARE (V50-V59)

Note: Categories V51-V58 are intended for use to indicate a reason for care in patients who may have already been treated for some disease or injury not now present, but who are receiving care to consolidate the treatment, to deal with residual states, or to prevent recurrence.

Excludes: *follow-up examination for medical surveillance following treatment (V67.0-V67.9)*

V50 Elective surgery for purposes other than remedying health states

V50.0 Hair transplant

V50.1 Other plastic surgery for unacceptable cosmetic appearance
Breast augmentation or reduction
Face-lift

Excludes: *encounter for breast reduction (611.1)*
plastic surgery following healed injury or operation (V51.0-V51.8)

V50.2 Routine or ritual circumcision
Circumcision in the absence of significant medical indication

V50.3 Ear piercing

⑤ **V50.4 Prophylactic organ removal**

Excludes: *organ donations (V59.0-V59.9)*
therapeutic organ removal—code to condition

V50.41 Breast

V50.42 Ovary

V50.49 Other

V50.8 Other

V50.9 Unspecified

V51 Aftercare involving the use of plastic surgery
Plastic surgery following healed injury or operation

Excludes: *cosmetic plastic surgery (V50.1)*
plastic surgery as treatment for current condition or injury—code to condition or injury
repair of scarred tissue—code to scar

V51.0 Encounter for breast reconstruction following mastectomy

Excludes: *deformity and disproportion of reconstructed breast (612.0-612.1)*

V51.8 Other aftercare involving the use of plastic surgery

V52 Fitting and adjustment of prosthetic device and implant
Includes: removal of device

Excludes: *malfunction or complication of prosthetic device (996.0-996.7)*
status only, without need for care (V43.0-V43.8)

● Code new
to this edition
▲ Revision of
existing code
④ ⑤ Fourth or fifth
digit required

V52.0 Artificial arm (complete) (partial)

V52.1 Artificial leg (complete) (partial)

V52.2 Artificial eye

V52.3 Dental prosthetic device

V52.4 Breast prosthesis and implant
Elective implant exchange (different material) (different size)
Removal of tissue expander without synchronous insertion of permanent implant

Excludes: admission for initial breast implant insertion for breast augmentation (V50.1)
complications of breast implant (996.54, 996.69, 996.79)
encounter for breast reconstruction following mastectomy (V51.0)

V52.8 Other specified prosthetic device

V52.9 Unspecified prosthetic device

V53 Fitting and adjustment of other device
Includes: removal of device
replacement of device

Excludes: status only, without need for care (V45.0-V45.8)

⑤ **V53.0 Devices related to nervous system and special senses**

V53.01 Fitting and adjustment of cerebral ventricular (communicating) shunt

V53.02 Neuropacemaker (brain) (peripheral nerve) (spinal cord)

V53.09 Fitting and adjustment of other devices related to nervous system and special senses
Auditory substitution device
Visual substitution device

V53.1 Spectacles and contact lenses

V53.2 Hearing aid

⑤ **V53.3 Cardiac device**
Reprogramming

V53.31 Cardiac pacemaker

Excludes: automatic implantable cardiac defibrillator with synchronous cardiac pacemaker (V53.32)
mechanical complication of cardiac pacemaker (996.01)

V53.32 Automatic implantable cardiac defibrillator
With synchronous cardiac pacemaker

V53.39 Other cardiac device

V53.4 Orthodontic devices

⑤ **V53.5 Other gastrointestinal appliance and device**

Excludes: colostomy (V55.3)
ileostomy (V55.2)
other artificial opening of digestive tract (V55.4)

V53.50 Fitting and adjustment of intestinal appliance and device

V53.51 Fitting and adjustment of gastric lap band

V53.59 Fitting and adjustment of other gastrointestinal appliance and device

V53.6 Urinary devices
Urinary catheter

Excludes: cystostomy (V55.5)
nephrostomy (V55.6)
ureterostomy (V55.6)
urethrostomy (V55.6)

V53.7 Orthopedic devices

Orthopedic:	Orthopedic:
brace	corset
cast	shoes

Excludes: other orthopedic aftercare (V54)

V53.8 Wheelchair

⑤ **V53.9 Other and unspecified device**

V53.90 Unspecified device

V53.91 Fitting and adjustment of insulin pump
Insulin pump titration

Add 4th or 5th digit	Nonspecific code	Unspecific code	Secondary Dx Only	Primary Dx Only

V53.99 Other device

V54 Other orthopedic aftercare

> *Excludes:* fitting and adjustment of orthopedic devices (V53.7)
> malfunction of internal orthopedic device (996.40-996.49)
> other complication of nonmechanical nature (996.60-996.79)

⑤ **V54.0 Aftercare involving internal fixation device**

> *Excludes:* malfunction of internal orthopedic device (996.40-996.49)
> removal of external fixation device (V54.89)

V54.01 Encounter for removal of internal fixation device

V54.02 Encounter for lengthening/adjustment of growth rod

V54.09 Other aftercare involving internal fixation device

⑤ **V54.1 Aftercare for healing traumatic fracture**

> *Excludes:* aftercare following joint replacement (V54.81)
> aftercare for amputation stump (V54.89)

V54.10 Aftercare for healing traumatic fracture of arm, unspecified

V54.11 Aftercare for healing traumatic fracture of upper arm

V54.12 Aftercare for healing traumatic fracture of lower arm

V54.13 Aftercare for healing traumatic fracture of hip

V54.14 Aftercare for healing traumatic fracture of leg, unspecified

V54.15 Aftercare for healing traumatic fracture of upper leg

> *Excludes:* aftercare for healing traumatic fracture of hip (V54.13)

V54.16 Aftercare for healing traumatic fracture of lower leg

V54.17 Aftercare for healing traumatic fracture of vertebrae

V54.19 Aftercare for healing traumatic fracture of other bone

⑤ **V54.2 Aftercare for healing pathologic fracture**

> *Excludes:* aftercare following joint replacement (V54.81)

V54.20 Aftercare for healing pathologic fracture of arm, unspecified

V54.21 Aftercare for healing pathologic fracture of upper arm

V54.22 Aftercare for healing pathologic fracture of lower arm

V54.23 Aftercare for healing pathologic fracture of hip

V54.24 Aftercare for healing pathologic fracture of leg, unspecified

V54.25 Aftercare for healing pathologic fracture of upper leg

> *Excludes:* aftercare for healing pathologic fracture of hip (V54.23)

V54.26 Aftercare for healing pathologic fracture of lower leg

V54.27 Aftercare for healing pathologic fracture of vertebrae

V54.29 Aftercare for healing pathologic fracture of other bone

⑤ **V54.8 Other orthopedic aftercare**

V54.81 Aftercare following joint replacement
Use additional code to identify joint replacement site (V43.60-V43.69)

● **V54.82** Aftercare following explantation of joint prosthesis
Aftercare following explantation of joint prosthesis, staged procedure
Encounter for joint prosthesis insertion following prior explantation of joint
prosthesis

V54.89 Other orthopedic aftercare
Aftercare for healing fracture NOS

V54.9 Unspecified orthopedic aftercare

V55 Attention to artificial openings

> Includes: adjustment or repositioning of catheter
> closure
> passage of sounds or bougies
> reforming
> removal or replacement of catheter
> toilet or cleansing

> *Excludes:* complications of external stoma (519.00-519.09, 569.60-569.69, 596.81-596.83,
> 997.49)
> status only, without need for care (V44.0-V44.9)

● Code new
to this edition

▲ Revision of
existing code

④ ⑤ Fourth or fifth
digit required

V55.0 Tracheostomy

V55.1 Gastrostomy

V55.2 Ileostomy

V55.3 Colostomy

V55.4 Other artificial opening of digestive tract

V55.5 Cystostomy

V55.6 Other artificial opening of urinary tract
   Nephrostomy   Urethrostomy
   Ureterostomy

V55.7 Artificial vagina

V55.8 Other specified artificial opening

V55.9 Unspecified artificial opening

V56 Encounter for dialysis and dialysis catheter care
   Use additional code to identify the associated condition

   Excludes: *dialysis preparation—code to condition*

   DEFINITION Dialysis is a medical procedure to remove wastes and additional fluid from the blood after the kidneys have stopped functioning.

V56.0 Extracorporeal dialysis
   Dialysis (renal) NOS

   Excludes: *dialysis status (V45.11)*

V56.1 Fitting and adjustment of extracorporeal dialysis catheter
   Removal or replacement of catheter
   Toilet or cleansing

   Use additional code for any concurrent extracorporeal dialysis (V56.0)

V56.2 Fitting and adjustment of peritoneal dialysis catheter
   Use additional code for any concurrent peritoneal dialysis (V56.8)

⑤ **V56.3 Encounter for adequacy testing for dialysis**

   V56.31 Encounter for adequacy testing for hemodialysis

   V56.32 Encounter for adequacy testing for peritoneal dialysis
      Peritoneal equilibration test

V56.8 Other dialysis
   Peritoneal dialysis

V57 Care involving use of rehabilitation procedures
   Use additional code to identify underlying condition

V57.0 Breathing exercises

V57.1 Other physical therapy
   Therapeutic and remedial exercises, except breathing

⑤ **V57.2 Occupational therapy and vocational rehabilitation**

   V57.21 Encounter for occupational therapy

   V57.22 Encounter for vocational therapy

V57.3 Speech-language therapy

V57.4 Orthoptic training

⑤ **V57.8 Other specified rehabilitation procedure**

   V57.81 Orthotic training
      Gait training in the use of artificial limbs

   V57.89 Other
      Multiple training or therapy

V57.9 Unspecified rehabilitation procedure

V58 Encounter for other and unspecified procedures and aftercare

   Excludes: *convalescence and palliative care (V66)*

V58.0 Radiotherapy
   Encounter or admission for radiotherapy

   Excludes: *encounter for radioactive implant—code to condition*
      radioactive iodine therapy—code to condition

⑤ **V58.1 Encounter for chemotherapy and immunotherapy for neoplastic conditions**
   Encounter or admission for chemotherapy

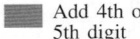
Add 4th or   Nonspecific   Unspecific   Secondary   Primary
5th digit   code   code   Dx Only   Dx Only

Excludes: *chemotherapy and immunotherapy for nonneoplastic conditions—code to condition*

V58.11 **Encounter for antineoplastic chemotherapy**

V58.12 **Encounter for antineoplastic immunotherapy**

V58.2 **Blood transfusion, without reported diagnosis**

⑤ **V58.3** **Attention to dressings and sutures**
Change or removal of wound packing

Excludes: *attention to drains (V58.49)*
planned postoperative wound closure (V58.41)

V58.30 **Encounter for change or removal of nonsurgical wound dressing**
Encounter for change or removal of wound dressing NOS

V58.31 **Encounter for change or removal of surgical wound dressing**

V58.32 **Encounter for removal of sutures**
Encounter for removal of staples

⑤ **V58.4** **Other aftercare following surgery**
Note: Codes from this subcategory should be used in conjunction with other aftercare codes to fully identify the reason for the aftercare encounter

Excludes: *aftercare following sterilization reversal surgery (V26.22)*
attention to artificial openings (V55.0-V55.9)
orthopedic aftercare (V54.0-V54.9)

V58.41 **Encounter for planned postoperative wound closure**

Excludes: *disruption of operative wound (998.31-998.32)*
encounter for dressings and suture aftercare (V58.30-V58.32)

V58.42 **Aftercare following surgery for neoplasm**
Conditions classifiable to 140-239

V58.43 **Aftercare following surgery for injury and trauma**
Conditions classifiable to 800-999

Excludes: *aftercare for healing traumatic fracture (V54.10-V54.19)*

V58.44 **Aftercare following organ transplant**
Use additional code to identify the organ transplanted (V42.0-V42.9)

V58.49 **Other specified aftercare following surgery**
Change or removal of drains

V58.5 **Orthodontics**

Excludes: *fitting and adjustment of orthodontic device (V53.4)*

⑤ **V58.6** **Long-term (current) drug use**
Long-term (current) prophylactic drug use

Excludes: *drug abuse (305.00-305.93)*
drug abuse and dependence complicating pregnancy (648.3-648.4)
drug dependence (304.00-304.93)
hormone replacement therapy (postmenopausal) (V07.4)
use of agents affecting estrogen receptors and estrogen levels (V07.51-V07.59)

ALERT! Assign a code from subcategory V58.6 if the patient is receiving a medication for an extended period as a prophylactic measure (such as for the prevention of deep vein thrombosis) or as treatment of a chronic condition (such as arthritis) or a disease requiring a lengthy course of treatment (such as cancer).

ALERT! Do not assign a code from subcategory V58.6 for medication being administered for a brief period of time to treat an acute illness or injury (such as a course of antibiotics to treat acute bronchitis).

V58.61 **Long-term (current) use of anticoagulants**
Excludes: *long-term (current) use of aspirin (V58.66)*

V58.62 **Long-term (current) use of antibiotics**

V58.63 **Long-term (current) use of antiplatelets/antithrombotics**
Excludes: *long-term (current) use of aspirin (V58.66)*

V58.64 **Long-term (current) use of non-steroidal anti-inflammatories (NSAID)**
Excludes: *long-term (current) use of aspirin (V58.66)*

V58.65 **Long-term (current) use of steroids**

V58.66 **Long-term (current) use of aspirin**

V58.67 **Long-term (current) use of insulin**

● Code new to this edition　　▲ Revision of existing code　　④ ⑤ Fourth or fifth digit required

● **V58.68** **Long term (current) use of bisphosphonates**

V58.69 **Long-term (current) use of other medications**
Long term current use of methadone for pain control
Long term current use of opiate analgesic
Other high-risk medications

Excludes: *methadone maintenance NOS (304.00)*
methadone use NOS (304.00)

⑤ **V58.7** **Aftercare following surgery to specified body systems, not elsewhere classified**
Note: Codes from this subcategory should be used in conjunction with other aftercare codes to
fully identify the reason for the aftercare encounter

Excludes: *aftercare following organ transplant (V58.44)*
aftercare following surgery for neoplasm (V58.42)

V58.71 **Aftercare following surgery of the sense organs, NEC**
Conditions classifiable to 360-379, 380-389

V58.72 **Aftercare following surgery of the nervous system, NEC**
Conditions classifiable to 320-359

Excludes: *aftercare following surgery of the sense organs, NEC (V58.71)*

V58.73 **Aftercare following surgery of the circulatory system, NEC**
Conditions classifiable to 390-459

V58.74 **Aftercare following surgery of the respiratory system, NEC**
Conditions classifiable to 460-519

V58.75 **Aftercare following surgery of the teeth, oral cavity and digestive system,
NEC**
Conditions classifiable to 520-579

V58.76 **Aftercare following surgery of the genitourinary system, NEC**
Conditions classifiable to 580-629

Excludes: *aftercare following sterilization reversal (V26.22)*

V58.77 **Aftercare following surgery of the skin and subcutaneous tissue, NEC**
Conditions classifiable to 680-709

V58.78 **Aftercare following surgery of the musculoskeletal system, NEC**
Conditions classifiable to 710-739

Excludes: *orthopedic aftercare (V54.01-V54.9)*

⑤ **V58.8** **Other specified procedures and aftercare**

V58.81 **Fitting and adjustment of vascular catheter**
Removal or replacement of catheter
Toilet or cleansing

Excludes: *complication of renal dialysis catheter (996.73)*
complication of vascular catheter (996.74)
dialysis preparation — code to condition
encounter for dialysis (V56.0-V56.8)
fitting and adjustment of dialysis catheter (V56.1)

V58.82 **Fitting and adjustment of non-vascular catheter NEC**
Removal or replacement of catheter
Toilet or cleansing

Excludes: *fitting and adjustment of peritoneal dialysis catheter (V56.2)*
fitting and adjustment of urinary catheter (V53.6)

V58.83 **Encounter for therapeutic drug monitoring**
Use additional code for any associated long-term (current) drug use (V58.61-V58.69)

Excludes: *blood-drug testing for medicolegal reasons (V70.4)*

V58.89 **Other specified aftercare**

V58.9 **Unspecified aftercare**

V59 **Donors**

Excludes: *examination of potential donor (V70.8)*
self-donation of organ or tissue—code to condition

ALERT! Category V59 donor codes are are used for living individuals who are donating blood
or other body tissue. These codes are only for individuals donating for others, not for self
donations. They are not for use to identify cadaveric donations

⑤ **V59.0** **Blood**

V59.01 **Whole blood**

Add 4th or 5th digit | Nonspecific code | Unspecific code | Secondary Dx Only | Primary Dx Only

V59.02 **Stem cells**

V59.09 **Other**

V59.1 **Skin**

V59.2 **Bone**

V59.3 **Bone marrow**

V59.4 **Kidney**

V59.5 **Cornea**

V59.6 **Liver**

⑤ **V59.7** **Egg (oocyte) (ovum)**

    V59.70 **Egg (oocyte) (ovum) donor, unspecified**

    V59.71 **Egg (oocyte) (ovum) donor, under age 35, anonymous recipient**
        Egg donor, under age 35 NOS

    V59.72 **Egg (oocyte) (ovum) donor, under age 35, designated recipient**

    V59.73 **Egg (oocyte) (ovum) donor, age 35 and over, anonymous recipient**
        Egg donor, age 35 and over NOS

    V59.74 **Egg (oocyte) (ovum) donor, age 35 and over, designated recipient**

V59.8 **Other specified organ or tissue**

V59.9 **Unspecified organ or tissue**

PERSONS ENCOUNTERING HEALTH SERVICES IN OTHER CIRCUMSTANCES (V60-V69)

V60 **Housing, household, and economic circumstances**

  V60.0 **Lack of housing**

Hobos	Transients
Social migrants	Vagabonds
Tramps	

  V60.1 **Inadequate housing**
      Lack of heating
      Restriction of space
      Technical defects in home preventing adequate care

  V60.2 **Inadequate material resources**
      Economic problem
      Poverty NOS

  V60.3 **Person living alone**

  V60.4 **No other household member able to render care**
      Person requiring care (has) (is):
        family member too handicapped, ill, or otherwise unsuited to render care
        partner temporarily away from home
        temporarily away from usual place of abode

    Excludes: holiday relief care (V60.5)

  V60.5 **Holiday relief care**
      Provision of health care facilities to a person normally cared for at home, to enable
        relatives to take a vacation

  V60.6 **Person living in residential institution**
      Boarding school resident

⑤ **V60.8** **Other specified housing or economic circumstances**

    V60.81 **Foster care (status)**

    V60.89 **Other specified housing or economic circumstances**

  V60.9 **Unspecified housing or economic circumstance**

V61 **Other family circumstances**
    Includes: when these circumstances or fear of them, affecting the person directly involved or
        others, are mentioned as the reason, justified or not, for seeking or receiving
        medical advice or care

⑤ **V61.0** **Family disruption**

    V61.01 **Family disruption due to family member on military deployment**
        Individual or family affected by other family member being on deployment

    Excludes: family disruption due to family member on non-military extended absence from
        home (V61.08)

● Code new to this edition	▲ Revision of existing code	④ ⑤ Fourth or fifth digit required

V61.02 **Family disruption due to return of family member from military deployment**
Individual or family affected by other family member having returned from deployment (current or past conflict)

V61.03 **Family disruption due to divorce or legal separation**

V61.04 **Family disruption due to parent-child estrangement**
Excludes: *other family estrangement (V61.09)*

V61.05 **Family disruption due to child in welfare custody**

V61.06 **Family disruption due to child in foster care or in care of non-parental family member**

V61.07 **Family disruption due to death of family member**
Excludes: *bereavement (V62.82)*

V61.08 **Family disruption due to other extended absence of family member**
Excludes: *family disruption due to family member on military deployment (V61.01)*

V61.09 **Other family disruption**
Family estrangement NOS

⑤ **V61.1 Counseling for marital and partner problems**
Excludes: *problems related to:*
psychosexual disorders (302.0-302.9)
sexual function (V41.7)

V61.10 **Counseling for marital and partner problems, unspecified**
Marital conflict
Marital relationship problem
Partner conflict
Partner relationship problem

V61.11 **Counseling for victim of spousal and partner abuse**
Excludes: *encounter for treatment of current injuries due to abuse (995.80-995.85)*

V61.12 **Counseling for perpetrator of spousal and partner abuse**

⑤ **V61.2 Parent-child problems**

V61.20 **Counseling for parent-child problem, unspecified**
Concern about behavior of child
Parent-child conflict
Parent-child relationship problem

V61.21 **Counseling for victim of child abuse**
Child battering
Child neglect
Excludes: *current injuries due to abuse (995.50-995.59)*

V61.22 **Counseling for perpetrator of parental child abuse**
Excludes: *counseling for non-parental abuser (V62.83)*

V61.23 **Counseling for parent-biological child problem**
Concern about behavior of biological child
Parent-biological child conflict
Parent-biological child relationship problem

V61.24 **Counseling for parent-adopted child problem**
Concern about behavior of adopted child
Parent-adopted child conflict
Parent-adopted child relationship problem

V61.25 **Counseling for parent (guardian)-foster child problem**
Concern about behavior of foster child
Parent (guardian)-foster child conflict
Parent (guardian)-foster child relationship problem

V61.29 **Other parent-child problems**

V61.3 Problems with aged parents or in-laws

⑤ **V61.4 Health problems within family**

V61.41 **Alcoholism in family**

V61.42 **Substance abuse in family**

V61.49 **Other**
Care of sick or handicapped person in family or household
Presence of sick or handicapped person in family or household

| Add 4th or 5th digit | Nonspecific code | Unspecific code | Secondary Dx Only | Primary Dx Only |

V61.5 Multiparity

V61.6 Illegitimacy or illegitimate pregnancy

V61.7 Other unwanted pregnancy

V61.8 Other specified family circumstances
Problems with family members NEC
Sibling relationship problem

V61.9 Unspecified family circumstance

V62 Other psychosocial circumstances
Includes: those circumstances or fear of them, affecting the person directly involved or others, mentioned as the reason, justified or not, for seeking or receiving medical advice or care

Excludes: *previous psychological trauma (V15.41-V15.49)*

V62.0 Unemployment

Excludes: *circumstances when main problem is economic inadequacy or poverty (V60.2)*

V62.1 Adverse effects of work environment

⑤ **V62.2** Other occupational circumstances or maladjustment

V62.21 Personal current military deployment status
Individual (civilian or military) currently deployed in theater or in support of military war, peacekeeping and humanitarian operations

V62.22 Personal history of return from military deployment
Individual (civilian or military) with past history of military war, peacekeeping and humanitarian deployment (current or past conflict)

V62.29 Other occupational circumstances or maladjustment
Career choice problem
Dissatisfaction with employment
Occupational problem

V62.3 Educational circumstances
Academic problem
Dissatisfaction with school environment
Educational handicap

V62.4 Social maladjustment
Acculturation problem
Cultural deprivation
Political, religious, or sex discrimination
Social:
isolation
persecution

V62.5 Legal circumstances
Imprisonment
Legal investigation
Litigation
Prosecution

V62.6 Refusal of treatment for reasons of religion or conscience

⑤ **V62.8** Other psychological or physical stress, not elsewhere classified

V62.81 Interpersonal problems, not elsewhere classified
Relational problem NOS

V62.82 Bereavement, uncomplicated

Excludes: *bereavement as adjustment reaction (309.0)*
family disruption due to death of family member (V61.07)

V62.83 Counseling for perpetrator of physical/sexual abuse

Excludes: *counseling for perpetrator of parental child abuse (V61.22)*
counseling for perpetrator of spousal and partner abuse (V61.12)

V62.84 Suicidal ideation

Excludes: *suicidal tendencies (300.9)*

V62.85 Homicidal ideation

V62.89 Other
Borderline intellectual functioning
Life circumstance problems
Phase of life problems
Religious or spiritual problem

V62.9 Unspecified psychosocial circumstance

V63 Unavailability of other medical facilities for care

V63.0 Residence remote from hospital or other health care facility

● Code new to this edition　▲ Revision of existing code　④ ⑤ Fourth or fifth digit required

V63.1 Medical services in home not available

> *Excludes:* no other household member able to render care (V60.4)

V63.2 Person awaiting admission to adequate facility elsewhere

V63.8 Other specified reasons for unavailability of medical facilities
Person on waiting list undergoing social agency investigation

V63.9 Unspecified reason for unavailability of medical facilities

V64 Persons encountering health services for specific procedures, not carried out

⑤ **V64.0 Vaccination not carried out**

V64.00 Vaccination not carried out, unspecified reason

V64.01 Vaccination not carried out because of acute illness

V64.02 Vaccination not carried out because of chronic illness or condition

V64.03 Vaccination not carried out because of immune compromised state

V64.04 Vaccination not carried out because of allergy to vaccine or component

V64.05 Vaccination not carried out because of caregiver refusal
Guardian refusal
Parent refusal

> *Excludes:* vaccination not carried out because of caregiver refusal for religious reasons (V64.07)

V64.06 Vaccination not carried out because of patient refusal

V64.07 Vaccination not carried out for religious reasons

V64.08 Vaccination not carried out because patient had disease being vaccinated against

V64.09 Vaccination not carried out for other reason

V64.1 Surgical or other procedure not carried out because of contraindication

V64.2 Surgical or other procedure not carried out because of patient's decision

V64.3 Procedure not carried out for other reasons

⑤ **V64.4 Closed surgical procedure converted to open procedure**

V64.41 Laparoscopic surgical procedure converted to open procedure

V64.42 Thoracoscopic surgical procedure converted to open procedure

V64.43 Arthroscopic surgical procedure converted to open procedure

V65 Other persons seeking consultation

V65.0 Healthy person accompanying sick person
Boarder

⑤ **V65.1 Person consulting on behalf of another person**
Advice or treatment for nonattending third party

> *Excludes:* concern (normal) about sick person in family (V61.41-V61.49)

V65.11 Pediatric pre-birth visit for expectant parent(s)
Pre-adoption visit for adoptive parent(s)

V65.19 Other person consulting on behalf of another person

V65.2 Person feigning illness
Malingerer
Peregrinating patient

V65.3 Dietary surveillance and counseling
Dietary surveillance and counseling (in):
 NOS
 colitis
 diabetes mellitus
 food allergies or intolerance
 gastritis
 hypercholesterolemia
 hypoglycemia
 obesity
Use additional code to identify Body Mass Index (BMI), if known (V85.0-V85.54)

▦ Add 4th or 5th digit	▦ Nonspecific code	▦ Unspecific code	▦ Secondary Dx Only	▦ Primary Dx Only

⑤ **V65.4 Other counseling, not elsewhere classified**
  Health:
    advice
    education
    instruction

  Excludes: *counseling (for):*
    contraception (V25.40-V25.49)
    genetic (V26.31-V26.39)
    on behalf of third party (V65.11, V65.19)
    procreative management (V26.41-V26.49)

  V65.40 Counseling NOS

  V65.41 Exercise counseling

  V65.42 Counseling on substance use and abuse

  V65.43 Counseling on injury prevention

  V65.44 Human immunodeficiency virus [HIV] counseling

  V65.45 Counseling on other sexually transmitted diseases

  V65.46 Encounter for insulin pump training

  V65.49 Other specified counseling

V65.5 Person with feared complaint in whom no diagnosis was made
  Feared condition not demonstrated
  Problem was normal state
  "Worried well"

V65.8 Other reasons for seeking consultation

  Excludes: *specified symptoms*

V65.9 Unspecified reason for consultation

V66 Convalescence and palliative care

V66.0 Following surgery

V66.1 Following radiotherapy

V66.2 Following chemotherapy

V66.3 Following psychotherapy and other treatment for mental disorder

V66.4 Following treatment of fracture

V66.5 Following other treatment

V66.6 Following combined treatment

V66.7 Encounter for palliative care
  End-of-life care
  Hospice care
  Terminal care

Code first underlying disease

V66.9 Unspecified convalescence

V67 Follow-up examination
  Includes: surveillance only following completed treatment

  Excludes: *surveillance of contraception (V25.40-V25.49)*

⑤ **V67.0 Following surgery**

  V67.00 Following surgery, unspecified

  V67.01 Follow-up vaginal pap smear
    Vaginal pap smear, status-post hysterectomy for malignant condition

  Use additional code to identify:
    acquired absence of uterus (V88.01-88.03)
    personal history of malignant neoplasm (V10.40-V10.44)

  Excludes: *vaginal pap smear status-post hysterectomy for non-malignant condition (V76.47)*

  V67.09 Following other surgery

  Excludes: *sperm count following sterilization reversal (V26.22)*
    sperm count for fertility testing (V26.21)

V67.1 Following radiotherapy

V67.2 Following chemotherapy
  Cancer chemotherapy follow-up

V67.3 Following psychotherapy and other treatment for mental disorder

● Code new
  to this edition

▲ Revision of
  existing code

④ ⑤ Fourth or fifth
  digit required

V67.4 Following treatment of healed fracture
    Excludes: *current (healing) fracture aftercare (V54.0-V54.9)*

⑤ **V67.5 Following other treatment**
    V67.51 Following completed treatment with high-risk medication, NEC
    Excludes: *long-term (current) drug use (V58.61-V58.69)*

    V67.59 Other

V67.6 Following combined treatment

V67.9 Unspecified follow-up examination

V68 Encounters for administrative purposes

⑤ **V68.0 Issue of medical certificates**
    Excludes: *encounter for general medical examination (V70.0-V70.9)*

    V68.01 Disability examination
    Use additional code(s) to identify:
        specific examination(s), screening and testing performed (V72.0-V82.9)

    V68.09 Other issue of medical certificates

V68.1 Issue of repeat prescriptions
    Issue of repeat prescription for:
      appliance
      glasses
      medications
    Excludes: *repeat prescription for contraceptives (V25.41-V25.49)*

V68.2 Request for expert evidence

⑤ **V68.8 Other specified administrative purpose**
    V68.81 Referral of patient without examination or treatment
    V68.89 Other

V68.9 Unspecified administrative purpose

V69 Problems related to lifestyle

V69.0 Lack of physical exercise

V69.1 Inappropriate diet and eating habits
    Excludes: *anorexia nervosa (307.1)*
        bulimia (783.6)
        malnutrition and other nutritional deficiencies (260-269.9)
        other and unspecified eating disorders (307.50-307.59)

V69.2 High-risk sexual behavior

V69.3 Gambling and betting
    Excludes: *pathological gambling (312.31)*

V69.4 Lack of adequate sleep
    Sleep deprivation
    Excludes: *insomnia (780.52)*

V69.5 Behavioral insomnia of childhood

V69.8 Other problems related to lifestyle
    Self-damaging behavior
    ALERT! Use this code as a secondary code if an asymptomatic patient is in a known high risk group for HIV

V69.9 Problem related to lifestyle, unspecified

PERSONS WITHOUT REPORTED DIAGNOSIS ENCOUNTERED DURING EXAMINATION AND INVESTIGATION OF INDIVIDUALS AND POPULATIONS (V70-V82)

    Note: Nonspecific abnormal findings disclosed at the time of these examinations are classifiable to categories 790-796.

V70 General medical examination
    Use additional code(s) to identify any special screening examination(s) performed (V73.0-V82.9)

| | Add 4th or 5th digit | | Nonspecific code | | Unspecific code | | Secondary Dx Only | | Primary Dx Only |

V70.0 **Routine general medical examination at a health care facility**
Health checkup

Excludes: *health checkup of infant or child over 28 days old (V20.2)*
health supervision of newborn 8 to 28 days old (V20.32)
health supervision of newborn under 8 days old (V20.31)
pre-procedural general physical examination (V72.83)

V70.1 **General psychiatric examination, requested by the authority**

V70.2 **General psychiatric examination, other and unspecified**

V70.3 **Other medical examination for administrative purposes**
General medical examination for:

admission to old age home	marriage
adoption	prison
camp	school admission
driving license	sports competition
immigration and naturalization	
insurance certification	

Excludes: *attendance for issue of medical certificates (V68.0)*
pre-employment screening (V70.5)

V70.4 **Examination for medicolegal reasons**
Blood-alcohol tests
Blood-drug tests
Paternity testing

Excludes: *examination and observation following:*
accidents (V71.3, V71.4)
assault (V71.6)
rape (V71.5)

V70.5 **Health examination of defined subpopulations**

Armed forces personnel	Preschool children
Inhabitants of institutions	Prisoners
Occupational health	Prostitutes
examinations	Refugees
Pre-employment screening	School children
	Students

V70.6 **Health examination in population surveys**

Excludes: *special screening (V73.0-V82.9)*

V70.7 **Examination of participant in clinical trial**
Examination of participant or control in clinical research

V70.8 **Other specified general medical examinations**
Examination of potential donor of organ or tissue

V70.9 **Unspecified general medical examination**

V71 **Observation and evaluation for suspected conditions not found**

Note: This category is to be used when persons without a diagnosis are suspected of having an abnormal condition, without signs or symptoms, which requires study, but after examination and observation, is found not to exist. This category is also for use for administrative and legal observation status.

Excludes: *suspected maternal and fetal conditions not found (V89.01-V89.09)*

⑤ **V71.0** **Observation for suspected mental condition**

V71.01 **Adult antisocial behavior**
Dyssocial behavior or gang activity in adult without manifest psychiatric disorder

V71.02 **Childhood or adolescent antisocial behavior**
Dyssocial behavior or gang activity in child or adolescent without manifest psychiatric disorder

V71.09 **Other suspected mental condition**

V71.1 **Observation for suspected malignant neoplasm**

V71.2 **Observation for suspected tuberculosis**

V71.3 **Observation following accident at work**

V71.4 **Observation following other accident**
Examination of individual involved in motor vehicle traffic accident

V71.5 **Observation following alleged rape or seduction**
Examination of victim or culprit

● Code new
to this edition

▲ Revision of
existing code

④ ⑤ Fourth or fifth
digit required

V71.6 Observation following other inflicted injury
Examination of victim or culprit

V71.7 Observation for suspected cardiovascular disease

⑤ **V71.8 Observation and evaluation for other specified suspected conditions**

Excludes: *contact with and (suspected) exposure to (potentially) hazardous substances (V15.84-V15.86, V87.0- V87.31)*

V71.81 Abuse and neglect

Excludes: *adult abuse and neglect (995.80-995.85)*
child abuse and neglect (995.50-995.59)

V71.82 Observation and evaluation for suspected exposure to anthrax

V71.83 Observation and evaluation for suspected exposure to other biological agent

V71.89 Other specified suspected conditions

V71.9 Observation for unspecified suspected condition

V72 Special investigations and examinations
Includes: routine examination of specific system

Excludes: *general medical examination (V70.0-V70.4)*
general screening examination of defined population groups (V70.5, V70.6, V70.7)
health supervision of newborn 8 to 28 days old (V20.32)
health supervision of newborn under 8 days old (V20.31)
routine examination of infant or child over 28 days old (V20.2)

Use additional code(s) to identify any special screening examination(s) performed (V73.0-V82.9)

V72.0 Examination of eyes and vision

⑤ **V72.1 Examination of ears and hearing**

V72.11 Encounter for hearing examination following failed hearing screening

V72.12 Encounter for hearing conservation and treatment

V72.19 Other examination of ears and hearing

V72.2 Dental examination

⑤ **V72.3 Gynecological examination**

Excludes: *cervical Papanicolaou smear without general gynecological examination (V76.2)*
routine examination in contraceptive management (V25.40-V25.49)

V72.31 Routine gynecological examination
General gynecological examination with or without Papanicolaou cervical smear
Pelvic examination (annual) (periodic)

Use additional code to identify routine:
human papillomavirus (HPV) screening (V73.81)
routine vaginal Papanicolaou smear (V76.47)

V72.32 Encounter for Papanicolaou cervical smear to confirm findings of recent normal smear following initial abnormal smear

⑤ **V72.4 Pregnancy examination or test**

V72.40 Pregnancy examination or test, pregnancy unconfirmed
Possible pregnancy, not (yet) confirmed

V72.41 Pregnancy examination or test, negative result

V72.42 Pregnancy examination or test, positive result

V72.5 Radiological examination, not elsewhere classified
Routine chest x-ray

Excludes: *radiologic examinations as part of pre-procedural testing (V72.81-V72.84)*

⑤ **V72.6 Laboratory examination**
Encounters for blood and urine testing

V72.60 Laboratory examination, unspecified

V72.61 Antibody response examination
Immunity status testing

Excludes: *encounter for allergy testing (V72.7)*

V72.62 Laboratory examination ordered as part of a routine general medical examination
Blood tests for routine general physical examination

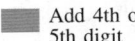
Add 4th or 5th digit   Nonspecific code   Unspecific code   Secondary Dx Only   Primary Dx Only

V72.63 Pre-procedural laboratory examination
Blood tests prior to treatment or procedure
Pre-operative laboratory examination

V72.69 Other laboratory examination

V72.7 Diagnostic skin and sensitization tests
Allergy tests
Skin tests for hypersensitivity

Excludes: *diagnostic skin tests for bacterial diseases (V74.0-V74.9)*

⑤ **V72.8 Other specified examinations**

Excludes: *pre-procedural laboratory examinations (V72.63)*

V72.81 Pre-operative cardiovascular examination
Pre-procedural cardiovascular examination

V72.82 Pre-operative respiratory examination
Pre-procedural respiratory examination

V72.83 Other specified pre-operative examination
Examination prior to chemotherapy
Other pre-procedural examination
Pre-procedural general physical examination

Excludes: *routine general medical examination (V70.0)*

V72.84 Pre-operative examination, unspecified
Pre-procedural examination, unspecified

V72.85 Other specified examination

V72.86 Encounter for blood typing

V72.9 Unspecified examination

V73 Special screening examination for viral and chlamydial diseases
DEFINITION Chlamydia is a type of bacteria one species of which causes an infection very similar to gonorrhea in the way that it is spread, the symptoms it produces, and the long-term consequences.

V73.0 Poliomyelitis

V73.1 Smallpox

V73.2 Measles

V73.3 Rubella

V73.4 Yellow fever

V73.5 Other arthropod-borne viral diseases
Dengue fever   Viral encephalitis:
Hemorrhagic fever   mosquito-borne
                                        tick-borne

V73.6 Trachoma

⑤ **V73.8 Other specified viral and chlamydial diseases**

V73.81 Human papillomavirus (HPV)

V73.88 Other specified chlamydial diseases

V73.89 Other specified viral diseases

ALERT! Use this code if a patient is being seen to determine his or her HIV status

⑤ **V73.9 Unspecified viral and chlamydial disease**

V73.98 Unspecified chlamydial disease

V73.99 Unspecified viral disease

V74 Special screening examination for bacterial and spirochetal diseases
Includes: diagnostic skin tests for these diseases

V74.0 Cholera

V74.1 Pulmonary tuberculosis

V74.2 Leprosy [Hansen's disease]

V74.3 Diphtheria

V74.4 Bacterial conjunctivitis

● Code new
   to this edition
▲ Revision of
   existing code
④ ⑤ Fourth or fifth
      digit required

V74.5 Venereal disease
Screening for bacterial and spirochetal sexually transmitted diseases
Screening for sexually transmitted diseases NOS

Excludes: special screening for nonbacterial sexually transmitted diseases (V73.81-V73.89, V75.4, V75.8)

V74.6 Yaws

V74.8 Other specified bacterial and spirochetal diseases
Brucellosis   Tetanus
Leptospirosis   Whooping cough
Plague

V74.9 Unspecified bacterial and spirochetal disease

V75 Special screening examination for other infectious diseases

V75.0 Rickettsial diseases

V75.1 Malaria

V75.2 Leishmaniasis

V75.3 Trypanosomiasis
Chagas' disease
Sleeping sickness

V75.4 Mycotic infections

V75.5 Schistosomiasis

V75.6 Filariasis

V75.7 Intestinal helminthiasis

V75.8 Other specified parasitic infections

V75.9 Unspecified infectious disease

V76 Special screening for malignant neoplasms

V76.0 Respiratory organs

⑤ **V76.1 Breast**

V76.10 Breast screening, unspecified

V76.11 Screening mammogram for high-risk patient

V76.12 Other screening mammogram

V76.19 Other screening breast examination

V76.2 Cervix
Routine cervical Papanicolaou smear

Excludes: special screening for human papillomavirus (V73.81)
            that as part of a general gynecological examination (V72.31)

V76.3 Bladder

⑤ **V76.4 Other sites**

V76.41 Rectum

V76.42 Oral cavity

V76.43 Skin

V76.44 Prostate

V76.45 Testis

V76.46 Ovary

V76.47 Vagina
Vaginal pap smear status-post hysterectomy for non-malignant condition
Use additional code to identify acquired absence of uterus (V88.01-V88.03)

Excludes: vaginal pap smear status-post hysterectomy for malignant condition (V67.01)

V76.49 Other sites

⑤ **V76.5 Intestine**

V76.50 Intestine, unspecified

V76.51 Colon
Screening colonoscopy NOS

Excludes: rectum (V76.41)

V76.52 Small intestine

⑤ **V76.8 Other neoplasm**

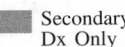 Add 4th or 5th digit   Nonspecific code   Unspecific code   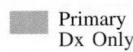 Secondary Dx Only   Primary Dx Only

V76.81 Nervous system

V76.89 Other neoplasm

V76.9 Unspecified

V77 Special screening for endocrine, nutritional, metabolic, and immunity disorders

V77.0 Thyroid disorders

V77.1 Diabetes mellitus

V77.2 Malnutrition

V77.3 Phenylketonuria [PKU]

V77.4 Galactosemia

V77.5 Gout

V77.6 Cystic fibrosis
        Screening for mucoviscidosis

V77.7 Other inborn errors of metabolism

V77.8 Obesity

⑤ V77.9 Other and unspecified endocrine, nutritional, metabolic, and immunity disorders

V77.91 Screening for lipoid disorders
        Screening cholesterol level
        Screening for hypercholesterolemia
        Screening for hyperlipidemia

V77.99 Other and unspecified endocrine, nutritional, metabolic, and immunity disorders

V78 Special screening for disorders of blood and blood-forming organs

V78.0 Iron deficiency anemia

V78.1 Other and unspecified deficiency anemia

V78.2 Sickle-cell disease or trait

V78.3 Other hemoglobinopathies

V78.8 Other disorders of blood and blood-forming organs

V78.9 Unspecified disorder of blood and blood-forming organs

V79 Special screening for mental disorders and developmental handicaps

V79.0 Depression

V79.1 Alcoholism

▲ V79.2 Intellectual disabilities

V79.3 Developmental handicaps in early childhood

V79.8 Other specified mental disorders and developmental handicaps

V79.9 Unspecified mental disorder and developmental handicap

V80 Special screening for neurological, eye, and ear diseases

⑤ V80.0 Neurological conditions

V80.01 Traumatic brain injury

V80.09 Other neurological conditions

V80.1 Glaucoma

V80.2 Other eye conditions
        Screening for:
            cataract
            congenital anomaly of eye
            senile macular lesions

        Excludes: general vision examination (V72.0)

V80.3 Ear diseases

        Excludes: general hearing examination (V72.11-V72.19)

V81 Special screening for cardiovascular, respiratory, and genitourinary diseases

V81.0 Ischemic heart disease

V81.1 Hypertension

V81.2 Other and unspecified cardiovascular conditions

V81.3 Chronic bronchitis and emphysema

● Code new   ▲ Revision of   ④ ⑤ Fourth or fifth
  to this edition   existing code   digit required

V81.4 Other and unspecified respiratory conditions

Excludes: *screening for:*
lung neoplasm (V76.0)
pulmonary tuberculosis (V74.1)

V81.5 Nephropathy
Screening for asymptomatic bacteriuria

V81.6 Other and unspecified genitourinary conditions

V82 Special screening for other conditions

V82.0 Skin conditions

V82.1 Rheumatoid arthritis

V82.2 Other rheumatic disorders

V82.3 Congenital dislocation of hip

V82.4 Maternal postnatal screening for chromosomal anomalies

Excludes: *antenatal screening by amniocentesis (V28.0)*

V82.5 Chemical poisoning and other contamination
Screening for:
heavy metal poisoning
ingestion of radioactive substance
poisoning from contaminated water supply
radiation exposure

V82.6 Multiphasic screening

⑤ **V82.7 Genetic screening**

Excludes: *genetic testing for procreative management (V26.31-V26.39)*

V82.71 Screening for genetic disease carrier status

V82.79 Other genetic screening

⑤ **V82.8 Other specified conditions**

V82.81 Osteoporosis
Use additional code to identify:
hormone replacement therapy (postmenopausal) status (V07.4)
postmenopausal (natural) status (V49.81)

V82.89 Other specified conditions

V82.9 Unspecified condition

GENETICS (V83-V84)

V83 Genetic carrier status

⑤ **V83.0 Hemophilia A carrier**

V83.01 Asymptomatic hemophilia A carrier

V83.02 Symptomatic hemophilia A carrier

⑤ **V83.8 Other genetic carrier status**

V83.81 Cystic fibrosis gene carrier

V83.89 Other genetic carrier status

V84 Genetic susceptibility to disease
Includes: Confirmed abnormal gene

Excludes: *chromosomal anomalies (758.0-758.9)*
Use additional code, if applicable, for any associated family history of the disease (V16-V19)

ALERT! Codes from category V84 should not be used as principal or first listed codes. If the patient has the condition to which he or she is susceptible, and that condition is the reason for the encounter, the code for the current condition should be sequenced first.

⑤ **V84.0 Genetic susceptibility to malignant neoplasm**
Code first, if applicable, any current malignant neoplasms (140.0-195.8, 200.0-208.9, 230.0-234.9)
Use additional code, if applicable, for any personal history of malignant neoplasm (V10.0-V10.9)

V84.01 Genetic susceptibility to malignant neoplasm of breast

V84.02 Genetic susceptibility to malignant neoplasm of ovary

V84.03 Genetic susceptibility to malignant neoplasm of prostate

V84.04 Genetic susceptibility to malignant neoplasm of endometrium

V84.09 Genetic susceptibility to other malignant neoplasm

Add 4th or 5th digit | Nonspecific code | Unspecific code | Secondary Dx Only | Primary Dx Only

⑤ **V84.8 Genetic susceptibility to other disease**

> **V84.81** **Genetic susceptibility to multiple endocrine neoplasia [MEN]**
>
> Excludes: *multiple endocrine neoplasia [MEN] syndromes (258.01-258.03)*

> **V84.89** **Genetic susceptibility to other disease**

BODY MASS INDEX (V85)

V85 Body Mass Index [BMI]

> Kilograms per meters squared
>
> Note: BMI adult codes are for use for persons over 20 years old
>
> **DEFINITION** Body mass index (BMI) is a measurement of the relative percentages of fat and muscle mass in the human body

V85.0 Body Mass Index less than 19, adult

V85.1 Body Mass Index between 19-24, adult

⑤ **V85.2 Body Mass Index between 25-29, adult**

> **V85.21** **Body Mass Index 25.0-25.9, adult**
>
> **V85.22** **Body Mass Index 26.0-26.9, adult**
>
> **V85.23** **Body Mass Index 27.0-27.9, adult**
>
> **V85.24** **Body Mass Index 28.0-28.9, adult**
>
> **V85.25** **Body Mass Index 29.0-29.9, adult**

⑤ **V85.3 Body Mass Index between 30-39, adult**

> **V85.30** **Body Mass Index 30.0-30.9, adult**
>
> **V85.31** **Body Mass Index 31.0-31.9, adult**
>
> **V85.32** **Body Mass Index 32.0-32.9, adult**
>
> **V85.33** **Body Mass Index 33.0-33.9, adult**
>
> **V85.34** **Body Mass Index 34.0-34.9, adult**
>
> **V85.35** **Body Mass Index 35.0-35.9, adult**
>
> **V85.36** **Body Mass Index 36.0-36.9, adult**
>
> **V85.37** **Body Mass Index 37.0-37.9, adult**
>
> **V85.38** **Body Mass Index 38.0-38.9, adult**
>
> **V85.39** **Body Mass Index 39.0-39.9, adult**

⑤ **V85.4 Body Mass Index 40 and over, adult**

> **V85.41** **Body Mass Index 40.0-44.9, adult**
>
> **V85.42** **Body Mass Index 45.0-49.9, adult**
>
> **V85.43** **Body Mass Index 50.0-59.9, adult**
>
> **V85.44** **Body Mass Index 60.0-69.9, adult**
>
> **V85.45** **Body Mass Index 70 and over, adult**

⑤ **V85.5 Body Mass Index, pediatric**

> Note:BMI pediatric codes are for use for persons age 2-20 years old. These percentiles are based on the growth charts published by the Centers for Disease Control and Prevention (CDC)
>
> **V85.51** **Body Mass Index, pediatric, less than 5th percentile for age**
>
> **V85.52** **Body Mass Index, pediatric, 5th percentile to less than 85th percentile for age**
>
> **V85.53** **Body Mass Index, pediatric, 85th percentile to less than 95th percentile for age**
>
> **V85.54** **Body Mass Index, pediatric, greater than or equal to 95th percentile for age**

ESTROGEN RECEPTOR STATUS (V86)

V86 Estrogen receptor status

> *Code first malignant neoplasm of breast (174.0-174.9, 175.0-175.9)*

V86.0 Estrogen receptor positive status (ER+)

V86.1 Estrogen receptor negative status (ER−)

● Code new to this edition   ▲ Revision of existing code   ④ ⑤ Fourth or fifth digit required

OTHER SPECIFIED PERSONAL EXPOSURES AND HISTORY PRESENTING HAZARDS TO HEALTH (V87)

V87 Other specified personal exposures and history presenting hazards to health

⑤ **V87.0** Contact with and (suspected) exposure to hazardous metals

> *Excludes:* *exposure to lead (V15.86)*
> *toxic effect of metals (984.0-985.9)*

V87.01 Arsenic

● **V87.02** Contact with and (suspected) exposure to uranium

> *Excludes:* *retained depleted uranium fragments (V90.01)*

V87.09 Other hazardous metals
Chromium compounds
Nickel dust

⑤ **V87.1** Contact with and (suspected) exposure to hazardous aromatic compounds

> *Excludes:* *toxic effects of aromatic compounds (982.0, 983.0)*

V87.11 Aromatic amines

V87.12 Benzene

V87.19 Other hazardous aromatic compounds
Aromatic dyes NOS
Polycyclic aromatic hydrocarbons

V87.2 Contact with and (suspected) exposure to other potentially hazardous chemicals
Dyes NOS

> *Excludes:* *exposure to asbestos (V15.84)*
> *toxic effect of chemicals (980-989)*

⑤ **V87.3** Contact with and (suspected) exposure to other potentially hazardous substances

> *Excludes:* *contact with and (suspected) exposure to potentially hazardous body fluids*
> *(V15.85)*
> *personal history of retained foreign body fully removed (V15.53)*
> *toxic effect of substances (980-989)*

V87.31 Exposure to mold

V87.32 Contact with and (suspected) exposure to algae bloom

V87.39 Contact with and (suspected) exposure to other potentially hazardous substances

⑤ **V87.4** Personal history of drug therapy

> *Excludes:* *long-term (current) drug use (V58.61-V58.69)*

V87.41 Personal history of antineoplastic chemotherapy

V87.42 Personal history of monoclonal drug therapy

V87.43 Personal history of estrogen therapy

V87.44 Personal history of inhaled steroid therapy

V87.45 Personal history of systemic steroid therapy
Personal history of steroid therapy NOS

V87.46 Personal history of immunosuppression therapy

> *Excludes:* *personal history of steroid therapy (V87.44, V87.45)*

V87.49 Personal history of other drug therapy

ACQUIRED ABSENCE OF OTHER ORGANS AND TISSUE (V88)

⑤ **V88** Acquired absence of other organs and tissue

⑤ **V88.0** Acquired absence of cervix and uterus

V88.01 Acquired absence of both cervix and uterus
Acquired absence of uterus NOS
Status post total hysterectomy

V88.02 Acquired absence of uterus with remaining cervical stump
Status post partial hysterectomy with remaining cervical stump

V88.03 Acquired absence of cervix with remaining uterus

⑤ **V88.1** Acquired absence of pancreas
Use additional code to identify any associated:
insulin use (V58.67)
secondary diabetes mellitus (249.00-249.91)

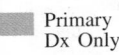

| | Add 4th or 5th digit | | Nonspecific code | | Unspecific code | | Secondary Dx Only | | Primary Dx Only |

V88.11 Acquired total absence of pancreas
Acquired absence of pancreas NOS

V88.12 Acquired partial absence of pancreas

● **V88.2 Acquired absence of joint**
Acquired absence of joint following prior explantation of joint prosthesis
Joint prosthesis explantation status

   ● **V88.21 Acquired absence of hip joint**
Acquired absence of hip joint following explantation of joint prosthesis, with
or without presence of antibiotic-impregnated cement spacer

   ● **V88.22 Acquired absence of knee joint**
Acquired absence of knee joint following explantation of joint prosthesis, with
or without presence of antibiotic-impregnated cement spacer

   ● **V88.29 Acquired absence of other joint**
Acquired absence of other joint following explantation of joint prosthesis, with
or without presence of antibiotic-impregnated cement spacer

OTHER SUSPECTED CONDITIONS NOT FOUND (V89)

⑤ **V89 Other suspected conditions not found**

   ⑤ **V89.0 Suspected maternal and fetal conditions not found**

   Excludes: *known or suspected fetal anomalies affecting management of mother, not ruled out*
(655.00, 655.93, 656.00-656.93, 657.00-657.03, 658.00-658.93)
newborn and perinatal conditions - code to condition

   V89.01 Suspected problem with amniotic cavity and membrane not found
Suspected oligohydramnios not found
Suspected polyhydramnios not found

   V89.02 Suspected placental problem not found

   V89.03 Suspected fetal anomaly not found

   V89.04 Suspected problem with fetal growth not found

   V89.05 Suspected cervical shortening not found

   V89.09 Other suspected maternal and fetal condition not found

RETAINED FOREIGN BODY (V90)

V90 Retained foreign body
Embedded fragment (status)
Embedded splinter (status)
Retained foreign body status

   Excludes: *artificial joint prosthesis status (V43.60-V43.69)*
foreign body accidentally left during a procedure (998.4)
foreign body entering through orifice (930.0-939.9)
in situ cardiac devices (V45.00-V45.09)
organ or tissue replaced by other means (V43.0-V43.89)
organ or tissue replaced by transplant (V42.0-V42.9)
personal history of retained foreign body removed (V15.53)
superficial foreign body (splinter) (categories 910-917 and 919 with 4th character
6 or 7, 918.0)

   ⑤ **V90.0 Retained radioactive fragment**

   V90.01 Retained depleted uranium fragments

   V90.09 Other retained radioactive fragments
Other retained depleted isotope fragments
Retained nontherapeutic radioactive fragments

   ⑤ **V90.1 Retained metal fragments**

   Excludes: *retained radioactive metal fragments (V90.01-V90.09)*

   V90.10 Retained metal fragments, unspecified
Retained metal fragment NOS

   V90.11 Retained magnetic metal fragments

   V90.12 Retained nonmagnetic metal fragments

   V90.2 Retained plastic fragments
Acrylics fragments
Diethylhexylphthalates fragments
Isocyanate fragments

   ⑤ **V90.3 Retained organic fragments**

   V90.31 Retained animal quills or spines

● Code new
to this edition

▲ Revision of
existing code

④ ⑤ Fourth or fifth
digit required

V90.32 Retained tooth

V90.33 Retained wood fragments

V90.39 Other retained organic fragments

⑤ V90.8 Other specified retained foreign body

V90.81 Retained glass fragments

V90.83 Retained stone or crystalline fragments
          Retained concrete or cement fragments

V90.89 Other specified retained foreign body

V90.9 Retained foreign body, unspecified material

MULTIPLE GESTATION PLACENTA STATUS (V91)

V91 Multiple gestation placenta status
      Code first multiple gestation (651.0-651.9)

⑤ V91.0 Twin gestation placenta status

V91.00 Twin gestation, unspecified number of placenta, unspecified number of amniotic sacs

V91.01 Twin gestation, monochorionic/monoamniotic (one placenta, one amniotic sac)

V91.02 Twin gestation, monochorionic/diamniotic (one placenta, two amniotic sacs)

V91.03 Twin gestation, dichorionic/diamniotic (two placentae, two amniotic sacs)

V91.09 Twin gestation, unable to determine number of placenta and number of amniotic sacs

⑤ V91.1 Triplet gestation placenta status

V91.10 Triplet gestation, unspecified number of placenta and unspecified number of amniotic sacs

V91.11 Triplet gestation, with two or more monochorionic fetuses

V91.12 Triplet gestation, with two or more monoamniotic fetuses

V91.19 Triplet gestation, unable to determine number of placenta and number of amniotic sacs

⑤ V91.2 Quadruplet gestation placenta status

V91.20 Quadruplet gestation, unspecified number of placenta and unspecified number of amniotic sacs

V91.21 Quadruplet gestation, with two or more monochorionic fetuses

V91.22 Quadruplet gestation, with two or more monoamniotic fetuses

V91.29 Quadruplet gestation, unable to determine number of placenta and number of amniotic sacs

⑤ V91.9 Other specified multiple gestation placenta status
          Placenta status for multiple gestations greater than quadruplets

V91.90 Other specified multiple gestation, unspecified number of placenta and unspecified number of amniotic sacs

V91.91 Other specified multiple gestation, with two or more monochorionic fetuses

V91.92 Other specified multiple gestation, with two or more monoamniotic fetuses

V91.99 Other specified multiple gestation, unable to determine number of placenta and number of amniotic sacs

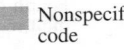 Add 4th or 5th digit

 Nonspecific code

Unspecific code

 Secondary Dx Only

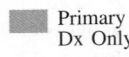 Primary Dx Only

This page intentionally left blank.

● Code new
to this edition

▲ Revision of
existing code

④ ⑤ Fourth or fifth
digit required

Chapter 19: Supplemental Classification of External Causes of Injury and Poisoning (E-codes, E800-E999)

DEFINITIONS AND CODING ALERTS

This chapter includes definitions of selected key words, terms and phrases and coding alerts for adding points to the clinical domain, references to coding late effects where appropriate, and references to personal history V-codes in situations where the acute or chronic condition is no longer active. An example from this chapter is as follows:

ACCIDENTAL FALLS (E880-E888)

> **ALERT!** For coding late effects of accidental fall see E929.3
> **ALERT!** For personal history of fall see V15.88

MULTIPLE CODING FOR A SINGLE CONDITION

In addition to the etiology or manifestation convention that requires two codes to fully describe a single condition that affects multiple body systems, there are other single conditions that also require more than one code. "Use additional code" notes are found in the tabular at codes that are not part of an etiology or manifestation pair where a secondary code is useful to fully describe a condition. The sequencing rule is the same as the etiology or manifestation pair - , "use additional code" indicates that a secondary code should be added.

"Code first" notes are also under certain codes that are not specifically manifestation codes but may be due to an underlying cause. When a "code first" note is present and an underlying condition is present the underlying condition should be sequenced first.

"Code, if applicable, any causal condition first", notes indicate that this code may be assigned as a principal diagnosis when the causal condition is unknown or not applicable. If a causal condition is known, then the code for that condition should be sequenced as the principal or first-listed diagnosis. Multiple codes may be needed for late effects, complication codes and obstetric codes to more fully describe a condition. See the specific guidelines for these conditions for further instruction.

COMBINATION CODE

A combination code is a single code used to classify: two diagnoses, or a diagnosis with an associated secondary process (manifestation) A diagnosis with an associated complication Combination codes are identified by referring to subterm entries in the Alphabetic Index and by reading the inclusion and exclusion notes in the Tabular List.

Assign only the combination code when that code fully identifies the diagnostic conditions involved or when the Alphabetic Index so directs. Multiple coding should not be used when the classification provides a combination code that clearly identifies all of the elements documented in the diagnosis. When the combination code lacks necessary specificity in describing the manifestation or complication, an additional code should be used as a secondary code.

CODING LATE EFFECTS

A late effect is the residual effect (condition produced) after the acute phase of an illness or injury has terminated. There is no time limit on when a late effect code can be used. The residual may be apparent early, such as in cerebrovascular accident cases, or it may occur months or years later, such as that due to a previous injury. Coding of late effects generally requires two codes sequenced in the following order: The condition or nature of the late effect is sequenced first. The late effect code is sequenced second.

An exception to the above guidelines are those instances where the code for late effect is followed by a manifestation code identified in the Tabular List and title, or the late effect code has been expanded (at the fourth and fifth-digit levels) to include the manifestation(s). The code for the acute phase of an illness or injury that led to the late effect is never used with a code for the late effect.

	Add 4th or 5th digit		Nonspecific code		Unspecified code		Manifestation code

INTRODUCTION

These guidelines are provided for those who are currently collecting E codes in order that there will be standardization in the process. If your institution plans to begin collecting E codes, these guidelines are to be applied. The use of E codes is supplemental to the application of ICD-9-CM diagnosis codes. E codes are never to be recorded as principal diagnoses (first-listed in non-inpatient setting) and are not required for reporting to CMS.

External causes of injury and poisoning codes (E codes) are intended to provide data for injury research and evaluation of injury prevention strategies. E codes capture how the injury or poisoning happened (cause), the intent (unintentional or accidental; or intentional, such as suicide or assault), and the place where the event occurred.

Some major categories of E codes include:

transport accidents poisoning and adverse effects of drugs, medicinal substances and biologicals accidental falls accidents caused by fire and flames accidents due to natural and environmental factors late effects of accidents, assaults or self injury assaults or purposely inflicted injury suicide or self inflicted injury

These guidelines apply for the coding and collection of E codes from records in hospitals, outpatient clinics, emergency departments, other ambulatory care settings and provider offices, and nonacute care settings, except when other specific guidelines apply.

GENERAL E CODE CODING GUIDELINES

An E code may be used with any code in the range of 001-V84.8, which indicates an injury, poisoning, or adverse effect due to an external cause.

Assign the appropriate E code for the initial encounter of an injury, poisoning, or adverse effect of drugs, not for subsequent treatment. External cause of injury codes (E-codes) may be assigned while the acute fracture codes are still applicable.

See Official Guidelines, Section I.C.17.b.1 for coding of acute fractures.

Use the full range of E codes to completely describe the cause, the intent and the place of occurrence, if applicable, for all injuries, poisonings, and adverse effects of drugs.

Assign as many E codes as necessary to fully explain each cause. If only one E code can be recorded, assign the E code most related to the principal diagnosis.

The selection of the appropriate E code is guided by the Index to External Causes, which is located after the alphabetical index to diseases and by Inclusion and Exclusion notes in the Tabular List.

An E code can never be a principal (first listed) diagnosis.

An external cause code is not appropriate with a code from subcategory 995.9, unless the patient also has an injury, poisoning, or adverse effect of drugs.

PLACE OF OCCURRENCE GUIDELINE

Use an additional code from category E849 to indicate the Place of Occurrence for injuries and poisonings. The Place of Occurrence describes the place where the event occurred and not the patient's activity at the time of the event.

Do not use E849.9 if the place of occurrence is not stated.

ADVERSE EFFECTS OF DRUGS, MEDICINAL AND BIOLOGICAL SUBSTANCES GUIDELINES

Do not code directly from the Table of Drugs and Chemicals. Always refer back to the Tabular List.

Use as many codes as necessary to describe completely all drugs, medicinal or biological substances.

If the same E code would describe the causative agent for more than one adverse reaction, assign the code only once.

If two or more drugs, medicinal or biological substances are reported, code each individually unless the combination code is listed in the Table of Drugs and Chemicals. In that case, assign the E code for the combination.

● Code new to this edition ▲ Revision of existing code ④ ⑤ Fourth or fifth digit required

When a reaction results from the interaction of a drug(s) and alcohol, use poisoning codes and E codes for both.

If the reporting format limits the number of E codes that can be used in reporting clinical data, code the one most related to the principal diagnosis. Include at least one from each category (cause, intent, place) if possible.

If there are different fourth digit codes in the same three digit category, use the code for "Other specified" of that category. If there is no "Other specified" code in that category, use the appropriate "Unspecified" code in that category.

If the codes are in different three digit categories, assign the appropriate E code for other multiple drugs and medicinal substances.

Codes from the E930-E949 series must be used to identify the causative substance for an adverse effect of drug, medicinal and biological substances, correctly prescribed and properly administered. The effect, such as tachycardia, delirium, gastrointestinal hemorrhaging, vomiting, hypokalemia, hepatitis, renal failure, or respiratory failure, is coded and followed by the appropriate code from the E930-E949 series.

MULTIPLE CAUSE E CODE CODING GUIDELINES

If two or more events cause separate injuries, an E code should be assigned for each cause. The first listed E code will be selected in the following order:

1. E codes for child and adult abuse take priority over all other E codes.

2. E codes for terrorism events take priority over all other E codes except child and adult abuse

3. E codes for cataclysmic events take priority over all other E codes except child and adult abuse and terrorism.

4. E codes for transport accidents take priority over all other E codes except cataclysmic events and child and adult abuse and terrorism.

5. The first-listed E code should correspond to the cause of the most serious diagnosis due to an assault, accident, or self-harm, following the order of hierarchy listed above.

CHILD AND ADULT ABUSE GUIDELINE

Intentional injury

When the cause of an injury or neglect is intentional child or adult abuse, the first listed E code should be assigned from categories E960-E968, Homicide and injury purposely inflicted by other persons, (except category E967.. An E code from category E967, Child and adult battering and other maltreatment, should be added as an additional code to identify the perpetrator, if known.

Accidental intent

In cases of neglect when the intent is determined to be accidental E code E904.0, Abandonment or neglect of infant and helpless person, should be the first listed E code.

UNKNOWN OR SUSPECTED INTENT GUIDELINE

If the intent (accident, self-harm, assault) of the cause of an injury or poisoning is unknown or unspecified, code the intent as undetermined E980-E989.

If the intent (accident, self-harm, assault) of the cause of an injury or poisoning is questionable, probable or suspected, code the intent as undetermined E980-E989.

UNDETERMINED CAUSE

When the intent of an injury or poisoning is known, but the cause is unknown, use codes: E928.9, Unspecified accident, E958.9, Suicide and self-inflicted injury by unspecified means, and E968.9, Assault by unspecified means.

These E codes should rarely be used, as the documentation in the medical record, in both the inpatient outpatient and other settings, should normally provide sufficient detail to determine the cause of the injury.

	Add 4th or 5th digit		Nonspecific code		Unspecified code		Manifestation code

LATE EFFECTS OF EXTERNAL CAUSE GUIDELINES

Late effect E codes exist for injuries and poisonings but not for adverse effects of drugs, misadventures and surgical complications.

A late effect E code (E929, E959, E969, E977, E989, or E999.1), should be used with any report of a late effect or sequela resulting from a previous injury or poisoning (905-909..

A late effect E code should never be used with a related current nature of injury code.

Use a late effect E code for subsequent visits when a late effect of the initial injury or poisoning is being treated. There is no late effect E code for adverse effects of drugs.
Do not use a late effect E code for subsequent visits for followup care (e.g., to assess healing, to receive rehabilitative therapy) of the injury or poisoning when no late effect of the injury has been documented.

MISADVENTURES AND COMPLICATIONS OF CARE GUIDELINES

Assign a code in the range of E870-E876 if misadventures are stated by the provider.

Assign a code in the range of E878-E879 if the provider attributes an abnormal reaction or later complication to a surgical or medical procedure, but does not mention misadventure at the time of the procedure as the cause of the reaction.

TERRORISM GUIDELINES

Cause of injury identified by the Federal Government (FBI) as terrorism

When the cause of an injury is identified by the Federal Government (FBI) as terrorism, the first-listed E-code should be a code from category E979, Terrorism. The definition of terrorism employed by the FBI is found at the inclusion note at E979. The terrorism E-code is the only E-code that should be assigned. Additional E codes from the assault categories should not be assigned.

Cause of an injury is suspected to be the result of terrorism

When the cause of an injury is suspected to be the result of terrorism a code from category E979 should not be assigned. Assign a code in the range of E codes based circumstances on the documentation of intent and mechanism.

Code E979.9, Terrorism, secondary effects

Assign code E979.9, Terrorism, secondary effects, for conditions occurring subsequent to the terrorist event. This code should not be assigned for conditions that are due to the initial terrorist act.

● Code new to this edition ▲ Revision of existing code ④ ⑤ Fourth or fifth digit required

SUPPLEMENTARY CLASSIFICATION OF EXTERNAL CAUSES OF INJURY AND POISONING (E000-E999)

This section is provided to permit the classification of environmental events, circumstances, and conditions as the cause of injury, poisoning, and other adverse effects. Where a code from this section is applicable, it is intended that it shall be used in addition to a code from one of the main chapters of *ICD-9-CM*, indicating the nature of the condition. Certain other conditions which may be stated to be due to external causes are classified in Chapters 1 to 16 of *ICD-9-CM*. For these, the "E" code classification should be used for more detailed analysis.

Machinery accidents [other than those connected with transport] are classifiable to category E919, in which the fourth-digit allows a broad classification of the type of machinery involved.

Categories for "late effects" of accidents and other external causes are to be found at E929, E959, E969, E977, E989, and E999.

EXTERNAL CAUSE STATUS (E000)

Note: A code from category E000 should be used in conjunction with the external cause code(s) assigned to a record to indicate the status of the person at the time the event occurred. A single code from category E000 should be assigned for an encounter.

E000 External cause status

E000.0 Civilian activity done for income or pay
Civilian activity done for financial or other compensation
Excludes: *military activity (E000.1)*

E000.1 Military activity
Excludes: *activity of off duty military personnel (E000.8)*

E000.2 Volunteer activity
Excludes: *activity of child or other family member assisting in compensated work of other family member (E000.8)*

E000.8 Other external cause status
Activity NEC
Activity of child or other family member assisting in compensated work of other family member
Hobby not done for income
Leisure activity
Off-duty activity of military personnel
Recreation or sport not for income or while a student
Student activity

E000.9 Unspecified external cause status

ACTIVITY (E001-E030)

Note: Categories E001 to E030 are provided for use to indicate the activity of the person seeking healthcare for an injury or health condition, such as a heart attack while shoveling snow, which resulted from, or was contributed to, by the activity. These codes are appropriate for use for both acute injuries, such as those from chapter 17, and conditions that are due to the long-term, cumulative effects of an activity, such as those from chapter 13. They are also appropriate for use with external cause codes for cause and intent if identifying the activity provides additional information on the event.

These codes should be used in conjunction with other external cause codes for external cause status (E000) and place of occurrence (E849).

This section contains the following broad activity categories:
E001 Activities involving walking and running
E002 Activities involving water and water craft
E003 Activities involving ice and snow
E004 Activities involving climbing, rappelling, and jumping off
E005 Activities involving dancing and other rhythmic movement
E006 Activities involving other sports and athletics played individually
E007 Activities involving other sports and athletics played as a team or group
E008 Activities involving other specified sports and athletics
E009 Activity involving other cardiorespiratory exercise
E010 Activity involving other muscle strengthening exercises
E011 Activities involving computer technology and electronic devices
E012 Activities involving arts and handcrafts
E013 Activities involving personal hygiene and household maintenance
E014 Activities involving person providing caregiving
E015 Activities involving food preparation, cooking and grilling

Add 4th or 5th digit   Nonspecific code   Unspecified code   Manifestation code

E016 Activities involving property and land maintenance, building and construction
E017 Activities involving roller coasters and other types of external motion
E018 Activities involving playing musical instrument
E019 Activities involving animal care
E029 Other activity
E030 Unspecified activity

E001 Activities involving walking and running

Excludes: walking an animal (E019.0)
walking or running on a treadmill (E009.0)

E001.0 Walking, marching and hiking
Walking, marching and hiking on level or elevated terrain
Excludes: mountain climbing (E004.0)

E001.1 Running

E002 Activities involving water and water craft

Excludes: activities involving ice (E003.0-E003.9)
boating and other watercraft transport accidents (E830-E838)

E002.0 Swimming

E002.1 Springboard and platform diving

E002.2 Water polo

E002.3 Water aerobics and water exercise

E002.4 Underwater diving and snorkeling
SCUBA diving

E002.5 Rowing, canoeing, kayaking, rafting and tubing
Canoeing, kayaking, rafting and tubing in calm and turbulent water

E002.6 Water skiing and wake boarding

E002.7 Surfing, windsurfing and boogie boarding

E002.8 Water sliding

E002.9 Other activity involving water and watercraft
Activity involving water NOS
Parasailing
Water survival training and testing

E003 Activities involving ice and snow

Excludes: shoveling ice and snow (E016.0)

E003.0 Ice skating
Figure skating (singles) (pairs)
Ice dancing
Excludes: ice hockey (E003.1)

E003.1 Ice hockey

E003.2 Snow (alpine) (downhill) skiing, snow boarding, sledding, tobogganing and snow tubing
Excludes: cross country skiing (E003.3)

E003.3 Cross country skiing
Nordic skiing

E003.9 Other activity involving ice and snow
Activity involving ice and snow NOS

E004 Activities involving climbing, rappelling and jumping off

Excludes: hiking on level or elevated terrain (E001.0)
jumping rope (E006.5)
sky diving (E840-E844)
trampoline jumping (E005.3)

E004.0 Mountain climbing, rock climbing and wall climbing

E004.1 Rappelling

E004.2 BASE jumping
Building, Antenna, Span, Earth jumping

E004.3 Bungee jumping

E004.4 Hang gliding

● Code new to this edition   ▲ Revision of existing code   ④ ⑤ Fourth or fifth digit required

E004.9   **Other activity involving climbing, rappelling and jumping off**

E005 **Activities involving dancing and other rhythmic movement**

    Excludes: *martial arts (E008.4)*

E005.0   **Dancing**

E005.1   **Yoga**

E005.2   **Gymnastics**
      Rhythmic gymnastics
    Excludes: *trampoline (E005.3)*

E005.3   **Trampoline**

E005.4   **Cheerleading**

E005.9   **Other activity involving dancing and other rhythmic movements**

E006 **Activities involving other sports and athletics played individually**

    Excludes: *dancing (E005.0)*
           gymnastic (E005.2)
           trampoline (E005.3)
           yoga (E005.1)

E006.0   **Roller skating (inline) and skateboarding**

E006.1   **Horseback riding**

E006.2   **Golf**

E006.3   **Bowling**

E006.4   **Bike riding**

    Excludes: *transport accident involving bike riding (E800-E829)*

E006.5   **Jumping rope**

E006.6   **Non-running track and field events**

    Excludes: *running (any form) (E001.1)*

E006.9   **Other activity involving other sports and athletics played individually**

    Excludes: *activities involving climbing, rappelling, and jumping (E004.0-E004.9)*
           activities involving ice and snow (E003.0-E003.9)
           activities involving walking and running (E001.0-E001.9)
           activities involving water and watercraft (E002.0-E002.9)

E007 **Activities involving other sports and athletics played as a team or group**

    Excludes: *ice hockey (E003.1)*
           water polo (E002.2)

E007.0   **American tackle football**
      Football NOS

E007.1   **American flag or touch football**

E007.2   **Rugby**

E007.3   **Baseball**
      Softball

E007.4   **Lacrosse and field hockey**

E007.5   **Soccer**

E007.6   **Basketball**

E007.7   **Volleyball (beach) (court)**

E007.8   **Physical games generally associated with school recess, summer camp and children**
      Capture the flag
      Dodge ball
      Four square
      Kickball

E007.9   **Other activity involving other sports and athletics played as a team or group**
      Cricket

E008 **Activities involving other specified sports and athletics**

E008.0   **Boxing**

E008.1   **Wrestling**

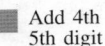 Add 4th or 5th digit   Nonspecific code   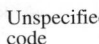 Unspecified code   Manifestation code

E008.2 **Racquet and hand sports**
Handball
Racquetball
Squash
Tennis

E008.3 **Frisbee**
Ultimate frisbee

E008.4 **Martial arts**
Combatives

E008.9 **Other specified sports and athletics activity**

Excludes: sports and athletics activities specified in categories E001-E007

E009 **Activity involving other cardiorespiratory exercise**
Activity involving physical training

E009.0 **Exercise machines primarily for cardiorespiratory conditioning**
Elliptical and stepper machines
Stationary bike
Treadmill

E009.1 **Calisthenics**
Jumping jacks
Warm up and cool down

E009.2 **Aerobic and step exercise**

E009.3 **Circuit training**

E009.4 **Obstacle course**
Challenge course
Confidence course

E009.5 **Grass drills**
Guerilla drills

E009.9 **Other activity involving other cardiorespiratory exercise**

Excludes: activities involving cardiorespiratory exercise specified in categories E001-E008

E010 **Activity involving other muscle strengthening exercises**

E010.0 **Exercise machines primarily for muscle strengthening**

E010.1 **Push-ups, pull-ups, sit-ups**

E010.2 **Free weights**
Barbells
Dumbbells

E010.3 **Pilates**

E010.9 **Other activity involving other muscle strengthening exercises**

Excludes: activities involving muscle strengthening specified in categories E001-E009

E011 **Activities involving computer technology and electronic devices**

Excludes: electronic musical keyboard or instruments (E018.0)

E011.0 **Computer keyboarding**
Electronic game playing using keyboard or other stationary device

E011.1 **Hand held interactive electronic device**
Cellular telephone and communication device
Electronic game playing using interactive device

Excludes: electronic game playing using keyboard or other stationary device (E011.0)

E011.9 **Other activity involving computer technology and electronic devices**

E012 **Activities involving arts and handcrafts**

Excludes: activities involving playing musical instrument (E018.0-E018.3)

E012.0 **Knitting and crocheting**

E012.1 **Sewing**

E012.2 **Furniture building and finishing**
Furniture repair

E012.9 **Activity involving other arts and handcrafts**

● Code new
to this edition
▲ Revision of
existing code
④ ⑤ Fourth or fifth
digit required

E013 Activities involving personal hygiene and household maintenance

Excludes: activities involving cooking and grilling (E015.0-E015.9)
activities involving property and land maintenance, building and construction (E016.0-E016.9)
activity involving persons providing caregiving (E014.0-E014.9)
dishwashing (E015.0)
food preparation (E015.0)
gardening (E016.1)

E013.0 **Personal bathing and showering**

E013.1 **Laundry**

E013.2 **Vacuuming**

E013.3 **Ironing**

E013.4 **Floor mopping and cleaning**

E013.5 **Residential relocation**
Packing up and unpacking involved in moving to a new residence

E013.8 **Other personal hygiene activity**

E013.9 **Other household maintenance**

E014 Activities involving person providing caregiving

E014.0 **Caregiving involving bathing**

E014.1 **Caregiving involving lifting**

E014.9 **Other activity involving person providing caregiving**

E015 Activities involving food preparation, cooking and grilling

E015.0 **Food preparation and clean up**
Dishwashing

E015.1 **Grilling and smoking food**

E015.2 **Cooking and baking**
Use of stove, oven and microwave oven

E015.9 **Other activity involving cooking and grilling**

E016 Activities involving property and land maintenance, building and construction

E016.0 **Digging, shoveling and raking**
Dirt digging
Raking leaves
Snow shoveling

E016.1 **Gardening and landscaping**
Pruning, trimming shrubs, weeding

E016.2 **Building and construction**

E016.9 **Other activity involving property and land maintenance, building and construction**

E017 Activities involving roller coasters and other types of external motion

E017.0 **Roller coaster riding**

E017.9 **Other activity involving external motion**

E018 Activities involving playing musical instrument
Activity involving playing electric musical instrument

E018.0 **Piano playing**
Musical keyboard (electronic) playing

E018.1 **Drum and other percussion instrument playing**

E018.2 **String instrument playing**

E018.3 **Wind and brass instrument playing**

E019 Activities involving animal care

Excludes: horseback riding (E006.1)

E019.0 **Walking an animal**

E019.1 **Milking an animal**

E019.2 **Grooming and shearing an animal**

E019.9 **Other activity involving animal care**

E029 Other activity

E029.0 **Refereeing a sports activity**

E029.1 **Spectator at an event**

Add 4th or
5th digit

Nonspecific
code

Unspecified
code

Manifestation
code

E029.2   **Rough housing and horseplay**

E029.9   **Other activity**

E030 Unspecified activity

TRANSPORT ACCIDENTS (E800-E848)

Definitions and examples related to transport accidents

(a) A **transport accident** (E800-E848) is any accident involving a device designed primarily for, or being used at the time primarily for, conveying persons or goods from one place to another.

Includes: accidents involving:

> aircraft and spacecraft (E840-E845)
> watercraft (E830-E838)
> motor vehicle (E810-E825)
> railway (E800-E807)
> other road vehicles (E826-E829)

In classifying accidents which involve more than one kind of transport, the above order of precedence of transport accidents should be used.

Accidents involving agriculture and construction machines, such as tractors, cranes, and bulldozers, are regarded as transport accidents only when these vehicles are under their own power on a highway [otherwise the vehicles are regarded as machinery]. Vehicles which can travel on land or water, such as hovercraft and other amphibious vehicles, are regarded as watercraft when on the water, as motor vehicles when on the highway, and as off-road motor vehicles when on land, but off the highway.

Excludes: *accidents:*

> *in sports which involve the use of transport but where the transport vehicle itself was not involved in the accident*
> *involving vehicles which are part of industrial equipment used entirely on industrial premises*
> *occurring during transportation but unrelated to the hazards associated with the means of transportation [e.g., injuries received in a fight on board ship; transport vehicle involved in a cataclysm such as an earthquake]*
> *to persons engaged in the maintenance or repair of transport equipment or vehicle not in motion, unless injured by another vehicle in motion*

(b) A **railway accident** is a transport accident involving a railway train or other railway vehicle operated on rails, whether in motion or not.

Excludes: *accidents:*

> *in repair shops*
> *in roundhouse or on turntable*
> *on railway premises but not involving a train or other railway vehicle*

(c) A **railway train** or **railway vehicle** is any device with or without cars coupled to it, designed for traffic on a railway.

Includes: interurban:

> electric car (operated chiefly on its own right-of-way, not open to other traffic)
> streetcar (operated chiefly on its own right-of-way, not open to other traffic)
> railway train, any power [diesel] [electric] [steam]
> funicular
> monorail or two-rail
> subterranean or elevated
> other vehicle designed to run on a railway track

Excludes: *interurban electric cars [streetcars] specified to be operating on a right-of-way that forms part of the public street or highway [definition (n)]*

(d) A **railway** or **railroad** is a right-of-way designed for traffic on rails, which is used by carriages or wagons transporting passengers or freight, and by other rolling stock, and which is not open to other public vehicular traffic.

(e) A **motor vehicle accident** is a transport accident involving a motor vehicle. It is defined as a motor vehicle traffic accident or as a motor vehicle nontraffic accident according to whether the accident occurs on a public highway or elsewhere.

Excludes: *injury or damage due to cataclysm*

> *injury or damage while a motor vehicle, not under its own power, is being loaded on, or unloaded from, another conveyance*

(f) A **motor vehicle traffic accident** is any motor vehicle accident occurring on a public highway [i.e., originating, terminating, or involving a vehicle partially on the highway]. A motor vehicle accident is assumed to have occurred on the highway unless another place is specified, except in the case of accidents involving only off-road motor vehicles which are classified as nontraffic accidents unless the contrary is stated.

(g) A **motor vehicle nontraffic accident** is any motor vehicle accident which occurs entirely in any place other than a public highway.

810   ● Code new   ▲ Revision of   ④ ⑤ Fourth or fifth
           to this edition   existing code   digit required

(h) A **public highway [trafficway]** or **street** is the entire width between property lines [or other boundary lines] of every way or place, of which any part is open to the use of the public for purposes of vehicular traffic as a matter of right or custom. A roadway is that part of the public highway designed, improved, and ordinarily used, for vehicular travel.

Includes: approaches (public) to:
>docks
>public building
>station

Excludes: *driveway (private)*
>*parking lot*
>*ramp*
>*roads in:*
>*airfield*
>*farm*
>*industrial premises*
>*mine*
>*private grounds*
>*quarry*

(i) A **motor vehicle** is any mechanically or electrically powered device, not operated on rails, upon which any person or property may be transported or drawn upon a highway. Any object such as a trailer, coaster, sled, or wagon being towed by a motor vehicle is considered a part of the motor vehicle.

Includes: automobile [any type]
>bus
>construction machinery, farm and industrial machinery, steam roller, tractor, army tank, highway grader, or similar vehicle on wheels or treads, while in transport under own power
>fire engine (motorized)
>motorcycle
>motorized bicycle [moped] or scooter
>trolley bus not operating on rails
>truck
>van

Excludes: *devices used solely to move persons or materials within the confines of a building and its premises, such as:*
>*building elevator*
>*coal car in mine*
>*electric baggage or mail truck used solely within a railroad station*
>*electric truck used solely within an industrial plant*
>*moving overhead crane*

(j) A **motorcycle** is a two-wheeled motor vehicle having one or two riding saddles and sometimes having a third wheel for the support of a sidecar. The sidecar is considered part of the motorcycle.

Includes: motorized:
>bicycle [moped]
>scooter
>tricycle

(k) An **off-road motor vehicle** is a motor vehicle of special design, to enable it to negotiate rough or soft terrain or snow. Examples of special design are high construction, special wheels and tires, driven by treads, or support on a cushion of air.

Includes: all terrain vehicle [ATV]
>army tank
>hovercraft, on land or swamp
>snowmobile

(l) A **driver** of a motor vehicle is the occupant of the motor vehicle operating it or intending to operate it. A **motorcyclist** is the driver of a motorcycle. Other authorized occupants of a motor vehicle are **passengers.**

(m) An **other road vehicle** is any device, except a motor vehicle, in, on, or by which any person or property may be transported on a highway.

Includes: animal carrying a person or goods
>animal-drawn vehicle
>animal harnessed to conveyance
>bicycle [pedal cycle]
>streetcar
>tricycle (pedal)

Excludes: *pedestrian conveyance [definition (q)]*

811

Add 4th or 5th digit	Nonspecific code	Unspecified code	Manifestation code

(n) A **streetcar** is a device designed and used primarily for transporting persons within a municipality, running on rails, usually subject to normal traffic control signals, and operated principally on a right-of-way that forms part of the traffic way. A trailer being towed by a streetcar is considered a part of the streetcar.

Includes: interurban or intraurban electric or streetcar, when specified to be operating on a street or public highway

tram (car)

trolley (car)

(o) A **pedal cycle** is any road transport vehicle operated solely by pedals.

Includes: bicycle

pedal cycle

tricycle

Excludes: *motorized bicycle [definition (i)]*

(p) A **pedal cyclist** is any person riding on a pedal cycle or in a sidecar attached to such a vehicle.

(q) A **pedestrian conveyance** is any human powered device by which a pedestrian may move other than by walking or by which a walking person may move another pedestrian.

Includes:

baby carriage	pushchair
coaster wagon	roller skates
heelies	scooter
ice skates	skateboard
motorized mobility	skis
scooter	sled
perambulator	wheelchair (electric)
pushcart	wheelies

(r) A **pedestrian** is any person involved in an accident who was not at the time of the accident riding in or on a motor vehicle, railroad train, streetcar, animal-drawn or other vehicle, or on a bicycle or animal.

Includes: person:

changing tire of vehicle

in or operating a pedestrian conveyance

making adjustment to motor of vehicle

on foot

(s) A **watercraft** is any device for transporting passengers or goods on the water.

(t) A **small boat** is any watercraft propelled by paddle, oars, or small motor, with a passenger capacity of less than ten.

Includes:

boat NOS	rowboat
canoe	rowing shell
coble	scull
dinghy	skiff
punt	small motorboat
raft	

Excludes: *barge*

lifeboat (used after abandoning ship)

raft (anchored) being used as diving platform

yacht

(u) An **aircraft** is any device for transporting passengers or goods in the air.

Includes: airplane [any type]

balloon

bomber

dirigible

glider (hang)

military aircraft

parachute

(v) A **commercial transport aircraft** is any device for collective passenger or freight transportation by air, whether run on commercial lines for profit or by government authorities, with the exception of military craft.

● Code new to this edition ▲ Revision of existing code ④ ⑤ Fourth or fifth digit required

RAILWAY ACCIDENTS (E800-E807)

Note: For definitions of railway accident and related terms see definitions (a) to (d).

Excludes: *accidents involving railway train and:*
> *aircraft (E840.0-E845.9)*
> *motor vehicle (E810.0-E825.9)*
> *watercraft (E830.0-E838.9)*

The following fourth-digit subdivisions are for use with categories E800-E807 to identify the injured person:

.0 Railway employee
Any person who by virtue of his employment in connection with a railway, whether by the railway company or not, is at increased risk of involvement in a railway accident, such as:
catering staff of train
driver
guard
porter
postal staff on train
railway fireman
shunter
sleeping car attendant

.1 Passenger on railway
Any authorized person traveling on a train, except a railway employee.

Excludes: *intending passenger waiting at station (.8)*
> *unauthorized rider on railway vehicle (.8)*

.2 Pedestrian
See definition (r)

.3 Pedal cyclist
See definition (p)

.8 Other specified person
Intending passenger or bystander waiting at station
Unauthorized rider on railway vehicle

.9 Unspecified person

④ **E800 Railway accident involving collision with rolling stock**
Includes: collision between railway trains or railway vehicles, any kind
collision NOS on railway
derailment with antecedent collision with rolling stock or NOS

④ **E801 Railway accident involving collision with other object**
Includes: collision of railway train with:
> buffers
> fallen tree on railway
> gates
> platform
> rock on railway
> streetcar
> other nonmotor vehicle
> other object

Excludes: *collision with:*
> *aircraft (E840.0-E842.9)*
> *motor vehicle (E810.0-E810.9, E820.0-E822.9)*

④ **E802 Railway accident involving derailment without antecedent collision**

④ **E803 Railway accident involving explosion, fire, or burning**

Excludes: *explosion or fire, with antecedent derailment (E802.0-E802.9)*
> *explosion or fire, with mention of antecedent collision (E800.0-E801.9)*

④ **E804 Fall in, on, or from railway train**
Includes: fall while alighting from or boarding railway train

Excludes: *fall related to collision, derailment, or explosion of railway train (E800.0-E803.9)*

Add 4th or 5th digit Nonspecific code Unspecified code Manifestation code

④ **E805** **Hit by rolling stock**
        Includes: crushed by railway train or part
                     injured by railway train or part
                     killed by railway train or part
                     knocked down by railway train or part
                     run over by railway train or part

        Excludes: *pedestrian hit by object set in motion by railway train (E806.0-E806.9)*

④ **E806** **Other specified railway accident**
        Includes: hit by object falling in railway train
                     injured by door or window on railway train
                     nonmotor road vehicle or pedestrian hit by object set in motion by railway train
                     railway train hit by falling:
                     earth NOS
                     rock
                     tree
                     other object

        Excludes: *railway accident due to cataclysm (E908-E909)*

④ **E807** **Railway accident of unspecified nature**
        Includes:
                     found dead on railway right-of-way NOS
                     injured on railway right-of-way NOS
                     railway accident NOS

MOTOR VEHICLE TRAFFIC ACCIDENTS (E810-E819)

      Note: For definitions of motor vehicle traffic accident, and related terms, see definitions (e) to (k).

      Excludes: *accidents involving motor vehicle and aircraft (E840.0-E845.9)*

      The following fourth-digit subdivisions are for use with categories E810-E819 to identify the
          injured person:

      .0 Driver of motor vehicle other than motorcycle
          See definition (l)

      .1 Passenger in motor vehicle other than motorcycle
          See definition (l)

      .2 Motorcyclist
          See definition (l)

      .3 Passenger on motorcycle
          See definition (l)

      .4 Occupant of streetcar

      .5 Rider of animal; occupant of animal-drawn vehicle

      .6 Pedal cyclist
          See definition (p)

      .7 Pedestrian
          See definition (r)

      .8 Other specified person
          Occupant of vehicle other than above
          Person in railway train involved in accident
          Unauthorized rider of motor vehicle

      .9 Unspecified person
      ALERT! For coding late effects of motor vehicle accident see E929.0

④ **E810** **Motor vehicle traffic accident involving collision with train**

      Excludes: *motor vehicle collision with object set in motion by railway train (E815.0-E815.9)*
                 railway train hit by object set in motion by motor vehicle (E818.0-E818.9)

④ **E811** **Motor vehicle traffic accident involving re-entrant collision with another motor vehicle**
        Includes: collision between motor vehicle which accidentally leaves the roadway then
                     re-enters the same roadway, or the opposite roadway on a divided highway, and
                     another motor vehicle

      Excludes: *collision on the same roadway when none of the motor vehicles involved have left*
                 and re-entered the roadway (E812.0-E812.9)

④ **E812** **Other motor vehicle traffic accident involving collision with motor vehicle**
        Includes: collision with another motor vehicle parked, stopped, stalled, disabled, or
                     abandoned on the highway
                     motor vehicle collision NOS

      Excludes: *collision with object set in motion by another motor vehicle (E815.0-E815.9)*
                 re-entrant collision with another motor vehicle (E811.0-E811.9)

● Code new
  to this edition
▲ Revision of
  existing code
④ ⑤ Fourth or fifth
     digit required

④ **E813** **Motor vehicle traffic accident involving collision with other vehicle**
    Includes: collision between motor vehicle, any kind, and:
            other road (nonmotor transport) vehicle, such as:
              animal carrying a person
              animal-drawn vehicle
              pedal cycle
              streetcar

    Excludes: *collision with:*
        object set in motion by nonmotor road vehicle (E815.0-E815.9)
        pedestrian (E814.0-E814.9)
        nonmotor road vehicle hit by object set in motion by motor vehicle
          (E818.0-E818.9)

④ **E814** **Motor vehicle traffic accident involving collision with pedestrian**
    Includes: collision between motor vehicle, any kind, and pedestrian
            pedestrian dragged, hit, or run over by motor vehicle, any kind

    Excludes: *pedestrian hit by object set in motion by motor vehicle (E818.0-E818.9)*

④ **E815** **Other motor vehicle traffic accident involving collision on the highway**
    Includes: collision (due to loss of control) (on highway) between motor vehicle, any kind, and:
            abutment (bridge) (overpass)
            animal (herded) (unattended)
            fallen stone, traffic sign, tree, utility pole
            guard rail or boundary fence
            interhighway divider
            landslide (not moving)
            object set in motion by railway train or road vehicle (motor) (nonmotor)
            object thrown in front of motor vehicle
            safety island
            temporary traffic sign or marker
            wall of cut made for road
            other object, fixed, movable, or moving

    Excludes: *collision with:*
        any object off the highway (resulting from loss of control) (E816.0-E816.9)
        any object which normally would have been off the highway and is not stated to
          have been on it (E816.0-E816.9)
        motor vehicle parked, stopped, stalled, disabled, or abandoned on highway
          (E812.0-E812.9)
        moving landslide (E909)
      motor vehicle hit by object:
        set in motion by railway train or road vehicle (motor) (nonmotor)
          (E818.0-E818.9)
         thrown into or on vehicle (E818.0-E818.9)

Add 4th or 5th digit   Nonspecific code   Unspecified code   Manifestation code

④ **E816** **Motor vehicle traffic accident due to loss of control, without collision on the highway**
  Includes: motor vehicle:
        failing to make curve and:
          colliding with object off the highway
          overturning
          stopping abruptly off the highway
        going out of control (due to):
          blowout and:
            colliding with object off the highway
            overturning
            stopping abruptly off the highway
          burst tire and:
            colliding with object off the highway
            overturning
            stopping abruptly off the highway
          driver falling asleep and:
            colliding with object off the highway
            overturning
            stopping abruptly off the highway
          driver inattention and:
            colliding with object off the highway
            overturning
            stopping abruptly off the highway
          excessive speed and:
            colliding with object off the highway
            overturning
            stopping abruptly off the highway
          failure of mechanical part and:
            colliding with object off the highway
            overturning
            stopping abruptly off the highway

  Excludes: *collision on highway following loss of control (E810.0-E815.9)*
        loss of control of motor vehicle following collision on the highway
          (E810.0-E815.9)

④ **E817** **Noncollision motor vehicle traffic accident while boarding or alighting**
  Includes: fall down stairs of motor bus while boarding or alighting
        fall from car in street while boarding or alighting
        injured by moving part of the vehicle while boarding or alighting
        trapped by door of motor bus while boarding or alighting

④ **E818** **Other noncollision motor vehicle traffic accident**
  Includes: accidental poisoning from exhaust gas generated by motor vehicle while in motion
        breakage of any part of motor vehicle while in motion
        explosion of any part of motor vehicle while in motion
        fall, jump, or being accidentally pushed from motor vehicle while in motion
        fire starting in motor vehicle while in motion
        hit by object thrown into or on motor vehicle while in motion
        injured by being thrown against some part of, or object in motor vehicle while in
          motion
        injury from moving part of motor vehicle while in motion
        object falling in or on motor vehicle while in motion
        object thrown on motor vehicle while in motion
        collision of railway train or road vehicle except motor vehicle, with object set in
          motion by motor vehicle
        motor vehicle hit by object set in motion by railway train or road vehicle (motor)
          (nonmotor)
        pedestrian, railway train, or road vehicle (motor) (nonmotor) hit by object set in
          motion by motor vehicle

  Excludes: *collision between motor vehicle and:*
        object set in motion by railway train or road vehicle (motor) (nonmotor)
          (E815.0-E815.9)
        object thrown towards the motor vehicle (E815.0-E815.9)
        person overcome by carbon monoxide generated by stationary motor vehicle off
          the roadway with motor running (E868.2)

④ **E819** **Motor vehicle traffic accident of unspecified nature**
  Includes: motor vehicle traffic accident NOS
        traffic accident NOS

● Code new
   to this edition
▲ Revision of
   existing code
④ ⑤ Fourth or fifth
   digit required

MOTOR VEHICLE NONTRAFFIC ACCIDENTS (E820-E825)

Note: For definitions of motor vehicle nontraffic accident and related terms see definitions (a) to (k).

Includes: accidents involving motor vehicles being used in recreational or sporting activities off the highway

collision and noncollision motor vehicle accidents occurring entirely off the highway

Excludes: *accidents involving motor vehicle and:*
aircraft (E840.0-E845.9)
watercraft (E830.0-E838.9)
accidents, not on the public highway, involving agricultural and construction machinery but not involving another motor vehicle (E919.0, E919.2, E919.7)

The following fourth-digit subdivisions are for use with categories E820-E825 to identify the injured person:

.0 Driver of motor vehicle other than motorcycle
See definition (l)

.1 Passenger in motor vehicle other than motorcycle
See definition (l)

.2 Motorcyclist
See definition (l)

.3 Passenger on motorcycle
See definition (l)

.4 Occupant of streetcar

.5 Rider of animal; occupant of animal-drawn vehicle

.6 Pedal cyclist
See definition (p)

.7 Pedestrian
See definition (r)

.8 Other specified person
Occupant of vehicle other than above
Person on railway train involved in accident
Unauthorized rider of motor vehicle

.9 Unspecified person

ALERT! For coding late effects of motor vehicle accident see E929.0

ALERT! For coding late effects of other transport accident see E929.1

④ **E820** **Nontraffic accident involving motor-driven snow vehicle**
Includes: breakage of part of motor-driven snow vehicle (not on public highway)
fall from motor-driven snow vehicle (not on public highway)
hit by motor-driven snow vehicle (not on public highway)
overturning of motor-driven snow vehicle (not on public highway)
run over or dragged by motor-driven snow vehicle (not on public highway)
collision of motor-driven snow vehicle with:
animal (being ridden) (-drawn vehicle)
another off-road motor vehicle
other motor vehicle, not on public highway
railway train
other object, fixed or movable
injury caused by rough landing of motor-driven snow vehicle (after leaving ground on rough terrain)

Excludes: *accident on the public highway involving motor driven snow vehicle (E810.0-E819.9)*

▨ Add 4th or 5th digit	▨ Nonspecific code	▨ Unspecified code	▨ Manifestation code

④ **E821** **Nontraffic accident involving other off-road motor vehicle**

Includes: breakage of part of off-road motor vehicle, except snow vehicle (not on public highway)
fall from off-road motor vehicle, except snow vehicle (not on public highway)
hit by off-road motor vehicle, except snow vehicle (not on public highway)
overturning of off-road motor vehicle, except snow vehicle (not on public highway)
run over or dragged by off-road motor vehicle, except snow vehicle (not on public highway)
thrown against some part of or object in off-road motor vehicle, except snow vehicle (not on public highway)
collision with:
  animal (being ridden) (-drawn vehicle)
  another off-road motor vehicle, except snow vehicle
  other motor vehicle, not on public highway
  other object, fixed or movable

Excludes: *accident on public highway involving off-road motor vehicle (E810.0-E819.9)*
collision between motor driven snow vehicle and other off-road motor vehicle (E820.0-E820.9)
hovercraft accident on water (E830.0-E838.9)

④ **E822** **Other motor vehicle nontraffic accident involving collision with moving object**

Includes: collision, not on public highway, between motor vehicle, except off-road motor vehicle and:
animal
nonmotor vehicle
other motor vehicle, except off-road motor vehicle
pedestrian
railway train
other moving object

Excludes: *collision with:*
motor-driven snow vehicle (E820.0-E820.9)
other off-road motor vehicle (E821.0-E821.9)

④ **E823** **Other motor vehicle nontraffic accident involving collision with stationary object**

Includes: collision, not on public highway, between motor vehicle, except off-road motor vehicle, and any object, fixed or movable, but not in motion

④ **E824** **Other motor vehicle nontraffic accident while boarding and alighting**

Includes: fall while boarding or alighting from motor vehicle, except off-road motor vehicle, not on public highway
injury from moving part of motor vehicle while boarding or alighting from motor vehicle, except off-road motor vehicle, not on public highway
trapped by door of motor vehicle while boarding or alighting from motor vehicle, except off-road motor vehicle, not on public highway

④ **E825** **Other motor vehicle nontraffic accident of other and unspecified nature**

Includes: accidental poisoning from carbon monoxide generated by motor vehicle while in motion, not on public highway
breakage of any part of motor vehicle while in motion, not on public highway
explosion of any part of motor vehicle while in motion, not on public highway
fall, jump, or being accidentally pushed from motor vehicle while in motion, not on public highway
fire starting in motor vehicle while in motion, not on public highway
hit by object thrown into, towards, or on motor vehicle while in motion, not on public highway
injured by being thrown against some part of, or object in motor vehicle while in motion, not on public highway
injury from moving part of motor vehicle while in motion, not on public highway
object falling in or on motor vehicle while in motion, not on public highway
motor vehicle nontraffic accident NOS

Excludes: *fall from or in stationary motor vehicle (E884.9, E885.9)*
overcome by carbon monoxide or exhaust gas generated by stationary motor vehicle off the roadway with motor running (E868.2)
struck by falling object from or in stationary motor vehicle (E916)

● Code new to this edition   ▲ Revision of existing code   ④ ⑤ Fourth or fifth digit required

OTHER ROAD VEHICLE ACCIDENTS (E826-E829)

Note: Other road vehicle accidents are transport accidents involving road vehicles other than motor vehicles. For definitions of other road vehicle and related terms see definitions (m) to (o).

Includes: accidents involving other road vehicles being used in recreational or sporting activities

Excludes: *collision of other road vehicle [any] with:*
> *aircraft (E840.0-E845.9)*
> *motor vehicle (E813.0-E813.9, E820.0-E822.9)*
> *railway train (E801.0-E801.9)*

The following fourth-digit subdivisions are for use with categories E826-E829 to identify the injured person:

.0 Pedestrian
See definition (r)

.1 Pedal cyclist
See definition (p)

.2 Rider of animal

.3 Occupant of animal-drawn vehicle

.4 Occupant of streetcar

.8 Other specified person

.9 Unspecified person

④ **E826 Pedal cycle accident**
[0-9]

Includes: breakage of any part of pedal cycle
collision between pedal cycle and:
> animal (being ridden) (herded) (unattended)
> another pedal cycle
> nonmotor road vehicle, any
> pedestrian
> other object, fixed, movable, or moving, not set in motion by motor vehicle, railway train, or aircraft
entanglement in wheel of pedal cycle
fall from pedal cycle
hit by object falling or thrown on the pedal cycle
pedal cycle accident NOS
pedal cycle overturned

④ **E827 Animal-drawn vehicle accident**
[0,2-4,8,9]

Includes: breakage of any part of vehicle
collision between animal-drawn vehicle and:
> animal (being ridden) (herded) (unattended)
> nonmotor road vehicle, except pedal cycle
> pedestrian, pedestrian conveyance, or pedestrian vehicle
> other object, fixed, movable, or moving, not set in motion by motor vehicle, railway train, or aircraft
fall from animal-drawn vehicle
knocked down by animal-drawn vehicle
overturning of animal-drawn vehicle
run over by animal-drawn vehicle
thrown from animal-drawn vehicle

Excludes: *collision of animal-drawn vehicle with pedal cycle (E826.0-E826.9)*

| | Add 4th or 5th digit | | Nonspecific code | | Unspecified code | | Manifestation code |

④ **E828** **Accident involving animal being ridden**
[0,2,4,8,9]

Includes: collision between animal being ridden and:
   another animal
   nonmotor road vehicle, except pedal cycle, and animal-drawn vehicle
   pedestrian, pedestrian conveyance, or pedestrian vehicle
   other object, fixed, movable, or moving, not set in motion by motor vehicle,
      railway train, or aircraft
   fall from animal being ridden
   knocked down by animal being ridden
   thrown from animal being ridden
   trampled by animal being ridden
   ridden animal stumbled and fell

Excludes: *collision of animal being ridden with:*
   animal-drawn vehicle (E827.0-E827.9)
   pedal cycle (E826.0-E826.9)

④ **E829** **Other road vehicle accidents**
[0,4,8,9]

Includes: accident while boarding or alighting from:
   streetcar
   nonmotor road vehicle not classifiable to E826-E828
   blow from object in:
   streetcar
   nonmotor road vehicle not classifiable to E826-E828
   breakage of any part of:
   streetcar
   nonmotor road vehicle not classifiable to E826-E828
   caught in door of:
   streetcar
   nonmotor road vehicle not classifiable to E826-E828
   derailment of:
   streetcar
   nonmotor road vehicle not classifiable to E826-E828
   fall in, on, or from:
   streetcar
   nonmotor road vehicle not classifiable to E826-E828
   fire in:
   streetcar
   nonmotor road vehicle not classifiable to E826-E828
   collision between streetcar or nonmotor road vehicle, except as in E826-E828, and:
   animal (not being ridden)
   another nonmotor road vehicle not classifiable to E826-E828
   pedestrian
   other object, fixed, movable, or moving, not set in motion by motor vehicle,
      railway train, or aircraft
   nonmotor road vehicle accident NOS
   streetcar accident NOS

Excludes: *collision with:*
   animal being ridden (E828.0-E828.9)
   animal-drawn vehicle (E827.0-E827.9)
   pedal cycle (E826.0-E826.9)

● Code new to this edition   ▲ Revision of existing code   ④ ⑤ Fourth or fifth digit required

WATER TRANSPORT ACCIDENTS (E830-E838)

Note: For definitions of water transport accident and related terms see definitions (a), (s), and (t).

Includes: watercraft accidents in the course of recreational activities

Excludes: *accidents involving both aircraft, including objects set in motion by aircraft, and watercraft (E840.0-E845.9)*

The following fourth-digit subdivisions are for use with categories E830-E838 to identify the injured person:

.0 **Occupant of small boat, unpowered**

.1 **Occupant of small boat, powered**
   See definition (t)

Excludes: *water skier (.4)*

.2 **Occupant of other watercraft—crew**
   Persons:
   engaged in operation of watercraft
   providing passenger services [cabin attendants, ship's physician, catering personnel]
   working on ship during voyage in other capacity [musician in band, operators of shops and beauty parlors]

.3 **Occupant of other watercraft—other than crew**
   Passenger
   Occupant of lifeboat, other than crew, after abandoning ship

.4 **Water skier**

.5 **Swimmer**

.6 **Dockers, stevedores**
   Longshoreman employed on the dock in loading and unloading ships

.7 **Occupant of military watercraft, any type**

.8 **Other specified person**
   Immigration and custom officials on board ship
   Person:
   accompanying passenger or member of crew
   visiting boat
   Pilot (guiding ship into port)

.9 **Unspecified person**

④ **E830** **Accident to watercraft causing submersion**
   Includes: submersion and drowning due to:
   boat overturning
   boat submerging
   falling or jumping from burning ship
   falling or jumping from crushed watercraft
   ship sinking
   other accident to watercraft

④ **E831** **Accident to watercraft causing other injury**
   Includes: any injury, except submersion and drowning, as a result of an accident to watercraft
   burned while ship on fire
   crushed between ships in collision
   crushed by lifeboat after abandoning ship
   fall due to collision or other accident to watercraft
   hit by falling object due to accident to watercraft
   injured in watercraft accident involving collision
   struck by boat or part thereof after fall or jump from damaged boat

Excludes: *burns from localized fire or explosion on board ship (E837.0-E837.9)*

④ **E832** **Other accidental submersion or drowning in water transport accident**
   Includes: submersion or drowning as a result of an accident other than accident to the watercraft, such as:
   fall:
   from gangplank
   from ship
   overboard
   thrown overboard by motion of ship
   washed overboard

Excludes: *submersion or drowning of swimmer or diver who voluntarily jumps from boat not involved in an accident (E910.0-E910.9)*

Add 4th or 5th digit	Nonspecific code	Unspecified code	Manifestation code

④ **E833** **Fall on stairs or ladders in water transport**
     Excludes: fall due to accident to watercraft (E831.0-E831.9)

④ **E834** **Other fall from one level to another in water transport**
     Excludes: fall due to accident to watercraft (E831.0-E831.9)

④ **E835** **Other and unspecified fall in water transport**
     Excludes: fall due to accident to watercraft (E831.0-E831.9)

④ **E836** **Machinery accident in water transport**
     Includes: injuries in water transport caused by:
               deck machinery
               engine room machinery
               galley machinery
               laundry machinery
               loading machinery

④ **E837** **Explosion, fire, or burning in watercraft**
     Includes: explosion of boiler on steamship
               localized fire on ship

     Excludes: burning ship (due to collision or explosion) resulting in:
          submersion or drowning (E830.0-E830.9)
          other injury (E831.0-E831.9)

④ **E838** **Other and unspecified water transport accident**
     Includes: accidental poisoning by gases or fumes on ship
               atomic power plant malfunction in watercraft
               crushed between ship and stationary object [wharf]
               crushed between ships without accident to watercraft
               crushed by falling object on ship or while loading or unloading
               hit by boat while water skiing
               struck by boat or part thereof (after fall from boat)
               watercraft accident NOS

AIR AND SPACE TRANSPORT ACCIDENTS (E840-E845)

Note: For definition of aircraft and related terms see definitions (u) and (v).

The following fourth-digit subdivisions are for use with categories E840-E845 to identify the injured person:

  .0 **Occupant of spacecraft**

  .1 **Occupant of military aircraft, any**
     Crew in military aircraft [air force] [army] [national guard] [navy]
     Passenger (civilian) (military) in military aircraft [air force] [army] [national guard] [navy]
     Troops in military aircraft [air force] [army] [national guard] [navy]

     Excludes: occupants of aircraft operated under jurisdiction of police departments (.5)
          parachutist (.7)

  .2 **Crew of commercial aircraft (powered) in surface to surface transport**

  .3 **Other occupant of commercial aircraft (powered) in surface to surface transport**
     Flight personnel:
       not part of crew
       on familiarization flight
     Passenger on aircraft (powered) NOS

  .4 **Occupant of commercial aircraft (powered) in surface to air transport**
     Occupant [crew] [passenger] of aircraft (powered) engaged in activities, such as:
       aerial spraying (crops) (fire retardants)
       air drops of emergency supplies
       air drops of parachutists, except from military craft
       crop dusting
       lowering of construction material [bridge or telephone pole]
       sky writing

  .5 **Occupant of other powered aircraft**
     Occupant [crew] [passenger] of aircraft [powered] engaged in activities, such as:
       aerobatic flying
       aircraft racing
       rescue operation
       storm surveillance
       traffic surveillance
     Occupant of private plane NOS

● Code new   ▲ Revision of   ④ ⑤ Fourth or fifth
   to this edition   existing code   digit required

.6 Occupant of unpowered aircraft, except parachutist
    Occupant of aircraft classifiable to E842

.7 Parachutist (military) (other)
    Person making voluntary descent

Excludes: *person making descent after accident to aircraft (.1-.6)*

.8 Ground crew, airline employee
    Persons employed at airfields (civil) (military) or launching pads, not occupants of aircraft

.9 Other person

④ **E840 Accident to powered aircraft at takeoff or landing**
    Includes: collision of aircraft with any object, fixed, movable, or moving while taking off or landing
                crash while taking off or landing
                explosion on aircraft while taking off or landing
                fire on aircraft while taking off or landing
                forced landing

④ **E841 Accident to powered aircraft, other and unspecified**
    Includes: aircraft accident NOS
                aircraft crash or wreck NOS
                any accident to powered aircraft while in transit or when not specified whether in transit, taking off, or landing
                collision of aircraft with another aircraft, bird, or any object, while in transit
                explosion on aircraft while in transit
                fire on aircraft while in transit

④ **E842 Accident to unpowered aircraft**
[6-9]
    Includes: any accident, except collision with powered aircraft, to:
                balloon
                glider
                hang glider
                kite carrying a person
                hit by object falling from unpowered aircraft

④ **E843 Fall in, on, or from aircraft**
[0-9]
    Includes: accident in boarding or alighting from aircraft, any kind
                fall in, on, or from aircraft [any kind], while in transit, taking off, or landing, except when as a result of an accident to aircraft

④ **E844 Other specified air transport accidents**
[0-9]
    Includes: hit by:
                    aircraft without accident to aircraft
                    object falling from aircraft without accident to aircraft
                injury by or from:
                    machinery on aircraft without accident to aircraft
                    rotating propeller without accident to aircraft
                    voluntary parachute descent without accident to aircraft
                poisoning by carbon monoxide from aircraft while in transit without accident to aircraft
                sucked into jet without accident to aircraft
                any accident involving other transport vehicle (motor) (nonmotor) due to being hit by object set in motion by aircraft (powered)

Excludes: *air sickness (E903)*
            effects of:
            high altitude (E902.0-E902.1)
            pressure change (E902.0-E902.1)
            injury in parachute descent due to accident to aircraft (840.0-E842.9)

④ **E845 Accident involving spacecraft**
[0,8,9]
    Includes: launching pad accident

Excludes: *effects of weightlessness in spacecraft (E928.0)*

	Add 4th or 5th digit		Nonspecific code		Unspecified code		Manifestation code

VEHICLE ACCIDENTS NOT ELSEWHERE CLASSIFIABLE (E846-E848)

E846 **Accidents involving powered vehicles used solely within the buildings and premises of industrial or commercial establishment**

Accident to, on, or involving:
  battery powered airport passenger vehicle
  battery powered trucks (baggage) (mail)
  coal car in mine
  logging car
  self propelled truck, industrial
  station baggage truck (powered)
  tram, truck, or tub (powered) in mine or quarry
Breakage of any part of vehicle
Collision with:
  pedestrian
  other vehicle or object within premises
Explosion of powered vehicle, industrial or commercial
Fall from powered vehicle, industrial or commercial
Overturning of powered vehicle, industrial or commercial
Struck by powered vehicle, industrial or commercial

> *Excludes:* *accidental poisoning by exhaust gas from vehicle not elsewhere classifiable (E868.2)*
> *injury by crane, lift (fork), or elevator (E919.2)*

E847 **Accidents involving cable cars not running on rails**

Accident to, on, or involving:
  cable car, not on rails
  ski chair-lift
  ski-lift with gondola
  téléférique
Breakage of cable
Caught or dragged by cable car, not on rails
Fall or jump from cable car, not on rails
Object thrown from or in cable car, not on rails

E848 **Accidents involving other vehicles, not elsewhere classifiable**

Accident to, on, or involving:
  ice yacht
  land yacht
  nonmotor, nonroad vehicle NOS

PLACE OF OCCURRENCE (E849)

E849 **Place of occurrence**

The following category is for use to denote the place where the injury or poisoning occurred.

E849.0 **Home**

Apartment	Private:
Boarding house	driveway
Farm house	garage
Home premises	garden
House (residential)	home
Noninstitutional place	walk
of residence	Swimming pool in private house or garden
	Yard of home

> *Excludes:* *home under construction but not yet occupied (E849.3)*
> *institutional place of residence (E849.7)*

E849.1 **Farm**

Farm:
  buildings
  land under cultivation

> *Excludes:* *farm house and home premises of farm (E849.0)*

E849.2 **Mine and quarry**

Gravel pit
Sand pit
Tunnel under construction

● Code new to this edition   ▲ Revision of existing code   ④ ⑤ Fourth or fifth digit required

E849.3 Industrial place and premises

Building under construction	Industrial yard
Dockyard	Loading platform (factory) (store)
Dry dock	Plant, industrial
Factory	Railway yard
building	Shop (place of work)
premises	Warehouse
Garage (place of work)	Workhouse

E849.4 Place for recreation and sport

Amusement park	Public park
Baseball field	Racecourse
Basketball court	Resort NOS
Beach resort	Riding school
Cricket ground	Rifle range
Fives court	Seashore resort
Football field	Skating rink
Golf course	Sports ground
Gymnasium	Sports palace
Hockey field	Stadium
Holiday camp	Swimming pool, public
Ice palace	Tennis court
Lake resort	Vacation resort
Mountain resort	
Playground, including school playground	

Excludes: *that in private house or garden (E849.0)*

E849.5 Street and highway

E849.6 Public building

Building (including adjacent grounds) used by the general public or by a particular group of the public, such as:

airport	nightclub
bank	office
café	office building
casino	opera house
church	post office
cinema	public hall
clubhouse	radio broadcasting station
courthouse	restaurant
dance hall	school (state) (public) (private)
garage building (for car storage)	shop, commercial
hotel	station (bus) (railway)
market (grocery or other commodity)	store
movie house	theater
music hall	

Excludes: *home garage (E849.0)*
industrial building or workplace (E849.3)

E849.7 Residential institution

Children's home	Old people's home
Dormitory	Orphanage
Hospital	Prison
Jail	Reform school

E849.8 Other specified places

Beach NOS	Pond or pool (natural)
Canal	Prairie
Caravan site NOS	Public place NOS
Derelict house	Railway line
Desert	Reservoir
Dock	River
Forest	Sea
Harbor	Seashore NOS
Hill	Stream
Lake NOS	Swamp
Mountain	Trailer court
Parking lot	Woods
Parking place	

▨ Add 4th or 5th digit	▨ Nonspecific code	▨ Unspecified code	▨ Manifestation code

E849.9   Unspecified place

ACCIDENTAL POISONING BY DRUGS, MEDICINAL SUBSTANCES, AND BIOLOGICALS (E850-E858)

Includes: accidental overdose of drug, wrong drug given or taken in error, and drug taken inadvertently

accidents in the use of drugs and biologicals in medical and surgical procedures

Excludes: *administration with suicidal or homicidal intent or intent to harm, or in circumstances classifiable to E980-E989 (E950.0-E950.5, E962.0, E980.0-E980.5)*

correct drug properly administered in therapeutic or prophylactic dosage, as the cause of adverse effect (E930.0-E949.9)

See Alphabetic Index for more complete list of specific drugs to be classified under the fourth-digit subdivisions. The American Hospital Formulary numbers can be used to classify new drugs listed by the American Hospital Formulary Service (AHFS). See appendix C.

ALERT! For coding late effects of accidental poisoning see E929.2

E850   Accidental poisoning by analgesics, antipyretics, and antirheumatics

E850.0   Heroin
Diacetylmorphine

E850.1   Methadone

E850.2   Other opiates and related narcotics
Codeine [methylmorphine]   Morphine
Meperidine [pethidine]   Opium (alkaloids)

E850.3   Salicylates
Acetylsalicylic acid [aspirin]
Amino derivatives of salicylic acid
Salicylic acid salts

E850.4   Aromatic analgesics, not elsewhere classified
Acetanilid
Paracetamol [acetaminophen]
Phenacetin [acetophenetidin]

E850.5   Pyrazole derivatives
Aminophenazone [amidopyrine]
Phenylbutazone

E850.6   Antirheumatics [antiphlogistics]
Gold salts   Indomethacin

Excludes: *salicylates (E850.3)*
steroids (E858.0)

E850.7   Other non-narcotic analgesics
Pyrabital

E850.8   Other specified analgesics and antipyretics
Pentazocine

E850.9   Unspecified analgesic or antipyretic

E851   Accidental poisoning by barbiturates
Amobarbital [amylobarbitone]
Barbital [barbitone]
Butabarbital [butabarbitone]
Pentobarbital [pentobarbitone]
Phenobarbital [phenobarbitone]
Secobarbital [quinalbarbitone]

Excludes: *thiobarbiturates (E855.1)*

E852   Accidental poisoning by other sedatives and hypnotics

E852.0   Chloral hydrate group

E852.1   Paraldehyde

E852.2   Bromine compounds
Bromides   Carbromal (derivatives)

E852.3   Methaqualone compounds

E852.4   Glutethimide group

E852.5   Mixed sedatives, not elsewhere classified

E852.8   Other specified sedatives and hypnotics

● Code new
   to this edition

▲ Revision of
   existing code

④ ⑤ Fourth or fifth
   digit required

E852.9 **Unspecified sedative or hypnotic**
Sleeping:
drug NOS
pill NOS
tablet NOS

E853 **Accidental poisoning by tranquilizers**

E853.0 **Phenothiazine-based tranquilizers**
Chlorpromazine   Prochlorperazine
Fluphenazine   Promazine

E853.1 **Butyrophenone-based tranquilizers**
Haloperidol   Trifluperidol
Spiperone

E853.2 **Benzodiazepine-based tranquilizers**
Chlordiazepoxide   Lorazepam
Diazepam   Medazepam
Flurazepam   Nitrazepam

E853.8 **Other specified tranquilizers**
Hydroxyzine   Meprobamate

E853.9 **Unspecified tranquilizer**

E854 **Accidental poisoning by other psychotropic agents**

E854.0 **Antidepressants**
Amitriptyline   Monoamine oxidase [MAO] inhibitors
Imipramine

E854.1 **Psychodysleptics [hallucinogens]**
Cannabis derivatives Mescaline
Lysergide [LSD]   Psilocin
marijuana (derivatives) Psilocybin

E854.2 **Psychostimulants**
Amphetamine   Caffeine

> Excludes: *central appetite depressants (E858.8)*

E854.3 **Central nervous system stimulants**
Analeptics   Opiate antagonists

E854.8 **Other psychotropic agents**

E855 **Accidental poisoning by other drugs acting on central and autonomic nervous system**

E855.0 **Anticonvulsant and anti-Parkinsonism drugs**
Amantadine
Hydantoin derivatives
Levodopa [L-dopa]
Oxazolidine derivatives [paramethadione] [trimethadione]
Succinimides

E855.1 **Other central nervous system depressants**
Ether   Intravenous anesthetics
Gaseous anesthetics   Thiobarbiturates, such as thiopental sodium
Halogenated hydrocarbon
  derivatives

E855.2 **Local anesthetics**
Cocaine   Procaine
Lidocaine [lignocaine] Tetracaine

E855.3 **Parasympathomimetics [cholinergics]**
Acetylcholine   Pilocarpine
Anticholinesterase:
  organophosphorus
  reversible

E855.4 **Parasympatholytics [anticholinergics and antimuscarinics] and spasmolytics**
Atropine   Hyoscine [scopolamine]
Homatropine   Quaternary ammonium derivatives

E855.5 **Sympathomimetics [adrenergics]**
Epinephrine [adrenalin]
Levarterenol [noradrenalin]

E855.6 **Sympatholytics [antiadrenergics]**
Phenoxybenzamine   Tolazoline hydrochloride

Add 4th or 5th digit   Nonspecific code   Unspecified code   Manifestation code

E855.8   Other specified drugs acting on central and autonomic nervous systems

E855.9   Unspecified drug acting on central and autonomic nervous systems

E856   Accidental poisoning by antibiotics

E857   Accidental poisoning by other anti-infectives

E858   Accidental poisoning by other drugs

    E858.0   Hormones and synthetic substitutes

    E858.1   Primarily systemic agents

    E858.2   Agents primarily affecting blood constituents

    E858.3   Agents primarily affecting cardiovascular system

    E858.4   Agents primarily affecting gastrointestinal system

    E858.5   Water, mineral, and uric acid metabolism drugs

    E858.6   Agents primarily acting on the smooth and skeletal muscles and respiratory system

    E858.7   Agents primarily affecting skin and mucous membrane, ophthalmological, otorhinolaryngological, and dental drugs

    E858.8   Other specified drugs
        Central appetite depressants

    E858.9   Unspecified drug

ACCIDENTAL POISONING BY OTHER SOLID AND LIQUID SUBSTANCES, GASES, AND VAPORS (E860-E869)

Note: Categories in this section are intended primarily to indicate the external cause of poisoning states classifiable to 980-989. They may also be used to indicate external causes of localized effects classifiable to 001-799.

ALERT! For coding late effects of accidental poisoning see E929.2

E860   Accidental poisoning by alcohol, not elsewhere classified

    E860.0   Alcoholic beverages
        Alcohol in preparations intended for consumption

    E860.1   Other and unspecified ethyl alcohol and its products
        Denatured alcohol   Grain alcohol NOS
        Ethanol NOS   Methylated spirit

    E860.2   Methyl alcohol
        Methanol   Wood alcohol

    E860.3   Isopropyl alcohol
        Dimethyl carbinol   Secondary propyl alcohol
        Isopropanol
        Rubbing alcohol substitute

    E860.4   Fusel oil
        Alcohol:
          amyl
          butyl
          propyl

    E860.8   Other specified alcohols

    E860.9   Unspecified alcohol

E861   Accidental poisoning by cleansing and polishing agents, disinfectants, paints, and varnishes

    E861.0   Synthetic detergents and shampoos

    E861.1   Soap products

    E861.2   Polishes

    E861.3   Other cleansing and polishing agents
        Scouring powders

    E861.4   Disinfectants
        Household and other disinfectants not ordinarily used on the person

        Excludes: carbolic acid or phenol (E864.0)

    E861.5   Lead paints

    ALERT! For personal history of contact with and (suspected) exposure to lead see V15.86

    E861.6   Other paints and varnishes
        Lacquers   Paints, other than lead
        Oil colors   White washes

● Code new to this edition   ▲ Revision of existing code   ④ ⑤ Fourth or fifth digit required

E861.9   Unspecified

E862   Accidental poisoning by petroleum products, other solvents and their vapors, not elsewhere classified

E862.0   Petroleum solvents
Petroleum:
ether
benzine
naphtha

E862.1   Petroleum fuels and cleaners
Antiknock additives to petroleum fuels
Gas oils
Gasoline or petrol
Kerosene

Excludes: kerosene insecticides (E863.4)

E862.2   Lubricating oils

E862.3   Petroleum solids
Paraffin wax

E862.4   Other specified solvents
Benzene

E862.9   Unspecified solvent

E863   Accidental poisoning by agricultural and horticultural chemical and pharmaceutical preparations other than plant foods and fertilizers

Excludes: plant foods and fertilizers (E866.5)

E863.0   Insecticides of organochlorine compounds

Benzene hexachloride	Dieldrin
Chlordane	Endrine
DDT	Toxaphene

E863.1   Insecticides of organophosphorus compounds

Demeton	Parathion
Diazinon	Phenylsulphthion
Dichlorvos	Phorate
Malathion	Phosdrin
Methyl parathion	

E863.2   Carbamates

Aldicarb	Propoxur
Carbaryl	

E863.3   Mixtures of insecticides

E863.4   Other and unspecified insecticides
Kerosene insecticides

E863.5   Herbicides
2, 4-Dichlorophenoxyacetic acid [2, 4-D]
2, 4, 5-Trichlorophenoxyacetic acid [2, 4, 5-T]
Chlorates
Diquat
Mixtures of plant food and fertilizers with herbicides
Paraquat

E863.6   Fungicides
Organic mercurials (used in seed dressing)
Pentachlorophenols

E863.7   Rodenticides

Fluoroacetates	Warfarin
Squill and derivatives	Zinc phosphide
Thallium	

E863.8   Fumigants

Cyanides	Phosphine
Methyl bromide	

E863.9   Other and unspecified

E864   Accidental poisoning by corrosives and caustics, not elsewhere classified

Excludes: those as components of disinfectants (E861.4)

E864.0   Corrosive aromatics
Carbolic acid or phenol

Add 4th or 5th digit	Nonspecific code	Unspecified code	Manifestation code

E864.1 Acids
Acid:
hydrochloric
nitric
sulfuric

E864.2 Caustic alkalis
Lye

E864.3 Other specified corrosives and caustics

E864.4 Unspecified corrosives and caustics

E865 Accidental poisoning from poisonous foodstuffs and poisonous plants
Includes: any meat, fish, or shellfish
plants, berries, and fungi eaten as, or in mistake for, food, or by a child

Excludes: *anaphylactic shock due to adverse food reaction (995.60-995.69)*
food poisoning (bacterial) (005.0-005.9)
poisoning and toxic reactions to venomous plants (E905.6-E905.7)

E865.0 Meat

E865.1 Shellfish

E865.2 Other fish

E865.3 Berries and seeds

E865.4 Other specified plants

E865.5 Mushrooms and other fungi

E865.8 Other specified foods

E865.9 Unspecified foodstuff or poisonous plant

E866 Accidental poisoning by other and unspecified solid and liquid substances

Excludes: *these substances as a component of:*
medicines (E850.0-E858.9)
paints (E861.5-E861.6)
pesticides (E863.0-E863.9)
petroleum fuels (E862.1)

E866.0 Lead and its compounds and fumes
ALERT! For personal history of contact with and (suspected) exposure to lead see V15.86

E866.1 Mercury and its compounds and fumes

E866.2 Antimony and its compounds and fumes

E866.3 Arsenic and its compounds and fumes

E866.4 Other metals and their compounds and fumes

Beryllium (compounds)	Iron (compounds)
Brass fumes	Manganese (compounds)
Cadmium (compounds)	Nickel (compounds)
Copper salts	Thallium (compounds)

E866.5 Plant foods and fertilizers

Excludes: *mixtures with herbicides (E863.5)*

E866.6 Glues and adhesives

E866.7 Cosmetics

E866.8 Other specified solid or liquid substances

E866.9 Unspecified solid or liquid substance

E867 Accidental poisoning by gas distributed by pipeline
Carbon monoxide from incomplete combustion of piped gas
Coal gas NOS
Liquefied petroleum gas distributed through pipes (pure or mixed with air)
Piped gas (natural) (manufactured)

E868 Accidental poisoning by other utility gas and other carbon monoxide

E868.0 Liquefied petroleum gas distributed in mobile containers
Butane or carbon monoxide from incomplete combustion of this gas
Liquefied hydrocarbon gas NOS or carbon monoxide from incomplete combustion of this gas
Propane or carbon monoxide from incomplete combustion of this gas

● Code new to this edition   ▲ Revision of existing code   ④ ⑤ Fourth or fifth digit required

E868.1 **Other and unspecified utility gas**
Acetylene or or carbon monoxide from incomplete combustion of these gases
Gas NOS used for lighting, heating, cooking, or carbon monoxide from incomplete combustion of these gases
Water gas or carbon monoxide from incomplete combustion of these gases

E868.2 **Motor vehicle exhaust gas**
Exhaust gas from:
   farm tractor, not in transit
   gas engine
   motor pump
   motor vehicle, not in transit
   any type of combustion engine not in watercraft

Excludes: *poisoning by carbon monoxide from:*
   aircraft while in transit (E844.0-E844.9)
   motor vehicle while in transit (E818.0-E818.9)
   watercraft whether or not in transit (E838.0-E838.9)

E868.3 **Carbon monoxide from incomplete combustion of other domestic fuels**
Carbon monoxide from incomplete combustion of:
   coal in domestic stove or fireplace
   coke in domestic stove or fireplace
   kerosene in domestic stove or fireplace
   wood in domestic stove or fireplace

Excludes: *carbon monoxide from smoke and fumes due to conflagration (E890.0-E893.9)*

E868.8 **Carbon monoxide from other sources**
Carbon monoxide from:
   blast furnace gas
   incomplete combustion of fuels in industrial use
   kiln vapor

E868.9 **Unspecified carbon monoxide**

E869 **Accidental poisoning by other gases and vapors**

Excludes: *effects of gases used as anesthetics (E855.1, E938.2)*
   fumes from heavy metals (E866.0-E866.4)
   smoke and fumes due to conflagration or explosion (E890.0-E899)

E869.0 **Nitrogen oxides**

E869.1 **Sulfur dioxide**

E869.2 **Freon**

E869.3 **Lacrimogenic gas [tear gas]**
Bromobenzyl cyanide   Ethyliodoacetate
Chloroacetophenone

E869.4 **Second-hand tobacco smoke**

E869.8 **Other specified gases and vapors**
Chlorine   Hydrocyanic acid gas

E869.9 **Unspecified gases and vapors**

MISADVENTURES TO PATIENTS DURING SURGICAL AND MEDICAL CARE (E870-E876)

Excludes: *accidental overdose of drug and wrong drug given in error (E850.0-E858.9)*
   surgical and medical procedures as the cause of abnormal reaction by the patient, without mention of misadventure at the time of procedure (E878.0-E879.9)

E870 **Accidental cut, puncture, perforation, or hemorrhage during medical care**

E870.0 **Surgical operation**

E870.1 **Infusion or transfusion**

E870.2 **Kidney dialysis or other perfusion**

E870.3 **Injection or vaccination**

E870.4 **Endoscopic examination**

E870.5 **Aspiration of fluid or tissue, puncture, and catheterization**
Abdominal paracentesis   Lumbar puncture
Aspirating needle biopsy   Thoracentesis
Blood sampling

Excludes: *heart catheterization (E870.6)*

E870.6 **Heart catheterization**

E870.7 **Administration of enema**

Add 4th or 5th digit   Nonspecific code   Unspecified code   Manifestation code

E870.8 Other specified medical care

E870.9 Unspecified medical care

E871 Foreign object left in body during procedure

E871.0 Surgical operation

E871.1 Infusion or transfusion

E871.2 Kidney dialysis or other perfusion

E871.3 Injection or vaccination

E871.4 Endoscopic examination

E871.5 Aspiration of fluid or tissue, puncture, and catheterization
   Abdominal paracentesis   Lumbar puncture
   Aspiration needle biopsy   Thoracentesis
   Blood sampling

   Excludes: heart catheterization (E871.6)

E871.6 Heart catheterization

E871.7 Removal of catheter or packing

E871.8 Other specified procedures

E871.9 Unspecified procedure

E872 Failure of sterile precautions during procedure

E872.0 Surgical operation

E872.1 Infusion or transfusion

E872.2 Kidney dialysis and other perfusion

E872.3 Injection or vaccination

E872.4 Endoscopic examination

E872.5 Aspiration of fluid or tissue, puncture, and catheterization
   Abdominal paracentesis   Lumbar puncture
   Aspirating needle biopsy   Thoracentesis
   Blood sampling

   Excludes: heart catheterization (E872.6)

E872.6 Heart catheterization

E872.8 Other specified procedures

E872.9 Unspecified procedure

E873 Failure in dosage

   Excludes: accidental overdose of drug, medicinal or biological substance (E850.0-E858.9)

E873.0 Excessive amount of blood or other fluid during transfusion or infusion

E873.1 Incorrect dilution of fluid during infusion

E873.2 Overdose of radiation in therapy

E873.3 Inadvertent exposure of patient to radiation during medical care

E873.4 Failure in dosage in electroshock or insulin-shock therapy

E873.5 Inappropriate [too hot or too cold] temperature in local application and packing

E873.6 Nonadministration of necessary drug or medicinal substance

E873.8 Other specified failure in dosage

E873.9 Unspecified failure in dosage

E874 Mechanical failure of instrument or apparatus during procedure

E874.0 Surgical operation

E874.1 Infusion and transfusion
   Air in system

E874.2 Kidney dialysis and other perfusion

E874.3 Endoscopic examination

E874.4 Aspiration of fluid or tissue, puncture, and catheterization
   Abdominal paracentesis   Lumbar puncture
   Aspirating needle biopsy   Thoracentesis
   Blood sampling

   Excludes: heart catheterization (E874.5)

E874.5 Heart catheterization

● Code new to this edition   ▲ Revision of existing code   ④ ⑤ Fourth or fifth digit required

E874.8   Other specified procedures

E874.9   Unspecified procedure

E875   Contaminated or infected blood, other fluid, drug, or biological substance

Includes: presence of:
         bacterial pyrogens
         endotoxin-producing bacteria
         serum hepatitis-producing agent

E875.0   Contaminated substance transfused or infused

E875.1   Contaminated substance injected or used for vaccination

E875.2   Contaminated drug or biological substance administered by other means

E875.8   Other

E875.9   Unspecified

E876   Other and unspecified misadventures during medical care

E876.0   Mismatched blood in transfusion

E876.1   Wrong fluid in infusion

E876.2   Failure in suture and ligature during surgical operation

E876.3   Endotracheal tube wrongly placed during anesthetic procedure

E876.4   Failure to introduce or to remove other tube or instrument

> *Excludes:*   *foreign object left in body during procedure (E871.0-E871.9)*

E876.5   Performance of wrong operation (procedure) on correct patient
       Wrong device implanted into correct surgical site

> *Excludes:*   *correct operation (procedure) performed on wrong body part (E876.7)*

E876.6   Performance of operation (procedure) on patient not scheduled for surgery
       Performance of operation (procedure) intended for another patient
       Performance of operation (procedure) on wrong patient

E876.7   Performance of correct operation (procedure) on wrong side/body part
       Performance of correct operation (procedure) on wrong side
       Performance of correct operation (procedure) on wrong site

E876.8   Other specified misadventures during medical care
       Performance of inappropriate treatment NEC

E876.9   Unspecified misadventure during medical care

SURGICAL AND MEDICAL PROCEDURES AS THE CAUSE OF ABNORMAL REACTION OF PATIENT OR LATER COMPLICATION, WITHOUT MENTION OF MISADVENTURE AT THE TIME OF PROCEDURE (E878-E879)

Includes: procedures as the cause of abnormal reaction, such as:
         displacement or malfunction of prosthetic device
         hepatorenal failure, postoperative
         malfunction of external stoma
         postoperative intestinal obstruction
         rejection of transplanted organ

> *Excludes:*   *anesthetic management properly carried out as the cause of adverse effect*
>   *(E937.0-E938.9)*
> *infusion and transfusion, without mention of misadventure in the technique of*
>   *procedure (E930.0-E949.9)*

E878   Surgical operation and other surgical procedures as the cause of abnormal reaction of patient, or of later complication, without mention of misadventure at the time of operation

E878.0   Surgical operation with transplant of whole organ
       Transplantation of:
       heart
       kidney
       liver

E878.1   Surgical operation with implant of artificial internal device
       Cardiac pacemaker   Heart valve prosthesis
       Electrodes implanted in brain   Internal orthopedic device

E878.2 **Surgical operation with anastomosis, bypass, or graft, with natural or artificial tissues used as implant**

Anastomosis: Graft of blood vessel, tendon, or skin
arteriovenous
gastrojejunal

Excludes: external stoma (E878.3)

E878.3 **Surgical operation with formation of external stoma**

Colostomy Gastrostomy
Cystostomy Ureterostomy
Duodenostomy

E878.4 **Other restorative surgery**

E878.5 **Amputation of limb(s)**

E878.6 **Removal of other organ (partial) (total)**

E878.8 **Other specified surgical operations and procedures**

E878.9 **Unspecified surgical operations and procedures**

E879 **Other procedures, without mention of misadventure at the time of procedure, as the cause of abnormal reaction of patient, or of later complication**

E879.0 **Cardiac catheterization**

E879.1 **Kidney dialysis**

E879.2 **Radiological procedure and radiotherapy**

Excludes: radio-opaque dyes for diagnostic x-ray procedures (E947.8)

E879.3 **Shock therapy**

Electroshock therapy Insulin-shock therapy

E879.4 **Aspiration of fluid**

Lumbar puncture Thoracentesis

E879.5 **Insertion of gastric or duodenal sound**

E879.6 **Urinary catheterization**

E879.7 **Blood sampling**

E879.8 **Other specified procedures**

Blood transfusion

E879.9 **Unspecified procedure**

ACCIDENTAL FALLS (E880-E888)

Excludes: falls (in or from):
burning building (E890.8, E891.8)
into fire (E890.0-E899)
into water (with submersion or drowning) (E910.0-E910.9)
machinery (in operation) (E919.0-E919.9)
on edged, pointed, or sharp object (E920.0-E920.9)
transport vehicle (E800.0-E845.9)
vehicle not elsewhere classifiable (E846-E848)

ALERT! For coding late effects of accidental fall see E929.3

ALERT! For personal history of fall see V15.88

E880 **Fall on or from stairs or steps**

E880.0 **Escalator**

E880.1 **Fall on or from sidewalk curb**

Excludes: fall from moving sidewalk (E885.9)

E880.9 **Other stairs or steps**

E881 **Fall on or from ladders or scaffolding**

E881.0 **Fall from ladder**

E881.1 **Fall from scaffolding**

● Code new to this edition ▲ Revision of existing code ④ ⑤ Fourth or fifth digit required

E882 Fall from or out of building or other structure

Fall from:	Fall from:
balcony	turret
bridge	viaduct
building	wall
flagpole	window
tower	Fall through roof

Excludes: *collapse of a building or structure (E916)*
fall or jump from burning building (E890.8, E891.8)

E883 Fall into hole or other opening in surface

Includes:

fall into:	fall into:
cavity	shaft
dock	swimming pool
hole	tank
pit	well
quarry	

Excludes: *fall into water NOS (E910.9)*
that resulting in drowning or submersion without mention of injury (E910.0-E910.9)

E883.0 Accident from diving or jumping into water [swimming pool]
Strike or hit:
against bottom when jumping or diving into water
wall or board of swimming pool
water surface

Excludes: *diving with insufficient air supply (E913.2)*
effects of air pressure from diving (E902.2)

E883.1 Accidental fall into well

E883.2 Accidental fall into storm drain or manhole

E883.9 Fall into other hole or other opening in surface

E884 Other fall from one level to another

E884.0 Fall from playground equipment

Excludes: *recreational machinery (E919.8)*

E884.1 Fall from cliff

E884.2 Fall from chair

E884.3 Fall from wheelchair
Fall from motorized mobility scooter
Fall from motorized wheelchair

E884.4 Fall from bed

E884.5 Fall from other furniture

E884.6 Fall from commode
Toilet

E884.9 Other fall from one level to another

Fall from:	Fall from:
embankment	stationary vehicle
haystack	tree

E885 Fall on same level from slipping, tripping, or stumbling

E885.0 Fall from (nonmotorized) scooter

Excludes: *fall from motorized mobility scooter (E884.3)*

E885.1 Fall from roller skates
Heelies
In-line skates
Wheelies

E885.2 Fall from skateboard

E885.3 Fall from skis

E885.4 Fall from snowboard

E885.9 Fall from other slipping, tripping or stumbling
Fall on moving sidewalk

E886 Fall on same level from collision, pushing, or shoving, by or with other person

Excludes: *crushed or pushed by a crowd or human stampede (E917.1, E917.6)*

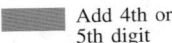 Add 4th or 5th digit

 Nonspecific code

 Unspecified code

 Manifestation code

E886.0   In sports
Tackles in sports

> *Excludes:* kicked, stepped on, struck by object, in sports (E917.0, E917.5)

E886.9   Other and unspecified
Fall from collision of pedestrian (conveyance) with another pedestrian (conveyance)

E887   Fracture, cause unspecified

E888   Other and unspecified fall
Accidental fall NOS
Fall on same level NOS

E888.0   Fall resulting in striking against sharp object
Use additional external cause code to identify object (E920)

E888.1   Fall resulting in striking against other object

E888.8   Other fall

E888.9   Unspecified fall
Fall NOS

ACCIDENTS CAUSED BY FIRE AND FLAMES (E890-E899)

Includes: asphyxia or poisoning due to conflagration or ignition
burning by fire
secondary fires resulting from explosion

> *Excludes:* arson (E968.0)
> *fire in or on:*
> *machinery (in operation) (E919.0-E919.9)*
> *transport vehicle other than stationary vehicle (E800.0-E845.9)*
> *vehicle not elsewhere classifiable (E846-E848)*

ALERT! For coding late effects of accident caused by fire see E929.4

E890   Conflagration in private dwelling
Includes: conflagration in:
apartment
boarding house
camping place
caravan
farmhouse
house
lodging house
mobile home
private garage
rooming house
tenement
conflagration originating from sources classifiable to E893-E898 in the above buildings

E890.0   Explosion caused by conflagration

E890.1   Fumes from combustion of polyvinylchloride [PVC] and similar material in conflagration

E890.2   Other smoke and fumes from conflagration
Carbon monoxide from conflagration in private building
Fumes NOS from conflagration in private building
Smoke NOS from conflagration in private building

E890.3   Burning caused by conflagration

E890.8   Other accident resulting from conflagration
Collapse of burning private building
Fall from burning private building
Hit by object falling from burning private building
Jump from burning private building

E890.9   Unspecified accident resulting from conflagration in private dwelling
ALERT! For coding late effects of unspecified accident see E929.9

● Code new   ▲ Revision of   ④ ⑤ Fourth or fifth
to this edition   existing code   digit required

E891 Conflagration in other and unspecified building or structure

Conflagration in:
  barn
  church
  convalescent and other
    residential home
  dormitory of educational
    institution
  factory

Conflagration in:
  farm outbuildings
  hospital
  hotel
  school
  store
  theater

Conflagration originating from sources classifiable to E893-E898, in the above buildings

E891.0 Explosion caused by conflagration

E891.1 Fumes from combustion of polyvinylchloride [PVC] and similar material in conflagration

E891.2 Other smoke and fumes from conflagration
  Carbon monoxide from conflagration in building or structure
  Fumes NOS from conflagration in building or structure
  Smoke NOS from conflagration in building or structure

E891.3 Burning caused by conflagration

E891.8 Other accident resulting from conflagration
  Collapse of burning building or structure
  Fall from burning building or structure
  Hit by object falling from burning building or structure
  Jump from burning building or structure

E891.9 Unspecified accident resulting from conflagration of other and unspecified building or structure

  ALERT! For coding late effects of unspecified accident see E929.9

E892 Conflagration not in building or structure
  Fire (uncontrolled) (in) (of):
    forest
    grass
    hay
    lumber
    mine
    prairie
    transport vehicle [any], except while in transit
    tunnel

E893 Accident caused by ignition of clothing

  Excludes: ignition of clothing:
      from highly inflammable material (E894)
      with conflagration (E890.0-E892)

E893.0 From controlled fire in private dwelling
  Ignition of clothing from:
    normal fire (charcoal) (coal) (electric) (gas) (wood) in:
      brazier in private dwelling (as listed in E890)
      fireplace in private dwelling (as listed in E890)
      furnace in private dwelling (as listed in E890)
      stove in private dwelling (as listed in E890)

E893.1 From controlled fire in other building or structure
  Ignition of clothing from:
    normal fire (charcoal) (coal) (electric) (gas) (wood) in:
      brazier in other building or structure (as listed in E891)
      fireplace in other building or structure (as listed in E891)
      furnace in other building or structure (as listed in E891)
      stove in other building or structure (as listed in E891)

E893.2 From controlled fire not in building or structure
  Ignition of clothing from:
    bonfire (controlled)
    brazier fire (controlled), not in building or structure
    trash fire (controlled)

  Excludes: conflagration not in building (E892)
      trash fire out of control (E892)

| | Add 4th or 5th digit | | Nonspecific code | | Unspecified code | | Manifestation code |

E893.8 From other specified sources

Ignition of clothing from:
- blowlamp
- blowtorch
- burning bedspread
- candle
- cigar

Ignition of clothing from:
- cigarette
- lighter
- matches
- pipe
- welding torch

E893.9 Unspecified source

Ignition of clothing (from controlled fire NOS) (in building NOS) NOS

E894 Ignition of highly inflammable material

Ignition of:
- benzine (with ignition of clothing)
- gasoline (with ignition of clothing)
- fat (with ignition of clothing)
- kerosene (with ignition of clothing)
- paraffin (with ignition of clothing)
- petrol (with ignition of clothing)

Excludes: *ignition of highly inflammable material with:*
  conflagration (E890.0-E892)
  explosion (E923.0-E923.9)

E895 Accident caused by controlled fire in private dwelling

Burning by (flame of) normal fire (charcoal) (coal) (electric) (gas) (wood) in:
- brazier in private dwelling (as listed in E890)
- fireplace in private dwelling (as listed in E890)
- furnace in private dwelling (as listed in E890)
- stove in private dwelling (as listed in E890)

Excludes: *burning by hot objects not producing fire or flames (E924.0-E924.9)*
  ignition of clothing from these sources (E893.0)
  poisoning by carbon monoxide from incomplete combustion of fuel (E867-E868.9)
  that with conflagration (E890.0-E890.9)

E896 Accident caused by controlled fire in other and unspecified building or structure

Burning by (flame of) normal fire (charcoal) (coal) (electric) (gas) (wood) in:
- brazier in other building or structure (as listed in E891)
- fireplace in other building or structure (as listed in E891)
- furnace in other building or structure (as listed in E891)
- stove in other building or structure (as listed in E891)

Excludes: *burning by hot objects not producing fire or flames (E924.0-E924.9)*
  ignition of clothing from these sources (E893.1)
  poisoning by carbon monoxide from incomplete combustion of fuel (E867-E868.9)
  that with conflagration (E891.0-E891.9)

E897 Accident caused by controlled fire not in building or structure

Burns from flame of:
- bonfire (controlled)
- brazier fire (controlled), not in building or structure
- trash fire (controlled)

Excludes: *ignition of clothing from these sources (E893.2)*
  trash fire out of control (E892)
  that with conflagration (E892)

E898 Accident caused by other specified fire and flames

Excludes: *conflagration (E890.0-E892)*
  that with ignition of:
  clothing (E893.0-E893.9)
  highly inflammable material (E894)

E898.0 Burning bedclothes

Bed set on fire NOS

E898.1 Other

Burning by:
- blowlamp
- blowtorch
- candle
- cigar
- cigarette
- fire in room NOS

Burning by:
- lamp
- lighter
- matches
- pipe
- welding torch

E899 Accident caused by unspecified fire

Burning NOS

● Code new
  to this edition

▲ Revision of
  existing code

④ ⑤ Fourth or fifth
  digit required

ACCIDENTS DUE TO NATURAL AND ENVIRONMENTAL FACTORS (E900-E909)

ALERT! For coding late effects of accident due to natural and environmental factors see E929.5

E900 Excessive heat

E900.0 Due to weather conditions
Excessive heat as the external cause of:
    ictus solaris
    siriasis
    sunstroke

E900.1 Of man-made origin
Heat (in):	Heat (in):
boiler room	generated in transport vehicle
drying room	kitchen
factory	
furnace room	

E900.9 Of unspecified origin

E901 Excessive cold

E901.0 Due to weather conditions
Excessive cold as the cause of:
    chilblains NOS
    immersion foot

E901.1 Of man-made origin
Contact with or inhalation of:
    dry ice
    liquid air
    liquid hydrogen
    liquid nitrogen
Prolonged exposure in:
    deep freeze unit
    refrigerator

E901.8 Other specified origin

E901.9 Of unspecified origin

E902 High and low air pressure and changes in air pressure

E902.0 Residence or prolonged visit at high altitude
Residence or prolonged visit at high altitude as the cause of:
    Acosta syndrome
    Alpine sickness
    altitude sickness
    Andes disease
    anoxia, hypoxia
    barotitis, barodontalgia, barosinusitis, otitic barotrauma
    hypobarism, hypobaropathy
    mountain sickness
    range disease

E902.1 In aircraft
Sudden change in air pressure in aircraft during ascent or descent as the cause of:
    aeroneurosis
    aviators' disease

E902.2 Due to diving
High air pressure from rapid descent in water as the cause of:
    caisson disease
    divers' disease
    divers' palsy or paralysis
Reduction in atmospheric pressure while surfacing from deep water diving as the cause of:
    caisson disease
    divers' disease
    divers' palsy or paralysis

E902.8 Due to other specified causes
Reduction in atmospheric pressure while surfacing from underground

E902.9 Unspecified cause

E903 Travel and motion

	Add 4th or 5th digit		Nonspecific code		Unspecified code		Manifestation code

E904 Hunger, thirst, exposure, and neglect

> *Excludes:* *any condition resulting from homicidal intent (E968.0-E968.9)*
>> *hunger, thirst, and exposure resulting from accidents connected with transport (E800.0-E848)*

E904.0 Abandonment or neglect of infants and helpless persons
  Exposure to weather conditions resulting from abandonment or neglect
  Hunger or thirst resulting from abandonment or neglect
  Desertion of newborn
  Inattention at or after birth
  Lack of care (helpless person) (infant)

> *Excludes:* *criminal [purposeful] neglect (E968.4)*

E904.1 Lack of food
  Lack of food as the cause of:
    inanition
    insufficient nourishment
    starvation

> *Excludes:* *hunger resulting from abandonment or neglect (E904.0)*

E904.2 Lack of water
  Lack of water as the cause of:
    dehydration
    inanition

> *Excludes:* *dehydration due to acute fluid loss (276.51)*

E904.3 Exposure (to weather conditions), not elsewhere classifiable
  Exposure NOS   Struck by hailstones
  Humidity

> *Excludes:* *struck by lightning (E907)*

E904.9 Privation, unqualified
  Destitution

E905 Venomous animals and plants as the cause of poisoning and toxic reactions
  Includes: chemical released by animal
       insects
       release of venom through fangs, hairs, spines, tentacles, and other venom
         apparatus

> *Excludes:* *eating of poisonous animals or plants (E865.0-E865.9)*

E905.0 Venomous snakes and lizards
  Cobra   Mamba
  Copperhead snake   Rattlesnake
  Coral snake   Sea snake
  Fer de lance   Snake (venomous)
  Gila monster   Viper
  Krait   Water moccasin

> *Excludes:* *bites of snakes and lizards known to be nonvenomous (E906.2)*

E905.1 Venomous spiders
  Black widow spider   Tarantula (venomous)
  Brown spider

E905.2 Scorpion

E905.3 Hornets, wasps, and bees
  Yellow jacket

E905.4 Centipede and venomous millipede (tropical)

E905.5 Other venomous arthropods
  Sting of:
    ant
    caterpillar

E905.6 Venomous marine animals and plants
  Puncture by sea urchin spine   Sting of:
  Sting of: nematocysts
    coral   sea anemone
    jelly fish   sea cucumber
                                   other marine animal or plant

> *Excludes:* *bites and other injuries caused by nonvenomous marine animal (E906.2-E906.8)*
>> *bite of sea snake (venomous) (E905.0)*

● Code new
  to this edition

▲ Revision of
  existing code

④ ⑤ Fourth or fifth
    digit required

E905.7 **Poisoning and toxic reactions caused by other plants**

Injection of poisons or toxins into or through skin by plant thorns, spines, or other mechanisms

Excludes: puncture wound NOS by plant thorns or spines (E920.8)

E905.8 **Other specified**

E905.9 **Unspecified**

Sting NOS   Venomous bite NOS

E906 Other injury caused by animals

Excludes: poisoning and toxic reactions caused by venomous animals and insects
(E905.0-E905.9)
road vehicle accident involving animals (E827.0-E828.9)
tripping or falling over an animal (E885.9)

E906.0 **Dog bite**

E906.1 **Rat bite**

E906.2 **Bite of nonvenomous snakes and lizards**

E906.3 **Bite of other animal except arthropod**

Cats   Rodents, except rats
Moray eel   Shark

E906.4 **Bite of nonvenomous arthropod**

Insect bite NOS

E906.5 **Bite by unspecified animal**

Animal bite NOS

E906.8 **Other specified injury caused by animal**

Butted by animal
Fallen on by horse or other animal, not being ridden
Gored by animal
Implantation of quills of porcupine
Pecked by bird
Run over by animal, not being ridden
Stepped on by animal, not being ridden

Excludes: injury by animal being ridden (E828.0-E828.9)

E906.9 **Unspecified injury caused by animal**

E907 Lightning

Excludes: injury from:

fall of tree or other object caused by lightning (E916)
fire caused by lightning (E890.0-E892)

E908 Cataclysmic storms, and floods resulting from storms

Excludes: collapse of dam or man-made structure causing flood (E909.3)

E908.0 **Hurricane**

Storm surge
"Tidal wave" caused by storm action
Typhoon

E908.1 **Tornado**

Cyclone
Twisters

E908.2 **Floods**

Torrential rainfall
Flash flood

Excludes: collapse of dam or man-made structure causing flood (909.3)

E908.3 **Blizzard (snow) (ice)**

E908.4 **Dust storm**

E908.8 **Other cataclysmic storms**

E908.9 **Unspecified cataclysmic storms, and floods resulting from storms**

Storm NOS

E909 Cataclysmic earth surface movements and eruptions

Excludes: "tidal wave" caused by storm action (E908.0)

transport accident involving collision with avalanche or landslide not in motion
(E800.0-E848)

| | Add 4th or 5th digit | | Nonspecific code | | Unspecified code | | Manifestation code |

E909.0 **Earthquakes**

E909.1 **Volcanic eruptions**
Burns from lava
Ash inhalation

E909.2 **Avalanche, landslide, or mudslide**

E909.3 **Collapse of dam or man-made structure**

E909.4 **Tidal wave caused by earthquake**
Tidal wave NOS
Tsunami

Excludes: *tidal wave caused by tropical storm (E908.0)*

E909.8 **Other cataclysmic earth surface movements and eruptions**

E909.9 **Unspecified cataclysmic earth surface movements and eruptions**

ACCIDENTS CAUSED BY SUBMERSION, SUFFOCATION, AND FOREIGN BODIES (E910-E915)

E910 **Accidental drowning and submersion**
Includes: immersion
swimmers' cramp

Excludes: *diving accident (NOS) (resulting in injury except drowning) (E883.0)*
diving with insufficient air supply (E913.2)
drowning and submersion due to:
cataclysm (E908-E909)
machinery accident (E919.0-E919.9)
transport accident (E800.0-E845.9)
effect of high and low air pressure (E902.2)
injury from striking against objects while in running water (E917.2)

E910.0 **While water-skiing**
Fall from water skis with submersion or drowning

Excludes: *accident to water-skier involving a watercraft and resulting in submersion or other*
injury (E830.4, E831.4)

E910.1 **While engaged in other sport or recreational activity with diving equipment**
Scuba diving NOS
Skin diving NOS
Underwater spear fishing NOS

E910.2 **While engaged in other sport or recreational activity without diving equipment**
Fishing or hunting, except from boat or with diving equipment
Ice skating
Playing in water
Surfboarding
Swimming NOS
Voluntarily jumping from boat, not involved in accident, for swim NOS
Wading in water

Excludes: *jumping into water to rescue another person (E910.3)*

E910.3 **While swimming or diving for purposes other than recreation or sport**
Marine salvage (with diving equipment)
Pearl diving (with diving equipment)
Placement of fishing nets (with diving equipment)
Rescue (attempt) of another person (with diving equipment)
Underwater construction or repairs (with diving equipment)

E910.4 **In bathtub**

E910.8 **Other accidental drowning or submersion**
Drowning in:
quenching tank
swimming pool

E910.9 **Unspecified accidental drowning or submersion**
Accidental fall into water NOS
Drowning NOS

● Code new
to this edition
▲ Revision of
existing code
④ ⑤ Fourth or fifth
digit required

E911 Inhalation and ingestion of food causing obstruction of respiratory tract or suffocation
>> Aspiration and inhalation of food [any] (into respiratory tract) NOS
>> Asphyxia by food [including bone, seed in food, regurgitated food]
>> Choked on food [including bone, seed in food, regurgitated food]
>> Suffocation by food [including bone, seed in food, regurgitated food]
>> Compression of trachea by food lodged in esophagus
>> Interruption of respiration by food lodged in esophagus
>> Obstruction of respiration by food lodged in esophagus
>> Obstruction of pharynx by food (bolus)

> Excludes: *injury, except asphyxia and obstruction of respiratory passage, caused by food*
>> *(E915)*
>> *obstruction of esophagus by food without mention of asphyxia or obstruction of*
>> *respiratory passage (E915)*

E912 Inhalation and ingestion of other object causing obstruction of respiratory tract or suffocation
>> Aspiration and inhalation of foreign body except food (into respiratory tract) NOS
>> Foreign object [bean] [marble] in nose
>> Obstruction of pharynx by foreign body
>> Compression by foreign body in esophagus
>> Interruption of respiration by foreign body in esophagus
>> Obstruction of respiration by foreign body in esophagus

> Excludes: *injury, except asphyxia and obstruction of respiratory passage, caused by foreign*
>> *body (E915)*
>> *obstruction of esophagus by foreign body without mention of asphyxia or*
>> *obstruction in respiratory passage (E915)*

E913 Accidental mechanical suffocation

> Excludes: *mechanical suffocation from or by:*
>> *accidental inhalation or ingestion of:*
>>> *food (E911)*
>>> *foreign object (E912)*
>> *cataclysm (E908-E909)*
>> *explosion (E921.0-E921.9, E923.0-E923.9)*
>> *machinery accident (E919.0-E919.9)*

E913.0 In bed or cradle

> Excludes: *suffocation by plastic bag (E913.1)*

E913.1 By plastic bag

E913.2 Due to lack of air (in closed place)
>> Accidentally closed up in refrigerator or other airtight enclosed space
>> Diving with insufficient air supply

> Excludes: *suffocation by plastic bag (E913.1)*

E913.3 By falling earth or other substance
>> Cave-in NOS

> Excludes: *cave-in caused by cataclysmic earth surface movements and eruptions (E909)*
>> *struck by cave-in without asphyxiation or suffocation (E916)*

E913.8 Other specified means
>> Accidental hanging, except in bed or cradle

E913.9 Unspecified means
>> Asphyxia, mechanical NOS
>> Strangulation NOS
>> Suffocation NOS

E914 Foreign body accidentally entering eye and adnexa

> Excludes: *corrosive liquid (E924.1)*

E915 Foreign body accidentally entering other orifice

> Excludes: *aspiration and inhalation of foreign body, any, (into respiratory tract) NOS*
>> *(E911-E912)*

Add 4th or
5th digit

Nonspecific
code

Unspecified
code

Manifestation
code

OTHER ACCIDENTS (E916-E928)

E916 Struck accidentally by falling object

Collapse of building, except on fire
Falling:
   rock
   snowslide NOS
   stone
   tree

Object falling from:
   machine, not in operation
   stationary vehicle

   Code first: collapse of building on fire (E890.0-E891.9)
         falling object in:
            cataclysm (E908-E909)
            machinery accidents (E919.0-E919.9)
            transport accidents (E800.0-E845.9)
            vehicle accidents not elsewhere classifiable (E846-E848)
         object set in motion by:
            explosion (E921.0-E921.9, E923.0-E923.9)
            firearm (E922.0-E922.9)
            projected object (E917.0-E917.9)

ALERT! For coding late effects of other accidents see E929.8

E917 Striking against or struck accidentally by objects or persons

Includes: bumping into or against:
            object (moving) (projected) (stationary)
            pedestrian conveyance
            person
         colliding with:
            object (moving) (projected) (stationary)
            pedestrian conveyance
            person
         kicking against:
            object (moving) (projected) (stationary)
            pedestrian conveyance
            person
         stepping on:
            object (moving) (projected) (stationary)
            pedestrian conveyance
            person
         struck by:
            object (moving) (projected) (stationary)
            pedestrian conveyance
            person

Excludes: *fall from collision with another person, except when caused by a crowd*
     (E886.0-E886.9)
   fall from stumbling over object (E885.9)
   fall resulting in striking against object (E888.0, E888.1)
   injury caused by:
     assault (E960.0-E960.1, E967.0-E967.9)
     cutting or piercing instrument (E920.0-E920.9)
     explosion (E921.0-E921.9, E923.0-E923.9)
     firearm (E922.0-E922.9)
     machinery (E919.0-E919.9)
     transport vehicle (E800.0-E845.9)
     vehicle not elsewhere classifiable (E846-E848)

E917.0 In sports without subsequent fall
   Kicked or stepped on during game (football) (rugby)
   Struck by hit or thrown ball
   Struck by hockey stick or puck

E917.1 Caused by a crowd, by collective fear or panic without subsequent fall
   Crushed by crown or human stampede
   Pushed by crown or human stampede
   Stepped on by crown or human stampede

E917.2 In running water without subsequent fall
Excludes: *drowning or submersion (E910.0-E910.9)*
     that in sports (E917.0, E917.5)

E917.3 Furniture without subsequent fall
Excludes: *fall from furniture (E884.2, E884.4-E884.5)*

● Code new
   to this edition
    ▲ Revision of
      existing code
    ④ ⑤ Fourth or fifth
         digit required

E917.4 **Other stationary object without subsequent fall**
Bath tub
Fence
Lamp-post

E917.5 **Object in sports with subsequent fall**
Knocked down while boxing

E917.6 **Caused by a crowd, by collective fear or panic with subsequent fall**

E917.7 **Furniture with subsequent fall**

Excludes: *fall from furniture (E884.2, E884.4-E884.5)*

E917.8 **Other stationary object with subsequent fall**
Bath tub
Fence
Lamp-post

E917.9 **Other striking against with or without subsequent fall**

E918 **Caught accidentally in or between objects**
Caught, crushed, jammed, or pinched in or between moving or stationary objects, such as:
escalator
folding object
hand tools, appliances, or implements
sliding door and door frame
under packing crate
washing machine wringer

Excludes: *injury caused by:*
cutting or piercing instrument (E920.0-E920.9)
machinery (E919.0-E919.9)
mechanism or component of firearm and air gun (E928.7)
transport vehicle (E800.0-E845.9)
vehicle not elsewhere classifiable (E846-E848)
struck accidentally by:
falling object (E916)
object (moving) (projected) (E917.0-E917.9)

E919 **Accidents caused by machinery**
Includes:
burned by machinery (accident)
caught in (moving parts of) machinery (accident)
collapse of machinery (accident)
crushed by machinery (accident)
cut or pierced by machinery (accident)
drowning or submersion caused by machinery (accident)
explosion of, on, in machinery (accident)
fall from or into moving part of machinery (accident)
fire starting in or on machinery (accident)
mechanical suffocation caused by machinery (accident)
object falling from, on, in motion by machinery (accident)
overturning of machinery (accident)
pinned under machinery (accident)
run over by machinery (accident)
struck by machinery (accident)
thrown from machinery (accident)
caught between machinery and other object
machinery accident NOS

Excludes: *accidents involving machinery, not in operation (E884.9, E916-E918)*
injury caused by:
electric current in connection with machinery (E925.0-E925.9)
escalator (E880.0, E918)
explosion of pressure vessel in connection with machinery (E921.0-E921.9)
mechanism or component of firearm and air gun (E928.7)
moving sidewalk (E885.9)
powered hand tools, appliances, and implements (E916-E918, E920.0-E921.9,
E923.0-E926.9)
transport vehicle accidents involving machinery (E800.0-E848.9)
poisoning by carbon monoxide generated by machine (E868.8)

Add 4th or 5th digit   Nonspecific code   Unspecified code   Manifestation code

E919.0 Agriculture machines

Animal-powered
  agricultural machine
Combine
Derrick, hay
Farm machinery NOS

Farm tractor
Harvester
Hay mower or rake
Reaper
Thresher

Excludes: *that in transport under own power on the highway (E810.0-E819.9)*
that being towed by another vehicle on the highway (E810.0-E819.9,
E827.0-E827.9, E829.0-E829.9)
that involved in accident classifiable to E820-E829 (E820.0-E829.9)

E919.1 Mining and earth-drilling machinery

Bore or drill (land)
(seabed)
Shaft hoist

Shaft lift
Under-cutter

Excludes: *coal car, tram, truck, and tub in mine (E846)*

E919.2 Lifting machines and appliances

Chain hoist except in agricultural or mining operations
Crane except in agricultural or mining operations
Derrick except in agricultural or mining operations
Elevator (building) (grain) except in agricultural or mining operations
Forklift truck except in agricultural or mining operations
Lift except in agricultural or mining operations
Pulley block except in agricultural or mining operations
Winch except in agricultural or mining operations

Excludes: *that being towed by another vehicle on the highway (E810.0-E819.9,*
E827.0-E827.9, E829.0-E829.9)
that in transport under own power on the highway (E810.0-E819.9)
that involved in accident classifiable to E820-E829 (E820.0-E829.9)

E919.3 Metalworking machines

Abrasive wheel
Forging machine
Lathe
Mechanical shears

Metal:
  drilling machine
  milling machine
  power press
  rolling-mill
  sawing machine

E919.4 Woodworking and forming machines

Band saw
Bench saw
Circular saw
Molding machine
Overhead plane

Powered saw
Radial saw
Sander

Excludes: *hand saw (E920.1)*

E919.5 Prime movers, except electrical motors

Gas turbine
Internal combustion engine

Steam engine
Water driven turbine

Excludes: *that being towed by other vehicle on the highway (E810.0-E819.9, E827.0-E827.9,*
E829.0-E829.9)
that in transport under own power on the highway (E810.0-E819.9)

E919.6 Transmission machinery

Transmission:
  belt
  cable
  chain
  gear

Transmission:
  pinion
  pulley
  shaft

E919.7 Earth moving, scraping, and other excavating machines

Bulldozer
Road scraper

Steam shovel

Excludes: *that being towed by other vehicle on the highway (E810.0-E819.9, E827.0-E827.9,*
E829.0-E829.9)
that in transport under own power on the highway (E810.0-E819.9)

● Code new
   to this edition
▲ Revision of
   existing code
④ ⑤ Fourth or fifth
   digit required

E919.8 Other specified machinery

Machines for manufacture of: Printing machine
    clothing   Recreational machinery
    foodstuffs and beverages   Spinning, weaving, and textile machines
    paper

E919.9 Unspecified machinery

E920 Accidents caused by cutting and piercing instruments or objects

Includes: accidental injury (by) object:
       edged
       pointed
       sharp

Excludes: *injury caused by mechanism or component of firearm and air gun (E928.7)*

E920.0 Powered lawn mower

E920.1 Other powered hand tools

Any powered hand tool [compressed air] [electric] [explosive cartridge] [hydraulic power], such as:
    drill   rivet gun
    hand saw   snow blower
    hedge clipper   staple gun

Excludes: *band saw (E919.4)*
           bench saw (E919.4)

E920.2 Powered household appliances and implements

Blender   Electric:
Electric: knife
   beater or mixer   sewing machine
   can opener   Garbage disposal appliance
   fan

E920.3 Knives, swords, and daggers

E920.4 Other hand tools and implements

Axe   Paper cutter
Can opener NOS   Pitchfork
Chisel   Rake
Fork   Scissors
Hand saw   Screwdriver
Hoe   Sewing machine, not powered
Ice pick   Shovel
Needle (sewing)

E920.5 Hypodermic needle

Contaminated needle
Needle stick

E920.8 Other specified cutting and piercing instruments or objects

Arrow   Nail
Broken glass   Plant thorn
Dart   Splinter
Edge of stiff paper   Tin can lid
Lathe turnings

Excludes: *animal spines or quills (E906.8)*
          flying glass due to explosion (E921.0-E923.9)

E920.9 Unspecified cutting and piercing instrument or object

E921 Accident caused by explosion of pressure vessel

Includes: accidental explosion of pressure vessels, whether or not part of machinery

Excludes: *explosion of pressure vessel on transport vehicle (E800.0-E845.9)*

E921.0 Boilers

E921.1 Gas cylinders

Air tank   Pressure gas tank

E921.8 Other specified pressure vessels

Aerosol can   Pressure cooker
Automobile tire

E921.9 Unspecified pressure vessel

	Add 4th or 5th digit		Nonspecific code		Unspecified code		Manifestation code

E922 **Accident caused by firearm and air gun missile**

> Excludes: *injury caused by mechanism or component of firearm and air gun (E928.7)*

E922.0 **Handgun**
    Pistol   Revolver

> Excludes: *Verey pistol (E922.8)*

E922.1 **Shotgun (automatic)**

E922.2 **Hunting rifle**

E922.3 **Military firearms**
    Army rifle   Machine gun

E922.4 **Air gun**
    BB gun   Pellet gun

E922.5 **Paintball gun**

E922.8 **Other specified firearm missile**
    Verey pistol [flare]

E922.9 **Unspecified firearm missile**
    Gunshot wound NOS   Shot NOS

E923 **Accident caused by explosive material**
    Includes: flash burns and other injuries resulting from explosion of explosive material
                 ignition of highly explosive material with explosion

> Excludes: *explosion:*
>
>   *in or on machinery (E919.0-E919.9)*
>   *on any transport vehicle, except stationary motor vehicle (E800.0-E848)*
>   *with conflagration (E890.0, E891.0, E892)*
>   *injury caused by mechanism or component of firearm and air gun (E928.7)*
>   *secondary fires resulting from explosion (E890.0-E899)*

E923.0 **Fireworks**

E923.1 **Blasting materials**
    Blasting cap   Explosive [any] used in blasting operations
    Detonator
    Dynamite

E923.2 **Explosive gases**
    Acetylene   Fire damp
    Butane   Gasoline fumes
    Coal gas   Methane
    Explosion in mine NOS   Propane

E923.8 **Other explosive materials**
    Bomb   Torpedo
    Explosive missile   Explosion in munitions:
    Grenade   dump
    Mine   factory
    Shell

E923.9 **Unspecified explosive material**
    Explosion NOS

E924 **Accident caused by hot substance or object, caustic or corrosive material, and steam**

> Excludes: *burning NOS (E899)*
>
>   *chemical burn resulting from swallowing a corrosive substance (E860.0-E864.4)*
>   *fire caused by these substances and objects (E890.0-E894)*
>   *radiation burns (E926.0-E926.9)*
>   *therapeutic misadventures (E870.0-E876.9)*

E924.0 **Hot liquids and vapors, including steam**
    Burning or scalding by:
       boiling water
       hot or boiling liquids not primarily caustic or corrosive
       liquid metal
       steam
       other hot vapor

> Excludes: *hot (boiling) tap water (E924.2)*

● Code new
   to this edition   ▲ Revision of   ④ ⑤ Fourth or fifth
                  existing code   digit required

E924.1 Caustic and corrosive substances
Burning by:
acid [any kind]
ammonia
caustic oven cleaner or other substance
corrosive substance
lye
vitriol

E924.2 Hot (boiling) tap water

E924.8 Other
Burning by:
heat from electric heating appliance
hot object NOS
light bulb
steam pipe

E924.9 Unspecified

E925 Accident caused by electric current
Includes: electric current from exposed wire, faulty appliance, high voltage cable, live rail, or open electric socket as the cause of:
burn
cardiac fibrillation
convulsion
electric shock
electrocution
puncture wound
respiratory paralysis

Excludes: *burn by heat from electrical appliance (E924.8)*
lightning (E907)

E925.0 Domestic wiring and appliances

E925.1 Electric power generating plants, distribution stations, transmission lines
Broken power line

E925.2 Industrial wiring, appliances, and electrical machinery
Conductors
Control apparatus
Electrical equipment and machinery
Transformers

E925.8 Other electric current
Wiring and appliances in or on:
farm [not farmhouse]
outdoors
public building
residential institutions
schools

E925.9 Unspecified electric current
Burns or other injury from electric current NOS
Electric shock NOS
Electrocution NOS

E926 Exposure to radiation

Excludes: *abnormal reaction to or complication of treatment without mention of misadventure (E879.2)*
atomic power plant malfunction in water transport (E838.0-E838.9)
misadventure to patient in surgical and medical procedures (E873.2-E873.3)
use of radiation in war operations (E996-E997.9)

Add 4th or 5th digit   Nonspecific code   Unspecified code   Manifestation code

E926.0 **Radiofrequency radiation**
  Overexposure to:
    microwave radiation from:
      high-powered radio and television transmitters
      industrial radiofrequency induction heaters
      radar installations
    radar radiation from:
      high-powered radio and television transmitters
      industrial radiofrequency induction heaters
      radar installations
    radiofrequency from:
      high-powered radio and television transmitters
      industrial radiofrequency induction heaters
      radar installations
    radiofrequency radiation [any] from:
      high-powered radio and television transmitters
      industrial radiofrequency induction heaters
      radar installations

E926.1 **Infra-red heaters and lamps**
  Exposure to infra-red radiation from heaters and lamps as the cause of:
    blistering
    burning
    charring
    inflammatory change

  Excludes: *physical contact with heater or lamp (E924.8)*

E926.2 **Visible and ultraviolet light sources**
  Arc lamps
  Black light sources
  Electrical welding arc
  Oxygas welding torch
  Sun rays
  Tanning bed

  Excludes: *excessive heat from these sources (E900.1-E900.9)*

E926.3 **X-rays and other electromagnetic ionizing radiation**
  Gamma rays   X-rays (hard) (soft)

E926.4 **Lasers**

E926.5 **Radioactive isotopes**
  Radiobiologicals   Radiopharmaceuticals

E926.8 **Other specified radiation**
  Artificially accelerated beams of ionized particles generated by:
    betatrons
    synchrotrons

E926.9 **Unspecified radiation**
  Radiation NOS

E927 **Overexertion and strenuous and repetitive movements or loads**
Use additional code to identify activity (E001-E030)

E927.0 **Overexertion from sudden strenuous movement**
  Sudden trauma from strenuous movement

E927.1 **Overexertion from prolonged static position**
  Overexertion from maintaining prolonged positions, such as:
    holding
    sitting
    standing

E927.2 **Excessive physical exertion from prolonged activity**

E927.3 **Cumulative trauma from repetitive motion**
  Cumulative trauma from repetitive movements

E927.4 **Cumulative trauma from repetitive impact**

E927.8 **Other overexertion and strenuous and repetitive movements or loads**

E927.9 **Unspecified overexertion and strenuous and repetitive movements or loads**

E928 **Other and unspecified environmental and accidental causes**

E928.0 **Prolonged stay in weightless environment**
  Weightlessness in spacecraft (simulator)

● Code new   ▲ Revision of   ④ ⑤ Fourth or fifth
      to this edition   existing code   digit required

E928.1 **Exposure to noise**
　　Noise (pollution)
　　Sound waves
　　Supersonic waves

E928.2 **Vibration**

E928.3 **Human bite**

E928.4 **External constriction caused by hair**

E928.5 **External constriction caused by other object**

E928.6 **Environmental exposure to harmful algae and toxins**
　　Algae bloom NOS
　　Blue-green algae bloom
　　Brown tide
　　Cyanobacteria bloom
　　Florida red tide
　　Harmful algae bloom
　　Pfiesteria piscicida
　　Red tide

E928.7 **Mechanism or component of firearm and air gun**
　　Injury due to:
　　　explosion of gun parts
　　　recoil
　　Pierced, cut, crushed, or pinched by slide trigger mechanism, scope or other gun part
　　Powder burn from firearm or air gun

　　Excludes: *accident caused by firearm and air gun missile (E922.0-E922.9)*

E928.8 **Other**

E928.9 **Unspecified accident**
　　Accident NOS stated as accidentally inflicted
　　Blow NOS stated as accidentally inflicted
　　Casualty (not due to war), stated as accidentally inflicted, but not otherwise specified
　　Decapitation, stated as accidentally inflicted, but not otherwise specified
　　Injury [any part of body, or unspecified], stated as accidentally inflicted, but not otherwise specified
　　Killed, stated as accidentally inflicted, but not otherwise specified
　　Knocked down, stated as accidentally inflicted, but not otherwise specified
　　Mangled, stated as accidentally inflicted, but not otherwise specified
　　Wound, stated as accidentally inflicted, but not otherwise specified

　　Excludes: *fracture, cause unspecified (E887)*
　　　　　　injuries undetermined whether accidentally or purposely inflicted (E980.0-E989)

　　ALERT! For coding late effects of unspecified accident see E929.9

LATE EFFECTS OF ACCIDENTAL INJURY (E929)

Note: This category is to be used to indicate accidental injury as the cause of death or disability from late effects, which are themselves classifiable elsewhere. The "late effects" include conditions reported as such or as sequelae which may occur at any time after the acute injury.

E929 **Late effects of accidental injury**
　　Excludes: *late effects of:*
　　　　　　surgical and medical procedures (E870.0-E879.9)
　　　　　　therapeutic use of drugs and medicines (E930.0-E949.9)

E929.0 **Late effects of motor vehicle accident**
　　Late effects of accidents classifiable to E810-E825

E929.1 **Late effects of other transport accident**
　　Late effects of accidents classifiable to E800-E807, E826-E838, E840-E848

E929.2 **Late effects of accidental poisoning**
　　Late effects of accidents classifiable to E850-E858, E860-E869

E929.3 **Late effects of accidental fall**
　　Late effects of accidents classifiable to E880-E888

E929.4 **Late effects of accident caused by fire**
　　Late effects of accidents classifiable to E890-E899

E929.5 **Late effects of accident due to natural and environmental factors**
　　Late effects of accidents classifiable to E900-E909

E929.8 **Late effects of other accidents**
　　Late effects of accidents classifiable to E910-E928.8

	Add 4th or 5th digit		Nonspecific code		Unspecified code		Manifestation code

E929.9 Late effects of unspecified accident
Late effects of accidents classifiable to E928.9

DRUGS, MEDICINAL AND BIOLOGICAL SUBSTANCES CAUSING ADVERSE EFFECTS IN THERAPEUTIC USE (E930-E949)

Includes: correct drug properly administered in therapeutic or prophylactic dosage, as the cause of any adverse effect including allergic or hypersensitivity reactions

Excludes: *accidental overdose of drug and wrong drug given or taken in error (E850.0-E858.9)*
accidents in the technique of administration of drug or biological substance, such as accidental puncture during injection, or contamination of drug (E870.0-E876.9)
administration with suicidal or homicidal intent or intent to harm, or in circumstances classifiable to E950.0-E950.5, E962.0, E980.0-E980.5

See Alphabetic Index for more complete list of specific drugs to be classified under the fourth-digit subdivisions. The American Hospital Formulary numbers can be used to classify new drugs listed by the American Hospital Formulary Service (AHFS). See appendix C.

E930 Antibiotics

Excludes: *that used as eye, ear, nose, and throat [ENT], and local anti-infectives (E946.0-E946.9)*

DEFINITION An antibiotic is any substance that can destroy or inhibit the growth of bacteria and similar microorganisms

E930.0 Penicillins
Natural
Synthetic
Semisynthetic, such as:
 ampicillin
 cloxacillin
 nafcillin
 oxacillin

E930.1 Antifungal antibiotics
Amphotericin B
Griseofulvin
Hachimycin [trichomycin]
Nystatin

E930.2 Chloramphenicol group
Chloramphenicol
Thiamphenicol

E930.3 Erythromycin and other macrolides
Oleandomycin
Spiramycin

E930.4 Tetracycline group
Doxycycline
Minocycline
Oxytetracycline

E930.5 Cephalosporin group
Cephalexin
Cephaloglycin
Cephaloridine
Cephalothin

E930.6 Antimycobacterial antibiotics
Cycloserine
Kanamycin
Rifampin
Streptomycin

E930.7 Antineoplastic antibiotics
Actinomycins, such as:
 Cactinomycin
 Dactinomycin
 Bleomycin
 Daunorubicin
 Mitomycin

Excludes: *other antineoplastic drugs (E933.1)*

● Code new
 to this edition

▲ Revision of
 existing code

④ ⑤ Fourth or fifth
 digit required

E930.8 Other specified antibiotics

E930.9 Unspecified antibiotic

E931 Other anti-infectives

> *Excludes:* ENT, and local anti-infectives (E946.0-E946.9)

E931.0 Sulfonamides
Sulfadiazine
Sulfafurazole
Sulfamethoxazole

E931.1 Arsenical anti-infectives

E931.2 Heavy metal anti-infectives
Compounds of:
antimony
bismuth
lead
mercury

> *Excludes:* mercurial diuretics (E944.0)

ALERT! For personal history of contact with and (suspected) exposure to lead see V15.86

E931.3 Quinoline and hydroxyquinoline derivatives
Chiniofon
Diiodohydroxyquin

> *Excludes:* antimalarial drugs (E931.4)

E931.4 Antimalarials and drugs acting on other blood protozoa
Chloroquine phosphate   Proguanil [chloroguanide]
Cycloguanil   Pyrimethamine
Primaquine   Quinine (sulphate)

E931.5 Other antiprotozoal drugs
Emetine

E931.6 Anthelmintics
Hexylresorcinol   Piperazine
Male fern oleoresin   Thiabendazole

E931.7 Antiviral drugs
Methisazone

> *Excludes:* amantadine (E936.4)
> cytarabine (E933.1)
> idoxuridine (E946.5)

E931.8 Other antimycobacterial drugs
Ethambutol   Para-aminosalicylic acid derivatives
Ethionamide   Sulfones
Isoniazid

E931.9 Other and unspecified anti-infectives
Flucytosine   Nitrofuran derivatives

E932 Hormones and synthetic substitutes

DEFINITION Hormones are chemical substances having a specific regulatory effect on the activity of a certain organ or organs.

E932.0 Adrenal cortical steroids
Cortisone derivatives
Desoxycorticosterone derivatives
Fluorinated corticosteroids

ALERT! For personal history of inhaled steroid therapy see V87.44

ALERT! For personal history of systemic steroid therapy see V87.45

E932.1 Androgens and anabolic congeners
Nandrolone phenpropionate
Oxymetholone
Testosterone and preparations

E932.2 Ovarian hormones and synthetic substitutes
Contraceptives, oral
Estrogens
Estrogens and progestogens combined
Progestogens

ALERT! For personal history of estrogen therapy see V87.43

| | Add 4th or 5th digit | | Nonspecific code | | Unspecified code | | Manifestation code |

E932.3 Insulins and antidiabetic agents

Acetohexamide	Insulin
Biguanide derivatives, oral	Phenformin
Chlorpropamide	Sulfonylurea derivatives, oral
Glucagon	Tolbutamide

Excludes: adverse effect of insulin administered for shock therapy (E879.3)

E932.4 Anterior pituitary hormones

Corticotropin	Somatotropin [growth hormone]
Gonadotropin	

E932.5 Posterior pituitary hormones
    Vasopressin

Excludes: oxytocic agents (E945.0)

E932.6 Parathyroid and parathyroid derivatives

E932.7 Thyroid and thyroid derivatives

Dextrothyroxine	Liothyronine
Levothyroxine sodium	Thyroglobulin

E932.8 Antithyroid agents

Iodides	Thiourea
Thiouracil	

E932.9 Other and unspecified hormones and synthetic substitutes

E933 Primarily systemic agents

E933.0 Antiallergic and antiemetic drugs

Antihistamines	Diphenylpyraline
Chlorpheniramine	Thonzylamine
Diphenhydramine	Tripelennamine

Excludes: phenothiazine-based tranquilizers (E939.1)

E933.1 Antineoplastic and immunosuppressive drugs

Azathioprine	Mechlorethamine hydrochloride
Busulfan	Mercaptopurine
Chlorambucil	Triethylenethiophosphoramide [thio-TEPA]
Cyclophosphamide	
Cytarabine	
Fluorouracil	

Excludes: antineoplastic antibiotics (E930.7)

ALERT! For personal history of antineoplastic chemotherapy see V87.41

ALERT! For personal history of immunosuppressive therapy see V87.46

E933.2 Acidifying agents

E933.3 Alkalizing agents

E933.4 Enzymes, not elsewhere classified
    Penicillinase

E933.5 Vitamins, not elsewhere classified
    Vitamin A
    Vitamin D

Excludes: nicotinic acid (E942.2)
         vitamin K (E934.3)

E933.6 Oral bisphosphonates

E933.7 Intravenous bisphosphonates

E933.8 Other systemic agents, not elsewhere classified
    Heavy metal antagonists

E933.9 Unspecified systemic agent

E934 Agents primarily affecting blood constituents

E934.0 Iron and its compounds
    Ferric salts
    Ferrous sulphate and other ferrous salts

E934.1 Liver preparations and other antianemic agents
    Folic acid

E934.2 Anticoagulants

Coumarin	Prothrombin synthesis inhibitor
Heparin	Warfarin sodium
Phenindione	

● Code new
   to this edition

▲ Revision of
   existing code

④ ⑤ Fourth or fifth
       digit required

E934.3 **Vitamin K [phytonadione]**

E934.4 **Fibrinolysis-affecting drugs**
Aminocaproic acid   Streptokinase
Streptodornase   Urokinase

E934.5 **Anticoagulant antagonists and other coagulants**
Hexadimethrine bromide   Protamine sulfate

E934.6 **Gamma globulin**

E934.7 **Natural blood and blood products**
Blood plasma   Packed red cells
Human fibrinogen   Whole blood

E934.8 **Other agents affecting blood constituents**
Macromolecular blood substitutes

E934.9 **Unspecified agent affecting blood constituents**

E935 **Analgesics, antipyretics, and antirheumatics**
DEFINITION Analgesics are drugs that reduce or eliminate pain. Antipyretics are drugs that reduce body temperature in situations such as fever. Antirheumatics are drugs that act against diseases with inflammation or pain in muscles or joints.

E935.0 **Heroin**
Diacetylmorphine

E935.1 **Methadone**

E935.2 **Other opiates and related narcotics**
Codeine [methylmorphine]   Opium (alkaloids)
Morphine   Meperidine [pethidine]

E935.3 **Salicylates**
Acetylsalicylic acid [aspirin]
Amino derivatives of salicylic acid
Salicylic acid salts

E935.4 **Aromatic analgesics, not elsewhere classified**
Acetanilid
Paracetamol [acetaminophen]
Phenacetin [acetophenetidin]

E935.5 **Pyrazole derivatives**
Aminophenazone [aminopyrine]
Phenylbutazone

E935.6 **Antirheumatics [antiphlogistics]**
Gold salts   Indomethacin

Excludes: salicylates (E935.3)
         steroids (E932.0)

E935.7 **Other non-narcotic analgesics**
Pyrabital

E935.8 **Other specified analgesics and antipyretics**
Pentazocine

E935.9 **Unspecified analgesic and antipyretic**

E936 **Anticonvulsants and anti-Parkinsonism drugs**
DEFINITION Anticonvulsants are drugs used to prevent or treat seizures.

E936.0 **Oxazolidine derivatives**
Paramethadione
Trimethadione

E936.1 **Hydantoin derivatives**
Phenytoin

E936.2 **Succinimides**
Ethosuximide
Phensuximide

E936.3 **Other and unspecified anticonvulsants**
Beclamide
Primidone

E936.4 **Anti-Parkinsonism drugs**
Amantadine
Ethopropazine [profenamine]
Levodopa [L-dopa]

| | Add 4th or 5th digit | | Nonspecific code | | Unspecified code | | Manifestation code |

E937 **Sedatives and hypnotics**

E937.0 **Barbiturates**
Amobarbital [amylobarbitone]
Barbital [barbitone]
Butabarbital [butabarbitone]
Pentobarbital [pentobarbitone]
Phenobarbital [phenobarbitone]
Secobarbital [quinalbarbitone]

Excludes: thiobarbiturates (E938.3)

E937.1 **Chloral hydrate group**

E937.2 **Paraldehyde**

E937.3 **Bromine compounds**
Bromide
Carbromal (derivatives)

E937.4 **Methaqualone compounds**

E937.5 **Glutethimide group**

E937.6 **Mixed sedatives, not elsewhere classified**

E937.8 **Other sedatives and hypnotics**

E937.9 **Unspecified**
Sleeping:
drug NOS
pill NOS
tablet NOS

E938 **Other central nervous system depressants and anesthetics**

E938.0 **Central nervous system muscle-tone depressants**
Chlorphenesin (carbamate)   Methocarbamol
Mephenesin

E938.1 **Halothane**

E938.2 **Other gaseous anesthetics**
Ether
Halogenated hydrocarbon derivatives, except halothane
Nitrous oxide

E938.3 **Intravenous anesthetics**
Ketamine   Thiobarbiturates, such as thiopental sodium
Methohexital
[methohexitone]

E938.4 **Other and unspecified general anesthetics**

E938.5 **Surface and infiltration anesthetics**
Cocaine   Procaine
Lidocaine [lignocaine]   Tetracaine

E938.6 **Peripheral nerve- and plexus-blocking anesthetics**

E938.7 **Spinal anesthetics**

E938.9 **Other and unspecified local anesthetics**

E939 **Psychotropic agents**
DEFINITION Psychotropic agents are drugs that act primarily upon the central nervous system resulting in altered brain function, changes in perception, mood, consciousness and behavior.

E939.0 **Antidepressants**
Amitriptyline   Monoamine oxidase [MAO] inhibitors
Imipramine

E939.1 **Phenothiazine-based tranquilizers**
Chlorpromazine   Prochlorperazine
Fluphenazine   Promazine
Phenothiazine

E939.2 **Butyrophenone-based tranquilizers**
Haloperidol   Trifluperidol
Spiperone

E939.3 **Other antipsychotics, neuroleptics, and major tranquilizers**

E939.4 **Benzodiazepine-based tranquilizers**
Chlordiazepoxide   Lorazepam
Diazepam   Medazepam
Flurazepam   Nitrazepam

● Code new
  to this edition
▲ Revision of
  existing code
④ ⑤ Fourth or fifth
    digit required

E939.5 **Other tranquilizers**
     Hydroxyzine   Meprobamate

E939.6 **Psychodysleptics [hallucinogens]**
     Cannabis (derivatives)   Mescaline
     Lysergide [LSD]   Psilocin
     Marijuana (derivatives)   Psilocybin

E939.7 **Psychostimulants**
     Amphetamine   Caffeine

     Excludes: central appetite depressants (E947.0)

E939.8 **Other psychotropic agents**

E939.9 **Unspecified psychotropic agent**

E940 **Central nervous system stimulants**

E940.0 **Analeptics**
     Lobeline
     Nikethamide

E940.1 **Opiate antagonists**
     Levallorphan
     Nalorphine
     Naloxone

E940.8 **Other specified central nervous system stimulants**

E940.9 **Unspecified central nervous system stimulant**

E941 **Drugs primarily affecting the autonomic nervous system**

E941.0 **Parasympathomimetics [cholinergics]**
     Acetylcholine   Pilocarpine
     Anticholinesterase:
       organophosphorus
       reversible

E941.1 **Parasympatholytics [anticholinergics and antimuscarinics] and spasmolytics**
     Atropine   Hyoscine [scopolamine]
     Homatropine   Quaternary ammonium derivatives

     Excludes: papaverine (E942.5)

E941.2 **Sympathomimetics [adrenergics]**
     Epinephrine [adrenalin]
     Levarterenol [noradrenalin]

E941.3 **Sympatholytics [antiadrenergics]**
     Phenoxybenzamine
     Tolazoline hydrochloride

E941.9 **Unspecified drug primarily affecting the autonomic nervous system**

E942 **Agents primarily affecting the cardiovascular system**

E942.0 **Cardiac rhythm regulators**
     Practolol   Propranolol
     Procainamide   Quinidine

E942.1 **Cardiotonic glycosides and drugs of similar action**
     Digitalis glycosides   Strophanthins
     Digoxin

E942.2 **Antilipemic and antiarteriosclerotic drugs**
     Cholestyramine   Nicotinic acid derivatives
     Clofibrate   Sitosterols

     Excludes: dextrothyroxine (E932.7)

E942.3 **Ganglion-blocking agents**
     Pentamethonium bromide

E942.4 **Coronary vasodilators**
     Dipyridamole   Nitrites
     Nitrates [nitroglycerin]   Prenylamine

E942.5 **Other vasodilators**
     Cyclandelate   Hydralazine
     Diazoxide   Papaverine

E942.6 **Other antihypertensive agents**
     Clonidine   Rauwolfia alkaloids
     Guanethidine   Reserpine

| | Add 4th or 5th digit | | Nonspecific code | | Unspecified code | | Manifestation code |

E942.7 Antivaricose drugs, including sclerosing agents
Monoethanolamine   Zinc salts

E942.8 Capillary-active drugs
Adrenochrome derivatives   Metaraminol
Bioflavonoids

E942.9 Other and unspecified agents primarily affecting the cardiovascular system

E943 Agents primarily affecting gastrointestinal system

E943.0 Antacids and antigastric secretion drugs
Aluminum hydroxide   Magnesium trisilicate

E943.1 Irritant cathartics
Bisacodyl   Phenolphthalein
Castor oil

E943.2 Emollient cathartics
Sodium dioctyl sulfosuccinate

E943.3 Other cathartics, including intestinal atonia drugs
Magnesium sulfate

E943.4 Digestants
Pancreatin   Pepsin
Papain

E943.5 Antidiarrheal drugs
Bismuth subcarbonate   Pectin
Kaolin

Excludes: anti-infectives (E930.0-E931.9)

E943.6 Emetics

E943.8 Other specified agents primarily affecting the gastrointestinal system

E943.9 Unspecified agent primarily affecting the gastrointestinal system

E944 Water, mineral, and uric acid metabolism drugs

E944.0 Mercurial diuretics
Chlormerodrin   Mercurophylline
Mercaptomerin   Mersalyl

E944.1 Purine derivative diuretics
Theobromine   Theophylline

Excludes: aminophylline [theophylline ethylenediamine] (E945.7)

E944.2 Carbonic acid anhydrase inhibitors
Acetazolamide

E944.3 Saluretics
Benzothiadiazides
Chlorothiazide group

E944.4 Other diuretics
Ethacrynic acid
Furosemide

E944.5 Electrolytic, caloric, and water-balance agents

E944.6 Other mineral salts, not elsewhere classified

E944.7 Uric acid metabolism drugs
Cinchophen and congeners   Phenoquin
Colchicine   Probenecid

E945 Agents primarily acting on the smooth and skeletal muscles and respiratory system

E945.0 Oxytocic agents
Ergot alkaloids
Prostaglandins

E945.1 Smooth muscle relaxants
Adiphenine
Metaproterenol [orciprenaline]

Excludes: papaverine (E942.5)

E945.2 Skeletal muscle relaxants
Alcuronium chloride
Suxamethonium chloride

E945.3 Other and unspecified drugs acting on muscles

● Code new to this edition   ▲ Revision of existing code   ④ ⑤ Fourth or fifth digit required

E945.4 Antitussives
Dextromethorphan
Pipazethate hydrochloride

E945.5 Expectorants
Acetylcysteine   Ipecacuanha
Cocillana   Terpin hydrate
Guaifenesin [glyceryl guaiacolate]

E945.6 Anti-common cold drugs

E945.7 Antiasthmatics
Aminophylline [theophylline ethylenediamine]

E945.8 Other and unspecified respiratory drugs

E946 Agents primarily affecting skin and mucous membrane, ophthalmological, otorhinolaryngological, and dental drugs

E946.0 Local anti-infectives and anti-inflammatory drugs

E946.1 Antipruritics

E946.2 Local astringents and local detergents

E946.3 Emollients, demulcents, and protectants

E946.4 Keratolytics, keratoplastics, other hair treatment drugs and preparations

E946.5 Eye anti-infectives and other eye drugs
Idoxuridine

E946.6 Anti-infectives and other drugs and preparations for ear, nose, and throat

E946.7 Dental drugs topically applied

E946.8 Other agents primarily affecting skin and mucous membrane
Spermicides

E946.9 Unspecified agent primarily affecting skin and mucous membrane

E947 Other and unspecified drugs and medicinal substances

E947.0 Dietetics

E947.1 Lipotropic drugs

E947.2 Antidotes and chelating agents, not elsewhere classified

E947.3 Alcohol deterrents

E947.4 Pharmaceutical excipients

E947.8 Other drugs and medicinal substances
Contrast media used for diagnostic x-ray procedures
Diagnostic agents and kits
ALERT! For personal history of allergy to radiographic dye see V15.08

E947.9 Unspecified drug or medicinal substance

E948 Bacterial vaccines

E948.0 BCG vaccine

E948.1 Typhoid and paratyphoid

E948.2 Cholera

E948.3 Plague

E948.4 Tetanus

E948.5 Diphtheria

E948.6 Pertussis vaccine, including combinations with a pertussis component

E948.8 Other and unspecified bacterial vaccines

E948.9 Mixed bacterial vaccines, except combinations with a pertussis component

E949 Other vaccines and biological substances
Excludes: gamma globulin (E934.6)

E949.0 Smallpox vaccine

E949.1 Rabies vaccine

E949.2 Typhus vaccine

E949.3 Yellow fever vaccine

E949.4 Measles vaccine

E949.5 Poliomyelitis vaccine

E949.6 Other and unspecified viral and rickettsial vaccines
Mumps vaccine

859

| | Add 4th or 5th digit | | Nonspecific code | | Unspecified code | | Manifestation code |

E949.7 **Mixed viral-rickettsial and bacterial vaccines, except combinations with a pertussis component**

Excludes: combinations with a pertussis component (E948.6)

E949.9 **Other and unspecified vaccines and biological substances**

SUICIDE AND SELF-INFLICTED INJURY (E950-E959)

Includes: injuries in suicide and attempted suicide
self-inflicted injuries specified as intentional

ALERT! For coding late effects of self-inflicted injury see E959

E950 **Suicide and self-inflicted poisoning by solid or liquid substances**

E950.0 **Analgesics, antipyretics, and antirheumatics**

E950.1 **Barbiturates**

E950.2 **Other sedatives and hypnotics**

E950.3 **Tranquilizers and other psychotropic agents**

E950.4 **Other specified drugs and medicinal substances**

E950.5 **Unspecified drug or medicinal substances**

E950.6 **Agricultural and horticultural chemical and pharmaceutical preparations other than plant foods and fertilizers**

E950.7 **Corrosive and caustic substances**
Suicide and self-inflicted poisoning by substances classifiable to E864

E950.8 **Arsenic and its compounds**

E950.9 **Other and unspecified solid and liquid substances**

E951 **Suicide and self-inflicted poisoning by gases in domestic use**

E951.0 **Gas distributed by pipeline**

E951.1 **Liquefied petroleum gas distributed in mobile containers**

E951.8 **Other utility gas**

E952 **Suicide and self-inflicted poisoning by other gases and vapors**

E952.0 **Motor vehicle exhaust gas**

E952.1 **Other carbon monoxide**

E952.8 **Other specified gases and vapors**

E952.9 **Unspecified gases and vapors**

E953 **Suicide and self-inflicted injury by hanging, strangulation, and suffocation**

E953.0 **Hanging**

E953.1 **Suffocation by plastic bag**

E953.8 **Other specified means**

E953.9 **Unspecified means**

E954 **Suicide and self-inflicted injury by submersion [drowning]**

E955 **Suicide and self-inflicted injury by firearms, air guns and explosives**

E955.0 **Handgun**

E955.1 **Shotgun**

E955.2 **Hunting rifle**

E955.3 **Military firearms**

E955.4 **Other and unspecified firearm**
Gunshot NOS
Shot NOS

E955.5 **Explosives**

E955.6 **Air gun**
BB gun
Pellet gun

E955.7 **Paintball gun**

E955.9 **Unspecified**

E956 **Suicide and self-inflicted injury by cutting and piercing instrument**

E957 **Suicide and self-inflicted injuries by jumping from high place**

E957.0 **Residential premises**

E957.1 **Other man-made structures**

● Code new
to this edition

▲ Revision of
existing code

④ ⑤ Fourth or fifth
digit required

E957.2   **Natural sites**

E957.9   **Unspecified**

E958   Suicide and self-inflicted injury by other and unspecified means

E958.0   **Jumping or lying before moving object**

E958.1   **Burns, fire**

E958.2   **Scald**

E958.3   **Extremes of cold**

E958.4   **Electrocution**

E958.5   **Crashing of motor vehicle**

E958.6   **Crashing of aircraft**

E958.7   **Caustic substances, except poisoning**

> Excludes: *poisoning by caustic substance (E950.7)*

E958.8   Other specified means

E958.9   Unspecified means

E959   **Late effects of self-inflicted injury**

> Note: This category is to be used to indicate circumstances classifiable to E950-E958 as the cause of death or disability from late effects, which are themselves classifiable elsewhere. The "late effects" include conditions reported as such or as sequelae which may occur at any time after the attempted suicide or self-inflicted injury.

HOMICIDE AND INJURY PURPOSELY INFLICTED BY OTHER PERSONS (E960-E969)

> Includes: injuries inflicted by another person with intent to injure or kill, by any means

> Excludes: *injuries due to:*
>> *legal intervention (E970-E978)*
>> *operations of war (E990-E999)*
>> *terrorism (E979)*

> **ALERT!** For coding late effects of injury purposely inflicted by other person see E969

E960   Fight, brawl, rape

E960.0   **Unarmed fight or brawl**
> Beatings NOS
> Brawl or fight with hands, fists, feet
> Injured or killed in fight NOS

> Excludes: *homicidal:*
>> *injury by weapons (E965.0-E966, E969)*
>> *strangulation (E963)*
>> *submersion (E964)*

E960.1   **Rape**

E961   **Assault by corrosive or caustic substance, except poisoning**
> Injury or death purposely caused by corrosive or caustic substance, such as:
>> acid [any]
>> corrosive substance
>> vitriol

> Excludes: *burns from hot liquid (E968.3)*
>> *chemical burns from swallowing a corrosive substance (E962.0-E962.9)*

E962   Assault by poisoning

E962.0   **Drugs and medicinal substances**
> Homicidal poisoning by any drug or medicinal substance

E962.1   Other solid and liquid substances

E962.2   Other gases and vapors

E962.9   Unspecified poisoning

E963   **Assault by hanging and strangulation**
> Homicidal (attempt):
>> garrotting or ligature
>> hanging
>> strangulation
>> suffocation

E964   **Assault by submersion [drowning]**

E965   Assault by firearms and explosives

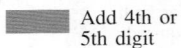 Add 4th or 5th digit   Nonspecific code   Unspecified code   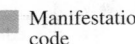 Manifestation code

E965.0 Handgun
    Pistol
    Revolver

E965.1 Shotgun

E965.2 Hunting rifle

E965.3 Military firearms

E965.4 Other and unspecified firearm

E965.5 Antipersonnel bomb

E965.6 Gasoline bomb

E965.7 Letter bomb

E965.8 Other specified explosive
    Bomb NOS (placed in) car
    Bomb NOS (placed in) house
    Dynamite

E965.9 Unspecified explosive

E966 Assault by cutting and piercing instrument
    Assassination (attempt), homicide (attempt) by any instrument classifiable under E920
    Homicidal cut, any part of the body
    Homicidal puncture, any part of the body
    Homicidal stab, any part of the body
    Stabbed, any part of the body

E967 Perpetrator of child and adult abuse
Note: selection of the correct perpetrator code is based on the relationship between the perpetrator and the victim

E967.0 By father, stepfather or boyfriend
    Male partner of child's parent or guardian

E967.1 By other specified person

E967.2 By mother, stepmother or girlfriend
    Female partner of child's parent or guardian

E967.3 By spouse or partner
    Abuse of spouse or partner by ex-spouse or ex-partner

E967.4 By child

E967.5 By sibling

E967.6 By grandparent

E967.7 By other relative

E967.8 By non-related caregiver

E967.9 By unspecified person

E968 Assault by other and unspecified means

E968.0 Fire
    Arson
    Homicidal burns NOS

    Excludes: burns from hot liquid (E968.3)

E968.1 Pushing from a high place

E968.2 Striking by blunt or thrown object

E968.3 Hot liquid
    Homicidal burns by scalding

E968.4 Criminal neglect
    Abandonment of child, infant, or other helpless person with intent to injure or kill

E968.5 Transport vehicle
    Being struck by other vehicle or run down with intent to injure
    Pushed in front of, thrown from, or dragged by moving vehicle with intent to injure

E968.6 Air gun
    BB gun
    Pellet gun

E968.7 Human bite

E968.8 Other specified means

● Code new to this edition   ▲ Revision of existing code   ④ ⑤ Fourth or fifth digit required

E968.9 Unspecified means

Assassination (attempt) NOS
Homicidal (attempt):
   injury NOS
   wound NOS

Manslaughter (nonaccidental)
Murder (attempt) NOS
Violence, non-accidental

E969 Late effects of injury purposely inflicted by other person

Note: This category is to be used to indicate circumstances classifiable to E960-E968 as the cause of death or disability from late effects, which are themselves classifiable elsewhere. The "late effects" include conditions reported as such, or as sequelae which may occur at any time after the acute injury.

LEGAL INTERVENTION (E970-E978)

Includes: injuries inflicted by the police or other law-enforcing agents, including military on duty, in the course of arresting or attempting to arrest lawbreakers, suppressing disturbances, maintaining order, and other legal action
legal execution

Excludes: *injuries caused by civil insurrections (E990.0-E999)*

ALERT! For coding late effects of injuries due to legal intervention see E977

E970 Injury due to legal intervention by firearms

Gunshot wound
Injury by:
   machine gun
   revolver
   rifle pellet or rubber bullet
   shot NOS

E971 Injury due to legal intervention by explosives

Injury by:
   dynamite
   explosive shell
   grenade
   mortar bomb

E972 Injury due to legal intervention by gas

Asphyxiation by gas
Injury by tear gas
Poisoning by gas

E973 Injury due to legal intervention by blunt object

Hit, struck by:
   baton (nightstick)
   blunt object
   stave

E974 Injury due to legal intervention by cutting and piercing instrument

Cut
Incised wound
Injured by bayonet
Stab wound

E975 Injury due to legal intervention by other specified means

Blow
Manhandling

E976 Injury due to legal intervention by unspecified means

E977 Late effects of injuries due to legal intervention

Note: This category is to be used to indicate circumstances classifiable to E970-E976 as the cause of death or disability from late effects, which are themselves classifiable elsewhere. The "late effects" include conditions reported as such, or as sequelae which may occur at any time after the acute injury due to legal intervention.

E978 Legal execution

All executions performed at the behest of the judiciary or ruling authority [whether permanent or temporary] as:

asphyxiation by gas
beheading, decapitation
   (by guillotine)
capital punishment
electrocution

hanging
poisoning
shooting
other specified means

Add 4th or 5th digit   Nonspecific code   Unspecified code   Manifestation code

TERRORISM (E979)

E979 **Terrorism**
Injuries resulting from the unlawful use of force or violence against persons or property to intimidate or coerce a Government, the civilian population, or any segment thereof, in furtherance of political or social objective

ALERT! For coding late effect of injury due to terrorism see E999.1

E979.0 **Terrorism involving explosion of marine weapons**
Depth-charge
Marine mine
Mine NOS, at sea or in harbor
Sea-based artillery shell
Torpedo
Underwater blast

E979.1 **Terrorism involving destruction of aircraft**
Aircraft used as a weapon
Aircraft:
 burned
 exploded
 shot down
Crushed by falling aircraft

E979.2 **Terrorism involving other explosions and fragments**
Antipersonnel bomb (fragments)
Blast NOS
Explosion (of):
 artillery shell
 breech-block
 cannon block
 mortar bomb
 munitions being used in terrorism
 NOS
Fragments from:
 artillery shell
 bomb
 grenade
 guided missile
 land-mine
 rocket
 shell
 shrapnel
Mine NOS

E979.3 **Terrorism involving fires, conflagration and hot substances**
Burning building or structure:
 collapse of
 fall from
 hit by falling object in
 jump from
Conflagration NOS
Fire (causing):
 asphyxia
 burns
 NOS
 other injury
Melting of fittings and furniture in burning
Petrol bomb
Smouldering building or structure

E979.4 **Terrorism involving firearms**
Bullet:
 carbine
 machine gun
 pistol
 rifle
 rubber (rifle)
Pellets (shotgun)

E979.5 **Terrorism involving nuclear weapons**
Blast effects
Exposure to ionizing radiation from nuclear weapon
Fireball effects
Heat from nuclear weapon
Other direct and secondary effects of nuclear weapons

● Code new to this edition   ▲ Revision of existing code   ④ ⑤ Fourth or fifth digit required

E979.6 Terrorism involving biological weapons
Anthrax
Cholera
Smallpox

E979.7 Terrorism involving chemical weapons
Gases, fumes, chemicals
Hydrogen cyanide
Phosgene
Sarin

E979.8 Terrorism involving other means
Drowning and submersion
Lasers
Piercing or stabbing instruments
Terrorism NOS

E979.9 Terrorism, secondary effects
Note: This code is for use to identify conditions occuring subsequent to a terrorist attack not those that are due to the intial terrorist act

Excludes: *late effect of terroist attack (E999.1)*

INJURY UNDETERMINED WHETHER ACCIDENTALLY OR PURPOSELY INFLICTED (E980-E989)

Note: Categories E980-E989 are for use when it is unspecified or it cannot be determined whether the injuries are accidental (unintentional), suicide (attempted), or assault.

ALERT! For coding late effects of injury undetermined whether accidentally or purposely inflicted see E989

E980 Poisoning by solid or liquid substances, undetermined whether accidentally or purposely inflicted

E980.0 Analgesics, antipyretics, and antirheumatics

E980.1 Barbiturates

E980.2 Other sedatives and hypnotics

E980.3 Tranquilizers and other psychotropic agents

E980.4 Other specified drugs and medicinal substances

E980.5 Unspecified drug or medicinal substance

E980.6 Corrosive and caustic substances
Poisoning, undetermined whether accidental or purposeful, by substances classifiable to E864

E980.7 Agricultural and horticultural chemical and pharmaceutical preparations other than plant foods and fertilizers

E980.8 Arsenic and its compounds

E980.9 Other and unspecified solid and liquid substances

E981 Poisoning by gases in domestic use, undetermined whether accidentally or purposely inflicted

E981.0 Gas distributed by pipeline

E981.1 Liquefied petroleum gas distributed in mobile containers

E981.8 Other utility gas

E982 Poisoning by other gases, undetermined whether accidentally or purposely inflicted

E982.0 Motor vehicle exhaust gas

E982.1 Other carbon monoxide

E982.8 Other specified gases and vapors

E982.9 Unspecified gases and vapors

E983 Hanging, strangulation, or suffocation, undetermined whether accidentally or purposely inflicted

E983.0 Hanging

E983.1 Suffocation by plastic bag

E983.8 Other specified means

E983.9 Unspecified means

E984 Submersion [drowning], undetermined whether accidentally or purposely inflicted

E985 Injury by firearms, air guns and explosives, undetermined whether accidentally or purposely inflicted

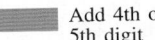 Add 4th or 5th digit

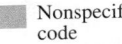 Nonspecific code

Unspecified code

Manifestation code

865

E985.0	Handgun
E985.1	Shotgun
E985.2	Hunting rifle
E985.3	Military firearms
E985.4	Other and unspecified firearm
E985.5	Explosives
E985.6	Air gun

       BB gun
       Pellet gun

E985.7	Paintball gun

E986 Injury by cutting and piercing instruments, undetermined whether accidentally or purposely inflicted

E987 Falling from high place, undetermined whether accidentally or purposely inflicted

E987.0	Residential premises
E987.1	Other man-made structures
E987.2	Natural sites
E987.9	Unspecified site

E988 Injury by other and unspecified means, undetermined whether accidentally or purposely inflicted

E988.0	Jumping or lying before moving object
E988.1	Burns, fire
E988.2	Scald
E988.3	Extremes of cold
E988.4	Electrocution
E988.5	Crashing of motor vehicle
E988.6	Crashing of aircraft
E988.7	Caustic substances, except poisoning
E988.8	Other specified means
E988.9	Unspecified means

E989 Late effects of injury, undetermined whether accidentally or purposely inflicted

    Note: This category is to be used to indicate circumstances classifiable to E980-E988 as the cause of death or disability from late effects, which are themselves classifiable elsewhere. The "late effects" include conditions reported as such or as sequelae which may occur at any time after the acute injury, undetermined whether accidentally or purposely inflicted.

INJURY RESULTING FROM OPERATIONS OF WAR (E990-E999)

    Includes: injuries to military personnel and civilians caused by war and civil insurrections and occurring during the time of war and insurrection, and peacekeeping missions.

    Excludes: *accidents during training of military personnel, manufacture of war material and transport, unless attributable to enemy action*

    ALERT! For coding late effect of injury due to war operations see E999.0

E990 Injury due to war operations by fires and conflagrations

    Includes: asphyxia, burns, or other injury originating from fire caused by a fire-producing device or indirectly by any conventional weapon

E990.0	From gasoline bomb

       Incendiary bomb

E990.1	From flamethrower
E990.2	From incendiary bullet
E990.3	From fire caused indirectly from conventional weapon

    Excludes: *fire aboard military aircraft (E994.3)*

E990.9	From other and unspecified source

E991 Injury due to war operations by bullets and fragments

    Excludes: *injury due to bullets and fragments due to war operations, but occurring after cessation of hostilities (E998.0)*
        injury due to explosion of artillery shells and mortars (E993.2)
        injury due to explosion of improvised explosive device [IED] (E993.3-E993.5)
        injury due to sea-based artillery shell (E992.3)

● Code new to this edition   ▲ Revision of existing code   ④ ⑤ Fourth or fifth digit required

E991.0   **Rubber bullets (rifle)**

E991.1   **Pellets (rifle)**

E991.2   **Other bullets**
  Bullet [any, except rubber bullets and pellets]
    carbine
    machine gun
    pistol
    rifle
    shotgun

E991.3   **Antipersonnel bomb (fragments)**

E991.4   **Fragments from munitions**
  Fragments from:
    artillery shell
    bombs, except antipersonnel
    detonation of unexploded ordnance [UXO]
    grenade
    guided missile
    land mine
    rockets
    shell

E991.5   **Fragments from person-borne improvised explosive device [IED]**

E991.6   **Fragments from vehicle-borne improvised explosive device [IED]**
  IED borne by land, air, or water transport vehicle

E991.7   **Fragments from other improvised explosive device [IED]**
  Roadside IED

E991.8   **Fragments from weapons**
  Fragments from:
    artillery
    autocannons
    automatic grenade launchers
    missile launchers
    mortars
    small arms

E991.9   **Other and unspecified fragments**
  Shrapnel NOS

E992   **Injury due to war operations by explosion of marine weapons**

E992.0   **Torpedo**

E992.1   **Depth charge**

E992.2   **Marine mines**
  Marine mines at sea or in harbor

E992.3   **Sea-based artillery shell**

E992.8   **Other by other marine weapons**

E992.9   **Unspecified marine weapon**
  Underwater blast NOS

E993   **Injury due to war operations by other explosion**
  Injuries due to direct or indirect pressure or air blast of an explosion occurring during war operations

  Excludes: _injury due to fragments resulting from an explosion (E991.0-E991.9)_
      injury due to detonation of unexploded ordnance but occurring after cessation of hostilities (E998.0-E998.9)
      injury due to nuclear weapons (E996.0-E996.9)

E993.0   **Aerial bomb**

E993.1   **Guided missile**

E993.2   **Mortar**
  Artillery shell

E993.3   **Person-borne improvised explosive device [IED]**

E993.4   **Vehicle-borne improvised explosive device [IED]**
  IED borne by land, air, or water transport vehicle

E993.5   **Other improvised explosive device [IED]**
  Roadside IED

E993.6   **Unintentional detonation of own munitions**
  Unintentional detonation of own ammunition (artillery) (mortars)

Add 4th or 5th digit   Nonspecific code   Unspecified code   Manifestation code

E993.7 Unintentional discharge of own munitions launch device
Unintentional explosion of own:
Autocannons
Automatic grenade launchers
Missile launchers
Small arms

E993.8 Other specified explosion
Bomb
Grenade
Land mine

E993.9 Unspecified explosion
Air blast NOS
Blast NOS
Blast wave NOS
Blast wind NOS
Explosion NOS

E994 Injury due to war operations by destruction of aircraft

E994.0 Destruction of aircraft due to enemy fire or explosives
Air to air missile
Explosive device placed on aircraft
Rocket propelled grenade [RPG]
Small arms fire
Surface to air missile

E994.1 Unintentional destruction of aircraft due to own onboard explosives

E994.2 Destruction of aircraft due to collision with other aircraft

E994.3 Destruction of aircraft due to onboard fire

E994.8 Other destruction of aircraft

E994.9 Unspecified destruction of aircraft

E995 Injury due to war operations by other and unspecified forms of conventional warfare

E995.0 Unarmed hand-to-hand combat
Excludes: *intentional restriction of airway (E995.3)*

E995.1 Struck by blunt object
Baton (nightstick)
Stave

E995.2 Piercing object
Bayonet
Knife
Sword

E995.3 Intentional restriction of air and airway
Intentional submersion
Strangulation
Suffocation

E995.4 Unintentional drowning due to inability to surface or obtain air
Submersion

E995.8 Other forms of conventional warfare

E995.9 Unspecified form of conventional warfare

E996 Injury due to war operations by nuclear weapons
Dirty bomb NOS
Excludes: *late effects of injury due to nuclear weapons (E999.1, E999.0)*

E996.0 Direct blast effect of nuclear weapon
Injury to bodily organs due to blast pressure

E996.1 Indirect blast effect of nuclear weapon
Injury due to being thrown by blast
Injury due to being struck or crushed by blast debris

E996.2 Thermal radiation effect of nuclear weapon
Burns due to thermal radiation
Fireball effects
Flash burns
Heat effects

● Code new   ▲ Revision of   ④ ⑤ Fourth or fifth
  to this edition   existing code   digit required

E996.3   Nuclear radiation effects
    Acute radiation exposure
    Beta burns
    Fallout exposure
    Radiation sickness
    Secondary effects of nuclear weapons

E996.8   Other effects of nuclear weapons

E996.9   Unspecified effect of nuclear weapon

E997   Injury due to war operations by other forms of unconventional warfare

E997.0   Lasers

E997.1   Biological warfare

E997.2   Gases, fumes, and chemicals

E997.3   Weapon of mass destruction [WMD], unspecified

E997.8   Other specified forms of unconventional warfare

E997.9   Unspecified form of unconventional warfare

E998   Injury due to war operations but occurring after cessation of hostilities
    Injuries due to operations of war but occurring after cessation of hostilities by any means classifiable under E990-E997
    Injuries by explosion of bombs or mines placed in the course of operations of war, if the explosion occurred after cessation of hostilities

E998.0   Explosion of mines

E998.1   Explosion of bombs

E998.8   Injury due to other war operations but occurring after cessation of hostilities

E998.9   Injury due to unspecified war operations but occurring after cessation of hostilities

E999   Late effect of injury due to war operations and terrorism
    Note: This category is to be used to indicate circumstances classifiable to E979, E990-E998 as the cause of death or disability from late effects, which are themselves classifiable elsewhere. The "late effects" include conditions reported as such or as sequelae which may occur at any time after the acute injury, resulting from operations of war or terrorism.

E999.0   Late effect of injury due to war operations

E999.1   Late effect of injury due to terrorism

| | Add 4th or 5th digit | | Nonspecific code | | Unspecified code | | Manifestation code |

This page intentionally left blank.

● Code new
to this edition

▲ Revision of
existing code

④ ⑤ Fourth or fifth
digit required

APPENDIX A:
MORPHOLOGY OF NEOPLASMS

The World Health Organization has published an adaptation of the International Classification of Diseases for oncology (ICD-O). It contains a coded nomenclature for the morphology of neoplasms, which is reproduced here for those who wish to use it in conjunction with Chapter 2 of the *International Classification of Diseases, 9th Revision, Clinical Modification*.

The morphology code numbers consist of five digits; the first four identify the histological type of the neoplasm and the fifth indicates its behavior. The one-digit behavior code is as follows:

/0 Benign

/1 Uncertain whether benign or malignant
    Borderline malignancy

/2 Carcinoma in situ
    Intraepithelial
    Noninfiltrating
    Noninvasive

/3 Malignant, primary site

/6 Malignant, metastatic site
    Secondary site

/9 Malignant, uncertain whether primary or metastatic site

In the nomenclature below, the morphology code numbers include the behavior code appropriate to the histological type of neoplasm, but this behavior code should be changed if other reported information makes this necessary. For example, "chordoma (M9370/3)" is assumed to be malignant; the term "benign chordoma" should be coded M9370/0. Similarly, "superficial spreading adenocarcinoma (M8143/3)" described as "noninvasive" should be coded M8143/2 and "melanoma (M8720/3)" described as "secondary" should be coded M8720/6.

The following table shows the correspondence between the morphology code and the different sections of Chapter 2:

Morphology code Histology/Behavior			ICD-9-CM Chapter 2
Any	0	210-229	Benign neoplasms
M8000-M8004	1	239	Neoplasms of unspecified nature
M8010+	1	235-238	Neoplasms of uncertain behavior
Any	2	230-234	Carcinoma in situ
Any	3	140-195 200-208	Malignant neoplasms, stated or presumed to be primary
Any	6	196-198	Malignant neoplasms, stated or presumed to be secondary

The ICD-O behavior digit /9 is inapplicable in an ICD context, since all malignant neoplasms are presumed to be primary (/3) or secondary (/6) according to other information on the medical record.

Only the first-listed term of the full ICD-O morphology nomenclature appears against each code number in the list below. The ICD-9-CM Alphabetical Index (Volume 2), however, includes all the ICD-O synonyms as well as a number of other morphological names still likely to be encountered on medical records but omitted from ICD-O as outdated or otherwise undesirable.

A coding difficulty sometimes arises where a morphological diagnosis contains two qualifying adjectives that have different code numbers. An example is "transitional cell epidermoid carcinoma." "Transitional cell carcinoma NOS" is M8120/3 and "epidermoid carcinoma NOS" is M8070/3. In such circumstances, the higher number (M8120/3 in this example) should be used, as it is usually more specific.

CODED NOMENCLATURE FOR MORPHOLOGY OF NEOPLASMS

M800   **Neoplasms NOS**
M8000/0   *Neoplasm, benign*
M8000/1   *Neoplasm, uncertain whether benign or malignant*
M8000/3   *Neoplasm, malignant*
M8000/6   *Neoplasm, metastatic*
M8000/9   *Neoplasm, malignant, uncertain whether primary or metastatic*
M8001/0   *Tumor cells, benign*
M8001/1   *Tumor cells, uncertain whether benign or malignant*
M8001/3   *Tumor cells, malignant*
M8002/3   *Malignant tumor, small cell type*
M8003/3   *Malignant tumor, giant cell type*
M8004/3   *Malignant tumor, fusiform cell type*

M801-M804   **Epithelial neoplasms NOS**
M8010/0   *Epithelial tumor, benign*
M8010/2   *Carcinoma in situ NOS*
M8010/3   *Carcinoma NOS*
M8010/6   *Carcinoma, metastatic NOS*
M8010/9   *Carcinomatosis*
M8011/0   *Epithelioma, benign*
M8011/3   *Epithelioma, malignant*
M8012/3   *Large cell carcinoma NOS*
M8020/3   *Carcinoma, undifferentiated type NOS*
M8021/3   *Carcinoma, anaplastic type NOS*
M8022/3   *Pleomorphic carcinoma*
M8030/3   *Giant cell and spindle cell carcinoma*
M8031/3   *Giant cell carcinoma*
M8032/3   *Spindle cell carcinoma*
M8033/3   *Pseudosarcomatous carcinoma*
M8034/3   *Polygonal cell carcinoma*
M8035/3   *Spheroidal cell carcinoma*
M8040/1   *Tumorlet*
M8041/3   *Small cell carcinoma NOS*
M8042/3   *Oat cell carcinoma*
M8043/3   *Small cell carcinoma, fusiform cell type*

M805-M808   **Papillary and squamous cell neoplasms**
M8050/0   *Papilloma NOS (except Papilloma of urinary bladder M8120/1)*
M8050/2   *Papillary carcinoma in situ*
M8050/3   *Papillary carcinoma NOS*
M8051/0   *Verrucous papilloma*
M8051/3   *Verrucous carcinoma NOS*
M8052/0   *Squamous cell papilloma*
M8052/3   *Papillary squamous cell carcinoma*
M8053/0   *Inverted papilloma*
M8060/0   *Papillomatosis NOS*
M8070/2   *Squamous cell carcinoma in situ NOS*
M8070/3   *Squamous cell carcinoma NOS*
M8070/6   *Squamous cell carcinoma, metastatic NOS*
M8071/3   *Squamous cell carcinoma, keratinizing type NOS*
M8072/3   *Squamous cell carcinoma, large cell, nonkeratinizing type*
M8073/3   *Squamous cell carcinoma, small cell, nonkeratinizing type*
M8074/3   *Squamous cell carcinoma, spindle cell type*
M8075/3   *Adenoid squamous cell carcinoma*
M8076/2   *Squamous cell carcinoma in situ with questionable stromal invasion*
M8076/3   *Squamous cell carcinoma, microinvasive*
M8080/2   *Queyrat's erythroplasia*
M8081/2   *Bowen's disease*
M8082/3   *Lymphoepithelial carcinoma*

M809-M811   **Basal cell neoplasms**
M8090/1   *Basal cell tumor*
M8090/3   *Basal cell carcinoma NOS*
M8091/3   *Multicentric basal cell carcinoma*
M8092/3   *Basal cell carcinoma, morphea type*
M8093/3   *Basal cell carcinoma, fibroepithelial type*
M8094/3   *Basosquamous carcinoma*
M8095/3   *Metatypical carcinoma*
M8096/0   *Intraepidermal epithelioma of Jadassohn*
M8100/0   *Trichoepithelioma*
M8101/0   *Trichofolliculoma*

M8102/0	*Tricholemmoma*
M8110/0	*Pilomatrixoma*

M812-M813 Transitional cell papillomas and carcinomas

M8120/0	*Transitional cell papilloma NOS*
M8120/1	*Urothelial papilloma*
M8120/2	*Transitional cell carcinoma in situ*
M8120/3	*Transitional cell carcinoma NOS*
M8121/0	*Schneiderian papilloma*
M8121/1	*Transitional cell papilloma, inverted type*
M8121/3	*Schneiderian carcinoma*
M8122/3	*Transitional cell carcinoma, spindle cell type*
M8123/3	*Basaloid carcinoma*
M8124/3	*Cloacogenic carcinoma*
M8130/3	*Papillary transitional cell carcinoma*

M814-M838 Adenomas and adenocarcinomas

M8140/0	*Adenoma NOS*
M8140/1	*Bronchial adenoma NOS*
M8140/2	*Adenocarcinoma in situ*
M8140/3	*Adenocarcinoma NOS*
M8140/6	*Adenocarcinoma, metastatic NOS*
M8141/3	*Scirrhous adenocarcinoma*
M8142/3	*Linitis plastica*
M8143/3	*Superficial spreading adenocarcinoma*
M8144/3	*Adenocarcinoma, intestinal type*
M8145/3	*Carcinoma, diffuse type*
M8146/0	*Monomorphic adenoma*
M8147/0	*Basal cell adenoma*
M8150/0	*Islet cell adenoma*
M8150/3	*Islet cell carcinoma*
M8151/0	*Insulinoma NOS*
M8151/3	*Insulinoma, malignant*
M8152/0	*Glucagonoma NOS*
M8152/3	*Glucagonoma, malignant*
M8153/1	*Gastrinoma NOS*
M8153/3	*Gastrinoma, malignant*
M8154/3	*Mixed islet cell and exocrine adenocarcinoma*
M8160/0	*Bile duct adenoma*
M8160/3	*Cholangiocarcinoma*
M8161/0	*Bile duct cystadenoma*
M8161/3	*Bile duct cystadenocarcinoma*
M8170/0	*Liver cell adenoma*
M8170/3	*Hepatocellular carcinoma NOS*
M8180/0	*Hepatocholangioma, benign*
M8180/3	*Combined hepatocellular carcinoma and cholangiocarcinoma*
M8190/0	*Trabecular adenoma*
M8190/3	*Trabecular adenocarcinoma*
M8191/0	*Embryonal adenoma*
M8200/0	*Eccrine dermal cylindroma*
M8200/3	*Adenoid cystic carcinoma*
M8201/3	*Cribriform carcinoma*
M8210/0	*Adenomatous polyp NOS*
M8210/3	*Adenocarcinoma in adenomatous polyp*
M8211/0	*Tubular adenoma NOS*
M8211/3	*Tubular adenocarcinoma*
M8220/0	*Adenomatous polyposis coli*
M8220/3	*Adenocarcinoma in adenomatous polyposis coli*
M8221/0	*Multiple adenomatous polyps*
M8230/3	*Solid carcinoma NOS*
M8231/3	*Carcinoma simplex*
M8240/1	*Carcinoid tumor NOS*
M8240/3	*Carcinoid tumor, malignant*
M8241/1	*Carcinoid tumor, argentaffin NOS*
M8241/3	*Carcinoid tumor, argentaffin, malignant*
M8242/1	*Carcinoid tumor, nonargentaffin NOS*
M8242/3	*Carcinoid tumor, nonargentaffin, malignant*
M8243/3	*Mucocarcinoid tumor, malignant*
M8244/3	*Composite carcinoid*
M8250/1	*Pulmonary adenomatosis*
M8250/3	*Bronchiolo-alveolar adenocarcinoma*
M8251/0	*Alveolar adenoma*

M8251/3	Alveolar adenocarcinoma
M8260/0	Papillary adenoma NOS
M8260/3	Papillary adenocarcinoma NOS
M8261/1	Villous adenoma NOS
M8261/3	Adenocarcinoma in villous adenoma
M8262/3	Villous adenocarcinoma
M8263/0	Tubulovillous adenoma
M8270/0	Chromophobe adenoma
M8270/3	Chromophobe carcinoma
M8280/0	Acidophil adenoma
M8280/3	Acidophil carcinoma
M8281/0	Mixed acidophil-basophil adenoma
M8281/3	Mixed acidophil-basophil carcinoma
M8290/0	Oxyphilic adenoma
M8290/3	Oxyphilic adenocarcinoma
M8300/0	Basophil adenoma
M8300/3	Basophil carcinoma
M8310/0	Clear cell adenoma
M8310/3	Clear cell adenocarcinoma NOS
M8311/1	Hypernephroid tumor
M8312/3	Renal cell carcinoma
M8313/0	Clear cell adenofibroma
M8320/3	Granular cell carcinoma
M8321/0	Chief cell adenoma
M8322/0	Water-clear cell adenoma
M8322/3	Water-clear cell adenocarcinoma
M8323/0	Mixed cell adenoma
M8323/3	Mixed cell adenocarcinoma
M8324/0	Lipoadenoma
M8330/0	Follicular adenoma
M8330/3	Follicular adenocarcinoma NOS
M8331/3	Follicular adenocarcinoma, well differentiated type
M8332/3	Follicular adenocarcinoma, trabecular type
M8333/0	Microfollicular adenoma
M8334/0	Macrofollicular adenoma
M8340/3	Papillary and follicular adenocarcinoma
M8350/3	Nonencapsulated sclerosing carcinoma
M8360/1	Multiple endocrine adenomas
M8361/1	Juxtaglomerular tumor
M8370/0	Adrenal cortical adenoma NOS
M8370/3	Adrenal cortical carcinoma
M8371/0	Adrenal cortical adenoma, compact cell type
M8372/0	Adrenal cortical adenoma, heavily pigmented variant
M8373/0	Adrenal cortical adenoma, clear cell type
M8374/0	Adrenal cortical adenoma, glomerulosa cell type
M8375/0	Adrenal cortical adenoma, mixed cell type
M8380/0	Endometrioid adenoma NOS
M8380/1	Endometrioid adenoma, borderline malignancy
M8380/3	Endometrioid carcinoma
M8381/0	Endometrioid adenofibroma NOS
M8381/1	Endometrioid adenofibroma, borderline malignancy
M8381/3	Endometrioid adenofibroma, malignant

M839-M842 Adnexal and skin appendage neoplasms

M8390/0	Skin appendage adenoma
M8390/3	Skin appendage carcinoma
M8400/0	Sweat gland adenoma
M8400/1	Sweat gland tumor NOS
M8400/3	Sweat gland adenocarcinoma
M8401/0	Apocrine adenoma
M8401/3	Apocrine adenocarcinoma
M8402/0	Eccrine acrospiroma
M8403/0	Eccrine spiradenoma
M8404/0	Hidrocystoma
M8405/0	Papillary hydradenoma
M8406/0	Papillary syringadenoma
M8407/0	Syringoma NOS
M8410/0	Sebaceous adenoma
M8410/3	Sebaceous adenocarcinoma
M8420/0	Ceruminous adenoma
M8420/3	Ceruminous adenocarcinoma

M843   **Mucoepidermoid neoplasms**
M8430/1   *Mucoepidermoid tumor*
M8430/3   *Mucoepidermoid carcinoma*

M844-M849 Cystic, mucinous, and serous neoplasms
M8440/0   *Cystadenoma NOS*
M8440/3   *Cystadenocarcinoma NOS*
M8441/0   *Serous cystadenoma NOS*
M8441/1   *Serous cystadenoma, borderline malignancy*
M8441/3   *Serous cystadenocarcinoma NOS*
M8450/0   *Papillary cystadenoma NOS*
M8450/1   *Papillary cystadenoma, borderline malignancy*
M8450/3   *Papillary cystadenocarcinoma NOS*
M8460/0   *Papillary serous cystadenoma NOS*
M8460/1   *Papillary serous cystadenoma, borderline malignancy*
M8460/3   *Papillary serous cystadenocarcinoma*
M8461/0   *Serous surface papilloma NOS*
M8461/1   *Serous surface papilloma, borderline malignancy*
M8461/3   *Serous surface papillary carcinoma*
M8470/0   *Mucinous cystadenoma NOS*
M8470/1   *Mucinous cystadenoma, borderline malignancy*
M8470/3   *Mucinous cystadenocarcinoma NOS*
M8471/0   *Papillary mucinous cystadenoma NOS*
M8471/1   *Papillary mucinous cystadenoma, borderline malignancy*
M8471/3   *Papillary mucinous cystadenocarcinoma*
M8480/0   *Mucinous adenoma*
M8480/3   *Mucinous adenocarcinoma*
M8480/6   *Pseudomyxoma peritonei*
M8481/3   *Mucin-producing adenocarcinoma*
M8490/3   *Signet ring cell carcinoma*
M8490/6   *Metastatic signet ring cell carcinoma*

M850-M854 Ductal, lobular, and medullary neoplasms
M8500/2   *Intraductal carcinoma, noninfiltrating NOS*
M8500/3   *Infiltrating duct carcinoma*
M8501/2   *Comedocarcinoma, noninfiltrating*
M8501/3   *Comedocarcinoma NOS*
M8502/3   *Juvenile carcinoma of the breast*
M8503/0   *Intraductal papilloma*
M8503/2   *Noninfiltrating intraductal papillary adenocarcinoma*
M8504/0   *Intracystic papillary adenoma*
M8504/2   *Noninfiltrating intracystic carcinoma*
M8505/0   *Intraductal papillomatosis NOS*
M8506/0   *Subareolar duct papillomatosis*
M8510/3   *Medullary carcinoma NOS*
M8511/3   *Medullary carcinoma with amyloid stroma*
M8512/3   *Medullary carcinoma with lymphoid stroma*
M8520/2   *Lobular carcinoma in situ*
M8520/3   *Lobular carcinoma NOS*
M8521/3   *Infiltrating ductular carcinoma*
M8530/3   *Inflammatory carcinoma*
M8540/3   *Paget's disease, mammary*
M8541/3   *Paget's disease and infiltrating duct carcinoma of breast*
M8542/3   *Paget's disease, extramammary (except Paget's disease of bone)*

M855   **Acinar cell neoplasms**
M8550/0   *Acinar cell adenoma*
M8550/1   *Acinar cell tumor*
M8550/3   *Acinar cell carcinoma*

M856-M858 Complex epithelial neoplasms
M8560/3   *Adenosquamous carcinoma*
M8561/0   *Adenolymphoma*
M8570/3   *Adenocarcinoma with squamous metaplasia*
M8571/3   *Adenocarcinoma with cartilaginous and osseous metaplasia*
M8572/3   *Adenocarcinoma with spindle cell metaplasia*
M8573/3   *Adenocarcinoma with apocrine metaplasia*
M8580/0   *Thymoma, benign*
M8580/3   *Thymoma, malignant*

M859-M867 Specialized gonadal neoplasms
M8590/1   *Sex cord-stromal tumor*
M8600/0   *Thecoma NOS*
M8600/3   *Theca cell carcinoma*

M8610/0	*Luteoma NOS*
M8620/1	*Granulosa cell tumor NOS*
M8620/3	*Granulosa cell tumor, malignant*
M8621/1	*Granulosa cell-theca cell tumor*
M8630/0	*Androblastoma, benign*
M8630/1	*Androblastoma NOS*
M8630/3	*Androblastoma, malignant*
M8631/0	*Sertoli-Leydig cell tumor*
M8632/1	*Gynandroblastoma*
M8640/0	*Tubular androblastoma NOS*
M8640/3	*Sertoli cell carcinoma*
M8641/0	*Tubular androblastoma with lipid storage*
M8650/0	*Leydig cell tumor, benign*
M8650/1	*Leydig cell tumor NOS*
M8650/3	*Leydig cell tumor, malignant*
M8660/0	*Hilar cell tumor*
M8670/0	*Lipid cell tumor of ovary*
M8671/0	*Adrenal rest tumor*

M868-M871 Paragangliomas and glomus tumors

M8680/1	*Paraganglioma NOS*
M8680/3	*Paraganglioma, malignant*
M8681/1	*Sympathetic paraganglioma*
M8682/1	*Parasympathetic paraganglioma*
M8690/1	*Glomus jugulare tumor*
M8691/1	*Aortic body tumor*
M8692/1	*Carotid body tumor*
M8693/1	*Extra-adrenal paraganglioma NOS*
M8693/3	*Extra-adrenal paraganglioma, malignant*
M8700/0	*Pheochromocytoma NOS*
M8700/3	*Pheochromocytoma, malignant*
M8710/3	*Glomangiosarcoma*
M8711/0	*Glomus tumor*
M8712/0	*Glomangioma*

M872-M879 Nevi and melanomas

M8720/0	*Pigmented nevus NOS*
M8720/3	*Malignant melanoma NOS*
M8721/3	*Nodular melanoma*
M8722/0	*Balloon cell nevus*
M8722/3	*Balloon cell melanoma*
M8723/0	*Halo nevus*
M8724/0	*Fibrous papule of the nose*
M8725/0	*Neuronevus*
M8726/0	*Magnocellular nevus*
M8730/0	*Nonpigmented nevus*
M8730/3	*Amelanotic melanoma*
M8740/0	*Junctional nevus*
M8740/3	*Malignant melanoma in junctional nevus*
M8741/2	*Precancerous melanosis NOS*
M8741/3	*Malignant melanoma in precancerous melanosis*
M8742/2	*Hutchinson's melanotic freckle*
M8742/3	*Malignant melanoma in Hutchinson's melanotic freckle*
M8743/3	*Superficial spreading melanoma*
M8750/0	*Intradermal nevus*
M8760/0	*Compound nevus*
M8761/1	*Giant pigmented nevus*
M8761/3	*Malignant melanoma in giant pigmented nevus*
M8770/0	*Epithelioid and spindle cell nevus*
M8771/3	*Epithelioid cell melanoma*
M8772/3	*Spindle cell melanoma NOS*
M8773/3	*Spindle cell melanoma, type A*
M8774/3	*Spindle cell melanoma, type B*
M8775/3	*Mixed epithelioid and spindle cell melanoma*
M8780/0	*Blue nevus NOS*
M8780/3	*Blue nevus, malignant*
M8790/0	*Cellular blue nevus*

M880 Soft tissue tumors and sarcomas NOS

M8800/0	*Soft tissue tumor, benign*
M8800/3	*Sarcoma NOS*
M8800/9	*Sarcomatosis NOS*
M8801/3	*Spindle cell sarcoma*

M8802/3	*Giant cell sarcoma (except of bone M9250/3)*
M8803/3	*Small cell sarcoma*
M8804/3	*Epithelioid cell sarcoma*

M881-M883 Fibromatous neoplasms

M8810/0	*Fibroma NOS*
M8810/3	*Fibrosarcoma NOS*
M8811/0	*Fibromyxoma*
M8811/3	*Fibromyxosarcoma*
M8812/0	*Periosteal fibroma*
M8812/3	*Periosteal fibrosarcoma*
M8813/0	*Fascial fibroma*
M8813/3	*Fascial fibrosarcoma*
M8814/3	*Infantile fibrosarcoma*
M8820/0	*Elastofibroma*
M8821/1	*Aggressive fibromatosis*
M8822/1	*Abdominal fibromatosis*
M8823/1	*Desmoplastic fibroma*
M8830/0	*Fibrous histiocytoma NOS*
M8830/1	*Atypical fibrous histiocytoma*
M8830/3	*Fibrous histiocytoma, malignant*
M8831/0	*Fibroxanthoma NOS*
M8831/1	*Atypical fibroxanthoma*
M8831/3	*Fibroxanthoma, malignant*
M8832/0	*Dermatofibroma NOS*
M8832/1	*Dermatofibroma protuberans*
M8832/3	*Dermatofibrosarcoma NOS*

M884   Myxomatous neoplasms

| M8840/0 | *Myxoma NOS* |
| M8840/3 | *Myxosarcoma* |

M885-M888 Lipomatous neoplasms

M8850/0	*Lipoma NOS*
M8850/3	*Liposarcoma NOS*
M8851/0	*Fibrolipoma*
M8851/3	*Liposarcoma, well differentiated type*
M8852/0	*Fibromyxolipoma*
M8852/3	*Myxoid liposarcoma*
M8853/3	*Round cell liposarcoma*
M8854/3	*Pleomorphic liposarcoma*
M8855/3	*Mixed type liposarcoma*
M8856/0	*Intramuscular lipoma*
M8857/0	*Spindle cell lipoma*
M8860/0	*Angiomyolipoma*
M8860/3	*Angiomyoliposarcoma*
M8861/0	*Angiolipoma NOS*
M8861/1	*Angiolipoma, infiltrating*
M8870/0	*Myelolipoma*
M8880/0	*Hibernoma*
M8881/0	*Lipoblastomatosis*

M889-M892 Myomatous neoplasms

M8890/0	*Leiomyoma NOS*
M8890/1	*Intravascular leiomyomatosis*
M8890/3	*Leiomyosarcoma NOS*
M8891/1	*Epithelioid leiomyoma*
M8891/3	*Epithelioid leiomyosarcoma*
M8892/1	*Cellular leiomyoma*
M8893/0	*Bizarre leiomyoma*
M8894/0	*Angiomyoma*
M8894/3	*Angiomyosarcoma*
M8895/0	*Myoma*
M8895/3	*Myosarcoma*
M8900/0	*Rhabdomyoma NOS*
M8900/3	*Rhabdomyosarcoma NOS*
M8901/3	*Pleomorphic rhabdomyosarcoma*
M8902/3	*Mixed type rhabdomyosarcoma*
M8903/0	*Fetal rhabdomyoma*
M8904/0	*Adult rhabdomyoma*
M8910/3	*Embryonal rhabdomyosarcoma*
M8920/3	*Alveolar rhabdomyosarcoma*

M893-M899 Complex mixed and stromal neoplasms

M8930/3	*Endometrial stromal sarcoma*
M8931/1	*Endolymphatic stromal myosis*
M8932/0	*Adenomyoma*
M8940/0	*Pleomorphic adenoma*
M8940/3	*Mixed tumor, malignant NOS*
M8950/3	*Mullerian mixed tumor*
M8951/3	*Mesodermal mixed tumor*
M8960/1	*Mesoblastic nephroma*
M8960/3	*Nephroblastoma NOS*
M8961/3	*Epithelial nephroblastoma*
M8962/3	*Mesenchymal nephroblastoma*
M8970/3	*Hepatoblastoma*
M8980/3	*Carcinosarcoma NOS*
M8981/3	*Carcinosarcoma, embryonal type*
M8982/0	*Myoepithelioma*
M8990/0	*Mesenchymoma, benign*
M8990/1	*Mesenchymoma, NOS*
M8990/3	*Mesenchymoma, malignant*
M8991/3	*Embryonal sarcoma*

M900-M903 Fibroepithelial neoplasms

M9000/0	*Brenner tumor NOS*
M9000/1	*Brenner tumor, borderline malignancy*
M9000/3	*Brenner tumor, malignant*
M9010/0	*Fibroadenoma NOS*
M9011/0	*Intracanalicular fibroadenoma NOS*
M9012/0	*Pericanalicular fibroadenoma*
M9013/0	*Adenofibroma NOS*
M9014/0	*Serous adenofibroma*
M9015/0	*Mucinous adenofibroma*
M9020/0	*Cellular intracanalicular fibroadenoma*
M9020/1	*Cystosarcoma phyllodes NOS*
M9020/3	*Cystosarcoma phyllodes, malignant*
M9030/0	*Juvenile fibroadenoma*

M904 Synovial neoplasms

M9040/0	*Synovioma, benign*
M9040/3	*Synovial sarcoma NOS*
M9041/3	*Synovial sarcoma, spindle cell type*
M9042/3	*Synovial sarcoma, epithelioid cell type*
M9043/3	*Synovial sarcoma, biphasic type*
M9044/3	*Clear cell sarcoma of tendons and aponeuroses*

M905 Mesothelial neoplasms

M9050/0	*Mesothelioma, benign*
M9050/3	*Mesothelioma, malignant*
M9051/0	*Fibrous mesothelioma, benign*
M9051/3	*Fibrous mesothelioma, malignant*
M9052/0	*Epithelioid mesothelioma, benign*
M9052/3	*Epithelioid mesothelioma, malignant*
M9053/0	*Mesothelioma, biphasic type, benign*
M9053/3	*Mesothelioma, biphasic type, malignant*
M9054/0	*Adenomatoid tumor NOS*

M906-M909 Germ cell neoplasms

M9060/3	*Dysgerminoma*
M9061/3	*Seminoma NOS*
M9062/3	*Seminoma, anaplastic type*
M9063/3	*Spermatocytic seminoma*
M9064/3	*Germinoma*
M9070/3	*Embryonal carcinoma NOS*
M9071/3	*Endodermal sinus tumor*
M9072/3	*Polyembryoma*
M9073/1	*Gonadoblastoma*
M9080/0	*Teratoma, benign*
M9080/1	*Teratoma NOS*
M9080/3	*Teratoma, malignant NOS*
M9081/3	*Teratocarcinoma*
M9082/3	*Malignant teratoma, undifferentiated type*
M9083/3	*Malignant teratoma, intermediate type*
M9084/0	*Dermoid cyst*
M9084/3	*Dermoid cyst with malignant transformation*

M9090/0	*Struma ovarii NOS*
M9090/3	*Struma ovarii, malignant*
M9091/1	*Strumal carcinoid*

M910   **Trophoblastic neoplasms**

M9100/0	*Hydatidiform mole NOS*
M9100/1	*Invasive hydatidiform mole*
M9100/3	*Choriocarcinoma*
M9101/3	*Choriocarcinoma combined with teratoma*
M9102/3	*Malignant teratoma, trophoblastic*

M911   **Mesonephromas**

M9110/0	*Mesonephroma, benign*
M9110/1	*Mesonephric tumor*
M9110/3	*Mesonephroma, malignant*
M9111/1	*Endosalpingioma*

M912-M916 **Blood vessel tumors**

M9120/0	*Hemangioma NOS*
M9120/3	*Hemangiosarcoma*
M9121/0	*Cavernous hemangioma*
M9122/0	*Venous hemangioma*
M9123/0	*Racemose hemangioma*
M9124/3	*Kupffer cell sarcoma*
M9130/0	*Hemangioendothelioma, benign*
M9130/1	*Hemangioendothelioma NOS*
M9130/3	*Hemangioendothelioma, malignant*
M9131/0	*Capillary hemangioma*
M9132/0	*Intramuscular hemangioma*
M9140/3	*Kaposi's sarcoma*
M9141/0	*Angiokeratoma*
M9142/0	*Verrucous keratotic hemangioma*
M9150/0	*Hemangiopericytoma, benign*
M9150/1	*Hemangiopericytoma NOS*
M9150/3	*Hemangiopericytoma, malignant*
M9160/0	*Angiofibroma NOS*
M9161/1	*Hemangioblastoma*

M917   **Lymphatic vessel tumors**

M9170/0	*Lymphangioma NOS*
M9170/3	*Lymphangiosarcoma*
M9171/0	*Capillary lymphangioma*
M9172/0	*Cavernous lymphangioma*
M9173/0	*Cystic lymphangioma*
M9174/0	*Lymphangiomyoma*
M9174/1	*Lymphangiomyomatosis*
M9175/0	*Hemolymphangioma*

M918-M920 **Osteomas and osteosarcomas**

M9180/0	*Osteoma NOS*
M9180/3	*Osteosarcoma NOS*
M9181/3	*Chondroblastic osteosarcoma*
M9182/3	*Fibroblastic osteosarcoma*
M9183/3	*Telangiectatic osteosarcoma*
M9184/3	*Osteosarcoma in Paget's disease of bone*
M9190/3	*Juxtacortical osteosarcoma*
M9191/0	*Osteoid osteoma NOS*
M9200/0	*Osteoblastoma*

M921-M924 **Chondromatous neoplasms**

M9210/0	*Osteochondroma*
M9210/1	*Osteochondromatosis NOS*
M9220/0	*Chondroma NOS*
M9220/1	*Chondromatosis NOS*
M9220/3	*Chondrosarcoma NOS*
M9221/0	*Juxtacortical chondroma*
M9221/3	*Juxtacortical chondrosarcoma*
M9230/0	*Chondroblastoma NOS*
M9230/3	*Chondroblastoma, malignant*
M9240/3	*Mesenchymal chondrosarcoma*
M9241/0	*Chondromyxoid fibroma*

M925   **Giant cell tumors**

M9250/1	*Giant cell tumor of bone NOS*
M9250/3	*Giant cell tumor of bone, malignant*

M9251/1	*Giant cell tumor of soft parts NOS*
M9251/3	*Malignant giant cell tumor of soft parts*

M926   **Miscellaneous bone tumors**
M9260/3	*Ewing's sarcoma*
M9261/3	*Adamantinoma of long bones*
M9262/0	*Ossifying fibroma*

M927-M934   **Odontogenic tumors**
M9270/0	*Odontogenic tumor, benign*
M9270/1	*Odontogenic tumor NOS*
M9270/3	*Odontogenic tumor, malignant*
M9271/0	*Dentinoma*
M9272/0	*Cementoma NOS*
M9273/0	*Cementoblastoma, benign*
M9274/0	*Cementifying fibroma*
M9275/0	*Gigantiform cementoma*
M9280/0	*Odontoma NOS*
M9281/0	*Compound odontoma*
M9282/0	*Complex odontoma*
M9290/0	*Ameloblastic fibro-odontoma*
M9290/3	*Ameloblastic odontosarcoma*
M9300/0	*Adenomatoid odontogenic tumor*
M9301/0	*Calcifying odontogenic cyst*
M9310/0	*Ameloblastoma NOS*
M9310/3	*Ameloblastoma, malignant*
M9311/0	*Odontoameloblastoma*
M9312/0	*Squamous odontogenic tumor*
M9320/0	*Odontogenic myxoma*
M9321/0	*Odontogenic fibroma NOS*
M9330/0	*Ameloblastic fibroma*
M9330/3	*Ameloblastic fibrosarcoma*
M9340/0	*Calcifying epithelial odontogenic tumor*

M935-M937   **Miscellaneous tumors**
M9350/1	*Craniopharyngioma*
M9360/1	*Pinealoma*
M9361/1	*Pineocytoma*
M9362/3	*Pineoblastoma*
M9363/0	*Melanotic neuroectodermal tumor*
M9370/3	*Chordoma*

M938-M948   **Gliomas**
M9380/3	*Glioma, malignant*
M9381/3	*Gliomatosis cerebri*
M9382/3	*Mixed glioma*
M9383/1	*Subependymal glioma*
M9384/1	*Subependymal giant cell astrocytoma*
M9390/0	*Choroid plexus papilloma NOS*
M9390/3	*Choroid plexus papilloma, malignant*
M9391/3	*Ependymoma NOS*
M9392/3	*Ependymoma, anaplastic type*
M9393/1	*Papillary ependymoma*
M9394/1	*Myxopapillary ependymoma*
M9400/3	*Astrocytoma NOS*
M9401/3	*Astrocytoma, anaplastic type*
M9410/3	*Protoplasmic astrocytoma*
M9411/3	*Gemistocytic astrocytoma*
M9420/3	*Fibrillary astrocytoma*
M9421/3	*Pilocytic astrocytoma*
M9422/3	*Spongioblastoma NOS*
M9423/3	*Spongioblastoma polare*
M9430/3	*Astroblastoma*
M9440/3	*Glioblastoma NOS*
M9441/3	*Giant cell glioblastoma*
M9442/3	*Glioblastoma with sarcomatous component*
M9443/3	*Primitive polar spongioblastoma*
M9450/3	*Oligodendroglioma NOS*
M9451/3	*Oligodendroglioma, anaplastic type*
M9460/3	*Oligodendroblastoma*
M9470/3	*Medulloblastoma NOS*
M9471/3	*Desmoplastic medulloblastoma*
M9472/3	*Medullomyoblastoma*

| M9480/3 | *Cerebellar sarcoma NOS* |
| M9481/3 | *Monstrocellular sarcoma* |

M949-M952 Neuroepitheliomatous neoplasms

M9490/0	*Ganglioneuroma*
M9490/3	*Ganglioneuroblastoma*
M9491/0	*Ganglioneuromatosis*
M9500/3	*Neuroblastoma NOS*
M9501/3	*Medulloepithelioma NOS*
M9502/3	*Teratoid medulloepithelioma*
M9503/3	*Neuroepithelioma NOS*
M9504/3	*Spongioneuroblastoma*
M9505/1	*Ganglioglioma*
M9506/0	*Neurocytoma*
M9507/0	*Pacinian tumor*
M9510/3	*Retinoblastoma NOS*
M9511/3	*Retinoblastoma, differentiated type*
M9512/3	*Retinoblastoma, undifferentiated type*
M9520/3	*Olfactory neurogenic tumor*
M9521/3	*Esthesioneurocytoma*
M9522/3	*Esthesioneuroblastoma*
M9523/3	*Esthesioneuroepithelioma*

M953 Meningiomas

M9530/0	*Meningioma NOS*
M9530/1	*Meningiomatosis NOS*
M9530/3	*Meningioma, malignant*
M9531/0	*Meningotheliomatous meningioma*
M9532/0	*Fibrous meningioma*
M9533/0	*Psammomatous meningioma*
M9534/0	*Angiomatous meningioma*
M9535/0	*Hemangioblastic meningioma*
M9536/0	*Hemangiopericytic meningioma*
M9537/0	*Transitional meningioma*
M9538/1	*Papillary meningioma*
M9539/3	*Meningeal sarcomatosis*

M954-M957 Nerve sheath tumor

M9540/0	*Neurofibroma NOS*
M9540/1	*Neurofibromatosis NOS*
M9540/3	*Neurofibrosarcoma*
M9541/0	*Melanotic neurofibroma*
M9550/0	*Plexiform neurofibroma*
M9560/0	*Neurilemmoma NOS*
M9560/1	*Neurinomatosis*
M9560/3	*Neurilemmoma, malignant*
M9570/0	*Neuroma NOS*

M958 Granular cell tumors and alveolar soft part sarcoma

M9580/0	*Granular cell tumor NOS*
M9580/3	*Granular cell tumor, malignant*
M9581/3	*Alveolar soft part sarcoma*

M959-M963 Lymphomas, NOS or diffuse

M9590/0	*Lymphomatous tumor, benign*
M9590/3	*Malignant lymphoma NOS*
M9591/3	*Malignant lymphoma, non Hodgkin's type*
M9600/3	*Malignant lymphoma, undifferentiated cell type NOS*
M9601/3	*Malignant lymphoma, stem cell type*
M9602/3	*Malignant lymphoma, convoluted cell type NOS*
M9610/3	*Lymphosarcoma NOS*
M9611/3	*Malignant lymphoma, lymphoplasmacytoid type*
M9612/3	*Malignant lymphoma, immunoblastic type*
M9613/3	*Malignant lymphoma, mixed lymphocytic-histiocytic NOS*
M9614/3	*Malignant lymphoma, centroblastic-centrocytic, diffuse*
M9615/3	*Malignant lymphoma, follicular center cell NOS*
M9620/3	*Malignant lymphoma, lymphocytic, well differentiated NOS*
M9621/3	*Malignant lymphoma, lymphocytic, intermediate differentiation NOS*
M9622/3	*Malignant lymphoma, centrocytic*
M9623/3	*Malignant lymphoma, follicular center cell, cleaved NOS*
M9630/3	*Malignant lymphoma, lymphocytic, poorly differentiated NOS*
M9631/3	*Prolymphocytic lymphosarcoma*
M9632/3	*Malignant lymphoma, centroblastic type NOS*
M9633/3	*Malignant lymphoma, follicular center cell, noncleaved NOS*

M964	**Reticulosarcomas**
M9640/3	*Reticulosarcoma NOS*
M9641/3	*Reticulosarcoma, pleomorphic cell type*
M9642/3	*Reticulosarcoma, nodular*

M965-M966 Hodgkin's disease

M9650/3	*Hodgkin's disease NOS*
M9651/3	*Hodgkin's disease, lymphocytic predominance*
M9652/3	*Hodgkin's disease, mixed cellularity*
M9653/3	*Hodgkin's disease, lymphocytic depletion NOS*
M9654/3	*Hodgkin's disease, lymphocytic depletion, diffuse fibrosis*
M9655/3	*Hodgkin's disease, lymphocytic depletion, reticular type*
M9656/3	*Hodgkin's disease, nodular sclerosis NOS*
M9657/3	*Hodgkin's disease, nodular sclerosis, cellular phase*
M9660/3	*Hodgkin's paragranuloma*
M9661/3	*Hodgkin's granuloma*
M9662/3	*Hodgkin's sarcoma*

M969	**Lymphomas, nodular or follicular**
M9690/3	*Malignant lymphoma, nodular NOS*
M9691/3	*Malignant lymphoma, mixed lymphocytic-histiocytic, nodular*
M9692/3	*Malignant lymphoma, centroblastic-centrocytic, follicular*
M9693/3	*Malignant lymphoma, lymphocytic, well differentiated, nodular*
M9694/3	*Malignant lymphoma, lymphocytic, intermediate differentiation, nodular*
M9695/3	*Malignant lymphoma, follicular center cell, cleaved, follicular*
M9696/3	*Malignant lymphoma, lymphocytic, poorly differentiated, nodular*
M9697/3	*Malignant lymphoma, centroblastic type, follicular*
M9698/3	*Malignant lymphoma, follicular center cell, noncleaved, follicular*

M970	**Mycosis fungoides**
M9700/3	*Mycosis fungoides*
M9701/3	*Sezary's disease*

M971-M972 Miscellaneous reticuloendothelial neoplasms

M9710/3	*Microglioma*
M9720/3	*Malignant histiocytosis*
M9721/3	*Histiocytic medullary reticulosis*
M9722/3	*Letterer-Siwe's disease*

M973	**Plasma cell tumors**
M9730/3	*Plasma cell myeloma*
M9731/0	*Plasma cell tumor, benign*
M9731/1	*Plasmacytoma NOS*
M9731/3	*Plasma cell tumor, malignant*

M974	**Mast cell tumors**
M9740/1	*Mastocytoma NOS*
M9740/3	*Mast cell sarcoma*
M9741/3	*Malignant mastocytosis*

M975	**Burkitt's tumor**
M9750/3	*Burkitt's tumor*

M980-M994 Leukemias

M980	**Leukemias NOS**
M9800/3	*Leukemia NOS*
M9801/3	*Acute leukemia NOS*
M9802/3	*Subacute leukemia NOS*
M9803/3	*Chronic leukemia NOS*
M9804/3	*Aleukemic leukemia NOS*

M981	**Compound leukemias**
M9810/3	*Compound leukemia*

M982	**Lymphoid leukemias**
M9820/3	*Lymphoid leukemia NOS*
M9821/3	*Acute lymphoid leukemia*
M9822/3	*Subacute lymphoid leukemia*
M9823/3	*Chronic lymphoid leukemia*
M9824/3	*Aleukemic lymphoid leukemia*
M9825/3	*Prolymphocytic leukemia*

M983	**Plasma cell leukemias**
M9830/3	*Plasma cell leukemia*

M984	**Erythroleukemias**
M9840/3	*Erythroleukemia*
M9841/3	*Acute erythremia*

M9842/3   *Chronic erythremia*

M985   **Lymphosarcoma cell leukemias**
M9850/3   *Lymphosarcoma cell leukemia*

M986   **Myeloid leukemias**
M9860/3   *Myeloid leukemia NOS*
M9861/3   *Acute myeloid leukemia*
M9862/3   *Subacute myeloid leukemia*
M9863/3   *Chronic myeloid leukemia*
M9864/3   *Aleukemic myeloid leukemia*
M9865/3   *Neutrophilic leukemia*
M9866/3   *Acute promyelocytic leukemia*

M987   **Basophilic leukemias**
M9870/3   *Basophilic leukemia*

M988   **Eosinophilic leukemias**
M9880/3   *Eosinophilic leukemia*

M989   **Monocytic leukemias**
M9890/3   *Monocytic leukemia NOS*
M9891/3   *Acute monocytic leukemia*
M9892/3   *Subacute monocytic leukemia*
M9893/3   *Chronic monocytic leukemia*
M9894/3   *Aleukemic monocytic leukemia*

M990-M994 Miscellaneous leukemias
M9900/3   *Mast cell leukemia*
M9910/3   *Megakaryocytic leukemia*
M9920/3   *Megakaryocytic myelosis*
M9930/3   *Myeloid sarcoma*
M9940/3   *Hairy cell leukemia*

M995-M997 Miscellaneous myeloproliferative and lymphoproliferative disorders
M9950/1   *Polycythemia vera*
M9951/1   *Acute panmyelosis*
M9960/1   *Chronic myeloproliferative disease*
M9961/1   *Myelosclerosis with myeloid metaplasia*
M9962/1   *Idiopathic thrombocythemia*
M9970/1   *Chronic lymphoproliferative disease*

This page intentionally left blank.

APPENDIX B:
GLOSSARY OF MENTAL DISORDERS

Note: *Appendix B Glossary of Mental Disorders* has been removed from the official ICD-9-CM CD-Rom effective with the FY2005 update.

This page intentionally left blank.

APPENDIX C:
CLASSIFICATION OF DRUGS BY AMERICAN HOSPITAL FORMULARY SERVICE LIST NUMBER AND THEIR ICD-9-CM EQUIVALENTS

The coding of adverse effects of drugs is keyed to the continually revised Hospital Formulary of the American Hospital Formulary Service (AHFS) published under the direction of the American Society of Hospital Pharmacists.

AHFS*LIST	ICD-9-CM Diagnosis Code

The following section gives the ICD-9-CM diagnosis code for each AHFS list.

4:00	**ANTIHISTAMINE DRUGS**	963.0
8:00	**ANTI-INFECTIVE AGENTS**	
8:04	Amebacides	961.5
	hydroxyquinoline derivatives	961.3
	arsenical anti-infectives	961.1
8:08	Anthelmintics	961.6
	quinoline derivatives	961.3
8:12.04	Antifungal Antibiotics	960.1
	nonantibiotics	961.9
8:12.06	Cephalosporins	960.5
8:12.08	Chloramphenicol	960.2
8:12.12	The Erythromycins	960.3
8:12.16	The Penicillins	960.0
8:12.20	The Streptomycins	960.6
8:12.24	The Tetracyclines	960.4
8:12.28	Other Antibiotics	960.8
	antimycobacterial antibiotics	960.6
	macrolides	960.3
8:16	Antituberculars	961.8
	antibiotics	960.6
8:18	Antivirals	961.7
8:20	Plasmodicides (antimalarials)	961.4
8:24	Sulfonamides	961.0
8:26	The Sulfones	961.8
8:28	Treponemicides	961.2
8:32	Trichomonacides	961.5
	hydroxyquinoline derivatives	961.3
	nitrofuran derivatives	961.9
8:36	Urinary Germicides	961.9
	quinoline derivatives	961.3
8:40	Other Anti-Infectives	961.9
10:00	**ANTINEOPLASTIC AGENTS**	963.1
	antibiotics	960.7
	progestogens	962.2
12:00	**AUTONOMIC DRUGS**	
12:04	Parasympathomimetic (Cholinergic) Agents	971.0
12:08	Parasympatholytic (Cholinergic Blocking) Agents	971.1
12:12	Sympathomimetic (Adrenergic) Agents	971.2
12:16	Sympatholytic (Adrenergic Blocking) Agents	971.3

	AHFS*LIST	ICD-9-CM Diagnosis Code
12:20	Skeletal Muscle Relaxants	975.2
	central nervous system muscle-tone depressants	968.0
16:00	**BLOOD DERIVATIVES**	964.7
20:00	**BLOOD FORMATION AND COAGULATION**	
20:04	Antianemia Drugs	964.1
20:04.04	Iron Preparations	964.0
20:04.08	Liver and Stomach Preparations	964.1
20:12.04	Anticoagulants	964.2
20:12.08	Antiheparin agents	964.5
20:12.12	Coagulants	964.5
20:12.16	Hemostatics	964.5
	capillary-active drugs	972.8
	fibrinolysis-affecting agents	964.4
	natural products	964.7
24:00	**CARDIOVASCULAR DRUGS**	
24:04	Cardiac Drugs	972.9
	cardiotonic agents	972.1
	rhythm regulators	972.0
24:06	Antilipemic Agents	972.2
	thyroid derivatives	962.7
24:08	Hypotensive Agents	972.6
	adrenergic blocking agents	971.3
	ganglion-blocking agents	972.3
	vasodilators	972.5
24:12	Vasodilating Agents	972.5
	coronary	972.4
	nicotinic acid derivatives	972.2
24:16	Sclerosing Agents	972.7
28:00	**CENTRAL NERVOUS SYSTEM DRUGS**	
28:04	General Anesthetics	968.4
	gaseous anesthetics	968.2
	halothane	968.1
	intravenous anesthetics	968.3
28:08	Analgesics and Antipyretics	965.9
	antirheumatics	965.6
	aromatic analgesics	965.4
	non-narcotics NEC	965.7
	opium alkaloids	965.00
	heroin	965.01
	methadone	965.02
	specified type NEC	965.09
	pyrazole derivatives	965.5
	salicylates	965.1
	specified type NEC	965.8
28:10	Narcotic Antagonists	970.1
28:12	Anticonvulsants	966.3
	barbiturates	967.0
	benzodiazepine-based tranquilizers	969.4
	bromides	967.3
	hydantoin derivatives	966.1
	oxazolidine derivative	966.0
	succinimides	966.2
28:16.04	Antidepressants	969.0

	AHFS*LIST	ICD-9-CM Diagnosis Code
28:16.08	Tranquilizers	969.5
	benzodiazepine-based	969.4
	butyrophenone-based	969.2
	major NEC	969.3
	phenothiazine-based	969.1
28:16.12	Other Psychotherapeutic Agents	969.8
28:20	Respiratory and Cerebral Stimulants	970.9
	analeptics	970.0
	anorexigenic agents	977.0
	psychostimulants	969.7
	specified type NEC	970.8
28:24	Sedatives and Hypnotics	967.9
	barbiturates	967.0
	benzodiazepine-based tranquilizers	969.4
	chloral hydrate group	967.1
	glutethamide group	967.5
	intravenous anesthetics	968.3
	methaqualone	967.4
	paraldehyde	967.2
	phenothiazine-based tranquilizers	969.1
	specified type NEC	967.8
	thiobarbiturates	968.3
	tranquilizer NEC	969.5
36:00	**DIAGNOSTIC AGENTS**	977.8
40:00	**ELECTROLYTE, CALORIC, AND WATER BALANCE AGENTS NEC**	974.5
40:04	Acidifying Agents	963.2
40:08	Alkalinizing Agents	963.3
40:10	Ammonia Detoxicants	974.5
40:12	Replacement Solutions NEC	974.5
	plasma volume expanders	964.8
40:16	Sodium-Removing Resins	974.5
40:18	Potassium-Removing Resins	974.5
40:20	Caloric Agents	974.5
40:24	Salt and Sugar Substitutes	974.5
40:28	Diuretics NEC	974.4
	carbonic acid anhydrase inhibitors	974.2
	mercurials	974.0
	purine derivatives	974.1
	saluretics	974.3
40:36	Irrigating Solutions	974.5
40:40	Uricosuric Agents	974.7
44:00	**ENZYMES NEC**	963.4
	fibrinolysis-affecting agents	964.4
	gastric agents	973.4
48:00	**EXPECTORANTS AND COUGH PREPARATIONS**	
	antihistamine agents	963.0
	antitussives	975.4
	codeine derivatives	965.09
	expectorants	975.5
	narcotic agents NEC	965.09

AHFS*LIST	ICD-9-CM Diagnosis Code

52:00   **EYE, EAR, NOSE, AND THROAT PREPARATIONS**

52:04	Anti-Infectives	
	ENT	976.6
	ophthalmic	976.5
52:04.04	Antibiotics	
	ENT	976.6
	ophthalmic	976.5
52:04.06	Antivirals	
	ENT	976.6
	ophthalmic	976.5
52:04.08	Sulfonamides	
	ENT	976.6
	ophthalmic	976.5
52:04.12	Miscellaneous Anti-Infectives	
	ENT	976.6
	ophthalmic	976.5
52:08	Anti-Inflammatory Agents	
	ENT	976.6
	ophthalmic	976.5
52:10	Carbonic Anhydrase Inhibitors	974.2
52:12	Contact Lens Solutions	976.5
52:16	Local Anesthetics	968.5
52:20	Miotics	971.0
52:24	Mydriatics	
	adrenergics	971.2
	anticholinergics	971.1
	antimuscarinics	971.1
	parasympatholytics	971.1
	spasmolytics	971.1
	sympathomimetics	971.2
52:28	Mouth Washes and Gargles	976.6
52:32	Vasoconstrictors	971.2
52:36	Unclassified Agents	
	ENT	976.6
	ophthalmic	976.5

56:00   **GASTROINTESTINAL DRUGS**

56:04	Antacids and Absorbants	973.0
56:08	Anti-Diarrhea Agents	973.5
56:10	Antiflatulents	973.8
56:12	Cathartics NEC	973.3
	emollients	973.2
	irritants	973.1
56:16	Digestants	973.4
56:20	Emetics and Antiemetics	
	antiemetics	963.0
	emetics	973.6
56:24	Lipotropic Agents	977.1

60:00   **GOLD COMPOUNDS**   965.6

64:00   **HEAVY METAL ANTAGONISTS**   963.8

68:00   **HORMONES AND SYNTHETIC SUBSTITUTES**

68:04	Adrenals	962.0
68:08	Androgens	962.1

AHFS*LIST		ICD-9-CM Diagnosis Code
68:12	Contraceptives	962.2
68:16	Estrogens	962.2
68:18	Gonadotropins	962.4
68:20	Insulins and Antidiabetic Agents	962.3
68:20.08	Insulins	962.3
68:24	Parathyroid	962.6
68:28	Pituitary	
	anterior	962.4
	posterior	962.5
68:32	Progestogens	962.2
68:34	Other Corpus Luteum Hormones	962.2
68:36	Thyroid and Antithyroid	
	antithyroid	962.8
	thyroid	962.7
72:00	**LOCAL ANESTHETICS NEC**	968.9
	topical (surface) agents	968.5
	infiltrating agents (intradermal) (subcutaneous)	
	(submucosal)	968.5
	nerve blocking agents (peripheral)	968.6
	(plexus)(regional)	
	spinal	968.7
76:00	**OXYTOCICS**	975.0
78:00	**RADIOACTIVE AGENTS**	990
80:00	**SERUMS, TOXOIDS, AND VACCINES**	
80:04	Serums	979.9
	immune globulin (gamma) (human)	964.6
80:08	Toxoids NEC	978.8
	diphtheria	978.5
	and tetanus	978.9
	with pertussis component	978.6
	tetanus	978.4
	and diphtheria	978.9
	with pertussis component	978.6
80:12	Vaccines NEC	979.9
	bacterial NEC	978.8
	with	
	other bacterial component	978.9
	pertussis component	978.6
	viral and rickettsial component	979.7
	rickettsial NEC	979.6
	with	
	bacterial component	979.7
	pertussis component	978.6
	viral component	979.7
	viral NEC	979.6
	with	
	bacterial component	979.7
	pertussis component	978.6
	rickettsial component	979.7
84:00	**SKIN AND MUCOUS MEMBRANE PREPARATIONS**	
84:04	Anti-Infectives	976.0
84:04.04	Antibiotics	976.0
84:04.08	Fungicides	976.0
84:04.12	Scabicides and Pediculicides	976.0
84:04.16	Miscellaneous Local Anti-Infectives	976.0

	AHFS*LIST	ICD-9-CM Diagnosis Code
84:06	Anti-Inflammatory Agents	976.0
84:08	Antipruritics and Local Anesthetics	
	antipruritics	976.1
	local anesthetics	968.5
84:12	Astringents	976.2
84:16	Cell Stimulants and Proliferants	976.8
84:20	Detergents	976.2
84:24	Emollients, Demulcents, and Protectants	976.3
84:28	Keratolytic Agents	976.4
84:32	Keratoplastic Agents	976.4
84:36	Miscellaneous Agents	976.8
86:00	**SPASMOLYTIC AGENTS**	975.1
	antiasthmatics	975.7
	papaverine	972.5
	theophyllin	974.1
88:00	**VITAMINS**	
88:04	Vitamin A	963.5
88:08	Vitamin B Complex	963.5
	hematopoietic vitamin	964.1
	nicotinic acid derivatives	972.2
88:12	Vitamin C	963.5
88:16	Vitamin D	963.5
88:20	Vitamin E	963.5
88:24	Vitamin K Activity	964.3
88:28	Multivitamin Preparations	963.5
92:00	**UNCLASSIFIED THERAPEUTIC AGENTS**	

APPENDIX D:
CLASSIFICATION OF INDUSTRIAL ACCIDENTS ACCORDING TO AGENCY

Annex B to the Resolution concerning Statistics of Employment Injuries adopted by the Tenth International Conference of Labor Statisticians on 12 October 1962

1 MACHINES

11 Prime-Movers, except Electrical Motors
111 Steam engines
112 Internal combustion engines
119 Others

12 Transmission Machinery
121 Transmission shafts
122 Transmission belts, cables, pulleys, pinions, chains, gears
129 Others

13 Metalworking Machines
131 Power presses
132 Lathes
133 Milling machines
134 Abrasive wheels
135 Mechanical shears
136 Forging machines
137 Rolling-mills
139 Others

14 Wood and Assimilated Machines
141 Circular saws
142 Other saws
143 Molding machines
144 Overhand planes
149 Others

15 Agricultural Machines
151 Reapers (including combine reapers)
152 Threshers
159 Others

16 Mining Machinery
161 Under-cutters
169 Others

19 Other Machines Not Elsewhere Classified
191 Earth-moving machines, excavating and scraping machines, except means of transport
192 Spinning, weaving and other textile machines
193 Machines for the manufacture of foodstuffs and beverages
194 Machines for the manufacture of paper
195 Printing machines
199 Others

2 MEANS OF TRANSPORT AND LIFTING EQUIPMENT

21 Lifting Machines and Appliances
211 Cranes
212 Lifts and elevators
213 Winches
214 Pulley blocks
219 Others

22 Means of Rail Transport
221 Inter-urban railways
222 Rail transport in mines, tunnels, quarries, industrial establishments, docks, etc.
229 Others

23 Other Wheeled Means of Transport, Excluding Rail Transport
231 Tractors
232 Lorries

2 MEANS OF TRANSPORT AND LIFTING EQUIPMENT *continued*

233 Trucks
234 Motor vehicles, not elsewhere classified
235 Animal-drawn vehicles
236 Hand-drawn vehicles
239 Others

24 Means of Air Transport

25 Means of Water Transport
251 Motorized means of water transport
252 Non-motorized means of water transport

26 Other Means of Transport
261 Cable-cars
262 Mechanical conveyors, except cable-cars
269 Others

3 OTHER EQUIPMENT

31 Pressure Vessels
311 Boilers
312 Pressurized containers
313 Pressurized piping and accessories
314 Gas cylinders
315 Caissons, diving equipment
319 Others

32 Furnaces, Ovens, Kilns
321 Blast furnaces
322 Refining furnaces
323 Other furnaces
324 Kilns
325 Ovens

33 Refrigerating Plants

34 Electrical Installations, Including Electric Motors, but Excluding Electric Hand Tools
341 Rotating machines
342 Conductors
343 Transformers
344 Control apparatus
349 Others

35 Electric Hand Tools

36 Tools, Implements, and Appliances, Except Electric Hand Tools
361 Power-driven hand tools, except electric hand tools
362 Hand tools, not power-driven
369 Others

37 Ladders, Mobile Ramps

38 Scaffolding

39 Other Equipment, Not Elsewhere Classified

4 MATERIALS, SUBSTANCES AND RADIATIONS

41 Explosives

42 Dusts, Gases, Liquids and Chemicals, Excluding Explosives
421 Dusts
422 Gases, vapors, fumes
423 Liquids, not elsewhere classified
424 Chemicals, not elsewhere classified

43 Flying Fragments

44 Radiations
441 Ionizing radiations
449 Others

49 Other Materials and Substances Not Elsewhere Classified

5 WORKING ENVIRONMENT

51 Outdoor
511 Weather
512 Traffic and working surfaces
513 Water
519 Others

52 Indoor
521 Floors
522 Confined quarters
523 Stairs
524 Other traffic and working surfaces
525 Floor openings and wall openings
526 Environmental factors (lighting, ventilation, temperature, noise, etc.)
529 Others

53 Underground
531 Roofs and faces of mine roads and tunnels, etc.
532 Floors of mine roads and tunnels, etc.
533 Working-faces of mines, tunnels, etc.
534 Mine shafts
535 Fire
536 Water
539 Others

6 OTHER AGENCIES, NOT ELSEWHERE CLASSIFIED

61 Animals
611 Live animals
612 Animals products

69 Other Agencies, Not Elsewhere Classified

7 AGENCIES NOT CLASSIFIED FOR LACK OF SUFFICIENT DATA

This page intentionally left blank.

APPENDIX E:
LIST OF THREE-DIGIT CATEGORIES

1. INFECTIOUS AND PARASITIC DISEASES

Intestinal infectious diseases (001-009)
- 001 Cholera
- 002 Typhoid and paratyphoid fevers
- 003 Other salmonella infections
- 004 Shigellosis
- 005 Other food poisoning (bacterial)
- 006 Amebiasis
- 007 Other protozoal intestinal diseases
- 008 Intestinal infections due to other organisms
- 009 Ill-defined intestinal infections

Tuberculosis (010-018)
- 010 Primary tuberculous infection
- 011 Pulmonary tuberculosis
- 012 Other respiratory tuberculosis
- 013 Tuberculosis of meninges and central nervous system
- 014 Tuberculosis of intestines, peritoneum, and mesenteric glands
- 015 Tuberculosis of bones and joints
- 016 Tuberculosis of genitourinary system
- 017 Tuberculosis of other organs
- 018 Miliary tuberculosis

Zoonotic bacterial diseases (020-027)
- 020 Plague
- 021 Tularemia
- 022 Anthrax
- 023 Brucellosis
- 024 Glanders
- 025 Melioidosis
- 026 Rat-bite fever
- 027 Other zoonotic bacterial diseases

Other bacterial diseases (030-041)
- 030 Leprosy
- 031 Diseases due to other mycobacteria
- 032 Diphtheria
- 033 Whooping cough
- 034 Streptococcal sore throat and scarlet fever
- 035 Erysipelas
- 036 Meningococcal infection
- 037 Tetanus
- 038 Septicemia
- 039 Actinomycotic infections
- 040 Other bacterial diseases
- 041 Bacterial infection in conditions classified elsewhere and of unspecified site

Human immunodeficiency virus (HIV) infection (042)
- 042 Human immunodeficiency virus [HIV] disease

Poliomyelitis and other non-arthropod-borne viral diseases of central nervous system (045-049)
- 045 Acute poliomyelitis
- 046 Slow virus infections and prion diseases of central nervous system
- 047 Meningitis due to enterovirus
- 048 Other enterovirus diseases of central nervous system
- 049 Other non-arthropod-borne viral diseases of central nervous system

Viral diseases generally accompanied by exanthem (050-059)
- 050 Smallpox
- 051 Cowpox and paravaccinia
- 052 Chickenpox
- 053 Herpes zoster
- 054 Herpes simplex
- 055 Measles
- 056 Rubella

1. INFECTIOUS AND PARASITIC DISEASES *continued*

057   Other viral exanthemata
058   Other human herpesviruses
059   Other poxvirus infections

Arthropod-borne viral diseases (060-066)
060   Yellow fever
061   Dengue
062   Mosquito-borne viral encephalitis
063   Tick-borne viral encephalitis
064   Viral encephalitis transmitted by other and unspecified arthropods
065   Arthropod-borne hemorrhagic fever
066   Other arthropod-borne viral diseases

Other diseases due to viruses and Chlamydiae (070-079)
070   Viral hepatitis
071   Rabies
072   Mumps
073   Ornithosis
074   Specific diseases due to Coxsackie virus
075   Infectious mononucleosis
076   Trachoma
077   Other diseases of conjunctiva due to viruses and Chlamydiae
078   Other diseases due to viruses and Chlamydiae
079   Viral and Chlamydial infection in conditions classified elsewhere and of unspecified
      site

Rickettsioses and other arthropod-borne diseases (080-088)
080   Louse-borne [epidemic] typhus
081   Other typhus
082   Tick-borne rickettsioses
083   Other rickettsioses
084   Malaria
085   Leishmaniasis
086   Trypanosomiasis
087   Relapsing fever
088   Other arthropod-borne diseases

Syphilis and other venereal diseases (090-099)
090   Congenital syphilis
091   Early syphilis, symptomatic
092   Early syphilis, latent
093   Cardiovascular syphilis
094   Neurosyphilis
095   Other forms of late syphilis, with symptoms
096   Late syphilis, latent
097   Other and unspecified syphilis
098   Gonococcal infections
099   Other venereal diseases

Other spirochetal diseases (100-104)
100   Leptospirosis
101   Vincent's angina
102   Yaws
103   Pinta
104   Other spirochetal infection

Mycoses (110-118)
110   Dermatophytosis
111   Dermatomycosis, other and unspecified
112   Candidiasis
114   Coccidioidomycosis
115   Histoplasmosis
116   Blastomycotic infection
117   Other mycoses
118   Opportunistic mycoses

Helminthiases (120-129)
120   Schistosomiasis [bilharziasis]
121   Other trematode infections

1. INFECTIOUS AND PARASITIC DISEASES *continued*

122 Echinococcosis
123 Other cestode infection
124 Trichinosis
125 Filarial infection and dracontiasis
126 Ancylostomiasis and necatoriasis
127 Other intestinal helminthiases
128 Other and unspecified helminthiases
129 Intestinal parasitism, unspecified

Other infectious and parasitic diseases (130-136)

130 Toxoplasmosis
131 Trichomoniasis
132 Pediculosis and phthirus infestation
133 Acariasis
134 Other infestation
135 Sarcoidosis
136 Other and unspecified infectious and parasitic diseases

Late effects of infectious and parasitic diseases (137-139)

137 Late effects of tuberculosis
138 Late effects of acute poliomyelitis
139 Late effects of other infectious and parasitic diseases

2. NEOPLASMS

Malignant neoplasm of lip, oral cavity, and pharynx (140-149)

140 Malignant neoplasm of lip
141 Malignant neoplasm of tongue
142 Malignant neoplasm of major salivary glands
143 Malignant neoplasm of gum
144 Malignant neoplasm of floor of mouth
145 Malignant neoplasm of other and unspecified parts of mouth
146 Malignant neoplasm of oropharynx
147 Malignant neoplasm of nasopharynx
148 Malignant neoplasm of hypopharynx
149 Malignant neoplasm of other and ill-defined sites within the lip, oral cavity, and pharynx

Malignant neoplasm of digestive organs and peritoneum (150-159)

150 Malignant neoplasm of esophagus
151 Malignant neoplasm of stomach
152 Malignant neoplasm of small intestine, including duodenum
153 Malignant neoplasm of colon
154 Malignant neoplasm of rectum, rectosigmoid junction, and anus
155 Malignant neoplasm of liver and intrahepatic bile ducts
156 Malignant neoplasm of gallbladder and extrahepatic bile ducts
157 Malignant neoplasm of pancreas
158 Malignant neoplasm of retroperitoneum and peritoneum
159 Malignant neoplasm of other and ill-defined sites within the digestive organs and peritoneum

Malignant neoplasm of respiratory and intrathoracic organs (160-165)

160 Malignant neoplasm of nasal cavities, middle ear, and accessory sinuses
161 Malignant neoplasm of larynx
162 Malignant neoplasm of trachea, bronchus, and lung
163 Malignant neoplasm of pleura
164 Malignant neoplasm of thymus, heart, and mediastinum
165 Malignant neoplasm of other and ill-defined sites within the respiratory system and intrathoracic organs

Malignant neoplasm of bone, connective tissue, skin, and breast (170-176)

170 Malignant neoplasm of bone and articular cartilage
171 Malignant neoplasm of connective and other soft tissue
172 Malignant melanoma of skin
173 Other and unspecified malignant neoplasm of skin
174 Malignant neoplasm of female breast
175 Malignant neoplasm of male breast
176 Kaposi's sarcoma

2. NEOPLASMS *continued*

Malignant neoplasm of genitourinary organs (179-189)
179 Malignant neoplasm of uterus, part unspecified
180 Malignant neoplasm of cervix uteri
181 Malignant neoplasm of placenta
182 Malignant neoplasm of body of uterus
183 Malignant neoplasm of ovary and other uterine adnexa
184 Malignant neoplasm of other and unspecified female genital organs
185 Malignant neoplasm of prostate
186 Malignant neoplasm of testis
187 Malignant neoplasm of penis and other male genital organs
188 Malignant neoplasm of bladder
189 Malignant neoplasm of kidney and other and unspecified urinary organs

Malignant neoplasm of other and unspecified sites (190-199)
190 Malignant neoplasm of eye
191 Malignant neoplasm of brain
192 Malignant neoplasm of other and unspecified parts of nervous system
193 Malignant neoplasm of thyroid gland
194 Malignant neoplasm of other endocrine glands and related structures
195 Malignant neoplasm of other and ill-defined sites
196 Secondary and unspecified malignant neoplasm of lymph nodes
197 Secondary malignant neoplasm of respiratory and digestive systems
198 Secondary malignant neoplasm of other specified sites
199 Malignant neoplasm without specification of site

Malignant neoplasm of lymphatic and hematopoietic tissue (200-208)
200 Lymphosarcoma and reticulosarcoma and other specified malignant tumors of lymphatic tissue
201 Hodgkin's disease
202 Other malignant neoplasm of lymphoid and histiocytic tissue
203 Multiple myeloma and immunoproliferative neoplasms
204 Lymphoid leukemia
205 Myeloid leukemia
206 Monocytic leukemia
207 Other specified leukemia
208 Leukemia of unspecified cell type

Neuroendocrine tumors (209)
209 Neuroendocrine tumors

Benign neoplasms (210-229)
210 Benign neoplasm of lip, oral cavity, and pharynx
211 Benign neoplasm of other parts of digestive system
212 Benign neoplasm of respiratory and intrathoracic organs
213 Benign neoplasm of bone and articular cartilage
214 Lipoma
215 Other benign neoplasm of connective and other soft tissue
216 Benign neoplasm of skin
217 Benign neoplasm of breast
218 Uterine leiomyoma
219 Other benign neoplasm of uterus
220 Benign neoplasm of ovary
221 Benign neoplasm of other female genital organs
222 Benign neoplasm of male genital organs
223 Benign neoplasm of kidney and other urinary organs
224 Benign neoplasm of eye
225 Benign neoplasm of brain and other parts of nervous system
226 Benign neoplasm of thyroid gland
227 Benign neoplasm of other endocrine glands and related structures
228 Hemangioma and lymphangioma, any site
229 Benign neoplasm of other and unspecified sites

Carcinoma in situ (230-234)
230 Carcinoma in situ of digestive organs
231 Carcinoma in situ of respiratory system
232 Carcinoma in situ of skin
233 Carcinoma in situ of breast and genitourinary system
234 Carcinoma in situ of other and unspecified sites

2. NEOPLASMS *continued*

Neoplasms of uncertain behavior (235-238)
- 235   Neoplasm of uncertain behavior of digestive and respiratory systems
- 236   Neoplasm of uncertain behavior of genitourinary organs
- 237   Neoplasm of uncertain behavior of endocrine glands and nervous system
- 238   Neoplasm of uncertain behavior of other and unspecified sites and tissues

Neoplasm of unspecified nature (239)
- 239   Neoplasm of unspecified nature

3. ENDOCRINE, NUTRITIONAL AND METABOLIC DISEASES, AND IMMUNITY DISORDERS

Disorders of thyroid gland (240-246)
- 240   Simple and unspecified goiter
- 241   Nontoxic nodular goiter
- 242   Thyrotoxicosis with or without goiter
- 243   Congenital hypothyroidism
- 244   Acquired hypothyroidism
- 245   Thyroiditis
- 246   Other disorders of thyroid

Diseases of other endocrine glands (249-259)
- 249   Secondary diabetes mellitus
- 250   Diabetes mellitus
- 251   Other disorders of pancreatic internal secretion
- 252   Disorders of parathyroid gland
- 253   Disorders of the pituitary gland and its hypothalamic control
- 254   Diseases of thymus gland
- 255   Disorders of adrenal glands
- 256   Ovarian dysfunction
- 257   Testicular dysfunction
- 258   Polyglandular dysfunction and related disorders
- 259   Other endocrine disorders

Nutritional deficiencies (260-269)
- 260   Kwashiorkor
- 261   Nutritional marasmus
- 262   Other severe protein-calorie malnutrition
- 263   Other and unspecified protein-calorie malnutrition
- 264   Vitamin A deficiency
- 265   Thiamine and niacin deficiency states
- 266   Deficiency of B-complex components
- 267   Ascorbic acid deficiency
- 268   Vitamin D deficiency
- 269   Other nutritional deficiencies

Other metabolic and immunity disorders (270-279)
- 270   Disorders of amino-acid transport and metabolism
- 271   Disorders of carbohydrate transport and metabolism
- 272   Disorders of lipoid metabolism
- 273   Disorders of plasma protein metabolism
- 274   Gout
- 275   Disorders of mineral metabolism
- 276   Disorders of fluid, electrolyte, and acid-base balance
- 277   Other and unspecified disorders of metabolism
- 278   Overweight, obesity and other hyperalimentation
- 279   Disorders involving the immune mechanism

4. DISEASES OF THE BLOOD AND BLOOD-FORMING ORGANS

Diseases of blood and blood-forming organs (280-289)
- 280   Iron deficiency anemias
- 281   Other deficiency anemias
- 282   Hereditary hemolytic anemias
- 283   Acquired hemolytic anemias
- 284   Aplastic anemia and other bone marrow failure syndromes
- 285   Other and unspecified anemias
- 286   Coagulation defects
- 287   Purpura and other hemorrhagic conditions

5. MENTAL DISORDERS
    288 Diseases of white blood cells
    289 Other diseases of blood and blood-forming organs

Organic psychotic conditions (290-294)
    290 Dementias
    291 Alcohol-induced mental disorders
    292 Drug-induced mental disorders
    293 Transient mental disorders due to conditions classified elsewhere
    294 Persistent mental disorders due to conditions classified elsewhere

Other psychoses (295-299)
    295 Schizophrenic disorders
    296 Episodic mood disorders
    297 Delusional disorders
    298 Other nonorganic psychoses
    299 Pervasive developmental disorders

Neurotic disorders, personality disorders, and other nonpsychotic mental disorders (300-316)
    300 Anxiety, dissociative and somatoform disorders
    301 Personality disorders
    302 Sexual and gender identity disorders
    303 Alcohol dependence syndrome
    304 Drug dependence
    305 Nondependent abuse of drugs
    306 Physiological malfunction arising from mental factors
    307 Special symptoms or syndromes, not elsewhere classified
    308 Acute reaction to stress
    309 Adjustment reaction
    310 Specific nonpsychotic mental disorders due to brain damage
    311 Depressive disorder, not elsewhere classified
    312 Disturbance of conduct, not elsewhere classified
    313 Disturbance of emotions specific to childhood and adolescence
    314 Hyperkinetic syndrome of childhood
    315 Specific delays in development
    316 Psychic factors associated with diseases classified elsewhere

Mental retardation (317-319)
    317 Mild intellectual disabilities
    318 Other specified intellectual disabilities
    319 Unspecified intellectual disabilities

6. DISEASES OF THE NERVOUS SYSTEM AND SENSE ORGANS
Inflammatory diseases of the central nervous system (320-326)
    320 Bacterial meningitis
    321 Meningitis due to other organisms
    322 Meningitis of unspecified cause
    323 Encephalitis, myelitis, and encephalomyelitis
    324 Intracranial and intraspinal abscess
    325 Phlebitis and thrombophlebitis of intracranial venous sinuses
    326 Late effects of intracranial abscess or pyogenic infection

Organic sleep disorders (327)
    327 Organic sleep disorders

Hereditary and degenerative diseases of the central nervous system (330-337)
    330 Cerebral degenerations usually manifest in childhood
    331 Other cerebral degenerations
    332 Parkinson's disease
    333 Other extrapyramidal disease and abnormal movement disorders
    334 Spinocerebellar disease
    335 Anterior horn cell disease
    336 Other diseases of spinal cord
    337 Disorders of the autonomic nervous system

Pain (338)
    338 Pain, not elsewhere classified

Other headache syndromes (339)
    339 Other headache syndromes

6. DISEASES OF THE NERVOUS SYSTEM AND SENSE ORGANS *continued*

Other disorders of the central nervous system (340-349)

340	Multiple sclerosis
341	Other demyelinating diseases of central nervous system
342	Hemiplegia and hemiparesis
343	Infantile cerebral palsy
344	Other paralytic syndromes
345	Epilepsy and recurrent seizures
346	Migraine
347	Cataplexy and narcolepsy
348	Other conditions of brain
349	Other and unspecified disorders of the nervous system

Disorders of the peripheral nervous system (350-359)

350	Trigeminal nerve disorders
351	Facial nerve disorders
352	Disorders of other cranial nerves
353	Nerve root and plexus disorders
354	Mononeuritis of upper limb and mononeuritis multiplex
355	Mononeuritis of lower limb and unspecified site
356	Hereditary and idiopathic peripheral neuropathy
357	Inflammatory and toxic neuropathy
358	Myoneural disorders
359	Muscular dystrophies and other myopathies

Disorders of the eye and adnexa (360-379)

360	Disorders of the globe
361	Retinal detachments and defects
362	Other retinal disorders
363	Chorioretinal inflammations, scars and other disorders of choroid
364	Disorders of iris and ciliary body
365	Glaucoma
366	Cataract
367	Disorders of refraction and accommodation
368	Visual disturbances
369	Blindness and low vision
370	Keratitis
371	Corneal opacity and other disorders of cornea
372	Disorders of conjunctiva
373	Inflammation of eyelids
374	Other disorders of eyelids
375	Disorders of lacrimal system
376	Disorders of the orbit
377	Disorders of optic nerve and visual pathways
378	Strabismus and other disorders of binocular eye movements
379	Other disorders of eye

Diseases of the ear and mastoid process (380-389)

380	Disorders of external ear
381	Nonsuppurative otitis media and Eustachian tube disorders
382	Suppurative and unspecified otitis media
383	Mastoiditis and related conditions
384	Other disorders of tympanic membrane
385	Other disorders of middle ear and mastoid
386	Vertiginous syndromes and other disorders of vestibular system
387	Otosclerosis
388	Other disorders of ear
389	Hearing loss

7. DISEASES OF THE CIRCULATORY SYSTEM

Acute rheumatic fever (390-392)

390	Rheumatic fever without mention of heart involvement
391	Rheumatic fever with heart involvement
392	Rheumatic chorea

Chronic rheumatic heart disease (393-398)

393	Chronic rheumatic pericarditis
394	Diseases of mitral valve

7. DISEASES OF THE CIRCULATORY SYSTEM *continued*

395   Diseases of aortic valve
396   Diseases of mitral and aortic valves
397   Diseases of other endocardial structures
398   Other rheumatic heart disease

Hypertensive disease (401-405)
401   Essential hypertension
402   Hypertensive heart disease
403   Hypertensive chronic kidney disease
404   Hypertensive heart and chronic kidney disease
405   Secondary hypertension

Ischemic heart disease (410-414)
410   Acute myocardial infarction
411   Other acute and subacute form of ischemic heart disease
412   Old myocardial infarction
413   Angina pectoris
414   Other forms of chronic ischemic heart disease

Diseases of pulmonary circulation (415-417)
415   Acute pulmonary heart disease
416   Chronic pulmonary heart disease
417   Other diseases of pulmonary circulation

Other forms of heart disease (420-429)
420   Acute pericarditis
421   Acute and subacute endocarditis
422   Acute myocarditis
423   Other diseases of pericardium
424   Other diseases of endocardium
425   Cardiomyopathy
426   Conduction disorders
427   Cardiac dysrhythmias
428   Heart failure
429   Ill-defined descriptions and complications of heart disease

Cerebrovascular disease (430-438)
430   Subarachnoid hemorrhage
431   Intracerebral hemorrhage
432   Other and unspecified intracranial hemorrhage
433   Occlusion and stenosis of precerebral arteries
434   Occlusion of cerebral arteries
435   Transient cerebral ischemia
436   Acute but ill-defined cerebrovascular disease
437   Other and ill-defined cerebrovascular disease
438   Late effects of cerebrovascular disease

Diseases of arteries, arterioles, and capillaries (440-449)
440   Atherosclerosis
441   Aortic aneurysm and dissection
442   Other aneurysm
443   Other peripheral vascular disease
444   Arterial embolism and thrombosis
445   Atheroembolism
446   Polyarteritis nodosa and allied conditions
447   Other disorders of arteries and arterioles
448   Diseases of capillaries
449   Septic arterial embolism

Diseases of veins and lymphatics, and other diseases of circulatory system (451-459)
451   Phlebitis and thrombophlebitis
452   Portal vein thrombosis
453   Other venous embolism and thrombosis
454   Varicose veins of lower extremities
455   Hemorrhoids
456   Varicose veins of other sites
457   Noninfective disorders of lymphatic channels
458   Hypotension
459   Other disorders of circulatory system

8. DISEASES OF THE RESPIRATORY SYSTEM

Acute respiratory infections (460-466)
- 460 Acute nasopharyngitis [common cold]
- 461 Acute sinusitis
- 462 Acute pharyngitis
- 463 Acute tonsillitis
- 464 Acute laryngitis and tracheitis
- 465 Acute upper respiratory infections of multiple or unspecified sites
- 466 Acute bronchitis and bronchiolitis

Other diseases of upper respiratory tract (470-478)
- 470 Deviated nasal septum
- 471 Nasal polyps
- 472 Chronic pharyngitis and nasopharyngitis
- 473 Chronic sinusitis
- 474 Chronic disease of tonsils and adenoids
- 475 Peritonsillar abscess
- 476 Chronic laryngitis and laryngotracheitis
- 477 Allergic rhinitis
- 478 Other diseases of upper respiratory tract

Pneumonia and influenza (480-488)
- 480 Viral pneumonia
- 481 Pneumococcal pneumonia [*Streptococcus pneumoniae* pneumonia]
- 482 Other bacterial pneumonia
- 483 Pneumonia due to other specified organism
- 484 Pneumonia in infectious diseases classified elsewhere
- 485 Bronchopneumonia, organism unspecified
- 486 Pneumonia, organism unspecified
- 487 Influenza
- 488 Influenza due to certain identified influenza viruses

Chronic obstructive pulmonary disease and allied conditions (490-496)
- 490 Bronchitis, not specified as acute or chronic
- 491 Chronic bronchitis
- 492 Emphysema
- 493 Asthma
- 494 Bronchiectasis
- 495 Extrinsic allergic alveolitis
- 496 Chronic airway obstruction, not elsewhere classified

Pneumoconioses and other lung diseases due to external agents (500-508)
- 500 Coal workers' pneumoconiosis
- 501 Asbestosis
- 502 Pneumoconiosis due to other silica or silicates
- 503 Pneumoconiosis due to other inorganic dust
- 504 Pneumopathy due to inhalation of other dust
- 505 Pneumoconiosis, unspecified
- 506 Respiratory conditions due to chemical fumes and vapors
- 507 Pneumonitis due to solids and liquids
- 508 Respiratory conditions due to other and unspecified external agents

Other diseases of respiratory system (510-519)
- 510 Empyema
- 511 Pleurisy
- 512 Pneumothorax and air leak
- 513 Abscess of lung and mediastinum
- 514 Pulmonary congestion and hypostasis
- 515 Postinflammatory pulmonary fibrosis
- 516 Other alveolar and parietoalveolar pneumopathy
- 517 Lung involvement in conditions classified elsewhere
- 518 Other diseases of lung
- 519 Other diseases of respiratory system

9. DISEASES OF THE DIGESTIVE SYSTEM

Diseases of oral cavity, salivary glands, and jaws (520-529)
- 520 Disorders of tooth development and eruption
- 521 Diseases of hard tissues of teeth
- 522 Diseases of pulp and periapical tissues

9. DISEASES OF THE DIGESTIVE SYSTEM *continued*

523 Gingival and periodontal diseases
524 Dentofacial anomalies, including malocclusion
525 Other diseases and conditions of the teeth and supporting structures
526 Diseases of the jaws
527 Diseases of the salivary glands
528 Diseases of the oral soft tissues, excluding lesions specific for gingiva and tongue
529 Diseases and other conditions of the tongue

Diseases of esophagus, stomach, and duodenum (530-538)

530 Diseases of esophagus
531 Gastric ulcer
532 Duodenal ulcer
533 Peptic ulcer, site unspecified
534 Gastrojejunal ulcer
535 Gastritis and duodenitis
536 Disorders of function of stomach
537 Other disorders of stomach and duodenum
538 Gastrointestinal mucositis (ulcerative)
539 Complications of bariatric procedures

Appendicitis (540-543)

540 Acute appendicitis
541 Appendicitis, unqualified
542 Other appendicitis
543 Other diseases of appendix

Hernia of abdominal cavity (550-553)

550 Inguinal hernia
551 Other hernia of abdominal cavity, with gangrene
552 Other hernia of abdominal cavity, with obstruction, but without mention of gangrene
553 Other hernia of abdominal cavity without mention of obstruction or gangrene

Noninfectious enteritis and colitis (555-558)

555 Regional enteritis
556 Ulcerative colitis
557 Vascular insufficiency of intestine
558 Other and unspecified noninfectious gastroenteritis and colitis

Other diseases of intestines and peritoneum (560-569)

560 Intestinal obstruction without mention of hernia
562 Diverticula of intestine
564 Functional digestive disorders, not elsewhere classified
565 Anal fissure and fistula
566 Abscess of anal and rectal regions
567 Peritonitis and retroperitoneal infections
568 Other disorders of peritoneum
569 Other disorders of intestine

Other diseases of digestive system (570-579)

570 Acute and subacute necrosis of liver
571 Chronic liver disease and cirrhosis
572 Liver abscess and sequelae of chronic liver disease
573 Other disorders of liver
574 Cholelithiasis
575 Other disorders of gallbladder
576 Other disorders of biliary tract
577 Diseases of pancreas
578 Gastrointestinal hemorrhage
579 Intestinal malabsorption

10. DISEASES OF THE GENITOURINARY SYSTEM

Nephritis, nephrotic syndrome, and nephrosis (580-589)

580 Acute glomerulonephritis
581 Nephrotic syndrome
582 Chronic glomerulonephritis
583 Nephritis and nephropathy, not specified as acute or chronic
584 Acute kidney failure
585 Chronic kidney disease (CKD)

10. DISEASES OF THE GENITOURINARY SYSTEM *continued*

586 Renal failure, unspecified
587 Renal sclerosis, unspecified
588 Disorders resulting from impaired renal function
589 Small kidney of unknown cause

Other diseases of urinary system (590-599)

590 Infections of kidney
591 Hydronephrosis
592 Calculus of kidney and ureter
593 Other disorders of kidney and ureter
594 Calculus of lower urinary tract
595 Cystitis
596 Other disorders of bladder
597 Urethritis, not sexually transmitted, and urethral syndrome
598 Urethral stricture
599 Other disorders of urethra and urinary tract

Diseases of male genital organs (600-608)

600 Hyperplasia of prostate
601 Inflammatory diseases of prostate
602 Other disorders of prostate
603 Hydrocele
604 Orchitis and epididymitis
605 Redundant prepuce and phimosis
606 Infertility, male
607 Disorders of penis
608 Other disorders of male genital organs

Disorders of breast (610-612)

610 Benign mammary dysplasias
611 Other disorders of breast
612 Deformity and disproportion of reconstructed breast

Inflammatory disease of female pelvic organs (614-616)

614 Inflammatory disease of ovary, fallopian tube, pelvic cellular tissue, and peritoneum
615 Inflammatory diseases of uterus, except cervix
616 Inflammatory disease of cervix, vagina, and vulva

Other disorders of female genital tract (617-629)

617 Endometriosis
618 Genital prolapse
619 Fistula involving female genital tract
620 Noninflammatory disorders of ovary, fallopian tube, and broad ligament
621 Disorders of uterus, not elsewhere classified
622 Noninflammatory disorders of cervix
623 Noninflammatory disorders of vagina
624 Noninflammatory disorders of vulva and perineum
625 Pain and other symptoms associated with female genital organs
626 Disorders of menstruation and other abnormal bleeding from female genital tract
627 Menopausal and postmenopausal disorders
628 Infertility, female
629 Other disorders of female genital organs

11. COMPLICATIONS OF PREGNANCY, CHILDBIRTH AND THE PUERPERIUM

Ectopic and molar pregnancy (630-633)

630 Hydatidiform mole
631 Other abnormal product of conception
632 Missed abortion
633 Ectopic pregnancy

Other pregnancy with abortive outcome (634-639)

634 Abortion
635 Legally induced abortion
636 Illegally induced abortion
637 Unspecified abortion
638 Failed attempted abortion
639 Complications following abortion and ectopic and molar pregnancies

11. COMPLICATIONS OF PREGNANCY, CHILDBIRTH AND THE PUERPERIUM *continued*

Complications mainly related to pregnancy (640-649)

- 640 Hemorrhage in early pregnancy
- 641 Antepartum hemorrhage, abruptio placentae, and placenta previa
- 642 Hypertension complicating pregnancy, childbirth, and the puerperium
- 643 Excessive vomiting in pregnancy
- 644 Early or threatened labor
- 645 Late pregnancy
- 646 Other complications of pregnancy, not elsewhere classified
- 647 Infectious and parasitic conditions in the mother classifiable elsewhere but complicating pregnancy, childbirth, and the puerperium
- 648 Other current conditions in the mother classifiable elsewhere but complicating pregnancy, childbirth, and the puerperium
- 649 Other conditions or status of the mother complicating pregnancy, childbirth or the puerperium

Normal delivery, and other indications for care in pregnancy, labor, and delivery (650-659)

- 650 Normal delivery
- 651 Multiple gestation
- 652 Malposition and malpresentation of fetus
- 653 Disproportion
- 654 Abnormality of organs and soft tissues of pelvis
- 655 Known or suspected fetal abnormality affecting management of mother
- 656 Other known or suspected fetal and placental problems affecting management of mother
- 657 Polyhydramnios
- 658 Other problems associated with amniotic cavity and membranes
- 659 Other indications for care or intervention related to labor and delivery and not elsewhere classified

Complications occurring mainly in the course of labor and delivery (660-669)

- 660 Obstructed labor
- 661 Abnormality of forces of labor
- 662 Long labor
- 663 Umbilical cord complications
- 664 Trauma to perineum and vulva during delivery
- 665 Other obstetrical trauma
- 666 Postpartum hemorrhage
- 667 Retained placenta or membranes, without hemorrhage
- 668 Complications of the administration of anesthetic or other sedation in labor and delivery
- 669 Other complications of labor and delivery, not elsewhere classified

Complications of the puerperium (670-677)

- 670 Major puerperal infection
- 671 Venous complications in pregnancy and the puerperium
- 672 Pyrexia of unknown origin during the puerperium
- 673 Obstetrical pulmonary embolism
- 674 Other and unspecified complications of the puerperium, not elsewhere classified
- 675 Infections of the breast and nipple associated with childbirth
- 676 Other disorders of the breast associated with childbirth, and disorders of lactation
- 677 Late effect of complication of pregnancy, childbirth, and the puerperium

Other maternal and fetal complications (678-679)

- 678 Other fetal conditions
- 679 Complications of in utero procedures

12. DISEASES OF THE SKIN AND SUBCUTANEOUS TISSUE

Infections of skin and subcutaneous tissue (680-686)

- 680 Carbuncle and furuncle
- 681 Cellulitis and abscess of finger and toe
- 682 Other cellulitis and abscess
- 683 Acute lymphadenitis
- 684 Impetigo
- 685 Pilonidal cyst
- 686 Other local infections of skin and subcutaneous tissue

Other inflammatory conditions of skin and subcutaneous tissue (690-698)

- 690 Erythematosquamous dermatosis
- 691 Atopic dermatitis and related conditions

12. DISEASES OF THE SKIN AND SUBCUTANEOUS TISSUE *continued*

692 Contact dermatitis and other eczema
693 Dermatitis due to substances taken internally
694 Bullous dermatoses
695 Erythematous conditions
696 Psoriasis and similar disorders
697 Lichen
698 Pruritus and related conditions

Other diseases of skin and subcutaneous tissue (700-709)

700 Corns and callosities
701 Other hypertrophic and atrophic conditions of skin
702 Other dermatoses
703 Diseases of nail
704 Diseases of hair and hair follicles
705 Disorders of sweat glands
706 Diseases of sebaceous glands
707 Chronic ulcer of skin
708 Urticaria
709 Other disorders of skin and subcutaneous tissue

13. DISEASES OF THE MUSCULOSKELETAL SYSTEM AND CONNECTIVE TISSUE

Arthropathies and related disorders (710-719)

710 Diffuse diseases of connective tissue
711 Arthropathy associated with infections
712 Crystal arthropathies
713 Arthropathy associated with other disorders classified elsewhere
714 Rheumatoid arthritis and other inflammatory polyarthropathies
715 Osteoarthrosis and allied disorders
716 Other and unspecified arthropathies
717 Internal derangement of knee
718 Other derangement of joint
719 Other and unspecified disorder of joint

Dorsopathies (720-724)

720 Ankylosing spondylitis and other inflammatory spondylopathies
721 Spondylosis and allied disorders
722 Intervertebral disc disorders
723 Other disorders of cervical region
724 Other and unspecified disorders of back

Rheumatism, excluding the back (725-729)

725 Polymyalgia rheumatica
726 Peripheral enthesopathies and allied syndromes
727 Other disorders of synovium, tendon, and bursa
728 Disorders of muscle, ligament, and fascia
729 Other disorders of soft tissues

Osteopathies, chondropathies, and acquired musculoskeletal deformities (730-739)

730 Osteomyelitis, periostitis, and other infections involving bone
731 Osteitis deformans and osteopathies associated with other disorders classified elsewhere
732 Osteochondropathies
733 Other disorders of bone and cartilage
734 Flat foot
735 Acquired deformities of toe
736 Other acquired deformities of limbs
737 Curvature of spine
738 Other acquired deformity
739 Nonallopathic lesions, not elsewhere classified

14. CONGENITAL ANOMALIES

740 Anencephalus and similar anomalies
741 Spina bifida
742 Other congenital anomalies of nervous system
743 Congenital anomalies of eye
744 Congenital anomalies of ear, face, and neck
745 Bulbus cordis anomalies and anomalies of cardiac septal closure

14. CONGENITAL ANOMALIES *continued*

746 Other congenital anomalies of heart
747 Other congenital anomalies of circulatory system
748 Congenital anomalies of respiratory system
749 Cleft palate and cleft lip
750 Other congenital anomalies of upper alimentary tract
751 Other congenital anomalies of digestive system
752 Congenital anomalies of genital organs
753 Congenital anomalies of urinary system
754 Certain congenital musculoskeletal deformities
755 Other congenital anomalies of limbs
756 Other congenital musculoskeletal anomalies
757 Congenital anomalies of the integument
758 Chromosomal anomalies
759 Other and unspecified congenital anomalies

15. CERTAIN CONDITIONS ORIGINATING IN THE PERINATAL PERIOD

Maternal causes of perinatal morbidity and mortality (760-763)

760 Fetus or newborn affected by maternal conditions which may be unrelated to present pregnancy
761 Fetus or newborn affected by maternal complications of pregnancy
762 Fetus or newborn affected by complications of placenta, cord, and membranes
763 Fetus or newborn affected by other complications of labor and delivery

Other conditions originating in the perinatal period (764-779)

764 Slow fetal growth and fetal malnutrition
765 Disorders relating to short gestation and low birthweight
766 Disorders relating to long gestation and high birthweight
767 Birth trauma
768 Intrauterine hypoxia and birth asphyxia
769 Respiratory distress syndrome
770 Other respiratory conditions of fetus and newborn
771 Infections specific to the perinatal period
772 Fetal and neonatal hemorrhage
773 Hemolytic disease of fetus or newborn, due to isoimmunization
774 Other perinatal jaundice
775 Endocrine and metabolic disturbances specific to the fetus and newborn
776 Hematological disorders of newborn
777 Perinatal disorders of digestive system
778 Conditions involving the integument and temperature regulation of fetus and newborn
779 Other and ill-defined conditions originating in the perinatal period

16. SYMPTOMS, SIGNS, AND ILL-DEFINED CONDITIONS

Symptoms (780-789)

780 General symptoms
781 Symptoms involving nervous and musculoskeletal systems
782 Symptoms involving skin and other integumentary tissue
783 Symptoms concerning nutrition, metabolism, and development
784 Symptoms involving head and neck
785 Symptoms involving cardiovascular system
786 Symptoms involving respiratory system and other chest symptoms
787 Symptoms involving digestive system
788 Symptoms involving urinary system
789 Other symptoms involving abdomen and pelvis

Nonspecific abnormal findings (790-796)

790 Nonspecific findings on examination of blood
791 Nonspecific findings on examination of urine
792 Nonspecific abnormal findings in other body substances
793 Nonspecific (abnormal) findings on radiological and other examination of body structure
794 Nonspecific abnormal results of function studies
795 Other and nonspecific abnormal cytological, histological, immunological and DNA test findings
796 Other nonspecific abnormal findings

Ill-defined and unknown causes of morbidity and mortality (797-799)

797 Senility without mention of psychosis

16. SYMPTOMS, SIGNS, AND ILL-DEFINED CONDITIONS *continued*

798   Sudden death, cause unknown
799   Other ill-defined and unknown causes of morbidity and mortality

17. INJURY AND POISONING

Fracture of skull (800-804)

800   Fracture of vault of skull
801   Fracture of base of skull
802   Fracture of face bones
803   Other and unqualified skull fractures
804   Multiple fractures involving skull or face with other bones

Fracture of neck and trunk (805-809)

805   Fracture of vertebral column without mention of spinal cord injury
806   Fracture of vertebral column with spinal cord injury
807   Fracture of rib(s), sternum, larynx, and trachea
808   Fracture of pelvis
809   Ill-defined fractures of bones of trunk

Fracture of upper limb (810-819)

810   Fracture of clavicle
811   Fracture of scapula
812   Fracture of humerus
813   Fracture of radius and ulna
814   Fracture of carpal bone(s)
815   Fracture of metacarpal bone(s)
816   Fracture of one or more phalanges of hand
817   Multiple fractures of hand bones
818   Ill-defined fractures of upper limb
819   Multiple fractures involving both upper limbs, and upper limb with rib(s) and sternum

Fracture of lower limb (820-829)

820   Fracture of neck of femur
821   Fracture of other and unspecified parts of femur
822   Fracture of patella
823   Fracture of tibia and fibula
824   Fracture of ankle
825   Fracture of one or more tarsal and metatarsal bones
826   Fracture of one or more phalanges of foot
827   Other, multiple, and ill-defined fractures of lower limb
828   Multiple fractures involving both lower limbs, lower with upper limb, and lower
       limb(s) with rib(s) and sternum
829   Fracture of unspecified bones

Dislocation (830-839)

830   Dislocation of jaw
831   Dislocation of shoulder
832   Dislocation of elbow
833   Dislocation of wrist
834   Dislocation of finger
835   Dislocation of hip
836   Dislocation of knee
837   Dislocation of ankle
838   Dislocation of foot
839   Other, multiple, and ill-defined dislocations

Sprains and strains of joints and adjacent muscles (840-848)

840   Sprains and strains of shoulder and upper arm
841   Sprains and strains of elbow and forearm
842   Sprains and strains of wrist and hand
843   Sprains and strains of hip and thigh
844   Sprains and strains of knee and leg
845   Sprains and strains of ankle and foot
846   Sprains and strains of sacroiliac region
847   Sprains and strains of other and unspecified parts of back
848   Other and ill-defined sprains and strains

Intracranial injury, excluding those with skull fracture (850-854)

850   Concussion
851   Cerebral laceration and contusion

17. INJURY AND POISONING *continued*

852 Subarachnoid, subdural, and extradural hemorrhage, following injury
853 Other and unspecified intracranial hemorrhage following injury
854 Intracranial injury of other and unspecified nature

Internal injury of thorax, abdomen, and pelvis (860-869)

860 Traumatic pneumothorax and hemothorax
861 Injury to heart and lung
862 Injury to other and unspecified intrathoracic organs
863 Injury to gastrointestinal tract
864 Injury to liver
865 Injury to spleen
866 Injury to kidney
867 Injury to pelvic organs
868 Injury to other intra-abdominal organs
869 Internal injury to unspecified or ill-defined organs

Open wound of head, neck, and trunk (870-879)

870 Open wound of ocular adnexa
871 Open wound of eyeball
872 Open wound of ear
873 Other open wound of head
874 Open wound of neck
875 Open wound of chest (wall)
876 Open wound of back
877 Open wound of buttock
878 Open wound of genital organs (external), including traumatic amputation
879 Open wound of other and unspecified sites, except limbs

Open wound of upper limb (880-887)

880 Open wound of shoulder and upper arm
881 Open wound of elbow, forearm, and wrist
882 Open wound of hand except finger(s) alone
883 Open wound of finger(s)
884 Multiple and unspecified open wound of upper limb
885 Traumatic amputation of thumb (complete) (partial)
886 Traumatic amputation of other finger(s) (complete) (partial)
887 Traumatic amputation of arm and hand (complete) (partial)

Open wound of lower limb (890-897)

890 Open wound of hip and thigh
891 Open wound of knee, leg [except thigh], and ankle
892 Open wound of foot except toe(s) alone
893 Open wound of toe(s)
894 Multiple and unspecified open wound of lower limb
895 Traumatic amputation of toe(s) (complete) (partial)
896 Traumatic amputation of foot (complete) (partial)
897 Traumatic amputation of leg(s) (complete) (partial)

Injury to blood vessels (900-904)

900 Injury to blood vessels of head and neck
901 Injury to blood vessels of thorax
902 Injury to blood vessels of abdomen and pelvis
903 Injury to blood vessels of upper extremity
904 Injury to blood vessels of lower extremity and unspecified sites

Late effects of injuries, poisonings, toxic effects, and other external causes (905-909)

905 Late effects of musculoskeletal and connective tissue injuries
906 Late effects of injuries to skin and subcutaneous tissues
907 Late effects of injuries to the nervous system
908 Late effects of other and unspecified injuries
909 Late effects of other and unspecified external causes

Superficial injury (910-919)

910 Superficial injury of face, neck, and scalp except eye
911 Superficial injury of trunk
912 Superficial injury of shoulder and upper arm
913 Superficial injury of elbow, forearm, and wrist
914 Superficial injury of hand(s) except finger(s) alone
915 Superficial injury of finger(s)

17. INJURY AND POISONING *continued*

916 Superficial injury of hip, thigh, leg, and ankle
917 Superficial injury of foot and toe(s)
918 Superficial injury of eye and adnexa
919 Superficial injury of other, multiple, and unspecified sites

Contusion with intact skin surface (920-924)
920 Contusion of face, scalp, and neck except eye(s)
921 Contusion of eye and adnexa
922 Contusion of trunk
923 Contusion of upper limb
924 Contusion of lower limb and of other and unspecified sites

Crushing injury (925-929)
925 Crushing injury of face, scalp, and neck
926 Crushing injury of trunk
927 Crushing injury of upper limb
928 Crushing injury of lower limb
929 Crushing injury of multiple and unspecified sites

Effects of foreign body entering through orifice (930-939)
930 Foreign body on external eye
931 Foreign body in ear
932 Foreign body in nose
933 Foreign body in pharynx and larynx
934 Foreign body in trachea, bronchus, and lung
935 Foreign body in mouth, esophagus, and stomach
936 Foreign body in intestine and colon
937 Foreign body in anus and rectum
938 Foreign body in digestive system, unspecified
939 Foreign body in genitourinary tract

Burns (940-949)
940 Burn confined to eye and adnexa
941 Burn of face, head, and neck
942 Burn of trunk
943 Burn of upper limb, except wrist and hand
944 Burn of wrist(s) and hand(s)
945 Burn of lower limb(s)
946 Burns of multiple specified sites
947 Burn of internal organs
948 Burns classified according to extent of body surface involved
949 Burn, unspecified

Injury to nerves and spinal cord (950-957)
950 Injury to optic nerve and pathways
951 Injury to other cranial nerve(s)
952 Spinal cord injury without evidence of spinal bone injury
953 Injury to nerve roots and spinal plexus
954 Injury to other nerve(s) of trunk excluding shoulder and pelvic girdles
955 Injury to peripheral nerve(s) of shoulder girdle and upper limb
956 Injury to peripheral nerve(s) of pelvic girdle and lower limb
957 Injury to other and unspecified nerves

Certain traumatic complications and unspecified injuries (958-959)
958 Certain early complications of trauma
959 Injury, other and unspecified

Poisoning by drugs, medicinal and biological substances (960-979)
960 Poisoning by antibiotics
961 Poisoning by other anti-infectives
962 Poisoning by hormones and synthetic substitutes
963 Poisoning by primarily systemic agents
964 Poisoning by agents primarily affecting blood constituents
965 Poisoning by analgesics, antipyretics, and antirheumatics
966 Poisoning by anticonvulsants and anti-Parkinsonism drugs
967 Poisoning by sedatives and hypnotics
968 Poisoning by other central nervous system depressants and anesthetics
969 Poisoning by psychotropic agents
970 Poisoning by central nervous system stimulants

17. INJURY AND POISONING *continued*

971 Poisoning by drugs primarily affecting the autonomic nervous system
972 Poisoning by agents primarily affecting the cardiovascular system
973 Poisoning by agents primarily affecting the gastrointestinal system
974 Poisoning by water, mineral, and uric acid metabolism drugs
975 Poisoning by agents primarily acting on the smooth and skeletal muscles and respiratory system
976 Poisoning by agents primarily affecting skin and mucous membrane, ophthalmological, otorhinolaryngological, and dental drugs
977 Poisoning by other and unspecified drugs and medicinals
978 Poisoning by bacterial vaccines
979 Poisoning by other vaccines and biological substances

Toxic effects of substances chiefly nonmedicinal as to source (980-989)

980 Toxic effect of alcohol
981 Toxic effect of petroleum products
982 Toxic effect of solvents other than petroleum-based
983 Toxic effect of corrosive aromatics, acids, and caustic alkalis
984 Toxic effect of lead and its compounds (including fumes)
985 Toxic effect of other metals
986 Toxic effect of carbon monoxide
987 Toxic effect of other gases, fumes, or vapors
988 Toxic effect of noxious substances eaten as food
989 Toxic effect of other substances, chiefly nonmedicinal as to source

Other and unspecified effects of external causes (990-995)

990 Effects of radiation, unspecified
991 Effects of reduced temperature
992 Effects of heat and light
993 Effects of air pressure
994 Effects of other external causes
995 Certain adverse effects, not elsewhere classified

Complications of surgical and medical care, not elsewhere classified (996-999)

996 Complications peculiar to certain specified procedures
997 Complications affecting specified body systems, not elsewhere classified
998 Other complications of procedures, not elsewhere classified
999 Complications of medical care, not elsewhere classified

SUPPLEMENTARY CLASSIFICATION OF FACTORS INFLUENCING HEALTH STATUS AND CONTACT WITH HEALTH SERVICES

Persons with potential health hazards related to communicable diseases (V01-V06)

V01 Contact with or exposure to communicable diseases
V02 Carrier or suspected carrier of infectious diseases
V03 Need for prophylactic vaccination and inoculation against bacterial diseases
V04 Need for prophylactic vaccination and inoculation against certain viral diseases
V05 Need for other prophylactic vaccination and inoculation against single diseases
V06 Need for prophylactic vaccination and inoculation against combinations of diseases

Persons with need for isolation, other potential health hazards and prophylactic measures (V07-V09)

V07 Need for isolation and other prophylactic or treatment measures
V08 Asymptomatic human immunodeficiency virus (HIV) infection status
V09 Infection with drug-resistant microorganisms

Persons with potential health hazards related to personal and family history (V10-V19)

V10 Personal history of malignant neoplasm
V11 Personal history of mental disorder
V12 Personal history of certain other diseases
V13 Personal history of other diseases
V14 Personal history of allergy to medicinal agents
V15 Other personal history presenting hazards to health
V16 Family history of malignant neoplasm
V17 Family history of certain chronic disabling diseases
V18 Family history of certain other specific conditions
V19 Family history of other conditions

Persons encountering health services in circumstances related to reproduction and development (V20-V29)

V20 Health supervision of infant or child
V21 Constitutional states in development

SUPPLEMENTARY CLASSIFICATION...HEALTH STATUS/HEALTH SERVICES *continued*

V22 Normal pregnancy
V23 Supervision of high-risk pregnancy
V24 Postpartum care and examination
V25 Encounter for contraceptive management
V26 Procreative management
V27 Outcome of delivery
V28 Encounter for antenatal screening of mother
V29 Observation and evaluation of newborns and infants for suspected condition not found

Liveborn infants according to type of birth (V30-V39)
V30 Single liveborn
V31 Twin, mate liveborn
V32 Twin, mate stillborn
V33 Twin, unspecified
V34 Other multiple, mates all liveborn
V35 Other multiple, mates all stillborn
V36 Other multiple, mates live- and stillborn
V37 Other multiple, unspecified
V39 Unspecified

Persons with a condition influencing their health status (V40-V49)
V40 Mental and behavioral problems
V41 Problems with special senses and other special functions
V42 Organ or tissue replaced by transplant
V43 Organ or tissue replaced by other means
V44 Artificial opening status
V45 Other postprocedural states
V46 Other dependence on machines and devices
V47 Other problems with internal organs
V48 Problems with head, neck, and trunk
V49 Other conditions influencing health status

Persons encountering health services for specific procedures and aftercare (V50-V59)
V50 Elective surgery for purposes other than remedying health states
V51 Aftercare involving the use of plastic surgery
V52 Fitting and adjustment of prosthetic device and implant
V53 Fitting and adjustment of other device
V54 Other orthopedic aftercare
V55 Attention to artificial openings
V56 Encounter for dialysis and dialysis catheter care
V57 Care involving use of rehabilitation procedures
V58 Encounter for other and unspecified procedures and aftercare
V59 Donors

Persons encountering health services in other circumstances (V60-V69)
V60 Housing, household, and economic circumstances
V61 Other family circumstances
V62 Other psychosocial circumstances
V63 Unavailability of other medical facilities for care
V64 Persons encountering health services for specific procedures, not carried out
V65 Other persons seeking consultation
V66 Convalescence and palliative care
V67 Follow-up examination
V68 Encounters for administrative purposes
V69 Problems related to lifestyle

Persons without reported diagnosis encountered during examination and investigation of individuals and populations (V70-V86)
V70 General medical examination
V71 Observation and evaluation for suspected conditions not found
V72 Special investigations and examinations
V73 Special screening examination for viral and chlamydial diseases
V74 Special screening examination for bacterial and spirochetal diseases
V75 Special screening examination for other infectious diseases
V76 Special screening for malignant neoplasms
V77 Special screening for endocrine, nutritional, metabolic, and immunity disorders
V78 Special screening for disorders of blood and blood-forming organs

SUPPLEMENTARY CLASSIFICATION...HEALTH STATUS/HEALTH SERVICES *continued*

V79 Special screening for mental disorders and developmental handicaps
V80 Special screening for neurological, eye, and ear diseases
V81 Special screening for cardiovascular, respiratory, and genitourinary diseases
V82 Special screening for other conditions
V83 Genetic carrier status
V84 Genetic susceptibility to disease
V85 Body mass index
V86 Estrogen receptor status
V87 Other specified personal exposures and history presenting hazards to health
V88 Acquired absence of other organs and tissue
V89 Other suspected conditions not found

Retained Foreign Body (V90)
V90 Retained foreign body

Multiple Gestation Placenta Status (V91)
V91 Multiple gestation placenta status

SUPPLEMENTARY CLASSIFICATION OF EXTERNAL CAUSES OF INJURY AND POISONING

External cause status (E000)
E000 External cause status

Activity (E001-E030)
E001 Activities involving walking and running
E002 Activities involving water and water craft
E003 Activities involving ice and snow
E004 Activities involving climbing, rappelling and jumping off
E005 Activities involving dancing and other rhythmic movement
E006 Activities involving other sports and athletics played individually
E007 Activities involving other sports and athletics played as a team or group
E008 Activities involving other specified sports and athletics
E009 Activities involving other cardiorespiratory exercise
E010 Activities involving other muscle strengthening exercises
E011 Activities involving computer technology and electronic devices
E012 Activities involving arts and handcrafts
E013 Activities involving personal hygiene and household maintenance
E014 Activities involving person providing caregiving
E015 Activities involving food preparation, cooking and grilling
E016 Activities involving property and land maintenance, building and construction
E017 Activities involving roller coasters and other types of external motion
E018 Activities involving playing musical instruments
E019 Activities involving animal care
E029 Other activity
E030 Unspecified activity

Railway accidents (E800-E807)
E800 Railway accident involving collision with rolling stock
E801 Railway accident involving collision with other object
E802 Railway accident involving derailment without antecedent collision
E803 Railway accident involving explosion, fire, or burning
E804 Fall in, on, or from railway train
E805 Hit by rolling stock
E806 Other specified railway accident
E807 Railway accident of unspecified nature

Motor vehicle traffic accidents (E810-E819)
E810 Motor vehicle traffic accident involving collision with train
E811 Motor vehicle traffic accident involving re-entrant collision with another motor vehicle
E812 Other motor vehicle traffic accident involving collision with another motor vehicle
E813 Motor vehicle traffic accident involving collision with other vehicle
E814 Motor vehicle traffic accident involving collision with pedestrian
E815 Other motor vehicle traffic accident involving collision on the highway
E816 Motor vehicle traffic accident due to loss of control, without collision on the highway
E817 Noncollision motor vehicle traffic accident while boarding or alighting
E818 Other noncollision motor vehicle traffic accident
E819 Motor vehicle traffic accident of unspecified nature

SUPPLEMENTARY CLASSIFICATION...INJURY AND POISONING *continued*

Motor vehicle nontraffic accidents (E820-E825)

E820 Nontraffic accident involving motor-driven snow vehicle
E821 Nontraffic accident involving other off-road motor vehicle
E822 Other motor vehicle nontraffic accident involving collision with moving object
E823 Other motor vehicle nontraffic accident involving collision with stationary object
E824 Other motor vehicle nontraffic accident while boarding and alighting
E825 Other motor vehicle nontraffic accident of other and unspecified nature

Other road vehicle accidents (E826-E829)

E826 Pedal cycle accident
E827 Animal-drawn vehicle accident
E828 Accident involving animal being ridden
E829 Other road vehicle accidents

Water transport accidents (E830-E838)

E830 Accident to watercraft causing submersion
E831 Accident to watercraft causing other injury
E832 Other accidental submersion or drowning in water transport accident
E833 Fall on stairs or ladders in water transport
E834 Other fall from one level to another in water transport
E835 Other and unspecified fall in water transport
E836 Machinery accident in water transport
E837 Explosion, fire, or burning in watercraft
E838 Other and unspecified water transport accident

Air and space transport accidents (E840-E845)

E840 Accident to powered aircraft at takeoff or landing
E841 Accident to powered aircraft, other and unspecified
E842 Accident to unpowered aircraft
E843 Fall in, on, or from aircraft
E844 Other specified air transport accidents
E845 Accident involving spacecraft

Vehicle accidents, not elsewhere classifiable (E846-E849)

E846 Accidents involving powered vehicles used solely within the buildings and premises of an industrial or commercial establishment
E847 Accidents involving cable cars not running on rails
E848 Accidents involving other vehicles, not elsewhere classifiable
E849 Place of occurrence

Accidental poisoning by drugs, medicinal substances, and biologicals (E850-E858)

E850 Accidental poisoning by analgesics, antipyretics, and antirheumatics
E851 Accidental poisoning by barbiturates
E852 Accidental poisoning by other sedatives and hypnotics
E853 Accidental poisoning by tranquilizers
E854 Accidental poisoning by other psychotropic agents
E855 Accidental poisoning by other drugs acting on central and autonomic nervous systems
E856 Accidental poisoning by antibiotics
E857 Accidental poisoning by other anti-infectives
E858 Accidental poisoning by other drugs

Accidental poisoning by other solid and liquid substances, gases, and vapors (E860-E869)

E860 Accidental poisoning by alcohol, not elsewhere classified
E861 Accidental poisoning by cleansing and polishing agents, disinfectants, paints, and varnishes
E862 Accidental poisoning by petroleum products, other solvents and their vapors, not elsewhere classified
E863 Accidental poisoning by agricultural and horticultural chemical and pharmaceutical preparations other than plant foods and fertilizers
E864 Accidental poisoning by corrosives and caustics, not elsewhere classified
E865 Accidental poisoning from poisonous foodstuffs and poisonous plants
E866 Accidental poisoning by other and unspecified solid and liquid substances
E867 Accidental poisoning by gas distributed by pipeline
E868 Accidental poisoning by other utility gas and other carbon monoxide
E869 Accidental poisoning by other gases and vapors

Misadventures to patients during surgical and medical care (E870-E876)

E870 Accidental cut, puncture, perforation, or hemorrhage during medical care
E871 Foreign object left in body during procedure
E872 Failure of sterile precautions during procedure

SUPPLEMENTARY CLASSIFICATION...INJURY AND POISONING *continued*

E873 Failure in dosage
E874 Mechanical failure of instrument or apparatus during procedure
E875 Contaminated or infected blood, other fluid, drug, or biological substance
E876 Other and unspecified misadventures during medical care

Surgical and medical procedures as the cause of abnormal reaction of patient or later complication, without mention of misadventure at the time of procedure (E878-E879)

E878 Surgical operation and other surgical procedures as the cause of abnormal reaction of patient, or of later complication, without mention of misadventure at the time of operation
E879 Other procedures, without mention of misadventure at the time of procedure, as the cause of abnormal reaction of patient, or of later complication

Accidental falls (E880-E888)

E880 Fall on or from stairs or steps
E881 Fall on or from ladders or scaffolding
E882 Fall from or out of building or other structure
E883 Fall into hole or other opening in surface
E884 Other fall from one level to another
E885 Fall on same level from slipping, tripping, or stumbling
E886 Fall on same level from collision, pushing or shoving, by or with other person
E887 Fracture, cause unspecified
E888 Other and unspecified fall

Accidents caused by fire and flames (E890-E899)

E890 Conflagration in private dwelling
E891 Conflagration in other and unspecified building or structure
E892 Conflagration not in building or structure
E893 Accident caused by ignition of clothing
E894 Ignition of highly inflammable material
E895 Accident caused by controlled fire in private dwelling
E896 Accident caused by controlled fire in other and unspecified building or structure
E897 Accident caused by controlled fire not in building or structure
E898 Accident caused by other specified fire and flames
E899 Accident caused by unspecified fire

Accidents due to natural and environmental factors (E900-E909)

E900 Excessive heat
E901 Excessive cold
E902 High and low air pressure and changes in air pressure
E903 Travel and motion
E904 Hunger, thirst, exposure, and neglect
E905 Venomous animals and plants as the cause of poisoning and toxic reactions
E906 Other injury caused by animals
E907 Lightning
E908 Cataclysmic storms, and floods resulting from storms
E909 Cataclysmic earth surface movements and eruptions

Accidents caused by submersion, suffocation, and foreign bodies (E910-E915)

E910 Accidental drowning and submersion
E911 Inhalation and ingestion of food causing obstruction of respiratory tract or suffocation
E912 Inhalation and ingestion of other object causing obstruction of respiratory tract or suffocation
E913 Accidental mechanical suffocation
E914 Foreign body accidentally entering eye and adnexa
E915 Foreign body accidentally entering other orifice

Other accidents (E916-E928)

E916 Struck accidentally by falling object
E917 Striking against or struck accidentally by objects or persons
E918 Caught accidentally in or between objects
E919 Accidents caused by machinery
E920 Accidents caused by cutting and piercing instruments or objects
E921 Accident caused by explosion of pressure vessel
E922 Accident caused by firearm and air gun missile
E923 Accident caused by explosive material
E924 Accident caused by hot substance or object, caustic or corrosive material, and steam
E925 Accident caused by electric current
E926 Exposure to radiation

SUPPLEMENTARY CLASSIFICATION...INJURY AND POISONING *continued*

    E927 Overexertion and strenuous and repetitive movements or loads
    E928 Other and unspecified environmental and accidental causes

Late effects of accidental injury (E929)

    E929 Late effects of accidental injury

Drugs, medicinal and biological substances causing adverse effects in therapeutic use (E930-E949)

    E930 Antibiotics
    E931 Other anti-infectives
    E932 Hormones and synthetic substitutes
    E933 Primarily systemic agents
    E934 Agents primarily affecting blood constituents
    E935 Analgesics, antipyretics, and antirheumatics
    E936 Anticonvulsants and anti-Parkinsonism drugs
    E937 Sedatives and hypnotics
    E938 Other central nervous system depressants and anesthetics
    E939 Psychotropic agents
    E940 Central nervous system stimulants
    E941 Drugs primarily affecting the autonomic nervous system
    E942 Agents primarily affecting the cardiovascular system
    E943 Agents primarily affecting gastrointestinal system
    E944 Water, mineral, and uric acid metabolism drugs
    E945 Agents primarily acting on the smooth and skeletal muscles and respiratory system
    E946 Agents primarily affecting skin and mucous membrane, ophthalmological, otorhinolaryngological, and dental drugs
    E947 Other and unspecified drugs and medicinal substances
    E948 Bacterial vaccines
    E949 Other vaccines and biological substances

Suicide and self-inflicted injury (E950-E959)

    E950 Suicide and self-inflicted poisoning by solid or liquid substances
    E951 Suicide and self-inflicted poisoning by gases in domestic use
    E952 Suicide and self-inflicted poisoning by other gases and vapors
    E953 Suicide and self-inflicted injury by hanging, strangulation, and suffocation
    E954 Suicide and self-inflicted injury by submersion [drowning]
    E955 Suicide and self-inflicted injury by firearms, air guns and explosives
    E956 Suicide and self-inflicted injury by cutting and piercing instruments
    E957 Suicide and self-inflicted injuries by jumping from high place
    E958 Suicide and self-inflicted injury by other and unspecified means
    E959 Late effects of self-inflicted injury

Homicide and injury purposely inflicted by other persons (E960-E969)

    E960 Fight, brawl, and rape
    E961 Assault by corrosive or caustic substance, except poisoning
    E962 Assault by poisoning
    E963 Assault by hanging and strangulation
    E964 Assault by submersion [drowning]
    E965 Assault by firearms and explosives
    E966 Assault by cutting and piercing instrument
    E967 Perpetrator of child and adult abuse
    E968 Assault by other and unspecified means
    E969 Late effects of injury purposely inflicted by other person

Legal intervention (E970-E978)

    E970 Injury due to legal intervention by firearms
    E971 Injury due to legal intervention by explosives
    E972 Injury due to legal intervention by gas
    E973 Injury due to legal intervention by blunt object
    E974 Injury due to legal intervention by cutting and piercing instruments
    E975 Injury due to legal intervention by other specified means
    E976 Injury due to legal intervention by unspecified means
    E977 Late effects of injuries due to legal intervention
    E978 Legal execution
    E979 Terrorism

SUPPLEMENTARY CLASSIFICATION...INJURY AND POISONING *continued*

Injury undetermined whether accidentally or purposely inflicted (E980-E989)

E980 Poisoning by solid or liquid substances, undetermined whether accidentally or purposely inflicted

E981 Poisoning by gases in domestic use, undetermined whether accidentally or purposely inflicted

E982 Poisoning by other gases, undetermined whether accidentally or purposely inflicted

E983 Hanging, strangulation, or suffocation, undetermined whether accidentally or purposely inflicted

E984 Submersion [drowning], undetermined whether accidentally or purposely inflicted

E985 Injury by firearms, air guns and explosives, undetermined whether accidentally or purposely inflicted

E986 Injury by cutting and piercing instruments, undetermined whether accidentally or purposely inflicted

E987 Falling from high place, undetermined whether accidentally or purposely inflicted

E988 Injury by other and unspecified means, undetermined whether accidentally or purposely inflicted

E989 Late effects of injury, undetermined whether accidentally or purposely inflicted

Injury resulting from operations of war (E990-E999)

E990 Injury due to war operations by fires and conflagrations

E991 Injury due to war operations by bullets and fragments

E992 Injury due to war operations by explosion of marine weapons

E993 Injury due to war operations by other explosion

E994 Injury due to war operations by destruction of aircraft

E995 Injury due to war operations by other and unspecified forms of conventional warfare

E996 Injury due to war operations by nuclear weapons

E997 Injury due to war operations by other forms of unconventional warfare

E998 Injury due to war operations but occurring after cessation of hostilities

E999 Late effects of injury due to war operations and terrorism

DISEASES: ALPHABETIC INDEX

VOLUME 2

A

AAT (alpha-1 antitrypsin) deficiency 273.4
AAV (disease) (illness) (infection)—*see* Human
  immunodeficiency virus (disease) (illness)
  (infection)
Abactio —*see* Abortion, induced
Abactus venter —*see* Abortion, induced
Abarognosis 781.99
Abasia (-astasia) 307.9
  atactica 781.3
  choreic 781.3
  hysterical 300.11
  paroxysmal trepidant 781.3
  spastic 781.3
  trembling 781.3
  trepidans 781.3
Abderhalden-Kaufmann-Lignac syndrome
  (cystinosis) 270.0
Abdomen, abdominal —*see also* condition
  accordion 306.4
  acute 789.0
  angina 557.1
  burst 868.00
  convulsive equivalent (*see also* Epilepsy) 345.5
  heart 746.87
  muscle deficiency syndrome 756.79
  obstipum 756.79
Abdominalgia 789.0
  periodic 277.31
Abduction contracture, hip or other joint —*see*
  Contraction, joint
Abercrombie's syndrome (amyloid
  degeneration) 277.39
Aberrant (congenital)—*see also* Malposition,
  congenital
  adrenal gland 759.1
  blood vessel NEC 747.60
    arteriovenous NEC 747.60
    cerebrovascular 747.81
    gastrointestinal 747.61
    lower limb 747.64
    renal 747.62
    spinal 747.82
    upper limb 747.63
  breast 757.6
  endocrine gland NEC 759.2
  gastrointestinal vessel (peripheral) 747.61
  hepatic duct 751.69
  lower limb vessel (peripheral) 747.64
  pancreas 751.7
  parathyroid gland 759.2
  peripheral vascular vessel NEC 747.60
  pituitary gland (pharyngeal) 759.2
  renal blood vessel 747.62
  sebaceous glands, mucous membrane, mouth
    750.26
  spinal vessel 747.82
  spleen 759.0
  testis (descent) 752.51
  thymus gland 759.2
  thyroid gland 759.2
  upper limb vessel (peripheral) 747.63
Aberratio
  lactis 757.6
  testis 752.51
Aberration —*see also* Anomaly
  chromosome—*see* Anomaly, chromosome(s)
  distantial 368.9

Aberration—*continued*
  mental (*see also* Disorder, mental,
    nonpsychotic) 300.9
Abetalipoproteinemia 272.5
Abionarce 780.79
Abiotrophy 799.89
Ablatio
  placentae—*see* Placenta, ablatio
  retinae (*see also* Detachment, retina) 361.9
Ablation
  pituitary (gland) (with hypofunction) 253.7
  placenta—*see* Placenta, ablatio
  uterus 621.8
Ablepharia, ablepharon, ablephary 743.62
Ablepsia —*see* Blindness
Ablepsy —*see* Blindness
Ablutomania 300.3
Abnormal, abnormality, abnormalities —*see
  also* Anomaly
  acid-base balance 276.4
    fetus or newborn—*see* Distress, fetal
  adaptation curve, dark 368.63
  alveolar ridge 525.9
  amnion 658.9
    affecting fetus or newborn 762.9
  anatomical relationship NEC 759.9
  apertures, congenital, diaphragm 756.6
  auditory perception NEC 388.40
  autosomes NEC 758.5
    13 758.1
    18 758.2
    21 or 22 758.0
    D_1 758.1
    E_3 758.2
    G 758.0
  ballistocardiogram 794.39
  basal metabolic rate (BMR) 794.7
  biosynthesis, testicular androgen 257.2
  blood level (of)
    cobalt 790.6
    copper 790.6
    iron 790.6
    lead 790.6
    lithium 790.6
    magnesium 790.6
    mineral 790.6
    zinc 790.6
  blood pressure
    elevated (without diagnosis of hypertension)
      796.2
    low (*see also* Hypotension) 458.9
      reading (incidental) (isolated) (nonspecific)
        796.3
  blood sugar 790.29
  bowel sounds 787.5
  breathing behavior—*see* Respiration
  caloric test 794.19
  cervix (acquired) NEC 622.9
    congenital 752.40
    in pregnancy or childbirth 654.6
      causing obstructed labor 660.2
        affecting fetus or newborn 763.1
  chemistry, blood NEC 790.6
  chest sounds 786.7
  chorion 658.9
    affecting fetus or newborn 762.9
  chromosomal NEC 758.89

Abnormal, abnormality—*continued*
  analysis, nonspecific result 795.2
  autosomes (*see also* Abnormal, autosomes
    NEC) 758.5
    fetal, (suspected) affecting management of
      pregnancy 655.1
    sex 758.81
  clinical findings NEC 796.4
  communication—*see* Fistula
  configuration of pupils 379.49
  coronary
    artery 746.85
    vein 746.9
  cortisol-binding globulin 255.8
  course, Eustachian tube 744.24
  creatinine clearance 794.4
  dentofacial NEC 524.9
    functional 524.50
    specified type NEC 524.89
  development, developmental NEC 759.9
    bone 756.9
    central nervous system 742.9
  direction, teeth 524.30
  Dynia (*see also* Defect, coagulation) 286.9
  Ebstein 746.2
  echocardiogram 793.2
  echoencephalogram 794.01
  echogram NEC—*see* Findings, abnormal,
    structure
  electrocardiogram (ECG) (EKG) 794.31
  electroencephalogram (EEG) 794.02
  electromyogram (EMG) 794.17
    ocular 794.14
  electro-oculogram (EOG) 794.12
  electroretinogram (ERG) 794.11
  erythrocytes 289.9
    congenital, with perinatal jaundice 282.9
      [774.0]
  Eustachian valve 746.9
  excitability under minor stress 301.9
  fat distribution 782.9
  feces 787.7
  fetal heart rate—*see* Distress, fetal
  fetus NEC
    affecting management of pregnancy—*see*
      Pregnancy, management affected by, fetal
    causing disproportion 653.7
      affecting fetus or newborn 763.1
      causing obstructed labor 660.1
        affecting fetus or newborn 763.1
  findings without manifest disease—*see*
    Findings, abnormal
  fluid
    amniotic 792.3
    cerebrospinal 792.0
    peritoneal 792.9
    pleural 792.9
    synovial 792.9
    vaginal 792.9
  forces of labor NEC 661.9
    affecting fetus or newborn 763.7
  form, teeth 520.2
  function studies
    auditory 794.15
    bladder 794.9
    brain 794.00
    cardiovascular 794.30
    endocrine NEC 794.6
    kidney 794.4
    liver 794.8
    nervous system
      central 794.00

Abnormal, abnormality—*continued*
    peripheral 794.19
    oculomotor 794.14
    pancreas 794.9
    placenta 794.9
    pulmonary 794.2
    retina 794.11
    special senses 794.19
    spleen 794.9
    thyroid 794.5
    vestibular 794.16
  gait 781.2
    hysterical 300.11
  gastrin secretion 251.5
  globulin
    cortisol-binding 255.8
    thyroid-binding 246.8
  glucagon secretion 251.4
  glucose 790.29
    in pregnancy, childbirth, or puerperium 648.8
      fetus or newborn 775.0
    non-fasting 790.29
  gravitational (G) forces or states 994.9
  hair NEC 704.2
  hard tissue formation in pulp 522.3
  head movement 781.0
  heart
    rate
      fetus, affecting liveborn infant
        before the onset of labor 763.81
        during labor 763.82
        unspecified as to time of onset 763.83
      intrauterine
        before the onset of labor 763.81
        during labor 763.82
        unspecified as to time of onset 763.83
      newborn
        before the onset of labor 763.81
        during labor 763.82
        unspecified as to time of onset 763.83
    shadow 793.2
    sounds NEC 785.3
  hemoglobin (*see also* Disease, hemoglobin)
    282.7
    trait—*see* Trait, hemoglobin, abnormal
  hemorrhage, uterus—*see* Hemorrhage, uterus
  histology NEC 795.4
  increase in
    appetite 783.6
    development 783.9
  involuntary movement 781.0
  jaw closure 524.51
  karyotype 795.2
  knee jerk 796.1
  labor NEC 661.9
    affecting fetus or newborn 763.7
  laboratory findings—*see* Findings, abnormal
  length, organ or site, congenital—*see* Distortion
  liver function test 790.6
  loss of height 781.91
  loss of weight 783.21
  lung shadow 793.19
  mammogram 793.80
    calcification 793.89
    calculus 793.89
    microcalcification 793.81
  Mantoux test 795.51
  membranes (fetal)
    affecting fetus or newborn 762.9
    complicating pregnancy 658.8
  menstruation—*see* Menstruation

Abnormal, abnormality —*continued*
  metabolism (*see also* condition) 783.9
  movement 781.0
    disorder, NEC 333.90
      sleep related, unspecified 780.58
      specified, NEC 333.99
    head 781.0
    involuntary 781.0
    specified type NEC 333.99
  muscle contraction, localized 728.85
  myoglobin (Aberdeen) (Annapolis) 289.9
  narrowness, eyelid 743.62
  optokinetic response 379.57
  organs or tissues of pelvis NEC
    in pregnancy or childbirth 654.9
      affecting fetus or newborn 763.89
      causing obstructed labor 660.2
        affecting fetus or newborn 763.1
  origin—*see* Malposition, congenital
  palmar creases 757.2
  Papanicolaou (smear)
    anus 796.70
      with
        atypical squamous cells
          cannot exclude high grade squamous
            intraepithelial lesion (ASC-H)
            796.72
          of undetermined significance (ASC-US)
            796.71
        cytologic evidence of malignancy 796.76
        high grade squamous intraepithelial lesion
          (HGSIL) 796.74
        low grade squamous intraepithelial lesion
          (LGSIL) 796.73
      glandular 796.70
      specified finding NEC 796.79
    cervix 795.00
      with
        atypical squamous cell
          cannot exclude high grade squamous
            intraepithelial lesion (ASC-H)
            795.02
          of undetermined significance (ASC-US)
            795.01
        cytologic evidence of malignancy 795.06
        favor benign (ASCUS favor benign)
          795.01
        favor dysplasia (ASCUS favor dysplasia)
          795.02
        high grade squamous intraepithelial lesion
          (HGSIL) 795.04
        low grade squamous intraepithelial lesion
          (LGSIL) 795.03
        nonspecific finding NEC 795.09
    other site 796.9
    vagina 795.10
      with
        atypical squamous cells
          cannot exclude high grade squamous
            intraepithelial lesion (ASC-H)
            795.12
          of undetermined significance (ASC-US)
            795.11
        cytologic evidence of malignancy 795.16
        high grade squamous intraepithelial lesion
          (HGSIL) 795.14
        low grade squamous intraepithelial lesion
          (LGSIL) 795.13
      glandular 795.10
      specified finding NEC 795.19

Abnormal, abnormality —*continued*
  parturition
    affecting fetus or newborn 763.9
    mother—*see* Delivery, complicated
  pelvis (bony)—*see* Deformity, pelvis
  percussion, chest 786.7
  periods (grossly) (*see also* Menstruation) 626.9
  phonocardiogram 794.39
  placenta—*see* Placenta, abnormal
  plantar reflex 796.1
  plasma protein—*see* Deficiency, plasma, protein
  pleural folds 748.8
  position—*see also* Malposition
    gravid uterus 654.4
      causing obstructed labor 660.2
        affecting fetus or newborn 763.1
  posture NEC 781.92
  presentation (fetus)—*see* Presentation, fetus,
    abnormal
  product of conception NEC 631.8
  puberty—*see* Puberty
  pulmonary
    artery 747.39
    function, newborn 770.89
    test results 794.2
    ventilation, newborn 770.89
      hyperventilation 786.01
  pulsations in neck 785.1
  pupil reflexes 379.40
  quality of milk 676.8
  radiological examination 793.99
    abdomen NEC 793.6
    biliary tract 793.3
    breast 793.89
      mammogram NOS 793.80
      mammographic
        calcification 793.89
        calculus 793.89
        microcalcification 793.81
    gastrointestinal tract 793.4
    genitourinary organs 793.5
    head 793.0
    image test inconclusive due to excess body fat
      793.91
    intrathoracic organ NEC 793.2
    lung (field) 793.19
    musculoskeletal system 793.7
    retroperitoneum 793.6
    skin and subcutaneous tissue 793.99
    skull 793.0
  red blood cells 790.09
    morphology 790.09
    volume 790.09
  reflex NEC 796.1
  renal function test 794.4
  respiration signs—*see* Respiration
  response to nerve stimulation 794.10
  retinal correspondence 368.34
  rhythm, heart—*see also* Arrhythmia fetus—*see*
    Distress, fetal
  saliva 792.4
  scan
    brain 794.09
    kidney 794.4
    liver 794.8
    lung 794.2
    thyroid 794.5
  secretion
    gastrin 251.5
    glucagon 251.4
  semen 792.2

Abnormal, abnormality —*continued*
  serum level (of)
    acid phosphatase 790.5
    alkaline phosphatase 790.5
    amylase 790.5
    enzymes NEC 790.5
    lipase 790.5
  shape
    cornea 743.41
    gallbladder 751.69
    gravid uterus 654.4
      affecting fetus or newborn 763.89
      causing obstructed labor 660.2
        affecting fetus or newborn 763.1
    head (*see also* Anomaly, skull) 756.0
    organ or site, congenital NEC—*see* Distortion
  sinus venosus 747.40
  size
    fetus, complicating delivery 653.5
      causing obstructed labor 660.1
    gallbladder 751.69
    head (*see also* Anomaly, skull) 756.0
    organ or site, congenital NEC—*see* Distortion
    teeth 520.2
  skin and appendages, congenital NEC 757.9
  soft parts of pelvis—*see* Abnormal, organs or tissues of pelvis
  spermatozoa 792.2
  sputum (amount) (color) (excessive) (odor) (purulent) 786.4
  stool NEC 787.7
    bloody 578.1
      occult 792.1
    bulky 787.7
    color (dark) (light) 792.1
    content (fat) (mucus) (pus) 792.1
    occult blood 792.1
  synchondrosis 756.9
  test results without manifest disease—*see* Findings, abnormal
  thebesian valve 746.9
  thermography—*see* Findings, abnormal, structure
  threshold, cones or rods (eye) 368.63
  thyroid-binding globulin 246.8
  thyroid product 246.8
  toxicology (findings) NEC 796.0
  tracheal cartilage (congenital) 748.3
  transport protein 273.8
  ultrasound results—*see* Findings, abnormal, structure
  umbilical cord
    affecting fetus or newborn 762.6
    complicating delivery 663.9
    specified NEC 663.8
  union
    cricoid cartilage and thyroid cartilage 748.3
    larynx and trachea 748.3
    thyroid cartilage and hyoid bone 748.3
  urination NEC 788.69
    psychogenic 306.53
    stream
      intermittent 788.61
      slowing 788.62
      splitting 788.61
      weak 788.62
    urgency 788.63
  urine (constituents) NEC 791.9

Abnormal, abnormality —*continued*
  uterine hemorrhage (*see also* Hemorrhage, uterus) 626.9
    climacteric 627.0
    postmenopausal 627.1
  vagina (acquired) (congenital)
    in pregnancy or childbirth 654.7
      affecting fetus or newborn 763.89
      causing obstructed labor 660.2
        affecting fetus or newborn 763.1
  vascular sounds 785.9
  vectorcardiogram 794.39
  visually evoked potential (VEP) 794.13
  vulva (acquired) (congenital)
    in pregnancy or childbirth 654.8
      affecting fetus or newborn 763.89
      causing obstructed labor 660.2
        affecting fetus or newborn 763.1
  weight
    gain 783.1
      of pregnancy 646.1
        with hypertension—*see* Toxemia, of pregnancy
    loss 783.21
  x-ray examination—*see* Abnormal, radiological examination

Abnormally formed uterus —*see* Anomaly, uterus

Abnormity (any organ or part)—*see* Anomaly

ABO
  hemolytic disease 773.1
  incompatibility (due to transfusion of blood or blood products)
    with hemolytic transfusion reaction (HTR)
      (not specified as acute or delayed) 999.61
      24 hours or more after transfusion 999.63
      acute 999.62
      delayed 999.63
      less than 24 hours after transfusion 999.62
      unspecified time after transfusion 999.61
    reaction 999.60
    specified NEC 999.69

Abocclusion 524.20

Abolition, language 784.69

Aborter, habitual or recurrent NEC
  without current pregnancy 629.81
  current abortion (*see also* Abortion, spontaneous) 634.9
  affecting fetus or newborn 761.8
  observation in current pregnancy 646.3

Abortion (complete) (incomplete) (inevitable) (with retained products of conception) 637.9

> *Note*—Use the following fifth-digit subclassification with categories 634-637:
>
> 0 unspecifhed
> 1 incomplete
> 2 complete

  with
    complication(s) (any) following previous abortion—*see* category 639
    damage to pelvic organ (laceration) (rupture) (tear) 637.2
    embolism (air) (amniotic fluid) (blood clot) (pulmonary) (pyemic) (septic) (soap) 637.6
    genital tract and pelvic infection 637.0
    hemorrhage, delayed or excessive 637.1
    metabolic disorder 637.4
    renal failure (acute) 637.3

Abortion—*continued*
  sepsis (genital tract) (pelvic organ) 637.0
    urinary tract 637.7
  shock (postoperative) (septic) 637.5
  specified complication NEC 637.7
  toxemia 637.3
  unspecified complication(s) 637.8
    urinary tract infection 637.7
  accidental—*see* Abortion, spontaneous
  artificial—*see* Abortion, induced
  attempted (failed)—*see* Abortion, failed
  criminal—*see* Abortion, illegal
  early—*see* Abortion, spontaneous
  elective—*see* Abortion, legal
  failed (legal) 638.9
    with
      damage to pelvic organ (laceration) (rupture) (tear) 638.2
      embolism (air) (amniotic fluid) (blood clot) (pulmonary) (pyemic) (septic) (soap) 638.6
      genital tract and pelvic infection 638.0
      hemorrhage, delayed or excessive 638.1
      metabolic disorder 638.4
      renal failure (acute) 638.3
      sepsis (genital tract) (pelvic organ) 638.0
        urinary tract 638.7
      shock (postoperative) (septic) 638.5
      specified complication NEC 638.7
      toxemia 638.3
      unspecified complication(s) 638.8
        urinary tract infection 638.7
  fetal indication—*see* Abortion, legal
  fetus 779.6
  following threatened abortion—*see* Abortion, by type
  habitual or recurrent (care during pregnancy) 646.3
    with current abortion (*see also* Abortion, spontaneous) 634.9
      affecting fetus or newborn 761.8
    without current pregnancy 629.81
  homicidal—*see* Abortion, illegal
  illegal 636.9
    with
      damage to pelvic organ (laceration) (rupture) (tear) 636.2
      embolism (air) (amniotic fluid) (blood clot) (pulmonary) (pyemic) (septic) (soap) 636.6
      genital tract and pelvic infection 636.0
      hemorrhage, delayed or excessive 636.1
      metabolic disorder 636.4
      renal failure 636.3
      sepsis (genital tract) (pelvic organ) 636.0
        urinary tract 636.7
      shock (postoperative) (septic) 636.5
      specified complication NEC 636.7
      toxemia 636.3
      unspecified complication(s) 636.8
        urinary tract infection 636.7
    fetus 779.6
  induced 637.9
    illegal—*see* Abortion, illegal
    legal indications—*see* Abortion, legal
    medical indications—*see* Abortion, legal
    therapeutic—*see* Abortion, legal
  late—*see* Abortion, spontaneous

Abortion—*continued*
  legal (legal indication) (medical indication) (under medical supervision) 635.9
    with
      damage to pelvic organ (laceration) (rupture) (tear) 635.2
      embolism (air) (amniotic fluid) (blood clot) (pulmonary) (pyemic) (soap) 635.6
      genital tract and pelvic infection 635.0
      hemorrhage, delayed or excessive 635.1
      metabolic disorder 635.4
      renal failure (acute) 635.3
      sepsis (genital tract) (pelvic organ) 635.0
        urinary tract 635.7
      shock (postoperative) (septic) 635.5
      specified complication NEC 635.7
      toxemia 635.3
      unspecified complication(s) 635.8
        urinary tract infection 635.7
    fetus 779.6
  medical indication—*see* Abortion, legal
  mental hygiene problem—*see* Abortion, legal
  missed 632
  operative—*see* Abortion, legal
  psychiatric indication—*see* Abortion, legal
  recurrent—*see* Abortion, spontaneous
  self-induced—*see* Abortion, illegal
  septic—*see* Abortion, by type, with sepsis
  spontaneous 634.9
    with
      damage to pelvic organ (laceration) (rupture) (tear) 634.2
      embolism (air) (amniotic fluid) (blood clot) (pulmonary) (pyemic) (septic) (soap) 634.6
      genital tract and pelvic infection 634.0
      hemorrhage, delayed or excessive 634.1
      metabolic disorder 634.4
      renal failure 634.3
      sepsis (genital tract) (pelvic organ) 634.0
        urinary tract 634.7
      shock (postoperative) (septic) 634.5
      specified complication NEC 634.7
      toxemia 634.3
      unspecified complication(s) 634.8
        urinary tract infection 634.7
    fetus 761.8
    threatened 640.0
      affecting fetus or newborn 762.1
  surgical—*see* Abortion, legal
  therapeutic—*see* Abortion, legal
  threatened 640.0
    affecting fetus or newborn 762.1
  tubal—*see* Pregnancy, tubal
  voluntary—*see* Abortion, legal
Abortus fever 023.9
Aboulomania 301.6
Abrachia 755.20
Abrachiatism 755.20
Abrachiocephalia 759.89
Abrachiocephalus 759.89
Abrami's disease (acquired hemolytic jaundice) 283.9
Abramov-Fiedler myocarditis (acute isolated myocarditis) 422.91
Abrasion —*see also* Injury, superficial, by site
  cornea 918.1

Abrasion—*continued*
  dental 521.20
    extending into
      dentine 521.22
      pulp 521.23
    generalized 521.25
    limited to enamel 521.21
    localized 521.24
  teeth, tooth (dentifrice) (habitual) (hard tissues)
    (occupational) (ritual) (traditional) (wedge
    defect) (*see also* Abrasion, dental) 521.20
Abrikossov's tumor (M9580/0)—*see also*
  Neoplasm, connective tissue, benign
  malignant (M9580/3)—*see* Neoplasm,
  connective tissue, malignant
Abrism 988.8
Abruption, placenta —*see* Placenta, abruptio
Abruptio placentae —*see* Placenta, abruptio
Abscess (acute) (chronic) (infectional)
  (lymphangitic) (metastatic) (multiple)
  (pyogenic) (septic) (with lymphangitis) (*see*
  also Cellulitis) 682.9
  abdomen, abdominal
    cavity 567.22
    wall 682.2
  abdominopelvic 567.22
  accessory sinus (chronic) (*see also* Sinusitis)
    473.9
  adrenal (capsule) (gland) 255.8
  alveolar 522.5
    with sinus 522.7
  amebic 006.3
    bladder 006.8
    brain (with liver or lung abscess) 006.5
    liver (without mention of brain or lung
      abscess) 006.3
      with
        brain abscess (and lung abscess) 006.5
        lung abscess 006.4
    lung (with liver abscess) 006.4
      with brain abscess 006.5
    seminal vesicle 006.8
    specified site NEC 006.8
    spleen 006.8
  anaerobic 040.0
  ankle 682.6
  anorectal 566
  antecubital space 682.3
  antrum (chronic) (Highmore) (*see also* Sinusitis,
    maxillary) 473.0
  anus 566
  apical (tooth) 522.5
    with sinus (alveolar) 522.7
  appendix 540.1
  areola (acute) (chronic) (nonpuerperal) 611.0
    puerperal, postpartum 675.1
  arm (any part, above wrist) 682.3
  artery (wall) 447.2
  atheromatous 447.2
  auditory canal (external) 380.10
  auricle (ear) (staphylococcal) (streptococcal)
    380.10
  axilla, axillary (region) 682.3
    lymph gland or node 683
  back (any part) 682.2

Abscess—*continued*
  Bartholin's gland 616.3
    with
      abortion—*see* Abortion, by type, with sepsis
      ectopic pregnancy (*see also* categories
        633.0-633.9) 639.0
      molar pregnancy (*see also* categories
        630-632) 639.0
    complicating pregnancy or puerperium 646.6
    following
      abortion 639.0
      ectopic or molar pregnancy 639.0
  bartholinian 616.3
  Bezold's 383.01
  bile, biliary, duct or tract (*see also* Cholecystitis)
    576.8
  bilharziasis 120.1
  bladder (wall) 595.89
    amebic 006.8
  bone (subperiosteal) (*see also* Osteomyelitis)
    730.0
    accessory sinus (chronic) (*see also* Sinusitis)
      473.9
    acute 730.0
    chronic or old 730.1
    jaw (lower) (upper) 526.4
    mastoid—*see* Mastoiditis, acute
    petrous (*see also* Petrositis) 383.20
    spinal (tuberculous) (*see also* Tuberculosis)
      015.0 *[730.88]*
      nontuberculous 730.08
  bowel 569.5
  brain (any part) 324.0
    amebic (with liver or lung abscess) 006.5
    cystic 324.0
    late effect—*see* category 326
    otogenic 324.0
    tuberculous (*see also* Tuberculosis) 013.3
  breast (acute) (chronic) (nonpuerperal) 611.0
    newborn 771.5
    puerperal, postpartum 675.1
    tuberculous (*see also* Tuberculosis) 017.9
  broad ligament (chronic) (*see also* Disease,
    pelvis, inflammatory) 614.4
    acute 614.3
  Brodie's (chronic) (localized) (*see also*
    Osteomyelitis) 730.1
  bronchus 519.19
  buccal cavity 528.3
  bulbourethral gland 597.0
  bursa 727.89
    pharyngeal 478.29
  buttock 682.5
  canaliculus, breast 611.0
  canthus 372.20
  cartilage 733.99
  cecum 569.5
    with appendicitis 540.1
  cerebellum, cerebellar 324.0
    late effect—*see* category 326
  cerebral (embolic) 324.0
    late effect—*see* category 326
  cervical (neck region) 682.1
    lymph gland or node 683
    stump (*see also* Cervicitis) 616.0
  cervix (stump) (uteri) (*see also* Cervicitis) 616.0
  cheek, external 682.0
    inner 528.3
  chest 510.9
    with fistula 510.0
    wall 682.2

Abscess—*continued*
chin 682.0
choroid 363.00
ciliary body 364.3
circumtonsillar 475
cold (tuberculous)—*see also* Tuberculosis,
    abscess
    articular—*see* Tuberculosis, joint
colon (wall) 569.5
colostomy or enterostomy 569.6
conjunctiva 372.00
connective tissue NEC 682.9
cornea 370.55
    with ulcer 370.00
corpus
    cavernosum 607.2
    luteum (*see also* Salpingo-oophoritis) 614.2
Cowper's gland 597.0
cranium 324.0
cul-de-sac (Douglas') (posterior) (*see also*
    Disease, pelvis, inflammatory) 614.4
    acute 614.3
dental 522.5
    with sinus (alveolar) 522.7
dentoalveolar 522.5
    with sinus (alveolar) 522.7
diaphragm, diaphragmatic 567.22
digit NEC 681.9
Douglas' cul-de-sac or pouch (*see also* Disease,
    pelvis, inflammatory) 614.4
    acute 614.3
Dubois' 090.5
ductless gland 259.8
ear
    acute 382.00
    external 380.10
    inner 386.30
    middle—*see* Otitis media
elbow 682.3
endamebic—*see* Abscess, amebic
entamebic—*see* Abscess, amebic
enterostomy 569.6
epididymis 604.0
epidural 324.9
    brain 324.0
    late effect—*see* category 326
    spinal cord 324.1
epiglottis 478.79
epiploon, epiploic 567.22
erysipelatous (*see also* Erysipelas) 035
esophagostomy 530.86
esophagus 530.19
ethmoid (bone) (chronic) (sinus) (*see also*
    Sinusitis, ethmoidal) 473.2
external auditory canal 380.10
extradural 324.9
    brain 324.0
    late effect—*see* category 326
    spinal cord 324.1
extraperitoneal—*see* Abscess, peritoneum
eye 360.00
eyelid 373.13
face (any part, except eye) 682.0
fallopian tube (*see also* Salpingo-oophoritis)
    614.2
fascia 728.89
fauces 478.29
fecal 569.5
femoral (region) 682.6
filaria, filarial (*see also* Infestation, filarial)
    125.9

Abscess—*continued*
finger (any) (intrathecal) (periosteal)
    (subcutaneous) (subcuticular) 681.00
fistulous NEC 682.9
flank 682.2
foot (except toe) 682.7
forearm 682.3
forehead 682.0
frontal (sinus) (chronic) (*see also* Sinusitis,
    frontal) 473.1
gallbladder (*see also* Cholecystitis, acute) 575.0
gastric 535.0
genital organ or tract NEC
    female 616.9
        with
            abortion—*see* Abortion, by type, with
                sepsis
            ectopic pregnancy (*see also* categories
                633.0-633.9) 639.0
            molar pregnancy (*see also* categories
                630-632) 639.0
        following
            abortion 639.0
            ectopic or molar pregnancy 639.0
        puerperal, postpartum, childbirth 670.8
    male 608.4
genitourinary system, tuberculous (*see also*
    Tuberculosis) 016.9
gingival 523.30
gland, glandular (lymph) (acute) NEC 683
glottis 478.79
gluteal (region) 682.5
gonorrheal NEC (*see also* Gonococcus) 098.0
groin 682.2
gum 523.30
hand (except finger or thumb) 682.4
head (except face) 682.8
heart 429.89
heel 682.7
helminthic (*see also* Infestation, by specific
    parasite) 128.9
hepatic 572.0
    amebic (*see also* Abscess, liver, amebic) 006.3
    duct 576.8
hip 682.6
    tuberculous (active) (*see also* Tuberculosis)
        015.1
ileocecal 540.1
ileostomy (bud) 569.6
iliac (region) 682.2
    fossa 540.1
iliopsoas 567.31
    tuberculous (see also Tuberculosis) 015.0
        [730.88]
infraclavicular (fossa) 682.3
inguinal (region) 682.2
    lymph gland or node 683
intersphincteric (anus) 566
intestine, intestinal 569.5
    rectal 566
intra-abdominal (*see also* Abscess, peritoneum)
    567.22
    postoperative 998.59
intracranial 324.0
    late effect—*see* category 326
intramammary—*see* Abscess, breast
intramastoid (*see also* Mastoiditis, acute) 383.00
intraorbital 376.01
intraperitoneal 567.22
intraspinal 324.1
    late effect—*see* category 326

Abscess—*continued*
  intratonsillar 475
  iris 364.3
  ischiorectal 566
  jaw (bone) (lower) (upper) 526.4
    skin 682.0
  joint (*see also* Arthritis, pyogenic) 711.0
    vertebral (tuberculous) (*see also* Tuberculosis)
      015.0 *[730.88]*
    nontuberculous 724.8
  kidney 590.2
    with
      abortion—*see* Abortion, by type, with
        urinary tract infection
      calculus 592.0
      ectopic pregnancy (*see also* categories
        633.0-633.9) 639.8
      molar pregnancy (*see also* categories
        630-632) 639.8
    complicating pregnancy or puerperium 646.6
      affecting fetus or newborn 760.1
    following
      abortion 639.8
      ectopic or molar pregnancy 639.8
  knee 682.6
    joint 711.06
    tuberculous (active) (*see also* Tuberculosis)
      015.2
  labium (majus) (minus) 616.4
    complicating pregnancy, childbirth, or
      puerperium 646.6
  lacrimal (passages) (sac) (*see also*
    Dacryocystitis) 375.30
    caruncle 375.30
    gland (*see also* Dacryoadenitis) 375.00
  lacunar 597.0
  larynx 478.79
  lateral (alveolar) 522.5
    with sinus 522.7
  leg, except foot 682.6
  lens 360.00
  lid 373.13
  lingual 529.0
    tonsil 475
  lip 528.5
  Littre's gland 597.0
  liver 572.0
    amebic 006.3
      with
        brain abscess (and lung abscess) 006.5
        lung abscess 006.4
      due to Entamoeba histolytica 006.3
    dysenteric (*see also* Abscess, liver, amebic)
      006.3
    pyogenic 572.0
    tropical (*see also* Abscess, liver, amebic)
      006.3
  loin (region) 682.2
  lumbar (tuberculous) (*see also* Tuberculosis)
    015.0 *[730.88]*
    nontuberculous 682.2
  lung (miliary) (putrid) 513.0
    amebic (with liver abscess) 006.4
      with brain abscess 006.5
  lymph, lymphatic, gland or node (acute) 683
    any site, except mesenteric 683
    mesentery 289.2
  lymphangitic, acute—*see* Cellulitis
  malar 526.4
  mammary gland—*see* Abscess, breast
  marginal (anus) 566

Abscess—*continued*
  mastoid (process) (*see also* Mastoiditis, acute)
    383.00
    subperiosteal 383.01
  maxilla, maxillary 526.4
    molar (tooth) 522.5
      with sinus 522.7
    premolar 522.5
    sinus (chronic) (*see also* Sinusitis, maxillary)
      473.0
  mediastinum 513.1
  meibomian gland 373.12
  meninges (*see also* Meningitis) 320.9
  mesentery, mesenteric 567.22
  mesosalpinx (*see also* Salpingo-oophoritis)
    614.2
  milk 675.1
  Monro's (psoriasis) 696.1
  mons pubis 682.2
  mouth (floor) 528.3
  multiple sites NEC 682.9
  mural 682.2
  muscle 728.89
    psoas 567.31
  myocardium 422.92
  nabothian (follicle) (*see also* Cervicitis) 616.0
  nail (chronic) (with lymphangitis) 681.9
    finger 681.02
    toe 681.11
  nasal (fossa) (septum) 478.19
    sinus (chronic) (*see also* Sinusitis) 473.9
  nasopharyngeal 478.29
  nates 682.5
  navel 682.2
    newborn NEC 771.4
  neck (region) 682.1
    lymph gland or node 683
  nephritic (*see also* Abscess, kidney) 590.2
  nipple 611.0
    puerperal, postpartum 675.0
  nose (septum) 478.19
    external 682.0
  omentum 567.22
  operative wound 998.59
  orbit, orbital 376.01
  ossifluent—*see* Abscess, bone
  ovary, ovarian (corpus luteum) (*see also*
    Salpingo-oophoritis) 614.2
  oviduct (*see also* Salpingo-oophoritis) 614.2
  palate (soft) 528.3
    hard 526.4
  palmar (space) 682.4
  pancreas (duct) 577.0
  paradontal 523.30
  parafrenal 607.2
  parametric, parametrium (chronic) (*see also*
    Disease, pelvis, inflammatory) 614.4
    acute 614.3
  paranephric 590.2
  parapancreatic 577.0
  parapharyngeal 478.22
  pararectal 566
  parasinus (*see also* Sinusitis) 473.9
  parauterine (*see also* Disease, pelvis,
    inflammatory) 614.4
    acute 614.3
  paravaginal (*see also* Vaginitis) 616.10
  parietal region 682.8
  parodontal 523.30
  parotid (duct) (gland) 527.3
    region 528.3

Abscess—*continued*
parumbilical 682.2
  newborn 771.4
pectoral (region) 682.2
pelvirectal 567.22
pelvis, pelvic
  female (chronic) (*see also* Disease, pelvis,
    inflammatory) 614.4
    acute 614.3
  male, peritoneal (cellular tissue)—*see*
    Abscess, peritoneum
  tuberculous (*see also* Tuberculosis) 016.9
penis 607.2
  gonococcal (acute) 098.0
    chronic or duration of 2 months or over
      098.2
perianal 566
periapical 522.5
  with sinus (alveolar) 522.7
periappendiceal 540.1
pericardial 420.99
pericecal 540.1
pericemental 523.30
pericholecystic (*see also* Cholecystitis, acute)
  575.0
pericoronal 523.30
peridental 523.30
perigastric 535.0
perimetric (*see also* Disease, pelvis,
  inflammatory) 614.4
  acute 614.3
perinephric, perinephritic (*see also* Abscess,
  kidney) 590.2
perineum, perineal (superficial) 682.2
  deep (with urethral involvement) 597.0
  urethra 597.0
periodontal (parietal) 523.31
  apical 522.5
periosteum, periosteal (*see also* Periostitis)
  730.3
  with osteomyelitis (*see also* Osteomyelitis)
    730.2
    acute or subacute 730.0
    chronic or old 730.1
peripleuritic 510.9
  with fistula 510.0
periproctic 566
periprostatic 601.2
perirectal (staphylococcal) 566
perirenal (tissue) (*see also* Abscess, kidney)
  590.2
perisinuous (nose) (*see also* Sinusitis) 473.9
peritoneum, peritoneal (perforated) (ruptured)
  567.22
  with
    abortion—*see* Abortion, by type, with sepsis
    appendicitis 540.1
    ectopic pregnancy (*see also* categories
      633.0-633.9) 639.0
    molar pregnancy (*see also* categories
      630-632) 639.0
  following
    abortion 639.0
    ectopic or molar pregnancy 639.0
  pelvic, female (*see also* Disease, pelvis,
    inflammatory) 614.4
    acute 614.3
  postoperative 998.59
  puerperal, postpartum, childbirth 670.8
  tuberculous (*see also* Tuberculosis) 014.0
peritonsillar 475

Abscess—*continued*
perityphlic 540.1
periureteral 593.89
periurethral 597.0
  gonococcal (acute) 098.0
    chronic or duration of 2 months or over
      098.2
  periuterine (*see also* Disease, pelvis,
    inflammatory) 614.4
    acute 614.3
perivesical 595.89
pernicious NEC 682.9
petrous bone—*see* Petrositis
phagedenic NEC 682.9
  chancroid 099.0
pharynx, pharyngeal (lateral) 478.29
phlegmonous NEC 682.9
pilonidal 685.0
pituitary (gland) 253.8
pleura 510.9
  with fistula 510.0
popliteal 682.6
postanal 566
postcecal 540.1
postlaryngeal 478.79
postnasal 478.19
postpharyngeal 478.24
posttonsillar 475
posttyphoid 002.0
Pott's (*see also* Tuberculosis) 015.0 *[730.88]*
pouch of Douglas (chronic) (*see also* Disease,
  pelvis, inflammatory) 614.4
premammary—*see* Abscess, breast
prepatellar 682.6
prostate (*see also* Prostatitis) 601.2
  gonococcal (acute) 098.12
    chronic or duration of 2 months or over 098.32
psoas 567.31
  tuberculous (*see also* Tuberculosis) 015.0
    [730.88]
pterygopalatine fossa 682.8
pubis 682.2
puerperal—Puerperal, abscess, by site
pulmonary—*see* Abscess, lung
pulp, pulpal (dental) 522.0
  finger 681.01
  toe 681.10
pyemic—*see* Septicemia
pyloric valve 535.0
rectovaginal septum 569.5
rectovesical 595.89
rectum 566
regional NEC 682.9
renal (*see also* Abscess, kidney) 590.2
retina 363.00
retrobulbar 376.01
retrocecal 567.22
retrolaryngeal 478.79
retromammary—*see* Abscess, breast
retroperineal 682.2
retroperitoneal 567.38
  postprocedural 998.59
retropharyngeal 478.24
  tuberculous (*see also* Tuberculosis) 012.8
retrorectal 566
retrouterine (*see also* Disease, pelvis,
  inflammatory) 614.4
  acute 614.3
retrovesical 595.89
root, tooth 522.5
  with sinus (alveolar) 522.7

Abscess—*continued*
  round ligament (*see also* Disease, pelvis,
      inflammatory) 614.4
    acute 614.3
  rupture (spontaneous) NEC 682.9
  sacrum (tuberculous) (*see also* Tuberculosis)
      015.0 *[730.88]*
    nontuberculous 730.08
  salivary duct or gland 527.3
  scalp (any part) 682.8
  scapular 730.01
  sclera 379.09
  scrofulous (*see also* Tuberculosis) 017.2
  scrotum 608.4
  seminal vesicle 608.0
    amebic 006.8
  septal, dental 522.5
    with sinus (alveolar) 522.7
  septum (nasal) 478.19
  serous (*see also* Periostitis) 730.3
  shoulder 682.3
  side 682.2
  sigmoid 569.5
  sinus (accessory) (chronic) (nasal) (*see also*
      Sinusitis) 473.9
    intracranial venous (any) 324.0
    late effect—*see* category 326
  Skene's duct or gland 597.0
  skin NEC 682.9
    tuberculous (primary) (*see also* Tuberculosis)
      017.0
  sloughing NEC 682.9
  specified site NEC 682.8
    amebic 006.8
  spermatic cord 608.4
  sphenoidal (sinus) (*see also* Sinusitis,
      sphenoidal) 473.3
  spinal
    cord (any part) (staphylococcal) 324.1
      tuberculous (*see also* Tuberculosis) 013.5
    epidural 324.1
  spine (column) (tuberculous) (*see also*
      Tuberculosis) 015.0 *[730.88]*
    nontuberculous 730.08
  spleen 289.59
    amebic 006.8
  staphylococcal NEC 682.9
  stitch 998.59
  stomach (wall) 535.0
  strumous (tuberculous) (*see also* Tuberculosis)
      017.2
  subarachnoid 324.9
    brain 324.0
    cerebral 324.0
    late effect—*see* category 326
    spinal cord 324.1
  subareolar—*see also* Abscess, breast
    puerperal, postpartum 675.1
  subcecal 540.1
  subcutaneous NEC 682.9
  subdiaphragmatic 567.22
  subdorsal 682.2
  subdural 324.9
    brain 324.0
    late effect—*see* category 326
    spinal cord 324.1
  subgaleal 682.8
  subhepatic 567.22
  sublingual 528.3
    gland 527.3
  submammary—*see* Abscess, breast

Abscess—*continued*
  submandibular (region) (space) (triangle) 682.0
    gland 527.3
  submaxillary (region) 682.0
    gland 527.3
  submental (pyogenic) 682.0
    gland 527.3
  subpectoral 682.2
  subperiosteal—*see* Abscess, bone
  subperitoneal 567.22
  subphrenic—*see also* Abscess, peritoneum
      567.22
    postoperative 998.59
  subscapular 682.2
  subungual 681.9
  suburethral 597.0
  sudoriparous 705.89
  suppurative NEC 682.9
  supraclavicular (fossa) 682.3
  suprahepatic 567.22
  suprapelvic (*see also* Disease, pelvis,
      inflammatory) 614.4
    acute 614.3
  suprapubic 682.2
  suprarenal (capsule) (gland) 255.8
  sweat gland 705.89
  syphilitic 095.8
  teeth, tooth (root) 522.5
    with sinus (alveolar) 522.7
    supporting structures NEC 523.30
  temple 682.0
  temporal region 682.0
  temporosphenoidal 324.0
    late effect—*see* category 326
  tendon (sheath) 727.89
  testicle—*see* Orchitis
  thecal 728.89
  thigh (acquired) 682.6
  thorax 510.9
    with fistula 510.0
  throat 478.29
  thumb (intrathecal) (periosteal) (subcutaneous)
      (subcuticular) 681.00
  thymus (gland) 254.1
  thyroid (gland) 245.0
  toe (any) (intrathecal) (periosteal)
      (subcutaneous) (subcuticular) 681.10
  tongue (staphylococcal) 529.0
  tonsil(s) (lingual) 475
  tonsillopharyngeal 475
  tooth, teeth (root) 522.5
    with sinus (alveolar) 522.7
    supporting structure NEC 523.30
  trachea 478.9
  trunk 682.2
  tubal (*see also* Salpingo-oophoritis) 614.2
  tuberculous—*see* Tuberculosis, abscess
  tubo-ovarian (*see also* Salpingo-oophoritis)
      614.2
  tunica vaginalis 608.4
  umbilicus NEC 682.2
    newborn 771.4
  upper arm 682.3
  upper respiratory 478.9
  urachus 682.2
  urethra (gland) 597.0
  urinary 597.0

Abscess—*continued*
  uterus, uterine (wall) (*see also* Endometritis)
    615.9
    ligament (*see also* Disease, pelvis,
      inflammatory) 614.4
      acute 614.3
    neck (*see also* Cervicitis) 616.0
  uvula 528.3
  vagina (wall) (*see also* Vaginitis) 616.10
  vaginorectal (*see also* Vaginitis) 616.10
  vas deferens 608.4
  vermiform appendix 540.1
  vertebra (column) (tuberculous) (*see also*
    Tuberculosis) 015.0 *[730.88]*
    nontuberculous 730.0
  vesical 595.89
  vesicouterine pouch (*see also* Disease, pelvis,
    inflammatory) 614.4
  vitreous (humor) (pneumococcal) 360.04
  vocal cord 478.5
  von Bezold's 383.01
  vulva 616.4
    complicating pregnancy, childbirth, or
      puerperium 646.6
  vulvovaginal gland (*see also* Vaginitis) 616.3
  web-space 682.4
  wrist 682.4
Absence (organ or part) (complete or partial)
  acoustic nerve 742.8
  adrenal (gland) (congenital) 759.1
    acquired V45.79
  albumin (blood) 273.8
  alimentary tract (complete) (congenital) (partial)
    751.8
    lower 751.5
    upper 750.8
  alpha-fucosidase 271.8
  alveolar process (acquired) 525.8
    congenital 750.26
  anus, anal (canal) (congenital) 751.2
  aorta (congenital) 747.22
  aortic valve (congenital) 746.89
  appendix, congenital 751.2
  arm (acquired) V49.60
    above elbow V49.66
    below elbow V49.65
    congenital (*see also* Deformity, reduction,
      upper limb) 755.20
      lower—*see* Absence, forearm, congenital
      upper (complete) (partial) (with absence of
        distal elements, incomplete) 755.24
        with
          complete absence of distal elements
            755.21
          forearm (incomplete) 755.23
  artery (congenital) (peripheral) NEC (*see also*
    Anomaly, peripheral vascular system)
    747.60
    brain 747.81
    cerebral 747.81
    coronary 746.85
    pulmonary 747.31
    umbilical 747.5
  atrial septum 745.69
  auditory canal (congenital) (external) 744.01
  auricle (ear) (with stenosis or atresia of auditory
    canal), congenital 744.01
  bile, biliary duct (common) or passage
    (congenital) 751.61
  bladder (acquired) V45.74
    congenital 753.8

Absence—*continued*
  bone (congenital) NEC 756.9
    marrow 284.9
      acquired (secondary) 284.89
      congenital 284.09
      hereditary 284.09
      idiopathic 284.9
    skull 756.0
  bowel sounds 787.5
  brain 740.0
    specified part 742.2
  breast(s) (acquired) V45.71
    congenital 757.6
  broad ligament (congenital) 752.19
  bronchus (congenital) 748.3
  calvarium, calvaria (skull) 756.0
  canaliculus lacrimalis, congenital 743.65
  carpal(s) (congenital) (complete) (partial) (with
    absence of distal elements, incomplete) (*see
    also* Deformity, reduction, upper limb)
    755.28
    with complete absence of distal elements
      755.21
  cartilage 756.9
  caudal spine 756.13
  cecum (acquired) (postoperative)
    (posttraumatic) V45.72
    congenital 751.2
  cementum 520.4
  cerebellum (congenital) (vermis) 742.2
  cervix (acquired) (uteri) V88.01
    with remaining uterus V88.03
    and uterus V88.01
    congenital 752.43
  chin, congenital 744.89
  cilia (congenital) 743.63
    acquired 374.89
  circulatory system, part NEC 747.89
  clavicle 755.51
  clitoris (congenital) 752.49
  coccyx, congenital 756.13
  cold sense (*see also* Disturbance, sensation)
    782.0
  colon (acquired) (postoperative) V45.72
    congenital 751.2
  congenital
    lumen—*see* Atresia
    organ or site NEC—*see* Agenesis
    septum—*see* Imperfect, closure
  corpus callosum (congenital) 742.2
  cricoid cartilage 748.3
  diaphragm (congenital) (with hernia) 756.6
    with obstruction 756.6
  digestive organ(s) or tract, congenital (complete)
    (partial) 751.8
    acquired V45.79
    lower 751.5
    upper 750.8
  ductus arteriosus 747.89
  duodenum (acquired) (postoperative) V45.72
    congenital 751.1
  ear, congenital 744.09
    acquired V45.79
    auricle 744.01
    external 744.01
    inner 744.05
    lobe, lobule 744.21
    middle, except ossicles 744.03
      ossicles 744.04
    ossicles 744.04
  ejaculatory duct (congenital) 752.89

Absence—*continued*
  endocrine gland NEC (congenital) 759.2
  epididymis (congenital) 752.89
    acquired V45.77
  epiglottis, congenital 748.3
  epileptic (atonic) (typical) (*see also* Epilepsy)
      345.0
  erythrocyte 284.9
  erythropoiesis 284.9
    congenital 284.01
  esophagus (congenital) 750.3
  Eustachian tube (congenital) 744.24
  extremity (acquired)
    congenital (*see also* Deformity, reduction)
        755.4
    lower V49.70
    upper V49.60
  extrinsic muscle, eye 743.69
  eye (acquired) V45.78
    adnexa (congenital) 743.69
    congenital 743.00
    muscle (congenital) 743.69
  eyelid (fold), congenital 743.62
    acquired 374.89
  face
    bones NEC 756.0
    specified part NEC 744.89
  fallopian tube(s) (acquired) V45.77
    congenital 752.19
  femur, congenital (complete) (partial) (with
      absence of distal elements, incomplete) (*see
      also* Deformity, reduction, lower limb)
      755.34
    with
      complete absence of distal elements 755.31
      tibia and fibula (incomplete) 755.33
  fibrin 790.92
    fibrinogen (congenital) 286.3
      acquired 286.6
  fibula, congenital (complete) (partial) (with
      absence of distal elements, incomplete) (*see
      also* Deformity, reduction, lower limb)
      755.37
    with
      complete absence of distal elements 755.31
      tibia 755.35
        with
          complete absence of distal elements
              755.31
          femur (incomplete) 755.33
            with complete absence of distal
                elements 755.31
  finger (acquired) V49.62
    congenital (complete) (partial) (*see also*
        Deformity, reduction, upper limb) 755.29
      meaning all fingers (complete) (partial)
          755.21
    transverse 755.21
  fissures of lungs (congenital) 748.5
  foot (acquired) V49.73
    congenital (complete) 755.31
  forearm (acquired) V49.65
    congenital (complete) (partial) (with absence
        of distal elements, incomplete) (*see also*
        Deformity, reduction, upper limb) 755.25
      with
        complete absence of distal elements (hand
            and fingers) 755.21
        humerus (incomplete) 755.23
  fovea centralis 743.55

Absence—*continued*
  fucosidase 271.8
    gallbladder (acquired) V45.79
    congenital 751.69
  gamma globulin (blood) 279.00
  genital organs
    acquired V45.77
    congenital
      female 752.89
        external 752.49
        internal NEC 752.89
      male 752.89
        penis 752.69
  genitourinary organs, congenital NEC 752.89
  glottis 748.3
  gonadal, congenital NEC 758.6
  hair (congenital) 757.4
    acquired—*see* Alopecia
  hand (acquired) V49.63
    congenital (complete) (*see also* Deformity,
        reduction, upper limb) 755.21
  heart (congenital) 759.89
    acquired—*see* Status, organ replacement
  heat sense (*see also* Disturbance, sensation)
      782.0
  humerus, congenital (complete) (partial) (with
      absence of distal elements, incomplete) (*see
      also* Deformity, reduction, upper limb)
      755.24
    with
      complete absence of distal elements 755.21
      radius and ulna (incomplete) 755.23
  hymen (congenital) 752.49
  ileum (acquired) (postoperative) (posttraumatic)
      V45.72
    congenital 751.1
  immunoglobulin, isolated NEC 279.03
    IgA 279.01
    IgG 279.03
    IgM 279.02
  incus (acquired) 385.24
    congenital 744.04
  internal ear (congenital) 744.05
  intestine (acquired) (small) V45.72
    congenital 751.1
      large 751.2
    large V45.72
      congenital 751.2
  iris (congenital) 743.45
  jaw—*see* Absence, mandible
  jejunum (acquired) V45.72
    congenital 751.1
  joint (acquired) (following prior explantation of
      joint prosthesis) (with or without presence of
      antibiotic-impregnated cement spacer) NEC
      V88.29
    congenital NEC 755.8
    hip V88.21
    knee V88.22
  kidney(s) (acquired) V45.73
    congenital 753.0
  labium (congenital) (majus) (minus) 752.49
  labyrinth, membranous 744.05
  lacrimal apparatus (congenital) 743.65
  larynx (congenital) 748.3
  leg (acquired) V49.70
    above knee V49.76
    below knee V49.75

Absence—*continued*
  congenital (partial) (unilateral) (*see also*
      Deformity, reduction, lower limb) 755.31
    lower (complete) (partial) (with absence of
        distal elements, incomplete) 755.35
      with
        complete absence of distal elements
            (foot and toes) 755.31
        thigh (incomplete) 755.33
          with complete absence of distal
              elements 755.31
      upper—*see* Absence, femur
  lens (congenital) 743.35
    acquired 379.31
  ligament, broad (congenital) 752.19
  limb (acquired)
    congenital (complete) (partial) (*see also*
        Deformity, reduction) 755.4
      lower 755.30
        complete 755.31
        incomplete 755.32
        longitudinal—*see* Deficiency, lower limb,
            longitudinal
        transverse 755.31
      upper 755.20
        complete 755.21
        incomplete 755.22
        longitudinal—*see* Deficiency, upper limb,
            longitudinal
        transverse 755.21
    lower NEC V49.70
    upper NEC V49.60
  lip 750.26
  liver (congenital) (lobe) 751.69
  lumbar (congenital) (vertebra) 756.13
    isthmus 756.11
    pars articularis 756.11
  lumen—*see* Atresia
  lung (bilateral) (congenital) (fissure) (lobe)
      (unilateral) 748.5
    acquired (any part) V45.76
  mandible (congenital) 524.09
  maxilla (congenital) 524.09
  menstruation 626.0
  metacarpal(s), congenital (complete) (partial)
      (with absence of distal elements,
      incomplete) (*see also* Deformity, reduction,
      upper limb) 755.28
    with all fingers, complete 755.21
  metatarsal(s), congenital (complete) (partial)
      (with absence of distal elements,
      incomplete) (*see also* Deformity, reduction,
      lower limb) 755.38
    with complete absence of distal elements
        755.31
  muscle (congenital) (pectoral) 756.81
    ocular 743.69
  musculoskeletal system (congenital) NEC 756.9
  nail(s) (congenital) 757.5
  neck, part 744.89
  nerve 742.8
  nervous system, part NEC 742.8
  neutrophil 288.00
  nipple (congenital) 757.6
    acquired V45.71
  nose (congenital) 748.1
    acquired 738.0
  nuclear 742.8
  ocular muscle (congenital) 743.69

Absence—*continued*
  organ
    of Corti (congenital) 744.05
    or site
      acquired V45.79
      congenital NEC 759.89
  osseous meatus (ear) 744.03
  ovary (acquired) V45.77
    congenital 752.0
  oviduct (acquired) V45.77
    congenital 752.19
  pancreas (congenital) 751.7
    acquired (postoperative) (posttraumatic)
        V88.11
      partial V88.12
      total V88.11
  parathyroid gland (congenital) 759.2
  parotid gland(s) (congenital) 750.21
  patella, congenital 755.64
  pelvic girdle (congenital) 755.69
  penis (congenital) 752.69
    acquired V45.77
  pericardium (congenital) 746.89
  perineal body (congenital) 756.81
  phalange(s), congenital 755.4
    lower limb (complete) (intercalary) (partial)
        (terminal) (*see also* Deformity, reduction,
        lower limb) 755.39
      meaning all toes (complete) (partial) 755.31
      transverse 755.31
    upper limb (complete) (intercalary) (partial)
        (terminal) (*see also* Deformity, reduction,
        upper limb) 755.29
      meaning all digits (complete) (partial)
          755.21
      transverse 755.21
  pituitary gland (congenital) 759.2
  postoperative—*see* Absence, by site, acquired
  prostate (congenital) 752.89
    acquired V45.77
  pulmonary
    artery 747.31
    trunk 747.31
    valve (congenital) 746.01
    vein 747.49
  punctum lacrimale (congenital) 743.65
  radius, congenital (complete) (partial) (with
      absence of distal elements, incomplete)
      755.26
    with
      complete absence of distal elements 755.21
      ulna 755.25
        with
          complete absence of distal elements
              755.21
          humerus (incomplete) 755.23
  ray, congenital 755.4
    lower limb (complete) (partial) (*see also*
        Deformity, reduction, lower limb) 755.38
      meaning all rays 755.31
      transverse 755.31
    upper limb (complete) (partial) (*see also*
        Deformity, reduction, upper limb) 755.28
      meaning all rays 755.21
      transverse 755.21
  rectum (congenital) 751.2
    acquired V45.79
  red cell 284.9
    acquired (secondary) 284.81
    congenital 284.01
    hereditary 284.01
    idiopathic 284.9

Absence—*continued*
respiratory organ (congenital) NEC 748.9
rib (acquired) 738.3
  congenital 756.3
roof of orbit (congenital) 742.0
round ligament (congenital) 752.89
sacrum, congenital 756.13
salivary gland(s) (congenital) 750.21
scapula 755.59
scrotum, congenital 752.89
seminal tract or duct (congenital) 752.89
  acquired V45.77
septum (congenital)—*see also* Imperfect,
  closure, septum
  atrial 745.69
  and ventricular 745.7
  between aorta and pulmonary artery 745.0
  ventricular 745.3
  and atrial 745.7
sex chromosomes 758.81
shoulder girdle, congenital (complete) (partial)
  755.59
skin (congenital) 757.39
skull bone 756.0
  with
    anencephalus 740.0
    encephalocele 742.0
    hydrocephalus 742.3
      with spina bifida (*see also* Spina bifida)
      741.0
    microcephalus 742.1
spermatic cord (congenital) 752.89
spinal cord 742.59
spine, congenital 756.13
spleen (congenital) 759.0
  acquired V45.79
sternum, congenital 756.3
stomach (acquired) (partial) (postoperative)
  V45.75
  congenital 750.7
  with postgastric surgery syndrome 564.2
submaxillary gland(s) (congenital) 750.21
superior vena cava (congenital) 747.49
tarsal(s), congenital (complete) (partial) (with
  absence of distal elements, incomplete) (*see
  also* Deformity, reduction, lower limb)
  755.38
teeth, tooth (congenital) 520.0
  with abnormal spacing 524.30
  acquired 525.10
    due to
      caries 525.13
      extraction 525.10
      periodontal disease 525.12
      trauma 525.11
    with malocclusion 524.30
tendon (congenital) 756.81
testis (congenital) 752.89
  acquired V45.77
thigh (acquired) 736.89
thumb (acquired) V49.61
  congenital 755.29
thymus gland (congenital) 759.2
thyroid (gland) (surgical) 246.8
  with hypothyroidism 244.0
  cartilage, congenital 748.3
  congenital 243

Absence—*continued*
tibia, congenital (complete) (partial) (with absence
  of distal elements, incomplete) (*see also*
  Deformity, reduction, lower limb) 755.36
  with
    complete absence of distal elements 755.31
    fibula 755.35
      with
        complete absence of distal elements
        755.31
      femur (incomplete) 755.33
        with complete absence of distal
        elements 755.31
toe (acquired) V49.72
  congenital (complete) (partial) 755.39
    meaning all toes 755.31
    transverse 755.31
  great V49.71
tongue (congenital) 750.11
tooth, teeth, (congenital) 520.0
  with abnormal spacing 524.30
  acquired 525.10
    due to
      caries 525.13
      extraction 525.10
      periodontal disease 525.12
      trauma 525.11
    with malocclusion 524.30
trachea (cartilage) (congenital) (rings) 748.3
transverse aortic arch (congenital) 747.21
tricuspid valve 746.1
ulna, congenital (complete) (partial) (with
  absence of distal elements, incomplete) (*see
  also* Deformity, reduction, upper limb)
  755.27
  with
    complete absence of distal elements 755.21
    radius 755.25
      with
        complete absence of distal elements
        755.21
      humerus (incomplete) 755.23
umbilical artery (congenital) 747.5
ureter (congenital) 753.4
  acquired V45.74
urethra, congenital 753.8
  acquired V45.74
urinary system, part NEC, congenital 753.8
  acquired V45.74
uterus (acquired) V88.01
  with remaining cervical stump V88.02
  and cervix V88.01
  congenital 752.31
uvula (congenital) 750.26
vagina, congenital 752.45
  acquired V45.77
vas deferens (congenital) 752.89
  acquired V45.77
vein (congenital) (peripheral) NEC (*see also*
  Anomaly, peripheral vascular system)
  747.60
  brain 747.81
  great 747.49
  portal 747.49
  pulmonary 747.49
vena cava (congenital) (inferior) (superior)
  747.49
ventral horn cell 742.59
ventricular septum 745.3
vermis of cerebellum 742.2
vertebra, congenital 756.13
vulva, congenital 752.49

Absentia epileptica (*see also* Epilepsy) 345.0
Absinthemia (*see also* Dependence) 304.6
Absinthism (*see also* Dependence) 304.6
Absorbent system disease 459.89
Absorption
  alcohol, through placenta or breast milk 760.71
  antibiotics, through placenta or breast milk
    760.74
  anticonvulsants, through placenta or breast milk
    760.77
  antifungals, through placenta or breast milk
    760.74
  anti-infective, through placenta or breast milk
    760.74
  antimetabolics, through placenta or breast milk
    760.78
  chemical NEC 989.9
    specified chemical or substance—*see* Table of
      drugs and chemicals
    through placenta or breast milk (fetus or
      newborn) 760.70
      alcohol 760.71
      anticonvulsants 760.77
      antifungals 760.74
      anti-infective agents 760.74
      antimetabolics 760.78
      cocaine 760.75
      "crack" 760.75
      diethylstilbestrol *[DES]* 760.76
      hallucinogenic agents 760.73
      medicinal agents NEC 760.79
      narcotics 760.72
      obstetric anesthetic or analgesic drug 763.5
      specified agent NEC 760.79
      suspected, affecting management of
        pregnancy 655.5
  cocaine, through placenta or breast milk 760.75
  drug NEC (*see also* Reaction, drug)
    through placenta or breast milk (fetus or
      newborn) 760.70
      alcohol 760.71
      anticonvulsants 760.77
      antifungals 760.74
      anti-infective agents 760.74
      antimetabolics 760.78
      cocaine 760.75
      "crack" 760.75
      diethylstilbestrol (DES) 760.76
      hallucinogenic agents 760.73
      medicinal agents NEC 760.79
      narcotics 760.72
      obstetric anesthetic or analgesic drug 763.5
      specified agent NEC 760.79
      suspected, affecting management of
        pregnancy 655.5
  fat, disturbance 579.8
  hallucinogenic agents, through placenta or
    breast milk 760.73
  immune sera, through placenta or breast milk
    760.79
  lactose defect 271.3
  medicinal agents NEC, through placenta or
    breast milk 760.79
  narcotics, through placenta or breast milk
    760.72
  noxious substance,—*see* Absorption, chemical
  protein, disturbance 579.8
  pus or septic, general—*see* Septicemia
  quinine, through placenta or breast milk 760.74
  toxic substance—*see* Absorption, chemical
  uremic—*see* Uremia

Abstinence symptoms or syndrome
  alcohol 291.81
  drug 292.0
  neonatal 779.5
Abt-Letterer-Siwe syndrome (acute
  histiocytosis X) (M9722/3) 202.5
Abulia 799.89
Abulomania 301.6
Abuse
  adult 995.80
    emotional 995.82
    multiple forms 995.85
    neglect (nutritional) 995.84
    physical 995.81
    psychological 995.82
    sexual 995.83
  alcohol (*see also* Alcoholism) 305.0
    dependent 303.9
    non-dependent 305.0
  child 995.50
    counseling
      perpetrator
        non-parent V62.83
        parent V61.22
      victim V61.21
    emotional 995.51
    multiple forms 995.59
    neglect (nutritional) 995.52
    physical 995.54
      shaken infant syndrome 995.55
    psychological 995.51
    sexual 995.53
  drugs, nondependent 305.9

> *Note—Use the following fifth-digit*
> *subclassification with the following codes:*
> *305.0, 305.2-305.9:*
>
> *0 unspecifidd*
> *1 continuous*
> *2 episodic*
> *3 in remission*

    amphetamine type 305.7
    antidepressants 305.8
    anxiolytic 305.4
    barbiturates 305.4
    caffeine 305.9
    cannabis 305.2
    cocaine type 305.6
    hallucinogens 305.3
    hashish 305.2
    hypnotic 305.4
    inhalant 305.9
    LSD 305.3
    marijuana 305.2
    mixed 305.9
    morphine type 305.5
    opioid type 305.5
    phencyclidine (PCP) 305.9
    sedative 305.4
    specified NEC 305.9
    tranquilizers 305.4
  spouse 995.80
  tobacco 305.1
Acalcerosis 275.40
Acalcicosis 275.40
Acalculia 784.69
  developmental 315.1
Acanthocheilonemiasis 125.4
Acanthocytosis 272.5
Acanthokeratodermia 701.1

Acantholysis 701.8
  bullosa 757.39
Acanthoma (benign) (M8070/0)—*see also*
    Neoplasm, by site, benign
  malignant (M8070/3)—*see* Neoplasm, by site,
    malignant
Acanthosis (acquired) (nigricans) 701.2
  adult 701.2
  benign (congenital) 757.39
  congenital 757.39
  glycogenic
    esophagus 530.8
  juvenile 701.2
  tongue 529.8
Acanthrocytosis 272.5
Acapnia 276.3
Acarbia 276.2
Acardia 759.89
Acardiacus amorphus 759.89
Acardiotrophia 429.1
Acardius 759.89
Acariasis 133.9
  sarcoptic 133.0
Acaridiasis 133.9
Acarinosis 133.9
Acariosis 133.9
Acarodermatitis 133.9
  urticarioides 133.9
Acarophobia 300.29
Acatalasemia 277.89
Acatalasia 277.89
Acatamathesia 784.69
Acataphasia 784.59
Acathisia 781.0
  due to drugs 333.99
Acceleration, accelerated
  atrioventricular conduction 426.7
  idioventricular rhythm 427.89
Accessory (congenital)
  adrenal gland 759.1
  anus 751.5
  appendix 751.5
  atrioventricular conduction 426.7
  auditory ossicles 744.04
  auricle (ear) 744.1
  autosome(s) NEC 758.5
    21 or 22 758.0
  biliary duct or passage 751.69
  bladder 753.8
  blood vessels (peripheral) (congenital) NEC (*see
    also* Anomaly, peripheral vascular system)
    747.60
    cerebral 747.81
    coronary 746.85
  bone NEC 756.9
    foot 755.67
  breast tissue, axilla 757.6
  carpal bones 755.56
  cecum 751.5
  cervix 752.44
  chromosome(s) NEC 758.5
    13-15 758.1
    16-18 758.2
    21 or 22 758.0
    autosome(s) NEC 758.5
    D_1 758.1
    E_3 758.2
    G 758.0
    sex 758.81
  coronary artery 746.85

Accessory—*continued*
  cusp(s), heart valve NEC 746.89
    pulmonary 746.09
  cystic duct 751.69
  digits 755.00
  ear (auricle) (lobe) 744.1
  endocrine gland NEC 759.2
  external os 752.44
  eyelid 743.62
  eye muscle 743.69
  face bone(s) 756.0
  fallopian tube (fimbria) (ostium) 752.19
  fingers 755.01
  foreskin 605
  frontonasal process 756.0
  gallbladder 751.69
  genital organ(s)
    female 752.89
      external 752.49
      internal NEC 752.89
    male NEC 752.89
      penis 752.69
  genitourinary organs NEC 752.89
  heart 746.89
    valve NEC 746.89
      pulmonary 746.09
  hepatic ducts 751.69
  hymen 752.49
  intestine (large) (small) 751.5
  kidney 753.3
  lacrimal canal 743.65
  leaflet, heart valve NEC 746.89
    pulmonary 746.09
  ligament, broad 752.19
  liver (duct) 751.69
  lobule (ear) 744.1
  lung (lobe) 748.69
  muscle 756.82
  navicular of carpus 755.56
  nervous system, part NEC 742.8
  nipple 757.6
  nose 748.1
  organ or site NEC—*see* Anomaly, specified type NEC
  ovary 752.0
  oviduct 752.19
  pancreas 751.7
  parathyroid gland 759.2
  parotid gland (and duct) 750.22
  pituitary gland 759.2
  placental lobe—*see* Placenta, abnormal
  preauricular appendage 744.1
  prepuce 605
  renal arteries (multiple) 747.62
  rib 756.3
    cervical 756.2
  roots (teeth) 520.2
  salivary gland 750.22
  sesamoids 755.8
  sinus—*see* condition
  skin tags 757.39
  spleen 759.0
  sternum 756.3
  submaxillary gland 750.22
  tarsal bones 755.67
  teeth, tooth 520.1
    causing crowding 524.31
  tendon 756.89
  thumb 755.01
  thymus gland 759.2
  thyroid gland 759.2
  toes 755.02

Accessory—*continued*
  tongue 750.13
  tragus 744.1
  ureter 753.4
  urethra 753.8
  urinary organ or tract NEC 753.8
  uterus 752.2
  vagina 752.49
  valve, heart NEC 746.89
    pulmonary 746.09
  vertebra 756.19
  vocal cords 748.3
  vulva 752.49
Accident, accidental —*see also* condition
  birth NEC 767.9
  cardiovascular (*see also* Disease,
    cardiovascular) 429.2
  cerebral (*see also* Disease, cerebrovascular,
    acute) 434.91
  cerebrovascular (current) (CVA) (*see also*
    Disease, cerebrovascular, acute) 434.91
    aborted 434.91
    embolic 434.11
    healed or old V12.54
    hemorrhagic—*see* Hemorrhage, brain
    impending 435.9
    ischemic 434.91
    late effect—*see* Late effect(s) (of)
      cerebrovascular disease
    postoperative 997.02
    thrombotic 434.01
  coronary (*see also* Infarct, myocardium) 410.9
  craniovascular (*see also* Disease,
    cerebrovascular, acute) 436
  during pregnancy, to mother
    affecting fetus or newborn 760.5
  heart, cardiac (*see also* Infarct, myocardium)
    410.9
  intrauterine 779.89
  vascular—*see* Disease, cerebrovascular, acute
Accommodation
  disorder of 367.51
    drug-induced 367.89
    toxic 367.89
  insufficiency of 367.4
  paralysis of 367.51
    hysterical 300.11
  spasm of 367.53
Accouchement —*see* Delivery
Accreta placenta (without hemorrhage) 667.0
  with hemorrhage 666.0
Accretio cordis (nonrheumatic) 423.1
Accretions on teeth 523.6
Accumulation secretion, prostate 602.8
Acephalia, acephalism, acephaly 740.0
Acephalic monster 740.0
Acephalobrachia monster 759.89
Acephalocardia 759.89
Acephalocardius 759.89
Acephalochiria 759.89
Acephalochirus monster 759.89
Acephalogaster 759.89
Acephalostomus monster 759.89
Acephalothorax 759.89
Acephalus 740.0
Acetonemia 790.6
  diabetic 250.1
    due to secondary diabetes 249.1
Acetonglycosuria 982.8
Acetonuria 791.6

Achalasia 530.0
  cardia 530.0
  digestive organs congenital NEC 751.8
  esophagus 530.0
  pelvirectal 751.3
  psychogenic 306.4
  pylorus 750.5
  sphincteral NEC 564.89
Achard-Thiers syndrome (adrenogenital) 255.2
Ache (s)—*see* Pain
Acheilia 750.26
Acheiria 755.21
Achillobursitis 726.71
Achillodynia 726.71
Achlorhydria, achlorhydric 536.0
  anemia 280.9
  diarrhea 536.0
  neurogenic 536.0
  postvagotomy 564.2
  psychogenic 306.4
  secondary to vagotomy 564.2
Achloroblepsia 368.52
Achloropsia 368.52
Acholia 575.8
Acholuric jaundice (familial) (splenomegalic)
  (*see also* Spherocytosis) 282.0
  acquired 283.9
Achondroplasia 756.4
Achrestic anemia 281.8
Achroacytosis, lacrimal gland 375.00
  tuberculous (*see also* Tuberculosis) 017.3
Achroma, cutis 709.00
Achromate (congenital) 368.54
Achromatopia 368.54
Achromatopsia (congenital) 368.54
Achromia
  congenital 270.2
  parasitica 111.0
  unguium 703.8
Achylia
  gastrica 536.8
    neurogenic 536.3
    psychogenic 306.4
  pancreatica 577.1
Achylosis 536.8
Acid
  burn—*see also* Burn, by site
    from swallowing acid—*see* Burn, internal
      organs
  deficiency
    amide nicotinic 265.2
    amino 270.9
    ascorbic 267
    folic 266.2
    nicotinic (amide) 265.2
    pantothenic 266.2
  intoxication 276.2
  peptic disease 536.8
  stomach 536.8
    psychogenic 306.4
Acidemia 276.2
  arginosuccinic 270.6
  fetal
    affecting management of pregnancy 656.3
    before onset of labor, in liveborn infant 768.2
    during labor and delivery, in liveborn infant
      768.3
    intrauterine—*see* Distress, fetal 656.3
    unspecified as to time of onset, in liveborn
      infant 768.4

Acidemia—*continued*
  newborn 775.81
  pipecolic 270.7
Acidity, gastric (high) (low) 536.8
  psychogenic 306.4
Acidocytopenia 288.59
Acidocytosis 288.3
Acidopenia 288.59
Acidosis 276.2
  diabetic 250.1
    due to secondary diabetes 249.1
  fetal, affecting management of pregnancy 656.8
  fetal, affecting newborn 775.81
  kidney tubular 588.89
  lactic 276.2
  metabolic NEC 276.2
    with respiratory acidosis 276.4
      of newborn 775.81
    late, of newborn 775.7
  newborn 775.81
  renal
    hyperchloremic 588.89
    tubular (distal) (proximal) 588.89
  respiratory 276.2
    complicated by
      metabolic acidosis 276.4
        of newborn 775.81
      metabolic alkalosis 276.4
Aciduria 791.9
  arginosuccinic 270.6
  beta-aminoisobutyric (BAIB) 277.2
  glutaric
    type I 270.7
    type II (type IIA, IIB, IIC) 277.85
    type III 277.86
  glycolic 271.8
  methylmalonic 270.3
    with glycinemia 270.7
  organic 270.9
  orotic (congenital) (hereditary) (pyrimidine
    deficiency) 281.4
Acladiosis 111.8
  skin 111.8
Aclasis
  diaphyseal 756.4
  tarsoepiphyseal 756.59
Acleistocardia 745.5
Aclusion 524.4
Acmesthesia 782.0
Acne (pustular) (vulgaris) 706.1
  agminata (*see also* Tuberculosis) 017.0
  artificialis 706.1
  atrophica 706.0
  cachecticorum (Hebra) 706.1
  conglobata 706.1
  conjunctiva 706.1
  cystic 706.1
  decalvans 704.09
  erythematosa 695.3
  eyelid 706.1
  frontalis 706.0
  indurata 706.1
  keloid 706.1
  lupoid 706.0
  necrotic, necrotica 706.0
    miliaris 704.8
  neonatal 706.1
  nodular 706.1
  occupational 706.1
  papulosa 706.1
  rodens 706.0

Acne—*continued*
  rosacea 695.3
  scorbutica 267
  scrofulosorum (Bazin) (*see also* Tuberculosis)
    017.0
  summer 692.72
  tropical 706.1
  varioliformis 706.0
Acneiform drug eruptions 692.3
Acnitis (primary) (*see also* Tuberculosis) 017.0
Acomia 704.00
Acontractile bladder 344.61
Aconuresis (*see also* Incontinence) 788.30
Acosta's disease 993.2
Acousma 780.1
Acoustic —*see* condition
Acousticophobia 300.29
Acquired —*see* condition
Acquired immunodeficiency syndrome —*see*
    Human immunodeficiency virus (disease)
    (illness) (infection)
Acragnosis 781.99
Acrania (monster) 740.0
Acroagnosis 781.99
Acroangiodermatitis 448.9
Acroasphyxia, chronic 443.89
Acrobrachycephaly 756.0
Acrobystiolith 608.89
Acrobystitis 607.2
Acrocephalopolysyndactyly 755.55
Acrocephalosyndactyly 755.55
Acrocephaly 756.0
Acrochondrohyperplasia 759.82
Acrocyanosis 443.89
  newborn 770.83
Acrodermatitis 686.8
  atrophicans (chronica) 701.8
  continua (Hallopeau) 696.1
  enteropathica 686.8
  Hallopeau's 696.1
  perstans 696.1
  pustulosa continua 696.1
  recalcitrant pustular 696.1
Acrodynia 985.0
Acrodysplasia 755.55
Acrohyperhidrosis (*see also* Hyperhidrosis)
    780.8
Acrokeratosis verruciformis 757.39
Acromastitis 611.0
Acromegaly, acromegalia (skin) 253.0
Acromelalgia 443.82
Acromicria, acromikria 756.59
Acronyx 703.0
Acropachy, thyroid (*see also* Thyrotoxicosis)
    242.9
Acropachyderma 757.39
Acroparesthesia 443.89
  simple (Schultz's type) 443.89
  vasomotor (Nothnagel's type) 443.89
Acropathy thyroid (*see also* Thyrotoxicosis) 242.9
Acrophobia 300.29
Acroposthitis 607.2
Acroscleriasis (*see also* Scleroderma) 710.1
Acroscleroderma (*see also* Scleroderma) 710.1
Acrosclerosis (*see also* Scleroderma) 710.1
Acrosphacelus 785.4
Acrosphenosyndactylia 755.55
Acrospiroma, eccrine (M8402/0)—*see*
    Neoplasm, skin, benign
Acrostealgia 732.9

Acrosyndactyly (*see also* Syndactylism) 755.10
Acrotrophodynia 991.4
Actinic —*see also* condition
   cheilitis (due to sun) 692.72
      chronic NEC 692.74
      due to radiation, except from sun 692.82
   conjunctivitis 370.24
   dermatitis (due to sun) (*see also* Dermatitis, actinic) 692.70
      due to
         roentgen rays or radioactive substance 692.82
         ultraviolet radiation, except from sun 692.82
         sun NEC 692.70
   elastosis solare 692.74
   granuloma 692.73
   keratitis 370.24
   ophthalmia 370.24
   reticuloid 692.73
Actinobacillosis, general 027.8
Actinobacillus
   lignieresii 027.8
   mallei 024
   muris 026.1
Actinocutitis NEC (*see also* Dermatitis, actinic) 692.70
Actinodermatitis NEC (*see also* Dermatitis, actinic) 692.70
Actinomyces
   israelii (infection)—*see* Actinomycosis
   muris-ratti (infection) 026.1
Actinomycosis actinomycotic 039.9
   with
      pneumonia 039.1
   abdominal 039.2
   cervicofacial 039.3
   cutaneous 039.0
   pulmonary 039.1
   specified site NEC 039.8
   thoracic 039.1
Actinoneuritis 357.89
Action, heart
   disorder 427.9
      postoperative 997.1
   irregular 427.9
      postoperative 997.1
      psychogenic 306.2
Active —*see* condition
Activity decrease, functional 780.99
Acute —*see also* condition
   abdomen NEC 789.0
   gallbladder (*see also* Cholecystitis, acute) 575.0
Acyanoblepsia 368.53
Acyanopsia 368.53
Acystia 753.8
Acystinervia —*see* Neurogenic, bladder
Acystineuria —*see* Neurogenic, bladder
Adactylia, adactyly (congenital) 755.4
   lower limb (complete) (intercalary) (partial) (terminal) (*see also* Deformity, reduction, lower limb) 755.39
      meaning all digits (complete) (partial) 755.31
      transverse (complete) (partial) 755.31
   upper limb (complete) (intercalary) (partial) (terminal) (*see also* Deformity, reduction, upper limb) 755.29
      meaning all digits (complete) (partial) 755.21
      transverse (complete) (partial) 755.21
Adair-Dighton syndrome (brittle bones and blue sclera, deafness) 756.51

Adamantinoblastoma (M9310/0)—*see* Ameloblastoma
Adamantinoma (M9310/0)—*see* Ameloblastoma
Adamantoblastoma (M9310/0)—*see* Ameloblastoma
Adams-Stokes (-Morgagni) disease or syndrome (syncope with heart block) 426.9
Adaptation reaction (*see also* Reaction, adjustment) 309.9
Addiction —*see also* Dependence
   absinthe 304.6
   alcoholic (ethyl) (methyl) (wood) 303.9
      complicating pregnancy, childbirth, or puerperium 648.4
         affecting fetus or newborn 760.71
      suspected damage to fetus affecting management of pregnancy 655.4
   drug (*see also* Dependence) 304.9
   ethyl alcohol 303.9
   heroin 304.0
   hospital 301.51
   methyl alcohol 303.9
   methylated spirit 303.9
   morphine (-like substances) 304.0
   nicotine 305.1
   opium 304.0
   tobacco 305.1
   wine 303.9
Addison's
   anemia (pernicious) 281.0
   disease (bronze) (primary adrenal insufficiency) 255.41
      tuberculous (*see also* Tuberculosis) 017.6
   keloid (morphea) 701.0
   melanoderma (adrenal cortical hypofunction) 255.41
Addison-Biermer anemia (pernicious) 281.0
Addison-Gull disease —*see* Xanthoma
Addisonian crisis or melanosis (acute adrenocortical insufficiency) 255.41
Additional —*see also* Accessory
   chromosome(s) 758.5
      13-15 758.1
      16-18 758.2
      21 758.0
      autosome(s) NEC 758.5
      sex 758.81
Adduction contracture, hip or other joint —*see* Contraction, joint
ADEM (acute disseminated encephalomyelitis) (postinfectious) 136.9 *[323.61]*
   infectious 136.9 *[323.61]*
   noninfectious 323.81
Adenasthenia gastrica 536.0
Aden fever 061
Adenitis (*see also* Lymphadenitis) 289.3
   acute, unspecified site 683
      epidemic infectious 075
   axillary 289.3
      acute 683
      chronic or subacute 289.1
   Bartholin's gland 616.89
   bulbourethral gland (*see also* Urethritis) 597.89
   cervical 289.3
      acute 683
      chronic or subacute 289.1
   chancroid (Ducrey's bacillus) 099.0
   chronic (any lymph node, except mesenteric) 289.1
      mesenteric 289.2
   Cowper's gland (*see also* Urethritis) 597.89

Adenitis——*continued*
  epidemic, acute 075
  gangrenous 683
  gonorrheal NEC 098.89
  groin 289.3
    acute 683
    chronic or subacute 289.1
  infectious 075
  inguinal (region) 289.3
    acute 683
    chronic or subacute 289.1
  lymph gland or node, except mesenteric 289.3
    acute 683
    chronic or subacute 289.1
    mesenteric (acute) (chronic) (nonspecific)
      (subacute) 289.2
    mesenteric (acute) (chronic) (nonspecific)
      (subacute) 289.2
    due to Pasteurella multocida (P. septica) 027.2
  parotid gland (suppurative) 527.2
  phlegmonous 683
  salivary duct or gland (any) (recurring)
    (suppurative) 527.2
  scrofulous (*see also* Tuberculosis) 017.2
  septic 289.3
  Skene's duct or gland (*see also* Urethritis)
    597.89
  strumous, tuberculous (*see also* Tuberculosis)
    017.2
  subacute, unspecified site 289.1
  sublingual gland (suppurative) 527.2
  submandibular gland (suppurative) 527.2
  submaxillary gland (suppurative) 527.2
  suppurative 683
  tuberculous—*see* Tuberculosis, lymph gland
  urethral gland (*see also* Urethritis) 597.89
  venereal NEC 099.8
  Wharton's duct (suppurative) 527.2
Adenoacanthoma (M8570/3)—*see* Neoplasm, by
  site, malignant
Adenoameloblastoma (M9300/0) 213.1
  upper jaw (bone) 213.0
Adenocarcinoma (M8140/3)—*see also*
  Neoplasm, by site, malignant

> *Note—The list of adjectival modifiers below is
> not exhaustive. A description of
> adenocarcinoma that does not appear in this list
> should be coded in the same manner as
> carcinoma with that description. Thus, "mixed
> acidophil-basophil adenocarcinoma," should be
> coded in the same manner as "mixed
> acidophil-basophil carcinoma," which appears
> in the list under "Carcinoma."*
>
> *Except where otherwise indicated, the
> morphological varieties of adenocarcinoma in
> the list below should be coded by site as for
> "Neoplasm, malignant."*

  with
    apocrine metaplasia (M8573/3)
    cartilaginous (and osseous) metaplasia
      (M8571/3)
    osseous (and cartilaginous) metaplasia
      (M8571/3)
    spindle cell metaplasia (M8572/3)
    squamous metaplasia (M8570/3)
  acidophil (M8280/3)
    specified site—*see* Neoplasm, by site,
      malignant
    unspecified site 194.3

Adenocarcinoma— *continued*
  acinar (M8550/3)
  acinic cell (M8550/3)
  adrenal cortical (M8370/3) 194.0
  alveolar (M8251/3)
  and
    epidermoid carcinoma, mixed (M8560/3)
    squamous cell carcinoma, mixed (M8560/3)
  apocrine (M8401/3)
    breast—*see* Neoplasm, breast, malignant
    specified site NEC—*see* Neoplasm, skin,
      malignant
    unspecified site 173.99
  basophil (M8300/3)
    specified site—*see* Neoplasm, by site,
      malignant
    unspecified site 194.3
    bile duct type (M8160/3)
    sliver 155.1
    specified site NEC—*see* Neoplasm, by site,
      malignant
    unspecified site 155.1
  bronchiolar (M8250/3)—*see* Neoplasm, lung,
    malignant
  ceruminous (M8420/3) 173.29
  chromophobe (M8270/3)
    specified site—*see* Neoplasm, by site,
      malignant
    unspecified site 194.3
  clear cell (mesonephroid type) (M8310/3)
  colloid (M8480/3)
  cylindroid type (M8200/3)
  diffuse type (M8145/3)
    pecified site—*see* Neoplasm, by site,
      malignant
    unspecified site 151.9
  duct (infiltrating) (M8500/3)
    with Paget's disease (M8541/3)—*see*
      Neoplasm, breast, malignant
    specified site—*see* Neoplasm, by site,
      malignant
    unspecified site 174.9
  embryonal (M9070/3)
  endometrioid (M8380/3)—*see* Neoplasm, by
    site, malignant
  eosinophil (M8280/3)
    specified site—*see* Neoplasm, by site,
      malignant
    unspecified site 194.3
  follicular (M8330/3)
    and papillary (M8340/3) 193
    moderately differentiated type (M8332/3) 193
    pure follicle type (M8331/3) 193
    specified site—*see* Neoplasm, by site,
      malignant
    trabecular type (M8332/3) 193
    unspecified type 193
    well differentiated type (M8331/3) 193
  gelatinous (M8480/3)
  granular cell (M8320/3)
  Hürthle cell (M8290/3) 193
  in
    adenomatous
      polyp (M8210/3)
      polyposis coli (M8220/3) 153.9
    polypoid adenoma (M8210/3)
    tubular adenoma (M8210/3)
    villous adenoma (M8261/3)
  infiltrating duct (M8500/3)
    with Paget's disease (M8541/3)—*see*
      Neoplasm, breast, malignant

Adenocarcinoma—*continued*
  specified site—*see* Neoplasm, by site,
    malignant
  unspecified site 174.9
  inflammatory (M8530/3)
  specified site—*see* Neoplasm, by site,
    malignant
  unspecified site 174.9
  in situ (M8140/2)—*see* Neoplasm, by site, in
    situ
  intestinal type (M8144/3)
  specified site—*see* Neoplasm, by site,
    malignant
  unspecified site 151.9
  intraductal (noninfiltrating) (M8500/2)
    papillary (M8503/2)
    specified site—*see* Neoplasm, by site, in situ
    unspecified site 233.0
  specified site—*see* Neoplasm, by site, in situ
  unspecified site 233.0
  islet cell (M8150/3)
    and exocrine, mixed (M8154/3)
    specified site—*see* Neoplasm, by site,
      malignant
    unspecified site 157.9
    pancreas 157.4
    specified site NEC—*see* Neoplasm, by site,
      malignant
    unspecified site 157.4
  lobular (M8520/3)
  specified site—*see* Neoplasm, by site,
    malignant
  unspecified site 174.9
  medullary (M8510/3)
  mesonephric (M9110/3)
  mixed cell (M8323/3)
  mucinous (M8480/3)
  mucin-producing (M8481/3)
  mucoid (M8480/3)—*see also* Neoplasm, by site,
    malignant
    cell (M8300/3)
    specified site—*see* Neoplasm, by site,
      malignant
    unspecified site 194.3
  nonencapsulated sclerosing (M8350/3) 193
  oncocytic (M8290/3)
  oxyphilic (M8290/3)
  papillary (M8260/3)
    and follicular (M8340/3) 193
    intraductal (noninfiltrating) (M8503/2)
    specified site—*see* Neoplasm, by site, in situ
    unspecified site 233.0
    serous (M8460/3)
    specified site—*see* Neoplasm, by site,
      malignant
    unspecified site 183.0
  papillocystic (M8450/3)
  specified site—*see* Neoplasm, by site,
    malignant
  unspecified site 183.0
  pseudomucinous (M8470/3)
  specified site—*see* Neoplasm, by site,
    malignant
  unspecified site 183.0
  renal cell (M8312/3) 189.0
  sebaceous (M8410/3)
  serous (M8441/3)—*see also* Neoplasm, by site,
    malignant
    papillary
    specified site—*see* Neoplasm, by site,
      malignant
    unspecified site 183.0

Adenocarcinoma—*continued*
  signet ring cell (M8490/3)
  superficial spreading (M8143/3)
  sweat gland (M8400/3)—*see* Neoplasm, skin,
    malignant
  trabecular (M8190/3)
  tubular (M8211/3)
  villous (M8262/3)
  water-clear cell (M8322/3) 194.1
Adenofibroma (M9013/0)
  clear cell (M8313/0)—*see* Neoplasm, by site,
    benign
  endometrioid (M8381/0) 220
    borderline malignancy (M8381/1) 236.2
    malignant (M8381/3) 183.0
  mucinous (M9015/0)
    specified site—*see* Neoplasm, by site, benign
    unspecified site 220
  prostate 600.20
    with other lower urinary tract symptoms
      (LUTS) 600.21
    with urinary
      obstruction 600.21
      retention 600.21
  serous (M9014/0)
    specified site—*see* Neoplasm, by site, benign
    unspecified site 220
  specified site—*see* Neoplasm, by site, benign
  unspecified site 220
Adenofibrosis
  breast 610.2
  endometrioid 617.0
Adenoiditis 474.01
  acute 463
  chronic 474.01
    with chronic tonsillitis 474.02
Adenoids (congenital) (of nasal fossa) 474.9
  hypertrophy 474.12
  vegetations 474.2
Adenolipomatosis (symmetrical) 272.8
Adenolymphoma (M8561/0)
  specified site—*see* Neoplasm, by site, benign
  unspecified site 210.2
Adenoma (sessile) (M8140/0)—*see also*
  Neoplasm, by site, benign

> *Note—Except where otherwise indicated, the morphological varieties of adenoma in the list below should be coded by site as for "Neoplasm, benign."*

  acidophil (M8280/0)
    specified site—*see* Neoplasm, by site, benign
    unspecified site 227.3
  acinar (cell) (M8550/0)
  acinic cell (M8550/0)
  adrenal (cortex) (cortical) (functioning)
    (M8370/0) 227.0
    clear cell type (M8373/0) 227.0
    compact cell type (M8371/0) 227.0
    glomerulosa cell type (M8374/0) 227.0
    heavily pigmented variant (M8372/0) 227.0
    mixed cell type (M8375/0) 227.0
  alpha cell (M8152/0)
    pancreas 211.7
    specified site NEC—*see* Neoplasm, by site,
      benign
    unspecified site 211.7
  alveolar (M8251/0)
  apocrine (M8401/0)
    breast 217

Adenoma—*continued*
   specified site NEC—*see* Neoplasm, skin,
      benign
   unspecified site 216.9
  basal cell (M8147/0)
  basophil (M8300/0)
   specified site—*see* Neoplasm, by site, benign
   unspecified site 227.3
  beta cell (M8151/0)
   pancreas 211.7
   specified site NEC—*see* Neoplasm, by site,
      benign
   unspecified site 211.7
  bile duct (M8160/0) 211.5
  black (M8372/0) 227.0
  bronchial (M8140/1) 235.7
   carcinoid type (M8240/3)—*see* Neoplasm,
      lung, malignant
   cylindroid type (M8200/3)—*see* Neoplasm,
      lung, malignant
  ceruminous (M8420/0) 216.2
  chief cell (M8321/0) 227.1
   chromophobe (M8270/0)
   (specified site—*see* Neoplasm, by site, benign
   unspecified site 227.3
  clear cell (M8310/0)
  colloid (M8334/0)
   specified site—*see* Neoplasm, by site, benign
   unspecified site 226
  cylindroid type, bronchus (M8200/3)—*see*
      Neoplasm, lung, malignant
  duct (M8503/0)
  embryonal (M8191/0)
  endocrine, multiple (M8360/1)
   single specified site—*see* Neoplasm, by site,
      uncertain behavior
   two or more specified sites 237.4
   unspecified site 237.4
  endometrioid (M8380/0)—*see also* Neoplasm,
      by site, benign
   borderline malignancy (M8380/1)—*see*
      Neoplasm, by site, uncertain behavior
  eosinophil (M8280/0)
   specified site—*see* Neoplasm, by site, benign
   unspecified site 227.3
  fetal (M8333/0)
   specified site—*see* Neoplasm, by site, benign
   unspecified site 226
  follicular (M8330/0)
   specified site—*see* Neoplasm, by site, benign
   unspecified site 226
  hepatocellular (M8170/0) 211.5
  Hürthle cell (M8290/0) 226
  intracystic papillary (M8504/0)
  islet cell (functioning) (M8150/0)
   pancreas 211.7
   specified site NEC—*see* Neoplasm, by site,
      benign
   unspecified site 211.7
  liver cell (M8170/0) 211.5
  macrofollicular (M8334/0)
   specified site NEC—*see* Neoplasm, by site,
      benign
   unspecified site 226
  malignant, malignum (M8140/3)—*see*
      Neoplasm, by site, malignant
  mesonephric (M9110/0)
  microfollicular (M8333/0)
   specified site—*see* Neoplasm, by site, benign
   unspecified site 226
  mixed cell (M8323/0)

Adenoma—*continued*
  monomorphic (M8146/0)
  mucinous (M8480/0)
  mucoid cell (M8300/0)
   specified site—*see* Neoplasm, by site, benign
   unspecified site 227.3
  multiple endocrine (M8360/1)
   single specified site—*see* Neoplasm, by site,
      uncertain behavior
   two or more specified sites 237.4
   unspecified site 237.4
  nipple (M8506/0) 217
  oncocytic (M8290/0)
  oxyphilic (M8290/0)
  papillary (M8260/0)—*see also* Neoplasm, by
      site, benign
   intracystic (M8504/0)
  papillotubular (M8263/0)
  Pick's tubular (M8640/0)
   specified site—*see* Neoplasm, by site, benign
   unspecified site
    female 220
    male 222.0
  pleomorphic (M8940/0)
  polypoid (M8210/0)
  prostate (benign) 600.20
   with
    other lower urinary tract symptoms (LUTS)
      600.21
    urinary
     obstruction 600.21
     retention 600.21
  rete cell 222.0
  sebaceous, sebaceum (gland) (senile)
    (M8410/0)—*see also* Neoplasm, skin,
    benign
   disseminata 759.5
  Sertoli cell (M8640/0)
   specified site—*see* Neoplasm, by site, benign
   unspecified site
    female 220
    male 222.0
  skin appendage (M8390/0)—*see* Neoplasm,
    skin, benign
  sudoriferous gland (M8400/0)—*see* Neoplasm,
    skin, benign
  sweat gland or duct (M8400/0)—*see* Neoplasm,
    skin, benign
  testicular (M8640/0)
   specified site—*see* Neoplasm, by site, benign
   unspecified site
    female 220
    male 222.0
  thyroid 226
  trabecular (M8190/0)
  tubular (M8211/0)—*see also* Neoplasm, by site,
    benign
   papillary (M8460/3)
   Pick's (M8640/0)
    specified site—*see* Neoplasm, by site, benign
    unspecified site
     female 220
     male 222.0
  tubulovillous (M8263/0)
  villoglandular (M8263/0)
  villous (M8261/1)—*see* Neoplasm, by site,
    uncertain behavior
  water-clear cell (M8322/0) 227.1
  wolffian duct (M9110/0)

Adenomatosis (M8220/0)
  endocrine (multiple) (M8360/1)
    single specified site—*see* Neoplasm, by site,
      uncertain behavior
    two or more specified sites 237.4
    unspecified site 237.4
  erosive of nipple (M8506/0) 217
  pluriendocrine—*see* Adenomatosis, endocrine
  pulmonary (M8250/1) 235.7
    malignant (M8250/3)—*see* Neoplasm, lung,
      malignant
  specified site—*see* Neoplasm, by site, benign
  unspecified site 211.3
Adenomatous
  cyst, thyroid (gland)—*see* Goiter, nodular
  goiter (nontoxic) (*see also* Goiter, nodular)
    241.9
  toxic or with hyperthyroidism 242.3
Adenomyoma (M8932/0)—*see also* Neoplasm,
  by site, benign
  prostate 600.20
    with
      other lower urinary tract symptoms (LUTS)
        600.21
      urinary
        obstruction 600.21
        retention 600.21
Adenomyometritis 617.0
Adenomyosis (uterus) (internal) 617.0
Adenopathy (lymph gland) 785.6
  inguinal 785.6
  mediastinal 785.6
  mesentery 785.6
  syphilitic (secondary) 091.4
    tracheobronchial 785.6
  tuberculous (*see also* Tuberculosis) 012.1
    primary, progressive 010.8
  tuberculous (*see also* Tuberculosis, lymph
    gland) 017.2
    tracheobronchial 012.1
    primary, progressive 010.8
Adenopharyngitis 462
Adenophlegmon 683
Adenosalpingitis 614.1
Adenosarcoma (M8960/3) 189.0
Adenosclerosis 289.3
Adenosis
  breast (sclerosing) 610.2
  vagina, congenital 752.49
Adentia (complete) (partial) (*see also* Absence,
  teeth) 520.0
Adherent
  labium (minus) 624.4
  pericardium (nonrheumatic) 423.1
    rheumatic 393
  placenta 667.0
    with hemorrhage 666.0
  prepuce 605
  scar (skin) NEC 709.2
  tendon in scar 709.2
Adhesion(s), adhesive
  (postinfectional)(postoperative)
  abdominal (wall) (*see also* Adhesions,
    peritoneum) 568.0
  amnion to fetus 658.8
    affecting fetus or newborn 762.8
  appendix 543.9
  arachnoiditis—*see* Meningitis
  auditory tube (Eustachian) 381.89
  bands—*see also* Adhesions, peritoneum
    cervix 622.3
    uterus 621.5

Adhesion(s)—*continued*
  bile duct (any) 576.8
  bladder (sphincter) 596.89
  bowel (*see also* Adhesions, peritoneum) 568.0
  cardiac 423.1
    rheumatic 398.99
  cecum (*see also* Adhesions, peritoneum) 568.0
  cervicovaginal 622.3
    congenital 752.49
    postpartal 674.8
    old 622.3
  cervix 622.3
  clitoris 624.4
  colon (*see also* Adhesions, peritoneum) 568.0
  common duct 576.8
  congenital—*see also* Anomaly, specified type
    NEC
    fingers (*see also* Syndactylism, fingers)
      755.11
    labium (majus) (minus) 752.49
    omental, anomalous 751.4
    ovary 752.0
    peritoneal 751.4
    toes (*see also* Syndactylism, toes) 755.13
    tongue (to gum or roof of mouth) 750.12
  conjunctiva (acquired) (localized) 372.62
    congenital 743.63
    extensive 372.63
  cornea—*see* Opacity, cornea
  cystic duct 575.8
  diaphragm (*see also* Adhesions, peritoneum)
    568.0
  due to foreign body—*see* Foreign body
  duodenum (*see also* Adhesions, peritoneum)
    568.0
    with obstruction 537.3
  ear, middle—*see* Adhesions, middle ear
  epididymis 608.89
  epidural—*see* Adhesions, meninges
  epiglottis 478.79
  Eustachian tube 381.89
  eyelid 374.46
    postoperative 997.99
      surgically created V45.69
  gallbladder (*see also* Disease, gallbladder) 575.8
  globe 360.89
  heart 423.1
    rheumatic 398.99
  ileocecal (coil) (*see also* Adhesions,
    peritoneum) 568.0
  ileum (*see also* Adhesions, peritoneum) 568.0
  intestine (postoperative) (*see also* Adhesions,
    peritoneum) 568.0
    with obstruction 560.81
      with hernia—*see also* Hernia, by site, with
        obstruction
      gangrenous—*see* Hernia, by site, with
        gangrene
  intra-abdominal (*see also* Adhesions,
    peritoneum) 568.0
  iris 364.70
    to corneal graft 996.79
  joint (*see also* Ankylosis) 718.5
  kidney 593.89
  labium (majus) (minus), congenital 752.49
  liver 572.8
  lung 511.0
  mediastinum 519.3
  meninges 349.2
    cerebral (any) 349.2
      congenital 742.4
    congenital 742.8

Adhesion(s)—*continued*
  spinal (any) 349.2
    congenital 742.59
    tuberculous (cerebral) (spinal) (*see also*
      Tuberculosis, meninges) 013.0
  mesenteric (*see also* Adhesions, peritoneum)
    568.0
  middle ear (fibrous) 385.10
    drum head 385.19
      to
        incus 385.11
        promontorium 385.13
        stapes 385.12
    specified NEC 385.19
  nasal (septum) (to turbinates) 478.19
  nerve NEC 355.9
    spinal 355.9
      root 724.9
        cervical NEC 723.4
        lumbar NEC 724.4
        lumbosacral 724.4
        thoracic 724.4
  ocular muscle 378.60
  omentum (*see also* Adhesions, peritoneum)
    568.0
  organ or site, congenital NEC—*see* Anomaly,
    specified type NEC
  ovary 614.6
    congenital (to cecum, kidney, or omentum)
      752.0
  parauterine 614.6
  parovarian 614.6
  pelvic (peritoneal)
    female 614.6
    male (*see also* Adhesions, peritoneum) 568.0
    postpartal (old) 614.6
    tuberculous (*see also* Tuberculosis) 016.9
  penis to scrotum (congenital) 752.69
  periappendiceal (*see also* Adhesions,
    peritoneum) 568.0
  pericardium (nonrheumatic) 423.1
    rheumatic 393
    tuberculous (*see also* Tuberculosis) 017.9
      [420.0]
  pericholecystic 575.8
  perigastric (*see also* Adhesions, peritoneum)
    568.0
  periovarian 614.6
  periprostatic 602.8
  perirectal (*see also* Adhesions, peritoneum)
    568.0
  perirenal 593.89
  peritoneum, peritoneal (fibrous) (postoperative)
    568.0
    with obstruction (intestinal) 560.81
      with hernia—*see also* Hernia, by site, with
        obstruction
        gangrenous—*see* Hernia, by site, with
          gangrene
    duodenum 537.3
    congenital 751.4
    female, (postoperative) (postinfective) 614.6
    pelvic, female 614.6
    pelvic, male 568.0
    postpartal, pelvic 614.6
    to uterus 614.6
  peritubal 614.6
  periureteral 593.89
  periuterine 621.5
  perivesical 596.89
  perivesicular (seminal vesicle) 608.89

Adhesion(s)—*continued*
  pleura, pleuritic 511.0
    tuberculous (*see also* Tuberculosis, pleura)
      012.0
  pleuropericardial 511.0
  postoperative (gastrointestinal tract) (*See also*
    Adhesions, peritoneum) 568.0
    eyelid 997.99
      surgically created V45.69
    urethra 598.2
  postpartal, old 624.4
  preputial, prepuce 605
  pulmonary 511.0
  pylorus (*see also* Adhesions, peritoneum) 568.0
  Rosenmüller's fossa 478.29
  sciatic nerve 355.0
  seminal vesicle 608.89
  shoulder (joint) 726.0
  sigmoid flexure (*see also* Adhesions,
    peritoneum) 568.0
  spermatic cord (acquired) 608.89
    congenital 752.89
  spinal canal 349.2
    nerve 355.9
      root 724.9
        cervical NEC 723.4
        lumbar NEC 724.4
        lumbosacral 724.4
        thoracic 724.4
  stomach (*see also* Adhesions, peritoneum) 568.0
  subscapular 726.2
  tendonitis 726.90
    shoulder 726.0
  testicle 608.89
  tongue (congenital) (to gum or roof of mouth)
    750.12
    acquired 529.8
  trachea 519.19
  tubo-ovarian 614.6
  tunica vaginalis 608.89
  ureter 593.89
  uterus 621.5
    to abdominal wall 614.6
      in pregnancy or childbirth 654.4
        affecting fetus or newborn 763.89
  vagina (chronic) (postoperative) (postradiation)
    623.2
  vaginitis (congenital) 752.49
  vesical 596.89
  vitreomacular adhesion 379.27
  vitreous 379.29
Adie (-Holmes) syndrome (tonic pupillary
  reaction) 379.46
Adiponecrosis neonatorum 778.1
Adiposa dolorosa 272.8
Adiposalgia 272.8
Adiposis 278.0
  cerebralis 253.8
  dolorosa 272.8
  tuberosa simplex 272.8
Adiposity 278.02
  heart (*see also* Degeneration, myocardial) 429.1
  localized 278.1
Adiposogenital dystrophy 253.8
Adjustment
  prosthesis or other device—*see* Fitting of
  reaction—*see* Reaction, adjustment
Administration, prophylactic
  antibiotics, long term V58.62
    short term use—*omit code*
  antitoxin, any V07.2

Administration—*continued*
  antivenin V07.2
  chemotherapeutic agent NEC V07.39
  chemotherapy NEC V07.39
  diphtheria antitoxin V07.2
  fluoride V07.31
  gamma globulin V07.2
  immune sera (gamma globulin) V07.2
  passive immunization agent V07.2
  RhoGAM V07.2
Admission (encounter)
  as organ donor—*see* Donor
  by mistake V68.9
  for
    adequacy testing (for)
      hemodialysis V56.31
      peritoneal dialysis V56.32
    adjustment (of)
      artificial
        arm (complete) (partial) V52.0
        eye V52.2
        leg (complete) (partial) V52.1
      brain neuropacemaker V53.02
      breast
        implant V52.4
          exchange (different material) (different
            size) V52.4
        prosthesis V52.4
      cardiac device V53.39
        defibrillator, automatic implantable (with
          synchronous cardiac pacemaker)
          V53.32
        pacemaker V53.31
          carotid sinus V53.39
      catheter
        non-vascular V58.82
        vascular V58.81
      cerebral ventricle (communicating) shunt
        V53.01
      colostomy belt V53.5
      contact lenses V53.1
      cystostomy device V53.6
      dental prosthesis V52.3
      device, unspecified type V53.90
        abdominal V53.59
        cardiac V53.39
          defibrillator, automatic implantable (with
            synchronous cardiac pacemaker)
            V53.32
          pacemaker V53.31
            carotid sinus V53.39
        cerebral ventricle (communicating) shunt
          V53.01
        gastrointestinal NEC V53.59
        insulin pump V53.91
        intestinal V53.50
        nervous system V53.09
        orthodontic V53.4
        other device V53.99
        prosthetic V52.9
          breast V52.4
          dental V52.3
          eye V52.2
          specified type NEC V52.8
        special senses V53.09
        substitution
          auditory V53.09
          nervous system V53.09
          visual V53.09
        urinary V53.6

Admission—*continued*
  for —*continued*
    adjustment (of)—*continued*
      dialysis catheter
        extracorporeal V56.1
        peritoneal V56.2
      diaphragm (contraceptive) V25.02
      gastric lap band V53.51
      gastrointestinal applicance and device NEC
        V53.59
      growth rod V54.02
      hearing aid V53.2
      ileostomy device V53.5
      intestinal appliance and device V53.50
      neuropacemaker (brain) (peripheral nerve)
        (spinal cord) V53.02
      orthodontic device V53.4
      orthopedic (device) V53.7
        brace V53.7
        cast V53.7
        shoes V53.7
      pacemaker
        brain V53.02
        cardiac V53.31
        carotid sinus V53.39
        peripheral nerve V53.02
        spinal cord V53.02
      prosthesis V52.9
        arm (complete) (partial) V52.0
        breast V52.4
        dental V52.3
        eye V52.2
        leg (complete) (partial) V52.1
        specified type NEC V52.8
      spectacles V53.1
      wheelchair V53.8
    adoption referral or proceedings V68.89
    aftercare (*see also* Aftercare) V58.9
      cardiac pacemaker V53.31
      chemotherapy (oral) (intravenous) V58.11
      dialysis
        extracorporeal (renal) V56.0
        peritoneal V56.8
        renal V56.0
      fracture (*see also* Aftercare, fracture) V54.9
      medical NEC V58.89
      organ transplant V58.44
      orthopedic V54.9
        following explantation of joint prosthesis
          (for joint prosthesis insertion) (staged
          procedure) V54.82
        specified type NEC V54.89
      pacemaker device
        brain V53.02
        cardiac V53.31
        carotid sinus V53.39
        nervous system V53.02
        spinal cord V53.02
      postoperative NEC V58.49
        wound closure, planned V58.41
      postpartum
        immediately after delivery V24.0
        routine follow-up V24.2
      postradiation V58.0
      radiation therapy V58.0
      removal of
        non-vascular catheter V58.82
        vascular catheter V58.81
      specified NEC V58.89
        removal of vascular catheter V58.81
      surgical NEC V58.49
        wound closure, planned V58.41

Admission—*continued*
  for —*continued*
  antineoplastic
    chemotherapy (oral) (intravenous) V58.11
    immunotherapy V58.12
  assisted reproductive fertility procedure cycle
    V26.81
  artificial insemination V26.1
  attention to artificial opening (of) V55.9
    artificial vagina V55.7
    colostomy V55.3
    cystostomy V55.5
    enterostomy V55.4
    gastrostomy V55.1
    ileostomy V55.2
    jejunostomy V55.4
    nephrostomy V55.6
    specified site NEC V55.8
      intestinal tract V55.4
      urinary tract V55.6
    tracheostomy V55.0
    ureterostomy V55.6
    urethrostomy V55.6
  battery replacement
    cardiac pacemaker V53.31
  blood typing V72.86
    Rh typing V72.86
  boarding V65.0
  breast
    augmentation or reduction V50.1
    implant exchange (different material)
      (different size) V52.4
    reconstruction following mastectomy V51.0
    removal
      prophylactic V50.41
      tissue expander without synchronous
        insertion of permanent implant V52.4
  change of
    cardiac pacemaker (battery) V53.31
    carotid sinus pacemaker V53.39
    catheter in artificial opening—*see* Attention
      to, artificial, opening
    drains V58.49
    dressing
      wound V58.30
        nonsurgical V58.30
        surgical V58.31
    fixation device
      external V54.89
      internal V54.01
    Kirschner wire V54.89
    neuropacemaker device (brain) (peripheral
      nerve) (spinal cord) V53.02
    nonsurgical wound dressing V58.30
    pacemaker device
      brain V53.02
      cardiac V53.31
      carotid sinus V53.39
      nervous system V53.02
    plaster cast V54.89
    splint, external V54.89
    Steinmann pin V54.89
    surgical wound dressing V58.31
    traction device V54.89
    wound packing V58.30
      nonsurgical V58.30
      surgical V58.31
  checkup only V70.0
  chemotherapy, (oral) (intravenous)
    antineoplastic V58.11
  circumcision, ritual or routine (in absence of
    medical indication) V50.2

Admission—*continued*
  for —*continued*
  clinical research investigation (control)
    (normal comparison) (participant) V70.7
  closure of artificial opening—*see* Attention to,
    artificial, opening
  contraceptive
    counseling V25.09
      emergency V25.03
      postcoital V25.03
    management V25.9
      specified type NEC V25.8
  convalescence following V66.9
    chemotherapy V66.2
    psychotherapy V66.3
    radiotherapy V66.1
    surgery V66.0
    treatment (for) V66.5
      combined V66.6
      fracture V66.4
      mental disorder NEC V66.3
      specified condition NEC V66.5
  cosmetic surgery NEC V50.1
    breast reconstruction following mastectomy
      V51.0
    following healed injury or operation V51.8
  counseling (*see also* Counseling) V65.40
    without complaint or sickness V65.49
    contraceptive management V25.09
      emergency V25.03
      postcoital V25.03
    dietary V65.3
    exercise V65.41
    fertility preservation (prior to cancer
      therapy) (prior to surgical removal of
      gonads) V26.42
    for
      nonattending third party V65.19
      pediatric
        pre-adoption visit for adoptive parent(s)
          V65.11
        pre-birth visit for expectant parent(s)
          V65.11
      victim of abuse
        child V61.21
        partner or spouse V61.11
    genetic V26.33
    gonorrhea V65.45
    HIV V65.44
    human immunodeficiency virus V65.44
    injury prevention V65.43
    insulin pump training V65.46
    natural family planning
      procreative V26.41
      to avoid pregnancy V25.04
    procreative management V26.49
      using natural family planning V26.41
    sexually transmitted disease NEC V65.45
      HIV V65.44
    specified reason NEC V65.49
    substance use and abuse V65.42
    syphilis V65.45
    victim of abuse
      child V61.21
      partner or spouse V61.11
  desensitization to allergens V07.1
  dialysis V56.0
    catheter
      fitting and adjustment
        extracorporeal V56.1
        peritoneal V56.2

Admission—*continued*
  for —*continued*
    dialysis—*continued*
      removal or replacement
        extracorporeal V56.1
        peritoneal V56.2
      extracorporeal (renal) V56.0
      peritoneal V56.8
      renal V56.0
    dietary surveillance and counseling V65.3
    drug monitoring, therapeutic V58.83
    ear piercing V50.3
    elective surgery V50.9
      breast
        augmentation or reduction V50.1
        removal, prophylactic V50.41
        reconstruction following mastectomy
          V51.0
      circumcision, ritual or routine (in absence of
        medical indication) V50.2
      cosmetic NEC V50.1
        breast reconstruction following mastecomy
          V51.0
        following healed injury or operation V51.8
      ear piercing V50.3
      face-lift V50.1
      hair transplant V50.0
      plastic
        breast reconstruction following mastecomy
          V51.0
        cosmetic NEC V50.1
        following healed injury or operation V51.8
      prophylactic organ removal V50.49
        breast V50.41
        ovary V50.42
      repair of scarred tissue (following healed
        injury or operation) V51.8
      specified type NEC V50.8
    end-of-life care V66.7
    examination (*see also* Examination) V70.9
      administrative purpose NEC V70.3
      adoption V70.3
      allergy V72.7
      antibody response V72.61
      at health care facility V70.0
      athletic team V70.3
      camp V70.3
      cardiovascular, preoperative V72.81
      clinical research investigation (control)
        (participant) V70.7
      dental V72.2
      developmental testing (child) (infant) V20.2
      donor (potential) V70.8
      driver's license V70.3
      ear V72.19
      employment V70.5
      eye V72.0
      follow-up (routine)—*see* Examination,
        follow-up
      for admission to
        old age home V70.3
        school V70.3
      general V70.9
        specified reason NEC V70.8
      gynecological V72.31
      health supervision
        child (over 28 days old) V20.2
        infant (over 28 days old) V20.2
        newborn
          8 to 28 days old V20.32
          under 8 days old V20.31

Admission—*continued*
  for —*continued*
    examination—*continued*
      hearing V72.19
        following failed hearing screening V72.11
      immigration V70.3
      infant
        8 to 28 days old V20.32
        over 28 days old, routine V20.2
        under 8 days old V20.31
      insurance certification V70.3
      laboratory V72.60
        ordered as part of a routine general
          medical examination V72.62
        pre-operative V72.63
        pre-procedural V72.63
        specified NEC V72.69
      marriage license V70.3
      medical (general) (*see also* Examination,
        medical) V70.9
      medicolegal reasons V70.4
      naturalization V70.3
      pelvic (annual) (periodic) V72.31
      postpartum checkup V24.2
      pregnancy (possible) (unconfirmed) V72.40
        negative result V72.41
        positive result V72.42
      preoperative V72.84
        cardiovascular V72.81
        respiratory V72.82
        specified NEC V72.83
      preprocedural V72.84
        cardiovascular V72.81
        general physical V72.83
        respiratory V72.82
        specified NEC V72.83
      prior to chemotherapy V72.83
      prison V70.3
      psychiatric (general) V70.2
        requested by authority V70.1
      radiological NEC V72.5
      respiratory, preoperative V72.82
      school V70.3
      screening—*see* Screening
      skin hypersensitivity V72.7
      specified type NEC V72.85
      sport competition V70.3
      vision V72.0
      well baby and child care V20.2
    exercise therapy V57.1
    face-lift, cosmetic reason V50.1
    fertility preservation (prior to cancer therapy)
      (prior to surgical removal of gonads)
      V26.82
    fitting (of)
      artificial
        arm (complete) (partial) V52.0
        eye V52.2
        leg (complete) (partial) V52.1
      biliary drainage tube V58.82
      brain neuropacemaker V53.02
      breast V52.4
        implant V50.1
        prosthesis V52.4
      cardiac pacemaker V53.31
      catheter
        non-vascular V58.82
        vascular V58.81
      cerebral ventricle (communicating) shunt
        V53.01
      chest tube V58.82

Admission—*continued*
 for —*continued*
  fitting (of)—*continued*
   colostomy belt V53.5
   contact lenses V53.1
   cystostomy device V53.6
   dental prosthesis V52.3
   device, unspecified type V53.90
    abdominal V53.59
    cerebral ventricle (communicating) shunt V53.01
    gastrointestinal NEC V53.59
    insulin pump V53.91
    intestinal V53.50
    intrauterine contraceptive
     insertion V25.11
     removal V25.12
      and reinsertion V25.13
     replacement V25.13
    nervous system V53.09
    orthodontic V53.4
    other device V53.99
    prosthetic V52.9
     breast V52.4
     dental V52.3
     eye V52.2
    special senses V53.09
    substitution
     auditory V53.09
     nervous system V53.09
     visual V53.09
   diaphragm (contraceptive) V25.02
   fistula (sinus tract) drainage tube V58.82
   gastric lap band V53.51
   gastrointestinal appliance and device NEC V53.59
   growth rod V54.02
   hearing aid V53.2
   ileostomy device V53.5
   intestinal appliance and device V53.50
   intrauterine contraceptive device
    insertion V25.11
    removal V25.12
     and reinsertion V25.13
    replacement V25.13
   neuropacemaker (brain) (peripheral nerve) (spinal cord) V53.02
   orthodontic device V53.4
   orthopedic (device) V53.7
    brace V53.7
    cast V53.7
    shoes V53.7
   pacemaker
    brain V53.02
    cardiac V53.31
    carotid sinus V53.39
    spinal cord V53.02
   pleural drainage tube V58.82
   portacath V58.81
   prosthesis V52.9
    arm (complete) (partial) V52.0
    breast V52.4
    dental V52.3
    eye V52.2
    leg (complete) (partial) V52.1
    specified type NEC V52.8
   spectacles V53.1
   wheelchair V53.8
  follow-up examination (routine) (following) V67.9
   cancer chemotherapy V67.2
   chemotherapy V67.2

Admission—*continued*
 for —*continued*
  follow-up examination—*continued*
   high-risk medication NEC V67.51
   injury NEC V67.59
   psychiatric V67.3
   psychotherapy V67.3
   radiotherapy V67.1
   specified surgery NEC V67.09
    surgery V67.00
   treatment (for) V67.9
    combined V67.6
    fracture V67.4
    involving high-risk medication NEC V67.51
    mental disorder V67.3
    specified NEC V67.59
   vaginal pap smear V67.01
  hair transplant, for cosmetic reason V50.0
  health advice, education, or instruction V65.4
  hearing conservation and treatment V72.12
  hormone replacement therapy (postmenopausal) V07.4
  hospice care V66.7
  immunizations (childhood) appropriate for age V20.2
  immunotherapy, antineoplastic V58.12
  in vitro fertilization cycle V26.81
  insertion (of)
   intrauterine contraceptive device V25.11
   subdermal implantable contraceptive V25.5
  insulin pump titration V53.91
  insulin pump training V65.46
  intrauterine device
   insertion V25.11
   removal V25.12
    and reinsertion V25.13
   management V25.42
   replacement V25.13
  investigation to determine further disposition V63.8
  isolation V07.0
  issue of
   disability examination certificate V68.01
   medical certificate NEC V68.09
   repeat prescription NEC V68.1
    contraceptive device NEC V25.49
  kidney dialysis V56.0
  lengthening of growth rod V54.02
  mental health evaluation V70.2
   requested by authority V70.1
  natural family planning counseling and advice
   procreative V26.41
   to avoid pregnancy V25.04
  nonmedical reason NEC V68.89
  nursing care evaluation V63.8
  observation (without need for further medical care) (*see also* Observation) V71.9
   accident V71.4
   alleged rape or seduction V71.5
   criminal assault V71.6
   following accident V71.4
    at work V71.3
   foreign body ingestion V71.89
   growth and development variations, childhood V21.0
   inflicted injury NEC V71.6
   ingestion of deleterious agent or foreign body V71.89
   injury V71.6
   malignant neoplasm V71.1
   mental disorder V71.09

Admission—*continued*
for —*continued*
  observation—*continued*
    newborn—*see* Observation, suspected
      condition, newborn
    rape V71.5
    specified NEC V71.89
    suspected
      abuse V71.81
      accident V71.4
        at work V71.3
      benign neoplasm V71.89
      cardiovascular V71.7
      disorder V71.9
      exposure
        anthrax V71.82
        biological agent NEC V71.83
        SARS V71.83
      heart V71.7
      inflicted injury NEC V71.6
      malignant neoplasm V71.1
      maternal and fetal problem not found
        amniotic cavity and membrane V89.01
        cervical shortening V89.05
        fetal anomaly V89.03
        fetal growth V89.04
        oligohydramnios V89.01
        other specified NEC V89.09
        placenta V89.02
        polyhydramnios V89.01
      mental NEC V71.09
      neglect V71.81
      specified condition NEC V71.89
      tuberculosis V71.2
    tuberculosis V71.2
  occupational therapy V57.21
  organ transplant, donor—*see* Donor
  ovary, ovarian removal, prophylactic V50.42
  palliative care V66.7
  Papanicolaou smear
    cervix V76.2
      for suspected malignant neoplasm V76.2
        no disease found V71.1
      routine, as part of gynecological
        examination V72.31
      to confirm findings of recent normal smear
        following initial abnormal smear
        V72.32
    vaginal V76.47
      following hysterectomy for malignant
        condition V67.01
  passage of sounds or bougie in artificial
    opening—*see* Attention to, artificial, opening
  paternity testing V70.4
  peritoneal dialysis V56.8
  physical therapy NEC V57.1
  plastic surgery
    breast reconstruction following mastectomy
      V51.0
    cosmetic NEC V50.1
    following healed injury or operation V51.8
  postmenopausal hormone replacement therapy
    V07.4
  postpartum observation
    immediately after delivery V24.0
    routine follow-up V24.2
  poststerilization (for restoration) V26.0
  procreative management V26.9
    assisted reproductive fertility procedure
      cycle V26.81
    in vitro fertilization cycle V26.81
    specified type NEC V26.89

Admission—*continued*
for —*continued*
  prophylactic
    administration of
      antibiotics, long-term V58.62
        short term use—*omit code*
      antitoxin, any V07.2
      antivenin V07.2
      chemotherapeutic agent NEC V07.39
      chemotherapy NEC V07.39
      diphtheria antitoxin V07.2
      fluoride V07.31
      gamma globulin V07.2
      immune sera (gamma globulin) V07.2
      RhoGAM V07.2
      tetanus antitoxin V07.2
    breathing exercises V57.0
    chemotherapy NEC V07.39
      fluoride V07.31
    measure V07.9
      specified type NEC V07.8
    organ removal V50.49
      breast V50.41
      ovary V50.42
  psychiatric examination (general) V70.2
    requested by authority V70.1
  radiation management V58.0
  radiotherapy V58.0
  reconstruction following mastectomy V51.0
  reforming of artificial opening—*see* Attention
    to, artificial, opening
  rehabilitation V57.9
    multiple types V57.89
    occupational V57.21
    orthoptic V57.4
    orthotic V57.81
    physical NEC V57.1
    specified type NEC V57.89
    speech (-language) V57.3
    vocational V57.22
  removal of
    breast tissue expander without synchronous
      insertion of permanent implant V52.4
    cardiac pacemaker V53.31
    cast (plaster) V54.89
    catheter from artificial opening—*see*
      Attention to, artificial, opening
    cerebral ventricle (communicating) shunt
      V53.01
    cystostomy catheter V55.5
    device
      cerebral ventricle (communicating) shunt
        V53.01
      fixation
        external V54.89
        internal V54.01
      intrauterine contraceptive V25.12
      traction, external V54.89
    drains V58.49
    dressing
      wound V58.30
        nonsurgical V58.30
        surgical V58.31
    fixation device
      external V54.89
      internal V54.01
    intrauterine contraceptive device V25.12
    Kirschner wire V54.89
    neuropacemaker (brain) (peripheral nerve)
      (spinal cord) V53.02
    nonsurgical wound dressing V58.30

Admission—*continued*
  for —*continued*
    removal of—*continued*
      orthopedic fixation device
        external V54.89
        internal V54.01
      pacemaker device
        brain V53.02
        cardiac V53.31
        carotid sinus V53.39
        nervous system V53.02
      plaster cast V54.89
      plate (fracture) V54.01
      rod V54.01
      screw (fracture) V54.01
      splint, traction V54.89
      staples V58.32
      Steinmann pin V54.89
      subdermal implantable contraceptive V25.43
      surgical wound dressing V58.31
      sutures V58.32
      traction device, external V54.89
      ureteral stent V53.6
      wound packing V58.30
        nonsurgical V58.30
        surgical V58.31
    repair of scarred tissue (following healed
      injury or operation) V51.8
    replacement of intrauterine contraceptive
      device V25.13
    reprogramming of cardiac pacemaker V53.31
    respirator (ventilator) dependence
      during
        mechanical failure V46.14
        power failure V46.12
      for weaning V46.13
    restoration of organ continuity
      (poststerilization) (tuboplasty) (vasoplasty)
      V26.0
    Rh typing V72.86
    routine infant and child vision and hearing
      testing V20.2
    sensitivity test—*see also* Test, skin
      allergy NEC V72.7
      bacterial disease NEC V74.9
      Dick V74.8
      Kveim V82.89
      Mantoux V74.1
      mycotic infection NEC V75.4
      parasitic disease NEC V75.8
      Schick V74.3
      Schultz-Charlton V74.8
    social service (agency) referral or evaluation
      V63.8
    speech(-language) therapy V57.3
    sterilization V25.2
    suspected disorder (ruled out) (without need
      for further care)—*see* Observation
    terminal care V66.7
    tests only—*see* Test
    therapeutic drug monitoring V58.83
    therapy
      blood transfusion, without reported
        diagnosis V58.2
      breathing exercises V57.0
      chemotherapy, antineoplastic V58.11
        prophylactic NEC V07.39
          fluoride V07.31

Admission—*continued*
  for —*continued*
    therapy—*continued*
      dialysis (intermittent) (treatment)
        extracorporeal V56.0
        peritoneal V56.8
        renal V56.0
        specified type NEC V56.8
      exercise (remedial) NEC V57.1
        breathing V57.0
      immunotherapy, antineoplastic V58.12
      long-term (current) (prophylactic) drug use
        NEC V58.69
        antibiotics V58.62
          short-term use—*omit code*
        anticoagulants V58.61
        anti-inflammatories, non-steroidal
          (NSAID) V58.64
        antiplatelets V58.63
        antithrombotics V58.63
        aspirin V58.66
        bisphosphonates V58.68
        high-risk medications NEC V58.69
        insulin V58.67
        methadone for pain control V58.69
        opiate analgesic V58.69
        steroids V58.65
      occupational V57.21
      orthoptic V57.4
      physical NEC V57.1
      radiation V58.0
      speech(-language) V57.3
      vocational V57.22
    toilet or cleaning
      of artificial opening — *see* Attention to,
        artificial, opening
      of non-vascular catheter V58.82
      of vascular catheter V58.81
    treatment
      measure V07.9
        specified type NEC V07.8
    tubal ligation V25.2
    tuboplasty for previous sterilization V26.0
    ultrasound, routine fetal V28.3
    vaccination, prophylactic (against)
      arthropod-borne virus, viral NEC V05.1
        disease NEC V05.1
        encephalitis V05.0
      Bacille Calmette Guérin (BCG) V03.2
      BCG V03.2
      chickenpox V05.4
      cholera alone V03.0
        with typhoid-paratyphoid (cholera + TAB)
          V06.0
      common cold V04.7
      dengue V05.1
      diphtheria alone V03.5
      diphtheria-tetanus-pertussis (DTP) (DTaP)
        V06.1
        with
          poliomyelitis (DTP + polio) V06.3
          typhoid-paratyphoid (DTP + TAB)
            V06.2
      diphtheria-tetanus [Td] [DT] without
        pertussis V06.5
      disease (single) NEC V05.9
        bacterial NEC V03.9
          specified type NEC V03.89
        combinations NEC V06.9
          specified type NEC V06.8
        specified type NEC V05.8
        viral NEC V04.89

Admission—*continued*
  for —*continued*
    vaccination—*continued*
      encephalitis, viral, arthropod-borne V05.0
      Hemophilus influenzae, type B [Hib]
        V03.81
      hepatitis, viral V05.3
      human papillomavirus (HPV) V04.89
      immune sera (gamma globulin) V07.2
      influenza V04.81
        with
          Streptococcus pneumoniae
            [pneumococcus] V06.6
      Leishmaniasis V05.2
      measles alone V04.2
      measles-mumps-rubella (MMR) V06.4
      mumps alone V04.6
        with measles and rubella (MMR) V06.4
      not done because of contraindication V64.09
      pertussis alone V03.6
      plague V03.3
      pneumonia V03.82
      poliomyelitis V04.0
        with diphtheria-tetanus-pertussis (DTP +
          polio) V06.3
      rabies V04.5
      respiratory syncytial virus (RSV) V04.82
      rubella alone V04.3
        with measles and mumps (MMR) V06.4
      smallpox V04.1
      specified type NEC V05.8
        Streptococcus pneumoniae
          [pneumococcus] V03.82
        with
          influenza V06.6
      tetanus toxoid alone V03.7
        with diphtheria [Td] [DT] V06.5
        and pertussis (DTP) (DTaP) V06.1
      tuberculosis (BCG) V03.2
      tularemia V03.4
      typhoid alone V03.1
        with diphtheria-tetanus-pertussis (TAB +
          DTP) V06.2
      typhoid-paratyphoid alone (TAB) V03.1
      typhus V05.8
      varicella V05.4
      viral encephalitis, arthropod-borne V05.0
      viral hepatitis V05.3
      yellow fever V04.4
    vasectomy V25.2
    vasoplasty for previous sterilization V26.0
    vision examination V72.0
    vocational therapy V57.22
    waiting period for admission to other facility
      V63.2
      undergoing social agency investigation
        V63.8
    well baby and child care V20.2
    x-ray of chest
      for suspected tuberculosis V71.2
      routine V72.5
Adnexitis (suppurative) (*see also*
  Salpingo-oophoritis) 614.2
Adolescence NEC V21.2
Adoption
  agency referral V68.89
  examination V70.3
  held for V68.89
Adrenal gland —*see* condition
Adrenalism 255.9
  tuberculous (*see also* Tuberculosis) 017.6

Adrenalitis, adrenitis 255.8
  meningococcal hemorrhagic 036.3
Adrenarche, precocious 259.1
Adrenocortical syndrome 255.2
Adrenogenital syndrome (acquired) (congenital)
  255.2
  iatrogenic, fetus or newborn 760.79
Adrenoleukodystrophy 277.86
  neonatal 277.86
  x-linked 277.86
Adrenomyeloneuropathy 277.86
Adventitious bursa —*see* Bursitis
Adynamia (episodica) (hereditary) (periodic)
  359.3
Adynamic
  ileus or intestine (*see also* ileus) 560.1
  ureter 753.22
Aeration lung imperfect, newborn 770.5
Aerobullosis 993.3
Aerocele —*see* Embolism, air
Aerodermectasia
  subcutaneous (traumatic) 958.7
    surgical 998.81
  surgical 998.81
Aerodontalgia 993.2
Aeroembolism 993.3
Aerogenes capsulatus infection (*see also*
  Gangrene, gas) 040.0
Aero-otitis media 993.0
Aerophagy, aerophagia 306.4
  psychogenic 306.4
Aerosinusitis 993.1
Aerotitis 993.0
Affection, affections —*see also* Disease
  sacroiliac (joint), old 724.6
  shoulder region NEC 726.2
Afibrinogenemia 286.3
  acquired 286.6
  congenital 286.3
  postpartum 666.3
African
  sleeping sickness 086.5
  tick fever 087.1
  trypanosomiasis 086.5
    Gambian 086.3
    Rhodesian 086.4
Aftercare V58.9
  amputation stump V54.89
  artificial openings—*see* Attention to, artificial,
    opening
  blood transfusion without reported diagnosis
    V58.2
  breathing exercise V57.0
  cardiac device V53.39
    defibrillator, automatic implantable (with
      synchronous cardiac pacemaker) V53.32
    pacemaker V53.31
      carotid sinus V53.39
  carotid sinus pacemaker V53.39
  cerebral ventricle (communicating) shunt
    V53.01
  chemotherapy (oral) (intravenous) session
    (adjunctive) (maintenance) V58.11
  defibrillator, automatic implantable cardiac
    (with synchronous cardiac pacemaker)
    V53.32
  exercise (remedial) (therapeutic) V57.1
    breathing V57.0
  extracorporeal dialysis (intermittent) (treatment)
    V56.0

Aftercare—*continued*
  following surgery NEC V58.49
    wound closure, planned V58.41
    for
      injury V58.43
      neoplasm V58.42
      organ transplant V58.44
      trauma V58.43
    joint
      explantation of prosthesis (staged procedure)
        V54.82
      replacement V54.81
    of
      circulatory system V58.73
      digestive system V58.75
      genital organs V58.76
      genitourinary system V58.76
      musculoskeletal system V58.78
      nervous system V58.72
      oral cavity V58.75
      respiratory system V58.74
      sense organs V58.71
      skin V58.77
      subcutaneous tissue V58.77
      teeth V58.75
      urinary system V58.76
    spinal —*see* Aftercare, following surgery, of,
      specified body system
  fracture V54.9
    healing V54.89
      pathologic
        ankle V54.29
        arm V54.20
          lower V54.22
          upper V54.21
        finger V54.29
        foot V54.29
        hand V54.29
        hip V54.23
        leg V54.24
          lower V54.26
          upper V54.25
        pelvis V54.29
        specified site NEC V54.29
        toe(s) V54.29
        vertebrae V54.27
        wrist V54.29
      traumatic
        ankle V54.19
        arm V54.10
          lower V54.12
          upper V54.11
        finger V54.19
        foot V54.19
        hand V54.19
        hip V54.13
        leg V54.14
          lower V54.16
          upper V54.15
        pelvis V54.19
        specified site NEC V54.19
        toe(s) V54.19
        vertebrae V54.17
        wrist V54.19
    removal of
      external fixation device V54.89
      internal fixation device V54.01
    specified care NEC V54.89
  gait training V57.1
    for use of artificial limb(s) V57.81
  internal fixation device V54.09

Aftercare—*continued*
  involving
    dialysis (intermittent) (treatment)
      extracorporeal V56.0
      peritoneal V56.8
      renal V56.0
    gait training V57.1
      for use of artificial limb(s) V57.81
    growth rod
      adjustment V54.02
      lengthening V54.02
    internal fixation device V54.09
    orthoptic training V57.4
    orthotic training V57.81
    radiotherapy session V58.0
    removal of
      drains V58.49
      dressings
        wound V58.30
          nonsurgical V58.30
          surgical V58.31
      fixation device
        external V54.89
        internal V54.01
      fracture plate V54.01
      nonsurgical wound dressing V58.30
      pins V54.01
      plaster cast V54.89
      rods V54.01
      screws V54.01
      staples V58.32
      surgical wound dressings V58.31
      sutures V58.32
      traction device, external V54.89
      wound packing V58.30
        nonsurgical V58.30
        surgical V58.31
  neuropacemaker (brain) (peripheral nerve)
    (spinal cord) V53.02
  occupational therapy V57.21
  orthodontic V58.5
  orthopedic V54.9
    change of external fixation or traction device
      V54.8
    following joint
      explantation of prosthesis (staged procedure)
        V54.82
      replacement V54.81
    internal fixation device V54.09
    removal of fixation device
      external V54.89
      internal V54.01
    specified care NEC V54.89
  orthoptic training V57.4
  orthotic training V57.81
  pacemaker
    brain V53.02
    cardiac V53.31
    carotid sinus V53.39
    peripheral nerve V53.02
    spinal cord V53.02
  peritoneal dialysis (intermittent) (treatment)
    V56.8
  physical therapy NEC V57.1
    breathing exercises V57.0
  radiotherapy session V58.0
  rehabilitation procedure V57.9
    breathing exercises V57.0
    multiple types V57.89
    occupational V57.21
    orthoptic V57.4

Aftercare—*continued*
  rehabilitation procedure—*continued*
    orthotic V57.81
    physical therapy NEC V57.1
    remedial exercises V57.1
    specified type NEC V57.89
    speech(-language) V57.3
    therapeutic exercises V57.1
    vocational V57.22
  renal dialysis (intermittent) (treatment) V56.0
  specified type NEC V58.89
    removal of non-vascular catheter V58.82
    removal of vascular catheter V58.81
  speech(-language) therapy V57.3
  stump, amputation V54.89
  vocational rehabilitation V57.22
After-cataract 366.50
  obscuring vision 366.53
  specified type, not obscuring vision 366.52
Agalactia 676.4
Agammaglobulinemia 279.00
  with lymphopenia 279.2
  acquired (primary) (secondary) 279.06
  Bruton's X-linked 279.04
  infantile sex-linked (Bruton's) (congenital) 279.04
  Swiss-type 279.2
Aganglionosis (bowel) (colon) 751.3
Age (old) (*see also* Senile) 797
Agenesis —*see also* Absence, by site, congenital
  acoustic nerve 742.8
  adrenal (gland) 759.1
  alimentary tract (complete) (partial) NEC 751.8
    lower 751.2
    upper 750.8
  anus, anal (canal) 751.2
  aorta 747.22
  appendix 751.2
  arm (complete) (partial) (*see also* Deformity, reduction, upper limb) 755.20
  artery (peripheral) NEC (*see also* Anomaly, peripheral vascular system) 747.60
    brain 747.81
    coronary 746.85
    pulmonary 747.31
    umbilical 747.5
  auditory (canal) (external) 744.01
  auricle (ear) 744.01
  bile, biliary duct or passage 751.61
  bone NEC 756.9
  brain 740.0
    specified part 742.2
  breast 757.6
  bronchus 748.3
  canaliculus lacrimalis 743.65
  carpus NEC (*see also* Deformity, reduction, upper limb) 755.28
  cartilage 756.9
  cecum 751.2
  cerebellum 742.2
  cervix 752.43
  chin 744.89
  cilia 743.63
  circulatory system, part NEC 747.89
  clavicle 755.51
  clitoris 752.49
  coccyx 756.13
  colon 751.2
  corpus callosum 742.2
  cricoid cartilage 748.3
  diaphragm (with hernia) 756.6

Agenesis—*continued*
  digestive organ(s) or tract (complete) (partial) NEC 751.8
    lower 751.2
    upper 750.8
  ductus arteriosus 747.89
  duodenum 751.1
  ear NEC 744.09
    auricle 744.01
    lobe 744.21
  ejaculatory duct 752.89
  endocrine (gland) NEC 759.2
  epiglottis 748.3
  esophagus 750.3
  Eustachian tube 744.24
  extrinsic muscle, eye 743.69
  eye 743.00
    adnexa 743.69
  eyelid (fold) 743.62
  face
    bones NEC 756.0
    specified part NEC 744.89
  fallopian tube 752.19
  femur NEC (*see also* Absence, femur, congenital) 755.34
  fibula NEC (*see also* Absence, fibula, congenital) 755.37
  finger NEC (*see also* Absence, finger, congenital) 755.29
  foot (complete) (*see also* Deformity, reduction, lower limb) 755.31
  gallbladder 751.69
  gastric 750.8
  genitalia, genital (organ)
    female 752.89
      external 752.49
      internal NEC 752.89
    male 752.89
      penis 752.69
  glottis 748.3
  gonadal 758.6
  hair 757.4
  hand (complete) (*see also* Deformity, reduction, upper limb) 755.21
  heart 746.89
    valve NEC 746.89
      aortic 746.89
      mitral 746.89
      pulmonary 746.01
  hepatic 751.69
  humerus NEC (*see also* Absence, humerus, congenital) 755.24
  hymen 752.49
  ileum 751.1
  incus 744.04
  intestine (small) 751.1
    large 751.2
  iris (dilator fibers) 743.45
  jaw 524.09
  jejunum 751.1
  kidney(s) (partial) (unilateral) 753.0
  labium (majus) (minus) 752.49
  labyrinth, membranous 744.05
  lacrimal apparatus (congenital) 743.65
  larynx 748.3
  leg NEC (*see also* Deformity, reduction, lower limb) 755.30
  lens 743.35
  limb (complete) (partial) (*see also* Deformity, reduction) 755.4
    lower NEC 755.30
    upper 755.20

Agenesis—*continued*
  lip 750.26
  liver 751.69
  lung (bilateral) (fissures) (lobe) (unilateral)
      748.5
  mandible 524.09
  maxilla 524.09
  metacarpus NEC 755.28
  metatarsus NEC 755.38
  muscle (any) 756.81
  musculoskeletal system NEC 756.9
  nail(s) 757.5
  neck, part 744.89
  nerve 742.8
  nervous system, part NEC 742.8
  nipple 757.6
  nose 748.1
  nuclear 742.8
  organ
    of Corti 744.05
    or site not listed—*see* Anomaly, specified type
        NEC
  osseous meatus (ear) 744.03
  ovary 752.0
  oviduct 752.19
  pancreas 751.7
  parathyroid (gland) 759.2
  patella 755.64
  pelvic girdle (complete) (partial) 755.69
  penis 752.69
  pericardium 746.89
  perineal body 756.81
  pituitary (gland) 759.2
  prostate 752.89
  pulmonary
    artery 747.31
    trunk 747.31
    vein 747.49
  punctum lacrimale 743.65
  radioulnar NEC (*see also* Absence, forearm,
      congenital) 755.25
  radius NEC (*see also* Absence, radius,
      congenital) 755.26
  rectum 751.2
  renal 753.0
  respiratory organ NEC 748.9
  rib 756.3
  roof of orbit 742.0
  round ligament 752.89
  sacrum 756.13
  salivary gland 750.21
  scapula 755.59
  scrotum 752.89
  seminal duct or tract 752.89
  septum
    atrial 745.69
    between aorta and pulmonary artery 745.0
    ventricular 745.3
  shoulder girdle (complete) (partial) 755.59
  skull (bone) 756.0
    with
      anencephalus 740.0
      encephalocele 742.0
      hydrocephalus 742.3
        with spina bifida (*see also* Spina bifida)
            741.0
      microcephalus 742.1
  spermatic cord 752.89
  spinal cord 742.59

Agenesis—*continued*
  spine 756.13
    lumbar 756.13
      isthmus 756.11
      pars articularis 756.11
  spleen 759.0
  sternum 756.3
  stomach 750.7
  tarsus NEC 755.38
  tendon 756.81
  testicular 752.89
  testis 752.89
  thymus (gland) 759.2
  thyroid (gland) 243
    cartilage 748.3
  tibia NEC (*see also* Absence, tibia, congenital)
      755.36
  tibiofibular NEC 755.35
  toe (complete) (partial) (*see also* Absence, toe,
      congenital) 755.39
  tongue 750.11
  trachea (cartilage) 748.3
  ulna NEC (*see also* Absence, ulna, congenital)
      755.27
  ureter 753.4
  urethra 753.8
  urinary tract NEC 753.8
  uterus 752.31
  uvula 750.26
  vagina (total) (partial) 752.45
  vas deferens 752.89
  vein(s) (peripheral) NEC (*see also* Anomaly,
      peripheral vascular system) 747.60
    brain 747.81
    great 747.49
    portal 747.49
    pulmonary 747.49
  vena cava (inferior) (superior) 747.49
  vermis of cerebellum 742.2
  vertebra 756.13
    lumbar 756.13
      isthmus 756.11
      pars articularis 756.11
  vulva 752.49
Ageusia (*see also* Disturbance, sensation) 781.1
Aggressiveness 301.3
Aggressive outburst (*see also* Disturbance,
    conduct) 312.0
  in children or adolescents 313.9
Aging skin 701.8
Agitated —*see* condition
Agitation 307.9
  catatonic (*see also* Schizophrenia) 295.2
Aglossia (congenital) 750.11
Aglycogenosis 271.0
Agnail (finger) (with lymphangitis) 681.02
Agnosia (body image) (tactile) 784.69
  verbal 784.69
    auditory 784.69
    developmental 315.8
    secondary to organic lesion 784.69
  visual 368.16
    object 368.16
Agoraphobia 300.22
  with panic disorder 300.21
Agrammatism 784.69
Agranulocytopenia (see also Agranulocytosis)
    288.09

Agranulocytosis (see also Neutropenia) 288.09
  chronic 288.09
  cyclical 288.02
  due to infection 288.04
  genetic 288.01
  infantile 288.01
  periodic 288.02
  pernicious 288.09
Agraphia (absolute) 784.69
  with alexia 784.61
  developmental 315.39
Agrypnia (*see also* Insomnia) 780.52
Ague (*see also* Malaria) 084.6
  brass-founders' 985.8
  dumb 084.6
  tertian 084.1
Agyria 742.2
AHTR (acute hemolytic transfusion reaction)
  —*see* Complications, transfusion
Ahumada-del Castillo syndrome (nonpuerperal
  galactorrhea and amenorrhea) 253.1
AIDS 042
AIDS-associated retrovirus (disease) (illness) 042
  infection—*see* Human immunodeficiency virus,
    infection
AIDS-associated virus (disease) (illness) 042
  infection—*see* Human immunodeficiency virus,
    infection
AIDS-like disease (illness) (syndrome) 042
AIDS-related complex 042
AIDS-related conditions 042
AIDS-related virus (disease) (illness) 042
  infection—*see* Human immunodeficiency virus,
    infection
AIDS virus (disease) (illness) 042
  infection—*see* Human immunodeficiency virus,
    infection
Ailment, heart —*see* Disease, heart
Ailurophobia 300.29
AIN I (anal intraepithelial neoplasia I)
  (histologically confirmed) 569.44
AIN II (anal intraepithelial neoplasia II)
  (histologically confirmed) 569.44
AIN III (anal intraepithelial neoplasia III)
  230.6
  anal canal 230.5
Ainhum (disease) 136.0
AIPHI (acute idiopathic pulmonary hemorrhage
  in infants (over 28 days old)) 786.31
Air
  anterior mediastinum 518.1
  compressed, disease 993.3
  embolism (any site) (artery) (cerebral) 958.0
    with
      abortion—*see* Abortion, by type, with
        embolism
      ectopic pregnancy (*see also* categories
        633.0-633.9) 639.6
      molar pregnancy (*see also* categories
        630-632) 639.6
    due to implanted device—*see* Complications,
      due to (presence of) any device, implant,
      or graft classified to 996.0-996.5 NEC
    following
      abortion 639.6
      ectopic or molar pregnancy 639.6
    infusion, perfusion, or transfusion 999.1
    in pregnancy, childbirth, or puerperium 673.0
    traumatic 958.0
  hunger 786.09
    psychogenic 306.1

Air —*continued*
  leak (lung) (pulmonary) (thorax) 512.84
    iatrogenic 512.1
    persistant 512.84
    postoperative 512.2
  rarefied, effects of—*see* Effect, adverse, high altitude
    sickness 994.6
Airplane sickness 994.6
Akathisia, acathisia 781.0
  due to drugs 333.99
  neuroleptic-induced acute 333.99
Akinesia algeria 352.6
Akiyami 100.89
Akureyri disease (epidemic neuromyasthenia) 049.8
Alacrima (congenital) 743.65
Alactasia (hereditary) 271.3
Alagille syndrome 759.89
Alalia 784.3
  developmental 315.31
    receptive-expressive 315.32
  secondary to organic lesion 784.3
Alaninemia 270.8
Alastrim 050.1
Albarrán's disease (colibacilluria) 791.9
Albers-Schönberg's disease (marble bones)
  756.52
Albert's disease 726.71
Albinism, albino (choroid) (cutaneous) (eye)
  (generalized) (isolated) (ocular)
  (oculocutaneous) (partial) 270.2
Albinismus 270.2
Albright (-Martin) (-Bantam) disease
  (pseudohypoparathyroidism) 275.49
Albright (-McCune) (-Sternberg) syndrome
  (osteitis fibrosa disseminata) 756.59
Albuminous —*see* condition
Albuminuria, albuminuric (acute) (chronic)
  (subacute) 791.0
  Bence-Jones 791.0
  cardiac 785.9
  complicating pregnancy, childbirth, or
    puerperium 646.2
    with hypertension—*see* Toxemia, of
      pregnancy
    affecting fetus or newborn 760.1
  cyclic 593.6
  gestational 646.2
  gravidarum 646.2
    with hypertension—*see* Toxemia, of
      pregnancy
    affecting fetus or newborn 760.1
  heart 785.9
  idiopathic 593.6
  orthostatic 593.6
  postural 593.6
  pre-eclamptic (mild) 642.4
    affecting fetus or newborn 760.0
    severe 642.5
      affecting fetus or newborn 760.0
  recurrent physiologic 593.6
  scarlatinal 034.1
Albumosuria 791.0
  Bence-Jones 791.0
  myelopathic (M9730/3) 203.0
Alcaptonuria 270.2
Alcohol, alcoholic
  abstinence 291.81
  acute intoxication 305.0
    with dependence 303.0

Alcohol, alcoholic—*continued*
  addiction (*see also* Alcoholism) 303.9
    maternal
      with suspected fetal damage affecting
        management of pregnancy 655.4
      affecting fetus or newborn 760.71
  amnestic disorder, persisting 291.1
  anxiety 291.89
  brain syndrome, chronic 291.2
  cardiopathy 425.5
  chronic (*see also* Alcoholism) 303.9
  cirrhosis (liver) 571.2
  delirium 291.0
    acute 291.0
    chronic 291.1
    tremens 291.0
    withdrawal 291.0
  dementia NEC 291.2
  deterioration 291.2
  drunkenness (simple) 305.0
  hallucinosis (acute) 291.3
  induced
    circadian rhythm sleep disorder 291.82
    hypersomnia 291.82
    insomnia 291.82
    mental disorder 291.9
      anxiety 291.89
      mood 291.89
      sexual 291.89
      sleep 291.82
      specified type 291.89
    parasomnia 291.82
    persisting
      amnestic disorder 291.1
      dementia 291.2
    psychotic disorder
      with
        delusions 291.5
        hallucinations 291.3
    sleep disorder 291.82
  insanity 291.9
  intoxication (acute) 305.0
    with dependence 303.0
    pathological 291.4
  jealousy 291.5
  Korsakoff's, Korsakov's, Korsakow's 291.1
  liver NEC 571.3
    acute 571.1
    chronic 571.2
  mania (acute) (chronic) 291.9
  mood 291.89
  paranoia 291.5
  paranoid (type) psychosis 291.5
  pellagra 265.2
  poisoning, accidental (acute) NEC 980.9
    specified type of alcohol—*see* Table of drugs
      and chemicals
  psychosis (*see also* Psychosis, alcoholic) 291.9
    Korsakoff's, Korsakov's, Korsakow's 291.1
    polyneuritic 291.1
    with
      delusions 291.5
      hallucinations 291.3
  related disorder 291.9
  withdrawal symptoms, syndrome NEC 291.81
    delirium 291.0
    hallucinosis 291.3

Alcoholism 303.9

Note—*Use the following fifth-digit*
subclassification with category 303:

0 *unspecified*
1 *continuous*
2 *episodic*
3 *in remission*

  with psychosis (*see also* Psychosis, alcoholic)
    291.9
  acute 303.0
  chronic 303.9
    with psychosis 291.9
  complicating pregnancy, childbirth, or
    puerperium 648.4
  affecting fetus or newborn 760.71
  history V11.3
  Korsakoff's, Korsakov's, Korsakow's 291.1
  suspected damage to fetus affecting
    management of pregnancy 655.4
Alder's anomaly or syndrome (leukocyte
    granulation anomaly) 288.2
Alder-Reilly anomaly (leukocyte granulation) 288.2
Aldosteronism (primary) 255.10
  congenital 255.10
  familial type I 255.11
  glucocorticoid-remediable 255.11
  secondary 255.14
Aldosteronoma (M8370/1) 237.2
Aldrich (-Wiskott) syndrome
    (eczema-thrombocytopenia) 279.12
Aleppo boil 085.1
Aleukemic —*see* condition
Aleukia
  congenital 288.09
  hemorrhagica 284.9
    acquired (secondary) 284.89
    congenital 284.09
    idiopathic 284.9
  splenica 289.4
Alexia (congenital) (developmental) 315.01
  secondary to organic lesion 784.61
Algoneurodystrophy 733.7
Algophobia 300.29
Alibert's disease (mycosis fungoides) (M9700/3)
    202.1
Alibert-Bazin disease (M9700/3) 202.1
Alice in Wonderland syndrome 293.89
Alienation, mental (*see also* Psychosis) 298.9
Alkalemia 276.3
Alkalosis 276.3
  metabolic 276.3
    with respiratory acidosis 276.4
  respiratory 276.3
Alkaptonuria 270.2
Allen-Masters syndrome 620.6
Allergic bronchopulmonary aspergillosis 518.6
Allergy, allergic (reaction) 995.3
  air-borne substance (*see also* Fever, hay) 477.9
    specified allergen NEC 477.8
  alveolitis (extrinsic) 495.9
    due to
      Aspergillus clavatus 495.4
      cryptostroma corticale 495.6
      organisms (fungal, thermophilic
        actinomycete, other) growing in
        ventilation (air conditioning systems)
        495.7
    specified type NEC 495.8

Allergy, allergic—*continued*
anaphylactic reaction or shock 995.0
  due to
    food—*see* Anaphylactic reaction or shock,
      due to, food
angioedema 995.1
angioneurotic edema 995.1
animal (cat) (dog) (epidermal) 477.8
  dander 477.2
  hair 477.2
arthritis (*see also* Arthritis, allergic) 716.2
asthma—*see* Asthma
bee sting (anaphylactic shock) 989.5
biological—*see* Allergy, drug
bronchial asthma—*see* Asthma
conjunctivitis (eczematous) 372.14
dander, animal (cat) (dog) 477.2
dandruff 477.8
dermatitis (venenata)—*see* Dermatitis
diathesis V15.09
drug, medicinal substance, and biological (any)
  (correct medicinal substance properly
    administered) (external) (internal) 995.27
  wrong substance given or taken NEC 977.9
    specified drug or substance—*see* Table of
      drugs and chemicals
dust (house) (stock) 477.8
eczema—*see* Eczema
endophthalmitis 360.19
epidermal (animal) 477.8
existing dental restorative material 525.66
feathers 477.8
food (any) (ingested) 693.1
  atopic 691.8
  in contact with skin 692.5
gastritis 535.4
gastroenteritis 558.3
gastrointestinal 558.3
grain 477.0
grass (pollen) 477.0
  asthma (*see also* Asthma) 493.0
  hay fever 477.0
hair, animal (cat) (dog) 477.2
hay fever (grass) (pollen) (ragweed) (tree) (*see
  also* Fever, hay) 477.9
history (of) V15.09
  to
    arachnid bite V15.06
    eggs V15.03
    food additives V15.05
    insect bite V15.06
    latex V15.07
    milk products V15.02
    nuts V15.05
      peanuts V15.01
    radiographic dye V15.08
    seafood V15.04
    specified food NEC V15.05
    spider bite V15.06
horse serum—*see* Allergy, serum
inhalant 477.9
  dust 477.8
  pollen 477.0
  specified allergen other than pollen 477.8
kapok 477.8
medicine—*see* Allergy, drug
migraine 339.00
milk protein 558.3
pannus 370.62
pneumonia 518.3

Allergy, allergic—*continued*
pollen (any) (hay fever) 477.0
  asthma (*see also* Asthma) 493.0
primrose 477.0
primula 477.0
purpura 287.0
ragweed (pollen) (Senecio jacobae) 477.0
  asthma (*see also* Asthma) 493.0
  hay fever 477.0
respiratory (*see also* Allergy, inhalant) 477.9
  due to
    drug—*see* Allergy, drug
    food—*see* Allergy, food
rhinitis (*see also* Fever, hay) 477.9
  due to food 477.1
rose 477.0
Senecio jacobae 477.0
serum (prophylactic) (therapeutic) 999.59
  anaphylactic reaction or shock 999.49
shock (anaphylactic)
  due to
    adverse effect of correct medicinal substance
      properly administered 995.0
    food—*see* Anaphylactic reaction or shock,
      due to, food
  from
    administration of blood products 999.41
    immunization 999.42
    serum NEC 999.49
sinusitis (*see also* Fever, hay) 477.9
skin reaction 692.9
  specified substance—*see* Dermatitis, due to
tree (any) (hay fever) (pollen) 477.0
  asthma (*see also* Asthma) 493.0
upper respiratory (*see also* Fever, hay) 477.9
urethritis 597.89
urticaria 708.0
vaccine—*see* Allergy, serum
Allescheriosis 117.6
Alligator skin disease (ichthyosis congenita) 757.1
acquired 701.1
Allocheiria, allochiria (*see also* Disturbance,
  sensation) 782.0
Almeida's disease (Brazilian blastomycosis) 116.1
Alopecia (atrophicans) (pregnancy) (premature)
  (senile) 704.00
adnata 757.4
areata 704.01
celsi 704.01
cicatrisata 704.09
circumscripta 704.01
congenital, congenitalis 757.4
disseminata 704.01
effluvium (telogen) 704.02
febrile 704.09
generalisata 704.09
hereditaria 704.09
marginalis 704.01
mucinosa 704.09
postinfectional 704.09
seborrheica 704.09
specific 091.82
syphilitic (secondary) 091.82
telogen effluvium 704.02
totalis 704.09
toxica 704.09
universalis 704.09
x-ray 704.09
Alper's disease 330.8
Alpha-lipoproteinemia 272.4
Alpha thalassemia 282.43
Alphos 696.1

Alpine sickness 993.2
Alport's syndrome (hereditary
 hematuria-nephropathy-deafness) 759.89
**ALPS (autoimmune lymphoproliferative
 syndrome)** 279.41
ALTE (apparent life threatening event) in
 newborn and infant 799.82
Alteration (of), altered
 awareness 780.09
  transient 780.02
 consciousness 780.09
  persistent vegetative state 780.03
  transient 780.02
 mental status 780.97
  amnesia (retrograde) 780.93
  memory loss 780.93
Alternaria (infection) 118
Alternating —*see* condition
Altitude, high (effects)—*see* Effect, adverse,
 high altitude
Aluminosis (of lung) 503
Alvarez syndrome (transient cerebral ischemia) 435.9
Alveolar capillary block syndrome 516.64
Alveolitis
 allergic (extrinsic) 495.9
  due to organisms (fungal, thermophilic
   actinomycete, other) growing in ventilation
   (air conditioning systems) 495.7
  specified type NEC 495.8
 due to
  Aspergillus clavatus 495.4
  Cryptostroma corticale 495.6
 fibrosing (chronic) (cryptogenic) (lung) 516.31
  idiopathic 516.30
  rheumatoid 714.81
 jaw 526.5
 sicca dolorosa 526.5
Alveolus, alveolar —*see* condition
Alymphocytosis (pure) 279.2
Alymphoplasia, thymic 279.2
Alzheimer's
 dementia (senile)
  with behavioral disturbance 331.0 *[294.11]*
  without behavioral disturbance 331.0 *[294.10]*
 disease or sclerosis 331.0
  with dementia—*see* Alzheimer's, dementia
Amastia (*see also* Absence, breast) 611.89
Amaurosis (acquired) (congenital) (*see also*
 Blindness) 369.00
 fugax 362.34
 hysterical 300.11
 Leber's (congenital) 362.76
 tobacco 377.34
 uremic—*see* Uremia
Amaurotic familial idiocy (infantile) (juvenile)
 (late) 330.1
Ambisexual 752.7
Amblyopia (acquired) (congenital) (partial) 368.00
 color 368.59
  acquired 368.55
 deprivation 368.02
 ex anopsia 368.00
 hysterical 300.11
 nocturnal 368.60
  vitamin A deficiency 264.5
 refractive 368.03
 strabismic 368.01
 suppression 368.01
 tobacco 377.34
 toxic NEC 377.34
 uremic—*see* Uremia

Ameba, amebic (histolytica)–*see also* Amebiasis
 abscess 006.3
  bladder 006.8
  brain (with liver and lung abscess) 006.5
  liver 006.3
   with brain abscess (and lung abscess) 006.5
   with lung abscess 006.4
  lung (with liver abscess) 006.4
   with brain abscess 006.5
  seminal vesicle 006.8
  spleen 006.8
 carrier (suspected of) V02.2
 meningoencephalitis
  due to Naegleria (gruberi) 136.29
  primary 136.29
Amebiasis NEC 006.9
 with
  brain abscess (with liver or lung abscess) 006.5
  liver abscess (without mention of brain or lung
   abscess) 006.3
  lung abscess (with liver abscess) 006.4
   with brain abscess 006.5
 acute 006.0
 bladder 006.8
 chronic 006.1
 cutaneous 006.6
 cutis 006.6
 due to organism other than Entamoeba
  histolytica 007.8
 hepatic (*see also* Abscess, liver, amebic) 006.3
 nondysenteric 006.2
 seminal vesicle 006.8
 specified
  organism NEC 007.8
  site NEC 006.8
Ameboma 006.8
Amelia 755.4
 lower limb 755.31
 upper limb 755.21
Ameloblastoma (M9310/0) 213.1
 jaw (bone) (lower) 213.1
  upper 213.0
 long bones (M9261/3)—*see* Neoplasm, bone,
  malignant
 malignant (M9310/3) 170.1
  jaw (bone) (lower) 170.1
   upper 170.0
 mandible 213.1
 tibial (M9261/3) 170.7
Amelogenesis imperfecta 520.5
 nonhereditaria (segmentalis) 520.4
Amenorrhea (primary) (secondary) 626.0
 due to ovarian dysfunction 256.8
 hyperhormonal 256.8
Amentia (*see also* Disability, intellectual) 319
 Meynert's (nonalcoholic) 294.0
  alcoholic 291.1
 nevoid 759.6
American
 leishmaniasis 085.5
 mountain tick fever 066.1
 trypanosomiasis—*see* Trypanosomiasis,
  American
Ametropia (*see also* Disorder, accommodation) 367.9
Amianthosis 501
Amimia 784.69
Amino acid
 deficiency 270.9
  anemia 281.4
 metabolic disorder (*see also* Disorder, amino
  acid) 270.9

Aminoaciduria 270.9
  imidazole 270.5
Amnesia (retrograde) 780.93
  auditory 784.69
    developmental 315.31
    secondary to organic lesion 784.69
  dissociative 300.12
  hysterical or dissociative type 300.12
  psychogenic 300.12
  transient global 437.7
Amnestic (confabulatory) syndrome 294.0
  alcohol-induced persisting 291.1
  drug-induced persisting 292.83
  posttraumatic 294.0
Amniocentesis screening (for) V28.2
  alphafetoprotein level, raised V28.1
  chromosomal anomalies V28.0
Amnion, amniotic —*see also* condition
  nodosum 658.8
Amnionitis (complicating pregnancy) 658.4
  affecting fetus or newborn 762.7
Amoral trends 301.7
Amotio retinae (*see also* Detachment, retina) 361.9
Ampulla
  lower esophagus 530.89
  phrenic 530.89
Amputation
  any part of fetus, to facilitate delivery 763.89
  cervix (supravaginal) (uteri) 622.8
    in pregnancy or childbirth 654.6
      affecting fetus or newborn 763.89
  clitoris—*see* Wound, open, clitoris
  congenital
    lower limb 755.31
    upper limb 755.21
  neuroma (traumatic)—*see also* Injury, nerve, by site
  surgical complications (late) 997.61
  penis—*see* Amputation, traumatic, penis
  status (without complication)—*see* Absence, by site, acquired
  stump (surgical)(posttraumatic)
    abnormal, painful, or with complication (late) 997.60
    healed or old NEC —*see also* Absence, by site, acquired
      lower V49.70
      upper V49.60
  traumatic (complete) (partial)

Note—"Complicated" includes traumatic amputation with delayed healing, delayed treatment, foreign body, or infection.

---

  arm 887.4
    at or above elbow 887.2
      complicated 887.3
    below elbow 887.0
      complicated 887.1
    both (bilateral) (any level(s)) 887.6
      complicated 887.7
    complicated 887.5
  finger(s) (one or both hands) 886.0
    with thumb(s) 885.0
      complicated 885.1
    complicated 886.1
  foot (except toe(s) only) 896.0
    and other leg 897.6
      complicated 897.7
    both (bilateral) 896.2
      complicated 896.3
    complicated 896.1

Amputation—*continued*
    toe(s) only (one or both feet) 895.0
      complicated 895.1
  genital organ(s) (external) NEC 878.8
    complicated 878.9
  hand (except finger(s) only) 887.0
    and other arm 887.6
      complicated 887.7
    both (bilateral) 887.6
      complicated 887.7
    complicated 887.1
    finger(s) (one or both hands) 886.0
      with thumb(s) 885.0
        complicated 885.1
      complicated 886.1
    thumb(s) (with fingers of either hand) 885.0
      complicated 885.1
  head 874.9
  late effect—*see* Late, effects (of), amputation
  leg 897.4
    and other foot 897.6
      complicated 897.7
    at or above knee 897.2
      complicated 897.3
    below knee 897.0
      complicated 897.1
    both (bilateral) 897.6
      complicated 897.7
    complicated 897.5
  lower limb(s) except toe(s)—*see* Amputation, traumatic, leg
  nose—*see* Wound, open, nose
  penis 878.0
    complicated 878.1
  sites other than limbs—*see* Wound, open, by site
  thumb(s) (with finger(s) of either hand) 885.0
    complicated 885.1
  toe(s) (one or both feet) 895.0
    complicated 895.1
  upper limb(s)—*see* Amputation, traumatic, arm
Amputee (bilateral) (old) —*see also* Absence, by site, acquired V49.70
Amusia 784.69
  developmental 315.39
  secondary to organic lesion 784.69
Amyelencephalus 740.0
Amyelia 742.59
Amygdalitis— *see* Tonsillitis
Amygdalolith 474.8
Amyloid disease or degeneration 277.30
  heart 277.39 *[425.7]*
Amyloidosis (familial) (general) (generalized) (genetic) (primary) 277.30
  with lung involvement 277.39 *[517.8]*
  cardiac, hereditary 277.39
  heart 277.39 *[425.7]*
  nephropathic 277.39 *[583.81]*
  neuropathic (Portuguese) (Swiss) 277.39 *[357.4]*
  pulmonary 277.39 *[517.8]*
  secondary 277.39
  systemic, inherited 277.39
Amylopectinosis (brancher enzyme deficiency) 271.0
Amylophagia 307.52
Amyoplasia, congenita 756.89
Amyotonia 728.2
  congenita 358.8

Amyotrophia, amyotrophy, amyotrophic 728.2
  congenita 756.89
  diabetic 250.6 *[353.5]*
    due to secondary diabetes 249.6 *[353.5]*
  lateral sclerosis (syndrome) 335.20
  neuralgic 353.5
  sclerosis (lateral) 335.20
  spinal progressive 335.21
Anacidity
  gastric 536.0
  psychogenic 306.4
Anaerosis of newborn 770.88
Analbuminemia 273.8
Analgesia (*see also* Anesthesia) 782.0
Analphalipoproteinemia 272.5
Anaphylactic reaction or shock (correct
  substance properly administered) 995.0
  due to
    administration of blood and blood products
      999.41
    chemical - *see* Table of Drugs and Chemicals
    correct medicinal substance properly
      administered 995.0
    drug or medicinal substance
      correct substance properly administered
        995.0
      overdose or wrong substance given or taken
        977.9
      specified drug - *see* Table of Drugs and
        Chemicals
    following sting(s) 989.5
    food 995.60
      additives 995.66
      crustaceans 995.62
      eggs 995.68
      fish 995.65
      fruits 995.63
      milk products 995.67
      nuts (tree) 995.64
      peanuts 995.61
      seeds 995.64
      specified NEC 995.69
      tree nuts 995.64
      vegetables 995.63
    immunization 999.42
    overdose or wrong substance given or taken
      977.9
    specified drug—*see* Table of drugs and
      chemicals
    serum NEC 999.49
  following sting(s) 989.5
  purpura 287.0
  serum NEC 999.49
Anaphylactoid reaction or shock —*see*
  Anaphylactic reaction or shock
Anaphylaxis —*see* Anaphylactic reaction or
  shock
Anaplasia, cervix 622.10
Anaplasmosis, human 082.49
Anarthria 784.51
Anarthritic rheumatoid disease 446.5
Anasarca 782.3
  cardiac (*see also* Failure, heart) 428.0
  fetus or newborn 778.0
  lung 514
  nutritional 262
  pulmonary 514
  renal (*see also* Nephrosis) 581.9
Anaspadias 752.62

Anastomosis
  aneurysmal—*see* Aneurysm
  arteriovenous, congenital NEC (*see also*
    Anomaly, arteriovenous) 747.60
    ruptured, of brain (*see also* Hemorrhage,
      subarachnoid) 430
  intestinal 569.89
    complicated NEC 997.49
      involving urinary tract 997.5
  retinal and choroidal vessels 743.58
    acquired 362.17
Anatomical narrow angle (glaucoma) 365.02
Ancylostoma (infection) (infestation) 126.9
  americanus 126.1
  braziliense 126.2
  caninum 126.8
  ceylanicum 126.3
  duodenale 126.0
  Necator americanus 126.1
Ancylostomiasis (intestinal) 126.9
  Ancylostoma
    americanus 126.1
    caninum 126.8
    ceylanicum 126.3
    duodenale 126.0
  braziliense 126.2
  Necator americanus 126.1
Anders' disease or syndrome (adiposis tuberosa
  simplex) 272.8
Andersen's glycogen storage disease 271.0
Anderson's disease 272.7
Andes disease 993.2
Andrews' disease (bacterid) 686.8
Androblastoma (M8630/1)
  benign (M8630/0)
    specified site—*see* Neoplasm, by site, benign
    unspecified site
      female 220
      male 222.0
  malignant (M8630/3)
    specified site—*see* Neoplasm, by site,
      malignant
    unspecified site
      female 183.0
      male 186.9
  specified site—*see* Neoplasm, by site, uncertain
    behavior
  tubular (M8640/0)
    with lipid storage (M8641/0)
      specified site—*see* Neoplasm, by site,
        benign
      unspecified site
        female 220
      male 222.0
    specified site—*see* Neoplasm, by site, benign
    unspecified site
      female 220
      male 222.0
  unspecified site
    female 236.2
    male 236.4
Android pelvis 755.69
  with disproportion (fetopelvic) 653.3
    affecting fetus or newborn 763.1
    causing obstructed labor 660.1
      affecting fetus or newborn 763.1
Anectasis, pulmonary (newborn or fetus) 770.5

Anemia 285.9
in
    chronic illness NEC 285.29
    chronic kidney disease 285.21
    end-stage renal disease 285.21
    neoplastic disease 285.22
with
    disorder of
        anaerobic glycolysis 282.3
        pentose phosphate pathway 282.2
    koilonychia 280.9
    6-phosphogluconic dehydrogenase deficiency
        282.2
achlorhydric 280.9
achrestic 281.8
Addison's (pernicious) 281.0
Addison-Biermer (pernicious) 281.0
agranulocytic 288.09
amino acid deficiency 281.4
antineoplastic chemotherapy induced 285.3
aplastic 284.9
    acquired (secondary) 284.89
    congenital 284.01
    constitutional 284.01
    due to
        antineoplastic chemotherapy 284.89
        chronic systemic disease 284.89
        drugs 284.89
        infection 284.89
        radiation 284.89
    idiopathic 284.9
    myxedema 244.9
    of or complicating pregnancy 648.2
    red cell (acquired) (adult) (with thymoma)
        284.81
        congenital 284.01
        pure 284.01
    specified type NEC 284.89
    toxic (paralytic) 284.89
aregenerative 284.9
    congenital 284.01
asiderotic 280.9
atypical (primary) 285.9
autohemolysis of Selwyn and Dacie (type I)
    282.2
autoimmune hemolytic 283.0
Baghdad Spring 282.2
Balantidium coli 007.0
Biermer's (pernicious) 281.0
blood loss (chronic) 280.0
    acute 285.1
bothriocephalus 123.4
brickmakers' (*see also* Ancylostomiasis) 126.9
cerebral 437.8
childhood 282.9
chlorotic 280.9
chronica congenita aregenerativa 284.01
chronic 285.9
    blood loss 280.0
    hemolytic 282.9
      idiopathic 283.9
    simple 281.9
combined system disease NEC 281.0 *[336.2]*
    due to dietary deficiency 281.1 *[336.2]*
complicating pregnancy or childbirth 648.2
congenital (following fetal blood loss) 776.5
    aplastic 284.01
    due to isoimmunization NEC 773.2
    Heinz-body 282.7
    hereditary hemolytic NEC 282.9

Anemia—*continued*
congenital—*continued*
    nonspherocytic
        Type I 282.2
        Type II 282.3
    pernicious 281.0
    spherocytic (*see also* Spherocytosis) 282.0
Cooley's (erythroblastic) 282.44
crescent—*see* Disease, sickle-cell
cytogenic 281.0
Dacie's (nonspherocytic)
    Type I 282.2
    Type II 282.3
Davidson's (refractory) 284.9
deficiency 281.9
    2, 3 diphosphoglycurate mutase 282.3
    2, 3 PG 282.3
    6-PGD 282.2
    6-phosphogluronic dehydrogenase 282.2
    amino acid 281.4
    combined B_{12} and folate 281.3
    enzyme, drug-induced (hemolytic) 282.2
    erythrocytic glutathione 282.2
    folate 281.2
        dietary 281.2
        drug-induced 281.2
    folic acid 281.2
        dietary 281.2
        drug-induced 281.2
    G-6-PD 282.2
    GGS-R 282.2
    glucose-6-phosphate dehydrogenase (G-6-PD)
        282.2
    glucose-phosphate isomerase 282.3
    glutathione peroxidase 282.2
    glutathione reductase 282.2
    glyceraldehyde phosphate dehydrogenase
        282.3
    GPI 282.3
    G SH 282.2
    hexokinase 282.3
    iron (Fe) 280.9
        specified NEC 280.8
    nutritional 281.9
        with
            poor iron absorption 280.9
            specified deficiency NEC 281.8
        due to inadequate dietary iron intake 280.1
        specified type NEC 281.8
    of or complicating pregnancy 648.2
    pentose phosphate pathway 282.2
    PFK 282.3
    phosphofructo-aldolase 282.3
    phosphofructokinase 282.3
    phosphoglycerate kinase 282.3
    PK 282.3
    protein 281.4
    pyruvate kinase (PK) 282.3
        TPI 282.3
        triosephosphate isomerase 282.3
        vitamin B_{12} NEC 281.1
            dietary 281.1
            pernicious 281.0
Diamond-Blackfan (congenital hypoplastic)
    284.01
dibothriocephalus 123.4
dimorphic 281.9
diphasic 281.8
diphtheritic 032.89
Diphyllobothrium 123.4

Anemia—*continued*
  drepanocytic (*see also* Disease, sickle-cell)
    282.60
  due to
    antineoplastic chemotherapy 285.3
    blood loss (chronic) 280.0
      acute 285.1
    chemotherapy, antineoplastic 285.3
    defect of Embden-Meyerhof pathway
      glycolysis 282.3
    disorder of glutathione metabolism 282.2
    drug - see Anemia, by type (see also Table of
      Drugs and Chemicals)
      chemotherapy, antineoplastic 285.3
    fetal blood loss 776.5
    fish tapeworm (D. latum) infestation 123.4
    glutathione metabolism disorder 282.2
    hemorrhage (chronic) 280.0
      acute 285.1
    hexose monophosphate (HMP) shunt
      deficiency 282.2
    impaired absorption 280.9
    loss of blood (chronic) 280.0
      acute 285.1
    myxedema 244.9
    Necator americanus 126.1
    prematurity 776.6
    selective vitamin B$_{12}$ malabsorption with
      proteinuria 281.1
  Dyke-Young type (secondary) (symptomatic)
    283.9
  dyserythropoietic (congenital) (types I, II, III)
    285.8
  dyshemopoietic (congenital) 285.8
  Egypt (*see also* Ancylostomiasis) 126.9
  elliptocytosis (*see also* Elliptocytosis) 282.1
  enzyme deficiency, drug-induced 282.2
  epidemic (*see also* Ancylostomiasis) 126.9
  EPO resistant 285.21
  erythroblastic
    familial 282.44
    fetus or newborn (*see also* Disease, hemolytic)
      773.2
      late 773.5
  erythrocytic glutathione deficiency 282.2
  erythropoietin-resistant (EPO resistant anemia)
    285.21
  essential 285.9
  Faber's (achlorhydric anemia) 280.9
  factitious (self-induced blood letting) 280.0
  familial erythroblastic (microcytic) 282.44
  Fanconi's (congenital pancytopenia) 284.09
  favism 282.2
  fetal 678.0
    following blood loss, affecting newborn 776.5
  fetus or newborn
    due to
      ABO
        antibodies 773.1
        incompatibility, maternal/fetal 773.1
        isoimmunization 773.1
      Rh
        antibodies 773.0
        incompatibility, maternal/fetal 773.0
        isoimmunization 773.0
    following fetal blood loss 776.5
  fish tapeworm (D. latum) infestation 123.4
  folate (folic acid) deficiency 281.2
    dietary 281.2
    drug-induced 281.2
  folate malabsorption, congenital 281.2

Anemia—*continued*
  folic acid deficiency 281.2
    dietary 281.2
    drug-induced 281.2
  G-6-PD 282.2
  general 285.9
  glucose-6-phosphate dehydrogenase deficiency
    282.2
  glutathione-reductase deficiency 282.2
  goat's milk 281.2
  granulocytic 288.09
  Heinz-body, congenital 282.7
  hemoglobin deficiency 285.9
  hemolytic 283.9
    acquired 283.9
      with hemoglobinuria NEC 283.2
      autoimmune (cold type) (idiopathic)
        (primary) (secondary) (symptomatic)
        (warm type) 283.0
      due to
        cold reactive antibodies 283.0
        drug exposure 283.0
        warm reactive antibodies 283.0
      fragmentation 283.19
      idiopathic (chronic) 283.9
      infectious 283.19
        autoimmune 283.0
      non-autoimmune NEC 283.10
      toxic 283.19
      traumatic cardiac 283.19
    acute 283.9
      due to enzyme deficiency NEC 282.3
      fetus or newborn (*see also* Disease,
        hemolytic) 773.2
        late 773.5
      Lederer's (acquired infectious hemolytic
        anemia) 283.19
    autoimmune (acquired) 283.0
    chronic 282.9
      idiopathic 283.9
    cold type (secondary) (symptomatic) 283.0
    congenital (spherocytic) (*see also*
      Spherocytosis) 282.0
    nonspherocytic—*see* Anemia, hemolytic,
      nonspherocytic, congenital
    drug-induced 283.0
      enzyme deficiency 282.2
    due to
      cardiac conditions 283.19
      drugs 283.0
      enzyme deficiency NEC 282.3
        drug-induced 282.2
      presence of shunt or other internal prosthetic
        device 283.19
      thrombotic thrombocytopenic purpura 446.6
    elliptocytotic (*see also* Elliptocytosis) 282.1
    familial 282.9
    hereditary 282.9
      due to enzyme deficiency NEC 282.3
      specified NEC 282.8
    idiopathic (chronic) 283.9
    infectious (acquired) 283.19
    mechanical 283.19
    microangiopathic 283.19
    non-autoimmune NEC 283.10
    nonspherocytic
      congenital or hereditary NEC 282.3
        glucose-6-phosphate dehydrogenase
          deficiency 282.2
        pyruvate kinase (PK) deficiency 282.3
        type I 282.2

Anemia—*continued*
hemolytic—*continued*
  type II 282.3
  type I 282.2
  type II 282.3
  of or complicating pregnancy 648.2
  resulting from presence of shunt or other
    internal prosthetic device 283.19
  secondary 283.19
    autoimmune 283.0
  sickle-cell—*see* Disease, sickle-cell
  Stransky-Regala type (Hb-E) (*see also*
    Disease, hemoglobin) 282.7
  symptomatic 283.19
    autoimmune 283.0
  toxic (acquired) 283.19
  uremic (adult) (child) 283.11
  warm type (secondary) (symptomatic) 283.0
hemorrhagic (chronic) 280.0
  acute 285.1
HEMPAS 285.8
hereditary erythroblast multinuclearity- positive
  acidified serum test 285.8
Herrick's (hemoglobin S disease) 282.61
hexokinase deficiency 282.3
high A$_2$ 282.46
hookworm (*see also* Ancylostomiasis) 126.9
hypochromic (idiopathic) (microcytic)
  (normoblastic) 280.9
  with iron loading 285.0
  due to blood loss (chronic) 280.0
    acute 285.1
  familial sex linked 285.0
  pyridoxine-responsive 285.0
hypoplasia, red blood cells 284.81
  congenital or familial 284.01
hypoplastic (idiopathic) 284.9
  congenital 284.01
  familial 284.01
  of childhood 284.09
idiopathic 285.9
  hemolytic, chronic 283.9
infantile 285.9
infective, infectional 285.9
intertropical (*see also* Ancylostomiasis) 126.9
iron (Fe) deficiency 280.9
  due to blood loss (chronic) 280.0
    acute 285.1
  of or complicating pregnancy 648.2
  specified NEC 280.8
Jaksch's (pseudoleukemia infantum) 285.8
Joseph-Diamond-Blackfan (congenital
  hypoplastic) 284.01
labyrinth 386.50
Lederer's (acquired infectious hemolytic
  anemia) 283.19
leptocytosis (hereditary) 282.40
leukoerythroblastic 284.2
macrocytic 281.9
  nutritional 281.2
  of or complicating pregnancy 648.2
  tropical 281.2
malabsorption (familial), selective B$_{12}$ with
  proteinuria 281.1
malarial (*see also* Malaria) 084.6
malignant (progressive) 281.0
malnutrition 281.9
marsh (*see also* Malaria) 084.6
Mediterranean 282.40
  with hemoglobinopathy 282.49

Anemia—*continued*
megaloblastic 281.9
  combined B$_{12}$ and folate deficiency 281.3
  nutritional (of infancy) 281.2
  of infancy 281.2
  of or complicating pregnancy 648.2
  refractory 281.3
  specified NEC 281.3
megalocytic 281.9
microangiopathic hemolytic 283.19
microcytic (hypochromic) 280.9
  due to blood loss (chronic) 280.0
    acute 285.1
  familial 282.49
  hypochromic 280.9
microdrepanocytosis 282.41
miners' (*see also* Ancylostomiasis) 126.9
myelopathic 285.8
myelophthisic (normocytic) 284.2
newborn (*see also* Disease, hemolytic) 773.2
  due to isoimmunization (*see also* Disease,
    hemolytic) 773.2
  late, due to isoimmunization 773.5
  posthemorrhagic 776.5
nonregenerative 284.9
nonspherocytic hemolytic—*see* Anemia,
  hemolytic, nonspherocytic
normocytic (infectional) (not due to blood loss)
  285.9
  due to blood loss (chronic) 280.0
    acute 285.1
  myelophthisic 284.2
nutritional (deficiency) 281.9
  with
    poor iron absorption 280.9
    specified deficiency NEC 281.8
  due to inadequate dietary iron intake 280.1
  megaloblastic (of infancy) 281.2
of childhood 282.9
of chronic
  disease NEC 285.29
  illness NEC 285.29
of or complicating pregnancy 648.2
  affecting fetus or newborn 760.8
of prematurity 776.6
orotic aciduric (congenital) (hereditary) 281.4
osteosclerotic 289.89
ovalocytosis (hereditary) (*see also*
  Elliptocytosis) 282.1
paludal (*see also* Malaria) 084.6
pentose phosphate pathway deficiency 282.2
pernicious (combined system disease)
  (congenital) (dorsolateral spinal
  degeneration) (juvenile) (myelopathy)
  (neuropathy) (posterior sclerosis) (primary)
  (progressive) (spleen) 281.0
  of or complicating pregnancy 648.2
pleochromic 285.9
  of sprue 281.8
portal 285.8
posthemorrhagic (chronic) 280.0
  acute 285.1
  newborn 776.5
postoperative
  due to (acute) blood loss 285.1
    chronic blood loss 280.0
  other 285.9
postpartum 648.2
pressure 285.9
primary 285.9
profound 285.9

Anemia—*continued*
  progressive 285.9
    malignant 281.0
    pernicious 281.0
  protein-deficiency 281.4
  pseudoleukemica infantum 285.8
  puerperal 648.2
  pure red cell 284.81
    congenital 284.01
  pyridoxine-responsive (hypochromic) 285.0
  pyruvate kinase (PK) deficiency 282.3
  refractoria sideroblastica 238.72
  refractory (primary) 238.72
    with
      excess
        blasts-1 (RAEB-1) 238.72
        blasts-2 (RAEB-2) 238.73
      hemochromatosis 238.72
      ringed sideroblasts (RARS) 238.72
    due to
      drug 285.0
      myelodysplastic syndrome 238.72
      toxin 285.0
    hereditary 285.0
    idiopathic 238.72
    megaloblastic 281.3
    sideroblastic 238.72
      hereditary 285.0
    sideropenic 280.9
  Rietti-Greppi-Micheli (thalassemia minor)
    282.46
  scorbutic 281.8
  secondary (to) 285.9
    blood loss (chronic) 280.0
      acute 285.1
    hemorrhage 280.0
      acute 285.1
    inadequate dietary iron intake 280.1
  semiplastic 284.9
  septic 285.9
  sickle-cell (*see also* Disease, sickle-cell) 282.60
  sideroachrestic 285.0
  sideroblastic (acquired) (any type) (congenital)
    (drug-induced) (due to disease) (hereditary)
    (primary) (secondary) (sex-linked
    hypochromic) (vitamin B_6 responsive) 285.0
    refractory 238.72
    congenital 285.0
    drug-induced 285.0
    hereditary 285.0
    sex-linked hypochromic 285.0
    vitamin B_6-responsive 285.0
  sideropenic (refractory) 280.9
    due to blood loss (chronic) 280.0
      acute 285.1
  simple chronic 281.9
  specified type NEC 285.8
  spherocytic (hereditary) (*see also* Spherocytosis)
    282.0
  splenic 285.8
    familial (Gaucher's) 272.7
  splenomegalic 285.8
  stomatocytosis 282.8
  syphilitic 095.8
  target cell (oval) 285.8
    with thalassemia —*see* Thalassemia
  thalassemia 282.40
  thrombocytopenic (*see also* Thrombocytopenia)
    287.5
  toxic 284.89
  triosephosphate isomerase deficiency 282.3

Anemia—*continued*
  tropical, macrocytic 281.2
  tuberculous (*see also* Tuberculosis) 017.9
  vegan's 281.1
  vitamin
    B_6-responsive 285.0
    B_{12} deficiency (dietary) 281.1
      pernicious 281.0
  von Jaksch's (pseudoleukemia infantum) 285.8
  Witts' (achlorhydric anemia) 280.9
  Zuelzer (-Ogden) (nutritional megaloblastic
    anemia) 281.2
Anencephalus, anencephaly 740.0
  fetal, affecting management of pregnancy 655.0
Anergasia (*see also* Psychosis, organic) 294.9
  senile 290.0
Anesthesia, anesthetic 782.0
  complication or reaction NEC 995.22
    due to
      correct substance properly administered
        995.22
      overdose or wrong substance given 968.4
        specified anesthetic—*see* Table of drugs
          and chemicals
  cornea 371.81
  death from
    correct substance properly administered 995.4
    during delivery 668.9
    overdose or wrong substance given 968.4
      specified anesthetic—*see* Table of drugs and
        chemicals
  eye 371.81
  functional 300.11
  hyperesthetic, thalamic 338.0
  hysterical 300.11
  local skin lesion 782.0
  olfactory 781.1
  sexual (psychogenic) 302.72
  shock
    due to
      correct substance properly administered 995.4
      overdose or wrong substance given 968.4
      specified anesthetic—*see* Table of drugs and
        chemicals
  skin 782.0
  tactile 782.0
  testicular 608.9
  thermal 782.0
Anetoderma (maculosum) 701.3
Aneuploidy NEC 758.5
Aneurin deficiency 265.1
Aneurysm (anastomotic) (artery) (cirsoid)
  (diffuse) (false) (fusiform) (multiple)
  (ruptured) (saccular) (varicose) 442.9
  abdominal (aorta) 441.4
    ruptured 441.3
    syphilitic 093.0
  aorta, aortic (nonsyphilitic) 441.9
    abdominal 441.4
      dissecting 441.02
      ruptured 441.3
      syphilitic 093.0
    arch 441.2
      ruptured 441.1
    arteriosclerotic NEC 441.9
      ruptured 441.5
    ascending 441.2
      ruptured 441.1
    congenital 747.29

Aneurysm—*continued*
aorta—*continued*
  descending 441.9
    abdominal 441.4
      ruptured 441.3
    ruptured 441.5
    thoracic 441.2
      ruptured 441.1
  dissecting 441.00
    abdominal 441.02
    thoracic 441.01
    thoracoabdominal 441.03
  due to coarctation (aorta) 747.10
  ruptured 441.5
  sinus, right 747.29
  syphilitic 093.0
  thoracoabdominal 441.7
    ruptured 441.6
  thorax, thoracic (arch) (nonsyphilitic) 441.2
    dissecting 441.01
    ruptured 441.1
    syphilitic 093.0
  transverse 441.2
    ruptured 441.1
  valve (heart) (*see also* Endocarditis, aortic)
    424.1
arteriosclerotic NEC 442.9
  cerebral 437.3
    ruptured (*see also* Hemorrhage,
      subarachnoid) 430
arteriovenous (congenital) (peripheral) NEC
  (*see also* Anomaly, arteriovenous) 747.32
  acquired NEC 447.0
    brain 437.3
      ruptured (*see also* Hemorrhage,
        subarachnoid) 430
    coronary 414.11
    pulmonary 417.0
  brain (cerebral) 747.81
    ruptured (*see also* Hemorrhage,
      subarachnoid) 430
  coronary 746.85
  pulmonary 747.3
  retina 743.58
  specified site NEC 747.89
    acquired 447.0
  traumatic (*see also* Injury, blood vessel, by
    site) 904.9
basal—*see* Aneurysm, brain
berry (congenital) (ruptured) (*see also*
  Hemorrhage, subarachnoid) 430
  nonruptured 437.3
brain 437.3
  arteriosclerotic 437.3
    ruptured (*see also* Hemorrhage,
      subarachnoid) 430
  arteriovenous 747.81
    acquired 437.3
      ruptured (*see also* Hemorrhage,
        subarachnoid) 430
    ruptured (*see also* Hemorrhage,
      subarachnoid) 430
  berry (congenital) (ruptured) (*see also*
    Hemorrhage, subarachnoid) 430
    nonruptured 437.3
  congenital 747.81
    ruptured (*see also* Hemorrhage,
      subarachnoid) 430
  meninges 437.3
    ruptured (*see also* Hemorrhage,
      subarachnoid) 430

Aneurysm—*continued*
brain—*continued*
  miliary (congenital) (ruptured) (*see also*
    Hemorrhage, subarachnoid) 430
  mycotic 421.0
    ruptured (*see also* Hemorrhage,
      subarachnoid) 430
  nonruptured 437.3
  ruptured (*see also* Hemorrhage, subarachnoid)
    430
  syphilitic 094.87
  syphilitic (hemorrhage) 094.87
  traumatic—*see* Injury, intracranial
cardiac (false) (*see also* Aneurysm, heart)
  414.10
carotid artery (common) (external) 442.81
  internal (intracranial portion) 437.3
    extracranial portion 442.81
    ruptured into brain (*see also* Hemorrhage,
      subarachnoid) 430
  syphilitic 093.89
  intracranial 094.87
cavernous sinus (*see also* Aneurysm, brain)
  437.3
  arteriovenous 747.81
    ruptured (*see also* Hemorrhage,
      subarachnoid) 430
  congenital 747.81
    ruptured (*see also* Hemorrhage,
      subarachnoid) 430
celiac 442.84
central nervous system, syphilitic 094.89
cerebral—*see* Aneurysm, brain
chest—*see* Aneurysm, thorax
circle of Willis (*see also* Aneurysm, brain)
  437.3
  congenital 747.81
    ruptured (*see also* Hemorrhage,
      subarachnoid) 430
  ruptured (*see also* Hemorrhage, subarachnoid)
    430
common iliac artery 442.2
congenital (peripheral) NEC 747.60
  brain 747.81
    ruptured (*see also* Hemorrhage,
      subarachnoid) 430
  cerebral—*see* Aneurysm, brain, congenital
  coronary 746.85
  gastrointestinal 747.61
  lower limb 747.64
  pulmonary 747.32
  renal 747.62
  retina 743.58
  specified site NEC 747.89
  spinal 747.82
  upper limb 747.63
conjunctiva 372.74
conus arteriosus (*see also* Aneurysm, heart) 414.10
coronary (arteriosclerotic) (artery) (vein) (*see
  also* Aneurysm, heart) 414.11
  arteriovenous 746.85
  congenital 746.85
  syphilitic 093.89
cylindrical 441.9
  ruptured 441.5
  syphilitic 093.9
dissecting 442.9
  aorta 441.00
    abdominal 441.02
    thoracic 441.01
    thoracoabdominal 441.03
  syphilitic 093.9

Aneurysm—*continued*
ductus arteriosus 747.0
embolic—*see* Embolism, artery
endocardial, infective (any valve) 421.0
femoral 442.3
gastroduodenal 442.84
gastroepiploic 442.84
heart (chronic or with a stated duration of over 8 weeks) (infectional) (wall) 414.10
  acute or with a stated duration of 8 weeks or less (*see also* Infarct, myocardium) 410.9
  congenital 746.89
  valve—*see* Endocarditis
hepatic 442.84
iliac (common) 442.2
infective (any valve) 421.0
innominate (nonsyphilitic) 442.89
  syphilitic 093.89
interauricular septum (*see also* Aneurysm, heart) 414.10
interventricular septum (*see also* Aneurysm, heart) 414.10
intracranial—*see* Aneurysm, brain
intrathoracic (nonsyphilitic) 441.2
  ruptured 441.1
  syphilitic 093.0
jugular vein (acute) 453.89
  chronic 453.76
lower extremity 442.3
lung (pulmonary artery) 417.1
malignant 093.9
mediastinal (nonsyphilitic) 442.89
  syphilitic 093.89
miliary (congenital) (ruptured) (*see also* Hemorrhage, subarachnoid) 430
mitral (heart) (valve) 424.0
mural (arteriovenous) (heart) (*see also* Aneurysm, heart) 414.10
mycotic, any site 421.0
  ruptured, brain (*see also* Hemorrhage, subarachnoid) 430
  without endocarditis —*see* Aneurysm, by site
myocardium (*see also* Aneurysm, heart) 414.10
neck 442.81
pancreaticoduodenal 442.84
patent ductus arteriosus 747.0
peripheral NEC 442.89
  congenital NEC (*see also* Aneurysm, congenital) 747.60
popliteal 442.3
pulmonary 417.1
  arteriovenous 747.32
    acquired 417.0
  syphilitic 093.89
  valve (heart) (*see also* Endocarditis, pulmonary) 424.3
racemose 442.9
  congenital (peripheral) NEC 747.60
radial 442.0
Rasmussen's (*see also* Tuberculosis) 011.2
renal 442.1
retinal (acquired) 362.17
  congenital 743.58
  diabetic 250.5 *[362.01]*
    due to secondary diabetes 249.5 *[362.01]*
sinus, aortic (of Valsalva) 747.29
specified site NEC 442.89
spinal (cord) 442.89
  congenital 747.82
  syphilitic (hemorrhage) 094.89
spleen, splenic 442.83

Aneurysm—*continued*
subclavian 442.82
  syphilitic 093.89
superior mesenteric 442.84
syphilitic 093.9
  aorta 093.0
  central nervous system 094.89
  congenital 090.5
  spine, spinal 094.89
thoracoabdominal 441.7
  ruptured 441.6
thorax, thoracic (arch) (nonsyphilitic) 441.2
  dissecting 441.01
  ruptured 441.1
  syphilitic 093.0
traumatic (complication) (early)—*see* Injury, blood vessel, by site
tricuspid (heart) (valve)—*see* Endocarditis, tricuspid
ulnar 442.0
upper extremity 442.0
valve, valvular—*see* Endocarditis
venous 456.8
  congenital NEC (*see also* Aneurysm, congenital) 747.60
ventricle (arteriovenous) (*see also* Aneurysm, heart) 414.10
visceral artery NEC 442.84
Angiectasis 459.89
Angiectopia 459.9
Angiitis 447.6
allergic granulomatous 446.4
hypersensitivity 446.20
  Goodpasture's syndrome 446.21
  specified NEC 446.29
necrotizing 446.0
Wegener's (necrotizing respiratory granulomatosis) 446.4
Angina (attack) (cardiac) (chest) (effort) (heart) (pectoris) (syndrome) (vasomotor) 413.9
abdominal 557.1
accelerated 411.1
agranulocytic 288.03
aphthous 074.0
catarrhal 462
crescendo 411.1
croupous 464.4
cruris 443.9
  due to atherosclerosis NEC (*see also* Arteriosclerosis, extremities) 440.20
decubitus 413.0
diphtheritic (membranous) 032.0
equivalent 413.9
erysipelatous 034.0
erythematous 462
exudative, chronic 476.0
faucium 478.29
gangrenous 462
  diphtheritic 032.0
infectious 462
initial 411.1
intestinal 557.1
ludovici 528.3
Ludwig's 528.3
malignant 462
  diphtheritic 032.0
membranous 464.4
  diphtheritic 032.0
mesenteric 557.1
monocytic 075
nocturnal 413.0

Angina—*continued*
 phlegmonous 475
  diphtheritic 032.0
 preinfarctional 411.1
 Prinzmetal's 413.1
 progressive 411.1
 pseudomembranous 101
 psychogenic 306.2
 pultaceous, diphtheritic 032.0
 scarlatinal 034.1
 septic 034.0
 simple 462
 stable NEC 413.9
 staphylococcal 462
 streptococcal 034.0
 stridulous, diphtheritic 032.3
 syphilitic 093.9
  congenital 090.5
 tonsil 475
 trachealis 464.4
 unstable 411.1
 variant 413.1
 Vincent's 101
Angioblastoma (M9161/1)—*see* Neoplasm,
  connective tissue, uncertain behavior
Angiocholecystitis (*see also* Cholecystitis, acute)
  575.0
Angiocholitis (*see also* Cholecystitis, acute) 576.1
Angiodysgensis spinalis 336.1
Angiodysplasia (intestinalis) (intestine) 569.84
 with hemorrhage 569.85
 duodenum 537.82
  with hemorrhage 537.83
 stomach 537.82
  with hemorrhage 537.83
Angioedema (allergic) (any site) (with urticaria)
  995.1
 hereditary 277.6
Angioendothelioma (M9130/1)—*see also*
  Neoplasm, by site, uncertain behavior
 benign (M9130/0) (*see also* Hemangioma, by
  site) 228.00
 bone (M9260/3)—*see* Neoplasm, bone, malignant
 Ewing's (M9260/3)—*see* Neoplasm, bone,
  malignant
 nervous system (M9130/0) 228.09
Angiofibroma (M9160/0)—*see also* Neoplasm,
  by site, benign
 juvenile (M9160/0) 210.7
  specified site—*see* Neoplasm, by site, benign
  unspecified site 210.7
Angiohemophilia (A) (B) 286.4
Angioid streaks (choroid) (retina) 363.43
Angiokeratoma (M9141/0)—*see also* Neoplasm,
  skin, benign
 corporis diffusum 272.7
Angiokeratosis
 diffuse 272.7
Angioleiomyoma (M8894/0)—*see* Neoplasm,
  connective tissue, benign
Angioleucitis 683
Angiolipoma (M8861/0) (*see also* Lipoma, by
  site) 214.9
 infiltrating (M8861/1)—*see* Neoplasm,
  connective tissue, uncertain behavior
Angioma (M9120/0) (*see also* Hemangioma, by
  site) 228.00
 capillary 448.1
 hemorrhagicum hereditaria 448.0
 malignant (M9120/3)—*see* Neoplasm,
  connective tissue, malignant

Angioma—*continued*
 pigmentosum et atrophicum 757.33
 placenta—*see* Placenta, abnormal
 plexiform (M9131/0)—*see* Hemangioma, by site
 senile 448.1
 serpiginosum 709.1
 spider 448.1
 stellate 448.1
Angiomatosis 757.32
 bacillary 083.8
 corporis diffusum universale 272.7
 cutaneocerebral 759.6
 encephalocutaneous 759.6
 encephalofacial 759.6
 encephalotrigeminal 759.6
 hemorrhagic familial 448.0
 hereditary familial 448.0
 heredofamilial 448.0
 meningo-oculofacial 759.6
 multiple sites 228.09
 neuro-oculocutaneous 759.6
 retina (Hippel's disease) 759.6
 retinocerebellosa 759.6
 retinocerebral 759.6
 systemic 228.09
Angiomyolipoma (M8860/0)
 specified site—*see* Neoplasm, connective tissue, benign
 unspecified site 223.0
Angiomyoliposarcoma (M8860/3)—*see*
  Neoplasm, connective tissue, malignant
Angiomyoma (M8894/0)—*see* Neoplasm,
  connective tissue, benign
Angiomyosarcoma (M8894/3)—*see* Neoplasm,
  connective tissue, malignant
Angioneurosis 306.2
Angioneurotic edema (allergic) (any site) (with
  urticaria) 995.1
 hereditary 277.6
Angiopathia, angiopathy 459.9
 diabetic (peripheral) 250.7 *[443.81]*
  due to secondary diabetes 249.7 [443.81]
 peripheral 443.9
  diabetic 250.7 *[443.81]*
   due to secondary diabetes 249.7 [443.81]
  specified type NEC 443.89
 retinae syphilitica 093.89
 retinalis (juvenilis) 362.18
  background 362.10
  diabetic 250.5 *[362.01]*
   due to secondary diabetes 249.5 [362.01]
  proliferative 362.29
  tuberculous (*see also* Tuberculosis) 017.3 *[362.18]*
Angiosarcoma (M9120/3)—*see* Neoplasm,
  connective tissue, malignant
Angiosclerosis —*see* Arteriosclerosis
Angioscotoma, enlarged 368.42
Angiospasm 443.9
 brachial plexus 353.0
 cerebral 435.9
 cervical plexus 353.2
 nerve
  arm 354.9
   axillary 353.0
   median 354.1
   ulnar 354.2
  autonomic (*see also* Neuropathy, peripheral,
   autonomic) 337.9
  axillary 353.0
  leg 355.8
   plantar 355.6
  lower extremity—*see* Angiospasm, nerve, leg

Angiospasm—*continued*
median 354.1
peripheral NEC 355.9
spinal NEC 355.9
sympathetic (*see also* Neuropathy, peripheral, autonomic) 337.9
ulnar 354.2
upper extremity—*see* Angiospasm, nerve, arm
peripheral NEC 443.9
traumatic 443.9
foot 443.9
leg 443.9
vessel 443.9
Angiospastic disease or edema 443.9
Angle's
class I 524.21
class II 524.22
class III 524.23
Anguillulosis 127.2
Angulation
cecum (*see also* Obstruction, intestine) 560.9
coccyx (acquired) 738.6
congenital 756.19
femur (acquired) 736.39
congenital 755.69
intestine (large) (small) (*see also* Obstruction, intestine) 560.9
sacrum (acquired) 738.5
congenital 756.19
sigmoid (flexure) (*see also* Obstruction, intestine) 560.9
spine (*see also* Curvature, spine) 737.9
tibia (acquired) 736.89
congenital 755.69
ureter 593.3
wrist (acquired) 736.09
congenital 755.59
Angulus infectiosus 686.8
Anhedonia 780.99
Anhidrosis (lid) (neurogenic) (thermogenic) 705.0
Anhydration 276.51
with
hypernatremia 276.0
hyponatremia 276.1
Anhydremia 276.52
with
hypernatremia 276.0
hyponatremia 276.1
Anidrosis 705.0
Aniridia (congenital) 743.45
Anisakiasis (infection) (infestation) 127.1
Anisakis larva infestation 127.1
Aniseikonia 367.32
Anisocoria (pupil) 379.41
congenital 743.46
Anisocytosis 790.09
Anisometropia (congenital) 367.31
Ankle —*see* condition
Ankyloblepharon (acquired) (eyelid) 374.46
filiforme (adnatum) (congenital) 743.62
total 743.62
Ankylodactly (*see also* Syndactylism) 755.10
Ankyloglossia 750.0
Ankylosis (fibrous) (osseous) 718.50
ankle 718.57
any joint, produced by surgical fusion V45.4
cricoarytenoid (cartilage) (joint) (larynx) 478.79
dental 521.6
ear ossicle NEC 385.22
malleus 385.21

Ankylosis—*continued*
elbow 718.52
finger 718.54
hip 718.55
incostapedial joint (infectional) 385.22
joint, produced by surgical fusion NEC V45.4
knee 718.56
lumbosacral (joint) 724.6
malleus 385.21
multiple sites 718.59
postoperative (status) V45.4
sacroiliac (joint) 724.6
shoulder 718.51
specified site NEC 718.58
spine NEC 724.9
surgical V45.4
teeth, tooth (hard tissues) 521.6
temporomandibular joint 524.61
wrist 718.53
Ankylostoma —*see* Ancylostoma
Ankylostomiasis (intestinal)—*see* Ancylostomiasis
Ankylurethria (*see also* Stricture, urethra) 598.9
Annular —*see also* condition
detachment, cervix 622.8
organ or site, congenital NEC—*see* Distortion
pancreas (congenital) 751.7
Anodontia (complete) (partial) (vera) 520.0
with abnormal spacing 524.30
acquired 525.10
causing malocclusion 524.30
due to
caries 525.13
extraction 525.10
periodontal disease 525.12
trauma 525.11
Anomaly, anomalous (congenital) (unspecified type) 759.9
abdomen 759.9
abdominal wall 756.70
acoustic nerve 742.9
adrenal (gland) 759.1
Alder (-Reilly) (leukocyte granulation) 288.2
alimentary tract 751.9
lower 751.5
specified type NEC 751.8
upper (any part, except tongue) 750.9
tongue 750.10
specified type NEC 750.19
alveolar 524.70
ridge (process) 525.8
specified NEC 524.79
ankle (joint) 755.69
anus, anal (canal) 751.5
aorta, aortic 747.20
arch 747.21
coarctation (postductal) (preductal) 747.10
cusp or valve NEC 746.9
septum 745.0
specified type NEC 747.29
aorticopulmonary septum 745.0
apertures, diaphragm 756.6
appendix 751.5
aqueduct of Sylvius 742.3
with spina bifida (*see also* Spina bifida) 741.0
arm 755.50
reduction (*see also* Deformity, reduction, upper limb) 755.20

Anomaly, anomalous—*continued*
  arteriovenous (congenital) (peripheral) NEC
    747.60
    brain 747.81
    cerebral 747.81
    coronary 746.85
    gastrointestinal 747.61
      acquired—*see* Angiodysplasia
    lower limb 747.64
    renal 747.62
    specified site NEC 747.69
    spinal 747.82
    upper limb 747.63
  artery (*see also* Anomaly, peripheral vascular
    system) NEC 747.60
    brain 747.81
    cerebral 747.81
    coronary 746.85
    eye 743.9
    pulmonary 747.39
    renal 747.62
    retina 743.9
    umbilical 747.5
  arytenoepiglottic folds 748.3
  atrial
    bands 746.9
    folds 746.9
    septa 745.5
  atrioventricular
    canal 745.69
    common 745.69
    conduction 426.7
    excitation 426.7
    septum 745.4
  atrium—*see* Anomaly, atrial
  auditory canal 744.3
    specified type NEC 744.29
      with hearing impairment 744.02
  auricle
    ear 744.3
      causing impairment of hearing 744.02
    heart 746.9
      septum 745.5
  autosomes, autosomal NEC 758.5
  Axenfeld's 743.44
  back 759.9
  band
    atrial 746.9
    heart 746.9
    ventricular 746.9
  Bartholin's duct 750.9
  biliary duct or passage 751.60
    atresia 751.61
  bladder (neck) (sphincter) (trigone) 753.9
    specified type NEC 753.8
  blood vessel 747.9
    artery—*see* Anomly, artery
    peripheral vascular—*see* Anomaly, peripheral
      vascular system
    vein—*see* Anomaly, vein
  bone NEC 756.9
    ankle 755.69
    arm 755.50
    chest 756.3
    cranium 756.0
    face 756.0
    finger 755.50
    foot 755.67
    forearm 755.50
    frontal 756.0
    head 756.0

Anomaly, anomalous—*continued*
  bone—*continued*
    hip 755.63
    leg 755.60
    lumbosacral 756.10
    nose 748.1
    pelvic girdle 755.60
    rachitic 756.4
    rib 756.3
    shoulder girdle 755.50
    skull 756.0
      with
        anencephalus 740.0
        encephalocele 742.0
        hydrocephalus 742.3
          with spina bifida (*see also* Spina bifida)
            741.0
        microcephalus 742.1
    toe 755.66
  brain 742.9
    multiple 742.4
    reduction 742.2
    specified type NEC 742.4
    vessel 747.81
  branchial cleft NEC 744.49
    cyst 744.42
    fistula 744.41
    persistent 744.41
    sinus (external) (internal) 744.41
  breast 757.6
  broad ligament 752.10
    specified type NEC 752.19
  bronchus 748.3
  bulbar septum 745.0
  bulbus cordis 745.9
    persistent (in left ventricle) 745.8
  bursa 756.9
  canal of Nuck 752.9
  canthus 743.9
  capillary NEC (*see also* Anomaly, peripheral
    vascular system) 747.60
  cardiac 746.9
    septal closure 745.9
      acquired 429.71
    valve NEC 746.9
      pulmonary 746.00
      specified type NEC 746.89
  cardiovascular system 746.9
    complicating pregnancy, childbirth, or
      puerperium 648.5
  carpus 755.50
  cartilage, trachea 748.3
  cartilaginous 756.9
  caruncle, lacrimal, lachrymal 743.9
  cascade stomach 750.7
  cauda equina 742.59
  cecum 751.5
  cerebral—*see also* Anomaly, brain
    vessels 747.81
  cerebrovascular system 747.81
  cervix (uterus) 752.40
    with doubling of vagina and uterus 752.2
    in pregnancy or childbirth 654.6
      affecting fetus or newborn 763.89
      causing obstructed labor 660.2
        affecting fetus or newborn 763.1
  Chédiak-Higashi (-Steinbrinck) (congenital
    gigantism of peroxidase granules) 288.2
  cheek 744.9
  chest (wall) 756.3

Anomaly, anomalous—*continued*
 chin 744.9
  specified type NEC 744.89
 chordae tendineae 746.9
 choroid 743.9
  plexus 742.9
 chromosomes, chromosomal 758.9
  13 (13-15) 758.1
  18 (16-18) 758.2
  21 or 22 758.0
  autosomes NEC (*see also* Abnormality,
    autosomes) 758.5
  deletion 758.39
  Christchurch 758.39
  D_1 758.1
  E_3 758.2
  G 758.0
  mitochondrial 758.9
  mosaics 758.89
  sex 758.81
   complement, XO 758.6
   complement, XXX 758.81
   complement, XYY 758.81
   gonadal dysgenesis 758.6
   Klinefelter's 758.7
   Turner's 758.6
  trisomy 21 758.0
 cilia 743.9
 circulatory system 747.9
  specified type NEC 747.89
 clavicle 755.51
 clitoris 752.40
 coccyx 756.10
 colon 751.5
 common duct 751.60
 communication
  coronary artery 746.85
  left ventricle with right atrium 745.4
 concha (ear) 744.3
 connection
  renal vessels with kidney 747.62
  total pulmonary venous 747.41
 connective tissue 756.9
  specified type NEC 756.89
 cornea 743.9
  shape 743.41
  size 743.41
  specified type NEC 743.49
 coronary
  artery 746.85
  vein 746.89
 cranium—*see* Anomaly, skull
 cricoid cartilage 748.3
 cushion, endocardial 745.60
  specified type NEC 745.69
 cystic duct 751.60
 dental arch 524.20
  specified NEC 524.29
 dental arch relationship 524.20
  angle's class I 524.21
  angle's class II 524.22
  angle's class III 524.23
  articulation
   anterior 524.27
   posterior 524.27
   reverse 524.27
  disto-occlusion 524.22
   division I 524.22
   division II 524.22
  excessive horizontal overlap 524.26
  interarch distance (excessive) (inadequate)
    524.28

Anomaly, anomalous—*continued*
 dental arch relationship—*continued*
  mesio-occlusion 524.23
  neutro-occlusion 524.21
  open
   anterior occlusal relationship 524.24
   posterior occlusal relationship 524.25
  specified NEC 524.29
 dentition 520.6
 dentofacial NEC 524.9
  functional 524.50
  specified type NEC 524.89
 dermatoglyphic 757.2
 Descemet's membrane 743.9
  specified type NEC 743.49
 development
  cervix 752.40
  vagina 752.40
  vulva 752.40
 diaphragm, diaphragmatic (apertures) NEC
   756.6
 digestive organ(s) or system 751.9
  lower 751.5
  specified type NEC 751.8
  upper 750.9
 distribution, coronary artery 746.85
 ductus
  arteriosus 747.0
  Botalli 747.0
 duodenum 751.5
 dura 742.9
  brain 742.4
  spinal cord 742.59
 ear 744.3
  causing impairment of hearing 744.00
   specified type NEC 744.09
  external 744.3
   causing impairment of hearing 744.02
   specified type NEC 744.29
  inner (causing impairment of hearing) 744.05
  middle, except ossicles (causing impairment
    of hearing) 744.03
   ossicles 744.04
  ossicles 744.04
  prominent auricle 744.29
  specified type NEC 744.29
   with hearing impairment 744.09
 Ebstein's (heart) 746.2
  tricuspid valve 746.2
 ectodermal 757.9
 Eisenmenger's (ventricular septal defect) 745.4
 ejaculatory duct 752.9
  specified type NEC 752.89
 elbow (joint) 755.50
 endocardial cushion 745.60
  specified type NEC 745.69
 endocrine gland NEC 759.2
 epididymis 752.9
 epiglottis 748.3
 esophagus 750.9
  specified type NEC 750.4
 Eustachian tube 744.3
  specified type NEC 744.24
 eye (any part) 743.9
  adnexa 743.9
   specified type NEC 743.69
  anophthalmos 743.00
  anterior
   chamber and related structures 743.9
    angle 743.9
     specified type NEC 743.44
    specified type NEC 743.44

Anomaly, anomalous—*continued*
  eye—*continued*
    segment 743.9
      combined 743.48
      multiple 743.48
      specified type NEC 743.49
    cataract (*see also* Cataract) 743.30
    glaucoma (*see also* Buphthalmia) 743.20
    lid 743.9
      specified type NEC 743.63
    microphthalmos (*see also* Microphthalmos) 743.10
    posterior segment 743.9
      specified type NEC 743.59
      vascular 743.58
      vitreous 743.9
        specified type NEC 743.51
    ptosis (eyelid) 743.61
    retina 743.9
      specified type NEC 743.59
    sclera 743.9
      specified type NEC 743.47
    specified type NEC 743.8
  eyebrow 744.89
  eyelid 743.9
    specified type NEC 743.63
  face (any part) 744.9
    bone(s) 756.0
    specified type NEC 744.89
  fallopian tube 752.10
    specified type NEC 752.19
  fascia 756.9
    specified type NEC 756.89
  femur 755.60
  fibula 755.60
  finger 755.50
    supernumerary 755.01
    webbed (*see also* Syndactylism, fingers) 755.11
  fixation, intestine 751.4
  flexion (joint) 755.9
    hip or thigh (*see also* Dislocation, hip,
      congenital) 754.30
  folds, heart 746.9
  foot 755.67
  foramen
    Botalli 745.5
    ovale 745.5
  forearm 755.50
  forehead (*see also* Anomaly, skull) 756.0
  form, teeth 520.2
  fovea centralis 743.9
  frontal bone (*see also* Anomaly, skull) 756.0
  gallbladder 751.60
  Gartner's duct 752.41
  gastrointestinal tract 751.9
    specified type NEC 751.8
    vessel 747.61
  genitalia, genital organ(s) or system
    female 752.9
      external 752.40
        specified type NEC 752.49
      internal NEC 752.9
    male (external and internal) 752.9
      epispadias 752.62
      hidden penis 752.65
      hydrocele, congenital 778.6
      hypospadias 752.61
      micropenis 752.64
      testis, undescended 752.51
        retractile 752.52
      specified type NEC 752.89
  genitourinary NEC 752.9

Anomaly, anomalous—*continued*
  Gerbode 745.4
  globe (eye) 743.9
  glottis 748.3
  granulation or granulocyte, genetic 288.2
    constitutional 288.2
    leukocyte 288.2
  gum 750.9
  gyri 742.9
  hair 757.9
    specified type NEC 757.4
  hand 755.50
  hard tissue formation in pulp 522.3
  head (*see also* Anomaly, skull) 756.0
  heart 746.9
    auricle 746.9
    bands 746.9
    fibroelastosis cordis 425.3
    folds 746.9
    malposition 746.87
    maternal, affecting fetus or newborn 760.3
    obstructive NEC 746.84
    patent ductus arteriosus (Botalli) 747.0
    septum 745.9
      acquired 429.71
      aortic 745.0
      aorticopulmonary 745.0
      atrial 745.5
      auricular 745.5
      between aorta and pulmonary artery 745.0
      endocardial cushion type 745.60
        specified type NEC 745.69
      interatrial 745.5
      interventricular 745.4
        with pulmonary stenosis or atresia,
          dextraposition of aorta, and
          hypertrophy of right ventricle 745.2
        acquired 429.71
      specified type NEC 745.8
      ventricular 745.4
        with pulmonary stenosis or atresia,
          dextraposition of aorta, and
          hypertrophy of right ventricle 745.2
        acquired 429.71
    specified type NEC 746.89
    tetralogy of Fallot 745.2
    valve NEC 746.9
      aortic 746.9
        atresia 746.89
        bicuspid valve 746.4
        insufficiency 746.4
        specified type NEC 746.89
        stenosis 746.3
          subaortic 746.81
          supravalvular 747.22
      mitral 746.9
        atresia 746.89
        insufficiency 746.6
        specified type NEC 746.89
        stenosis 746.5
      pulmonary 746.00
        atresia 746.01
        insufficiency 746.09
        stenosis 746.02
          infundibular 746.83
          subvalvular 746.83
      tricuspid 746.9
        atresia 746.1
        stenosis 746.1
    ventricle 746.9
  heel 755.67

Anomaly, anomalous—*continued*
Hegglin's 288.2
hemianencephaly 740.0
hemicephaly 740.0
hemicrania 740.0
hepatic duct 751.60
hip (joint) 755.63
hourglass
  bladder 753.8
  gallbladder 751.69
  stomach 750.7
humerus 755.50
hymen 752.40
hypersegmentation of neutrophils, hereditary
  288.2
hypophyseal 759.2
ileocecal (coil) (valve) 751.5
ileum (intestine) 751.5
ilium 755.60
integument 757.9
  specified type NEC 757.8
interarch distance (excessive) (inadequate)
  524.28
intervertebral cartilage or disc 756.10
intestine (large) (small) 751.5
  fixational type 751.4
iris 743.9
  specified type NEC 743.46
ischium 755.60
jaw NEC 524.9
  closure 524.51
  size NEC 524.00
  specified type NEC 524.89
jaw-cranial base relationship 524.10
  specified NEC 524.19
jejunum 751.5
joint 755.9
  hip
    dislocation (*see also* Dislocation, hip,
      congenital) 754.30
    predislocation (*see also* Subluxation,
      congenital, hip) 754.32
    preluxation (*see also* Subluxation,
      congenital, hip) 754.32
    subluxation (*see also* Subluxation,
      congenital, hip) 754.32
  lumbosacral 756.10
    spondylolisthesis 756.12
    spondylosis 756.11
  multiple arthrogryposis 754.89
  sacroiliac 755.69
Jordan's 288.2
kidney(s) (calyx) (pelvis) 753.9
  vessel 747.62
Klippel-Feil (brevicollis) 756.16
knee (joint) 755.64
labium (majus) (minus) 752.40
labyrinth, membranous (causing impairment of
  hearing) 744.05
lacrimal
  apparatus, duct or passage 743.9
    specified type NEC 743.65
  gland 743.9
    specified type NEC 743.64
Langdon Down (mongolism) 758.0
larynx, laryngeal (muscle) 748.3
  web, webbed 748.2
leg (lower) (upper) 755.60
  reduction NEC (*see also* Deformity, reduction,
    lower limb) 755.30

Anomaly, anomalous—*continued*
lens 743.9
  shape 743.36
  specified type NEC 743.39
leukocytes, genetic 288.2
  granulation (constitutional) 288.2
lid (fold) 743.9
ligament 756.9
  broad 752.10
  round 752.9
limb, except reduction deformity 755.9
  lower 755.60
    reduction deformity (*see also* Deformity,
      reduction, lower limb) 755.30
    specified type NEC 755.69
  upper 755.50
    reduction deformity (*see also* Deformity,
      reduction, upper limb) 755.20
    specified type NEC 755.59
lip 750.9
  harelip (*see also* Cleft, lip) 749.10
  specified type NEC 750.26
liver (duct) 751.60
  atresia 751.69
lower extremity 755.60
  vessel 747.64
lumbosacral (joint) (region) 756.10
lung (fissure) (lobe) NEC 748.60
  agenesis 748.5
  specified type NEC 748.69
lymphatic system 759.9
Madelung's (radius) 755.54
mandible 524.9
  size NEC 524.00
maxilla 524.9
  size NEC 524.00
May (-Hegglin) 288.2
meatus urinarius 753.9
  specified type NEC 753.8
meningeal bands or folds, constriction of 742.8
meninges 742.9
  brain 742.4
  spinal 742.59
meningocele (*see also* Spina bifida) 741.9
mesentery 751.9
metacarpus 755.50
metatarsus 755.67
middle ear, except ossicles (causing impairment
  of hearing) 744.03
  ossicles 744.04
mitral (leaflets) (valve) 746.9
  atresia 746.89
  insufficiency 746.6
  specified type NEC 746.89
  stenosis 746.5
mouth 750.9
  specified type NEC 750.26
multiple NEC 759.7
  specified type NEC 759.89
muscle 756.9
  eye 743.9
    specified type NEC 743.69
  specified type NEC 756.89
musculoskeletal system, except limbs 756.9
  specified type NEC 756.9
nail 757.9
  specified type NEC 757.5
narrowness, eyelid 743.62
nasal sinus or septum 748.1
neck (any part) 744.9
  specified type NEC 744.89

Anomaly, anomalous—*continued*
  nerve 742.9
    acoustic 742.9
      specified type NEC 742.8
    optic 742.9
    specified type NEC 742.8
    specified type NEC 742.8
  nervous system NEC 742.9
    brain 742.9
      specified type NEC 742.4
    specified type NEC 742.8
  neurological 742.9
  nipple 757.6
  nonteratogenic NEC 754.89
  nose, nasal (bone) (cartilage) (septum) (sinus)
      748.1
  ocular muscle 743.9
  omphalomesenteric duct 751.0
  opening, pulmonary veins 747.49
  optic
    disc 743.9
      specified type NEC 743.57
    nerve 742.9
  opticociliary vessels 743.9
  orbit (eye) 743.9
    specified type NEC 743.66
  organ
    of Corti (causing impairment of hearing)
      744.05
    or site 759.9
      specified type NEC 759.89
  origin
    both great arteries from same ventricle 745.11
    coronary artery 746.85
    innominate artery 747.69
    left coronary artery from pulmonary artery
      746.85
    pulmonary artery 747.39
    renal vessels 747.62
    subclavian artery (left) (right) 747.21
  osseous meatus (ear) 744.03
  ovary 752.0
  oviduct 752.10
  palate (hard) (soft) 750.9
    cleft (*see also* Cleft, palate) 749.00
  pancreas (duct) 751.7
  papillary muscles 746.9
  parathyroid gland 759.2
  paraurethral ducts 753.9
  parotid (gland) 750.9
  patella 755.64
  Pelger-Huët (hereditary hyposegmentation)
      288.2
  pelvic girdle 755.60
    specified type NEC 755.69
  pelvis (bony) 755.60
    complicating delivery 653.0
    rachitic 268.1
      fetal 756.4
  penis (glans) 752.69
  pericardium 746.89
  peripheral vascular system NEC 747.60
    gastrointestinal 747.61
    lower limb 747.64
    renal 747.62
    specified site NEC 747.69
    spinal 747.82
    upper limb 747.63
  Peter's 743.44
  pharynx 750.9
    branchial cleft 744.41
    specified type NEC 750.29

Anomaly, anomalous—*continued*
  Pierre Robin 756.0
  pigmentation NEC 709.00
    congenital 757.33
  pituitary (gland) 759.2
  pleural folds 748.8
  portal vein 747.40
  position tooth, teeth 524.30
    crowding 524.31
    displacement 524.30
      horizontal 524.33
      vertical 524.34
    distance
      interocclusal
        excessive 524.37
        insufficient 524.36
    excessive spacing 524.32
    rotation 524.35
    specified NEC 524.39
  preauricular sinus 744.46
  prepuce 752.9
  prostate 752.9
  pulmonary 748.60
    artery 747.39
    circulation 747.39
    specified type NEC 748.69
    valve 746.00
      atresia 746.01
      insufficiency 746.09
      specified type NEC 746.09
      stenosis 746.02
        infundibular 746.83
        subvalvular 746.83
    vein 747.40
    venous
      connection 747.49
        partial 747.42
        total 747.41
      return 747.49
        partial 747.42
        total (TAPVR) (complete)
          (subdiaphragmatic)
          (supradiaphragmatic) 747.41
  pupil 743.9
  pylorus 750.9
    hypertrophy 750.5
    stenosis 750.5
  rachitic, fetal 756.4
  radius 755.50
  rectovaginal (septum) 752.40
  rectum 751.5
  refraction 367.9
  renal 753.9
    vessel 747.62
  respiratory system 748.9
    specified type NEC 748.8
  rib 756.3
    cervical 756.2
  Rieger's 743.44
  rings, trachea 748.3
  rotation—*see also* Malrotation
    hip or thigh (*see also* Subluxation, congenital,
      hip) 754.32
  round ligament 752.9
  sacroiliac (joint) 755.69
  sacrum 756.10
  saddle
    back 754.2
    nose 754.0
      syphilitic 090.5
  salivary gland or duct 750.9
    specified type NEC 750.26

Anomaly, anomalous—*continued*
  scapula 755.50
  sclera 743.9
    specified type NEC 743.47
  scrotum 752.9
  sebaceous gland 757.9
  seminal duct or tract 752.9
  sense organs 742.9
    specified type NEC 742.8
  septum
    heart—*see* Anomaly, heart, septum
    nasal 748.1
  sex chromosomes NEC (*see also* Anomaly,
    chromosomes) 758.81
    shoulder (girdle) (joint) 755.50
    specified type NEC 755.59
  sigmoid (flexure) 751.5
  sinus of Valsalva 747.29
  site NEC 759.9
  skeleton generalized NEC 756.50
  skin (appendage) 757.9
    specified type NEC 757.39
  skull (bone) 756.0
    with
      anencephalus 740.0
      encephalocele 742.0
      hydrocephalus 742.3
        with spina bifida (*see also* Spina bifida)
          741.0
      microcephalus 742.1
  specified type NEC
    adrenal (gland) 759.1
    alimentary tract (complete) (partial) 751.8
      lower 751.5
      upper 750.8
    ankle 755.69
    anus, anal (canal) 751.5
    aorta, aortic 747.29
      arch 747.21
    appendix 751.5
    arm 755.59
    artery (peripheral) NEC (*see also* Anomaly,
      peripheral vascular system) 747.60
      brain 747.81
      coronary 746.85
      eye 743.58
      pulmonary 747.39
      retinal 743.58
      umbilical 747.5
    auditory canal 744.29
      causing impairment of hearing 744.02
    bile duct or passage 751.69
    bladder 753.8
      neck 753.8
    bone(s) 756.9
      arm 755.59
      face 756.0
      leg 755.69
      pelvic girdle 755.69
      shoulder girdle 755.59
      skull 756.0
        with
          anencephalus 740.0
          encephalocele 742.0
          hydrocephalus 742.3
            with spina bifida (*see also* Spina
              bifida) 741.0
          microcephalus 742.1
    brain 742.4
    breast 757.6
    broad ligament 752.19
    bronchus 748.3

Anomaly, anomalous—*continued*
  specified type NEC—*continued*
    canal of Nuck 752.89
    cardiac septal closure 745.8
    carpus 755.59
    cartilaginous 756.9
    cecum 751.5
    cervix 752.49
    chest (wall) 756.3
    chin 744.89
    ciliary body 743.46
    circulatory system 747.89
    clavicle 755.51
    clitoris 752.49
    coccyx 756.19
    colon 751.5
    common duct 751.69
    connective tissue 756.89
    cricoid cartilage 748.3
    cystic duct 751.69
    diaphragm 756.6
    digestive organ(s) or tract 751.8
      lower 751.5
      upper 750.8
    duodenum 751.5
    ear 744.29
      auricle 744.29
        causing impairment of hearing 744.02
      causing impairment of hearing 744.09
      inner (causing impairment of hearing)
        744.05
      middle, except ossicles 744.03
        ossicles 744.04
    ejaculatory duct 752.89
    endocrine 759.2
    epiglottis 748.3
    esophagus 750.4
    Eustachian tube 744.24
    eye 743.8
      lid 743.63
      muscle 743.69
    face 744.89
      bone(s) 756.0
    fallopian tube 752.19
    fascia 756.89
    femur 755.69
    fibula 755.69
    finger 755.59
    foot 755.67
    fovea centralis 743.55
    gallbladder 751.69
    Gartner's duct 752.89
    gastrointestinal tract 751.8
    genitalia, genital organ(s)
      female 752.89
        external 752.49
        internal NEC 752.89
      male 752.89
        penis 752.69
        scrotal transposition 752.81
    genitourinary tract NEC 752.89
    glottis 748.3
    hair 757.4
    hand 755.59
    heart 746.89
      valve NEC 746.89
        pulmonary 746.09
    hepatic duct 751.69
    hydatid of Morgagni 752.89
    hymen 752.49
    integument 757.8

Anomaly, anomalous—*continued*
  specified type NEC—*continued*
    intestine (large) (small) 751.5
      fixational type 751.4
    iris 743.46
    jejunum 751.5
    joint 755.8
    kidney 753.3
    knee 755.64
    labium (majus) (minus) 752.49
    labyrinth, membranous 744.05
    larynx 748.3
    leg 755.69
    lens 743.39
    limb, except reduction deformity 755.8
      lower 755.69
        reduction deformity (*see also* Deformity,
          reduction, lower limb) 755.30
      upper 755.59
        reduction deformity (*see also* Deformity,
          reduction, upper limb) 755.20
    lip 750.26
    liver 751.69
    lung (fissure) (lobe) 748.69
    meatus urinarius 753.8
    metacarpus 755.59
    mouth 750.26
    Müllerian
      cervix 752.49
      uterus 752.39
      vagina 752.49
    muscle 756.89
      eye 743.69
    musculoskeletal system, except limbs 756.9
    nail 757.5
    neck 744.89
    nerve 742.8
      acoustic 742.8
      optic 742.8
    nervous system 742.8
    nipple 757.6
    nose 748.1
    organ NEC 759.89
      of Corti 744.05
    osseous meatus (ear) 744.03
    ovary 752.0
    oviduct 752.19
    pancreas 751.7
    parathyroid 759.2
    patella 755.64
    pelvic girdle 755.69
    penis 752.69
    pericardium 746.89
    peripheral vascular system NEC (*see also*
      Anomaly, peripheral vascular system)
      747.60
    pharynx 750.29
    pituitary 759.2
    prostate 752.89
    radius 755.59
    rectum 751.5
    respiratory system 748.8
    rib 756.3
    round ligament 752.89
    sacrum 756.19
    salivary duct or gland 750.26
    scapula 755.59
    sclera 743.47
    scrotum 752.89
      transposition 752.81
    seminal duct or tract 752.89

Anomaly, anomalous—*continued*
  specified type NEC—*continued*
    shoulder girdle 755.59
    site NEC 759.89
    skin 757.39
    skull (bone(s)) 756.0
      with
        anencephalus 740.0
        encephalocele 742.0
        hydrocephalus 742.3
          with spina bifida (*see also* Spina bifida)
            741.0
        microcephalus 742.1
    specified organ or site NEC 759.89
    spermatic cord 752.89
    spinal cord 742.59
    spine 756.19
    spleen 759.0
    sternum 756.3
    stomach 750.7
    tarsus 755.67
    tendon 756.89
    testis 752.89
    thorax (wall) 756.3
    thymus 759.2
    thyroid (gland) 759.2
      cartilage 748.3
    tibia 755.69
    toe 755.66
    tongue 750.19
    trachea (cartilage) 748.3
    ulna 755.59
    urachus 753.7
    ureter 753.4
      obstructive 753.29
    urethra 753.8
      obstructive 753.6
    urinary tract 753.8
    uterus (Müllerian) 752.39
    uvula 750.26
    vagina 752.49
    vascular NEC (*see also* Anomaly, peripheral
      vascular system) 747.60
      brain 747.81
    vas deferens 752.89
    vein(s) (peripheral) NEC (*see also* Anomaly,
      peripheral vascular system) 747.60
      brain 747.81
      great 747.49
      portal 747.49
      pulmonary 747.49
    vena cava (inferior) (superior) 747.49
    vertebra 756.19
    vulva 752.49
  spermatic cord 752.9
  spine, spinal 756.10
    column 756.10
    cord 742.9
      meningocele (*see also* Spina bifida) 741.9
      specified type NEC 742.59
      spina bifida (*see also* Spina bifida) 741.9
      vessel 747.82
    meninges 742.59
    nerve root 742.9
  spleen 759.0
  Sprengel's 755.52
  sternum 756.3
  stomach 750.9
    specified type NEC 750.7
  submaxillary gland 750.9
  superior vena cava 747.40

Anomaly, anomalous—*continued*
  talipes—*see* Talipes
  tarsus 755.67
    with complete absence of distal elements
      755.31
  teeth, tooth NEC 520.9
    position 524.30
      crowding 524.31
      displacement 524.30
        horizontal 524.33
        vertical 524.34
      distance
        interocclusal
          excessive 524.37
          insufficient 524.36
      excessive spacing 524.32
      rotation 524.35
      specified NEC 524.39
    spacing 524.30
  tendon 756.9
    specified type NEC 756.89
  termination
    coronary artery 746.85
  testis 752.9
  thebesian valve 746.9
  thigh 755.60
    flexion (*see also* Subluxation, congenital, hip)
      754.32
  thorax (wall) 756.3
  throat 750.9
  thumb 755.50
    supernumerary 755.01
  thymus gland 759.2
  thyroid (gland) 759.2
    cartilage 748.3
  tibia 755.60
    saber 090.5
  toe 755.66
    supernumerary 755.02
    webbed (*see also* Syndactylism, toes) 755.13
  tongue 750.10
    specified type NEC 750.19
  trachea, tracheal 748.3
    cartilage 748.3
    rings 748.3
  tragus 744.3
  transverse aortic arch 747.21
  trichromata 368.59
  trichromatopsia 368.59
  tricuspid (leaflet) (valve) 746.9
    atresia 746.1
    Ebstein's 746.2
    specified type NEC 746.89
    stenosis 746.1
  trunk 759.9
  Uhl's (hypoplasia of myocardium, right
    ventricle) 746.84
  ulna 755.50
  umbilicus 759.9
    artery 747.5
  union, trachea with larynx 748.3
  unspecified site 759.9
  upper extremity 755.50
    vessel 747.63
  urachus 753.7
    specified type NEC 753.7
  ureter 753.9
    obstructive 753.20
    specified type NEC 753.4
      obstructive 753.29

Anomaly, anomalous—*continued*
  urethra (valve) 753.9
    obstructive 753.6
    specified type NEC 753.8
  urinary tract or system (any part, except
    urachus) 753.9
    specified type NEC 753.8
    urachus 753.7
  uterus 752.39
    with only one functioning horn 752.33
    in pregnancy or childbirth 654.0
      affecting fetus or newborn 763.89
      causing obstructed labor 660.2
        affecting fetus or newborn 763.1
  uvula 750.9
  vagina 752.40
  valleculae 748.3
  valve (heart) NEC 746.9
    formation, ureter 753.29
    pulmonary 746.00
    specified type NEC 746.89
  vascular NEC (*see also* Anomaly, peripheral
    vascular system) 747.60
    ring 747.21
  vas deferens 752.9
  vein(s) (peripheral) NEC (*see also* Anomaly,
    peripheral vascular system) 747.60
    brain 747.81
    cerebral 747.81
    coronary 746.89
    great 747.40
      specified type NEC 747.49
    portal 747.40
    pulmonary 747.40
    retina 743.9
  vena cava (inferior) (superior) 747.40
  venous—*see* Anomaly, vein
  venous return (pulmonary) 747.49
    partial 747.42
    total 747.41
  ventricle, ventricular (heart) 746.9
    bands 746.9
    folds 746.9
    septa 745.4
  vertebra 756.10
  vesicourethral orifice 753.9
  vessels NEC (*see also* Anomaly, peripheral
    vascular system) 747.60
    optic papilla 743.9
  vitelline duct 751.0
  vitreous humor 743.9
    specified type NEC 743.51
  vulva 752.40
  wrist (joint) 755.50
Anomia 784.69
Anonychia 757.5
  acquired 703.8
Anophthalmos, anophthalmus (clinical)
  (congenital) (globe) 743.00
  acquired V45.78
Anopsia (altitudinal) (quadrant) 368.46
Anorchia 752.89
Anorchism, anorchidism 752.89
Anorexia 783.0
  hysterical 300.11
  nervosa 307.1
Anosmia (*see also* Disturbance, sensation) 781.1
  hysterical 300.11
  postinfectional 478.9
  psychogenic 306.7
  traumatic 951.8
Anosognosia 780.99

Anosphrasia 781.1
Anosteoplasia 756.50
Anotia 744.09
Anovulatory cycle 628.0
Anoxemia 799.02
  newborn 770.88
Anoxia 799.02
  altitude 993.2
  cerebral 348.1
    with
      abortion—*see* Abortion, by type,
        with specified complication NEC
      ectopic pregnancy (*see also* categories
        633.0-633.9) 639.8
      molar pregnancy (*see also* categories
        630-632) 639.8
    complicating
      delivery (cesarean) (instrumental) 669.4
      ectopic or molar pregnancy 639.8
      obstetric anesthesia or sedation 668.2
    during or resulting from a procedure 997.01
    following
      abortion 639.8
      ectopic or molar pregnancy 639.8
    newborn (*see also* Distress, fetal, liveborn
      infant) 770.88
  due to drowning 994.1
  fetal, affecting newborn 770.88
  heart—*see* Insufficiency, coronary
  high altitude 993.2
  intrauterine
    fetal death (before onset of labor) 768.0
      during labor 768.1
    liveborn infant—*see* Distress, fetal, liveborn
      infant
  myocardial—*see* Insufficiency, coronary
  newborn 768.9
    mild or moderate 768.6
    severe 768.5
  pathological 799.02
Anteflexion —*see* Anteversion
Antenatal
  care, normal pregnancy V22.1
    first V22.0
  sampling
    chorionic villus V28.89
  screening of mother (for) V28.9
    based on amniocentesis NEC V28.2
      chromosomal anomalies V28.0
      raised alphafetoprotein levels V28.1
    chromosomal anomalies V28.0
    fetal growth retardation using ultrasonics
      V28.4
    genomic V28.89
    isoimmunization V28.5
    malformations using ultrasonics V28.3
    proteomic V28.89
    raised alphafetoprotein levels in amniotic fluid
      V28.1
    risk
      pre-term labor V28.82
    specified condition NEC V28.89
    Streptococcus B V28.6
    survey
      fetal anatomic V28.81
    testing
      nuchal translucency V28.89
Antepartum —*see* condition
Anterior —*see also* condition
  spinal artery compression syndrome 721.1
Antero-occlusion 524.24

Anteversion
  cervix (—*see* Anteversion, uterus)
  femur (neck), congenital 755.63
  uterus, uterine (cervix) (postinfectional)
    (postpartal, old) 621.6
    congenital 752.39
    in pregnancy or childbirth 654.4
      affecting fetus or newborn 763.89
      causing obstructed labor 660.2
        affecting fetus or newborn 763.1
Anthracosilicosis (occupational) 500
Anthracosis (lung) (occupational) 500
  lingua 529.3
Anthrax 022.9
  with pneumonia 022.1 *[484.5]*
  colitis 022.2
  cutaneous 022.0
  gastrointestinal 022.2
  intestinal 022.2
  pulmonary 022.1
  respiratory 022.1
  septicemia 022.3
  specified manifestation NEC 022.8
Anthropoid pelvis 755.69
  with disproportion (fetopelvic) 653.2
    affecting fetus or newborn 763.1
    causing obstructed labor 660.1
      affecting fetus or newborn 763.1
Anthropophobia 300.29
Antibioma, breast 611.0
Antibodies
  maternal (blood group) (*see also*
    Incompatibility) 656.2
    anti-D, cord blood 656.1
    fetus or newborn 773.0
Antibody
  anticardiolipin 795.79
    with
      hemorrhagic disorder 286.53
      hypercoagulable state 289.81
  antiphosphatidylglycerol 795.79
    with
      hemorrhagic disorder 286.53
      hypercoagulable state 289.81
  antiphosphatidylinositol 795.79
    with
      hemorrhagic disorder 286.53
      hypercoagulable state 289.81
  antiphosphatidylserine 795.79
    with
      hemorrhagic disorder 286.53
      hypercoagulable state 289.81
  antiphospholipid 795.79
    with
      hemorrhagic disorder 286.53
      hypercoagulable state 289.81
  deficiency syndrome
    agammaglobulinemic 279.00
    congenital 279.04
    hypogammaglobulinemic 279.00
Anticoagulant
  intrinsic, circulating, causing hemorrhagic
    disorder (see also Circulating,
    anticoagulants) 286.59
  lupus (LAC) 795.79
    with
      hemorrhagic disorder 286.53
      hypercoagulable state 289.81
Antimongolism syndrome 758.39
Antimonial cholera 985.4
Antisocial personality 301.7

Antithrombinemia (*see also* Circulating
  anticoagulants) 286.59
Antithromboplastinemia (*see also* Circulating
  anticoagulants) 286.59
Antithromboplastinogenemia (*see also*
  Circulating anticoagulants) 286.59
Antitoxin complication or reaction —*see*
  Complications, vaccination
Anton (-Babinski) syndrome
  (hemiasomatognosia) 307.9
Antritis (chronic) 473.0
  maxilla 473.0
    acute 461.0
  stomach 535.4
Antrum, antral —*see* condition
Anuria 788.5
  with
    abortion—*see* Abortion, by type, with renal failure
    ectopic pregnancy (*see also* categories
      633.0-633.9) 639.3
    molar pregnancy (*see also* categories 630-632)
      639.3
  calculus (impacted) (recurrent) 592.9
    kidney 592.0
    ureter 592.1
  congenital 753.3
  due to a procedure 997.5
  following
    abortion 639.3
    ectopic or molar pregnancy 639.3
  newborn 753.3
  postrenal 593.4
  puerperal, postpartum, childbirth 669.3
  specified as due to a procedure 997.5
  sulfonamide
    correct substance properly administered 788.5
    overdose or wrong substance given or taken
      961.0
  traumatic (following crushing) 958.5
Anus, anal —*see also* condition
  high risk human papillomavirus (HPV) DNA
    test positive 796.75
  low risk human papillomavirus (HPV) DNA test
    positive 796.79
Anusitis 569.49
Anxiety (neurosis) (reaction) (state) 300.00
  alcohol-induced 291.89
  depression 300.4
  drug-induced 292.89
  due to or associated with physical condition 293.84
  generalized 300.02
  hysteria 300.20
  in
    acute stress reaction 308.0
    transient adjustment reaction 309.24
  panic type 300.01
  separation, abnormal 309.21
  syndrome (organic) (transient) 293.84
Aorta, aortic —*see* condition
Aortectasia (*see also* Ectasia, aortic) 447.70
  with aneurysm 441.9
Aortitis (nonsyphilitic) 447.6
  arteriosclerotic 440.0
  calcific 447.6
  Döhle-Heller 093.1
  luetic 093.1
  rheumatic (*see also* Endocarditis, acute,
    rheumatic) 391.1
  rheumatoid—*see* Arthritis, rheumatoid
  specific 093.1
  syphilitic 093.1
    congenital 090.5

Apathetic 799.25
  thyroid storm (*see also* Thyrotoxicosis) 242.9
Apathy 799.25
Apepsia 536.8
  achlorhydric 536.0
  psychogenic 306.4
Aperistalsis, esophagus 530.0
Apert's syndrome (acrocephalosyndactyly)
  755.55
Apert-Gallais syndrome (adrenogenital) 255.2
Apertognathia 524.20
Aphagia 787.20
  psychogenic 307.1
Aphakia (acquired) (bilateral) (postoperative)
  (unilateral) 379.31
  congenital 743.35
Aphalangia (congenital) 755.4
  lower limb (complete) (intercalary) (partial)
    (terminal) 755.39
    meaning all digits (complete) (partial) 755.31
    transverse 755.31
  upper limb (complete) (intercalary) (partial)
    (terminal) 755.29
    meaning all digits (complete) (partial) 755.21
    transverse 755.21
Aphasia (amnestic) (ataxic) (auditory) (Broca's)
  (choreatic) (classic) (expressive) (global)
  (ideational) (ideokinetic) (ideomotor) (jargon)
  (motor) (nominal) (receptive) (semantic)
  (sensory) (syntactic) (verbal) (visual)
  (Wernicke's) 784.3
  developmental 315.31
  syphilis, tertiary 094.89
  uremic—*see* Uremia
Aphemia 784.3
  uremic—*see* Uremia
Aphonia 784.41
  clericorum 784.49
  hysterical 300.11
  organic 784.41
  psychogenic 306.1
Aphthae, aphthous —*see also* condition
  Bednar's 528.2
  cachectic 529.0
  epizootic 078.4
  fever 078.4
  oral 528.2
  stomatitis 528.2
  thrush 112.0
  ulcer (oral) (recurrent) 528.2
    genital organ(s) NEC
      female 616.50
      male 608.89
    larynx 478.79
Apical —*see* condition
Apical ballooning syndrome 429.83
Aplasia —*see also* Agenesis
  alveolar process (acquired) 525.8
    congenital 750.26
  aorta (congenital) 747.22
  aortic valve (congenital) 746.89
  axialis extracorticalis (congenital) 330.0
  bone marrow (myeloid) 284.9
    acquired (secondary) 284.89
    congenital 284.01
    idiopathic 284.9
  brain 740.0
    specified part 742.2
  breast 757.6
  bronchus 748.3
  cementum 520.4

Aplasia—*continued*
  cerebellar 742.2
  congenital (pure) red cell 284.01
  corpus callosum 742.2
  erythrocyte 284.81
    congenital 284.01
  extracortical axial 330.0
  eye (congenital) 743.00
  fovea centralis (congenital) 743.55
  germinal (cell) 606.0
  iris 743.45
  labyrinth, membranous 744.05
  limb (congenital) 755.4
    lower NEC 755.30
    upper NEC 755.20
  lung (bilateral) (congenital) (unilateral) 748.5
  nervous system NEC 742.8
  nuclear 742.8
  ovary 752.0
  Pelizaeus-Merzbacher 330.0
  prostate (congenital) 752.89
  red cell (with thymoma) 284.81
    acquired (secondary) 284.81
      due to drugs 284.81
    adult 284.81
    congenital 284.01
    hereditary 284.01
    of infants 284.01
    primary 284.01
    pure 284.01
      due to drugs 284.81
  round ligament (congenital) 752.89
  salivary gland 750.21
  skin (congenital) 757.39
  spinal cord 742.59
  spleen 759.0
  testis (congenital) 752.89
  thymic, with immunodeficiency 279.2
  thyroid 243
  uterus 752.39
  ventral horn cell 742.59
Apleuria 756.3
Apnea, apneic (spells) 786.03
  newborn, neonatorum 770.81
    essential 770.81
    obstructive 770.82
    primary 770.81
    sleep 770.81
    specified NEC 770.82
  psychogenic 306.1
  sleep, unspecified 780.57
    with
      hypersomnia, unspecified 780.53
      hyposomnia, unspecified 780.51
      insomnia, unspecified 780.51
      sleep disturbance 780.57
    central, in conditions classified elsewhere 327.27
    obstructive (adult) (pediatric) 327.23
    organic 327.20
    other 327.29
    primary central 327.21
Apneumatosis newborn 770.4
Apodia 755.31
Apophysitis (bone) (*see also* Osteochondrosis) 732.9
  calcaneus 732.5
  juvenile 732.6
Apoplectiform convulsions (*see also* Disease, cerebrovascular, acute) 436

Apoplexia, apoplexy, apoplectic (*see also* Disease, cerebrovascular, acute) 436
  abdominal 569.89
  adrenal 036.3
  attack 436
  basilar (*see also* Disease, cerebrovascular, acute) 436
  brain (*see also* Disease, cerebrovascular, acute) 436
  bulbar (*see also* Disease, cerebrovascular, acute) 436
  capillary (*see also* Disease, cerebrovascular, acute) 436
  cardiac (*see also* Infarct, myocardium) 410.9
  cerebral (*see also* Disease, cerebrovascular, acute) 436
  chorea (*see also* Disease, cerebrovascular, acute) 436
  congestive (*see also* Disease, cerebrovascular, acute) 436
    newborn 767.4
  embolic (*see also* Embolism, brain) 434.1
  fetus 767.0
  fit (*see also* Disease, cerebrovascular, acute) 436
  healed or old V12.54
  heart (auricle) (ventricle) (*see also* Infarct, myocardium) 410.9
  heat 992.0
  hemiplegia (*see also* Disease, cerebrovascular, acute) 436
  hemorrhagic (stroke) (*see also* Hemorrhage, brain) 432.9
  ingravescent (*see also* Disease, cerebrovascular, acute) 436
  late effect—*see* Late effect(s) (of) cerebrovascular disease
  lung—*see* Embolism, pulmonary
  meninges, hemorrhagic (*see also* Hemorrhage, subarachnoid) 430
  neonatorum 767.0
  newborn 767.0
  pancreatitis 577.0
  placenta 641.2
  progressive (*see also* Disease, cerebrovascular, acute) 436
  pulmonary (artery) (vein)—*see* Embolism, pulmonary
  sanguineous (*see also* Disease, cerebrovascular, acute) 436
  seizure (*see also* Disease, cerebrovascular, acute) 436
  serous (*see also* Disease, cerebrovascular, acute) 436
  spleen 289.59
  stroke (*see also* Disease, cerebrovascular, acute) 436
  thrombotic (*see also* Thrombosis, brain) 434.0
  uremic—*see* Uremia
  uteroplacental 641.2
Appendage
  fallopian tube (cyst of Morgagni) 752.11
  intestine (epiploic) 751.5
  preauricular 744.1
  testicular (organ of Morgagni) 752.89
Appendicitis 541
  with
    perforation, peritonitis (generalized), or rupture 540.0
      with peritoneal abscess 540.1
    peritoneal abscess 540.1

Apendicitis—*continued*
  acute (catarrhal) (fulminating) (gangrenous)
      (inflammatory) (obstructive) (retrocecal)
      (suppurative) 540.9
    with
      perforation, peritonitis, or rupture 540.0
        with peritoneal abscess 540.1
      peritoneal abscess 540.1
    amebic 006.8
    chronic (recurrent) 542
    exacerbation—*see* Appendicitis, acute
    fulminating—*see* Appendicitis, acute
    gangrenous—*see* Appendicitis, acute
    healed (obliterative) 542
    interval 542
    neurogenic 542
    obstructive 542
    pneumococcal 541
    recurrent 542
    relapsing 542
    retrocecal 541
    subacute (adhesive) 542
    subsiding 542
    suppurative—*see* Appendicitis, acute
    tuberculous (*see also* Tuberculosis) 014.8
Appendiclausis 543.9
Appendicolithiasis 543.9
Appendicopathia oxyurica 127.4
Appendix, appendicular —*see also* condition
    Morgagni (male) 752.89
      fallopian tube 752.11
Appetite
    depraved 307.52
    excessive 783.6
      psychogenic 307.51
    lack or loss (*see also* Anorexia) 783.0
      nonorganic origin 307.59
    perverted 307.52
      hysterical 300.11
Apprehension, apprehensiveness (abnormal)
    (state) 300.00
    specified type NEC 300.09
Approximal wear 521.10
Apraxia (classic) (ideational) (ideokinetic)
    (ideomotor) (motor) 784.69
    oculomotor, congenital 379.51
    verbal 784.69
Aptyalism 527.7
Aqueous misdirection 365.83
Arabicum elephantiasis (*see also* Infestation,
    filarial) 125.9
Arachnidism 989.5
Arachnitis —*see* Meningitis
Arachnodactyly 759.82
Arachnoidism 989.5
Arachnoiditis (acute) (adhesive) (basic) (brain)
    (cerebrospinal) (chiasmal) (chronic) (spinal)
    (*see also* Meningitis) 322.9
    meningococcal (chronic) 036.0
    syphilitic 094.2
    tuberculous (*see also* Tuberculosis, meninges)
      013.0
Araneism 989.5
Arboencephalitis, Australian 062.4
Arborization block (heart) 426.6
Arbor virus, arbovirus (infection) NEC 066.9
ARC 042
Arches —*see* condition
Arcuate uterus 752.36
Arcuatus uterus 752.36

Arcus (cornea)
    juvenilis 743.43
      interfering with vision 743.42
    senilis 371.41
Arc-welders' lung 503
Arc-welders' syndrome (photokeratitis) 370.24
Areflexia 796.1
Areola —*see* condition
Argentaffinoma (M8241/1)—*see also* Neoplasm,
    by site, uncertain behavior
    benign (M8241/0)—*see* Neoplasm, by site,
      benign
    malignant (M8241/3)—*see* Neoplasm, by site,
      malignant
    syndrome 259.2
Argentinian hemorrhagic fever 078.7
Arginosuccinicaciduria 270.6
Argonz-Del Castillo syndrome (nonpuerperal
    galactorrhea and amenorrhea) 253.1
**Argyll-Robertson phenomenon pupil, or
    syndrome** (syphilitic) 094.89
    atypical 379.45
    nonluetic 379.45
    nonsyphilitic 379.45
    reversed 379.45
Argyria, argyriasis NEC 985.8
    conjunctiva 372.55
    cornea 371.16
    from drug or medicinal agent
      correct substance properly administered 709.09
      overdose or wrong substance given or taken 961.2
Arhinencephaly 742.2
Arias-Stella phenomenon 621.30
Ariboflavinosis 266.0
Arizona enteritis 008.1
Arm —*see* condition
Armenian disease 277.31
Arnold-Chiari obstruction or syndrome (*see
    also* Spina bifida) 741.0
    type I 348.4
    type II (*see also* Spina bifida) 741.0
    type III 742.0
    type IV 742.2
Arousals
    confusional 327.41
Arrest, arrested
    active phase of labor 661.1
      affecting fetus or newborn 763.7
    any plane in pelvis
      complicating delivery 660.1
        affecting fetus or newborn 763.1
    bone marrow (*see also* Anemia, aplastic) 284.9
    cardiac 427.5
      with
        abortion—*see* Abortion, by type, with
          specified complication NEC
        ectopic pregnancy (*see also* categories
          633.0-633.9) 639.8
        molar pregnancy (*see also* categories
          630-632) 639.8
      complicating
        anesthesia
          correct substance properly administered 427.5
            obstetric 668.1
          overdose or wrong substance given 968.4
            specified anesthetic—*see* Table of drugs
              and chemicals
        delivery (cesarean) (instrumental) 669.4
        ectopic or molar pregnancy 639.8
        surgery (nontherapeutic) (therapeutic) 997.1
      fetus or newborn 779.85

Arrest, arrested—*continued*
  cardiac—*continued*
    following
      abortion 639.8
      ectopic or molar pregnancy 639.8
    personal history, successfully rescucitated
      V12.53
    postoperative (immediate) 997.1
      long-term effect of cardiac surgery 429.4
  cardiorespiratory (*see also* Arrest, cardiac) 427.5
  deep transverse 660.3
    affecting fetus or newborn 763.1
  development or growth
    bone 733.91
    child 783.40
    fetus 764.9
      affecting management of pregnancy 656.5
    tracheal rings 748.3
  epiphyseal 733.91
  granulopoiesis 288.09
  heart—*see* Arrest, cardiac
  respiratory 799.1
    newborn 770.87
  sinus 426.6
  transverse (deep) 660.3
    affecting fetus or newborn 763.1
Arrhenoblastoma (M8630.1)
  benign (M8630/0)
    specified site—*see* Neoplasm, by site, benign
    unspecified site
      female 220
      male 222.0
  malignant (M8630/3)
    specified site— *see* Neoplasm, by site,
      malignant
    unspecified site
      female 183.0
      male 186.9
  specified site—*see* Neoplasm, by site, uncertain
    behavior
  unspecified site
    female 236.2
    male 236.4
Arrhinencephaly 742.2
  due to
    trisomy 13 (13-15) 758.1
    trisomy 18 (16-18) 758.2
Arrhythmia (auricle) (cardiac) (cordis) (gallop
  rhythm) (juvenile) (nodal) (reflex) (sinus)
  (supraventricular) (transitory) (ventricle) 427.9
  bigeminal rhythm 427.89
  block 426.9
  bradycardia 427.89
  contractions, premature 427.60
  coronary sinus 427.89
  ectopic 427.89
  extrasystolic 427.60
  postoperative 997.1
  psychogenic 306.2
  vagal 780.2
Arrillaga-Ayerza syndrome (pulmonary artery
  sclerosis with pulmonary hypertension) 416.0
Arsenical
  dermatitis 692.4
  keratosis 692.4
  pigmentation 985.1
    from drug or medicinal agent
      correct substance properly administered
        709.09
      overdose or wrong substance given or taken
        961.1

Arsenism 985.1
  from drug or medicinal agent
    correct substance properly administered 692.4
    overdose or wrong substance given or taken
      961.1
Arterial —*see* condition
Arteriectasis 447.8
Arteriofibrosis —*see* Arteriosclerosis
Arteriolar sclerosis —*see* Arteriosclerosis
Arteriolith —*see* Arteriosclerosis
Arteriolitis 447.6
  necrotizing, kidney 447.5
  renal—*see* Hypertension, kidney
Arteriolosclerosis —*see* Arteriosclerosis
Arterionephrosclerosis (*see also* Hypertension,
  kidney) 403.90
Arteriopathy 447.9
Arteriosclerosis, arteriosclerotic (artery)
  (deformans) (diffuse) (disease) (endarteritis)
  (general) (obliterans) (obliterative) (occlusive)
  (senile) (with calcification) 440.9
  with
    gangrene 440.24
    psychosis (*see also* Psychosis, arteriosclerotic)
      290.40
    ulceration 440.23
  aorta 440.0
  arteries of extremities NEC — *see*
    Arteriosclerosis, extremities
  basilar (artery) (*see also* Occlusion, artery,
    basilar) 433.0
  brain 437.0
  bypass graft
    coronary artery 414.05
      autologous artery (gastroepiploic) (internal
        mammary) 414.04
      autologous vein 414.02
      nonautologous biological 414.03
      of transplanted heart 414.07
    extremity 440.30
      autologous vein 440.31
      nonautologous biological 440.32
  cardiac — *see* Arteriosclerosis, coronary
  cardiopathy — *see* Arteriosclerosis, coronary
  cardiorenal (*see also* Hypertension, cardiorenal)
    404.90
  cardiovascular (*see also* Disease,
    cardiovascular) 429.2
  carotid (artery) (common) (internal) (*see also*
    Occlusion, artery, carotid) 433.1
  central nervous system 437.0
  cerebral 437.0
    late effect—*see* Late effect(s) (of)
      cerebrovascular disease
  cerebrospinal 437.0
  cerebrovascular 437.0
  coronary (artery) 414.00
    due to
      calcified coronary lesion (severely) 414.4
      lipid rich plaque 414.3
    graft—*see* Arteriosclerosis, bypass graft
    native artery 414.01
      of transplanted heart 414.06
    of transplanted heart 414.06
  extremities (native artery) 440.20
    bypass graft 440.30
      autologous vein 440.31
      nonautologous biological 440.32

Arteriosclerosis, arteriosclerotic—*continued*
  extremities—*continued*
    claudication (intermittent) 440.21
      and
        gangrene 440.24
        rest pain 440.22
          and
            gangrene 440.24
            ulceration 440.23
              and gangrene 440.24
          ulceration 440.23
            and gangrene 440.24
      gangrene 440.24
      rest pain 440.22
        and gangrene 440.24
        and ulceration 440.23
          and gangrene 440.24
      specified site NEC 440.29
      ulceration 440.23
        and gangrene 440.24
  heart (disease) — *see also* Arteriosclerosis, coronary
    valve 424.99
      aortic 424.1
      mitral 424.0
      pulmonary 424.3
      tricuspid 424.2
  iliac 440.8
  kidney (*see also* Hypertension, kidney) 403.90
  labyrinth, labyrinthine 388.00
  medial NEC 440.20
  mesentery (artery) 557.1
  Mönckeberg's 440.20
  myocarditis 429.0
  nephrosclerosis (*see also* Hypertension, kidney) 403.90
  peripheral (of extremities) *see* Arteriosclerosis, extremities
  precerebral 433.9
    specified artery NEC 433.8
  pulmonary (idiopathic) 416.0
  renal (*see also* Hypertension, kidney) 403.90
    arterioles (*see also* Hypertension, kidney) 403.90
    artery 440.1
  retinal (vascular) 440.8 *[362.13]*
  specified artery NEC 440.8
    with gangrene 440.8 *[785.4]*
  spinal (cord) 437.0
  vertebral (artery) (*see also* Occlusion, artery, vertebral) 433.2
Arteriospasm 443.9
Arteriovenous —*see* condition
Arteritis 447.6
  allergic (*see also* Angiitis, hypersensitivity) 446.20
  aorta (nonsyphilitic) 447.6
    syphilitic 093.1
  aortic arch 446.7
  brachiocephalica 446.7
  brain 437.4
    syphilitic 094.89
  branchial 446.7
  cerebral 437.4
    late effect—*see* Late effect(s) (of) cerebrovascular disease
    syphilitic 094.89
  coronary (artery) —*see also* Arteriosclerosis, coronary
    rheumatic 391.9
      chronic 398.99
    syphilitic 093.89

Arteritis—*continued*
  cranial (left) (right) 446.5
  deformans—*see* Arteriosclerosis
  giant cell 446.5
  necrosing or necrotizing 446.0
  nodosa 446.0
  obliterans—*see also* Arteriosclerosis
    subclaviocarotica 446.7
  pulmonary 417.8
  retina 362.18
  rheumatic—*see* Fever, rheumatic
  senile—*see* Arteriosclerosis
  suppurative 447.2
  syphilitic (general) 093.89
    brain 094.89
    coronary 093.89
    spinal 094.89
  temporal 446.5
  young female, syndrome 446.7
Artery, arterial —*see* condition
Arthralgia (*see also* Pain, joint) 719.4
  allergic (*see also* Pain, joint) 719.4
  in caisson disease 993.3
  psychogenic 307.89
  rubella 056.71
  Salmonella 003.23
  temporomandibular joint 524.62
Arthritis, arthritic (acute) (chronic) (subacute) 716.9

Note—Use the following fifth-digit subclassification with categories 711-712, 715-716:

0 *site unspecified*
1 *shoulder region*
2 *upper arm*
3 *forearm*
4 *hand*
5 *pelvic region and thigh*
6 *lower leg*
7 *ankle and foot*
8 *other specified sites*
9 *multiple sites*

  allergic 716.2
  ankylosing (crippling) (spine) 720.0
    sites other than spine 716.9
  atrophic 714.0
    spine 720.9
  back (*see also* Arthritis, spine) 721.90
  Bechterew's (ankylosing spondylitis) 720.0
  blennorrhagic 098.50
  cervical, cervicodorsal (*see also* Spondylosis, cervical) 721.0
  Charcot's 094.0 *[713.5]*
    diabetic 250.6 *[713.5]*
      due to secondary diabetes 249.6 *[713.5]*
    syringomyelic 336.0 *[713.5]*
    tabetic 094.0 *[713.5]*
  chylous (*see also* Filariasis) 125.9 *[711.7]*
  climacteric NEC 716.3
  coccyx 721.8
  cricoarytenoid 478.79
  crystal (-induced)—*see* Arthritis, due to crystals
  deformans (*see also* Osteoarthrosis) 715.9
    spine 721.90
      with myelopathy 721.91
  degenerative (*see also* Osteoarthrosis) 715.9
    idiopathic 715.09
    polyarticular 715.09
    spine 721.90
      with myelopathy 721.91

Arthritis, arthritic—*continued*
 dermatoarthritis, lipoid 272.8 *[713.0]*
 due to or associated with
  acromegaly 253.0 *[713.0]*
  actinomycosis 039.8 *[711.4]*
  amyloidosis 277.39 *[713.7]*
  bacterial disease NEC 040.89 *[711.4]*
  Behçet's syndrome 136.1 *[711.2]*
  blastomycosis 116.0 *[711.6]*
  brucellosis (*see also* Brucellosis) 023.9
    [711.4]
  caisson disease 993.3
  coccidioidomycosis 114.3 *[711.6]*
  coliform (Escherichia coli) 711.0
  colitis, ulcerative (*see also* Colitis, ulcerative)
    556.9 *[713.1]*
  cowpox 051.01 *[711.5]*
  crystals (*see also* Gout)
   dicalcium phosphate 275.49 *[712.1]*
   pyrophosphate 275.49 *[712.2]*
   specified NEC 275.49 *[712.8]*
  dermatoarthritis, lipoid 272.8 *[713.0]*
  dermatological disorder NEC 709.9 *[713.3]*
  diabetes 250.6 *[713.5]*
   due to secondary diabetes 249.6 *[713.5]*
  diphtheria 032.89 *[711.4]*
  dracontiasis 125.7 *[711.7]*
  dysentery 009.0 *[711.3]*
  endocrine disorder NEC 259.9 *[713.0]*
  enteritis NEC 009.1 *[711.3]*
   infectious (*see also* Enteritis, infectious)
     009.0 *[711.3]*
    specified organism NEC 008.8 *[711.3]*
   regional (*see also* Enteritis, regional) 555.9
     [713.1]
    specified organism NEC 008.8 *[711.3]*
  epiphyseal slip, nontraumatic (old) 716.8
  erysipelas 035 *[711.4]*
  erythema
   epidemic 026.1
   multiforme 695.10 *[713.3]*
   nodosum 695.2 *[713.3]*
  Escherichia coli 711.0
  filariasis NEC 125.9 *[711.7]*
  gastrointestinal condition NEC 569.9 *[713.1]*
  glanders 024 *[711.4]*
  Gonococcus 098.50
  gout 274.00
  H. influenzae 711.0
  helminthiasis NEC 128.9 *[711.7]*
  hematological disorder NEC 289.9 *[713.2]*
  hemochromatosis 275.03 *[713.0]*
  hemoglobinopathy NEC (*see also* Disease,
    hemoglobin) 282.7 *[713.2]*
  hemophilia (*see also* Hemophilia) 286.0
    [713.2]
  Hemophilus influenzae (H. influenzae) 711.0
  Henoch (-Schönlein) purpura 287.0 *[713.6]*
  histoplasmosis NEC (*see also* Histoplasmosis)
    115.99 *[711.6]*
  human parvovirus 079.83 *[711.5]*
  hyperparathyroidism 252.00 *[713.0]*
  hypersensitivity reaction NEC 995.3 *[713.6]*
  hypogammaglobulinemia (*see also*
    Hypogammaglobulinemia) 279.00 *[713.0]*
  hypothyroidism NEC 244.9 *[713.0]*
  infection (*see also* Arthritis, infectious) 711.9
  infectious disease NEC 136.9 *[711.8]*
  leprosy (*see also* Leprosy) 030.9 *[711.4]*
  leukemia NEC (M9800/3) 208.9 *[713.2]*
  lipoid dermatoarthritis 272.8 *[713.0]*

Arthritis, arthritic—*continued*
 due to or associated with—*continued*
  Lyme disease 088.81 *[711.8]*
  meaning Osteoarthritis—*see* Osteoarthrosis
  Mediterranean fever, familial 277.31 *[713.7]*
  meningococcal infection 036.82
  metabolic disorder NEC 277.9 *[713.0]*
  multiple myelomatosis (M9730/3) 203.0
    [713.2]
  mumps 072.79 *[711.5]*
  mycobacteria 031.8 *[711.4]*
  mycosis NEC 117.9 *[711.6]*
  neurological disorder NEC 349.9 *[713.5]*
  ochronosis 270.2 *[713.0]*
  O'Nyong Nyong 066.3 *[711.5]*
  parasitic disease NEC 136.9 *[711.8]*
  paratyphoid fever (*see also* Fever,
    paratyphoid) 002.9 *[711.3]*
  parvovirus B19 079.83 *[711.5]*
  Pneumococcus 711.0
  poliomyelitis (*see also* Poliomyelitis) 045.9
    [711.5]
  Pseudomonas 711.0
  psoriasis 696.0
  pyogenic organism (E. coli) (H. influenzae)
    (Pseudomonas) (Streptococcus) 711.0
  rat-bite fever 026.1 *[711.4]*
  regional enteritis (*see also* Enteritis, regional)
    555.9 *[713.1]*
  Reiter's disease 099.3 *[711.1]*
  respiratory disorder NEC 519.9 *[713.4]*
  reticulosis, malignant (M9720/3) 202.3
    [713.2]
  rubella 056.71
  salmonellosis 003.23
  sarcoidosis 135 *[713.7]*
  serum sickness 999.59 *[713.6]*
  Staphylococcus 711.0
  Streptococcus 711.0
  syphilis (*see also* Syphilis) 094.0 *[711.4]*
  syringomyelia 336.0 *[713.5]*
  thalassemia (*see also* Thalassemia) 282.40
    [713.2]
  tuberculosis (*see also* Tuberculosis, arthritis)
    015.9 *[711.4]*
  typhoid fever 002.0 *[711.3]*
  ulcerative colitis (*see also* Colitis, ulcerative)
    556.9 *[713.1]*
  urethritis
   nongonococcal (*see also* Urethritis,
     nongonococcal) 099.40 *[711.1]*
   nonspecific (*see also* Urethritis,
     nongonococcal) 099.40 *[711.1]*
   Reiter's 099.3 *[711.1]*
  viral disease NEC 079.99 *[711.5]*
 erythema epidemic 026.1
 gonococcal 098.50
 gouty 274.00
  acute 274.01
 hypertrophic (*see also* Osteoarthrosis) 715.9
  spine 721.90
   with myelopathy 721.91
 idiopathic, blennorrheal 099.3
 in caisson disease 993.3 *[713.8]*
 infectious or infective (acute) (chronic)
    (subacute) NEC 711.9
  nonpyogenic 711.9
  spine 720.9
 inflammatory NEC 714.9

Arthritis, arthritic—*continued*
  juvenile rheumatoid (chronic) (polyarticular)
      714.30
    acute 714.31
    monoarticular 714.33
    pauciarticular 714.32
  lumbar (*see also* Spondylosis, lumbar) 721.3
  meningococcal 036.82
  menopausal NEC 716.3
  migratory—*see* Fever, rheumatic
  neuropathic (Charcot's) 094.0 *[713.5]*
    diabetic 250.6 *[713.5]*
      due to secondary diabetes 249.6 *[713.5]*
    nonsyphilitic NEC 349.9 *[713.5]*
    syringomyelic 336.0 *[713.5]*
    tabetic 094.0 *[713.5]*
  nodosa (*see also* Osteoarthrosis) 715.9
    spine 721.90
      with myelopathy 721.91
  nonpyogenic NEC 716.9
    spine 721.90
      with myelopathy 721.91
  ochronotic 270.2 *[713.0]*
  palindromic (*see also* Rheumatism,
      palindromic) 719.3
  pneumococcal 711.0
  postdysenteric 009.0 *[711.3]*
  postrheumatic, chronic (Jaccoud's) 714.4
  primary progressive 714.0
    spine 720.9
  proliferative 714.0
    spine 720.0
  psoriatic 696.0
  purulent 711.0
  pyogenic or pyemic 711.0
  reactive 099.3
  rheumatic 714.0
    acute or subacute—*see* Fever, rheumatic
    chronic 714.0
    spine 720.9
  rheumatoid (nodular) 714.0
    with
      splenoadenomegaly and leukopenia 714.1
      visceral or systemic involvement 714.2
    aortitis 714.89
    carditis 714.2
    heart disease 714.2
    juvenile (chronic) (polyarticular) 714.30
      acute 714.31
      monoarticular 714.33
      pauciarticular 714.32
    spine 720.0
  rubella 056.71
  sacral, sacroiliac, sacrococcygeal (*see also*
      Spondylosis, sacral) 721.3
  scorbutic 267
  senile or senescent (*see also* Osteoarthrosis)
      715.9
    spine 721.90
      with myelopathy 721.91
  septic 711.0
  serum (nontherapeutic) (therapeutic) 999.59
      [713.6]
  specified form NEC 716.8
  spine 721.90
    with myelopathy 721.91
    atrophic 720.9
    degenerative 721.90
      with myelopathy 721.91
    hypertrophic (with deformity) 721.90
      with myelopathy 721.91

Arthritis, arthritic—*continued*
  spine—*continued*
    infectious or infective NEC 720.9
    Marie-Strümpell 720.0
    nonpyogenic 721.90
      with myelopathy 721.91
    pyogenic 720.9
    rheumatoid 720.0
    traumatic (old) 721.7
    tuberculous (*see also* Tuberculosis) 015.0
        [720.81]
  staphylococcal 711.0
  streptococcal 711.0
  suppurative 711.0
  syphilitic 094.0 *[713.5]*
    congenital 090.49 *[713.5]*
  syphilitica deformans (Charcot) 094.0 *[713.5]*
  temporomandibular joint 524.69
  thoracic (*see also* Spondylosis, thoracic) 721.2
  toxic of menopause 716.3
  transient 716.4
  traumatic (chronic) (old) (post) 716.1
    current injury—*see* nature of injury
  tuberculous (*see also* Tuberculosis, arthritis)
        015.9 *[711.4]*
  urethritica 099.3 *[711.1]*
  urica, uratic 274.00
  venereal 099.3 *[711.1]*
  vertebral (*see also* Arthritis, spine) 721.90
  villous 716.8
  von Bechterew's 720.0
Arthrocele (*see also* Effusion, joint) 719.0
Arthrochondritis —*see* Arthritis
Arthrodesis status V45.4
Arthrodynia (*see also* Pain, joint) 719.4
  psychogenic 307.89
Arthrodysplasia 755.9
Arthrofibrosis, joint (*see also* Ankylosis) 718.5
Arthrogryposis 728.3
  multiplex, congenita 754.89
Arthrokatadysis 715.35
Arthrolithiasis 274.00
Arthro-onychodysplasia 756.89
Arthro-osteo-onychodysplasia 756.89
Arthropathy (*see also* Arthritis) 716.9

> *Note*—*Use the following fifth-digit
> subclassification with categories 711-712, 716:*
>
> 0 *site unspecified*
> 1 *shoulder region*
> 2 *upper arm*
> 3 *forearm*
> 4 *hand*
> 5 *pelvic region and thigh*
> 6 *lower leg*
> 7 *ankle and foot*
> 8 *other specified sites*
> 9 *multiple sites*

  Behçet's 136.1 *[711.2]*
  Charcot's 094.0 *[713.5]*
    diabetic 250.6 *[713.5]*
      due to secondary diabetes 249.6 *[713.5]*
    syringomyelic 336.0 *[713.5]*
    tabetic 094.0 *[713.5]*
  crystal (-induced)—*see* Arthritis, due to crystals

Arthropathy—*continued*
gouty 274.00
  acute 274.01
  chronic (without mention of tophus (tophi)) 274.02
    with tophus (tophi) 274.03
neurogenic, neuropathic (Charcot's) (tabetic) 094.0 *[713.5]*
  diabetic 250.6 *[713.5]*
    due to secondary diabetes 249.6 *[713.5]*
  nonsyphilitic NEC 349.9 *[713.5]*
  syringomyelic 336.0 *[713.5]*
postdysenteric NEC 009.0 *[711.3]*
postrheumatic, chronic (Jaccoud's) 714.4
psoriatic 696.0
pulmonary 731.2
specified NEC 716.8
syringomyelia 336.0 *[713.5]*
tabes dorsalis 094.0 *[713.5]*
tabetic 094.0 *[713.5]*
transient 716.4
traumatic 716.1
uric acid 274.00
Arthrophyte (*see also* Loose, body, joint) 718.1
Arthrophytis 719.80
ankle 719.87
elbow 719.82
foot 719.87
hand 719.84
hip 719.85
knee 719.86
multiple sites 719.89
pelvic region 719.85
shoulder (region) 719.81
specified site NEC 719.88
wrist 719.83
Arthropyosis (*see also* Arthritis, pyogenic) 711.0
Arthroscopic surgical procedure converted to open procedure V64.43
Arthrosis (deformans) (degenerative) (*see also* Osteoarthrosis) 715.9
Charcot's 094.0 *[713.5]*
polyarticular 715.09
spine (*see also* Spondylosis) 721.90
Arthus' phenomenon 995.21
due to
  correct substance properly administered 995.21
  overdose or wrong substance given or taken 977.9
    specified drug—*see* Table of drugs and chemicals
serum 999.59
Articular —*see also* condition
disc disorder (reducing or non-reducing) 524.63
spondylolisthesis 756.12
Articulation
anterior 524.27
posterior 524.27
reverse 524.27
Artificial
device (prosthetic)—*see* Fitting, device
insemination V26.1
menopause (states) (symptoms) (syndrome) 627.4
opening status (functioning) (without complication) V44.9
  anus (colostomy) V44.3
  colostomy V44.3
  cystostomy V44.50
    appendico-vesicostomy V44.52
    cutaneous-vesicostomy V44.51
    specified type NEC V44.59

Artificial—*continued*
opening status—*continued*
  enterostomy V44.4
  gastrostomy V44.1
  ileostomy V44.2
  intestinal tract NEC V44.4
  jejunostomy V44.4
  nephrostomy V44.6
  specified site NEC V44.8
  tracheostomy V44.0
  ureterostomy V44.6
  urethrostomy V44.6
  urinary tract NEC V44.6
  vagina V44.7
  vagina status V44.7
ARV (disease) (illness) (infection)—*see* Human immunodeficiency virus (disease) (illness) (infection)
Arytenoid —*see* condition
Asbestosis (occupational) 501
Asboe-Hansen's disease (incontinentia pigmenti) 757.33
Ascariasis (intestinal) (lung) 127.0
Ascaridiasis 127.0
Ascaridosis 127.0
Ascaris 127.0
lumbricoides (infestation) 127.0
pneumonia 127.0
Ascending —*see* condition
ASC-H (atypical squamous cells cannot exclude high grade squamous intraepithelial lesion)
anus 796.72
cervix 795.02
vagina 795.12
Aschoff's bodies (*see also* Myocarditis, rheumatic) 398.0
Ascites 789.59
abdominal NEC 789.59
cancerous (M8000/6) 789.51
cardiac 428.0
chylous (nonfilarial) 457.8
  filarial (*see also* Infestation, filarial) 125.9
congenital 778.0
due to S. japonicum 120.2
fetal, causing fetopelvic disproportion 653.7
heart 428.0
joint (*see also* Effusion, joint) 719.0
malignant (M8000/6) 789.51
pseudochylous 789.59
syphilitic 095.2
tuberculous (*see also* Tuberculosis) 014.0
Ascorbic acid (vitamin C) deficiency (scurvy) 267
ASC-US (atypical squamous cells of undetermined significance)
anus 796.71
cervix 795.01
vagina 795.11
ASCVD (arteriosclerotic cardiovascular disease) 429.2
Aseptic —*see* condition
Asherman's syndrome 621.5
Asialia 527.7
Asiatic cholera (*see also* Cholera) 001.9
Asocial personality or trends 301.7
Asomatognosia 781.8
Aspergillosis 117.3
with pneumonia 117.3 *[484.6]*
allergic bronchopulmonary 518.6
nonsyphilitic NEC 117.3

Aspergillus (flavus) (fumigatus) (infection)
  (terreus) 117.3
Aspermatogenesis 606.0
Aspermia (testis) 606.0
Asphyxia, asphyxiation (by) 799.01
  antenatal—*see* Distress, fetal
  bedclothes 994.7
  birth (*see also* Asphyxia, newborn) 768.9
  bunny bag 994.7
  carbon monoxide 986
  caul (*see also* Asphyxia, newborn) 768.9
  cave-in 994.7
    crushing—*see* Injury, internal, intrathoracic
      organs
  constriction 994.7
  crushing—*see* Injury, internal, intrathoracic
    organs
  drowning 994.1
  fetal, affecting newborn 768.9
  food or foreign body (in larynx) 933.1
    bronchioles 934.8
    bronchus (main) 934.1
    lung 934.8
    nasopharynx 933.0
    nose, nasal passages 932
    pharynx 933.0
    respiratory tract 934.9
      specified part NEC 934.8
    throat 933.0
    trachea 934.0
  gas, fumes, or vapor NEC 987.9
    specified—*see* Table of drugs and chemicals
  gravitational changes 994.7
  hanging 994.7
  inhalation—*see* Inhalation
  intrauterine
    fetal death (before onset of labor) 768.0
      during labor 768.1
    liveborn infant—*see* Distress, fetal, liveborn
      infant
  local 443.0
  mechanical 994.7
    during birth (*see also* Distress, fetal) 768.9
  mucus 933.1
    bronchus (main) 934.1
    larynx 933.1
    lung 934.8
    nasal passages 932
    newborn 770.18
    pharynx 933.0
    respiratory tract 934.9
      specified part NEC 934.8
    throat 933.0
    trachea 934.0
    vaginal (fetus or newborn) 770.18
  newborn 768.9
    blue 768.6
    livida 768.6
    mild or moderate 768.6
    pallida 768.5
    severe 768.5
    white 768.5
    with neurologic involvement 768.5
  pathological 799.01
  plastic bag 994.7
  postnatal (*see also* Asphyxia, newborn) 768.9
    mechanical 994.7
  pressure 994.7
  reticularis 782.61
  strangulation 994.7
  submersion 994.1

Asphyxia, asphyxiation—*continued*
  traumatic NEC—*see* Injury, internal,
    intrathoracic organs
  vomiting, vomitus—*see* Asphyxia, food or
    foreign body
Aspiration
  acid pulmonary (syndrome) 997.39
    obstetric 668.0
  amniotic fluid 770.13
    with respiratory symptoms 770.14
  bronchitis 507.0
  clear amniotic fluid 770.13
    with
      pneumonia 770.14
      pneumonitis 770.14
      respiratory symptoms 770.14
  contents of birth canal 770.17
    with respiratory symptoms 770.18
  fetal 770.10
    blood 770.15
      with
        pneumonia 770.16
        pneumonitis 770.16
      pneumonitis 770.18
  food, foreign body, or gasoline (with
    asphyxiation)—*see* Asphyxia, food or
    foreign body
  meconium 770.11
    with
      pneumonia 770.12
      pneumonitis 770.12
      respiratory symptoms 770.12
    below vocal cords 770.11
      with respiratory symptoms 770.12
  mucus 933.1
    into
      bronchus (main) 934.1
      lung 934.8
      respiratory tract 934.9
        specified part NEC 934.8
      trachea 934.0
    newborn 770.17
    vaginal (fetus or newborn) 770.17
  newborn 770.10
    with respiratory symptoms 770.18
    blood 770.15
      with
        pneumonia 770.16
        pneumonitis 770.16
        respiratory symptoms 770.16
  pneumonia 507.0
    fetus or newborn 770.18
      meconium 770.12
  pneumonitis 507.0
    fetus or newborn 770.18
      meconium 770.12
    obstetric 668.0
  postnatal stomach contents 770.85
    with
      pneumonia 770.86
      pneumonitis 770.86
      respiratory symptoms 770.86
  syndrome of newborn (massive) 770.18
    meconium 770.12
  vernix caseosa 770.17
Asplenia 759.0
  with mesocardia 746.87
Assam fever 085.0

Assimilation, pelvis
  with disproportion 653.2
    affecting fetus or newborn 763.1
    causing obstructed labor 660.1
      affecting fetus or newborn 763.1
Assmann's focus (*see also* Tuberculosis) 011.0
Astasia (-abasia) 307.9
  hysterical 300.11
Asteatosis 706.8
  cutis 706.8
Astereognosis 780.99
Asterixis 781.3
  in liver disease 572.8
Asteroid hyalitis 379.22
Asthenia, asthenic 780.79
  cardiac (*see also* Failure, heart) 428.9
    psychogenic 306.2
  cardiovascular (*see also* Failure, heart) 428.9
    psychogenic 306.2
  heart (*see also* Failure, heart) 428.9
    psychogenic 306.2
  hysterical 300.11
  myocardial (*see also* Failure, heart) 428.9
    psychogenic 306.2
  nervous 300.5
  neurocirculatory 306.2
  neurotic 300.5
  psychogenic 300.5
  psychoneurotic 300.5
  psychophysiologic 300.5
  reaction, psychoneurotic 300.5
  senile 797
  Stiller's 780.79
  tropical anhidrotic 705.1
Asthenopia 368.13
  accommodative 367.4
  hysterical (muscular) 300.11
  psychogenic 306.7
Asthenospermia 792.2
Asthma, asthmatic (bronchial) (catarrh) (spasmodic) 493.9

Note—The following fifth digit subclassification is for use with codes 493.0-493.2, 493.9:

0 unspecified
1 with status asthmaticus
2 with (acute) exacerbation

---

  with
    chronic obstructive pulmonary disease (COPD) 493.2
    hay fever 493.0
    rhinitis, allergic 493.0
  allergic 493.9
    stated cause (external allergen) 493.0
  atopic 493.0
  cardiac (*see also* Failure, ventricular, left) 428.1
  cardiobronchial (*see also* Failure, ventricular, left) 428.1
  cardiorenal (*see also* Hypertension, cardiorenal) 404.90
  childhood 493.0
  colliers' 500
  cough variant 493.82
  croup 493.9
  detergent 507.8
  due to
    detergent 507.8
    inhalation of fumes 506.3
    internal immunological process 493.0

Asthma, asthmatic—*continued*
  endogenous (intrinsic) 493.1
  eosinophilic 518.3
  exercise induced bronchospasm 493.81
  exogenous (cosmetics) (dander or dust) (drugs) (dust) (feathers) (food) (hay) (platinum) (pollen) 493.0
  extrinsic 493.0
  grinders' 502
  hay 493.0
  heart (*see also* Failure, ventricular, left) 428.1
  IgE 493.0
  infective 493.1
  intrinsic 493.1
  Kopp's 254.8
  late-onset 493.1
  meat-wrappers' 506.9
  Millar's (laryngismus stridulus) 478.75
  millstone makers' 502
  miners' 500
  Monday morning 504
  New Orleans (epidemic) 493.0
  platinum 493.0
  pneumoconiotic (occupational) NEC 505
  potters' 502
  psychogenic 316 [493.9]
  pulmonary eosinophilic 518.3
  red cedar 495.8
  Rostan's (*see also* Failure, ventricular, left) 428.1
  sandblasters' 502
  sequoiosis 495.8
  stonemasons' 502
  thymic 254.8
  tuberculous (*see also* Tuberculosis, pulmonary) 011.9
  Wichmann's (laryngismus stridulus) 478.75
  wood 495.8
Astigmatism (compound) (congenital) 367.20
  irregular 367.22
  regular 367.21
Astroblastoma (M9430/3)
  nose 748.1
  specified site—*see* Neoplasm, by site, malignant
  unspecified site 191.9
Astrocytoma (cystic) (M9400/3)
  anaplastic type (M9401/3)
    specified site—*see* Neoplasm, by site, malignant
    unspecified site 191.9
  fibrillary (M9420/3)
    specified site—*see* Neoplasm, by site, malignant
    unspecified site 191.9
  fibrous (M9420/3)
    specified site—*see* Neoplasm, by site, malignant
    unspecified site 191.9
  gemistocytic (M9411/3)
    specified site—*see* Neoplasm, by site, malignant
    unspecified site 191.9
  juvenile (M9421/3)
    specified site—*see* Neoplasm, by site, malignant
    unspecified site 191.9
  nose 748.1
  pilocytic (M9421/3)
    specified site—*see* Neoplasm, by site, malignant
    unspecified site 191.9

Astrocytoma—*continued*
piloid (M9421/3)
   specified site—*see* Neoplasm, by site, malignant
   unspecified site 191.9
protoplasmic (M9410/3)
   specified site—*see* Neoplasm, by site,
      malignant
   unspecified site 191.9
specified site—*see* Neoplasm, by site, malignant
subependymal (M9383/1) 237.5
   giant cell (M9384/1) 237.5
unspecified site 191.9
Astroglioma (M9400/3)
nose 748.1
specified site—*see* Neoplasm, by site, malignant
unspecified site 191.9
Asymbolia 784.60
Asymmetrical breathing 786.09
Asymmetry —*see also* Distortion
breast, between native and reconstructed 612.1
chest 786.9
face 754.0
jaw NEC 524.12
   maxillary 524.11
pelvis with disproportion 653.0
   affecting fetus or newborn 763.1
   causing obstructed labor 660.1
      affecting fetus or newborn 763.1
Asynergia 781.3
Asynergy 781.3
ventricular 429.89
Asystole (heart) (*see also* Arrest, cardiac) 427.5
At risk for falling V15.88
Ataxia, ataxy, ataxic 781.3
acute 781.3
brain 331.89
cerebellar 334.3
   hereditary (Marie's) 334.2
   in
      alcoholism 303.9 *[334.4]*
      myxedema (*see also* Myxedema) 244.9
         [334.4]
      neoplastic disease NEC 239.9 *[334.4]*
cerebral 331.89
family, familial 334.2
   cerebral (Marie's) 334.2
   spinal (Friedreich's) 334.0
   Friedreich's (heredofamilial) (spinal) 334.0
frontal lobe 781.3
gait 781.2
   hysterical 300.11
general 781.3
hereditary NEC 334.2
   cerebellar 334.2
   spastic 334.1
   spinal 334.0
heredofamilial (Marie's) 334.2
hysterical 300.11
locomotor (progressive) 094.0
   diabetic 250.6 *[337.1]*
      due to secondary diabetes 249.6 *[337.1]*
Marie's (cerebellar) (heredofamilial) 334.2
nonorganic origin 307.9
partial 094.0
postchickenpox 052.7
progressive locomotor 094.0
psychogenic 307.9
Sanger-Brown's 334.2
spastic 094.0
   hereditary 334.1
   syphilitic 094.0

Ataxia, ataxy, ataxic—*continued*
spinal
   hereditary 334.0
   progressive locomotor 094.0
telangiectasia 334.8
Ataxia-telangiectasia 334.8
Atelectasis (absorption collapse) (complete)
   (compression) (massive) (partial)
   (postinfective) (pressure collapse)
   (pulmonary) (relaxation) 518.0
newborn (congenital) (partial) 770.5
   primary 770.4
primary 770.4
tuberculous (*see also* Tuberculosis, pulmonary)
   011.9
Ateleiosis, ateliosis 253.3
Atelia —*see* Distortion
Ateliosis 253.3
Atelocardia 746.9
Atelomyelia 742.59
Athelia 757.6
Atheroembolism
extremity
   lower 445.02
   upper 445.01
kidney 445.81
specified site NEC 445.89
Atheroma, atheromatous (*see also*
   Arteriosclerosis) 440.9
aorta, aortic 440.0
   valve (*see also* Endocarditis, aortic) 424.1
artery—*see* Arteriosclerosis
basilar, (artery) (*see also* Occlusion, artery,
   basilar) 433.0
carotid (artery) (common) (internal) (*see also*
   Occlusion, artery, carotid) 433.1
cerebral (arteries) 437.0
coronary (artery)—*see* Arteriosclerosis, coronary
degeneration—*see* Arteriosclerosis
heart, cardiac —*see* Arteriosclerosis, coronary
mitral (valve) 424.0
myocardium, myocardial —*see* Arteriosclerosis,
   coronary
pulmonary valve (heart) (*see also* Endocarditis,
   pulmonary) 424.3
skin 706.2
tricuspid (heart) (valve) 424.2
valve, valvular—*see* Endocarditis
vertebral (artery) (*see also* Occlusion, artery,
   vertebral) 433.2
Atheromatosis —*see also* Arteriosclerosis
arterial, congenital 272.8
Atherosclerosis —*see* Arteriosclerosis
Athetosis (acquired) 781.0
bilateral 333.79
congenital (bilateral) 333.6
double 333.71
unilateral 781.0
Athlete's
foot 110.4
heart 429.3
Athletic team examination V70.3
Athrepsia 261
Athyrea (acquired) (*see also* Hypothyroidism) 244.9
congenital 243
Athyreosis (congenital) 243
acquired—*see* Hypothyroidism
Athyroidism (acquired) (*see also*
   Hypothyroidism) 244.9
congenital 243
Atmospheric pyrexia 992.0

Atonia, atony, atonic
abdominal wall 728.2
bladder (sphincter) 596.4
  neurogenic NEC 596.54
    with cauda equina syndrome 344.61
capillary 448.9
cecum 564.89
  psychogenic 306.4
colon 564.89
  psychogenic 306.4
congenital 779.89
dyspepsia 536.3
  psychogenic 306.4
intestine 564.89
  psychogenic 306.4
stomach 536.3
  neurotic or psychogenic 306.4
  psychogenic 306.4
uterus 661.2
  affecting fetus or newborn 763.7
  with hemorrhage (postpartum) 666.1
  without hemorrhage
    intrapartum 661.2
    postpartum 669.8
vesical 596.4
Atopy NEC V15.09
Atransferrinemia, congenital 273.8
Atresia, atretic (congenital) 759.89
alimentary organ or tract NEC 751.8
  lower 751.2
  upper 750.8
ani, anus, anal (canal) 751.2
aorta 747.22
  with hypoplasia of ascending aorta and
    defective development of left ventricle
    (with mitral valve atresia) 746.7
  arch 747.11
  ring 747.21
aortic (orifice) (valve) 746.89
  arch 747.11
aqueduct of Sylvius 742.3
  with spina bifida (*see also* Spina bifida) 741.0
artery NEC (*see also* Atresia, blood vessel)
  747.60
  cerebral 747.81
  coronary 746.85
  eye 743.58
  pulmonary 747.31
  umbilical 747.5
auditory canal (external) 744.02
bile, biliary duct (common) or passage 751.61
  acquired (*see also* Obstruction, biliary) 576.2
bladder (neck) 753.6
blood vessel (peripheral) NEC 747.60
  cerebral 747.81
  gastrointestinal 747.61
  lower limb 747.64
  pulmonary (artery) 747.31
  renal 747.62
  spinal 747.82
  upper limb 747.63
bronchus 748.3
canal, ear 744.02
cardiac
  valve 746.89
    aortic 746.89
    mitral 746.89
    pulmonary 746.01
    tricuspid 746.1
cecum 751.2

Atresia, atretic—*continued*
cervix (acquired) 622.4
  congenital 752.43
  in pregnancy or childbirth 654.6
    affecting fetus or newborn 763.89
    causing obstructed labor 660.2
      affecting fetus or newborn 763.1
choana 748.0
colon 751.2
cystic duct 751.61
  acquired 575.8
    with obstruction (*see also* Obstruction,
      gallbladder) 575.2
digestive organs NEC 751.8
duodenum 751.1
ear canal 744.02
ejaculatory duct 752.89
epiglottis 748.3
esophagus 750.3
Eustachian tube 744.24
fallopian tube (acquired) 628.2
  congenital 752.19
follicular cyst 620.0
foramen of
  Luschka 742.3
    with spina bifida (*see also* Spina bifida) 741.0
  Magendie 742.3
    with spina bifida (*see also* Spina bifida)
      741.0
gallbladder 751.69
genital organ
  external
    female 752.49
    male NEC 752.89
      penis 752.69
  internal
    female 752.89
    male 752.89
glottis 748.3
gullet 750.3
heart
  valve NEC 746.89
    aortic 746.89
    mitral 746.89
    pulmonary 746.01
    tricuspid 746.1
hymen 752.42
  acquired 623.3
  postinfective 623.3
ileum 751.1
intestine (small) 751.1
  large 751.2
iris, filtration angle (*see also* Buphthalmia)
  743.20
jejunum 751.1
kidney 753.3
lacrimal, apparatus 743.65
  acquired—*see* Stenosis, lacrimal
larynx 748.3
ligament, broad 752.19
lung 748.5
meatus urinarius 753.6
mitral valve 746.89
  with atresia or hypoplasia of aortic orifice or
    valve, with hypoplasia of ascending aorta
    and defective development of left ventricle
    746.7
nares (anterior) (posterior) 748.0
nasolacrimal duct 743.65
nasopharynx 748.8

Atresia, atretic—*continued*
  nose, nostril 748.0
    acquired 738.0
    organ or site NEC—*see* Anomaly, specified
      type NEC
  osseous meatus (ear) 744.03
  oviduct (acquired) 628.2
    congenital 752.19
  parotid duct 750.23
    acquired 527.8
  pulmonary (artery) 747.31
    valve 746.01
    vein 747.49
  pulmonic 746.01
  pupil 743.46
  rectum 751.2
  salivary duct or gland 750.23
    acquired 527.8
  sublingual duct 750.23
    acquired 527.8
  submaxillary duct or gland 750.23
    acquired 527.8
  trachea 748.3
  tricuspid valve 746.1
  ureter 753.29
  ureteropelvic junction 753.21
  ureterovesical orifice 753.22
  urethra (valvular) 753.6
  urinary tract NEC 753.29
  uterus 752.31
    acquired 621.8
  vagina (acquired) 623.2
    congenital (total) (partial) 752.45
    postgonococcal (old) 098.2
    postinfectional 623.2
    senile 623.2
  vascular NEC (*see also* Atresia, blood vessel)
      747.60
    cerebral 747.81
  vas deferens 752.89
  vein NEC (*see also* Atresia, blood vessel)
      747.60
    cardiac 746.89
    great 747.49
    portal 747.49
    pulmonary 747.49
  vena cava (inferior) (superior) 747.49
  vesicourethral orifice 753.6
  vulva 752.49
    acquired 624.8
Atrichia, atrichosis 704.00
  congenital (universal) 757.4
Atrioventricularis commune 745.69
Atrophia —*see also* Atrophy
  alba 709.09
  cutis 701.8
    idiopathica progressiva 701.8
    senilis 701.8
  dermatological, diffuse (idiopathic) 701.8
  flava hepatis (acuta) (subacuta) (*see also*
      Necrosis, liver) 570
  gyrata of choroid and retina (central) 363.54
    generalized 363.57
  senilis 797
    dermatological 701.8
  unguium 703.8
    congenita 757.5

Atrophoderma, atrophodermia 701.9
  diffusum (idiopathic) 701.8
  maculatum 701.3
    et striatum 701.3
      due to syphilis 095.8
    syphilitic 091.3
  neuriticum 701.8
  pigmentosum 757.33
  reticulatum symmetricum faciei 701.8
  senile 701.8
  symmetrical 701.8
  vermiculata 701.8
Atrophy, atrophic
  adrenal (autoimmune) (capsule) (cortex) (gland) 255.41
    with hypofunction 255.41
  alveolar process or ridge (edentulous) 525.20
    mandible 525.20
      minimal 525.21
      moderate 525.22
      severe 525.23
    maxilla 525.20
      minimal 525.24
      moderate 525.25
      severe 525.26
  appendix 543.9
  Aran-Duchenne muscular 335.21
  arm 728.2
  arteriosclerotic—*see* Arteriosclerosis
  arthritis 714.0
    spine 720.9
  bile duct (any) 576.8
  bladder 596.89
  blanche (of Milian) 701.3
  bone (senile) 733.99
    due to
      disuse 733.7
      infection 733.99
      tabes dorsalis (neurogenic) 094.0
    posttraumatic 733.99
  brain (cortex) (progressive) 331.9
    with dementia 290.10
    Alzheimer's 331.0
      with dementia—*see* Alzheimer's dementia
    circumscribed (Pick's) 331.11
      with dementia
        with behavioral disturbance 331.11
          [294.11]
        without behavioral disturbance 331.11
          [294.10]
    congenital 742.4
    hereditary 331.9
    senile 331.2
  breast 611.4
    puerperal, postpartum 676.3
  buccal cavity 528.9
  cardiac (brown) (senile) (*see also* Degeneration,
      myocardial) 429.1
  cartilage (infectional) (joint) 733.99
  cast, plaster of Paris 728.2
  cerebellar—*see* Atrophy, brain
  cerebral—*see* Atrophy, brain
  cervix (endometrium) (mucosa) (myometrium)
      (senile) (uteri) 622.8
    menopausal 627.8
  Charcot-Marie-Tooth 356.1

Atrophy, atrophic—*continued*
 choroid 363.40
  diffuse secondary 363.42
  hereditary (*see also* Dystrophy, choroid)
    363.50
   gyrate
    central 363.54
    diffuse 363.57
    generalized 363.57
  senile 363.41
 ciliary body 364.57
 colloid, degenerative 701.3
 conjunctiva (senile) 372.89
 corpus cavernosum 607.89
 cortical (*see also* Atrophy, brain) 331.9
 Cruveilhier's 335.21
 cystic duct 576.8
 dacryosialadenopathy 710.2
 degenerative
  colloid 701.3
  senile 701.3
 Déjérine-Thomas 333.0
 diffuse idiopathic, dermatological 701.8
 disuse
  bone 733.7
  muscle 728.2
  pelvic muscles and anal sphincter 618.83
 Duchenne-Aran 335.21
 ear 388.9
 edentulous alveolar ridge 525.20
  mandible 525.20
   minimal 525.21
   moderate 525.22
   severe 525.23
  maxilla 525.20
   minimal 525.24
   moderate 525.25
   severe 525.26
 emphysema, lung 492.8
 endometrium (senile) 621.8
  cervix 622.8
 enteric 569.89
 epididymis 608.3
 eyeball, cause unknown 360.41
 eyelid (senile) 374.50
 facial (skin) 701.9
 facioscapulohumeral (Landouzy-Déjérine) 359.1
 fallopian tube (senile), acquired 620.3
 fatty, thymus (gland) 254.8
 gallbladder 575.8
 gastric 537.89
 gastritis (chronic) 535.1
 gastrointestinal 569.89
 genital organ, male 608.89
 glandular 289.3
 globe (phthisis bulbi) 360.41
 gum (*see also* Recession, gingival) 523.20
 hair 704.2
 heart (brown) (senile) (*see also* Degeneration,
    myocardial) 429.1
 hemifacial 754.0
  Romberg 349.89
 hydronephrosis 591
 infantile 261
  paralysis, acute (*see also* Poliomyelitis, with
    paralysis) 045.1
 intestine 569.89
 iris (generalized) (postinfectional) (sector
    shaped) 364.59
  essential 364.51
  progressive 364.51
  sphincter 364.54

Atrophy, atrophic—*continued*
 kidney (senile) (*see also* Sclerosis, renal) 587
  with hypertension (*see also* Hypertension,
    kidney) 403.90
  congenital 753.0
  hydronephrotic 591
  infantile 753.0
 lacrimal apparatus (primary) 375.13
  secondary 375.14
 Landouzy-Déjérine 359.1
 laryngitis, infection 476.0
 larynx 478.79
 Leber's optic 377.16
 lip 528.5
 liver (acute) (subacute) (*see also* Necrosis, liver)
    570
  chronic (yellow) 571.8
  yellow (congenital) 570
   with
    abortion—*see* Abortion, by type, with
      specified complication NEC
    ectopic pregnancy (*see also* categories
      633.0-633.9) 639.8
    molar pregnancy (*see also* categories
      630-632) 639.8
   chronic 571.8
   complicating pregnancy 646.7
   following
    abortion 639.8
    ectopic or molar pregnancy 639.8
   from injection, inoculation or transfusion
     (onset within 8 months after
     administration)—*see* Hepatitis, viral
   healed 571.5
   obstetric 646.7
   postabortal 639.8
   postimmunization—*see* Hepatitis, viral
   posttransfusion—*see* Hepatitis, viral
   puerperal, postpartum 674.8
 lung (senile) 518.89
  congenital 748.69
 macular (dermatological) 701.3
  syphilitic, skin 091.3
   striated 095.8
 muscle, muscular 728.2
  disuse 728.2
  Duchenne-Aran 335.21
  extremity (lower) (upper) 728.2
  familial spinal 335.11
  general 728.2
  idiopathic 728.2
  infantile spinal 335.0
  myelopathic (progressive) 335.10
  myotonic 359.21
  neuritic 356.1
  neuropathic (peroneal) (progressive) 356.1
  peroneal 356.1
  primary (idiopathic) 728.2
  progressive (familial) (hereditary) (pure)
    335.21
   adult (spinal) 335.19
   infantile (spinal) 335.0
   juvenile (spinal) 335.11
   spinal 335.10
    adult 335.19
    hereditary or familial 335.11
    infantile 335.0
  pseudohypertrophic 359.1
   spinal (progressive) 335.10
    adult 335.19
    Aran-Duchenne 335.21
    familial 335.11

Atrophy, atrophic—*continued*
  muscle, muscular—*continued*
    pseudohypertrophic —*continued*
      hereditary 335.11
      infantile 335.0
        juvenile 335.11
     syphilitic 095.6
  myocardium (*see also* Degeneration,
    myocardial) 429.1
  myometrium (senile) 621.8
    cervix 622.8
  myotatic 728.2
  myotonia 359.21
  nail 703.8
    congenital 757.5
  nasopharynx 472.2
    abducens 378.54
    accessory 352.4
    acoustic or auditory 388.5
    cranial 352.9
     first (olfactory) 352.0
     second (optic) (*see also* Atrophy, optic
      nerve) 377.10
     third (oculomotor) (partial) 378.51
      total 378.52
     fourth (trochlear) 378.53
     fifth (trigeminal) 350.8
     sixth (abducens) 378.54
     seventh (facial) 351.8
     eighth (auditory) 388.5
     ninth (glossopharyngeal) 352.2
     tenth (pneumogastric) (vagus) 352.3
     eleventh (accessory) 352.4
     twelfth (hypoglossal) 352.5
    facial 351.8
    glossopharyngeal 352.2
    hypoglossal 352.5
    oculomotor (partial) 378.51
     total 378.52
    olfactory 352.0
    peripheral 355.9
    pneumogastric 352.3
    trigeminal 350.8
    trochlear 378.53
    vagus (pneumogastric) 352.3
  nervous system, congenital 742.8
  neuritic (*see also* Disorder, nerve) 355.9
  neurogenic NEC 355.9
    bone
     tabetic 094.0
  nutritional 261
  old age 797
  olivopontocerebellar 333.0
  optic nerve (ascending) (descending)
    (infectional) (nonfamilial) (papillomacular
    bundle) (postretinal) (secondary NEC)
    (simple) 377.10
    associated with retinal dystrophy 377.13
    dominant hereditary 377.16
    glaucomatous 377.14
    hereditary (dominant) (Leber's) 377.16
    Leber's (hereditary) 377.16
    partial 377.15
    postinflammatory 377.12
    primary 377.11
    syphilitic 094.84
     congenital 090.49
     tabes dorsalis 094.0
  orbit 376.45
  ovary (senile), acquired 620.3
  oviduct (senile), acquired 620.3

Atrophy, atrophic—*continued*
  palsy, diffuse 335.20
  pancreas (duct) (senile) 577.8
  papillary muscle 429.81
  paralysis 355.9
  parotid gland 527.0
  patches skin 701.3
    senile 701.8
  penis 607.89
  pharyngitis 472.1
  pharynx 478.29
  pluriglandular 258.8
  polyarthritis 714.0
  prostate 602.2
  pseudohypertrophic 359.1
  renal (*see also* Sclerosis, renal) 587
  reticulata 701.8
  retina (*see also* Degeneration, retina) 362.60
    hereditary (*see also* Dystrophy, retina) 362.70
  rhinitis 472.0
  salivary duct or gland 527.0
  scar NEC 709.2
  sclerosis, lobar (of brain) 331.0
    with dementia
     with behavioral disturbance 331.0 *[294.11]*
     without behavioral disturbance 331.0
      [294.10]
  scrotum 608.89
  seminal vesicle 608.89
  senile 797
    degenerative, of skin 701.3
  skin (patches) (senile) 701.8
  spermatic cord 608.89
  spinal (cord) 336.8
    acute 336.8
    muscular (chronic) 335.10
     adult 335.19
     familial 335.11
     juvenile 335.10
    paralysis 335.10
     acute (*see also* Poliomyelitis, with paralysis)
      045.1
  spine (column) 733.99
  spleen (senile) 289.59
  spots (skin) 701.3
    senile 701.8
  stomach 537.89
  striate and macular 701.3
    syphilitic 095.8
  subcutaneous 701.9
    due to injection 999.9
  sublingual gland 527.0
  submaxillary gland 527.0
  Sudeck's 733.7
  suprarenal (autoimmune) (capsule) (gland)
    255.41
    with hypofunction 255.41
  tarso-orbital fascia, congenital 743.66
  testis 608.3
  thenar, partial 354.0
  throat 478.29
  thymus (fat) 254.8
  thyroid (gland) 246.8
    with
     cretinism 243
     myxedema 244.9
    congenital 243
  tongue (senile) 529.8
    papillae 529.4
    smooth 529.4
  trachea 519.19

Atrophy, atrophic—*continued*
tunica vaginalis 608.89
turbinate 733.99
tympanic membrane (nonflaccid) 384.82
    flaccid 384.81
ulcer (*see also* Ulcer, skin) 707.9
upper respiratory tract 478.9
uterus, uterine (acquired) (senile) 621.8
    cervix 622.8
    due to radiation (intended effect) 621.8
vagina (senile) 627.3
vascular 459.89
vas deferens 608.89
vertebra (senile) 733.99
vulva (primary) (senile) 624.1
Werdnig-Hoffmann 335.0
yellow (acute) (congenital) (liver) (subacute)
    (*see also* Necrosis, liver) 570
    chronic 571.8
    resulting from administration of blood,
        plasma, serum, or other biological
        substance (within 8 months of
        administration)—*see* Hepatitis, viral
Attack
akinetic (*see also* Epilepsy) 345.0
angina—*see* Angina
apoplectic (*see also* Disease, cerebrovascular,
    acute) 436
benign shuddering 333.93
bilious—*see* Vomiting
cataleptic 300.11
cerebral (*see also* Disease, cerebrovascular,
    acute) 436
coronary (*see also* Infarct, myocardium) 410.9
cyanotic, newborn 770.83
epileptic (*see also* Epilepsy) 345.9
epileptiform 780.39
heart (*see also* Infarct, myocardium) 410.9
hemiplegia (*see also* Disease, cerebrovascular,
    acute) 436
hysterical 300.11
jacksonian (*see also* Epilepsy) 345.5
myocardium, myocardial (*see also* Infarct,
    myocardium) 410.9
myoclonic (*see also* Epilepsy) 345.1
panic 300.01
paralysis (*see also* Disease, cerebrovascular,
    acute) 436
paroxysmal 780.39
psychomotor (*see also* Epilepsy) 345.4
salaam (*see also* Epilepsy) 345.6
schizophreniform (*see also* Schizophrenia)
    295.4
sensory and motor 780.39
syncope 780.2
toxic, cerebral 780.39
transient ischemic (TIA) 435.9
unconsciousness 780.2
    hysterical 300.11
vasomotor 780.2
vasovagal (idiopathic) (paroxysmal) 780.2
Attention to
artificial
    opening (of) V55.9
        digestive tract NEC V55.4
        specified site NEC V55.8
        urinary tract NEC V55.6
    vagina V55.7
colostomy V55.3
cystostomy V55.5

Attention to—*continued*
dressing
    wound V58.30
        nonsurgical V58.30
        surgical V58.31
gastrostomy V55.1
ileostomy V55.2
jejunostomy V55.4
nephrostomy V55.6
surgical dressings V58.31
sutures V58.32
tracheostomy V55.0
ureterostomy V55.6
urethrostomy V55.6
Attrition
gum (*see also* Recession, gingival) 523.20
teeth (hard tissues) 521.10
    excessive 521.10
        extending into
            dentine 521.12
            pulp 521.13
        generalized 521.15
        limited to enamel 521.11
        localized 521.14
Atypical —*see also* condition
cells
    endocervical 795.00
    endometrial 795.00
    glandular
        anus 796.70
        cervical 795.00
        vaginal 795.10
    distribution, vessel (congenital) (peripheral)
        NEC 747.60
    endometrium 621.9
    kidney 593.89
Atypism, cervix 622.10
Audible tinnitus (*see also* Tinnitus) 388.30
Auditory —*see* condition
Audry's syndrome (acropachyderma) 757.39
Aujeszky's disease 078.89
Aura
jacksonian (*see also* Epilepsy) 345.5
persistent migraine 346.5
    with cerebral infarction 346.6
    without cerebral infarction 346.5
Aurantiasis, cutis 278.3
Auricle, auricular —*see* condition
Auriculotemporal syndrome 350.8
Australian
Q fever 083.0
X disease 062.4
Autism, autistic (child) (infantile) 299.0
Autodigestion 799.89
Autoerythrocyte sensitization 287.2
Autographism 708.3
Autoimmune
cold sensitivity 283.0
disease NEC 279.49
hemolytic anemia 283.0
inhibitors to clotting factors 286.52
lymphoproliferative syndrome (ALPS) 279.41
thyroiditis 245.2
Autoinfection, septic —*see* Septicemia
Autointoxication 799.89
Automatism 348.89
epileptic (*see also* Epilepsy) 345.4
paroxysmal, idiopathic (*see also* Epilepsy) 345.4
    with temporal sclerosis 348.81

Autonomic, autonomous
  bladder 596.54
    neurogenic 596.54
      with cauda equine 344.61
  dysreflexia 337.3
  faciocephalalgia (*see also* Neuropathy,
    peripheral, autonomic) 337.9
  hysterical seizure 300.11
  imbalance (*see also* Neuropathy, peripheral,
    autonomic) 337.9
Autophony 388.40
Autosensitivity, erythrocyte 287.2
Autotopagnosia 780.99
Autotoxemia 799.89
Autumn —*see* condition
Avellis' syndrome 344.89
Aversion
  oral 783.3
    newborn 779.31
    nonorganic origin 307.59
Aviators
  disease or sickness (*see also* Effect, adverse,
    high altitude) 993.2
  ear 993.0
  effort syndrome 306.2
Avitaminosis (multiple NEC) (*see also*
  Deficiency, vitamin) 269.2
  A 264.9
  B 266.9
    with
      beriberi 265.0
      pellagra 265.2
  B$_1$ 265.1
  B$_2$ 266.0
  B$_6$ 266.1
  B$_{12}$ 266.2
  C (with scurvy) 267
  D 268.9
    with
      osteomalacia 268.2
      rickets 268.0
  E 269.1
  G 266.0
  H 269.1
  K 269.0
  multiple 269.2
  nicotinic acid 265.2
  P 269.1
Avulsion (traumatic) 879.8
  blood vessel—*see* Injury, blood vessel, by site
  cartilage—*see also* Dislocation, by site
    knee, current (*see also* Tear, meniscus) 836.2
    symphyseal (inner), complicating delivery 665.6
  complicated 879.9
  diaphragm—*see* Injury, internal, diaphragm
  ear—*see* Wound, open, ear
  epiphysis of bone—*see* Fracture, by site
  external site other than limb—*see* Wound, open,
    by site
  eye 871.3
  fingernail—*see* Wound, open, finger
  fracture—*see* Fracture, by site
  genital organs, external—*see* Wound, open,
    genital organs
  head (intracranial) NEC—*see also* Injury,
    intracranial, with open intracranial wound
    complete 874.9
    external site NEC 873.8
      complicated 873.9
  internal organ or site—*see* Injury, internal, by site

Avulsion—*continued*
  joint—*see also* Dislocation, by site
    capsule—*see* Sprain, by site
  ligament—*see* Sprain, by site
  limb—*see also* Amputation, traumatic, by site
    skin and subcutaneous tissue—*see* Wound,
      open, by site
  muscle—*see* Sprain, by site
  nerve (root)—*see* Injury, nerve, by site
  scalp—*see* Wound, open, scalp
  skin and subcutaneous tissue—*see* Wound,
    open, by site
  symphyseal cartilage (inner), complicating
    delivery 665.6
  tendon—*see also* Sprain, by site
    with open wound—*see* Wound, open, by site
  toenail—*see* Wound, open, toe(s)
  tooth 873.63
    complicated 873.73
Awaiting organ transplant status V49.83
Awareness of heart beat 785.1
Axe grinders' disease 502
Axenfeld's anomaly or syndrome 743.44
Axilla, axillary —*see also* condition
  breast 757.6
Axonotmesis —*see* Injury, nerve, by site
Ayala's disease 756.89
Ayerza's disease or syndrome (pulmonary
  artery sclerosis with pulmonary hypertension)
  416.0
Azoospermia 606.0
Azorean disease (of the nervous system) 334.8
Azotemia 790.6
  meaning uremia (*see also* Uremia) 586
Aztec ear 744.29
Azygos lobe, lung (fissure) 748.69

B

Baader's syndrome (erythema multiforme exudativum) 695.19
Baastrup's syndrome 721.5
Babesiasis 088.82
Babesiosis 088.82
Babington's disease (familial hemorrhagic telangiectasia) 448.0
Babinski's syndrome (cardiovascular syphilis) 093.89
Babinski-Fröhlich syndrome (adiposogenital dystrophy) 253.8
Babinski-Nageotte syndrome 344.89
Bacillary —*see* condition
Bacilluria 791.9
  asymptomatic, in pregnancy or puerperium 646.5
  tuberculous (*see also* Tuberculosis) 016.9
Bacillus —*see also* Infection, bacillus
  abortus infection 023.1
  anthracis infection 022.9
  coli
    infection 041.49
      generalized 038.42
      intestinal 008.00
    pyemia 038.42
    septicemia 038.42
  Flexner's 004.1
  fusiformis infestation 101
  mallei infection 024
  Shiga's 004.0
  suipestifer infection (*see also* Infection, Salmonella) 003.9
Back —*see* condition
Backache (postural) 724.5
  psychogenic 307.89
  sacroiliac 724.6
Backflow (pyelovenous) (*see also* Disease, renal) 593.9
Backknee (*see also* Genu, recurvatum) 736.5
Bacteremia (*see also* Infection, bacillus) 790.7
  newborn 771.83
Bacteria
  in blood (*see also* Bacteremia) 790.7
  in urine (*see also* Bacteriuria) 599.0
Bacterial —*see* condition
Bactericholia (*see also* Cholecystitis, acute) 575.0
Bacterid, bacteride (Andrews' pustular) 686.8
Bacteriuria, bacteruria 791.9
  with
    urinary tract infection 599.0
  asymptomatic 791.9
    in pregnancy or puerperium 646.5
      affecting fetus or newborn 760.1
Bad
  breath 784.99
  heart—*see* Disease, heart
  trip (*see also* Abuse, drugs, nondependent) 305.3
Baehr-Schiffrin disease (thrombotic thrombocytopenic purpura) 446.6
Baelz's disease (cheilitis glandularis apostematosa) 528.5
Baerensprung's disease (eczema marginatum) 110.3
Bagassosis (occupational) 495.1
Baghdad boil 085.1

Bagratuni's syndrome (temporal arteritis) 446.5
Baker's
  cyst (knee) 727.51
    tuberculous (*see also* Tuberculosis) 015.2
  itch 692.89
Bakwin-Krida syndrome (craniometaphyseal dysplasia) 756.89
Balanitis (circinata) (gangraenosa) (infectious) (vulgaris) 607.1
  amebic 006.8
  candidal 112.2
  chlamydial 099.53
  due to Ducrey's bacillus 099.0
  erosiva circinata et gangraenosa 607.1
  gangrenous 607.1
  gonococcal (acute) 098.0
    chronic or duration of 2 months or over 098.2
  nongonococcal 607.1
  phagedenic 607.1
  venereal NEC 099.8
  xerotica obliterans 607.81
Balanoposthitis 607.1
  chlamydial 099.53
  gonococcal (acute) 098.0
    chronic or duration of 2 months or over 098.2
  ulcerative NEC 099.8
Balanorrhagia —*see* Balanitis
Balantidiasis 007.0
Balantidiosis 007.0
Balbuties, balbutio (*see also* Disorder, fluency) 315.35
Bald
  patches on scalp 704.00
  tongue 529.4
Baldness (*see also* Alopecia) 704.00
Balfour's disease (chloroma) 205.3
Balint's syndrome (psychic paralysis of visual fixation) 368.16
Balkan grippe 083.0
Ball
  food 938
  hair 938
Ballantyne (-Runge) syndrome (postmaturity) 766.22
Balloon disease (*see also* Effect, adverse, high altitude) 993.2
Ballooning posterior leaflet syndrome 424.0
Baló's disease or concentric sclerosis 341.1
Bamberger's disease (hypertrophic pulmonary osteoarthropathy) 731.2
Bamberger-Marie disease (hypertrophic pulmonary osteoarthropathy) 731.2
Bamboo spine 720.0
Bancroft's filariasis 125.0
Band(s)
  adhesive (*see also* Adhesions, peritoneum) 568.0
  amniotic 658.8
    affecting fetus or newborn 762.8
  anomalous or congenital—*see also* Anomaly, specified type NEC
    atrial 746.9
    heart 746.9
    intestine 751.4
    omentum 751.4
    ventricular 746.9
  cervix 622.3
  gallbladder (congenital) 751.69

Band(s)—*continued*
  intestinal (adhesive) (*see also* Adhesions,
    peritoneum) 568.0
    congenital 751.4
  obstructive (*see also* Obstruction, intestine)
    560.81
  periappendiceal (congenital) 751.4
  peritoneal (adhesive) (*see also* Adhesions,
    peritoneum) 568.0
    with intestinal obstruction 560.81
    congenital 751.4
  uterus 621.5
  vagina 623.2
Bandemia (without diagnosis of specific
    infection) 288.66
Bandl's ring (contraction)
  complicating delivery 661.4
    affecting fetus or newborn 763.7
Bang's disease (Brucella abortus) 023.1
Bangkok hemorrhagic fever 065.4
Bannister's disease 995.1
Bantam-Albright-Martin disease
    (pseudohypoparathyroidism) 275.49
Banti's disease or syndrome (with cirrhosis)
    (with portal hypertension)—*see* Cirrhosis, liver
Bar
  calcaneocuboid 755.67
  calcaneonavicular 755.67
  cubonavicular 755.67
  prostate 600.90
    with
      other lower urinary tract symptoms (LUTS)
        600.91
      urinary
        obstruction 600.91
        retention 600.91
  talocalcaneal 755.67
Baragnosis 780.99
Barasheh, barashek 266.2
Barcoo disease or rot (*see also* Ulcer, skin) 707.9
Bard-Pic syndrome (carcinoma, head of
    pancreas) 157.0
Bärensprung's disease (eczema marginatum)
    110.3
Baritosis 503
Barium lung disease 503
Barlow's syndrome (meaning mitral valve
    prolapse) 424.0
Barlow (-Möller) disease or syndrome (meaning
    infantile scurvy) 267
Barodontalgia 993.2
Baron Münchausen syndrome 301.51
Barosinusitis 993.1
Barotitis 993.0
Barotrauma 993.2
  odontalgia 993.2
  otitic 993.0
  sinus 993.1
Barraquer's disease or syndrome (progressive
    lipodystrophy) 272.6
Barré-Guillain syndrome 357.0
Barré-Liéou syndrome (posterior cervical
    sympathetic) 723.2
Barrel chest 738.3
Barrett's esophagus 530.85
Barrett's syndrome or ulcer (chronic peptic
    ulcer of esophagus) 530.85
Bársony-Polgár syndrome (corkscrew
    esophagus) 530.5
Bársony-Teschendorf syndrome (corkscrew
    esophagus) 530.5

Barth syndrome 759.89
Bartholin's
  adenitis (*see also* Bartholinitis) 616.89
  gland—*see* condition
Bartholinitis (suppurating) 616.89
  gonococcal (acute) 098.0
    chronic or duration of 2 months or over 098.2
Bartonellosis 088.0
Bartter's syndrome (secondary
    hyperaldosteronism with juxtaglomerular
    hyperplasia) 255.13
Basal—*see* condition
Basan's (hidrotic) ectodermal dysplasia 757.31
Baseball finger 842.13
Basedow's disease or syndrome (exophthalmic
    goiter) 242.0
Basic —*see* condition
Basilar —*see* condition
Bason's (hidrotic) ectodermal dysplasia 757.31
Basopenia 288.59
Basophilia 288.65
Basophilism (corticoadrenal) (Cushing's)
    (pituitary) (thymic) 255.0
Bassen-Kornzweig syndrome
    (abetalipoproteinemia) 272.5
Bat ear 744.29
Bateman's
  disease 078.0
  purpura (senile) 287.2
Bathing cramp 994.1
Bathophobia 300.23
Batten's disease, retina 330.1 *[362.71]*
Batten-Mayou disease 330.1 *[362.71]*
Batten-Steinert syndrome 359.21
Battered
  adult (syndrome) 995.81
  baby or child (syndrome) 995.54
  spouse (syndrome) 995.81
Battey mycobacterium infection 031.0
Battledore placenta —*see* Placenta, abnormal
Battle exhaustion (*see also* Reaction, stress,
    acute) 308.9
Baumgarten-Cruveilhier (cirrhosis) disease, or
    syndrome 571.5
Bauxite
  fibrosis (of lung) 503
  workers' disease 503
Bayle's disease (dementia paralytica) 094.1
Bazin's disease (primary) (*see also* Tuberculosis)
    017.1
Beach ear 380.12
Beaded hair (congenital) 757.4
Beals syndrome 759.82
Beard's disease (neurasthenia) 300.5
Bearn-Kunkel (-Slater) syndrome (lupoid
    hepatitis) 571.49
Beat
  elbow 727.2
  hand 727.2
  knee 727.2
Beats
  ectopic 427.60
  escaped, heart 427.60
    postoperative 997.1
  premature (nodal) 427.60
    atrial 427.61
    auricular 427.61
    postoperative 997.1
    specified type NEC 427.69
    supraventricular 427.61
    ventricular 427.69

Beau's
  disease or syndrome (*see also* Degeneration, myocardial) 429.1
  lines (transverse furrows on fingernails) 703.8
Bechterew's disease (ankylosing spondylitis) 720.0
Bechterew-Strümpell-Marie syndrome (ankylosing spondylitis) 720.0
Beck's syndrome (anterior spinal artery occlusion) 433.8
Becker's
  disease
    idiopathic mural endomyocardial disease 425.2
    myotonia congenita, recessive form 359.22
  dystrophy 359.22
Beckwith (-Wiedemann) syndrome 759.89
Bedbugs bite(s) —*see* Injury, superfiical, by site
Bed confinement status V49.84
Bedclothes, asphyxiation or suffocation by 994.7
Bednar's aphthae 528.2
Bedsore (*see also* Ulcer, pressure) 707.00
  with gangrene 707.00 *[785.4]*
Bedwetting (*see also* Enuresis) 788.36
Beer-drinkers' heart (disease) 425.5
Bee sting (with allergic or anaphylactic shock) 989.5
Begbie's disease (exophthalmic goiter) 242.0
Behavior disorder, disturbance —*see also* Disturbance, conduct
  antisocial, without manifest psychiatric disorder
    adolescent V71.02
    adult V71.01
    child V71.02
  dyssocial, without manifest psychiatric disorder
    adolescent V71.02
    adult V71.01
    child V71.02
  high-risk—*see* Problem
Behçet's syndrome 136.1
Behr's disease 362.50
Beigel's disease or morbus (white piedra) 111.2
Bejel 104.0
Bekhterev's disease (ankylosing spondylitis) 720.0
Bekhterev-Strümpell-Marie syndrome (ankylosing spondylitis) 720.0
Belching (*see also* Eructation) 787.3
Bell's
  disease (*see also* Psychosis, affective) 296.0
  mania (*see also* Psychosis, affective) 296.0
  palsy, paralysis 351.0
    infant 767.5
    newborn 767.5
    syphilitic 094.89
  spasm 351.0
Bence-Jones albuminuria, albuminosuria, or proteinuria 791.0
Bends 993.3
Benedikt's syndrome (paralysis) 344.89
Benign —*see also* condition
  cellular changes, cervix 795.09
  prostate
    hyperplasia 600.20
      with urinary retention 600.21
    neoplasm 222.2
    with
      other lower urinary tract symptoms (LUTS) 600.21
      urinary
        obstruction 600.21
        retention 600.21

Bennett's
  disease (leukemia) 208.9
  fracture (closed) 815.01
    open 815.11
Benson's disease 379.22
Bent
  back (hysterical) 300.11
  nose 738.0
    congenital 754.0
Bereavement V62.82
  as adjustment reaction 309.0
Berger's paresthesia (lower limb) 782.0
Bergeron's disease (hysteroepilepsy) 300.11
Beriberi (acute) (atrophic) (chronic) (dry) (subacute) (wet) 265.0
  with polyneuropathy 265.0 *[357.4]*
  heart (disease) 265.0 *[425.7]*
  leprosy 030.1
  neuritis 265.0 *[357.4]*
Berlin's disease or edema (traumatic) 921.3
Berloque dermatitis 692.72
Bernard-Horner syndrome (*see also* Neuropathy, peripheral, autonomic) 337.9
Bernard-Sergent syndrome (acute adrenocortical insufficiency) 255.41
Bernard-Soulier disease or thrombopathy 287.1
Bernhardt's disease or paresthesia 355.1
Bernhardt-Roth disease or syndrome (paresthesia) 355.1
Bernheim's syndrome (*see also* Failure, heart) 428.0
Bertielliasis 123.8
Bertolotti's syndrome (sacralization of fifth lumbar vertebra) 756.15
Berylliosis (acute) (chronic) (lung) (occupational) 503
Besnier's
  lupus pernio 135
  prurigo (atopic dermatitis) (infantile eczema) 691.8
Besnier-Boeck disease or sarcoid 135
Besnier-Boeck-Schaumann disease (sarcoidosis) 135
Best's disease 362.76
Bestiality 302.1
Beta-adrenergic hyperdynamic circulatory state 429.82
Beta-aminoisobutyric aciduria 277.2
Beta-mercaptolactate-cysteine disulfiduria 270.0
Beta thalassemia (mixed) 282.46
  major 282.44
  minor 282.46
Beurmann's disease (sporotrichosis) 117.1
Bezoar 938
  intestine 936
  stomach 935.2
Bezold's abscess (*see also* Mastoiditis) 383.01
Bianchi's syndrome (aphasia-apraxia-alexia) 784.69
Bicornuate or bicornis uterus (complete) (partial) 752.34
  in pregnancy or childbirth 654.0
    with obstructed labor 660.2
      affecting fetus or newborn 763.1
    affecting fetus or newborn 763.89
Bicuspid aortic valve 746.4
Biedl-Bardet syndrome 759.89
Bielschowsky's disease 330.1

Bielschowsky-Jansky
 amaurotic familial idiocy 330.1
 disease 330.1
Biemond's syndrome (obesity, polydactyly, and
  intellectual disabilities) 759.89
Biermer's anemia or disease (pernicious
  anemia) 281.0
Biett's disease 695.4
Bifid (congenital)—see also Imperfect, closure
 apex, heart 746.89
 clitoris 752.49
 epiglottis 748.3
 kidney 753.3
 nose 748.1
 patella 755.64
 scrotum 752.89
 toe 755.66
 tongue 750.13
 ureter 753.4
 uterus 752.34
 uvula 749.02
  with cleft lip (see also Cleft, palate, with cleft
   lip) 749.20
Biforis uterus (suprasimplex) 752.34
Bifurcation (congenital)—see also Imperfect,
  closure
 gallbladder 751.69
 kidney pelvis 753.3
 renal pelvis 753.3
 rib 756.3
 tongue 750.13
 trachea 748.3
 ureter 753.4
 urethra 753.8
 uvula 749.02
  with cleft lip (see also Cleft, palate, with cleft
   lip) 749.20
 vertebra 756.19
Bigeminal pulse 427.89
Bigeminy 427.89
Big spleen syndrome 289.4
Bilateral —see condition
Bile duct —see condition
Bile pigments in urine 791.4
Bilharziasis (see also Schistosomiasis) 120.9
 chyluria 120.0
 cutaneous 120.3
 galacturia 120.0
 hematochyluria 120.0
 intestinal 120.1
 lipemia 120.9
 lipuria 120.0
 Oriental 120.2
 piarhemia 120.9
 pulmonary 120.2
 tropical hematuria 120.0
 vesical 120.0
Biliary —see condition
Bilious (attack)—see also Vomiting
 fever, hemoglobinuric 084.8
Bilirubinuria 791.4
Biliuria 791.4
Billroth's disease
 meningocele (see also Spina bifida) 741.9
Bilobate placenta —see Placenta, abnormal
Bilocular
 heart 745.7
 stomach 536.8
Bing-Horton syndrome (histamine cephalgia)
 339.00

Binswanger's disease or dementia 290.12
Biörck (-Thorson) syndrome (malignant
  carcinoid) 259.2
Biparta, bipartite —see also Imperfect, closure
 carpal scaphoid 755.59
 patella 755.64
 placenta—see Placenta, abnormal
 vagina 752.49
Bird
 face 756.0
 fanciers' lung or disease 495.2
 flu (see also Influenza, avian) 488.02
Bird's disease (oxaluria) 271.8
Birth
 abnormal fetus or newborn 763.9
 accident, fetus or newborn—see Birth, injury
 complications in mother—see Delivery,
  complicated
 compression during NEC 767.9
 defect—see Anomaly
 delayed, fetus 763.9
 difficult NEC, affecting fetus or newborn 763.9
 dry, affecting fetus or newborn 761.1
 forced, NEC, affecting fetus or newborn 763.89
 forceps, affecting fetus or newborn 763.2
 hematoma of sternomastoid 767.8
 immature 765.1
  extremely 765.0
 inattention, after or at 995.52
 induced, affecting fetus or newborn 763.89
 infant—see Newborn
 injury NEC 767.9
  adrenal gland 767.8
  basal ganglia 767.0
  brachial plexus (paralysis) 767.6
  brain (compression) (pressure) 767.0
  cerebellum 767.0
  cerebral hemorrhage 767.0
  conjunctiva 767.8
  eye 767.8
  fracture
   bone, any except clavicle or spine 767.3
   clavicle 767.2
   femur 767.3
   humerus 767.3
   long bone 767.3
   radius and ulna 767.3
   skeleton NEC 767.3
   skull 767.3
   spine 767.4
   tibia and fibula 767.3
  hematoma 767.8
   liver (subcapsular) 767.8
   mastoid 767.8
   skull 767.19
   sternomastoid 767.8
   testes 767.8
   vulva 767.8
  intracranial (edema) 767.0
  laceration
   brain 767.0
   by scalpel 767.8
   peripheral nerve 767.7
  liver 767.8
  meninges
   brain 767.0
   spinal cord 767.4
  nerves (cranial, peripheral) 767.7
   brachial plexus 767.6
   facial 767.5

Birth—*continued*
  injury—*continued*
    paralysis 767.7
      brachial plexus 767.6
      Erb (-Duchenne) 767.6
      facial nerve 767.5
      Klumpke (-Déjérine) 767.6
      radial nerve 767.6
      spinal (cord) (hemorrhage) (laceration)
        (rupture) 767.4
    rupture
      intracranial 767.0
      liver 767.8
      spinal cord 767.4
      spleen 767.8
      viscera 767.8
    scalp 767.19
    scalpel wound 767.8
    skeleton NEC 767.3
    specified NEC 767.8
    spinal cord 767.4
    spleen 767.8
    subdural hemorrhage 767.0
    tentorial, tear 767.0
    testes 767.8
    vulva 767.8
  instrumental, NEC, affecting fetus or newborn
    763.2
  lack of care, after or at 995.52
  multiple
    affected by maternal complications of
      pregnancy 761.5
    healthy liveborn—*see* Newborn, multiple
  neglect, after or at 995.52
  newborn—*see* Newborn
  palsy or paralysis NEC 767.7
  precipitate, fetus or newborn 763.6
  premature (infant) 765.1
  prolonged, affecting fetus or newborn 763.9
  retarded, fetus or newborn 763.9
  shock, newborn 779.89
  strangulation or suffocation
    due to aspiration of clear amniotic fluid 770.13
      with respiratory symptoms 770.14
    mechanical 767.8
  trauma NEC 767.9
  triplet
    affected by maternal complications of
      pregnancy 761.5
    healthy liveborn—*see* Newborn, multiple
  twin
    affected by maternal complications of
      pregnancy 761.5
    healthy liveborn—*see* Newborn, twin
  ventouse, affecting fetus or newborn 763.3
Birt-Hogg-Dube syndrome 759.89
Birthmark 757.32
Bisalbuminemia 273.8
Biskra button 085.1
Bite(s)
  with intact skin surface—*see* Contusion
  animal—*see* Wound, open, by site
    intact skin surface—*see* Contusion
  bedbug—*see* Injury, superficial, by site
  centipede 989.5
  chigger 133.8
  fire ant 989.5
  flea—*see* Injury, superficial, by site
  human (open wound)—*see also* Wound, open,
    by site
    intact skin surface—*see* Contusion

Bite(s)—*continued*
  insect
    nonvenomous—*see* Injury, superficial, by site
    venomous 989.5
  mad dog (death from) 071
  open
    anterior 524.24
    posterior 524.25
  poisonous 989.5
  red bug 133.8
  reptile 989.5
    nonvenomous—*see* Wound, open, by site
  snake 989.5
    nonvenomous—*see* Wound, open, by site
  spider (venomous) 989.5
    nonvenomous—*see* Injury, superficial, by site
    venomous 989.5
Biting
  cheek or lip 528.9
  nail 307.9
Black
  death 020.9
  eye NEC 921.0
  hairy tongue 529.3
  heel 924.20
  lung disease 500
  palm 923.20
Blackfan-Diamond anemia or syndrome
  (congenital hypoplastic anemia) 284.01
Blackhead 706.1
Blackout 780.2
Blackwater fever 084.8
Bladder —*see* Condition
Blast
  blindness 921.3
  concussion—*see* Blast, injury
  injury 869.0
    with open wound into cavity 869.1
    abdomen or thorax—*see* Injury, internal, by
      site
    brain (*see also* Concussion, brain) 850.9
      with skull fracture—*see* Fracture, skull
    ear (acoustic nerve trauma) 951.5
      with perforation, tympanic membrane—*see*
        Wound, open, ear, drum
    lung (*see also* Injury, internal, lung) 861.20
    otitic (explosive) 388.11
Blastomycosis, blastomycotic (chronic)
  (cutaneous) (disseminated) (lung) (pulmonary)
  (systemic) 116.0
  Brazilian 116.1
  European 117.5
  keloidal 116.2
  North American 116.0
  primary pulmonary 116.0
  South American 116.1
Bleb(s) 709.8
  emphysematous (bullous) (diffuse) (lung)
    (ruptured) (solitary) 492.0
  filtering, eye (postglaucoma) (status) V45.69
    with complication 997.99
    postcataract extraction (complication) 997.99
  lung (ruptured) 492.0
    congenital 770.5
  subpleural (emphysematous) 492.0
Bleeder (familial) (hereditary) (*see also* Defect,
  coagulation) 286.9
  nonfamilial 286.9

Bleeding (*see also* Hemorrhage) 459.0
  anal 569.3
  anovulatory 628.0
  atonic, following delivery 666.1
  capillary 448.9
  due to subinvolution 621.1
    puerperal 666.2
  ear 388.69
  excessive, associated with menopausal onset
    627.0
  familial (*see also* Defect, coagulation) 286.9
  following intercourse 626.7
  gastrointestinal 578.9
  gums 523.8
  hemorrhoids—*see* Hemorrhoids, bleeding
  intermenstrual
    irregular 626.6
    regular 626.5
  intraoperative 998.11
  irregular NEC 626.4
  menopausal 627.0
  mouth 528.9
  nipple 611.79
  nose 784.7
  ovulation 626.5
  postclimacteric 627.1
  postcoital 626.7
  postmenopausal 627.1
    following induced menopause 627.4
  postoperative 998.11
  preclimacteric 627.0
  puberty 626.3
    excessive, with onset of menstrual periods
      626.3
  rectum, rectal 569.3
  tendencies (*see also* Defect, coagulation) 286.9
  throat 784.8
  umbilical stump 772.3
  umbilicus 789.9
  unrelated to menstrual cycle 626.6
  uterus, uterine 626.9
    climacteric 627.0
    dysfunctional 626.8
    functional 626.8
    unrelated to menstrual cycle 626.6
  vagina, vaginal 623.8
    functional 626.8
  vicarious 625.8
Blennorrhagia, blennorrhagic —*see*
    Blennorrhea
Blennorrhea (acute) 098.0
  adultorum 098.40
  alveolaris 523.40
  chronic or duration of 2 months or over 098.2
  gonococcal (neonatorum) 098.40
  inclusion (neonatal) (newborn) 771.6
  neonatorum 098.40
Blepharelosis (*see also* Entropion) 374.00
Blepharitis (eyelid) 373.00
  angularis 373.01
  ciliaris 373.00
    with ulcer 373.01
  marginal 373.00
    with ulcer 373.01
  scrofulous (*see also* Tuberculosis) 017.3
    [373.00]
  squamous 373.02
  ulcerative 373.01
Blepharochalasis 374.34
  congenital 743.62
Blepharoclonus 333.81

Blepharoconjunctivitis (*see also* Conjunctivitis)
    372.20
  angular 372.21
  contact 372.22
Blepharophimosis (eyelid) 374.46
  congenital 743.62
Blepharoplegia 374.89
Blepharoptosis 374.30
  congenital 743.61
Blepharopyorrhea 098.49
Blepharospasm 333.81
  due to drugs 333.85
Blessig's cyst 362.62
Blighted ovum 631.8
Blind
  bronchus (congenital) 748.3
  eye—*see also* Blindness
    hypertensive 360.42
    hypotensive 360.41
  loop syndrome (postoperative) 579.2
  sac, fallopian tube (congenital) 752.19
  spot, enlarged 368.42
  tract or tube (congenital) NEC—*see* Atresia
Blindness (acquired) (congenital) (both eyes) 369.00
  with deafness V49.85
  blast 921.3
    with nerve injury—*see* Injury, nerve, optic
  Bright's—*see* Uremia
  color (congenital) 368.59
    acquired 368.55
    blue 368.53
    green 368.52
    red 368.51
    total 368.54
  concussion 950.9
  cortical 377.75
  day 368.10
    acquired 368.10
    congenital 368.10
    hereditary 368.10
    specified type NEC 368.10
  due to
    injury NEC 950.9
    refractive error—*see* Error, refractive
  eclipse (total) 363.31
  emotional 300.11
  face 368.16
  hysterical 300.11
  legal (both eyes) (USA definition) 369.4
    with impairment of better (less impaired) eye
      near-total 369.02
        with
          lesser eye impairment 369.02
            near-total 369.04
            total 369.03
      profound 369.05
        with
          lesser eye impairment 369.05
            near-total 369.07
            profound 369.08
            total 369.06
      severe 369.21
        with
          lesser eye impairment 369.21
            blind 369.11
            near-total 369.13
            profound 369.14
            severe 369.22
            total 369.12
      total
        with lesser eye impairment total 369.01

Blindness—*continued*
  mind 784.69
  moderate
    both eyes 369.25
      with impairment of lesser eye (specified as)
        blind, not further specified 369.15
        low vision, not further specified 369.23
        near-total 369.17
        profound 369.18
        severe 369.24
        total 369.16
    one eye 369.74
      with vision of other eye (specified as)
        near-normal 369.75
        normal 369.76
  near-total
    both eyes 369.04
      with impairment of lesser eye (specified as)
        blind, not further specified 369.02
        total 369.03
    one eye 369.64
      with vision of other eye (specified as)
        near-normal 369.65
        normal 369.66
  night 368.60
    acquired 368.62
    congenital (Japanese) 368.61
    hereditary 368.61
    specified type NEC 368.69
    vitamin A deficiency 264.5
  nocturnal—*see* Blindness, night
  one eye 369.60
    with low vision of other eye 369.10
  profound
    both eyes 369.08
      with impairment of lesser eye (specified as)
        blind, not further specified 369.05
        near-total 369.07
        total 369.06
    one eye 369.67
      with vision of other eye (specified as)
        near-normal 369.68
        normal 369.69
  psychic 784.69
  severe
    both eyes 369.22
      with impairment of lesser eye (specified as)
        blind, not further specified 369.11
        low vision, not further specified 369.21
        near-total 369.13
        profound 369.14
        total 369.12
    one eye 369.71
      with vision of other eye (specified as)
        near-normal 369.72
        normal 369.73
  snow 370.24
  sun 363.31
  temporary 368.12
  total
    both eyes 369.01
    one eye 369.61
      with vision of other eye (specified as)
        near-normal 369.62
        normal 369.63
  transient 368.12
  traumatic NEC 950.9
  word (developmental) 315.01
    acquired 784.61
    secondary to organic lesion 784.61

Blister —*see also* Injury, superficial, by site
  beetle dermatitis 692.89
  due to burn—*see* Burn, by site, second degree
  fever 054.9
  fracture—*omit code*
  multiple, skin, nontraumatic 709.8
Bloating 787.3
Bloch-Siemens syndrome (incontinentia
  pigmenti) 757.33
Bloch-Stauffer dyshormonal dermatosis 757.33
Bloch-Sulzberger disease or syndrome
  (incontinentia pigmenti) (melanoblastosis) 757.33
Block
  alveolar capillary 516.8
  arborization (heart) 426.6
  arrhythmic 426.9
  atrioventricular (AV) (incomplete) (partial)
    426.10
    with
      2:1 atrioventricular response block 426.13
      atrioventricular dissociation 426.0
    first degree (incomplete) 426.11
    second degree (Mobitz type I) 426.13
      Mobitz (type) II 426.12
    third degree 426.0
    complete 426.0
      congenital 746.86
    congenital 746.86
    Mobitz (incomplete)
      type I (Wenckebach's) 426.13
      type II 426.12
    partial 426.13
  auriculoventricular (*see also* Block,
    atrioventricular) 426.10
    complete 426.0
      congenital 746.86
    congenital 746.86
  bifascicular (cardiac) 426.53
  bundle branch (complete) (false) (incomplete)
    426.50
    bilateral 426.53
    left (complete) (main stem) 426.3
      with right bundle branch block 426.53
      anterior fascicular 426.2
        with
          posterior fascicular block 426.3
          right bundle branch block 426.52
      hemiblock 426.2
      incomplete 426.2
        with right bundle branch block 426.53
      posterior fascicular 426.2
        with
          anterior fascicular block 426.3
          right bundle branch block 426.51
    right 426.4
      with
        left bundle branch block (incomplete)
          (main stem) 426.53
        left fascicular block 426.53
          anterior 426.52
          posterior 426.51
    Wilson's type 426.4
  cardiac 426.9
  conduction 426.9
    complete 426.0
  Eustachian tube (*see also* Obstruction,
    Eustachian tube) 381.60
  fascicular (left anterior) (left posterior) 426.2

Block—*continued*
  foramen Magendie (acquired) 331.3
    congenital 742.3
      with spina bifida (*see also* Spina bifida) 741.0
  heart 426.9
    first degree (atrioventricular) 426.11
    second degree (atrioventricular) 426.13
    third degree (atrioventricular) 426.0
    bundle branch (complete) (false) (incomplete)
      426.50
      bilateral 426.53
      left (*see also* Block, bundle branch, left)
        426.3
      right (*see also* Block, bundle branch, right)
        426.4
    complete (atrioventricular) 426.0
    congenital 746.86
    incomplete 426.13
    intra-atrial 426.6
    intraventricular NEC 426.6
    sinoatrial 426.6
    specified type NEC 426.6
  hepatic vein 453.0
  intraventricular (diffuse) (myofibrillar) 426.6
    bundle branch (complete) (false) (incomplete)
      426.50
      bilateral 426.53
      left (*see also* Block, bundle branch, left)
        426.3
      right (*see also* Block, bundle branch, right)
        426.4
  kidney (*see also* Disease, renal) 593.9
    postcystoscopic 997.5
  myocardial (*see also* Block, heart) 426.9
  nodal 426.10
  optic nerve 377.49
  organ or site (congenital) NEC—*see* Atresia
  parietal 426.6
  peri-infarction 426.6
  portal (vein) 452
  sinoatrial 426.6
  sinoauricular 426.6
  spinal cord 336.9
  trifascicular 426.54
  tubal 628.2
  vein NEC 453.9
Blocq's disease or syndrome (astasia-abasia)
  307.9
Blood
  constituents, abnormal NEC 790.6
  disease 289.9
    specified NEC 289.89
  donor V59.01
    other blood components V59.09
    stem cells V59.02
    whole blood V59.01
  dyscrasia 289.9
    with
      abortion—*see* Abortion, by type, with
        hemorrhage, delayed or excessive
      ectopic pregnancy (*see also* categories
        633.0-633.9) 639.1
      molar pregnancy (*see also* categories
        630-632) 639.1
    following
      abortion 639.1
      ectopic or molar pregnancy 639.1
    newborn NEC 776.9
    puerperal, postpartum 666.3
  flukes NEC (*see also* Infestation, Schistosoma)
    120.9

Blood—*continued*
  in
    feces (*see also* Melena) 578.1
      occult 792.1
    urine (*see also* Hematuria) 599.70
  mole 631.8
  occult 792.1
  poisoning (*see also* Septicemia) 038.9
  pressure
    decreased, due to shock following injury 958.4
    fluctuating 796.4
    high (*see also* Hypertension) 401.9
      borderline 796.2
      incidental reading (isolated) (nonspecific),
        without diagnosis of hypertension 796.2
    low (*see also* Hypotension) 458.9
      incidental reading (isolated) (nonspecific),
        without diagnosis of hypotension 796.3
  spitting (*see also* Hemoptysis) 786.30
  staining cornea 371.12
  transfusion
    without reported diagnosis V58.2
    donor V59.01
      stem cells V59.02
    reaction or complication—*see* Complications,
      transfusion
  tumor—*see* Hematoma
  vessel rupture—*see* Hemorrhage
  vomiting (*see also* Hematemesis) 578.0
Blood-forming organ disease 289.9
Bloodgood's disease 610.1
Bloodshot eye 379.93
Bloom (-Machacek) (-Torre) syndrome 757.39
Blotch, palpebral 372.55
Blount's disease (tibia vara) 732.4
Blount-Barber syndrome (tibia vara) 732.4
Blue
  baby 746.9
  bloater 491.20
    with acute bronchitis 491.22
    with exacerbation (acute) 491.21
  diaper syndrome 270.0
  disease 746.9
  dome cyst 610.0
  drum syndrome 381.02
  sclera 743.47
    with fragility of bone and deafness 756.51
  toe syndrome 445.02
Blueness (cyanosis) 782.5
Blurred vision 368.8
Blushing (abnormal) (excessive) 782.62
BMI (body mass index)
  adult
    25.0-25.9 V85.21
    26.0-26.9 V85.22
    27.0-27.9 V85.23
    28.0-28.9 V85.24
    29.0-29.9 V85.25
    30.0-30.9 V85.30
    31.0-31.9 V85.31
    32.0-32.9 V85.32
    33.0-33.9 V85.33
    34.0-34.9 V85.34
    35.0-35.9 V85.35
    36.0-36.9 V85.36
    37.0-37.9 V85.37
    38.0-38.9 V85.38
    39.0-39.9 V85.39
    40.0-44.9 V85.41
    45.0-49.9 V85.42
    50.0-59.9 V85.43

BMI (body mass index)—*continued*
  60.0-69.9 V85.44
  70 and over V85.45
  between 19-24 V85.1
  less than 19 V85.0
  pediatric
    5th percentile to less than 85th percentile for age V85.52
    85th percentile to less than 95th percentile for age V85.53
    greater than or equal to 95th percentile for age V85.54
    less than 5th percentile for age V85.51
Boarder, hospital V65.0
  infant V65.0
Bockhart's impetigo (superficial folliculitis) 704.8
Bodechtel-Guttmann disease (subacute sclerosing panencephalitis) 046.2
Boder-Sedgwick syndrome (ataxia-telangiectasia) 334.8
Body, bodies
  Aschoff (*see also* Myocarditis, rheumatic) 398.0
  asteroid, vitreous 379.22
  choroid, colloid (degenerative) 362.57
    hereditary 362.77
  cytoid (retina) 362.82
  drusen (retina) (*see also* Drusen) 362.57
    optic disc 377.21
  fibrin, pleura 511.0
  foreign—*see* Foreign body
  Hassall-Henle 371.41
  loose
    joint (*see also* Loose, body, joint) 718.1
      knee 717.6
    knee 717.6
    sheath, tendon 727.82
  Mallory's 034.1
  mass index (BMI)
    adult
      25.0-25.9 V85.21
      26.0-26.9 V85.22
      27.0-27.9 V85.23
      28.0-28.9 V85.24
      29.0-29.9 V85.25
      30.0-30.9 V85.30
      31.0-31.9 V85.31
      32.0-32.9 V85.32
      33.0-33.9 V85.33
      34.0-34.9 V85.34
      35.0-35.9 V85.35
      36.0-36.9 V85.36
      37.0-37.9 V85.37
      38.0-38.9 V85.38
      39.0-39.9 V85.39
      40.0-44.9 V85.41
      45.0-49.9 V85.42
      50.0-59.9 V85.43
      60.0-69.9 V85.44
      70 and over V85.45
      between 19-24 V85.1
      less than 19 V85.0
    pediatric
      5th percentile to less than 85th percentile for age V85.52
      85th percentile to less than 95th percentile for age V85.53
      greater than or equal to 95th percentile for age V85.54
      less than 5th percentile for age V85.51
  Mooser 081.0
  Negri 071

Body, bodies—*continued*
  rice (joint) (*see also* Loose, body, joint) 718.1
    knee 717.6
  rocking 307.3
Boeck's
  disease (sarcoidosis) 135
  lupoid (miliary) 135
  sarcoid 135
Boerhaave's syndrome (spontaneous esophageal rupture) 530.4
Boggy
  cervix 622.8
  uterus 621.8
Boil (*see also* Carbuncle) 680.9
  abdominal wall 680.2
  Aleppo 085.1
  ankle 680.6
  anus 680.5
  arm (any part, above wrist) 680.3
  auditory canal, external 680.0
  axilla 680.3
  back (any part) 680.2
  Baghdad 085.1
  breast 680.2
  buttock 680.5
  chest wall 680.2
  corpus cavernosum 607.2
  Delhi 085.1
  ear (any part) 680.0
  eyelid 373.13
  face (any part, except eye) 680.0
  finger (any) 680.4
  flank 680.2
  foot (any part) 680.7
  forearm 680.3
  Gafsa 085.1
  genital organ, male 608.4
  gluteal (region) 680.5
  groin 680.2
  hand (any part) 680.4
  head (any part, except face) 680.8
  heel 680.7
  hip 680.6
  knee 680.6
  labia 616.4
  lacrimal (*see also* Dacryocystitis) 375.30
    gland (*see also* Dacryoadenitis) 375.00
    passages (duct) (sac) (*see also* Dacryocystitis) 375.30
  leg, any part except foot 680.6
  multiple sites 680.9
  Natal 085.1
  neck 680.1
  nose (external) (septum) 680.0
  orbit, orbital 376.01
  partes posteriores 680.5
  pectoral region 680.2
  penis 607.2
  perineum 680.2
  pinna 680.0
  scalp (any part) 680.8
  scrotum 608.4
  seminal vesicle 608.0
  shoulder 680.3
  skin NEC 680.9
  specified site NEC 680.8
  spermatic cord 608.4
  temple (region) 680.0
  testis 608.4
  thigh 680.6
  thumb 680.4
  toe (any) 680.7

Boil —*continued*
tropical 085.1
trunk 680.2
tunica vaginalis 608.4
umbilicus 680.2
upper arm 680.3
vas deferens 608.4
vulva 616.4
wrist 680.4
Bold hives (*see also* Urticaria) 708.9
Bolivian hemorrhagic fever 078.7
Bombé, iris 364.74
Bomford-Rhoads anemia (refractory) 238.72
Bone —*see* condition
Bonnevie-Ullrich syndrome 758.6
Bonnier's syndrome 386.19
Bonvale Dam fever 780.79
Bony block of joint 718.80
ankle 718.87
elbow 718.82
foot 718.87
hand 718.84
hip 718.85
knee 718.86
multiple sites 718.89
pelvic region 718.85
shoulder (region) 718.81
specified site NEC 718.88
wrist 718.83
BOOP (bronchiolitis obliterans organized
penumonia) 516.8
Borderline
diabetes mellitus 790.29
hypertension 796.2
intellectual functioning V62.89
osteopenia 733.90
pelvis 653.1
with obstruction during labor 660.1
affecting fetus or newborn 763.1
psychosis (*see also* Schizophrenia) 295.5
of childhood (*see also* Psychosis, childhood)
299.8
schizophrenia (*see also* Schizophrenia) 295.5
Borna disease 062.9
Bornholm disease (epidemic pleurodynia) 074.1
Borrelia vincentii (mouth) (pharynx) (tonsils) 101
Bostock's catarrh (*see also* Fever, hay) 477.9
Boston exanthem 048
Botalli, ductus (patent) (persistent) 747.0
Bothriocephalus latus infestation 123.4
Botulism 005.1
food poisoning 005.1
infant 040.41
non-foodborne 040.42
wound 040.42
Bouba (*see also* Yaws) 102.9
Bouffée délirante 298.3
Bouillaud's disease or syndrome (rheumatic
heart disease) 391.9
Bourneville's disease (tuberous sclerosis) 759.5
Boutonneuse fever 082.1
Boutonniere
deformity (finger) 736.21
hand (intrinsic) 736.21
Bouveret (-Hoffmann) disease or syndrome
(paroxysmal tachycardia) 427.2
Bovine heart —*see* Hypertrophy, cardiac
Bowel —*see* condition
Bowen's
dermatosis (precancerous) (M8081/2)—*see*
Neoplasm, skin, in situ

Bowen's—*continued*
disease (M8081/2)—*see* Neoplasm, skin, in situ
epithelioma (M8081/2)—*see* Neoplasm, skin, in
situ
type
epidermoid carcinoma in situ (M8081/2)—*see*
Neoplasm, skin, in situ
intraepidermal squamous cell carcinoma
(M8081/2)—*see* Neoplasm, skin, in situ
Bowing
femur 736.89
congenital 754.42
fibula 736.89
congenital 754.43
forearm 736.09
away from midline (cubitus valgus) 736.01
toward midline (cubitus varus) 736.02
leg(s), long bones, congenital 754.44
radius 736.09
away from midline (cubitus valgus) 736.01
toward midline (cubitus varus) 736.02
tibia 736.89
congenital 754.43
Bowleg (s) 736.42
congenital 754.44
rachitic 268.1
Boyd's dysentery 004.2
Brachial —*see* condition
Brachman-de Lange syndrome (Amsterdam
dwarf, intellectual disabilities, and
brachycephaly) 759.89
Brachycardia 427.89
Brachycephaly 756.0
Brachymorphism and ectopia lentis 759.89
Bradley's disease (epidemic vomiting) 078.82
Bradycardia 427.89
chronic (sinus) 427.81
newborn 779.81
nodal 427.89
postoperative 997.1
reflex 337.09
sinoatrial 427.89
with paroxysmal tachyarrhythmia or
tachycardia 427.81
chronic 427.81
sinus 427.89
with paroxysmal tachyarrhythmia or
tachycardia 427.81
chronic 427.81
persistent 427.81
severe 427.81
tachycardia syndrome 427.81
vagal 427.89
Bradykinesia 781.0
Bradypnea 786.09
Brailsford's disease 732.3
radial head 732.3
tarsal scaphoid 732.5
Brailsford-Morquio disease or syndrome
(mucopolysaccharidosis IV) 277.5
Brain —*see also* condition
death 348.82
syndrome (acute) (chronic) (nonpsychotic)
(organic) (with neurotic reaction) (with
behavioral reaction) (*see also* Syndrome,
brain) 310.9
with
presenile brain disease 290.10
psychosis, psychotic reaction (*see also*
Psychosis, organic) 294.9
congenital (*see also* Disability, intellectual) 319

Branched-chain amino-acid disease 270.3
Branchial —*see* condition
Brandt's syndrome (acrodermatitis
   enteropathica) 686.8
Brash (water) 787.1
Brass-founders' ague 985.8
Bravais-Jacksonian epilepsy (*see also* Epilepsy)
   345.5
Braxton Hicks contractions 644.1
Braziers' disease 985.8
Brazilian
   blastomycosis 116.1
   leishmaniasis 085.5
BRBPR (bright red blood per rectum) 569.3
Break
   cardiorenal—*see* Hypertension, cardiorenal
   retina (*see also* Defect, retina) 361.30
Breakbone fever 061
Breakdown
   device, implant, or graft—*see* Complications,
      mechanical
   nervous (*see also* Disorder, mental,
      nonpsychotic) 300.9
   perineum 674.2
Breast —*see also* condition
   buds 259.1
      in newborn 779.89
   dense 793.82
   nodule 793.89
Breast feeding difficulties 676.8
Breath
   foul 784.99
   holder, child 312.81
   holding spells 786.9
   shortness 786.05
Breathing
   asymmetrical 786.09
   bronchial 786.09
   exercises V57.0
   labored 786.09
   mouth 784.99
      causing malocclusion 524.59
   periodic 786.09
      high altitude 327.22
   tic 307.20
Breathlessness 786.09
Breda's disease (*see also* Yaws) 102.9
Breech
   delivery, affecting fetus or newborn 763.0
   extraction, affecting fetus or newborn 763.0
   presentation (buttocks) (complete) (frank) 652.2
      with successful version 652.1
      before labor, affecting fetus or newborn 761.7
      during labor, affecting fetus or newborn 763.0
Breisky's disease (kraurosis vulvae) 624.09
Brennemann's syndrome (acute mesenteric
   lymphadenitis) 289.2
Brenner's
   tumor (benign) (M9000/0) 220
      borderline malignancy (M9000/1) 236.2
      malignant (M9000/3) 183.0
      proliferating (M9000/1) 236.2
Bretonneau's disease (diphtheritic malignant
   angina) 032.0
Breus' mole 631.8
Brevicollis 756.16
Bricklayers' itch 692.89
Brickmakers' anemia 126.9
Bridge
   myocardial 746.85

Bright's
   blindness—*see* Uremia
   disease (*see also* Nephritis) 583.9
      arteriosclerotic (*see also* Hypertension,
         kidney) 403.90
Bright red blood per rectum (BRBPR) 569.3
Brill's disease (recrudescent typhus) 081.1
   flea-borne 081.0
   louse-borne 081.1
Brill-Symmers disease (follicular lymphoma)
   (M9690/3) 202.0
Brill-Zinsser disease (recrudescent typhus) 081.1
Brinton's disease (linitis plastica) (M8142/3) 151.9
Brion-Kayser disease (*see also* Fever,
   paratyphoid) 002.9
Briquet's disorder or syndrome 300.81
Brissaud's
   infantilism (infantile myxedema) 244.9
   motor-verbal tic 307.23
Brissaud-Meige syndrome (infantile myxedema)
   244.9
Brittle
   bones (congenital) 756.51
   nails 703.8
      congenital 757.5
Broad —*see also* condition
   beta disease 272.2
   ligament laceration syndrome 620.6
Brock's syndrome (atelectasis due to enlarged
   lymph nodes) 518.0
Brocq's disease 691.8
   atopic (diffuse) neurodermatitis 691.8
   lichen simplex chronicus 698.3
   parakeratosis psoriasiformis 696.2
   parapsoriasis 696.2
Brocq-Duhring disease (dermatitis
   herpetiformis) 694.0
Brodie's
   abscess (localized) (chronic) (*see also*
      Osteomyelitis) 730.1
   disease (joint) (*see also* Osteomyelitis) 730.1
Broken
   arches 734
      congenital 755.67
   back—*see* Fracture, vertebra, by site
   bone—*see* Fracture, by site
   compensation—*see* Disease, heart
   heart syndrome 429.83
   implant or internal device—*see* listing under
      Complications, mechanical
   neck—*see* Fracture, vertebra, cervical
   nose 802.0
      open 802.1
   tooth, teeth 873.63
      complicated 873.73
Bromhidrosis 705.89
Bromidism, bromism
   acute 967.3
      correct substance properly administered 349.82
      overdose or wrong substance given or taken
         967.3
   chronic (*see also* Dependence) 304.1
Bromidrosiphobia 300.23
Bromidrosis 705.89
Bronchi, bronchial —*see* condition
Bronchiectasis (cylindrical) (diffuse) (fusiform)
      (localized) (moniliform) (postinfectious)
      (recurrent) (saccular) 494.0
   with acute exacerbation 494.1
   congenital 748.61
   tuberculosis (*see also* Tuberculosis) 011.5

Bronchiolectasis —*see* Bronchiectasis
Bronchiolitis (acute) (infectious) (subacute)
466.19
with
bronchospasm or obstruction 466.19
influenza, flu, or grippe (*see also* Influenza)
487.1
catarrhal (acute) (subacute) 466.19
chemical 506.0
chronic 506.4
chronic (obliterative) 491.8
due to external agent—*see* Bronchitis, acute,
due to
fibrosa obliterans 491.8
influenzal (*see also* Influenza) 487.1
obliterans 491.8
status post lung transplant 996.84
with organizing pneumonia (BOOP) 516.8
obliterative (chronic) (diffuse) (subacute) 491.8
due to fumes or vapors 506.4
respiratory syncytial virus 466.11
vesicular—*see* Pneumonia, broncho-
Bronchitis (diffuse) (hypostatic) (infectious)
(inflammatory) (simple) 490
with
emphysema—*see* Emphysema
influenza, flu, or grippe(*see also* Influenza)
487.1
obstruction airway, chronic 491.20
with
acute bronchitis 491.22
exacerbation (acute) 491.21
tracheitis 490
acute or subacute 466.0
with bronchospasm or obstruction 466.0
chronic 491.8
acute or subacute 466.0
with
bronchiectasis 494.1
bronchospasm 466.0
obstruction 466.0
tracheitis 466.0
chemical (due to fumes or vapors) 506.0
due to
fumes or vapors 506.0
radiation 508.8
allergic (acute) (*see also* Asthma) 493.9
arachidic 934.1
aspiration 507.0
due to fumes or vapors 506.0
asthmatic (acute) 493.90
with
acute exacerbation 493.92
status asthmaticus 493.91
chronic 493.2
capillary 466.19
with bronchospasm or obstruction 466.19
chronic 491.8
caseous (*see also* Tuberculosis) 011.3
Castellani's 104.8
catarrhal 490
acute—*see* Bronchitis, acute
chronic 491.0
chemical (acute) (subacute) 506.0
chronic 506.4
due to fumes or vapors (acute) (subacute)
506.0
chronic 506.4
chronic 491.9
with
tracheitis (chronic) 491.8
asthmatic 493.2

Bronchitis—*continued*
chronic—*continued*
catarrhal 491.0
chemical (due to fumes and vapors) 506.4
due to
fumes or vapors (chemical) (inhalation) 506.4
radiation 508.8
tobacco smoking 491.0
mucopurulent 491.1
obstructive 491.20
with
acute bronchitis 491.22
exacerbation (acute) 491.21
purulent 491.1
simple 491.0
specified type NEC 491.8
croupous 466.0
with bronchospasm or obstruction 466.0
due to fumes or vapors 506.0
emphysematous 491.20
with
acute bronchitis 491.22
exacerbation (acute) 491.21
exudative 466.0
fetid (chronic) (recurrent) 491.1
fibrinous, acute or subacute 466.0
with bronchospasm or obstruction 466.0
grippal (*see also* Influenza) 487.1
influenzal (*see also* Influenza) 487.1
membranous, acute or subacute 466.0
with bronchospasm or obstruction 466.0
moulders' 502
mucopurulent (chronic) (recurrent) 491.1
acute or subacute 466.0
non-obstructive 491.0
obliterans 491.8
obstructive (chronic) 491.20
with
acute bronchitis 491.22
exacerbation (acute) 491.21
pituitous 491.1
plastic (inflammatory) 466.0
pneumococcal, acute or subacute 466.0
with bronchospasm or obstruction 466.0
pseudomembranous 466.0
purulent (chronic) (recurrent) 491.1
acute or subacute 466.0
with bronchospasm or obstruction 466.0
putrid 491.1
scrofulous (*see also* Tuberculosis) 011.3
senile 491.9
septic, acute or subacute 466.0
with bronchospasm or obstruction 466.0
smokers' 491.0
spirochetal 104.8
suffocative, acute or subacute 466.0
summer (*see also* Asthma) 493.9
suppurative (chronic) 491.1
acute or subacute 466.0
tuberculous (*see also* Tuberculosis) 011.3
ulcerative 491.8
Vincent's 101
Vincent's 101
viral, acute or subacute 466.0
with bronchospasm or obstruction 466.0
Bronchoalveolitis 485
Bronchoaspergillosis 117.3
Bronchocele
meaning
dilatation of bronchus 519.19
goiter 240.9
Bronchogenic carcinoma 162.9

Bronchohemisporosis 117.9
Broncholithiasis 518.89
  tuberculous (*see also* Tuberculosis) 011.3
Bronchomalacia 748.3
Bronchomoniliasis 112.89
Bronchomycosis 112.89
Bronchonocardiosis 039.1
Bronchopleuropneumonia —*see* Pneumonia,
  broncho-
Bronchopneumonia —*see* Pneumonia, broncho-
Bronchopneumonitis —*see* Pneumonia, broncho-
Bronchopulmonary —*see* condition
Bronchopulmonitis —*see* Pneumonia, broncho-
Bronchorrhagia 786.30
  newborn 770.3
  tuberculous (*see also* Tuberculosis) 011.3
Bronchorrhea (chronic) (purulent) 491.0
  acute 466.0
Bronchospasm 519.11
  with
    asthma—*see* Asthma
    bronchiolitis, acute 466.19
      due to respiratory syncytial virus 466.11
    bronchitis—*see* Bronchitis
    chronic obstructive pulmonary disease
      (COPD) 496
    emphysema—*see* Emphysema
      due to external agent—*see* Condition,
        respiratory, acture, due to
  acute 519.11
  due to external agent—*see* Condition,
    respiratory, acute, due to
  exercise induced 493.81
Bronchospirochetosis 104.8
Bronchostenosis 519.19
Bronchus —*see* condition
Bronze, bronzed
  diabetes 275.01
  disease (Addison's) (skin) 255.41
    tuberculous (*see also* Tuberculosis) 017.6
Brooke's disease or tumor (M8100/0)—*see*
  Neoplasm, skin, benign
Brow presentation complicating delivery 652.4
Brown's tendon sheath syndrome 378.61
Brown enamel of teeth (hereditary) 520.5
Brown-Séquard's paralysis (syndrome) 344.89
Brucella, brucellosis (infection) 023.9
  abortus 023.1
  canis 023.3
  dermatitis, skin 023.9
  melitensis 023.0
  mixed 023.8
  suis 023.2
Bruck's disease 733.99
Bruck-de Lange disease or syndrome
    (Amsterdam dwarf, intellectual disabilities,
    and brachycephaly) 759.89
Brugada syndrome 746.89
Brug's filariasis 125.1
Brugsch's syndrome (acropachyderma) 757.39
Bruhl's disease (splenic anemia with fever) 285.8
Bruise (skin surface intact)—*see also* Contusion
  with
    fracture—*see* Fracture, by site
    open wound—*see* Wound, open, by site
    internal organ (abdomen, chest, or pelvis)—*see*
      Injury, internal, by site
  umbilical cord 663.6
    affecting fetus or newborn 762.6

Bruit 785.9
  arterial (abdominal) (carotid) 785.9
  supraclavicular 785.9
Brushburn —*see* Injury, superficial, by site
Bruton's X-linked agammaglobulinemia 279.04
Bruxism 306.8
  sleep related 327.53
Bubbly lung syndrome 770.7
Bubo 289.3
  blennorrhagic 098.89
  chancroidal 099.0
  climatic 099.1
  due to Hemophilus ducreyi 099.0
  gonococcal 098.89
  indolent NEC 099.8
  inguinal NEC 099.8
    chancroidal 099.0
    climatic 099.1
    due to H. ducreyi 099.0
  scrofulous (*see also* Tuberculosis) 017.2
  soft chancre 099.0
  suppurating 683
  syphilitic 091.0
    congenital 090.0
  tropical 099.1
  venereal NEC 099.8
  virulent 099.0
Bubonic plague 020.0
Bubonocele —*see* Hernia, inguinal
Buccal —*see* condition
Buchanan's disease (juvenile osteochondrosis of
    iliac crest) 732.1
Buchem's syndrome (hyperostosis corticalis) 733.3
Buchman's disease (osteochondrosis, juvenile)
    732.1
Bucket handle fracture (semilunar cartilage)
    (*see also* Tear, meniscus) 836.2
Budd-Chiari syndrome (hepatic vein
    thrombosis) 453.0
Budgerigar-fanciers' disease or lung 495.2
Büdinger-Ludloff-Läwen disease 717.89
Buds
  breast 259.1
  in newborn 779.89
Buerger's disease (thromboangiitis obliterans)
    443.1
Bulbar —*see* condition
Bulbus cordis 745.9
  persistent (in left ventricle) 745.8
Bulging fontanels (congenital) 756.0
Bulimia 783.6
  nervosa 307.51
  nonorganic origin 307.51
Bulky uterus 621.2
Bulla(e) 709.8
  lung (emphysematous) (solitary) 492.0
Bullet wound —*see also* Wound, open, by site
  fracture—*see* Fracture, by site, open
  internal organ (abdomen, chest, or pelvis)—*see*
    Injury, internal, by site, with open wound
  intracranial—*see* Laceration, brain, with open
    wound
Bullis fever 082.8
Bullying (*see also* Disturbance, conduct) 312.0
Bundle
  branch block (complete) (false) (incomplete)
    426.50
    bilateral 426.53
    left (*see also* Block, bundle branch, left) 426.3
      hemiblock 426.2
    right (*see also* Block, bundle branch, right) 426.4

Bundle—*continued*
of His—*see* condition
of Kent syndrome (anomalous atrioventricular
excitation) 426.7
Bungpagga 040.81
Bunion 727.1
Bunionette 727.1
Bunyamwera fever 066.3
Buphthalmia, buphthalmos (congenital) 743.20
associated with
keratoglobus, congenital 743.22
megalocornea 743.22
ocular anomalies NEC 743.22
isolated 743.21
simple 743.21
Bürger-Grütz disease or syndrome (essential
familial hyperlipemia) 272.3
Buried roots 525.3
Burke's syndrome 577.8
Burkitt's
tumor (M9750/3) 200.2
type malignant, lymphoma, lymphoblastic, or
undifferentiated (M9750/3) 200.2
Burn (acid) (cathode ray) (caustic) (chemical)
(electric heating appliance) (electricity) (fire)
(flame) (hot liquid or object) (irradiation)
(lime) (radiation) (steam) (thermal) (x-ray)
949.0

*Note—Use the following fifth-digit
subclassification with category 948 to indicate
the percent of body surface with third degree
burn:*

0　*less than 10% or unspecified*
1　*10-19%*
2　*20-29%*
3　*30-39%*
4　*40-49%*
5　*50-59%*
6　*60-69%*
7　*70-79%*
8　*80-89%*
9　*90% or more of body surface*

with
blisters—*see* Burn, by site, second degree
erythema—*see* Burn, by site, first degree
skin loss (epidermal)—*see also* Burn, by site,
second degree
full thickness—*see also* Burn, by site, third
degree
with necrosis of underlying tissues—*see*
Burn, by site, third degree, deep
first degree—*see* Burn, by site, first degree
second degree—*see* Burn, by site, second degree
third degree—*see also* Burn, by site, third degree
deep—*see* Burn, by site, third degree, deep
abdomen, abdominal (muscle) (wall) 942.03
with
trunk—*see* Burn, trunk, multiple sites
first degree 942.13
second degree 942.23
third degree 942.33
deep 942.43
with loss of body part 942.53
ankle 945.03
with
lower limb(s)—*see* Burn, leg, multiple sites
first degree 945.13
second degree 945.23

Burn—*continued*
ankle—*continued*
third degree 945.33
deep 945.43
with loss of body part 945.53
anus—*see* Burn, trunk, specified site NEC
arm(s) 943.00
first degree 943.10
second degree 943.20
third degree 943.30
deep 943.40
with loss of body part 943.50
lower—*see* Burn, forearm(s)
multiple sites, except hand(s) or wrist(s) 943.09
first degree 943.19
second degree 943.29
third degree 943.39
deep 943.49
with loss of body part 943.59
upper 943.03
first degree 943.13
second degree 943.23
third degree 943.33
deep 943.43
with loss of body part 943.53
auditory canal (external)—*see* Burn, ear
auricle (ear)—*see* Burn, ear
axilla 943.04
with
upper limb(s) except hand(s) or wrist(s)—*see*
Burn, arm(s), multiple sites
first degree 943.14
second degree 943.24
third degree 943.34
deep 943.44
with loss of body part 943.54
back 942.04
with
trunk—*see* Burn, trunk, multiple sites
first degree 942.14
second degree 942.24
third degree 942.34
deep 942.44
with loss of body part 942.54
biceps
brachii—*see* Burn, arm(s), upper
femoris—*see* Burn, thigh
breast(s) 942.01
with
trunk—*see* Burn, trunk, multiple sites
first degree 942.11
second degree 942.21
third degree 942.31
deep 942.41
with loss of body part 942.51
brow—*see* Burn, forehead
buttock(s)—*see* Burn, back
canthus (eye) 940.1
chemical 940.0
cervix (uteri) 947.4
cheek (cutaneous) 941.07
with
face or head—*see* Burn, head, multiple sites
first degree 941.17
second degree 941.27
third degree 941.37
deep 941.47
with loss of body part 941.57

Burn—*continued*
  chest wall (anterior) 942.02
    with
      trunk—*see* Burn, trunk, multiple sites
    first degree 942.12
    second degree 942.22
    third degree 942.32
      deep 942.42
        with loss of body part 942.52
  chin 941.04
    with
      face or head—*see* Burn, head, multiple sites
    first degree 941.14
    second degree 941.24
    third degree 941.34
      deep 941.44
        with loss of body part 941.54
  clitoris—*see* Burn, genitourinary organs, external
  colon 947.3
  conjunctiva (and cornea) 940.4
    chemical
      acid 940.3
      alkaline 940.2
  cornea (and conjunctiva) 940.4
    chemical
      acid 940.3
      alkaline 940.2
  costal region—*see* Burn, chest wall
  due to ingested chemical agent—*see* Burn, internal organs
  ear (auricle) (canal) (drum) (external) 941.01
    with
      face or head—*see* Burn, head, multiple sites
    first degree 941.11
    second degree 941.21
    third degree 941.31
      deep 941.41
        with loss of a body part 941.51
  elbow 943.02
    with
      hand(s) and wrist(s)—*see* Burn, multiple specified sites
      upper limb(s) except hand(s) or wrist(s)—*see also* Burn, arm(s), multiple sites
    first degree 943.12
    second degree 943.22
    third degree 943.32
      deep 943.42
        with loss of body part 943.52
  electricity, electric current—*see* Burn, by site
  entire body—*see* Burn, multiple, specified sites
  epididymis—*see* Burn, genitourinary organs, external
  epigastric region—*see* Burn, abdomen
  epiglottis 947.1
  esophagus 947.2
  extent (percent of body surface)
    less than 10 percent 948.0
    10-19 percent 948.1
    20-29 percent 948.2
    30-39 percent 948.3
    40-49 percent 948.4
    50-59 percent 948.5
    60-69 percent 948.6
    70-79 percent 948.7
    80-89 percent 948.8
    90 percent or more 948.9

Burn—*continued*
  extremity
    lower—*see* Burn, leg
    upper—*see* Burn, arm(s)
  eye(s) (and adnexa) (only) 940.9
    with
      face, head, or neck 941.02
        first degree 941.12
        second degree 941.22
        third degree 941.32
          deep 941.42
            with loss of body part 941.52
      other sites (classifiable to more than one category in 940-945)—*see* Burn, multiple, specified sites
      resulting rupture and destruction of eyeball 940.5
    specified part—*see* Burn, by site
  eyeball—*see also* Burn, eye
    with resulting rupture and destruction of eyeball 940.5
  eyelid(s) 940.1
    chemical 940.0
  face—*see* Burn, head
  finger (nail) (subungual) 944.01
    with
      hand(s)—*see* Burn, hand(s), multiple sites
      other sites—*see* Burn, multiple, specified sites
    thumb 944.04
      first degree 944.14
      second degree 944.24
      third degree 944.34
        deep 944.44
          with loss of body part 944.54
    first degree 944.11
    second degree 944.21
    third degree 944.31
      deep 944.41
        with loss of body part 944.51
    multiple (digits) 944.03
      with thumb—*see* Burn, finger, with thumb
      first degree 944.13
      second degree 944.23
      third degree 944.33
        deep 944.43
          with loss of body part 944.53
  flank—*see* Burn, abdomen
  foot 945.02
    with
      lower limb(s)—*see* Burn, leg, multiple sites
    first degree 945.12
    second degree 945.22
    third degree 945.32
      deep 945.42
        with loss of body part 945.52
  forearm(s) 943.01
    with
      upper limb(s) except hand(s) or wrist(s)—*see* Burn, arm(s), multiple sites
    first degree 943.11
    second degree 943.21
    third degree 943.31
      deep 943.41
        with loss of body part 943.51
  forehead 941.07
    with
      face or head—*see* Burn, head, multiple sites
    first degree 941.17
    second degree 941.27

Burn—*continued*
  forehead—*continued*
    third degree 941.37
      deep 941.47
        with loss of body part 941.57
  fourth degree—*see* Burn, by site, third degree,
    deep
  friction—*see* Injury, superficial, by site
  from swallowing caustic or corrosive substance
    NEC—*see* Burn, internal organs
  full thickness—*see* Burn, by site, third degree
  gastrointestinal tract 947.3
  genitourinary organs
    external 942.05
      with
        trunk—*see* Burn, trunk, multiple sites
      first degree 942.15
      second degree 942.25
      third degree 942.35
        deep 942.45
          with loss of body part 942.55
    internal 947.8
  globe (eye)—*see* Burn, eyeball
  groin—*see* Burn, abdomen
  gum 947.0
  hand(s) (phalanges) (and wrist) 944.00
    first degree 944.10
    second degree 944.20
    third degree 944.30
      deep 944.40
        with loss of body part 944.50
    back (dorsal surface) 944.06
      first degree 944.16
      second degree 944.26
      third degree 944.36
        deep 944.46
          with loss of body part 944.56
    multiple sites 944.08
      first degree 944.18
      second degree 944.28
      third degree 944.38
        deep 944.48
          with loss of body part 944.58
  head (and face) 941.00
    eye(s) only 940.9
      specified part—*see* Burn, by site
    first degree 941.10
    second degree 941.20
    third degree 941.30
      deep 941.40
        with loss of body part 941.50
    multiple sites 941.09
      with eyes—*see* Burn, eyes, with face, head,
        or neck
      first degree 941.19
      second degree 941.29
      third degree 941.39
        deep 941.49
          with loss of body part 941.59
  heel—*see* Burn, foot
  hip—*see* Burn, trunk, specified site NEC
  iliac region—*see* Burn, trunk, specified site
    NEC
  infected 958.3
  inhalation (*see also* Burn, internal organs) 947.9
  internal organs 947.9
    from caustic or corrosive substance
      (swallowing) NEC 947.9
    specified NEC (*see also* Burn, by site) 947.8
  interscapular region—*see* Burn, back
  intestine (large) (small) 947.3

Burn—*continued*
  iris—*see* Burn, eyeball
  knee 945.05
    with
      lower limb(s)—*see* Burn, leg, multiple sites
    first degree 945.15
    second degree 945.25
    third degree 945.35
      deep 945.45
        with loss of body part 945.55
  labium (majus) (minus)—*see* Burn,
    genitourinary organs, external
  lacrimal apparatus, duct, gland, or sac 940.1
    chemical 940.0
  larynx 947.1
  late effect—*see* Late, effects (of), burn
  leg 945.00
    first degree 945.10
    second degree 945.20
    third degree 945.30
      deep 945.40
        with loss of body part 945.50
    lower 945.04
      with other part(s) of lower limb(s)—*see*
        Burn, leg, multiple sites
      first degree 945.14
      second degree 945.24
      third degree 945.34
        deep 945.44
          with loss of body part 945.54
    multiple sites 945.09
      first degree 945.19
      second degree 945.29
      third degree 945.39
        deep 945.49
          with loss of body part 945.59
    upper—*see* Burn, thigh
  lightning—*see* Burn, by site
  limb(s)
    lower (including foot or toe(s))—*see* Burn, leg
    upper (except wrist and hand)—*see* Burn,
      arm(s)
  lip(s) 941.03
    with
      face or head—*see* Burn, head, multiple sites
    first degree 941.13
    second degree 941.23
    third degree 941.33
      deep 941.43
        with loss of body part 941.53
  lumbar region—*see* Burn, back
  lung 947.1
  malar region—*see* Burn, cheek
  mastoid region—*see* Burn, scalp
  membrane, tympanic—*see* Burn, ear
  midthoracic region—*see* Burn, chest wall
  mouth 947.0
  multiple (*see also* Burn, unspecified) 949.0
    specified sites (classifiable to more than one
      category in 940-945) 946.0
      first degree 946.1
      second degree 946.2
      third degree 946.3
        deep 946.4
          with loss of body part 946.5
  muscle, abdominal—*see* Burn, abdomen
  nasal (septum)—*see* Burn, nose
  neck 941.08
    with
      face or head—*see* Burn, head, multiple sites
    first degree 941.18

Burn—*continued*
  neck—*continued*
    second degree 941.28
    third degree 941.38
      deep 941.48
        with loss of body part 941.58
  nose (septum) 941.05
    with
      face or head—*see* Burn, head, multiple sites
    first degree 941.15
    second degree 941.25
    third degree 941.35
      deep 941.45
        with loss of body part 941.55
  occipital region—*see* Burn, scalp
  orbit region 940.1
    chemical 940.0
  oronasopharynx 947.0
  palate 947.0
  palm(s) 944.05
    with
      hand(s) and wrist(s)—*see* Burn, hand(s),
        multiple sites
    first degree 944.15
    second degree 944.25
    third degree 944.35
      deep 944.45
        with loss of a body part 944.55
  parietal region—*see* Burn, scalp
  penis–*see* Burn, genitourinary organs, external
  perineum—*see* Burn, genitourinary organs,
    external
  periocular area 940.1
    chemical 940.0
  pharynx 947.0
  pleura 947.1
  popliteal space—*see* Burn, knee
  prepuce—*see* Burn, genitourinary organs,
    external
  pubic region—*see* Burn, genitourinary organs,
    external
  pudenda—*see* Burn, genitourinary organs,
    external
  rectum 947.3
  sac, lacrimal 940.1
    chemical 940.0
  sacral region—*see* Burn, back
  salivary (ducts) (glands) 947.0
  scalp 941.06
    with
      face or neck—*see* Burn, head, multiple sites
    first degree 941.16
    second degree 941.26
    third degree 941.36
      deep 941.46
        with loss of body part 941.56
  scapular region 943.06
    with
      upper limb(s), except hand(s) or
        wrist(s)—*see* Burn, arm(s), multiple sites
    first degree 943.16
    second degree 943.26
    third degree 943.36
      deep 943.46
        with loss of body part 943.56
  sclera—*see* Burn, eyeball
  scrotum—*see* Burn, genitourinary organs,
    external
  septum, nasal—*see* Burn, nose

Burn—*continued*
  shoulder(s) 943.05
    with
      hand(s) and wrist(s)—*see* Burn, multiple,
        specified sites
      upper limb(s), except hand(s) or
        wrist(s)—*see* Burn, arm(s), multiple sites
    first degree 943.15
    second degree 943.25
    third degree 943.35
      deep 943.45
        with loss of body part 943.55
  skin NEC (*see also* Burn, unspecified) 949.0
  skull—*see* Burn, head
  small intestine 947.3
  sternal region—*see* Burn, chest wall
  stomach 947.3
  subconjunctival—*see* Burn, conjunctiva
  subcutaneous—*see* Burn, by site, third degree
  submaxillary region—*see* Burn, head
  submental region—*see* Burn, chin
  sun—*see* Sunburn
  supraclavicular fossa—*see* Burn, neck
  supraorbital—*see* Burn, forehead
  temple—*see* Burn, scalp
  temporal region—*see* Burn, scalp
  testicle—*see* Burn, genitourinary organs,
    external
  testis—*see* Burn, genitourinary organs, external
  thigh 945.06
    with
      lower limb(s)–*see* Burn, leg, multiple sites
    first degree 945.16
    second degree 945.26
    third degree 945.36
      deep 945.46
        with loss of body part 945.56
  thorax (external)—*see* Burn, chest wall
  throat 947.0
  thumb(s) (nail) (subungual) 944.02
    with
      finger(s)—*see* Burn, finger, with other sites,
        thumb
      hand(s) and wrist(s)—*see* Burn, hand(s),
        multiple sites
    first degree 944.12
    second degree 944.22
    third degree 944.32
      deep 944.42
        with loss of body part 944.52
  toe (nail) (subungual) 945.01
    with
      lower limb(s)—*see* Burn, leg, multiple sites
    first degree 945.11
    second degree 945.21
    third degree 945.31
      deep 945.41
        with loss of body part 945.51
  tongue 947.0
  tonsil 947.0
  trachea 947.1
  trunk 942.00
    first degree 942.10
    second degree 942.20
    third degree 942.30
      deep 942.40
        with loss of body part 942.50

Burn—*continued*
  trunk—*continued*
    multiple sites 942.09
      first degree 942.19
      second degree 942.29
      third degree 942.39
        deep 942.49
          with loss of body part 942.59
    specified site NEC 942.09
      first degree 942.19
      second degree 942.29
      third degree 942.39
        deep 942.49
          with loss of body part 942.59
  tunica vaginalis—*see* Burn, genitourinary
    organs, external
  tympanic membrane—*see* Burn, ear
  tympanum—*see* Burn, ear
  ultraviolet 692.82
  unspecified site (multiple) 949.0
    with extent of body surface involved specified
      less than 10 percent 948.0
      10-19 percent 948.1
      20-29 percent 948.2
      30-39 percent 948.3
      40-49 percent 948.4
      50-59 percent 948.5
      60-69 percent 948.6
      70-79 percent 948.7
      80-89 percent 948.8
      90 percent or more 948.9
    first degree 949.1
    second degree 949.2
    third degree 949.3
      deep 949.4
        with loss of body part 949.5
  uterus 947.4
  uvula 947.0
  vagina 947.4
  vulva—*see* Burn, genitourinary organs, external
  wrist(s) 944.07
    with
      hand(s)—*see* Burn, hand(s), multiple sites
    first degree 944.17
    second degree 944.27
    third degree 944.37
      deep 944.47
        with loss of body part 944.57
Burnett's syndrome (milk-alkali) 275.42
Burnier's syndrome (hypophyseal dwarfism)
  253.3
Burning
  feet syndrome 266.2
  sensation (*see also* Disturbance, sensation)
    782.0
  tongue 529.6
Burns' disease (osteochondrosis, lower ulna)
  732.3
Bursa —*see also* condition
  pharynx 478.29
Bursitis NEC 727.3
  Achilles tendon 726.71
  adhesive 726.90
    shoulder 726.0
  ankle 726.79
  buttock 726.5
  calcaneal 726.79
  collateral ligament
    fibular 726.63
    tibial 726.62
  Duplay's 726.2

Bursitis—*continued*
  elbow 726.33
  finger 726.8
  foot 726.79
  gonococcal 098.52
  hand 726.4
  hip 726.5
  infrapatellar 726.69
  ischiogluteal 726.5
  knee 726.60
  occupational NEC 727.2
  olecranon 726.33
  pes anserinus 726.61
  pharyngeal 478.29
  popliteal 727.51
  prepatellar 726.65
  radiohumeral 727.3
  scapulohumeral 726.19
    adhesive 726.0
  shoulder 726.10
    adhesive 726.0
  subacromial 726.19
    adhesive 726.0
  subcoracoid 726.19
  subdeltoid 726.19
    adhesive 726.0
  subpatellar 726.69
  syphilitic 095.7
  Thornwaldt's, Tornwaldt's (pharyngeal) 478.29
  toe 726.79
  trochanteric area 726.5
  wrist 726.4
Burst stitches or sutures (complication of
  surgery) (external) (*see also* Dehiscence)
  998.32
  internal 998.31
Buruli ulcer 031.1
Bury's disease (erythema elevatum diutinum)
  695.89
Buschke's disease or scleredema (adultorum)
  710.1
Busquet's disease (osteoperiostitis) (*see also*
  Osteomyelitis) 730.1
Busse-Buschke disease (cryptococcosis) 117.5
Buttock —*see* condition
Button
  Biskra 085.1
  Delhi 085.1
  oriental 085.1
Buttonhole hand (intrinsic) 736.21
Bwamba fever (encephalitis) 066.3
Byssinosis (occupational) 504
Bywaters' syndrome 958.5

C

Cacergasia 300.9
Cachexia 799.4
  cancerous —*see also* Neoplasm, by site,
    malignant 799.4
  cardiac—*see* Disease, heart
  dehydration 276.51
    with
      hypernatremia 276.0
      hyponatremia 276.1
    due to malnutrition 799.4
  exophthalmic 242.0
  heart—*see* Disease, heart
  hypophyseal 253.2
  hypopituitary 253.2
  lead 984.9
    specified type of lead—*see* Table of drugs and
      chemicals
  malaria 084.9
  malignant —*see also* Neoplasm, by site,
    malignant 799.4
  marsh 084.9
  nervous 300.5
  old age 797
  pachydermic—*see* Hypothyroidism
  paludal 084.9
  pituitary (postpartum) 253.2
  renal (*see also* Disease, renal) 593.9
  saturnine 984.9
    specified type of lead—*see* Table of drugs and
      chemicals
  senile 797
  Simmonds' (pituitary cachexia) 253.2
  splenica 289.59
  strumipriva (*see also* Hypothyroidism) 244.9
  tuberculous NEC (*see also* Tuberculosis) 011.9
café au lait spots 709.09
Caffey's disease or syndrome (infantile cortical
    hyperostosis) 756.59
Caisson disease 993.3
Caked breast (puerperal, postpartum) 676.2
Cake kidney 753.3
Calabar swelling 125.2
Calcaneal spur 726.73
Calcaneoapophysitis 732.5
Calcaneonavicular bar 755.67
Calcareous —*see* condition
Calcicosis (occupational) 502
Calciferol (vitamin D) deficiency 268.9
  with
    osteomalacia 268.2
    rickets (*see also* Rickets) 268.0
Calcification
  adrenal (capsule) (gland) 255.41
    tuberculous (*see also* Tuberculosis) 017.6
  aorta 440.0
  artery (annular)—*see* Arteriosclerosis
  auricle (ear) 380.89
  bladder 596.98
    due to S. hematobium 120.0
  brain (cortex)—*see* Calcification, cerebral
  bronchus 519.19
  bursa 727.82
  cardiac (*see also* Degeneration, myocardial) 429.1
  cartilage (postinfectional) 733.99
  cerebral (cortex) 348.89
    artery 437.0
  cervix (uteri) 622.8

Calcification—*continued*
  choroid plexus 349.2
  conjunctiva 372.54
  corpora cavernosa (penis) 607.89
  cortex (brain)—*see* Calcification, cerebral
  dental pulp (nodular) 522.2
  dentinal papilla 520.4
  disc, intervertebral 722.90
    cervical, cervicothoracic 722.91
    lumbar, lumbosacral 722.93
    thoracic, thoracolumbar 722.92
  fallopian tube 620.8
  falx cerebri—*see* Calcification, cerebral
  fascia 728.89
  gallbladder 575.8
  general 275.40
  heart (*see also* Degeneration, myocardial) 429.1
    valve—*see* Endocarditis
  intervertebral cartilage or disc (postinfectional)
      722.90
    cervical, cervicothoracic 722.91
    lumbar, lumbosacral 722.93
    thoracic, thoracolumbar 722.92
  intracranial—*see* Calcification, cerebral
  intraspinal ligament 728.89
  joint 719.80
    ankle 719.87
    elbow 719.82
    foot 719.87
    hand 719.84
    hip 719.85
    knee 719.86
    multiple sites 719.89
    pelvic region 719.85
    shoulder (region) 719.81
    specified site NEC 719.88
    wrist 719.83
  kidney 593.89
    tuberculous (*see also* Tuberculosis) 016.0
  larynx (senile) 478.79
  lens 366.8
  ligament 728.89
    intraspinal 728.89
    knee (medial collateral) 717.89
  lung 518.89
    active 518.89
    postinfectional 518.89
    tuberculous (*see also* Tuberculosis,
        pulmonary) 011.9
  lymph gland or node (postinfectional) 289.3
    tuberculous (*see also* Tuberculosis, lymph
        gland) 017.2
  mammographic 793.89
  massive (paraplegic) 728.10
  medial NEC (*see also* Arteriosclerosis,
      extremities) 440.20
  meninges (cerebral) 349.2
  metastatic 275.40
  Mönckeberg's—*see* Arteriosclerosis
  muscle 728.10
    heterotopic, postoperative 728.13
  myocardium, myocardial (*see also*
      Degeneration, myocardial) 429.1
  ovary 620.8
  pancreas 577.8
  penis 607.99
  periarticular 728.89
  pericardium (*see also* Pericarditis) 423.8

Calcification—*continued*
pineal gland 259.8
pleura 511.0
  postinfectional 518.89
  tuberculous (*see also* Tuberculosis, pleura)
    012.0
pulp (dental) (nodular) 522.2
renal 593.89
rider's bone 733.99
sclera 379.16
semilunar cartilage 717.89
spleen 289.59
subcutaneous 709.3
suprarenal (capsule) (gland) 255.41
tendon (sheath) 727.82
  with bursitis, synovitis or tenosynovitis 727.82
trachea 519.19
ureter 593.89
uterus 621.8
vitreous 379.29
Calcified —*see also* Calcification
hematoma NEC 959.9
Calcinosis (generalized) (interstitial) (tumoral)
    (universalis) 275.49
circumscripta 709.3
cutis 709.3
intervertebralis 275.49 [722.90]
Raynaud's
    phenomenonsclerodactylytelangiectasis
    (CRST) 710.1
Calciphylaxis (*see also* Calcification, by site)
    275.49
Calcium
blood
  high (*see also* Hypercalcemia) 275.42
  low (*see also* Hypocalcemia) 275.41
deposits—*see also* Calcification, by site
  in bursa 727.82
  in tendon (sheath) 727.82
    with bursitis, synovitis or tenosynovitis
    727.82
salts or soaps in vitreous 379.22
Calciuria 791.9
Calculi —*see* Calculus
Calculosis, intrahepatic —*see*
    Choledocholithiasis
Calculus, calculi, calculous 592.9
ampulla of Vater—*see* Choledocholithiasis
anuria (impacted) (recurrent) 592.0
appendix 543.9
bile duct (any)—*see* Choledocholithiasis
biliary—*see* Cholelithiasis
bilirubin, multiple—*see* Cholelithiasis
bladder (encysted) (impacted) (urinary) 594.1
  diverticulum 594.0
bronchus 518.89
calyx (kidney) (renal) 592.0
  congenital 753.3
cholesterol (pure) (solitary)—*see* Cholelithiasis
common duct (bile)—*see* Choledocholithiasis
conjunctiva 372.54
cystic 594.1
  duct—*see* Cholelithiasis
dental 523.6
  subgingival 523.6
  supragingival 523.6
epididymis 608.89

Calculus, calculi, calculous—*continued*
gallbladder—*see also* Cholelithiasis
  congenital 751.69
hepatic (duct)—*see* Choledocholithiasis
intestine (impaction) (obstruction) 560.39
kidney (impacted) (multiple) (pelvis) (recurrent)
    (staghorn) 592.0
  congenital 753.3
lacrimal (passages) 375.57
liver (impacted)—*see* Choledocholithiasis
lung 518.89
mammographic 793.89
nephritic (impacted) (recurrent) 592.0
nose 478.19
pancreas (duct) 577.8
parotid gland 527.5
pelvis, encysted 592.0
prostate 602.0
pulmonary 518.89
renal (impacted) (recurrent) 592.0
  congenital 753.3
salivary (duct) (gland) 527.5
seminal vesicle 608.89
staghorn 592.0
Stensen's duct 527.5
sublingual duct or gland 527.5
  congenital 750.26
submaxillary duct, gland, or region 527.5
suburethral 594.8
tonsil 474.8
tooth, teeth 523.6
tunica vaginalis 608.89
ureter (impacted) (recurrent) 592.1
urethra (impacted) 594.2
urinary (duct) (impacted) (passage) (tract) 592.9
  lower tract NEC 594.9
    specified site 594.8
vagina 623.8
vesical (impacted) 594.1
Wharton's duct 527.5
Caliectasis 593.89
California
disease 114.0
encephalitis 062.5
Caligo cornea 371.03
Callositas, callosity (infected) 700
Callus (infected) 700
bone 726.91
excessive, following fracture—*see also* Late,
    effect (of), fracture
Calvé (-Perthes) disease (osteochondrosis,
    femoral capital) 732.1
Calvities (*see also* Alopecia) 704.00
Cameroon fever (*see also* Malaria) 084.6
Camptocormia 300.11
Camptodactyly (congenital) 755.59
Camurati-Engelmann disease (diaphyseal
    sclerosis) 756.59
Canal —*see* condition
Canaliculitis (lacrimal) (acute) 375.31
Actinomyces 039.8
chronic 375.41
Canavan's disease 330.0

Cancer (M8000/3)—*see also* Neoplasm, by site, malignant

Note—The term "cancer" when modified by an adjective or adjectival phrase indicating a morphological type should be coded in the same manner as "carcinoma" with that adjective or phrase. Thus, "squamous-cell cancer" should be coded in the same manner as "squamous-cell carcinoma," which appears in the list under "Carcinoma."

  bile duct type (M8160/3), liver 155.1
  hepatocellular (M8170/3) 155.0
Cancerous (M8000/3)—*see* Neoplasm, by site, malignant
Cancerphobia 300.29
Cancrum oris 528.1
Candidiasis, candidal 112.9
  with pneumonia 112.4
  balanitis 112.2
  congenital 771.7
  disseminated 112.5
  endocarditis 112.81
  esophagus 112.84
  intertrigo 112.3
  intestine 112.85
  lung 112.4
  meningitis 112.83
  mouth 112.0
  nails 112.3
  neonatal 771.7
  onychia 112.3
  otitis externa 112.82
  otomycosis 112.82
  paronychia 112.3
  perionyxis 112.3
  pneumonia 112.4
  pneumonitis 112.4
  skin 112.3
  specified site NEC 112.89
  systemic 112.5
  urogenital site NEC 112.2
  vagina 112.1
  vulva 112.1
  vulvovaginitis 112.1
Candidiosis —*see* Candidiasis
Candiru infection or infestation 136.8
Canities (premature) 704.3
  congenital 757.4
Canker (mouth) (sore) 528.2
  rash 034.1
Cannabinosis 504
Canton fever 081.9
Cap
  cradle 690.11
Capillariasis 127.5
Capillary —*see* condition
Caplan's syndrome 714.81
Caplan-Colinet syndrome 714.81
Capsule —*see* condition
Capsulitis (joint) 726.90
  adhesive (shoulder) 726.0
  hip 726.5
  knee 726.60
  labyrinthine 387.8
  thyroid 245.9
  wrist 726.4
Caput
  crepitus 756.0
  medusae 456.8
  succedaneum 767.19

Carapata disease 087.1
Carate —*see* Pinta
Carbohydrate-deficient glycoprotein syndrome (CDGS) 271.8
Carboxyhemoglobinemia 986
Carbuncle 680.9
  abdominal wall 680.2
  ankle 680.6
  anus 680.5
  arm (any part, above wrist) 680.3
  auditory canal, external 680.0
  axilla 680.3
  back (any part) 680.2
  breast 680.2
  buttock 680.5
  chest wall 680.2
  corpus cavernosum 607.2
  ear (any part) (external) 680.0
  eyelid 373.13
  face (any part, except eye) 680.0
  finger (any) 680.4
  flank 680.2
  foot (any part) 680.7
  forearm 680.3
  genital organ (male) 608.4
  gluteal (region) 680.5
  groin 680.2
  hand (any part) 680.4
  head (any part, except face) 680.8
  heel 680.7
  hip 680.6
  kidney (*see also* Abscess, kidney) 590.2
  knee 680.6
  labia 616.4
  lacrimal
    gland (*see also* Dacryoadenitis) 375.00
    passages (duct) (sac) (*see also* Dacryocystitis) 375.30
  leg, any part except foot 680.6
  lower extremity, any part except foot 680.6
  malignant 022.0
  multiple sites 680.9
  neck 680.1
  nose (external) (septum) 680.0
  orbit, orbital 376.01
  partes posteriores 680.5
  pectoral region 680.2
  penis 607.2
  perineum 680.2
  pinna 680.0
  scalp (any part) 680.8
  scrotum 608.4
  seminal vesicle 608.0
  shoulder 680.3
  skin NEC 680.9
  specified site NEC 680.8
  spermatic cord 608.4
  temple (region) 680.0
  testis 608.4
  thigh 680.6
  thumb 680.4
  toe (any part) 680.7
  trunk 680.2
  tunica vaginalis 608.4
  umbilicus 680.2
  upper arm 680.3
  urethra 597.0
  vas deferens 608.4
  vulva 616.4
  wrist 680.4
Carbunculus (*see also* Carbuncle) 680.9

Carcinoid (tumor) (M8240/1)—*see* Tumor, carcinoid
Carcinoidosis 259.2
Carcinoma (M8010/3)—*see also* Neoplasm, by site, malignant

> *Note—Except where otherwise indicated, the morphological varieties of carcinoma in the list below should be coded by site as for "Neoplasm, malignant."*

with
  apocrine metaplasia (M8573/3)
  cartilaginous (and osseous) metaplasia (M8571/3)
  osseous (and cartilaginous) metaplasia (M8571/3)
  productive fibrosis (M8141/3)
  spindle cell metaplasia (M8572/3)
  squamous metaplasia (M8570/3)
acidophil (M8280/3)
  specified site—*see* Neoplasm, by site, malignant
  unspecified site 194.3
acidophil-basophil, mixed (M8281/3)
  specified site—*see* Neoplasm, by site, malignant
  unspecified site 194.3
acinar (cell) (M8550/3)
acinic cell (M8550/3)
adenocystic (M8200/3)
adenoid
  cystic (M8200/3)
  squamous cell (M8075/3)
adenosquamous (M8560/3)
adnexal (skin) (M8390/3)—*see* Neoplasm, skin, malignant
adrenal cortical (M8370/3) 194.0
alveolar (M8251/3)
  cell (M8250/3)—*see* Neoplasm, lung, malignant
anaplastic type (M8021/3)
apocrine (M8401/3)
  breast—*see* Neoplasm, breast, malignant
  specified site NEC—*see* Neoplasm, skin, malignant
  unspecified site 173.99
basal cell (pigmented) (M8090/3) (*see also* Neoplasm, skin, malignant) 173.91
  fibro-epithelial type (M8093/3)—*see* Neoplasm, skin, malignant
  morphea type (M8092/3)—*see* Neoplasm, skin, malignant
  multicentric (M8091/3)—*see* Neoplasm, skin, malignant
basaloid (M8123/3)
basal-squamous cell, mixed (M8094/3)—*see* Neoplasm, skin, malignant
basophil (M8300/3)
  specified site—*see* Neoplasm, by site, malignant
  unspecified site 194.3
basophil-acidophil, mixed (M8281/3)
  specified site—*see* Neoplasm, by site, malignant
  unspecified site 194.3
basosquamous (M8094/3)—*see* Neoplasm, skin, malignant

Carcinoma—*continued*
bile duct type (M8160/3)
  and hepatocellular, mixed (M8180/3) 155.0
  liver 155.1
  specified site NEC—*see* Neoplasm, by site, malignant
  unspecified site 155.1
branchial or branchiogenic 146.8
bronchial or bronchogenic—*see* Neoplasm, lung, malignant
bronchiolar (terminal) (M8250/3)—*see* Neoplasm, lung, malignant
bronchiolo-alveolar (M8250/3)—*see* Neoplasm, lung, malignant
bronchogenic (epidermoid) 162.9
C cell (M8510/3)
  specified site—*see* Neoplasm, by site, malignant
  unspecified site 193
ceruminous (M8420/3) 173.29
chorionic (M9100/3)
  specified site—*see* Neoplasm, by site, malignant
  unspecified site
    female 181
    male 186.9
chromophobe (M8270/3)
  specified site—*see* Neoplasm, by site, malignant
  unspecified site 194.3
clear cell (mesonephroid type) (M8310/3)
cloacogenic (M8124/3)
  specified site—*see* Neoplasm, by site, malignant
  unspecified site 154.8
colloid (M8480/3)
cribriform (M8201/3)
cylindroid type (M8200/3)
diffuse type (M8145/3)
  specified site—*see* Neoplasm, by site, malignant
  unspecified site 151.9
duct (cell) (M8500/3)
  with Paget's disease (M8541/3)—*see* Neoplasm, breast, malignant
  infiltrating (M8500/3)
    specified site—*see* Neoplasm, by site, malignant
    unspecified site 174.9
ductal (M8500/3)
ductular, infiltrating (M8521/3)
embryonal (M9070/3)
  and teratoma, mixed (M9081/3)
  combined with choriocarcinoma (M9101/3)—*see* Neoplasm, by site, malignant
  infantile type (M9071/3)
  liver 155.0
  polyembryonal type (M9072/3)
endometrioid (M8380/3)
eosinophil (M8280/3)
  specified site—*see* Neoplasm, by site, malignant
  unspecified site 194.3
epidermoid (M8070/3)—*see also* Carcinoma, squamous cell
  and adenocarcinoma, mixed (M8560/3)
  in situ, Bowen's type (M8081/2)—*see* Neoplasm, skin, in situ
  intradermal—*see* Neoplasm, skin, in situ

Carcinoma—*continued*

fibroepithelial type basal cell (M8093/3)—*see* Neoplasm, skin, malignant

follicular (M8330/3)
  and papillary (mixed) (M8340/3) 193
  moderately differentiated type (M8332/3) 193
  pure follicle type (M8331/3) 193
  specified site—*see* Neoplasm, by site, malignant
  trabecular type (M8332/3) 193
  unspecified site 193
  well differentiated type (M8331/3) 193

gelatinous (M8480/3)

giant cell (M8031/3)
  and spindle cell (M8030/3)

granular cell (M8320/3)

granulosa cell (M8620/3) 183.0

hepatic cell (M8170/3) 155.0

hepatocellular (M8170/3) 155.0
  and bile duct, mixed (M8180/3) 155.0

hepatocholangiolitic (M8180/3) 155.0

Hurthle cell (thyroid) 193

hypernephroid (M8311/3)

in
  adenomatous
    polyp (M8210/3)
    polyposis coli (M8220/3) 153.9
  pleomorphic adenoma (M8940/3)
  polypoid adenoma (M8210/3)
  situ (M8010/3)—*see* Carcinoma, in situ
  tubular adenoma (M8210/3)
  villous adenoma (M8261/3)

infiltrating duct (M8500/3)
  with Paget's disease (M8541/3)—*see* Neoplasm, breast, malignant
  specified site—*see* Neoplasm, by site, malignant
  unspecified site 174.9

inflammatory (M8530/3)
  specified site—*see* Neoplasm, by site, malignant
  unspecified site 174.9

in situ (M8010/2)—*see also* Neoplasm, by site, in situ
  epidermoid (M8070/2)—*see also* Neoplasm, by site, in situ
    with questionable stromal invasion (M8076/2)
      specified site—*see* Neoplasm, by site, in situ
      unspecified site 233.1
    Bowen's type (M8081/2)—*see* Neoplasm, skin, in situ
  intraductal (M8500/2)
    specified site—*see* Neoplasm, by site, in situ
    unspecified site 233.0
  lobular (M8520/2)
    specified site—*see* Neoplasm, by site, in situ
    unspecified site 233.0
  papillary (M8050/2)—*see* Neoplasm, by site, in situ
  squamous cell (M8070/2)—*see also* Neoplasm, by site, in situ
    with questionable stromal invasion (M8076/2)
  specified site—*see* Neoplasm, by site, in situ
    unspecified site 233.1
  transitional cell (M8120/2)—*see* Neoplasm, by site, in situ

Carcinoma—*continued*

intestinal type (M8144/3)
  specified site—*see* Neoplasm, by site, malignant
  unspecified site 151.9

intraductal (noninfiltrating) (M8500/2)
  papillary (M8503/2)
    specified site—*see* Neoplasm, by site, in situ
    unspecified site 233.0
  specified site—*see* Neoplasm, by site, in situ
  unspecified site 233.0

intraepidermal (M8070/2)—*see also* Neoplasm, skin, in situ
  squamous cell, Bowen's type (M8081/2)—*see* Neoplasm, skin, in situ

intraepithelial (M8010/2)—*see also* Neoplasm, by site, in situ
  squamous cell (M8072/2)—*see* Neoplasm, by site, in situ

intraosseous (M9270/3) 170.1
  upper jaw (bone) 170.0

islet cell (M8150/3)
  and exocrine, mixed (M8154/3)
    specified site—*see* Neoplasm, by site, malignant
    unspecified site 157.9
  pancreas 157.4
  specified site NEC—*see* Neoplasm, by site, malignant
  unspecified site 157.4

juvenile, breast (M8502/3)—*see* Neoplasm, breast, malignant

Kulchitsky's cell (carcinoid tumor of intestine) 259.2

large cell (M8012/3)
  squamous cell, nonkeratinizing type (M8072/3)

Leydig cell (testis) (M8650/3)
  specified site—*see* Neoplasm, by site, malignant
  unspecified site 186.9
    female 183.0
    male 186.9

liver cell (M8170/3) 155.0

lobular (infiltrating) (M8520/3)
  non-infiltrating (M8520/3)
    specified site—*see* Neoplasm, by site, in situ
    unspecified site 233.0
  specified site—*see* Neoplasm, by site, malignant
  unspecified site 174.9

lymphoepithelial (M8082/3)

medullary (M8510/3)
  with
    amyloid stroma (M8511/3)
      specified site—*see* Neoplasm, by site, malignant
      unspecified site 193
    lymphoid stroma (M8512/3)
      specified site—*see* Neoplasm, by site, malignant
      unspecified site 174.9

Carcinoma—*continued*
  Merkel cell 209.36
    buttock 209.36
    ear 209.31
    eyelid, including canthus 209.31
    face 209.31
    genitals 209.36
    lip 209.31
    lower limb 209.34
    neck 209.32
    nodal presentation 209.75
    scalp 209.32
    secondary (any site) 209.75
    specified site NEC 209.36
    trunk 209.35
    unknown primary site 209.75
    upper limb 209.33
    visceral metastatic presentation 209.75
  mesometanephric (M9110/3)
  mesonephric (M9110/3)
  metastatic (M8010/6)—*see* Metastasis, cancer
  metatypical (M8095/3)—*see* Neoplasm, skin,
    malignant
  morphea type basal cell (M8092/3)—*see*
    Neoplasm, skin, malignant
  mucinous (M8480/3)
  mucin-producing (M8481/3)
  mucin-secreting (M8481/3)
  mucoepidermoid (M8430/3)
  mucoid (M8480/3)
    cell (M8300/3)
      specified site—*see* Neoplasm, by site,
        malignant
      unspecified site 194.3
  mucous (M8480/3)
  neuroendocrine
    high grade (M8240/3) 209.30
    malignant poorly differentiated (M8240/3)
      209.30
  nonencapsulated sclerosing (M8350/3) 193
  noninfiltrating
    intracystic (M8504/2)—*see* Neoplasm, by site,
      in situ
    intraductal (M8500/2)
      papillary (M8503/2)
        specified site—*see* Neoplasm, by site, in
          situ
        unspecified site 233.0
      specified site—*see* Neoplasm, by site, in situ
      unspecified site 233.0
    lobular (M8520/2)
      specified site—*see* Neoplasm, by site, in situ
      unspecified site 233.0
  oat cell (M8042/3)
    specified site—*see* Neoplasm, by site,
      malignant
    unspecified site 162.9
  odontogenic (M9270/3) 170.1
    upper jaw (bone) 170.0
  onocytic (M8290/3)
  oxyphilic (M8290/3)
  papillary (M8050/3)
    and follicular (mixed) (M8340/3) 193
    epidermoid (M8052/3)
    intraductal (noninfiltrating) (M8503/2)
      specified site—*see* Neoplasm, by site, in situ
      unspecified site 233.0

Carcinoma—*continued*
  papillary—*continued*
    serous (M8460/3)
      specified site—*see* Neoplasm, by site,
        malignant
      surface (M8461/3)
        specified site—*see* Neoplasm, by site,
          malignant
        unspecified site 183.0
      unspecified site 183.0
    squamous cell (M8052/3)
    transitional cell (M8130/3)
  papillocystic (M8450/3)
    specified site—*see* Neoplasm, by site,
      malignant
    unspecified site 183.0
  parafollicular cell (M8510/3)
    specified site—*see* Neoplasm, by site,
      malignant
    unspecified site 193
  pleomorphic (M8022/3)
  polygonal cell (M8034/3)
  prickle cell (M8070/3)
  pseudoglandular, squamous cell (M8075/3)
  pseudomucinous (M8470/3)
    specified site—*see* Neoplasm, by site,
      malignant
    unspecified site 183.0
  pseudosarcomatous (M8033/3)
  regaud type (M8082/3)—*see* Neoplasm,
    nasopharynx, malignant
  renal cell (M8312/3) 189.0
  reserve cell (M8041/3)
  round cell (M8041/3)
  Schmincke (M8082/3)—*see* Neoplasm,
    nasopharynx, malignant
  Schneiderian (M8121/3)
    specified site—*see* Neoplasm, by site,
      malignant
    unspecified site 160.0
  scirrhous (M8141/3)
  sebaceous (M8410/3)—*see* Neoplasm, skin,
    malignant
  secondary (M8010/6)—*see* Neoplasm, by site,
    malignant, secondary
  secretory, breast (M8502/3)—*see* Neoplasm,
    breast, malignant
  serous (M8441/3)
    papillary (M8460/3)
      specified site—*see* Neoplasm, by site,
        malignant
      unspecified site 183.0
    surface, papillary (M8461/3)
      specified site—*see* Neoplasm, by site,
        malignant
      unspecified site 183.0
  Sertoli cell (M8640/3)
    specified site—*see* Neoplasm, by site,
      malignant
    unspecified site 186.9
  signet ring cell (M8490/3)
    metastatic (M8490/6)—*see* Neoplasm, by site,
      secondary
  simplex (M8231/3)
  skin appendage (M8390/3)—*see* Neoplasm,
    skin, malignant
  small cell (M8041/3)
    fusiform cell type (M8043/3)
    squamous cell, non-keratinizing type
      (M8073/3)

Carcinoma—*continued*
  solid (M8230/3)
    with amyloid stroma (M8511/3)
      specified site—*see* Neoplasm, by site,
        malignant
      unspecified site 193
  spheroidal cell (M8035/3)
  spindle cell (M8032/3)
    and giant cell (M8030/3)
  spinous cell (M8070/3)
  squamous (cell) (M8070/3)
    adenoid type (M8075/3)
    and adenocarcinoma, mixed (M8560/3)
    intraepidermal, Bowen's type—*see* Neoplasm,
      skin, in situ
    keratinizing type (large cell) (M8071/3)
    large cell, non-keratinizing type (M8072/3)
    microinvasive (M8076/3)
      specified site—*see* Neoplasm, by site,
        malignant
      unspecified site 180.9
    non-keratinizing type (M8072/3)
    papillary (M8052/3)
    pseudoglandular (M8075/3)
    skin (see also Neoplasm, skin, malignant) 173.92
    small cell, non-keratinizing type (M8073/3)
    spindle cell type (M8074/3)
    verrucous (M8051/3)
  superficial spreading (M8143/3)
  sweat gland (M8400/3)—*see* Neoplasm, skin,
    malignant
  theca cell (M8600/3) 183.0
  thymic (M8580/3) 164.0
  trabecular (M8190/3)
  transitional (cell) (M8120/3)
    papillary (M8130/3)
    spindle cell type (M8122/3)
  tubular (M8211/3)
  undifferentiated type (M8020/3)
  urothelial (M8120/3)
  ventriculi 151.9
  verrucous (epidermoid) (squamous cell)
    (M8051/3)
  villous (M8262/3)
  water-clear cell (M8322/3) 194.1
  wolffian duct (M9110/3)
Carcinomaphobia 300.29
Carcinomatosis
  peritonei (M8010/6) 197.6
  specified site NEC (M8010/3)—*see* Neoplasm,
    by site, malignant
  unspecified site (M8010/6) 199.0
Carcinosarcoma (M8980/3)—*see also*
  Neoplasm, by site, malignant
  embryonal type (M8981/3)—*see* Neoplasm, by
    site, malignant
Cardia, cardial —*see* condition
Cardiac —*see also* condition
  death—*see* Disease, heart
  device
    defibrillator, automatic implantable (with
      synchronous cardiac pacemaker) V45.02
    in situ NEC V45.00
    pacemaker
      cardiac
        fitting or adjustment V53.3
        in situ V45.01
      carotid sinus
        fitting or adjustment V53.3
        in situ V45.09
  pacemaker—*see* Cardiac, device, pacemaker
  tamponade 423.3

Cardialgia (*see also* Pain, precordial) 786.51
Cardiectasis —*see* Hypertrophy, cardiac
Cardiochalasia 530.81
Cardiomalacia (*see also* Degeneration,
  myocardial) 429.1
Cardiomegalia glycogenica diffusa 271.0
Cardiomegaly (*see also* Hypertrophy, cardiac)
  429.3
  congenital 746.89
  glycogen 271.0
  hypertensive (*see also* Hypertension, heart)
    402.90
  idiopathic 429.3
Cardiomyoliposis (*see also* Degeneration,
  myocardial) 429.1
Cardiomyopathy (congestive) (constrictive)
  (familial) (infiltrative) (obstructive)
  (restrictive) (sporadic) 425.4
  alcoholic 425.5
  amyloid 277.39 *[425.7]*
  beriberi 265.0 *[425.7]*
  cobalt-beer 425.5
  congenital 425.3
  due to
    amyloidosis 277.39 *[425.7]*
    beriberi 265.0 *[425.7]*
    cardiac glycogenesis 271.0 *[425.7]*
    Chagas' disease 086.0
    Friedreich's ataxia 334.0 *[425.8]*
    mucopolysaccharidosis 277.5 *[425.7]*
    myotonia atrophica 359.21 *[425.8]*
    progressive muscular dystrophy 359.1 *[425.8]*
    sarcoidosis 135 *[425.8]*
  glycogen storage 271.0 *[425.7]*
  hypertensive—*see* Hypertension, with, heart
    involvement
  hypertrophic 425.18
    nonobstructive 425.18
    obstructive 425.11
      congenital 746.84
  idiopathic (concentric) 425.4
  in
    Chagas' disease 086.0
    sarcoidosis 135 *[425.8]*
  ischemic 414.8
  metabolic NEC 277.9 *[425.7]*
    amyloid 277.39 *[425.7]*
    thyrotoxic (*see also* Thyrotoxicosis) 242.9
      [425.7]
    thyrotoxicosis (*see also* Thyrotoxicosis) 242.9
      [425.7]
  newborn 425.4
    congenital 425.3
  nutritional 269.9 *[425.7]*
    beriberi 265.0 *[425.7]*
  obscure of Africa 425.2
  peripartum 674.5
  postpartum 674.5
  primary 425.4
  secondary 425.9
  stress induced 429.83
  takotsubo 429.83
  thyrotoxic (*see also* Thyrotoxicosis) 242.9 *[425.7]*
  toxic NEC 425.9
  tuberculous (*see also* Tuberculosis) 017.9 *[425.8]*
Cardionephritis —*see* Hypertension, cardiorenal
Cardionephropathy —*see* Hypertension,
  cardiorenal
Cardionephrosis —*see* Hypertension,
  cardiorenal
Cardioneurosis 306.2
Cardiopathia nigra 416.0

Cardiopathy (*see also* Disease, heart) 429.9
  hypertensive (*see also* Hypertension, heart) 402.90
  idiopathic 425.4
  mucopolysaccharidosis 277.5 *[425.7]*
Cardiopericarditis (*see also* Pericarditis) 423.9
Cardiophobia 300.29
Cardioptosis 746.87
Cardiorenal —*see* condition
Cardiorrhexis (*see also* Infarct, myocardium) 410.9
Cardiosclerosis —*see* Arteriosclerosis, coronary
Cardiosis —*see* Disease, heart
Cardiospasm (esophagus) (reflex) (stomach) 530.0
  congenital 750.7
Cardiostenosis —*see* Disease, heart
Cardiosymphysis 423.1
Cardiothyrotoxicosis —*see* Hyperthyroidism
Cardiovascular —*see* condition
Carditis (acute) (bacterial) (chronic) (subacute) 429.89
  Coxsackie 074.20
  hypertensive (*see also* Hypertension, heart) 402.90
  meningococcal 036.40
  rheumatic—*see* Disease, heart, rheumatic
  rheumatoid 714.2
Care (of)
  child (routine) V20.1
  convalescent following V66.9
    chemotherapy V66.2
    medical NEC V66.5
    psychotherapy V66.3
    radiotherapy V66.1
    surgery V66.0
    surgical NEC V66.0
    treatment (for) V66.5
      combined V66.6
      fracture V66.4
      mental disorder NEC V66.3
      specified type NEC V66.5
  end-of-life care V66.7
  family member (handicapped) (sick)
    creating problem for family V61.49
    provided away from home for holiday relief V60.5
    unavailable, due to
      absence (person rendering care) (sufferer) V60.4
      inability (any reason) of person rendering care V60.4
  holiday relief V60.5
  hospice V66.7
  lack of (at or after birth) (infant) (child) 995.52
    adult 995.84
  lactation of mother V24.1
  palliative V66.7
  postpartum
    immediately after delivery V24.0
    routine follow-up V24.2
  prenatal V22.1
    first pregnancy V22.0
    high risk pregnancy V23.9
      inconclusive fetal viability V23.87
      specified problem NEC V23.8
  terminal V66.7
  unavailable, due to
    absence of person rendering care V60.4
    inability (any reason) of person rendering care V60.4
  well baby V20.1

Caries (bone) (*see also* Tuberculosis, bone) 015.9 *[730.8]*
  arrested 521.04
  cementum 521.03
  cerebrospinal (tuberculous) 015.0 *[730.88]*
  dental (acute) (chronic) (incipient) (infected) 521.00
    with pulp exposure 521.03
    extending to
      dentine 521.02
      pulp 521.03
    other specified NEC 521.09
    pit and fissure 521.06
    primary
      pit and fissure origin 521.06
      root surface 521.08
      smooth surface origin 521.07
    root surface 521.08
    smooth surface 521.07
  dentin (acute) (chronic) 521.02
  enamel (acute) (chronic) (incipient) 521.01
  external meatus 380.89
  hip (*see also* Tuberculosis) 015.1 *[730.85]*
  initial 521.01
  knee 015.2 *[730.86]*
  labyrinth 386.8
  limb NEC 015.7 *[730.88]*
  mastoid (chronic) (process) 383.1
  middle ear 385.89
  nose 015.7 *[730.88]*
  orbit 015.7 *[730.88]*
  ossicle 385.24
  petrous bone 383.20
  sacrum (tuberculous) 015.0 *[730.88]*
  spine, spinal (column) (tuberculous) 015.0 *[730.88]*
  syphilitic 095.5
    congenital 090.0 *[730.8]*
  teeth (internal) 521.00
    initial 521.01
  vertebra (column) (tuberculous) 015.0 *[730.88]*
Carini's syndrome (ichthyosis congenita) 757.1
Carious teeth 521.00
Carneous mole 631.8
Carnosinemia 270.5
Carotid body or sinus syndrome 337.01
Carotidynia 337.01
Carotinemia (dietary) 278.3
Carotinosis (cutis) (skin) 278.3
Carpal tunnel syndrome 354.0
Carpenter's syndrome 759.89
Carpopedal spasm (*see also* Tetany) 781.7
Carpoptosis 736.05
Carrier (suspected) of
  amebiasis V02.2
  bacterial disease (meningococcal, staphylococcal, streptococcal) NEC V02.59
  cholera V02.0
  cystic fibrosis gene V83.81
  defective gene V83.89
  diphtheria V02.4
  dysentery (bacillary) V02.3
    amebic V02.2
  Endamoeba histolytica V02.2
  gastrointestinal pathogens NEC V02.3
  genetic defect V83.89
  gonorrhea V02.7
  group B streptococcus V02.51
  HAA (hepatitis Australian-antigen) V02.61
  hemophilia A (asymptomatic) V83.01
    symptomatic V83.02

Carrier—*continued*
  hepatitis V02.60
    Australian-antigen (HAA) V02.61
    B V02.61
    C V02.62
    serum V02.61
    specified type NEC V02.69
    viral V02.60
  infective organism NEC V02.9
  malaria V02.9
  paratyphoid V02.3
  Salmonella V02.3
    typhosa V02.1
  serum hepatitis V02.61
  Shigella V02.3
  Staphylococcus NEC V02.59
    methicillin
      resistant Staphylococcus aureus V02.54
      susceptible Staphylococcus aureus V02.53
  Streptococcus NEC V02.52
    group B V02.51
  typhoid V02.1
  venereal disease NEC V02.8
Carrión's disease (Bartonellosis) 088.0
Car sickness 994.6
Carter's
  relapsing fever (Asiatic) 087.0
Cartilage —*see* condition
Caruncle (inflamed)
  abscess, lacrimal (*see also* Dacryocystitis) 375.30
  conjunctiva 372.00
    acute 372.00
  eyelid 373.00
  labium (majus) (minus) 616.89
  lacrimal 375.30
  urethra (benign) 599.3
  vagina (wall) 616.89
Cascade stomach 537.6
Caseation lymphatic gland (*see also*
    Tuberculosis) 017.2
Caseous
  bronchitis—*see* Tuberculosis, pulmonary
  meningitis 013.0
  pneumonia—*see* Tuberculosis, pulmonary
Cassidy (-Scholte) syndrome (malignant
    carcinoid) 259.2
Castellani's bronchitis 104.8
Castleman's tumor or lymphoma (mediastinal
    lymph node hyperplasia) 785.6
Castration, traumatic 878.2
  complicated 878.3
Casts in urine 791.7
Cat's ear 744.29
Catalepsy 300.11
  catatonic (acute) (*see also* Schizophrenia) 295.2
  hysterical 300.11
  schizophrenic (*see also* Schizophrenia) 295.2
Cataphasia (*see also* Disorder, fluency) 315.35
Cataplexy (idiopathic) *see also* Narcolepsy
Cataract (anterior cortical) (anterior polar)
    (black) (capsular) (central) (cortical)
    (hypermature) (immature) (incipient) (mature)
    366.9
  anterior
    and posterior axial embryonal 743.33
    pyramidal 743.31
    subcapsular polar
      infantile, juvenile, or presenile 366.01
      senile 366.13

Cataract—*continued*
  associated with
    calcinosis 275.40 [366.42]
    craniofacial dysostosis 756.0 [366.44]
    galactosemia 271.1 [366.44]
    hypoparathyroidism 252.1 [366.42]
    myotonic disorders 359.21 [366.43]
    neovascularization 366.33
  blue dot 743.39
  cerulean 743.39
  complicated NEC 366.30
  congenital 743.30
    capsular or subcapsular 743.31
    cortical 743.32
    nuclear 743.33
    specified type NEC 743.39
    total or subtotal 743.34
    zonular 743.32
  coronary (congenital) 743.39
    acquired 366.12
  cupuliform 366.14
  diabetic 250.5 [366.41]
    due to secondary diabetes 249.5 [366.41]
  drug-induced 366.45
  due to
    chalcosis 360.24 [366.34]
    chronic choroiditis (*see also* Choroiditis)
      363.20 [366.32]
    degenerative myopia 360.21 [366.34]
    glaucoma (*see also* Glaucoma) 365.9 [366.31]
    infection, intraocular NEC 366.32
    inflammatory ocular disorder NEC 366.32
    iridocyclitis, chronic 364.10 [366.33]
    pigmentary retinal dystrophy 362.74 [366.34]
    radiation 366.46
  electric 366.46
  glassblowers' 366.46
  heat ray 366.46
  heterochromic 366.33
  in eye disease NEC 366.30
  infantile (*see also* Cataract, juvenile) 366.00
  intumescent 366.12
  irradiational 366.46
  juvenile 366.00
    anterior subcapsular polar 366.01
    combined forms 366.09
    cortical 366.03
    lamellar 366.03
    nuclear 366.04
    posterior subcapsular polar 366.02
    specified NEC 366.09
    zonular 366.03
  lamellar 743.32
    infantile, juvenile, or presenile 366.03
  morgagnian 366.18
  myotonic 359.21 [366.43]
  myxedema 244.9 [366.44]
  nuclear 366.16
  posterior, polar (capsular) 743.31
    infantile, juvenile, or presenile 366.02
    senile 366.14
  presenile (*see also* Cataract, juvenile) 366.00
  punctate
    acquired 366.12
    congenital 743.39
  secondary (membrane) 366.50
    obscuring vision 366.53
    specified type, not obscuring vision 366.52

Cataract—*continued*
  senile 366.10
    anterior subcapsular polar 366.13
    combined forms 366.19
    cortical 366.15
    hypermature 366.18
    immature 366.12
    incipient 366.12
    mature 366.17
    nuclear 366.16
    posterior subcapsular polar 366.14
    specified NEC 366.19
    total or subtotal 366.17
  snowflake 250.5 *[366.41]*
    due to secondary diabetes 249.5 *[366.41]*
  specified NEC 366.8
  subtotal (senile) 366.17
    congenital 743.34
  sunflower 360.24 *[366.34]*
  tetanic NEC 252.1 *[366.42]*
  total (mature) (senile) 366.17
    congenital 743.34
    localized 366.21
    traumatic 366.22
  toxic 366.45
  traumatic 366.20
    partially resolved 366.23
    total 366.22
  zonular (perinuclear) 743.32
    infantile, juvenile, or presenile 366.03
Cataracta 366.10
  brunescens 366.16
  cerulea 743.39
  complicata 366.30
  congenita 743.30
  coralliformis 743.39
  coronaria (congenital) 743.39
    acquired 366.12
  diabetic 250.5 *[366.41]*
    due to secondary diabetes 249.5 *[366.41]*
  floriformis 360.24 *[366.34]*
  membranacea
    accreta 366.50
    congenita 743.39
  nigra 366.16
Catarrh, catarrhal (inflammation) (*see also*
    condition) 460
  acute 460
  asthma, asthmatic (*see also* Asthma) 493.9
  Bostock's (*see also* Fever, hay) 477.9
  bowel—*see* Enteritis
  bronchial 490
    acute 466.0
    chronic 491.0
    subacute 466.0
  cervix, cervical (canal) (uteri)—*see* Cervicitis
  chest (*see also* Bronchitis) 490
  chronic 472.0
  congestion 472.0
  conjunctivitis 372.03
  due to syphilis 095.9
    congenital 090.0
  enteric—*see* Enteritis
  epidemic (*see also* Influenza) 487.1
  Eustachian 381.50
  eye (acute) (vernal) 372.03
  fauces (*see also* Pharyngitis) 462
  febrile 460
  fibrinous acute 466.0
  gastroenteric—*see* Enteritis
  gastrointestinal—*see* Enteritis

Catarrh, catarrhal—*continued*
  gingivitis 523.00
  hay (*see also* Fever, hay) 477.9
  infectious 460
  intestinal—*see* Enteritis
  larynx (*see also* Laryngitis, chronic) 476.0
  liver 070.1
    with hepatic coma 070.0
  lung (*see also* Bronchitis) 490
    acute 466.0
    chronic 491.0
  middle ear (chronic)—*see* Otitis media, chronic
  mouth 528.00
  nasal (chronic) (*see also* Rhinitis) 472.0
    acute 460
  nasobronchial 472.2
  nasopharyngeal (chronic) 472.2
    acute 460
  nose—*see* Catarrh, nasal
  ophthalmia 372.03
  pneumococcal, acute 466.0
  pulmonary (*see also* Bronchitis) 490
    acute 466.0
    chronic 491.0
  spring (eye) 372.13
  suffocating (*see also* Asthma) 493.9
  summer (hay) (*see also* Fever, hay) 477.9
  throat 472.1
  tracheitis 464.10
    with obstruction 464.11
  tubotympanal 381.4
    acute (*see also* Otitis media, acute,
        nonsuppurative) 381.00
    chronic 381.10
  vasomotor (*see also* Fever, hay) 477.9
  vesical (bladder)—*see* Cystitis
Catarrhus aestivus (*see also* Fever, hay) 477.9
Catastrophe, cerebral (*see also* Disease,
    cerebrovascular, acute) 436
Catatonia, catatonic (acute) 781.99
  agitation 295.2
  dementia (praecox) 295.2
  due to or associated with physical condition 293.89
  excitation 295.2
  excited type 295.2
  in conditions classified elsewhere 293.89
  schizophrenia 295.2
  stupor 295.2
  with
    affective psychosis —*see* Psychosis, affective
Cat-scratch —*see also* Injury, superficial
  disease or fever 078.3
Cauda equina —*see also* condition syndrome
    344.60
Cauliflower ear 738.7
Caul over face 768.9
Causalgia 355.9
  lower limb 355.71
  upper limb 354.4
Cause
  external, general effects NEC 994.9
  not stated 799.9
  unknown 799.9
Caustic burn —*see also* Burn, by site
  from swallowing caustic or corrosive
    substance—*see* Burn, internal organs
Cavare's disease (familial periodic paralysis) 359.3
Cave-in, injury
  crushing (severe) (*see also* Crush, by site) 869.1
  suffocation 994.7
Cavernitis (penis) 607.2
  lymph vessel—*see* Lymphangioma

Cavernositis 607.2
Cavernous —*see* condition
Cavitation of lung (*see also* Tuberculosis) 011.2
  nontuberculous 518.89
  primary, progressive 010.8
Cavity
  lung—*see* Cavitation of lung
  optic papilla 743.57
  pulmonary—*see* Cavitation of lung
  teeth 521.00
  vitreous (humor) 379.21
Cavovarus foot, congenital 754.59
Cavus foot (congenital) 754.71
  acquired 736.73
Cazenave's
  disease (pemphigus) NEC 694.4
  lupus (erythematosus) 695.4
CDGS (carbohydrate-deficient glycoprotein syndrome) 271.8
Cecitis —*see* Appendicitis
Cecocele —*see* Hernia
Cecum —*see* condition
Celiac
  artery compression syndrome 447.4
  disease 579.0
  infantilism 579.0
Cell, cellular —*see also* condition
  anterior chamber (eye) (positive aqueous ray) 364.04
Cellulitis (diffuse) (with lymphangitis) (*see also* Abscess) 682.9
  abdominal wall 682.2
  anaerobic (*see also* Gas gangrene) 040.0
  ankle 682.6
  anus 566
  areola 611.0
  arm (any part, above wrist) 682.3
  auditory canal (external) 380.10
  axilla 682.3
  back (any part) 682.2
  breast 611.0
    postpartum 675.1
  broad ligament (*see also* Disease, pelvis, inflammatory) 614.4
    acute 614.3
  buttock 682.5
  cervical (neck region) 682.1
  cervix (uteri) (*see also* Cervicitis) 616.0
  cheek, external 682.0
    internal 528.3
  chest wall 682.2
  chronic NEC 682.9
  colostomy 569.61
  corpus cavernosum 607.2
  digit 681.9
  Douglas' cul-de-sac or pouch (chronic) (*see also* Disease, pelvis, inflammatory) 614.4
    acute 614.3
  drainage site (following operation) 998.59
  ear, external 380.10
  enterostomy 569.61
  erysipelar (*see also* Erysipelas) 035
  esophagostomy 530.86
  eyelid 373.13
  face (any part, except eye) 682.0
  finger (intrathecal) (periosteal) (subcutaneous) (subcuticular) 681.00
  flank 682.2
  foot (except toe) 682.7
  forearm 682.3
  gangrenous (*see also* Gangrene) 785.4

Cellulitis—*continued*
  genital organ NEC
    female—*see* Abscess, genital organ, female
    male 608.4
  glottis 478.71
  gluteal (region) 682.5
  gonococcal NEC 098.0
  groin 682.2
  hand (except finger or thumb) 682.4
  head (except face) NEC 682.8
  heel 682.7
  hip 682.6
  jaw (region) 682.0
  knee 682.6
  labium (majus) (minus) (*see also* Vulvitis) 616.10
  larynx 478.71
  leg, except foot 682.6
  lip 528.5
  mammary gland 611.0
  mouth (floor) 528.3
  multiple sites NEC 682.9
  nasopharynx 478.21
  navel 682.2
    newborn NEC 771.4
  neck (region) 682.1
  nipple 611.0
  nose 478.19
    external 682.0
  orbit, orbital 376.01
  palate (soft) 528.3
  pectoral (region) 682.2
  pelvis, pelvic
    with
      abortion—*see* Abortion, by type, with sepsis
      ectopic pregnancy (*see also* categories 633.0-633.9) 639.0
      molar pregnancy (*see also* categories 630-632) 639.0
    female (*see also* Disease, pelvis, inflammatory) 614.4
      acute 614.3
    following
      abortion 639.0
      ectopic or molar pregnancy 639.0
    male 567.21
    puerperal, postpartum, childbirth 670.8
  penis 607.2
  perineal, perineum 682.2
  perirectal 566
  peritonsillar 475
  periurethral 597.0
  periuterine (*see also* Disease, pelvis, inflammatory) 614.4
    acute 614.3
  pharynx 478.21
  phlegmonous NEC 682.9
  rectum 566
  retromammary 611.0
  retroperitoneal (*see also* Peritonitis) 567.238
  round ligament (*see also* Disease, pelvis, inflammatory) 614.4
    acute 614.3
  scalp (any part) 682.8
    dissecting 704.8
  scrotum 608.4
  seminal vesicle 608.0
  septic NEC 682.9
  shoulder 682.3
  specified sites NEC 682.8
  spermatic cord 608.4

Cellulitis—*continued*
  submandibular (region) (space) (triangle) 682.0
    gland 527.3
  submaxillary 528.3
    gland 527.3
  submental (pyogenic) 682.0
    gland 527.3
  suppurative NEC 682.9
  testis 608.4
  thigh 682.6
  thumb (intrathecal) (periosteal) (subcutaneous) (subcuticular) 681.00
  toe (intrathecal) (periosteal) (subcutaneous) (subcuticular) 681.10
  tonsil 475
  trunk 682.2
  tuberculous (primary) (*see also* Tuberculosis) 017.0
  tunica vaginalis 608.4
  umbilical 682.2
    newborn NEC 771.4
  vaccinal 999.39
  vagina—*see* Vaginitis
  vas deferens 608.4
  vocal cords 478.5
  vulva (*see also* Vulvitis) 616.10
  wrist 682.4
Cementoblastoma, benign (M9273/0) 213.1
  upper jaw (bone) 213.0
Cementoma (M9273/0) 213.1
  gigantiform (M9275/0) 213.1
    upper jaw (bone) 213.0
  upper jaw (bone) 213.0
Cementoperiostitis 523.40
  acute 523.33
  apical 523.40
Cephalgia, cephalalgia (*see also* Headache) 784.0
  histamine 339.00
  nonorganic origin 307.81
  other trigeminal autonomic (TACS) 339.09
  psychogenic 307.81
  tension 307.81
Cephalhematocele, cephalematocele
  due to birth injury 767.19
  fetus or newborn 767.19
  traumatic (*see also* Contusion, head) 920
Cephalhematoma, cephalematoma (calcified)
  due to birth injury 767.19
  fetus or newborn 767.19
  traumatic (*see also* Contusion, head) 920
Cephalic —*see* condition
Cephalitis —*see* Encephalitis
Cephalocele 742.0
Cephaloma —*see* Neoplasm, by site, malignant
Cephalomenia 625.8
Cephalopelvic —*see* condition
Cercomoniasis 007.3
Cerebellitis —*see* Encephalitis
Cerebellum (cerebellar)—*see* condition
Cerebral —*see* condition
Cerebritis —*see* Encephalitis
Cerebrohepatorenal syndrome 759.89
Cerebromacular degeneration 330.1
Cerebromalacia (*see also* Softening, brain) 348.89
  due to cerebrovascular accident 438.89
Cerebrosidosis 272.7
Cerebrospasticity —*see* Palsy, cerebral
Cerebrospinal —*see* condition
Cerebrum —*see* condition
Ceroid storage disease 272.7
Cerumen (accumulation) (impacted) 380.4

Cervical —*see also* condition
  auricle 744.43
  high risk human papillomavirus (HPV) DNA test positive 795.05
  intraepithelial glandular neoplasia 233.1
  low rish human papillomavirus (Hpv) DNA test positive 795.09
  rib 756.2
  shortening —*see* Short, cervical
Cervicalgia 723.1
Cervicitis (acute) (chronic) (nonvenereal) (subacute) (with erosion or ectropion) 616.0
  with
    abortion—*see* Abortion, by type, with sepsis
    ectopic pregnancy (*see also* categories 633.0-633.9) 639.0
    molar pregnancy (*see also* categories 630-632) 639.0
    ulceration 616.0
  chlamydial 099.53
  complicating pregnancy or puerperium 646.6
    affecting fetus or newborn 760.8
  following
    abortion 639.0
    ectopic or molar pregnancy 639.0
  gonococcal (acute) 098.15
    chronic or duration of 2 months or more 098.35
  senile (atrophic) 616.0
  syphilitic 095.8
  trichomonal 131.09
  tuberculous (*see also* Tuberculosis) 016.7
Cervicoaural fistula 744.49
Cervicocolpitis (emphysematosa) (*see also* Cervicitis) 616.0
Cervix —*see* condition
Cesarean delivery, operation or section NEC 669.7
  affecting fetus or newborn 763.4
  (planned) occurring after 37 completed weeks of gestation but before 39 completed weeks gestation due to (spontaneous) onset of labor 649.8
  post mortem, affecting fetus or newborn 761.6
  previous, affecting management of pregnancy 654.2
Céstan's syndrome 344.89
Céstan-Chenais paralysis 344.89
Céstan-Raymond syndrome 433.8
Cestode infestation NEC 123.9
  specified type NEC 123.8
Cestodiasis 123.9
CGF (congenital generalized fibromatosis) 759.89
Chaberts' disease 022.9
Chacaleh 266.2
Chafing 709.8
Chagas' disease (*see also* Trypanosomiasis, American) 086.2
  with heart involvement 086.0
Chagres fever 084.0
Chalasia (cardiac sphincter) 530.81
Chalazion 373.2
Chalazoderma 757.39
Chalcosis 360.24
  cornea 371.15
  crystalline lens 360.24 *[366.34]*
  retina 360.24
Chalicosis (occupational) (pulmonum) 502
Chancre (any genital site) (hard) (indurated) (infecting) (primary) (recurrent) 091.0
  congenital 090.0
  conjunctiva 091.2

Chancre—*continued*
Ducrey's 099.0
extragenital 091.2
eyelid 091.2
Hunterian 091.0
lip (syphilis) 091.2
mixed 099.8
nipple 091.2
Nisbet's 099.0
of
 carate 103.0
 pinta 103.0
 yaws 102.0
palate, soft 091.2
phagedenic 099.0
Ricord's 091.0
Rollet's (syphilitic) 091.0
seronegative 091.0
seropositive 091.0
simple 099.0
soft 099.0
 bubo 099.0
urethra 091.0
yaws 102.0
Chancriform syndrome 114.1
Chancroid 099.0
anus 099.0
penis (Ducrey's bacillus) 099.0
perineum 099.0
rectum 099.0
scrotum 099.0
urethra 099.0
vulva 099.0
Chandipura fever 066.8
Chandler's disease (osteochondritis dissecans, hip) 732.7
Change(s) (of)—*see also* Removal of
arteriosclerotic—*see* Arteriosclerosis
battery
 cardiac pacemaker V53.31
bone 733.90
 diabetic 250.8 *[731.8]*
 due to secondary diabetes 249.8 [731.8]
 in disease, unknown cause 733.90
bowel habits 787.99
cardiorenal (vascular) (*see also* Hypertension, cardiorenal) 404.90
cardiovascular—*see* Disease, cardiovascular
circulatory 459.9
cognitive or personality change of other type, nonpsychotic 310.1
color, teeth, tooth
 during formation 520.8
 extrinsic 523.6
 intrinsic posteruptive 521.7
contraceptive device V25.42
cornea, corneal
 degenerative NEC 371.40
 membrane NEC 371.30
 senile 371.41
coronary (*see also* Ischemia, heart) 414.9
degenerative
 chamber angle (anterior) (iris) 364.56
 ciliary body 364.57
 spine or vertebra (*see also* Spondylosis) 721.90
dental pulp, regressive 522.2
drains V58.49
dressing
 wound V58.30
  nonsurgical V58.30
  surgical V58.31

Change(s) (of)—*continued*
fixation device V54.89
 external V54.89
 internal V54.01
heart—*see also* Disease, heart
hip joint 718.95
hyperplastic larynx 478.79
hypertrophic
 nasal sinus (*see also* Sinusitis) 473.9
 turbinate, nasal 478.0
 upper respiratory tract 478.9
inflammatory—*see* Inflammation
joint (*see also* Derangement, joint) 718.90
 sacroiliac 724.6
Kirschner wire V54.89
knee 717.9
macular, congenital 743.55
malignant (M——/3)—*see also* Neoplasm, by site, malignant

Note—for malignant change occurring in a neoplasm, use the appropriate M code with behavior digit /3 e.g., malignant change in uterine fibroid—M8890/3. For malignant change occurring in a nonneoplastic condition (e.g., gastric ulcer) use the M code M8000/3.

---

mental (status) NEC 780.97
 due to or associated with physical condition—*see* Syndrome, brain
myocardium, myocardial—*see* Degeneration, myocardial
of life (*see also* Menopause) 627.2
pacemaker battery (cardiac) V53.31
peripheral nerve 355.9
personality (nonpsychotic) NEC 310.1
plaster cast V54.89
refractive, transient 367.81
regressive, dental pulp 522.2
retina 362.9
 myopic (degenerative) (malignant) 360.21
 vascular appearance 362.13
sacroiliac joint 724.6
scleral 379.19
 degenerative 379.16
senile (*see also* Senility) 797
sensory (*see also* Disturbance, sensation) 782.0
skin texture 782.8
spinal cord 336.9
splint, external V54.89
subdermal implantable contraceptive V25.5
suture V58.32
traction device V54.89
trophic 355.9
 arm NEC 354.9
 leg NEC 355.8
 lower extremity NEC 355.8
 upper extremity NEC 354.9
vascular 459.9
vasomotor 443.9
voice 784.49
 psychogenic 306.1
wound packing V58.30
 nonsurgical V58.30
 surgical V58.31
Changing sleep-work schedule, affecting sleep 327.36
Changuinola fever 066.0
Chapping skin 709.8
Character
depressive 301.12
Charcot's
arthropathy 094.0 *[713.5]*
cirrhosis—*see* Cirrhosis, biliary

Charcot's—*continued*
 disease 094.0
  spinal cord 094.0
 fever (biliary) (hepatic) (intermittent)—*see*
  Choledocholithiasis
 joint (disease) 094.0 *[713.5]*
  diabetic 250.6 *[713.5]*
   due to secondary diabetes 249.6 [713.5]
  syringomyelic 336.0 *[713.5]*
 syndrome (intermittent claudication) 443.9
  due to atherosclerosis 440.21
Charcot-Marie-Tooth disease paralysis, or
  syndrome 356.1
CHARGE association (syndrome) 759.89
Charleyhorse (quadriceps) 843.8
 muscle, except quadriceps—*see* Sprain, by site
Charlouis' disease (*see also* Yaws) 102.9
Chauffeur's fracture —*see* Fracture, ulna, lower
  end
Cheadle (-Möller) (-Barlow) disease or syndrome
  (infantile scurvy) 267
Checking (of)
 contraceptive device (intrauterine) V25.42
 device
  fixation V54.89
   external V54.89
   internal V54.09
  traction V54.89
  Kirschner wire V54.89
  plaster cast V54.89
  splint, external V54.89
Checkup
 following treatment—*see* Examination
 health V70.0
 infant (over 28 days old) (not sick) V20.2
 newborn, routine
  8 to 28 days old V20.32
  over 28 days old, routine V20.2
  under 8 days old V20.31
  weight V20.32
 pregnancy (normal) V22.1
  first V22.0
  high risk pregnancy V23.9
   inconclusive fetal viability V23.87
   specified problem NEC V23.8
Chédiak-Higashi (-Steinbrinck) anomaly,
  disease, or syndrome (congenital gigantism of
  peroxidase granules) 288.2
Cheek —*see also* condition
 biting 528.9
Cheese itch 133.8
Cheese washers' lung 495.8
Cheilitis 528.5
 actinic (due to sun) 692.72
  chronic NEC 692.74
   due to radiation, except from sun 692.82
  due to radiation, except from sun 692.82
 acute 528.5
 angular 528.5
 catarrhal 528.5
 chronic 528.5
 exfoliative 528.5
 gangrenous 528.5
 glandularis apostematosa 528.5
 granulomatosa 351.8
 infectional 528.5
 membranous 528.5
 Miescher's 351.8
 suppurative 528.5
 ulcerative 528.5
 vesicular 528.5
Cheilodynia 528.5

Cheilopalatoschisis (*see also* Cleft, palate, with
  cleft lip) 749.20
Cheilophagia 528.9
Cheiloschisis (*see also* Cleft, lip) 749.10
Cheilosis 528.5
 with pellagra 265.2
 angular 528.5
 due to
  dietary deficiency 266.0
  vitamin deficiency 266.0
Cheiromegaly 729.89
Cheiropompholyx 705.81
Cheloid (*see also* Keloid) 701.4
Chemical burn —*see also* Burn, by site
 from swallowing chemical—*see* Burn, internal
  organs
Chemodectoma (M8693/1)—*see* Paraganglioma,
  nonchromaffin
Chemoprophylaxis NEC V07.39
Chemosis, conjunctiva 372.73
Chemotherapy
 convalescence V66.2
 encounter (for) (oral) (intravenous) V58.11
 maintenance (oral) (intravenous) V58.11
 prophylactic NEC V07.39
  fluoride V07.31
Cherubism 526.89
Chest —*see* condition
Cheyne-Stokes respiration (periodic) 786.04
Chiari's
 disease or syndrome (hepatic vein thrombosis)
  453.0
 malformation
  type I 348.4
  type II (*see also* Spina bifida) 741.0
  type III 742.0
  type IV 742.2
 network 746.89
Chiari-Frommel syndrome 676.6
Chicago disease (North American blastomycosis)
  116.0
Chickenpox (*see also* Varicella) 052.9
 exposure to V01.71
 vaccination and inoculation (prophylactic) V05.4
Chiclero ulcer 085.4
Chiggers 133.8
Chignon 111.2
 fetus or newborn (from vacuum extraction)
  767.19
Chigoe disease 134.1
Chikungunya fever 066.3
Chilaiditi's syndrome (subphrenic displacement,
  colon) 751.4
Chilblains 991.5
 lupus 991.5
Child
 behavior causing concern V61.20
  adopted child V61.24
  biological child V61.23
  foster child V61.25
Childbed fever 670.8
Childbirth —*see also* Delivery
 puerperal complications—*see* Puerperal
Childhood, period of rapid growth V21.0
Chill (s) 780.64
 with fever 780.60
 without fever 780.64
 congestive 780.99
  in malarial regions 084.6
 septic—*see* Septicemia
 urethral 599.84

Chilomastigiasis 007.8
Chin —*see* condition
Chinese dysentery 004.9
Chiropractic dislocation (*see also* Lesion, nonallopathic, by site) 739.9
Chitral fever 066.0
Chlamydia, chlamydial -*see* **condition**
Chloasma 709.09
  cachecticorum 709.09
  eyelid 374.52
   congenital 757.33
   hyperthyroid 242.0
  gravidarum 646.8
  idiopathic 709.09
  skin 709.09
  symptomatic 709.09
Chloroma (M9930/3) 205.3
Chlorosis 280.9
  Egyptian (*see also* Ancylostomiasis) 126.9
  miners' (*see also* Ancylostomiasis) 126.9
Chlorotic anemia 280.9
Chocolate cyst (ovary) 617.1
Choked
  disk or disc—*see* Papilledema
  on food, phlegm, or vomitus NEC (*see also* Asphyxia, food) 933.1
  phlegm 933.1
  while vomiting NEC (*see also* Asphyxia, food) 933.1
Chokes (resulting from bends) 993.3
Choking sensation 784.99
Cholangiectasis (*see also* Disease, gallbladder) 575.8
Cholangiocarcinoma (M8160/3)
  and hepatocellular carcinoma, combined (M8180/3) 155.0
  liver 155.1
  specified site NEC—*see* Neoplasm, by site, malignant
  unspecified site 155.1
Cholangiohepatitis 575.8
  due to fluke infestation 121.1
Cholangiohepatoma (M8180/3) 155.0
Cholangiolitis (acute) (chronic) (extrahepatic) (gangrenous) 576.1
  intrahepatic 575.8
  paratyphoidal (*see also* Fever, paratyphoid) 002.9
  typhoidal 002.0
Cholangioma (M8160/0) 211.5
  malignant—*see* Cholangiocarcinoma
Cholangitis (acute) (ascending) (catarrhal) (chronic) (infective) (malignant) (primary) (recurrent) (sclerosing) (secondary) (stenosing) (suppurative) 576.1
  chronic nonsuppurative destructive 571.6
  nonsuppurative destructive (chronic) 571.6
Cholecystdocholithiasis —*see* Choledocholithiasis
Cholecystitis 575.10
  with
   calculus, stones in
    bile duct (common) (hepatic)—*see* Choledocholithiasis
    gallbladder—*see* Cholelithiasis
  acute 575.0
  acute and chronic 575.12
  chronic 575.11
  emphysematous (acute) (*see also* Cholecystitis, acute) 575.0
  gangrenous (*see also* Cholecystitis, acute) 575.0
  paratyphoidal, current (*see also* Fever, paratyphoid) 002.9
  suppurative (*see also* Cholecystitis, acute) 575.0
  typhoidal 002.0

Choledochitis (suppurative) 576.1
Choledocholith —*see* Choledocholithiasis
Choledocholithiasis 574.5

> *Note*—Use the following fifth-digit subclassification with category 574:
>
> 0 without mention of obstruction
> 1 with obstruction

  with
   cholecystitis 574.4
    acute 574.3
    chronic 574.4
   cholelithiasis 574.9
    with
     cholecystitis 574.7
      acute 574.6
      and chronic 574.8
     chronic 574.7
Cholelithiasis (impacted) (multiple) 574.2

> *Note*—Use the following fifth-digit subclassification with category 574:
>
> 0 without mention of obstruction
> 1 with obstruction

  with
   cholecystitis 574.1
    acute 574.0
    chronic 574.1
   choledocholithiasis 574.9
    with
     cholecystitis 574.7
      acute 574.6
      and chronic 574.8
     chronic cholecystitis 574.7
Cholemia (*see also* Jaundice) 782.4
  familial 277.4
  Gilbert's (familial nonhemolytic) 277.4
Cholemic gallstone —*see* Cholelithiasis
Choleperitoneum, choleperitonitis (*see also* Disease, gallbladder) 567.81
Cholera (algid) (Asiatic) (asphyctic) (epidemic) (gravis) (Indian) (malignant) (morbus) (pestilential) (spasmodic) 001.9
  antimonial 985.4
  carrier (suspected) of V02.0
  classical 001.0
  contact V01.0
  due to
   Vibrio
    cholerae (Inaba, Ogawa, Hikojima serotypes) 001.0
    El Tor 001.1
  El Tor 001.1
  exposure to V01.0
  vaccination, prophylactic (against) V03.0
Cholerine (*see also* Cholera) 001.9
Cholestasis 576.8
  due to total parenteral nutrition (TPN) 573.8
Cholesteatoma (ear) 385.30
  attic (primary) 385.31
  diffuse 385.35
  external ear (canal) 380.21
  marginal (middle ear) 385.32
   with involvement of mastoid cavity 385.33
   secondary (with middle ear involvement) 385.33
  mastoid cavity 385.30

Cholesteatoma—*continued*
  middle ear (secondary) 385.32
    with involvement of mastoid cavity 385.33
  postmastoidectomy cavity (recurrent) 383.32
  primary 385.31
  recurrent, postmastoidectomy cavity 383.32
  secondary (middle ear) 385.32
    with involvement of mastoid cavity 385.33
Cholesteatosis (middle ear) (*see also*
    Cholesteatoma) 385.30
  diffuse 385.35
Cholesteremia 272.0
Cholesterin
  granuloma, middle ear 385.82
  in vitreous 379.22
Cholesterol
  deposit
    retina 362.82
    vitreous 379.22
  elevated (high) 272.0
    with elevated (high) triglycerides 272.2
  imbibition of gallbladder (*see also* Disease,
    gallbladder) 575.6
Cholesterolemia 272.0
  essential 272.0
  familial 272.0
  hereditary 272.0
Cholesterosis, cholesterolosis (gallbladder) 575.6
  middle ear (*see also* Cholesteatoma) 385.30
  with
    cholecystitis—*see* Cholecystitis
    cholelithiasis—*see* Cholelithiasis
Cholocolic fistula (*see also* Fistula, gallbladder)
  575.5
Choluria 791.4
Chondritis (purulent) 733.99
  auricle 380.03
  costal 733.6
    Tietze's 733.6
  patella, posttraumatic 717.7
  pinna 380.03
  posttraumatica patellae 717.7
  tuberculous (active) (*see also* Tuberculosis) 015.9
    intervertebral 015.0 *[730.88]*
Chondroangiopathia calcarea seu punctate
  756.59
Chondroblastoma (M9230/0)—*see also*
  Neoplasm, bone, benign
  malignant (M9230/3)—*see* Neoplasm, bone,
    malignant
Chondrocalcinosis (articular) (crystal deposition)
  (dihydrate) (*see also* Arthritis, due to, crystals)
  275.49 *[712.3]*
  due to
    calcium pyrophosphate 275.49 *[712.2]*
    dicalcium phosphate crystals 275.49 *[712.1]*
    pyrophosphate crystals 275.4 *[712.2]*
Chondrodermatitis nodularis helicis 380.00
Chondrodysplasia 756.4
  angiomatose 756.4
  calcificans congenita 756.59
  epiphysialis punctata 756.59
  hereditary deforming 756.4
  rhizomelic punctata 277.86
Chondrodystrophia (fetalis) 756.4
  calcarea 756.4
  calcificans congenita 756.59
  fetalis hypoplastica 756.59
  hypoplastica calcinosa 756.59
  punctata 756.59
  tarda 277.5

Chondrodystrophy (familial) (hypoplastic) 756.4
  myotonic (congenital) 359.23
Chondroectodermal dysplasia 756.55
Chondrolysis 733.99
Chondroma (M9220/0)—*see also* Neoplasm
  cartilage, benign
  juxtacortical (M9221/0)—*see* Neoplasm, bone,
    benign
  periosteal (M9221/0)—*see* Neoplasm, bone,
    benign
Chondromalacia 733.92
  epiglottis (congenital) 748.3
  generalized 733.92
  knee 717.7
  larynx (congenital) 748.3
  localized, except patella 733.92
  patella, patellae 717.7
  systemic 733.92
  tibial plateau 733.92
  trachea (congenital) 748.3
Chondromatosis (M9220/1)—*see* Neoplasm,
  cartilage, uncertain behavior
Chondromyxosarcoma (M9220/3)—*see*
  Neoplasm, cartilage, malignant
Chondro-osteodysplasia (Morquio-Brailsford
  type) 277.5
Chondro-osteodystrophy 277.5
Chondro-osteodystrophy 277.5
Chondro-osteoma (M9210/0)—*see* Neoplasm,
  bone, benign
Chondropathia tuberosa 733.6
Chondrosarcoma (M9220/3)—*see also*
  Neoplasm, cartilage, malignant
  juxtacortical (M9221/3)—*see* Neoplasm, bone,
    malignant
  mesenchymal (M9240/3)—*see* Neoplasm,
    connective tissue, malignant
Chordae tendineae rupture (chronic) 429.5
Chordee (nonvenereal) 607.89
  congenital 752.63
  gonococcal 098.2
Chorditis (fibrinous) (nodosa) (tuberosa) 478.5
Chordoma (M9370/3)—*see* Neoplasm, by site,
  malignant
Chorea (gravis) (minor) (spasmodic) 333.5
  with
    heart involvement—*see* Chorea with
      rheumatic heart disease
    rheumatic heart disease (chronic, inactive, or
      quiescent) (conditions classifiable to
      393-398)—*see also* Rheumatic heart
      condition involved
      active or acute (conditions classifiable to
        391) 392.0
  acute—*see* Chorea, Sydenham's
  apoplectic (*see also* Disease, cerebrovascular,
    acute) 436
  chronic 333.4
  electric 049.8
  gravidarum—*see* Eclampsia, pregnancy
  habit 307.22
  hereditary 333.4
  Huntington's 333.4
  posthemiplegic 344.89
  pregnancy—*see* Eclampsia, pregnancy
  progressive 333.4
    chronic 333.4
    hereditary 333.4
  rheumatic (chronic) 392.9
    with heart disease or involvement—*see*
      Chorea, with rheumatic heart disease

Chorea—*continued*
  senile 333.5
  Sydenham's 392.9
    with heart involvement—*see* Chorea, with
      rheumatic heart disease
    nonrheumatic 333.5
  variabilis 307.23
Choreoathetosis (paroxysmal) 333.5
Chorioadenoma (destruens) (M9100/1) 236.1
Chorioamnionitis 658.4
  affecting fetus or newborn 762.7
Chorioangioma (M9120/0) 219.8
Choriocarcinoma (M9100/3)
  combined with
    embryonal carcinoma (M9101/3)—*see*
      Neoplasm, by site, malignant
    teratoma (M9101/3)—*see* Neoplasm, by site,
      malignant
  specified site—*see* Neoplasm, by site, malignant
  unspecified site
    female 181
    male 186.9
Chorioencephalitis, lymphocytic (acute)
    (serous) 049.0
Chorioepithelioma (M9100/3)—*see*
    Choriocarcinoma
Choriomeningitis (acute) (benign) (lymphocytic)
    (serous) 049.0
Chorionepithelioma (M9100/3)—*see*
    Choriocarcinoma
Chorionitis (*see also* Scleroderma) 710.1
Chorioretinitis 363.20
  disseminated 363.10
    generalized 363.13
    in
      neurosyphilis 094.83
      secondary syphilis 091.51
    peripheral 363.12
    posterior pole 363.11
    tuberculous (*see also* Tuberculosis) 017.3
      [363.13]
  due to
    histoplasmosis (*see also* Histoplasmosis) 115.92
    toxoplasmosis (acquired) 130.2
      congenital (active) 771.2
  focal 363.00
    juxtapapillary 363.01
    peripheral 363.04
    posterior pole NEC 363.03
  juxtapapillaris, juxtapapillary 363.01
  progressive myopia (degeneration) 360.21
  syphilitic (secondary) 091.51
    congenital (early) 090.0 *[363.13]*
      late 090.5 *[363.13]*
    late 095.8 *[363.13]*
  tuberculous (*see also* Tuberculosis) 017.3 *[363.13]*
Choristoma —*see* Neoplasm, by site, benign
Choroid —*see* condition
Choroideremia, choroidermia (initial stage)
    (late stage) (partial or total atrophy) 363.55
Choroiditis (*see also* Chorioretinitis) 363.20
  leprous 030.9 *[363.13]*
  senile guttate 363.41
  sympathetic 360.11
  syphilitic (secondary) 091.51
    congenital (early) 090.0 *[363.13]*
      late 090.5 *[363.13]*
    late 095.8 *[363.13]*
  Tay's 363.41
  tuberculous (*see also* Tuberculosis) 017.3
    [363.13]

Choroidopathy NEC 363.9
  degenerative (*see also* Degeneration, choroid)
    363.40
  hereditary (*see also* Dystrophy, choroid) 363.50
  specified type NEC 363.8
Choroidoretinitis —*see* Chorioretinitis
Choroidosis, central serous 362.41
Choroidretinopathy, serous 362.41
Christian's syndrome (chronic histiocytosis X)
    277.89
Christian-Weber disease (nodular
    nonsuppurative panniculitis) 729.30
Christmas disease 286.1
Chromaffinoma (M8700/0)—*see also*
    Neoplasm, by site, benign
  malignant (M8700/3)—*see* Neoplasm, by site,
    malignant
Chromatopsia 368.59
Chromhidrosis, chromidrosis 705.89
Chromoblastomycosis 117.2
Chromomycosis 117.2
Chromophytosis 111.0
Chromotrichomycosis 111.8
Chronic —*see* condition
Churg-Strauss syndrome 446.4
Chyle cyst, mesentery 457.8
Chylocele (nonfilarial) 457.8
  filarial (*see also* Infestation, filarial) 125.9
  tunica vaginalis (nonfilarial) 608.84
    filarial (*see also* Infestation, filarial) 125.9
Chylomicronemia (fasting) (with
    hyperprebetalipoproteinemia) 272.3
Chylopericardium (acute) 420.90
Chylothorax (nonfilarial) 457.8
  filarial (*see also* Infestation, filarial) 125.9
Chylous
  ascites 457.8
  cyst of peritoneum 457.8
  hydrocele 603.9
  hydrothorax (nonfilarial) 457.8
    filarial (*see also* Infestation, filarial) 125.9
Chyluria 791.1
  bilharziasis 120.0
  due to
    Brugia (malayi) 125.1
    Wuchereria (bancrofti) 125.0
      malayi 125.1
  filarial (*see also* Infestation, filarial) 125.9
  filariasis (*see also* Infestation, filarial) 125.9
  nonfilarial 791.1
Cicatricial (deformity)—*see* Cicatrix
Cicatrix (adherent) (contracted) (painful)
    (vicious) 709.2
  adenoid 474.8
  alveolar process 525.8
  anus 569.49
  auricle 380.89
  bile duct (*see also* Disease, biliary) 576.8
  bladder 596.89
  bone 733.99
  brain 348.89
  cervix (postoperative) (postpartal) 622.3
    in pregnancy or childbirth 654.6
      causing obstructed labor 660.2
  chorioretinal 363.30
    disseminated 363.35
    macular 363.32
    peripheral 363.34
    posterior pole NEC 363.33
  choroid—*see* Cicatrix, chorioretinal

Cicatrix—*continued*
  common duct (*see also* Disease, biliary) 576.8
  congenital 757.39
  conjunctiva 372.64
  cornea 371.00
    tuberculous (*see also* Tuberculosis) 017.3 *[371.05]*
  duodenum (bulb) 537.3
  esophagus 530.3
  eyelid 374.46
    with
      ectropion—*see* Ectropion
      entropion—*see* Entropion
  hypopharynx 478.29
  knee, semilunar cartilage 717.5
  lacrimal
    canaliculi 375.53
    duct
      acquired 375.56
      neonatal 375.55
    punctum 375.52
    sac 375.54
  larynx 478.79
  limbus (cystoid) 372.64
  lung 518.89
  macular 363.32
    disseminated 363.35
    peripheral 363.34
  middle ear 385.89
  mouth 528.9
  muscle 728.89
  nasolacrimal duct
    acquired 375.56
    neonatal 375.55
  nasopharynx 478.29
  palate (soft) 528.9
  penis 607.89
  prostate 602.8
  rectum 569.49
  retina 363.30
    disseminated 363.35
    macular 363.32
    peripheral 363.34
    posterior pole NEC 363.33
  semilunar cartilage—*see* Derangement,
    meniscus
  seminal vesicle 608.89
  skin 709.2
    infected 686.8
    postinfectional 709.2
    tuberculous (*see also* Tuberculosis) 017.0
  specified site NEC 709.2
  throat 478.29
  tongue 529.8
  tonsil (and adenoid) 474.8
  trachea 478.9
  tuberculous NEC (*see also* Tuberculosis) 011.9
  ureter 593.89
  urethra 599.84
  uterus 621.8
  vagina 623.4
    in pregnancy or childbirth 654.7
      causing obstructed labor 660.2
  vocal cord 478.5
  wrist, constricting (annular) 709.2
CIDP (chronic inflammatory demyelinating
  polyneuropathy) 357.81
CIN I (cervical intraepithelial neoplasia I) 622.11
CIN II (cervical intraepithelial neoplasia II) 622.12
CIN III (cervical intraepithelial neoplasia III) 233.1

Cinchonism
  correct substance properly administered 386.9
  overdose or wrong substance given or taken
    961.4
Circine herpes 110.5
Circle of Willis —*see* condition
Circular —*see also* condition
  hymen 752.49
Circulating anticoagulants, antibodies or
  inhibitors (*see also* Anticoagulants) 286.59
  extrinsic 287.8
  following childbirth 666.3
  intrinsic, causing hemorrhagic disorder 286.59
    with
      acquired hemophilia 286.52
      antiphospholipid antibody 286.53
  postpartum 666.3
Circulation
  collateral (venous), any site 459.89
  defective 459.9
    congenital 747.9
    lower extremity 459.89
  embryonic 747.9
  failure 799.89
    fetus or newborn 779.89
    peripheral 785.59
  fetal, persistent 747.83
  heart, incomplete 747.9
Circulatory system —*see* condition
Circulus senilis 371.41
Circumcision
  in absence of medical indication V50.2
  ritual V50.2
  routine V50.2
Circumscribed —*see* condition
Circumvallata placenta —*see* Placenta,
  abnormal
Cirrhosis, cirrhotic 571.5
  with alcoholism 571.2
  alcoholic (liver) 571.2
  atrophic (of liver)—*see* Cirrhosis, portal
  Baumgarten-Cruveilhier 571.5
  biliary (cholangiolitic) (cholangitic)
    (cholestatic) (extrahepatic) (hypertrophic)
    (intrahepatic) (nonobstructive) (obstructive)
    (pericholangiolitic) (posthepatic) (primary)
    (secondary) (xanthomatous) 571.6
    due to
      clonorchiasis 121.1
      flukes 121.3
  brain 331.9
  capsular—*see* Cirrhosis, portal
  cardiac 571.5
    alcoholic 571.2
  central (liver)—*see* Cirrhosis, liver
  Charcot's 571.6
  cholangiolitic—*see* Cirrhosis, biliary
  cholangitic—*see* Cirrhosis, biliary
  cholestatic—*see* Cirrhosis, biliary
  clitoris (hypertrophic) 624.2
  coarsely nodular 571.5
  congestive (liver)—*see* Cirrhosis, cardiac
  Cruveilhier-Baumgarten 571.5
  cryptogenic (of liver) 571.5
    alcoholic 571.2
  dietary (*see also* Cirrhosis, portal) 571.5
  due to
    bronzed diabetes 275.01
    congestive hepatomegaly—*see* Cirrhosis, cardiac
    cystic fibrosis 277.00

Cirrhosis, cirrhotic—*continued*
  due to—*continued*
    hemochromatosis (*see also* Hemochromatosis) 275.03
    hepatolenticular degeneration 275.1
    passive congestion (chronic)—*see* Cirrhosis, cardiac
    Wilson's disease 275.1
    xanthomatosis 272.2
  extrahepatic (obstructive)—*see* Cirrhosis, biliary
  fatty 571.8
    alcoholic 571.0
  florid 571.2
  Glisson's—*see* Cirrhosis, portal
  Hanot's (hypertrophic)—*see* Cirrhosis, biliary
  hepatic—*see* Cirrhosis, liver
  hepatolienal—*see* Cirrhosis, liver
  hobnail—*see* Cirrhosis, portal
  hypertrophic—*see also* Cirrhosis, liver
    biliary—*see* Cirrhosis, biliary
    Hanot's—*see* Cirrhosis, biliary
  infectious NEC—*see* Cirrhosis, portal
  insular—*see* Cirrhosis, portal
  intrahepatic (obstructive) (primary) (secondary)—*see* Cirrhosis, biliary
  juvenile (*see also* Cirrhosis, portal) 571.5
  kidney (*see also* Sclerosis, renal) 587
  Laennec's (of liver) 571.2
    nonalcoholic 571.5
  liver (chronic) (hepatolienal) (hypertrophic) (nodular) (splenomegalic) (unilobar) 571.5
    with alcoholism 571.2
    alcoholic 571.2
    congenital (due to failure of obliteration of umbilical vein) 777.8
    cryptogenic 571.5
      alcoholic 571.2
    fatty 571.8
      alcoholic 571.0
    macronodular 571.5
      alcoholic 571.2
    micronodular 571.5
      alcoholic 571.2
    nodular, diffuse 571.5
      alcoholic 571.2
    pigmentary 275.01
    portal 571.5
      alcoholic 571.2
    postnecrotic 571.5
      alcoholic 571.2
    syphilitic 095.3
  lung (chronic) (*see also* Fibrosis, lung) 515
  macronodular (of liver) 571.5
    alcoholic 571.2
  malarial 084.9
  metabolic NEC 571.5
  micronodular (of liver) 571.5
    alcoholic 571.2
  monolobular—*see* Cirrhosis, portal
  multilobular—*see* Cirrhosis, portal
  nephritis (*see also* Sclerosis, renal) 587
  nodular—*see* Cirrhosis, liver
  nutritional (fatty) 571.5
  obstructive (biliary) (extrahepatic) (intrahepatic)—*see* Cirrhosis, biliary
  ovarian 620.8
  paludal 084.9
  pancreas (duct) 577.8
  pericholangiolitic—*see* Cirrhosis, biliary
  periportal—*see* Cirrhosis, portal
  pigment, pigmentary (of liver) 275.01

Cirrhosis, cirrhotic—*continued*
  portal (of liver) 571.5
    alcoholic 571.2
  posthepatitic (*see also* Cirrhosis, postnecrotic) 571.5
  postnecrotic (of liver) 571.5
    alcoholic 571.2
  primary (intrahepatic)—*see* Cirrhosis, biliary
  pulmonary (*see also* Fibrosis, lung) 515
  renal (*see also* Sclerosis, renal) 587
  septal (*see also* Cirrhosis, postnecrotic) 571.5
  spleen 289.51
  splenomegalic (of liver)—*see* Cirrhosis, liver
  stasis (liver)—*see* Cirrhosis, liver
  stomach 535.4
  Todd's (*see also* Cirrhosis, biliary) 571.6
  toxic (nodular)—*see* Cirrhosis, postnecrotic
  trabecular—*see* Cirrhosis, postnecrotic
  unilobar—*see* Cirrhosis, liver
  vascular (of liver)—*see* Cirrhosis, liver
  xanthomatous (biliary) (*see also* Cirrhosis, biliary) 571.6
    due to xanthomatosis (familial) (metabolic) (primary) 272.2
Cistern, subarachnoid 793.0
Citrullinemia 270.6
Citrullinuria 270.6
Ciuffini-Pancoast tumor (M8010/3) (carcinoma, pulmonary apex) 162.3
Civatte's disease or poikiloderma 709.09
CJD (Creutzfeldt-Jakob disease) 046.19
  variant (vCJD) 046.11
CLABSI (central line-associated bloodstream infection) 999.32
Clam diggers' itch 120.3
Clap —*see* Gonorrhea
Clark's paralysis 343.9
Clarke-Hadfield syndrome (pancreatic infantilism) 577.8
Clastothrix 704.2
Claude's syndrome 352.6
Claude Bernard-Horner syndrome (*see also* Neuropathy, peripheral, autonomic) 337.9
Claudication, intermittent 443.9
  cerebral (artery) (*see also* Ischemia, cerebral, transient) 435.9
  due to atherosclerosis 440.21
  spinal cord (arteriosclerotic) 435.1
    syphilitic 094.89
  spinalis 435.1
  venous (axillary) 453.89
Claudicatio venosa intermittens 453.89
Claustrophobia 300.29
Clavus (infected) 700
Claw foot (congenital) 754.71
  acquired 736.74
Claw hand (acquired) 736.06
  congenital 755.59
Clawtoe (congenital) 754.71
  acquired 735.5
Clay eating 307.52
Clay shovelers' fracture —*see* Fracture, vertebra, cervical
Cleansing of artificial opening (*see also* Attention to artificial opening) V55.9
Cleft (congenital)—*see also* Imperfect, closure
  alveolar process 525.8
  branchial (persistent) 744.41
    cyst 744.42
  clitoris 752.49
  cricoid cartilage, posterior 748.3
  facial (*see also* Cleft, lip) 749.10

Cleft—*continued*
lip 749.10
  with cleft palate 749.20
    bilateral (lip and palate) 749.24
      with unilateral lip or palate 749.25
      complete 749.23
      incomplete 749.24
    unilateral (lip and palate) 749.22
      with bilateral lip or palate 749.25
      complete 749.21
      incomplete 749.22
  bilateral 749.14
    with cleft palate, unilateral 749.25
    complete 749.13
    incomplete 749.14
  unilateral 749.12
    with cleft palate, bilateral 749.25
    complete 749.11
    incomplete 749.12
nose 748.1
palate 749.00
  with cleft lip 749.20
    bilateral (lip and palate) 749.24
      with unilateral lip or palate 749.25
      complete 749.23
      incomplete 749.24
    unilateral (lip and palate) 749.22
      with bilateral lip or palate 749.25
      complete 749.21
      incomplete 749.22
  bilateral 749.04
    with cleft lip, unilateral 749.25
    complete 749.03
    incomplete 749.04
  unilateral 749.02
    with cleft lip, bilateral 749.25
    complete 749.01
    incomplete 749.02
penis 752.69
posterior, cricoid cartilage 748.3
scrotum 752.89
sternum (congenital) 756.3
thyroid cartilage (congenital) 748.3
tongue 750.13
uvula 749.02
  with cleft lip (*see also* Cleft, lip, with cleft palate) 749.20
water 366.12
Cleft hand (congenital) 755.58
Cleidocranial dysostosis 755.59
Cleidotomy, fetal 763.89
Cleptomania 312.32
Clérambault's syndrome 297.8
erotomania 302.89
Clergyman's sore throat 784.49
Click, clicking
systolic syndrome 785.2
Clifford's syndrome (postmaturity) 766.22
Climacteric (*see also* Menopause) 627.2
arthritis NEC (*see also* Arthritis, climacteric) 716.3
depression (*see also* Psychosis, affective) 296.2
disease 627.2
  recurrent episode 296.3
  single episode 296.2
female (symptoms) 627.2
male (symptoms) (syndrome) 608.89
melancholia (*see also* Psychosis, affective) 296.2
  recurrent episode 296.3
  single episode 296.2
paranoid state 297.2

Climacteric—*continued*
paraphrenia 297.2
polyarthritis NEC 716.39
  male 608.89
symptoms (female) 627.2
Clinical research investigation (control) (participant) V70.7
Clinodactyly 755.59
Clitoris —*see* condition
Cloaca, persistent 751.5
Clonorchiasis 121.1
Clonorchiosis 121.1
Clonorchis infection, liver 121.1
Clonus 781.0
Closed bite 524.20
Closed surgical procedure converted to open procedure
arthroscopic V64.43
laparoscopic V64.41
thoracoscopic V64.42
Closure
artificial opening (*see also* Attention to artificial opening) V55.9
congenital, nose 748.0
cranial sutures, premature 756.0
defective or imperfect NEC—*see* Imperfect, closure
fistula, delayed—*see* Fistula
fontanelle, delayed 756.0
foramen ovale, imperfect 745.5
hymen 623.3
interauricular septum, defective 745.5
interventricular septum, defective 745.4
lacrimal duct 375.56
  congenital 743.65
  neonatal 375.55
nose (congenital) 748.0
  acquired 738.0
primary angle without glaucoma damage 365.06
vagina 623.2
valve—*see* Endocarditis
vulva 624.8
Clot (blood)
artery (obstruction) (occlusion) (*see also* Embolism) 444.9
atrial appendage 429.89
bladder 596.7
brain (extradural or intradural) (*see also* Thrombosis, brain) 434.0
  late effect—*see* Late effect(s) (of) cerebrovascular disease
circulation 444.9
heart (*see also* Infarct, myocardium) 410.9
  without myocardial infarction 429.89
vein (*see also* Thrombosis) 453.9
Clotting defect NEC (*see also* Defect, coagulation) 286.9
Clouded state 780.09
epileptic (*see also* Epilepsy) 345.9
paroxysmal (idiopathic) (*see also* Epilepsy) 345.9
Clouding
corneal graft 996.51
Cloudy
antrum, antra 473.0
dialysis effluent 792.5
Clouston's (hidrotic) ectodermal dysplasia 757.31
Clubbing of fingers 781.5
Clubfinger 736.29
acquired 736.29
congenital 754.89

Clubfoot (congenital) 754.70
  acquired 736.71
  equinovarus 754.51
  paralytic 736.71
Club hand (congenital) 754.89
  acquired 736.07
Clubnail (acquired) 703.8
  congenital 757.5
Clump kidney 753.3
Clumsiness 781.3
  syndrome 315.4
Cluttering (see also Disorder, fluency) 315.35
Clutton's joints 090.5
Coagulation, intravascular (diffuse)
    (disseminated) (see also Fibrinolysis) 286.6
  newborn 776.2
Coagulopathy (see also Defect, coagulation) 286.9
  consumption 286.6
  intravascular (disseminated) NEC 286.6
    newborn 776.2
Coalition
  calcaneoscaphoid 755.67
  calcaneus 755.67
  tarsal 755.67
Coal miners'
  elbow 727.2
  lung 500
Coal workers' lung or pneumoconiosis 500
Coarctation
  aorta (postductal) (preductal) 747.10
  pulmonary artery 747.31
Coated tongue 529.3
Coats' disease 362.12
Cocainism (see also Dependence) 304.2
Coccidioidal granuloma 114.3
Coccidioidomycosis 114.9
  with pneumonia 114.0
  cutaneous (primary) 114.1
  disseminated 114.3
  extrapulmonary (primary) 114.1
  lung 114.5
    acute 114.0
    chronic 114.4
    primary 114.0
  meninges 114.2
  primary (pulmonary) 114.0
    acute 114.0
  prostate 114.3
  pulmonary 114.5
    acute 114.0
    chronic 114.4
    primary 114.0
  specified site NEC 114.3
Coccidioidosis 114.9
  lung 114.5
    acute 114.0
    chronic 114.4
    primary 114.0
  meninges 114.2
Coccidiosis (colitis) (diarrhea) (dysentery) 007.2
Cocciuria 791.9
Coccus in urine 791.9
Coccydynia 724.79
Coccygodynia 724.79
Coccyx —see condition
Cochin-China
  diarrhea 579.1
    anguilluliasis 127.2
  ulcer 085.1
Cock's peculiar tumor 706.2
Cockayne's disease or syndrome (microcephaly
    and dwarfism) 759.89

Cockayne-Weber syndrome (epidermolysis
    bullosa) 757.39
Cocked-up toe 735.2
Codman's tumor (benign chondroblastoma)
    (M9230/0)—see Neoplasm, bone, benign
Coenurosis 123.8
Coffee workers' lung 495.8
Cogan's syndrome 370.52
  congenital oculomotor apraxia 379.51
  nonsyphilitic interstitial keratitis 370.52
Coiling, umbilical cord —see Complications,
    umbilical cord
Coitus, painful (female) 625.0
  male 608.89
  psychogenic 302.76
Cold 460
  with influenza, flu, or grippe (see also
      Influenza) 487.1
  abscess—see also Tuberculosis, abscess
    articular—see Tuberculosis, joint
  agglutinin
    disease (chronic) or syndrome 283.0
    hemoglobinuria 283.0
      paroxysmal (cold) (nocturnal) 283.2
  allergic (see also Fever, hay) 477.9
  bronchus or chest—see Bronchitis
    with grippe or influenza (see also Influenza)
      487.1
  common (head) 460
    vaccination, prophylactic (against) V04.7
  deep 464.10
  effects of 991.9
    specified effect NEC 991.8
  excessive 991.9
    specified effect NEC 991.8
  exhaustion from 991.8
  exposure to 991.9
    specified effect NEC 991.8
  grippy (see also Influenza) 487.1
  head 460
  injury syndrome (newborn) 778.2
  intolerance 780.99
  on lung—see Bronchitis
  rose 477.0
  sensitivity, autoimmune 283.0
  virus 460
Coldsore (see also Herpes, simplex) 054.9
Colibacillosis 041.49
  generalized 038.42
Colibacilluria 791.9
Colic (recurrent) 789.7
  abdomen 789.7
    (recurrent)psychogenic 307.89
  appendicular 543.9
  appendix 543.9
  bile duct—see Choledocholithiasis
  biliary—see Cholelithiasis
  bilious—see Cholelithiasis
  common duct—see Choledocholithiasis
  Devonshire NEC 984.9
    specified type of lead—see Table of drugs and
      chemicals
  flatulent 787.3
  gallbladder or gallstone—see Cholelithiasis
  gastric 536.8
  hepatic (duct)—see Choledocholithiasis
  hysterical 300.11
  in
    adult 789.0
    child over 12 months old 789.0
    infant 789.7

Colic—*continued*
  infantile 789.7
  intestinal 789.7
  kidney 788.0
  lead NEC 984.9
    specified type of lead—*see* Table of drugs and
      chemicals
  liver (duct)—*see* Choledocholithiasis
  mucous 564.9
    psychogenic 316 *[564.9]*
  nephritic 788.0
  painter's NEC 984.9
  pancreas 577.8
  psychogenic 306.4
  renal 788.0
  saturnine NEC 984.9
    specified type of lead—*see* Table of drugs and
      chemicals
  spasmodic 789.7
  ureter 788.0
  urethral 599.84
    due to calculus 594.2
  uterus 625.8
    menstrual 625.3
  vermicular 543.9
  virus 460
  worm NEC 128.9
Colicystitis (*see also* Cystitis) 595.9
Colitis (acute) (catarrhal) (croupous) (cystica
  superficialis) (exudative) (hemorrhagic)
  (noninfectious) (phlegmonous) (presumed
  noninfectious) 558.9
  adaptive 564.9
  allergic 558.3
  amebic (*see also* Amebiasis) 006.9
    nondysenteric 006.2
  anthrax 022.2
  bacillary (*see also* Infection, Shigella) 004.9
  balantidial 007.0
  chronic 558.9
    ulcerative (*see also* Colitis, ulcerative) 556.9
  coccidial 007.2
  dietetic 558.9
  due to radiation 558.1
  eosinophilic 558.42
  functional 558.9
  gangrenous 009.0
  giardial 007.1
  granulomatous 555.1
  gravis (*see also* Colitis, ulcerative) 556.9
  infectious (*see also* Enteritis, due to, specific
    organism) 009.0
    presumed 009.1
  ischemic 557.9
    acute 557.0
    chronic 557.1
    due to mesenteric artery insufficiency 557.1
  membranous 564.9
    psychogenic 316 *[564.9]*
  mucous 564.9
    psychogenic 316 *[564.9]*
  necrotic 009.0
  polyposa (*see also* Colitis, ulcerative) 556.9
  protozoal NEC 007.9
  pseudomembranous 008.45
  pseudomucinous 564.9
  regional 555.1
  segmental 555.1
  septic (*see also* Enteritis, due to, specific
    organism) 009.0
  spastic 564.9
    psychogenic 316 *[564.9]*

Colitis—*continued*
  staphylococcus 008.41
    food 005.0
  thromboulcerative 557.0
  toxic 558.2
  transmural 555.1
  trichomonal 007.3
  tuberculous (ulcerative) 014.8
  ulcerative (chronic) (idiopathic) (nonspecific)
    556.9
    entero- 556.0
    fulminant 557.0
    ileo- 556.1
    left-sided 556.5
    procto- 556.2
    proctosigmoid 556.3
    psychogenic 316 *[556]*
    specified NEC 556.8
    universal 556.6
Collagen disease NEC 710.9
  nonvascular 710.9
  vascular (allergic) (*see also* Angiitis,
    hypersensitivity) 446.20
Collagenosis (*see also* Collagen disease) 710.9
  cardiovascular 425.4
  mediastinal 519.3
Collapse 780.2
  adrenal 255.8
  cardiorenal (*see also* Hypertension, cardiorenal)
    404.90
  cardiorespiratory 785.51
    fetus or newborn 779.85
  cardiovascular (*see also* Disease, heart) 785.51
    fetus or newborn 779.85
  circulatory (peripheral) 785.59
    with
      abortion—*see* Abortion, by type, with shock
      ectopic pregnancy (*see also* categories
        633.0-633.9) 639.5
      molar pregnancy (*see also* categories
        630-632) 639.5
    during or after labor and delivery 669.1
    fetus or newborn 779.85
    following
      abortion 639.5
      ectopic or molar pregnancy 639.5
    during or after labor and delivery 669.1
    fetus or newborn 779.89
    during or resulting from a surgical procedure
      998.00
  external ear canal 380.50
    secondary to
      inflammation 380.53
      surgery 380.52
      trauma 380.51
  general 780.2
  heart—*see* Disease, heart
  heat 992.1
  hysterical 300.11
  labyrinth, membranous (congenital) 744.05
  lung (massive) (*see also* Atelectasis) 518.0
    pressure, during labor 668.0
  myocardial—*see* Disease, heart
  nervous (*see also* Disorder, mental,
    nonpsychotic) 300.9
  neurocirculatory 306.2
  nose 738.0
  postoperative (cardiovascular) 998.09
  pulmonary (*see also* Atelectasis) 518.0
    fetus or newborn 770.5
      partial 770.5
      primary 770.4

Collapse—*continued*
  thorax 512.89
    iatrogenic 512.1
    postoperative 512.1
  trachea 519.19
  valvular—*see* Endocarditis
  vascular (peripheral) 785.59
    with
      abortion—*see* Abortion, by type, with shock
      ectopic pregnancy (*see also* categories
        633.0-633.9) 639.5
      molar pregnancy (*see also* categories
        630-632) 639.5
    cerebral (*see also* Disease, cerebrovascular,
      acute) 436
    during or after labor and delivery 669.1
    fetus or newborn 779.89
    following
      abortion 639.5
      ectopic or molar pregnancy 639.5
    vasomotor 785.59
    vertebra 733.13
Collateral —*see also* condition
  circulation (venous) 459.89
  dilation, veins 459.89
Colles' fracture (closed) (reversed) (separation)
  813.41
  open 813.51
Collet's syndrome 352.6
Collet-Sicard syndrome 352.6
Colliculitis urethralis (*see also* Urethritis) 597.89
Colliers'
  asthma 500
  lung 500
  phthisis (*see also* Tuberculosis) 011.4
Collodion baby (ichthyosis congenita) 757.1
Colloid milium 709.3
Coloboma NEC 743.49
  choroid 743.59
  fundus 743.52
  iris 743.46
  lens 743.36
  lids 743.62
  optic disc (congenital) 743.57
    acquired 377.23
  retina 743.56
  sclera 743.47
Coloenteritis —*see* Enteritis
Colon —*see* condition
Colonization
  MRSA (methicillin resistant Staphylococcus
    aureus) V02.54
  MSSA (methicillin susceptible Staphylococcus
    aureus) V02.53
Coloptosis 569.89
Color
  amblyopia NEC 368.59
    acquired 368.55
  blindness NEC (congenital) 368.59
    acquired 368.55
Colostomy
  attention to V55.3
  fitting or adjustment V53.5
  malfunctioning 569.62
  status V44.3
Colpitis (*see also* Vaginitis) 616.10
Colpocele 618.6
Colpocystitis (*see also* Vaginitis) 616.10
Colporrhexis 665.4
Colpospasm 625.1
Column, spinal, vertebral —*see* condition

Coma 780.01
  apoplectic (*see also* Disease, cerebrovascular,
    acute) 436
  diabetic (with ketoacidosis) 250.3
    due to secondary diabetes 249.3
    hyperosmolar 250.2
      due to secondary diabetes 249.2
  eclamptic (*see also* Eclampsia) 780.39
  epileptic 345.3
  hepatic 572.2
  hyperglycemic 250.2
    due to secondary diabetes 249.2
  hyperosmolar (diabetic) (nonketotic) 250.2
    due to secondary diabetes 249.2
  hypoglycemic 251.0
    diabetic 250.3
      due to secondary diabetes 249.3
  insulin 250.3
    due to secondary diabetes 249.3
    hyperosmolar 250.2
      due to secondary diabetes 249.2
    non-diabetic 251.0
    organic hyperinsulinism 251.0
  Kussmaul's (diabetic) 250.3
    due to secondary diabetes 249.3
  liver 572.2
  newborn 779.2
  prediabetic 250.2
    due to secondary diabetes 249.2
  uremic—*see* Uremia
Combat fatigue (*see also* Reaction, stress, acute)
  308.9
Combined —*see* condition
Comedo 706.1
Comedocarcinoma (M8501/3)—*see also*
  Neoplasm, breast, malignant
  noninfiltrating (M8501/2)
    specified site—*see* Neoplasm, by site, in situ
    unspecified site 233.0
Comedomastitis 610.4
Comedones 706.1
  lanugo 757.4
Comma bacillus, carrier (suspected) of V02.3
Comminuted fracture —*see* Fracture, by site
Common
  aortopulmonary trunk 745.0
  atrioventricular canal (defect) 745.69
  atrium 745.69
  cold (head) 460
    vaccination, prophylactic (against) V04.7
  truncus (arteriosus) 745.0
  ventricle 745.3
Commotio (current)
  cerebri (*see also* Concussion, brain) 850.9
    with skull fracture—*see* Fracture, skull, by site
  retinae 921.3
  spinalis—*see* Injury, spinal, by site
Commotion (current)
  brain (without skull fracture) (*see also*
    Concussion, brain) 850.9
    with skull fracture—*see* Fracture, skull, by site
  spinal cord—*see* Injury, spinal, by site
Communication
  abnormal—*see also* Fistula
    between
      base of aorta and pulmonary artery 745.0
      left ventricle and right atrium 745.4
      pericardial sac and pleural sac 748.8
      pulmonary artery and pulmonary vein
        747.39

Communication—*continued*
  congenital, between uterus and
    anterior abdominal wall 752.39
    bladder 752.39
    intestine 752.39
    rectum 752.39
  left ventricular-right atrial 745.4
  pulmonary artery-pulmonary vein 747.39
Compartment syndrome —*see* Syndrome,
  compartment
Compensation
  broken—*see* Failure, heart
  failure—*see* Failure, heart
  neurosis, psychoneurosis 300.11
Complaint —*see also* Disease
  bowel, functional 564.9
    psychogenic 306.4
  intestine, functional 564.9
    psychogenic 306.4
  kidney (*see also* Disease, renal) 593.9
  liver 573.9
  miners' 500
Complete —*see* condition
Complex
  cardiorenal (*see also* Hypertension, cardiorenal)
    404.90
  castration 300.9
  Costen's 524.60
  ego-dystonic homosexuality 302.0
  Eisenmenger's (ventricular septal defect) 745.4
  homosexual, ego-dystonic 302.0
  hypersexual 302.89
  inferiority 301.9
  jumped process
    spine—*see* Dislocation, vertebra
  primary, tuberculosis (*see also* Tuberculosis) 010.0
  regional pain syndrome 355.9
    type I 337.20
      lower limb 337.22
      specified site NEC 337.29
      upper limb 337.21
    type II
      lower limb 355.71
      upper limb 354.4
  Taussig-Bing (transposition, aorta and
    overriding pulmonary artery) 745.11
Complications
  abortion NEC—*see* categories 634-639
  accidental puncture or laceration during a
    procedure 998.2
  amniocentesis, fetal 679.1
  amputation stump (late) (surgical) 997.60
    traumatic—*see* Amputation, traumatic
  anastomosis (and bypass)—*see also*
    Complications, due to (presence of) any
    device, implant, or graft classified to
    996.0-996.5 NEC
    hemorrhage NEC 998.11
    intestinal (internal) NEC 997.49
      involving urinary tract 997.5
    mechanical—*see* Complications, mechanical,
      graft
    urinary tract (involving intestinal tract) 997.5
  anesthesia, anesthetic NEC (*see also* Anesthesia,
    complication) 995.22
    in labor and delivery 668.9
      affecting fetus or newborn 763.5
      cardiac 668.1
      central nervous system 668.2
      pulmonary 668.0
      specified type NEC 668.8

Complications—*continued*
  aortocoronary (bypass) graft 996.03
    atherosclerosis —*see* Arteriosclerosis,
      coronary
    embolism 996.72
    occlusion NEC 996.72
    thrombus 996.72
  arthroplasty (*see also* Complications, prosthetic
    joint) 996.49
  artificial opening
    cecostomy 569.60
    colostomy 569.6
    cystostomy 596.83
      infection 596.81
      mechanical 596.82
      specified complication NEC 596.83
    enterostomy 569.60
    esophagostomy 530.87
      infection 530.86
      mechanical 530.87
    gastrostomy 536.40
    ileostomy 569.60
    jejunostomy 569.60
    nephrostomy 997.5
    tracheostomy 519.00
    ureterostomy 997.5
    urethrostomy 997.5
  bariatric surgery
    gastric band procedure 539.09
      infection 539.01
    specified procedure NEC 539.89
      infection 539.81
  bile duct implant (prosthetic) NEC 996.79
    infection or inflammation 996.69
    mechanical 996.59
  bleeding (intraoperative) (postoperative) 998.11
  blood vessel graft 996.1
    aortocoronary 996.03
      atherosclerosis —*see* Arteriosclerosis,
        coronary
      embolism 996.72
      occlusion NEC 996.72
      thrombus 996.72
    atherosclerosis —*see* Arteriosclerosis,
      extremities
    embolism 996.74
    occlusion NEC 996.74
    thrombus 996.74
  bone growth stimulator NEC 996.78
    infection or inflammation 996.67
  bone marrow transplant 996.85
  breast implant (prosthetic) NEC 996.79
    infection or inflammation 996.69
    mechanical 996.54
  bypass—*see also* Complications, anastomosis
    aortocoronary 996.03
      atherosclerosis —*see* Arteriosclerosis,
        coronary
      embolism 996.72
      occlusion NEC 996.72
      thrombus 996.72
    carotid artery 996.1
      atherosclerosis —*see* Arteriosclerosis,
        extremities
      embolism 996.74
      occlusion NEC 996.74
      thrombus 996.74
  cardiac (*see also* Disease, heart) 429.9
    device, implant, or graft NEC 996.72
      infection or inflammation 996.61
      long-term effect 429.4

Complications—*continued*
  cardiac—*continued*
    device—*continued*
      mechanical (*see also* Complications,
        mechanical, by type) 996.00
      valve prosthesis 996.71
        infection or inflammation 996.61
      postoperative NEC 997.1
        long-term effect 429.4
  cardiorenal (*see also* Hypertension, cardiorenal)
    404.90
  carotid artery bypass graft 996.1
    atherosclerosis —*see* Arteriosclerosis,
      extremities
    embolism 996.74
    occlusion NEC 996.74
    thrombus 996.74
  cataract fragments in eye 998.82
  catheter device—*see also* Complications, due to
    (presence of) any device, implant, or graft
    classified to 996.0-996.5 NEC
    mechanical—*see* Complications, mechanical,
      catheter
  cecostomy 569.60
  cesarean section wound 674.3
  chemotherapy (antineoplastic) 995.29
  chin implant (prosthetic) NEC 996.79
    infection or inflammation 996.69
    mechanical 996.59
  colostomy (enterostomy) 569.60
    specified type NEC 569.69
  contraceptive device, intrauterine NEC 996.76
    infection 996.65
    inflammation 996.65
    mechanical 996.32
  cord (umbilical)—*see* Complications, umbilical cord
  cornea
    due to contact lens 371.82
  coronary (artery) bypass (graft) NEC 996.03
    atherosclerosis —*see* Arteriosclerosis, coronary
    embolism 996.72
    infection or inflammation 996.61
    mechanical 996.03
    occlusion NEC 996.72
    specified type NEC 996.72
    thrombus 996.72
  cystostomy 596.83
    infection 596.81
    mechanical 596.82
    specified complication NEC 596.83
  delivery 669.9
    procedure (instrumental) (manual) (surgical) 669.4
    specified type NEC 669.8
  dialysis (hemodialysis) (peritoneal) (renal) NEC
    999.9
    catheter NEC—*see also* Complications, due to
      (presence of) any device, implant or graft
      classified to 996.0-996.5 NEC
      infection or inflammation 996.62
        peritoneal 996.68
      mechanical 996.1
        peritoneal 996.56
  drug NEC 995.29
  due to (presence of) any device, implant, or graft
    classified to 996.0-996.5 NEC 996.70
    with infection or inflammation—*see*
      Complications, infection or inflammation,
      due to (presence of) any device, implant,
      or graft classified to 996.0-996.5 NEC

Complications—*continued*
  due to—*continued*
    arterial NEC 996.74
      coronary NEC 996.03
        atherosclerosis —*see* Arteriosclerosis,
          coronary
        embolism 996.72
        occlusion NEC 996.72
        specified type NEC 996.72
        thrombus 996.72
      renal dialysis 996.73
    arteriovenous fistula or shunt NEC 996.74
    bone growth stimulator 996.78
    breast NEC 996.79
    cardiac NEC 996.72
      defibrillator 996.72
      pacemaker 996.72
      valve prosthesis 996.71
    catheter NEC 996.79
      spinal 996.75
      urinary, indwelling 996.76
      vascular NEC 996.74
        renal dialysis 996.73
      ventricular shunt 996.75
    coronary (artery) bypass (graft) NEC 996.03
      atherosclerosis —*see* Arteriosclerosis,
        coronary
      embolism 996.72
      occlusion NEC 996.72
      thrombus 996.72
    electrodes
      brain 996.75
      heart 996.72
    esophagostomy 530.87
    gastrointestinal NEC 996.79
    genitourinary NEC 996.76
    heart valve prosthesis NEC 996.71
    infusion pump 996.74
    insulin pump 996.57
    internal
      joint prosthesis 996.77
      orthopedic NEC 996.78
      specified type NEC 996.79
    intrauterine contraceptive device NEC 996.76
    joint prosthesis, internal NEC 996.77
    mechanical—*see* Complications, mechanical
    nervous system NEC 996.75
    ocular lens NEC 996.79
    orbital NEC 996.79
    orthopedic NEC 996.78
      joint, internal 996.77
    renal dialysis 996.73
    specified type NEC 996.79
    urinary catheter, indwelling 996.76
    vascular NEC 996.74
    ventricular shunt 996.75
  during dialysis NEC 999.9
  ectopic or molar pregnancy NEC 639.9
  electroshock therapy NEC 999.9
  enterostomy 569.60
    specified type NEC 569.69
  esophagostomy 530.87
    infection 530.86
    mechanical 530.87
  external (fixation) device with internal
    component(s) NEC 996.78
    infection or inflammation 996.67
    mechanical 996.49
  extracorporeal circulation NEC 999.9

Complications—*continued*
  eye implant (prosthetic) NEC 996.79
    infection or inflammation 996.69
    mechanical
      ocular lens 996.53
      orbital globe 996.59
  fetal, from amniocentesis 679.1
  gastrointestinal, postoperative NEC (*see also*
      Complications, surgical procedures) 997.49
  gastrostomy 536.40
    specified type NEC 536.49
  genitourinary device, implant or graft NEC
      996.76
    erosion of implanted vaginal mesh 629.31
    exposure of implanted vaginal mesh 629.32
    infection or inflammation 996.65
      urinary catheter, indwelling 996.64
    mechanical (*see also* Complications,
        mechanical, by type) 996.30
      specified NEC 996.39
  graft (bypass) (patch)—*see also* Complications,
      due to (presence of) any device, implant, or
      graft classified to 996.0-996.5 NEC
    bone marrow 996.85
    corneal NEC 996.79
      infection or inflammation 996.69
      rejection or reaction 996.51
      retroprosthetic membrane 996.51
    mechanical—*see* Complications, mechanical,
        graft
    organ (immune or nonimmune cause) (partial)
        (total) 996.80
      bone marrow 996.85
      heart 996.83
      intestines 996.87
      kidney 996.81
      liver 996.82
      lung 996.84
      pancreas 996.86
      specified NEC 996.89
    skin NEC 996.79
      infection or inflammation 996.69
      rejection 996.52
        artificial 996.55
        decellularized allodermis 996.55
  heart—*see also* Disease, heart
    transplant (immune or nonimmune cause)
        996.83
  hematoma (intraoperative) (postoperative)
      998.12
  hemorrhage (intraoperative) (postoperative)
      998.11
  hyperalimentation therapy NEC 999.9
  immunization (procedure)—*see* Complications,
      vaccination
  implant—*see also* Complications, due to
      (presence of) any device, implant, or graft
      classified to 996.0-996.5 NEC
    dental placement, hemorrhagic 525.71
    mechanical—*see* Complications, mechanical,
        implant
  infection and inflammation
    due to (presence of) any device, implant, or
        graft classified to 996.0-996.5 NEC 996.60
      arterial NEC 996.62
        coronary 996.61
        renal dialysis 996.62
      arteriovenous fistula or shunt 996.62
      artificial heart 996.61
      bone growth stimulator 996.67
      breast 996.69
      cardiac 996.61

Complications—*continued*
  infection and inflammation—*continued*
    due to—*continued*
      catheter NEC 996.69
        central venous 999.31
          bloodstream 999.32
          localized 999.33
        Hickman 999.31
          bloodstream 999.32
          localized 999.33
        peripherally inserted central (PICC) 999.31
          bloodstream 999.32
          localized 999.33
        peritoneal 996.68
        portacath (port-a-cath) 999.31
          bloodstream 999.32
          localized 999.33
        spinal 996.63
        triple lumen 999.31
          bloodstream 999.32
          localized 999.33
        umbilical venous 999.31
          bloodstream 999.32
          localized 999.33
        urinary, indwelling 996.64
        vascular (arterial) (dialysis) (peripheral
            venous) NEC 996.62
        ventricular shunt 996.63
      central venous catheter 999.31
        bloodstream 999.32
        localized 999.33
      coronary artery bypass 996.61
      electrodes
        brain 996.63
        heart 996.61
      gastrointestinal NEC 996.69
      genitourinary NEC 996.65
        indwelling urinary catheter 996.64
      heart assist device 996.61
      heart valve 996.61
      Hickman catheter 999.31
        bloodstream 999.32
        localized 999.33
      infusion pump 996.62
      insulin pump 996.69
      intrauterine contraceptive device 996.65
      joint prosthesis, internal 996.66
      ocular lens 996.69
      orbital (implant) 996.69
      orthopedic NEC 996.67
        joint, internal 996.66
      peripherally inserted central catheter (PICC)
          999.31
        bloodstream 999.32
        localized 999.33
      portacath (port-a-cath) 999.31
        bloodstream 999.32
        localized 999.33
      specified type NEC 996.69
      triple lumen catheter 999.31
        bloodstream 999.32
        localized 999.33
      umbilical venous catheter 999.31
        bloodstream 999.32
        localized 999.33
      urinary catheter, indwelling 996.64
      ventricular shunt 996.63
    infusion (procedure) 999.88
      blood—*see* Complications, transfusion
      infection NEC 999.39
      sepsis NEC 999.39

Complications—*continued*
  inhalation therapy NEC 999.9
  injection (procedure) 999.9
    drug reaction (*see also* Reaction, drug) 995.27
    infection NEC 999.39
    sepsis NEC 999.39
    serum (prophylactic) (therapeutic)—*see*
      Complications, vaccination
    vaccine (any)—*see* Complications,
      vaccination
  inoculation (any)—*see* Complications, vaccination
  insulin pump 996.57
  internal device (catheter) (electronic) (fixation)
    (prosthetic) NEC—*see also* Complications,
    due to (presence of) any device, implant, or
    graft classified to 996.0-996.5 NEC
    mechanical—*see* Complications, mechanical
  intestinal pouch, specified NEC 569.79
  intestinal transplant (immune or nonimmune
    cause) 996.87
  intraoperative bleeding or hemorrhage 998.11
  intrauterine contraceptive device (*see also*
    Complications, contraceptive device) 996.76
    infection or inflammation 996.65
    with fetal damage affecting management of
      pregnancy 655.8
  in utero procedure
    fetal 679.1
    maternal 679.0
  jejunostomy 569.60
  kidney transplant (immune or nonimmune
    cause) 996.81
  labor 669.9
    specified condition NEC 669.8
  liver transplant (immune or nonimmune cause)
    996.82
  lumbar puncture 349.0
  mechanical
    anastomosis—*see* Complications, mechanical,
      graft
    artificial heart 996.09
    bypass—*see* Complications, mechanical, graft
    catheter NEC 996.59
      cardiac 996.09
      cystostomy 596.82
      dialysis (hemodialysis) 996.1
        peritoneal 996.56
      during a procedure 998.2
      urethral, indwelling 996.31
    colostomy 569.62
    device NEC 996.59
      balloon (counterpulsation), intra-aortic 996.1
      cardiac 996.00
        automatic implantable defibrillator 996.04
        long-term effect 429.4
        specified NEC 996.09
      contraceptive, intrauterine 996.32
      counterpulsation, intra-aortic 996.1
      fixation, external, with internal components
        996.49
      fixation, internal (nail, rod, plate) 996.40
      genitourinary 996.30
        specified NEC 996.39
      insulin pump 996.57
      nervous system 996.2
      orthopedic, internal 996.40
        prosthetic joint (*see also* Complications,
          mechanical device, orthopedic,
          prosthetic, joint) 996.47

Complications—*continued*
  mechanical—*continued*
    device—*continued*
      prosthetic NEC 996.59
        joint 996.47
          articular bearing surface wear 996.46
          aseptic loosening 996.41
          breakage 996.43
          dislocation 996.42
          failure 996.47
          fracture 996.43
            around prosthetic 996.44
            peri-prosthetic 996.44
          instability 996.42
          loosening 996.41
          peri-prosthetic osteolysis 996.45
          subluxation 996.42
          wear 996.46
      umbrella, vena cava 996.1
      vascular 996.1
    dorsal column stimulator 996.2
    electrode NEC 996.59
      brain 996.2
      cardiac 996.01
      spinal column 996.2
    enterostomy 569.62
    esophagostomy 530.87
    fistula, arteriovenous, surgically created 996.1
    gastrostomy 536.42
    graft NEC 996.52
      aortic (bifurcation) 996.1
      aortocoronary bypass 996.03
      blood vessel NEC 996.1
      bone 996.49
      cardiac 996.00
      carotid artery bypass 996.1
      cartilage 996.49
      corneal 996.51
      coronary bypass 996.03
      decellularized allodermis 996.55
      genitourinary 996.30
        specified NEC 996.39
      muscle 996.49
      nervous system 996.2
      organ (immune or nonimmune cause) 996.80
        heart 996.83
        intestines 996.87
        kidney 996.81
        liver 996.82
        lung 996.84
        pancreas 996.86
        specified NEC 996.89
      orthopedic, internal 996.49
      peripheral nerve 996.2
      prosthetic NEC 996.59
      skin 996.52
        artificial 996.55
        specified NEC 996.59
      tendon 996.49
      tissue NEC 996.52
      tooth 996.59
      ureter, without mention of resection 996.39
      vascular 996.1
    heart valve prosthesis 996.02
      long-term effect 429.4
    implant NEC 996.59
      cardiac 996.00
        automatic implantable defibrillator 996.04
        long-term effect 429.4
        specified NEC 996.09

Complications—*continued*
  mechanical—*continued*
    implant—*continued*
      electrode NEC 996.59
        brain 996.2
        cardiac 996.01
        spinal column 996.2
      genitourinary 996.30
      nervous system 996.2
      orthopedic, internal 996.49
      prosthetic NEC 996.59
        in
          bile duct 996.59
          breast 996.54
          chin 996.59
          eye
            ocular lens 996.53
            orbital globe 996.59
        vascular 996.1
      insulin pump 996.57
      nonabsorbable surgical material 996.59
      pacemaker NEC 996.59
        brain 996.2
        cardiac 996.01
        nerve (phrenic) 996.2
      patch—*see* Complications, mechanical, graft
      prosthesis NEC 996.59
        bile duct 996.59
        breast 996.54
        chin 996.59
        ocular lens 996.53
        reconstruction, vas deferens 996.39
      reimplant NEC 996.59
        extremity (*see also* Complications,
          reattached, extremity) 996.90
        organ (*see also* Complications, transplant,
          organ, by site) 996.80
      repair—*see* Complications, mechanical, graft
      respirator (ventilator) V46.14
      shunt NEC 996.59
        arteriovenous, surgically created 996.1
        ventricular (communicating) 996.2
      stent NEC 996.59
      tracheostomy 519.02
      vas deferens reconstruction 996.39
      ventilator (respirator) V46.14
  medical care NEC 999.9
    cardiac NEC 997.1
    gastrointestinal NEC 997.49
    nervous system NEC 997.00
    peripheral vascular NEC 997.2
    respiratory NEC 997.39
    urinary NEC 997.5
    vascular
      mesenteric artery 997.71
      other vessels 997.79
      peripheral vessels 997.2
      renal artery 997.72
  nephrostomy 997.5
  nervous system
    device, implant, or graft NEC 349.1
      mechanical 996.2
    postoperative NEC 997.00
  obstetric 669.9
    procedure (instrumental) (manual) (surgical)
      669.4
    specified NEC 669.8
    surgical wound 674.3
  ocular lens implant NEC 996.79
    infection or inflammation 996.69
    mechanical 996.53

Complications—*continued*
  organ transplant—*see* Complications, transplant,
    organ, by site
  orthopedic device, implant, or graft
    internal (fixation) (nail) (plate) (rod) NEC
      996.78
    infection or inflammation 996.67
    joint prosthesis 996.77
      infection or inflammation 996.66
    mechanical 996.40
  pacemaker (cardiac) 996.72
    infection or inflammation 996.61
    mechanical 996.01
  pancreas transplant (immune or nonimmune
    cause) 996.86
  perfusion NEC 999.9
  perineal repair (obstetrical) 674.3
    disruption 674.2
  pessary (uterus) (vagina)—*see* Complications,
    contraceptive device
  phototherapy 990
  postcystoscopic 997.5
  postmastoidectomy NEC 383.30
  postoperative—*see* Complications, surgical
    procedures
  pregnancy NEC 646.9
    affecting fetus or newborn 761.9
  prosthetic device, internal—*see also*
    Complications, due to (presence of) any
    device, implant, or graft classified to
    996.0-996.5 NEC
    mechanical NEC (*see also* Complications,
      mechanical) 996.59
  puerperium NEC (*see also* Puerperal) 674.9
  puncture, spinal 349.0
  pyelogram 997.5
  radiation 990
  radiotherapy 990
  reattached
    body part, except extremity 996.99
    extremity (infection) (rejection) 996.90
      arm(s) 996.94
      digit(s) (hand) 996.93
        foot 996.95
      finger(s) 996.93
      foot 996.95
      forearm 996.91
      hand 996.92
      leg 996.96
      lower NEC 996.96
      toe(s) 996.95
      upper NEC 996.94
  reimplant—*see also* Complications, due to
    (presence of) any device, implant, or graft
    classified to 996.0-996.5 NEC
    bone marrow 996.85
    extremity (*see also* Complications, reattached,
      extremity) 996.90
      due to infection 996.90
    mechanical—*see* Complications, mechanical,
      reimplant
    organ (immune or nonimmune cause) (partial)
      (total) (*see also* Complications, transplant,
      organ, by site) 996.80
  renal allograft 996.81
  renal dialysis—*see* Complications, dialysis
  respirator (ventilator), mechanical V46.14
  respiratory 519.9
    device, implant or graft NEC 996.79
      infection or inflammation 996.69
      mechanical 996.59

Complications—*continued*
  respiratory—*continued*
    distress syndrome, adult, following trauma and
      surgery 518.52
    insufficiency, acute, postoperative 518.52
    postoperative NEC 997.39
    therapy NEC 999.9
  sedation during labor and delivery 668.9
    affecting fetus or newborn 763.5
    cardiac 668.1
    central nervous system 668.2
    pulmonary 668.0
    specified type NEC 668.8
  seroma (intraoperative) (postoperative)
    (noninfected) 998.13
    infected 998.51
  shunt—*see also* Complications, due to (presence
    of) any device, implant, or graft classified to
    996.0-996.5 NEC
    mechanical—*see* Complications, mechanical,
      shunt
  specified body system NEC
    device, implant, or graft—*see* Complications,
      due to (presence of) any device, implant,
      or graft classified to 996.0-996.5 NEC
    postoperative NEC 997.99
  spinal puncture or tap 349.0
  stoma, external
    gastrointestinal tract
      colostomy 569.60
      enterostomy 569.60
      esophagostomy 530.87
        infection 530.86
        mechanical 530.87
      gastrostomy 536.40
    urinary tract 997.5
  stomach banding 539.09
  stomach stapling 539.89
  surgical procedures 998.9
    accidental puncture or laceration 998.2
    amputation stump (late) 997.60
    anastomosis—*see* Complications, anastomosis
    burst stitches or sutures (external) (*see also*
      Dehiscence) 998.32
      internal 998.31
    cardiac 997.1
      long-term effect following cardiac surgery
        429.4
    cataract fragments in eye 998.82
    catheter device—*see* Complications, catheter
      device
    cecostomy malfunction 569.62
    colostomy malfunction 569.62
    cystostomy malfunction 596.82
      infection 596.81
      mechanical 596.82
      specified complication NEC 596.83
    dehiscence (of incision) (external) (*see also*
      Dehiscence) 998.32
      internal 998.31
    dialysis NEC (*see also* Complications,
      dialysis) 999.9
    disruption (*see also* Dehiscence)
      anastomosis (internal)—*see* Complications,
        mechanical, graft
      internal suture (line) 998.31
      wound (external) 998.32
        internal 998.31
    dumping syndrome (postgastrectomy) 564.2
    elephantiasis or lymphedema 997.99
      postmastectomy 457.0

Complications—*continued*
  surgical procedures—*continued*
    emphysema (surgical) 998.81
    enterostomy malfunction 569.62
    esophagostomy malfunction 530.87
    evisceration 998.32
    fistula (persistent postoperative) 998.6
    foreign body inadvertently left in wound
      (sponge) (suture) (swab) 998.4
    from nonabsorbable surgical material
      (Dacron) (mesh) (permanent suture)
      (reinforcing) (Teflon)—*see* Complications,
      due to (presence of) any device, implant,
      or graft classified to 996.0-996.5 NEC
    gastrointestinal NEC 997.49
    gastrostomy malfunction 536.42
    hematoma 998.12
    hemorrhage 998.11
    ileostomy malfunction 569.62
    internal prosthetic device NEC (*see also*
      Complications, internal device) 996.70
      hemolytic anemia 283.19
      infection or inflammation 996.60
      malfunction—*see* Complications,
        mechanical
      mechanical complication—*see*
        Complications, mechanical
      thrombus 996.70
    jejunostomy malfunction 569.62
    nervous system NEC 997.00
    obstruction, internal anastomosis—*see*
      Complications, mechanical, graft
    other body system NEC 997.99
    peripheral vascular NEC 997.2
    postcardiotomy syndrome 429.4
    postcholecystectomy syndrome 576.0
    postcommissurotomy syndrome 429.4
    postgastrectomy dumping syndrome 564.2
    postmastectomy lymphedema syndrome 457.0
    postmastoidectomy 383.30
      cholesteatoma, recurrent 383.32
      cyst, mucosal 383.31
      granulation 383.33
      inflammation, chronic 383.33
    postvagotomy syndrome 564.2
    postvalvulotomy syndrome 429.4
    reattached extremity (infection) (rejection)
      (*see also* Complications, reattached,
      extremity) 996.90
    respiratory NEC 997.39
    seroma 998.13
    shock (endotoxic) (septic) 998.02
      hypovolemic 998.09
    shunt, prosthetic (thrombus)—*see also*
      Complications, due to (presence of) any
      device, implant, or graft classified to
      996.0-996.5 NEC
      hemolytic anemia 283.19
    specified complication NEC 998.89
    stitch abscess 998.59
    transplant—*see* Complications, graft
    ureterostomy malfunction 997.5
    urethrostomy malfunction 997.5
    urinary NEC 997.5
    vascular
      mesenteric artery 997.71
      other vessels 997.79
      peripheral vessels 997.2
      renal artery 997.72
    wound infection 998.59

Complications—*continued*
 therapeutic misadventure NEC 999.9
  surgical treatment 998.9
 tracheostomy 519.00
 transfusion (blood) (lymphocytes) (plasma)
   999.80
  acute lung injury (TRALI) 518.7
  atrophy, liver, yellow, subacute (within 8
    months of administration)—*see* Hepatitis,
    viral
  bone marrow 996.85
  embolism
   air 999.1
   thrombus 999.2
  febrile nonhemolytic reaction (FNHTR)780.66
  hemolysis NEC 999.89
   bone marrow 996.85
  hemolytic reaction, incompatibility
    unspecified 999.83
   acute 999.84
   delayed 999.85
  hepatitis (serum) (type B) (within 8 months
    after administration) *see* Hepatitis, viral
  incompatibility reaction
   ABO 999.60
    with hemolytic transfusion reaction (HTR)
     (not specified as acute or delayed)
     999.61
    acute 999.62
    delayed 999.63
    specified type NEC 999.69
   minor blood group 999.89
   non-ABO (minor antigens) (Duffy) (Kell)
     (Kidd) (Lewis) (M) (N) (P) (S) 999.75
    with hemolytic transfusion reaction (HTR)
     (not specified as acute or delayed)
     999.76
    acute 999.77
    delayed 999.78
    specified type NEC 999.79
   Rh antigen (C) (c) (D) (E) (e) (factor) 999.70
    with hemolytic transfusion reaction (HTR)
     (not specified as acute or delayed)
     999.71
    acute 999.72
    delayed 999.73
    specified type NEC 999.74
  infection 999.39
   acute 999.34
  jaundice (serum) (within 8 months after
    administration) *see* Hepatitis, viral
  sepsis 999.39
  shock or reaction NEC 999.89
   bone marrow 996.85
  specified reaction NEC 999.89
  subacute yellow atrophy of liver (within 8 months
    after administration) *see* Hepatitis, viral
  thromboembolism 999.2
 transplant—*see also* Complications, due to
   (presence of) any device, implant, or graft
   classified to 996.0-996.5 NEC
  bone marrow 996.85
  organ (immune or nonimmune cause) (partial)
    (total) 996.80
   bone marrow 996.85
   heart 996.83
   intestines 996.87
   kidney 996.81
   liver 996.82
   lung 996.84
   pancreas 996.86
   specified NEC 996.89

Complications—*continued*
 transplant—*continued*
  stem cell(s) 996.88
   from
    peripheral blood 996.88
    umbilical cord 996.88
 trauma NEC (early) 958.8
 ultrasound therapy NEC 999.9
 umbilical cord
  affecting fetus or newborn 762.6
  complicating delivery 663.9
   affecting fetus or newborn 762.6
   specified type NEC 663.8
 urethral catheter NEC 996.76
  infection or inflammation 996.64
  mechanical 996.31
 urinary, postoperative NEC 997.5
 vaccination 999.9
  anaphylaxis NEC 999.42
  cellulitis 999.39
  encephalitis or encephalomyelitis 323.51
  hepatitis (serum) (type B) (within 8 months
    after administration) *see* Hepatitis, viral
  infection (general) (local) NEC 999.39
  jaundice (serum) (within 8 months after
    administration) *see* Hepatitis, viral
  meningitis 997.09 *[321.8]*
  myelitis 323.52
  protein sickness 999.52
  reaction (allergic) 999.52
   serum 999.52
  sepsis 999.39
  serum intoxication, sickness, rash, or other
    serum reaction NEC 999.52
  shock (allergic) (anaphylactic) 999.49
  subacute yellow atrophy of liver (within 8 months
    after administration) *see* Hepatitis, viral
  vaccinia (generalized) 999.0
   localized 999.39
 vascular
  device, implant, or graft NEC 996.74
   infection or inflammation 996.62
   mechanical NEC 996.1
    cardiac (*see also* Complications,
      mechanical, by type) 996.00
  following infusion, perfusion, or transfusion
    999.2
  postoperative NEC 997.2
   mesenteric artery 997.71
   other vessels 997.79
   peripheral vessels 997.2
   renal artery 997.72
 ventilation therapy NEC 999.9
 ventilator (respirator), mechanical V46.14
Compound presentation complicating delivery
  652.8
 causing obstructed labor 660.0
Compressed air disease 993.3
Compression
 with injury—*see* specific injury
 arm NEC 354.9
 artery 447.1
  celiac, syndrome 447.4
 brachial plexus 353.0
 brain (stem) 348.4
  due to
   contusion, brain—*see* Contusion, brain
   injury NEC—*see also* Hemorrhage, brain,
     traumatic
    birth—*see* Birth, injury, brain
   laceration, brain—*see* Laceration, brain
  osteopathic 739.0

Compression—*continued*
  bronchus 519.19
  by cicatrix—*see* Cicatrix
  cardiac 423.9
  cauda equina 344.60
    with neurogenic bladder 344.61
  celiac (artery) (axis) 447.4
  cerebral—*see* Compression, brain
  cervical plexus 353.2
  cord (umbilical)—*see* Compression, umbilical
      cord
  cranial nerve 352.9
    second 377.49
    third (partial) 378.51
      total 378.52
    fourth 378.53
    fifth 350.8
    sixth 378.54
    seventh 351.8
  divers' squeeze 993.3
  duodenum (external) (*see also* Obstruction,
      duodenum) 537.3
  during birth 767.9
  esophagus 530.3
    congenital, external 750.3
  Eustachian tube 381.63
  facies (congenital) 754.0
  fracture—*see* Fracture, by site
  heart—*see* Disease, heart
  intestine (*see also* Obstruction, intestine) 560.9
    with hernia—*see* Hernia, by site, with
        obstruction
  laryngeal nerve, recurrent 478.79
  leg NEC 355.8
  lower extremity NEC 355.8
  lumbosacral plexus 353.1
  lung 518.89
  lymphatic vessel 457.1
  medulla—*see* Compression, brain
  nerve NEC—*see also* Disorder, nerve
    arm NEC 354.9
    autonomic nervous system (*see also*
        Neuropathy, peripheral, autonomic) 337.9
    axillary 353.0
    cranial NEC 352.9
    due to displacement of intervertebral disc
        722.2
      with myelopathy 722.70
      cervical 722.0
        with myelopathy 722.71
      lumbar, lumbosacral 722.10
        with myelopathy 722.73
      thoracic, thoracolumbar 722.11
        with myelopathy 722.72
    iliohypogastric 355.79
    ilioinguinal 355.79
    leg NEC 355.8
    lower extremity NEC 355.8
    median (in carpal tunnel) 354.0
    obturator 355.79
    optic 377.49
    plantar 355.6
    posterior tibial (in tarsal tunnel) 355.5
    root (by scar tissue) NEC 724.9
      cervical NEC 723.4
      lumbar NEC 724.4
      lumbosacral 724.4
      thoracic 724.4
    saphenous 355.79
    sciatic (acute) 355.0
    sympathetic 337.9

Compression—*continued*
  nerve—*continued*
    traumatic—*see* Injury, nerve
    ulnar 354.2
    upper extremity NEC 354.9
  peripheral—*see* Compression, nerve
  spinal (cord) (old or nontraumatic) 336.9
    by displacement of intervertebral disc—*see*
        Displacement, intervertebral disc
    nerve
      root NEC 724.9
        postoperative 722.80
          cervical region 722.81
          lumbar region 722.83
          thoracic region 722.82
        traumatic—*see* Injury, nerve, spinal
      traumatic—*see* Injury, nerve, spinal
    spondylogenic 721.91
      cervical 721.1
      lumbar, lumbosacral 721.42
      thoracic 721.41
    traumatic—*see also* Injury, spinal, by site
      with fracture, vertebra—*see* Fracture,
          vertebra, by site, with spinal cord injury
  spondylogenic—*see* Compression, spinal cord,
      spondylogenic
  subcostal nerve (syndrome) 354.8
  sympathetic nerve NEC 337.9
  syndrome 958.5
  thorax 512.89
    iatrogenic 512.1
    postoperative 512.1
  trachea 519.19
    congenital 748.3
  ulnar nerve (by scar tissue) 354.2
  umbilical cord
    affecting fetus or newborn 762.5
      cord prolapsed 762.4
    complicating delivery 663.2
      cord around neck 663.1
      cord prolapsed 663.0
  upper extremity NEC 354.9
  ureter 593.3
  urethra—*see* Stricture, urethra
  vein 459.2
  vena cava (inferior) (superior) 459.2
  vertebral NEC—*see* Compression, spinal (cord)
Compulsion, compulsive
  eating 307.51
  neurosis (obsessive) 300.3
  personality 301.4
  states (mixed) 300.3
  swearing 300.3
    in Gilles de la Tourette's syndrome 307.23
  tics and spasms 307.22
  water drinking NEC (syndrome) 307.9
Concato's disease (pericardial polyserositis) 423.2
  peritoneal 568.82
  pleural—*see* Pleurisy
Concavity, chest wall 738.3
Concealed
  hemorrhage NEC 459.0
  penis 752.65
Concentric fading 368.12
Concern (normal) about sick person in family
    V61.49
Concrescence (teeth) 520.2
Concretio cordis 423.1
  rheumatic 393

Concretion —*see also* Calculus
  appendicular 543.9
  canaliculus 375.57
  clitoris 624.8
  conjunctiva 372.54
  eyelid 374.56
  intestine (impaction) (obstruction) 560.39
  lacrimal (passages) 375.57
  prepuce (male) 605
    female (clitoris) 624.8
  salivary gland (any) 527.5
  seminal vesicle 608.89
  stomach 537.89
  tonsil 474.8
Concussion (current) 850.9
  with
    loss of consciousness 850.5
      brief (less than one hour)
        30 minutes or less 850.11
        31-59 minutes 850.12
      moderate (1-24 hours) 850.2
      prolonged (more than 24 hours) (with
        complete recovery) (with return to
        pre-existing conscious level) 850.3
        without return to pre-existing conscious
          level 850.4
    mental confusion or disorientation (without
      loss of consciousness) 850.0
      with loss of consciousness—*see* Concussion,
        with, loss of consciousness
  without loss of consciousness 850.0
  blast (air) (hydraulic) (immersion) (underwater)
    869.0
    with open wound into cavity 869.1
    abdomen or thorax—*see* Injury, internal, by site
    brain—*see* Concussion, brain
    ear (acoustic nerve trauma) 951.5
      with perforation, tympanic membrane—*see*
        Wound, open, ear drum
    thorax—*see* Injury, internal, intrathoracic
      organs NEC
  brain or cerebral (without skull fracture) 850.9
    with
      loss of consciousness 850.5
        brief (less than one hour)
          30 minutes or less 850.11
          31-59 minutes 850.12
        moderate (1-24 hours) 850.2
        prolonged (more than 24 hours) (with
          complete recovery) (with return to
          pre-existing conscious level) 850.3
          without return to pre-existing conscious
            level 850.4
      mental confusion or disorientation (without
        loss of consciousness) 850.0
        with loss of consciousness—*see*
          Concussion, brain, with, loss of
          consciousness
      skull fracture—*see* Fracture, skull, by site
    without loss of consciousness 850.0
  cauda equina 952.4
  cerebral—*see* Concussion, brain
  conus medullaris (spine) 952.4
  hydraulic—*see* Concussion, blast
  internal organs—*see* Injury, internal, by site
  labyrinth—*see* Injury, intracranial
  ocular 921.3
  osseous labyrinth—*see* Injury, intracranial

Concussion—*continued*
  spinal (cord)—*see also* Injury, spinal, by site
    due to
      broken
        back—*see* Fracture, vertebra, by site, with
          spinal cord injury
        neck—*see* Fracture, vertebra, cervical,
          with spinal cord injury
      fracture, fracture dislocation, or compression
        fracture of spine or vertebra—*see*
          Fracture, vertebra, by site, with spinal
          cord injury
    syndrome 310.2
    underwater blast—*see* Concussion, blast
Condition —*see also* Disease
  fetal hematologic 678.0
  psychiatric 298.9
  respiratory NEC 519.9
    acute or subacute NEC 519.9
      due to
        external agent 508.9
          specified type NEC 508.8
        fumes or vapors (chemical) (inhalation) 506.3
        radiation 508.0
        smoke inhalation 508.2
    chronic NEC 519.9
      due to
        external agent 508.9
          specified type NEC 508.8
        fumes or vapors (chemical) (inhalation) 506.4
        radiation 508.1
    due to
      external agent 508.9
        specified type NEC 508.8
      fumes or vapors (chemical) (inhalation)
        506.9
Conduct disturbance (*see also* Disturbance,
    conduct) 312.9
  adjustment reaction 309.3
  hyperkinetic 314.2
Condyloma NEC 078.11
  acuminatum 078.11
  gonorrheal 098.0
  latum 091.3
  syphilitic 091.3
    congenital 090.0
  venereal, syphilitic 091.3
Confinement —*see* Delivery
Conflagration —*see also* Burn, by site
  asphyxia (by inhalation of gases, fumes, or
    vapors) 987.9
    specified agent—*see* Table of drugs and
      chemicals
Conflict
  family V61.9
    specified circumstance NEC V61.8
  interpersonal NEC V62.81
  marital V61.10
    involving
      divorce V61.03
      estrangement V61.09
  parent(guardian)-child V61.20
    adopted child V61.24
    biological child V61.23
    foster child V61.25
  partner V61.10
Confluent —*see* condition
Confusion, confused (mental) (state) (*see also*
    State, confusional) 298.9
  acute 293.0
  epileptic 293.0

Confusion, confused—*continued*
  postoperative 293.9
  psychogenic 298.2
  reactive (from emotional stress, psychological
    trauma) 298.2
  subacute 293.1
Confusional arousals 327.41
Congelation 991.9
Congenital —*see also* condition
  aortic septum 747.29
  generalized fibromatosis (CGF) 759.89
  intrinsic factor deficiency 281.0
  malformation—*see* Anomaly
Congestion, congestive
  asphyxia, newborn 768.9
  bladder 596.89
  bowel 569.89
  brain (*see also* Disease, cerebrovascular NEC)
    437.8
    malarial 084.9
  breast 611.79
  bronchi 519.19
  bronchial tube 519.19
  catarrhal 472.0
  cerebral—*see* Congestion, brain
  cerebrospinal—*see* Congestion, brain
  chest 786.9
  chill 780.99
    malarial (*see also* Malaria) 084.6
  circulatory NEC 459.9
  conjunctiva 372.71
  due to disturbance of circulation 459.9
  duodenum 537.3
  enteritis—*see* Enteritis
  eye 372.71
  fibrosis syndrome (pelvic) 625.5
  gastroenteritis—*see* Enteritis
  general 799.89
  glottis 476.0
  heart (*see also* Failure, heart) 428.0
  hepatic 573.0
  hypostatic (lung) 514
  intestine 569.89
  intracranial—*see* Congestion, brain
  kidney 593.89
  labyrinth 386.50
  larynx 476.0
  liver 573.0
  lung 786.9
    active or acute (*see also* Pneumonia) 486
      congenital 770.0
    chronic 514
    hypostatic 514
    idiopathic, acute 518.52
    passive 514
  malaria, malarial (brain) (fever) (*see also*
    Malaria) 084.6
  medulla—*see* Congestion, brain
  nasal 478.19
  nose 478.19
  orbit, orbital 376.33
    inflammatory (chronic) 376.10
      acute 376.00
  ovary 620.8
  pancreas 577.8
  pelvic, female 625.5
  pleural 511.0
  prostate (active) 602.1
  pulmonary—*see* Congestion, lung
  renal 593.89
  retina 362.89

Congestion, congestive—*continued*
  seminal vesicle 608.89
  spinal cord 336.1
  spleen 289.51
    chronic 289.51
  stomach 537.89
  trachea 464.11
  urethra 599.84
  uterus 625.5
    with subinvolution 621.1
  viscera 799.89
Congestive —*see* Congestion
Conical
  cervix 622.6
  cornea 371.60
  teeth 520.2
Conjoined twins 759.4
  causing disproportion (fetopelvic) 678.1
  fetal 678.1
Conjugal maladjustment V61.10
  involving
    divorce V61.03
    estrangement V61.09
Conjunctiva —*see* condition
Conjunctivitis (exposure) (infectious)
    (nondiphtheritic) (pneumococcal) (pustular)
    (staphylococcal) (streptococcal) NEC 372.30
  actinic 370.24
  acute 372.00
    atopic 372.05
    chemical 372.06
    contagious 372.03
    follicular 372.02
    hemorrhagic (viral) 077.4
    toxic 372.06
  adenoviral (acute) 077.3
  allergic (chronic) 372.14
    with hay fever 372.05
  anaphylactic 372.05
  angular 372.03
  Apollo (viral) 077.4
  atopic 372.05
  blennorrhagic (neonatorum) 098.40
  catarrhal 372.03
  chemical 372.06
    allergic 372.05
    meaning corrosion, *see* Burn, conjunctiva
  chlamydial 077.98
    due to
      Chlamydial trachomatis—*see* Trachoma
      paratrachoma 077.0
  chronic 372.10
    allergic 372.14
    follicular 372.12
    simple 372.11
    specified type NEC 372.14
    vernal 372.13
  diphtheritic 032.81
  due to
    dust 372.05
    enterovirus type 70 077.4
    erythema multiforme 695.10 *[372.33]*
    filariasis (*see also* Filariasis) 125.9 *[372.15]*
    mucocutaneous
      disease NEC 372.33
      leishmaniasis 085.5 *[372.15]*
    Reiter's disease 099.3 *[372.33]*
    syphilis 095.8 *[372.10]*
    toxoplasmosis (acquired) 130.1
      congenital (active) 771.2
    trachoma—*see* Trachoma

Conjunctivitis—*continued*
  dust 372.05
  eczematous 370.31
  epidemic 077.1
    hemorrhagic 077.4
  follicular (acute) 372.02
    adenoviral (acute) 077.3
  chronic 372.12
  glare 370.24
  gonococcal (neonatorum) 098.40
  granular (trachomatous) 076.1
    late effect 139.1
  hemorrhagic (acute) (epidemic) 077.4
  herpetic (simplex) 054.43
    zoster 053.21
  inclusion 077.0
  infantile 771.6
  influenzal 372.03
  Koch-Weeks 372.03
  light 372.05
  medicamentosa 372.05
  membranous 372.04
  meningococcic 036.89
  Morax-Axenfeld 372.02
  mucopurulent NEC 372.03
  neonatal 771.6
    gonococcal 098.40
  Newcastle's 077.8
  nodosa 360.14
  of Beal 077.3
  parasitic 372.15
    filariasis (*see also* Filariasis) 125.9 *[372.15]*
    mucocutaneous leishmaniasis 085.5 *[372.15]*
  Parinaud's 372.02
  petrificans 372.39
  phlyctenular 370.31
  pseudomembranous 372.04
    diphtheritic 032.81
  purulent 372.03
  Reiter's 099.3 *[372.33]*
  rosacea 695.3 *[372.31]*
  serous 372.01
    viral 077.99
  simple chronic 372.11
  specified NEC 372.39
  sunlamp 372.04
  swimming pool 077.0
  toxic 372.06
  trachomatous (follicular) 076.1
    acute 076.0
    late effect 139.1
  traumatic NEC 372.39
  tuberculous (*see also* Tuberculosis) 017.3 *[370.31]*
  tularemic 021.3
  tularensis 021.3
  vernal 372.13
    limbar 372.13 *[370.32]*
  viral 077.99
    acute hemorrhagic 077.4
    specified NEC 077.8
Conjunctivochalasis 372.81
Conjunctoblepharitis —*see* Conjunctivitis
Conn (-Louis) syndrome (primary aldosteronism) 255.12
Connective tissue —*see* condition
Conradi (-Hünermann) syndrome or disease (chondrodysplasia calcificans congenita) 756.59
Consanguinity V19.7
Consecutive —*see* condition
Consolidated lung (base)—*see* Pneumonia, lobar

Constipation 564.00
  atonic 564.09
  drug induced
    correct substance properly administered 564.09
    overdose or wrong substance given or taken 977.9
      specified drug—*see* Table of drugs and chemicals
  neurogenic 564.09
  other specified NEC 564.09
  outlet dysfunction 564.02
  psychogenic 306.4
  simple 564.00
  slow transit 564.01
  spastic 564.09
Constitutional —*see also* condition
  arterial hypotension (*see also* Hypotension) 458.9
  obesity 278.00
    morbid 278.01
  psychopathic state 301.9
  short stature in childhood 783.43
  state, developmental V21.9
    specified development NEC V21.8
  substandard 301.6
Constitutionally substandard 301.6
Constriction
  anomalous, meningeal bands or folds 742.8
  aortic arch (congenital) 747.10
  asphyxiation or suffocation by 994.7
  bronchus 519.19
  canal, ear (*see also* Stricture, ear canal, acquired) 380.50
  duodenum 537.3
  gallbladder (*see also* Obstruction, gallbladder) 575.2
    congenital 751.69
  intestine (*see also* Obstruction, intestine) 560.9
  larynx 478.74
    congenital 748.3
  meningeal bands or folds, anomalous 742.8
  organ or site, congenital NEC—*see* Atresia
  prepuce (congenital) 605
  pylorus 537.0
    adult hypertrophic 537.0
    congenital or infantile 750.5
    newborn 750.5
  ring (uterus) 661.4
    affecting fetus or newborn 763.7
  spastic—*see also* Spasm
    ureter 593.3
    urethra—*see* Stricture, urethra
  stomach 537.89
  ureter 593.3
  urethra—*see* Stricture, urethra
  visual field (functional) (peripheral) 368.45
Constrictive —*see* condition
Consultation V65.9
  medical—*see also* Counseling, medical
  specified reason NEC V65.8
  without complaint or sickness V65.9
    feared complaint unfounded V65.5
    specified reason NEC V65.8
Consumption —*see* Tuberculosis
Contact —*see also* Exposure (suspected)
  with
    AIDS virus V01.79
    anthrax V01.81
    asbestos V15.84
    cholera V01.0
    communicable disease V01.9
      specified type NEC V01.89
      viral NEC V01.79
    Escherichia coli (E. coli) V01.83

Contact—*continued*
  with—*continued*
    German measles V01.4
    gonorrhea V01.6
    HIV V01.79
    human immunodeficiency virus V01.79
    lead V15.86
    meningococcus V01.84
    parasitic disease NEC V01.89
    poliomyelitis V01.2
    potentially hazardous body fluids V15.85
    rabies V01.5
    rubella V01.4
    SARS-associated coronavirus V01.82
    smallpox V01.3
    syphilis V01.6
    tuberculosis V01.1
    varicella V01.71
    venereal disease V01.6
    viral disease NEC V01.79
  dermatitis—*see* Dermatitis
Contamination, food (*see also* Poisoning, food) 005.9
Contraception, contraceptive
  advice NEC V25.09
    family planning V25.09
    fitting of diaphragm V25.02
    prescribing or use of
      oral contraceptive agent V25.01
      specified agent NEC V25.02
  counseling NEC V25.09
    emergency V25.03
    family planning V25.09
    fitting of diaphragm V25.02
    prescribing or use of
      oral contraceptive agent V25.01
        emergency V25.03
        postcoital V25.03
      specified agent NEC V25.02
  device (in situ) V45.59
    causing menorrhagia 996.76
    checking V25.42
    complications 996.32
    insertion V25.11
    intrauterine V45.51
    reinsertion V25.13
    removal V25.12
      and reinsertion V25.13
    replacement V25.13
    subdermal V45.52
  fitting of diaphragm V25.02
  insertion
    intrauterine contraceptive device V25.11
    subdermal implantable V25.5
  maintenance V25.40
    examination V25.40
      intrauterine device V25.42
      oral contraceptive V25.41
      specified method NEC V25.49
      subdermal implantable V25.43
    intrauterine device V25.42
    oral contraceptive V25.41
    specified method NEC V25.49
    subdermal implantable V25.43
  management NEC V25.49
  prescription
    oral contraceptive agent V25.01
      emergency V25.03
      postcoital V25.03
      repeat V25.41
    specified agent NEC V25.02
      repeat V25.49

Contraception, contraceptive—*continued*
    sterilization V25.2
    surveillance V25.40
      intrauterine device V25.42
      oral contraceptive agent V25.41
      specified method NEC V25.49
      subdermal implantable V25.43
Contraction, contracture, contracted
  Achilles tendon (*see also* Short, tendon,
      Achilles) 727.81
  anus 564.89
  axilla 729.90
  bile duct (*see also* Disease, biliary) 576.8
  bladder 596.89
    neck or sphincter 596.0
  bowel (*see also* Obstruction, intestine) 560.9
  Braxton Hicks 644.1
  breast implant, capsular 611.83
  bronchus 519.19
  burn (old)—*see* Cicatrix
  capsular, of breast implant 611.83
  cecum (*see also* Obstruction, intestine) 560.9
  cervix (*see also* Stricture, cervix) 622.4
    congenital 752.49
  cicatricial—*see* Cicatrix
  colon (*see also* Obstruction, intestine) 560.9
  conjunctiva trachomatous, active 076.1
    late effect 139.1
  Dupuytren's 728.6
  eyelid 374.41
  eye socket (after enucleation) 372.64
  face 729.90
  fascia (lata) (postural) 728.89
    Dupuytren's 728.6
    palmar 728.6
    plantar 728.71
  finger NEC 736.29
    congenital 755.59
    joint (*see also* Contraction, joint) 718.44
  flaccid, paralytic
    joint (*see also* Contraction, joint) 718.4
    muscle 728.85
      ocular 378.50
  gallbladder (*see also* Obstruction, gallbladder)
      575.2
  hamstring 728.89
    tendon 727.81
  heart valve—*see* Endocarditis
  Hicks' 644.1
  hip (*see also* Contraction, joint) 718.4
  hourglass
    bladder 596.89
      congenital 753.8
    gallbladder (*see also* Obstruction, gallbladder)
      575.2
      congenital 751.69
    stomach 536.8
      congenital 750.7
      psychogenic 306.4
    uterus 661.4
      affecting fetus or newborn 763.7
      hysterical 300.11
  infantile (*see also* Epilepsy) 345.6
  internal os (*see also* Stricture, cervix) 622.4
  intestine (*see also* Obstruction, intestine) 560.9
  joint (abduction) (acquired) (adduction)
      (flexion) (rotation) 718.40
    ankle 718.47
    congenital NEC 755.8
      generalized or multiple 754.89
        lower limb joints 754.89

Contraction—*continued*
  hip (*see also* Subluxation, congenital, hip)
    754.32
  lower limb (including pelvic girdle) not
    involving hip 754.89
  upper limb (including shoulder girdle)
    755.59
  elbow 718.42
  foot 718.47
  hand 718.44
  hip 718.45
  hysterical 300.11
  knee 718.46
  multiple sites 718.49
  pelvic region 718.45
  shoulder (region) 718.41
  specified site NEC 718.48
  wrist 718.43
  kidney (granular) (secondary) (*see also*
    Sclerosis, renal) 587
  congenital 753.3
  hydronephritic 591
  pyelonephritic (*see also* Pyelitis, chronic)
    590.00
  tuberculous (*see also* Tuberculosis) 016.0
  ligament 728.89
  congenital 756.89
  liver—*see* Cirrhosis, liver
  muscle (postinfectional) (postural) NEC 728.85
  congenital 756.89
    sternocleidomastoid 754.1
  extraocular 378.60
  eye (extrinsic) (*see also* Strabismus) 378.9
    paralytic (*see also* Strabismus, paralytic)
     378.50
  flaccid 728.85
  hysterical 300.11
  ischemic (Volkmann's) 958.6
  paralytic 728.85
  posttraumatic 958.6
  psychogenic 306.0
    specified as conversion reaction 300.11
  myotonic 728.85
  neck (*see also* Torticollis) 723.5
  congenital 754.1
  psychogenic 306.0
  ocular muscle (*see also* Strabismus) 378.9
  paralytic (*see also* Strabismus, paralytic) 378.50
  organ or site, congenital NEC—*see* Atresia
  outlet (pelvis)—*see* Contraction, pelvis
  palmar fascia 728.6
  paralytic
    joint (*see also* Contraction, joint) 718.4
    muscle 728.85
     ocular (*see also* Strabismus, paralytic) 378.50
  pelvis (acquired) (general) 738.6
  affecting fetus or newborn 763.1
  complicating delivery 653.1
    causing obstructed labor 660.1
    generally contracted 653.1
     causing obstructed labor 660.1
    inlet 653.2
     causing obstructed labor 660.1
    midpelvic 653.8
     causing obstructed labor 660.1
    midplane 653.8
     causing obstructed labor 660.1
    outlet 653.3
     causing obstructed labor 660.1
  plantar fascia 728.71

Contraction—*continued*
  premature
    atrial 427.61
    auricular 427.61
    auriculoventricular 427.61
    heart (junctional) (nodal) 427.60
    supraventricular 427.61
    ventricular 427.69
  prostate 602.8
  pylorus (*see also* Pylorospasm) 537.81
  rectosigmoid (*see also* Obstruction, intestine) 560.9
  rectum, rectal (sphincter) 564.89
    psychogenic 306.4
  ring (Bandl's) 661.4
    affecting fetus or newborn 763.7
  scar—*see* Cicatrix
  sigmoid (*see also* Obstruction, intestine) 560.9
  socket, eye 372.64
  spine (*see also* Curvature, spine) 737.9
  stomach 536.8
    hourglass 536.8
     congenital 750.7
     psychogenic 306.4
    psychogenic 306.4
  tendon (sheath) (*see also* Short, tendon) 727.81
  toe 735.8
  ureterovesical orifice (postinfectional) 593.3
  urethra 599.84
  uterus 621.8
    abnormal 661.9
     affecting fetus or newborn 763.7
    clonic, hourglass or tetanic 661.4
     affecting fetus or newborn 763.7
    dyscoordinate 661.4
     affecting fetus or newborn 763.7
    hourglass 661.4
     affecting fetus or newborn 763.7
    hypotonic NEC 661.2
     affecting fetus or newborn 763.7
    incoordinate 661.4
     affecting fetus or newborn 763.7
    inefficient or poor 661.2
     affecting fetus or newborn 763.7
    irregular 661.2
     affecting fetus or newborn 763.7
    tetanic 661.4
     affecting fetus or newborn 763.7
  vagina (outlet) 623.2
  vesical 596.89
    neck or urethral orifice 596.0
  visual field, generalized 368.45
  Volkmann's (ischemic) 958.6
Contusion (skin surface intact) 924.9
  with
    crush injury—*see* Crush
    dislocation—*see* Dislocation, by site
    fracture—*see* Fracture, by site
    internal injury—*see also* Injury, internal, by
     site
     heart—*see* Contusion, cardiac
     kidney—*see* Contusion, kidney
     liver—*see* Contusion, liver
     lung—*see* Contusion, lung
     spleen—*see* Contusion, spleen
    intracranial injury—*see* Injury, intracranial
    nerve injury—*see* Injury, nerve
    open wound—*see* Wound, open, by site
  abdomen, abdominal (muscle) (wall) 922.2
    organ(s) NEC 868.00
  adnexa, eye NEC 921.9

Contusion—*continued*

ankle 924.21
  with other parts of foot 924.20
arm 923.9
  lower (with elbow) 923.10
  upper 923.03
    with shoulder or axillary region 923.09
auditory canal (external) (meatus) (and other
    part(s) of neck, scalp, or face, except eye)
    920
auricle, ear (and other part(s) of neck, scalp, or
    face except eye) 920
axilla 923.02
  with shoulder or upper arm 923.09
back 922.31
bone NEC 924.9
brain (cerebral) (membrane) (with hemorrhage)
    851.8

---

*Note—Use the following fifth-digit
subclassification with categories 851-854:*

0 unspecified state of consciousness
1 with no loss of consciousness
*2 with brief [less than one hour] loss
    of consciousness*
*3 with moderate [1-24 hours] loss of
    consciousness*
*4 with prolonged [more than 24 hours] loss of
    consciousness and return to pre-existing
    conscious level*
*5 with prolonged [more than 24 hours] loss of
    consciousness, without return to pre-existing
    conscious level*
*Use fifth-digit 5 to designate when a patient is
unconscious and dies before regaining
conciousness, regardless of the duration of the
loss of conciousness*
*6 with loss of consciousness of unspecified
    duration*
9 with concussion, unspecified

---

  with
    open intracranial wound 851.9
    skull fracture—*see* Fracture, skull, by site
  cerebellum 851.4
    with open intracranial wound 851.5
  cortex 851.0
    with open intracranial wound 851.1
  occipital lobe 851.4
    with open intracranial wound 851.5
  stem 851.4
    with open intracranial wound 851.5
breast 922.0
brow (and other part(s) of neck, scalp, or face,
    except eye) 920
buttock 922.32
canthus 921.1
cardiac 861.01
  with open wound into thorax 861.11
cauda equina (spine) 952.4
cerebellum—*see* Contusion, brain, cerebellum
cerebral—*see* Contusion, brain
cheek(s) (and other part(s) of neck, scalp, or
    face, except eye) 920
chest (wall) 922.1
chin (and other part(s) of neck, scalp, or face,
    except eye) 920
clitoris 922.4
conjunctiva 921.1
conus medullaris (spine) 952.4
cornea 921.3

Contusion—*continued*

corpus cavernosum 922.4
cortex (brain) (cerebral)—*see* Contusion, brain,
    cortex
costal region 922.1
ear (and other part(s) of neck, scalp, or face
    except eye) 920
elbow 923.11
  with forearm 923.10
epididymis 922.4
epigastric region 922.2
eye NEC 921.9
eyeball 921.3
eyelid(s) (and periocular area) 921.1
face (and neck, or scalp any part, except eye)
    920
femoral triangle 922.2
fetus or newborn 772.6
finger(s) (nail) (subungual) 923.3
flank 922.2
foot (with ankle) (excluding toe(s)) 924.20
forearm (and elbow) 923.10
forehead (and other part(s) of neck, scalp, or
    face, except eye) 920
genital organs, external 922.4
globe (eye) 921.3
groin 922.2
gum(s) (and other part(s) of neck, scalp, or face,
    except eye) 920
hand(s) (except fingers alone) 923.20
head (any part, except eye) (and face) (and neck)
    920
heart—*see* Contusion, cardiac
heel 924.20
hip 924.01
  with thigh 924.00
iliac region 922.2
inguinal region 922.2
internal organs (abdomen, chest, or pelvis)
    NEC—*see* Injury, internal, by site
interscapular region 922.33
iris (eye) 921.3
kidney 866.01
  with open wound into cavity 866.11
knee 924.11
  with lower leg 924.10
labium (majus) (minus) 922.4
lacrimal apparatus, gland, or sac 921.1
larynx (and other part(s) of neck, scalp, or face,
    except eye) 920
late effect—*see* Late, effects (of), contusion
leg 924.5
  lower (with knee) 924.10
lens 921.3
lingual (and other part(s) of neck, scalp, or face,
    except eye) 920
lip(s) (and other part(s) of neck, scalp, or face,
    except eye) 920
liver 864.01
  with
    laceration—*see* Laceration, liver
    open wound into cavity 864.11
lower extremity 924.5
  multiple sites 924.4
lumbar region 922.31
lung 861.21
  with open wound into thorax 861.31
malar region (and other part(s) of neck, scalp, or
    face, except eye) 920
mandibular joint (and other part(s) of neck,
    scalp, or face, except eye) 920

Contusion—*continued*
mastoid region (and other part(s) of neck, scalp, or face, except eye) 920
membrane, brain—*see* Contusion, brain
midthoracic region 922.1
mouth (and other part(s) of neck, scalp, or face, except eye) 920
multiple sites (not classifiable to same three-digit category) 924.8
　lower limb 924.4
　trunk 922.8
　upper limb 923.8
muscle NEC 924.9
myocardium—*see* Contusion, cardiac
nasal (septum) (and other part(s) of neck, scalp, or face, except eye) 920
neck (and scalp, or face any part, except eye) 920
nerve—*see* Injury, nerve, by site
nose (and other part(s) of neck, scalp, or face, except eye) 920
occipital region (scalp) (and neck or face, except eye) 920
　lobe—*see* Contusion, brain, occipital lobe
orbit (region) (tissues) 921.2
palate (soft) (and other part(s) of neck, scalp, or face, except eye) 920
parietal region (scalp) (and neck, or face, except eye) 920
　lobe—*see* Contusion, brain
penis 922.4
pericardium—*see* Contusion, cardiac
perineum 922.4
periocular area 921.1
pharynx (and other part(s) of neck, scalp, or face, except eye) 920
popliteal space (*see also* Contusion, knee) 924.11
prepuce 922.4
pubic region 922.4
pudenda 922.4
pulmonary—*see* Contusion, lung
quadriceps femoralis 924.00
rib cage 922.1
sacral region 922.32
salivary ducts or glands (and other part(s) of neck, scalp, or face, except eye) 920
scalp (and neck, or face any part, except eye) 920
scapular region 923.01
　with shoulder or upper arm 923.09
sclera (eye) 921.3
scrotum 922.4
shoulder 923.00
　with upper arm or axillar regions 923.09
skin NEC 924.9
skull 920
spermatic cord 922.4
spinal cord—*see also* Injury, spinal, by site
　cauda equina 952.4
　conus medullaris 952.4
spleen 865.01
　with open wound into cavity 865.11
sternal region 922.1
stomach—*see* Injury, internal, stomach
subconjunctival 921.1
subcutaneous NEC 924.9
submaxillary region (and other part(s) of neck, scalp, or face, except eye) 920
submental region (and other part(s) of neck, scalp, or face, except eye) 920

Contusion—*continued*
subperiosteal NEC 924.9
supraclavicular fossa (and other part(s) of neck, scalp, or face, except eye) 920
supraorbital (and other part(s) of neck, scalp, or face, except eye) 920
temple (region) (and other part(s) of neck, scalp, or face, except eye) 920
testis 922.4
thigh (and hip) 924.00
thorax 922.1
　organ—*see* Injury, internal, intrathoracic
throat (and other part(s) of neck, scalp, or face, except eye) 920
thumb(s) (nail) (subungual) 923.3
toe(s) (nail) (subungual) 924.3
tongue (and other part(s) of neck, scalp, or face, except eye) 920
trunk 922.9
　multiple sites 922.8
　specified site—*see* Contusion, by site
tunica vaginalis 922.4
tympanum (membrane) (and other part(s) of neck, scalp, or face, except eye) 920
upper extremity 923.9
　multiple sites 923.8
uvula (and other part(s) of neck, scalp, or face, except eye) 920
vagina 922.4
vocal cord(s) (and other part(s) of neck, scalp, or face, except eye) 920
vulva 922.4
wrist 923.21
　with hand(s), except finger(s) alone 923.20
Conus (any type) (congenital) 743.57
acquired 371.60
medullaris syndrome 336.8
Convalescence (following) V66.9
chemotherapy V66.2
medical NEC V66.5
psychotherapy V66.3
radiotherapy V66.1
surgery NEC V66.0
treatment (for) NEC V66.5
　combined V66.6
　fracture V66.4
　mental disorder NEC V66.3
　specified disorder NEC V66.5
Conversion
closed surgical procedure to open procedure
　arthroscopic V64.43
　laparoscopic V64.41
　thoracoscopic V64.42
hysteria, hysterical, any type 300.11
neurosis, any 300.11
reaction, any 300.11
Converter, tuberculosis (test reaction) 795.51
Convulsions (idiopathic) 780.39
apoplectiform (*see also* Disease, cerebrovascular, acute) 436
brain 780.39
cerebral 780.39
cerebrospinal 780.39
due to trauma NEC—*see* Injury, intracranial
eclamptic (*see also* Eclampsia) 780.39
epileptic (*see also* Epilepsy) 345.9
epileptiform (*see also* Seizure, epileptiform) 780.39
epileptoid (*see also* Seizure, epileptiform) 780.39

Convulsions—*continued*
  ether
    anesthetic
      correct substance properly administered
        780.39
      overdose or wrong substance given 968.2
    other specified type—*see* Table of drugs and
      chemicals
  febrile (simple) 780.31
    complex 780.32
  generalized 780.39
  hysterical 300.11
  infantile 780.39
    epilepsy—*see* Epilepsy
  internal 780.39
  jacksonian (*see also* Epilepsy) 345.5
  myoclonic 333.2
  newborn 779.0
  paretic 094.1
  pregnancy (nephritic) (uremic)—*see* Eclampsia,
    pregnancy
  psychomotor (*see also* Epilepsy) 345.4
  puerperal, postpartum—*see* Eclampsia,
    pregnancy
  recurrent 780.39
    epileptic—*see* Epilepsy
  reflex 781.0
  repetitive 780.39
    epileptic—*see* Epilepsy
  salaam (*see also* Epilepsy) 345.6
  scarlatinal 034.1
  spasmodic 780.39
  tetanus, tetanic (*see also* Tetanus) 037
  thymic 254.8
  uncinate 780.39
  uremic 586
Convulsive —*see also* Convulsions
  disorder or state 780.39
    epileptic—*see* Epilepsy
  equivalent, abdominal (*see also* Epilepsy) 345.5
Cooke-Apert-Gallais syndrome (adrenogenital)
  255.2
Cooley's anemia (erythroblastic) 282.44
Coolie itch 126.9
Cooper's
  disease 610.1
  hernia—*see* Hernia, Cooper's
Coordination disturbance 781.3
Copper wire arteries, retina 362.13
Copra itch 133.8
Coprolith 560.39
Coprophilia 302.89
Coproporphyria, hereditary 277.1
Coprostasis 560.32
  with hernia—*see also* Hernia, by site, with
    obstruction
  gangrenous—*see* Hernia, by site, with gangrene
Cor
  biloculare 745.7
  bovinum—*see* Hypertrophy, cardiac
  bovis—*see also* Hypertrophy, cardiac
  pulmonale (chronic) 416.9
    acute 415.0
  triatriatum, triatrium 746.82
  triloculare 745.8
    biatriatum 745.3
    biventriculare 745.69
Corbus' disease 607.1

Cord —*see also* condition
  around neck (tightly) (with compression)
    affecting fetus or newborn 762.5
    complicating delivery 663.1
      without compression 663.3
        affecting fetus or newborn 762.6
  bladder NEC 344.61
    tabetic 094.0
  prolapse
    affecting fetus or newborn 762.4
    complicating delivery 663.0
Cord's angiopathy (*see also* Tuberculosis) 017.3
  [362.18]
Cordis ectopia 746.87
Corditis (spermatic) 608.4
Corectopia 743.46
Cori type glycogen storage disease —*see*
  Disease, glycogen storage
Cork-handlers' disease or lung 495.3
Corkscrew esophagus 530.5
Corlett's pyosis (impetigo) 684
Corn (infected) 700
Cornea—*see also* condition
  donor V59.5
  guttata (dystrophy) 371.57
  plana 743.41
Cornelia de Lange's syndrome (Amsterdam
  dwarf, intellectual disabilities, and
  brachycephaly) 759.89
Cornual gestation or pregnancy —*see*
  Pregnancy, cornual
Cornu cutaneum 702.8
Coronary (artery)—*see also* condition
  arising from aorta or pulmonary trunk 746.85
Corpora —*see also* condition
  amylacea (prostate) 602.8
  cavernosa—*see* condition
Corpulence (*see also* Obesity) 278.0
Corpus —*see* condition
Corrigan's disease —*see* Insufficiency, aortic
Corrosive burn —*see* Burn, by site
Corsican fever (*see also* Malaria) 084.6
Cortical —*see also* condition
  blindness 377.75
  necrosis, kidney (bilateral) 583.6
Corticoadrenal —*see* condition
Corticosexual syndrome 255.2
Coryza (acute) 460
  with grippe or influenza (*see also* Influenza)
    487.1
  syphilitic 095.8
    congenital (chronic) 090.0
Costen's syndrome or complex 524.60
Costiveness (*see also* Constipation) 564.00
Costochondritis 733.6
Cotard's syndrome (paranoia) 297.1
Cot death 798.0
Cotia virus 059.8
Cotungo's disease 724.3
Cough 786.2
  with hemorrhage (*see also* Hemoptysis) 786.39
  affected 786.2
  bronchial 786.2
    with grippe or influenza (*see also* Influenza)
      487.1
  chronic 786.2
  epidemic 786.2
  functional 306.1
  hemorrhagic 786.39

Cough—*continued*
　hysterical 300.11
　laryngeal, spasmodic 786.2
　nervous 786.2
　psychogenic 306.1
　smokers' 491.0
　tea tasters' 112.89
Counseling NEC V65.40
　without complaint or sickness V65.49
　abuse victim NEC V62.89
　　child V61.21
　　partner V61.11
　　spouse V61.11
　child abuse, maltreatment, or neglect V61.21
　contraceptive NEC V25.09
　　device (intrauterine) V25.02
　　maintenance V25.40
　　　intrauterine contraceptive device V25.42
　　　oral contraceptive (pill) V25.41
　　　specified type NEC V25.49
　　　subdermal implantable V25.43
　　management NEC V25.9
　　oral contraceptive (pill) V25.01
　　　emergency V25.03
　　　postcoital V25.03
　　prescription NEC V25.02
　　　oral contraceptive (pill) V25.01
　　　　emergency V25.03
　　　　postcoital V25.03
　　　　repeat prescription V25.41
　　　repeat prescription V25.40
　　subdermal implantable V25.43
　　surveillance V25.40
　dietary V65.3
　exercise V65.41
　expectant parents(s)
　　pediatric pre-adoption visit V65.11
　　pediatric pre-birth visit V65.11
　explanation of
　　investigation finding NEC V65.49
　　medication NEC V65.49
　family planning V25.09
　　natural
　　　procreative V26.41
　　　to avoid pregnancy V25.04
　for nonattending third party V65.19
　genetic V26.33
　gonorrhea V65.45
　health (advice) (education) (instruction) NEC
　　V65.49
　HIV V65.44
　human immunodeficiency virus V65.44
　injury prevention V65.43
　insulin pump training V65.46
　marital V61.10
　medical (for) V65.9
　　boarding school resident V60.6
　　condition not demonstrated V65.5
　　feared complaint and no disease found V65.5
　　institutional resident V60.6
　　on behalf of another V65.19
　　person living alone V60.3
　natural family planning
　　procreative V26.41
　　to avoid pregnancy V25.04
　parent(guardian)-child conflict V61.20
　　adopted child V61.24
　　biological child V61.23
　　foster child V61.25
　　specified problem NEC V61.29

Counseling—*continued*
　partner abuse
　　perpetrator V61.12
　　victim V61.11
　pediatric
　　pre-adoption visit for adoptive parent(s)
　　　V65.11
　　pre-birth visit for expectant parent(s) V65.11
　perpetrator of
　　child abuse V62.83
　　　parental V61.22
　　partner abuse V61.12
　　spouse abuse V61.12
　procreative V65.49
　sex NEC V65.49
　　transmitted disease NEC V65.45
　　　HIV V65.44
　specified reason NEC V65.49
　spousal abuse
　　perpetrator V61.12
　　victim V61.11
　substance use and abuse V65.42
　syphilis V65.45
　victim (of)
　　abuse NEC V62.89
　　child abuse V61.21
　　partner abuse V61.11
　　spousal abuse V61.11
Coupled rhythm 427.89
Couvelaire uterus (complicating delivery)—*see*
　Placenta, separation
Cowper's gland —*see* condition
Cowperitis (*see also* Urethritis) 597.89
　gonorrheal (acute) 098.0
　　chronic or duration of 2 months or over 098.2
Cowpox (abortive) 051.01
　due to vaccination 999.0
　eyelid 051.01 *[373.5]*
　　postvaccination 999.0 *[373.5]*
Coxa
　plana 732.1
　valga (acquired) 736.31
　　congenital 755.61
　　late effect of rickets 268.1
　vara (acquired) 736.32
　　congenital 755.62
　　late effect of rickets 268.1
Coxae malum senilis 715.25
Coxalgia (nontuberculous) 719.45
　tuberculous (*see also* Tuberculosis) 015.1 *[730.85]*
Coxalgic pelvis 736.30
Coxitis 716.65
Coxsackie (infection) (virus) 079.2
　central nervous system NEC 048
　endocarditis 074.22
　enteritis 008.67
　meningitis (aseptic) 047.0
　myocarditis 074.23
　pericarditis 074.21
　pharyngitis 074.0
　pleurodynia 074.1
　specific disease NEC 074.8
Crabs, meaning pubic lice 132.2
Crack baby 760.75
Cracked
　nipple 611.2
　　puerperal, postpartum 676.1
　puerperal, postpartum 676.1
　tooth 521.81
Cradle cap 690.11
Craft neurosis 300.89

Craigiasis 007.8
Cramp(s) 729.82
  abdominal 789.0
  bathing 994.1
  colic 789.7
    infantile 789.7
    psychogenic 306.4
  due to immersion 994.1
  extremity (lower) (upper) NEC 729.82
  fireman 992.2
  heat 992.2
  hysterical 300.11
  immersion 994.1
  intestinal 789.0
    psychogenic 306.4
  linotypist's 300.89
    organic 333.84
  muscle (extremity) (general) 729.82
    due to immersion 994.1
    hysterical 300.11
  occupational (hand) 300.89
    organic 333.84
  psychogenic 307.89
  salt depletion 276.1
  sleep related leg 327.52
  stoker 992.2
  stomach 789.0
  telegraphers' 300.89
    organic 333.84
  typists' 300.89
    organic 333.84
  uterus 625.8
    menstrual 625.3
  writers' 333.84
    organic 333.84
    psychogenic 300.89
Cranial —*see* condition
Cranioclasis, fetal 763.89
Craniocleidodysostosis 755.59
Craniofenestria (skull) 756.0
Craniolacunia (skull) 756.0
Craniopagus 759.4
Craniopathy, metabolic 733.3
Craniopharyngeal —*see* condition
Craniopharyngioma (M9350/1) 237.0
Craniorachischisis (totalis) 740.1
Cranioschisis 756.0
Craniostenosis 756.0
Craniosynostosis 756.0
Craniotabes (cause unknown) 733.3
  rachitic 268.1
  syphilitic 090.5
Craniotomy, fetal 763.89
Cranium —*see* condition
Craw-craw 125.3
CRBSI (catheter-related bloodstream infection) 999.31
Creaking joint 719.60
  ankle 719.67
  elbow 719.62
  foot 719.67
  hand 719.64
  hip 719.65
  knee 719.66
  multiple sites 719.69
  pelvic region 719.65
  shoulder (region) 719.61
  specified site NEC 719.68
  wrist 719.63

Creeping
  eruption 126.9
  palsy 335.21
  paralysis 335.21
Crenated tongue 529.8
Creotoxism 005.9
Crepitus
  caput 756.0
  joint 719.60
    ankle 719.67
    elbow 719.62
    foot 719.67
    hand 719.64
    hip 719.65
    knee 719.66
    multiple sites 719.69
    pelvic region 719.65
    shoulder (region) 719.61
    specified site NEC 719.68
    wrist 719.63
Crescent or conus choroid, congenital 743.57
Cretin, cretinism (athyrotic) (congenital) (endemic) (metabolic) (nongoitrous) (sporadic) 243
  goitrous (sporadic) 246.1
  pelvis (dwarf type) (male type) 243
    with disproportion (fetopelvic) 653.1
      affecting fetus or newborn 763.1
      causing obstructed labor 660.1
        affecting fetus or newborn 763.1
  pituitary 253.3
Cretinoid degeneration 243
Creutzfeldt-Jakob disease (CJD) (syndrome) 046.19
  with dementia
    with behavioral disturbance 046.19 *[294.11]*
    without behavioral disturbance 046.19 *[294.10]*
  familial 046.19
  iatrogenic 046.19
  specified NEC 046.19
  sporadic 046.19
  variant (vCJD) 046.11
    with dementia
      with behavioral disturbance 046.11 *[294.11]*
      without behavioral disturbance 046.11 *[294.10]*
Crib death 798.0
Cribriform hymen 752.49
Cri-du-chat syndrome 758.31
Crigler-Najjar disease or syndrome (congenital hyperbilirubinemia) 277.4
Crimean hemorrhagic fever 065.0
Criminalism 301.7
Crisis
  abdomen 789.0
  addisonian (acute adrenocortical insufficiency) 255.41
  adrenal (cortical) 255.41
  asthmatic—*see* Asthma
  brain, cerebral (*see also* Disease, cerebrovascular, acute) 436
  celiac 579.0
  Dietl's 593.4
  emotional NEC 309.29
    acute reaction to stress 308.0
    adjustment reaction 309.9
    specific to childhood or adolescence 313.9
  gastric (tabetic) 094.0
  glaucomatocyclitic 364.22
  heart (*see also* Failure, heart) 428.9

Crisis—*continued*
hypertensive—*see* Hypertension
nitritoid
 correct substance properly administered 458.29
 overdose or wrong substance given or taken 961.1
oculogyric 378.87
 psychogenic 306.7
Pel's 094.0
psychosexual identity 302.6
rectum 094.0
renal 593.81
sickle cell 282.62
stomach (tabetic) 094.0
tabetic 094.0
thyroid (*see also* Thyrotoxicosis) 242.9
thyrotoxic (*see also* Thyrotoxicosis) 242.9
vascular—*see* Disease, cerebrovascular, acute
Crocq's disease (acrocyanosis) 443.89
Crohn's disease (*see also* Enteritis, regional) 555.9
Cronkhite-Canada syndrome 211.3
Crooked septum, nasal 470
Cross
birth (of fetus) complicating delivery 652.3
 with successful version 652.1
 causing obstructed labor 660.0
bite, anterior or posterior 524.27
eye (*see also* Esotropia) 378.00
Crossed ectopia of kidney 753.3
Crossfoot 754.50
Croup, croupus (acute) (angina) (catarrhal) (infective) (inflammatory) (laryngeal) (membranous) (nondiphtheritic) (pseudomembranous) 464.4
asthmatic (*see also* Asthma) 493.9
bronchial 466.0
diphtheritic (membranous) 032.3
false 478.75
spasmodic 478.75
 diphtheritic 032.3
stridulous 478.75
 diphtheritic 032.3
Crouzon's disease (craniofacial dysostosis) 756.0
Crowding, teeth 524.31
CRST syndrome (cutaneous systemic sclerosis) 710.1
Cruchet's disease (encephalitis lethargica) 049.8
Cruelty in children (*see also* Disturbance, conduct) 312.9
Crural ulcer (*see also* Ulcer, lower extremity) 707.10
Crush, crushed, crushing (injury) 929.9
abdomen 926.19
 internal—*see* Injury, internal, abdomen
ankle 928.21
 with other parts of foot 928.20
arm 927.9
 lower (and elbow) 927.10
 upper 927.03
  with shoulder or axillary region 927.09
axilla 927.02
 with shoulder or upper arm 927.09
back 926.11
breast 926.19
buttock 926.12
cheek 925.1
chest—*see* Injury, internal, chest
ear 925.1

Crush, crushed, crushing—*continued*
elbow 927.11
 with forearm 927.10
face 925.1
finger(s) 927.3
 with hand(s) 927.20
  and wrist(s) 927.21
flank 926.19
foot, excluding toe(s) alone (with ankle) 928.20
forearm (and elbow) 927.10
genitalia, external (female) (male) 926.0
 internal—*see* Injury, internal, genital organ NEC
hand, except finger(s) alone (and wrist) 927.20
head—*see* Fracture, skull, by site
heel 928.20
hip 928.01
 with thigh 928.00
internal organ (abdomen, chest, or pelvis)—*see* Injury, internal, by site
knee 928.11
 with leg, lower 928.10
labium (majus) (minus) 926.0
larynx 925.2
late effect—*see* Late, effects (of), crushing
leg 928.9
 lower 928.10
  and knee 928.11
 upper 928.00
limb
 lower 928.9
  multiple sites 928.8
 upper 927.9
  multiple sites 927.8
multiple sites NEC 929.0
neck 925.2
nerve—*see* Injury, nerve, by site
nose 802.0
 open 802.1
penis 926.0
pharynx 925.2
scalp 925.2
scapular region 927.01
 with shoulder or upper arm 927.09
scrotum 926.0
shoulder 927.00
 with upper arm or axillary region 927.09
skull or cranium—*see* Fracture, skull, by site
spinal cord—*see* Injury, spinal, by site
syndrome (complication of trauma) 958.5
testis 926.0
thigh (with hip) 928.00
throat 925.2
thumb(s) (and fingers) 927.3
toe(s) 928.3
 with foot 928.20
  and ankle 928.21
tonsil 925.2
trunk 926.9
 chest—*see* Injury, internal, intrathoracic organs NEC
 internal organ—*see* Injury, internal, by site
 multiple sites 926.8
 specified site NEC 926.19
vulva 926.0
wrist 927.21
 with hand(s), except fingers alone 927.20
Crusta lactea 690.11
Crusts 782.8
Crutch paralysis 953.4
Cruveilhier's disease 335.21
Cruveilhier-Baumgarten cirrhosis, disease, or syndrome 571.5

Cruz-Chagas disease (*see also* Trypanosomiasis)
    086.2
Crying
  constant, continuous
    adolescent 780.95
    adult 780.95
    baby 780.92
    child 780.95
    infant 780.92
    newborn 780.92
  excessive
    adolescent 780.95
    adult 780.95
    baby 780.92
    child 780.95
    infant 780.92
    newborn 780.92
Cryofibrinogenemia 273.2
Cryoglobulinemia (mixed) 273.2
Crypt (anal) (rectal) 569.49
Cryptitis (anal) (rectal) 569.49
Cryptococcosis (European) (pulmonary)
    (systemic) 117.5
Cryptococcus 117.5
  epidermicus 117.5
  neoformans, infection by 117.5
Cryptopapillitis (anus) 569.49
Cryptophthalmos (eyelid) 743.06
Cryptorchid, cryptorchism, cryptorchidism
    752.51
Cryptosporidiosis 007.4
  hepatobiliary 136.8
  respiratory 136.8
Cryptotia 744.29
Crystallopathy
  calcium pyrophosphate (*see also* Arthritis)
    275.49 *[712.2]*
  dicalcium phosphate (*see also* Arthritis) 275.49
    [712.1]
  gouty 274.00
  pyrophosphate NEC (*see also* Arthritis) 275.49
    [712.2]
  uric acid 274.00
Crystalluria 791.9
Csillag's disease (lichen sclerosus et atrophicus)
    701.0
Cuban itch 050.1
Cubitus
  valgus (acquired) 736.01
    congenital 755.59
    late effect of rickets 268.1
  varus (acquired) 736.02
    congenital 755.59
    late effect of rickets 268.1
Cultural deprivation V62.4
Cupping of optic disc 377.14
Curling's ulcer —*see* Ulcer, duodenum
Curling esophagus 530.5
Curschmann (-Batten) (-Steinert) disease or
    syndrome 359.21
Curvature
  organ or site, congenital NEC—*see* Distortion
  penis (lateral) 752.69
  Pott's (spinal) (*see also* Tuberculosis) 015.0
    [737.43]
  radius, idiopathic, progressive (congenital) 755.54

Curvature—*continued*
  spine (acquired) (angular) (idiopathic)
      (incorrect) (postural) 737.9
    congenital 754.2
    due to or associated with
      Charcot-Marie-Tooth disease 356.1 *[737.40]*
      mucopolysaccharidosis 277.5 *[737.40]*
      neurofibromatosis 237.71 *[737.40]*
      osteitis
        deformans 731.0 *[737.40]*
        fibrosa cystica 252.01 *[737.40]*
      osteoporosis (*see also* Osteoporosis) 733.00
          [737.40]
      poliomyelitis (*see also* Poliomyelitis) 138
          [737.40]
      tuberculosis (Pott's curvature) (*see also*
          Tuberculosis) 015.0 *[737.43]*
    kyphoscoliotic (*see also* Kyphoscoliosis)
        737.30
    kyphotic (*see also* Kyphosis) 737.10
    late effect of rickets 268.1 *[737.40]*
    Pott's 015.0 *[737.40]*
    scoliotic (*see also* Scoliosis) 737.30
    specified NEC 737.8
    tuberculous 015.0 *[737.40]*
Cushing's
  basophilism, disease, or syndrome (iatrogenic)
      (idiopathic) (pituitary basophilism) (pituitary
      dependent) 255.0
  ulcer—*see* Ulcer, peptic
Cushingoid due to steroid therapy
  correct substance properly administered 255.0
  overdose or wrong substance given or taken
      962.0
Cut (external)—*see* Wound, open, by site
Cutaneous —*see also* condition
  hemorrhage 782.7
  horn (cheek) (eyelid) (mouth) 702.8
  larva migrans 126.9
Cutis —*see also* condition
  hyperelastic 756.83
    acquired 701.8
  laxa 756.83
    senilis 701.8
  marmorata 782.61
  osteosis 709.3
  pendula 756.83
    acquired 701.8
  rhomboidalis nuchae 701.8
  verticis gyrata 757.39
    acquired 701.8
Cyanopathy, newborn 770.83
Cyanosis 782.5
  autotoxic 289.7
  common atrioventricular canal 745.69
  congenital 770.83
  conjunctiva 372.71
  due to
    endocardial cushion defect 745.60
    nonclosure, foramen botalli 745.5
    patent foramen botalli 745.5
    persistent foramen ovale 745.5
  enterogenous 289.7
  fetus or newborn 770.83
  ostium primum defect 745.61
  paroxysmal digital 443.0
  retina, retinal 362.10
Cycle
  anovulatory 628.0
  menstrual, irregular 626.4
Cyclencephaly 759.89

Cyclical vomiting 536.2
  associated with migraine 346.2
  psychogenic 306.4
Cyclitic membrane 364.74
Cyclitis (*see also* Iridocyclitis) 364.3
  acute 364.00
    primary 364.01
    recurrent 364.02
  chronic 364.10
    in
      sarcoidosis 135 *[364.11]*
      tuberculosis (*see also* Tuberculosis) 017.3
        [364.11]
  Fuchs' heterochromic 364.21
  granulomatous 364.10
  lens induced 364.23
  nongranulomatous 364.00
  posterior 363.21
  primary 364.01
  recurrent 364.02
  secondary (noninfectious) 364.04
    infectious 364.03
  subacute 364.00
    primary 364.01
    recurrent 364.02
Cyclokeratitis —*see* Keratitis
Cyclophoria 378.44
Cyclopia, cyclops 759.89
Cycloplegia 367.51
Cyclospasm 367.53
Cyclosporiasis 007.5
Cyclothymia 301.13
Cyclothymic personality 301.13
Cyclotropia 378.33
Cyesis —*see* Pregnancy
Cylindroma (M8200/3)—*see also* Neoplasm, by
  site, malignant
  eccrine dermal (M8200/0)—*see* Neoplasm, skin, benign
  skin (M8200/0)—*see* Neoplasm, skin, benign
Cylindruria 791.7
Cyllosoma 759.89
Cynanche
  diphtheritic 032.3
  tonsillaris 475
Cynorexia 783.6
Cyphosis —*see* Kyphosis
Cyprus fever (*see also* Brucellosis) 023.9
Cyriax's syndrome (slipping rib) 733.99
Cyst (mucus) (retention) (serous) (simple)

Note—*In general, cysts are not neoplastic and
are classified to the appropriate category for
disease of the specified anatomical site. This
generalization does not apply to certain types of
cysts which are neoplastic in nature, for
example, dermoid, nor does it apply to cysts of
certain structures, for example, branchial cleft,
which are classified as developmental
anomalies. The following listing includes some
of the most frequently reported sites of cysts as
well as qualifiers which indicate the type of cyst.
The latter qualifiers usually are not repeated
under the anatomical sites. Since the code
assignment for a given site may vary depending
upon the type of cyst, the coder should refer to
the listings under the specified type of cyst
before consideration is given to the site.*

---

  accessory, fallopian tube 752.11
  adenoid (infected) 474.8
  adrenal gland 255.8
    congenital 759.1

Cyst —*continued*
  air, lung 518.89
  allantoic 753.7
  alveolar process (jaw bone) 526.2
  amnion, amniotic 658.8
  anterior chamber (eye) 364.60
    exudative 364.62
    implantation (surgical) (traumatic) 364.61
    parasitic 360.13
  anterior nasopalatine 526.1
  antrum 478.19
  anus 569.49
  apical (periodontal) (tooth) 522.8
  appendix 543.9
  arachnoid, brain 348.0
  arytenoid 478.79
  auricle 706.2
  Baker's (knee) 727.51
    tuberculous (*see also* Tuberculosis) 015.2
  Bartholin's gland or duct 616.2
  bile duct (*see also* Disease, biliary) 576.8
  bladder (multiple) (trigone) 596.89
  Blessig's 362.62
  blood, endocardial (*see also* Endocarditis)
    424.90
  blue dome 610.0
  bone (local) 733.20
    aneurysmal 733.22
    jaw 526.2
      developmental (odontogenic) 526.0
      fissural 526.1
      latent 526.89
    solitary 733.21
    unicameral 733.21
  brain 348.0
    congenital 742.4
    hydatid (*see also* Echinococcus) 122.9
    third ventricle (colloid) 742.4
  branchial (cleft) 744.42
  branchiogenic 744.42
  breast (benign) (blue dome) (pedunculated)
    (solitary) (traumatic) 610.0
    involution 610.4
    sebaceous 610.8
  broad ligament (benign) 620.8
    embryonic 752.11
  bronchogenic (mediastinal) (sequestration)
    518.89
    congenital 748.4
  buccal 528.4
  bulbourethral gland (Cowper's) 599.89
  bursa, bursal 727.49
    pharyngeal 478.26
  calcifying odontogenic (M9301/0) 213.1
    upper jaw (bone) 213.0
  canal of Nuck (acquired) (serous) 629.1
    congenital 752.41
  canthus 372.75
  carcinomatous (M8010/3)—*see* Neoplasm, by
    site, malignant
  cartilage (joint)—*see* Derangement, joint
  cauda equina 336.8
  cavum septi pellucidi NEC 348.0
  celomic (pericardium) 746.89
  cerebellopontine (angle)—*see* Cyst, brain
  cerebellum—*see* Cyst, brain
  cerebral—*see* Cyst, brain
  cervical lateral 744.42
  cervix 622.8
    embryonal 752.41
    nabothian (gland) 616.0

Cyst —*continued*
  chamber, anterior (eye) 364.60
    exudative 364.62
    implantation (surgical) (traumatic) 364.61
    parasitic 360.13
  chiasmal, optic NEC (*see also* Lesion, chiasmal)
      377.54
  chocolate (ovary) 617.1
  choledochal (congenital) 751.69
    acquired 576.8
  choledochus 751.69
  chorion 658.8
  choroid plexus 348.0
  chyle, mesentery 457.8
  ciliary body 364.60
    exudative 364.64
    implantation 364.61
    primary 364.63
  clitoris 624.8
  coccyx (*see also* Cyst, bone) 733.20
  colloid
    third ventricle (brain) 742.4
    thyroid gland—*see* Goiter
  colon 569.89
  common (bile) duct (*see also* Disease, biliary)
      576.8
  congenital NEC 759.89
    adrenal glands 759.1
    epiglottis 748.3
    esophagus 750.4
    fallopian tube 752.11
    kidney 753.10
      multiple 753.19
      single 753.11
    larynx 748.3
    liver 751.62
    lung 748.4
    mediastinum 748.8
    ovary 752.0
    oviduct 752.11
    pancreas 751.7
    periurethral (tissue) 753.8
    prepuce NEC 752.69
      penis 752.69
    sublingual 750.26
    submaxillary gland 750.26
    thymus (gland) 759.2
    tongue 750.19
    ureterovesical orifice 753.4
    vulva 752.41
  conjunctiva 372.75
  cornea 371.23
  corpora quadrigemina 348.0
  corpus
    albicans (ovary) 620.2
    luteum (ruptured) 620.1
  Cowper's gland (benign) (infected) 599.89
  cranial meninges 348.0
  craniobuccal pouch 253.8
  craniopharyngeal pouch 253.8
  cystic duct (*see also* Disease, gallbladder) 575.8
  Cysticercus (any site) 123.1
  Dandy-Walker 742.3
    with spina bifida (*see also* Spina bifida) 741.0
  dental 522.8
    developmental 526.0
    eruption 526.0
    lateral periodontal 526.0
    primordial (keratocyst) 526.0
    root 522.8

Cyst —*continued*
  dentigerous 526.0
    mandible 526.0
    maxilla 526.0
  dermoid (M9084/0)—*see also* Neoplasm, by
      site, benign
    with malignant transformation (M9084/3)
        183.0
    implantation
      external area or site (skin) NEC 709.8
      iris 364.61
      skin 709.8
      vagina 623.8
      vulva 624.8
    mouth 528.4
    oral soft tissue 528.4
    sacrococcygeal 685.1
      with abscess 685.0
  developmental of ovary, ovarian 752.0
  dura (cerebral) 348.0
    spinal 349.2
  ear (external) 706.2
  echinococcal (*see also* Echinococcus) 122.9
  embryonal
    cervix uteri 752.41
    genitalia, female external 752.41
    uterus 752.39
    vagina 752.41
  endometrial 621.8
    ectopic 617.9
  endometrium (uterus) 621.8
    ectopic—*see* Endometriosis
  enteric 751.5
  enterogenous 751.5
  epidermal (inclusion) (*see also* Cyst, skin) 706.2
  epidermoid (inclusion) (*see also* Cyst, skin)
      706.2
    mouth 528.4
    not of skin—*see* Cyst, by site
    oral soft tissue 528.4
  epididymis 608.89
  epiglottis 478.79
  epiphysis cerebri 259.8
  epithelial (inclusion) (*see also* Cyst, skin) 706.2
  epoophoron 752.11
  eruption 526.0
  esophagus 530.89
  ethmoid sinus 478.19
  eye (retention) 379.8
    congenital 743.03
    posterior segment, congenital 743.54
  eyebrow 706.2
  eyelid (sebaceous) 374.84
    infected 373.13
    sweat glands or ducts 374.84
  falciform ligament (inflammatory) 573.8
  fallopian tube 620.8
    congenital 752.11
  female genital organs NEC 629.89
  fimbrial (congenital) 752.11
  fissural (oral region) 526.1
  follicle (atretic) (graafian) (ovarian) 620.0
    nabothian (gland) 616.0
  follicular (atretic) (ovarian) 620.0
    dentigerous 526.0
  frontal sinus 478.19
  gallbladder or duct 575.8
  ganglion 727.43
  Gartner's duct 752.41
  gas, of mesentery 568.89
  gingiva 523.8

Cyst —*continued*
  gland of moll 374.84
  globulomaxillary 526.1
  graafian follicle 620.0
  granulosal lutein 620.2
  hemangiomatous (M9121/0) (*see also*
    Hemangioma) 228.00
  hydatid (*see also* Echinococcus) 122.9
    fallopian tube (Morgagni) 752.11
    liver NEC 122.8
    lung NEC 122.9
    Morgagni 752.89
     fallopian tube 752.11
    specified site NEC 122.9
  hymen 623.8
    embryonal 752.41
  hypopharynx 478.26
  hypophysis, hypophyseal (duct) (recurrent)
    253.8
    cerebri 253.8
  implantation (dermoid)
    anterior chamber (eye) 364.61
    external area or site (skin) NEC 709.8
    iris 364.61
    vagina 623.8
    vulva 624.8
  incisor, incisive canal 526.1
  inclusion (epidermal) (epithelial) (epidermoid)
    (mucous) (squamous) (*see also* Cyst, skin)
    706.2
    not of skin—*see* Neoplasm, by site, benign
  intestine (large) (small) 569.89
  intracranial—*see* Cyst, brain
  intraligamentous 728.89
    knee 717.89
  intrasellar 253.8
  iris (idiopathic) 364.60
    exudative 364.62
    implantation (surgical) (traumatic) 364.61
    miotic pupillary 364.55
    parasitic 360.13
  Iwanoff's 362.62
  jaw (bone) (aneurysmal) (extravasation)
    (hemorrhagic) (traumatic) 526.2
    developmental (odontogenic) 526.0
    fissural 526.1
  keratin 706.2
  kidney (congenital) 753.10
    acquired 593.2
    calyceal (*see also* Hydronephrosis) 591
    multiple 753.19
    pyelogenic (*see also* Hydronephrosis) 591
    simple 593.2
    single 753.11
    solitary (not congenital) 593.2
  labium (majus) (minus) 624.8
    sebaceous 624.8
  lacrimal
    apparatus 375.43
    gland or sac 375.12
  larynx 478.79
  lens 379.39
    congenital 743.39
  lip (gland) 528.5
  liver 573.8
    congenital 751.62
    hydatid (*see also* Echinococcus) 122.8
     granulosis 122.0
     multilocularis 122.5

Cyst —*continued*
  lung 518.89
    congenital 748.4
    giant bullous 492.0
  lutein 620.1
  lymphangiomatous (M9173/0) 228.1
  lymphoepithelial
    mouth 528.4
    oral soft tissue 528.4
  macula 362.54
  malignant (M8000/3)—*see* Neoplasm, by site,
    malignant
  mammary gland (sweat gland) (*see also* Cyst,
    breast) 610.0
  mandible 526.2
    dentigerous 526.0
    radicular 522.8
  maxilla 526.2
    dentigerous 526.0
    radicular 522.8
  median
    anterior maxillary 526.1
    palatal 526.1
  mediastinum (congenital) 748.8
  meibomian (gland) (retention) 373.2
    infected 373.12
  membrane, brain 348.0
  meninges (cerebral) 348.0
    spinal 349.2
  meniscus knee 717.5
  mesentery, mesenteric (gas) 568.89
    chyle 457.8
    gas 568.89
  mesonephric duct 752.89
  mesothelial
    peritoneum 568.89
    pleura (peritoneal) 568.89
  milk 611.5
  miotic pupillary (iris) 364.55
  Morgagni (hydatid) 752.89
    fallopian tube 752.11
  mouth 528.4
  Müllerian duct 752.89
    appendix testis 608.89
    cervix (embryonal) 752.41
    fallopian tube 752.11
    prostatic utricle 599.89
    vagina (embryonal) 752.41
  multilocular (ovary) (M8000/1) 239.5
  myometrium 621.8
  nabothian (follicle) (ruptured) 616.0
  nasal sinus 478.19
  nasoalveolar 528.4
  nasolabial 528.4
  nasopalatine (duct) 526.1
    anterior 526.1
  nasopharynx 478.26
  neoplastic (M8000/1)—*see also* Neoplasm, by
    site, unspecified nature
    benign (M8000/0)—*see* Neoplasm, by site, benign
    uterus 621.8
  nervous system—*see* Cyst, brain
  neuroenteric 742.59
  neuroepithelial ventricle 348.0
  nipple 610.0
  nose 478.19
    skin of 706.2
  odontogenic, developmental 526.0
  omentum (lesser) 568.89
    congenital 751.8

Cyst —*continued*
oral soft tissue (dermoid) (epidermoid)
    (lymphoepithelial) 528.4
ora serrata 361.19
orbit 376.81
ovary, ovarian (twisted) 620.2
    adherent 620.2
    chocolate 617.1
    corpus
        albicans 620.2
        luteum 620.1
    dermoid (M9084/0) 220
    developmental 752.0
    due to failure of involution NEC 620.2
    endometrial 617.1
    follicular (atretic) (graafian) (hemorrhagic)
        620.0
    hemorrhagic 620.2
    in pregnancy or childbirth 654.4
        affecting fetus or newborn 763.89
        causing obstructed labor 660.2
            affecting fetus or newborn 763.1
    multilocular (M8000/1) 239.5
    pseudomucinous (M8470/0) 220
    retention 620.2
    serous 620.2
    theca lutein 620.2
    tuberculous (*see also* Tuberculosis) 016.6
    unspecified 620.2
oviduct 620.8
palatal papilla (jaw) 526.1
palate 526.1
    fissural 526.1
    median (fissural) 526.1
palatine, of papilla 526.1
pancreas, pancreatic 577.2
    congenital 751.7
    false 577.2
    hemorrhagic 577.2
    true 577.2
paralabral
    hip 718.85
    shoulder 840.7
paramesonephric duct - see Cyst, Müllerian duct
paranephric 593.2
para ovarian 752.11
paraphysis, cerebri 742.4
parasitic NEC 136.9
parathyroid (gland) 252.8
paratubal (fallopian) 620.8
paraurethral duct 599.89
paroophoron 752.11
parotid gland 527.6
    mucous extravasation or retention 527.6
parovarian 752.11
pars planus 364.60
    exudative 364.64
    primary 364.63
pelvis, female
    in pregnancy or childbirth 654.4
        affecting fetus or newborn 763.89
        causing obstructed labor 660.2
            affecting fetus or newborn 763.1
penis (sebaceous) 607.89
periapical 522.8
pericardial (congenital) 746.89
    acquired (secondary) 423.8
pericoronal 526.0
perineural (Tarlov's) 355.9
periodontal 522.8
    lateral 526.0

Cyst —*continued*
peripancreatic 577.2
peripelvic (lymphatic) 593.2
peritoneum 568.89
    chylous 457.8
pharynx (wall) 478.26
pilar 704.41
pilonidal (infected) (rectum) 685.1
    with abscess 685.0
    malignant (M9084/3) 173.59
pituitary (duct) (gland) 253.8
placenta (amniotic)—*see* Placenta, abnormal
pleura 519.8
popliteal 727.51
porencephalic 742.4
    acquired 348.0
postanal (infected) 685.1
    with abscess 685.0
posterior segment of eye, congenital 743.54
postmastoidectomy cavity 383.31
preauricular 744.47
prepuce 607.89
    congenital 752.69
primordial (jaw) 526.0
prostate 600.3
pseudomucinous (ovary) (M8470/0) 220
pudenda (sweat glands) 624.8
pupillary, miotic 364.55
    sebaceous 624.8
radicular (residual) 522.8
radiculodental 522.8
ranular 527.6
Rathke's pouch 253.8
rectum (epithelium) (mucous) 569.49
renal—*see* Cyst, kidney
residual (radicular) 522.8
retention (ovary) 620.2
retina 361.19
    macular 362.54
    parasitic 360.13
    primary 361.13
    secondary 361.14
retroperitoneal 568.89
sacrococcygeal (dermoid) 685.1
    with abscess 685.0
salivary gland or duct 527.6
    mucous extravasation or retention 527.6
Sampson's 617.1
sclera 379.19
scrotum (sebaceous) 706.2
    sweat glands 706.2
sebaceous (duct) (gland) 706.2
    breast 610.8
    eyelid 374.84
    genital organ NEC
        female 629.89
        male 608.89
    scrotum 706.2
semilunar cartilage (knee) (multiple) 717.5
seminal vesicle 608.89
serous (ovary) 620.2
sinus (antral) (ethmoidal) (frontal) (maxillary)
    (nasal) (sphenoidal) 478.19
Skene's gland 599.89
skin (epidermal) (epidermoid, inclusion)
    (epithelial) (inclusion) (retention)
    (sebaceous) 706.2
    breast 610.8
    eyelid 374.84
    genital organ NEC
        female 629.89
        male 608.89

Cyst —*continued*
neoplastic 216.3
scrotum 706.2
sweat gland or duct 705.89
solitary
bone 733.21
kidney 593.2
spermatic cord 608.89
sphenoid sinus 478.19
spinal meninges 349.2
spine (*see also* Cyst, bone) 733.20
spleen NEC 289.59
congenital 759.0
hydatid (*see also* Echinococcus) 122.9
spring water (pericardium) 746.89
subarachnoid 348.0
intrasellar 793.0
subdural (cerebral) 348.0
spinal cord 349.2
sublingual gland 527.6
mucous extravasation or retention 527.6
submaxillary gland 527.6
mucous extravasation or retention 527.6
suburethral 599.89
suprarenal gland 255.8
suprasellar—*see* Cyst, brain
sweat gland or duct 705.89
sympathetic nervous system 337.9
synovial 727.40
popliteal space 727.51
Tarlov's 355.9
tarsal 373.2
tendon (sheath) 727.42
testis 608.89
theca-lutein (ovary) 620.2
Thornwaldt's, Tornwaldt's 478.26
thymus (gland) 254.8
thyroglossal (duct) (infected) (persistent) 759.2
thyroid (gland) 246.2
adenomatous—*see* Goiter, nodular
colloid (*see also* Goiter) 240.9
thyrolingual duct (infected) (persistent) 759.2
tongue (mucous) 529.8
tonsil 474.8
tooth (dental root) 522.8
trichilemmal (proliferating) 704.42
tubo-ovarian 620.8
inflammatory 614.1
tunica vaginalis 608.89
turbinate (nose) (*see also* Cyst, bone) 733.20
Tyson's gland (benign) (infected) 607.89
umbilicus 759.89
urachus 753.7
ureter 593.89
ureterovesical orifice 593.89
congenital 753.4
urethra 599.84
urethral gland (Cowper's) 599.89
uterine
ligament 620.8
embryonic 752.11
tube 620.8
uterus (body) (corpus) (recurrent) 621.8
embryonal 752.39
utricle (ear) 386.8
prostatic 599.89
utriculus masculinus 599.89
vagina, vaginal (squamous cell) (wall) 623.8
embryonal 752.41
implantation 623.8
inclusion 623.8

Cyst —*continued*
vallecula, vallecular 478.79
ventricle, neuroepithelial 348.0
verumontanum 599.89
vesical (orifice) 596.89
vitreous humor 379.29
vulva (sweat glands) 624.8
congenital 752.41
implantation 624.8
inclusion 624.8
sebaceous gland 624.8
vulvovaginal gland 624.8
wolffian 752.89
Cystadenocarcinoma (M8440/3)—*see also*
Neoplasm, by site, malignant
bile duct type (M8161/3) 155.1
endometrioid (M8380/3)—*see* Neoplasm, by
site, malignant
mucinous (M8470/3)
papillary (M8471/3)
specified site—*see* Neoplasm, by site,
malignant
unspecified site 183.0
specified site—*see* Neoplasm, by site,
malignant
unspecified site 183.0
papillary (M8450/3)
mucinous (M8471/3)
specified site—*see* Neoplasm, by site,
malignant
unspecified site 183.0
pseudomucinous (M8471/3)
specified site—*see* Neoplasm, by site,
malignant
unspecified site 183.0
serous (M8460/3)
specified site—*see* Neoplasm, by site,
malignant
unspecified site 183.0
specified site—*see* Neoplasm, by site,
malignant
unspecified 183.0
pseudomucinous (M8470/3)
papillary (M8471/3)
specified site—*see* Neoplasm, by site,
malignant
unspecified site 183.0
specified site—*see* Neoplasm, by site,
malignant
unspecified site 183.0
serous (M8441/3)
papillary (M8460/3)
specified site—*see* Neoplasm, by site,
malignant
unspecified site 183.0
specified site—*see* Neoplasm, by site,
malignant
unspecified site 183.0
Cystadenofibroma (M9013/0)
clear cell (M8313/0)—*see* Neoplasm, by site,
benign
endometrioid (M8381/0) 220
borderline malignancy (M8381/1) 236.2
malignant (M8381/3) 183.0
mucinous (M9015/0)
specified site—*see* Neoplasm, by site, benign
unspecified site 220
serous (M9014/0)
specified site—*see* Neoplasm, by site, benign
unspecified site 220
specified site—*see* Neoplasm, by site, benign
unspecified site 220

Cystadenoma (M8440/0)—*see also* Neoplasm,
  by site, benign
  bile duct (M8161/0) 211.5
  endometrioid (M8380/0)—*see also* Neoplasm,
    by site, benign
    borderline malignancy (M8380/1)—*see*
      Neoplasm, by site, uncertain behavior
  malignant (M8440/3)—*see* Neoplasm, by site,
    malignant
  mucinous (M8470/0)
    borderline malignancy (M8470/1)
      specified site—*see* Neoplasm, uncertain
        behavior
      unspecified site 236.2
    papillary (M8471/0)
      borderline malignancy (M8471/1)
        specified site—*see* Neoplasm, by site,
          uncertain behavior
        unspecified site 236.2
      specified site—*see* Neoplasm, by site,
        benign
      unspecified site 220
    specified site—*see* Neoplasm, by site, benign
    unspecified site 220
  papillary (M8450/0)
    borderline malignancy (M8450/1)
      specified site—*see* Neoplasm, by site,
        uncertain behavior
      unspecified site 236.2
    lymphomatosum (M8561/0) 210.2
    mucinous (M8471/0)
      borderline malignancy (M8471/1)
        specified site—*see* Neoplasm, by site,
          uncertain behavior
        unspecified site 236.2
      specified site—*see* Neoplasm, by site,
        benign
      unspecified site 220
    pseudomucinous (M8471/0)
      borderline malignancy (M8471/1)
        specified site—*see* Neoplasm, by site,
          uncertain behavior
        unspecified site 236.2
      specified site—*see* Neoplasm, by site,
        benign
      unspecified site 220
    serous (M8460/0)
      borderline malignancy (M8460/1)
        specified site—*see* Neoplasm, by site,
          uncertain behavior
        unspecified site 236.2
      specified site—*see* Neoplasm, by site,
        benign
      unspecified site 220
    specified site—*see* Neoplasm, by site, benign
    unspecified site 220
  pseudomucinous (M8470/0)
    borderline malignancy (M8470/1)
      specified site—*see* Neoplasm, by site,
        uncertain behavior
      unspecified site 236.2
    papillary (M8471/0)
      borderline malignancy (M8471/1)
        specified site—*see* Neoplasm, by site,
          uncertain behavior
        unspecified site 236.2
      specified site—*see* Neoplasm, by site,
        benign
      unspecified site 220
    specified site—*see* Neoplasm, by site, benign
    unspecified site 220

Cystadenoma—*continued*
  serous (M8441/0)
    borderline malignancy (M8441/1)
      specified site—*see* Neoplasm, by site,
        uncertain behavior
      unspecified site 236.2
    papillary (M8460/0)
      borderline malignancy (M8460/1)
        specified site—*see* Neoplasm, by site,
          uncertain behavior
        unspecified site 236.2
      specified site—*see* Neoplasm, by site,
        benign
      unspecified site 220
    specified site—*see* Neoplasm, by site, benign
    unspecified site 220
  thyroid 226
Cystathioninemia 270.4
Cystathioninuria 270.4
Cystic —*see also* condition
  breast, chronic 610.1
  corpora lutea 620.1
  degeneration, congenital
    brain 742.4
    kidney (*see also* Cystic, disease, kidney)
      753.10
  disease
    breast, chronic 610.1
    kidney, congenital 753.10
      medullary 753.16
      multiple 753.19
      polycystic—*see* Polycystic, kidney
      single 753.11
      specified NEC 753.19
    liver, congenital 751.62
    lung 518.89
      congenital 748.4
    pancreas, congenital 751.7
    semilunar cartilage 717.5
  duct—*see* condition
  eyeball, congenital 743.03
  fibrosis (pancreas) 277.00
    with
      manifestations
        gastrointestinal 277.03
        pulmonary 277.02
        specified NEC 277.09
      meconium ileus 277.01
      pulmonary exacerbation 277.02
  hygroma (M9173/0) 228.1
  kidney, congenital 753.10
    medullary 753.16
    multiple 753.19
    polycystic—*see* Polycystic, kidney
    single 753.11
    specified NEC 753.19
  liver, congenital 751.62
  lung 518.89
    congenital 748.4
  mass—*see* Cyst
  mastitis, chronic 610.1
  ovary 620.2
  pancreas, congenital 751.7
Cysticerciasis 123.1
Cysticercosis (mammary) (subretinal) 123.1
Cysticercus 123.1
  cellulosae infestation 123.1
Cystinosis (malignant) 270.0
Cystinuria 270.0

Cystitis (bacillary) (colli) (diffuse) (exudative) (hemorrhagic) (purulent) (recurrent) (septic) (suppurative) (ulcerative) 595.9
  with
    abortion—*see* Abortion, by type, with urinary tract infection
    ectopic pregnancy (*see also* categories 633.0-633.9) 639.8
    fibrosis 595.1
    leukoplakia 595.1
    malakoplakia 595.1
    metaplasia 595.1
    molar pregnancy (*see also* categories 630-632) 639.8
  actinomycotic 039.8 *[595.4]*
  acute 595.0
    of trigone 595.3
  allergic 595.89
  amebic 006.8 *[595.4]*
  bilharzial 120.9 *[595.4]*
  blennorrhagic (acute) 098.11
    chronic or duration of 2 months or more 098.31
  bullous 595.89
  calculous 594.1
  chlamydial 099.53
  chronic 595.2
    interstitial 595.1
    of trigone 595.3
  complicating pregnancy, childbirth, or puerperium 646.6
    affecting fetus or newborn 760.1
  cystic(a) 595.81
  diphtheritic 032.84
  echinococcal
    granulosus 122.3 *[595.4]*
    multilocularis 122.6 *[595.4]*
  emphysematous 595.89
  encysted 595.81
  follicular 595.3
  following
    abortion 639.8
    ectopic or molar pregnancy 639.8
  gangrenous 595.89
  glandularis 595.89
  gonococcal (acute) 098.11
    chronic or duration of 2 months or more 098.31
  incrusted 595.89
  interstitial 595.1
  irradiation 595.82
  irritation 595.89
  malignant 595.89
  monilial 112.2
  of trigone 595.3
  panmural 595.1
  polyposa 595.89
  prostatic 601.3
  radiation 595.82
  Reiter's (abacterial) 099.3
  specified NEC 595.89
  subacute 595.2
  submucous 595.1
  syphilitic 095.8
  trichomoniasis 131.09
  tuberculous (*see also* Tuberculosis) 016.1
  ulcerative 595.1

Cystocele
  female (without uterine prolapse) 618.01
    with uterine prolapse 618.4
      complete 618.3
      incomplete 618.2
    lateral 618.02
    midline 618.01
    paravaginal 618.02
  in pregnancy or childbirth 654.4
    affecting fetus or newborn 763.89
    causing obstructed labor 660.2
      affecting fetus or newborn 763.1
  male 596.89
Cystoid
  cicatrix limbus 372.64
  degeneration macula 362.53
Cystolithiasis 594.1
Cystoma (M8440/0)—*see also* Neoplasm, by site, benign
  endometrial, ovary 617.1
  mucinous (M8470/0)
    specified site—*see* Neoplasm, by site, benign
    unspecified site 220
  serous (M8441/0)
    specified site—*see* Neoplasm, by site, benign
    unspecified site 220
  simple (ovary) 620.2
Cystoplegia 596.53
Cystoptosis 596.89
Cystopyelitis (*see also* Pyelitis) 590.80
Cystorrhagia 596.89
Cystosarcoma phyllodes (M9020/1) 238.3
  benign (M9020/0) 217
  malignant (M9020/3)—*see* Neoplasm, breast, malignant
Cystostomy status V44.50
  appendico-vesicostomy V44.52
  cutaneous-vesicostomy V44.51
  specified type NEC V44.59
  with complication 596.83
    infection 596.81
    mechanical 596.82
    specified complication NEC 596.83
Cystourethritis (*see also* Urethritis) 597.89
Cystourethrocele (*see also* Cystocele)
  female (without uterine prolapse) 618.09
    with uterine prolapse 618.4
      complete 618.3
      incomplete 618.2
  male 596.89
Cytomegalic inclusion disease 078.5
  congenital 771.1
Cytomycosis, reticuloendothelial (*see also* Histoplasmosis, American) 115.00
Cytopenia 289.9
  refractory
    with
      multilineage dysplasia (RCMD) 238.72
      and ringed sideroblasts (RCMD-RS) 238.72

D

Daae (-Finsen) disease (epidemic pleurodynia) 074.1
Dabney's grip 074.1
Da Costa's syndrome (neurocirculatory asthenia) 306.2
Dacryoadenitis, dacryadenitis 375.00
  acute 375.01
  chronic 375.02
Dacryocystitis 375.30
  acute 375.32
  chronic 375.42
  neonatal 771.6
  phlegmonous 375.33
  syphilitic 095.8
    congenital 090.0
  trachomatous, active 076.1
    late effect 139.1
  tuberculous (see also Tuberculosis) 017.3
Dacryocystoblennorrhea 375.42
Dacryocystocele 375.43
Dacryolith, dacryolithiasis 375.57
Dacryoma 375.43
Dacryopericystitis (acute) (subacute) 375.32
  chronic 375.42
Dacryops 375.11
Dacryosialadenopathy, atrophic 710.2
Dacryostenosis 375.56
  congenital 743.65
Dactylitis
  bone (see also Osteomyelitis) 730.2
  sickle-cell 282.62
    Hb-C 282.64
    Hb-SS 282.62
    specified NEC 282.69
  syphilitic 095.5
  tuberculous (see also Tuberculosis) 015.5
Dactylolysis spontanea 136.0
Dactylosymphysis (see also Syndactylism) 755.10
Damage
  arteriosclerotic—see Arteriosclerosis
  brain 348.9
    anoxic, hypoxic 348.1
      during or resulting from a procedure 997.01
    ischemic, in newborn 768.70
      mild 768.71
      moderate 768.72
      severe 768.73
    child NEC 343.9
    due to birth injury 767.0
    minimal (child) (see also Hyperkinesia) 314.9
    newborn 767.0
  cardiac—see also Disease, heart
  cardiorenal (vascular) (see also Hypertension, cardiorenal) 404.90
  central nervous system—see Damage, brain
  cerebral NEC—see Damage, brain
  coccyx, complicating delivery 665.6
  coronary (see also Ischemia, heart) 414.9
  eye, birth injury 767.8
  heart—see also Disease, heart
    valve—see Endocarditis
  hypothalamus NEC 348.9
  liver 571.9
    alcoholic 571.3
  medication 995.20

Damage—continued
  myocardium (see also Degeneration, myocardial) 429.1
  pelvic
    joint or ligament, during delivery 665.6
    organ NEC
      with
        abortion—see Abortion, by type, with damage to pelvic organs
        ectopic pregnancy (see also categories 633.0-633.9) 639.2
        molar pregnancy (see also categories 630-632) 639.2
      during delivery 665.5
      following
        abortion 639.2
        ectopic or molar pregnancy 639.2
  renal (see also Disease, renal) 593.9
  skin, solar 692.79
    acute 692.72
    chronic 692.74
  subendocardium, subendocardial (see also Degeneration, myocardial) 429.1
  vascular 459.9
Dameshek's syndrome (erythroblastic anemia) 282.49
Dana-Putnam syndrome (subacute combined sclerosis with pernicious anemia) 281.0 *[336.2]*
Danbolt (-Closs) syndrome (acrodermatitis enteropathica) 686.8
Dandruff 690.18
Dandy fever 061
Dandy-Walker deformity or syndrome (atresia, foramen of Magendie) 742.3
  with spina bifida (see also Spina bifida) 741.0
Dangle foot 736.79
Danielssen's disease (anesthetic leprosy) 030.1
Danlos' syndrome 756.83
Darier's disease (congenital) (keratosis follicularis) 757.39
  due to vitamin A deficiency 264.8
  meaning erythema annulare centrifugum 695.0
Darier-Roussy sarcoid 135
Dark area on retina 239.81
Darling's
  disease (see also Histoplasmosis, American) 115.00
  histoplasmosis (see also Histoplasmosis, American) 115.00
Dartre 054.9
Darwin's tubercle 744.29
Davidson's anemia (refractory) 284.9
Davies' disease 425.0
Davies-Colley syndrome (slipping rib) 733.99
Dawson's encephalitis 046.2
Day blindness (see also Blindness, day) 368.60
Dead
  fetus
    retained (in utero) 656.4
      early pregnancy (death before 22 completed weeks gestation) 632
      late (death after 22 completed weeks gestation) 656.4
    syndrome 641.3
  labyrinth 386.50
  ovum, retained 631.8

Deaf and dumb NEC 389.7
Deaf mutism (acquired) (congenital) NEC 389.7
  endemic 243
  hysterical 300.11
  syphilitic, congenital 090.0
Deafness (acquired) (complete) (congenital)
  (hereditary) (middle ear) (partial) 389.9
  with
    blindness V49.85
    blue sclera and fragility of bone 756.51
  auditory fatigue 389.9
  aviation 993.0
    nerve injury 951.5
  boilermakers' 951.5
  central 389.14
    with conductive hearing loss 389.20
      bilateral 389.22
      unilateral 389.21
  conductive (air) 389.00
    with sensorineural hearing loss 389.20
      bilateral 389.22
      unilateral 389.21
    bilateral 389.06
    combined types 389.08
    external ear 389.01
    inner ear 389.04
    middle ear 389.03
    multiple types 389.08
    tympanic membrane 389.02
    unilateral 389.05
  emotional (complete) 300.11
  functional (complete) 300.11
  high frequency 389.8
  hysterical (complete) 300.11
  injury 951.5
  low frequency 389.8
  mental 784.69
  mixed conductive and sensorineural 389.20
    bilateral 389.22
    unilateral 389.21
  nerve
    with conductive hearing loss 389.20
      bilateral 389.22
      unilateral 389.21
    bilateral 389.12
    unilateral 389.13
  neural
    with conductive hearing loss 389.20
      bilateral 389.22
      unilateral 389.21
    bilateral 389.12
    unilateral 389.13
  noise-induced 388.12
    nerve injury 951.5
  nonspeaking 389.7
  perceptive 389.10
    with conductive hearing loss 389.20
      bilateral 389.22
      unilateral 389.21
    central 389.14
    neural
      bilateral 389.12
      unilateral 389.13
    sensorineural 389.10
      asymmetrical 389.16
      bilateral 389.18
      unilateral 389.15
    sensory
      bilateral 389.11
      unilateral 389.17
  psychogenic (complete) 306.7

Deafness—*continued*
  sensorineural (*see also* Deafness, perceptive)
    389.10
    asymmetrical 389.16
    bilateral 389.18
    unilateral 389.15
  sensory
    with conductive hearing loss 389.20
      bilateral 389.22
      unilateral 389.21
    bilateral 389.11
    unilateral 389.17
  specified type NEC 389.8
  sudden NEC 388.2
  syphilitic 094.89
  transient ischemic 388.02
  transmission—*see* Deafness, conductive
  traumatic 951.5
  word (secondary to organic lesion) 784.69
    developmental 315.31
Death
  after delivery (cause not stated) (sudden) 674.9
  anesthetic
    due to
      correct substance properly administered
        995.4
      overdose or wrong substance given 968.4
        specified anesthetic—*see* Table of drugs
          and chemicals
    during delivery 668.9
  brain 348.82
  cardiac (sudden) (SCD)—code to underlying
    condition
    family history of V17.41
    personal history of, successfully resuscitated
      V12.53
  cause unknown 798.2
  cot (infant) 798.0
  crib (infant) 798.0
  fetus, fetal (cause not stated) (intrauterine) 779.9
    early, with retention (before 22 completed
      weeks gestation) 632
    from asphyxia or anoxia (before labor) 768.0
      during labor 768.1
    late, affecting management of pregnancy (after
      22 completed weeks gestation) 656.4
  from pregnancy NEC 646.9
  instantaneous 798.1
  intrauterine (*see also* Death, fetus) 779.9
    complicating pregnancy 656.4
  maternal, affecting fetus or newborn 761.6
  neonatal NEC 779.9
  sudden (cause unknown) 798.1
    cardiac (SCD)
      family history of V17.41
      personal history of, successfully resuscitated
        V12.53
    during delivery 669.9
      under anesthesia NEC 668.9
    infant, syndrome (SIDS) 798.0
    puerperal, during puerperium 674.9
  unattended (cause unknown) 798.9
  under anesthesia NEC
    due to
      correct substance properly administered
        995.4
      overdose or wrong substance given 968.4
        specified anesthetic—*see* Table of drugs
          and chemicals
    during delivery 668.9
  violent 798.1

de Beurmann-Gougerot disease (sporotrichosis)
117.1
Debility (general) (infantile) (postinfectional)
799.3
  with nutritional difficulty 269.9
  congenital or neonatal NEC 779.9
  nervous 300.5
  old age 797
  senile 797
Débove's disease (splenomegaly) 789.2
Decalcification
  bone (*see also* Osteoporosis) 733.00
  teeth 521.89
Decapitation 874.9
  fetal (to facilitate delivery) 763.89
Decapsulation, kidney 593.89
Decay
  dental 521.00
  senile 797
  tooth, teeth 521.00
Decensus, uterus —*see* Prolapse, uterus
Deciduitis (acute)
  with
    abortion—*see* Abortion, by type, with sepsis
    ectopic pregnancy (*see also* categories
      633.0-633.9) 639.0
    molar pregnancy (*see also* categories 630-632)
      639.0
  affecting fetus or newborn 760.8
  following
    abortion 639.0
    ectopic or molar pregnancy 639.0
  in pregnancy 646.6
  puerperal, postpartum 670.1
Deciduoma malignum (M9100/3) 181
Deciduous tooth (retained) 520.6
Decline (general) (*see also* Debility) 799.3
Decompensation
  cardiac (acute) (chronic) (*see also* Disease,
    heart) 429.9
    failure—*see* Failure, heart
  cardiorenal (*see also* Hypertension, cardiorenal)
    404.90
  cardiovascular (*see also* Disease,
    cardiovascular) 429.2
  heart (*see also* Disease, heart) 429.9
    failure—*see* Failure, heart
  hepatic 572.2
  myocardial (acute) (chronic) (*see also* Disease,
    heart) 429.9
    failure—*see* Failure, heart
  respiratory 519.9
Decompression sickness 993.3
Decrease, decreased
  blood
    platelets (*see also* Thrombocytopenia) 287.5
    pressure 796.3
      due to shock following
        injury 958.4
        operation 998.00
    white cell count 288.50
      specified NEC 288.59
  cardiac reserve—*see* Disease, heart
  estrogen 256.39
    postablative 256.2
  fetal movements 655.7
  fragility of erythrocytes 289.89
  function
    adrenal (cortex) 255.41
      medulla 255.5
    ovary in hypopituitarism 253.4

Decrease, decreased—*continued*
    parenchyma of pancreas 577.8
    pituitary (gland) (lobe) (anterior) 253.2
      posterior (lobe) 253.8
  functional activity 780.99
  glucose 790.29
  haptoglobin (serum) NEC 273.8
  leukocytes 288.50
  libido 799.81
  lymphocytes 288.51
  platelets (*see also* Thrombocytopenia) 287.5
  pulse pressure 785.9
  respiration due to shock following injury 958.4
  sexual desire 799.81
  tear secretion NEC 375.15
  tolerance
    fat 579.8
    salt and water 276.9
  vision NEC 369.9
  white blood cell count 288.50
Decubital gangrene (*see also* Ulcer, pressure)
  707.00 *[785.4]*
Decubiti (*see also* Ulcer, pressure) 707.00
Decubitus (ulcer) (*see also* Ulcer, pressure)
  707.00
  with gangrene 707.00 *[785.4]*
  ankle 707.06
  back
    lower 707.03
    upper 707.02
  buttock 707.05
  coccyx 707.03
  elbow 707.01
  head 707.09
  heel 707.07
  hip 707.04
  other site 707.09
  sacrum 707.03
  shoulder blades 707.02
Deepening acetabulum 718.85
Defect, defective 759.9
  3-beta-hydroxysteroid dehydrogenase 255.2
  11-hydroxylase 255.2
  21-hydroxylase 255.2
  abdominal wall, congenital 756.70
  aorticopulmonary septum 745.0
  aortic septal 745.0
  atrial septal (ostium secundum type) 745.5
    acquired 429.71
    ostium primum type 745.61
    sinus venosus 745.8
  atrioventricular
    canal 745.69
    septum 745.4
      acquired 429.71
  atrium secundum 745.5
    acquired 429.71
  auricular septal 745.5
    acquired 429.71
  bilirubin excretion 277.4
  biosynthesis, testicular androgen 257.2
  bridge 525.60
  bulbar septum 745.0
  butanol-insoluble iodide 246.1
  chromosome—*see* Anomaly, chromosome
  circulation (acquired) 459.9
    congenital 747.9
    newborn 747.9
  clotting NEC (*see also* Defect, coagulation)
    286.9

Defect, defective—*continued*
coagulation (factor) (*see also* Deficiency,
coagulation factor) 286.9
with
abortion—*see* Abortion, by type, with
hemorrhage
ectopic pregnancy (*see also* categories
634-638) 639.1
molar pregnancy (*see also* categories
630-632) 639.1
acquired (any) 286.7
antepartum or intrapartum 641.3
affecting fetus or newborn 762.1
causing hemorrhage of pregnancy or delivery
641.3
complicating pregnancy, childbirth, or the
puerperium 649.3
due to
liver disease 286.7
vitamin K deficiency 286.7
newborn, transient 776.3
postpartum 666.3
specified type NEC 286.9
conduction (heart) 426.9
bone (*see also* Deafness, conductive) 389.00
congenital, organ or site NEC—*see also*
Anomaly
circulation 747.9
Descemet's membrane 743.9
specified type NEC 743.49
diaphragm 756.6
ectodermal 757.9
esophagus 750.9
pulmonic cusps—*see* Anomaly, heart valve
respiratory system 748.9
specified type NEC 748.8
crown 525.60
cushion endocardial 745.60
dental restoration 525.60
dentin (hereditary) 520.5
Descemet's membrane (congenital) 743.9
acquired 371.30
specific type NEC 743.49
deutan 368.52
developmental—*see also* Anomaly, by site
cauda equina 742.59
left ventricle 746.9
with atresia or hypoplasia of aortic orifice or
valve, with hypoplasia of ascending
aorta 746.7
in hypoplastic left heart syndrome 746.7
testis 752.9
vessel 747.9
diaphragm
with elevation, eventration, or hernia—*see*
Hernia, diaphragm
congenital 756.6
with elevation, eventration, or hernia 756.6
gross (with elevation, eventration, or hernia)
756.6
ectodermal, congenital 757.9
Eisenmenger's (ventricular septal defect) 745.4
endocardial cushion 745.60
specified type NEC 745.69
esophagus, congenital 750.9
extensor retinaculum 728.9
fibrin polymerization (*see also* Defect,
coagulation) 286.3

Defect, defective—*continued*
filling
biliary tract 793.3
bladder 793.5
dental 525.60
gallbladder 793.3
kidney 793.5
stomach 793.4
ureter 793.5
fossa ovalis 745.5
gene, carrier (suspected) of V83.89
Gerbode 745.4
glaucomatous, without elevated tension 365.89
Hageman (factor) (*see also* Defect, coagulation)
286.3
hearing (*see also* Deafness) 389.9
high grade 317
homogentisic acid 270.2
interatrial septal 745.5
acquired 429.71
interauricular septal 745.5
acquired 429.71
interventricular septal 745.4
with pulmonary stenosis or atresia,
dextroposition of aorta, and hypertrophy of
right ventricle 745.2
acquired 429.71
in tetralogy of Fallot 745.2
iodide trapping 246.1
iodotyrosine dehalogenase 246.1
kynureninase 270.2
learning, specific 315.2
major osseous 731.3
mental (*see also* Disability, intellectual) 319
osseous, major 731.3
osteochondral NEC 738.8
ostium
primum 745.61
secundum 745.5
pericardium 746.89
peroxidase-binding 246.1
placental blood supply—*see* Placenta,
insufficiency
platelet (qualitative) 287.1
constitutional 286.4
postural, spine 737.9
protan 368.51
pulmonic cusps, congenital 746.00
renal pelvis 753.9
obstructive 753.29
specified type NEC 753.3
respiratory system, congenital 748.9
specified type NEC 748.8
retina, retinal 361.30
with detachment (*see also* Detachment, retina,
with retinal defect) 361.00
multiple 361.33
with detachment 361.02
nerve fiber bundle 362.85
single 361.30
with detachment 361.01
septal (closure) (heart) NEC 745.9
acquired 429.71
atrial 745.5
specified type NEC 745.8
speech NEC 784.59
developmental 315.39
late effect of cerebrovascular disease — *see*
Late effect(s) (of) cerebrovascular disease,
speech and language deficit
secondary to organic lesion 784.59

Defect, defective—*continued*
Taussig-Bing (transposition, aorta and
overriding pulmonary artery) 745.11
teeth, wedge 521.20
thyroid hormone synthesis 246.1
tritan 368.53
ureter 753.9
obstructive 753.29
vascular (acquired) (local) 459.9
congenital (peripheral) NEC 747.60
gastrointestinal 747.61
lower limb 747.64
renal 747.62
specified NEC 747.69
spinal 747.82
upper limb 747.63
ventricular septal 745.4
with pulmonary stenosis or atresia,
dextraposition of aorta, and hypertrophy of
right ventricle 745.2
acquired 429.71
atrioventricular canal type 745.69
between infundibulum and anterior portion
745.4
in tetralogy of Fallot 745.2
isolated anterior 745.4
vision NEC 369.9
visual field 368.40
arcuate 368.43
heteronymous, bilateral 368.47
homonymous, bilateral 368.46
localized NEC 368.44
nasal step 368.44
peripheral 368.44
sector 368.43
voice and resonance 784.40
wedge, teeth (abrasion) 521.20
Defeminization syndrome 255.2
Deferentitis 608.4
gonorrheal (acute) 098.14
chronic or duration of 2 months or over 098.34
Defibrination syndrome (*see also* Fibrinolysis)
286.6
Deficiency, deficient
3-beta-hydroxysteroid dehydrogenase 255.2
6-phosphogluconic dehydrogenase (anemia)
282.2
11-beta-hydroxylase 255.2
17-alpha-hydroxylase 255.2
18-hydroxysteroid dehydrogenase 255.2
20-alpha-hydroxylase 255.2
21-hydroxylase 255.2
AAT (alpha-1 antitrypsin) 273.4
abdominal muscle syndrome 756.79
accelerator globulin (Ac G) (blood) (*see also*
Defect, coagulation) 286.3
AC globulin (congenital) (*see also* Defect,
coagulation) 286.3
acquired 286.7
activating factor (blood) (*see also* Defect,
coagulation) 286.3
adenohypophyseal 253.2
adenosine deaminase 277.2
aldolase (hereditary) 271.2
alpha-1-antitrypsin 273.4
alpha-1-trypsin inhibitor 273.4
alpha-fucosidase 271.8
alpha-lipoprotein 272.5
alpha-mannosidase 271.8
amino acid 270.9
anemia—*see* Anemia, deficiency

Deficiency, deficient—*continued*
aneurin 265.1
with beriberi 265.0
antibody NEC 279.00
antidiuretic hormone 253.5
antihemophilic
factor (A) 286.0
B 286.1
C 286.2
globulin (AHG) NEC 286.0
antithrombin III 289.81
antitrypsin 273.4
argininosuccinate synthetase or lyase 270.6
ascorbic acid (with scurvy) 267
autoprothrombin
I (*see also* Defect, coagulation) 286.3
II 286.1
C (*see also* Defect, coagulation) 286.3
bile salt 579.8
biotin 266.2
biotinidase 277.6
bradykinase-1 277.6
brancher enzyme (amylopectinosis) 271.0
calciferol 268.9
with
osteomalacia 268.2
rickets (*see also* Rickets) 268.0
calcium 275.40
dietary 269.3
calorie, severe 261
carbamyl phosphate synthetase 270.6
cardiac (*see also* Insufficiency, myocardial)
428.0
carnitine 277.81
due to
hemodialysis 277.83
inborn errors of metabolism 277.82
valproic acid therapy 277.83
iatrogenic 277.83
palmitoyltransferase (CPT1, CPT2) 277.85
palmityl transferase (CPT1, CPT2) 277.85
primary 277.81
secondary 277.84
carotene 264.9
Carr factor (*see also* Defect, coagulation) 286.9
central nervous system 349.9
ceruloplasmin 275.1
cevitamic acid (with scurvy) 267
choline 266.2
Christmas factor 286.1
chromium 269.3
citrin 269.1
clotting (blood) (*see also* Defect, coagulation)
286.9
coagulation factor NEC 286.9
with
abortion—*see* Abortion, by type, with
hemorrhage
ectopic pregnancy (*see also* categories
634-638) 639.1
molar pregnancy (*see also* categories
630-632) 639.1
acquired (any) 286.7
antepartum or intrapartum 641.3
affecting fetus or newborn 762.1
complicating pregnancy, childbirth, or the
puerperium 649.3
due to
liver disease 286.7
vitamin K deficiency 286.7
newborn, transient 776.3

Deficiency, deficient—*continued*
  coagulation factor —*continued*
    postpartum 666.3
    specified type NEC 286.3
  color vision (congenital) 368.59
    acquired 368.55
  combined glucocorticoid and mineralocorticoid
    255.41
  combined, two or more coagulation factors (*see
    also* Defect, coagulation) 286.9
  complement factor NEC 279.8
  contact factor (*see also* Defect, coagulation)
    286.3
  copper NEC 275.1
  corticoadrenal 255.41
  craniofacial axis 756.0
  cyanocobalamin (vitamin B$_{12}$) 266.2
  debrancher enzyme (limit dextrinosis) 271.0
  desmolase 255.2
  diet 269.9
  dihydrofolate reductase 281.2
  dihydropteridine reductase 270.1
  dihydropyrimidine dehydrogenase (DPD) 277.6
  disaccharidase (intestinal) 271.3
  disease NEC 269.9
  ear(s) V48.8
  edema 262
  endocrine 259.9
  enzymes, circulating NEC (*see also* Deficiency,
    by specific enzyme) 277.6
  ergosterol 268.9
    with
      osteomalacia 268.2
      rickets (*see also* Rickets) 268.0
  erythrocytic glutathione (anemia) 282.2
  eyelid(s) V48.8
  factor (*see also* Defect, coagulation) 286.9
    I (congenital) (fibrinogen) 286.3
      antepartum or intrapartum 641.3
        affecting fetus or newborn 762.1
      newborn, transient 776.3
      postpartum 666.3
    II (congenital) (prothrombin) 286.3
    V (congenital) (labile) 286.3
    VII (congenital) (stable) 286.3
    VIII (congenital) (functional) 286.0
      with
        functional defect 286.0
        vascular defect 286.4
    IX (Christmas) (congenital) (functional) 286.1
    X (congenital) (Stuart-Prower) 286.3
    XI (congenital) (plasma thromboplastin
      antecedent) 286.2
    XII (congenital) (Hageman) 286.3
    XIII (congenital) (fibrin stabilizing) 286.3
    Hageman 286.3
    multiple (congenital) 286.9
      acquired 286.7
  fibrinase (*see also* Defect, coagulation) 286.3
  fibrinogen (congenital) (*see also* Defect,
    coagulation) 286.3
    acquired 286.6
  fibrin stabilizing factor (congenital) (*see also*
    Defect, coagulation) 286.3
    acquired 286.7
  finger—*see* Absence, finger
  Fletcher factor (*see also* Defect, coagulation)
    286.9
  fluorine 269.3
  folate, anemia 281.2
  folic acid (vitamin B$_c$) 266.2
    anemia 281.2

Deficiency, deficient—*continued*
  follicle-stimulating hormone (FSH) 253.4
  fructokinase 271.2
  fructose-1, 6-diphosphate 271.2
  fructose-1-phosphate aldolase 271.2
  FSH (follicle-stimulating hormone) 253.4
  fucosidase 271.8
  galactokinase 271.1
  galactose-1-phosphate uridyl transferase 271.1
  gamma globulin in blood 279.00
  glass factor (*see also* Defect, coagulation) 286.3
  glucocorticoid 255.41
  glucose-6-phosphatase 271.0
  glucose-6-phosphate dehydrogenase anemia 282.2
  glucuronyl transferase 277.4
  glutathione-reductase (anemia) 282.2
  glycogen synthetase 271.0
  growth hormone 253.3
  Hageman factor (congenital) (*see also* Defect,
    coagulation) 286.3
  head V48.0
  hemoglobin (*see also* Anemia) 285.9
  hepatophosphorylase 271.0
  hexose monophosphate (HMP) shunt 282.2
  HGH (human growth hormone) 253.3
  HG-PRT 277.2
  homogentisic acid oxidase 270.2
  hormone—*see also* Deficiency, by specific
    hormone
    anterior pituitary (isolated) (partial) NEC
      253.4
      growth (human) 253.3
    follicle-stimulating 253.4
    growth (human) (isolated) 253.3
    human growth 253.3
    interstitial cell-stimulating 253.4
    luteinizing 253.4
    melanocyte-stimulating 253.4
    testicular 257.2
  human growth hormone 253.3
  humoral 279.00
    with
      hyper-IgM 279.05
        autosomal recessive 279.05
        X-linked 279.05
      increased IgM 279.05
      congenital hypogammaglobulinemia 279.04
      non-sex-linked 279.06
    selective immunoglobulin NEC 279.03
      IgA 279.01
      IgG 279.03
      IgM 279.02
        increased 279.05
    specified NEC 279.09
  hydroxylase 255.2
  hypoxanthine-guanine
    phosphoribosyltransferase (HG-PRT) 277.2
  ICSH (interstitial cell-stimulating hormone)
    253.4
  immunity NEC 279.3
    cell-mediated 279.10
      with
        hyperimmunoglobulinemia 279.2
        thrombocytopenia and eczema 279.12
      specified NEC 279.19
    combined (severe) 279.2
      syndrome 279.2
    common variable 279.06
    humoral NEC 279.00
    IgA (secretory) 279.01
    IgG 279.03
    IgM 279.02

Deficiency, deficient—*continued*
immunoglobulin, selective NEC 279.03
  IgA 279.01
  IgG 279.03
  IgM 279.02
inositol (B complex) 266.2
interferon 279.49
internal organ V47.0
interstitial cell-stimulating hormone (ICSH)
  253.4
intrinsic (urethral) sphincter (ISD) 599.82
intrinsic factor (Castle's) (congenital) 281.0
invertase 271.3
iodine 269.3
iron, anemia 280.9
labile factor (congenital) (*see also* Defect,
  coagulation) 286.3
  acquired 286.7
lacrimal fluid (acquired) 375.15
  congenital 743.64
lactase 271.3
Laki-Lorand factor (*see also* Defect,
  coagulation) 286.3
lecithin-cholesterol acyltranferase 272.5
LH (luteinizing hormone) 253.4
limb V49.0
  lower V49.0
    congenital (*see also* Deficiency, lower limb,
      congenital) 755.30
  upper V49.0
    congenital (*see also* Deficiency, upper limb,
      congenital) 755.20
lipocaic 577.8
lipoid (high-density) 272.5
lipoprotein (familial) (high density) 272.5
liver phosphorylase 271.0
long chain 3-hydroxyacyl CoA dehydrogenase
  (LCHAD) 277.85
long chain/very long chain acyl CoA
  dehydrogenase (LCAD, VLCAD) 277.85
lower limb V49.0
  congenital 755.30
    with complete absence of distal elements
      755.31
    longitudinal (complete) (partial) (with distal
      deficiencies, incomplete) 755.32
      with complete absence of distal elements
        755.31
      combined femoral, tibial, fibular
        (incomplete) 755.33
      femoral 755.34
      fibular 755.37
      metatarsal(s) 755.38
      phalange(s) 755.39
        meaning all digits 755.31
      tarsal(s) 755.38
      tibia 755.36
      tibiofibular 755.35
      transverse 755.31
luteinizing hormone (LH) 253.4
lysosomal alpha-1, 4 glucosidase 271.0
magnesium 275.2
mannosidase 271.8
medium chain acyl CoA dehydrogenase
  (MCAD) 277.85
melanocyte-stimulating hormone (MSH) 253.4
menadione (vitamin K) 269.0
  newborn 776.0
mental (familial) (hereditary) (*see also*
  Disability, intellectual) 319

Deficiency, deficient—*continued*
methylenetetrahydrofolate reductase (MTHFR)
  270.4
mineral NEC 269.3
mineralocorticoid 255.42
molybdenum 269.3
moral 301.7
multiple, syndrome 260
myocardial (*see also* Insufficiency myocardial)
  428.0
myophosphorylase 271.0
NADH (DPNH) -methemoglobin-reductase
  (congenital) 289.7
NADH diaphorase or reductase (congenital)
  289.7
neck V48.1
niacin (amide) (-tryptophan) 265.2
nicotinamide 265.2
nicotinic acid (amide) 265.2
nose V48.8
number of teeth (*see also* Anodontia) 520.0
nutrition, nutritional 269.9
  specified NEC 269.8
ornithine transcarbamylase 270.6
ovarian 256.39
oxygen (*see also* Anoxia) 799.02
pantothenic acid 266.2
parathyroid (gland) 252.1
phenylalanine hydroxylase 270.1
phosphoenolpyruvate carboxykinase 271.8
phosphofructokinase 271.2
phosphoglucomutase 271.0
phosphohexosisomerase 271.0
phosphomannomutase 271.8
phosphomannose isomerase 271.8
phosphomannosyl mutase 271.8
phosphorylase kinase, liver 271.0
pituitary (anterior) 253.2
  posterior 253.5
placenta—*see* Placenta, insufficiency
plasma
  cell 279.00
  protein (paraproteinemia) (pyroglobulinemia)
    273.8
    gamma globulin 279.00
  thromboplastin
    antecedent (PTA) 286.2
    component (PTC) 286.1
platelet NEC 287.1
  constitutional 286.4
polyglandular 258.9
potassium (K) 276.8
proaccelerin (congenital) (*see also* Defect,
  congenital) 286.3
  acquired 286.7
proconvertin factor (congenital) (*see also*
  Defect, coagulation) 286.3
  acquired 286.7
prolactin 253.4
protein 260
  anemia 281.4
  C 289.81
  plasma—*see* Deficiency, plasma, protein
  S 289.81
prothrombin (congenital) (*see also* Defect,
  coagulation) 286.3
  acquired 286.7
Prower factor (*see also* Defect, coagulation)
  286.3
PRT 277.2
pseudocholinesterase 289.89

Deficiency, deficient—*continued*
  psychobiological 301.6
  PTA 286.2
  PTC 286.1
  purine nucleoside phosphorylase 277.2
  pyracin (alpha) (beta) 266.1
  pyridoxal 266.1
  pyridoxamine 266.1
  pyridoxine (derivatives) 266.1
  pyruvate carboxylase 271.8
  pyruvate dehydrogenase 271.8
  pyruvate kinase (PK) 282.3
  riboflavin (vitamin B$_2$) 266.0
  saccadic eye movements 379.57
  salivation 527.7
  salt 276.1
  secretion
    ovary 256.39
    salivary gland (any) 527.7
    urine 788.5
  selenium 269.3
  serum
    antitrypsin, familial 273.4
    protein (congenital) 273.8
  short chain acyl CoA dehydrogenase (SCAD)
    277.85
  short stature homeobox gene (SHOX)
    with
      dyschondrosteosis 756.89
      short stature (idiopathic) 783.43
      Turner's syndrome 758.6
  smooth pursuit movements (eye) 379.58
  sodium (Na) 276.1
  SPCA (*see also* Defect, coagulation) 286.3
  specified NEC 269.8
  stable factor (congenital) (*see also* Defect,
    coagulation) 286.3
    acquired 286.7
  Stuart (-Prower) factor (*see also* Defect,
    coagulation) 286.3
  sucrase 271.3
  sucrase-isomaltase 271.3
  sulfite oxidase 270.0
  syndrome, multiple 260
  thiamine, thiaminic (chloride) 265.1
  thrombokinase (*see also* Defect, coagulation) 286.3
    newborn 776.0
  thrombopoieten 287.39
  thymolymphatic 279.2
  thyroid (gland) 244.9
  tocopherol 269.1
  toe—*see* Absence, toe
  tooth bud (*see also* Anodontia) 520.0
  trunk V48.1
  UDPG-glycogen transferase 271.0
  upper limb V49.0
    congenital 755.20
      with complete absence of distal elements
        755.21
      longitudinal (complete) (partial) (with distal
        deficiencies, incomplete) 755.22
        carpal(s) 755.28
        combined humeral, radial, ulnar
          (incomplete) 755.23
        humeral 755.24
        metacarpal(s) 755.28
        phalange(s) 755.29
          meaning all digits 755.21
        radial 755.26
        radioulnar 755.25
        ulnar 755.27
      transverse (complete) (partial) 755.21

Deficiency, deficient—*continued*
  vascular 459.9
  vasopressin 253.5
  viosterol (*see also* Deficiency, calciferol) 268.9
  vitamin (multiple) NEC 269.2
    A 264.9
      with
        Bitôt's spot 264.1
          corneal 264.2
            with corneal ulceration 264.3
        keratomalacia 264.4
        keratosis, follicular 264.8
        night blindness 264.5
        scar of cornea, xerophthalmic 264.6
        specified manifestation NEC 264.8
          ocular 264.7
        xeroderma 264.8
        xerophthalmia 264.7
        xerosis
          conjunctival 264.0
            with Bitôt's spot 264.1
          corneal 264.2
            with corneal ulceration 264.3
    B (complex) NEC 266.9
      with
        beriberi 265.0
        pellagra 265.2
        specified type NEC 266.2
    B$_1$ NEC 265.1
      beriberi 265.0
    B$_2$ 266.0
    B$_6$ 266.1
    B$_{12}$ 266.2
    B$_c$ (folic acid) 266.2
    C (ascorbic acid) (with scurvy) 267
    D (calciferol) (ergosterol) 268.9
      with
        osteomalacia 268.2
        rickets (*see also* Rickets) 268.0
    E 269.1
    folic acid 266.2
    G 266.0
    H 266.2
    K 269.0
      of newborn 776.0
    nicotinic acid 265.2
    P 269.1
    PP 265.2
    specified NEC 269.1
    zinc 269.3
Deficient —*see also* Deficiency
  blink reflex 374.45
  craniofacial axis 756.0
  number of teeth (*see also* Anodontia) 520.0
  secretion of urine 788.5
Deficit
  attention 799.51
  cognitive communication 799.52
  concentration 799.51
  executive function 799.55
  frontal lobe 799.55
  neurologic NEC 781.99
    due to
      cerebrovascular lesion (*see also* Disease,
        cerebrovascular, acute) 436
      late effect—*see* Late effect(s) (of)
        cerebrovascular disease
      transient ischemic attack 435.9

Deficit—*continued*
neurologic—*continued*
ischemic
reversible (RIND) 434.91
history of (personal) V12.54
prolonged (PRIND) 434.91
history of (personal) V12.54
oxygen 799.02
psychomotor 799.54
visuospatial 799.53
Deflection
radius 736.09
septum (acquired) (nasal) (nose) 470
spine—*see* Curvature, spine
turbinate (nose) 470
Defluvium
capillorum (*see also* Alopecia) 704.00
ciliorum 374.55
unguium 703.8
Deformity 738.9
abdomen, congenital 759.9
abdominal wall
acquired 738.8
congenital 756.70
muscle deficiency syndrome 756.79
acquired (unspecified site) 738.9
specified site NEC 738.8
adrenal gland (congenital) 759.1
alimentary tract, congenital 751.9
lower 751.5
specified type NEC 751.8
upper (any part, except tongue) 750.9
specified type NEC 750.8
tongue 750.10
specified type NEC 750.19
ankle (joint) (acquired) 736.70
abduction 718.47
congenital 755.69
contraction 718.47
specified NEC 736.79
anus (congenital) 751.5
acquired 569.49
aorta (congenital) 747.20
acquired 447.8
arch 747.21
acquired 447.8
coarctation 747.10
aortic
arch 747.21
acquired 447.8
cusp or valve (congenital) 746.9
acquired (*see also* Endocarditis, aortic)
424.1
ring 747.21
appendix 751.5
arm (acquired) 736.89
congenital 755.50
arteriovenous (congenital) (peripheral) NEC
747.60
gastrointestinal 747.61
lower limb 747.64
renal 747.62
specified NEC 747.69
spinal 747.82
upper limb 747.63
artery (congenital) (peripheral) NEC (*see also*
Deformity, vascular) 747.60
acquired 447.8
cerebral 747.81
coronary (congenital) 746.85
acquired (*see also* Ischemia, heart) 414.9

Deformity—*continued*
artery—*continued*
retinal 743.9
umbilical 747.5
atrial septal (congenital) (heart) 745.5
auditory canal (congenital) (external) (*see also*
Deformity, ear) 744.3
acquired 380.50
auricle
ear (congenital) (*see also* Deformity, ear)
744.3
acquired 380.32
heart (congenital) 746.9
back (acquired)—*see* Deformity, spine
Bartholin's duct (congenital) 750.9
bile duct (congenital) 751.60
acquired 576.8
with calculus, choledocholithiasis, or
stones—*see* Choledocholithiasis
biliary duct or passage (congenital) 751.60
acquired 576.8
with calculus, choledocholithiasis, or
stones—*see* Choledocholithiasis
bladder (neck) (sphincter) (trigone) (acquired)
596.89
congenital 753.9
bone (acquired) NEC 738.9
congenital 756.9
turbinate 738.0
boutonniere (finger) 736.21
brain (congenital) 742.9
acquired 348.89
multiple 742.4
reduction 742.2
vessel (congenital) 747.81
breast (acquired) 611.89
congenital 757.6
reconstructed 612.0
bronchus (congenital) 748.3
acquired 519.19
bursa, congenital 756.9
canal of Nuck 752.9
canthus (congenital) 743.9
acquired 374.89
capillary (acquired) 448.9
congenital NEC (*see also* Deformity, vascular)
747.60
cardiac—*see* Deformity, heart
cardiovascular system (congenital) 746.9
caruncle, lacrimal (congenital) 743.9
acquired 375.69
cascade, stomach 537.6
cecum (congenital) 751.5
acquired 569.89
cerebral (congenital) 742.9
acquired 348.89
cervix (acquired) (uterus) 622.8
congenital 752.40
cheek (acquired) 738.19
congenital 744.9
chest (wall) (acquired) 738.3
congenital 754.89
late effect of rickets 268.1
chin (acquired) 738.19
congenital 744.9
choroid (congenital) 743.9
acquired 363.8
plexus (congenital) 742.9
acquired 349.2
cicatricial—*see* Cicatrix

Deformity—*continued*
  cilia (congenital) 743.9
    acquired 374.89
  circulatory system (congenital) 747.9
  clavicle (acquired) 738.8
    congenital 755.51
  clitoris (congenital) 752.40
    acquired 624.8
  clubfoot—*see* Clubfoot
  coccyx (acquired) 738.6
    congenital 756.10
  colon (congenital) 751.5
    acquired 569.89
  concha (ear) (congenital) (*see also* Deformity,
    ear) 744.3
    acquired 380.32
  congenital, organ or site not listed (*see also*
    Anomaly) 759.9
  cornea (congenital) 743.9
    acquired 371.70
  coronary artery (congenital) 746.85
    acquired (*see also* Ischemia, heart) 414.9
  cranium (acquired) 738.19
    congenital (*see also* Deformity, skull,
      congenital) 756.0
  cricoid cartilage (congenital) 748.3
    acquired 478.79
  cystic duct (congenital) 751.60
    acquired 575.8
  Dandy-Walker 742.3
    with spina bifida (*see also* Spina bifida) 741.0
  diaphragm (congenital) 756.6
    acquired 738.8
  digestive organ(s) or system (congenital) NEC
    751.9
    specified type NEC 751.8
  ductus arteriosus 747.0
  duodenal bulb 537.89
  duodenum (congenital) 751.5
    acquired 537.89
  dura (congenital) 742.9
    brain 742.4
      acquired 349.2
    spinal 742.59
      acquired 349.2
  ear (congenital) 744.3
    acquired 380.32
    auricle 744.3
      causing impairment of hearing 744.02
    causing impairment of hearing 744.00
    external 744.3
      causing impairment of hearing 744.02
    internal 744.05
    lobule 744.3
    middle 744.03
      ossicles 744.04
    ossicles 744.04
  ectodermal (congenital) NEC 757.9
    specified type NEC 757.8
  ejaculatory duct (congenital) 752.9
    acquired 608.89
  elbow (joint) (acquired) 736.00
    congenital 755.50
    contraction 718.42
  endocrine gland NEC 759.2
  epididymis (congenital) 752.9
    acquired 608.89
    torsion 608.24
  epiglottis (congenital) 748.3
    acquired 478.79
  esophagus (congenital) 750.9
    acquired 530.89

Deformity—*continued*
  Eustachian tube (congenital) NEC 744.3
    specified type NEC 744.24
  extremity (acquired) 736.9
    congenital, except reduction deformity 755.9
      lower 755.60
      upper 755.50
    reduction—*see* Deformity, reduction
  eye (congenital) 743.9
    acquired 379.8
    muscle 743.9
  eyebrow (congenital) 744.89
  eyelid (congenital) 743.9
    acquired 374.89
    specified type NEC 743.62
  face (acquired) 738.19
    congenital (any part) 744.9
      due to intrauterine malposition and pressure 754.0
  fallopian tube (congenital) 752.10
    acquired 620.8
  femur (acquired) 736.89
    congenital 755.60
  fetal
    with fetopelvic disproportion 653.7
      affecting fetus or newborn 763.1
    causing obstructed labor 660.1
      affecting fetus or newborn 763.1
    known or suspected, affecting management of
      pregnancy 655.9
  finger (acquired) 736.20
    boutonniere type 736.21
    congenital 755.50
    flexion contracture 718.44
    swan neck 736.22
  flexion (joint) (acquired) 736.9
    congenital NEC 755.9
    hip or thigh (acquired) 736.39
      congenital (*see also* Subluxation, congenital,
        hip) 754.32
  foot (acquired) 736.70
    cavovarus 736.75
      congenital 754.59
    congenital NEC 754.70
      specified type NEC 754.79
    valgus (acquired) 736.79
      congenital 754.60
        specified type NEC 754.69
    varus (acquired) 736.79
      congenital 754.50
        specified type NEC 754.59
  forearm (acquired) 736.00
    congenital 755.50
  forehead (acquired) 738.19
    congenital (*see also* Deformity, skull,
      congenital) 756.0
  frontal bone (acquired) 738.19
    congenital (*see also* Deformity, skull,
      congenital) 756.0
  gallbladder (congenital) 751.60
    acquired 575.8
  gastrointestinal tract (congenital) NEC 751.9
    acquired 569.89
    specified type NEC 751.8
  genitalia, genital organ(s) or system NEC
    congenital 752.9
    female (congenital) 752.9
      acquired 629.89
      external 752.40
      internal 752.9
    male (congenital) 752.9
      acquired 608.89

Deformity—*continued*
globe (eye) (congenital) 743.9
  acquired 360.89
gum (congenital) 750.9
  acquired 523.9
gunstock 736.02
hand (acquired) 736.00
  claw 736.06
  congenital 755.50
  minus (and plus) (intrinsic) 736.09
  pill roller (intrinsic) 736.09
  plus (and minus) (intrinsic) 736.09
  swan neck (intrinsic) 736.09
head (acquired) 738.10
  congenital (*see also* Deformity, skull,
    congenital) 756.0
  specified NEC 738.19
heart (congenital) 746.9
  auricle (congenital) 746.9
  septum 745.9
    auricular 745.5
    specified type NEC 745.8
    ventricular 745.4
  valve (congenital) NEC 746.9
    acquired—*see* Endocarditis
    pulmonary (congenital) 746.00
    specified type NEC 746.89
  ventricle (congenital) 746.9
heel (acquired) 736.76
  congenital 755.67
hepatic duct (congenital) 751.60
  acquired 576.8
    with calculus, choledocholithiasis, or
      stones—*see* Choledocholithiasis
hip (joint) (acquired) 736.30
  congenital NEC 755.63
  flexion 718.45
    congenital (*see also* Subluxation, congenital,
      hip) 754.32
hourglass—*see* Contraction, hourglass
humerus (acquired) 736.89
  congenital 755.50
hymen (congenital) 752.40
hypophyseal (congenital) 759.2
ileocecal (coil) (valve) (congenital) 751.5
  acquired 569.89
ileum (intestine) (congenital) 751.5
  acquired 569.89
ilium (acquired) 738.6
  congenital 755.60
integument (congenital) 757.9
intervertebral cartilage or disc (acquired)—*see
  also* Displacement, intervertebral disc
  congenital 756.10
intestine (large) (small) (congenital) 751.5
  acquired 569.89
iris (acquired) 364.75
  congenital 743.9
  prolapse 364.89
ischium (acquired) 738.6
  congenital 755.60
jaw (acquired) (congenital) NEC 524.9
  due to intrauterine malposition and pressure
    754.0
joint (acquired) NEC 738.8
  congenital 755.9
  contraction (abduction) (adduction) (extension)
    (flexion)—*see* Contraction, joint
kidney(s) (calyx) (pelvis) (congenital) 753.9
  acquired 593.89
  vessel 747.62
    acquired 459.9

Deformity—*continued*
Klippel-Feil (brevicollis) 756.16
knee (acquired) NEC 736.6
  congenital 755.64
labium (majus) (minus) (congenital) 752.40
  acquired 624.8
lacrimal apparatus or duct (congenital) 743.9
  acquired 375.69
larynx (muscle) (congenital) 748.3
  acquired 478.79
  web (glottic) (subglottic) 748.2
leg (lower) (upper) (acquired) NEC 736.89
  congenital 755.60
  reduction—*see* Deformity, reduction, lower limb
lens (congenital) 743.9
  acquired 379.39
lid (fold) (congenital) 743.9
  acquired 374.89
ligament (acquired) 728.9
  congenital 756.9
limb (acquired) 736.9
  congenital, except reduction deformity 755.9
    lower 755.60
      reduction (*see also* Deformity, reduction,
        lower limb) 755.30
    upper 755.50
      reduction (*see also* Deformity, reduction,
        lower limb) 755.20
  specified NEC 736.89
lip (congenital) NEC 750.9
  acquired 528.5
  specified type NEC 750.26
liver (congenital) 751.60
  acquired 573.8
  duct (congenital) 751.60
    acquired 576.8
      with calculus, choledocholithiasis, or
        stones—*see* Choledocholithiasis
lower extremity—*see* Deformity, leg
lumbosacral (joint) (region) (congenital) 756.10
  acquired 738.5
lung (congenital) 748.60
  acquired 518.89
  specified type NEC 748.69
lymphatic system, congenital 759.9
Madelung's (radius) 755.54
maxilla (acquired) (congenital) 524.9
meninges or membrane (congenital) 742.9
  brain 742.4
    acquired 349.2
  spinal (cord) 742.59
    acquired 349.2
mesentery (congenital) 751.9
  acquired 568.89
metacarpus (acquired) 736.00
  congenital 755.50
metatarsus (acquired) 736.70
  congenital 754.70
middle ear, except ossicles (congenital) 744.03
  ossicles 744.04
mitral (leaflets) (valve) (congenital) 746.9
  acquired—*see* Endocarditis, mitral
  Ebstein's 746.89
  parachute 746.5
  specified type NEC 746.89
  stenosis, congenital 746.5
mouth (acquired) 528.9
  congenital NEC 750.9
    specified type NEC 750.26
multiple, congenital NEC 759.7
  specified type NEC 759.89

Deformity—*continued*
  muscle (acquired) 728.9
    congenital 756.9
      specified type NEC 756.89
      sternocleidomastoid (due to intrauterine
        malposition and pressure) 754.1
  musculoskeletal system, congenital NEC 756.9
    specified type NEC 756.9
  nail (acquired) 703.9
    congenital 757.9
  nasal—*see* Deformity, nose
  neck (acquired) NEC 738.2
    congenital (any part) 744.9
      sternocleidomastoid 754.1
  nervous system (congenital) 742.9
  nipple (congenital) 757.6
    acquired 611.89
  nose, nasal (cartilage) (acquired) 738.0
    bone (turbinate) 738.0
    congenital 748.1
      bent 754.0
      squashed 754.0
    saddle 738.0
      syphilitic 090.5
    septum 470
      congenital 748.1
    sinus (wall) (congenital) 748.1
      acquired 738.0
    syphilitic (congenital) 090.5
      late 095.8
  ocular muscle (congenital) 743.9
    acquired 378.60
  opticociliary vessels (congenital) 743.9
  orbit (congenital) (eye) 743.9
    acquired NEC 376.40
      associated with craniofacial deformities 376.44
      due to
        bone disease 376.43
        surgery 376.47
        trauma 376.47
  organ of Corti (congenital) 744.05
  ovary (congenital) 752.0
    acquired 620.8
  oviduct (congenital) 752.10
    acquired 620.8
  palate (congenital) 750.9
    acquired 526.89
    cleft (congenital) (*see also* Cleft, palate) 749.00
    hard, acquired 526.89
    soft, acquired 528.9
  pancreas (congenital) 751.7
    acquired 577.8
  parachute, mitral valve 746.5
  parathyroid (gland) 759.2
  parotid (gland) (congenital) 750.9
    acquired 527.8
  patella (acquired) 736.6
    congenital 755.64
  pelvis, pelvic (acquired) (bony) 738.6
    with disproportion (fetopelvic) 653.0
      affecting fetus or newborn 763.1
      causing obstructed labor 660.1
        affecting fetus or newborn 763.1
    congenital 755.60
    rachitic (late effect) 268.1
  penis (glans) (congenital) 752.9
    acquired 607.89
  pericardium (congenital) 746.9
    acquired—*see* Pericarditis
  pharynx (congenital) 750.9
    acquired 478.29

Deformity—*continued*
  Pierre Robin (congenital) 756.0
  pinna (acquired) 380.32
    congenital 744.3
  pituitary (congenital) 759.2
  pleural folds (congenital) 748.8
  portal vein (congenital) 747.40
  posture—*see* Curvature, spine
  prepuce (congenital) 752.9
    acquired 607.89
  prostate (congenital) 752.9
    acquired 602.8
  pulmonary valve—*see* Endocarditis, pulmonary
  pupil (congenital) 743.9
    acquired 364.75
  pylorus (congenital) 750.9
    acquired 537.89
  rachitic (acquired), healed or old 268.1
  radius (acquired) 736.00
    congenital 755.50
      reduction—*see* Deformity, reduction, upper
        limb
  rectovaginal septum (congenital) 752.40
    acquired 623.8
  rectum (congenital) 751.5
    acquired 569.49
  reduction (extremity) (limb) 755.4
    brain 742.2
    lower limb 755.30
      with complete absence of distal elements
        755.31
      longitudinal (complete) (partial) (with distal
        deficiencies, incomplete) 755.32
        with complete absence of distal elements
          755.31
        combined femoral, tibial, fibular
          (incomplete) 755.33
        femoral 755.34
        fibular 755.37
        metatarsal(s) 755.38
        phalange(s) 755.39
          meaning all digits 755.31
        tarsal(s) 755.38
        tibia 755.36
        tibiofibular 755.35
        transverse 755.31
    upper limb 755.20
      with complete absence of distal elements 755.21
      longitudinal (complete) (partial) (with distal
        deficiencies, incomplete) 755.22
      with complete absence of distal elements
        755.21
      carpal(s) 755.28
      combined humeral, radial, ulnar
        (incomplete) 755.23
      humeral 755.24
      metacarpal(s) 755.28
      phalange(s) 755.29
        meaning all digits 755.21
      radial 755.26
      radioulnar 755.25
      ulnar 755.27
    transverse (complete) (partial) 755.21
  renal—*see* Deformity, kidney
  respiratory system (congenital) 748.9
    specified type NEC 748.8
  rib (acquired) 738.3
    congenital 756.3
      cervical 756.2

Deformity—*continued*
rotation (joint) (acquired) 736.9
  congenital 755.9
  hip or thigh 736.39
    congenital (*see also* Subluxation, congenital,
      hip) 754.32
sacroiliac joint (congenital) 755.69
  acquired 738.5
sacrum (acquired) 738.5
  congenital 756.10
saddle
  back 737.8
  nose 738.0
    syphilitic 090.5
salivary gland or duct (congenital) 750.9
  acquired 527.8
scapula (acquired) 736.89
  congenital 755.50
scrotum (congenital) 752.9
  acquired 608.89
sebaceous gland, acquired 706.8
seminal tract or duct (congenital) 752.9
  acquired 608.89
septum (nasal) (acquired) 470
  congenital 748.1
shoulder (joint) (acquired) 736.89
  congenital 755.50
    specified type NEC 755.59
  contraction 718.41
sigmoid (flexure) (congenital) 751.5
  acquired 569.89
sinus of Valsalva 747.29
skin (congenital) 757.9
  acquired NEC 709.8
skull (acquired) 738.19
  congenital 756.0
    with
      anencephalus 740.0
      encephalocele 742.0
      hydrocephalus 742.3
        with spina bifida (*see also* Spina bifida)
          741.0
      microcephalus 742.1
      due to intrauterine malposition and pressure
        754.0
soft parts, organs or tissues (of pelvis)
  in pregnancy or childbirth NEC 654.9
    affecting fetus or newborn 763.89
    causing obstructed labor 660.2
      affecting fetus or newborn 763.1
spermatic cord (congenital) 752.9
  acquired 608.89
    torsion 608.22
      extravaginal 608.21
      intravaginal 608.22
spinal
  column—*see* Deformity, spine
  cord (congenital) 742.9
    acquired 336.8
    vessel (congenital) 747.82
  nerve root (congenital) 742.9
    acquired 724.9
    vessel 747.82
spine (acquired) NEC 738.5
  congenital 756.10
    due to intrauterine malposition and pressure
      754.2
  kyphoscoliotic (*see also* Kyphoscoliosis) 737.30
  kyphotic (*see also* Kyphosis) 737.10
  lordotic (*see also* Lordosis) 737.20
  rachitic 268.1
  scoliotic (*see also* Scoliosis) 737.30

Deformity—*continued*
spleen
  acquired 289.59
  congenital 759.0
Sprengel's (congenital) 755.52
sternum (acquired) 738.3
  congenital 756.3
stomach (congenital) 750.9
  acquired 537.89
submaxillary gland (congenital) 750.9
  acquired 527.8
swan neck (acquired)
  finger 736.22
  hand 736.09
talipes—*see* Talipes
teeth, tooth NEC 520.9
testis (congenital) 752.9
  acquired 608.89
    torsion 608.20
thigh (acquired) 736.89
  congenital 755.60
thorax (acquired) (wall) 738.3
  congenital 754.89
  late effect of rickets 268.1
thumb (acquired) 736.20
  congenital 755.50
thymus (tissue) (congenital) 759.2
thyroid (gland) (congenital) 759.2
  cartilage 748.3
    acquired 478.79
tibia (acquired) 736.89
  congenital 755.60
  saber 090.5
toe (acquired) 735.9
  congenital 755.66
  specified NEC 735.8
tongue (congenital) 750.10
  acquired 529.8
tooth, teeth NEC 520.9
trachea (rings) (congenital) 748.3
  acquired 519.19
transverse aortic arch (congenital) 747.21
tricuspid (leaflets) (valve) (congenital) 746.9
  acquired—*see* Endocarditis, tricuspid
  atresia or stenosis 746.1
  specified type NEC 746.89
trunk (acquired) 738.3
  congenital 759.9
ulna (acquired) 736.00
  congenital 755.50
upper extremity—*see* Deformity, arm
urachus (congenital) 753.7
ureter (opening) (congenital) 753.9
  acquired 593.89
urethra (valve) (congenital) 753.9
  acquired 599.84
urinary tract or system (congenital) 753.9
  urachus 753.7
uterus (congenital) 752.39
  acquired 621.8
uvula (congenital) 750.9
  acquired 528.9
vagina (congenital) 752.40
  acquired 623.8
valve, valvular (heart) (congenital) 746.9
  acquired—*see* Endocarditis
  pulmonary 746.00
  specified type NEC 746.89
vascular (congenital) (peripheral) NEC 747.60
  acquired 459.9
  gastrointestinal 747.61
  lower limb 747.64

Deformity—*continued*
  vascular—*continued*
    renal 747.62
    specified site NEC 747.69
    spinal 747.82
    upper limb 747.63
  vas deferens (congenital) 752.9
    acquired 608.89
  vein (congenital) NEC (*see also* Deformity,
    vascular) 747.60
    brain 747.81
    coronary 746.9
    great 747.40
  vena cava (inferior) (superior) (congenital)
    747.40
  vertebra—*see* Deformity, spine
  vesicourethral orifice (acquired) 596.89
    congenital NEC 753.9
      specified type NEC 753.8
  vessels of optic papilla (congenital) 743.9
  visual field (contraction) 368.45
  vitreous humor (congenital) 743.9
    acquired 379.29
  vulva (congenital) 752.40
    acquired 624.8
  wrist (joint) (acquired) 736.00
    congenital 755.50
    contraction 718.43
    valgus 736.03
      congenital 755.59
    varus 736.04
      congenital 755.59
Degeneration, degenerative
  adrenal (capsule) (gland) 255.8
    with hypofunction 255.41
    fatty 255.8
    hyaline 255.8
    infectional 255.8
    lardaceous 277.39
  amyloid (any site) (general) 277.39
  anterior cornua, spinal cord 336.8
  anterior labral 840.8
  aorta, aortic 440.0
    fatty 447.8
    valve (heart) (*see also* Endocarditis, aortic)
      424.1
  arteriovascular—*see* Arteriosclerosis
  artery, arterial (atheromatous) (calcareous)—*see*
    also Arteriosclerosis
    amyloid 277.39
    lardaceous 277.39
    medial NEC (*see also* Arteriosclerosis,
      extremities) 440.20
  articular cartilage NEC (*see also* Disorder,
    cartilage, articular) 718.0
    elbow 718.02
    knee 717.5
    patella 717.7
    shoulder 718.01
    spine (*see also* Spondylosis) 721.90
  atheromatous—*see* Arteriosclerosis
  bacony (any site) 277.39
  basal nuclei or ganglia NEC 333.0
  bone 733.90
  brachial plexus 353.0
  brain (cortical) (progressive) 331.9
    arteriosclerotic 437.0
    childhood 330.9
      specified type NEC 330.8
    congenital 742.4

Degeneration, degenerative—*continued*
  brain—*continued*
    cystic 348.0
      congenital 742.4
    familial NEC 331.89
    grey matter 330.8
    heredofamilial NEC 331.89
    in
      alcoholism 303.9 *[331.7]*
      beriberi 265.0 *[331.7]*
      cerebrovascular disease 437.9 *[331.7]*
      congenital hydrocephalus 742.3 *[331.7]*
        with spina bifida (*see also* Spina bifida)
          741.0 *[331.7]*
      Fabry's disease 272.7 *[330.2]*
      Gaucher's disease 272.7 *[330.2]*
      Hunter's disease or syndrome 277.5 *[330.3]*
      lipidosis
        cerebral 330.1
        generalized 272.7 *[330.2]*
      mucopolysaccharidosis 277.5 *[330.3]*
      myxedema (*see also* Myxedema) 244.9
        [331.7]
      neoplastic disease NEC (M8000/1) 239.9
        [331.7]
      Niemann-Pick disease 272.7 *[330.2]*
      sphingolipidosis 272.7 *[330.2]*
      vitamin B$_{12}$ deficiency 266.2 *[331.7]*
    motor centers 331.89
    senile 331.2
    specified type NEC 331.89
  breast—*see* Disease, breast
  Bruch's membrane 363.40
  bundle of His 426.50
    left 426.3
    right 426.4
  calcareous NEC 275.49
  capillaries 448.9
    amyloid 277.39
    fatty 448.9
    lardaceous 277.39
  cardiac (brown) (calcareous) (fatty) (fibrous)
    (hyaline) (mural) (muscular) (pigmentary)
    (senile) (with arteriosclerosis) (*see also*
    Degeneration, myocardial) 429.1
    valve, valvular—*see* Endocarditis
  cardiorenal (*see also* Hypertension, cardiorenal)
    404.90
  cardiovascular (*see also* Disease, cardiovascular)
    429.2
    renal (*see also* Hypertension, cardiorenal) 404.90
  cartilage (joint)—*see* Derangement, joint
  cerebellar NEC 334.9
    primary (hereditary) (sporadic) 334.2
  cerebral—*see* Degeneration, brain
  cerebromacular 330.1
  cerebrovascular 437.1
    due to hypertension 437.2
    late effect—*see* Late effect(s) (of)
      cerebrovascular disease
  cervical plexus 353.2
  cervix 622.8
    due to radiation (intended effect) 622.8
      adverse effect or misadventure 622.8
  changes, spine or vertebra (*see also*
    Spondylosis) 721.90
  chitinous 277.39
  chorioretinal 363.40
    congenital 743.53
    hereditary 363.50

Degeneration, degenerative—*continued*
choroid (colloid) (drusen) 363.40
  hereditary 363.50
  senile 363.41
    diffuse secondary 363.42
cochlear 386.8
collateral ligament (knee) (medial) 717.82
  lateral 717.81
combined (spinal cord) (subacute) 266.2 *[336.2]*
  with anemia (pernicious) 281.0 *[336.2]*
    due to dietary deficiency 281.1 *[336.2]*
  due to vitamin B$_{12}$ deficiency anemia (dietary)
    281.1 *[336.2]*
conjunctiva 372.50
  amyloid 277.39 *[372.50]*
cornea 371.40
  calcerous 371.44
  familial (hereditary) (*see also* Dystrophy,
    cornea) 371.50
    macular 371.55
    reticular 371.54
  hyaline (of old scars) 371.41
  marginal (Terrien's) 371.48
  mosaic (shagreen) 371.41
  nodular 371.46
  peripheral 371.48
  senile 371.41
cortical (cerebellar) (parenchymatous) 334.2
  alcoholic 303.9 *[334.4]*
  diffuse, due to arteriopathy 437.0
corticobasal 331.6
corticostriatal-spinal 334.8
cretinoid 243
cruciate ligament (knee) (posterior) 717.84
  anterior 717.83
cutis 709.3
  amyloid 277.39
dental pulp 522.2
disc disease—*see* Degeneration, intervertebral
  disc
dorsolateral (spinal cord)—*see* Degeneration,
  combined
endocardial 424.90
extrapyramidal NEC 333.90
eye NEC 360.40
  macular (*see also* Degeneration, macula) 362.50
    congenital 362.75
    hereditary 362.76
fatty (diffuse) (general) 272.8
  liver 571.8
    alcoholic 571.0
  localized site—*see* Degeneration, by site, fatty
  placenta—*see* Placenta, abnormal
globe (eye) NEC 360.40
  macular—*see* Degeneration, macula
grey matter 330.8
heart (brown) (calcareous) (fatty) (fibrous)
  (hyaline) (mural) (muscular) (pigmentary)
  (senile) (with arteriosclerosis) (*see also*
  Degeneration, myocardial) 429.1
  amyloid 277.39 *[425.7]*
  atheromatous —*see* Arteriosclerosis, coronary
  gouty 274.82
  hypertensive (*see also* Hypertension, heart)
    402.90
  ischemic 414.9
  valve, valvular—*see* Endocarditis
hepatolenticular (Wilson's) 275.1
hepatorenal 572.4
heredofamilial
  brain NEC 331.89
  spinal cord NEC 336.8

Degeneration, degenerative—*continued*
hyaline (diffuse) (generalized) 728.9
  localized—*see also* Degeneration, by site
    cornea 371.41
    keratitis 371.41
hypertensive vascular—*see* Hypertension
infrapatellar fat pad 729.31
internal semilunar cartilage 717.3
intervertebral disc 722.6
  with myelopathy 722.70
  cervical, cervicothoracic 722.4
    with myelopathy 722.71
  lumbar, lumbosacral 722.52
    with myelopathy 722.73
  thoracic, thoracolumbar 722.51
    with myelopathy 722.72
intestine 569.89
  amyloid 277.39
  lardaceous 277.39
iris (generalized) (*see also* Atrophy, iris) 364.59
  pigmentary 364.53
  pupillary margin 364.54
ischemic—*see* Ischemia
joint disease (*see also* Osteoarthrosis) 715.9
  multiple sites 715.09
  spine (*see also* Spondylosis) 721.90
kidney (*see also* Sclerosis, renal) 587
  amyloid 277.39 *[583.81]*
  cyst, cystic (multiple) (solitary) 593.2
    congenital (*see also* Cystic, disease, kidney)
      753.10
  fatty 593.89
  fibrocystic (congenital) 753.19
  lardaceous 277.39 *[583.81]*
  polycystic (congenital) 753.12
    adult type (APKD) 753.13
    autosomal dominant 753.13
    autosomal recessive 753.14
    childhood type (CPKD) 753.14
    infantile type 753.14
  waxy 277.39 *[583.81]*
Kuhnt-Junius (retina) 362.52
labyrinth, osseous 386.8
lacrimal passages, cystic 375.12
lardaceous (any site) 277.39
lateral column (posterior), spinal cord (*see also*
  Degeneration, combined) 266.2 *[336.2]*
lattice 362.63
lens 366.9
  infantile, juvenile, or presenile 366.00
  senile 366.10
lenticular (familial) (progressive) (Wilson's)
  (with cirrhosis of liver) 275.1
  striate artery 437.0
lethal ball, prosthetic heart valve 996.02
ligament
  collateral (knee) (medial) 717.82
    lateral 717.81
  cruciate (knee) (posterior) 717.84
    anterior 717.83
liver (diffuse) 572.8
  amyloid 277.39
  congenital (cystic) 751.62
  cystic 572.8
    congenital 751.62
  fatty 571.8
    alcoholic 571.0
  hypertrophic 572.8
  lardaceous 277.39
  parenchymatous, acute or subacute (*see also*
    Necrosis, liver) 570

Degeneration, degenerative—*continued*
  liver—*continued*
    pigmentary 572.8
    toxic (acute) 573.8
    waxy 277.39
  lung 518.8
  lymph gland 289.3
    hyaline 289.3
    lardaceous 277.39
  macula (acquired) (senile) 362.50
    atrophic 362.51
    Best's 362.76
    congenital 362.75
    cystic 362.54
    cystoid 362.53
    disciform 362.52
    dry 362.51
    exudative 362.52
    familial pseudoinflammatory 362.77
    hereditary 362.76
    hole 362.54
    juvenile (Stargardt's) 362.75
    nonexudative 362.51
    pseudohole 362.54
    wet 362.52
  medullary—*see* Degeneration, brain
  membranous labyrinth, congenital (causing
    impairment of hearing) 744.05
  meniscus—*see* Derangement, joint
  microcystoid 362.62
  mitral—*see* Insufficiency, mitral
  Mönckeberg's (*see also* Arteriosclerosis,
    extremities) 440.20
  moral 301.7
  motor centers, senile 331.2
  mural (*see also* Degeneration, myocardial) 429.1
    heart, cardiac (*see also* Degeneration,
      myocardial) 429.1
    myocardium, myocardial (*see also*
      Degeneration, myocardial) 429.1
  muscle 728.9
    fatty 728.9
    fibrous 728.9
    heart (*see also* Degeneration, myocardial)
      429.1
    hyaline 728.9
  muscular progressive 728.2
  myelin, central nervous system NEC 341.9
  myocardium, myocardial (brown) (calcareous)
    (fatty) (fibrous) (hyaline) (mural) (muscular)
    (pigmentary) (senile) (with arteriosclerosis)
    429.1
    with rheumatic fever (conditions classifiable
      to 390) 398.0
      active, acute, or subacute 391.2
        with chorea 392.0
      inactive or quiescent (with chorea) 398.0
    amyloid 277.39 *[425.7]*
    congenital 746.89
    fetus or newborn 779.89
    gouty 274.82
    hypertensive (*see also* Hypertension, heart)
      402.90
    ischemic 414.8
    rheumatic (*see also* Degeneration,
      myocardium, with rheumatic fever) 398.0
    syphilitic 093.82
  nasal sinus (mucosa) (*see also* Sinusitis) 473.9
    frontal 473.1
    maxillary 473.0
  nerve—*see* Disorder, nerve

Degeneration, degenerative—*continued*
  nervous system 349.89
    amyloid 277.39 *[357.4]*
    autonomic (*see also* Neuropathy, peripheral,
      autonomic) 337.9
    fatty 349.89
    peripheral autonomic NEC (*see also*
      Neuropathy, peripheral, autonomic) 337.9
  nipple 611.9
  nose 478.19
  oculoacousticocerebral, congenital (progressive)
    743.8
  olivopontocerebellar (familial) (hereditary) 333.0
  osseous labyrinth 386.8
  ovary 620.8
    cystic 620.2
    microcystic 620.2
  pallidal, pigmentary (progressive) 333.0
  pancreas 577.8
    tuberculous (*see also* Tuberculosis) 017.9
  papillary muscle 429.81
  paving stone 362.61
  penis 607.89
  peritoneum 568.89
  pigmentary (diffuse) (general)
    localized—*see* Degeneration, by site
    pallidal (progressive) 333.0
    secondary 362.65
  pineal gland 259.8
  pituitary (gland) 253.8
  placenta (fatty) (fibrinoid) (fibroid)—*see*
    Placenta, abnormal
  popliteal fat pad 729.31
  posterolateral (spinal cord) (*see also*
    Degeneration, combined) 266.2 *[336.2]*
  pulmonary valve (heart) (*see also* Endocarditis,
    pulmonary) 424.3
  pulp (tooth) 522.2
  pupillary margin 364.54
  renal (*see also* Sclerosis, renal) 587
    fibrocystic 753.19
    polycystic 753.12
      adult type (APKD) 753.13
      autosomal dominant 753.13
      autosomal recessive 753.14
      childhood type (CPKD) 753.14
      infantile type 753.14
  reticuloendothelial system 289.89
  retina (peripheral) 362.60
    with retinal defect (*see also* Detachment,
      retina, with retinal defect) 361.00
    cystic (senile) 362.50
    cystoid 362.53
    hereditary (*see also* Dystrophy, retina) 362.70
      cerebroretinal 362.71
      congenital 362.75
      juvenile (Stargardt's) 362.75
      macula 362.76
    Kuhnt-Junius 362.52
    lattice 362.63
    macular (*see also* Degeneration, macula) 362.50
    microcystoid 362.62
    palisade 362.63
    paving stone 362.61
    pigmentary (primary) 362.74
      secondary 362.65
    posterior pole (*see also* Degeneration, macula)
      362.50
    secondary 362.66
    senile 362.60
      cystic 362.53
      reticular 362.64

Degeneration, degenerative—*continued*
saccule, congenital (causing impairment of hearing) 744.05
sacculocochlear 386.8
senile 797
  brain 331.2
  cardiac, heart, or myocardium (*see also* Degeneration, myocardial) 429.1
  motor centers 331.2
  reticule 362.64
  retina, cystic 362.50
  vascular—*see* Arteriosclerosis
silicone rubber poppet (prosthetic valve) 996.02
sinus (cystic) (*see also* Sinusitis) 473.9
  polypoid 471.1
skin 709.3
  amyloid 277.39
  colloid 709.3
spinal (cord) 336.8
  amyloid 277.39
  column 733.90
  combined (subacute) (*see also* Degeneration, combined) 266.2 *[336.2]*
    with anemia (pernicious) 281.0 *[336.2]*
  dorsolateral (*see also* Degeneration, combined) 266.2 *[336.2]*
  familial NEC 336.8
  fatty 336.8
  funicular (*see also* Degeneration, combined) 266.2 *[336.2]*
  heredofamilial NEC 336.8
  posterolateral (*see also* Degeneration, combined) 266.2 *[336.2]*
  subacute combined—*see* Degeneration, combined
  tuberculous (*see also* Tuberculosis) 013.8
spine 733.90
spleen 289.59
  amyloid 277.39
  lardaceous 277.39
stomach 537.89
  lardaceous 277.39
strionigral 333.0
sudoriparous (cystic) 705.89
suprarenal (capsule) (gland) 255.8
  with hypofunction 255.41
sweat gland 705.89
synovial membrane (pulpy) 727.9
tapetoretinal 362.74
  adult or presenile form 362.50
testis (postinfectional) 608.89
thymus (gland) 254.8
  fatty 254.8
  lardaceous 277.39
thyroid (gland) 246.8
tricuspid (heart) (valve)—*see* Endocarditis, tricuspid
tuberculous NEC (*see also* Tuberculosis) 011.9
turbinate 733.90
uterus 621.8
  cystic 621.8
vascular (senile)—*see also* Arteriosclerosis
  hypertensive—*see* Hypertension
vitreoretinal (primary) 362.73
  secondary 362.66
vitreous humor (with infiltration) 379.21
wallerian NEC—*see* Disorder, nerve
waxy (any site) 277.39
Wilson's hepatolenticular 275.1

Deglutition
paralysis 784.99
  hysterical 300.11
pneumonia 507.0
Degos' disease or syndrome 447.8
Degradation disorder, branched-chain amino-acid 270.3
Dehiscence
anastomosis—*see* Complications, anastomosis
cesarean wound 674.1
closure of
  cornea 998.32
  fascia, superficial or muscular 998.31
  internal organ 998.31
  mucosa 998.32
  muscle or muscle flap 998.31
  ribs or rib cage 998.31
  skin 998.32
  skull or craniotomy 998.31
  sternum or sternotomy 998.31
  subcutaneous tissue 998.32
  tendon or ligament 998.31
  traumatic laceration (external) (internal) 998.33
episiotomy 674.2
operation wound 998.32
  deep 998.31
  external 998.32
  internal 998.31
  superficial 998.32
perineal wound (postpartum) 674.2
postoperative 998.32
  abdomen 998.32
    internal 998.31
  internal 998.31
traumatic injury wound repair 998.33
uterine wound 674.1
Dehydration (cachexia) 276.51
newborn 775.5
with
  hypernatremia 276.0
  hyponatremia 276.1
Deiters' nucleus syndrome 386.19
Déjérine's disease 356.0
Déjérine-Klumpke paralysis 767.6
Déjérine-Roussy syndrome 338.0
Déjérine-Sottas disease or neuropathy (hypertrophic) 356.0
Déjérine-Thomas atrophy or syndrome 333.0
de Lange's syndrome (Amsterdam dwarf, intellectual disabilities, and brachycephaly) 759.89
Delay, delayed
adaptation, cones or rods 368.63
any plane in pelvis
  affecting fetus or newborn 763.1
  complicating delivery 660.1
birth or delivery NEC 662.1
  affecting fetus or newborn 763.9
  second twin, triplet, or multiple mate 662.3
closure—*see also* Fistula
  cranial suture 756.0
  fontanel 756.0
coagulation NEC 790.92
conduction (cardiac) (ventricular) 426.9
delivery NEC 662.1
  second twin, triplet, etc. 662.3
    affecting fetus or newborn 763.89
development
  in childhood 783.40
    physiological 783.40
  intellectual NEC 315.9
  learning NEC 315.2

Delay, delayed—*continued*
  development—*continued*
    reading 315.00
    sexual 259.0
    speech 315.39
      and language due to hearing loss 315.34
      associated with hyperkinesis 314.1
      spelling 315.09
    gastric emptying 536.8
    menarche 256.39
      due to pituitary hypofunction 253.4
    menstruation (cause unknown) 626.8
    milestone in childhood 783.42
    motility—*see* Hypomotility
    passage of meconium (newborn) 777.1
    primary respiration 768.9
    puberty 259.0
    separation of umbilical cord 779.83
    sexual maturation, female 259.0
    vaccination V64.00
Del Castillo's syndrome (germinal aplasia) 606.0
Deleage's disease 359.89
Deletion syndrome
  5p 758.31
  22q11.2 758.32
  autosomal NEC 758.39
  constitutional 5q deletion 758.39
Delhi (boil) (button) (sore) 085.1
Delinquency (juvenile) 312.9
  group (*see also* Disturbance, conduct) 312.2
  neurotic 312.4
Delirium, delirious 780.09
  acute 780.09
    due to conditions classified elsewhere 293.0
  alcoholic 291.0
    acute 291.0
    chronic 291.1
  alcoholicum 291.0
  chronic (*see also* Psychosis) 293.89
    due to or associated with physical
      condition—*see* Psychosis, organic
    due to conditions classified elsewhere 293.0
  drug-induced 292.81
  eclamptic (*see also* Eclampsia) 780.39
  exhaustion (*see also* Reaction, stress, acute)
    308.9
  hysterical 300.11
  in
    presenile dementia 290.11
    senile dementia 290.3
  induced by drug 292.81
  manic, maniacal (acute) (*see also* Psychosis,
    affective) 296.0
    recurrent episode 296.1
    single episode 296.0
  puerperal 293.9
  senile 290.3
  subacute (psychotic) 293.1
  thyroid (*see also* Thyrotoxicosis) 242.9
  traumatic—*see also* Injury, intracranial
    with
      lesion, spinal cord—*see* Injury, spinal, by
        site
      shock, spinal—*see* Injury, spinal, by site
  tremens (impending) 291.0
  uremic—*see* Uremia
  withdrawal
    alcoholic (acute) 291.0
      chronic 291.1
    drug 292.0

Delivery

Note—Use the following fifth-digit
subclassification with categories
640-649, 651-676:

0 unspecified as to episode of care
1 delivered, with or without mention of
  antepartum condition
2 delivered, with mention of
  postpartum complication
3 antepartum condition or complication
4 postpartum condition or
  complication

  breech (assisted) (spontaneous) 652.2
    affecting fetus or newborn 763.0
    extraction NEC 669.6
  cesarean (for) 669.7
    abnormal
      cervix 654.6
      pelvic organs or tissues 654.9
      pelvis (bony) (major) NEC 653.0
      presentation or position 652.9
        in multiple gestation 652.6
      size, fetus 653.5
      soft parts (of pelvis) 654.9
      uterus, congenital 654.0
      vagina 654.7
      vulva 654.8
    abruptio placentae 641.2
    acromion presentation 652.8
    affecting fetus or newborn 763.4
    anteversion, cervix or uterus 654.4
    atony, uterus 661.2
      with hemorrhage 666.1
    bicornis or bicornuate uterus 654.0
    breech presentation 652.2
    brow presentation 652.4
    cephalopelvic disproportion (normally formed
      fetus) 653.4
    chin presentation 652.4
    cicatrix of cervix 654.6
    contracted pelvis (general) 653.1
      inlet 653.2
      outlet 653.3
    cord presentation or prolapse 663.0
    cystocele 654.4
    deformity (acquired) (congenital)
      pelvic organs or tissues NEC 654.9
      pelvis (bony) NEC 653.0
    displacement, uterus NEC 654.4
    disproportion NEC 653.9
    distress
      fetal 656.8
      maternal 669.0
    eclampsia 642.6
    face presentation 652.4
    failed
      forceps 660.7
      trial of labor NEC 660.6
      vacuum extraction 660.7
      ventouse 660.7
    fetal deformity 653.7
    fetal-maternal hemorrhage 656.0
    fetus, fetal
      distress 656.8
      prematurity 656.8
    fibroid (tumor) (uterus) 654.1
    footling 652.8
      with successful version 652.1

Delivery—*continued*
  cesarean—*continued*
    hemorrhage (antepartum) (intrapartum) NEC
      641.9
    hydrocephalic fetus 653.6
    incarceration of uterus 654.3
    incoordinate uterine action 661.4
    inertia, uterus 661.2
      primary 661.0
      secondary 661.1
    lateroversion, uterus or cervix 654.4
    mal lie 652.9
    malposition
      fetus 652.9
        in multiple gestation 652.6
      pelvic organs or tissues NEC 654.9
      uterus NEC or cervix 654.4
    malpresentation NEC 652.9
      in multiple gestation 652.6
    maternal
      diabetes mellitus (conditions classifiable to
        249 and 250) 648.0
      heart disease NEC 648.6
    meconium in liquor 656.8
      staining only 792.3
    oblique presentation 652.3
    oversize fetus 653.5
    pelvic tumor NEC 654.9
    placental insufficiency 656.5
    placenta previa 641.0
      with hemorrhage 641.1
    (planned) occurring after 37 completed weeks
      of gestation but before 39 completed
      weeks gestation due to (spontaneous) onset
      of labor 649.8
    poor dilation, cervix 661.0
    pre-eclampsia 642.4
      severe 642.5
    previous
      cesarean delivery 654.2
      surgery (to)
        cervix 654.6
        gynecological NEC 654.9
        rectum 654.8
        uterus NEC 654.9
          from previous cesarean delivery 654.2
        vagina 654.7
    prolapse
      arm or hand 652.7
      uterus 654.4
    prolonged labor 662.1
    rectocele 654.4
    retroversion, uterus or cervix 654.3
    rigid
      cervix 654.6
      pelvic floor 654.4
      perineum 654.8
      vagina 654.7
      vulva 654.8
    sacculation, pregnant uterus 654.4
    scar(s)
      cervix 654.6
      cesarean delivery 654.2
      uterus NEC 654.9
        due to previous cesarean delivery 654.2
    Shirodkar suture in situ 654.5
    shoulder presentation 652.8
    stenosis or stricture, cervix 654.6
    transverse presentation or lie 652.3
    tumor, pelvic organs or tissues NEC 654.4
    umbilical cord presentation or prolapse 663.0

Delivery—*continued*
  completely normal case—*see* category 650
  complicated (by) NEC 669.9
    abdominal tumor, fetal 653.7
      causing obstructed labor 660.1
    abnormal, abnormality of
      cervix 654.6
        causing obstructed labor 660.2
      forces of labor 661.9
      formation of uterus 654.0
      pelvic organs or tissues 654.9
        causing obstructed labor 660.2
      pelvis (bony) (major) NEC 653.0
        causing obstructed labor 660.1
      presentation or position NEC 652.9
        causing obstructed labor 660.0
      size, fetus 653.5
        causing obstructed labor 660.1
      soft parts (of pelvis) 654.9
        causing obstructed labor 660.2
      uterine contractions NEC 661.9
      uterus (formation) 654.0
        causing obstructed labor 660.2
      vagina 654.7
        causing obstructed labor 660.2
    abnormally formed uterus (any type)
      (congenital) 654.0
      causing obstructed labor 660.2
    acromion presentation 652.8
      causing obstructed labor 660.0
    adherent placenta 667.0
      with hemorrhage 666.0
    adhesions, uterus (to abdominal wall) 654.4
    advanced maternal age NEC 659.6
      multigravida 659.6
      primigravida 659.5
    air embolism 673.0
    amnionitis 658.4
    amniotic fluid embolism 673.1
    anesthetic death 668.9
    annular detachment, cervix 665.3
    antepartum hemorrhage—*see* Delivery,
      complicated, hemorrhage
    anteversion, cervix or uterus 654.4
      causing obstructed labor 660.2
    apoplexy 674.0
      placenta 641.2
    arrested active phase 661.1
    asymmetrical pelvis bone 653.0
      causing obstructed labor 660.1
    atony, uterus with hemorrhage (hypotonic)
      (inertia) 666.1
      hypertonic 661.4
    Bandl's ring 661.4
    battledore placenta—*see* Placenta, abnormal
    bicornis or bicornuate uterus 654.0
      causing obstructed labor 660.2
    birth injury to mother NEC 665.9
    bleeding (*see also* Delivery, complicated,
      hemorrhage) 641.9
    breech presentation (assisted) (buttocks)
      (complete) (frank) (spontaneous) 652.2
      with successful version 652.1
    brow presentation 652.4
    cephalopelvic disproportion (normally formed
      fetus) 653.4
      causing obstructed labor 660.1
    cerebral hemorrhage 674.0
    cervical dystocia 661.2
    chin presentation 652.4
      causing obstructed labor 660.0

Delivery—*continued*
  complicated by—*continued*
    cicatrix
      cervix 654.6
        causing obstructed labor 660.2
      vagina 654.7
        causing obstructed labor 660.2
    coagulation defect 649.3
    colporrhexis 665.4
      with perineal laceration 664.0
    compound presentation 652.8
      causing obstructed labor 660.0
    compression of cord (umbilical) 663.2
      around neck 663.1
      cord prolapsed 663.0
    contraction, contracted pelvis 653.1
      causing obstructed labor 660.1
      general 653.1
        causing obstructed labor 660.1
      inlet 653.2
        causing obstructed labor 660.1
      midpelvic 653.8
        causing obstructed labor 660.1
      midplane 653.8
        causing obstructed labor 660.1
      outlet 653.3
        causing obstructed labor 660.1
    contraction ring 661.4
    cord (umbilical) 663.9
      around neck, tightly or with compression 663.1
        without compression 663.3
      bruising 663.6
      complication NEC 663.9
        specified type NEC 663.8
      compression NEC 663.2
      entanglement NEC 663.3
        with compression 663.2
      forelying 663.0
      hematoma 663.6
      marginal attachment 663.8
      presentation 663.0
      prolapse (complete) (occult) (partial) 663.0
      short 663.4
      specified complication NEC 663.8
      thrombosis (vessels) 663.6
      vascular lesion 663.6
      velamentous insertion 663.8
    Couvelaire uterus 641.2
    cretin pelvis (dwarf type) (male type) 653.1
      causing obstructed labor 660.1
    crossbirth 652.3
      with successful version 652.1
      causing obstructed labor 660.0
    cyst (Gartner's duct) 654.7
    cystocele 654.4
      causing obstructed labor 660.2
    death of fetus (near term) 656.4
      early (before 22 completed weeks'
        gestation) 632
    deformity (acquired) (congenital)
      fetus 653.7
        causing obstructed labor 660.1
      pelvic organs or tissues NEC 654.9
        causing obstructed labor 660.2
      pelvis (bony) NEC 653.0
        causing obstructed labor 660.1
    delay, delayed
      delivery in multiple pregnancy 662.3
        due to locked mates 660.5
      following rupture of membranes
        (spontaneous) 658.2
        artificial 658.3

Delivery—*continued*
  complicated by—*continued*
    depressed fetal heart tones 659.7
    diastasis recti 665.8
    dilatation
      bladder 654.4
        causing obstructed labor 660.2
      cervix, incomplete, poor or slow 661.0
    diseased placenta 656.7
    displacement uterus NEC 654.4
      causing obstructed labor 660.2
    disproportion NEC 653.9
      causing obstructed labor 660.1
    disruptio uteri—*see* Delivery, complicated,
        rupture, uterus
    distress
      fetal 656.8
      maternal 669.0
    double uterus (congenital) 654.0
      causing obstructed labor 660.2
    dropsy amnion 657
    dysfunction, uterus 661.9
      hypertonic 661.4
      hypotonic 661.2
        primary 661.0
        secondary 661.1
      incoordinate 661.4
    dystocia
      cervical 661.2
      fetal—*see* Delivery, complicated, abnormal,
          presentation
      maternal—*see* Delivery, complicated,
          prolonged labor
      pelvic—*see* Delivery, complicated,
          contraction pelvis
      positional 652.8
      shoulder girdle 660.4
    eclampsia 642.6
    ectopic kidney 654.4
      causing obstructed labor 660.2
    edema, cervix 654.6
      causing obstructed labor 660.2
    effusion, amniotic fluid 658.1
    elderly multigravida 659.6
    elderly primigravida 659.5
    embolism (pulmonary) 673.2
      air 673.0
      amniotic fluid 673.1
      blood-clot 673.2
      cerebral 674.0
      fat 673.8
      pyemic 673.3
      septic 673.3
    entanglement, umbilical cord 663.3
      with compression 663.2
      around neck (with compression) 663.1
    eversion, cervix or uterus 665.2
    excessive
      fetal growth 653.5
        causing obstructed labor 660.1
      size of fetus 653.5
        causing obstructed labor 660.1
    face presentation 652.4
      causing obstructed labor 660.0
      to pubes 660.3
    failure, fetal head to enter pelvic brim 652.5
      causing obstructed labor 660.0
    female genital mutilation 660.8

Delivery—*continued*
complicated by—*continued*
fetal
acid-base balance 656.8
death (near term) NEC 656.4
early (before 22 completed weeks'
gestation) 632
deformity 653.7
causing obstructed labor 660.1
distress 656.8
heart rate or rhythm 659.7
reduction of multiple fetuses reduced to
single fetus 651.7
fetopelvic disproportion 653.4
causing obstructed labor 660.1
fever during labor 659.2
fibroid (tumor) (uterus) 654.1
causing obstructed labor 660.2
fibromyomata 654.1
causing obstructed labor 660.2
forelying umbilical cord 663.0
fracture of coccyx 665.6
hematoma 664.5
broad ligament 665.7
ischial spine 665.7
pelvic 665.7
perineum 664.5
soft tissues 665.7
subdural 674.0
umbilical cord 663.6
vagina 665.7
vulva or perineum 664.5
hemorrhage (uterine) (antepartum)
(intrapartum) (pregnancy) 641.9
accidental 641.2
associated with
afibrinogenemia 641.3
coagulation defect 641.3
hyperfibrinolysis 641.3
hypofibrinogenemia 641.3
cerebral 674.0
due to
low-lying placenta 641.1
placenta previa 641.1
premature separation of placenta (normally
implanted) 641.2
retained placenta 666.0
trauma 641.8
uterine leiomyoma 641.8
marginal sinus rupture 641.2
placenta NEC 641.9
postpartum (atonic) (immediate) (within 24
hours) 666.1
with retained or trapped placenta 666.0
third stage 666.0
delayed 666.2
secondary 666.2
hourglass contraction, uterus 661.4
hydramnios 657
hydrocephalic fetus 653.6
causing obstructed labor 660.1
hydrops fetalis 653.7
causing obstructed labor 660.1
hypertension—*see* Hypertension, complicating
pregnancy
hypertonic uterine dysfunction 661.4
hypotonic uterine dysfunction 661.2
impacted shoulders 660.4
incarceration, uterus 654.3
causing obstructed labor 660.2
incomplete dilation (cervix) 661.0
incoordinate uterus 661.4

Delivery—*continued*
complicated by—*continued*
indication NEC 659.9
specified type NEC 659.8
inertia, uterus 661.2
hypertonic 661.4
hypotonic 661.2
primary 661.0
secondary 661.1
infantile
genitalia 654.4
causing obstructed labor 660.2
uterus (os) 654.4
causing obstructed labor 660.2
injury (to mother) NEC 665.9
intrauterine fetal death (near term) NEC 656.4
early (before 22 completed weeks'
gestation) 632
inversion, uterus 665.2
kidney, ectopic 654.4
causing obstructed labor 660.2
knot (true), umbilical cord 663.2
labor
onset (spontaneous) after 37 completed
weeks of gestation but before 39
completed weeks gestation with delivery
by (planned) cesarean section 649.8
premature (before 37 completed weeks
gestation) 644.2
laceration 664.9
anus (sphincter) (healed) (old) 654.8
not associated with third-degree perineal
laceration 664.6
with mucosa 664.3
bladder (urinary) 665.5
bowel 665.5
central 664.4
cervix (uteri) 665.3
fourchette 664.0
hymen 664.0
labia (majora) (minora) 664.0
pelvic
floor 664.1
organ NEC 665.5
perineum, perineal 664.4
first degree 664.0
second degree 664.1
third degree 664.2
fourth degree 664.3
central 664.4
extensive NEC 664.4
muscles 664.1
skin 664.0
slight 664.0
peritoneum (pelvic) 665.5
periurethral tissue 664.8
rectovaginal (septum) (without perineal
laceration) 665.4
with perineum 664.2
with anal or rectal mucosa 664.3
skin (perineum) 664.0
specified site or type NEC 664.8
sphincter ani (healed) (old) 654.8
not associated with third-degree perineal
laceration 664.6
with mucosa 664.3
urethra 665.5
uterus 665.1
before labor 665.0

Delivery—*continued*
  complicated by—*continued*
   laceration—*continued*
    vagina, vaginal (deep) (high) (sulcus) (wall)
     (without perineal laceration) 665.4
     with perineum 664.0
      muscles, with perineum 664.1
     vulva 664.0
    lateroversion, uterus or cervix 654.4
     causing obstructed labor 660.2
    locked mates 660.5
    low implantation of placenta—*see* Delivery,
     complicated, placenta, previa
    mal lie 652.9
    malposition
     fetus NEC 652.9
      causing obstructed labor 660.0
     pelvic organs or tissues NEC 654.9
      causing obstructed labor 660.2
     placenta 641.1
      without hemorrhage 641.0
     uterus NEC or cervix 654.4
      causing obstructed labor 660.2
    malpresentation 652.9
     causing obstructed labor 660.0
    marginal sinus (bleeding) (rupture) 641.2
    maternal hypotension syndrome 669.2
    meconium in liquor 656.8
    membranes, retained—*see* Delivery,
     complicated, placenta, retained
    mentum presentation 652.4
     causing obstructed labor 660.0
    metrorrhagia (myopathia)—*see* Delivery,
     complicated, hemorrhage
    metrorrhexis—*see* Delivery, complicated,
     rupture, uterus
    multiparity (grand) 659.4
    myelomeningocele, fetus 653.7
     causing obstructed labor 660.1
    Nägele's pelvis 653.0
     causing obstructed labor 660.1
    nonengagement, fetal head 652.5
     causing obstructed labor 660.0
    oblique presentation 652.3
     causing obstructed labor 660.0
    obstetric
     shock 669.1
     trauma NEC 665.9
    obstructed labor 660.9
     due to
      abnormality pelvic organs or tissues
       (conditions classifiable to 654.0-654.9)
       660.2
      deep transverse arrest 660.3
      impacted shoulders 660.4
      locked twins 660.5
      malposition and malpresentation of fetus
       (conditions classifiable to 652.0-652.9)
       660.0
      persistent occipitoposterior 660.3
      shoulder dystocia 660.4
    occult prolapse of umbilical cord 663.0
    oversize fetus 653.5
     causing obstructed labor 660.1
    pathological retraction ring, uterus 661.4
    pelvic
     arrest (deep) (high) (of fetal head)
      (transverse) 660.3
     deformity (bone)—*see also* Deformity,
      pelvis, with disproportion
      soft tissue 654.9
       causing obstructed labor 660.2

Delivery—*continued*
  complicated by—*continued*
   pelvic—*continued*
    tumor NEC 654.9
     causing obstructed labor 660.2
   penetration, pregnant uterus by instrument 665.1
   perforation—*see* Delivery, complicated,
    laceration
   persistent
    hymen 654.8
     causing obstructed labor 660.2
    occipitoposterior 660.3
   placenta, placental
    ablatio 641.2
    abnormality 656.7
     with hemorrhage 641.2
    abruptio 641.2
    accreta 667.0
     with hemorrhage 666.0
    adherent (without hemorrhage) 667.0
     with hemorrhage 666.0
    apoplexy 641.2
    battledore 663.8
    detachment (premature) 641.2
    disease 656.7
    hemorrhage NEC 641.9
    increta (without hemorrhage) 667.0
     with hemorrhage 666.0
    low (implantation) 641.1
     without hemorrhage 641.0
    malformation 656.7
     with hemorrhage 641.2
    malposition 641.1
     without hemorrhage 641.0
    marginal sinus rupture 641.2
    percreta 667.0
     with hemorrhage 666.0
    premature separation 641.2
    previa (central) (lateral) (marginal) (partial)
     641.1
     without hemorrhage 641.0
    retained (with hemorrhage) 666.0
     without hemorrhage 667.0
    rupture of marginal sinus 641.2
    separation (premature) 641.2
    trapped 666.0
     without hemorrhage 667.0
    vicious insertion 641.1
   polyhydramnios 657
   polyp, cervix 654.6
    causing obstructed labor 660.2
   precipitate labor 661.3
   premature
    labor (before 37 completed weeks gestation)
     644.2
    rupture, membranes 658.1
     delayed delivery following 658.2
   presenting umbilical cord 663.0
   previous
    cesarean delivery 654.2
    surgery
     cervix 654.6
      causing obstructed labor 660.2
     gynecological NEC 654.9
      causing obstructed labor 660.2
     perineum 654.8
     rectum 654.8
     uterus NEC 654.9
      due to previous cesarean delivery 654.2
     vagina 654.7
      causing obstructed labor 660.2
     vulva 654.8

Delivery—*continued*
  complicated by—*continued*
    primary uterine inertia 661.0
    primipara, elderly or old 659.5
    prolapse
      arm or hand 652.7
        causing obstructed labor 660.0
      cord (umbilical) 663.0
      fetal extremity 652.8
      foot or leg 652.8
        causing obstructed labor 660.0
      umbilical cord (complete) (occult) (partial)
        663.0
      uterus 654.4
        causing obstructed labor 660.2
    prolonged labor 662.1
      active phase 661.2
      due to
        cervical dystocia 661.2
        contraction ring 661.4
        tetanic uterus 661.4
        uterine inertia 661.2
          primary 661.0
          secondary 661.1
      first stage 662.0
      latent phase 661.0
      second stage 662.2
    pyrexia during labor 659.2
    rachitic pelvis 653.2
      causing obstructed labor 660.1
    rectocele 654.4
      causing obstructed labor 660.2
    retained membranes or portions of placenta
      666.2
      without hemorrhage 667.1
    retarded (prolonged) birth 662.1
    retention secundines (with hemorrhage) 666.2
      without hemorrhage 667.1
    retroversion, uterus or cervix 654.3
      causing obstructed labor 660.2
    rigid
      cervix 654.6
        causing obstructed labor 660.2
      pelvic floor 654.4
        causing obstructed labor 660.2
      perineum or vulva 654.8
        causing obstructed labor 660.2
      vagina 654.7
        causing obstructed labor 660.2
    Robert's pelvis 653.0
      causing obstructed labor 660.1
    rupture—*see also* Delivery, complicated,
      laceration
      bladder (urinary) 665.5
      cervix 665.3
      marginal sinus 641.2
      membranes, premature 658.1
      pelvic organ NEC 665.5
      perineum (without mention of other
        laceration)—*see* Delivery, complicated,
        laceration, perineum
      peritoneum (pelvic) 665.5
      urethra 665.5
      uterus (during labor) 665.1
        before labor 665.0
    sacculation, pregnant uterus 654.4
    sacral teratomas, fetal 653.7
      causing obstructed labor 660.1

Delivery—*continued*
  complicated by—*continued*
    scar(s)
      cervix 654.6
        causing obstructed labor 660.2
      cesarean delivery 654.2
        causing obstructed labor 660.2
      perineum 654.8
        causing obstructed labor 660.2
      uterus NEC 654.9
        causing obstructed labor 660.2
        due to previous cesarean delivery 654.2
      vagina 654.7
        causing obstructed labor 660.2
      vulva 654.8
        causing obstructed labor 660.2
    scoliotic pelvis 653.0
      causing obstructed labor 660.1
    secondary uterine inertia 661.1
    secundines, retained—*see* Delivery,
      complicated, placenta, retained
    separation
      placenta (premature) 641.2
      pubic bone 665.6
      symphysis pubis 665.6
    septate vagina 654.7
      causing obstructed labor 660.2
    shock (birth) (obstetric) (puerperal) 669.1
    short cord syndrome 663.4
    shoulder
      girdle dystocia 660.4
      presentation 652.8
        causing obstructed labor 660.0
    Siamese twins 678.1
    slow slope active phase 661.2
    spasm
      cervix 661.4
      uterus 661.4
    spondylolisthesis, pelvis 653.3
      causing obstructed labor 660.1
    spondylolysis (lumbosacral) 653.3
      causing obstructed labor 660.1
    spondylosis 653.0
      causing obstructed labor 660.1
    stenosis or stricture
      cervix 654.6
        causing obstructed labor 660.2
      vagina 654.7
        causing obstructed labor 660.2
    sudden death, unknown cause 669.9
    tear (pelvic organ) (*see also* Delivery,
      complicated, laceration) 664.9
      anal sphincter (healed) (old) 654.8
        not associated with third-degree perineal
          laceration 664.6
    teratomas, sacral, fetal 653.7
      causing obstructed labor 660.1
    tetanic uterus 661.4
    tipping pelvis 653.0
      causing obstructed labor 660.1
    transverse
      arrest (deep) 660.3
      presentation or lie 652.3
        with successful version 652.1
        causing obstructed labor 660.0
    trauma (obstetrical) NEC 665.9
      periurethral 664.8

Delivery—*continued*
  complicated by—*continued*
    tumor
      abdominal, fetal 653.7
        causing obstructed labor 660.1
      pelvic organs or tissues NEC 654.9
        causing obstructed labor 660.2
    umbilical cord (*see also* Delivery,
        complicated, cord) 663.9
      around neck tightly, or with compression
        663.1
      entanglement NEC 663.3
        with compression 663.2
      prolapse (complete) (occult) (partial) 663.0
    unstable lie 652.0
      causing obstructed labor 660.0
    uterine
      inertia (*see also* Delivery, complicated,
        inertia, uterus) 661.2
      spasm 661.4
    vasa previa 663.5
    velamentous insertion of cord 663.8
    young maternal age 659.8
  delayed NEC 662.1
    following rupture of membranes (spontaneous)
      658.2
      artificial 658.3
    second twin, triplet, etc. 662.3
  difficult NEC 669.9
    previous, affecting management of pregnancy
      or childbirth V23.49
    specified type NEC 669.8
  early onset (spontaneous) 644.2
  forceps NEC 669.5
    affecting fetus or newborn 763.2
  footling 652.8
    with successful version 652.1
  missed (at or near term) 656.4
  multiple gestation NEC 651.9
    with fetal loss and retention of one or more
      fetus(es) 651.6
    following (elective) fetal reduction 651.7
    specified type NEC 651.8
      with fetal loss and retention of one or more
        fetus(es) 651.6
      following (elective) fetal reduction 651.7
  nonviable infant 656.4
  normal—*see* category 650
  precipitate 661.3
    affecting fetus or newborn 763.6
  premature NEC (before 37 completed weeks
      gestation) 644.2
    previous, affecting management of pregnancy
      V23.41
  quadruplet NEC 651.2
    with fetal loss and retention of one or more
      fetus(es) 651.5
    following (elective) fetal reduction 651.7
  quintuplet NEC 651.8
    with fetal loss and retention of one or more
      fetus(es) 651.6
    following (elective) fetal reduction 651.7
  sextuplet NEC 651.8
    with fetal loss and retention of one or more
      fetus(es) 651.6
    following (elective) fetal reduction 651.7
  specified complication NEC 669.8
  stillbirth (near term) NEC 656.4
    early (before 22 completed weeks' gestation)
      632

Delivery—*continued*
  term pregnancy (live birth) NEC—*see* category
    650
    stillbirth NEC 656.4
  threatened premature 644.2
  triplets NEC 651.1
    with fetal loss and retention of one or more
      fetus(es) 651.4
    delayed delivery (one or more mates) 662.3
    following (elective) fetal reduction 651.7
    locked mates 660.5
  twins NEC 651.0
    with fetal loss and retention of one or more
      fetus(es) 651.3
    delayed delivery (one or more mates) 662.3
    following (elective) fetal reduction 651.7
    locked mates 660.5
  uncomplicated—*see* category 650
  vacuum extractor NEC 669.5
    affecting fetus or newborn 763.3
  ventouse NEC 669.5
    affecting fetus or newborn 763.3
Dellen, cornea 371.41
Delusions (paranoid) 297.9
  grandiose 297.1
  parasitosis 300.29
  systematized 297.1
Dementia 294.20
  with behavioral disturbance (aggressive)
    (combative) (violent) 294.21
  alcohol-induced persisting (*see also* Psychosis,
    alcoholic) 291.2
  Alzheimer's—*see* Alzheimer's dementia
  arteriosclerotic (simple type) (uncomplicated)
    290.40
    with
      acute confusional state 290.41
      delirium 290.41
      delusions 290.42
      depressed mood 290.43
    depressed type 290.43
    paranoid type 290.42
  Binswanger's 290.12
  catatonic (acute) (*see also* Schizophrenia) 295.2
  congenital (*see also* Disability, intellectual) 319
  degenerative 290.9
    presenile-onset—*see* Dementia, presenile
    senile-onset—*see* Dementia, senile
  developmental (*see also* Schizophrenia) 295.9
  dialysis 294.8
    transient 293.9
  drug-induced persisting (*see also* Psychosis,
    drug) 292.82
  due to or associated with condition(s) classified
      elsewhere
    Alzheimer's
      with behavioral disturbance 331.0 *[294.11]*
      without behavioral disturbance 331.0
        [294.10]
    cerebral lipidoses
      with behavioral disturbance 330.1 *[294.11]*
      without behavioral disturbance 330.1
        [294.10]
    epilepsy
      with behavioral disturbance 345.9 *[294.11]*
      without behavioral disturbance 345.9
        [294.10]
    hepatolenticular degeneration
      with behavioral disturbance 275.1 *[294.11]*
      without behavioral disturbance 275.1
        [294.10]

Dementia—*continued*
  due to or associated with—*continued*
    HIV
      with behavioral disturbance 042 *[294.11]*
      without behavioral disturbance 042 *[294.10]*
    Huntington's chorea
      with behavioral disturbance 333.4 *[294.11]*
      without behavioral disturbance 333.4
        [294.10]
    Jakob-Creutzfeldt disease (CJD)
      with behavioral disturbance 046.19 *[294.11]*
      without behavioral disturbance 046.19
        [294.10]
      variant (vCJD) 046.11
        with dementia
          with behavioral disturbance 046.11
            [294.11]
          without behavioral disturbance 046.11
            [294.10]
    Lewy bodies
      with behavioral disturbance 331.82 *[294.11]*
      without behavioral disturbance 331.82
        [294.10]
    multiple sclerosis
      with behavioral disturbance 340 *[294.11]*
      without behavioral disturbance 340 *[294.10]*
    neurosyphilis
      with behavioral disturbance 094.9 *[294.11]*
      without behavioral disturbance 094.9
        [294.10]
    Parkinsonism
      with behavioral disturbance 331.82 *[294.11]*
      without behavioral disturbance 331.82
        [294.10]
    Parkinson's disease
      with behavioral disturbance 332.0 *[294.11]*
      without behavioral disturbance 332.0
        [294.10]
    Pelizaeus-Merzbacher disease
      with behavioral disturbance 333.0 *[294.11]*
      without behavioral disturbance 333.0
        [294.10]
    Pick's disease
      with behavioral disturbance 331.11 *[294.11]*
      without behavioral disturbance 331.11
        [294.10]
    polyarteritis nodosa
      with behavioral disturbance 446.0 *[294.11]*
      without behavioral disturbance 446.0
        [294.10]
    syphilis
      with behavioral disturbance 094.1 *[294.11]*
      without behavioral disturbance 094.1
        [294.10]
    Wilson's disease
      with behavioral disturbance 275.1 *[294.11]*
      without behavioral disturbance 275.1
        [294.10]
  frontal 331.19
    with behavioral disturbance 331.19 *[294.11]*
    without behavioral disturbance 331.19
      [294.10]
  frontotemporal 331.19
    with behavioral disturbance 331.19 *[294.11]*
    without behavioral disturbance 331.19
      [294.10]
  hebephrenic (acute) 295.1
  Heller's (infantile psychosis) (*see also*
    Psychosis, childhood) 299.1
  idiopathic 290.9
    presenile-onset—*see* Dementia, presenile
    senile-onset—*see* Dementia, senile

Dementia—*continued*
  in
    arteriosclerotic brain disease 290.40
    senility 290.0
  induced by drug 292.82
  infantile, infantilia (*see also* Psychosis,
    childhood) 299.0
  Lewy body 331.82
    with behavioral disturbance 331.82 *[294.11]*
    without behavioral disturbance 331.82 *[294.10]*
  multi-infarct (cerebrovascular) (*see also*
    Dementia, arteriosclerotic) 290.40
  old age 290.0
  paralytica, paralytic 094.1
    juvenilis 090.40
    syphilitic 094.1
      congenital 090.40
    tabetic form 094.1
  paranoid (*see also* Schizophrenia) 295.3
  paraphrenic (*see also* Schizophrenia) 295.3
  paretic 094.1
  praecox (*see also* Schizophrenia) 295.9
  presenile 290.10
    with
      acute confusional state 290.11
      delirium 290.11
      delusional features 290.12
      depressive features 290.13
    depressed type 290.13
    paranoid type 290.12
    simple type 290.10
    uncomplicated 290.10
  primary (acute) (*see also* Schizophrenia) 295.0
  progressive, syphilitic 094.1
  puerperal—*see* Psychosis, puerperal
  schizophrenic (*see also* Schizophrenia) 295.9
  senile 290.0
    with
      acute confusional state 290.3
      delirium 290.3
      delusional features 290.20
      depressive features 290.21
    depressed type 290.21
    exhaustion 290.0
    paranoid type 290.20
  simple type (acute) (*see also* Schizophrenia) 295.0
  simplex (acute) (*see also* Schizophrenia) 295.0
  syphilitic 094.1
  uremic—*see* Uremia
  vascular 290.40
    with
      delirium 290.41
      delusions 290.42
      depressed mood 290.43
Demerol dependence (*see also* Dependence)
  304.0
Demineralization, ankle (*see also* Osteoporosis)
  733.00
Demodex folliculorum (infestation) 133.8
Demoralization 799.25
de Morgan's spots (senile angiomas) 448.1
Demyelinating
  polyneuritis, chronic inflammatory 357.81
Demyelination, demyelinization
  central nervous system 341.9
    specified NEC 341.8
  corpus callosum (central) 341.8
  global 340
Dengue (fever) 061
  sandfly 061
  vaccination, prophylactic (against) V05.1
  virus hemorrhagic fever 065.4

Dens
  evaginatus 520.2
  in dente 520.2
  invaginatus 520.2
Dense breast(s) 793.82
Density
  increased, bone (disseminated) (generalized)
    (spotted) 733.99
  lung (nodular) 518.89
Dental —*see also* condition
  examination only V72.2
Dentia praecox 520.6
Denticles (in pulp) 522.2
Dentigerous cyst 526.0
Dentin
  irregular (in pulp) 522.3
  opalescent 520.5
  secondary (in pulp) 522.3
  sensitive 521.89
Dentinogenesis imperfecta 520.5
Dentinoma (M9271/0) 213.1
  upper jaw (bone) 213.0
Dentition 520.7
  abnormal 520.6
  anomaly 520.6
  delayed 520.6
  difficult 520.7
  disorder of 520.6
  precocious 520.6
  retarded 520.6
Denture sore (mouth) 528.9
Dependence

> *Note—Use the following fifth-digit*
> *subclassification with category 304:*
>
> *0 unspecified*
> *1 continuous*
> *2 episodic*
> *3 in remission*

  with
    withdrawal symptoms
      alcohol 291.81
      drug 292.0
  14-hydroxy-dihydromorphinone 304.0
  absinthe 304.6
  acemorphan 304.0
  acetanilid(e) 304.6
  acetophenetidin 304.6
  acetorphine 304.0
  acetyldihydrocodeine 304.0
  acetyldihydrocodeinone 304.0
  Adalin 304.1
  Afghanistan black 304.3
  agrypnal 304.1
  alcohol, alcoholic (ethyl) (methyl) (wood) 303.9
    maternal, with suspected fetal damage
      affecting management of pregnancy 655.4
  allobarbitone 304.1
  allonal 304.1
  allylisopropylacetylurea 304.1
  alphaprodine (hydrochloride) 304.0
  Alurate 304.1
  Alvodine 304.0
  amethocaine 304.6
  amidone 304.0
  amidopyrine 304.6
  aminopyrine 304.6
  amobarbital 304.1
  amphetamine(s) (type) (drugs classifiable to
    969.7) 304.4

Dependence—*continued*
  amylene hydrate 304.6
  amylobarbitone 304.1
  amylocaine 304.6
  Amytal (sodium) 304.1
  analgesic (drug) NEC 304.6
    synthetic with morphine-like effect 304.0
  anesthetic (agent) (drug) (gas) (general) (local)
    NEC 304.6
  Angel dust 304.6
  anileridine 304.0
  antipyrine 304.6
  anxiolytic 304.1
  aprobarbital 304.1
  aprobarbitone 304.1
  atropine 304.6
  Avertin (bromide) 304.6
  barbenyl 304.1
  barbital(s) 304.1
  barbitone 304.1
  barbiturate(s) (compounds) (drugs classifiable to
    967.0) 304.1
  barbituric acid (and compounds) 304.1
  benzedrine 304.4
  benzylmorphine 304.0
  Beta-chlor 304.1
  bhang 304.3
  blue velvet 304.0
  Brevital 304.1
  bromal (hydrate) 304.1
  bromide(s) NEC 304.1
  bromine compounds NEC 304.1
  bromisovalum 304.1
  bromoform 304.1
  Bromo-seltzer 304.1
  bromural 304.1
  butabarbital (sodium) 304.1
  butabarpal 304.1
  butallylonal 304.1
  butethal 304.1
  buthalitone (sodium) 304.1
  Butisol 304.1
  butobarbitone 304.1
  butyl chloral (hydrate) 304.1
  caffeine 304.4
  cannabis (indica) (sativa) (resin) (derivatives)
    (type) 304.3
  carbamazepine 304.6
  Carbrital 304.1
  carbromal 304.1
  carisoprodol 304.6
  Catha (edulis) 304.4
  chloral (betaine) (hydrate) 304.1
  chloralamide 304.1
  chloralformamide 304.1
  chloralose 304.1
  chlordiazepoxide 304.1
  Chloretone 304.1
  chlorobutanol 304.1
  chlorodyne 304.1
  chloroform 304.6
  Cliradon 304.0
  coca (leaf) and derivatives 304.2
  cocaine 304.2
    hydrochloride 304.2
    salt (any) 304.2
  codeine 304.0
  combination of drugs (excluding morphine or
    opioid type drug) NEC 304.8
    morphine or opioid type drug with any other
      drug 304.7

Dependence—*continued*
  croton-chloral 304.1
  cyclobarbital 304.1
  cyclobarbitone 304.1
  dagga 304.3
  Delvinal 304.1
  Demerol 304.0
  desocodeine 304.0
  desomorphine 304.0
  desoxyephedrine 304.4
  DET 304.5
  dexamphetamine 304.4
  dexedrine 304.4
  dextromethorphan 304.0
  dextromoramide 304.0
  dextronorpseudophedrine 304.4
  dextrorphan 304.0
  diacetylmorphine 304.0
  Dial 304.1
  diallylbarbituric acid 304.1
  diamorphine 304.0
  diazepam 304.1
  dibucaine 304.6
  dichloroethane 304.6
  diethyl barbituric acid 304.1
  diethylsulfone-diethylmethane 304.1
  difencloxazine 304.0
  dihydrocodeine 304.0
  dihydrocodeinone 304.0
  dihydrohydroxycodeinone 304.0
  dihydroisocodeine 304.0
  dihydromorphine 304.0
  dihydromorphinone 304.0
  dihydroxcodeinone 304.0
  Dilaudid 304.0
  dimenhydrinate 304.6
  dimethylmeperidine 304.0
  dimethyltriptamine 304.5
  Dionin 304.0
  diphenoxylate 304.6
  dipipanone 304.0
  d-lysergic acid diethylamide 304.5
  DMT 304.5
  Dolophine 304.0
  DOM 304.2
  Doriden 304.1
  dormiral 304.1
  Dormison 304.1
  Dromoran 304.0
  drug NEC 304.9
    analgesic NEC 304.6
    combination (excluding morphine or opioid
        type drug) NEC 304.8
      morphine or opioid type drug with any other
          drug 304.7
    complicating pregnancy, childbirth, or
        puerperium 648.3
      affecting fetus or newborn 779.5
    hallucinogenic 304.5
    hypnotic NEC 304.1
    narcotic NEC 304.9
    psychostimulant NEC 304.4
    sedative 304.1
    soporific NEC 304.1
    specified type NEC 304.6
    suspected damage to fetus affecting
        management of pregnancy 655.5
    synthetic, with morphine-like effect 304.0
    tranquilizing 304.1
  duboisine 304.6

Dependence—*continued*
  ectylurea 304.1
  Endocaine 304.6
  Equanil 304.1
  Eskabarb 304.1
  ethchlorvynol 304.1
  ether (ethyl) (liquid) (vapor) (vinyl) 304.6
  ethidene 304.6
  ethinamate 304.1
  ethoheptazine 304.6
  ethyl
    alcohol 303.9
    bromide 304.6
    carbamate 304.6
    chloride 304.6
    morphine 304.0
  ethylene (gas) 304.6
    dichloride 304.6
  ethylidene chloride 304.6
  etilfen 304.1
  etorphine 304.0
  etoval 304.1
  eucodal 304.0
  euneryl 304.1
  Evipal 304.1
  Evipan 304.1
  fentanyl 304.0
  ganja 304.3
  gardenal 304.1
  gardenpanyl 304.1
  gelsemine 304.6
  Gelsemium 304.6
  Gemonil 304.1
  glucochloral 304.1
  glue (airplane) (sniffing) 304.6
  glutethimide 304.1
  hallucinogenics 304.5
  hashish 304.3
  headache powder NEC 304.6
  Heavenly Blue 304.5
  hedonal 304.1
  hemp 304.3
  heptabarbital 304.1
  Heptalgin 304.0
  heptobarbitone 304.1
  heroin 304.0
    salt (any) 304.0
  hexethal (sodium) 304.1
  hexobarbital 304.1
  Hycodan 304.0
  hydrocodone 304.0
  hydromorphinol 304.0
  hydromorphinone 304.0
  hydromorphone 304.0
  hydroxycodeine 304.0
  hypnotic NEC 304.1
  Indian hemp 304.3
  inhalant 304.6
  intranarcon 304.1
  Kemithal 304.1
  ketobemidone 304.0
  khat 304.4
  kif 304.3
  Lactuca (virosa) extract 304.1
  lactucarium 304.1
  laudanum 304.0
  Lebanese red 304.3
  Leritine 304.0

Dependence—*continued*
  lettuce opium 304.1
  Levanil 304.1
  Levo-Dromoran 304.0
  levo-iso-methadone 304.0
  levorphanol 304.0
  Librium 304.1
  Lomotil 304.6
  Lotusate 304.1
  LSD (-25) (and derivatives) 304.5
  Luminal 304.1
  lysergic acid 304.5
    amide 304.5
  maconha 304.3
  magic mushroom 304.5
  marijuana 304.3
  MDA (methylene dioxyamphetamine) 304.4
  Mebaral 304.1
  Medinal 304.1
  Medomin 304.1
  megahallucinogenics 304.5
  meperidine 304.0
  mephobarbital 304.1
  meprobamate 304.1
  mescaline 304.5
  methadone 304.0
  methamphetamine(s) 304.4
  methaqualone 304.1
  metharbital 304.1
  methitural 304.1
  methobarbitone 304.1
  methohexital 304.1
  methopholine 304.6
  methyl
    alcohol 303.9
    bromide 304.6
    morphine 304.0
    sulfonal 304.1
  methylated spirit 303.9
  methylbutinol 304.6
  methyldihydromorphinone 304.0
  methylene
    chloride 304.6
    dichloride 304.6
    dioxyamphetamine (MDA) 304.4
  methylparafynol 304.1
  methylphenidate 304.4
  methyprylone 304.1
  metopon 304.0
  Miltown 304.1
  morning glory *seeds* 304.5
  morphinan(s) 304.0
  morphine (sulfate) (sulfite) (type) (drugs
    classifiable to 965.00-965.09) 304.0
  morphine or opioid type drug (drugs classifiable
    to 965.00-965.09) with any other drug 304.7
  morphinol(s) 304.0
  morphinon 304.0
  morpholinylethylmorphine 304.0
  mylomide 304.1
  myristicin 304.5
  narcotic (drug) NEC 304.9
  nealbarbital 304.1
  nealbarbitone 304.1
  Nembutal 304.1
  Neonal 304.1
  Neraval 304.1
  Neravan 304.1
  neurobarb 304.1
  nicotine 305.1
  Nisentil 304.0

Dependence—*continued*
  nitrous oxide 304.6
  Noctec 304.1
  Noludar 304.1
  nonbarbiturate sedatives and tranquilizers with
    similar effect 304.1
  noptil 304.1
  normorphine 304.0
  noscapine 304.0
  Novocaine 304.6
  Numorphan 304.0
  nunol 304.1
  Nupercaine 304.6
  Oblivon 304.1
  on
    aspirator V46.0
    hemodialysis V45.11
    hyperbaric chamber V46.8
    iron lung V46.11
    machine (enabling) V46.9
      specified type NEC V46.8
    peritoneal dialysis V45.11
    Possum (Patient-Operated-Selector-
      Mechanism) V46.8
    renal dialysis machine V45.11
    respirator (ventilator) V46.11
      encounter
        during
          mechanical failure V46.14
          power failure V46.12
        for weaning V46.13
    supplemental oxygen V46.2
    wheelchair V46.3
  opiate 304.0
  opioids 304.0
  opioid type drug 304.0
    with any other drug 304.7
  opium (alkaloids) (derivatives) (tincture) 304.0
  ortal 304.1
  Oxazepam 304.1
  oxycodone 304.0
  oxymorphone 304.0
  Palfium 304.0
  Panadol 304.6
  pantopium 304.0
  pantopon 304.0
  papaverine 304.0
  paracetamol 304.6
  paracodin 304.0
  paraldehyde 304.1
  paregoric 304.0
  Parzone 304.0
  PCP (phencyclidine) 304.6
  Pearly Gates 304.5
  pentazocine 304.0
  pentobarbital 304.1
  pentobarbitone (sodium) 304.1
  Pentothal 304.1
  Percaine 304.6
  Percodan 304.0
  Perichlor 304.1
  Pernocton 304.1
  Pernoston 304.1
  peronine 304.0
  pethidine (hydrochloride) 304.0
  petrichloral 304.1
  peyote 304.5
  Phanodorn 304.1
  phenacetin 304.6
  phenadoxone 304.0
  phenaglycodol 304.1
  phenazocine 304.0

Dependence—*continued*
  phencyclidine 304.6
  phenmetrazine 304.4
  phenobal 304.1
  phenobarbital 304.1
  phenobarbitone 304.1
  phenomorphan 304.0
  phenonyl 304.1
  phenoperidine 304.0
  pholcodine 304.0
  piminodine 304.0
  Pipadone 304.0
  Pitkin's solution 304.6
  Placidyl 304.1
  polysubstance 304.8
  Pontocaine 304.6
  pot 304.3
  potassium bromide 304.1
  Preludin 304.4
  Prinadol 304.0
  probarbital 304.1
  procaine 304.6
  propanal 304.1
  propoxyphene 304.6
  psilocibin 304.5
  psilocin 304.5
  psilocybin 304.5
  psilocyline 304.5
  psilocyn 304.5
  psychedelic agents 304.5
  psychostimulant NEC 304.4
  psychotomimetic agents 304.5
  pyrahexyl 304.3
  Pyramidon 304.6
  quinalbarbitone 304.1
  racemoramide 304.0
  racemorphan 304.0
  Rela 304.6
  scopolamine 304.6
  secobarbital 304.1
  Seconal 304.1
  sedative NEC 304.1
    nonbarbiturate with barbiturate effect 304.1
  Sedormid 304.1
  sernyl 304.1
  sodium bromide 304.1
  Soma 304.6
  Somnal 304.1
  Somnos 304.1
  Soneryl 304.1
  soporific (drug) NEC 304.1
  specified drug NEC 304.6
  speed 304.4
  spinocaine 304.6
  Stovaine 304.6
  STP 304.5
  stramonium 304.6
  Sulfonal 304.1
  sulfonethylmethane 304.1
  sulfonmethane 304.1
  Surital 304.1
  synthetic drug with morphine-like effect 304.0
  talbutal 304.1
  tetracaine 304.6
  tetrahydrocannabinol 304.3
  tetronal 304.1
  THC 304.3
  thebacon 304.0
  thebaine 304.0
  thiamil 304.1
  thiamylal 304.1

Dependence—*continued*
  thiopental 304.1
  tobacco 305.1
  toluene, toluol 304.6
  tranquilizer NEC 304.1
    nonbarbiturate with barbiturate effect 304.1
  tribromacetaldehyde 304.6
  tribromethanol 304.6
  tribromomethane 304.6
  trichloroethanol 304.6
  trichoroethyl phosphate 304.1
  triclofos 304.1
  Trional 304.1
  Tuinal 304.1
  Turkish Green 304.3
  urethan(e) 304.6
  Valium 304.1
  Valmid 304.1
  veganin 304.0
  veramon 304.1
  Veronal 304.1
  versidyne 304.6
  vinbarbital 304.1
  vinbarbitone 304.1
  vinyl bitone 304.1
  vitamin B_6 266.1
  wine 303.9
  Zactane 304.6
Dependency
  passive 301.6
  reactions 301.6
Depersonalization (episode, in neurotic state)
  (neurotic) (syndrome) 300.6
Depletion
  carbohydrates 271.9
  complement factor 279.8
  extracellular fluid 276.52
  plasma 276.52
  potassium 276.8
    nephropathy 588.89
  salt or sodium 276.1
    causing heat exhaustion or prostration 992.4
    nephropathy 593.9
  volume 276.50
    extracellular fluid 276.52
    plasma 276.52
Deployment (military)
  personal history of V62.22
  returned from V62.22
  status V62.21
Deposit
  argentous, cornea 371.16
  bone, in Boeck's sarcoid 135
  calcareous, calcium—*see* Calcification
  cholesterol
    retina 362.82
    skin 709.3
    vitreous (humor) 379.22
  conjunctival 372.56
  cornea, corneal NEC 371.10
    argentous 371.16
    in
      cystinosis 270.0 *[371.15]*
      mucopolysaccharidosis 277.5 *[371.15]*
  crystalline, vitreous (humor) 379.22
  hemosiderin, in old scars of cornea 371.11
  metallic, in lens 366.45
  skin 709.3
  teeth, tooth (betel) (black) (green) (materia alba)
    (orange) (soft) (tobacco) 523.6
  urate, in kidney (*see also* Disease, renal) 593.9
Depraved appetite 307.52

Depression 311
  acute (*see also* Psychosis, affective) 296.2
    recurrent episode 296.3
    single episode 296.2
  agitated (*see also* Psychosis, affective) 296.2
    recurrent episode 296.3
    single episode 296.2
  anaclitic 309.21
  anxiety 300.4
  arches 734
    congenital 754.61
  autogenous (*see also* Psychosis, affective) 296.2
    recurrent episode 296.3
    single episode 296.2
  basal metabolic rate (BMR) 794.7
  bone marrow 289.9
  central nervous system 799.1
    newborn 779.2
  cerebral 331.9
    newborn 779.2
  cerebrovascular 437.8
    newborn 779.2
  chest wall 738.3
  endogenous (*see also* Psychosis, affective) 296.2
    recurrent episode 296.3
    single episode 296.2
  functional activity 780.99
  hysterical 300.11
  involutional, climacteric, or menopausal (*see also* Psychosis, affective) 296.2
    recurrent episode 296.3
    single episode 296.2
  major 296.2
    recurrent episode 296.3
    single episode 296.2
  manic (*see also* Psychosis, affective) 296.80
  medullary 348.89
    newborn 779.2
  mental 300.4
  metatarsal heads—*see* Depression, arches
  metatarsus—*see* Depression, arches
  monopolar (*see also* Psychosis, affective) 296.2
    recurrent episode 296.3
    single episode 296.2
  nervous 300.4
  neurotic 300.4
  nose 738.0
  postpartum 648.4
  psychogenic 300.4
    reactive 298.0
  psychoneurotic 300.4
  psychotic (*see also* Psychosis, affective) 296.2
    reactive 298.0
    recurrent episode 296.3
    single episode 296.2
  reactive 300.4
    neurotic 300.4
    psychogenic 298.0
    psychoneurotic 300.4
    psychotic 298.0
  recurrent 296.3
  respiratory center 348.89
    newborn 770.89
  scapula 736.89
  senile 290.21
  situational (acute) (brief) 309.0
    prolonged 309.1
  skull 754.0
  sternum 738.3
  visual field 368.40

Depressive reaction —*see also* Reaction, depressive
  acute (transient) 309.0
    with anxiety 309.28
  prolonged 309.1
  situational (acute) 309.0
    prolonged 309.1
Deprivation
  cultural V62.4
  emotional V62.89
    affecting
      adult 995.82
      infant or child 995.51
  food 994.2
    specific substance NEC 269.8
  protein (familial) (kwashiorkor) 260
  sleep V69.4
  social V62.4
    affecting
      adult 995.82
      infant or child 995.51
  symptoms, syndrome
    alcohol 291.81
    drug 292.0
  vitamins (*see also* Deficiency, vitamin) 269.2
  water 994.3
de Quervain's
  disease (tendon sheath) 727.04
  thyroiditis (subacute granulomatous thyroiditis) 245.1
  syndrome 259.51
Derangement
  ankle (internal) 718.97
    current injury (*see also* Dislocation, ankle) 837.0
    recurrent 718.37
  cartilage (articular) NEC (*see also* Disorder, cartilage, articular) 718.0
    knee 717.9
      recurrent 718.36
    recurrent 718.3
  collateral ligament (knee) (medial) (tibial) 717.82
    current injury 844.1
      lateral (fibular) 844.0
    lateral (fibular) 717.81
      current injury 844.0
  cruciate ligament (knee) (posterior) 717.84
    anterior 717.83
      current injury 844.2
    current injury 844.2
  elbow (internal) 718.92
    current injury (*see also* Dislocation, elbow) 832.00
    recurrent 718.32
  gastrointestinal 536.9
  heart—*see* Disease, heart
  hip (joint) (internal) (old) 718.95
    current injury (*see also* Dislocation, hip) 835.00
    recurrent 718.35
  intervertebral disc—*see* Displacement, intervertebral disc
  joint (internal) 718.90
    ankle 718.97
    current injury—*see also* Dislocation, by site
      knee, meniscus or cartilage (*see also* Tear, meniscus) 836.2
    elbow 718.92
    foot 718.97
    hand 718.94
    hip 718.95

Derangement—*continued*
joint—*continued*
knee 717.9
multiple sites 718.99
pelvic region 718.95
recurrent 718.30
ankle 718.37
elbow 718.32
foot 718.37
hand 718.34
hip 718.35
knee 718.36
multiple sites 718.39
pelvic region 718.35
shoulder (region) 718.31
specified site NEC 718.38
temporomandibular (old) 524.69
wrist 718.33
shoulder (region) 718.91
specified site NEC 718.98
spine NEC 724.9
temporomandibular 524.69
wrist 718.93
knee (cartilage) (internal) 717.9
current injury (*see also* Tear, meniscus) 836.2
ligament 717.89
capsular 717.85
collateral—*see* Derangement, collateral
ligament
cruciate—*see* Derangement, cruciate
ligament
specified NEC 717.85
recurrent 718.36
low back NEC 724.9
meniscus NEC (knee) 717.5
current injury (*see also* Tear, meniscus) 836.2
lateral 717.40
anterior horn 717.42
posterior horn 717.43
specified NEC 717.49
medial 717.3
anterior horn 717.1
posterior horn 717.2
recurrent 718.3
site other than knee—*see* Disorder, cartilage,
articular
mental (*see also* Psychosis) 298.9
rotator cuff (recurrent) (tear) 726.10
current 840.4
sacroiliac (old) 724.6
current—*see* Dislocation, sacroiliac
semilunar cartilage (knee) 717.5
current injury 836.2
lateral 836.1
medial 836.0
recurrent 718.3
shoulder (internal) 718.91
current injury (*see also* Dislocation, shoulder)
831.00
recurrent 718.31
spine (recurrent) NEC 724.9
current—*see* Dislocation, spine
temporomandibular (internal) (joint) (old)
524.69
current—*see* Dislocation, jaw
Dercum's disease or syndrome (adiposis
dolorosa) 272.8
Derealization (neurotic) 300.6
Dermal —*see* condition
Dermaphytid —*see* Dermatophytosis
Dermatergosis —*see* Dermatitis

Dermatitis (allergic) (contact) (occupational)
(venenata) 692.9
ab igne 692.82
acneiform 692.9
actinic (due to sun) 692.70
acute 692.72
chronic NEC 692.74
other than from sun NEC 692.82
ambustionis
due to
burn or scald—*see* Burn, by site
sunburn (*see also* Sunburn) 692.71
amebic 006.6
ammonia 691.0
anaphylactoid NEC 692.9
arsenical 692.4
artefacta 698.4
psychogenic 316 *[698.4]*
asthmatic 691.8
atopic (allergic) (intrinsic) 691.8
psychogenic 316 *[691.8]*
atrophicans 701.8
diffusa 701.8
maculosa 701.3
autoimmune progesterone 279.49
berlock, berloque 692.72
blastomycetic 116.0
blister beetle 692.89
Brucella NEC 023.9
bullosa 694.9
striata pratensis 692.6
bullous 694.9
mucosynechial, atrophic 694.60
with ocular involvement 694.61
seasonal 694.8
calorica
due to
burn or scald—*see* Burn, by site
cold 692.89
sunburn (*see also* Sunburn) 692.71
caterpillar 692.89
cercarial 120.3
combustionis
due to
burn or scald—*see* Burn, by site
sunburn (*see also* Sunburn) 692.71
congelationis 991.5
contusiformis 695.2
diabetic 250.8
diaper 691.0
diphtheritica 032.85
due to
acetone 692.2
acids 692.4
adhesive plaster 692.4
alcohol (skin contact) (substances classifiable
to 980.0-980.9) 692.4
taken internally 693.8
alkalis 692.4
allergy NEC 692.9
ammonia (household) (liquid) 692.4
animal
dander (cat) (dog) 692.84
hair (cat) (dog) 692.84
arnica 692.3
arsenic 692.4
taken internally 693.8
blister beetle 692.89
cantharides 692.3
carbon disulphide 692.2
caterpillar 692.89

Dermatitis—*continued*
  due to—*continued*
    caustics 692.4
    cereal (ingested) 693.1
      contact with skin 692.5
    chemical(s) NEC 692.4
      internal 693.8
      irritant NEC 692.4
      taken internally 693.8
    chlorocompounds 692.2
    coffee (ingested) 693.1
      contact with skin 692.5
    cold weather 692.89
    cosmetics 692.81
    cyclohexanes 692.2
    dander, animal (cat) (dog) 692.84
    deodorant 692.81
    detergents 692.0
    dichromate 692.4
    drugs and medicinals (correct substance
        properly administered) (internal use) 693.0
      external (in contact with skin) 692.3
        wrong substance given or taken 976.9
          specified substance—*see* Table of drugs
              and chemicals
      wrong substance given or taken 977.9
        specified substance—*see* Table of drugs
            and chemicals
    dyes 692.89
      hair 692.89
    epidermophytosis—*see* Dermatophytosis
    esters 692.2
    external irritant NEC 692.9
      specified agent NEC 692.89
    eye shadow 692.81
    fish (ingested) 693.1
      contact with skin 692.5
    flour (ingested) 693.1
      contact with skin 692.5
    food (ingested) 693.1
      in contact with skin 692.5
    fruit (ingested) 693.1
      contact with skin 692.5
    fungicides 692.3
    furs 692.84
    glycols 692.2
    greases NEC 692.1
    hair, animal (cat) (dog) 692.84
    hair dyes 692.89
    hot
      objects and materials—*see* Burn, by site
      weather or places 692.89
    hydrocarbons 692.2
    infrared rays, except from sun 692.82
      solar NEC (*see also* Dermatitis, due to, sun)
          692.70
    ingested substance 693.9
      drugs and medicinals (*see also* Dermatitis,
          due to, drugs and medicinals) 693.0
      food 693.1
      specified substance NEC 693.8
    ingestion or injection of
      chemical 693.8
      drug (correct substance properly
          administered) 693.0
        wrong substance given or taken 977.9
          specified substance—*see* Table of drugs
              and chemicals
    insecticides 692.4

Dermatitis—*continued*
  due to—*continued*
    internal agent 693.9
      drugs and medicinals (*see also* Dermatitis,
          due to, drugs and medicinals) 693.0
      food (ingested) 693.1
        in contact with skin 692.5
      specified agent NEC 693.8
    iodine 692.3
    iodoform 692.3
    irradiation 692.82
    jewelry 692.83
    keratolytics 692.3
    ketones 692.2
    lacquer tree (Rhus verniciflua) 692.6
    light (sun) NEC (*see also* Dermatitis, due to,
        sun) 692.70
      other 692.82
    low temperature 692.89
    mascara 692.81
    meat (ingested) 693.1
      contact with skin 692.5
    mercury, mercurials 692.3
    metals 692.83
    milk (ingested) 693.1
      contact with skin 692.5
    Neomycin 692.3
    nylon 692.4
    oils NEC 692.1
    paint solvent 692.2
    pediculocides 692.3
    petroleum products (substances classifiable to
        981) 692.4
    phenol 692.3
    photosensitiveness, photosensitivity (sun)
        692.72
      other light 692.82
    plants NEC 692.6
    plasters, medicated (any) 692.3
    plastic 692.4
    poison
      ivy (Rhus toxicodendron) 692.6
      oak (Rhus diversiloba) 692.6
      plant or vine 692.6
      sumac (Rhus venenata) 692.6
      vine (Rhus radicans) 692.6
    preservatives 692.89
    primrose (primula) 692.6
    primula 692.6
    radiation 692.82
      sun NEC (*see also* Dermatitis, due to, sun)
          692.70
      tanning bed 692.82
    radioactive substance 692.82
    radium 692.82
    ragweed (Senecio jacobae) 692.6
    Rhus (diversiloba) (radicans) (toxicodendron)
        (venenata) (verniciflua) 692.6
    rubber 692.4
    scabicides 692.3
    Senecio jacobae 692.6
    solar radiation—*see* Dermatitis, due to, sun
    solvents (any) (substances classifiable to
        982.0-982.8) 692.2
      chlorocompound group 692.2
      cyclohexane group 692.2
      ester group 692.2
      glycol group 692.2
      hydrocarbon group 692.2
      ketone group 692.2
      paint 692.2

Dermatitis—*continued*
  due to—*continued*
   specified agent NEC 692.89
   sun 692.70
    acute 692.72
    chronic NEC 692.74
    specified NEC 692.79
   sunburn (*see also* Sunburn) 692.71
   sunshine NEC (*see also* Dermatitis, due to,
     sun) 692.70
   tanning bed 692.82
   tetrachlorethylene 692.2
   toluene 692.2
   topical medications 692.3
   turpentine 692.2
   ultraviolet rays, except from sun 692.82
    sun NEC (*see also* Dermatitis, due to, sun)
      692.70
   vaccine or vaccination (correct substance
     properly administered) 693.0
    wrong substance given or taken
     bacterial vaccine 978.8
      specified—*see* Table of drugs and
        chemicals
     other vaccines NEC 979.9
      specified—*see* Table of drugs and
        chemicals
   varicose veins (*see also* Varicose, vein,
     inflamed or infected) 454.1
   x-rays 692.82
  dyshydrotic 705.81
  dysmenorrheica 625.8
  eczematoid NEC 692.9
   infectious 690.8
  eczematous NEC 692.9
  epidemica 695.89
  erysipelatosa 695.81
  escharotica—*see* Burn, by site
  exfoliativa, exfoliative 695.89
   generalized 695.89
   infantum 695.81
   neonatorum 695.81
  eyelid 373.31
   allergic 373.32
   contact 373.32
   eczematous 373.31
   herpes (zoster) 053.20
    simplex 054.41
   infective 373.5
    due to
     actinomycosis 039.3 *[373.5]*
     herpes
      simplex 054.41
      zoster 053.20
     impetigo 684 *[373.5]*
     leprosy (*see also* Leprosy) 030.0 *[373.4]*
     lupus vulgaris (tuberculous) (*see also*
       Tuberculosis) 017.0 *[373.4]*
     mycotic dermatitis (*see also*
       Dermatomycosis) 111.9 *[373.5]*
     vaccinia 051.02 *[373.5]*
      postvaccination 999.0 *[373.5]*
     yaws (*see also* Yaws) 102.9 *[373.4]*
  facta, factitia 698.4
   psychogenic 316 *[698.4]*
  ficta 698.4
   psychogenic 316 *[698.4]*
  flexural 691.8
  follicularis 704.8
  friction 709.8

Dermatitis—*continued*
  fungus 111.9
   specified type NEC 111.8
  gangrenosa, gangrenous (infantum) (*see also*
    Gangrene) 785.4
  gestationis 646.8
  gonococcal 098.89
  gouty 274.89
  harvest mite 133.8
  heat 692.89
  herpetiformis (bullous) (erythematous)
    (pustular) (vesicular) 694.0
   juvenile 694.2
   senile 694.5
  hiemalis 692.89
  hypostatic, hypostatica 454.1
   with ulcer 454.2
  impetiginous 684
  infantile (acute) (chronic) (intertriginous)
    (intrinsic) (seborrheic) 690.12
  infectiosa eczematoides 690.8
  infectious (staphylococcal) (streptococcal) 686.9
   eczematoid 690.8
  infective eczematoid 690.8
  Jacquet's (diaper dermatitis) 691.0
  leptus 133.8
  lichenified NEC 692.9
  lichenoid, chronic 701.0
  lichenoides purpurica pigmentosa 709.1
  meadow 692.6
  medicamentosa (correct substance properly
    administered) (internal use) (*see also*
    Dermatitis, due to, drugs or medicinals)
    693.0
   due to contact with skin 692.3
  mite 133.8
  multiformis 694.0
   juvenile 694.2
   senile 694.5
  napkin 691.0
  neuro 698.3
  neurotica 694.0
  nummular NEC 692.9
  osteatosis, osteatotic 706.8
  papillaris capillitii 706.1
  pellagrous 265.2
  perioral 695.3
  perstans 696.1
  photosensitivity (sun) 692.72
   other light 692.82
  pigmented purpuric lichenoid 709.1
  polymorpha dolorosa 694.0
  primary irritant 692.9
  pruriginosa 694.0
  pruritic NEC 692.9
  psoriasiform nodularis 696.2
  psychogenic 316
  purulent 686.00
  pustular contagious 051.2
  pyococcal 686.00
  pyocyaneus 686.09
  pyogenica 686.00
  radiation 692.82
  repens 696.1
  Ritter's (exfoliativa) 695.81
  Schamberg's (progressive pigmentary
    dermatosis) 709.09
  schistosome 120.3
  seasonal bullous 694.8
  seborrheic 690.10
   infantile 690.12

Dermatitis—*continued*
  sensitization NEC 692.9
  septic (*see also* Septicemia) 686.00
    gonococcal 098.89
  solar, solare NEC (*see also* Dermatitis, due to, sun) 692.70
  stasis 454.1
    due to
      postphlebitic syndrome 459.12
        with ulcer 459.13
      varicose veins—*see* Varicose
    ulcerated or with ulcer (varicose) 454.2
  sunburn (*see also* Sunburn) 692.71
  suppurative 686.00
  traumatic NEC 709.8
  trophoneurotica 694.0
  ultraviolet, except from sun 692.82
    due to sun NEC (*see also* Dermatitis, due to, sun) 692.70
  varicose 454.1
    with ulcer 454.2
  vegetans 686.8
  verrucosa 117.2
  xerotic 706.8
Dermatoarthritis, lipoid 272.8 *[713.0]*
Dermatochalasia, dermatochalasis 374.87
Dermatofibroma (lenticulare) (M8832/0)—*see also* Neoplasm, skin, benign
  protuberans (M8832/1)—*see* Neoplasm, skin, uncertain behavior
Dermatofibrosarcoma (protuberans) (M8832/3) *see* Neoplasm, skin, malignant
Dermatographia 708.3
Dermatolysis (congenital) (exfoliativa) 757.39
  acquired 701.8
  eyelids 374.34
  palpebrarum 374.34
  senile 701.8
Dermatomegaly NEC 701.8
Dermatomucomyositis 710.3
Dermatomycosis 111.9
  furfuracea 111.0
  specified type NEC 111.8
Dermatomyositis (acute) (chronic) 710.3
Dermatoneuritis of children 985.0
Dermatophiliasis 134.1
Dermatophytide —*see* Dermatophytosis
Dermatophytosis (Epidermophyton) (infection) (microsporum) (tinea) (Trichophyton) 110.9
  beard 110.0
  body 110.5
  deep seated 110.6
  fingernails 110.1
  foot 110.4
  groin 110.3
  hand 110.2
  nail 110.1
  perianal (area) 110.3
  scalp 110.0
  scrotal 110.8
  specified site NEC 110.8
  toenails 110.1
  vulva 110.8
Dermatopolyneuritis 985.0
Dermatorrhexis 756.83
  acquired 701.8
Dermatosclerosis (*see also* Scleroderma) 710.1
  localized 701.0
Dermatosis 709.9
  Andrews' 686.8
  atopic 691.8

Dermatosis— *continued*
  Bowen's (M8081/2)—*see* Neoplasm, skin, in situ
  bullous 694.9
    specified type NEC 694.8
  erythematosquamous 690.8
  exfoliativa 695.89
  factitial 698.4
  gonococcal 098.89
  herpetiformis 694.0
    juvenile 694.2
    senile 694.5
  hysterical 300.11
  linear IgA 694.8
  menstrual NEC 709.8
  neutrophilic, acute febrile 695.89
  occupational (*see also* Dermatitis) 692.9
  papulosa nigra 709.8
  pigmentary NEC 709.00
    progressive 709.09
    Schamberg's 709.09
    Siemens-Bloch 757.33
  progressive pigmentary 709.09
  psychogenic 316
  pustular subcorneal 694.1
  Schamberg's (progressive pigmentary) 709.09
  senile NEC 709.3
  Unna's (seborrheic dermatitis) 690.10
Dermographia 708.3
Dermographism 708.3
Dermoid (cyst) (M9084/0)—*see also* Neoplasm, by site, benign
  with malignant transformation (M9084/3) 183.0
Dermopathy
  infiltrative, with thyrotoxicosis 242.0
  nephrogenic fibrosing 701.8
  senile NEC 709.3
Dermophytosis —*see* Dermatophytosis
Descemet's membrane —*see* condition
Descemetocele 371.72
Descending —*see* condition
Descensus uteri (complete) (incomplete) (partial) (without vaginal wall prolapse) 618.1
  with mention of vaginal wall prolapse—*see* Prolapse, uterovaginal
Desensitization to allergens V07.1
Desert
  rheumatism 114.0
  sore (*see also* Ulcer, skin) 707.9
Desertion (child) (newborn) 995.52
  adult 995.84
Desmoid (extra-abdominal) (tumor) (M8821/1)—*see also* Neoplasm, connective tissue, uncertain behavior
  abdominal (M8822/1)—*see* Neoplasm, connective tissue, uncertain behavior
Despondency 300.4
Desquamative dermatitis NEC 695.89
Destruction
  articular facet (*see also* Derangement, joint) 718.9
    vertebra 724.9
  bone 733.90
    syphilitic 095.5
  joint (*see also* Derangement, joint) 718.9
    sacroiliac 724.6
  kidney 593.89
  live fetus to facilitate birth NEC 763.89
  ossicles (ear) 385.24
  rectal sphincter 569.49
  septum (nasal) 478.19
  tuberculous NEC (*see also* Tuberculosis) 011.9
  tympanic membrane 384.82
  tympanum 385.89
  vertebral disc—*see* Degeneration, intervertebral disc

Destructiveness (*see also* Disturbance, conduct) 312.9
  adjustment reaction 309.3
Detachment
  cartilage—*see also* Sprain, by site
    knee—*see* Tear, meniscus
  cervix, annular 622.8
    complicating delivery 665.3
  choroid (old) (postinfectional) (simple) (spontaneous) 363.70
    hemorrhagic 363.72
    serous 363.71
  knee, medial meniscus (old) 717.3
    current injury 836.0
  ligament—*see* Sprain, by site
  placenta (premature)—*see* Placenta, separation
  retina (recent) 361.9
    with retinal defect (rhegmatogenous) 361.00
      giant tear 361.03
      multiple 361.02
      partial
        with
          giant tear 361.03
          multiple defects 361.02
          retinal dialysis (juvenile) 361.04
          single defect 361.01
        retinal dialysis (juvenile) 361.04
        single 361.01
        subtotal 361.05
        total 361.05
    delimited (old) (partial) 361.06
    old
      delimited 361.06
      partial 361.06
      total or subtotal 361.07
    pigment epithelium (RPE) (serous) 362.42
      exudative 362.42
      hemorrhagic 362.43
    rhegmatogenous (*see also* Detachment, retina, with retinal defect) 361.00
    serous (without retinal defect) 361.2
    specified type NEC 361.89
    traction (with vitreoretinal organization) 361.81
  vitreous humor 379.21
Detergent asthma 507.8
Deterioration
  epileptic
    with behavioral disturbance 345.9 *[294.11]*
    without behavioral disturbance 345.9 *[294.10]*
  heart, cardiac (*see also* Degeneration, myocardial) 429.1
  mental (*see also* Psychosis) 298.9
  myocardium, myocardial (*see also* Degeneration, myocardial) 429.1
  senile (simple) 797
  transplanted organ—*see* Complications, transplant, organ, by site
de Toni-Fanconi syndrome (cystinosis) 270.0
Deuteranomaly 368.52
Deuteranopia (anomalous trichromat) (complete) (incomplete) 368.52
Deutschländer's disease —*see* Fracture, foot
Development
  abnormal, bone 756.9
  arrested 783.40
    bone 733.91
    child 783.40
    due to malnutrition (protein-calorie) 263.2
    fetus or newborn 764.9
    tracheal rings (congenital) 748.3

Development—*continued*
  defective, congenital—*see also* Anomaly
    cauda equina 742.59
    left ventricle 746.9
      with atresia or hypoplasia of aortic orifice or valve with hypoplasia of ascending aorta 746.7
      in hypoplastic left heart syndrome 746.7
  delayed (*see also* Delay, development) 783.40
    arithmetical skills 315.1
    language (skills) 315.31
      and speech due to hearing loss 315.34
      expressive 315.31
      mixed receptive-expressive 315.32
    learning skill, specified NEC 315.2
    mixed skills 315.5
    motor coordination 315.4
    reading 315.00
    specified
      learning skill NEC 315.2
      type NEC, except learning 315.8
    speech 315.39
      and language due to hearing loss 315.34
      associated with hyperkinesia 314.1
      phonological 315.39
    spelling 315.09
    written expression 315.2
  imperfect, congenital—*see also* Anomaly
    heart 746.9
    lungs 748.60
  improper (fetus or newborn) 764.9
  incomplete (fetus or newborn) 764.9
    affecting management of pregnancy 656.5
    bronchial tree 748.3
    organ or site not listed—*see* Hypoplasia
    respiratory system 748.9
  sexual, precocious NEC 259.1
  tardy, mental (*see also* Disability, intellectual) 319
Developmental —*see* condition
Devergie's disease (pityriasis rubra pilaris) 696.4
Deviation
  conjugate (eye) 378.87
    palsy 378.81
    spasm, spastic 378.82
  esophagus 530.89
  eye, skew 378.87
  mandible, opening and closing 524.53
  midline (jaw) (teeth) 524.29
    specified site NEC—*see* Malposition
  occlusal plane 524.76
  organ or site, congenital NEC—*see* Malposition, congenital
  septum (acquired) (nasal) 470
    congenital 754.0
  sexual 302.9
    bestiality 302.1
    coprophilia 302.89
    ego-dystonic
      homosexuality 302.0
      lesbianism 302.0
    erotomania 302.89
      Clérambault's 297.8
    exhibitionism (sexual) 302.4
    fetishism 302.81
      transvestic 302.3
    frotteurism 302.89
    homosexuality, ego-dystonic 302.0
      pedophilic 302.2
    lesbianism, ego-dystonic 302.0
    masochism 302.83
    narcissism 302.89
    necrophilia 302.89

Deviation—*continued*
  sexual—*continued*
    nymphomania 302.89
    pederosis 302.2
    pedophilia 302.2
    sadism 302.84
    sadomasochism 302.84
    satyriasis 302.89
    specified type NEC 302.89
    transvestic fetishism 302.3
    transvestism 302.3
    voyeurism 302.82
    zoophilia (erotica) 302.1
  teeth, midline 524.29
  trachea 519.19
  ureter (congenital) 753.4
Devic's disease 341.0
Device
  cerebral ventricle (communicating) in situ V45.2
  contraceptive—*see* Contraceptive, device
  drainage, cerebrospinal fluid V45.2
Devil's
  grip 074.1
  pinches (purpura simplex) 287.2
Devitalized tooth 522.9
Devonshire colic 984.9
  specified type of lead—*see* Table of drugs and chemicals
Dextraposition, aorta 747.21
  with ventricular septal defect, pulmonary stenosis or atresia, and hypertrophy of right ventricle 745.2
  in tetralogy of Fallot 745.2
Dextratransposition, aorta 745.11
Dextrinosis, limit (debrancher enzyme deficiency) 271.0
Dextrocardia (corrected) (false) (isolated) (secondary) (true) 746.87
  with
    complete transposition of viscera 759.3
    situs inversus 759.3
Dextroversion, kidney (left) 753.3
Dhobie itch 110.3
DHTR (delayed hemolytic transfusion reaction) - *see* Complications, transfusion
Diabetes, diabetic (brittle) (congenital) (familial) (mellitus) (severe) (slight) (without complication) 250.0

Note—Use the following fifth-digit subclassification with category 250:

0 type II or unspecified type, not stated as uncontrolled
   Fifth-digit 0 is for use for type II patients, even if the patient requires insulin
1 type I [juvenile type], not stated as uncontrolled
2 type II or unspecified type, uncontrolled
   Fifth-digit 2 is for use for type II patients, even if the paiten requires insulin
3 type I [juvenile type], uncontrolled

---

  with
    coma (with ketoacidosis) 250.3
      due to secondary diabetes 249.3
      hyperosmolar (nonketotic) 250.2
        due to secondary diabetes 249.2
    complication NEC 250.9
      due to secondary diabetes 249.9
    specified NEC 250.8
      due to secondary diabetes 249.8

Diabetes, diabetic—*continued*
  with—*continued*
    gangrene 250.7 *[785.4]*
      due to secondary diabetes 249.7 *[785.4]*
    hyperglycemia — code to Diabetes, by type, with 5th digit for not stated as uncontrolled
    hyperosmolarity 250.2
      due to secondary diabetes 249.2
    ketosis, ketoacidosis 250.1
      due to secondary diabetes 249.1
    loss of protective sensation (LOPS) - *see* Diabetes, neuropathy
    osteomyelitis 250.8 *[731.8]*
      due to secondary diabetes 249.8 *[731.8]*
    specified manifestations NEC 250.8
      due to secondary diabetes 249.8
  acetonemia 250.1
    due to secondary diabetes 249.1
  acidosis 250.1
    due to secondary diabetes 249.1
  amyotrophy 250.6 *[353.5]*
    due to secondary diabetes 249.6 *[353.5]*
  angiopathy, peripheral 250.7 *[443.81]*
    due to secondary diabetes 249.7 *[443.81]*
  asymptomatic 790.29
  autonomic neuropathy (peripheral) 250.6 *[337.1]*
    due to secondary diabetes 249.6 *[337.1]*
  bone change 250.8 *[731.8]*
    due to secondary diabetes 249.8 *[731.8]*
  borderline 790.29
  bronze, bronzed 275.01
  cataract 250.5 *[366.41]*
    due to secondary diabetes 249.5 *[366.41]*
  chemical induced—see Diabetes, secondary
  complicating pregnancy, childbirth, or puerperium 648.0
  coma (with ketoacidosis) 250.3
    due to secondary diabetes 249.3
    hyperglycemic 250.3
      due to secondary diabetes 249.3
    hyperosmolar (nonketotic) 250.2
      due to secondary diabetes 249.2
    hypoglycemic 250.3
      due to secondary diabetes 249.3
    insulin 250.3
      due to secondary diabetes 249.3
  complicating pregnancy, childbirth, or puerperium (maternal) (conditions classifiable to 249 and 250) 648.0
    affecting fetus or newborn 775.0
  complication NEC 250.9
    due to secondary diabetes 249.9
    specified NEC 250.8
      due to secondary diabetes 249.8
  dorsal sclerosis 250.6 *[340]*
    due to secondary diabetes 249.6 *[340]*
  drug induced—*see also* Diabetes, secondary
    overdose or wrong substance given or taken — *see* Table of Drugs and Chemicals
  due to
    cystic fibrosis — *see* Diabetes, secondary
    infection — *see* Diabetes, secondary
  dwarfism-obesity syndrome 258.1
  gangrene 250.7 *[785.4]*
    due to secondary diabetes 249.7 *[785.4]*
  gastroparesis 250.6 *[536.3]*
    due to secondary diabetes 249.6 *[536.3]*
  gestational 648.8
    complicating pregnancy, childbirth, or puerperium 648.8
  glaucoma 250.5 *[365.44]*
    due to secondary diabetes 249.5 *[365.44]*

Diabetes, diabetic—*continued*
  glomerulosclerosis (intercapillary) 250.4 *[581.81]*
    due to secondary diabetes 249.4 *[581.81]*
  glycogenosis, secondary 250.8 *[259.8]*
    due to secondary diabetes 249.8 *[259.8]*
  hemochromatosis (*see also* Hemochromatosis)
    275.03
  hyperosmolar coma 250.2
    due to secondary diabetes 249.2
  hyperosmolarity 250.2
    due to secondary diabetes 249.2
  hypertension-nephrosis syndrome 250.4 *[581.81]*
    due to secondary diabetes 249.4 *[581.81]*
  hypoglycemia 250.8
    due to secondary diabetes 249.8
  hypoglycemic shock 250.8
    due to secondary diabetes 249.8
  inadequately controlled—code to Diabetes, by
    type, with 5th digit for not stated as
    uncontrolled
  insipidus 253.5
    nephrogenic 588.1
    pituitary 253.5
    vasopressin-resistant 588.1
  intercapillary glomerulosclerosis 250.4 *[581.81]*
    due to secondary diabetes 249.4 *[581.81]*
  iritis 250.5 *[364.42]*
    due to secondary diabetes 249.5 *[364.42]*
  ketosis, ketoacidosis 250.1
    due to secondary diabetes 249.1
  Kimmelstiel (-Wilson) disease or syndrome
    (intercapillary glomerulosclerosis) 250.4
    [581.81]
    due to secondary diabetes 249.4 *[581.81]*
  Lancereaux's (diabetes mellitus with marked
    emaciation) 250.8 *[261]*
    due to secondary diabetes 249.8 *[261]*
  latent (chemical)—*see* Diabetes, secondary
  complicating pregnancy, childbirth, or
    puerperium 648.0
  lipoidosis 250.8 *[272.7]*
    due to secondary diabetes 249.8 *[272.7]*
  macular edema 250.5 *[362.07]*
    due to secondary diabetes 249.5 *[362.07]*
  maternal
    with manifest disease in the infant 775.1
    affecting fetus or newborn 775.0
  microaneurysms, retinal 250.5 *[362.01]*
    due to secondary diabetes 249.5 *[362.01]*
  mononeuropathy 250.6 *[355.9]*
    due to secondary diabetes 249.6 *[355.9]*
  neonatal, transient 775.1
  nephropathy 250.4 *[583.81]*
    due to secondary diabetes 249.4 *[583.81]*
  nephrosis (syndrome) 250.4 *[581.81]*
    due to secondary diabetes 249.4 *[581.81]*
  neuralgia 250.6 *[357.2]*
    due to secondary diabetes 249.6 *[357.2]*
  neuritis 250.6 *[357.2]*
    due to secondary diabetes 249.6 *[357.2]*
  neurogenic arthropathy 250.6 *[713.5]*
    due to secondary diabetes 249.6 *[713.5]*
  neuropathy 250.6 *[357.2]*
    autonomic (peripheral) 250.6 *[337.1]*
      due to secondary diabetes 249.6 *[337.1]*
    due to secondary diabetes 249.6 *[357.2]*
  nonclinical 790.29
  osteomyelitis 250.8 *[731.8]*
    due to secondary diabetes 249.8 *[731.8]*
  out of control—code to Diabetes, by type, with
    5th digit for uncontrolled

Diabetes, diabetic—*continued*
  peripheral autonomic neuropathy 250.6 *[337.1]*
    due to secondary diabetes 249.6 *[337.1]*
  phosphate 275.3
  polyneuropathy 250.6 *[357.2]*
    due to secondary diabetes 249.6 *[357.2]*
  poorly controlled—code to Diabetes, by type,
    with 5th digit for not stated as uncontrolled
  renal (true) 271.4
  retinal
    edema 250.5 *[362.07]*
      due to secondary diabetes 249.5 *[362.07]*
    hemorrhage 250.5 *[362.01]*
      due to secondary diabetes 249.5 *[362.01]*
    microaneurysms 250.5 *[362.01]*
      due to secondary diabetes 249.5 *[362.01]*
  retinitis 250.5 *[362.01]*
    due to secondary diabetes 249.5 *[362.01]*
  retinopathy 250.5 *[362.01]*
    due to secondary diabetes 249.5 *[362.01]*
    background 250.5 *[362.01]*
      due to secondary diabetes 249.5 *[362.01]*
    nonproliferative 250.5 *[362.03]*
      due to secondary diabetes 249.5 *[362.03]*
      mild 250.5 *[362.04]*
        due to secondary diabetes 249.5 *[362.04]*
      moderate 250.5 *[362.05]*
        due to secondary diabetes 249.5 *[362.05]*
      severe 250.5 *[362.06]*
        due to secondary diabetes 249.5 *[362.06]*
    proliferative 250.5 *[362.02]*
      due to secondary diabetes 249.5 *[362.02]*
  secondary (chemical-induced) (due to chronic
    condition) (due to infection) (drug-induced)
    249.0
    with
      coma (with ketoacidosis) 249.3
        hyperosmolar (nonketotic) 249.2
      complication NEC 249.9
        specified NEC 249.8
      gangrene 249.7 *[785.4]*
      hyperosmolarity 249.2
      ketosis, ketoacidosis 249.1
      osteomyelitis 249.8 *[731.8]*
      specified manifestations NEC 249.8
    acetonemia 249.1
    acidosis 249.1
    amyotrophy 249.6 *[353.5]*
    angiopathy, peripheral 249.7 *[443.81]*
    autonomic neuropathy (peripheral) 249.6 *[337.1]*
    bone change 249.8 *[731.8]*
    cataract 249.5 *[366.41]*
    coma (with ketoacidosis) 249.3
      hyperglycemic 249.3
      hyperosmolar (nonketotic) 249.2
      hypoglycemic 249.3
      insulin 249.3
    complicating pregnancy, childbirth, or
      puerperium (maternal) 648.0
      affecting fetus or newborn 775.0
    complication NEC 249.9
      specified NEC 249.8
    dorsal sclerosis 249.6 *[340]*
    due to overdose or wrong substance given or
      taken — *see* Table of Drugs and
      Chemicals
    gangrene 249.7 *[785.4]*
    gastroparesis 249.6 *[536.3]*
    glaucoma 249.5 *[365.44]*
    glomerulosclerosis (intercapillary) 249.4 *[581.81]*
    glycogenosis, secondary 249.8 *[259.8]*
    hyperosmolar coma 249.2

Diabetes, diabetic—*continued*
secondary—*continued*
hyperosmolarity 249.2
hypertension-nephrosis syndrome 249.4 *[581.81]*
hypoglycemia 249.8
hypoglycemic shock 249.8
intercapillary glomerulosclerosis 249.4 *[581.81]*
iritis 249.5 *[364.42]*
ketosis, ketoacidosis 249.1
Kimmelstiel (-Wilson) disease or syndrome
(intercapillary glomerulosclerosis) 249.4
[581.81]
Lancereaux's (diabetes mellitus with marked
emaciation) 249.8 *[261]*
lipoidosis 249.8 *[272.7]*
macular edema 249.5 *[362.07]*
maternal
with manifest disease in the infant 775.1
affecting fetus or newborn 775.0
microaneurysms, retinal 249.5 *[362.01]*
mononeuropathy 249.6 *[355.9]*
nephropathy 249.4 *[583.81]*
nephrosis (syndrome) 249.4 *[581.81]*
neuralgia 249.6 *[357.2]*
neuritis 249.6 *[357.2]*
neurogenic arthropathy 249.6 *[713.5]*
neuropathy 249.6 *[357.2]*
autonomic (peripheral) 249.6 *[337.1]*
osteomyelitis 249.8 *[731.8]*
peripheral autonomic neuropathy 249.6 *[337.1]*
polyneuropathy 249.6 *[357.2]*
retinal
edema 249.5 *[362.07]*
hemorrhage 249.5 *[362.01]*
microaneurysms 249.5 *[362.01]*
retinitis 249.5 *[362.01]*
retinopathy 249.5 *[362.01]*
background 249.5 *[362.01]*
nonproliferative 249.5 *[362.03]*
mild 249.5 *[362.04]*
moderate 249.5 *[362.05]*
severe 249.5 *[362.06]*
proliferative 249.5 *[362.02]*
ulcer (skin) 249.8 *[707.9]*
lower extremity 249.8 *[707.10]*
ankle 249.8 *[707.13]*
calf 249.8 *[707.12]*
foot 249.8 *[707.15]*
heel 249.8 *[707.14]*
knee 249.8 *[707.19]*
specified site NEC 249.8 *[707.19]*
thigh 249.8 *[707.11]*
toes 249.8 *[707.15]*
specified site NEC 249.8 *[707.8]*
xanthoma 249.8 [272.2]
steroid induced—*see also* Diabetes, secondary
overdose or wrong substance given or taken
962.0
stress 790.29
subclinical 790.29
subliminal 790.29
sugar 250.0
ulcer (skin) 250.8 *[707.9]*
due to secondary diabetes 249.8 *[707.9]*
lower extremity 250.8 *[707.10]*
due to secondary diabetes 249.8 *[707.10]*
ankle 250.8 *[707.13]*
due to secondary diabetes 249.8 *[707.13]*
calf 250.8 *[707.12]*
due to secondary diabetes 249.8 *[707.12]*

Diabetes, diabetic—*continued*
ulcer—*continued*
lower extremity—*continued*
foot 250.8 *[707.15]*
due to secondary diabetes 249.8 *[707.15]*
heel 250.8 *[707.14]*
due to secondary diabetes 249.8 *[707.14]*
knee 250.8 *[707.19]*
due to secondary diabetes 249.8 *[707.19]*
specified site NEC 250.8 *[707.19]*
due to secondary diabetes 249.8 *[707.19]*
thigh 250.8 *[707.11]*
due to secondary diabetes 249.8 *[707.11]*
toes 250.8 *[707.15]*
due to secondary diabetes 249.8 *[707.15]*
specified site NEC 250.8 *[707.8]*
due to secondary diabetes 249.8 *[707.8]*
xanthoma 250.8 *[272.2]*
due to secondary diabetes 249.8 *[272.2]*
Diacyclothrombopathia 287.1
Diagnosis deferred 799.9
Dialysis (intermittent) (treatment)
anterior retinal (juvenile) (with detachment)
361.04
extracorporeal V56.0
hemodialysis V56.0
status only V45.11
peritoneal V56.8
status only V45.11
renal V56.0
status only V45.11
specified type NEC V56.8
Diamond-Blackfan anemia or syndrome
(congenital hypoplastic anemia) 284.01
Diamond-Gardener syndrome (autoerythrocyte
sensitization) 287.2
Diaper rash 691.0
Diaphoresis (excessive) NEC (*see also*
Hyperhidrosis) 780.8
Diaphragm —*see* condition
Diaphragmalgia 786.52
Diaphragmitis 519.4
Diaphyseal aclasis 756.4
Diaphysitis 733.99
Diarrhea, diarrheal (acute) (autumn) (bilious)
(bloody) (catarrhal) (choleraic) (chronic)
(gravis) (green) (infantile) (lienteric)
(noninfectious) (presumed noninfectious)
(putrefactive) (secondary) (sporadic)
(summer) (symptomatic) (thermic) 787.91
achlorhydric 536.0
allergic 558.3
amebic (*see also* Amebiasis) 006.9
with abscess—*see* Abscess, amebic
acute 006.0
chronic 006.1
nondysenteric 006.2
bacillary—*see* Dysentery, bacillary
bacterial NEC 008.5
balantidial 007.0
bile salt-induced 579.8
cachectic NEC 787.91
chilomastix 007.8
choleriformis 001.1
coccidial 007.2
Cochin-China 579.1
anguilluliasis 127.2
psilosis 579.1
Dientamoeba 007.8
dietetic 787.91

Diarrhea, diarrheal—*continued*
due to
achylia gastrica 536.8
Aerobacter aerogenes 008.2
Bacillus coli—*see* Enteritis, E. coli
bacteria NEC 008.5
bile salts 579.8
Capillaria
hepatica 128.8
philippinensis 127.5
Clostridium perfringens (C) (F) 008.46
Enterobacter aerogenes 008.2
enterococci 008.49
Escherichia coli—*see* Enteritis, E. coli
Giardia lamblia 007.1
Heterophyes heterophyes 121.6
irritating foods 787.91
Metagonimus yokogawai 121.5
Necator americanus 126.1
Paracolobactrum arizonae 008.1
Paracolon bacillus NEC 008.47
Arizona 008.1
Proteus (bacillus) (mirabilis) (Morganii) 008.3
Pseudomonas aeruginosa 008.42
S. japonicum 120.2
specified organism NEC 008.8
bacterial 008.49
viral NEC 008.69
Staphylococcus 008.41
Streptococcus 008.49
anaerobic 008.46
Strongyloides stercoralis 127.2
Trichuris trichiuria 127.3
virus NEC (*see also* Enteritis, viral) 008.69
dysenteric 009.2
due to specified organism NEC 008.8
dyspeptic 787.91
endemic 009.3
epidemic 009.3
fermentative 787.91
flagellate 007.9
Flexner's (ulcerative) 004.1
functional 564.5
following gastrointestinal surgery 564.4
psychogenic 306.4
giardial 007.1
Giardia lamblia 007.1
hill 579.1
hyperperistalsis (nervous) 306.4
infectious 009.2
presumed 009.3
inflammatory 787.91
due to specified organism NEC 008.8
malarial (*see also* Malaria) 084.6
mite 133.8
mycotic 117.9
nervous 306.4
neurogenic 564.5
parenteral NEC 009.2
postgastrectomy 564.4
postvagotomy 564.4
prostaglandin induced 579.8
protozoal NEC 007.9
psychogenic 306.4
septic 009.2
due to specified organism NEC 008.8
specified organism NEC 008.8
bacterial 008.49
viral NEC 008.69
Staphylococcus 008.41

Diarrhea, diarrheal—*continued*
Streptococcus 008.49
anaerobic 088.46
toxic 558.2
travelers' 009.2
due to specified organism NEC 008.8
trichomonal 007.3
tropical 579.1
tuberculous 014.8
ulcerative (chronic) (*see also* Colitis, ulcerative)
556.9
viral (*see also* Enteritis, viral) 008.8
zymotic NEC 009.2
Diastasis
cranial bones 733.99
congenital 756.0
joint (traumatic)—*see* Dislocation, by site
muscle 728.84
congenital 756.89
recti (abdomen) 728.84
complicating delivery 665.8
congenital 756.79
Diastema, teeth, tooth 524.30
Diastematomyelia 742.51
Diataxia, cerebral, infantile 343.0
Diathesis
allergic V15.09
bleeding (familial) 287.9
cystine (familial) 270.0
gouty 274.9
hemorrhagic (familial) 287.9
newborn NEC 776.0
oxalic 271.8
scrofulous (*see also* Tuberculosis) 017.2
spasmophilic (*see also* Tetany) 781.7
ulcer 536.9
uric acid 274.9
Diaz's disease or osteochondrosis 732.5
Dibothriocephaliasis 123.4
larval 123.5
Dibothriocephalus (infection) (infestation)
(latus) 123.4
larval 123.5
Dicephalus 759.4
Dichotomy, teeth 520.2
Dichromat, dichromata (congenital) 368.59
Dichromatopsia (congenital) 368.59
Dichuchwa 104.0
Dicroceliasis 121.8
Didelphys, didelphic (*see also* Double uterus)
752.2
Didymitis (*see also* Epididymitis) 604.90
Died —*see also* Death
without
medical attention (cause unknown) 798.9
sign of disease 798.2
Dientamoeba diarrhea 007.8
Dietary
inadequacy or deficiency 269.9
surveillance and counseling V65.3
Dietl's crisis 593.4
Dieulafoy lesion (hemorrhagic) of
duodenum 537.84
esophagus 530.82
intestine 569.86
stomach 537.84
Dieulafoy's ulcer —*see* Ulcer, stomach
Difficult
birth, affecting fetus or newborn 763.9
delivery NEC 669.9

Difficulty
  feeding 783.3
    adult 783.3
    breast 676.8
    child 783.3
    elderly 783.3
    infant 783.3
    newborn 779.31
  nonorganic (infant) NEC 307.59
  mechanical, gastroduodenal stoma 537.89
  reading 315.00
  specific, spelling 315.09
  swallowing (*see also* Dysphagia) 787.20
  walking 719.7
Diffuse —*see* condition
Diffused ganglion 727.42
DiGeorge's syndrome (thymic hypoplasia) 279.11
Digestive —*see* condition
Di Guglielmo's disease or syndrome (M9841/3) 207.0
Dihydropyrimidine dehydrogenase disease (DPD) 277.6
Diktyoma (M9051/3)—*see* Neoplasm, by site, malignant
Dilaceration, tooth 520.4
Dilatation
  anus 564.89
    venule—*see* Hemorrhoids
  aorta (focal) (general) (*see also* Ectasia, aortic) 447.70
    with aneurysm 441.9
    congenital 747.29
    infectional 093.0
    ruptured 441.5
    syphilitic 093.0
  appendix (cystic) 543.9
  artery 447.8
  bile duct (common) (congenital) 751.69
    acquired 576.8
  bladder (sphincter) 596.89
    congenital 753.8
    in pregnancy or childbirth 654.4
      causing obstructed labor 660.2
        affecting fetus or newborn 763.1
  blood vessel 459.89
  bronchus, bronchi 494.0
    with acute exacerbation 494.1
  calyx (due to obstruction) 593.89
  capillaries 448.9
  cardiac (acute) (chronic) (*see also* Hypertrophy, cardiac) 429.3
    congenital 746.89
      valve NEC 746.89
        pulmonary 746.09
    hypertensive (*see also* Hypertension, heart) 402.90
  cavum septi pellucidi 742.4
  cecum 564.89
    psychogenic 306.4
  cervix (uteri)—*see also* Incompetency, cervix
    incomplete, poor, slow
      affecting fetus or newborn 763.7
      complicating delivery 661.0
        affecting fetus or newborn 763.7
  colon 564.7
    congenital 751.3
    due to mechanical obstruction 560.89
    psychogenic 306.4

Dilatation—*continued*
  common bile duct (congenital) 751.69
    acquired 576.8
      with calculus, choledocholithiasis, or stones—*see* Choledocholithiasis
  cystic duct 751.69
    acquired (any bile duct) 575.8
  duct, mammary 610.4
  duodenum 564.89
  esophagus 530.89
    congenital 750.4
    due to
      achalasia 530.0
      cardiospasm 530.0
  Eustachian tube, congenital 744.24
  fontanel 756.0
  gallbladder 575.8
    congenital 751.69
  gastric 536.8
    acute 536.1
    psychogenic 306.4
  heart (acute) (chronic) (*see also* Hypertrophy, cardiac) 429.3
    congenital 746.89
    hypertensive (*see also* Hypertension, heart) 402.90
    valve—*see also* Endocarditis
      congenital 746.89
  ileum 564.89
    psychogenic 306.4
  inguinal rings—*see* Hernia, inguinal
  jejunum 564.89
    psychogenic 306.4
  kidney (calyx) (collecting structures) (cystic) (parenchyma) (pelvis) 593.89
  lacrimal passages 375.69
  lymphatic vessel 457.1
  mammary duct 610.4
  Meckel's diverticulum (congenital) 751.0
  meningeal vessels, congenital 742.8
  myocardium (acute) (chronic) (*see also* Hypertrophy, cardiac) 429.3
  organ or site, congenital NEC—*see* Distortion
  pancreatic duct 577.8
  pelvis, kidney 593.89
  pericardium—*see* Pericarditis
  pharynx 478.29
  prostate 602.8
  pulmonary
    artery (idiopathic) 417.8
      congenital 747.39
    valve, congenital 746.09
  pupil 379.43
  rectum 564.89
  renal 593.89
  saccule vestibularis, congenital 744.05
  salivary gland (duct) 527.8
  sphincter ani 564.89
  stomach 536.8
    acute 536.1
    psychogenic 306.4
  submaxillary duct 527.8
  trachea, congenital 748.3
  ureter (idiopathic) 593.89
    congenital 753.20
    due to obstruction 593.5
  urethra (acquired) 599.84
  vasomotor 443.9
  vein 459.89

Dilatation—*continued*
 ventricular, ventricle (acute) (chronic) (*see also*
   Hypertrophy, cardiac) 429.3
   cerebral, congenital 742.4
   hypertensive (*see also* Hypertension, heart) 402.90
 venule 459.89
 anus—*see* Hemorrhoids
 vesical orifice 596.89
Dilated, dilation —*see* Dilatation
Diminished
 hearing (acuity) (*see also* Deafness) 389.9
 pulse pressure 785.9
 vision NEC 369.9
 vital capacity 794.2
Diminuta taenia 123.6
Diminution, sense or sensation (cold) (heat)
 (tactile) (vibratory) (*see also* Disturbance,
 sensation) 782.0
Dimitri-Sturge-Weber disease
 (encephalocutaneous angiomatosis) 759.6
Dimple
 parasacral 685.1
   with abscess 685.0
 pilonidal 685.1
   with abscess 685.0
 postanal 685.1
   with abscess 685.0
Dioctophyma renale (infection) (infestation) 128.8
Dipetalonemiasis 125.4
Diphallus 752.69
Diphtheria, diphtheritic (gangrenous)
 (hemorrhagic) 032.9
 carrier (suspected) of V02.4
 cutaneous 032.85
 cystitis 032.84
 faucial 032.0
 infection of wound 032.85
 inoculation (anti) (not sick) V03.5
 laryngeal 032.3
 myocarditis 032.82
 nasal anterior 032.2
 nasopharyngeal 032.1
 neurological complication 032.89
 peritonitis 032.83
 specified site NEC 032.89
Diphyllobothriasis (intestine) 123.4
 larval 123.5
Diplacusis 388.41
Diplegia (upper limbs) 344.2
 brain or cerebral 437.8
 congenital 343.0
 facial 351.0
   congenital 352.6
 infantile or congenital (cerebral) (spastic)
   (spinal) 343.0
 lower limbs 344.1
 syphilitic, congenital 090.49
Diplococcus, diplococcal —*see* condition
Diplomyelia 742.59
Diplopia 368.2
 refractive 368.15
Dipsomania (*see also* Alcoholism) 303.9
 with psychosis (*see also* Psychosis, alcoholic) 291.9
Dipylidiasis 123.8
 intestine 123.8
Direction, teeth, abnormal 524.30
Dirt-eating child 307.52

Disability, disabilities
 heart—*see* Disease, heart
 intellectual 319
   borderline V62.89
   mild, IQ 50-70 317⁻
   moderate, IQ 35-49 318.0
   profound, IQ under 20 318.2
   severe, IQ 20-34 318.1
 learning NEC 315.2
 special spelling 315.09
Disarticulation (*see also* Derangement, joint) 718.9
 meaning
   amputation
     status—*see* Absence, by site
     traumatic —*see* Amputation, traumatic
   dislocation, traumatic or congenital—*see*
     Dislocation
Disaster, cerebrovascular (*see also* Disease,
 cerebrovascular, acute) 436
Discharge
 anal NEC 787.99
 breast (female) (male) 611.79
 conjunctiva 372.89
 continued locomotor idiopathic (*see also*
   Epilepsy) 345.5
 diencephalic autonomic idiopathic (*see also*
   Epilepsy) 345.5
 ear 388.60
   blood 388.69
   cerebrospinal fluid 388.61
 excessive urine 788.42
 eye 379.93
 nasal 478.19
 nipple 611.79
 patterned motor idiopathic (*see also* Epilepsy) 345.5
 penile 788.7
 postnasal—*see* Sinusitis
 sinus, from mediastinum 510.0
 umbilicus 789.9
 urethral 788.7
   bloody 599.84
 vaginal 623.5
Discitis 722.90
 cervical, cervicothoracic 722.91
 lumbar, lumbosacral 722.93
 thoracic, thoracolumbar 722.92
Discogenic syndrome —*see* Displacement,
 intervertebral disc
Discoid
 kidney 753.3
 meniscus, congenital 717.5
 semilunar cartilage 717.5
Discoloration
 mouth 528.9
 nails 703.8
 teeth 521.7
   due to
     drugs 521.7
     metals (copper) (silver) 521.7
     pulpal bleeding 521.7
   during formation 520.8
   extrinsic 523.6
   intrinsic posteruptive 521.7
Discomfort
 chest 786.59
 visual 368.13
Discomycosis —*see* Actinomycosis
Discontinuity, ossicles, ossicular chain 385.23

Discrepancy
　centric occlusion
　　maximum intercuspation 524.55
　　of teeth 524.55
　leg length (acquired) 736.81
　　congenital 755.30
　uterine size-date 649.6
Discrimination
　political V62.4
　racial V62.4
　religious V62.4
　sex V62.4
Disease, diseased —*see also* Syndrome
　Abrami's (acquired hemolytic jaundice) 283.9
　absorbent system 459.89
　accumulation—*see* Thesaurismosis
　acid-peptic 536.8
　Acosta's 993.2
　Adams-Stokes (-Morgagni) (syncope with heart
　　block) 426.9
　Addison's (bronze) (primary adrenal
　　insufficiency) 255.41
　　anemia (pernicious) 281.0
　　tuberculous (*see also* Tuberculosis) 017.6
　Addison-Gull—*see* Xanthoma
　adenoids (and tonsils) (chronic) 474.9
　adrenal (gland) (capsule) (cortex) 255.9
　　hyperfunction 255.3
　　hypofunction 255.41
　　specified type NEC 255.8
　ainhum (dactylolysis spontanea) 136.0
　akamushi (scrub typhus) 081.2
　Akureyri (epidemic neuromyasthenia) 049.8
　Albarrán's (colibacilluria) 791.9
　Albers-Schönberg's (marble bones) 756.52
　Albert's 726.71
　Albright (-Martin) (-Bantam) 275.49
　Alibert's (mycosis fungoides) (M9700/3) 202.1
　Alibert-Bazin (M9700/3) 202.1
　alimentary canal 569.9
　alligator skin (ichthyosis congenital) 757.1
　　acquired 701.1
　Almeida's (Brazilian blastomycosis) 116.1
　Alpers' 330.8
　alpine 993.2
　altitude 993.2
　alveoli, teeth 525.9
　Alzheimer's—*see* Alzheimer's
　amyloid (any site) 277.30
　anarthritic rheumatoid 446.5
　Anders' (adiposis tuberosa simplex) 272.8
　Andersen's (glycogenosis IV) 271.0
　Anderson's (angiokeratoma corporis diffusum)
　　272.7
　Andes 993.2
　Andrews' (bacterid) 686.8
　angiospastic, angiospasmodic 443.9
　　cerebral 435.9
　　　with transient neurologic deficit 435.9
　　vein 459.89
　anterior
　　chamber 364.9
　　horn cell 335.9
　　　specified type NEC 335.8
　antral (chronic) 473.0
　　acute 461.0
　anus NEC 569.49
　aorta (nonsyphilitic) 447.9
　　syphilitic NEC 093.89
　aortic (heart) (valve) (*see also* Endocarditis,
　　aortic) 424.1

Disease, diseased—*continued*
　apollo 077.4
　aponeurosis 726.90
　appendix 543.9
　aqueous (chamber) 364.9
　arc-welders' lung 503
　Armenian 277.31
　Arnold-Chiari (*see also* Spina bifida) 741.0
　arterial 447.9
　　occlusive (*see also* Occlusion, by site) 444.22
　　　with embolus or thrombus—*see* Occlusion,
　　　　by site
　　due to stricture or stenosis 447.1
　　specified type NEC 447.8
　arteriocardiorenal (*see also* Hypertension,
　　cardiorenal) 404.90
　arteriolar (generalized) (obliterative) 447.9
　　specified type NEC 447.8
　arteriorenal—*see* Hypertension, kidney
　arteriosclerotic—*see also* Arteriosclerosis
　　cardiovascular 429.2
　　coronary —*see* Arteriosclerosis, coronary
　　heart —*see* Arteriosclerosis, coronary
　artery 447.9
　　cerebral 437.9
　　coronary —*see* Arteriosclerosis, coronary
　　specified type NEC 447.8
　arthropod-borne NEC 088.9
　　specified type NEC 088.89
　Asboe-Hansen's (incontinentia pigmenti) 757.33
　atticoantral, chronic (with posterior or superior
　　marginal perforation of ear drum) 382.2
　auditory canal, ear 380.9
　Aujeszky's 078.89
　auricle, ear NEC 380.30
　Australian X 062.4
　autoimmune NEC 279.49
　　hemolytic (cold type) (warm type) 283.0
　　parathyroid 252.1
　　thyroid 245.2
　aviators' (*see also* Effect, adverse, high altitude)
　　993.2
　ax(e)-grinders' 502
　Ayala's 756.89
　Ayerza's (pulmonary artery sclerosis with
　　pulmonary hypertension) 416.0
　Azorean (of the nervous system) 334.8
　Babington's (familial hemorrhagic
　　telangiectasia) 448.0
　back bone NEC 733.90
　bacterial NEC 040.89
　　zoonotic NEC 027.9
　　specified type NEC 027.8
　Baehr-Schiffrin (thrombotic thrombocytopenic
　　purpura) 446.6
　Baelz's (cheilitis glandularis apostematosa)
　　528.5
　Baerensprung's (eczema marginatum) 110.3
　Balfour's (chloroma) 205.3
　balloon (*see also* Effect, adverse, high altitude)
　　993.2
　Baló's 341.1
　Bamberger (-Marie) (hypertrophic pulmonary
　　osteoarthropathy) 731.2
　Bang's (Brucella abortus) 023.1
　Bannister's 995.1
　Banti's (with cirrhosis) (with portal
　　hypertension)—*see* Cirrhosis, liver
　Barcoo (*see also* Ulcer, skin) 707.9
　barium lung 503
　Barlow (-Möller) (infantile scurvy) 267

Disease, diseased—*continued*

barometer makers' 985.0

Barraquer (-Simons) (progressive lipodystrophy) 272.6

basal ganglia 333.90
  degenerative NEC 333.0
  specified NEC 333.89

Basedow's (exophthalmic goiter) 242.0

basement membrane NEC 583.89
  with
    pulmonary hemorrhage (Goodpasture's syndrome) 446.21 *[583.81]*

Bateman's 078.0
  purpura (senile) 287.2

Batten's 330.1 *[362.71]*

Batten-Mayou (retina) 330.1 *[362.71]*

Batten-Steinert 359.21

Battey 031.0

Baumgarten-Cruveilhier (cirrhosis of liver) 571.5

bauxite-workers' 503

Bayle's (dementia paralytica) 094.1

Bazin's (primary) (*see also* Tuberculosis) 017.1

Beard's (neurasthenia) 300.5

Beau's (*see also* Degeneration, myocardial) 429.1

Bechterew's (ankylosing spondylitis) 720.0

Becker's
  idiopathic mural endomyocardial disease 425.2
  myotonia congenita, recessive form 359.22

Begbie's (exophthalmic goiter) 242.0

Behr's 362.50

Beigel's (white piedra) 111.2

Bekhterev's (ankylosing spondylitis) 720.0

Bell's (*see also* Psychosis, affective) 296.0

Bennett's (leukemia) 208.9

Benson's 379.22

Bergeron's (hysteroepilepsy) 300.11

Berlin's 921.3

Bernard-Soulier (thrombopathy) 287.1

Bernhardt (-Roth) 355.1

beryllium 503

Besnier-Boeck (-Schaumann) (sarcoidosis) 135

Best's 362.76

Beurmann's (sporotrichosis) 117.1

Bielschowsky (-Jansky) 330.1

Biermer's (pernicious anemia) 281.0

Biett's (discoid lupus erythematosus) 695.4

bile duct (*see also* Disease, biliary) 576.9

biliary (duct) (tract) 576.9
  with calculus, choledocholithiasis, or stones—*see* Choledocholithiasis

Billroth's (meningocele) (*see also* Spina bifida) 741.9

Binswanger's 290.12

Bird's (oxaluria) 271.8

bird fanciers' 495.2

black lung 500

bladder 596.9
  specified NEC 596.89

bleeder's 286.0

Bloch-Sulzberger (incontinentia pigmenti) 757.33

Blocq's (astasia-abasia) 307.9

blood (-forming organs) 289.9
  specified NEC 289.89
  vessel 459.9

Bloodgood's 610.1

Blount's (tibia vara) 732.4

blue 746.9

Bodechtel-Guttmann (subacute sclerosing panencephalitis) 046.2

Boeck's (sarcoidosis) 135

Disease, diseased—*continued*

bone 733.90
  fibrocystic NEC 733.29
    jaw 526.2
  marrow 289.9
  Paget's (osteitis deformans) 731.0
  specified type NEC 733.99
  von Recklinghausen's (osteitis fibrosa cystica) 252.01

Bonfils'—*see* Disease, Hodgkin's

Borna 062.9

Bornholm (epidemic pleurodynia) 074.1

Bostock's (*see also* Fever, hay) 477.9

Bouchard's (myopathic dilatation of the stomach) 536.1

Bouillaud's (rheumatic heart disease) 391.9

Bourneville (-Brissaud) (tuberous sclerosis) 759.5

Bouveret (-Hoffmann) (paroxysmal tachycardia) 427.2

bowel 569.9
  functional 564.9
    psychogenic 306.4

Bowen's (M8081/2)—*see* Neoplasm, skin, in situ

Bozzolo's (multiple myeloma) (M9730/3) 203.0

Bradley's (epidemic vomiting) 078.82

Brailsford's 732.3
  radius, head 732.3
  tarsal, scaphoid 732.5

Brailsford-Morquio (mucopolysaccharidosis IV) 277.5

brain 348.9
  Alzheimer's 331.0
    with dementia—*see* Alzheimer's, dementia
  arterial, artery 437.9
  arteriosclerotic 437.0
  congenital 742.9
  degenerative—*see* Degeneration, brain
  inflammatory—*see also* Encephalitis
  late effect—*see* category 326
  organic 348.9
    arteriosclerotic 437.0
  parasitic NEC 123.9
  Pick's 331.11
    with dementia
      with behavioral disturbance 331.11 *[294.11]*
      without behavioral disturbance 331.11 *[294.10]*
  senile 331.2

braziers' 985.8

breast 611.9
  cystic (chronic) 610.1
  fibrocystic 610.1
  inflammatory 611.0
  Paget's (M8540/3) 174.0
  puerperal, postpartum NEC 676.3
  specified NEC 611.89

Breda's (*see also* Yaws) 102.9

Breisky's (kraurosis vulvae) 624.09

Bretonneau's (diphtheritic malignant angina) 032.0

Bright's (*see also* Nephritis) 583.9
  arteriosclerotic (*see also* Hypertension, kidney) 403.90

Brill's (recrudescent typhus) 081.1
  flea-borne 081.0
  louse-borne 081.1

Brill-Symmers (follicular lymphoma) (M9690/3) 202.0

Brill-Zinsser (recrudescent typhus) 081.1

Disease, diseased—*continued*
Brinton's (leather bottle stomach) (M8142/3) 151.9
Brion-Kayser (*see also* Fever, paratyphoid) 002.9
broad
  beta 272.2
  ligament, noninflammatory 620.9
    specified NEC 620.8
Brocq's 691.8
  meaning
    atopic (diffuse) neurodermatitis 691.8
    dermatitis herpetiformis 694.0
    lichen simplex chronicus 698.3
    parapsoriasis 696.2
    prurigo 698.2
Brocq-Duhring (dermatitis herpetiformis) 694.0
Brodie's (joint) (*see also* Osteomyelitis) 730.1
bronchi 519.19
bronchopulmonary 519.19
bronze (Addison's) 255.41
  tuberculous (*see also* Tuberculosis) 017.6
Brown-Séquard 344.89
Bruck's 733.99
Bruck-de Lange (Amsterdam dwarf, intellectual disabilities, and brachycephaly) 759.89
Bruhl's (splenic anemia with fever) 285.8
Bruton's (X-linked agammaglobulinemia) 279.04
buccal cavity 528.9
Buchanan's (juvenile osteochondrosis, iliac crest) 732.1
Buchman's (osteochondrosis juvenile) 732.1
Budgerigar-fanciers' 495.2
Büdinger-Ludloff-Läwen 717.89
Buerger's (thromboangiitis obliterans) 443.1
Bürger-Grütz (essential familial hyperlipemia) 272.3
Burns' (lower ulna) 732.3
bursa 727.9
Bury's (erythema elevatum diutinum) 695.89
Buschke's 710.1
Busquet's (*see also* Osteomyelitis) 730.1
Busse-Buschke (cryptococcosis) 117.5
C2 (*see also* Alcoholism) 303.9
Caffey's (infantile cortical hyperostosis) 756.59
caisson 993.3
calculous 592.9
California 114.0
Calvé (-Perthes) (osteochondrosis, femoral capital) 732.1
Camurati-Engelmann (diaphyseal sclerosis) 756.59
Canavan's 330.0
capillaries 448.9
Carapata 087.1
cardiac-*see* Disease, heart
cardiopulmonary, chronic 416.9
cardiorenal (arteriosclerotic) (hepatic) (hypertensive) (vascular) (*see also* Hypertension, cardiorenal) 404.90
cardiovascular (arteriosclerotic) 429.2
  congenital 746.9
  hypertensive (*see also* Hypertension, heart) 402.90
    benign 402.10
    malignant 402.00
  renal (*see also* Hypertension, cardiorenal) 404.90
  syphilitic (asymptomatic) 093.9
carotid gland 259.8

Disease, diseased—*continued*
Carrión's (Bartonellosis) 088.0
cartilage NEC 733.90
  specified NEC 733.99
Castellani's 104.8
cat-scratch 078.3
Cavare's (familial periodic paralysis) 359.3
Cazenave's (pemphigus) 694.4
cecum 569.9
celiac (adult) 579.0
  infantile 579.0
cellular tissue NEC 709.9
central core 359.0
cerebellar, cerebellum—*see* Disease, brain
cerebral (*see also* Disease, brain) 348.9
  arterial, artery 437.9
  degenerative—*see* Degeneration, brain
cerebrospinal 349.9
cerebrovascular NEC 437.9
  acute 436
    embolic—*see* Embolism, brain
    late effect—*see* Late effect(s) (of) cerebrovascular disease
    puerperal, postpartum, childbirth 674.0
    thrombotic—*see* Thrombosis, brain
  arteriosclerotic 437.0
  embolic—*see* Embolism, brain
  ischemic, generalized NEC 437.1
  late effect—*see* Late effect(s) (of) cerebrovascular disease
  occlusive 437.1
  puerperal, postpartum, childbirth 674.0
  specified type NEC 437.8
  thrombotic—*see* Thrombosis, brain
ceroid storage 272.7
cervix (uteri)
  inflammatory 616.0
  noninflammatory 622.9
    specified NEC 622.8
Chabert's 022.9
Chagas' (*see also* Trypanosomiasis, American) 086.2
Chandler's (osteochondritis dissecans, hip) 732.7
Charcot's (joint) 094.0 *[713.5]*
  spinal cord 094.0
Charcot-Marie-Tooth 356.1
Charlouis' (*see also* Yaws) 102.9
Cheadle (-Möller) (-Barlow) (infantile scurvy) 267
Chédiak-Steinbrinck (-Higashi) (congenital gigantism of peroxidase granules) 288.2
cheek, inner 528.9
chest 519.9
Chiari's (hepatic vein thrombosis) 453.0
Chicago (North American blastomycosis) 116.0
chignon (white piedra) 111.2
chigoe, chigo (jigger) 134.1
childhood granulomatous 288.1
Chinese liver fluke 121.1
chlamydial NEC 078.88
cholecystic (*see also* Disease, gallbladder) 575.9
choroid 363.9
  degenerative (*see also* Degeneration, choroid) 363.40
  hereditary (*see also* Dystrophy, choroid) 363.50
  specified type NEC 363.8
Christian's (chronic histiocytosis X) 277.89
Christian-Weber (nodular nonsuppurative panniculitis) 729.30

Disease, diseased—*continued*

Christmas 286.1
ciliary body 364.9
  specified NEC 364.89
circulatory (system) NEC 459.9
  chronic, maternal, affecting fetus or newborn
    760.3
  specified NEC 459.89
  syphilitic 093.9
    congenital 090.5
Civatte's (poikiloderma) 709.09
climacteric 627.2
  male 608.89
coagulation factor deficiency (congenital) (*see
  also* Defect, coagulation) 286.9
Coats' 362.12
coccidioidal pulmonary 114.5
  acute 114.0
  chronic 114.4
  primary 114.0
  residual 114.4
Cockayne's (microcephaly and dwarfism)
  759.89
Cogan's 370.52
cold
  agglutinin 283.0
    or hemoglobinuria 283.0
      paroxysmal (cold) (nocturnal) 283.2
  hemagglutinin (chronic) 283.0
collagen NEC 710.9
  nonvascular 710.9
  specified NEC 710.8
  vascular (allergic) (*see also* Angiitis,
    hypersensitivity) 446.20
colon 569.9
  functional 564.9
    congenital 751.3
  ischemic 557.0
combined system (of spinal cord) 266.2 *[336.2]*
  with anemia (pernicious) 281.0 *[336.2]*
compressed air 993.3
Concato's (pericardial polyserositis) 423.2
  peritoneal 568.82
  pleural—*see* Pleurisy
congenital NEC 799.89
conjunctiva 372.9
  chlamydial 077.98
    specified NEC 077.8
  specified type NEC 372.89
  viral 077.99
    specified NEC 077.8
connective tissue, diffuse (*see also* Disease,
  collagen) 710.9
Conor and Bruch's (boutonneuse fever) 082.1
Conradi (-Hünermann) 756.59
Cooley's (erythroblastic anemia) 282.44
Cooper's 610.1
Corbus' 607.1
cork-handlers' 495.3
cornea (*see also* Keratopathy) 371.9
coronary (*see also* Ischemia, heart) 414.9
  congenital 746.85
  ostial, syphilitic 093.20
    aortic 093.22
    mitral 093.21
    pulmonary 093.24
    tricuspid 093.23
Corrigan's—*see* Insufficiency, aortic
Cotugno's 724.3
Coxsackie (virus) NEC 074.8
cranial nerve NEC 352.9

Disease, diseased—*continued*

Creutzfeldt-Jakob (CJD) 046.19
  with dementia
    with behavioral disturbance 046.19 *[294.11]*
    without behavioral disturbance 046.19
      [294.10]
  familial 046.19
  iatrogenic 046.19
  specified NEC 046.19
  sporadic 046.19
  variant (vCJD) 046.11
    with dementia
      with behavioral disturbance 046.11
        [294.11]
      without behavioral disturbance 046.11
        [294.10]
Crigler-Najjar (congenital hyperbilirubinemia)
  277.4
Crocq's (acrocyanosis) 443.89
Crohn's (intestine) (*see also* Enteritis, regional)
  555.9
Crouzon's (craniofacial dysostosis) 756.0
Cruchet's (encephalitis lethargica) 049.8
Cruveilhier's 335.21
Cruz-Chagas (*see also* Trypanosomiasis,
  American) 086.2
crystal deposition (*see also* Arthritis, due to,
  crystals) 712.9
Csillag's (lichen sclerosus et atrophicus) 701.0
Curschmann's 359.21
Cushing's (pituitary basophilism) 255.0
cystic
  breast (chronic) 610.1
  kidney, congenital (*see also* Cystic, disease,
    kidney) 753.10
  liver, congenital 751.62
  lung 518.89
    congenital 748.4
  pancreas 577.2
    congenital 751.7
  renal, congenital (*see also* Cystic, disease,
    kidney) 753.10
  semilunar cartilage 717.5
cysticercus 123.1
cystine storage (with renal sclerosis) 270.0
cytomegalic inclusion (generalized) 078.5
  with
    pneumonia 078.5 *[484.1]*
  congenital 771.1
Daae (-Finsen) (epidemic pleurodynia) 074.1
dancing 297.8
Danielssen's (anesthetic leprosy) 030.1
Darier's (congenital) (keratosis follicularis)
  757.39
  erythema annulare centrifugum 695.0
  vitamin A deficiency 264.8
Darling's (histoplasmosis) (*see also*
  Histoplasmosis, American) 115.00
Davies' 425.0
de Beurmann-Gougerot (sporotrichosis) 117.1
Débove's (splenomegaly) 789.2
deer fly (*see also* Tularemia) 021.9
deficiency 269.9
degenerative—*see also* Degeneration
  disc—*see* Degeneration, intervertebral disc
Degos' 447.8
Déjérine (-Sottas) 356.0
Deleage's 359.89
demyelinating, demyelinizating (brain stem)
  (central nervous system) 341.9
  multiple sclerosis 340
  specified NEC 341.8

Disease, diseased—*continued*
de Quervain's (tendon sheath) 727.04
  thyroid (subacute granulomatous thyroiditis) 245.1
Dercum's (adiposis dolorosa) 272.8
Deutschländer's—*see* Fracture, foot
Devergie's (pityriasis rubra pilaris) 696.4
Devic's 341.0
diaphorase deficiency 289.7
diaphragm 519.4
diarrheal, infectious 009.2
diatomaceous earth 502
Diaz's (osteochondrosis astragalus) 732.5
digestive system 569.9
Di Guglielmo's (erythemic myelosis) (M9841/3) 207.0
Dimitri-Sturge-Weber (encephalocutaneous angiomatosis) 759.6
disc, degenerative—*see* Degeneration, intervertebral disc
discogenic (*see also* Disease, intervertebral disc) 722.90
diverticular—*see* Diverticula
Down's (mongolism) 758.0
Dubini's (electric chorea) 049.8
Dubois' (thymus gland) 090.5
Duchenne's 094.0
  locomotor ataxia 094.0
  muscular dystrophy 359.1
  paralysis 335.22
  pseudohypertrophy, muscles 359.1
Duchenne-Griesinger 359.1
ductless glands 259.9
Duhring's (dermatitis herpetiformis) 694.0
Dukes (-Filatov) 057.8
duodenum NEC 537.9
  specified NEC 537.89
Duplay's 726.2
Dupré's (meningism) 781.6
Dupuytren's (muscle contracture) 728.6
Durand-Nicolas-Favre (climatic bubo) 099.1
Duroziez's (congenital mitral stenosis) 746.5
Dutton's (trypanosomiasis) 086.9
Eales' 362.18
ear (chronic) (inner) NEC 388.9
  middle 385.9
    adhesive (*see also* Adhesions, middle ear) 385.10
    specified NEC 385.89
Eberth's (typhoid fever) 002.0
Ebstein's
  heart 746.2
  meaning diabetes 250.4 *[581.81]*
    due to secondary diabetes 249.4 *[581.81]*
Echinococcus (*see also* Echinococcus) 122.9
ECHO virus NEC 078.89
Economo's (encephalitis lethargica) 049.8
Eddowes' (brittle bones and blue sclera) 756.51
Edsall's 992.2
Eichstedt's (pityriasis versicolor) 111.0
Ellis-van Creveld (chondroectodermal dysplasia) 756.55
endocardium—*see* Endocarditis
endocrine glands or system NEC 259.9
  specified NEC 259.8
endomyocardial, idiopathic mural 425.2
Engel-von Recklinghausen (osteitis fibrosa cystica) 252.01
Engelmann's (diaphyseal sclerosis) 756.59
English (rickets) 268.0
Engman's (infectious eczematoid dermatitis) 690.8

Disease, diseased—*continued*
enteroviral, enterovirus NEC 078.89
  central nervous system NEC 048
epidemic NEC 136.9
epididymis 608.9
epigastric, functional 536.9
  psychogenic 306.4
Erb (-Landouzy) 359.1
Erb-Goldflam 358.00
Erdheim-Chester (ECD) 277.89
Erichsen's (railway spine) 300.16
esophagus 530.9
  functional 530.5
  psychogenic 306.4
Eulenburg's (congenital paramyotonia) 359.29
Eustachian tube 381.9
Evans' (thrombocytopenic purpura) 287.32
external auditory canal 380.9
extrapyramidal NEC 333.90
eye 379.90
  anterior chamber 364.9
  inflammatory NEC 364.3
  muscle 378.9
eyeball 360.9
eyelid 374.9
eyeworm of Africa 125.2
Fabry's (angiokeratoma corporis diffusum) 272.7
facial nerve (seventh) 351.9
  newborn 767.5
Fahr-Volhard (malignant nephrosclerosis) 403.00
fallopian tube, noninflammatory 620.9
  specified NEC 620.8
familial periodic 277.31
  paralysis 359.3
Fanconi's (congenital pancytopenia) 284.09
Farber's (disseminated lipogranulomatosis) 272.8
fascia 728.9
  inflammatory 728.9
Fauchard's (periodontitis) 523.40
Favre-Durand-Nicolas (climatic bubo) 099.1
Favre-Racouchot (elastoidosis cutanea nodularis) 701.8
Fede's 529.0
Feer's 985.0
Felix's (juvenile osteochondrosis, hip) 732.1
Fenwick's (gastric atrophy) 537.89
Fernels' (aortic aneurysm) 441.9
fibrocaseous, of lung (*see also* Tuberculosis, pulmonary) 011.9
fibrocystic—*see also* Fibrocystic, disease
  newborn 277.01
Fiedler's (leptospiral jaundice) 100.0
fifth 057.0
Filatoff's (infectious mononucleosis) 075
Filatov's (infectious mononucleosis) 075
file-cutters' 984.9
  specified type of lead—*see* Table of drugs and chemicals
filterable virus NEC 078.89
fish skin 757.1
  acquired 701.1
Flajani (-Basedow) (exophthalmic goiter) 242.0
Flatau-Schilder 341.1
flax-dressers' 504
Fleischner's 732.3
flint 502
fluke—*see* Infestation, fluke
Følling's (phenylketonuria) 270.1
foot and mouth 078.4

Disease, diseased—*continued*
foot process 581.3
Forbes' (glycogenosis III) 271.0
Fordyce's (ectopic sebaceous glands) (mouth)
  750.26
Fordyce-Fox (apocrine miliaria) 705.82
Fothergill's
  meaning scarlatina anginosa 034.1
  neuralgia (*see also* Neuralgia, trigeminal)
    350.1
Fournier's 608.83
  female 616.89
fourth 057.8
Fox (-Fordyce) (apocrine miliaria) 705.82
Francis' (*see also* Tularemia) 021.9
Franklin's (heavy chain) 273.2
Frei's (climatic bubo) 099.1
Freiberg's (flattening metatarsal) 732.5
Friedländer's (endarteritis obliterans)—*see*
  Arteriosclerosis
Friedreich's
  combined systemic or ataxia 334.0
  facial hemihypertrophy 756.0
  myoclonia 333.2
Fröhlich's (adiposogenital dystrophy) 253.8
Frommel's 676.6
frontal sinus (chronic) 473.1
  acute 461.1
Fuller's earth 502
fungus, fungous NEC 117.9
Gaisböck's (polycythemia hypertonica) 289.0
gallbladder 575.9
  congenital 751.60
Gamna's (siderotic splenomegaly) 289.51
Gamstorp's (adynamia episodica hereditaria)
  359.3
Gandy-Nanta (siderotic splenomegaly) 289.51
gannister (occupational) 502
Garré's (*see also* Osteomyelitis) 730.1
gastric (*see also* Disease, stomach) 537.9
gastroesophageal reflux (GERD) 530.81
gastrointestinal (tract) 569.9
  amyloid 277.39
  functional 536.9
    psychogenic 306.4
Gaucher's (adult) (cerebroside lipidosis)
  (infantile) 272.7
Gayet's (superior hemorrhagic
  polioencephalitis) 265.1
Gee (-Herter) (-Heubner) (-Thaysen)
  (nontropical sprue) 579.0
generalized neoplastic (M8000/6) 199.0
genital organs NEC
  female 629.9
    specified NEC 629.89
  male 608.9
Gerhardt's (erythromelalgia) 443.82
Gerlier's (epidemic vertigo) 078.81
Gibert's (pityriasis rosea) 696.3
Gibney's (perispondylitis) 720.9
Gierke's (glycogenosis I) 271.0
Gilbert's (familial nonhemolytic jaundice) 277.4
Gilchrist's (North American blastomycosis)
  116.0
Gilford (-Hutchinson) (progeria) 259.8
Gilles de la Tourette's (motor-verbal tic) 307.23
Giovannini's 117.9
gland (lymph) 289.9
Glanzmann's (hereditary hemorrhagic
  thrombasthenia) 287.1
glassblowers' 527.1

Disease, diseased—*continued*
Glénard's (enteroptosis) 569.89
Glisson's (*see also* Rickets) 268.0
glomerular
  membranous, idiopathic 581.1
  minimal change 581.3
glycogen storage (Andersen's) (Cori types 1-7)
  (Forbes') (McArdle-Schmid-Pearson)
  (Pompe's) (types I-VII) 271.0
  cardiac 271.0 *[425.7]*
  generalized 271.0
  glucose-6-phosphatase deficiency 271.0
  heart 271.0 *[425.7]*
  hepatorenal 271.0
  liver and kidneys 271.0
  myocardium 271.0 *[425.7]*
  von Gierke's (glycogenosis I) 271.0
Goldflam-Erb 358.00
Goldscheider's (epidermolysis bullosa) 757.39
Goldstein's (familial hemorrhagic
  telangiectasia) 448.0
gonococcal NEC 098.0
Goodall's (epidemic vomiting) 078.82
Gordon's (exudative enteropathy) 579.8
Gougerot's (trisymptomatic) 709.1
Gougerot-Carteaud (confluent reticulate
  papillomatosis) 701.8
Gougerot-Hailey-Hailey (benign familial
  chronic pemphigus) 757.39
graft-versus-host 279.50
  acute 279.51
    on chronic 279.53
  chronic 279.52
grain-handlers' 495.8
Grancher's (splenopneumonia)—*see* Pneumonia
granulomatous (childhood) (chronic) 288.1
graphite lung 503
Graves' (exophthalmic goiter) 242.0
Greenfield's 330.0
green monkey 078.89
Griesinger's (*see also* Ancylostomiasis) 126.9
grinders' 502
Grisel's 723.5
Gruby's (tinea tonsurans) 110.0
Guertin's (electric chorea) 049.8
Guillain-Barré 357.0
Guinon's (motor-verbal tic) 307.23
Gull's (thyroid atrophy with myxedema) 244.8
Gull and Sutton's—*see* Hypertension, kidney
gum NEC 523.9
Günther's (congenital erythropoietic porphyria)
  277.1
gynecological 629.9
  specified NEC 629.89
H 270.0
Haas' 732.3
Habermann's (acute parapsoriasis varioliformis)
  696.2
Haff 985.1
Hageman (congenital factor XII deficiency) (*see
  also* Defect, congenital) 286.3
Haglund's (osteochondrosis os tibiale externum)
  732.5
Hagner's (hypertrophic pulmonary
  osteoarthropathy) 731.2
Hailey-Hailey (benign familial chronic
  pemphigus) 757.39
hair (follicles) NEC 704.9
  specified type NEC 704.8
Hallervorden-Spatz 333.0

Disease, diseased—*continued*
  Hallopeau's (lichen sclerosus et atrophicus)
    701.0
  Hamman's (spontaneous mediastinal
    emphysema) 518.1
  hand, foot, and mouth 074.3
  Hand-Schüller-Christian (chronic histiocytosis
    X) 277.89
  Hanot's—*see* Cirrhosis, biliary
  Hansen's (leprosy) 030.9
    benign form 030.1
    malignant form 030.0
  Harada's 363.22
  Harley's (intermittent hemoglobinuria) 283.2
  Hart's (pellagra-cerebellar ataxia renal
    aminoaciduria) 270.0
  Hartnup (pellagra-cerebellar ataxia-renal
    aminoaciduria) 270.0
  Hashimoto's (struma lymphomatosa) 245.2
  Hb—*see* Disease, hemoglobin
  heart (organic) 429.9
    with
      acute pulmonary edema (*see also* Failure,
        ventricular, left) 428.1
      hypertensive 402.91
        with renal failure 404.92
        benign 402.11
          with renal failure 404.12
        malignant 402.01
          with renal failure 404.02
      kidney disease—*see* Hypertension,
        cardiorenal
      rheumatic fever (conditions classifiable to
        390)
        active 391.9
          with chorea 392.0
        inactive or quiescent (with chorea) 398.90
    amyloid 277.39 *[425.7]*
    aortic (valve) (*see also* Endocarditis, aortic)
      424.1
    arteriosclerotic or sclerotic (minimal)
      (senile)—*see* Arteriosclerosis, coronary
    artery, arterial —*see* Arteriosclerosis,
      coronary
    atherosclerotic —*see* Arteriosclerosis,
      coronary
    beer drinkers' 425.5
    beriberi 265.0 *[425.7]*
    black 416.0
    congenital NEC 746.9
      cyanotic 746.9
      maternal, affecting fetus or newborn 760.3
      specified type NEC 746.89
    congestive (*see also* Failure, heart) 428.0
    coronary 414.9
    cryptogenic 429.9
    due to
      amyloidosis 277.39 *[425.7]*
      beriberi 265.0 *[425.7]*
      cardiac glycogenosis 271.0 *[425.7]*
      Friedreich's ataxia 334.0 *[425.8]*
      gout 274.82
      mucopolysaccharidosis 277.5 *[425.7]*
      myotonia atrophica 359.21 *[425.8]*
      progressive muscular dystrophy 359.1
        [425.8]
      sarcoidosis 135 *[425.8]*
    fetal 746.9
      inflammatory 746.89
    fibroid (*see also* Myocarditis) 429.0

Disease, diseased—*continued*
  heart—*continued*
    functional 427.9
      postoperative 997.1
      psychogenic 306.2
    glycogen storage 271.0 *[425.7]*
    gonococcal NEC 098.85
    gouty 274.82
    hypertensive (*see also* Hypertension, heart)
      402.90
      benign 402.10
      malignant 402.00
    hyperthyroid (*see also* Hyperthyroidism)
      242.9 *[425.7]*
    incompletely diagnosed—*see* Disease, heart
    ischemic (chronic) (*see also* Ischemia, heart)
      414.9
      acute (*see also* Infarct, myocardium) 410.9
        without myocardial infarction 411.89
          with coronary (artery) occlusion 411.81
      asymptomatic 412
      diagnosed on ECG or other special
        investigation but currently presenting no
        symptoms 412
    kyphoscoliotic 416.1
    mitral (*see also* Endocarditis, mitral) 394.9
    muscular (*see also* Degeneration, myocardial)
      429.1
    postpartum 674.8
    psychogenic (functional) 306.2
    pulmonary (chronic) 416.9
      acute 415.0
      specified NEC 416.8
    rheumatic (chronic) (inactive) (old)
      (quiescent) (with chorea) 398.90
      active or acute 391.9
        with chorea (active) (rheumatic)
          (Sydenham's) 392.0
      specified type NEC 391.8
      maternal, affecting fetus or newborn 760.3
    rheumatoid—*see* Arthritis, rheumatoid
    sclerotic —*see* Arteriosclerosis, coronary
    senile (*see also* Myocarditis) 429.0
    specified type NEC 429.89
    syphilitic 093.89
      aortic 093.1
        aneurysm 093.0
      asymptomatic 093.89
      congenital 090.5
    thyroid (gland) (*see also* Hyperthyroidism)
      242.9 *[425.7]*
    thyrotoxic (*see also* Thyrotoxicosis) 242.9
      [425.7]
    tuberculous (*see also* Tuberculosis) 017.9
      [425.8]
    valve, valvular (obstructive)
      (regurgitant)—*see also* Endocarditis
      congenital NEC (*see also* Anomaly, heart,
        valve) 746.9
      pulmonary 746.00
      specified type NEC 746.89
    vascular—*see* Disease, cardiovascular
  heavy-chain (gamma G) 273.2
  Heberden's 715.04
  Hebra's
    dermatitis exfoliativa 695.89
    erythema multiforme exudativum 695.19
    pityriasis
      maculata et circinata 696.3
      rubra 695.89
        pilaris 696.4
    prurigo 698.2

Disease, diseased—*continued*
Heerfordt's (uveoparotitis) 135
Heidenhain's 290.10
  with dementia 290.10
Heilmeyer-Schöner (M9842/3) 207.1
Heine-Medin (*see also* Poliomyelitis) 045.9
Heller's (*see also* Psychosis, childhood) 299.1
Heller-Döhle (syphilitic aortitis) 093.1
hematopoietic organs 289.9
hemoglobin (Hb) 282.7
  with thalassemia 282.49
  abnormal (mixed) NEC 282.7
    with thalassemia 282.49
  AS genotype 282.5
  Bart's 282.43
  C (Hb-C) 282.7
    with other abnormal hemoglobin NEC 282.7
    elliptocytosis 282.7
    Hb-S (without crisis) 282.63
      with
        crisis 282.64
        vaso-occlusive pain 282.64
    sickle-cell (without crisis) 282.63
      with
        crisis 282.64
        vaso-occlusive pain 282.64
    thalassemia 282.49
  constant spring 282.7
  D (Hb-D) 282.7
    with other abnormal hemoglobin NEC 282.7
    Hb-S (without crisis) 282.68
      with crisis 282.69
    sickle-cell (without crisis) 282.68
      with crisis 282.69
    thalassemia 282.49
  E (Hb-E) 282.7
    with other abnormal hemoglobin NEC 282.7
    Hb-S (without crisis) 282.68
      with crisis 282.69
    sickle-cell (without crisis) 282.68
      with crisis 282.69
    thalassemia 282.47
  elliptocytosis 282.7
  F (Hb-F) 282.7
  G (Hb-G) 282.7
  H (Hb-H) 282.43
  hereditary persistence, fetal (HPFH) ("Swiss variety") 282.7
  high fetal gene 282.7
  I thalassemia 282.49
  M 289.7
  S—*see also* Disease, sickle-cell, Hb-S
    thalassemia (without crisis) 282.41
      with
        crisis 282.42
        vaso-occlusive pain 282.42
  spherocytosis 282.7
  unstable, hemolytic 282.7
  Zurich (Hb-Zurich) 282.7
hemolytic (fetus) (newborn) 773.2
  autoimmune (cold type) (warm type) 283.0
  due to or with
    incompatibility
      ABO (blood group) 773.1
      blood (group) (Duffy) (Kell) (Kidd) (Lewis) (M) (S) NEC 773.2
      Rh (blood group) (factor) 773.0
      Rh negative mother 773.0
  unstable hemoglobin 282.7
hemorrhagic 287.9
  newborn 776.0

Disease, diseased—*continued*
Henoch (-Schönlein) (purpura nervosa) 287.0
hepatic—*see* Disease, liver
hepatolenticular 275.1
heredodegenerative NEC
  brain 331.89
  spinal cord 336.8
Hers' (glycogenosis VI) 271.0
Herter (-Gee) (-Heubner) (nontropical sprue) 579.0
Herxheimer's (diffuse idiopathic cutaneous atrophy) 701.8
Heubner's 094.89
Heubner-Herter (nontropical sprue) 579.0
high fetal gene or hemoglobin thalassemia (*see also* Thalassemia) 282.40
Hildenbrand's (typhus) 081.9
hip (joint) NEC 719.95
  congenital 755.63
  suppurative 711.05
  tuberculous (*see also* Tuberculosis) 015.1 [730.85]
Hippel's (retinocerebral angiomatosis) 759.6
Hirschfeld's (acute diabetes mellitus) (*see also* Diabetes) 250.0
  due to secondary diabetes 249.0
Hirschsprung's (congenital megacolon) 751.3
His (-Werner) (trench fever) 083.1
HIV 042
Hodgkin's (M9650/3) 201.9

Note—Use the following fifth-digit subclassification with categories 201:

0 *unspecified site*
1 *lymph nodes of head, face, and neck*
2 *intrathoracic lymph nodes*
3 *intra-abdominal lymph nodes*
4 *lymph nodes of axilla and upper limb*
5 *lymph nodes of inguinal region and lower limb*
6 *intrapelvic lymph nodes*
7 *spleen*
8 *lymph nodes of multiple sites*

---

  lymphocytic
    depletion (M9653/3) 201.7
      diffuse fibrosis (M9654/3) 201.7
      reticular type (M9655/3) 201.7
    predominance (M9651/3) 201.4
  lymphocytic-histiocytic predominance (M9651/3) 201.4
  mixed cellularity (M9652/3) 201.6
  nodular sclerosis (M9656/3) 201.5
    cellular phase (M9657/3) 201.5
Hodgson's 441.9
  ruptured 441.5
Hoffa (-Kastert) (liposynovitis prepatellaris) 272.8
Holla (*see also* Spherocytosis) 282.0
homozygous-Hb-S 282.61
hoof and mouth 078.4
hookworm (*see also* Ancylostomiasis) 126.9
Horton's (temporal arteritis) 446.5
host-versus-graft (immune or nonimmune cause) 279.50
HPFH (hereditary persistence of fetal hemoglobin) ("Swiss variety") 282.7
Huchard's (continued arterial hypertension) 401.9
Huguier's (uterine fibroma) 218.9
human immunodeficiency (virus) 042
hunger 251.1

Disease, diseased—*continued*
Hunt's
  dyssynergia cerebellaris myoclonica 334.2
  herpetic geniculate ganglionitis 053.11
Huntington's 333.4
Huppert's (multiple myeloma) (M9730/3) 203.0
Hurler's (mucopolysaccharidosis I) 277.5
Hutchinson's, meaning
  angioma serpiginosum 709.1
  cheiropompholyx 705.81
  prurigo estivalis 692.72
Hutchinson-Boeck (sarcoidosis) 135
Hutchinson-Gilford (progeria) 259.8
hyaline (diffuse) (generalized) 728.9
  membrane (lung) (newborn) 769
hydatid (*see also* Echinococcus) 122.9
Hyde's (prurigo nodularis) 698.3
hyperkinetic (*see also* Hyperkinesia) 314.9
  heart 429.82
hypertensive (*see also* Hypertension) 401.9
hypophysis 253.9
  hyperfunction 253.1
  hypofunction 253.2
Iceland (epidemic neuromyasthenia) 049.8
I cell 272.7
ill-defined 799.89
immunologic NEC 279.9
immunoproliferative 203.8
inclusion 078.5
  salivary gland 078.5
infancy, early NEC 779.9
infective NEC 136.9
inguinal gland 289.9
internal semilunar cartilage, cystic 717.5
intervertebral disc 722.90
  with myelopathy 722.70
  cervical, cervicothoracic 722.91
    with myelopathy 722.71
  lumbar, lumbosacral 722.93
    with myelopathy 722.73
  thoracic, thoracolumbar 722.92
    with myelopathy 722.72
intestine 569.9
  functional 564.9
    congenital 751.3
    psychogenic 306.4
  lardaceous 277.39
  organic 569.9
  protozoal NEC 007.9
iris 364.9
  specified NEC 364.89
iron
  metabolism (*see also* Hemochromatosis) 275.09
  storage (*see also* Hemochromatosis) 275.03
Isambert's (*see also* Tuberculosis, larynx) 012.3
Iselin's (osteochondrosis, fifth metatarsal) 732.5
Island (scrub typhus) 081.2
itai-itai 985.5
Jadassohn's (maculopapular erythroderma) 696.2
Jadassohn-Pellizari's (anetoderma) 701.3
Jakob-Creutzfeldt (CJD) 046.19
  with dementia
    with behavioral disturbance 046.19 *[294.11]*
    without behavioral disturbance 046.19
      [294.10]
  familial 046.19
  iatrogenic 046.19
  specified NEC 046.19
  sporadic 046.19

Disease, diseased—*continued*
  variant (vCJD) 046.11
    with dementia
      with behavioral disturbance 046.11 *[294.11]*
      without behavioral disturbance 046.11
        [294.10]
Jaksch (-Luzet) (pseudoleukemia infantum) 285.8
Janet's 300.89
Jansky-Bielschowsky 330.1
jaw NEC 526.9
  fibrocystic 526.2
Jensen's 363.05
Jeune's (asphyxiating thoracic dystrophy) 756.4
jigger 134.1
Johnson-Stevens (erythema multiforme
  exudativum) 695.13
joint NEC 719.9
  ankle 719.97
  Charcot 094.0 *[713.5]*
  degenerative (*see also* Osteoarthrosis) 715.9
    multiple 715.09
    spine (*see also* Spondylosis) 721.90
  elbow 719.92
  foot 719.97
  hand 719.94
  hip 719.95
  hypertrophic (chronic) (degenerative) (*see also*
    Osteoarthrosis) 715.9
    spine (*see also* Spondylosis) 721.90
  knee 719.96
  Luschka 721.90
  multiple sites 719.99
  pelvic region 719.95
  sacroiliac 724.6
  shoulder (region) 719.91
  specified site NEC 719.98
  spine NEC 724.9
    pseudarthrosis following fusion 733.82
    sacroiliac 724.6
  wrist 719.93
Jourdain's (acute gingivitis) 523.00
Jüngling's (sarcoidosis) 135
Kahler (-Bozzolo) (multiple myeloma)
  (M9730/3) 203.0
Kalischer's 759.6
Kaposi's 757.33
  lichen ruber 697.8
    acuminatus 696.4
    moniliformis 697.8
  xeroderma pigmentosum 757.33
Kaschin-Beck (endemic polyarthritis) 716.00
  ankle 716.07
  arm 716.02
    lower (and wrist) 716.03
    upper (and elbow) 716.02
  foot (and ankle) 716.07
  forearm (and wrist) 716.03
  hand 716.04
  leg 716.06
    lower 716.06
    upper 716.05
  multiple sites 716.09
  pelvic region (hip) (thigh) 716.05
  shoulder region 716.01
  specified site NEC 716.08
Katayama 120.2
Kawasaki 446.1
Kedani (scrub typhus) 081.2

Disease, diseased—*continued*
kidney (functional) (pelvis) (*see also* Disease, renal) 593.9
  chronic 585.9
    requiring chronic dialysis 585.6
    stage
      I 585.1
      II (mild) 585.2
      III (moderate) 585.3
      IV (severe) 585.4
      V 585.5
  cystic (congenital) 753.10
    multiple 753.19
    single 753.11
    specified NEC 753.19
  fibrocystic (congenital) 753.19
  in gout 274.10
  polycystic (congenital) 753.12
    adult type (APKD) 753.13
    autosomal dominant 753.13
    autosomal recessive 753.14
    childhood type (CPKD) 753.14
    infantile type 753.14
Kienböck's (carpal lunate) (wrist) 732.3
Kimmelstiel (-Wilson) (intercapillary glomerulosclerosis) 250.4 *[581.81]*
  due to secondary diabetes 249.4 *[581.81]*
Kinnier Wilson's (hepatolenticular degeneration) 275.1
kissing 075
Kleb's (*see also* Nephritis) 583.9
Klinger's 446.4
Klippel's 723.8
Klippel-Feil (brevicollis) 756.16
knight's 911.1
Köbner's (epidermolysis bullosa) 757.39
Koenig-Wichmann (pemphigus) 694.4
Köhler's
  first (osteoarthrosis juvenilis) 732.5
  second (Freiberg's infraction, metatarsal head) 732.5
  patellar 732.4
  tarsal navicular (bone) (osteoarthrosis juvenilis) 732.5
Köhler-Freiberg (infraction, metatarsal head) 732.5
Köhler-Mouchet (osteoarthrosis juvenilis) 732.5
Köhler-Pellegrini-Stieda (calcification, knee joint) 726.62
Kok 759.89
König's (osteochondritis dissecans) 732.7
Korsakoff's (nonalcoholic) 294.0
  alcoholic 291.1
Kostmann's (infantile genetic agranulocytosis) 288.01
Krabbe's 330.0
Kraepelin-Morel (*see also* Schizophrenia) 295.9
Kraft-Weber-Dimitri 759.6
Kufs' 330.1
Kugelberg-Welander 335.11
Kuhnt-Junius 362.52
Kümmell's (-Verneuil) (spondylitis) 721.7
Kundrat's (lymphosarcoma) 200.1
kuru 046.0
Kussmaul (-Meier) (polyarteritis nodosa) 446.0
Kyasanur Forest 065.2
Kyrle's (hyperkeratosis follicularis in cutem penetrans) 701.1
labia
  inflammatory 616.10
  noninflammatory 624.9
    specified NEC 624.8

Disease, diseased—*continued*
labyrinth, ear 386.8
lacrimal system (apparatus) (passages) 375.9
  gland 375.00
  specified NEC 375.89
Lafora's 333.2
Lagleyze-von Hippel (retinocerebral angiomatosis) 759.6
Lancereaux-Mathieu (leptospiral jaundice) 100.0
Landry's 357.0
Lane's 569.89
lardaceous (any site) 277.39
Larrey-Weil (leptospiral jaundice) 100.0
Larsen (-Johansson) (juvenile osteopathia patellae) 732.4
larynx 478.70
Lasègue's (persecution mania) 297.9
Leber's 377.16
Lederer's (acquired infectious hemolytic anemia) 283.19
Legg's (capital femoral osteochondrosis) 732.1
Legg-Calvé-Perthes (capital femoral osteochondrosis) 732.1
Legg-Calvé-Waldenström (femoral capital osteochondrosis) 732.1
Legg-Perthes (femoral capital osteochondrosis) 732.1
Legionnaires' 482.84
Leigh's 330.8
Leiner's (exfoliative dermatitis) 695.89
Leloir's (lupus erythematosus) 695.4
Lenegre's 426.0
lens (eye) 379.39
Leriche's (osteoporosis, posttraumatic) 733.7
Letterer-Siwe (acute histiocytosis X) (M9722/3) 202.5
Lev's (acquired complete heart block) 426.0
Lewandowski's (*see also* Tuberculosis) 017.0
Lewandowski-Lutz (epidermodysplasia verruciformis) 078.19
Lewy body 331.82
  with dementia
    with behavioral disturbance 331.82 *[294.11]*
    without behavioral disturbance 331.82 *[294.10]*
Leyden's (periodic vomiting) 536.2
Libman-Sacks (verrucous endocarditis) 710.0 *[424.91]*
Lichtheim's (subacute combined sclerosis with pernicious anemia) 281.0 *[336.2]*
ligament 728.9
light chain 203.0
Lightwood's (renal tubular acidosis) 588.89
Lignac's (cystinosis) 270.0
Lindau's (retinocerebral angiomatosis) 759.6
Lindau-von Hippel (angiomatosis retinocerebellosa) 759.6
lip NEC 528.5
lipidosis 272.7
lipoid storage NEC 272.7
Lipschütz's 616.50
Little's—*see* Palsy, cerebral
liver 573.9
  alcoholic 571.3
    acute 571.1
    chronic 571.3
  chronic 571.9
    alcoholic 571.3
  cystic, congenital 751.62
  drug-induced 573.3

Disease, diseased—*continued*
  liver—*continued*
    due to
      chemicals 573.3
      fluorinated agents 573.3
      hypersensitivity drugs 573.3
      isoniazids 573.3
    end stage NEC 572.8
      due to hepatitis —*see* Hepatitis
    fibrocystic (congenital) 751.62
    glycogen storage 271.0
    organic 573.9
    polycystic (congenital) 751.62
  Lobo's (keloid blastomycosis) 116.2
  Lobstein's (brittle bones and blue sclera) 756.61
  locomotor system 334.9
  Lorain's (pituitary dwarfism) 253.3
  Lou Gehrig's 335.20
  Lucas-Championnière (fibrinous bronchitis) 466.0
  Ludwig's (submaxillary cellulitis) 528.3
  luetic—*see* Syphilis
  lumbosacral region 724.6
  lung NEC 518.89
    black 500
    congenital 748.60
    cystic 518.89
      congenital 748.4
    fibroid (chronic) (*see also* Fibrosis, lung) 515
    fluke 121.2
      Oriental 121.2
    in
      amyloidosis 277.39 *[517.8]*
      polymyositis 710.4 *[517.8]*
      sarcoidosis 135 *[517.8]*
      Sjögren's syndrome 710.2 *[517.8]*
      syphilis 095.1
      systemic lupus erythematosus 710.0 *[517.8]*
      systemic sclerosis 710.1 *[517.2]*
    interstitial (chronic) 515
      acute 136.3
      respiratory bronchiolitis 516.34
    nonspecific, chronic 496
    obstructive (chronic) (COPD) 496
      with
        acute
          bronchitis 491.22
          exacerbation NEC 491.21
        alveolitis, allergic (*see also* Alveolitis, allergic) 495.9
        asthma (chronic) (obstructive) 493.2
        bronchiectasis 494.0
          with exacerbation (acute) 494.1
        bronchitis (chronic) 491.20
          with
            acute bronchitis 491.22
            exacerbation (acute) 491.21
          decompensated 491.21
            with exacerbation 491.21
        emphysema NEC 492.8
      diffuse (with fibrosis) 496
    of childhood, specified NEC 516.69
    polycystic 518.89
      asthma (chronic) (obstructive) 493.2
      congenital 748.4
    purulent (cavitary) 513.0
    restrictive 518.89
    rheumatoid 714.81
      diffuse interstitial 714.81
    specified NEC 518.89
  Lutembacher's (atrial septal defect with mitral stenosis) 745.5

Disease, diseased—*continued*
  Lutz-Miescher (elastosis perforans serpiginosa) 701.1
  Lutz-Splendore-de Almeida (Brazilian blastomycosis) 116.1
  Lyell's (toxic epidermal necrolysis) 695.15
    due to drug
      correct substance properly administered 695.15
      overdose or wrong substance given or taken 977.9
        specific drug—*see* Table of drugs and chemicals
  Lyme 088.81
  lymphatic (gland) (system) 289.9
    channel (noninfective) 457.9
    vessel (noninfective) 457.9
      specified NEC 457.8
  lymphoproliferative (chronic) (M9970/1) 238.79
    X linked 759.89
  Machado-Joseph 334.8
  Madelung's (lipomatosis) 272.8
  Madura (actinomycotic) 039.9
    mycotic 117.4
  Magitot's 526.4
  Majocchi's (purpura annularis telangiectodes) 709.1
  malarial (*see also* Malaria) 084.6
  Malassez's (cystic) 608.89
  Malibu 919.8
    infected 919.9
  malignant (M8000/3)—*see also* Neoplasm, by site, malignant
    previous, affecting management of pregnancy V23.8
  Manson's 120.1
  maple bark 495.6
  maple syrup (urine) 270.3
  Marburg (virus) 078.89
  Marchiafava (-Bignami) 341.8
  Marfan's 090.49
    congenital syphilis 090.49
    meaning Marfan's syndrome 759.82
  Marie-Bamberger (hypertrophic pulmonary osteoarthropathy) (secondary) 731.2
    primary or idiopathic (acropachyderma) 757.39
    pulmonary (hypertrophic osteoarthropathy) 731.2
  Marie-Strümpell (ankylosing spondylitis) 720.0
  Marion's (bladder neck obstruction) 596.0
  Marsh's (exophthalmic goiter) 242.0
  Martin's 715.27
  mast cell 757.33
    systemic (M9741/3) 202.6
  mastoid (*see also* Mastoiditis) 383.9
    process 385.9
  maternal, unrelated to pregnancy NEC, affecting fetus or newborn 760.9
  Mathieu's (leptospiral jaundice) 100.0
  Mauclaire's 732.3
  Mauriac's (erythema nodosum syphiliticum) 091.3
  Maxcy's 081.0
  McArdle (-Schmid-Pearson) (glycogenosis V) 271.0
  mediastinum NEC 519.3
  Medin's (*see also* Poliomyelitis) 045.9
  Mediterranean 282.40
    with hemoglobinopathy 282.49
  medullary center (idiopathic) (respiratory) 348.89

Disease, diseased—*continued*
Meige's (chronic hereditary edema) 757.0
Meleda 757.39
Ménétrier's (hypertrophic gastritis) 535.2
Ménière's (active) 386.00
  cochlear 386.02
  cochleovestibular 386.01
  inactive 386.04
  in remission 386.04
  vestibular 386.03
meningeal—*see* Meningitis
mental (*see also* Psychosis) 298.9
Merzbacher-Pelizaeus 330.0
mesenchymal 710.9
mesenteric embolic 557.0
metabolic NEC 277.9
metal polishers' 502
metastatic—*see* Metastasis
Mibelli's 757.39
microdrepanocytic 282.41
microvascular —*code to condition*
microvillus
  atrophy 751.5
  inclusion (MVD) 751.5
Miescher's 709.3
Mikulicz's (dryness of mouth, absent or
  decreased lacrimation) 527.1
Milkman (-Looser) (osteomalacia with
  pseudofractures) 268.2
Miller's (osteomalacia) 268.2
Mills' 335.29
Milroy's (chronic hereditary edema) 757.0
Minamata 985.0
Minor's 336.1
Minot's (hemorrhagic disease, newborn) 776.0
Minot-von Willebrand-Jürgens
  (angiohemophilia) 286.4
Mitchell's (erythromelalgia) 443.82
mitral—*see* Endocarditis, mitral
Mljet (mal de Meleda) 757.39
Möbius', Moebius' 346.2
Moeller's 267
Möller (-Barlow) (infantile scurvy) 267
Mönckeberg's (*see also* arteriosclerosis,
  extremities) 440.20
Mondor's (thrombophlebitis of breast) 451.89
Monge's 993.2
Morel-Kraepelin (*see also* Schizophrenia) 295.9
Morgagni's (syndrome) (hyperostosis frontalis
  interna) 733.3
Morgagni-Adams-Stokes (syncope with heart
  block) 426.9
Morquio (-Brailsford) (-Ullrich)
  (mucopolysaccharidosis IV) 277.5
Morton's (with metatarsalgia) 355.6
Morvan's 336.0
motor neuron (bulbar) (mixed type) 335.20
Mouchet's (juvenile osteochondrosis, foot)
  732.5
mouth 528.9
Moyamoya 437.5
Mucha's (acute parapsoriasis varioliformis)
  696.2
mu-chain 273.2
mucolipidosis (I) (II) (III) 272.7
Münchmeyer's (exostosis luxurians) 728.11
Murri's (intermittent hemoglobinuria) 283.2
muscle 359.9
  inflammatory 728.9
  ocular 378.9
musculoskeletal system 729.90

Disease, diseased—*continued*
mushroom workers' 495.5
Myà's (congenital dilation, colon) 751.3
mycotic 117.9
myeloproliferative (chronic) (M9960/1) 238.79
myocardium, myocardial (*see also*
  Degeneration, myocardial) 429.1
  hypertensive (*see also* Hypertension, heart)
    402.90
  primary (idiopathic) 425.4
myoneural 358.9
Naegeli's 287.1
nail 703.9
  specified type NEC 703.8
Nairobi sheep 066.1
nasal 478.19
  cavity NEC 478.19
  sinus (chronic)—*see* Sinusitis
navel (newborn) NEC 779.89
  delayed separation of umbilical cord 779.83
nemaline body 359.0
neoplastic, generalized (M8000/6) 199.0
nerve—*see* Disorder, nerve
nervous system (central) 349.9
  autonomic, peripheral (*see also* Neuropathy,
    peripheral, autonomic) 337.9
  congenital 742.9
  inflammatory—*see* Encephalitis
  parasympathetic (*see also* Neuropathy,
    peripheral, autonomic) 337.9
  peripheral NEC 355.9
  prion NEC 046.79
  specified NEC 349.89
  sympathetic (*see also* Neuropathy, peripheral,
    autonomic) 337.9
  vegetative (*see also* Neuropathy, peripheral,
    autonomic) 337.9
Nettleship's (urticaria pigmentosa) 757.33
Neumann's (pemphigus vegetans) 694.4
neurologic (central) NEC (*see also* Disease,
  nervous system) 349.9
  peripheral NEC 355.9
neuromuscular system NEC 358.9
Newcastle 077.8
Nicolas (-Durand) -Favre (climatic bubo) 099.1
Niemann-Pick (lipid histiocytosis) 272.7
nipple 611.9
  Paget's (M8540/3) 174.0
Nishimoto (-Takeuchi) 437.5
nonarthropod-borne NEC 078.89
  central nervous system NEC 049.9
  enterovirus NEC 078.89
non-autoimmune hemolytic NEC 283.10
Nonne-Milroy-Meige (chronic hereditary
  edema) 757.0
Norrie's (congenital progressive
  oculoacousticocerebral degeneration) 743.8
nose 478.19
nucleus pulposus—*see* Disease, intervertebral
  disc
nutritional 269.9
  maternal, affecting fetus or newborn 760.4
oasthouse, urine 270.2
obliterative vascular 447.1
Odelberg's (juvenile osteochondrosis) 732.1
Oguchi's (retina) 368.61
Ohara's (*see also* Tularemia) 021.9
Ollier's (chondrodysplasia) 756.4
Opitz's (congestive splenomegaly) 289.51
Oppenheim's 358.8

Disease, diseased—*continued*
Oppenheim-Urbach (necrobiosis lipoidica
   diabeticorum) 250.8 *[709.3]*
   due to secondary diabetes 249.8 *[709.3]*
optic nerve NEC 377.49
orbit 376.9
   specified NEC 376.89
Oriental liver fluke 121.1
Oriental lung fluke 121.2
Ormond's 593.4
Osgood's tibia (tubercle) 732.4
Osgood-Schlatter 732.4
Osler (-Vaquez) (polycythemia vera) (M9950/1)
   238.4
Osler-Rendu (familial hemorrhagic
   telangiectasia) 448.0
osteofibrocystic 252.01
Otto's 715.35
outer ear 380.9
ovary (noninflammatory) NEC 620.9
   cystic 620.2
   polycystic 256.4
   specified NEC 620.8
Owren's (congenital) (*see also* Defect,
   coagulation) 286.3
Paas' 756.59
Paget's (osteitis deformans) 731.0
   with infiltrating duct carcinoma of the breast
      (M8541/3)—*see* Neoplasm, breast, malignant
   bone 731.0
      osteosarcoma in (M9184/3)—*see* Neoplasm,
         bone, malignant
   breast (M8540/3) 174.0
   extramammary (M8542/3)—*see also*
      Neoplasm, skin, malignant
      anus 154.3
      skin 173.59
   malignant (M8540/3)
      breast 174.0
      specified site NEC (M8542/3)—*see*
         Neoplasm, skin, malignant
      unspecified site 174.0
   mammary (M8540/3) 174.0
   nipple (M8540/3) 174.0
palate (soft) 528.9
Paltauf-Sternberg 201.9
pancreas 577.9
   cystic 577.2
      congenital 751.7
   fibrocystic 277.00
Panner's 732.3
   capitellum humeri 732.3
   head of humerus 732.3
   tarsal navicular (bone) (osteochondrosis) 732.5
panvalvular—*see* Endocarditis, mitral
parametrium 629.9
parasitic NEC 136.9
   cerebral NEC 123.9
   intestinal NEC 129
   mouth 112.0
   skin NEC 134.9
   specified type—*see* Infestation
   tongue 112.0
parathyroid (gland) 252.9
   specified NEC 252.8
Parkinson's 332.0
parodontal 523.9
Parrot's (syphilitic osteochondritis) 090.0
Parry's (exophthalmic goiter) 242.0
Parson's (exophthalmic goiter) 242.0
Pavy's 593.6

Disease, diseased—*continued*
Paxton's (white piedra) 111.2
Payr's (splenic flexure syndrome) 569.89
pearl-workers' (chronic osteomyelitis) (*see also*
   Osteomyelitis) 730.1
Pel-Ebstein—*see* Disease, Hodgkin's
Pelizaeus-Merzbacher 330.0
   with dementia
      with behavioral disturbance 330.0 *[294.11]*
      without behavioral disturbance 330.0
         [294.10]
Pellegrini-Stieda (calcification, knee joint) 726.62
pelvis, pelvic
   female NEC 629.9
      specified NEC 629.89
   gonococcal (acute) 098.19
      chronic or duration of 2 months or over 098.39
   infection (*see also* Disease, pelvis, inflammatory)
      614.9
   inflammatory (female) (PID) 614.9
      with
         abortion—*see* Abortion, by type, with sepsis
         ectopic pregnancy (*see also* categories
            633.0-633.9) 639.0
         molar pregnancy (*see also* categories
            630-632) 639.0
      acute 614.3
      chronic 614.4
      complicating pregnancy 646.6
         affecting fetus or newborn 760.8
      following
         abortion 639.0
         ectopic or molar pregnancy 639.0
      peritonitis (acute) 614.5
         chronic NEC 614.7
      puerperal, postpartum, childbirth 670.8
      specified NEC 614.8
   organ, female NEC 629.9
      specified NEC 629.89
   peritoneum, female NEC 629.9
      specified NEC 629.89
   penis 607.9
      inflammatory 607.2
peptic NEC 536.9
   acid 536.8
periapical tissues NEC 522.9
pericardium 423.9
   specified type NEC 423.8
perineum
   female
      inflammatory 616.9
         specified NEC 616.89
      noninflammatory 624.9
         specified NEC 624.8
   male (inflammatory) 682.2
periodic (familial) (Reimann's) NEC 277.31
   paralysis 359.3
periodontal NEC 523.9
   specified NEC 523.8
periosteum 733.90
peripheral
   arterial 443.9
   autonomic nervous system (*see also*
      Neuropathy, autonomic) 337.9
   nerve NEC (*see also* Neuropathy) 356.9
      multiple—*see* Polyneuropathy
   vascular 443.9
      specified type NEC 443.89
peritoneum 568.9
   pelvic, female 629.9
      specified NEC 629.89

Disease, diseased—*continued*
Perrin-Ferraton (snapping hip) 719.65
persistent mucosal (middle ear) (with posterior or superior marginal perforation of ear drum) 382.2
Perthes' (capital femoral osteochondrosis) 732.1
Petit's (*see also* Hernia, lumbar) 553.8
Peutz-Jeghers 759.6
Peyronie's 607.85
Pfeiffer's (infectious mononucleosis) 075
pharynx 478.20
Phocas' 610.1
photochromogenic (acid-fast bacilli) (pulmonary) 031.0
   nonpulmonary 031.9
Pick's
   brain 331.11
      with dementia
         with behavioral disturbance 331.11 *[294.11]*
         without behavioral disturbance 331.11 *[294.10]*
   cerebral atrophy 331.11
      with dementia
         with behavioral disturbance 331.11 *[294.11]*
         without behavioral disturbance 331.11 *[294.10]*
   lipid histiocytosis 272.7
   liver (pericardial pseudocirrhosis of liver) 423.2
   pericardium (pericardial pseudocirrhosis of liver) 423.2
   polyserositis (pericardial pseudocirrhosis of liver) 423.2
Pierson's (osteochondrosis) 732.1
pigeon fancier's or breeders' 495.2
pineal gland 259.8
pink 985.0
Pinkus' (lichen nitidus) 697.1
pinworm 127.4
pituitary (gland) 253.9
   hyperfunction 253.1
   hypofunction 253.2
pituitary snuff-takers' 495.8
placenta
   affecting fetus or newborn 762.2
   complicating pregnancy or childbirth 656.7
pleura (cavity) (*see also* Pleurisy) 511.0
Plummer's (toxic nodular goiter) 242.3
pneumatic
   drill 994.9
   hammer 994.9
policeman's 729.2
Pollitzer's (hidradenitis suppurativa) 705.83
polycystic (congenital) 759.89
   kidney or renal 753.12
      adult type (APKD) 753.13
      autosomal dominant 753.13
      autosomal recessive 753.14
      childhood type (CPKD) 753.14
      infantile type 753.14
   liver or hepatic 751.62
   lung or pulmonary 518.89
      congenital 748.4
   ovary, ovaries 256.4
   spleen 759.0
polyethylene 996.45
Pompe's (glycogenosis II) 271.0
Poncet's (tuberculous rheumatism) (*see also* Tuberculosis) 015.9
Posada-Wernicke 114.9

Disease, diseased—*continued*
Potain's (pulmonary edema) 514
Pott's (*see also* Tuberculosis) 015.0 *[730.88]*
   osteomyelitis 015.0 *[730.88]*
   paraplegia 015.0 *[730.88]*
   spinal curvature 015.0 *[737.43]*
   spondylitis 015.0 *[720.81]*
Potter's 753.0
Poulet's 714.2
pregnancy NEC (*see also* Pregnancy) 646.9
Preiser's (osteoporosis) 733.09
Pringle's (tuberous sclerosis) 759.5
Profichet's 729.90
prostate 602.9
   specified type NEC 602.8
protozoal NEC 136.8
   intestine, intestinal NEC 007.9
pseudo-Hurler's (mucolipidosis III) 272.7
psychiatric (*see also* Psychosis) 298.9
psychotic (*see also* Psychosis) 298.9
Puente's (simple glandular cheilitis) 528.5
puerperal NEC (*see also* Puerperal) 674.9
pulmonary—*see also* Disease, lung
   amyloid 277.39 *[517.8]*
   artery 417.9
   circulation, circulatory 417.9
      specified NEC 417.8
   diffuse obstructive (chronic) 496
      with
         acute bronchitis 491.22
         asthma (chronic) (obstructive) 493.2
         bronchitis (chronic) 491.20
            with exacerbation (acute) 491.21
         exacerbation NEC (acute) 491.21
   heart (chronic) 416.9
      specified NEC 416.8
   hypertensive (vascular) 416.0
      cardiovascular 416.0
   obstructive diffuse (chronic) 496
      decompensated 491.21
         with exacerbation 491.21
      with
         acute bronchitis 491.22
         asthma (chronic) (obstructive) 493.2
         bronchitis (chronic) 491.20
            with
               exacerbation (acute) 491.21
            acute 491.22
         exacerbation NEC (acute) 491.21
   valve (*see also* Endocarditis, pulmonary) 424.3
pulp (dental) NEC 522.9
pulseless 446.7
Putnam's (subacute combined sclerosis with pernicious anemia) 281.0 *[336.2]*
Pyle (-Cohn) (craniometaphyseal dysplasia) 756.89
pyramidal tract 333.90
Quervain's
   tendon sheath 727.04
   thyroid (subacute granulomatous thyroiditis) 245.1
Quincke's—*see* Edema, angioneurotic
Quinquaud (acne decalvans) 704.09
rag sorters' 022.1
Raynaud's (Paroxysmal digital cyanosis) 443.0
reactive airway—*see* Asthma
Recklinghausen's (M9540/1) 237.71
   bone (osteitis fibrosa cystica) 252.01
Recklinghausen-Applebaum (hemochromatosis) (*see also* Hemochromatosis) 275.03
Reclus' (cystic) 610.1

Disease, diseased—*continued*
rectum NEC 569.49
Refsum's (heredopathia atactica
    polyneuritiformis) 356.3
Reichmann's (gastrosuccorrhea) 536.8
Reimann's (periodic) 277.31
Reiter's 099.3
renal (functional) (pelvis) (*see also* Disease,
    kidney) 593.9
  with
    edema (*see also* Nephrosis) 581.9
    exudative nephritis 583.89
    lesion of interstitial nephritis 583.89
    stated generalized cause—*see* Nephritis
  acute 593.9
  basement membrane NEC 583.89
    with
      pulmonary hemorrhage (Goodpasture's
        syndrome) 446.21 *[583.81]*
  chronic (*see also* Disease, kidney, chronic)
    585.9
  complicating pregnancy or puerperium NEC
    646.2
    with hypertension—*see* Toxemia, of
      pregnancy
    affecting fetus or newborn 760.1
  cystic, congenital (*see also* Cystic, disease,
    kidney) 753.10
  diabetic 250.4 *[583.81]*
    due to secondary diabetes 249.4 *[581.81]*
  due to
    amyloidosis 277.39 *[583.81]*
    diabetes mellitus 250.4 *[583.81]*
      due to secondary diabetes 249.4 *[581.81]*
    systemic lupus erythematosis 710.0 *[583.81]*
  end-stage 585.6
  exudative 583.89
  fibrocystic (congenital) 753.19
  gonococcal 098.19 *[583.81]*
  gouty 274.10
  hypertensive (*see also* Hypertension, kidney)
    403.90
  immune complex NEC 583.89
  interstitial (diffuse) (focal) 583.89
  lupus 710.0 *[583.81]*
  maternal, affecting fetus or newborn 760.1
    hypertensive 760.0
  phosphate-losing (tubular) 588.0
  polycystic (congenital) 753.12
    adult type (APKD) 753.13
    autosomal dominant 753.13
    autosomal recessive 753.14
    childhood type (CPKD) 753.14
    infantile type 753.14
  specified lesion or cause NEC (*see also*
    Glomerulonephritis) 583.89
  subacute 581.9
  syphilitic 095.4
  tuberculous (*see also* Tuberculosis) 016.0
    [583.81]
  tubular (*see also* Nephrosis, tubular) 584.5
Rendu-Olser-Weber (familial hemorrhagic
    telangiectasia) 448.0
renovascular (arteriosclerotic) (*see also*
    Hypertension, kidney) 403.90
respiratory (tract) 519.9
  acute or subacute (upper) NEC 465.9
    due to fumes or vapors 506.3
    multiple sites NEC 465.8
    noninfectious 478.9
    streptococcal 034.0

Disease, diseased—*continued*
  respiratory (tract)—*continued*
    chronic 519.9
      arising in the perinatal period 770.7
      due to fumes or vapors 506.4
    due to
      aspiration of liquids or solids 508.9
      external agents NEC 508.9
        specified NEC 508.8
      fumes or vapors 506.9
        acute or subacute NEC 506.3
        chronic 506.4
    fetus or newborn NEC 770.9
    obstructive 496
    smoke inhalation 508.2
    specified type NEC 519.8
    upper (acute) (infectious) NEC 465.9
      multiple sites NEC 465.8
      noninfectious NEC 478.9
      streptococcal 034.0
  retina, retinal NEC 362.9
    Batten's or Batten-Mayou 330.1 *[362.71]*
    degeneration 362.89
    vascular lesion 362.17
  rheumatic (*see also* Arthritis) 716.8
    heart—*see* Disease, heart, rheumatic
  rheumatoid (heart)—*see* Arthritis, rheumatoid
  rickettsial NEC 083.9
    specified type NEC 083.8
  Riedel's (ligneous thyroiditis) 245.3
  Riga (-Fede) (cachectic aphthae) 529.0
  Riggs' (compound periodontitis) 523.40
  Ritter's 695.81
  Rivalta's (cervicofacial actinomycosis) 039.3
  Robles' (onchocerciasis) 125.3 *[360.13]*
  Roger's (congenital interventricular septal
    defect) 745.4
  Rokitansky's (*see also* Necrosis, liver) 570
  Romberg's 349.89
  Rosenthal's (factor XI deficiency) 286.2
  Rossbach's (hyperchlorhydria) 536.8
    psychogenic 306.4
  Roth (-Bernhardt) 355.1
  Runeberg's (progressive pernicious anemia)
    281.0
  Rust's (tuberculous spondylitis) (*see also*
    Tuberculosis) 015.0 *[720.81]*
  Rustitskii's (multiple myeloma) (M9730/3)
    203.0
  Ruysch's (Hirschsprung's disease) 751.3
  Sachs (-Tay) 330.1
  sacroiliac NEC 724.6
  salivary gland or duct NEC 527.9
    inclusion 078.5
      streptococcal 034.0
    virus 078.5
  Sander's (paranoia) 297.1
  Sandhoff's 330.1
  sandworm 126.9
  Savill's (epidemic exfoliative dermatitis) 695.89
  Schamberg's (progressive pigmentary
    dermatosis) 709.09
  Schaumann's (sarcoidosis) 135
  Schenck's (sporotrichosis) 117.1
  Scheuermann's (osteochondrosis) 732.0
  Schilder (-Flatau) 341.1
  Schimmelbusch's 610.1
  Schlatter's tibia (tubercle) 732.4
  Schlatter-Osgood 732.4

Disease, diseased—*continued*
Schmorl's 722.30
  cervical 722.39
  lumbar, lumbosacral 722.32
  specified region NEC 722.39
  thoracic, thoracolumbar 722.31
Scholz's 330.0
Schönlein (-Henoch) (purpura rheumatica) 287.0
Schottmüller's (*see also* Fever, paratyphoid)
  002.9
Schüller-Christian (chronic histiocytosis X)
  277.89
Schultz's (agranulocytosis) 288.09
Schwalbe-Ziehen-Oppenheimer 333.6
Schwartz-Jampel 359.23
Schweninger-Buzzi (macular atrophy) 701.3
sclera 379.19
scrofulous (*see also* Tuberculosis) 017.2
scrotum 608.9
sebaceous glands NEC 706.9
Secretan's (posttraumatic edema) 782.3
semilunar cartilage, cystic 717.5
seminal vesicle 608.9
Senear-Usher (pemphigus erythematosus) 694.4
serum NEC 999.59
Sever's (osteochondrosis calcaneum) 732.5
sexually transmitted —*see* Disease, venereal
Sézary's (reticulosis) (M9701/3) 202.2
Shaver's (bauxite pneumoconiosis) 503
Sheehan's (postpartum pituitary necrosis) 253.2
shimamushi (scrub typhus) 081.2
shipyard 077.1
sickle-cell 282.60
  with
    crisis 282.62
    Hb-S disease 282.61
    other abnormal hemoglobin (Hb-D) (Hb-E)
      (Hb-G) (Hb-J) (Hb-K) (Hb-O) (Hb-P)
      (high fetal gene) (without crisis) 282.68
      with crisis 282.69
  elliptocytosis 282.60
  Hb-C (without crisis) 282.63
    with
      crisis 282.64
      vaso-occlusive pain 282.64
  Hb-S 282.61
    with
      crisis 282.62
      Hb-C (without crisis) 282.63
        with
          crisis 282.64
          vaso-occlusive pain 282.64
      other abnormal hemoglobin (Hb-D) (Hb-E)
        (Hb-G) (Hb-J) (Hb-K) (Hb-O) (Hb-P)
        (high fetal gene) (without crisis) 282.68
        with crisis 282.69
  spherocytosis 282.60
  thalassemia (without crisis) 282.41
    with
      crisis 282.42
      vaso-occlusive pain 282.42
Siegal-Cattan-Mamou (periodic) 277.31
silo fillers' 506.9
Simian B 054.3
Simmonds' (pituitary cachexia) 253.2
Simons' (progressive lipodystrophy) 272.6
Sinding-Larsen (juvenile osteopathia patellae)
  732.4
sinus—*see also* Sinusitis
  brain 437.9
  specified NEC 478.19

Disease, diseased—*continued*
Sirkari's 085.0
sixth (*see also* Exanthem subitum) 058.10
Sjögren (-Gougerot) 710.2
  with lung involvement 710.2 *[517.8]*
Skevas-Zerfus 989.5
skin NEC 709.9
  due to metabolic disorder 277.9
  specified type NEC 709.8
sleeping (*see also* Narcolepsy) 347.00
  meaning sleeping sickness (*see also*
    Trypanosomiasis) 086.5
small vessel 443.9
Smith-Strang (oasthouse urine) 270.2
Sneddon-Wilkinson (subcorneal pustular
  dermatosis) 694.1
South African creeping 133.8
Spencer's (epidemic vomiting) 078.82
Spielmeyer-Stock 330.1
Spielmeyer-Vogt 330.1
spine, spinal 733.90
  combined system (*see also* Degeneration,
    combined) 266.2 *[336.2]*
    with pernicious anemia 281.0 *[336.2]*
  cord NEC 336.9
    congenital 742.9
  demyelinating NEC 341.8
  joint (*see also* Disease, joint, spine) 724.9
  tuberculous 015.0 *[730.8]*
spinocerebellar 334.9
  specified NEC 334.8
spleen (organic) (postinfectional) 289.50
  amyloid 277.39
  lardaceous 277.39
  polycystic 759.0
  specified NEC 289.59
sponge divers' 989.5
Stanton's (melioidosis) 025
Stargardt's 362.75
Startle 759.89
Steinert's 359.21
Sternberg's—*see* Disease, Hodgkin's
Stevens-Johnson (erythema multiforme
  exudativum) 695.13
Sticker's (erythema infectiosum) 057.0
Stieda's (calcification, knee joint) 726.62
Still's (juvenile rheumatoid arthritis) 714.30
  adult onset 714.2
Stiller's (asthenia) 780.79
Stokes' (exophthalmic goiter) 242.0
Stokes-Adams (syncope with heart block) 426.9
Stokvis (-Talma) (enterogenous cyanosis) 289.7
stomach NEC (organic) 537.9
  functional 536.9
    psychogenic 306.4
  lardaceous 277.39
stonemasons' 502
storage
  glycogen (*see also* Disease, glycogen storage)
    271.0
  lipid 272.7
  mucopolysaccharide 277.5
striatopallidal system 333.90
  specified NEC 333.89
Strümpell-Marie (ankylosing spondylitis) 720.0
Stuart's (congenital factor X deficiency) (*see
  also* Defect, coagulation) 286.3
Stuart-Prower (congenital factor X deficiency)
  (*see also* Defect, coagulation) 286.3
Sturge (-Weber) (-Dimitri) (encephalocutaneous
  angiomatosis) 759.6

Disease, diseased—*continued*
  Stuttgart 100.89
  Sudeck's 733.7
  supporting structures of teeth NEC 525.9
  suprarenal (gland) (capsule) 255.9
    hyperfunction 255.3
    hypofunction 255.41
  Sutton's 709.09
  Sutton and Gull's—*see* Hypertension, kidney
  sweat glands NEC 705.9
    specified type NEC 705.89
  sweating 078.2
  Sweeley-Klionsky 272.7
  Swift (-Feer) 985.0
  swimming pool (bacillus) 031.1
  swineherd's 100.89
  Sylvest's (epidemic pleurodynia) 074.1
  Symmers (follicular lymphoma) (M9690/3)
    202.0
  sympathetic nervous system (*see also*
    Neuropathy, peripheral, autonomic) 337.9
  synovium 727.9
  syphilitic—*see* Syphilis
  systemic tissue mast cell (M9741/3) 202.6
  Taenzer's 757.4
  Takayasu's (pulseless) 446.7
  Talma's 728.85
  Tangier (familial high-density lipoprotein
    deficiency) 272.5
  Tarral-Besnier (pityriasis rubra pilaris) 696.4
  Tay-Sachs 330.1
  Taylor's 701.8
  tear duct 375.69
  teeth, tooth 525.9
    hard tissues 521.9
      specified NEC 521.89
    pulp NEC 522.9
  tendon 727.9
    inflammatory NEC 727.9
  terminal vessel 443.9
  testis 608.9
  Thaysen-Gee (nontropical sprue) 579.0
  Thomsen's 359.22
  Thomson's (congenital poikiloderma) 757.33
  Thornwaldt's, Tornwaldt's (pharyngeal bursitis)
    478.29
  throat 478.20
    septic 034.0
  thromboembolic (*see also* Embolism) 444.9
  thymus (gland) 254.9
    specified NEC 254.8
  thyroid (gland) NEC 246.9
    heart (*see also* Hyperthyroidism) 242.9
      [425.7]
    lardaceous 277.39
    specified NEC 246.8
  Tietze's 733.6
  Tommaselli's
    correct substance properly administered
      599.70
    overdose or wrong substance given or taken
      961.4
  tongue 529.9
  tonsils, tonsillar (and adenoids) (chronic) 474.9
    specified NEC 474.8
  tooth, teeth 525.9
    hard tissues 521.9
      specified NEC 521.89
    pulp NEC 522.9
  Tornwaldt's (pharyngeal bursitis) 478.29
  Tourette's 307.23

Disease, diseased—*continued*
  trachea 519.19
  tricuspid—*see* Endocarditis, tricuspid
  triglyceride-storage, type I, II, III 272.7
  triple vessel (coronary arteries) —*see*
    Arteriosclerosis, coronary
  trisymptomatic, Gougerot's 709.1
  trophoblastic (*see also* Hydatidiform mole) 630
    previous, affecting management of pregnancy
      V23.1
  tsutsugamushi (scrub typhus) 081.2
  tube (fallopian), noninflammatory 620.9
    specified NEC 620.8
  tuberculous NEC (*see also* Tuberculosis) 011.9
  tubo-ovarian
    inflammatory (*see also* Salpingo-oophoritis)
      614.2
    noninflammatory 620.9
      specified NEC 620.8
  tubotympanic, chronic (with anterior perforation
    of ear drum) 382.1
  tympanum 385.9
  Uhl's 746.84
  umbilicus (newborn) NEC 779.89
    delayed separation 779.83
  Underwood's (sclerema neonatorum) 778.1
  undiagnosed 799.9
  Unna's (seborrheic dermatitis) 690.18
  unstable hemoglobin hemolytic 282.7
  Unverricht (-Lundborg) 345.1
  Urbach-Oppenheim (necrobiosis lipoidica
    diabeticorum) 250.8 [709.3]
    due to secondary diabetes 249.8 [709.3]
  Urbach-Wiethe (lipoid proteinosis) 272.8
  ureter 593.9
  urethra 599.9
    specified type NEC 599.84
  urinary (tract) 599.9
    bladder 596.9
      specified NEC 596.89
    maternal, affecting fetus or newborn 760.1
  Usher-Senear (pemphigus erythematosus) 694.4
  uterus (organic) 621.9
    infective (*see also* Endometritis) 615.9
    inflammatory (*see also* Endometritis) 615.9
    noninflammatory 621.9
      specified type NEC 621.8
  uveal tract
    anterior 364.9
    posterior 363.9
  vagabonds' 132.1
  vagina, vaginal
    inflammatory 616.10
    noninflammatory 623.9
      specified NEC 623.8
  Valsuani's (progressive pernicious anemia,
    puerperal) 648.2
    complicating pregnancy or puerperium 648.2
  valve, valvular—*see also* Endocarditis
    congenital NEC (*see also* Anomaly, heart,
      valve) 746.9
    pulmonary 746.00
      specified type NEC 746.89
  van Bogaert-Nijssen (-Peiffer) 330.0
  van Creveld-von Gierke (glycogenosis I) 271.0
  van den Bergh's (enterogenous cyanosis) 289.7
  van Neck's (juvenile osteochondrosis) 732.1
  Vaquez (-Osler) (polycythemia vera) (M9950/1)
    238.4

Disease, diseased—*continued*

vascular 459.9
  arteriosclerotic—*see* Arteriosclerosis
  hypertensive—*see* Hypertension
  obliterative 447.1
    peripheral 443.9
  occlusive 459.9
  peripheral (occlusive) 443.9
    in (due to) (with) diabetes mellitus 250.7
     [443.81]
      in (due to) (with) secondary diabetes 249.7
       [443.81]
    specified type NEC 443.89
vas deferens 608.9
vasomotor 443.9
vasospastic 443.9
vein 459.9
venereal 099.9
  fifth 099.1
  sixth 099.1
  chlamydial NEC 099.50
    anus 099.52
    bladder 099.53
    cervix 099.53
    epididymis 099.54
    genitourinary NEC 099.55
      lower 099.53
      specified NEC 099.54
    pelvic inflammatory disease 099.54
    perihepatic 099.56
    peritoneum 099.56
    pharynx 099.51
    rectum 099.52
    specified site NEC 099.59
    testis 099.54
    vagina 099.53
    vulva 099.53
  complicating pregnancy, childbirth, or
    puerperium 647.2
  specified nature or type NEC 099.8
    chlamydial—*see* Disease, venereal,
      chlamydial
Verneuil's (syphilitic bursitis) 095.7
Verse's (calcinosis intervertebralis) 275.49
  [722.90]
vertebra, vertebral NEC 733.90
  disc—*see* Disease, Intervertebral disc
vibration NEC 994.9
Vidal's (lichen simplex chronicus) 698.3
Vincent's (trench mouth) 101
Virchow's 733.99
virus (filterable) NEC 078.89
  arbovirus NEC 066.9
  arthropod-borne NEC 066.9
  central nervous system NEC 049.9
    specified type NEC 049.8
  complicating pregnancy, childbirth, or
    puerperium 647.6
  contact (with) V01.79
    varicella V01.71
  exposure to V01.79
    varicella V01.71
  Marburg 078.89
  maternal
    with fetal damage affecting management of
      pregnancy 655.3
  nonarthropod-borne NEC 078.89
    central nervous system NEC 049.9
      specified NEC 049.8
  vaccination, prophylactic (against) V04.89
vitreous 379.29

Disease, diseased—*continued*

vocal cords NEC 478.5
Vogt's (Cecile) 333.71
Vogt-Spielmeyer 330.1
Volhard-Fahr (malignant nephrosclerosis)
  403.00
Volkmann's
  acquired 958.6
von Bechterew's (ankylosing spondylitis) 720.0
von Economo's (encephalitis lethargica) 049.8
von Eulenburg's (congenital paramyotonia)
  359.29
von Gierke's (glycogenosis I) 271.0
von Graefe's 378.72
von Hippel's (retinocerebral angiomatosis)
  759.6
von Hippel-Lindau (angiomatosis
  retinocerebellosa) 759.6
von Jaksch's (pseudoleukemia infantum) 285.8
von Recklinghausen's (M9540/1) 237.71
  bone (osteitis fibrosa cystica) 252.01
von Recklinghausen-Applebaum (hemochromatosis)
  (see also Hemochromatosis) 275.03
von Willebrand (-Jürgens) (angiohemophilia)
  286.4
von Zambusch's (lichen sclerosus et atrophicus)
  701.0
Voorhoeve's (dyschondroplasia) 756.4
Vrolik's (osteogenesis imperfecta) 756.51
vulva
  inflammatory 616.10
  noninflammatory 624.9
    specified NEC 624.8
Wagner's (colloid milium) 709.3
Waldenström's (osteochondrosis capital
  femoral) 732.1
Wallgren's (obstruction of splenic vein with
  collateral circulation) 459.89
Wardrop's (with lymphangitis) 681.9
  finger 681.02
  toe 681.11
Wassilieff's (leptospiral jaundice) 100.0
wasting NEC 799.4
  due to malnutrition 261
  paralysis 335.21
Waterhouse-Friderichsen 036.3
waxy (any site) 277.39
Weber-Christian (nodular nonsuppurative
  panniculitis) 729.30
Wegner's (syphilitic osteochondritis) 090.0
Weil's (leptospiral jaundice) 100.0
  of lung 100.0
Weir Mitchell's (erythromelalgia) 443.82
Werdnig-Hoffmann 335.0
Werlhof's *(see also* Purpura, thrombocytopenic)
  287.39
Wermer's 258.01
Werner's (progeria adultorum) 259.8
Werner-His (trench fever) 083.1
Werner-Schultz (agranulocytosis) 288.09
Wernicke's (superior hemorrhagic
  polioencephalitis) 265.1
Wernicke-Posadas 114.9
Whipple's (intestinal lipodystrophy) 040.2
whipworm 127.3
white
  blood cell 288.9
    specified NEC 288.8
  spot 701.0
White's (congenital) (keratosis follicularis)
  757.39

Disease, diseased—*continued*
  Whitmore's (melioidosis) 025
  Widal-Abrami (acquired hemolytic jaundice)
    283.9
  Wilkie's 557.1
  Wilkinson-Sneddon (subcorneal pustular
    dermatosis) 694.1
  Willis' (diabetes mellitus) (*see also* Diabetes)
    250.0
    due to secondary diabetes 249.0
  Wilson's (hepatolenticular degeneration) 275.1
  Wilson-Brocq (dermatitis exfoliativa) 695.89
  winter vomiting 078.82
  Wise's 696.2
  Wohlfart-Kugelberg-Welander 335.11
  Woillez's (acute idiopathic pulmonary
    congestion) 518.52
  Wolman's (primary familial xanthomatosis)
    272.7
  wool-sorters' 022.1
  Zagari's (xerostomia) 527.7
  Zahorsky's (exanthem subitum) 058.10
  Ziehen-Oppenheim 333.6
  zoonotic, bacterial NEC 027.9
    specified type NEC 027.8
Disfigurement (due to scar) 709.2
  head V48.6
  limb V49.4
  neck V48.7
  trunk V48.7
Disgerminoma —*see* Dysgerminoma
Disinsertion, retina 361.04
Disintegration, complete, of the body 799.89
  traumatic 869.1
Disk kidney 753.3
Dislocatable hip, congenita l (*see also*
  Dislocation, hip, congenital) 754.30
Dislocation (articulation) (closed) (displacement)
  (simple) (subluxation) 839.8

*Note—"Closed" includes simple, complete,
partial, uncomplicated, and unspecified
dislocation. "Open" includes dislocation
specified as infected or compound and
dislocation with foreign body. "Chronic,"
"habitual," "old," or "recurrent" dislocations
should be coded as indicated under the entry
"Dislocation, recurrent"; and "pathological"
as indicated under the entry "Dislocation,
pathological." For late effect of dislocation see
Late, effect, dislocation.*

  with fracture—*see* Fracture, by site
  acromioclavicular (joint) (closed) 831.04
    open 831.14
  anatomical site (closed)
    specified NEC 839.69
      open 839.79
    unspecified or ill-defined 839.8
      open 839.9
  ankle (scaphoid bone) (closed) 837.0
    open 837.1
  arm (closed) 839.8
    open 839.9
  astragalus (closed) 837.0
    open 837.1
  atlanto-axial (closed) 839.01
    open 839.11
  atlas (closed) 839.01
    open 839.11
  axis (closed) 839.02
    open 839.12

Dislocation—*continued*
  back (closed) 839.8
    open 839.9
  Bell-Daly 723.8
  breast bone (closed) 839.61
    open 839.71
  capsule, joint—*see* Dislocation, by site
  carpal (bone)—*see* Dislocation, wrist
  carpometacarpal (joint) (closed) 833.04
    open 833.14
  cartilage (joint)—*see also* Dislocation, by site
    knee—*see* Tear, meniscus
  cervical, cervicodorsal, or cervicothoracic
    (spine) (vertebra)—*see* Dislocation,
    vertebra, cervical
  chiropractic (*see also* Lesion, nonallopathic)
    739.9
  chondrocostal—*see* Dislocation, costochondral
  chronic—*see* Dislocation, recurrent
  clavicle (closed) 831.04
    open 831.14
  coccyx (closed) 839.41
    open 839.51
  collar bone (closed) 831.04
    open 831.14
  compound (open) NEC 839.9
  congenital NEC 755.8
    hip (*see also* Dislocation, hip, congenital)
      754.30
    lens 743.37
    rib 756.3
    sacroiliac 755.69
    spine NEC 756.19
    vertebra 756.19
  coracoid (closed) 831.09
    open 831.19
  costal cartilage (closed) 839.69
    open 839.79
  costochondral (closed) 839.69
    open 839.79
  cricoarytenoid articulation (closed) 839.69
    open 839.79
  cricothyroid (cartilage) articulation (closed)
    839.69
    open 839.79
  dorsal vertebrae (closed) 839.21
    open 839.31
  ear ossicle 385.23
  elbow (closed) 832.00
    anterior (closed) 832.01
      open 832.11
    congenital 754.89
    divergent (closed) 832.09
      open 832.19
    lateral (closed) 832.04
      open 832.14
    medial (closed) 832.03
      open 832.13
    open 832.10
    posterior (closed) 832.02
      open 832.12
    recurrent 718.32
    specified type NEC 832.09
      open 832.19
  eye 360.81
    lateral 376.36
  eyeball 360.81
    lateral 376.36

Dislocation—*continued*
  femur
    distal end (closed) 836.50
      anterior 836.52
        open 836.62
      lateral 836.54
        open 836.64
      medial 836.53
        open 836.63
      open 836.60
      posterior 836.51
        open 836.61
    proximal end (closed) 835.00
      anterior (pubic) 835.03
        open 835.13
      obturator 835.02
        open 835.12
      open 835.10
      posterior 835.01
        open 835.11
  fibula
    distal end (closed) 837.0
      open 837.1
    proximal end (closed) 836.59
      open 836.69
  finger(s) (phalanx) (thumb) (closed) 834.00
    interphalangeal (joint) 834.02
      open 834.12
    metacarpal (bone), distal end 834.01
      open 834.11
    metacarpophalangeal (joint) 834.01
      open 834.11
    open 834.10
    recurrent 718.34
  foot (closed) 838.00
    open 838.10
    recurrent 718.37
  forearm (closed) 839.8
    open 839.9
  fracture—*see* Fracture, by site
  glenoid (closed) 831.09
    open 831.19
  habitual—*see* Dislocation, recurrent
  hand (closed) 839.8
    open 839.9
  hip (closed) 835.00
    anterior 835.03
      obturator 835.02
        open 835.12
      open 835.13
    congenital (unilateral) 754.30
      with subluxation of other hip 754.35
      bilateral 754.31
    developmental 718.75
    open 835.10
    posterior 835.01
      open 835.11
    recurrent 718.35
  humerus (closed) 831.00
    distal end (*see also* Dislocation, elbow) 832.00
    open 831.10
    proximal end (closed) 831.00
      anterior (subclavicular) (subcoracoid)
          (subglenoid) (closed) 831.01
        open 831.11
      inferior (closed) 831.03
        open 831.13
      open 831.10
      posterior (closed) 831.02
        open 831.12
  implant—*see* Complications, mechanical

Dislocation—*continued*
  incus 385.23
  infracoracoid (closed) 831.01
    open 831.11
  innominate (pubic junction) (sacral junction)
      (closed) 839.69
    acetabulum (*see also* Dislocation, hip) 835.00
    open 839.79
  interphalangeal (joint)
    finger or hand (closed) 834.02
      open 834.12
    foot or toe (closed) 838.06
      open 838.16
  jaw (cartilage) (meniscus) (closed) 830.0
    open 830.1
    recurrent 524.69
  joint NEC (closed) 839.8
    developmental 718.7
    open 839.9
    pathological—*see* Dislocation, pathological
    recurrent—*see* Dislocation, recurrent
  knee (closed) 836.50
    anterior 836.51
      open 836.61
    congenital (with genu recurvatum) 754.41
    habitual 718.36
    lateral 836.54
      open 836.64
    medial 836.53
      open 836.63
    old 718.36
    open 836.60
    posterior 836.52
      open 836.62
    recurrent 718.36
    rotatory 836.59
      open 836.69
  lacrimal gland 375.16
  leg (closed) 839.8
    open 839.9
  lens (crystalline) (complete) (partial) 379.32
    anterior 379.33
    congenital 743.37
    ocular implant 996.53
    posterior 379.34
    traumatic 921.3
  ligament—*see* Dislocation, by site
  lumbar (vertebrae) (closed) 839.20
    open 839.30
  lumbosacral (vertebrae) (closed) 839.20
    congenital 756.19
    open 839.30
  mandible (closed) 830.0
    open 830.1
  maxilla (inferior) (closed) 830.0
    open 830.1
  meniscus (knee)—*see also* Tear, meniscus
    other sites—*see* Dislocation, by site
  metacarpal (bone)
    distal end (closed) 834.01
      open 834.11
    proximal end (closed) 833.05
      open 833.15
  metacarpophalangeal (joint) (closed) 834.01
    open 834.11
  metatarsal (bone) (closed) 838.04
    open 838.14
  metatarsophalangeal (joint) (closed) 838.05
    open 838.15
  midcarpal (joint) (closed) 833.03
    open 833.13

Dislocation—*continued*
  midtarsal (joint) (closed) 838.02
    open 838.12
  Monteggia's—*see* Dislocation, hip
  multiple locations (except fingers only or toes
      only) (closed) 839.8
    open 839.9
  navicular (bone) foot (closed) 837.0
    open 837.1
  neck (*see also* Dislocation, vertebra, cervical)
      839.00
  Nélaton's—*see* Dislocation, ankle
  nontraumatic (joint)—*see* Dislocation,
      pathological
  nose (closed) 839.69
    open 839.79
  not recurrent, not current injury—*see*
      Dislocation, pathological
  occiput from atlas (closed) 839.01
    open 839.11
  old—*see* Dislocation, recurrent
  open (compound) NEC 839.9
  ossicle, ear 385.23
  paralytic (flaccid) (spastic)—*see* Dislocation,
      pathological
  patella (closed) 836.3
    congenital 755.64
    open 836.4
  pathological NEC 718.20
    ankle 718.27
    elbow 718.22
    foot 718.27
    hand 718.24
    hip 718.25
    knee 718.26
    lumbosacral joint 724.6
    multiple sites 718.29
    pelvic region 718.25
    sacroiliac 724.6
    shoulder (region) 718.21
    specified site NEC 718.28
    spine 724.8
      sacroiliac 724.6
    wrist 718.23
  pelvis (closed) 839.69
    acetabulum (*see also* Dislocation, hip) 835.00
    open 839.79
  phalanx
    foot or toe (closed) 838.09
      open 838.19
    hand or finger (*see also* Dislocation, finger)
        834.00
  postpoliomyelitic—*see* Dislocation,
      pathological
  prosthesis, internal—*see* Complications,
      mechanical
  radiocarpal (joint) (closed) 833.02
    open 833.12
  radioulnar (joint)
    distal end (closed) 833.01
      open 833.11
    proximal end (*see also* Dislocation, elbow)
        832.00
  radius
    distal end (closed) 833.00
      open 833.10
    proximal end (closed) 832.01
      open 832.11

Dislocation—*continued*
  recurrent (*see also* Derangement, joint,
      recurrent) 718.3
    elbow 718.32
    hip 718.35
    joint NEC 718.38
    knee 718.36
    lumbosacral (joint) 724.6
    patella 718.36
    sacroiliac 724.6
    shoulder 718.31
    temporomandibular 524.69
  rib (cartilage) (closed) 839.69
    congenital 756.3
    open 839.79
  sacrococcygeal (closed) 839.42
    open 839.52
  sacroiliac (joint) (ligament) (closed) 839.42
    congenital 755.69
    open 839.52
    recurrent 724.6
  sacrum (closed) 839.42
    open 839.52
  scaphoid (bone)
    ankle or foot (closed) 837.0
      open 837.1
    wrist (closed) (*see also* Dislocation, wrist)
        833.00
      open 833.10
  scapula (closed) 831.09
    open 831.19
  semilunar cartilage, knee—*see* Tear, meniscus
  septal cartilage (nose) (closed) 839.69
    open 839.79
  septum (nasal) (old) 470
  sesamoid bone—*see* Dislocation, by site
  shoulder (blade) (ligament) (closed) 831.00
    anterior (subclavicular) (subcoracoid)
        (subglenoid) (closed) 831.01
      open 831.11
    chronic 718.31
    inferior 831.03
      open 831.13
    open 831.10
    posterior (closed) 831.02
      open 831.12
    recurrent 718.31
  skull—*see* Injury, intracranial
  Smith's—*see* Dislocation, foot
  spine (articular process) (*see also* Dislocation,
      vertebra) (closed) 839.40
    atlanto-axial (closed) 839.01
      open 839.11
      recurrent 723.8
    cervical, cervicodorsal, cervicothoracic
        (closed) (*see also* Dislocation, vertebrae,
        cervical) 839.00
      open 839.10
      recurrent 723.8
    coccyx 839.41
      open 839.51
    congenital 756.19
    due to birth trauma 767.4
    open 839.50
    recurrent 724.9
    sacroiliac 839.42
      recurrent 724.6
    sacrum (sacrococcygeal) (sacroiliac) 839.42
      open 839.52
  spontaneous—*see* Dislocation, pathological

Dislocation—*continued*
  sternoclavicular (joint) (closed) 839.61
    open 839.71
  sternum (closed) 839.61
    open 839.71
  subastragalar—*see* Dislocation, foot
  subglenoid (closed) 831.01
    open 831.11
  symphysis
    jaw (closed) 830.0
      open 830.1
    mandibular (closed) 830.0
      open 830.1
    pubis (closed) 839.69
      open 839.79
  tarsal (bone) (joint) 838.01
    open 838.11
  tarsometatarsal (joint) 838.03
    open 838.13
  temporomandibular (joint) (closed) 830.0
    open 830.1
    recurrent 524.69
  thigh
    distal end (*see also* Dislocation, femur, distal
      end) 836.50
    proximal end (*see also* Dislocation, hip) 835.00
  thoracic (vertebrae) (closed) 839.21
    open 839.31
  thumb(s) (*see also* Dislocation, finger) 834.00
  thyroid cartilage (closed) 839.69
    open 839.79
  tibia
    distal end (closed) 837.0
      open 837.1
    proximal end (closed) 836.50
      anterior 836.51
        open 836.61
      lateral 836.54
        open 836.64
      medial 836.53
        open 836.63
      open 836.60
      posterior 836.52
        open 836.62
      rotatory 836.59
        open 836.69
  tibiofibular
    distal (closed) 837.0
      open 837.1
    superior (closed) 836.59
      open 836.69
  toe(s) (closed) 838.09
    open 838.19
  trachea (closed) 839.69
    open 839.79
  ulna
    distal end (closed) 833.09
      open 833.19
    proximal end—*see* Dislocation, elbow
  vertebra (articular process) (body) (closed)
    (traumatic) 839.40
    cervical, cervicodorsal or cervicothoracic
      (closed) 839.00
      first (atlas) 839.01
        open 839.11
      second (axis) 839.02
        open 839.12
      third 839.03
        open 839.13
      fourth 839.04
        open 839.14

Dislocation—*continued*
  vertebra—*continued*
    cervical—*continued*
      fifth 839.05
        open 839.15
      sixth 839.06
        open 839.16
      seventh 839.07
        open 839.17
      congenital 756.19
      multiple sites 839.08
        open 839.18
      open 839.10
    congenital 756.19
    dorsal 839.21
      open 839.31
      recurrent 724.9
    lumbar, lumbosacral 839.20
      open 839.30
    non-traumatic —*see* Displacement,
      intervertebral disc
    open NEC 839.50
    recurrent 724.9
    specified region NEC 839.49
      open 839.59
    thoracic 839.21
      open 839.31
  wrist (carpal bone) (scaphoid) (semilunar)
    (closed) 833.00
    carpometacarpal (joint) 833.04
      open 833.14
    metacarpal bone, proximal end 833.05
      open 833.15
    midcarpal (joint) 833.03
      open 833.13
    open 833.10
    radiocarpal (joint) 833.02
      open 833.12
    radioulnar (joint) 833.01
      open 833.11
    recurrent 718.33
    specified site NEC 833.09
      open 833.19
  xiphoid cartilage (closed) 839.61
    open 839.71
Dislodgement
  artificial skin graft 996.55
  decellularized allodermis graft 996.55
Disobedience, hostile (covert) (overt) (*see also*
  Disturbance, conduct) 312.0
Disorder —*see also* Disease
  academic underachievement, childhood and
    adolescence 313.83
  accommodation 367.51
    drug-induced 367.89
    toxic 367.89
  adjustment (*see also* Reaction, adjustment) 309.9
    with
      anxiety 309.24
      anxiety and depressed mood 309.28
      depressed mood 309.0
      disturbance of conduct 309.3
      disturbance of emotions and conduct 309.4
  adrenal (capsule) (cortex) (gland) 255.9
    specified type NEC 255.8
  adrenogenital 255.2
  affective (*see also* Psychosis, affective) 296.90
    atypical 296.81
  aggressive, unsocialized (*see also* Disturbance,
    conduct) 312.0

Disorder—*continued*
  alcohol, alcoholic (*see also* Alcohol) 291.9
    induced mood 291.89
  allergic—*see* Allergy
  amino acid (metabolic) (*see also* Disturbance,
    metabolism, amino acid) 270.9
    albinism 270.2
    alkaptonuria 270.2
    argininosuccinicaciduria 270.6
    beta-amino-isobutyricaciduria 277.2
    cystathioninuria 270.4
    cystinosis 270.0
    cystinuria 270.0
    glycinuria 270.0
    homocystinuria 270.4
    imidazole 270.5
    maple syrup (urine) disease 270.3
    neonatal, transitory 775.89
    oasthouse urine disease 270.2
    ochronosis 270.2
    phenylketonuria 270.1
    phenylpyruvic oligophrenia 270.1
    purine NEC 277.2
    pyrimidine NEC 277.2
    renal transport NEC 270.0
    specified type NEC 270.8
    transport NEC 270.0
      renal 270.0
    xanthinuria 277.2
  amnestic (*see also* Amnestic syndrome) 294.08
    alcohol-induced persisting 291.1
    drug-induced persisting 292.83
    in conditions classified elsewhere 294.0
  anaerobic glycolysis with anemia 282.3
  anxiety (*see also* Anxiety) 300.00
    due to or associated with physical condition
      293.84
  arteriole 447.9
    specified type NEC 447.8
  artery 447.9
    specified type NEC 447.8
  articulation—*see* Disorder, joint
  Asperger's 299.8
  attachment of infancy or early childhood 313.89
  attention deficit 314.00
    with hyperactivity 314.01
    predominantly
      combined hyperactive/inattentive 314.01
      hyperactive/impulsive 314.01
      inattentive 314.00
    residual type 314.8
  auditory processing disorder 388.45
    acquired 388.45
    developmental 315.32
  autistic 299.0
  autoimmune NEC 279.49
    hemolytic (cold type) (warm type) 283.0
    parathyroid 252.1
    thyroid 245.2
  avoidant, childhood or adolescence 313.21
  balance
    acid-base 276.9
      mixed (with hypercapnia) 276.4
    electrolyte 276.9
    fluid 276.9
  behavior NEC (*see also* Disturbance, conduct)
    312.9
    disruptive 312.9
  bilirubin excretion 277.4

Disorder—*continued*
  bipolar (affective) (alternating) 296.80

> *Note*—Use the following fifth-digit
> subclassification with categories 296.0-296.6:
>
> 0   unspecified
> 1   mild
> 2   moderate
> 3   severe, without mention of psychotic
>   behavior
> 4   severe, specified as with psychotic
>   behavior
> 5   in partial or unspecified remission
> 6   in full remission

    atypical 296.7
    currently
      depressed 296.5
      hypomanic 296.4
      manic 296.4
    mixed 296.6
    specified type NEC 296.89
    type I 296.7
      most recent episode (or current)
        depressed 296.5
        hypomanic 296.4
        manic 296.4
        mixed 296.6
        unspecified 296.7
      single manic episode 296.0
    type II (recurrent major depressive episodes
      with hypomania) 296.89
  bladder 596.9
    functional NEC 596.59
    specified NEC 596.89
  bleeding 286.9
  bone NEC 733.90
    specified NEC 733.99
  brachial plexus 353.0
  branched-chain amino-acid degradation 270.3
  breast 611.9
    puerperal, postpartum 676.3
    specified NEC 611.89
  Briquet's 300.81
  bursa 727.9
    shoulder region 726.10
  carbohydrate metabolism, congenital 271.9
  cardiac, functional 427.9
    postoperative 997.1
    psychogenic 306.2
  cardiovascular, psychogenic 306.2
  cartilage NEC 733.90
    articular 718.00
      ankle 718.07
      elbow 718.02
      foot 718.07
      hand 718.04
      hip 718.05
      knee 717.9
      multiple sites 718.09
      pelvic region 718.05
      shoulder region 718.01
      specified
        site NEC 718.08
        type NEC 733.99
      wrist 718.03
  catatonic—*see* Catatonia
  central auditory processing 315.32
    acquired 388.45
    developmental 315.32
  cervical region NEC 723.9

Disorder—*continued*
cervical root (nerve) NEC 353.2
character NEC (*see also* Disorder, personality)
301.9
ciliary body 364.9
specified NEC 364.89
coagulation (factor) (*see also* Defect,
coagulation) 286.9
factor VIII (congenital) (functional) 286.0
factor IX (congenital) (functional) 286.1
neonatal, transitory 776.3
coccyx 724.70
specified NEC 724.79
cognitive 294.9
colon 569.9
functional 564.9
congenital 751.3
communication 307.9
conduct (*see also* Disturbance, conduct) 312.9
adjustment reaction 309.3
adolescent onset type 312.82
childhood onset type 312.81
compulsive 312.30
specified type NEC 312.39
hyperkinetic 314.2
onset unspecified 312.89
socialized (type) 312.20
aggressive 312.23
unaggressive 312.21
specified NEC 312.89
conduction, heart 426.9
specified NEC 426.89
conflict
sexual orientation 302.0
congenital
glycosylation (CDG) 271.8
convulsive (secondary) (*see also* Convulsions)
780.39
due to injury at birth 767.0
idiopathic 780.39
coordination 781.3
cornea NEC 371.89
due to contact lens 371.82
corticosteroid metabolism NEC 255.2
cranial nerve—*see* Disorder, nerve, cranial
cyclothymic 301.13
degradation, branched-chain amino acid 270.3
delusional 297.1
dentition 520.6
depersonalization 300.6
depressive NEC 311
atypical 296.82
major (*see also* Psychosis, affective) 296.2
recurrent episode 296.3
single episode 296.2
development, specific 315.9
associated with hyperkinesia 314.1
coordination 315.4
language 315.31
and speech due to hearing loss 315.34
learning 315.2
arithmetical 315.1
reading 315.00
mixed 315.5
motor coordination 315.4
specified type NEC 315.8
speech 315.39
and language due to hearing loss 315.34
diaphragm 519.4

Disorder—*continued*
digestive 536.9
fetus or newborn 777.9
specified NEC 777.8
psychogenic 306.4
disintegrative, childhood 299.1
dissociative 300.15
identity 300.14
nocturnal 307.47
drug-related 292.9
dysmorphic body 300.7
dysthymic 300.4
ear 388.9
degenerative NEC 388.00
external 380.9
specified 380.89
pinna 380.30
specified type NEC 388.8
vascular NEC 388.00
eating NEC 307.50
electrolyte NEC 276.9
with
abortion—*see* Abortion, by type, with
metabolic disorder
ectopic pregnancy (*see also* categories
633.0-633.9) 639.4
molar pregnancy (*see also* categories
630-632) 639.4
acidosis 276.2
metabolic 276.2
respiratory 276.2
alkalosis 276.3
metabolic 276.3
respiratory 276.3
following
abortion 639.4
ectopic or molar pregnancy 639.4
neonatal, transitory NEC 775.5
emancipation as adjustment reaction 309.22
emotional (*see also* Disorder, mental,
nonpsychotic) V40.9
endocrine 259.9
specified type NEC 259.8
esophagus 530.9
functional 530.5
psychogenic 306.4
explosive
intermittent 312.34
isolated 312.35
expressive language 315.31
eye 379.90
globe—*see* Disorder, globe
ill-defined NEC 379.99
limited duction NEC 378.63
specified NEC 379.8
eyelid 374.9
degenerative 374.50
sensory 374.44
specified type NEC 374.89
vascular 374.85
factitious (with combined psychological and
physical signs and symptoms) (with
predominantly physical signs and
symptoms) 300.19
with predominantly psychological signs and
symptoms 300.16
factor, coafulation (*see also* Defect, coagulation)
286.9
VIII (congenital) (functional) 286.0
IX (congenital) (functional) 286.1
fascia 728.9

Disorder—*continued*
fatty acid oxidation 277.85
feeding —*see* Feeding
female sexual arousal 302.72
fluency 315.35
  adult onset 307.0
  childhood onset 315.35
  due to late effect of cerebrovascular accident
    438.14
  in conditions classified elsewhere 784.52
fluid NEC 276.9
gastric (functional) 536.9
  motility 536.8
  psychogenic 306.4
  secretion 536.8
gastrointestinal (functional) NEC 536.9
  newborn (neonatal) 777.9
    specified NEC 777.8
  psychogenic 306.4
gender (child) 302.6
  adult 302.85
gender identity (childhood) 302.6
  adolescents 302.85
  adults (-life) 302.85
genitourinary system, psychogenic 306.50
globe 360.9
  degenerative 360.20
    specified NEC 360.29
  specified type NEC 360.89
hearing—*see also* Deafness
  conductive type (air) (*see also* Deafness,
    conductive) 389.00
  mixed conductive and sensorineural 389.20
    bilateral 389.22
    unilateral 389.21
  nerve
    bilateral 389.12
    unilateral 389.13
  perceptive (*see also* Deafness, perceptive)
    389.10
  sensorineural type NEC (*see also* Deafness,
    sensorineural) 389.10
heart action 427.9
  postoperative 997.1
hematological, transient neonatal 776.9
  specified type NEC 776.8
hematopoietic organs 289.9
hemorrhagic NEC 287.9
  due to intrinsic circulating anticoagulants,
    antibodies or inhibitors 286.59
    with
      acquired hemophilia 286.52
      antiphospholipid antibody 286.53
  specified type NEC 287.8
hemostasis (*see also* Defect, coagulation) 286.9
homosexual conflict 302.0
hypomanic (chronic) 301.11
identity
  childhood and adolescence 313.82
    gender 302.6
  gender 302.6
immune mechanism (immunity) 279.9
  single complement (C_1-C_9) 279.8
  specified type NEC 279.8
impulse control (*see also* Disturbance, conduct,
  compulsive) 312.30
infant sialic acid storage 271.8
integument, fetus or newborn 778.9
  specified type NEC 778.8
interactional psychotic (childhood) (*see also*
  Psychosis, childhood) 299.1

Disorder—*continued*
intermittent explosive 312.34
intervertebral disc 722.90
  cervical, cervicothoracic 722.91
  lumbar, lumbosacral 722.93
  thoracic, thoracolumbar 722.92
intestinal 569.9
  functional NEC 564.9
    congenital 751.3
    postoperative 564.4
  psychogenic 306.4
introverted, of childhood and adolescence
  313.22
involuntary emotional expression (IEED) 310.81
iris 364.9
  specified NEC 364.89
iron, metabolism 275.09
  specified type NEC 275.09
isolated explosive 312.35
joint NEC 719.90
  ankle 719.97
  elbow 719.92
  foot 719.97
  hand 719.94
  hip 719.95
  knee 719.96
  multiple sites 719.99
  pelvic region 719.95
  psychogenic 306.0
  shoulder (region) 719.91
  specified site NEC 719.98
  temporomandibular 524.60
    sounds on opening or closing 524.64
    specified NEC 524.69
  wrist 719.93
kidney 593.9
  functional 588.9
    specified NEC 588.89
labyrinth, labyrinthine 386.9
  specified type NEC 386.8
lactation 676.9
language (developmental) (expressive) 315.31
  mixed receptive-expressive 315.32
learning 315.9
ligament 728.9
ligamentous attachments, peripheral—*see also*
  Enthesopathy
  spine 720.1
limb NEC 729.90
  psychogenic 306.0
lipid
  metabolism, congenital 272.9
  storage 272.7
lipoprotein deficiency (familial) 272.5
low back NEC 724.9
  psychogenic 306.0
lumbosacral
  plexus 353.1
  root (nerve) NEC 353.4
lymphoproliferative (chronic) NEC (M9970/1)
  238.79
  post-transplant (PTLD) 238.77
major depressive (*see also* Psychosis, affective)
  296.2
  recurrent episode 296.3
  single episode 296.2
male erectile 607.84
  nonorganic origin 302.72
manic (*see also* Psychosis, affective) 296.0
  atypical 296.81
mathematics 315.1

Disorder—*continued*

  meniscus NEC (*see also* Disorder, cartilage, articular) 718.0

  menopausal 627.9

    specified NEC 627.8

  menstrual 626.9

    psychogenic 306.52

    specified NEC 626.8

  mental (nonpsychotic) 300.9

    affecting management of pregnancy, childbirth, or puerperium 648.4

    drug-induced 292.9

      hallucinogen persistent perception 292.89

      specified type NEC 292.89

    due to or associated with

      alcoholism 291.9

      drug consumption NEC 292.9

        specified type NEC 292.89

      physical condition NEC 293.9

    induced by drug 292.9

      specified type NEC 292.89

    neurotic (*see also* Neurosis) 300.9

    of infancy, childhood or adolescence 313.9

    persistent

      other

        due to conditions classified elsewhere 294.8

      unspecified

        due to conditions classified elsewhere 294.9

    presenile 310.1

      psychotic NEC 290.10

    previous, affecting management of pregnancy V23.8

    psychoneurotic (*see also* Neurosis) 300.9

    psychotic (*see also* Psychosis) 298.9

      brief 298.8

      senile 290.20

    specific, following organic brain damage 310.9

      cognitive or personality change of other type 310.1

      frontal lobe syndrome 310.0

      postconcussional syndrome 310.2

      specified type NEC 310.89

    transient

      in conditions classified elsewhere 293.9

  metabolism NEC 277.9

    with

      abortion—*see* Abortion, by type, with metabolic disorder

      ectopic pregnancy (*see also* categories 633.0-633.9) 639.4

      molar pregnancy (*see also* categories 630-632) 639.4

    alkaptonuria 270.2

    amino acid (*see also* Disorder, amino acid) 270.9

      specified type NEC 270.8

    ammonia 270.6

    arginine 270.6

    argininosuccinic acid 270.6

    basal 794.7

    bilirubin 277.4

    calcium 275.40

    carbohydrate 271.9

      specified type NEC 271.8

    cholesterol 272.9

    citrulline 270.6

    copper 275.1

    corticosteroid 255.2

    cystine storage 270.0

    cystinuria 270.0

    fat 272.9

    fatty acid oxidation 277.85

Disorder—*continued*

  metabolism—*continued*

    following

      abortion 639.4

      ectopic or molar pregnancy 639.4

    fructosemia 271.2

    fructosuria 271.2

    fucosidosis 271.8

    due to conditions classified elsewhere 294.8

    galactose-1-phosphate uridyl transferase 271.1

    glutamine 270.7

    glycine 270.7

    glycogen storage NEC 271.0

      hepatorenal 271.0

    hemochromatosis (*see also* Hemochromatosis) 275.03

    in labor and delivery 669.0

    iron 275.09

    lactose 271.3

    lipid 272.9

      specified type NEC 272.8

      storage 272.7

    lipoprotein—*see also* Hyperlipemia deficiency (familial) 272.5

    lysine 270.7

    magnesium 275.2

    mannosidosis 271.8

    mineral 275.9

      specified type NEC 275.8

    mitochondrial 277.87

    mucopolysaccharide 277.5

    nitrogen 270.9

    ornithine 270.6

    oxalosis 271.8

    pentosuria 271.8

    phenylketonuria 270.1

    phosphate 275.3

    phosphorus 275.3

    plasma protein 273.9

      specified type NEC 273.8

    porphyrin 277.1

    purine 277.2

    pyrimidine 277.2

    serine 270.7

    sodium 276.9

    specified type NEC 277.89

    steroid 255.2

    threonine 270.7

    urea cycle 270.6

    xylose 271.8

  micturition NEC 788.69

    psychogenic 306.53

  misery and unhappiness, of childhood and adolescence 313.1

  mitochondrial metabolism 277.87

  mitral valve 424.0

  mood (*see also* Disorder, bipolar) 296.90

    alcohol-induced 291.89

    episodic 296.90

      specified NEC 296.99

    in conditions classified elsewhere 293.83

  motor tic 307.20

    chronic 307.22

    transient (childhood) 307.21

  movement NEC 333.90

    hysterical 300.11

    medication-induced 333.90

    periodic limb 327.51

    sleep related, unspecified 780.58

      other organic 327.59

    specified type NEC 333.99

    stereotypic 307.3

Disorder—*continued*
  mucopolysaccharide 277.5
  muscle 728.9
    psychogenic 306.0
    specified type NEC 728.3
  muscular attachments, peripheral—*see also*
    Enthesopathy
    spine 720.1
  musculoskeletal system NEC 729.90
    psychogenic 306.0
  myeloproliferative (chronic) NEC (M9960/1)
    238.79
  myoneural 358.9
    due to lead 358.2
    specified type NEC 358.8
    toxic 358.2
  myotonic 359.29
  neck region NEC 723.9
  nerve 349.9
    abducens NEC 378.54
    accessory 352.4
    acoustic 388.5
    auditory 388.5
    auriculotemporal 350.8
    axillary 353.0
    cerebral—*see* Disorder, nerve, cranial
    cranial 352.9
      first 352.0
      second 377.49
      third
        partial 378.51
        total 378.52
      fourth 378.53
      fifth 350.9
      sixth 378.54
      seventh NEC 351.9
      eighth 388.5
      ninth 352.2
      tenth 352.3
      eleventh 352.4
      twelfth 352.5
      multiple 352.6
    entrapment—*see* Neuropathy, entrapment
    facial 351.9
      specified NEC 351.8
    femoral 355.2
    glossopharyngeal NEC 352.2
    hypoglossal 352.5
    iliohypogastric 355.79
    ilioinguinal 355.79
    intercostal 353.8
    lateral
      cutaneous of thigh 355.1
      popliteal 355.3
    lower limb NEC 355.8
    medial, popliteal 355.4
    median NEC 354.1
    obturator 355.79
    oculomotor
      partial 378.51
      total 378.52
    olfactory 352.0
    optic 377.49
      hypoplasia 377.43
      ischemic 377.41
      nutritional 377.33
      toxic 377.34
    peroneal 355.3
    phrenic 354.8
    plantar 355.6
    pneumogastric 352.3

Disorder—*continued*
  nerve—*continued*
    posterior tibial 355.5
    radial 354.3
    recurrent laryngeal 352.3
    root 353.9
      specified NEC 353.8
    saphenous 355.79
    sciatic NEC 355.0
    specified NEC 355.9
      lower limb 355.79
      upper limb 354.8
    spinal 355.9
    sympathetic NEC 337.9
    trigeminal 350.9
      specified NEC 350.8
    trochlear 378.53
    ulnar 354.2
    upper limb NEC 354.9
    vagus 352.3
  nervous system NEC 349.9
    autonomic (peripheral) (*see also* Neuropathy,
      peripheral, autonomic) 337.9
    cranial 352.9
    parasympathetic (*see also* Neuropathy,
      peripheral, autonomic) 337.9
    specified type NEC 349.89
    sympathetic (*see also* Neuropathy, peripheral,
      autonomic) 337.9
    vegetative (*see also* Neuropathy, peripheral,
      autonomic) 337.9
  neurohypophysis NEC 253.6
  neurological NEC 781.99
    peripheral NEC 355.9
  neuromuscular NEC 358.9
    hereditary NEC 359.1
    specified NEC 358.8
    toxic 358.2
  neurotic 300.9
    specified type NEC 300.89
  neutrophil, polymorphonuclear (functional) 288.1
  nightmare 307.47
  night terror 307.46
  obsessive-compulsive 300.3
  oppositional defiant, childhood and adolescence
    313.81
  optic
    chiasm 377.54
      associated with
        inflammatory disorders 377.54
        neoplasm NEC 377.52
          pituitary 377.51
        pituitary disorders 377.51
        vascular disorders 377.53
    nerve 377.49
    radiations 377.63
    tracts 377.63
  orbit 376.9
    specified NEC 376.89
  orgasmic
    female 302.73
    male 302.74
  overanxious, of childhood and adolescence
    313.0
  oxidation, fatty acid 277.85
  pancreas, internal secretion (other than diabetes
    mellitus) 251.9
    specified type NEC 251.8
  panic 300.01
    with agoraphobia 300.21
  papillary muscle NEC 429.81

Disorder—*continued*
  paranoid 297.9
    induced 297.3
    shared 297.3
  parathyroid 252.9
    specified type NEC 252.8
  paroxysmal, mixed 780.39
  pentose phosphate pathway with anemia 282.2
  periodic limb movement 327.51
  peroxisomal 277.86
  personality 301.9
    affective 301.10
    aggressive 301.3
    amoral 301.7
    anancastic, anankastic 301.4
    antisocial 301.7
    asocial 301.7
    asthenic 301.6
    avoidant 301.82
    borderline 301.83
    compulsive 301.4
    cyclothymic 301.13
    dependent-passive 301.6
    dyssocial 301.7
    emotional instability 301.59
    epileptoid 301.3
    explosive 301.3
    following organic brain damage 310.1
    histrionic 301.50
    hyperthymic 301.11
    hypomanic (chronic) 301.11
    hypothymic 301.12
    hysterical 301.50
    immature 301.89
    inadequate 301.6
    introverted 301.21
    labile 301.59
    moral deficiency 301.7
    narcissistic 301.81
    obsessional 301.4
    obsessive-compulsive 301.4
    overconscientious 301.4
    paranoid 301.0
    passive (-dependent) 301.6
    passive-aggressive 301.84
    pathological NEC 301.9
    pseudosocial 301.7
    psychopathic 301.9
    schizoid 301.20
      introverted 301.21
      schizotypal 301.22
    schizotypal 301.22
    seductive 301.59
    type A 301.4
    unstable 301.59
  pervasive developmental 299.9
    childhood-onset 299.8
    specified NEC 299.8
  phonological 315.39
  pigmentation, choroid (congenital) 743.53
  pinna 380.30
    specified type NEC 380.39
  pituitary, thalamic 253.9
    anterior NEC 253.4
    iatrogenic 253.7
    postablative 253.7
    specified NEC 253.8
  pityriasis-like NEC 696.8
  platelets (blood) 287.1
  polymorphonuclear neutrophils (functional) 288.1
  porphyrin metabolism 277.1

Disorder—*continued*
  postmenopausal 627.9
    specified type NEC 627.8
  post-transplant lymphoproliferative (PTLD) 238.77
  post-traumatic stress (PTSD) 309.81
    acute 309.81
    brief 309.81
    chronic 309.81
  premenstrual dysphoric (PMDD) 625.4
  psoriatic-like NEC 696.8
  psychic, with diseases classified elsewhere 316
  psychogenic NEC (*see also* condition) 300.9
    allergic NEC
      respiratory 306.1
    anxiety 300.00
      atypical 300.00
      generalized 300.02
    appetite 307.59
    articulation, joint 306.0
    asthenic 300.5
    blood 306.8
    cardiovascular (system) 306.2
    compulsive 300.3
    cutaneous 306.3
    depressive 300.4
    digestive (system) 306.4
    dysmenorrheic 306.52
    dyspneic 306.1
    eczematous 306.3
    endocrine (system) 306.6
    eye 306.7
    feeding 307.59
    functional NEC 306.9
    gastric 306.4
    gastrointestinal (system) 306.4
    genitourinary (system) 306.50
    heart (function) (rhythm) 306.2
    hemic 306.8
    hyperventilatory 306.1
    hypochondriacal 300.7
    hysterical 300.10
    intestinal 306.4
    joint 306.0
    learning 315.2
    limb 306.0
    lymphatic (system) 306.8
    menstrual 306.52
    micturition 306.53
    monoplegic NEC 306.0
    motor 307.9
    muscle 306.0
    musculoskeletal 306.0
    neurocirculatory 306.2
    obsessive 300.3
    occupational 300.89
    organ or part of body NEC 306.9
    organs of special sense 306.7
    paralytic NEC 306.0
    phobic 300.20
    physical NEC 306.9
    pruritic 306.3
    rectal 306.4
    respiratory (system) 306.1
    rheumatic 306.0
    sexual (function) 302.70
      specified type NEC 302.79
    sexual orientation conflict 302.0
    skin (allergic) (eczematous) (pruritic) 306.3

Disorder—*continued*
  psychogenic—*continued*
    sleep 307.40
      initiation or maintenance 307.41
        persistent 307.42
        transient 307.41
      movement 780.58
      sleep terror 307.46
      specified type NEC 307.49
    specified part of body NEC 306.8
    stomach 306.4
  psychomotor NEC 307.9
    hysterical 300.11
  psychoneurotic (*see also* Neurosis) 300.9
    mixed NEC 300.89
  psychophysiologic (*see also* Disorder, psychosomatic) 306.9
  psychosexual identity (childhood) 302.6
    adult-life 302.85
  psychosomatic NEC 306.9
    allergic NEC
      respiratory 306.1
    articulation, joint 306.0
    cardiovascular (system) 306.2
    cutaneous 306.3
    digestive (system) 306.4
    dysmenorrheic 306.52
    dyspneic 306.1
    endocrine (system) 306.6
    eye 306.7
    gastric 306.4
    gastrointestinal (system) 306.4
    genitourinary (system) 306.50
    heart (functional) (rhythm) 306.2
    hyperventilatory 306.1
    intestinal 306.4
    joint 306.0
    limb 306.0
    lymphatic (system) 306.8
    menstrual 306.52
    micturition 306.53
    monoplegic NEC 306.0
    muscle 306.0
    musculoskeletal 306.0
    neurocirculatory 306.2
    organs of special sense 306.7
    paralytic NEC 306.0
    pruritic 306.3
    rectal 306.4
    respiratory (system) 306.1
    rheumatic 306.0
    sexual (function) 302.70
      specified type NEC 302.79
    skin 306.3
    specified part of body NEC 306.8
    stomach 306.4
  psychotic (*see also* Psychosis) 298.9
    brief 298.8
  PTSD (post-traumatic stress disorder) 309.81
  purine metabolism NEC 277.2
  pyrimidine metabolism NEC 277.2
  reactive attachment of infancy or early childhood 313.89
  reading, developmental 315.00
  reflex 796.1
  REM sleep behavior 327.42
  renal function, impaired 588.9
    specified type NEC 588.89
  renal transport NEC 588.89

Disorder—*continued*
  respiration, respiratory NEC 519.9
    due to
      aspiration of liquids or solids 508.9
      inhalation of fumes or vapors 506.9
      smoke inhalation 508.2
    psychogenic 306.1
  retina 362.9
    specified type NEC 362.89
  rumination 307.53
  sacroiliac joint NEC 724.6
  sacrum 724.6
  schizo-affective (*see also* Schizophrenia) 295.7
  schizoid, childhood or adolescence 313.22
  schizophreniform 295.4
  schizotypal personality 301.22
  secretion, thyrocalcitonin 246.0
  seizure 345.9
    recurrent 345.9
      epileptic—*see* Epilepsy
  semantic pragmatic 315.39
    with autism 299.0
  sense of smell 781.1
    psychogenic 306.7
  separation anxiety 309.21
  sexual (*see also* Deviation, sexual) 302.9
    aversion 302.79
    desire, hypoactive 302.71
    function, psychogenic 302.70
  shyness, of childhood and adolescence 313.21
  single complement (C_1-C_9) 279.8
  skin NEC 709.9
    fetus or newborn 778.9
      specified type 778.8
    psychogenic (allergic) (eczematous) (pruritic) 306.3
    specified type NEC 709.8
    vascular 709.1
  sleep 780.50
    alcohol induced 291.82
    arousal 307.46
      confusional 327.41
    circadian rhythm 327.30
      advanced sleep phase type 327.32
      alcohol induced 291.82
      delayed sleep phase type 327.31
      drug induced 292.85
      free running type 327.34
      in conditions classified elsewhere 327.37
      irregular sleep-wake type 327.33
      jet lag type 327.35
      other 327.39
      shift work type 327.36
    drug induced 292.85
    initiation or maintenance (*see also* Insomnia) 780.52
      nonorganic origin (transient) 307.41
        persistent 307.42
    nonorganic origin 307.40
      specified type NEC 307.49
    organic specified type NEC 327.8
    periodic limb movement 327.51
    specified NEC 780.59
    wake
      cycle—*see* Disorder, sleep, circadian rhythm
      schedule—*see* Disorder, sleep, circadian rhythm
    with apnea—*see* Apnea, sleep
  social, of childhood and adolescence 313.22
  soft tissue 729.90
    specified type NEC 729.99

Disorder—*continued*

somatization 300.81
somatoform (atypical) (undifferentiated) 300.82
  severe 300.81
  specified type NEC 300.89
speech NEC 784.59
  nonorganic origin 307.9
spine NEC 724.9
  ligamentous or muscular attachments,
    peripheral 720.1
steroid metabolism NEC 255.2
stomach (functional) (*see also* Disorder, gastric) 536.9
  psychogenic 306.4
storage, iron 275.09
stress (*see also* Reaction, stress, acute) 308.3
  posttraumatic
    acute 309.81
    brief 309.81
    chronic 309.81
substitution 300.11
suspected—*see* Observation
synovium 727.9
temperature regulation, fetus or newborn 778.4
temporomandibular joint NEC 524.60
  sounds on opening or closing 524.64
  specified NEC 524.69
tendon 727.9
  shoulder region 726.10
thoracic root (nerve) NEC 353.3
thyrocalcitonin secretion 246.0
thyroid (gland) NEC 246.9
  specified type NEC 246.8
tic 307.20
  chronic (motor or vocal) 307.22
  motor-verbal 307.23
  organic origin 333.1
  transient (of childhood) 307.21
tooth NEC 525.9
  development NEC 520.9
    specified type NEC 520.8
  eruption 520.6
  specified type NEC 525.8
Tourette's 307.23
transport, carbohydrate 271.9
  specified type NEC 271.8
tubular, phosphate-losing 588.0
tympanic membrane 384.9
unaggressive, unsocialized (*see also*
  Disturbance, conduct) 312.1
undersocialized, unsocialized—*see also*
  Disturbance, conduct
  aggressive (type) 312.0
  unaggressive (type) 312.1
vision, visual NEC 368.9
  binocular NEC 368.30
  cortex 377.73
    associated with
      inflammatory disorders 377.73
      neoplasms 377.71
      vascular disorders 377.72
    pathway NEC 377.63
    associated with
      inflammatory disorders 377.63
      neoplasms 377.61
      vascular disorders 377.62
vocal tic
  chronic 307.22
wakefulness (*see also* Hypersomnia) 780.54
  nonorganic origin (transient) 307.43
  persistent 307.44
written expression 315.2

Disorganized globe 360.29
Displacement, displaced

> *Note—For acquired displacement of bones,
> cartilage, joints, tendons, due to injury, see also
> Dislocation. Displacements at ages under one
> year should be considered congenital, provided
> there is no indication the condition was
> acquired after birth.*

acquired traumatic of bond, cartilage, joint,
  tendon NEC (without fracture) (*see also*
  Dislocation) 839.8
  with fracture—*see* Fracture, by site
adrenal gland (congenital) 759.1
alveolus and teeth, vertical 524.75
appendix, retrocecal (congenital) 751.5
auricle (congenital) 744.29
bladder (acquired) 596.89
  congenital 753.8
brachial plexus (congenital) 742.8
brain stem, caudal 742.4
canaliculus lacrimalis 743.65
cardia, through esophageal hiatus 750.6
cerebellum, caudal 742.4
cervix —*see* Displacement, uterus
colon (congenital) 751.4
device, implant, or graft—*see* Complications,
  mechanical
epithelium
  columnar of cervix 622.10
  cuboidal, beyond limits of external os (uterus)
    752.49
esophageal mucosa into cardia of stomach,
  congenital 750.4
esophagus (acquired) 530.89
  congenital 750.4
eyeball (acquired) (old) 376.36
  congenital 743.8
  current injury 871.3
  lateral 376.36
fallopian tube (acquired) 620.4
  congenital 752.19
  opening (congenital) 752.19
gallbladder (congenital) 751.69
gastric mucosa 750.7
  into
    duodenum 750.7
    esophagus 750.7
    Meckel's diverticulum, congenital 750.7
globe (acquired) (lateral) (old) 376.36
  current injury 871.3
graft
  artificial skin graft 996.55
  decellularized allodermis graft 996.55
heart (congenital) 746.87
  acquired 429.89
hymen (congenital) (upward) 752.49
internal prosthesis NEC—*see* Complications,
  mechanical
intervertebral disc (with neuritis, radiculitis,
  sciatica, or other pain) 722.2
  with myelopathy 722.70
  cervical, cervicodorsal, cervicothoracic 722.0
    with myelopathy 722.71
    due to major trauma—*see* Dislocation,
      vertebra, cervical
  due to trauma—*see* Dislocation, vertebra
  lumbar, lumbosacral 722.10
    with myelopathy 722.73
    due to major trauma—*see* Dislocation,
      vertebra, lumbar

Displacement, displaced—*continued*
 intervertebral disc—*continued*
  thoracic, thoracolumbar 722.11
   with myelopathy 722.72
   due to major trauma—*see* Dislocation,
    vertebra, thoracic
 intrauterine device 996.32
 kidney (acquired) 593.0
  congenital 753.3
 lacrimal apparatus or duct (congenital) 743.65
 macula (congenital) 743.55
 Meckel's diverticulum (congenital) 751.0
 nail (congenital) 757.5
  acquired 703.8
 opening of Wharton's duct in mouth 750.26
 organ or site, congenital NEC—*see* Malposition,
  congenital
 ovary (acquired) 620.4
  congenital 752.0
  free in peritoneal cavity (congenital) 752.0
  into hernial sac 620.4
 oviduct (acquired) 620.4
  congenital 752.19
 parathyroid (gland) 252.8
 parotid gland (congenital) 750.26
 punctum lacrimale (congenital) 743.65
 sacroiliac (congenital) (joint) 755.69
  current injury—*see* Dislocation, sacroiliac
  old 724.6
 spine (congenital) 756.19
 spleen, congenital 759.0
 stomach (congenital) 750.7
  acquired 537.89
 subglenoid (closed) 831.01
 sublingual duct (congenital) 750.26
 teeth, tooth 524.30
  horizontal 524.33
  vertical 524.34
 tongue (congenital) (downward) 750.19
 trachea (congenital) 748.3
 ureter or ureteric opening or orifice (congenital)
  753.4
 uterine opening of oviducts or fallopian tubes
  752.19
 uterus, uterine (*see also* Malposition, uterus) 621.6
  congenital 752.39
 ventricular septum 746.89
  with rudimentary ventricle 746.89
 xyphoid bone (process) 738.3
Disproportion 653.9
 affecting fetus or newborn 763.1
 breast, reconstructed 612.1
  between native and reconstructed 612.1
 caused by
  conjoined twins 678.1
  contraction, pelvis (general) 653.1
   inlet 653.2
   midpelvic 653.8
   midplane 653.8
   outlet 653.3
  fetal
   ascites 653.7
   hydrocephalus 653.6
   hydrops 653.7
   meningomyelocele 653.7
   sacral teratoma 653.7
   tumor 653.7
  hydrocephalic fetus 653.6
  pelvis, pelvic, abnormality (bony) NEC 653.0
  unusually large fetus 653.5
 causing obstructed labor 660.1

Disproportion—*continued*
 cephalopelvic, normally formed fetus 653.4
  causing obstructed labor 660.1
 fetal NEC 653.5
  causing obstructed labor 660.1
 fetopelvic, normally formed fetus 653.4
  causing obstructed labor 660.1
 mixed maternal and fetal origin, normally
  formed fetus 653.4
 pelvis, pelvic (bony) NEC 653.1
  causing obstructed labor 660.1
 specified type NEC 653.8
Disruption
 cesarean wound 674.1
 family V61.09
  due to
   child in
    care of non-parental family member
     V61.06
    foster care V61.06
    welfare custody V61.05
   death of family member V61.07
   divorce V61.03
   estrangement V61.09
    parent-child V61.04
   extended absence of family member NEC
    V61.08
   family member
    on military deployment V61.01
    return from military deployment V61.02
   legal separation V61.03
 gastrointestinal anastomosis 997.49
 ligament(s)—*see also* Sprain
  knee
   current injury—*see* Dislocation, knee
   old 717.89
    capsular 717.85
    collateral (medial) 717.82
     lateral 717.81
    cruciate (posterior) 717.84
     anterior 717.83
    specified site NEC 717.85
 marital V61.10
  involving
   divorce V61.03
   estrangement V61.09
 operation wound (external) (*see also*
  Dehiscence) 998.32
  internal 998.31
 organ transplant, anastomosis site—*see*
  Complications, transplant, organ, by site
 ossicles, ossicular chain 385.23
  traumatic—*see* Fracture, skull, base
 parenchyma
  liver (hepatic)—*see* Laceration, liver, major
  spleen—*see* Laceration, spleen, parenchyma,
   massive
 phase-shift, of 24 hour sleep wake cycle,
  unspecified 780.55
  nonorganic origin 307.45
 sleep wake cycle (24 hour), unspecified 780.55
  circadian rhythm 327.33
  nonorganic origin 307.45
 suture line (external) (*see also* Dehiscence)
  998.32
  internal 998.31
 wound 998.30
  cesarean operation 674.1
  episiotomy 674.2
  operation (surgical) 998.32
   cesarean 674.1
   internal 998.31

Disruption—*continued*
  wound—*continued*
    perineal (obstetric) 674.2
    uterine 674.1
Disruptio uteri —*see also* Rupture, uterus
  complicating delivery—*see* Delivery,
    complicated, rupture, uterus
Dissatisfaction with
  employment V62.29
  school environment V62.3
Dissecting —*see* condition
Dissection
  aorta 441.00
    abdominal 441.02
    thoracic 441.01
    thoracoabdominal 441.03
  artery, arterial
    carotid 443.21
    coronary 414.12
    iliac 443.22
    renal 443.23
    specified NEC 443.29
    vertebral 443.24
  vascular 459.9
  wound—*see* Wound, open, by site
Disseminated —*see* condition
Dissociated personality NEC 300.15
Dissociation
  auriculoventricular or atrioventricular (any
    degree) (AV) 426.89
    with heart block 426.0
  interference 426.89
  isorhythmic 426.89
  rhythm
    atrioventricular (AV) 426.89
    interference 426.89
Dissociative
  identity disorder 300.14
  reaction NEC 300.15
Dissolution, vertebra (*see also* Osteoporosis)
  733.00
Distention
  abdomen (gaseous) 787.3
  bladder 596.89
  cecum 569.89
  colon 569.89
  gallbladder 575.8
  gaseous (abdomen) 787.3
  intestine 569.89
  kidney 593.89
  liver 573.9
  seminal vesicle 608.89
  stomach 536.8
    acute 536.1
    psychogenic 306.4
  ureter 593.5
  uterus 621.8
Distichia, distichiasis (eyelid) 743.63
Distoma hepaticum infestation 121.3
Distomiasis 121.9
  bile passages 121.3
    due to Clonorchis sinensis 121.1
  hemic 120.9
  hepatic (liver) 121.3
    due to Clonorchis sinensis (clonorchiasis) 121.1
  intestinal 121.4
  liver 121.3
    due to Clonorchis sinensis 121.1
  lung 121.2
  pulmonary 121.2
Distomolar (fourth molar) 520.1
  causing crowding 524.31

Disto-occlusion (division I) (division II) 524.22
Distortion (congenital)
  adrenal (gland) 759.1
  ankle (joint) 755.69
  anus 751.5
  aorta 747.29
  appendix 751.5
  arm 755.59
  artery (peripheral) NEC (*see also* Distortion,
    peripheral vascular system) 747.60
    cerebral 747.81
    coronary 746.85
    pulmonary 747.39
    retinal 743.58
    umbilical 747.5
  auditory canal 744.29
    causing impairment of hearing 744.02
  bile duct or passage 751.69
  bladder 753.8
  brain 742.4
  bronchus 748.3
  cecum 751.5
  cervix (uteri) 752.49
  chest (wall) 756.3
  clavicle 755.51
  clitoris 752.49
  coccyx 756.19
  colon 751.5
  common duct 751.69
  cornea 743.41
  cricoid cartilage 748.3
  cystic duct 751.69
  duodenum 751.5
  ear 744.29
    auricle 744.29
      causing impairment of hearing 744.02
    causing impairment of hearing 744.09
    external 744.29
      causing impairment of hearing 744.02
    inner 744.05
    middle, except ossicles 744.03
      ossicles 744.04
    ossicles 744.04
  endocrine (gland) NEC 759.2
  epiglottis 748.3
  Eustachian tube 744.24
  eye 743.8
    adnexa 743.69
  face bone(s) 756.0
  fallopian tube 752.19
  femur 755.69
  fibula 755.69
  finger(s) 755.59
  foot 755.67
  gallbladder 751.69
  genitalia, genital organ(s)
    female 752.89
      external 752.49
      internal NEC 752.89
    male 752.89
      penis 752.69
  glottis 748.3
  gyri 742.4
  hand bone(s) 755.59
  heart (auricle) (ventricle) 746.89
    valve (cusp) 746.89
  hepatic duct 751.69
  humerus 755.59
  hymen 752.49
  ileum 751.5

Distortion—*continued*
  intestine (large) (small) 751.5
    with anomalous adhesions, fixation or
        malrotation 751.4
  jaw NEC 524.89
  jejunum 751.5
  kidney 753.3
  knee (joint) 755.64
  labium (majus) (minus) 752.49
  larynx 748.3
  leg 755.69
  lens 743.36
  liver 751.69
  lumbar spine 756.19
    with disproportion (fetopelvic) 653.0
      affecting fetus or newborn 763.1
      causing obstructed labor 660.1
  lumbosacral (joint) (region) 756.19
  lung (fissures) (lobe) 748.69
  nerve 742.8
  nose 748.1
  organ
    of Corti 744.05
    or site not listed—*see* Anomaly, specified type NEC
  ossicles, ear 744.04
  ovary 752.0
  oviduct 752.19
  pancreas 751.7
  parathyroid (gland) 759.2
  patella 755.64
  peripheral vascular system NEC 747.60
    gastrointestinal 747.61
    lower limb 747.64
    renal 747.62
    spinal 747.82
    upper limb 747.63
  pituitary (gland) 759.2
  radius 755.59
  rectum 751.5
  rib 756.3
  sacroiliac joint 755.69
  sacrum 756.19
  scapula 755.59
  shoulder girdle 755.59
  site not listed—*see* Anomaly, specified type NEC
  skull bone(s) 756.0
    with
      anencephalus 740.0
      encephalocele 742.0
      hydrocephalus 742.3
        with spina bifida (*see also* Spina bifida) 741.0
      microcephalus 742.1
  spinal cord 742.59
  spine 756.19
  spleen 759.0
  sternum 756.3
  thorax (wall) 756.3
  thymus (gland) 759.2
  thyroid (gland) 759.2
    cartilage 748.3
  tibia 755.69
  toe(s) 755.66
  tongue 750.19
  trachea (cartilage) 748.3
  ulna 755.59
  ureter 753.4
    causing obstruction 753.20
  urethra 753.8
    causing obstruction 753.6
  uterus 752.39
  vagina 752.49

Distortion—*continued*
  vein (peripheral) NEC (*see also* Distortion,
      peripheral vascular system) 747.60
    great 747.49
    portal 747.49
    pulmonary 747.49
  vena cava (inferior) (superior) 747.49
  vertebra 756.19
  visual NEC 368.15
    shape or size 368.14
  vulva 752.49
  wrist (bones) (joint) 755.59
Distress
  abdomen 789.0
  colon 789.0
  emotional V40.9
  epigastric 789.0
  fetal (syndrome) 768.4
    affecting management of pregnancy or
        childbirth 656.8
    liveborn infant 768.4
      first noted
        before onset of labor 768.2
        during labor and delivery 768.3
    stillborn infant (death before onset of labor)
        768.0
      death during labor 768.1
  gastrointestinal (functional) 536.9
    psychogenic 306.4
  intestinal (functional) NEC 564.9
    psychogenic 306.4
  intrauterine (*see* Distress, fetal)
  leg 729.5
  maternal 669.0
  mental V40.9
  respiratory 786.09
    acute (adult) 518.82
    adult syndrome (following trauma and
        surgery) 518.52
      specified NEC 518.82
    fetus or newborn 770.89
    syndrome (idiopathic) (newborn) 769
  stomach 536.9
    psychogenic 306.4
Distribution vessel, atypical NEC 747.60
  coronary artery 746.85
  spinal 747.82
Districhiasis 704.2
Disturbance —*see also* Disease
  absorption NEC 579.9
    calcium 269.3
    carbohydrate 579.8
    fat 579.8
    protein 579.8
    specified type NEC 579.8
    vitamin (*see also* Deficiency, vitamin) 269.2
  acid-base equilibrium 276.9
  activity and attention, simple, with hyperkinesis
      314.01
  amino acid (metabolic) (*see also* Disorder,
      amino acid) 270.9
    imidazole 270.5
    maple syrup (urine) disease 270.3
    transport 270.0
  assimilation, food 579.9
  attention, simple 314.00
    with hyperactivity 314.01
  auditory, nerve, except deafness 388.5
  behavior (*see also* Disturbance, conduct) 312.9
  blood clotting (hypoproteinemia) (mechanism)
      (*see also* Defect, coagulation) 286.9

Disturbance—*continued*
  central nervous system NEC 349.9
  cerebral nerve NEC 352.9
  circulatory 459.9
  conduct 312.9

---

*Note—Use the following fifth-digit
subclassification with categories 312.0-312.2:*

0 *unspecified*
1 *mild*
2 *moderate*
3 *severe*

---

    adjustment reaction 309.3
    adolescent onset type 312.82
    childhood onset type 312.81
    compulsive 312.30
      intermittent explosive disorder 312.34
      isolated explosive disorder 312.35
      kleptomania 312.32
      pathological gambling 312.31
      pyromania 312.33
    hyperkinetic 314.2
    intermittent explosive 312.34
    isolated explosive 312.35
    memory (*see also* Amnesia) 780.99
    mixed with emotions 312.4
    socialized (type) 312.20
      aggressive 312.23
      unaggressive 312.21
    specified type NEC 312.89
    undersocialized, unsocialized
      aggressive (type) 312.0
      unaggressive (type) 312.1
  coordination 781.3
  cranial nerve NEC 352.9
  deep sensibility—*see* Disturbance, sensation
  digestive 536.9
    psychogenic 306.4
  electrolyte—*see* Imbalance, electrolyte
  emotions specific to childhood or adolescence
    313.9
    with
      academic underachievement 313.83
      anxiety and fearfulness 313.0
      elective mutism 313.23
      identity disorder 313.82
      jealousy 313.3
      misery and unhappiness 313.1
      oppositional defiant disorder 313.81
      overanxiousness 313.0
      sensitivity 313.21
      shyness 313.21
      social withdrawal 313.22
      withdrawal reaction 313.22
      involving relationship problems 313.3
    mixed 313.89
    specified type NEC 313.89
  endocrine (gland) 259.9
    neonatal, transitory 775.9
      specified NEC 775.89
  equilibrium 780.4
  feeding (elderly) (infant) 783.3
    newborn 779.31
    nonorganic origin NEC 307.59
    psychogenic NEC 307.59
  fructose metabolism 271.2
  gait 781.2
    hysterical 300.11

Disturbance—*continued*
  gastric (functional) 536.9
    motility 536.8
    psychogenic 306.4
    secretion 536.8
  gastrointestinal (functional) 536.9
    psychogenic 306.4
  habit, child 307.9
  hearing, except deafness 388.40
  heart, functional (conditions classifiable to 426,
    427, 428)
    due to presence of (cardiac) prosthesis 429.4
    postoperative (immediate) 997.1
      long-term effect of cardiac surgery 429.4
    psychogenic 306.2
  hormone 259.9
  innervation uterus, sympathetic,
    parasympathetic 621.8
  keratinization NEC
    gingiva 523.10
    lip 528.5
    oral (mucosa) (soft tissue) 528.79
      residual ridge mucosa
        excessive 528.72
        minimal 528.71
    tongue 528.79
  labyrinth, labyrinthine (vestibule) 386.9
  learning, specific NEC 315.2
  memory (*see also* Amnesia) 780.93
    mild, following organic brain damage 310.89
  mental (*see also* Disorder, mental) 300.9
    associated with diseases classified elsewhere
      316
  metabolism (acquired) (congenital) (*see also*
    Disorder, metabolism) 277.9
    with
      abortion—*see* Abortion, by type, with
        metabolic disorder
      ectopic pregnancy (*see also* categories
        633.0-633.9) 639.4
      molar pregnancy (*see also* categories
        630-632) 639.4
    amino acid (*see also* Disorder, amino acid)
      270.9
      aromatic NEC 270.2
      branched-chain 270.3
      specified type NEC 270.8
      straight-chain NEC 270.7
      sulfur-bearing 270.4
      transport 270.0
    ammonia 270.6
    arginine 270.6
    argininosuccinic acid 270.6
    carbohydrate NEC 271.9
    cholesterol 272.9
    citrulline 270.6
    cystathionine 270.4
    fat 272.9
    following
      abortion 639.4
      ectopic or molar pregnancy 639.4
    general 277.9
      carbohydrate 271.9
      iron 275.09
      phosphate 275.3
      sodium 276.9
    glutamine 270.7
    glycine 270.7
    histidine 270.5
    homocystine 270.4
    in labor or delivery 669.0

Disturbance—*continued*
  metabolism—*continued*
    iron 275.09
    isoleucine 270.3
    leucine 270.3
    lipoid 272.9
      specified type NEC 272.8
    lysine 270.7
    methionine 270.4
    neonatal, transitory 775.9
      specified type NEC 775.89
    nitrogen 788.99
    ornithine 270.6
    phosphate 275.3
    phosphatides 272.7
    serine 270.7
    sodium NEC 276.9
    threonine 270.7
    tryptophan 270.2
    tyrosine 270.2
    urea cycle 270.6
    valine 270.3
  motor 796.1
  nervous functional 799.21
  neuromuscular mechanism (eye) due to syphilis
    094.84
  nutritional 269.9
    nail 703.8
  ocular motion 378.87
    psychogenic 306.7
  oculogyric 378.87
    psychogenic 306.7
  oculomotor NEC 378.87
    psychogenic 306.7
  olfactory nerve 781.1
  optic nerve NEC 377.49
  oral epithelium, including tongue 528.79
    residual ridge mucosa
      excessive 528.72
      minimal 528.71
  personality (pattern) (trait) (*see also* Disorder,
    personality) 301.9
    following organic brain damage 310.1
  polyglandular 258.9
  psychomotor 307.9
  pupillary 379.49
  reflex 796.1
  rhythm, heart 427.9
    postoperative (immediate) 997.1
      long-term effect of cardiac surgery 429.4
    psychogenic 306.2
  salivary secretion 527.7
  sensation (cold) (heat) (localization) (tactile
    discrimination localization) (texture)
    (vibratory) NEC 782.0
    hysterical 300.11
    skin 782.0
    smell 781.1
    taste 781.1
  sensory (*see also* Disturbance, sensation) 782.0
    innervation 782.0
  situational (transient) (*see also* Reaction,
    adjustment) 309.9
    acute 308.3
  sleep 780.50
    initiation or maintenance (*see also* Insomnia)
      780.52
      nonorganic origin 307.41
    nonorganic origin 307.40
      specified type NEC 307.49
    specified NEC 780.59
      nonorganic origin 307.49

Disturbance—*continued*
  sleep—*continued*
    wakefulness (*see also* Hypersomnia) 780.54
      nonorganic origin 307.43
    with apnea—*see* Apnea, sleep
  sociopathic 301.7
  speech NEC 784.59
    developmental 315.39
      associated with hyperkinesis 314.1
    secondary to organic lesion 784.59
  stomach (functional) (*see also* Disturbance,
    gastric) 536.9
  sympathetic (nerve) (*see also* Neuropathy,
    peripheral, autonomic) 337.9
  temperature sense 782.0
    hysterical 300.11
  tooth
    eruption 520.6
    formation 520.4
    structure, hereditary NEC 520.5
  touch (*see also* Disturbance, sensation) 782.0
  vascular 459.9
    arteriosclerotic—*see* Arteriosclerosis
    vasomotor 443.9
    vasospastic 443.9
  vestibular labyrinth 386.9
  vision, visual NEC 368.9
    psychophysical 368.16
    specified NEC 368.8
    subjective 368.10
  voice and resonance784.40
  wakefulness (initiation or maintenance) (*see
    also* Hypersomnia) 780.54
    nonorganic origin 307.43
Disulfiduria, beta-mercaptolactate-cysteine 270.0
Disuse atrophy, bone 733.7
Ditthomska syndrome 307.81
Diuresis 788.42
Divers'
  palsy or paralysis 993.3
  squeeze 993.3
Diverticula, diverticulosis, diverticulum (acute)
  (multiple) (perforated) (ruptured) 562.10
  with diverticulitis 562.11
  aorta (Kommerell's) 747.21
  appendix (noninflammatory) 543.9
  bladder (acquired) (sphincter) 596.3
    congenital 753.8
  broad ligament 620.8
  bronchus (congenital) 748.3
    acquired 494.0
      with acute exacerbation 494.1
  calyx, calyceal (kidney) 593.89
  cardia (stomach) 537.1
  cecum 562.10
    with
      diverticulitis 562.11
        with hemorrhage 562.13
      hemorrhage 562.12
    congenital 751.5
  colon (acquired) 562.10
    with
      diverticulitis 562.11
        with hemorrhage 562.13
      hemorrhage 562.12
    congenital 751.5
  duodenum 562.00
    with
      diverticulitis 562.01
        with hemorrhage 562.03
      hemorrhage 562.02
    congenital 751.5

Diverticula, diverticulosis—*continued*
  epiphrenic (esophagus) 530.6
  esophagus (congenital) 750.4
    acquired 530.6
    epiphrenic 530.6
    pulsion 530.6
    traction 530.6
    Zenker's 530.6
  Eustachian tube 381.89
  fallopian tube 620.8
  gallbladder (congenital) 751.69
  gastric 537.1
  heart (congenital) 746.89
  ileum 562.00
    with
      diverticulitis 562.01
        with hemorrhage 562.03
      hemorrhage 562.02
  intestine (large) 562.10
    with
      diverticulitis 562.11
        with hemorrhage 562.13
      hemorrhage 562.12
    congenital 751.5
    small 562.00
      with
        diverticulitis 562.01
          with hemorrhage 562.03
        hemorrhage 562.02
      congenital 751.5
  jejunum 562.00
    with
      diverticulitis 562.01
        with hemorrhage 562.03
      hemorrhage 562.02
  kidney (calyx) (pelvis) 593.89
    with calculus 592.0
  Kommerell's 747.21
  laryngeal ventricle (congenital) 748.3
  Meckel's (displaced) (hypertrophic) 751.0
  midthoracic 530.6
  organ or site, congenital NEC—*see* Distortion
  pericardium (congenital) (cyst) 746.89
    acquired (true) 423.8
  pharyngoesophageal (pulsion) 530.6
  pharynx (congenital) 750.27
  pulsion (esophagus) 530.6
  rectosigmoid 562.10
    with
      diverticulitis 562.11
        with hemorrhage 562.13
      hemorrhage 562.12
    congenital 751.5
  rectum 562.10
    with
      diverticulitis 562.11
        with hemorrhage 562.13
      hemorrhage 562.12
  renal (calyces) (pelvis) 593.89
    with calculus 592.0
  Rokitansky's 530.6
  seminal vesicle 608.0
  sigmoid 562.10
    with
      diverticulitis 562.11
        with hemorrhage 562.13
      hemorrhage 562.12
    congenital 751.5
  small intestine 562.00
    with
      diverticulitis 562.01
        with hemorrhage 562.03

Diverticula, diverticulosis—*continued*
    hemorrhage 562.02
  stomach (cardia) (juxtacardia) (juxtapyloric)
      (acquired) 537.1
    congenital 750.7
  subdiaphragmatic 530.6
  trachea (congenital) 748.3
    acquired 519.19
  traction (esophagus) 530.6
  ureter (acquired) 593.89
    congenital 753.4
  ureterovesical orifice 593.89
  urethra (acquired) 599.2
    congenital 753.8
  ventricle, left (congenital) 746.89
  vesical (urinary) 596.3
    congenital 753.8
  Zenker's (esophagus) 530.6
Diverticulitis (acute) (*see also* Diverticula) 562.11
  with hemorrhage 562.13
  bladder (urinary) 596.3
  cecum (perforated) 562.11
    with hemorrhage 562.13
  colon (perforated) 562.11
    with hemorrhage 562.13
  duodenum 562.01
    with hemorrhage 562.03
  esophagus 530.6
  ileum (perforated) 562.01
    with hemorrhage 562.03
  intestine (large) (perforated) 562.11
    with hemorrhage 562.13
    small 562.01
      with hemorrhage 562.03
  jejunum (perforated) 562.01
    with hemorrhage 562.03
  Meckel's (perforated) 751.0
  pharyngoesophageal 530.6
  rectosigmoid (perforated) 562.11
    with hemorrhage 562.13
  rectum 562.11
    with hemorrhage 562.13
  sigmoid (old) (perforated) 562.11
    with hemorrhage 562.13
  small intestine (perforated) 562.01
    with hemorrhage 562.03
  vesical (urinary) 596.3
Diverticulosis —*see* Diverticula
Division
  cervix uteri 622.8
    external os into two openings by frenum 752.44
  external (cervical) into two openings by frenum
      752.44
  glans penis 752.69
  hymen 752.49
  labia minora (congenital) 752.49
  ligament (partial or complete) (current)—*see
      also* Sprain, by site
    with open wound—*see* Wound, open, by site
  muscle (partial or complete) (current)—*see also*
      Sprain, by site
    with open wound—*see* Wound, open, by site
  nerve—*see* Injury, nerve, by site
  penis glans 752.69
  spinal cord—*see* Injury, spinal, by site
  vein 459.9
    traumatic—*see* Injury, vascular, by site
Divorce V61.03
Dix-Hallpike neurolabyrinthitis 386.12
Dizziness 780.4
  hysterical 300.11
  psychogenic 306.9

Doan-Wiseman syndrome (primary splenic neutropenia) 289.53
Dog bite —*see* Wound, open, by site
Döhle-Heller aortitis 093.1
Döhle body-panmyelopathic syndrome 288.2
Dolichocephaly, dolichocephalus 754.0
Dolichocolon 751.5
Dolichostenomelia 759.82
Donohue's syndrome (leprechaunism) 259.8
Donor
 blood V59.01
  other blood components V59.09
  stem cells V59.02
  whole blood V59.01
 bone V59.2
  marrow V59.3
 cornea V59.5
 egg (oocyte) (ovum) V59.70
  age 35 and over V59.73
   anonymous recipient V59.73
   designated recipient V59.74
  under age 35 V59.71
   anonymous recipient V59.71
   designated recipient V59.72
 heart V59.8
 kidney V59.4
 liver V59.6
 lung V59.8
 lymphocyte V59.8
 organ V59.9
  specified NEC V59.8
 potential, examination of V70.8
 skin V59.1
 specified organ or tissue NEC V59.8
 sperm V59.8
 stem cells V59.02
 tissue V59.9
  specified type NEC V59.8
Donovanosis (granuloma venereum) 099.2
DOPS (diffuse obstructive pulmonary syndrome) 496
Double
 albumin 273.8
 aortic arch 747.21
 auditory canal 744.29
 auricle (heart) 746.82
 bladder 753.8
 external (cervical) os 752.44
 kidney with double pelvis (renal) 753.3
 larynx 748.3
 meatus urinarius 753.8
 organ or site NEC—*see* Accessory
 orifice
  heart valve NEC 746.89
   pulmonary 746.09
 outlet, right ventricle 745.11
 pelvis (renal) with double ureter 753.4
 penis 752.69
 tongue 750.13
 ureter (one or both sides) 753.4
  with double pelvis (renal) 753.4
 urethra 753.8
 urinary meatus 753.8
 uterus (any degree) 752.2
  with doubling of cervix and vagina 752.2
  in pregnancy or childbirth 654.0
   affecting fetus or newborn 763.89
 vagina 752.47
  with doubling of cervix and uterus 752.2
 vision 368.2
 vocal cords 748.3
 vulva 752.49
 whammy (syndrome) 360.81

Douglas' pouch, cul-de-sac —*see* condition
Down's disease or syndrome (mongolism) 758.0
Down-growth, epithelial (anterior chamber) 364.61
DPD (dihydropyrimidine dehydrogenase deficiency) 277.6
Dracontiasis 125.7
Dracunculiasis 125.7
Dracunculosis 125.7
Drainage
 abscess (spontaneous)—*see* Abscess
 anomalous pulmonary veins to hepatic veins or right atrium 747.41
 stump (amputation) (surgical) 997.62
 suprapubic, bladder 596.89
Dream state, hysterical 300.13
Drepanocytic anemia (*see also* Disease, sickle cell) 282.60
Dresbach's syndrome (elliptocytosis) 282.1
Dreschlera (infection) 118
 hawaiiensis 117.8
Dressler's syndrome (postmyocardial infarction) 411.0
Dribbling (post-void) **788.35**
Drift, ulnar 736.09
Drinking (alcohol)—*see also* Alcoholism
 excessive, to excess NEC (*see also* Abuse, drugs, nondependent) 305.0
  bouts, periodic 305.0
  continual 303.9
  episodic 305.0
  habitual 303.9
  periodic 305.0
Drip, postnasal (chronic) 784.91
 due to
  allergic rhinitis —*see* Rhinitis, allergic
  common cold 460
  gastroesophageal reflux —*see* Reflux, gastroesophageal
  nasopharyngitis —*see* Nasopharyngitis
  other known condition —*code to condition*
  sinusitis —*see* Sinusitis
Drivers' license examination V70.3
Droop
 Cooper's 611.81
 facial 781.94
Drop
 finger 736.29
 foot 736.79
 hematocrit (precipitous) 790.01
 hemoglobin 790.01
 toe 735.8
 wrist 736.05
Dropped
 dead 798.1
 heart beats 426.6
Dropsy, dropsical (*see also* Edema) 782.3
 abdomen 789.59
 amnion (*see also* Hydramnios) 657
 brain—*see* Hydrocephalus
 cardiac (*see also* Failure, heart) 428.0
 cardiorenal (*see also* Hypertension, cardiorenal) 404.90
 chest 511.9
 fetus or newborn 778.0
  due to isoimmunization 773.3
 gangrenous (*see also* Gangrene) 785.4
 heart (*see also* Failure, heart) 428.0
 hepatic—*see* Cirrhosis, liver
 infantile—*see* Hydrops, fetalis
 kidney (*see also* Nephrosis) 581.9
 liver—*see* Cirrhosis, liver

Dropsy, dropsical—*continued*
  lung 514
  malarial (*see also* Malaria) 084.9
  neonatorum—*see* Hydrops, fetalis
  nephritic 581.9
  newborn—*see* Hydrops, fetalis
  nutritional 269.9
  ovary 620.8
  pericardium (*see also* Pericarditis) 423.9
  renal (*see also* Nephrosis) 581.9
  uremic—*see* Uremia
Drowned, drowning (near) 994.1
  lung 518.52
Drowsiness 780.09
Drug —*see also* condition
  addiction (*see also* listing under Dependence) 304.9
  adverse effect, correct substance properly
    administered 995.20
  allergy 995.27
  dependence (*see also* listing under Dependence) 304.9
  habit (*see also* listing under Dependence) 304.9
  hypersensitivity 995.27
  induced
    circadian rhythm sleep disorder 292.85
    hypersomnia 292.85
    insomnia 292.85
    mental disorder 292.9
      anxiety 292.89
      mood 292.84
      sexual 292.89
      sleep 292.85
      specified type 292.89
    parasomnia 292.85
    persisting
      amnestic disorder 292.83
      dementia 292.82
    psychotic disorder
      with
        delusions 292.11
        hallucinations 292.12
    sleep disorder 292.85
  intoxication 292.89
  overdose—*see* Table of drugs and chemicals
  poisoning—*see* Table of drugs and chemicals
  therapy (maintenance) status NEC
    chemotherapy, antineoplastic V58.11
    immunotherapy, antineoplastic V58.12
    long-term (current) (prophylactic) use V58.69
      antibiotics V58.62
      anticoagulants V58.61
      anti-inflammatories, non-steroidal (NSAID)
        V58.64
      antiplatelets V58.63
      antithrombotics V58.63
      aspirin V58.66
      bisphosphonates V58.68
      high-risk medications NEC V58.69
      insulin V58.67
      methadone for pain control V58.69
      opiate analgesic V58.69
      steroids V58.65
    methadone 304.00
  wrong substance given or taken in error—*see*
    Table of drugs and chemicals
Drunkenness (*see also* Abuse, drugs,
  nondependent) 305.0
  acute in alcoholism (*see also* Alcoholism) 303.0
  chronic (*see also* Alcoholism) 303.9
  pathologic 291.4
  simple (acute) 305.0
    in alcoholism 303.0
  sleep 307.47

Drusen
  optic disc or papilla 377.21
  retina (colloid) (hyaloid degeneration) 362.57
    hereditary 362.77
Drusenfieber 075
Dry, dryness —*see also* condition
  eye 375.15
    syndrome 375.15
  larynx 478.79
  mouth 527.7
  nose 478.19
  skin syndrome 701.1
  socket (teeth) 526.5
  throat 478.29
DSAP (disseminated superficial actinic
  porokeratosis) 692.75
DSTR (delayed serologic transfusion reaction)
  due to or resulting from incompatibility
    ABO 999.69
    non-ABO antigen (minor) (Duffy) (Kell)
      (Kidd) (Lewis) (M) (N) (P) (S) 999.79
    Rh antigen (C) (c) (D) (E) (e) 999.74
Duane's retraction syndrome 378.71
Duane-Stilling-Turk syndrome (ocular
  retraction syndrome) 378.71
Dubin-Johnson disease or syndrome 277.4
Dubini's disease (electric chorea) 049.8
Dubois' abscess or disease 090.5
Duchenne's
  disease 094.0
    locomotor ataxia 094.0
    muscular dystrophy 359.1
    pseudohypertrophy, muscles 359.1
  paralysis 335.22
  syndrome 335.22
Duchenne-Aran myelopathic muscular atrophy
  (nonprogressive) (progressive) 335.21
Duchenne-Griesinger disease 359.1
Ducrey's
  bacillus 099.0
  chancre 099.0
  disease (chancroid) 099.0
Duct, ductus —*see* condition
Duengero 061
Duhring's disease (dermatitis herpetiformis) 694.0
Dukes (-Filatov) disease 057.8
Dullness
  cardiac (decreased) (increased) 785.3
Dumb ague (*see also* Malaria) 084.6
Dumbness (*see also* Aphasia) 784.3
Dumdum fever 085.0
Dumping syndrome (postgastrectomy) 564.2
  nonsurgical 536.8
Duodenitis (nonspecific) (peptic) 535.60
  due to
    Strongyloides stercoralis 127.2
  with hemorrhage 535.61
Duodenocholangitis 575.8
Duodenum, duodenal —*see* condition
Duplay's disease, periarthritis, or syndrome
  726.2
Duplex —*see also* Accessory
  kidney 753.3
  placenta—*see* Placenta, abnormal
  uterus 752.2
Duplication —*see also* Accessory
  anus 751.5
  aortic arch 747.21
  appendix 751.5
  biliary duct (any) 751.69
  bladder 753.8

Duplication—*continued*
 cecum 751.5
  and appendix 751.5
 cervical, cervix 752.44
 clitoris 752.49
 cystic duct 751.69
 digestive organs 751.8
 duodenum 751.5
 esophagus 750.4
 fallopian tube 752.19
 frontonasal process 756.0
 gallbladder 751.69
 ileum 751.5
 intestine (large) (small) 751.5
 jejunum 751.5
 kidney 753.3
 liver 751.69
 nose 748.1
 pancreas 751.7
 penis 752.69
 respiratory organs NEC 748.9
 salivary duct 750.22
 spinal cord (incomplete) 742.51
 stomach 750.7
 ureter 753.4
 vagina 752.47
 vas deferens 752.89
 vocal cords 748.3
Dupré's disease or syndrome (meningism) 781.6
Dupuytren's
 contraction 728.6
 disease (muscle contracture) 728.6
 fracture (closed) 824.4
  ankle (closed) 824.4
   open 824.5
  fibula (closed) 824.4
   open 824.5
   open 824.5
  radius (closed) 813.42
   open 813.52
 muscle contracture 728.6
Durand-Nicolas-Favre disease (climatic bubo) 099.1
Durotomy incidental (inadvertent) (*see also* Tear, dural) 349.31
Duroziez's disease (congenital mitral stenosis) 746.5
Dust
 conjunctivitis 372.05
 reticulation (occupational) 504
Dutton's
 disease (trypanosomiasis) 086.9
 relapsing fever (West African) 087.1
Dwarf, dwarfism 259.4
 with infantilism (hypophyseal) 253.3
 achondroplastic 756.4
 Amsterdam 759.89
 bird-headed 759.89
 congenital 259.4
 constitutional 259.4
 hypophyseal 253.3
 infantile 259.4
 Levi type 253.3
 Lorain-Levi (pituitary) 253.3
 Lorain type (pituitary) 253.3
 metatropic 756.4
 nephrotic-glycosuric, with hypophosphatemic rickets 270.0
 nutritional 263.2
 ovarian 758.6
 pancreatic 577.8
 pituitary 253.3
 polydystrophic 277.5

Dwarf, dwarfism—*continued*
 primordial 253.3
 psychosocial 259.4
 renal 588.0
  with hypertension—*see* Hypertension, kidney
 Russell's (uterine dwarfism and craniofacial dysostosis) 759.89
Dyke-Young anemia or syndrome (acquired macrocytic hemolytic anemia) (secondary) (symptomatic) 283.9
Dynia abnormality (*see also* Defect, coagulation) 286.9
Dysacousis 388.40
Dysadrenocortism 255.9
 hyperfunction 255.3
 hypofunction 255.41
Dysarthria 784.51
 due to late effect of cerebrovascular disease (*see also* Late effect(s) (of) cerebrovascular disease) 438.13
Dysautonomia (*see also* Neuropathy, peripheral, autonomic) 337.9
 familial 742.8
Dysbarism 993.3
Dysbasia 719.7
 angiosclerotica intermittens 443.9
  due to atherosclerosis 440.21
 hysterical 300.11
 lordotica (progressiva) 333.6
 nonorganic origin 307.9
 psychogenic 307.9
Dysbetalipoproteinemia (familial) 272.2
Dyscalculia 315.1
Dyschezia (*see also* Constipation) 564.00
Dyschondroplasia (with hemangiomata) 756.4
 Voorhoeve's 756.4
Dyschondrosteosis 756.59
Dyschromia 709.00
Dyscollagenosis 710.9
Dyscoria 743.41
Dyscraniopyophalangy 759.89
Dyscrasia
 blood 289.9
  with antepartum hemorrhage 641.3
  hemorrhage, subungual 287.8
  puerperal, postpartum 666.3
 ovary 256.8
 plasma cell 273.9
 pluriglandular 258.9
 polyglandular 258.9
Dysdiadochokinesia 781.3
Dysectasia, vesical neck 596.89
Dysendocrinism 259.9
Dysentery, dysenteric (bilious) (catarrhal) (diarrhea) (epidemic) (gangrenous) (hemorrhagic) (infectious) (sporadic) (tropical) (ulcerative) 009.0
 abscess, liver (*see also* Abscess, amebic) 006.3
 amebic (*see also* Amebiasis) 006.9
  with abscess—*see* Abscess, amebic
  acute 006.0
  carrier (suspected) of V02.2
  chronic 006.1
 arthritis (*see also* Arthritis, due to, dysentery) 009.0 *[711.3]*
  bacillary 004.9 *[711.3]*
 asylum 004.9
 bacillary 004.9
  arthritis 004.9 *[711.3]*
  Boyd 004.2
  Flexner 004.1

Dysentery, dysenteric—*continued*
  bacillary—*continued*
    Schmitz (-Stutzer) 004.0
    Shiga 004.0
    Shigella 004.9
      group A 004.0
      group B 004.1
      group C 004.2
      group D 004.3
      specified type NEC 004.8
    Sonne 004.3
    specified type NEC 004.8
  bacterium 004.9
  balantidial 007.0
  Balantidium coli 007.0
  Boyd's 004.2
  Chilomastix 007.8
  Chinese 004.9
  choleriform 001.1
  coccidial 007.2
  Dientamoeba fragilis 007.8
  due to specified organism NEC—*see* Enteritis,
    due to, by organism
  Embadomonas 007.8
  Endolimax nana—*see* Dysentery, amebic
  Entamoba, entamebic—*see* Dysentery, amebic
  Flexner's 004.1
  Flexner-Boyd 004.2
  giardial 007.1
  Giardia lamblia 007.1
  Hiss-Russell 004.1
  lamblia 007.1
  leishmanial 085.0
  malarial (*see also* Malaria) 084.6
  metazoal 127.9
  Monilia 112.89
  protozoal NEC 007.9
  Russell's 004.8
  salmonella 003.0
  schistosomal 120.1
  Schmitz (-Stutzer) 004.0
  Shiga 004.0
  Shigella NEC (*see also* Dysentery, bacillary)
    004.9
    boydii 004.2
    dysenteriae 004.0
      Schmitz 004.0
      Shiga 004.0
    flexneri 004.1
    Group A 004.0
    Group B 004.1
    Group C 004.2
    Group D 004.3
    Schmitz 004.0
    Shiga 004.0
    Sonnei 004.3
  Sonne 004.3
  strongyloidiasis 127.2
  trichomonal 007.3
  tuberculous (*see also* Tuberculosis) 014.8
  viral (*see also* Enteritis, viral) 008.8
Dysequilibrium 780.4
Dysesthesia 782.0
  hysterical 300.11
Dysfibrinogenemia (congenital) (*see also* Defect,
  coagulation) 286.3
Dysfunction
  adrenal (cortical) 255.9
    hyperfunction 255.3
    hypofunction 255.41

Dysfunction—*continued*
  associated with sleep stages or arousal from
    sleep 780.56
    nonorganic origin 307.47
  bladder NEC 596.59
  bleeding, uterus 626.8
  brain, minimal (*see also* Hyperkinesia) 314.9
  cerebral 348.30
  colon 564.9
    psychogenic 306.4
  colostomy or enterostomy 569.62
  cystic duct 575.8
  diastolic 429.9
    with heart failure—*see* Failure, heart
    due to
      cardiomyopathy—*see* Cardiomyopathy
      hypertension—*see* Hypertension, heart
  endocrine NEC 259.9
  endometrium 621.8
  enteric stoma 569.62
  enterostomy 569.62
  erectile 607.84
    nonorganic origin 302.72
  esophagostomy 530.87
  Eustachian tube 381.81
  gallbladder 575.8
  gastrointestinal 536.9
  gland, glandular NEC 259.9
  heart 427.9
    postoperative (immediate) 997.1
      long-term effect of cardiac surgery 429.4
  hemoglobin 289.89
  hepatic 573.9
  hepatocellular NEC 573.9
  hypophysis 253.9
    hyperfunction 253.1
    hypofunction 253.2
    posterior lobe 253.6
      hypofunction 253.5
  kidney (*see also* Disease, renal) 593.9
  labyrinthine 386.50
    specified NEC 386.58
  liver 573.9
    constitutional 277.4
  minimal brain (child) (*see also* Hyperkinesia)
    314.9
  ovary, ovarian 256.9
    hyperfunction 256.1
      estrogen 256.0
    hypofunction 256.39
      postablative 256.2
    postablative 256.2
    specified NEC 256.8
  papillary muscle 429.81
    with myocardial infarction 410.8
  parathyroid 252.8
    hyperfunction 252.00
    hypofunction 252.1
  pineal gland 259.8
  pituitary (gland) 253.9
    hyperfunction 253.1
    hypofunction 253.2
    posterior 253.6
      hypofunction 253.5
  placental—*see* Placenta, insufficiency
  platelets (blood) 287.1
  polyglandular 258.9
    specified NEC 258.8

Dysfunction—*continued*
　psychosexual 302.70
　　with
　　　dyspareunia (functional) (psychogenic)
　　　　302.76
　　　frigidity 302.72
　　　impotence 302.72
　　　inhibition
　　　　orgasm
　　　　　female 302.73
　　　　　male 302.74
　　　　sexual
　　　　　desire 302.71
　　　　　excitement 302.72
　　　premature ejaculation 302.75
　　　sexual aversion 302.79
　　　specified disorder NEC 302.79
　　　vaginismus 306.51
　pylorus 537.9
　rectum 564.9
　　psychogenic 306.4
　segmental (*see also* Dysfunction, somatic) 739.9
　senile 797
　sexual 302.70
　sinoatrial node 427.81
　somatic 739.9
　　abdomen 739.9
　　acromioclavicular 739.7
　　cervical 739.1
　　cervicothoracic 739.1
　　costochondral 739.8
　　costovertebral 739.8
　　extremities
　　　lower 739.6
　　　upper 739.7
　　head 739.0
　　hip 739.5
　　umbar, lumbosacral 739.3
　　occipitocervical 739.0
　　pelvic 739.5
　　pubic 739.5
　　rib cage 739.8
　　sacral 739.4
　　sacrococcygeal 739.4
　　sacroiliac 739.4
　　specified site NEC 739.9
　　sternochondral 739.8
　　sternoclavicular 739.7
　　temporomandibular 739.0
　　thoracic, thoracolumbar 739.2
　stomach 536.9
　　psychogenic 306.4
　suprarenal 255.9
　　hyperfunction 255.3
　　hypofunction 255.41
　symbolic NEC 784.60
　　specified type NEC 784.69
　systolic 429.9
　　with heart failure—*see* Failure, heart
　temporomandibular (joint)
　　(joint-pain-syndrome) NEC 524.60
　　sounds on opening or closing 524.64
　　specified NEC 524.69
　testicular 257.9
　　hyperfunction 257.0
　　hypofunction 257.2
　　specified type NEC 257.8
　thymus 254.9

Dysfunction—*continued*
　thyroid 246.9
　　complicating pregnancy, childbirth, or
　　　puerperium 648.1
　　hyperfunction—*see* Hyperthyroidism
　　hypofunction—*see* Hypothyroidism
　uterus, complicating delivery 661.9
　　affecting fetus or newborn 763.7
　　hypertonic 661.4
　　hypotonic 661.2
　　　primary 661.0
　　　secondary 661.1
　velopharyngeal (acquired) 528.9
　　congenital 750.29
　ventricular 429.9
　　with congestive heart failure (*see also* Failure,
　　　heart) 428.0
　　due to
　　　cardiomyopathy—*see* Cardiomyopathy
　　　hypertension—*see* Hypertension, heart
　　left, reversible following sudden emotional
　　　stress 429.83
　vesicourethral NEC 596.59
　vestibular 386.50
　　specified type NEC 386.58
Dysgammaglobulinemia 279.06
Dysgenesis
　gonadal (due to chromosomal anomaly) 758.6
　　pure 752.7
　kidney(s) 753.0
　ovarian 758.6
　renal 753.0
　reticular 279.2
　seminiferous tubules 758.6
　tidal platelet 287.31
Dysgerminoma (M9060/3)
　specified site—*see* Neoplasm, by site, malignant
　unspecified site
　　female 183.0
　　male 186.9
Dysgeusia 781.1
Dysgraphia 781.3
Dyshidrosis 705.81
Dysidrosis 705.81
Dysinsulinism 251.8
Dyskaryotic cervical smear 795.09
Dyskeratosis (*see also* Keratosis) 701.1
　bullosa hereditaria 757.39
　cervix 622.10
　congenital 757.39
　follicularis 757.39
　　vitamin A deficiency 264.8
　gingiva 523.8
　oral soft tissue NEC 528.79
　tongue 528.79
　uterus NEC 621.8
Dyskinesia 781.3
　biliary 575.8
　esophagus 530.5
　hysterical 300.11
　intestinal 564.89
　neuroleptic-induced tardive 333.85
　nonorganic origin 307.9
　orofacial 333.82
　　due to drugs 333.85
　psychogenic 307.9
　subacute, due to drugs 333.85
　tardive (oral) 333.85
Dyslalia 784.59
　developmental 315.39

Dyslexia 784.61
  developmental 315.02
  secondary to organic lesion 784.61
Dyslipidemia 272.4
Dysmaturity *(see also* Immaturity) 765.1
  lung 770.4
  pulmonary 770.4
Dysmenorrhea (essential) (exfoliative)
  (functional) (intrinsic) (membranous)
  (primary) (secondary) 625.3
  psychogenic 306.52
Dysmetabolic syndrome X 277.7
Dysmetria 781.3
Dysmorodystrophia mesodermalis congenita
  759.82
Dysnomia 784.3
Dysorexia 783.0
  hysterical 300.11
Dysostosis
  cleidocranial, cleidocranialis 755.59
  craniofacial 756.0
  Fairbank's (idiopathic familial generalized
    osteophytosis) 756.50
  mandibularis 756.0
  mandibulofacial, incomplete 756.0
  multiplex 277.5
  orodigitofacial 759.89
Dyspareunia (female) 625.0
  male 608.89
  psychogenic 302.76
Dyspepsia (allergic) (congenital) (fermentative)
  (flatulent) (functional) (gastric) (gastrointestinal)
  (neurogenic) (occupational) (reflex) 536.8
  acid 536.8
  atonic 536.3
    psychogenic 306.4
  diarrhea 787.91
    psychogenic 306.4
  intestinal 564.89
    psychogenic 306.4
  nervous 306.4
  neurotic 306.4
  psychogenic 306.4
Dysphagia 787.20
  cervical 787.29
  functional 300.11
  hysterical 300.11
  nervous 300.11
  neurogenic 787.29
  oral phase 787.21
  oropharyngeal phase 787.22
  pharyngeal phase 787.23
  pharyngoesophageal phase 787.24
  psychogenic 306.4
  sideropenic 280.8
  spastica 530.5
  specified NEC 787.29
Dysphagocytosis, congenital 288.1
Dysphasia 784.59
Dysphonia 784.42
  clericorum 784.49
  functional 300.11
  hysterical 300.11
  psychogenic 306.1
  spastica 478.79
Dyspigmentation *—see also* Pigmentation
  eyelid (acquired) 374.52
Dyspituitarism 253.9
  hyperfunction 253.1
  hypofunction 253.2
  posterior lobe 253.6

Dysplasia *—see also* Anomaly
  alveolar capillary, with vein misalignment
    516.64
  anus 569.44
    intraepithelial neoplasia I (AIN I)
      (histologically confirmed) 569.44
    intraepithelial neoplasia II (AIN II)
      (histologically confirmed) 569.44
    intraepithelial neoplasia III (AIN III) 230.6
      anal canal 230.5
    mild (histologically confirmed) 569.44
    moderate (histologically confirmed) 569.44
    severe 230.6
      anal canal 230.5
  artery
    fibromuscular NEC 447.8
      carotid 447.8
      renal 447.3
  bladder 596.89
  bone (fibrous) NEC 733.29
    diaphyseal, progressive 756.59
    jaw 526.89
    monostotic 733.29
    polyostotic 756.54
    solitary 733.29
  brain 742.9
  bronchopulmonary, fetus or newborn 770.7
  cervix (uteri) 622.10
    cervical intraepithelial neoplasia I (CIN 1)
      622.11
    cervical intraepithelial neoplasia II (CIN II)
      622.12
    cervical intraepithelial neoplasia III (CIN III)
      233.1
    CIN I 622.11
    CIN II 622.12
    CIN III 233.1
    mild 622.11
    moderate 622.12
    severe 233.1
  chondroectodermal 756.55
  chondromatose 756.4
  colon 211.3
  craniocarpotarsal 759.89
  craniometaphyseal 756.89
  dentinal 520.5
  diaphyseal, progressive 756.59
  ectodermal (anhidrotic) (Bason) (Clouston's)
    (congenital) (Feinmesser) (hereditary)
    (hidrotic) (Marshall) (Robinson's) 757.31
  epiphysealis 756.9
    multiplex 756.56
    punctata 756.59
  epiphysis 756.9
    multiple 756.56
  epithelial
    epiglottis 478.79
    uterine cervix 622.10
  erythroid NEC 289.89
  eye *(see also* Microphthalmos) 743.10
  familial metaphyseal 756.89
  fibromuscular, artery NEC 447.8
    carotid 447.8
    renal 447.3
  fibrous
    bone NEC 733.29
    diaphyseal, progressive 756.59
    jaw 526.89
    monostotic 733.29
    polyostotic 756.54
    solitary 733.29

Dysplasia—*continued*
high grade, focal—*see* Neoplasm, by site, benign
hip (congenital) 755.63
  with dislocation (*see also* Dislocation, hip,
    congenital) 754.30
hypohidrotic ectodermal 757.31
joint 755.8
kidney 753.15
leg 755.69
linguofacialis 759.89
lung 748.5
macular 743.55
mammary (benign) (gland) 610.9
  cystic 610.1
  specified type NEC 610.8
metaphyseal 756.9
  familial 756.89
monostotic fibrous 733.29
muscle 756.89
myeloid NEC 289.89
nervous system (general) 742.9
neuroectodermal 759.6
oculoauriculovertebral 756.0
oculodentodigital 759.89
olfactogenital 253.4
osteo-onycho-arthro (hereditary) 756.89
periosteum 733.99
polyostotic fibrous 756.54
progressive diaphyseal 756.59
prostate 602.3
  intraepithelial neoplasia I (PIN I) 602.3
  intraepithelial neoplasia II (PIN II) 602.3
  intraepithelial neoplasia III (PIN III) 233.4
renal 753.15
renofacialis 753.0
retinal NEC 743.56
retrolental (*see also* Retinopathy of prematurity)
    362.21
skin 709.8
spinal cord 742.9
thymic, with immunodeficiency 279.2
vagina 623.0
  mild 623.0
  moderate 623.0
  severe 233.31
vocal cord 478.5
vulva 624.8
  intraepithelial neoplasia I (VIN I) 624.01
  intraepithelial neoplasia II (VIN II) 624.02
  intraepithelial neoplasia III (VIN III) 233.32
  mild 624.01
  moderate 624.02
  severe 233.32
  VIN I 624.01
  VIN II 624.02
  VIN III 233.32
Dyspnea (nocturnal) (paroxysmal) 786.09
asthmatic (bronchial) (*see also* Asthma) 493.9
  with bronchitis (*see also* Asthma) 493.9
    chronic 493.2
cardiac (*see also* Failure, ventricular, left) 428.1
cardiac (*see also* Failure, ventricular, left) 428.1
functional 300.11
hyperventilation 786.01
hysterical 300.11
Monday morning 504
newborn 770.89
psychogenic 306.1
uremic—*see* Uremia
Dyspraxia 781.3
syndrome 315.4

Dysproteinemia 273.8
transient with copper deficiency 281.4
Dysprothrombinemia (constitutional) (*see also*
  Defect, coagulation) 286.3
Dysreflexia, autonomic 337.3
Dysrhythmia
cardiac 427.9
  postoperative (immediate) 997.1
    long-term effect of cardiac surgery 429.4
  specified type NEC 427.89
cerebral or cortical 348.30
Dyssecretosis, mucoserous 710.2
**Dyssocial reaction without manifest psychiatric
  disorder**
adolescent V71.02
adult V71.01
child V71.02
Dyssomnia NEC 780.56
nonorganic origin 307.47
Dyssplenism 289.4
Dyssynergia
biliary (*see also* Disease, biliary) 576.8
cerebellaris myoclonica 334.2
detrusor sphincter (bladder) 596.55
ventricular 429.89
Dystasia, hereditary areflexic 334.3
Dysthymia 300.4
Dysthymic disorder 300.4
Dysthyroidism 246.9
Dystocia 660.9
affecting fetus or newborn 763.1
cervical 661.2
  affecting fetus or newborn 763.7
contraction ring 661.4
  affecting fetus or newborn 763.7
fetal 660.9
  abnormal size 653.5
  affecting fetus or newborn 763.1
  deformity 653.7
maternal 660.9
  affecting fetus or newborn 763.1
positional 660.0
  affecting fetus or newborn 763.1
shoulder (girdle) 660.4
  affecting fetus or newborn 763.1
uterine NEC 661.4
  affecting fetus or newborn 763.7
Dystonia
acute
  due to drugs 333.72
    neuroleptic-induced acute 333.72
deformans progressiva 333.6
lenticularis 333.6
musculorum deformans 333.6
torsion (idiopathic) 333.6
  acquired 333.79
  fragments (of) 333.89
  genetic 333.6
  symptomatic 333.79
Dystonic
movements 781.0
Dystopia kidney 753.3
Dystrophy, dystrophia 783.9
adiposogenital 253.8
asphyxiating thoracic 756.4
Becker's type 359.22
brevicollis 756.16
Bruch's membrane 362.77
cervical (sympathetic) NEC 337.09
chondro-osseus with punctate epiphyseal
    dysplasia 756.59

Dystrophy, dystrophia—*continued*
choroid (hereditary) 363.50
  central (areolar) (partial) 363.53
    total (gyrate) 363.54
  circinate 363.53
  circumpapillary (partial) 363.51
    total 363.52
  diffuse
    partial 363.56
    total 363.57
  generalized
    partial 363.56
    total 363.57
  gyrate
    central 363.54
    generalized 363.57
  helicoid 363.52
  peripapillary—*see* Dystrophy, choroid,
    circumpapillary
  serpiginous 363.54
cornea (hereditary) 371.50
  anterior NEC 371.52
  Cogan's 371.52
  combined 371.57
  crystalline 371.56
  endothelial (Fuchs') 371.57
  epithelial 371.50
    juvenile 371.51
    microscopic cystic 371.52
  granular 371.53
  lattice 371.54
  macular 371.55
  marginal (Terrien's) 371.48
  Meesman's 371.51
  microscopic cystic (epithelial) 371.52
  nodular, Salzmann's 371.46
  polymorphous 371.58
  posterior NEC 371.58
  ring-like 371.52
  Salzmann's nodular 371.46
  stromal NEC 371.56
dermatochondrocorneal 371.50
Duchenne's 359.1
due to malnutrition 263.9
Erb's 359.1
familial
  hyperplastic periosteal 756.59
  osseous 277.5
foveal 362.77
Fuchs', cornea 371.57
Gowers' muscular 359.1
hair 704.2
hereditary, progressive muscular 359.1
hypogenital, with diabetic tendency 759.81
Landouzy-Déjérine 359.1
Leyden-Möbius 359.1
mesodermalis congenita 759.82
muscular 359.1
  congenital (hereditary) 359.0
    myotonic 359.22
  distal 359.1
  Duchenne's 359.1
  Erb's 359.1
  fascioscapulohumeral 359.1
  Gowers' 359.1
  hereditary (progressive) 359.1
  Landouzy-Déjérine 359.1
  limb-girdle 359.1
  myotonic 359.21
  progressive (hereditary) 359.1
    Charcot-Marie-Tooth 356.1
  pseudohypertrophic (infantile) 359.1

Dystrophy, dystrophia—*continued*
myocardium, myocardial (*see also*
  Degeneration, myocardial) 429.1
myotonic 359.21
myotonica 359.21
nail 703.8
  congenital 757.5
neurovascular (traumatic) (*see also* Neuropathy,
  peripheral, autonomic) 337.9
nutritional 263.9
ocular 359.1
oculocerebrorenal 270.8
oculopharyngeal 359.1
ovarian 620.8
papillary (and pigmentary) 701.1
pelvicrural atrophic 359.1
pigmentary (*see also* Acanthosis) 701.2
pituitary (gland) 253.8
polyglandular 258.8
posttraumatic sympathetic—*see* Dystrophy,
  sympathetic
progressive ophthalmoplegic 359.1
reflex neuromuscular—*see* Dystrophy,
  sympathetic
retina, retinal (hereditary) 362.70
  albipunctate 362.74
  Bruch's membrane 362.77
  cone, progressive 362.75
  hyaline 362.77
  in
    Bassen-Kornzweig syndrome 272.5
      [362.72]
    cerebroretinal lipidosis 330.1 *[362.71]*
    Refsum's disease 356.3 *[362.72]*
    systemic lipidosis 272.7 *[362.71]*
  juvenile (Stargardt's) 362.75
  pigmentary 362.74
  pigment epithelium 362.76
  progressive cone (-rod) 362.75
  pseudoinflammatory foveal 362.77
  rod, progressive 362.75
  sensory 362.75
  vitelliform 362.76
Salzmann's nodular 371.46
scapuloperoneal 359.1
skin NEC 709.9
sympathetic (posttraumatic) (reflex) 337.20
  lower limb 337.22
  specified NEC 337.29
  upper limb 337.21
tapetoretinal NEC 362.74
thoracic asphyxiating 756.4
unguium 703.8
  congenital 757.5
vitreoretinal (primary) 362.73
  secondary 362.66
vulva 624.09
Dysuria 788.1
psychogenic 306.53

E

Eagle-Barrett syndrome 756.71
Eales' disease (syndrome) 362.18
Ear —*see also* condition
    ache 388.70
        otogenic 388.71
        referred 388.72
    lop 744.29
    piercing V50.3
    swimmers' acute 380.12
    tank 380.12
    tropical 111.8 *[380.15]*
    wax 380.4
Earache 388.70
    otogenic 388.71
    referred 388.72
Early satiety 780.94
Eaton-Lambert syndrome (*see also* Syndrome,
    Lambert-Eaton) 358.30
Eberth's disease (typhoid fever) 002.0
Ebstein's
    anomaly or syndrome (downward displacement,
        tricuspid valve into right ventricle) 746.2
    disease (diabetes) 250.4 *[581.81]*
        due to secondary diabetes 249.4 *[581.81]*
Eccentro-osteochondrodysplasia 277.5
Ecchondroma (M9210/0)—*see* Neoplasm, bone,
    benign
Ecchondrosis (M9210/1) 238.0
Ecchordosis physaliphora 756.0
Ecchymosis (multiple) 459.89
    conjunctiva 372.72
    eye (traumatic) 921.0
    eyelids (traumatic) 921.1
    newborn 772.6
    spontaneous 782.7
    traumatic—*see* Contusion
ECD (Erdheim-Chester disease) 277.89
Echinococciasis —*see* Echinococcus
Echinococcosis —*see* Echinococcus
Echinococcus (infection) 122.9
    granulosus 122.4
        liver 122.0
        lung 122.1
        orbit 122.3 *[376.13]*
        specified site NEC 122.3
        thyroid 122.2
    liver NEC 122.8
        granulosus 122.0
        multilocularis 122.5
    lung NEC 122.9
        granulosus 122.1
        multilocularis 122.6
    multilocularis 122.7
        liver 122.5
        specified site NEC 122.6
    orbit 122.9 *[376.13]*
        granulosus 122.3 *[376.13]*
        multilocularis 122.6 *[376.13]*
    specified site NEC 122.9
        granulosus 122.3
        multilocularis 122.6 *[376.13]*
    thyroid NEC 122.9
        granulosus 122.2
        multilocularis 122.6
Echinorhynchiasis 127.7
Echinostomiasis 121.8
Echolalia 784.69
ECHO virus infection NEC 079.1

Eclampsia, eclamptic (coma) (convulsions)
    (delirium) 780.39
    female, child-bearing age NEC—*see* Eclampsia,
        pregnancy
    gravidarum—*see* Eclampsia, pregnancy
    male 780.39
    not associated with pregnancy or childbirth
        780.39
    pregnancy, childbirth or puerperium 642.6
        with pre-existing hypertension 642.7
        affecting fetus or newborn 760.0
    uremic 586
Eclipse blindness (total) 363.31
Economic circumstance affecting care V60.9
    specified type NEC V60.89
Economo's disease (encephalitis lethargica) 049.8
Ectasia, ectasis
    annuloaortic 424.1
    aorta (*see also* Ectasia, aortic) 447.70
        with aneurysm 441.9
        ruptured 441.5
    aortic 447.70
        with aneurysm 441.9
        abdominal 447.72
        thoracic 447.71
        thoracoabdominal 447.73
    breast 610.4
    capillary 448.9
    cornea (marginal) (postinfectional) 371.71
    duct (mammary) 610.4
    gastric antral vascular (GAVE) 537.82
        with hemorrhage 537.83
        without hemorrhage 537.82
    kidney 593.89
    mammary duct (gland) 610.4
    papillary 448.9
    renal 593.89
    salivary gland (duct) 527.8
    scar, cornea 371.71
    sclera 379.11
Ecthyma 686.8
    contagiosum 051.2
    gangrenosum 686.09
    infectiosum 051.2
Ectocardia 746.87
Ectodermal dysplasia, congenital 757.31
Ectodermosis erosiva pluriorificialis 695.19
Ectopic, ectopia (congenital) 759.89
    abdominal viscera 751.8
        due to defect in anterior abdominal wall
            756.79
    ACTH syndrome 255.0
    adrenal gland 759.1
    anus 751.5
    auricular beats 427.61
    beats 427.60
    bladder 753.5
    bone and cartilage in lung 748.69
    brain 742.4
    breast tissue 757.6
    cardiac 746.87
    cerebral 742.4
    cordis 746.87
    endometrium 617.9
    gallbladder 751.69
    gastric mucosa 750.7
    gestation—*see* Pregnancy, ectopic
    heart 746.87

Ectopic, ectopia—*continued*
  hormone secretion NEC 259.3
  hyperparathyroidism 259.3
  kidney (crossed) (intrathoracic) (pelvis) 753.3
    in pregnancy or childbirth 654.4
      causing obstructed labor 660.2
  lens 743.37
  lentis 743.37
  mole—*see* Pregnancy, ectopic
  organ or site NEC—*see* Malposition, congenital
  ovary 752.0
  pancreas, pancreatic tissue 751.7
  pregnancy—*see* Pregnancy, ectopic
  pupil 364.75
  renal 753.3
  sebaceous glands of mouth 750.26
  secretion
    ACTH 255.0
    adrenal hormone 259.3
    adrenalin 259.3
    adrenocorticotropin 255.0
    antidiuretic hormone (ADH) 259.3
    epinephrine 259.3
    hormone NEC 259.3
    norepinephrine 259.3
    pituitary (posterior) 259.3
  spleen 759.0
  testis 752.51
  thyroid 759.2
  ureter 753.4
  ventricular beats 427.69
  vesicae 753.5
Ectrodactyly 755.4
  finger (*see also* Absence, finger, congenital) 755.29
  toe (*see also* Absence, toe, congenital) 755.39
Ectromelia 755.4
  lower limb 755.30
  upper limb 755.20
Ectropion 374.10
  anus 569.49
  cervix 622.0
    with mention of cervicitis 616.0
  cicatricial 374.14
  congenital 743.62
  eyelid 374.10
    cicatricial 374.14
    congenital 743.62
    mechanical 374.12
    paralytic 374.12
    senile 374.11
    spastic 374.13
  iris (pigment epithelium) 364.54
  lip (congenital) 750.26
    acquired 528.5
  mechanical 374.12
  paralytic 374.12
  rectum 569.49
  senile 374.11
  spastic 374.13
  urethra 599.84
  uvea 364.54
Eczema (acute) (allergic) (chronic)
    (erythematous) (fissum) (occupational)
    (rubrum) (squamous) 692.9
  asteatotic 706.8
  atopic 691.8
  contact NEC 692.9
  dermatitis NEC 692.9
  due to specified cause—*see* Dermatitis, due to
  dyshidrotic 705.81
  external ear 380.22
  flexural 691.8

Eczema—*continued*
  gouty 274.89
  herpeticum 054.0
  hypertrophicum 701.8
  hypostatic—*see* Varicose, vein
  impetiginous 684
  infantile (acute) (chronic) (due to any substance)
    (intertriginous) (seborrheic) 690.12
  intertriginous NEC 692.9
    infantile 690.12
  intrinsic 691.8
  lichenified NEC 692.9
  marginatum 110.3
  nummular 692.9
  pustular 686.8
  seborrheic 690.18
    infantile 690.12
  solare 692.72
  stasis (lower extremity) 454.1
    ulcerated 454.2
  vaccination, vaccinatum 999.0
  varicose (lower extremity)—*see* Varicose, vein
  verrucosum callosum 698.3
Eczematoid, exudative 691.8
Eddowes' syndrome (brittle bones and blue
    sclera) 756.51
Edema, edematous 782.3
  with nephritis (*see also* Nephrosis) 581.9
  allergic 995.1
  angioneurotic (allergic) (any site) (with
    urticaria) 995.1
    hereditary 277.6
  angiospastic 443.9
  Berlin's (traumatic) 921.3
  brain (cytotoxic) (vasogenic) 348.5
    due to birth injury 767.8
    fetus or newborn 767.8
  cardiac (*see also* Failure, heart) 428.0
  cardiovascular (*see also* Failure, heart) 428.0
  cerebral—*see* Edema, brain
  cerebrospinal vessel—*see* Edema, brain
  cervix (acute) (uteri) 622.8
    puerperal, postpartum 674.8
  chronic hereditary 757.0
  circumscribed, acute 995.1
    hereditary 277.6
  complicating pregnancy (gestational) 646.1
    with hypertension—*see* Toxemia, of pregnancy
  conjunctiva 372.73
  connective tissue 782.3
  cornea 371.20
    due to contact lenses 371.24
    idiopathic 371.21
    secondary 371.22
  due to
    lymphatic obstruction—*see* Edema, lymphatic
    salt retention 276.0
  epiglottis—*see* Edema, glottis
  essential, acute 995.1
    hereditary 277.6
  extremities, lower—*see* Edema, legs
  eyelid NEC 374.82
  familial, hereditary (legs) 757.0
  famine 262
  fetus or newborn 778.5
  genital organs
    female 629.89
    male 608.86
  gestational 646.1
    with hypertension—*see* Toxemia, of pregnancy

Edema, edematous—*continued*
glottis, glottic, glottides (obstructive) (passive) 478.6
  allergic 995.1
    hereditary 277.6
  due to external agent—*see* Condition, respiratory, acute, due to specified agent
heart (*see also* Failure, heart) 428.0
  newborn 779.89
heat 992.7
hereditary (legs) 757.0
inanition 262
infectious 782.3
intracranial 348.5
  due to injury at birth 767.8
iris 364.89
joint (*see also* Effusion, joint) 719.0
larynx (*see also* Edema, glottis) 478.6
legs 782.3
  due to venous obstruction 459.2
  hereditary 757.0
localized 782.3
  due to venous obstruction 459.2
    lower extremity 459.2
lower extremities—*see* Edema, legs
lungs 514
  acute 518.4
    with heart disease or failure (*see also* Failure, ventricular, left) 428.1
      congestive 428.0
    chemical (due to fumes or vapors) 506.1
    due to
      external agent(s) NEC 508.9
        specified NEC 508.8
      fumes and vapors (chemical) (inhalation) 506.1
      radiation 508.0
  chemical (acute) 506.1
    chronic 506.4
  chronic 514
    chemical (due to fumes or vapors) 506.4
    due to
      external agent(s) NEC 508.9
        specified NEC 508.8
      fumes or vapors (chemical) (inhalation) 506.4
      radiation 508.1
  due to
    external agent 508.9
      specified NEC 508.8
    high altitude 993.2
    near drowning 994.1
  postoperative 518.4
  terminal 514
lymphatic 457.1
  due to mastectomy operation 457.0
macula 362.83
  cystoid 362.53
  diabetic 250.5 *[362.07]*
    due to secondary diabetes 249.5 *[362.07]*
malignant (*see also* Gangrene, gas) 040.0
Milroy's 757.0
nasopharynx 478.25
neonatorum 778.5
nutritional (newborn) 262
  with dyspigmentation, skin and hair 260
optic disc or nerve—*see* Papilledema
orbit 376.33
  circulatory 459.89
palate (soft) (hard) 528.9
pancreas 577.8

Edema, edematous—*continued*
penis 607.83
periodic 995.1
  hereditary 277.6
pharynx 478.25
pitting 782.3
pulmonary—*see* Edema, lung
Quincke's 995.1
  hereditary 277.6
renal (*see also* Nephrosis) 581.9
retina (localized) (macular) (peripheral) 362.83
  cystoid 362.53
  diabetic 250.5 *[362.07]*
    due to secondary diabetes 249.5 *[362.07]*
salt 276.0
scrotum 608.86
seminal vesicle 608.86
spermatic cord 608.86
spinal cord 336.1
starvation 262
stasis (*see also* Hypertension, venous) 459.30
subconjunctival 372.73
subglottic (*see also* Edema, glottis) 478.6
supraglottic (*see also* Edema, glottis) 478.6
testis 608.86
toxic NEC 782.3
traumatic NEC 782.3
tunica vaginalis 608.86
vas deferens 608.86
vocal cord—*see* Edema, glottis
vulva (acute) 624.8
Edentia (complete) (partial) (*see also* Absence, tooth) 520.0
acquired (*see also* Edentulism) 525.40
  due to
    caries 525.13
    extraction 525.10
    periodontal disease 525.12
    specified NEC 525.19
    trauma 525.11
causing malocclusion 524.30
congenital (deficiency of tooth buds) 520.0
Edentulism 525.40
complete 525.40
  class I 525.41
  class II 525.42
  class III 525.43
  class IV 525.44
partial 525.50
  class I 525.51
  class II 525.52
  class III 525.53
  class IV 525.54
Edsall's disease 992.2
Educational handicap V62.3
Edwards' syndrome 758.2
Effect, adverse NEC
abnormal gravitational (G) forces or states 994.9
air pressure—*see* Effect, adverse, atmospheric pressure
altitude (high)—*see* Effect, adverse, high altitude
anesthetic
  in labor and delivery NEC 668.9
    affecting fetus or newborn 763.5
antitoxin—*see* Complications, vaccination
atmospheric pressure 993.9
  due to explosion 993.4
  high 993.3
  low—*see* Effect, adverse, high altitude
  specified effect NEC 993.8

Effect, adverse—*continued*
biological, correct substance properly
administered (*see also* Effect, adverse, drug)
995.20
blood (derivatives) (serum) (transfusion)—*see*
Complications, transfusion
chemical substance NEC 989.9
specified—*see* Table of drugs and chemicals
cobalt, radioactive (*see also* Effect, adverse,
radioactive substance) 990
cold (temperature) (weather) 991.9
chilblains 991.5
frostbite—*see* Frostbite
specified effect NEC 991.8
drugs and medicinals 995.20
correct substance properly administered
995.20
overdose or wrong substance given or taken
977.9
specified drug—*see* Table of drugs and
chemicals
electric current (shock) 994.8
burn—*see* Burn, by site
electricity (electrocution) (shock) 994.8
burn—*see* Burn, by site
exertion (excessive) 994.5
exposure 994.9
exhaustion 994.4
external cause NEC 994.9
fallout (radioactive) NEC 990
fluoroscopy NEC 990
foodstuffs
allergic reaction (*see also* Allergy, food) 693.1
anaphylactic reaction or shock due to food
NEC—*see* Anaphylactic reaction or shock,
due to food
noxious 988.9
specified type NEC (*see also* Poisoning, by
name of noxious foodstuff) 988.8
gases, fumes, or vapors—*see* Table of drugs and
chemicals
glue (airplane) sniffing 304.6
heat—*see* Heat
high altitude NEC 993.2
anoxia 993.2
on
fears 993.0
sinuses 993.1
polycythemia 289.0
hot weather—*see* Heat
hunger 994.2
immersion, foot 991.4
immunization—*see* Complications, vaccination
immunological agents—*see* Complications,
vaccination
implantation (removable) of isotope or radium
NEC 990
infrared (radiation) (rays) NEC 990
burn—*see* Burn, by site
dermatitis or eczema 692.82
infusion—*see* Complications, infusion
ingestion or injection of isotope (therapeutic)
NEC 990
irradiation NEC (*see also* Effect, adverse,
radiation) 990
isotope (radioactive) NEC 990
lack of care (child) (infant) (newborn) 995.52
adult 995.84
lightning 994.0
burn—*see* Burn, by site
Lirugin—*see* Complications, vaccination

Effect, adverse—*continued*
medicinal substance, correct, properly
administered (*see also* Effect, adverse,
drugs) 995.20
mesothorium NEC 990
motion 994.6
noise, inner ear 388.10
other drug, medicinal and biological substance
995.29
overheated places—*see* Heat
polonium NEC 990
psychosocial, of work environment V62.1
radiation (diagnostic) (fallout) (infrared) (natural
source) (therapeutic) (tracer) (ultraviolet)
(x-ray) NEC 990
with pulmonary manifestations
acute 508.0
chronic 508.1
dermatitis or eczema 692.82
due to sun NEC (*see also* Dermatitis, due to,
sun) 692.70
fibrosis of lungs 508.1
maternal with suspected damage to fetus
affecting management of pregnancy 655.6
pneumonitis 508.0
radioactive substance NEC 990
dermatitis or eczema 692.82
radioactivity NEC 990
radiotherapy NEC 990
dermatitis or eczema 692.82
radium NEC 990
reduced temperature 991.9
frostbite—*see* Frostbite
immersion, foot (hand) 991.4
specified effect NEC 991.8
roentgenography NEC 990
roentgenoscopy NEC 990
roentgen rays NEC 990
serum (prophylactic) (therapeutic) NEC 999.59
specified NEC 995.89
external cause NEC 994.9
strangulation 994.7
submersion 994.1
teletherapy NEC 990
thirst 994.3
transfusion—*see* Complications, transfusion
ultraviolet (radiation) (rays) NEC 990
burn—*see also* Burn, by site
from sun (*see also* Sunburn) 692.71
dermatitis or eczema 692.82
due to sun NEC (*see also* Dermatitis, due to,
sun) 692.70
uranium NEC 990
vaccine (any)—*see* Complications, vaccination
weightlessness 994.9
whole blood—*see also* Complications,
transfusion
overdose or wrong substance given (*see also*
Table of drugs and chemicals) 964.7
working environment V62.1
x-rays NEC 990
dermatitis or eczema 692.82
Effect, remote
of cancer —*see* condition
Effects, late—*see* Late, effect (of)
Effluvium, telogen 704.02
Effort
intolerance 306.2
syndrome (aviators) (psychogenic) 306.2

Effusion
  Amniotic fluid (*see also* Rupture, membranes, premature) 658.1
  brain (serous) 348.5
  bronchial (*see also* Bronchitis) 490
  cerebral 348.5
  cerebrospinal (*see also* Meningitis) 322.9
    vessel 348.5
  chest—*see* Effusion, pleura
  intracranial 348.5
  joint 719.00
    ankle 719.07
    elbow 719.02
    foot 719.07
    hand 719.04
    hip 719.05
    knee 719.06
    multiple sites 719.09
    pelvic region 719.05
    shoulder (region) 719.01
    specified site NEC 719.08
    wrist 719.03
  meninges (*see also* Meningitis) 322.9
  pericardium, pericardial (*see also* Pericarditis) 423.9
    acute 420.90
  peritoneal (chronic) 568.82
  pleura, pleurisy, pleuritic, pleuropericardial 511.9
    bacterial, nontuberculous 511.1
    fetus or newborn 511.9
    malignant 511.81
    nontuberculous 511.9
      bacterial 511.1
    pneumococcal 511.1
    staphylococcal 511.1
    streptococcal 511.1
    tuberculous (*see also* Tuberculosis, pleura) 012.0
      primary progressive 010.1
    traumatic 862.29
      with open wound 862.39
  pulmonary—*see* Effusion, pleura
  spinal (*see also* Meningitis) 322.9
  thorax, thoracic—*see* Effusion, pleura
Egg (oocyte) (ovum)
  donor V59.70
    age 35 and over V59.73
      anonymous recipient V59.73
      designated recipient V59.74
    under age 35 V59.71
      anonymous recipient V59.71
      designated recipient V59.72
Eggshell nails 703.8
  congenital 757.5
Ego-dystonic
  homosexuality 302.0
  lesbianism 302.0
  sexual orientation 302.0
Egyptian splenomegaly 120.1
Ehlers-Danlos syndrome 756.83
Ehrlichiosis 082.40
  chaffeensis 082.41
  specified type NEC 082.49
Eichstedt's disease (pityriasis versicolor) 111.0
EIN (endometrial intraepithelial neoplasia) 621.35
Eisenmenger's complex or syndrome
  (ventricular septal defect) 745.4
Ejaculation, semen
  painful 608.89
    psychogenic 306.59
  premature 302.75
  retrograde 608.87
Ekbom syndrome (restless legs) 333.94

Ekman's syndrome (brittle bones and blue sclera) 756.51
Elastic skin 756.83
  acquired 701.8
Elastofibroma (M8820/0)—*see* Neoplasm, connective tissue, benign
Elastoidosis
  cutanea nodularis 701.8
  cutis cystica et comedonica 701.8
Elastoma 757.39
  juvenile 757.39
  Miescher's (elastosis perforans serpiginosa) 701.1
Elastomyofibrosis 425.3
Elastosis 701.8
  atrophicans 701.8
  perforans serpiginosa 701.1
  reactive perforating 701.1
  senilis 701.8
  solar (actinic) 692.74
Elbow —*see* condition
Electric
  current, electricity, effects (concussion) (fatal) (nonfatal) (shock) 994.8
  burn—*see* Burn, by site
  feet (foot) syndrome 266.2
  shock from electroshock gun (taser) 994.8
Electrocution 994.8
Electrolyte imbalance 276.9
  with
    abortion—*see* Abortion, by type, with metabolic disorder
    ectopic pregnancy (*see also* categories 633.0-633.9) 639.4
    hyperemesis gravidarum (before 22 completed weeks gestation) 643.1
    molar pregnancy (*see also* categories 630-632) 639.4
  following
    abortion 639.4
    ectopic or molar pregnancy 639.4
Elephant man syndrome 237.71
Elephantiasis (nonfilarial) 457.1
  arabicum (*see also* Infestation, filarial) 125.9
  congenita hereditaria 757.0
  congenital (any site) 757.0
  due to
    Brugia (malayi) 125.1
    mastectomy operation 457.0
    Wuchereria (bancrofti) 125.0
      malayi 125.1
  eyelid 374.83
  filarial (*see also* Infestation, filarial) 125.9
  filariensis (*see also* Infestation, filarial) 125.9
  gingival 523.8
  glandular 457.1
  graecorum 030.9
  lymphangiectatic 457.1
  lymphatic vessel 457.1
    due to mastectomy operation 457.0
  neuromatosa 237.71
  postmastectomy 457.0
  scrotum 457.1
  streptococcal 457.1
  surgical 997.99
    postmastectomy 457.0
  telangiectodes 457.1
  vulva (nonfilarial) 624.8
Elevated —*see also* Elevation
  findings on laboratory examination — see Findings, abnormal, without diagnosis (examination) (laboratory test)

Elevated—*continued*
 GFR (glomerular filtration rate) — see Findings,
  abnormal, without diagnosis (examination)
  (laboratory test)
Elevation
 17-ketosteroids 791.9
 acid phosphatase 790.5
 alkaline phosphatase 790.5
 amylase 790.5
 antibody titers 795.79
 basal metabolic rate (BMR) 794.7
 blood pressure (*see also* Hypertension) 401.9
  reading (incidental) (isolated) (nonspecific),
   no diagnosis of hypertension 796.2
 blood sugar 790.29
 body temperature (of unknown origin) (*see also*
  Pyrexia) 780.60
 C-reactive protein (CRP) 790.95
 cancer antigen 125 [CA 125] 795.82
 carcinoembryonic antigen [CEA] 795.81
 cholesterol 272.0
  with high triglycerides 272.2
 conjugate, eye 378.81
 CRP (C-reactive protein) 790.95
 diaphragm, congenital 756.6
 GFR (glomerular filtration rate) — see Findings,
  abnormal, without diagnosis (examination)
  (laboratory test)
 glucose
  fasting 790.21
  tolerance test 790.22
 immunoglobulin level 795.79
 indolacetic acid 791.9
 lactic acid dehydrogenase (LDH) level 790.4
 leukocytes 288.60
 lipase 790.5
 lipoprotein a level 272.8
 liver function test (LFT) 790.6
  alkaline phosphatase 790.5
  aminotransferase 790.4
  bilirubin 782.4
  hepatic enzyme NEC 790.5
  lactate dehydrogenase 790.4
 lymphocytes 288.61
 prostate specific antigen (PSA) 790.93
 renin 790.99
  in hypertension (*see also* Hypertension,
   renovascular) 405.91
 Rh titer (see also Complications, transfusion)
  999.70
 scapula, congenital 755.52
 sedimentation rate 790.1
 SGOT 790.4
 SGPT 790.4
 transaminase 790.4
 triglycerides 272.1
  with high cholesterol 272.2
 vanillylmandelic acid 791.9
 venous pressure 459.89
 VMA 791.9
 white blood cell count 288.60
  specified NEC 288.69
Elliptocytosis (congenital) (hereditary) 282.1
 Hb-C (disease) 282.7
 hemoglobin disease 282.7
 sickle-cell (disease) 282.60
  trait 282.5
Ellis-van Creveld disease or syndrome
 (chondroectodermal dysplasia) 756.55
Ellison-Zollinger syndrome (gastric
 hypersecretion with pancreatic islet cell
 tumor) 251.5

Elongation, elongated (congenital)—*see also*
 Distortion
 bone 756.9
 cervix (uteri) 752.49
  acquired 622.6
  hypertrophic 622.6
 colon 751.5
 common bile duct 751.69
 cystic duct 751.69
 frenulum, penis 752.69
 labia minora, acquired 624.8
 ligamentum patellae 756.89
 petiolus (epiglottidis) 748.3
 styloid bone (process) 733.99
 tooth, teeth 520.2
 uvula 750.26
  acquired 528.9
Elschnig bodies or pearls 366.51
El Tor cholera 001.1
Emaciation (due to malnutrition) 261
Emancipation disorder 309.22
Embadomoniasis 007.8
Embarrassment heart, cardiac —*see* Disease,
 heart
Embedded
 fragment (status) - *see* Foreign body, retained
 splinter (status) - *see* Foreign body, retained
 tooth, teeth 520.6
  root only 525.3
Embolic —*see* condition
Embolism 444.9
 with
  abortion—*see* Abortion, by type, with
   embolism
  ectopic pregnancy (*see also* categories
   633.0-633.9) 639.6
  molar pregnancy (*see also* categories 630-632)
   639.6
 air (any site) 958.0
  with
   abortion—*see* Abortion, by type, with
    embolism
   ectopic pregnancy (*see also* categories
    633.0-633.9) 639.6
   molar pregnancy (*see also* categories
    630-632) 639.6
  due to implanted device—*see* Complications,
   due to (presence of) any device, implant,
   or graft classified to 996.0-996.5 NEC
  following
   abortion 639.6
   ectopic or molar pregnancy 639.6
   infusion, perfusion, or transfusion 999.1
  in pregnancy, childbirth, or puerperium 673.0
  traumatic 958.0
 amniotic fluid (pulmonary) 673.1
  with
   abortion—*see* Abortion, by type, with
    embolism
   ectopic pregnancy (*see also* categories
    633.0-633.9) 639.6
   molar pregnancy (*see also* categories
    630-632) 639.6
  following
   abortion 639.6
   ectopic or molar pregnancy 639.6
 aorta, aortic 444.1
  abdominal 444.09
   saddle 444.01
  bifurcation 444.09
  saddle 444.01
  thoracic 444.1

Embolism—*continued*
artery 444.9
  auditory, internal 433.8
  basilar (*see also* Occlusion, artery, basilar)
    433.0
  bladder 444.89
  carotid (common) (internal) (*see also*
    Occlusion, artery, carotid) 433.1
  cerebellar (anterior inferior) (posterior
    inferior) (superior) 433.8
  cerebral (*see also* Embolism, brain) 434.1
  choroidal (anterior) 433.8
  communicating posterior 433.8
  coronary (*see also* Infarct, myocardium) 410.9
    without myocardial infarction 411.81
  extremity 444.22
    lower 444.22
    upper 444.21
  hypophyseal 433.8
  mesenteric (with gangrene) 557.0
  ophthalmic (*see also* Occlusion, retina) 362.30
  peripheral 444.22
  pontine 433.8
  precerebral NEC—*see* Occlusion, artery,
    precerebral
  pulmonary—*see* Embolism, pulmonary
  pyemic 449
    pulmonary 415.12
  renal 593.81
  retinal (*see also* Occlusion, retina) 362.30
  septic 449
    pulmonary 415.12
  specified site NEC 444.89
  vertebral (*see also* Occlusion, artery,
    vertebral) 433.2
auditory, internal 433.8
basilar (artery) (*see also* Occlusion, artery,
  basilar) 433.0
birth, mother—*see* Embolism, obstetrical
blood-clot
  with
    abortion—*see* Abortion, by type, with embolism
    ectopic pregnancy (*see also* categories
      633.0-633.9) 639.6
    molar pregnancy (*see also* categories
      630-632) 639.6
  following
    abortion 639.6
    ectopic or molar pregnancy 639.6
  in pregnancy, childbirth, or puerperium 673.2
brain 434.1
  with
    abortion—*see* Abortion, by type, with embolism
    ectopic pregnancy (*see also* categories
      633.0-633.9) 639.6
    molar pregnancy (*see also* categories
      630-632) 639.6
  following
    abortion 639.6
    ectopic or molar pregnancy 639.6
  late effect—*see* Late effect(s) (of)
    cerebrovascular disease
  puerperal, postpartum, childbirth 674.0
capillary 448.9
cardiac (*see also* Infarct, myocardium) 410.9
carotid (artery) (common) (internal) (*see also*
  Occlusion, artery, carotid) 433.1
cavernous sinus (venous)—*see* Embolism,
  intracranial venous sinus
cerebral (*see also* Embolism, brain) 434.1
cholesterol—*see* Atheroembolism
choroidal (anterior) (artery) 433.8

Embolism—*continued*
coronary (artery or vein) (systemic) (*see also*
  Infarct, myocardium) 410.9
  without myocardial infarction 411.81
due to (presence of) any device, implant, or graft
  classifiable to 996.0-996.5 —*see*
  Complications, due to (presence of) any
  device, implant, or graft classified to
  996.0-996.5 NEC
encephalomalacia (*see also* Embolism, brain) 434.1
extremities 444.22
  lower 444.22
  upper 444.21
eye 362.30
fat (cerebral) (pulmonary) (systemic) 958.1
  with
    abortion—*see* Abortion, by type, with embolism
    ectopic pregnancy (*see also* categories
      633.0-633.9) 639.6
    molar pregnancy (*see also* categories
      630-632) 639.6
  complicating delivery or puerperium 673.8
  following
    abortion 639.6
    ectopic or molar pregnancy 639.6
  in pregnancy, childbirth, or the puerperium 673.8
femoral (artery) 444.22
  vein 453.6
    deep 453.41
following
  abortion 639.6
  ectopic or molar pregnancy 639.6
  infusion, perfusion, or transfusion
    air 999.1
    thrombus 999.2
heart (fatty) (*see also* Infarct, myocardium) 410.9
hepatic (vein) 453.0
iliac (artery) 444.81
iliofemoral 444.81
in pregnancy, childbirth, or puerperium
  (pulmonary)—*see* Embolism, obstetrical
intestine (artery) (vein) (with gangrene) 557.0
intracranial (*see also* Embolism, brain) 434.1
  venous sinus (any) 325
    late effect—*see* category 326
    nonpyogenic 437.6
      in pregnancy or puerperium 671.5
kidney (artery) 593.81
lateral sinus (venous)—*see* Embolism,
  intracranial venous sinus
longitudinal sinus (venous)—*see* Embolism,
  intracranial venous sinus
lower extremity 444.22
lung (massive)—*see* Embolism, pulmonary
meninges (*see also* Embolism, brain) 434.1
mesenteric (artery) (with gangrene) 557.0
multiple NEC 444.9
obstetrical (pulmonary) 673.2
  air 673.0
  amniotic fluid (pulmonary) 673.1
  blood-clot 673.2
  cardiac 674.8
  fat 673.8
  heart 674.8
  pyemic 673.3
  septic 673.3
  specified NEC 674.8
ophthalmic (*see also* Occlusion, retina) 362.30
paradoxical NEC 444.9
penis 607.82

Embolism—*continued*
  peripheral arteries NEC 444.22
    lower 444.22
    upper 444.21
  pituitary 253.8
  popliteal (artery) 444.22
  portal (vein) 452
  postoperative NEC 997.2
    cerebral 997.02
    mesenteric artery 997.71
    other vessels 997.79
    peripheral vascular 997.2
    pulmonary 415.11
      septic 415.11
    renal artery 997.72
  precerebral artery (*see also* Occlusion, artery,
    precerebral) 433.9
  puerperal—*see* Embolism, obstetrical
  pulmonary (acute) (artery) (vein) 415.19
    with
      abortion—*see* Abortion, by type, with
        embolism
      ectopic pregnancy (*see also* categories
        633.0-633.9) 639.6
      molar pregnancy (*see also* categories
        630-632) 639.6
    chronic 416.2
    following
      abortion 639.6
      ectopic or molar pregnancy 639.6
    healed or old V12.55
    iatrogenic 415.11
    in pregnancy, childbirth, or puerperium—*see*
      Embolism, obstetrical
    personal history of V12.55
    postoperative 415.11
    septic 415.12
  pyemic (multiple) (*see also* Septicemia) 415.12
    with
      abortion—*see* Abortion, by type, with embolism
      ectopic pregnancy (*see also* categories
        633.0-633.9) 639.6
      molar pregnancy (*see also* categories
        630-632) 639.6
    Aerobacter aerogenes 415.12
    enteric gram-negative bacilli 415.12
    Enterobacter aerogenes 415.12
    Escherichia coli 415.12
    following
      abortion 639.6
      ectopic or molar pregnancy 639.6
    Hemophilus influenzae 415.12
    pneumococcal 415.12
    Proteus vulgaris 415.12
    Pseudomonas (aeruginosa) 415.12
    puerperal, postpartum, childbirth (any
      organism) 673.3
    Serratia 415.12
    specified organism NEC 415.12
    staphylococcal 415.12
      aureus 415.12
      specified organism NEC 415.12
    streptococcal 415.12
  renal (artery) 593.81
    vein 453.3
  retina, retinal (*see also* Occlusion, retina) 362.30
  saddle
    abdominal aorta 444.01
    pulmonary artery 415.13
  septic 415.12
    arterial 449
  septicemic—*see* Embolism, pyemic

Embolism—*continued*
  sinus—*see* Embolism, intracranial venous sinus
  soap
    with
      abortion—*see* Abortion, by type, with embolism
      ectopic pregnancy (*see also* categories
        633.0-633.9) 639.6
      molar pregnancy (*see also* categories
        630-632) 639.6
    following
      abortion 639.6
      ectopic or molar pregnancy 639.6
  spinal cord (nonpyogenic) 336.1
    in pregnancy or puerperium 671.5
    pyogenic origin 324.1
    late effect—*see* category 326
  spleen, splenic (artery) 444.89
  thrombus (thromboembolism) following
    infusion, perfusion, or transfusion 999.2
  upper extremity 444.21
  vein 453.9
    with inflammation or phlebitis—*see*
      Thrombophlebitis
    antecubital (acute) 453.81
      chronic 453.71
    axillary (acute) 453.84
      chronic 453.74
    basilic (acute) 453.81
      chronic 453.71
    brachial (acute) 453.82
      chronic 453.72
    brachiocephalic (acute) (innominate) 453.87
      chronic 453.77
    cephalic (acute) 453.81
      chronic 453.71
    cerebral (*see also* Embolism, brain) 434.1
    coronary (*see also* Infarct, myocardium) 410.9
      without myocardial infarction 411.81
    hepatic 453.0
    internal jugular (acute) 453.86
      chronic 453.76
    lower extremity (superficial) 453.6
      deep 453.40
        acute 453.40
          calf 453.42
          distal (lower leg) 453.42
          femoral 453.41
          iliac 453.41
          lower leg 453.42
          peroneal 453.42
          popliteal 453.41
          proximal (upper leg) 453.41
          thigh 453.41
          tibial 453.42
        chronic 453.50
          calf 453.52
          distal (lower leg) 453.52
          femoral 453.51
          iliac 453.51
          lower leg 453.52
          peroneal 453.52
          popliteal 453.51
          proximal (upper leg) 453.51
          thigh 453.51
          tibial 453.52
      saphenous (greater) (lesser) 453.6
      superficial 453.6
    mesenteric (with gangrene) 557.0
    portal 452
    pulmonary—*see* Embolism, pulmonary
    radial (acute) 453.82
      chronic 453.72

Embolism—*continued*
  vein—*continued*
    renal 453.3
    saphenous (greater) (lesser) 453.6
    specified NEC (acute) 453.89
      chronic 453.79
      with inflammation or phlebitis—*see*
        Thrombophlebitis
    subclavian (acute) 453.85
      chronic 453.75
    superior vena cava (acute) 453.87
      chronic 453.77
    thoracic (acute) 453.87
      chronic 453.77
    ulnar (acute(453.82
      chronic 453.72
    upper extremity (acute) 453.83
      chronic 453.73
        deep 453.72
        superficial 453.71
      deep 453.82
      superficial 453.81
  vena cava
    inferior 453.2
    superior (acute) 453.87
      chronic 453.77
  vessels of brain (*see also* Embolism, brain)
    434.1
Embolization —*see* Embolism
Embolus —*see* Embolism
Embryoma (M9080/1)—*see also* Neoplasm, by
  site, uncertain behavior
  benign (M9080/0)—*see* Neoplasm, by site, benign
  kidney (M8960/3) 189.0
  liver (M8970/3) 155.0
  malignant (M9080/3)—*see also* Neoplasm, by
    site, malignant
    kidney (M8960/3) 189.0
    liver (M8970/3) 155.0
    testis (M9070/3) 186.9
      undescended 186.0
  testis (M9070/3) 186.9
    undescended 186.0
Embryonic
  circulation 747.9
  heart 747.9
  vas deferens 752.89
Embryopathia NEC 759.9
Embryotomy, fetal 763.89
Embryotoxon 743.43
  interfering with vision 743.42
Emesis —*see also* Vomiting
  bilious 787.04
  gravidarum—*see* Hyperemesis, gravidarum
Emissions, nocturnal (semen) 608.89
Emotional
  crisis—*see* Crisis, emotional
  disorder (*see also* Disorder, mental) 300.9
  instability (excessive) 301.3
  lability 799.24
  overlay—*see* Reaction, adjustment
  upset 300.9
Emotionality, pathological 301.3
Emotogenic disease (*see also* Disorder,
  psychogenic) 306.9

Emphysema (atrophic) (centriacinar)
  (centrilobular) (chronic) (diffuse) (essential)
  (hypertrophic) (interlobular) (lung)
  (obstructive) (panlobular) (paracicatricial)
  (paracinar) (postural) (pulmonary) (senile)
  (subpleural) (traction) (unilateral) (unilobular)
  (vesicular) 492.8
  with bronchitis
    chronic 491.20
      with
        acute bronchitis 491.22
        exacerbation (acute) 491.21
  bullous (giant) 492.0
  cellular tissue 958.7
    surgical 998.81
  compensatory 518.2
  congenital 770.2
  conjunctiva 372.89
  connective tissue 958.7
    surgical 998.81
  due to fumes or vapors 506.4
  eye 376.89
  eyelid 374.85
    surgical 998.81
    traumatic 958.7
  fetus or newborn (interstitial) (mediastinal)
    (unilobular) 770.2
  heart 416.9
  interstitial 518.1
    congenital 770.2
    fetus or newborn 770.2
  laminated tissue 958.7
    surgical 998.81
  mediastinal 518.1
    fetus or newborn 770.2
  newborn (interstitial) (mediastinal) (unilobular)
    770.2
  obstructive diffuse with fibrosis 492.8
  orbit 376.89
  subcutaneous 958.7
    due to trauma 958.7
    nontraumatic 518.1
    surgical 998.81
  surgical 998.81
  thymus (gland) (congenital) 254.8
  traumatic 958.7
  tuberculous (*see also* Tuberculosis, pulmonary)
    011.9
Employment examination (certification) V70.5
Empty sella (turcica) syndrome 253.8
Empyema (chest) (diaphragmatic) (double)
  (encapsulated) (general) (interlobar) (lung)
  (medial) (necessitatis) (perforating chest wall)
  (pleura) (pneumococcal) (residual) (sacculated)
  (streptococcal) (supradiaphragmatic) 510.9
  with fistula 510.0
  accessory sinus (chronic) (*see also* Sinusitis) 473.9
  acute 510.9
    with fistula 510.0
  antrum (chronic) (*see also* Sinusitis, maxillary)
    473.0
  brain (any part) (*see also* Abscess, brain) 324.0
  ethmoidal (sinus) (chronic) (*see also* Sinusitis,
    ethmoidal) 473.2
  extradural (*see also* Abscess, extradural) 324.9
  frontal (sinus) (chronic) (*see also* Sinusitis,
    frontal) 473.1
  gallbladder (*see also* Cholecystitis, acute) 575.0
  mastoid (process) (acute) (*see also* Mastoiditis,
    acute) 383.00

Empyema—*continued*
maxilla, maxillary 526.4
  sinus (chronic) (*see also* Sinusitis, maxillary) 473.0
nasal sinus (chronic) (*see also* Sinusitis) 473.9
sinus (accessory) (nasal) (*see also* Sinusitis) 473.9
sphenoidal (chronic) (sinus) (*see also* Sinusitis, sphenoidal) 473.3
subarachnoid (*see also* Abscess, extradural) 324.9
subdural (*see also* Abscess, extradural) 324.9
tuberculous (*see also* Tuberculosis, pleura) 012.0
ureter (*see also* Ureteritis) 593.89
ventricular (*see also* Abscess, brain) 324.0
Enameloma 520.2
Encephalitis (bacterial) (chronic) (hemorrhagic) (idiopathic) (nonepidemic) (spurious) (subacute) 323.9
acute—*see also* Encephalitis, viral
  disseminated (postinfectious) NEC 136.9 *[323.61]*
    postimmunization or postvaccination 323.51
  inclusional 049.8
  inclusion body 049.8
  necrotizing 049.8
arboviral, arbovirus NEC 064
arthropod-borne (*see also* Encephalitis, viral, arthropod-borne) 064
Australian X 062.4
Bwamba fever 066.3
California (virus) 062.5
Central European 063.2
Czechoslovakian 063.2
Dawson's (inclusion body) 046.2
diffuse sclerosing 046.2
due to
  actinomycosis 039.8 *[323.41]*
  cat-scratch disease 078.3 *[323.01]*
  human herpesvirus 6 058.21
  human herpesvirus 7 058.29
  human herpesvirus NEC 058.29
  human immunodeficiency virus [HIV] disease 042 *[323.01]*
  infectious mononucleosis 075 *[323.01]*
  malaria (*see also* Malaria) 084.6 *[323.2]*
  Negishi virus 064
  ornithosis 073.7 *[323.01]*
  other infection classified elsewhere 136.9 *[323.41]*
  prophylactic inoculation against smallpox 323.51
  rickettsiosis (*see also* Rickettsiosis) 083.9 *[323.1]*
  rubella 056.01
  toxoplasmosis (acquired) 130.0
    congenital (active) 771.2 *[323.41]*
  typhus (fever) (*see also* Typhus) 081.9 *[323.1]*
  vaccination (smallpox) 323.51
Eastern equine 062.2
endemic 049.8
epidemic 049.8
equine (acute) (infectious) (viral) 062.9
  Eastern 062.2
  Venezuelan 066.2
  Western 062.1
Far Eastern 063.0
following vaccination or other immunization procedure 323.51
herpes 054.3
human herpesvirus 6 058.21
human herpesvirus 7 058.29
human herpesvirus NEC 058.29
Ilheus (virus) 062.8
inclusion body 046.2
infectious (acute) (virus) NEC 049.8

Encephalitis—*continued*
influenzal (*see also* Influenza) 487.8 *[323.41]*
  lethargic 049.8
Japanese (B type) 062.0
La Crosse 062.5
Langat 063.8
late effect—*see* Late, effect, encephalitis
lead 984.9 *[323.71]*
lethargic (acute) (infectious) (influenzal) 049.8
lethargica 049.8
louping ill 063.1
lupus 710.0 *[323.81]*
lymphatica 049.0
Mengo 049.8
meningococcal 036.1
mumps 072.2
Murray Valley 062.4
myoclonic 049.8
Negishi virus 064
otitic NEC 382.4 *[323.41]*
parasitic NEC 123.9 *[323.41]*
periaxialis (concentrica) (diffusa) 341.1
postchickenpox 052.0
postexanthematous NEC 057.9 *[323.62]*
postimmunization 323.51
postinfectious NEC 136.9 *[323.62]*
postmeasles 055.0
posttraumatic 323.81
postvaccinal (smallpox) 323.51
postvaricella 052.0
postviral NEC 079.99 *[323.62]*
  postexanthematous 057.9 *[323.62]*
    specified NEC 057.8 *[323.62]*
Powassan 063.8
progressive subcortical (Binswanger's) 290.12
Rasmussen 323.81
Rio Bravo 049.8
rubella 056.01
Russian
  autumnal 062.0
  spring-summer type (taiga) 063.0
saturnine 984.9 *[323.71]*
Semliki Forest 062.8
serous 048
slow-acting virus NEC 046.8
specified cause NEC 323.81
St. Louis type 062.3
subacute sclerosing 046.2
subcorticalis chronica 290.12
summer 062.0
suppurative 324.0
syphilitic 094.81
  congenital 090.41
tick-borne 063.9
torula, torular 117.5 *[323.41]*
toxic NEC 989.9 *[323.71]*
toxoplasmic (acquired) 130.0
  congenital (active) 771.2 *[323.41]*
trichinosis 124 *[323.41]*
Trypanosomiasis (*see also* Trypanosomiasis) 086.9 *[323.2]*
tuberculous (*see also* Tuberculosis) 013.6
type B (Japanese) 062.0
type C 062.3
van Bogaert's 046.2
Venezuelan 066.2
Vienna type 049.8

Encephalitis—*continued*
viral, virus 049.9
  arthropod-borne NEC 064
    mosquito-borne 062.9
      Australian X disease 062.4
      California virus 062.5
      Eastern equine 062.2
      Ilheus virus 062.8
      Japanese (B type) 062.0
      Murray Valley 062.4
      specified type NEC 062.8
      St. Louis 062.3
      type B 062.0
      type C 062.3
      Western equine 062.1
    tick-borne 063.9
      biundulant 063.2
      Central European 063.2
      Czechoslovakian 063.2
      diphasic meningoencephalitis 063.2
      Far Eastern 063.0
      Langat 063.8
      louping ill 063.1
      Powassan 063.8
      Russian spring-summer (taiga) 063.0
      specified type NEC 063.8
    vector unknown 064
  slow acting NEC 046.8
  specified type NEC 049.8
  vaccination, prophylactic (against) V05.0
  von Economo's 049.8
  Western equine 062.1
  West Nile type 066.41
Encephalocele 742.0
  orbit 376.81
Encephalocystocele 742.0
Encephaloduroarteriomyosynangiosis (EDAMS) 437.5
Encephalomalacia (brain) (cerebellar) (cerebral) (cerebrospinal) (*see also* Softening, brain) 348.89
  due to
    hemorrhage (*see also* Hemorrhage, brain) 431
    recurrent spasm of artery 435.9
  embolic (cerebral) (*see also* Embolism, brain) 434.1
  subcorticalis chronicus arteriosclerotica 290.12
  thrombotic (*see also* Thrombosis, brain) 434.0
Encephalomeningitis —*see* Meningoencephalitis
Encephalomeningocele 742.0
Encephalomeningomyelitis —*see* Meningoencephalitis
Encephalomeningopathy (*see also* Meningoencephalitis) 349.9
Encephalomyelitis (chronic) (granulomatous) (myalgic, benign) (*see also* Encephalitis) 323.9
  abortive disseminated 049.8
  acute disseminated (ADEM) (postinfectious) 136.9 *[323.61]*
    infectious 136.9 *[323.61]*
    noninfectious 323.81
    postimmunization 323.51
  due to
    cat-scratch disease 078.3 *[323.01]*
    infectious mononucleosis 075 *[323.01]*
    ornithosis 073.7 *[323.01]*
    vaccination (any) 323.51
  equine (acute) (infectious) 062.9
    Eastern 062.2
    Venezuelan 066.2
    Western 062.1

Encephalomyelitis—*continued*
  funicularis infectiosa 049.8
  late effect—*see* Late, effect, encephalitis
  Munch-Peterson's 049.8
  postchickenpox 052.0
  postimmunization 323.51
  postmeasles 055.0
  postvaccinal (smallpox) 323.51
  rubella 056.01
  specified cause NEC 323.81
  syphilitic 094.81
  West Nile 066.41
Encephalomyelocele 742.0
Encephalomyelomeningitis —*see* Meningoencephalitis
Encephalomyeloneuropathy 349.9
Encephalomyelopathy 349.9
  subacute necrotizing (infantile) 330.8
Encephalomyeloradiculitis (acute) 357.0
Encephalomyeloradiculoneuritis (acute) 357.0
Encephalomyeloradiculopathy 349.9
Encephalomyocarditis 074.23
Encephalopathia hyperbilirubinemica newborn 774.7
  due to isoimmunization (conditions classifiable to 773.0-773.2) 773.4
Encephalopathy (acute) 348.30
  alcoholic 291.2
  anoxic—*see* Damage, brain, anoxic
  arteriosclerotic 437.0
    late effect—*see* Late effect(s) (of) cerebrovascular disease
  bilirubin, newborn 774.7
    due to isoimmunization 773.4
  congenital 742.9
  demyelinating (callosal) 341.8
  due to
    birth injury (intracranial) 767.8
    dialysis 294.8
      transient 293.9
    drugs (—*see also* Table of Drugs and Chemicals) 349.82
    hyperinsulinism—*see* Hyperinsulinism
    influenza (virus) (*see also* Influenza) 487.8
      identified
        avian 488.09
        (novel) 2009 H1N1 488.19
    lack of vitamin (*see also* Deficiency, vitamin) 269.2
    nicotinic acid deficiency 291.2
    serum (nontherapeutic) (therapeutic) 999.59
    syphilis 094.81
    trauma (postconcussional) 310.2
      current (*see also* Concussion, brain) 850.9
      with skull fracture—*see* Fracture, skull, by site, with intracranial injury
    vaccination 323.51
  hepatic 572.2
  hyperbilirubinemic, newborn 774.7
    due to isoimmunization (conditions classifiable to 773.0-773.2) 773.4
  hypertensive 437.2
  hypoglycemic 251.2
  hypoxic—*see also* Damage, brain, anoxic
    ischemic (HIE) 768.70
      mild 768.71
      moderate 768.72
      severe 768.73
  infantile cystic necrotizing (congenital) 341.8
  lead 984.9 *[323.71]*
  leukopolio 330.0

Encephalopathy—*continued*
  metabolic (*see also* Delirium) 348.31
    drug induced 349.82
    toxic 349.82
  necrotizing
    hemorrhagic (acute) 323.61
    subacute 330.8
  other specified type NEC 348.39
  pellagrous 265.2
  portal-systemic 572.2
  postcontusional 310.2
  posttraumatic 310.2
  saturnine 984.9 *[323.71]*
  septic 348.31
  spongioform, subacute (viral) 046.19
  subacute
    necrotizing 330.8
    spongioform 046.19
    viral, spongioform 046.19
  subcortical progressive (Schilder) 341.1
    chronic (Binswanger's) 290.12
  toxic 349.82
    metabolic 349.82
  traumatic (postconcussional) 310.2
    current (*see also* Concussion, brain) 850.9
      with skull fracture—*see* Fracture, skull, by
        site, with intracranial injury
  vitamin B deficiency NEC 266.9
  Wernicke's (superior hemorrhagic
    polioencephalitis) 265.1
Enchephalorrhagia (*see also* Hemorrhage,
  brain) 432.9
  healed or old V12.54
  late effect—*see* Late effect(s) (of)
    cerebrovascular disease
Encephalosis, posttraumatic 310.2
Enchondroma (M9220/0)—*see also* Neoplasm,
  bone, benign
  multiple, congenital 756.4
Enchondromatosis (cartilaginous) (congenital)
  (multiple) 756.4
Enchondroses, multiple (cartilaginous)
  (congenital) 756.4
Encopresis (*see also* Incontinence, feces) 787.60
  nonorganic origin 307.7
Encounter for —*see also* Admission for
  administrative purpose only V68.9
    referral of patient without examination or
      treatment V68.81
    specified purpose NEC V68.89
  chemotherapy, (oral) (intravenous)
    antineoplastic V58.11
  determination of fetal viability of pregnancy
    V23.87
  disability examination V68.01
  end-of-life care V66.7
  hospice care V66.7
  immunizations (childhood) appropriate for age V20.2
  immunotherapy, antineoplastic V58.12
  joint prosthesis insertion following prior
    explantation of joint prosthesis V54.82
  palliative care V66.7
  radiotherapy V58.0
  respirator (ventilator) dependence
    during
      mechanical failure V46.14
      power failure V46.12
    for weaning V46.13
  routine infant and child vision and hearing
    testing V20.2

Encounter for—*continued*
  school examination V70.3
    following surgery V67.09
  screening mammogram NEC V76.12
    for high-risk patient V76.11
  paternity testing V70.4
  terminal care V66.7
  weaning from respirator (ventilator) V46.13
Encystment —*see* Cyst
End-of-life care V66.7
Endamebiasis —*see* Amebiasis
Endamoeba —*see* Amebiasis
Endarteritis (bacterial, subacute) (infective)
  (septic) 447.6
  brain, cerebral or cerebrospinal 437.4
    late effect—*see* Late effect(s) (of)
      cerebrovascular disease
  coronary (artery) —*see* Arteriosclerosis,
    coronary
  deformans—*see* Arteriosclerosis
  embolic (*see also* Embolism) 444.9
  obliterans—*see also* Arteriosclerosis
    pulmonary 417.8
  pulmonary 417.8
  retina 362.18
  senile—*see* Arteriosclerosis
  syphilitic 093.89
    brain or cerebral 094.89
    congenital 090.5
    spinal 094.89
  tuberculous (*see also* Tuberculosis) 017.9
Endemic —*see* condition
Endocarditis (chronic) (indeterminate)
  (interstitial) (marantic) (nonbacterial
  thrombotic) (residual) (sclerotic) (sclerous)
  (senile) (valvular) 424.90
  with
    rheumatic fever (conditions classifiable to
      390)
      active—*see* Endocarditis, acute, rheumatic
      inactive or quiescent (with chorea) 397.9
  acute or subacute 421.9
    rheumatic (aortic) (mitral) (pulmonary)
      (tricuspid) 391.1
      with chorea (acute) (rheumatic)
        (Sydenham's) 392.0
  aortic (heart) (nonrheumatic) (valve) 424.1
    with
      mitral (valve) disease 396.9
        active or acute 391.1
          with chorea (acute) (rheumatic)
            (Sydenham's) 392.0
      rheumatic fever (conditions classifiable to
        390)
        active—*see* Endocarditis, acute, rheumatic
        inactive or quiescent (with chorea) 395.9
          with mitral disease 396.9
    acute or subacute 421.9
    arteriosclerotic 424.1
    congenital 746.89
    hypertensive 424.1
    rheumatic (chronic) (inactive) 395.9
      with mitral (valve) disease 396.9
        active or acute 391.1
          with chorea (acute) (rheumatic)
            (Sydenham's) 392.0
      active or acute 391.1
        with chorea (acute) (rheumatic)
          (Sydenham's) 392.0
    specified cause, except rheumatic 424.1
    syphilitic 093.22

Endocarditis—*continued*
  arteriosclerotic or due to arteriosclerosis 424.99
  atypical verrucous (Libman-Sacks) 710.0
    [424.91]
  bacterial (acute) (any valve) (chronic) (subacute)
    421.0
  blastomycotic 116.0 *[421.1]*
  candidal 112.81
  congenital 425.3
  constrictive 421.0
  Coxsackie 074.22
  due to
    blastomycosis 116.0 *[421.1]*
    candidiasis 112.81
    Coxsackie (virus) 074.22
    disseminated lupus erythematosus 710.0
      [424.91]
    histoplasmosis (*see also* Histoplasmosis) 115.94
    hypertension (benign) 424.99
    moniliasis 112.81
    prosthetic cardiac valve 996.61
    Q fever 083.0 *[421.1]*
    serratia marcescens 421.0
    typhoid (fever) 002.0 *[421.1]*
  fetal 425.3
  gonococcal 098.84
  hypertensive 424.99
  infectious or infective (acute) (any valve)
    (chronic) (subacute) 421.0
  lenta (acute) (any valve) (chronic) (subacute)
    421.0
  Libman-Sacks 710.0 *[424.91]*
  Loeffler's (parietal fibroplastic) 421.0
  malignant (acute) (any valve) (chronic)
    (subacute) 421.0
  meningococcal 036.42
  mitral (chronic) (double) (fibroid) (heart)
    (inactive) (valve) (with chorea) 394.9
    with
      aortic (valve) disease 396.9
        active or acute 391.1
          with chorea (acute) (rheumatic)
            (Sydenham's) 392.0
      rheumatic fever (conditions classifiable to
        390)
        active—*see* Endocarditis, acute, rheumatic
        inactive or quiescent (with chorea) 394.9
          with aortic valve disease 396.9
    active or acute 391.1
      bacterial 421.0
      with chorea (acute) (rheumatic)
        (Sydenham's) 392.0
    arteriosclerotic 424.0
    congenital 746.89
    hypertensive 424.0
    nonrheumatic 424.0
      acute or subacute 421.9
    syphilitic 093.21
  monilial 112.81
  mycotic (acute) (any valve) (chronic) (subacute)
    421.0
  pneumococcic (acute) (any valve) (chronic)
    (subacute) 421.0
  pulmonary (chronic) (heart) (valve) 424.3
    with
      rheumatic fever (conditions classifiable to 390)
        active—*see* Endocarditis, acute, rheumatic
        inactive or quiescent (with chorea) 397.1
    acute or subacute 421.9
      rheumatic 391.1
        with chorea (acute) (rheumatic)
          (Sydenham's) 392.0

Endocarditis—*continued*
  pulmonary—*continued*
    arteriosclerotic or due to arteriosclerosis 424.3
    congenital 746.09
    hypertensive or due to hypertension (benign)
      424.3
    rheumatic (chronic) (inactive) (with chorea)
      397.1
      active or acute 391.1
        with chorea (acute) (rheumatic)
          (Sydenham's) 392.0
    syphilitic 093.24
  purulent (acute) (any valve) (chronic) (subacute)
    421.0
  rheumatic (chronic) (inactive) (with chorea)
    397.9
    active or acute (aortic) (mitral) (pulmonary)
      (tricuspid) 391.1
      with chorea (acute) (rheumatic)
        (Sydenham's) 392.0
  septic (acute) (any valve) (chronic) (subacute)
    421.0
  specified cause, except rheumatic 424.99
  streptococcal (acute) (any valve) (chronic)
    (subacute) 421.0
  subacute—*see* Endocarditis, acute
  suppurative (any valve) (acute) (chronic)
    (subacute) 421.0
  syphilitic NEC 093.20
  toxic (*see also* Endocarditis, acute) 421.9
  tricuspid (chronic) (heart) (inactive) (rheumatic)
    (valve) (with chorea) 397.0
    with
      rheumatic fever (conditions classifiable to
        390)
        active—*see* Endocarditis, acute, rheumatic
        inactive or quiescent (with chorea) 397.0
    active or acute 391.1
      with chorea (acute) (rheumatic)
        (Sydenham's) 392.0
    arteriosclerotic 424.2
    congenital 746.89
    hypertensive 424.2
    nonrheumatic 424.2
      acute or subacute 421.9
    specified cause, except rheumatic 424.2
    syphilitic 093.23
  tuberculous (*see also* Tuberculosis) 017.9
    [424.91]
  typhoid 002.0 *[421.1]*
  ulcerative (acute) (any valve) (chronic)
    (subacute) 421.0
  vegetative (acute) (any valve) (chronic)
    (subacute) 421.0
  verrucous (acute) (any valve) (chronic)
    (subacute) NEC 710.0 *[424.91]*
    nonbacterial 710.0 *[424.91]*
    nonrheumatic 710.0 *[424.91]*
Endocardium, endocardial —*see also* condition
  cushion defect 745.60
    specified type NEC 745.69
Endocervicitis (*see also* Cervicitis) 616.0
  due to
    intrauterine (contraceptive) device 996.65
    gonorrheal (acute) 098.15
      chronic or duration of 2 months or over 098.35
  hyperplastic 616.0
  syphilitic 095.8
  trichomonal 131.09
  tuberculous (*see also* Tuberculosis) 016.7
Endocrine —*see* condition
Endocrinopathy, pluriglandular 258.9

Endodontitis 522.0
Endomastoiditis (*see also* Mastoiditis) 383.9
Endometrioma 617.9
Endometriosis 617.9
  appendix 617.5
  bladder 617.8
  bowel 617.5
  broad ligament 617.3
  cervix 617.0
  colon 617.5
  cul-de-sac (Douglas') 617.3
  exocervix 617.0
  fallopian tube 617.2
  female genital organ NEC 617.8
  gallbladder 617.8
  in scar of skin 617.6
  internal 617.0
  intestine 617.5
  lung 617.8
  myometrium 617.0
  ovary 617.1
  parametrium 617.3
  pelvic peritoneum 617.3
  peritoneal (pelvic) 617.3
  rectovaginal septum 617.4
  rectum 617.5
  round ligament 617.3
  skin 617.6
  specified site NEC 617.8
  stromal (M8931/1) 236.0
  umbilicus 617.8
  uterus 617.0
    internal 617.0
  vagina 617.4
  vulva 617.8
Endometritis (nonspecific) (purulent) (septic)
    (suppurative) 615.9
  with
    abortion—*see* Abortion, by type, with sepsis
    ectopic pregnancy (*see also* categories
       633.0-633.9) 639.0
    molar pregnancy (*see also* categories 630-632)
       639.0
  acute 615.0
  blennorrhagic 098.16
    acute 098.16
    chronic or duration of 2 months or over 098.36
  cervix, cervical (*see also* Cervicitis) 616.0
    hyperplastic 616.0
  chronic 615.1
  complicating pregnancy 670.1
    affecting fetus or newborn 760.8
    septic 670.2
  decidual 615.9
  following
    abortion 639.0
    ectopic or molar pregnancy 639.0
  gonorrheal (acute) 098.16
    chronic or duration of 2 months or over 098.36
  hyperplastic (*see also* Hyperplasia,
       endometrium) 621.30
    cervix 616.0
  polypoid—*see* Endometritis, hyperplastic
  puerperal, postpartum, childbirth 670.1
    septic 670.2
  senile (atrophic) 615.9
  subacute 615.0
  tuberculous (*see also* Tuberculosis) 016.7
Endometrium —*see* condition
Endomyocardiopathy, South African 425.2

Endomyocarditis —*see* Endocarditis
Endomyofibrosis 425.0
Endomyometritis (*see also* Endometritis) 615.9
Endopericarditis —*see* Endocarditis
Endoperineuritis —*see* Disorder, nerve
Endophlebitis (*see also* Phlebitis) 451.9
  leg 451.2
    deep (vessels) 451.19
    superficial (vessels) 451.0
  portal (vein) 572.1
  retina 362.18
  specified site NEC 451.89
  syphilitic 093.89
Endophthalmia (*see also* Endophthalmitis) 360.00
  gonorrheal 098.42
Endophthalmitis (globe) (infective) (metastatic)
    (purulent) (subacute) 360.00
  acute 360.01
  bleb associated 379.63
  chronic 360.03
  parasitic 360.13
  phacoanaphylactic 360.19
  specified type NEC 360.19
  sympathetic 360.11
Endosalpingioma (M9111/1) 236.2
Endosalpingiosis 629.89
Endosteitis —*see* Osteomyelitis
Endothelioma, bone (M9260/3)—*see* Neoplasm,
    bone, malignant
Endotheliosis 287.8
  hemorrhagic infectional 287.8
Endotoxemia —*code to condition*
Endotoxic shock 785.52
  postoperative 998.02
Endotrachelitis (*see also* Cervicitis) 616.0
Enema rash 692.89
**Engel-von Recklinghausen disease or
    syndrome** (osteitis fibrosa cystica) 252.01
Engelmann's disease (diaphyseal sclerosis)
    756.59
English disease (*see also* Rickets) 268.0
Engman's disease (infectious eczematoid
    dermatitis) 690.8
Engorgement
  breast 611.79
    newborn 778.7
    puerperal, postpartum 676.2
  liver 573.9
  lung 514
  pulmonary 514
  retina, venous 362.37
  stomach 536.8
  venous, retina 362.37
Enlargement, enlarged —*see also* Hypertrophy
  abdomen 789.3
  adenoids 474.12
    and tonsils 474.10
  alveolar process or ridge 525.8
  apertures of diaphragm (congenital) 756.6
  blind spot, visual field 368.42
  gingival 523.8
  heart, cardiac (*see also* Hypertrophy, cardiac) 429.3
  lacrimal gland, chronic 375.03
  liver (*see also* Hypertrophy, liver) 789.1
  lymph gland or node 785.6
  orbit 376.46
  organ or site, congenital NEC—*see* Anomaly,
       specified type NEC
  parathyroid (gland) 252.01
  pituitary fossa 793.0

Enlargement, enlarged—*continued*
prostate (simple) (soft) 600.00
with
other lower urinary tract symptoms (LUTS) 600.01
urinary
obstruction 600.01
retention 600.01
sella turcica 793.0
spleen (*see also* Splenomegaly) 789.2
congenital 759.0
thymus (congenital) (gland) 254.0
thyroid (gland) (*see also* Goiter) 240.9
tongue 529.8
tonsils 474.11
and adenoids 474.10
uterus 621.2
Enophthalmos 376.50
due to
atrophy of orbital tissue 376.51
surgery 376.52
trauma 376.52
Enostosis 526.89
Entamebiasis —*see* Amebiasis
Entamebic —*see* Amebiasis
Entanglement, umbilical cord (s) 663.3
with compression 663.2
affecting fetus or newborn 762.5
around neck with compression 663.1
twins in monoamniotic sac 663.2
Enteralgia 789.0
Enteric —*see* condition
Enteritis (acute) (catarrhal) (choleraic) (chronic)
(congestive) (diarrheal) (exudative) (follicular)
(hemorrhagic) (infantile) (lienteric)
(noninfectious) (perforative) (phlegmonous)
(presumed noninfectious)
(pseudomembranous) 558.9
adaptive 564.9
aertrycke infection 003.0
allergic 558.3
amebic (*see also* Amebiasis) 006.9
with abscess—*see* Abscess, amebic
acute 006.0
with abscess—*see* Abscess, amebic
nondysenteric 006.2
chronic 006.1
with abscess—*see* Abscess, amebic
nondysenteric 006.2
nondysenteric 006.2
anaerobic (cocci) (gram-negative)
(gram-positive) (mixed) NEC 008.46
bacillary NEC 004.9
bacterial NEC 008.5
specified NEC 008.49
Bacteroides (fragilis) (melaninogeniscus)
(oralis) 008.46
Butyrivibrio (fibriosolvens) 008.46
Campylobacter 008.43
Candida 112.85
Chilomastix 007.8
choleriformis 001.1
chronic 558.9
ulcerative (*see also* Colitis, ulcerative) 556.9
cicatrizing (chronic) 555.0
Clostridium
botulinum 005.1
difficile 008.45
haemolyticum 008.46
novyi 008.46
perfringens (C) (F) 008.46
specified type NEC 008.46

Enteritis—*continued*
coccidial 007.2
dietetic 558.9
due to
achylia gastrica 536.8
adenovirus 008.62
Aerobacter aerogenes 008.2
anaerobes—*see* Enteritis, anaerobic 008.46
Arizona (bacillus) 008.1
astrovirus 008.66
Bacillus coli—*see* Enteritis, E. coli 008.0
bacteria NEC 008.5
specified NEC 008.49
Bacteroides 008.46
Butyrivibrio (fibriosolvens) 008.46
calicivirus 008.65
Campylobacter 008.43
Clostridium—*see* Enteritis, Clostridium
Cockle agent 008.64
Coxsackie (virus) 008.67
Ditchling agent 008.64
ECHO virus 008.67
Enterobacter aerogenes 008.2
enterococci 008.49
enterovirus NEC 008.67
Escherichia coli—*see* Enteritis, E. coli
Eubacterium 008.46
Fusobacterium (nucleatum) 008.46
gram-negative bacteria NEC 008.47
anaerobic NEC 008.46
Hawaii agent 008.63
irritating foods 558.9
Klebsiella aerogenes 008.47
Marin County agent 008.66
Montgomery County agent 008.63
norovirus 008.63
Norwalk-like agent 008.63
Norwalk virus 008.63
Otofuke agent 008.63
Paracolobactrum arizonae 008.1
paracolon bacillus NEC 008.47
Arizona 008.1
Paramatta agent 008.64
Peptococcus 008.46
Peptostreptococcus 008.46
Propionibacterium 008.46
Proteus (bacillus) (mirabilis) (morganii) 008.3
Pseudomonas aeruginosa 008.42
radiation 558.1
Rotavirus 008.61
Sapporo agent 008.63
small round virus (SRV) NEC 008.64
featureless NEC 008.63
structured NEC 008.63
Snow Mountain (SM) agent 008.63
specified
bacteria NEC 008.49
organism, nonbacterial NEC 008.8
virus NEC 008.69
Staphylococcus 008.41
Streptococcus 008.49
anaerobic 008.46
Taunton agent 008.63
Torovirus 008.69
Treponema 008.46
Veillonella 008.46
virus 008.8
specified type NEC 008.69
Wollan (W) agent 008.64
Yersinia enterocolitica 008.44
dysentery—*see* Dysentery

Enteritis—*continued*
E. coli 008.00
  enterohemorrhagic 008.04
  enteroinvasive 008.03
  enteropathogenic 008.01
  enterotoxigenic 008.02
  specified type NEC 008.09
el tor 001.1
embadomonial 007.8
eosinophilic 558.41
epidemic 009.0
Eubacterium 008.46
fermentative 558.9
fulminant 557.0
Fusobacterium (nucleatum) 008.46
gangrenous (*see also* Enteritis, due to, by organism) 009.0
giardial 007.1
gram-negative bacteria NEC 008.47
  anaerobic NEC 008.46
infectious NEC (*see also* Enteritis, due to, by organism) 009.0
  presumed 009.1
influenzal (*see also* Influenza) 487.8
ischemic 557.9
  acute 557.0
  chronic 557.1
  due to mesenteric artery insufficiency 557.1
membranous 564.9
mucous 564.9
myxomembranous 564.9
necrotic (*see also* Enteritis, due to, by organism) 009.0
necroticans 005.2
necrotizing of fetus or newborn (*see also* Enterocolitis, necrotizing, newborn) 777.50
neurogenic 564.9
newborn 777.8
  necrotizing (*see also* Enterocolitis, necrotizing, newborn) 777.50
parasitic NEC 129
paratyphoid (fever) (*see also* Fever, paratyphoid) 002.9
Peptococcus 008.46
Peptostreptococcus 008.46
Propionibacterium 008.46
protozoal NEC 007.9
radiation 558.1
regional (of) 555.9
  intestine
    large (bowel, colon, or rectum) 555.1
      with small intestine 555.2
    small (duodenum, ileum, or jejunum) 555.0
      with large intestine 555.2
Salmonella infection 003.0
salmonellosis 003.0
segmental (*see also* Enteritis, regional) 555.9
septic (*see also* Enteritis, due to, by organism) 009.0
Shigella 004.9
simple 558.9
spasmodic 564.9
spastic 564.9
staphylococcal 008.41
  due to food 005.0
streptococcal 008.49
  anaerobic 008.46
toxic 558.2
Treponema (denticola) (macrodentium) 008.46
trichomonal 007.3
tuberculous (*see also* Tuberculosis) 014.8
typhosa 002.0

Enteritis—*continued*
ulcerative (chronic) (*see also* Colitis, ulcerative) 556.9
Veillonella 008.46
viral 008.8
  adenovirus 008.62
  enterovirus 008.67
  specified virus NEC 008.69
Yersinia enterocolitica 008.44
zymotic 009.0
Enteroarticular syndrome 099.3
Enterobiasis 127.4
Enterobius vermicularis 127.4
Enterocele (*see also* Hernia) 553.9
pelvis, pelvic (acquired) (congenital) 618.6
vagina, vaginal (acquired) (congenital) 618.6
Enterocolitis —*see also* Enteritis
fetus or newborn (*see also* Enterocolitis, necrotizing, newborn) 777.8
  necrotizing 777.50
fulminant 557.0
granulomatous 555.2
hemorrhagic (acute) 557.0
  chronic 557.1
necrotizing (acute) (membranous) 557.0
  newborn 777.50
    with
      perforation 777.53
      pneumatosis without perforation 777.52
      pneumatosis and perforation 777.53
    stage I 777.51
    stage II 777.52
    stage III 777.53
    without pneumatosis, without perforation 777.51
primary necrotizing (*see also* Enterocolitis, necrotizing, newborn) 777.50
pseudomembranous 008.45
  newborn 008.45
radiation 558.1
  newborn (*see also* Enterocolitis, necrotizing, newborn) 777.50
ulcerative 556.0
Enterocystoma 751.5
Enterogastritis —*see* Enteritis
Enterogenous cyanosis 289.7
Enterolith, enterolithiasis (impaction) 560.39
with hernia—*see also* Hernia, by site, with obstruction
  gangrenous—*see* Hernia, by site, with gangrene
Enteropathy 569.9
exudative (of Gordon) 579.8
gluten 579.0
hemorrhagic, terminal 557.0
protein-losing 579.8
Enteroperitonitis (*see also* Peritonitis) 567.9
Enteroptosis 569.89
Enterorrhagia 578.9
Enterospasm 564.9
psychogenic 306.4
Enterostenosis (*see also* Obstruction, intestine) 560.9
Enterostomy status V44.4
with complication 569.60
Enthesopathy 726.39
ankle and tarsus 726.70
elbow region 726.30
  specified NEC 726.39
hip 726.5

Enthesopathy—*continued*
  knee 726.60
  peripheral NEC 726.8
  shoulder region 726.10
    adhesive 726.0
  spinal 720.1
  wrist and carpus 726.4
Entrance, air into vein —*see* Embolism, air
Entrapment, nerve —*see* Neuropathy,
    entrapment
Entropion (eyelid) 374.00
  cicatricial 374.04
  congenital 743.62
  late effect of trachoma (healed) 139.1
  mechanical 374.02
  paralytic 374.02
  senile 374.01
  spastic 374.03
Enucleation of eye (current) (traumatic) 871.3
Enuresis 788.30
  habit disturbance 307.6
  nocturnal 788.36
    psychogenic 307.6
  nonorganic origin 307.6
  psychogenic 307.6
Enzymopathy 277.9
Eosinopenia 288.59
Eosinophilia 288.3
  with
    angiolymphoid hyperplasia (ALHE) 228.01
  allergic 288.3
  hereditary 288.3
  idiopathic 288.3
  infiltrative 518.3
  Loeffler's 518.3
  myalgia syndrome 710.5
  pulmonary (tropical) 518.3
  secondary 288.3
  tropical 518.3
Eosinophilic —*see also* condition
  fasciitis 728.89
  granuloma (bone) 277.89
  infiltration lung 518.3
Ependymitis (acute) (cerebral) (chronic)
    (granular) (*see also* Meningitis) 322.9
Ependymoblastoma (M9392/3)
  specified site—*see* Neoplasm, by site, malignant
  unspecified site 191.9
Ependymoma (epithelial) (malignant) (M9391/3)
  anaplastic type (M9392/3)
    specified site—*see* Neoplasm, by site, malignant
    unspecified site 191.9
  benign (M9391/0)
    specified site—*see* Neoplasm, by site, benign
    unspecified site 225.0
  myxopapillary (M9394/1) 237.5
  papillary (M9393/1) 237.5
  specified site—*see* Neoplasm, by site, malignant
  unspecified site 191.9
Ependymopathy 349.2
  spinal cord 349.2
Ephelides, ephelis 709.09
Ephemeral fever (*see also* Pyrexia) 780.60
Epiblepharon (congenital) 743.62
Epicanthus, epicanthic fold (congenital) (eyelid)
    743.63
Epicondylitis (elbow) (lateral) 726.32
  medial 726.31

Epicystitis (*see also* Cystitis) 595.9
Epidemic —*see* condition
Epidermidalization, cervix —*see* condition
Epidermidization, cervix —*see* condition
Epidermis, epidermal —*see* condition
Epidermization, cervix —*see* condition
Epidermodysplasia verruciformis 078.19
Epidermoid
  cholesteatoma—*see* Cholesteatoma
  inclusion (*see also* Cyst, skin) 706.2
Epidermolysis
  acuta (combustiformis) (toxica) 695.15
  bullosa 757.39
  necroticans combustiformis 695.15
    due to drug
      correct substance properly administered 695.15
      overdose or wrong substance given or taken
        977.9
      specified drug—*see* Table of drugs and
        chemicals
Epidermophytid —*see* Dermatophytosis
Epidermophytosis (infected)—*see*
    Dermatophytosis
Epidermosis, ear (middle) (*see also*
    Cholesteatoma) 385.30
Epididymis —*see* condition
Epididymitis (nonvenereal) 604.90
  with abscess 604.0
  acute 604.99
  blennorrhagic (acute) 098.0
    chronic or duration of 2 months or over 098.2
  caseous (*see also* Tuberculosis) 016.4
  chlamydial 099.54
  diphtheritic 032.89 *[604.91]*
  filarial 125.9 *[604.91]*
  gonococcal (acute) 098.0
    chronic or duration of 2 months or over 098.2
  recurrent 604.99
  residual 604.99
  syphilitic 095.8 *[604.91]*
  tuberculous (*see also* Tuberculosis) 016.4
Epididymo-orchitis (*see also* Epididymitis)
    604.90
  with abscess 604.0
  chlamydial 099.54
  gonococcal (acute) 098.13
    chronic or duration of 2 months or over 098.33
Epidural —*see* condition
Epigastritis (*see also* Gastritis) 535.5
Epigastrium, epigastric —*see* condition
Epigastrocele (*see also* Hernia, epigastric) 553.29
Epiglottiditis (acute) 464.30
  with obstruction 464.31
  chronic 476.1
  viral 464.30
    with obstruction 464.31
Epiglottis —*see* condition
Epiglottitis (acute) 464.30
  with obstruction 464.31
  chronic 476.1
  viral 464.30
    with obstruction 464.31
Epignathus 759.4
Epilepsia
  partialis continua (*see also* Epilepsy) 345.7
  procursiva (*see also* Epilepsy) 345.8

Epilepsy, epileptic (idiopathic) 345.9

Note—use the following fifth-digit subclassification with categories 345.0, 345.1, 345.4-345.9

0 without mention of intractable epilepsy
1 with intractable epilepsy
      pharmacoresistant (pharmacologically resistant)
      poorly controlled
      refractory (medically)
      treatment resistant

abdominal 345.5
absence (attack) 345.0
akinetic 345.0
  psychomotor 345.4
automatism 345.4
autonomic diencephalic 345.5
brain 345.9
Bravais-Jacksonian 345.5
cerebral 345.9
climacteric 345.9
clonic 345.1
clouded state 345.9
coma 345.3
communicating 345.4
complicating pregnancy, childbirth or the
  puerperium 649.4
congenital 345.9
convulsions 345.9
cortical (focal) (motor) 345.5
cursive (running) 345.8
cysticercosis 123.1
deterioration
  with behavioral disturbance 345.9 *[294.11]*
  without behavioral disturbance 345.9 *[294.10]*
due to syphilis 094.89
equivalent 345.5
fit 345.9
focal (motor) 345.5
gelastic 345.8
generalized 345.9
  convulsive 345.1
  flexion 345.1
  nonconvulsive 345.0
grand mal (idiopathic) 345.1
Jacksonian (motor) (sensory) 345.5
Kojevnikoff's, Kojevnikov's, Kojewnikoff's
  345.7
laryngeal 786.2
limbic system 345.4
localization related (focal) (partial) and epileptic
  syndromes
  with
    complex partial seizures 345.4
    simple partial seizures 345.5
major (motor) 345.1
minor 345.0
mixed (type) 345.9
motor partial 345.5
musicogenic 345.1
myoclonus, myoclonic 345.1
  progressive (familial) 345.1
nonconvulsive, generalized 345.0
parasitic NEC 123.9

Epilepsy, epileptic—*continued*
partial (focalized) 345.5
  with
    impairment of consciousness 345.4
    memory and ideational disturbances 345.4
  abdominal type 345.5
  motor type 345.5
  psychomotor type 345.4
  psychosensory type 345.4
  secondarily generalized 345.4
  sensory type 345.5
  somatomotor type 345.5
  somatosensory type 345.5
  temporal lobe type 345.4
  visceral type 345.5
  visual type 345.5
  without impairment of consciousness 345.5
peripheral 345.9
petit mal 345.0
photokinetic 345.8
progressive myoclonic (familial) 345.1
psychic equivalent 345.5
psychomotor 345.4
psychosensory 345.4
reflex 345.1
seizure 345.9
senile 345.9
sensory-induced 345.5
sleep (*see also* Narcolepsy) 347.00
somatomotor type 345.5
somatosensory 345.5
specified type NEC 345.8
status (grand mal) 345.3
  focal motor 345.7
  petit mal 345.2
  psychomotor 345.7
  temporal lobe 345.7
symptomatic 345.9
temporal lobe 345.4
tonic (-clonic) 345.1
traumatic (injury unspecified) 907.0
  injury specified—*see* Late, effect (of)
    specified injury
twilight 293.0
uncinate (gyrus) 345.4
Unverricht (-Lundborg) (familial myoclonic)
  345.1
visceral 345.5
visual 345.5
Epileptiform
  convulsions 780.39
  seizure 780.39
Epiloia 759.5
Epimenorrhea 626.2
Epipharyngitis (*see also* Nasopharyngitis) 460
Epiphora 375.20
  due to
    excess lacrimation 375.21
    insufficient drainage 375.22
Epiphyseal arrest 733.91
  femoral head 732.2
Epiphyseolysis, epiphysiolysis (*see also* Osteochondrosis) 732.9
Epiphysitis (*see also* Osteochondrosis) 732.9
  juvenile 732.6
  marginal (Scheuermann's) 732.0
  os calcis 732.5
  syphilitic (congenital) 090.0
  vertebral (Scheuermann's) 732.0
Epiplocele (*see also* Hernia) 553.9
Epiploitis (*see also* Peritonitis) 567.9

Epiplosarcomphalocele (*see also* Hernia, umbilicus) 553.1
Episcleritis 379.00
  gouty 274.89 *[379.09]*
  nodular 379.02
  periodica fugax 379.01
    angioneurotic—*see* Edema, angioneurotic
  specified NEC 379.09
  staphylococcal 379.00
  suppurative 379.00
  syphilitic 095.0
  tuberculous (*see also* Tuberculosis) 017.3
    [379.09]
Episode
  brain (*see also* Disease, cerebrovascular, acute) 436
  cerebral (*see also* Disease, cerebrovascular, acute) 436
  depersonalization (in neurotic state) 300.6
  hyporesponsive 780.09
  psychotic (*see also* Psychosis) 298.9
    organic, transient 293.9
  schizophrenic (acute) NEC (*see also* Schizophrenia) 295.4
Epispadias
  female 753.8
  male 752.62
Episplenitis 289.59
Epistaxis (multiple) 784.7
  hereditary 448.0
  vicarious menstruation 625.8
Epithelioma (malignant) (M8011/3)—*see also* Neoplasm, by site, malignant
  adenoides cysticum (M8100/0)—*see* Neoplasm, skin, benign
  basal cell (M8090/3)—*see* Neoplasm, skin, malignant
  benign (M8011/0)—*see* Neoplasm, by site, benign
  Bowen's (M8081/2)—*see* Neoplasm, skin, in situ
  calcifying (benign) (Malherbe's) (M8110/0)—*see* Neoplasm, skin, benign
  external site—*see* Neoplasm, skin, malignant
  intraepidermal, Jadassohn (M8096/0)—*see* Neoplasm, skin, benign
  squamous cell (M8070/3)—*see* Neoplasm, by site, malignant
Epitheliopathy
  pigment, retina 363.15
  posterior multifocal placoid (acute) 363.15
Epithelium, epithelial —*see* condition
Epituberculosis (allergic) (with atelectasis) (*see also* Tuberculosis) 010.8
Eponychia 757.5
Epstein's
  nephrosis or syndrome (*see also* Nephrosis) 581.9
  pearl (mouth) 528.4
Epstein-Barr infection (viral) 075
  chronic 780.79 *[139.8]*
Epulis (giant cell) (gingiva) 523.8
Equinia 024
Equinovarus (congenital) 754.51
  acquired 736.71
Equivalent
  angina 413.9
  convulsive (abdominal) (*see also* Epilepsy) 345.5
  epileptic (psychic) (*see also* Epilepsy) 345.5

Erb's
  disease 359.1
  palsy, paralysis (birth) (brachial) (newborn) 767.6
    spinal (spastic) syphilitic 094.89
  pseudohypertrophic muscular dystrophy 359.1
Erb (-Duchenne) paralysis (birth injury) (newborn) 767.6
Erb-Goldflam disease or syndrome 358.00
Erdheim-Chester disease (ECD) 277.89
Erdheim's syndrome (acromegalic macrospondylitis) 253.0
Erection, painful (persistent) 607.3
Ergosterol deficiency (vitamin D) 268.9
  with
    osteomalacia 268.2
    rickets (*see also* Rickets) 268.0
Ergotism (ergotized grain) 988.2
  from ergot used as drug (migraine therapy)
    correct substance properly administered 349.82
    overdose or wrong substance given or taken 975.0
Erichsen's disease (railway spine) 300.16
Erlacher-Blount syndrome (tibia vara) 732.4
Erosio interdigitalis blastomycetica 112.3
Erosion
  arteriosclerotic plaque—*see* Arteriosclerosis, by site
  artery NEC 447.2
    without rupture 447.8
  bone 733.99
  bronchus 519.19
  cartilage (joint) 733.99
  cervix (uteri) (acquired) (chronic) (congenital) 622.0
    with mention of cervicitis 616.0
  cornea (recurrent) (*see also* Keratitis) 371.42
    traumatic 918.1
  dental (idiopathic) (occupational) 521.30
    extending into
      dentine 521.32
      pulp 521.33
    generalized 521.35
    limited to enamel 521.31
    localized 521.34
  duodenum, postpyloric—*see* Ulcer, duodenum
  esophagus 530.89
  gastric 535.4
  implanted vaginal mesh
    in, into
      pelvic floor muscles 629.31
      surrounding organ(s) or tissue 629.31
  intestine 569.89
  lymphatic vessel 457.8
  pylorus, pyloric (ulcer) 535.4
  sclera 379.16
  spine, aneurysmal 094.89
  spleen 289.59
  stomach 535.4
  teeth (idiopathic) (occupational) (*see also* Erosion, dental) 521.30
    due to
      medicine 521.30
      persistent vomiting 521.30
  urethra 599.84
  uterus 621.8
  vaginal prosthetic materials NEC
    in, into
      pelvic floor muscles 629.31
      surrounding organ(s) or tissue 629.31
  vertebra 733.99
Erotomania 302.89
  Clérambault's 297.8

Error
in diet 269.9
refractive 367.9
astigmatism (*see also* Astigmatism) 367.20
drug-induced 367.89
hypermetropia 367.0
hyperopia 367.0
myopia 367.1
presbyopia 367.4
toxic 367.89
Eructation 787.3
nervous 306.4
psychogenic 306.4
Eruption
creeping 126.9
drug—*see* Dermatitis, due to, drug
Hutchinson, summer 692.72
Kaposi's varicelliform 054.0
napkin (psoriasiform) 691.0
polymorphous
light (sun) 692.72
other source 692.82
psoriasiform, napkin 691.0
recalcitrant pustular 694.8
ringed 695.89
skin (*see also* Dermatitis) 782.1
creeping (meaning hookworm) 126.9
due to
chemical(s) NEC 692.4
internal use 693.8
drug—*see* Dermatitis, due to, drug
prophylactic inoculation or vaccination
against disease—*see* Dermatitis, due to,
vaccine
smallpox vaccination NEC—*see* Dermatitis,
due to, vaccine
erysipeloid 027.1
feigned 698.4
Hutchinson, summer 692.72
Kaposi's, varicelliform 054.0
vaccinia 999.0
lichenoid, axilla 698.3
polymorphous, due to light 692.72
toxic NEC 695.0
vesicular 709.8
teeth, tooth
accelerated 520.6
delayed 520.6
difficult 520.6
disturbance of 520.6
in abnormal sequence 520.6
incomplete 520.6
late 520.6
natal 520.6
neonatal 520.6
obstructed 520.6
partial 520.6
persistent primary 520.6
premature 520.6
prenatal 520.6
vesicular 709.8
Erysipelas (gangrenous) (infantile) (newborn)
(phlegmonous) (suppurative) 035
external ear 035 *[380.13]*
puerperal, postpartum, childbirth 670.8
Erysipelatoid (Rosenbach's) 027.1
Erysipeloid (Rosenbach's) 027.1

Erythema, erythematous (generalized) 695.9
ab igne—*see* Burn, by site, first degree
annulare (centrifugum) (rheumaticum) 695.0
arthriticum epidemicum 026.1
brucellum (*see also* Brucellosis) 023.9
bullosum 695.19
caloricum—*see* Burn, by site, first degree
chronicum migrans 088.81
chronicum 088.81
circinatum 695.19
diaper 691.0
due to
chemical (contact) NEC 692.4
internal 693.8
drug (internal use) 693.0
contact 692.3
elevatum diutinum 695.89
endemic 265.2
epidemic, arthritic 026.1
figuratum perstans 695.0
gluteal 691.0
gyratum (perstans) (repens) 695.19
heat—*see* Burn, by site, first degree
ichthyosiforme congenitum 757.1
induratum (primary) (scrofulosorum) (*see also*
Tuberculosis) 017.1
nontuberculous 695.2
infantum febrile 057.8
infectional NEC 695.9
infectiosum 057.0
inflammation NEC 695.9
intertrigo 695.89
iris 695.10
lupus (discoid) (localized) (*see also* Lupus,
erythematosus) 695.4
marginatum 695.0
rheumaticum—*see* Fever, rheumatic
medicamentosum—*see* Dermatitis, due to, drug
migrans 529.1
multiforme 695.10
bullosum 695.19
conjunctiva 695.19
exudativum (Hebra) 695.19
major 695.12
minor 695.11
pemphigoides 694.5
napkin 691.0
neonatorum 778.8
nodosum 695.2
tuberculous (*see also* Tuberculosis) 017.1
nummular, nummulare 695.19
palmar 695.0
palmaris hereditarium 695.0
pernio 991.5
perstans solare 692.72
rash, newborn 778.8
scarlatiniform (exfoliative) (recurrent) 695.0
simplex marginatum 057.8
solare (*see also* Sunburn) 692.71
streptogenes 696.5
toxic, toxicum NEC 695.0
newborn 778.8
tuberculous (primary) (*see also* Tuberculosis)
017.0
venenatum 695.0
Erythematosus —*see* condition
Erythematous —*see* condition
Erythermalgia (primary) 443.82
Erythralgia 443.82
Erythrasma 039.0

Erythredema 985.0
  polyneuritica 985.0
  polyneuropathy 985.0
Erythremia (acute) (M9841/3) 207.0
  chronic (M9842/3) 207.1
  secondary 289.0
Erythroblastopenia (acquired) 284.89
  congenital 284.01
Erythroblastophthisis 284.01
Erythroblastosis (fetalis) (newborn) 773.2
  due to
    ABO
      antibodies 773.1
      incompatibility, maternal/fetal 773.1
      isoimmunization 773.1
    Rh
      antibodies 773.0
      incompatibility, maternal/fetal 773.0
      isoimmunization 773.0
Erythrocyanosis (crurum) 443.89
Erythrocythemia —*see* Erythremia
Erythrocytopenia 285.9
Erythrocytosis (megalosplenic)
  familial 289.6
  oval, hereditary (*see also* Elliptocytosis) 282.1
  secondary 289.0
  stress 289.0
Erythroderma (*see also* Erythema) 695.9
  desquamativa (in infants) 695.89
  exfoliative 695.89
  ichthyosiform, congenital 757.1
  infantum 695.89
  maculopapular 696.2
  neonatorum 778.8
  psoriaticum 696.1
  secondary 695.9
Erythrodysesthesia, palmar plantar (PPE) 693.0
Erythrogenesis imperfecta 284.09
Erythroleukemia (M9840/3) 207.0
Erythromelalgia 443.82
Erythromelia 701.8
Erythropenia 285.9
Erythrophagocytosis 289.9
Erythrophobia 300.23
Erythroplakia
  oral mucosa 528.79
  tongue 528.79
Erythroplasia (Queyrat) (M8080/2)
  specified site—*see* Neoplasm, skin, in situ
  unspecified site 233.5
Erythropoiesis, idiopathic ineffective 285.0
Escaped beats, heart 427.60
  postoperative 997.1
Escherichia coli (E. coli) —*see* Infection,
    Escherichia coli
Esoenteritis —*see* Enteritis
Esophagalgia 530.89
Esophagectasis 530.89
  due to cardiospasm 530.0
Esophagismus 530.5
Esophagitis (alkaline) (chemical) (chronic)
    (infectional) (necrotic) (postoperative) 530.10
  acute 530.12
  candidal 112.84
  eosinophilic 530.13
  reflux 530.11
  specified NEC 530.19
  tuberculous (*see also* Tuberculosis) 017.8
  ulcerative 530.19
Esophagocele 530.6
Esophagodynia 530.89

Esophagomalacia 530.89
Esophagoptosis 530.89
Esophagospasm 530.5
Esophagostenosis 530.3
Esophagostomiasis 127.7
Esophagostomy
  complication 530.87
    infection 530.86
    malfunctioning 530.87
    mechanical 530.87
Esophagotracheal —*see* condition
Esophagus —*see* condition
Esophoria 378.41
  convergence, excess 378.84
  divergence, insufficiency 378.85
Esotropia (nonaccommodative) 378.00
  accommodative 378.35
  alternating 378.05
    with
      A pattern 378.06
      specified noncomitancy NEC 378.08
      V pattern 378.07
      X pattern 378.08
      Y pattern 378.08
    intermittent 378.22
  intermittent 378.20
    alternating 378.22
    monocular 378.21
  monocular 378.01
    with
      A pattern 378.02
      specified noncomitancy NEC 378.04
      V pattern 378.03
      X pattern 378.04
      Y pattern 378.04
    intermittent 378.21
Espundia 085.5
Essential —*see* condition
Esterapenia 289.89
Esthesioneuroblastoma (M9522/3) 160.0
Esthesioneurocytoma (M9521/3) 160.0
Esthesioneuroepithelioma (M9523/3) 160.0
Esthiomene 099.1
Estivo-autumnal
  fever 084.0
  malaria 084.0
Estrangement V61.09
Estriasis 134.0
Ethanolaminuria 270.8
Ethanolism (*see also* Alcoholism) 303.9
Ether dependence, dependency (*see also*
    Dependence) 304.6
Etherism (*see also* Dependence) 304.6
Ethmoid, ethmoidal —*see* condition
Ethmoiditis (chronic) (nonpurulent) (purulent)
    (*see also* Sinusitis, ethmoidal) 473.2
  influenzal (*see also* Influenza) 487.1
  Woakes' 471.1
Ethylism (*see also* Alcoholism) 303.9
Eulenburg's disease (congenital paramyotonia)
    359.29
Eunuchism 257.2
Eunuchoidism 257.2
  hypogonadotropic 257.2
European blastomycosis 117.5
Eustachian —*see* condition
Euthyroid sick syndrome 790.94
Euthyroidism 244.9

Evaluation
　fetal lung maturity 659.8
　for suspected condition (*see also* Observation) V71.9
　　abuse V71.81
　　exposure
　　　antrax V71.82
　　　biologic agent NEC V71.83
　　　SARS V71.83
　　neglect V71.81
　　newborn—*see* Observation, suspected,
　　　condition, newborn
　　specified condition NEC V71.89
　mental health V70.2
　　requested by authority V70.1
　nursing care V63.8
　social service V63.8
Evans' syndrome (thrombocytopenic purpura) 287.32
**Event, apparent life threatening in newborn
　and infant (ALTE)** 799.82
Eventration
　colon into chest—*see* Hernia, diaphragm
　diaphragm (congenital) 756.6
Eversion
　bladder 596.89
　cervix (uteri) 622.0
　　with mention of cervicitis 616.0
　foot NEC 736.79
　　congenital 755.67
　lacrimal punctum 375.51
　punctum lacrimale (postinfectional) (senile) 375.51
　ureter (meatus) 593.89
　urethra (meatus) 599.84
　uterus 618.1
　　complicating delivery 665.2
　　　affecting fetus or newborn 763.89
　　puerperal, postpartum 674.8
Evidence
　of malignancy
　　cytologic
　　　without histologic confirmation
　　　　anus 796.76
　　　　cervix 795.06
　　　　vagina 795.16
Evisceration
　birth injury 767.8
　bowel (congenital)—*see* Hernia, ventral
　congenital (*see also* Hernia, ventral) 553.29
　operative wound 998.32
　traumatic NEC 869.1
　　eye 871.3
Evulsion —*see* Avulsion
Ewing's
　angioendothelioma (M9260/3)—*see* Neoplasm,
　　bone, malignant
　sarcoma (M9260/3)—*see* Neoplasm, bone,
　　malignant
　tumor (M9260/3)—*see* Neoplasm, bone, malignant
Exaggerated lumbosacral angle (with impinging
　spine) 756.12
Examination (general) (routine) (of) (for) V70.9
　allergy V72.7
　annual V70.0
　cardiovascular preoperative V72.81
　cervical Papanicolaou smear V76.2
　　as a part of routine gynecological examination
　　　V72.31
　　　to confirm findings of recent normal smear
　　　　following initial abnormal smear V72.32
　child care (routine) V20.2
　clinical research investigation (normal control
　　patient) (participant) V70.7

Examination—*continued*
　dental V72.2
　developmental testing (child) (infant) V20.2
　donor (potential) V70.8
　ear V72.19
　eye V72.0
　following
　　accident (motor vehicle) V71.4
　　alleged rape or seduction (victim or culprit) V71.5
　　inflicted injury (victim or culprit) NEC V71.6
　　rape or seduction, alleged (victim or culprit) V71.5
　　treatment (for) V67.9
　　　combined V67.6
　　　fracture V67.4
　　　involving high-risk medication NEC V67.51
　　　mental disorder V67.3
　　　specified condition NEC V67.59
　follow-up (routine) (following) V67.9
　　cancer chemotherapy V67.2
　　chemotherapy V67.2
　　disease NEC V67.59
　　high-risk medication NEC V67.51
　　injury NEC V67.59
　　population survey V70.6
　　postpartum V24.2
　　psychiatric V67.3
　　psychotherapy V67.3
　　radiotherapy V67.1
　　specified surgery NEC V67.09
　　surgery V67.00
　　vaginal pap smear V67.01
　gynecological V72.31
　　for contraceptive maintenance V25.40
　　　intrauterine device V25.42
　　　pill V25.41
　　　specified method NEC V25.49
　health (of)
　　armed forces personnel V70.5
　　checkup V70.0
　　child, routine V20.2
　　defined subpopulation NEC V70.5
　　inhabitants of institutions V70.5
　　occupational V70.5
　　pre-employment screening V70.5
　　preschool children V70.5
　　　for admission to school V70.3
　　prisoners V70.5
　　　for entrance into prison V70.3
　　prostitutes V70.5
　　refugees V70.5
　　school children V70.5
　　students V70.5
　hearing V72.19
　　following failed hearing screening V72.11
　infant
　　8 to 28 days old V20.32
　　over 28 days old, routine V20.2
　　under 8 days old V20.31
　laboratory V72.60
　　ordered as part of a routine general medical
　　　examination V72.62
　　pre-operative V72.63
　　pre-procedural V72.63
　　specified NEC V72.69
　lactating mother V24.1
　medical (for) (of) V70.9
　　administrative purpose NEC V70.3
　　admission to
　　　old age home V70.3
　　　prison V70.3
　　　school V70.3
　　adoption V70.3

Examination—*continued*
medical (for) (of)—*continued*
armed forces personnel V70.5
at health care facility V70.0
camp V70.3
child, routine V20.2
clinical research investigation (control)
(normal comparison) (participant) V70.7
defined subpopulation NEC V70.5
donor (potential) V70.8
driving license V70.3
general V70.9
routine V70.0
specified reason NEC V70.8
immigration V70.3
inhabitants of institutions V70.5
insurance certification V70.3
marriage V70.3
medicolegal reasons V70.4
naturalization V70.3
occupational V70.5
population survey V70.6
pre-employment V70.5
preschool children V70.5
for admission to school V70.3
prison V70.3
prisoners V70.5
for entrance into prison V70.3
prostitutes V70.5
refugees V70.5
school children V70.5
specified reason NEC V70.8
sport competition V70.3
students V70.5
medicolegal reason V70.4
pelvic (annual) (periodic) V72.31
periodic (annual) (routine) V70.0
postpartum
immediately after delivery V24.0
routine follow-up V24.2
pregnancy (unconfirmed) (possible) V72.40
negative result V72.41
positive result V72.42
prenatal V22.1
first pregnancy V22.0
high-risk pregnancy V23.9
specified problem NEC V23.8
to determine fetal viability V23.87
preoperative V72.84
cardiovascular V72.81
respiratory V72.82
specified NEC V72.83
preprocedural V72.84
cardiovascular V72.81
general physical V72.83
respiratory V72.82
specified NEC V72.83
prior to chemotherapy V72.83
psychiatric V70.2
follow-up not needing further care V67.3
requested by authority V70.1
radiological NEC V72.5
respiratory preoperative V72.82
screening—*see* Screening
sensitization V72.7
skin V72.7
hypersensitivity V72.7
special V72.9
specified type or reason NEC V72.85
preoperative V72.83
specified NEC V72.83

Examination—*continued*
teeth V72.2
vaginal Papanicolaou smear V76.47
following hysterectomy for malignant
condition V67.01
victim or culprit following
alleged rape or seduction V71.5
inflicted injury NEC V71.6
vision V72.0
well baby V20.2
Exanthem, exanthema (*see also* Rash) 782.1
Boston 048
epidemic, with meningitis 048
lichenoid psoriasiform 696.2
subitum 058.10
due to
human herpesvirus 6 058.11
human herpesvirus 7 058.12
viral, virus NEC 057.9
specified type NEC 057.8
Excess, excessive, excessively
alcohol level in blood 790.3
carbohydrate tissue, localized 278.1
carotene (dietary) 278.3
cold 991.9
specified effect NEC 991.8
convergence 378.84
crying 780.95
of
adolescent 780.95
adult 780.95
baby 780.92
child 780.95
infant (baby) 780.92
newborn 780.92
development, breast 611.1
diaphoresis (*see also* Hyperhidrosis) 780.8
distance, interarch 524.28
divergence 378.85
drinking (alcohol) NEC (*see also* Abuse, drugs,
nondependent) 305.0
continual (*see also* Alcoholism) 303.9
habitual (*see also* Alcoholism) 303.9
eating 783.6
eyelid fold (congenital) 743.62
fat 278.02
in heart (*see also* Degeneration, myocardial) 429.1
tissue, localized 278.1
foreskin 605
gas 787.3
gastrin 251.5
glucagon 251.4
heat (*see also* Heat) 992.9
horizontal
overjet 524.26
overlap 524.26
interarch distance 524.28
intermaxillary vertical dimension 524.37
interocclusal distance of teeth 524.37
large
colon 564.7
congenital 751.3
fetus or infant 766.0
with obstructed labor 660.1
affecting management of pregnancy 656.6
causing disproportion 653.5
newborn (weight of 4500 grams or more) 766.0

Excess, excessive, excessively—*continued*
long
  colon 751.5
  organ or site, congenital NEC—*see* Anomaly, specified type NEC
  umbilical cord (entangled)
    affecting fetus or newborn 762.5
    in pregnancy or childbirth 663.3
      with compression 663.2
menstruation 626.2
number of teeth 520.1
  causing crowding 524.31
nutrients (dietary) NEC 783.6
potassium (K) 276.7
salivation (*see also* Ptyalism) 527.7
secretion—*see also* Hypersecretion
  milk 676.6
  sputum 786.4
  sweat (*see also* Hyperhidrosis) 780.8
short
  organ or site, congenital NEC—*see* Anomaly, specified type NEC
  umbilical cord
    affecting fetus or newborn 762.6
    in pregnancy or childbirth 663.4
skin NEC 701.9
  eyelid 743.62
    acquired 374.30
sodium (Na) 276.0
spacing of teeth 524.32
sputum 786.4
sweating (*see also* Hyperhidrosis) 780.8
tearing (ducts) (eye) (*see also* Epiphora) 375.20
thirst 783.5
  due to deprivation of water 994.3
tissue in reconstructed breast 612.0
tuberosity 524.07
vitamin
  A (dietary) 278.2
    administered as drug (chronic) (prolonged excessive intake) 278.2
      reaction to sudden overdose 963.5
  D (dietary) 278.4
    administered as drug (chronic) (prolonged excessive intake) 278.4
      reaction to sudden overdose 963.5
weight 278.02
  gain 783.1
    of pregnancy 646.1
  loss 783.21
Excitability, abnormal, under minor stress 309.29
Excitation
catatonic (*see also* Schizophrenia) 295.2
psychogenic 298.1
reactive (from emotional stress, psychological trauma) 298.1
Excitement
manic (*see also* Psychosis, affective) 296.0
  recurrent episode 296.1
  single episode 296.0
mental, reactive (from emotional stress, psychological trauma) 298.1
state, reactive (from emotional stress, psychological trauma) 298.1
Excluded pupils 364.76
Excoriation (traumatic) (*see also* Injury, superficial, by site) 919.8
neurotic 698.4
Excyclophoria 378.44
Excyclotropia 378.33
Exencephalus, exencephaly 742.0

Exercise
breathing V57.0
remedial NEC V57.1
therapeutic NEC V57.1
Exfoliation
skin
  due to erythematous condition 695.50
    involving (percent of body surface)
      less than 10 percent 695.50
      10-19 percent 695.51
      20-29 percent 695.52
      30-39 percent 695.53
      40-49 percent 695.54
      50-59 percent 695.55
      60-69 percent 695.56
      70-79 percent 695.57
      80-89 percent 695.58
      90 percent or more 695.59
teeth
  due to systemic causes 525.0
Exfoliative —*see also* condition
dermatitis 695.89
Exhaustion, exhaustive (physical NEC) 780.79
battle (*see also* Reaction, stress, acute) 308.9
cardiac (*see also* Failure, heart) 428.9
delirium (*see also* Reaction, stress, acute) 308.9
due to
  cold 991.8
  excessive exertion 994.5
  exposure 994.4
  overexertion 994.5
fetus or newborn 779.89
heart (*see also* Failure, heart) 428.9
heat 992.5
  due to
    salt depletion 992.4
    water depletion 992.3
manic (*see also* Psychosis, affective) 296.0
  recurrent episode 296.1
  single episode 296.0
maternal, complicating delivery 669.8
  affecting fetus or newborn 763.89
mental 300.5
myocardium, myocardial (*see also* Failure, heart) 428.9
nervous 300.5
old age 797
postinfectional NEC 780.79
psychogenic 300.5
psychosis (*see also* Reaction, stress, acute) 308.9
senile 797
  dementia 290.0
Exhibitionism (sexual) 302.4
Exomphalos 756.72
Exophoria 378.42
convergence, insufficiency 378.83
divergence, excess 378.85
Exophthalmic
cachexia 242.0
goiter 242.0
ophthalmoplegia 242.0 *[376.22]*
Exophthalmos 376.30
congenital 743.66
constant 376.31
endocrine NEC 259.9 *[376.22]*
hyperthyroidism 242.0 *[376.21]*
intermittent NEC 376.34
malignant 242.0 *[376.21]*
pulsating 376.35
  endocrine NEC 259.9 *[376.22]*
thyrotoxic 242.0 *[376.21]*

Exostosis 726.91
 cartilaginous (M9210/0)—*see* Neoplasm, bone,
   benign
 congenital 756.4
 ear canal, external 380.81
 gonococcal 098.89
 hip 726.5
 intracranial 733.3
 jaw (bone) 526.81
 luxurians 728.11
 multiple (cancellous) (congenital) (hereditary) 756.4
 nasal bones 726.91
 orbit, orbital 376.42
 osteocartilaginous (M9210/0)—*see* Neoplasm,
   bone, benign
 spine 721.8
   with spondylosis—*see* Spondylosis
 syphilitic 095.5
 wrist 726.4
Exotropia 378.10
 alternating 378.15
   with
     A pattern 378.16
     specified noncomitancy 378.18
     V pattern 378.17
     X pattern 378.18
     Y pattern 378.18
   intermittent 378.24
 intermittent 378.20
   alternating 378.24
   monocular 378.23
 monocular 378.11
   with
     A pattern 378.12
     specified noncomitancy NEC 378.14
     V pattern 378.13
     X pattern 378.14
     Y pattern 378.14
   intermittent 378.23
Explanation of
 investigation finding V65.4
 medication V65.4
Exposure (suspected) 994.9
 algae bloom V87.32
 cold 991.9
   specified effect NEC 991.8
 effects of 994.9
 exhaustion due to 994.4
 implanted vaginal mesh
   into vagina 629.32
   through vaginal wall 629.32
 to
   AIDS virus V01.79
   anthrax V01.81
   aromatic
     amines V87.11
     dyes V87.19
   arsenic V87.01
   asbestos V15.84
   benzene V87.12
   body fluids (hazardous) V15.85
   cholera V01.0
   communicable disease V01.9
     specified type NEC V01.89
   chromium compounds V87.09
   dyes V87.2
     aromatic V87.19
   Escherichia coli (E. coli) V01.83
   German measles V01.4
   gonorrhea V01.6

Exposure—*continued*
 to —*continued*
   hazardous
     aromatic compounds NEC V87.19
     body fluids V15.85
     chemicals NEC V87.2
     metals V87.09
     substances V87.39
   HIV V01.79
   human immunodeficiency virus V01.79
   lead V15.86
   meningococcus V01.84
   mold V87.31
   nickel dust V87.09
   parasitic disease V01.89
   poliomyelitis V01.2
   polycyclic aromatic hydrocarbons V87.19
   potentially hazardous body fluids V15.85
   rabies V01.5
   rubella V01.4
   SARS-associated coronavirus V01.82
   smallpox V01.3
   syphilis V01.6
   tuberculosis V01.1
   uranium V87.02
   varicella V01.71
   venereal disease V01.6
   viral disease NEC V01.79
     varicella V01.71
   vaginal prosthetic materials NEC
     into vagina 629.32
     through vaginal wall 629.32
Exsanguination, fetal 772.0
Exstrophy
 abdominal content 751.8
 bladder (urinary) 753.5
Extensive —*see* condition
Extra —*see also* Accessory
 rib 756.3
   cervical 756.2
Extraction
 with hook 763.89
 breech NEC 669.6
   affecting fetus or newborn 763.0
 cataract postsurgical V45.61
 manual NEC 669.8
   affecting fetus or newborn 763.89
Extrasystole 427.60
 atrial 427.61
 postoperative 997.1
 ventricular 427.69
Extrauterine gestation or pregnancy —*see*
 Pregnancy, ectopic
Extravasation
 blood 459.0
   lower extremity 459.0
 chemotherapy, vesicant 999.81
 chyle into mesentery 457.8
 pelvicalyceal 593.4
 pyelosinus 593.4
 urine 788.8
   from ureter 788.8
 vesicant
   agent NEC 999.82
   chemotherapy 999.81
Extremity —*see* condition
Extrophy —*see* Exstrophy

Extroversion
    bladder 753.5
    uterus 618.1
        complicating delivery 665.2
            affecting fetus or newborn 763.89
        postpartal (old) 618.1
Extruded tooth 524.34
Extrusion
    alveolus and teeth 524.75
    breast implant (prosthetic) 996.54
    device, implant, or graft—*see* Complications,
        mechanical
    eye implant (ball) (globe) 996.59
    intervertebral disc—*see* Displacement,
        intervertebral disc
    lacrimal gland 375.43
    mesh (reinforcing) 996.59
    ocular lens implant 996.53
    prosthetic device NEC—*see* Complications,
        mechanical
    vitreous 379.26
Exudate, pleura —*see* Effusion, pleura
Exudates, retina 362.82
Exudative —*see* condition
Eye, eyeball, eyelid—*see* condition
Eyestrain 368.13
Eyeworm disease of Africa 125.2

F

Faber's anemia or syndrome (achlorhydric anemia) 280.9
Fabry's disease (angiokeratoma corporis diffusum) 272.7
Face, facial —*see* condition
Facet of cornea 371.44
Faciocephalalgia, autonomic (*see also* Neuropathy, peripheral, autonomic) 337.9
Facioscapulohumeral myopathy 359.1
Factitious disorder, illness —*see* Illness, factitious
Factor
    deficiency—*see* Deficiency, factor
    psychic, associated with diseases classified elsewhere 316
    risk—*see* Problem
    V Leiden mutation 289.81
Fahr-Volhard disease (malignant nephrosclerosis) 403.00
Failure, failed
    adenohypophyseal 253.2
    attempted abortion (legal) (*see also* Abortion, failed) 638.9
    bone marrow (anemia) 284.9
        acquired (secondary) 284.89
        congenital 284.09
        idiopathic 284.9
    cardiac (*see also* Failure, heart) 428.9
        newborn 779.89
    cardiorenal (chronic) 428.9
        hypertensive (*see also* Hypertension, cardiorenal) 404.93
    cardiorespiratory 799.1
        specified during or due to a procedure 997.1
            long-term effect of cardiac surgery 429.4
    cardiovascular (chronic) 428.9
    cerebrovascular 437.8
    cervical dilatation in labor 661.0
        affecting fetus or newborn 763.7
    circulation, circulatory 799.89
        fetus or newborn 779.89
        peripheral 785.50
            postoperative 998.00
    compensation—*see* Disease, heart
    conscious sedation, during procedure 995.24
    congestive (*see also* Failure, heart) 428.0
    coronary (*see also* Insufficiency, coronary) 411.89
    dental implant 525.79
        due to
            infection 525.71
            lack of attached gingiva 525.72
            occlusal trauma (caused by poor prosthetic design) 525.72
            parafunctional habits 525.72
            periodontal infection (peri-implantitis) 525.72
            poor oral hygiene 525.72
            unintentional loading 525.71
        endosseous NEC 525.79
        mechanical 525.73
        osseointegration 525.71
            due to
                complications of systemic disease 525.71
                poor bone quality 525.71
                premature loading 525.71
            iatrogenic 525.71
            prior to intentional prosthetic loading 525.71

Failure, failed—*continued*
    dental implant—*continued*
        post-osseointegration
            biological 525.72
                iatrogenic 525.72
                due to complications of systemic disease 525.72
            mechanical 525.73
        pre-integration 525.71
        pre-osseointegration 525.71
    dental prosthesis causing loss of dental implant 525.73
    dental restoration
        marginal integrity 525.61
        periodontal anatomical integrity 525.65
    descent of head (at term) 652.5
        affecting fetus or newborn 763.1
        in labor 660.0
            affecting fetus or newborn 763.1
    device, implant, or graft—*see* Complications, mechanical
    engagement of head NEC 652.5
        in labor 660.0
    extrarenal 788.99
    fetal head to enter pelvic brim 652.5
        affecting fetus or newborn 763.1
        in labor 660.0
            affecting fetus or newborn 763.1
    forceps NEC 660.7
        affecting fetus or newborn 763.1
    fusion (joint) (spinal) 996.49
    growth in childhood 783.43
    heart (acute) (sudden) 428.9
        with
            abortion—*see* Abortion, by type, with specified complication NEC
            acute pulmonary edema (*see also* Failure, ventricular, left) 428.1
                with congestion (*see also* Failure, heart) 428.0
            decompensation (*see also* Failure, heart) 428.0
            dilation—*see* Disease, heart
            ectopic pregnancy (*see also* categories 633.0-633.9) 639.8
            molar pregnancy (*see also* categories 630-632) 639.8
        arteriosclerotic 440.9
        combined left-right sided 428.0
        combined systolic and diastolic 428.40
            acute 428.41
            acute on chronic 428.43
            chronic 428.42
        compensated (*see also* Failure, heart) 428.0
        complicating
            abortion—*see* Abortion, by type, with specified complication NEC
            delivery (cesarean) (instrumental) 669.4
            ectopic pregnancy (*see also* categories 633.0-633.9) 639.8
            molar pregnancy (*see also* categories 630-632) 639.8
            obstetric anesthesia or sedation 668.1
            surgery 997.1
        congestive (compensated) (decompensated) (*see also* Failure, heart) 428.0
            with rheumatic fever (conditions classifiable to 390)
                active 391.8
                inactive or quiescent (with chorea) 398.91

Failure, failed—*continued*
  heart—*continued*
    congestive—*continued*
      fetus or newborn 779.89
      hypertensive (*see also* Hypertension, heart)
          402.91
        with renal disease (*see also* Hypertension,
            cardiorenal) 404.91
          with renal failure 404.93
        benign 402.11
        malignant 402.01
      rheumatic (chronic) (inactive) (with chorea)
          398.91
        active or acute 391.8
          with chorea (Sydenham's) 392.0
      decompensated (*see also* Failure, heart) 428.0
      degenerative (*see also* Degeneration,
          myocardial) 429.1
      diastolic 428.30
        acute 428.31
        acute or chronic 428.33
        chronic 428.32
      due to presence of (cardiac) prosthesis 429.4
      fetus or newborn 779.89
      following
        abortion 639.8
        cardiac surgery 429.4
        ectopic or molar pregnancy 639.8
      high output NEC 428.9
      hypertensive (*see also* Hypertension, heart) 402.91
        with renal disease (*see also* Hypertension,
            cardiorenal) 404.91
          with renal failure 404.93
        benign 402.11
        malignant 402.01
      left (ventricular) (*see also* Failure, ventricular,
          left) 428.1
        with right-sided failure (*see also* Failure,
            heart) 428.0
      low output (syndrome) NEC 428.9
      organic—*see* Disease, heart
      postoperative (immediate) 997.1
        long term effect of cardiac surgery 429.4
      rheumatic (chronic) (congestive) (inactive) 398.91
      right (secondary to left heart failure,
          conditions classifiable to 428.1)
          (ventricular) (*see also* Failure, heart) 428.0
      senile 797
      specified during or due to a procedure 997.1
        long-term effect of cardiac surgery 429.4
      systolic 428.20
        acute 428.21
        acute on chronic 428.23
        chronic 428.22
      thyrotoxic (*see also* Thyrotoxicosis) 242.9 *[425.7]*
      valvular—*see* Endocarditis
    hepatic 572.8
      acute 570
      due to a procedure 997.49
    hepatorenal 572.4
    hypertensive heart (*see also* Hypertension,
        heart) 402.91
      benign 402.11
      malignant 402.01
    induction (of labor) 659.1
      abortion (legal) (*see also* Abortion, failed)
          638.9
      affecting fetus or newborn 763.89
      by oxytocic drugs 659.1
      instrumental 659.0
      mechanical 659.0

Failure, failed—*continued*
    induction (of labor)—*continued*
      medical 659.1
      surgical 659.0
    initial alveolar expansion, newborn 770.4
    involution, thymus (gland) 254.8
    kidney—*see* Failure, renal
    lactation 676.4
    Leydig's cell, adult 257.2
    liver 572.8
      acute 570
    medullary 799.89
    mitral—*see* Endocarditis, mitral
    moderate sedation, during procedure 995.24
    myocardium, myocardial (*see also* Failure,
        heart) 428.9
      chronic (*see also* Failure, heart) 428.0
      congestive (*see also* Failure, heart) 428.0
    ovarian (primary) 256.39
      iatrogenic 256.2
      postablative 256.2
      postirradiation 256.2
      postsurgical 256.2
    ovulation 628.0
    prerenal 788.99
    renal (kidney) 586
      with
        abortion—*see* Abortion, by type, with renal
            failure
        ectopic pregnancy (*see also* categories
            633.0-633.9) 639.3
        edema (*see also* Nephrosis) 581.9
        hypertension (*see also* Hypertension,
            kidney) 403.91
        hypertensive heart disease (conditions
            classifiable to 402) 404.92
          with heart failure 404.93
          benign 404.12
            with heart failure 404.13
          malignant 404.02
            with heart failure 404.03
        molar pregnancy (*see also* categories
            630-632) 639.3
        tubular necrosis (acute) 584.5
      acute 584.9
        with lesion of
          necrosis
            cortical (renal) 584.6
            medullary (renal) (papillary) 584.7
            tubular 584.5
          specified pathology NEC 584.8
      chronic 585.9
        hypertensive or with hypertension (*see also*
            Hypertension, kidney) 403.91
      due to a procedure 997.5
      following
        abortion 639.3
        crushing 958.5
        ectopic or molar pregnancy 639.3
        labor and delivery (acute) 669.3
      hypertensive (*see also* Hypertension, kidney)
          403.91
      puerperal, postpartum 669.3
    respiration, respiratory 518.81
      acute 518.81
        following trauma and surgery 518.51
      acute and chronic 518.84
        following trauma and surgery 518.53
      center 348.89
        newborn 770.84
      chronic 518.83

Failure, failed—*continued*
respiration, respiratory—*continued*
following trauma and surgery or shock 518.51
newborn 770.84
rotation
cecum 751.4
colon 751.4
intestine 751.4
kidney 753.3
sedation, during procedure
conscious 995.24
moderate 995.24
segmentation—*see also* Fusion
fingers (*see also* Syndactylism, fingers) 755.11
toes (*see also* Syndactylism, toes) 755.13
seminiferous tubule, adult 257.2
senile (general) 797
with psychosis 290.20
testis, primary (seminal) 257.2
to progress 661.2
to thrive
adult 783.7
child 783.41
newborn 779.34
transplant 996.80
bone marrow 996.85
organ (immune or nonimmune cause) 996.80
bone marrow 996.85
heart 996.83
intestines 996.87
kidney 996.81
liver 996.82
lung 996.84
pancreas 996.86
specified NEC 996.89
skin 996.52
artificial 996.55
decellularized allodermis 996.55
temporary allograft or pigskin graft—*omit code*
stem cell(s) 996.88
from
peripheral blood 996.88
umbilical blood 996.88
trial of labor NEC 660.6
affecting fetus or newborn 763.1
tubal ligation 998.89
urinary 586
vacuum extraction
abortion—*see* Abortion, failed
delivery NEC 660.7
affecting fetus or newborn 763.1
vasectomy 998.89
ventouse NEC 660.7
affecting fetus or newborn 763.1
ventricular (*see also* Failure, heart) 428.9
left 428.1
with rheumatic fever (conditions classifiable to 390)
active 391.8
with chorea 392.0
inactive or quiescent (with chorea) 398.91
hypertensive (*see also* Hypertension, heart) 402.91
benign 402.11
malignant 402.01
rheumatic (chronic) (inactive) (with chorea) 398.91
active or acute 391.8
with chorea 392.0
right (*see also* Failure, heart) 428.0
vital centers, fetus or newborn 779.8
weight gain in childhood 783.41

Fainting (fit) (spell) 780.2
Falciform hymen 752.49
Fall, maternal, affecting fetus or newborn 760.5
Fallen arches 734
Falling, any organ or part —*see* Prolapse
Fallopian
insufflation
fertility testing V26.21
following sterilization reversal V26.22
tube—*see* condition
Fallot's
pentalogy 745.2
tetrad or tetralogy 745.2
triad or trilogy 746.09
Fallout, radioactive (adverse effect) NEC 990
False —*see also* condition
bundle branch block 426.50
bursa 727.89
croup 478.75
joint 733.82
labor (pains) 644.1
opening, urinary, male 752.69
passage, urethra (prostatic) 599.4
positive
serological test for syphilis 795.6
Wassermann reaction 795.6
pregnancy 300.11
Family, familial —*see also* condition
affected by
family member
currently on deployment (military) V61.01
returned from deployment (military) (current or past conflict) V61.02
disruption (*see also* Disruption, family) V61.09
estrangement V61.09
hemophagocytic
lymphohistiocytosis 288.4
reticulosis 288.4
Li-fraumeni (syndrome) V84.01
planning advice V25.09
natural
procreative V26.41
to avoid pregnancy V25.04
problem V61.9
specified circumstance NEC V61.8
retinoblastoma (syndrome) 190.5
Famine 994.2
edema 262
Fanconi's anemia (congenital pancytopenia) 284.09
Fanconi (-de Toni) (-Debré) syndrome (cystinosis) 270.0
Farber (-Uzman) syndrome or disease (disseminated lipogranulomatosis) 272.8
Farcin 024
Farcy 024
Farmers'
lung 495.0
skin 692.74
Farsightedness 367.0
Fascia —*see* condition
Fasciculation 781.0
Fasciculitis optica 377.32
Fasciitis 729.4
eosinophilic 728.89
necrotizing 728.86
nodular 728.79
perirenal 593.4
plantar 728.71
pseudosarcomatous 728.79
traumatic (old) NEC 728.79
current—*see* Sprain, by site

Fasciola hepatica infestation 121.3
Fascioliasis 121.3
Fasciolopsiasis (small intestine) 121.4
Fasciolopsis (small intestine) 121.4
Fast pulse 785.0
Fat
  embolism (cerebral) (pulmonary) (systemic) 958.1
    with
      abortion—*see* Abortion, by type, with embolism
      ectopic pregnancy (*see also* categories 633.0-633.9) 639.6
      molar pregnancy (*see also* categories 630-632) 639.6
    complicating delivery or puerperium 673.8
    following
      abortion 639.6
      ectopic or molar pregnancy 639.6
    in pregnancy, childbirth, or the puerperium 673.8
  excessive 278.02
    in heart (*see also* Degeneration, myocardial) 429.1
  general 278.02
  hernia, herniation 729.30
    eyelid 374.34
    knee 729.31
    orbit 374.34
    retro-orbital 374.34
    retropatellar 729.31
    specified site NEC 729.39
  indigestion 579.8
  in stool 792.1
  localized (pad) 278.1
    heart (*see also* Degeneration, myocardial) 429.1
    knee 729.31
    retropatellar 729.31
  necrosis—*see also* Fatty, degeneration
    breast (aseptic) (segmental) 611.3
    mesentery 567.82
    omentum 567.82
    peritoneum 567.82
  pad 278.1
Fatal familial insomnia (FFI) 046.72
Fatal syncope 798.1
Fatigue 780.79
  auditory deafness (*see also* Deafness) 389.9
  chronic, syndrome 780.71
  combat (*see also* Reaction, stress, acute) 308.9
  during pregnancy 646.8
  general 780.79
    psychogenic 300.5
  heat (transient) 992.6
  muscle 729.89
  myocardium (*see also* Failure, heart) 428.9
  nervous 300.5
  neurosis 300.5
  operational 300.89
  postural 729.89
  posture 729.89
  psychogenic (general) 300.5
  senile 797
  syndrome NEC 300.5
    chronic 780.71
  undue 780.79
  voice 784.49
Fatness 278.02

Fatty —*see also* condition
  apron 278.1
  degeneration (diffuse) (general) NEC 272.8
    localized—*see* Degeneration, by site, fatty
    placenta—*see* Placenta, abnormal
    heart (enlarged) (*see also* Degeneration, myocardial) 429.1
  infiltration (diffuse) (general) (*see also* Degeneration, by site, fatty) 272.8
    heart (enlarged) (*see also* Degeneration, myocardial) 429.1
  liver 571.8
    alcoholic 571.0
  necrosis—*see* Degeneration, fatty
  phanerosis 272.8
Fauces —*see* condition
Fauchard's disease (periodontitis) 523.40
Faucitis 478.29
Faulty —*see also* condition
  position of teeth 524.30
Favism (anemia) 282.2
Favre-Racouchot disease (elastoidosis cutanea nodularis) 701.8
Favus 110.9
  beard 110.0
  capitis 110.0
  corporis 110.5
  eyelid 110.8
  foot 110.4
  hand 110.2
  scalp 110.0
  specified site NEC 110.8
Fear, fearfulness (complex) (reaction) 300.20
  child 313.0
  of
    animals 300.29
    closed spaces 300.29
    crowds 300.29
    eating in public 300.23
    heights 300.29
    open spaces 300.22
      with panic attacks 300.21
    public speaking 300.23
    streets 300.22
      with panic attacks 300.21
    travel 300.22
      with panic attacks 300.21
    washing in public 300.23
  transient 308.0
Feared complaint unfounded V65.5
Febricula (continued) (simple) (*see also* Pyrexia) 780.60
Febrile (*see also* Pyrexia) 780.60
  convulsion (simple) 780.31
    complex 780.32
  nonhemolytic transfusion reaction (FNHTR) 780.66
  seizure (simple) 780.31
    atypical 780.32
    complex 780.32
    complicated 780.32
Febris (*see also* Fever) 780.60
  aestiva (*see also* Fever, hay) 477.9
  flava (*see also* Fever, yellow) 060.9
  melitensis 023.0
  pestis (*see also* Plague) 020.9
  puerperalis 672
  recurrens (*see also* Fever, relapsing) 087.9
    pediculo vestimenti 087.0
  rubra 034.1
  typhoidea 002.0
  typhosa 002.0

Fecal —*see* condition
Fecalith (impaction) 560.32
  with hernia—*see also* Hernia, by site, with
    obstruction
    gangrenous—*see* Hernia, by site, with gangrene
  appendix 543.9
  congenital 777.1
Fede's disease 529.0
Feeble-minded 317
Feeble rapid pulse due to shock following
  injury 958.4
Feeding
  faulty (elderly) (infant) 783.3
    newborn 779.31
  formula check V20.2
  improper (elderly) (infant) 783.3
    newborn 779.31
  problem (elderly) (infant) 783.3
    newborn 779.31
    nonorganic origin 307.59
Feeling of foreign body in throat 784.99
Feer's disease 985.0
Feet —*see* condition
Feigned illness V65.2
Feil-Klippel syndrome (brevicollis) 756.16
Feinmesser's (hidrotic) ectodermal dysplasia
  757.31
Felix's disease (juvenile osteochondrosis, hip)
  732.1
Felon (any digit) (with lymphangitis) 681.01
  herpetic 054.6
Felty's syndrome (rheumatoid arthritis with
  splenomegaly and leukopenia) 714.1
Feminism in boys 302.6
Feminization, testicular 259.51
  with pseudohermaphroditism, male 259.51
Femoral hernia —*see* Hernia, femoral
Femora vara 736.32
Femur, femoral —*see* condition
Fenestrata placenta —*see* Placenta, abnormal
Fenestration, fenestrated —*see also* Imperfect,
  closure
  aorta-pulmonary 745.0
  aorticopulmonary 745.0
  aortopulmonary 745.0
  cusps, heart valve NEC 746.89
    pulmonary 746.09
  hymen 752.49
  pulmonic cusps 746.09
Fenwick's disease 537.89
Fermentation (gastric) (gastrointestinal)
  (stomach) 536.8
  intestine 564.89
    psychogenic 306.4
  psychogenic 306.4
Fernell's disease (aortic aneurysm) 441.9
Fertile eunuch syndrome 257.2
Fertility, meaning multiparity—*see* Multiparity
Fetal
  alcohol syndrome 760.71
  anemia 678.0
  thrombocytopenia 678.0
  twin to twin transfusion 678.0
Fetalis uterus 752.39
Fetid
  breath 784.99
  sweat 705.89
Fetishism 302.81
  transvestic 302.3

Fetomaternal hemorrhage
  affecting management of pregnancy 656.0
  fetus or newborn 772.0
Fetus, fetal —*see also* condition
  papyraceous 779.89
  type lung tissue 770.4
Fever 780.60
  with chills 780.60
    in malarial regions (*see also* Malaria) 084.6
  abortus NEC 023.9
  Aden 061
  African tick-borne 087.1
  American
    mountain tick 066.1
    spotted 082.0
  and ague (*see also* Malaria) 084.6
  aphthous 078.4
  arbovirus hemorrhagic 065.9
  Assam 085.0
  Australian A or Q 083.0
  Bangkok hemorrhagic 065.4
  biliary, Charcot's intermittent—*see*
    Choledocholithiasis
  bilious, hemoglobinuric 084.8
  blackwater 084.8
  blister 054.9
  Bonvale Dam 780.79
  boutonneuse 082.1
  brain 323.9
    late effect—*see* category 326
  breakbone 061
  Bullis 082.8
  Bunyamwera 066.3
  Burdwan 085.0
  Bwamba (encephalitis) 066.3
  Cameroon (*see also* Malaria) 084.6
  Canton 081.9
  catarrhal (acute) 460
    chronic 472.0
  cat-scratch 078.3
  cerebral 323.9
    late effect—*see* category 326
  cerebrospinal (meningococcal) (*see also*
    Meningitis, cerebrospinal) 036.0
  Chagres 084.0
  Chandipura 066.8
  changuinola 066.0
  Charcot's (biliary) (hepatic) (intermittent)—*see*
    Choledocholithiasis
  Chikungunya (viral) 066.3
    hemorrhagic 065.4
  childbed 670.8
  Chitral 066.0
  Colombo (*see also* Fever, paratyphoid) 002.9
  Colorado tick (virus) 066.1
  congestive
    malarial (*see also* Malaria) 084.6
    remittent (*see also* Malaria) 084.6
  Congo virus 065.0
  continued 780.60
    malarial 084.0
  Corsican (*see also* Malaria) 084.6
  Crimean hemorrhagic 065.0
  Cyprus (*see also* Brucellosis) 023.9
  dandy 061
  deer fly (*see also* Tularemia) 021.9
  dehydration, newborn 778.4
  dengue (virus) 061
    hemorrhagic 065.4
  desert 114.0
  due to heat 992.0
  Dumdum 085.0

Fever—*continued*
enteric 002.0
ephemeral (of unknown origin) (*see also*
Pyrexia) 780.60
epidemic, hemorrhagic of the Far East 065.0
erysipelatous (*see also* Erysipelas) 035
estivo-autumnal (malarial) 084.0
etiocholanolone 277.31
famine—*see also* Fever, relapsing
meaning typhus—*see* Typhus
Far Eastern hemorrhagic 065.0
five day 083.1
Fort Bragg 100.89
gastroenteric 002.0
gastromalarial (*see also* Malaria) 084.6
Gibraltar (*see also* Brucellosis) 023.9
glandular 075
Guama (viral) 066.3
Haverhill 026.1
hay (allergic) (with rhinitis) 477.9
with
asthma (bronchial) (*see also* Asthma) 493.0
due to
dander, animal (cat) (dog) 477.2
dust 477.8
fowl 477.8
hair, animal (cat) (dog) 477.2
pollen, any plant or tree 477.0
specified allergen other than pollen 477.8
heat (effects) 992.0
hematuric, bilious 084.8
hemoglobinuric (malarial) 084.8
bilious 084.8
hemorrhagic (arthropod-borne) NEC 065.9
with renal syndrome 078.6
arenaviral 078.7
Argentine 078.7
Bangkok 065.4
Bolivian 078.7
Central Asian 065.0
chikungunya 065.4
Crimean 065.0
dengue (virus) 065.4
Ebola 065.8
epidemic 078.6
of Far East 065.0
Far Eastern 065.0
Junin virus 078.7
Korean 078.6
Kyasanur forest 065.2
Machupo virus 078.7
mite-borne NEC 065.8
mosquito-borne 065.4
Omsk 065.1
Philippine 065.4
Russian (Yaroslav) 078.6
Singapore 065.4
Southeast Asia 065.4
Thailand 065.4
tick-borne NEC 065.3
hepatic (*see also* Cholecystitis) 575.8
intermittent (Charcot's)—*see*
Choledocholithiasis
herpetic (*see also* Herpes) 054.9
Hyalomma tick 065.0
icterohemorrhagic 100.0
inanition 780.60
newborn 778.4
in conditions classified elsewhere 780.61
infective NEC 136.9

Fever—*continued*
intermittent (bilious) (*see also* Malaria) 084.6
hepatic (Charcot)—*see* Choledocholithiasis
of unknown origin (*see also* Pyrexia) 780.60
pernicious 084.0
iodide
correct substance properly administered
780.60
overdose or wrong substance given or taken
975.5
Japanese river 081.2
jungle yellow 060.0
Junin virus, hemorrhagic 078.7
Katayama 120.2
Kedani 081.2
Kenya 082.1
Korean hemorrhagic 078.6
Lassa 078.89
Lone Star 082.8
lung—*see* Pneumonia
Machupo virus, hemorrhagic 078.7
malaria, malarial (*see also* Malaria) 084.6
Malta (*see also* Brucellosis) 023.9
Marseilles 082.1
marsh (*see also* Malaria) 084.6
Mayaro (viral) 066.3
Mediterranean (*see also* Brucellosis) 023.9
familial 277.31
tick 082.1
meningeal—*see* Meningitis
metal fumes NEC 985.8
Meuse 083.1
Mexican—*see* Typhus, Mexican
Mianeh 087.1
miasmatic (*see also* Malaria) 084.6
miliary 078.2
milk, female 672
mill 504
mite-borne hemorrhagic 065.8
Monday 504
mosquito-borne NEC 066.3
hemorrhagic NEC 065.4
mountain 066.1
meaning
Rocky Mountain spotted 082.0
undulant fever (*see also* Brucellosis) 023.9
tick (American) 066.1
Mucambo (viral) 066.3
mud 100.89
Neapolitan (*see also* Brucellosis) 023.9
neutropenic 288.00
newborn (environmentally induced) 778.4
nine-mile 083.0
nonexanthematous tick 066.1
North Asian tick-borne typhus 082.2
Omsk hemorrhagic 065.1
O'nyong-nyong (viral) 066.3
Oropouche (viral) 066.3
Oroya 088.0
paludal (*see also* Malaria) 084.6
Panama 084.0
pappataci 066.0
paratyphoid 002.9
A 002.1
B (Schottmüller's) 002.2
C (Hirschfeld) 002.3
parrot 073.9
periodic 277.31
pernicious, acute 084.0
persistent (of unknown origin) (*see also*
Pyrexia) 780.60

Fever—*continued*
petechial 036.0
pharyngoconjunctival 077.2
   adenoviral type 3 077.2
Philippine hemorrhagic 065.4
phlebotomus 066.0
Piry 066.8
Pixuna (viral) 066.3
Plasmodium ovale 084.3
pleural (*see also* Pleurisy) 511.0
pneumonic—*see* Pneumonia
polymer fume 987.8
postimmunization 780.63
postoperative 780.62
   due to infection 998.59
posttransfusion 780.66
postvaccination 780.63
pretibial 100.89
puerperal, postpartum 672
putrid—*see* Septicemia
pyemic—*see* Septicemia
Q 083.0
   with pneumonia 083.0 *[484.8]*
quadrilateral 083.0
quartan (malaria) 084.2
Queensland (coastal) 083.0
   seven-day 100.89
Quintan (A) 083.1
quotidian 084.0
rabbit (*see also* Tularemia) 021.9
rat-bite 026.9
   due to
      Spirillum minor or minus 026.0
      Spirochaeta morsus muris 026.0
      Streptobacillus moniliformis 026.1
recurrent—*see* Fever, relapsing
relapsing 087.9
   Carter's (Asiatic) 087.0
   Dutton's (West African) 087.1
   Koch's 087.9
   louse-borne (epidemic) 087.0
   Novy's (American) 087.1
   Obermeyer's (European) 087.0
   spirillum NEC 087.9
   tick-borne (endemic) 087.1
remittent (bilious) (congestive) (gastric) (*see also* Malaria) 084.6
rheumatic (active) (acute) (chronic) (subacute) 390
   with heart involvement 391.9
      carditis 391.9
      endocarditis (aortic) (mitral) (pulmonary) (tricuspid) 391.1
      multiple sites 391.8
      myocarditis 391.2
      pancarditis, acute 391.8
      pericarditis 391.0
      specified type NEC 391.8
      valvulitis 391.1
   inactive or quiescent with cardiac hypertrophy 398.99
      carditis 398.90
      endocarditis 397.9
         aortic (valve) 395.9
            with mitral (valve) disease 396.9
         mitral (valve) 394.9
            with aortic (valve) disease 396.9
         pulmonary (valve) 397.1
         tricuspid (valve) 397.0
      heart conditions (classifiable to 429.3, 429.6, 429.9) 398.99
         failure (congestive) (conditions classifiable to 428.0, 428.9) 398.91

Fever—*continued*
rheumatic—*continued*
   inactive—*continued*
      left ventricular failure (conditions classifiable to 428.1) 398.91
      myocardial degeneration (conditions classifiable to 429.1) 398.0
      myocarditis (conditions classifiable to 429.0) 398.0
      pancarditis 398.99
      pericarditis 393
Rift Valley (viral) 066.3
Rocky Mountain spotted 082.0
rose 477.0
Ross river (viral) 066.3
Russian hemorrhagic 078.6
sandfly 066.0
San Joaquin (valley) 114.0
São Paulo 082.0
scarlet 034.1
septic—*see* Septicemia
seven-day 061
   Japan 100.89
   Queensland 100.89
shin bone 083.1
Singapore hemorrhagic 065.4
solar 061
sore 054.9
South African tick-bite 087.1
Southeast Asia hemorrhagic 065.4
spinal—*see* Meningitis
spirillary 026.0
splenic (*see also* Anthrax) 022.9
spotted (Rocky Mountain) 082.0
   American 082.0
   Brazilian 082.0
   Colombian 082.0
   meaning
      cerebrospinal meningitis 036.0
      typhus 082.9
spring 309.23
steroid
   correct substance properly administered 780.60
   overdose or wrong substance given or taken 962.0
streptobacillary 026.1
subtertian 084.0
Sumatran mite 081.2
sun 061
swamp 100.89
sweating 078.2
swine 003.8
sylvatic yellow 060.0
Tahyna 062.5
tertian—*see* Malaria, tertian
Thailand hemorrhagic 065.4
thermic 992.0
three day 066.0
   with Coxsackie exanthem 074.8
tick
   American mountain 066.1
   Colorado 066.1
   Kemerovo 066.1
   Mediterranean 082.1
   mountain 066.1
   nonexanthematous 066.1
   Quaranfil 066.1
tick-bite NEC 066.1
tick-borne NEC 066.1
   hemorrhagic NEC 065.3
transitory of newborn 778.4

Fever—*continued*
trench 083.1
tsutsugamushi 081.2
typhogastric 002.0
typhoid (abortive) (ambulant) (any site)
(hemorrhagic) (infection) (intermittent)
(malignant) (rheumatic) 002.0
typhomalarial (*see also* Malaria) 084.6
typhus—*see* Typhus
undulant (*see also* Brucellosis) 023.9
unknown origin (*see also* Pyrexia) 780.60
uremic—*see* Uremia
uveoparotid 135
valley (Coccidioidomycosis) 114.0
Venezuelan equine 066.2
Volhynian 083.1
Wesselsbron (viral) 066.3
West
African 084.8
Nile (viral) 066.40
with
cranial nerve disorders 066.42
encephalitis 066.41
optic neuritis 066.42
other complications 066.49
other neurologic manifestations 066.42
polyradiculitis 066.42
Whitmore's 025
Wolhynian 083.1
worm 128.9
Yaroslav hemorrhagic 078.6
yellow 060.9
jungle 060.0
sylvatic 060.0
urban 060.1
vaccination, prophylactic (against) V04.4
Zika (viral) 066.3
Fibrillation
atrial (established) (paroxysmal) 427.31
auricular (atrial) (established) 427.31
cardiac (ventricular) 427.41
coronary (*see also* Infarct, myocardium) 410.9
heart (ventricular) 427.41
muscular 728.9
postoperative 997.1
ventricular 427.41
Fibrin
ball or bodies, pleural (sac) 511.0
chamber, anterior (eye) (gelatinous exudate)
364.04
Fibrinogenolysis (hemorrhagic)—*see*
Fibrinolysis
Fibrinogenopenia (congenital) (hereditary) (*see
also* Defect, coagulation) 286.3
acquired 286.6
Fibrinolysis (acquired) (hemorrhagic)
(pathologic) 286.6
with
abortion—*see* Abortion, by type, with
hemorrhage, delayed or excessive
ectopic pregnancy (*see also* categories
633.0-633.9) 639.1
molar pregnancy (*see also* categories 630-632)
639.1
antepartum or intrapartum 641.3
affecting fetus or newborn 762.1
following
abortion 639.1
ectopic or molar pregnancy 639.1
newborn, transient 776.2
postpartum 666.3

Fibrinopenia (hereditary) (*see also* Defect,
coagulation) 286.3
acquired 286.6
Fibrinopurulent —*see* condition
Fibrinous —*see* condition
Fibroadenoma (M9010/0)
cellular intracanalicular (M9020/0) 217
giant (intracanalicular) (M9020/0) 217
intracanalicular (M9011/0)
cellular (M9020/0) 217
giant (M9020/0) 217
specified site—*see* Neoplasm, by site, benign
unspecified site 217
juvenile (M9030/0) 217
pericanalicular (M9012/0)
specified site—*see* Neoplasm, by site, benign
unspecified site 217
phyllodes (M9020/0) 217
prostate 600.20
with
other lower urinary tract symptoms (LUTS)
600.21
urinary
obstruction 600.21
retention 600.21
specified site—*see* Neoplasm, by site, benign
unspecified site 217
Fibroadenosis, breast (chronic) (cystic) (diffuse)
(periodic) (segmental) 610.2
Fibroangioma (M9160/0)—*see also* Neoplasm,
by site, benign
juvenile (M9160/0)
specified site—*see* Neoplasm, by site, benign
unspecified site 210.7
Fibrocellulitis progressiva ossificans 728.11
Fibrochondrosarcoma (M9220/3)—*see*
Neoplasm, cartilage, malignant
Fibrocystic
disease 277.00
bone NEC 733.29
breast 610.1
jaw 526.2
kidney (congenital) 753.19
liver 751.62
lung 518.89
congenital 748.4
pancreas 277.00
kidney (congenital) 753.19
Fibrodysplasia ossificans multiplex
(progressiva) 728.11
Fibroelastosis (cordis) (endocardial)
(endomyocardial) 425.3
Fibroid (tumor) (M8890/0)—*see also* Neoplasm,
connective tissue, benign
disease, lung (chronic) (*see also* Fibrosis, lung)
515
heart (disease) (*see also* Myocarditis) 429.0
induration, lung (chronic) (*see also* Fibrosis,
lung) 515
in pregnancy or childbirth 654.1
affecting fetus or newborn 763.89
causing obstructed labor 660.2
affecting fetus or newborn 763.1
liver—*see* Cirrhosis, liver
lung (*see also* Fibrosis, lung) 515
pneumonia (chronic) (*see also* Fibrosis, lung)
515
uterus (M8890/0) (*see also* Leiomyoma, uterus)
218.9
Fibrolipoma (M8851/0) (*see also* Lipoma, by
site) 214.9

Fibroliposarcoma (M8850/3)—*see* Neoplasm, connective tissue, malignant
Fibroma (M8810/0)—*see also* Neoplasm, connective tissue, benign
  ameloblastic (M9330/0) 213.1
    upper jaw (bone) 213.0
  bone (nonossifying) 733.99
    ossifying (M9262/0)—*see* Neoplasm, bone, benign
    cementifying (M9274/0)—*see* Neoplasm, bone, benign
    chondromyxoid (M9241/0)—*see* Neoplasm, bone, benign
    desmoplastic (M8823/1)—*see* Neoplasm, connective tissue, uncertain behavior
    facial (M8813/0)—*see* Neoplasm, connective tissue, benign
    invasive (M8821/1)—*see* Neoplasm, connective tissue, uncertain behavior
    molle (M8851/0) (*see also* Lipoma, by site) 214.9
    myxoid (M8811/0)—*see* Neoplasm, connective tissue, benign
    nasopharynx, nasopharyngeal (juvenile) (M9160/0) 210.7
    nonosteogenic (nonossifying)—*see* Dysplasia, fibrous
    odontogenic (M9321/0) 213.1
      upper jaw (bone) 213.0
    ossifying (M9262/0)—*see* Neoplasm, bone, benign
    periosteal (M8812/0)—*see* Neoplasm, bone, benign
  prostate 600.20
    with
      other lower urinary tract symptoms (LUTS) 600.21
      urinary
        obstruction 600.21
        retention 600.21
  soft (M8851/0) (*see also* Lipoma, by site) 214.9
Fibromatosis 728.79
  abdominal (M8822/1)—*see* Neoplasm, connective tissue, uncertain behavior
  aggressive (M8821/1)—*see* Neoplasm, connective tissue, uncertain behavior
  congenital generalized (CGF) 759.89
  Dupuytren's 728.6
  gingival 523.8
  plantar fascia 728.71
  proliferative 728.79
  pseudosarcomatous (proliferative) (subcutaneous) 728.79
  subcutaneous pseudosarcomatous (proliferative) 728.79
Fibromyalgia 729.1
Fibromyoma (M8890/0)—*see also* Neoplasm, connective tissue, benign
  uterus (corpus) (*see also* Leiomyoma, uterus) 218.9
    in pregnancy or childbirth 654.1
      affecting fetus or newborn 763.89
      causing obstructed labor 660.2
        affecting fetus or newborn 763.1
Fibromyositis (*see also* Myositis) 729.1
  scapulohumeral 726.2
Fibromyxolipoma (M8852/0) (*see also* Lipoma, by site) 214.9
Fibromyxoma (M8811/0)—*see* Neoplasm, connective tissue, benign
Fibromyxosarcoma (M8811/3)—*see* Neoplasm, connective tissue, malignant
Fibro-odontoma, ameloblastic (M9290/0) 213.1
  upper jaw (bone) 213.0

Fibro-osteoma (M9262/0)—*see* Neoplasm, bone, benign
Fibroplasia, retrolental (*see also* Retinopathy of prematurity) 362.21
Fibropurulent —*see* condition
Fibrosarcoma (M8810/3)—*see also* Neoplasm, connective tissue, malignant
  ameloblastic (M9330/3) 170.1
    upper jaw (bone) 170.0
  congenital (M8814/3)—*see* Neoplasm, connective tissue, malignant
  fascial (M8813/3)—*see* Neoplasm, connective tissue, malignant
  infantile (M8814/3)—*see* Neoplasm, connective tissue, malignant
  odontogenic (M9330/3) 170.1
    upper jaw (bone) 170.0
  periosteal (M8812/3)—*see* Neoplasm, bone, malignant
Fibrosclerosis
  breast 610.3
  corpora cavernosa (penis) 607.89
  familial multifocal NEC 710.8
  multifocal (idiopathic) NEC 710.8
  penis (corpora cavernosa) 607.89
Fibrosis, fibrotic
  adrenal (gland) 255.8
  alveolar (diffuse) 516.31
  amnion 658.8
  anal papillae 569.49
  anus 569.49
  appendix, appendiceal, noninflammatory 543.9
  arteriocapillary—*see* Arteriosclerosis
  bauxite (of lung) 503
  biliary 576.8
    due to Clonorchis sinensis 121.1
  bladder 596.89
    interstitial 595.1
    localized submucosal 595.1
    panmural 595.1
  bone, diffuse 756.59
  breast 610.3
  capillary—*see also* Arteriosclerosis
    lung (chronic) (*see also* Fibrosis, lung) 515
  cardiac (*see also* Myocarditis) 429.0
  cervix 622.8
  chorion 658.8
  corpus cavernosum 607.89
  cystic (of pancreas) 277.00
    with
      manifestations
        gastrointestinal 277.03
        pulmonary 277.02
        specified NEC 277.09
      meconium ileus 277.01
      pulmonary exacerbation 277.02
  due to (presence of) any device, implant, or graft—*see* Complications, due to (presence of) any device, implant, or graft classified to 996.0-996.5 NEC
  ejaculatory duct 608.89
  endocardium (*see also* Endocarditis) 424.90
  endomyocardial (African) 425.0
  epididymis 608.89
  eye muscle 378.62
  graphite (of lung) 503
  heart (*see also* Myocarditis) 429.0
  hepatic—*see also* Cirrhosis, liver
    due to Clonorchis sinensis 121.1
  hepatolienal—*see* Cirrhosis, liver
  hepatosplenic—*see* Cirrhosis, liver

Fibrosis, fibrotic—*continued*
  infrapatellar fat pad 729.31
  interstitial pulmonary, newborn 770.7
  intrascrotal 608.89
  kidney (*see also* Sclerosis, renal) 587
  liver—*see* Cirrhosis, liver
  lung (atrophic) (capillary) (chronic) (confluent)
    (massive) (perialveolar) (peribronchial) 515
    with
      anthracosilicosis (occupational) 500
      anthracosis (occupational) 500
      asbestosis (occupational) 501
      bagassosis (occupational) 495.1
      bauxite 503
      berylliosis (occupational) 503
      byssinosis (occupational) 504
      calcicosis (occupational) 502
      chalicosis (occupational) 502
      dust reticulation (occupational) 504
      farmers' lung 495.0
      gannister disease (occupational) 502
      graphite 503
      pneumonoconiosis (occupational) 505
      pneumosiderosis (occupational) 503
      siderosis (occupational) 503
      silicosis (occupational) 502
      tuberculosis (*see also* Tuberculosis) 011.4
    diffuse (idiopathic) (interstitial) 516.31
    due to
      bauxite 503
      fumes or vapors (chemical) (inhalation) 506.4
      graphite 503
    following radiation 508.1
    postinflammatory 515
    silicotic (massive) (occupational) 502
    tuberculous (*see also* Tuberculosis) 011.4
  lymphatic gland 289.3
  median bar 600.90
    with
      other lower urinary tract symptoms (LUTS)
        600.91
      urinary
        obstruction 600.91
        retention 600.91
  mediastinum (idiopathic) 519.3
  meninges 349.2
  muscle NEC 728.2
    iatrogenic (from injection) 999.9
  myocardium, myocardial (*see also* Myocarditis)
    429.0
  oral submucous 528.8
  ovary 620.8
  oviduct 620.8
  pancreas 577.8
    cystic 277.00
      with
        manifestations
          gastrointestinal 277.03
          pulmonary 277.02
          specified NEC 277.09
        meconium ileus 277.01
        pulmonary exacerbation 277.02
  penis 607.89
  periappendiceal 543.9
  periarticular (*see also* Ankylosis) 718.5
  pericardium 423.1
  perineum, in pregnancy or childbirth 654.8
    affecting fetus or newborn 763.89
    causing obstructed labor 660.2
      affecting fetus or newborn 763.1

Fibrosis, fibrotic—*continued*
  perineural NEC 355.9
    foot 355.6
  periureteral 593.89
  placenta—*see* Placenta, abnormal
  pleura 511.0
  popliteal fat pad 729.31
  preretinal 362.56
  prostate (chronic) 600.90
    with
      other lower urinary tract symptoms (LUTS)
        600.91
      urinary
        obstruction 600.91
        retention 600.91
  pulmonary (chronic) (*see also* Fibrosis, lung)
    515
    alveolar capillary block 516.8
    idiopathic 516.31
    interstitial
      diffuse (idiopathic) 516.31
      newborn 770.7
  radiation—*see* Effect, adverse, radiation
  rectal sphincter 569.49
  retroperitoneal, idiopathic 593.4
  sclerosing mesenteric (idiopathic) 567.82
  scrotum 608.89
  seminal vesicle 608.89
  senile 797
  skin NEC 709.2
  spermatic cord 608.89
  spleen 289.59
    bilharzial (*see also* Schistosomiasis) 120.9
  subepidermal nodular (M8832/0)—*see*
    Neoplasm, skin, benign
  submucous NEC 709.2
    oral 528.8
    tongue 528.8
  syncytium—*see* Placenta, abnormal
  testis 608.89
    chronic, due to syphilis 095.8
  thymus (gland) 254.8
  tunica vaginalis 608.89
  ureter 593.89
  urethra 599.84
  uterus (nonneoplastic) 621.8
    bilharzial (*see also* Schistosomiasis) 120.9
    neoplastic (*see also* Leiomyoma, uterus) 218.9
  vagina 623.8
  valve, heart (*see also* Endocarditis) 424.90
  vas deferens 608.89
  vein 459.89
    lower extremities 459.89
  vesical 595.1
Fibrositis (periarticular) (rheumatoid) 729.0
  humeroscapular region 726.2
  nodular, chronic
    Jaccoud's 714.4
    rheumatoid 714.4
  ossificans 728.11
  scapulohumeral 726.2
Fibrothorax 511.0
Fibrotic —*see* Fibrosis
Fibrous —*see* condition
Fibroxanthoma (M8831/0)—*see also* Neoplasm,
  connective tissue, benign
  atypical (M8831/1)—*see* Neoplasm, connective
    tissue, uncertain behavior
  malignant (M8831/3)—*see* Neoplasm,
    connective tissue, malignant
Fibroxanthosarcoma (M8831/3)—*see*
  Neoplasm, connective tissue, malignant

Fiedler's
  disease (leptospiral jaundice) 100.0
  myocarditis or syndrome (acute isolated
    myocarditis) 422.91
Fiessinger-Leroy (-Reiter) syndrome 099.3
Fiessinger-Rendu syndrome (erythema
  muliforme exudativum) 695.19
Fifth disease (eruptive) 057.0
  venereal 099.1
Filaria, filarial —*see* Infestation, filarial
Filariasis (*see also* Infestation, filarial) 125.9
  bancroftian 125.0
  Brug's 125.1
  due to
    bancrofti 125.0
    Brugia (Wuchereria) (malayi) 125.1
    Loa loa 125.2
    malayi 125.1
    organism NEC 125.6
    Wuchereria (bancrofti) 125.0
      malayi 125.1
  Malayan 125.1
  ozzardi 125.5
  specified type NEC 125.6
Filatoff's, Filatov's, Filatow's disease
  (infectious mononucleosis) 075
File-cutters' disease 984.9
  specified type of lead—*see* Table of drugs and
    chemicals
Filling defect
  biliary tract 793.3
  bladder 793.5
  duodenum 793.4
  gallbladder 793.3
  gastrointestinal tract 793.4
  intestine 793.4
  kidney 793.5
  stomach 793.4
  ureter 793.5
Filtering bleb, eye (postglaucoma) (status)
  V45.69
  with complication or rupture 997.99
  postcataract extraction (complication) 997.99
Fimbrial cyst (congenital) 752.11
Fimbriated hymen 752.49
Financial problem affecting care V60.2
Findings (abnormal), without diagnosis
  (examination) (laboratory test) 796.4
  17-ketosteroids, elevated 791.9
  acetonuria 791.6
  acid phosphatase 790.5
  albumin-globulin ratio 790.99
  albuminuria 791.0
  alcohol in blood 790.3
  alkaline phosphatase 790.5
  amniotic fluid 792.3
  amylase 790.5
  anisocytosis 790.09
  antenatal screening 796.5
  anthrax positive 795.31
  antibody titers, elevated 795.79
  anticardiolipin antibody 795.79
  antigen-antibody reaction 795.79
  antiphosphatidylglycerol antibody 795.79
  antiphosphatidylinositol antibody 795.79
  antiphosphatidylserine antibody 795.79
  antiphospholipid antibody 795.79
  bacteriuria 791.9
  ballistocardiogram 794.39
  bicarbonate 276.9
  bile in urine 791.4

Findings —*continued*
  bilirubin 277.4
  bleeding time (prolonged) 790.92
  blood culture, positive 790.7
  blood gas level 790.91
  blood sugar level 790.29
    high 790.29
      fasting glucose 790.21
      glucose tolerance test 790.22
    low 251.2
  C-reactive protein (CRP) 790.95
  calcium 275.40
  cancer antigen 125 [CA 125] 795.82
  carbonate 276.9
  carcinoembryonic antigen [CEA] 795.81
  casts, urine 791.7
  catecholamines 791.9
  cells, urine 791.7
  cerebrospinal fluid (color) (content) (pressure)
    792.0
  cervical
    high risk human papillomavirus (HPV) DNA
      test positive 795.05
    low risk human papillomavirus (HPV) DNA
      test positive 795.09
    non-atypical endometrial cells 795.09
  chloride 276.9
  cholesterol 272.9
    high 272.0
      with high triglycerides 272.2
  chromosome analysis 795.2
  chyluria 791.1
  circulation time 794.39
  cloudy dialysis effluent 792.5
  cloudy urine 791.9
  coagulation study 790.92
  cobalt, blood 790.6
  color of urine (unusual) NEC 791.9
  copper, blood 790.6
  creatinine clearance 794.4
  crystals, urine 791.9
  culture, positive NEC 795.39
    blood 790.7
    HIV V08
    human immunodeficiency virus V08
    nose 795.39
      Staphylococcus — *see* Carrier (suspected)
        of, Staphylococcus
    skin lesion NEC 795.39
    spinal fluid 792.0
    sputum 795.39
    stool 792.1
    throat 795.39
    urine 791.9
    viral
      human immunodeficiency V08
    wound 795.39
  cytology specified site NEC 796.9
  echocardiogram 793.2
  echoencephalogram 794.01
  echogram NEC—*see* Findings, abnormal,
    structure
  electrocardiogram (ECG) (EKG) 794.31
  electroencephalogram (EEG) 794.02
  electrolyte level, urinary 791.9
  electromyogram (EMG) 794.17
    ocular 794.14
  electro-oculogram (EOG) 794.12
  electroretinogram (ERG) 794.11
  enzymes, serum NEC 790.5
  fibrinogen titer coagulation study 790.92

Findings—*continued*
  filling defect—*see* Filling defect
  function study NEC 794.9
    auditory 794.15
    bladder 794.9
    brain 794.00
    cardiac 794.30
    endocrine NEC 794.6
      thyroid 794.5
    kidney 794.4
    liver 794.8
    nervous system
      central 794.00
      peripheral 794.19
    oculomotor 794.14
    pancreas 794.9
    placenta 794.9
    pulmonary 794.2
    retina 794.11
    special senses 794.19
    spleen 794.9
    vestibular 794.16
  gallbladder, nonvisualization 793.3
  glucose 790.29
    elevated
      fasting 790.21
      tolerance test 790.22
  glycosuria 791.5
  heart
    shadow 793.2
    sounds 785.3
  hematinuria 791.2
  hematocrit
    drop (precipitous) 790.01
    elevated 282.7
    low 285.9
  hematologic NEC 790.99
  hematuria 599.70
  hemoglobin
    drop 790.01
    elevated 282.7
    low 285.9
  hemoglobinuria 791.2
  histological NEC 795.4
  hormones 259.9
  immunoglobulins, elevated 795.79
  indolacetic acid, elevated 791.9
  iron 790.6
  karyotype 795.2
  ketonuria 791.6
  lactic acid dehydrogenase (LDH) 790.4
  lead 790.6
  lipase 790.5
  lipids NEC 272.9
  lithium, blood 790.6
  liver function test 790.6
  lung field (shadow) 793.19
    coin lesion 793.11
  magnesium, blood 790.6
  mammogram 793.80
    calcification 793.89
    caclulus 793.89
    dense breasts 793.82
    inconclusive 793.82
      due to dense breasts 793.82
    microcalcification 793.81
  mediastinal shift 793.2
  melanin, urine 791.9
  microbiologic NEC 795.39
  mineral, blood NEC 790.6
  myoglobinuria 791.3
  nasal swab, anthrax 795.31

Findings—*continued*
  neonatal screening 796.6
  nitrogen derivatives, blood 790.6
  nonvisualization of gallbladder 793.3
  nose culture, positive 795.39
  odor of urine (unusual) NEC 791.9
  oxygen saturation 790.91
  Papanicolaou (smear) 796.9
    anus 796.70
      with
        atypical squamous cells
          cannot exclude high grade squamous
            intraepithelial lesion (ASC-H)
            796.72
          of undetermined significance (ASC-US)
            796.71
        cytologic evidence of malignancy 796.76
        high grade squamous intraepithelial lesion
          (HGSIL) 796.74
        low grade squamous intraepithelial lesion
          (LGSIL) 796.73
      glandular 796.70
      specified finding NEC 796.79
    cervix 795.00
      with
        atypical squamous cells
          cannot exclude high grade squamous
            intrepithelial lesion (ASC-H) 795.02
          of undetermined significance (ASC-US)
            795.01
        cytologic evidence of malignancy 795.06
        high grade squamous intraepithelial lesion
          (HGSIL) 795.04
        low grade squamous intraepithelial lesion
          (LGSIL) 795.03
        non-atypical endometrial cells 795.09
      dyskaryotic 795.09
      non-atypical endometrial cells 795.09
      nonspecific finding NEC 795.09
    other site 796.9
    vagina 795.10
      with
        atypical squamous cells
          cannot exclude high grade squamous
            intraepithelial lesion (ASC-H)
            795.12
          of undetermined significance (ASC-US)
            795.11
        cytologic evidence of malignancy 795.16
        high grade squamous intraepithelial lesion
          (HGSIL) 795.14
        low grade squamous intraepithelial lesion
          (LGSIL) 795.13
      glandular 795.10
      specified NEC 795.19
  peritoneal fluid 792.9
  phonocardiogram 794.39
  phosphorus 275.3
  pleural fluid 792.9
  pneumoencephalogram 793.0
  PO$_2$-oxygen ratio 790.91
  poikilocytosis 790.09
  potassium
    deficiency 276.8
    excess 276.7
  PPD 795.51
  prostate specific antigen (PSA) 790.93
  protein, serum NEC 790.99
  proteinuria 791.0
  prothrombin time (partial) (prolonged) (PT)
    (PTT) 790.92
  pyuria 791.9

Findings —*continued*
　radiologic (x-ray) 793.99
　　abdomen 793.6
　　biliary tract 793.3
　　breast 793.89
　　　abnormal mammogram NOS 793.80
　　　mammographic
　　　　calcification 793.89
　　　　calculus 793.89
　　　　microcalcification 793.81
　　gastrointestinal tract 793.4
　　genitourinary organs 793.5
　　head 793.0
　　image test inconclusive due to excess body fat
　　　793.91
　　intrathoracic organs NEC 793.2
　　lung 793.19
　　musculoskeletal 793.7
　　placenta 793.99
　　retroperitoneum 793.6
　　skin 793.99
　　skull 793.0
　　subcutaneous tissue 793.99
　red blood cell 790.09
　　count 790.09
　　morphology 790.09
　　sickling 790.09
　　volume 790.09
　saliva 792.4
　scan NEC 794.9
　　bladder 794.9
　　bone 794.9
　　brain 794.09
　　kidney 794.4
　　liver 794.8
　　lung 794.2
　　pancreas 794.9
　　placental 794.9
　　spleen 794.9
　　thyroid 794.5
　sedimentation rate, elevated 790.1
　semen 792.2
　serological (for)
　　human immunodeficiency virus (HIV)
　　　inconclusive 795.71
　　　positive V08
　　syphilis—*see* Findings, serology for syphilis
　serology for syphilis
　　false positive 795.6
　　positive 097.1
　　　false 795.6
　　　follow-up of latent syphilis—*see* Syphilis,
　　　　latent
　　　only finding—*see* Syphilis, latent
　serum 790.99
　　blood NEC 790.99
　　enzymes NEC 790.5
　　proteins 790.99
　SGOT 790.4
　SGPT 790.4
　sickling of red blood cells 790.09
　skin test, positive 795.79
　　tuberculin (without active tuberculosis) 795.51
　sodium 790.6
　　deficiency 276.1
　　excess 276.0
　specified NEC 796.9
　spermatozoa 792.2
　spinal fluid 792.0
　　culture, positive 792.0
　sputum culture, positive 795.39

Findings —*continued*
　for acid-fast bacilli 795.39
　stool NEC 792.1
　　bloody 578.1
　　　occult 792.1
　　color 792.1
　　culture, positive 792.1
　　occult blood 792.1
　stress test 794.39
　structure, body (echogram) (thermogram)
　　(ultrasound) (x-ray) NEC 793.99
　　abdomen 793.6
　　breast 793.89
　　　abnormal mammogram 793.80
　　　mammographic
　　　　calcification 793.89
　　　　calculus 793.89
　　　　microcalcification 793.81
　　gastrointestinal tract 793.4
　　genitourinary organs 793.5
　　head 793.0
　　　echogram (ultrasound) 794.01
　　intrathoracic organs NEC 793.2
　　lung 793.19
　　musculoskeletal 793.7
　　placenta 793.99
　　retroperitoneum 793.6
　　skin 793.99
　　subcutaneous tissue NEC 793.99
　synovial fluid 792.9
　thermogram—*see* Finding, abnormal, structure
　throat culture, positive 795.39
　thyroid (function) 794.5
　　metabolism (rate) 794.5
　　scan 794.5
　　uptake 794.5
　total proteins 790.99
　toxicology (drugs) (heavy metals) 796.0
　transaminase (level) 790.4
　triglycerides 272.9
　　high 272.1
　　　with high cholesterol 272.2
　tuberculin skin test (without active tuberculosis)
　　795.51
　tumor markers NEC 795.89
　ultrasound—*see also* Finding, abnormal,
　　structure
　　cardiogram 793.2
　uric acid, blood 790.6
　urine, urinary constituents 791.9
　　acetone 791.6
　　albumin 791.0
　　bacteria 791.9
　　bile 791.4
　　blood 599.70
　　casts or cells 791.7
　　chyle 791.1
　　culture, positive 791.9
　　glucose 791.5
　　hemoglobin 791.2
　　ketone 791.6
　　protein 791.0
　　pus 791.9
　　sugar 791.5
　vaginal
　　fluid 792.9
　　high risk human papillomavirus (HPV) DNA
　　　test positive 795.15
　　low risk human papillomavirus (HPV) DNA
　　　test positive 795.19
　vanillylmandelic acid, elevated 791.9

Findings —*continued*
vectorcardiogram (VCG) 794.39
ventriculogram (cerebral) 793.0
VMA, elevated 791.9
Wassermann reaction
false positive 795.6
positive 097.1
follow-up of latent syphilis—*see* Syphilis, latent
only finding—*see* Syphilis, latent
white blood cell 288.9
count 288.9
elevated 288.60
low 288.50
differential 288.9
morphology 288.9
wound culture 795.39
xerography 793.89
zinc, blood 790.6
Finger —*see* condition
Finnish type nephrosis (congenital) 759.89
Fire, St. Anthony's (*see also* Erysipelas) 035
Fish
hook stomach 537.89
meal workers' lung 495.8
Fisher's syndrome 357.0
Fissure, fissured
abdominal wall (congenital) 756.79
anus, anal 565.0
congenital 751.5
buccal cavity 528.9
clitoris (congenital) 752.49
ear, lobule (congenital) 744.29
epiglottis (congenital) 748.3
larynx 478.79
congenital 748.3
lip 528.5
congenital (*see also* Cleft, lip) 749.10
nipple 611.2
puerperal, postpartum 676.1
palate (congenital) (*see also* Cleft, palate) 749.00
postanal 565.0
rectum 565.0
skin 709.8
streptococcal 686.9
spine (congenital) (*see also* Spina bifida) 741.9
sternum (congenital) 756.3
tongue (acquired) 529.5
congenital 750.13
Fistula (sinus) 686.9
abdomen (wall) 569.81
bladder 596.2
intestine 569.81
ureter 593.82
uterus 619.2
abdominorectal 569.81
abdominosigmoidal 569.81
abdominothoracic 510.0
abdominouterine 619.2
congenital 752.39
abdominovesical 596.2
accessory sinuses (*see also* Sinusitis) 473.9
actinomycotic—*see* Actinomycosis
alveolar
antrum (*see also* Sinusitis, maxillary) 473.0
process 522.7
anorectal 565.1
antrobuccal (*see also* Sinusitis, maxillary) 473.0
antrum (*see also* Sinusitis, maxillary) 473.0

Fistula—*continued*
anus, anal (infectional) (recurrent) 565.1
congenital 751.5
tuberculous (*see also* Tuberculosis) 014.8
aortic sinus 747.29
aortoduodenal 447.2
appendix, appendicular 543.9
arteriovenous (acquired) 447.0
brain 437.3
congenital 747.81
ruptured (*see also* Hemorrhage, subarachnoid) 430
ruptured (*see also* Hemorrhage, subarachnoid) 430
cerebral 437.3
congenital 747.81
congenital (peripheral) 747.60
brain—*see* Fistula, arteriovenous, brain, congenital
coronary 746.85
gastrointestinal 747.61
lower limb 747.64
pulmonary 747.39
renal 747.62
specified NEC 747.69
upper limb 747.63
coronary 414.19
congenital 746.85
heart 414.19
pulmonary (vessels) 417.0
congenital 747.39
surgically created (for dialysis) V45.11
complication NEC 996.73
atherosclerosis —*see* Arteriosclerosis, extremities
embolism 996.74
infection or inflammation 996.62
mechanical 996.1
occlusion NEC 996.74
thrombus 996.74
traumatic—*see* Injury, blood vessel, by site
artery 447.2
aural 383.81
congenital 744.49
auricle 383.81
congenital 744.49
Bartholin's gland 619.8
bile duct (*see also* Fistula, biliary) 576.4
biliary (duct) (tract) 576.4
congenital 751.69
bladder (neck) (sphincter) 596.2
into seminal vesicle 596.2
bone 733.99
brain 348.8
arteriovenous—*see* Fistula, arteriovenous, brain
branchial (cleft) 744.41
branchiogenous 744.41
breast 611.0
puerperal, postpartum 675.1
bronchial 510.0
bronchocutaneous, bronchomediastinal, bronchopleural, bronchopleuromediastinal (infective) 510.0
tuberculous (*see also* Tuberculosis) 011.3
bronchoesophageal 530.89
congenital 750.3
buccal cavity (infective) 528.3
canal, ear 380.89

Fistula—*continued*
carotid-cavernous
  congenital 747.81
    with hemorrhage 430
  traumatic 900.82
    with hemorrhage (*see also* Hemorrhage,
      brain, traumatic) 853.0
    late effect 908.3
cecosigmoidal 569.81
cecum 569.81
cerebrospinal (fluid) 349.81
cervical, lateral (congenital) 744.41
cervicoaural (congenital) 744.49
cervicosigmoidal 619.1
cervicovesical 619.0
cervix 619.8
chest (wall) 510.0
cholecystocolic (*see also* Fistula, gallbladder)
  575.5
cholecystocolonic (*see also* Fistula, gallbladder)
  575.5
cholecystoduodenal (*see also* Fistula,
  gallbladder) 575.5
cholecystoenteric (*see also* Fistula, gallbladder)
  575.5
cholecystogastric (*see also* Fistula, gallbladder)
  575.5
cholecystointestinal (*see also* Fistula,
  gallbladder) 575.5
choledochoduodenal 576.4
cholocolic (*see also* Fistula, gallbladder) 575.5
coccyx 685.1
  with abscess 685.0
colon 569.81
colostomy 569.69
colovaginal (acquired) 619.1
common duct (bile duct) 576.4
congenital, NEC—*see* Anomaly, specified type
  NEC
cornea, causing hypotony 360.32
coronary, arteriovenous 414.19
  congenital 746.85
costal region 510.0
cul-de-sac, Douglas' 619.8
cutaneous 686.9
cystic duct (*see also* Fistula, gallbladder) 575.5
  congenital 751.69
cystostomy 596.83
dental 522.7
diaphragm 510.0
  bronchovisceral 510.0
  pleuroperitoneal 510.0
  pulmonoperitoneal 510.0
duodenum 537.4
ear (canal) (external) 380.89
enterocolic 569.81
enterocutaneous 569.81
enteroenteric 569.81
entero-uterine 619.1
  congenital 752.39
enterovaginal 619.1
  congenital 752.49
enterovesical 596.1
epididymis 608.89
  tuberculous (*see also* Tuberculosis) 016.4
esophagobronchial 530.89
  congenital 750.3
esophagocutaneous 530.89
esophagopleurocutaneous 530.89
esophagotracheal 530.84
  congenital 750.3

Fistula—*continued*
esophagus 530.89
  congenital 750.4
ethmoid (*see also* Sinusitis, ethmoidal) 473.2
eyeball (cornea) (sclera) 360.32
eyelid 373.11
fallopian tube (external) 619.2
fecal 569.81
  congenital 751.5
from periapical lesion 522.7
frontal sinus (*see also* Sinusitis, frontal) 473.1
gallbladder 575.5
  with calculus, cholelithiasis, stones (*see also*
    Cholelithiasis) 574.2
  congenital 751.69
gastric 537.4
gastrocolic 537.4
  congenital 750.7
  tuberculous (*see also* Tuberculosis) 014.8
gastroenterocolic 537.4
gastroesophageal 537.4
gastrojejunal 537.4
gastrojejunocolic 537.4
genital
  organs
    female 619.9
      specified site NEC 619.8
    male 608.89
  tract-skin (female) 619.2
hepatopleural 510.0
hepatopulmonary 510.0
horseshoe 565.1
ileorectal 569.81
ileosigmoidal 569.81
ileostomy 569.69
ileovesical 596.1
ileum 569.81
in ano 565.1
  tuberculous (*see also* Tuberculosis) 014.8
inner ear (*see also* Fistula, labyrinth) 386.40
intestine 569.81
intestinocolonic (abdominal) 569.81
intestinoureteral 593.82
intestinouterine 619.1
intestinovaginal 619.1
  congenital 752.49
intestinovesical 596.1
involving female genital tract 619.9
  digestive-genital 619.1
  genital tract-skin 619.2
  specified site NEC 619.8
  urinary-genital 619.0
ischiorectal (fossa) 566
jejunostomy 569.69
jejunum 569.81
joint 719.80
  ankle 719.87
  elbow 719.82
  foot 719.87
  hand 719.84
  hip 719.85
  knee 719.86
  multiple sites 719.89
  pelvic region 719.85
  shoulder (region) 719.81
  specified site NEC 719.88
  tuberculous—*see* Tuberculosis, joint
  wrist 719.83
kidney 593.89
labium (majus) (minus) 619.8

Fistula—*continued*
  labyrinth, labyrinthine NEC 386.40
    combined sites 386.48
    multiple sites 386.48
    oval window 386.42
    round window 386.41
    semicircular canal 386.43
  lacrimal, lachrymal (duct) (gland) (sac) 375.61
  lacrimonasal duct 375.61
  laryngotracheal 748.3
  larynx 478.79
  lip 528.5
    congenital 750.25
  lumbar, tuberculous (*see also* Tuberculosis)
    015.0 *[730.8]*
  lung 510.0
  lymphatic (node) (vessel) 457.8
  mamillary 611.0
  mammary (gland) 611.0
    puerperal, postpartum 675.1
  mastoid (process) (region) 383.1
  maxillary (*see also* Sinusitis, maxillary) 473.0
  mediastinal 510.0
  mediastinobronchial 510.0
  mediastinocutaneous 510.0
  middle ear 385.89
  mouth 528.3
  nasal 478.19
    sinus (*see also* Sinusitis) 473.9
  nasopharynx 478.29
  nipple—*see* Fistula, breast
  nose 478.19
  oral (cutaneous) 528.3
    maxillary (*see also* Sinusitis, maxillary) 473.0
    nasal (with cleft palate) (*see also* Cleft, palate)
      749.00
  orbit, orbital 376.10
  oro-antral (*see also* Sinusitis, maxillary) 473.0
  oval window (internal ear) 386.42
  oviduct (external) 619.2
  palate (hard) 526.89
    soft 528.9
  pancreatic 577.8
  pancreaticoduodenal 577.8
  parotid (gland) 527.4
    region 528.3
  pelvoabdominointestinal 569.81
  penis 607.89
  perianal 565.1
  pericardium (pleura) (sac) (*see also* Pericarditis)
    423.8
  pericecal 569.81
  perineal—*see* Fistula, perineum
  perineorectal 569.81
  perineosigmoidal 569.81
  perineo-urethroscrotal 608.89
  perineum, perineal (with urethral involvement)
    NEC 599.1
    tuberculous (*see also* Tuberculosis) 017.9
    ureter 593.82
  perirectal 565.1
    tuberculous (*see also* Tuberculosis) 014.8
  peritoneum (*see also* Peritonitis) 567.22
  periurethral 599.1
  pharyngo-esophageal 478.29
  pharynx 478.29
    branchial cleft (congenital) 744.41
  pilonidal (infected) (rectum) 685.1
    with abscess 685.0

Fistula—*continued*
  pleura, pleural, pleurocutaneous,
    pleuroperitoneal 510.0
    stomach 510.0
    tuberculous (*see also* Tuberculosis) 012.0
  pleuropericardial 423.8
  postauricular 383.81
  postoperative, persistent 998.6
  preauricular (congenital) 744.46
  prostate 602.8
  pulmonary 510.0
    arteriovenous 417.0
      congenital 747.39
    tuberculous (*see also* Tuberculosis,
      pulmonary) 011.9
  pulmonoperitoneal 510.0
  rectolabial 619.1
  rectosigmoid (intercommunicating) 569.81
  rectoureteral 593.82
  rectourethral 599.1
    congenital 753.8
  rectouterine 619.1
    congenital 752.39
  rectovaginal 619.1
    congenital 752.49
    old, postpartal 619.1
    tuberculous (*see also* Tuberculosis) 014.8
  rectovesical 596.1
    congenital 753.8
  rectovesicovaginal 619.1
  rectovulvar 619.1
    congenital 752.49
  rectum (to skin) 565.1
    tuberculous (*see also* Tuberculosis) 014.8
  renal 593.89
  retroauricular 383.81
  round window (internal ear) 386.41
  salivary duct or gland 527.4
    congenital 750.24
  sclera 360.32
  scrotum (urinary) 608.89
    tuberculous (*see also* Tuberculosis) 016.5
  semicircular canals (internal ear) 386.43
  sigmoid 569.81
    vesicoabdominal 596.1
  sigmoidovaginal 619.1
    congenital 752.49
  skin 686.9
    ureter 593.82
    vagina 619.2
  sphenoidal sinus (*see also* Sinusitis, sphenoidal)
    473.3
  splenocolic 289.59
  stercoral 569.81
  stomach 537.4
  sublingual gland 527.4
    congenital 750.24
  submaxillary
    gland 527.4
      congenital 750.24
    region 528.3
  thoracic 510.0
    duct 457.8
  thoracicoabdominal 510.0
  thoracicogastric 510.0
  thoracicointestinal 510.0
  thoracoabdominal 510.0
  thoracogastric 510.0
  thorax 510.0
  thyroglossal duct 759.2
  thyroid 246.8
  trachea (congenital) (external) (internal) 748.3

Fistula—*continued*
tracheoesophageal 530.84
  congenital 750.3
  following tracheostomy 519.09
  traumatic
    arteriovenous (*see also* Injury, blood vessel,
      by site) 904.9
    brain—*see* Injury, intracranial
tuberculous—*see* Tuberculosis, by site
typhoid 002.0
umbilical 759.89
umbilico-urinary 753.8
urachal, urachus 753.7
ureter (persistent) 593.82
ureteroabdominal 593.82
ureterocervical 593.82
ureterorectal 593.82
ureterosigmoido-abdominal 593.82
ureterovaginal 619.0
ureterovesical 596.2
urethra 599.1
  congenital 753.8
  tuberculous (*see also* Tuberculosis) 016.3
urethroperineal 599.1
urethroperineovesical 596.2
urethrorectal 599.1
  congenital 753.8
urethroscrotal 608.89
urethrovaginal 619.0
urethrovesical 596.2
urethrovesicovaginal 619.0
urinary (persistent) (recurrent) 599.1
uteroabdominal (anterior wall) 619.2
  congenital 752.39
uteroenteric 619.1
uterofecal 619.1
uterointestinal 619.1
  congenital 752.39
uterorectal 619.1
  congenital 752.39
uteroureteric 619.0
uterovaginal 619.8
uterovesical 619.0
  congenital 752.39
uterus 619.8
vagina (wall) 619.8
  postpartal, old 619.8
vaginocutaneous (postpartal) 619.2
vaginoileal (acquired) 619.1
vaginoperineal 619.2
vesical NEC 596.2
vesicoabdominal 596.2
vesicocervicovaginal 619.0
vesicocolic 596.1
vesicocutaneous 596.2
vesicoenteric 596.1
vesicointestinal 596.1
vesicometrorectal 619.1
vesicoperineal 596.2
vesicorectal 596.1
  congenital 753.8
vesicosigmoidal 596.1
vesicosigmoidovaginal 619.1
vesicoureteral 596.2
vesicoureterovaginal 619.0
vesicourethral 596.2
vesicourethrorectal 596.1
vesicouterine 619.0
  congenital 752.39
vesicovaginal 619.0
vulvorectal 619.1
  congenital 752.49

Fit 780.39
apoplectic (*see also* Disease, cerebrovascular,
  acute) 436
  late effect—*see* Late effect(s) (of)
    cerebrovascular disease
epileptic (*see also* Epilepsy) 345.9
fainting 780.2
hysterical 300.11
newborn 779.0
Fitting (of)
artificial
  arm (complete) (partial) V52.0
  breast V52.4
    implant exchange (different material)
      (different size) V52.4
  eye(s) V52.2
  leg(s) (complete) (partial) V52.1
brain neuropacemaker V53.02
cardiac pacemaker V53.31
carotid sinus pacemaker V53.39
cerebral ventricle (communicating) shunt V53.01
colostomy belt V53.5
contact lenses V53.1
cystostomy device V53.6
defibrillator, automatic implantable (with
  synchronous cardiac pacemaker) V53.32
dentures V52.3
device, unspecified type V53.90
  abdominal V53.59
  cardiac
    defibrillator, automatic implantable (with
      synchronous cardiac pacemaker) V53.32
    pacemaker V53.31
    specified NEC V53.39
  cerebral ventricle (communicating) shunt
    V53.01
  gastrointestinal NEC V53.59
  insulin pump V53.91
  intestinal V53.50
  intrauterine contraceptive
    insertion V25.11
    removal V25.12
      and reinsertion V25.13
    replacement V25.13
  nervous system V53.09
  orthodontic V53.4
  orthoptic V53.1
  other device V53.99
  prosthetic V52.9
    breast V52.4
    dental V52.3
    eye V52.2
    specified type NEC V52.8
  special senses V53.09
  substitution
    auditory V53.09
    nervous system V53.09
    visual V53.09
  urinary V53.6
diaphragm (contraceptive) V25.02
gastric lap band V53.51
gastrointestinal appliance and device NEC V53.59
glasses (reading) V53.1
growth rod V54.02
hearing aid V53.2
ileostomy device V53.5
intestinal appliance and device V53.50
intrauterine contraceptive device
  insertion V25.11
  removal V25.12
    and reinsertion V25.13
  replacement V25.13

Fitting—*continued*
　neuropacemaker (brain) (peripheral nerve)
　　(spinal cord) V53.02
　orthodontic device V53.4
　orthopedic (device) V53.7
　　brace V53.7
　　cast V53.7
　　corset V53.7
　　shoes V53.7
　pacemaker (cardiac) V53.31
　　brain V53.02
　　carotid sinus V53.39
　　peripheral nerve V53.02
　　spinal cord V53.02
　prosthesis V52.9
　　arm (complete) (partial) V52.0
　　breast V52.4
　　　implant exchange (different material)
　　　　(different size) V52.4
　　dental V52.3
　　eye V52.2
　　leg (complete) (partial) V52.1
　　specified type NEC V52.8
　spectacles V53.1
　wheelchair V53.8
Fitz's syndrome (acute hemorrhagic pancreatitis)
　577.0
Fitz-Hugh and Curtis syndrome 098.86
　due to
　　Chlamydia trachomatis 099.56
　　Neisseria gonorrhoeae (gonococcal peritonitis)
　　　098.86
Fixation
　joint—*see* Ankylosis
　larynx 478.79
　pupil 364.76
　stapes 385.22
　　deafness (*see also* Deafness, conductive) 389.04
　uterus (acquired)—*see* Malposition, uterus
　vocal cord 478.5
Flaccid —*see* condition
　foot 736.79
　forearm 736.09
　palate, congenital 750.26
Flail
　chest 807.4
　　newborn 767.3
　joint (paralytic) 718.80
　　ankle 718.87
　　elbow 718.82
　　foot 718.87
　　hand 718.84
　　hip 718.85
　　knee 718.86
　　multiple sites 718.89
　　pelvic region 718.85
　　shoulder (region) 718.81
　　specified site NEC 718.88
　　wrist 718.83
Flajani (-Basedow) syndrome or disease
　(exophthalmic goiter) 242.0
Flap, liver 572.8
Flare, anterior chamber (aqueous) (eye) 364.04
Flashback phenomena (drug) (hallucinogenic) 292.89
Flat
　chamber (anterior) (eye) 360.34
　chest, congenital 754.89
　electroencephalogram (EEG) 348.89

Flat —*continued*
　foot (acquired) (fixed type) (painful) (postural)
　　(spastic) 734
　　congenital 754.61
　　　rocker bottom 754.61
　　　vertical talus 754.61
　　rachitic 268.1
　　rocker bottom (congenital) 754.61
　　vertical talus, congenital 754.61
　organ or site, congenital NEC—*see* Anomaly,
　　specified type NEC
　pelvis 738.6
　　with disproportion (fetopelvic) 653.2
　　　affecting fetus or newborn 763.1
　　　causing obstructed labor 660.1
　　　　affecting fetus or newborn 763.1
　　congenital 755.69
Flatau-Schilder disease 341.1
Flattening
　head, femur 736.39
　hip 736.39
　lip (congenital) 744.89
　nose (congenital) 754.0
　　acquired 738.0
Flatulence 787.3
Flatus 787.3
　vaginalis 629.89
Flax dressers' disease 504
Flea bite —*see* Injury, superficial, by site
Fleischer (-Kayser) ring (corneal pigmentation)
　275.1 *[371.14]*
Fleischner's disease 732.3
Fleshy mole 631.8
Flexibilitas cerea (*see also* Catalepsy) 300.11
Flexion
　cervix —*see* Flexion, uterus
　contracture, joint (*see also* Contraction, joint) 718.4
　deformity, joint (*see also* Contraction, joint) 736.9
　　hip, congenital (*see also* Subluxation,
　　　congenital, hip) 754.32
　uterus (*see also* Malposition, uterus) 621.6
Flexner's
　bacillus 004.1
　diarrhea (ulcerative) 004.1
　dysentery 004.1
Flexner-Boyd dysentery 004.2
Flexure —*see* condition
Floater, vitreous 379.24
Floating
　cartilage (joint) (*see also* Disorder, cartilage,
　　articular) 718.0
　　knee 717.6
　gallbladder (congenital) 751.69
　kidney 593.0
　　congenital 753.3
　liver (congenital) 751.69
　rib 756.3
　spleen 289.59
Flooding 626.2
Floor —*see* condition
Floppy
　infant NEC 781.99
　iris syndrome 364.81
　valve syndrome (mitral) 424.0
Flu —*see also* Influenza
　bird (*see also* Influenza, avian) 488.02
　gastric NEC 008.8
　swine —*see* Influenza, (novel) 2009 H1N1
Fluctuating blood pressure 796.4

Fluid
abdomen 789.59
chest (*see also* Pleurisy, with effusion) 511.9
heart (*see also* Failure, heart) 428.0
joint (*see also* Effusion, joint) 719.0
loss (acute) 276.50
with
hypernatremia 276.0
hyponatremia 276.1
lung—*see also* Edema, lung
encysted 511.89
peritoneal cavity 789.59
malignant 789.51
pleural cavity (*see also* Pleurisy, with effusion) 511.9
retention 276.69
Flukes NEC (*see also* Infestation, fluke) 121.9
blood NEC (*see also* Infestation, Schistosoma) 120.9
liver 121.3
Fluor (albus) (vaginalis) 623.5
trichomonal (Trichomonas vaginalis) 131.00
Fluorosis (dental) (chronic) 520.3
Flushing 782.62
menopausal 627.2
Flush syndrome 259.2
Flutter
atrial or auricular 427.32
heart (ventricular) 427.42
atrial 427.32
impure 427.32
postoperative 997.1
ventricular 427.42
Flux (bloody) (serosanguineous) 009.0
FNHTR (febrile hemolytic transfusion reaction) 780.66
Focal —*see* condition
Fochier's abscess —*see* Abscess, by site
Focus, Assmann's (*see also* Tuberculosis) 011.0
Fogo selvagem 694.4
Foix-Alajouanine syndrome 336.1
Folds, anomalous —*see also* Anomaly, specified type NEC
Bowman's membrane 371.31
Descemet's membrane 371.32
epicanthic 743.63
heart 746.89
posterior segment of eye, congenital 743.54
Folie à deux 297.3
Follicle
cervix (nabothian) (ruptured) 616.0
graafian, ruptured, with hemorrhage 620.0
nabothian 616.0
Folliclis (primary) (*see also* Tuberculosis) 017.0
Follicular —*see also* condition
cyst (atretic) 620.0
Folliculitis 704.8
abscedens et suffodiens 704.8
decalvans 704.09
gonorrheal (acute) 098.0
chronic or duration of 2 months or more 098.2
keloid, keloidalis 706.1
pustular 704.8
ulerythematosa reticulata 701.8
Folliculosis, conjunctival 372.02
Folling's disease (phenylketonuria) 270.1
Follow-up (examination) (routine) (following) V67.9
cancer chemotherapy V67.2
chemotherapy V67.2
fracture V67.4
high-risk medication V67.51

Follow-upt—*continued*
injury NEC V67.59
postpartum
immediately after delivery V24.0
routine V24.2
psychiatric V67.3
psychotherapy V67.3
radiotherapy V67.1
specified condition NEC V67.59
specified surgery NEC V67.09
surgery V67.00
vaginal pap smear V67.01
treatment V67.9
combined NEC V67.6
fracture V67.4
involving high-risk medication NEC V67.51
mental disorder V67.3
specified NEC V67.59
Fong's syndrome (hereditary osteoonychodysplasia) 756.89
Food
allergy 693.1
anaphylactic shock—*see* Anaphylactic reaction or shock, due to, food
asphyxia (from aspiration or inhalation) (*see also* Asphyxia, food) 933.1
choked on (*see also* Asphyxia, food) 933.1
deprivation 994.2
specified kind of food NEC 269.8
intoxication (*see also* Poisoning, food) 005.9
lack of 994.2
poisoning (*see also* Poisoning, food) 005.9
refusal or rejection NEC 307.59
strangulation or suffocation (*see also* Asphyxia, food) 933.1
toxemia (*see also* Poisoning, food) 005.9
Foot —*see also* condition
and mouth disease 078.4
process disease 581.3
Foramen ovale (nonclosure) (patent) (persistent) 745.5
Forbes' (glycogen storage) disease 271.0
Forbes-Albright syndrome (nonpuerperal amenorrhea and lactation associated with pituitary tumor) 253.1
Forced birth or delivery NEC 669.8
affecting fetus or newborn NEC 763.89
Forceps
delivery NEC 669.5
affecting fetus or newborn 763.2
Fordyce's disease (ectopic sebaceous glands) (mouth) 750.26
Fordyce-Fox disease (apocrine miliaria) 705.82
Forearm —*see* condition
Foreign body

Note—*For foreign body with open wound or other injury, see Wound, open, or the type of injury specified.*

accidentally left during a procedure 998.4
anterior chamber (eye) 871.6
magnetic 871.5
retained or old 360.51
retained or old 360.61
ciliary body (eye) 871.6
magnetic 871.5
retained or old 360.52
retained or old 360.62

Foreign body—*continued*
  entering through orifice (current) (old)
    accessory sinus 932
    air passage (upper) 933.0
      lower 934.8
    alimentary canal 938
    alveolar process 935.0
    antrum (Highmore) 932
    anus 937
    appendix 936
    asphyxia due to (*see also* Asphyxia, food)
      933.1
    auditory canal 931
    auricle 931
    bladder 939.0
    bronchioles 934.8
    bronchus (main) 934.1
    buccal cavity 935.0
    canthus (inner) 930.1
    cecum 936
    cervix (canal) uterine 939.1
    coil, ileocecal 936
    colon 936
    conjunctiva 930.1
    conjunctival sac 930.1
    cornea 930.0
    digestive organ or tract NEC 938
    duodenum 936
    ear (external) 931
    esophagus 935.1
    eye (external) 930.9
      combined sites 930.8
      intraocular—*see* Foreign body, by site
      specified site NEC 930.8
    eyeball 930.8
      intraocular—*see* Foreign body, intraocular
    eyelid 930.1
      retained or old 374.86
    frontal sinus 932
    gastrointestinal tract 938
    genitourinary tract 939.9
    globe 930.8
      penetrating 871.6
        magnetic 871.5
          retained or old 360.50
        retained or old 360.60
    gum 935.0
    Highmore's antrum 932
    hypopharynx 933.0
    ileocecal coil 936
    ileum 936
    inspiration (of) 933.1
    intestine (large) (small) 936
    lacrimal apparatus, duct, gland, or sac 930.2
    larynx 933.1
    lung 934.8
    maxillary sinus 932
    mouth 935.0
    nasal sinus 932
    nasopharynx 933.0
    nose (passage) 932
    nostril 932
    oral cavity 935.0
    palate 935.0
    penis 939.3
    pharynx 933.0
    pyriform sinus 933.0
    rectosigmoid 937
      junction 937
    rectum 937

Foreign body—*continued*
  entering through—*continued*
    respiratory tract 934.9
      specified part NEC 934.8
    sclera 930.1
    sinus 932
      accessory 932
      frontal 932
      maxillary 932
      nasal 932
      pyriform 933.0
    small intestine 936
    stomach (hairball) 935.2
    suffocation by (*see also* Asphyxia, food) 933.1
    swallowed 938
      tongue 933.0
    tear ducts or glands 930.2
    throat 933.0
    tongue 935.0
      swallowed 933.0
    tonsil, tonsillar 933.0
      fossa 933.0
    trachea 934.0
    ureter 939.0
    urethra 939.0
    uterus (any part) 939.1
    vagina 939.2
    vulva 939.2
    wind pipe 934.0
  feeling of, in throat 784.99
  granuloma (old) 728.82
    bone 733.99
    in operative wound (inadvertently left) 998.4
      due to surgical material intentionally
        left—*see* Complications, due to
        (presence of) any device, implant, or
        graft classified to 996.0-996.5 NEC
    muscle 728.82
    skin 709.4
    soft tissue 709.1
    subcutaneous tissue 709.4
  in
    bone (residual) 733.99
    open wound—*see* Wound, open, by site
      complicated
    soft tissue (residual) 729.6
  inadvertently left in operation wound (causing
    adhesions, obstruction, or perforation) 998.4
  ingestion, ingested NEC 938
  inhalation or inspiration (*see also* Asphyxia,
    food) 933.1
  internal organ, not entering through an
    orifice—*see* Injury, internal, by site, with
    open wound
  intraocular (nonmagnetic) 871.6
    combined sites 871.6
      magnetic 871.5
        retained or old 360.59
      retained or old 360.69
    magnetic 871.5
      retained or old 360.50
    retained or old 360.60
    specified site NEC 871.6
      magnetic 871.5
        retained or old 360.59
      retained or old 360.69
  iris (nonmagnetic) 871.6
    magnetic 871.5
      retained or old 360.52
    retained or old 360.62

Foreign body—*continued*
   lens (nonmagnetic) 871.6
      magnetic 871.5
         retained or old 360.53
      retained or old 360.63
   lid, eye 930.1
   ocular muscle 870.4
      retained or old 376.6
   old or residual
      bone 733.99
      eyelid 374.86
      middle ear 385.83
      muscle 729.6
         ocular 376.6
      retrobulbar 376.6
      skin 729.6
         with granuloma 709.4
      soft tissue 729.6
         with granuloma 709.4
      subcutaneous tissue 729.6
         with granuloma 709.4
   operation wound, left accidentally 998.4
   orbit 870.4
      retained or old 376.6
   posterior wall, eye 871.6
      magnetic 871.5
         retained or old 360.55
      retained or old 360.65
   respiratory tree 934.9
      specified site NEC 934.8
   retained (old) (nonmagnetic) (in) V90.9
      anterior chamber (eye) 360.61
         magnetic 360.51
      ciliary body 360.62
         magnetic 360.52
      eyelid 374.86
      fragment(s)
         acrylics V90.2
         animal quills V90.31
         animal spines V90.31
         cement V90.83
         concrete V90.83
         crystalline V90.83
         depleted
            isotope V90.09
            uranium V90.01
         diethylhexylphthalates V90.2
         glass V90.81
         isocyanate V90.2
         metal V90.10
            magnetic V90.11
            nonmagnetic V90.12
         organic NEC V90.39
         plastic V90.2
         radioactive
            nontherapeutic V90.09
            specified NEC V90.09
         stone V90.83
         tooth V90.32
         wood V90.33
      globe 360.60
         magnetic 360.50
      intraocular 360.60
         magnetic 360.50
         specified site NEC 360.69
            magnetic 360.59
      iris 360.62
         magnetic 360.52
      lens 360.63
         magnetic 360.53
      muscle 729.6

Foreign body—*continued*
   retained—*continued*
      orbit 376.6
      posterior wall of globe 360.65
         magnetic 360.55
      retina 360.65
         magnetic 360.55
      retrobulbar 376.6
      skin 729.6
         with granuloma 709.4
      soft tissue 729.6
         with granuloma 709.4
      specified NEC V90.89
      subcutaneous tissue 729.6
         with granuloma 709.4
      vitreous 360.64
         magnetic 360.54
   retina 871.6
      magnetic 871.5
         retained or old 360.55
      retained or old 360.65
   superficial, without major open wound (*see also*
         Injury, superficial, by site) 919.6
   swallowed NEC 938
   throat, feeling of 784.99
   vitreous (humor) 871.6
      magnetic 871.5
         retained or old 360.54
      retained or old 360.64
Forking, aqueduct of Sylvius 742.3
   with spina bifida (*see also* Spina bifida) 741.0
Formation
   bone in scar tissue (skin) 709.3
   connective tissue in vitreous 379.25
   Elschnig pearls (postcataract extraction) 366.51
   hyaline in cornea 371.49
   sequestrum in bone (due to infection) (*see also*
         Osteomyelitis) 730.1
   valve
      colon, congenital 751.5
      ureter (congenital) 753.29
Formication 782.0
Fort Bragg fever 100.89
Fossa —*see also* condition
   pyriform—*see* condition
Foster care (status) V60.81
Foster-Kennedy syndrome 377.04
Fothergill's
   disease, meaning scarlatina anginosa 034.1
   neuralgia (*see also* Neuralgia, trigeminal) 350.1
Foul breath 784.99
Found dead (cause unknown) 798.9
Foundling V20.0
Fournier's disease (idiopathic gangrene) 608.83
   female 616.89
Fourth
   cranial nerve—*see* condition
   disease 057.8
   molar 520.1
Foville's syndrome 344.89
Fox's
   disease (apocrine miliaria) 705.82
   impetigo (contagiosa) 684
Fox-Fordyce disease (apocrine miliaria) 705.82

Fracture (abduction) (adduction) (avulsion) (compression) (crush) (dislocation) (oblique) (separation) (closed) 829.0

> *Note—For fracture of any of the following sites with fracture of other bones—see Fracture, multiple.*
>
> *"Closed" includes the following descriptions of fractures, with or without delayed healing, unless they are specified as open or compound:*
>
>   comminuted
>   depressed
>   elevated
>   fissured
>   greenstick
>   impacted
>   linear
>   simple
>   slipped epiphysis
>   spiral
>   unspecified
>
> *"Open" includes the following descriptions of fractures, with or without delayed healing:*
>
>   compound
>   infected
>   missile
>   puncture
>   with foreign body
>
> *For late effect of fracture, see Late, effect, fracture, by site.*

with
    internal injuries in same region (conditions classifiable to 860-869)—*see also* Injury, internal, by site
        pelvic region—*see* Fracture, pelvis
acetabulum (with visceral injury) (closed) 808.0
    open 808.1
acromion (process) (closed) 811.01
    open 811.11
alveolus (closed) 802.8
    open 802.9
ankle (malleolus) (closed) 824.8
    bimalleolar (Dupuytren's) (Pott's) 824.4
        open 824.5
    bone 825.21
        open 825.31
    lateral malleolus only (fibular) 824.2
        open 824.3
    medial malleolus only (tibial) 824.0
        open 824.1
    open 824.9
    pathologic 733.16
    talus 825.21
        open 825.31
    trimalleolar 824.6
        open 824.7
antrum—*see* Fracture, skull, base
arm (closed) 818.0
    and leg(s) (any bones) 828.0
        open 828.1
    both (any bones) (with rib(s)) (with sternum) 819.0
        open 819.1
    lower 813.80
        open 813.90
    open 818.1
    upper—*see* Fracture, humerus

Fracture—*continued*
astragalus (closed) 825.21
    open 825.31
atlas—*see* Fracture, vertebra, cervical, first
axis—*see* Fracture, vertebra, cervical, second
back—*see* Fracture, vertebra, by site
Barton's—*see* Fracture, radius, lower end
basal (skull)—*see* Fracture, skull, base
Bennett's (closed) 815.01
    open 815.11
bimalleolar (closed) 824.4
    open 824.5
bone (closed) NEC 829.0
    birth injury NEC 767.3
    open 829.1
    pathologic NEC (*see also* Fracture, pathologic) 733.10
    stress NEC (*see also* Fracture, stress) 733.95
boot top—*see* Fracture, fibula
boxers'—*see* Fracture, metacarpal bone(s)
breast bone—*see* Fracture, sternum
bucket handle (semilunar cartilage)—*see* Tear, meniscus
buckle — see Fracture, torus
burst—*see* Fracture, traumatic, by site
bursting—*see* Fracture, phalanx, hand, distal
calcaneus (closed) 825.0
    open 825.1
capitate (bone) (closed) 814.07
    open 814.17
capitellum (humerus) (closed) 812.49
    open 812.59
carpal bone(s) (wrist NEC) (closed) 814.00
    open 814.10
    specified site NEC 814.09
        open 814.19
cartilage, knee (semilunar)—*see* Tear, meniscus
cervical—*see* Fracture, vertebra, cervical
chauffeur's—*see* Fracture, ulna, lower end
chisel—*see* Fracture, radius, upper end
chronic — see Fracture, pathologic
clavicle (interligamentous part) (closed) 810.00
    acromial end 810.03
        open 810.13
    due to birth trauma 767.2
    open 810.10
    shaft (middle third) 810.02
        open 810.12
    sternal end 810.01
        open 810.11
clayshovelers'—*see* Fracture, vertebra, cervical
coccyx—*see also* Fracture, vertebra, coccyx
    complicating delivery 665.6
collar bone—*see* Fracture, clavicle
Colles' (reversed) (closed) 813.41
    open 813.51
comminuted—*see* Fracture, by site
compression—*see also* Fracture, by site
    nontraumatic—*see* Fracture, pathologic
congenital 756.9
coracoid process (closed) 811.02
    open 811.12
coronoid process (ulna) (closed) 813.02
    mandible (closed) 802.23
        open 802.33
    open 813.12
corpus cavernosum penis 959.13
costochondral junction—*see* Fracture, rib
costosternal junction—*see* Fracture, rib
cranium—*see* Fracture, skull, by site

Fracture—*continued*
  cricoid cartilage (closed) 807.5
    open 807.6
  cuboid (ankle) (closed) 825.23
    open 825.33
  cuneiform
    foot (closed) 825.24
      open 825.34
    wrist (closed) 814.03
      open 814.13
  dental implant 525.73
  dental restorative material
    with loss of material 525.64
    without loss of material 525.63
  due to
    birth injury—*see* Birth injury, fracture
    gunshot—*see* Fracture, by site, open
    neoplasm—*see* Fracture, pathologic
    osteoporosis—*see* Fracture, pathologic
  Dupuytren's (ankle) (fibula) (closed) 824.4
    open 824.5
    radius 813.42
      open 813.52
  Duverney's—*see* Fracture, ilium
  elbow—*see also* Fracture, humerus, lower end
    olecranon (process) (closed) 813.01
      open 813.11
    supracondylar (closed) 812.41
      open 812.51
  ethmoid (bone) (sinus)—*see* Fracture, skull, base
  face bone(s) (closed) NEC 802.8
    with
      other bone(s)—*see also* Fracture, multiple, skull
      skull—*see also* Fracture, skull
        involving other bones—*see* Fracture,
          multiple, skull
    open 802.9
  fatigue—*see* Fracture, march
  femur, femoral (closed) 821.00
    cervicotrochanteric 820.03
      open 820.13
    condyles, epicondyles 821.21
      open 821.31
    distal end—*see* Fracture, femur, lower end
    epiphysis (separation)
      capital 820.01
        open 820.11
      head 820.01
        open 820.11
      lower 821.22
        open 821.32
      trochanteric 820.01
        open 820.11
      upper 820.01
        open 820.11
    head 820.09
      open 820.19
    lower end or extremity (distal end) (closed)
        821.20
      condyles, epicondyles 821.21
        open 821.31
      epiphysis (separation) 821.22
        open 821.32
      multiple sites 821.29
        open 821.39
      open 821.30
      specified site NEC 821.29
        open 821.39
      supracondylar 821.23
        open 821.33
      T-shaped 821.21
        open 821.31

Fracture—*continued*
  femur—*continued*
    neck (closed) 820.8
      base (cervicotrochanteric) 820.03
        open 820.13
      extracapsular 820.20
        open 820.30
      intertrochanteric (section) 820.21
        open 820.31
      intracapsular 820.00
        open 820.10
      intratrochanteric 820.21
        open 821.31
      midcervical 820.02
        open 820.12
      open 820.9
      pathologic 733.14
        specified part NEC 733.15
      specified site NEC 820.09
        open 820.19
      stress 733.96
      transcervical 820.02
        open 820.12
      transtrochanteric 820.20
        open 820.30
    open 821.10
    pathologic 733.14
      specified part NEC 733.15
    peritrochanteric (section) 820.20
      open 820.30
    shaft (lower third) (middle third) (upper third)
        821.01
      open 821.11
      stress 733.97
    subcapital 820.09
      open 820.19
    subtrochanteric (region) (section) 820.22
      open 820.32
    supracondylar 821.23
      open 821.33
    transepiphyseal 820.01
      open 820.11
    trochanter (greater) (lesser) (*see also* Fracture,
        femur, neck, by site) 820.20
      open 820.30
    T-shaped, into knee joint 821.21
      open 821.31
    upper end 820.8
      open 820.9
  fibula (closed) 823.81
    with tibia 823.82
      open 823.92
    distal end 824.8
      open 824.9
    epiphysis
      lower 824.8
        open 824.9
      upper—*see* Fracture, fibula, upper end
    head—*see* Fracture, fibula, upper end
    involving ankle 824.2
      open 824.3
    lower end or extremity 824.8
      open 824.9
    malleolus (external) (lateral) 824.2
      open 824.3
    open NEC 823.91
    pathologic 733.16
    proximal end—*see* Fracture, fibula, upper end
    shaft 823.21
      with tibia 823.22
        open 823.32
      open 823.31

Fracture—*continued*
 fibula—*continued*
  stress 733.93
  torus 853.41
   with tibia 823.42
  upper end or extremity (epiphysis) (head)
    (proximal end) (styloid) 823.01
   with tibia 823.02
    open 823.12
   open 823.11
 finger(s), of one hand (closed) (*see also*
   Fracture, phalanx, hand) 816.00
  with
   metacarpal bone(s), of same hand 817.0
    open 817.1
   thumb of same hand 816.03
    open 816.13
  open 816.10
 foot, except toe(s) alone (closed) 825.20
  open 825.30
 forearm (closed) NEC 813.80
  lower end (distal end) (lower epiphysis)
    813.40
   open 813.50
  open 813.90
  shaft 813.20
   open 813.30
  upper end (proximal end) (upper epiphysis)
    813.00
   open 813.10
 fossa, anterior, middle, or posterior—*see*
   Fracture, skull, base
 frontal (bone)—*see also* Fracture, skull, vault
  sinus—*see* Fracture, skull base
 Galeazzi's—*see* Fracture, radius, lower end
 glenoid (cavity) (fossa) (scapula) (closed)
    811.03
  open 811.13
 Gosselin's—*see* Fracture, ankle
 greenstick—*see* Fracture, by site
 grenade-throwers'—*see* Fracture, humerus,
   shaft
 gutter—*see* Fracture, skull, vault
 hamate (closed) 814.08
  open 814.18
 hand, one (closed) 815.00
  carpals 814.00
   open 814.10
   specified site NEC 814.09
    open 814.19
  metacarpals 815.00
   open 815.10
  multiple, bones of one hand 817.0
   open 817.1
  open 815.10
  phalanges (*see also* Fracture, phalanx, hand)
    816.00
   open 816.10
 healing
  aftercare (*see also* Aftercare, fracture) V54.89
  change of cast V54.89
  complications—*see* condition
  convalescence V66.4
  removal of
   cast V54.89
   fixation device
    external V54.89
    internal V54.01
 heel bone (closed) 825.0
  open 825.1
 Hill-Sachs 812.09

Fracture—*continued*
 hip (closed) (*see also* Fracture, femur, neck)
    820.8
  open 820.9
  pathologic 733.14
 humerus (closed) 812.20
  anatomical neck 812.02
   open 812.12
  articular process (*see also* Fracture, humerus,
    condyle(s)) 812.44
   open 812.54
  capitellum 812.49
   open 812.59
  condyle(s) 812.44
   lateral (external) 812.42
    open 812.52
   medial (internal epicondyle) 812.43
    open 812.53
   open 812.54
  distal end—*see* Fracture, humerus, lower end
  epiphysis
   lower (*see also* Fracture, humerus,
     condyle(s)) 812.44
    open 812.54
   upper 812.09
    open 812.19
  external condyle 812.42
   open 812.52
  great tuberosity 812.03
   open 812.13
  head 812.09
   open 812.19
  internal epicondyle 812.43
   open 812.53
  lesser tuberosity 812.09
   open 812.19
  lower end or extremity (distal end) (*see also*
    Fracture, humerus, by site) 812.40
   multiple sites NEC 812.49
    open 812.59
   open 812.50
   specified site NEC 812.49
    open 812.59
  neck 812.01
   open 812.11
  open 812.30
  pathologic 733.11
  proximal end—*see* Fracture, humerus, upper
    end
  shaft 812.21
   open 812.31
  supracondylar 812.41
   open 812.51
  surgical neck 812.01
   open 812.11
  trochlea 812.49
   open 812.59
  T-shaped 812.44
   open 812.54
  tuberosity—*see* Fracture, humerus, upper end
  upper end or extremity (proximal end) (*see
    also* Fracture, humerus, by site) 812.00
   open 812.10
   specified site NEC 812.09
    open 812.19
 hyoid bone (closed) 807.5
  open 807.6
 hyperextension—*see* Fracture, radius, lower end
 ilium (with visceral injury) (closed) 808.41
  open 808.51
 impaction, impacted—*see* Fracture, by site
 incus—*see* Fracture, skull, base

Fracture—*continued*
  innominate bone (with visceral injury) (closed)
    808.49
    open 808.59
  instep, of one foot (closed) 825.20
    with toe(s) of same foot 827.0
      open 827.1
    open 825.30
  insufficiency—*see* Fracture, pathologic, by site
  internal
    ear—*see* Fracture, skull, base
    semilunar cartilage, knee—*see* Tear,
      meniscus, medial
  intertrochanteric—*see* Fracture, femur, neck,
    intertrochanteric
  ischium (with visceral injury) (closed) 808.42
    open 808.52
  jaw (bone) (lower) (closed) (*see also* Fracture,
    mandible) 802.20
    angle 802.25
      open 802.35
    open 802.30
    upper—*see* Fracture, maxilla
  knee
    cap (closed) 822.0
      open 822.1
    cartilage (semilunar)—*see* Tear, meniscus
  labyrinth (osseous)—*see* Fracture, skull, base
  larynx (closed) 807.5
    open 807.6
  late effect—*see* Late, effects (of), fracture
  Le Fort's—*see* Fracture, maxilla
  leg (closed) 827.0
    with rib(s) or sternum 828.0
      open 828.1
    both (any bones) 828.0
      open 828.1
    lower—*see* Fracture, tibia
      open 827.1
    upper—*see* Fracture, femur
  limb
    lower (multiple) (closed) NEC 827.0
      open 827.1
    upper (multiple) (closed) NEC 818.0
      open 818.1
  long bones, due to birth trauma—*see* Birth
    injury, fracture
  lumbar—*see* Fracture, vertebra, lumbar
  lunate bone (closed) 814.02
    open 814.12
  malar bone (closed) 802.4
    open 802.5
  Malgaigne's (closed) 808.43
    open 808.53
  malleolus (closed)0 824.8
    bimalleolar 824.4
      open 824.5
    lateral 824.2
      and medial—*see also* Fracture, malleolus,
        bimalleolar
        with lip of tibia—*see* Fracture, malleolus,
          trimalleolar
      open 824.3
    medial (closed) 824.0
      and lateral—*see also* Fracture, malleolus,
        bimalleolar
        with lip of tibia—*see* Fracture, malleolus,
          trimalleolar
      open 824.1
    open 824.9
    trimalleolar (closed) 824.6
      open 824.7

Fracture—*continued*
  malleus—*see* Fracture, skull, base
  malunion 733.81
  mandible (closed) 802.20
    angle 802.25
      open 802.35
    body 802.28
      alveolar border 802.27
        open 802.37
      open 802.38
      symphysis 802.26
        open 802.36
    condylar process 802.21
      open 802.31
    coronoid process 802.23
      open 802.33
    multiple sites 802.29
      open 802.39
    open 802.30
    ramus NEC 802.24
      open 802.34
    subcondylar 802.22
      open 802.32
  manubrium—*see* Fracture, sternum
  march 733.95
    femoral neck 733.96
    fibula 733.93
    metatarsals 733.94
    pelvis 733.98
    shaft of femur 733.97
    tibia 733.93
  maxilla, maxillary (superior) (upper jaw)
    (closed) 802.4
    inferior—*see* Fracture, mandible
    open 802.5
  meniscus, knee—*see* Tear, meniscus
  metacarpus, metacarpal (bone(s)), of one hand
    (closed) 815.00
    with phalanx, phalanges, hand (finger(s))
      (thumb) of same hand 817.0
      open 817.1
    base 815.02
      first metacarpal 815.01
        open 815.11
      open 815.12
      thumb 815.01
        open 815.11
    multiple sites 815.09
      open 815.19
    neck 815.04
      open 815.14
    open 815.10
    shaft 815.03
      open 815.13
  metatarsus, metatarsal (bone(s)), of one foot
    (closed) 825.25
    with tarsal bone(s) 825.29
      open 825.39
    open 825.35
  Monteggia's (closed) 813.03
    open 813.13
  Moore's—*see* Fracture, radius, lower end
  multangular bone (closed)
    larger 814.05
      open 814.15
    smaller 814.06
      open 814.16

Fracture—*continued*
  multiple (closed) 829.0

Note—Multiple fractures of sites classifiable to the same three- or four-digit category are coded to that category, except for sites classifiable to 810-818 or 820-827 in different limbs.

Multiple fractures of sites classifiable to different fourth-digit subdivisions within the same three-digit category should be dealt with according to coding rules.

Multiple fractures of sites classifiable to different three-digit categories (identifiable from the listing under "Fracture"), and of sites classifiable to 810-818 or 820-827 in different limbs should be coded according to the following list, which should be referred to in the following priority order: skull or face bones, pelvis or vertebral column, legs, arms.

---

  arm (multiple bones in same arm except in hand alone) (sites classifiable to 810-817 with sites classifiable to a different three-digit category in 810-817 in same arm) (closed) 818.0
    open 818.1
  arms, both or arm(s) with rib(s) or sternum (sites classifiable to 810-818 with sites classifiable to same range of categories in other limb or to 807) (closed) 819.0
    open 819.1
  bones of trunk NEC (closed) 809.0
    open 809.1
  hand, metacarpal bone(s) with phalanx or phalanges of same hand (sites classifiable to 815 with sites classifiable to 816 in same hand) (closed) 817.0
    open 817.1
  leg (multiple bones in same leg) (sites classifiable to 820-826 with sites classifiable to a different three-digit category in that range in same leg) (closed) 827.0
    open 827.1
  legs, both or leg(s) with arm(s), rib(s), or sternum (sites classifiable to 820-827 with sites classifiable to same range of categories in other leg or to 807 or 810-819) (closed) 828.0
    open 828.1
  open 829.1
  pelvis with other bones except skull or face bones (sites classifiable to 808 with sites classifiable to 805-807 or 810-829) (closed) 809.0
    open 809.1
  skull, specified or unspecified bones, or face bone(s) with any other bone(s) (sites classifiable to 800-803 with sites classifiable to 805-829) (closed) 804.0

Fracture—*continued*
  multiple—*continued*

Note—Use the following fifth-digit subclassification with categories 800, 801, 803, and 804:

0 unspecified state of consciousness
1 with no loss of consciousness
2 with brief [less than one hour] loss of consciousness
3 with moderate [1-24 hours] loss of consciousness
4 with prolonged [more than 24 hours] loss of consciousness and return to pre-existing conscious level
5 with prolonged [more than 24 hours] loss of consciousness, without return to pre-existing conscious level
Use fifth-digit 5 to designate when a patient is unconcious and dies before regaining conciousness, regardless of the duration of the loss of conciousness
6 with loss of consciousness of unspecified duration
9 with concussion, unspecified

---

  with
    contusion, cerebral 804.1
    epidural hemorrhage 804.2
    extradural hemorrhage 804.2
    hemorrhage (intracranial) NEC 804.3
    intracranial injury NEC 804.4
    laceration, cerebral 804.1
    subarachnoid hemorrhage 804.2
    subdural hemorrhage 804.2
  open 804.5
    with
      contusion, cerebral 804.6
      epidural hemorrhage 804.7
      extradural hemorrhage 804.7
      hemorrhage (intracranial) NEC 804.8
      intracranial injury NEC 804.9
      laceration, cerebral 804.6
      subarachnoid hemorrhage 804.7
      subdural hemorrhage 804.7
  vertebral column with other bones, except skull or face bones (sites classifiable to 805 or 806 with sites classifiable to 807-808 or 810-829) (closed) 809.0
    open 809.1
  nasal (bone(s)) (closed) 802.0
    open 802.1
  sinus—Fracture, skull, base
  navicular
    carpal (wrist) (closed) 814.01
      open 814.11
    tarsal (ankle) (closed) 825.22
      open 825.32
  neck—*see* Fracture, vertebra, cervical
  neural arch—*see* Fracture, vertebra, by site
  nonunion 733.82
  nose, nasal (bone) (septum) (closed) 802.0
    open 802.1
  occiput—*see* Fracture, skull, base
  odontoid process—*see* Fracture, vertebra, cervical

Fracture—*continued*

olecranon (process) (ulna) (closed) 813.01
  open 813.11
open 829.1
orbit, orbital (bone) (region) (closed) 802.8
  floor (blow-out) 802.6
    open 802.7
  open 802.9
  roof—*see* Fracture, skull, base
  specified part NEC 802.8
    open 802.9
os
  calcis (closed) 825.0
    open 825.1
  magnum (closed) 814.07
    open 814.17
  pubis (with visceral injury) (closed) 808.2
    open 808.3
  triquetrum (closed) 814.03
    open 814.13
osseous
  auditory meatus—*see* Fracture, skull, base
  labyrinth—*see* Fracture, skull, base
  ossicles, auditory (incus) (malleus)
    (stapes)—*see* Fracture, skull, base
osteoporotic—*see* Fracture, pathologic
palate (closed) 802.8
  open 802.9
paratrooper—*see* Fracture, tibia, lower end
parietal bone—*see* Fracture, skull, vault
parry—*see* Fracture, Monteggia's
patella (closed) 822.0
  open 822.1
pathologic (cause unknown) 733.10
  ankle 733.16
  femur (neck) 733.14
    specified NEC 733.15
  fibula 733.16
  hip 733.14
  humerus 733.11
  radius 733.12
  specified site NEC 733.19
  tibia 733.16
  ulna 733.12
  vertebrae (collapse) 733.13
  wrist 733.12
pedicle (of vertebral arch)—*see* Fracture,
  vertebra, by site
pelvis, pelvic (bone(s)) (with visceral injury)
  (closed) 808.8
  multiple
    with
      disruption of pelvic circle 808.43
        open 808.53
      disruption of pelvic ring 808.43
        open 808.53
    without
      disruption of pelvic circle 808.44
        open 808.54
      disruption of pelvic ring 808.44
        open 808.54
  open 808.9
  rim (closed) 808.49
    open 808.59
  stress 733.98
peritrochanteric (closed) 820.20
  open 820.30
phalanx, phalanges, of one
  foot (closed) 826.0
    with bone(s) of same lower limb 827.0
      open 827.1
    open 826.1

Fracture—*continued*

phalanx, phalanges—*continued*
  hand (closed) 816.00
    with metacarpal bone(s) of same hand 817.0
      open 817.1
    distal 816.02
      open 816.12
    middle 816.01
      open 816.11
    multiple sites NEC 816.03
      open 816.13
    open 816.10
    proximal 816.01
      open 816.11
pisiform (closed) 814.04
  open 814.14
pond—Fracture, skull, vault
Pott's (closed) 824.4
  open 824.5
prosthetic device, internal—*see* Complications,
  mechanical
pubis (with visceral injury) (closed) 808.2
  open 808.3
Quervain's (closed) 814.01
  open 814.11
radius (alone) (closed) 813.81
  with ulna NEC 813.83
    open 813.93
  distal end—*see* Fracture, radius, lower end
  epiphysis
    lower—*see* Fracture, radius, lower end
    upper—*see* Fracture, radius, upper end
  head—*see* Fracture, radius, upper end
  lower end or extremity (distal end) (lower
    epiphysis) 813.42
    with ulna (lower end) 813.44
      open 813.54
    open 813.52
    torus 813.45
      with ulna 813.47
  neck—*see* Fracture, radius, upper end
  open NEC 813.91
  pathologic 733.12
  proximal end—*see* Fracture, radius, upper end
  shaft (closed) 813.21
    with ulna (shaft) 813.23
      open 813.33
    open 813.31
  upper end 813.07
    with ulna (upper end) 813.08
      open 813.18
    epiphysis 813.05
      open 813.15
    head 813.05
      open 813.15
    multiple sites 813.07
      open 813.17
    neck 813.06
      open 813.16
    open 813.17
    specified site NEC 813.07
      open 813.17
ramus
  inferior or superior (with visceral injury)
    (closed) 808.2
    open 808.3
  ischium—*see* Fracture, ischium
  mandible 802.24
    open 802.34

Fracture—*continued*
rib(s) (closed) 807.0

*Note—Use the following fifth-digit
subclassification with categories 807.0-807.1:*

0 *rib(s), unspecified*
1 *one rib*
2 *two ribs*
3 *three ribs*
4 *four ribs*
5 *five ribs*
6 *six ribs*
7 *seven ribs*
8 *eight or more ribs*
9 *multiple ribs, unspecified*

    with flail chest (open) 807.4
    open 807.1
  root, tooth 873.63
    complicated 873.73
  sacrum—*see* Fracture, vertebra, sacrum
  scaphoid
    ankle (closed) 825.22
      open 825.32
    wrist (closed) 814.01
      open 814.11
  scapula (closed) 811.00
    acromial, acromion (process) 811.01
      open 811.11
    body 811.09
      open 811.19
    coracoid process 811.02
      open 811.12
    glenoid (cavity) (fossa) 811.03
      open 811.13
    neck 811.03
      open 811.13
    open 811.10
  semilunar
    bone, wrist (closed) 814.02
      open 814.12
    cartilage (interior) (knee)—*see* Tear, meniscus
  sesamoid bone—*see* Fracture, by site
  Shepherd's (closed) 825.21
    open 825.31
  shoulder—*see also* Fracture, humerus, upper
    end
    blade—*see* Fracture, scapula
  silverfork—*see* Fracture, radius, lower end
  sinus (ethmoid) (frontal) (maxillary) (nasal)
    (sphenoidal)—*see* Fracture, skull, base
    maxillary—*see* Fracture, maxilla
  Skillern's—*see* Fracture, radius, shaft

Fracture—*continued*
skull (multiple NEC) (with face bones) (closed)
  803.0

*Note—Use the following fifth-digit
subclassification with categories 800, 801, 803,
and 804:*

0 *unspecified state of consciousness*
1 *with no loss of consciousness*
2 *with brief [less than one hour] loss of
   consciousness*
3 *with moderate [1-24 hours] loss of
   consciousness*
4 *with prolonged [more than 24 hours] loss of
   consciousness and return to pre-existing
   conscious level*
5 *with prolonged [more than 24 hours] loss of
   consciousness, without return to pre-existing
   conscious level*
*Use fifth-digit 5 to designate when a patient is
unconscious and dies before regaining
consciousness, regardless of the duration of the
loss of consciousness*
6 *with loss of consciousness of unspecified
   duration*
9 *with concussion, unspecified*

    with
      contusion, cerebral 803.1
      epidural hemorrhage 803.2
      extradural hemorrhage 803.2
      hemorrhage (intracranial) NEC 803.3
      intracranial injury NEC 803.4
      laceration, cerebral 803.1
      other bones—*see* Fracture, multiple, skull
      subarachnoid hemorrhage 803.2
      subdural hemorrhage 803.2
    base (antrum) (ethmoid bone) (fossa) (internal
      ear) (nasal sinus) (occiput) (sphenoid)
      (temporal bone) (closed) 801.0
    with
      contusion, cerebral 801.1
      epidural hemorrhage 801.2
      extradural hemorrhage 801.2
      hemorrhage (intracranial) NEC 801.3
      intracranial injury NEC 801.4
      laceration, cerebral 801.1
      subarachnoid hemorrhage 801.2
      subdural hemorrhage 801.2
    open 801.5
      with
        contusion, cerebral 801.6
        epidural hemorrhage 801.7
        extradural hemorrhage 801.7
        hemorrhage (intracranial) NEC 801.8
        intracranial injury NEC 801.9
        laceration, cerebral 801.6
        subarachnoid hemorrhage 801.7
        subdural hemorrhage 801.7
    birth injury 767.3
    face bones—*see* Fracture, face bones
    open 803.5
      with
        contusion, cerebral 803.6
        epidural hemorrhage 803.7
        extradural hemorrhage 803.7
        hemorrhage (intracranial) NEC 803.8
        intracranial injury NEC 803.9
        laceration, cerebral 803.6
        subarachnoid hemorrhage 803.7
        subdural hemorrhage 803.7

Fracture—*continued*
 skull—*continued*
  vault (frontal bone) (parietal bone) (vertex)
   (closed) 800.0
   with
    contusion, cerebral 800.1
    epidural hemorrhage 800.2
    extradural hemorrhage 800.2
    hemorrhage (intracranial) NEC 800.3
    intracranial injury NEC 800.4
    laceration, cerebral 800.1
    subarachnoid hemorrhage 800.2
    subdural hemorrhage 800.2
   open 800.5
    with
     contusion, cerebral 800.6
     epidural hemorrhage 800.7
     extradural hemorrhage 800.7
     hemorrhage (intracranial) NEC 800.8
     intracranial injury NEC 800.9
     laceration, cerebral 800.6
     subarachnoid hemorrhage 800.7
     subdural hemorrhage 800.7
 Smith's 813.41
  open 813.51
 sphenoid (bone) (sinus)—*see* Fracture, skull,
  base
 spine—*see also* Fracture, vertebra, by site
  due to birth trauma 767.4
 spinous process—*see* Fracture, vertebra, by site
 spontaneous—*see* Fracture, pathologic
 sprinters'—*see* Fracture, ilium
 stapes—*see* Fracture, skull, base
 stave—*see also* Fracture, metacarpus,
  metacarpal bone(s)
 spine—*see* Fracture, tibia, upper end
 sternum (closed) 807.2
  with flail chest (open) 807.4
  open 807.3
 Stieda's—*see* Fracture, femur, lower end
 stress 733.95
  femoral neck 733.96
  fibula 733.93
  metatarsals 733.94
  pelvis 733.98
  shaft of femur 733.97
  specified site NEC 733.95
  tibia 733.93
 styloid process
  metacarpal (closed) 815.02
   open 815.12
  radius—*see* Fracture, radius, lower end
  temporal bone—*see* Fracture, skull, base
  ulna—*see* Fracture, ulna, lower end
 supracondylar, elbow 812.41
  open 812.51
 symphysis pubis (with visceral injury) (closed)
  808.2
  open 808.3
 talus (ankle bone) (closed) 825.21
  open 825.31
 tarsus, tarsal bone(s) (with metatarsus) of one
  foot (closed) NEC 825.29
  open 825.39
 temporal bone (styloid)—*see* Fracture, skull,
  base
 tendon—*see* Sprain, by site
 thigh—*see* Fracture, femur, shaft
 thumb (and finger(s)) of one hand (closed) (*see
  also* Fracture, phalanx, hand) 816.00
  with metacarpal bone(s) of same hand 817.0
   open 817.1

Fracture—*continued*
 thumb—*continued*
  metacarpal(s)—*see* Fracture, metacarpus
  open 816.10
 thyroid cartilage (closed) 807.5
  open 807.6
 tibia (closed) 823.80
  with fibula 823.82
   open 823.92
  condyles—*see* Fracture, tibia, upper end
  distal end 824.8
   open 824.9
  epiphysis
   lower 824.8
    open 824.9
   upper—*see* Fracture, tibia, upper end
  head (involving knee joint)—*see* Fracture,
   tibia, upper end
  intercondyloid eminence—*see* Fracture, tibia,
   upper end
  involving ankle 824.0
   open 824.1
  lower end or extremity (anterior lip) (posterior
   lip) 824.8
   open 824.9
  malleolus (internal) (medial) 824.0
   open 824.1
  open NEC 823.90
  pathologic 733.16
  proximal end—*see* Fracture, tibia, upper end
  shaft 823.20
   with fibula 823.22
    open 823.32
   open 823.30
  spine—*see* Fracture, tibia, upper end
  stress 733.93
  torus 823.40
   with tibia 823.42
  tuberosity—*see* Fracture, tibia, upper end
  upper end or extremity (condyle) (epiphysis)
   (head) (spine) (proximal end) (tuberosity)
   823.00
   with fibula 823.02
    open 823.12
   open 823.10
 toe(s), of one foot (closed) 826.0
  with bone(s) of same lower limb 827.0
   open 827.1
  open 826.1
 tooth (root) 873.63
  complicated 873.73
 torus
  fibula 823.41
   with tibia 823.42
  humerus 812.49
  radius (alone) 813.45
   with ulna 813.47
  tibia 823.40
   with fibula 823.42
  ulna (alone) 813.46
   with radius 813.47
 trachea (closed) 807.5
  open 807.6
 transverse process—*see* Fracture, vertebra, by
  site
 trapezium (closed) 814.05
  open 814.15
 trapezoid bone (closed) 814.06
  open 814.16
 trimalleolar (closed) 824.6
  open 824.7

Fracture—*continued*

triquetral (bone) (closed) 814.03
  open 814.13
trochanter (greater) (lesser) (closed) (*see also* Fracture, femur, neck, by site) 820.20
  open 820.30
trunk (bones) (closed) 809.0
  open 809.1
tuberosity (external)—*see* Fracture, by site
ulna (alone) (closed) 813.82
  with radius NEC 813.83
    open 813.93
  coronoid process (closed) 813.02
    open 813.12
  distal end—*see* Fracture, ulna, lower end
  epiphysis
    lower—*see* Fracture, ulna, lower end
    upper—*see* Fracture, ulna, upper, end
  head—*see* Fracture, ulna, lower end
  lower end (distal end) (head) (lower epiphysis) (styloid process) 813.43
    with radius (lower end) 813.44
      open 813.54
    open 813.53
  olecranon process (closed) 813.01
    open 813.11
  open NEC 813.92
  pathologic 733.12
  proximal end—*see* Fracture, ulna, upper end
  shaft 813.22
    with radius (shaft) 813.23
      open 813.33
    open 813.32
  styloid process—*see* Fracture, ulna, lower end
  torus 813.46
    with radius 813.47
  transverse—*see* Fracture, ulna, by site
  upper end (epiphysis) 813.04
    with radius (upper end) 813.08
      open 813.18
    multiple sites 813.04
      open 813.14
    open 813.14
    specified site NEC 813.04
      open 813.14
unciform (closed) 814.08
  open 814.18
vertebra, vertebral (back) (body) (column) (neural arch) (pedicle) (spine) (spinous process) (transverse process) (closed) 805.8
  with
    hematomyelia—*see* Fracture, vertebra, by site, with spinal cord injury
    injury to
      cauda equina—*see* Fracture, vertebra, sacrum, with spinal cord injury
      nerve—*see* Fracture, vertebra, by site, with spinal cord injury
      paralysis—*see* Fracture, vertebra, by site, with spinal cord injury
      paraplegia—*see* Fracture, vertebra, by site, with spinal cord injury
      quadriplegia—*see* Fracture, vertebra, by site, with spinal cord injury
      spinal concussion—*see* Fracture, vertebra, by site, with spinal cord injury

Fracture—*continued*

vertebra—*continued*
  with—*continued*
    spinal cord injury (closed) NEC 806.8

Note—Use the following fifth-digit subclassification with categories 806.0-806.3:

C_1-C_4 *or unspecified level and* D_1-D_6 *(T_1-T_6) or unspecified level with:*

0 *unspecified spinal cord injury*
1 *complete lesion of cord*
2 *anterior cord syndrome*
3 *central cord syndrome*
4 *specified injury NEC*

C_5-C_7 *level and* D_7-D_{12} *level with:*

5 *unspecified spinal cord injury*
6 *complete lesion of cord*
7 *anterior cord syndrome*
8 *central cord syndrome*
9 *specified injury NEC*

      cervical 806.0
        open 806.1
      dorsal, dorsolumbar 806.2
        open 806.3
      open 806.9
      thoracic, thoracolumbar 806.2
        open 806.3
  atlanto-axial—*see* Fracture, vertebra, cervical
  cervical (hangman) (teardrop) (closed) 805.00
    with spinal cord injury—*see* Fracture, vertebra, with spinal cord injury, cervical
    first (atlas) 805.01
      open 805.11
    second (axis) 805.02
      open 805.12
    third 805.03
      open 805.13
    fourth 805.04
      open 805.14
    fifth 805.05
      open 805.15
    sixth 805.06
      open 805.16
    seventh 805.07
      open 805.17
    multiple sites 805.08
      open 805.18
    open 805.10
  chronic 733.13
  coccyx (closed) 805.6
    with spinal cord injury (closed) 806.60
      cauda equina injury 806.62
        complete lesion 806.61
          open 806.71
        open 806.72
      open 806.70
      specified type NEC 806.69
        open 806.79
    open 805.7
  collapsed 733.13
  compression, not due to trauma 733.13
  dorsal (closed) 805.2
    with spinal cord injury—*see* Fracture, vertebra, with spinal cord injury, dorsal
    open 805.3

Fracture—*continued*
 vertebra—*continued*
  dorsolumbar (closed) 805.2
   with spinal cord injury—*see* Fracture,
    vertebra, with spinal cord injury, dorsal
   open 805.3
  due to osteoporosis 733.13
  fetus or newborn 767.4
  lumbar (closed) 805.4
   with spinal cord injury (closed) 806.4
    open 806.5
   open 805.5
  nontraumatic 733.13
  open NEC 805.9
  pathologic 733.13
  sacrum (closed) 805.6
   with spinal cord injury 806.60
    cauda equina injury 806.62
     complete lesion 806.61
      open 806.71
     open 806.72
    open 806.70
    specified type NEC 806.69
     open 806.79
   open 805.7
  site unspecified (closed) 805.8
   with spinal cord injury (closed) 806.8
    open 806.9
   open 805.9
  stress (any site) 733.95
  thoracic (closed) 805.2
   with spinal cord injury—*see* Fracture,
    vertebra, with spinal cord injury,
    thoracic
   open 805.3
 vertex—*see* Fracture, skull, vault
 vomer (bone) 802.0
  open 802.1
 Wagstaffe's—*see* Fracture, ankle
 wrist (closed) 814.00
  open 814.10
  pathologic 733.12
 xiphoid (process)—*see* Fracture, sternum
 zygoma (zygomatic arch) (closed) 802.4
  open 802.5
Fragile X syndrome 759.83
Fragilitas
 crinium 704.2
 hair 704.2
 ossium 756.51
  with blue sclera 756.51
 unguium 703.8
  congenital 757.5
Fragility
 bone 756.51
  with deafness and blue sclera 756.51
 capillary (hereditary) 287.8
 hair 704.2
 nails 703.8
Fragmentation —*see* Fracture, by site
Frailty 797
Frambesia, frambesial (tropica) (*see also* Yaws)
  102.9
 initial lesion or ulcer 102.0
 primary 102.0
Frambeside
 gummatous 102.4
 of early yaws 102.2
Frambesioma 102.1
Franceschetti's syndrome (mandibulofacial
  dysostosis) 756.0
Francis' disease (*see also* Tularemia) 021.9

Frank's essential thrombocytopenia (*see also*
  Purpura, thrombocytopenic) 287.39
Franklin's disease (heavy chain) 273.2
Fraser's syndrome 759.89
Freckle 709.09
 malignant melanoma in (M8742/3)—*see*
  Melanoma
 melanotic (of Hutchinson) (M8742/2)—*see*
  Neoplasm, skin, in situ
 retinal 239.81
Freeman-Sheldon syndrome 759.89
Freezing 991.9
 specified effect NEC 991.8
Frei's disease (climatic bubo) 099.1
Freiberg's
 disease (osteochondrosis, second metatarsal) 732.5
 infraction of metatarsal head 732.5
 osteochondrosis 732.5
Fremitus, friction, cardiac 785.3
Frenulum lingua 750.0
Frenum
 external os 752.44
 tongue 750.0
Frequency (urinary) NEC 788.41
 micturition 788.41
 nocturnal 788.43
 psychogenic 306.53
Frey's syndrome (auriculotemporal syndrome)
  705.22
Friction
 burn (*see also* Injury, superficial, by site) 919.0
 fremitus, cardiac 785.3
 precordial 785.3
 sounds, chest 786.7
Friderichsen-Waterhouse syndrome or disease
  036.3
Friedländer's
 B (bacillus) NEC (*see also* condition) 041.3
  sepsis or septicemia 038.49
 disease (endarteritis obliterans)—*see*
  Arteriosclerosis
Friedreich's
 ataxia 334.0
 combined systemic disease 334.0
 disease 333.2
  combined systemic 334.0
 myoclonia 333.2
 sclerosis (spinal cord) 334.0
Friedrich-Erb-Arnold syndrome
  (acropachyderma) 757.39
Frigidity 302.72
 psychic or psychogenic 302.72
Fröhlich's disease or syndrome (adiposogenital
  dystrophy) 253.8
Froin's syndrome 336.8
Frommel's disease 676.6
Frommel-Chiari syndrome 676.6
Frontal —*see also* condition
 lobe syndrome 310.0
Frostbite 991.3
 face 991.0
 foot 991.2
 hand 991.1
 specified site NEC 991.3
Frotteurism 302.89
Frozen 991.9
 pelvis 620.8
 shoulder 726.0
Fructosemia 271.2
Fructosuria (benign) (essential) 271.2

Fuchs'
 black spot (myopic) 360.21
 corneal dystrophy (endothelial) 371.57
 heterochromic cyclitis 364.21
Fucosidosis 271.8
Fugue 780.99
 dissociative 300.13
 hysterical (dissociative) 300.13
 reaction to exceptional stress (transient) 308.1
Fukuhara syndrome 277.87
Fuller Albright's syndrome (osteitis fibrosa
   disseminata) 756.59
Fuller's earth disease 502
Fulminant, fulminating —*see* condition
Functional —*see* condition
Functioning
 borderline intellectual V62.89
Fundus —*see also* condition
 flavimaculatus 362.76
Fungemia 117.9
Fungus, fungous
 cerebral 348.89
 disease NEC 117.9
 infection—*see* Infection, fungus
 testis (*see also* Tuberculosis) 016.5 *[608.81]*
Funiculitis (acute) 608.4
 chronic 608.4
 endemic 608.4
 gonococcal (acute) 098.14
  chronic or duration of 2 months or over 098.34
 tuberculous (*see also* Tuberculosis) 016.5
FUO (fever of unknown origin) (*see also* Pyrexia)
   780.60
Funnel
 breast (acquired) 738.3
  congenital 754.81
  late effect of rickets 268.1
 chest (acquired) 738.3
  congenital 754.81
  late effect of rickets 268.1
 pelvis (acquired) 738.6
  with disproportion (fetopelvic) 653.3
   affecting fetus or newborn 763.1
   causing obstructed labor 660.1
    affecting fetus or newborn 763.1
  congenital 755.69
  tuberculous (*see also* Tuberculosis) 016.9
Furfur 690.18
 microsporon 111.0
Furor, paroxysmal (idiopathic) (*see also*
   Epilepsy) 345.8
Furriers' lung 495.8
Furrowed tongue 529.5
 congenital 750.13
Furrowing nail (s) (transverse) 703.8
 congenital 757.5
Furuncle 680.9
 abdominal wall 680.2
 ankle 680.6
 anus 680.5
 arm (any part, above wrist) 680.3
 auditory canal, external 680.0
 axilla 680.3
 back (any part) 680.2
 breast 680.2
 buttock 680.5
 chest wall 680.2
 corpus cavernosum 607.2
 ear (any part) 680.0
 eyelid 373.13

Furuncle—*continued*
 face (any part, except eye) 680.0
 finger (any) 680.4
 flank 680.2
 foot (any part) 680.7
 forearm 680.3
 gluteal (region) 680.5
 groin 680.2
 hand (any part) 680.4
 head (any part, except face) 680.8
 heel 680.7
 hip 680.6
 kidney (*see also* Abscess, kidney) 590.2
 knee 680.6
 labium (majus) (minus) 616.4
 lacrimal
  gland (*see also* Dacryoadenitis) 375.00
  passages (duct) (sac) (*see also* Dacryocystitis)
    375.30
 leg, any part except foot 680.6
 malignant 022.0
 multiple sites 680.9
 neck 680.1
 nose (external) (septum) 680.0
 orbit 376.01
 partes posteriores 680.5
 pectoral region 680.2
 penis 607.2
 perineum 680.2
 pinna 680.0
 scalp (any part) 680.8
 scrotum 608.4
 seminal vesicle 608.0
 shoulder 680.3
 skin NEC 680.9
 specified site NEC 680.8
 spermatic cord 608.4
 temple (region) 680.0
 testis 604.90
 thigh 680.6
 thumb 680.4
 toe (any) 680.7
 trunk 680.2
 tunica vaginalis 608.4
 umbilicus 680.2
 upper arm 680.3
 vas deferens 608.4
 vulva 616.4
 wrist 680.4
Furunculosis (*see also* Furuncle) 680.9
 external auditory meatus 680.0 *[380.13]*
Fusarium (infection) 118
Fusion, fused (congenital)
 anal (with urogenital canal) 751.5
 aorta and pulmonary artery 745.0
 astragaloscaphoid 755.67
 atria 745.5
 atrium and ventricle 745.69
 auditory canal 744.02
 auricles, heart 745.5
 binocular, with defective stereopsis 368.33
 bone 756.9
 cervical spine—*see* Fusion, spine
 choanal 748.0
 commissure, mitral valve 746.5
 cranial sutures, premature 756.0
 cusps, heart valve NEC 746.89
  mitral 746.5
  tricuspid 746.89
 ear ossicles 744.04
 fingers (*see also* Syndactylism, fingers) 755.11

Fusion, fused—*continued*
  hymen 752.42
  hymeno-urethral 599.89
    causing obstructed labor 660.1
      affecting fetus or newborn 763.1
  joint (acquired)—*see also* Ankylosis
    congenital 755.8
  kidneys (incomplete) 753.3
  labium (majus) (minus) 752.49
  larynx and trachea 748.3
  limb 755.8
    lower 755.69
    upper 755.59
  lobe, lung 748.5
  lumbosacral (acquired) 724.6
    congenital 756.15
    surgical V45.4
  nares (anterior) (posterior) 748.0
  nose, nasal 748.0
  nostril(s) 748.0
  organ or site NEC—*see* Anomaly, specified
      type NEC
  ossicles 756.9
    auditory 744.04
  pulmonary valve segment 746.02
  pulmonic cusps 746.02
  ribs 756.3
  sacroiliac (acquired) (joint) 724.6
    congenital 755.69
    surgical V45.4
  skull, imperfect 756.0
  spine (acquired) 724.9
    arthrodesis status V45.4
    congenital (vertebra) 756.15
    postoperative status V45.4
  sublingual duct with submaxillary duct at
      opening in mouth 750.26
  talonavicular (bar) 755.67
  teeth, tooth 520.2
  testes 752.89
  toes (*see also* Syndactylism, toes) 755.13
  trachea and esophagus 750.3
  twins 759.4
  urethral-hymenal 599.89
  vagina 752.49
  valve cusps—*see* Fusion, cusps, heart valve
  ventricles, heart 745.4
  vertebra (arch)—*see* Fusion, spine
  vulva 752.49
Fusospirillosis (mouth) (tongue) (tonsil) 101
Fussy infant (baby) 780.91

Gafsa boil 085.1
Gain, weight (abnormal) (excessive) (see also
   Weight, gain) 783.1
Gaisböck's disease or syndrome (polycythemia
   hypertonica) 289.0
Gait
   abnormality 781.2
      hysterical 300.11
   ataxic 781.2
      hysterical 300.11
   disturbance 781.2
      hysterical 300.11
   paralytic 781.2
   scissor 781.2
   spastic 781.2
   staggering 781.2
      hysterical 300.11
Galactocele (breast) (infected) 611.5
   puerperal, postpartum 676.8
Galactophoritis 611.0
   puerperal, postpartum 675.2
Galactorrhea 676.6
   not associated with childbirth 611.6
Galactosemia (classic) (congenital) 271.1
Galactosuria 271.1
Galacturia 791.1
   bilharziasis 120.0
Galen's vein —*see* condition
Gallbladder —*see also* condition
   acute (*see also* Disease, gallbladder) 575.0
Gall duct —*see* condition
Gallop rhythm 427.89
Gallstone (cholemic) (colic) (impacted)—*see
   also* Cholelithiasis
   causing intestinal obstruction 560.31
Gambling, pathological 312.31
Gammaloidosis 277.39
Gammopathy 273.9
   macroglobulinemia 273.3
   monoclonal (benign) (essential) (idiopathic)
      (with lymphoplasmacytic dyscrasia) 273.1
Gamna's disease (siderotic splenomegaly)
   289.51
Gampsodactylia (congenital) 754.71
Gamstorp's disease (adynamia episodica
   hereditaria) 359.3
Gandy-Nanta disease (siderotic splenomegaly)
   289.51
**Gang activity without manifest psychiatric
   disorder** V71.09
   adolescent V71.02
   adult V71.01
   child V71.02
Gangliocytoma (M9490/0)—*see* Neoplasm,
   connective tissue, benign
Ganglioglioma (M9505/1)—*see* Neoplasm, by
   site, uncertain behavior
Ganglion 727.43
   joint 727.41
   of yaws (early) (late) 102.6
   periosteal (*see also* Periostitis) 730.3
   tendon sheath (compound) (diffuse) 727.42
   tuberculous (*see also* Tuberculosis) 015.9
Ganglioneuroblastoma (M9490/3)—*see*
   Neoplasm, connective tissue, malignant
Ganglioneuroma (M9490/0)—*see also*
   Neoplasm, connective tissue, benign

Ganglioneuroma—*continued*
   malignant (M9490/3)—*see* Neoplasm,
      connective tissue, malignant
Ganglioneuromatosis (M9491/0)—*see*
   Neoplasm, connective tissue, benign
Ganglionitis
   fifth nerve (*see also* Neuralgia, trigeminal)
      350.1
   gasserian 350.1
   geniculate 351.1
      herpetic 053.11
      newborn 767.5
   herpes zoster 053.11
   herpetic geniculate (Hunt's syndrome) 053.11
Gangliosidosis 330.1
Gangosa 102.5
Gangrene, gangrenous (anemia) (artery)
   (cellulitis) (dermatitis) (dry) (infective)
   (moist) (pemphigus) (septic) (skin) (stasis)
   (ulcer) 785.4
   with
      arteriosclerosis (native artery) 440.24
         bypass graft 440.30
            autologous vein 440.31
            nonautologous biological 440.32
      diabetes (mellitus) 250.7 *[785.4]*
         due to secondary diabetes 249.7 *[785.4]*
   abdomen (wall) 785.4
   adenitis 683
   alveolar 526.5
   angina 462
      diphtheritic 032.0
   anus 569.49
   appendices epiploicae—*see* Gangrene,
      mesentery
   appendix—*see* Appendicitis, acute
   arteriosclerotic —*see* Arteriosclerosis, with,
      gangrene
   auricle 785.4
   Bacillus welchii (*see also* Gangrene, gas) 040.0
   bile duct (*see also* Cholangitis) 576.8
   bladder 595.89
   bowel—*see* Gangrene, intestine
   cecum—*see* Gangrene, intestine
   Clostridium perfringens or welchii (*see also*
      Gangrene, gas) 040.0
   colon—*see* Gangrene, intestine
   connective tissue 785.4
   cornea 371.40
   corpora cavernosa (infective) 607.2
      noninfective 607.89
   cutaneous, spreading 785.4
   decubital (*see also* Ulcer, pressure) 707.00
      [785.4]
   diabetic (any site) 250.7 *[785.4]*
      due to secondary diabetes 249.7 *[785.4]*
   dropsical 785.4
   emphysematous (*see also* Gangrene, gas) 040.0
   epidemic (ergotized grain) 988.2
   epididymis (infectional) (*see also* Epididymitis)
      604.99
   erysipelas (*see also* Erysipelas) 035
   extremity (lower) (upper) 785.4
   gallbladder or duct (*see also* Cholecystitis,
      acute) 575.0

Gangrene, gangrenous—*continued*
gas (bacillus) 040.0
　with
　　abortion—*see* Abortion, by type, with sepsis
　　ectopic pregnancy (*see also* categories
　　　633.0-633.9) 639.0
　　molar pregnancy (*see also* categories
　　　630-632) 639.0
　following
　　abortion 639.0
　　ectopic or molar pregnancy 639.0
　puerperal, postpartum, childbirth 670.8
glossitis 529.0
gum 523.8
hernia—*see* Hernia, by site, with gangrene
hospital noma 528.1
intestine, intestinal (acute) (hemorrhagic)
　(massive) 557.0
　with
　　hernia—*see* Hernia, by site, with gangrene
　　mesenteric embolism or infarction 557.0
　　obstruction (*see also* Obstruction, intestine)
　　　560.9
laryngitis 464.00
　with obstruction 464.01
liver 573.8
lung 513.0
　spirochetal 104.8
lymphangitis 457.2
Meleney's (cutaneous) 686.09
mesentery 557.0
　with
　　embolism or infarction 557.0
　　intestinal obstruction (*see also* Obstruction,
　　　intestine) 560.9
mouth 528.1
noma 528.1
orchitis 604.90
ovary (*see also* Salpingo-oophoritis) 614.2
pancreas 577.0
penis (infectional) 607.2
　noninfective 607.89
perineum 785.4
pharynx 462
　septic 034.0
pneumonia 513.0
Pott's 440.24
presenile 443.1
pulmonary 513.0
pulp, tooth 522.1
quinsy 475
Raynaud's (symmetric gangrene) 443.0 *[785.4]*
rectum 569.49
retropharyngeal 478.24
rupture—*see* Hernia, by site, with gangrene
scrotum 608.4
　noninfective 608.83
senile 440.24
sore throat 462
spermatic cord 608.4
　noninfective 608.89
spine 785.4
spirochetal NEC 104.8
spreading cutaneous 785.4
stomach 537.89
stomatitis 528.1
symmetrical 443.0 *[785.4]*
testis (infectional) (*see also* Orchitis) 604.99
　noninfective 608.89
throat 462
　diphtheritic 032.0

Gangrene, gangrenous—*continued*
thyroid (gland) 246.8
tonsillitis (acute) 463
tooth (pulp) 522.1
tuberculous NEC (*see also* Tuberculosis) 011.9
tunica vaginalis 608.4
　noninfective 608.89
umbilicus 785.4
uterus (*see also* Endometritis) 615.9
uvulitis 528.3
vas deferens 608.4
　noninfective 608.89
vulva (*see also* Vulvitis) 616.10
Gannister disease (occupational) 502
　with tuberculosis—*see* Tuberculosis, pulmonary
Ganser's syndrome, hysterical 300.16
Gardner-Diamond syndrome (autoerythrocyte
　sensitization) 287.2
Gargoylism 277.5
Garré's
　disease (*see also* Osteomyelitis) 730.1
　osteitis (sclerosing) (*see also* Osteomyelitis)
　　730.1
　osteomyelitis (*see also* Osteomyelitis) 730.1
Garrod's pads, knuckle 728.79
Gartner's duct
　cyst 752.41
　persistent 752.41
Gas 787.3
　asphyxia, asphyxiation, inhalation, poisoning,
　　suffocation NEC 987.9
　　specified gas—*see* Table of drugs and
　　　chemicals
　bacillus gangrene or infection—*see* Gas,
　　gangrene
　cyst, mesentery 568.89
　excessive 787.3
　gangrene 040.0
　　with
　　　abortion—*see* Abortion, by type, with sepsis
　　　ectopic pregnancy (*see also* categories
　　　　633.0-633.9) 639.0
　　　molar pregnancy (*see also* categories
　　　　630-632) 639.0
　　following
　　　abortion 639.0
　　　ectopic or molar pregnancy 639.0
　　puerperal, postpartum, childbirth 670.8
　on stomach 787.3
　pains 787.3
Gastradenitis 535.0
Gastralgia 536.8
　psychogenic 307.89
Gastrectasis, gastrectasia 536.1
　psychogenic 306.4
Gastric —*see* condition
Gastrinoma (M8153/1)
　malignant (M8153/3)
　　pancreas 157.4
　　specified site NEC—*see* Neoplasm, by site,
　　　malignant
　　unspecified site 157.4
　specified site—*see* Neoplasm, by site,
　　uncertain behavior
　unspecified site 235.5

Gastritis 535.5

Note—*Use the following fifth-digit subclassification for category 535:*

0 *without mention of hemorrhage*
1 *with hemorrhage*

  acute 535.0
  alcoholic 535.3
  allergic 535.4
  antral 535.4
  atrophic 535.1
  atrophic-hyperplastic 535.1
  bile-induced 535.4
  catarrhal 535.0
  chronic (atrophic) 535.1
  cirrhotic 535.4
  corrosive (acute) 535.4
  dietetic 535.4
  due to diet deficiency 269.9 [535.4]
  eosinophilic 535.7
  erosive 535.4
  follicular 535.4
    chronic 535.1
  giant hypertrophic 535.2
  glandular 535.4
    chronic 535.1
  hypertrophic (mucosa) 535.2
    chronic giant 211.1
  irritant 535.4
  nervous 306.4
  phlegmonous 535.0
  psychogenic 306.4
  sclerotic 535.4
  spastic 536.8
  subacute 535.0
  superficial 535.4
  suppurative 535.0
  toxic 535.4
  tuberculous (*see also* Tuberculosis) 017.9
Gastrocarcinoma (M8010/3) 151.9
Gastrocolic —*see* condition
Gastrocolitis —*see* Enteritis
Gastrodisciasis 121.8
Gastroduodenitis (*see also* Gastritis) 535.5
  catarrhal 535.0
  infectional 535.0
  virus, viral 008.8
    specified type NEC 008.69
Gastrodynia 536.8
Gastroenteritis (acute) (catarrhal) (congestive)
    (hemorrhagic) (noninfectious) (*see also*
    Enteritis) 558.9
  aertrycke infection 003.0
  allergic 558.3
  chronic 558.9
    ulcerative (*see also* Colitis, ulcerative) 556.9
  dietetic 558.9
  due to
    antineoplastic chemotherapy 558.9
    food poisoning (*see also* Poisoning, food) 005.9
    radiation 558.1
  eosinophilic 558.41
  epidemic 009.0
  functional 558.9
  infectious (*see also* Enteritis, due to, by
    organism) 009.0
    presumed 009.1
  salmonella 003.0
  septic (*see also* Enteritis, due to, by organism)
    009.0

Gastroenteritis—*continued*
  toxic 558.2
  tuberculous (*see also* Tuberculosis) 014.8
  ulcerative (*see also* Colitis, ulcerative) 556.9
  viral NEC 008.8
    specified type NEC 008.69
  zymotic 009.0
Gastroenterocolitis —*see* Enteritis
Gastroenteropathy, protein-losing 579.8
Gastroenteroptosis 569.89
**Gastroesophageal laceration-hemorrhage
    syndrome** 530.7
Gastroesophagitis 530.19
Gastrohepatitis (*see also* Gastritis) 535.5
Gastrointestinal —*see* condition
Gastrojejunal —*see* condition
Gastrojejunitis (*see also* Gastritis) 535.5
Gastrojejunocolic —*see* condition
Gastroliths 537.89
Gastromalacia 537.89
Gastroparalysis 536.3
  diabetic 250.6 [536.3]
    due to secondary diabetes 249.6 [536.3]
Gastroparesis 536.3
  diabetic 250.6 [536.3]
    due to secondary diabetes 249.6 [536.3]
Gastropathy 537.9
  congestive portal 537.89
  erythematous 535.5
  exudative 579.8
  portal hypertension 537.89
Gastroptosis 537.5
Gastrorrhagia 578.0
Gastrorrhea 536.8
  psychogenic 306.4
Gastroschisis (congenital) 756.73
  acquired 569.89
Gastrospasm (neurogenic) (reflex) 536.8
  neurotic 306.4
  psychogenic 306.4
Gastrostaxis 578.0
Gastrostenosis 537.89
Gastrostomy
  attention to V55.1
  complication 536.40
    specified type 536.49
  infection 536.41
  malfunctioning 536.42
  status V44.1
Gastrosuccorrhea (continuous) (intermittent) 536.8
  neurotic 306.4
  psychogenic 306.4
Gaucher's
  disease (adult) (cerebroside lipidosis) (infantile)
    272.7
  hepatomegaly 272.7
  splenomegaly (cerebroside lipidosis) 272.7
GAVE (gastric antral vascular ectasia) 537.82
  with hemorrhage 537.83
  without hemorrhage 537.82
Gayet's disease (superior hemorrhagic
    polioencephalitis) 265.1
Gayet-Wernicke's syndrome (superior
    hemorrhagic polioencephalitis) 265.1
Gee (-Herter) (-Heubner) (-Thaysen) disease or
    syndrome (nontropical sprue) 579.0
Gélineau's syndrome (*see also* Narcolepsy) 347.00
Gemination, teeth 520.2
Gemistocytoma (M9411/3)
  specified site—*see* Neoplasm, by site, malignant
  unspecified site 191.9

General, generalized —*see* condition
Genetic
  susceptibility to
    MEN (multiple endocrine neoplasia) V84.81
    neoplasia
      multiple endocrine (MEN) V84.81
    neoplasm
      malignant, of
        breast V84.01
        endometrium V84.04
        other V84.09
        ovary V84.02
        prostate V84.03
      specified disease NEC V84.89
Genital —*see* condition
  warts 078.11
Genito-anorectal syndrome 099.1
Genitourinary system —*see* condition
Genu
  congenital 755.64
  extrorsum (acquired) 736.42
    congenital 755.64
    late effects of rickets 268.1
  introrsum (acquired) 736.41
    congenital 755.64
    late effects of rickets 268.1
  rachitic (old) 268.1
  recurvatum (acquired) 736.5
    congenital 754.40
      with dislocation of knee 754.41
    late effects of rickets 268.1
  valgum (acquired) (knock-knee) 736.41
    congenital 755.64
    late effects of rickets 268.1
  varum (acquired) (bowleg) 736.42
    congenital 755.64
    late effects of rickets 268.1
Geographic tongue 529.1
Geophagia 307.52
Geotrichosis 117.9
  intestine 117.9
  lung 117.9
  mouth 117.9
Gephyrophobia 300.29
Gerbode defect 745.4
GERD (gastroesophageal reflux disease) 530.81
Gerhardt's
  disease (erythromelalgia) 443.82
  syndrome (vocal cord paralysis) 478.30
Gerlier's disease (epidemic vertigo) 078.81
German measles 056.9
  exposure to V01.4
Germinoblastoma (diffuse) (M9614/3) 202.8
  follicular (M9692/3) 202.0
Germinoma (M9064/3)—*see* Neoplasm, by site,
  malignant
Gerontoxon 371.41
Gerstmann's syndrome (finger agnosia) 784.69
Gerstmann-Sträussler-Scheinker syndrome
  (GSS) 046.71
Gestation (period)—*see also* Pregnancy
  ectopic NEC (*see also* Pregnancy, ectopic) 633.90
    with intrauterine pregnancy 633.91

Gestation (period)—*continued*
  multiple
    placenta status
      quadruplet
        two or more monoamniotic fetuses V91.22
        two or more monochorionic fetuses
          V91.21
        unable to determine number of placenta
          and number of amniotic sacs V91.29
        unspecified number of placenta and
          unspecified number of amniotic sacs
          V91.20
      specified (greater than quadruplets) NEC
        two or more monoamniotic fetuses V91.92
        two or more monochorionic fetuses
          V91.91
        unable to determine number of placenta
          and number of amniotic sacs V91.99
        unspecified number of placenta and
          unspecified number of amniotic sacs
          V91.90
      triplet
        two or more monoamniotic fetuses V91.12
        two or more monochorionic fetuses
          V91.11
        unable to determine number of placenta
          and number of amniotic sacs V91.19
        unspecified number of placenta,
          unspecified number of amniotic sacs
          V91.10
      twin
        dichorionic/diamniotic (two placentae, two
          amniotic sacs) V91.03
        monochorionic/diamniotic (one placenta,
          two amniotic sacs) V91.02
        monochorionic/monoamniotic (one
          placenta, one amniotic sac) V91.01
        unable to determine number of placenta
          and number of amniotic sacs V91.09
        unspecified number of placenta,
          unspecified number of amniotic sacs
          V91.00
Gestational proteinuria 646.2
  with hypertension—*see* Toxemia, of pregnancy
Ghon tubercle primary infection (*see also*
  Tuberculosis) 010.0
Ghost
  teeth 520.4
  vessels, cornea 370.64
Ghoul hand 102.3
Gianotti Crosti syndrome 057.8
  due to known virus—*see* Infection, virus
  due to unknown virus 057.8
Giant
  cell
    epulis 523.8
    peripheral (gingiva) 523.8
    tumor, tendon sheath 727.02
  colon (congenital) 751.3
  esophagus (congenital) 750.4
  kidney 753.3
  urticaria 995.1
    hereditary 277.6
Giardia lamblia infestation 007.1
Giardiasis 007.1
Gibert's disease (pityriasis rosea) 696.3
Gibraltar fever —*see* Brucellosis
Giddiness 780.4
  hysterical 300.11
  psychogenic 306.9
Gierke's disease (glycogenosis I) 271.0

Gigantism (cerebral) (hypophyseal) (pituitary) 253.0
Gilbert's disease or cholemia (familial nonhemolytic jaundice) 277.4
Gilchrist's disease (North American blastomycosis) 116.0
Gilford (-Hutchinson) disease or syndrome (progeria) 259.8
Gilles de la Tourette's disease (motor-verbal tic) 307.23
Gillespie's syndrome (dysplasia oculodentodigitalis) 759.89
Gingivitis 523.10
  acute 523.00
    necrotizing 101
    non-plaque induced 523.01
    plaque induced 523.00
  catarrhal 523.00
  chronic 523.10
    non-plaque induced 523.11
  desquamative 523.10
  expulsiva 523.40
  hyperplastic 523.10
  marginal, simple 523.10
  necrotizing, acute 101
  non-plaque induced 523.11
  pellagrous 265.2
  plaque induced 523.10
  ulcerative 523.10
    acute necrotizing 101
  Vincent's 101
Gingivoglossitis 529.0
Gingivopericementitis 523.40
Gingivosis 523.10
Gingivostomatitis 523.10
  herpetic 054.2
Giovannini's disease 117.9
GISA (glycopeptide intermediate staphylococcus aureus) V09.8
Gland, glandular —*see* condition
Glanders 024
Glanzmann (-Naegeli) disease or thrombasthenia 287.1
Glassblowers' disease 527.1
Glaucoma (capsular) (inflammatory) (noninflammatory) (primary) 365.9
  with increased episcleral venous pressure 365.82
  absolute 360.42
  acute 365.22
    narrow angle 365.22
    secondary 365.60
  angle closure 365.20
    acute 365.22
    attack 365.22
    chronic 365.23
    crisis 365.22
    intermittent 365.21
    interval 365.21
    primary 365.20
      chronic 365.23
    residual stage 365.24
    subacute 365.21
  angle recession 365.65
  border line 365.00
  chronic 365.11
    noncongestive 365.11
    open angle 365.11
    simple 365.11
  closed angle—*see* Glaucoma, angle closure

Glaucoma—*continued*
  congenital 743.20
    associated with other eye anomalies 743.22
    simple 743.21
  congestive—*see* Glaucoma, narrow angle
  corticosteroid-induced (glaucomatous stage) 365.31
    residual stage 365.32
  exfoliation 365.52
  hemorrhagic 365.60
  hypersecretion 365.81
  in or with
    aniridia 365.42
    Axenfeld's anomaly 365.41
    congenital syndromes NEC 759.89 *[365.44]*
    disorder of lens NEC 365.59
    inflammation, ocular 365.62
    iris
      anomalies NEC 365.42
      atrophy, essential 365.42
      bombé 365.61
    microcornea 365.43
    neurofibromatosis 237.71 *[365.44]*
    ocular
      cysts NEC 365.64
      disorders NEC 365.60
      trauma 365.65
      tumors NEC 365.64
    pupillary block or seclusion 365.61
    Rieger's anomaly or syndrome 365.41
    seclusion of pupil 365.61
    Sturge-Weber (-Dimitri) syndrome 759.6 *[365.44]*
    systemic syndrome NEC 365.44
    tumor of globe 365.64
    vascular disorders NEC 365.63
  infantile 365.14
    congenital 743.20
      associated with other eye anomalies 743.22
      simple 743.21
  inflammatory 365.62
  juvenile 365.14
  low tension 365.12
  malignant 365.83
  narrow angle (primary) 365.20
    acute 365.22
    chronic 365.23
    intermittent 365.21
    interval 365.21
    residual stage 365.24
    subacute 365.21
  neovascular 365.63
  newborn 743.20
    associated with other eye anomalies 743.22
    simple 743.21
  noncongestive (chronic) 365.11
  nonobstructive (chronic) 365.11
  normal tension 365.12
  obstructive 365.60
    due to lens changes 365.59
  open angle 365.10
    with
      abnormal optic disc appearance or asymmetry 365.01
      borderline findings
        high risk 365.05
        intraocular pressure 365.01
        low risk 365.01
      cupping of optic discs 365.01
      thin central corneal thickness (pachymetry) 365.01

Glaucoma—*continued*
  open angle—*continued*
    high risk 365.05
    low risk 365.01
    primary 365.11
    residual stage 365.15
  phacoanaphylactic 365.59
  phacolytic 365.51
  phacomorphic
    acute 365.22
    borderline 365.06
  pigment dispersion 365.13
  pigmentary 365.13
  postinfectious 365.60
  pseudoexfoliation 365.52
  secondary NEC 365.60
    due to
      steroids 365.31
      surgery 365.60
  simple (chronic) 365.11
  simplex 365.11
  stage
    advanced 365.73
    early 365.71
    end-stage 365.73
    indeterminate 365.74
    mild 365.71
    moderate 365.72
    severe 365.73
    unspecified 365.70
  steroid
    induced 365.31
    responders 365.03
  suspect 365.00
    primary angle closure 365.02
  syphilitic 095.8
  traumatic NEC 365.65
    newborn 767.8
  uveitic 365.62
  wide angle (*see also* Glaucoma, open angle)
    365.10
Glaucomatous flecks (subcapsular) 366.31
Glazed tongue 529.4
Gleet 098.2
Glénard's disease or syndrome (enteroptosis)
  569.89
Glinski-Simmonds syndrome (pituitary
  cachexia) 253.2
Glioblastoma (multiforme) (M9440/3)
  with sarcomatous component (M9442/3)
    specified site—*see* Neoplasm, by site,
      malignant
    unspecified site 191.9
  giant cell (M9441/3)
    specified site—*see* Neoplasm, by site, malignant
    unspecified site 191.9
  specified site—*see* Neoplasm, by site, malignant
  unspecified site 191.9
Glioma (malignant) (M9380/3)
  astrocytic (M9400/3)
    specified site—*see* Neoplasm, by site,
      malignant
    unspecified site 191.9
  mixed (M9382/3)
    specified site—*see* Neoplasm, by site,
      malignant
    unspecified site 191.9
  nose 748.1
  specified site NEC—*see* Neoplasm, by site,
    malignant
  subependymal (M9383/1) 237.5
  unspecified site 191.9

Gliomatosis cerebri (M9381/3) 191.0
Glioneuroma (M9505/1)—*see* Neoplasm, by
  site, uncertain behavior
Gliosarcoma (M9380/3)
  specified site—*see* Neoplasm, by site, malignant
  unspecified site 191.9
Gliosis (cerebral) 349.89
  spinal 336.0
Glisson's
  cirrhosis—*see* Cirrhosis, portal
  disease (*see also* Rickets) 268.0
Glissonitis 573.3
Globinuria 791.2
Globus 306.4
  hystericus 300.11
Glomangioma (M8712/0) (*see also*
  Hemangioma) 228.00
Glomangiosarcoma (M8710/3)—*see* Neoplasm,
  connective tissue, malignant
Glomerular nephritis (*see also* Nephritis) 583.9
Glomerulitis (*see also* Nephritis) 583.9
Glomerulonephritis (*see also* Nephritis) 583.9
  with
    edema (*see also* Nephrosis) 581.9
    lesion of
      exudative nephritis 583.89
      interstitial nephritis (diffuse) (focal) 583.89
      necrotizing glomerulitis 583.4
        acute 580.4
      chronic 582.4
      renal necrosis 583.9
        cortical 583.6
        medullary 583.7
      specified pathology NEC 583.89
        acute 580.89
        chronic 582.89
    necrosis, renal 583.9
      cortical 583.6
      medullary (papillary) 583.7
    specified pathology or lesion NEC 583.89
  acute 580.9
    with
      exudative nephritis 580.89
      interstitial nephritis (diffuse) (focal) 580.89
      necrotizing glomerulitis 580.4
    extracapillary with epithelial crescents 580.4
    poststreptococcal 580.0
    proliferative (diffuse) 580.0
    rapidly progressive 580.4
    specified pathology NEC 580.89
  arteriolar (*see also* Hypertension, kidney) 403.90
  arteriosclerotic (*see also* Hypertension, kidney)
    403.90
  ascending (*see also* Pyelitis) 590.80
  basement membrane NEC 583.89
    with
      pulmonary hemorrhage (Goodpasture's
        syndrome) 446.21 *[583.81]*
  chronic 582.9
    with
      exudative nephritis 582.89
      interstitial nephritis (diffuse) (focal) 582.89
      necrotizing glomerulitis 582.4
      specified pathology or lesion NEC 582.89
    endothelial 582.2
    extracapillary with epithelial crescents 582.4
    hypocomplementemic persistent 582.2
    lobular 582.2
    membranoproliferative 582.2
    membranous 582.1
      and proliferative (mixed) 582.2
      sclerosing 582.1

Glomerulonephritis—*continued*
  chronic—*continued*
    mesangiocapillary 582.2
    mixed membranous and proliferative 582.2
    proliferative (diffuse) 582.0
    rapidly progressive 582.4
    sclerosing 582.1
  cirrhotic—*see* Sclerosis, renal
  desquamative—*see* Nephrosis
  due to or associated with
    amyloidosis 277.39 *[583.81]*
      with nephrotic syndrome 277.39 *[581.81]*
      chronic 277.39 *[582.81]*
    diabetes mellitus 250.4 *[583.81]*
      due to secondary diabetes 249.4 *[581.81]*
      with nephrotic syndrome 250.4 *[581.81]*
        due to secondary diabetes 249.4 *[581.81]*
    diphtheria 032.89 *[580.81]*
    gonococcal infection (acute) 098.19 *[583.81]*
      chronic or duration or 2 months or over
        098.39 *[583.81]*
    infectious hepatitis 070.9 *[580.81]*
    malaria (with nephrotic syndrome) 084.9
      [581.81]
    mumps 072.79 *[580.81]*
    polyarteritis (nodosa) (with nephrotic
      syndrome) 446.0 *[581.81]*
    specified pathology NEC 583.89
      acute 580.89
      chronic 582.89
    streptotrichosis 039.8 *[583.81]*
    subacute bacterial endocarditis 421.0 *[580.81]*
    syphilis (late) 095.4
      congenital 090.5 *[583.81]*
      early 091.69 *[583.81]*
    systemic lupus erythematosus 710.0 *[583.81]*
      with nephrotic syndrome 710.0 *[581.81]*
      chronic 710.0 *[582.81]*
    tuberculosis (*see also* Tuberculosis) 016.0
      [583.81]
    typhoid fever 002.0 *[580.81]*
  extracapillary with epithelial crescents 583.4
    acute 580.4
    chronic 582.4
  exudative 583.89
    acute 580.89
    chronic 582.89
  focal (*see also* Nephritis) 583.9
    embolic 580.4
  granular 582.89
  granulomatous 582.89
  hydremic (*see also* Nephrosis) 581.9
  hypocomplementemic persistent 583.2
    with nephrotic syndrome 581.2
    chronic 582.2
  immune complex NEC 583.89
  infective (*see also* Pyelitis) 590.80
  interstitial (diffuse) (focal) 583.89
    with nephrotic syndrome 581.89
    acute 580.89
    chronic 582.89
  latent or quiescent 582.9
  lobular 583.2
    with nephrotic syndrome 581.2
    chronic 582.2
  membranoproliferative 583.2
    with nephrotic syndrome 581.2
    chronic 582.2

Glomerulonephritis—*continued*
  membranous 583.1
    with nephrotic syndrome 581.1
    and proliferative (mixed) 583.2
      with nephrotic syndrome 581.2
      chronic 582.2
    chronic 582.1
    sclerosing 582.1
      with nephrotic syndrome 581.1
  mesangiocapillary 583.2
    with nephrotic syndrome 581.2
    chronic 582.2
  minimal change 581.3
  mixed membranous and proliferative 583.2
    with nephrotic syndrome 581.2
    chronic 582.2
  necrotizing 583.4
    acute 580.4
    chronic 582.4
  nephrotic (*see also* Nephrosis) 581.9
  old—*see* Glomerulonephritis, chronic
  parenchymatous 581.89
  poststreptococcal 580.0
  proliferative (diffuse) 583.0
    with nephrotic syndrome 581.0
    acute 580.0
    chronic 582.0
  purulent (*see also* Pyelitis) 590.80
  quiescent—*see* Nephritis, chronic
  rapidly progressive 583.4
    acute 580.4
    chronic 582.4
  sclerosing membranous (chronic) 582.1
    with nephrotic syndrome 581.1
  septic (*see also* Pyelitis) 590.80
  specified pathology or lesion NEC 583.89
    with nephrotic syndrome 581.89
    acute 580.89
    chronic 582.89
  suppurative (acute) (disseminated) (*see also*
    Pyelitis) 590.80
  toxic—*see* Nephritis, acute
  tubal, tubular—*see* Nephrosis, tubular
  type II (Ellis)—*see* Nephrosis
  vascular—*see* Hypertension, kidney
Glomerulosclerosis (*see also* Sclerosis, renal) 587
  focal 582.1
    with nephrotic syndrome 581.1
    intercapillary (nodular) (with diabetes) 250.4
      [581.81]
      due to secondary diabetes 249.4 *[581.81]*
Glossagra 529.6
Glossalgia 529.6
Glossitis 529.0
  areata exfoliativa 529.1
  atrophic 529.4
  benign migratory 529.1
  gangrenous 529.0
  Hunter's 529.4
  median rhomboid 529.2
  Moeller's 529.4
  pellagrous 265.2
Glossocele 529.8
Glossodynia 529.6
  exfoliativa 529.4
Glossoncus 529.8
Glossophytia 529.3
Glossoplegia 529.8
Glossoptosis 529.8
Glossopyrosis 529.6

Glossotrichia 529.3
Glossy skin 701.9
Glottis —*see* condition
Glottitis —*see* Glossitis
Glucagonoma (M8152/0)
  malignant (M8152/3)
    pancreas 157.4
    specified site NEC—*see* Neoplasm, by site,
      malignant
    unspecified site 157.4
  pancreas 211.7
  specified site NEC—*see* Neoplasm, by site, benign
  unspecified site 211.7
Glucoglycinuria 270.7
Glue ear syndrome 381.20
Glue sniffing (airplane glue) (*see also*
  Dependence) 304.6
Glycinemia (with methylmalonic acidemia) 270.7
Glycinuria (renal) (with ketosis) 270.0
Glycogen
  infiltration (*see also* Disease, glycogen storage)
    271.0
  storage disease (*see also* Disease, glycogen
    storage) 271.0
Glycogenosis (*see also* Disease, glycogen
    storage) 271.0
  cardiac 271.0 *[425.7]*
  Cori, types I-VII 271.0
  diabetic, secondary 250.8 *[259.8]*
    due to secondary diabetes 249.8 *[259.8]*
  diffuse (with hepatic cirrhosis) 271.0
  generalized 271.0
  glucose-6-phosphatase deficiency 271.0
  hepatophosphorylase deficiency 271.0
  hepatorenal 271.0
  myophosphorylase deficiency 271.0
  pulmonary interstitial 516.62
Glycopenia 251.2
Glycopeptide
  intermediate staphylococcus aureus (GISA) V09.8
  resistent
    enterococcus V09.8
    staphylococcus aureus (GRSA) V09.8
Glycoprolinuria 270.8
Glycosuria 791.5
  renal 271.4
Gnathostoma (spinigerum) (infection)
    (infestation) 128.1
  wandering swellings from 128.1
Gnathostomiasis 128.1
Goiter (adolescent) (colloid) (diffuse) (dipping)
    (due to iodine deficiency) (endemic)
    (euthyroid) (heart) (hyperplastic) (internal)
    (intrathoracic) (juvenile) (mixed type)
    (nonendemic) (parenchymatous) (plunging)
    (sporadic) (subclavicular) (substernal) 240.9
  with
    hyperthyroidism (recurrent) (*see also* Goiter,
      toxic) 242.0
    thyrotoxicosis (*see also* Goiter, toxic) 242.0
  adenomatous (*see also* Goiter, nodular) 241.9
  cancerous (M8000/3) 193
  complicating pregnancy, childbirth, or
    puerperium 648.1
  congenital 246.1
  cystic (*see also* Goiter, nodular) 241.9
  due to enzyme defect in synthesis of thyroid
    hormone (butane-insoluble iodine)
    (coupling) (deiodinase) (iodide trapping or
    organification) (iodotyrosine dehalogenase)
    (peroxidase) 246.1

Goiter—*continued*
  dyshormonogenic 246.1
  exophthalmic (*see also* Goiter, toxic) 242.0
  familial (with deaf-mutism) 243
  fibrous 245.3
  lingual 759.2
  lymphadenoid 245.2
  malignant (M8000/3) 193
  multinodular (nontoxic) 241.1
    toxic or with hyperthyroidism (*see also* Goiter,
      toxic) 242.2
  nodular (nontoxic) 241.9
    with
      hyperthyroidism (*see also* Goiter, toxic)
        242.3
      thyrotoxicosis (*see also* Goiter, toxic) 242.3
    endemic 241.9
    exophthalmic (diffuse) (*see also* Goiter, toxic)
      242.0
    multinodular (nontoxic) 241.1
    sporadic 241.9
    toxic (*see also* Goiter, toxic) 242.3
    uninodular (nontoxic) 241.0
  nontoxic (nodular) 241.9
    multinodular 241.1
    uninodular 241.0
  pulsating (*see also* Goiter, toxic) 242.0
  simple 240.0
  toxic 242.0

> *Note—Use the following fifth-digit*
> *subclassification with category 242:*
>
> 0   *without mention of thyrotoxic crisis*
>   *or storm*
> 1   *with mention of thyrotoxic crisis or storm*

    adenomatous 242.3
      multinodular 242.2
      uninodular 242.1
    multinodular 242.2
    nodular 242.3
      multinodular 242.2
      uninodular 242.1
    uninodular 242.1
  uninodular (nontoxic) 241.0
    toxic or with hyperthyroidism (*see also* Goiter,
      toxic) 242.1
Goldberg (-Maxwell) (-Morris) syndrome
    (testicular feminization) 259.51
Goldblatt's
  hypertension 440.1
  kidney 440.1
Goldenhar's syndrome (oculoauriculovertebral
    dysplasia) 756.0
Goldflam-Erb disease or syndrome 358.00
Goldscheider's disease (epidermolysis bullosa)
    757.39
Goldstein's disease (familial hemorrhagic
    telangiectasia) 448.0
Golfer's elbow 726.32
Goltz-Gorlin syndrome (dermal hypoplasia)
    757.39
Gonadoblastoma (M9073/1)
  specified site—*see* Neoplasm, by site uncertain
    behavior
  unspecified site
    female 236.2
    male 236.4
Gonecystitis (*see also* Vesiculitis) 608.0
Gongylonemiasis 125.6
  mouth 125.6

Goniosynechiae 364.73
Gonococcemia 098.89
Gonococcus, gonococcal (disease) (infection)
   (*see also* condition) 098.0
  anus 098.7
  bursa 098.52
  chronic NEC 098.2
  complicating pregnancy, childbirth, or
    puerperium 647.1
    affecting fetus or newborn 760.2
  conjunctiva, conjunctivitis (neonatorum) 098.40
  dermatosis 098.89
  endocardium 098.84
  epididymo-orchitis 098.13
    chronic or duration of 2 months or over 098.33
  eye (newborn) 098.40
  fallopian tube (chronic) 098.37
    acute 098.17
  genitourinary (acute) (organ) (system) (tract)
    (*see also* Gonorrhea) 098.0
    lower 098.0
      chronic 098.2
    upper 098.10
      chronic 098.30
  heart NEC 098.85
  joint 098.50
  keratoderma 098.81
  keratosis (blennorrhagica) 098.81
  lymphatic (gland) (node) 098.89
  meninges 098.82
  orchitis (acute) 098.13
    chronic or duration of 2 months or over 098.33
  pelvis (acute) 098.19
    chronic or duration of 2 months or over 098.39
  pericarditis 098.83
  peritonitis 098.86
  pharyngitis 098.6
  pharynx 098.6
  proctitis 098.7
  pyosalpinx (chronic) 098.37
    acute 098.17
  rectum 098.7
  septicemia 098.89
  skin 098.89
  specified site NEC 098.89
  synovitis 098.51
  tendon sheath 098.51
  throat 098.6
  urethra (acute) 098.0
    chronic or duration of 2 months or over 098.2
  vulva (acute) 098.0
    chronic or duration of 2 months or over 098.2
Gonocytoma (M9073/1)
  specified site—*see* Neoplasm, by site, uncertain
    behavior
  unspecified site
    female 236.2
    male 236.4
Gonorrhea 098.0
  acute 098.0
  Bartholin's gland (acute) 098.0
    chronic or duration of 2 months or over 098.2
  bladder (acute) 098.11
    chronic or duration of 2 months or over 098.31
  carrier (suspected of) V02.7
  cervix (acute) 098.15
    chronic or duration of 2 months or over 098.35
  chronic 098.2
  complicating pregnancy, childbirth, or
    puerperium 647.1
    affecting fetus or newborn 760.2

Gonorrhea—*continued*
  conjunctiva, conjunctivitis (neonatorum) 098.40
  contact V01.6
  Cowper's gland (acute) 098.0
    chronic or duration of 2 months or over 098.2
    duration of two months or over 098.2
  exposure to V01.6
  fallopian tube (chronic) 098.37
    acute 098.17
  genitourinary (acute) (organ) (system) (tract)
    098.0
    chronic 098.2
    duration of two months or over 098.2
  kidney (acute) 098.19
    chronic or duration of 2 months or over 098.39
  ovary (acute) 098.19
    chronic or duration of 2 months or over 098.39
  pelvis (acute) 098.19
    chronic or duration of 2 months or over 098.39
  penis (acute) 098.0
    chronic or duration of 2 months or over 098.2
  prostate (acute) 098.12
    chronic or duration of 2 months or over 098.32
  seminal vesicle (acute) 098.14
    chronic or duration of 2 months or over 098.34
  specified site NEC—*see* Gonococcus
  spermatic cord (acute) 098.14
    chronic or duration of 2 months or over 098.34
  urethra (acute) 098.0
    chronic or duration of 2 months or over 098.2
  vagina (acute) 098.0
    chronic or duration of 2 months or over 098.2
  vas deferens (acute) 098.14
    chronic or duration of 2 months or over 098.34
  vulva (acute) 098.0
    chronic or duration of 2 months or over 098.2
Goodpasture's syndrome (pneumorenal) 446.21
Good's syndrome 279.06
Gopalan's syndrome (burning feet) 266.2
Gordon's disease (exudative enteropathy) 579.8
Gorlin-Chaudhry-Moss syndrome 759.89
Gougerot's syndrome (trisymptomatic) 709.1
Gougerot-Blum syndrome (pigmented purpuric
  lichenoid dermatitis) 709.1
Gougerot-Carteaud disease or syndrome
  (confluent reticulate papillomatosis) 701.8
Gougerot-Hailey-Hailey disease (benign familial
  chronic pemphigus) 757.39
Gougerot (-Houwer) -Sjögren syndrome
  (keratoconjunctivitis sicca) 710.2
Gouley's syndrome (constrictive pericarditis)
  423.2
Goundou 102.6
Gout, gouty 274.9
  with
    specified manifestations NEC 274.89
    tophi (tophus) 274.03
  acute 274.01
  arthritis 274.00
    acute 274.01
  arthropathy 274.00
    acute 274.01
    chronic (without mention of tophus (tophi))
      274.02
      with tophus (tophi) 274.03
  attack 274.01
  chronic 274.02
    tophaceous 274.03
  degeneration, heart 274.82
  diathesis 274.9
  eczema 274.89

Gout, gouty—*continued*
  episcleritis 274.89 *[379.09]*
  external ear (tophus) 274.81
  flare 274.01
  glomerulonephritis 274.10
  iritis 274.89 *[364.11]*
  joint 274.00
  kidney 274.10
  lead 984.9
    specified type of lead—*see* Table of drugs and chemicals
  nephritis 274.10
  neuritis 274.89 *[357.4]*
  phlebitis 274.89 *[451.9]*
  rheumatic 714.0
  saturnine 984.9
    specified type of lead—*see* Table of drugs and chemicals
  spondylitis 274.00
  synovitis 274.00
  syphilitic 095.8
  tophi 274.03
    ear 274.81
    heart 274.82
    specified site NEC 274.82
Gowers'
  muscular dystrophy 359.1
  syndrome (vasovagal attack) 780.2
Gowers-Paton-Kennedy syndrome 377.04
Gradenigo's syndrome 383.02
Graft-versus-host disease 279.50
  due to organ transplant NEC—*see* Complications, transplant, organ
Graham Steell's murmur (pulmonic regurgitation) (*see also* Endocarditis, pulmonary) 424.3
Grain-handlers' disease or lung 495.8
Grain mite (itch) 133.8
Grand
  mal (idiopathic) (*see also* Epilepsy) 345.1
    hysteria of Charcot 300.11
    nonrecurrent or isolated 780.39
  multipara
    affecting management of labor and delivery 659.4
    status only (not pregnant) V61.5
Granite workers' lung 502
Granular —*see also* condition
  inflammation, pharynx 472.1
  kidney (contracting) (*see also* Sclerosis, renal) 587
  liver—*see* Cirrhosis, liver
  nephritis—*see* Nephritis
Granulation tissue, abnormal —*see also* Granuloma
  abnormal or excessive 701.5
  postmastoidectomy cavity 383.33
  postoperative 701.5
  skin 701.5
Granulocytopenia, granulocytopenic (primary) 288.00
  malignant 288.09
Granuloma NEC 686.1
  abdomen (wall) 568.89
    skin (pyogenicum) 686.1
      from residual foreign body 709.4
  annulare 695.89
  anus 569.49
  apical 522.6
  appendix 543.9
  aural 380.23

Granuloma—*continued*
  beryllium (skin) 709.4
    lung 503
  bone (*see also* Osteomyelitis) 730.1
    eosinophilic 277.89
    from residual foreign body 733.99
  canaliculus lacrimalis 375.81
  cerebral 348.89
  cholesterin, middle ear 385.82
  coccidioidal (progressive) 114.3
    lung 114.4
    meninges 114.2
    primary (lung) 114.0
  colon 569.89
  conjunctiva 372.61
  dental 522.6
  ear, middle (cholesterin) 385.82
    with otitis media—*see* Otitis media
  eosinophilic 277.89
    bone 277.89
    lung 277.89
    oral mucosa 528.9
  exuberant 701.5
  eyelid 374.89
  facial
    lethal midline 446.3
    malignant 446.3
  faciale 701.8
  fissuratum (gum) 523.8
  foot NEC 686.1
  foreign body (in soft tissue) NEC 728.82
    bone 733.99
    in operative wound 998.4
    muscle 728.82
    skin 709.4
    subcutaneous tissue 709.4
  fungoides 202.1
  gangraenescens 446.3
  giant cell (central) (jaw) (reparative) 526.3
    gingiva 523.8
    peripheral (gingiva) 523.8
  gland (lymph) 289.3
  Hodgkin's (M9661/3) 201.1
  ileum 569.89
  infectious NEC 136.9
  inguinale (Donovan) 099.2
    venereal 099.2
  intestine 569.89
  iridocyclitis 364.10
  jaw (bone) 526.3
    reparative giant cell 526.3
  kidney (*see also* Infection, kidney) 590.9
  lacrimal sac 375.81
  larynx 478.79
  lethal midline 446.3
  lipid 277.89
  lipoid 277.89
  liver 572.8
  lung (infectious) (*see also* Fibrosis, lung) 515
    coccidioidal 114.4
    eosinophilic 277.89
  lymph gland 289.3
  Majocchi's 110.6
  malignant, face 446.3
  mandible 526.3
  mediastinum 519.3
  midline 446.3
  monilial 112.3
  muscle 728.82
    from residual foreign body 728.82
  nasal sinus (*see also* Sinusitis) 473.9

Granuloma—*continued*
 operation wound 998.59
  foreign body 998.4
  stitch (external) 998.89
   internal organ 998.89
  talc 998.7
 oral mucosa, eosinophilic or pyogenic 528.9
 orbit, orbital 376.11
 paracoccidioidal 116.1
 penis, venereal 099.2
 periapical 522.6
 peritoneum 568.89
  due to ova of helminths NEC (*see also*
    Helminthiasis) 128.9
 postmastoidectomy cavity 383.33
 postoperative–*see* Granuloma, operation wound
 prostate 601.8
 pudendi (ulcerating) 099.2
 pudendorum (ulcerative) 099.2
 pulp, internal (tooth) 521.49
 pyogenic, pyogenicum (skin) 686.1
  maxillary alveolar ridge 522.6
  oral mucosa 528.9
 rectum 569.49
 reticulohistiocytic 277.89
 rubrum nasi 705.89
 sarcoid 135
 Schistosoma 120.9
 septic (skin) 686.1
 silica (skin) 709.4
 sinus (accessory) (infectional) (nasal) (*see also*
    Sinusitis) 473.9
 skin (pyogenicum) 686.1
  from foreign body or material 709.4
 sperm 608.89
 spine
  syphilitic (epidural) 094.89
  tuberculous (*see also* Tuberculosis) 015.0
    [730.88]
 stitch (postoperative) 998.89
  internal wound 998.89
 suppurative (skin) 686.1
 suture (postoperative) 998.89
  internal wound 998.89
 swimming pool 031.1
 talc 728.82
  in operation wound 998.7
 telangiectaticum (skin) 686.1
 tracheostomy 519.09
 trichophyticum 110.6
 tropicum 102.4
 umbilicus 686.1
  newborn 771.4
 urethra 599.84
 uveitis 364.10
 vagina 099.2
 venereum 099.2
 vocal cords 478.5
 Wegener's (necrotizing respiratory
    granulomatosis) 446.4
Granulomatosis NEC 686.1
 disciformis chronica et progressiva 709.3
 infantiseptica 771.2
 lipoid 277.89
 lipophagic, intestinal 040.2
 miliary 027.0
 necrotizing, respiratory 446.4
 progressive, septic 288.1
 Wegener's (necrotizing respiratory) 446.4
Granulomatous tissue —*see* Granuloma
Granulosis rubra nasi 705.89
Graphite fibrosis (of lung) 503

Graphospasm 300.89
 organic 333.84
Grating scapula 733.99
Gravel (urinary) (*see also* Calculus) 592.9
Graves' disease (exophthalmic goiter) (*see also*
    Goiter, toxic) 242.0
Gravis —*see* condition
Grawitz's tumor (hypernephroma) (M8312/3)
    189.0
Grayness, hair (premature) 704.3
 congenital 757.4
Gray or grey syndrome (chloramphenicol)
    (newborn) 779.4
Greenfield's disease 330.0
Green sickness 280.9
Greenstick fracture —*see* Fracture, by site
Greig's syndrome (hypertelorism) 756.0
Grief 309.0
Griesinger's disease (*see also* Ancylostomiasis)
    126.9
Grinder's
 asthma 502
 lung 502
 phthisis (*see also* Tuberculosis) 011.4
Grinding, teeth 306.8
Grip
 Dabney's 074.1
 devil's 074.1
Grippe, grippal —*see also* Influenza
 Balkan 083.0
 intestinal (*see also* Influenza) 487.8
 summer 074.8
Grippy cold (*see also* Influenza) 487.1
Grisel's disease 723.5
Groin —*see* condition
Grooved
 nails (transverse) 703.8
 tongue 529.5
  congenital 750.13
Ground itch 126.9
Growing pains, children 781.99
Growth (fungoid) (neoplastic) (new)
    (M8000/1)—*see also* Neoplasm, by site,
    unspecified nature
 adenoid (vegetative) 474.12
 benign (M8000/0)—*see* Neoplasm, by site,
    benign
 fetal, poor 764.9
  affecting management of pregnancy 656.5
 malignant (M8000/3)—*see* Neoplasm, by site
    malignant
 rapid, childhood V21.0
 secondary (M8000/6)—*see* Neoplasm, by site,
    malignant, secondary
GRSA (glycopeptide resistant staphylococcus
    aureus) V09.8
Gruber's hernia —*see* Hernia, Gruber's
Gruby's disease (tinea tonsurans) 110.0
GSS (Gerstmann-Straussler-Scheinker syndrome)
    046.71
G-trisomy 758.0
Guama fever 066.3
Gubler (-Millard) paralysis or syndrome 344.89
Guérin-Stern syndrome (arthrogryposis
    multiplex congenita) 754.89
Guertin's disease (electric chorea) 049.8
Guillain-Barré disease or syndrome 357.0
Guinea worms (infection) (infestation) 125.7
Guinon's disease (motor-verbal tic) 307.23
Gull's disease (thyroid atrophy with myxedema)
    244.8

Gull and Sutton's disease —*see* Hypertension, kidney
Gum —*see* condition
Gumboil 522.7
Gumma (syphilitic) 095.9
  artery 093.89
    cerebral or spinal 094.89
  bone 095.5
    of yaws (late) 102.6
  brain 094.89
  cauda equina 094.89
  central nervous system NEC 094.9
  ciliary body 095.8 *[364.11]*
  congenital 090.5
    testis 090.5
  eyelid 095.8 *[373.5]*
  heart 093.89
  intracranial 094.89
  iris 095.8 *[364.11]*
  kidney 095.4
  larynx 095.8
  leptomeninges 094.2
  liver 095.3
  meninges 094.2
  myocardium 093.82
  nasopharynx 095.8
  neurosyphilitic 094.9
  nose 095.8
  orbit 095.8
  palate (soft) 095.8
  penis 095.8
  pericardium 093.81
  pharynx 095.8
  pituitary 095.8
  scrofulous (*see also* Tuberculosis) 017.0
  skin 095.8
  specified site NEC 095.8
  spinal cord 094.89
  tongue 095.8
  tonsil 095.8
  trachea 095.8
  tuberculous (*see also* Tuberculosis) 017.0
  ulcerative due to yaws 102.4
  ureter 095.8
  yaws 102.4
    bone 102.6
Gunn's syndrome (jaw-winking syndrome) 742.8
Gunshot wound —*see also* Wound, open, by site
  fracture—*see* Fracture, by site, open
  internal organs (abdomen, chest, or pelvis)—*see* Injury, internal, by site, with open wound
  intracranial—*see* Laceration, brain, with open intracranial wound
Günther's disease or syndrome (congenital erythropoietic porphyria) 277.1
Gustatory hallucination 780.1
Gynandrism 752.7
Gynandroblastoma (M8632/1)
  specified site—*see* Neoplasm, by site, uncertain behavior
  unspecified site
    female 236.2
    male 236.4
Gynandromorphism 752.7
Gynatresia (congenital) 752.49
Gynecoid pelvis, male 738.6
Gynecological examination V72.31
  for contraceptive maintenance V25.40
Gynecomastia 611.1
Gynephobia 300.29

Gyrate scalp 757.39

H

Haas' disease (osteochondrosis head of humerus) 732.3
Habermann's disease (acute parapsoriasis varioliformis) 696.2
Habit, habituation
chorea 307.22
disturbance, child 307.9
drug (*see also* Dependence) 304.9
laxative (*see also* Abuse, drugs, nondependent) 305.9
spasm 307.20
chronic 307.22
transient (of childhood) 307.21
tic 307.20
chronic 307.22
transient (of childhood) 307.21
use of
nonprescribed drugs (*see also* Abuse, drugs, nondependent) 305.9
patent medicines (*see also* Abuse, drugs, nondependent) 305.9
vomiting 536.2
Hadfield-Clarke syndrome (pancreatic infantilism) 577.8
Haff disease 985.1
Hageman factor defect, deficiency, or disease (*see also* Defect, coagulation) *286.3*
Haglund's disease (osteochondrosis os tibiale externum) 732.5
Haglund-Läwen-Fründ syndrome 717.89
Hagner's disease (hypertrophic pulmonary osteoarthropathy) 731.2
Hag teeth, tooth 524.39
Hailey-Hailey disease (benign familial chronic pemphigus) 757.39
Hair —*see also* condition
plucking 307.9
Hairball in stomach 935.2
Hairy black tongue 529.3
Half vertebra 756.14
Halitosis 784.99
Hallermann-Streiff syndrome 756.0
Hallervorden-Spatz disease or syndrome 333.0
Hallopeau's
acrodermatitis (continua) 696.1
disease (lichen sclerosis et atrophicus) 701.0
Hallucination (auditory) (gustatory) (olfactory) (tactile) 780.1
alcohol-induced 291.3
drug-induced 292.12
visual 368.16
Hallucinosis 298.9
alcohol-induced (acute) 291.3
drug-induced 292.12
Hallus —*see* Hallux
Hallux 735.9
limitus 735.8
malleus (acquired) 735.3
rigidus (acquired) 735.2
congenital 755.66
late effects of rickets 268.1
valgus (acquired) 735.0
congenital 755.66
varus (acquired) 735.1
congenital 755.66
Halo, visual 368.15
Hamartoblastoma 759.6

Hamartoma 759.6
epithelial (gingival), odontogenic, central, or peripheral (M9321/0) 213.1
upper jaw (bone) 213.0
vascular 757.32
Hamartosis, hamartoses NEC 759.6
Hamman's disease or syndrome (spontaneous mediastinal emphysema) 518.1
Hamman-Rich syndrome (diffuse interstitial pulmonary fibrosis) 516.33
Hammer toe (acquired) 735.4
congenital 755.66
late effects of rickets 268.1
Hand —*see* condition
Hand-Schüller-Christian disease or syndrome (chronic histiocytosis x) 277.89
Hand-foot syndrome 693.0
Hanging (asphyxia) (strangulation) (suffocation) 994.7
Hangnail (finger) (with lymphangitis) 681.02
Hangover (alcohol) (*see also* Abuse, drugs, nondependent) 305.0
Hanot's cirrhosis or disease —*see* Cirrhosis, biliary
Hanot-Chauffard (-Troisier) syndrome (bronze diabetes) 275.01
Hansen's disease (leprosy) 030.9
benign form 030.1
malignant form 030.0
Harada's disease or syndrome 363.22
Hard chancre 091.0
Hard firm prostate 600.10
with
urinary
obstruction 600.11
retention 600.11
Hardening
artery—*see* Arteriosclerosis
brain 348.89
liver 571.8
Hare's syndrome (M8010/3) (carcinoma, pulmonary apex) 162.3
Harelip (*see also* Cleft, lip) 749.10
Harkavy's syndrome 446.0
Harlequin (fetus) 757.1
color change syndrome 779.89
Harley's disease (intermittent hemoglobinuria) 283.2
Harris'
lines 733.91
syndrome (organic hyperinsulinism) 251.1
Hart's disease or syndrome (pellagra-cerebellar ataxia-renal aminoaciduria) 270.0
Hartmann's pouch (abnormal sacculation of gallbladder neck) 575.8
of intestine V44.3
attention to V55.3
Hartnup disease (pellagra-cerebellar ataxia-renal aminoaciduria) 270.0
Harvester lung 495.0
Hashimoto's disease or struma (struma lymphomatosa) 245.2
Hassall-Henle bodies (corneal warts) 371.41
Haut mal (*see also* Epilepsy) 345.1
Haverhill fever 026.1
Hawaiian wood rose dependence 304.5
Hawkins' keloid 701.4

Hay
  asthma (*see also* Asthma) 493.0
    fever (allergic) (with rhinitis) 477.9with
        asthma (bronchial) (*see also* Asthma) 493.0
    allergic, due to grass, pollen, ragweed, or tree
        477.0
    conjunctivitis 372.05
    due to
      dander, animal (cat) (dog) 477.2
      dust 477.8
      fowl 477.8
      hair, animal (cat) (dog) 477.2
      pollen 477.0
      specified allergen other than pollen 477.8
Hayem-Faber syndrome (achlorhydric anemia)
    280.9
Hayem-Widal syndrome (acquired hemolytic
    jaundice) 283.9
Haygarth's nodosities 715.04
Hazard-Crile tumor (M8350/3) 193
Hb (abnormal)
  disease—*see* Disease, hemoglobin
  trait—*see* Trait
H disease 270.0
Head —*see also* condition
  banging 307.3
Headache 784.0
  allergic 339.00
  associated with sexual activity 339.82
  cluster 339.00
    chronic 339.02
    episodic 339.01
  daily
    chronic 784.0
    new persistent (NPDH) 339.42
  drug induced 339.3
  due to
    loss, spinal fluid 349.0
    lumbar puncture 349.0
    saddle block 349.0
  emotional 307.81
  histamine 339.00
  hypnic 339.81
  lumbar puncture 349.0
  medication overuse 339.3
  menopausal 627.2
  menstrual 346.4
  migraine 346.9
  nasal septum 784.0
  nonorganic origin 307.81
  orgasmic 339.82
  postspinal 349.0
  post-traumatic 339.20
    acute 339.21
    chronic 339.22
  premenstrual 346.4
  preorgasmic 339.82
  primary
    cough 339.83
    exertional 339.84
    stabbing 339.85
    thunderclap 339.43
  psychogenic 307.81
  psychophysiologic 307.81
  rebound 339.3
  short lasting unilateral neuralgiform with
      conjunctival injection and tearing (SUNCT)
      339.05
  sick 346.9

Headache—*continued*
  spinal 349.0
    complicating labor and delivery 668.8
    postpartum 668.8
  spinal fluid loss 349.0
  syndrome
    cluster 339.00
    complicated NEC 339.44
    periodic in child or adolescent 346.2
    specified NEC 339.89
  tension 307.81
    type 339.10
      chronic 339.12
      episodic 339.11
  vascular 784.0
    migraine type 346.9
  vasomotor 346.9
Health
  advice V65.4
  audit V70.0
  checkup V70.0
  education V65.4
  hazard (*see also* History of) V15.9
    falling V15.88
    specified cause NEC V15.89
  instruction V65.4
  services provided because of (of)
    boarding school residence V60.6
    holiday relief for person providing home care
        V60.5
    inadequate
      housing V60.1
      resources V60.2
    lack of housing V60.0
    no care available in home V60.4
    person living alone V60.3
    poverty V60.3
    residence in institution V60.6
    specified cause NEC V60.89
    vacation relief for person providing home care
        V60.5
Healthy
  donor (*see also* Donor) V59.9
  infant or child
    accompanying sick mother V65.0
    receiving care V20.1
  person
    accompanying sick relative V65.0
    admitted for sterilization V25.2
    receiving prophylactic inoculation or
        vaccination (*see also* Vaccination,
        prophylactic) V05.9
Hearing
  conservation and treatment V72.12
  examination V72.19
    following failed hearing screening V72.11
Heart —*see* condition
Heartburn 787.1
  psychogenic 306.4
Heat (effects) 992.9
  apoplexy 992.0
  burn—*see* Burn, by site
    from sun (*see also* Sunburn) 692.71
  collapse 992.1
  cramps 992.2
  dermatitis or eczema 692.89
  edema 992.7
  erythema—*see* Burn, by site
  excessive 992.9
    specified effect NEC 992.8

Heat —*continued*
exhaustion 992.5
  anhydrotic 992.3
  due to
    salt (and water) depletion 992.4
    water depletion 992.3
fatigue (transient) 992.6
fever 992.0
hyperpyrexia 992.0
prickly 705.1
prostration—*see* Heat, exhaustion
pyrexia 992.0
rash 705.1
specified effect NEC 992.8
stroke 992.0
sunburn (*see also* Sunburn) 692.71
syncope 992.1
Heavy-chain disease 273.2
Heavy-for-dates (fetus or infant) 766.1
4500 grams or more 766.0
exceptionally 766.0
Hebephrenia, hebephrenic (acute) (*see also*
  Schizophrenia) 295.1
dementia (praecox) (*see also* Schizophrenia)
  295.1
schizophrenia (*see also* Schizophrenia) 295.1
Heberden's
disease or nodes 715.04
syndrome (angina pectoris) 413.9
Hebra's disease
dermatitis exfoliativa 695.89
erythema multiforme exudativum 695.19
pityriasis 695.89
  maculata et circinata 696.3
  rubra 695.89
    pilaris 696.4
prurigo 698.2
Hebra, nose 040.1
Hedinger's syndrome (malignant carcinoid)
  259.2
Heel —*see* condition
Heerfordt's disease or syndrome (uveoparotitis)
  135
Hegglin's anomaly or syndrome 288.2
Heidenhain's disease 290.10
with dementia 290.10
Heilmeyer-Schöner disease (M9842/3) 207.1
Heine-Medin disease (*see also* Poliomyelitis)
  045.9
Heinz-body anemia, congenital 282.7
Heller's disease or syndrome (infantile
  psychosis) (*see also* Psychosis, childhood) 299.1
H.E.L.L.P. 642.5
Helminthiasis (*see also* Infestation, by specific
  parasite) 128.9
Ancylostoma (*see also* Ancylostoma) 126.9
intestinal 127.9
  mixed types (types classifiable to more than
    one of the titles 120.0-127.7) 127.8
  specified type 127.7
mixed types (intestinal) (types classifiable to
  more than one of the titles 120.0-127.7) 127.8
Necator americanus 126.1
specified type NEC 128.8
Trichinella 124
Heloma 700
Hemangioblastoma (M9161/1)—*see also*
  Neoplasm, connective tissue, uncertain
  behavior
malignant (M9161//3)—*see* Neoplasm,
  connective tissue, malignant

Hemangioblastomatosis, cerebelloretinal 759.6
Hemangioendothelioma (M9130/1)—*see also*
  Neoplasm, by site, uncertain behavior
benign (M9130/0) 228.00
bone (diffuse) (M9130/3)—*see* Neoplasm, bone,
  malignant
malignant (M9130/3)—*see* Neoplasm,
  connective tissue, malignant
nervous system (M9130/0) 228.09
Hemangioendotheliosarcoma (M9130/3)—*see*
  Neoplasm, connective tissue, malignant
Hemangiofibroma (M9160/0)—*see* Neoplasm,
  by site, benign
Hemangiolipoma (M8861/0)—*see* Lipoma
Hemangioma (M9120/0) 228.00
arteriovenous (M9123/0)—*see* Hemangioma, by
  site
brain 228.02
capillary (M9131/0)—*see* Hemangioma, by site
cavernous (M9121/0)—*see* Hemangioma, by
  site
central nervous system NEC 228.09
choroid 228.09
heart 228.09
infantile (M9131/0)—*see* Hemangioma, by site
intra-abdominal structures 228.04
intracranial structures 228.02
intramuscular (M9132/0)—*see* Hemangioma, by site
iris 228.09
juvenile (M9131/0)—*see* Hemangioma, by site
malignant (M9120/3)—*see* Neoplasm,
  connective tissue, malignant
meninges 228.09
  brain 228.02
  spinal cord 228.09
peritoneum 228.04
placenta—*see* Placenta, abnormal
plexiform (M9131/0)—*see* Hemangioma, by
  site
racemose (M9123/0)—*see* Hemangioma, by site
retina 228.03
retroperitoneal tissue 228.04
sclerosing (M8832/0)—*see* Neoplasm, skin,
  benign
simplex (M9131/0)—*see* Hemangioma, by site
skin and subcutaneous tissue 228.01
specified site NEC 228.09
spinal cord 228.09
venous (M9122/0)—*see* Hemangioma, by site
verrucous keratotic (M9142/0)—*see*
  Hemangioma, by site
Hemangiomatosis (systemic) 757.32
involving single site—*see* Hemangioma
Hemangiopericytoma (M9150/1)—*see also*
  Neoplasm, connective tissue, uncertain
  behavior
benign (M9150/0)—*see* Neoplasm, connective
  tissue, benign
malignant (M9150/3)—*see* Neoplasm,
  connective tissue, malignant
Hemangiosarcoma (M9120/3)—*see* Neoplasm,
  connective tissue, malignant
Hemarthrosis (nontraumatic) 719.0
ankle 719.17
elbow 719.12
foot 719.17
hand 719.14
hip 719.15
knee 719.16
multiple sites 719.19
pelvic region 719.15
shoulder (region) 719.11

Hemarthrosis—*continued*
specified site NEC 719.18
traumatic—*see* Sprain, by site
wrist 719.13
Hematemesis 578.0
with ulcer—*see* Ulcer, by site, with hemorrhage
due to S. japonicum 120.2
Goldstein's (familial hemorrhagic
telangiectasia) 448.0
newborn 772.4
due to swallowed maternal blood 777.3
Hematidrosis 705.89
Hematinuria (*see also* Hemoglobinuria) 791.2
malarial 084.8
paroxysmal 283.2
Hematite miners' lung 503
Hematobilia 576.8
Hematocele (congenital) (diffuse) (idiopathic)
608.83
broad ligament 620.7
canal of Nuck 629.0
cord, male 608.83
fallopian tube 620.8
female NEC 629.0
ischiorectal 569.89
male NEC 608.83
ovary 629.0
pelvis, pelvic
female 629.0
with ectopic pregnancy (*see also* Pregnancy,
ectopic) 633.90
with intrauterine pregnancy 633.91
male 608.83
periuterine 629.0
retrouterine 629.0
scrotum 608.83
spermatic cord (diffuse) 608.83
testis 608.84
traumatic—*see* Injury, internal, pelvis
tunica vaginalis 608.83
uterine ligament 629.0
uterus 621.4
vagina 623.6
vulva 624.5
Hematocephalus 742.4
Hematochezia (*see also* Melena) 578.1
Hematochyluria (*see also* Infestation, filarial)
125.9
Hematocolpos 626.8
Hematocornea 371.12
Hematogenous —*see* condition
Hematoma (skin surface intact) (traumatic)—*see*
also Contusion

Note—*Hematomas are coded according to*
origin and the nature and site of the hematoma
or the accompanying injury. Hematomas of
unspecified origin are coded as injuries of the
sites involved, except:
(a) *hematomas of genital organs which are*
coded as diseases of the organ involved
unless they complicate pregnancy or
delivery
(b) *hematomas of the eye which are coded as*
diseases of the eye.

For late effect of hematoma classifiable to
920-924 see Late, effect, contusion

Hematoma—*continued*
with
crush injury—*see* Crush
fracture—*see* Fracture, by site
injury of internal organs—*see also* Injury,
internal, by site
kidney—*see* Hematoma, kidney, traumatic
liver—*see* Hematoma, liver, traumatic
spleen—*see* Hematoma, spleen
nerve injury—*see* Injury, nerve
open wound—*see* Wound, open, by site
skin surface intact—*see* Contusion
abdomen (wall)—*see* Contusion, abdomen
amnion 658.8
aorta, dissecting 441.00
abdominal 441.02
thoracic 441.01
thoracoabdominal 441.03
aortic intramural—*see* Dissection, aorta
arterial (complicating trauma) 904.9
specified site—*see* Injury, blood vessel, by site
auricle (ear) 380.31
birth injury 767.8
skull 767.19
brain (traumatic) 853.0

Note—*Use the following fifth-digit*
subclassification with categories 851-854:

0 *unspecified state of consciousness*
1 *with no loss of consciousness*
2 *with brief [less than one hour] loss of*
consciousness
3 *with moderate [1-24 hours] loss of*
consciousness
4 *with prolonged [more than 24 hours] loss of*
consciousness and return to pre-existing
conscious level
5 *with prolonged [more than 24 hours] loss of*
consciousness, without return to pre-existing
conscious level
Use *fifth-digit 5 to designate when a patient is*
unconscious and dies before regaining
consciousness, regardless of the duration of the
loss of consciousness
6 *with loss of consciousness of unspecified*
duration
9 *with concussion, unspecified*

with
cerebral
contusion—*see* Contusion, brain
laceration—*see* Laceration, brain
open intracranial wound 853.1
skull fracture—*see* Fracture, skull, by site
extradural or epidural 852.4
with open intracranial wound 852.5
fetus or newborn 767.0
nontraumatic 432.0
fetus or newborn NEC 767.0
nontraumatic (*see also* Hemorrhage, brain) 431
epidural or extradural 432.0
newborn NEC 772.8
subarachnoid, arachnoid, or meningeal (*see*
also Hemorrhage, subarachnoid) 430
subdural (*see also* Hemorrhage, subdural)
432.1
subarachnoid, arachnoid, or meningeal 852.0
with open intracranial wound 852.1
fetus or newborn 772.2
nontraumatic (*see also* Hemorrhage,
subarachnoid) 430

Hematoma—*continued*
  brain—*continued*
    subdural 852.2
      with open intracranial wound 852.3
      fetus or newborn (localized) 767.0
      nontraumatic (*see also* Hemorrhage,
        subdural) 432.1
  breast (nontraumatic) 611.89
  broad ligament (nontraumatic) 620.7
    complicating delivery 665.7
    traumatic—*see* Injury, internal, broad
      ligament
  calcified NEC 959.9
  capitis 920
    due to birth injury 767.19
    newborn 767.19
  cerebral—*see* Hematoma, brain
  cesarean section wound 674.3
  chorion—*see* Placenta, abnormal
  complicating delivery (perineum) (vulva) 664.5
    pelvic 665.7
    vagina 665.7
  corpus
    cavernosum (nontraumatic) 607.82
    luteum (nontraumatic) (ruptured) 620.1
  dura (mater)—*see* Hematoma, brain, subdural
  epididymis (nontraumatic) 608.83
  epidural (traumatic)—*see also* Hematoma,
    brain, extradural
    spinal—*see* Injury, spinal, by site
  episiotomy 674.3
  external ear 380.31
  extradural—*see also* Hematoma, brain,
    extradural
    fetus or newborn 767.0
    nontraumatic 432.0
      fetus or newborn 767.0
  fallopian tube 620.8
  genital organ (nontraumatic)
    female NEC 629.89
    male NEC 608.83
    traumatic (external site) 922.4
    internal—*see* Injury, internal, genital organ
  graafian follicle (ruptured) 620.0
  internal organs (abdomen, chest, or pelvis)—*see
    also* Injury, internal, by site
    kidney—*see* Hematoma, kidney, traumatic
    liver—*see* Hematoma, liver, traumatic
    spleen—*see* Hematoma, spleen
  intracranial—*see* Hematoma, brain
  kidney, cystic 593.81
    traumatic 866.01
      with open wound into cavity 866.11
  labia (nontraumatic) 624.5
  lingual (and other parts of neck, scalp, or face,
    except eye) 920
  liver (subcapsular) 573.8
    birth injury 767.8
    fetus or newborn 767.8
    traumatic NEC 864.01
      with
        laceration—*see* Laceration, liver
        open wound into cavity 864.11
  mediastinum—*see* Injury, internal, mediastinum
  meninges, meningeal (brain)—*see also*
    Hematoma, brain, subarachnoid
    spinal—*see* Injury, spinal, by site
  mesosalpinx (nontraumatic) 620.8
    traumatic—*see* Injury, internal, pelvis
  muscle (traumatic)—*see* Contusion, by site
    nontraumatic 729.92

Hematoma—*continued*
  nasal (septum) (and other part(s) of neck, scalp,
    or face, except eye) 920
  obstetrical surgical wound 674.3
  orbit, orbital (nontraumatic) 376.32
    traumatic 921.2
  ovary (corpus luteum) (nontraumatic) 620.1
    traumatic—*see* Injury, internal, ovary
  pelvis (female) (nontraumatic) 629.89
    complicating delivery 665.7
    male 608.83
    traumatic—*see also* Injury, internal, pelvis
      specified organ NEC (*see also* Injury,
        internal, pelvis) 867.6
  penis (nontraumatic) 607.82
  pericranial (and neck, or face any part, except
    eye) 920
    due to injury at birth 767.19
  perineal wound (obstetrical) 674.3
    complicating delivery 664.5
  perirenal, cystic 593.81
  pinna 380.31
  placenta—*see* Placenta, abnormal
  postoperative 998.12
  retroperitoneal (nontraumatic) 568.81
    traumatic—*see* Injury, internal,
      retroperitoneum
  retropubic, male 568.81
  scalp (and neck, or face any part, except eye)
    920
    fetus or newborn 767.19
  scrotum (nontraumatic) 608.83
    traumatic 922.4
  seminal vesicle (nontraumatic) 608.83
    traumatic—*see* Injury, internal, seminal
      vesicle
  soft tissue 729.92
  spermatic cord—*see also* Injury, internal,
    spermatic cord
    nontraumatic 608.83
  spinal (cord) (meninges)—*see also* Injury,
    spinal, by site
    fetus or newborn 767.4
    nontraumatic 336.1
  spleen 865.01
    with
      laceration—*see* Laceration, spleen
      open wound into cavity 865.11
  sternocleidomastoid, birth injury 767.8
  sternomastoid, birth injury 767.8
  subarachnoid—*see also* Hematoma, brain,
    subarachnoid
    fetus or newborn 772.2
    nontraumatic (*see also* Hemorrhage,
      subarachnoid) 430
    newborn 772.2
  subdural—*see also* Hematoma, brain, subdural
    fetus or newborn (localized) 767.0
    nontraumatic (*see also* Hemorrhage, subdural)
      432.1
  subperiosteal (syndrome) 267
    traumatic—*see* Hematoma, by site
  superficial, fetus or newborn 772.6
  syncytium—*see* Placenta, abnormal
  testis (nontraumatic) 608.83
    birth injury 767.8
    traumatic 922.4
  tunica vaginalis (nontraumatic) 608.83
  umbilical cord 663.6
    affecting fetus or newborn 762.6
  uterine ligament (nontraumatic) 620.7
    traumatic—*see* Injury, internal, pelvis

Hematoma—*continued*
  uterus 621.4
    traumatic—*see* Injury, internal, pelvis
  vagina (nontraumatic) (ruptured) 623.6
    complicating delivery 665.7
    traumatic 922.4
  vas deferens (nontraumatic) 608.83
    traumatic—*see* Injury, internal, vas deferens
  vitreous 379.23
  vocal cord 920
  vulva (nontraumatic) 624.5
    complicating delivery 664.5
    fetus or newborn 767.8
    traumatic 922.4
Hematometra 621.4
Hematomyelia 336.1
  with fracture of vertebra (*see also* Fracture,
    vertebra, by site, with spinal cord injury)
    806.8
  fetus or newborn 767.4
Hematomyelitis 323.9
  late effect—*see* category 326
Hematoperitoneum (*see also* Hemoperitoneum)
    568.81
Hematopneumothorax (*see also* Hemothorax)
    511.89
Hematopoiesis, cyclic 288.02
Hematoporphyria (acquired) (congenital) 277.1
Hematoporphyrinuria (acquired) (congenital)
    277.1
Hematorachis, hematorrhachis 336.1
  fetus or newborn 767.4
Hematosalpinx 620.8
  with
    ectopic pregnancy (*see also* categories
      633.0-633.9) 639.2
    molar pregnancy (*see also* categories 630-632)
      639.2
  infectional (*see also* Salpingo-oophoritis) 614.2
Hematospermia 608.82
Hematothorax (*see also* Hemothorax) 511.89
Hematotympanum 381.03
Hematuria (benign) (essential) (idiopathic)
    599.70
  due to S. hematobium 120.0
  endemic 120.0
  gross 599.71
  intermittent 599.70
  malarial 084.8
  microscopic 599.72
  paroxysmal 599.70
  sulfonamide
    correct substance properly administered
      599.70
    overdose or wrong substance given or taken
      961.0
  tropical (bilharziasis) 120.0
  tuberculous (*see also* Tuberculosis) 016.9
Hematuric bilious fever 084.8
Hemeralopia 368.10
  acquired 286.5
Hemiabiotrophy 799.89
Hemi-akinesia 781.8
Hemianalgesia (*see also* Disturbance, sensation)
    782.0
Hemianencephaly 740.0
Hemianesthesia (*see also* Disturbance, sensation)
    782.0

Hemianopia, hemianopsia (altitudinal)
    (homonymous) 368.46
  binasal 368.47
  bitemporal 368.47
  heteronymous 368.47
  syphilitic 095.8
Hemiasomatognosia 307.9
Hemiathetosis 781.0
Hemiatrophy 799.89
  cerebellar 334.8
  face 349.89
    progressive 349.89
  fascia 728.9
  leg 728.2
  tongue 529.8
Hemiballism (us) 333.5
Hemiblock (cardiac) (heart) (left) 426.2
Hemicardia 746.89
Hemicephalus, hemicephaly 740.0
Hemichorea 333.5
Hemicrania 346.9
  congenital malformation 740.0
  continua 339.41
  paroxysmal 339.03
    chronic 339.04
    episodic 339.03
Hemidystrophy —*see* Hemiatrophy
Hemiectromelia 755.4
Hemihypalgesia (*see also* Disturbance,
    sensation) 782.0
Hemihypertrophy (congenital) 759.89
  cranial 756.0
Hemihypesthesia (*see also* Disturbance,
    sensation) 782.0
Hemi-inattention 781.8
Hemimelia 755.4
  lower limb 755.30
    paraxial (complete) (incomplete) (intercalary)
      (terminal) 755.32
      fibula 755.37
      tibia 755.36
    transverse (complete) (partial) 755.31
  upper limb 755.20
    paraxial (complete) (incomplete) (intercalary)
      (terminal) 755.22
      radial 755.26
      ulnar 755.27
    transverse (complete) (partial) 755.21
Hemiparalysis (*see also* Hemiplegia) 342.9
Hemiparesis (*see also* Hemiplegia) 342.9
Hemiparesthesia (*see also* Disturbance,
    sensation) 782.0
Hemiplegia 342.9
  acute (*see also* Disease, cerebrovascular, acute)
    436
  alternans facialis 344.89
  apoplectic (*see also* Disease, cerebrovascular,
    acute) 436
    late effect or residual
      affecting
        dominant side 438.21
        nondominant side 438.22
        unspecified side 438.20
  arteriosclerotic 437.0
    late effect or residual
      affecting
        dominant side 438.21
        nondominant side 438.22
        unspecified side 438.20
  ascending (spinal) NEC 344.89

Hemiplegia—*continued*
  attack (*see also* Disease, cerebrovascular, acute)
    436
  brain, cerebral (current episode) 437.8
    congenital 343.1
  cerebral—*see* Hemiplegia, brain
  congenital (cerebral) (spastic) (spinal) 343.1
  conversion neurosis (hysterical) 300.11
  cortical—*see* Hemiplegia, brain
  due to
    arteriosclerosis 437.0
      late effect or residual
        affecting
          dominant side 438.21
          nondominant side 438.22
          unspecified side 438.20
    cerebrovascular lesion (*see also* Disease,
      cerebrovascular, acute) 436
      late effect
        affecting
          dominant side 438.21
          nondominant side 438.22
          unspecified side 438.20
    embolic (current) (*see also* Embolism, brain)
      434.1
      late effect
        affecting
          dominant side 438.21
          nondominant side 438.22
          unspecified side 438.20
  flaccid 342.0
  hypertensive (current episode) 437.8
  infantile (postnatal) 343.4
  late effect
    birth injury, intracranial or spinal 343.4
    cerebrovascular lesion—*see* Late effect(s) (of)
      cerebrovascular disease
    viral encephalitis 139.0
  middle alternating NEC 344.89
  newborn NEC 767.0
  seizure (current episode) (*see also* Disease,
    cerebrovascular, acute) 436
  spastic 342.1
    congenital or infantile 343.1
  specified NEC 342.8
  thrombotic (current) (*see also* Thrombosis,
    brain) 434.0
    late effect—*see* late effect(s) (of)
      cerebrovascular disease
Hemisection, spinal cord —*see* Fracture,
  vertebra, by site, with spinal cord injury
Hemispasm 781.0
  facial 781.0
Hemispatial neglect 781.8
Hemisporosis 117.9
Hemitremor 781.0
Hemivertebra 756.14
Hemobilia 576.8
Hemocholecyst 575.8
Hemochromatosis (acquired) (liver)
  (myocardium) (secondary) 275.03
  diabetic 275.03
  due to repeated red blood cell transfusions
    275.02
  hereditary 275.01
  primary idiopathic 275.01
  specified NEC 275.03
  transfusion associated (red blood cell) 275.02
    with refractory anemia 238.72
Hemodialysis V56.0

Hemoglobin —*see also* condition
  abnormal (disease)—*see* Disease, hemoglobin
  AS genotype 282.5
  fetal, hereditary persistence 282.7
  H Constant Spring 282.43
  H disease 282.43
  high-oxygen-affinity 289.0
  low NEC 285.9
  S (Hb-S), heterozygous 282.5
Hemoglobinemia 283.2
  due to blood transfusion NEC 999.89
    bone marrow 996.85
  paroxysmal 283.2
Hemoglobinopathy (mixed) (*see also* Disease,
  hemoglobin) 282.7
  with thalassemia 282.49
  sickle-cell 282.60
    with thalassemia (without crisis) 282.41
      with
        crisis 282.42
        vaso-occlusive pain 282.42
Hemoglobinuria, hemoglobinuric 791.2
  with anemia, hemolytic, acquired (chronic) NEC
    283.2
  cold (agglutinin) (paroxysmal) (with Raynaud's
    syndrome) 283.2
  due to
    exertion 283.2
    hemolysis (from external causes) NEC 283.2
  exercise 283.2
  fever (malaria) 084.8
  infantile 791.2
  intermittent 283.2
  malarial 084.8
  march 283.2
  nocturnal (paroxysmal) 283.2
  paroxysmal (cold) (nocturnal) 283.2
Hemolymphangioma (M9175/0) 228.1
Hemolysis
  fetal—*see* Jaundice, fetus or newborn
  intravascular (disseminated) NEC 286.6
    with
      abortion—*see* Abortion, by type, with
        hemorrhage, delayed or excessive
      ectopic pregnancy (*see also* categories
        633.0-633.9) 639.1
      hemorrhage of pregnancy 641.3
        affecting fetus or newborn 762.1
      molar pregnancy (*see also* categories
        630-632) 639.1
    acute 283.2
    following
      abortion 639.1
      ectopic or molar pregnancy 639.1
  neonatal—*see* Jaundice, fetus or newborn
  transfusion NEC 999.89
    bone marrow 996.85
Hemolytic —*see also* condition
  anemia—*see* Anemia, hemolytic
  uremic syndrome 283.11
Hemometra 621.4
Hemopericardium (with effusion) 423.0
  newborn 772.8
  traumatic (*see also* Hemothorax, traumatic) 860.2
    with open wound into thorax 860.3
Hemoperitoneum 568.81
  infectional (*see also* Peritonitis) 567.29
  traumatic—*see* Injury, internal, peritoneum
Hemophagocytic syndrome 288.4
  infection-associated 288.4

Hemophilia (familial) (hereditary) 286.0
  A 286.0
    carrier (asymptomatic) V83.01
      symptomatic V83.02
  acquired 286.52
  autoimmune 286.52
  B (Leyden) 286.1
  C 286.2
  calcipriva (*see also* Fibrinolysis) 286.7
  classical 286.0
  nonfamilial 286.7
  secondary 286.52
  vascular 286.4
Hemophilus influenzae NEC 041.5
  arachnoiditis (basic) (brain) (spinal) 320.0
    late effect—*see* category 326
  bronchopneumonia 482.2
  cerebral ventriculitis 320.0
    late effect—*see* category 326
  cerebrospinal inflammation 320.0
    late effect—*see* category 326
  infection NEC 041.5
  leptomeningitis 320.0
    late effect—*see* category 326
  meningitis (cerebral) (cerebrospinal) (spinal) 320.0
    late effect—*see* category 326
  meningomyelitis 320.0
    late effect—*see* category 326
  pachymeningitis (adhesive) (fibrous) (hemorrhagic) (hypertrophic) (spinal) 320.0
    late effect—*see* category 326
  pneumonia (broncho-) 482.2
Hemophthalmos 360.43
Hemopneumothorax (*see also* Hemothorax) 511.89
  traumatic 860.4
    with open wound into thorax 860.5
Hemoptysis 786.30
  due to Paragonimus (westermani) 121.2
  newborn 770.3
  specified NEC 786.39
  tuberculous (*see also* Tuberculosis, pulmonary) 011.9
Hemorrhage, hemorrhagic (nontraumatic) 459.0
  abdomen 459.0
  accidental (antepartum) 641.2
    affecting fetus or newborn 762.1
  adenoid 474.8
  adrenal (capsule) (gland) (medulla) 255.41
    newborn 772.5
  after labor—*see* Hemorrhage, postpartum
  alveolar
    lung, newborn 770.3
    process 525.8
  alveolus 525.8
  amputation stump (surgical) 998.11
    secondary, delayed 997.69
  anemia (chronic) 280.0
    acute 285.1
  antepartum—*see* Hemorrhage, pregnancy
  anus (sphincter) 569.3
  apoplexy (stroke) 432.9
  arachnoid—*see* Hemorrhage, subarachnoid
  artery NEC 459.0
    brain (*see also* Hemorrhage, brain) 431
    middle meningeal—*see* Hemorrhage, subarachnoid
  basilar (ganglion) (*see also* Hemorrhage, brain) 431
  bladder 596.89
  blood dyscrasia 289.9

Hemorrhage, hemorrhagic—*continued*
  bowel 578.9
    newborn 772.4
  brain (miliary) (nontraumatic) 431
    with
      birth injury 767.0
    arachnoid—*see* Hemorrhage, subarachnoid
    due to
      birth injury 767.0
      rupture of aneurysm (congenital) (*see also* Hemorrhage, subarachnoid) 430
      mycotic 431
      syphilis 094.89
    epidural or extradural—*see* Hemorrhage, extradural
    fetus or newborn (anoxic) (hypoxic) (due to birth trauma) (nontraumatic) 767.0
    intraventricular 772.10
      grade I 772.11
      grade II 772.12
      grade III 772.13
      grade IV 772.14
    iatrogenic 997.02
    postoperative 997.02
    puerperal, postpartum, childbirth 674.0
    stem 431
    subarachnoid, arachnoid or meningeal—*see* Hemorrhage, subarachnoid
    subdural—*see* Hemorrhage, subdural
    traumatic NEC 853.0

Note—Use the following fifth-digit subclassification with categories 851-854:

0 unspecified state of consciousness
1 with no loss of consciousness
2 with brief [less than one hour] loss of consciousness
3 with moderate [1-24 hours] loss of consciousness
4 with prolonged [more than 24 hours] loss of consciousness and return to pre-existing conscious level
5 with prolonged [more than 24 hours] loss of consciousness, without return to pre-existing conscious level
Use fifth-digit 5 to designate when a patient is unconscious and dies before regaining consciousness, regardless of the duration of the loss of consciousness
6 with loss of consciousness of unspecified duration
9 with concussion, unspecified

    with
      cerebral
        contusion—*see* Contusion, brain
        laceration—*see* Laceration, brain
      open intracranial wound 853.1
      skull fracture—*see* Fracture, skull, by site
    extradural or epidural 852.4
      with open intracranial wound 852.5
    subarachnoid 852.0
      with open intracranial wound 852.1
    subdural 852.2
      with open intracranial wound 852.3
  breast 611.79
  bronchial tube—*see* Hemorrhage, lung
  bronchopulmonary—*see* Hemorrhage, lung
  bronchus (cause unknown) (*see also* Hemorrhage, lung) 786.30
  bulbar (*see also* Hemorrhage, brain) 431

Hemorrhage, hemorrhagic—*continued*
  bursa 727.89
  capillary 448.9
    primary 287.8
  capsular—*see* Hemorrhage, brain
  cardiovascular 429.89
  cecum 578.9
  cephalic (*see also* Hemorrhage, brain) 431
  cerebellar (*see also* Hemorrhage, brain) 431
  cerebellum (*see also* Hemorrhage, brain) 431
  cerebral (*see also* Hemorrhage, brain) 431
    fetus or newborn (anoxic) (traumatic) 767.0
  cerebromeningeal (*see also* Hemorrhage, brain) 431
  cerebrospinal (*see also* Hemorrhage, brain) 431
  cerebrovascular accident—*see* Hemorrhage, brain
  cerebrum (*see also* Hemorrhage, brain) 431
  cervix (stump) (uteri) 622.8
  cesarean section wound 674.3
  chamber, anterior (eye) 364.41
  childbirth—*see* Hemorrhage, complicating, delivery
  choroid 363.61
    expulsive 363.62
  ciliary body 364.41
  cochlea 386.8
  colon—*see* Hemorrhage, intestine
  complicating
    delivery 641.9
      affecting fetus or newborn 762.1
      associated with
        afibrinogenemia 641.3
          affecting fetus or newborn 763.89
        coagulation defect 641.3
          affecting fetus or newborn 763.89
        hyperfibrinolysis 641.3
          affecting fetus or newborn 763.89
        hypofibrinogenemia 641.3
          affecting fetus or newborn 763.89
      due to
        low-lying placenta 641.1
          affecting fetus or newborn 762.0
        placenta previa 641.1
          affecting fetus or newborn 762.0
        premature separation of placenta 641.2
          affecting fetus or newborn 762.1
        retained
          placenta 666.0
          secundines 666.2
        trauma 641.8
          affecting fetus or newborn 763.89
        uterine leiomyoma 641.8
          affecting fetus or newborn 763.89
    surgical procedure 998.11
  complication(s)
    of dental implant placement 525.71
  concealed NEC 459.0
  congenital 772.9
  conjunctiva 372.72
    newborn 772.8
  cord, newborn 772.0
    slipped ligature 772.3
    stump 772.3
  corpus luteum (ruptured) 620.1
  cortical (*see also* Hemorrhage, brain) 431
  cranial 432.9
  cutaneous 782.7
    newborn 772.6

Hemorrhage, hemorrhagic—*continued*
  cyst, pancreas 577.2
  cystitis—*see* Cystitis
  delayed
    with
      abortion—*see* Abortion, by type, with hemorrhage, delayed or excessive
      ectopic pregnancy (*see also* categories 633.0-633.9) 639.1
      molar pregnancy (*see also* categories 630-632) 639.1
    following
      abortion 639.1
      ectopic or molar pregnancy 639.1
    postpartum 666.2
  diathesis (familial) 287.9
    newborn 776.0
  disease 287.9
    newborn 776.0
    specified type NEC 287.8
  disorder 287.9
    due to intrinsic circulating anticoagulants, antibodies, or inhibitors 286.59
    with
      acquired hemophilia 286.52
      antiphospholipid antibody 286.53
    specified type NEC 287.8
  due to
    any device, implant, or graft (presence of) classifiable to 996.0-996.5—*see* Complications, due to (presence of) any device, implant, or graft classified to 996.0—996.5 NEC
    intrinsic circulating anticoagulant, antibodies, or inhibitors 286.59
    with
      acquired hemophilia 286.52
      antiphospholipid antibody 286.53
  duodenum, duodenal 537.89
    ulcer—*see* Ulcer, duodenum, with hemorrhage
  dura mater—*see* Hemorrhage, subdural
  endotracheal—*see* Hemorrhage, lung
  epicranial subaponeurotic (massive) 767.11
  epidural—*see* Hemorrhage, extradural
  episiotomy 674.3
  esophagus 530.82
    varix (*see also* Varix, esophagus, bleeding) 456.0
  excessive
    with
      abortion—*see* Abortion, by type, with hemorrhage, delayed or excessive
      ectopic pregnancy (*see also* categories 633.0-633.9) 639.1
      molar pregnancy (*see also* categories 630-632) 639.1
    following
      abortion 639.1
      ectopic or molar pregnancy 639.1
  external 459.0
  extradural (traumatic)—*see also* Hemorrhage, brain, traumatic, extradural
    birth injury 767.0
    fetus or newborn (anoxic) (traumatic) 767.0
    nontraumatic 432.0
  eye 360.43
    chamber (anterior) (aqueous) 364.41
    fundus 362.81
  eyelid 374.81
  fallopian tube 620.8

Hemorrhage, hemorrhagic—*continued*
fetomaternal 772.0
  affecting management of pregnancy or
    puerperium 656.0
fetus, fetal, affecting newborn772.0
  from
    cut end of co-twin's cord 772.0
    placenta 772.0
    ruptured cord 772.0
    vasa previa 772.0
  into
    co-twin 772.0
    mother's circulation 772.0
      affecting management of pregnancy or
        puerperium 656.0
fever (*see also* Fever, hemorrhagic) 065.9
  with renal syndrome 078.6
  arthropod-borne NEC 065.9
  Bangkok 065.4
  Crimean 065.0
  dengue virus 065.4
  epidemic 078.6
  Junin virus 078.7
  Korean 078.6
  Machupo virus 078.7
  mite-borne 065.8
  mosquito-borne 065.4
  Philippine 065.4
  Russian (Yaroslav) 078.6
  Singapore 065.4
  southeast Asia 065.4
  Thailand 065.4
  tick-borne NEC 065.3
fibrinogenolysis (*see also* Fibrinolysis) 286.6
fibrinolytic (acquired) (*see also* Fibrinolysis)
  286.6
fontanel 767.19
from tracheostomy stoma 519.09
fundus, eye 362.81
funis
  affecting fetus or newborn 772.0
  complicating delivery 663.8
gastric (*see also* Hemorrhage, stomach) 578.9
gastroenteric 578.9
  newborn 772.4
gastrointestinal (tract) 578.9
  newborn 772.4
genitourinary (tract) NEC 599.89
gingiva 523.8
globe 360.43
gravidarum—*see* Hemorrhage, pregnancy
gum 523.8
heart 429.89
hypopharyngeal (throat) 784.8
intermenstrual 626.6
  irregular 626.6
  regular 626.5
internal (organs) 459.0
  capsule (*see also* Hemorrhage, brain) 431
  ear 386.8
  newborn 772.8
  intestine 578.9
  congenital 772.4
  newborn 772.4
into
  bladder wall 596.7
  bursa 727.89
  corpus luysii (*see also* Hemorrhage, brain) 431
intra-abdominal 459.0
  during or following surgery 998.11
intra-alveolar, newborn (lung) 770.3
intracerebral (*see also* Hemorrhage, brain) 431

Hemorrhage, hemorrhagic—*continued*
intracranial NEC 432.9
  puerperal, postpartum, childbirth 674.0
  traumatic—*see* Hemorrhage, brain, traumatic
intramedullary NEC 336.1
intraocular 360.43
intraoperative 998.11
intrapartum—*see* Hemorrhage, complicating,
  delivery
intrapelvic
  female 629.89
  male 459.0
intraperitoneal 459.0
intrapontine (*see also* Hemorrhage, brain) 431
intrauterine 621.4
  complicating delivery—*see* Hemorrhage,
    complicating, delivery
  in pregnancy or childbirth—*see* Hemorrhage,
    pregnancy
  postpartum (*see also* Hemorrhage,
    postpartum) 666.1
intraventricular (*see also* Hemorrhage, brain) 431
  fetus or newborn (anoxic) (traumatic) 772.10
    grade I 772.11
    grade II 772.12
    grade III 772.13
    grade IV 772.14
intravesical 596.7
iris (postinfectional) (postinflammatory) (toxic)
  364.41
joint (nontraumatic) 719.10
  ankle 719.17
  elbow 719.12
  foot 719.17
  forearm 719.13
  hand 719.14
  hip 719.15
  knee 719.16
  lower leg 719.16
  multiple sites 719.19
  pelvic region 719.15
  shoulder (region) 719.11
  specified site NEC 719.18
  thigh 719.15
  upper arm 719.12
  wrist 719.13
kidney 593.81
knee (joint) 719.16
labyrinth 386.8
leg NEC 459.0
lenticular striate artery (*see also* Hemorrhage,
  brain) 431
ligature, vessel 998.11
liver 573.8
lower extremity NEC 459.0
lung 786.30
  newborn 770.3
  tuberculous (*see also* Tuberculosis,
    pulmonary) 011.9
malaria 084.8
marginal sinus 641.2
massive subaponeurotic, birth injury 767.11
maternal, affecting fetus or newborn 762.1
mediastinum 786.30
medulla (*see also* Hemorrhage, brain) 431
membrane (brain) (*see also* Hemorrhage,
  subarachnoid) 430
  spinal cord—*see* Hemorrhage, spinal cord
meninges, meningeal (brain) (middle) (*see also*
  Hemorrhage, subarachnoid) 430
  spinal cord—*see* Hemorrhage, spinal cord
mesentery 568.81

Hemorrhage, hemorrhagic—*continued*
  metritis 626.8
  midbrain (*see also* Hemorrhage, brain) 431
  mole 631.8
  mouth 528.9
  mucous membrane NEC 459.0
    newborn 772.8
  muscle 728.89
  nail (subungual) 703.8
  nasal turbinate 784.7
    newborn 772.8
  nasopharynx 478.29
  navel, newborn 772.3
  newborn 772.9
    adrenal 772.5
    alveolar (lung) 770.3
    brain (anoxic) (hypoxic) (due to birth trauma) 767.0
    cerebral (anoxic) (hypoxic) (due to birth
      trauma) 767.0
    conjunctiva 772.8
    cutaneous 772.6
    diathesis 776.0
    due to vitamin K deficiency 776.0
    epicranial subaponeurotic (massive) 767.11
    gastrointestinal 772.4
    internal (organs) 772.8
    intestines 772.4
    intra-alveolar (lung) 770.3
    intracranial (from any perinatal cause) 767.0
    intraventricular (from any perinatal cause) 772.10
      grade I 772.11
      grade II 772.12
      grade III 772.13
      grade IV 772.14
    lung 770.3
    pulmonary (massive) 770.3
    spinal cord, traumatic 767.4
    stomach 772.4
    subaponeurotic (massive) 767.11
    subarachnoid (from any perinatal cause) 772.2
    subconjunctival 772.8
    subgaleal 767.11
    umbilicus 772.0
      slipped ligature 772.3
      vasa previa 772.0
  nipple 611.79
  nose 784.7
    newborn 772.8
  obstetrical surgical wound 674.3
  omentum 568.89
    newborn 772.4
  optic nerve (sheath) 377.42
  orbit 376.32
  ovary 620.1
  oviduct 620.8
  pancreas 577.8
  parathyroid (gland) (spontaneous) 252.8
  parturition—*see* Hemorrhage, complicating,
    delivery
  penis 607.82
  pericardium, pericarditis 423.0
  perineal wound (obstetrical) 674.3
  peritoneum, peritoneal 459.0
  peritonsillar tissue 474.8
    after operation on tonsils 998.11
    due to infection 475
  petechial 782.7
  pituitary (gland) 253.8
  placenta NEC 641.9
    affecting fetus or newborn 762.1
    from surgical or instrumental damage 641.8
      affecting fetus or newborn 762.1

Hemorrhage, hemorrhagic—*continued*
  placenta previa 641.1
    affecting fetus or newborn 762.0
  pleura—*see* Hemorrhage, lung
  polioencephalitis, superior 265.1
  polymyositis—*see* Polymyositis
  pons (*see also* Hemorrhage, brain) 431
  pontine (*see also* Hemorrhage, brain) 431
  popliteal 459.0
  postcoital 626.7
  postextraction (dental) 998.11
  postmenopausal 627.1
  postnasal 784.7
  postoperative 998.11
  postpartum (atonic) (following delivery of
    placenta) 666.1
    delayed or secondary (after 24 hours) 666.2
    retained placenta 666.0
    third stage 666.0
  pregnancy (concealed) 641.9
    accidental 641.2
      affecting fetus or newborn 762.1
    affecting fetus or newborn 762.1
    before 22 completed weeks gestation 640.9
      affecting fetus or newborn 762.1
    due to
      abruptio placenta 641.2
        affecting fetus or newborn 762.1
      afibrinogenemia or other coagulation defect
        (conditions classifiable to 286.0-286.9)
        641.3
        affecting fetus or newborn 762.1
      coagulation defect 641.3
        affecting fetus or newborn 762.1
      hyperfibrinolysis 641.3
        affecting fetus or newborn 762.1
      hypofibrinogenemia 641.3
        affecting fetus or newborn 762.1
      leiomyoma, uterus 641.8
        affecting fetus or newborn 762.1
      low-lying placenta 641.1
        affecting fetus or newborn 762.1
      marginal sinus (rupture) 641.2
        affecting fetus or newborn 762.1
      placenta previa 641.1
        affecting fetus or newborn 762.0
      premature separation of placenta (normally
        implanted) 641.2
        affecting fetus or newborn 762.1
      threatened abortion 640.0
        affecting fetus or newborn 762.1
      trauma 641.8
        affecting fetus or newborn 762.1
    early (before 22 completed weeks gestation)
      640.9
      affecting fetus or newborn 762.1
    previous, affecting management of pregnancy
      or childbirth V23.49
    unavoidable—*see* Hemorrhage, pregnancy,
      due to placenta previa
  prepartum (mother)—*see* Hemorrhage,
    pregnancy
  preretinal, cause unspecified 362.81
  prostate 602.1
  puerperal (*see also* Hemorrhage, postpartum)
    666.1
  pulmonary (*see also* Hemorrhage, lung) 786.30
    acute idiopathic in infants (AIPHI) (over 28
      days old) 786.31
    newborn (massive) 770.3
    renal syndrome 446.21

Hemorrhage, hemorrhagic—*continued*
purpura (primary) (*see also* Purpura,
    thrombocytopenic) 287.39
rectum (sphincter) 569.3
recurring, following initial hemorrhage at time
    of injury 958.2
renal 593.81
    pulmonary syndrome 446.21
respiratory tract (*see also* Hemorrhage, lung)
    786.30
retina, retinal (deep) (superficial) (vessels) 362.81
    diabetic 250.5 *[362.01]*
        due to secondary diabetes 249.5 *[362.01]*
    due to birth injury 772.8
retrobulbar 376.89
retroperitoneal 459.0
retroplacental (*see also* Placenta, separation) 641.2
scalp 459.0
    due to injury at birth 767.19
scrotum 608.83
secondary (nontraumatic) 459.0
    following initial hemorrhage at time of injury
        958.2
seminal vesicle 608.83
skin 782.7
    newborn 772.6
spermatic cord 608.83
spinal (cord) 336.1
    aneurysm (ruptured) 336.1
        syphilitic 094.89
    due to birth injury 767.4
    fetus or newborn 767.4
spleen 289.59
spontaneous NEC 459.0
    petechial 782.7
stomach 578.9
    newborn 772.4
    ulcer—*see* Ulcer, stomach, with hemorrhage
subaponeurotic, newborn 767.11
    massive (birth injury) 767.11
subarachnoid (nontraumatic) 430
    fetus or newborn (anoxic) (traumatic) 772.2
    puerperal, postpartum, childbirth 674.0
    traumatic—*see* Hemorrhage, brain, traumatic,
        subarachnoid
subconjunctival 372.72
    due to birth injury 772.8
    newborn 772.8
subcortical (*see also* Hemorrhage, brain) 431
subcutaneous 782.7
subdiaphragmatic 459.0
subdural (nontraumatic) 432.1
    due to birth injury 767.0
    fetus or newborn (anoxic) (hypoxic) (due to
        birth trauma) 767.0
    puerperal, postpartum, childbirth 674.0
    spinal 336.1
    traumatic—*see* Hemorrhage, brain, traumatic,
        subdural
subgaleal 767.11
subhyaloid 362.81
subperiosteal 733.99
subretinal 362.81
subtentorial (*see also* Hemorrhage, subdural) 432.1
subungual 703.8
    due to blood dyscrasia 287.8
suprarenal (capsule) (gland) 255.41
    fetus or newborn 772.5
tentorium (traumatic)—*see also* Hemorrhage,
    brain, traumatic
    fetus or newborn 767.0
    nontraumatic—*see* Hemorrhage, subdural

Hemorrhage, hemorrhagic—*continued*
testis 608.83
thigh 459.0
third stage 666.0
thorax—*see* Hemorrhage, lung
throat 784.8
thrombocythemia 238.71
thymus (gland) 254.8
thyroid (gland) 246.3
    cyst 246.3
tongue 529.8
tonsil 474.8
    postoperative 998.11
tooth socket (postextraction) 998.11
trachea—*see* Hemorrhage, lung
traumatic—*see also* nature of injury
    brain—*see* Hemorrhage, brain, traumatic
    recurring or secondary (following initial
        hemorrhage at time of injury) 958.2
tuberculous NEC (*see also* Tuberculosis,
    pulmonary) 011.9
tunica vaginalis 608.83
ulcer—*see* Ulcer, by site, with hemorrhage
umbilicus, umbilical cord 772.0
    after birth, newborn 772.3
    complicating delivery 663.8
        affecting fetus or newborn 772.0
    slipped ligature 772.3
    stump 772.3
unavoidable (due to placenta previa) 641.1
    affecting fetus or newborn 762.0
upper extremity 459.0
urethra (idiopathic) 599.84
uterus, uterine (abnormal) 626.9
    climacteric 627.0
    complicating delivery—*see* Hemorrhage,
        complicating, delivery
    due to
        intrauterine contraceptive device 996.76
            perforating uterus 996.32
    functional or dysfunctional 626.8
    in pregnancy—*see* Hemorrhage, pregnancy
    intermenstrual 626.6
        irregular 626.6
        regular 626.5
    postmenopausal 627.1
    postpartum (*see also* Hemorrhage,
        postpartum) 666.1
    prepubertal 626.8
    pubertal 626.3
    puerperal (immediate) 666.1
vagina 623.8
vasa previa 663.5
    affecting fetus or newborn 772.0
vas deferens 608.83
ventricular (*see also* Hemorrhage, brain) 431
vesical 596.89
viscera 459.0
    newborn 772.8
vitreous (humor) (intraocular) 379.23
vocal cord 478.5
vulva 624.8
Hemorrhoids (anus) (rectum) (without
    complication) 455.6
bleeding, prolapsed, strangulated, or ulcerated
    NEC 455.8
    external 455.5
    internal 455.2
complicated NEC 455.8
complicating pregnancy and puerperium 671.8

Hemorrhoids—*continued*
external 455.3
  with complication NEC 455.5
  bleeding, prolapsed, strangulated, or ulcerated
    455.5
  thrombosed 455.4
internal 455.0
  with complication NEC 455.2
  bleeding, prolapsed, strangulated, or ulcerated
    455.2
  thrombosed 455.1
residual skin tag 455.9
sentinel pile 455.9
thrombosed NEC 455.7
  external 455.4
  internal 455.1
Hemosalpinx 620.8
Hemosiderosis 275.09
dietary 275.09
pulmonary (idiopathic) 275.09 *[516.1]*
transfusion NEC 275.02
  bone marrow 996.85
Hemospermia 608.82
Hemothorax 511.89
bacterial, nontuberculous 511.1
newborn 772.8
nontuberculous 511.89
  bacterial 511.1
pneumococcal 511.1
postoperative 998.11
staphylococcal 511.1
streptococcal 511.1
traumatic 860.2
  with
    open wound into thorax 860.3
    pneumothorax 860.4
      with open wound into thorax 860.5
tuberculous (*see also* Tuberculosis, pleura) 012.0
Hemotympanum 385.89
Hench-Rosenberg syndrome (palindromic
  arthritis) (*see also* Rheumatism, palindromic)
  719.3
Henle's warts 371.41
Henoch (-Schönlein)
disease or syndrome (allergic purpura) 287.0
purpura (allergic) 287.0
Henpue, henpuye 102.6
Heparitinuria 277.5
Hepar lobatum 095.3
Heparin-induced thrombocytopenia (HIT)
  289.84
Hepatalgia 573.8
Hepatic —*see also* condition
flexure syndrome 569.89
Hepatitis 573.3
acute (*see also* Necrosis, liver) 570
  alcoholic 571.1
  infective 070.1
    with hepatic coma 070.0
alcoholic 571.1
amebic—*see* Abscess, liver, amebic
anicteric (acute)—*see* Hepatitis, viral
antigen-associated (HAA) *see* Hepatitis, viral,
  type B
Australian antigen (positive) *see* Hepatitis, viral,
  type B
autoimmune 571.42

Hepatitis—*continued*
catarrhal (acute) 070.1
  with hepatic coma 070.0
  chronic 571.40
  newborn 070.1
    with hepatic coma 070.0
chemical 573.3
cholangiolitic 573.8
cholestatic 573.8
chronic 571.40
  active 571.49
    viral—*see* Hepatitis, viral
  aggressive 571.49
  persistent 571.41
  viral—*see* Hepatitis, viral
cytomegalic inclusion virus 078.5 *[573.1]*
diffuse 573.3
"dirty needle"—*see* Hepatitis, viral
  with hepatic coma 070.2
drug-induced 573.3
due to
  Coxsackie 074.8 *[573.1]*
  cytomegalic inclusion virus 078.5 *[573.1]*
  infectious mononucleosis 075 *[573.1]*
  malaria 084.9 *[573.2]*
  mumps 072.71
  secondary syphilis 091.62
  toxoplasmosis (acquired) 130.5
    congenital (active) 771.2
epidemic—*see* Hepatitis, viral, type A
fetus or newborn 774.4
fibrous (chronic) 571.49
  acute 570
from injection, inoculation, or transfusion
  (blood) (other substance) (plasma) (serum)
  (onset within 8 months after administration)
  see Hepatitis, viral
fulminant (viral) (*see also* Hepatitis, viral) 070.9
  with hepatic coma 070.6
  type A 070.1
    with hepatic coma 070.0
  type B—*see* Hepatitis, viral, Type B
giant cell (neonatal) 774.4
hemorrhagic 573.8
history of
  B V12.09
  C V12.09
homologous serum—*see* Hepatitis, viral
hypertrophic (chronic) 571.49
  acute 570
nfectious, infective (acute) (chronic) (subacute)
  070.1
  with hepatic coma 070.0
inoculation—*see* Hepatitis, viral
interstitial (chronic) 571.49
  acute 570
lupoid 571.49
malarial 084.9 *[573.2]*
malignant (*see also* Necrosis, liver) 570
neonatal (toxic) 774.4
newborn 774.4
parenchymatous (acute) (*see also* Necrosis,
  liver) 570
peliosis 573.3
persistent, chronic 571.41
plasma cell 571.49
postimmunization—*see* Hepatitis, viral
postnecrotic 571.49
posttransfusion—*see* Hepatitis, viral
recurrent 571.49

Hepatitis—*continued*
septic 573.3
serum—*see* Hepatitis, viral
  carrier (suspected) of V02.61
subacute (*see also* Necrosis, liver) 570
suppurative (diffuse) 572.0
syphilitic (late) 095.3
  congenital (early) 090.0 *[573.2]*
    late 090.5 *[573.2]*
  secondary 091.62
toxic (noninfectious) 573.3
  fetus or newborn 774.4
tuberculous (*see also* Tuberculosis) 017.9
viral (acute) (anicteric) (cholangiolitic)
    (cholestatic) (chronic) (subacute) 070.9
  with hepatic coma 070.6
  AU-SH type virus—*see* Hepatitis, viral, type
      B
  Australian antigen—*see* Hepatitis, viral, type
      B
  B-antigen—*see* Hepatitis, viral, type B
  Coxsackie 074.8 *[573.1]*
  cytomegalic inclusion 078.5 *[573.1]*
  IH (virus)—*see* Hepatitis, viral, type A
  infectious hepatitis virus—*see* Hepatitis, viral,
      type A
  serum hepatitis virus—*see* Hepatitis, viral,
      type B
  SH—*see* Hepatitis, viral, type B
  specified type NEC 070.59
    with hepatic coma 070.49
  type A 070.1
    with hepatic coma 070.0
  type B (acute) 070.30
    with
      hepatic coma 070.20
        with hepatitis delta 070.21
      hepatitis delta 070.31
        with hepatic coma 070.21
    carrier status V02.61
    chronic 070.32
      with
        hepatic coma 070.22
          with hepatitis delta 070.23
        hepatitis delta 070.33
          with hepatic coma 070.23
  type C
    with hepatic coma 070.41
    acute 070.51
      with hepatic coma 070.41
    carrier status V02.62
    chronic 070.54
      with hepatic coma 070.44
    in remission 070.54
    unspecified 070.70
      with hepatic coma 070.71
  type delta (with hepatitis B carrier state)
      070.52
    with
      active hepatitis B disease—*see* Hepatitis,
          viral, type B
      hepatic coma 070.42
  type E 070.53
    with hepatic coma 070.43
  vaccination and inoculation (prophylactic)
      V05.3
Waldenström's (lupoid hepatitis) 571.49
Hepatization, lung (acute)—*see also* Pneumonia,
    lobar
chronic (*see also* Fibrosis, lung) 515
Hepatoblastoma (M8970/3) 155.0
Hepatocarcinoma (M8170/3) 155.0

Hepatocholangiocarcinoma (M8180/3) 155.0
Hepatocholangioma, benign (M8180/0) 211.5
Hepatocholangitis 573.8
Hepatocystitis (*see also* Cholecystitis) 575.10
Hepatodystrophy 570
Hepatolenticular degeneration 275.1
Hepatolithiasis —*see* Choledocholithiasis
Hepatoma (malignant) (M8170/3) 155.0
  benign (M8170/0) 211.5
  congenital (M8970/3) 155.0
  embryonal (M8970/3) 155.0
Hepatomegalia glycogenica diffusa 271.0
Hepatomegaly (*see also* Hypertrophy, liver)
    789.1
  congenital 751.69
    syphilitic 090.0
  due to Clonorchis sinensis 121.1
  Gaucher's 272.7
  syphilitic (congenital) 090.0
Hepatoptosis 573.8
Hepatorrhexis 573.8
Hepatosis, toxic 573.8
Hepatosplenomegaly 571.8
  due to S. japonicum 120.2
  hyperlipemic (Burger-Grutz type) 272.3
Herald patch 696.3
Hereditary —*see* condition
Heredodegeneration 330.9
  macular 362.70
Heredopathia atactica polyneuritiformis 356.3
Heredosyphilis (*see also* Syphilis, congenital)
    090.9
Hermaphroditism (true) 752.7
  with specified chromosomal anomaly—*see*
      Anomaly, chromosomes, sex
Hernia, hernial (acquired) (recurrent) 553.9
  with
    gangrene (obstructed) NEC 551.9
    obstruction NEC 552.9
      and gangrene 551.9
  abdomen (wall)—*see* Hernia, ventral
  abdominal, specified site NEC 553.8
    with
      gangrene (obstructed) 551.8
      obstruction 552.8
        and gangrene 551.8
  appendix 553.8
    with
      gangrene (obstructed) 551.8
      obstruction 552.8
        and gangrene 551.8
  bilateral (inguinal)—*see* Hernia, inguinal
  bladder (sphincter)
    congenital (female) (male) 756.71
    female (*see also* Cystocele, female) 618.01
    male 596.89
  brain 348.4
    congenital 742.0
  broad ligament 553.8
  cartilage, vertebral—*see* Displacement,
      intervertebral disc
  cerebral 348.4
    congenital 742.0
    endaural 742.0
  ciliary body 364.89
    traumatic 871.1
  colic 553.9
    with
      gangrene (obstructed) 551.9
      obstruction 552.9
        and gangrene 551.9

Hernia, hernial—*continued*
  colon 553.9
    with
      gangrene (obstructed) 551.9
      obstruction 552.9
        and gangrene 551.9
  colostomy (stoma) 569.69
  Cooper's (retroperitoneal) 553.8
    with
      gangrene (obstructed) 551.8
      obstruction 552.8
        and gangrene 551.8
  crural—*see* Hernia, femoral
  cystostomy 596.83
  diaphragm, diaphragmatic 553.3
    with
      gangrene (obstructed) 551.3
      obstruction 552.3
        and gangrene 551.3
    congenital 756.6
    due to gross defect of diaphragm 756.6
    traumatic 862.0
      with open wound into cavity 862.1
  direct (inguinal)—*see* Hernia, inguinal
  disc, intervertebral—*see* Displacement,
      intervertebral disc
  diverticulum, intestine 553.9
    with
      gangrene (obstructed) 551.9
      obstruction 552.9
        and gangrene 551.9
  double (inguinal)—*see* Hernia, inguinal
  due to adhesion with obstruction 552.9
  duodenojejunal 553.8
    with
      gangrene (obstructed) 551.8
      obstruction 552.8
        and gangrene 551.8
  en glissade—*see* Hernia, inguinal
  enterostomy (stoma) 569.69
  epigastric 553.29
    with
      gangrene (obstruction) 551.29
      obstruction 552.29
        and gangrene 551.29
    recurrent 553.21
      with
        gangrene (obstructed) 551.21
        obstruction 552.21
          and gangrene 551.21
  esophageal hiatus (sliding) 553.3
    with
      gangrene (obstructed) 551.3
      obstruction 552.3
        and gangrene 551.3
    congenital 750.6
  external (inguinal)—*see* Hernia, inguinal
  fallopian tube 620.4
  fascia 728.89
  fat 729.30
    eyelid 374.34
    orbital 374.34
    pad 729.30
      eye, eyelid 374.34
      knee 729.31
      orbit 374.34
      popliteal (space) 729.31
      specified site NEC 729.39

Hernia, hernial—*continued*
  femoral (unilateral) 553.00
    with
      gangrene (obstructed) 551.00
      obstruction 552.00
        with gangrene 551.00
    bilateral 553.02
      gangrenous (obstructed) 551.02
      obstructed 552.02
        with gangrene 551.02
      recurrent 553.03
        gangrenous (obstructed) 551.03
        obstructed 552.03
          with gangrene 551.03
    recurrent (unilateral) 553.01
      bilateral 553.03
        gangrenous (obstructed) 551.03
        obstructed 552.03
          with gangrene 551.03
      gangrenous (obstructed) 551.01
      obstructed 552.01
        with gangrene 551.01
  foramen
    Bochdalek 553.3
      with
        gangrene (obstructed) 551.3
        obstruction 552.3
          and gangrene 551.3
      congenital 756.6
    magnum 348.4
    Morgagni, morgagnian 553.3
      with
        gangrene 551.3
        obstruction 552.3
          and gangrene 551.3
      congenital 756.6
  funicular (umbilical) 553.1
    with
      gangrene (obstructed) 551.1
      obstruction 552.1
        and gangrene 551.1
  spermatic cord—*see* Hernia, inguinal
  gangrenous—*see* Hernia, by site, with gangrene
  gastrointestinal tract 553.9
    with
      gangrene (obstructed) 551.9
      obstruction 552.9
        and gangrene 551.9
  gluteal—*see* Hernia, femoral
  Gruber's (internal mesogastric) 553.8
    with
      gangrene (obstructed) 551.8
      obstruction 552.8
        and gangrene 551.8
  Hesselbach's 553.8
    with
      gangrene (obstructed) 551.8
      obstruction 552.8
        and gangrene 551.8
  hiatal (esophageal) (sliding) 553.3
    with
      gangrene (obstructed) 551.3
      obstruction 552.3
        and gangrene 551.3
    congenital 750.6
  incarcerated (*see also* Hernia, by site, with
      obstruction) 552.9
    gangrenous (*see also* Hernia, by site, with
        gangrene) 551.9

Hernia, hernial—*continued*
incisional 553.21
  with
    gangrene (obstructed) 551.21
    obstruction 552.21
      and gangrene 551.21
  lumbar—*see* Hernia, lumbar
  recurrent 553.21
    with
      gangrene (obstructed) 551.21
      obstruction 552.21
        and gangrene 551.21
indirect (inguinal)—*see* Hernia, inguinal
infantile—*see* Hernia, inguinal
infrapatellar fat pad 729.31
inguinal (direct) (double) (encysted) (external)
  (funicular) (indirect) (infantile) (internal)
  (interstitial) (oblique) (scrotal) (sliding)
  550.9

Note—*Use the following fifth-digit subclassification with category 550:*

0 *unilateral or unspecified (not specified as recurrent)*
1 *unilateral or unspecified, recurrent*
2 *bilateral (not specified as recurrent)*
3 *bilateral, recurrent*

---

  with
    gangrene (obstructed) 550.0
    obstruction 550.1
      and gangrene 550.0
internal 553.8
  with
    gangrene (obstructed) 551.8
    obstruction 552.8
      and gangrene 551.8
  inguinal—*see* Hernia, inguinal
interstitial 553.9
  with
    gangrene (obstructed) 551.9
    obstruction 552.9
      and gangrene 551.9
  inguinal—*see* Hernia, inguinal
intervertebral cartilage or disc—*see*
  Displacement, intervertebral disc
intestine, intestinal 553.9
  with
    gangrene (obstructed) 551.9
    obstruction 552.9
      and gangrene 551.9
intra-abdominal 553.9
  with
    gangrene (obstructed) 551.9
    obstruction 552.9
      and gangrene 551.9
intraparietal 553.9
  with
    gangrene (obstructed) 551.9
    obstruction 552.9
      and gangrene 551.9
iris 364.89
  traumatic 871.1
irreducible (*see also* Hernia, by site, with
  obstruction) 552.9
  gangrenous (with obstruction) (*see also*
    Hernia, by site, with gangrene) 551.9
ischiatic 553.8
  with
    gangrene (obstructed) 551.8
    obstruction 552.8
      and gangrene 551.8

Hernia, hernial—*continued*
ischiorectal 553.8
  with
    gangrene (obstructed) 551.8
    obstruction 552.8
      and gangrene 551.8
lens 379.32
  traumatic 871.1
linea
  alba—*see* Hernia, epigastric
  semilunaris—*see* Hernia, spigelian
Littre's (diverticular) 553.9
  with
    gangrene (obstructed) 551.9
    obstruction 552.9
      and gangrene 551.9
lumbar 553.8
  with
    gangrene (obstructed) 551.8
    obstruction 552.8
      and gangrene 551.8
  intervertebral disc 722.10
lung (subcutaneous) 518.89
  congenital 748.69
mediastinum 519.3
mesenteric (internal) 553.8
  with
    gangrene (obstructed) 551.8
    obstruction 552.8
      and gangrene 551.8
mesocolon 553.8
  with
    gangrene (obstructed) 551.8
    obstruction 552.8
      and gangrene 551.8
muscle (sheath) 728.89
nucleus pulposus—*see* Displacement,
  intervertebral disc
oblique (inguinal)—*see* Hernia, inguinal
obstructive (*see also* Hernia, by site, with
  obstruction) 552.9
  gangrenous (with obstruction) (*see also*
    Hernia, by site, with gangrene) 551.9
obturator 553.8
  with
    gangrene (obstructed) 551.8
    obstruction 552.8
      and gangrene 551.8
omental 553.8
  with
    gangrene (obstructed) 551.8
    obstruction 552.8
      and gangrene 551.8
orbital fat (pad) 374.34
ovary 620.4
oviduct 620.4
paracolostomy (stoma) 569.69
paraduodenal 553.8
  with
    gangrene (obstructed) 551.8
    obstruction 552.8
      and gangrene 551.8
paraesophageal 553.3
  with
    gangrene (obstructed) 551.3
    obstruction 552.3
      and gangrene 551.3
  congenital 750.6

Hernia, hernial—*continued*
parahiatal 553.3
with
gangrene (obstructed) 551.3
obstruction 552.3
and gangrene 551.3
paraumbilical 553.1
with
gangrene (obstructed) 551.1
obstruction 552.1
and gangrene 551.1
parietal 553.9
with
gangrene (obstructed) 551.9
obstruction 552.9
and gangrene 551.9
perineal 553.8
with
gangrene (obstructed) 551.8
obstruction 552.8
and gangrene 551.8
peritoneal sac, lesser 553.8
with
gangrene (obstructed) 551.8
obstruction 552.8
and gangrene 551.8
popliteal fat pad 729.31
postoperative 553.21
with
gangrene (obstructed) 551.21
obstruction 552.21
and gangrene 551.21
pregnant uterus 654.4
prevesical 596.89
properitoneal 553.8
with
gangrene (obstructed) 551.8
obstruction 552.8
and gangrene 551.8
pudendal 553.8
with
gangrene (obstructed) 551.8
obstruction 552.8
and gangrene 551.8
rectovaginal 618.6
retroperitoneal 553.8
with
gangrene (obstructed) 551.8
obstruction 552.8
and gangrene 551.8
Richter's (parietal) 553.9
with
gangrene (obstructed) 551.9
obstruction 552.9
and gangrene 551.9
Rieux's, Riex's (retrocecal) 553.8
with
gangrene (obstructed) 551.8
obstruction 552.8
and gangrene 551.8
sciatic 553.8
with
gangrene (obstructed) 551.8
obstruction 552.8
and gangrene 551.8
scrotum, scrotal—*see* Hernia, inguinal
sliding (inguinal)—*see also* Hernia, inguinal
hiatus—*see* Hernia, hiatal

Hernia, hernial—*continued*
spigelian 553.29
with
gangrene (obstructed) 551.29
obstruction 552.29
and gangrene 551.29
spinal (*see also* Spina bifida) 741.9
with hydrocephalus 741.0
strangulated (*see also* Hernia, by site, with
obstruction) 552.9
gangrenous (with obstruction) (*see also*
Hernia, by site, with gangrene) 551.9
supraumbilicus (linea alba)—*see* Hernia,
epigastric
tendon 727.9
testis (nontraumatic) 550.9
meaning
scrotal hernia 550.9
symptomatic late syphilis 095.8
Treitz's (fossa) 553.8
with
gangrene (obstructed) 551.8
obstruction 552.8
and gangrene 551.8
tunica
albuginea 608.89
vaginalis 752.89
umbilicus, umbilical 553.1
with
gangrene (obstructed) 551.1
obstruction 552.1
and gangrene 551.1
ureter 593.89
with obstruction 593.4
uterus 621.8
pregnant 654.4
vaginal (posterior) 618.6
Velpeau's (femoral) (*see also* Hernia, femoral)
553.00
ventral 553.20
with
gangrene (obstructed) 551.20
obstruction 552.20
and gangrene 551.20
recurrent 553.21
with
gangrene (obstructed) 551.21
obstruction 552.21
and gangrene 551.21
vesical
congenital (female) (male) 756.71
female (*see also* Cystocele, female) 618.01
male 596.89
vitreous (into anterior chamber) 379.21
traumatic 871.1
Herniation —*see also* Hernia
brain (stem) 348.4
cerebral 348.4
gastric mucosa (into duodenal bulb) 537.89
mediastinum 519.3
nucleus pulposus—*see* Displacement,
intervertebral disc
Herpangina 074.0
Herpes, herpetic 054.9
auricularis (zoster) 053.71
simplex 054.73
blepharitis (zoster) 053.20
simplex 054.41
circinate 110.5
circinatus 110.5
bullous 694.5

Herpes, herpetic—*continued*
  conjunctiva (simplex) 054.43
    zoster 053.21
  cornea (simplex) 054.43
    disciform (simplex) 054.43
    zoster 053.21
  encephalitis 054.3
  eye (zoster) 053.29
    simplex 054.40
  eyelid (zoster) 053.20
    simplex 054.41
  febrilis 054.9
  fever 054.9
  geniculate ganglionitis 053.11
  genital, genitalis 054.10
    specified site NEC 054.19
  gestationis 646.8
  gingivostomatitis 054.2
  iridocyclitis (simplex) 054.44
    zoster 053.22
  iris (any site) 695.10
  iritis (simplex) 054.44
  keratitis (simplex) 054.43
    dendritic 054.42
    disciform 054.43
    interstitial 054.43
      zoster 053.21
  keratoconjunctivitis (simplex) 054.43
    zoster 053.21
  labialis 054.9
    meningococcal 036.89
  lip 054.9
  meningitis (simplex) 054.72
    zoster 053.0
  ophthalmicus (zoster) 053.20
    simplex 054.40
  otitis externa (zoster) 053.71
    simplex 054.73
  penis 054.13
  perianal 054.10
  pharyngitis 054.79
  progenitalis 054.10
  scrotum 054.19
  septicemia 054.5
  simplex 054.9
    complicated 054.8
      ophthalmic 054.40
        specified NEC 054.49
      specified NEC 054.79
    congenital 771.2
    external ear 054.73
    keratitis 054.43
      dendritic 054.42
    meningitis 054.72
    myelitis 054.74
    neuritis 054.79
    specified complication NEC 054.79
      ophthalmic 054.49
    visceral 054.71
  stomatitis 054.2
  tonsurans 110.0
    maculosus (of Hebra) 696.3
  visceral 054.71
  vulva 054.12
  vulvovaginitis 054.11
  whitlow 054.6

Herpes, herpetic—*continued*
  zoster 053.9
    auricularis 053.71
    complicated 053.8
      specified NEC 053.79
    conjunctiva 053.21
    cornea 053.21
    ear 053.71
    eye 053.29
    geniculate 053.11
    keratitis 053.21
      interstitial 053.21
    myelitis 053.14
    neuritis 053.10
    ophthalmicus(a) 053.20
    oticus 053.71
    otitis externa 053.71
    specified complication NEC 053.79
    specified site NEC 053.9
  zosteriform, intermediate type 053.9
Herrick's
  anemia (hemoglobin S disease) 282.61
  syndrome (hemoglobin S disease) 282.61
Hers' disease (glycogenosis VI) 271.0
Herter's infantilism (nontropical sprue) 579.0
Herter (-Gee) disease or syndrome (nontropical sprue) 579.0
Herxheimer's disease (diffuse idiopathic cutaneous atrophy) 701.8
Herxheimer's reaction 995.91
Hesitancy, urinary 788.64
Hesselbach's hernia —*see* Hernia, Hesselbach's
Heterochromia (congenital) 743.46
  acquired 364.53
  cataract 366.33
  cyclitis 364.21
  hair 704.3
  iritis 364.21
  retained metallic foreign body 360.62
    magnetic 360.52
  uveitis 364.21
Heterophoria 378.40
  alternating 378.45
  vertical 378.43
Heterophyes, small intestine 121.6
Heterophyiasis 121.6
Heteropsia 368.8
Heterotopia, heterotopic —*see also* Malposition, congenital
  cerebralis 742.4
  pancreas, pancreatic 751.7
  spinalis 742.59
Heterotropia 378.30
  intermittent 378.20
    vertical 378.31
  vertical (constant) (intermittent) 378.31
Heubner's disease 094.89
Heubner-Herter disease or syndrome (nontropical sprue) 579.0
Hexadactylism 755.00
Heyd's syndrome (hepatorenal) 572.4
HGSIL (high grade squamous intrepithelial lesion) (cytologic finding) (Pap smear finding)
  anus 796.74
  cervix 795.04
    biopsy finding —code to CIN II or CIN III
  vagina 795.14
Hibernoma (M8880/0)—*see* Lipoma
Hiccough 786.8
  epidemic 078.89
  psychogenic 306.1

Hiccup (*see also* Hiccough) 786.8
Hicks (-Braxton) contractures 644.1
Hidden penis 752.65
Hidradenitis (axillaris) (suppurative) 705.83
Hidradenoma (nodular) (M8400/0)—*see also*
   Neoplasm, skin, benign
  clear cell (M8402/0)—*see* Neoplasm, skin,
    benign
  papillary (M8405/0)—*see* Neoplasm, skin,
    benign
Hidrocystoma (M8404/0)—*see* Neoplasm, skin,
   benign
HIE (hypoxic-ischemic encephalopathy) 768.70
  mild 768.71
  moderate 768.72
  severe 768.73
High
  A$_2$ anemia 282.46
  altitude effects 993.2
    anoxia 993.2
    on
      ears 993.0
      sinuses 993.1
    polycythemia 289.0
  arch
    foot 755.67
    palate 750.26
  artery (arterial) tension (*see also* Hypertension)
    401.9
    without diagnosis of hypertension 796.2
  basal metabolic rate (BMR) 794.7
  blood pressure (*see also* Hypertension) 401.9
    borderline 796.2
    incidental reading (isolated) (nonspecific), no
      diagnosis of hypertension 796.2
  cholesterol 272.0
    with high triglycerides 272.2
  compliance bladder 596.4
  diaphragm (congenital) 756.6
  frequency deafness (congenital) (regional) 389.8
  head at term 652.5
  output failure (cardiac) (*see also* Failure, heart)
    428.9
  oxygen-affinity hemoglobin 289.0
  palate 750.26
  risk
    behavior —*see* Problem
    family situation V61.9
      specified circumstance NEC V61.8
    human papillomavirus (HPV) DNA test
      positive
      anal 796.75
      cervical 795.05
      vaginal 795.15
    individual NEC V62.89
    infant NEC V20.1
    patient taking drugs (prescribed) V67.51
      nonprescribed (*see also* Abuse, drugs,
        nondependent) 305.9
    pregnancy V23.9
      inadequate prenatal care V23.7
      inconclusive fetal viability V23.87
      specified problem NEC V23.8
  temperature (of unknown origin) (*see also*
    Pyrexia) 780.60
  thoracic rib 756.3
  triglycerides 272.1
    with high cholesterol 272.2
Hildenbrand's disease (typhus) 081.9
Hilger's syndrome 337.09

Hill diarrhea 579.1
Hilliard's lupus (*see also* Tuberculosis) 017.0
Hilum —*see* condition
Hip —*see* condition
Hippel's disease (retinocerebral angiomatosis) 759.6
Hippus 379.49
Hirschfeld's disease (acute diabetes mellitus) (*see*
  also Diabetes) 250.0
  due to secondary diabetes 249.0
Hirschsprung's disease or megacolon
  (congenital) 751.3
Hirsuties (*see also* Hypertrichosis) 704.1
Hirsutism (*see also* Hypertrichosis) 704.1
Hirudiniasis (external) (internal) 134.2
His-Werner disease (trench fever) 083.1
Hiss-Russell dysentery 004.1
Histamine cephalgia 339.00
Histidinemia 270.5
Histidinuria 270.5
Histiocytic syndromes 288.4
Histiocytoma (M8832/0)—*see also* Neoplasm,
  skin, benign
  fibrous (M8830/0)—*see also* Neoplasm, skin,
    benign
    atypical (M8830/1)—*see* Neoplasm,
      connective tissue, uncertain behavior
    malignant (M8830/0)—*see* Neoplasm,
      connective tissue, malignant
Histiocytosis (acute) (chronic) (subacute) 277.89
  acute differentiated progressive (M9722/3) 202.5
  adult pulmonary Langerhans cell (PLCH) 516.5
  cholesterol 277.89
  essential 277.89
  lipid, lipoid (essential) 272.7
  lipochrome (familial) 288.1
  malignant (M9720/3) 202.3
  non-Langerhans cell 277.89
  polyostotic sclerosing 277.89
  X (chronic) 277.89
    acute (progressive) (M9722/3) 202.5
Histoplasmosis 115.90
  with
    endocarditis 115.94
    meningitis 115.91
    pericarditis 115.93
    pneumonia 115.95
    retinitis 115.92
    specified manifestation NEC 115.99
  African (due to Histoplasma duboisii) 115.10
    with
      endocarditis 115.14
      meningitis 115.11
      pericarditis 115.13
      pneumonia 115.15
      retinitis 115.12
      specified manifestation NEC 115.19
  American (due to Histoplasma capsulatum) 115.00
    with
      endocarditis 115.04
      meningitis 115.01
      pericarditis 115.03
      pneumonia 115.05
      retinitis 115.02
      specified manifestation NEC 115.09
  Darling's—*see* Histoplasmosis, American
  large form (*see also* Histoplasmosis, African) 115.10
  lung 115.05
  small form (*see also* Histoplasmosis, American)
    115.00

History (personal) of
 abuse
  emotional V15.42
  neglect V15.42
  physical V15.41
  sexual V15.41
 affective psychosis V11.1
 alcoholism V11.3
  specified as drinking problem (*see also* Abuse,
   drugs, nondependent) 305.0
 allergy (to) V15.09
  analgesic agent NEC V14.6
  anesthetic NEC V14.4
  antibiotic agent NEC V14.1
   penicillin V14.0
  anti-infective agent NEC V14.3
  arachnid bite V15.06
  diathesis V15.09
  drug V14.9
   specified type NEC V14.8
  eggs V15.03
  food additives V15.05
  insect bite V15.06
  latex V15.07
  medicinal agents V14.9
   specified type NEC V14.8
  milk products V15.02
  narcotic agent NEC V14.5
  nuts V15.05
   peanuts V15.01
  penicillin V14.0
  radiographic dye V15.08
  seafood V15.04
  serum V14.7
  specified food NEC V15.05
  specified nonmedicinal agents NEC V15.09
  spider bite V15.06
  sulfa V14.2
  sulfonamides V14.2
  therapeutic agent NEC V15.09
  vaccine V14.7
 anaphylactic reaction or shock V13.81
 anaphylaxis V13.81
 anemia V12.3
 arrest, sudden cardiac V12.53
 arthritis V13.4
 attack, transient ischemic (TIA) V12.54
 benign neoplasm of brain V12.41
 blood disease V12.3
 calculi, urinary V13.01
 cardiovascular disease V12.50
  myocardial infarction 412
 chemotherapy, antineoplastic V87.41
 child abuse V15.41
 cigarette smoking V15.82
 circulatory system disease V12.50
  myocardial infarction 412
 cleft lip and palate, corrected V13.64
 combat and operational stress reaction V11.4
 congenital malformation (corrected)
  circulatory system V13.65
  digestive system V13.67
  ear V13.64
  eye V13.64
  face V13.64
  genitourinary system V13.62
  heart V13.65
  integument V13.68
  limbs V13.68
  musculoskeletal V13.68
  neck V13.64

History—*continued*
 congenital malformation—*continued*
  nervous system V13.63
  respiratory system V13.66
  specified type NEC V13.69
 contraception V15.7
 death, sudden, successfully resuscitated V12.53
 deficit
  prolonged reversible ischemic neurologic
   (PRIND) V12.54
  reversible ischemic neurologic (RIND) V12.54
 diathesis, allergic V15.09
 digestive system disease V12.70
  peptic ulcer V12.71
  polyps, colonic V12.72
  specified NEC V12.79
 disease (of) V13.9
  blood V12.3
  blood-forming organs V12.3
  cardiovascular system V12.50
  circulatory system V12.50
   specified NEC V12.59
  digestive system V12.70
   peptic ulcer V12.71
   polyps, colonic V12.72
   specified NEC V12.79
  infectious V12.00
   malaria V12.03
   methicillin resistant Staphylococcus aureus
    (MRSA) V12.04
   MRSA (methicillin resistant Staphylococcus
    aureus) V12.04
   poliomyelitis V12.02
   specified NEC V12.09
   tuberculosis V12.01
  parasitic V12.00
   specified NEC V12.09
  respiratory system V12.60
   pneumonia V12.61
   specified NEC V12.69
  skin V13.3
  specified site NEC V13.89
  subcutaneous tissue V13.3
  trophoblastic V13.1
   affecting management of pregnancy V23.1
 disorder (of) V13.9
  endocrine V12.29
   gestational diabetes V12.21
  genital system V13.29
  hematological V12.3
  immunity V12.29
  mental V11.9
   affective type V11.1
   manic-depressive V11.1
   neurosis V11.2
   schizophrenia V11.0
   specified type NEC V11.8
  metabolic V12.29
  musculoskeletal NEC V13.59
  nervous system V12.40
   specified type NEC V12.49
  obstetric V13.29
   affecting management of current pregnancy
    V23.49
    ectopic pregnancy V23.42
    pre-term labor V13.21
  sense organs V12.40
   specified type NEC V12.49
  specified site NEC V13.89

History—*continued*
  disorder—*continued*
    urinary system V13.00
      calculi V13.01
      infection V13.02
      nephrotic syndrome V13.03
      specified NEC V13.09
    drug use
      nonprescribed (*see also* Abuse, drugs,
        nondependent) 305.9
      patent (*see also* Abuse, drugs, nondependent)
        305.9
    dysplasia
      cervical (conditions classifiable to 622.10-
        622.12) V13.22
      vaginal (conditions classifiable to 623.0)
        V13.23
      vulvar (conditions classifiable to
        624.01-624.02) V13.24
    effect NEC of external cause V15.89
    embolism V12.51
      pulmonary V12.55
    emotional abuse V15.42
    encephalitis V12.42
    endocrine disorder V12.29
      gestational diabetes V12.21
    estrogen therapy V87.43
    extracorporeal membrane oxygenation (ECMO)
      V15.87
    failed
      conscious sedation V15.80
      moderate sedation V15.80
    falling V15.88
    family
      allergy V19.6
      anemia V18.2
      arteriosclerosis V17.49
      arthritis V17.7
      asthma V17.5
      blindness V19.0
      blood disorder NEC V18.3
      cardiovascular disease V17.49
      carrier, genetic disease V18.9
      cerebrovascular disease V17.1
      chronic respiratory condition NEC V17.6
      colonic polyps V18.51
      congenital anomalies V19.5
      consanguinity V19.7
      coronary artery disease V17.3
      cystic fibrosis V18.19
      deafness V19.2
      diabetes mellitus V18.0
      digestive disorders V18.59
      disabilities, intellectual V18.4
      disease or disorder (of)
        allergic V19.6
        blood NEC V18.3
        cardiovascular NEC V17.49
        cerebrovascular V17.1
        colonic polyps V18.51
        coronary artery V17.3
        death, sudden cardiac (SCD) V17.41
        digestive V18.59
        ear NEC V19.3
        endocrine V18.19
          multiple neoplasia (MEN) syndrome
            V18.11
        eye NEC V19.19
          glaucoma V19.11
        genitourinary NEC V18.7
        glaucoma V19.11

History—*continued*
  family—*continued*
    disease or disorder—*continued*
      hypertensive V17.49
      infectious V18.8
      ischemic heart V17.3
      kidney V18.69
        polycystic V18.61
      mental V17.0
      metabolic V18.19
      musculoskeletal NEC V17.89
        osteoporosis V17.81
      neurological NEC V17.2
      parasitic V18.8
      psychiatric condition V17.0
      skin condition V19.4
    ear disorder NEC V19.3
    endocrine disease V18.19
      multiple neoplasia (MEN) syndrome V18.11
    epilepsy V17.2
    eye disorder NEC V19.19
      glaucoma V19.11
    genetic disease carrier V18.9
    genitourinary disease NEC V18.7
    glaucoma V19.11
    glomerulonephritis V18.69
    gout V18.19
    hay fever V17.6
    hearing loss V19.2
    hematopoietic neoplasia V16.7
    Hodgkin's disease V16.7
    Huntington's chorea V17.2
    hydrocephalus V19.5
    hypertension V17.49
    infarction, myocardial V17.3
    infectious disease V18.8
    intellectual disabilities V18.4
    ischemic heart disease V17.3
    kidney disease V18.69
      polycystic V18.61
    leukemia V16.6
    lymphatic malignant neoplasia NEC V16.7
    malignant neoplasm (of) NEC V16.9
      anorectal V16.0
      anus V16.0
      appendix V16.0
      bladder V16.52
      bone V16.8
      brain V16.8
      breast V16.3
        male V16.8
      bronchus V16.1
      cecum V16.0
      cervix V16.49
      colon V16.0
      duodenum V16.0
      esophagus V16.0
      eye V16.8
      gallbladder V16.0
      gastrointestinal tract V16.0
      genital organs V16.40
      hemopoietic NEC V16.7
      ileum V16.0
      ilium V16.8
      intestine V16.0
      intrathoracic organs NEC V16.2
      kidney V16.51
      larynx V16.2
      liver V16.0
      lung V16.1
      lymphatic NEC V16.7

History—*continued*
  family—*continued*
    malignant neoplasm—*continued*
      ovary V16.41
      oviduct V16.41
      pancreas V16.0
      penis V16.49
      prostate V16.42
      rectum V16.0
      respiratory organs NEC V16.2
      skin V16.8
      specified site NEC V16.8
      stomach V16.0
      testis V16.43
      trachea V16.1
      ureter V16.59
      urethra V16.59
      urinary organs V16.59
      uterus V16.49
      vagina V16.49
      vulva V16.49
    MEN (multiple endocrine neoplasia
      syndrome) V18.11
    mental retardation—see History, family,
      intellectual disabilities
    metabolic disease NEC V18.19
    mongolism V19.5
    multiple
      endocrine neoplasia (MEN) syndrome
        V18.11
      myeloma V16.7
    musculoskeletal disease NEC V17.89
      osteoporosis V17.81
    myocardial infarction V17.3
    nephritis V18.69
    nephrosis V18.69
    osteoporosis V17.81
    parasitic disease V18.8
    polycystic kidney disease V18.61
    psychiatric disorder V17.0
    psychosis V17.0
    retinitis pigmentosa V19.19
    schizophrenia V17.0
    skin conditions V19.4
    specified condition NEC V19.8
    stroke (cerebrovascular) V17.1
    sudden cardiac death (SCD) V17.41
    visual loss V19.0
  foreign body fully removed V15.53
  fracture, healed
    pathologic V13.51
    stress V13.52
    traumatic V15.51
  genital system disorder V13.29
    pre-term labor V13.21
  gestational diabetes V12.21
  health hazard V15.9
    falling V15.88
    specified cause NEC V15.89
  hepatitis
    B V12.09
    C V12.09
  Hodgkin's disease V10.72
  hypospadias (corrected) V13.61
  immunity disorder V12.29
  immunosuppression therapy V87.46
  infarction, cerebral, without residual deficits
    V12.54
  infection
    central nervous system V12.42
    urinary (tract) V13.02

History—*continued*
  infectious disease V12.00
    malaria V12.03
    methicillin resistant Staphylococcus aureus
      (MRSA) V12.04
    MRSA (methicillin resistant Staphylococcus
      aureus) V12.04
    poliomyelitis V12.02
    specified NEC V12.09
    tuberculosis V12.01
  injury NEC V15.59
    traumatic brain V15.52
  insufficient prenatal care V23.7
  in utero procedure
    during pregnancy V15.21
    while a fetus V15.22
  irradiation V15.3
  leukemia V10.60
    lymphoid V10.61
    monocytic V10.63
    myeloid V10.62
    specified type NEC V10.69
  little or no prenatal care V23.7
  low birth weight (*see also* Status, low birth
    weight) V21.30
  lymphosarcoma V10.71
  malaria V12.03
  malignant carcinoid tumor V10.91
  malignant neuroendocrine tumor V10.91
  malignant neoplasm (of) V10.90
    accessory sinus V10.22
    adrenal V10.88
    anus V10.06
    bile duct V10.09
    bladder V10.51
    bone V10.81
    brain V10.85
    breast V10.3
    bronchus V10.11
    cervix uteri V10.41
    colon V10.05
    connective tissue NEC V10.89
    corpus uteri V10.42
    digestive system V10.00
      specified part NEC V10.09
    duodenum V10.09
    endocrine gland NEC V10.88
    epididymis V10.48
    esophagus V10.03
    eye V10.84
    fallopian tube V10.44
    female genital organ V10.40
      specified site NEC V10.44
    gallbladder V10.09
    gastrointestinal tract V10.00
    gum V10.02
    hematopoietic NEC V10.79
    hypopharynx V10.02
    ileum V10.09
    intrathoracic organs NEC V10.20
    jejunum V10.09
    kidney V10.52
    large intestine V10.05
    larynx V10.21
    lip V10.02
    liver V10.07
    lung V10.11
    lymphatic NEC V10.79
    lymph glands or nodes NEC V10.79
    male genital organ V10.45
      specified site NEC V10.49

History—*continued*
  malignant neoplasm—*continued*
    mediastinum V10.29
    melanoma (of skin) V10.82
    middle ear V10.22
    mouth V10.02
      specified part NEC V10.02
    nasal cavities V10.22
    nasopharynx V10.02
    nervous system NEC V10.86
    nose V10.22
    oropharynx V10.02
    ovary V10.43
    pancreas V10.09
    parathyroid V10.88
    penis V10.49
    pharynx V10.02
    pineal V10.88
    pituitary V10.88
    placenta V10.44
    pleura V10.29
    prostate V10.46
    rectosigmoid junction V10.06
    rectum V10.06
    renal pelvis V10.53
    respiratory organs NEC V10.20
    salivary gland V10.02
    skin V10.83
      melanoma V10.82
    small intestine NEC V10.09
    soft tissue NEC V10.89
    specified site NEC V10.89
    stomach V10.04
    testis V10.47
    thymus V10.29
    thyroid V10.87
    tongue V10.01
    trachea V10.12
    ureter V10.59
    urethra V10.59
    urinary organ V10.50
    uterine adnexa V10.44
    uterus V10.42
    vagina V10.44
    vulva V10.44
  manic-depressive psychosis V11.1
  meningitis V12.42
  mental disorder V11.9
    affective type V11.1
    manic-depressive V11.1
    neurosis V11.2
    schizophrenia V11.0
    specified type NEC V11.8
  Merkel cell carcinoma V10.91
  metabolic disorder V12.29
  methicillin resistant Staphylococcus aureus
    (MRSA) V12.04
  MRSA (methicillin resistant Staphylococcus
    aureus) V12.04
  musculoskeletal disorder NEC V13.59
  myocardial infarction 412
  neglect (emotional) V15.42
  nephrotic syndrome V13.03
  nervous system disorder V12.40
    specified type NEC V12.49
  neurosis V11.2
  noncompliance with medical treatment V15.81
  nutritional deficiency V12.1

History—*continued*
  obstetric disorder V13.29
    affecting management of current pregnancy
      V23.49
      ectopic pregnancy 23.42
      pre-term labor V23.41
    pre-term labor V13.41
  parasitic disease V12.00
    specified NEC V12.09
  perinatal problems V13.7
    low birth weight (*see also* Status, low birth
      weight) V21.30
  physical abuse V15.41
  poisoning V15.6
  poliomyelitis V12.02
  polyps, colonic V12.72
  poor obstetric V23.49
    affecting management of current pregnancy
      V23.49
      ectopic pregnancy 23.42
      pre-term labor V23.41
    pre-term labor V13.41
  prolonged reversible ischemic neurologic
    deficits (PRIND) V12.54
  psychiatric disorder V11.9
    affective type V11.1
    manic-depressive V11.1
    neurosis V11.2
    schizophrenia V11.0
    specified type NEC V11.8
  psychological trauma V15.49
    emotional abuse V15.42
    neglect V15.42
    physical abuse V15.41
    rape V15.41
  psychoneurosis V11.2
  radiation therapy V15.3
  rape V15.41
  respiratory system disease V12.60
    pneumonia V12.61
    specified NEC V12.69
  reticulosarcoma V10.71
  return from military deployment V62.22
  reversible ischemic neurologic deficit (RIND)
    V12.54
  schizophrenia V11.0
  skin disease V13.3
  smoking (tobacco) V15.82
  steroid therapy V87.45
    inhaled V87.44
    systemic V87.45
  stroke without residual deficits V12.54
  subcutaneous tissue disease V13.3
  sudden
    cardiac
      arrest V12.53
      death (successfully resuscitated) V12.53
  surgery (to)
    great vessels V15.1
    heart V15.1
    in utero
      during pregnancy V15.21
      while a fetus V15.22
    organs NEC V15.29
  syndrome, nephrotic V13.03
  therapy
    antineoplastic drug V87.41
    drug NEC V87.49
    estrogen V87.43
    immunosuppression V87.46
    monoclonal drug V87.42

History—*continued*
  therapy—*continued*
    steroid V87.45
      inhaled V87.44
      systemic V87.45
    thrombophlebitis V12.52
    thrombosis V12.51
      pulmonary V12.55
    tobacco use V15.82
    trophoblastic disease V13.1
    affecting management of pregnancy V23.1
    tuberculosis V12.01
    ulcer, peptic V12.71
    urinary system disorder V13.00
      calculi V13.01
      infection V13.02
      nephrotic syndrome V13.03
      specified NEC V13.09
HIT (heparin-induced thrombocytopenia) 289.84
HIV infection (disease) (illness)—*see* Human
  immunodeficiency virus (disease) (illness)
  (infection)
Hives (bold) (*see also* Urticaria) 708.9
Hoarseness 784.42
Hobnail liver —*see* Cirrhosis, portal
Hobo, hoboism V60.0
Hodgkin's
  disease (M9650/3) 201.9
    lymphocytic
      depletion (M9653/3) 201.7
        diffuse fibrosis (M9654/3) 201.7
        reticular type (M9655/3) 201.7
      predominance (M9651/3) 201.4
      lymphocytic-histiocytic predominance
        (M9651/3) 201.4
      mixed cellularity (M9652/3) 201.6
      nodular sclerosis (M9656/3) 201.5
        cellular phase (M9657/3) 201.5
    granuloma (M9661/3) 201.1
    lymphogranulomatosis (M9650/3) 201.9
    lymphoma (M9650/3) 201.9
    lymphosarcoma (M9650/3) 201.9
    paragranuloma (M9660/3) 201.0
    sarcoma (M9662/3) 201.2
Hodgson's disease (aneurysmal dilatation of
  aorta) 441.9
  ruptured 441.5
Hodi-potsy 111.0
Hoffa -(Kastert) disease or syndrome
  (liposynovitis prepatellaris) 272.8
Hoffmann's syndrome 244.9 *[359.5]*
Hoffmann-Bouveret syndrome (paroxysmal
  tachycardia) 427.2
Hole
  macula 362.54
  optic disc, crater-like 377.22
  retina (macula) 362.54
    round 361.31
      with detachment 361.01
Holla disease (*see also* Spherocytosis) 282.0
Holländer-Simons syndrome (progressive
  lipodystrophy) 272.6
Hollow foot (congenital) 754.71
  acquired 736.73
Holmes' syndrome (visual disorientation) 368.16
Holoprosencephaly 742.2
  due to
    trisomy 13 758.1
    trisomy 18 758.2

Holthouse's hernia —*see* Hernia, inguinal
Homesickness 309.89
Homicidal ideation V62.85
Homocystinemia 270.4
Homocystinuria 270.4
Homologous serum jaundice (prophylactic)
  (therapeutic)—*see* Hepatitis, viral
Homosexuality —*omit code*
  ego-dystonic 302.0
  pedophilic 302.2
  problems with 302.0
Homozygous Hb-S disease 282.61
Honeycomb lung 518.89
  congenital 748.4
Hong Kong ear 117.3
HOOD (hereditary osteo-onychodysplasia) 756.89
Hooded
  clitoris 752.49
  penis 752.69
Hookworm (anemia) (disease) (infestation)—*see*
  Ancylostomiasis
Hoppe-Goldflam syndrome 358.00
Hordeolum (external) (eyelid) 373.11
  internal 373.12
Horn
  cutaneous 702.8
    cheek 702.8
    eyelid 702.8
    penis 702.8
  iliac 756.89
  nail 703.8
    congenital 757.5
  papillary 700
Horner's
  syndrome (*see also* Neuropathy, peripheral,
    autonomic) 337.9
    traumatic 954.0
  teeth 520.4
Horseshoe kidney (congenital) 753.3
Horton's
  disease (temporal arteritis) 446.5
  headache or neuralgia 339.00
Hospice care V66.7
Hospitalism (in children) NEC 309.83
Hourglass contraction, contracture
  bladder 596.89
  gallbladder 575.2
    congenital 751.69
  stomach 536.8
    congenital 750.7
    psychogenic 306.4
  uterus 661.4
    affecting fetus or newborn 763.7
Household circumstance affecting care V60.9
  specified type NEC V60.89
Housemaid's knee 727.2
Housing circumstance affecting care V60.9
  specified type NEC V60.89
HTLV-I infection 079.51
HTLV-II infection 079.52
HTLV-III (disease) (illness) (infection)—*see*
  Human immunodeficiency virus (disease)
  (illness) (infection)
HTLV-III/LAV
  (disease) (illness) (infection)—*see* Human
    immunodeficiency virus (disease) (illness)
    (infection)

HTR (hemolytic transfusion reaction)
due to or resulting from
  incompatibility
    ABO 999.61
      acute 999.62
      delayed 999.63
    non-ABO antigen (minor) (Duffy) (Kell)
      (Kidd) (Lewis) (M) (N) (P) (S) 999.76
      acute 999.77
      delayed 999.78
    Rh antigen (C) (c) (D) (E) (e) 999.71
      acture 999.72
      delayed 999.73
Huchard's disease (continued arterial
  hypertension) 401.9
Hudson-Stähli lines 371.11
Huguier's disease (uterine fibroma) 218.9
Hum, venous —*omit code*
Human bite (open wound)—*see also* Wound,
  open, by site
  intact skin surface—*see* Contusion
Human immunodeficiency virus (disease)
  (illness) 042
  infection V08
    with symptoms, symptomatic 042
Human immunodeficiency virus-2 infection
  079.53
Human immunovirus (disease) (illness)
  (infection)—*see* Human immunodeficiency
  virus (disease) (illness) (infection)
Human papillomavirus 079.4
  high risk, DNA test positive
    anal 796.75
    cervical 795.05
    vaginal 795.15
  low risk, DNA test positive
    anal 796.79
    cervical 795.09
    vaginal 795.19
Human parovirus 079.83
Human T-cell lymphotrophic virus I infection
  079.51
Human T-cell lymphotrophic virus II infection
  079.52
Human T-cell lymphotropic virus-III (disease)
  (illness) (infection)—*see* Human
  immunodeficiency virus (disease) (illness)
  (infection)
Hungry bone syndrome 275.5
Humpback (acquired) 737.9
  congenital 756.19
Hunchback (acquired) 737.9
  congenital 756.19
Hunger 994.2
  air, psychogenic 306.1
  disease 251.1
Hunner's ulcer (*see also* Cystitis) 595.1
Hunt's
  neuralgia 053.11
  syndrome (herpetic geniculate ganglionitis)
    053.11
    dyssynergia cerebellaris myoclonica 334.2
Hunter's glossitis 529.4
Hunter (-Hurler) syndrome
  (mucopolysaccharidosis II) 277.5
Hunterian chancre 091.0
Huntington's
  chorea 333.4
  disease 333.4
Huppert's disease (multiple myeloma)
  (M9730/3) 203.0

Hurler (-Hunter) disease or syndrome
  (mucopolysaccharidosis II) 277.5
Hürthle cell
  adenocarcinoma (M8290/3) 193
  adenoma (M8290/0) 226
  carcinoma (M8290/3) 193
  tumor (M8290/0) 226
Hutchinson's
  disease meaning
    angioma serpiginosum 709.1
    cheiropompholyx 705.81
    prurigo estivalis 692.72
    summer eruption, or summer prurigo 692.72
  incisors 090.5
  melanotic freckle (M8742/2)—*see also*
    Neoplasm, skin, in situ
    malignant melanoma in (M8742/3)—*see*
      Melanoma
  teeth or incisors (congenital syphilis) 090.5
Hutchinson-Boeck disease or syndrome
  (sarcoidosis) 135
Hutchinson-Gilford disease or syndrome
  (progeria) 259.8
Hyaline
  degeneration (diffuse) (generalized) 728.9
    localized—*see* Degeneration, by site
  membrane (disease) (lung) (newborn) 769
Hyalinosis cutis et mucosae 272.8
Hyalin plaque, sclera, senile 379.16
Hyalitis (asteroid) 379.22
  syphilitic 095.8
Hydatid
  cyst or tumor—*see also* Echinococcus
    fallopian tube 752.11
    mole—*see* Hydatidiform mole
    Morgagni (congenital) 752.89
      fallopian tube 752.11
Hydatidiform mole (benign) (complicating
  pregnancy) (delivered) (undelivered) 630
  invasive (M9100/1) 236.1
  malignant (M9100/1) 236.1
  previous, affecting management of pregnancy
    V23.1
Hydatidosis —*see* Echinococcus
Hyde's disease (prurigo nodularis) 698.3
Hydradenitis 705.83
Hydradenoma (M8400/0)—*see* Hidradenoma
Hydralazine lupus or syndrome
  correct substance properly administered 695.4
  overdose or wrong substance given or taken
    972.6
Hydramnios 657
  affecting fetus or newborn 761.3
Hydrancephaly 742.3
  with spina bifida (*see also* Spina bifida) 741.0
Hydranencephaly 742.3
  with spina bifida (*see also* Spina bifida) 741.0
Hydrargyrism NEC 985.0
Hydrarthrosis (*see also* Effusion, joint) 719.0
  gonococcal 098.50
  intermittent (*see also* Rheumatism, palindromic)
    719.3
  of yaws (early) (late) 102.6
  syphilitic 095.8
    congenital 090.5
Hydremia 285.9
Hydrencephalocele (congenital) 742.0
Hydrencephalomeningocele (congenital) 742.0

Hydroa 694.0
  aestivale 692.72
  gestationis 646.8
  herpetiformis 694.0
  pruriginosa 694.0
  vacciniforme 692.72
Hydroadenitis 705.83
Hydrocalycosis (*see also* Hydronephrosis) 591
  congenital 753.29
Hydrocalyx (*see also* Hydronephrosis) 591
Hydrocele (calcified) (chylous) (idiopathic)
    (infantile) (inguinal canal) (recurrent) (senile)
    (spermatic cord) (testis) (tunica vaginalis) 603.9
  canal of Nuck (female) 629.1
    male 603.9
  congenital 778.6
  encysted 603.0
    congenital 778.6
  female NEC 629.89
  infected 603.1
  round ligament 629.89
  specified type NEC 603.8
    congenital 778.6
  spinalis (*see also* Spina bifida) 741.9
  vulva 624.8
Hydrocephalic fetus
  affecting management of pregnancy 655.0
  causing disproportion 653.6
    with obstructed labor 660.1
      affecting fetus or newborn 763.1
Hydrocephalus (acquired) (external) (internal)
    (malignant) (noncommunicating) (obstructive)
    (recurrent) 331.4
  aqueduct of Sylvius stricture 742.3
    with spina bifida (*see also* Spina bifida) 741.0
  chronic 742.3
    with spina bifida (*see also* Spina bifida) 741.0
  communicating 331.3
  congenital (external) (internal) 742.3
    with spina bifida (*see also* Spina bifida) 741.0
  due to
    stricture of aqueduct of Sylvius 742.3
      with spina bifida (*see also* Spina bifida)
        741.0
    toxoplasmosis (congenital) 771.2
  fetal affecting management of pregnancy 655.0
  foramen Magendie block (acquired) 331.3
    congenital 742.3
      with spina bifida (*see also* Spina bifida)
        741.0
  newborn 742.3
    with spina bifida (*see also* Spina bifida) 741.0
  normal pressure 331.5
    idiopathic (INPH) 331.5
    secondary 331.3
  otitic 348.2
  syphilitic, congenital 090.49
  tuberculous (*see also* Tuberculosis) 013.8
Hydrocolpos (congenital) 623.8
Hydrocystoma (M8404/0)—*see* Neoplasm, skin,
    benign
Hydroencephalocele (congenital) 742.0
Hydroencephalomeningocele (congenital) 742.0
Hydrohematopneumothorax (*see also*
    Hemothorax) 511.89
Hydromeningitis —*see* Meningitis
Hydromeningocele (spinal) (*see also* Spina
    bifida) 741.9
  cranial 742.0
Hydrometra 621.8
Hydrometrocolpos 623.8

Hydromicrocephaly 742.1
Hydromphalus (congenital) (since birth) 757.39
Hydromyelia 742.53
Hydromyelocele (*see also* Spina bifida) 741.9
Hydronephrosis 591
  atrophic 591
  congenital 753.29
  due to S. hematobium 120.0
  early 591
  functionless (infected) 591
  infected 591
  intermittent 591
  primary 591
  secondary 591
  tuberculous (*see also* Tuberculosis) 016.0
Hydropericarditis (*see also* Pericarditis) 423.9
Hydropericardium (*see also* Pericarditis) 423.9
Hydroperitoneum 789.59
Hydrophobia 071
Hydrophthalmos (*see also* Buphthalmia) 743.20
Hydropneumohemothorax (*see also*
    Hemothorax) 511.89
Hydropneumopericarditis (*see also* Pericarditis)
    423.9
Hydropneumopericardium (*see also*
    Pericarditis) 423.9
Hydropneumothorax 511.89
  nontuberculous 511.89
    bacterial 511.1
  pneumococcal 511.1
  staphylococcal 511.1
  streptococcal 511.1
  traumatic 860.0
    with open wound into thorax 860.1
  tuberculous (*see also* Tuberculosis, pleural) 012.0
Hydrops 782.3
  abdominis 789.59
  amnii (complicating pregnancy) (*see also*
    Hydramnios) 657
  articulorum intermittens (*see also* Rheumatism,
    palindromic) 719.3
  cardiac (*see also* Failure, heart) 428.0
  congenital—*see* Hydrops, fetalis
  endolymphatic (*see also* Disease, Ménière's)
    386.00
  fetal, fetalis or newborn 778.0
    due to
      alpha thalassemia 282.43
      isoimmunization 773.3
    not due to isoimmunization 778.0
  gallbladder 575.3
  idiopathic (fetus or newborn) 778.0
  joint (*see also* Effusion, joint) 719.0
  labyrinth (*see also* Disease, Ménière's) 386.00
  meningeal NEC 331.4
  nutritional 262
  pericardium—*see* Pericarditis
  pleura (*see also* Hydrothorax) 511.89
  renal (*see also* Nephrosis) 581.9
  spermatic cord (*see also* Hydrocele) 603.9
Hydropyonephrosis (*see also* Pyelitis) 590.80
  chronic 590.00
Hydrorachis 742.53
Hydrorrhea (nasal) 478.19
  gravidarum 658.1
  pregnancy 658.1
Hydrosadenitis 705.83
Hydrosalpinx (fallopian tube) (follicularis) 614.1

Hydrothorax (double) (pleural) 511.89
  chylous (nonfilarial) 457.8
    filaria (*see also* Infestation, filarial) 125.9
  nontuberculous 511.89
    bacterial 511.1
  pneumococcal 511.1
  staphylococcal 511.1
  streptococcal 511.1
  traumatic 862.29
    with open wound into thorax 862.39
  tuberculous (*see also* Tuberculosis, pleura) 012.0
Hydroureter 593.5
  congenital 753.22
Hydroureteronephrosis (*see also*
    Hydronephrosis) 591
Hydrourethra 599.84
Hydroxykynureninuria 270.2
Hydroxyprolinemia 270.8
Hydroxyprolinuria 270.8
Hygroma (congenital) (cystic) (M9173/0) 228.1
  prepatellar 727.3
  subdural—*see* Hematoma, subdural
Hymen —*see* condition
Hymenolepiasis (diminuta) (infection)
    (infestation) (nana) 123.6
Hymenolepis (diminuta) (infection) (infestation)
    (nana) 123.6
Hypalgesia (*see also* Disturbance, sensation)
    782.0
Hyperabduction syndrome 447.8
Hyperacidity, gastric 536.8
  psychogenic 306.4
Hyperactive, hyperactivity 314.01
  basal cell, uterine cervix 622.10
  bladder 596.51
  bowel (syndrome) 564.9
    sounds 787.5
  cervix epithelial (basal) 622.10
  child 314.01
  colon 564.9
  gastrointestinal 536.8
    psychogenic 306.4
  intestine 564.9
  labyrinth (unilateral) 386.51
    with loss of labyrinthine reactivity 386.58
    bilateral 386.52
  nasal mucous membrane 478.19
  stomach 536.8
  thyroid (gland) (*see also* Thyrotoxicosis) 242.9
Hyperacusis 388.42
Hyperadrenalism (cortical) 255.3
  medullary 255.6
Hyperadrenocorticism 255.3
  congenital 255.2
  iatrogenic
    correct substance properly administered 255.3
    overdose or wrong substance given or taken 962.0
Hyperaffectivity 301.11
Hyperaldosteronism (atypical) (hyperplastic)
    (normoaldosteronal) (normotensive) (primary)
    255.10
  secondary 255.14
Hyperalgesia (*see also* Disturbance, sensation)
    782.0
Hyperalimentation 783.6
  carotene 278.3
  specified NEC 278.8
  vitamin A 278.2
  vitamin D 278.4

Hyperaminoaciduria 270.9
  arginine 270.6
  citrulline 270.6
  cystine 270.0
  glycine 270.0
  lysine 270.7
  ornithine 270.6
  renal (types I, II, III) 270.0
Hyperammonemia (congenital) 270.6
Hyperamnesia 780.99
Hyperamylasemia 790.5
Hyperaphia 782.0
Hyperazotemia 791.9
Hyperbetalipoproteinemia (acquired) (essential)
    (familial) (hereditary) (primary) (secondary)
    272.0
  with pre-betalipoproteinemia 272.2
Hyperbilirubinemia 782.4
  congenital 277.4
  constitutional 277.4
  neonatal (transient) (*see also* Jaundice, fetus or
    newborn) 774.6
  of prematurity 774.2
Hyperbilirubinemica encephalopathia,
  newborn 774.7
  due to isoimmunization 773.4
Hypercalcemia, hypercalcemic (idiopathic) 275.42
  nephropathy 588.89
Hypercalcinuria 275.40
Hypercapnia 786.09
  with mixed acid-base disorder 276.4
  fetal, affecting newborn 770.89
Hypercarotinemia 278.3
Hypercementosis 521.5
Hyperchloremia 276.9
Hyperchlorhydria 536.8
  neurotic 306.4
  psychogenic 306.4
Hypercholesterinemia —*see*
    Hypercholesterolemia
Hypercholesterolemia 272.0
  with hyperglyceridemia, endogenous 272.2
  essential 272.0
  familial 272.0
  hereditary 272.0
  primary 272.0
  pure 272.0
Hypercholesterolosis 272.0
Hyperchylia gastricsa 536.8
  psychogenic 306.4
Hyperchylomicronemia (familial) (with
    hyperbetalipoproteinemia) 272.3
Hypercoagulation syndrome (primary) 289.81
  secondary 289.82
Hypercorticosteronism
  correct substance properly administered 255.3
  overdose or wrong substance given or taken
    962.0
Hypercortisonism
  correct substance properly administered 255.3
  overdose or wrong substance given or taken
    962.0
Hyperdynamic beta-adrenergic state or
  syndrome (circulatory) 429.82
Hyperekplexia 759.89
Hyperelectrolytemia 276.9

Hyperemesis 536.2
arising during pregnancy—*see* Hyperemesis, gravidarum
gravidarum (mild) (before 22 completed weeks gestation) 643.0
with
carbohydrate depletion 643.1
dehydration 643.1
electrolyte imbalance 643.1
metabolic disturbance 643.1
affecting fetus or newborn 761.8
severe (with metabolic disturbance) 643.1
psychogenic 306.4
Hyperemia (acute) 780.99
anal mucosa 569.49
bladder 596.7
cerebral 437.8
conjunctiva 372.71
ear, internal, acute 386.30
enteric 564.89
eye 372.71
eyelid (active) (passive) 374.82
intestine 564.89
iris 364.41
kidney 593.81
labyrinth 386.30
liver (active) (passive) 573.8
lung 514
ovary 620.8
passive 780.99
pulmonary 514
renal 593.81
retina 362.89
spleen 289.59
stomach 537.89
Hyperesthesia (body surface) (*see also* Disturbance, sensation) 782.0
larynx (reflex) 478.79
hysterical 300.11
pharynx (reflex) 478.29
Hyperestrinism 256.0
Hyperestrogenism 256.0
Hyperestrogenosis 256.0
Hyperexplexia 759.89
Hyperextension, joint 718.80
ankle 718.87
elbow 718.82
foot 718.87
hand 718.84
hip 718.85
knee 718.86
multiple sites 718.89
pelvic region 718.85
shoulder (region) 718.81
specified site NEC 718.88
wrist 718.83
Hyperfibrinolysis —*see* Fibrinolysis
Hyperfolliculinism 256.0
Hyperfructosemia 271.2
Hyperfunction
adrenal (cortex) 255.3
androgenic, acquired benign 255.3
medulla 255.6
virilism 255.2
corticoadrenal NEC 255.3
labyrinth—*see* Hyperactive, labyrinth
medulloadrenal 255.6
ovary 256.1
estrogen 256.0
pancreas 577.8
parathyroid (gland) 252.00

Hyperfunction—*continued*
pituitary (anterior) (gland) (lobe) 253.1
testicular 257.0
Hypergammaglobulinemia 289.89
monoclonal, benign (BMH) 273.1
polyclonal 273.0
Waldenström's 273.0
Hyperglobulinemia 273.8
Hyperglycemia 790.29
maternal
affecting fetus or newborn 775.0
manifest diabetes in infant 775.1
postpancreatectomy (complete) (partial) 251.3
Hyperglyceridemia 272.1
endogenous 272.1
essential 272.1
familial 272.1
hereditary 272.1
mixed 272.3
pure 272.1
Hyperglycinemia 270.7
Hypergonadism
ovarian 256.1
testicular (infantile) (primary) 257.0
Hyperheparinemia (*see also* Circulating, intrinsic anticoagulants) 287.5
Hyperhidrosis, hyperidrosis 705.21
axilla 705.21
face 705.21
focal (localized) 705.21
primary 705.21
axilla 705.21
face 705.21
palms 705.21
soles 705.21
secondary 705.22
axilla 705.22
face 705.22
palms 705.22
soles 705.22
generalized 780.8
palms 705.21
psychogenic 306.3
secondary 780.8
soles 705.21
Hyperhistidinemia 270.5
Hyperinsulinism (ectopic) (functional) (organic) NEC 251.1
iatrogenic 251.0
reactive 251.2
spontaneous 251.2
therapeutic misadventure (from administration of insulin) 962.3
Hyperiodemia 276.9
Hyperirritability (cerebral), in newborn 779.1
Hyperkalemia 276.7
Hyperkeratosis (*see also* Keratosis) 701.1
cervix 622.2
congenital 757.39
cornea 371.89
due to yaws (early) (late) (palmar or plantar) 102.3
eccentrica 757.39
figurata centrifuga atrophica 757.39
follicularis 757.39
in cutem penetrans 701.1
limbic (cornea) 371.89
palmoplantaris climacterica 701.1
pinta (carate) 103.1
senile (with pruritus) 702.0
tongue 528.79
universalis congenita 757.1

Hyperkeratosis—*continued*
vagina 623.1
vocal cord 478.5
vulva 624.09
Hyperkinesia, hyperkinetic (disease) (reaction)
(syndrome) 314.9
with
attention deficit —*see* Disorder, attention deficit
conduct disorder 314.2
developmental delay 314.1
simple disturbance of activity and attention
314.01
specified manifestation NEC 314.8
heart (disease) 429.82
of childhood or adolescence NEC 314.9
Hyperlacrimation (*see also* Epiphora) 375.20
Hyperlipemia (*see also* Hyperlipidemia) 272.4
Hyperlipidemia 272.4
carbohydrate-induced 272.1
combined 272.2
endogenous 272.1
exogenous 272.3
fat-induced 272.3
group
A 272.0
B 272.1
C 272.2
D 272.3
mixed 272.2
specified type NEC 272.4
Hyperlipidosis 272.7
hereditary 272.7
Hyperlipoproteinemia (acquired) (essential)
(familial) (hereditary) (primary) (secondary)
272.4
Fredrickson type
I 272.3
IIa 272.0
IIb 272.2
III 272.2
IV 272.1
V 272.3
low-density-lipoid-type (LDL) 272.0
very-low-density-lipoid-type [VLDL] 272.1
Hyperlucent lung, unilateral 492.8
Hyperluteinization 256.1
Hyperlysinemia 270.7
Hypermagnesemia 275.2
neonatal 775.5
Hypermaturity (fetus or newborn)
post-term infant 766.21
prolonged gestation infant 766.22
Hypermenorrhea 626.2
Hypermetabolism 794.7
Hypermethioninemia 270.4
Hypermetropia (congenital) 367.0
Hypermobility
cecum 564.9
coccyx 724.71
colon 564.9
psychogenic 306.4
ileum 564.89
joint (acquired) 718.80
ankle 718.87
elbow 718.82
foot 718.87
hand 718.84
hip 718.85
knee 718.86
multiple sites 718.89

Hypermobility—*continued*
pelvic region 718.85
shoulder (region) 718.81
specified site NEC 718.88
wrist 718.83
kidney, congenital 753.3
meniscus (knee) 717.5
scapula 718.81
stomach 536.8
psychogenic 306.4
syndrome 728.5
testis, congenital 752.52
urethral 599.81
Hypermotility
gastrointestinal 536.8
intestine 564.9
psychogenic 306.4
stomach 536.8
Hypernasality 784.43
Hypernatremia 276.0
with water depletion 276.0
Hypernephroma (M8312/3) 189.0
Hyperopia 367.0
Hyperorexia 783.6
Hyperornithinemia 270.6
Hyperosmia (*see also* Disturbance, sensation)
781.1
Hyperosmolality 276.0
Hyperosteogenesis 733.99
Hyperostosis 733.99
calvarial 733.3
cortical 733.3
infantile 756.59
frontal, internal of skull 733.3
interna frontalis 733.3
monomelic 733.99
skull 733.3
congenital 756.0
vertebral 721.8
with spondylosis—*see* Spondylosis
ankylosing 721.6
Hyperovarianism 256.1
Hyperovarism, hyperovaria 256.1
Hyperoxaluria (primary) 271.8
Hyperoxia 987.8
Hyperparathyroidism 252.00
ectopic 259.3
other 252.08
primary 252.01
secondary (of renal origin) 588.81
non-renal 252.02
tertiary 252.08
Hyperpathia (*see also* Disturbance, sensation)
782.0
psychogenic 307.80
Hyperperistalsis 787.4
psychogenic 306.4
Hyperpermeability, capillary 448.9
Hyperphagia 783.6
Hyperphenylalaninemia 270.1
Hyperphoria 378.40
alternating 378.45
Hyperphosphatemia 275.3
Hyperpiesia (*see also* Hypertension) 401.9
Hyperpiesis (*see also* Hypertension) 401.9
Hyperpigmentation —*see* Pigmentation
Hyperpinealism 259.8
Hyperpipecolatemia 270.7
Hyperpituitarism 253.1

Hyperplasia, hyperplastic
  adenoids (lymphoid tissue) 474.12
    and tonsils 474.10
  adrenal (capsule) (cortex) (gland) 255.8
    with
      sexual precocity (male) 255.2
      virilism, adrenal 255.2
      virilization (female) 255.2
    congenital 255.2
    due to excess ACTH (ectopic) (pituitary) 255.0
    medulla 255.8
  alpha cells (pancreatic)
    with
      gastrin excess 251.5
      glucagon excess 251.4
  angiolymphoid, with eosinophilia (ALHE)
      228.01
  appendix (lymphoid) 543.0
  artery, fibromuscular NEC 447.8
    carotid 447.8
    renal 447.3
  bone 733.99
    marrow 289.9
  breast (see also Hypertrophy, breast) 611.1
    ductal 610.8
      atypical 610.8
  carotid artery 447.8
  cementation, cementum (teeth) (tooth) 521.5
  cervical gland 785.6
  cervix (uteri) 622.10
    basal cell 622.10
    congenital 752.49
    endometrium 622.10
    polypoid 622.10
  chin 524.05
  clitoris, congenital 752.49
  dentin 521.5
  endocervicitis 616.0
  endometrium, endometrial (adenomatous)
      (atypical) (cystic) (glandular) (polypoid)
      (uterus) 621.30
    with atypia 621.33
    without atypia
      complex 621.32
      simple 621.31
    benign 621.34
    cervix 622.10
  epithelial 709.8
    focal, oral, including tongue 528.79
    mouth (focal) 528.79
    nipple 611.89
    skin 709.8
    tongue (focal) 528.79
    vaginal wall 623.0
  erythroid 289.9
  fascialis ossificans (progressiva) 728.11
  fibromuscular, artery NEC 447.8
    carotid 447.8
    renal 447.3
  genital
    female 629.89
    male 608.89
  gingiva 523.8
  glandularis
    cystica uteri 621.30
    endometrium (uterus) 621.30
    interstitialis uteri 621.30
  granulocytic 288.69
  gum 523.8
  hymen, congenital 752.49
  islands of Langerhans 251.1

Hyperplasia, hyperplastic—*continued*
  islet cell (pancreatic) 251.9
    alpha cells
      with excess
        gastrin 251.5
        glucagon 251.4
    beta cells 251.1
  juxtaglomerular (complex) (kidney) 593.89
  kidney (congenital) 753.3
  liver (congenital) 751.69
  lymph node (gland) 785.6
  lymphoid (diffuse) (nodular) 785.6
    appendix 543.0
    intestine 569.89
  mandibular 524.02
    alveolar 524.72
    unilateral condylar 526.89
  Marchand multiple nodular (liver)—*see*
      Cirrhosis, postnecrotic
  maxillary 524.01
    alveolar 524.71
  medulla, adrenal 255.8
  myometrium, myometrial 621.2
  neuroendocrine cell, of infancy 516.61
  nose (lymphoid) (polypoid) 478.19
  oral soft tissue (inflammatory) (irritative)
      (mucosa) NEC 528.9
    gingiva 523.8
    tongue 529.8
  organ or site, congenital NEC—*see* Anomaly,
      specified type NEC
  ovary 620.8
  palate, papillary 528.9
  pancreatic islet cells 251.9
    alpha
      with excess
        gastrin 251.5
        glucagon 251.4
    beta 251.1
  parathyroid (gland) 252.01
  persistent, vitreous (primary) 743.51
  pharynx (lymphoid) 478.29
  prostate 600.90
    with
      other lower urinary tract symptoms (LUTS)
        600.91
      urinary
        obstruction 600.91
        retention 600.91
    adenofibromatous 600.20
      with
        other lower urinary tract symptoms
          (LUTS) 600.21
        urinary
          obstruction 600.21
          retention 600.21
    nodular 600.10
      with
        urinary
          obstruction 600.11
          retention 600.11
  renal artery (fibromuscular) 447.3
  reticuloendothelial (cell) 289.9
  salivary gland (any) 527.1
  Schimmelbusch's 610.1
  suprarenal (capsule) (gland) 255.8
  thymus (gland) (persistent) 254.0
  thyroid (see also Goiter) 240.9
    primary 242.0
    secondary 242.2

Hyperplasia, hyperplastic—*continued*
  tonsil (lymphoid tissue) 474.11
    and adenoids 474.10
  urethrovaginal 599.89
  uterus, uterine (myometrium) 621.2
    endometrium (*see also* Hyperplasia,
      endometrium) 621.30
  vitreous (humor), primary persistent 743.51
  vulva 624.3
  zygoma 738.11
Hyperpnea (*see also* Hyperventilation) 786.01
Hyperpotassemia 276.7
Hyperprebetalipoproteinemia 272.1
  with chylomicronemia 272.3
  familial 272.1
Hyperprolactinemia 253.1
Hyperprolinemia 270.8
Hyperproteinemia 273.8
Hyperprothrombinemia 289.89
Hyperpselaphesia 782.0
Hyperpyrexia 780.60
  heat (effects of) 992.0
  malarial (*see also* Malaria) 084.6
  malignant, due to anesthetic 995.86
  rheumatic—*see* Fever, rheumatic
  unknown origin (*see also* Pyrexia) 780.60
Hyperreactor, vascular 780.2
Hyperreflexia 796.1
  bladder, autonomic 596.54
    with cauda equina 344.61
  detrusor 344.61
Hypersalivation (*see also* Ptyalism) 527.7
Hypersarcosinemia 270.8
Hypersecretion
  ACTH 255.3
  androgens (ovarian) 256.1
  calcitonin 246.0
  corticoadrenal 255.3
  cortisol 255.0
  estrogen 256.0
  gastric 536.8
    psychogenic 306.4
  gastrin 251.5
  glucagon 251.4
  hormone
    ACTH 255.3
    anterior pituitary 253.1
    growth NEC 253.0
    ovarian androgen 256.1
    testicular 257.0
    thyroid stimulating 242.8
  insulin—*see* Hyperinsulinism
  lacrimal glands (*see also* Epiphora) 375.20
  medulloadrenal 255.6
  milk 676.6
  ovarian androgens 256.1
  pituitary (anterior) 253.1
  salivary gland (any) 527.7
  testicular hormones 257.0
  thyrocalcitonin 246.0
  upper respiratory 478.9
Hypersegmentation, hereditary 288.2
  eosinophils 288.2
  neutrophil nuclei 288.2
Hypersensitive, hypersensitiveness,
  hypersensitivity —*see also* Allergy
  angiitis 446.20
    specified NEC 446.29
  carotid sinus 337.01
  colon 564.9
    psychogenic 306.4

Hypersensitive, hypersensitivity—*continued*
  DNA (deoxyribonucleic acid) NEC 287.2
  drug (*see also* Allergy, drug) 995.27
  due to correct medicinal substance properly
    administered 995.27
  esophagus 530.89
  insect bites—*see* Injury, superficial, by site
  labyrinth 386.58
  pain (*see also* Disturbance, sensation) 782.0
  pneumonitis NEC 495.9
  reaction (*see also* Allergy) 995.3
    upper respiratory tract NEC 478.8
  stomach (allergic) (nonallergic) 536.8
    psychogenic 306.4
Hypersomatotropism (classic) 253.0
Hypersomnia, unspecified 780.54
  with sleep apnea, unspecified 780.53
  alcohol induced 291.82
  drug induced 291.85
  due to
    medical condition classified elsewhere 327.14
    mental disorder 327.15
  idiopathic
    with long sleep time 327.11
    without long sleep time 327.12
  menstrual related 327.13
  nonorganic origin 307.43
    persistent (primary) 307.44
    transient 307.43
  organic 327.10
    other 327.19
  primary 307.44
  recurrent 327.13
Hypersplenia 289.4
Hypersplenism 289.4
Hypersteatosis 706.3
Hyperstimulation, ovarian 256.1
Hypersuprarenalism 255.3
Hypersusceptibility —*see* Allergy
Hyper-TBG-nemia 246.8
Hypertelorism 756.0
  orbit, orbital 376.41

"H" listing resumes after
Hypertension table...

Hypertension, hypertensive

	Malignant	Benign	Unspecified
(arterial) (arteriolar) (crisis) (degeneration) (disease) (essential) (fluctuating) (idiopathic) (intermittent) (labile) (low renin) (orthostatic) (paroxysmal) (primary) (systemic) (uncontrolled) (vascular)	401.0	401.1	401.9
with			
chronic kidney disease			
stage I through stage IV, or unspecified	403.00	403.10	403.90
stage V or end stage renal disease	403.01	403.11	403.91
heart involvement (conditions classifiable to 429.0-429.3, 429.8, 429.9 due to hypertension) (see also Hypertension, heart)	402.00	402.10	402.90
with kidney involvement—see Hypertension, cardiorenal			
renal (kidney) involvement (only conditions classifiable to 585, 587) (excludes conditions classifiable to 584) (see also Hypertension, kidney)	403.00	403.10	403.90
with heart involvement—see Hypertension, cardiorenal			
failure (and sclerosis) (see also Hypertension, kidney) . .	403.01	403.11	403.91
sclerosis without failure (see also Hypertension, kidney) .	403.00	403.10	403.90
accelerated (see also Hypertension, by type, malignant)	401.0	—	—
antepartum—see Hypertension complicating pregnancy, childbirth, or the puerperium			
borderline	—	—	796.2
cardiorenal (disease)	404.00	404.10	404.90
with			
chronic kidney disease			
stage I through stage IV, or unspecified	404.00	404.10	404.90
and heart failure	404.01	404.11	404.91
stage V or end stage renal disease	404.02	404.12	404.92
and heart failure	404.03	404.13	404.93
heart failure.	404.01	404.11	404.91
and chronic kidney disease.	404.01	404.11	404.91
stage I through stage IV or unspecified	404.01	404.11	404.91
stage V or end stage renal disease	404.03	404.13	404.93
cardiovascular disease (arteriosclerotic) (sclerotic)	402.00	402.10	402.90
with			
heart failure.	402.01	402.11	402.91
renal involvement (conditions classifiable to 403) (see also Hypertension, cardiorenal)	404.00	404.10	404.90
cardiovascular renal (disease) (sclerosis) (see also Hypertension cardiorenal)	404.00	404.10	404.90
cerebrovascular disease NEC	437.2	437.2	437.2
complicating pregnancy, childbirth, or the puerperium	642.2	642.0	642.9
with			
albuminuria (and edema) (mild)	—	—	642.4
severe			642.5
chronic kidney disease	642.2	642.2	642.2
and heart disease	642.2	642.2	642.2
edema (mild)	—	—	642.4
severe	—	—	642.5
heart disease	642.2	642.2	642.2
and chronic kidney disease.	642.2	642.2	642.2
renal disease	642.2	642.2	642.2
and heart disease	642.2	642.2	642.2
chronic	642.2	642.0	642.0
with pre-eclampsia or eclampsia	642.7	642.7	642.7
fetus or newborn	760.0	760.0	760.0
essential.	—	642.0	642.0
with pre-eclampsia or eclampsia	—	642.7	642.7
fetus or newborn	760.0	760.0	760.0
fetus or newborn	760.0	760.0	760.0
gestational	—	—	642.3
pre-existing	642.2	642.0	642.0
with pre-eclampsia or eclampsia	642.7	642.7	642.7
fetus or newborn	760.0	760.0	760.0
secondary to renal disease	642.1	642.1	642.1
with pre-eclampsia or eclampsia	642.7	642.7	642.7
fetus or newborn	760.0	760.0	760.0
transient.	—	—	642.3
due to			
aldosteronism, primary.	405.09	405.19	405.99
brain tumor.	405.09	405.19	405.99
bulbar poliomyelitis	405.09	405.19	405.99
calculus			
kidney	405.09	405.19	405.99
ureter.	405.09	405.19	405.99
coarctation, aorta.	405.09	405.19	405.99
Cushing's disease	405.09	405.19	405.99

	Malignant	Benign	Unspecified
glomerulosclerosis (*see also* Hypertension, kidney)	403.00	403.10	403.90
periarteritis nodosa	405.09	405.19	405.99
pheochromocytoma.	405.09	405.19	405.99
polycystic kidney(s)	405.09	405.19	405.99
polycythemia	405.09	405.19	405.99
porphyria	405.09	405.19	405.99
pyelonephritis	405.09	405.19	405.99
renal (artery)			
aneurysm	405.01	405.11	405.91
anomaly	405.01	405.11	405.91
embolism	405.01	405.11	405.91
fibromuscular hyperplasia	405.01	405.11	405.91
occlusion	405.01	405.11	405.91
stenosis	405.01	405.11	405.91
thrombosis	405.01	405.11	405.91
encephalopathy	437.2	437.2	437.2
gestational (transient) NEC	—	—	642.3
Goldblatt's	440.1	440.1	440.1
heart (disease) (conditions classifiable to 429.0-429.3, 429.8, 429.9 due to hypertension)	402.00	402.10	402.90
with			
heart failure.	402.01	402.11	402.91
hypertensive kidney disease (conditions classifiable to 403) (*see also* Hypertension, cardiorenal)	404.00	404.10	404.90
renal sclerosis (*see also* Hypertension, cardiorenal)	404.00	404.10	404.90
intracranial, benign	—	348.2	—
intraocular.	—	—	365.04
kidney.	403.00	403.10	403.90
with			
chronic kidney disease			
stage I through stage IV, or unspecified	403.00	403.10	403.90
stage V or end stage renal disease	403.01	403.11	403.91
heart involvement (conditions classifiable to 429.0-429.3, 429.8, 429.9 due to hypertension) (*see also* Hypertension cardiorenal)	404.00	404.10	404.90
hypertensive heart (disease) (conditions classifiable to 402) (*see also* Hypertension, cardiorenal)	404.00	404.10	404.90
lesser circulation	—	—	416.0
necrotizing	401.0	—	—
ocular	—	—	365.04
pancreatic duct—code to underlying condition			
with chronic pancreatitis	—	—	577.1
portal (due to chronic liver disease)	—	—	572.3
postoperative	—	—	997.91
psychogenic	—	—	306.2
puerperal, postpartum—*see* Hypertension, complicating pregnancy, childbirth, or the puerperium			
pulmonary (artery) (secondary)	—	—	416.8
idiopathic	—	—	416.0
primary	—	—	416.0
of newborn	—	—	747.83
with			
cor pulmonale (chronic)	—	—	416.8
acute	—	—	415.0
right heart ventricular strain/failure	—	—	416.8
acute	—	—	415.0
secondary	—	—	416.8
renal (disease) (*see also* Hypertension, kidney).	403.00	403.10	403.90
renovascular NEC.	405.01	405.11	405.91
secondary NEC	405.09	405.19	405.99
due to			
aldosteronism, primary	405.09	405.19	405.99
brain tumor	405.09	405.19	405.99
bulbar poliomyelitis	405.09	405.19	405.99
calculus			
kidney	405.09	405.19	405.99
ureter.	405.09	405.19	405.99
coarctation, aorta	405.09	405.19	405.99
Cushing's disease	405.09	405.19	405.99
glomerulosclerosis (*see also* Hypertension, kidney)	403.00	403.10	403.90
periarteritis nodosa	405.09	405.19	405.99
pheochromocytoma.	405.09	405.19	405.99
polycystic kidney(s)	405.09	405.19	405.99
polycythemia	405.09	405.19	405.99
porphyria	405.09	405.19	405.99
pyelonephritis	405.09	405.19	405.99
renal (artery)			
aneurysm	405.01	405.11	405.91
anomaly	405.01	405.11	405.91

	Malignant	Benign	Unspecified
embolism	405.01	405.11	405.91
fibromuscular hyperplasia	405.01	405.11	405.91
occlusion	405.01	405.11	405.91
stenosis	405.01	405.11	405.91
thrombosis	405.01	405.11	405.91
transient	—	—	796.2
of pregnancy	—	—	642.3
venous, chronic (asymptomatic) (idiopathic)	—	—	459.30
with			
complication, NEC	—	—	459.39
due to			
deep vein thrombosis (see also Syndrome, postphlebetic)	—	—	459.10
inflammation	—	—	459.32
with ulcer	—	—	459.33
ulcer	—	—	459.31
with inflammation	—	—	459.33

Hypertensive urgency —*see* Hypertension
Hyperthecosis, ovary 256.8
Hyperthermia (of unknown origin) (*see also* Pyrexia) 780.60
  malignant (due to anesthesia) 995.86
  newborn 778.4
Hyperthymergasia (*see also* Psychosis, affective) 296.0
  reactive (from emotional stress, psychological trauma) 298.1
  recurrent episode 296.1
  single episode 296.0
Hyperthymism 254.8
Hyperthyroid (recurrent)—*see* Hyperthyroidism
Hyperthyroidism (latent) (preadult) (recurrent) (without goiter) 242.9

Note—Use the following fifth-digit subclassification with category 242:

0 without mention of thyrotoxic crisis or storm
1 with mention of thyrotoxic crisis or storm

---

  with
    goiter (diffuse) 242.0
      adenomatous 242.3
        multinodular 242.2
        uninodular 242.1
      nodular 242.3
        multinodular 242.2
        uninodular 242.1
      thyroid nodule 242.1
  complicating pregnancy, childbirth, or puerperium 648.1
  neonatal (transient) 775.3
Hypertonia —Hypertonicity
Hypertonicity
  bladder 596.51
  fetus or newborn 779.89
  gastrointestinal (tract) 536.8
  infancy 779.89
    due to electrolyte imbalance 779.89
  muscle 728.85
  stomach 536.8
    psychogenic 306.4
  uterus, uterine (contractions) 661.4
    affecting fetus or newborn 763.7
Hypertony —*see* Hypertonicity
Hypertransaminemia 790.4
Hypertrichosis 704.1
  congenital 757.4
  eyelid 374.54
  lanuginosa 757.4
    acquired 704.1
Hypertriglyceridemia, essential 272.1
Hypertrophy, hypertrophic
  adenoids (infectional) 474.12
    and tonsils (faucial) (infective) (lingual) (lymphoid) 474.10
  adrenal 255.8
  alveolar process or ridge 525.8
  anal papillae 569.49
  apocrine gland 705.82
  artery NEC 447.8
    carotid 447.8
    congenital (peripheral) NEC 747.60
    gastrointestinal 747.61
    lower limb 747.64
    renal 747.62
    specified NEC 747.69
    spinal 747.82

Hypertrophy, hypertrophic—*continued*
  arthritis (chronic) (*see also* Osteoarthrosis) 715.9
    spine (*see also* Spondylosis) 721.90
  arytenoid 478.79
  asymmetrical (heart) 429.9
  auricular—*see* Hypertrophy, cardiac
  Bartholin's gland 624.8
  bile duct 576.8
  bladder (sphincter) (trigone) 596.89
  blind spot, visual field 368.42
  bone 733.99
  brain 348.89
  breast 611.1
    cystic 610.1
    fetus or newborn 778.7
    fibrocystic 610.1
    massive pubertal 611.1
    puerperal, postpartum 676.3
    senile (parenchymatous) 611.1
  cardiac (chronic) (idiopathic) 429.3
    with
      rheumatic fever (conditions classifiable to 390)
        active 391.8
          with chorea 392.0
        inactive or quiescent (with chorea) 398.99
    congenital NEC 746.89
    fatty (*see also* Degeneration, myocardial) 429.1
    hypertensive (*see also* Hypertension, heart) 402.90
    rheumatic (with chorea) 398.99
      active or acute 391.8
        with chorea 392.0
    valve (*see also* Endocarditis) 424.90
      congenital NEC 746.89
  cartilage 733.99
  cecum 569.89
  cervix (uteri) 622.6
    congenital 752.49
    elongation 622.6
  clitoris (cirrhotic) 624.2
    congenital 752.49
  colon 569.89
    congenital 751.3
  conjunctiva, lymphoid 372.73
  cornea 371.89
  corpora cavernosa 607.89
  duodenum 537.89
  endometrium (uterus) (*see also* Hyperplasia, endometrium) 621.30
    cervix 622.6
  epididymis 608.89
  esophageal hiatus (congenital) 756.6
    with hernia—*see* Hernia, diaphragm
  eyelid 374.30
  falx, skull 733.99
  fat pad 729.30
    infrapatellar 729.31
    knee 729.31
    orbital 374.34
    popliteal 729.31
    prepatellar 729.31
    retropatellar 729.31
    specified site NEC 729.39
  foot (congenital) 755.67
  frenum, frenulum (tongue) 529.8
    linguae 529.8
    lip 528.5
  gallbladder or cystic duct 575.8
  gastric mucosa 535.2

Hypertrophy, hypertrophic—*continued*
gingiva 523.8
gland, glandular (general) NEC 785.6
gum (mucous membrane) 523.8
heart (idiopathic)—*see also* Hypertrophy,
  cardiac
  valve—*see also* Endocarditis
    congenital NEC 746.89
hemifacial 754.0
hepatic—*see* Hypertrophy, liver
hiatus (esophageal) 756.6
hilus gland 785.6
hymen, congenital 752.49
ileum 569.89
infrapatellar fat pad 729.31
intestine 569.89
jejunum 569.89
kidney (compensatory) 593.1
  congenital 753.3
labial frenulum 528.5
labium (majus) (minus) 624.3
lacrimal gland, chronic 375.03
ligament 728.9
  spinal 724.8
linguae frenulum 529.8
lingual tonsil (infectional) 474.11
lip (frenum) 528.5
  congenital 744.81
liver 789.1
  acute 573.8
  cirrhotic—*see* Cirrhosis, liver
  congenital 751.69
  fatty—*see* Fatty, liver
lymph gland 785.6
  tuberculous—*see* Tuberculosis, lymph gland
mammary gland—*see* Hypertrophy, breast
maxillary frenulum 528.5
Meckel's diverticulum (congenital) 751.0
medial meniscus, acquired 717.3
median bar 600.90
  with
    other lower urinary tract symptoms (LUTS)
      600.91
    urinary
      obstruction 600.91
      retention 600.91
mediastinum 519.3
meibomian gland 373.2
meniscus, knee, congenital 755.64
metatarsal head 733.99
metatarsus 733.99
mouth 528.9
mucous membrane
  alveolar process 523.8
  nose 478.19
  turbinate (nasal) 478.0
muscle 728.9
muscular coat, artery NEC 447.8
  carotid 447.8
  renal 447.3
myocardium (*see also* Hypertrophy, cardiac)
  429.3
  idiopathic 425.18
myometrium 621.2
nail 703.8
  congenital 757.5
nasal 478.19
  alae 478.19
  bone 738.0
  cartilage 478.19
  mucous membrane (septum) 478.19
  sinus (*see also* Sinusitis) 473.9

Hypertrophy, hypertrophic—*continued*
nasal—*continued*
  turbinate 478.0
nasopharynx, lymphoid (infectional) (tissue)
  (wall) 478.29
neck, uterus 622.6
nipple 611.1
normal aperture diaphragm (congenital) 756.6
nose (*see also* Hypertrophy, nasal) 478.19
orbit 376.46
organ or site, congenital NEC—*see* Anomaly,
  specified type NEC
osteoarthropathy (pulmonary) 731.2
ovary 620.8
palate (hard) 526.89
  soft 528.9
pancreas (congenital) 751.7
papillae
  anal 569.49
  tongue 529.3
parathyroid (gland) 252.01
parotid gland 527.1
penis 607.89
phallus 607.89
  female (clitoris) 624.2
pharyngeal tonsil 474.12
pharyngitis 472.1
pharynx 478.29
  lymphoid (infectional) (tissue) (wall) 478.29
pituitary (fossa) (gland) 253.8
popliteal fat pad 729.31
preauricular (lymph) gland (Hampstead) 785.6
prepuce (congenital) 605
  female 624.2
prostate (asymptomatic) (early) (recurrent) 600.90
  with
    other lower urinary tract symptoms (LUTS)
      600.91
    urinary
      obstruction 600.91
      retention 600.91
  adenofibromatous 600.20
    with
      other lower urinary tract symptoms
        (LUTS) 600.21
      urinary
        obstruction 600.21
        retention 600.21
  benign 600.00
    with
      other lower urinary tract symptoms
        (LUTS) 600.01
      urinary
        obstruction 600.01
        retention 600.01
  congenital 752.89
psuedoedematous hypodermal 757.0
pseudomuscular 359.1
pylorus (muscle) (sphincter) 537.0
  congenital 750.5
  infantile 750.5
rectal sphincter 569.49
rectum 569.49
renal 593.1
rhinitis (turbinate) 472.0
salivary duct or gland 527.1
  congenital 750.26
scaphoid (tarsal) 733.99
scar 701.4
scrotum 608.89
sella turcica 253.8

Hypertrophy, hypertrophic—*continued*
  seminal vesicle 608.89
  sigmoid 569.89
  skin condition NEC 701.9
  spermatic cord 608.89
  spinal ligament 724.8
  spleen—*see* Splenomegaly
  spondylitis (spine) (*see also* Spondylosis) 721.90
  stomach 537.89
  subaortic stenosis (idiopathic) 425.11
  sublingual gland 527.1
    congenital 750.26
  submaxillary gland 527.1
  suprarenal (gland) 255.8
  tendon 727.9
  testis 608.89
    congenital 752.89
  thymic, thymus (congenital) (gland) 254.0
  thyroid (gland) (*see also* Goiter) 240.9
    primary 242.0
    secondary 242.2
  toe (congenital) 755.65
    acquired 735.8
  tongue 529.8
    congenital 750.15
    frenum 529.8
    papillae (foliate) 529.3
  tonsil (faucial) (infective) (lingual) (lymphoid)
      474.11
    and adenoids 474.10
    with
      adenoiditis 474.01
      tonsillitis 474.00
        and adenoiditis 474.02
  tunica vaginalis 608.89
  turbinate (mucous membrane) 478.0
  ureter 593.89
  urethra 599.84
  uterus 621.2
    puerperal, postpartum 674.8
  uvula 528.9
  vagina 623.8
  vas deferens 608.89
  vein 459.89
  ventricle, ventricular (heart) (left) (right)—*see
      also* Hypertrophy, cardiac
    congenital 746.89
    due to hypertension (left) (right) (*see also*
        Hypertension, heart) 402.90
      benign 402.10
      malignant 402.00
    right with ventricular septal defect, pulmonary
        stenosis or atresia, and dextraposition of
        aorta 745.2
  verumontanum 599.89
  vesical 596.89
  vocal cord 478.5
  vulva 624.3
    stasis (nonfilarial) 624.3
Hypertropia (intermittent) (periodic) 378.31
Hypertyrosinemia 270.2
Hyperuricemia 790.6
Hypervalinemia 270.3
Hyperventilation (tetany) 786.01
  hysterical 300.11
  psychogenic 306.1
  syndrome 306.1
Hyperviscidosis 277.00
Hyperviscosity (of serum) (syndrome) NEC
    273.3
  polycythemic 289.0
  sclerocythemic 282.8

Hypervitaminosis (dietary) NEC 278.8
  A (dietary) 278.2
  D (dietary) 278.4
  from excessive administration or use of vitamin
      preparations (chronic) 278.8
    reaction to sudden overdose 963.5
  vitamin A 278.2
    reaction to sudden overdose 963.5
  vitamin D 278.4
    reaction to sudden overdose 963.5
  vitamin K
    correct substance properly administered 278.8
    overdose or wrong substance given or taken
        964.3
Hypervolemia 276.69
Hypesthesia (*see also* Disturbance, sensation)
    782.0
  cornea 371.81
Hyphema (anterior chamber) (ciliary body) (iris)
    364.41
  traumatic 921.3
Hyphemia —*see* Hyphema
Hypoacidity, gastric 536.8
  psychogenic 306.4
Hypoactive labyrinth (function)—*see*
    Hypofunction, labyrinth
Hypoadrenalism 255.41
  tuberculous (*see also* Tuberculosis) 017.6
Hypoadrenocorticism 255.41
  pituitary 253.4
Hypoalbuminemia 273.8
Hypoaldosteronism 255.42
Hypoalphalipoproteinemia 272.5
Hypobarism 993.2
Hypobaropathy 993.2
Hypobetalipoproteinemia (familial) 272.5
Hypocalcemia 275.41
  cow's milk 775.4
  dietary 269.3
  neonatal 775.4
  phosphate-loading 775.4
Hypocalcification, teeth 520.4
Hypochloremia 276.9
Hypochlorhydria 536.8
  neurotic 306.4
  psychogenic 306.4
Hypocholesteremia 272.5
Hypochondria (reaction) 300.7
Hypochondriac 300.7
Hypochondriasis 300.7
Hypochromasia blood cells 280.9
Hypochromic anemia 280.9
  due to blood loss (chronic) 280.0
    acute 285.1
  microcytic 280.9
Hypocoagulability (*see also* Defect, coagulation)
    286.9
Hypocomplementemia 279.8
Hypocythemia (progressive) 284.9
Hypodontia (*see also* Anodontia) 520.0
Hypoeosinophilia 288.59
Hypoesthesia (*see also* Disturbance, sensation)
    782.0
  cornea 371.81
  tactile 782.0
Hypoestrinism 256.39
Hypoestrogenism 256.39
Hypoferremia 280.9
  due to blood loss (chronic) 280.0

Hypofertility
female 628.9
male 606.1
Hypofibrinogenemia 286.3
acquired 286.6
congenital 286.3
Hypofunction
adrenal (gland) 255.41
cortex 255.41
medulla 255.5
specified NEC 255.5
cerebral 331.9
corticoadrenal NEC 255.41
intestinal 564.89
labyrinth (unilateral) 386.53
with loss of labyrinthine reactivity 386.55
bilateral 386.54
with loss of labyrinthine reactivity 386.56
Leydig cell 257.2
ovary 256.39
postablative 256.2
pituitary (anterior) (gland) (lobe) 253.2
posterior 253.5
testicular 257.2
iatrogenic 257.1
postablative 257.1
postirradiation 257.1
postsurgical 257.1
Hypogammaglobulinemia 279.00
acquired primary 279.06
non-sex-linked, congenital 279.06
sporadic 279.06
transient of infancy 279.09
Hypogenitalism (congenital) (female) (male)
752.89
penis 752.69
Hypoglycemia (spontaneous) 251.2
coma 251.0
diabetic 250.3
due to secondary diabetes 249.3
diabetic 250.8
due to secondary diabetes 249.8
due to insulin 251.0
therapeutic misadventure 962.3
familial (idiopathic) 251.2
following gastrointestinal surgery 579.3
infantile (idiopathic) 251.2
in infant of diabetic mother 775.0
leucine-induced 270.3
neonatal 775.6
reactive 251.2
specified NEC 251.1
Hypoglycemic shock 251.0
diabetic 250.8
due to secondary diabetes 249.8
due to insulin 251.0
functional (syndrome) 251.1
Hypogonadism
female 256.39
gonadotrophic (isolated) 253.4
hypogonadotropic (isolated) (with anosmia) 253.4
isolated 253.4
male 257.2
hereditary familial (Reifenstein's syndrome)
259.52
ovarian (primary) 256.39
pituitary (secondary) 253.4
testicular (primary) (secondary) 257.2
Hypohidrosis 705.0
Hypohidrotic ectodermal dysplasia 757.31
Hypoidrosis 705.0

Hypoinsulinemia, postsurgical 251.3
postpancreatectomy (complete) (partial) 251.3
Hypokalemia 276.8
Hypokinesia 780.99
Hypoleukia splenica 289.4
Hypoleukocytosis 288.50
Hypolipidemia 272.5
Hypolipoproteinemia 272.5
Hypomagnesemia 275.2
neonatal 775.4
Hypomania, hypomanic reaction (*see also*
Psychosis, affective) 296.0
recurrent episode 296.1
single episode 296.0
Hypomastia (congenital) 611.82
Hypomenorrhea 626.1
Hypometabolism 783.9
Hypomotility
gastrointestinal tract 536.8
psychogenic 306.4
intestine 564.89
psychogenic 306.4
stomach 536.8
psychogenic 306.4
Hyponasality 784.44
Hyponatremia 276.1
Hypo-ovarianism 256.39
Hypo-ovarism 256.39
Hypoparathyroidism (idiopathic) (surgically
induced) 252.1
neonatal 775.4
Hypoperfusion (in)
newborn 779.89
Hypopharyngitis 462
Hypophoria 378.40
Hypophosphatasia 275.3
Hypophosphatemia (acquired) (congenital)
(familial) 275.3
renal 275.3
Hypophyseal, hypophysis —*see also* condition
dwarfism 253.3
gigantism 253.0
syndrome 253.8
Hypophyseothalamic syndrome 253.8
Hypopiesis —*see* Hypotension
Hypopigmentation 709.00
eyelid 374.53
Hypopinealism 259.8
Hypopituitarism (juvenile) (syndrome) 253.2
due to
hormone therapy 253.7
hypophysectomy 253.7
radiotherapy 253.7
postablative 253.7
postpartum hemorrhage 253.2
Hypoplasia, hypoplasis 759.89
adrenal (gland) 759.1
alimentary tract 751.8
lower 751.2
upper 750.8
angiolymphoid, with eosinophilia (ALHE) 228.01
anus, anal (canal) 751.2
aorta 747.22
aortic
arch (tubular) 747.10
orifice or valve with hypoplasia of ascending
aorta and defective development of left
ventricle (with mitral valve atresia) 746.7
appendix 751.2
areola 757.6
arm (*see also* Absence, arm, congenital) 755.20

Hypoplasia, hypoplasis—*continued*
artery (congenital) (peripheral) NEC 747.60
  brain 747.81
  cerebral 747.81
  coronary 746.85
  gastrointestinal 747.61
  lower limb 747.64
  pulmonary 747.31
  renal 747.62
  retinal 743.58
  specified NEC 747.69
  spinal 747.82
  umbilical 747.5
  upper limb 747.63
auditory canal 744.29
  causing impairment of hearing 744.02
biliary duct (common) or passage 751.61
bladder 753.8
bone NEC 756.9
  face 756.0
  malar 756.0
  mandible 524.04
    alveolar 524.74
  marrow 284.9
    acquired (secondary) 284.89
    congenital 284.09
    idiopathic 284.9
  maxilla 524.03
    alveolar 524.73
  skull (*see also* Hypoplasia, skull) 756.0
brain 742.1
  gyri 742.2
  specified part 742.2
breast (areola) 611.82
bronchus (tree) 748.3
cardiac 746.89
  valve—*see* Hypoplasia, heart, valve
  vein 746.89
carpus (*see also* Absence, carpal, congenital)
  755.28
cartilaginous 756.9
cecum 751.2
cementum 520.4
  hereditary 520.5
cephalic 742.1
cerebellum 742.2
cervix (uteri) 752.43
chin 524.06
clavicle 755.51
coccyx 756.19
colon 751.2
corpus callosum 742.2
cricoid cartilage 748.3
dermal, focal (Goltz) 757.39
digestive organ(s) or tract NEC 751.8
  lower 751.2
  upper 750.8
ear 744.29
  auricle 744.23
  lobe 744.29
  middle, except ossicles 744.03
    ossicles 744.04
  ossicles 744.04
enamel of teeth (neonatal) (postnatal) (prenatal)
  520.4
  hereditary 520.5
endocrine (gland) NEC 759.2
endometrium 621.8
epididymis 752.89
epiglottis 748.3
erythroid, congenital 284.01

Hypoplasia, hypoplasis—*continued*
erythropoietic, chronic acquired 284.81
esophagus 750.3
Eustachian tube 744.24
eye (*see also* Microphthalmos) 743.10
  lid 743.62
face 744.89
  bone(s) 756.0
fallopian tube 752.19
femur (*see also* Absence, femur, congenital)
  755.34
fibula (*see also* Absence, fibula, congenital)
  755.37
finger (*see also* Absence, finger, congenital)
  755.29
focal dermal 757.39
foot 755.31
gallbladder 751.69
genitalia, genital organ(s)
  female 752.89
    external 752.49
    internal NEC 752.89
  in adiposogenital dystrophy 253.8
  male 752.89
    penis 752.69
glottis 748.3
hair 757.4
hand 755.21
heart 746.89
  left (complex) (syndrome) 746.7
  valve NEC 746.89
    pulmonary 746.01
humerus (*see also* Absence, humerus,
  congenital) 755.24
hymen 752.49
intestine (small) 751.1
  large 751.2
iris 743.46
jaw 524.09
kidney(s) 753.0
labium (majus) (minus) 752.49
labyrinth, membranous 744.05
lacrimal duct (apparatus) 743.65
larynx 748.3
leg (*see also* Absence, limb, congenital, lower)
  755.30
limb 755.4
  lower (*see also* Absence, limb, congenital,
    lower) 755.30
  upper (*see also* Absence, limb, congenital,
    upper) 755.20
liver 751.69
lung (lobe) 748.5
mammary (areolar) 611.82
mandibular 524.04
  alveolar 524.74
  unilateral condylar 526.89
maxillary 524.03
  alveolar 524.73
medullary 284.9
megakaryocytic 287.30
metacarpus (*see also* Absence, metacarpal,
  congenital) 755.28
metatarsus (*see also* Absence, metatarsal,
  congenital) 755.38
muscle 756.89
  eye 743.69
myocardium (congenital) (Uhl's anomaly)
  746.84
nail(s) 757.5
nasolacrimal duct 743.65

Hypoplasia, hypoplasis—*continued*
  nervous system NEC 742.8
  neural 742.8
  nose, nasal 748.1
  ophthalmic (*see also* Microphthalmos) 743.10
  optic nerve 377.43
  organ
    of Corti 744.05
    or site NEC—*see* Anomaly, by site
  osseous meatus (ear) 744.03
  ovary 752.0
  oviduct 752.19
  pancreas 751.7
  parathyroid (gland) 759.2
  parotid gland 750.26
  patella 755.64
  pelvis, pelvic girdle 755.69
  penis 752.69
  peripheral vascular system (congenital) NEC 747.60
    gastrointestinal 747.61
    lower limb 747.64
    renal 747.62
    specified NEC 747.69
    spinal 747.82
    upper limb 747.63
  pituitary (gland) 759.2
  pulmonary 748.5
    arteriovenous 747.32
    artery 747.31
    valve 746.01
  punctum lacrimale 743.65
  radioulnar (*see also* Absence, radius, congenital, with ulna) 755.25
  radius (*see also* Absence, radius, congenital) 755.26
  rectum 751.2
  respiratory system NEC 748.9
  rib 756.3
  sacrum 756.19
  scapula 755.59
  shoulder girdle 755.59
  skin 757.39
  skull (bone) 756.0
    with
      anencephalus 740.0
      encephalocele 742.0
      hydrocephalus 742.3
        with spina bifida (*see also* Spina bifida) 741.0
      microcephalus 742.1
  spinal (cord) (ventral horn cell) 742.59
    vessel 747.82
  spine 756.19
  spleen 759.0
  sternum 756.3
  tarsus (*see also* Absence, tarsal, congenital) 755.38
  testis, testicle 752.89
  thymus (gland) 279.11
  thyroid (gland) 243
    cartilage 748.3
  tibiofibular (*see also* Absence, tibia, congenital, with fibula) 755.35
  toe (*see also* Absence, toe, congenital) 755.39
  tongue 750.16
  trachea (cartilage) (rings) 748.3
  Turner's (tooth) 520.4
  ulna (*see also* Absence, ulna, congenital) 755.27
  umbilical artery 747.5
  ureter 753.29
  uterus 752.32
  vagina 752.45
  vascular (peripheral) NEC (*see also* Hypoplasia, peripheral vascular system) 747.60
    brain 747.81

Hypoplasia, hypoplasis—*continued*
  vein(s) (peripheral) NEC (*see also* Hypoplasia, peripheral vascular system 747.60
    brain 747.81
    cardiac 746.89
    great 747.49
    portal 747.49
    pulmonary 747.49
  vena cava (inferior) (superior) 747.49
  vertebra 756.19
  vulva 752.49
  zonule (ciliary) 743.39
  zygoma 738.12
Hypopotassemia 276.8
Hypoproaccelerinemia (*see also* Defect, coagulation) 286.3
Hypoproconvertinemia (congenital) (*see also* Defect, coagulation) 286.3
Hypoproteinemia (essential) (hypermetabolic) (idiopathic) 273.8
Hypoproteinosis 260
Hypoprothrombinemia (congenital) (hereditary) (idiopathic) (*see also* Defect, coagulation) 286.3
  acquired 286.7
  newborn 776.3
Hypopselaphesia 782.0
Hypopyon (anterior chamber) (eye) 364.05
  iritis 364.05
  ulcer (cornea) 370.04
Hypopyrexia 780.99
Hyporeflex 796.1
Hyporeninemia, extreme 790.99
  in primary aldosteronism 255.10
Hyporesponsive episode 780.09
Hyposecretion
  ACTH 253.4
    ovary 256.39
    postablative 256.2
  salivary gland (any) 527.7
Hyposegmentation of neutrophils, hereditary 288.2
Hyposiderinemia 280.9
Hyposmolality 276.1
  syndrome 276.1
Hyposomatotropism 253.3
Hyposomnia, unspecified (*see also* Insomnia) 780.52
  with sleep apnea, unspecified 780.51
Hypospadias (male) 752.61
  female 753.8
Hypospermatogenesis 606.1
Hyposphagma 372.72
Hyposplenism 289.59
Hypostasis, pulmonary 514
Hypostatic —*see* condition
Hyposthenuria 593.89
Hyposuprarenalism 255.41
Hypo-TBG-nemia 246.8
Hypotension (arterial) (constitutional) 458.9
  chronic 458.1
  iatrogenic 458.29
  maternal, syndrome (following labor and delivery) 669.2
  of hemodialysis 458.21
  orthostatic (chronic) 458.0
    dysautonomic-dyskinetic syndrome 333.0
  permanent idiopathic 458.1
  postoperative 458.29

Hypotension—*continued*
  postural 458.0
  specified type NEC 458.8
  transient 796.3
Hypothermia (accidental) 991.6
  anesthetic 995.89
  associated with low environmental temperature
    991.6
  newborn NEC 778.3
  not associated with low environmental
    temperature 780.65
Hypothymergasia (*see also* Psychosis, affective)
    296.2
  recurrent episode 296.3
  single episode 296.2
Hypothyroidism (acquired) 244.9
  complicating pregnancy, childbirth, or
    puerperium 648.1
  congenital 243
  due to
    ablation 244.1
      radioactive iodine 244.1
      surgical 244.0
    iodine (administration) (ingestion) 244.2
      radioactive 244.1
    irradiation therapy 244.1
    p-aminosalicylic acid (PAS) 244.3
    phenylbutazone 244.3
    resorcinol 244.3
    specified cause NEC 244.8
    surgery 244.0
  goitrous (sporadic) 246.1
  iatrogenic NEC 244.3
  iodine 244.2
  pituitary 244.8
  postablative NEC 244.1
  postsurgical 244.0
  primary 244.9
  secondary NEC 244.8
  specified cause NEC 244.8
  sporadic goitrous 246.1
Hypotonia, hypotonicity, hypotony 781.3
  benign congenital 358.8
  bladder 596.4
  congenital 779.89
    benign 358.8
  eye 360.30
    due to
      fistula 360.32
      ocular disorder NEC 360.33
    following loss of aqueous or vitreous 360.33
    primary 360.31
  infantile muscular (benign) 359.0
  muscle 728.9
  uterus, uterine (contractions)—*see* Inertia,
    uterus
Hypotrichosis 704.09
  congenital 757.4
  lid (congenital) 757.4
    acquired 374.55
  postinfectional NEC 704.09
Hypotropia 378.32
Hypoventilation 786.09
  congenital central alveolar syndrome 327.25
  idiopathic sleep related nonobstructive alveolar
    327.24
  obesity 278.03
  sleep related, in conditions classifiable
    elsewhere 327.26
Hypovitaminosis (*see also* Deficiency, vitamin)
    269.2

Hypovolemia 276.52
  surgical shock 998.09
  traumatic (shock) 958.4
Hypoxemia (*see also* Anoxia) 799.02
  sleep related, in conditions classifiable
    elsewhere 327.26
Hypoxia (*see also* Anoxia) 799.02
  cerebral 348.1
    during or resulting from a procedure 997.01
  newborn 770.88
    mild or moderate 768.6
    severe 768.5
  fetal, affecting newborn 770.88
  intrauterine—*see* Distress, fetal
  myocardial (*see also* Insufficiency, coronary)
    411.89
    arteriosclerotic —*see* Arteriosclerosis,
      coronary
  newborn 770.88
  sleep related 327.24
Hypoxic-ischemic encephalopathy (HIE) 768.70
  mild 768.71
  moderate 768.72
  severe 768.73
Hypsarrhythmia (*see also* Epilepsy) 345.6
Hysteralgia, pregnant uterus 646.8
Hysteria, hysterical 300.10
  anxiety 300.20
  Charcot's gland 300.11
  conversion (any manifestation) 300.11
  dissociative type NEC 300.15
  psychosis, acute 298.1
Hysteroepilepsy 300.11
Hysterotomy, affecting fetus or newborn
    763.89

I

Iatrogenic syndrome of excess cortisol 255.0
IBM (inclusion body myositis) 359.71
Iceland disease (epidemic neuromyasthenia) 049.8
Ichthyosis (congenita) 757.1
  acquired 701.1
  fetalis gravior 757.1
  follicularis 757.1
  hystrix 757.39
  lamellar 757.1
  lingual 528.6
  palmaris and plantaris 757.39
  simplex 757.1
  vera 757.1
  vulgaris 757.1
Ichthyotoxism 988.0
  bacterial (*see also* Poisoning, food) 005.9
Icteroanemia, hemolytic (acquired) 283.9
  congenital (*see also* Spherocytosis) 282.0
Icterus (*see also* Jaundice) 782.4
  catarrhal—*see* Icterus, infectious
  conjunctiva 782.4
    newborn 774.6
  epidemic—*see* Icterus, infectious
  febrilis—*see* Icterus, infectious
  fetus or newborn—*see* Jaundice, fetus or newborn
  gravis (*see also* Necrosis, liver) 570
    complicating pregnancy 646.7
      affecting fetus or newborn 760.8
    fetus or newborn NEC 773.0
    obstetrical 646.7
      affecting fetus or newborn 760.8
  hematogenous (acquired) 283.9
  hemolytic (acquired) 283.9
    congenital (*see also* Spherocytosis) 282.0
  hemorrhagic (acute) 100.0
    leptospiral 100.0
    newborn 776.0
    spirochetal 100.0
  infectious 070.1
    with hepatic coma 070.0
    leptospiral 100.0
    spirochetal 100.0
  intermittens juvenilis 277.4
  malignant (*see also* Necrosis, liver) 570
  neonatorum (*see also* Jaundice, fetus or
    newborn) 774.6
  pernicious (*see also* Necrosis, liver) 570
  spirochetal 100.0
Ictus solaris, solis 992.0
Ideation
  homicidal V62.85
  suicidal V62.84
Identity disorder 313.82
  dissociative 300.14
  gender role (child) 302.6
    adult 302.85
  psychosexual (child) 302.6
    adult 302.85
Idioglossia 307.9
Idiopathic —*see* condition
Idiosyncrasy (*see also* Allergy) 995.3
  drug, medicinal substance, and biological—*see*
    Allergy, drug

Idiot, idiocy (congenital) 318.2
  amaurotic (Bielschowsky) (-Jansky) (family)
    (infantile (late)) (juvenile (late))
    (Vogt-Spielmeyer) 330.1
  microcephalic 742.1
  Mongolian 758.0
  oxycephalic 756.0
Id reaction (due to bacteria) 692.89
**IEED (involuntary emotional expression
  disorder)** 310.81
IFIS (intraoperative floppy iris syndrome)
  364.81
IgE asthma 493.0
Ileitis (chronic) (*see also* Enteritis) 558.9
  infectious 009.0
  noninfectious 558.9
  regional (ulcerative) 555.0
    with large intestine 555.2
  segmental 555.0
    with large intestine 555.2
  terminal (ulcerative) 555.0
    with large intestine 555.2
Ileocolitis (*see also* Enteritis) 558.9
  infectious 009.0
  regional 555.2
  ulcerative 556.1
Ileostomy status V44.2
  with complication 569.60
Ileotyphus 002.0
Ileum —*see* condition
Ileus (adynamic) (bowel) (colon) (inhibitory)
  (intestine) (neurogenic) (paralytic) 560.1
  arteriomesenteric duodenal 537.2
  due to gallstone (in intestine) 560.31
  duodenal, chronic 537.2
  following gastrointestinal surgery 997.49
  gallstone 560.31
  mechanical (*see also* Obstruction, intestine) 560.9
  meconium 777.1
    due to cystic fibrosis 277.01
  myxedema 564.89
  postoperative 997.49
  transitory, newborn 777.4
Iliac —*see* condition
Iliotibial band friction syndrome 728.89
Ill, louping 063.1
Illegitimacy V61.6
Illness —*see also* Disease
  factitious 300.19
    with
      combined psychological and physical signs
        and symptoms 300.19
      physical symptoms 300.19
      predominantly
        physical signs and symptoms 300.19
        psychological symptoms 300.16
    chronic (with physical symptoms) 301.51
  heart—*see* Disease, heart
  manic-depressive (*see also* Psychosis, affective)
    296.80
  mental (*see also* Disorder, mental) 300.9
Imbalance 781.2
  autonomic (*see also* Neuropathy, peripheral,
    autonomic) 337.9

Imbalance—*continued*
electrolyte 276.9
  with
    abortion—*see* Abortion, by type, with
      metabolic disorder
    ectopic pregnancy (*see also* categories
      633.0-633.9) 639.4
    hyperemesis gravidarum (before 22
      completed weeks gestation) 643.1
    molar pregnancy (*see also* categories
      630-632) 639.4
  following
    abortion 639.4
    ectopic or molar pregnancy 639.4
  neonatal, transitory NEC 775.5
endocrine 259.9
eye muscle NEC 378.9
  heterophoria—*see* Heterophoria
glomerulotubular NEC 593.89
hormone 259.9
hysterical (*see also* Hysteria) 300.10
labyrinth NEC 386.50
posture 729.90
sympathetic (*see also* Neuropathy, peripheral,
  autonomic) 337.9
Imbecile, imbecility 318.0
moral 301.7
old age 290.9
senile 290.9
specified IQ—*see* IQ
unspecified IQ 318.0
Imbedding, intrauterine device 996.32
Imbibition, cholesterol (gallbladder) 575.6
Imerslund (-Gräsbeck) syndrome (anemia due to
  familial selective vitamin B$_{12}$ malabsorption)
  281.1
Iminoacidopathy 270.8
Iminoglycinuria, familial 270.8
Immature —*see also* Immaturity
personality 301.89
Immaturity 765.1
extreme 765.0
fetus or infant light-for-dates—*see*
  Light-for-dates
lung, fetus or newborn 770.4
organ or site NEC—*see* Hypoplasia
pulmonary, fetus or newborn 770.4
reaction 301.89
sexual (female) (male) 259.0
Immersion 994.1
foot 991.4
hand 991.4
Immobile, immobility
complete
  due to severe physical disability or frality
    780.72
intestine 564.89
joint—*see* Ankylosis
syndrome (paraplegic) 728.3
Immunization
ABO
  affecting management of pregnancy 656.2
  fetus or newborn 773.1
complication—*see* Complications, vaccination
Rh factor
  affecting management of pregnancy 656.1
  fetus or newborn 773.0
  from transfusion (*see also* Complications,
    transfusion) 999.70

Immunodeficiency 279.3
with
  adenosine-deaminase deficiency 279.2
  defect, predominant
    B-cell 279.00
    T-cell 279.10
  hyperimmunoglobulinemia 279.2
  lymphopenia, hereditary 279.2
  thrombocytopenia and eczema 279.12
  thymic
    aplasia 279.2
    dysplasia 279.2
autosomal recessive, Swiss-type 279.2
common variable 279.06
severe combined (SCID) 279.2
to Rh factor
  affecting management of pregnancy 656.1
  fetus or newborn 773.0
X-linked, with increased IgM 279.05
Immunotherapy, prophylactic V07.2
antineoplastic V58.12
Impaction, impacted
bowel, colon, rectum 560.30
  with hernia—*see also* Hernia, by site, with
    obstruction
    gangrenous—*see* Hernia, by site, with
      gangrene
  by
    calculus 560.32
    gallstone 560.31
    fecal 560.32
    specified type NEC 560.32
calculus—*see* Calculus
cerumen (ear) (external) 380.4
cuspid 520.6
dental 520.6
fecal, feces 560.32
  with hernia—*see also* Hernia, by site, with
    obstruction
    gangrenous—*see* Hernia, by site, with
      gangrene
fracture—*see* Fracture, by site
gallbladder—*see* Cholelithiasis
gallstone(s)—*see* Cholelithiasis
  in intestine (any part) 560.31
intestine(s) 560.30
  with hernia—*see also* Hernia, by site, with
    obstruction
    gangrenous—*see* Hernia, by site, with
      gangrene
  by
    calculus 560.32
    gallstone 560.31
    fecal 560.32
    specified type NEC 560.32
intrauterine device (IUD) 996.32
molar 520.6
shoulder 660.4
  affecting fetus or newborn 763.1
tooth, teeth 520.6
turbinate 733.99
Impaired, impairment (function)
arm V49.1
  movement, involving
    musculoskeletal system V49.1
    nervous system V49.2
auditory discrimination 388.43
back V48.3
body (entire) V49.89
cognitive, mild, so stated 331.83
combined visual hearing V49.85

Impaired, impairment—*continued*
  dual sensory V49.85
  glucose
    fasting 790.21
    tolerance test (oral) 790.22
  hearing (*see also* Deafness) 389.9
    combined with visual impairment V49.85
  heart—*see* Disease, heart
  kidney (*see also* Disease, renal) 593.9
    disorder resulting from 588.9
      specified NEC 588.89
  leg V49.1
    movement, involving
      musculoskeletal system V49.1
      nervous system V49.2
  limb V49.1
    movement, involving
      musculoskeletal system V49.1
      nervous system V49.2
  liver 573.8
  mastication 524.9
  mild cognitive, so stated 331.83
  mobility
    ear ossicles NEC 385.22
    incostapedial joint 385.22
    malleus 385.21
  myocardium, myocardial (*see also*
    Insufficiency, myocardial) 428.0
  neuromusculoskeletal NEC V49.89
    back V48.3
    head V48.2
    limb V49.2
    neck V48.3
    spine V48.3
    trunk V48.3
  rectal sphincter 787.99
  renal (*see also* Disease, renal) 593.9
    disorder resulting from 588.9
      specified NEC 588.89
  spine V48.3
  vision NEC 369.9
    both eyes NEC 369.3
    combined with hearing impairment V49.85
    moderate 369.74
      both eyes 369.25
        with impairment of lesser eye (specified
          as)
        blind, not further specified 369.15
        low vision, not further specified 369.23
        near-total 369.17
        profound 369.18
        severe 369.24
        total 369.16
      one eye 369.74
        with vision of other eye (specified as)
        near-normal 369.75
        normal 369.76
    near-total 369.64
      both eyes 369.04
        with impairment of lesser eye (specified
          as)
        blind, not further specified 369.02
        total 369.03
      one eye 369.64
        with vision of other eye (specified as)
        near-normal 369.65
        normal 369.66
    one eye 369.60
      with low vision of other eye 369.10

Impaired, impairment—*continued*
  vision—*continued*
    profound 369.67
      both eyes 369.08
        with impairment of lesser eye (specified
          as)
        blind, not further specified 369.05
        near-total 369.07
        total 369.06
      one eye 369.67
        with vision of other eye (specified as)
        near-normal 369.68
        normal 369.69
    severe 369.71
      both eyes 369.22
        with impairment of lesser eye (specified as)
        blind, not further specified 369.11
        low vision, not further specified 369.21
        near-total 369.13
        profound 369.14
        total 369.12
      one eye 369.71
        with vision of other eye (specified as)
        near-normal 369.72
        normal 369.73
    total
      both eyes 369.01
      one eye 369.61
        with vision of other eye (specified as)
        near-normal 369.62
        normal 369.63
Impaludism —*see* Malaria
Impediment, speech NEC 784.59
  psychogenic 307.9
  secondary to organic lesion 784.59
Impending
  cerebrovascular accident or attack 435.9
  coronary syndrome 411.1
  delirium tremens 291.0
  myocardial infarction 411.1
Imperception, auditory (acquired) (congenital)
  389.9
Imperfect
  aeration, lung (newborn) 770.5
  closure (congenital)
    alimentary tract NEC 751.8
      lower 751.5
      upper 750.8
    atrioventricular ostium 745.69
    atrium (secundum) 745.5
      primum 745.61
    branchial cleft or sinus 744.41
    choroid 743.59
    cricoid cartilage 748.3
    cusps, heart valve NEC 746.89
      pulmonary 746.09
    ductus
      arteriosus 747.0
      Botalli 747.0
    ear drum 744.29
      causing impairment of hearing 744.03
    endocardial cushion 745.60
    epiglottis 748.3
    esophagus with communication to bronchus or
      trachea 750.3
    Eustachian valve 746.89
    eyelid 743.62
    face, facial (*see also* Cleft, lip) 749.10
    foramen
      Botalli 745.5
      ovale 745.5

Imperfect—*continued*
  closure (congenital)—*continued*
    genitalia, genital organ(s) or system
      female 752.89
        external 752.49
        internal NEC 752.89
        uterus 752.39
      male 752.89
        penis 752.69
    glottis 748.3
    heart valve (cusps) NEC 746.89
    interatrial ostium or septum 745.5
    interauricular ostium or septum 745.5
    interventricular ostium or septum 745.4
    iris 743.46
    kidney 753.3
    larynx 748.3
    lens 743.36
    lip (*see also* Cleft, lip) 749.10
    nasal septum or sinus 748.1
    nose 748.1
    omphalomesenteric duct 751.0
    optic nerve entry 743.57
    organ or site NEC—*see* Anomaly, specified
      type, by site
    ostium
      interatrial 745.5
      interauricular 745.5
      interventricular 745.4
    palate (*see also* Cleft, palate) 749.00
    preauricular sinus 744.46
    retina 743.56
    roof of orbit 742.0
    sclera 743.47
    septum
      aortic 745.0
      aorticopulmonary 745.0
      atrial (secundum) 745.5
        primum 745.61
      between aorta and pulmonary artery 745.0
      heart 745.9
      interatrial (secundum) 745.5
        primum 745.61
      interauricular (secundum) 745.5
        primum 745.61
      interventricular 745.4
        with pulmonary stenosis or atresia,
          dextraposition of aorta, and
          hypertrophy of right ventricle 745.2
        in tetralogy of Fallot 745.2
      nasal 748.1
      ventricular 745.4
        with pulmonary stenosis or atresia,
          dextraposition of aorta, and
          hypertrophy of right ventricle 745.2
        in tetralogy of Fallot 745.2
    skull 756.0
      with
        anencephalus 740.0
        encephalocele 742.0
        hydrocephalus 742.3
          with spina bifida (*see also* Spina bifida)
            741.0
        microcephalus 742.1
    spine (with meningocele) (*see also* Spina
      bifida) 741.90
    thyroid cartilage 748.3
    trachea 748.3
    tympanic membrane 744.29
      causing impairment of hearing 744.03
    uterus (with communication to bladder,
      intestine, or rectum) 752.39

Imperfect—*continued*
  closure (congenital)—*continued*
    uvula 749.02
      with cleft lip (*see also* Cleft, palate, with
        cleft lip) 749.20
    vitelline duct 751.0
  development—*see* Anomaly, by site
  erection 607.84
  fusion—*see* Imperfect, closure
  inflation lung (newborn) 770.5
  intestinal canal 751.5
  poise 729.90
  rotation—*see* Malrotation
  septum, ventricular 745.4
Imperfectly descended testis 752.51
Imperforate (congenital)—*see also* Atresia
  anus 751.2
  bile duct 751.61
  cervix (uteri) 752.49
  esophagus 750.3
  hymen 752.42
  intestine (small) 751.1
    large 751.2
  jejunum 751.1
  pharynx 750.29
  rectum 751.2
  salivary duct 750.23
  urethra 753.6
  urinary meatus 753.6
  vagina 752.49
Impervious (congenital)—*see also* Atresia
  anus 751.2
  bile duct 751.61
  esophagus 750.3
  intestine (small) 751.1
    large 751.2
  rectum 751.2
  urethra 753.6
Impetiginization of other dermatoses 684
Impetigo (any organism) (any site) (bullous)
  (circinate) (contagiosa) (neonatorum)
  (simplex) 684
  Bockhart's (superficial folliculitis) 704.8
  external ear 684 *[380.13]*
  eyelid 684 *[373.5]*
  Fox's (contagiosa) 684
  furfuracea 696.5
  herpetiformis 694.3
    nonobstetrical 694.3
  staphylococcal infection 684
  ulcerative 686.8
  vulgaris 684
Impingement, soft tissue between teeth 524.89
  anterior 524.81
  posterior 524.82
Implant, endometrial 617.9
Implantation
  anomalous—*see also* Anomaly, specified type,
    by site
    ureter 753.4
  cyst
    external area or site (skin) NEC 709.8
    iris 364.61
    vagina 623.8
    vulva 624.8
  dermoid (cyst)
    external area or site (skin) NEC 709.8
    iris 364.61
    vagina 623.8
    vulva 624.8
  placenta, low or marginal—*see* Placenta previa

Impotence (sexual) 607.84
  organic origin NEC 607.84
  psychogenic 302.72
Impoverished blood 285.9
Impression, basilar 756.0
Imprisonment V62.5
Improper
  development, infant 764.9
Improperly tied umbilical cord (causing
  hemorrhage) 772.3
Impulses, obsessional 300.3
Impulsive 799.23
  neurosis 300.3
Impulsiveness 799.23
Inaction, kidney (*see also* Disease, renal) 593.9
Inactive —*see* condition
Inadequate, inadequacy
  aesthetics of dental restoration 525.67
  biologic 301.6
  cardiac and renal—*see* Hypertension, cardiorenal
  constitutional 301.6
  development
    child 783.40
    fetus 764.9
      affecting management of pregnancy 656.5
    genitalia
      after puberty NEC 259.0
      congenital—*see* Hypoplasia, genitalia
    lungs 748.5
    organ or site NEC—*see* Hypoplasia, by site
  dietary 269.9
  distance, interarch 524.28
  education V62.3
  environment
    economic problem V60.2
    household condition NEC V60.1
    poverty V60.2
    unemployment V62.0
  functional 301.6
  household care, due to
    family member
      handicapped or ill V60.4
      temporarily away from home V60.4
        on vacation V60.5
    technical defects in home V60.1
    temporary absence from home of person
      rendering care V60.4
  housing (heating) (space) V60.1
  interarch distance 524.28
  material resources V60.2
  mental (*see also* Disability, intellectual) 319
  nervous system 799.29
  personality 301.6
  prenatal care in current pregnancy V23.7
  pulmonary
    function 786.09
      newborn 770.89
    ventilation, newborn 770.89
  respiration 786.09
    newborn 770.89
  sample
    cytology
      anal 796.78
      cervical 795.08
      vaginal 795.18
  social 301.6
Inanition 263.9
  with edema 262
  due to
    deprivation of food 994.2
    malnutrition 263.9
  fever 780.60

Inappropriate
  change in quantitative human chorionic
    gonadotropin (hCG) in early pregnancy
    631.0
  level of quantitative human chorionic
    gonadotropin (hCG) for gestational age in
    early pregnancy 631.0
  secretion
    ACTH 255.0
    antidiuretic hormone (ADH) (excessive) 253.6
      deficiency 253.5
    ectopic hormone NEC 259.3
    pituitary (posterior) 253.6
Inattention after or at birth 995.52
Inborn errors of metabolism —*see* Disorder,
  metabolism
Incarceration, incarcerated
  bubonocele—*see also* Hernia, inguinal, with
    obstruction
    gangrenous—*see* Hernia, inguinal, with
      gangrene
  colon (by hernia)—*see also* Hernia, by site, with
    obstruction
    gangrenous—*see* Hernia, by site, with
      gangrene
  enterocele 552.9
    gangrenous 551.9
  epigastrocele 552.29
    gangrenous 551.29
  epiplocele 552.9
    gangrenous 551.9
  exomphalos 552.1
    gangrenous 551.1
  fallopian tube 620.8
  hernia—*see also* Hernia, by site, with
    obstruction
    gangrenous—*see* Hernia, by site, with
      gangrene
  iris, in wound 871.1
  lens, in wound 871.1
  merocele (*see also* Hernia, femoral, with
    obstruction) 552.00
  Omentum (by hernia)—*see also* Hernia, by site,
    with obstruction
    gangrenous—*see* Hernia, by site, with
      gangrene
  omphalocele 756.72
  rupture (meaning hernia) (*see also* Hernia, by
    site, with obstruction) 552.9
    gangrenous (*see also* Hernia, by site, with
      gangrene) 551.9
  sarcoepiplocele 552.9
    gangrenous 551.9
  sarcoepiplomphalocele 552.1
    with gangrene 551.1
  uterus 621.8
    gravid 654.3
      causing obstructed labor 660.2
        affecting fetus or newborn 763.1
Incident, cerebrovascular (*see also* Disease,
  cerebrovascular, acute) 436
Incineration (entire body) (from fire,
  conflagration, electricity, or lightning)—*see*
  Burn, multiple, specified sites
Incised wound
  external—*see* Wound, open, by site
  internal organs (abdomen, chest, or pelvis)—*see*
    Injury, internal, by site, with open wound
Incision, incisional
  hernia—*see* Hernia, incisional
  surgical, complication—*see* Complications,
    surgical procedures

Incision, incisional—*continued*
  traumatic
    external—*see* Wound, open, by site
    internal organs (abdomen, chest or
      pelvis)—*see* Injury, internal, by site, with
      open wound
Inclusion
  azurophilic leukocytic 288.2
  blennorrhea (neonatal) (newborn) 771.6
  cyst—*see* Cyst, skin
  gallbladder in liver (congenital) 751.69
Incompatibility
  ABO
    affecting management of pregnancy 656.2
    fetus or newborn 773.1
    infusion or transfusion reaction (*see also*
      Complications, transfusion) 999.60
  blood (group) (Duffy) (E) (K(ell)) (Kidd)
    (Lewis) (M) (N) (P) (S) NEC
    affecting management of pregnancy 656.2
    fetus or newborn 773.2
    infusion or transfusion reaction (*see also*
      Complications, transfusion) 999.75
  contour of existing restoration of tooth
    with oral health 525.65
  marital V61.10
    involving
      divorce V61.03
      estrangement V61.09
  non-ABO (*see also* Complications, transfusion)
    999.75
  Rh (antigen) (C) (c) (D) (E) (e) (blood group)
    (factor)
    affecting management of pregnancy 656.1
    fetus or newborn 773.0
    infusion or transfusion reaction (*see also*
      Complications, transfusion) 999.70
  Rhesus—*see* Incompatibility, Rh
Incompetency, incompetence, incompetent
  annular
    aortic (valve) (*see also* Insufficiency, aortic)
      424.1
    mitral (valve)—(*see also* Insufficiency, mitral)
      424.0
    pulmonary valve (heart) (*see also*
      Endocarditis, pulmonary) 424.3
  aortic (valve) (*see also* Insufficiency, aortic)
    424.1
    syphilitic 093.22
  cardiac (orifice) 530.0
    valve—*see* Endocarditis
  cervix, cervical (os) 622.5
    in pregnancy 654.5
      affecting fetus or newborn 761.0
  chronotropic 426.89
    with
      autonomic dysfunction 337.9
      ischemic heart disease 414.9
      left ventricular dysfunction 429.89
      sinus node dysfunction 427.81
  esophagogastric (junction) (sphincter) 530.0
  heart valve, congenital 746.89
  mitral (valve)—*see* Insufficiency, mitral
  papillary muscle (heart) 429.81
  pelvic fundus
    pubocervical tissue 618.81
    rectovaginal tissue 618.82
  pulmonary valve (heart) (*see also* Endocarditis,
    pulmonary) 424.3
    congenital 746.09

Incompetency, incompetence—*continued*
  tricuspid (annular) (rheumatic) (valve) (*see also*
    Endocarditis, tricuspid) 397.0
  valvular—*see* Endocarditis
  vein, venous (saphenous) (varicose) (*see also*
    Varicose, vein) 454.9
  velopharyngeal (closure)
    acquired 528.9
    congenital 750.29
Incomplete —*see also* condition
  bladder emptying 788.21
  defecation 787.61
  expansion lungs (newborn) 770.5
  gestation (liveborn)—*see* Immaturity
  rotation—*see* Malrotation
Inconclusive
  image test due to excess body fat 793.91
  mammogram, mammography 793.82
    due to dense breasts 793.82
Incontinence 788.30
  without sensory awareness 788.34
  anal sphincter 787.60
  continuous leakage 788.37
  feces, fecal 787.60
    due to hysteria 300.11
    nonorganic origin 307.7
  hysterical 300.11
  mixed (male) (female) (urge and stress) 788.33
  overflow 788.38
  paradoxical 788.39
  rectal 787.60
  specified NEC 788.39
  stress (female) 625.6
    male NEC 788.32
  urethral sphincter 599.84
  urge 788.31
    and stress (male) (female) 788.33
  urine 788.30
    active 788.30
    due to
      cognitive impairment 788.91
      severe physical disability 788.91
      immobility 788.91
    functional 788.91
    male 788.30
      stress 788.32
        and urge 788.33
    neurogenic 788.39
    nonorganic origin 307.6
    stress (female) 625.6
      male NEC 788.32
    urge 788.31
      and stress 788.33
Incontinentia pigmenti 757.33
Incoordinate
  uterus (action) (contractions) 661.4
    affecting fetus or newborn 763.7
Incoordination
  esophageal-pharyngeal (newborn) 787.24
  muscular 781.3
  papillary muscle 429.81
Increase, increased
  abnormal, in development 783.9
  androgens (ovarian) 256.1
  anticoagulants (antithrombin) (anti-II)
    (anti-VIIIa) (anti-IXa) (anti-XIa)
    (prothrombin) (*see also* Anticoagulants)
    286.59
    anti-IIa 287.8
    anti-Xa 287.8
    extrinsic 287.8
    postpartum 666.3

Increase, increased—*continued*
  cold sense (*see also* Disturbance, sensation)
    782.0
  estrogen 256.0
  function
    adrenal (cortex) 255.3
      medulla 255.6
    pituitary (anterior) (gland) (lobe) 253.1
      posterior 253.6
  heat sense (*see also* Disturbance, sensation) 782.0
  intracranial pressure 781.99
    injury at birth 767.8
  light reflex of retina 362.13
  permeability, capillary 448.9
  pressure
    intracranial 781.99
      injury at birth 767.8
    intraocular 365.00
  pulsations 785.9
  pulse pressure 785.9
  sphericity, lens 743.36
  splenic activity 289.4
  venous pressure 459.89
    portal 572.3
Incrustation, cornea, lead or zinc 930.0
Incyclophoria 378.44
Incyclotropia 378.33
Indeterminate sex 752.7
India rubber skin 756.83
Indicanuria 270.2
Indigestion (bilious) (functional) 536.8
  acid 536.8
  catarrhal 536.8
  due to decomposed food NEC 005.9
  fat 579.8
  nervous 306.4
  psychogenic 306.4
Indirect —*see* condition
Indolent bubo NEC 099.8
Induced
  abortion—*see* Abortion, induced
  birth, affecting fetus or newborn 763.89
  delivery—*see* Delivery
  labor—*see* Delivery
Induration, indurated
  brain 348.89
  breast (fibrous) 611.79
    puerperal, postpartum 676.3
  broad ligament 620.8
  chancre 091.0
    anus 091.1
    congenital 090.0
    extragenital NEC 091.2
  corpora cavernosa (penis) (plastic) 607.89
  liver (chronic) 573.8
    acute 573.8
  lung (black) (brown) (chronic) (fibroid) (*see also* Fibrosis, lung) 515
    essential brown 275.09 [516.1]
  penile 607.89
  phlebitic—*see* Phlebitis
  skin 782.8
  stomach 537.89
Induratio penis plastica 607.89
Industrial —*see* condition
Inebriety (*see also* Abuse, drugs, nondependent) 305.0
Inefficiency
  kidney (*see also* Disease, renal) 593.9
  thyroid (acquired) (gland) 244.9

Inelasticity, skin 782.8
Inequality, leg (acquired) (length) 736.81
  congenital 755.30
Inertia
  bladder 596.4
    neurogenic 596.54
      with cauda equina syndrome 344.61
  stomach 536.8
    psychogenic 306.4
  uterus, uterine 661.2
    affecting fetus or newborn 763.7
    primary 661.0
    secondary 661.1
  vesical 596.4
    neurogenic 596.54
      with cauda equina 344.61
Infant —*see also* condition
  excessive crying of 780.92
  fussy (baby) 780.91
  held for adoption V68.89
  newborn—*see* Newborn
  post-term (gestation period over 40 completed weeks to 42 completed weeks) 766.21
  prolonged gestation of (period over 42 completed weeks) 766.22
  syndrome of diabetic mother 775.0
"Infant Hercules" syndrome 255.2
Infantile —*see also* condition
  genitalia, genitals 259.0
    in pregnancy or childbirth NEC 654.4
      affecting fetus or newborn 763.89
      causing obstructed labor 660.2
        affecting fetus or newborn 763.1
  heart 746.9
  kidney 753.3
  lack of care 995.52
  macula degeneration 362.75
  melanodontia 521.05
  os, uterus (*see also* Infantile, genitalia) 259.0
  pelvis 738.6
    with disproportion (fetopelvic) 653.1
      affecting fetus or newborn 763.1
      causing obstructed labor 660.1
        affecting fetus or newborn 763.1
  penis 259.0
  testis 257.2
  uterus (*see also* Infantile, genitalia) 259.0
  vulva 752.49
Infantilism 259.9
  with dwarfism (hypophyseal) 253.3
  Brissaud's (infantile myxedema) 244.9
  celiac 579.0
  Herter's (nontropical sprue) 579.0
  hypophyseal 253.3
  hypothalamic (with obesity) 253.8
  idiopathic 259.9
  intestinal 579.0
  pancreatic 577.8
  pituitary 253.3
  renal 588.0
  sexual (with obesity) 259.0
Infants, healthy liveborn —*see* Newborn
Infarct, infarction
  adrenal (capsule) (gland) 255.41
  amnion 658.8
  anterior (with contiguous portion of intraventricular septum) NEC (*see also* Infarct, myocardium) 410.1
  appendices epiploicae 557.0
  bowel 557.0

Infarct, infarction—*continued*
- brain (stem) 434.91
  - embolic (*see also* Embolism, brain) 434.11
  - healed or old, without residuals V12.54
    - iatrogenic 997.02
    - postoperative 997.02
  - puerperal, postpartum, childbirth 674.0
  - thrombotic (*see also* Thrombosis, brain) 434.01
- breast 611.89
- Brewer's (kidney) 593.81
- cardiac (*see also* Infarct, myocardium) 410.9
- cerebellar (*see also* Infarct, brain) 434.91
  - embolic (*see also* Embolism, brain) 434.11
- cerebral (*see also* Infarct, brain) 434.91
  - aborted 434.91
  - embolic (*see also* Embolism, brain) 434.11
  - thrombotic (*see also* Infarct, brain) 434.01
- chorion 658.8
- colon (acute) (agnogenic) (embolic) (hemorrhagic) (nonocclusive) (nonthrombotic) (occlusive) (segmental) (thrombotic) (with gangrene) 557.0
- coronary artery (*see also* Infarct, myocardium) 410.9
- cortical 434.91
- embolic (*see also* Embolism) 444.9
- fallopian tube 620.8
- gallbladder 575.8
- heart (*see also* Infarct, myocardium) 410.9
- hepatic 573.4
- hypophysis (anterior lobe) 253.8
- impending (myocardium) 411.1
- intestine (acute) (agnogenic) (embolic) (hemorrhagic) (nonocclusive) (nonthrombotic) (occlusive) (thrombotic) (with gangrene) 557.0
- kidney 593.81
- liver 573.4
- lung (embolic) (thrombotic) 415.19
  - with
    - abortion—*see* Abortion, by type, with, embolism
    - ectopic pregnancy (*see also* categories 633.0-633.9) 639.6
    - molar pregnancy (*see also* categories 630-632) 639.6
  - following
    - abortion 639.6
    - ectopic or molar pregnancy 639.6
  - iatrogenic 415.11
  - in pregnancy, childbirth, or puerperium—*see* Embolism, obstetrical
  - postoperative 415.11
  - septic 415.12
- lymph node or vessel 457.8
- medullary (brain)—*see* Infarct, brain
- meibomian gland (eyelid) 374.85
- mesentery, mesenteric (embolic) (thrombotic) (with gangrene) 557.0
- midbrain—*see* Infarct, brain
- myocardium, myocardial (acute or with a stated duration of 8 weeks or less) (with hypertension) 410.9

Note—use the following fifth-digit subclassification with category 410

0 *episode unspecified*
1 *initial episode*
2 *subsequent episode without recurrence*

Infarct, infarction—*continued*
- myocardium—*continued*
  - with symptoms after 8 weeks from date of infarction 414.8
  - anterior (wall) (with contiguous portion of intraventricular septum) NEC 410.1
  - anteroapical (with contiguous portion of intraventricular septum) 410.1
  - anterolateral (wall) 410.0
  - anteroseptal (with contiguous portion of intraventricular septum) 410.1
  - apical-lateral 410.5
  - atrial 410.8
  - basal-lateral 410.5
  - chronic (with symptoms after 8 weeks from date of infarction) 414.8
  - diagnosed on ECG, but presenting no symptoms 412
  - diaphragmatic wall (with contiguous portion of intraventricular septum) 410.4
  - healed or old, currently presenting no symptoms 412
  - high lateral 410.5
  - impending 411.1
  - inferior (wall) (with contiguous portion of intraventricular septum) 410.4
  - inferolateral (wall) 410.2
  - inferoposterior wall 410.3
  - intraoperative 997.1
  - lateral wall 410.5
  - non-Q wave 410.7
  - non-ST elevation (NSTEMI) 410.7
  - nontransmural 410.7
  - papillary muscle 410.8
  - past (diagnosed on ECG or other special investigation, but currently presenting no symptoms) 412
    - with symptoms NEC 414.8
  - posterior (strictly) (true) (wall) 410.6
  - posterobasal 410.6
  - posteroinferior 410.3
  - posterolateral 410.5
  - postprocedural 997.1
  - previous, currently presenting no symptoms 412
  - Q-wave (see also Infarct, myocardium, by site) 410.9
  - septal 410.8
  - specified site NEC 410.8
  - ST elevation (STEMI) 410.9
    - anterior (wall) 410.1
    - anterolateral (wall) 410.0
    - inferior (wall) 410.4
    - inferolateral (wall) 410.2
    - inferoposterior (wall) 410.3
    - lateral (wall) 410.5
    - posterior (strictly) (true) (wall) 410.6
    - specified site NEC 410.8
  - subendocardial 410.7
  - syphilitic 093.82
- non-ST elevation myocardial infarction (NSTEMI) 410.7
- nontransmural 410.7
- omentum 557.0
- ovary 620.8
- pancreas 577.8
- papillary muscle (*see also* Infarct, myocardium) 410.8
- parathyroid gland 252.8
- pituitary (gland) 253.8

Infarct, infarction—*continued*
placenta (complicating pregnancy) 656.7
  affecting fetus or newborn 762.2
pontine—*see* Infarct, brain
posterior NEC (*see also* Infarct, myocardium) 410.6
prostate 602.8
pulmonary (artery) (hemorrhagic) (vein) 415.19
with
  abortion—*see* Abortion, by type, with embolism
  ectopic pregnancy (*see also* categories 633.0-633.9) 639.6
  molar pregnancy (*see also* categories 630-632) 639.6
following
  abortion 639.6
  ectopic or molar pregnancy 639.6
iatrogenic 415.11
in pregnancy, childbirth, or puerperium—*see* Embolism, obstetrical
postoperative 415.11
septic 415.12
renal 593.81
  embolic or thrombotic 593.81
retina, retinal 362.84
  with occlusion—*see* Occlusion, retina
spinal (acute) (cord) (embolic) (nonembolic) 336.1
spleen 289.59
  embolic or thrombotic 444.89
subchorionic—*see* Infarct, placenta
subendocardial (*see also* Infarct, myocardium) 410.7
suprarenal (capsule) (gland) 255.41
syncytium—*see* Infarct, placenta
testis 608.83
thrombotic (*see also* Thrombosis) 453.9
  artery, arterial—*see* Embolism
thyroid (gland) 246.3
ventricle (heart) (*see also* Infarct, myocardium) 410.9

Infecting —*see*. condition
Infection, infected, infective (opportunistic) 136.9
with
  influenza viruses occurring in pigs or other animals - *see* Influenza, due to identified, novel influenza A virus
  lymphangitis - *see* Lymphangitis
abortion—*see* Abortion, by type, with sepsis
abscess (skin)—*see* Abscess, by site
Absidia 117.7
Acanthocheilonema (perstans) 125.4
  streptocerca 125.6
acanthamoeba 136.21
accessory sinus (chronic) (*see also* Sinusitis) 473.9
Achorion—*see* Dermatophytosis
Acremonium falciforme 117.4
acromioclavicular (joint) 711.91
actinobacillus
  lignieresii 027.8
  mallei 024
  muris 026.1
actinomadura—*see* Actinomycosis
Actinomyces (israelii)—*see also* Actinomycosis
  muris-ratti 026.1
Actinomycetales (actinomadura) (Actinomyces) (Nocardia) (Streptomyces)—*see* Actinomycosis
actinomycotic NEC (*see also* Actinomycosis) 039.9

Infection, infected, infective—*continued*
adenoid (chronic) 474.01
  acute 463
  and tonsil (chronic) 474.02
  acute or subacute 463
adenovirus NEC 079.0
  in diseases classified elsewhere—*see* category 079
  unspecified nature or site 079.0
Aerobacter aerogenes NEC 041.85
  enteritis 008.2
aerogenes capsulatus (*see also* Gangrene, gas) 040.0
aertrycke (*see also* Infection, Salmonella) 003.9
ajellomyces dermatitidis 116.0
alimentary canal NEC (*see also* Enteritis, due to, by organism) 009.0
Allescheria boydii 117.6
Alternaria 118
alveolus, alveolar (process) (pulpal origin) 522.4
ameba, amebic (histolytica) (*see also* Amebiasis) 006.9
  acute 006.0
  chronic 006.1
  free-living 136.29
  hartmanni 007.8
  specified
    site NEC 006.8
    type NEC 007.8
amniotic fluid or cavity 658.4
  affecting fetus or newborn 762.7
anaerobes (cocci) (gram-negative) (gram positive) (mixed) NEC 041.84
anal canal 569.49
Ancylostoma braziliense 126.2
Angiostrongylus cantonensis 128.8
anisakiasis 127.1
Anisakis larva 127.1
anthrax (*see also* Anthrax) 022.9
antrum (chronic) (*see also* Sinusitis, maxillary) 473.0
anus (papillae) (sphincter) 569.49
arbor virus NEC 066.9
arbovirus NEC 066.9
argentophil-rod 027.0
Ascaris lumbricoides 127.0
ascomycetes 117.4
Aspergillus (flavus) (fumigatus) (terreus) 117.3
atypical
  acid-fast (bacilli) (*see also* Mycobacterium, atypical) 031.9
  mycobacteria (*see also* Mycobacterium, atypical) 031.9
auditory meatus (circumscribed) (diffuse) (external) (*see also* Otitis, externa) 380.10
auricle (ear) (*see also* Otitis, externa) 380.10
axillary gland 683
Babesiasis 088.82
Babesiosis 088.82
Bacillus NEC 041.89
  abortus 023.1
  anthracis (*see also* Anthrax) 022.9
  cereus (food poisoning) 005.89
  coli—*see* Infection, Escherichia coli
  coliform NEC 041.85
  Ducrey's (any location) 099.0
  Flexner's 004.1
  Friedländer's NEC 041.3
  fusiformis 101
  gas (gangrene) (*see also* Gangrene, gas) 040.0
  mallei 024
  melitensis 023.0

Infection, infected, infective—*continued*
  Bacillus—*continued*
    paratyphoid, paratyphosus 002.9
      A 002.1
      B 002.2
      C 002.3
    Schmorl's 040.3
    Shiga 004.0
    suipestifer (*see also* Infection, Salmonella)
      003.9
    swimming pool 031.1
    typhosa 002.0
    welchii (*see also* Gangrene, gas) 040.0
    Whitmore's 025
  bacterial NEC 041.9
    specified NEC 041.89
      anaerobic NEC 041.84
      gram-negative NEC 041.85
        anaerobic NEC 041.84
  Bacterium
    paratyphosum 002.9
      A 002.1
      B 002.2
      C 002.3
    typhosum 002.0
  Bacteroides (fragilis) (melaninogenicus) (oralis)
    NEC 041.82
  balantidium coli 007.0
  Bartholin's gland 616.89
  Basidiobolus 117.7
  Bedsonia 079.98
    specified NEC 079.88
  bile duct 576.1
  bladder (*see also* Cystitis) 595.9
  Blastomyces, blastomycotic 116.0
    brasiliensis 116.1
    dermatitidis 116.0
    European 117.5
    Loboi 116.2
    North American 116.0
    South American 116.1
  bleb
    postprocedural 379.60
      stage 1 379.61
      stage 2 379.62
      stage 3 379.63
  blood stream—*see also* Septicemia
    catheter-related (CRBSI) 999.31
    central line-associated (CLABSI) 999.32
    due to central venous catheter 999.32
  bone 730.9
    specified—*see* Osteomyelitis
  Bordetella 033.9
    bronchiseptica 033.8
    parapertussis 033.1
    pertussis 033.0
  Borrelia
    bergdorfi 088.81
    vincentii (mouth) (pharynx) (tonsil) 101
  bovine stomatitis 059.11
  brain (*see also* Encephalitis) 323.9
    late effect—*see* category 326
    membranes—(*see also* Meningitis) 322.9
    septic 324.0
      late effect—*see* category 326
    meninges (*see also* Meningitis) 320.9
  branchial cyst 744.42

Infection, infected, infective—*continued*
  breast 611.0
    puerperal, postpartum 675.2
      with nipple 675.9
        specified type NEC 675.8
      nonpurulent 675.2
      purulent 675.1
  bronchus (*see also* Bronchitis) 490
    fungus NEC 117.9
  Brucella 023.9
    abortus 023.1
    canis 023.3
    melitensis 023.0
    mixed 023.8
    suis 023.2
  Brugia (Wuchereria) malayi 125.1
  bursa—*see* Bursitis
  buttocks (skin) 686.9
  Candida (albicans) (tropicalis) (*see also*
    Candidiasis) 112.9
    congenital 771.7
  Candiru 136.8
  Capillaria
    hepatica 128.8
    philippinensis 127.5
  cartilage 733.99
  cat liver fluke 121.0
  catheter-related bloodstream (CRBSI) 999.31
  cellulitis—*see* Cellulitis, by site
  central line-associated 999.31
    bloodstream 999.32
  Cephalosporum falciforme 117.4
  Cercomonas hominis (intestinal) 007.3
  cerebrospinal (*see also* Meningitis) 322.9
    late effect—*see* category 326
  cervical gland 683
  cervix (*see also* Cervicitis) 616.0
  cesarean section wound 674.3
  Chilomastix (intestinal) 007.8
  Chlamydia 079.98
    specified NEC 079.88
  Cholera (*see also* Cholera) 001.9
  chorionic plate 658.8
  Cladosporium
    bantianum 117.8
    carrionii 117.2
    mansoni 111.1
    trichoides 117.8
    wernecki 111.1
  Clonorchis (sinensis) (liver) 121.1
  Clostridium (haemolyticum) (novyi) NEC
    041.84
    botulinum 005.1
    histolyticum (*see also* Gangrene, gas) 040.0
    oedematiens (*see also* Gangrene, gas) 040.0
    perfringens 041.83
      due to food 005.2
    septicum (*see also* Gangrene, gas) 040.0
    sordelii (*see also* Gangrene, gas) 040.0
    welchii (*see also* Gangrene, gas) 040.0
      due to food 005.2
  Coccidioides (immitis) (*see also*
    Coccidioidomycosis) 114.9
  coccus NEC 041.89
  colon (*see also* Enteritis, due to, by organism) 009.0
    bacillus—*see* Infection, Escherichia coli
  colostomy or enterostomy 569.61
  common duct 576.1
  complicating pregnancy, childbirth, or
    puerperium NEC 647.9
    affecting fetus or newborn 760.2

Infection, infected, infective—*continued*
  Condiobolus 117.7
  congenital NEC 771.89
    Candida albicans 771.7
    chronic 771.2
    Cytomegalovirus 771.1
    hepatitis, viral 771.2
    Herpes simplex 771.2
    listeriosis 771.2
    malaria 771.2
    poliomyelitis 771.2
    rubella 771.0
    toxoplasmosis 771.2
    tuberculosis 771.2
    urinary (tract) 771.82
    vaccinia 771.2
  coronavirus 079.89
    SARS-associated 079.82
  corpus luteum (*see also* Salpingo-oophoritis)
      614.2
  Corynebacterium diphtheriae—*see* Diphtheria
  cotia virus 059.8
  Coxsackie (*see also* Coxsackie) 079.2
    endocardium 074.22
    heart NEC 074.20
    in diseases classified elsewhere—*see* category 079
    meninges 047.0
    myocardium 074.23
    pericardium 074.21
    pharynx 074.0
    specified disease NEC 074.8
    unspecified nature or site 079.2
  Cryptococcus neoformans 117.5
  Cryptosporidia 007.4
  Cunninghamella 117.7
  cyst—*see* Cyst
  Cysticercus cellulosae 123.1
  cystostomy 596.83
  cytomegalovirus 078.5
    congenital 771.1
  dental (pulpal origin) 522.4
  deuteromycetes 117.4
  Dicrocoelium dendriticum 121.8
  Dipetalonema (perstans) 125.4
    streptocerca 125.6
  diphtherial—*see* Diphtheria
  Diphyllobothrium (adult) (latum) (pacificum)
      123.4
    larval 123.5
  Diplogonoporus (grandis) 123.8
  Dipylidium (caninum) 123.8
  Dirofilaria 125.6
  dog tapeworm 123.8
  Dracunculus medinensis 125.7
  Dreschlera 118
    hawaiiensis 117.8
  Ducrey's bacillus (any site) 099.0
  due to or resulting from
    central venous catheter (*see also*
        Complications, due to, catheter, central
        venous) 999.31
      bloodstream 999.32
      localized 999.33
    device, implant, or graft (any) (presence
        of)—*see* Complications, infection and
        inflammation, due to (presence of) any
        device, implant, or graft classified to
        996.0-996.5 NEC

Infection, infected, infective—*continued*
  due to or resulting from—*continued*
    injection, inoculation, infusion, transfusion, or
        vaccination (prophylactic) (therapeutic)
        999.39
      blood and blood products
        acute 999.34
    injury NEC—*see* Wound, open, by site,
        complicated
    surgery 998.59
  duodenum 535.6
  ear—*see also* Otitis
    external (*see also* Otitis, externa) 380.10
    inner (*see also* Labyrinthitis) 386.30
    middle —*see* Otitis, media
  Eaton's agent NEC 041.81
  Eberthella typhosa 002.0
  Ebola 078.89
  echinococcosis 122.9
  Echinococcus (*see also* Echinococcus) 122.9
  Echinostoma 121.8
  ECHO virus 079.1
    in diseases classified elsewhere—*see* category
        079
    unspecified nature or site 079.1
  Ehrlichiosis 082.40
    chaffeensis 082.41
    specified type NEC 082.49
  Endamoeba—*see* Infection, ameba
  endocardium (*see also* Endocarditis) 421.0
  endocervix (*see also* Cervicitis) 616.0
  Entamoeba—*see* Infection, ameba
  enteric (*see also* Enteritis, due to, by organism)
      009.0
  Enterobacter aerogenes NEC 041.85
  Enterobacter sakazakii 041.85
  Enterobius vermicularis 127.4
  enterococcus NEC 041.04
  enterovirus NEC 079.89
    central nervous system NEC 048
    enteritis 008.67
    meningitis 047.9
  Entomophthora 117.7
  Epidermophyton—*see* Dermatophytosis
  epidermophytosis—*see* Dermatophytosis
  episiotomy 674.3
  Epstein-Barr virus 075
    chronic 780.79 *[139.8]*
  erysipeloid 027.1
  Erysipelothrix (insidiosa) (rhusiopathiae) 027.1
  erythema infectiosum 057.0
  Escherichia coli (E. coli) 041.49
    enteritis—*see* Enteritis, E. coli
    generalized 038.42
    intestinal—*see* Enteritis, E. coli
    non-Shiga toxin-producing 041.49
    Shiga toxin-producing (STEC) 041.43
      with
        unspecified O group 041.43
      non-O157 (with known O group) 041.42
      O157 (with confirmation of Shiga toxin
          when H antigen is unknown, or is not
          H7) 041.41
      O157:H- (nonmotile) with confirmation of
          Shiga toxin 041.41
      O157:H7 with or without confirmation of
          Shiga toxin-production 041.41
      specified NEC 041.42
  esophagostomy 530.86
  ethmoidal (chronic) (sinus) (*see also* Sinusitis,
      ethmoidal) 473.2

Infection, infected, infective—*continued*
  Eubacterium 041.84
  Eustachian tube (ear) 381.50
    acute 381.51
    chronic 381.52
  exanthema subitum (*see also* Exanthem
    subitum) 058.10
  exit site 999.33
  external auditory canal (meatus) (*see also* Otitis,
    externa) 380.10
  eye NEC 360.00
  eyelid 373.9
    specified NEC 373.8
  fallopian tube (*see also* Salpingo-oophoritis)
    614.2
  fascia 728.89
  Fasciola
    gigantica 121.3
    hepatica 121.3
  Fasciolopsis (buski) 121.4
  fetus (intra-amniotic)—*see* Infection, congenital
  filarial—*see* Infestation, filarial
  finger (skin) 686.9
    abscess (with lymphangitis) 681.00
      pulp 681.01
    cellulitis (with lymphangitis) 681.00
    distal closed space (with lymphangitis) 681.00
    nail 681.02
      fungus 110.1
  fish tapeworm 123.4
    larval 123.5
  flagellate, intestinal 007.9
  fluke—*see* Infestation, fluke
  focal
    teeth (pulpal origin) 522.4
    tonsils 474.00
      and adenoids 474.02
  Fonsecaea
    compactum 117.2
    pedrosoi 117.2
  food (*see also* Poisoning, food) 005.9
  foot (skin) 686.9
    fungus 110.4
  Francisella tularensis (*see also* Tularemia) 021.9
  frontal sinus (chronic) (*see also* Sinusitis,
    frontal) 473.1
  fungus NEC 117.9
    beard 110.0
    body 110.5
    dermatiacious NEC 117.8
    foot 110.4
    groin 110.3
    hand 110.2
    nail 110.1
    pathogenic to compromised host only 118
    perianal (area) 110.3
    scalp 110.0
    scrotum 110.8
    skin 111.9
      foot 110.4
      hand 110.2
    toenails 110.1
    trachea 117.9
  Fusarium 118
  Fusobacterium 041.84
  gallbladder (*see also* Cholecystitis, acute) 575.0
  Gardnerella vaginalis 041.89
  gas bacillus (*see also* Gas, gangrene) 040.0
  gastric (*see also* Gastritis) 535.5
  Gastrodiscoides hominis 121.8
  gastroenteric (*see also* Enteritis, due to, by
    organism) 009.0

Infection, infected, infective—*continued*
  gastrointestinal (*see also* Enteritis, due to, by
    organism) 009.0
  gastrostomy 536.41
  generalized NEC (*see also* Septicemia) 038.9
  genital organ or tract NEC
    female 614.9
      with
        abortion—*see* Abortion, by type, with sepsis
        ectopic pregnancy (*see also* categories
          633.0-633.9) 639.0
        molar pregnancy (*see also* categories
          630-632) 639.0
      complicating pregnancy 646.6
        affecting fetus or newborn 760.8
      following
        abortion 639.0
        ectopic or molar pregnancy 639.0
      puerperal, postpartum, childbirth 670.8
      minor or localized 646.6
        affecting fetus or newborn 760.8
    male 608.4
  genitourinary tract NEC 599.0
  Ghon tubercle, primary (*see also* Tuberculosis)
    010.0
  Giardia lamblia 007.1
  gingival (chronic) 523.10
    acute 523.00
    Vincent's 101
  glanders 024
  Glenosporopsis amazonica 116.2
  Gnathostoma spinigerum 128.1
  Gongylonema 125.6
  gonococcal NEC (*see also* Gonococcus) 098.0
  gram-negative bacilli NEC 041.85
    anaerobic 041.84
  guinea worm 125.7
  gum (*see also* Infection, gingival) 523.10
  Hantavirus 079.81
  heart 429.89
  Helicobacter pylori [*H. pylori*] 041.86
  helminths NEC 128.9
    intestinal 127.9
      mixed (types classifiable to more than one
        category in 120.0-127.7) 127.8
      specified type NEC 127.7
    specified type NEC 128.8
  Hemophilus influenzae NEC 041.5
    generalized 038.41
  Herpes (simplex) (*see also* Herpes, simplex)
    054.9
    congenital 771.2
    zoster (*see also* Herpes, zoster) 053.9
      eye NEC 053.29
  Heterophyes heterophyes 121.6
  Histoplasma (*see also* Histoplasmosis) 115.90
    capsulatum (*see also* Histoplasmosis,
      American) 115.00
    duboisii (*see also* Histoplasmosis, African)
      115.10
  HIV V08
    with symptoms, symptomatic 042
  hookworm (*see also* Ancylostomiasis) 126.9
  human herpesvirus 6 058.81
  human herpesvirus 7 058.82
  human herpesvirus 8 058.89
  human herpesvirus NEC 058.89
  human immunodeficiency virus V08
    with symptoms, symptomatic 042
  human papillomavirus 079.4
  hydrocele 603.1
  hydronephrosis 591

Infection, infected, infective—*continued*
  Hymenolepis 123.6
  hypopharynx 478.29
  inguinal glands 683
    due to soft chancre 099.0
  insertion site 999.33
  intestine, intestinal (*see also* Enteritis, due to, by
    organism) 009.0
  intrauterine (*see also* Endometritis) 615.9
    complicating delivery 646.6
  isospora belli or hominis 007.2
  Japanese B encephalitis 062.0
  jaw (bone) (acute) (chronic) (lower) (subacute)
    (upper) 526.4
  joint—*see* Arthritis, infectious or infective
  Kaposi's sarcoma-associated herpesvirus 058.89
  kidney (cortex) (hematogenous) 590.9
    with
      abortion—*see* Abortion, by type, with
        urinary tract infection
      calculus 592.0
      ectopic pregnancy (*see also* categories
        633.0-633.9) 639.8
      molar pregnancy (*see also* categories
        630-632) 639.8
    complicating pregnancy or puerperium 646.6
      affecting fetus or newborn 760.1
    following
      abortion 639.8
      ectopic or molar pregnancy 639.8
    pelvis and ureter 590.3
  Klebsiella pneumoniae NEC 041.3
  knee (skin) NEC 686.9
    joint—*see* Arthritis, infectious
  Koch's (*see also* Tuberculosis, pulmonary) 011.9
  labia (majora) (minora) (*see also* Vulvitis)
    616.10
  lacrimal
    gland (*see also* Dacryoadenitis) 375.00
    passages (duct) (sac) (*see also* Dacryocystitis)
      375.30
  larynx NEC 478.79
  leg (skin) NEC 686.9
  Leishmania (*see also* Leishmaniasis) 085.9
    braziliensis 085.5
    donovani 085.0
    Ethiopica 085.3
    furunculosa 085.1
    infantum 085.0
    mexicana 085.4
    tropica (minor) 085.1
      major 085.2
  Leptosphaeria senegalensis 117.4
  leptospira (*see also* Leptospirosis) 100.9
    Australis 100.89
    Bataviae 100.89
    pyrogenes 100.89
    specified type NEC 100.89
  leptospirochetal NEC (*see also* Leptospirosis)
    100.9
  Leptothrix—*see* Actinomycosis
  Listeria monocytogenes (listeriosis) 027.0
    congenital 771.2
  liver fluke—*see* Infestation, fluke, liver
  Loa loa 125.2
    eyelid 125.2 *[373.6]*
  Loboa loboi 116.2
  local, skin (staphylococcal) (streptococcal) NEC
    686.9
    abscess—*see* Abscess, by site
    cellulitis—*see* Cellulitis, by site
    ulcer (*see also* Ulcer, skin) 707.9

Infection, infected, infective—*continued*
  Loefflerella
    mallei 024
    whitmori 025
  lung 518.89
    atypical Mycobacterium 031.0
      tuberculous (*see also* Tuberculosis,
        pulmonary) 011.9
    basilar 518.89
    chronic 518.89
    fungus NEC 117.9
    spirochetal 104.8
    virus—*see* Pneumonia, virus
  lymph gland (axillary) (cervical) (inguinal) 683
    mesenteric 289.2
  lymphoid tissue, base of tongue or posterior
    pharynx, NEC 474.00
  madurella
    grisea 117.4
    mycetomii 117.4
  major
    with
      abortion—*see* Abortion, by type, with sepsis
      ectopic pregnancy (*see also* categories
        633.0-633.9) 639.0
      molar pregnancy (*see also* categories
        630-632) 639.0
    following
      abortion 639.0
      ectopic or molar pregnancy 639.0
    puerperal, postpartum, childbirth 670.0
  malarial—*see* Malaria
  Malassezia furfur 111.0
  Malleomyces
    mallei 024
    pseudomallei 025
  mammary gland 611.0
    puerperal, postpartum 675.2
  Mansonella (ozzardi) 125.5
  mastoid (suppurative)—*see* Mastoiditis
  maxilla, maxillary 526.4
    sinus (chronic) (*see also* Sinusitis, maxillary)
      473.0
  mediastinum 519.2
  medina 125.7
  meibomian
    cyst 373.12
    gland 373.12
  melioidosis 025
  meninges (*see also* Meningitis) 320.9
  meningococcal (*see also* condition) 036.9
    brain 036.1
    cerebrospinal 036.0
    endocardium 036.42
    generalized 036.2
    meninges 036.0
    meningococcemia 036.2
    specified site NEC 036.89
  mesenteric lymph nodes or glands NEC 289.2
  Metagonimus 121.5
  metatarsophalangeal 711.97
  methicillin
    resistant Staphylococcus aureus (MRSA) 041.12
    susceptible Staphylococcus aureus (MSSA)
      041.11
  microorganism resistant to drugs—*see*
    Resistance (to), drugs by microorganisms
  Microsporidia 136.8
  microsporum, microsporic—*see*
    Dermatophytosis
  Mima polymorpha NEC 041.85
  mixed flora NEC 041.89

Infection, infected, infective—*continued*
Monilia (*see also* Candidiasis) 112.9
  neonatal 771.7
monkeypox 059.01
Monosporium apiospermum 117.6
mouth (focus) NEC 528.9
  parasitic 112.0
MRSA (methicillin resistant Staphylococcus
  aureus) 041.12
MSSA (methicillin susceptible Staphylococcus
  aureus) 041.11
Mucor 117.7
muscle NEC 728.89
mycelium NEC 117.9
mycetoma
  actinomycotic NEC (*see also* Actinomycosis) 039.9
  mycotic NEC 117.4
Mycobacterium, mycobacterial (*see also*
  Mycobacterium) 031.9
mycoplasma NEC 041.81
mycotic NEC 117.9
  pathogenic to compromised host only 118
  skin NEC 111.9
  systemic 117.9
myocardium NEC 422.90
nail (chronic) (with lymphangitis) 681.9
  finger 681.02
    fungus 110.1
    ingrowing 703.0
  toe 681.11
    fungus 110.1
nasal sinus (chronic) (*see also* Sinusitis) 473.9
nasopharynx (chronic) 478.29
  acute 460
navel 686.9
  newborn 771.4
Neisserian—*see* Gonococcus
Neotestudina rosatii 117.4
newborn, generalized 771.89
nipple 611.0
  puerperal, postpartum 675.0
    with breast 675.9
      specified type NEC 675.8
Nocardia—*see* Actinomycosis
nose 478.19
nostril 478.19
obstetrical surgical wound 674.3
Oesophagostomum (apiostomum) 127.7
Oestrus ovis 134.0
Oidium albicans (*see also* Candidiasis) 112.9
Onchocerca (volvulus) 125.3
  eye 125.3 *[360.13]*
  eyelid 125.3 *[373.6]*
operation wound 998.59
Opisthorchis (felineus) (tenuicollis) (viverrini)
  121.0
orbit 376.00
  chronic 376.10
orthopoxvirus 059.00
  specified NEC 059.09
ovary (*see also* Salpingo-oophoritis) 614.2
Oxyuris vermicularis 127.4
pancreas 577.0
Paracoccidioides brasiliensis 116.1
Paragonimus (westermani) 121.2
parainfluenza virus 079.89
parameningococcus NEC 036.9
  with meningitis 036.0
parapoxvirus 059.10
  specified NEC 059.19
parasitic NEC 136.9

Infection, infected, infective—*continued*
paratyphoid 002.9
  Type A 002.1
  Type B 002.2
  Type C 002.3
paraurethral ducts 597.89
parotid gland 527.2
Pasteurella NEC 027.2
  multocida (cat-bite) (dog-bite) 027.2
  pestis (*see also* Plague) 020.9
  pseudotuberculosis 027.2
  septica (cat-bite) (dog-bite) 027.2
  tularensis (*see also* Tularemia) 021.9
pelvic, female (*see also* Disease, pelvis,
  inflammatory) 614.9
penis (glans) (retention) NEC 607.2
  herpetic 054.13
Peptococcus 041.84
Peptostreptococcus 041.84
periapical (pulpal origin) 522.4
peridental 523.30
perineal wound (obstetrical) 674.3
periodontal 523.31
periorbital 376.00
  chronic 376.10
perirectal 569.49
perirenal (*see also* Infection, kidney) 590.9
peritoneal (*see also* Peritonitis) 567.9
periureteral 593.89
periurethral 597.89
Petriellidium boydii 117.6
pharynx 478.29
  Coxsackie virus 074.0
  phlegmonous 462
  posterior, lymphoid 474.00
Phialophora
  gougerotii 117.8
  jeanselmei 117.8
  verrucosa 117.2
Piedraia hortai 111.3
pinna, acute 380.11
pinta 103.9
  intermediate 103.1
  late 103.2
  mixed 103.3
  primary 103.0
pinworm 127.4
pityrosporum furfur 111.0
pleuropneumonia-like organisms NEC (PPLO)
  041.81
pneumococcal NEC 041.2
  generalized (purulent) 038.2
Pneumococcus NEC 041.2
port 999.33
postoperative wound 998.59
posttraumatic NEC 958.3
postvaccinal 999.39
poxvirus 059.9
  specified NEC 059.8
prepuce NEC 607.1
Propionibacterium 041.84
prostate (capsule) (*see also* Prostatitis) 601.9
Proteus (mirabilis) (morganii) (vulgaris) NEC
  041.6
  enteritis 008.3
protozoal NEC 136.8
  intestinal NEC 007.9
Pseudomonas NEC 041.7
  mallei 024
  pneumonia 482.1
  pseudomallei 025

Infection, infected, infective—*continued*
  psittacosis 073.9
  puerperal, postpartum (major) 670.0
    minor 646.6
  pulmonary—*see* Infection, lung
  purulent—*see* Abscess
  putrid, generalized—*see* Septicemia
  pyemic—*see* Septicemia
  Pyrenochaeta romeroi 117.4
  Q fever 083.0
  rabies 071
  rectum (sphincter) 569.49
  renal (*see also* Infection, kidney) 590.9
    pelvis and ureter 590.3
  reservoir 999.33
  resistant to drugs—*see* Resistance (to), drugs by
    microorganisms
  respiratory 519.8
    chronic 519.8
    influenzal (acute) (upper) (*see also* Influenza)
      487.1
    lung 518.89
    rhinovirus 460
    syncytial virus 079.6
    upper (acute) (infectious) NEC 465.9
      with flu, grippe, or influenza (*see also*
        Influenza) 487.1
      influenzal (*see also* Influenza) 487.1
      multiple sites NEC 465.8
      streptococcal 034.0
      viral NEC 465.9
  respiratory syncytial virus (RSV) 079.6
  resulting from presence of shunt or other
      internal prosthetic device—*see*
      Complications, infection and inflammation,
      due to (presence of) any device, implant, or
      graft classified to 996.0-996.5 NEC
  retroperitoneal 567.39
  retrovirus 079.50
    human immunodeficiency virus type 2
      (HIV-2) 079.53
    human T-cell lymphotrophic virus type I
      (HTLV-I) 079.51
    human T-cell lymphotrophic virus type II
      (HTLV-II) 079.52
    specified NEC 079.59
  Rhinocladium 117.1
  Rhinosporidium (*see*beri) 117.0
  rhinovirus
    in diseases classified elsewhere—*see* category
      079
    unspecified nature or site 079.3
  Rhizopus 117.7
  rickettsial 083.9
  rickettsialpox 083.2
  rubella (*see also* Rubella) 056.9
    congenital 771.0
  Saccharomyces (*see also* Candidiasis) 112.9
  Saksenaea 117.7
  salivary duct or gland (any) 527.2
  Salmonella (aertrycke) (callinarum)
    (choleraesuis) (enteritidis) (suipestifer)
    (typhimurium) 003.9
    with
      arthritis 003.23
      gastroenteritis 003.0
      localized infection 003.20
        specified type NEC 003.29
      meningitis 003.21
      osteomyelitis 003.24
      pneumonia 003.22

Infection, infected, infective—*continued*
    septicemia 003.1
      specified manifestation NEC 003.8
    due to food (poisoning) (any serotype) (*see*
      also Poisoning, food, due to, Salmonella)
    hirschfeldii 002.3
    localized 003.20
      specified type NEC 003.29
    paratyphi 002.9
      A 002.1
      B 002.2
      C 002.3
    schottmuelleri 002.2
    specified type NEC 003.8
    typhi 002.0
    typhosa 002.0
  saprophytic 136.8
  Sarcocystis, lindemanni 136.5
  SARS-associated coronavirus 079.82
  scabies 133.0
  Schistosoma—*see* Infestation, Schistosoma
  Schmorl's bacillus 040.3
  scratch or other superficial injury—*see* Injury,
    superficial, by site
  scrotum (acute) NEC 608.4
  sealpox 059.12
  secondary, burn or open wound (dislocation)
    (fracture) 958.3
  seminal vesicle (*see also* Vesiculitis) 608.0
  septic
    generalized—*see* Septicemia
    localized, skin (*see also* Abscess) 682.9
  septicemic—*see* Septicemia
  seroma 998.51
  Serratia (marcescens) 041.85
    generalized 038.44
  sheep liver fluke 121.3
  Shigella 004.9
    boydii 004.2
    dysenteriae 004.0
    Flexneri 004.1
    group
      A 004.0
      B 004.1
      C 004.2
      D 004.3
    Schmitz (-Stutzer) 004.0
    Schmitzii 004.0
    Shiga 004.0
    Sonnei 004.3
    specified type NEC 004.8
  Sin Nombre virus 079.81
  sinus (*see also* Sinusitis) 473.9
    pilonidal 685.1
      with abscess 685.0
    skin NEC 686.9
  Skene's duct or gland (*see also* Urethritis) 597.89
  skin (local) (staphylococcal) (streptococcal)
    NEC 686.9
    abscess—*see* Abscess, by site
    cellulitis—*see* Cellulitis, by site
    due to fungus 111.9
      specified type NEC 111.8
    mycotic 111.9
      specified type NEC 111.8
    ulcer (*see also* Ulcer, skin) 707.9
  slow virus 046.9
    specified condition NEC 046.8
  Sparganum (mansoni) (proliferum) 123.5
  spermatic cord NEC 608.4

Infection, infected, infective—*continued*
  sphenoidal (chronic) (sinus) (*see also* Sinusitis,
    sphenoidal) 473.3
  Spherophorus necrophorus 040.3
  spinal cord NEC (*see also* Encephalitis) 323.9
    abscess 324.1
      late effect—*see* category 326
    late effect—*see* category 326
    meninges—*see* Meningitis
    streptococcal 320.2
  Spirillum
    minus or minor 026.0
    morsus muris 026.0
    obermeieri 087.0
  spirochetal NEC 104.9
    lung 104.8
    specified nature or site NEC 104.8
  spleen 289.59
  Sporothrix schenckii 117.1
  Sporotrichum (schenckii) 117.1
  Sporozoa 136.8
  staphylococcal NEC 041.10
    aureus 041.11
      methicillin
        resistant (MRSA) 041.12
        susceptible MSSA 041.11
    food poisoning 005.0
    generalized (purulent) 038.10
      aureus 038.11
        methicillin
          resistant 038.12
          susceptible 038.11
      specified organism NEC 038.19
    pneumonia 482.40
      aureus 482.41
        methicillin
          resistant (MRSA) 482.42
          susceptible (MSSA) 482.41
      MRSA (methicillin resistant staphylococcus
        aureus) 482.42
      MSSA (methicillin susceptible
        staphylococcus aureus) 482.41
      specified type NEC 482.49
    septicemia 038.10
      aureus 038.11
        methicillin
          resistant (MRSA) 038.12
          susceptible (MSSA) 038.11
      MRSA (methicillin resistant staphylococcus
        aureus) 038.12
      MSSA (methicillin susceptible
        staphylococcus aureus) 038.11
      specified organism NEC 038.19
    specified NEC 041.19
  steatoma 706.2
  Stellantchasmus falcatus 121.6
  Streptobacillus moniliformis 026.1
  streptococcal NEC 041.00
    generalized (purulent) 038.0
    group
      A 041.01
      B 041.02
      C 041.03
      D [enterococcus] 041.04
      G 041.05
    pneumonia—*see* Pneumonia, streptococcal
      482.3
    septicemia 038.0
    sore throat 034.0
    specified NEC 041.09
  Streptomyces—*see* Actinomycosis

Infection, infected, infective—*continued*
  streptotrichosis—*see* Actinomycosis
  Strongyloides (stercoralis) 127.2
  stump (amputation) (posttraumatic) (surgical)
    997.62
    traumatic—*see* Amputation, traumatic, by site,
      complicated
  subcutaneous tissue, local NEC 686.9
  submaxillary region 528.9
  suipestifer (*see also* Infection, Salmonella) 003.9
  swimming pool bacillus 031.1
  syphilitic—*see* Syphilis
  systemic—*see* Septicemia
  Taenia—*see* Infestation, Taenia
  Taeniarhynchus saginatus 123.2
  tanapox 059.21
  tapeworm—*see* Infestation, tapeworm
  tendon (sheath) 727.89
  Ternidens diminutus 127.7
  testis (*see also* Orchitis) 604.90
  thigh (skin) 686.9
  threadworm 127.4
  throat 478.29
    pneumococcal 462
    staphylococcal 462
    streptococcal 034.0
    viral NEC (*see also* Pharyngitis) 462
  thumb (skin) 686.9
    abscess (with lymphangitis) 681.00
      pulp 681.01
    cellulitis (with lymphangitis) 681.00
    nail 681.02
  thyroglossal duct 529.8
  toe (skin) 686.9
    abscess (with lymphangitis) 681.10
    cellulitis (with lymphangitis) 681.10
    nail 681.11
      fungus 110.1
  tongue NEC 529.0
    parasitic 112.0
  tonsil (faucial) (lingual) (pharyngeal) 474.00
    acute or subacute 463
    and adenoid 474.02
    tag 474.00
  tooth, teeth 522.4
    periapical (pulpal origin) 522.4
    peridental 523.30
    periodontal 523.31
    pulp 522.0
    socket 526.5
  TORCH - see Infection, congenital NEC
    without active infection 760.2
  Torula histolytica 117.5
  Toxocara (cani) (cati) (felis) 128.0
  Toxoplasma gondii (*see also* Toxoplasmosis) 130.9
  trachea, chronic 491.8
    fungus 117.9
  traumatic NEC 958.3
  trematode NEC 121.9
  trench fever 083.1
  Treponema
    denticola 041.84
    macrodenticum 041.84
    pallidum (*see also* Syphilis) 097.9
  Trichinella (spiralis) 124
  Trichomonas 131.9
    bladder 131.09
    cervix 131.09
    hominis 007.3
    intestine 007.3
    prostate 131.03
    specified site NEC 131.8

Infection, infected, infective—*continued*
  urethra 131.02
  urogenitalis 131.00
  vagina 131.01
  vulva 131.01
  Trichophyton, trichophytid—*see*
    Dermatophytosis
  Trichosporon (beigelii) cutaneum 111.2
  Trichostrongylus 127.6
  Trichuris (trichiuria) 127.3
  Trombicula (irritans) 133.8
  Trypanosoma (*see also* Trypanosomiasis) 086.9
    cruzi 086.2
  tubal (*see also* Salpingo-oophoritis) 614.2
  tuberculous NEC (*see also* Tuberculosis) 011.9
  tubo-ovarian (*see also* Salpingo-oophoritis)
    614.2
  tunica vaginalis 608.4
  tunnel 999.33
  tympanic membrane—*see* Myringitis
  typhoid (abortive) (ambulant) (bacillus) 002.0
  typhus 081.9
    flea-borne (endemic) 081.0
    louse-borne (epidemic) 080
    mite-borne 081.2
    recrudescent 081.1
    tick-borne 082.9
      African 082.1
      North Asian 082.2
  umbilicus (septic) 686.9
    newborn NEC 771.4
  ureter 593.89
  urethra (*see also* Urethritis) 597.80
  urinary (tract) NEC 599.0
    with
      abortion—*see* Abortion, by type, with
        urinary tract infection
      ectopic pregnancy (*see also* categories
        633.0-633.9) 639.8
      molar pregnancy (*see also* categories
        630-632) 639.8
    candidal 112.2
    complicating pregnancy, childbirth, or
      puerperium 646.6
      affecting fetus or newborn 760.1
      asymptomatic 646.5
        affecting fetus or newborn 760.1
    diplococcal (acute) 098.0
      chronic 098.2
    due to Trichomonas (vaginalis) 131.00
    following
      abortion 639.8
      ectopic or molar pregnancy 639.8
    gonococcal (acute) 098.0
      chronic or duration of 2 months or over
        098.2
    newborn 771.82
    trichomonal 131.00
    tuberculous (*see also* Tuberculosis) 016.3
  uterus, uterine (*see also* Endometritis) 615.9
  utriculus masculinus NEC 597.89
  vaccination 999.39
  vagina (granulation tissue) (wall) (*see also*
    Vaginitis) 616.10
  varicella 052.9
  varicose veins—*see* Varicose, veins
  variola 050.9
    major 050.0
    minor 050.1
  vas deferens NEC 608.4
  Veillonella 041.84

Infection, infected, infective—*continued*
  verumontanum 597.89
  vesical (*see also* Cystitis) 595.9
  Vibrio
    cholerae 001.0
      El Tor 001.1
    parahaemolyticus (food poisoning) 005.4
    vulnificus 041.85
  Vincent's (gums) (mouth) (tonsil) 101
  virus, viral 079.99
    adenovirus
      in diseases classified elsewhere—*see*
        category 079
      unspecified nature or site 079.0
    central nervous system NEC 049.9
      enterovirus 048
        meningitis 047.9
          specified type NEC 047.8
      slow virus 046.9
        specified condition NEC 046.8
    chest 519.8
    conjunctivitis 077.99
      specified type NEC 077.8
    coronavirus 079.89
      SARS-associated 079.82
    Coxsackie (*see also* Infection, Coxsackie) 079.2
    Ebola 065.8
    ECHO
      in diseases classified elsewhere—*see*
        category 079
      unspecified nature or site 079.1
    encephalitis 049.9
      arthropod-borne NEC 064
      tick-borne 063.9
        specified type NEC 063.8
    enteritis NEC (*see also* Enteritis, viral) 008.8
    exanthem NEC 057.9
    Hantavirus 079.81
    human papilloma 079.4
    in diseases classified elsewhere—*see* category 079
    intestine (*see also* Enteritis, viral) 008.8
    lung—*see* Pneumonia, viral
    respiratory syncytial virus (RSV) 079.6
    rhinovirus
      in diseases classified elsewhere—*see*
        category 079
      unspecified nature or site 079.3
    salivary gland disease 078.5
    slow 046.9
      specified condition NEC 046.8
    specified type NEC 079.89
      in diseases classified elsewhere—*see*
        category 079
      unspecified nature or site 079.99
    warts 078.10
      specified NEC 078.19
    yaba monkey tumor 059.22
  vulva (*see also* Vulvitis) 616.10
  whipworm 127.3
  Whitmore's bacillus 025
  wound (local) (posttraumatic) NEC 958.3
    with
      dislocation—*see* Dislocation, by site, open
      fracture—*see* Fracture, by site, open
      open wound—*see* Wound, open, by site,
        complicated
    postoperative 998.59
    surgical 998.59
  Wuchereria 125.0
    bancrofti 125.0
    malayi 125.1

Infection, infected, infective—*continued*
  yaba monkey tumor virus 059.22
  yatapoxvirus 059.20
  yaws—*see* Yaws
  yeast (*see also* Candidiasis) 112.9
  yellow fever (*see also* Fever, yellow) 060.9
  Yersinia pestis (*see also* Plague) 020.9
  Zeis' gland 373.12
  zoonotic bacterial NEC 027.9
  Zopfia senegalensis 117.4
Infective, infectious —*see* condition
Inferiority complex 301.9
  constitutional psychopathic 301.9
Infertility
  female 628.9
    age related 628.8
    associated with
      adhesions, peritubal 614.6 *[628.2]*
      anomaly
        cervical mucus 628.4
        congenital
          cervix 628.4
          fallopian tube 628.2
          uterus 628.3
          vagina 628.4
      anovulation 628.0
      dysmucorrhea 628.4
      endometritis, tuberculous (*see also*
        Tuberculosis) 016.7 *[628.3]*
      Stein-Leventhal syndrome 256.4 *[628.0]*
    due to
      adiposogenital dystrophy 253.8 *[628.1]*
      anterior pituitary disorder NEC 253.4
        [628.1]
        hyperfunction 253.1 *[628.1]*
      cervical anomaly 628.4
      fallopian tube anomaly 628.2
      ovarian failure 256.39 *[628.0]*
      Stein-Leventhal syndrome 256.4 *[628.0]*
      uterine anomaly 628.3
      vaginal anomaly 628.4
    nonimplantation 628.3
    origin
      cervical 628.4
      pituitary-hypothalamus NEC 253.8 *[628.1]*
        anterior pituitary NEC 253.4 *[628.1]*
        hyperfunction NEC 253.1 *[628.1]*
        dwarfism 253.3 *[628.1]*
        panhypopituitarism 253.2 *[628.1]*
      specified NEC 628.8
      tubal (block) (occlusion) (stenosis) 628.2
        adhesions 614.6 *[628.2]*
      uterine 628.3
      vaginal 628.4
    previous, requiring supervision of pregnancy
      V23.0
  male 606.9
    absolute 606.0
    due to
      azoospermia 606.0
      drug therapy 606.8
      extratesticular cause NEC 606.8
      germinal cell
        aplasia 606.0
        desquamation 606.1
      hypospermatogenesis 606.1
      infection 606.8
      obstruction, afferent ducts 606.8
      oligospermia 606.1
      radiation 606.8

Infertility—*continued*
  male—*continued*
    due to—*continued*
      spermatogenic arrest (complete) 606.0
        incomplete 606.1
      systemic disease 606.8
Infestation 134.9
  Acanthocheilonema (perstans) 125.4
    streptocerca 125.6
  Acariasis 133.9
    demodex folliculorum 133.8
    Sarcoptes scabiei 133.0
    trombiculae 133.8
  Agamofilaria streptocerca 125.6
  Ancylostoma, Ankylostoma 126.9
    americanum 126.1
    braziliense 126.2
    canium 126.8
    ceylanicum 126.3
    duodenale 126.0
    new world 126.1
    old world 126.0
  Angiostrongylus cantonensis 128.8
  anisakiasis 127.1
  Anisakis larva 127.1
  arthropod NEC 134.1
  Ascaris lumbricoides 127.0
  Bacillus fusiformis 101
  Balantidium coli 007.0
  beef tapeworm 123.2
  Bothriocephalus (latus) 123.4
    larval 123.5
  broad tapeworm 123.4
    larval 123.5
  Brugia malayi 125.1
  Candiru 136.8
  Capillaria
    hepatica 128.8
    philippinensis 127.5
  cat liver fluke 121.0
  Cercomonas hominis (intestinal) 007.3
  cestodes 123.9
    specified type NEC 123.8
  chigger 133.8
  chigoe 134.1
  Chilomastix 007.8
  Clonorchis (sinensis) (liver) 121.1
  coccidia 007.2
  complicating pregnancy, childbirth, or
      puerperium 647.9
    affecting fetus or newborn 760.8
  Cysticercus cellulosae 123.1
  Demodex folliculorum 133.8
  Dermatobia (hominis) 134.0
  Dibothriocephalus (latus) 123.4
    larval 123.5
  Dicrocoelium dendriticum 121.8
  Diphyllobothrium (adult) (intestinal) (latum)
      (pacificum) 123.4
    larval 123.5
  Diplogonoporus (grandis) 123.8
  Dipylidium (caninum) 123.8
  Distoma hepaticum 121.3
  dog tapeworm 123.8
  Dracunculus medinensis 125.7
  dragon worm 125.7
  dwarf tapeworm 123.6
  Echinococcus (*see also* Echinococcus) 122.9
  Echinostoma ilocanum 121.8
  Embadomonas 007.8
  Endamoeba (histolytica)—*see* Infection, ameba
  Entamoeba (histolytica)—*see* Infection, ameba

Infestation—*continued*
  Enterobius vermicularis 127.4
  Epidermophyton—*see* Dermatophytosis
  eyeworm 125.2
  Fasciola
    gigantica 121.3
    hepatica 121.3
  Fasciolopsis (buski) (small intestine) 121.4
  filarial 125.9
    due to
      Acanthocheilonema (perstans) 125.4
        streptocerca 125.6
      Brugia (Wuchereria) malayi 125.1
      Dracunculus medinensis 125.7
      guinea worms 125.7
      Mansonella (ozzardi) 125.5
      Onchocerca volvulus 125.3
        eye 125.3 *[360.13]*
        eyelid 125.3 *[373.6]*
      Wuchereria (bancrofti) 125.0
        malayi 125.1
    specified type NEC 125.6
  fish tapeworm 123.4
    larval 123.5
  fluke 121.9
    blood NEC (*see also* Schistosomiasis) 120.9
    cat liver 121.0
    intestinal (giant) 121.4
    liver (sheep) 121.3
      cat 121.0
      Chinese 121.1
      clonorchiasis 121.1
      fascioliasis 121.3
      Oriental 121.1
    lung (oriental) 121.2
    sheep liver 121.3
  fly larva 134.0
  Gasterophilus (intestinalis) 134.0
  Gastrodiscoides hominis 121.8
  Giardia lamblia 007.1
  Gnathostoma (spinigerum) 128.1
  Gongylonema 125.6
  guinea worm 125.7
  helminth NEC 128.9
    intestinal 127.9
      mixed (types classifiable to more than one
        category in 120.0-127.7) 127.8
      specified type NEC 127.7
    specified type NEC 128.8
  Heterophyes heterophyes (small intestine) 121.6
  hookworm (*see also* Infestation, ancylostoma)
    126.9
  Hymenolepis (diminuta) (nana) 123.6
  intestinal NEC 129
  leeches (aquatic) (land) 134.2
  Leishmania—*see* Leishmaniasis
  lice (*see also* infestation, pediculus) 132.9
  Linguatulidae, linguatula (pentastoma) (serrata)
    134.1
  Loa loa 125.2
    eyelid 125.2 *[373.6]*
  louse (*see also* Infestation, pediculus) 132.9
    body 132.1
    head 132.0
    pubic 132.2
  maggots 134.0
  Mansonella (ozzardi) 125.5
  medina 125.7
  Metagonimus yokogawai (small intestine) 121.5
  Microfilaria streptocerca 125.3
    eye 125.3 *[360.13]*
    eyelid 125.3 *[373.6]*

Infestation—*continued*
  Microsporon furfur 111.0
  microsporum—*see* Dermatophytosis
  mites 133.9
    scabic 133.0
    specified type NEC 133.8
  Monilia (albicans) (*see also* Candidiasis) 112.9
    vagina 112.1
    vulva 112.1
  mouth 112.0
  Necator americanus 126.1
  nematode (intestinal) 127.9
    Ancylostoma (*see also* Ancylostoma) 126.9
    Ascaris lumbricoides 127.0
    conjunctiva NEC 128.9
    Dioctophyma 128.8
    Enterobius vermicularis 127.4
    Gnathostoma spinigerum 128.1
    Oesophagostomum (apiostomum) 127.7
    Physaloptera 127.4
    specified type NEC 127.7
    Strongyloides stercoralis 127.2
    Ternidens diminutus 127.7
    Trichinella spiralis 124
    Trichostrongylus 127.6
    Trichuris (trichiuria) 127.3
  Oesophagostomum (apiostomum) 127.7
  Oestrus ovis 134.0
  Onchocerca (volvulus) 125.3
    eye 125.3 *[360.13]*
    eyelid 125.3 *[373.6]*
  Opisthorchis (felineus) (tenuicollis) (viverrini)
    121.0
  Oxyuris vermicularis 127.4
  Paragonimus (westermani) 121.2
  parasite, parasitic NEC 136.9
    eyelid 134.9 *[373.6]*
    intestinal 129
    mouth 112.0
    orbit 376.13
    skin 134.9
    tongue 112.0
  pediculus 132.9
    capitis (humanus) (any site) 132.0
    corporis (humanus) (any site) 132.1
    eyelid 132.0 *[373.6]*
    mixed (classifiable to more than one category
      in 132.0-132.2) 132.3
    pubis (any site) 132.2
  phthirus (pubis) (any site) 132.2
    with any infestation classifiable to 132.0 and
      132.1 132.3
  pinworm 127.4
  pork tapeworm (adult) 123.0
  protozoal NEC 136.8
  pubic louse 132.2
  rat tapeworm 123.6
  red bug 133.8
  roundworm (large) NEC 127.0
  sand flea 134.1
  saprophytic NEC 136.8
  Sarcoptes scabiei 133.0
  scabies 133.0
  Schistosoma 120.9
    bovis 120.8
    cercariae 120.3
    hematobium 120.0
    intercalatum 120.8
    japonicum 120.2
    mansoni 120.1
    mattheii 120.8

Infestation—*continued*
  Schistosoma —*continued*
    specified
      site—*see* Schistosomiasis
      type NEC 120.8
    spindale 120.8
  screw worms 134.0
  skin NEC 134.9
  Sparganum (mansoni) (proliferum) 123.5
    larval 123.5
  specified type NEC 134.8
  Spirometra larvae 123.5
  Sporozoa NEC 136.8
  Stellantchasmus falcatus 121.6
  Strongyloides 127.2
  Strongylus (gibsoni) 127.7
  Taenia 123.3
    diminuta 123.6
    Echinococcus (*see also* Echinococcus) 122.9
    mediocanellata 123.2
    nana 123.6
    saginata (mediocanellata) 123.2
    solium (intestinal form) 123.0
      larval form 123.1
  Taeniarhynchus saginatus 123.2
  tapeworm 123.9
    beef 123.2
    broad 123.4
      larval 123.5
    dog 123.8
    dwarf 123.6
    fish 123.4
      larval 123.5
    pork 123.0
    rat 123.6
  Ternidens diminutus 127.7
  Tetranychus molestissimus 133.8
  threadworm 127.4
  tongue 112.0
  Toxocara (cani) (cati) (felis) 128.0
  trematode(s) NEC 121.9
  Trichina spiralis 124
  Trichinella spiralis 124
  Trichocephalus 127.3
  Trichomonas 131.9
    bladder 131.09
    cervix 131.09
    intestine 007.3
    prostate 131.03
    specified site NEC 131.8
    urethra (female) (male) 131.02
    urogenital 131.00
    vagina 131.01
    vulva 131.01
  Trichophyton—*see* Dermatophytosis
  Trichostrongylus instabilis 127.6
  Trichuris (trichiuria) 127.3
  Trombicula (irritans) 133.8
  Trypanosoma—*see* Trypanosomiasis
  Tunga penetrans 134.1
  Uncinaria americana 126.1
  whipworm 127.3
  worms NEC 128.9
    intestinal 127.9
  Wuchereria 125.0
    bancrofti 125.0
    malayi 125.1
Infiltrate, infiltration
  with an iron compound 275.09
  amyloid (any site) (generalized) 277.39
  calcareous (muscle) NEC 275.49
    localized—*see* Degeneration, by site

Infiltrate, infiltration—*continued*
  calcium salt (muscle) 275.49
  chemotherapy, vesicant 999.81
  corneal (*see also* Edema, cornea) 371.20
  eyelid 373.9
  fatty (diffuse) (generalized) 272.8
    localized—*see* Degeneration, by site, fatty
  glycogen, glycogenic (*see also* Disease, glycogen storage) 271.10
  heart, cardiac
    fatty (*see also* Degeneration, myocardial) 429.1
    glycogenic 271.0 *[425.7]*
  inflammatory in vitreous 379.29
  kidney (*see also* Disease, renal) 593.9
  leukemic (M9800/3)—*see* Leukemia
  liver 573.8
    fatty—*see* Fatty, liver
    glycogen (*see also* Disease, glycogen storage) 271.0
  lung (*see also* Infiltrate, pulmonary) 793.19
    eosinophilic 518.3
    x-ray finding only 793.19
  lymphatic (*see also* Leukemia, lymphatic) 204.9
    gland, pigmentary 289.3
  muscle, fatty 728.9
  myelogenous (*see also* Leukemia, myeloid) 205.9
  myocardium, myocardial
    fatty (*see also* Degeneration, myocardial) 429.1
    glycogenic 271.0 *[425.7]*
  pulmonary 793.19
    with
      eosinophilia 518.3
      pneumonia—*see* Pneumonia, by type
    x-ray finding only 793.19
  Ranke's primary (*see also* Tuberculosis) 010.0
  skin, lymphocyctic (benign) 709.8
  thymus (gland) (fatty) 254.8
  urine 788.8
  vesicant
    agent NEC 999.82
    chemotherapy 999.81
  vitreous humor 379.29
Infirmity 799.89
  senile 797
Inflammation, inflamed, inflammatory (with exudation)
  abducens (nerve) 378.54
  accessory sinus (chronic) (*see also* Sinusitis) 473.9
  adrenal (gland) 255.8
  alimentary canal—*see* Enteritis
  alveoli (teeth) 526.5
    scorbutic 267
  amnion—*see* Amnionitis
  anal canal 569.49
  antrum (chronic) (*see also* Sinusitis, maxillary) 473.0
  anus 569.49
  appendix (*see also* Appendicitis) 541
  arachnoid—*see* Meningitis
  areola 611.0
    puerperal, postpartum 675.0
  areolar tissue NEC 686.9
  artery—*see* Arteritis
  auditory meatus (external) (*see also* Otitis, externa) 380.10
  Bartholin's gland 616.89
  bile duct or passage 576.1
  bladder (*see also* Cystitis) 595.9

Inflammation—*continued*
bleb
postprocedural 379.60
stage 1 379.61
stage 2 379.62
stage 3 379.63
bone—*see* Osteomyelitis
bowel (*see also* Enteritis) 558.9
brain (*see also* Encephalitis) 323.9
late effect—*see* category 326
membrane—*see* Meningitis
breast 611.0
puerperal, postpartum 675.2
broad ligament (*see also* Disease, pelvis,
inflammatory) 614.4
acute 614.3
bronchus—*see* Bronchitis
bursa—*see* Bursitis
capsule
liver 573.3
spleen 289.59
catarrhal (*see also* Catarrh) 460
vagina 616.10
cecum (*see also* Appendicitis) 541
cerebral (*see also* Encephalitis) 323.9
late effect—*see* category 326
membrane—*see* Meningitis
cerebrospinal (*see also* Meningitis) 322.9
late effect—*see* category 326
meningococcal 036.0
tuberculous (*see also* Tuberculosis) 013.6
cervix (uteri) (*see also* Cervicitis) 616.0
chest 519.9
choroid NEC (*see also* Choroiditis) 363.20
cicatrix (tissue)—*see* Cicatrix
colon (*see also* Enteritis) 558.9
granulomatous 555.1
newborn 558.9
connective tissue (diffuse) NEC 728.9
cornea (*see also* Keratitis) 370.9
with ulcer (*see also* Ulcer, cornea) 370.00
corpora cavernosa (penis) 607.2
cranial nerve—*see* Disorder, nerve, cranial
diarrhea—*see* Diarrhea
disc (intervertebral) (space) 722.90
cervical, cervicothoracic 722.91
lumbar, lumbosacral 722.93
thoracic, thoracolumbar 722.93
Douglas' cul-de-sac or pouch (chronic) (*see also*
Disease, pelvis, inflammatory) 614.4
acute 614.3
due to (presence of) any device, implant, or graft
classifiable to 996.0-996.5—*see*
Complications, infection and inflammation,
due to (presence of) any device, implant, or
graft classified to 996.0-996.5 NEC
duodenum 535.6
dura mater—*see* Meningitis
ear—*see also* Otitis
external (*see also* Otitis, externa) 380.10
inner (*see also* Labyrinthitis) 386.30
middle—*see* Otitis media
esophagus 530.10
ethmoidal (chronic) (sinus) (*see also* Sinusitis,
ethmoidal) 473.2
Eustachian tube (catarrhal) 381.50
acute 381.51
chronic 381.52
extrarectal 569.49
eye 379.99
eyelid 373.9
specified NEC 373.8

Inflammation—*continued*
fallopian tube (*see also* Salpingo-oophoritis)
614.2
fascia 728.9
fetal membranes (acute) 658.4
affecting fetus or newborn 762.7
follicular, pharynx 472.1
frontal (chronic) (sinus) (*see also* Sinusitis,
frontal) 473.1
gallbladder (*see also* Cholecystitis, acute) 575.0
gall duct (*see also* Cholecystitis) 575.10
gastrointestinal (*see also* Enteritis) 558.9
genital organ (diffuse) (internal)
female 614.9
with
abortion—*see* Abortion, by type, with
sepsis
ectopic pregnancy (*see also* categories
633.0-633.9) 639.0
molar pregnancy (*see also* categories
630-632) 639.0
complicating pregnancy, childbirth, or
puerperium 646.6
affecting fetus or newborn 760.8
following
abortion 639.0
ectopic or molar pregnancy 639.0
male 608.4
gland (lymph) (*see also* Lymphadenitis) 289.3
glottis (*see also* Laryngitis) 464.00
with obstruction 464.01
granular, pharynx 472.1
gum 523.10
heart (*see also* Carditis) 429.89
hepatic duct 576.8
hernial sac—*see* Hernia, by site
ileum (*see also* Enteritis) 558.9
terminal or regional 555.0
with large intestine 555.2
intervertebral disc 722.90
cervical, cervicothoracic 722.91
lumbar, lumbosacral 722.93
thoracic, thoracolumbar 722.92
intestine (*see also* Enteritis) 558.9
jaw (acute) (bone) (chronic) (lower)
(suppurative) (upper) 526.4
jejunum—*see* Enteritis
joint NEC (*see also* Arthritis) 716.9
sacroiliac 720.2
kidney (*see also* Nephritis) 583.9
knee (joint) 716.66
tuberculous (active) (*see also* Tuberculosis)
015.2
labium (majus) (minus) (*see also* Vulvitis) 616.10
lacrimal
gland (*see also* Dacryoadenitis) 375.00
passages (duct) (sac) (*see also* Dacryocystitis)
375.30
larynx (*see also* Laryngitis) 464.00
with obstruction 464.01
diphtheritic 032.3
leg NEC 686.9
lip 528.5
liver (capsule) (*see also* Hepatitis) 573.3
acute 570
chronic 571.40
suppurative 572.0
lung (acute) (*see also* Pneumonia) 486
chronic (interstitial) 518.89
lymphatic vessel (*see also* Lymphangitis) 457.2
lymph node or gland (*see also* Lymphadenitis)
289.3

Inflammation—*continued*
mammary gland 611.0
puerperal, postpartum 675.2
maxilla, maxillary 526.4
sinus (chronic) (*see also* Sinusitis, maxillary)
473.0
membranes of brain or spinal cord—*see*
Meningitis
meninges—*see* Meningitis
mouth 528.00
muscle 728.9
myocardium (*see also* Myocarditis) 429.0
nasal sinus (chronic) (*see also* Sinusitis) 473.9
nasopharynx—*see* Nasopharyngitis
navel 686.9
newborn NEC 771.4
nerve NEC 729.2
nipple 611.0
puerperal, postpartum 675.0
nose 478.19
suppurative 472.0
oculomotor nerve 378.51
optic nerve 377.30
orbit (chronic) 376.10
acute 376.00
chronic 376.10
ovary (*see also* Salpingo-oophoritis) 614.2
oviduct (*see also* Salpingo-oophoritis) 614.2
pancreas—*see* Pancreatitis
parametrium (chronic) (*see also* Disease, pelvis,
inflammatory) 614.4
acute 614.3
parotid region 686.9
gland 527.2
pelvis, female (*see also* Disease, pelvis,
inflammatory) 614.9
penis (corpora cavernosa) 607.2
perianal 569.49
pericardium (*see also* Pericarditis) 423.9
perineum (female) (male) 686.9
perirectal 569.49
peritoneum (*see also* Peritonitis) 567.9
periuterine (*see also* Disease, pelvis,
inflammatory) 614.9
perivesical (*see also* Cystitis) 595.9
petrous bone (*see also* Petrositis) 383.20
pharynx (*see also* Pharyngitis) 462
follicular 472.1
granular 472.1
pia mater—*see* Meningitis
pleura—*see* Pleurisy
postmastoidectomy cavity 383.30
chronic 383.33
pouch, internal ileoanal 569.71
prostate (*see also* Prostatitis) 601.9
rectosigmoid—*see* Rectosigmoiditis
rectum (*see also* Proctitis) 569.49
respiratory, upper (*see also* Infection,
respiratory, upper) 465.9
chronic, due to external agent—*see* Condition,
respiratory, chronic, due to, external agent
due to
fumes or vapors (chemical) (inhalation)
506.2
radiation 508.1
retina (*see also* Retinitis) 363.20
retrocecal (*see also* Appendicitis) 541
retroperitoneal (*see also* Peritonitis) 567.9
salivary duct or gland (any) (suppurative) 527.2
scorbutic, alveoli, teeth 267
scrotum 608.4
sigmoid—*see* Enteritis

Inflammation—*continued*
sinus (*see also* Sinusitis) 473.9
Skene's duct or gland (*see also* Urethritis)
597.89
skin 686.9
spermatic cord 608.4
sphenoidal (sinus) (*see also* Sinusitis,
sphenoidal) 473.3
spinal
cord (*see also* Encephalitis) 323.9
late effect—*see* category 326
membrane—*see* Meningitis
nerve—*see* Disorder, nerve
spine (*see also* Spondylitis) 720.9
spleen (capsule) 289.59
stomach—*see* Gastritis
stricture, rectum 569.49
subcutaneous tissue NEC 686.9
suprarenal (gland) 255.8
synovial (fringe) (membrane)—*see* Bursitis
tendon (sheath) NEC 726.90
testis (*see also* Orchitis) 604.90
thigh 686.9
throat (*see also* Sore throat) 462
thymus (gland) 254.8
thyroid (gland) (*see also* Thyroiditis) 245.9
tongue 529.0
tonsil—*see* Tonsillitis
trachea—*see* Tracheitis
trochlear nerve 378.53
tubal (*see also* Salpingo-oophoritis) 614.2
tuberculous NEC (*see also* Tuberculosis) 011.9
tubo-ovarian (*see also* Salpingo-oophoritis)
614.2
tunica vaginalis 608.4
tympanic membrane—*see* Myringitis
umbilicus, umbilical 686.9
newborn NEC 771.4
uterine ligament (*see also* Disease, pelvis,
inflammatory) 614.4
acute 614.3
uterus (catarrhal) (*see also* Endometritis) 615.9
uveal tract (anterior) (*see also* Iridocyclitis)
364.3
posterior—*see* Chorioretinitis
sympathetic 360.11
vagina (*see also* Vaginitis) 616.10
vas deferens 608.4
vein (*see also* Phlebitis) 451.9
thrombotic 451.9
cerebral (*see also* Thrombosis, brain) 434.0
leg 451.2
deep (vessels) NEC 451.19
superficial (vessels) 451.0
lower extremity 451.2
deep (vessels) NEC 451.19
superficial (vessels) 451.0
vocal cord 478.5
vulva (*see also* Vulvitis) 616.10
Inflation, lung imperfect (newborn) 770.5
Influenza, influenzal 487.1
with
bronchitis 487.1
bronchopneumonia 487.0
cold (any type) 487.1
digestive manifestations 487.8
hemoptysis 487.1
involvement of
gastrointestinal tract 487.8
nervous system 487.8
laryngitis 487.1

Influenza—*continued*
with—*continued*
  manifestations NEC 487.8
    respiratory 487.1
      pneumonia 487.0
    pharyngitis 487.1
    pneumonia (any form classifiable to 480-483, 485-486) 487.0
    respiratory manifestations NEC 487.1
    sinusitis 487.1
    sore throat 487.1
    tonsillitis 487.1
    tracheitis 487.1
    upper respiratory infection (acute) 487.1
  A/H5N1 see also Influenza, avian) 488.02
  abdominal 487.8
  Asian 487.1
  avian 488.02
    with involvement of gastrointestinal tract 488.09
    bronchopneumonia 488.01
    laryngitis 488.02
    manifestations NEC 488.09
    respiratory 488.02
    pharyngitis 488.02
    pneumonia (any form classifiable to 480-483, 485-486) 488.01
    respiratory infection (acute) (upper) 488.02
  bronchial 487.1
  bronchopneumonia 487.0
  catarrhal 487.1
  due to identified
    animal origin influenza virus - see Influenza, due to identified, novel influenza A virus
    avian influenza virus 488.02
      with
        manifestations NEC 488.09
          respiratory 488.02
        pneumonia (any form classifiable to 480-483, 485-486) 488.01
    (novel) 2009 H1N1 influenza virus 488.12
      with
        manifestations NEC 488.19
          respiratory 488.12
        pneumonia 488.11
    novel influenza A virus 488.82
      with
        encephalopathy 488.89
        involvement of gastrointestinal tract 488.89
        laryngitis 488.82
        manifestations NEC 488.89
          respiratory (acute) (upper) 488.82
        pharyngitis 488.82
        pneumonia 488.81
  epidemic 487.1
  gastric 487.8
  intestinal 487.8
  laryngitis 487.1
  maternal affecting fetus or newborn 760.2
    manifest influenza in infant 771.2
  (novel) 2009 H1N1 488.12
    with involvement of gastrointestinal tract 488.19
    bronchopneumonia 488.11
    laryngitis 488.12
    manifestations NEC 488.19
      respiratory 488.12
    pharyngitis 488.12
    pneumonia (any form classifiable to 480-483, 485-486) 488.11
    respiratory infection (acute) (upper) 488.12

Influenza—*continued*
  novel A/H1N1 (*see also* Influenza, (novel) 2009 H1N1) 488.12
  novel influenza A viruses not previously found in humans — *see* Influenza, due to identified, novel influenza A virus
  pharyngitis 487.1
  pneumonia (any form) 487.0
  respiratory (upper) 487.1
  specified NEC 487.1
  stomach 487.8
  vaccination, prophylactic (against) V04.81
Influenza-like disease (*see also* Influenza) 487.1
Infraction, Freiberg's (metatarsal head) 732.5
Infraeruption, teeth 524.34
Infusion complication, misadventure or reaction —*see* Complication, infusion
Ingestion
  chemical—*see* Table of drugs and chemicals
  drug or medicinal substance
    overdose or wrong substance given or taken 977.9
      specified drug—*see* Table of drugs and chemicals
  foreign body NEC (*see also* Foreign body) 938
Ingrowing
  hair 704.8
  nail (finger) (toe) (infected) 703.0
Inguinal —*see also* condition
  testis 752.51
Inhalation
  carbon monoxide 986
  flame
    mouth 947.0
    lung 947.1
  food or foreign body (*see also* Asphyxia, food or foreign body) 933.1
  gas, fumes, or vapor (noxious) 987.9
    specified agent—*see* Table of drugs and chemicals
  liquid or vomitus (*see also* Asphyxia, food or foreign body) 933.1
  lower respiratory tract NEC 934.9
  meconium (fetus or newborn) 770.11
    with respiratory symptoms 770.12
  mucus (*see also* Asphyxia, mucus) 933.1
  oil (causing suffocation) (*see also* Asphyxia, food or foreign body) 933.1
  pneumonia—*see* Pneumonia, aspiration
  smoke 508.2
  steam 987.9
  stomach contents or secretions (*see also* Asphyxia, food or foreign body) 933.1
    in labor and deliver 668.0
Inhibition, inhibited
  academic as adjustment reaction 309.23
  orgasm
    female 302.73
    male 302.74
  sexual
    desire 302.71
    excitement 302.72
  work as adjustment reaction 309.23
Inhibitor
  autoimmune, to clotting factors 286.52
  systemic lupus erythematosus (presence of) 795.79
    with
      hemorrhagic disorder 286.53
      hypercoagulable state 289.81
Iniencephalus, iniencephaly 740.2

Injected eye 372.74
Injury 959.9

> *Note—For abrasion, insect bite (nonvenomous),
> blister, or scratch, see Injury, superficial. For
> laceration, traumatic rupture, tear, or
> penetrating wound of internal organs, such as
> heart, lung, liver, kidney, pelvic organs, whether
> or not accompanied by open wound in the same
> region, see Injury, internal. For nerve injury,
> see Injury, nerve. For late effect of injuries
> classifiable to 850-854, 860-869, 900-919,
> 950-959, see Late, effect, injury, by type.*

abdomen, abdominal (viscera)—*see also* Injury,
    internal, abdomen
  muscle or wall 959.12
acoustic, resulting in deafness 951.5
adenoid 959.09
adrenal (gland)—*see* Injury, internal, adrenal
alveolar (process) 959.09
ankle (and foot) (and knee) (and leg, except
    thigh) 959.7
anterior chamber, eye 921.3
anus 959.19
aorta (thoracic) 901.0
  abdominal 902.0
appendix—*see* Injury, internal, appendix
arm, upper (and shoulder) 959.2
artery (complicating trauma) (*see also* Injury,
    blood vessel, by site) 904.9
  cerebral or meningeal (*see also* Hemorrhage,
    brain, traumatic, subarachnoid) 852.0
auditory canal (external) (meatus) 959.09
auricle, auris, ear 959.09
axilla 959.2
back 959.19
bile duct—*see* Injury, internal, bile duct
birth—*see also* Birth, injury
  canal NEC, complicating delivery 665.9
bladder (sphincter)—*see* Injury, internal,
    bladder
blast (air) (hydraulic) (immersion) (underwater)
    NEC 869.0
  with open wound into cavity NEC 869.1
  abdomen or thorax—*see* Injury, internal, by
    site
  brain—*see* Concussion, brain
  ear (acoustic nerve trauma) 951.5
    with perforation of tympanic
      membrane—*see* Wound, open, ear, drum
blood vessel NEC 904.9
  abdomen 902.9
    multiple 902.87
    specified NEC 902.89
  aorta (thoracic) 901.0
    abdominal 902.0
  arm NEC 903.9
  axillary 903.00
    artery 903.01
    vein 903.02
  azygos vein 901.89
  basilic vein 903.1
  brachial (artery) (vein) 903.1
  bronchial 901.89
  carotid artery 900.00
    common 900.01
    external 900.02
    internal 900.03
  celiac artery 902.20
    specified branch NEC 902.24
  cephalic vein (arm) 903.1
  colica dextra 902.26

Injury—*continued*
  blood vessel—*continued*
    cystic
      artery 902.24
      vein 902.39
    deep plantar 904.6
    digital (artery) (vein) 903.5
    due to accidental puncture or laceration during
      procedure 998.2
    extremity
      lower 904.8
        multiple 904.7
        specified NEC 904.7
      upper 903.9
        multiple 903.8
        specified NEC 903.8
    femoral
      artery (superficial) 904.1
        above profunda origin 904.0
        common 904.0
      vein 904.2
    gastric
      artery 902.21
      vein 902.39
    head 900.9
      intracranial—*see* Injury, intracranial
      multiple 900.82
      specified NEC 900.89
    hemiazygos vein 901.89
    hepatic
      artery 902.22
      vein 902.11
    hypogastric 902.59
      artery 902.51
      vein 902.52
    ileocolic
      artery 902.26
      vein 902.31
    iliac 902.50
      artery 902.53
      specified branch NEC 902.59
      vein 902.54
    innominate
      artery 901.1
      vein 901.3
    intercostal (artery) (vein) 901.81
    jugular vein (external) 900.81
      internal 900.1
    leg NEC 904.8
    mammary (artery) (vein) 901.82
    mesenteric
      artery 902.20
        inferior 902.27
        specified branch NEC 902.29
        superior (trunk) 902.25
          branches, primary 902.26
      vein 902.39
        inferior 902.32
        superior (and primary subdivisions) 902.31
    neck 900.9
      multiple 900.82
      specified NEC 900.89
    ovarian 902.89
      artery 902.81
      vein 902.82
    palmar artery 903.4
    pelvis 902.9
      multiple 902.87
      specified NEC 902.89
    plantar (deep) (artery) (vein) 904.6

Injury—*continued*
  blood vessel—*continued*
    popliteal 904.40
      artery 904.41
      vein 904.42
    portal 902.33
    pulmonary 901.40
      artery 901.41
      vein 901.42
    radial (artery) (vein) 903.2
    renal 902.40
      artery 902.41
      specified NEC 902.49
      vein 902.42
    saphenous
      artery 904.7
      vein (greater) (lesser) 904.3
    splenic
      artery 902.23
      vein 902.34
    subclavian
      artery 901.1
      vein 901.3
    suprarenal 902.49
    thoracic 901.9
      multiple 901.83
      specified NEC 901.89
    tibial 904.50
      artery 904.50
        anterior 904.51
        posterior 904.53
      vein 904.50
        anterior 904.52
        posterior 904.54
    ulnar (artery) (vein) 903.3
    uterine 902.59
      artery 902.55
      vein 902.56
    vena cava
      inferior 902.10
        specified branches NEC 902.19
      superior 901.2
  brachial plexus 953.4
    newborn 767.6
  brain (traumatic) NEC (*see also* Injury,
      intracranial) 854.0
    due to fracture of skull—see Fracture, skull,
      by site
  breast 959.19
  broad ligament—*see* Injury, internal, broad
      ligament
  bronchus, bronchi—*see* Injury, internal, bronchus
  brow 959.09
  buttock 959.19
  canthus, eye 921.1
  cathode ray 990
  cauda equina 952.4
    with fracture, vertebra—*see* Fracture, vertebra,
      sacrum
  cavernous sinus (*see also* Injury, intracranial)
      854.0
  cecum—*see* Injury, internal, cecum
  celiac ganglion or plexus 954.1
  cerebellum (*see also* Injury, intracranial) 854.0
  cervix (uteri)—*see* Injury, internal, cervix
  cheek 959.09
  chest—*see* Injury, internal, chest
    wall 959.11
  childbirth—*see also* Birth, injury
    maternal NEC 665.9
  chin 959.09

Injury—*continued*
  choroid (eye) 921.3
  clitoris 959.14
  coccyx 959.19
    complicating delivery 665.6
  colon—*see* Injury, internal, colon
  common duct—*see* Injury, internal, common
      duct
  conjunctiva 921.1
    superficial 918.2
  cord
    spermatic—*see* Injury, internal, spermatic
      cord
    spinal—*see* Injury, spinal, by site
  cornea 921.3
    abrasion 918.1
    due to contact lens 371.82
    penetrating—*see* Injury, eyeball, penetrating
    superficial 918.1
      due to contact lens 371.82
  cortex (cerebral) (*see also* Injury, intracranial)
      854.0
    visual 950.3
  costal region 959.11
  costochondral 959.11
  cranial
    bones—*see* Fracture, skull, by site
    cavity (*see also* Injury, intracranial) 854.0
    nerve—*see* Injury, nerve, cranial
  crushing—*see* Crush
  cutaneous sensory nerve
    lower limb 956.4
    upper limb 955.5
  deep tissue—*see* Contusion, by site
    meaning pressure ulcer 707.25
  delivery—*see also* Birth, injury
    maternal NEC 665.9
  Descemet's membrane—*see* Injury, eyeball,
      penetrating
  diaphragm—*see* Injury, internal, diaphragm
  diffuse axonal—*see* Injury, intracranial
  duodenum—*see* Injury, internal, duodenum
  ear (auricle) (canal) (drum) (external) 959.09
  elbow (and forearm) (and wrist) 959.3
  epididymis 959.14
  epigastric region 959.12
  epiglottis 959.09
  epiphyseal, current—*see* Fracture, by site
  esophagus—*see* Injury, internal, esophagus
  Eustachian tube 959.09
  extremity (lower) (upper) NEC 959.8
  eye 921.9
    penetrating eyeball—*see* Injury, eyeball,
      penetrating
    superficial 918.9
  eyeball 921.3
    penetrating 871.7
      with
        partial loss (of intraocular tissue) 871.12
        prolapse or exposure (of intraocular tissue)
          871.1
        without prolapse 871.0
      foreign body (nonmagnetic) 871.6
        magnetic 871.5
    superficial 918.9
  eyebrow 959.09
  eyelid(s) 921.1
    laceration—*see* Laceration, eyelid
    superficial 918.0
  face (and neck) 959.09
  fallopian tube—*see* Injury, internal, fallopian tube

Injury—*continued*
  finger(s) (nail) 959.5
  flank 959.19
  foot (and ankle) (and knee) (and leg except
    thigh) 959.7
  forceps NEC 767.9
    scalp 767.19
  forearm (and elbow) (and wrist) 959.3
  forehead 959.09
  gallbladder—*see* Injury, internal, gallbladder
  gasserian ganglion 951.2
  gastrointestinal tract—*see* Injury, internal,
    gastrointestinal tract
  genital organ(s)
    with
      abortion—*see* Abortion, by type, with,
        damage to pelvic organs
      ectopic pregnancy (*see also* categories
        633.0-633.9) 639.2
      molar pregnancy (*see also* categories
        630-632) 639.2
    external 959.14
      fracture of corpus cavernosum penis 959.13
    following
      abortion 639.2
      ectopic or molar pregnancy 639.2
    internal—*see* Injury, internal, genital organs
    obstetrical trauma NEC 665.9
      affecting fetus or newborn 763.89
  gland
    lacrimal 921.1
      laceration 870.8
    parathyroid 959.09
    salivary 959.09
    thyroid 959.09
  globe (eye) (*see also* Injury, eyeball) 921.3
  grease gun—*see* Wound, open, by site,
    complicated
  groin 959.19
  gum 959.09
  hand(s) (except fingers) 959.4
  head NEC 959.01
    with
      loss of consciousness 850.5
      skull fracture—*see* Fracture, skull, by site
  heart—*see* Injury, internal, heart
  heel 959.7
  hip (and thigh) 959.6
  hymen 959.14
  hyperextension (cervical) (vertebra) 847.0
  ileum—*see* Injury, internal, ileum
  iliac region 959.19
  infrared rays NEC 990
  instrumental (during surgery) 998.2
    birth injury—*see* Birth, injury
    nonsurgical (*see also* Injury, by site) 959.9
    obstetrical 665.9
      affecting fetus or newborn 763.89
      bladder 665.5
      cervix 665.3
      high vaginal 665.4
      perineal NEC 664.9
      urethra 665.5
      uterus 665.5

Injury—*continued*
  internal 869.0

  Note—*For injury of internal organ(s) by foreign
  body entering through a natural orifice (e.g.,
  inhaled, ingested, or swallowed)—see Foreign
  body, entering through orifice.*

  *For internal injury of any of the following sites
  with internal injury of any other of the sites—
  see Injury, internal, multiple.*

    with
      fracture
        pelvis—*see* Fracture, pelvis
        specified site, except pelvis—*see* Injury,
          internal, by site
        open wound into cavity 869.1
    abdomen, abdominal (viscera) NEC 868.00
      with
        fracture, pelvis—*see* Fracture, pelvis
        open wound into cavity 868.10
      specified site NEC 868.09
        with open wound into cavity 868.19
    adrenal (gland) 868.01
      with open wound into cavity 868.11
    aorta (thoracic) 901.0
      abdominal 902.0
    appendix 863.85
      with open wound into cavity 863.95
    bile duct 868.02
      with open wound into cavity 868.12
    bladder (sphincter) 867.0
      with
        abortion—*see* Abortion, by type, with,
          damage to pelvic organs
        ectopic pregnancy (*see also* categories
          633.0-633.9) 639.2
        molar pregnancy (*see also* categories
          630-632) 639.2
        open wound into cavity 867.1
      following
        abortion 639.2
        ectopic or molar pregnancy 639.2
      obstetrical trauma 665.5
        affecting fetus or newborn 763.89
    blood vessel—*see* Injury, blood vessel, by site
    broad ligament 867.6
      with open wound into cavity 867.7
    bronchus, bronchi 862.21
      with open wound into cavity 862.31
    cecum 863.89
      with open wound into cavity 863.99
    cervix (uteri) 867.4
      with
        abortion—*see* Abortion, by type, with
          damage to pelvic organs
        ectopic pregnancy (*see also* categories
          633.0-633.9) 639.2
        molar pregnancy (*see also* categories
          630-632) 639.2
        open wound into cavity 867.5
      following
        abortion 639.2
        ectopic or molar pregnancy 639.2
      obstetrical trauma 665.3
        affecting fetus or newborn 763.89
    chest (*see also* Injury, internal, intrathoracic
      organs) 862.8
      with open wound into cavity 862.9

Injury—*continued*
  internal—*continued*
    colon 863.40
      with
        open wound into cavity 863.50
        rectum 863.46
          with open wound into cavity 863.56
      ascending (right) 863.41
        with open wound into cavity 863.51
      descending (left) 863.43
        with open wound into cavity 863.53
      multiple sites 863.46
        with open wound into cavity 863.56
      sigmoid 863.44
        with open wound into cavity 863.54
      specified site NEC 863.49
        with open wound into cavity 863.59
      transverse 863.42
        with open wound into cavity 863.52
    common duct 868.02
      with open wound into cavity 868.12
    complicating delivery 665.9
      affecting fetus or newborn 763.89
    diaphragm 862.0
      with open wound into cavity 862.1
    duodenum 863.21
      with open wound into cavity 863.31
    esophagus (intrathoracic) 862.22
      with open wound into cavity 862.32
      cervical region 874.4
        complicated 874.5
    fallopian tube 867.6
      with open wound into cavity 867.7
    gallbladder 868.02
      with open wound into cavity 868.12
    gastrointestinal tract NEC 863.80
      with open wound into cavity 863.90
    genital organ NEC 867.6
      with open wound into cavity 867.7
    heart 861.00
      with open wound into thorax 861.10
    ileum 863.29
      with open wound into cavity 863.39
    intestine NEC 863.89
      with open wound into cavity 863.99
      large NEC 863.40
        with open wound into cavity 863.50
      small NEC 863.20
        with open wound into cavity 863.30
    intra-abdominal (organ) 868.00
      with open wound into cavity 868.10
      multiple sites 868.09
        with open wound into cavity 868.19
      specified site NEC 868.09
        with open wound into cavity 868.19
    intrathoracic organs (multiple) 862.8
      with open wound into cavity 862.9
      diaphragm (only)—*see* Injury, internal,
        diaphragm
      heart (only)—*see* Injury, internal, heart
      lung (only)—*see* Injury, internal, lung
      specified site NEC 862.29
        with open wound into cavity 862.39
    intrauterine (*see also* Injury, internal, uterus)
      867.4
      with open wound into cavity 867.5
    jejunum 863.29
      with open wound into cavity 863.39

Injury—*continued*
  internal—*continued*
    kidney (subcapsular) 866.00
      with
        disruption of parenchyma (complete)
          866.03
          with open wound into cavity 866.13
        hematoma (without rupture of capsule)
          866.01
          with open wound into cavity 866.11
        laceration 866.02
          with open wound into cavity 866.12
        open wound into cavity 866.10
    liver 864.00
      with
        contusion 864.01
          with open wound into cavity 864.11
        hematoma 864.01
          with open wound into cavity 864.11
        laceration 864.05
          with open wound into cavity 864.15
        major (disruption of hepatic
          parenchyma) 864.04
          with open wound into cavity 864.14
        minor (capsule only) 864.02
          with open wound into cavity 864.12
        moderate (involving parenchyma) 864.03
          with open wound into cavity 864.13
        multiple 864.04
        stellate 864.04
          with open wound in cavity 864.14
      open wound into cavity 864.10
    lung 861.20
      with open wound into thorax 861.30
      aspiration 507.0
      hemopneumothorax—*see*
        Hemopneumothorax, traumatic
      hemothorax—*see* Hemothorax, traumatic
      pneumohemothorax—*see*
        Pneumohemothorax, traumatic
      pneumothorax—*see* Pneumothorax,
        traumatic
      transfusion related, acute (TRALI) 518.7
    mediastinum 862.29
      with open wound into cavity 862.39
    mesentery 863.89
      with open wound into cavity 863.99
    mesosalpinx 867.6
      with open wound into cavity 867.7
    multiple 869.0

    Note—Multiple internal injuries of sites
    classifiable to the same three- or four-digit
    category should be classified to that category.
    Multiple injuries classifiable to different
    fourth-digit subdivisions of 861 (heart and lung
    injuries) should be dealt with according to
    coding rules.

      with open wound into cavity 869.1
      intra-abdominal organ (sites classifiable to
        863-868)
        with
          intrathoracic organ(s) (sites classifiable
            to 861-862) 869.0
            with open wound into cavity 869.1
          other intra-abdominal organ(s) (sites
            classifiable to 863-868, except where
            classifiable to the same three-digit
            category) 868.09
            with open wound into cavity 868.19

Injury—*continued*
  internal—*continued*
    multiple—*continued*
      intrathoracic organ (sites classifiable to
        861-862)
        with
          intra-abdominal organ(s) (sites
            classifiable to 863-868) 869.0
            with open wound into cavity 869.1
          other intrathoracic organ(s) (sites
            classifiable to 861-862, except where
            classifiable to the same three-digit
            category) 862.8
            with open wound into cavity 862.9
      myocardium—*see* Injury, internal, heart
      ovary 867.6
        with open wound into cavity 867.7
      pancreas (multiple sites) 863.84
        with open wound into cavity 863.94
        body 863.82
          with open wound into cavity 863.92
        head 863.81
          with open wound into cavity 863.91
        tail 863.83
          with open wound into cavity 863.93
      pelvis, pelvic (organs) (viscera) 867.8
        with
          fracture, pelvis—*see* Fracture, pelvis
          open wound into cavity 867.9
        specified site NEC 867.6
          with open wound into cavity 867.7
      peritoneum 868.03
        with open wound into cavity 868.13
      pleura 862.29
        with open wound into cavity 862.39
      prostate 867.6
        with open wound into cavity 867.7
      rectum 863.45
        with
          colon 863.46
            with open wound into cavity 863.56
          open wound into cavity 863.55
      retroperitoneum 868.04
        with open wound into cavity 868.14
      round ligament 867.6
        with open wound into cavity 867.7
      seminal vesicle 867.6
        with open wound into cavity 867.7
      spermatic cord 867.6
        with open wound into cavity 867.7
        scrotal—*see* Wound, open, spermatic cord
      spleen 865.00
        with
          disruption of parenchyma (massive)
            865.04
            with open wound into cavity 865.14
          hematoma (without rupture of capsule)
            865.01
            with open wound into cavity 865.11
          open wound into cavity 865.10
          tear, capsular 865.02
            with open wound into cavity 865.12
            extending into parenchyma 865.03
              with open wound into cavity 865.13
      stomach 863.0
        with open wound into cavity 863.1

Injury—*continued*
  internal—*continued*
    suprarenal gland (multiple) 868.01
      with open wound into cavity 868.11
    thorax, thoracic (cavity) (organs) (multiple)
      (*see also* Injury, internal, intrathoracic
      organs) 862.8
      with open wound into cavity 862.9
    thymus (gland) 862.29
      with open wound into cavity 862.39
    trachea (intrathoracic) 862.29
      with open wound into cavity 862.39
      cervical region (*see also* Wound, open,
        trachea) 874.02
    ureter 867.2
      with open wound into cavity 867.3
    urethra (sphincter) 867.0
      with
        abortion—*see* Abortion, by type, with,
          damage to pelvic organs
        ectopic pregnancy (*see also* categories
          633.0-633.9) 639.2
        molar pregnancy (*see also* categories
          630-632) 639.2
        open wound into cavity 867.1
      following
        abortion 639.2
        ectopic or molar pregnancy 639.2
      obstetrical trauma 665.5
        affecting fetus or newborn 763.89
    uterus 867.4
      with
        abortion—*see* Abortion, by type, with,
          damage to pelvic organs
        ectopic pregnancy (*see also* categories
          633.0-633.9) 639.2
        molar pregnancy (*see also* categories
          630-632) 639.2
        open wound into cavity 867.5
      following
        abortion 639.2
        ectopic or molar pregnancy 639.2
      obstetrical trauma NEC 665.5
        affecting fetus or newborn 763.89
    vas deferens 867.6
      with open wound into cavity 867.7
    vesical (sphincter) 867.0
      with open wound into cavity 867.1
    viscera (abdominal) (*see also* Injury, internal,
      multiple) 868.00
      with
        fracture, pelvis—*see* Fracture, pelvis
        open wound into cavity 868.10
      thoracic NEC (*see also* Injury, internal,
        intrathoracic organs) 862.8
      with open wound into cavity 862.9
  interscapular region 959.19
  intervertebral disc 959.19
  intestine—*see* Injury, internal, intestine
  intra-abdominal (organs) NEC—*see* Injury,
    internal, intra-abdominal

Injury—*continued*
  intracranial (traumatic) 854.0

Note—Use the following fifth-digit subclassification with categories 851-854:

0 *unspecifidd state of consciousness*
1 *with no loss of consciousness*
2 *with brief [less than one hour] loss of consciousness*
3 *with moderate [1-24 hours] loss of consciousness*
4 *with prolonged [more than 24 hours] loss of consciousness and return to pre-existing conscious level*
5 *with prolonged [more than 24 hours] loss of consciousness, without return to pre-existing conscious level*
Use fifth-digit 5 to designate when a patient is unconscious and dies before regaining consciousness, regardless of the duration of the loss of consciousness
6 *with loss of consciousness of unspecified duration*
9 *with concussion, unspecified*

---

  with
    open intracranial wound 854.1
    skull fracture—*see* Fracture, skull, by site
  contusion 851.8
    with open intracranial wound 851.9
    brain stem 851.4
      with open intracranial wound 851.5
    cerebellum 851.4
      with open intracranial wound 851.5
    cortex (cerebral) 851.0
      with open intracranial wound 851.2
  hematoma—*see* Injury, intracranial, hemorrhage
  hemorrhage 853.0
    with
      laceration—*see* Injury, intracranial, laceration
      open intracranial wound 853.1
    extradural 852.4
      with open intracranial wound 852.5
    subarachnoid 852.0
      with open intracranial wound 852.1
    subdural 852.2
      with open intracranial wound 852.3
  laceration 851.8
    with open intracranial wound 851.9
    brain stem 851.6
      with open intracranial wound 851.7
    cerebellum 851.6
      with open intracranial wound 851.7
    cortex (cerebral) 851.2
      with open intracranial wound 851.3
  intraocular—*see* Injury, eyeball, penetrating
  intrathoracic organs (multiple)—*see* Injury, internal, intrathoracic organs
  intrauterine—*see* Injury, internal, intrauterine
  iris 921.3
    penetrating—*see* Injury, eyeball, penetrating
  jaw 959.09
  jejunum—*see* Injury, internal, jejunum

Injury—*continued*
  joint NEC 959.9
    old or residual 718.80
      ankle 718.87
      elbow 718.82
      foot 718.87
      hand 718.84
      hip 718.85
      knee 718.86
      multiple sites 718.89
      pelvic region 718.85
      shoulder (region) 718.81
      specified site NEC 718.88
      wrist 718.83
  kidney—*see* Injury, internal, kidney
    acute (nontraumatic) 584.9
  knee (and ankle) (and foot) (and leg, except thigh) 959.7
  labium (majus) (minus) 959.14
  labyrinth, ear 959.09
  lacrimal apparatus, gland, or sac 921.1
    laceration 870.8
  larynx 959.09
  late effect—*see* Late, effects (of), injury
  leg except thigh (and ankle) (and foot) (and knee) 959.7
    upper or thigh 959.6
  lens, eye 921.3
    penetrating—*see* Injury, eyeball, penetrating
  lid, eye—*see* Injury, eyelid
  lip 959.09
  liver—*see* Injury, internal, liver
  lobe, parietal—*see* Injury, intracranial
  lumbar (region) 959.19
    plexus 953.5
  lumbosacral (region) 959.19
    plexus 953.5
  lung—*see* Injury, internal, lung
  malar region 959.09
  mastoid region 959.09
  maternal, during pregnancy, affecting fetus or newborn 760.5
  maxilla 959.09
  mediastinum—*see* Injury, internal, mediastinum
  membrane
    brain (*see also* Injury, intracranial) 854.0
    tympanic 959.09
  meningeal artery—*see* Hemorrhage, brain, traumatic, subarachnoid
  meninges (cerebral)—*see* Injury, intracranial
  mesenteric
    artery—*see* Injury, blood vessel, mesenteric, artery
    plexus, inferior 954.1
    vein—*see* Injury, blood vessel, mesenteric, vein
  mesentery—*see* Injury, internal, mesentery
  mesosalpinx—*see* Injury, internal, mesosalpinx
  middle ear 959.09
  midthoracic region 959.11
  mouth 959.09
  multiple (sites not classifiable to the same four-digit category in 959.0-959.7) 959.8
    internal 869.0
      with open wound into cavity 869.1
  musculocutaneous nerve 955.4
  nail
    finger 959.5
    toe 959.7

Injury—*continued*
  nasal (septum) (sinus) 959.09
  nasopharynx 959.09
  neck (and face) 959.09
  nerve 957.9
    abducens 951.3
    abducent 951.3
    accessory 951.6
    acoustic 951.5
    ankle and foot 956.9
    anterior crural, femoral 956.1
    arm (*see also* Injury, nerve, upper limb) 955.9
    auditory 951.5
    axillary 955.0
    brachial plexus 953.4
    cervical sympathetic 954.0
    cranial 951.9
      first or olfactory 951.8
      second or optic 950.0
      third or oculomotor 951.0
      fourth or trochlear 951.1
      fifth or trigeminal 951.2
      sixth or abducens 951.3
      seventh or facial 951.4
      eighth, acoustic, or auditory 951.5
      ninth or glossopharyngeal 951.8
      tenth, pneumogastric, or vagus 951.8
      eleventh or accessory 951.6
      twelfth or hypoglossal 951.7
      newborn 767.7
    cutaneous sensory
      lower limb 956.4
      upper limb 955.5
    digital (finger) 955.6
      toe 956.5
    facial 951.4
      newborn 767.5
    femoral 956.1
    finger 955.9
    foot and ankle 956.9
    forearm 955.9
    glossopharyngeal 951.8
    hand and wrist 955.9
    head and neck, superficial 957.0
    hypoglossal 951.7
    involving several parts of body 957.8
    leg (*see also* Injury, nerve, lower limb) 956.9
    lower limb 956.9
      multiple 956.8
      specified site NEC 956.5
    lumbar plexus 953.5
    lumbosacral plexus 953.5
    median 955.1
      forearm 955.1
      wrist and hand 955.1
    multiple (in several parts of body) (sites not classifiable to the same three-digit category) 957.8
    musculocutaneous 955.4
    musculospiral 955.3
      upper arm 955.3
    oculomotor 951.0
    olfactory 951.8
    optic 950.0
    pelvic girdle 956.9
      multiple sites 956.8
      specified site NEC 956.5
    peripheral 957.9
      multiple (in several regions) (sites not classifiable to the same three-digit category) 957.8
      specified site NEC 957.1

Injury—*continued*
  nerve—*continued*
    peroneal 956.3
      ankle and foot 956.3
      lower leg 956.3
    plantar 956.5
    plexus 957.9
      celiac 954.1
      mesenteric, inferior 954.1
      spinal 953.9
        brachial 953.4
        lumbosacral 953.5
        multiple sites 953.8
      sympathetic NEC 954.1
    pneumogastric 951.8
    radial 955.3
      wrist and hand 955.3
    sacral plexus 953.5
    sciatic 956.0
      thigh 956.0
    shoulder girdle 955.9
      multiple 955.8
      specified site NEC 955.7
    specified site NEC 957.1
    spinal 953.9
      plexus—*see* Injury, nerve, plexus, spinal
      root 953.9
        cervical 953.0
        dorsal 953.1
        lumbar 953.2
        multiple sites 953.8
        sacral 953.3
    splanchnic 954.1
    sympathetic NEC 954.1
      cervical 954.0
    thigh 956.9
    tibial 956.5
      ankle and foot 956.2
      lower leg 956.5
      posterior 956.2
    toe 956.9
    trigeminal 951.2
    trochlear 951.1
    trunk, excluding shoulder and pelvic girdles 954.9
      specified site NEC 954.8
      sympathetic NEC 954.1
    ulnar 955.2
      forearm 955.2
      wrist (and hand) 955.2
    upper limb 955.9
      multiple 955.8
      specified site NEC 955.7
    vagus 951.8
    wrist and hand 955.9
  nervous system, diffuse 957.8
  nose (septum) 959.09
  obstetrical NEC 665.9
    affecting fetus or newborn 763.89
  occipital (region) (scalp) 959.09
    lobe (*see also* Injury, intracranial) 854.0
  optic 950.9
    chiasm 950.1
    cortex 950.3
    nerve 950.0
    pathways 950.2
  orbit, orbital (region) 921.2
    penetrating 870.3
      with foreign body 870.4
  ovary—*see* Injury, internal, ovary
  paint-gun—*see* Wound, open, by site, complicated

Injury—*continued*
palate (soft) 959.09
pancreas—*see* Injury, internal, pancreas
parathyroid (gland) 959.09
parietal (region) (scalp) 959.09
lobe—*see* Injury, intracranial
pelvic
floor 959.19
complicating delivery 664.1
affecting fetus or newborn 763.89
joint or ligament, complicating delivery 665.6
affecting fetus or newborn 763.89
organs—*see also* Injury, internal, pelvis
with
abortion—*see* Abortion, by type, with
damage to pelvic organs
ectopic pregnancy (*see also* categories
633.0-633.9) 639.2
molar pregnancy (*see also* categories
633.0-633.9) 639.2
following
abortion 639.2
ectopic or molar pregnancy 639.2
obstetrical trauma 665.5
affecting fetus or newborn 763.89
pelvis 959.19
penis 959.14
fracture of corpus cavernosum 959.13
perineum 959.14
peritoneum—*see* Injury, internal, peritoneum
periurethral tissue
with
abortion—*see* Abortion, by type, with
damage to pelvic organs
ectopic pregnancy (*see also* categories
633.0-633.9) 639.2
molar pregnancy (*see also* categories
630-632) 639.2
complicating delivery 664.8
affecting fetus or newborn 763.89
following
abortion 639.2
ectopic or molar pregnancy 639.2
phalanges
foot 959.7
hand 959.5
pharynx 959.09
pleura—*see* Injury, internal, pleura
popliteal space 959.7
post-cardiac surgery (syndrome) 429.4
prepuce 959.14
prostate—*see* Injury, internal, prostate
pubic region 959.19
pudenda 959.14
radiation NEC 990
radioactive substance or radium NEC 990
rectovaginal septum 959.14
rectum—*see* Injury, internal, rectum
retina 921.3
penetrating—*see* Injury, eyeball, penetrating
retroperitoneal—*see* Injury, internal,
retroperitoneum
roentgen rays NEC 990
round ligament—*see* Injury, internal, round
ligament
sacral (region) 959.19
plexus 953.5
sacroiliac ligament NEC 959.19
sacrum 959.19
salivary ducts or glands 959.09

Injury—*continued*
scalp 959.09
due to birth trauma 767.19
fetus or newborn 767.19
scapular region 959.2
sclera 921.3
penetrating—*see* Injury, eyeball, penetrating
superficial 918.2
scrotum 959.14
seminal vesicle—*see* Injury, internal, seminal
vesicle
shoulder (and upper arm) 959.2
sinus
cavernous (*see also* Injury, intracranial) 854.0
nasal 959.09
skeleton NEC, birth injury 767.3
skin NEC 959.9
skull—*see* Fracture, skull, by site
soft tissue (of external sites) (severe)—*see*
Wound, open, by site
specified site NEC 959.8
spermatic cord—*see* Injury, internal, spermatic
cord
spinal (cord) 952.9
with fracture, vertebra—*see* Fracture, vertebra,
by site, with spinal cord injury
cervical (C_1-C_4) 952.00
with
anterior cord syndrome 952.02
central cord syndrome 952.03
complete lesion of cord 952.01
incomplete lesion NEC 952.04
posterior cord syndrome 952.04
C_5-C_7 level 952.05
with
anterior cord syndrome 952.07
central cord syndrome 952.08
complete lesion of cord 952.06
incomplete lesion NEC 952.09
posterior cord syndrome 952.09
specified type NEC 952.09
specified type NEC 952.04
dorsal (D_1-D_6) (T_1-T_6) (thoracic) 952.10
with
anterior cord syndrome 952.12
central cord syndrome 952.13
complete lesion of cord 952.11
incomplete lesion NEC 952.14
posterior cord syndrome 952.14
D_7-D_{12} level (T_7-T_{12}) 952.15
with
anterior cord syndrome 952.17
central cord syndrome 952.18
complete lesion of cord 952.16
incomplete lesion NEC 952.19
posterior cord syndrome 952.19
specified type NEC 952.19
specified type NEC 952.14
lumbar 952.2
multiple sites 952.8
nerve (root) NEC—*see* Injury, nerve, spinal,
root
plexus 953.9
brachial 953.4
lumbosacral 953.5
multiple sites 953.8
sacral 952.3
thoracic (*see also* Injury, spinal, dorsal)
952.10
spleen—*see* Injury, internal, spleen
stellate ganglion 954.1

Injury—*continued*
  sternal region 959.11
  stomach—*see* Injury, internal, stomach
  subconjunctival 921.1
  subcutaneous 959.9
  subdural—*see* Injury, intracranial
  submaxillary region 959.09
  submental region 959.09
  subungual
    fingers 959.5
    toes 959.7
  superficial 919

Note—Use the following fourth-digit
subdivisions with categories 910-919:

.0 *Abrasion or friction burn without mention of*
   infection
.1 *Abrasion or friction burn, infected*
.2 *Blister without mention of infection*
.3 *Blister, infected*
.4 *Insect bite, nonvenomous, without mention*
   of infection
.5 *Insect bite, nonvenomous, infected*
.6 *Superficial foreign body (splinter) without*
   major open wound and without mention of
   infection
.7 *Superficial foreign body (splinter) without*
   major open wound, infected
.8 *Other and unspecified superficial injury*
   without mention of infection
.9 *Other and unspecified superficial injury,*
   infected

For late effects of superficial injury, see
category 906.2.

---

    abdomen, abdominal (muscle) (wall) (and
      other part(s) of trunk) 911
    ankle (and hip, knee, leg, or thigh) 916
    anus (and other part(s) of trunk) 911
    arm 913
      upper (and shoulder) 912
    auditory canal (external) (meatus) (and other
      part(s) of face, neck, or scalp, except eye)
      910
    axilla (and upper arm) 912
    back (and other part(s) of trunk) 911
    breast (and other part(s) of trunk) 911
    brow (and other part(s) of face, neck or scalp,
      except eye) 910
    buttock (and other part(s) of trunk) 911
    canthus, eye 918.0
    cheek(s) (and other part(s) of face, neck, or
      scalp, except eye) 910
    chest wall (and other part(s) of trunk) 911
    chin (and other part(s) of face, neck, or scalp,
      except eye) 910
    clitoris (and other part(s) of trunk) 911
    conjunctiva 918.2
    cornea 918.1
      due to contact lens 371.82
    costal region (and other part(s) of trunk) 911
    ear(s) (auricle) (canal) (drum) (external) (and
      other part(s) of face, neck, or scalp, except
      eye) 910
    elbow (and forearm) (and wrist) 913
    epididymis (and other part(s) of trunk) 911
    epigastric region (and other part(s) of trunk)
      911
    epiglottis (and other part(s) of face, neck, or
      scalp, except eye) 910

Injury—*continued*
  superficial—*continued*
    eye(s) (and adnexa) NEC 918.9
    eyelid(s) (and periocular area) 918.0
    face (any part(s), except eye) (and neck or
      scalp) 910
    finger(s) (nail) (any) 915
    flank (and other part(s) of trunk) 911
    foot (phalanges) (and toe(s)) 917
    forearm (and elbow) (and wrist) 913
    forehead (and other part(s) of face, neck, or
      scalp, except eye) 910
    globe (eye) 918.9
    groin (and other part(s) of trunk) 911
    gum(s) (and other part(s) of face, neck, or
      scalp, except eye) 910
    hand(s) (except fingers alone) 914
    head (and other part(s) of face, neck, or scalp,
      except eye) 910
    heel (and foot or toe) 917
    hip (and ankle, knee, leg, or thigh) 916
    iliac region (and other part(s) of trunk) 911
    interscapular region (and other part(s) of
      trunk) 911
    iris 918.9
    knee (and ankle, hip, leg, or thigh) 916
    labium (majus) (minus) (and other part(s) of
      trunk) 911
    lacrimal (apparatus) (gland) (sac) 918.0
    leg (lower) (upper) (and ankle, hip, knee, or
      thigh) 916
    lip(s) (and other part(s) of face, neck, or scalp,
      except eye) 910
    lower extremity (except foot) 916
    lumbar region (and other part(s) of trunk) 911
    malar region (and other part(s) of face, neck,
      or scalp, except eye) 910
    mastoid region (and other part(s) of face, neck,
      or scalp, except eye) 910
    midthoracic region (and other part(s) of trunk)
      911
    mouth (and other part(s) of face, neck, or
      scalp, except eye) 910
    multiple sites (not classifiable to the same
      three-digit category) 919
    nasal (septum) (and other part(s) of face, neck,
      or scalp, except eye) 910
    neck (and face or scalp, any part(s), except
      eye) 910
    nose (septum) (and other part(s) of face, neck,
      or scalp, except eye) 910
    occipital region (and other part(s) of face,
      neck, or scalp, except eye) 910
    orbital region 918.0
    palate (soft) (and other part(s) of face, neck, or
      scalp, except eye) 910
    parietal region (and other part(s) of face, neck,
      or scalp, except eye) 910
    penis (and other part(s) of trunk) 911
    perineum (and other part(s) of trunk) 911
    periocular area 918.0
    pharynx (and other part(s) of face, neck, or
      scalp, except eye) 910
    popliteal space (and ankle, hip, leg, or thigh)
      916
    prepuce (and other part(s) of trunk) 911
    pubic region (and other part(s) of trunk) 911
    pudenda (and other part(s) of trunk) 911
    sacral region (and other part(s) of trunk) 911
    salivary (ducts) (glands) (and other part(s) of
      face, neck, or scalp, except eye) 910

Injury—*continued*
  superficial—*continued*
    scalp (and other part(s) of face or neck, except eye) 910
    scapular region (and upper arm) 912
    sclera 918.2
    scrotum (and other part(s) of trunk) 911
    shoulder (and upper arm) 912
    skin NEC 919
    specified site(s) NEC 919
    sternal region (and other part(s) of trunk) 911
    subconjunctival 918.2
    subcutaneous NEC 919
    submaxillary region (and other part(s) of face, neck, or scalp, except eye) 910
    submental region (and other part(s) of face, neck, or scalp, except eye) 910
    supraclavicular fossa (and other part(s) of face, neck or scalp, except eye) 910
    supraorbital 918.0
    temple (and other part(s) of face, neck, or scalp, except eye) 910
    temporal region (and other part(s) of face, neck, or scalp, except eye) 910
    testis (and other part(s) of trunk) 911
    thigh (and ankle, hip, knee, or leg) 916
    thorax, thoracic (external) (and other part(s) of trunk) 911
    throat (and other part(s) of face, neck, or scalp, except eye) 910
    thumb(s) (nail) 915
    toe(s) (nail) (subungual) (and foot) 917
    tongue (and other part(s) of face, neck, or scalp, except eye) 910
    tooth, teeth (*see also* Abrasion, dental) 521.20
    trunk (any part(s)) 911
    tunica vaginalis (and other part(s) of trunk) 911
    tympanum, tympanic membrane (and other part(s) of face, neck, or scalp, except eye) 910
    upper extremity NEC 913
    uvula (and other part(s) of face, neck, or scalp, except eye) 910
    vagina (and other part(s) of trunk) 911
    vulva (and other part(s) of trunk) 911
    wrist (and elbow) (and forearm) 913
  supraclavicular fossa 959.19
  supraorbital 959.09
  surgical complication (external or internal site) 998.2
  symphysis pubis 959.19
    complicating delivery 665.6
      affecting fetus or newborn 763.89
  temple 959.09
  temporal region 959.09
  testis 959.14
  thigh (and hip) 959.6
  thorax, thoracic (external) 959.11
    cavity—*see* Injury, internal, thorax
    internal—*see* Injury, internal, intrathoracic organs
  throat 959.09
  thumb(s) (nail) 959.5
  thymus—*see* Injury, internal, thymus
  thyroid (gland) 959.09
  toe (nail) (any) 959.7
  tongue 959.09
  tonsil 959.09
  tooth NEC 873.63
    complicated 873.73

Injury—*continued*
  trachea—*see* Injury, internal, trachea
  trunk 959.19
  tunica vaginalis 959.14
  tympanum, tympanic membrane 959.09
  ultraviolet rays NEC 990
  ureter—*see* Injury, internal, ureter
  urethra (sphincter)—*see* Injury, internal, urethra
  uterus—*see* Injury, internal, uterus
  uvula 959.09
  vagina 959.14
  vascular—*see* Injury, blood vessel
  vas deferens—*see* Injury, internal, vas deferens
  vein (*see also* Injury, blood vessel, by site) 904.9
  vena cava
    inferior 902.10
    superior 901.2
  vesical (sphincter)—*see* Injury, internal, vesical
  viscera (abdominal)—*see* Injury, internal, viscera
    with fracture, pelvis—*see* Fracture, pelvis
  visual 950.9
    cortex 950.3
  vitreous (humor) 871.2
  vulva 959.14
  whiplash (cervical spine) 847.0
  wringer—*see* Crush, by site
  wrist (and elbow) (and forearm) 959.3
  x-ray NEC 990
Inoculation —*see also* Vaccination
  complication or reaction—*see* Complication, vaccination
INPH (idiopathic normal pressure hydrocephalus) 331.5
Insanity, insane (*see also* Psychosis) 298.9
  adolescent (*see also* Schizophrenia) 295.9
  alternating (*see also* Psychosis, affective, circular) 296.7
  confusional 298.9
    acute 293.0
    subacute 293.1
  delusional 298.9
  paralysis, general 094.1
    progressive 094.1
  paresis, general 094.1
  senile 290.20
Insect
  bite—*see* Injury, superficial, by site
  venomous, poisoning by 989.5
Insemination, artificial V26.1
Insensitivity
  adrenocorticotropin hormone (ACTH) 255.41
  androgen 259.50
    complete 259.51
    partial 259.52
Insertion
  cord (umbilical) lateral or velamentous 663.8
    affecting fetus or newborn 762.6
  intrauterine contraceptive device V25.11
  placenta, vicious—*see* Placenta, previa
  subdermal implantable contraceptive V25.5
  velamentous, umbilical cord 663.8
    affecting fetus or newborn 762.6
Insolation 992.0
  meaning sunstroke 992.0
Insomnia, unspecified 780.52
  with sleep apnea, unspecified 780.51
  adjustment 307.41
  alcohol induced 291.82
  behavioral, of childhood V69.5

Insomnia—*continued*
  drug induced 292.85
  due to
    medical condition classified elsewhere 327.01
    mental disorder 327.02
  fatal familial (FFI) 046.72
  idiopathic 307.42
  nonorganic origin 307.41
    persistent (primary) 307.42
    transient 307.41
  organic 327.00
  other 327.09
  paradoxical 307.42
  primary 307.42
  psychophysiological 307.42
  subjective complaint 307.49
Inspiration
  food or foreign body (*see also* Asphyxia, food or
    foreign body) 933.1
  mucus (*see also* Asphyxia, mucus) 933.1
Inspissated bile syndrome, newborn 774.4
Instability
  detrusor 596.59
  emotional (excessive) 301.3
  joint (posttraumatic) 718.80
    ankle 718.87
    elbow 718.82
    foot 718.87
    hand 718.84
    hip 718.85
    knee 718.86
    lumbosacral 724.6
    multiple sites 718.89
    pelvic region 718.85
    sacroiliac 724.6
    shoulder (region) 718.81
    specified site NEC 718.88
    wrist 718.83
  lumbosacral 724.6
  nervous 301.89
  personality (emotional) 301.59
  thyroid, paroxysmal 242.9
  urethral 599.83
  vasomotor 780.2
Insufficiency, insufficient
  accommodation 367.4
  adrenal (gland) (acute) (chronic) 255.41
    medulla 255.5
    primary 255.41
    specified NEC 255.5
  adrenocortical 255.41
  anterior (occlusal) guidance 524.54
  anus 569.49
  aortic (valve) 424.1
    with
      mitral (valve) disease 396.1
        insufficiency, incompetence, or
          regurgitation 396.3
        stenosis or obstruction 396.1
      stenosis or obstruction 424.1
        with mitral (valve) disease 396.8
    congenital 746.4
    rheumatic 395.1
      with
        mitral (valve) disease 396.1
          insufficiency, incompetence, or
            regurgitation 396.3
          stenosis or obstruction 396.1
        stenosis or obstruction 395.2
          with mitral (valve) disease 396.8
    specified cause NEC 424.1
    syphilitic 093.22

Insufficiency, insufficient—*continued*
  arterial 447.1
    basilar artery 435.0
    carotid artery 435.8
    cerebral 437.1
    coronary (acute or subacute) 411.89
    mesenteric 557.1
    peripheral 443.9
    precerebral 435.9
    vertebral artery 435.1
    vertibrobasilar 435.3
  arteriovenous 459.9
  basilar artery 435.0
  biliary 575.8
  cardiac (*see also* Insufficiency, myocardial)
    428.0
    complicating surgery 997.1
    due to presence of (cardiac) prosthesis 429.4
    postoperative 997.1
      long-term effect of cardiac surgery 429.4
    specified during or due to a procedure 997.1
      long-term effect of cardiac surgery 429.4
  cardiorenal (*see also* Hypertension, cardiorenal)
    404.90
  cardiovascular (*see also* Disease,
    cardiovascular) 429.2
    renal (*see also* Hypertension, cardiorenal)
      404.90
  carotid artery 435.8
  cerebral (vascular) 437.9
  cerebrovascular 437.9
    with transient focal neurological signs and
      symptoms 435.9
    acute 437.1
      with transient focal neurological signs and
        symptoms 435.9
  circulatory NEC 459.9
    fetus or newborn 779.89
  convergence 378.83
  coronary (acute or subacute) 411.89
    chronic or with a stated duration of over 8
      weeks 414.8
  corticoadrenal 255.41
  dietary 269.9
  divergence 378.85
  food 994.2
  gastroesophageal 530.89
  gonadal
    ovary 256.39
    testis 257.2
  gonadotropic hormone secretion 253.4
  heart—*see also* Insufficiency, myocardial
    fetus or newborn 779.89
    valve (*see also* Endocarditis) 424.90
      congenital NEC 746.89
  hepatic 573.8
  idiopathic autonomic 333.0
  interocclusal distance of teeth (ridge) 524.36
  kidney
    acute 593.9
    chronic 585.9
  labyrinth, labyrinthine (function) 386.53
    bilateral 386.54
    unilateral 386.53
  lacrimal 375.15
  liver 573.8
  lung (acute) (*see also* Insufficiency, pulmonary)
    518.82
    following trauma and surgery 518.25
    newborn 770.89
  mental (congenital) (*see also* Disability,
    intellectual) 319

Insufficiency, insufficient—*continued*
  mesenteric 557.1
  mitral (valve) 424.0
    with
      aortic (valve) disease 396.3
        insufficiency, incompetence, or
          regurgitation 396.3
        stenosis or obstruction 396.2
      obstruction or stenosis 394.2
        with aortic valve disease 396.8
    congenital 746.6
    rheumatic 394.1
      with
        aortic (valve) disease 396.3
          insufficiency, incompetence, or
            regurgitation 396.3
          stenosis or obstruction 396.2
        obstruction or stenosis 394.2
          with aortic valve disease 396.8
      active or acute 391.1
        with chorea, rheumatic (Sydenham's)
          392.0
    specified cause, except rheumatic 424.0
  muscle
    heart—*see* Insufficiency, myocardial
    ocular (*see also* Strabismus) 378.9
  myocardial, myocardium (with arteriosclerosis)
    428.0
    with rheumatic fever (conditions classifiable
      to 390)
      active, acute, or subacute 391.2
        with chorea 392.0
      inactive or quiescent (with chorea) 398.0
    congenital 746.89
    due to presence of (cardiac) prosthesis 429.4
    fetus or newborn 779.89
    following cardiac surgery 429.4
    hypertensive (*see also* Hypertension, heart)
      402.91
      benign 402.11
      malignant 402.01
    postoperative 997.1
      long-term effect of cardiac surgery 429.4
    rheumatic 398.0
      active, acute, or subacute 391.2
        with chorea (Sydenham's) 392.0
    syphilitic 093.82
  nourishment 994.2
  organic 799.89
  ovary 256.39
    postablative 256.2
  pancreatic 577.8
  parathyroid (gland) 252.1
  peripheral vascular (arterial) 443.9
  pituitary (anterior) 253.2
    posterior 253.5
  placental—*see* Placenta, insufficiency
  platelets 287.5
  prenatal care in current pregnancy V23.7
  progressive pluriglandular 258.9
  pseudocholinesterase 289.89
  pulmonary (acute) 518.82
    following
      shock 518.52
      surgery 518.52
      trauma 518.52
    newborn 770.89
    valve (*see also* Endocarditis, pulmonary)
      424.3
      congenital 746.09
  pyloric 537.0

Insufficiency, insufficient—*continued*
  renal 593.9
    acute 593.9
    chronic 585.9
    due to a procedure 997.5
  respiratory 786.09
    acute 518.82
      following trauma and surgery 518.52
    newborn 770.89
  rotation—*see* Malrotation
  suprarenal 255.41
    medulla 255.5
  tarso-orbital fascia, congenital 743.66
  tear film 375.15
  testis 257.2
  thyroid (gland) (acquired)—*see also*
    Hypothyroidism
    congenital 243
  tricuspid (*see also* Endocarditis, tricuspid) 397.0
    congenital 746.89
    syphilitic 093.23
  urethral sphincter 599.84
  valve, valvular (heart) (*see also* Endocarditis)
    424.90
  vascular 459.9
    intestine NEC 557.9
    mesenteric 557.1
    peripheral 443.9
    renal (*see also* Hypertension, kidney) 403.90
  velopharyngeal
    acquired 528.9
    congenital 750.29
  venous (peripheral) 459.81
  ventricular—*see* Insufficiency, myocardial
  vertebral artery 435.1
  vertibrobasilar artery 435.3
  weight gain during pregnancy 646.8
  zinc 269.3
Insufflation
  fallopian
    fertility testing V26.21
    following sterilization reversal V26.22
  meconium 770.11
    with respiratory symptoms 770.12
Insular —*see* condition
Insulinoma (M8151/0)
  malignant (M8151/3)
    pancreas 157.4
    specified site—*see* Neoplasm, by site,
      malignant
    unspecified site 157.4
  pancreas 211.7
  specified site—*see* Neoplasm, by site, benign
  unspecified site 211.7
Insuloma —*see* Insulinoma
Insult
  brain 437.9
    acute 436
  cerebral 437.9
    acute 436
  cerebrovascular 437.9
    acute 436
  vascular NEC 437.9
    acute 436
Insurance examination (certification) V70.3
Intemperance (*see also* Alcoholism) 303.9
Interception of pregnancy (menstrual
  extraction) V25.3
Interference
  balancing side 524.56
  non-working side 524.56

Intermenstrual
  bleeding 626.6
    irregular 626.6
    regular 626.5
  hemorrhage 626.6
    irregular 626.6
    regular 626.5
  ain(s) 625.2
Intermittent— *see* condition
Internal —*see* condition
Interproximal wear 521.10
Interrogation
  cardiac defibrillator (automatic) (implantable)
      V53.32
  cardiac pacemaker V53.31
  cardiac (event) (loop) recorder V53.39
  infusion pump (implanted) (intrathecal) V53.09
  neurostimulator V53.02
Interruption
  aortic arch 747.11
  bundle of His 426.50
  fallopian tube (for sterilization) V25.2
  phase-shift, sleep cycle 307.45
  repeated REM-sleep 307.48
  sleep
    due to perceived environmental disturbances
        307.48
    phase-shift, of 24-hour sleep-wake cycle
        307.45
    repeated REM-sleep type 307.48
  vas deferens (for sterilization) V25.2
Intersexuality 752.7
Interstitial —*see* condition
Intertrigo 695.89
  labialis 528.5
Intervertebral disc —*see* condition
Intestine, intestinal —*see also* condition
  flu 487.8
Intolerance
  carbohydrate NEC 579.8
  cardiovascular exercise, with pain (at rest) (with
      less than ordinary activity) (with ordinary
      activity) V47.2
  cold 780.99
  disaccharide (hereditary) 271.3
  drug
    correct substance properly administered 995.27
    wrong substance given or taken in error 977.9
      specified drug—*see* Table of drugs and
          chemicals
  effort 306.2
  fat NEC 579.8
  foods NEC 579.8
  fructose (hereditary) 271.2
  glucose (-galactose) (congenital) 271.3
  gluten 579.0
  lactose (hereditary) (infantile) 271.3
  lysine (congenital) 270.7
  milk NEC 579.8
  protein (familial) 270.7
  starch NEC 579.8
  sucrose (-isomaltose) (congenital) 271.3
Intoxicated NEC (*see also* Alcoholism) 305.0
Intoxication
  acid 276.2
  acute
    alcoholic 305.0
      with alcoholism 303.0
      hangover effects 305.0
    caffeine 305.9
    hallucinogenic (*see also* Abuse, drugs,
        nondependent) 305.3

Intoxication—*continued*
  alcohol (acute) 305.0
    with alcoholism 303.0
    hangover effects 305.0
    idiosyncratic 291.4
    pathological 291.4
  alimentary canal 558.2
  ammonia (hepatic) 572.2
  caffeine 305.9
  chemical—*see also* Table of drugs and chemicals
    via placenta or breast milk 760.70
      alcohol 760.71
      anticonvulsants 760.77
      antifungals 760.74
      anti-infective agents 760.74
      antimetabolics 760.78
      cocaine 760.75
      "crack" 760.75
      hallucinogenic agents NEC 760.73
      medicinal agents NEC 760.79
      narcotics 760.72
      obstetric anesthetic or analgesic drug 763.5
      specified agent NEC 760.79
      suspected, affecting management of
          pregnancy 655.5
  cocaine, through placenta or breast milk 760.75
  delirium
    alcohol 291.0
    drug 292.81
  drug 292.89
    with delirium 292.81
    correct substance properly administered (*see
        also* Allergy, drug) 995.27
    newborn 779.4
    obstetric anesthetic or sedation 668.9
      affecting fetus or newborn 763.5
    overdose or wrong substance given or
        taken—*see* Table of drugs and chemicals
    pathologic 292.2
    specific to newborn 779.4
    via placenta or breast milk 760.70
      alcohol 760.71
      anticonvulsants 760.77
      antifungals 760.74
      anti-infective agents 760.74
      antimetabolics 760.78
      cocaine 760.75
      "crack" 760.75
      hallucinogenic agents 760.73
      medicinal agents NEC 760.79
      narcotics 760.72
      obstetric anesthetic or analgesic drug 763.5
      specified agent NEC 760.79
      suspected, affecting management of
          pregnancy 655.5
  enteric—*see* Intoxication, intestinal
  fetus or newborn, via placenta or breast milk
      760.70
    alcohol 760.71
    anticonvulsants 760.77
    antifungals 760.74
    anti-infective agents 760.74
    antimetabolics 760.78
    cocaine 760.75
    "crack" 760.75
    hallucinogenic agents 760.73
    medicinal agents NEC 760.79
    narcotics 760.72
    obstetric anesthetic or analgesic drug 763.5
    specified agent NEC 760.79
    suspected, affecting management of pregnancy
        655.5

Intoxication—*continued*
  food—*see* Poisoning, food
  gastrointestinal 558.2
  hallucinogenic (acute) 305.3
  hepatocerebral 572.2
  idiosyncratic alcohol 291.4
  intestinal 569.89
    due to putrefaction of food 005.9
  methyl alcohol (*see also* Alcoholism) 305.0
    with alcoholism 303.0
  non-foodborne due to toxins of Clostridium
    botulinum [*C. botulinum*] —*see* Botulism
  pathologic 291.4
    drug 292.2
  potassium (K) 276.7
  septic
    with
      abortion—*see* Abortion, by type, with sepsis
      ectopic pregnancy (*see also* categories
        633.0-633.9) 639.0
      molar pregnancy (*see also* categories
        630-632) 639.0
    during labor 659.3
    following
      abortion 639.0
      ectopic or molar pregnancy 639.0
    generalized—*see* Septicemia
    puerperal, postpartum, childbirth 670.2
  serum (prophylactic) (therapeutic) 999.59
  uremic—*see* Uremia
  water 276.69
Intracranial —*see* condition
Intrahepatic gallbladder 751.69
Intraligamentous —*see also* condition
  pregnancy—*see* Pregnancy, cornual
Intraocular —*see also* condition
  sepsis 360.00
Intrathoracic —*see also* condition
  kidney 753.3
  stomach—*see* Hernia, diaphragm
Intrauterine contraceptive device
  checking V25.42
  insertion V25.11
  in situ V45.51
  management V25.42
  prescription V25.02
    repeat V25.42
  reinsertion V25.13
  removal V25.12
    and reinsertion V25.13
  replacement V25.13
Intraventricular —*see* condition
Intrinsic deformity —*see* Deformity
Intruded tooth 524.34
Intrusion, repetitive, of sleep (due to
  environmental disturbances) (with atypical
  polysomnographic features) 307.48
Intumescent, lens (eye) NEC 366.9
  senile 366.12
Intussusception (colon) (enteric) (intestine)
  (rectum) 560.0
  appendix 543.9
  congenital 751.5
  fallopian tube 620.8
  ileocecal 560.0
  ileocolic 560.0
  ureter (with obstruction) 593.4
Invagination
  basilar 756.0
  colon or intestine 560.0
Invalid (since birth) 799.89
Invalidism (chronic) 799.89

Inversion
  albumin-globulin (A-G) ratio 273.8
  bladder 596.89
  cecum (*see also* Intussusception) 560.0
  cervix 622.8
  nipple 611.79
    congenital 757.6
    puerperal, postpartum 676.3
  optic papilla 743.57
  organ or site, congenital NEC—*see* Anomaly,
    specified type NEC
  sleep rhythm 327.39
    nonorganic origin 307.45
  testis (congenital) 752.51
  uterus (postinfectional) (postpartal, old) 621.7
    chronic 621.7
    complicating delivery 665.2
      affecting fetus or newborn 763.89
  vagina—*see* Prolapse, vagina
Investigation
  allergens V72.7
  clinical research (control) (normal comparison)
    (participant) V70.7
Inviability —*see* Immaturity
Involuntary movement, abnormal 781.0
Involution, involutional —*see also* condition
  breast, cystic or fibrocystic 610.1
  depression (*see also* Psychosis, affective) 296.2
    recurrent episode 296.3
    single episode 296.2
  melancholia (*see also* Psychosis, affective) 296.2
    recurrent episode 296.3
    single episode 296.2
  ovary, senile 620.3
  paranoid state (reaction) 297.2
  paraphrenia (climacteric) (menopause) 297.2
  psychosis 298.8
  thymus failure 254.8
IQ
  under 20 318.2
  20-34 318.1
  35-49 318.0
  50-70 317
IRDS 769
Irideremia 743.45
Iridis rubeosis 364.42
  diabetic 250.5 *[364.42]*
  due to secondary diabetes 249.5 *[364.42]*
Iridochoroiditis (panuveitis) 360.12
Iridocyclitis NEC 364.3
  acute 364.00
    primary 364.01
    recurrent 364.02
  chronic 364.10
    in
      lepromatous leprosy 030.0 *[364.11]*
      sarcoidosis 135 *[364.11]*
      tuberculosis (*see also* Tuberculosis) 017.3
        [364.11]
  due to allergy 364.04
  endogenous 364.01
  gonococcal 098.41
  granulomatous 364.10
  herpetic (simplex) 054.44
    zoster 053.22
  hypopyon 364.05
  lens induced 364.23
  nongranulomatous 364.00
    primary 364.01
    recurrent 364.02
  rheumatic 364.10

Iridocyclitis—*continued*
  secondary 364.04
    infectious 364.03
    noninfectious 364.04
  subacute 364.00
    primary 364.01
    recurrent 364.02
  sympathetic 360.11
  syphilitic (secondary) 091.52
  tuberculous (chronic) (*see also* Tuberculosis)
    017.3 *[364.11]*
Iridocyclochoroiditis (panuveitis) 360.12
Iridodialysis 364.76
Iridodonesis 364.89
Iridoplegia (complete) (partial) (reflex) 379.49
Iridoschisis 364.52
IRIS (Immune Reconstitution Inflammatory
  Syndrome) 995.90
Iris —*see* condition
Iritis 364.3
  acute 364.00
    primary 364.01
    recurrent 364.02
  chronic 364.10
    in
      sarcoidosis 135 *[364.11]*
      tuberculosis (*see also* Tuberculosis) 017.3
        [364.11]
  diabetic 250.5 *[364.42]*
    due to secondary diabetes 249.5 *[364.42]*
  due to
    allergy 364.04
    herpes simplex 054.44
    leprosy 030.0 *[364.11]*
  endogenous 364.01
  gonococcal 098.41
  gouty 274.89 *[364.11]*
  granulomatous 364.10
  hypopyon 364.05
  lens induced 364.23
  nongranulomatous 364.00
  papulosa 095.8 *[364.11]*
  primary 364.01
  recurrent 364.02
  rheumatic 364.10
  secondary 364.04
    infectious 364.03
    noninfectious 364.04
  subacute 364.00
    primary 364.01
    recurrent 364.02
  sympathetic 360.11
  syphilitic (secondary) 091.52
    congenital 090.0 *[364.11]*
    late 095.8 *[364.11]*
  tuberculous (*see also* Tuberculosis) 017.3 *[364.11]*
  uratic 274.89 *[364.11]*
Iron
  deficiency anemia 280.9
  metabolism disease 275.09
  storage disease 275.09
Iron-miners' lung 503
Irradiated enamel (tooth, teeth) 521.89
Irradiation
  burn—*see* Burn, by site
  effects, adverse 990
Irreducible, irreducibility —*see* condition
Irregular, irregularity
  action, heart 427.9
  alveolar process 525.8
  bleeding NEC 626.4

Irregular, irregularity—*continued*
  breathing 786.09
  colon 569.89
  contour
    of cornea 743.41
      acquired 371.70
    reconstructed breast 612.0
  dentin in pulp 522.3
  eye movements NEC 379.59
  menstruation (cause unknown) 626.4
  periods 626.4
  prostate 602.9
  pupil 364.75
  respiratory 786.09
  septum (nasal) 470
  shape, organ or site, congenital NEC—*see*
    Distortion
  sleep-wake rhythm (non-24-hour) 327.39
    nonorganic origin 307.45
  vertebra 733.99
Irritability 799.22
  bladder 596.89
    neurogenic 596.54
      with cauda equina syndrome 344.61
  bowel (syndrome) 564.1
  bronchial (*see also* Bronchitis) 490
  cerebral, newborn 779.1
  colon 564.1
    psychogenic 306.4
  duodenum 564.89
  heart (psychogenic) 306.2
  ileum 564.89
  jejunum 564.89
  myocardium 306.2
  nervousness 799.21
  rectum 564.89
  stomach 536.9
    psychogenic 306.4
  sympathetic (nervous system) (*see also*
    Neuropathy, peripheral, autonomic) 337.9
  urethra 599.84
  ventricular (heart) (psychogenic) 306.2
Irritable —(*see also* Irritability) 799.22
Irritation
  anus 569.49
  axillary nerve 353.0
  bladder 596.89
  brachial plexus 353.0
  brain (traumatic) (*see also* Injury, intracranial)
    854.0
    nontraumatic—*see* Encephalitis
  bronchial (*see also* Bronchitis) 490
  cerebral (traumatic) (*see also* Injury,
    intracranial) 854.0
    nontraumatic—*see* Encephalitis
  cervical plexus 353.2
  cervix (*see also* Cervicitis) 616.0
  choroid, sympathetic 360.11
  cranial nerve—*see* Disorder, nerve, cranial
  digestive tract 536.9
    psychogenic 306.4
  gastric 536.9
    psychogenic 306.4
  gastrointestinal (tract) 536.9
    functional 536.9
    psychogenic 306.4
  globe, sympathetic 360.11
  intestinal (bowel) 564.9
  labyrinth 386.50
  lumbosacral plexus 353.1

Irritation—*continued*
  meninges (traumatic) (*see also* Injury,
    intracranial) 854.0
    nontraumatic—*see* Meningitis
  myocardium 306.2
  nerve—*see* Disorder, nerve
  nervous 799.21
  nose 478.19
  penis 607.89
  perineum 709.9
  peripheral
    autonomic nervous system (*see also*
      Neuropathy, peripheral, autonomic) 337.9
    nerve—*see* Disorder, nerve
  peritoneum (*see also* Peritonitis) 567.9
  pharynx 478.29
  plantar nerve 355.6
  spinal (cord) (traumatic)—*see also* Injury,
    spinal, by site
    nerve—*see also* Disorder, nerve
      root NEC 724.9
      traumatic—*see* Injury, nerve, spinal
    nontraumatic—*see* Myelitis
  stomach 536.9
    psychogenic 306.4
  sympathetic nerve NEC (*see also* Neuropathy,
    peripheral, autonomic) 337.9
  ulnar nerve 354.2
  vagina 623.9
Isambert's disease 012.3
Ischemia, ischemic 459.9
  basilar artery (with transient neurologic deficit)
    435.0
  bone NEC 733.40
  bowel (transient) 557.9
    acute 557.0
    chronic 557.1
    due to mesenteric artery insufficiency 557.1
  brain—*see also* Ischemia, cerebral
    recurrent focal 435.9
  cardiac (*see also* Ischemia, heart) 414.9
  cardiomyopathy 414.8
  carotid artery (with transient neurologic deficit)
    435.8
  cerebral (chronic) (generalized) 437.1
    arteriosclerotic 437.0
    intermittent (with transient neurologic deficit)
      435.9
    newborn 779.2
    puerperal, postpartum, childbirth 674.0
    recurrent focal (with transient neurologic
      deficit) 435.9
    transient (with transient neurologic deficit)
      435.9
  colon 557.9
    acute 557.0
    chronic 557.1
    due to mesenteric artery insufficiency 557.1
  coronary (chronic) (*see also* Ischemia, heart)
    414.9
  demand 411.89
  heart (chronic or with a stated duration of over 8
    weeks) 414.9
    acute or with a stated duration of 8 weeks or
      less (*see also* Infarct, myocardium) 410.9
      without myocardial infarction 411.89
        with coronary (artery) occlusion 411.81
    subacute 411.89
  intestine (transient) 557.9
    acute 557.0
    chronic 557.1
    due to mesenteric artery insufficiency 557.1

Ischemia, ischemic—*continued*
  kidney 593.81
  labyrinth 386.50
  muscles, leg 728.89
  myocardium, myocardial (chronic or with a
    stated duration of over 8 weeks) 414.8
    acute (*see also* Infarct, myocardium) 410.9
      without myocardial infarction 411.89
        with coronary (artery) occlusion 411.81
  renal 593.81
  retina, retinal 362.84
  small bowel 557.9
    acute 557.0
    chronic 557.1
    due to mesenteric artery insufficiency 557.1
  spinal cord 336.1
  subendocardial (*see also* Insufficiency,
    coronary) 411.89
  supply (*see also* Angina) 414.9
  vertebral artery (with transient neurologic
    deficit) 435.1
Ischialgia (*see also* Sciatica) 724.3
Ischiopagus 759.4
Ischium, ischial —*see* condition
Ischomenia 626.8
Ischuria 788.5
Iselin's disease or osteochondrosis 732.5
Islands of
  parotid tissue in
    lymph nodes 750.26
    neck structures 750.26
  submaxillary glands in
    fascia 750.26
    lymph nodes 750.26
    neck muscles 750.26
Islet cell tumor, pancreas (M8150/0) 211.7
Isoimmunization NEC (*see also* Incompatibility)
  656.2
  anti-E 656.2
  fetus or newborn 773.2
    ABO blood groups 773.1
    Rhesus (Rh) factor 773.0
Isolation V07.0
  social V62.4
Isosporosis 007.2
Issue
  medical certificate NEC V68.09
    cause of death V68.09
    disability examination V68.01
    fitness V68.09
    incapacity V68.09
  repeat prescription NEC V68.1
    appliance V68.1
    contraceptive V25.40
      device NEC V25.49
        intrauterine V25.42
        specified type NEC V25.49
      pill V25.41
    glasses V68.1
    medicinal substance V68.1
Itch (*see also* Pruritus) 698.9
  bakers' 692.89
  barbers' 110.0
  bricklayers' 692.89
  cheese 133.8
  clam diggers' 120.3
  coolie 126.9
  copra 133.8
  Cuban 050.1
  dew 126.9
  dhobie 110.3

Itch —*continued*
eye 379.99
filarial (*see also* Infestation, filarial) 125.9
grain 133.8
grocers' 133.8
ground 126.9
harvest 133.8
jock 110.3
Malabar 110.9
  beard 110.0
  foot 110.4
  scalp 110.0
meaning scabies 133.0
Norwegian 133.0
perianal 698.0
poultrymen's 133.8
sarcoptic 133.0
scrub 134.1
seven year V61.10
  meaning scabies 133.0
straw 133.8
swimmers' 120.3
washerwoman's 692.4
water 120.3
winter 698.8
Itsenko-Cushing syndrome (pituitary
  basophilism) 255.0
Ivemark's syndrome (asplenia with congenital
  heart disease) 759.0
Ivory bones 756.52
Ixodes 134.8
Ixodiasis 134.8

J

Jaccoud's nodular fibrositis, chronic (Jaccoud's syndrome) 714.4
Jackson's
  membrane 751.4
  paralysis or syndrome 344.89
  veil 751.4
Jacksonian
  epilepsy (*see also* Epilepsy) 345.5
  seizures (focal) (*see also* Epilepsy) 345.5
Jacob's ulcer (M8090/3)—*see* Neoplasm, skin, malignant, by site
Jacquet's dermatitis (diaper dermatitis) 691.0
Jadassohn's
  blue nevus (M8780/0)—*see* Neoplasm, skin, benign
  disease (maculopapular erythroderma) 696.2
  intraepidermal epithelioma (M8096/0)—*see* Neoplasm, skin, benign
Jadassohn-Lewandowski syndrome (pachyonychia congenita) 757.5
Jadassohn-Pellizari's disease (anetoderma) 701.3
Jadassohn-Tièche nevus (M8780/0)—*see* Neoplasm, skin, benign
Jaffe-Lichtenstein (-Uehlinger) syndrome 252.01
Jahnke's syndrome (encephalocutaneous angiomatosis) 759.6
Jakob-Creutzfeldt disease (CJD) (syndrome) 046.19
  with dementia
    with behavioral disturbance 046.19 *[294.11]*
    without behavioral disturbance 046.19 *[294.10]*
  familial 046.19
  iatrogenic 046.19
  specified NEC 046.19
  sporadic 046.19
  variant (vCJD) 046.11
    with dementia
      with behavioral disturbance 046.11 *[294.11]*
      without behavioral disturbance 046.11 *[294.10]*
Jaksch (-Luzet) disease or syndrome (pseudoleukemia infantum) 285.8
Jamaican
  neuropathy 349.82
  paraplegic tropical ataxic-spastic syndrome 349.82
Janet's disease (psychasthenia) 300.89
Janiceps 759.4
Jansky-Bielschowsky amaurotic familial idiocy 330.1
Japanese
  B type encephalitis 062.0
  river fever 081.2
  seven-day fever 100.89
Jaundice (yellow) 782.4
  acholuric (familial) (splenomegalic) (*see also* Spherocytosis) 282.0
    acquired 283.9
  breast milk 774.39
  catarrhal (acute) 070.1
    with hepatic coma 070.0
    chronic 571.9
    epidemic—*see* Jaundice, epidemic
  cholestatic (benign) 782.4
  chronic idiopathic 277.4
  epidemic (catarrhal) 070.1

Jaundice—*continued*
  with hepatic coma 070.0
  leptospiral 100.0
  spirochetal 100.0
  febrile (acute) 070.1
    with hepatic coma 070.0
    leptospiral 100.0
    spirochetal 100.0
  fetus or newborn 774.6
    due to or associated with
      ABO
        antibodies 773.1
        incompatibility, maternal/fetal 773.1
        isoimmunization 773.1
      absence or deficiency of enzyme system for bilirubin conjugation (congenital) 774.39
      blood group incompatibility NEC 773.2
      breast milk inhibitors to conjugation 774.39
        associated with preterm delivery 774.2
      bruising 774.1
      Crigler-Najjar syndrome 277.4 *[774.31]*
      delayed conjugation 774.30
        associated with preterm delivery 774.2
      development 774.39
      drugs or toxins transmitted from mother 774.1
      G-6-PD deficiency 282.2 *[774.0]*
      galactosemia 271.1 *[774.5]*
      Gilbert's syndrome 277.4 *[774.31]*
      hepatocellular damage 774.4
      hereditary hemolytic anemia (*see also* Anemia, hemolytic) 282.9 *[774.0]*
      hypothyroidism, congenital 243 *[774.31]*
      incompatibility, maternal/fetal NEC 773.2
      infection 774.1
      inspissated bile syndrome 774.4
      isoimmunization NEC 773.2
      mucoviscidosis 277.01 *[774.5]*
      obliteration of bile duct, congenital 751.61 *[774.5]*
      polycythemia 774.1
      preterm delivery 774.2
      red cell defect 282.9 *[774.0]*
      Rh
        antibodies 773.0
        incompatibility, maternal/fetal 773.0
        isoimmunization 773.0
      spherocytosis (congenital) 282.0 *[774.0]*
      swallowed maternal blood 774.1
    physiological NEC 774.6
  from injection, inoculation, infusion, or transfusion (blood) (plasma) (serum) (other substance) (onset within 8 months after administration)—*see* Hepatitis, viral
  Gilbert's (familial nonhemolytic) 277.4
  hematogenous 283.9
  hemolytic (acquired) 283.9
    congenital (*see also* Spherocytosis) 282.0
  hemorrhagic (acute) 100.0
    leptospiral 100.0
    newborn 776.0
    spirochetal 100.0
  hepatocellular 573.8
  homologous (serum)—*see* Hepatitis, viral
  idiopathic, chronic 277.4
  infectious (acute) (subacute) 070.1
    with hepatic coma 070.0
    leptospiral 100.0
    spirochetal 100.0

Jaundice—*continued*
  leptospiral 100.0
  malignant (*see also* Necrosis, liver) 570
  newborn (physiological) (*see also* Jaundice,
    fetus or newborn) 774.6
  nonhemolytic, congenital familial (Gilbert's)
    277.4
  nuclear, newborn (*see also* Kernicterus of
    newborn) 774.7
  obstructive NEC (*see also* Obstruction, biliary)
    576.8
  postimmunization—*see* Hepatitis, viral
  posttransfusion—*see* Hepatitis, viral
  regurgitation (*see also* Obstruction, biliary)
    576.8
  serum (homologous) (prophylactic)
    (therapeutic)—*see* Hepatitis, viral
  spirochetal (hemorrhagic) 100.0
  symptomatic 782.4
    newborn 774.6
Jaw —*see* condition
Jaw-blinking 374.43
  congenital 742.8
Jaw-winking phenomenon or syndrome 742.8
Jealousy
  alcoholic 291.5
  childhood 313.3
  sibling 313.3
Jejunitis (*see also* Enteritis) 558.9
Jejunostomy status V44.4
Jejunum, jejunal —*see* condition
Jensen's disease 363.05
Jericho boil 085.1
Jerks, myoclonic 333.2
Jervell-Lange-Nielsen syndrome 426.82
Jeune's disease or syndrome (asphyxiating
    thoracic dystrophy) 756.4
Jigger disease 134.1
Job's syndrome (chronic granulomatous disease)
    288.1
Jod-Basedow phenomenon 242.8
Johnson-Stevens disease (erythema multiforme
    exudativum) 695.13
Joint —*see also* condition
  Charcot's 094.0 *[713.5]*
  false 733.82
  flail—*see* Flail, joint
  mice—*see* Loose, body, joint, by site
  sinus to bone 730.9
  von Gies' 095.8
Jordan's anomaly or syndrome 288.2
Josephs-Diamond-Blackfan anemia (congenital
    hypoplastic) 284.01
Joubert syndrome 759.89
Jumpers' knee 727.2
Jungle yellow fever 060.0
Jüngling's disease (sarcoidosis) 135
Junin virus hemorrhagic fever 078.7
Juvenile —*see also* condition
  delinquent 312.9
    group (*see also* Disturbance, conduct) 312.2
    neurotic 312.4

K

Kabuki syndrome 759.89
Kahler (-Bozzolo) disease (multiple myeloma)
    (M9730/3) 203.0
Kakergasia 300.9
Kakke 265.0
Kala-azar (Indian) (infantile) (Mediterranean)
    (Sudanese) 085.0
Kalischer's syndrome (encephalocutaneous
    angiomatosis) 759.6
Kallmann's syndrome (hypogonadotropic
    hypogonadism with anosmia) 253.4
Kanner's syndrome (autism) (see also
    Psychosis, childhood) 299.0
Kaolinosis 502
Kaposi's
  disease 757.33
    lichen ruber 696.4
      acuminatus 696.4
      moniliformis 697.8
    xeroderma pigmentosum 757.33
  sarcoma (M9140/3) 176.9
    adipose tissue 176.1
    aponeurosis 176.1
    artery 176.1
    associated herpesvirus infection 058.89
    blood vessel 176.1
    bursa 176.1
    connective tissue 176.1
    external genitalia 176.8
    fascia 176.1
    fatty tissue 176.1
    fibrous tissue 176.1
    gastrointestinal tract NEC 176.3
    ligament 176.1
    lung 176.4
    lymph
      gland(s) 176.5
      node(s) 176.5
    lymphatic(s) NEC 176.1
    muscle (skeletal) 176.1
    oral cavity NEC 176.8
    palate 176.2
    scrotum 176.8
    skin 176.0
    soft tissue 176.1
    specified site NEC 176.8
    subcutaneous tissue 176.1
    synovia 176.1
    tendon (sheath) 176.1
    vein 176.1
    vessel 176.1
    viscera NEC 176.9
    vulva 176.8
  varicelliform eruption 054.0
  vaccinia 999.0
Kartagener's syndrome or triad (sinusitis,
    bronchiectasis, situs inversus) 759.3
Kasabach-Merritt syndrome (capillary
    hemangioma associated with
    thrombocytopenic purpura) 287.39
Kaschin-Beck disease (endemic
    polyarthritis)—see Disease, Kaschin-Beck
Kast's syndrome (dyschondroplasia with
    hemangiomas) 756.4
Katatonia (see also Schizophrenia) 295.2
Katayama disease or fever 120.2
Kathisophobia 781.0
Kawasaki disease 446.1

Kayser-Fleischer ring (cornea) (pseudosclerosis)
    275.1 [371.14]
Kaznelson's syndrome (congenital hypoplastic
    anemia) 284.01
Kearns-Sayre syndrome 277.87
Kedani fever 081.2
Kelis 701.4
Kelly (-Patterson) syndrome (sideropenic
    dysphagia) 280.8
Keloid, cheloid 701.4
  Addison's (morphea) 701.0
  cornea 371.00
  Hawkins' 701.4
  scar 701.4
Keloma 701.4
Kenya fever 082.1
Keratectasia 371.71
  congenital 743.41
Keratinization NEC
  alveolar ridge mucosa
    excessive 528.72
    minimal 528.71
Keratitis (nodular) (nonulcerative) (simple)
    (zonular) NEC 370.9
  with ulceration (see also Ulcer, cornea) 370.00
  actinic 370.24
  arborescens 054.42
  areolar 370.22
  bullosa 370.8
  deep—see Keratitis, interstitial
  dendritic(a) 054.42
  desiccation 370.34
  diffuse interstitial 370.52
  disciform(is) 054.43
    varicella 052.7 [370.44]
  epithelialis vernalis 372.13 [370.32]
  exposure 370.34
  filamentary 370.23
  gonococcal (congenital) (prenatal) 098.43
  herpes, herpetic (simplex) NEC 054.43
    zoster 053.21
  hypopyon 370.04
  in
    chickenpox 052.7 [370.44]
    exanthema (see also Exanthem) 057.9
        [370.44]
    paravaccinia (see also Paravaccinia) 051.9
        [370.44]
    smallpox (see also Smallpox) 050.9 [370.44]
    vernal conjunctivitis 372.13 [370.32]
  interstitial (nonsyphilitic) 370.50
    with ulcer (see also Ulcer, cornea) 370.00
    diffuse 370.52
    herpes, herpetic (simplex) 054.43
      zoster 053.21
    syphilitic (congenital) (hereditary) 090.3
    tuberculous (see also Tuberculosis) 017.3
        [370.59]
  lagophthalmic 370.34
  macular 370.22
  neuroparalytic 370.35
  neurotrophic 370.35
  nummular 370.22
  oyster-shuckers' 370.8
  parenchymatous—see Keratitis, interstitial
  petrificans 370.8
  phlyctenular 370.31

Keratitis—*continued*
postmeasles 055.71
punctata, punctate 370.21
leprosa 030.0 *[370.21]*
profunda 090.3
superficial (Thygeson's) 370.21
purulent 370.8
pustuliformis profunda 090.3
rosacea 695.3 *[370.49]*
sclerosing 370.54
specified type NEC 370.8
stellate 370.22
striate 370.22
superficial 370.20
with conjunctivitis (*see also*
Keratoconjunctivitis) 370.40
punctate (Thygeson's) 370.21
suppurative 370.8
syphilitic (congenital) (prenatal) 090.3
trachomatous 076.1
late effect 139.1
tuberculous (phlyctenular) (*see also*
Tuberculosis) 017.3 *[370.31]*
ulcerated (*see also* Ulcer, cornea) 370.00
vesicular 370.8
welders' 370.24
xerotic (*see also* Keratomalacia) 371.45
vitamin A deficiency 264.4
Keratoacanthoma 238.2
Keratocele 371.72
Keratoconjunctivitis (*see also* Keratitis) 370.40
adenovirus type 8 077.1
epidemic 077.1
exposure 370.34
gonococcal 098.43
herpetic (simplex) 054.43
zoster 053.21
in
chickenpox 052.7 *[370.44]*
exanthema (*see also* Exanthem) 057.9
[370.44]
paravaccinia (*see also* Paravaccinia) 051.9
[370.44]
smallpox (*see also* Smallpox) 050.9 *[370.44]*
infectious 077.1
neurotrophic 370.35
phlyctenular 370.31
postmeasles 055.71
shipyard 077.1
sicca (Sjögren's syndrome) 710.2
not in Sjögren's syndrome 370.33
specified type NEC 370.49
tuberculous (phlyctenular) (*see also*
Tuberculosis) 017.3 *[370.31]*
Keratoconus 371.60
acute hydrops 371.62
congenital 743.41
stable 371.61
Keratocyst (dental) 526.0
Keratoderma, keratodermia (congenital)
(palmaris et plantaris) (symmetrical) 757.39
acquired 701.1
blennorrhagica 701.1
gonococcal 098.81
climacterium 701.1
eccentrica 757.39
gonorrheal 098.81
punctata 701.1
tylodes, progressive 701.1
Keratodermatocele 371.72

Keratoglobus 371.70
congenital 743.41
associated with buphthalmos 743.22
Keratohemia 371.12
Keratoiritis (*see also* Iridocyclitis) 364.3
syphilitic 090.3
tuberculous (*see also* Tuberculosis) 017.3
[364.11]
Keratolysis exfoliativa (congenital) 757.39
acquired 695.89
neonatorum 757.39
Keratoma 701.1
congenital 757.39
malignum congenitale 757.1
palmaris et plantaris hereditarium 757.39
senile 702.0
Keratomalacia 371.45
vitamin A deficiency 264.4
Keratomegaly 743.41
Keratomycosis 111.1
nigricans (palmaris) 111.1
Keratopathy 371.40
band (*see also* Keratitis) 371.43
bullous (*see also* Keratitis) 371.23
degenerative (*see also* Degeneration, cornea)
371.40
hereditary (*see also* Dystrophy, cornea) 371.50
discrete colliquative 371.49
Keratoscleritis, tuberculous (*see also*
Tuberculosis) 017.3 *[370.31]*
Keratosis 701.1
actinic 702.0
arsenical 692.4
blennorrhagica 701.1
gonococcal 098.81
congenital (any type) 757.39
ear (middle) (*see also* Cholesteatoma) 385.30
female genital (external) 629.89
follicular, vitamin A deficiency 264.8
follicularis 757.39
acquired 701.1
congenital (acneiformis) (Siemens') 757.39
spinulosa (decalvans) 757.39
vitamin A deficiency 264.8
gonococcal 098.81
larynx, laryngeal 478.79
male genital (external) 608.89
middle ear (*see also* Cholesteatoma) 385.30
nigricans 701.2
congenital 757.39
obturans 380.21
oral epithelium
residual ridge mucosa
excessive 528.72
minimal 528.71
palmaris et plantaris (symmetrical) 757.39
penile 607.89
pharyngeus 478.29
pilaris 757.39
acquired 701.1
punctata (palmaris et plantaris) 701.1
scrotal 608.89
seborrheic 702.19
inflamed 702.11
senilis 702.0
solar 702.0
suprafollicularis 757.39
tonsillaris 478.29
vagina 623.1
vegetans 757.39
vitamin A deficiency 264.8
Kerato-uveitis (*see also* Iridocyclitis) 364.3

Keraunoparalysis 994.0
Kerion (celsi) 110.0
Kernicterus of newborn (not due to
  isoimmunization) 774.7
  due to isoimmunization (conditions classifiable
    to 773.0-773.2) 773.4
Ketoacidosis 276.2
  diabetic 250.1
  due to secondary diabetes 249.1
Ketonuria 791.6
  branched-chain, intermittent 270.3
Ketosis 276.2
  diabetic 250.1
  due to secondary diabetes 249.1
Kidney —*see* condition
Kienböck's
  disease 732.3
  adult 732.8
  osteochondrosis 732.3
Kimmelstiel (-Wilson) disease or syndrome
  (intercapillary glomerulosclerosis) 250.4
  [581.81]
  due to secondary diabetes 249.4 *[581.81]*
Kink, kinking
  appendix 543.9
  artery 447.1
  cystic duct, congenital 751.61
  hair (acquired) 704.2
  ileum or intestine (*see also* Obstruction,
    intestine) 560.9
  Lane's (*see also* Obstruction, intestine) 560.9
  organ or site, congenital NEC—*see* Anomaly,
    specified type NEC, by site
  ureter (pelvic junction) 593.3
    congenital 753.20
  vein(s) 459.2
    caval 459.2
    peripheral 459.2
Kinnier Wilson's disease (hepatolenticular
  degeneration) 275.1
Kissing
  osteophytes 721.5
  spine 721.5
  vertebra 721.5
Klauder's syndrome (erythema multiforme
  exudativum) 695.19
Kleb's disease (*see also* Nephritis) 583.9
Klein-Waardenburg syndrome
  (ptosisepicanthus) 270.2
Kleine-Levin syndrome 327.13
Kleptomania 312.32
Klinefelter's syndrome 758.7
Klinger's disease 446.4
Klippel's disease 723.8
Klippel-Feil disease or syndrome (brevicollis)
  756.16
Klippel-Trenaunay syndrome 759.89
Klumpke (-Déjérine) palsy, paralysis (birth)
  (newborn) 767.6
Klüver-Bucy (-Terzian) syndrome 310.0
Knee —*see* condition
Knifegrinders' rot (*see also* Tuberculosis) 011.4
Knock-knee (acquired) 736.41
  congenital 755.64
Knot
  intestinal, syndrome (volvulus) 560.2
  umbilical cord (true) 663.2
    affecting fetus or newborn 762.5
Knots, surfer 919.8
  infected 919.9

Knotting (of)
  hair 704.2
  intestine 560.2
Knuckle pads (Garrod's) 728.79
Köbner's disease (epidermolysis bullosa) 757.39
Koch's
  infection (*see also* Tuberculosis, pulmonary)
    011.9
  relapsing fever 087.9
Koch-Weeks conjunctivitis 372.03
Koenig-Wichman disease (pemphigus) 694.4
Köhler's disease (osteochondrosis) 732.5
  first (osteochondrosis juvenilis) 732.5
  second (Freiburg's infarction, metatarsal head)
    732.5
  patellar 732.4
  tarsal navicular (bone) (osteoarthosis juvenilis)
    732.5
Köhler-Mouchet disease (osteoarthrosis
  juvenilis) 732.5
Köhler-Pellegrini-Stieda disease or syndrome
  (calcification, knee joint) 726.62
Koilonychia 703.8
  congenital 757.5
Kojevnikov's, Kojewnikoff's epilepsy (*see also*
  Epilepsy) 345.7
König's
  disease (osteochondritis dissecans) 732.7
  syndrome 564.89
Koniophthisis (*see also* Tuberculosis) 011.4
Koplik's spots 055.9
Kopp's asthma 254.8
Korean hemorrhagic fever 078.6
Korsakoff (-Wernicke) disease, psychosis, or
  syndrome (nonalcoholic) 294.0
  alcoholic 291.1
Korsakov's disease —*see* Korsakoff's disease
Korsakow's disease —*see* Korsakoff's disease
Kostmann's disease or syndrome (infantile
  genetic agranulocytosis) 288.01
Krabbe's
  disease (leukodystrophy) 330.0
  syndrome
    congenital muscle hypoplasia 756.89
    cutaneocerebral angioma 759.6
Kraepelin-Morel disease (*see also*
  Schizophrenia) 295.9
Kraft-Weber-Dimitri disease 759.6
Kraurosis
  ani 569.49
  penis 607.0
  vagina 623.8
  vulva 624.09
Kreotoxism 005.9
Krukenberg's
  spindle 371.13
  tumor (M8490/6) 198.6
Kufs' disease 330.1
Kugelberg-Welander disease 335.11
Kuhnt-Junius degeneration or disease 362.52
Kulchitsky's cell carcinoma (carcinoid tumor of
  intestine) 259.2
Kümmell's disease or spondylitis 721.7
Kundrat's disease (lymphosarcoma) 200.1
Kunekune —*see* Dermatophytosis
Kunkel syndrome (lupoid hepatitis) 571.49
Kupffer cell sarcoma (M9124/3) 155.0
Kuru 046.0

Kussmaul's
 coma (diabetic) 250.3
  due to secondary diabetes 249.3
 disease (polyarteritis nodosa) 446.0
 respiration (air hunger) 786.09
Kwashiorkor (marasmus type) 260
Kyasanur Forest disease 065.2
Kyphoscoliosis, kyphoscoliotic (acquired) (*see
   also* Scoliosis) 737.30
 congenital 756.19
 due to radiation 737.33
 heart (disease) 416.1
 idiopathic 737.30
  infantile
    progressive 737.32
    resolving 737.31
 late effect of rickets 268.1 *[737.43]*
 specified NEC 737.39
 thoracogenic 737.34
 tuberculous (*see also* Tuberculosis) 015.0
   [737.43]
Kyphosis, kyphotic (acquired) (postural) 737.10
 adolescent postural 737.0
 congenital 756.19
 dorsalis juvenilis 732.0
 due to or associated with
   Charcot-Marie-Tooth disease 356.1 *[737.41]*
   mucopolysaccharidosis 277.5 *[737.41]*
   neurofibromatosis 237.71 *[737.41]*
   osteitis
     deformans 731.0 *[737.41]*
     fibrosa cystica 252.01 *[737.41]*
   osteoporosis (*see also* Osteoporosis) 733.0
     [737.41]
   poliomyelitis (*see also* Poliomyelitis) 138
     [737.41]
   radiation 737.11
   tuberculosis (*see also* Tuberculosis) 015.0
     [737.41]
 Kümmell's 721.7
 late effect of rickets 268.1 *[737.41]*
 Morquio-Brailsford type (spinal) 277.5 *[737.41]*
 pelvis 738.6
 postlaminectomy 737.12
 specified cause NEC 737.19
 syphilitic, congenital 090.5 *[737.41]*
 tuberculous (*see also* Tuberculosis) 015.0
   [737.41]
Kyrle's disease (hyperkeratosis follicularis in
   cutem penetrans) 701.1

L

Labia, labium —*see* condition
Labiated hymen 752.49
Labile
  blood pressure 796.2
  emotions, emotionality 301.3
  vasomotor system 443.9
Lability, emotional 799.24
Labioglossal paralysis 335.22
Labium leporinum (*see also* Cleft, lip) 749.10
Labor (*see also* Delivery)
  with complications—*see* Delivery, complicated
  abnormal NEC 661.9
    affecting fetus or newborn 763.7
  arrested active phase 661.1
    affecting fetus or newborn 763.7
  desultory 661.2
    affecting fetus or newborn 763.7
  dyscoordinate 661.4
    affecting fetus or newborn 763.7
  early onset (22-36 weeks gestation) 644.2
  failed
    induction 659.1
      mechanical 659.0
      medical 659.1
      surgical 659.0
    trial (vaginal delivery) 660.6
  false 644.1
  forced or induced, affecting fetus or newborn
    763.89
  hypertonic 661.4
    affecting fetus or newborn 763.7
  hypotonic 661.2
    affecting fetus or newborn 763.7
    primary 661.0
      affecting fetus or newborn 763.7
    secondary 661.1
      affecting fetus or newborn 763.7
  incoordinate 661.4
    affecting fetus or newborn 763.7
  irregular 661.2
    affecting fetus or newborn 763.7
  long—*see* Labor, prolonged
  missed (at or near term) 656.4
  obstructed NEC 660.9
    affecting fetus or newborn 763.1
    due to female genital mutilation 660.8
    specified cause NEC 660.8
      affecting fetus or newborn 763.1
  pains, spurious 644.1
  precipitate 661.3
    affecting fetus or newborn 763.6
  premature 644.2
    threatened 644.0
  prolonged or protracted 662.1
    affecting fetus or newborn 763.89
    first stage 662.0
      affecting fetus or newborn 763.89
    second stage 662.2
      affecting fetus or newborn 763.89
  threatened NEC 644.1
  undelivered 644.1
Labored breathing (*see also* Hyperventilation)
  786.09

Labyrinthitis (inner ear) (destructive) (latent)
    386.30
  circumscribed 386.32
  diffuse 386.31
  focal 386.32
  purulent 386.33
  serous 386.31
  suppurative 386.33
  syphilitic 095.8
  toxic 386.34
  viral 386.35
Laceration —*see also* Wound, open, by site
  accidental, complicating surgery 998.2
  Achilles tendon 845.09
    with open wound 892.2
  anus (sphincter) 879.6
    with
      abortion—*see* Abortion, by type, with
        damage to pelvic organs
      ectopic pregnancy (*see also* categories
        633.0-633.9) 639.2
      molar pregnancy (*see also* categories
        630-632) 639.2
    complicated 879.7
    complicating delivery (healed) (old) 654.8
      with laceration of anal or rectal mucosa
        664.3
      not associated with third-degree perineal
        laceration 664.6
    following
      abortion 639.2
      ectopic or molar pregnancy 639.2
    nontraumatic, nonpuerperal (healed) (old)
      569.43
  bladder (urinary)
    with
      abortion—*see* Abortion, by type, with
        damage to pelvic organs
      ectopic pregnancy (*see also* categories
        633.0-633.9) 639.2
      molar pregnancy (*see also* categories
        630-632) 639.2
    following
      abortion 639.2
      ectopic or molar pregnancy 639.2
    obstetrical trauma 665.5
  blood vessel—*see* Injury, blood vessel, by site
  bowel
    with
      abortion—*see* Abortion, by type, with
        damage to pelvic organs
      ectopic pregnancy (*see also* categories
        633.0-633.9) 639.2
      molar pregnancy (*see also* categories
        630-632) 639.2
    following
      abortion 639.2
      ectopic or molar pregnancy 639.2
    obstetrical trauma 665.5
  brain (with hemorrhage) (cerebral) (membrane)
    851.8

Laceration—*continued*

> *Note—Use the following fifth-digit*
> *subclassification with categories 851-854:*
>
> 0 *unspecified state of consciousness*
> 1 *with no loss of consciousness*
> 2 *with brief [less than one hour] loss of*
>   *consciousness*
> 3 *with moderate [1-24 hours] loss of*
>   *consciousness*
> 4 *with prolonged [more than 24 hours] loss of*
>   *consciousness and return to pre-existing*
>   *conscious level*
> 5 *with prolonged [more than 24 hours] loss of*
>   *consciousness, without return to pre-existing*
>   *conscious level*
> *Use fifth-digit 5 to designate when a patient is*
> *unconscious and dies before regaining*
> *consciousness, regardless of the duration of the*
> *loss of consciousness*
> 6 *with loss of consciousness of unspecified*
>   *duration*
> 9 *with concussion, unspecified*

with
   open intracranial wound 851.9
   skull fracture—*see* Fracture, skull, by site
cerebellum 851.6
   with open intracranial wound 851.7
cortex 851.2
   with open intracranial wound 851.3
   during birth 767.0
stem 851.6
   with open intracranial wound 851.7
broad ligament
   with
      abortion—*see* Abortion, by type, with
         damage to pelvic organs
      ectopic pregnancy (*see also* categories
         633.0-633.9) 639.2
      molar pregnancy (*see also* categories
         630-632) 639.2
   following
      abortion 639.2
      ectopic or molar pregnancy 639.2
   nontraumatic 620.6
   obstetrical trauma 665.6
   syndrome (nontraumatic) 620.6
capsule, joint—*see* Sprain, by site
cardiac—*see* Laceration, heart
causing eversion of cervix uteri (old) 622.0
central, complicating delivery 664.4
cerebellum—*see* Laceration, brain, cerebellum
cerebral—*see also* Laceration, brain
   during birth 767.0
cervix (uteri)
   with
      abortion—*see* Abortion, by type, with
         damage to pelvic organs
      ectopic pregnancy (*see also* categories
         633.0-633.9) 639.2
      molar pregnancy (*see also* categories
         630-632) 639.2
   following
      abortion 639.2
      ectopic or molar pregnancy 639.2
   nonpuerperal, nontraumatic 622.3
   obstetrical trauma (current) 665.3
   old (postpartal) 622.3
   traumatic—*see* Injury, internal, cervix
chordae heart 429.5

Laceration—*continued*
complicated 879.9
cornea—*see* Laceration, eyeball
   superficial 918.1
cortex (cerebral)—*see* Laceration, brain, cortex
esophagus 530.89
eye(s)—*see* Laceration, ocular
eyeball NEC 871.4
   with prolapse or exposure of intraocular tissue
      871.1
   penetrating—*see* Penetrating wound, eyeball
   specified as without prolapse of intraocular
      tissue 871.0
eyelid NEC 870.8
   full thickness 870.1
      involving lacrimal passages 870.2
   skin (and periocular area) 870.0
   penetrating—*see* Penetrating wound, orbit
fourchette
   with
      abortion—*see* Abortion, by type, with
         damage to pelvic organs
      ectopic pregnancy (*see also* categories
         633.0-633.9) 639.2
      molar pregnancy (*see also* categories
         630-632) 639.2
   complicating delivery 664.0
   following
      abortion 639.2
      ectopic or molar pregnancy 639.2
heart (without penetration of heart chambers)
   861.02
   with
      open wound into thorax 861.12
      penetration of heart chambers 861.03
         with open wound into thorax 861.13
hernial sac—*see* Hernia, by site
internal organ (abdomen) (chest) (pelvis)
   NEC—*see* Injury, internal, by site
kidney (parenchyma) 866.02
   with
      complete disruption of parenchyma (rupture)
         866.03
         with open wound into cavity 866.13
      open wound into cavity 866.12
labia
   complicating delivery 664.0
ligament—*see also* Sprain, by site
   with open wound—*see* Wound, open, by site
liver 864.05
   with open wound into cavity 864.15
   major (disruption of hepatic parenchyma)
      864.04
      with open wound into cavity 864.14
   minor (capsule only) 864.02
      with open wound into cavity 864.12
   moderate (involving parenchyma without
      major disruption) 864.03
      with open wound into cavity 864.13
   multiple 864.04
      with open wound into cavity 864.14
   stellate 864.04
      with open wound into cavity 864.14
lung 861.22
   with open wound into thorax 861.32
meninges—*see* Laceration, brain
meniscus (knee) (*see also* Tear, meniscus) 836.2
   old 717.5
   site other than knee—*see also* Sprain, by site
      old NEC (*see also* Disorder, cartilage,
         articular) 718.0

Laceration—*continued*
  muscle—*see also* Sprain, by site
    with open wound—*see* Wound, open, by site
  myocardium—*see* Laceration, heart
  nerve—*see* Injury, nerve, by site
  ocular NEC (*see also* Laceration, eyeball) 871.4
    adnexa NEC 870.8
      penetrating 870.3
        with foreign body 870.4
  orbit (eye) 870.8
    penetrating 870.3
      with foreign body 870.4
  pelvic
    floor (muscles)
      with
        abortion—*see* Abortion, by type, with
          damage to pelvic organs
        ectopic pregnancy (*see also* categories
          633.0-633.9) 639.2
        molar pregnancy (*see also* categories
          630-632) 639.2
      complicating delivery 664.1
      following
        abortion 639.2
        ectopic or molar pregnancy 639.2
      nonpuerperal 618.7
      old (postpartal) 618.7
    organ NEC
      with
        abortion—*see* Abortion, by type, with
          damage to pelvic organs
        ectopic pregnancy (*see also* categories
          633.0-633.9) 639.2
        molar pregnancy (*see also* categories
          630-632) 639.2
      complicating delivery 665.5
        affecting fetus or newborn 763.89
      following
        abortion 639.2
        ectopic or molar pregnancy 639.2
      obstetrical trauma 665.5
  perineum, perineal (old) (postpartal) 618.7
    with
      abortion—*see* Abortion, by type, with
        damage to pelvic floor
      ectopic pregnancy (*see also* categories
        633.0-633.9) 639.2
      molar pregnancy (*see also* categories
        630-632) 639.2
    complicating delivery 664.4
      first degree 664.0
      second degree 664.1
      third degree 664.2
      fourth degree 664.3
      central 664.4
      involving
        anal sphincter (healed) (old) 654.8
          not associated with third-degree perineal
            laceration 664.6
        fourchette 664.0
        hymen 664.0
        labia 664.0
        pelvic floor 664.1
        perineal muscles 664.1
        rectovaginal septum 664.2
          with anal mucosa 664.3
        skin 664.0
        sphincter (anal) (healed) (old) 654.8
          not associated with third-degree perineal
            laceration 664.6
          with anal mucosa 664.3

Laceration—*continued*
    vagina 664.0
    vaginal muscles 664.1
    vulva 664.0
    secondary 674.2
    following
      abortion 639.2
      ectopic or molar pregnancy 639.2
    male 879.6
      complicated 879.7
    muscles, complicating delivery 664.1
    nonpuerperal, current injury 879.6
      complicated 879.7
    secondary (postpartal) 674.2
  peritoneum
    with
      abortion—*see* Abortion, by type, with
        damage to pelvic organs
      ectopic pregnancy (*see also* categories
        633.0-633.9) 639.2
      molar pregnancy (*see also* categories
        630-632) 639.2
    following
      abortion 639.2
      ectopic or molar pregnancy 639.2
    obstetrical trauma 665.5
  periurethral tissue
    with
      abortion—*see* Abortion, by type, with
        damage to pelvic organs
      ectopic pregnancy (*see also* categories
        633.0-633.9) 639.2
      molar pregnancy (*see also* categories
        630-632) 639.2
    following
      abortion 639.2
      ectopic or molar pregnancy 639.2
    obstetrical trauma 664.8
  rectovaginal (septum)
    with
      abortion—*see* Abortion, by type, with
        damage to pelvic organs
      ectopic pregnancy (*see also* categories
        633.0-633.9) 639.2
      molar pregnancy (*see also* categories
        630-632) 639.2
    complicating delivery 665.4
      with perineum 664.2
        involving anal or rectal mucosa 664.3
    following
      abortion 639.2
      ectopic or molar pregnancy 639.2
    nonpuerperal 623.4
    old (postpartal) 623.4
  spinal cord (meninges)—*see also* Injury, spinal,
    by site
    due to injury at birth 767.4
    fetus or newborn 767.4
  spleen 865.09
    with
      disruption of parenchyma (massive) 865.04
        with open wound into cavity 865.14
      open wound into cavity 865.19
    capsule (without disruption of parenchyma)
      865.02
      with open wound into cavity 865.12
    parenchyma 865.03
      with open wound into cavity 865.13
      massive disruption (rupture) 865.04
        with open wound into cavity 865.14

Laceration—*continued*
tendon 848.9
with open wound–*see* Wound, open, by site
Achilles 845.09
with open wound 892.2
lower limb NEC 844.9
with open wound NEC 894.2
upper limb NEC 840.9
with open wound NEC 884.2
tentorium cerebelli—*see* Laceration, brain,
cerebellum
tongue 873.64
complicated 873.74
urethra
with
abortion—*see* Abortion, by type, with
damage to pelvic organs
ectopic pregnancy (*see also* categories
633.0- 633.9) 639.2
molar pregnancy (*see also* categories
630-632) 639.2
following
abortion 639.2
ectopic or molar pregnancy 639.2
nonpuerperal, nontraumatic 599.84
obstetrical trauma 665.5
uterus
with
abortion—*see* Abortion, by type, with
damage to pelvic organs
ectopic pregnancy (*see also* categories
633.0-633.9) 639.2
molar pregnancy (*see also* categories
630-632) 639.2
following
abortion 639.2
ectopic or molar pregnancy 639.2
nonpuerperal, nontraumatic 621.8
obstetrical trauma NEC 665.5
old (postpartal) 621.8
vagina
with
abortion—*see* Abortion, by type, with
damage to pelvic organs
ectopic pregnancy (*see also* categories
633.0-633.9) 639.2
molar pregnancy (*see also* categories
630-632) 639.2
perineal involvement, complicating delivery
664.0
complicating delivery 665.4
first degree 664.0
second degree 664.1
third degree 664.2
fourth degree 664.3
high 665.4
muscles 664.1
sulcus 665.4
wall 665.4
following
abortion 639.2
ectopic or molar pregnancy 639.2
nonpuerperal, nontraumatic 623.4
old (postpartal) 623.4
valve, heart—*see* Endocarditis
vulva
with
abortion—*see* Abortion, by type, with
damage to pelvic organs
ectopic pregnancy (*see also* categories
633.0-633.9) 639.2

Laceration—*continued*
molar pregnancy (*see also* categories
630-632) 639.2
complicating delivery 664.0
following
abortion 639.2
ectopic or molar pregnancy 639.2
nonpuerperal, nontraumatic 624.4
old (postpartal) 624.4
Lachrymal —*see* condition
Lachrymonasal duct —*see* condition
Lack of
adequate intermaxillary vertical dimension 524.36
appetite (*see also* Anorexia) 783.0
care
in home V60.4
of adult 995.84
of infant (at or after birth) 995.52
coordination 781.3
development—*see also* Hypoplasia
physiological in childhood 783.40
education V62.3
energy 780.79
financial resources V60.2
food 994.2
in environment V60.89
growth in childhood 783.43
heating V60.1
housing (permanent) (temporary) V60.0
adequate V60.1
material resources V60.2
medical attention 799.89
memory (*see also* Amnesia) 780.93
mild, following organic brain damage 310.89
ovulation 628.0
person able to render necessary care V60.4
physical exercise V69.0
physiologic development in childhood 783.40
posterior occlusal support 524.57
prenatal care in current pregnancy V23.7
shelter V60.0
sleep V69.4
water 994.3
Lacrimal —*see* condition
Lacrimation, abnormal (*see also* Epiphora) 375.20
Lacrimonasal duct —*see* condition
Lactation, lactating (breast) (puerperal)
(postpartum)
defective 676.4
disorder 676.9
specified type NEC 676.8
excessive 676.6
failed 676.4
mastitis NEC 675.2
mother (care and/or examination) V24.1
nonpuerperal 611.6
suppressed 676.5
Lacticemia 271.3
excessive 276.2
Lactosuria 271.3
Lacunar skull 756.0
Laennec's cirrhosis (alcoholic) 571.2
nonalcoholic 571.5
Lafora's disease 333.2
Lag, lid (nervous) 374.41
Lagleyze-von Hippel disease (retinocerebral
angiomatosis) 759.6

Lagophthalmos (eyelid) (nervous) 374.20
  cicatricial 374.23
  keratitis (*see also* Keratitis) 370.34
  mechanical 374.22
  paralytic 374.21
La grippe *—see* Influenza
Lahore sore 085.1
Lakes, venous (cerebral) 437.8
Laki-Lorand factor deficiency (*see also* Defect,
  coagulation) 286.3
Lalling 307.9
Lambliasis 007.1
Lame back 724.5
Lancereaux's diabetes (diabetes mellitus with
  marked emaciation) 250.8 *[261]*
  due to secondary diabetes 249.8 *[261]*
Landau-Kleffner syndrome 345.8
Landouzy-Déjérine dystrophy
  (fascioscapulohumeral atrophy) 359.1
Landry's disease or paralysis 357.0
Landry-Guillain-Barré syndrome 357.0
Lane's
  band 751.4
  disease 569.89
  kink (*see also* Obstruction, intestine) 560.9
Langdon Down's syndrome (mongolism) 758.0
Language abolition 784.69
Lanugo (persistent) 757.4
Laparoscopic surgical procedure converted to
  open procedure V64.41
Lardaceous
  degeneration (any site) 277.39
  disease 277.39
  kidney 277.39 *[583.81]*
  liver 277.39
Large
  baby (regardless of gestational age) 766.1
    exceptionally (weight of 4500 grams or more)
      766.0
    of diabetic mother 775.0
  ear 744.22
  fetus—*see also* Oversize, fetus
    causing disproportion 653.5
      with obstructed labor 660.1
  for dates
    fetus or newborn (regardless of gestational
      age) 766.1
      affecting management of pregnancy 656.6
      exceptionally (weight of 4500 grams or
        more) 766.0
  physiological cup 743.57
  stature 783.9
  waxy liver 277.39
  white kidney—*see* Nephrosis
Larsen's syndrome (flattened facies and multiple
  congenital dislocations) 755.8
Larsen-Johansson disease (juvenile osteopathia
  patellae) 732.4
Larva migrans
  cutaneous NEC 126.9
    ancylostoma 126.9
  of Diptera in vitreous 128.0
  visceral NEC 128.0
Laryngeal *—see also* condition
  syncope 786.2
Laryngismus (acute) (infectious) (stridulous)
  478.75
  congenital 748.3
  diphtheritic 032.3

Laryngitis (acute) (edematous) (fibrinous)
  (gangrenous) (infective) (infiltrative)
  (malignant) (membranous) (phlegmonous)
  (pneumococcal) (pseudomembranous) (septic)
  (subglottic) (suppurative) (ulcerative) (viral)
  464.00
  with
    influenza, flu, or grippe (*see also* Influenza)
      487.1
    obstruction 464.01
    tracheitis (*see also* Laryngotracheitis) 464.20
      with obstruction 464.21
      acute 464.20
        with obstruction 464.21
      chronic 476.1
  atrophic 476.0
  Borrelia vincentii 101
  catarrhal 476.0
  chronic 476.0
    with tracheitis (chronic) 476.1
    due to external agent—*see* Condition,
      respiratory, chronic, due to
  diphtheritic (membranous) 032.3
  due to external agent—*see* Inflammation,
    respiratory, upper, due to
  H. influenzae 464.00
    with obstruction 464.01
  Hemophilus influenzae 464.00
    with obstruction 464.01
  hypertrophic 476.0
  influenzal (*see also* Influenza) 487.1
  pachydermic 478.79
  sicca 476.0
  spasmodic 478.75
    acute 464.00
      with obstruction 464.01
  streptococcal 034.0
  stridulous 478.75
  syphilitic 095.8
    congenital 090.5
  tuberculous (*see also* Tuberculosis, larynx)
    012.3
  Vincent's 101
Laryngocele (congenital) (ventricular) 748.3
Laryngofissure 478.79
  congenital 748.3
Laryngomalacia (congenital) 748.3
Laryngopharyngitis (acute) 465.0
  chronic 478.9
  due to external agent—*see* Condition,
    respiratory, chronic, due to
  due to external agent—*see* Inflammation,
    respiratory, upper, due to
  septic 034.0
Laryngoplegia (*see also* Paralysis, vocal cord)
  478.30
Laryngoptosis 478.79
Laryngospasm 478.75
  due to external agent—*see* Condition,
    respiratory, acute, due to
Laryngostenosis 478.74
  congenital 748.3
Laryngotracheitis (acute) (infectional) (viral)
  (*see also* Laryngitis) 464.20
  with obstruction 464.21
  atrophic 476.1
  Borrelia vincentii 101
  catarrhal 476.1
  chronic 476.1
    due to external agent—*see* Condition,
      respiratory, chronic, due to

Laryngotracheitis—*continued*
  diphtheritic (membranous) 032.3
  due to external agent—*see* Inflammation,
    respiratory, upper, due to
  H. influenzae 464.20
    with obstruction 464.21
  hypertrophic 476.1
  influenzal (*see also* Influenza) 487.1
  pachydermic 478.75
  sicca 476.1
  spasmodic 478.75
    acute 464.20
      with obstruction 464.21
  streptococcal 034.0
  stridulous 478.75
  syphilitic 095.8
    congenital 090.5
  tuberculous (*see also* Tuberculosis, larynx)
    012.3
  Vincent's 101
Laryngotracheobronchitis (*see also* Bronchitis)
  490
  acute 466.0
  chronic 491.8
  viral 466.0
Laryngotracheobronchopneumonitis —*see*
  Pneumonia, broncho-
Larynx, laryngeal —*see* condition
Lasègue's disease (persecution mania) 297.9
Lassa fever 078.89
Lassitude (*see also* Weakness) 780.79
Late —*see also* condition
  infant
    post-term (gestation period over 40
      completed weeks to 42 completed
      weeks) 766.21
    prolonged gestation (period over 42
      completed weeks) 766.22
Late effect(s) (of) —*see also* condition
  abscess
    intracranial or intraspinal (conditions
      classifiable to 324)–*see* category 326
  adverse effect of drug, medicinal or biological
    substance 909.5
  allergic reaction 909.9
  amputation
    postoperative (late) 997.60
    traumatic (injury classifiable to 885-887 and
      895-897) 905.9
  burn (injury classifiable to 948-949) 906.9
    extremities NEC (injury classifiable to 943 or
      945) 906.7
      hand or wrist (injury classifiable to 944)
        906.6
    eye (injury classifiable to 940) 906.5
    face, head, and neck (injury classifiable to
      941) 906.5
    specified site NEC (injury classifiable to 942
      and 946-947) 906.8
  cerebrovascular disease (conditions classifiable
    to 430-437) 438.9
    with
      alterations of sensations 438.6
      aphasia 438.11
      apraxia 438.81
      ataxia 438.84
      cognitive deficits 438.0
      disturbances of vision 438.7
      dysarthria 438.13
      dysphagia 438.82
      dysphasia 438.12
      facial droop 438.83

Late effect(s) (of)—*continued*
  cerebrovascular disease—*continued*
    with—*continued*
      facial weakness 438.83
      fluency disorder 438.14
      hemiplegia/hemiparesis
        affecting
          dominant side 438.21
          nondominant side 438.22
          unspecified side 438.20
      monoplegia of lower limb
        affecting
          dominant side 438.41
          nondominant side 438.42
          unspecified side 438.40
      monoplegia of upper limb
        affecting
          dominant side 438.31
          nondominant side 438.32
          unspecified side 438.30
      paralytic syndrome NEC
        affecting
          bilateral 438.53
          dominant side 438.51
          nondominant side 438.52
          unspecified side 438.50
      speech and language deficit 438.10
        specified type NEC 438.19
      stuttering 438.14
      vertigo 438.85
    specified type NEC 438.89
  childbirth complication(s) 677
  complication(s) of
    childbirth 677
    delivery 677
    pregnancy 677
    puerperium 677
    surgical and medical care (conditions
      classifiable to 996-999) 909.3
    trauma (conditions classifiable to 958) 908.6
  contusion (injury classifiable to 920-924) 906.3
  crushing (injury classifiable to 925-929) 906.4
  delivery complication(s) 677
  dislocation (injury classifiable to 830-839) 905.6
  encephalitis or encephalomyelitis (conditions
    classifiable to 323)—*see* category 326
    in infectious diseases 139.8
      viral (conditions classifiable to 049.8, 049.9,
        062-064) 139.0
  external cause NEC (conditions classifiable to
    995) 909.9
    certain conditions classifiable to categories
      991-994 909.4
  foreign body in orifice (injury classifiable to
    930-939) 908.5
  fracture (multiple) (injury classifiable to
    828-829) 905.5
    extremity
      lower (injury classifiable to 821-827) 905.4
        neck of femur (injury classifiable to 820)
          905.3
      upper (injury classifiable to 810-819) 905.2
    face and skull (injury classifiable to 800-804)
      905.0
    skull and face (injury classifiable to 800-804)
      905.0
    spine and trunk (injury classifiable to 805 and
      807-809) 905.1
      with spinal cord lesion (injury classifiable to
        806) 907.2

Late effect(s) (of)—*continued*
infection
pyogenic, intracranial—*see* category 326
infectious diseases (conditions classifiable to
001-136) NEC 139.8
injury (injury classifiable to 959) 908.9
blood vessel 908.3
abdomen and pelvis (injury classifiable to
902) 908.4
extremity (injury classifiable to 903-904)
908.3
head and neck (injury classifiable to 900)
908.3
intracranial (injury classifiable to 850-854)
907.0
with skull fracture 905.0
thorax (injury classifiable to 901) 908.4
internal organ NEC (injury classifiable to 867
and 869) 908.2
abdomen (injury classifiable to 863-866 and
868) 908.1
thorax (injury classifiable to 860-862) 908.0
intracranial (injury classifiable to 850-854)
907.0
with skull fracture (injury classifiable to
800-801 and 803-804) 905.0
nerve NEC (injury classifiable to 957) 907.9
cranial (injury classifiable to 950-951) 907.1
peripheral NEC (injury classifiable to 957)
907.9
lower limb and pelvic girdle (injury
classifiable to 956) 907.5
upper limb and shoulder girdle (injury
classifiable to 955) 907.4
roots and plexus(es), spinal (injury
classifiable to 953) 907.3
trunk (injury classifiable to 954) 907.3
pregnancy complication(s) 677
puerperal complication(s) 677
spinal
cord (injury classifiable to 806 and 952)
907.2
nerve root(s) and plexus(es) (injury
classifiable to 953) 907.3
superficial (injury classifiable to 910-919)
906.2
tendon (tendon injury classifiable to 840-848,
880-884 with .2, and 890-894 with .2)
905.8
meningitis
bacterial (conditions classifiable to 320)—*see*
category 326
unspecified cause (conditions classifiable to
322)—*see* category 326
myelitis (*see also* Late, effect(s) (of),
encephalitis)—*see* category 326
parasitic diseases (conditions classifiable to
001-136 NEC) 139.8
phlebitis or thrombophlebitis of intracranial
venous sinuses (conditions classifiable to
325)—*see* category 326
poisoning due to drug, medicinal or biological
substance (conditions classifiable to
960-979) 909.0
poliomyelitis, acute (conditions classifiable to
045) 138
radiation (conditions classifiable to 990) 909.2
rickets 268.1
sprain and strain without mention of tendon
injury (injury classifiable to 840-848, except
tendon injury) 905.7
tendon involvement 905.8

Late effect(s) (of)—*continued*
toxic effect of
drug, medicinal or biological substance
(conditions classifiable to 960-979) 909.0
nonmedical substance (conditions classifiable
to 980-989) 909.1
trachoma (conditions classifiable to 076) 139.1
tuberculosis 137.0
bones and joints (conditions classifiable to
015) 137.3
central nervous system (conditions classifiable
to 013) 137.1
genitourinary (conditions classifiable to 016)
137.2
pulmonary (conditions classifiable to 010-012)
137.0
specified organs NEC (conditions classifiable
to 014, 017-018) 137.4
viral encephalitis (conditions classifiable to
049.8, 049.9, 062-064) 139.0
wound, open
extremity (injury classifiable to 880-884 and
890-894, except .2) 906.1
tendon (injury classifiable to 880-884 with
.2 and 890-894 with .2) 905.8
head, neck, and trunk (injury classifiable to
870-879) 906.0
Latent —*see* condition
Lateral —*see* condition
Laterocession —*see* Lateroversion
Lateroflexion —*see* Lateroversion
Lateroversion
cervix—*see* Lateroversion, uterus
uterus, uterine (cervix) (postinfectional)
(postpartal, old) 621.6
congenital 752.39
in pregnancy or childbirth 654.4
affecting fetus or newborn 763.89
Lathyrism 988.2
Launois' syndrome (pituitary gigantism) 253.0
Launois-Bensaude's lipomatosis 272.8
Launois-Cléret syndrome (adiposogenital
dystrophy) 253.8
Laurence-Moon-Biedl syndrome (obesity,
polydactyly, and intellectual disabilities)
759.89
LAV (disease) (illness) (infection)—*see* Human
immunodeficiency virus (disease) (illness)
(infection)
LAV/HTLV-III (disease) (illness)
(infection)—*see* Human immunodeficiency
virus (disease) (illness) (infection)
Lawford's syndrome (encephalocutaneous
angiomatosis) 759.6
Lax, laxity —*see also* Relaxation
ligament 728.4
skin (acquired) 701.8
congenital 756.83
Laxative habit (*see also* Abuse, drugs,
nondependent) 305.9
Lazy leukocyte syndrome 288.09
LCAD (long chain/very long chain acyl CoA
dehydrogenase deficiency, VLCAD) 277.85
LCHAD (long chain 3-hydroxyacyl CoA
dehydrogenase deficiency) 277.85
Lead —*see also* condition
exposure (suspected) to V15.86
incrustation of cornea 371.15
poisoning 984.9
specified type of lead—*see* Table of drugs and
chemicals

Lead miner's lung 503
Leakage
  amniotic fluid 658.1
    with delayed delivery 658.2
    affecting fetus or newborn 761.1
  bile from drainage tube (T tube) 997.49
  blood (microscopic), fetal, into maternal
    circulation 656.0
    affecting management of pregnancy or
      puerperium 656.0
  device, implant, or graft—*see* Complications,
    mechanical
  spinal fluid at lumbar puncture site 997.09
  urine, continuous 788.37
Leaky heart —*see* Endocarditis
Learning defect, specific NEC
  (strephosymbolia) 315.2
Leather bottle stomach (M8142/3) 151.9
Leber's
  congenital amaurosis 362.76
  optic atrophy (hereditary) 377.16
Lederer's anemia or disease (acquired
  infectious hemolytic anemia) 283.19
Lederer-Brill syndrome (acquired infectious
  hemolytic anemia) 283.19
Leeches (aquatic) (land) 134.2
Left-sided neglect 781.8
Leg —*see* condition
Legal investigation V62.5
Legg (-Calvé) -Perthes disease or syndrome
  (osteochondrosis, femoral capital) 732.1
Legionnaires' disease 482.84
Leigh's disease 330.8
Leiner's disease (exfoliative dermatitis) 695.89
Leiofibromyoma (M8890/0)—*see also*
  Leiomyoma
  uterus (cervix) (corpus) (*see also* Leiomyoma,
    uterus) 218.9
Leiomyoblastoma (M8891/1)—*see* Neoplasm,
  connective tissue, uncertain behavior
Leiomyofibroma (M8890/0)—*see also*
  Neoplasm, connective tissue, benign
  uterus (cervix) (corpus) (*see also* Leiomyoma,
    uterus) 218.9
Leiomyoma (M8890/0)—*see also* Neoplasm,
  connective tissue, benign
  bizarre (M8893/0)—*see* Neoplasm, connective
    tissue, benign
  cellular (M8892/1)—*see* Neoplasm, connective
    tissue, uncertain behavior
  epithelioid (M8891/1)—*see* Neoplasm,
    connective tissue, uncertain behavior
  prostate (polypoid) 600.20
    with
      other lower urinary tract symptoms (LUTS)
        600.21
      urinary
        obstruction 600.21
        retention 600.21
  uterus (cervix) (corpus) 218.9
    interstitial 218.1
    intramural 218.1
    submucous 218.0
    subperitoneal 218.2
    subserous 218.2
    vascular (M8894/0)—*see* Neoplasm,
      connective tissue, benign
Leiomyomatosis (intravascular) (M8890/1)—*see*
  Neoplasm, connective tissue, uncertain
  behavior

Leiomyosarcoma (M8890/3)—*see also*
  Neoplasm, connective tissue, malignant
  epithelioid (M8891/3)—*see* Neoplasm,
    connective tissue, malignant
Leishmaniasis 085.9
  American 085.5
    cutaneous 085.4
    mucocutaneous 085.5
  Asian desert 085.2
  Brazilian 085.5
  cutaneous 085.9
    acute necrotizing 085.2
    American 085.4
    Asian desert 085.2
    diffuse 085.3
    dry form 085.1
    Ethiopian 085.3
    eyelid 085.5 *[373.6]*
    late 085.1
    lepromatous 085.3
    recurrent 085.1
    rural 085.2
    ulcerating 085.1
    urban 085.1
    wet form 085.2
    zoonotic form 085.2
  dermal—*see also* Leishmaniasis, cutaneous
    post kala-azar 085.0
  eyelid 085.5 *[373.6]*
  infantile 085.0
  Mediterranean 085.0
  mucocutaneous (American) 085.5
  naso-oral 085.5
  nasopharyngeal 085.5
  Old World 085.1
  tegumentaria diffusa 085.4
  vaccination, prophylactic (against) V05.2
  visceral (Indian) 085.0
Leishmanoid, dermal —*see also* Leishmaniasis,
  cutaneous
  post kala-azar 085.0
Leloir's disease 695.4
Lemiere syndrome 451.89
Lenegre's disease 426.0
Lengthening, leg 736.81
Lennox-Gastaut syndrome 345.0
  with tonic seizures 345.1
Lennox's syndrome (*see also* Epilepsy) 345.0
Lens —*see* condition
Lenticonus (anterior) (posterior) (congenital)
  743.36
Lenticular degeneration, progressive 275.1
Lentiglobus (posterior) (congenital) 743.36
Lentigo (congenital) 709.09
  juvenile 709.09
  Maligna (M8742/2)—*see also* Neoplasm, skin,
    in situ
    melanoma (M8742/3)—*see* Melanoma
  senile 709.09
Leonine leprosy 030.0
Leontiasis
  ossium 733.3
  syphilitic 095.8
    congenital 090.5
Léopold-Lévi's syndrome (paroxysmal thyroid
  instability) 242.9
Lepore hemoglobin syndrome 282.45
Lepothrix 039.0
Lepra 030.9
  Willan's 696.1
Leprechaunism 259.8

Lepromatous leprosy 030.0
Leprosy 030.9
  anesthetic 030.1
  beriberi 030.1
  borderline (group B) (infiltrated) (neuritic) 030.3
  cornea (*see also* Leprosy, by type) 030.9
    [371.89]
  dimorphous (group B) (infiltrated)
    (lepromatous) (neuritic) (tuberculoid) 030.3
  eyelid 030.0 *[373.4]*
  indeterminate (group I) (macular) (neuritic)
    (uncharacteristic) 030.2
  leonine 030.0
  lepromatous (diffuse) (infiltrated) (macular)
    (neuritic) (nodular) (type L) 030.0
  macular (early) (neuritic) (simple) 030.2
  maculoanesthetic 030.1
  mixed 030.0
  neuro 030.1
  nodular 030.0
  primary neuritic 030.3
  specified type or group NEC 030.8
  tubercular 030.1
  tuberculoid (macular) (maculoanesthetic)
    (major) (minor) (neuritic) (type T) 030.1
Leptocytosis, hereditary 282.40
Leptomeningitis (chronic) (circumscribed)
  (hemorrhagic) (nonsuppurative) (*see also*
  Meningitis) 322.9
  aseptic 047.9
    adenovirus 049.1
    Coxsackie virus 047.0
    ECHO virus 047.1
    enterovirus 047.9
    lymphocytic choriomeningitis 049.0
  epidemic 036.0
  late effect—*see* category 326
  meningococcal 036.0
  pneumococcal 320.1
  syphilitic 094.2
  tuberculous (*see also* Tuberculosis, meninges)
    013.0
Leptomeningopathy (*see also* Meningitis) 322.9
Leptospiral —*see* condition
Leptospirochetal —*see* condition
Leptospirosis 100.9
  autumnalis 100.89
  canicula 100.89
  grippotyphosa 100.89
  hebdomidis 100.89
  icterohemorrhagica 100.0
  nanukayami 100.89
  pomona 100.89
  Weil's disease 100.0
Leptothricosis —*see* Actinomycosis
Leptothrix infestation —*see* Actinomycosis
Leptotricosis —*see* Actinomycosis
Leptus dermatitis 133.8
Léri's pleonosteosis 756.89
Léri-Weill syndrome 756.59
Leriche syndrome (aortic bifurcation occlusion)
  444.09
Lermoyez's syndrome (*see also* Disease,
  Ménière's) 386.00
Lesbianism —*omit code*
  egodystonic 302.0
  problems with 302.0
Lesch-Nyhan syndrome (hypoxanthine-guanine-
  phosphoriboxyltransferase deficiency) 277.2

Lesion(s)
  abducens nerve 378.54
  alveolar process 525.8
  anorectal 569.49
  aortic (valve)—*see* Endocarditis, aortic
  auditory nerve 388.5
  basal ganglion 333.90
  bile duct (*see also* Disease, biliary) 576.8
  bladder 596.9
  bone 733.90
  brachial plexus 353.0
  brain 348.89
    congenital 742.9
    vascular (*see also* Lesion, cerebrovascular)
      437.9
      degenerative 437.1
      healed or old without residuals V12.54
      hypertensive 437.2
      late effect—*see* Late effect(s) (of)
        cerebrovascular disease
  buccal 528.9
  calcified—*see* Calcification
  canthus 373.9
  carate—*see* Pinta, lesions
  cardia 537.89
  cardiac—*see also* Disease, heart congenital 746.9
    valvular—*see* Endocarditis
  cauda equina 344.60
    with neurogenic bladder 344.61
  cecum 569.89
  cerebral—*see* Lesion, brain
  cerebrovascular (*see also* Disease,
    cerebrovascular NEC) 437.9
    degenerative 437.1
    healed or old without residuals V12.54
    hypertensive 437.2
    specified type NEC 437.8
  cervical root (nerve) NEC 353.2
  chiasmal 377.54
    associated with
      inflammatory disorders 377.54
      neoplasm NEC 377.52
      pituitary 377.51
      pituitary disorders 377.51
      vascular disorders 377.53
  chorda tympani 351.8
  coin, lung 793.11
  colon 569.89
  congenital—*see* Anomaly
  conjunctiva 372.9
  coronary artery (*see also* Ischemia, heart) 414.9
  cranial nerve 352.9
    first 352.0
    second 377.49
    third
      partial 378.51
      total 378.52
    fourth 378.53
    fifth 350.9
    sixth 378.54
    seventh 351.9
    eighth 388.5
    ninth 352.2
    tenth 352.3
    eleventh 352.4
    twelfth 352.5
  cystic—*see* Cyst
  degenerative—*see* Degeneration
  dermal (skin) 709.9

Lesion(s)—*continued*
  Dieulafoy (hemorrhagic)
    of
      duodenum 537.84
      intestine 569.86
      stomach 537.84
    duodenum 537.89
      with obstruction 537.3
    eyelid 373.9
    gasserian ganglion 350.8
    gastric 537.89
    gastroduodenal 537.89
    gastrointestinal 569.89
    glossopharyngeal nerve 352.2
    heart (organic)—*see also* Disease, heart
      vascular—*see* Disease, cardiovascular
    helix (ear) 709.9
    high grade myelodysplastic syndrome 238.73
    hyperchromic, due to pinta (carate) 103.1
    hyperkeratotic (*see also* Hyperkeratosis) 701.1
    hypoglossal nerve 352.5
    hypopharynx 478.29
    hypothalamic 253.9
    ileocecal coil 569.89
    ileum 569.89
    iliohypogastric nerve 355.79
    ilioinguinal nerve 355.79
    in continuity—*see* Injury, nerve, by site
    inflammatory—*see* Inflammation
    intestine 569.89
    intracerebral—*see* Lesion, brain
    intrachiasmal (optic) (*see also* Lesion, chiasmal)
        377.54
    intracranial, space-occupying NEC 784.2
    joint 719.90
      ankle 719.97
      elbow 719.92
      foot 719.97
      hand 719.94
      hip 719.95
      knee 719.96
      multiple sites 719.99
      pelvic region 719.95
      sacroiliac (old) 724.6
      shoulder (region) 719.91
      specified site NEC 719.98
      wrist 719.93
    keratotic (*see also* Keratosis) 701.1
    kidney (*see also* Disease, renal) 593.9
    laryngeal nerve (recurrent) 352.3
    leonine 030.0
    lip 528.5
    liver 573.8
    low grade myelodysplastic syndrome 238.72
    lumbosacral
      plexus 353.1
      root (nerve) NEC 353.4
    lung 518.89
      coin 793.11
    maxillary sinus 473.0
    mitral—*see* Endocarditis, mitral
    Morel Lavallée — see Hematoma, by site
    motor cortex 348.89
    nerve (*see also* Disorder, nerve) 355.9
    nervous system 349.9
      congenital 742.9

Lesion(s)—*continued*
  nonallopathic NEC 739.9
    in region (of)
      abdomen 739.9
      acromioclavicular 739.7
      cervical, cervicothoracic 739.1
      costochondral 739.8
      costovertebral 739.8
      extremity
        lower 739.6
        upper 739.7
      head 739.0
      hip 739.5
      lower extremity 739.6
      lumbar, lumbosacral 739.3
      occipitocervical 739.0
      pelvic 739.5
      pubic 739.5
      rib cage 739.8
      sacral, sacrococcygeal, sacroiliac 739.4
      sternochondral 739.8
      sternoclavicular 739.7
      thoracic, thoracolumbar 739.2
      upper extremity 739.7
  nose (internal) 478.19
  obstructive—*see* Obstruction
  obturator nerve 355.79
  occlusive
    artery—*see* Embolism, artery
  organ or site NEC—*see* Disease, by site
  osteolytic 733.90
  paramacular, of retina 363.32
  peptic 537.89
  periodontal, due to traumatic occlusion 523.8
  perirectal 569.49
  peritoneum (granulomatous) 568.89
  pigmented (skin) 709.00
  pinta—*see* Pinta, lesions
  polypoid—*see* Polyp
  prechiasmal (optic) (*see also* Lesion, chiasmal)
      377.54
  primary—*see also* Syphilis, primary
    carate 103.0
    pinta 103.0
    yaws 102.0
  pulmonary 518.89
    valve (*see also* Endocarditis, pulmonary)
        424.3
  pylorus 537.89
  radiation NEC 990
  radium NEC 990
  rectosigmoid 569.89
  retina, retinal—*see also* Retinopathy
    vascular 362.17
  retroperitoneal 568.89
  romanus 720.1
  sacroiliac (joint) 724.6
  salivary gland 527.8
    benign lymphoepithelial 527.8
  saphenous nerve 355.79
  secondary—*see* Syphilis, secondary
  sigmoid 569.89
  sinus (accessory) (nasal) (*see also* Sinusitis)
      473.9
  skin 709.9
    suppurative 686.00
  SLAP (superior glenoid labrum) 840.7
  space-occupying, intracranial NEC 784.2

Lesion(s)—*continued*
  spinal cord 336.9
    congenital 742.9
    traumatic (complete) (incomplete)
      (transverse)—*see also* Injury, spinal, by
      site
      with
        broken
          back—*see* Fracture, vertebra, by site,
            with spinal cord injury
          neck—*see* Fracture, vertebra, cervical,
            with spinal cord injury
        fracture, vertebra—*see* Fracture, vertebra,
          by site, with spinal cord injury
  spleen 289.50
  stomach 537.89
  superior glenoid labrum (SLAP) 840.7
  syphilitic—*see* Syphilis
  tertiary—*see* Syphilis, tertiary
  thoracic root (nerve) 353.3
  tonsillar fossa 474.9
  tooth, teeth 525.8
    white spot 521.01
  traumatic NEC (*see also* nature and site of
    injury) 959.9
  tricuspid (valve)—*see* Endocarditis, tricuspid
  trigeminal nerve 350.9
  ulcerated or ulcerative—*see* Ulcer
  uterus NEC 621.9
  vagina 623.8
  vagus nerve 352.3
  valvular—*see* Endocarditis
  vascular 459.9
    affecting central nervous system (*see also*
      Lesion, cerebrovascular) 437.9
    following trauma (*see also* Injury, blood
      vessel, by site) 904.9
    retina 362.17
    traumatic—*see* Injury, blood vessel, by site
    umbilical cord 663.6
      affecting fetus or newborn 762.6
  visual
    cortex NEC (*see also* Disorder, visual, cortex)
      377.73
    pathway NEC (*see also* Disorder, visual,
      pathway) 377.63
  warty—*see* Verruca
  white spot, on teeth 521.01
  x-ray NEC 990
Lethargic —*see* condition
Lethargy 780.79
Letterer-Siwe disease (acute histiocytosis X)
  (M9722/3) 202.5
Leucinosis 270.3
Leucocoria 360.44
Leucosarcoma (M9850/3) 207.8
Leukasmus 270.2
Leukemia, leukemic (congenital) (M9800/3) 208.9

Note—Use the following fifth-digit
subclassification for categories 203-208:

0 without mention of having achieved
  remission, failed remission
1 in remission
2 in relapse

---

  acute NEC (M9801/3) 208.0
  aleukemic NEC (M9804/3) 208.8
    granulocytic (M9864/3) 205.8
  basophilic (M9870/3) 205.1
  blast (cell) (M9801/3) 208.0

Leukemia, leukemic—*continued*
  blastic (M9801/3) 208.0
    granulocytic (M9861/3) 205.0
  chronic NEC (M9803/3) 208.1
  compound (M9810/3) 207.8
  eosinophilic (M9880/3) 205.1
  giant cell (M9910/3) 207.2
  granulocytic (M9860/3) 205.9
    acute (M9861/3) 205.0
    aleukemic (M9864/3) 205.8
    blastic (M9861/3) 205.0
    chronic (M9863/3) 205.1
    subacute (M9862/3) 205.2
    subleukemic (M9864/3) 205.8
  hairy cell (M9940/3) 202.4
  hemoblastic (M9801/3) 208.0
  histiocytic (M9890/3) 206.9
  lymphatic (M9820/3) 204.9
    acute (M9821/3) 204.0
    aleukemic (M9824/3) 204.8
    chronic (M9823/3) 204.1
    subacute (M9822/3) 204.2
    subleukemic (M9824/3) 204.8
  lymphoblastic (M9821/3) 204.0
  lymphocytic (M9820/3) 204.9
    acute (M9821/3) 204.0
    aleukemic (M9824/3) 204.8
    chronic (M9823/3) 204.1
    granular
      large T-cell 204.8
    subacute (M9822/3) 204.2
    subleukemic (M9824/3) 204.8
  lymphogenous (M9820/3)—*see* Leukemia,
    lymphoid
  lymphoid (M9820/3) 204.9
    acute (M9821/3) 204.0
    aleukemic (M9824/3) 204.8
    blastic (M9821/3) 204.0
    chronic (M9823/3) 204.1
    subacute (M9822/3) 204.2
    subleukemic (M9824/3) 204.8
  lymphosarcoma cell (M9850/3) 207.8
  mast cell (M9900/3) 207.8
  megakaryocytic (M9910/3) 207.2
  megakaryocytoid (M9910/3) 207.2
  mixed (cell) (M9810/3) 207.8
  monoblastic (M9891/3) 206.0
  monocytic (Schilling-type) (M9890/3) 206.9
    acute (M9891/3) 206.0
    aleukemic (M9894/3) 206.8
    chronic (M9893/3) 206.1
    Naegeli-type (M9863/3) 205.1
    subacute (M9892/3) 206.2
    subleukemic (M9894/3) 206.8
  monocytoid (M9890/3) 206.9
    acute (M9891/3) 206.0
    aleukemic (M9894/3) 206.8
    chronic (M9893/3) 206.1
    myelogenous (M9863/3) 205.1
    subacute (M9892/3) 206.2
    subleukemic (M9894/3) 206.8
  monomyelocytic (M9860/3)—*see* Leukemia,
    myelomonocytic
  myeloblastic (M9861/3) 205.0
  myelocytic (M9863/3) 205.1
    acute (M9861/3) 205.0
  myelogenous (M9860/3) 205.9
    acute (M9861/3) 205.0
    aleukemic (M9864/3) 205.8
    chronic (M9863/3) 205.1
    monocytoid (M9863/3) 205.1

Leukemia, leukemic—*continued*
myelogenous—*continued*
  subacute (M9862/3) 205.2
  subleukemic (M9864) 205.8
  myeloid (M9860/3) 205.9
   acute (M9861/3) 205.0
   aleukemic (M9864/3) 205.8
   chronic (M9863/3) 205.1
   subacute (M9862/3) 205.2
   subleukemic (M9864/3) 205.8
  myelomonocytic (M9860/3) 205.9
   acute (M9861/3) 205.0
   chronic (M9863/3) 205.1
 Naegeli-type monocytic (M9863/3) 205.1
 neutrophilic (M9865/3) 205.1
 plasma cell (M9830/3) 203.1
 plasmacytic (M9830/3) 203.1
 prolymphocytic (M9825/3)—*see* Leukemia,
   lymphoid
 promyelocytic, acute (M9866/3) 205.0
 Schilling-type monocytic (M9890/3)—*see*
   Leukemia, monocytic
 stem cell (M9801/3) 208.0
 subacute NEC (M9802/3) 208.2
 subleukemic NEC (M9804/3) 208.8
 thrombocytic (M9910/3) 207.2
 undifferentiated (M9801/3) 208.0
Leukemoid reaction (basophilic) (lymphocytic)
  (monocytic) (myelocytic) (neutrophilic) 288.62
Leukoaraiosis (hypertensive) 437.1
Leukoariosis —*see* Leukoaraiosis
Leukoclastic vasculitis 446.29
Leukocoria 360.44
Leukocythemia —*see* Leukemia
Leukocytopenia 288.50
Leukocytosis 288.60
 basophilic 288.8
 eosinophilic 288.3
 lymphocytic 288.8
 monocytic 288.8
 neutrophilic 288.8
Leukoderma 709.09
 syphilitic 091.3
  late 095.8
Leukodermia (*see also* Leukoderma) 709.09
Leukodystrophy (cerebral) (globoid cell)
  (metachromatic) (progressive) (sudanophilic)
  330.0
Leukoedema, mouth or tongue 528.79
Leukoencephalitis
 acute hemorrhagic (postinfectious) NEC 136.9
   [323.61]
 postimmunization or postvaccinal 323.51
 subacute sclerosing 046.2
  van Bogaert's 046.2
 van Bogaert's (sclerosing) 046.2
Leukoencephalopathy (*see also* Encephalitis) 323.9
 acute necrotizing hemorrhagic (postinfectious)
   136.9 *[323.61]*
 postimmunization or postvaccinal 323.51
 arteriosclerotic 437.0
 Binswanger's 290.12
 metachromatic 330.0
 multifocal (progressive) 046.3
 progressive multifocal 046.3
 reversible, posterior 348.5
Leukoerythroblastosis 289.9
Leukoerythrosis 289.0

Leukokeratosis (*see also* Leukoplakia) 702.8
 mouth 528.6
 nicotina palati 528.79
 tongue 528.6
Leukokoria 360.44
Leukokraurosis vulva, vulvae 624.09
Leukolymphosarcoma (M9850/3) 207.8
Leukoma (cornea) (interfering with central
  vision) 371.03
 adherent 371.04
Leukomalacia, periventricular 779.7
Leukomelanopathy, hereditary 288.2
Leukonychia (punctata) (striata) 703.8
 congenital 757.5
Leukopathia
 unguium 703.8
  congenital 757.5
Leukopenia 288.50
 basophilic 288.59
 cyclic 288.02
 eosinophilic 288.59
 familial 288.59
 malignant (see also Agranulocytosis) 288.09
 periodic 288.02
 transitory neonatal 776.7
Leukopenic —*see* condition
Leukoplakia 702.8
 anus 569.49
 bladder (postinfectional) 596.89
 buccal 528.6
 cervix (uteri) 622.2
 esophagus 530.83
 gingiva 528.6
 kidney (pelvis) 593.89
 larynx 478.79
 lip 528.6
 mouth 528.6
 oral soft tissue (including tongue) (mucosa) 528.6
 palate 528.6
 pelvis (kidney) 593.89
 penis (infectional) 607.0
 rectum 569.49
 syphilitic 095.8
 tongue 528.6
 tonsil 478.29
 ureter (postinfectional) 593.89
 urethra (postinfectional) 599.84
 uterus 621.8
 vagina 623.1
 vesical 596.89
 vocal cords 478.5
 vulva 624.09
Leukopolioencephalopathy 330.0
Leukorrhea (vagina) 623.5
 due to trichomonas (vaginalis) 131.00
 trichomonal (Trichomonas vaginalis) 131.00
Leukosarcoma (M9850/3) 207.8
Leukosis (M9800/3)—*see* Leukemia
Lev's disease or syndrome (acquired complete
  heart block) 426.0
Levi's syndrome (pituitary dwarfism) 253.3
Levocardia (isolated) 746.87
 with situs inversus 759.3
Levulosuria 271.2
Lewandowski's disease (primary) (*see also*
  Tuberculosis) 017.0
Lewandowski-Lutz disease (epidermodysplasia
  verruciformis) 078.19
Lewy body dementia 331.82
Lewy body disease 331.82
Leyden's disease (periodic vomiting) 536.2
Leyden's-Möbius dystrophy 359.1

Leydig cell
carcinoma (M8650/3)
specified site—*see* Neoplasm, by site, malignant
unspecified site
female 183.0
male 186.9
tumor (M8650/1)
benign (M8650/0)
specified site—*see* Neoplasm, by site, benign
unspecified site
female 220
male 222.0
malignant (M8650/3)
specified site—*see* Neoplasm, by site, malignant
unspecified site
female 183.0
male 186.9
specified site—*see* Neoplasm, by site, uncertain behavior
unspecified site
female 236.2
male 236.4
Leydig-Sertoli cell tumor (M8631/0)
specified site—*see* Neoplasm, by site, benign
unspecified site
female 220
male 222.0
LGSIL (low grade squamous intraepithelial lesion)
anus 796.73
cervix 795.03
vagina 795.13
Liar, pathologic 301.7
Libman-Sacks disease or syndrome 710.0 *[424.91]*
Lice (infestation) 132.9
body (pediculus corporis) 132.1
crab 132.2
head (pediculus capitis) 132.0
mixed (classifiable to more than one of the categories 132.0-132.2) 132.3
pubic (pediculus pubis) 132.2
Lichen 697.9
albus 701.0
annularis 695.89
atrophicus 701.0
corneus obtusus 698.3
myxedematous 701.8
nitidus 697.1
pilaris 757.39
acquired 701.1
planopilaris 697.0
planus (acute) (chronicus) (hypertrophic) (verrucous) 697.0
morphoeicus 701.0
sclerosus (et atrophicus) 701.0
ruber 696.4
acuminatus 696.4
moniliformis 697.8
obtusus corneus 698.3
of Wilson 697.0
planus 697.0
sclerosus (et atrophicus) 701.0
scrofulosus (primary) (*see also* Tuberculosis) 017.0
simplex (Vidal's) 698.3
chronicus 698.3
circumscriptus 698.3
spinulosus 757.39
mycotic 117.9
striata 697.8
urticatus 698.2

Lichenification 698.3
nodular 698.3
Lichenoides tuberculosis (primary) (*see also* Tuberculosis) 017.0
Lichtheim's disease or syndrome (subacute combined sclerosis with pernicious anemia) 281.0 *[336.2]*
Lien migrans 289.59
Lientery (*see also* Diarrhea) 787.91
infectious 009.2
Life circumstance problem NEC V62.89
Li-Fraumeni cancer syndrome V84.01
Ligament —*see* condition
Light-for-dates (infant) 764.0
with signs of fetal malnutrition 764.1
affecting management of pregnancy 656.5
Light-headedness 780.4
Lightning (effects) (shock) (stroke) (struck by) 994.0
burn—*see* Burn, by site
foot 266.2
Lightwood's disease or syndrome (renal tubular acidosis) 588.89
Lignac's disease (cystinosis) 270.0
Lignac (-de Toni) (-Fanconi) (-Debré) syndrome (cystinosis) 270.0
Lignac (-Fanconi) syndrome (cystinosis) 270.0
Ligneous thyroiditis 245.3
Likoff's syndrome (angina in menopausal women) 413.9
Limb —*see* condition
Limitation of joint motion (*see also* Stiffness, joint) 719.5
sacroiliac 724.6
Limit dextrinosis 271.0
Limited
cardiac reserve—*see* Disease, heart
duction, eye NEC 378.63
mandibular range of motion 524.52
Lindau's disease (retinocerebral angiomatosis) 759.6
Lindau (-von Hippel) disease (angiomatosis retinocerebellosa) 759.6
Linea corneae senilis 371.41
Lines
Beau's (transverse furrows on fingernails) 703.8
Harris' 733.91
Hudson-Stähli 371.11
Stähli's 371.11
Lingua
geographical 529.1
nigra (villosa) 529.3
plicata 529.5
congenital 750.13
tylosis 528.6
Lingual (tongue)—*see also* condition
thyroid 759.2
Linitis (gastric) 535.4
plastica (M8142/3) 151.9
Lioderma essentialis (cum melanosis et telangiectasia) 757.33
Lip —*see also* condition
biting 528.9
Lipalgia 272.8
Lipedema —*see* Edema
Lipemia (*see also* Hyperlipidemia) 272.4
retina, retinalis 272.3
Lipidosis 272.7
cephalin 272.7
cerebral (infantile) (juvenile) (late) 330.1
cerebroretinal 330.1 *[362.71]*
cerebroside 272.7

Lipidosis—*continued*
  cerebrospinal 272.7
  chemically-induced 272.7
  cholesterol 272.7
  diabetic 250.8 *[272.7]*
    due to secondary diabetes 249.8 *[272.7]*
  dystopic (hereditary) 272.7
  glycolipid 272.7
  hepatosplenomegalic 272.3
  hereditary, dystopic 272.7
  sulfatide 330.0
Lipoadenoma (M8324/0)—*see* Neoplasm, by
    site, benign
Lipoblastoma (M8881/0)—*see* Lipoma, by site
Lipoblastomatosis (M8881/0)—*see* Lipoma, by
    site
Lipochondrodystrophy 277.5
Lipochrome histiocytosis (familial) 288.1
Lipodermatosclerosis 729.39
Lipodystrophia progressiva 272.6
Lipodystrophy (progressive) 272.6
  insulin 272.6
  intestinal 040.2
  mesenteric 567.82
Lipofibroma (M8851/0)—*see* Lipoma, by site
Lipoglycoproteinosis 272.8
Lipogranuloma, sclerosing 709.8
Lipogranulomatosis (disseminated) 272.8
  kidney 272.8
Lipoid —*see* condition
  histiocytosis 272.7
    essential 272.7
  nephrosis (*see also* Nephrosis) 581.3
  proteinosis of Urbach 272.8
Lipoidemia (*see also* Hyperlipidemia) 272.4
Lipoidosis (*see also* Lipidosis) 272.7
Lipoma (M8850/0) 214.9
  breast (skin) 214.1
  face 214.0
  fetal (M8881/0)—*see also* Lipoma, by site
    fat cell (M8880/0)—*see* Lipoma, by site
  infiltrating (M8856/0)—*see* Lipoma, by site
  intra-abdominal 214.3
  intramuscular (M8856/0)—*see* Lipoma, by site
  intrathoracic 214.2
  kidney 214.3
  mediastinum 214.2
  muscle 214.8
  peritoneum 214.3
  retroperitoneum 214.3
  skin 214.1
    face 214.0
  spermatic cord 214.4
  spindle cell (M8857/0)—*see* Lipoma, by site
  stomach 214.3
  subcutaneous tissue 214.1
    face 214.0
  thymus 214.2
  thyroid gland 214.2
Lipomatosis (dolorosa) 272.8
  epidural 214.8
  fetal (M8881/0)—*see* Lipoma, by site
  Launois-Bensaude's 272.8
Lipomyohemangioma (M8860/0)
  specified site—*see* Neoplasm, connective tissue,
    benign
  unspecified site 223.0
Lipomyoma (M8860/0)
  specified site—*see* Neoplasm, connective tissue,
    benign
  unspecified site 223.0

Lipomyxoma (M8852/0)—*see* Lipoma, by site
Lipomyxosarcoma (M8852/3)—*see* Neoplasm,
    connective tissue, malignant
Lipophagocytosis 289.89
Lipoproteinemia (alpha) 272.4
  broad-beta 272.2
  floating-beta 272.2
  hyper-pre-beta 272.1
Lipoproteinosis (Rössle-Urbach-Wiethe) 272.8
Liposarcoma (M8850/3)—*see also* Neoplasm,
    connective tissue, malignant
  differentiated type (M8851/3)—*see* Neoplasm,
    connective tissue, malignant
  embryonal (M8852/3)—*see* Neoplasm,
    connective tissue, malignant
  mixed type (M8855/3)—*see* Neoplasm,
    connective tissue, malignant
  myxoid (M8852/3)—*see* Neoplasm, connective
    tissue, malignant
  pleomorphic (M8854/3)—*see* Neoplasm,
    connective tissue, malignant
  round cell (M8853/3)—*see* Neoplasm,
    connective tissue, malignant
  well differentiated type (M8851/3)—*see*
    Neoplasm, connective tissue, malignant
Liposynovitis prepatellaris 272.8
Lipping
  cervix 622.0
  spine (*see also* Spondylosis) 721.90
  vertebra (*see also* Spondylosis) 721.90
Lip pits (mucus), congenital 750.25
Lipschütz disease or ulcer 616.50
Lipuria 791.1
  bilharziasis 120.0
Liquefaction, vitreous humor 379.21
Lisping 307.9
Lissauer's paralysis 094.1
Lissencephalia, lissencephaly 742.2
Listerellose 027.0
Listeriose 027.0
Listeriosis 027.0
  congenital 771.2
  fetal 771.2
  suspected fetal damage affecting management of
    pregnancy 655.4
Listlessness 780.79
Lithemia 790.6
Lithiasis —*see also* Calculus
  hepatic (duct)—*see* Choledocholithiasis
  urinary 592.9
Lithopedion 779.9
  affecting management of pregnancy 656.8
Lithosis (occupational) 502
  with tuberculosis—*see* Tuberculosis, pulmonary
Lithuria 791.9
Litigation V62.5
Little
  league elbow 718.82
  stroke syndrome 435.9
Little's disease —*see* Palsy, cerebral
Littre's
  gland—*see* condition
  hernia—*see* Hernia, Littre's
Littritis (*see also* Urethritis) 597.89
Livedo 782.61
  annularis 782.61
  racemose 782.61
  reticularis 782.61
Live flesh 781.0
Liver —*see also* condition
  donor V59.6

Livida, asphyxia
newborn 768.6
Living
alone V60.3
with handicapped person V60.4
Lloyd's syndrome 258.1
Loa loa 125.2
Loasis 125.2
Lobe, lobar —*see* condition
Lobo's disease or blastomycosis 116.2
Lobomycosis 116.2
Lobotomy syndrome 310.0
Lobstein's disease (brittle bones and blue sclera)
756.51
Lobster-claw hand 755.58
Lobulation (congenital)—*see also* Anomaly,
specified type NEC, by site
kidney, fetal 753.3
liver, abnormal 751.69
spleen 759.0
Lobule, lobular —*see* condition
Local, localized —*see* condition
Locked bowel or intestine (*see also* Obstruction,
intestine) 560.9
Locked twins 660.5
affecting fetus or newborn 763.1
Locked-in state 344.81
Locking
joint (*see also* Derangement, joint) 718.90
knee 717.9
Lockjaw (*see also* Tetanus) 037
Locomotor ataxia (progressive) 094.0
Löffler's
endocarditis 421.0
eosinophilia or syndrome 518.3
pneumonia 518.3
syndrome (eosinophilic pneumonitis) 518.3
Löfgren's syndrome (sarcoidosis) 135
Loiasis 125.2
eyelid 125.2 *[373.6]*
Loneliness V62.89
Lone star fever 082.8
Long labor 662.1
affecting fetus or newborn 763.89
first stage 662.0
second stage 662.2
Long-term (current) (prophylactic) drug use
V58.69
antibiotics V58.62
anticoagulants V58.61
anti-inflammatories, non-steroidal (NSAID) V58.64
antiplatelets/antithrombotics V58.63
aspirin V58.66
bisphosphonates V58.68
high-risk medications NEC V58.69
insulin V58.67
methadone for pain control V58.69
opiate analgesic V58.69
pain killers V58.69
anti-inflammatory non-steroidal (NSAID)
V58.64
aspirin V58.66
steroids V58.65
tamoxifen V07.51
Longitudinal stripes or grooves, nails 703.8
congenital 757.5
Loop
intestine (*see also* Volvulus) 560.2
intrascleral nerve 379.29
vascular on papilla (optic) 743.57

Loose —*see also* condition
body
in tendon sheath 727.82
joint 718.10
ankle 718.17
elbow 718.12
foot 718.17
hand 718.14
hip 718.15
knee 717.6
multiple sites 718.19
pelvic region 718.15
prosthetic implant—*see* Complications,
mechanical
shoulder (region) 718.11
specified site NEC 718.18
wrist 718.13
cartilage (joint) (*see also* Loose, body, joint)
718.1
knee 717.6
facet (vertebral) 724.9
prosthetic implant—*see* Complications,
mechanical
sesamoid, joint (*see also* Loose, body, joint)
718.1
tooth, teeth 525.8
Loosening epiphysis 732.9
Looser (-Debray) -Milkman syndrome
(osteomalacia with pseudofractures) 268.2
Lop ear (deformity) 744.29
Lorain's disease or syndrome (pituitary
dwarfism) 253.3
Lorain-Levi syndrome (pituitary dwarfism)
253.3
Lordosis (acquired) (postural) 737.20
congenital 754.2
due to or associated with
Charcot-Marie-Tooth disease 356.1 *[737.42]*
mucopolysaccharidosis 277.5 *[737.42]*
neurofibromatosis 237.71 *[737.42]*
osteitis
deformans 731.0 *[737.42]*
fibrosa cystica 252.01 *[737.42]*
osteoporosis (*see also* Osteoporosis) 733.00
[737.42]
poliomyelitis (*see also* Poliomyelitis) 138
[737.42]
tuberculosis (*see also* Tuberculosis) 015.0
[737.42]
late effect of rickets 268.1 *[737.42]*
postlaminectomy 737.21
postsurgical NEC 737.22
rachitic 268.1 *[737.42]*
specified NEC 737.29
tuberculous (*see also* Tuberculosis) 015.0 *[737.42]*
Loss
appetite 783.0
hysterical 300.11
nonorganic origin 307.59
psychogenic 307.59
blood—*see* Hemorrhage
central vision 368.41
consciousness 780.09
transient 780.2
control, sphincter, rectum 787.60
nonorganic origin 307.7
ear ossicle, partial 385.24
elasticity, skin 782.8
extremity or member, traumatic, current—*see*
Amputation, traumatic

Loss —*continued*
  fluid (acute) 276.50
    with
      hypernatremia 276.0
      hyponatremia 276.1
    fetus or newborn 775.5
  hair 704.00
  hearing—*see also* Deafness
    central 389.14
    conductive (air) 389.00
      with sensorineural hearing loss 389.20
        bilateral 389.22
        unilateral 389.21
      bilateral 389.06
      combined types 389.08
      external ear 389.01
      inner ear 389.04
      middle ear 389.03
      multiple types 389.08
      tympanic membrane 389.02
      unilateral 389.05
    mixed conductive and sensorineural 389.20
      bilateral 389.22
      unilateral 389.21
    mixed type 389.20
      bilateral 389.22
      unilateral 389.21
    nerve
      bilateral 389.12
      unilateral 389.13
    neural
      bilateral 389.12
      unilateral 389.13
    noise-induced 388.12
    perceptive NEC (*see also* Loss, hearing,
      sensorineural) 389.10
    sensorineural 389.10
      with conductive hearing loss 389.20
        bilateral 389.22
        unilateral 389.21
      asymmetrical 389.16
      bilateral 389.18
      central 389.14
      neural
        bilateral 389.12
        unilateral 389.13
      sensory
        bilateral 389.11
        unilateral 389.17
      unilateral 389.15
    sensory
      bilateral 389.11
      unilateral 389.17
    specified type NEC 389.8
    sudden NEC 388.2
  height 781.91
  labyrinthine reactivity (unilateral) 386.55
    bilateral 386.56
  memory (*see also* Amnesia) 780.93
    mild, following organic brain damage 310.89
  mind (*see also* Psychosis) 298.9
  occusal vertical dimension 524.37
  organ or part—*see* Absence, by site, acquired
  recurrent pregnancy—*see* Pregnancy,
    management affected by, abortion, habitual
  sensation 782.0
  sense of
    smell (*see also* Disturbance, sensation) 781.1
    taste (*see also* Disturbance, sensation) 781.1
    touch (*see also* Disturbance, sensation) 781.1
  sight (acquired) (complete) (congenital)—*see*
    Blindness

Loss —*continued*
  spinal fluid
    headache 349.0
  substance of
    bone (*see also* Osteoporosis) 733.00
    cartilage 733.99
      ear 380.32
    vitreous (humor) 379.26
  tooth, teeth
    acquired 525.10
      due to
        caries 525.13
        extraction 525.10
        periodontal disease 525.12
        specified NEC 525.19
        trauma 525.11
  vision, visual (*see also* Blindness) 369.9
    both eyes (*see also* Blindness, both eyes)
      369.3
    complete (*see also* Blindness, both eyes) 369.00
    one eye 369.8
    sudden 368.11
    transient 368.12
  vitreous 379.26
  voice (*see also* Aphonia) 784.41
  weight (cause unknown) 783.21
Lou Gehrig's disease 335.20
Louis-Bar syndrome (ataxia-telangiectasia) 334.8
Louping ill 063.1
Lousiness —*see* Lice
Low
  back syndrome 724.2
  basal metabolic rate (BMR) 794.7
  birthweight 765.1
    extreme (less than 1000 grams) 765.0
    for gestational age 764.0
    status (*see also* Status, low birth weight)
      V21.30
  bladder compliance 596.52
  blood pressure (*see also* Hypotension) 458.9
    reading (incidental) (isolated) (nonspecific)
      796.3
  cardiac reserve—*see* Disease, heart
  compliance bladder 596.52
  frequency deafness—*see* Disorder, hearing
  function—*see also* Hypofunction
    kidney (*see also* Disease, renal) 593.9
    liver 573.9
  hemoglobin 285.9
  implantation, placenta—*see* Placenta, previa
  insertion, placenta—*see* Placenta, previa
  lying
    kidney 593.0
    organ or site, congenital—*see* Malposition,
      congenital
    placenta—*see* Placenta, previa
  output syndrome (cardiac) (*see also* Failure,
    heart) 428.9
  platelets (blood) (*see also* Thrombocytopenia)
    287.5
  reserve, kidney (*see also* Disease, renal) 593.9
  risk
    human papillomavirus (HPV) DNA test
      positive
      anal 796.79
      cervical 795.09
      vaginal 795.19
  salt syndrome 593.9
  tension glaucoma 365.12
  vision 369.9
    both eyes 369.20
    one eye 369.70

Lowe (-Terrey-MacLachlan) syndrome (oculocerebrorenal dystrophy) 270.8
Lower extremity —*see* condition
Lown (-Ganong)-Levine syndrome (short P-R interval, normal QRS complex, and paroxysmal supraventricular tachycardia) 426.81
LSD reaction (*see also* Abuse, drugs, nondependent) 305.3
L-shaped kidney 753.3
Lucas-Championnière disease (fibrinous bronchitis) 466.0
Lucey-Driscoll syndrome (jaundice due to delayed conjugation) 774.30
Ludwig's
  angina 528.3
  disease (submaxillary cellulitis) 528.3
Lues (venerea), luetic—*see* Syphilis
Luetscher's syndrome (dehydration) 276.51
Lumbago 724.2
  due to displacement, intervertebral disc 722.10
Lumbalgia 724.2
  due to displacement, intervertebral disc 722.10
Lumbar —*see* condition
Lumbarization, vertebra 756.15
Lumbermen's itch 133.8
Lump —*see also* Mass
  abdominal 789.3
  breast 611.72
  chest 786.6
  epigastric 789.3
  head 784.2
  kidney 753.3
  liver 789.1
  lung 786.6
  mediastinal 786.6
  neck 784.2
  nose or sinus 784.2
  pelvic 789.3
  skin 782.2
  substernal 786.6
  throat 784.2
  umbilicus 789.3
Lunacy (*see also* Psychosis) 298.9
Lunatomalacia 732.3
Lung —*see also* condition
  donor V59.8
  drug addict's 417.8
  mainliners' 417.8
  vanishing 492.0
Lupoid (miliary) of Boeck 135
Lupus 710.0
  anticoagulant 795.79
  with
    hemorrhagic disorder 286.53
    hypercoagulable state 289.81
  Cazenave's (erythematosus) 695.4
  discoid (local) 695.4
  disseminated 710.0
  erythematodes (discoid) (local) 695.4
  erythematosus (discoid) (local) 695.4
    disseminated 710.0
    eyelid 373.34
    systemic 710.0
    with
      encephalitis 710.0 *[323.81]*
      lung involvement 710.0 *[517.8]*
    inhibitor (presence of) 795.79
      with hypercoagulable state 289.81
  exedens 017.0

Lupus—*continued*
  eyelid (*see also* Tuberculosis) 017.0 *[373.4]*
  Hilliard's 017.0
  hydralazine
    correct substance properly administered 695.4
    overdose or wrong substance given or taken 972.6
  miliaris disseminatus faciei 017.0
  nephritis 710.0 *[583.81]*
    acute 710.0 *[580.81]*
    chronic 710.0 *[582.81]*
  nontuberculous, not disseminated 695.4
  pernio (Besnier) 135
  tuberculous (*see also* Tuberculosis) 017.0
    eyelid (*see also* Tuberculosis) 017.0 *[373.4]*
  vulgaris 017.0
Luschka's joint disease 721.90
Luteinoma (M8610/0) 220
Lutembacher's disease or syndrome (atrial septal defect with mitral stenosis) 745.5
Luteoma (M8610/0) 220
Lutz-Miescher disease (elastosis perforans serpiginosa) 701.1
Lutz-Splendore-de Almeida disease (Brazilian blastomycosis) 116.1
Luxatio
  bulbi due to birth injury 767.8
  coxae congenita (*see also* Dislocation, hip, congenital) 754.30
  erecta—*see* Dislocation, shoulder
  imperfecta—*see* Sprain, by site
  perinealis—*see* Dislocation, hip
Luxation —*see also* Dislocation, by site
  eyeball 360.81
    due to birth injury 767.8
    lateral 376.36
  genital organs (external) NEC—*see* Wound, open, genital organs
  globe (eye) 360.81
    lateral 376.36
  lacrimal gland (postinfectional) 375.16
  lens (old) (partial) 379.32
    congenital 743.37
      syphilitic 090.49 *[379.32]*
    Marfan's disease 090.49
    spontaneous 379.32
  penis—*see* Wound, open, penis
  scrotum—*see* Wound, open, scrotum
  testis—*see* Wound, open, testis
L-xyloketosuria 271.8
Lycanthropy (*see also* Psychosis) 298.9
Lyell's disease or syndrome (toxic epidermal necrolysis) 695.15
  due to drug
    correct substance properly administered 695.15
    overdose or wrong substance given or taken 977.9
      specified drug—*see* Table of drugs and chemicals
Lyme disease 088.81
Lymph
  gland or node—*see* condition
  scrotum (*see also* Infestation, filarial) 125.9
Lymphadenitis 289.3
  with
    abortion—*see* Abortion, by type, with sepsis
    ectopic pregnancy (*see also* categories 633.0-633.9) 639.0
    molar pregnancy (*see also* categories 630-632) 639.0

Lymphadenitis—*continued*
acute 683
  mesenteric 289.2
any site, except mesenteric 289.3
  acute 683
  chronic 289.1
  mesenteric (acute) (chronic) (nonspecific)
    (subacute) 289.2
  subacute 289.1
    mesenteric 289.2
breast, puerperal, postpartum 675.2
chancroidal (congenital) 099.0
chronic 289.1
  mesenteric 289.2
dermatopathic 695.89
due to
  anthracosis (occupational) 500
  Brugia (Wuchereria) malayi 125.1
  diphtheria (toxin) 032.89
  lymphogranuloma venereum 099.1
  Wuchereria bancrofti 125.0
following
  abortion 639.0
  ectopic or molar pregnancy 639.0
generalized 289.3
gonorrheal 098.89
granulomatous 289.1
infectional 683
mesenteric (acute) (chronic) (nonspecific)
    (subacute) 289.2
  due to Bacillus typhi 002.0
tuberculous (*see also* Tuberculosis) 014.8
mycobacterial 031.8
purulent 683
pyogenic 683
regional 078.3
septic 683
streptococcal 683
subacute, unspecified site 289.1
suppurative 683
syphilitic (early) (secondary) 091.4
  late 095.8
tuberculous—*see* Tuberculosis, lymph gland
venereal 099.1
Lymphadenoid goiter 245.2
Lymphadenopathy (general) 785.6
due to toxoplasmosis (acquired) 130.7
  congenital (active) 771.2
Lymphadenopathy-associated virus (disease)
  (illness) (infection)—*see* Human Immunodeficiency virus (disease) (illness) (infection)
Lymphadenosis 785.6
acute 075
Lymphangiectasis 457.1
conjunctiva 372.89
postinfectional 457.1
scrotum 457.1
Lymphangiectatic elephantiasis , nonfilarial
  457.1
Lymphangioendothelioma (M9170/0) 228.1
malignant (M9170/3)—*see* Neoplasm,
  connective tissue, malignant
Lymphangioleiomyomatosis 516.4
Lymphangioma (M9170/0) 228.1
capillary (M9171/0) 228.1
cavernous (M9172/0) 228.1
cystic (M9173/0) 228.1
malignant (M9170/3)—*see* Neoplasm,
  connective tissue, malignant
Lymphangiomyoma (M9174/0) 228.1
Lymphangiomyomatosis 516.4

Lymphangiosarcoma (M9170/3)—*see*
  Neoplasm, connective tissue, malignant
Lymphangitis 457.2
with
  abortion—*see* Abortion, by type, with sepsis
  abscess—*see* Abscess, by site
  cellulitis—*see* Abscess, by site
  ectopic pregnancy (*see also* categories
    633.0-633.9) 639.0
  molar pregnancy (*see also* categories 630-632)
    639.0
acute (with abscess or cellulitis) 682.9
  specified site—*see* Abscess, by site
breast, puerperal, postpartum 675.2
chancroidal 099.0
chronic (any site) 457.2
due to
  Brugia (Wuchereria) malayi 125.1
  Wuchereria bancrofti 125.0
following
  abortion 639.0
  ectopic or molar pregnancy 639.0
gangrenous 457.2
penis
  acute 607.2
  gonococcal (acute) 098.0
    chronic or duration of 2 months or more 098.2
puerperal, postpartum, childbirth 670.8
strumous, tuberculous (*see also* Tuberculosis)
  017.2
subacute (any site) 457.2
tuberculous—*see* Tuberculosis, lymph gland
Lymphatic (vessel)—*see* condition
Lymphatism 254.8
scrofulous (*see also* Tuberculosis) 017.2
Lymphectasia 457.1
Lymphedema (*see also* Elephantiasis) 457.1
acquired (chronic) 457.1
chronic hereditary 757.0
congenital 757.0
idiopathic hereditary 757.0
praecox 457.1
secondary 457.1
surgical NEC 997.99
  postmastectomy (syndrome) 457.0
Lymph-hemangioma (M9120/0)—*see*
  Hemangioma, by site
Lymphoblastic —*see* condition
Lymphoblastoma (diffuse) (M9630/3) 200.1
giant follicular (M9690/3) 202.0
macrofollicular (M9690/3) 202.0
Lymphoblastosis, acute benign 075
Lymphocele 457.8
Lymphocythemia 288.51
Lymphocytic —*see also* condition
chorioencephalitis (acute) (serous) 049.0
choriomeningitis (acute) (serous) 049.0
Lymphocytoma (diffuse) (malignant) (M9620/3)
  200.1
Lymphocytomatosis (M9620/3) 200.1
Lymphocytopenia 288.51
Lymphocytosis (symptomatic) 288.61
infectious (acute) 078.89
Lymphoepithelioma (M8082/3)—*see* Neoplasm,
  by site, malignant
Lymphogranuloma (malignant) (M9650/3) 201.9
inguinale 099.1
venereal (any site) 099.1
  with stricture of rectum 099.1
venereum 099.1

Lymphogranulomatosis (malignant) (M9650/3)
201.9
 benign (Boeck's sarcoid) (Schaumann's) 135
 Hodgkin's (M9650/3) 201.9
Lymphohistiocytosis, familial hemophagocytic
288.4
Lymphoid —*see* condition
Lympholeukoblastoma (M9850/3) 207.8
Lympholeukosarcoma (M9850/3) 207.8
Lymphoma (malignant) (M9590/3) 202.8

> *Note—Use the following fifth-digit*
> *subclassification with categories 200-202:*
>
> 0 *unspecifidd site*
> 1 *lymph nodes of head, face and neck*
> 2 *intrathoracic lymph nodes*
> 3 *intra-abdominal lymph nodes*
> 4 *lymph nodes of axilla and upper limb*
> 5 *lymph nodes of inguinal region and*
>   *lower limb*
> 6 *intrapelvic lymph nodes*
> 7 *spleen*
> 8 *lymph nodes of multiple sites*

 wenign (M9580/0)—*see* Neoplasm, by site, benign
 Burkitt's type (lymphoblastic) (undifferentiated)
  (M9750/3) 200.2
 Castleman's (mediastinal lymph node hyperplasia)
  785.6
 centroblastic-centrocytic
  diffuse (M9614/3) 202.8
  follicular (M9692/3) 202.0
 centroblastic type (diffuse) (M9632/3) 202.8
  follicular (M9697/3) 202.0
 centrocytic (M9622/3) 202.8
 compound (M9613/3) 200.8
 convoluted cell type (lymphoblastic) (M9602/3)
  202.8
 diffuse NEC (M9590/3) 202.8
  large B cell 202.8
 follicular (giant) (M9690/3) 202.0
  center cell (diffuse) (M9615/3) 202.8
   cleaved (diffuse) (M9623/3) 202.8
    follicular (M9695/3) 202.0
   non-cleaved (diffuse) (M9633/3) 202.8
    follicular (M9698/3) 202.0
  centroblastic-centrocytic (M9692/3) 202.0
  centroblastic type (M9697/3) 202.0
  large cell 202.0
  lymphocytic
   intermediate differentiation (M9694/3) 202.0
   poorly differentiated (M9696/3) 202.0
  mixed (cell type) (lymphocytic-histiocytic)
   (small cell and large cell) (M9691/3) 202.0
 germinocytic (M9622/3) 202.8
 giant, follicular or follicle (M9690/3) 202.0
 histiocytic (diffuse) (M9640/3) 200.0
  nodular (M9642/3) 200.0
  pleomorphic cell type (M9641/3) 200.0
 Hodgkin's (M9650/3) (*see also* Disease,
  Hodgkin's) 201.9
 immunoblastic (type) (M9612/3) 200.8
 large cell (M9640/3) 200.7
  anaplastic 200.6
  nodular (M9642/3) 202.0
  pleomorphic cell type (M9641/3) 200.0
 lymphoblastic (diffuse) (M9630/3) 200.1
  Burkitt's type (M9750/3) 200.2
  convoluted cell type (M9602/3) 202.8

Lymphoma—*continued*
 lymphocytic (cell type) (diffuse) (M9620/3) 200.1
  with plasmacytoid differentiation, diffuse
   (M9611/3) 200.8
  intermediate differentiation (diffuse)
   (M9621/3) 200.1
   follicular (M9694/3) 202.0
   nodular (M9694/3) 202.0
  nodular (M9690/3) 202.0
  poorly differentiated (diffuse) (M9630/3) 200.1
   follicular (M9696/3) 202.0
   nodular (M9696/3) 202.0
  well differentiated (diffuse) (M9620/3) 200.1
   follicular (M9693/3) 202.0
   nodular (M9693/3) 202.0
 lymphocytic-histiocytic, mixed (diffuse)
  (M9613/3) 200.8
  follicular (M9691/3) 202.0
  nodular (M9691/3) 202.0
 lymphoplasmacytoid type (M9611/3) 200.8
 lymphosarcoma type (M9610/3) 200.1
 macrofollicular (M9690/3) 202.0
 mantle cell 200.4
 marginal zone 200.3
  extranodal B-cell 200.3
  nodal B-cell 200.3
  splenic B-cell 200.3
 mixed cell type (diffuse) (M9613/3) 200.8
  follicular (M9691/3) 202.0
  nodular (M9691/3) 202.0
 nodular (M9690/3) 202.0
  histiocytic (M9642/3) 200.0
  lymphocytic (M9690.3) 202.0
   intermediate differentiation (M9694/3) 202.0
   poorly differentiated (M9696/3) 202.0
  mixed (cell type) (lymphocytic-histiocytic)
   (small cell and large cell) (M9691/3) 202.0
 non-Hodgkin's type NEC (M9591/3) 202.8
 peripheral T-cell 202.7
 primary central nervous system 200.5
 reticulum cell (type) (M9640/3) 200.0
 small cell and large cell, mixed (diffuse)
  (M9613/3) 200.8
  follicular (M9691/3) 202.0
  nodular (M9691/3) 202.0
 stem cell (type) (M9601/3) 202.8
 T-cell 202.1
  peripheral 202.7
 undifferentiated (cell type) (non-Burkitt's)
  (M9600/3) 202.8
  Burkitt's type (M9750/3) 200.2
Lymphomatosis (M9590/3)—*see also*
 Lymphoma
 granulomatous 099.1
Lymphopathia
 venereum 099.1
 veneris 099.1
Lymphopenia 288.51
 familial 279.2
Lymphoreticulosis, benign (of inoculation)
 078.3
Lymphorrhea 457.8
Lymphosarcoma (M9610/3) 200.1
 diffuse (M9610/3) 200.1
  with plasmacytoid differentiation (M9611/3)
   200.8
  lymphoplasmacytic (M9611/3) 200.8
 follicular (giant) (M9690/3) 202.0
  lymphoblastic (M9696/3) 202.0
  lymphocytic, intermediate differentiation
   (M9694/3) 202.0
  mixed cell type (M9691/3) 202.0

Lymphosarcoma—*continued*
  giant follicular (M9690/3) 202.0
  Hodgkin's (M9650/3) 201.9
  immunoblastic (M9612/3) 200.8
  lymphoblastic (diffuse) (M9630/3) 200.1
    follicular (M9696/3) 202.0
    nodular (M9696/3) 202.0
  lymphocytic (diffuse) (M9620/3) 200.1
    intermediate differentiation (diffuse)
      (M9621/3) 200.1
      follicular (M9694/3) 202.0
      nodular (M9694/3) 202.0
  mixed cell type (diffuse) (M9613/3) 200.8
    follicular (M9691/3) 202.0
    nodular (M9691/3) 202.0
  nodular (M9690/3) 202.0
    lymphoblastic (M9696/3) 202.0
    lymphocytic, intermediate differentiation
      (M9694/3) 202.0
    mixed cell type (M9691/3) 202.0
  prolymphocytic (M9631/3) 200.1
  reticulum cell (M9640/3) 200.0
Lymphostasis 457.8
Lypemania (*see also* Melancholia) 296.2
Lyssa 071

M

Macacus ear 744.29
Maceration
fetus (cause not stated) 779.9
wet feet, tropical (syndrome) 991.4
Machado-Joseph disease 334.8
Machupo virus hemorrhagic fever 078.7
Macleod's syndrome (abnormal transradiancy, one lung) 492.8
Macrocephalia, macrocephaly 756.0
Macrocheilia (congenital) 744.81
Macrochilia (congenital) 744.81
Macrocolon (congenital) 751.3
Macrocornea 743.41
associated with buphthalmos 743.22
Macrocytic —*see* condition
Macrocytosis 289.89
Macrodactylia, macrodactylism (fingers) (thumbs) 755.57
toes 755.65
Macrodontia 520.2
Macroencephaly 742.4
Macrogenia 524.05
Macrogenitosomia (female) (male) (praecox) 255.2
Macrogingivae 523.8
Macroglobulinemia (essential) (idiopathic) (monoclonal) (primary) (syndrome) (Waldenström's) 273.3
Macroglossia (congenital) 750.15
acquired 529.8
Macrognathia, macrognathism (congenital) 524.00
mandibular 524.02
alveolar 524.72
maxillary 524.01
alveolar 524.71
Macrogyria (congenital) 742.4
Macrohydrocephalus (*see also* Hydrocephalus) 331.4
Macromastia (*see also* Hypertrophy, breast) 611.1
Macrophage activation syndrome 288.4
Macropsia 368.14
Macrosigmoid 564.7
congenital 751.3
Macrospondylitis, acromegalic 253.0
Macrostomia (congenital) 744.83
Macrotia (external ear) (congenital) 744.22
Macula
cornea, corneal
congenital 743.43
interfering with vision 743.42
interfering with central vision 371.03
not interfering with central vision 371.02
degeneration (*see also* Degeneration, macula) 362.50
hereditary (*see also* Dystrophy, retina) 362.70
edema, cystoid 362.53
Maculae ceruleae 132.1
Macules and papules 709.8
Maculopathy, toxic 362.55
Madarosis 374.55
Madelung's
deformity (radius) 755.54
disease (lipomatosis) 272.8
lipomatosis 272.8

Madness (*see also* Psychosis) 298.9
myxedema (acute) 293.0
subacute 293.1
Madura
disease (actinomycotic) 039.9
mycotic 117.4
foot (actinomycotic) 039.4
mycotic 117.4
Maduromycosis (actinomycotic) 039.9
mycotic 117.4
Maffucci's syndrome (dyschondroplasia with hemangiomas) 756.4
Magenblase syndrome 306.4
Main en griffe (acquired) 736.06
congenital 755.59
Maintenance
chemotherapy regimen or treatment V58.11
dialysis regimen or treatment
extracorporeal (renal) V56.0
peritoneal V56.8
renal V56.0
drug therapy or regimen
chemotherapy, antineoplastic V58.11
immunotherapy, antineoplastic V58.12
external fixation NEC V54.89
methadone 304.00
radiotherapy V58.0
traction NEC V54.89
Majocchi's
disease (purpura annularis telangiectodes) 709.1
granuloma 110.6
Major —*see* condition
Mal
cerebral (idiopathic) (*see also* Epilepsy) 345.9
comital (*see also* Epilepsy) 345.9
de los pintos (*see also* Pinta) 103.9
de Meleda 757.39
de mer 994.6
lie—*see* Presentation, fetal
perforant (*see also* Ulcer, lower extremity) 707.15
Malabar itch 110.9
beard 110.0
foot 110.4
scalp 110.0
Malabsorption 579.9
calcium 579.8
carbohydrate 579.8
disaccharide 271.3
drug-induced 579.8
due to bacterial overgrowth 579.8
fat 579.8
folate, congenital 281.2
galactose 271.1
glucose-galactose (congenital) 271.3
intestinal 579.9
isomaltose 271.3
lactose (hereditary) 271.3
methionine 270.4
monosaccharide 271.8
postgastrectomy 579.3
postsurgical 579.3
protein 579.8
sucrose (-isomaltose) (congenital) 271.3
syndrome 579.9
postgastrectomy 579.3
postsurgical 579.3

Malacia, bone 268.2
  juvenile (*see also* Rickets) 268.0
  Kienböck's (juvenile) (lunate) (wrist) 732.3
    adult 732.8
Malacoplakia
  bladder 596.89
  colon 569.89
  pelvis (kidney) 593.89
  ureter 593.89
  urethra 599.84
Malacosteon 268.2
  juvenile (*see also* Rickets) 268.0
Maladaptation —*see* Maladjustment
Maladie de Roger 745.4
Maladjustment
  conjugal V61.10
    involving
      divorce V61.03
      estrangement V61.09
  educational V62.3
  family V61.9
    specified circumstance NEC V61.8
  marital V61.10
    involving
      divorce V61.03
      estrangement V61.09
  occupational V62.29
    current military deployment status V62.21
  simple, adult (*see also* Reaction, adjustment)
    309.9
  situational acute (*see also* Reaction, adjustment)
    309.9
  social V62.4
Malaise 780.79
Malakoplakia —*see* Malacoplakia
Malaria, malarial (fever) 084.6
  algid 084.9
  any type, with
    algid malaria 084.9
    blackwater fever 084.8
    fever
      blackwater 084.8
      hemoglobinuric (bilious) 084.8
    hemoglobinuria, malarial 084.8
    hepatitis 084.9 *[573.2]*
    nephrosis 084.9 *[581.81]*
    pernicious complication NEC 084.9
      cardiac 084.9
      cerebral 084.9
  cardiac 084.9
  carrier (suspected) of V02.9
  cerebral 084.9
  complicating pregnancy, childbirth, or
    puerperium 647.4
  congenital 771.2
  congestion, congestive 084.6
    brain 084.9
  continued 084.0
  estivo-autumnal 084.0
  falciparum (malignant tertian) 084.0
  hematinuria 084.8
  hematuria 084.8
  hemoglobinuria 084.8
  hemorrhagic 084.6
  induced (therapeutically) 084.7
    accidental—*see* Malaria, by type
  liver 084.9 *[573.2]*
  malariae (quartan) 084.2
  malignant (tertian) 084.0
  mixed infections 084.5
  monkey 084.4
  ovale 084.3

Malaria, malarial—*continued*
  pernicious, acute 084.0
  Plasmodium, P.
    falciparum 084.0
    malariae 084.2
    ovale 084.3
    vivax 084.1
  quartan 084.2
  quotidian 084.0
  recurrent 084.6
    induced (therapeutically) 084.7
      accidental—*see* Malaria, by type
  remittent 084.6
  specified types NEC 084.4
  spleen 084.6
  subtertian 084.0
  tertian (benign) 084.1
    malignant 084.0
  tropical 084.0
  typhoid 084.6
  vivax (benign tertian) 084.1
Malassez's disease (testicular cyst) 608.89
Malassimilation 579.9
Maldescent, testis 752.51
Maldevelopment —*see also* Anomaly, by site
  brain 742.9
  colon 751.5
  hip (joint) 755.63
    congenital dislocation (*see also* Dislocation,
      hip, congenital) 754.30
  mastoid process 756.0
  middle ear, except ossicles 744.03
    ossicles 744.04
  newborn (not malformation) 764.9
  ossicles, ear 744.04
  spine 756.10
  toe 755.66
Male type pelvis 755.69
  with disproportion (fetopelvic) 653.2
    affecting fetus or newborn 763.1
    causing obstructed labor 660.1
      affecting fetus or newborn 763.1
Malformation (congenital)—*see also* Anomaly
  arteriovenous
    pulmonary 747.32
  bone 756.9
  bursa 756.9
  Chiari
    type I 348.4
    type II (*see also* Spina bifida) 741.0
    type III 742.0
    type IV 742.2
  circulatory system NEC 747.9
    specified type NEC 747.89
  cochlea 744.05
  digestive system NEC 751.9
    lower 751.5
    specified type NEC 751.8
    upper 750.9
  eye 743.9
  gum 750.9
  heart NEC 746.9
    specified type NEC 746.89
    valve 746.9
  internal ear 744.05
  joint NEC 755.9
    specified type NEC 755.8
  Mondini's (congenital) (malformation, cochlea)
    744.05
  muscle 756.9
  nervous system (central) 742.9

Malformation—*continued*
pelvic organs or tissues
  in pregnancy or childbirth 654.9
    affecting fetus or newborn 763.89
    causing obstructed labor 660.2
      affecting fetus or newborn 763.1
placenta (*see also* Placenta, abnormal) 656.7
respiratory organs 748.9
  specified type NEC 748.8
Rieger's 743.44
sense organs NEC 742.9
  specified type NEC 742.8
skin 757.9
  specified type NEC 757.8
spinal cord 742.9
teeth, tooth NEC 520.9
tendon 756.9
throat 750.9
umbilical cord (complicating delivery) 663.9
  affecting fetus or newborn 762.6
umbilicus 759.9
urinary system NEC 753.9
  specified type NEC 753.8
venous —*see* Anomaly, vein
Malfunction —*see also* Dysfunction
arterial graft 996.1
cardiac pacemaker 996.01
catheter device—*see* Complications,
  mechanical, catheter
colostomy 569.62
  valve 569.62
cystostomy 596.82
  infection 596.81
  mechanical 596.82
  specified complication NEC 596.83
device, implant, or graft NEC—*see*
  Complications, mechanical
enteric stoma 569.62
enterostomy 569.62
esophagostomy 530.87
gastroenteric 536.8
gastrostomy 536.42
ileostomy
  valve 569.62
nephrostomy 997.5
pacemaker—*see* Complications, mechanical,
  pacemaker
prosthetic device, internal—*see* Complications,
  mechanical
tracheostomy 519.02
valve
  colostomy 569.62
  ileostomy 569.62
vascular graft or shunt 996.1
Malgaigne's fracture (closed) 808.43
open 808.53
Malherbe's
calcifying epithelioma (M8110/0)—*see*
  Neoplasm, skin, benign
tumor (M8110/0)—*see* Neoplasm, skin, benign
Malibu disease 919.8
infected 919.9
Malignancy (M8000/3)—*see* Neoplasm, by site,
  malignant
Malignant —*see* condition
Malingerer, malingering V65.2
Mallet, finger (acquired) 736.1
congenital 755.59
late effect of rickets 268.1
Malleus 024
Mallory's bodies 034.1
Mallory-Weiss syndrome 530.7

Malnutrition (calorie) 263.9
complicating pregnancy 648.9
degree
  first 263.1
  second 263.0
  third 262
  mild (protein) 263.1
  moderate (protein) 263.0
  severe 261
    protein-calorie 262
fetus 764.2
  "light-for-dates" 764.1
following gastrointestinal surgery 579.3
intrauterine or fetal 764.2
  fetus or infant "light-for-dates" 764.1
lack of care, or neglect (child) (infant) 995.52
  adult 995.84
malignant 260
mild (protein) 263.1
moderate (protein) 263.0
protein 260
protein-calorie 263.9
  mild 263.1
  moderate 263.0
  severe 262
  specified type NEC 263.8
severe 261
  protein-calorie NEC 262
Malocclusion (teeth) 524.4
angle's class I 524.21
angle's class II 524.22
angle's class III 524.23
due to
  abnormal swallowing 524.59
  accessory teeth (causing crowding) 524.31
  dentofacial abnormality NEC 524.89
  impacted teeth (causing crowding) 520.6
  missing teeth 524.30
  mouth breathing 524.59
  sleep posture 524.59
  supernumerary teeth (causing crowding)
    524.31
  thumb sucking 524.59
  tongue, lip, or finger habits 524.59
temporomandibular (joint) 524.69
Malposition
cardiac apex (congenital) 746.87
cervix—*see* Malposition, uterus
congenital
  adrenal (gland) 759.1
  alimentary tract 751.8
    lower 751.5
    upper 750.8
  aorta 747.21
  appendix 751.5
  arterial trunk 747.29
  artery (peripheral) NEC (*see also* Malposition,
    congenital, peripheral vascular system)
    747.60
    coronary 746.85
    pulmonary 747.39
  auditory canal 744.29
    causing impairment of hearing 744.02
  auricle (ear) 744.29
    causing impairment of hearing 744.02
  cervical 744.43
  biliary duct or passage 751.69
  bladder (mucosa) 753.8
    exteriorized or extroverted 753.5
  brachial plexus 742.8
  brain tissue 742.4

Malposition—*continued*
  congenital—*continued*
    breast 757.6
    bronchus 748.3
    cardiac apex 746.87
    cecum 751.5
    clavicle 755.51
    colon 751.5
    digestive organ or tract NEC 751.8
      lower 751.5
      upper 750.8
    ear (auricle) (external) 744.29
      ossicles 744.04
    endocrine (gland) NEC 759.2
    epiglottis 748.3
    Eustachian tube 744.24
    eye 743.8
    facial features 744.89
    fallopian tube 752.19
    finger(s) 755.59
      supernumerary 755.01
    foot 755.67
    gallbladder 751.69
    gastrointestinal tract 751.8
    genitalia, genital organ(s) or tract
      female 752.89
        external 752.49
        internal NEC 752.89
      male 752.89
        penis 752.69
        scrotal transposition 752.81
    glottis 748.3
    hand 755.59
    heart 746.87
      dextrocardia 746.87
        with complete transposition of viscera 759.3
    hepatic duct 751.69
    hip (joint) (*see also* Dislocation, hip, congenital) 754.30
    intestine (large) (small) 751.5
      with anomalous adhesions, fixation, or malrotation 751.4
    joint NEC 755.8
    kidney 753.3
    larynx 748.3
    limb 755.8
      lower 755.69
      upper 755.59
    liver 751.69
    lung (lobe) 748.69
    nail(s) 757.5
    nerve 742.8
    nervous system NEC 742.8
    nose, nasal (septum) 748.1
    organ or site NEC—*see* Anomaly, specified type NEC, by site
    ovary 752.0
    pancreas 751.7
    parathyroid (gland) 759.2
    patella 755.64
    peripheral vascular system 747.60
      gastrointestinal 747.61
      lower limb 747.64
      renal 747.62
      specified NEC 747.69
      spinal 747.82
      upper limb 747.63
    pituitary (gland) 759.2
    respiratory organ or system NEC 748.9

Malposition—*continued*
  congenital—*continued*
    rib (cage) 756.3
      supernumerary in cervical region 756.2
    scapula 755.59
    shoulder 755.59
    spinal cord 742.59
    spine 756.19
    spleen 759.0
    sternum 756.3
    stomach 750.7
    symphysis pubis 755.69
    testis (undescended) 752.51
    thymus (gland) 759.2
    thyroid (gland) (tissue) 759.2
      cartilage 748.3
    toe(s) 755.66
      supernumerary 755.02
    tongue 750.19
    trachea 748.3
    uterus 752.39
    vein(s) (peripheral) NEC (*see also* Malposition, congenital, peripheral vascular system) 747.60
      great 747.49
      portal 747.49
      pulmonary 747.49
    vena cava (inferior) (superior) 747.49
  device, implant, or graft—*see* Complications, mechanical
  fetus NEC (*see also* Presentation, fetal) 652.9
    with successful version 652.1
    affecting fetus or newborn 763.1
    before labor, affecting fetus or newborn 761.7
    causing obstructed labor 660.0
    in multiple gestation (one fetus or more) 652.6
      with locking 660.5
      causing obstructed labor 660.0
  gallbladder (*see also* Disease, gallbladder) 575.8
  gastrointestinal tract 569.89
    congenital 751.8
  heart (*see also* Malposition, congenital, heart) 746.87
  intestine 569.89
    congenital 751.5
  pelvic organs or tissues
    in pregnancy or childbirth 654.4
      affecting fetus or newborn 763.89
      causing obstructed labor 660.2
        affecting fetus or newborn 763.1
  placenta—*see* Placenta, previa
  stomach 537.89
    congenital 750.7
  tooth, teeth 524.30
    with impaction 520.6
  uterus (acquired) (acute) (adherent) (any degree) (asymptomatic) (postinfectional) (postpartal, old) 621.6
    anteflexion or anteversion (*see also* Anteversion, uterus) 621.6
    congenital 752.39
    flexion 621.6
      lateral (*see also* Lateroversion, uterus) 621.6
    in pregnancy or childbirth 654.4
      affecting fetus or newborn 763.89
      causing obstructed labor 660.2
        affecting fetus or newborn 763.1
    inversion 621.6
    lateral (flexion) (version) (*see also* Lateroversion, uterus) 621.6
    lateroflexion (*see also* Lateroversion, uterus) 621.6

Malposition—*continued*
  uterus—*continued*
    lateroversion (*see also* Lateroversion, uterus)
      621.6
    retroflexion or retroversion (*see also*
      Retroversion, uterus) 621.6
Malposture 729.90
Malpresentation, fetus (*see also* Presentation,
  fetal) 652.9
Malrotation
  cecum 751.4
  colon 751.4
  intestine 751.4
  kidney 753.3
MALT (mucosa associated lymphoid tissue) 200.3
Malt workers' lung 495.4
Malta fever (*see also* Brucellosis) 023.9
Maltosuria 271.3
Maltreatment (of)
  adult 995.80
    emotional 995.82
    multiple forms 995.85
    neglect (nutritional) 995.84
    physical 995.81
    psychological 995.82
    sexual 995.83
  child 995.50
    emotional 995.51
    multiple forms 995.59
    neglect (nutritional) 995.52
    psychological 995.51
    physical 995.54
      shaken infant syndrome 995.55
    sexual 995.53
  spouse (*see also* Maltreatment, adult) 995.80
Malum coxae senilis 715.25
Malunion, fracture 733.81
Mammillitis (*see also* Mastitis) 611.0
  puerperal, postpartum 675.2
Mammitis (*see also* Mastitis) 611.0
  puerperal, postpartum 675.2
Mammographic
  calcification 793.89
  calculus 793.89
  microcalcification 793.81
Mammoplasia 611.1
Management
  contraceptive V25.9
    specified type NEC V25.8
  procreative V26.9
    specified type NEC V26.89
Mangled NEC (*see also* nature and site of injury)
  959.9
Mania (monopolar) (*see also* Psychosis,
  affective) 296.0
  alcoholic (acute) (chronic) 291.9
  Bell's—*see* Mania, chronic
  chronic 296.0
    recurrent episode 296.1
    single episode 296.0
  compulsive 300.3
  delirious (acute) 296.0
    recurrent episode 296.1
    single episode 296.0
  epileptic (*see also* Epilepsy) 345.4
  hysterical 300.10
  inhibited 296.89
  puerperal (after delivery) 296.0
    recurrent episode 296.1
    single episode 296.0

Mania—*continued*
  recurrent episode 296.1
  senile 290.8
  single episode 296.0
  stupor 296.89
  stuporous 296.89
  unproductive 296.89
Manic-depressive insanity, psychosis reaction, or
  syndrome (*see also* Psychosis, affective) 296.80
  circular (alternating) 296.7
    currently
      depressed 296.5
      episode unspecified 296.7
      hypomanic, previously depressed 296.4
      manic 296.4
    mixed 296.6
  depressed (type), depressive 296.2
    atypical 296.82
    recurrent episode 296.3
    single episode 296.2
  hypomanic 296.0
    recurrent episode 296.1
    single episode 296.0
  manic 296.0
    atypical 296.81
    recurrent episode 296.1
    single episode 296.0
  mixed NEC 296.89
  perplexed 296.89
  stuporous 296.89
Manifestations, rheumatoid
  lungs 714.81
  pannus—*see* Arthritis, rheumatoid
  subcutaneous nodules—*see* Arthritis, rheumatoid
Mankowsky's syndrome (familial dysplastic
  osteopathy) 731.2
Mannoheptulosuria 271.8
Mannosidosis 271.8
Manson's
  disease (schistosomiasis) 120.1
  pyosis (pemphigus contagiosus) 684
  schistosomiasis 120.1
Mansonellosis 125.5
Manual —*see* condition
Maple bark disease 495.6
Maple bark-strippers' lung 495.6
Maple syrup (urine) disease or syndrome 270.3
Marable's syndrome (celiac artery compression)
  447.4
Marasmus 261
  brain 331.9
  due to malnutrition 261
  intestinal 569.89
  nutritional 261
  senile 797
  tuberculous NEC (*see also* Tuberculosis) 011.9
Marble
  bones 756.52
  skin 782.61
Marburg disease (virus) 078.89
March
  foot 733.94
  hemoglobinuria 283.2
Marchand multiple nodular hyperplasia (liver)
  571.5
Marchesani (-Weill) syndrome
  (brachymorphism and ectopia lentis) 759.89
Marchiafava (-Bignami) disease or syndrome 341.8
Marchiafava-Micheli syndrome (paroxysmal
  nocturnal hemoglobinuria) 283.2

Marcus Gunn's syndrome (jaw-winking syndrome) 742.8

Marfan's
 congenital syphilis 090.49
 disease 090.49
 syndrome (arachnodactyly) 759.82
  meaning congenital syphilis 090.49
   with luxation of lens 090.49 [379.32]

Marginal
 implantation, placenta—see Placenta, previa
 placenta—see Placenta, previa
 sinus (hemorrhage) (rupture) 641.2
  affecting fetus or newborn 762.1

Marie's
 cerebellar ataxia 334.2
 syndrome (acromegaly) 253.0

Marie-Bamberger disease or syndrome
  (hypertrophic) (pulmonary) (secondary) 731.2
 idiopathic (acropachyderma) 757.39
 primary (acropachyderma) 757.39

Marie-Charcot-Tooth neuropathic atrophy, muscle 356.1

Marie-Strümpell arthritis or disease
  (ankylosing spondylitis) 720.0

Marihuana, marijuana
 abuse (see also Abuse, drugs, nondependent) 305.2
 dependence (see also Dependence) 304.3

Marion's disease (bladder neck obstruction) 596.0

Marital conflict V61.10

Mark
 port wine 757.32
 raspberry 757.32
 strawberry 757.32
 stretch 701.3
 tattoo 709.09

Maroteaux-Lamy syndrome
  (mucopolysaccharidosis VI) 277.5

Marriage license examination V70.3

Marrow (bone)
 arrest 284.9
 megakaryocytic 287.30
 poor function 289.9

Marseilles fever 082.1

Marsh's disease (exophthalmic goiter) 242.0

Marshall's (hidrotic) ectodermal dysplasia 757.31

Marsh fever (see also Malaria) 084.6

Martin's disease 715.27

Martin-Albright syndrome
  (pseudohypoparathyroidism) 275.49

Martorell-Fabre syndrome (pulseless disease) 446.7

Masculinization, female with adrenal hyperplasia 255.2

Masculinovoblastoma (M8670/0) 220

Masochism 302.83

Masons' lung 502

Mass
 abdominal 789.3
 anus 787.99
 bone 733.90
 breast 611.72
 cheek 784.2
 chest 786.6
 cystic—see Cyst
 ear 388.8
 epigastric 789.3
 eye 379.92
 female genital organ 625.8
 gum 784.2
 head 784.2

Mass—continued
 intracranial 784.2
 joint 719.60
  ankle 719.67
  elbow 719.62
  foot 719.67
  hand 719.64
  hip 719.65
  knee 719.66
  multiple sites 719.69
  pelvic region 719.65
  shoulder (region) 719.61
  specified site NEC 719.68
  wrist 719.63
 kidney (see also Disease, kidney) 593.9
 lung 786.6
 lymph node 785.6
 malignant (M8000/3)—see Neoplasm, by site, malignant
 mediastinal 786.6
 mouth 784.2
 muscle (limb) 729.89
 neck 784.2
 nose or sinus 784.2
 palate 784.2
 pelvis, pelvic 789.3
 penis 607.89
 perineum 625.8
 rectum 787.99
 scrotum 608.89
 skin 782.2
 specified organ NEC—see Disease of specified organ or site
 splenic 789.2
 substernal 786.6
  thyroid (see also Goiter) 240.9
 superficial (localized) 782.2
 testes 608.89
 throat 784.2
 tongue 784.2
 umbilicus 789.3
 uterus 625.8
 vagina 625.8
 vulva 625.8

Massive —see condition

Mastalgia 611.71
 psychogenic 307.89

Mast cell
 disease 757.33
  systemic (M9741/3) 202.6
 leukemia (M9900/3) 207.8
 sarcoma (M9740/3) 202.6
 tumor (M9740/1) 238.5
  malignant (M9740/3) 202.6

Masters-Allen syndrome 620.6

Mastitis (acute) (adolescent) (diffuse) (interstitial) (lobular) (nonpuerperal) (nonsuppurative) (parenchymatous) (phlegmonous) (simple) (subacute) (suppurative) 611.0
 chronic (cystic) (fibrocystic) 610.1
 cystic 610.1
  Schimmelbusch's type 610.1
 fibrocystic 610.1
 infective 611.0
 lactational 675.2
 lymphangitis 611.0
 neonatal (noninfective) 778.7
  infective 771.5
 periductal 610.4
 plasma cell 610.4

Mastitis—*continued*
puerperal, postpartum, (interstitial)
(nonpurulent) (parenchymatous) 675.2
purulent 675.1
stagnation 676.2
puerperalis 675.2
retromammary 611.0
puerperal, postpartum 675.1
submammary 611.0
puerperal, postpartum 675.1
Mastocytoma (M9740/1) 238.5
malignant (M9740/3) 202.6
Mastocytosis 757.33
malignant (M9741/3) 202.6
systemic (M9741/3) 202.6
Mastodynia 611.71
psychogenic 307.89
Mastoid —*see* condition
Mastoidalgia (*see also* Otalgia) 388.70
Mastoiditis (coalescent) (hemorrhagic)
(pneumococcal) (streptococcal) (suppurative)
383.9
acute or subacute 383.00
with
Gradenigo's syndrome 383.02
petrositis 383.02
specified complication NEC 383.02
subperiosteal abscess 383.01
chronic (necrotic) (recurrent) 383.1
tuberculous (*see also* Tuberculosis) 015.6
Mastopathy, mastopathia 611.9
chronica cystica 610.1
diffuse cystic 610.1
estrogenic 611.89
ovarian origin 611.89
Mastoplasia 611.1
Masturbation 307.9
Maternal condition, affecting fetus or newborn
acute yellow atrophy of liver 760.8
albuminuria 760.1
anesthesia or analgesia 763.5
blood loss 762.1
chorioamnionitis 762.7
circulatory disease, chronic (conditions
classifiable to 390-459, 745-747) 760.3
congenital heart disease (conditions classifiable
to 745-746) 760.3
cortical necrosis of kidney 760.1
death 761.6
diabetes mellitus 775.0
manifest diabetes in the infant 775.1
disease NEC 760.9
circulatory system, chronic (conditions
classifiable to 390-459, 745-747) 760.3
genitourinary system (conditions classifiable
to 580-599) 760.1
respiratory (conditions classifiable to 490-519,
748) 760.3
eclampsia 760.0
hemorrhage NEC 762.1
hepatitis acute, malignant, or subacute 760.8
hyperemesis (gravidarum) 761.8
hypertension (arising during pregnancy)
(conditions classifiable to 642) 760.0
infection
disease classifiable to 001-136 760.2
genital tract NEC 760.8
urinary tract 760.1
influenza 760.2
manifest influenza in the infant 771.2

Maternal condition—*continued*
injury (conditions classifiable to 800-996) 760.5
malaria 760.2
manifest malaria in infant or fetus 771.2
malnutrition 760.4
necrosis of liver 760.8
nephritis (conditions classifiable to 580-583)
760.1
nephrosis (conditions classifiable to 581) 760.1
noxious substance transmitted via breast milk or
placenta 760.70
alcohol 760.71
anticonvulsants 760.77
antifungals 760.74
anti-infective agents 760.74
antimetabolics 760.78
cocaine 760.75
"crack" 760.75
diethylstilbestrol [DES] 760.76
hallucinogenic agents 760.73
medicinal agents NEC 760.79
narcotics 760.72
obstetric anesthetic or analgesic drug 760.72
specified agent NEC 760.79
nutritional disorder (conditions classifiable to
260-269) 760.4
operation unrelated to current delivery (*see also*
Newborn, affected by) 760.64
pre-eclampsia 760.04
pyelitis or pyelonephritis, arising during
pregnancy (conditions classifiable to 590)
760.1
renal disease or failure 760.1
respiratory disease, chronic (conditions
classifiable to 490-519, 748) 760.3
rheumatic heart disease (chronic) (conditions
classifiable to 393-398) 760.3
rubella (conditions classifiable to 056) 760.2
manifest rubella in the infant or fetus 771.0
surgery unrelated to current delivery (*see also*
Newborn, affected by) 760.6
to uterus or pelvic organs 760.64
syphilis (conditions classifiable to 090-097)
760.2
manifest syphilis in the infant or fetus 090.0
thrombophlebitis 760.3
toxemia (of pregnancy) 760.0
pre-eclamptic 760.0
toxoplasmosis (conditions classifiable to 130)
760.2
manifest toxoplasmosis in the infant or fetus
771.2
transmission of chemical substance through the
placenta 760.70
alcohol 760.71
anticonvulsants 760.77
antifungals 760.74
anti-infective agents 760.74
antimetabolics 760.78
cocaine 760.75
"crack" 760.75
diethylstilbestrol [DES] 760.76
hallucinogenic agents 760.73
narcotics 760.72
specified substance NEC 760.79
uremia 760.1
urinary tract conditions (conditions classifiable
to 580-599) 760.1
vomiting (pernicious) (persistent) (vicious) 761.8
Maternity —*see* Delivery
Matheiu's disease (leptospiral jaundice) 100.0
Mauclaire's disease or osteochondrosis 732.3

Maxcy's disease 081.0
Maxilla, maxillary —*see* condition
May (-Hegglin) anomaly or syndrome 288.2
Mayaro fever 066.3
Mazoplasia 610.8
MBD (minimal brain dysfunction), child (*see also* Hyperkinesia) 314.9
MCAD (medium chain acyl CoA dehydrogenase deficiency) 277.85
McArdle (-Schmid-Pearson) disease or syndrome (glycogenosis V) 271.0
McCune-Albright syndrome (osteitis fibrosa disseminata) 756.59
MCLS (mucocutaneous lymph node syndrome) 446.1
McQuarrie's syndrome (idiopathic familial hypoglycemia) 251.2
Measles (black) (hemorrhagic) (suppressed) 055.9
  with
    encephalitis 055.0
    keratitis 055.71
    keratoconjunctivitis 055.71
    otitis media 055.2
    pneumonia 055.1
    complication 055.8
      specified type NEC 055.79
    encephalitis 055.0
    French 056.9
    German 056.9
    keratitis 055.71
    keratoconjunctivitis 055.71
    liberty 056.9
    otitis media 055.2
    pneumonia 055.1
    specified complications NEC 055.79
    vaccination, prophylactic (against) V04.2
Meatitis, urethral (*see also* Urethritis) 597.89
Meat poisoning —*see* Poisoning, food
Meatus, meatal —*see* condition
Meat-wrappers' asthma 506.9
Meckel's
  diverticulitis 751.0
  diverticulum (displaced) (hypertrophic) 751.0
Meconium
  aspiration 770.11
    with
      pneumonia 770.12
      pneumonitis 770.12
      respiratory symptoms 770.12
    below vocal cords 770.11
      with respiratory symptoms 770.12
    syndrome 770.12
  delayed passage in newborn 777.1
  ileus 777.1
    due to cystic fibrosis 277.01
  in liquor 792.3
    noted during delivery 656.8
  insufflation 770.11
    with respiratory symptoms 770.12
  obstruction
    fetus or newborn 777.1
      in mucoviscidosis 277.01
  passage of 792.3
    noted during delivery 763.84
  peritonitis 777.6
  plug syndrome (newborn) NEC 777.1
  staining 779.84

Median —*see also* condition
  arcuate ligament syndrome 447.4
  bar (prostate) 600.90
    with
      other lower urinary tract symptoms (LUTS) 600.91
      urinary
        obstruction 600.91
        retention 600.91
  vesical orifice 600.90
    with
      other lower urinary tract symptoms (LUTS) 600.91
      urinary
        obstruction 600.91
        retention 600.91
  rhomboid glossitis 529.2
Mediastinal shift 793.2
Mediastinitis (acute) (chronic) 519.2
  actinomycotic 039.8
  syphilitic 095.8
  tuberculous (*see also* Tuberculosis) 012.8
Mediastinopericarditis (*see also* Pericarditis) 423.9
  acute 420.90
  chronic 423.8
    rheumatic 393
  rheumatic, chronic 393
Mediastinum, mediastinal —*see* condition
Medical services provided for —*see* Health, services provided because (of)
Medicine poisoning (by overdose) (wrong substance given or taken in error) 977.9
  specified drug or substance—*see* Table of drugs and chemicals
Medin's disease (poliomyelitis) 045.9
Mediterranean
  anemia 282.40
    with other hemoglobinopathy 282.49
  disease or syndrome (hemopathic) 282.40
    with other hemoglobinopathy 282.49
  fever (*see also* Brucellosis) 023.9
    familial 277.31
    kala-azar 085.0
    leishmaniasis 085.0
    tick fever 082.1
Medulla —*see* condition
Medullary
  cystic kidney 753.16
  sponge kidney 753.17
Medullated fibers
  optic (nerve) 743.57
  retina 362.85
Medulloblastoma (M9470/3)
  desmoplastic (M9471/3) 191.6
  specified site—*see* Neoplasm, by site, malignant
  unspecified site 191.6
Medulloepithelioma (M9501/3)—*see also* Neoplasm, by site, malignant
  teratoid (M9502/3)—*see* Neoplasm, by site, malignant
Medullomyoblastoma (M9472/3)
  specified site—*see* Neoplasm, by site, malignant
  unspecified site 191.6
Meekeren-Ehlers-Danlos syndrome 756.83
Megacaryocytic —*see* condition
Megacolon (acquired) (functional) (not Hirschsprung's disease) 564.7
  aganglionic 751.3
  congenital, congenitum 751.3
  Hirschsprung's (disease) 751.3

Megacolon—*continued*
  psychogenic 306.4
  toxic (*see also* Colitis, ulcerative) 556.9
Megaduodenum 537.3
Megaesophagus (functional) 530.0
  congenital 750.4
Megakaryocytic —*see* condition
Megalencephaly 742.4
Megalerythema (epidermicum) (infectiosum)
  057.0
Megalia, cutis et ossium 757.39
Megaloappendix 751.5
Megalocephalus, megalocephaly NEC 756.0
Megalocornea 743.41
  associated with buphthalmos 743.22
Megalocytic anemia 281.9
Megalodactylia (fingers) (thumbs) 755.57
  toes 755.65
Megaloduodenum 751.5
Megaloesophagus (functional) 530.0
  congenital 750.4
Megalogastria (congenital) 750.7
Megalomania 307.9
Megalophthalmos 743.8
Megalopsia 368.14
Megalosplenia (*see also* Splenomegaly) 789.2
Megaloureter 593.89
  congenital 753.22
Megarectum 569.49
Megasigmoid 564.7
  congenital 751.3
Megaureter 593.89
  congenital 753.22
Megrim 346.9
Meibomian
  cyst 373.2
    infected 373.12
  gland—*see* condition
  infarct (eyelid) 374.85
  stye 373.11
Meibomitis 373.12
Meige
  Milroy disease (chronic hereditary edema) 757.0
  syndrome (blepharospasm-oromandibular
    dystonia) 333.82
Melalgia, nutritional 266.2
Melancholia (*see also* Psychosis, affective)
  296.90
  climacteric 296.2
    recurrent episode 296.3
    single episode 296.2
  hypochondriac 300.7
  intermittent 296.2
    recurrent episode 296.3
    single episode 296.2
  involutional 296.2
    recurrent episode 296.3
    single episode 296.2
  menopausal 296.2
    recurrent episode 296.3
    single episode 296.2
  puerperal 296.2
  reactive (from emotional stress, psychological
    trauma) 298.0
  recurrent 296.3
  senile 290.21
  stuporous 296.2
    recurrent episode 296.3
    single episode 296.2
Melanemia 275.0

Melanoameloblastoma (M9363/0)—*see*
  Neoplasm, bone, benign
Melanoblastoma (M8720/3)—*see* Melanoma
Melanoblastosis
  Block-Sulzberger 757.33
  cutis linearis sive systematisata 757.33
Melanocarcinoma (M8720/3)—*see* Melanoma
Melanocytoma, eyeball (M8726/0) 224.0
Melanocytosis, neurocutaneous 757.33
Melanoderma, melanodermia 709.09
  Addison's (primary adrenal insufficiency) 255.41
Melanodontia, infantile 521.05
Melanodontoclasia 521.05
Melanoepithelioma (M8720/3)—*see* Melanoma
Melanoma (malignant) (M8720/3) 172.9

*Note—Except where otherwise indicated, the
morphological varieties of melanoma in the list
below should be coded by site as for
"Melanoma (malignant)." Internal sites should
be coded to malignant neoplasm of those sites.*

  abdominal wall 172.5
  ala nasi 172.3
  amelanotic (M8730/3)—*see* Melanoma, by site
  ankle 172.7
  anus, anal 154.3
    canal 154.2
  arm 172.6
  auditory canal (external) 172.2
  auricle (ear) 172.2
  auricular canal (external) 172.2
  axilla 172.5
  axillary fold 172.5
  back 172.5
  balloon cell (M8722/3)—*see* Melanoma, by site
  benign (M8720/0)—*see* Neoplasm, skin, benign
  breast (female) (male) 172.5
  brow 172.3
  buttock 172.5
  canthus (eye) 172.1
  cheek (external) 172.3
  chest wall 172.5
  chin 172.3
  choroid 190.6
  conjunctiva 190.3
  ear (external) 172.2
  epithelioid cell (M8771/3)—*see also* Melanoma,
    by site
    and spindle cell, mixed (M8775/3)—*see*
      Melanoma, by site
  external meatus (ear) 172.2
  eye 190.9
  eyebrow 172.3
  eyelid (lower) (upper) 172.1
  face NEC 172.3
  female genital organ (external) NEC 184.4
  finger 172.6
  flank 172.5
  foot 172.7
  forearm 172.6
  forehead 172.3
  foreskin 187.1
  gluteal region 172.5
  groin 172.5
  hand 172.6
  heel 172.7
  helix 172.2
  hip 172.7

Melanoma—*continued*
in
  giant pigmented nevus (M8761/3)—*see*
    Melanoma, by site
  Hutchinson's melanotic freckle
    (M8742/3)—*see* Melanoma, by site
  junctional nevus (M8740/3)—*see* Melanoma,
    by site
  precancerous melanosis (M8741/3)—*see*
    Melanoma, by site
in situ—*see* Melanoma, by site
  skin 172.9
interscapular region 172.5
iris 190.0
jaw 172.3
juvenile (M8770/0)—*see* Neoplasm, skin, benign
knee 172.7
labium
  majus 184.1
  minus 184.2
lacrimal gland 190.2
leg 172.7
lip (lower) (upper) 172.0
liver 197.7
lower limb NEC 172.7
male genital organ (external) NEC 187.9
meatus, acoustic (external) 172.2
meibomian gland 172.1
metastatic
  of or from specified site—*see* Melanoma, by site
  site not of skin—*see* Neoplasm, by site,
    malignant, secondary
  to specified site—*see* Neoplasm, by site,
    malignant, secondary
  unspecified site 172.9
nail 172.9
  finger 172.6
  toe 172.7
neck 172.4
nodular (M8721/3)—*see* Melanoma, by site
nose, external 172.3
orbit 190.1
penis 187.4
perianal skin 172.5
perineum 172.5
pinna 172.2
popliteal (fossa) (space) 172.7
prepuce 187.1
pubes 172.5
pudendum 184.4
retina 190.5
scalp 172.4
scrotum 187.7
septum nasal (skin) 172.3
shoulder 172.6
skin NEC 172.8
  in situ 172.9
spindle cell (M8772/3)—*see also* Melanoma, by
  site
  type A (M8773/3) 190.0
  type B (M8774/3) 190.0
submammary fold 172.5
superficial spreading (M8743/3)—*see*
  Melanoma, by site
temple 172.3
thigh 172.7
toe 172.7
trunk NEC 172.5
umbilicus 172.5
upper limb NEC 172.6
vagina vault 184.0
vulva 184.4

Melanoplakia 528.9
Melanosarcoma (M8720/3)—*see also* Melanoma
  epithelioid cell (M8771/3)—*see* Melanoma
Melanosis 709.09
  addisonian (primary adrenal insufficiency)
    255.41
    tuberculous (*see also* Tuberculosis) 017.6
  adrenal 255.41
  colon 569.89
  conjunctiva 372.55
    congenital 743.49
  corii degenerativa 757.33
  cornea (presenile) (senile) 371.12
    congenital 743.43
      interfering with vision 743.42
    prenatal 743.43
      interfering with vision 743.42
  eye 372.55
    congenital 743.49
  jute spinners' 709.09
  lenticularis progressiva 757.33
  liver 573.8
  precancerous (M8741/2)—*see also* Neoplasm,
    skin, in situ
    malignant melanoma in (M8741/3)—*see* Melanoma
  Riehl's 709.09
  sclera 379.19
    congenital 743.47
  suprarenal 255.41
  tar 709.09
  toxic 709.09
Melanuria 791.9
MELAS syndrome (mitochondrial
  encephalopathy, lactic acidosis and stroke-like
  episodes) 277.87
Melasma 709.09
  adrenal (gland) 255.41
  suprarenal (gland) 255.41
Melena 578.1
  due to
    swallowed maternal blood 777.3
    ulcer—*see* Ulcer, by site, with hemorrhage
  newborn 772.4
    due to swallowed maternal blood 777.3
Meleney's
  gangrene (cutaneous) 686.09
  ulcer (chronic undermining) 686.09
Melioidosis 025
Melitensis, febris 023.0
Melitococcosis 023.0
Melkersson (-Rosenthal) syndrome 351.8
Mellitus, diabetes —*see* Diabetes
Melorheostosis (bone) (leri) 733.99
Meloschisis 744.83
Melotia 744.29
Membrana
  capsularis lentis posterior 743.39
  epipapillaris 743.57
Membranacea placenta —*see* Placenta,
  abnormal
Membranaceous uterus 621.8
Membrane, membranous —*see also* condition
  folds, congenital—*see* Web
  Jackson's 751.4
  over face (causing asphyxia), fetus or newborn
    768.9
  premature rupture—*see* Rupture, membranes,
    premature
  pupillary 364.74
    persistent 743.46

Membrane, membranous—*continued*
  retained (complicating delivery) (with
    hemorrhage) 666.2
    without hemorrhage 667.1
  secondary (eye) 366.50
  unruptured (causing asphyxia) 768.9
  vitreous humor 379.25
Membranitis, fetal 658.4
  affecting fetus or newborn 762.7
Memory disturbance, loss or lack (*see also*
  Amnesia) 780.93
  mild, following organic brain damage 310.89
MEN (multiple endocrine neoplasia) syndrome
  type 1 258.01
  type IIA 258.02
  type IIB 258.03
Menadione (vitamin K) deficiency 269.0
Menarche, precocious 259.1
Mendacity, pathologic 301.7
Mende's syndrome (ptosis-epicanthus) 270.2
Mendelson's syndrome (resulting from a
  procedure) 997.32
  obstetric 668.0
Ménétrier's disease or syndrome (hypertrophic
  gastritis) 535.2
Ménière's disease, syndrome, or vertigo 386.00
  cochlear 386.02
  cochleovestibular 386.01
  inactive 386.04
  in remission 386.04
  vestibular 386.03
Meninges, meningeal —*see* condition
Meningioma (M9530/0)—*see also* Neoplasm,
  meninges, benign
  angioblastic (M9535/0)—*see* Neoplasm,
    meninges, benign
  angiomatous (M9534/0)—*see* Neoplasm,
    meninges, benign
  endotheliomatous (M9531/0)—*see* Neoplasm,
    meninges, benign
  fibroblastic (M9532/0)—*see* Neoplasm,
    meninges, benign
  fibrous (M9532/0)—*see* Neoplasm, meninges,
    benign
  hemangioblastic (M9535/0)—*see* Neoplasm,
    meninges, benign
  hemangiopericytic (M9536/0)—*see* Neoplasm,
    meninges, benign
  malignant (M9530/3)—*see* Neoplasm,
    meninges, malignant
  meningiothelial (M9531/0)—*see* Neoplasm,
    meninges, benign
  meningotheliomatous (M9531/0)—*see*
    Neoplasm, meninges, benign
  mixed (M9537/0)—*see* Neoplasm, meninges,
    benign
  multiple (M9530/1) 237.6
  papillary (M9538/1) 237.6
  psammomatous (M9533/0)—*see* Neoplasm,
    meninges, benign
  syncytial (M9531/0)—*see* Neoplasm, meninges,
    benign
  transitional (M9537/0)—*see* Neoplasm,
    meninges, benign
Meningiomatosis (diffuse) (M9530/1) 237.6
Meningism (*see also* Meningismus) 781.6
Meningismus (infectional) (pneumococcal) 781.6
  due to serum or vaccine 997.09 *[321.8]*
  influenzal NEC (*see also* Influenza) 487.8

Meningitis (basal) (basic) (basilar) (brain) (cerebral)
  (cervical) (congestive) (diffuse) (hemorrhagic)
  (infantile) (membranous) (metastatic)
  (nonspecific) (pontine) (progressive) (simple)
  (spinal) (subacute) (sympathetica) (toxic) 322.9
  abacterial NEC (*see also* Meningitis, aseptic) 047.9
  actinomycotic 039.8 *[320.7]*
  adenoviral 049.1
  Aerobacter aerogenes 320.82
  anaerobes (cocci) (gram-negative)
    (gram-positive) (mixed) (NEC) 320.81
  arbovirus NEC 066.9 *[321.2]*
    specified type NEC 066.8 *[321.2]*
  aseptic (acute) NEC 047.9
    adenovirus 049.1
    Coxsackie virus 047.0
    due to
      adenovirus 049.1
      Coxsackie virus 047.0
      ECHO virus 047.1
      enterovirus 047.9
      mumps 072.1
      poliovirus (*see also* Poliomyelitis) 045.2 *[321.2]*
    ECHO virus 047.1
    herpes (simplex) virus 054.72
      zoster 053.0
    leptospiral 100.81
    lymphocytic choriomeningitis 049.0
    noninfective 322.0
  Bacillus pyocyaneus 320.89
  bacterial NEC 320.9
    anaerobic 320.81
    gram-negative 320.82
      anaerobic 320.81
  Bacteroides (fragilis) (oralis) (melaninogenicus)
    320.81
  cancerous (M8000/6) 198.4
  candidal 112.83
  carcinomatous (M8010/6) 198.4
  caseous (*see also* Tuberculosis, meninges) 013.0
  cerebrospinal (acute) (chronic) (diplococcal)
    (endemic) (epidemic) (fulminant) (infectious)
    (malignant) (meningococcal) (sporadic) 036.0
    carrier (suspected) of V02.59
  chronic NEC 322.2
  clear cerebrospinal fluid NEC 322.0
  Clostridium (haemolyticum) (novyi) NEC 320.81
  coccidioidomycosis 114.2
  Coxsackie virus 047.0
  cryptococcal 117.5 *[321.0]*
  diplococcal 036.0
    gram-negative 036.0
    gram-positive 320.1
  Diplococcus pneumoniae 320.1
  due to
    actinomycosis 039.8 *[320.7]*
    adenovirus 049.1
    coccidiomycosis 114.2
    enterovirus 047.9
      specified NEC 047.8
    histoplasmosis (*see also* Histoplasmosis) 115.91
    Listerosis 027.0 *[320.7]*
    Lyme disease 088.81 *[320.7]*
    moniliasis 112.83
    mumps 072.1
    neurosyphilis 094.2
    nonbacterial organisms NEC 321.8
    oidiomycosis 112.83
    poliovirus (*see also* Poliomyelitis) 045.2
      [321.2]

Meningitis—*continued*
 due to—*continued*
  preventive immunization, inoculation, or
    vaccination 997.09 *[321.8]*
  sarcoidosis 135 *[321.4]*
  sporotrichosis 117.1 *[321.1]*
  syphilis 094.2
   acute 091.81
   congenital 090.42
   secondary 091.81
  trypanosomiasis (*see also* Trypanosomiasis)
    086.9 *[321.3]*
  whooping cough 033.9 *[320.7]*
 E. coli 320.82
 ECHO virus 047.1
 endothelial-leukocytic, benign, recurrent 047.9
 Enterobacter aerogenes 320.82
 enteroviral 047.9
  specified type NEC 047.8
 enterovirus 047.9
  specified NEC 047.8
 eosinophilic 322.1
 epidemic NEC 036.0
 Escherichia coli (E. coli) 320.82
 Eubacterium 320.81
 fibrinopurulent NEC 320.9
  specified type NEC 320.89
 Friedländer (bacillus) 320.82
 fungal NEC 117.9 *[321.1]*
 Fusobacterium 320.81
 gonococcal 098.82
 gram-negative bacteria NEC 320.82
  anaerobic 320.81
  cocci 036.0
   specified NEC 320.82
 gram-negative cocci NEC 036.0
  specified NEC 320.82
 gram-positive cocci NEC 320.9
 H. influenzae 320.0
 herpes (simplex) virus 054.72
  zoster 053.0
 infectious NEC 320.9
 influenzal 320.0
 Klebsiella pneumoniae 320.82
 late effect—*see* Late, effect, meningitis
 leptospiral (aseptic) 100.81
 Listerella (monocytogenes) 027.0 *[320.7]*
 Listeria monocytogenes 027.0 *[320.7]*
 lymphocytic (acute) (benign) (serous) 049.0
  choriomeningitis virus 049.0
 meningococcal (chronic) 036.0
 Mima polymorpha 320.82
 Mollaret's 047.9
 monilial 112.83
 mumps (virus) 072.1
 mycotic NEC 117.9 *[321.1]*
 Neisseria 036.0
 neurosyphilis 094.2
 nonbacterial NEC (*see also* Meningitis, aseptic) 047.9
 nonpyogenic NEC 322.0
 oidiomycosis 112.83
 ossificans 349.2
 Peptococcus 320.81
 Peptostreptococcus 320.81
 pneumococcal 320.1
 poliovirus (*see also* Poliomyelitis) 045.2 *[321.2]*
 Proprionibacterium 320.81
 Proteus morganii 320.82
 Pseudomonas (aeruginosa) (pyocyaneus) 320.82
 purulent NEC 320.9
  specified organism NEC 320.89

Meningitis—*continued*
 pyogenic NEC 320.9
  specified organism NEC 320.89
 Salmonella 003.21
 septic NEC 320.9
  specified organism NEC 320.89
 serosa circumscripta NEC 322.0
 serous NEC (*see also* Meningitis, aseptic) 047.9
  lymphocytic 049.0
  syndrome 348.2
 Serratia (marcescens) 320.82
  specified organism NEC 320.89
 sporadic cerebrospinal 036.0
 sporotrichosis 117.1 *[321.1]*
 staphylococcal 320.3
 sterile 997.09
 streptococcal (acute) 320.2
 suppurative 320.9
  specified organism NEC 320.89
 syphilitic 094.2
  acute 091.81
  congenital 090.42
  secondary 091.81
 torula 117.5 *[321.0]*
 traumatic (complication of injury) 958.8
 Treponema (denticola) (macrodenticum) 320.81
 trypanosomiasis 086.1 *[321.3]*
 tuberculous (*see also* Tuberculosis, meninges) 013.0
 typhoid 002.0 *[320.7]*
 Veillonella 320.81
 Vibrio vulnificus 320.82
 viral, virus NEC (*see also* Meningitis, aseptic)
    047.9
 Wallgren's (*see also* Meningitis, aseptic) 047.9
Meningocele (congenital) (spinal) (*see also* Spina
    bifida) 741.9
 acquired (traumatic) 349.2
 cerebral 742.0
 cranial 742.0
Meningocerebritis —*see* Meningoencephalitis
Meningococcemia (acute) (chronic) 036.2
Meningococcus, meningococcal (*see also*
    condition) 036.9
 adrenalitis, hemorrhagic 036.3
 carditis 036.40
 carrier (suspected) of V02.59
 cerebrospinal fever 036.0
 encephalitis 036.1
 endocarditis 036.42
 exposure to V01.84
 infection NEC 036.9
 meningitis (cerebrospinal) 036.0
 myocarditis 036.43
 optic neuritis 036.81
 pericarditis 036.41
 septicemia (chronic) 036.2
Meningoencephalitis (*see also* Encephalitis)
    323.9
 acute NEC 048
 bacterial, purulent, pyogenic, or septic—*see*
    Meningitis
 chronic NEC 094.1
 diffuse NEC 094.1
 diphasic 063.2
 due to
  actinomycosis 039.8 *[320.7]*
  blastomycosis NEC (*see also* Blastomycosis)
    116.0 *[323.41]*
  free-living amebae 136.29
  Listeria monocytogenes 027.0 *[320.7]*
  Lyme disease 088.81 *[320.7]*

Meningoencephalitis—*continued*
due to—*continued*
mumps 072.2
Naegleria (amebae) (gruberi) (organisms) 136.29
rubella 056.01
sporotrichosis 117.1 *[321.1]*
toxoplasmosis (acquired) 130.0
congenital (active) 771.2 *[323.41]*
Trypanosoma 086.1 *[323.2]*
epidemic 036.0
herpes 054.3
herpetic 054.3
H. influenzae 320.0
infectious (acute) 048
influenzal 320.0
late effect—*see* category 326
Listeria monocytogenes 027.0 *[320.7]*
lymphocytic (serous) 049.0
mumps 072.2
parasitic NEC 123.9 *[323.41]*
pneumococcal 320.1
primary amebic 136.29
rubella 056.01
serous 048
lymphocytic 049.0
specific 094.2
staphylococcal 320.3
streptococcal 320.2
syphilitic 094.2
toxic NEC 989.9 *[323.71]*
due to
carbon tetrachloride (vapor) 987.8 *[323.71]*
hydroxyquinoline derivatives poisoning 961.3 *[323.71]*
lead 984.9 *[323.71]*
mercury 985.0 *[323.71]*
thallium 985.8 *[323.71]*
toxoplasmosis (acquired) 130.0
trypanosomic 086.1 *[323.2]*
tuberculous (*see also* Tuberculosis, meninges) 013.0
virus NEC 048
Meningoencephalocele 742.0
syphilitic 094.89
congenital 090.49
Meningoencephalomyelitis (*see also* Meningoencephalitis) 323.9
acute NEC 048
disseminated (postinfectious) 136.9 *[323.61]*
postimmunization or postvaccination 323.51
due to
actinomycosis 039.8 *[320.7]*
torula 117.5 *[323.41]*
toxoplasma or toxoplasmosis (acquired) 130.0
congenital (active) 771.2 *[323.41]*
late effect—*see* category 326
Meningoencephalomyelopathy (*see also* Meningoencephalomyelitis) 349.9
Meningoencephalopathy (*see also* Meningoencephalitis) 348.39
Meningoencephalopoliomyelitis (*see also* Poliomyelitis, bulbar) 045.0
late effect 138
Meningomyelitis (*see also* Meningoencephalitis) 323.9
blastomycotic NEC (*see also* Blastomycosis) 116.0 *[323.41]*

Meningomyelitis—*continued*
due to
actinomycosis 039.8 *[320.7]*
blastomycosis (*see also* Blastomycosis) 116.0 *[323.41]*
Meningococcus 036.0
sporotrichosis 117.1 *[323.41]*
torula 117.5 *[323.41]*
late effect—*see* category 326
lethargic 049.8
meningococcal 036.0
syphilitic 094.2
tuberculous (*see* Tuberculosis, meninges) 013.0
Meningomyelocele (*see also* Spina bifida) 741.9
syphilitic 094.89
Meningomyeloneuritis —*see* Meningoencephalitis
Meningoradiculitis —*see* Meningitis
Meningovascular —*see* condition
Meniscocytosis 282.60
Menkes' syndrome —*see* Syndrome, Menkes'
Menolipsis 626.0
Menometrorrhagia 626.2
Menopause, menopausal (symptoms) (syndrome) 627.2
arthritis (any site) NEC 716.3
artificial 627.4
bleeding 627.0
crisis 627.2
depression (*see also* Psychosis, affective) 296.2
agitated 296.2
recurrent episode 296.3
single episode 296.2
psychotic 296.2
recurrent episode 296.3
single episode 296.2
recurrent episode 296.3
single episode 296.2
melancholia (*see also* Psychosis, affective) 296.2
recurrent episode 296.3
single episode 296.2
paranoid state 297.2
paraphrenia 297.2
postsurgical 627.4
premature 256.31
postirradiation 256.2
postsurgical 256.2
psychoneurosis 627.2
psychosis NEC 298.8
surgical 627.4
toxic polyarthritis NEC 716.39
Menorrhagia (primary) 626.2
climacteric 627.0
menopausal 627.0
postclimacteric 627.1
postmenopausal 627.1
preclimacteric 627.0
premenopausal 627.0
puberty (menses retained) 626.3
Menorrhalgia 625.3
Menoschesis 626.8
Menostaxis 626.2
Menses, retention 626.8
Menstrual —*see* Menstruation
cycle, irregular 626.4
disorders NEC 626.9
extraction V25.3
fluid, retained 626.8
molimen 625.4
period, normal V65.5
regulation V25.3

Menstruation
absent 626.0
anovulatory 628.0
delayed 626.8
difficult 625.3
disorder 626.9
    psychogenic 306.52
    specified NEC 626.8
during pregnancy 640.8
excessive 626.2
frequent 626.2
infrequent 626.1
irregular 626.4
latent 626.8
membranous 626.8
painful (primary) (secondary) 625.3
    psychogenic 306.52
passage of clots 626.2
precocious 259.1
protracted 626.8
retained 626.8
retrograde 626.8
scanty 626.1
suppression 626.8
vicarious (nasal) 625.8
Mentagra (*see also* Sycosis) 704.8
Mental —*see also* condition
deficiency (*see also* Disability, intellectual) 319
deterioration (*see also* Psychosis) 298.9
disorder (*see also* Disorder, mental) 300.9
exhaustion 300.5
insufficiency (congenital) (*see also* Disability,
    intellectual) 319
observation without need for further medical
    care NEC V71.09
retardation —*see* Disability, intellectual
subnormality (*see also* Disability, intellectual)
    319
    mild 317
    moderate 318.0
    profound 318.2
    severe 318.1
upset (*see also* Disorder, mental) 300.9
Meralgia paresthetica 355.1
Mercurial —*see* condition
Mercurialism NEC 985.0
Merergasia 300.9
Merkel cell tumor —*see* Carcinoma, Merkel cell
Merocele (*see also* Hernia, femoral) 553.00
Meromelia 755.4
lower limb 755.30
    intercalary 755.32
        femur 755.34
            tibiofibular (complete) (incomplete)
                755.33
        fibula 755.37
        metatarsal(s) 755.38
        tibia 755.36
        tibiofibular 755.35
    terminal (complete) (partial) (transverse)
        755.31
        longitudinal 755.32
            metatarsal(s) 755.38
            phalange(s) 755.39
            tarsal(s) 755.38
        transverse 755.31

Meromelia—*continued*
upper limb 755.20
    intercalary 755.22
        carpal(s) 755.28
        humeral 755.24
            radioulnar (complete) (incomplete) 755.23
        metacarpal(s) 755.28
        phalange(s) 755.29
        radial 755.26
        radioulnar 755.25
        ulnar 755.27
    terminal (complete) (partial) (transverse) 755.21
        longitudinal 755.22
            carpal(s) 755.28
            metacarpal(s) 755.28
            phalange(s) 755.29
        transverse 755.21
Merosmia 781.1
MERRF syndrome (myoclonus with epilepsy
    and with ragged red fibers) 277.87
Merycism (*see also* Rumination)—*see also*
    Vomiting
    psychogenic 307.53
Merzbacher-Pelizaeus disease 330.0
Mesaortitis —*see* Aortitis
Mesarteritis —*see* Arteritis
Mesencephalitis (*see also* Encephalitis) 323.9
    late effect—*see* category 326
Mesenchymoma (M8990/1)—*see also*
    Neoplasm, connective tissue, uncertain
    behavior
    benign (M8990/0)—*see* Neoplasm, connective
        tissue, benign
    malignant (M8990/3)—*see* Neoplasm,
        connective tissue, malignant
Mesenteritis
retractile 567.82
sclerosing 567.82
Mesentery, mesenteric —*see* condition
Mesiodens, mesiodentes 520.1
causing crowding 524.31
Mesio-occlusion 524.23
Mesocardia (with asplenia) 746.87
Mesocolon —*see* condition
Mesonephroma (malignant) (M9110/3)—*see*
    also Neoplasm, by site, malignant
    benign (M9110/0)—*see* Neoplasm, by site, benign
Mesophlebitis —*see* Phlebitis
Mesostromal dysgenesis 743.51
Mesothelioma (malignant) (M9050/3)—*see also*
    Neoplasm, by site, malignant
    benign (M9050/0)—*see* Neoplasm, by site, benign
    biphasic type (M9053/3)—*see also* Neoplasm,
        by site, malignant
        benign (M9053/0)—*see* Neoplasm, by site,
            benign
    epithelioid (M9052/3)—*see also* Neoplasm, by
        site, malignant
        benign (M9052/0)—*see* Neoplasm, by site,
            benign
    fibrous (M9051/3)—*see also* Neoplasm, by site,
        malignant
        benign (M9051/0)—*see* Neoplasm, by site,
            benign
Metabolic syndrome 277.7
Metabolism disorder 277.9
specified type NEC 277.89
Metagonimiasis 121.5
Metagonimus infestation (small intestine) 121.5

Metal
  pigmentation (skin) 709.00
  polishers' disease 502
Metalliferous miners' lung 503
Metamorphopsia 368.14
Metaplasia
  bone, in skin 709.3
  breast 611.89
  cervix—*omit code*
  endometrium (squamous) 621.8
  esophagus 530.85
  intestinal, of gastric mucosa 537.89
  kidney (pelvis) (squamous) (*see also* Disease,
    renal) 593.89
  myelogenous 289.89
  myeloid 289.89
    agnogenic 238.76
    megakaryocytic 238.76
  spleen 289.59
  squamous cell
    amnion 658.8
    bladder 596.89
    cervix—*see* condition
    trachea 519.19
    tracheobronchial tree 519.19
    uterus 621.8
      cervix—*see* condition
Metastasis, metastatic
  abscess—*see* Abscess
  calcification 275.40
  cancer, neoplasm, or disease
    from specified site (M8000/3)—*see*
      Neoplasm, by site, malignant
    to specified site (M8000/6)—*see* Neoplasm,
      by site, secondary
  deposits (in) (M8000/6)—*see* Neoplasm, by site,
    secondary
  mesentery, of neuroendocrine tumor 209.74
  pneumonia 038.8 *[484.8]*
  spread (to) (M8000/6)—*see* Neoplasm, by site,
    secondary
Metatarsalgia 726.70
  anterior 355.6
  due to Freiberg's disease 732.5
  Morton's 355.6
Metatarsus, metatarsal —*see also* condition
  adductus varus (congenital) 754.53
  abductus valgus (congenital) 764.60
  primus varus 754.52
  valgus (adductus) (congenital) 754.60
  varus (abductus) (congenital) 754.53
    primus 754.52
Methadone use 304.00
Methemoglobinemia 289.7
  acquired (with sulfhemoglobinemia) 289.7
  congenital 289.7
  enzymatic 289.7
  Hb-M disease 289.7
  hereditary 289.7
  toxic 289.7
Methemoglobinuria (*see also* Hemoglobinuria)
  791.2
Methicillin
  resistant staphylococcus aureus (MRSA) 041.12
    colonization V02.54
    personal history of V12.04
  susceptible staphylococcus aureus (MSSA)
    041.11
    colonization V02.53
Methioninemia 270.4

Metritis (catarrhal) (septic) (suppurative) (*see
    also* Endometritis) 615.9
  blennorrhagic 098.16
    chronic or duration of 2 months or over 098.36
  cervical (*see also* Cervicitis) 616.0
  gonococcal 098.16
    chronic or duration of 2 months or over 098.36
  hemorrhagic 626.8
  puerperal, postpartum, childbirth 670.1
    septic 670.2
  tuberculous (*see also* Tuberculosis) 016.7
Metropathia hemorrhagica 626.8
Metroperitonitis (*see also* Peritonitis, pelvic,
    female) 614.5
Metrorrhagia 626.6
  arising during pregnancy—*see* Hemorrhage,
    pregnancy
  postpartum NEC 666.2
  primary 626.6
  psychogenic 306.59
  puerperal 666.2
Metrorrhexis —*see* Rupture, uterus
Metrosalpingitis (*see also* Salpingo-oophoritis)
  614.2
Metrostaxis 626.6
Metrovaginitis (*see also* Endometritis) 615.9
  gonococcal (acute) 098.16
    chronic or duration of 2 months or over 098.36
Mexican fever —*see* Typhus, Mexican
Meyenburg-Altherr-Uehlinger syndrome
  733.99
Meyer-Schwickerath and Weyers syndrome
  (dysplasia oculodentodigitalis) 759.89
Meynert's amentia (nonalcoholic) 294.0
  alcoholic 291.1
Mibelli's disease 757.39
Mice, joint (*see also* Loose, body, joint) 718.1
  knee 717.6
Micheli-Rietti syndrome (thalassemia minor)
  282.46
Michotte's syndrome 721.5
Micrencephalon, micrencephaly 742.1
Microalbuminuria 791.0
Microaneurysm, retina 362.14
  diabetic 250.5 *[362.01]*
    due to secondary diabetes 249.5 *[362.01]*
Microangiopathy 443.9
  diabetic (peripheral) 250.7 *[443.81]*
    due to secondary diabetes 249.7 *[443.81]*
    retinal 250.5 *[362.01]*
      due to secondary diabetes 249.5 *[362.01]*
  peripheral 443.9
    diabetic 250.7 *[443.81]*
      due to secondary diabetes 249.7 *[443.81]*
  retinal 362.18
    diabetic 250.5 *[362.01]*
      due to secondary diabetes 249.5 *[362.01]*
  thrombotic 446.6
    Moschcowitz's (thrombotic thrombocytopenic
      purpura) 446.6
Microcalcification, mammographic 793.81
Microcephalus, microcephalic, microcephaly
  742.1
  due to toxoplasmosis (congenital) 771.2
Microcheilia 744.82
Microcolon (congenital) 751.5
Microcornea (congenital) 743.41
Microcytic —*see* condition
Microdeletions NEC 758.33
Microdontia 520.2

Microdrepanocytosis (thalassemia-Hb-S disease) 282.41
with sickle cell crisis 282.42
Microembolism
atherothrombotic—*see also* Atheroembolism
retina 362.33
Microencephalon 742.1
Microfilaria streptocerca infestation 125.3
Microgastria (congenital) 750.7
Microgenia 524.06
Microgenitalia (congenital) 752.89
penis 752.64
Microglioma (M9710/3)
specified site—*see* Neoplasm, by site, malignant
unspecified site 191.9
Microglossia (congenital) 750.16
Micrognathia, micrognathism (congenital) 524.00
mandibular 524.04
alveolar 524.74
maxillary 524.03
alveolar 524.73
Microgyria (congenital) 742.2
Microinfarct, heart (*see also* Insufficiency, coronary) 411.89
Microlithiasis, alveolar, pulmonary 516.2
Micromastia 611.82
Micromyelia (congenital) 742.59
Micropenis 752.64
Microphakia (congenital) 743.36
Microphthalmia (congenital) (*see also* Microphthalmos) 743.10
Microphthalmos (congenital) 743.10
associated with eye and adnexal anomalies NEC 743.12
due to toxoplasmosis (congenital) 771.2
isolated 743.11
simple 743.11
syndrome 759.89
Micropsia 368.14
Microsporidiosis 136.8
Microsporon furfur infestation 111.0
Microsporosis (*see also* Dermatophytosis) 110.9
nigra 111.1
Microstomia (congenital) 744.84
Microthelia 757.6
Microthromboembolism —*see* Embolism
Microtia (congenital) (external ear) 744.23
Microtropia 378.34
Microvillus inclusion disease (MVD) 751.5
Micturition
disorder NEC 788.69
psychogenic 306.53
frequency 788.41
psychogenic 306.53
nocturnal 788.43
painful 788.1
psychogenic 306.53
Middle
ear—*see* condition
lobe (right) syndrome 518.0
Midplane —*see* condition
Miescher's disease 709.3
cheilitis 351.8
granulomatosis disciformis 709.3
Miescher-Leder syndrome or granulomatosis 709.3
Mieten's syndrome 759.89

Migraine (idiopathic) 346.9

Note: The following fifth digit subclassification is for use with category 346

0 without mention of intractable migraine
without mention of status migrainosus
without mention of refractory migraine
without mention of status migrainosus
1 with intractable migraine, so stated, without mention of status migrainosus
with refractory migraine, so stated, without mention of status migrainosus
2 without mention of intractable migraine with status migrainosus
without mention of refractory migraine with status migrainosus
3 with intractable migraine, so stated, with status migrainosus
with refractory migraine, so stated, with status migrainosus

with aura (acute-onset) (without headache) (prolonged) (typical) 346.0
without aura 346.1
chronic 346.7
transformed 346.7
abdominal (syndrome) 346.2
allergic (histamine) 346.2
atypical 346.8
basilar 346.0
chronic without aura 346.7
classic(al) 346.0
common 346.1
comlicated 346.0
hemiplegic 346.3
familial 346.3
sporadic 346.3
lower-half 339.00
menstrual 346.4
menstrually related 346.4
ophthalmic 346.8
ophthalmoplegic 346.2
premenstrual 346.4
pure menstrual 346.4
retinal 346.0
specified form NEC 346.8
transformed without aura 346.7
variant 346.2
Migrant, social V60.0
Migratory, migrating —*see also* condition
person V60.0
testis, congenital 752.52
Mikulicz's disease or syndrome (dryness of mouth, absent or decreased lacrimation) 527.1
Milian atrophia blanche 701.3
Miliaria (crystallina) (rubra) (tropicalis) 705.1
apocrine 705.82
Miliary —*see* condition
Milium (*see also* Cyst, sebaceous) 706.2
colloid 709.3
eyelid 374.84
Milk
crust 690.11
excess secretion 676.6
fever, female 672
poisoning 988.8
retention 676.2
sickness 988.8
spots 423.1
Milkers' nodes 051.1

Milk-leg (deep vessels) 671.4
  complicating pregnancy 671.3
  nonpuerperal 451.19
  puerperal, postpartum, childbirth 671.4
Milkman (-Looser) disease or syndrome
  (osteomalacia with pseudofractures) 268.2
Milky urine (*see also* Chyluria) 791.1
Millar's asthma (laryngismus stridulus) 478.75
Millard-Gubler paralysis or syndrome 344.89
Millard-Gubler-Foville paralysis 344.89
Miller-Dieker syndrome 758.33
Miller's disease (osteomalacia) 268.2
Miller Fisher's syndrome 357.0
Milles' syndrome (encephalocutaneous
  angiomatosis) 759.6
Mills' disease 335.29
Millstone makers' asthma or lung 502
Milroy's disease (chronic hereditary edema) 757.0
Miners' —*see also* condition
  asthma 500
  elbow 727.2
  knee 727.2
  lung 500
  nystagmus 300.89
  phthisis (*see also* Tuberculosis) 011.4
  tuberculosis (*see also* Tuberculosis) 011.4
Minkowski-Chauffard syndrome (*see also*
  Spherocytosis) 282.0
Minor —*see* condition
Minor's disease 336.1
Minot's disease (hemorrhagic disease, newborn)
  776.0
Minot-von Willebrand (-Jürgens) disease or
  syndrome (angiohemophilia) 286.4
Minus (and plus) hand (intrinsic) 736.09
Miosis (persistent) (pupil) 379.42
Mirizzi's syndrome (hepatic duct stenosis) (*see
  also* Obstruction, biliary) 576.2
  with calculus, cholelithiasis, or stones—*see*
    Choledocholithiasis
Mirror writing 315.09
  secondary to organic lesion 784.69
Misadventure (prophylactic) (therapeutic) (*see
  also* Complications) 999.9
  administration of insulin 962.3
  infusion—*see* Complications, infusion
  local applications (of fomentations, plasters,
    etc.) 999.9
    burn or scald—*see* Burn, by site
  medical care (early) (late) NEC 999.9
    adverse effect of drugs or chemicals—*see*
      Table of drugs and chemicals
    burn or scald—*see* Burn, by site
  radiation NEC 990
  radiotherapy NEC 990
  surgical procedure (early) (late)—*see*
    Complications, surgical procedure
  transfusion—*see* Complications, transfusion
  vaccination or other immunological
    procedure—*see* Complications, vaccination
Misanthropy 301.7
Miscarriage —*see* Abortion, spontaneous
Mischief, malicious, child (*see also* Disturbance,
  conduct) 312.0
Misdirection
  aqueous 365.83
Mismanagement, feeding 783.3

Misplaced, misplacement
  kidney (*see also* Disease, renal) 593.0
    congenital 753.3
  organ or site, congenital NEC—*see* Malposition,
    congenital
Missed
  abortion 632
  delivery (at or near term) 656.4
  labor (at or near term) 656.4
Misshapen reconstructed breast 612.0
Missing —*see also* Absence
  teeth (acquired) 525.10
    congenital (*see also* Anodontia) 520.0
    due to
      caries 525.13
      extraction 525.10
      periodontal disease 525.12
      trauma 525.11
      specified NEC 525.19
  vertebrae (congenital) 756.13
Misuse of drugs NEC (*see also* Abuse, drug,
  nondependent) 305.9
Mitchell's disease (erythromelalgia) 443.82
Mite (s)
  diarrhea 133.8
  grain (itch) 133.8
  hair follicle (itch) 133.8
  in sputum 133.8
**Mitochondrial encephalopathy, lactic acidosis
  and stroke-like episodes** (MELAS
  syndrome) 277.87
**Mitochondrial neurogastrointestinal
  encephalopathy syndrome (MNGIE)** 277.87
Mitral —*see* condition
Mittelschmerz 625.2
Mixed —*see* condition
Mljet disease (mal de Meleda) 757.39
Mobile, mobility
  cecum 751.4
  coccyx 733.99
  excessive—*see* Hypermobility
  gallbladder 751.69
  kidney 593.0
    congenital 753.3
  organ or site, congenital NEC—*see* Malposition,
    congenital
  spleen 289.59
Mobitz heart block (atrioventricular) 426.10
  type I (Wenckebach's) 426.13
  type II 426.12
Möbius'
  disease 346.2
  syndrome
    congenital oculofacial paralysis 352.6
    ophthalmoplegic migraine 346.2
Moeller (-Barlow) disease (infantile scurvy) 267
  glossitis 529.4
Mohr's syndrome (Types I and II) 759.89
Mola destruens (M9100/1) 236.1
Molarization, premolars 520.2
Molar pregnancy 631.8
  hydatidiform (delivered) (undelivered) 630
Mold (s) in vitreous 117.9
Molding, head (during birth)—*omit code*
Mole (pigmented) (M8720/0)—*see also*
  Neoplasm, skin, benign
  blood 631.8
  Breus' 631.8
  cancerous (M8720/3)—*see* Melanoma
  carneous 631.8
  destructive (M9100/1) 236.1

Mole—*continued*
  ectopic—*see* Pregnancy, ectopic
  fleshy 631.8
  hemorrhagic 631.8
  hydatid, hydatidiform (benign) (complicating
    pregnancy) (delivered) (undelivered) (*see*
    also Hydatidiform mole) 630
    invasive (M9100/1) 236.1
    malignant (M9100/1) 236.1
    previous, affecting management of pregnancy
      V23.1
  invasive (hydatidiform) (M9100/1) 236.1
  malignant
    meaning
      malignant hydatidiform mole (M9100/1) 236.1
      melanoma (M8720/3)—*see* Melanoma
  nonpigmented (M8730/0)—*see* Neoplasm, skin,
    benign
  pregnancy NEC 631.8
  skin (M8720/0)—*see* Neoplasm, skin, benign
  stone 631.8
  tubal—*see* Pregnancy, tubal
  vesicular (*see also* Hydatidiform mole) 630
Molimen, molimina (menstrual) 625.4
Mollaret's meningitis 047.9
Mollities (cerebellar) (cerebral) 437.8
  ossium 268.2
Molluscum
  contagiosum 078.0
  epitheliale 078.0
  fibrosum (M8851/0)—*see* Lipoma, by site
  pendulum (M8851/0)—*see* Lipoma, by site
**Mönckeberg's arteriosclerosis, degeneration
  disease, or sclerosis** (*see also*
  Arteriosclerosis, extremities) 440.20
Monday fever 504
Monday morning dyspnea or asthma 504
Mondini's malformation (cochlea) 744.05
Mondor's disease (thrombophlebitis of breast)
  451.89
**Mongolian, mongolianism, mongolism
  mongoloid** 758.0
  spot 757.33
Monilethrix (congenital) 757.4
Monilia infestation —*see* Candidiasis
Moniliasis —*see also* Candidiasis
  neonatal 771.7
  vulvovaginitis 112.1
Monkeypox 059.01
Monoarthritis 716.60
  ankle 716.67
  arm 716.62
    lower (and wrist) 716.63
    upper (and elbow) 716.62
  foot (and ankle) 716.67
  forearm (and wrist) 716.63
  hand 716.64
  leg 716.66
    lower 716.66
    upper 716.65
  pelvic region (hip) (thigh) 716.65
  shoulder (region) 716.61
  specified site NEC 716.68
Monoblastic —*see* condition
Monochromatism (cone) (rod) 368.54
Monocytic —*see* condition
Monocytopenia 288.59
Monocytosis (symptomatic) 288.63
Monofixation syndrome 378.34
Monomania (*see also* Psychosis) 298.9

Mononeuritis 355.9
  cranial nerve—*see* Disorder, nerve, cranial
  femoral nerve 355.2
  lateral
    cutaneous nerve of thigh 355.1
    popliteal nerve 355.3
  lower limb 355.8
    specified nerve NEC 355.79
  medial popliteal nerve 355.4
  median nerve 354.1
  multiplex 354.5
  plantar nerve 355.6
  posterior tibial nerve 355.5
  radial nerve 354.3
  sciatic nerve 355.0
  ulnar nerve 354.2
  upper limb 354.9
    specified nerve NEC 354.8
  vestibular 388.5
Mononeuropathy (*see also* Mononeuritis) 355.9
  diabetic NEC 250.6 *[355.9]*
    due to secondary diabetes 249.6 *[355.9]*
    lower limb 250.6 *[355.8]*
      due to secondary diabetes 249.6 *[355.8]*
    upper limb 250.6 *[354.9]*
      due to secondary diabetes 249.6 *[354.9]*
  iliohypogastric nerve 355.79
  ilioinguinal nerve 355.79
  obturator nerve 355.79
  saphenous nerve 355.79
Mononucleosis, infectious 075
  with hepatitis 075 *[573.1]*
Monoplegia 344.5
  brain (current episode) (*see also* Paralysis,
    brain) 437.8
  fetus or newborn 767.8
  cerebral (current episode) (*see also* Paralysis,
    brain) 437.8
  congenital or infantile (cerebral) (spastic)
    (spinal) 343.3
  embolic (current) (*see also* Embolism, brain)
    434.1
    late effect—*see* Late effect(s) (of)
      cerebrovascular disease
  infantile (cerebral) (spastic) (spinal) 343.3
  lower limb 344.30
    affecting
      dominant side 344.31
      nondominant side 344.32
    due to late effect of cerebrovascular accident
      —*see* Late effect(s) (of) cerebrovascular
      accident
  newborn 767.8
  psychogenic 306.0
    specified as conversion reaction 300.11
  thrombotic (current) (*see also* Thrombosis,
    brain) 434.0
    late effect—*see* Late effect(s) (of)
      cerebrovascular disease
  transient 781.4
  upper limb 344.40
    affecting
      dominant side 344.41
      nondominant side 344.42
    due to late effect of cerebrovascular accident
      —*see* Late effect(s) (of) cerebrovascular
      accident
Monorchism, monorchidism 752.89
Monteggia's fracture (closed) 813.03
  open 813.13

Mood swings
brief compensatory 296.99
rebound 296.99
Moore's syndrome (*see also* Epilepsy) 345.5
Mooren's ulcer (cornea) 370.07
Mooser-Neill reaction 081.0
Mooser bodies 081.0
Moral
deficiency 301.7
imbecility 301.7
Morax-Axenfeld conjunctivitis 372.03
Morbilli (*see also* Measles) 055.9
Morbus
anglicus, anglorum 268.0
Beigel 111.2
caducus (*see also* Epilepsy) 345.9
caeruleus 746.89
celiacus 579.0
comitialis (*see also* Epilepsy) 345.9
cordis—*see also* Disease, heart
valvulorum—*see* Endocarditis
coxae 719.95
tuberculous (*see also* Tuberculosis) 015.1
hemorrhagicus neonatorum 776.0
maculosus neonatorum 772.6
renum 593.0
senilis (*see also* Osteoarthrosis) 715.9
Morel-Kraepelin disease (*see also*
Schizophrenia) 295.9
Morel-Moore syndrome (hyperostosis frontalis
interna) 733.3
Morel-Morgagni syndrome (hyperostosis
frontalis interna) 733.3
Morgagni
cyst, organ, hydatid, or appendage 752.89
fallopian tube 752.11
disease or syndrome (hyperostosis frontalis
interna) 733.3
Morgagni-Adams-Stokes syndrome (syncope
with heart block) 426.9
Morgagni-Stewart-Morel syndrome
(hyperostosis frontalis interna) 733.3
Moria (*see also* Psychosis) 298.9
Morning sickness 643.0
Moron 317
Morphea (guttate) (linear) 701.0
Morphine dependence (*see also* Dependence)
304.0
Morphinism (*see also* Dependence) 304.0
Morphinomania (*see also* Dependence) 304.0
Morphoea 701.0
Morquio (-Brailsford) (-Ullrich) disease or
syndrome (mucopolysaccharidosis IV) 277.5
kyphosis 277.5
Morris syndrome (testicular feminization)
259.51
Morsus humanus (open wound)—*see also*
Wound, open, by site
skin surface intact—*see* Contusion
Mortification (dry) (moist) (*see also* Gangrene)
785.4
Morton's
disease 355.6
foot 355.6
metatarsalgia (syndrome) 355.6
neuralgia 355.6
neuroma 355.6
syndrome (metatarsalgia) (neuralgia) 355.6
toe 355.6
Morvan's disease 336.0

Mosaicism, mosaic (chromosomal) 758.9
autosomal 758.5
sex 758.81
Moschcowitz's syndrome (thrombotic
thrombocytopenic purpura) 446.6
Mother yaw 102.0
Motion sickness (from travel, any vehicle) (from
roundabouts or swings) 994.6
Mottled teeth (enamel) (endemic) (nonendemic)
520.3
Mottling enamel (endemic) (nonendemic) (teeth)
520.3
Mouchet's disease 732.5
Mould (s) (in vitreous) 117.9
Moulders'
bronchitis 502
tuberculosis (*see also* Tuberculosis) 011.4
Mounier-Kuhn syndrome 748.3
with
acute exacerbation 494.1
bronchiectasis 494.0
with (acute) exacerbation 494.1
acquired 519.19
with bronchiectasis 494.0
with (acute) exacerbation 494.1
Mountain
fever—*see* Fever, mountain
sickness 993.2
with polycythemia, acquired 289.0
acute 289.0
tick fever 066.1
Mouse, joint (*see also* Loose, body, joint) 718.1
knee 717.6
Mouth —*see* condition
Movable
coccyx 724.71
kidney (*see also* Disease, renal) 593.0
congenital 753.3
organ or site, congenital NEC—*see* Malposition,
congenital
spleen 289.59
Movement
abnormal (dystonic) (involuntary) 781.0
decreased fetal 655.7
paradoxical facial 374.43
Moya Moya disease 437.5
Mozart's ear 744.29
MRSA (methicillin resistant staphylococcus
aureus) 041.12
colonization V02.54
personal history of V12.04
MSSA (methicillin susceptible staphylococcus
aureus) 041.11
colonization V02.53
Mucha's disease (acute parapsoriasis
varioliformis) 696.2
Mucha-Haberman syndrome (acute
parapsoriasis varioliformis) 696.2
Mu-chain disease 273.2
Mucinosis (cutaneous) (papular) 701.8
Mucocele
appendix 543.9
buccal cavity 528.9
gallbladder (*see also* Disease, gallbladder) 575.3
lacrimal sac 375.43
orbit (eye) 376.81
salivary gland (any) 527.6
sinus (accessory) (nasal) 478.19
turbinate (bone) (middle) (nasal) 478.19
uterus 621.8

Mucocutaneous lymph node syndrome (acute) (febrile) (infantile) 446.1
Mucoenteritis 564.9
Mucolipidosis I, II, III 272.7
Mucopolysaccharidosis (types 1-6) 277.5
  cardiopathy 277.5 *[425.7]*
Mucormycosis (lung) 117.7
Mucosa associated lymphoid tissue (MALT) 200.3
Mucositis —*see also* Inflammation, by site 528.00
  cervix (ulcerative) 616.81
  due to
    antineoplastic therapy (ulcerative) 528.01
    other drugs (ulcerative) 528.02
    specified NEC 528.09
  gastrointestinal (ulcerative) 538
  nasal (ulcerative) 478.11
  necroticans agranulocytica (*see also* Agranulocytosis) 288.09
  ulcerative 528.00
  vagina (ulcerative) 616.81
  vulva (ulcerative) 616.81
Mucous —*see also* condition
  patches (syphilitic) 091.3
    congenital 090.0
Mucoviscidosis 277.00
  with meconium obstruction 277.01
Mucus
  asphyxia or suffocation (*see also* Asphyxia, mucus) 933.1
    newborn 770.18
  in stool 792.1
  plug (*see also* Asphyxia, mucus) 933.1
    aspiration, of newborn 770.17
    tracheobronchial 519.19
    newborn 770.18
Muguet 112.0
Mulberry molars 090.5
Müllerian mixed tumor (M8950/3)—*see* Neoplasm, by site, malignant
Multicystic kidney 753.19
Multilobed placenta —*see* Placenta, abnormal
Multinodular prostate 600.10
  with
    urinary
      obstruction 600.11
      retention 600.11
Multiparity V61.5
  affecting
    fetus or newborn 763.89
    management of
      labor and delivery 659.4
      pregnancy V23.3
  requiring contraceptive management (*see also* Contraception) V25.9
Multipartita placenta —*see* Placenta, abnormal
Multiple, multiplex —*see also* condition
  birth
    affecting fetus or newborn 761.5
    healthy liveborn—*see* Newborn, multiple
  digits (congenital) 755.00
    fingers 755.01
    toes 755.02
  organ or site NEC—*see* Accessory
  personality 300.14
  renal arteries 747.62
Mumps 072.9
  with complication 072.8
    specified type NEC 072.79
  encephalitis 072.2
  hepatitis 072.71

Mumps—*continued*
  meningitis (aseptic) 072.1
  meningoencephalitis 072.2
  oophoritis 072.79
  orchitis 072.0
  pancreatitis 072.3
  polyneuropathy 072.72
  vaccination, prophylactic (against) V04.6
Mumu (*see also* Infestation, filarial) 125.9
Münchausen syndrome 301.51
Münchmeyer's disease or syndrome (exostosis luxurians) 728.11
Mural —*see* condition
Murmur (cardiac) (heart) (nonorganic) (organic) 785.2
  abdominal 787.5
  aortic (valve) (*see also* Endocarditis, aortic) 424.1
  benign—*omit code*
  cardiorespiratory 785.2
  diastolic—*see* condition
  Flint (*see also* Endocarditis, aortic) 424.1
  functional—*omit code*
  Graham Steell (pulmonic regurgitation) (*see also* Endocarditis, pulmonary) 424.3
  innocent—*omit code*
  insignificant—*omit code*
  midsystolic 785.2
  mitral (valve)—*see* stenosis, mitral
  physiologic—*see* condition
  presystolic, mitral—*see* Insufficiency, mitral
  pulmonic (valve) (*see also* Endocarditis, pulmonary) 424.3
  Still's (vibratory)—*omit code*
  systolic (valvular)—*see* condition
  tricuspid (valve)—*see* Endocarditis, tricuspid
  valvular—*see* condition
  vibratory—*omit code*
  undiagnosed 785.2
Murri's disease (intermittent hemoglobinuria) 283.2
Muscae volitantes 379.24
Muscle, muscular —*see* condition
Musculoneuralgia 729.1
Mushrooming hip 718.95
Mushroom workers' (pickers') lung 495.5
Mutation(s)
  factor V Leiden 289.81
  prothrombin gene 289.81
  surfactant, of lung 516.63
Mutism (*see also* Aphasia) 784.3
  akinetic 784.3
  deaf (acquired) (congenital) 389.7
  hysterical 300.11
  selective (elective) 313.23
    adjustment reaction 309.83
MVD (microvillus inclusion disease) 751.5
MVID (microvillus inclusion disease) 751.5
Myà's disease (congenital dilation, colon) 751.3
Myalgia (intercostal) 729.1
  eosinophilia syndrome 710.5
  epidemic 074.1
    cervical 078.89
  psychogenic 307.89
  traumatic NEC 959.9
Myasthenia 358.00
  cordis—*see* Failure, heart
  gravis 358.00
    with exacerbation (acute) 358.01
    in crisis 358.01
    neonatal 775.2
    pseudoparalytica 358.00

Myasthenia—*continued*
  stomach 536.8
    psychogenic 306.4
  syndrome in
    botulism 005.1 *[358.1]*
    diabetes mellitus 250.6 *[358.1]*
      due to secondary diabetes 249.6 *[358.1]*
    hypothyroidism (*see also* Hypothyroidism)
      244.9 *[358.1]*
    malignant neoplasm NEC 199.1 *[358.1]*
    pernicious anemia 281.0 *[358.1]*
    thyrotoxicosis (*see also* Thyrotoxicosis) 242.9
      [358.1]
Myasthenic 728.87
Mycelium infection NEC 117.9
Mycetismus 988.1
Mycetoma (actinomycotic) 039.9
  bone 039.8
    mycotic 117.4
  foot 039.4
    mycotic 117.4
  madurae 039.9
    mycotic 117.4
  maduromycotic 039.9
    mycotic 117.4
  mycotic 117.4
  nocardial 039.9
Mycobacteriosis —*see* Mycobacterium
Mycobacterium, mycobacterial (infection) 031.9
  acid-fast (bacilli) 031.9
  anonymous (*see also* Mycobacterium, atypical)
    031.9
  atypical (acid-fast bacilli) 031.9
    cutaneous 031.1
    pulmonary 031.0
      tuberculous (*see also* Tuberculosis,
        pulmonary) 011.9
    specified site NEC 031.8
  avium 031.0
    intracellulare complex bacteremia (MAC) 031.2
  balnei 031.1
  Battey 031.0
  cutaneous 031.1
  disseminated 031.2
    avium-intracellulare complex (DMAC) 031.2
  fortuitum 031.0
  intracellulare (battey bacillus) 031.0
  kakerifu 031.8
  kansasii 031.0
  kasongo 031.8
  leprae—*see* Leprosy
  luciflavum 031.0
  marinum 031.1
  pulmonary 031.0
    tuberculous (*see also* Tuberculosis,
      pulmonary) 011.9
  scrofulaceum 031.1
  tuberculosis (human, bovine)—*see also* Tuberculosis
    avian type 031.0
  ulcerans 031.1
  xenopi 031.0
Mycosis, mycotic 117.9
  cutaneous NEC 111.9
  ear 111.8 *[380.15]*
  fungoides (M9700/3) 202.1
  mouth 112.0
  pharynx 117.9
  skin NEC 111.9
  stomatitis 112.0
  systemic NEC 117.9
  tonsil 117.9
  vagina, vaginitis 112.1

Mydriasis (persistent) (pupil) 379.43
Myelatelia 742.59
Myelinoclasis, perivascular, acute
    (postinfectious) NEC 136.9 *[323.61]*
  postimmunization or postvaccinal 323.51
Myelinosis, central pontine 341.8
Myelitis (ascending) (cerebellar) (childhood)
    (chronic) (descending) (diffuse) (disseminated)
    (pressure) (progressive) (spinal cord) (subacute)
    (*see also* Encephalitis) 323.9
  acute (transverse) 341.20
    idiopathic 341.22
    in conditions classified elsewhere 341.21
  due to
    other infection classified elsewhere 136.9
      [323.42]
    specified cause NEC 323.82
    vaccination (any) 323.52
    viral diseases classified elsewhere 323.02
  herpes simplex 054.74
  herpes zoster 053.14
  late effect—*see* category 326
  optic neuritis in 341.0
  postchickenpox 052.2
  postimmunization 323.52
  postinfectious 136.9 *[323.63]*
  postvaccinal 323.52
  postvaricella 052.2
  syphilitic (transverse) 094.89
  toxic 989.9 *[323.72]*
  transverse 323.82
    acute 341.20
      idiopathic 341.22
      in conditions classified elsewhere 341.21
    idiopathic 341.22
  tuberculous (*see also* Tuberculosis) 013.6
  virus 049.9
Myeloblastic —*see* condition
Myelocele (*see also* Spina bifida) 741.9
  with hydrocephalus 741.0
Myelocystocele (*see also* Spina bifida) 741.9
Myelocytic —*see* condition
Myelocytoma 205.1
Myelodysplasia (spinal cord) 742.59
  meaning myelodysplastic syndrome—*see*
    Syndrome, myelodysplastic
Myeloencephalitis —*see* Encephalitis
Myelofibrosis 289.83
  with myeloid metaplasia 238.76
  idiopathic (chronic) 238.76
  megakaryocytic 238.79
  primary 238.76
  secondary 289.83
Myelogenous —*see* condition
Myeloid —*see* condition
Myelokathexis 288.09
Myeloleukodystrophy 330.0
Myelolipoma (M8870/0)—*see* Neoplasm, by site,
    benign
Myeloma (multiple) (plasma cell) (plasmacytic)
    (M9730/3) 203.0
  monostotic (M9731/1) 238.6
  solitary (M9731/1) 238.6
Myelomalacia 336.8
Myelomata, multiple (M9730/3) 203.0
Myelomatosis (M9730/3) 203.0
Myelomeningitis —*see* Meningoencephalitis
Myelomeningocele (spinal cord) (*see also* Spina
    bifida) 741.9
  fetal, causing fetopelvic disproportion 653.7

Myelo-osteo-musculodysplasia hereditaria
  756.89
Myelopathic —*see* condition
Myelopathy (spinal cord) 336.9
  cervical 721.1
  diabetic 250.6 *[336.3]*
    due to secondary diabetes 249.6 *[336.3]*
  drug-induced 336.8
  due to or with
    carbon tetrachloride 987.8 *[323.72]*
    degeneration or displacement, intervertebral
      disc 722.70
      cervical, cervicothoracic 722.71
      lumbar, lumbosacral 722.73
      thoracic, thoracolumbar 722.72
    hydroxyquinoline derivatives 961.3 *[323.72]*
    infection—*see* Encephalitis
    intervertebral disc disorder 722.70
      cervical, cervicothoracic 722.71
      lumbar, lumbosacral 722.73
      thoracic, thoracolumbar 722.72
    lead 984.9 *[323.72]*
    mercury 985.0 *[323.72]*
    neoplastic disease (*see also* Neoplasm, by site)
      239.9 *[336.3]*
    pernicious anemia 281.0 *[336.3]*
    spondylosis 721.91
      cervical 721.1
      lumbar, lumbosacral 721.42
      thoracic 721.41
    thallium 985.8 *[323.72]*
  lumbar, lumbosacral 721.42
  necrotic (subacute) 336.1
  radiation-induced 336.8
  spondylogenic NEC 721.91
    cervical 721.1
    lumbar, lumbosacral 721.42
    thoracic 721.41
  thoracic 721.41
  toxic NEC 989.9 *[323.72]*
  transverse (*see also* Myelitis) 323.82
  vascular 336.1
Myelophthisis 284.2
Myeloproliferative disease (M9960/1) 238.79
Myeloradiculitis (*see also* Polyneuropathy) 357.0
Myeloradiculodysplasia (spinal) 742.59
Myelosarcoma (M9930/3) 205.3
Myelosclerosis 289.89
  with myeloid metaplasia (M9961/1) 238.76
  disseminated, of nervous system 340
  megakaryocytic (M9961/1) 238.79
Myelosis (M9860/3) (*see also* Leukemia,
  myeloid) 205.9
  acute (M9861/3) 205.0
  aleukemic (M9864/3) 205.8
  chronic (M9863/3) 205.1
  erythremic (M9840/3) 207.0
    acute (M9841/3) 207.0
  megakaryocytic (M9920/3) 207.2
  nonleukemic (chronic) 288.8
  subacute (M9862/3) 205.2
Myesthenia —*see* Myasthenia
Myiasis (cavernous) 134.0
  orbit 134.0 *[376.13]*
Myoadenoma, prostate 600.20
  with
    other lower urinary tract symptoms (LUTS)
      600.21
    urinary
      obstruction 600.21
      retention 600.21

Myoblastoma
  granular cell (M9580/0)—*see also* Neoplasm,
    connective tissue, benign
    malignant (M9580/3)—*see* Neoplasm,
      connective tissue, malignant
    tongue (M9580/0) 210.1
Myocardial —*see* condition
Myocardiopathy (congestive) (constrictive)
  (familial) (idiopathic) (infiltrative)
  (obstructive) (primary) (restrictive) (sporadic)
  425.4
  alcoholic 425.5
  amyloid 277.39 *[425.7]*
  beriberi 265.0 *[425.7]*
  cobalt-beer 425.5
  due to
    amyloidosis 277.39 *[425.7]*
    beriberi 265.0 *[425.7]*
    cardiac glycogenosis 271.0 *[425.7]*
    Chagas' disease 086.0
    Friedreich's ataxia 334.0 *[425.8]*
    influenza (*see also* Influenza) 487.8 *[425.8]*
    mucopolysaccharidosis 277.5 *[425.7]*
    myotonia atrophica 359.21 *[425.8]*
    progressive muscular dystrophy 359.1 *[425.8]*
    sarcoidosis 135 *[425.8]*
  glycogen storage 271.0 *[425.7]*
  hypertrophic 425.18
    nonobstructive 425.18
    obstructive 425.11
  metabolic NEC 277.9 *[425.7]*
  nutritional 269.9 *[425.7]*
  obscure (African) 425.2
  peripartum 674.5
  postpartum 674.5
  secondary 425.9
  thyrotoxic (*see also* Thyrotoxicosis) 242.9
    [425.7]
  toxic NEC 425.9
Myocarditis (fibroid) (interstitial) (old)
  (progressive) (senile) (with arteriosclerosis)
  429.0
  with
    rheumatic fever (conditions classifiable to
      390) 398.0
      active (*see also* Myocarditis, acute,
        rheumatic) 391.2
      inactive or quiescent (with chorea) 398.0
  active (nonrheumatic) 422.90
    rheumatic 391.2
      with chorea (acute) (rheumatic)
        (Sydenham's) 392.0
  acute or subacute (interstitial) 422.90
    due to Streptococcus (beta-hemolytic) 391.2
    idiopathic 422.91
    rheumatic 391.2
      with chorea (acute) (rheumatic)
        (Sydenham's) 392.0
    specified type NEC 422.99
  aseptic of newborn 074.23
  bacterial (acute) 422.92
  chagasic 086.0
  chronic (interstitial) 429.0
  congenital 746.89
  constrictive 425.4
  Coxsackie (virus) 074.23
  diphtheritic 032.82

Myocarditis—*continued*
  due to or in
    Coxsackie (virus) 074.23
    diphtheria 032.82
    epidemic louse-borne typhus 080 *[422.0]*
    influenza (*see also* Influenza) 487.8 *[422.0]*
    Lyme disease 088.81 *[422.0]*
    scarlet fever 034.1 *[422.0]*
    toxoplasmosis (acquired) 130.3
    tuberculosis (*see also* Tuberculosis) 017.9
      [422.0]
    typhoid 002.0 *[422.0]*
    typhus NEC 081.9 *[422.0]*
  eosinophilic 422.91
  epidemic of newborn 074.23
  Fiedler's (acute) (isolated) (subacute) 422.91
  giant cell (acute) (subacute) 422.91
  gonococcal 098.85
  granulomatous (idiopathic) (isolated)
    (nonspecific) 422.91
  hypertensive (*see also* Hypertension, heart)
    402.90
  idiopathic 422.91
    granulomatous 422.91
  infective 422.92
  influenzal (*see also* Influenza) 487.8 *[422.0]*
  isolated (diffuse) (granulomatous) 422.91
  malignant 422.99
  meningococcal 036.43
  nonrheumatic, active 422.90
  parenchymatous 422.90
  pneumococcal (acute) (subacute) 422.92
  rheumatic (chronic) (inactive) (with chorea)
    398.0
    active or acute 391.2
      with chorea (acute) (rheumatic)
        (Sydenham's) 392.0
  septic 422.92
  specific (giant cell) (productive) 422.91
  staphylococcal (acute) (subacute) 422.92
  suppurative 422.92
  syphilitic (chronic) 093.82
  toxic 422.93
    rheumatic (*see also* Myocarditis, acute
      rheumatic) 391.2
  tuberculous (*see also* Tuberculosis) 017.9
    [422.0]
  typhoid 002.0 *[422.0]*
  valvular—*see* Endocarditis
  viral, except Coxsackie 422.91
    Coxsackie 074.23
    of newborn (Coxsackie) 074.23
Myocardium, myocardial —*see* condition
Myocardosis (*see also* Cardiomyopathy) 425.4
Myoclonia (essential) 333.2
  epileptica 345.1
  Friedrich's 333.2
  massive 333.2
Myoclonic
  epilepsy, familial (progressive) 345.1
  jerks 333.2
Myoclonus (familial essential) (multifocal)
    (simplex) 333.2
  with epilepsy and with ragged red fibers
    (MERRF syndrome) 277.87
  facial 351.8
  massive (infantile) 333.2
  palatal 333.2
  pharyngeal 333.2

Myocytolysis 429.1
Myodiastasis 728.84
Myoendocarditis —*see also* Endocarditis
  acute or subacute 421.9
Myoepithelioma (M8982/0)—*see* Neoplasm, by
    site, benign
Myofascitis (acute) 729.1
  low back 724.2
Myofibroma (M8890/0)—*see also* Neoplasm,
    connective tissue, benign
  uterus (cervix) (corpus) (*see also* Leiomyoma)
    218.9
Myofibromatosis
  infantile 759.89
Myofibrosis 728.2
  heart (*see also* Myocarditis) 429.0
  humeroscapular region 726.2
  scapulohumeral 726.2
Myofibrositis (*see also* Myositis) 729.1
  scapulohumeral 726.2
Myogelosis (occupational) 728.89
Myoglobinuria 791.3
Myoglobulinuria, primary 791.3
Myokymia —*see also* Myoclonus
  facial 351.8
Myolipoma (M8860/0)
  specified site—*see* Neoplasm, connective tissue,
    benign
  unspecified site 223.0
Myoma (M8895/0)—*see also* Neoplasm,
    connective tissue, benign
  cervix (stump) (uterus) (*see also* Leiomyoma)
    218.9
  malignant (M8895/3)—*see* Neoplasm,
    connective tissue, malignant
  prostate 600.20
    with
      other lower urinary tract symptoms (LUTS)
        600.21
      urinary
        obstruction 600.21
        retention 600.21
  uterus (cervix) (corpus) (*see also* Leiomyoma)
    218.9
    in pregnancy or childbirth 654.1
      affecting fetus or newborn 763.89
      causing obstructed labor 660.2
        affecting fetus or newborn 763.1
Myomalacia 728.9
  cordis, heart (*see also* Degeneration,
    myocardial) 429.1
Myometritis (*see also* Endometritis) 615.9
Myometrium —*see* condition
Myonecrosis, clostridial 040.0
Myopathy 359.9
  alcoholic 359.4
  amyloid 277.39 *[359.6]*
  benign congenital 359.0
  central core 359.0
  centronuclear 359.0
  congenital (benign) 359.0
  critical illness 359.81
  distal 359.1
  due to drugs 359.4
  endocrine 259.9 *[359.5]*
    specified type NEC 259.8 *[359.5]*
  extraocular muscles 376.82
  facioscapulohumeral 359.1

Myopathy—*continued*
in
  Addison's disease 255.41 *[359.5]*
  amyloidosis 277.39 *[359.6]*
  cretinism 243 *[359.5]*
  Cushing's syndrome 255.0 *[359.5]*
  disseminated lupus erythematosus 710.0 *[359.6]*
  giant cell arteritis 446.5 *[359.6]*
  hyperadrenocorticism NEC 255.3 *[359.5]*
  hyperparathyroidism 252.01 *[359.5]*
  hypopituitarism 253.2 *[359.5]*
  hypothyroidism (*see also* Hypothyroidism) 244.9 *[359.5]*
  malignant neoplasm NEC (M8000/3) 199.1 *[359.6]*
  myxedema (*see also* Myxedema) 244.9 *[359.5]*
  polyarteritis nodosa 446.0 *[359.6]*
  rheumatoid arthritis 714.0 *[359.6]*
  sarcoidosis 135 *[359.6]*
  scleroderma 710.1 *[359.6]*
  Sjögren's disease 710.2 *[359.6]*
  thyrotoxicosis (*see also* Thyrotoxicosis) 242.9 *[359.5]*
inflammatory 359.79
  immune NEC 359.79
  specified NEC 359.79
intensive care (ICU) 359.81
limb-girdle 359.1
myotubular 359.0
necrotizing, acute 359.81
nemaline 359.0
ocular 359.1
oculopharyngeal 359.1
of critical illness 359.81
primary 359.89
progressive NEC 359.89
proximal myotonic (PROMM) 359.21
quadriplegic, acute 359.81
rod body 359.0
scapulohumeral 359.1
specified type NEC 359.89
toxic 359.4
Myopericarditis (*see also* Pericarditis) 423.9
Myopia (axial) (congenital) (increased curvature or refraction, nucleus of lens) 367.1
degenerative, malignant 360.21
malignant 360.21
progressive high (degenerative) 360.21
Myosarcoma (M8895/3)—*see* Neoplasm, connective tissue, malignant
Myosis (persistent) 379.42
stromal (endolymphatic) (M8931/1) 236.0
Myositis 729.1
clostridial 040.0
due to posture 729.1
epidemic 074.1
fibrosa or fibrous (chronic) 728.2
  Volkmann's (complicating trauma) 958.6
inclusion body (IBM) 359.71
infective 728.0
interstitial 728.81
multiple—*see* Polymyositis
occupational 729.1
orbital, chronic 376.12
ossificans 728.12
  circumscribed 728.12
  progressive 728.11
  traumatic 728.12
progressive fibrosing 728.11

Mpurulent 728.0
rheumatic 729.1
rheumatoid 729.1
suppurative 728.0
syphilitic 095.6
traumatic (old) 729.1
Myospasia impulsiva 307.23
Myotonia (acquisita) (intermittens) 728.85
atrophica 359.21
congenita 359.22
  acetazolamide responsive 359.22
  dominant form 359.22
  recessive form 359.22
drug-induced 359.24
dystrophica 359.21
fluctuans 359.29
levior 359.22
permanens 359.29
Myotonic pupil 379.46
Myriapodiasis 134.1
Myringitis
with otitis media—*see* Otitis media
acute 384.00
  specified type NEC 384.09
bullosa hemorrhagica 384.01
bullous 384.01
chronic 384.1
Mysophobia 300.29
Mytilotoxism 988.0
Myxadenitis labialis 528.5
Myxedema (adult) (idiocy) (infantile) (juvenile) (thyroid gland) (*see also* Hypothyroidism) 244.9
circumscribed 242.9
congenital 243
cutis 701.8
localized (pretibial) 242.9
madness (acute) 293.0
  subacute 293.1
papular 701.8
pituitary 244.8
postpartum 674.8
pretibial 242.9
primary 244.9
Myxochondrosarcoma (M9220/3)—*see* Neoplasm, cartilage, malignant
Myxofibroma (M8811/0)—*see also* Neoplasm, connective tissue, benign
odontogenic (M9320/0) 213.1
  upper jaw (bone) 213.0
Myxofibrosarcoma (M8811/3)—*see* Neoplasm, connective tissue, malignant
Myxolipoma (M8852/0) (*see also* Lipoma, by site) 214.9
Myxoliposarcoma (M8852/3)—*see* Neoplasm, connective tissue, malignant
Myxoma (M8840/0)—*see also* Neoplasm, connective tissue, benign
odontogenic (M9320/0) 213.1
  upper jaw (bone) 213.0
Myxosarcoma (M8840/3)—*see* Neoplasm, connective tissue, malignant

N

Naegeli's
  disease (hereditary hemorrhagic
    thrombasthenia) 287.1
  leukemia, monocytic (M9863/3) 205.1
  syndrome (incontinentia pigmenti) 757.33
Naffziger's syndrome 353.0
Naga sore (*see also* Ulcer, skin) 707.9
Nägele's pelvis 738.6
  with disproportion (fetopelvic) 653.0
    affecting fetus or newborn 763.1
    causing obstructed labor 660.1
      affecting fetus or newborn 763.1
Nager-de Reynier syndrome (dysostosis
    mandibularis) 756.0
Nail —*see also* condition
  biting 307.9
  patella syndrome (hereditary
    osteo-onychodysplasia) 756.89
Nanism, nanosomia (*see also* Dwarfism) 259.4
  hypophyseal 253.3
  pituitary 253.3
  renis, renalis 588.0
Nanukayami 100.89
Napkin rash 691.0
Narcissism 301.81
Narcolepsy 347.00
  with cataplexy 347.01
  in conditions classified elsewhere 347.10
    with cataplexy 347.11
Narcosis
  carbon dioxide (respiratory) 786.09
  due to drug
    correct substance properly administered 780.09
    overdose or wrong substance given or taken
      977.9
      specified drug—*see* Table of drugs and
        chemicals
Narcotism (chronic) (*see also* listing under
    Dependence) 304.9
  acute
    correct substance properly administered 349.82
    overdose or wrong substance given or taken
      967.8
      specified drug—*see* Table of drugs and
        chemicals
NARP syndrome (Neuropathy, ataxia and
    retinitis pigmentosa) 277.87
Narrow
  anterior chamber angle 365.02
  pelvis (inlet) (outlet)—*see* Contraction, pelvis
Narrowing
  artery NEC 447.1
    auditory, internal 433.8
    basilar 433.0
      with other precerebral artery 433.3
      bilateral 433.3
    carotid 433.1
      with other precerebral artery 433.3
      bilateral 433.3
    cerebellar 433.8
    choroidal 433.8
    communicating posterior 433.8
    coronary —*see also* Arteriosclerosis, coronary
      congenital 746.85
        due to syphilis 090.5
    hypophyseal 433.8
    pontine 433.8

Narrowing—*continued*
    precerebral NEC 433.9
      multiple or bilateral 433.3
      specified NEC 433.8
    vertebral 433.2
      with other precerebral artery 433.3
      bilateral 433.3
  auditory canal (external) (*see also* Stricture, ear
    canal, acquired) 380.50
  cerebral arteries 437.0
  cicatricial—*see* Cicatrix
  congenital—*see* Anomaly, congenital
  coronary artery—*see* Narrowing, artery,
    coronary
  ear, middle 385.22
  Eustachian tube (*see also* Obstruction,
    Eustachian tube) 381.60
  eyelid 374.46
    congenital 743.62
  intervertebral disc or space NEC—*see*
    Degeneration, intervertebral disc
  joint space, hip 719.85
  larynx 478.74
  lids 374.46
    congenital 743.62
  mesenteric artery (with gangrene) 557.0
  palate 524.89
  palpebral fissure 374.46
  retinal artery 362.13
  ureter 593.3
  urethra (*see also* Stricture, urethra) 598.9
Narrowness, abnormal, eyelid 743.62
Nasal —*see* condition
Nasolacrimal —*see* condition
Nasopharyngeal —*see also* condition
  bursa 478.29
  pituitary gland 759.2
  torticollis 723.5
Nasopharyngitis (acute) (infective) (subacute) 460
  chronic 472.2
    due to external agent—*see* Condition,
      respiratory, chronic, due to
    due to external agent—*see* Condition,
      respiratory, due to
  septic 034.0
  streptococcal 034.0
  suppurative (chronic) 472.2
  ulcerative (chronic) 472.2
Nasopharynx, nasopharyngeal —*see* condition
Natal tooth, teeth 520.6
Nausea (*see also* Vomiting) 787.02
  epidemic 078.82
  gravidarum—*see* Hyperemesis, gravidarum
  marina 994.6
  with vomiting 787.01
Naval —*see* condition
Neapolitan fever (*see also* Brucellosis) 023.9
Near drowning 994.1
Nearsightedness 367.1
Near-syncope 780.2
Nebécourt's syndrome 253.3
Nebula, cornea (eye) 371.01
  congenital 743.43
    interfering with vision 743.42
Necator americanus infestation 126.1
Necatoriasis 126.1
Neck —*see* condition
Necrencephalus (*see also* Softening, brain) 437.8

Necrobacillosis 040.3
Necrobiosis 799.89
  brain or cerebral (*see also* Softening, brain) 437.8
  lipoidica 709.3
    diabeticorum 250.8 *[709.3]*
    due to secondary diabetes 249.8 *[709.3]*
Necrodermolysis 695.15
Necrolysis, toxic epidermal 695.15
  due to drug
    correct substance properly administered 695.15
    overdose or wrong substance given or taken
      977.9
    specified drug—*see* Table of drugs and
      chemicals
  Stevens-Johnson syndrome overlap (SJS-TEN
    overlap syndrome) 695.14
Necrophilia 302.89
Necrosis, necrotic
  adrenal (capsule) (gland) 255.8
  antrum, nasal sinus 478.19
  aorta (hyaline) (*see also* Aneurysm, aorta) 441.9
    cystic medial 441.00
      abdominal 441.02
      thoracic 441.01
      thoracoabdominal 441.03
    ruptured 441.5
  arteritis 446.0
  artery 447.5
  aseptic, bone 733.40
    femur (head) (neck) 733.42
      medial condyle 733.43
    humoral head 733.41
    jaw 733.45
    medial femoral condyle 733.43
    specified site NEC 733.49
    talus 733.44
  avascular, bone NEC (*see also* Necrosis, aseptic,
    bone) 733.40
  bladder (aseptic) (sphincter) 596.89
  bone (*see also* Osteomyelitis) 730.1
    acute 730.0
    aseptic or avascular 733.40
      femur (head) (neck) 733.42
        medial condyle 733.43
      humoral head 733.41
      jaw 733.45
      medial femoral condyle 733.43
      specified site NEC 733.49
      talus 733.44
    ethmoid 478.19
    ischemic 733.40
    jaw 526.4
      aseptic 733.45
    marrow 289.89
    Paget's (osteitis deformans) 731.0
    tuberculous—*see* Tuberculosis, bone
  brain (softening) (*see also* Softening, brain) 437.8
  breast (aseptic) (fat) (segmental) 611.3
  bronchus, bronchi 519.19
  central nervous system NEC (*see also*
    Softening, brain) 437.8
  cerebellar (*see also* Softening, brain) 437.8
  cerebral (softening) (*see also* Softening, brain) 437.8
  cerebrospinal (softening) (*see also* Softening,
    brain) 437.8
  colon 557.0
  cornea (*see also* Keratitis) 371.40
  cortical, kidney 583.6
  cystic medial (aorta) 441.00
    abdominal 441.02
    thoracic 441.01
    thoracoabdominal 441.03

Necrosis, necrotic—*continued*
  dental 521.09
    pulp 522.1
  due to swallowing corrosive substance—*see*
    Burn, by site
  ear (ossicle) 385.24
  esophagus 530.89
  ethmoid (bone) 478.19
  eyelid 374.50
  fat, fatty (generalized) (*see also* Degeneration,
    fatty) 272.8
    abdominal wall 567.82
    breast (aseptic) (segmental) 611.3
    intestine 569.89
    localized—*see* Degeneration, by site, fatty
    mesentery 567.82
    omentum 567.82
    pancreas 577.8
    peritoneum 567.82
    skin (subcutaneous) 709.3
      newborn 778.1
  femur (aseptic) (avascular) 733.42
    head 733.42
    medial condyle 733.43
    neck 733.42
  gallbladder (*see also* Cholecystitis, acute) 575.0
  gangrenous 785.4
  gastric 537.89
  glottis 478.79
  heart (myocardium)—*see* Infarct, myocardium
  hepatic (*see also* Necrosis, liver) 570
  hip (aseptic) (avascular) 733.42
  intestine (acute) (hemorrhagic) (massive) 557.0
  ischemic 785.4
  jaw 526.4
    aseptic 733.45
  kidney (bilateral) 583.9
    acute 584.9
    cortical 583.6
      acute 584.6
        with
          abortion—*see* Abortion, by type, with
            renal failure
          ectopic pregnancy (*see also* categories
            633.0-633.9) 639.3
          molar pregnancy (*see also* categories
            630-632) 639.3
          complicating pregnancy 646.2
            affecting fetus or newborn 760.1
          following labor and delivery 669.3
    medullary (papillary) (*see also* Pyelitis) 590.80
      in
        acute renal failure 584.7
        nephritis, nephropathy 583.7
    papillary (*see also* Pyelitis) 590.80
      in
        acute renal failure 584.7
        nephritis, nephropathy 583.7
    tubular 584.5
      with
        abortion—*see* Abortion, by type, with
          renal failure
        ectopic pregnancy (*see also* categories
          633.0-633.9) 639.3
        molar pregnancy (*see also* categories
          630-632) 639.3
      complicating
        abortion 639.3
        ectopic or molar pregnancy 639.3
        pregnancy 646.2
          affecting fetus or newborn 760.1

Necrosis, necrotic—*continued*
  kidney—*continued*
    tubular—*continued*
      following labor and delivery 669.3
      traumatic 958.5
  larynx 478.79
  liver (acute) (congenital) (diffuse) (massive)
    (subacute) 570
    with
      abortion—*see* Abortion, by type, with
        specified complication NEC
      ectopic pregnancy (*see also* categories
        633.0-633.9) 639.8
      molar pregnancy (*see also* categories
        630-632) 639.8
    complicating pregnancy 646.7
      affecting fetus or newborn 760.8
    following
      abortion 639.8
      ectopic or molar pregnancy 639.8
    obstetrical 646.7
    postabortal 639.8
    puerperal, postpartum 674.8
    toxic 573.3
  lung 513.0
  lymphatic gland 683
  mammary gland 611.3
  mastoid (chronic) 383.1
  mesentery 557.0
    fat 567.82
  mitral valve—*see* Insufficiency, mitral
  myocardium, myocardial—*see* Infarct,
    myocardium
  nose (septum) 478.19
  omentum 557.0
    with mesenteric infarction 557.0
    fat 567.82
  orbit, orbital 376.10
  ossicles, ear (aseptic) 385.24
  ovary (*see also* Salpingo-oophoritis) 614.2
  pancreas (aseptic) (duct) (fat) 577.8
    acute 577.0
    infective 577.0
  papillary, kidney (*see also* Pyelitis) 590.80
  perineum 624.8
  peritoneum 557.0
    with mesenteric infarction 557.0
    fat 567.82
  pharynx 462
    in granulocytopenia 288.09
  phosphorus 983.9
  pituitary (gland) (postpartum) (Sheehan) 253.2
  placenta (*see also* Placenta, abnormal) 656.7
  pneumonia 513.0
  pulmonary 513.0
  pulp (dental) 522.1
  pylorus 537.89
  radiation—*see* Necrosis, by site
  radium—*see* Necrosis, by site
  renal—*see* Necrosis, kidney
  sclera 379.19
  scrotum 608.89
  skin or subcutaneous tissue 709.8
    due to burn—*see* Burn, by site
    gangrenous 785.4
  spine, spinal (column) 730.18
    acute 730.18
    cord 336.1
  spleen 289.59
  stomach 537.89
  stomatitis 528.1

Necrosis, necrotic—*continued*
  subcutaneous fat 709.3
    fetus or newborn 778.1
  subendocardial—*see* Infarct, myocardium
  suprarenal (capsule) (gland) 255.8
  teeth, tooth 521.09
  testis 608.89
  thymus (gland) 254.8
  tonsil 474.8
  trachea 519.19
  tuberculous NEC—*see* Tuberculosis
  tubular (acute) (anoxic) (toxic) 584.5
    due to a procedure 997.5
  umbilical cord, affecting fetus or newborn 762.6
  vagina 623.8
  vertebra (lumbar) 730.18
    acute 730.18
    tuberculous (*see also* Tuberculosis) 015.0 *[730.8]*
  vesical (aseptic) (bladder) 596.89
  vulva 624.8
  x-ray—*see* Necrosis, by site
Necrospermia 606.0
Necrotizing angiitis 446.0
Negativism 301.7
Neglect (child) (newborn) NEC 995.52
  adult 995.84
  after or at birth 995.52
  hemispatial 781.8
  left-sided 781.8
  sensory 781.8
  visuospatial 781.8
Negri bodies 071
Neill-Dingwall syndrome (microcephaly and
  dwarfism) 759.89
Neisserian infection NEC—*see* Gonococcus
Nematodiasis NEC (*see also* Infestation,
  Nematode) 127.9
  ancylostoma (*see also* Ancylostomiasis) 126.9
Neoformans cryptococcus infection 117.5
Neonatal —*see also* condition
  abstinence syndrome 779.5
  adrenoleukodystrophy 277.86
  teeth, tooth 520.6
Neonatorum —*see* condition
Neoplasia
  anal intraepithelial I (AIN I) (histologically
    confirmed) 569.44
  anal intraepithelial II (AIN II) (histologically
    confirmed) 569.44
  anal intraepithelial III (AIN III) 230.6
    anal canal 230.5
  endometrial intraepithelial (EIN) 621.35
  multiple endocine (MEN)
    type I 258.01
    type II A 258.02
    type II B 258.03
  vaginal intraepithelial I (VAIN I) 623.0
  vaginal intraepithelial II (VAIN II) 623.0
  vaginal intraepithelial III (VAIN III) 233.31
  vulvar intraepithelial I (VIN I) 624.01
  vulvar intraepithelial II (VIN II) 624.02
  vulvar intraepithelial III (VIN III) 233.32

  "N" listing resumes after
  "Neoplasm, neoplastic" table...

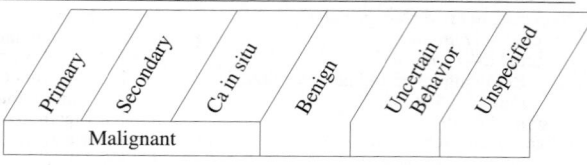

	Malignant — Primary	Malignant — Secondary	Ca in situ	Benign	Uncertain Behavior	Unspecified
Neoplasm, neoplastic	199.1	199.1	234.9	229.9	238.9	239.9

> *Note—1. The list below gives the code numbers for neoplasms by anatomical site. For each site there are six possible code numbers according to whether the neoplasm in question is malignant, benign, in situ, of uncertain behavior, or of unspecified nature. The description of the neoplasm will often indicate which of the six columns is appropriate; e.g., malignant melanoma of skin, benign fibroadenoma of breast, carcinoma in situ of cervix uteri.*
>
> *Where such descriptors are not present, the remainder of the Index should be consulted where guidance is given to the appropriate column for each morphological (histological) variety listed; e.g., Mesonephroma—see Neoplasm, malignant; Embryoma—see also Neoplasm, uncertain behavior; Disease, Bowen's—see Neoplasm, skin, in situ. However, the guidance in the Index can be overridden if one of the descriptors mentioned above is present; e.g., malignant adenoma of colon is coded to 153.9 and not to 211.3 as the adjective "malignant" overrides the Index entry "Adenoma—see also Neoplasm, benign."*
>
> *Note—2. Sites marked with the sign * (e.g., face NEC*) should be classified to malignant neoplasm of skin of these sites if the variety of neoplasm is a squamous cell carcinoma or an epidermoid carcinoma and to benign neoplasm of skin of these sites if the variety of neoplasm is a papilloma (any type).*

	Primary	Secondary	Ca in situ	Benign	Uncertain Behavior	Unspecified
abdomen, abdominal	195.2	198.89	234.8	229.8	238.8	239.89
cavity	195.2	198.89	234.8	229.8	238.8	239.89
organ	195.2	198.89	234.8	229.8	238.8	239.89
viscera	195.2	198.89	234.8	229.8	238.8	239.89
wall	173.50	198.2	232.5	216.5	238.2	239.2
basal cell carcinoma	173.51	—	—	—	—	—
connective tissue	171.5	198.89	—	215.5	238.1	239.2
specified type NEC.	173.59	—	—	—	—	—
squamous cell carcinoma	173.52	—	—	—	—	—
abdominopelvic	195.8	198.89	234.8	229.8	238.8	239.89
accessory sinus—*see* Neoplasm, sinus						
acoustic nerve	192.0	198.4	—	225.1	237.9	239.7
acromion (process)	170.4	198.5	—	213.4	238.0	239.2
adenoid (pharynx) (tissue)	147.1	198.89	230.0	210.7	235.1	239.0
adipose tissue (*see also* Neoplasm,						
connective tissue)	171.9	198.89	—	215.9	238.1	239.2
adnexa (uterine)	183.9	198.82	233.39	221.8	236.3	239.5
adrenal (cortex) (gland)						
(medulla)	194.0	198.7	234.8	227.0	237.2	239.7
ala nasi (external)	173.30	198.2	232.3	216.3	238.2	239.2
alimentary canal or						
tract NEC	159.9	197.8	230.9	211.9	235.5	239.0
alveolar	143.9	198.89	230.0	210.4	235.1	239.0
mucosa	143.9	198.89	230.0	210.4	235.1	239.0
lower	143.1	198.89	230.0	210.4	235.1	239.0
upper	143.0	198.89	230.0	210.4	235.1	239.0
ridge or process	170.1	198.5	—	213.1	238.0	239.2
carcinoma	143.9	—	—	—	—	—
lower	143.1	—	—	—	—	—
upper	143.0	—	—	—	—	—
lower	170.1	198.5	—	213.1	238.0	239.2
mucosa	143.9	198.89	230.0	210.4	235.1	239.0
lower	143.1	198.89	230.0	210.4	235.1	239.0
upper	143.0	198.89	230.0	210.4	235.1	239.0
upper	170.0	198.5	—	213.0	238.0	239.2
sulcus	145.1	198.89	230.0	210.4	235.1	239.0
alveolus	143.9	198.89	230.0	210.4	235.1	239.0
lower	143.1	198.89	230.0	210.4	235.1	239.0
upper	143.0	198.89	230.0	210.4	235.1	239.0
ampulla of Vater	156.2	197.8	230.8	211.5	235.3	239.0
ankle NEC*	195.5	198.89	232.7	229.8	238.8	239.89
anorectum, anorectal						
(junction)	154.8	197.5	230.7	211.4	235.2	239.0

	Malignant			Benign	Uncertain Behavior	Unspecified
	Primary	Secondary	Ca in situ			
antecubital fossa or space*......	195.4	198.89	232.6	229.8	238.8	239.89
antrum (Highmore)						
(maxillary)	160.2	197.3	231.8	212.0	235.9	239.1
pyloric	151.2	197.8	230.2	211.1	235.2	239.0
tympanicum	160.1	197.3	231.8	212.0	235.9	239.1
anus, anal...............	154.3	197.5	230.6	211.4	235.5	239.0
canal	154.2	197.5	230.5	211.4	235.5	239.0
contiguous sites with rectosigmoid						
junction or rectum	154.8	—	—	—	—	—
margin (*see also* Neoplasm, anus,						
skin)	173.50	198.2	232.5	216.5	238.2	239.2
skin.................	173.50	198.2	232.5	216.5	238.2	239.2
basal cell carcinoma	173.51	—	—	—	—	—
specified type NEC........	173.59	—	—	—	—	—
squamous cell carcinoma	173.52	—	—	—	—	—
sphincter	154.2	197.5	230.5	211.4	235.5	239.0
aorta (thoracic)............	171.4	198.89	—	215.4	238.1	239.2
abdominal	171.5	198.89	—	215.5	238.1	239.2
aortic body	194.6	198.89	—	227.6	237.3	239.7
aponeurosis.............	171.9	198.89	—	215.9	238.1	239.2
palmar	171.2	198.89	—	215.2	238.1	239.2
plantar	171.3	198.89	—	215.3	238.1	239.2
appendix	153.5	197.5	230.3	211.3	235.2	239.0
arachnoid (cerebral)	192.1	198.4	—	225.2	237.6	239.7
spinal.............	192.3	198.4	—	225.4	237.6	239.7
areola (female)............	174.0	198.81	233.0	217	238.3	239.3
male	175.0	198.81	233.0	217	238.3	239.3
arm NEC*	195.4	198.89	232.6	229.8	238.8	239.89
artery—*see* Neoplasm, connective tissue						
aryepiglottic fold..........	148.2	198.89	230.0	210.8	235.1	239.0
hypopharyngeal aspect.......	148.2	198.89	230.0	210.8	235.1	239.0
laryngeal aspect	161.1	197.3	231.0	212.1	235.6	239.1
marginal zone	148.2	198.89	230.0	210.8	235.1	239.0
arytenoid (cartilage)	161.3	197.3	231.0	212.1	235.6	239.1
fold—*see* Neoplasm, aryepiglottic						
associated with transplanted organ. .	199.2	—	—	—	—	—
atlas...............	170.2	198.5	—	213.2	238.0	239.2
atrium, cardiac	164.1	198.89	—	212.7	238.8	239.89
auditory						
canal (external) (skin) (*see also*						
Neoplasm, skin, ear)......	173.20	198.2	232.2	216.2	238.2	239.2
internal...............	160.1	197.3	231.8	212.0	235.9	239.1
nerve...............	192.0	198.4	—	225.1	237.9	239.7
tube................	160.1	197.3	231.8	212.0	235.9	239.1
opening...........	147.2	198.89	230.0	210.7	235.1	239.0
auricle, ear (*see also* Neoplasm,						
skin, ear)	173.20	198.2	232.2	216.2	238.2	239.2
cartilage	171.0	198.89	—	215.0	238.1	239.2
auricular canal (external) (*see also*						
Neoplasm, skin, ear)	173.20	198.2	232.2	216.2	238.2	239.2
internal	160.1	197.3	231.8	212.0	235.9	239.1
autonomic nerve or nervous						
system NEC..........	171.9	198.89	—	215.9	238.1	239.2
axilla, axillary	195.1	198.89	234.8	229.8	238.8	239.89
fold (*see also* Neoplasm, skin,						
trunk)..............	173.50	198.2	232.5	216.5	238.2	239.2
back NEC*..............	195.8	198.89	232.5	229.8	238.8	239.89
Bartholin's gland...........	184.1	198.82	233.32	221.2	236.3	239.5
basal ganglia	191.0	198.3	—	225.0	237.5	239.6
basis pedunculi...........	191.7	198.3	—	225.0	237.5	239.6
bile or biliary (tract)	156.9	197.8	230.8	211.5	235.3	239.0
canaliculi (biliferi)						
(intrahepatic)	155.1	197.8	230.8	211.5	235.3	239.0

	Primary	Secondary	Ca in situ	Benign	Uncertain Behavior	Unspecified
		Malignant				
canals, interlobular	155.1	197.8	230.8	211.5	235.3	239.0
contiguous sites	156.8	—	—	—	—	—
duct or passage (common) (cyst)						
(extrahepatic)	156.1	197.8	230.8	211.5	235.3	239.0
contiguous sites with						
gallbladder	156.8	—	—	—	—	—
interlobular	155.1	197.8	230.8	211.5	235.3	239.0
intrahepatic	155.1	197.8	230.8	211.5	235.3	239.0
and extrahepatic	156.9	197.8	230.8	211.5	235.3	239.0
bladder (urinary)	188.9	198.1	233.7	223.3	236.7	239.4
contiguous sites	188.8	—	—	—	—	—
dome	188.1	198.1	233.7	223.3	236.7	239.4
neck	188.5	198.1	233.7	223.3	236.7	239.4
orifice	188.9	198.1	233.7	223.3	236.7	239.4
ureteric	188.6	198.1	233.7	223.3	236.7	239.4
urethral	188.5	198.1	233.7	223.3	236.7	239.4
sphincter	188.8	198.1	233.7	223.3	236.7	239.4
trigone	188.0	198.1	233.7	223.3	236.7	239.4
urachus	188.7	—	233.7	223.3	236.7	239.4
wall	188.9	198.1	233.7	223.3	236.7	239.4
anterior	188.3	198.1	233.7	223.3	236.7	239.4
lateral	188.2	198.1	233.7	223.3	236.7	239.4
posterior	188.4	198.1	233.7	223.3	236.7	239.4
blood vessel—*see* Neoplasm, connective tissue						
bone (periosteum)	170.9	198.5	—	213.9	238.0	239.2

Note—Carcinomas and adenocarcinomas, of any type other than intraosseous or odontogenic, of the sites listed under "Neoplasm, bone" should be considered as constituting metastatic spread from an unspecified primary site and coded to 198.5 for morbidity coding .

	Primary	Secondary	Ca in situ	Benign	Uncertain Behavior	Unspecified
acetabulum	170.6	198.5	—	213.6	238.0	239.2
acromion (process)	170.4	198.5	—	213.4	238.0	239.2
ankle	170.8	198.5	—	213.8	238.0	239.2
arm NEC	170.4	198.5	—	213.4	238.0	239.2
astragalus	170.8	198.5	—	213.8	238.0	239.2
atlas	170.2	198.5	—	213.2	238.0	239.2
axis	170.2	198.5	—	213.2	238.0	239.2
back NEC	170.2	198.5	—	213.2	238.0	239.2
calcaneus	170.8	198.5	—	213.8	238.0	239.2
calvarium	170.0	198.5	—	213.0	238.0	239.2
carpus (any)	170.5	198.5	—	213.5	238.0	239.2
cartilage NEC	170.9	198.5	—	213.9	238.0	239.2
clavicle	170.3	198.5	—	213.3	238.0	239.2
clivus	170.0	198.5	—	213.0	238.0	239.2
coccygeal vertebra	170.6	198.5	—	213.6	238.0	239.2
coccyx	170.6	198.5	—	213.6	238.0	239.2
costal cartilage	170.3	198.5	—	213.3	238.0	239.2
costovertebral joint	170.3	198.5	—	213.3	238.0	239.2
cranial	170.0	198.5	—	213.0	238.0	239.2
cuboid	170.8	198.5	—	213.8	238.0	239.2
cuneiform	170.9	198.5	—	213.9	238.0	239.2
ankle	170.8	198.5	—	213.8	238.0	239.2
wrist	170.5	198.5	—	213.5	238.0	239.2
digital	170.9	198.5	—	213.9	238.0	239.2
finger	170.5	198.5	—	213.5	238.0	239.2
toe	170.8	198.5	—	213.8	238.0	239.2
elbow	170.4	198.5	—	213.4	238.0	239.2
ethmoid (labyrinth)	170.0	198.5	—	213.0	238.0	239.2
face	170.0	198.5	—	213.0	238.0	239.2
lower jaw	170.1	198.5	—	213.1	238.0	239.2
femur (any part)	170.7	198.5	—	213.7	238.0	239.2
fibula (any part)	170.7	198.5	—	213.7	238.0	239.2
finger (any)	170.5	198.5	—	213.5	238.0	239.2
foot	170.8	198.5	—	213.8	238.0	239.2

	Malignant			Benign	Uncertain Behavior	Unspecified
	Primary	Secondary	Ca in situ			
forearm	170.4	198.5	—	213.4	238.0	239.2
frontal	170.0	198.5	—	213.0	238.0	239.2
hand	170.5	198.5	—	213.5	238.0	239.2
heel	170.8	198.5	—	213.8	238.0	239.2
hip	170.6	198.5	—	213.6	238.0	239.2
humerus (any part)	170.4	198.5	—	213.4	238.0	239.2
hyoid	170.0	198.5	—	213.0	238.0	239.2
ilium	170.6	198.5	—	213.6	238.0	239.2
innominate	170.6	198.5	—	213.6	238.0	239.2
intervertebral cartilage or disc	170.2	198.5	—	213.2	238.0	239.2
ischium	170.6	198.5	—	213.6	238.0	239.2
jaw (lower)	170.1	198.5	—	213.1	238.0	239.2
upper	170.0	198.5	—	213.0	238.0	239.2
knee	170.7	198.5	—	213.7	238.0	239.2
leg NEC	170.7	198.5	—	213.7	238.0	239.2
limb NEC	170.9	198.5	—	213.9	238.0	239.2
lower (long bones)	170.7	198.5	—	213.7	238.0	239.2
short bones	170.8	198.5	—	213.8	238.0	239.2
upper (long bones)	170.4	198.5	—	213.4	238.0	239.2
short bones	170.5	198.5	—	213.5	238.0	239.2
long	170.9	198.5	—	213.9	238.0	239.2
lower limbs NEC	170.7	198.5	—	213.7	238.0	239.2
upper limbs NEC	170.4	198.5	—	213.4	238.0	239.2
malar	170.0	198.5	—	213.0	238.0	239.2
mandible	170.1	198.5	—	213.1	238.0	239.2
marrow NEC	202.9	198.5	—	—	—	238.79
mastoid	170.0	198.5	—	213.0	238.0	239.2
maxilla, maxillary (superior)	170.0	198.5	—	213.0	238.0	239.2
inferior	170.1	198.5	—	213.1	238.0	239.2
metacarpus (any)	170.5	198.5	—	213.5	238.0	239.2
metatarsus (any)	170.8	198.5	—	213.8	238.0	239.2
navicular (ankle)	170.8	198.5	—	213.8	238.0	239.2
hand	170.5	198.5	—	213.5	238.0	239.2
nose, nasal	170.0	198.5	—	213.0	238.0	239.2
occipital	170.0	198.5	—	213.0	238.0	239.2
orbit	170.0	198.5	—	213.0	238.0	239.2
parietal	170.0	198.5	—	213.0	238.0	239.2
patella	170.8	198.5	—	213.8	238.0	239.2
pelvic	170.6	198.5	—	213.6	238.0	239.2
phalanges	170.9	198.5	—	213.9	238.0	239.2
foot	170.8	198.5	—	213.8	238.0	239.2
hand	170.5	198.5	—	213.5	238.0	239.2
pubic	170.6	198.5	—	213.6	238.0	239.2
radius (any part)	170.4	198.5	—	213.4	238.0	239.2
rib	170.3	198.5	—	213.3	238.0	239.2
sacral vertebra	170.6	198.5	—	213.6	238.0	239.2
sacrum	170.6	198.5	—	213.6	238.0	239.2
scaphoid (of hand)	170.5	198.5	—	213.5	238.0	239.2
of ankle	170.8	198.5	—	213.8	238.0	239.2
scapula (any part)	170.4	198.5	—	213.4	238.0	239.2
sella turcica	170.0	198.5	—	213.0	238.0	239.2
short	170.9	198.5	—	213.9	238.0	239.2
lower limb	170.8	198.5	—	213.8	238.0	239.2
upper limb	170.5	198.5	—	213.5	238.0	239.2
shoulder	170.4	198.5	—	213.4	238.0	239.2
skeleton, skeletal NEC	170.9	198.5	—	213.9	238.0	239.2
skull	170.0	198.5	—	213.0	238.0	239.2
sphenoid	170.0	198.5	—	213.0	238.0	239.2
spine, spinal (column)	170.2	198.5	—	213.2	238.0	239.2
coccyx	170.6	198.5	—	213.6	238.0	239.2
sacrum	170.6	198.5	—	213.6	238.0	239.2

	Malignant					
	Primary	Secondary	Ca in situ	Benign	Uncertain Behavior	Unspecified
sternum	170.3	198.5	—	213.3	238.0	239.2
tarsus (any)	170.8	198.5	—	213.8	238.0	239.2
temporal	170.0	198.5	—	213.0	238.0	239.2
thumb	170.5	198.5	—	213.5	238.0	239.2
tibia (any part)	170.7	198.5	—	213.7	238.0	239.2
toe (any)	170.8	198.5	—	213.8	238.0	239.2
trapezium	170.5	198.5	—	213.5	238.0	239.2
trapezoid	170.5	198.5	—	213.5	238.0	239.2
turbinate	170.0	198.5	—	213.0	238.0	239.2
ulna (any part)	170.4	198.5	—	213.4	238.0	239.2
unciform	170.5	198.5	—	213.5	238.0	239.2
vertebra (column)	170.2	198.5	—	213.2	238.0	239.2
coccyx	170.6	198.5	—	213.6	238.0	239.2
sacrum	170.6	198.5	—	213.6	238.0	239.2
vomer	170.0	198.5	—	213.0	238.0	239.2
wrist	170.5	198.5	—	213.5	238.0	239.2
xiphoid process	170.3	198.5	—	213.3	238.0	239.2
zygomatic	170.0	198.5	—	213.0	238.0	239.2
book-leaf (mouth)	145.8	198.89	230.0	210.4	235.1	239.0
bowel—*see* Neoplasm, intestine						
brachial plexus	171.2	198.89	—	215.2	238.1	239.2
brain NEC	191.9	198.3	—	225.0	237.5	239.6
basal ganglia	191.0	198.3	—	225.0	237.5	239.6
cerebellopontine angle	191.6	198.3	—	225.0	237.5	239.6
cerebellum NOS	191.6	198.3	—	225.0	237.5	239.6
cerebrum	191.0	198.3	—	225.0	237.5	239.6
choroid plexus	191.5	198.3	—	225.0	237.5	239.6
contiguous sites	191.8	—	—	—	—	—
corpus callosum	191.8	198.3	—	225.0	237.5	239.6
corpus striatum	191.0	198.3	—	225.0	237.5	239.6
cortex (cerebral)	191.0	198.3	—	225.0	237.5	239.6
frontal lobe	191.1	198.3	—	225.0	237.5	239.6
globus pallidus	191.0	198.3	—	225.0	237.5	239.6
hippocampus	191.2	198.3	—	225.0	237.5	239.6
hypothalamus	191.0	198.3	—	225.0	237.5	239.6
internal capsule	191.0	198.3	—	225.0	237.5	239.6
medulla oblongata	191.7	198.3	—	225.0	237.5	239.6
meninges	192.1	198.4	—	225.2	237.6	239.7
midbrain	191.7	198.3	—	225.0	237.5	239.6
occipital lobe	191.4	198.3	—	225.0	237.5	239.6
parietal lobe	191.3	198.3	—	225.0	237.5	239.6
peduncle	191.7	198.3	—	225.0	237.5	239.6
pons	191.7	198.3	—	225.0	237.5	239.6
stem	191.7	198.3	—	225.0	237.5	239.6
tapetum	191.8	198.3	—	225.0	237.5	239.6
temporal lobe	191.2	198.3	—	225.0	237.5	239.6
thalamus	191.0	198.3	—	225.0	237.5	239.6
uncus	191.2	198.3	—	225.0	237.5	239.6
ventricle (floor)	191.5	198.3	—	225.0	237.5	239.6
branchial (cleft) (vestiges)	146.8	198.89	230.0	210.6	235.1	239.0
breast (connective tissue) (female) (glandular tissue) (soft parts)	174.9	198.81	233.0	217	238.3	239.3
areola	174.0	198.81	233.0	217	238.3	239.3
male	175.0	198.81	233.0	217	238.3	239.3
axillary tail	174.6	198.81	233.0	217	238.3	239.3
central portion	174.1	198.81	233.0	217	238.3	239.3
contiguous sites	174.8	—	—	—	—	—
ectopic sites	174.8	198.81	233.0	217	238.3	239.3
inner	174.8	198.81	233.0	217	238.3	239.3
lower	174.8	198.81	233.0	217	238.3	239.3
lower-inner quadrant	174.3	198.81	233.0	217	238.3	239.3
lower-outer quadrant	174.5	198.81	233.0	217	238.3	239.3

	Malignant					
	Primary	Secondary	Ca in situ	Benign	Uncertain Behavior	Unspecified
male	175.9	198.81	233.0	217	238.3	239.3
areola	175.0	198.81	233.0	217	238.3	239.3
ectopic tissue	175.9	198.81	233.0	217	238.3	239.3
nipple	175.0	198.81	233.0	217	238.3	239.3
mastectomy site (skin) (*see also* Neoplasm, mastectomy site)	173.50	198.2	—	—	—	—
specified as breast tissue	174.8	198.81	—	—	—	—
midline	174.8	198.81	233.0	217	238.3	239.3
nipple	174.0	198.81	233.0	217	238.3	239.3
male	175.0	198.81	233.0	217	238.3	239.3
outer	174.8	198.81	233.0	217	238.3	239.3
skin (*see also* Neoplasm, mastectomy site)	173.50	198.2	232.5	216.5	238.2	239.2
tail (axillary)	174.6	198.81	233.0	217	238.3	239.3
upper	174.8	198.81	233.0	217	238.3	239.3
upper-inner quadrant	174.2	198.81	233.0	217	238.3	239.3
upper-outer quadrant	174.4	198.81	233.0	217	238.3	239.3
broad ligament	183.3	198.82	233.39	221.0	236.3	239.5
bronchiogenic, bronchogenic (lung)	162.9	197.0	231.2	212.3	235.7	239.1
bronchiole	162.9	197.0	231.2	212.3	235.7	239.1
bronchus	162.9	197.0	231.2	212.3	235.7	239.1
carina	162.2	197.0	231.2	212.3	235.7	239.1
contiguous sites with lung or trachea	162.8	—	—	—	—	—
lower lobe of lung	162.5	197.0	231.2	212.3	235.7	239.1
main	162.2	197.0	231.2	212.3	235.7	239.1
middle lobe of lung	162.4	197.0	231.2	212.3	235.7	239.1
upper lobe of lung	162.3	197.0	231.2	212.3	235.7	239.1
brow	173.30	198.2	232.3	216.3	238.2	239.2
basal cell carcinoma	173.31	—	—	—	—	—
specified type NEC	173.39	—	—	—	—	—
squamous cell carcinoma	173.32	—	—	—	—	—
buccal (cavity)	145.9	198.89	230.0	210.4	235.1	239.0
commissure	145.0	198.89	230.0	210.4	235.1	239.0
groove (lower) (upper)	145.1	198.89	230.0	210.4	235.1	239.0
mucosa	145.0	198.89	230.0	210.4	235.1	239.0
sulcus (lower) (upper)	145.1	198.89	230.0	210.4	235.1	239.0
bulbourethral gland	189.3	198.1	233.9	223.81	236.99	239.5
bursa—*see* Neoplasm, connective tissue						
buttock NEC*	195.3	198.89	232.5	229.8	238.8	239.89
calf*	195.5	198.89	232.7	229.8	238.8	239.89
calvarium	170.0	198.5	—	213.0	238.0	239.2
calyx, renal	189.1	198.0	233.9	223.1	236.91	239.5
canal						
anal	154.2	197.5	230.5	211.4	235.5	239.0
auditory (external) (*see also* Neoplasm, skin, ear)	173.20	198.2	232.2	216.2	238.2	239.2
auricular (external) (*see also* Neoplasm, skin, ear)	173.20	198.2	232.2	216.2	238.2	239.2
canaliculi, biliary (biliferi) (intrahepatic)	155.1	197.8	230.8	211.5	235.3	239.0
canthus (eye) (inner) (outer)	173.10	198.2	232.1	216.1	238.2	239.2
basal cell carcinoma	173.11	—	—	—	—	—
specified type NEC	173.19	—	—	—	—	—
squamous cell carcinoma	173.12	—	—	—	—	—
capillary—*see* Neoplasm, connective tissue						
caput coli	153.4	197.5	230.3	211.3	235.2	239.0
cardia (gastric)	151.0	197.8	230.2	211.1	235.2	239.0
cardiac orifice (stomach)	151.0	197.8	230.2	211.1	235.2	239.0
cardio-esophageal junction	151.0	197.8	230.2	211.1	235.2	239.0

	Malignant			Benign	Uncertain Behavior	Unspecified
	Primary	Secondary	Ca in situ			
cardio-esophagus	151.0	197.8	230.2	211.1	235.2	239.0
carina (bronchus)	162.2	197.0	231.2	212.3	235.7	239.1
carotid (artery)	171.0	198.89	—	215.0	238.1	239.2
body	194.5	198.89	—	227.5	237.3	239.7
carpus (any bone)	170.5	198.5	—	213.5	238.0	239.2
cartilage (articular) (joint) NEC—*see also*						
Neoplasm, bone	170.9	198.5	—	213.9	238.0	239.2
arytenoid	161.3	197.3	231.0	212.1	235.6	239.1
auricular	171.0	198.89	—	215.0	238.1	239.2
bronchi	162.2	197.3	—	212.3	235.7	239.1
connective tissue—*see* Neoplasm,						
connective tissue						
costal	170.3	198.5	—	213.3	238.0	239.2
cricoid	161.3	197.3	231.0	212.1	235.6	239.1
cuneiform	161.3	197.3	231.0	212.1	235.6	239.1
ear (external)	171.0	198.89	—	215.0	238.1	239.2
ensiform	170.3	198.5	—	213.3	238.0	239.2
epiglottis	161.1	197.3	231.0	212.1	235.6	239.1
anterior surface	146.4	198.89	230.0	210.6	235.1	239.0
eyelid	171.0	198.89	—	215.0	238.1	239.2
intervertebral	170.2	198.5	—	213.2	238.0	239.2
larynx, laryngeal	161.3	197.3	231.0	212.1	235.6	239.1
nose, nasal	160.0	197.3	231.8	212.0	235.9	239.1
pinna	171.0	198.89	—	215.0	238.1	239.2
rib	170.3	198.5	—	213.3	238.0	239.2
semilunar (knee)	170.7	198.5	—	213.7	238.0	239.2
thyroid	161.3	197.3	231.0	212.1	235.6	239.1
trachea	162.0	197.3	231.1	212.2	235.7	239.1
cauda equina	192.2	198.3	—	225.3	237.5	239.7
cavity						
buccal	145.9	198.89	230.0	210.4	235.1	239.0
nasal	160.0	197.3	231.8	212.0	235.9	239.1
oral	145.9	198.89	230.0	210.4	235.1	239.0
peritoneal	158.9	197.6	—	211.8	235.4	239.0
tympanic	160.1	197.3	231.8	212.0	235.9	239.1
cecum	153.4	197.5	230.3	211.3	235.2	239.0
central						
nervous system—*see*						
Neoplasm, nervous system						
white matter	191.0	198.3	—	225.0	237.5	239.6
cerebellopontine (angle)	191.6	198.3	—	225.0	237.5	239.6
cerebellum, cerebellar	191.6	198.3	—	225.0	237.5	239.6
cerebrum, cerebral (cortex)						
(hemisphere)						
(white matter)	191.0	198.3	—	225.0	237.5	239.6
meninges	192.1	198.4	—	225.2	237.6	239.7
peduncle	191.7	198.3	—	225.0	237.5	239.6
ventricle (any)	191.5	198.3	—	225.0	237.5	239.6
cervical region	195.0	198.89	234.8	229.8	238.8	239.89
cervix (cervical) (uteri)						
(uterus)	180.9	198.82	233.1	219.0	236.0	239.5
canal	180.0	198.82	233.1	219.0	236.0	239.5
contiguous sites	180.8	—	—	—	—	—
endocervix (canal) (gland)	180.0	198.82	233.1	219.0	236.0	239.5
exocervix	180.1	198.82	233.1	219.0	236.0	239.5
external os	180.1	198.82	233.1	219.0	236.0	239.5
internal os	180.0	198.82	233.1	219.0	236.0	239.5
nabothian gland	180.0	198.82	233.1	219.0	236.0	239.5
squamocolumnar junction	180.8	198.82	233.1	219.0	236.0	239.5
stump	180.8	198.82	233.1	219.0	236.0	239.5
cheek	195.0	198.89	234.8	229.8	238.8	239.89
external	173.30	198.2	232.3	216.3	238.2	239.2
basal cell carcinoma	173.31	—	—	—	—	—

| | Malignant | | | | | |
	Primary	Secondary	Ca in situ	Benign	Uncertain Behavior	Unspecified
specified type NEC.	173.39	—	—	—	—	—
squamous cell carcinoma	173.32	—	—	—	—	—
inner aspect.	145.0	198.89	230.0	210.4	235.1	239.0
internal	145.0	198.89	230.0	210.4	235.1	239.0
mucosa	145.0	198.89	230.0	210.4	235.1	239.0
chest (wall) NEC.	195.1	198.89	234.8	229.8	238.8	239.89
chiasma opticum	192.0	198.4	—	225.1	237.9	239.7
chin.	173.30	198.2	232.3	216.3	238.2	239.2
basal cell carcinoma	173.31	—	—	—	—	—
specified type NEC.	173.39	—	—	—	—	—
squamous cell carcinoma	173.32	—	—	—	—	—
choana	147.3	198.89	230.0	210.7	235.1	239.0
cholangiole	155.1	197.8	230.8	211.5	235.3	239.0
choledochal duct	156.1	197.8	230.8	211.5	235.3	239.0
choroid	190.6	198.4	234.0	224.6	238.8	239.81
plexus.	191.5	198.3	—	225.0	237.5	239.6
ciliary body.	190.0	198.4	234.0	224.0	238.8	239.89
clavicle	170.3	198.5	—	213.3	238.0	239.2
clitoris	184.3	198.82	233.32	221.2	236.3	239.5
clivus	170.0	198.5	—	213.0	238.0	239.2
cloacogenic zone.	154.8	197.5	230.7	211.4	235.5	239.0
coccygeal						
body or glomus.	194.6	198.89	—	227.6	237.3	239.7
vertebra.	170.6	198.5	—	213.6	238.0	239.2
coccyx	170.6	198.5	—	213.6	238.0	239.2
colon—see also Neoplasm,						
intestine, large	153.9	197.5	230.3	211.3	235.2	239.0
with rectum.	154.0	197.5	230.4	211.4	235.2	239.0
column, spinal—see Neoplasm, spine						
columnella (see also Neoplasm,						
skin, face)	173.30	198.2	232.3	216.3	238.2	239.2
commissure						
labial, lip	140.6	198.89	230.0	210.4	235.1	239.0
laryngeal	161.0	197.3	231.0	212.1	235.6	239.1
common (bile) duct	156.1	197.8	230.8	211.5	235.3	239.0
concha (see also Neoplasm, skin,						
ear).	173.20	198.2	232.2	216.2	238.2	239.2
nose	160.0	197.3	231.8	212.0	235.9	239.1
conjunctiva	190.3	198.4	234.0	224.3	238.8	239.89
connective tissue NEC.	171.9	198.89	—	215.9	238.1	239.2

Note—For neoplasms of connective tissue (blood vessel, bursa, fasica, ligament, muscle, peripheral nerves, sympathetic and parasympathetic nerves, and ganglia, synovia, tendon, etc.) or of morphological types that indicate connective tissue, code according to the list under "Neoplasm, connective tissue;" for sites that do not appear in this list, code to neoplasm of that site; e.g.: liposarcoma, shoulder 171.2; leiomyosarcoma, stomach 151.9; neurofibroma, chest wall 215.4.
Morphological types that indicate connective tissue appear in their proper palce in the alphabetic index with the instruction "see Neoplasm, connective tissue..."

	Primary	Secondary	Ca in situ	Benign	Uncertain Behavior	Unspecified
abdomen	171.5	198.89	—	215.5	238.1	239.2
abdominal wall.	171.5	198.89	—	215.5	238.1	239.2
ankle	171.3	198.89	—	215.3	238.1	239.2
antecubital fossa or space	171.2	198.89	—	215.2	238.1	239.2
arm	171.2	198.89	—	215.2	238.1	239.2
auricle (ear).	171.0	198.89	—	215.0	238.1	239.2
axilla	171.4	198.89	—	215.4	238.1	239.2
back	171.7	198.89	—	215.7	238.1	239.2
breast (female) (see also						
Neoplasm, breast).	174.9	198.81	233.0	217	238.3	239.3
male	175.9	198.81	233.0	217	238.3	239.3
buttock	171.6	198.89	—	215.6	238.1	239.2
calf	171.3	198.89	—	215.3	238.1	239.2
cervical region	171.0	198.89	—	215.0	238.1	239.2
cheek	171.0	198.89	—	215.0	238.1	239.2

	Malignant			Benign	Uncertain Behavior	Unspecified
	Primary	Secondary	Ca in situ			
chest (wall)	171.4	198.89	—	215.4	238.1	239.2
chin	171.0	198.89	—	215.0	238.1	239.2
contiguous sites	171.8	—	—	—	—	—
diaphragm	171.4	198.89	—	215.4	238.1	239.2
ear (external)	171.0	198.89	—	215.0	238.1	239.2
elbow	171.2	198.89	—	215.2	238.1	239.2
extrarectal	171.6	198.89	—	215.6	238.1	239.2
extremity	171.8	198.89	—	215.8	238.1	239.2
lower	171.3	198.89	—	215.3	238.1	239.2
upper	171.2	198.89	—	215.2	238.1	239.2
eyelid	171.0	198.89	—	215.0	238.1	239.2
face	171.0	198.89	—	215.0	238.1	239.2
finger	171.2	198.89	—	215.2	238.1	239.2
flank	171.7	198.89	—	215.7	238.1	239.2
foot	171.3	198.89	—	215.3	238.1	239.2
forearm	171.2	198.89	—	215.2	238.1	239.2
forehead	171.0	198.89	—	215.0	238.1	239.2
gastric	171.5	198.89	—	215.5	238.1	—
gastrointestinal	171.5	198.89	—	215.5	238.1	—
gluteal region	171.6	198.89	—	215.6	238.1	239.2
great vessels NEC	171.4	198.89	—	215.4	238.1	239.2
groin	171.6	198.89	—	215.6	238.1	239.2
hand	171.2	198.89	—	215.2	238.1	239.2
head	171.0	198.89	—	215.0	238.1	239.2
heel	171.3	198.89	—	215.3	238.1	239.2
hip	171.3	198.89	—	215.3	238.1	239.2
hypochondrium	171.5	198.89	—	215.5	238.1	239.2
iliopsoas muscle	171.6	198.89	—	215.5	238.1	239.2
infraclavicular region	171.4	198.89	—	215.4	238.1	239.2
inguinal (canal) (region)	171.6	198.89	—	215.6	238.1	239.2
intestine	171.5	198.89	—	215.5	238.1	—
intrathoracic	171.4	198.89	—	215.4	238.1	239.2
ischorectal fossa	171.6	198.89	—	215.6	238.1	239.2
jaw	143.9	198.89	230.0	210.4	235.1	239.0
knee	171.3	198.89	—	215.3	238.1	239.2
leg	171.3	198.89	—	215.3	238.1	239.2
limb NEC	171.9	198.89	—	215.8	238.1	239.2
lower	171.3	198.89	—	215.3	238.1	239.2
upper	171.2	198.89	—	215.2	238.1	239.2
nates	171.6	198.89	—	215.6	238.1	239.2
neck	171.0	198.89	—	215.0	238.1	239.2
orbit	190.1	198.4	234.0	224.1	238.8	239.89
pararectal	171.6	198.89	—	215.6	238.1	239.2
para-urethral	171.6	198.89	—	215.6	238.1	239.2
paravaginal	171.6	198.89	—	215.6	238.1	239.2
pelvis (floor)	171.6	198.89	—	215.6	238.1	239.2
pelvo-abdominal	171.8	198.89	—	215.8	238.1	239.2
perineum	171.6	198.89	—	215.6	238.1	239.2
perirectal (tissue)	171.6	198.89	—	215.6	238.1	239.2
periurethral (tissue)	171.6	198.89	—	215.6	238.1	239.2
popliteal fossa or space	171.3	198.89	—	215.3	238.1	239.2
presacral	171.6	198.89	—	215.6	238.1	239.2
psoas muscle	171.5	198.89	—	215.5	238.1	239.2
pterygoid fossa	171.0	198.89	—	215.0	238.1	239.2
rectovaginal septum or wall	171.6	198.89	—	215.6	238.1	239.2
rectovesical	171.6	198.89	—	215.6	238.1	239.2
retroperitoneum	158.0	197.6	—	211.8	235.4	239.0
sacrococcygeal region	171.6	198.89	—	215.6	238.1	239.2
scalp	171.0	198.89	—	215.0	238.1	239.2
scapular region	171.4	198.89	—	215.4	238.1	239.2
shoulder	171.2	198.89	—	215.2	238.1	239.2
skin (dermis) NEC	173.90	198.2	232.9	216.9	238.2	239.2

	Malignant			Benign	Uncertain Behavior	Unspecified
	Primary	Secondary	Ca in situ			
stomach	171.5	198.89	—	215.5	238.1	—
submental	171.0	198.89	—	215.0	238.1	239.2
supraclavicular region	171.0	198.89	—	215.0	238.1	239.2
temple	171.0	198.89	—	215.0	238.1	239.2
temporal region	171.0	198.89	—	215.0	238.1	239.2
thigh	171.3	198.89	—	215.3	238.1	239.2
thoracic (duct) (wall)	171.4	198.89	—	215.4	238.1	239.2
thorax	171.4	198.89	—	215.4	238.1	239.2
thumb	171.2	198.89	—	215.2	238.1	239.2
toe	171.3	198.89	—	215.3	238.1	239.2
trunk	171.7	198.89	—	215.7	238.1	239.2
umbilicus	171.5	198.89	—	215.5	238.1	239.2
vesicorectal	171.6	198.89	—	215.6	238.1	239.2
wrist	171.2	198.89	—	215.2	238.1	239.2
conus medullaris	192.2	198.3	—	225.3	237.5	239.7
cord (true) (vocal)	161.0	197.3	231.0	212.1	235.6	239.1
false	161.1	197.3	231.0	212.1	235.6	239.1
spermatic	187.6	198.82	233.6	222.8	236.6	239.5
spinal (cervical) (lumbar)						
(thoracic)	192.2	198.3	—	225.3	237.5	239.7
cornea (limbus)	190.4	198.4	234.0	224.4	238.8	239.89
corpus						
albicans	183.0	198.6	233.39	220	236.2	239.5
callosum, brain	191.8	198.3	—	225.0	237.5	239.6
cavernosum	187.3	198.82	233.5	222.1	236.6	239.5
gastric	151.4	197.8	230.2	211.1	235.2	239.0
penis	187.3	198.82	233.5	222.1	236.6	239.5
striatum, cerebrum	191.0	198.3	—	225.0	237.5	239.6
uteri	182.0	198.82	233.2	219.1	236.0	239.5
isthmus	182.1	198.82	233.2	219.1	236.0	239.5
cortex						
adrenal	194.0	198.7	234.8	227.0	237.2	239.7
cerebral	191.0	198.3	—	225.0	237.5	239.6
costal cartilage	170.3	198.5	—	213.3	238.0	239.2
costovertebral joint	170.3	198.5	—	213.3	238.0	239.2
Cowper's gland	189.3	198.1	233.9	223.81	236.99	239.5
cranial (fossa, any)	191.9	198.3	—	225.0	237.5	239.6
meninges	192.1	198.4	—	225.2	237.6	239.7
nerve (any)	192.0	198.4	—	225.1	237.9	239.7
craniobuccal pouch	194.3	198.89	234.8	227.3	237.0	239.7
craniopharyngeal (duct)						
(pouch)	194.3	198.89	234.8	227.3	237.0	239.7
cricoid	148.0	198.89	230.0	210.8	235.1	239.0
cartilage	161.3	197.3	231.0	212.1	235.6	239.1
cricopharynx	148.0	198.89	230.0	210.8	235.1	239.0
crypt of Morgagni	154.8	197.5	230.7	211.4	235.2	239.0
crystalline lens	190.0	198.4	234.0	224.0	238.8	239.89
cul-de-sac (Douglas')	158.8	197.6	—	211.8	235.4	239.0
cuneiform cartilage	161.3	197.3	231.0	212.1	235.6	239.1
cutaneous—*see* Neoplasm, skin						
cutis—*see* Neoplasm, skin						
cystic (bile) duct (common)	156.1	197.8	230.8	211.5	235.3	239.0
dermis—*see* Neoplasm, skin						
diaphragm	171.4	198.89	—	215.4	238.1	239.2
digestive organs, system,						
tube, tract NEC	159.9	197.8	230.9	211.9	235.5	239.0
contiguous sites with						
peritoneum	159.8	—	—	—	—	—
disc, intervertebral	170.2	198.5	—	213.2	238.0	239.2
disease, generalized	199.0	199.0	234.9	229.9	238.9	199.0
disseminated	199.0	199.0	234.9	229.9	238.9	199.0
Douglas' cul-de-sac or pouch	158.8	197.6	—	211.8	235.4	239.0
duodenojejunal junction	152.8	197.4	230.7	211.2	235.2	239.0

	Malignant			Benign	Uncertain Behavior	Unspecified
	Primary	Secondary	Ca in situ			
duodenum	152.0	197.4	230.7	211.2	235.2	239.0
dura (cranial) (mater)	192.1	198.4	—	225.2	237.6	239.7
cerebral	192.1	198.4	—	225.2	237.6	239.7
spinal	192.3	198.4	—	225.4	237.6	239.7
ear (external) (see also Neoplasm, ear, skin)	173.20	198.2	232.2	216.2	238.2	239.2
auricle or auris (see also Neoplasm, ear, skin)	173.20	198.2	232.2	216.2	238.2	239.2
canal, external (see also Neoplasm, ear, skin)	173.20	198.2	232.2	216.2	238.2	239.2
cartilage	171.0	198.89	—	215.0	238.1	239.2
external meatus (see also Neoplasm, ear, skin)	173.20	198.2	232.2	216.2	238.2	239.2
inner	160.1	197.3	231.8	212.0	235.9	239.89
lobule (see also Neoplasm, ear, skin)	173.20	198.2	232.2	216.2	238.2	239.2
middle	160.1	197.3	231.8	212.0	235.9	239.89
contiguous sites with accessory sinuses or nasal cavities	160.8	—	—	—	—	—
skin	173.20	198.2	232.2	216.2	238.2	239.2
basal cell carcinoma	173.21	—	—	—	—	—
specified type NEC	173.29	—	—	—	—	—
squamous cell carcinoma	173.22	—	—	—	—	—
earlobe	173.20	198.2	232.2	216.2	238.2	239.2
basal cell carcinoma	173.21	—	—	—	—	—
specified type NEC	173.29	—	—	—	—	—
squamous cell carcinoma	173.22	—	—	—	—	—
ejaculatory duct	187.8	198.82	233.6	222.8	236.6	239.5
elbow NEC*	195.4	198.89	232.6	229.8	238.8	239.89
endocardium	164.1	198.89	—	212.7	238.8	239.89
endocervix (canal) (gland)	180.0	198.82	233.1	219.0	236.0	239.5
endocrine gland NEC	194.9	198.89	—	227.9	237.4	239.7
pluriglandular NEC	194.8	198.89	234.8	227.8	237.4	239.7
endometrium (gland) (stroma)	182.0	198.82	233.2	219.1	236.0	239.5
ensiform cartilage	170.3	198.5	—	213.3	238.0	239.2
enteric—see Neoplasm, intestine						
ependyma (brain)	191.5	198.3	—	225.0	237.5	239.6
epicardium	164.1	198.89	—	212.7	238.8	239.89
epididymis	187.5	198.82	233.6	222.3	236.6	239.5
epidural	192.9	198.4	—	225.9	237.9	239.7
epiglottis	161.1	197.3	231.0	212.1	235.6	239.1
anterior aspect or surface	146.4	198.89	230.0	210.6	235.1	239.0
cartilage	161.3	197.3	231.0	212.1	235.6	239.1
free border (margin)	146.4	198.89	230.0	210.6	235.1	239.0
junctional region	146.5	198.89	230.0	210.6	235.1	239.0
posterior (laryngeal) surface	161.1	197.3	231.0	212.1	235.6	239.1
suprahyoid portion	161.1	197.3	231.0	212.1	235.6	239.1
esophagogastric junction	151.0	197.8	230.2	211.1	235.2	239.0
esophagus	150.9	197.8	230.1	211.0	235.5	239.0
abdominal	150.2	197.8	230.1	211.0	235.5	239.0
cervical	150.0	197.8	230.1	211.0	235.5	239.0
contiguous sites	150.8	—	—	—	—	—
distal (third)	150.5	197.8	230.1	211.0	235.5	239.0
lower (third)	150.5	197.8	230.1	211.0	235.5	239.0
middle (third)	150.4	197.8	230.1	211.0	235.5	239.0
proximal (third)	150.3	197.8	230.1	211.0	235.5	239.0
specified part NEC	150.8	197.8	230.1	211.0	235.5	239.0
thoracic	150.1	197.8	230.1	211.0	235.5	239.0
upper (third)	150.3	197.8	230.1	211.0	235.5	239.0
ethmoid (sinus)	160.3	197.3	231.8	212.0	235.9	239.1

	Malignant Primary	Malignant Secondary	Malignant Ca in situ	Benign	Uncertain Behavior	Unspecified
bone or labyrinth	170.0	198.5	—	213.0	238.0	239.2
Eustachian tube	160.1	197.3	231.8	212.0	235.9	239.1
exocervix	180.1	198.82	233.1	219.0	236.0	239.5
external						
meatus (ear) (*see also* Neoplasm,						
skin, ear)	173.20	198.2	232.2	216.2	238.2	239.2
os, cervix uteri	180.1	198.82	233.1	219.0	236.0	239.5
extradural	192.9	198.4	—	225.9	237.9	239.7
extrahepatic (bile) duct	156.1	197.8	230.8	211.5	235.3	239.0
contiguous sites with						
gallbladder	156.8	—	—	—	—	—
extraocular muscle	190.1	198.4	234.0	224.1	238.8	239.89
extrarectal	195.3	198.89	234.8	229.8	238.8	239.89
extremity*	195.8	198.89	232.8	229.8	238.8	239.89
lower*	195.5	198.89	232.7	229.8	238.8	239.89
upper*	195.4	198.89	232.6	229.8	238.8	239.89
eye NEC	190.9	198.4	234.0	224.9	238.8	239.89
contiguous sites	190.8	—	—	—	—	—
specified sites NEC	190.8	198.4	234.0	224.8	238.8	239.89
eyeball	190.0	198.4	234.0	224.0	238.8	239.89
eyebrow	173.30	198.2	232.3	216.3	238.2	239.2
basal cell carcinoma	173.31	—	—	—	—	—
specified type NEC	173.39	—	—	—	—	—
squamous cell carcinoma	173.32	—	—	—	—	—
eyelid (lower) (skin) (upper)	173.10	198.2	232.1	216.1	238.2	239.2
basal cell carcinoma	173.11	—	—	—	—	—
cartilage	171.0	198.89	—	215.0	238.1	239.2
specified type NEC	173.19	—	—	—	—	—
squamous cell carcinoma	173.12	—	—	—	—	—
face NEC*	195.0	198.89	232.3	229.8	238.8	239.89
fallopian tube (accessory)	183.2	198.82	233.39	221.0	236.3	239.5
falx (cerebelli) (cerebri)	192.1	198.4	—	225.2	237.6	239.7
fascia—*see also* Neoplasm, connective tissue						
palmar	171.2	198.89	—	215.2	238.1	239.2
plantar	171.3	198.89	—	215.3	238.1	239.2
fatty tissue—*see* Neoplasm, connective tissue						
fauces, faucial NEC	146.9	198.89	230.0	210.6	235.1	239.0
pillars	146.2	198.89	230.0	210.6	235.1	239.0
tonsil	146.0	198.89	230.0	210.5	235.1	239.0
femur (any part)	170.7	198.5	—	213.7	238.0	239.2
fetal membrane	181	198.82	233.2	219.8	236.1	239.5
fibrous tissue—*see* Neoplasm, connective tissue						
fibula (any part)	170.7	198.5	—	213.7	238.0	239.2
filum terminale	192.2	198.3	—	225.3	237.5	239.7
finger NEC*	195.4	198.89	232.6	229.8	238.8	239.89
flank NEC*	195.8	198.89	232.5	229.8	238.8	239.89
follicle, nabothian	180.0	198.82	233.1	219.0	236.0	239.5
foot NEC*	195.5	198.89	232.7	229.8	238.8	239.89
forearm NEC*	195.4	198.89	232.6	229.8	238.8	239.89
forehead (skin)	173.30	198.2	232.3	216.3	238.2	239.2
basal cell carcinoma	173.31	—	—	—	—	—
specified type NEC	173.39	—	—	—	—	—
squamous cell carcinoma	173.32	—	—	—	—	—
foreskin	187.1	198.82	233.5	222.1	236.6	239.5
fornix						
pharyngeal	147.3	198.89	230.0	210.7	235.1	239.0
vagina	184.0	198.82	233.31	221.1	236.3	239.5
fossa (of)						
anterior (cranial)	191.9	198.3	—	225.0	237.5	239.6
cranial	191.9	198.3	—	225.0	237.5	239.6
ischiorectal	195.3	198.89	234.8	229.8	238.8	239.89
middle (cranial)	191.9	198.3	—	225.0	237.5	239.6
pituitary	194.3	198.89	234.8	227.3	237.0	239.7

	Malignant			Benign	Uncertain Behavior	Unspecified
	Primary	Secondary	Ca in situ			
posterior (cranial)	191.9	198.3	—	225.0	237.5	239.6
pterygoid	171.0	198.89	—	215.0	238.1	239.2
pyriform	148.1	198.89	230.0	210.8	235.1	239.0
Rosenmüller	147.2	198.89	230.0	210.7	235.1	239.0
tonsillar.	146.1	198.89	230.0	210.6	235.1	239.0
fourchette.	184.4	198.82	233.32	221.2	236.3	239.5
frenulum						
labii—see Neoplasm, lip, internal						
linguae	141.3	198.89	230.0	210.1	235.1	239.0
frontal						
bone	170.0	198.5	—	213.0	238.0	239.2
lobe, brain	191.1	198.3	—	225.0	237.5	239.6
meninges	192.1	198.4	—	225.2	237.6	239.7
pole	191.1	198.3	—	225.0	237.5	239.6
sinus	160.4	197.3	231.8	212.0	235.9	239.1
fundus						
stomach.	151.3	197.8	230.2	211.1	235.2	239.0
uterus	182.0	198.82	233.2	219.1	236.0	239.5
gall duct (extrahepatic).	156.1	197.8	230.8	211.5	235.3	239.0
intrahepatic	155.1	197.8	230.8	211.5	235.3	239.0
gallbladder	156.0	197.8	230.8	211.5	235.3	239.0
contiguous sites with						
extrahepatic bile ducts	156.8	—	—	—	—	—
ganglia (see also Neoplasm,						
connective tissue)	171.9	198.89	—	215.9	238.1	239.2
basal	191.0	198.3	—	225.0	237.5	239.6
ganglion (see also Neoplasm,						
connective tissue)	171.9	198.89	—	215.9	238.1	239.2
cranial nerve	192.0	198.4	—	225.1	237.9	239.7
Gartner's duct	184.0	198.82	233.31	221.1	236.3	239.5
gastric—see Neoplasm, stomach						
gastrocolic	159.8	197.8	230.9	211.9	235.5	239.0
gastroesophageal junction	151.0	197.8	230.2	211.1	235.2	239.0
gastrointestinal (tract) NEC	159.9	197.8	230.9	211.9	235.5	239.0
generalized	199.0	199.0	234.9	229.9	238.9	199.0
genital organ or tract						
female NEC	184.9	198.82	233.39	221.9	236.3	239.5
contiguous sites	184.8	—	—	—	—	—
specified site NEC	184.8	198.82	233.39	221.8	236.3	239.5
male NEC	187.9	198.82	233.6	222.9	236.6	239.5
contiguous sites	187.8	—	—	—	—	—
specified site NEC	187.8	198.82	233.6	222.8	236.6	239.5
genitourinary tract						
female	184.9	198.82	233.39	221.9	236.3	239.5
male	187.9	198.82	233.6	222.9	236.6	239.5
gingiva (alveolar) (marginal).	143.9	198.89	230.0	210.4	235.1	239.0
lower	143.1	198.89	230.0	210.4	235.1	239.0
mandibular	143.1	198.89	230.0	210.4	235.1	239.0
maxillary	143.0	198.89	230.0	210.4	235.1	239.0
upper	143.0	198.89	230.0	210.4	235.1	239.0
gland, glandular (lymphatic)						
(system)—see also Neoplasm,						
lymph gland						
endocrine NEC.	194.9	198.89	—	227.9	237.4	239.7
salivary—see Neoplasm,						
salivary, gland						
glans penis	187.2	198.82	233.5	222.1	236.6	239.5
globus pallidus	191.0	198.3	—	225.0	237.5	239.6
glomus						
coccygeal.	194.6	198.89	—	227.6	237.3	239.7
jugularis	194.6	198.89	—	227.6	237.3	239.7
glosso-epiglottic fold(s)	146.4	198.89	230.0	210.6	235.1	239.0
glossopalatine fold	146.2	198.89	230.0	210.6	235.1	239.0

	Malignant					
	Primary	Secondary	Ca in situ	Benign	Uncertain Behavior	Unspecified
glossopharyngeal sulcus	146.1	198.89	230.0	210.6	235.1	239.0
glottis	161.0	197.3	231.0	212.1	235.6	239.1
gluteal region*	195.3	198.89	232.5	229.8	238.8	239.89
great vessels NEC	171.4	198.89	—	215.4	238.1	239.2
groin NEC*	195.3	198.89	232.5	229.8	238.8	239.89
gum	143.9	198.89	230.0	210.4	235.1	239.0
contiguous sites	143.8	—	—	—	—	—
lower	143.1	198.89	230.0	210.4	235.1	239.0
upper	143.0	198.89	230.0	210.4	235.1	239.0
hand NEC*	195.4	198.89	232.6	229.8	238.8	239.89
head NEC*	195.0	198.89	232.4	229.8	238.8	239.89
heart	164.1	198.89	—	212.7	238.8	239.89
contiguous sites with mediastinum or thymus	164.8	—	—	—	—	—
heel NEC*	195.5	198.89	232.7	229.8	238.8	239.89
helix (*see also* Neoplasm, skin, ear) .	173.20	198.2	232.2	216.2	238.2	239.2
hematopoietic, hemopoietic tissue NEC	202.8	198.89	—	—	—	238.79
hemisphere, cerebral	191.0	198.3	—	225.0	237.5	239.6
hemorrhoidal zone	154.2	197.5	230.5	211.4	235.5	239.0
hepatic	155.2	197.7	230.8	211.5	235.3	239.0
duct (bile)	156.1	197.8	230.8	211.5	235.3	239.0
flexure (colon)	153.0	197.5	230.3	211.3	235.2	239.0
primary	155.0	—	—	—	—	—
hilus of lung	162.2	197.0	231.2	212.3	235.7	239.1
hip NEC*	195.5	198.89	232.7	229.8	238.8	239.89
hippocampus, brain	191.2	198.3	—	225.0	237.5	239.6
humerus (any part)	170.4	198.5	—	213.4	238.0	239.2
hymen	184.0	198.82	233.31	221.1	236.3	239.5
hypopharynx, hypopharyngeal NEC	148.9	198.89	230.0	210.8	235.1	239.0
contiguous sites	148.8	—	—	—	—	—
postcricoid region	148.0	198.89	230.0	210.8	235.1	239.0
posterior wall	148.3	198.89	230.0	210.8	235.1	239.0
pyriform fossa (sinus)	148.1	198.89	230.0	210.8	235.1	239.0
specified site NEC	148.8	198.89	230.0	210.8	235.1	239.0
wall	148.9	198.89	230.0	210.8	235.1	239.0
posterior	148.3	198.89	230.0	210.8	235.1	239.0
hypophysis	194.3	198.89	234.8	227.3	237.0	239.7
hypothalamus	191.0	198.3	—	225.0	237.5	239.6
ileocecum, ileocecal (coil, junction, valve)	153.4	197.5	230.3	211.3	235.2	239.0
ileum	152.2	197.4	230.7	211.2	235.2	239.0
ilium	170.6	198.5	—	213.6	238.0	239.2
immunoproliferative NEC	203.8	—	—	—	—	—
infraclavicular (region)*	195.1	198.89	232.5	229.8	238.8	239.89
inguinal (region)*	195.3	198.89	232.5	229.8	238.8	239.89
insula	191.0	198.3	—	225.0	237.5	239.6
insular tissue (pancreas)	157.4	197.8	230.9	211.7	235.5	239.0
brain	191.0	198.3	—	225.0	237.5	239.6
interarytenoid fold	148.2	198.89	230.0	210.8	235.1	239.0
hypopharyngeal aspect	148.2	198.89	230.0	210.8	235.1	239.0
laryngeal aspect	161.1	197.3	231.0	212.1	235.6	239.1
marginal zone	148.2	198.89	230.0	210.8	235.1	239.0
interdental papillae	143.9	198.89	230.0	210.4	235.1	239.0
lower	143.1	198.89	230.0	210.4	235.1	239.0
upper	143.0	198.89	230.0	210.4	235.1	239.0
internal						
capsule	191.0	198.3	—	225.0	237.5	239.6
os (cervix)	180.0	198.82	233.1	219.0	236.0	239.5
intervertebral cartilage or disc	170.2	198.5	—	213.2	238.0	239.2

	Malignant					
	Primary	Secondary	Ca in situ	Benign	Uncertain Behavior	Unspecified
intestine, intestinal	159.0	197.8	230.7	211.9	235.2	239.0
large	153.9	197.5	230.3	211.3	235.2	239.0
appendix	153.5	197.5	230.3	211.3	235.2	239.0
caput coli	153.4	197.5	230.3	211.3	235.2	239.0
cecum	153.4	197.5	230.3	211.3	235.2	239.0
colon	153.9	197.5	230.3	211.3	235.2	239.0
and rectum	154.0	197.5	230.4	211.4	235.2	239.0
ascending	153.6	197.5	230.3	211.3	235.2	239.0
caput	153.4	197.5	230.3	211.3	235.2	239.0
contiguous sites	153.8	—	—	—	—	—
descending	153.2	197.5	230.3	211.3	235.2	239.0
distal	153.2	197.5	230.3	211.3	235.2	239.0
left	153.2	197.5	230.3	211.3	235.2	239.0
pelvic	153.3	197.5	230.3	211.3	235.2	239.0
right	153.6	197.5	230.3	211.3	235.2	239.0
sigmoid (flexure)	153.3	197.5	230.3	211.3	235.2	239.0
transverse	153.1	197.5	230.3	211.3	235.2	239.0
contiguous sites	153.8	—	—	—	—	—
hepatic flexure	153.0	197.5	230.3	211.3	235.2	239.0
ileocecum,ileocecal						
(coil, valve)	153.4	197.5	230.3	211.3	235.2	239.0
sigmoid flexure (lower)						
(upper)	153.3	197.5	230.3	211.3	235.2	239.0
splenic flexure	153.7	197.5	230.3	211.3	235.2	239.0
small	152.9	197.4	230.7	211.2	235.2	239.0
contiguous sites	152.8	—	—	—	—	—
duodenum	152.0	197.4	230.7	211.2	235.2	239.0
ileum	152.2	197.4	230.7	211.2	235.2	239.0
jejunum	152.1	197.4	230.7	211.2	235.2	239.0
tract NEC	159.0	197.8	230.7	211.9	235.2	239.0
intra-abdominal	195.2	198.89	234.8	229.8	238.8	239.89
intracranial NEC	191.9	198.3	—	225.0	237.5	239.6
intrahepatic (bile) duct	155.1	197.8	230.8	211.5	235.3	239.0
intraocular	190.0	198.4	234.0	224.0	238.8	239.89
intraorbital	190.1	198.4	234.0	224.1	238.8	239.89
intrasellar	194.3	198.89	234.8	227.3	237.0	239.7
intrathoracic (cavity)						
(organs NEC)	195.1	198.89	234.8	229.8	238.8	239.89
contiguous sites with respiratory						
organs	165.8	—	—	—	—	—
iris	190.0	198.4	234.0	224.0	238.8	239.89
ischiorectal (fossa)	195.3	198.89	234.8	229.8	238.8	239.89
ischium	170.6	198.5	—	213.6	238.0	239.2
island of Reil	191.0	198.3	—	225.0	237.5	239.6
islands or islets of Langerhans	157.4	197.8	230.9	211.7	235.5	239.0
isthmus uteri	182.1	198.82	233.2	219.1	236.0	239.5
jaw	195.0	198.89	234.8	229.8	238.8	239.89
bone	170.1	198.5	—	213.1	238.0	239.2
carcinoma	143.9	—	—	—	—	—
lower	143.1	—	—	—	—	—
upper	143.0	—	—	—	—	—
lower	170.1	198.5	—	213.1	238.0	239.2
upper	170.0	198.5	—	213.0	238.0	239.2
carcinoma (any type)						
(lower) (upper)	195.0	—	—	—	—	—
skin (*see also* Neoplasm, skin						
face)	173.30	198.2	232.3	216.3	238.2	239.2
soft tissues	143.9	198.89	230.0	210.4	235.1	239.0
lower	143.1	198.89	230.0	210.4	235.1	239.0
upper	143.0	198.89	230.0	210.4	235.1	239.0
jejunum	152.1	197.4	230.7	211.2	235.2	239.0
joint NEC (*see also*						
Neoplasm, bone)	170.9	198.5	—	213.9	238.0	239.2

	Malignant					
	Primary	Secondary	Ca in situ	Benign	Uncertain Behavior	Unspecified
acromioclavicular	170.4	198.5	—	213.4	238.0	239.2
bursa or synovial membrane—*see* Neoplasm, connective tissue						
costovertebral	170.3	198.5	—	213.3	238.0	239.2
sternocostal	170.3	198.5	—	213.3	238.0	239.2
temporomandibular	170.1	198.5	—	213.1	238.0	239.2
junction						
anorectal	154.8	197.5	230.7	211.4	235.5	239.0
cardioesophageal	151.0	197.8	230.2	211.1	235.2	239.0
esophagogastric	151.0	197.8	230.2	211.1	235.2	239.0
gastroesophageal	151.0	197.8	230.2	211.1	235.2	239.0
hard and soft palate	145.5	198.89	230.0	210.4	235.1	239.0
ileocecal	153.4	197.5	230.3	211.3	235.2	239.0
pelvirectal	154.0	197.5	230.4	211.4	235.2	239.0
pelviureteric	189.1	198.0	233.9	223.1	236.91	239.5
rectosigmoid	154.0	197.5	230.4	211.4	235.2	239.0
squamocolumnar, of cervix	180.8	198.82	233.1	219.0	236.0	239.5
kidney (parenchyma)	189.0	198.0	233.9	223.0	236.91	239.5
calyx	189.1	198.0	233.9	223.1	236.91	239.5
hilus	189.1	198.0	233.9	223.1	236.91	239.5
pelvis	189.1	198.0	233.9	223.1	236.91	239.5
knee NEC*	195.5	198.89	232.7	229.8	238.8	239.89
labia (skin)	184.4	198.82	233.32	221.2	236.3	239.5
majora	184.1	198.82	233.32	221.2	236.3	239.5
minora	184.2	198.82	233.32	221.2	236.3	239.5
labial—*see also* Neoplasm, lip						
sulcus (lower) (upper)	145.1	198.89	230.0	210.4	235.1	239.0
labium (skin)	184.4	198.82	233.32	221.2	236.3	239.5
majus	184.1	198.82	233.32	221.2	236.3	239.5
minus	184.2	198.82	233.32	221.2	236.3	239.5
lacrimal						
canaliculi	190.7	198.4	234.0	224.7	238.8	239.89
duct (nasal)	190.7	198.4	234.0	224.7	238.8	239.89
gland	190.2	198.4	234.0	224.2	238.8	239.89
punctum	190.7	198.4	234.0	224.7	238.8	239.89
sac	190.7	198.4	234.0	224.7	238.8	239.89
Langerhans, islands or islets	157.4	197.8	230.9	211.7	235.5	239.0
laryngopharynx	148.9	198.89	230.0	210.8	235.1	239.0
larynx, laryngeal NEC	161.9	197.3	231.0	212.1	235.6	239.1
aryepiglottic fold	161.1	197.3	231.0	212.1	235.6	239.1
cartilage (arytenoid) (cricoid) (cuneiform) (thyroid)	161.3	197.3	231.0	212.1	235.6	239.1
commissure (anterior) (posterior)	161.0	197.3	231.0	212.1	235.6	239.1
contiguous sites	161.8	—	—	—	—	—
extrinsic NEC	161.1	197.3	231.0	212.1	235.6	239.1
meaning hypopharynx	148.9	198.89	230.0	210.8	235.1	239.0
interarytenoid fold	161.1	197.3	231.0	212.1	235.6	239.1
intrinsic	161.0	197.3	231.0	212.1	235.6	239.1
ventricular band	161.1	197.3	231.0	212.1	235.6	239.1
leg NEC*	195.5	198.89	232.7	229.8	238.8	239.89
lens, crystalline	190.0	198.4	234.0	224.0	238.8	239.89
lid (lower) (upper)	173.10	198.2	232.1	216.1	238.2	239.2
basal cell carcinoma	173.11	—	—	—	—	—
specified type NEC	173.19	—	—	—	—	—
squamous cell carcinoma	173.12	—	—	—	—	—
ligament—*see also* Neoplasm, connective tissue						
broad	183.3	198.82	233.39	221.0	236.3	239.5
Mackenrodt's	183.8	198.82	233.39	221.8	236.3	239.5
non-uterine—*see* Neoplasm, connective tissue						

	Malignant			Benign	Uncertain Behavior	Unspecified
	Primary	Secondary	Ca in situ			
round	183.5	198.82	—	221.0	236.3	239.5
sacro-uterine	183.4	198.82	—	221.0	236.3	239.5
uterine	183.4	198.82	—	221.0	236.3	239.5
utero-ovarian	183.8	198.82	233.39	221.8	236.3	239.5
uterosacral	183.4	198.82	—	221.0	236.3	239.5
limb*	195.8	198.89	232.8	229.8	238.8	239.89
lower*	195.5	198.89	232.7	229.8	238.8	239.89
upper*	195.4	198.89	232.6	229.8	238.8	239.89
limbus of cornea	190.4	198.4	234.0	224.4	238.8	239.89
lingual NEC (*see also* Neoplasm, tongue)	141.9	198.89	230.0	210.1	235.1	239.0
lingula, lung	162.3	197.0	231.2	212.3	235.7	239.1
lip (external) (lipstick area) (vermillion border)	140.9	198.89	230.0	210.0	235.1	239.0
buccal aspect—*see* Neoplasm, lip, internal						
commissure	140.6	198.89	230.0	210.4	235.1	239.0
contiguous sites	140.8	—	—	—	—	—
with oral cavity or pharynx	149.8	—	—	—	—	—
frenulum—*see* Neoplasm, lip, internal						
inner aspect—*see* Neoplasm, lip, internal						
internal (buccal) (frenulum) (mucosa) (oral)	140.5	198.89	230.0	210.0	235.1	239.0
lower	140.4	198.89	230.0	210.0	235.1	239.0
upper	140.3	198.89	230.0	210.0	235.1	239.0
lower	140.1	198.89	230.0	210.0	235.1	239.0
internal (buccal) (frenulum) (mucosa) (oral)	140.4	198.89	230.0	210.0	235.1	239.0
mucosa—*see* Neoplasm, lip, internal						
oral aspect—*see* Neoplasm, lip, internal						
skin (commissure) (lower)(upper)	173.00	198.2	232.0	216.0	238.2	239.2
basal cell carcinoma	173.01	—	—	—	—	—
specified type NEC	173.09	—	—	—	—	—
squamous cell carcinoma	173.02	—	—	—	—	—
upper	140.0	198.89	230.0	210.0	235.1	239.0
internal (buccal) (frenulum) (mucosa) (oral)	140.3	198.89	230.0	210.0	235.1	239.0
liver	155.2	197.7	230.8	211.5	235.3	239.0
primary	155.0	—	—	—	—	—
lobe						
azygos	162.3	197.0	231.2	212.3	235.7	239.1
frontal	191.1	198.3	—	225.0	237.5	239.6
lower	162.5	197.0	231.2	212.3	235.7	239.1
middle	162.4	197.0	231.2	212.3	235.7	239.1
occipital	191.4	198.3	—	225.0	237.5	239.6
parietal	191.3	198.3	—	225.0	237.5	239.6
temporal	191.2	198.3	—	225.0	237.5	239.6
upper	162.3	197.0	231.2	212.3	235.7	239.1
lumbosacral plexus	171.6	198.4	—	215.6	238.1	239.2
lung	162.9	197.0	231.2	212.3	235.7	239.1
azygos lobe	162.3	197.0	231.2	212.3	235.7	239.1
carina	162.2	197.0	231.2	212.3	235.7	239.1
contiguous sites with bronchus or trachea	162.8	—	—	—	—	—
hilus	162.2	197.0	231.2	212.3	235.7	239.1
lingula	162.3	197.0	231.2	212.3	235.7	239.1
lobe NEC	162.9	197.0	231.2	212.3	235.7	239.1
lower lobe	162.5	197.0	231.2	212.3	235.7	239.1
main bronchus	162.2	197.0	231.2	212.3	235.7	239.1
middle lobe	162.4	197.0	231.2	212.3	235.7	239.1
upper lobe	162.3	197.0	231.2	212.3	235.7	239.1
lymph, lymphatic						

| | Malignant | | | | | |
---	Primary	Secondary	Ca in situ	Benign	Uncertain Behavior	Unspecified
channel NEC (*see also* Neoplasm, connective tissue)	171.9	198.89	—	215.9	238.1	239.2
gland (secondary)	—	196.9	—	229.0	238.8	239.89
abdominal	—	196.2	—	229.0	238.8	239.89
aortic	—	196.2	—	229.0	238.8	239.89
arm	—	196.3	—	229.0	238.8	239.89
auricular (anterior) (posterior)	—	196.0	—	229.0	238.8	239.89
axilla, axillary	—	196.3	—	229.0	238.8	239.89
brachial	—	196.3	—	229.0	238.8	239.89
bronchial	—	196.1	—	229.0	238.8	239.89
bronchopulmonary	—	196.1	—	229.0	238.8	239.89
celiac	—	196.2	—	229.0	238.8	239.89
cervical	—	196.0	—	229.0	238.8	239.89
cervicofacial	—	196.0	—	229.0	238.8	239.89
Cloquet	—	196.5	—	229.0	238.8	239.89
colic	—	196.2	—	229.0	238.8	239.89
common duct	—	196.2	—	229.0	238.8	239.89
cubital	—	196.3	—	229.0	238.8	239.89
diaphragmatic	—	196.1	—	229.0	238.8	239.89
epigastric, inferior	—	196.6	—	229.0	238.8	239.89
epitrochlear	—	196.3	—	229.0	238.8	239.89
esophageal	—	196.1	—	229.0	238.8	239.89
face	—	196.0	—	229.0	238.8	239.89
femoral	—	196.5	—	229.0	238.8	239.89
gastric	—	196.2	—	229.0	238.8	239.89
groin	—	196.5	—	229.0	238.8	239.89
head	—	196.0	—	229.0	238.8	239.89
hepatic	—	196.2	—	229.0	238.8	239.89
hilar (pulmonary)	—	196.1	—	229.0	238.8	239.89
splenic	—	196.2	—	229.0	238.8	239.89
hypogastric	—	196.6	—	229.0	238.8	239.89
ileocolic	—	196.2	—	229.0	238.8	239.89
iliac	—	196.6	—	229.0	238.8	239.89
infraclavicular	—	196.3	—	229.0	238.8	239.89
inguina, inguinal	—	196.5	—	229.0	238.8	239.89
innominate	—	196.1	—	229.0	238.8	239.89
intercostal	—	196.1	—	229.0	238.8	239.89
intestinal	—	196.2	—	229.0	238.8	239.89
intrabdominal	—	196.2	—	229.0	238.8	239.89
intrapelvic	—	196.6	—	229.0	238.8	239.89
intrathoracic	—	196.1	—	229.0	238.8	239.9
jugular	—	196.0	—	229.0	238.8	239.89
leg	—	196.5	—	229.0	238.8	239.89
limb						
lower	—	196.5	—	229.0	238.8	239.9
upper	—	196.3	—	229.0	238.8	239.89
lower limb	—	196.5	—	229.0	238.8	238.9
lumbar	—	196.2	—	229.0	238.8	239.89
mandibular	—	196.0	—	229.0	238.8	239.89
mediastinal	—	196.1	—	229.0	238.8	239.89
mesenteric (inferior) (superior)	—	196.2	—	229.0	238.8	239.89
midcolic	—	196.2	—	229.0	238.8	239.89
multiple sites in categories 196.0-196.6	—	196.8	—	229.0	238.8	239.89
neck	—	196.0	—	229.0	238.8	239.89
obturator	—	196.6	—	229.0	238.8	239.89
occipital	—	196.0	—	229.0	238.8	239.89
pancreatic	—	196.2	—	229.0	238.8	239.89
para-aortic	—	196.2	—	229.0	238.8	239.89
paracervical	—	196.6	—	229.0	238.8	239.89
parametrial	—	196.6	—	229.0	238.8	239.89

	Malignant Primary	Malignant Secondary	Malignant Ca in situ	Benign	Uncertain Behavior	Unspecified
parasternal	—	196.1	—	229.0	238.8	239.89
parotid	—	196.0	—	229.0	238.8	239.89
pectoral	—	196.3	—	229.0	238.8	239.89
pelvic	—	196.6	—	229.0	238.8	239.89
peri-aortic	—	196.2	—	229.0	238.8	239.89
peripancreatic	—	196.2	—	229.0	238.8	239.89
popliteal	—	196.5	—	229.0	238.8	239.89
porta hepatis	—	196.2	—	229.0	238.8	239.89
portal	—	196.2	—	229.0	238.8	239.89
preauricular	—	196.0	—	229.0	238.8	239.89
prelaryngeal	—	196.0	—	229.0	238.8	239.89
presymphysial	—	196.6	—	229.0	238.8	239.89
pretracheal	—	196.0	—	229.0	238.8	239.89
primary (any site) NEC	202.9	—	—	—	—	—
pulmonary (hiler)	—	196.1	—	229.0	238.8	239.89
pyloric	—	196.2	—	229.0	238.8	239.89
retroperitoneal	—	196.2	—	229.0	238.8	239.89
retropharyngeal	—	196.0	—	229.0	238.8	239.89
Rosenmüller's	—	196.5	—	229.0	238.8	239.89
sacral	—	196.6	—	229.0	238.8	239.89
scalene	—	196.0	—	229.0	238.8	239.89
site NEC	—	196.9	—	229.0	238.8	239.89
splenic (hilar)	—	196.2	—	229.0	238.8	239.89
subclavicular	—	196.3	—	229.0	238.8	239.89
subinguinal	—	196.5	—	229.0	238.8	239.89
sublingual	—	196.0	—	229.0	238.8	239.89
submandibular	—	196.0	—	229.0	238.8	239.89
submaxillary	—	196.0	—	229.0	238.8	239.89
submental	—	196.0	—	229.0	238.8	239.89
subscapular	—	196.3	—	229.0	238.8	239.89
supraclavicular	—	196.0	—	229.0	238.8	239.89
thoracic	—	196.1	—	229.0	238.8	239.89
tibial	—	196.5	—	229.0	238.8	239.89
tracheal	—	196.1	—	229.0	238.8	239.89
tracheobronchial	—	196.1	—	229.0	238.8	239.89
upper limb	—	196.3	—	229.0	238.8	239.89
Virchow's	—	196.0	—	229.0	238.8	239.89
node—*see also* Neoplasm, lymph gland						
primary NEC	202.9	—	—	—	—	—
vessel (*see also* Neoplasm, connective tissue)	171.9	198.89	—	215.9	238.1	239.2
Mackenrodt's ligament	183.8	198.82	233.39	221.8	236.3	239.5
malar	170.0	198.5	—	213.0	238.0	239.2
region—*see* Neoplasm, cheek						
mammary gland—*see* Neoplasm, breast						
mandible	170.1	198.5	—	213.1	238.0	239.2
alveolar						
mucosa	143.1	198.89	230.0	210.4	235.1	239.0
ridge or process	170.1	198.5	—	213.1	238.0	239.2
carcinoma	143.1	—	—	—	—	—
carcinoma	143.1	—	—	—	—	—
marrow (bone) NEC	202.9	198.5	—	—	—	238.79
mastectomy site (skin)	173.50	198.2	—	—	—	—
basal cell carcinoma	173.51	—	—	—	—	—
specified as breast tissue	174.8	198.81	—	—	—	—
specified type NEC	173.59	—	—	—	—	—
squamous cell carcinoma	173.52	—	—	—	—	—
mastoid (air cells) (antrum) (cavity)	160.1	197.3	231.8	212.0	235.9	239.1
bone or process	170.0	198.5	—	213.0	238.0	239.2
maxilla, maxillary (superior)	170.0	198.5	—	213.0	238.0	239.2

| | Malignant | | | | | |
	Primary	Secondary	Ca in situ	Benign	Uncertain Behavior	Unspecified
alveolar						
mucosa	143.0	198.89	230.0	210.4	235.1	239.0
ridge or process	170.0	198.5	—	213.0	238.0	239.2
carcinoma	143.0	—	—	—	—	—
antrum	160.2	197.3	231.8	212.0	235.9	239.1
carcinoma	143.0	—	—	—	—	—
inferior—see Neoplasm, mandible						
sinus	160.2	197.3	231.8	212.0	235.9	239.1
meatus						
external (ear) (see also Neoplasm,						
skin, ear)	173.20	198.2	232.2	216.2	238.2	239.2
Meckel's diverticulum	152.3	197.4	230.7	211.2	235.2	239.0
mediastinum, mediastinal	164.9	197.1	—	212.5	235.8	239.89
anterior	164.2	197.1	—	212.5	235.8	239.89
contiguous sites with heart						
and thymus	164.8	—	—	—	—	—
posterior	164.3	197.1	—	212.5	235.8	239.89
medulla						
adrenal	194.0	198.7	234.8	227.0	237.2	239.7
oblongata	191.7	198.3	—	225.0	237.5	239.6
meibomian gland	173.10	198.2	232.1	216.1	238.2	239.2
basal cell carcinoma	173.11					
specified type NEC	173.19	—	—	—	—	—
squamous cell carcinoma	173.12	—	—	—	—	—
melanoma —see Melanoma						
meninges (brain) (cerebral)						
(cranial) (intracranial)	192.1	198.4	—	225.2	237.6	239.7
spinal (cord)	192.3	198.4	—	225.4	237.6	239.7
meniscus, knee joint						
(lateral) (medial)	170.7	198.5	—	213.7	238.0	239.2
mesentery, mesenteric	158.8	197.6	—	211.8	235.4	239.0
mesoappendix	158.8	197.6	—	211.8	235.4	239.0
mesocolon	158.8	197.6	—	211.8	235.4	239.0
mesopharynx—see Neoplasm, oropharynx						
mesosalpinx	183.3	198.82	233.39	221.0	236.3	239.5
mesovarium	183.3	198.82	233.39	221.0	236.3	239.5
metacarpus (any bone)	170.5	198.5	—	213.5	238.0	239.2
metastatic NEC—see also Neoplasm,						
by site, secondary	—	199.1	—	—	—	—
metatarsus (any bone)	170.8	198.5	—	213.8	238.0	239.2
midbrain	191.7	198.3	—	225.0	237.5	239.6
milk duct—see Neoplasm, breast						
mons						
pubis	184.4	198.82	233.32	221.2	236.3	239.5
veneris	184.4	198.82	233.32	221.2	236.3	239.5
motor tract	192.9	198.4	—	225.9	237.9	239.7
brain	191.9	198.3	—	225.0	237.5	239.6
spinal	192.2	198.3	—	225.3	237.5	239.7
mouth	145.9	198.89	230.0	210.4	235.1	239.0
contiguous sites	145.8	—	—	—	—	—
floor	144.9	198.89	230.0	210.3	235.1	239.0
anterior portion	144.0	198.89	230.0	210.3	235.1	239.0
contiguous sites	144.8	—	—	—	—	—
lateral portion	144.1	198.89	230.0	210.3	235.1	239.0
roof	145.5	198.89	230.0	210.4	235.1	239.0
specified part NEC	145.8	198.89	230.0	210.4	235.1	239.0
vestibule	145.1	198.89	230.0	210.4	235.1	239.0
mucosa						
alveolar (ridge or process)	143.9	198.89	230.0	210.4	235.1	239.0
lower	143.1	198.89	230.0	210.4	235.1	239.0
upper	143.0	198.89	230.0	210.4	235.1	239.0
buccal	145.0	198.89	230.0	210.4	235.1	239.0
cheek	145.0	198.89	230.0	210.4	235.1	239.0

1377

	Malignant			Benign	Uncertain Behavior	Unspecified
	Primary	Secondary	Ca in situ			
lip—*see* Neoplasm, lip, internal						
nasal	160.0	197.3	231.8	212.0	235.9	239.1
oral	145.0	198.89	230.0	210.4	235.1	239.0
Müllerian duct						
female	184.8	198.82	233.39	221.8	236.3	239.5
male	187.8	198.82	233.6	222.8	236.6	239.5
multiple sites NEC	199.0	199.0	234.9	229.9	238.9	199.0
muscle—*see also* Neoplasm, connective tissue						
extraocular	190.1	198.4	234.0	224.1	238.8	239.89
myocardium	164.1	198.89	—	212.7	238.8	239.89
myometrium	182.0	198.82	233.2	219.1	236.0	239.5
myopericardium	164.1	198.89	—	212.7	238.8	239.89
nabothian gland (follicle)	180.0	198.82	233.1	219.0	236.0	239.5
nail	173.90	198.2	232.9	216.9	238.2	239.2
finger (see also Neoplasm, skin, limb, upper)	173.60	198.2	232.6	216.6	238.2	239.2
toe (see also Neoplasm, skin, limb, lower)	173.70	198.2	232.7	216.7	238.2	239.2
nares, naris (anterior) (posterior)	160.0	197.3	231.8	212.0	235.9	239.1
nasal—*see* Neoplasm, nose						
nasolabial groove (*see also* Neoplasm, skin, face)	173.30	198.2	232.3	216.3	238.2	239.2
nasolacrimal duct	190.7	198.4	234.0	224.7	238.8	239.89
nasopharynx, nasopharyngeal	147.9	198.89	230.0	210.7	235.1	239.0
contiguous sites	147.8	—	—	—	—	—
floor	147.3	198.89	230.0	210.7	235.1	239.0
roof	147.0	198.89	230.0	210.7	235.1	239.0
specified site NEC	147.8	198.89	230.0	210.7	235.1	239.0
wall	147.9	198.89	230.0	210.7	235.1	239.0
anterior	147.3	198.89	230.0	210.7	235.1	239.0
lateral	147.2	198.89	230.0	210.7	235.1	239.0
posterior	147.1	198.89	230.0	210.7	235.1	239.0
superior	147.0	198.89	230.0	210.7	235.1	239.0
nates (*see also* Neoplasm, skin, trunk)	173.50	198.2	232.5	216.5	238.2	239.2
neck NEC*	195.0	198.89	234.8	229.8	238.8	239.89
skin	173.40	198.2	232.4	216.4	238.2	239.2
basal cell carcinoma	173.41	—	—	—	—	—
specified type NEC	173.49	—	—	—	—	—
squamous cell carcinoma	173.42	—	—	—	—	—
nerve (autonomic) (ganglion) (parasympathetic) (peripheral) (sympathetic)—*see also* Neoplasm, connective tissue						
abducens	192.0	198.4	—	225.1	237.9	239.7
accessory (spinal)	192.0	198.4	—	225.1	237.9	239.7
acoustic	192.0	198.4	—	225.1	237.9	239.7
auditory	192.0	198.4	—	225.1	237.9	239.7
brachial	171.2	198.89	—	215.2	238.1	239.2
cranial (any)	192.0	198.4	—	225.1	237.9	239.7
facial	192.0	198.4	—	225.1	237.9	239.7
femoral	171.3	198.89	—	215.3	238.1	239.2
glossopharyngeal	192.0	198.4	—	225.1	237.9	239.7
hypoglossal	192.0	198.4	—	225.1	237.9	239.7
intercostal	171.4	198.89	—	215.4	238.1	239.2
lumbar	171.7	198.89	—	215.7	238.1	239.2
median	171.2	198.89	—	215.2	238.1	239.2
obturator	171.3	198.89	—	215.3	238.1	239.2
oculomotor	192.0	198.4	—	225.1	237.9	239.7
olfactory	192.0	198.4	—	225.1	237.9	239.7
optic	192.0	198.4	—	225.1	237.9	239.7

	Malignant			Benign	Uncertain Behavior	Unspecified
	Primary	Secondary	Ca in situ			
peripheral NEC	171.9	198.89	—	215.9	238.1	239.2
radial	171.2	198.89	—	215.2	238.1	239.2
sacral	171.6	198.89	—	215.6	238.1	239.2
sciatic	171.3	198.89	—	215.3	238.1	239.2
spinal NEC	171.9	198.89	—	215.9	238.1	239.2
trigeminal	192.0	198.4	—	225.1	237.9	239.7
trochlear	192.0	198.4	—	225.1	237.9	239.7
ulnar	171.2	198.89	—	215.2	238.1	239.2
vagus	192.0	198.4	—	225.1	237.9	239.7
nervous system (central)						
NEC	192.9	198.4	—	225.9	237.9	239.7
autonomic NEC	171.9	198.89	—	215.9	238.1	239.2
brain—*see also* Neoplasm, brain						
membrane or meninges	192.1	198.4	—	225.2	237.6	239.7
contiguous sites	192.8	—	—	—	—	—
parasympathetic NEC	171.9	198.89	—	215.9	238.1	239.2
sympathetic NEC	171.9	198.89	—	215.9	238.1	239.2
nipple (female)	174.0	198.81	233.0	217	238.3	239.3
male	175.0	198.81	233.0	217	238.3	239.3
nose, nasal	195.0	198.89	234.8	229.8	238.8	239.89
ala (external) (*see also* Neoplasm, nose, skin)	173.30	198.2	232.3	216.3	238.2	239.2
bone	170.0	198.5	—	213.0	238.0	239.2
cartilage	160.0	197.3	231.8	212.0	235.9	239.1
cavity	160.0	197.3	231.8	212.0	235.9	239.1
contiguous sites with accessory sinuses or middle ear	160.8	—	—	—	—	—
choana	147.3	198.89	230.0	210.7	235.1	239.0
external (skin) (*see also* Neoplasm, nose, skin)	173.30	198.2	232.3	216.3	238.2	239.2
fossa	160.0	197.3	231.8	212.0	235.9	239.1
internal	160.0	197.3	231.8	212.0	235.9	239.1
mucosa	160.0	197.3	231.8	212.0	235.9	239.1
septum	160.0	197.3	231.8	212.0	235.9	239.1
posterior margin	147.3	198.89	230.0	210.7	235.1	239.0
sinus—*see* Neoplasm, sinus						
skin	173.30	198.2	232.3	216.3	238.2	239.2
basal cell carcinoma	173.31	—	—	—	—	—
specified type NEC	173.39	—	—	—	—	—
squamous cell carcinoma	173.32	—	—	—	—	—
turbinate (mucosa)	160.0	197.3	231.8	212.0	235.9	239.1
bone	170.0	198.5	—	213.0	238.0	239.2
vestibule	160.0	197.3	231.8	212.0	235.9	239.1
nostril	160.0	197.3	231.8	212.0	235.9	239.1
nucleus pulposus	170.2	198.5	—	213.2	238.0	239.2
occipital						
bone	170.0	198.5	—	213.0	238.0	239.2
lobe or pole, brain	191.4	198.3	—	225.0	237.5	239.6
odontogenic—*see* Neoplasm, jaw bone						
oesophagus—*see* Neoplasm, esophagus						
olfactory nerve or bulb	192.0	198.4	—	225.1	237.9	239.7
olive (brain)	191.7	198.3	—	225.0	237.5	239.6
omentum	158.8	197.6	—	211.8	235.4	239.0
operculum (brain)	191.0	198.3	—	225.0	237.5	239.6
optic nerve, chiasm, or tract	192.0	198.4	—	225.1	237.9	239.7
oral (cavity)	145.9	198.89	230.0	210.4	235.1	239.0
contiguous sites with lip or pharynx	149.8	—	—	—	—	—
ill-defined	149.9	198.89	230.0	210.4	235.1	239.0
mucosa	145.9	198.89	230.0	210.4	235.1	239.0
orbit	190.1	198.4	234.0	224.1	238.8	239.89

	Malignant			Benign	Uncertain Behavior	Unspecified
	Primary	Secondary	Ca in situ			
bone	170.0	198.5	—	213.0	238.0	239.2
eye	190.1	198.4	234.0	224.1	238.8	239.89
soft parts	190.1	198.4	234.0	224.1	238.8	239.89
organ of Zuckerkandl	194.6	198.89	—	227.6	237.3	239.7
oropharynx	146.9	198.89	230.0	210.6	235.1	239.0
branchial cleft (vestige)	146.8	198.89	230.0	210.6	235.1	239.0
contiguous sites	146.8	—	—	—	—	—
junctional region	146.5	198.89	230.0	210.6	235.1	239.0
lateral wall	146.6	198.89	230.0	210.6	235.1	239.0
pillars of fauces	146.2	198.89	230.0	210.6	235.1	239.0
posterior wall	146.7	198.89	230.0	210.6	235.1	239.0
specified part NEC	146.8	198.89	230.0	210.6	235.1	239.0
vallecula	146.3	198.89	230.0	210.6	235.1	239.0
os						
external	180.1	198.82	233.1	219.0	236.0	239.5
internal	180.0	198.82	233.1	219.0	236.0	239.5
ovary	183.0	198.6	233.39	220	236.2	239.5
oviduct	183.2	198.82	233.39	221.0	236.3	239.5
palate	145.5	198.89	230.0	210.4	235.1	239.0
hard	145.2	198.89	230.0	210.4	235.1	239.0
junction of hard and soft palate	145.5	198.89	230.0	210.4	235.1	239.0
soft	145.3	198.89	230.0	210.4	235.1	239.0
nasopharyngeal surface	147.3	198.89	230.0	210.7	235.1	239.0
posterior surface	147.3	198.89	230.0	210.7	235.1	239.0
superior surface	147.3	198.89	230.0	210.7	235.1	239.0
palatoglossal arch	146.2	198.89	230.0	210.6	235.1	239.0
palatopharyngeal arch	146.2	198.89	230.0	210.6	235.1	239.0
pallium	191.0	198.3	—	225.0	237.5	239.6
palpebra	173.10	198.2	232.1	216.1	238.2	239.2
basal cell carcinoma	173.11	—	—	—	—	—
specified type NEC	173.19	—	—	—	—	—
squamous cell carcinoma	173.12	—	—	—	—	—
pancreas	157.9	197.8	230.9	211.6	235.5	239.0
body	157.1	197.8	230.9	211.6	235.5	239.0
contiguous sites	157.8	—	—	—	—	—
duct (of Santorini) (of Wirsung)	157.3	197.8	230.9	211.6	235.5	239.0
ectopic tissue	157.8	197.8	230.9	211.6	235.5	239.0
head	157.0	197.8	230.9	211.6	235.5	239.0
islet cells	157.4	197.8	230.9	211.7	235.5	239.0
neck	157.8	197.8	230.9	211.6	235.5	239.0
tail	157.2	197.8	230.9	211.6	235.5	239.0
para-aortic body	194.6	198.89	—	227.6	237.3	239.7
paraganglion NEC	194.6	198.89	—	227.6	237.3	239.7
parametrium	183.4	198.82	—	221.0	236.3	239.5
paranephric	158.0	197.6	—	211.8	235.4	239.0
pararectal	195.3	198.89	—	229.8	238.8	239.89
parasagittal (region)	195.0	198.89	234.8	229.8	238.8	239.89
parasellar	192.9	198.4	—	225.9	237.9	239.7
parathyroid (gland)	194.1	198.89	234.8	227.1	237.4	239.7
paraurethral	195.3	198.89	—	229.8	238.8	239.89
gland	189.4	198.1	233.9	223.89	236.99	239.5
paravaginal	195.3	198.89	—	229.8	238.8	239.89
parenchyma, kidney	189.0	198.0	233.9	223.0	236.91	239.5
parietal						
bone	170.0	198.5	—	213.0	238.0	239.2
lobe, brain	191.3	198.3	—	225.0	237.5	239.6
parophoron	183.3	198.82	233.39	221.0	236.3	239.5
parotid (duct) (gland)	142.0	198.89	230.0	210.2	235.0	239.0
parovarium	183.3	198.82	233.39	221.0	236.3	239.5
patella	170.8	198.5	—	213.8	238.0	239.2
peduncle, cerebral	191.7	198.3	—	225.0	237.5	239.6

	Malignant			Benign	Uncertain Behavior	Unspecified
	Primary	Secondary	Ca in situ			
pelvirectal junction	154.0	197.5	230.4	211.4	235.2	239.0
pelvis, pelvic	195.3	198.89	234.8	229.8	238.8	239.89
bone	170.6	198.5	—	213.6	238.0	239.2
floor	195.3	198.89	234.8	229.8	238.8	239.89
renal	189.1	198.0	233.9	223.1	236.91	239.5
viscera	195.3	198.89	234.8	229.8	238.8	239.89
wall	195.3	198.89	234.8	229.8	238.8	239.89
pelvo-abdominal	195.8	198.89	234.8	229.8	238.8	239.89
penis	187.4	198.82	233.5	222.1	236.6	239.5
body	187.3	198.82	233.5	222.1	236.6	239.5
corpus (cavernosum)	187.3	198.82	233.5	222.1	236.6	239.5
glans	187.2	198.82	233.5	222.1	236.6	239.5
skin NEC	187.4	198.82	233.5	222.1	236.6	239.5
periadrenal (tissue)	158.0	197.6	—	211.8	235.4	239.0
perianal (skin) (*see also* Neoplasm, skin, anus)	173.50	198.2	232.5	216.5	238.2	239.2
pericardium	164.1	198.89	—	212.7	238.8	239.89
perinephric	158.0	197.6	—	211.8	235.4	239.0
perineum	195.3	198.89	234.8	229.8	238.8	239.89
periodontal tissue NEC	143.9	198.89	230.0	210.4	235.1	239.0
periosteum—*see* Neoplasm, bone						
peripancreatic	158.0	197.6	—	211.8	235.4	239.0
peripheral nerve NEC	171.9	198.89	—	215.9	238.1	239.2
perirectal (tissue)	195.3	198.89	—	229.8	238.8	239.89
perirenal (tissue)	158.0	197.6	—	211.8	235.4	239.0
peritoneum, peritoneal (cavity)	158.9	197.6	—	211.8	235.4	239.0
contiguous sites	158.8	—	—	—	—	—
with digestive organs	159.8	—	—	—	—	—
parietal	158.8	197.6	—	211.8	235.4	239.0
pelvic	158.8	197.6	—	211.8	235.4	239.0
specified part NEC	158.8	197.6	—	211.8	235.4	239.0
peritonsillar (tissue)	195.0	198.89	234.8	229.8	238.8	239.89
periurethral tissue	195.3	198.89	—	229.8	238.8	239.89
phalanges	170.9	198.5	—	213.9	238.0	239.2
foot	170.8	198.5	—	213.8	238.0	239.2
hand	170.5	198.5	—	213.5	238.0	239.2
pharynx, pharyngeal	149.0	198.89	230.0	210.9	235.1	239.0
bursa	147.1	198.89	230.0	210.7	235.1	239.0
fornix	147.3	198.89	230.0	210.7	235.1	239.0
recess	147.2	198.89	230.0	210.7	235.1	239.0
region	149.0	198.89	230.0	210.9	235.1	239.0
tonsil	147.1	198.89	230.0	210.7	235.1	239.0
wall (lateral) (posterior)	149.0	198.89	230.0	210.9	235.1	239.0
pia mater (cerebral) (cranial)	192.1	198.4	—	225.2	237.6	239.7
spinal	192.3	198.4	—	225.4	237.6	239.7
pillars of fauces	146.2	198.89	230.0	210.6	235.1	239.0
pineal (body) (gland)	194.4	198.89	234.8	227.4	237.1	239.7
pinna (ear) NEC (*see also* Neoplasm, skin, ear)	173.20	198.2	232.2	216.2	238.2	239.2
cartilage	171.0	198.89	—	215.0	238.1	239.2
piriform fossa or sinus	148.1	198.89	230.0	210.8	235.1	239.0
pituitary (body) (fossa) (gland) (lobe)	194.3	198.89	234.8	227.3	237.0	239.7
placenta	181	198.82	233.2	219.8	236.1	239.5
pleura, pleural (cavity)	163.9	197.2	—	212.4	235.8	239.1
contiguous sites	163.8	—	—	—	—	—
parietal	163.0	197.2	—	212.4	235.8	239.1
visceral	163.1	197.2	—	212.4	235.8	239.1
plexus						
brachial	171.2	198.89	—	215.2	238.1	239.2
cervical	171.0	198.89	—	215.0	238.1	239.2
choroid	191.5	198.3	—	225.0	237.5	239.6

	Malignant			Benign	Uncertain Behavior	Unspecified
	Primary	Secondary	Ca in situ			
lumbosacral	171.6	198.89	—	215.6	238.1	239.2
sacral	171.6	198.89	—	215.6	238.1	239.2
pluri-endocrine	194.8	198.89	234.8	227.8	237.4	239.7
pole						
frontal	191.1	198.3	—	225.0	237.5	239.6
occipital	191.4	198.3	—	225.0	237.5	239.6
pons (varolii)	191.7	198.3	—	225.0	237.5	239.6
popliteal fossa or space*	195.5	198.89	234.8	229.8	238.8	239.89
postcricoid (region)	148.0	198.89	230.0	210.8	235.1	239.0
posterior fossa (cranial)	191.9	198.3	—	225.0	237.5	239.6
postnasal space	147.9	198.89	230.0	210.7	235.1	239.0
prepuce	187.1	198.82	233.5	222.1	236.6	239.5
prepylorus	151.1	197.8	230.2	211.1	235.2	239.0
presacral (region)	195.3	198.89	—	229.8	238.8	239.89
prostate (gland)	185	198.82	233.4	222.2	236.5	239.5
utricle	189.3	198.1	233.9	223.81	236.99	239.5
pterygoid fossa	171.0	198.89	—	215.0	238.1	239.2
pubic bone	170.6	198.5	—	213.6	238.0	239.2
pudenda, pudendum (female)	184.4	198.82	233.32	221.2	236.3	239.5
pulmonary	162.9	197.0	231.2	212.3	235.7	239.1
putamen	191.0	198.3	—	225.0	237.5	239.6
pyloric						
antrum	151.2	197.8	230.2	211.1	235.2	239.0
canal	151.1	197.8	230.2	211.1	235.2	239.0
pylorus	151.1	197.8	230.2	211.1	235.2	239.0
pyramid (brain)	191.7	198.3	—	225.0	237.5	239.6
pyriform fossa or sinus	148.1	198.89	230.0	210.8	235.1	239.0
radius (any part)	170.4	198.5	—	213.4	238.0	239.2
Rathke's pouch	194.3	198.89	234.8	227.3	237.0	239.7
rectosigmoid (colon)						
(junction)	154.0	197.5	230.4	211.4	235.2	239.0
contiguous sites with						
anus or rectum	154.8	—	—	—	—	—
rectouterine pouch	158.8	197.6	—	211.8	235.4	239.0
rectovaginal septum or wall	195.3	198.89	234.8	229.8	238.8	239.89
rectovesical septum	195.3	198.89	234.8	229.8	238.8	239.89
rectum (ampulla)	154.1	197.5	230.4	211.4	235.2	239.0
and colon	154.0	197.5	230.4	211.4	235.2	239.0
contiguous sites with anus or						
rectosigmoid junction	154.8	—	—	—	—	—
renal	189.0	198.0	233.9	223.0	236.91	239.5
calyx	189.1	198.0	233.9	223.1	236.91	239.5
hilus	189.1	198.0	233.9	223.1	236.91	239.5
parenchyma	189.0	198.0	233.9	223.0	236.91	239.5
pelvis	189.1	198.0	233.9	223.1	236.91	239.5
respiratory						
organs or system NEC	165.9	197.3	231.9	212.9	235.9	239.1
contiguous sites with						
intrathoracic organs	165.8	—	—	—	—	—
specified sites NEC	165.8	197.3	231.8	212.8	235.9	239.1
tract NEC	165.9	197.3	231.9	212.9	235.9	239.1
upper	165.0	197.3	231.9	212.9	235.9	239.1
retina	190.5	198.4	234.0	224.5	238.8	239.81
retrobulbar	190.1	198.4	—	224.1	238.8	239.89
retrocecal	158.0	197.6	—	211.8	235.4	239.0
retromolar (area) (triangle)						
(trigone)	145.6	198.89	230.0	210.4	235.1	239.0
retro-orbital	195.0	198.89	234.8	229.8	238.8	239.89
retroperitoneal (space)						
(tissue)	158.0	197.6	—	211.8	235.4	239.0
contiguous sites	158.8	—	—	—	—	—
retroperitoneum	158.0	197.6	—	211.8	235.4	239.0
contiguous sites	158.8	—	—	—	—	—

| | Malignant | | | Benign | Uncertain Behavior | Unspecified |
	Primary	Secondary	Ca in situ			
retropharyngeal	149.0	198.89	230.0	210.9	235.1	239.0
retrovesical (septum)	195.3	198.89	234.8	229.8	238.8	239.89
rhinencephalon	191.0	198.3	—	225.0	237.5	239.6
rib	170.3	198.5	—	213.3	238.0	239.2
Rosenmüller's fossa	147.2	198.89	230.0	210.7	235.1	239.0
round ligament	183.5	198.82	—	221.0	236.3	239.5
sacrococcyx, sacrococcygeal	170.6	198.5	—	213.6	238.0	239.2
region	195.3	198.89	234.8	229.8	238.8	239.89
sacrouterine ligament	183.4	198.82	—	221.0	236.3	239.5
sacrum, sacral (vertebra)	170.6	198.5	—	213.6	238.0	239.2
salivary gland or duct						
(major)	142.9	198.89	230.0	210.2	235.0	239.0
contiguous sites	142.8	—	—	—	—	—
minor NEC	145.9	198.89	230.0	210.4	235.1	239.0
parotid	142.0	198.89	230.0	210.2	235.0	239.0
pluriglandular	142.8	198.89	230.0	210.2	235.0	239.0
sublingual	142.2	198.89	230.0	210.2	235.0	239.0
submandibular	142.1	198.89	230.0	210.2	235.0	239.0
submaxillary	142.1	198.89	230.0	210.2	235.0	239.0
salpinx (uterine)	183.2	198.82	233.39	221.0	236.3	239.5
Santorini's duct	157.3	197.8	230.9	211.6	235.5	239.0
scalp	173.40	198.2	232.4	216.4	238.2	239.2
basal cell carcinoma	173.41	—	—	—	—	—
specified type NEC	173.49	—	—	—	—	—
squamous cell carcinoma	173.42	—	—	—	—	—
scapula (any part)	170.4	198.5	—	213.4	238.0	239.2
scapular region	195.1	198.89	234.8	229.8	238.8	239.89
scar NEC (see also						
Neoplasm, skin)	173.90	198.2	232.9	216.9	238.2	239.2
sciatic nerve	171.3	198.89	—	215.3	238.1	239.2
sclera	190.0	198.4	234.0	224.0	238.8	239.89
scrotum (skin)	187.7	198.82	233.6	222.4	236.6	239.5
sebaceous gland—see Neoplasm, skin						
sella turcica	194.3	198.89	234.8	227.3	237.0	239.7
bone	170.0	198.5	—	213.0	238.0	239.2
semilunar cartilage (knee)	170.7	198.5	—	213.7	238.0	239.2
seminal vesicle	187.8	198.82	233.6	222.8	236.6	239.5
septum						
nasal	160.0	197.3	231.8	212.0	235.9	239.1
posterior margin	147.3	198.89	230.0	210.7	235.1	239.0
rectovaginal	195.3	198.89	234.8	229.8	238.8	239.89
rectovesical	195.3	198.89	234.8	229.8	238.8	239.89
urethrovaginal	184.9	198.82	233.39	221.9	236.3	239.5
vesicovaginal	184.9	198.82	233.39	221.9	236.3	239.5
shoulder NEC*	195.4	198.89	232.6	229.8	238.8	239.89
sigmoid flexure (lower)						
(upper)	153.3	197.5	230.3	211.3	235.2	239.0
sinus (accessory)	160.9	197.3	231.8	212.0	235.9	239.1
bone (any)	170.0	198.5	—	213.0	238.0	239.2
contiguous sites with middle ear or						
nasal cavities	160.8	—	—	—	—	—
ethmoidal	160.3	197.3	231.8	212.0	235.9	239.1
frontal	160.4	197.3	231.8	212.0	235.9	239.1
maxillary	160.2	197.3	231.8	212.0	235.9	239.1
nasal, paranasal NEC	160.9	197.3	231.8	212.0	235.9	239.1
pyriform	148.1	198.89	230.0	210.8	235.1	239.0
sphenoidal	160.5	197.3	231.8	212.0	235.9	239.1
skeleton, skeletal NEC	170.9	198.5	—	213.9	238.0	239.2
Skene's gland	189.4	198.1	233.9	223.89	236.99	239.5
skin NOS	173.90	198.2	232.9	216.9	238.2	239.2
abdominal wall	173.50	198.2	232.5	216.5	238.2	239.2
basal cell carcinoma	173.51	—	—	—	—	—
specified type NEC	173.59	—	—	—	—	—

	Malignant			Benign	Uncertain Behavior	Unspecified
	Primary	Secondary	Ca in situ			
squamous cell carcinoma	173.52	—	—	—	—	—
ala nasi (*see also* Neoplasm, skin, face)	173.30	198.2	232.3	216.3	238.2	239.2
ankle (*see also* Neoplasm, skin, limb, lower)	173.70	198.2	232.7	216.7	238.2	239.2
antecubital space (*see also* Neoplasm skin, limb, upper)	173.60	198.2	232.6	216.6	238.2	239.2
anus	173.50	198.2	232.5	216.5	238.2	239.2
basal cell carcinoma	173.51	—	—	—	—	—
specified type NEC	173.59	—	—	—	—	—
squamous cell carcinoma	173.52	—	—	—	—	—
arm (see also Neoplasm, skin limb, upper)	173.60	198.2	232.6	216.6	238.2	239.2
auditory canal (external) (*see also* Neoplasm, skin, ear)	173.20	198.2	232.2	216.2	238.2	239.2
auricle (ear) (*see also*Neoplasm, skin, ear)	173.20	198.2	232.2	216.2	238.2	239.2
auricular canal (external) (*see also* Neoplasm, skin, ear)	173.20	198.2	232.2	216.2	238.2	239.2
axilla, axillary fold (*see also* Neoplasm, skin, trunk)	173.50	198.2	232.5	216.5	238.2	239.2
back	173.50	198.2	232.5	216.5	238.2	239.2
basal cell carcinoma	173.51	—	—	—	—	—
specified type NEC	173.59	—	—	—	—	—
squamous cell carcinoma	173.52	—	—	—	—	—
basal cell carcinoma, unspecified site	173.91	—	—	—	—	—
breast (*see also* Neoplasm, skin, trunk)	173.50	198.2	232.5	216.5	238.2	239.2
brow (*see also* Neoplasm, skin, face)	173.30	198.2	232.3	216.3	238.2	239.2
buttock (*see also* Neoplasm, skin, trunk)	173.50	198.2	232.5	216.5	238.2	239.2
calf (*see also* Neoplasm, skin, limb, lower)	173.70	198.2	232.7	216.7	238.2	239.2
canthus (eye) (inner)(outer)	173.10	198.2	232.1	216.1	238.2	239.2
basal cell carcinoma	173.11	—	—	—	—	—
specified type NEC	173.19	—	—	—	—	—
squamous cell carcinoma	173.12	—	—	—	—	—
cervical region (*see also* Neoplasm, skin, neck)	173.40	198.2	232.4	216.4	238.2	239.2
cheek (external) (*see also* Neoplasm, skin, face)	173.30	198.2	232.3	216.3	238.2	239.2
chest (wall) (*see also* Neoplasm, skin, trunk)	173.50	198.2	232.5	216.5	238.2	239.2
chin (*see also* Neoplasm, skin, face)	173.30	198.2	232.3	216.3	238.2	239.2
clavicular area (*see also* Neoplasm, skin, trunk)	173.50	198.2	232.5	216.5	238.2	239.2
clitoris	184.3	198.82	233.32	221.2	236.3	239.5
columnella (*see also* Neoplasm, skin, face)	173.30	198.2	232.3	216.3	238.2	239.2
concha (*see also* Neoplasm, skin ear)	173.20	198.2	232.2	216.2	238.2	239.2
contiguous sites	173.80	—	—	—	—	—
basal cell carcinoma	173.81	—	—	—	—	—
specified type NEC	173.89	—	—	—	—	—
squamous cell carcinoma	173.82	—	—	—	—	—
ear (external)	173.20	198.2	232.2	216.2	238.2	239.2
basal cell carcinoma	173.21	—	—	—	—	—
specified type NEC	173.29	—	—	—	—	—
squamous cell carcinoma	173.22	—	—	—	—	—

	Malignant					
	Primary	Secondary	Ca in situ	Benign	Uncertain Behavior	Unspecified
elbow (*see also* Neoplasm, skin, limb, upper)	173.60	198.2	232.6	216.6	238.2	239.2
eyebrow (*see also* Neoplasm, skin, face)	173.30	198.2	232.3	216.3	238.2	239.2
eyelid	173.10	198.2	232.1	216.1	238.2	239.2
basal cell carcinoma	173.11	—	—	—	—	—
specified type NEC	173.19	—	—	—	—	—
squamous cell carcinoma	173.12	—	—	—	—	—
face NEC	173.30	198.2	232.3	216.3	238.2	239.2
basal cell carcinoma	173.31	—	—	—	—	—
specified type NEC	173.39	—	—	—	—	—
squamous cell carcinoma	173.32	—	—	—	—	—
female genital organs (external)	184.4	198.82	233.30	221.2	236.3	239.5
clitoris	184.3	198.82	233.32	221.2	236.3	239.5
labium NEC	184.4	198.82	233.32	221.2	236.3	239.5
majus	184.1	198.82	233.32	221.2	236.3	239.5
minus	184.2	198.82	233.32	221.2	236.3	239.5
pudendum	184.4	198.82	233.32	221.2	236.3	239.5
vulva	184.4	198.82	233.32	221.2	236.3	239.5
finger (*see also* Neoplasm, skin, limb, upper)	173.60	198.2	232.6	216.6	238.2	239.2
flank (*see also* Neoplasm, skin, trunk)	173.50	198.2	232.5	216.5	238.2	239.2
foot (*see also* Neoplasm, skin, limb, lower)	173.70	198.2	232.7	216.7	238.2	239.2
forearm (*see also* Neoplasm, skin, limb, upper)	173.60	198.2	232.6	216.6	238.2	239.2
forehead (*see also* Neoplasm, skin, face)	173.30	198.2	232.3	216.3	238.2	239.2
glabella (*see also* Neoplasm, skin, face)	173.30	198.2	232.3	216.3	238.2	239.2
gluteal region (*see also* Neoplasm, skin, trunk)	173.50	198.2	232.5	216.5	238.2	239.2
groin (*see also* Neoplasm, skin, trunk)	173.50	198.2	232.5	216.5	238.2	239.2
hand (*see also* Neoplasm, skin, limb, upper)	173.60	198.2	232.6	216.6	238.2	239.2
head NEC (*see also* Neoplasm, skin, scalp)	173.40	198.2	232.4	216.4	238.2	239.2
heel (*see also* Neoplasm, skin, limb, lower)	173.70	198.2	232.7	216.7	238.2	239.2
helix (*see also* Neoplasm, skin, ear)	173.20	198.2	232.2	216.2	238.2	239.2
hip	173.70	198.2	232.7	216.7	238.2	239.2
basal cell carcinoma	173.71	—	—	—	—	—
specified type NEC	173.79	—	—	—	—	—
squamous cell carcinoma	173.72	—	—	—	—	—
infraclavicular region (*see also* Neoplasm, skin, trunk)	173.50	198.2	232.5	216.5	238.2	239.2
inguinal region (*see also* Neoplasm, skin, trunk)	173.50	198.2	232.5	216.5	238.2	239.2
jaw (*see also* Neoplasm, skin, face)	173.30	198.2	232.3	216.3	238.2	239.2
knee (*see also* Neoplasm, skin, limb, lower)	173.70	198.2	232.7	216.7	238.2	239.2
labia						
majora	184.1	198.82	233.32	221.2	236.3	239.5
minora	184.2	198.82	233.32	221.2	236.3	239.5
leg (*see also* Neoplasm, skin, limb, lower)	173.70	198.2	232.7	216.7	238.2	239.2
lid (lower) (upper)	173.10	198.2	232.1	216.1	238.2	239.2
basal cell carcinoma	173.11	—	—	—	—	—
specified type NEC	173.19	—	—	—	—	—

	Malignant					
	Primary	Secondary	Ca in situ	Benign	Uncertain Behavior	Unspecified
squamous cell carcinoma 173.12	—	—	—	—	—
limb NEC. 173.90	198.2	232.9	216.9	238.2	239.5
lower 173.70	198.2	232.7	216.7	238.2	239.2
basal cell carcinoma 173.71	—	—	—	—	—
specified type NEC. 173.79	—	—	—	—	—
squamous cell carcinoma . . . 173.72	—	—	—	—	—
upper 173.60	198.2	232.6	216.6	238.2	239.2
basal cell carcinoma 173.61	—	—	—	—	—
specified type NEC. 173.69	—	—	—	—	—
squamous cell carcinoma . . . 173.62	—	—	—	—	—
lip (lower) (upper) 173.00	198.2	232.0	216.0	238.2	239.2
basal cell carcinoma 173.01	—	—	—	—	—
specified type NEC. 173.09	—	—	—	—	—
squamous cell carcinoma 173.02	—	—	—	—	—
male genital organs. 187.9	198.82	233.6	222.9	236.6	239.5
penis 187.4	198.82	233.5	222.1	236.6	239.5
prepuce 187.1	198.82	233.5	222.1	236.6	239.5
scrotum. 187.7	198.82	233.6	222.4	236.6	239.5
mastectomy site (*see also* Neoplasm, skin, trunk) 173.50	198.2	—	—	—	—
specified as breast tissue 174.8	198.81	—	—	—	
meatus, acoustic (external) (*see also* Neoplasm, skin, ear) 173.20	198.2	232.2	216.2	238.2	239.2
melanoma —*see* Melanoma						
nates (*see also* Neoplasm, skin, trunk). 173.50	198.2	232.5	216.5	238.2	239.2
neck 173.40	198.2	232.4	216.4	238.2	239.2
basal cell carcinoma 173.41	—	—	—	—	—
specified type NEC. 173.49	—	—	—	—	—
squamous cell carcinoma . . . 173.42	—	—	—	—	—
nose (external) (*see also* Neoplasm, skin, face) 173.30	198.2	232.3	216.3	238.2	239.2
palm (*see also* Neoplasm, skin, limb, upper) 173.60	198.2	232.6	216.6	238.2	239.2
palpebra 173.10	198.2	232.1	216.1	238.2	239.2
basal cell carcinoma 173.11	—	—	—	—	—
specified type NEC. 173.19	—	—	—	—	—
squamous cell carcinoma 173.12	—	—	—	—	—
penis NEC 187.4	198.82	233.5	222.1	236.6	239.5
perianal (*see also* Neoplasm, skin, anus) 173.50	198.2	232.5	216.5	238.2	239.2
perineum (*see also* Neoplasm, skin, anus) 173.50	198.2	232.5	216.5	238.2	239.2
pinna (*see also* Neoplasm, skin, ear) 173.20	198.2	232.2	216.2	238.2	239.2
plantar (*see also* Neoplasm, skin, limb, lower) 173.70	198.2	232.7	216.7	238.2	239.2
popliteal fossa or space (*see also* Neoplasm, skin, limb, lower) . 173.70	198.2	232.7	216.7	238.2	239.2
prepuce. 187.1	198.82	233.5	222.1	236.6	239.5
pubes (*see also* Neoplasm, skin, trunk). 173.50	198.2	232.5	216.5	238.2	239.2
sacrococcygeal region (*see also* Neoplasm, skin, trunk). 173.50	198.2	232.5	216.5	238.2	239.2
scalp 173.40	198.2	232.4	216.4	238.2	239.2
basal cell carcinoma 173.41	—	—	—	—	—
specified type NEC. 173.49	—	—	—	—	—
squamous cell carcinoma . . . 173.42	—	—	—	—	—
scapular region (*see also* Neoplasm, skin, trunk). 173.50	198.2	232.5	216.5	238.2	239.2
scrotum. 187.7	198.82	233.6	222.4	236.6	239.5
shoulder 173.60	198.2	232.6	216.6	238.2	239.2
basal cell carcinoma 173.61	—	—	—	—	—
specified type NEC. 173.69	—	—	—	—	—

	Malignant					
	Primary	Secondary	Ca in situ	Benign	Uncertain Behavior	Unspecified
squamous cell carcinoma	173.62	—	—	—	—	—
sole (foot) (see also Neoplasm, skin, limb, lower)	173.70	198.2	232.7	216.7	238.2	239.2
specified sites NEC	173.80	198.2	232.8	216.8	232.8	239.2
basal cell carcinoma	173.81	—	—	—	—	—
specified type NEC	173.89	—	—	—	—	—
squamous cell carcinoma	173.82	—	—	—	—	—
specified type NEC, unspecified site	173.99	—	—	—	—	—
squamous cell carcinoma, unspecified site	173.92	—	—	—	—	—
submammary fold (see also Neoplasm, skin, turnk)	173.50	198.2	232.5	216.5	238.2	239.2
supraclavicular region (see also Neoplasm, skin, neck)	173.40	198.2	232.4	216.4	238.2	239.2
temple (see also Neoplasm, skin, face)	173.30	198.2	232.3	216.3	238.2	239.2
thigh (see also Neoplasm, skin, limb, lower)	173.70	198.2	232.7	216.7	238.2	239.2
thoracic wall (see also Neoplasm, skin, trunk)	173.50	198.2	232.5	216.5	238.2	239.2
thumb (see also Neoplasm, skin, limb, upper)	173.60	198.2	232.6	216.6	238.2	239.2
toe (see also Neoplasm, skin, limb, lower)	173.70	198.2	232.7	216.7	238.2	239.2
tragus (see also Neoplasm, skin, ear)	173.20	198.2	232.2	216.2	238.2	239.2
trunk	173.50	198.2	232.5	216.5	238.2	239.2
basal cell carcinoma	173.51	—	—	—	—	—
specified type NEC	173.59	—	—	—	—	—
squamous cell carcinoma	173.52	—	—	—	—	—
umbilicus (see also Neoplasm, skin, trunk)	173.50	198.2	232.5	216.5	238.2	239.2
vulva	184.4	198.82	233.32	221.2	236.3	239.5
wrist (see also Neoplasm, skin, limb, upper)	173.60	198.2	232.6	216.6	238.2	239.2
skull	170.0	198.5	—	213.0	238.0	239.2
soft parts or tissues—see Neoplasm, connective tissue						
specified site NEC	195.8	198.89	234.8	229.8	238.8	239.89
spermatic cord	187.6	198.82	233.6	222.8	236.6	239.5
sphenoid	160.5	197.3	231.8	212.0	235.9	239.1
bone	170.0	198.5	—	213.0	238.0	239.2
sinus	160.5	197.3	231.8	212.0	235.9	239.1
sphincter						
anal	154.2	197.5	230.5	211.4	235.5	239.0
of Oddi	156.1	197.8	230.8	211.5	235.3	239.0
spine, spinal (column)	170.2	198.5	—	213.2	238.0	239.2
bulb	191.7	198.3	—	225.0	237.5	239.6
coccyx	170.6	198.5	—	213.6	238.0	239.2
cord (cervical) (lumbar) (sacral) (thoracic)	192.2	198.3	—	225.3	237.5	239.7
dura mater	192.3	198.4	—	225.4	237.6	239.7
lumbosacral	170.2	198.5	—	213.2	238.0	239.2
membrane	192.3	198.4	—	225.4	237.6	239.7
meninges	192.3	198.4	—	225.4	237.6	239.7
nerve (root)	171.9	198.89	—	215.9	238.1	239.2
pia mater	192.3	198.4	—	225.4	237.6	239.7
root	171.9	198.89	—	215.9	238.1	239.2
sacrum	170.6	198.5	—	213.6	238.0	239.2
spleen, splenic NEC	159.1	197.8	230.9	211.9	235.5	239.0
flexure (colon)	153.7	197.5	230.3	211.3	235.2	239.0
stem, brain	191.7	198.3	—	225.0	237.5	239.6

	Malignant				
	Primary	Secondary	Ca in situ	Benign	Uncertain Behavior	Unspecified
Stensen's duct	142.0	198.89	230.0	210.2	235.0	239.0
sternum.	170.3	198.5	—	213.3	238.0	239.2
stomach.	151.9	197.8	230.2	211.1	235.2	239.0
antrum (pyloric)	151.2	197.8	230.2	211.1	235.2	239.0
body	151.4	197.8	230.2	211.1	235.2	239.0
cardia.	151.0	197.8	230.2	211.1	235.2	239.0
cardiac orifice	151.0	197.8	230.2	211.1	235.2	239.0
contiguous sites	151.8	—	—	—	—	—
corpus	151.4	197.8	230.2	211.1	235.2	239.0
fundus	151.3	197.8	230.2	211.1	235.2	239.0
greater curvature NEC	151.6	197.8	230.2	211.1	235.2	239.0
lesser curvature NEC.	151.5	197.8	230.2	211.1	235.2	239.0
prepylorus	151.1	197.8	230.2	211.1	235.2	239.0
pylorus	151.1	197.8	230.2	211.1	235.2	239.0
wall NEC.	151.9	197.8	230.2	211.1	235.2	239.0
anterior NEC.	151.8	197.8	230.2	211.1	235.2	239.0
posterior NEC	151.8	197.8	230.2	211.1	235.2	239.0
stroma, endometrial	182.0	198.82	233.2	219.1	236.0	239.5
stump, cervical	180.8	198.82	233.1	219.0	236.0	239.5
subcutaneous (nodule) (tissue) NEC—*see* Neoplasm, connective tissue						
subdural	192.1	198.4	—	225.2	237.6	239.7
subglottis, subglottic	161.2	197.3	231.0	212.1	235.6	239.1
sublingual	144.9	198.89	230.0	210.3	235.1	239.0
gland or duct	142.2	198.89	230.0	210.2	235.0	239.0
submandibular gland.	142.1	198.89	230.0	210.2	235.0	239.0
submaxillary gland or duct.	142.1	198.89	230.0	210.2	235.0	239.0
submental.	195.0	198.89	234.8	229.8	238.8	239.89
subpleural	162.9	197.0	—	212.3	235.7	239.1
substernal.	164.2	197.1	—	212.5	235.8	239.89
sudoriferous, sudoriparous gland, site unspecified.	173.90	198.2	232.9	216.9	238.2	239.2
specified site—*see* Neoplasm, skin						
supraclavicular region	195.0	198.89	234.8	229.8	238.8	239.89
supraglottis.	161.1	197.3	231.0	212.1	235.6	239.1
suprarenal (capsule) (cortex) (gland) (medulla)	194.0	198.7	234.8	227.0	237.2	239.7
suprasellar (region).	191.9	198.3	—	225.0	237.5	239.6
sweat gland (apocrine) (eccrine), site unspecified	173.90	198.2	232.9	216.9	238.2	239.2
specified site—*see* Neoplasm, skin						
sympathetic nerve or nervous system NEC.	171.9	198.89	—	215.9	238.1	239.2
symphysis pubis	170.6	198.5	—	213.6	238.0	239.2
synovial membrane—*see* Neoplasm, connective tissue						
tapetum, brain	191.8	198.3	—	225.0	237.5	239.6
tarsus (any bone)	170.8	198.5	—	213.8	238.0	239.2
temple (skin) (*see also* Neoplasm, skin, face)	173.30	198.2	232.3	216.3	238.2	239.2
temporal						
bone	170.0	198.5	—	213.0	238.0	239.2
lobe or pole.	191.2	198.3	—	225.0	237.5	239.6
region.	195.0	198.89	234.8	229.8	238.8	239.89
skin (see also Neoplasm, skin, face)	173.30	198.2	232.3	216.3	238.2	239.2
tendon (sheath)—*see* Neoplasm, connective tissue						
tentorium (cerebelli)	192.1	198.4	—	225.2	237.6	239.7
testis, testes (descended) (scrotal)	186.9	198.82	233.6	222.0	236.4	239.5
ectopic	186.0	198.82	233.6	222.0	236.4	239.5

	Malignant			Benign	Uncertain Behavior	Unspecified
	Primary	Secondary	Ca in situ			
retained	186.0	198.82	233.6	222.0	236.4	239.5
undescended	186.0	198.82	233.6	222.0	236.4	239.5
thalamus	191.0	198.3	—	225.0	237.5	239.6
thigh NEC*	195.5	198.89	234.8	229.8	238.8	239.89
thorax, thoracic (cavity)						
(organs NEC)	195.1	198.89	234.8	229.8	238.8	239.89
duct	171.4	198.89	—	215.4	238.1	239.2
wall NEC	195.1	198.89	234.8	229.8	238.8	239.89
throat	149.0	198.89	230.0	210.9	235.1	239.0
thumb NEC*	195.4	198.89	232.6	229.8	238.8	239.89
thymus (gland)	164.0	198.89	—	212.6	235.8	239.89
contiguous sites with heart and						
mediastinum	164.8	—	—	—	—	—
thyroglossal duct	193	198.89	234.8	226	237.4	239.7
thyroid (gland)	193	198.89	234.8	226	237.4	239.7
cartilage	161.3	197.3	231.0	212.1	235.6	239.1
tibia (any part)	170.7	198.5	—	213.7	238.0	239.2
toe NEC*	195.5	198.89	232.7	229.8	238.8	239.89
tongue	141.9	198.89	230.0	210.1	235.1	239.0
anterior (two-thirds) NEC	141.4	198.89	230.0	210.1	235.1	239.0
dorsal surface	141.1	198.89	230.0	210.1	235.1	239.0
ventral surface	141.3	198.89	230.0	210.1	235.1	239.0
base (dorsal surface)	141.0	198.89	230.0	210.1	235.1	239.0
border (lateral)	141.2	198.89	230.0	210.1	235.1	239.0
contiguous sites	141.8	—	—	—	—	—
dorsal surface NEC	141.1	198.89	230.0	210.1	235.1	239.0
fixed part NEC	141.0	198.89	230.0	210.1	235.1	239.0
foramen cecum	141.1	198.89	230.0	210.1	235.1	239.0
frenulum linguae	141.3	198.89	230.0	210.1	235.1	239.0
junctional zone	141.5	198.89	230.0	210.1	235.1	239.0
margin (lateral)	141.2	198.89	230.0	210.1	235.1	239.0
midline NEC	141.1	198.89	230.0	210.1	235.1	239.0
mobile part NEC	141.4	198.89	230.0	210.1	235.1	239.0
posterior (third)	141.0	198.89	230.0	210.1	235.1	239.0
root	141.0	198.89	230.0	210.1	235.1	239.0
surface (dorsal)	141.1	198.89	230.0	210.1	235.1	239.0
base	141.0	198.89	230.0	210.1	235.1	239.0
ventral	141.3	198.89	230.0	210.1	235.1	239.0
tip	141.2	198.89	230.0	210.1	235.1	239.0
tonsil	141.6	198.89	230.0	210.1	235.1	239.0
tonsil	146.0	198.89	230.0	210.5	235.1	239.0
fauces, faucial	146.0	198.89	230.0	210.5	235.1	239.0
lingual	141.6	198.89	230.0	210.1	235.1	239.0
palatine	146.0	198.89	230.0	210.5	235.1	239.0
pharyngeal	147.1	198.89	230.0	210.7	235.1	239.0
pillar (anterior) (posterior)	146.2	198.89	230.0	210.6	235.1	239.0
tonsillar fossa	146.1	198.89	230.0	210.6	235.1	239.0
tooth socket NEC	143.9	198.89	230.0	210.4	235.1	239.0
trachea (cartilage) (mucosa)	162.0	197.3	231.1	212.2	235.7	239.1
contiguous sites with						
bronchus or lung	162.8	—	—	—	—	—
tracheobronchial	162.8	197.3	231.1	212.2	235.7	239.1
contiguous sites with lung	162.8	—	—	—	—	—
tragus (see also Neoplasm, skin, ear)	173.20	198.2	232.2	216.2	238.2	239.2
trunk NEC*	195.8	198.89	232.5	229.8	238.8	239.89
tubo-ovarian	183.8	198.82	233.39	221.8	236.3	239.5
tunica vaginalis	187.8	198.82	233.6	222.8	236.6	239.5
turbinate (bone)	170.0	198.5	—	213.0	238.0	239.2
nasal	160.0	197.3	231.8	212.0	235.9	239.1
tympanic cavity	160.1	197.3	231.8	212.0	235.9	239.1
ulna (any part)	170.4	198.5	—	213.4	238.0	239.2
umbilicus, umbilical (see also						
Neoplasm, skin, trunk)	173.50	198.2	232.5	216.5	238.2	239.2

	Malignant			Benign	Uncertain Behavior	Unspecified
	Primary	Secondary	Ca in situ			
uncus, brain	191.2	198.3	—	225.0	237.5	239.6
unknown site or unspecified	199.1	199.1	234.9	229.9	238.9	239.9
urachus	188.7	198.1	233.7	223.3	236.7	239.4
ureter, ureteral	189.2	198.1	233.9	223.2	236.91	239.5
orifice (bladder)	188.6	198.1	233.7	223.3	236.7	239.4
ureter-bladder (junction)	188.6	198.1	233.7	223.3	236.7	239.4
urethra, urethral (gland)	189.3	198.1	233.9	223.81	236.99	239.5
orifice, internal	188.5	198.1	233.7	223.3	236.7	239.4
urethrovaginal (septum)	184.9	198.82	233.39	221.9	236.3	239.5
urinary organ or system NEC	189.9	198.1	233.9	223.9	236.99	239.5
bladder—*see* Neoplasm, bladder						
contiguous sites	189.8	—	—	—	—	—
specified sites NEC	189.8	198.1	233.9	223.89	236.99	239.5
utero-ovarian	183.8	198.82	233.39	221.8	236.3	239.5
ligament	183.3	198.82	—	221.0	236.3	239.5
uterosacral ligament	183.4	198.82	—	221.0	236.3	239.5
uterus, uteri, uterine	179	198.82	233.2	219.9	236.0	239.5
adnexa NEC	183.9	198.82	233.39	221.8	236.3	239.5
contiguous sites	183.8	—	—	—	—	—
body	182.0	198.82	233.2	219.1	236.0	239.5
contiguous sites	182.8	—	—	—	—	—
cervix	180.9	198.82	233.1	219.0	236.0	239.5
cornu	182.0	198.82	233.2	219.1	236.0	239.5
corpus	182.0	198.82	233.2	219.1	236.0	239.5
endocervix (canal) (gland)	180.0	198.82	233.1	219.0	236.0	239.5
endometrium	182.0	198.82	233.2	219.1	236.0	239.5
exocervix	180.1	198.82	233.1	219.0	236.0	239.5
external os	180.1	198.82	233.1	219.0	236.0	239.5
fundus	182.0	198.82	233.2	219.1	236.0	239.5
internal os	180.0	198.82	233.1	219.0	236.0	239.5
isthmus	182.1	198.82	233.2	219.1	236.0	239.5
ligament	183.4	198.82	—	221.0	236.3	239.5
broad	183.3	198.82	233.39	221.0	236.3	239.5
round	183.5	198.82	—	221.0	236.3	239.5
lower segment	182.1	198.82	233.2	219.1	236.0	239.5
myometrium	182.0	198.82	233.2	219.1	236.0	239.5
squamocolumnar junction	180.8	198.82	233.1	219.0	236.0	239.5
tube	183.2	198.82	233.39	221.0	236.3	239.5
utricle, prostatic	189.3	198.1	233.9	223.81	236.99	239.5
uveal tract	190.0	198.4	234.0	224.0	238.8	239.89
uvula	145.4	198.89	230.0	210.4	235.1	239.0
vagina, vaginal (fornix) (vault) (wall)	184.0	198.82	233.31	221.1	236.3	239.5
vaginovesical	184.9	198.82	233.39	221.9	236.3	239.5
septum	184.9	198.82	233.39	221.9	236.3	239.5
vallecula (epiglottis)	146.3	198.89	230.0	210.6	235.1	239.0
vascular—*see* Neoplasm, connective tissue						
vas deferens	187.6	198.82	233.6	222.8	236.6	239.5
Vater's ampulla	156.2	197.8	230.8	211.5	235.3	239.0
vein, venous—*see* Neoplasm, connective tissue						
vena cava (abdominal) (inferior)	171.5	198.89	—	215.5	238.1	239.2
superior	171.4	198.89	—	215.4	238.1	239.2
ventricle (cerebral) (floor) (fourth) (lateral) (third)	191.5	198.3	—	225.0	237.5	239.6
cardiac (left) (right)	164.1	198.89	—	212.7	238.8	239.89
ventricular band of larynx	161.1	197.3	231.0	212.1	235.6	239.1
ventriculus—*see* Neoplasm, stomach						
vermillion border—*see* Neoplasm, lip						

	Malignant			Benign	Uncertain Behavior	Unspecified
	Primary	Secondary	Ca in situ			
vermis, cerebellum	191.6	198.3	—	225.0	237.5	239.6
vertebra (column)	170.2	198.5	—	213.2	238.0	239.2
coccyx	170.6	198.5	—	213.6	238.0	239.2
sacrum	170.6	198.5	—	213.6	238.0	239.2
vesical—*see* Neoplasm, bladder						
vesicle, seminal	187.8	198.82	233.6	222.8	236.6	239.5
vesicocervical tissue	184.9	198.82	233.39	221.9	236.3	239.5
vesicorectal	195.3	198.89	234.8	229.8	238.8	239.89
vesicovaginal	184.9	198.82	233.39	221.9	236.3	239.5
septum	184.9	198.82	233.39	221.9	236.3	239.5
vessel (blood)—*see* Neoplasm, connective tissue						
vestibular gland, greater	184.1	198.82	233.32	221.2	236.3	239.5
vestibule						
mouth	145.1	198.89	230.0	210.4	235.1	239.0
nose	160.0	197.3	231.8	212.0	235.9	239.1
Virchow's gland	—	196.0	—	229.0	238.8	239.89
viscera NEC	195.8	198.89	234.8	229.8	238.8	239.89
vocal cords (true)	161.0	197.3	231.0	212.1	235.6	239.1
false	161.1	197.3	231.0	212.1	235.6	239.1
vomer	170.0	198.5	—	213.0	238.0	239.2
vulva	184.4	198.82	233.32	221.2	236.3	239.5
vulvovaginal gland	184.4	198.82	233.32	221.2	236.3	239.5
Waldeyer's ring	149.1	198.89	230.0	210.9	235.1	239.0
Wharton's duct	142.1	198.89	230.0	210.2	235.0	239.0
white matter (central)						
(cerebral)	191.0	198.3	—	225.0	237.5	239.6
windpipe	162.0	197.3	231.1	212.2	235.7	239.1
Wirsung's duct	157.3	197.8	230.9	211.6	235.5	239.0
wolffian (body) (duct)						
female	184.8	198.82	233.39	221.8	236.3	239.5
male	187.8	198.82	233.6	222.8	236.6	239.5
womb—*see* Neoplasm, uterus						
wrist NEC*	195.4	198.89	232.6	229.8	238.8	239.89
xiphoid process	170.3	198.5	—	213.3	238.0	239.2
Zuckerkandl's organ	194.6	198.89	—	227.6	237.3	239.7

Neovascularization
  choroid 362.16
  ciliary body 364.42
  cornea 370.60
    deep 370.63
    localized 370.61
  iris 364.42
  retina 362.16
  subretinal 362.16
Nephralgia 788.0
Nephritis, nephritic (albuminuric) (azotemic)
    (congenital) (degenerative) (diffuse)
    (disseminated) (epithelial) (familial) (focal)
    (granulomatous) (hemorrhagic) (infantile)
    (nonsuppurative, excretory) (uremic) 583.9
  with
    edema—*see* Nephrosis
    lesion of
      glomerulonephritis
        hypocomplementemic persistent 583.2
          with nephrotic syndrome 581.2
            chronic 582.2
        lobular 583.2
          with nephrotic syndrome 581.2
            chronic 582.2
        membranoproliferative 583.2
          with nephrotic syndrome 581.2
            chronic 582.2
        membranous 583.1
          with nephrotic syndrome 581.1
            chronic 582.1
        mesangiocapillary 583.2
          with nephrotic syndrome 581.2
            chronic 582.2
        mixed membranous and proliferative 583.2
          with nephrotic syndrome 581.2
            chronic 582.2
        proliferative (diffuse) 583.0
          with nephrotic syndrome 581.0
            acute 580.0
            chronic 582.0
        rapidly progressive 583.4
          acute 580.4
          chronic 582.4
      interstitial nephritis (diffuse) (focal) 583.89
        with nephrotic syndrome 581.89
        acute 580.89
        chronic 582.89
      necrotizing glomerulitis 583.4
        acute 580.4
        chronic 582.4
      renal necrosis 583.9
        cortical 583.6
        medullary 583.7
      specified pathology NEC 583.89
        with nephrotic syndrome 581.89
        acute 580.89
        chronic 582.89
    necrosis, renal 583.9
      cortical 583.6
      medullary (papillary) 583.7
    nephrotic syndrome (*see also* Nephrosis) 581.9
    papillary necrosis 583.7
    specified pathology NEC 583.89
  acute 580.9
    extracapillary with epithelial crescents 580.4
    hypertensive (*see also* Hypertension, kidney)
        403.90
    necrotizing 580.4
    poststreptococcal 580.0
    proliferative (diffuse) 580.0

Nephritis, nephritic—*continued*
  acute—*continued*
    rapidly progressive 580.4
    specified pathology NEC 580.89
  amyloid 277.39 *[583.81]*
    chronic 277.39 *[582.81]*
  arteriolar (*see also* Hypertension, kidney)
      403.90
  arteriosclerotic (*see also* Hypertension, kidney)
      403.90
  ascending (*see also* Pyelitis) 590.80
  atrophic 582.9
  basement membrane NEC 583.89
    with
      pulmonary hemorrhage (Goodpasture's
          syndrome) 446.21 *[583.81]*
  calculous, calculus 592.0
  cardiac (*see also* Hypertension, kidney) 403.90
  cardiovascular (*see also* Hypertension, kidney)
      403.90
  chronic 582.9
    arteriosclerotic (*see also* Hypertension,
        kidney) 403.90
    hypertensive (*see also* Hypertension, kidney)
        403.90
  cirrhotic (*see also* Sclerosis, renal) 587
  complicating pregnancy, childbirth, or
      puerperium 646.2
    with hypertension 642.1
      affecting fetus or newborn 760.0
    affecting fetus or newborn 760.1
  croupous 580.9
  desquamative—*see* Nephrosis
  due to
    amyloidosis 277.39 *[583.81]*
      chronic 277.39 *[582.81]*
    arteriosclerosis (*see also* Hypertension,
        kidney) 403.90
    diabetes mellitus 250.4 *[583.81]*
      due to secondary diabetes 249.4 *[583.81]*
      with nephrotic syndrome 250.4 *[581.81]*
        due to secondary diabetes 249.4 *[581.81]*
    diphtheria 032.89 *[580.81]*
    gonococcal infection (acute) 098.19 *[583.81]*
      chronic or duration of 2 months or over
          098.39 *[583.81]*
    gout 274.10
    infectious hepatitis 070.9 *[580.81]*
    mumps 072.79 *[580.81]*
    specified kidney pathology NEC 583.89
      acute 580.89
      chronic 582.89
    streptotrichosis 039.8 *[583.81]*
    subacute bacterial endocarditis 421.0 *[580.81]*
    systemic lupus erythematosus 710.0 *[583.81]*
      chronic 710.0 *[582.81]*
    typhoid fever 002.0 *[580.81]*
  endothelial 582.2
  end stage (chronic) (terminal) NEC 585.6
  epimembranous 581.1
  exudative 583.89
    with nephrotic syndrome 581.89
    acute 580.89
    chronic 582.89
  gonococcal (acute) 098.19 *[583.81]*
    chronic or duration of 2 months or over 098.39
        [583.81]
  gouty 274.10
  hereditary (Alport's syndrome) 759.89
  hydremic—*see* Nephrosis
  hypertensive (*see also* Hypertension, kidney) 403.90

Nephritis, nephritic—*continued*
  hypocomplementemic persistent 583.2
    with nephrotic syndrome 581.2
    chronic 582.2
  immune complex NEC 583.89
  infective (*see also* Pyelitis) 590.80
  interstitial (diffuse) (focal) 583.89
    with nephrotic syndrome 581.89
    acute 580.89
    chronic 582.89
  latent or quiescent—*see* Nephritis, chronic
  lead 984.9
    specified type of lead—*see* Table of drugs and
      chemicals
  lobular 583.2
    with nephrotic syndrome 581.2
    chronic 582.2
  lupus 710.0 *[583.81]*
    acute 710.0 *[580.81]*
    chronic 710.0 *[582.81]*
  membranoproliferative 583.2
    with nephrotic syndrome 581.2
    chronic 582.2
  membranous 583.1
    with nephrotic syndrome 581.1
    chronic 582.1
  mesangiocapillary 583.2
    with nephrotic syndrome 581.2
    chronic 582.2
  minimal change 581.3
  mixed membranous and proliferative 583.2
    with nephrotic syndrome 581.2
    chronic 582.2
  necrotic, necrotizing 583.4
    acute 580.4
    chronic 582.4
  nephrotic—*see* Nephrosis
  old—*see* Nephritis, chronic
  parenchymatous 581.89
  polycystic 753.12
    adult type (APKD) 753.13
    autosomal dominant 753.13
    autosomal recessive 753.14
    childhood type (CPKD) 753.14
    infantile type 753.14
  poststreptococcal 580.0
  pregnancy—*see* Nephritis, complicating
    pregnancy
  proliferative 583.0
    with nephrotic syndrome 581.0
    acute 580.0
    chronic 582.0
  purulent (*see also* Pyelitis) 590.80
  rapidly progressive 583.4
    acute 580.4
    chronic 582.4
  salt-losing or salt-wasting (*see also* Disease,
    renal) 593.9
  saturnine 984.9
    specified type of lead—*see* Table of drugs and
      chemicals
  septic (*see also* Pyelitis) 590.80
  specified pathology NEC 583.89
    acute 580.89
    chronic 582.89
  staphylococcal (*see also* Pyelitis) 590.80
  streptotrichosis 039.8 *[583.81]*
  subacute (*see also* Nephrosis) 581.9
  suppurative (*see also* Pyelitis) 590.80
  syphilitic (late) 095.4
    congenital 090.5 *[583.81]*
    early 091.69 *[583.81]*

Nephritis, nephritic—*continued*
  terminal (chronic) (end-stage) NEC 585.6
  toxic—*see* Nephritis, acute
  tubal, tubular—*see* Nephrosis, tubular
  tuberculous (*see also* Tuberculosis) 016.0 *[583.81]*
  type II (Ellis)—*see* Nephrosis
  vascular—*see* Hypertension, kidney
  war 580.9
Nephroblastoma (M8960/3) 189.0
  epithelial (M8961/3) 189.0
  mesenchymal (M8962/3) 189.0
Nephrocalcinosis 275.49
Nephrocystitis, pustular (*see also* Pyelitis) 590.80
Nephrolithiasis (congenital) (pelvis) (recurrent)
    592.0
  uric acid 274.11
Nephroma (M8960/3) 189.0
  mesoblastic (M8960/1) 236.9
Nephronephritis (*see also* Nephrosis) 581.9
Nephronopthisis 753.16
Nephropathy (*see also* Nephritis) 583.9
  with
    exudative nephritis 583.89
    interstitial nephritis (diffuse) (focal) 583.89
    medullary necrosis 583.7
    necrosis 583.9
      cortical 583.6
      medullary or papillary 583.7
    papillary necrosis 583.7
    specified lesion or cause NEC 583.89
  analgesic 583.89
    with medullary necrosis, acute 584.7
  arteriolar (*see also* Hypertension, kidney)
    403.90
  arteriosclerotic (*see also* Hypertension, kidney)
    403.90
  complicating pregnancy 646.2
  diabetic 250.4 *[583.81]*
    due to secondary diabetes 249.4 *[583.81]*
  gouty 274.10
    specified type NEC 274.19
  hereditary amyloid 277.31
  hypercalcemic 588.89
  hypertensive (*see also* Hypertension, kidney)
    403.90
  hypokalemic (vacuolar) 588.89
  IgA 583.9
  obstructive 593.89
    congenital 753.20
  phenacetin 584.7
  phosphate-losing 588.0
  potassium depletion 588.89
  proliferative (*see also* Nephritis, proliferative) 583.0
  protein-losing 588.89
  salt-losing or salt-wasting (*see also* Disease,
    renal) 593.9
  sickle-cell (*see also* Disease, sickle-cell) 282.60
    [583.81]
  toxic 584.5
  vasomotor 584.5
  water-losing 588.89
Nephroptosis (*see also* Disease, renal) 593.0
  congenital (displaced) 753.3
Nephropyosis (*see also* Abscess, kidney) 590.2
Nephrorrhagia 593.81
Nephrosclerosis (arteriolar) (arteriosclerotic)
    (chronic) (hyaline) (*see also* Hypertension,
    kidney) 403.90
  gouty 274.10
  hyperplastic (arteriolar) (*see also* Hypertension,
    kidney) 403.90
  senile (*see also* Sclerosis, renal) 587

Nephrosis, nephrotic (Epstein's) (syndrome) 581.9
  with
    lesion of
      focal glomerulosclerosis 581.1
      glomerulonephritis
        endothelial 581.2
        hypocomplementemic persistent 581.2
        lobular 581.2
        membranoproliferative 581.2
        membranous 581.1
        mesangiocapillary 581.2
        minimal change 581.3
        mixed membranous and proliferative 581.2
        proliferative 581.0
      segmental hyalinosis 581.1
      specified pathology NEC 581.89
  acute—*see* Nephrosis, tubular
  anoxic—*see* Nephrosis, tubular
  arteriosclerotic (*see also* Hypertension, kidney)
      403.90
  chemical—*see* Nephrosis, tubular
  cholemic 572.4
  complicating pregnancy, childbirth, or
      puerperium—*see* Nephritis, complicating
      pregnancy
  diabetic 250.4 *[581.81]*
      due to secondary diabetes 249.4 *[581.81]*
  Finnish type (congenital) 759.89
  hemoglobinuric—*see* Nephrosis, tubular
  in
    amyloidosis 277.39 *[581.81]*
    diabetes mellitus 250.4 *[581.81]*
      due to secondary diabetes 249.4 *[581.81]*
    epidemic hemorrhagic fever 078.6
    malaria 084.9 *[581.81]*
    polyarteritis 446.0 *[581.81]*
    systemic lupus erythematosus 710.0 *[581.81]*
  ischemic—*see* Nephrosis, tubular
  lipoid 581.3
  lower nephron—*see* Nephrosis, tubular
  lupoid 710.0 *[581.81]*
  lupus 710.0 *[581.81]*
  malarial 084.9 *[581.81]*
  minimal change 581.3
  necrotizing—*see* Nephrosis, tubular
  osmotic (sucrose) 588.89
  polyarteritic 446.0 *[581.81]*
  radiation 581.9
  specified lesion or cause NEC 581.89
  syphilitic 095.4
  toxic—*see* Nephrosis, tubular
  tubular (acute) 584.5
    due to a procedure 997.5
    radiation 581.9
Nephrosonephritis hemorrhagic (endemic)
      078.6
Nephrostomy status V44.6
  with complication 997.5
Nerve —*see* condition
Nerves 799.21
Nervous (*see also* condition) 799.21
  breakdown 300.9
  heart 306.2
  stomach 306.4
  tension 799.21
Nervousness 799.21
Nesidioblastoma (M8150/0)
  pancreas 211.7
  specified site NEC—*see* Neoplasm, by site, benign
  unspecified site 211.7
Netherton's syndrome (ichthyosiform
      erythroderma) 757.1

Nettle rash 708.8
Nettleship's disease (urticaria pigmentosa) 757.33
Neumann's disease (pemphigus vegetans) 694.4
Neuralgia, neuralgic (acute) (*see also* Neuritis)
      729.2
  accessory (nerve) 352.4
  acoustic (nerve) 388.5
  ankle 355.8
  anterior crural 355.8
  anus 787.99
  arm 723.4
  auditory (nerve) 388.5
  axilla 353.0
  bladder 788.1
  brachial 723.4
  brain—*see* Disorder, nerve, cranial
  broad ligament 625.9
  cerebral—*see* Disorder, nerve, cranial
  ciliary 339.00
  cranial nerve—*see also* Disorder, nerve, cranial
    fifth or trigeminal (*see also* Neuralgia,
        trigeminal) 350.1
  ear 388.71
    middle 352.1
  facial 351.8
  finger 354.9
  flank 355.8
  foot 355.8
  forearm 354.9
  Fothergill's (*see also* Neuralgia, trigeminal)
      350.1
    postherpetic 053.12
  glossopharyngeal (nerve) 352.1
  groin 355.8
  hand 354.9
  heel 355.8
  Horton's 339.00
  Hunt's 053.11
  hypoglossal (nerve) 352.5
  iliac region 355.8
  infraorbital (*see also* Neuralgia, trigeminal)
      350.1
  inguinal 355.8
  intercostal (nerve) 353.8
    postherpetic 053.19
  jaw 352.1
  kidney 788.0
  knee 355.8
  loin 355.8
  malarial (*see also* Malaria) 084.6
  mastoid 385.89
  maxilla 352.1
  median thenar 354.1
  metatarsal 355.6
  middle ear 352.1
  migrainous 339.00
  Morton's 355.6
  nerve, cranial—*see* Disorder, nerve, cranial
  nose 352.0
  occipital 723.8
  olfactory (nerve) 352.0
  ophthalmic 377.30
    postherpetic 053.19
  optic (nerve) 377.30
  penis 607.9
  perineum 355.8
  pleura 511.0
  postherpetic NEC 053.19
    geniculate ganglion 053.11
    ophthalmic 053.19
    trifacial 053.12
    trigeminal 053.12

Neuralgia, neuralgic—*continued*
pubic region 355.8
radial (nerve) 723.4
rectum 787.99
sacroiliac joint 724.3
sciatic (nerve) 724.3
scrotum 608.9
seminal vesicle 608.9
shoulder 354.9
Sluder's 337.09
specified nerve NEC—*see* Disorder, nerve
spermatic cord 608.9
sphenopalatine (ganglion) 337.09
subscapular (nerve) 723.4
suprascapular (nerve) 723.4
testis 608.89
thenar (median) 354.1
thigh 355.8
tongue 352.5
trifacial (nerve) (*see also* Neuralgia, trigeminal)
    350.1
trigeminal (nerve) 350.1
    postherpetic 053.12
tympanic plexus 388.71
ulnar (nerve) 723.4
vagus (nerve) 352.3
wrist 354.9
writers' 300.89
    organic 333.84
Neurapraxia —*see* Injury, nerve
Neurasthenia 300.5
cardiac 306.2
gastric 306.4
heart 306.2
postfebrile 780.79
postviral 780.79
Neurilemmoma (M9560/0)—*see also* Neoplasm,
    connective tissue, benign
    acoustic (nerve) 225.1
malignant (M9560/3)—*see also* Neoplasm,
    connective tissue, malignant
    acoustic (nerve) 192.0
Neurilemmosarcoma (M9560/3)—*see*
    Neoplasm, connective tissue, malignant
Neurilemoma —*see* Neurilemmoma
Neurinoma (M9560/0)—*see* Neurilemmoma
Neurinomatosis (M9560/1)—*see also* Neoplasm,
    connective tissue, uncertain behavior
centralis 759.5
Neuritis (*see also* Neuralgia) 729.2
abducens (nerve) 378.54
accessory (nerve) 352.4
acoustic (nerve) 388.5
    syphilitic 094.86
alcoholic 357.5
    with psychosis 291.1
amyloid, any site 277.39 *[357.4]*
anterior crural 355.8
arising during pregnancy 646.4
arm 723.4
ascending 355.2
auditory (nerve) 388.5
brachial (nerve) NEC 723.4
    due to displacement, intervertebral disc 722.0
cervical 723.4
chest (wall) 353.8
costal region 353.8
cranial nerve—*see also* Disorder, nerve, cranial
    first or olfactory 352.0
    second or optic 377.30
    third or oculomotor 378.52
    fourth or trochlear 378.53

Neuritis—*continued*
cranial nerve—*continued*
    fifth or trigeminal (*see also* Neuralgia,
        trigeminal) 350.1
    sixth or abducens 378.54
    seventh or facial 351.8
        newborn 767.5
    eighth or acoustic 388.5
    ninth or glossopharyngeal 352.1
    tenth or vagus 352.3
    eleventh or accessory 352.4
    twelfth or hypoglossal 352.5
Déjérine-Sottas 356.0
diabetic 250.6 *[357.2]*
    due to secondary diabetes 249.6 *[357.2]*
diphtheritic 032.89 *[357.4]*
due to
    beriberi 265.0 *[357.4]*
    displacement, prolapse, protrusion, or rupture
        of intervertebral disc 722.2
        cervical 722.0
        lumbar, lumbosacral 722.10
        thoracic, thoracolumbar 722.11
    herniation, nucleus pulposus 722.2
        cervical 722.0
        lumbar, lumbosacral 722.10
        thoracic, thoracolumbar 722.11
endemic 265.0 *[357.4]*
facial (nerve) 351.8
    newborn 767.5
general—*see* Polyneuropathy
geniculate ganglion 351.1
    due to herpes 053.11
glossopharyngeal (nerve) 352.1
gouty 274.89 *[357.4]*
hypoglossal (nerve) 352.5
ilioinguinal (nerve) 355.8
in diseases classified elsewhere—*see*
    Polyneuropathy, in
infectious (multiple) 357.0
intercostal (nerve) 353.8
interstitial hypertrophic progressive NEC 356.9
leg 355.8
lumbosacral NEC 724.4
median (nerve) 354.1
    thenar 354.1
multiple (acute) (infective) 356.9
    endemic 265.0 *[357.4]*
multiplex endemica 265.0 *[357.4]*
nerve root (*see also* Radiculitis) 729.2
oculomotor (nerve) 378.52
olfactory (nerve) 352.0
optic (nerve) 377.30
    in myelitis 341.0
    meningococcal 036.81
pelvic 355.8
peripheral (nerve)—*see also* Neuropathy,
    peripheral
    complicating pregnancy or puerperium 646.4
    specified nerve NEC—*see* Mononeuritis
pneumogastric (nerve) 352.3
postchickenpox 052.7
postherpetic 053.19
progressive hypertrophic interstitial NEC 356.9
puerperal, postpartum 646.4
radial (nerve) 723.4
retrobulbar 377.32
    syphilitic 094.85
rheumatic (chronic) 729.2
sacral region 355.8
sciatic (nerve) 724.3
    due to displacement of intervertebral disc 722.10

Neuritis—*continued*
 serum 999.59
 specified nerve NEC—*see* Disorder, nerve
 spinal (nerve) 355.9
  root (*see also* Radiculitis) 729.2
 subscapular (nerve) 723.4
 suprascapular (nerve) 723.4
 syphilitic 095.8
 thenar (median) 354.1
 thoracic NEC 724.4
 toxic NEC 357.7
 trochlear (nerve) 378.53
 ulnar (nerve) 723.4
 vagus (nerve) 352.3
Neuroangiomatosis, encephalofacial 759.6
Neuroastrocytoma (M9505/1)—*see* Neoplasm,
 by site, uncertain behavior
Neuro-avitaminosis 269.2
Neuroblastoma (M9500/3)
 olfactory (M9522/3) 160.0
 specified site—*see* Neoplasm, by site, malignant
 unspecified site 194.0
Neurochorioretinitis (*see also* Chorioretinitis)
 363.20
Neurocirculatory asthenia 306.2
Neurocytoma (M9506/0)—*see* Neoplasm, by
 site, benign
Neurodermatitis (circumscribed) (circumscripta)
 (local) 698.3
 atopic 691.8
 diffuse (Brocq) 691.8
 disseminated 691.8
 nodulosa 698.3
Neuroencephalomyelopathy, optic 341.0
Neuroendocrine tumor —see Tumor,
 neuroendocrine
Neuroepithelioma (M9503/3)—*see also*
 Neoplasm, by site, malignant
 olfactory (M9521/3) 160.0
Neurofibroma (M9540/0)—*see also* Neoplasm,
 connective tissue, benign
 melanotic (M9541/0)—*see* Neoplasm,
  connective tissue, benign
 multiple (M9540/1) 237.70
  Type 1 237.71
  Type 2 237.72
 plexiform (M9550/0)—*see* Neoplasm,
  connective tissue, benign
Neurofibromatosis (multiple) (M9540/1) 237.70
 acoustic 237.72
 malignant (M9540/3)—*see* Neoplasm,
  connective tissue, malignant
 Schwannomatosis 237.73
 specified type NEC 237.79
 Type 1 237.71
 Type 2 237.72
 von Recklinghausen's 237.71
Neurofibrosarcoma (M9540/3)—*see* Neoplasm,
 connective tissue, malignant
Neurogenic —*see also* condition
 bladder (atonic) (automatic) (autonomic)
  (flaccid) (hypertonic) (hypotonic) (inertia)
  (infranuclear) (irritable) (motor) (nonreflex)
  (nuclear) (paralysis) (reflex) (sensory)
  (spastic) (supranuclear) (uninhibited) 596.54
  with cauda equina syndrome 344.61
 bowel 564.81
 heart 306.2
Neuroglioma (M9505/1)—*see* Neoplasm, by site,
 uncertain behavior
Neurolabyrinthitis (of Dix and Hallpike) 386.12

Neurolathyrism 988.2
Neuroleprosy 030.1
Neuroleptic malignant syndrome 333.92
Neurolipomatosis 272.8
Neuroma (M9570/0)—*see also* Neoplasm,
 connective tissue, benign
 acoustic (nerve) (M9560/0) 225.1
 amputation (traumatic)—*see also* Injury, nerve,
  by site
  surgical complication (late) 997.61
 appendix 211.3
 auditory nerve 225.1
 digital 355.6
  toe 355.6
 interdigital (toe) 355.6
 intermetatarsal 355.6
 Morton's 355.6
 multiple 237.70
  Type 1 237.71
  Type 2 237.72
 nonneoplastic 355.9
  arm NEC 354.9
  leg NEC 355.8
  lower extremity NEC 355.8
  specified site NEC—*see* Mononeuritis, by site
  upper extremity NEC 354.9
 optic (nerve) 225.1
 plantar 355.6
 plexiform (M9550/0)—*see* Neoplasm,
  connective tissue, benign
 surgical (nonneoplastic) 355.9
  arm NEC 354.9
  leg NEC 355.8
  lower extremity NEC 355.8
  upper extremity NEC 354.9
 traumatic—*see also* Injury, nerve, by site
  old—*see* Neuroma, nonneoplastic
Neuromyalgia 729.1
Neuromyasthenia (epidemic) 049.8
Neuromyelitis 341.8
 ascending 357.0
 optica 341.0
Neuromyopathy NEC 358.9
Neuromyositis 729.1
Neuronevus (M8725/0)—*see* Neoplasm, skin,
 benign
Neuronitis 357.0
 ascending (acute) 355.2
 vestibular 386.12
Neuroparalytic —*see* condition
Neuropathy, axtaxia and retinitis pigmentosa
 (NARP syndrome) 277.87
Neuropathy, neuropathic (*see also* Disorder,
 nerve) 355.9
 acute motor 357.82
 alcoholic 357.5
  with psychosis 291.1
 arm NEC 354.9
 ataxia and retinitis pigmentosa (NARP
  syndrome) 277.87
 autonomic (peripheral)—*see* Neuropathy,
  peripheral, autonomic
 axillary nerve 353.0
 brachial plexus 353.0
 cervical plexus 353.2
 chronic
  progressive segmentally demyelinating 357.89
  relapsing demyelinating 357.89
 congenital sensory 356.2
 Déjérine-Sottas 356.0

Neuropathy, neuropathic—*continued*
diabetic 250.6 *[357.2]*
  autonomic (peripheral) 250.6 *[337.1]*
  due to secondary diabetes 249.6 *[357.2]*
    autonomic (peripheral) 249.6 *[337.1]*
entrapment 355.9
  iliohypogastric nerve 355.79
  ilioinguinal nerve 355.79
  lateral cutaneous nerve of thigh 355.1
  median nerve 354.0
  obturator nerve 355.79
  peroneal nerve 355.3
  posterior tibial nerve 355.5
  saphenous nerve 355.79
  ulnar nerve 354.2
facial nerve 351.9
hereditary 356.9
  peripheral 356.0
  sensory (radicular) 356.2
hypertrophic
  Charcot-Marie-Tooth 356.1
  Déjérine-Sottas 356.0
  interstitial 356.9
  Refsum 356.3
intercostal nerve 354.8
ischemic—*see* Disorder, nerve
Jamaican (ginger) 357.7
leg NEC 355.8
lower extremity NEC 355.8
lumbar plexus 353.1
median nerve 354.1
motor
  acute 357.82
multiple (acute) (chronic) (*see also*
  Polyneuropathy) 356.9
optic 377.39
  ischemic 377.41
  nutritional 377.33
  toxic 377.34
peripheral (nerve) (*see also* Polyneuropathy) 356.9
  arm NEC 354.9
  autonomic 337.9
    amyloid 277.39 *[337.1]*
    idiopathic 337.00
    in
      amyloidosis 277.39 *[337.1]*
      diabetes (mellitus) 250.6 *[337.1]*
        due to secondary diabetes 249.6 *[337.1]*
      diseases classified elsewhere 337.1
      gout 274.89 *[337.1]*
      hyperthyroidism 242.9 *[337.1]*
  due to
    antitetanus serum 357.6
    arsenic 357.7
    drugs 357.6
    lead 357.7
    organophosphate compounds 357.7
    toxic agent NEC 357.7
  hereditary 356.0
  idiopathic 356.9
    progressive 356.4
    specified type NEC 356.8
  in diseases classified elsewhere—*see*
    Polyneuropathy, in
  leg NEC 355.8
  lower extremity NEC 355.8
  upper extremity NEC 354.9
plantar nerves 355.6
progressive
  hypertrophic interstitial 356.9
  inflammatory 357.89

Neuropathy, neuropathic—*continued*
radicular NEC 729.2
  brachial 723.4
  cervical NEC 723.4
  hereditary sensory 356.2
  lumbar 724.4
  lumbosacral 724.4
  thoracic NEC 724.4
sacral plexus 353.1
sciatic 355.0
spinal nerve NEC 355.9
  root (*see also* Radiculitis) 729.2
toxic 357.7
trigeminal sensory 350.8
ulnar nerve 354.2
upper extremity NEC 354.9
uremic 585.9 *[357.4]*
vitamin B$_{12}$ 266.2 *[357.4]*
  with anemia (pernicious) 281.0 *[357.4]*
    due to dietary deficiency 281.1 *[357.4]*
Neurophthisis —*see also* Disorder, nerve
peripheral 356.9
  diabetic 250.6 *[357.2]*
    due to secondary diabetes 249.6 *[357.2]*
Neuropraxia —*see* Injury,nerve
Neuroretinitis 363.05
syphilitic 094.85
Neurosarcoma 9M9540/3)—sde Neoplasm,
  connective tissue, malignant
Neurosclerosis —*see* Disorder, nerve
Neurosis, neurotic 300.9
accident 300.16
anancastic, anankastic 300.3
anxiety (state) 300.00
  generalized 300.02
  panic type 300.01
asthenic 300.5
bladder 306.53
cardiac (reflex) 306.2
cardiovascular 306.2
climacteric, unspecified type 627.2
colon 306.4
compensation 300.16
compulsive, compulsion 300.3
conversion 300.11
craft 300.89
cutaneous 306.3
depersonalization 300.6
depressive (reaction) (type) 300.4
endocrine 306.6
environmental 300.89
fatigue 300.5
functional (*see also* Disorder, psychosomatic)
  306.9
gastric 306.4
gastrointestinal 306.4
genitourinary 306.50
heart 306.2
hypochondriacal 300.7
hysterical 300.10
  conversion type 300.11
  dissociative type 300.15
impulsive 300.3
incoordination 306.0
  larynx 306.1
  vocal cord 306.1
intestine 306.4
larynx 306.1
  hysterical 300.11
  sensory 306.1
menopause, unspecified type 627.2

Neurosis, neurotic—*continued*
  mixed NEC 300.89
  musculoskeletal 306.0
  obsessional 300.3
    phobia 300.3
  obsessive-compulsive 300.3
  occupational 300.89
  ocular 306.7
  oral (*see also* Disorder, fluency) 315.35
  organ (*see also* Disorder, psychosomatic) 306.9
  pharynx 306.1
  phobic 300.20
  posttraumatic (acute) (situational) 309.81
    chronic 309.81
  psychasthenic (type) 300.89
  railroad 300.16
  rectum 306.4
  respiratory 306.1
  rumination 306.4
  senile 300.89
  sexual 302.70
  situational 300.89
  specified type NEC 300.89
  state 300.9
    with depersonalization episode 300.6
  stomach 306.4
  vasomotor 306.2
  visceral 306.4
  war 300.16
Neurospongioblastosis diffusa 759.5
Neurosyphilis (arrested) (early) (inactive) (late)
  (latent) (recurrent) 094.9
  with ataxia (cerebellar) (locomotor) (spastic)
    (spinal) 094.0
  acute meningitis 094.2
  aneurysm 094.89
  arachnoid (adhesive) 094.2
  arteritis (any artery) 094.89
  asymptomatic 094.3
  congenital 090.40
  dura (mater) 094.89
  general paresis 094.1
  gumma 094.9
  hemorrhagic 094.9
  juvenile (asymptomatic) (meningeal) 090.40
  leptomeninges (aseptic) 094.2
  meningeal 094.2
  meninges (adhesive) 094.2
  meningovascular (diffuse) 094.2
  optic atrophy 094.84
  parenchymatous (degenerative) 094.1
  paresis (*see also* Paresis, general) 094.1
  paretic (*see also* Paresis, general) 094.1
  relapse 094.9
  remission in (sustained) 094.9
  serological 094.3
  specified nature or site NEC 094.89
  tabes (dorsalis) 094.0
    juvenile 090.40
  tabetic 094.0
    juvenile 090.40
  taboparesis 094.1
    juvenile 090.40
  thrombosis 094.89
  vascular 094.89
Neurotic (*see also* Neurosis) 300.9
  excoriation 698.4
    psychogenic 306.3
Neurotmesis —*see* Injury, nerve, by site
Neurotoxemia —*see* Toxemia
Neutro-oclusion 524.21

Neutropenia, neutropenic (idiopathic)
  (pernicious) (primary) 288.00
  chronic 288.09
    hypoplastic 288.09
  congenital (nontransient) 288.01
  cyclic 288.02
  drug induced 288.03
  due to infection 288.04
  fever 288.00
  genetic 288.01
  immune 288.09
  infantile 288.01
  malignant 288.09
  neonatal, transitory (isoimmune) (maternal
    transfer) 776.7
  periodic 288.02
  splenic 289.53
  splenomegaly 289.53
  toxic 288.09
Neutrophilia, hereditary giant 288.2
Nevocarcinoma (M8720/3)—*see* Melanoma
Nevus (M8720/0)—*see also* Neoplasm, skin,
  benign

> *Note*—*Except where otherwise indicated, the
> varieties of nevus in the list below that are
> followed by a morphology code number (M----
> -/0) should be coded by site as for "Neoplasm,
> skin, benign."*

  acanthotic 702.8
  achromic (M8730/0)
  amelanotic (M8730/0)
  anemic, anemicus 709.09
  angiomatous (M9120/0) (*see also* Hemangioma)
    228.00
  araneus 448.1
  avasculosus 709.09
  balloon cell (M8722/0)
  bathing trunk (M8761/1) 238.2
  blue (M8780/0)
    cellular (M8790/0)
    giant (M8790/0)
    Jadassohn's (M8780/0)
    malignant (M8780/3)—*see* Melanoma
  capillary (M9131/0) (*see also* Hemangioma)
    228.00
  cavernous (M9121/0) (*see also* Hemangioma)
    228.00
  cellular (M8720/0)
    blue (M8790/0)
  comedonicus 757.33
  compound (M8760/0)
  conjunctiva (M8720/0) 224.3
  dermal (M8750/0)
    and epidermal (M8760/0)
  epithelioid cell (and spindle cell) (M8770/0)
  flammeus 757.32
    osteohypertrophic 759.89
  hairy (M8720/0)
  halo (M8723/0)
  hemangiomatous (M9120/0) (*see also*
    Hemangioma) 228.00
  intradermal (M8750/0)
  intraepidermal (M8740/0)
  involuting (M8724/0)
  Jadassohn's (blue) (M8780/0)
  junction, junctional (M8740/0)
    malignant melanoma in (M8740/3)—*see*
    Melanoma
  juvenile (M8770/0)
  lymphatic (M9170/0) 228.1

Nevus—*continued*
  magnocellular (M8726/0)
    specified site—*see* Neoplasm, by site, benign
    unspecified site 224.0
  malignant (M8720/3)—*see* Melanoma
  meaning hemangioma (M9120/0) (*see also*
    Hemangioma) 228.00
  melanotic (pigmented) (M8720/0)
  multiplex 759.5
  nonneoplastic 448.1
  nonpigmented (M8730/0)
  nonvascular (M8720/0)
  oral mucosa, white sponge 750.26
  osteohypertrophic, flammeus 759.89
  papillaris (M8720/0)
  papillomatosus (M8720/0)
  pigmented (M8720/0)
    giant (M8761/1)—*see also* Neoplasm, skin,
      uncertain behavior
      malignant melanoma in (M8761/3)—*see*
        Melanoma
  systematicus 757.33
  pilosus (M8720/0)
  port wine 757.32
  sanguineous 757.32
  sebaceous (senile) 702.8
  senile 448.1
  spider 448.1
  spindle cell (and epithelioid cell) (M8770/0)
  stellar 448.1
  strawberry 757.32
  syringocystadenomatous papilliferous
    (M8406/0)
  unius lateris 757.33
  Unna's 757.32
  vascular 757.32
  verrucous 757.33
  white sponge (oral mucosa) 750.26
Newborn (infant) (liveborn)
  abstinence syndrome 779.5
  affected by
    amniocentesis 760.61
    maternal abuse of drugs (gestational) (via
      placenta) (via breast milk) (see also
      Noxious, substances transmitted through
      placenta or breast milk (affecting fetus or
      newborn)) 760.70
      methamphetamine(s) 760.72
    procedure
      amniocentesis 760.61
      in utero NEC 760.62
      surgical on mother
        during pregnancy NEC 760.63
        previous not associated with pregnancy
          760.64
  apnea 770.81
    obstructive 770.82
    specified NEC 770.82
  breast buds 779.89
  cardiomyopathy 425.4
    congenital 425.3
  convulsion 779.0
  electrolyte imbalance NEC (transitory) 775.5
  fever (environmentally-induced) 778.4
  gestation
    24 completed weeks 765.22
    25-26 completed weeks 765.23
    27-28 completed weeks 765.24
    29-30 completed weeks 765.25
    31-32 completed weeks 765.26
    33-34 completed weeks 765.27

Newborn—*continued*
  gestation—*continued*
    35-36 completed weeks 765.28
    37 or more completed weeks 765.29
    less than 24 completed weeks 765.21
    unspecified completed weeks 765.20
  infection 771.89
    candida 771.7
    mastitis 771.5
    specified NEC 771.89
    urinary tract 771.82
  mastitis 771.5
  multiple NEC
    born in hospital (without mention of cesarean
      delivery or section) V37.00
      with cesarean delivery or section V37.01
    born outside hospital
      hospitalized V37.1
      not hospitalized V37.2
    mates all liveborn
      born in hospital (without mention of
        cesarean delivery or section) V34.00
        with cesarean delivery or section V34.01
      born outside hospital
        hospitalized V34.1
        not hospitalized V34.2
    mates all stillborn
      born in hospital (without mention of
        cesarean delivery or section) V35.00
        with cesarean delivery or section V35.01
      born outside hospital
        hospitalized V35.1
        not hospitalized V35.2
    mates liveborn and stillborn
      born in hospital (without mention of
        cesarean delivery or section) V36.00
        with cesarean delivery or section V36.01
      born outside hospital
        hospitalized V36.1
        not hospitalized V36.2
  omphalitis 771.4
  seizure 779.0
  sepsis 771.81
  single
    born in hospital (without mention of cesarean
      delivery or section) V30.00
      with cesarean delivery or section V30.01
    born outside hospital
      hospitalized V30.1
      not hospitalized V30.2
  specified condition NEC 779.89
  twin NEC
    born in hospital (without mention of cesarean
      delivery or section) V33.00
      with cesarean delivery or section V33.01
    born outside hospital
      hospitalized V33.1
      not hospitalized V33.2
    mate liveborn
      born in hospital V31.0
      born outside hospital
        hospitalized V31.1
        not hospitalized V31.2
    mate stillborn
      born in hospital V32.0
      born outside hospital
        hospitalized V32.1
        not hospitalized V32.2

Newborn—*continued*
  unspecified as to single or multiple birth
    born in hospital (without mention of cesarean
        delivery or section) V39.00
      with cesarean delivery or section V39.01
    born outside hospital
      hospitalized V39.1
      not hospitalized V39.2
    weight check V20.32
Newcastle's conjunctivitis or disease 077.8
Nezelof's syndrome (pure alymphocytosis) 279.13
Niacin (amide) deficiency 265.2
Nicolas-Durand-Favre disease (climatic bubo)
    099.1
Nicolas-Favre disease (climatic bubo) 099.1
Nicotinic acid (amide) deficiency 265.2
Niemann-Pick disease (lipid histiocytosis)
    (splenomegaly) 272.7
Night
  blindness (*see also* Blindness, night) 368.60
    congenital 368.61
    vitamin A deficiency 264.5
  cramps 729.82
  sweats 780.8
  terrors, child 307.46
Nightmare 307.47
  REM-sleep type 307.47
Nipple —*see* condition
Nisbet's chancre 099.0
Nishimoto (-Takeuchi) disease 437.5
Nitritoid crisis or reaction —*see* Crisis, nitritoid
Nitrogen retention, extrarenal 788.99
Nitrosohemoglobinemia 289.89
Njovera 104.0
No
  diagnosis 799.9
  disease (found) V71.9
  room at the inn V65.0
Nocardiasis —*see* Nocardiosis
Nocardiosis 039.9
  with pneumonia 039.1
  lung 039.1
  specified type NEC 039.8
Nocturia 788.43
  psychogenic 306.53
Nocturnal —*see also* condition
  dyspnea (paroxysmal) 786.09
  emissions 608.89
  enuresis 788.36
    psychogenic 307.6
  frequency (micturition) 788.43
    psychogenic 306.53
Nodal rhythm disorder 427.89
Nodding of head 781.0
Node (s)—*see also* Nodule
  Heberden's 715.04
  larynx 478.79
  lymph—*see* condition
  milkers' 051.1
  Osler's 421.0
  rheumatic 729.89
  Schmorl's 722.30
    lumbar, lumbosacral 722.32
    specified region NEC 722.39
    thoracic, thoracolumbar 722.31
  singers' 478.5
  skin NEC 782.2
  tuberculous—*see* Tuberculosis, lymph gland
  vocal cords 478.5
Nodosities, Haygarth's 715.04

Nodule(s), nodular
  actinomycotic (*see also* Actinomycosis) 039.9
  arthritic—*see* Arthritis, nodosa
  breast 793.89
  cutaneous 782.2
  Haygarth's 715.04
  inflammatory—*see* Inflammation
  juxta-articular 102.7
    syphilitic 095.7
    yaws 102.7
  larynx 478.79
  lung
    emphysematous 492.8
    solitary 793.11
  milkers' 051.1
  prostate 600.10
    with
      urinary
        obstruction 600.11
        retention 600.11
  pulmonary, solitary (subsegmental branch of the
      bronchial tree) 793.11
    multiple 793.19
  retrocardiac 785.9
  rheumatic 729.89
  rheumatoid—*see* Arthritis rheumatoid
  scrotum (inflammatory) 608.4
  singers' 478.5
  skin NEC 782.2
  solitary, lung 518.89
    emphysematous 492.8
  subcutaneous 782.2
  thyroid (gland) (nontoxic) (uninodular) 241.0
    with
      hyperthyroidism 242.1
      thyrotoxicosis 242.1
    toxic or with hyperthyroidism 242.1
  vocal cords 478.5
Noma (gangrenous) (hospital) (infective) 528.1
  auricle (*see also* Gangrene) 785.4
  mouth 528.1
  pudendi (*see also* Vulvitis) 616.10
  vulvae (*see also* Vulvitis) 616.10
Nomadism V60.0
Non-adherence
  artificial skin graft 996.55
  decellularized allodermis graft 996.55
Non-autoimmune hemolytic anemia NEC 283.10
Nonclosure —*see also* Imperfect, closure
  ductus
    arteriosus 747.0
    Botalli 747.0
  Eustachian valve 746.89
  foramen
    Botalli 745.5
    ovale 745.5
Noncompliance with medical treatment V15.81
  renal dialysis V45.12
Nondescent (congenital)—*see also* Malposition,
    congenital
  cecum 751.4
  colon 751.4
  testis 752.51
Nondevelopment
  brain 742.1
    specified part 742.2
  heart 746.89
  organ or site, congenital NEC—*see* Hypoplasia
Nonengagement
  head NEC 652.5
    in labor 660.1
      affecting fetus or newborn 763.1

Nonexanthematous tick fever 066.1
Nonexpansion, lung (newborn) NEC 770.4
Nonfunctioning
   cystic duct (*see also* Disease, gallbladder) 575.8
   gallbladder (*see also* Disease, gallbladder) 575.8
   kidney (*see also* Disease, renal) 593.9
   labyrinth 386.58
Nonhealing
   stump (surgical) 997.60
   wound, surgical 998.83
Nonimplantation of ovum, causing infertility
   628.3
Noninsufflation, fallopian tube 628.2
Nonne-Milroy-Meige syndrome (chronic
   hereditary edema) 757.0
Nonovulation 628.0
Nonpatent fallopian tube 628.2
Nonpneumatization, lung NEC 770.4
Nonreflex bladder 596.54
   with cauda equina 344.61
Nonretention of food —*see also* Vomiting
Nonrotation —*see* Malrotation
Nonsecretion, urine (*see also* Anuria) 788.5
   newborn 753.3
Nonunion
   fracture 733.82
   organ or site, congenital NEC—*see* Imperfect,
      closure
   symphysis pubis, congenital 755.69
   top sacrum, congenital 756.19
Nonviability 765.0
Nonvisualization, gallbladder 793.3
Nonvitalized tooth 522.9
Non-working side interference 524.56
Normal
   delivery—*see* category 650
   menses V65.5
   state (feared complaint unfounded) V65.5
Normoblastosis 289.89
Normocytic anemia (infectional) 285.9
   due to blood loss (chronic) 280.0
      acute 285.1
Norrie's disease (congenital) (progressive
   oculoacousticocerebral degeneration) 743.8
North American blastomycosis 116.0
Norwegian itch 133.0
Nose, nasal —*see* condition
Nosebleed 784.7
Nosomania 298.9
Nosophobia 300.29
Nostalgia 309.89
Notch of iris 743.46
Notched lip, congenital (*see also* Cleft, lip) 749.10
Notching nose, congenital (tip) 748.1
Nothnagel's
   syndrome 378.52
   vasomotor acroparesthesia 443.89
Novy's relapsing fever (American) 087.1
Noxious
   foodstuffs, poisoning by
      fish 988.0
      fungi 988.1
      mushrooms 988.1
      plants (food) 988.2
      shellfish 988.0
      specified type NEC 988.8
      toadstool 988.1

Noxious—*continued*
   substances transmitted through placenta or
      breast milk (affecting fetus or newborn)
      760.70
      acetretin 760.78
      alcohol 760.71
      aminopterin 760.78
      antiandrogens 760.79
      anticonvulsant 760.77
      antifungal 760.74
      anti-infective agents 760.74
      antimetabolic 760.78
      atorvastatin 760.78
      carbamazepine 760.77
      cocaine 760.75
      "crack" 760.75
      diethylstilbestrol (DES) 760.76
      divalproex sodium 760.77
      endocrine disrupting chemicals 760.79
      estrogens 760.79
      etretinate 760.78
      fluconazole 760.74
      fluvastatin 760.78
      hallucinogenic agents NEC 760.73
      hormones 760.79
      lithium 760.79
      lovastatin 760.78
      medicinal agents NEC 760.79
      methotrexate 760.78
      misoprostil 760.79
      narcotics 760.72
      obstetric anesthetic or analgesic 763.5
      phenobarbital 760.77
      phenytoin 760.77
      pravastatin 760.78
      progestins 760.79
      retinoic acid 760.78
      simvastatin 760.78
      solvents 760.79
      specified agent NEC 760.79
      statins 760.78
      suspected, affecting management of pregnancy
         655.5
      tetracycline 760.74
      thalidomide 760.79
      trimethadione 760.77
      valproate 760.77
      valproic acid 760.77
      vitamin A 760.78
NPDH (new persistent daily headache) 339.42
Nuchal hitch (arm) 652.8
Nucleus pulposus —*see* condition
Numbness 782.0
Nuns' knee 727.2
Nursemaid's
   elbow 832.2
   shoulder 831.0
Nutmeg liver 573.8
Nutrition, deficient or insufficient (particular
   kind of food) 269.9
   due to
      insufficient food 994.2
      lack of
         care (child) (infant) 995.52
            adult 995.84
         food 994.2
Nyctalopia (*see also* Blindness, night) 368.60
   vitamin A deficiency 264.5

Nycturia 788.43
  psychogenic 306.53
Nymphomania 302.89
Nystagmus 379.50
  associated with vestibular system disorders
    379.54
  benign paroxysmal positional 386.11
  central positional 386.2
  congenital 379.51
  deprivation 379.53
  dissociated 379.55
  latent 379.52
  miners' 300.89
  positional
    benign paroxysmal 386.11
    central 386.2
  specified NEC 379.56
  vestibular 379.54
  visual deprivation 379.53

O

Oasthouse urine disease 270.2
Obermeyer's relapsing fever (European) 087.0
Obesity (constitutional) (exogenous) (familial)
  (nutritional) (simple) 278.00
  adrenal 255.8
  complicating pregnancy, childbirth, or the
    puerperium 649.1
  due to hyperalimentation 278.00
  endocrine NEC 259.9
  endogenous 259.9
  Fröhlich's (adiposogenital dystrophy) 253.8
  glandular NEC 259.9
  hypothyroid (see also Hypothyroidism) 244.9
  hypoventilation syndrome 278.03
  morbid 278.01
  of pregnancy 649.1
  pituitary 253.8
  severe 278.01
  thyroid (see also Hypothyroidism) 244.9
Oblique —see also condition
  lie before labor, affecting fetus or newborn 761.7
Obliquity, pelvis 738.6
Obliteration
  abdominal aorta 446.7
  appendix (lumen) 543.9
  artery 447.1
  ascending aorta 446.7
  bile ducts 576.8
    with calculus, choledocholithiasis, or
      stones—see Choledocholithiasis
    congenital 751.61
      jaundice from 751.61 [774.5]
  common duct 576.8
    with calculus, choledocholithiasis, or
      stones—see Choledocholithiasis
    congenital 751.61
  cystic duct 575.8
    with calculus, choledocholithiasis, or
      stones—see Choledocholithiasis
  disease, arteriolar 447.1
  endometrium 621.8
  eye, anterior chamber 360.34
  fallopian tube 628.2
  lymphatic vessel 457.1
    postmastectomy 457.0
  organ or site, congenital NEC—see Atresia
  placental blood vessels—see Placenta, abnormal
  supra-aortic branches 446.7
  ureter 593.89
  urethra 599.84
  vein 459.9
  vestibule (oral) 525.8
Observation (for) V71.9
  without need for further medical care V71.9
  accident NEC V71.4
    at work V71.3
  criminal assault V71.6
  deleterious agent ingestion V71.89
  disease V71.9
    cardiovascular V71.7
    heart V71.7
    mental V71.09
    specified condition NEC V71.89
  foreign body ingestion V71.89
  growth and development variations V21.8
  injuries (accidental) V71.4
    inflicted NEC V71.6
      during alleged rape or seduction V71.5

Observation—continued
  malignant neoplasm, suspected V71.1
  postpartum
    immediately after delivery V24.0
    routine follow-up V24.2
  pregnancy
    high-risk V23.9
      inconclusive fetal viability V23.87
      specified problem NEC V23.8
    normal (without complication) V22.1
      with nonobstetric complication V22.2
      first V22.0
  rape or seduction, alleged V71.5
    injury during V71.5
  suicide attempt, alleged V71.89
  suspected (undiagnosed) (unproven)
    abuse V71.81
    cardiovascular disease V71.7
    child or wife battering victim V71.6
    concussion (cerebral) V71.6
    condition NEC V71.89
      infant—see Observation, suspected,
        condition, newborn
      maternal and fetal
        amniotic cavity and membrane problem
          V89.01
        cervical shortening V89.05
        fetal anomaly V89.03
        fetal growth problem V89.04
        oligohydramnios V89.01
        other specified problem NEC V89.09
        placental problem V89.02
        polyhydramnios V89.01
      newborn V29.9
        cardiovascular disease V29.8
        congenital anomaly V29.8
        genetic V29.3
        infectious V29.0
        ingestion foreign object V29.8
        injury V29.8
        metabolic V29.3
        neoplasm V29.8
        neurological V29.1
        poison, poisoning V29.8
        respiratory V29.2
        specified NEC V29.8
    exposure
      anthrax V71.82
      biological agent NEC V71.83
      SARS V71.83
    infectious disease not requiring isolation V71.89
    malignant neoplasm V71.1
    mental disorder V71.09
    neglect V71.81
    neoplasm
      benign V71.89
      malignant V71.1
    specified condition NEC V71.89
    tuberculosis V71.2
  tuberculosis, suspected V71.2
Obsession, obsessional 300.3
  ideas and mental images 300.3
  impulses 300.3
  neurosis 300.3
  phobia 300.3
  psychasthenia 300.3
  ruminations 300.3
  state 300.3
  syndrome 300.3

Obsessive-compulsive 300.3
  neurosis 300.3
  personality 301.4
  reaction 300.3
Obstetrical trauma NEC (complicating delivery)
  665.9
  with
    abortion—*see* Abortion, by type, with damage
      to pelvic organs
    ectopic pregnancy (*see also* categories
      633.0-633.9) 639.2
    molar pregnancy (*see also* categories 630-632)
      639.2
  affecting fetus or newborn 763.89
  following
    abortion 639.2
    ectopic or molar pregnancy 639.2
Obstipation (*see also* Constipation) 564.00
  psychogenic 306.4
Obstruction, obstructed, obstructive
  airway NEC 519.8
    with
      allergic alveolitis NEC 495.9
      asthma NEC (*see also* Asthma) 493.9
      bronchiectasis 494.0
        with acute exacerbation 494.1
      bronchitis (*see also* Bronchitis, with,
        obstruction) 491.20
      emphysema NEC 492.8
    chronic 496
      with
        allergic alveolitis NEC 495.5
        asthma NEC (*see also* Asthma) 493.2
        bronchiectasis 494.0
          with acute exacerbation 494.1
        bronchitis (*see also* Bronchitis, chronic,
          obstructive) 491.20
        emphysema NEC 492.8
    due to
      bronchospasm 519.11
      foreign body 934.9
      inhalation of fumes or vapors 506.9
      laryngospasm 478.75
  alimentary canal (*see also* Obstruction,
    intestine) 560.9
  ampulla of Vater 576.2
    with calculus, cholelithiasis, or stones—*see*
      Choledocholithiasis
  aortic (heart) (valve) (*see also* Stenosis, aortic) 424.1
    rheumatic (*see also* Stenosis, aortic,
      rheumatic) 395.0
  aortoiliac 444.09
  aqueduct of Sylvius 331.4
    congenital 742.3
      with spina bifida (*see also* Spina bifida) 741.0
  Arnold-Chiari (*see also* Spina bifida) 741.0
  artery (*see also* Embolism, artery) 444.9
    basilar (complete) (partial) (*see also*
      Occlusion, artery, basilar) 433.0
    carotid (complete) (partial) (*see also*
      Occlusion, artery, carotid) 433.1
    precerebral—*see* Occlusion, artery,
      precerebral NEC
    retinal (central) (*see also* Occlusion, retina)
      362.30
    vertebral (complete) (partial) (*see also*
      Occlusion, artery, vertebral) 433.2
  asthma (chronic) (with obstructive pulmonary
    disease) 493.2
  band (intestinal) 560.81

Obstruction, obstructed—*continued*
  bile duct or passage (*see also* Obstruction,
    biliary) 576.2
    congenital 751.61
      jaundice from 751.61 *[774.5]*
  biliary (duct) (tract) 576.2
    with calculus 574.51
      with cholecystitis (chronic) 574.41
        acute 574.31
    congenital 751.61
      jaundice from 751.61 *[774.5]*
    gallbladder 575.2
      with calculus 574.21
        with cholecystitis (chronic) 574.11
          acute 574.01
  bladder neck (acquired) 596.0
    congenital 753.6
  bowel (*see also* Obstruction, intestine) 560.9
  bronchus 519.19
  canal, ear (*see also* Stricture, ear canal,
    acquired) 380.50
  cardia 537.89
  caval veins (inferior) (superior) 459.2
  cecum (*see also* Obstruction, intestine) 560.9
  circulatory 459.9
  colon (*see also* Obstruction, intestine) 560.9
    sympathicotonic 560.89
  common duct (*see also* Obstruction, biliary)
    576.2
    congenital 751.61
  coronary (*see also* Arteriosclerosis, coronary)
    acute (*see also* Infarct, myocardium) 410.9
      without myocardial infarction 411.81
  cystic duct (*see also* Obstruction, gallbladder)
    575.2
    congenital 751.61
  device, implant, or graft—*see* Complications,
    due to (presence of) any device, implant, or
    graft classified to 996.0-996.5 NEC
  due to foreign body accidentally left in operation
    wound 998.4
  duodenum 537.3
    congenital 751.1
    due to
      compression NEC 537.3
      cyst 537.3
      intrinsic lesion or disease NEC 537.3
      scarring 537.3
      torsion 537.3
      ulcer 532.91
      volvulus 537.3
  ejaculatory duct 608.89
  endocardium 424.90
    arteriosclerotic 424.99
    specified cause, except rheumatic 424.99
  esophagus 530.3
  Eustachian tube (complete) (partial) 381.60
    cartilaginous
      extrinsic 381.63
      intrinsic 381.62
    due to
      cholesteatoma 381.61
      osseous lesion NEC 381.61
      polyp 381.61
    osseous 381.61
  fallopian tube (bilateral) 628.2
  fecal 560.32
    with hernia—*see also* Hernia, by site, with
      obstruction
      gangrenous—*see* Hernia, by site, with
        gangrene

Obstruction, obstructed—*continued*
  foramen of Monro (congenital) 742.3
    with spina bifida (*see also* Spina bifida) 741.0
  foreign body—*see* Foreign body
  gallbladder 575.2
    with calculus, cholelithiasis, or stones 574.21
      with cholecystitis (chronic) 574.11
        acute 574.01
    congenital 751.69
      jaundice from 751.69 *[774.5]*
  gastric outlet 537.0
  gastrointestinal (*see also* Obstruction, intestine) 560.9
  glottis 478.79
  hepatic 573.8
    duct (*see also* Obstruction, biliary) 576.2
      congenital 751.61
    icterus (*see also* Obstruction, biliary) 576.8
      congenital 751.61
  ileocecal coil (*see also* Obstruction, intestine) 560.9
  ileum (*see also* Obstruction, intestine) 560.9
  iliofemoral (artery) 444.81
  internal anastomosis—*see* Complications, mechanical, graft
  intestine (mechanical) (neurogenic) (paroxysmal) (postinfectional) (reflex) 560.9
    with
      adhesions (intestinal) (peritoneal) 560.81
      hernia—*see also* Hernia, by site, with obstruction
        gangrenous—*see* Hernia, by site, with gangrene
    adynamic (*see also* Ileus) 560.1
    by gallstone 560.31
    congenital or infantile (small) 751.1
      large 751.2
    due to
      Ascaris lumbricoides 127.0
      mural thickening 560.89
      procedure 997.49
        involving urinary tract 997.5
    impaction 560.32
    infantile—*see* Obstruction, intestine, congenital
    newborn
      due to
        fecaliths 777.1
        inspissated milk 777.2
        meconium (plug) 777.1
          in mucoviscidosis 277.01
        transitory 777.4
    specified cause NEC 560.89
    transitory, newborn 777.4
    volvulus 560.2
  intracardiac ball valve prosthesis 996.02
  jaundice (*see also* Obstruction, biliary) 576.8
    congenital 751.61
  jejunum (*see also* Obstruction, intestine) 560.9
  kidney 593.89
  labor 660.9
    affecting fetus or newborn 763.1
    by
      bony pelvis (conditions classifiable to 653.0-653.9) 660.1
      deep transverse arrest 660.3
      impacted shoulder 660.4
      locked twins 660.5
      malposition (fetus) (conditions classifiable to 652.0-652.9) 660.0
        head during labor 660.3

Obstruction, obstructed—*continued*
    persistent occipitoposterior position 660.3
    soft tissue, pelvic (conditions classifiable to 654.0-654.9) 660.2
  lacrimal
    canaliculi 375.53
    congenital 743.65
    punctum 375.52
    sac 375.54
  lacrimonasal duct 375.56
    congenital 743.65
    neonatal 375.55
  lacteal, with steatorrhea 579.2
  laryngitis (*see also* Laryngitis) 464.01
  larynx 478.79
    congenital 748.3
  liver 573.8
    cirrhotic (*see also* Cirrhosis, liver) 571.5
  lung 518.89
    with
      asthma—*see* Asthma
      bronchitis (chronic) 491.20
      emphysema NEC 492.8
    airway, chronic 496
    chronic NEC 496
      with
        asthma (chronic) (obstructive) 493.2
    disease, chronic 496
      with
        asthma (chronic) (obstructive) 493.2
    emphysematous 492.8
  lymphatic 457.1
  meconium
    fetus or newborn 777.1
      in mucoviscidosis 277.01
    newborn due to fecaliths 777.1
  mediastinum 519.3
  mitral (rheumatic)—*see* Stenosis, mitral
  nasal 478.19
    duct 375.56
      neonatal 375.55
    sinus—*see* Sinusitis
  nasolacrimal duct 375.56
    congenital 743.65
    neonatal 375.55
  nasopharynx 478.29
  nose 478.19
  organ or site, congenital NEC—*see* Atresia
  pancreatic duct 577.8
  parotid gland 527.8
  pelviureteral junction (*see also* Obstruction, ureter) 593.4
  pharynx 478.29
  portal (circulation) (vein) 452
  prostate 600.90
    with
      other lower urinary tract symptoms (LUTS) 600.91
      urinary
        obstruction 600.91
        retention 600.91
    valve (urinary) 596.0
  pulmonary
    valve (heart) (*see also* Endocarditis, pulmonary) 424.3
    vein, isolated 747.49
  pyemic—*see* Septicemia
  pylorus (acquired) 537.0
    congenital 750.5
    infantile 750.5
  rectosigmoid (*see also* Obstruction, intestine) 560.9

Obstruction, obstructed—*continued*
rectum 569.49
renal 593.89
respiratory 519.8
chronic 496
retinal (artery) (vein) (central) (*see also*
Occlusion, retina) 362.30
salivary duct (any) 527.8
with calculus 527.5
sigmoid (*see also* Obstruction, intestine) 560.9
sinus (accessory) (nasal) (*see also* Sinusitis)
473.9
Stensen's duct 527.8
stomach 537.89
acute 536.1
congenital 750.7
submaxillary gland 527.8
with calculus 527.5
thoracic duct 457.1
thrombotic—*see* Thrombosis
tooth eruption 520.6
trachea 519.19
tracheostomy airway 519.09
tricuspid—*see* Endocarditis, tricuspid
upper respiratory, congenital 748.8
ureter (functional) 593.4
congenital 753.20
due to calculus 592.1
ureteropelvic junction, congenital 753.21
ureterovesical junction, congenital 753.22
urethra 599.60
congenital 753.6
urinary (moderate) 599.60
organ or tract (lower) 599.60
due to
benign prostatic hypertrophy (BPH)—*see*
category 600
specified NEC 599.69
due to
benign prostatic hypertrophy
(BPH)—*see* category 600
prostatic valve 596.0
specified NEC 599.69
due to
benign prostatic hypertrophy (BPH)—*see*
category 600
uropathy 599.60
uterus 621.8
vagina 623.2
valvular—*see* Endocarditis
vascular graft or shunt 996.1
atherosclerosis —*see* Arteriosclerosis,
coronary
embolism 996.74
occlusion NEC 996.74
thrombus 996.74
vein, venous 459.2
caval (inferior) (superior) 459.2
thrombotic—*see* Thrombosis
vena cava (inferior) (superior) 459.2
ventricular shunt 996.2
vesical 596.0
vesicourethral orifice 596.0
vessel NEC 459.9
Obturator —*see* condition
Occlusal
plane deviation 524.76
wear, teeth 521.10

Occlusion
anus 569.49
congenital 751.2
infantile 751.2
aortoiliac (chronic) 444.09
aqueduct of Sylvius 331.4
congenital 742.3
with spina bifida (*see also* Spina bifida) 741.0
arteries of extremities, lower 444.22
without thrombus or embolus (*see also*
Arteriosclerosis, extremities) 440.20
due to stricture or stenosis 447.1
upper 444.21
without thrombus or embolus (*see also*
Arteriosclerosis, extremities) 440.20
due to stricture or stenosis 447.1
artery NEC (*see also* Embolism, artery) 444.9
auditory, internal 433.8
basilar 433.0
with other precerebral artery 433.3
bilateral 433.3
brain or cerebral (*see also* Infarct, brain) 434.9
carotid 433.1
with other precerebral artery 433.3
bilateral 433.3
cerebellar (anterior inferior) (posterior
inferior) (superior) 433.8
cerebral (*see also* Infarct, brain) 434.9
choroidal (anterior) 433.8
chronic total
coronary 414.2
extremity(ies) 440.4
complete
coronary 414.2
extremity(ies) 440.4
communicating posterior 433.8
coronary (thrombotic) (*see also* Infarct,
myocardium) 410.9
acute 410.9
without myocardial infarction 411.81
chronic total 414.2
complete 414.2
healed or old 412
total 414.2
extremity(ies)
chronic total 440.4
complete 440.4
total 440.4
hypophyseal 433.8
iliac 444.81
mesenteric (embolic) (thrombotic) (with
gangrene) 557.0
pontine 433.8
precerebral NEC 433.9
late effect—*see* Late effect(s) (of)
cerebrovascular disease
multiple or bilateral 433.3
puerperal, postpartum, childbirth 674.0
specified NEC 433.8
renal 593.81
retinal—*see* Occlusion, retina, artery
spinal 433.8
vertebral 433.2
with other precerebral artery 433.3
bilateral 433.3
basilar (artery)—*see* Occlusion, artery, basilar
bile duct (any) (*see also* Obstruction, biliary)
576.2
bowel (*see also* Obstruction, intestine) 560.9
brain (artery) (vascular) (*see also* Infarct, brain)
434.9

Occlusion—*continued*
  breast (duct) 611.89
  carotid (artery) (common) (internal)—*see*
    Occlusion, artery, carotid
  cerebellar (anterior inferior) (artery) (posterior
    inferior) (superior) 433.8
  cerebral (artery) (*see also* Infarct, brain) 434.9
  cerebrovascular (*see also* Infarct, brain) 434.9
    diffuse 437.0
  cervical canal (*see also* Stricture, cervix) 622.4
    by falciparum malaria 084.0
  cervix (uteri) (*see also* Stricture, cervix) 622.4
  choanal 748.0
  choroidal (artery) 433.8
  colon (*see also* Obstruction, intestine) 560.9
  communicating posterior artery 433.8
  coronary (artery) (thrombotic) (*see also* Infarct,
    myocardium) 410.9
    acute 410.9
      without myocardial infarction 411.81
    healed or old 412
      without myocardial infarction 411.81
  cystic duct (*see also* Obstruction, gallbladder)
    575.2
    congenital 751.69
  disto
    division I 524.22
    division II 524.22
  embolic—*see* Embolism
  fallopian tube 628.2
    congenital 752.19
  gallbladder (*see also* Obstruction, gallbladder)
    575.2
    congenital 751.69
      jaundice from 751.69 *[774.5]*
  gingiva, traumatic 523.8
  hymen 623.3
    congenital 752.42
  hypophyseal (artery) 433.8
  iliac artery 444.81
  intestine (*see also* Obstruction, intestine) 560.9
  kidney 593.89
  lacrimal apparatus—*see* Stenosis, lacrimal
  lung 518.89
  lymph or lymphatic channel 457.1
  mammary duct 611.89
  mesenteric artery (embolic) (thrombotic) (with
    gangrene) 557.0
  nose 478.1
    congenital 748.0
  organ or site, congenital NEC—*see* Atresia
  oviduct 628.2
    congenital 752.19
    periodontal, traumatic 523.8
  peripheral arteries (lower extremity) 444.22
    without thrombus or embolus (*see also*
      Arteriosclerosis, extremities) 440.20
    due to stricture or stenosis 447.1
    upper extremity 444.21
      without thrombus or embolus (*see also*
        Arteriosclerosis, extremities) 440.20
      due to stricture or stenosis 447.1
  pontine (artery) 433.8
  posterior lingual, of mandibular teeth 524.29
  precerebral artery—*see* Occlusion, artery,
    precerebral NEC
  puncta lacrimalia 375.52
  pupil 364.74
  pylorus (*see also* Stricture, pylorus) 537.0
  renal artery 593.81

Occlusion—*continued*
  retina, retinal (vascular) 362.30
    artery, arterial 362.30
      branch 362.32
      central (total) 362.31
      partial 362.33
      transient 362.34
      tributary 362.32
    vein 362.30
      branch 362.36
      central (total) 362.35
      incipient 362.37
      partial 362.37
      tributary 362.36
  spinal artery 433.8
  stent
    coronary 996.72
  teeth (mandibular) (posterior lingual) 524.29
  thoracic duct 457.1
  tubal 628.2
  ureter (complete) (partial) 593.4
    congenital 753.29
  urethra (*see also* Stricture, urethra) 598.9
    congenital 753.6
  uterus 621.8
  vagina 623.2
  vascular NEC 459.9
  vein—*see* Thrombosis
  vena cava
    inferior 453.2
    superior (acute) 453.87
      chronic 453.77
  ventricle (brain) NEC 331.4
  vertebral (artery)—*see* Occlusion, artery,
    vertebral
  vessel (blood) NEC 459.9
  vulva 624.8
Occlusio pupillae 364.74
Occupational
  problems NEC V62.29
  therapy V57.21
Ochlophobia 300.29
Ochronosis (alkaptonuric) (congenital)
    (endogenous) 270.2
  with chloasma of eyelid 270.2
Ocular muscle —*see also* condition
  myopathy 359.1
  torticollis 781.93
Oculoauriculovertebral dysplasia 756.0
Oculogyric
  crisis or disturbance 378.87
    psychogenic 306.7
Oculomotor syndrome 378.81
Oddi's sphincter spasm 576.5
Odelberg's disease (juvenile osteochondrosis)
    732.1
Odontalgia 525.9
Odontoameloblastoma (M9311/0) 213.1
  upper jaw (bone) 213.0
Odontoclasia 521.05
Odontoclasis 873.63
  complicated 873.73
Odontodysplasia, regional 520.4
Odontogenesis imperfecta 520.5
Odontoma (M9280/0) 213.1
  ameloblastic (M9311/0) 213.1
    upper jaw (bone) 213.0
  calcified (M9280/0) 213.1
    upper jaw (bone) 213.0

Odontoma—*continued*
  complex (M9282/0) 213.1
    upper jaw (bone) 213.0
  compound (M9281/0) 213.1
    upper jaw (bone) 213.0
  fibroameloblastic (M9290/0) 213.1
    upper jaw (bone) 213.0
  follicular 526.0
  upper jaw (bone) 213.0
Odontomyelitis (closed) (open) 522.0
Odontonecrosis 521.09
Odontorrhagia 525.8
Odontosarcoma, ameloblastic (M9290/3) 170.1
  upper jaw (bone) 170.0
Odynophagia 787.20
Oesophagostomiasis 127.7
Oesophagostomum infestation 127.7
Oestriasis 134.0
Ogilvie's syndrome (sympathicotonic colon
    obstruction) 560.89
Oguchi's disease (retina) 368.61
Ohara's disease (*see also* Tularemia) 021.9
Oidiomycosis (*see also* Candidiasis) 112.9
Oidiomycotic meningitis 112.83
Oidium albicans infection (*see also* Candidiasis)
    112.9
Old age 797
  dementia (of) 290.0
Olfactory —*see* condition
Oligemia 285.9
Oligergasia (*see also* Disability, intellectual) 319
Oligoamnios 658.0
  affecting fetus or newborn 761.2
Oligoastrocytoma, mixed (M9382/3)
  specified site—*see* Neoplasm, by site, malignant
  unspecified site 191.9
Oligocythemia 285.9
Oligodendroblastoma (M9460/3)
  specified site—*see* Neoplasm, by site, malignant
  unspecified site 191.9
Oligodendroglioma (M9450/3)
  anaplastic type (M9451/3)
    specified site—*see* Neoplasm, by site, malignant
    unspecified site 191.9
  specified site—*see* Neoplasm, by site, malignant
  unspecified site 191.9
Oligodendroma —*see* Oligodendroglioma
Oligodontia (*see also* Anodontia) 520.0
Oligoencephalon 742.1
Oligohydramnios 658.0
  affecting fetus or newborn 761.2
  due to premature rupture of membranes 658.1
    affecting fetus or newborn 761.2
Oligohydrosis 705.0
Oligomenorrhea 626.1
Oligophrenia (*see also* Disability, intellectual)
    319
  phenylpyruvic 270.1
Oligospermia 606.1
Oligotrichia 704.09
  congenita 757.4
Oliguria 788.5
  with
    abortion—*see* Abortion, by type, with renal failure
    ectopic pregnancy (*see also* categories
      633.0-633.9) 639.3
    molar pregnancy (*see also* categories 630-632)
      639.3

Oliguria—*continued*
  complicating
    abortion 639.3
    ectopic or molar pregnancy 639.3
    pregnancy 646.2
      with hypertension—*see* Toxemia, of
        pregnancy
  due to a procedure 997.5
  following labor and delivery 669.3
  heart or cardiac—*see* Failure, heart
  puerperal, postpartum 669.3
  specified due to a procedure 997.5
Ollier's disease (chondrodysplasia) 756.4
Omentitis (*see also* Peritonitis) 567.9
Omentocele (*see also* Hernia, omental) 553.8
Omentum, omental —*see* condition
Omphalitis (congenital) (newborn) 771.4
  not of newborn 686.9
  tetanus 771.3
Omphalocele 756.72
Omphalomesenteric duct, persistent 751.0
Omphalorrhagia, newborn 772.3
Omsk hemorrhagic fever 065.1
Onanism 307.9
Onchocerciasis 125.3
  eye 125.3 *[360.13]*
Onchocercosis 125.3
Oncocytoma (M8290/0)—*see* Neoplasm, by site,
    benign
Ondine's curse 348.89
Oneirophrenia (*see also* Schizophrenia) 295.4
Onychauxis 703.8
  congenital 757.5
Onychia (with lymphangitis) 681.9
  dermatophytic 110.1
  finger 681.02
  toe 681.11
Onychitis (with lymphangitis) 681.9
  finger 681.02
  toe 681.11
Onychocryptosis 703.0
Onychodystrophy 703.8
  congenital 757.5
Onychogryphosis 703.8
Onychogryposis 703.8
Onycholysis 703.8
Onychomadesis 703.8
Onychomalacia 703.8
Onychomycosis 110.1
  finger 110.1
  toe 110.1
Onycho-osteodysplasia 756.89
Onychophagy 307.9
Onychoptosis 703.8
Onychorrhexis 703.8
  congenital 757.5
Onychoschizia 703.8
Onychotrophia (*see also* Atrophy, nail) 703.8
O'nyong-nyong fever 066.3
Onyxis (finger) (toe) 703.0
Onyxitis (with lymphangitis) 681.9
  finger 681.02
  toe 681.11
Oocyte (egg) (ovum)
  donor V59.70
    age 35 and over V59.73
      anonymous recipient V59.73
      designated recipient V59.74
    under age 35 V59.71
      anonymous recipient V59.71
      designated recipient V59.72

Oophoritis (cystic) (infectional) (interstitial) (*see also* Salpingo-oophoritis) 614.2
  complicating pregnancy 646.6
  fetal (acute) 752.0
  gonococcal (acute) 098.19
    chronic or duration of 2 months or over 098.39
  tuberculous (*see also* Tuberculosis) 016.6
Opacity, opacities
  cornea 371.00
    central 371.03
    congenital 743.43
      interfering with vision 743.42
    degenerative (*see also* Degeneration, cornea) 371.40
    hereditary (*see also* Dystrophy, cornea) 371.50
    inflammatory (*see also* Keratitis) 370.9
    late effect of trachoma (healed) 139.1
    minor 371.01
    peripheral 371.02
  enamel (fluoride) (nonfluoride) (teeth) 520.3
  lens (*see also* Cataract) 366.9
  snowball 379.22
  vitreous (humor) 379.24
    congenital 743.51
Opalescent dentin (hereditary) 520.5
Open, opening
  abnormal, organ or site, congenital—*see* Imperfect, closure
  angle
    with
      borderline findings
        high risk 365.05
        intraocular pressure 365.01
        low risk 365.01
      cupping of discs 365.01
    high risk 365.05
    low risk 365.01
  bite
    anterior 524.24
    posterior 524.25
  false—*see* Imperfect, closure
  margin on tooth restoration 525.61
  restoration margins 525.61
  wound—*see* Wound, open, by site
Operation
  causing mutilation of fetus 763.89
  destructive, on live fetus, to facilitate birth 763.89
  for delivery, fetus or newborn 763.89
  maternal, unrelated to current delivery, affecting fetus or newborn (*see also* Newborn, affected by) 760.64
Operational fatigue 300.89
Operative —*see* condition
Operculitis (chronic) 523.40
  acute 523.30
Operculum, retina 361.32
  with detachment 361.01
Ophiasis 704.01
Ophthalmia (*see also* Conjunctivitis) 372.30
  actinic rays 370.24
  allergic (acute) 372.05
    chronic 372.14
  blennorrhagic (neonatorum) 098.40
  catarrhal 372.03
  diphtheritic 032.81
  Egyptian 076.1
  electric, electrica 370.24
  gonococcal (neonatorum) 098.40
  metastatic 360.11
  migraine 346.8

Ophthalmia—*continued*
  neonatorum, newborn 771.6
    gonococcal 098.40
  nodosa 360.14
  phlyctenular 370.31
    with ulcer (*see also* Ulcer, cornea) 370.00
  sympathetic 360.11
Ophthalmitis —*see* Ophthalmia
Ophthalmocele (congenital) 743.66
Ophthalmoneuromyelitis 341.0
Ophthalmopathy, infiltrative with thyrotoxicosis 242.0
Ophthalmoplegia (*see also* Strabismus) 378.9
  anterior internuclear 378.86
  ataxia-areflexia syndrome 357.0
  bilateral 378.9
  diabetic 250.5 *[378.86]*
    due to secondary diabetes 249.5 *[378.86]*
  exophthalmic 242.0 *[376.22]*
  external 378.55
    progressive 378.72
    total 378.56
  interna(l) (complete) (total) 367.52
  internuclear 378.86
  migraine 346.2
  painful 378.55
  Parinaud's 378.81
  progressive external 378.72
  supranuclear, progressive 333.0
  total (external) 378.56
    internal 367.52
  unilateral 378.9
Opisthognathism 524.00
Opisthorchiasis (felineus) (tenuicollis) (viverrini) 121.0
Opisthotonos, opisthotonus 781.0
Opitz's disease (congestive splenomegaly) 289.51
Opiumism (*see also* Dependence) 304.0
Oppenheim's disease 358.8
Oppenheim-Urbach disease or syndrome (necrobiosis lipoidica diabeticorum) 250.8 *[709.3]*
  due to secondary diabetes 249.8 *[709.3]*
Opsoclonia 379.59
Optic nerve —*see* condition
Orbit —*see* condition
Orchioblastoma (M9071/3) 186.9
Orchitis (nonspecific) (septic) 604.90
  with abscess 604.0
  blennorrhagic (acute) 098.13
    chronic or duration of 2 months or over 098.33
  diphtheritic 032.89 *[604.91]*
  filarial 125.9 *[604.91]*
  gangrenous 604.99
  gonococcal (acute) 098.13
    chronic or duration of 2 months or over 098.33
  mumps 072.0
  parotidea 072.0
  suppurative 604.99
  syphilitic 095.8 *[604.91]*
  tuberculous (*see also* Tuberculosis) 016.5 *[608.81]*
Orf 051.2
Organic —*see also* condition
  heart—*see* Disease, heart
  insufficiency 799.89
Oriental
  bilharziasis 120.2
  schistosomiasis 120.2
  sore 085.1
Orientation
  ego-dystonic sexual 302.0

Orifice —*see* condition
Origin, both great vessels from right ventricle 745.11
Ormond's disease or syndrome 593.4
Ornithosis 073.9
  with
    complication 073.8
      specified NEC 073.7
    pneumonia 073.0
    pneumonitis (lobular) 073.0
Orodigitofacial dysostosis 759.89
Oropouche fever 066.3
Orotaciduria, oroticaciduria (congenital)
  (hereditary) (pyrimidine deficiency) 281.4
Oroya fever 088.0
Orthodontics V58.5
  adjustment V53.4
  aftercare V58.5
  fitting V53.4
Orthopnea 786.02
Orthoptic training V57.4
Os, uterus —*see* condition
Osgood-Schlatter
  disease 732.4
  osteochondrosis 732.4
Osler's
  disease (M9950/1) (polycythemia vera) 238.4
  nodes 421.0
Osler-Rendu disease (familial hemorrhagic
  telangiectasia) 448.0
Osler-Vaquez disease (M9950/1) (polycythemia
  vera) 238.4
Osler-Weber-Rendu syndrome (familial
  hemorrhagic telangiectasia) 448.0
Osmidrosis 705.89
Osseous —*see* condition
Ossification
  artery—*see* Arteriosclerosis
  auricle (ear) 380.39
  bronchus 519.19
  cardiac (*see also* Degeneration, myocardial) 429.1
  cartilage (senile) 733.99
  coronary —*see* Arteriosclerosis, coronary
  diaphragm 728.10
  ear 380.39
    middle (*see also* Otosclerosis) 387.9
  falx cerebri 349.2
  fascia 728.10
  fontanel
    defective or delayed 756.0
    premature 756.0
  heart (*see also* Degeneration, myocardial) 429.1
    valve—*see* Endocarditis
  larynx 478.79
  ligament
    posterior longitudinal 724.8
      cervical 723.7
  meninges (cerebral) 349.2
    spinal 336.8
  multiple, eccentric centers 733.99
  muscle 728.10
    heterotopic, postoperative 728.13
  myocardium, myocardial (*see also*
    Degeneration, myocardial) 429.1
  penis 607.81
  periarticular 728.89
  sclera 379.16
  tendon 727.82
  trachea 519.19
  tympanic membrane (*see also*
    Tympanosclerosis) 385.00
  vitreous (humor) 360.44

Osteitis (*see also* Osteomyelitis) 730.2
  acute 730.0
  alveolar 526.5
  chronic 730.1
  condensans (ilii) 733.5
  deformans (Paget's) 731.0
    due to or associated with malignant neoplasm
      (*see also* Neoplasm, bone, malignant)
      170.9 [*731.1*]
  due to yaws 102.6
  fibrosa NEC 733.29
    cystica (generalisata) 252.01
    disseminata 756.59
    osteoplastica 252.01
  fragilitans 756.51
  Garré's (sclerosing) 730.1
  infectious (acute) (subacute) 730.0
    chronic or old 730.1
  jaw (acute) (chronic) (lower) (neonatal)
    (suppurative) (upper) 526.4
  parathyroid 252.01
  petrous bone (*see also* Petrositis) 383.20
  pubis 733.5
  sclerotic, nonsuppurative 730.1
  syphilitic 095.5
  tuberculosa
    cystica (of Jüngling) 135
    multiplex cystoides 135
Osteoarthritica spondylitis (spine) (*see also*
  Spondylosis) 721.90
Osteoarthritis (*see also* Osteoarthrosis) 715.9
  distal interphalangeal 715.9
  hyperplastic 731.2
  interspinalis (*see also* Spondylosis) 721.90
  spine, spinal NEC (*see also* Spondylosis) 721.90
Osteoarthropathy (*see also* Osteoarthrosis) 715.9
  chronic idiopathic hypertrophic 757.39
  familial idiopathic 757.39
  hypertrophic pulmonary 731.2
    secondary 731.2
  idiopathic hypertrophic 757.39
  primary hypertrophic 731.2
  pulmonary hypertrophic 731.2
  secondary hypertrophic 731.2
Osteoarthrosis (degenerative) (hypertrophic)
  (rheumatoid) 715.9

> *Note*—Use the following fifth-digit
> subclassification with category 715:
>
> 0 *site unspecified*
> 1 *shoulder region*
> 2 *upper arm*
> 3 *forearm*
> 4 *hand*
> 5 *pelvic region and thigh*
> 6 *lower leg*
> 7 *ankle and foot*
> 8 *other specified sites except spine*
> 9 *multiple sites*

  deformans alkaptonurica 270.2
  generalized 715.09
  juvenilis (Köhler's) 732.5
  localized 715.3
    idiopathic 715.1
    primary 715.1
    secondary 715.2
  multiple sites, not specified as generalized 715.89
  polyarticular 715.09
  spine (*see also* Spondylosis) 721.90
  temperomandibular joint 524.69

Osteoblastoma (M9200/0)—*see* Neoplasm, bone,
  benign
Osteochondritis (*see also* Osteochondrosis) 732.9
  dissecans 732.7
  hip 732.7
  ischiopubica 732.1
  multiple 756.59
  syphilitic (congenital) 090.0
Osteochondrodermodysplasia 756.59
Osteochondrodystrophy 277.5
  deformans 277.5
  familial 277.5
  fetalis 756.4
Osteochondrolysis 732.7
Osteochondroma (M9210/0)—*see also*
  Neoplasm, bone, benign
  multiple, congenital 756.4
Osteochondromatosis (M9210/1) 238.0
  synovial 727.82
Osteochondromyxosarcoma (M9180/3)—*see*
  Neoplasm, bone, malignant
Osteochondropathy NEC 732.9
Osteochondrosarcoma (M9180/3)—*see*
  Neoplasm, bone, malignant
Osteochondrosis 732.9
  acetabulum 732.1
  adult spine 732.8
  astragalus 732.5
  Blount's 732.4
  Buchanan's (juvenile osteochondrosis of iliac
    crest) 732.1
  Buchman's (juvenile osteochondrosis) 732.1
  Burns' 732.3
  calcaneus 732.5
  capitular epiphysis (femur) 732.1
  carpal
    lunate (wrist) 732.3
    scaphoid 732.3
  coxae juvenilis 732.1
  deformans juvenilis (coxae) (hip) 732.1
    Scheuermann's 732.0
    spine 732.0
    tibia 732.4
    vertebra 732.0
  Diaz's (astragalus) 732.5
  dissecans (knee) (shoulder) 732.7
  femoral capital epiphysis 732.1
  femur (head) (juvenile) 732.1
  foot (juvenile) 732.5
  Freiberg's (disease) (second metatarsal) 732.5
  Haas' 732.3
  Haglund's (os tibiale externum) 732.5
  hand (juvenile) 732.3
  head of
    femur 732.1
    humerus (juvenile) 732.3
  hip (juvenile) 732.1
  humerus (juvenile) 732.3
  iliac crest (juvenile) 732.1
  ilium (juvenile) 732.1
  ischiopubic synchondrosis 732.1
  Iselin's (osteochondrosis fifth metatarsal) 732.5
  juvenile, juvenilis 732.6
    arm 732.3
    capital femoral epiphysis 732.1
    capitellum humeri 732.3
    capitular epiphysis 732.1
    carpal scaphoid 732.3
    clavicle, sternal epiphysis 732.6
    coxae 732.1
    deformans 732.1

Osteochondrosis—*continued*
  juvenile—*continued*
    foot 732.5
    hand 732.3
    hip and pelvis 732.1
    lower extremity, except foot 732.4
    lunate, wrist 732.3
    medial cuneiform bone 732.5
    metatarsal (head) 732.5
    metatarsophalangeal 732.5
    navicular, ankle 732.5
    patella 732.4
    primary patellar center (of Köhler) 732.4
    specified site NEC 732.6
    spine 732.0
    tarsal scaphoid 732.5
    tibia (epiphysis) (tuberosity) 732.4
    upper extremity 732.3
    vertebra (body) (Calvé) 732.0
      epiphyseal plates (of Scheuermann) 732.0
  Kienböck's (disease) 732.3
  Köhler's (disease) (navicular, ankle) 732.5
    patellar 732.4
    tarsal navicular 732.5
  Legg-Calvé-Perthes (disease) 732.1
  lower extremity (juvenile) 732.4
  lunate bone 732.3
  Mauclaire's 732.3
  metacarpal heads (of Mauclaire) 732.3
  metatarsal (fifth) (head) (second) 732.5
  navicular, ankle 732.5
  os calcis 732.5
  Osgood-Schlatter 732.4
  os tibiale externum 732.5
  Panner's 732.3
  patella (juvenile) 732.4
  patellar center
    primary (of Köhler) 732.4
    secondary (of Sinding-Larsen) 732.4
  pelvis (juvenile) 732.1
  Pierson's 732.1
  radial head (juvenile) 732.3
  Scheuermann's 732.0
  Sever's (calcaneum) 732.5
  Sinding-Larsen (secondary patellar center) 732.4
  spine (juvenile) 732.0
    adult 732.8
  symphysis pubis (of Pierson) (juvenile) 732.1
  syphilitic (congenital) 090.0
  tarsal (navicular) (scaphoid) 732.5
  tibia (proximal) (tubercle) 732.4
  tuberculous—*see* Tuberculosis, bone
  ulna 732.3
  upper extremity (juvenile) 732.3
  van Neck's (juvenile osteochondrosis) 732.1
  vertebral (juvenile) 732.0
    adult 732.8
Osteoclastoma (M9250/1) 238.0
  malignant (M9250/3)—*see* Neoplasm, bone,
    malignant
Osteocopic pain 733.90
Osteodynia 733.90
Osteodystrophy
  azotemic 588.0
  chronica deformans hypertrophica 731.0
  congenital 756.50
    specified type NEC 756.59
  deformans 731.0
  fibrosa localisata 731.0
  parathyroid 252.01
  renal 588.0

Osteofibroma (M9262/0)—*see* Neoplasm, bone, benign
Osteofibrosarcoma (M9182/3)—*see* Neoplasm, bone, malignant
Osteogenesis imperfecta 756.51
Osteogenic —*see* condition
Osteoma (M9180/0)—*see also* Neoplasm, bone, benign
   osteoid (M9191/0)—*see also* Neoplasm, bone, benign
   giant (M9200/0)—*see* Neoplasm, bone, benign
Osteomalacia 268.2
   chronica deformans hypertrophica 731.0
   due to vitamin D deficiency 268.2
   infantile (*see also* Rickets) 268.0
   juvenile (*see also* Rickets) 268.0
   oncogenic 275.8
   pelvis 268.2
   vitamin D-resistant 275.3
Osteomalacic bone 268.2
Osteomalacosis 268.2
Osteomyelitis (general) (infective) (localized) (neonatal) (purulent) (pyogenic) (septic) (staphylococcal) (streptococcal) (suppurative) (with periostitis) 730.2

Note—Use the following fifth-digit subclassification with category 730:

0 *site unspecified*
1 *shoulder region*
2 *upper arm*
3 *forearm*
4 *hand*
5 *pelvic region and thigh*
6 *lower leg*
7 *ankle and foot*
8 *other specified sites*
9 *multiple sites*

---

   acute or subacute 730.0
   chronic or old 730.1
   due to or associated with
      diabetes mellitus 250.8 *[731.8]*
         due to secondary diabetes 249.8 *[731.8]*
      tuberculosis (*see also* Tuberculosis, bone) 015.9 *[730.8]*
         limb bones 015.5 *[730.8]*
         specified bones NEC 015.7 *[730.8]*
         spine 015.0 *[730.8]*
      typhoid 002.0 *[730.8]*
   Garré's 730.1
   jaw (acute) (chronic) (lower) (neonatal) (suppurative) (upper) 526.4
   nonsuppurating 730.1
   orbital 376.03
   petrous bone (*see also* Petrositis) 383.20
   Salmonella 003.24
   sclerosing, nonsuppurative 730.1
   sicca 730.1
   syphilitic 095.5
      congenital 090.0 *[730.8]*
   tuberculous—*see* Tuberculosis, bone
   typhoid 002.0 *[730.8]*
Osteomyelofibrosis 289.89
Osteomyelosclerosis 289.89
Osteonecrosis 733.40
   meaning osteomyelitis 730.1
Osteo-onycho-arthro dysplasia 756.89
Osteo-onychodysplasia, hereditary 756.89

Osteopathia
   condensans disseminata 756.53
   hyperostotica multiplex infantilis 756.59
   hypertrophica toxica 731.2
   striata 756.4
Osteopathy resulting from poliomyelitis (*see also* Poliomyelitis) 045.9 *[730.7]*
   familial dysplastic 731.2
Osteopecilia 756.53
Osteopenia 733.90
   borderline 733.90
Osteoperiostitis (*see also* Osteomyelitis) 730.2
   ossificans toxica 731.2
   toxica ossificans 731.2
Osteopetrosis (familial) 756.52
Osteophyte —*see* Exostosis
Osteophytosis —*see* Exostosis
Osteopoikilosis 756.53
Osteoporosis (generalized) 733.00
   circumscripta 731.0
   disuse 733.03
   drug-induced 733.09
   idiopathic 733.02
   postmenopausal 733.01
   posttraumatic 733.7
   screening V82.81
   senile 733.01
   specified type NEC 733.09
Osteoporosis-osteomalacia syndrome 268.2
Osteopsathyrosis 756.51
Osteoradionecrosis, jaw 526.89
Osteosarcoma (M9180/3)—*see also* Neoplasm, bone, malignant
   chondroblastic (M9181/3)—*see* Neoplasm, bone, malignant
   fibroblastic (M9182/3)—*see* Neoplasm, bone, malignant
   in Paget's disease of bone (M9184/3)—*see* Neoplasm, bone, malignant
   juxtacortical (M9190/3)—*see* Neoplasm, bone, malignant
   parosteal (M9190/3)—*see* Neoplasm, bone, malignant
   telangiectatic (M9183/3)—*see* Neoplasm, bone, malignant
Osteosclerosis 756.52
   fragilis (generalisata) 756.52
Osteosclerotic anemia 289.89
Osteosis
   acromegaloid 757.39
   cutis 709.3
   parathyroid 252.01
   renal fibrocystic 588.0
Österreicher-Turner syndrome 756.89
Ostium
   atrioventriculare commune 745.69
   primum (arteriosum) (defect) (persistent) 745.61
   secundum (arteriosum) (defect) (patent) (persistent) 745.5
Ostrum-Furst syndrome 756.59
Otalgia 388.70
   otogenic 388.71
   referred 388.72
Othematoma 380.31
Otitic hydrocephalus 348.2
Otitis 382.9
   with effusion 381.4
      purulent 382.4
      secretory 381.4
      serous 381.4
      suppurative 382.4

Otitis—*continued*
  acute 382.9
  adhesive (*see also* Adhesions, middle ear)
      385.10
  chronic 382.9
    with effusion 381.3
    mucoid, mucous (simple) 381.20
    purulent 382.3
    secretory 381.3
    serous 381.10
    suppurative 382.3
  diffuse parasitic 136.8
  externa (acute) (diffuse) (hemorrhagica) 380.10
    actinic 380.22
    candidal 112.82
    chemical 380.22
    chronic 380.23
      mycotic—*see* Otitis, externa, mycotic
      specified type NEC 380.23
    circumscribed 380.10
    contact 380.22
    due to
      erysipelas 035 *[380.13]*
      impetigo 684 *[380.13]*
      seborrheic dermatitis 690.10 *[380.13]*
    eczematoid 380.22
    furuncular 680.0 *[380.13]*
    infective 380.10
      chronic 380.16
    malignant 380.14
    mycotic (chronic) 380.15
      due to
        aspergillosis 117.3 *[380.15]*
        moniliasis 112.82
        otomycosis 111.8 *[380.15]*
    reactive 380.22
    specified type NEC 380.22
    tropical 111.8 *[380.15]*
  insidiosa (*see also* Otosclerosis) 387.9
  interna (*see also* Labyrinthitis) 386.30
  media (hemorrhagic) (staphylococcal)
      (streptococcal) 382.9
    acute 382.9
      with effusion 381.00
      allergic 381.04
        mucoid 381.05
        sanguineous 381.06
        serous 381.04
      catarrhal 381.00
      exudative 381.00
      mucoid 381.02
        allergic 381.05
      necrotizing 382.00
        with spontaneous rupture of ear drum
            382.01
        in
          influenza (*see also* Influenza) 487.8
              [382.02]
          measles 055.2
          scarlet fever 034.1 *[382.02]*
      nonsuppurative 381.00
      purulent 382.00
        with spontaneous rupture of ear drum
            382.01
      sanguineous 381.03
        allergic 381.06
      secretory 381.01
      seromucinous 381.02
      serous 381.01
        allergic 381.04

Otitis—*continued*
  media—*continued*
    acute—*continued*
      suppurative 382.00
        with spontaneous rupture of ear drum
            382.01
      due to
        influenza (*see also* Influenza) 487.8
            [382.02]
        scarlet fever 034.1 *[382.02]*
      transudative 381.00
    adhesive (*see also* Adhesions, middle ear) 385.10
    allergic 381.4
      acute 381.04
        mucoid 381.05
        sanguineous 381.06
        serous 381.04
      chronic 381.3
    catarrhal 381.4
      acute 381.00
      chronic (simple) 381.10
    chronic 382.9
      with effusion 381.3
      adhesive (*see also* Adhesions, middle ear)
          385.10
      allergic 381.3
      atticoantral, suppurative (with posterior or
          superior marginal perforation of ear
          drum) 382.2
      benign suppurative (with anterior perforation
          of ear drum) 382.1
      catarrhal 381.10
      exudative 381.3
      mucinous 381.20
      mucoid, mucous (simple) 381.20
      mucosanguineous 381.29
      nonsuppurative 381.3
      purulent 382.3
      secretory 381.3
      seromucinous 381.3
      serosanguineous 381.19
      serous (simple) 381.10
      suppurative 382.3
        atticoantral (with posterior or superior
            marginal perforation of ear drum)
            382.2
        benign (with anterior perforation of ear
            drum) 382.1
        tuberculous (*see also* Tuberculosis) 017.4
        tubotympanic 382.1
      transudative 381.3
    exudative 381.4
      acute 381.00
      chronic 381.3
    fibrotic (*see also* Adhesions, middle ear)
        385.10
    mucoid, mucous 381.4
      acute 381.02
      chronic (simple) 381.20
    mucosanguineous, chronic 381.29
    nonsuppurative 381.4
      acute 381.00
      chronic 381.3
    postmeasles 055.2
    purulent 382.4
      acute 382.00
        with spontaneous rupture of ear drum
            382.01
      chronic 382.3
    sanguineous, acute 381.03
      allergic 381.06

Otitis—*continued*
　media—*continued*
　　secretory 381.4
　　　acute or subacute 381.01
　　　chronic 381.3
　　seromucinous 381.4
　　　acute or subacute 381.02
　　　chronic 381.3
　　serosanguineous, chronic 381.19
　　serous 381.4
　　　acute or subacute 381.01
　　　chronic (simple) 381.10
　　subacute—*see* Otitis, media, acute
　　suppurative 382.4
　　　acute 382.00
　　　　with spontaneous rupture of ear drum 382.01
　　　chronic 382.3
　　　　atticoantral 382.2
　　　　benign 382.1
　　　　tuberculous (*see also* Tuberculosis) 017.4
　　　　tubotympanic 382.1
　　transudative 381.4
　　　acute 381.00
　　　chronic 381.3
　　tuberculous (*see also* Tuberculosis) 017.4
　postmeasles 055.2
Otoconia 386.8
Otolith syndrome 386.19
Otomycosis 111.8 *[380.15]*
　in
　　aspergillosis 117.3 *[380.15]*
　　moniliasis 112.82
Otopathy 388.9
Otoporosis (*see also* Otosclerosis) 387.9
Otorrhagia 388.69
　traumatic—*see* nature of injury
Otorrhea 388.60
　blood 388.69
　cerebrospinal (fluid) 388.61
Otosclerosis (general) 387.9
　cochlear (endosteal) 387.2
　involving
　　otic capsule 387.2
　　oval window
　　　nonobliterative 387.0
　　　obliterative 387.1
　　round window 387.2
　nonobliterative 387.0
　obliterative 387.1
　specified type NEC 387.8
Otospongiosis (*see also* Otosclerosis) 387.9
Otto's disease or pelvis 715.35
Outburst, aggressive (*see also* Disturbance, conduct) 312.0
　in children or adolescents 313.9
Outcome of delivery
　multiple birth NEC V27.9
　　all liveborn V27.5
　　all stillborn V27.7
　　some liveborn V27.6
　　unspecified V27.9
　single V27.9
　　liveborn V27.0
　　stillborn V27.1
　twins V27.9
　　both liveborn V27.2
　　both stillborn V27.4
　　one liveborn, one stillborn V27.3
Outlet —*see also* condition
　syndrome (thoracic) 353.0
Outstanding ears (bilateral) 744.29

Ovalocytosis (congenital) (hereditary) (*see also* Elliptocytosis) 282.1
Ovarian —*see also* condition
　pregnancy—*see* Pregnancy, ovarian
　remnant syndrome 620.8
　vein syndrome 593.4
Ovaritis (cystic) (*see also* Salpingo-oophoritis) 614.2
Ovary, ovarian —*see* condition
Overactive —*see also* Hyperfunction
　bladder 596.51
　eye muscle (*see also* Strabismus) 378.9
　hypothalamus 253.8
　thyroid (*see also* Thyrotoxicosis) 242.9
Overactivity, child 314.01
Overbite (deep) (excessive) (horizontal) (vertical) 524.29
Overbreathing (*see also* Hyperventilation) 786.01
Overconscientious personality 301.4
Overdevelopment —*see also* Hypertrophy
　breast (female) (male) 611.1
　nasal bones 738.0
　prostate, congenital 752.89
Overdistention —*see* Distention
Overdose overdosage (drug) 977.9
　specified drug or substance—*see* Table of drugs and chemicals
Overeating 783.6
　with obesity 278.0
　nonorganic origin 307.51
Overexertion (effects) (exhaustion) 994.5
Overexposure (effects) 994.9
　exhaustion 994.4
Overfeeding (*see also* Overeating) 783.6
Overfill, endodontic 526.62
Overgrowth, bone NEC 733.99
Overhanging
　tooth restoration 525.62
　unrepairable, dental restorative materials 525.62
Overheated (effects) (places)—*see* Heat
Overinhibited child 313.0
Overjet 524.29
　excessive horizontal 524.26
Overlaid, overlying (suffocation) 994.7
Overlap
　excessive horizontal 524.26
Overlapping toe (acquired) 735.8
　congenital (fifth toe) 755.66
Overload
　fluid 276.69
　　due to transfusion (blood) (blood components) 276.61
　iron, due to repeated red blood cell transfusions 275.02
　potassium (K) 276.7
　sodium (Na) 276.0
　transfusion associated circulatory (TACO) 276.61
Overnutrition (*see also* Hyperalimentation) 783.6
Overproduction —*see also* Hypersecretion
　ACTH 255.3
　cortisol 255.0
　growth hormone 253.0
　thyroid-stimulating hormone (TSH) 242.8
Overriding
　aorta 747.21
　finger (acquired) 736.29
　　congenital 755.59
　toe (acquired) 735.8
　　congenital 755.66

Oversize
fetus (weight of 4500 grams or more) 766.0
affecting management of pregnancy 656.6
causing disproportion 653.5
with obstructed labor 660.1
affecting fetus or newborn 763.1
Overstimulation, ovarian 256.1
Overstrained 780.79
heart—*see* Hypertrophy, cardiac
Overweight (*see also* Obesity) 278.02
Overwork 780.79
Oviduct —*see* condition
Ovotestis 752.7
Ovulation (cycle)
failure or lack of 628.0
pain 625.2
Ovum
blighted 631.8
donor V59.70
age 35 and over V59.73
anonymous recipient V59.73
designated recipient V59.74
under age 35 V59.71
anonymous recipient V59.71
designated recipient V59.72
dropsical 631.8
pathologic 631.8
Owren's disease or syndrome (parahemophilia)
(*see also* Defect, coagulation) 286.3
Oxalosis 271.8
Oxaluria 271.8
Ox heart —*see* Hypertrophy, cardiac
OX syndrome 758.6
Oxycephaly, oxycephalic 756.0
syphilitic, congenital 090.0
Oxyuriasis 127.4
Oxyuris vermicularis (infestation) 127.4
Ozena 472.0

789.0

P

Pacemaker syndrome 429.4
Pachyderma, pachydermia 701.8
  laryngis 478.5
  laryngitis 478.79
  larynx (verrucosa) 478.79
Pachydermatitis 701.8
Pachydermatocele (congenital) 757.39
  acquired 701.8
Pachydermatosis 701.8
Pachydermoperiostitis
  secondary 731.2
Pachydermoperiostosis
  primary idiopathic 757.39
  secondary 731.2
Pachymeningitis (adhesive) (basal) (brain)
    (cerebral) (cervical) (chronic) (circumscribed)
    (external) (fibrous) (hemorrhagic)
    (hypertrophic) (internal) (purulent) (spinal)
    (suppurative) (*see also* Meningitis) 322.9
  gonococcal 098.82
Pachyonychia (congenital) 757.5
  acquired 703.8
Pachyperiosteodermia
  primary or idiopathic 757.39
  secondary 731.2
Pachyperiostosis
  primary or idiopathic 757.39
  secondary 731.2
Pacinian tumor (M9507/0)—*see* Neoplasm,
    skin, benign
Pads, knuckle or Garrod's 728.79
Paget's disease (osteitis deformans) 731.0
  with infiltrating duct carcinoma of the breast
    (M8541/3)—*see* Neoplasm, breast,
    malignant
  bone 731.0
    osteosarcoma in (M9184/3)—*see* Neoplasm,
      bone, malignant
  breast (M8540/3) 174.0
  extramammary (M8542/3)—*see also* Neoplasm,
      skin, malignant
    anus 154.3
      skin 173.59
  malignant (M8540/3)
    breast 174.0
    specified site NEC (M8542/3)—*see*
      Neoplasm, skin, malignant
    unspecified site 174.0
  mammary (M8540/3) 174.0
  necrosis of bone 731.0
  nipple (M8540/3) 174.0
  osteitis deformans 731.0
Paget-Schroetter syndrome (intermittent venous
    claudication) 453.89
Pain(s) (*see also* Painful) 780.96
  abdominal 789.0
  acute 338.19
    due to trauma 338.11
    postoperative 338.18
      post-thoracotomy 338.12
  adnexa (uteri) 625.9
  alimentary, due to vascular insufficiency 557.9
  anginoid (*see also* Pain, precordial) 786.51
  anus 569.42
  arch 729.5
  arm 729.5
  axillary 729.5

Pain(s)—*continued*
  back (postural) 724.5
    low 724.2
    psychogenic 307.89
  bile duct 576.9
  bladder 788.99
  bone 733.90
  breast 611.71
    psychogenic 307.89
  broad ligament 625.9
  cancer associated 338.3
  cartilage NEC 733.90
  cecum 789.0
  cervicobrachial 723.3
  chest (central) 786.50
    atypical 786.59
    midsternal 786.51
    musculoskeletal 786.59
    noncardiac 786.59
    substernal 786.51
    wall (anterior) 786.52
  chronic 338.29
    associated with significant psychosocial
      dysfunction 338.4
    due to trauma 338.21
    postoperative 338.28
      post-thoracotomy 338.22
    syndrome 338.4
  coccyx 724.79
  colon 789.0
  common duct 576.9
  coronary—*see* Angina
  costochondral 786.52
  diaphragm 786.52
  due to (presence of) any device, implant, or graft
      classifiable to 996.0-996.5—*see*
      Complications, due to (presence of) any
      device, implant, or graft classified to
      996.0-996.5 NEC
    malignancy (primary) (secondary) 338.3
  ear (*see also* Otalgia) 388.70
  epigastric, epigastrium 789.0
  extremity (lower) (upper) 729.5
  eye 379.91
  face, facial 784.0
    atypical 350.2
    nerve 351.8
  false (labor) 644.1
  female genital organ NEC 625.9
    psychogenic 307.89
  finger 729.5
  flank 789.0
  foot 729.5
  gallbladder 575.9
  gas (intestinal) 787.3
  gastric 536.8
  generalized 780.96
  genital organ
    female 625.9
    male 608.9
    psychogenic 307.89
  groin 789.0
  growing 781.99
  hand 729.5
  head (*see also* Headache) 784.0
  heart (*see also* Pain, precordial) 786.51
  infraorbital (*see also* Neuralgia, trigeminal)
    350.1

PQR

Pain(s)—*continued*
  intermenstrual 625.2
  jaw 784.92
  joint 719.40
    ankle 719.47
    elbow 719.42
    foot 719.47
    hand 719.44
    hip 719.45
    knee 719.46
    multiple sites 719.49
    pelvic region 719.45
    psychogenic 307.89
    shoulder (region) 719.41
    specified site NEC 719.48
    wrist 719.43
  kidney 788.0
  labor, false or spurious 644.1
  laryngeal 784.1
  leg 729.5
  limb 729.5
  low back 724.2
  lumbar region 724.2
  mandible, mandibular 784.92
  mastoid (*see also* Otalgia) 388.70
  maxilla 784.92
  menstrual 625.3
  metacarpophalangeal (joint) 719.44
  metatarsophalangeal (joint) 719.47
  mouth 528.9
  muscle 729.1
    intercostal 786.59
  musculoskeletal (*see also* Pain, by site) 729.1
  nasal 478.19
  nasopharynx 478.29
  neck NEC 723.1
    psychogenic 307.89
  neoplasm related (acute) (chronic) 338.3
  nerve NEC 729.2
  neuromuscular 729.1
  nose 478.19
  ocular 379.91
  ophthalmic 379.91
  orbital region 379.91
  osteocopic 733.90
  ovary 625.9
    psychogenic 307.89
  over heart (*see also* Pain, precordial) 786.51
  ovulation 625.2
  pelvic (female) 625.9
    male NEC 789.0
      psychogenic 307.89
    psychogenic 307.89
  penis 607.9
    psychogenic 307.89
  pericardial (*see also* Pain, precordial) 786.51
  perineum
    female 625.9
    male 608.9
  pharynx 478.29
  pleura, pleural, pleuritic 786.52
  post-operative 338.18
    acute 338.18
    chronic 338.28
  post-thoracotomy 338.12
    acute 338.12
    chronic 338.22
  preauricular 388.70
  precordial (region) 786.51
    psychogenic 307.89
  premenstrual 625.4
  psychogenic 307.80

Pain(s)—*continued*
  cardiovascular system 307.89
  gastrointestinal system 307.89
  genitourinary system 307.89
  heart 307.89
  musculoskeletal system 307.89
  respiratory system 307.89
  skin 306.3
  radicular (spinal) (*see also* Radiculitis) 729.2
  rectum 569.42
  respiration 786.52
  retrosternal 786.51
  rheumatic NEC 729.0
    muscular 729.1
  rib 786.50
  root (spinal) (*see also* Radiculitis) 729.2
  round ligament (stretch) 625.9
  sacroiliac 724.6
  sciatic 724.3
  scrotum 608.9
    psychogenic 307.89
  seminal vesicle 608.9
  sinus 478.19
  skin 782.0
  spermatic cord 608.9
  spinal root (*see also* Radiculitis) 729.2
  stomach 536.8
    psychogenic 307.89
  substernal 786.51
  temporomandibular (joint) 524.62
  testis 608.9
    psychogenic 307.89
  thoracic spine 724.1
    with radicular and visceral pain 724.4
  throat 784.1
  tibia 733.90
  toe 729.5
  tongue 529.6
  tooth 525.9
  total hip replacement 996.77
  total knee replacement 996.77
  trigeminal (*see also* Neuralgia, trigeminal) 350.1
  tumor associated 338.3
  umbilicus 789.0
  ureter 788.0
  urinary (organ) (system) 788.0
  uterus 625.9
    psychogenic 307.89
  vagina 625.9
  vertebrogenic (syndrome) 724.5
  vesical 788.99
  vulva 625.9
  xiphoid 733.90
Painful —*see also* Pain
  arc syndrome 726.19
  coitus
    female 625.0
    male 608.89
    psychogenic 302.76
  ejaculation (semen) 608.89
    psychogenic 302.79
  erection 607.3
  feet syndrome 266.2
  menstruation 625.3
    psychogenic 306.52
  micturition 788.1
  ophthalmoplegia 378.55
  respiration 786.52
  scar NEC 709.2
  urination 788.1
  wire sutures 998.89

Painters' colic 984.9
  specified type of lead—*see* Table of drugs and
    chemicals
Palate —*see* condition
Palatoplegia 528.9
Palatoschisis (*see also* Cleft, palate) 749.00
Palilalia 784.69
Palindromic arthritis (*see also* Rheumatism,
    palindromic) 719.3
Palliative care V66.7
Pallor 782.61
  temporal, optic disc 377.15
Palmar —*see also* condition
  fascia—*see* condition
Palpable
  cecum 569.89
  kidney 593.89
  liver 573.9
  lymph nodes 785.6
  ovary 620.8
  prostate 602.9
  spleen (*see also* Splenomegaly) 789.2
  uterus 625.8
Palpitation (heart) 785.1
  psychogenic 306.2
Palsy (*see also* Paralysis) 344.9
  atrophic diffuse 335.20
  Bell's 351.0
    newborn 767.5
  birth 767.7
  brachial plexus 353.0
    fetus or newborn 767.6
  brain—*see also* Palsy, cerebral
    noncongenital or noninfantile 344.89
      due to vascular lesion—*see* category 438
      late effect—*see* Late effect(s) (of)
        cerebrovascular disease
    syphilitic 094.89
      congenital 090.49
  bulbar (chronic) (progressive) 335.22
    pseudo NEC 335.23
    supranuclear NEC 344.89
  cerebral (congenital) (infantile) (spastic) 343.9
    athetoid 333.71
    diplegic 343.0
      mue to prevhous vascular lesion—*see*
        category 438
      late effect—*see* Late effect(s) (of)
        cerebrovascular disease
    hemiplegic 343.1
    monoplegic 343.3
    noncongenital or noninfantile 437.8
      mue to prevhous vascular lesion—*see*
        category 438
      late effect—*see* Late effect(s) (of)
        cerebrovascular disease
    paraplegic 343.0
    quadriplegic 343.2
    spastic, not congenital or infantile 344.89
    syphilitic 094.89
      congenital 090.49
    tetraplegic 343.2
  cranial nerve—*see also* Disorder, nerve, cranial
    multiple 352.6
  creeping 335.21
  divers' 993.3
  Erb's (birth injury) 767.6
  facial 351.0
    newborn 767.5
  glossopharyngeal 352.2
  Klumpke (-Déjérine) 767.6

Palsy—*continued*
  lead 984.9
    specified type of lead—*see* Table of drugs and
      chemicals
  median nerve (tardy) 354.0
  peroneal nerve (acute) (tardy) 355.3
  progressive supranuclear 333.0
  pseudobulbar NEC 335.23
  radial nerve (acute) 354.3
  seventh nerve 351.0
    newborn 767.5
  shaking (*see also* Parkinsonism) 332.0
  spastic (cerebral) (spinal) 343.9
    hemiplegic 343.1
  specified nerve NEC—*see* Disorder, nerve
  supranuclear NEC 356.8
    progressive 333.0
  ulnar nerve (tardy) 354.2
  wasting 335.21
Paltauf-Sternberg disease 201.9
Paludism —*see* Malaria
Panama fever 084.0
Panaris (with lymphangitis) 681.9
  finger 681.02
  toe 681.11
Panaritium (with lymphangitis) 681.9
  finger 681.02
  toe 681.11
Panarteritis (nodosa) 446.0
  brain or cerebral 437.4
Pancake heart 793.2
  with cor pulmonale (chronic) 416.9
Pancarditis (acute) (chronic) 429.89
  with
    rheumatic fever (active) (acute) (chronic)
      (subacute) 391.8
    inactive or quiescent 398.99
  rheumatic, acute 391.8
    chronic or inactive 398.99
Pancoast's syndrome or tumor (carcinoma,
    pulmonary apex) (M8010/3) 162.3
Pancoast-Tobias syndrome (M8010/3)
    (carcinoma, pulmonary apex) 162.3
Pancolitis 556.6
Pancreas, pancreatic —*see* condition
Pancreatitis 577.0
  acute (edematous) (hemorrhagic) (recurrent) 577.0
  annular 577.0
  apoplectic 577.0
  calcereous 577.0
  chronic (infectious) 577.1
    recurrent 577.1
  cystic 577.2
  fibrous 577.8
  gangrenous 577.0
  hemorrhagic (acute) 577.0
  interstitial (chronic) 577.1
    acute 577.0
  malignant 577.0
  mumps 072.3
  painless 577.1
  recurrent 577.1
  relapsing 577.1
  subacute 577.0
  suppurative 577.0
  syphilitic 095.8
Pancreatolithiasis 577.8
Pancytolysis 289.9

Pancytopenia (acquired) 284.19
with
  malformations 284.09
  myelodysplastic syndrome — *see* Syndrome, myelodysplastic
congenital 284.09
due to
  antineoplastic chemotherapy 284.11
  drug, specified NEC 284.12
specified NEC 284.19
Panencephalitis —*see also* Encephalitis
subacute, sclerosing 046.2
Panhematopenia 284.81
  congenital 284.09
  constitutional 284.09
  splenic, primary 289.4
Panhemocytopenia 284.81
  congenital 284.09
  constitutional 284.09
Panhypogonadism 257.2
Panhypopituitarism 253.2
  prepubertal 253.3
Panic (attack) (state) 300.01
  reaction to exceptional stress (transient) 308.0
Panmyelopathy, familial constitutional 284.09
Panmyelophthisis 284.2
  acquired (secondary) 284.81
  congenital 284.2
  idiopathic 284.9
Panmyelosis (acute) (M9951/1) 238.79
Panner's disease 732.3
  capitellum humeri 732.3
  head of humerus 732.3
  tarsal navicular (bone) (osteochondrosis) 732.5
Panneuritis endemica 265.0 *[357.4]*
Panniculitis 729.30
  back 724.8
  knee 729.31
  mesenteric 567.82
  neck 723.6
  nodular, nonsuppurative 729.30
  sacral 724.8
  specified site NEC 729.39
Panniculus adiposus (abdominal) 278.1
Pannus (corneal) 370.62
  abdominal (symptomatic) 278.1
  allergic eczematous 370.62
  degenerativus 370.62
  keratic 370.62
  rheumatoid—*see* Arthritis, rheumatoid
  trachomatosus, trachomatous (active) 076.1
    [370.62]
    late effect 139.1
Panophthalmitis 360.02
Panotitis —*see* Otitis media
Pansinusitis (chronic) (hyperplastic) (nonpurulent) (purulent) 473.8
  acute 461.8
  due to fungus NEC 117.9
  tuberculous (*see also* Tuberculosis) 012.8
Panuveitis 360.12
  sympathetic 360.11
Panvalvular disease —*see* Endocarditis, mitral
Papageienkrankheit 073.9

Papanicolaou smear
anus 796.70
with
  atypical squamous cells
    cannot exclude high grade squamous intraepithelial lesion (ASC-H) 796.72
    of undetermined significance (ASC-US) 796.71
  cytologic evidence of malignancy 796.76
  high grade squamous intraepithelial lesion (HGSIL) 796.74
  low grade squamous intraepithelial lesion (LGSIL) 796.73
glandular 796.70
specified finding NEC 796.79
unsatisfactory cytology 796.78
cervix (screening test) V76.2
  as part of gynecological examination V72.31
  for suspected malignant neoplasm V76.2
    no disease found V71.1
  inadequate cytology sample 795.08
  nonspecific abnormal finding 795.00
    with
      atypical squamous cells—changes of undetermined significance
        cannot exclude high grade squamous intraepithelial lesion (ASC-H) 795.02
        of undetermined significance (ASC-US) 795.01
      cytologic evidence of malignancy 795.06
      high grade squamous intraepithelial lesion (HGSIL) 795.04
      low grade squamous intraepithelial lesion (LGSIL) 795.03
    nonspecific finding NEC 795.09
    satisfactory smear but lacking transformation zone 795.07
  to confirm findings of recent normal smear following initial abnormal smear V72.32
  unsatisfactory cervical cytology 795.08
other specified site—*see also* Screening, malignant neoplasm
for suspected malignant neoplasm—*see also* Screening, malignant neoplasm
  no disease found V71.1
nonspecific abnormal finding 796.9
vagina V76.47
with
  atypical squamous cells
    cannot exclude high grade squamous intraepithelial lesion (ASC-H) 795.12
    of undetermined significance (ASC-US) 795.11
  cytologic evidence of malignancy 795.16
  high grade squamous intraepithelial lesion (HGSIL) 795.14
  low grade squamous intraepithelial lesion (LGSIL) 795.13
abnormal NEC 795.19
following hysterectomy for malignant condition V67.01
inadequate cytology sample 795.18
unsatisfactory cytology 795.18
Papilledema 377.00
associated with
  decreased ocular pressure 377.02
  increased intracranial pressure 377.01
  retinal disorder 377.03
choked disc 377.00
infectional 377.00

Papillitis 377.31
  anus 569.49
  chronic lingual 529.4
  necrotizing, kidney 584.7
  optic 377.31
  rectum 569.49
  renal, necrotizing 584.7
  tongue 529.0
Papilloma (M8050/0)—*see also* Neoplasm, by
  site, benign

> *Note—Except where otherwise indicated, the*
> *morphological varieties of papilloma in the list*
> *below should be coded by site as for*
> *"Neoplasm, benign."*

  acuminatum (female) (male) 078.11
  bladder (urinary) (transitional cell) (M8120/1)
    236.7
    benign (M8120/0) 223.3
  choroid plexus (M9390/0) 225.0
    anaplastic type (M9390/3) 191.5
    malignant (M9390/3) 191.5
  ductal (M8503/0)
  dyskeratotic (M8052/0)
  epidermoid (M8052/0)
  hyperkeratotic (M8052/0)
  intracystic (M8504/0)
  intraductal (M8503/0)
  inverted (M8053/0)
  keratotic (M8052/0)
  parakeratotic (M8052/0)
  pinta (primary) 103.0
  renal pelvis (transitional cell) (M8120/1) 236.99
    benign (M8120/0) 223.1
  Schneiderian (M8121/0)
    specified site—*see* Neoplasm, by site, benign
    unspecified site 212.0
  serous surface (M8461/0)
    borderline malignancy (M8461/1)
      specified site—*see* Neoplasm, by site,
        uncertain behavior
      unspecified site 236.2
    specified site—*see* Neoplasm, by site, benign
    unspecified site 220
  squamous (cell) (M8052/0)
  transitional (cell) (M8120/0)
    bladder (urinary) (M8120/1) 236.7
    inverted type (M8121/1)—*see* Neoplasm, by
      site, uncertain behavior
    renal pelvis (M8120/1) 236.91
    ureter (M8120/1) 236.91
  ureter (transitional cell) (M8120/1) 236.91
    benign (M8120/0) 223.2
  urothelial (M8120/1)—*see* Neoplasm, by site,
    uncertain behavior
  verrucous (M8051/0)
  villous (M8261/1)—*see* Neoplasm, by site,
    uncertain behavior
  yaws, plantar or palmar 102.1
Papillomata, multiple, of yaws 102.1
Papillomatosis (M8060/0)—*see also* Neoplasm,
  by site, benign
  confluent and reticulate 701.8
  cutaneous 701.8
  ductal, breast 610.1
  Gougerot-Carteaud (confluent reticulate) 701.8
  intraductal (diffuse) (M8505/0)—*see* Neoplasm,
    by site, benign
  subareolar duct (M8506/0) 217
Papillon-Léage and Psaume syndrome
  (orodigitofacial dysostosis) 759.89

Papule 709.8
  carate (primary) 103.0
  fibrous, of nose (M8724/0) 216.3
  pinta (primary) 103.0
Papulosis
  lymphomatoid 709.8
  malignant 447.8
Papyraceous fetus 779.89
  complicating pregnancy 646.0
Paracephalus 759.7
Parachute mitral valve 746.5
Paracoccidioidomycosis 116.1
  mucocutaneous-lymphangitic 116.1
  pulmonary 116.1
  visceral 116.1
Paracoccidiomycosis —*see*
  Paracoccidioidomycosis
Paracusis 388.40
Paradentosis 523.5
Paradoxical facial movements 374.43
Paraffinoma 999.9
Paraganglioma (M8680/1)
  adrenal (M8700/0) 227.0
    malignant (M8700/3) 194.0
  aortic body (M8691/1) 237.3
    malignant (M8691/3) 194.6
  carotid body (M8692/1) 237.3
    malignant (M8692/3) 194.5
  chromaffin (M8700/0)—*see also* Neoplasm, by
    site, benign
    malignant (M8700/3)—*see* Neoplasm, by site,
      malignant
  extra-adrenal (M8693/1)
    malignant (M8693/3)
      specified site—*see* Neoplasm, by site,
        malignant
      unspecified site 194.6
    specified site—*see* Neoplasm, by site,
      uncertain behavior
    unspecified site 237.3
  glomus jugulare (M8690/1) 237.3
    malignant (M8690/3) 194.6
  jugular (M8690/1) 237.3
    malignant (M8680/3)
      specified site—*see* Neoplasm, by site,
        malignant
      unspecified site 194.6
  nonchromaffin (M8693/1)
    malignant (M8693/3)
      specified site—*see* Neoplasm, by site,
        malignant
      unspecified site 194.6
    specified site—*see* Neoplasm, by site,
      uncertain behavior
    unspecified site 237.3
  parasympathetic (M8682/1)
    specified site—*see* Neoplasm, by site,
      uncertain behavior
    unspecified site 237.3
  specified site—*see* Neoplasm, by site, uncertain
    behavior
  sympathetic (M8681/1)
    specified site—*see* Neoplasm, by site,
      uncertain behavior
    unspecified site 237.3
  unspecified site 237.3
Parageusia 781.1
  psychogenic 306.7
Paragonimiasis 121.2
Paragranuloma, Hodgkin's (M9660/3) 201.0

Parahemophilia (*see also* Defect, coagulation) 286.3
Parakeratosis 690.8
  psoriasiformis 696.2
  variegata 696.2
Paralysis, paralytic (complete) (incomplete) 344.9
  with
    broken
      back—*see* Fracture, vertebra, by site, with spinal cord injury
      neck—*see* Fracture, vertebra, cervical, with spinal cord injury
    fracture, vertebra—*see* Fracture, vertebra, by site, with spinal cord injury
    syphilis 094.89
  abdomen and back muscles 355.9
  abdominal muscles 355.9
  abducens (nerve) 378.54
  abductor 355.9
    lower extremity 355.8
    upper extremity 354.9
  accessory nerve 352.4
  accommodation 367.51
    hysterical 300.11
  acoustic nerve 388.5
  agitans 332.0
    arteriosclerotic 332.0
  alternating 344.89
    oculomotor 344.89
  amyotrophic 335.20
  ankle 355.8
  anterior serratus 355.9
  anus (sphincter) 569.49
  apoplectic (current episode) (*see also* Disease, cerebrovascular, acute) 436
    late effect—*see* Late effect(s) (of) cerebrovascular disease category 438
  arm 344.40
    affecting
      dominant side 344.41
      nondominant side 344.42
    both 344.2
    due to old CVA—*see* Category 438
    hysterical 300.11
    late effect—*see* Late effect(s) (of) cerebrovascular disease
    psychogenic 306.0
    transient 781.4
    traumatic NDC (*see also* Injury, nerve, upper limb) 955.9
  arteriosclerotic (current episode) 437.0
    late effect—*see* Late effect(s) (of) cerebrovascular disease
  ascending (spinal), acute 357.0
  associated, nuclear 344.89
  asthenic bulbar 358.00
  ataxic NEC 334.9
    general 094.1
  athetoid 333.71
  atrophic 356.9
    infantile, acute (*see also* Poliomyelitis, with paralysis) 045.1
    muscle NEC 355.9
    progressive 335.21
    spinal (acute) (*see also* Poliomyelitis, with paralysis) 045.1
  attack (*see also* Disease, cerebrovascular, acute) 436
  axillary 353.0
  Babinski-Nageotte's 344.89

Paralysis, paralytic—*continued*
  Bell's 351.0
    newborn 767.5
  Benedikt's 344.89
  birth (injury) 767.7
    brain 767.0
      intracranial 767.0
    spinal cord 767.4
  bladder (sphincter) 596.53
    neurogenic 596.54
      with cauda equina syndrome 344.61
    puerperal, postpartum, childbirth 665.5
    sensory 596.54
      with cauda equina 344.61
    spastic 596.54
      with cauda equina 344.61
  bowel, colon, or intestine (*see also* Ileus) 560.1
  brachial plexus 353.0
    due to birth injury 767.6
    newborn 767.6
  brain
    congenital—*see* Palsy, cerebral
    current episode 437.8
    diplegia 344.2
    due to previous vascular lesion—*see* category 438
    hemiplegia 342.9
      due to previous vascular lesion—*see* category 438
      late effect—*see* Late effect(s) (of) cerebrovascular disease
    infantile—*see* Palsy, cerebral
    late effect—*see* Late effect(s) (of) cerebrovascular disease
    monoplegia—*see also* Monoplegia
      due to previous vascular lesion—*see* category 438
      late effect—*see* Late effect(s) (of) cerebrovascular disease
    paraplegia 344.1
    quadriplegia —*see* Quadriplegia
    syphilitic, congenital 090.49
    triplegia 344.89
  bronchi 519.19
  Brown-Séquard's 344.89
  bulbar (chronic) (progressive) 335.22
    infantile (*see also* Poliomyelitis, bulbar) 045.0
    poliomyelitic (*see also* Poliomyelitis, bulbar) 045.0
    pseudo 335.23
    supranuclear 344.89
  bulbospinal 358.00
  cardiac (*see also* Failure, heart) 428.9
  cerebral
    current episode 437.8
    spastic, infantile—*see* Palsy, cerebral
  cerebrocerebellar 437.8
    diplegic infantile 343.0
  cervical
    plexus 353.2
    sympathetic NEC 337.09
  Céstan-Chenais 344.89
  Charcot-Marie-Tooth type 356.1
  childhood—*see* Palsy, cerebral
  Clark's 343.9
  colon (*see also* Ileus) 560.1
  compressed air 993.3
  compression
    arm NEC 354.9
    cerebral—*see* Paralysis, brain
    leg NEC 355.8
    lower extremity NEC 355.8
    upper extremity NEC 354.9

Paralysis, paralytic—*continued*
  congenital (cerebral) (spastic) (spinal)—*see*
    Palsy, cerebral
  conjugate movement (of eye) 378.81
    cortical (nuclear) (supranuclear) 378.81
  convergence 378.83
  cordis (*see also* Failure, heart) 428.9
  cortical (*see also* Paralysis, brain) 437.8
  cranial or cerebral nerve (*see also* Disorder,
    nerve, cranial) 352.9
  creeping 335.21
  crossed leg 344.89
  crutch 953.4
  deglutition 784.99
    hysterical 300.11
  dementia 094.1
  descending (spinal) NEC 335.9
  diaphragm (flaccid) 519.4
    due to accidental section of phrenic nerve
      during procedure 998.2
  digestive organs NEC 564.89
  diplegic—*see* Diplegia
  divergence (nuclear) 378.85
  divers' 993.3
  Duchenne's 335.22
  due to intracranial or spinal birth injury—*see*
    Palsy, cerebral
  embolic (current episode) (*see also* Embolism,
    brain) 434.1
    late effect —*see* Late effect(s) (of)
      cerebrovascular disease
  enteric (*see also* Ileus) 560.1
    with hernia—*see* Hernia, by site, with
      obstruction
  Erb's syphilitic spastic spinal 094.89
  Erb (-Duchenne) (birth) (newborn) 767.6
  esophagus 530.89
  essential, infancy (*see also* Poliomyelitis) 045.9
  extremity
    lower —*see* Paralysis, leg
      spastic (hereditary) 343.3
        noncongenital or noninfantile 344.1
      transient (cause unknown) 781.4
    upper —*see* Paralysis, arm
  eye muscle (extrinsic) 378.55
    intrinsic 367.51
  facial (nerve) 351.0
    birth injury 767.5
    congenital 767.5
    following operation NEC 998.2
    newborn 767.5
  familial 359.3
    periodic 359.3
    spastic 334.1
  fauces 478.29
  finger NEC 354.9
  foot NEC 355.8
  gait 781.2
  gastric nerve 352.3
  gaze 378.81
  general 094.1
    ataxic 094.1
    insane 094.1
    juvenile 090.40
    progressive 094.1
    tabetic 094.1
  glossopharyngeal (nerve) 352.2
  glottis (*see also* Paralysis, vocal cord) 478.30
  gluteal 353.4
  Gubler (-Millard) 344.89

Paralysis, paralytic—*continued*
  hand 354.9
    hysterical 300.11
    psychogenic 306.0
  heart (*see also* Failure, heart) 428.9
  hemifacial, progressive 349.89
  hemiplegic—*see* Hemiplegia
  hyperkalemic periodic (familial) 359.3
  hypertensive (current episode) 437.8
  hypoglossal (nerve) 352.5
  hypokalemic periodic 359.3
  Hyrtl's sphincter (rectum) 569.49
  hysterical 300.11
  ileus (*see also* Ileus) 560.1
  infantile (*see also* Poliomyelitis) 045.9
    atrophic acute 045.1
    bulbar 045.0
    cerebral—*see* Palsy, cerebral
    paralytic 045.1
    progressive acute 045.9
    spastic—*see* Palsy, cerebral
    spinal 045.9
  infective (*see also* Poliomyelitis) 045.9
  inferior nuclear 344.9
  insane, general or progressive 094.1
  internuclear 378.86
  interosseous 355.9
  intestine (*see also* Ileus) 560.1
  intracranial (current episode) (*see also* Paralysis,
    brain) 437.8
    due to birth injury 767.0
  iris 379.49
    due to diphtheria (toxin) 032.81 *[379.49]*
  ischemic, Volkmann's (complicating trauma)
    958.6
  isolated sleep, recurrent 327.43
  Jackson's 344.89
  jake 357.7
  Jamaica ginger (jake) 357.7
  juvenile general 090.40
  Klumpke (-Déjérine) (birth) (newborn) 767.6
  labioglossal (laryngeal) (pharyngeal) 335.22
  Landry's 357.0
  laryngeal nerve (recurrent) (superior) (*see also*
    Paralysis, vocal cord) 478.30
  larynx (*see also* Paralysis, vocal cord) 478.30
    due to diphtheria (toxin) 032.3
  late effect
    due to
      birth injury, brain or spinal (cord)—*see*
        Palsy, cerebral
      edema, brain or cerebral—*see* Paralysis,
        brain
      lesion
        cerebrovascular—*see* category 438
        late effect—*see* Late effect(s) (of)
          cerebrovascular disease
        spinal (cord)—*see* Paralysis, spinal
  lateral 335.24
  lead 984.9
    specified type of lead—*see* Table of drugs and
      chemicals
  left side—*see* Hemiplegia
  leg 344.30
    affecting
      dominant side 344.31
      nondominant side 344.32
    both (*see also* Paraplegia) 344.1
    crossed 344.89
    hysterical 300.11
    psychogenic 306.0
    transient or transitory 781.4

Paralysis, paralytic—*continued*
  leg —*continued*
      traumatic NEC (*see also* Injury, nerve, lower
          limb) 956.9
  levator palpebrae superioris 374.31
  limb NEC 344.5
      all four—*see* Quadriplegia
      quadriplegia—*see* Quadriplegia
  lip 528.5
  Lissauer's 094.1
  local 355.9
  lower limb—*see also* Paralysis, leg
      both (*see also* Paraplegia) 344.1
  lung 518.89
      newborn 770.89
  median nerve 354.1
  medullary (tegmental) 344.89
  mesencephalic NEC 344.89
      tegmental 344.89
  middle alternating 344.89
  Millard-Gubler-Foville 344.89
  monoplegic—*see* Monoplegia
  motor NEC 344.9
      cerebral—*see* Paralysis, brain
      spinal—*see* Paralysis, spinal
  multiple
      cerebral—*see* Paralysis, brain
      spinal—*see* Paralysis, spinal
  muscle (flaccid) 359.9
      due to nerve lesion NEC 355.9
      eye (extrinsic) 378.55
          intrinsic 367.51
          oblique 378.51
      iris sphincter 364.89
      ischemic (complicating trauma) (Volkmann's)
          958.6
      pseudohypertrophic 359.1
  muscular (atrophic) 359.9
      progressive 335.21
  musculocutaneous nerve 354.9
  musculospiral 354.9
  nerve—*see also* Disorder, nerve
      third or oculomotor (partial) 378.51
          total 378.52
      fourth or trochlear 378.53
      sixth or abducens 378.54
      seventh or facial 351.0
          birth injury 767.5
          due to
              injection NEC 999.9
              operation NEC 997.09
          newborn 767.5
      accessory 352.4
      auditory 388.5
      birth injury 767.7
      cranial or cerebral (*see also* Disorder, nerve,
          cranial) 352.9
      facial 351.0
          birth injury 767.5
          newborn 767.5
      laryngeal (*see also* Paralysis, vocal cord) 478.30
          newborn 767.7
      phrenic 354.8
          newborn 767.7
      radial 354.3
          birth injury 767.6
          newborn 767.6
      syphilitic 094.89
      traumatic NEC (*see also* Injury, nerve, by site)
          957.9
      trigeminal 350.9
      ulnar 354.2

Paralysis, paralytic—*continued*
  newborn NEC 767.0
  normokalemic periodic 359.3
  obstetrical, newborn 767.7
  ocular 378.9
  oculofacial, congenital 352.6
  oculomotor (nerve) (partial) 378.51
      alternating 344.89
      external bilateral 378.55
      total 378.52
  olfactory nerve 352.0
  palate 528.9
  palatopharyngolaryngeal 352.6
  paratrigeminal 350.9
  periodic (familial) (hyperkalemic) (hypokalemic)
      (normokalemic) (potassium sensitive)
      (secondary) 359.3
  peripheral
      autonomic nervous system—*see* Neuropathy,
          peripheral, autonomic
      nerve NEC 355.9
  peroneal (nerve) 355.3
  pharynx 478.29
  phrenic nerve 354.8
  plantar nerves 355.6
  pneumogastric nerve 352.3
  poliomyelitis (current) (*see also* Poliomyelitis,
      with paralysis) 045.1
      bulbar 045.0
  popliteal nerve 355.3
  pressure (*see also* Neuropathy, entrapment)
      355.9
  progressive 335.21
      atrophic 335.21
      bulbar 335.22
      general 094.1
      hemifacial 349.89
      infantile, acute (*see also* Poliomyelitis) 045.9
      multiple 335.20
  pseudobulbar 335.23
  pseudohypertrophic 359.1
      muscle 359.1
  psychogenic 306.0
  pupil, pupillary 379.49
  quadriceps 355.8
  quadriplegic (*see also* Quadriplegia) 344.0
  radial nerve 354.3
      birth injury 767.6
  rectum (sphincter) 569.49
  rectus muscle (eye) 378.55
  recurrent
      isolated sleep 327.43
      laryngeal nerve (*see also* Paralysis, vocal
          cord) 478.30
  respiratory (muscle) (system) (tract) 786.09
      center NEC 344.89
          fetus or newborn 770.87
      congenital 768.9
      newborn 768.9
  right side—*see* Hemiplegia
  Saturday night 354.3
  saturnine 984.9
      specified type of lead—*see* Table of drugs and
          chemicals
  sciatic nerve 355.0
  secondary—*see* Paralysis, late effect
  seizure (cerebral) (current episode) (*see also*
      Disease, cerebrovascular, acute) 436
      late effect—*see* Late effect(s) (of)
          cerebrovascular disease
  senile NEC 344.9

Paralysis, paralytic—*continued*
  serratus magnus 355.9
  shaking (*see also* Parkinsonism) 332.0
  shock (*see also* Disease, cerebrovascular, acute)
    436
    late effect—*see* Late effect(s) (of)
      cerebrovascular disease
  shoulder 354.9
  soft palate 528.9
  spasmodic—*see* Paralysis, spastic
  spastic 344.9
    cerebral infantile—*see* Palsy, cerebral
    congenital (cerebral)—*see* Palsy, cerebral
    familial 334.1
    hereditary 334.1
    infantile 343.9
    noncongenital or noninfantile, cerebral 344.9
    syphilitic 094.0
      spinal 094.89
  sphincter, bladder (*see also* Paralysis, bladder)
    596.53
  spinal (cord) NEC 344.1
    accessory nerve 352.4
    acute (*see also* Poliomyelitis) 045.9
    ascending acute 357.0
    atrophic (acute) (*see also* Poliomyelitis, with
      paralysis) 045.1
      spastic, syphilitic 094.89
    congenital NEC 343.9
    hemiplegic —*see* Hemiplegia
    hereditary 336.8
    infantile (*see also* Poliomyelitis) 045.9
    late effect NEC 344.89
    monoplegic—*see* Monoplegia
    nerve 355.9
    progressive 335.10
    quadriplegic —*see* Quadriplegia
    spastic NEC 343.9
    traumatic—*see* Injury, spinal, by site
  sternomastoid 352.4
  stomach 536.3
    diabetic 250.6 *[536.3]*
      due to secondary diabetes 249.6 *[536.3]*
    nerve (nondiabetic) 352.3
  stroke (current episode) *see* Infarct, brain
    late effect—*see* Late effect(s) (of)
      cerebrovascular disease
  subscapularis 354.8
  superior nuclear NEC 334.9
  supranuclear 356.8
  sympathetic
    cervical NEC 337.09
    nerve NEC (*see also* Neuropathy, peripheral,
      autonomic) 337.9
    nervous system—*see* Neuropathy, peripheral,
      autonomic
  syndrome 344.9
    specified NEC 344.89
  syphilitic spastic spinal (Erb's) 094.89
  tabetic general 094.1
  thigh 355.8
  throat 478.29
    diphtheritic 032.0
    muscle 478.29
  thrombotic (current episode) (*see also*
    Thrombosis, brain) 434.0
    late effect—*see* Late effect(s) (of)
      cerebrovascular disease
  thumb NEC 354.9
  tick (-bite) 989.5

Paralysis, paralytic—*continued*
  Todd's (postepileptic transitory paralysis)
    344.89
  toe 355.6
  tongue 529.8
  transient
    arm or leg NEC 781.4
    traumatic NEC (*see also* Injury, nerve, by site)
      957.9
  trapezius 352.4
  traumatic, transient NEC (*see also* Injury, nerve,
    by site) 957.9
  trembling (*see also* Parkinsonism) 332.0
  triceps brachii 354.9
  trigeminal nerve 350.9
  trochlear nerve 378.53
  ulnar nerve 354.2
  upper limb —*see also* Paralysis, arm
    both (*see also* Diplegia) 344.2
  uremic—*see* Uremia
  uveoparotitic 135
  uvula 528.9
    hysterical 300.11
    postdiphtheritic 032.0
  vagus nerve 352.3
  vasomotor NEC 337.9
  velum palati 528.9
  vesical (*see also* Paralysis, bladder) 596.53
  vestibular nerve 388.5
  visual field, psychic 368.16
  vocal cord 478.30
    bilateral (partial) 478.33
      complete 478.34
    complete (bilateral) 478.34
    unilateral (partial) 478.31
      complete 478.32
  Volkmann's (complicating trauma) 958.6
  wasting 335.21
  Weber's 344.89
  wrist NEC 354.9
Paramedial orifice, urethrovesical 753.8
Paramenia 626.9
Parametritis (chronic) (*see also* Disease, pelvis,
    inflammatory) 614.4
  acute 614.3
  puerperal, postpartum, childbirth 670.8
Parametrium, parametric —*see* condition
Paramnesia (*see also* Amnesia) 780.93
Paramolar 520.1
  causing crowding 524.31
Paramyloidosis 277.30
Paramyoclonus multiplex 333.2
Paramyotonia 359.29
  congenita (of von Eulenburg) 359.29
Paraneoplastic syndrome —*see* condition
Parangi (*see also* Yaws) 102.9
Paranoia 297.1
  alcoholic 291.5
  querulans 297.8
  senile 290.20
Paranoid
  dementia (*see also* Schizophrenia) 295.3
    praecox (acute) 295.3
    senile 290.20
  personality 301.0
  psychosis 297.9
    alcoholic 291.5
    climacteric 297.2
    drug-induced 292.11
    involutional 297.2

Paranoid—*continued*
  psychosis—*continued*
    menopausal 297.2
    protracted reactive 298.4
    psychogenic 298.4
      acute 298.3
    senile 290.20
  reaction (chronic) 297.9
    acute 298.3
  schizophrenia (acute) (*see also* Schizophrenia)
    295.3
  state 297.9
    alcohol-induced 291.5
    climacteric 297.2
    drug-induced 292.11
    due to or associated with
      arteriosclerosis (cerebrovascular) 290.42
      presenile brain disease 290.12
      senile brain disease 290.20
    involutional 297.2
    menopausal 297.2
    senile 290.20
    simple 297.0
    specified type NEC 297.8
  tendencies 301.0
  traits 301.0
  trends 301.0
  type, psychopathic personality 301.0
Paraparesis (*see also* Paraplegia) 344.1
Paraphasia 784.3
Paraphilia (*see also* Deviation, sexual) 302.9
Paraphimosis (congenital) 605
  chancroidal 099.0
Paraphrenia, paraphrenic (late) 297.2
  climacteric 297.2
  dementia (*see also* Schizophrenia) 295.3
  involutional 297.2
  menopausal 297.2
  schizophrenia (acute) (*see also* Schizophrenia)
    295.3
Paraplegia 344.1
  with
    broken back—*see* Fracture, vertebra, by site,
      with spinal cord injury
    fracture, vertebra—*see* Fracture, vertebra, by
      site, with spinal cord injury
  ataxic—*see* Degeneration, combined, spinal
    cord
  brain (current episode) (*see also* Paralysis,
    brain) 437.8
  cerebral (current episode) (*see also* Paralysis,
    brain) 437.8
  congenital or infantile (cerebral) (spastic)
    (spinal) 343.0
  cortical—*see* Paralysis, brain
  familial spastic 334.1
  functional (hysterical) 300.11
  hysterical 300.11
  infantile 343.0
  late effect 344.1
  Pott's (*see also* Tuberculosis) 015.0 *[730.88]*
  psychogenic 306.0
  spastic
    Erb's spinal 094.89
    hereditary 334.1
    not infantile or congenital 344.1
  spinal (cord)
    traumatic NEC—*see* Injury, spinal, by site
  syphilitic (spastic) 094.89
  traumatic NEC—*see* Injury, spinal, by site

Paraproteinemia 273.2
  benign (familial) 273.1
  monoclonal 273.1
  secondary to malignant or inflammatory disease
    273.1
Parapsoriasis 696.2
  en plaques 696.2
  guttata 696.2
  lichenoides chronica 696.2
  retiformis 696.2
  varioliformis (acuta) 696.2
Parascarlatina 057.8
Parasitic —*see also* condition
  disease NEC (*see also* Infestation, parasitic)
    136.9
    contact V01.89
    exposure to V01.89
    intestinal NEC 129
    skin NEC 134.9
  stomatitis 112.0
  sycosis 110.0
    beard 110.0
    scalp 110.0
  twin 759.4
Parasitism NEC 136.9
  intestinal NEC 129
  skin NEC 134.9
  specified—*see* Infestation
Parasitophobia 300.29
Parasomnia 307.47
  alcohol induced 291.82
  drug induced 292.85
  nonorganic origin 307.47
  organic 327.40
    in conditions classified elsewhere 327.44
    other 327.49
Paraspadias 752.69
Paraspasm facialis 351.8
Parathyroid gland —*see* condition
Parathyroiditis (autoimmune) 252.1
Parathyroprival tetany 252.1
Paratrachoma 077.0
Paratyphilitis (*see also* Appendicitis) 541
Paratyphoid (fever)—*see* Fever, paratyphoid
Paratyphus —*see* Fever, paratyphoid
Paraurethral duct 753.8
Para-urethritis 597.89
  gonococcal (acute) 098.0
    chronic or duration of 2 months or over 098.2
Paravaccinia NEC 051.9
  milkers' node 051.1
Paravaginitis (*see also* Vaginitis) 616.10
Parencephalitis (*see also* Encephalitis) 323.9
  late effect—*see* category 326
Parergasia 298.9
Paresis (*see also* Paralysis) 344.9
  accommodation 367.51
  bladder (spastic) (sphincter) (*see also* Paralysis,
    bladder) 596.53
    tabetic 094.0
  bowel, colon, or intestine (*see also* Ileus) 560.1
  brain or cerebral—*see* Paralysis, brain
  extrinsic muscle, eye 378.55
  general 094.1
    arrested 094.1
    brain 094.1
    cerebral 094.1
    insane 094.1
    juvenile 090.40
      remission 090.49

Paresis—*continued*
  general—*continued*
    progressive 094.1
    remission (sustained) 094.1
    tabetic 094.1
  heart (*see also* Failure, heart) 428.9
  infantile (*see also* Poliomyelitis) 045.9
  insane 094.1
  juvenile 090.40
  late effect—*see* Paralysis, late effect
  luetic (general) 094.1
  peripheral progressive 356.9
  pseudohypertrophic 359.1
  senile NEC 344.9
  stomach 536.3
    diabetic 250.6 *[536.3]*
      due to secondary diabetes 249.6 *[536.3]*
  syphilitic (general) 094.1
    congenital 090.40
  transient, limb 781.4
  vesical (sphincter) NEC 596.53
Paresthesia (*see also* Disturbance, sensation) 782.0
  Berger's (paresthesia of lower limb) 782.0
  Bernhardt 355.1
  Magnan's 782.0
Paretic —*see* condition
Parinaud's
  conjunctivitis 372.02
  oculoglandular syndrome 372.02
  ophthalmoplegia 378.81
  syndrome (paralysis of conjugate upward gaze) 378.81
Parkes Weber and Dimitri syndrome (encephalocutaneous angiomatosis) 759.6
Parkinson's disease, syndrome, or tremor —*see* Parkinsonism
Parkinsonism (arteriosclerotic) (idiopathic) (primary) 332.0
  associated with orthostatic hypotension (idiopathic) (symptomatic) 333.0
  due to drugs 332.1
  neuroleptic-induced 332.1
  secondary 332.1
  syphilitic 094.82
Parodontitis 523.40
Parodontosis 523.5
Paronychia (with lymphangitis) 681.9
  candidal (chronic) 112.3
  chronic 681.9
    candidal 112.3
    finger 681.02
    toe 681.11
  finger 681.02
  toe 681.11
  tuberculous (primary) (*see also* Tuberculosis) 017.0
Parorexia NEC 307.52
  hysterical 300.11
Parosmia 781.1
  psychogenic 306.7
Parotid gland —*see* condition
Parotiditis (*see also* Parotitis) 527.2
  epidemic 072.9
  infectious 072.9
Parotitis 527.2
  allergic 527.2
  chronic 527.2
  epidemic (*see also* Mumps) 072.9
  infectious (*see also* Mumps) 072.9
  noninfectious 527.2

Parotitis—*continued*
  nonspecific toxic 527.2
  not mumps 527.2
  postoperative 527.2
  purulent 527.2
  septic 527.2
  suppurative (acute) 527.2
  surgical 527.2
  toxic 527.2
Paroxysmal —*see also* condition
  dyspnea (nocturnal) 786.09
Parrot's disease (syphilitic osteochondritis) 090.0
Parrot fever 073.9
Parry's disease or syndrome (exophthalmic goiter) 242.0
Parry-Romberg syndrome 349.89
Parson's disease (exophthalmic goiter) 242.0
Parsonage-Aldren-Turner syndrome 353.5
Parsonage-Turner syndrome 353.5
Pars planitis 363.21
Particolored infant 757.39
Parturition —*see* Delivery
Parvovirus 079.83
  B19 079.83
  human 079.83
Passage
  false, urethra 599.4
  meconium noted during delivery 763.84
  of sounds or bougies (*see also* Attention to artificial opening) V55.9
Passive —*see* condition
Pasteurella septica 027.2
Pasteurellosis (*see also* Infection, Pasteurella) 027.2
PAT (paroxysmal atrial tachycardia) 427.0
Patau's syndrome (trisomy D_1) 758.1
Patch
  herald 696.3
Patches
  mucous (syphilitic) 091.3
    congenital 090.0
  smokers' (mouth) 528.6
Patellar —*see* condition
Patellofemoral syndrome 719.46
Patent —*see also* Imperfect closure
  atrioventricular ostium 745.69
  canal of Nuck 752.41
  cervix 622.5
    complicating pregnancy 654.5
      affecting fetus or newborn 761.0
  ductus arteriosus or Botalli 747.0
  Eustachian
    tube 381.7
    valve 746.89
  foramen
    Botalli 745.5
    ovale 745.5
  interauricular septum 745.5
  interventricular septum 745.4
  omphalomesenteric duct 751.0
  os (uteri)—*see* Patent, cervix
  ostium secundum 745.5
  urachus 753.7
  vitelline duct 751.0
Paternity testing V70.4
Paterson's syndrome (sideropenic dysphagia) 280.8
Paterson (-Brown) (-Kelly) syndrome (sideropenic dysphagia) 280.8

Paterson-Kelly syndrome or web (sideropenic dysphagia) 280.8
Pathologic, pathological —*see also* condition
asphyxia 799.01
drunkenness 291.4
emotionality 301.3
liar 301.7
personality 301.9
resorption, tooth 521.40
external 521.42
internal 521.41
specified NEC 521.49
sexuality (*see also* Deviation, sexual) 302.9
Pathology (of)—*see also* Disease
periradicular, associated with previous endodontic treatment 526.69
Patterned motor discharges, idiopathic (*see also* Epilepsy) 345.5
Patulous —*see also* Patent
anus 569.49
Eustachian tube 381.7
Pause, sinoatrial 427.81
Pavor nocturnus 307.46
Pavy's disease 593.6
Paxton's disease (white piedra) 111.2
Payr's disease or syndrome (splenic flexure syndrome) 569.89
PBA (pseudobulbar affect) 310.81
Pearls
Elschnig 366.51
enamel 520.2
Pearl-workers' disease (chronic osteomyelitis) (*see also* Osteomyelitis) 730.1
Pectenitis 569.49
Pectenosis 569.49
Pectoral —*see* condition
Pectus
carinatum (congenital) 754.82
acquired 738.3
rachitic (*see also* Rickets) 268.0
excavatum (congenital) 754.81
acquired 738.3
rachitic (*see also* Rickets) 268.0
recurvatum (congenital) 754.81
acquired 738.3
Pedatrophia 261
Pederosis 302.2
Pediculosis (infestation) 132.9
capitis (head louse) (any site) 132.0
corporis (body louse) (any site) 132.1
eyelid 132.0 *[373.6]*
mixed (classifiable to more than one category in 132.0-132.2) 132.3
pubis (pubic louse) (any site) 132.2
vestimenti 132.1
vulvae 132.2
Pediculus (infestation)—*see* Pediculosis
Pedophilia 302.2
Peg-shaped teeth 520.2
Pel's crisis 094.0
Pel-Ebstein disease —*see* Disease, Hodgkin's
Pelade 704.01
Pelger-Huët anomaly or syndrome (hereditary hyposegmentation) 288.2
Peliosis (rheumatica) 287.0
Pelizaeus-Merzbacher
disease 330.0
sclerosis, diffuse cerebral 330.0
Pellagra (alcoholic or with alcoholism) 265.2
with polyneuropathy 265.2 *[357.4]*

Pellagra-cerebellar-ataxia-renal aminoaciduria syndrome 270.0
Pellegrini's disease (calcification, knee joint) 726.62
Pellegrini (-Stieda) disease or syndrome (calcification, knee joint) 726.62
Pellizzi's syndrome (pineal) 259.8
Pelvic —*see also* condition
congestion-fibrosis syndrome 625.5
kidney 753.3
Pelvioectasis 591
Pelviolithiasis 592.0
Pelviperitonitis
female (*see also* Peritonitis, pelvic, female) 614.5
male (*see also* Peritonitis) 567.21
Pelvis, pelvic —*see also* condition or type
infantile 738.6
Nägele's 738.6
obliquity 738.6
Robert's 755.69
Pemphigoid 694.5
benign, mucous membrane 694.60
with ocular involvement 694.61
bullous 694.5
cicatricial 694.60
with ocular involvement 694.61
juvenile 694.2
Pemphigus 694.4
benign 694.5
chronic familial 757.39
Brazilian 694.4
circinatus 694.0
congenital, traumatic 757.39
conjunctiva 694.61
contagiosus 684
erythematodes 694.4
erythematosus 694.4
foliaceus 694.4
frambesiodes 694.4
gangrenous (*see also* Gangrene) 785.4
malignant 694.4
neonatorum, newborn 684
ocular 694.61
papillaris 694.4
seborrheic 694.4
South American 694.4
syphilitic (congenital) 090.0
vegetans 694.4
vulgaris 694.4
wildfire 694.4
Pendred's syndrome (familial goiter with deaf-mutism) 243
Pendulous
abdomen 701.9
in pregnancy or childbirth 654.4
affecting fetus or newborn 763.89
breast 611.89
Penetrating wound —*see also* Wound, open, by site
with internal injury—*see* Injury, internal, by site, with open wound
eyeball 871.7
with foreign body (nonmagnetic) 871.6
magnetic 871.5
ocular (*see also* Penetrating wound, eyeball) 871.7
adnexa 870.3
with foreign body 870.4
orbit 870.3
with foreign body 870.4

Penetration, pregnant uterus by instrument
with
  abortion—*see* Abortion, by type, with damage
    to pelvic organs
  ectopic pregnancy (*see also* categories
    633.0-633.9) 639.2
  molar pregnancy (*see also* categories 630-632)
    639.2
complication of delivery 665.1
  affecting fetus or newborn 763.89
following
  abortion 639.2
  ectopic or molar pregnancy 639.2
Penfield's syndrome (*see also* Epilepsy) 345.5
Penicilliosis of lung 117.3
Penis —*see* condition
Penitis 607.2
Penta X syndrome 758.81
Pentalogy (of Fallot) 745.2
Pentosuria (benign) (essential) 271.8
Peptic acid disease 536.8
Peregrinating patient V65.2
Perforated —*see* Perforation
Perforation, perforative (nontraumatic)
antrum (*see also* Sinusitis, maxillary) 473.0
appendix 540.0
  with peritoneal abscess 540.1
atrial septum, multiple 745.5
attic, ear 384.22
  healed 384.81
bile duct, except cystic (*see also* Disease,
  biliary) 576.3
  cystic 575.4
bladder (urinary) 596.6
with
  abortion—*see* Abortion, by type, with
    damage to pelvic organs
  ectopic pregnancy (*see also* categories
    633.0-633.9) 639.2
  molar pregnancy (*see also* categories
    630-632) 639.2
following
  abortion 639.2
  ectopic or molar pregnancy 639.2
  obstetrical trauma 665.5
bowel 569.83
with
  abortion—*see* Abortion, by type, with
    damage to pelvic organs
  ectopic pregnancy (*see also* categories
    633.0-633.9) 639.2
  molar pregnancy (*see also* categories
    630-632) 639.2
fetus or newborn 777.6
following
  abortion 639.2
  ectopic or molar pregnancy 639.2
  obstetrical trauma 665.5
broad ligament
with
  abortion—*see* Abortion, by type, with
    damage to pelvic organs
  ectopic pregnancy (*see also* categories
    633.0-633.9) 639.2
  molar pregnancy (*see also* categories
    630-632) 639.2
following
  abortion 639.2
  ectopic or molar pregnancy 639.2
  obstetrical trauma 665.6

Perforation, perforative—*continued*
by
  device, implant, or graft—*see* Complications,
    mechanical
  foreign body left accidentally in operation
    wound 998.4
  instrument (any) during a procedure,
    accidental 998.2
cecum 540.0
  with peritoneal abscess 540.1
cervix (uteri)—*see also* Injury, internal, cervix
with
  abortion—*see* Abortion, by type, with
    damage to pelvic organs
  ectopic pregnancy (*see also* categories
    633.0-633.9) 639.2
  molar pregnancy (*see also* categories
    630-632) 639.2
following
  abortion 639.2
  ectopic or molar pregnancy 639.2
  obstetrical trauma 665.3
colon 569.83
common duct (bile) 576.3
cornea (*see also* Ulcer, cornea) 370.00
  due to ulceration 370.06
cystic duct 575.4
diverticulum (*see also* Diverticula) 562.10
  small intestine 562.00
duodenum, duodenal (ulcer)—*see* Ulcer,
  duodenum, with perforation
ear drum—*see* Perforation, tympanum
enteritis—*see* Enteritis
esophagus 530.4
ethmoidal sinus (*see also* Sinusitis, ethmoidal)
  473.2
foreign body (external site)—*see also* Wound,
  open, by site, complicated
  internal site, by ingested object—*see* Foreign
    body
frontal sinus (*see also* Sinusitis, frontal) 473.1
gallbladder or duct (*see also* Disease,
  gallbladder) 575.4
gastric (ulcer)—*see* Ulcer, stomach, with
  perforation
heart valve—*see* Endocarditis
ileum (*see also* Perforation, intestine) 569.83
instrumental
  external—*see* Wound, open, by site
  pregnant uterus, complicating delivery 665.9
  surgical (accidental) (blood vessel) (nerve)
    (organ) 998.2
intestine 569.83
with
  abortion—*see* Abortion, by type, with
    damage to pelvic organs
  ectopic pregnancy (*see also* categories
    633.0-633.9) 639.2
  molar pregnancy (*see also* categories
    630-632) 639.2
fetus or newborn 777.6
obstetrical trauma 665.5
ulcerative NEC 569.83
jejunum, jejunal 569.83
  ulcer—*see* Ulcer, gastrojejunal, with
    perforation
mastoid (antrum) (cell) 383.89
maxillary sinus (*see also* Sinusitis, maxillary)
  473.0
membrana tympani—*see* Perforation, tympanum

Perforation, perforative—*continued*
  nasal
    septum 478.19
      congenital 748.1
      syphilitic 095.8
    sinus (*see also* Sinusitis) 473.9
      congenital 748.1
  palate (hard) 526.89
    soft 528.9
      syphilitic 095.8
    syphilitic 095.8
  palatine vault 526.89
    syphilitic 095.8
      congenital 090.5
  pelvic
    floor
      with
        abortion—*see* Abortion, by type, with
          damage to pelvic organs
        ectopic pregnancy (*see also* categories
          633.0-633.9) 639.2
        molar pregnancy (*see also* categories
          630-632) 639.2
        obstetrical trauma 664.1
    organ
      with
        abortion—*see* Abortion, by type, with
          damage to pelvic organs
        ectopic pregnancy (*see also* categories
          633.0-633.9) 639.2
        molar pregnancy (*see also* categories
          630-632) 639.2
      following
        abortion 639.2
        ectopic or molar pregnancy 639.2
        obstetrical trauma 665.5
  perineum—*see* Laceration, perineum
  periurethral tissue
    with
      abortion—*see* Abortion, by type, with
        damage to pelvic organs
      ectopic pregnancy (*see also* categories
        630-632) 639.2
      molar pregnancy (*see also* categories
        630-632) 639.2
  pharynx 478.29
  pylorus, pyloric (ulcer)—*see* Ulcer, stomach,
    with perforation
  rectum 569.49
  root canal space 526.61
  sigmoid 569.83
  sinus (accessory) (chronic) (nasal) (*see also*
    Sinusitis) 473.9
  sphenoidal sinus (*see also* Sinusitis, sphenoidal)
    473.3
  stomach (due to ulcer)—*see* Ulcer, stomach,
    with perforation
  surgical (accidental) (by instrument) (blood
    vessel) (nerve) (organ) 998.2
  traumatic
    external—*see* Wound, open, by site
    eye (*see also* Penetrating wound, ocular) 871.7
    internal organ—*see* Injury, internal, by site
  tympanum (membrane) (persistent
    posttraumatic) (postinflammatory) 384.20
    with
      otitis media—*see* Otitis media
    attic 384.22
    central 384.21
    healed 384.81
    marginal NEC 384.23

Perforation, perforative—*continued*
  tympanum—*continued*
    multiple 384.24
    pars flaccida 384.22
    total 384.25
    traumatic—*see* Wound, open, ear, drum
  typhoid, gastrointestinal 002.0
  ulcer—*see* Ulcer, by site, with perforation
  ureter 593.89
  urethra
    with
      abortion—*see* Abortion, by type, with
        damage to pelvic organs
      ectopic pregnancy (*see also* categories
        633.0-633.9) 639.2
      molar pregnancy (*see also* categories
        630-632) 639.2
    following
      abortion 639.2
      ectopic or molar pregnancy 639.2
      obstetrical trauma 665.5
  uterus—*see also* Injury, internal, uterus
    with
      abortion—*see* Abortion, by type, with
        damage to pelvic organs
      ectopic pregnancy (*see also* categories
        633.0-633.9) 639.2
      molar pregnancy (*see also* categories
        630-632) 639.2
      by intrauterine contraceptive device 996.32
    following
      abortion 639.2
      ectopic or molar pregnancy 639.2
      obstetrical trauma—*see* Injury, internal,
        uterus, obstetrical trauma
  uvula 528.9
    syphilitic 095.8
  vagina—*see* Laceration, vagina
  viscus NEC 799.89
    traumatic 868.00
    with open wound into cavity 868.10
Periadenitis mucosa necrotica recurrens 528.2
Periangiitis 446.0
Periantritis 535.4
Periappendicitis (acute) (*see also* Appendicitis)
  541
Periarteritis (disseminated) (infectious)
  (necrotizing) (nodosa) 446.0
Periarthritis (joint) 726.90
  Duplay's 726.2
  gonococcal 098.50
  humeroscapularis 726.2
  scapulohumeral 726.2
  shoulder 726.2
  wrist 726.4
Periarthrosis (angioneural)—*see* Periarthritis
Peribronchitis 491.9
  tuberculous (*see also* Tuberculosis) 011.3
Pericapsulitis, adhesive (shoulder) 726.0
Pericarditis (granular) (with decompensation)
  (with effusion) 423.9
  with
    rheumatic fever (conditions classifiable to
      390)
      active (*see also* Pericarditis, rheumatic)
        391.0
      inactive or quiescent 393
  actinomycotic 039.8 *[420.0]*

Pericarditis—*continued*
  acute (nonrheumatic) 420.90
    with chorea (acute) (rheumatic) (Sydenham's)
        392.0
    bacterial 420.99
    benign 420.91
    hemorrhagic 420.90
    idiopathic 420.91
    infective 420.90
    nonspecific 420.91
    rheumatic 391.0
      with chorea (acute) (rheumatic)
          (Sydenham's) 392.0
    sicca 420.90
    viral 420.91
  adhesive or adherent (external) (internal) 423.1
    acute—*see* Pericarditis, acute
    rheumatic (external) (internal) 393
  amebic 006.8 *[420.0]*
  bacterial (acute) (subacute) (with serous or
      seropurulent effusion) 420.99
  calcareous 423.2
  cholesterol (chronic) 423.8
    acute 420.90
  chronic (nonrheumatic) 423.8
    rheumatic 393
  constrictive 423.2
  Coxsackie 074.21
  due to
    actinomycosis 039.8 *[420.0]*
    amebiasis 006.8 *[420.0]*
    Coxsackie (virus) 074.21
    histoplasmosis (*see also* Histoplasmosis) 115.93
    nocardiosis 039.8 *[420.0]*
    tuberculosis (*see also* Tuberculosis) 017.9
        [420.0]
  fibrinocaseous (*see also* Tuberculosis) 017.9
      [420.0]
  fibrinopurulent 420.99
  fibrinous—*see* Pericarditis, rheumatic
  fibropurulent 420.99
  fibrous 423.1
  gonococcal 098.83
  hemorrhagic 423.0
  idiopathic (acute) 420.91
  infective (acute) 420.90
  meningococcal 036.41
  neoplastic (chronic) 423.8
    acute 420.90
  nonspecific 420.91
  obliterans, obliterating 423.1
  plastic 423.1
  pneumococcal (acute) 420.99
  postinfarction 411.0
  purulent (acute) 420.99
  rheumatic (active) (acute) (with effusion) (with
      pneumonia) 391.0
    with chorea (acute) (rheumatic) (Sydenham's)
        392.0
    chronic or inactive (with chorea) 393
  septic (acute) 420.99
  serofibrinous—*see* Pericarditis, rheumatic
  staphylococcal (acute) 420.99
  streptococcal (acute) 420.99
  suppurative (acute) 420.99
  syphilitic 093.81
  tuberculous (acute) (chronic) (*see also*
      Tuberculosis) 017.9 *[420.0]*
  uremic 585.9 *[420.0]*
  viral (acute) 420.91
Pericardium, pericardial —*see* condition
Pericellulitis (*see also* Cellulitis) 682.9

Pericementitis 523.40
  acute 523.30
  chronic (suppurative) 523.40
Pericholecystitis (*see also* Cholecystitis) 575.10
Perichondritis
  auricle 380.00
    acute 380.01
    chronic 380.02
  bronchus 491.9
  ear (external) 380.00
    acute 380.01
    chronic 380.02
  larynx 478.71
    syphilitic 095.8
    typhoid 002.0 *[478.71]*
  nose 478.19
  pinna 380.00
    acute 380.01
    chronic 380.02
  trachea 478.9
Periclasia 523.5
Pericolitis 569.89
Pericoronitis (chronic) 523.40
  acute 523.33
Pericystitis (*see also* Cystitis) 595.9
Pericytoma (M9150/1)—*see also* Neoplasm,
    connective tissue, uncertain behavior
  benign (M9150/0)—*see* Neoplasm, connective
      tissue, benign
  malignant (M9150/3)—*see* Neoplasm,
      connective tissue, malignant
Peridacryocystitis, acute 375.32
Peridiverticulitis (*see also* Diverticulitis) 562.11
Periduodenitis 535.6
Periendocarditis (*see also* Endocarditis) 424.90
  acute or subacute 421.9
Periepididymitis (*see also* Epididymitis) 604.90
Perifolliculitis (abscedens) 704.8
  capitis, abscedens et suffodiens 704.8
  dissecting, scalp 704.8
  scalp 704.8
  superficial pustular 704.8
Perigastritis (acute) 535.0
Perigastrojejunitis (acute) 535.0
Perihepatitis (acute) 573.3
  chlamydial 099.56
  gonococcal 098.86
Peri-ileitis (subacute) 569.89
Perilabyrinthitis (acute)—*see* Labyrinthitis
Perimeningitis —*see* Meningitis
Perimetritis (*see also* Endometritis) 615.9
Perimetrosalpingitis (*see also*
    Salpingo-oophoritis) 614.2
Perineocele 618.05
Perinephric —*see* condition
Perinephritic —*see* condition
Perinephritis (*see also* Infection, kidney) 590.9
  purulent (*see also* Abscess, kidney) 590.2
Perineum, perineal —*see* condition
Perineuritis NEC 729.2
Periodic —*see also* condition
  disease (familial) 277.31
  edema 995.1
    hereditary 277.6
  fever 277.31
  headache syndrome in child or adolescent 346.2
  limb movement disorder 327.51
  paralysis (familial) 359.3
  peritonitis 277.31
  polyserositis 277.31
  somnolence (*see also* Narcolepsy) 347.00

Periodontal
  cyst 522.8
  pocket 523.8
Periodontitis (chronic) (complex) (compound)
  (simplex) 523.40
  acute 523.33
  aggressive 523.30
    generalized 523.32
    localized 523.31
  apical 522.6
    acute (pulpal origin) 522.4
  generalized 523.42
  localized 523.41
Periodontoclasia 523.5
Periodontosis 523.5
Periods —*see also* Menstruation
  heavy 626.2
  irregular 626.4
Perionychia (with lymphangitis) 681.9
  finger 681.02
  toe 681.11
Perioophoritis (*see also* Salpingo-oophoritis) 614.2
Periorchitis (*see also* Orchitis) 604.90
Periosteum, periosteal —*see* condition
Periostitis (circumscribed) (diffuse) (infective) 730.3

Note—Use the following fifth-digit
subclassification with category 730:
0 site unspdcified
1 shoulder region
2 upper arm
3 forearm
4 hand
5 pelvic region and thigh
6 lower leg
7 ankle and foot
8 other specified sites
9 multiple sites

---

  with osteomyelitis (*see also* Osteomyelitis) 730.2
    acute or subacute 730.0
    chronic or old 730.1
  albuminosa, albuminosus 730.3
  alveolar 526.5
  alveolodental 526.5
  dental 526.5
  gonorrheal 098.89
  hyperplastica, generalized 731.2
  jaw (lower) (upper) 526.4
  monomelic 733.99
  orbital 376.02
  syphilitic 095.5
    congenital 090.0 *[730.8]*
    secondary 091.61
  tuberculous (*see also* Tuberculosis, bone) 015.9
    [730.8]
  yaws (early) (hypertrophic) (late) 102.6
Periostosis (*see also* Periostitis) 730.3
  with osteomyelitis (*see also* Osteomyelitis) 730.2
    acute or subacute 730.0
    chronic or old 730.1
  hyperplastic 756.59
Peripartum cardiomyopathy 674.5
Periphlebitis (*see also* Phlebitis) 451.9
  lower extremity 451.2
    deep (vessels) 451.19
    superficial (vessels) 451.0
  portal 572.1
  retina 362.18
  superficial (vessels) 451.0
  tuberculous (*see also* Tuberculosis) 017.9
    retina 017.3 *[362.18]*

Peripneumonia —*see* Pneumonia
Periproctitis 569.49
Periprostatitis (*see also* Prostatitis) 601.9
Perirectal —*see* condition
Perirenal —*see* condition
Perisalpingitis (*see also* Salpingo-oophoritis)
  614.2
Perisigmoiditis 569.89
Perisplenitis (infectional) 289.59
Perispondylitis —*see* Spondylitis
Peristalsis reversed or visible 787.4
Peritendinitis (*see also* Tenosynovitis) 726.90
  adhesive (shoulder) 726.0
Perithelioma (M9150/1)—*see* Pericytoma
Peritoneum, peritoneal —*see also* condition
  equilibration test V56.32
Peritonitis (acute) (adhesive) (fibrinous)
  (hemorrhagic) (idiopathic) (localized)
  (perforative) (primary) (with adhesions) (with
  effusion) 567.9
  with or following
    abortion—*see* Abortion, by type, with sepsis
    abscess 567.21
    appendicitis 540.0
      with peritoneal abscess 540.1
    ectopic pregnancy (*see also* categories
      633.0-633.9) 639.0
    molar pregnancy (*see also* categories 630-632)
      639.0
  aseptic 998.7
  bacterial 567.29
    spontaneous 567.23
  bile, biliary 567.81
  chemical 998.7
  chlamydial 099.56
  chronic proliferative 567.89
  congenital NEC 777.6
  diaphragmatic 567.22
  diffuse NEC 567.29
  diphtheritic 032.83
  disseminated NEC 567.29
  due to
    bile 567.81
    foreign
      body or object accidentally left during a
        procedure (instrument) (sponge) (swab)
        998.4
      substance accidentally left during a procedure
        (chemical) (powder) (talc) 998.7
    talc 998.7
    urine 567.89
  fibrinopurulent 567.29
  fibrinous 567.29
  fibrocaseous (*see also* Tuberculosis) 014.0
  fibropurulent 567.29
  general, generalized (acute) 567.21
  gonococcal 098.86
  in infective disease NEC 136.9 *[567.0]*
  meconium (newborn) 777.6
  pancreatic 577.8
  paroxysmal, benign 277.31
  pelvic
    female (acute) 614.5
      chronic NEC 614.7
        with adhesions 614.6
      puerperal, postpartum, childbirth 670.8
    male (acute) 567.21
  periodic (familial) 277.31
  phlegmonous 567.29
  pneumococcal 567.1
  postabortal 639.0

Peritonitis—*continued*
  proliferative, chronic 567.89
  puerperal, postpartum, childbirth 670.8
  purulent 567.29
  septic 567.29
  spontaneous bacterial 567.23
  staphylococcal 567.29
  streptococcal 567.29
  subdiaphragmatic 567.29
  subphrenic 567.29
  suppurative 567.29
  syphilitic 095.2
    congenital 090.0 *[567.0]*
  talc 998.7
  tuberculous (*see also* Tuberculosis) 014.0
  urine 567.89
Peritonsillar —*see* condition
Peritonsillitis 475
Perityphlitis (*see also* Appendicitis) 541
Periureteritis 593.89
Periurethral —*see* condition
Periurethritis (gangrenous) 597.89
Periuterine —*see* condition
Perivaginitis (*see also* Vaginitis) 616.10
Perivasculitis, retinal 362.18
Perivasitis (chronic) 608.4
Periventricular leukomalacia 779.7
Perivesiculitis (seminal) (*see also* Vesiculitis) 608.0
Perlèche 686.8
  due to
    moniliasis 112.0
    riboflavin deficiency 266.0
Pernicious —*see* condition
Pernio, perniosis 991.5
Persecution
  delusion 297.9
  social V62.4
Perseveration (tonic) 784.69
Persistence, persistent (congenital) 759.89
  anal membrane 751.2
  arteria stapedia 744.04
  atrioventricular canal 745.69
  bloody ejaculate 792.2
  branchial cleft 744.41
  bulbus cordis in left ventricle 745.8
  canal of Cloquet 743.51
  capsule (opaque) 743.51
  cilioretinal artery or vein 743.51
  cloaca 751.5
  communication—*see* Fistula, congenital
  convolutions
    aortic arch 747.21
    fallopian tube 752.19
    oviduct 752.19
    uterine tube 752.19
  double aortic arch 747.21
  ductus
    arteriosus 747.0
    Botalli 747.0
  fetal
    circulation 747.83
    form of cervix (uteri) 752.49
    hemoglobin (hereditary) ("Swiss variety") 282.7
    pulmonary hypertension 747.83
  foramen
    Botalli 745.5
    ovale 745.5
  Gartner's duct 752.41

Persistence, persistent—*continued*
  hemoglobin, fetal (hereditary) (HPFH) 282.7
  hyaloid
    artery (generally incomplete) 743.51
    system 743.51
  hymen (tag)
    in pregnancy or childbirth 654.8
      causing obstructed labor 660.2
  lanugo 757.4
  left
    posterior cardinal vein 747.49
    root with right arch of aorta 747.21
    superior vena cava 747.49
  Meckel's diverticulum 751.0
  mesonephric duct 752.89
    fallopian tube 752.11
  mucosal disease (middle ear) (with posterior or superior marginal perforation of ear drum) 382.2
  nail(s), anomalous 757.5
  occiput, anterior or posterior 660.3
    fetus or newborn 763.1
  omphalomesenteric duct 751.0
  organ or site NEC—*see* Anomaly, specified type NEC
  ostium
    atrioventriculare commune 745.69
    primum 745.61
    secundum 745.5
  ovarian rests in fallopian tube 752.19
  pancreatic tissue in intestinal tract 751.5
  primary (deciduous)
    teeth 520.6
    vitreous hyperplasia 743.51
  pulmonary hypertension 747.83
  pupillary membrane 743.46
    iris 743.46
  Rhesus (Rh) titer (*see also* Complications, transfusion) 999.70
  right aortic arch 747.21
  sinus
    urogenitalis 752.89
    venosus with imperfect incorporation in right auricle 747.49
  thymus (gland) 254.8
    hyperplasia 254.0
  thyroglossal duct 759.2
  thyrolingual duct 759.2
  truncus arteriosus or communis 745.0
  tunica vasculosa lentis 743.39
  umbilical sinus 753.7
  urachus 753.7
  vegetative state 780.03
  vitelline duct 751.0
  wolffian duct 752.89
Person (with)
  admitted for clinical research, as participant or control subject V70.7
  affected by
    family member
      currently on deployment (military) V61.01
      returned from deployment (military) (current or past conflict) V61.02
  awaiting admission to adequate facility elsewhere V63.2
    undergoing social agency investigation V63.8
  concern (normal) about sick person in family V61.49

Person—*continued*
consulting on behalf of another V65.19
  pediatric
    pre-adoption visit for adoptive parents V65.11
    pre-birth visit for expectant parents V65.11
currently deployed in theater or in support of
    military war, peacekeeping and
    humanitarian operations V62.21
feared
  complaint in whom no diagnosis was made
    V65.5
  condition not demonstrated V65.5
feigning illness V65.2
healthy, accompanying sick person V65.0
history of military war, peacekeeping and
    humanitarian deployment (current or past
    conflict) V62.22
living (in)
  alone V60.3
  boarding school V60.6
  residence remote from hospital or medical
    care facility V63.0
  residential institution V60.6
  without
    adequate
      financial resources V60.2
      housing (heating) (space) V60.1
    housing (permanent) (temporary) V60.0
    material resources V60.2
    person able to render necessary care V60.4
    shelter V60.0
medical services in home not available V63.1
on waiting list V63.2
  undergoing social agency investigation V63.8
sick or handicapped in family V61.49
"worried well" V65.5
Personality
affective 301.10
aggressive 301.3
amoral 301.7
anancastic, anankastic 301.4
antisocial 301.7
asocial 301.7
asthenic 301.6
avoidant 301.82
borderline 301.83
change 310.1
compulsive 301.4
cycloid 301.13
cyclothymic 301.13
dependent 301.6
depressive (chronic) 301.12
disorder, disturbance NEC 301.9
  with
    antisocial disturbance 301.7
    pattern disturbance NEC 301.9
    sociopathic disturbance 301.7
    trait disturbance 301.9
dual 300.14
dyssocial 301.7
eccentric 301.89
  "haltlose" type 301.89
emotionally unstable 301.59
epileptoid 301.3
explosive 301.3
fanatic 301.0
histrionic 301.50
hyperthymic 301.11
hypomanic 301.11
hypothymic 301.12
hysterical 301.50

Personality—*continued*
immature 301.89
inadequate 301.6
labile 301.59
masochistic 301.89
morally defective 301.7
multiple 300.14
narcissistic 301.81
obsessional 301.4
obsessive-compulsive 301.4
overconscientious 301.4
paranoid 301.0
passive (-dependent) 301.6
passive-aggressive 301.84
pathologic NEC 301.9
pattern defect or disturbance 301.9
pseudosocial 301.7
psychoinfantile 301.59
psychoneurotic NEC 301.89
psychopathic 301.9
  with
    amoral trend 301.7
    antisocial trend 301.7
    asocial trend 301.7
    pathologic sexuality (*see also* Deviation,
      sexual) 302.9
  mixed types 301.9
schizoid 301.20
  introverted 301.21
  schizotypal 301.22
type A 301.4
unstable (emotional) 301.59
Perthes' disease (capital femoral
    osteochondrosis) 732.1
Pertussis (*see also* Whooping cough) 033.9
vaccination, prophylactic (against) V03.6
Peruvian wart 088.0
Perversion, perverted
appetite 307.52
  hysterical 300.11
function
  pineal gland 259.8
  pituitary gland 253.9
    anterior lobe
      deficient 253.2
      excessive 253.1
    posterior lobe 253.6
  placenta—*see* Placenta, abnormal
sense of smell or taste 781.1
  psychogenic 306.7
sexual (*see also* Deviation, sexual) 302.9
Pervious, congenital —*see also* Imperfect,
    closure
ductus arteriosus 747.0
Pes (congenital) (*see also* Talipes) 754.70
abductus (congenital) 754.60
  acquired 736.79
acquired NEC 736.79
  planus 734
adductus (congenital) 754.79
  acquired 736.79
cavus 754.71
  acquired 736.73
planovalgus (congenital) 754.69
  acquired 736.79
planus (acquired) (any degree) 734
  congenital 754.61
  rachitic 268.1
valgus (congenital) 754.61
  acquired 736.79
varus (congenital) 754.50
  acquired 736.79

Pest (*see also* Plague) 020.9
Pestis (*see also* Plague) 020.9
  bubonica 020.0
  fulminans 020.0
  minor 020.8
  pneumonica—*see* Plague, pneumonic
Petechia, petechiae 782.7
  fetus or newborn 772.6
Petechial
  fever 036.0
  typhus 081.9
Petges-Cléjat or Petges-Clégat syndrome
  (poikilodermatomyositis) 710.3
Petit's
  disease (*see also* Hernia, lumbar) 553.8
Petit mal (idiopathic) (*see also* Epilepsy) 345.0
  status 345.2
Petrellidosis 117.6
Petrositis 383.20
  acute 383.21
  chronic 383.22
Peutz-Jeghers disease or syndrome 759.6
Peyronie's disease 607.85
Pfeiffer's disease 075
Phacentocele 379.32
  traumatic 921.3
Phacoanaphylaxis 360.19
Phacocele (old) 379.32
  traumatic 921.3
Phaehyphomycosis 117.8
Phagedena (dry) (moist) (*see also* Gangrene)
  785.4
  arteriosclerotic 440.24
  geometric 686.09
  penis 607.89
  senile 440.24
  sloughing 785.4
  tropical (*see also* Ulcer, skin) 707.9
  vulva 616.50
Phagedenic —*see also* condition
  abscess—*see also* Abscess
    chancroid 099.0
  bubo NEC 099.8
  chancre 099.0
  ulcer (tropical) (*see also* Ulcer, skin) 707.9
Phagomania 307.52
Phakoma 362.89
Phantom limb (syndrome) 353.6
Pharyngeal —*see also* condition
  arch remnant 744.41
  pouch syndrome 279.11
Pharyngitis (acute) (catarrhal) (gangrenous)
  (infective) (malignant) (membranous)
  (phlegmonous) (pneumococcal)
  (pseudomembranous) (simple)
  (staphylococcal) (subacute) (suppurative)
  (ulcerative) (viral) 462
  with influenza, flu, or grippe (*see also*
    Influenza) 487.1
  aphthous 074.0
  atrophic 472.1
  chlamydial 099.51
  chronic 472.1
  Coxsackie virus 074.0
  diphtheritic (membranous) 032.0
  follicular 472.1
  fusospirochetal 101
  gonococcal 098.6
  granular (chronic) 472.1
  herpetic 054.79

Pharyngitis—*continued*
  hypertrophic 472.1
  infectional, chronic 472.1
  influenzal (*see also* Influenza) 487.1
  lymphonodular, acute 074.8
  septic 034.0
  streptococcal 034.0
  tuberculous (*see also* Tuberculosis) 012.8
  vesicular 074.0
Pharyngoconjunctival fever 077.2
Pharyngoconjunctivitis, viral 077.2
Pharyngolaryngitis (acute) 465.0
  chronic 478.9
  septic 034.0
Pharyngoplegia 478.29
Pharyngotonsillitis 465.8
  tuberculous 012.8
Pharyngotracheitis (acute) 465.8
  chronic 478.9
Pharynx, pharyngeal —*see* condition
Phase of life problem NEC V62.89
Phenomenon
  Arthus' 995.21
  flashback (drug) 292.89
  jaw-winking 742.8
  Jod-Basedow 242.8
  L. E. cell 710.0
  lupus erythematosus cell 710.0
  Pelger-Huët (hereditary hyposegmentation) 288.2
  Raynaud's (paroxysmal digital cyanosis)
    (secondary) 443.0
  Reilly's (*see also* Neuropathy, peripheral,
    autonomic) 337.9
  vasomotor 780.2
  vasospastic 443.9
  vasovagal 780.2
  Wenckebach's, heart block (second degree) 426.13
Phenylketonuria (PKU) 270.1
Phenylpyruvicaciduria 270.1
Pheochromoblastoma (M8700/3)
  specified site—*see* Neoplasm, by site, malignant
  unspecified site 194.0
Pheochromocytoma (M8700/0)
  malignant (M8700/3)
    specified site—*see* Neoplasm, by site,
      malignant
    unspecified site 194.0
  specified site—*see* Neoplasm, by site, benign
  unspecified site 227.0
Phimosis (congenital) 605
  chancroidal 099.0
  due to infection 605
Phlebectasia (*see also* Varicose, vein) 454.9
  congenital NEC 747.60
  esophagus (*see also* Varix, esophagus) 456.1
    with hemorrhage (*see also* Varix, esophagus,
      bleeding) 456.0
Phlebitis (infective) (pyemic) (septic)
  (suppurative) 451.9
  antecubital vein 451.82
  arm NEC 451.84
    axillary vein 451.89
    basilic vein 451.82
    deep 451.83
    superficial 451.82
  basilic vein 451.82
  blue 451.19
  brachial vein 451.83
  breast, superficial 451.89

Phlebitis—*continued*
  cavernous (venous) sinus—*see* Phlebitis,
    intracranial sinus
  cephalic vein 451.82
  cerebral (venous) sinus—*see* Phlebitis,
    intracranial sinus
  chest wall, superficial 451.89
  complicating pregnancy or puerperium 671.2
    affecting fetus or newborn 760.3
  cranial (venous) sinus—*see* Phlebitis,
    intracranial sinus
  deep (vessels) 451.19
    femoral vein 451.11
    specified vessel NEC 451.19
  due to implanted device—*see* Complications,
    due to (presence of) any device, implant, or
    graft classified to 996.0-996.5 NEC
  during or resulting from a procedure 997.2
  femoral vein (deep) (superficial) 451.11
  femoropopliteal 451.19
  following infusion, perfusion, or transfusion
    999.2
  gouty 274.89 *[451.9]*
  hepatic veins 451.89
  iliac vein 451.81
  iliofemoral 451.11
  intracranial sinus (any) (venous) 325
    late effect—*see* category 326
    nonpyogenic 437.6
    in pregnancy or puerperium 671.5
  jugular vein 451.89
  lateral (venous) sinus—*see* Phlebitis,
    intracranial sinus
  leg 451.2
    deep (vessels) 451.19
      femoral vein 451.11
      specified vessel NEC 451.19
    superficial (vessels) 451.0
      femoral vein 451.11
  longitudinal sinus—*see* Phlebitis, intracranial
    sinus
  lower extremity 451.2
    deep (vessels) 451.19
      femoral vein 451.11
      specified vessel NEC 451.19
    superficial (vessels) 451.0
      femoral vein 451.11
  migrans, migrating (superficial) 453.1
  pelvic
    with
      abortion—*see* Abortion, by type, with sepsis
      ectopic pregnancy (*see also* categories
        633.0-633.9) 639.0
      molar pregnancy (*see also* categories
        630-632) 639.0
    following
      abortion 639.0
      ectopic or molar pregnancy 639.0
    puerperal, postpartum 671.4
  popliteal vein 451.19
  portal (vein) 572.1
  postoperative 997.2
  pregnancy 671.2
    deep 671.3
    specified type NEC 671.5
    superficial 671.2
  puerperal, postpartum, childbirth 671.2
    deep 671.4
    lower extremities 671.2
    pelvis 671.4
    specified site NEC 671.5
    superficial 671.2

Phlebitis—*continued*
  radial vein 451.83
  retina 362.18
  saphenous (great) (long) 451.0
    accessory or small 451.0
  sinus (meninges)—*see* Phlebitis, intracranial
    sinus
  specified site NEC 451.89
  subclavian vein 451.89
  syphilitic 093.89
  tibial vein 451.19
  ulcer, ulcerative 451.9
    leg 451.2
      deep (vessels) 451.19
        femoral vein 451.11
        specified vessel NEC 451.19
      superficial (vessels) 451.0
        femoral vein 451.11
    lower extremity 451.2
      deep (vessels) 451.19
        femoral vein 451.11
        specified vessel NEC 451.19
      superficial (vessels) 451.0
  ulnar vein 451.83
  umbilicus 451.89
  upper extremity—*see* Phlebitis, arm
  uterus (septic) (*see also* Endometritis) 615.9
  varicose (leg) (lower extremity) (*see also*
    Varicose, vein) 454.1
Phlebofibrosis 459.89
Phleboliths 459.89
Phlebosclerosis 459.89
Phlebothrombosis —*see* Thrombosis
Phlebotomus fever 066.0
Phlegm, choked on 933.1
Phlegmasia
  alba dolens (deep vessels) 451.19
    complicating pregnancy 671.3
    nonpuerperal 451.19
    puerperal, postpartum, childbirth 671.4
  cerulea dolens 451.19
Phlegmon (*see also* Abscess) 682.9
  erysipelatous (*see also* Erysipelas) 035
  iliac 682.2
    fossa 540.1
  throat 478.29
Phlegmonous —*see* condition
Phlyctenulosis (allergic) (keratoconjunctivitis)
  (nontuberculous) 370.31
  cornea 370.31
    with ulcer (*see also* Ulcer, cornea) 370.00
  tuberculous (*see also* Tuberculosis) 017.3
    [370.31]
Phobia, phobic (reaction) 300.20
  animal 300.29
  isolated NEC 300.29
  obsessional 300.3
  simple NEC 300.29
  social 300.23
  specified NEC 300.29
  state 300.20
Phocas' disease 610.1
Phocomelia 755.4
  lower limb 755.32
    complete 755.33
    distal 755.35
    proximal 755.34
  upper limb 755.22
    complete 755.23
    distal 755.25
    proximal 755.24
Phoria (*see also* Heterophoria) 378.40

Phosphate-losing tubular disorder 588.0
Phosphatemia 275.3
Phosphaturia 275.3
Photoallergic response **692.72**
Photocoproporphyria 277.1
Photodermatitis (sun) 692.72
  light other than sun 692.82
Photokeratitis 370.24
Photo-ophthalmia 370.24
Photophobia 368.13
Photopsia 368.15
Photoretinitis 363.31
Photoretinopathy 363.31
Photosensitiveness (sun) 692.72
  light other than sun 692.82
Photosensitization (sun) skin 692.72
  light other than sun 692.82
Phototoxic response **692.72**
Phrenitis 323.9
Phrynoderma 264.8
Phthiriasis (pubis) (any site) 132.2
  with any infestation classifiable to 132.0
    and 132.1 132.3
Phthirus infestation —*see* Phthiriasis
Phthisis (*see also* Tuberculosis) 011.9
  bulbi (infectional) 360.41
  colliers' 011.4
  cornea 371.05
  eyeball (due to infection) 360.41
  millstone makers' 011.4
  miners' 011.4
  potters' 011.4
  sandblasters' 011.4
  stonemasons' 011.4
Phycomycosis 117.7
Physalopteriasis 127.7
Physical therapy NEC V57.1
  breathing exercises V57.0
Physiological cup, optic papilla
  borderline, glaucoma suspect 365.00
  enlarged 377.14
  glaucomatous 377.14
Phytobezoar 938
  intestine 936
  stomach 935.2
Pian (*see also* Yaws) 102.9
Pianoma 102.1
Piarhemia, piarrhemia (*see also* Hyperlipemia)
  272.4
  bilharziasis 120.9
Pica 307.52
  hysterical 300.11
Pick's
  cerebral atrophy 331.11
    with dementia
      with behavioral disturbance 331.11 *[294.11]*
      without behavioral disturbance 331.11
        [294.10]
  disease
    brain 331.11
      dementia in
        with behavioral disturbance 331.11
          [294.11]
        without behavioral disturbance 331.11
          [294.10]
    lipid histiocytosis 272.7
    liver (pericardial pseudocirrhosis of liver)
      423.2
    pericardium (pericardial pseudocirrhosis of
      liver) 423.2

Pick's—*continued*
  polyserositis (pericardial pseudocirrhosis of
    liver) 423.2
  syndrome
    heart (pericardial pseudocirrhosis of liver)
      423.2
    liver (pericardial pseudocirrhosis of liver)
      423.2
  tubular adenoma (M8640/0)
    specified site—*see* Neoplasm, by site, benign
    unspecified site
      female 220
      male 222.0
Pick-Herxheimer syndrome (diffuse idiopathic
  cutaneous atrophy) 701.8
Pick-Niemann disease (lipid histiocytosis) 272.7
Pickwickian syndrome (cardiopulmonary
  obesity) 278.03
Piebaldism, classic 709.09
Piedra 111.2
  beard 111.2
    black 111.3
    white 111.2
  black 111.3
  scalp 111.3
    black 111.3
    white 111.2
  white 111.2
Pierre Marie's syndrome (pulmonary
  hypertrophic osteoarthropathy) 731.2
Pierre Marie-Bamberger syndrome
  (hypertrophic pulmonary osteoarthropathy)
  731.2
Pierre Mauriac's syndrome
  (diabetes-dwarfism-obesity) 258.1
Pierre Robin deformity or syndrome
  (congenital) 756.0
Pierson's disease or osteochondrosis 732.1
Pigeon
  breast or chest (acquired) 738.3
    congenital 754.82
    rachitic (*see also* Rickets) 268.0
  breeders' disease or lung 495.2
  fanciers' disease or lung 495.2
  toe 735.8
Pigmentation (abnormal) 709.00
  anomaly 709.00
    congenital 757.33
    specified NEC 709.09
  conjunctiva 372.55
  cornea 371.10
    anterior 371.11
    posterior 371.13
    stromal 371.12
  lids (congenital) 757.33
    acquired 374.52
  limbus corneae 371.10
  metals 709.00
  optic papilla, congenital 743.57
  retina (congenital) (grouped) (nevoid) 743.53
    acquired 362.74
  scrotum, congenital 757.33
Piles —*see* Hemorrhoids
Pili
  annulati or torti (congenital) 757.4
  incarnati 704.8
Pill roller hand (intrinsic) 736.09
Pilomatrixoma (M8110/0)—*see* Neoplasm, skin,
  benign
Pilonidal —*see* condition
Pimple 709.8

PIN I (prostatic intraepithelial neoplasia I)
　602.3
PIN II (prostatic intraepithelial neoplasia II)
　602.3
PIN III (prostatic intraepithelial neoplasia III)
　233.4
Pinched nerve —*see* Neuropathy, entrapment
Pineal body or gland —*see* condition
Pinealoblastoma (M9362/3) 194.4
Pinealoma (M9360/1) 237.1
　malignant (M9360/3) 194.4
Pineoblastoma (M9362/3) 194.4
Pineocytoma (M9361/1) 237.1
Pinguecula 372.51
Pingueculitis 372.34
Pinhole meatus (*see also* Stricture, urethra) 598.9
Pink
　disease 985.0
　eye 372.03
　puffer 492.8
Pinkus' disease (lichen nitidus) 697.1
Pinpoint
　meatus (*see also* Stricture, urethra) 598.9
　os (uteri) (*see also* Stricture, cervix) 622.4
Pinselhaare (congenital) 757.4
Pinta 103.9
　cardiovascular lesions 103.2
　chancre (primary) 103.0
　erythematous plaques 103.1
　hyperchromic lesions 103.1
　hyperkeratosis 103.1
　lesions 103.9
　　cardiovascular 103.2
　　hyperchromic 103.1
　　intermediate 103.1
　　late 103.2
　　mixed 103.3
　　primary 103.0
　　skin (achromic) (cicatricial) (dyschromic)
　　　103.2
　　　hyperchromic 103.1
　　　mixed (achromic and hyperchromic) 103.3
　papule (primary) 103.0
　skin lesions (achromic) (cicatricial)
　　(dyschromic) 103.2
　　hyperchromic 103.1
　　mixed (achromic and hyperchromic) 103.3
　vitiligo 103.2
Pintid 103.0
Pinworms (disease) (infection) (infestation)
　127.4
Piry fever 066.8
Pistol wound —*see* Gunshot wound
Pit, lip (mucus), congenital 750.25
Pitchers' elbow 718.82
Pithecoid pelvis 755.69
　with disproportion (fetopelvic) 653.2
　　affecting fetus or newborn 763.1
　　causing obstructed labor 660.1
Pithiatism 300.11
Pitted —*see also* Pitting
　teeth 520.4
Pitting (edema) (*see also* Edema) 782.3
　lip 782.3
　nail 703.8
　　congenital 757.5
Pituitary gland —*see* condition
Pituitary snuff-takers' disease 495.8

Pityriasis 696.5
　alba 696.5
　capitis 690.11
　circinata (et maculata) 696.3
　Hebra's (exfoliative dermatitis) 695.89
　lichenoides et varioliformis 696.2
　maculata (et circinata) 696.3
　nigra 111.1
　pilaris 757.39
　　acquired 701.1
　　Hebra's 696.4
　rosea 696.3
　rotunda 696.3
　rubra (Hebra) 695.89
　　pilaris 696.4
　sicca 690.18
　simplex 690.18
　specified type NEC 696.5
　streptogenes 696.5
　versicolor 111.0
　　scrotal 111.0
Placenta, placental
　ablatio 641.2
　　affecting fetus or newborn 762.1
　abnormal, abnormality 656.7
　　with hemorrhage 641.8
　　　affecting fetus or newborn 762.1
　　affecting fetus or newborn 762.2
　abruptio 641.2
　　affecting fetus or newborn 762.1
　accessory lobe—*see* Placenta, abnormal
　accreta (without hemorrhage) 667.0
　　with hemorrhage 666.0
　adherent (without hemorrhage) 667.0
　　with hemorrhage 666.0
　apoplexy—*see* Placenta, separation
　battledore—*see* Placenta, abnormal
　bilobate—*see* Placenta, abnormal
　bipartita—*see* Placenta, abnormal
　carneous mole 631.8
　centralis—*see* Placenta, previa
　circumvallata—*see* Placenta, abnormal
　cyst (amniotic)—*see* Placenta, abnormal
　deficiency—*see* Placenta, insufficiency
　degeneration—*see* Placenta, insufficiency
　detachment (partial) (premature) (with
　　hemorrhage) 641.2
　　affecting fetus or newborn 762.1
　dimidiata—*see* Placenta, abnormal
　disease 656.7
　　affecting fetus or newborn 762.2
　duplex—*see* Placenta, abnormal
　dysfunction—*see* Placenta, insufficiency
　fenestrata—*see* Placenta, abnormal
　fibrosis—*see* Placenta, abnormal
　fleshy mole 631.8
　hematoma—*see* Placenta, abnormal
　hemorrhage NEC—*see* Placenta, separation
　hormone disturbance or malfunction—*see*
　　Placenta, abnormal
　hyperplasia—*see* Placenta, abnormal
　increta (without hemorrhage) 667.0
　　with hemorrhage 666.0
　infarction 656.7
　　affecting fetus or newborn 762.2
　insertion, vicious—*see* Placenta, previa
　insufficiency
　　affecting
　　　fetus or newborn 762.2
　　　management of pregnancy 656.5
　lateral—*see* Placenta, previa

Placenta, placental—*continued*
  low implantation or insertion—*see* Placenta, previa
  low-lying—*see* Placenta, previa
  malformation—*see* Placenta, abnormal
  malposition—*see* Placenta, previa
  marginalis, marginata—*see* Placenta, previa
  marginal sinus (hemorrhage) (rupture) 641.2
    affecting fetus or newborn 762.1
  membranacea—*see* Placenta, abnormal
  multilobed—*see* Placenta, abnormal
  multipartita—*see* Placenta, abnormal
  necrosis—*see* Placenta, abnormal
  percreta (without hemorrhage) 667.0
    with hemorrhage 666.0
  polyp 674.4
  previa (central) (centralis) (complete) (lateral) (marginal) (marginalis) (partial) (partialis) (total) (with hemorrhage) 641.1
    affecting fetus or newborn 762.0
    noted
      before labor, without hemorrhage (with cesarean delivery) 641.0
      during pregnancy (without hemorrhage) 641.0
    without hemorrhage (before labor and delivery) (during pregnancy) 641.0
  retention (with hemorrhage) 666.0
    fragments, complicating puerperium (delayed hemorrhage) 666.2
      without hemorrhage 667.1
    postpartum, puerperal 666.2
      without hemorrhage 667.0
  separation (normally implanted) (partial) (premature) (with hemorrhage) 641.2
    affecting fetus or newborn 762.1
  septuplex—*see* Placenta, abnormal
  small—*see* Placenta, insufficiency
  softening (premature)—*see* Placenta, abnormal
  spuria—*see* Placenta, abnormal
  succenturiata—*see* Placenta, abnormal
  syphilitic 095.8
  transfusion syndromes 762.3
  transmission of chemical substance—*see* Absorption, chemical, through placenta
  trapped (with hemorrhage) 666.0
    without hemorrhage 667.0
  trilobate—*see* Placenta, abnormal
  tripartita—*see* Placenta, abnormal
  triplex—*see* Placenta, abnormal
  varicose vessel—*see* Placenta, abnormal
  vicious insertion—*see* Placenta, previa
Placentitis
  affecting fetus or newborn 762.7
  complicating pregnancy 658.4
Plagiocephaly (skull) 754.0
Plague 020.9
  abortive 020.8
  ambulatory 020.8
  bubonic 020.0
  cellulocutaneous 020.1
  lymphatic gland 020.0
  pneumonic 020.5
    primary 020.3
    secondary 020.4
  pulmonary—*see* Plague, pneumonic
  pulmonic—*see* Plague, pneumonic
  septicemic 020.2
  tonsillar 020.9
    septicemic 020.2
  vaccination, prophylactic (against) V03.3

Planning, family V25.09
  contraception V25.9
  natural
    procreative V26.41
    to avoid pregnancy V25.04
  procreation V26.49
    natural V26.41
Plaque
  artery, arterial—*see* Arteriosclerosis
  calcareous—*see* Calcification
  Hollenhorst's (retinal) 362.33
  tongue 528.6
Plasma cell myeloma 203.0
Plasmacytoma, plasmocytoma (solitary) (M9731/1) 238.6
  benign (M9731/0)—*see* Neoplasm, by site, benign
  malignant (M9731/3) 203.8
Plasmacytopenia 288.59
Plasmacytosis 288.64
Plaster ulcer (*see also* Ulcer, pressure) 707.00
Plateau iris syndrome (without glaucoma) 364.82
  with glaucoma 365.23
Platybasia 756.0
Platyonychia (congenital) 757.5
  acquired 703.8
Platypelloid pelvis 738.6
  with disproportion (fetopelvic) 653.2
    affecting fetus or newborn 763.1
    causing obstructed labor 660.1
      affecting fetus or newborn 763.1
  congenital 755.69
Platyspondylia 756.19
Plethora 782.62
  newborn 776.4
Pleura, pleural —*see* condition
Pleuralgia 786.52
Pleurisy (acute) (adhesive) (chronic) (costal) (diaphragmatic) (double) (dry) (fetid) (fibrinous) (fibrous) (interlobar) (latent) (lung) (old) (plastic) (primary) (residual) (sicca) (sterile) (subacute) (unresolved) (with adherent pleura) 511.0
  with
    effusion (without mention of cause) 511.9
      bacterial, nontuberculous 511.1
      nontuberculous NEC 511.9
        bacterial 511.1
      pneumococcal 511.1
      specified type NEC 511.89
      staphylococcal 511.1
      streptococcal 511.1
      tuberculous (*see also* Tuberculosis, pleura) 012.0
        primary, progressive 010.1
    influenza, flu, or grippe (*see also* Influenza) 487.1
    tuberculosis—*see* Pleurisy, tuberculous
  encysted 511.89
  exudative (*see also* Pleurisy, with effusion) 511.9
    bacterial, nontuberculous 511.1
  fibrinopurulent 510.9
    with fistula 510.0
  fibropurulent 510.9
    with fistula 510.0
  hemorrhagic 511.89
  influenzal (*see also* Influenza) 487.1
  pneumococcal 511.0
    with effusion 511.1

Pleurisy—*continued*
  purulent 510.9
    with fistula 510.0
  septic 510.9
    with fistula 510.0
  serofibrinous (*see also* Pleurisy, with effusion) 511.9
    bacterial, nontuberculous 511.1
  seropurulent 510.9
    with fistula 510.0
  serous (*see also* Pleurisy, with effusion) 511.9
    bacterial, nontuberculous 511.1
  staphylococcal 511.0
    with effusion 511.1
  streptococcal 511.0
    with effusion 511.1
  suppurative 510.9
    with fistula 510.0
  traumatic (post) (current) 862.29
    with open wound into cavity 862.39
  tuberculous (with effusion) (*see also*
      Tuberculosis, pleura) 012.0
    primary, progressive 010.1
Pleuritis sicca —*see* Pleurisy
Pleurobronchopneumonia (*see also* Pneumonia,
    broncho-) 485
Pleurodynia 786.52
  epidemic 074.1
  viral 074.1
Pleurohepatitis 573.8
Pleuropericarditis (*see also* Pericarditis) 423.9
  acute 420.90
Pleuropneumonia (acute) (bilateral) (double)
    (septic) (*see also* Pneumonia) 486
  chronic (*see also* Fibrosis, lung) 515
Pleurorrhea (*see also* Hydrothorax) 511.89
Plexitis, brachial 353.0
Plica
  knee 727.83
  polonica 132.0
  tonsil 474.8
Plicae dysphonia ventricularis 784.49
Plicated tongue 529.5
  congenital 750.13
Plug
  bronchus NEC 519.19
  meconium (newborn) NEC 777.1
  mucus—*see* Mucus, plug
Plumbism 984.9
  specified type of lead—*see* Table of drugs and
    chemicals
Plummer's disease (toxic nodular goiter) 242.3
Plummer-Vinson syndrome (sideropenic
    dysphagia) 280.8
Pluricarential syndrome of infancy 260
Plurideficiency syndrome of infancy 260
Plus (and minus) hand (intrinsic) 736.09
PMDD (premenstrual dysphoric disorder)
    625.4
PMS 625.4
Pneumathemia —*see* Air, embolism, by type
Pneumatic drill or hammer disease 994.9
Pneumatocele (lung) 518.89
  intracranial 348.89
  tension 492.0
Pneumatosis
  cystoides intestinalis 569.89
  peritonei 568.89
  pulmonum 492.8
Pneumaturia 599.84
Pneumoblastoma (M8981/3)—*see* Neoplasm,
    lung, malignant

Pneumocephalus 348.89
Pneumococcemia 038.2
Pneumococcus, pneumococcal —*see* condition
Pneumoconiosis (due to) (inhalation of) 505
  aluminum 503
  asbestos 501
  bagasse 495.1
  bauxite 503
  beryllium 503
  carbon electrode makers' 503
  coal
    miners' (simple) 500
    workers' (simple) 500
  cotton dust 504
  diatomite fibrosis 502
  dust NEC 504
    inorganic 503
    lime 502
    marble 502
    organic NEC 504
  fumes or vapors (from silo) 506.9
  graphite 503
  hard metal 503
  mica 502
  moldy hay 495.0
  rheumatoid 714.81
  silica NEC 502
    and carbon 500
  silicate NEC 502
  talc 502
Pneumocystis carinii pneumonia 136.3
Pneumocystis jiroveci pneumonia 136.3
Pneumocystosis 136.3
  with pneumonia 136.3
Pneumoenteritis 025
Pneumohemopericardium (*see also* Pericarditis)
    423.9
Pneumohemothorax (*see also* Hemothorax)
    511.89
  traumatic 860.4
    with open wound into thorax 860.5
Pneumohydropericardium (*see also*
    Pericarditis) 423.9
Pneumohydrothorax (*see also* Hydrothorax)
    511.89
Pneumomediastinum 518.1
  congenital 770.2
  fetus or newborn 770.2
Pneumomycosis 117.9
Pneumonia (acute) (Alpenstich) (benign)
    (bilateral) (brain) (cerebral) (circumscribed)
    (congestive) (creeping) (delayed resolution)
    (double) (epidemic) (fever) (flash) (fulminant)
    (fungoid) (granulomatous) (hemorrhagic)
    (incipient) (infantile) (infectious) (infiltration)
    (insular) (intermittent) (latent) (lobe)
    (migratory) (newborn) (organized)
    (overwhelming) (primary) (progressive)
    (pseudolobar) (purulent) (resolved)
    (secondary) (senile) (septic) (suppurative)
    (terminal) (true) (unresolved) (vesicular) 486
  with influenza, flu, or grippe 487.0
    due to
      identified (virus)
        avian 488.01
        (novel) 2009 H1N1 488.11
      novel influenza A 488.81
  adenoviral 480.0
  adynamic 514
  alba 090.0
  allergic 518.3

Pneumonia—*continued*
  alveolar—*see* Pneumonia, lobar
  anaerobes 482.81
  anthrax 022.1 *[484.5]*
  apex, apical—*see* Pneumonia, lobar
  ascaris 127.0 *[484.8]*
  aspiration 507.0
    due to
      aspiration of microorganisms
        bacterial 482.9
          specified type NEC 482.89
        specified organism NEC 483.8
          bacterial NEC 482.89
        viral 480.9
          specified type NEC 480.8
      food (regurgitated) 507.0
      gastric secretions 507.0
      milk 507.0
      oils, essences 507.1
      solids, liquids NEC 507.8
      vomitus 507.0
    fetal 770.18
      due to
        blood 770.16
        clear amniotic fluid 770.14
        meconium 770.12
        postnatal stomach contents 770.86
    newborn 770.18
      due to
        blood 770.16
        clear amniotic fluid 770.14
        meconium 770.12
        postnatal stomach contents 770.86
  asthenic 514
  atypical (disseminated, focal) (primary) 486
    with influenza (*see also* Influenza) 487.0
  bacillus 482.9
    specified type NEC 482.89
  bacterial 482.9
    specified type NEC 482.89
  Bacteroides (fragilis) (oralis) (melaninogenicus)
    482.81
  basal, basic, basilar—*see* Pneumonia, by type
  bronchiolitis obliterans organized (BOOP) 516.8
  broncho-, bronchial (confluent) (croupous)
    (diffuse) (disseminated) (hemorrhagic)
    (involving lobes) (lobar) (terminal) 485
    with influenza 487.0
    due to
      identified (virus)
        avian 488.01
        (novel) 2009 H1N1 488.11
      novel influenza A 488.81
    allergic 518.3
    aspiration (*see also* Pneumonia, aspiration)
      507.0
    bacterial 482.9
      specified type NEC 482.89
    capillary 466.19
      with bronchospasm or obstruction 466.19
    chronic (*see also* Fibrosis, lung) 515
    congenital (infective) 770.0
    diplococcal 481
    Eaton's agent 483.0
    Escherichia coli (E. coli) 482.82
    Friedländer's bacillus 482.0
    Hemophilus influenzae 482.2
    hiberno-vernal 083.0 *[484.8]*
    hypostatic 514
    influenzal (*see also* Influenza) 487.0
    inhalation (*see also* Pneumonia, aspiration) 507.0
      due to fumes or vapors (chemical) 506.0

Pneumonia—*continued*
  broncho, bronchial—*continued*
    Klebsiella 482.0
    lipid 507.1
      endogenous 516.8
    Mycoplasma (pneumoniae) 483.0
    ornithosis 073.0
    pleuropneumonia-like organisms (PPLO) 483.0
    pneumococcal 481
    Proteus 482.83
    pseudomonas 482.1
    specified organism NEC 483.8
      bacterial NEC 482.89
    staphylococcal 482.40
      aureus 482.41
        methicillin
          resistant (MRSA) 482.42
          susceptible (MSSA) 482.41
      specified type NEC 482.49
    streptococcal—*see* Pneumonia, streptococcal
    typhoid 002.0 *[484.8]*
    viral, virus (*see also* Pneumonia, viral) 480.9
  Butyrivibrio (fibrisolvens) 482.81
  Candida 112.4
  capillary 466.19
    with bronchospasm or obstruction 466.19
  caseous (*see also* Tuberculosis) 011.6
  catarrhal—*see* Pneumonia, broncho-
  central—*see* Pneumonia, lobar
  Chlamydia, chlamydial 483.1
    pneumoniae 483.1
    psittaci 073.0
    specified type NEC 483.1
    trachomatis 483.1
  cholesterol 516.8
  chronic (*see also* Fibrosis, lung) 515
  cirrhotic (chronic) (*see also* Fibrosis, lung) 515
  Clostridium (haemolyticum) (novyi) NEC
    482.81
  confluent—*see* Pneumonia, broncho-
  congenital (infective) 770.0
    aspiration 770.18
  croupous—*see* Pneumonia, lobar
  cryptogenic organizing 516.36
  cytomegalic inclusion 078.5 *[484.1]*
  deglutition (*see also* Pneumonia, aspiration)
    507.0
  desquamative interstitial 516.37
  diffuse—*see* Pneumonia, broncho-
  diplococcal, diplococcus (broncho-) (lobar) 481
  disseminated (focal)—*see* Pneumonia, broncho-
  due to
    adenovirus 480.0
    Bacterium anitratum 482.83
    Chlamydia, chlamydial 483.1
      pneumoniae 483.1
      psittaci 073.0
      specified type NEC 483.1
      trachomatis 483.1
    coccidioidomycosis 114.0
    Diplococcus (pneumoniae) 481
    Eaton's agent 483.0
    Escherichia coli (E. coli) 482.82
    Friedländer's bacillus 482.0
    fumes or vapors (chemical) (inhalation) 506.0
    fungus NEC 117.9 *[484.7]*
      coccidioidomycosis 114.0
    Hemophilus influenzae (H. influenzae) 482.2
    Herellea 482.83
    influenza (*see also* Influenza) 487.0
    Klebsiella pneumoniae 482.0
    Mycoplasma (pneumoniae) 483.0

Pneumonia—*continued*
  due to—*continued*
    parainfluenza virus 480.2
    pleuropneumonia-like organism (PPLO) 483.0
    Pneumococcus 481
    Pneumocystis carinii 136.3
    Pneumocystis jiroveci 136.3
    Proteus 482.83
    pseudomonas 482.1
    respiratory syncytial virus 480.1
    rickettsia 083.9 *[484.8]*
    SARS-associated coronavirus 480.3
    specified
      bacteria NEC 482.89
      organism NEC 483.8
      virus NEC 480.8
    Staphylococcus 482.40
      aureus 482.41
        methicillin
          resistant (MRSA) 482.42
          susceptible (MSSA) 482.41
      specified type NEC 482.49
    Streptococcus—*see also* Pneumonia,
      streptococcal
    pneumoniae 481
    virus (*see also* Pneumonia, viral) 480.9
  Eaton's agent 483.0
  embolic, embolism (*see also* Embolism,
    pulmonary) 415.1
  eosinophilic 518.3
  Escherichia coli (E. coli) 482.82
  Eubacterium 482.81
  fibrinous—*see* Pneumonia, lobar
  fibroid (chronic) (*see also* Fibrosis, lung) 515
  fibrous (*see also* Fibrosis, lung) 515
  Friedländer's bacillus 482.0
  Fusobacterium (nucleatum) 482.81
  gangrenous 513.0
  giant cell (*see also* Pneumonia, viral) 480.9
  gram-negative bacteria NEC 482.83
    anaerobic 482.81
  grippal (*see also* Influenza) 487.0
  Hemophilus influenzae (bronchial) (lobar) 482.2
  hypostatic (broncho-) (lobar) 514
  in
    actinomycosis 039.1
    anthrax 022.1 *[484.5]*
    aspergillosis 117.3 *[484.6]*
    candidiasis 112.4
    coccidioidomycosis 114.0
    cytomegalic inclusion disease 078.5 *[484.1]*
    histoplasmosis (*see also* Histoplasmosis)
      115.95
    infectious disease NEC 136.9 *[484.8]*
    measles 055.1
    mycosis, systemic NEC 117.9 *[484.7]*
    nocardiasis, nocardiosis 039.1
    ornithosis 073.0
    pneumocystosis 136.3
    psittacosis 073.0
    Q fever 083.0 *[484.8]*
    salmonellosis 003.22
    toxoplasmosis 130.4
    tularemia 021.2
    typhoid (fever) 002.0 *[484.8]*
    varicella 052.1
    whooping cough (*see also* Whooping cough)
      033.9 *[484.3]*
  infective, acquired prenatally 770.0
  influenzal (broncho) (lobar) (virus) (*see also*
    Influenza) 487.0

Pneumonia—*continued*
  inhalation (*see also* Pneumonia, aspiration) 507.0
    fumes or vapors (chemical) 506.0
  interstitial 516.8
    with influenzal (*see also* Influenza) 487.0
    acute
      due to Pneumocystis (carinii) (jiroveci)
        136.3
      meaning:
        acute interstitial pneumonitis 516.33
        atypical pneumonia—*see* Pneumonia,
          atypical
        bacterial pneumonia—*see* Pneumonia,
          bacterial
    chronic (*see also* Fibrosis, lung) 515
    desquamative 516.37
    hypostatic 514
    idiopathic 516.30
      lymphoid 516.35
    lipoid 507.1
    lymphoid (due to known underlying cause) 516.8
    non-specific (due to known underlying cause)
      516.8
    organizing (due to known underlying cause)
      516.8
    plasma cell 136.3
    pseudomonas 482.1
  intrauterine (infective) 770.0
    aspiration 770.18
      blood 770.16
      clear amniotic fluid 770.14
      meconium 770.12
      postnatal stomach contents 770.86
  Klebsiella pneumoniae 482.0
  Legionnaires' 482.84
  lipid, lipoid (exogenous) (interstitial) 507.1
    endogenous 516.8
  lobar (diplococcal) (disseminated) (double)
    (interstitial) (pneumococcal, any type) 481
    with influenza (*see also* Influenza) 487.0
    bacterial 482.9
      specified type NEC 482.89
    chronic (*see also* Fibrosis, lung) 515
    Escherichia coli (E. coli) 482.82
    Friedländer's bacillus 482.0
    Hemophilus influenzae (H. influenzae) 482.2
    hypostatic 514
    influenzal (*see also* Influenza) 487.0
    Klebsiella 482.0
    ornithosis 073.0
    Proteus 482.83
    pseudomonas 482.1
    psittacosis 073.0
    specified organism NEC 483.8
      bacterial NEC 482.89
    staphylococcal 482.40
      aureus 482.41
        methicillin
          resistant (MRSA) 482.42
          susceptible (MSSA) 482.41
      specified type NEC 482.49
    streptococcal—*see* Pneumonia, streptococcal
    viral, virus (*see also* Pneumonia, viral) 480.9
  lobular (confluent)—*see* Pneumonia, broncho-
  Löffler's 518.3
  massive—*see* Pneumonia, lobar
  meconium aspiration 770.12
  metastatic NEC 038.8 *[484.8]*
  methicillin resistant Staphylococcus aureus
    (MRSA) 482.42
  methicillin susceptible Staphylococcus aureus
    (MSSA) 482.41

Pneumonia—*continued*
  MRSA (methicillin resistant Staphylococcus
    aureus) 482.42
  MSSA (methicillin susceptible Staphylococcus
    aureus) 482.41
  multilobar —*see* Pneumonia, by type
  Mycoplasma (pneumoniae) 483.0
  necrotic 513.0
  nitrogen dioxide 506.9
  orthostatic 514
  parainfluenza virus 480.2
  parenchymatous (*see also* Fibrosis, lung) 515
  passive 514
  patchy—*see* Pneumonia, broncho
  Peptococcus 482.81
  Peptostreptococcus 482.81
  plasma cell 136.3
  pleurolobar—*see* Pneumonia, lobar
  pleuropneumonia-like organism (PPLO) 483.0
  pneumococcal (broncho) (lobar) 481
  Pneumocystis (carinii) (jiroveci) 136.3
  postinfectional NEC 136.9 *[484.8]*
  postmeasles 055.1
  postoperative 997.39
    aspiration 997.32
  primary atypical 486
  Proprionibacterium 482.81
  Proteus 482.83
  pseudomonas 482.1
  psittacosis 073.0
  radiation 508.0
  respiratory syncytial virus 480.1
  resulting from a procedure 997.39
    aspiration 997.32
  rheumatic 390 *[517.1]*
  Salmonella 003.22
  SARS-associated coronavirus 480.3
  segmented, segmental—*see* Pneumonia,
    broncho-
  Serratia (marcescens) 482.83
  specified
    bacteria NEC 482.89
    organism NEC 483.8
    virus NEC 480.8
  spirochetal 104.8 *[484.8]*
  staphylococcal (broncho) (lobar) 482.40
    aureus 482.41
      methicillin
        resistant (MRSA) 482.42
        susceptible (MSSA) 482.41
    specified type NEC 482.49
  static, stasis 514
  streptococcal (broncho) (lobar) NEC 482.30
    Group
      A 482.31
      B 482.32
      specified NEC 482.39
    pneumoniae 481
    specified type NEC 482.39
  Streptococcus pneumoniae 481
  traumatic (complication) (early) (secondary) 958.8
  tuberculous (any) (*see also* Tuberculosis) 011.6
  tularemic 021.2
  TWAR agent 483.1
  varicella 052.1
  Veillonella 482.81
  ventilator associated 997.31

Pneumonia—*continued*
  viral, virus (broncho) (interstitial) (lobar) 480.9
    with influenza, flu, or grippe (*see also*
      Influenza) 487.0
    adenoviral 480.0
    parainfluenza 480.2
    respiratory syncytial 480.1
    SARS-associated coronavirus 480.3
    specified type NEC 480.8
  white (congenital) 090.0
Pneumonic —*see* condition
Pneumonitis (acute) (primary) (*see also*
    Pneumonia) 486
  allergic 495.9
    specified type NEC 495.8
  aspiration 507.0
    due to fumes or gases 506.0
    fetal 770.18
      due to
        blood 770.16
        clear amniotic fluid 770.14
        meconium 770.12
        postnatal stomach contents 770.86
    newborn 770.18
      due to
        blood 770.16
        clear amniotic fluid 770.14
        meconium 770.12
        postnatal stomach contents 770.86
    obstetric 668.0
  chemical 506.0
    due to fumes or gases 506.0
    resulting from a procedure 997.32
  cholesterol 516.8
  chronic (*see also* Fibrosis, lung) 515
  congenital rubella 771.0
  crack 506.0
  due to
    crack (cocaine) 506.0
    fumes or vapors 506.0
    inhalation
      food (regurgitated), milk, vomitus 507.0
      oils, essences 507.1
      saliva 507.0
      solids, liquids NEC 507.8
    toxoplasmosis (acquired) 130.4
      congenital (active) 771.2 *[484.8]*
  eosinophilic 518.3
  fetal aspiration 770.18
    due to
      blood 770.16
      clear amniotic fluid 770.14
      meconium 770.12
      postnatal stomach contents 770.86
  hypersensitivity 495.9
  interstitial (chronic) (*see also* Fibrosis, lung) 515
    acute 516.33
    idiopathic
      lymphocytic 516.35
      non-specific 516.32
    lymphoid 516.8
  lymphoid, interstitial 516.8
  meconium aspiration 770.12
  postanesthetic
    correct substance properly administered 507.0
    obstetric 668.0
    overdose or wrong substance given 968.4
      specified anesthetic—*see* Table of drugs and
        chemicals
  postoperative 997.3
    aspiration 997.32
    obstetric 668.0

Pneumonitis—*continued*
  radiation 508.0
  rubella, congenital 771.0
  "ventilation" 495.7
  ventilator associated 997.31
  wood-dust 495.8
Pneumonoconiosis —*see* Pneumoconiosis
Pneumoparotid 527.8
Pneumopathy NEC 518.89
  alveolar 516.9
    specified NEC 516.8
  due to dust NEC 504
  parietoalveolar 516.9
    specified condition NEC 516.8
Pneumopericarditis (*see also* Pericarditis) 423.9
  acute 420.90
Pneumopericardium —*see also* Pericarditis
  congenital 770.2
  fetus or newborn 770.2
  traumatic (post) (*see also* Pneumothorax,
    traumatic) 860.0
    with open wound into thorax 860.1
Pneumoperitoneum 568.89
  fetus or newborn 770.2
Pneumophagia (psychogenic) 306.4
Pneumopleurisy, pneumopleuritis (*see also*
  Pneumonia) 486
Pneumopyopericardium 420.99
Pneumopyothorax (*see also* Pyopneumothorax)
  510.9
  with fistula 510.0
Pneumorrhagia 786.30
  newborn 770.3
  tuberculous (*see also* Tuberculosis, pulmonary)
    011.9
Pneumosiderosis (occupational) 503
Pneumothorax 512.89
  acute 512.89
  chronic 512.83
  congenital 770.2
  due to operative injury of chest wall or lung 512.1
    accidental puncture or laceration 512.1
  fetus or newborn 770.2
  iatrogenic 512.1
  postoperative 512.1
  specified type NEC 512.89
  spontaneous 512.89
    fetus or newborn 770.2
    primary 512.81
    secondary 512.82
    tension 512.0
  sucking 512.89
    iatrogenic 512.1
    postoperative 512.1
  tense valvular, infectional 512.0
  tension 512.0
    iatrogenic 512.1
    postoperative 512.1
    spontaneous 512.0
  traumatic 860.0
    with
      hemothorax 860.4
        with open wound into thorax 860.5
      open wound into thorax 860.1
  tuberculous (*see also* Tuberculosis) 011.7
Pocket(s)
  endocardial (*see also* Endocarditis) 424.90
  periodontal 523.8
Podagra 274.01
Podencephalus 759.89
Poikilocytosis 790.09

Poikiloderma 709.09
  Civatte's 709.09
  congenital 757.33
  vasculare atrophicans 696.2
Poikilodermatomyositis 710.3
Pointed ear 744.29
Poise imperfect 729.90
Poisoned —*see* Poisoning
Poisoning (acute)—*see also* Table of Drugs and
  Chemicals
  Bacillus, B.
    aertrycke (*see also* Infection, Salmonella) 003.9
    botulinus 005.1
    cholerae (suis) (*see also* Infection,
      Salmonella) 003.9
    paratyphosus (*see also* Infection, Salmonella)
      003.9
    suipestifer (*see also* Infection, Salmonella) 003.9
  bacterial toxins NEC 005.9
  berries, noxious 988.2
  blood (general)—*see* Septicemia
  botulism 005.1
  bread, moldy, mouldy—*see* Poisoning, food
  Ciguatera 988.0
  damaged meat—*see* Poisoning, food
  death-cap (Amanita phalloides) (Amanita verna)
    988.1
  decomposed food—*see* Poisoning, food
  diseased food—*see* Poisoning, food
  drug—*see* Table of drugs and chemicals
  epidemic, fish, meat, or other food—*see*
    Poisoning, food
  fava bean 282.2
  fish (bacterial)—*see also* Poisoning, food
    noxious 988.0
  food (acute) (bacterial) (diseased) (infected)
    NEC 005.9
    due to
      Bacillus
        aertrycke (*see also* Poisoning, food, due to
          Salmonella) 003.9
        botulinus 005.1
        cereus 005.89
        choleraesuis (*see also* Poisoning, food, due
          to Salmonella) 003.9
        paratyphosus (*see also* Poisoning, food,
          due to Salmonella) 003.9
        suipestifer (*see also* Poisoning, food, due
          to Salmonella) 003.9
      Clostridium 005.3
        botulinum 005.1
        perfringens 005.2
        welchii 005.2
      Salmonella (aertrycke) (callinarum)
        (choleraesuis) (enteritidis) (paratyphi)
        (suipestifer) 003.9
        with
          gastroenteritis 003.0
          localized infection(s) (*see also* Infection,
            Salmonella) 003.20
          septicemia 003.1
          specified manifestation NEC 003.8
      specified bacterium NEC 005.89
      Staphylococcus 005.0
      Streptococcus 005.8
      Vibrio parahaemolyticus 005.4
      Vibrio vulnificus 005.81
    noxious or naturally toxic 988.0
      berries 988.2
      fish 988.0
      mushroom 988.1
      plants NEC 988.2

Poisoning—*continued*
  ice cream—*see* Poisoning, food
  ichthyotoxism (bacterial) 005.9
  kreotoxism, food 005.9
  malarial—*see* Malaria
  meat—*see* Poisoning, food
  mushroom (noxious) 988.1
  mussel—*see also* Poisoning, food
    noxious 988.0
  noxious foodstuffs (*see also* Poisoning, food, noxious) 988.9
    specified type NEC 988.8
  plants, noxious 988.2
  pork—*see also* Poisoning, food
    specified NEC 988.8
    Trichinosis 124
  ptomaine—*see* Poisoning, food
  putrefaction, food—*see* Poisoning, food
  radiation 508.0
  Salmonella (*see also* Infection, Salmonella) 003.9
  sausage—*see also* Poisoning, food
    Trichinosis 124
  saxitoxin 988.0
  shellfish—*see also* Poisoning, food
    noxious (amnesic) (azaspiracid) (diarrheic) (neurotoxic) (paralytic) 988.0
  Staphylococcus, food 005.0
  toxic, from disease NEC 799.89
  truffles—*see* Poisoning, food
  uremic—*see* Uremia
  uric acid 274.9
  water 276.69
Poison ivy, oak, sumac or other plant dermatitis 692.6
Poker spine 720.0
Policeman's disease 729.2
Polioencephalitis (acute) (bulbar) (*see also* Poliomyelitis, bulbar) 045.0
  inferior 335.22
  influenzal (*see also* Influenza) 487.8
  superior hemorrhagic (acute) (Wernicke's) 265.1
  Wernicke's (superior hemorrhagic) 265.1
Polioencephalomyelitis (acute) (anterior) (bulbar) (*see also* Polioencephalitis) 045.0
Polioencephalopathy, superior hemorrhagic 265.1
  with
    beriberi 265.0
    pellagra 265.2
Poliomeningoencephalitis —*see* Meningoencephalitis
Poliomyelitis (acute) (anterior) (epidemic) 045.9

Note—Use the following fifth-digit subclassification with category 045:

0 poliovirus, unspecified type
1 poliovirus, type I
2 poliovirus, type II
3 poliovirus, type III

  with
    paralysis 045.1
      bulbar 045.0
  abortive 045.2
  ascending 045.9
    progressive 045.9
  bulbar 045.0
  cerebral 045.0
  chronic 335.21

Poliomyelitis—*continued*
  congenital 771.2
  contact V01.2
  deformities 138
  exposure to V01.2
  late effect 138
  nonepidemic 045.9
  nonparalytic 045.2
  old with deformity 138
  posterior, acute 053.19
  residual 138
  sequelae 138
  spinal, acute 045.9
  syphilitic (chronic) 094.89
  vaccination, prophylactic (against) V04.0
Poliosis (eyebrow) (eyelashes) 704.3
  circumscripta (congenital) 757.4
    acquired 704.3
  congenital 757.4
Pollakiuria 788.41
  psychogenic 306.53
Pollinosis 477.0
Pollitzer's disease (hidradenitis suppurativa) 705.83
Polyadenitis (*see also* Adenitis) 289.3
  malignant 020.0
Polyalgia 729.99
Polyangiitis (essential) 446.0
Polyarteritis (nodosa) (renal) 446.0
Polyarthralgia 719.49
  psychogenic 306.0
Polyarthritis, polyarthropathy NEC 716.59
  due to or associated with other specified conditions—*see* Arthritis, due to or associated with
  endemic (*see also* Disease, Kaschin-Beck) 716.0
  inflammatory 714.9
    specified type NEC 714.89
  juvenile (chronic) 714.30
    acute 714.31
  migratory—*see* Fever, rheumatic
  rheumatic 714.0
    fever (acute)—*see* Fever, rheumatic
Polycarential syndrome of infancy 260
Polychondritis (atrophic) (chronic) (relapsing) 733.99
Polycoria 743.46
Polycystic (congenital) (disease) 759.89
  degeneration, kidney—*see* Polycystic, kidney
  kidney (congenital) 753.12
    adult type (APKD) 753.13
    autosomal dominant 753.13
    autosomal recessive 753.14
    childhood type (CPKD) 753.14
    infantile type 753.14
  liver 751.62
  lung 518.89
    congenital 748.4
  ovary, ovaries 256.4
  spleen 759.0
Polycythemia (primary) (rubra) (vera) (M9950/1) 238.4
  acquired 289.0
  benign 289.0
    familial 289.6
  due to
    donor twin 776.4
    fall in plasma volume 289.0
    high altitude 289.0
    maternal-fetal transfusion 776.4
    stress 289.0

Polycythemia—*continued*
  emotional 289.0
  erythropoietin 289.0
  familial (benign) 289.6
  Gaisböck's (hypertonica) 289.0
  high altitude 289.0
  hypertonica 289.0
  hypoxemic 289.0
  neonatorum 776.4
  nephrogenous 289.0
  relative 289.0
  secondary 289.0
  spurious 289.0
  stress 289.0
Polycytosis cryptogenica 289.0
Polydactylism, polydactyly 755.00
  fingers 755.01
  toes 755.02
Polydipsia 783.5
Polydystrophic oligophrenia 277.5
Polyembryoma (M9072/3)—*see* Neoplasm, by
  site, malignant
Polygalactia 676.6
Polyglandular
  deficiency 258.9
  dyscrasia 258.9
  dysfunction 258.9
  syndrome 258.8
Polyhydramnios (*see also* Hydramnios) 657
Polymastia 757.6
Polymenorrhea 626.2
Polymicrogyria 742.2
Polymyalgia 725
  arteritica 446.5
  rheumatica 725
Polymyositis (acute) (chronic) (hemorrhagic) 710.4
  with involvement of
    lung 710.4 *[517.8]*
    skin 710.3
  ossificans (generalisata) (progressiva) 728.19
  Wagner's (dermatomyositis) 710.3
Polyneuritis, polyneuritic (*see also*
  Polyneuropathy) 356.9
  alcoholic 357.5
    with psychosis 291.1
  cranialis 352.6
  demyelinating, chronic inflammatory (CIDP)
    357.81
  diabetic 250.6 *[357.2]*
    due to secondary diabetes 249.6 *[357.2]*
  due to lack of vitamin NEC 269.2 *[357.4]*
  endemic 265.0 *[357.4]*
  erythredema 985.0
  febrile 357.0
  hereditary ataxic 356.3
  idiopathic, acute 357.0
  infective (acute) 357.0
  nutritional 269.9 *[357.4]*
  postinfectious 357.0
Polyneuropathy (peripheral) 356.9
  alcoholic 357.5
  amyloid 277.39 *[357.4]*
  arsenical 357.7
  critical illness 357.82
  demyelinating, chronic inflammatory (CIDP)
    357.81
  diabetic 250.6 *[357.2]*
    due to secondary diabetes 249.6 *[357.2]*

Polyneuropathy—*continued*
  due to
    antitetanus serum 357.6
    arsenic 357.7
    drug or medicinal substance 357.6
      correct substance properly administered 357.6
      overdose or wrong substance given or taken
        977.9
      specified drug—*see* Table of drugs and
        chemicals
    lack of vitamin NEC 269.2 *[357.4]*
    lead 357.7
    organophosphate compounds 357.7
    pellagra 265.2 *[357.4]*
    porphyria 277.1 *[357.4]*
    serum 357.6
    toxic agent NEC 357.7
  hereditary 356.0
  idiopathic 356.9
    progressive 356.4
  in
    amyloidosis 277.39 *[357.4]*
    avitaminosis 269.2 *[357.4]*
      specified NEC 269.1 *[357.4]*
    beriberi 265.0 *[357.4]*
    collagen vascular disease NEC 710.9 *[357.1]*
    deficiency
      B-complex NEC 266.2 *[357.4]*
      vitamin B 266.9 *[357.4]*
      vitamin B_6 266.1 *[357.4]*
    diabetes 250.6 *[357.2]*
      due to secondary diabetes 249.6 *[357.2]*
    diphtheria (*see also* Diphtheria) 032.89 *[357.4]*
    disseminated lupus erythematosus 710.0 *[357.1]*
    herpes zoster 053.13
    hypoglycemia 251.2 *[357.4]*
    malignant neoplasm (M8000/3) NEC 199.1
      [357.3]
    mumps 072.72
    pellagra 265.2 *[357.4]*
    polyarteritis nodosa 446.0 *[357.1]*
    porphyria 277.1 *[357.4]*
    rheumatoid arthritis 714.0 *[357.1]*
    sarcoidosis 135 *[357.4]*
    uremia 585.9 *[357.4]*
  lead 357.7
  nutritional 269.9 *[357.4]*
    specified NEC 269.8 *[357.4]*
  postherpetic 053.13
  progressive 356.4
  sensory (hereditary) 356.2
  specified NEC 356.8
Polyonychia 757.5
Polyopia 368.2
  refractive 368.15
Polyorchism, polyorchidism (three testes)
  752.89
Polyorrhymenitis (peritoneal) (*see also*
  Polyserositis) 568.82
  pericardial 423.2
Polyostotic fibrous dysplasia 756.54
Polyotia 744.1
Polyp, polypus

> *Note*—*Polyps of organs or sites that do not
> appear in the list below should be coded to the
> residual category for diseases of the organ or
> site concerned.*

  accessory sinus 471.8
  adenoid tissue 471.0

Polyp, polypus—*continued*
  adenomatous (M8210/0)—*see also* Neoplasm,
    by site, benign
    adenocarcinoma in (M8210/3)—*see*
      Neoplasm, by site, malignant
    carcinoma in (M8210/3)—*see* Neoplasm, by
      site, malignant
    multiple (M8221/0)—*see* Neoplasm, by site,
      benign
  antrum 471.8
  anus, anal (canal) (nonadenomatous) 569.0
    adenomatous 211.4
  Bartholin's gland 624.6
  bladder (M8120/1) 236.7
  broad ligament 620.8
  cervix (uteri) 622.7
    adenomatous 219.0
    in pregnancy or childbirth 654.6
      affecting fetus or newborn 763.89
      causing obstructed labor 660.2
    mucous 622.7
    nonneoplastic 622.7
  choanal 471.0
  cholesterol 575.6
  clitoris 624.6
  colon (M8210/0) (*see also* Polyp, adenomatous)
    211.3
  corpus uteri 621.0
  dental 522.0
  ear (middle) 385.30
  endometrium 621.0
  ethmoidal (sinus) 471.8
  fallopian tube 620.8
  female genital organs NEC 624.8
  frontal (sinus) 471.8
  gallbladder 575.6
  gingiva 523.8
  gum 523.8
  labia 624.6
  larynx (mucous) 478.4
  malignant (M8000/3)—*see* Neoplasm, by site,
    malignant
  maxillary (sinus) 471.8
  middle ear 385.30
  myometrium 621.0
  nares
    anterior 471.9
    posterior 471.0
  nasal (mucous) 471.9
    cavity 471.0
    septum 471.9
  nasopharyngeal 471.0
  neoplastic (M8210/0)—*see* Neoplasm, by site,
    benign
  nose (mucous) 471.9
  oviduct 620.8
  paratubal 620.8
  pharynx 478.29
    congenital 750.29
  placenta, placental 674.4
  prostate 600.20
    with
      other lower urinary tract symptoms (LUTS)
        600.21
      urinary
        obstruction 600.21
        retention 600.21
  pudenda 624.6
  pulp (dental) 522.0
  rectosigmoid 211.4

Polyp, polypus—*continued*
  rectum (nonadenomatous) 569.0
    adenomatous 211.4
  septum (nasal) 471.9
  sinus (accessory) (ethmoidal) (frontal)
    (maxillary) (sphenoidal) 471.8
  sphenoidal (sinus) 471.8
  stomach (M8210/0) 211.1
  tube, fallopian 620.8
  turbinate, mucous membrane 471.8
  ureter 593.89
  urethra 599.3
  uterine
    ligament 620.8
    tube 620.8
  uterus (body) (corpus) (mucous) 621.0
    in pregnancy or childbirth 654.1
      affecting fetus or newborn 763.89
      causing obstructed labor 660.2
  vagina 623.7
  vocal cord (mucous) 478.4
  vulva 624.6
Polyphagia 783.6
Polypoid —*see* condition
Polyposis —*see also* Polyp
  coli (adenomatous) (M8220/0) 211.3
    adenocarcinoma in (M8220/3) 153.9
    carcinoma in (M8220/3) 153.9
  familial (M8220/0) 211.3
  intestinal (adenomatous) (M8220/0) 211.3
  multiple (M8221/0)—*see* Neoplasm, by site,
    benign
Polyradiculitis (acute) 357.0
Polyradiculoneuropathy (acute) (segmentally
  demyelinating) 357.0
Polysarcia 278.00
Polyserositis (peritoneal) 568.82
  due to pericarditis 423.2
  paroxysmal (familial) 277.31
  pericardial 423.2
  periodic (familial) 277.31
  pleural—*see* Pleurisy
  recurrent 277.31
  tuberculous (*see also* Tuberculosis,
    polyserositis) 018.9
Polysialia 527.7
Polysplenia syndrome 759.0
Polythelia 757.6
Polytrichia (*see also* Hypertrichosis) 704.1
Polyunguia (congenital) 757.5
  acquired 703.8
Polyuria 788.42
Pompe's disease (glycogenosis II) 271.0
Pompholyx 705.81
Poncet's disease (tuberculous rheumatism) (*see
  also* Tuberculosis) 015.9
Pond fracture —*see* Fracture, skull, vault
Ponos 085.0
Pons, pontine —*see* condition
Poor
  aesthetics of existing restoration of tooth 525.67
  contractions, labor 661.2
    affecting fetus or newborn 763.7
  fetal growth NEC 764.9
    affecting management of pregnancy 656.5
  incorporation
    artificial skin graft 996.55
    decellularized allodermis graft 996.55

Poor—*continued*
obstetrical history V13.49
affecting management of current pregnancy V23.49
ectopic pregnancy V23.42
pre-term labor V23.41
pre-term labor V13.41
sucking reflex (newborn) 796.1
vision NEC 369.9
Poradenitis, nostras 099.1
Porencephaly (congenital) (development) (true)
742.4
acquired 348.0
nondevelopmental 348.0
traumatic (post) 310.2
Porocephaliasis 134.1
Porokeratosis 757.39
disseminated superficial actinic (DSAP) 692.75
Poroma, eccrine (M8402/0)—*see* Neoplasm,
skin, benign
Porphyria (acute) (congenital) (constitutional)
(erythropoietic) (familial) (hepatica)
(idiopathic) (idiosyncratic) (intermittent)
(latent) (mixed hepatic) (photosensitive)
(South African genetic) (Swedish) 277.1
acquired 277.1
cutaneatarda
hereditaria 277.1
symptomatica 277.1
due to drugs
correct substance properly administered 277.1
overdose or wrong substance given or taken 977.9
specified drug—*see* Table of drugs and
chemicals
secondary 277.1
toxic NEC 277.1
variegata 277.1
Porphyrinuria (acquired) (congenital)
(secondary) 277.1
Porphyruria (acquired) (congenital) 277.1
Portal —*see* condition
Port wine nevus or mark 757.32
Posadas-Wernicke disease 114.9
Position
fetus, abnormal (*see also* Presentation, fetal) 652.9
teeth, faulty (*see also* Anomaly, position tooth)
524.30
Positive
culture (nonspecific) 795.39
AIDS virus V08
blood 790.7
HIV V08
human immunodeficiency virus V08
nose 795.39
Staphylococcus — *see* Carrier (suspected)
of, Staphylococcus
skin lesion NEC 795.39
spinal fluid 792.0
sputum 795.39
stool 792.1
throat 795.39
urine 791.9
wound 795.39
findings, anthrax 795.31
HIV V08
human immunodeficiency virus (HIV) V08
PPD 795.51
serology
AIDS virus V08
inconclusive 795.71

Positive—*continued*
serology—*continued*
HIV V08
inconclusive 795.71
human immunodeficiency virus V08
inconclusive 795.71
syphilis 097.1
with signs or symptoms—*see* Syphilis, by
site and stage
false 795.6
skin test 795.7
tuberculin (without active tuberculosis) 795.51
VDRL 097.1
with signs or symptoms—*see* Syphilis, by site
and stage
false 795.6
Wassermann reaction 097.1
false 795.6
Postcardiotomy syndrome 429.4
Postcaval ureter 753.4
Postcholecystectomy syndrome 576.0
Postclimacteric bleeding 627.1
Postcommissurotomy syndrome 429.4
Postconcussional syndrome 310.2
Postcontusional syndrome 310.2
Postcricoid region —*see* condition
Post-dates (pregnancy) —*see* Pregnancy
Postencephalitic —*see also* condition
syndrome 310.89
Posterior —*see* condition
Posterolateral sclerosis (spinal cord)—*see*
Degeneration, combined
Postexanthematous —*see* condition
Postfebrile —*see* condition
Postgastrectomy dumping syndrome 564.2
Posthemiplegic chorea 344.89
Posthemorrhagic anemia (chronic) 280.0
acute 285.1
newborn 776.5
Posthepatitis syndrome 780.79
Postherpetic neuralgia (intercostal) (syndrome)
(zoster) 053.19
geniculate ganglion 053.11
ophthalmica 053.19
trigeminal 053.12
Posthitis 607.1
Postimmunization complication or reaction
—*see* Complications, vaccination
Postinfectious —*see* condition
Postinfluenzal syndrome 780.79
Postlaminectomy syndrome 722.80
cervical, cervicothoracic 722.81
kyphosis 737.12
lumbar, lumbosacral 722.83
thoracic, thoracolumbar 722.82
Postleukotomy syndrome 310.0
Postlobectomy syndrome 310.0
Postmastectomy lymphedema (syndrome) 457.0
Postmaturity, postmature (fetus or newborn)
(gestation period over 42 completed weeks)
766.22
affecting management of pregnancy
post-term pregnancy 645.1
prolonged pregnancy 645.2
syndrome 766.22
Postmeasles —*see also* condition
complication 055.8
specified NEC 055.79

Postmenopausal
  endometrium (atrophic) 627.8
    suppurative (*see also* Endometritis) 615.9
  hormone replacement therapy V07.4
  status (age related) (natural) V49.81
Postnasal drip 784.91
Postnatal —*see* condition
Postoperative —*see also* condition
  confusion state 293.9
  psychosis 293.9
  status NEC (*see also* Status (post)) V45.89
Postpancreatectomy hyperglycemia 251.3
Postpartum —*see also* condition
  anemia 648.2
  cardiomyopathy 674.5
  observation
    immediately after delivery V24.0
    routine follow-up V24.2
Postperfusion syndrome NEC 999.89
  bone marrow 996.85
Postpoliomyelitic —*see* condition
Postsurgery status NEC (*see also* Status (post))
  V45.89
Post-term (pregnancy) 645.1
  infant (gestation period over 40 completed
    weeks to 42 completed weeks) 766.21
**Post-transplant lymphoproliferative disorder
  (PTLD)** 238.77
Posttraumatic —*see* condition
Posttraumatic brain syndrome, nonpsychotic
  310.2
Post-Traumatic Stress Disorder (PTSD) 309.81
Post-typhoid abscess 002.0
Postures, hysterical 300.11
Postvaccinal reaction or complication —*see*
  Complications, vaccination
Postvagotomy syndrome 564.2
Postvalvulotomy syndrome 429.4
Postvasectomy sperm count V25.8
Potain's disease (pulmonary edema) 514
Potain's syndrome (gastrectasis with dyspepsia)
  536.1
Pott's
  curvature (spinal) (*see also* Tuberculosis) 015.0
    [737.43]
  disease or paraplegia (*see also* Tuberculosis)
    015.0 *[730.88]*
  fracture (closed) 824.4
    open 824.5
  gangrene 440.24
  osteomyelitis (*see also* Tuberculosis) 015.0 *[730.88]*
  spinal curvature (*see also* Tuberculosis) 015.0
    [737.43]
  tumor, puffy (*see also* Osteomyelitis) 730.2
Potter's
  asthma 502
  disease 753.0
  facies 754.0
  lung 502
  syndrome (with renal agenesis) 753.0
Pouch
  bronchus 748.3
  Douglas'—*see* condition
  esophagus, esophageal (congenital) 750.4
    acquired 530.6
  gastric 537.1
  Hartmann's (abnormal sacculation of
    gallbladder neck) 575.8
    of intestine V44.3
      attention to V55.3
  pharynx, pharyngeal (congenital) 750.27

Pouchitis 569.71
Poulet's disease 714.2
Poultrymen's itch 133.8
Poverty V60.2
PPE (plamar plantar erythrodysesthesia) 693.0
Prader-Labhart-Willi-Fanconi syndrome
  (hypogenital dystrophy with diabetic
  tendency) 759.81
Prader-Willi syndrome (hypogenital dystrophy
  with diabetic tendency) 759.81
Preachers' voice 784.49
Pre-AIDS —*see* Human immunodeficiency virus
  (disease) (illness) (infection)
Preauricular appendage 744.1
Prebetalipoproteinemia (acquired) (essential)
  (familial) (hereditary) (primary) (secondary)
  272.1
  with chylomicronemia 272.3
Precipitate labor 661.3
  affecting fetus or newborn 763.6
Preclimacteric bleeding 627.0
  menorrhagia 627.0
Precocious
  adrenarche 259.1
  menarche 259.1
  menstruation 259.1
  pubarche 259.1
  puberty NEC 259.1
  sexual development NEC 259.1
  thelarche 259.1
Precocity, sexual (constitutional) (cryptogenic)
  (female) (idiopathic) (male) NEC 259.1
  with adrenal hyperplasia 255.2
Precordial pain 786.51
  psychogenic 307.89
Predeciduous teeth 520.2
Prediabetes, prediabetic 790.29
  complicating pregnancy, childbirth, or
    puerperium 648.8
  fetus or newborn 775.89
Predislocation status of hip, at birth (*see also*
  Subluxation, congenital, hip) 754.32
Pre-eclampsia (mild) 642.4
  with pre-existing hypertension 642.7
  affecting fetus or newborn 760.0
  severe 642.5
  superimposed on pre-existing hypertensive
    disease 642.7
Preeruptive color change, teeth, tooth 520.8
Preexcitation 426.7
  atrioventricular conduction 426.7
  ventricular 426.7
Preglaucoma 365.00
Pregnancy (single) (uterine) (without sickness)
  V22.2

---

*Note—Use the following fifth-digit
subclassification with categories 640-649,
651-679:*

0 unspecified as to episode of care
*1 delivered, with or without mention of
    antepartum condition*
*2 delivered, with mention of postpartum
    complication*
3 antepartum condition or complication
4 postpartum condition or complication

---

  abdominal (ectopic) 633.00
    affecting fetus or newborn 761.4
    with intrauterine pregnancy 633.01

Pregnancy—*continued*
  abnormal NEC 646.9
  ampullar—*see* Pregnancy, tubal
  biochemical 631.0
  broad ligament—*see* Pregnancy, cornual
  cervical—*see* Pregnancy, cornual
  chemical 631.0
  combined (extrauterine and intrauterine)—*see*
      Pregnancy, cornual
  complicated (by) 646.9
    abnormal, abnormality NEC 646.9
      cervix 654.6
      cord (umbilical) 663.9
      glucose tolerance (conditions classifiable to
          790.21-790.29) 648.8
      pelvic organs or tissues NEC 654.9
      pelvis (bony) 653.0
      perineum or vulva 654.8
      placenta, placental (vessel) 656.7
      position
        cervix 654.4
        placenta 641.1
          without hemorrhage 641.0
        uterus 654.4
      size, fetus 653.5
      uterus (congenital) 654.0
    abscess or cellulitis
      bladder 646.6
      genitourinary tract (conditions classifiable to
          590, 595, 597, 599.0, 614.0-614.5,
          614.7-614.9, 615) 646.6
      kidney 646.6
      urinary tract NEC 646.6
    adhesion, pelvic peritoneal 648.9
    air embolism 673.0
    albuminuria 646.2
      with hypertension—*see* Toxemia, of
          pregnancy
    amnionitis 658.4
    amniotic fluid embolism 673.1
    anemia (conditions classifiable to 280-285)
        648.2
    appendicitis 648.9
    atrophy, yellow (acute) (liver) (subacute) 646.7
    bacilluria, asymptomatic 646.5
    bacteriuria, asymptomatic 646.5
    bariatric surgery status 649.2
    bicornis or bicornuate uterus 654.0
    biliary problems 646.8
    bone and joint disorders (conditions
        classifiable to 720-724 or conditions
        affecting lower limbs classifiable to
        711-719, 725-738) 648.7
    breech presentation 652.2
      with successful version 652.1
    cardiovascular disease (conditions classifiable
        to 390-398, 410-429) 648.6
      congenital (conditions classifiable to
          745-747) 648.5
    cerebrovascular disorders conditions
        (classifiable to 430-434, 436-437) 674.0
    cervicitis (conditions classifiable to 616.0)
        646.6
    chloasma (gravidarum) 646.8
    cholelithiasis 646.8
    cholestasis 646.7
    chorea (gravidarum)—*see* Eclampsia,
        pregnancy
    coagulation defect 649.3
    conjoined twins 678.1

Pregnancy—*continued*
  complicated by—*continued*
    contraction, pelvis (general) 653.1
      inlet 653.2
      outlet 653.3
    convulsions (eclamptic) (uremic) 642.6
      with pre-existing hypertension 642.7
    current disease or condition (nonobstetric)
      abnormal glucose tolerance 648.8
      anemia 648.2
      biliary tract 646.7
      bone and joint (lower limb) 648.7
      cardiovascular 648.6
        congenital 648.5
      cerebrovascular 674.0
      diabetes (conditions classifiable to 249 and
          250) 648.0
      drug dependence 648.3
      female genital mutilation 648.9
      genital organ or tract 646.6
      gonorrheal 647.1
      hypertensive 642.2
        chronic kidney 642.2
        renal 642.1
      infectious 647.9
        specified type NEC 647.8
      liver 646.7
      malarial 647.4
      nutritional deficiency 648.9
      parasitic NEC 647.8
      periodontal disease 648.9
      renal 646.2
        hypertensive 642.1
      rubella 647.5
      specified condition NEC 648.9
      syphilitic 647.0
      thyroid 648.1
      tuberculous 647.3
      urinary 646.6
      venereal 647.2
      viral NEC 647.6
    cystitis 646.6
    cystocele 654.4
    death of fetus (near term) 656.4
      early pregnancy (before 22 completed weeks
          gestation) 632
    deciduitis 646.6
    decreased fetal movements 655.7
    diabetes (mellitus) (conditions classifiable to
        249 and 250) 648.0
    disorders of liver and biliary tract 646.7
    displacement, uterus NEC 654.4
    disproportion—*see* Disproportion
    double uterus 654.0
    drug dependence (conditions classifiable to
        304) 648.3
    dysplasia, cervix 654.6
    early onset of delivery (spontaneous) 644.2
    eclampsia, eclamptic (coma) (convulsions)
        (delirium) (nephritis) (uremia) 642.6
      with pre-existing hypertension 642.7
    edema 646.1
      with hypertension—*see* Toxemia, of
          pregnancy
    effusion, amniotic fluid 658.1
      delayed delivery following 658.2
    embolism
      air 673.0
      amniotic fluid 673.1
      blood-clot 673.2
      cerebral 674.0

Pregnancy—*continued*
  complicated by—*continued*
    embolism—*continued*
      pulmonary NEC 673.2
      pyemic 673.3
      septic 673.3
    emesis (gravidarum)—*see* Pregnancy,
        complicated, vomiting
    endometritis (conditions classifiable to
        615.0-615.9) 670.1
      decidual 646.6
    epilepsy 649.4
    excessive weight gain NEC 646.1
    face presentation 652.4
    failure, fetal head to enter pelvic brim 652.5
    false labor (pains) 644.1
    fatigue 646.8
    fatty metamorphosis of liver 646.7
    female genital mutilation 648.9
    fetal
      anemia 678.0
      complications from in utero procedure 679.1
      conjoined twins 678.1
      death (near term) 656.4
        early (before 22 completed weeks
            gestation) 632
      deformity 653.7
      distress 656.8
      hematologic conditions 678.0
      reduction of multiple fetuses reduced to
          single fetus 651.7
      thrombocytopenia 678.0
      twin to twin transfusion 678.0
    fibroid (tumor) (uterus) 654.1
    footling presentation 652.8
      with successful version 652.1
    gallbladder disease 646.8
    gastric banding status 649.2
    gastric bypass status for obesity 649.2
    genital herpes (asymptomatic) (history of)
        (inactive) 647.6
    goiter 648.1
    gonococcal infection (conditions classifiable
        to 098) 647.1
    gonorrhea (conditions classifiable to 098)
        647.1
    hemorrhage 641.9
      accidental 641.2
      before 22 completed weeks gestation NEC
          640.9
      cerebrovascular 674.0
      due to
        afibrinogenemia or other coagulation
            defect (conditions classifiable to
            286.0-286.9) 641.3
        leiomyoma, uterine 641.8
        marginal sinus (rupture) 641.2
        premature separation, placenta 641.2
        trauma 641.8
      early (before 22 completed weeks gestation)
          640.9
      threatened abortion 640.0
      unavoidable 641.1
    hepatitis (acute) (malignant) (subacute) 646.7
      viral 647.6
    herniation of uterus 654.4
    high head at term 652.5
    hydatidiform mole (delivered) (undelivered)
        630
    hydramnios 657
    hydrocephalic fetus 653.6

Pregnancy—*continued*
  complicated by—*continued*
    hydrops amnii 657
    hydrorrhea 658.1
    hyperemesis (gravidarum)—*see* Hyperemesis,
        gravidarum
    hypertension—*see* Hypertension, complicating
        pregnancy
    hypertensive heart and chronic kidney disease
        642.2
    hypertensive
      chronic kidney disease 642.2
      heart and chronic kidney disease 642.2
      heart and renal disease 642.2
      heart disease 642.2
      renal disease 642.2
    hyperthyroidism 648.1
    hypothyroidism 648.1
    hysteralgia 646.8
    icterus gravis 646.7
    incarceration, uterus 654.3
    incompetent cervix (os) 654.5
    infection 647.9
      amniotic fluid 658.4
      bladder 646.6
      genital organ (conditions classifiable to
          614.0-614.5, 614.7-614.9, 615) 646.6
      kidney (conditions classifiable to
          590.0-590.9) 646.6
      urinary (tract) 646.6
        asymptomatic 646.5
    infective and parasitic diseases NEC 647.8
    inflammation
      bladder 646.6
      genital organ (conditions classifiable to
          614.0-614.5, 614.7-614.9, 615) 646.6
      urinary tract NEC 646.6
    injury 648.9
      obstetrical NEC 665.9
    insufficient weight gain 646.8
    insulin resistance 648.8
    intrauterine fetal death (near term) NEC 656.4
      early (before 22 completed weeks'
          gestation) 632
    malaria (conditions classifiable to 084) 647.4
    malformation, uterus (congenital) 654.0
    malnutrition (conditions classifiable to
        260-269) 648.9
    malposition
      fetus—*see* Pregnancy, complicated,
          malpresentation
      uterus or cervix 654.4
    malpresentation 652.9
      with successful version 652.1
      in multiple gestation 652.6
      specified type NEC 652.8
    marginal sinus hemorrhage or rupture 641.2
    maternal complications from in utero
        procedure 679.0
    maternal drug abuse 648.4
    maternal obesity syndrome 646.1
    menstruation 640.8
    mental disorders (conditions classifiable to
        290-303, 305.0, 305.2-305.9, 306-316,
        317-319) 648.4
    mentum presentation 652.4
    missed
      abortion 632
      delivery (at or near term) 656.4
      labor (at or near term) 656.4

Pregnancy—*continued*
  complicated by—*continued*
    necrosis
      genital organ or tract (conditions classifiable
        to 614.0-614.5, 614.7-614.9, 615) 646.6
      liver (conditions classifiable to 570) 646.7
      renal, cortical 646.2
    nephritis or nephrosis (conditions classifiable
      to 580-589) 646.2
      with hypertension 642.1
    nephropathy NEC 646.2
    neuritis (peripheral) 646.4
    nutritional deficiency (conditions classifiable
      to 260-269) 648.9
    obesity 649.1
      surgery status 649.2
    oblique lie or presentation 652.3
      with successful version 652.1
    obstetrical trauma NEC 665.9
    oligohydramnios NEC 658.0
    onset of contractions before 37 weeks 644.0
    oversize fetus 653.5
    papyraceous fetus 646.0
    patent cervix 654.5
    pelvic inflammatory disease (conditions
      classifiable to 614.0-614.5, 614.7-614.9,
      615) 646.6
    pelvic peritoneal adhesion 648.9
    placenta, placental
      abnormality 656.7
      abruptio or ablatio 641.2
      detachment 641.2
      disease 656.7
      infarct 656.7
      low implantation 641.1
        without hemorrhage 641.0
      malformation 656.7
      malposition 641.1
        without hemorrhage 641.0
      marginal sinus hemorrhage 641.2
      previa 641.1
        without hemorrhage 641.0
      separation (premature) (undelivered) 641.2
    placentitis 658.4
    pneumonia 648.9
    polyhydramnios 657
    postmaturity
      post-term 645.1
      prolonged 645.2
    prediabetes 648.8
    pre-eclampsia (mild) 642.4
      severe 642.5
      superimposed on pre-existing hypertensive
        disease 642.7
    premature rupture of membranes 658.1
      with delayed delivery 658.2
    previous
      ectopic pregnancy V23.42
      infertility V23.0
      in utero procedure during previous
        pregnancy V23.86
      nonobstetric condition V23.8
      poor obstetrical history V23.49
      premature delivery V23.41
      trophoblastic disease (conditions classifiable
        to 630) V23.1
    prolapse, uterus 654.4
    proteinuria (gestational) 646.2
      with hypertension—*see* Toxemia, of
        pregnancy
    pruritus (neurogenic) 646.8

Pregnancy—*continued*
  complicated by—*continued*
    psychosis or psychoneurosis 648.4
    ptyalism 646.8
    pyelitis (conditions classifiable to
      590.0-590.9) 646.6
    renal disease or failure NEC 646.2
      with secondary hypertension 642.1
      hypertensive 642.2
    retention, retained dead ovum 631.8
    retroversion, uterus 654.3
    Rh immunization, incompatibility, or
      sensitization 656.1
    rubella (conditions classifiable to 056) 647.5
    rupture
      amnion (premature) 658.1
        with delayed delivery 658.2
      marginal sinus (hemorrhage) 641.2
      membranes (premature) 658.1
        with delayed delivery 658.2
      uterus (before onset of labor) 665.0
    salivation (excessive) 646.8
    salpingo-oophoritis (conditions classifiable to
      614.0-614.2) 646.6
    septicemia (conditions classifiable to
      038.0-038.9) 647.8
      postpartum 670.2
      puerperal 670.2
    smoking 649.0
    spasms, uterus (abnormal) 646.8
    specified condition NEC 646.8
    spotting 649.5
    spurious labor pains 644.1
    status post
      bariatric surgery 649.2
      gastric banding 649.2
      gastric bypass for obesity 649.2
      obesity surgery 649.2
    superfecundation 651.9
    superfetation 651.9
    syphilis (conditions classifiable to 090-097)
      647.0
    threatened
      abortion 640.0
      premature delivery 644.2
      premature labor 644.0
    thrombophlebitis (superficial) 671.2
      deep 671.3
      septic 670.3
    thrombosis 671.2
      venous (superficial) 671.2
      deep 671.3
    thyroid dysfunction (conditions classifiable to
      240-246) 648.1
    thyroiditis 648.1
    thyrotoxicosis 648.1
    tobacco use disorder 649.0
    torsion of uterus 654.4
    toxemia—*see* Toxemia, of pregnancy
    transverse lie or presentation 652.3
      with successful version 652.1
    trauma 648.9
      obstetrical 665.9
    tuberculosis (conditions classifiable to
      010-018) 647.3
    tumor
      cervix 654.6
      ovary 654.4
      pelvic organs or tissue NEC 654.4
      uterus (body) 654.1
        cervix 654.6

Pregnancy—*continued*
  complicated by—*continued*
    tumor—*continued*
      vagina 654.7
      vulva 654.8
    unstable lie 652.0
    uremia—*see* Pregnancy, complicated, renal disease
    urethritis 646.6
    vaginitis or vulvitis (conditions classifiable to 616.1) 646.6
    varicose
      placental vessels 656.7
      veins (legs) 671.0
        perineum 671.1
        vulva 671.1
    varicosity, labia or vulva 671.1
    venereal disease NEC (conditions classifiable to 099) 647.2
    venous complication 671.9
    viral disease NEC (conditions classifiable to 042, 050-055, 057-079, 795.05, 795.15, 796.75) 647.6
    vomiting (incoercible) (pernicious) (persistent) (uncontrollable) (vicious) 643.9
      due to organic disease or other cause 643.8
      early—*see* Hyperemesis, gravidarum
      late (after 22 completed weeks gestation) 643.2
    young maternal age 659.8
  complications NEC 646.9
  cornual 633.80
    affecting fetus or newborn 761.4
    with intrauterine pregnancy 633.81
  death, maternal NEC 646.9
  delivered—*see* Delivery
  ectopic (ruptured) NEC 633.90
    with intrauterine pregnancy 633.91
    abdominal—*see* Pregnancy, abdominal
    affecting fetus or newborn 761.4
    combined (extrauterine and intrauterine)—*see* Pregnancy, cornual
    ovarian—*see* Pregnancy, ovarian
    specified type NEC 633.80
      affecting fetus or newborn 761.4
      with intrauterine pregnancy 633.81
    tubal—*see* Pregnancy, tubal
  examination, pregnancy
    negative result V72.41
    not confirmed V72.40
    positive result V72.42
  extrauterine—*see* Pregnancy, ectopic
  fallopian—*see* Pregnancy, tubal
  false 300.11
    labor (pains) 644.1
  fatigue 646.8
  illegitimate V61.6
  incidental finding V22.2
  in double uterus 654.0
  interstitial—*see* Pregnancy, cornual
  intraligamentous—*see* Pregnancy, cornual
  intramural—*see* Pregnancy, cornual
  intraperitoneal—*see* Pregnancy, abdominal
  isthmian—*see* Pregnancy, tubal
  management affected by
    abnormal, abnormality
      fetus (suspected) 655.9
        specified NEC 655.8
      placenta 656.7
    advanced maternal age NEC 659.6
      multigravida 659.6
      primigravida 659.5

Pregnancy—*continued*
  management affected by—*continued*
    antibodies (maternal)
      anti-c 656.1
      anti-d 656.1
      anti-e 656.1
      blood group (ABO) 656.2
        Rh(esus) 656.1
    appendicitis 648.9
    bariatric surgery status 649.2
    coagulation defect 649.3
    elderly multigravida 659.6
    elderly primigravida 659.5
    epilepsy 649.4
    fetal (suspected)
      abnormality 655.9
        abdominal 655.8
        acid-base balance 656.8
        cardiovascular 655.8
        facial 655.8
        gastrointestinal 655.8
        genitourinary 655.8
        heart rate or rhythm 659.7
        limb 655.8
        specified NEC 655.8
      acidemia 656.3
      anencephaly 655.0
      aneuploidy 655.1
      bradycardia 659.7
      central nervous system malformation 655.0
      chromosomal abnormalities (conditions classifiable to 758.0-758.9) 655.1
      damage from
        drugs 655.5
          obstetric, anesthetic, or sedative 655.5
        environmental toxins 655.8
        intrauterine contraceptive device 655.8
        maternal
          alcohol addiction 655.4
          disease NEC 655.4
          drug use 655.5
          listeriosis 655.4
          rubella 655.3
          toxoplasmosis 655.4
          viral infection 655.3
        radiation 655.6
      death (near term) 656.4
        early (before 22 completed weeks gestation) 632
      distress 656.8
      excessive growth 656.6
      growth retardation 656.5
      hereditary disease 655.2
      hydrocephalus 655.0
      intrauterine death 656.4
      poor growth 656.5
      spina bifida (with myelomeningocele) 655.0
    fetal-maternal hemorrhage 656.0
    gastric banding status 649.2
    gastric bypass status for obesity 649.2
    hereditary disease in family (possibly) affecting fetus 655.2
    incompatibility, blood groups (ABO) 656.2
      rh(esus) 656.1
    insufficient prenatal care V23.7
    insulin resistance 648.8
    intrauterine death 656.4
    isoimmunization (ABO) 656.2
      rh(esus) 656.1
    large-for-dates fetus 656.6
    light-for-dates fetus 656.5

Pregnancy—*continued*
  management affected by—*continued*
    meconium in liquor 656.8
    mental disorder (conditions classifiable to
        290-303, 305.0, 305.2-305.9, 306-316,
        317-319) 648.4
    multiparity (grand) 659.4
    obesity 649.1
      surgery status 649.2
    poor obstetric history V23.49
      pre-term labor V23.41
    postmaturity
      post-term 645.1
      prolonged 645.2
    post-term pregnancy 645.1
    previous
      abortion V23.2
        habitual 646.3
      cesarean delivery 654.2
      difficult delivery V23.49
      ectopic pregnancy V23.42
      forceps delivery V23.49
      habitual abortions 646.3
      hemorrhage, antepartum or postpartum
          V23.49
      hydatidiform mole V23.1
      infertility V23.0
      in utero procedure during previous
          pregnancy V23.86
      malignancy NEC V23.8
      nonobstetrical conditions V23.8
      premature delivery V23.41
      recurrent pregnancy loss 646.3
      trophoblastic disease (conditions in 630)
          V23.1
      vesicular mole V23.1
    prolonged pregnancy 645.2
    recurrent pregnancy loss 646.3
    small-for-dates fetus 656.5
    smoking 649.0
    spotting 649.5
    suspected conditions not found
      amniotic cavity and membrane problem
          V89.01
      cervical shortening V89.05
      fetal anomaly V89.03
      fetal growth problem V89.04
      oligohydramnios V89.01
      other specified problem NEC V89.09
      placental problem V89.02
      polyhydramnios V89.01
    tobacco use disorder 649.0
    venous complication 671.9
    young maternal age 659.8
  maternal death NEC 646.9
  mesometric (mural)—*see* Pregnancy, cornual
  molar 631.8
    hydatidiform (*see also* Hydatidiform mole)
        630
      previous, affecting management of
          pregnancy V23.1
    previous, affecting management of pregnancy
        V23.49
  multiple NEC 651.9
    with fetal loss and retention of one or more
        fetus(es) 651.6
    affecting fetus or newborn 761.5
    following (elective) fetal reduction 651.7
    specified type NEC 651.8
      with fetal loss and retention of one or more
          fetus(es) 651.6
      following (elective) fetal reduction 651.7

Pregnancy—*continued*
  mural—*see* Pregnancy, cornual
  observation NEC V22.1
    first pregnancy V22.0
    high-risk V23.9
      inconclusive fetal viability V23.87
      specified problem NEC V23.8
  ovarian 633.20
    affecting fetus or newborn 761.4
    with intrauterine pregnancy 633.21
  possible, not (yet) confirmed V72.40
  postmature
    post-term 645.1
    prolonged 645.2
  post-term 645.1
  prenatal care only V22.1
    first pregnancy V22.0
    high-risk V23.9
      inconclusive fetal viability V23.87
      specified problem NEC V23.8
  prolonged 645.2
  resulting from
    assisted reproductive technology V23.85
    in vitro fertilization V23.85
  quadruplet NEC 651.2
    with fetal loss and retention of one or more
        fetus(es) 651.5
    affecting fetus or newborn 761.5
    following (elective) fetal reduction 651.7
  quintuplet NEC 651.8
    with fetal loss and retention of one or more
        fetus(es) 651.6
    affecting fetus or newborn 761.5
    following (elective) fetal reduction 651.7
  sextuplet NEC 651.8
    with fetal loss and retention of one or more
        fetus(es) 651.6
    affecting fetus or newborn 761.5
    following (elective) fetal reduction 651.7
  spurious 300.11
  superfecundation NEC 651.9
    with fetal loss and retention of one or more
        fetus(es) 651.6
    following (elective) fetal reduction 651.7
  superfetation NEC 651.9
    with fetal loss and retention of one or more
        fetus(es) 651.6
    following (elective) fetal reduction 651.7
  supervision (of) (for)—*see also* Pregnancy,
      management affected by
    elderly
      multigravida V23.82
      primigravida V23.81
    high-risk V23.9
      inconclusive fetal viability V23.87
      insufficient prenatal care V23.7
      specified problem NEC V23.8
    inconclusive fetal viability V23.87
    multiparity V23.3
    normal NEC V22.1
      first V22.0
    poor
      obstetric history V23.49
        ectopic pregnancy V23.42
        pre-term labor V23.41
      reproductive history V23.5
    previous
      abortion V23.2
      hydatidiform mole V23.1
      infertility V23.0
      neonatal death V23.5
      stillbirth V23.5

Pregnancy—*continued*
  supervision—*continued*
    trophoblastic disease V23.1
      vesicular mole V23.1
    specified problem NEC V23.8
    young
      multigravida V23.84
      primigravida V23.83
  triplet NEC 651.1
    with fetal loss and retention of one or more
      fetus(es) 651.4
    affecting fetus or newborn 761.5
    following (elective) fetal reduction 651.7
  tubal (with rupture) 633.10
    affecting fetus or newborn 761.4
    with intrauterine pregnancy 633.11
  twin NEC 651.0
    with fetal loss and retention of one or more
      fetus(es) 651.3
    affecting fetus or newborn 761.5
    conjoined 678.1
    following (elective) fetal reduction 651.7
  unconfirmed V72.40
  undelivered (no other diagnosis) V22.2
    with false labor 644.1
    high-risk V23.9
      specified problem NEC V23.8
  unwanted NEC V61.7
Pregnant uterus —*see* condition
Preiser's disease (osteoporosis) 733.09
Prekwashiorkor 260
Preleukemia 238.75
Preluxation of hip, congenital (*see also*
  Subluxation, congenital, hip) 754.32
Premature —*see also* condition
  beats (nodal) 427.60
    atrial 427.61
    auricular 427.61
    postoperative 997.1
    specified type NEC 427.69
    supraventricular 427.61
    ventricular 427.69
  birth NEC 765.1
  closure
    cranial suture 756.0
    fontanel 756.0
    foramen ovale 745.8
  contractions 427.60
    atrial 427.61
    auricular 427.61
    auriculoventricular 427.61
    heart (extrasystole) 427.60
    junctional 427.60
    nodal 427.60
    postoperative 997.1
    ventricular 427.69
  ejaculation 302.75
  infant NEC 765.1
    excessive 765.0
    light-for-dates—*see* Light-for-dates
  labor 644.2
    threatened 644.0
  lungs 770.4
  menopause 256.31
  puberty 259.1
  rupture of membranes or amnion 658.1
    affecting fetus or newborn 761.1
    delayed delivery following 658.2
  senility (syndrome) 259.8
  separation, placenta (partial)—*see* Placenta,
    separation
  ventricular systole 427.69

Prematurity NEC 765.1
  extreme 765.0
Premenstrual syndrome 625.4
Premenstrual tension 625.4
Premolarization, cuspids 520.2
Premyeloma 273.1
Prenatal
  care, normal pregnancy V22.1
    first V22.0
  death, cause unknown—*see* Death, fetus
  screening—*see* Antenatal, screening
  teeth 520.6
Prepartum —*see* condition
Preponderance, left or right ventricular 429.3
Prepuce —*see* condition
PRES (posterior reversible encephalopathy
  syndrome) 348.39
Presbycardia 797
  hypertensive (*see also* Hypertension, heart) 402.90
Presbycusis 388.01
Presbyesophagus 530.89
Presbyophrenia 310.1
Presbyopia 367.4
Prescription of contraceptives NEC V25.02
  diaphragm V25.02
  oral (pill) V25.01
    emergency V25.03
    postcoital V25.03
    repeat V25.41
  repeat V25.40
  oral (pill) V25.41
Presenile —*see also* condition
  aging 259.8
  dementia (*see also* Dementia, presenile) 290.10
Presenility 259.8
Presentation, fetal
  abnormal 652.9
    with successful version 652.1
    before labor, affecting fetus or newborn 761.7
    causing obstructed labor 660.0
      affecting fetus or newborn, any, except
        breech 763.1
    in multiple gestation (one or more) 652.6
    specified NEC 652.8
  arm 652.7
    causing obstructed labor 660.0
  breech (buttocks) (complete) (frank) 652.2
    with successful version 652.1
      before labor, affecting fetus or newborn
        761.7
    before labor, affecting fetus or newborn 761.7
  brow 652.4
    causing obstructed labor 660.0
  buttocks 652.2
  chin 652.4
  complete 652.2
  compound 652.8
  cord 663.0
  extended head 652.4
  face 652.4
    to pubes 652.8
  footling 652.8
  frank 652.2
  hand, leg, or foot NEC 652.8
  incomplete 652.8
  mentum 652.4
  multiple gestation (one fetus or more) 652.6
  oblique 652.3
    with successful version 652.1
  shoulder 652.8
    affecting fetus or newborn 763.1

Presentation, fetal—*continued*
transverse 652.3
  with successful version 652.1
  umbilical cord 663.0
  unstable 652.0
Prespondylolisthesis (congenital) (lumbosacral)
  756.11
Pressure
area, skin ulcer (*see also* Ulcer, pressure) 707.00
atrophy, spine 733.99
birth, fetus or newborn NEC 767.9
brachial plexus 353.0
brain 348.4
  injury at birth 767.0
cerebral—*see* Pressure, brain
chest 786.59
cone, tentorial 348.4
  injury at birth 767.0
funis—*see* Compression, umbilical cord
hyposystolic (*see also* Hypotension) 458.9
increased
  intracranial 781.99
    due to
      benign intracranial hypertension 348.2
      hydrocephalus—*see* hydrocephalus
      injury at birth 767.8
  intraocular 365.00
lumbosacral plexus 353.1
mediastinum 519.3
necrosis (chronic) (skin) (*see also* Decubitus)
  707.00
nerve—*see* Compression, nerve
paralysis (*see also* Neuropathy, entrapment) 355.9
pre-ulcer skin changes limited to persistent focal
  erythema (*see also* Ulcer, pressure) 707.21
sore (chronic) (*see also* Ulcer, pressure) 707.00
spinal cord 336.9
ulcer (chronic) (*see also* Ulcer, pressure) 707.00
umbilical cord—*see* Compression, umbilical cord
venous, increased 459.89
Pre-syncope 780.2
Preterm infant NEC 765.1
extreme 765.0
Priapism (penis) 607.3
Prickling sensation (*see also* Disturbance,
  sensation) 782.0
Prickly heat 705.1
Primary —*see also* condition
angle closure suspect 365.02
Primigravida, elderly
affecting
  fetus or newborn 763.89
  management of pregnancy, labor, and delivery
    659.5
Primipara, old
affecting
  fetus or newborn 763.89
  management of pregnancy, labor, and delivery
    659.5
Primula dermatitis 692.6
Primus varus (bilateral) (metatarsus) 754.52
**PRIND (prolonged reversible ischemic
  neurologic deficit)** 434.91
history of personal V12.54
Pringle's disease (tuberous sclerosis) 759.5
Prinzmetal's angina 413.1
Prinzmetal-Massumi syndrome (anterior chest
  wall) 786.52
Prizefighter ear 738.7

Problem (with) V49.9
academic V62.3
acculturation V62.4
adopted child V61.24
aged
  in-law V61.3
  parent V61.3
  person NEC V61.8
alcoholism in family V61.41
anger reaction (*see also* Disturbance, conduct)
  312.0
behavior, child 312.9
behavioral V40.9
  specified NEC V40.39
betting V69.3
biological child V61.23
cardiorespiratory NEC V47.2
care of sick or handicapped person in family or
  household V61.49
career choice V62.29
communication V40.1
conscience regarding medical care V62.6
delinquency (juvenile) 312.9
diet, inappropriate V69.1
digestive NEC V47.3
ear NEC V41.3
eating habits, inappropriate V69.1
economic V60.2
  affecting care V60.9
    specified type NEC V60.89
educational V62.3
enuresis, child 307.6
exercise, lack of V69.0
eye NEC V41.1
family V61.9
  specified circumstance NEC V61.8
fear reaction, child 313.0
feeding (elderly) (infant) 783.3
  newborn 779.31
  nonorganic 307.59
fetal, affecting management of pregnancy 656.9
  specified type NEC 656.8
financial V60.2
foster child V61.25
functional V41.9
  specified type NEC V41.8
gambling V69.3
genital NEC V47.5
head V48.9
  deficiency V48.0
  disfigurement V48.6
  mechanical V48.2
  motor V48.2
  movement of V48.2
  sensory V48.4
  specified condition NEC V48.8
hearing V41.2
high-risk sexual behavior V69.2
identity 313.82
influencing health status NEC V49.89
internal organ NEC V47.9
  deficiency V47.0
  mechanical or motor V47.1
interpersonal NEC V62.81
jealousy, child 313.3
learning V40.0
legal V62.5
life circumstance NEC V62.89
lifestyle V69.9
  specified NEC V69.8

Problem—*continued*
limb V49.9
　deficiency V49.0
　disfigurement V49.4
　mechanical V49.1
　motor V49.2
　movement, involving
　　musculoskeletal system V49.1
　　nervous system V49.2
　sensory V49.3
　specified condition NEC V49.5
litigation V62.5
living alone V60.3
loneliness NEC V62.89
marital V61.10
　involving
　　divorce V61.03
　　estrangement V61.09
　　psychosexual disorder 302.9
　　sexual function V41.7
　relationship V61.10
mastication V41.6
medical care, within family V61.49
mental V40.9
　specified NEC V40.2
mental hygiene, adult V40.9
multiparity V61.5
nail biting, child 307.9
neck V48.9
　deficiency V48.1
　disfigurement V48.7
　mechanical V48.3
　motor V48.3
　movement V48.3
　sensory V48.5
　specified condition NEC V48.8
neurological NEC 781.99
none (feared complaint unfounded) V65.5
occupational V62.29
parent-child V61.20
　adopted child V61.24
　biological child V61.23
　foster child V61.25
　relationship V61.20
partner V61.10
　relationship V61.10
personal NEC V62.89
　interpersonal conflict NEC V62.81
personality (*see also* Disorder, personality)
　301.9
phase of life V62.89
placenta, affecting management of pregnancy
　656.9
　specified type NEC 656.8
poverty V60.2
presence of sick or handicapped person in
　family or household V61.49
psychiatric 300.9
psychosocial V62.9
　specified type NEC V62.89
relational NEC V62.81
relationship, childhood 313.3
religious or spiritual belief
　other than medical care V62.89
　regarding medical care V62.6
self-damaging behavior V69.8
sexual
　behavior, high-risk V69.2
　function NEC V41.7

Problem—*continued*
sibling
　relational V61.8
　relationship V61.8
sight V41.0
sleep disorder, child 307.40
sleep, lack of V69.4
smell V41.5
speech V40.1
spite reaction, child (*see also* Disturbance,
　conduct) 312.0
spoiled child reaction (*see also* Disturbance,
　conduct) 312.1
substance abuse in family V61.42
swallowing V41.6
tantrum, child (*see also* Disturbance, conduct)
　312.1
taste V41.5
thumb sucking, child 307.9
tic (child) 307.21
trunk V48.9
　deficiency V48.1
　disfigurement V48.7
　mechanical V48.3
　motor V48.3
　movement V48.3
　sensory V48.5
　specified condition NEC V48.8
unemployment V62.0
urinary NEC V47.4
voice production V41.4
Procedure (surgical) not done NEC V64.3
because of
　contraindication V64.1
　patient's decision V64.2
　　for reasons of conscience or religion V62.6
　specified reason NEC V64.3
Procidentia
anus (sphincter) 569.1
rectum (sphincter) 569.1
stomach 537.89
uteri 618.1
Proctalgia 569.42
fugax 564.6
spasmodic 564.6
　psychogenic 307.89
Proctitis 569.49
amebic 006.8
chlamydial 099.52
gonococcal 098.7
granulomatous 555.1
idiopathic 556.2
　with ulcerative sigmoiditis 556.3
tuberculous (*see also* Tuberculosis) 014.8
ulcerative (chronic) (nonspecific) 556.2
　with ulcerative sigmoiditis 556.3
Proctocele
female (without uterine prolapse) 618.04
　with uterine prolapse 618.4
　　complete 618.3
　　incomplete 618.2
male 569.49
Proctocolitis, idiopathic 556.2
with ulcerative sigmoiditis 556.3
Proctoptosis 569.1
Proctosigmoiditis 569.89
ulcerative (chronic) 556.3
Proctospasm 564.6
psychogenic 306.4
Prodromal-AIDS —*see* Human
　immunodeficiency virus (disease) (illness)
　(infection)

Profichet's disease or syndrome 729.90
Progeria (adultorum) (syndrome) 259.8
Prognathism (mandibular) (maxillary) 524.10
Progonoma (melanotic) (M9363/0)—*see*
    Neoplasm, by site, benign
Progressive —*see* condition
Prolapse, prolapsed
  anus, anal (canal) (sphincter) 569.1
  arm or hand, complicating delivery 652.7
    causing obstructed labor 660.0
      affecting fetus or newborn 763.1
    fetus or newborn 763.1
  bladder (acquired) (mucosa) (sphincter)
    congenital (female) (male) 756.71
    female (*see also* Cystocele, female) 618.01
    male 596.89
  breast implant (prosthetic) 996.54
  cecostomy 569.69
  cecum 569.89
  cervix, cervical (hypertrophied) 618.1
    anterior lip, obstructing labor 660.2
      affecting fetus or newborn 763.1
    congenital 752.49
    postpartal (old) 618.1
    stump 618.84
  ciliary body 871.1
  colon (pedunculated) 569.89
  colostomy 569.69
  conjunctiva 372.73
  cord—*see* Prolapse, umbilical cord
  cystostomy 596.83
  disc (intervertebral)—*see* Displacement,
    intervertebral disc
  duodenum 537.89
  eye implant (orbital) 996.59
    lens (ocular) 996.53
  fallopian tube 620.4
  fetal extremity, complicating delivery 652.8
    causing obstructed labor 660.0
    fetus or newborn 763.1
  funis—*see* Prolapse, umbilical cord
  gastric (mucosa) 537.89
  genital, female 618.9
    specified NEC 618.89
  globe 360 81
  ileostomy bud 569.69
  intervertebral disc—*see* Displacement,
    intervertebral disc
  intestine (small) 569.89
  iris 364.89
    traumatic 871.1
  kidney (*see also* Disease, renal) 593.0
    congenital 753.3
  laryngeal muscles or ventricle 478.79
  leg, complicating delivery 652.8
    causing obstructed labor 660.0
    fetus or newborn 763.1
  liver 573.8
  meatus urinarius 599.5
  mitral valve 424.0
  ocular lens implant 996.53
  organ or site, congenital NEC—*see* Malposition,
    congenital
  ovary 620.4
  pelvic (floor), female 618.89
  perineum, female 618.89
  pregnant uterus 654.4
  rectum (mucosa) (sphincter) 569.1
    due to Trichuris trichiuria 127.3
  spleen 289.59
  stomach 537.89

Prolapse, prolapsed—*continued*
  umbilical cord
    affecting fetus or newborn 762.4
    complicating delivery 663.0
  ureter 593.89
    with obstruction 593.4
  ureterovesical orifice 593.89
  urethra (acquired) (infected) (mucosa) 599.5
    congenital 753.8
  uterovaginal 618.4
    complete 618.3
    incomplete 618.2
    specified NEC 618.89
  uterus (first degree) (second degree) (third
    degree) (complete) (without vaginal wall
    prolapse) 618.1
    with mention of vaginal wall prolapse—*see*
      Prolapse, uterovaginal
    congenital 752.39
    in pregnancy or childbirth 654.4
      affecting fetus or newborn 763.1
      causing obstructed labor 660.2
        affecting fetus or newborn 763.1
    postpartal (old) 618.1
  uveal 871.1
  vagina (anterior) (posterior) (vault) (wall)
    (without uterine prolapse) 618.00
    with uterine prolapse 618.4
      complete 618.3
      incomplete 618.2
    paravaginal 618.02
    posthysterectomy 618.5
    specified NEC 618.09
  vitreous (humor) 379.26
    traumatic 871.1
  womb—*see* Prolapse, uterus
Prolapsus, female 618.9
Proliferative —*see* condition
Prolinemia 270.8
Prolinuria 270.8
Prolonged, prolongation
  bleeding time (*see also* Defect, coagulation) 790.92
    "idiopathic" (in von Willebrand's disease) 286.4
  coagulation time (*see also* Defect, coagulation)
    790.92
  gestation syndrome 766.22
  labor 662.1
    affecting fetus or newborn 763.89
    first stage 662.0
    second stage 662.2
  PR interval 426.11
  pregnancy 645.2
  prothrombin time (*see also* Defect, coagulation)
    790.92
  QT interval 794.31
    syndrome 426.82
  rupture of membranes (24 hours or more prior to
    onset of labor) 658.2
  uterine contractions in labor 661.4
    affecting fetus or newborn 763.7
Prominauris 744.29
Prominence
  auricle (ear) (congenital) 744.29
    acquired 380.32
  ischial spine or sacral promontory
    with disproportion (fetopelvic) 653.3
      affecting fetus or newborn 763.1
      causing obstructed labor 660.1
        affecting fetus or newborn 763.1
  nose (congenital) 748.1
    acquired 738.0
PROMM (proximal myotonic myotonia) 359.21

Pronation
ankle 736.79
foot 736.79
congenital 755.67
Prophylactic
administration of
antibiotics, long-term V58.62
short-term—omit code
antitoxin, any V07.2
antivenin V07.2
chemotherapeutic agent NEC V07.39
fluoride V07.31
diphtheria antitoxin V07.2
drug V07.39
gamma globulin V07.2
immune sera (gamma globulin) V07.2
RhoGAM V07.2
tetanus antitoxin V07.2
chemotherapy NEC V07.39
fluoride V07.31
hormone replacement (postmenopausal) V07.4
immunotherapy V07.2
measure V07.9
specified type NEC V07.8
medication V07.39
postmenopausal hormone replacement V07.4
sterilization V25.2
Proptosis (ocular) (*see also* Exophthalmos)
376.30
thyroid 242.0
Propulsion
eyeball 360.81
Prosecution, anxiety concerning V62.5
Prosopagnosia 368.16
Prostate, prostatic —*see* condition
Prostatism 600.90
with
other lower urinary tract symptoms (LUTS) 600.91
urinary
obstruction 600.91
retention 600.91
Prostatitis (congestive) (suppurative) 601.9
acute 601.0
cavitary 601.8
chlamydial 099.54
chronic 601.1
diverticular 601.8
due to Trichomonas (vaginalis) 131.03
fibrous 600.90
with
other lower urinary tract symptoms (LUTS)
600.91
urinary
obstruction 600.91
retention 600.91
gonococcal (acute) 098.12
chronic or duration of 2 months or over 098.32
granulomatous 601.8
hypertrophic 600.00
with
other lower urinary tract symptoms (LUTS)
600.01
urinary
obstruction 600.01
retention 600.01
specified type NEC 601.8
subacute 601.1
trichomonal 131.03
tuberculous (*see also* Tuberculosis) 016.5 *[601.4]*
Prostatocystitis 601.3
Prostatorrhea 602.8
Prostatoseminovesiculitis, trichomonal 131.03

Prostration 780.79
heat 992.5
anhydrotic 992.3
due to
salt (and water) depletion 992.4
water depletion 992.3
nervous 300.5
newborn 779.89
senile 797
Protanomaly 368.51
Protanopia (anomalous trichromat) (complete)
(incomplete) 368.51
Protection (against) (from) —*see* Prophylactic
Protein
deficiency 260
malnutrition 260
sickness (prophylactic) (therapeutic) 999.59
Proteinemia 790.99
Proteinosis
alveolar, lung or pulmonary 516.0
lipid 272.8
Proteinosis
lipoid (of Urbach) 272.8
Proteinuria (*see also* Albuminuria) 791.0
Bence-Jones NEC 791.0
gestational 646.2
with hypertension—*see* Toxemia, of
pregnancy
orthostatic 593.6
postural 593.6
Proteolysis, pathologic 286.6
Protocoproporphyria 277.1
Protoporphyria (erythrohepatic) (erythropoietic)
277.1
Protrusio acetabuli 718.65
Protrusion
acetabulum (into pelvis) 718.65
device, implant, or graft—*see* Complications,
mechanical
ear, congenital 744.29
intervertebral disc—*see* Displacement,
intervertebral disc
nucleus pulposus—*see* Displacement,
intervertebral disc
Proud flesh 701.5
Prune belly (syndrome) 756.71
Prurigo (ferox) (gravis) (Hebra's) (hebrae)
(mitis) (simplex) 698.2
agria 698.3
asthma syndrome 691.8
Besnier's (atopic dermatitis) (infantile eczema)
691.8
eczematodes allergicum 691.8
estivalis (Hutchinson's) 692.72
Hutchinson's 692.72
nodularis 698.3
psychogenic 306.3
Pruritus, pruritic 698.9
ani 698.0
psychogenic 306.3
conditions NEC 698.9
psychogenic 306.3
due to Onchocerca volvulus 125.3
ear 698.9
essential 698.9
genital organ(s) 698.1
psychogenic 306.3
gravidarum 646.8
hiemalis 698.8
neurogenic (any site) 306.3
perianal 698.0

Pruritus, pruritic—*continued*
  psychogenic (any site) 306.3
  scrotum 698.1
    psychogenic 306.3
  senile, senilis 698.8
  Trichomonas 131.9
  vulva, vulvae 698.1
    psychogenic 306.3
Psammocarcinoma (M8140/3)—*see* Neoplasm,
  by site, malignant
Pseudarthrosis, pseudoarthrosis (bone) 733.82
  joint following fusion V45.4
Pseudoacanthosis
  nigricans 701.8
Pseudoaneurysm —*see* Aneurysm
Pseudoangina (pectoris)—*see* Angina
Pseudoangioma 452
Pseudo-Argyll-Robertson pupil 379.45
Pseudoarteriosus 747.89
Pseudoarthrosis —*see* Pseudarthrosis
Pseudoataxia 799.89
Pseudobulbar affect (PBA) 310.81
Pseudobursa 727.89
Pseudocholera 025
Pseudochromidrosis 705.89
Pseudocirrhosis, liver, pericardial 423.2
Pseudocoarctation 747.21
Pseudocowpox 051.1
Pseudocoxalgia 732.1
Pseudocroup 478.75
Pseudocyesis 300.11
Pseudocyst
  lung 518.89
  pancreas 577.2
  retina 361.19
Pseudodementia 300.16
Pseudoelephantiasis neuroarthritica 757.0
Pseudoemphysema 518.89
Pseudoencephalitis
  superior (acute) hemorrhagic 265.1
Pseudoerosion cervix, congenital 752.49
Pseudoexfoliation, lens capsule 366.11
Pseudofracture (idiopathic) (multiple)
  (spontaneous) (symmetrical) 268.2
Pseudoglanders 025
Pseudoglioma 360.44
Pseudogout —*see* Chondrocalcinosis
Pseudohallucination 780.1
Pseudohemianesthesia 782.0
Pseudohemophilia (Bernuth's) (hereditary) (type
  B) 286.4
  type A 287.8
  vascular 287.8
Pseudohermaphroditism 752.7
  with chromosomal anomaly—*see* Anomaly,
    chromosomal
  adrenal 255.2
  female (without adrenocortical disorder) 752.7
    with adrenocortical disorder 255.2
    adrenal 255.2
  male (without gonadal disorder) 752.7
    with
      adrenocortical disorder 255.2
      cleft scrotum 752.7
      feminizing testis 259.51
      gonadal disorder 257.9
      adrenal 255.2
Pseudohole, macula 362.54
Pseudo-Hurler's disease (mucolipidosis III)
  272.7
Pseudohydrocephalus 348.2

Pseudohypertrophic muscular dystrophy
  (Erb's) 359.1
Pseudohypertrophy, muscle 359.1
Pseudohypoparathyroidism 275.49
Psuedopseudohypoparathyroidism 275.49
Pseudoinfluenza (*see also* Influenza) 487.1
Pseudoinsomnia 307.49
Pseudoleukemia 288.8
  infantile 285.8
Pseudomembranous —*see* condition
Pseudomeningocele (cerebral) (infective) 349.2
  postprocedural 997.01
  spinal 349.2
Pseudomenstruation 626.8
Pseudomucinous
  cyst (ovary) (M8470/0) 220
  peritoneum 568.89
Pseudomyeloma 273.1
Pseudomyxoma peritonei (M8480/6) 197.6
Pseudoneuritis optic (nerve) 377.24
  papilla 377.24
  congenital 743.57
Pseudoneuroma —*see* Injury, nerve, by site
Pseudo-obstruction
  intestine (chronic) (idiopathic) (intermittent
    secondary) (primary) 564.89
  acute 560.89
Pseudopapilledema 377.24
Pseudoparalysis
  arm or leg 781.4
  atonic, congenital 358.8
Pseudopelade 704.09
Pseudophakia V43.1
Pseudopolycythemia 289.0
Pseudopolyposis, colon 556.4
Pseudoporencephaly 348.0
Pseudopseudohypoparathyroidism 275.49
Pseudopsychosis 300.16
Pseudopterygium 372.52
Pseudoptosis (eyelid) 374.34
Pseudorabies 078.89
Pseudoretinitis, pigmentosa 362.65
Pseudorickets 588.0
  senile (Pozzi's) 731.0
Pseudorubella 057.8
Pseudoscarlatina 057.8
Pseudosclerema 778.1
Pseudosclerosis (brain)
  Jakob's 046.19
  of Westphal (-Strümpell) (hepatolenticular
    degeneration) 275.1
  spastic 046.19
    with behavioral disturbance 046.19 *[294.11]*
    without behavioral disturbance 046.19
      [294.10]
Pseudoseizure 780.39
  non-psychiatric 780.39
  psychiatric 300.11
Pseudotabes 799.89
  diabetic 250.6 *[337.1]*
    due to secondary diabetes 249.6 *[337.1]*
Pseudotetanus (*see also* Convulsions) 780.39
Pseudotetany 781.7
  hysterical 300.11
Pseudothalassemia 285.0
Pseudotrichinosis 710.3
Pseudotruncus arteriosus 747.29
Pseudotuberculosis, pasteurella (infection) 027.2

Pseudotumor
 cerebri 348.2
 orbit (inflammatory) 376.11
Pseudo-Turner's syndrome 759.89
Pseudoxanthoma elasticum 757.39
Psilosis (sprue) (tropical) 579.1
 Monilia 112.89
 nontropical 579.0
 not sprue 704.00
Psittacosis 073.9
Psoitis 728.89
Psora NEC 696.1
Psoriasis 696.1
 any type, except arthropathic 696.1
 arthritic, arthropathic 696.0
 buccal 528.6
 flexural 696.1
 follicularis 696.1
 guttate 696.1
 inverse 696.1
 mouth 528.6
 nummularis 696.1
 psychogenic 316 *[696.1]*
 punctata 696.1
 pustular 696.1
 rupioides 696.1
 vulgaris 696.1
Psorospermiasis 136.4
Psorospermosis 136.4
 follicularis (vegetans) 757.39
Psychalgia 307.80
Psychasthenia 300.89
 compulsive 300.3
 mixed compulsive states 300.3
 obsession 300.3
Psychiatric disorder or problem NEC 300.9
Psychogenic *—see also* condition
 factors associated with physical conditions 316
Psychoneurosis, psychoneurotic *(see also*
  Neurosis) 300.9
 anxiety (state) 300.00
 climacteric 627.2
 compensation 300.16
 compulsion 300.3
 conversion hysteria 300.11
 depersonalization 300.6
 depressive type 300.4
 dissociative hysteria 300.15
 hypochondriacal 300.7
 hysteria 300.10
  conversion type 300.11
  dissociative type 300.15
 mixed NEC 300.89
 neurasthenic 300.5
 obsessional 300.3
 obsessive-compulsive 300.3
 occupational 300.89
 personality NEC 301.89
 phobia 300.20
 senile NEC 300.89
Psychopathic *—see also* condition
 constitution, posttraumatic 310.2
  with psychosis 293.9
 personality 301.9
  amoral trends 301.7
  antisocial trends 301.7
  asocial trends 301.7
  mixed types 301.7
 state 301.9
Psychopathy, sexual *(see also* Deviation, sexual)
  302.9

Psychophysiologic, psychophysiological
  condition—*see* Reaction, psychophysiologic
Psychose passionelle 297.8
Psychosexual identity disorder 302.6
 adult-life 302.85
 childhood 302.6
Psychosis 298.9
 acute hysterical 298.1
 affecting management of pregnancy, childbirth,
  or puerperium 648.4
 affective *(see also* Disorder, mood) 296.90
  drug induced 292.84
  due to or associated with physical condition
   293.83

---

*Note—Use the following fifth-digit
subclassification with categories 296.0-296.6:*

0 unspecified
1 mild
2 moderate
*3 severe, without mention of psychotic
   behavior*
4 severe, specified as with psychotic behavior
5 in partial or unspecified remission
6 in full remission

---

 involutional 296.2
  recurrent episode 296.3
  single episode 296.2
 manic-depressive 296.80
  circular (alternating) 296.7
   currently depressed 296.5
   currently manic 296.4
  depressed type 296.2
   atypical 296.82
   recurrent episode 296.3
   single episode 296.2
  manic 296.0
   atypical 296.81
   recurrent episode 296.1
   single episode 296.0
  mixed type NEC 296.89
  specified type NEC 296.89
 senile 290.21
 specified type NEC 296.99
 alcoholic 291.9
  with
   anxiety 291.89
   delirium tremens 291.0
   delusions 291.5
   dementia 291.2
   hallucinosis 291.3
   jealousy 291.5
   mood disturbance 291.89
   paranoia 291.5
   persisting amnesia 291.1
   sexual dysfunction 291.89
   sleep disturbance 291.89
  amnestic confabulatory 291.1
  delirium tremens 291.0
  hallucinosis 291.3
  Korsakoff's, Korsakov's, Korsakow's 291.1
  paranoid type 291.5
  pathological intoxication 291.4
  polyneuritic 291.1
  specified type NEC 291.89
 alternating *(see also* Psychosis,
   manic-depressive, circular) 296.7
 anergastic *(see also* Psychosis, organic) 294.9

Psychosis—*continued*
  arteriosclerotic 290.40
    with
      acute confusional state 290.41
      delirium 290.41
      delusions 290.42
      depressed mood 290.43
    depressed type 290.43
    paranoid type 290.42
    simple type 290.40
    uncomplicated 290.40
  atypical 298.9
    depressive 296.82
    manic 296.81
  borderline (schizophrenia) (*see also*
    Schizophrenia) 295.5
  of childhood (*see also* Psychosis, childhood)
    299.8
    prepubertal 299.8
  brief reactive 298.8
  childhood, with origin specific to 299.9

> *Note—Use the following fifth-digit*
> *subclassification with category 299:*
>
> 0 *current or active state*
> 1 *residual state*

  atypical 299.8
  specified type NEC 299.8
  circular (*see also* Psychosis, manic-depressive,
    circular) 296.7
  climacteric (*see also* Psychosis, involutional)
    298.8
  confusional 298.9
    acute 293.0
    reactive 298.2
    subacute 293.1
  depressive (*see also* Psychosis, affective) 296.2
    atypical 296.82
    involutional 296.2
      recurrent episode 296.3
      single episode 296.2
    psychogenic 298.0
    reactive (emotional stress) (psychological
      trauma) 298.0
    recurrent episode 296.3
      with hypomania (bipolar II) 296.89
    single episode 296.2
  disintegrative, childhood (*see also* Psychosis,
    childhood) 299.1
  drug 292.9
    with
      affective syndrome 292.84
      amnestic syndrome 292.83
      anxiety 292.89
      delirium 292.81
        withdrawal 292.0
      delusions 292.11
      dementia 292.82
      depressive state 292.84
      hallucinations 292.12
      hallucinosis 292.12
      mood disorder 292.84
      mood disturbance 292.84
      organic personality syndrome NEC 292.89
      sexual dysfunction 292.89
      sleep disturbance 292.89
      withdrawal syndrome (and delirium) 292.0
    affective syndrome 292.84
    delusions 292.11
    hallucinatory state 292.12

Psychosis—*continued*
  drug—*continued*
    hallucinosis 292.12
    paranoid state 292.11
    specified type NEC 292.89
    withdrawal syndrome (and delirium) 292.0
  due to or associated with physical condition (*see*
    also Psychosis, organic) 293.9
  epileptic NEC 294.8
  excitation (psychogenic) (reactive) 298.1
  exhaustive (*see also* Reaction, stress, acute) 308.9
  hypomanic (*see also* Psychosis, affective) 296.0
    recurrent episode 296.1
    single episode 296.0
  hysterical 298.8
    acute 298.1
  incipient 298.8
    schizophrenic (*see also* Schizophrenia) 295.5
  induced 297.3
  infantile (*see also* Psychosis, childhood) 299.0
  infective 293.9
    acute 293.0
    subacute 293.1
  in
    conditions classified elsewhere
      with
        delusions 293.81
        hallucinations 293.82
    pregnancy, childbirth, or puerperium 648.4
  interactional (childhood) (*see also* Psychosis,
    childhood) 299.1
  involutional 298.8
    depressive (*see also* Psychosis, affective)
      296.2
      recurrent episode 296.3
      single episode 296.2
    melancholic 296.2
      recurrent episode 296.3
      single episode 296.2
    paranoid state 297.2
    paraphrenia 297.2
  Korsakoff's, Korakov's, Korsakow's
    (nonalcoholic) 294.0
    alcoholic 291.1
  mania (phase) (*see also* Psychosis, affective)
    296.0
    recurrent episode 296.1
    single episode 296.0
  manic (*see also* Psychosis, affective) 296.0
    atypical 296.81
    recurrent episode 296.1
    single episode 296.0
  manic-depressive 296.80
    circular 296.7
      currently
        depressed 296.5
        manic 296.4
      mixed 296.6
    depressive 296.2
      recurrent episode 296.3
        with hypomania (bipolar II) 296.89
      single episode 296.2
    hypomanic 296.0
      recurrent episode 296.1
      single episode 296.0
    manic 296.0
      atypical 296.81
      recurrent episode 296.1
      single episode 296.0
    mixed NEC 296.89
    perplexed 296.89
    stuporous 296.89

Psychosis—*continued*
  menopausal (*see also* Psychosis, involutional) 298.8
  mixed schizophrenic and affective (*see also* Schizophrenia) 295.7
  multi-infarct (cerebrovascular) (*see also* Psychosis, arteriosclerotic) 290.40
  organic NEC 294.9
    due to or associated with
      addiction
        alcohol (*see also* Psychosis, alcoholic) 291.9
        drug (*see also* Psychosis, drug) 292.9
      alcohol intoxication, acute (*see also* Psychosis, alcoholic) 291.9
      alcoholism (*see also* Psychosis, alcoholic) 291.9
      arteriosclerosis (cerebral) (*see also* Psychosis, arteriosclerotic) 290.40
      cerebrovascular disease
        acute (psychosis) 293.0
        arteriosclerotic (*see also* Psychosis, arteriosclerotic) 290.40
      childbirth—*see* Psychosis, puerperal
      dependence
        alcohol (*see also* Psychosis, alcoholic) 291.9
        drug 292.9
      disease
        alcoholic liver (*see also* Psychosis, alcoholic) 291.9
        brain
          arteriosclerotic (*see also* Psychosis, arteriosclerotic) 290.40
          cerebrovascular
            acute (psychosis) 293.0
            arteriosclerotic (*see also* Psychosis, arteriosclerotic) 290.40
        endocrine or metabolic 293.9
          acute (psychosis) 293.0
          subacute (psychosis) 293.1
        Jakob-Creutzfeldt 046.19
          with behavioral disturbance 046.19 *[294.11]*
          without behavioral disturbance 046.19 *[294.10]*
          familial 046.19
          iatrogenic 046.19
          specified NEC 046.19
          sporadic 046.19
          variant 046.11
            with dementia
              with behavioral disturbance 046.11 *[294.11]*
              without behavioral disturbance 046.11 *[294.10]*
        liver, alcoholic (*see also* Psychosis, alcoholic) 291.9
      disorder
        cerebrovascular
          acute (psychosis) 293.0
        endocrine or metabolic 293.9
          acute (psychosis) 293.0
          subacute (psychosis) 293.1
      epilepsy
        with behavioral disturbance 345.9 *[294.11]*
        without behavioral disturbance 345.9 *[294.10]*
        transient (acute) 293.0

Psychosis—*continued*
  organic—*continued*
    due to—*continued*
      Huntington's chorea
        with behavioral disturbance 333.4 *[294.11]*
        without behavioral disturbance 333.4 *[294.10]*
      infection
        brain 293.9
          acute (psychosis) 293.0
          chronic 294.8
          subacute (psychosis) 293.1
        intracranial NEC 293.9
          acute (psychosis) 293.0
          chronic 294.8
          subacute (psychosis) 293.1
      intoxication
        alcoholic (acute) (*see also* Psychosis, alcoholic) 291.9
        pathological 291.4
        drug (*see also* Psychosis, drug) 292.9
      ischemia
        cerebrovascular (generalized) (*see also* Psychosis, arteriosclerotic) 290.40
      Jakob-Creutzfeldt disease (syndrome) 046.19
        with behavioral disturbance 046.19 *[294.11]*
        without behavioral disturbance 046.19 *[294.10]*
        variant 046.11
          with dementia
            with behavioral disturbance 046.11 *[294.11]*
            without behavioral disturbance 046.11 *[294.10]*
      multiple sclerosis
        with behavioral disturbance 340 *[294.11]*
        without behavioral disturbance 340 *[294.10]*
      physical condition NEC 293.9
        with
          delusions 293.81
          hallucinations 293.82
      presenility 290.10
      puerperium—*see* Psychosis, puerperal
      sclerosis, multiple
        with behavioral disturbance 340 *[294.11]*
        without behavioral disturbance 340 *[294.10]*
      senility 290.20
      status epilepticus
        with behavioral disturbance 345.3 *[294.11]*
        without behavioral disturbance 345.3 *[294.10]*
      trauma
        brain (birth) (from electrical current) (surgical) 293.9
          acute (psychosis) 293.0
          chronic 294.8
          subacute (psychosis) 293.1
      unspecified physical condition 293.9
        with
          delusions 293.81
          hallucinations 293.82
  infective 293.9
    acute (psychosis) 293.0
    subacute 293.1

Psychosis—*continued*
organic—*continued*
posttraumatic 293.9
acute 293.0
subacute 293.1
specified type NEC 294.8
transient 293.9
with
anxiety 293.84
delusions 293.81
depression 293.83
hallucinations 293.82
depressive type 293.83
hallucinatory type 293.82
paranoid type 293.81
specified type NEC 293.89
paranoic 297.1
paranoid (chronic) 297.9
alcoholic 291.5
chronic 297.1
climacteric 297.2
involutional 297.2
menopausal 297.2
protracted reactive 298.4
psychogenic 298.4
acute 298.3
schizophrenic (*see also* Schizophrenia) 295.3
senile 290.20
paroxysmal 298.9
senile 290.20
polyneuritic, alcoholic 291.1
postoperative 293.9
postpartum—*see* Psychosis, puerperal
prepsychotic (*see also* Schizophrenia) 295.5
presbyophrenic (type) 290.8
presenile (*see also* Dementia, presenile) 290.10
prison 300.16
psychogenic 298.8
depressive 298.0
paranoid 298.4
acute 298.3
puerperal
specified type—*see* categories 295-298
unspecified type 293.89
acute 293.0
chronic 293.89
subacute 293.1
reactive (emotional stress) (psychological trauma) 298.8
brief 298.8
confusion 298.2
depressive 298.0
excitation 298.1
schizo-affective (depressed) (excited) (*see also* Schizophrenia) 295.7
schizophrenia, schizophrenic (*see also* Schizophrenia) 295.9
borderline type 295.5
of childhood (*see also* Psychosis, childhood) 299.8
catatonic (excited) (withdrawn) 295.2
childhood type (*see also* Psychosis, childhood) 299.9
hebephrenic 295.1
incipient 295.5
latent 295.5
paranoid 295.3
prepsychotic 295.5
prodromal 295.5
pseudoneurotic 295.5
pseudopsychopathic 295.5

Psychosis—*continued*
schizophrenic—*continued*
schizophreniform 295.4
simple 295.0
undifferentiated type 295.9
schizophreniform 295.4
senile NEC 290.20
with
delusional features 290.20
depressive features 290.21
depressed type 290.21
paranoid type 290.20
simple deterioration 290.20
specified type—*see* categories 295-298
shared 297.3
situational (reactive) 298.8
symbiotic (childhood) (*see also* Psychosis, childhood) 299.1
toxic (acute) 293.9
Psychotic (*see also* condition) 298.9
episode 298.9
due to or associated with physical conditions (*see also* Psychosis, organic) 293.9
Pterygium (eye) 372.40
central 372.43
colli 744.5
double 372.44
peripheral (stationary) 372.41
progressive 372.42
recurrent 372.45
Ptilosis 374.55
PTLD (post-transplant lymphoproliferative disorder) 238.77
Ptomaine (poisoning) (*see also* Poisoning, food) 005.9
Ptosis (adiposa) 374.30
breast 611.81
cecum 569.89
colon 569.89
congenital (eyelid) 743.61
specified site NEC—*see* Anomaly, specified type NEC
epicanthus syndrome 270.2
eyelid 374.30
congenital 743.61
mechanical 374.33
myogenic 374.32
paralytic 374.31
gastric 537.5
intestine 569.89
kidney (*see also* Disease, renal) 593.0
congenital 753.3
liver 573.8
renal (*see also* Disease, renal) 593.0
congenital 753.3
splanchnic 569.89
spleen 289.59
stomach 537.5
viscera 569.89
PTP (posttransfusion purpura) 287.41
PTSD (Post-Traumatic Stress Disorder) 309.81
Ptyalism 527.7
hysterical 300.11
periodic 527.2
pregnancy 646.8
psychogenic 306.4
Ptyalolithiasis 527.5
Pubalgia 848.8
Pubarche, precocious 259.1
Pubertas praecox 259.1

Puberty V21.1
abnormal 259.9
bleeding 626.3
delayed 259.0
precocious (constitutional) (cryptogenic)
    (idiopathic) NEC 259.1
    due to
        adrenal
            cortical hyperfunction 255.2
            hyperplasia 255.2
        cortical hyperfunction 255.2
        ovarian hyperfunction 256.1
            estrogen 256.0
        pineal tumor 259.8
        testicular hyperfunction 257.0
premature 259.1
    due to
        adrenal cortical hyperfunction 255.2
        pineal tumor 259.8
        pituitary (anterior) hyperfunction 253.1
Puckering, macula 362.56
Pudenda, pudendum —*see* condition
Puente's disease (simple glandular cheilitis)
    528.5
Puerperal
abscess
    areola 675.1
    Bartholin's gland 646.6
    breast 675.1
    cervix (uteri) 670.8
    fallopian tube 670.8
    genital organ 670.8
    kidney 646.6
    mammary 675.1
    mesosalpinx 670.8
    nabothian 646.6
    nipple 675.0
    ovary, ovarian 670.8
    oviduct 670.8
    parametric 670.8
    para-uterine 670.8
    pelvic 670.8
    perimetric 670
    periuterine 670.8
    retro-uterine 670.8
    subareolar 675.1
    suprapelvic 670.8
    tubal (ruptured) 670.8
    tubo-ovarian 670.8
    urinary tract NEC 646.6
    uterine, uterus 670.8
    vagina (wall) 646.6
    vaginorectal 646.6
    vulvovaginal gland 646.6
accident 674.9
adnexitis 670.8
afibrinogenemia, or other coagulation defect
    666.3
albuminuria (acute) (subacute) 646.2
    pre-eclamptic 642.4
anemia (conditions classifiable to 280-285)
    648.2
anuria 669.3
apoplexy 674.0
asymptomatic bacteriuria 646.5
atrophy, breast 676.3
blood dyscrasia 666.3
caked breast 676.2
cardiomyopathy 674.5
cellulitis—*see* Puerperal, abscess

Puerperal—*continued*
cerebrovascular disorder (conditions classifiable
    to 430-434, 436-437) 674.0
cervicitis (conditions classifiable to 616.0) 646.6
coagulopathy (any) 666.3
complications 674.9
    specified type NEC 674.8
convulsions (eclamptic) (uremic) 642.6
    with pre-existing hypertension 642.7
cracked nipple 676.1
cystitis 646.6
cystopyelitis 646.6
deciduitis (acute) 670.8
delirium NEC 293.9
diabetes (mellitus) (conditions classifiable to
    249 and 250) 648.0
disease 674.9
    breast NEC 676.3
    cerebrovascular (acute) 674.0
    nonobstetric NEC (*see also* Pregnancy,
        complicated, current disease or condition)
        648.9
    pelvis inflammatory 670.8
    renal NEC 646.2
    tubo-ovarian 670.8
    Valsuani's (progressive pernicious anemia) 648.2
disorder
    lactation 676.9
        specified type NEC 676.8
    nonobstetric NEC (*see also* Pregnancy,
        complicated, current disease or condition)
        648.9
disruption
    cesarean wound 674.1
    episiotomy wound 674.2
    perineal laceration wound 674.2
drug dependence (conditions classifiable to 304)
    648.3
eclampsia 642.6
    with pre-existing hypertension 642.7
embolism (pulmonary) 673.2
    air 673.0
    amniotic fluid 673.1
    blood-clot 673.2
    brain or cerebral 674.0
    cardiac 674.8
    fat 673.8
    intracranial sinus (venous) 671.5
    pyemic 673.3
    septic 673.3
    spinal cord 671.5
endometritis (conditions classifiable to
    615.0-615.9) 670.1
endophlebitis—*see* Puerperal, phlebitis
endotrachelitis 646.6
engorgement, breasts 676.2
erysipelas 670.8
failure
    lactation 676.4
    renal, acute 669.3
fever 672
    meaning pyrexia (of unknown origin) 672
    meaning sepsis 670.2
fissure, nipple 676.1
fistula
    breast 675.1
    mammary gland 675.1
    nipple 675.0
galactophoritis 675.2
galactorrhea 676.6

Puerperal—*continued*
  gangrene
    gas 670.8
      with sepsis 670.2
    uterus 670.8
  gonorrhea (conditions classifiable to 098) 647.1
  hematoma, subdural 674.0
  hematosalpinx, infectional 670.8
  hemiplegia, cerebral 674.0
  hemorrhage 666.1
    brain 674.0
    bulbar 674.0
    cerebellar 674.0
    cerebral 674.0
    cortical 674.0
    delayed (after 24 hours) (uterine) 666.2
    extradural 674.0
    internal capsule 674.0
    intracranial 674.0
    intrapontine 674.0
    meningeal 674.0
    pontine 674.0
    subarachnoid 674.0
    subcortical 674.0
    subdural 674.0
    uterine, delayed 666.2
    ventricular 674.0
  hemorrhoids 671.8
  hepatorenal syndrome 674.8
  hypertrophy
    breast 676.3
    mammary gland 676.3
  induration breast (fibrous) 676.3
  infarction
    lung—*see* Puerperal, embolism
    pulmonary—*see* Puerperal, embolism
  infection
    Bartholin's gland 646.6
    breast 675.2
      with nipple 675.9
        specified type NEC 675.8
    cervix 646.6
    endocervix 646.6
    fallopian tube 670.8
    generalized 670.0
    genital tract (major) 670.0
      minor or localized 646.6
    kidney (bacillus coli) 646.6
    mammary gland 675.2
      with nipple 675.9
        specified type NEC 675.8
    nipple 675.0
      with breast 675.9
        specified type NEC 675.8
    ovary 670.8
    pelvic 670.8
    peritoneum 670.8
    renal 646.6
    tubo-ovarian 670.8
    urinary (tract) NEC 646.6
      asymptomatic 646.5
    uterus, uterine 670.8
    vagina 646.6
  inflammation—*see also* Puerperal, infection
    areola 675.1
    Bartholin's gland 646.6
    breast 675.2
    broad ligament 670.8
    cervix (uteri) 646.6
    fallopian tube 670.8

Puerperal—*continued*
  inflammation—*continued*
    genital organs 670.8
      localized 646.6
    mammary gland 675.2
    nipple 675.0
    ovary 670.8
    oviduct 670.8
    pelvis 670.8
    periuterine 670.8
    tubal 670.8
    vagina 646.6
    vein—*see* Puerperal, phlebitis
  inversion, nipple 676.3
  ischemia, cerebral 674.0
  lymphangitis 670.8
    breast 675.2
  malaria (conditions classifiable to 084) 647.4
  malnutrition 648.9
  mammillitis 675.0
  mammitis 675.2
  mania 296.0
    recurrent episode 296.1
    single episode 296.0
  mastitis 675.2
    purulent 675.1
    retromammary 675.1
    submammary 675.1
  melancholia 296.2
    recurrent episode 296.3
    single episode 296.2
  mental disorder (conditions classifiable to
    290-303, 305.0, 305.2-305.9, 306-316,
    317-319) 648.4
  metritis (suppurative) 670.1
    septic 670.2
  metroperitonitis 670.8
  metrorrhagia 666.2
  metrosalpingitis 670.8
  metrovaginitis 670.8
  milk leg 671.4
  monoplegia, cerebral 674.0
  necrosis
    kidney, tubular 669.3
    liver (acute) (subacute) (conditions classifiable
      to 570) 674.8
    ovary 670.8
    renal cortex 669.3
  nephritis or nephrosis (conditions classifiable to
    580-589) 646.2
    with hypertension 642.1
  nutritional deficiency (conditions classifiable to
    260-269) 648.9
  occlusion, precerebral artery 674.0
  oliguria 669.3
  oophoritis 670.8
  ovaritis 670.8
  paralysis
    bladder (sphincter) 665.5
    cerebral 674.0
  paralytic stroke 674.0
  parametritis 670.8
  paravaginitis 646.6
  pelviperitonitis 670.8
  perimetritis 670.8
  perimetrosalpingitis 670.8
  perinephritis 646.6
  perioophoritis 670.8
  periphlebitis—*see* Puerperal, phlebitis
  perisalpingitis 670.8
  peritoneal infection 670.8

Puerperal—*continued*
  peritonitis (pelvic) 670.8
  perivaginitis 646.6
  phlebitis 671.2
    deep 671.4
    intracranial sinus (venous) 671.5
    pelvic 671.4
    specified site NEC 671.5
    superficial 671.2
  phlegmasia alba dolens 671.4
  placental polyp 674.4
  pneumonia, embolic—*see* Puerperal, embolism
  prediabetes 648.8
  pre-eclampsia (mild) 642.4
    with pre-existing hypertension 642.7
    severe 642.5
  psychosis, unspecified (*see also* Psychosis,
    puerperal) 293.89
  pyelitis 646.6
  pyelocystitis 646.6
  pyelohydronephrosis 646.6
  pyelonephritis 646.6
  pyelonephrosis 646.6
  pyemia 670.2
  pyocystitis 646.6
  pyohemia 670.2
  pyometra 670.8
  pyonephritis 646.6
  pyonephrosis 646.6
  pyo-oophoritis 670.8
  pyosalpingitis 670.8
  pyosalpinx 670.8
  pyrexia (of unknown origin) 672
  renal
    disease NEC 646.2
    failure, acute 669.3
  retention
    decidua (fragments) (with delayed
      hemorrhage) 666.2
      without hemorrhage 667.1
    placenta (fragments) (with delayed
      hemorrhage) 666.2
      without hemorrhage 667.1
    secundines (fragments) (with delayed
      hemorrhage) 666.2
      without hemorrhage 667.1
  retracted nipple 676.0
  rubella (conditions classifiable to 056) 647.5
  salpingitis 670.8
  salpingo-oophoritis 670.8
  salpingo-ovaritis 670.8
  salpingoperitonitis 670.8
  sapremia 670.2
  secondary perineal tear 674.2
  sepsis (pelvic) 670.2
  septicemia 670.2
  subinvolution (uterus) 674.8
  sudden death (cause unknown) 674.9
  suppuration—*see* Puerperal, abscess
  syphilis (conditions classifiable to 090-097)
    647.0
  tetanus 670.8
  thelitis 675.0
  thrombocytopenia 666.3
  thrombophlebitis (superficial) 671.2
    deep 671.4
    pelvic 671.4
    septic 670.3
    specified site NEC 671.5
  thrombosis (venous)—*see* Thrombosis,
    puerperal

Puerperal—*continued*
  thyroid dysfunction (conditions classifiable to
    240-246) 648.1
  toxemia (*see also* Toxemia, of pregnancy) 642.4
    eclamptic 642.6
      with pre-existing hypertension 642.7
    pre-eclamptic (mild) 642.4
      with
        convulsions 642.6
        pre-existing hypertension 642.7
      severe 642.5
  tuberculosis (conditions classifiable to 010-018)
    647.3
  uremia 669.3
  vaginitis (conditions classifiable to 616.1) 646.6
  varicose veins (legs) 671.0
    vulva or perineum 671.1
  venous complication 671.9
  vulvitis (conditions classifiable to 616.1) 646.6
  vulvovaginitis (conditions classifiable to 616.1)
    646.6
  white leg 671.4
Pulled muscle —*see* Sprain, by site
Pulmolithiasis 518.89
Pulmonary —*see* condition
Pulmonitis (unknown etiology) 486
Pulpitis (acute) (anachoretic) (chronic)
  (hyperplastic) (putrescent) (suppurative)
  (ulcerative) 522.0
Pulpless tooth 522.9
Pulse
  alternating 427.89
    psychogenic 306.2
  bigeminal 427.89
  fast 785.0
  feeble, rapid, due to shock following injury
    958.4
  rapid 785.0
  slow 427.89
  strong 785.9
  trigeminal 427.89
  water-hammer (*see also* Insufficiency, aortic)
    424.1
  weak 785.9
Pulseless disease 446.7
Pulsus
  alternans or trigeminy 427.89
    psychogenic 306.2
Punch drunk 310.2
Puncta lacrimalia occlusion 375.52
Punctiform hymen 752.49
Puncture (traumatic)—*see also* Wound, open, by
  site
  accidental, complicating surgery 998.2
  bladder, nontraumatic 596.6
  by
    device, implant, or graft—*see* Complications,
      mechanical
    foreign body
      internal organs—*see also* Injury, internal, by
        site
        by ingested object—*see* Foreign body
      left accidentally in operation wound 998.4
    instrument (any) during a procedure,
      accidental 998.2
  internal organs, abdomen, chest, or pelvis—*see*
    Injury, internal, by site
  kidney, nontraumatic 593.89
Pupil —*see* condition
Pupillary membrane 364.74
  persistent 743.46

Pupillotonia 379.46
  pseudotabetic 379.46
Purpura 287.2
  abdominal 287.0
  allergic 287.0
  anaphylactoid 287.0
  annularis telangiectodes 709.1
  arthritic 287.0
  autoerythrocyte sensitization 287.2
  autoimmune 287.0
  bacterial 287.0
  Bateman's (senile) 287.2
  capillary fragility (hereditary) (idiopathic) 287.8
  cryoglobulinemic 273.2
  devil's pinches 287.2
  fibrinolytic (see also Fibrinolysis) 286.6
  fulminans, fulminous 286.6
  gangrenous 287.0
  hemorrhagic (see also Purpura,
      thrombocytopenic) 287.39
    nodular 272.7
    nonthrombocytopenic 287.0
    thrombocytopenic 287.39
  Henoch's (purpura nervosa) 287.0
  Henoch-Schönlein (allergic) 287.0
  hypergammaglobulinemic (benign primary)
      (Waldenström's) 273.0
  idiopathic 287.31
    nonthrombocytopenic 287.0
    thrombocytopenic 287.31
  immune thrombocytopenic 287.31
  infectious 287.0
  malignant 287.0
  neonatorum 772.6
  nervosa 287.0
  newborn NEC 772.6
  nonthrombocytopenic 287.2
    hemorrhagic 287.0
    idiopathic 287.0
  nonthrombopenic 287.2
  peliosis rheumatica 287.0
  pigmentaria, progressiva 709.09
  posttransfusion (PTP) 287.41
    from whole blood (fresh) or blood products
      287.41
  primary 287.0
  primitive 287.0
  red cell membrane sensitivity 287.2
  rheumatica 287.0
  Schönlein (-Henoch) (allergic) 287.0
  scorbutic 267
  senile 287.2
  simplex 287.2
  symptomatica 287.0
  telangiectasia annularis 709.1
  thrombocytopenic (see also Thrombocytopenia)
      287.30
    congenital 287.33
    essential 287.30
    hereditary 287.31
    idiopathic 287.31
    immune 287.31
    neonatal, transitory (see also
        Thrombocytopenia, neonatal transitory)
        776.1
    primary 287.30
    puerperal, postpartum 666.3
    thrombotic 446.6
  thrombohemolytic (see also Fibrinolysis) 286.6

Purpura—continued
  thrombopenic (see also Thrombocytopenia)
      287.30
    congenital 287.33
    essential 287.30
  thrombotic 446.6
    thrombocytic 446.6
    thrombocytopenic 446.6
  toxic 287.0
  variolosa 050.0
  vascular 287.0
  visceral symptoms 287.0
  Werlhof's (see also Purpura, thrombocytopenic)
      287.39
Purpuric spots 782.7
Purulent —see condition
Pus
  absorption, general—see Septicemia
  in
    stool 792.1
    urine 791.9
  tube (rupture) (see also Salpingo-oophoritis)
      614.2
Pustular rash 782.1
Pustule 686.9
  malignant 022.0
  nonmalignant 686.9
Putnam's disease (subacute combined sclerosis
    with pernicious anemia) 281.0 [336.2]
Putnam-Dana syndrome (subacute combined
    sclerosis with pernicious anemia) 281.0
    [336.2]
Putrefaction, intestinal 569.89
Putrescent pulp (dental) 522.1
Pyarthritis —see Pyarthrosis
Pyarthrosis (see also Arthritis, pyogenic) 711.0
  tuberculous—see Tuberculosis, joint
Pycnoepilepsy, pycnolepsy (idiopathic) (see also
    Epilepsy) 345.0
Pyelectasia 593.89
Pyelectasis 593.89
Pyelitis (congenital) (uremic) 590.80
  with
    abortion—see Abortion, by type, with
        specified complication NEC
    contracted kidney 590.00
    ectopic pregnancy (see also categories
        633.0-633.9) 639.8
    molar pregnancy (see also categories 630-632)
        639.8
  acute 590.10
    with renal medullary necrosis 590.11
  chronic 590.00
    with
      renal medullary necrosis 590.01
  complicating pregnancy, childbirth, or
      puerperium 646.6
    affecting fetus or newborn 760.1
  cystica 590.3
  following
    abortion 639.8
    ectopic or molar pregnancy 639.8
  gonococcal 098.19
    chronic or duration of 2 months or over 098.39
  tuberculous (see also Tuberculosis) 016.0 [590.81]
Pyelocaliectasis 593.89
Pyelocystitis (see also Pyelitis) 590.80
Pyelohydronephrosis 591

Pyelonephritis (*see also* Pyelitis) 590.80
   acute 590.10
      with renal medullary necrosis 590.11
   chronic 590.00
   syphilitic (late) 095.4
   tuberculous (*see also* Tuberculosis) 016.0
      [590.81]
Pyelonephrosis (*see also* Pyelitis) 590.80
   chronic 590.00
Pyelophlebitis 451.89
Pyelo-ureteritis cystica 590.3
Pyemia, pyemic (purulent) (*see also* Septicemia)
   038.9
   abscess—*see* Abscess
   arthritis (*see also* Arthritis, pyogenic) 711.0
   Bacillus coli 038.42
   embolism—(*see also* Septicemia) 415.12
   fever 038.9
   infection 038.9
   joint (*see also* Arthritis, pyogenic) 711.0
   liver 572.1
   meningococcal 036.2
   newborn 771.81
   phlebitis—*see* Phlebitis
   pneumococcal 038.2
   portal 572.1
   postvaccinal 999.39
   puerperal 670.2
   specified organism NEC 038.8
   staphylococcal 038.10
      aureus 038.11
         methicillin
            resistant 038.12
            susceptible 038.11
      specified organism NEC 038.19
   streptococcal 038.0
   tuberculous—*see* Tuberculosis, miliary
Pygopagus 759.4
Pykno-epilepsy, pyknolepsy (idiopathic) (*see
   also* Epilepsy) 345.0
Pyle (-Cohn) disease (craniometaphyseal
   dysplasia) 756.89
Pylephlebitis (suppurative) 572.1
Pylethrombophlebitis 572.1
Pylethrombosis 572.1
Pyloritis (*see also* Gastritis) 535.5
Pylorospasm (reflex) 537.81
   congenital or infantile 750.5
   neurotic 306.4
   newborn 750.5
   psychogenic 306.4
Pylorus, pyloric —*see* condition
Pyoarthrosis —*see* Pyarthrosis
Pyocele
   mastoid 383.00
   sinus (accessory) (nasal) (*see also* Sinusitis)
      473.9
   turbinate (bone) 473.9
   urethra (*see also* Urethritis) 597.0
Pyococcal dermatitis 686.00
Pyococcide, skin 686.00
Pyocolpos (*see also* Vaginitis) 616.10
Pyocyaneus dermatitis 686.09
Pyocystitis (*see also* Cystitis) 595.9
Pyoderma, pyodermia NEC 686.00
   gangrenosum 686.01
   specified type NEC 686.09
   vegetans 686.8
Pyodermatitis 686.00
   vegetans 686.8
Pyogenic —*see* condition

Pyohemia —*see* Septicemia
Pyohydronephrosis (*see also* Pyelitis) 590.80
Pyometra 615.9
Pyometritis (*see also* Endometritis) 615.9
Pyometrium (*see also* Endometritis) 615.9
Pyomyositis 728.0
   ossificans 728.19
   tropical (bungpagga) 040.81
Pyonephritis (*see also* Pyelitis) 590.80
   chronic 590.00
Pyonephrosis (congenital) (*see also* Pyelitis)
   590.80
   acute 590.10
Pyo-oophoritis (*see also* Salpingo-oophoritis)
   614.2
Pyo-ovarium (*see also* Salpingo-oophoritis)
   614.2
Pyopericarditis 420.99
Pyopericardium 420.99
Pyophlebitis —*see* Phlebitis
Pyopneumopericardium 420.99
Pyopneumothorax (infectional) 510.9
   with fistula 510.0
   subdiaphragmatic (*see also* Peritonitis) 567.29
   subphrenic (*see also* Peritonitis) 567.29
   tuberculous (*see also* Tuberculosis, pleura) 012.0
Pyorrhea (alveolar) (alveolaris) 523.40
   degenerative 523.5
Pyosalpingitis (*see also* Salpingo-oophoritis) 614.2
Pyosalpinx (*see also* Salpingo-oophoritis) 614.2
Pyosepticemia —*see* Septicemia
Pyosis
   Corlett's (impetigo) 684
   Manson's (pemphigus contagiosus) 684
Pyothorax 510.9
   with fistula 510.0
   tuberculous (*see also* Tuberculosis, pleura)
      012.0
Pyoureter 593.89
   tuberculous (*see also* Tuberculosis) 016.2
Pyramidopallidonigral syndrome 332.0
Pyrexia (of unknown origin) (P.U.O.) 780.60
   atmospheric 992.0
   during labor 659.2
   environmentally-induced
      newborn 778.4
   heat 992.0
   newborn, environmentally-induced 778.4
   puerperal 672
Pyroglobulinemia 273.8
Pyromania 312.33
Pyrosis 787.1
Pyrroloporphyria 277.1
Pyuria (bacterial) 791.9

Q

Q fever 083.0
  with pneumonia 083.0 *[484.8]*
Quadricuspid aortic valve 746.89
Quadrilateral fever 083.0
Quadriparesis —*see* Quadriplegia
  meaning muscle weakness 728.87
Quadriplegia 344.00
  with fracture, vertebra (process)—*see* Fracture,
    vertebra, cervical, with spinal cord injury
  brain (current episode) 437.8
  cerebral (current episode) 437.8
  C1-C4
    complete 344.01
    incomplete 344.02
  C5-C7
    complete 344.03
    incomplete 344.04
  congenital or infantile (cerebral) (spastic)
    (spinal) 343.2
  cortical 437.8
  embolic (current episode) (*see also* Embolism,
    brain) 434.1
  functional 780.72
  infantile (cerebral) (spastic) (spinal) 343.2
  newborn NEC 767.0
  specified NEC 344.09
  thrombotic (current episode) (*see also*
    Thrombosis, brain) 434.0
  traumatic—*see* Injury, spinal, cervical
Quadruplet
  affected by maternal complications of pregnancy
    761.5
  healthy liveborn—*see* Newborn, multiple
  pregnancy (complicating delivery) NEC 651.8
    with fetal loss and retention of one or more
      fetus(es) 651.5
    following (elective) fetal reduction 651.7
Quarrelsomeness 301.3
Quartan
  fever 084.2
  malaria (fever) 084.2
Queensland fever 083.0
  coastal 083.0
  seven-day 100.89
Quervain's disease 727.04
  thyroid (subacute granulomatous thyroiditis)
    245.1
Queyrat's erythroplasia (M8080/2)
  specified site—*see* Neoplasm, skin, in situ
  unspecified site 233.5
Quincke's disease or edema —*see* Edema,
  angioneurotic
Quinquaud's disease (acne decalvans) 704.09
Quinsy (gangrenous) 475
Quintan fever 083.1
Quintuplet
  affected by maternal complications of pregnancy
    761.5
  healthy liveborn—*see* Newborn, multiple
  pregnancy (complicating delivery) NEC 651.2
    with fetal loss and retention of one or more
      fetus(es) 651.6
    following (elective) fetal reduction 651.7
Quotidian
  fever 084.0
  malaria (fever) 084.0

R

Rabbia 071
Rabbit fever (*see also* Tularemia) 021.9
Rabies 071
  contact V01.5
  exposure to V01.5
  inoculation V04.5
    reaction—*see* Complications, vaccination
  vaccination, prophylactic (against) V04.5
Rachischisis (*see also* Spina bifida) 741.9
Rachitic —*see also* condition
  deformities of spine 268.1
  pelvis 268.1
    with disproportion (fetopelvic) 653.2
      affecting fetus or newborn 763.1
      causing obstructed labor 660.1
        affecting fetus or newborn 763.1
Rachitis, rachitism —*see also* Rickets
  acute 268.0
  fetalis 756.4
  renalis 588.0
  tarda 268.0
Racket nail 757.5
Radial nerve —*see* condition
Radiation effects or sickness —*see also* Effect,
  adverse, radiation
  cataract 366.46
  dermatitis 692.82
  sunburn (*see also* Sunburn) 692.71
Radiculitis (pressure) (vertebrogenic) 729.2
  accessory nerve 723.4
  anterior crural 724.4
  arm 723.4
  brachial 723.4
  cervical NEC 723.4
  due to displacement of intervertebral disc—*see*
    Neuritis, due to, displacement intervertebral
    disc
  leg 724.4
  lumbar NEC 724.4
  lumbosacral 724.4
  rheumatic 729.2
  syphilitic 094.89
  thoracic (with visceral pain) 724.4
Radiculomyelitis 357.0
  toxic, due to
    Clostridium tetani 037
    Corynebacterium diphtheriae 032.89
Radiculopathy (*see also* Radiculitis) 729.2
Radioactive substances, adverse effect —*see*
  Effect, adverse, radioactive substance
Radiodermal burns (acute) (chronic)
  (occupational)—*see* Burn, by site
Radiodermatitis 692.82
Radionecrosis —*see* Effect, adverse, radiation
Radiotherapy session V58.0
Radium, adverse effect —*see* Effect, adverse,
  radioactive substance
Raeder-Harbitz syndrome (pulseless disease) 446.7
Rage (*see also* Disturbance, conduct) 312.0
  meaning rabies 071
Rag sorters' disease 022.1
Raillietiniasis 123.8
Railroad neurosis 300.16
Railway spine 300.16
Raised —*see* Elevation
Raiva 071
Rake teeth, tooth 524.39
Rales 786.7

Ramifying renal pelvis 753.3
Ramsay Hunt syndrome (herpetic geniculate ganglionitis) 053.11
  meaning dyssynergia cerebellaris myoclonica 334.2
Ranke's primary infiltration (*see also* Tuberculosis) 010.0
Ranula 527.6
  congenital 750.26
Rape
  adult 995.83
  alleged, observation or examination V71.5
  child 995.53
Rapid
  feeble pulse, due to shock, following injury 958.4
  heart (beat) 785.0
    psychogenic 306.2
  respiration 786.06
    psychogenic 306.1
  second stage (delivery) 661.3
    affecting fetus or newborn 763.6
  time-zone change syndrome 327.35
Rarefaction, bone 733.99
Rash 782.1
  canker 034.1
  diaper 691.0
  drug (internal use) 693.0
    contact 692.3
  ECHO 9 virus 078.89
  enema 692.89
  food (*see also* Allergy, food) 693.1
  heat 705.1
  napkin 691.0
  nettle 708.8
  pustular 782.1
  rose 782.1
    epidemic 056.9
    of infants 057.8
  scarlet 034.1
  serum (prophylactic) (therapeutic) 999.59
  toxic 782.1
  wandering tongue 529.1
Rasmussen's aneurysm (*see also* Tuberculosis) 011.2
Rat-bite fever 026.9
  due to Streptobacillus moniliformis 026.1
  spirochetal (morsus muris) 026.0
Rathke's pouch tumor (M9350/1) 237.0
Raymond (-Céstan) syndrome 433.8
Raynaud's
  disease or syndrome (paroxysmal digital cyanosis) 443.0
  gangrene (symmetric) 443.0 *[785.4]*
  phenomenon (paroxysmal digital cyanosis) (secondary) 443.0
RDS 769
Reaction
  acute situational maladjustment (*see also* Reaction, adjustment) 309.9
  adaptation (*see also* Reaction, adjustment) 309.9
  adjustment 309.9
    with
      anxious mood 309.24
        with depressed mood 309.28
      conduct disturbance 309.3
        combined with disturbance of emotions 309.4
      depressed mood 309.0
        brief 309.0
          with anxious mood 309.28
        prolonged 309.1
      elective mutism 309.83
      mixed emotions and conduct 309.4

Reaction—*continued*
  adjustment—*continued*
    with—*continued*
      mutism, elective 309.83
      physical symptoms 309.82
      predominant disturbance (of)
        conduct 309.3
        emotions NEC 309.29
          mixed 309.28
        mixed, emotions and conduct 309.4
        specified type NEC 309.89
        specific academic or work inhibition 309.23
      withdrawal 309.83
    depressive 309.0
      with conduct disturbance 309.4
      brief 309.0
      prolonged 309.1
    specified type NEC 309.89
  adverse food NEC 995.7
  affective (*see also* Psychosis, affective) 296.90
    specified type NEC 296.99
  aggressive 301.3
    unsocialized (*see also* Disturbance, conduct) 312.0
  allergic (*see also* Allergy) 995.3
    drug, medicinal substance, and biological—*see* Allergy, drug
    due to correct medical substance properly administered 995.27
    food—*see* Allergy, food
    serum 999.59
  anaphylactic—*see* Anaphylactic reaction
  anesthesia—*see* Anesthesia, complication
  anger 312.0
  antisocial 301.7
  antitoxin (prophylactic) (therapeutic)—*see* Complications, vaccination
  anxiety 300.00
  Arthus 995.21
  asthenic 300.5
  compulsive 300.3
  conversion (anesthetic) (autonomic) (hyperkinetic) (mixed paralytic) (paresthetic) 300.11
  deoxyribonuclease (DNA) (DNase) hypersensitivity NEC 287.2
  depressive 300.4
    acute 309.0
    affective (*see also* Psychosis, affective) 296.2
      recurrent episode 296.3
      single episode 296.2
    brief 309.0
    manic (*see also* Psychosis, affective) 296.80
    neurotic 300.4
    psychoneurotic 300.4
    psychotic 298.0
  dissociative 300.15
  drug NEC (*see also* Table of Drugs and Chemicals) 995.20
    allergic—*see also* Allergy, drug 995.27
    correct substance properly administered 995.20
    obstetric anesthetic or analgesic NEC 668.9
      affecting fetus or newborn 763.5
    specified drug—*see* Table of drugs and chemicals
    overdose or poisoning 977.9
      specified drug—*see* Table of drugs and chemicals
    specific to newborn 779.4
    transmitted via placenta or breast milk—*see* Absorption, drug, through placenta

Reaction—*continued*
  drug—*continued*
    withdrawal NEC 292.0
      infant of dependent mother 779.5
    wrong substance given or taken in error 977.9
      specified drug—*see* Table of drugs and
        chemicals
  dyssocial 301.7
  dystonic, acute, due to drugs 333.72
  erysipeloid 027.1
  fear 300.20
    child 313.0
  fluid loss, cerebrospinal 349.0
  food—*see also* Allergy, food
    adverse NEC 995.7
    anaphylactic shock—*see* Anaphylactic
      reaction or shock, due to food
  foreign
    body NEC 728.82
      in operative wound (inadvertently left) 998.4
      due to surgical material intentionally
        left—*see* Complications, due to
        (presence of) any device, implant, or
        graft classified to 996.0-996.5 NEC
    substance accidentally left during a procedure
      (chemical) (powder) (talc) 998.7
      body or object (instrument) (sponge) (swab)
        998.4
  graft-versus-host (GVH) 279.50
  grief (acute) (brief) 309.0
    prolonged 309.1
  gross stress (*see also* Reaction, stress, acute)
    308.9
  group delinquent (*see also* Disturbance,
    conduct) 312.2
  Herxheimer's 995.91
  hyperkinetic (*see also* Hyperkinesia) 314.9
  hypochondriacal 300.7
  hypoglycemic, due to insulin 251.0
    therapeutic misadventure 962.3
  hypomanic (*see also* Psychosis, affective) 296.0
    recurrent episode 296.1
    single episode 296.0
  hysterical 300.10
    conversion type 300.11
    dissociative 300.15
  id (bacterial cause) 692.89
  immaturity NEC 301.89
    aggressive 301.3
    emotional instability 301.59
  immunization—*see* Complications, vaccination
  incompatibility
    blood group (*see also* Complications,
      transfusion) 999.80
    ABO (due to transfusion of blood or blood
      products) (*see also* Complications,
      transfusion) 999.60
    minor blood group 999.89
    non-ABO (*see also* Complications,
      transfusion) 999.75
    Rh antigen (C) (c) (D) (E) (e) (factor)
      (infusion) (transfusion) (*see also*
      Complications, transfusion) 999.70
  inflammatory—*see* Infection
  infusion—*see* Complications, infusion
  inoculation (immune serum)—*see*
    Complications, vaccination
  insulin 995.23

Reaction—*continued*
  involutional
    paranoid 297.2
    psychotic (*see also* Psychosis, affective,
      depressive) 296.2
  leukemoid (basophilic) (lymphocytic)
    (monocytic) (myelocytic) (neutrophilic)
    288.62
  LSD (*see also* Abuse, drugs, nondependent) 305.3
  lumbar puncture 349.0
  manic-depressive (*see also* Psychosis, affective)
    296.80
    depressed 296.2
      recurrent episode 296.3
      single episode 296.2
    hypomanic 296.0
  neurasthenic 300.5
  neurogenic (*see also* Neurosis) 300.9
  neurotic NEC 300.9
  neurotic-depressive 300.4
  nitritoid—*see* Crisis, nitritoid
  nonspecific
    to
      cell mediated immunity measurement of
        gamma interferon antigen response
        without active tuberculosis 795.52
      QuantiFERON-TB test (QFT) without active
        tuberculosis 795.52
      tuberculin test (*see also* Reaction, tuberculin
        skin test) 795.51
  obsessive-compulsive 300.3
  organic 293.9
    acute 293.0
    subacute 293.1
  overanxious, child or adolescent 313.0
  paranoid (chronic) 297.9
    acute 298.3
    climacteric 297.2
    involutional 297.2
    menopausal 297.2
    senile 290.20
    simple 297.0
  passive
    aggressive 301.84
    dependency 301.6
  personality (*see also* Disorder, personality)
    301.9
  phobic 300.20
  postradiation—*see* Effect, adverse, radiation
  psychogenic NEC 300.9
  psychoneurotic (*see also* Neurosis) 300.9
    anxiety 300.00
    compulsive 300.3
    conversion 300.11
    depersonalization 300.6
    depressive 300.4
    dissociative 300.15
    hypochondriacal 300.7
    hysterical 300.10
      conversion type 300.11
      dissociative type 300.15
    neurasthenic 300.5
    obsessive 300.3
    obsessive-compulsive 300.3
    phobic 300.20
    tension state 300.9
  psychophysiologic NEC (*see also* Disorder,
    psychosomatic) 306.9
    cardiovascular 306.2
    digestive 306.4
    endocrine 306.6

Reaction—*continued*
 psychophysiologic —*continued*
  gastrointestinal 306.4
  genitourinary 306.50
  heart 306.2
  hemic 306.8
  intestinal (large) (small) 306.4
  laryngeal 306.1
  lymphatic 306.8
  musculoskeletal 306.0
  pharyngeal 306.1
  respiratory 306.1
  skin 306.3
  special sense organs 306.7
 psychosomatic (*see also* Disorder,
   psychosomatic) 306.9
 psychotic (*see also* Psychosis) 298.9
  depressive 298.0
  due to or associated with physical condition
    (*see also* Psychosis, organic) 293.9
  involutional (*see also* Psychosis, affective)
    296.2
   recurrent episode 296.3
   single episode 296.2
 pupillary (myotonic) (tonic) 379.46
 radiation—*see* Effect, adverse, radiation
 runaway—*see also* Disturbance, conduct
  socialized 312.2
  undersocialized, unsocialized 312.1
 scarlet fever toxin—*see* Complications,
   vaccination
 schizophrenic (*see also* Schizophrenia) 295.9
  latent 295.5
 serological for syphilis—*see* Serology for
   syphilis
 serum (prophylactic) (therapeutic) 999.59
  anaphylactic 999.49
  due to
   administration of blood and blood products
     999.51
    anaphylactic 999.41
   vaccination 999.52
    anaphylactic 999.41
  immediate 999.49
 situational (*see also* Reaction, adjustment) 309.9
  acute, to stress 308.3
  adjustment (*see also* Reaction, adjustment) 309.9
 somatization (*see also* Disorder, psychosomatic)
   306.9
 spinal puncture 349.0
 spite, child (*see also* Disturbance, conduct) 312.0
 stress, acute 308.9
  bone or cartilage —*see* Fracture, stress
  with predominant disturbance (of)
   consciousness 308.1
   emotions 308.0
   mixed 308.4
   psychomotor 308.2
   specified type NEC 308.3
 surgical procedure—*see* Complications, surgical
   procedure
 tetanus antitoxin—*see* Complications,
   vaccination
 toxin-antitoxin—*see* Complications, vaccination
 transfusion (blood) (bone marrow)
   (lymphocytes) (allergic) (see also
   Complications, transfusion) 999.80
 tuberculin skin test, nonspecific (without active
   tuberculosis) 795.51
  positive (without active tuberculosis) 795.51

Reaction—*continued*
 ultraviolet—*see* Effect, adverse, ultraviolet
 undersocialized, unsocialized—*see also*
   Disturbance, conduct
  aggressive (type) 312.0
  unaggressive (type) 312.1
 vaccination (any)—*see* Complications,
   vaccination
 white graft (skin) 996.52
 withdrawing, child or adolescent 313.22
 x-ray—*see* Effect, adverse, x-rays
Reactive depression (*see also* Reaction,
   depressive) 300.4
 neurotic 300.4
 psychoneurotic 300.4
 psychotic 298.0
Rebound tenderness 789.6
Recalcitrant patient V15.81
Recanalization, thrombus —*see* Thrombosis
Recession, receding
 chamber angle (eye) 364.77
 chin 524.06
 gingival (postinfective) (postoperative) 523.20
  generalized 523.25
  localized 523.24
  minimal 523.21
  moderate 523.22
  servere 523.23
Recklinghausen's disease (M9540/1) 237.71
 bones (osteitis fibrosa cystica) 252.01
Recklinghausen-Applebaum disease
   (hemochromatosis) 275.03
Reclus' disease (cystic) 610.1
Recrudescent typhus (fever) 081.1
Recruitment, auditory 388.44
Rectalgia 569.42
Rectitis 569.49
Rectocele
 female (without uterine prolapse) 618.04
  with uterine prolapse 618.4
   complete 618.3
   incomplete 618.2
 in pregnancy or childbirth 654.4
  causing obstructed labor 660.2
   affecting fetus or newborn 763.1
 male 569.49
 vagina, vaginal (outlet) 618.04
Rectosigmoiditis 569.89
 ulcerative (chronic) 556.3
Rectosigmoid junction —*see* condition
Rectourethral —*see* condition
Rectovaginal —*see* condition
Rectovesical —*see* condition
Rectum, rectal —*see* condition
Recurrent —*see* condition
 pregnancy loss - *see* Pregnancy, management
   affected by, abortion, habitual
Red bugs 133.8
Red cedar asthma 495.8
Redness
 conjunctiva 379.93
 eye 379.93
 nose 478.19
Reduced ventilatory or vital capacity 794.2
Reduction
 function
  kidney (*see also* Disease, renal) 593.9
  liver 573.8
 ventilatory capacity 794.2
 vital capacity 794.2

Redundant, redundancy
abdomen 701.9
anus 751.5
cardia 537.89
clitoris 624.2
colon (congenital) 751.5
foreskin (congenital) 605
intestine 751.5
labia 624.3
organ or site, congenital NEC—*see* Accessory
panniculus (abdominal) 278.1
prepuce (congenital) 605
pylorus 537.89
rectum 751.5
scrotum 608.89
sigmoid 751.5
skin (of face) 701.9
  eyelids 374.30
stomach 537.89
uvula 528.9
vagina 623.8
Reduplication —*see* Duplication
Referral
adoption (agency) V68.89
nursing care V63.8
patient without examination or treatment V68.81
social services V63.8
Reflex —*see also* condition
blink, deficient 374.45
hyperactive gag 478.29
neurogenic bladder NEC 596.54
  atonic 596.54
    with cauda equina syndrome 344.61
vasoconstriction 443.9
Reflux 530.81
acid 530.81
esophageal 530.81
esophagitis 530.11
gastroesophageal 530.81
mitral—*see* Insufficiency, mitral
ureteral —*see* Reflux, vesicoureteral
vasovagal 780.2
vesicoureteral 593.70
  with
    reflux nephropathy 593.73
      bilateral 593.72
      unilateral 593.71
Reformed gallbladder 576.0
Reforming, artificial openings (*see also*
  Attention to, artificial, opening) V55.9
Refractive error (*see also* Error, refractive) 367.9
Refsum's disease or syndrome (heredopathia
  atactica polyneuritiformis) 356.3
Refusal of
food 307.59
  hysterical 300.11
treatment because of, due to
  patient's decision NEC V64.2
  reason of conscience or religion V62.6
Regaud
tumor (M8082/3)—*see* Neoplasm, nasopharynx,
  malignant
type carcinoma (M8082/3)—*see* Neoplasm,
  nasopharynx, malignant
Regional —*see* condition
Regulation feeding (elderly) (infant) 783.3
newborn 779.31
Regurgitated
food, choked on 933.1
stomach contents, choked on 933.1

Regurgitation 787.03
aortic (valve) (*see also* Insufficiency, aortic) 424.1
  congenital 746.4
  syphilitic 093.22
food—*see also* Vomiting
  with reswallowing—*see* Rumination
  newborn 779.33
gastric contents—*see* Vomiting
heart—*see* Endocarditis
mitral (valve)—*see also* Insufficiency, mitral
  congenital 746.6
myocardial—*see* Endocarditis
pulmonary (heart) (valve) (*see also*
  Endocarditis, pulmonary) 424.3
stomach—*see* Vomiting
tricuspid—*see* Endocarditis, tricuspid
valve, valvular—*see* Endocarditis
vesicoureteral —*see* Reflux, vesicoureteral
Rehabilitation V57.9
multiple types V57.89
occupational V57.21
specified type NEC V57.89
speech(-language) V57.3
vocational V57.22
Reichmann's disease or syndrome
  (gastrosuccorrhea) 536.8
Reifenstein's syndrome (hereditary familial
  hypogonadism, male) 259.52
Reilly's syndrome or phenomenon (*see also*
  Neuropathy, peripheral, autonomic) 337.9
Reimann's periodic disease 277.31
Reinsertion, contraceptive device V25.42
intrauterine V25.13
Reiter's disease, syndrome, or urethritis 099.3
  [711.1]
Rejection
food, hysterical 300.11
transplant 996.80
  bone marrow 996.85
  corneal 996.51
  organ (immune or nonimmune cause) 996.80
    bone marrow 996.85
    heart 996.83
    intestines 996.87
    kidney 996.81
    liver 996.82
    lung 996.84
    pancreas 996.86
    specified NEC 996.89
  skin 996.52
    artificial 996.55
    decellularized allodermis 996.55
  stem cell(s) 996.88
    from
      peripheral blood 996.88
      umbilical cord 996.88
Relapsing fever 087.9
Carter's (Asiatic) 087.0
Dutton's (West African) 087.1
Koch's 087.9
louse-borne (epidemic) 087.0
Novy's (American) 087.1
Obermeyer's (European) 087.0
Spirillum 087.9
tick-borne (endemic) 087.1
Relaxation
anus (sphincter) 569.49
  due to hysteria 300.11
arch (foot) 734
  congenital 754.61
back ligaments 728.4

Relaxation—*continued*
  bladder (sphincter) 596.59
  cardio-esophageal 530.89
  cervix (*see also* Incompetency, cervix) 622.5
  diaphragm 519.4
  inguinal rings—*see* Hernia, inguinal
  joint (capsule) (ligament) (paralytic) (*see also*
      Derangement, joint) 718.90
    congenital 755.8
  lumbosacral joint 724.6
  pelvic floor 618.89
  pelvis 618.89
  perineum 618.89
  posture 729.90
  rectum (sphincter) 569.49
  sacroiliac (joint) 724.6
  scrotum 608.89
  urethra (sphincter) 599.84
  uterus (outlet) 618.89
  vagina (outlet) 618.89
  vesical 596.59
Remains
  canal of Cloquet 743.51
  capsule (opaque) 743.51
Remittent fever (malarial) 084.6
Remnant
  canal of Cloquet 743.51
  capsule (opaque) 743.51
  cervix, cervical stump (acquired) (postoperative)
      622.8
  cystic duct, postcholecystectomy 576.0
  fingernail 703.8
    congenital 757.5
  meniscus, knee 717.5
  thyroglossal duct 759.2
  tonsil 474.8
    infected 474.00
  urachus 753.7
Remote effect of cancer —*see* Condition
Removal (of)
  catheter (urinary) (indwelling) V53.6
    from artificial opening—*see* Attention to,
        artificial, opening
    non-vascular V58.82
    vascular V58.81
  cerebral ventricle (communicating) shunt V53.01
  device—*see also* Fitting (of)
    contraceptive V25.12
      with reinsertion V25.13
    fixation
      external V54.89
      internal V54.01
      traction V54.89
  drains V58.49
  dressing
    wound V58.30
      nonsurgical V58.30
      surgical V58.31
  ileostomy V55.2
  Kirschner wire V54.89
  non-vascular catheter V58.82
  pin V54.01
  plaster cast V54.89
  plate (fracture) V54.01
  rod V54.01
  screw V54.01
  splint, external V54.89
  subdermal implantable contraceptive V25.43
  staples V58.32
  sutures V58.32
  traction device, external V54.89

Removal (of)—*continued*
  vascular catheter V58.81
  wound packing V58.30
    nonsurgical V58.30
    surgical V58.31
Ren
  arcuatus 753.3
  mobile, mobilis (*see also* Disease, renal) 593.0
    congenital 753.3
  unguliformis 753.3
Renal —*see also* condition
  glomerulohyalinosis-diabetic syndrome 250.4
      [581.81]
    due to secondary diabetes 249.4 *[581.81]*
Rendu-Osler-Weber disease or syndrome
  (familial hemorrhagic telangiectasia) 448.0
Reninoma (M8361/1) 236.91
Rénon-Delille syndrome 253.8
Repair
  pelvic floor, previous, in pregnancy or childbirth
      654.4
    affecting fetus or newborn 763.89
  scarred tissue V51.8
Replacement by artificial or mechanical device
  or prosthesis of (*see also* Fitting (of))
  artificial skin V43.83
  bladder V43.5
  blood vessel V43.4
  breast V43.82
  eye globe V43.0
  heart
    with
      assist device V43.21
      fully implantable artificial heart V43.22
    valve V43.3
  intestine V43.89
  joint V43.60
    ankle 43.66
    elbow V43.62
    finger V43.69
    hip (partial) (total) V43.64
    knee V43.65
    shoulder V43.61
    specified NEC V43.69
    wrist V43.63
  kidney V43.89
  larynx V43.81
  lens V43.1
  limb(s) V43.7
  liver V43.89
  lung V43.89
  organ NEC V43.89
  pancreas V43.89
  skin (artificial) V43.83
  tissue NEC V43.89
Reprogramming
  cardiac pacemaker V53.31
Request for expert evidence V68.2
Reserve, decreased or low
  cardiac—*see* Disease, heart
  kidney (*see also* Disease, renal) 593.9
Residual —*see also* condition
  bladder 596.89
  foreign body—*see* Retention, foreign body
  state, schizophrenic (*see also* Schizophrenia)
      295.6
  urine 788.69

Resistance, resistant (to)

> *Note—Use the following subclassification for categories V09.5, V09.7, V09.8, V09.9.:*
>
> 0 *without mention of resistance to multiple drugs*
> 1 *with resistance to multiple drugs*
>
> V09.5 *quinolones and fluoroquinolones*
> V09.7 *antimycobacterial agents*
> V09.8 *specified drugs NEC*
> V09.9 *unspecified drugs*
>
> 9 *multiple sites*

activated protein C 289.81
drugs by microorganisms V09.90
   Amikacin V09.4
   aminoglycosides V09.4
   Amodiaquine V09.5
   Amoxicillin V09.0
   Ampicillin V09.0
   antimycobacterial agents V09.7
   Azithromycin V09.2
   Azlocillin V09.0
   Aztreonam V09.1
   B-lactam antibiotics V09.1
   Bacampicillin V09.0
   Bacitracin V09.8
   Benznidazole V09.8
   Capreomycin V09.7
   Carbenicillin V09.0
   Cefaclor V09.1
   Cefadroxil V09.1
   Cefamandole V09.1
   Cefatetan V09.1
   Cefazolin V09.1
   Cefixime V09.1
   Cefonicid V09.1
   Cefoperazone V09.1
   Ceforanide V09.1
   Cefotaxime V09.1
   Cefoxitin V09.1
   Ceftazidine V09.1
   Ceftizoxime V09.1
   Ceftriaxone V09.1
   Cefuroxime V09.1
   Cephalexin V09.1
   Cephaloglycin V09.1
   Cephaloridine V09.1
   cephalosporins V09.1
   Cephalothin V09.1
   Cephapirin V09.1
   Cephradine V09.1
   Chloramphenicol V09.8
   Chloraquine V09.5
   Chlorguanide V09.8
   Chlorproguanil V09.8
   Chlortetracycline V09.3
   Cinoxacin V09.5
   Ciprofloxacin V09.5
   Clarithromycin V09.2
   Clindamycin V09.8
   Clioquinol V09.5
   Clofazimine V09.7
   Cloxacillin V09.0
   Cyclacillin V09.0
   Cycloserine V09.7
   Dapsone [DZ] V09.7
   Demeclocycline V09.3
   Dicloxacillin V09.0

Resistance, resistant (to)—*continued*
drugs by microorganisms—*continued*
   Doxycycline V09.3
   Enoxacin V09.5
   Erythromycin V09.2
   Ethambutol [EMB] V09.7
   Ethionamide [ETA] V09.7
   fluoroquinolones NEC V09.5
   Gentamicin V09.4
   Halofantrine V09.8
   ImipenemV09.1
   Iodoquinol V09.5
   Isoniazid [INH] V09.7
   Kanamycin V09.4
   macrolides V09.2
   Mafenide V09.6
   MDRO (multiple drug resistant organisms) NOS V09.91
   Mefloquine V09.8
   Melassoprol V09.8
   Methacycline V09.3
   Methenamine V09.8
   Methicillin—*see* Infection, methicillin
   Metronidazole V09.8
   Mezlocillin V09.0
   Minocycline V09.3
   multiple drug resistant organisms NOS V09.91
   Nafcillin V09.0
   Nalidixic Acid V09.5
   Natamycin V09.2
   Neomycin V09.4
   Netilmicin V09.4
   Nimorazole V09.8
   Nitrofurantoin V09.8
   Nitrofurtimox V09.8
   Norfloxacin V09.5
   Nystatin V09.2
   Ofloxacin V09.5
   Oleandomycin V09.2
   Oxacillin V09.0
   Oxytetracycline V09.3
   Para-amino salicylic acid [PAS] V09.7
   Paromomycin V09.4
   Penicillin (G)(V)(VK) V09.0
   penicillins V09.0
   Pentamidine V09.8
   Piperacillin V09.0
   Primaquine V09.5
   Proguanil V09.8
   Pyrazinamide [PZA] V09.7
   Pyrimethamine/Sulfalene V09.8
   Pyrimethamine/Sulfodoxine V09.8
   Quinacrine V09.5
   Quinidine V09.8
   Quinine V09.8
   quinolones V09.5
   Rifabutin V09.7
   Rifampin [RIF] V09.7
   Rifamycin V09.7
   Rolitetracycline V09.3
   specified drugs NEC V09.8
   Spectinomycin V09.8
   Spiramycin V09.2
   Streptomycin [SM] V09.4
   Sulfacetamide V09.6
   Sulfacytine V90.6
   Sulfadiazine V09.6
   Sulfadoxine V09.6
   Sulfamethoxazole V09.6
   Sulfapyridine V09.6
   Sulfasalizine V09.6

Resistance, resistant (to)—*continued*
  drugs by microorganisms—*continued*
    Sulfasoxazole V09.6
    sulfonamides V09.6
    Sulfoxone V09.7
    Tetracycline V09.3
    tetracyclines V09.3
    Thiamphenicol V09.8
    Ticarcillin V09.0
    Tinidazole V09.8
    Tobramycin V09.4
    Triamphenicol V09.8
    Trimethoprim V09.8
    Vancomycin V09.8
  insulin 277.7
    complicating pregnancy 648.8
  thyroid hormone 246.8
Resorption
  biliary 576.8
    purulent or putrid (*see also* Cholecystitis)
      576.8
  dental (roots) 521.40
    alveoli 525.8
    pathological
      external 521.42
      internal 521.41
      specified NEC 521.49
  septic—*see* Septicemia
  teeth (roots) 521.40
    pathological
      external 521.42
      internal 521.41
      specified NEC 521.49
Respiration
  asymmetrical 786.09
  bronchial 786.09
  Cheyne-Stokes (periodic respiration) 786.04
  decreased, due to shock following injury 958.4
  disorder of 786.00
    psychogenic 306.1
    specified NEC 786.09
  failure 518.81
    acute 518.81
      following trauma and surgery 518.51
    acute and chronic 518.84
      following trauma and surgery 518.53
    chronic 518.83
    following trauma and surgery 518.51
    newborn 770.84
  insufficiency 786.09
    acute 518.82
    newborn NEC 770.89
  Kussmaul (air hunger) 786.09
  painful 786.52
  periodic 786.09
    high altitude 327.22
  poor 786.09
    newborn NEC 770.89
  sighing 786.7
    psychogenic 306.1
  wheezing 786.07
Respiratory —*see also* condition
  distress 786.09
    acute 518.82
    fetus or newborn NEC 770.89
    syndrome (newborn) 769
      adult (following trauma and surgery) 518.52
      specified NEC 518.82

Respiratory—*continued*
  failure 518.81
    acute 518.81
      following trauma and surgery 518.51
    acute and chronic 518.84
      following trauma and surgery 518.53
    chronic 518.83
    following trauma and surgery 518.51
Respiratory syncytial virus (RSV) 079.6
  bronchiolitis 466.11
  pneumonia 480.1
  vaccination, prophylactic (against) V04.82
Response
  photoallergic 692.72
  phototoxic 692.72
Rest, rests
  mesonephric duct 752.89
    fallopian tube 752.11
  ovarian, in fallopian tubes 752.19
  wolffian duct 752.89
Restless legs syndrome (RLS) 333.94
Restlessness 799.29
Restoration of organ continuity from previous
  sterilization (tuboplasty) (vasoplasty) V26.0
Restriction of housing space V60.1
Restzustand, schizophrenic (*see also*
  Schizophrenia) 295.6
Retained —*see* Retention
Retardation
  development, developmental, specific (*see also*
    Disorder, development, specific) 315.9
    learning, specific 315.2
      arithmetical 315.1
      language (skills) 315.31
        expressive 315.31
        mixed receptive-expressive 315.32
      mathematics 315.1
      reading 315.00
        phonological 315.39
      written expression 315.2
    motor 315.4
  endochondral bone growth 733.91
  growth (physical) in childhood 783.43
    due to malnutrition 263.2
    fetal (intrauterine) 764.9
      affecting management of pregnancy 656.5
  intrauterine growth 764.9
    affecting management of pregnancy 656.5
  mental—see Disability, intellectual
  motor, specific 315.4
  physical 783.43
    child 783.43
    due to malnutrition 263.2
    fetus (intrauterine) 764.9
      affecting management of pregnancy 656.5
  psychomotor NEC 307.9
  reading 315.00
Retching —*see* Vomiting
Retention, retained
  bladder NEC (*see also* Retention, urine) 788.20
    psychogenic 306.53
  carbon dioxide 276.2
  cholelithiasis, following cholecystectomy
    997.41
  cyst—*see* Cyst
  dead
    fetus (after 22 completed weeks gestation) 656.4
      early fetal death (before 22 completed weeks
        gestation) 632
    ovum 631.8

Retention, retained—*continued*
  decidua (following delivery) (fragments) (with
      hemorrhage) 666.2
    without hemorrhage 667.1
  deciduous tooth 520.6
  dental root 525.3
  fecal (*see also* Constipation) 564.00
  fluid 276.69
  foreign body—*see also* Foreign body, retained
    bone 733.99
    current trauma—*see* Foreign body, by site or type
    middle ear 385.83
    muscle 729.6
    soft tissue NEC 729.6
  gallstones, following cholecystectomy 997.41
  gastric 536.8
  membranes (following delivery) (with
      hemorrhage) 666.2
    with abortion—*see* Abortion, by type
    without hemorrhage 667.1
  menses 626.8
  milk (puerperal) 676.2
  nitrogen, extrarenal 788.99
  placenta (total) (with hemorrhage) 666.0
    with abortion—*see* Abortion, by type
    portions or fragments 666.2
      without hemorrhage 667.1
    without hemorrhage 667.0
  products of conception
    early pregnancy (fetal death before 22
        completed weeks gestation) 632
    following
      abortion—*see* Abortion, by type
      delivery 666.2
        with hemorrhage 666.2
        without hemorrhage 667.1
  secundines (following delivery) (with
      hemorrhage) 666.2
    with abortion—*see* Abortion, by type
    complicating puerperium (delayed
        hemorrhage) 666.2
    without hemorrhage 667.1
  smegma, clitoris 624.8
  urine NEC 788.20
    bladder, incomplete emptying 788.21
    due to benign prostatic hypertrophy
        (BPH)—*see* category 600
    due to benign prostatic hypertrophy
        (BPH)—*see* category 600
    psychogenic 306.53
    specified NEC 788.29
  water (in tissue) (*see also* Edema) 782.3
Reticulation, dust (occupational) 504
Reticulocytosis NEC 790.99
Reticuloendotheliosis
  acute infantile (M9722/3) 202.5
  leukemic (M9940/3) 202.4
  malignant (M9720/3) 202.3
  nonlipid (M9722/3) 202.5
Reticulohistiocytoma (giant cell) 277.89
Reticulohistiocytosis, multicentric 272.8
Reticulolymphosarcoma (diffuse) (M9613/3)
    200.8
  follicular (M9691/3) 202.0
  nodular (M9691/3) 202.0
Reticulosarcoma (M9640/3) 200.0
  odular (M9642/3) 200.0
  pleomorphic cell type (M9641/3) 200.0

Reticulosis (skin)
  acute of infancy (M9722/3) 202.5
  familial hemophagocytic 288.4
  histiocytic medullary (M9721/3) 202.3
  lipomelanotic 695.89
  malignant (M9720/3) 202.3
  Sézary's (M9701/3) 202.2
Retina, retinal —*see* condition
Retinitis (*see also* Chorioretinitis) 363.20
  albuminurica 585.9 *[363.10]*
  arteriosclerotic 440.8 *[362.13]*
  central angiospastic 362.41
  Coat's 362.12
  diabetic 250.5 *[362.01]*
    due to secondary diabetes 249.5 *[362.01]*
  disciformis 362.52
  disseminated 363.10
    metastatic 363.14
    neurosyphilitic 094.83
    pigment epitheliopathy 363.15
  exudative 362.12
  focal 363.00
    in histoplasmosis 115.92
      capsulatum 115.02
      duboisii 115.12
    juxtapapillary 363.05
    macular 363.06
    paramacular 363.06
    peripheral 363.08
    posterior pole NEC 363.07
  gravidarum 646.8
  hemorrhagica externa 362.12
  juxtapapillary (Jensen's) 363.05
  luetic—*see* Retinitis, syphilitic
  metastatic 363.14
  pigmentosa 362.74
  proliferans 362.29
  proliferating 362.29
  punctata albescens 362.76
  renal 585.9 *[363.13]*
  syphilitic (secondary) 091.51
    congenital 090.0 *[363.13]*
    early 091.51
    late 095.8 *[363.13]*
  syphilitica, central, recurrent 095.8 *[363.13]*
  tuberculous (*see also* Tuberculous) 017.3 *[363.13]*
Retinoblastoma (M9510/3) 190.5
  differentiated type (M9511/3) 190.5
  undifferentiated type (M9512/3) 190.5
Retinochoroiditis (*see also* Chorioretinitis) 363.20
  central angiospastic 362.41
  disseminated 363.10
    metastatic 363.14
    neurosyphilitic 094.83
    pigment epitheliopathy 363.15
    syphilitic 094.83
  due to toxoplasmosis (acquired) (focal) 130.2
  focal 363.00
    in histoplasmosis 115.92
      capsulatum 115.02
      duboisii 115.12
    juxtapapillary (Jensen's) 363.05
    macular 363.06
    paramacular 363.06
    peripheral 363.08
    posterior pole NEC 363.07
  juxtapapillaris 363.05
  syphilitic (disseminated) 094.83

Retinopathy (background) 362.10
  arteriosclerotic 440.8 *[362.13]*
  atherosclerotic 440.8 *[362.13]*
  central serous 362.41
  circinate 362.10
  Coat's 362.12
  diabetic 250.5 *[362.01]*
    due to secondary diabetes 249.5 *[362.01]*
    nonproliferative 250.5 *[362.03]*
      due to secondary diabetes 249.5 *[362.03]*
      mild 250.5 *[362.04]*
        due to secondary diabetes 249.5 *[362.04]*
      moderate 250.5 *[362.05]*
        due to secondary diabetes 249.5 *[362.05]*
      severe 250.5 *[362.06]*
        due to secondary diabetes 249.5 *[362.06]*
    proliferative 250.5 *[362.02]*
      due to secondary diabetes 249.5 *[362.02]*
  exudative 362.12
  hypertensive 362.11
  of prematurity 362.20
    cicatricial 362.21
    stage
      0 362.22
      1 362.23
      2 362.24
      3 362.25
      4 362.26
      5 362.27
  nonproliferative
    diabetic 250.5 *[362.03]*
      due to secondary diabetes 249.5 *[362.03]*
      mild 250.5 *[362.04]*
        due to secondary diabetes 249.5 *[362.04]*
      moderate 250.5 *[362.05]*
        due to secondary diabetes 249.5 *[362.05]*
      severe 250.5 *[362.06]*
        due to secondary diabetes 249.5 *[362.06]*
  pigmentary, congenital 362.74
  proliferative 362.29
    diabetic 250.5 *[362.02]*
      due to secondary diabetes 249.5 *[362.02]*
    sickle-cell 282.60 *[362.29]*
  solar 363.31
Retinoschisis 361.10
  bullous 361.12
  congenital 743.56
  flat 361.11
  juvenile 362.73
Retractile testis 752.52
Retraction
  cervix *see* Retraction, uterus
  drum (membrane) 384.82
  eyelid 374.41
  finger 736.29
  head 781.0
  lid 374.41
  lung 518.89
  mediastinum 519.3
  nipple 611.79
    congenital 757.6
    puerperal, postpartum 676.0
  palmar fascia 728.6
  pleura (*see also* Pleurisy) 511.0
  ring, uterus (Bandl's) (pathological) 661.4
    affecting fetus or newborn 763.7
  sternum (congenital) 756.3
    acquired 738.3
    during respiration 786.9
  substernal 738.3
  supraclavicular 738.8

Retraction—*continued*
  syndrome (Duane's) 378.71
  uterus 621.6
  valve (heart)—*see* Endocarditis
Retrobulbar —*see* condition
Retrocaval ureter 753.4
Retrocecal —*see also* condition
  appendix (congenital) 751.5
Retrocession —*see* Retroversion
Retrodisplacement —*see* Retroversion
Retroflection, retroflexion —*see* Retroversion
Retrognathia, retrognathism (mandibular)
  (maxillary) 524.06
Retrograde
  ejaculation 608.87
  menstruation 626.8
Retroiliac ureter 753.4
Retroperineal —*see* condition
Retroperitoneal —*see* condition
Retroperitonitis 567.39
Retropharyngeal —*see* condition
Retroplacental —*see* condition
Retroposition —*see* Retroversion
Retroprosthetic membrane 996.51
Retrosternal thyroid (congenital) 759.2
Retroversion, retroverted
  cervix *see* Retroversion, uterus
  female NEC (*see also* Retroversion, uterus) 621.6
  iris 364.70
  testis (congenital) 752.51
  uterus, uterine (acquired) (acute) (adherent) (any
    degree) (asymptomatic) (cervix)
    (postinfectional) (postpartal, old) 621.6
  congenital 752.39
  in pregnancy or childbirth 654.3
    affecting fetus or newborn 763.89
    causing obstructed labor 660.2
      affecting fetus or newborn 763.1
Retrusion, premaxilla (developmental) 524.04
Rett's syndrome 330.8
Reverse, reversed
  peristalsis 787.4
Reye's syndrome 331.81
Reye-Sheehan syndrome (postpartum pituitary
  necrosis) 253.2
Rh antigen (C) (c) (D) (E) (e) (factor)
  hemolytic disease 773.0
  incompatibility, immunization, or sensitization
    affecting management of pregnancy 656.1
    fetus or newborn 773.0
    transfusion reaction (*see also* Complications,
      transfusion) 999.70
  negative mother, affecting fetus or newborn
    773.0
  titer elevated (*see also* Complications,
    transfusion) 999.70
  transfusion reaction (*see also* Complications,
    transfusion) 999.70
Rhabdomyolysis (idiopathic) 728.88
Rhabdomyoma (M8900/0)—*see also* Neoplasm,
  connective tissue, benign
  adult (M8904/0)—*see* Neoplasm, connective
    tissue, benign
  fetal (M8903/0)—*see* Neoplasm, connective
    tissue, benign
  glycogenic (M8904/0)—*see* Neoplasm,
    connective tissue, benign

Rhabdomyosarcoma (M8900/3)—*see also*
  Neoplasm connective tissue, malignant
  alveolar (M8920/3)—*see* Neoplasm, connective
    tissue, malignant
  embryonal (M8910/3)—*see* Neoplasm,
    connective tissue malignant
  mixed type (M8902/3)—*see* Neoplasm,
    connective tissue, malignant
  pleomorphic (M8901/3)—*see* Neoplasm,
    connective tissue, malignant
Rhabdosarcoma (M8900/3)—*see*
  Rhabdomyosarcoma
Rhesus (factor) (Rh) incompatibility—*see* Rh,
  incompatibility
Rheumaticosis —*see* Rheumatism
Rheumatism, rheumatic (acute NEC) 729.0
  adherent pericardium 393
  arthritis
    acute or subacute—*see* Fever, rheumatic
    chronic 714.0
      spine 720.0
  articular (chronic) NEC (*see also* Arthritis)
    716.9
    acute or subacute—*see* Fever, rheumatic
  back 724.9
  blennorrhagic 098.59
  carditis—*see* Disease, heart, rheumatic
  cerebral—*see* Fever, rheumatic
  chorea (acute)—*see* Chorea, rheumatic
  chronic NEC 729.0
  coronary arteritis 391.9
    chronic 398.99
  degeneration, myocardium (*see also*
    Degeneration, myocardium, with rheumatic
    fever) 398.0
  desert 114.0
  febrile—*see* Fever, rheumatic
  fever—*see* Fever, rheumatic
  gonococcal 098.59
  gout 714.00
  heart
    disease (*see also* Disease, heart, rheumatic)
      398.90
    failure (chronic) (congestive) (inactive) 398.91
    hemopericardium—*see* Rheumatic, pericarditis
    hydropericardium—*see* Rheumatic, pericarditis
    inflammatory (acute) (chronic) (subacute)—*see*
      Fever, rheumatic
  intercostal 729.0
    meaning Tietze's disease 733.6
  joint (chronic) NEC (*see also* Arthritis) 716.9
    acute—*see* Fever, rheumatic
  mediastinopericarditis—*see* Rheumatic,
    pericarditis
  muscular 729.0
  myocardial degeneration (*see also*
    Degeneration, myocardium, with rheumatic
    fever) 398.0
  myocarditis (chronic) (inactive) (with chorea)
    398.0
    active or acute 391.2
      with chorea (acute) (rheumatic)
        (Sydenham's) 392.0
  myositis 729.1
  neck 724.9
  neuralgic 729.0
  neuritis (acute) (chronic) 729.2
  neuromuscular 729.0
  nodose—*see* Arthritis, nodosa
  nonarticular 729.0

Rheumatism, rheumatic—*continued*
  palindromic 719.30
    ankle 719.37
    elbow 719.32
    foot 719.37
    hand 719.34
    hip 719.35
    knee 719.36
    multiple sites 719.39
    pelvic region 719.35
    shoulder (region) 719.31
    specified site NEC 719.38
    wrist 719.33
  pancarditis, acute 391.8
    with chorea (acute) (rheumatic) (Sydenham's)
      392.0
    chronic or inactive 398.99
  pericarditis (active) (acute) (with effusion) (with
    pneumonia) 391.0
    with chorea (acute) (rheumatic) (Sydenham's)
      392.0
    chronic or inactive 393
  pericardium—*see* Rheumatic, pericarditis
  pleuropericarditis—*see* Rheumatic, pericarditis
  pneumonia 390 [517.1]
  pneumonitis 390 [517.1]
  pneumopericarditis—*see* Rheumatic,
    pericarditis
  polyarthritis
    acute or subacute—*see* Fever, rheumatic
    chronic 714.0
  polyarticular NEC (*see also* Arthritis) 716.9
  psychogenic 306.0
  radiculitis 729.2
  sciatic 724.3
  septic—*see* Fever, rheumatic
  spine 724.9
  subacute NEC 729.0
  torticollis 723.5
  tuberculous NEC (*see also* Tuberculosis) 015.9
  typhoid fever 002.0
Rheumatoid —*see also* condition
  lungs 714.81
Rhinitis (atrophic) (catarrhal) (chronic)
    (croupous) (fibrinous) (hyperplastic)
    (hypertrophic) (membranous) (purulent)
    (suppurative) (ulcerative) 472.0
  with
    hay fever (*see also* Fever, hay) 477.9
      with asthma (bronchial) 493.0
    sore throat—*see* Nasopharyngitis
  acute 460
  allergic (nonseasonal) (seasonal) (*see also*
    Fever, hay) 477.9
    due to food 477.1
    with asthma (*see also* Asthma) 493.0
  granulomatous 472.0
  infective 460
  obstructive 472.0
  pneumococcal 460
  syphilitic 095.8
    congenital 090.0
  tuberculous (*see also* Tuberculosis) 012.8
  vasomotor (*see also* Fever, hay) 477.9
Rhinoantritis (chronic) 473.0
  acute 461.0
Rhinodacryolith 375.57
Rhinolalia (aperta) (clausa) (open) 784.43
Rhinolith 478.19
  nasal sinus (*see also* Sinusitis) 473.9
Rhinomegaly 478.19

Rhinopharyngitis (acute) (subacute) (*see also*
   Nasopharyngitis) 460
  chronic 472.2
  destructive ulcerating 102.5
  mutilans 102.5
Rhinophyma 695.3
Rhinorrhea 478.19
  cerebrospinal (fluid) 349.81
  paroxysmal (*see also* Fever, hay) 477.9
  spasmodic (*see also* Fever, hay) 477.9
Rhinosalpingitis 381.50
  acute 381.51
  chronic 381.52
Rhinoscleroma 040.1
Rhinosporidiosis 117.0
Rhinovirus infection 079.3
Rhizomelic chrondrodysplasia punctata 277.86
Rhizomelique, pseudopolyarthritic 446.5
Rhoads and Bomford anemia (refractory)
  238.72
Rhus
  diversiloba dermatitis 692.6
  radicans dermatitis 692.6
  toxicodendron dermatitis 692.6
  venenata dermatitis 692.6
  verniciflua dermatitis 692.6
Rhythm
  atrioventricular nodal 427.89
  disorder 427.9
    coronary sinus 427.89
    ectopic 427.89
    nodal 427.89
  escape 427.89
  heart, abnormal 427.9
    fetus or newborn—*see* Abnormal, heart rate
  idioventricular 426.89
    accelerated 427.89
  nodal 427.89
  sleep, inversion 327.39
    nonorganic origin 307.45
Rhytidosis facialis 701.8
Rib —*see also* condition
  cervical 756.2
Riboflavin deficiency 266.0
Rice bodies (*see also* Loose, body, joint) 718.1
  knee 717.6
Richter's hernia —*see* Hernia, Richter's
Ricinism 988.2
Rickets (active) (acute) (adolescent) (adult)
  (chest wall) (congenital) (current) (infantile)
  (intestinal) 268.0
  celiac 579.0
  fetal 756.4
  hemorrhagic 267
  hypophosphatemic with nephrotic-glycosuric
    dwarfism 270.0
  kidney 588.0
  late effect 268.1
  renal 588.0
  scurvy 267
  vitamin D-resistant 275.3
Rickettsial disease 083.9
  specified type NEC 083.8
Rickettsialpox 083.2
Rickettsiosis NEC 083.9
  specified type NEC 083.8
  tick-borne 082.9
    specified type NEC 082.8
  vesicular 083.2
Ricord's chancre 091.0
Riddoch's syndrome (visual disorientation) 368.16

Rider's
  bone 733.99
  chancre 091.0
Ridge, alveolus —*see also* condition
  edentulous
    atrophy 525.20
      mandible 525.20
        minimal 525.21
        moderate 525.22
        severe 525.23
      maxilla 525.20
        minimal 525.24
        moderate 525.25
        severe 525.26
    flabby 525.20
Ridged ear 744.29
Riedel's
  disease (ligneous thyroiditis) 245.3
  lobe, liver 751.69
  struma (ligneous thyroiditis) 245.3
  thyroiditis (ligneous) 245.3
Rieger's anomaly or syndrome (mesodermal
  dysgenesis, anterior ocular segment) 743.44
Riehl's melanosis 709.09
Rietti-Greppi-Micheli anemia or syndrome 282.46
Rieux's hernia —*see* Hernia, Rieux's
Rift Valley fever 066.3
Riga's disease (cachectic aphthae) 529.0
Riga-Fede disease (cachectic aphthae) 529.0
Riggs' disease (compound periodontitis) 523.40
Right middle lobe syndrome 518.0
Rigid, rigidity —*see also* condition
  abdominal 789.4
  articular, multiple congenital 754.89
  back 724.8
  cervix uteri
    in pregnancy or childbirth 654.6
      affecting fetus or newborn 763.89
      causing obstructed labor 660.2
        affecting fetus or newborn 763.1
  hymen (acquired) (congenital) 623.3
  nuchal 781.6
  pelvic floor
    in pregnancy or childbirth 654.4
      affecting fetus or newborn 763.89
      causing obstructed labor 660.2
        affecting fetus or newborn 763.1
  perineum or vulva
    in pregnancy or childbirth 654.8
      affecting fetus or newborn 763.89
      causing obstructed labor 660.2
        affecting fetus or newborn 763.1
  spine 724.8
  vagina
    in pregnancy or childbirth 654.7
      affecting fetus or newborn 763.89
      causing obstructed labor 660.2
        affecting fetus or newborn 763.1
Rigors 780.99
Riley-Day syndrome (familial dysautonomia) 742.8
RIND (reversible ischemic neurological deficit)
  434.91
  history of personal V12.54
Ring(s)
  aorta 747.21
  Bandl's, complicating delivery 661.4
    affecting fetus or newborn 763.7
  contraction, complicating delivery 661.4
    affecting fetus or newborn 763.7
  esophageal (congenital) 750.3

Ring(s)—*continued*
Fleischer (-Kayser) (cornea) 275.1 *[371.14]*
hymenal, tight (acquired) (congenital) 623.3
Kayser-Fleischer (cornea) 275.1 *[371.14]*
retraction, uterus, pathological 661.4
  affecting fetus or newborn 763.7
Schatzki's (esophagus) (congenital) (lower) 750.3
  acquired 530.3
Soemmering's 366.51
trachea, abnormal 748.3
vascular (congenital) 747.21
Vossius' 921.3
  late effect 366.21
Ringed hair (congenital) 757.4
Ringing in the ear (*see also* Tinnitus) 388.30
Ringworm 110.9
beard 110.0
body 110.5
Burmese 110.9
corporeal 110.5
foot 110.4
groin 110.3
hand 110.2
honeycomb 110.0
nails 110.1
perianal (area) 110.3
scalp 110.0
specified site NEC 110.8
Tokelau 110.5
Rise, venous pressure 459.89
Risk
factor —*see* Problem
falling V15.88
suicidal 300.9
Ritter's disease (dermatitis exfoliativa
  neonatorum) 695.81
Rivalry, sibling 313.3
Rivalta's disease (cervicofacial actinomycosis)
  039.3
River blindness 125.3 *[360.13]*
Robert's pelvis 755.69
with disproportion (fetopelvic) 653.0
  affecting fetus or newborn 763.1
  causing obstructed labor 660.1
    affecting fetus or newborn 763.1
Robin's syndrome 756.0
Robinson's (hidrotic) ectodermal dysplasia 757.31
Robles' disease (onchocerciasis) 125.3 *[360.13]*
Rochalimea —*see* Rickettsial disease
Rocky Mountain fever (spotted) 082.0
Rodent ulcer 9M8090/3)—*see also* Neoplasm,
  skin, malignant
cornea 370.07
Roentgen ray, adverse effect —*see* Effect,
  adverse, x-ray
Roetheln 056.9
Roger's disease (congenital interventricular
  septal defect) 745.4
Rokitansky's
disease (*see also* Necrosis, liver) 570
tumor 620.2
Rokitansky-Aschoff sinuses (mucosal
  outpouching of gallbladder) (*see also* Disease,
  gallbladder) 575.8
Rokitansky-Kuster-Hauser syndrome
  (congenital absence vagina) 752.45
Rollet's chancre (syphilitic) 091.0
Rolling of head 781.0

Romano-Ward syndrome (prolonged QT
  interval syndrome) 426.82
Romanus lesion 720.1
Romberg's disease or syndrome 349.89
Roof, mouth —*see* condition
Rosacea 695.3
acne 695.3
keratitis 695.3 *[370.49]*
Rosary, rachitic 268.0
Rose
cold 477.0
fever 477.0
rash 782.1
  epidemic 056.9
  of infants 057.8
Rosen-Castleman-Liebow syndrome
  (pulmonary proteinosis) 516.0
Rosenbach's erysipelatoid or erysipeloid 027.1
Rosenthal's disease (factor XI deficiency) 286.2
Roseola 057.8
infantum, infantilis (*see also* Exanthem subitum)
  058.10
Rossbach's disease (hyperchlorhydria) 536.8
psychogenic 306.4
Rössle-Urbach-Wiethe lipoproteinosis 272.8
Ross river fever 066.3
Rostan's asthma (cardiac) (*see also* Failure,
  ventricular, left) 428.1
Rot
Barcoo (*see also* Ulcer, skin) 707.9
knife-grinders' (*see also* Tuberculosis) 011.4
Rot-Bernhardt disease 355.1
Rotation
anomalous, incomplete or insufficient—*see*
  Malrotation
cecum (congenital) 751.4
colon (congenital) 751.4
manual, affecting fetus or newborn 763.89
spine, incomplete or insufficient 737.8
tooth, teeth 524.35
vertebra, incomplete or insufficient 737.8
Röteln 056.9
Roth's disease or meralgia 355.1
Roth-Bernhardt disease or syndrome 355.1
Rothmund (-Thomson) syndrome 757.33
Rotor's disease or syndrome (idiopathic
  hyperbilirubinemia) 277.4
Rotundum ulcus —*see* Ulcer, stomach
Round
back (with wedging of vertebrae) 737.10
  late effect of rickets 268.1
hole, retina 361.31
  with detachment 361.01
ulcer (stomach)—*see* Ulcer, stomach
worms (infestation) (large) NEC 127.0
Roussy-Lévy syndrome 334.3
Routine postpartum follow-up V24.2
Roy (-Jutras) syndrome (acropachyderma) 757.39
Rubella (German measles) 056.9
complicating pregnancy, childbirth, or
  puerperium 647.5
complication 056.8
  neurological 056.00
    encephalomyelitis 056.01
    specified type NEC 056.09
  specified type NEC 056.79
congenital 771.0
contact V01.4
exposure to V01.4

Rubella—*continued*
maternal
with suspected fetal damage affecting
management of pregnancy 655.3
affecting fetus or newborn 760.2
manifest rubella in infant 771.0
specified complications NEC 056.79
vaccination, prophylactic (against) V04.3
Rubeola (measles) (*see also* Measles) 055.9
complicated 055.8
meaning rubella (*see also* Rubella) 056.9
scarlatinosis 057.8
Rubeosis iridis 364.42
diabetica 250.5 *[364.42]*
due to secondary diabetes 249.5 *[364.42]*
Rubinstein-Taybi's syndrome (brachydactylia,
short stature and intellectual disabilities)
759.89
Rud's syndrome (mental deficiency, epilepsy,
and infantilism) 759.89
Rudimentary (congenital)—*see also* Agenesis
arm 755.22
bone 756.9
cervix uteri 752.43
eye (*see also* Microphthalmos) 743.10
fallopian tube 752.19
leg 755.32
lobule of ear 744.21
patella 755.64
respiratory organs in thoracopagus 759.4
tracheal bronchus 748.3
uterine horn 752.39
uterus 752.39
in male 752.7
solid or with cavity 752.39
vagina 752.45
Ruiter-Pompen (-Wyers) syndrome
(angiokeratoma corporis diffusum) 272.7
Ruled out condition (*see also* Observation,
suspected) V71.9
Rumination —*see also* Vomiting
disorder 307.53
neurotic 300.3
obsessional 300.3
psychogenic 307.53
Runaway reaction —*see also* Disturbance,
conduct
socialized 312.2
undersocialized, unsocialized 312.1
Runeberg's disease (progressive pernicious
anemia) 281.0
Runge's syndrome (postmaturity) 766.22
Runny nose 784.99
Rupia 091.3
congenital 090.0
tertiary 095.9
Rupture, ruptured 553.9
abdominal viscera NEC 799.89
obstetrical trauma 665.5
abscess (spontaneous)—*see* Abscess, by site
amnion—*see* Rupture, membranes
aneurysm—*see* Aneurysm
anus (sphincter)—*see* Laceration, anus
aorta, aortic 441.5
abdominal 441.3
arch 441.1
ascending 441.1
descending 441.5
abdominal 441.3
thoracic 441.1

Rupture, ruptured—*continued*
aorta, aortic—*continued*
syphilitic 093.0
thoracoabdominal 441.6
thorax, thoracic 441.1
transverse 441.1
traumatic (thoracic) 901.0
abdominal 902.0
valve or cusp (*see also* Endocarditis, aortic) 424.1
appendix (with peritonitis) 540.0
traumatic—*see* Injury, internal,
gastrointestinal tract
with peritoneal abscess 540.1
arteriovenous fistula, brain (congenital) 430
artery 447.2
brain (*see also* Hemorrhage, brain) 431
coronary (*see also* Infarct, myocardium) 410.9
heart (*see also* Infarct, myocardium) 410.9
pulmonary 417.8
traumatic (complication) (*see also* Injury,
blood vessel, by site) 904.9
bile duct, except cystic (*see also* Disease,
biliary) 576.3
cystic 575.4
traumatic—*see* Injury, internal,
intra-abdominal
bladder (sphincter) 596.6
with
abortion—*see* Abortion, by type, with
damage to pelvic organs
ectopic pregnancy (*see also* categories
633.0-633.9) 639.2
molar pregnancy (*see also* categories
630-632) 639.2
following
abortion 639.2
ectopic or molar pregnancy 639.2
nontraumatic 596.6
obstetrical trauma 665.5
spontaneous 596.6
traumatic—*see* Injury, internal, bladder
blood vessel (*see also* Hemorrhage) 459.0
brain (*see also* Hemorrhage, brain) 431
heart (*see also* Infarct, myocardium) 410.9
traumatic (complication) (*see also* Injury,
blood vessel, by site) 904.9
bone—*see* Fracture, by site
bowel 569.89
traumatic—*see* Injury, internal, intestine
Bowman's membrane 371.31
brain
aneurysm (congenital) (*see also* Hemorrhage,
subarachnoid) 430
late effect—*see* Late effect(s) (of)
cerebrovascular disease
syphilitic 094.87
hemorrhagic (*see also* Hemorrhage, brain) 431
injury at birth 767.0
syphilitic 094.89
capillaries 448.9
cardiac (*see also* Infarct, myocardium) 410.9
cartilage (articular) (current)—*see also* Sprain,
by site
knee—*see* Tear, meniscus
semilunar—*see* Tear, meniscus
cecum (with peritonitis) 540.0
traumatic 863.89
with open wound into cavity 863.99
with peritoneal abscess 540.1

Rupture, ruptured—*continued*
  cerebral aneurysm (congenital) (*see also*
    Hemorrhage, subarachnoid) 430
    late effect—*see* Late effect(s) (of)
      cerebrovascular disease
  cervix (uteri)
    with
      abortion—*see* Abortion, by type, with
        damage to pelvic organs
      ectopic pregnancy (*see also* categories
        633.0-633.9) 639.2
      molar pregnancy (*see also* categories
        630-632) 639.2
    following
      abortion 639.2
      ectopic or molar pregnancy 639.2
    obstetrical trauma 665.3
    traumatic—*see* Injury, internal, cervix
  chordae tendineae 429.5
  choroid (direct) (indirect) (traumatic) 363.63
  circle of Willis (*see also* Hemorrhage,
    subarachnoid) 430
    late effect—*see* Late effect(s) (of)
      cerebrovascular disease
  colon 569.89
    traumatic—*see* Injury, internal, colon
  cornea (traumatic)—*see also* Rupture, eye
    due to ulcer 370.00
  coronary (artery) (thrombotic) (*see also* Infarct,
    myocardium) 410.9
  corpus luteum (infected) (ovary) 620.1
  cyst—*see* Cyst
  cystic duct (*see also* Disease, gallbladder) 575.4
  Descemet's membrane 371.33
    traumatic—*see* Rupture, eye
  diaphragm—*see also* Hernia, diaphragm
    traumatic—*see* Injury, internal, diaphragm
  diverticulum
    bladder 596.3
    intestine (large) (*see also* Diverticula) 562.10
      small 562.00
  duodenal stump 537.89
  duodenum (ulcer)—*see* Ulcer, duodenum, with
    perforation
  ear drum (*see also* Perforation, tympanum) 384.20
    with otitis media—*see* Otitis media
    traumatic—*see* Wound, open, ear
  esophagus 530.4
    traumatic 862.22
      with open wound into cavity 862.32
      cervical region—*see* Wound, open,
        esophagus
  eye (without prolapse of intraocular tissue) 871.0
    with
      exposure of intraocular tissue 871.1
      partial loss of intraocular tissue 871.2
      prolapse of intraocular tissue 871.1
    due to burn 940.5
  fallopian tube 620.8
    due to pregnancy—*see* Pregnancy, tubal
    traumatic—*see* Injury, internal, fallopian tube
  fontanel 767.3
  free wall (ventricle) (*see also* Infarct,
    myocardium) 410.9
  gallbladder or duct (*see also* Disease,
    gallbladder) 575.4
    traumatic—*see* Injury, internal, gallbladder
  gastric (*see also* Rupture, stomach) 537.89
    vessel 459.0
  globe (eye) (traumatic)—*see* Rupture, eye

Rupture, ruptured—*continued*
  graafian follicle (hematoma) 620.0
  heart (auricle) (ventricle) (*see also* Infarct,
    myocardium) 410.9
    infectional 422.90
    traumatic—*see* Rupture, myocardium,
      traumatic
  hymen 623.8
  internal
    organ, traumatic—*see also* Injury, internal, by
      site
      heart—*see* Rupture, myocardium, traumatic
      kidney—*see* Rupture, kidney
      liver—*see* Rupture, liver
      spleen—*see* Rupture, spleen, traumatic
      semilunar cartilage—*see* Tear, meniscus
  intervertebral disc—*see* Displacement,
    intervertebral disc
    traumatic (current)—*see* Dislocation, vertebra
  intestine 569.89
    traumatic—*see* Injury, internal, intestine
  intracranial, birth injury 767.0
  iris 364.76
    traumatic—*see* Rupture, eye
  joint capsule—*see* Sprain, by site
  kidney (traumatic) 866.03
    with open wound into cavity 866.13
    due to birth injury 767.8
    nontraumatic 593.89
  lacrimal apparatus (traumatic) 870.2
  lens (traumatic) 366.20
  ligament—*see also* Sprain, by site
    with open wound—*see* Wound, open, by site
    old (*see also* Disorder, cartilage, articular)
      718.0
  liver (traumatic) 864.04
    with open wound into cavity 864.14
    due to birth injury 767.8
    nontraumatic 573.8
  lymphatic (node) (vessel) 457.8
  marginal sinus (placental) (with hemorrhage) 641.2
    affecting fetus or newborn 762.1
  meaning hernia—*see* Hernia
  membrana tympani (*see also* Perforation,
    tympanum) 384.20
    with otitis media—*see* Otitis media
    traumatic—*see* Wound, open, ear
  membranes (spontaneous)
    artificial
      delayed delivery following 658.3
        affecting fetus or newborn 761.1
      fetus or newborn 761.1
    delayed delivery following 658.2
      affecting fetus or newborn 761.1
    premature (less than 24 hours prior to onset of
      labor) 658.1
      affecting fetus or newborn 761.1
      delayed delivery following 658.2
        affecting fetus or newborn 761.1
  meningeal artery (*see also* Hemorrhage,
    subarachnoid) 430
    late effect—*see* Late effect(s) (of)
      cerebrovascular disease
  meniscus (knee)—*see also* Tear, meniscus
    old (*see also* Derangement, meniscus) 717.5
    site other than knee—*see* Disorder, cartilage,
      articular
    site other than knee—*see* Sprain, by site
  mesentery 568.89
    traumatic—*see* Injury, internal, mesentery
  mitral—*see* Insufficiency, mitral

Rupture, ruptured—*continued*
muscle (traumatic) NEC—*see also* Sprain, by
site
with open wound—*see* Wound, open, by site
nontraumatic 728.83
musculotendinous cuff (nontraumatic)
(shoulder) 840.4
mycotic aneurysm, causing cerebral hemorrhage
(*see also* Hemorrhage, subarachnoid) 430
late effect—*see* Late effect(s) (of)
cerebrovascular disease
myocardium, myocardial (*see also* Infarct,
myocardium) 410.9
traumatic 861.03
with open wound into thorax 861.13
nontraumatic (meaning hernia) (*see also* Hernia,
by site) 553.9
obstructed (*see also* Hernia, by site, with
obstruction) 552.9
gangrenous (*see also* Hernia, by site, with
gangrene) 551.9
operation wound (*see also* Dehiscence) 998.32
internal 998.31
ovary, ovarian 620.8
corpus luteum 620.1
follicle (graafian) 620.0
oviduct 620.8
due to pregnancy—*see* Pregnancy, tubal
pancreas 577.8
traumatic—*see* Injury, internal, pancreas
papillary muscle (ventricular) 429.6
pelvic
floor, complicating delivery 664.1
organ NEC—*see* Injury, pelvic, organs
penis (traumatic)—*see* Wound, open, penis
perineum 624.8
during delivery (*see also* Laceration,
perineum, complicating delivery) 664.4
pharynx (nontraumatic) (spontaneous) 478.29
pregnant uterus (before onset of labor) 665.0
prostate (traumatic)—*see* Injury, internal,
prostate
pulmonary
artery 417.8
valve (heart) (*see also* Endocarditis,
pulmonary) 424.3
vein 417.8
vessel 417.8
pupil, sphincter 364.75
pus tube (*see also* Salpingo-oophoritis) 614.2
pyosalpinx (*see also* Salpingo-oophoritis) 614.2
rectum 569.49
traumatic—*see* Injury, internal, rectum
retina, retinal (traumatic) (without detachment)
361.30
with detachment (*see also* Detachment, retina,
with retinal defect) 361.00
rotator cuff (capsule) (traumatic) 840.4
nontraumatic (complete) 727.61
partial 726.13
sclera 871.0
semilunar cartilage, knee (*see also* Tear,
meniscus) 836.2
old (*see also* Derangement, meniscus) 717.5
septum (cardiac) 410.8
sigmoid 569.89
traumatic—*see* Injury, internal, colon, sigmoid
sinus of Valsalva 747.29

Rupture, ruptured—*continued*
spinal cord—*see also* Injury, spinal, by site
due to injury at birth 767.4
fetus or newborn 767.4
syphilitic 094.89
traumatic—*see also* Injury, spinal, by site
with fracture—*see* Fracture, vertebra, by
site, with spinal cord injury
spleen 289.59
congenital 767.8
due to injury at birth 767.8
malarial 084.9
nontraumatic 289.59
spontaneous 289.59
traumatic 865.04
with open wound into cavity 865.14
splenic vein 459.0
stomach 537.89
due to injury at birth 767.8
traumatic—*see* Injury, internal, stomach
ulcer—*see* Ulcer, stomach, with perforation
synovium 727.50
specified site NEC 727.59
tendon (traumatic)—*see also* Sprain, by site
with open wound—*see* Wound, open, by site
Achilles 845.09
nontraumatic 727.67
ankle 845.09
nontraumatic 727.68
biceps (long bead) 840.8
nontraumatic 727.62
foot 845.10
interphalangeal (joint) 845.13
metatarsophalangeal (joint) 845.12
nontraumatic 727.68
specified site NEC 845.19
tarsometatarsal (joint) 845.11
hand 842.10
carpometacarpal (joint) 842.11
interphalangeal (joint) 842.13
metacarpophalangeal (joint) 842.12
nontraumatic 727.63
extensors 727.63
flexors 727.64
specified site NEC 842.19
nontraumatic 727.60
specified site NEC 727.69
patellar 844.8
nontraumatic 727.66
quadriceps 844.8
nontraumatic 727.65
rotator cuff (capsule) 840.4
nontraumatic (complete) 727.61
partial 726.13
wrist 842.00
carpal (joint) 842.01
nontraumatic 727.63
extensors 727.63
flexors 727.64
radiocarpal (joint) (ligament) 842.02
radioulnar (joint), distal 842.09
specified site NEC 842.09
testis (traumatic) 878.2
complicated 878.3
due to syphilis 095.8
thoracic duct 457.8
tonsil 474.8
traumatic
with open wound—*see* Wound, open, by site
aorta—*see* Rupture, aorta, traumatic
ear drum—*see* Wound, open, ear, drum

Rupture, ruptured—*continued*

traumatic—*continued*

external site—*see* Wound, open, by site

eye 871.2

globe (eye)—*see* Wound, open, eyeball

internal organ (abdomen, chest, or

pelvis)—*see also* Injury, internal, by site

heart—*see* Rupture, myocardium, traumatic

kidney—*see* Rupture, kidney

liver—*see* Rupture, liver

spleen—*see* Rupture, spleen, traumatic

ligament, muscle, or tendon—*see also* Sprain,

by site

with open wound—*see* Wound, open, by site

meaning hernia—*see* Hernia

tricuspid (heart) (valve)—*see* Endocarditis,

tricuspid

tube, tubal 620.8

abscess (*see also* Salpingo-oophoritis) 614.2

due to pregnancy—*see* Pregnancy, tubal

tympanum, tympanic (membrane) (*see also*

Perforation, tympanum) 384.20

with otitis media—*see* Otitis media

traumatic—*see* Wound, open, ear, drum

umbilical cord 663.8

fetus or newborn 772.0

ureter (traumatic) (*see also* Injury, internal,

ureter) 867.2

nontraumatic 593.89

urethra 599.84

with

abortion—*see* Abortion, by type, with

damage to pelvic organs

ectopic pregnancy (*see also* categories

633.0-633.9) 639.2

molar pregnancy (*see also* categories

630-632) 639.2

following

abortion 639.2

ectopic or molar pregnancy 639.2

obstetrical trauma 665.5

traumatic—*see* Injury, internal urethra

uterosacral ligament 620.8

uterus (traumatic)—*see also* Injury, internal

uterus

affecting fetus or newborn 763.89

during labor 665.1

nonpuerperal, nontraumatic 621.8

nontraumatic 621.8

pregnant (during labor) 665.1

before labor 665.0

vaginal 878.6

complicated 878.7

complicating delivery—*see* Laceration,

vagina, complicating delivery

valve, valvular (heart)—*see* Endocarditis

varicose vein—*see* Varicose, vein

varix—*see* Varix

vena cava 459.0

ventricle (free wall) (left) (*see also* Infarct,

myocardium) 410.9

vesical (urinary) 596.6

traumatic—*see* Injury, internal, bladder

vessel (blood) 459.0

pulmonary 417.8

viscus 799.89

vulva 878.4

complicated 878.5

complicating delivery 664.0

Russell's dwarf (uterine dwarfism and

craniofacial dysostosis) 759.89

Russell's dysentery 004.8

Russell (-Silver) syndrome (congenital

hemihypertrophy and short stature) 759.89

Russian spring-summer type encephalitis 063.0

Rust's disease (tuberculous spondylitis) 015.0

[720.81]

Rustitskii's disease (multiple myeloma)

(M9730/3) 203.0

Ruysch's disease (Hirschsprung's disease) 751.3

Rytand-Lipsitch syndrome (complete

atrioventricular block) 426.0

S

Saber
shin 090.5
tibia 090.5
Sac, lacrimal —*see* condition
Saccharomyces infection (*see also* Candidiasis)
112.9
Saccharopinuria 270.7
Saccular —*see* condition
Sacculation
aorta (nonsyphilitic) (*see also* Aneurysm, aorta)
441.9
ruptured 441.5
syphilitic 093.0
bladder 596.3
colon 569.89
intralaryngeal (congenital) (ventricular) 748.3
larynx (congenital) (ventricular) 748.3
organ or site, congenital—*see* Distortion
pregnant uterus, complicating delivery 654.4
affecting fetus or newborn 763.1
causing obstructed labor 660.2
affecting fetus or newborn 763.1
rectosigmoid 569.89
sigmoid 569.89
ureter 593.89
urethra 599.2
vesical 596.3
Sachs (-Tay) disease (amaurotic familial idiocy)
330.1
Sacks-Libman disease 710.0 *[424.91]*
Sacralgia 724.6
Sacralization
fifth lumbar vertebra 756.15
incomplete (vertebra) 756.15
Sacrodynia 724.6
Sacroiliac joint —*see* condition
Sacroiliitis NEC 720.2
Sacrum —*see* condition
Saddle
back 737.8
embolus
abdominal aorta 444.01
pulmonary artery 415.13
injury—code to condition
nose 738.0
congenital 754.0
due to syphilis 090.5
Sadism (sexual) 302.84
Saemisch's ulcer 370.04
Saenger's syndrome 379.46
Sago spleen 277.39
Sailors' skin 692.74
Saint
Anthony's fire (*see also* Erysipelas) 035
Guy's dance—*see* Chorea
Louis-type encephalitis 062.3
triad (*see also* Hernia, diaphragm) 553.3
Vitus' dance—*see* Chorea
Salicylism
correct substance properly administered 535.4
overdose or wrong substance given or taken 965.1
Salivary duct or gland —*see also* condition
virus disease 078.5
Salivation (excessive) (*see also* Ptyalism) 527.7

Salmonella (aertrycke) (choleraesuis) (enteritidis)
(gallinarum) (suipestifer) (typhimurium) (*see
also* Infection, Salmonella) 003.9
arthritis 003.23
carrier (suspected) of V02.3
meningitis 003.21
osteomyelitis 003.24
pneumonia 003.22
septicemia 003.1
typhosa 002.0
carrier (suspected) of V02.1
Salmonellosis 003.0
with pneumonia 003.22
Salpingitis (catarrhal) (fallopian tube) (nodular)
(pseudofollicular) (purulent) (septic) (*see also*
Salpingo-oophoritis) 614.2
ear 381.50
acute 381.51
chronic 381.52
Eustachian (tube) 381.50
acute 381.51
chronic 381.52
follicularis 614.1
gonococcal (chronic) 098.37
acute 098.17
interstitial, chronic 614.1
isthmica nodosa 614.1
old—*see* Salpingo-oophoritis, chronic
puerperal, postpartum, childbirth 670.8
specific (chronic) 098.37
acute 098.17
tuberculous (acute) (chronic) (*see also*
Tuberculosis) 016.6
venereal (chronic) 098.37
acute 098.17
Salpingocele 620.4
Salpingo-oophoritis (catarrhal) (purulent)
(ruptured) (septic) (suppurative) 614.2
acute 614.0
with
abortion—*see* Abortion, by type, with sepsis
ectopic pregnancy (*see also* categories
633.0-633.9) 639.0
molar pregnancy (*see also* categories
630-632) 639.0
following
abortion 639.0
ectopic or molar pregnancy 639.0
gonococcal 098.17
puerperal, postpartum, childbirth 670.8
tuberculous (*see also* Tuberculosis) 016.6
chronic 614.1
gonococcal 098.37
tuberculous (*see also* Tuberculosis) 016.6
complicating pregnancy 646.6
affecting fetus or newborn 760.8
gonococcal (chronic) 098.37
acute 098.17
old—*see* Salpingo-oophoritis, chronic
puerperal 670.8
specific—*see* Salpingo-oophoritis, gonococcal
subacute (*see also* Salpingo-oophoritis, acute)
614.0
tuberculous (acute) (chronic) (*see also*
Tuberculosis) 016.6
venereal—*see* Salpingo-oophoritis, gonococcal
Salpingo-ovaritis (*see also* Salpingo-oophoritis)
614.2

STUV

Salpingoperitonitis (*see also*
Salpingo-oophoritis) 614.2
Salt-losing
nephritis (*see also* Disease, renal) 593.9
syndrome (*see also* Disease, renal) 593.9
Salt-rheum (*see also* Eczema) 692.9
Salzmann's nodular dystrophy 371.46
Sampling chorionic villus V28.89
Sampson's cyst or tumor 617.1
Sandblasters'
asthma 502
lung 502
Sander's disease (paranoia) 297.1
Sandfly fever 066.0
Sandhoff's disease 330.1
Sanfilippo's syndrome (mucopolysaccharidosis
III) 277.5
Sanger-Brown's ataxia 334.2
San Joaquin Valley fever 114.0
São Paulo fever or typhus 082.0
Saponification, mesenteric 567.89
Sapremia —*see* Septicemia
Sarcocele (benign)
syphilitic 095.8
congenital 090.5
Sarcoepiplocele (*see also* Hernia) 553.9
Sarcoepiplomphalocele (*see also* Hernia,
umbilicus) 553.1
Sarcoid (any site) 135
with lung involvement 135 *[517.8]*
Boeck's 135
Darier-Roussy 135
Spiegler-Fendt 686.8
Sarcoidosis 135
cardiac 135 *[425.8]*
lung 135 *[517.8]*
Sarcoma (M8800/3)—*see also* Neoplasm,
connective tissue, malignant
alveolar soft part (M9581/3)—*see* Neoplasm,
connective tissue, malignant
ameloblastic (M9330/3) 170.1
upper jaw (bone) 170.0
botryoid (M8910/3)—*see* Neoplasm, connective
tissue, malignant
botryoides (M8910/3)—*see* Neoplasm,
connective tissue, malignant
cerebellar (M9480/3) 191.6
circumscribed (arachnoidal) (M9471/3) 191.6
circumscribed (arachnoidal) cerebellar
(M9471/3) 191.6
clear cell, of tendons and aponeuroses
(M9044/3)—*see* Neoplasm, connective
tissue, malignant
embryonal (M8991/3)—*see* Neoplasm,
connective tissue, malignant
endometrial (stromal) (M8930/3) 182.0
isthmus 182.1
endothelial (M9130/3)—*see also* Neoplasm,
connective tissue, malignant
bone (M9260/3)—*see* Neoplasm, bone,
malignant
epithelioid cell (M8804/3)—*see* Neoplasm,
connective tissue, malignant
Ewing's (M9260/3)—*see* Neoplasm, bone,
malignant
follicular dendritic cell 202.9
germinoblastic (diffuse) (M9632/3) 202.8
follicular (M9697/3) 202.0

Sarcoma—*continued*
giant cell (M8802/3)—*see also* Neoplasm,
connective tissue, malignant
bone (M9250/3)—*see* Neoplasm, bone,
malignant
glomoid (M8710/3)—*see* Neoplasm, connective
tissue, malignant
granulocytic (M9930/3) 205.3
hemangioendothelial (M9130/3)—*see*
Neoplasm, connective tissue, malignant
hemorrhagic, multiple (M9140/3)—*see*
Kaposi's, sarcoma
Hodgkin's (M9662/3) 201.2
immunoblastic (M9612/3) 200.8
interdigitating dendritic cell 202.9
Kaposi's (M9140/3)—*see* Kaposi's, sarcoma
Kupffer cell (M9124/3) 155.0
Langerhans cell 202.9
leptomeningeal (M9530/3)—*see* Neoplasm,
meninges, malignant
lymphangioendothelial (M9170/3)—*see*
Neoplasm, connective tissue, malignant
lymphoblastic (M9630/3) 200.1
lymphocytic (M9620/3) 200.1
mast cell (M9740/3) 202.6
melanotic (M8720/3)—*see* Melanoma
meningeal (M9530/3)—*see* Neoplasm,
meninges, malignant
meningothelial (M9530/3)—*see* Neoplasm,
meninges, malignant
mesenchymal (M8800/3)—*see also* Neoplasm,
connective tissue, malignant
mixed (M8990/3)—*see* Neoplasm, connective
tissue, malignant
mesothelial (M9050/3)—*see* Neoplasm, by site,
malignant
monstrocellular (M9481/3)
specified site—*see* Neoplasm, by site, malignant
unspecified site 191.9
myeloid (M9930/3) 205.3
neurogenic (M9540/3)—*see* Neoplasm,
connective tissue, malignant
odontogenic (M9270/3) 170.1
upper jaw (bone) 170.0
osteoblastic (M9180/3)—*see* Neoplasm, bone,
malignant
osteogenic (M9180/3)—*see also* Neoplasm,
bone, malignant
juxtacortical (M9190/3)—*see* Neoplasm,
bone, malignant
periosteal (M9190/3)—*see* Neoplasm, bone,
malignant
periosteal (M8812/3)—*see also* Neoplasm,
bone, malignant
osteogenic (M9190/3)—*see* Neoplasm, bone,
malignant
plasma cell (M9731/3) 203.8
pleomorphic cell (M8802/3)—*see* Neoplasm,
connective tissue, malignant
reticuloendothelial (M9720/3) 202.3
reticulum cell (M9640/3) 200.0
nodular (M9642/3) 200.0
pleomorphic cell type (M9641/3) 200.0
round cell (M8803/3)—*see* Neoplasm,
connective tissue, malignant
small cell (M8803/3)—*see* Neoplasm,
connective tissue, malignant
spindle cell (M8801/3)—*see* Neoplasm,
connective tissue, malignant

Sarcoma—*continued*
  stromal (endometrial) (M8930/3) 182.0
    isthmus 182.1
  synovial (M9040/3)—*see also* Neoplasm,
    connective tissue, malignant
    biphasic type (M9043/3)—*see* Neoplasm,
      connective tissue, malignant
    epithelioid cell type (M9042/3)—*see*
      Neoplasm, connective tissue, malignant
    spindle cell type (M9041/3)—*see* Neoplasm,
      connective tissue, malignant
Sarcomatosis
  meningeal (M9539/3)—*see* Neoplasm,
    meninges, malignant
  specified site NEC (M8800/3)—*see* Neoplasm,
    connective tissue, malignant
  unspecified site (M8800/6) 171.9
Sarcosinemia 270.8
Sarcosporidiosis 136.5
Satiety, early 780.94
Satisfactory smear but lacking transformation
  zone
  anal 796.77
  cervical 795.07
Saturnine —*see* condition
Saturnism 984.9
  specified type of lead—*see* Table of drugs and
    chemicals
Satyriasis 302.89
Sauriasis —*see* Ichthyosis
Sauriderma 757.39
Sauriosis —*see* Ichthyosis
Savill's disease (epidemic exfoliative dermatitis)
  695.89
SBE (subacute bacterial endocarditis) 421.0
Scabies (any site) 133.0
Scabs 782.8
Scaglietti-Dagnini syndrome (acromegalic
  macrospondylitis) 253.0
Scald, scalded —*see also* Burn, by site
  skin syndrome 695.81
Scalenus anticus (anterior) syndrome 353.0
Scales 782.8
Scalp —*see* condition
Scaphocephaly 756.0
Scaphoiditis, tarsal 732.5
Scapulalgia 733.90
Scapulohumeral myopathy 359.1
Scar, scarring (*see also* Cicatrix) 709.2
  adherent 709.2
  atrophic 709.2
  cervix
    in pregnancy or childbirth 654.6
      affecting fetus or newborn 763.89
      causing obstructed labor 660.2
        affecting fetus or newborn 763.1
  cheloid 701.4
  chorioretinal 363.30
    disseminated 363.35
    macular 363.32
    peripheral 363.34
    posterior pole NEC 363.33
  choroid (*see also* Scar, chorioretinal) 363.30
  compression, pericardial 423.9
  congenital 757.39
  conjunctiva 372.64
  cornea 371.00
    xerophthalmic 264.6

Scar, scarring—*continued*
  due to previous cesarean delivery, complicating
    pregnancy or childbirth 654.2
    affecting fetus or newborn 763.89
  duodenal (bulb) (cap) 537.3
  hypertrophic 701.4
  keloid 701.4
  labia 624.4
  lung (base) 518.89
  macula 363.32
    disseminated 363.35
    peripheral 363.34
  muscle 728.89
  myocardium, myocardial 412
  painful 709.2
  papillary muscle 429.81
  posterior pole NEC 363.33
    macular—*see* Scar, macula
  postnecrotic (hepatic) (liver) 571.9
  psychic V15.49
  retina (*see also* Scar, chorioretinal) 363.30
  trachea 478.9
  uterus 621.8
    in pregnancy or childbirth NEC 654.9
      affecting fetus or newborn 763.89
      due to previous cesarean delivery 654.2
  vulva 624.4
Scarabiasis 134.1
Scarlatina 034.1
  anginosa 034.1
  maligna 034.1
  myocarditis, acute 034.1 *[422.0]*
    old (*see also* Myocarditis) 429.0
  otitis media 034.1 *[382.02]*
  ulcerosa 034.1
Scarlatinella 057.8
Scarlet fever (albuminuria) (angina)
  (convulsions) (lesions of lid) (rash) 034.1
Schamberg's disease, dermatitis, or dermatosis
  (progressive pigmentary dermatosis) 709.09
Schatzki's ring (esophagus) (lower) (congenital)
  750.3
  acquired 530.3
Schaufenster krankheit 413.9
Schaumann's
  benign lymphogranulomatosis 135
  disease (sarcoidosis) 135
  syndrome (sarcoidosis) 135
Scheie's syndrome (mucopolysaccharidosis IS)
  277.5
Schenck's disease (sporotrichosis) 117.1
Scheuermann's disease or osteochondrosis
  732.0
Scheuthauer-Marie-Sainton syndrome
  (cleidocranialis dysostosis) 755.59
Schilder (-Flatau) disease 341.1
Schilling-type monocytic leukemia (M9890/3)
  206.9
Schimmelbusch's disease, cystic mastitis, or
  hyperplasia 610.1
Schirmer's syndrome (encephalocutaneous
  angiomatosis) 759.6
Schistocelia 756.79
Schistoglossia 750.13
Schistosoma infestation —*see* Infestation,
  Schistosoma
Schistosomiasis 120.9
  Asiatic 120.2
  bladder 120.0
  chestermani 120.8

Schistosomiasis— *continued*
  colon 120.1
  cutaneous 120.3
  due to
    S. hematobium 120.0
    S. japonicum 120.2
    S. mansoni 120.1
    S. mattheii 120.8
  eastern 120.2
  genitourinary tract 120.0
  intestinal 120.1
  lung 120.2
  Manson's (intestinal) 120.1
  Oriental 120.2
  pulmonary 120.2
  specified type NEC 120.8
  vesical 120.0
Schizencephaly 742.4
Schizo-affective psychosis (*see also*
  Schizophrenia) 295.7
Schizodontia 520.2
Schizoid personality 301.20
  introverted 301.21
  schizotypal 301.22
Schizophrenia, schizophrenic (reaction) 295.9

> *Note—Use the following fifth-digit*
> *subclassification with category 295:*
>
> *0 unspecified*
> *1 subchronic*
> *2 chronic*
> *3 subchronic with acute exacerbation*
> *4 chronic with acute exacerbation*
> *5 in remission*

  acute (attack) NEC 295.8
    episode 295.4
  atypical form 295.8
  borderline 295.5
  catalepsy 295.2
  catatonic (type) (acute) (excited) (withdrawn) 295.2
  childhood (type) (*see also* Psychosis, childhood)
    299.9
  chronic NEC 295.6
  coenesthesiopathic 295.8
  cyclic (type) 295.7
  disorganized (type) 295.1
  flexibilitas cerea 295.2
  hebephrenic (type) (acute) 295.1
  incipient 295.5
  latent 295.5
  paranoid (type) (acute) 295.3
  paraphrenic (acute) 295.3
  prepsychotic 295.5
  primary (acute) 295.0
  prodromal 295.5
  pseudoneurotic 295.5
  pseudopsychopathic 295.5
  reaction 295.9
  residual type (state) 295.6
  restzustand 295.6
  schizo-affective (type) (depressed) (excited)
    295.7
  schizophreniform type 295.4
  simple (type) (acute) 295.0
  simplex (acute) 295.0
  specified type NEC 295.8
  syndrome of childhood NEC (*see also*
    Psychosis, childhood) 299.9
  undifferentiated type 295.9
    acute 295.8
    chronic 295.6

Schizothymia 301.20
  introverted 301.21
  schizotypal 301.22
Schlafkrankheit 086.5
Schlatter's tibia (osteochondrosis) 732.4
Schlatter-Osgood disease (osteochondrosis,
  tibial tubercle) 732.4
Schloffer's tumor (*see also* Peritonitis) 567.29
Schmidt's syndrome
  sphallo-pharyngo-laryngeal hemiplegia 352.6
  thyroid-adrenocortical insufficiency 258.1
  vagoaccessory 352.6
Schmincke
  carcinoma (M8082/3)—*see* Neoplasm,
    nasopharynx, malignant
  tumor (M8082/3)—*see* Neoplasm, nasopharynx,
    malignant
Schmitz (-Stutzer) dysentery 004.0
Schmorl's disease or nodes 722.30
  lumbar, lumbosacral 722.32
  specified region NEC 722.39
  thoracic, thoracolumbar 722.31
Schneider's syndrome 047.9
Schneiderian
  carcinoma (M8121/3)
    specified site—*see* Neoplasm, by site, malignant
    unspecified site 160.0
  papilloma (M8121/0)
    specified site—*see* Neoplasm, by site, benign
    unspecified site 212.0
Schnitzler syndrome 273.1
Schoffer's tumor (*see also* Peritonitis) 567.29
Scholte's syndrome (malignant carcinoid) 259.2
Scholz's disease 330.0
Scholz (-Bielschowsky-Henneberg) syndrome 330.0
Schönlein (-Henoch) disease (primary) (purpura)
  (rheumatic) 287.0
School examination V70.3
  following surgery V67.09
Schottmüller's disease (*see also* Fever,
  paratyphoid) 002.9
Schroeder's syndrome (endocrine-hypertensive) 255.3
Schüller-Christian disease or syndrome
  (chronic histiocytosis X) 277.89
Schultz's disease or syndrome (agranulocytosis)
  288.09
Schultze's acroparesthesia, simple 443.89
Schwalbe-Ziehen-Oppenheimer disease 333.6
Schwannoma (M9560/0)—*see also* Neoplasm,
  connective tissue, benign
  malignant (M9560/3)—*see* Neoplasm,
    connective tissue, malignant
Schwannomatosis 237.73
Schwartz (-Jampel) syndrome 359.23
Schwartz-Bartter syndrome (inappropriate
  secretion of antidiuretic hormone) 253.6
Schweninger-Buzzi disease (macular atrophy) 701.3
Sciatic —*see* condition
Sciatica (infectional) 724.3
  due to
    displacement of intervertebral disc 722.10
    herniation, nucleus pulposus 722.10
  wallet 724.3
Scimitar syndrome (anomalous venous drainage,
  right lung to inferior vena cava) 747.49
Sclera —*see* condition
Sclerectasia 379.11
Scleredema
  adultorum 710.1
  Buschke's 710.1
  newborn 778.1

Sclerema
  adiposum (newborn) 778.1
  adultorum 710.1
  edematosum (newborn) 778.1
  neonatorum 778.1
  newborn 778.1
Scleriasis —*see* Scleroderma
Scleritis 379.00
  with corneal involvement 379.05
  anterior (annular) (localized) 379.03
  brawny 379.06
  granulomatous 379.09
  posterior 379.07
  specified NEC 379.09
  suppurative 379.09
  syphilitic 095.0
  tuberculous (nodular) (*see also* Tuberculosis)
    017.3 *[379.09]*
Sclerochoroiditis (*see also* Scleritis) 379.00
Scleroconjunctivitis (*see also* Scleritis) 379.00
Sclerocystic ovary (syndrome) 256.4
Sclerodactylia 701.0
Scleroderma, sclerodermia (acrosclerotic)
    (diffuse) (generalized) (progressive)
    (pulmonary) 710.1
  circumscribed 701.0
  linear 701.0
  localized (linear) 701.0
  newborn 778.1
Sclerokeratitis 379.05
  meaning sclerosing keratitis 370.54
  tuberculous (*see also* Tuberculosis) 017.3
    [379.09]
Scleroma, trachea 040.1
Scleromalacia
  multiple 731.0
  perforans 379.04
Scleromyxedema 701.8
Scleroperikeratitis 379.05
Sclerose en plaques 340
Sclerosis, sclerotic
  adrenal (gland) 255.8
  Alzheimer's 331.0
    with dementia—*see* Alzheimer's, dementia
  amyotrophic (lateral) 335.20
  annularis fibrosi
    aortic 424.1
    mitral 424.0
  aorta, aortic 440.0
    valve (*see also* Endocarditis, aortic) 424.1
  artery, arterial, arteriolar, arteriovascular—*see*
    Arteriosclerosis
  ascending multiple 340
  Baló's (concentric) 341.1
  basilar—*see* Sclerosis, brain
  bone (localized) NEC 733.99
  brain (general) (lobular) 348.89
    Alzheimer's—*see* Alzheimer's dementia
    artery, arterial 437.0
    atrophic lobar 331.0
      with dementia
        with behavioral disturbance 331.0
          [294.11]
        without behavioral disturbance 331.0
          [294.10]
    diffuse 341.1
      familial (chronic) (infantile) 330.0
      infantile (chronic) (familial) 330.0
      Pelizaeus-Merzbacher type 330.0
    disseminated 340
    hereditary 334.2

Sclerosis, sclerotic—*continued*
  brain—*continued*
    hippocampal 348.81
    infantile, (degenerative) (diffuse) 330.0
    insular 340
    Krabbe's 330.0
    mesial temporal 348.81
    miliary 340
    multiple 340
    Pelizaeus-Merzbacher 330.0
    progressive familial 330.0
    senile 437.0
    temporal 348.81
      mesial 348.81
    tuberous 759.5
  bulbar, progressive 340
  bundle of His 426.50
    left 426.3
    right 426.4
  cardiac —*see* Arteriosclerosis, coronary
  cardiorenal (*see also* Hypertension, cardiorenal)
    404.90
  cardiovascular (*see also* Disease,
    cardiovascular) 429.2
    renal (*see also* Hypertension, cardiorenal)
      404.90
  centrolobar, familial 330.0
  cerebellar—*see* Sclerosis, brain
  cerebral—*see* Sclerosis, brain
  cerebrospinal 340
    disseminated 340
    multiple 340
  cerebrovascular 437.0
  choroid 363.40
    diffuse 363.56
  combined (spinal cord)—*see also* Degeneration,
    combined
    multiple 340
  concentric, Baló's 341.1
  cornea 370.54
  coronary (artery) —*see* Arteriosclerosis,
    coronary
  corpus cavernosum
    female 624.8
    male 607.89
  Dewitzky's
    aortic 424.1
    mitral 424.0
  diffuse NEC 341.1
  disease, heart —*see* Arteriosclerosis, coronary
  disseminated 340
  dorsal 340
  dorsolateral (spinal cord)—*see* Degeneration,
    combined
  endometrium 621.8
  extrapyramidal 333.90
  eye, nuclear (senile) 366.16
  Friedreich's (spinal cord) 334.0
  funicular (spermatic cord) 608.89
  gastritis 535.4
  general (vascular)—*see* Arteriosclerosis
  gland (lymphatic) 457.8
  hepatic 571.9
  hereditary
    cerebellar 334.2
    spinal 334.0
  hippocampal 348.81
  idiopathic cortical (Garré's) (*see also*
    Osteomyelitis) 730.1
  ilium, piriform 733.5

Sclerosis, sclerotic—*continued*
  insular 340
    pancreas 251.8
  Islands of Langerhans 251.8
  kidney—*see* Sclerosis, renal
  larynx 478.79
  lateral 335.24
    amyotrophic 335.20
    descending 335.24
    primary 335.24
    spinal 335.24
  liver 571.9
  lobar, atrophic (of brain) 331.0
    with dementia
      with behavioral disturbance 331.0 *[294.11]*
      without behavioral disturbance 331.0 *[294.10]*
  lung (*see also* Fibrosis, lung) 515
  mastoid 383.1
  mesial temporal 348.81
  mitral—*see* Endocarditis, mitral
  Mönckeberg's (medial) (*see also*
      Arteriosclerosis, extremities) 440.20
  multiple (brain stem) (cerebral) (generalized)
      (spinal cord) 340
  myocardium, myocardial —*see*
      Arteriosclerosis, coronary
  nuclear (senile), eye 366.16
  ovary 620.8
  pancreas 577.8
  penis 607.89
  peripheral arteries NEC (*see also*
      Arteriosclerosis, extremities) 440.20
  plaques 340
  pluriglandular 258.8
  polyglandular 258.8
  posterior (spinal cord) (syphilitic) 094.0
  posterolateral (spinal cord)—*see* Degeneration,
      combined
  prepuce 607.89
  primary lateral 335.24
  progressive systemic 710.1
  pulmonary (*see also* Fibrosis, lung) 515
    artery 416.0
    valve (heart) (*see also* Endocarditis,
        pulmonary) 424.3
  renal 587
    with
      cystine storage disease 270.0
      hypertension (*see also* Hypertension,
          kidney) 403.90
      hypertensive heart disease (conditions
          classifiable to 402) (*see also*
          Hypertension, cardiorenal) 404.90
      arteriolar (hyaline) (*see also* Hypertension,
          kidney) 403.90
      hyperplastic (*see also* Hypertension, kidney)
          403.90
  retina (senile) (vascular) 362.17
  rheumatic
    aortic valve 395.9
    mitral valve 394.9
  Schilder's 341.1
  senile—*see* Arteriosclerosis
  spinal (cord) (general) (progressive) (transverse)
      336.8
    ascending 357.0
    combined—*see also* Degeneration, combined
      multiple 340
      syphilitic 094.89
    disseminated 340
    dorsolateral—*see* Degeneration, combined

Sclerosis, sclerotic—*continued*
  hereditary (Friedreich's) (mixed form) 334.0
  lateral (amyotrophic) 335.24
  multiple 340
  posterior (syphilitic) 094.0
  stomach 537.89
  subendocardial, congenital 425.3
  systemic (progressive) 710.1
    with lung involvement 710.1 *[517.2]*
  temporal 348.81
    mesial 348.81
  tricuspid (heart) (valve)—*see* Endocarditis,
      tricuspid
  tuberous (brain) 759.5
  tympanic membrane (*see also*
      Tympanosclerosis) 385.00
  valve, valvular (heart)—*see* Endocarditis
  vascular—*see* Arteriosclerosis
  vein 459.89
Sclerotenonitis 379.07
Sclerotitis (*see also* Scleritis) 379.00
  syphilitic 095.0
  tuberculous (*see also* Tuberculosis) 017.3 *[379.09]*
Scoliosis (acquired) (postural) 737.30
  congenital 754.2
  due to or associated with
    Charcot-Marie-Tooth disease 356.1 *[737.43]*
    mucopolysaccharidosis 277.5 *[737.43]*
    neurofibromatosis 237.71 *[737.43]*
    osteitis
      deformans 731.0 *[737.43]*
      fibrosa cystica 252.01 *[737.43]*
    osteoporosis (*see also* Osteoporosis) 733.00
        [737.43]
    poliomyelitis 138 *[737.43]*
    radiation 737.33
    tuberculosis (*see also* Tuberculosis) 015.0
        [737.43]
  idiopathic 737.30
    infantile
      progressive 737.32
      resolving 737.31
  paralytic 737.39
  rachitic 268.1
  sciatic 724.3
  specified NEC 737.39
  thoracogenic 737.34
  tuberculous (*see also* Tuberculosis) 015.0 *[737.43]*
Scoliotic pelvis 738.6
  with disproportion (fetopelvic) 653.0
    affecting fetus or newborn 763.1
    causing obstructed labor 660.1
      affecting fetus or newborn 763.1
Scorbutus, scorbutic 267
  anemia 281.8
Scotoma (ring) 368.44
  arcuate 368.43
  Bjerrum 368.43
  blind spot area 368.42
  central 368.41
  centrocecal 368.41
  paracecal 368.42
  paracentral 368.41
  scintillating 368.12
  Seidel 368.43
Scratch —*see* Injury, superficial, by site
Scratchy throat 784.99
Screening (for) V82.9
  alcoholism V79.1
  anemia, deficiency NEC V78.1
    iron V78.0

Screening (for)—*continued*
 anomaly, congenital V82.89
 antenatal, of mother V28.9
  alphafetoprotein levels, raised V28.1
  based on amniocentesis V28.2
   chromosomal anomalies V28.0
   raised alphafetoprotein levels V28.1
  fetal growth retardation using ultrasonics V28.4
  genomic V28.89
  isoimmunization V28.5
  malformations using ultrasonics V28.3
  proteomic V28.89
  raised alphafetoprotein levels V28.1
  risk
   pre-term labor V28.82
  specified condition NEC V28.89
  Streptococcus B V28.6
 arterial hypertension V81.1
 arthropod-borne viral disease NEC V73.5
 asymptomatic bacteriuria V81.5
 bacterial
  and spirochetal sexually transmitted diseases V74.5
  conjunctivitis V74.4
  disease V74.9
   sexually transmitted V74.5
   specified condition NEC V74.8
 bacteriuria, asymptomatic V81.5
 blood disorder NEC V78.9
  specified type NEC V78.8
 bronchitis, chronic V81.3
 brucellosis V74.8
 cancer—*see* Screening, malignant neoplasm
 cardiovascular disease NEC V81.2
 cataract V80.2
 Chagas' disease V75.3
 chemical poisoning V82.5
 cholera V74.0
 cholesterol level V77.91
 chromosomal
  anomalies
   by amniocentesis, antenatal V28.0
   maternal postnatal V82.4
  athletes V70.3
 colonoscopy V76.51
 condition
  cardiovascular NEC V81.2
  eye NEC V80.2
  genitourinary NEC V81.6
  neurological NEC V80.09
  respiratory NEC V81.4
  skin V82.0
  specified NEC V82.89
 congenital
  anomaly V82.89
   eye V80.2
  dislocation of hip V82.3
  eye condition or disease V80.2
 conjunctivitis, bacterial V74.4
 contamination NEC (*see also* Poisoning) V82.5
 coronary artery disease V81.0
 cystic fibrosis V77.6
 deficiency anemia NEC V78.1
  iron V78.0
 dengue fever V73.5
 depression V79.0
 developmental handicap V79.9
  in early childhood V79.3
  specified type NEC V79.8
 diabetes mellitus V77.1
 diphtheria V74.3

Screening (for)—*continued*
 disease or disorder V82.9
  bacterial V74.9
   specified NEC V74.8
  blood V78.9
   specified type NEC V78.8
  blood-forming organ V78.9
   specified type NEC V78.8
  cardiovascular NEC V81.2
   hypertensive V81.1
   ischemic V81.0
  Chagas' V75.3
  chlamydial V73.98
   specified NEC V73.88
  ear NEC V80.3
  endocrine NEC V77.99
  eye NEC V80.2
  genitourinary NEC V81.6
  heart NEC V81.2
   hypertensive V81.1
   ischemic V81.0
  HPV (human papillomvirus) V73.81
  human papillomavirus (HPV) V73.81
  immunity NEC V77.99
  infectious NEC V75.9
  lipoid NEC V77.91
  mental V79.9
   specified type NEC V79.8
  metabolic NEC V77.99
   inborn NEC V77.7
  neurological NEC V80.09
  nutritional NEC V77.99
  rheumatic NEC V82.2
  rickettsial V75.0
  sexually transmitted V74.5
   bacterial V74.5
   spirochetal V74.5
  sickle-cell V78.2
   trait V78.2
  specified type NEC V82.89
  thyroid V77.0
  vascular NEC V81.2
   ischemic V81.0
  venereal V74.5
  viral V73.99
   arthropod-borne NEC V73.5
   specified type NEC V73.89
 dislocation of hip, congenital V82.3
 drugs in athletes V70.3
 elevated titer V82.9
 emphysema (chronic) V81.3
 encephalitis, viral (mosquito or tick borne) V73.5
 endocrine disorder NEC V77.99
 eye disorder NEC V80.2
  congenital V80.2
 fever
  dengue V73.5
  hemorrhagic V73.5
  yellow V73.4
 filariasis V75.6
 galactosemia V77.4
 genetic V82.79
  disease carrier status V82.71
 genitourinary condition NEC V81.6
 glaucoma V80.1
 gonorrhea V74.5
 gout V77.5
 Hansen's disease V74.2
 heart disease NEC V81.2
  hypertensive V81.1
  ischemic V81.0

Screening (for)—*continued*
  heavy metal poisoning V82.5
  helminthiasis, intestinal V75.7
  hematopoietic malignancy V76.89
  hemoglobinopathies NEC V78.3
  hemorrhagic fever V73.5
  Hodgkin's disease V76.89
  hormones in athletes V70.3
  HPV (human papillomavirus) V73.81
  human papillomavirus (HPV) V73.81
  hypercholesterolemia V77.91
  hyperlipidemia V77.91
  hypertension V81.1
  immunity disorder NEC V77.99
  inborn errors of metabolism NEC V77.7
  infection
    bacterial V74.9
     specified type NEC V74.8
    mycotic V75.4
    parasitic NEC V75.8
  infectious disease V75.9
    specified type NEC V75.8
  ingestion of radioactive substance V82.5
  intellectual disabilities V79.2
  intestinal helminthiasis V75.7
  iron deficiency anemia V78.0
  ischemic heart disease V81.0
  lead poisoning V82.5
  leishmaniasis V75.2
  leprosy V74.2
  leptospirosis V74.8
  leukemia V76.89
  lipoid disorder NEC V77.91
  lymphoma V76.89
  malaria V75.1
  malignant neoplasm (of) V76.9
    bladder V76.3
    blood V76.89
    breast V76.10
     mammogram NEC V76.12
      for high-risk patient V76.11
     specified type NEC V76.19
    cervix V76.2
    colon V76.51
    colorectal V76.51
    hematopoietic system V76.89
    intestine V76.50
     colon V76.51
     small V76.52
    lung V76.0
    lymph (glands) V76.89
    nervous system V76.81
    oral cavity V76.42
    other specified neoplasm NEC V76.89
    ovary V76.46
    prostate V76.44
    rectum V76.41
    respiratory organs V76.0
    skin V76.43
    specified sites NEC V76.49
    testis V76.45
    vagina V76.47
     following hysterectomy for malignant
      condition V67.01
  malnutrition V77.2
  mammogram NEC V76.12
    for high-risk patient V76.11
  maternal postnatal chromosomal anomalies V82.4
  measles V73.2

Screening (for)—*continued*
  mental
    disorder V79.9
     specified type NEC V79.8
    retardation — *see* Screening, intellectual
     disabilities
  metabolic errors, inborn V77.7
  metabolic disorder NEC V77.99
  mucoviscidosis V77.6
  multiphasic V82.6
  mycosis V75.4
  mycotic infection V75.4
  nephropathy V81.5
  neurological condition NEC V80.09
  nutritional disorder V77.99
    obesity V77.8
  obesity V77.8
  osteoporosis V82.81
  parasitic infection NEC V75.8
  phenylketonuria V77.3
  plague V74.8
  poisoning
    chemical NEC V82.5
    contaminated water supply V82.5
    heavy metal V82.5
  poliomyelitis V73.0
  postnatal chromosomal anomalies, maternal V82.4
  prenatal—*see* Screening, antenatal
  pulmonary tuberculosis V74.1
  radiation exposure V82.5
  renal disease V81.5
  respiratory condition NEC V81.4
  rheumatic disorder NEC V82.2
  rheumatoid arthritis V82.1
  rickettsial disease V75.0
  rubella V73.3
  schistosomiasis V75.5
  senile macular lesions of eye V80.2
  sexually transmitted diseases V74.5
    bacterial V74.5
    spirochetal V74.5
  sickle-cell anemia, disease, or trait V78.2
  skin condition V82.0
  sleeping sickness V75.3
  smallpox V73.1
  special V82.9
    specified condition NEC V82.89
  specified type NEC V82.89
  spirochetal disease V74.9
    sexually transmitted V74.5
    specified type NEC V74.8
  stimulants in athletes V70.3
  syphilis V74.5
  tetanus V74.8
  thyroid disorder V77.0
  trachoma V73.6
  traumatic brain injury V80.01
  trypanosomiasis V75.3
  tuberculosis, pulmonary V74.1
  venereal disease V74.5
  viral encephalitis
    mosquito-borne V73.5
    tick-borne V73.5
  whooping cough V74.8
  worms, intestinal V75.7
  yaws V74.6
  yellow fever V73.4
Scrofula (*see also* Tuberculosis) 017.2
Scrofulide (primary) (*see also* Tuberculosis) 017.0
Scrofuloderma, scrofulodermia (any site)
  (primary) (*see also* Tuberculosis) 017.0

Scrofulosis (universal) (*see also* Tuberculosis) 017.2
Scrofulosis lichen (primary) (*see also* Tuberculosis) 017.0
Scrofulous —*see* condition
Scrotal tongue 529.5
  congenital 750.13
Scrotum —*see* condition
Scurvy (gum) (infantile) (rickets) (scorbutic) 267
Sea-blue histiocyte syndrome 272.7
Seabright-Bantam syndrome (pseudohypoparathyroidism) 275.49
Sealpox 059.12
Seasickness 994.6
Seatworm 127.4
Sebaceous
  cyst (*see also* Cyst, sebaceous) 706.2
  gland disease NEC 706.9
Sebocystomatosis 706.2
Seborrhea, seborrheic 706.3
  adiposa 706.3
  capitis 690.11
  congestiva 695.4
  corporis 706.3
  dermatitis 690.10
    infantile 690.12
  diathesis in infants 695.89
  eczema 690.18
    infantile 690.12
  keratosis 702.19
    inflamed 702.11
  nigricans 705.89
  sicca 690.18
  wart 702.19
    inflamed 702.11
Seckel's syndrome 759.89
Seclusion pupil 364.74
Seclusiveness, child 313.22
Secondary —*see also* condition
  neoplasm—*see* Neoplasm, by site, malignant, secondary
Secretan's disease or syndrome (posttraumatic edema) 782.3
Secretion
  antidiuretic hormone, inappropriate (syndrome) 253.6
  catecholamine, by pheochromocytoma 255.6
  hormone
    antidiuretic, inappropriate (syndrome) 253.6
    by
      carcinoid tumor 259.2
      pheochromocytoma 255.6
    ectopic NEC 259.3
  urinary
    excessive 788.42
    suppression 788.5
Section
  cesarean
    affecting fetus or newborn 763.4
    post mortem, affecting fetus or newborn 761.6
    previous, in pregnancy or childbirth 654.2
      affecting fetus or newborn 763.89
  nerve, traumatic—*see* Injury, nerve, by site
Seeligmann's syndrome (ichthyosis congenita) 757.1
Segmentation, incomplete (congenital)—*see also* Fusion
  bone NEC 756.9
  lumbosacral (joint) 756.15
  vertebra 756.15
    lumbosacral 756.15

Seizure(s) 780.39
  akinetic (idiopathic) (*see also* Epilepsy) 345.0
    psychomotor 345.4
  apoplexy, apoplectic (*see also* Disease, cerebrovascular, acute) 436
  atonic (*see also* Epilepsy) 345.0
  autonomic 300.11
  brain or cerebral (*see also* Disease, cerebrovascular, acute) 436
  convulsive (*see also* Convulsions) 780.39
  cortical (focal) (motor) (*see also* Epilepsy) 345.5
  disorder (see also Epilepsy) 345.9
  due to stroke 438.89
  epilepsy, epileptic (cryptogenic) (*see also* Epilepsy) 345.9
  epileptiform, epileptoid 780.39
    focal (*see also* Epilepsy) 345.5
  febrile (simple) 780.31
    atypical 780.32
    complex 780.32
    complicated 780.32
    with status epilepticus 345.3
  heart—*see* Disease, heart
  hysterical 300.11
  Jacksonian (focal) (*see also* Epilepsy) 345.5
    motor type 345.5
    sensory type 345.5
  migraine triggered 346.0
  newborn 779.0
  paralysis (*see also* Disease, cerebrovascular, acute) 436
  post traumatic 780.33
  recurrent 345.8
    epileptic—*see* Epilepsy
  repetitive 780.39
    epileptic—*see* Epilepsy
  salaam (*see also* Epilepsy) 345.6
  uncinate (*see also* Epilepsy) 345.4
Self-mutilation 300.9
Semicoma 780.09
Semiconsciousness 780.09
Seminal
  vesicle—*see* condition
  vesiculitis (*see also* Vesiculitis) 608.0
Seminoma (M9061/3)
  anaplastic type (M9062/3)
    specified site—*see* Neoplasm, by site, malignant
    unspecified site 186.9
  specified site—*see* Neoplasm, by site, malignant
  spermatocytic (M9063/3)
    specified site—*see* Neoplasm, by site, malignant
    unspecified site 186.9
  unspecified site 186.9
Semliki Forest encephalitis 062.8
Senear-Usher disease or syndrome (pemphigus erythematosus) 694.4
Senecio jacobae dermatitis 692.6
Senectus 797
Senescence 797
Senile (*see also* condition) 797
  cervix (atrophic) 622.8
  degenerative atrophy, skin 701.3
  endometrium (atrophic) 621.8
  fallopian tube (atrophic) 620.3
  heart (failure) 797
  lung 492.8
  ovary (atrophic) 620.3
  syndrome 259.8
  vagina, vaginitis (atrophic) 627.3
  wart 702.0

Senility 797
  with
    acute confusional state 290.3
    delirium 290.3
    mental changes 290.9
    psychosis NEC (*see also* Psychosis, senile) 290.20
  premature (syndrome) 259.8
Sensation
  burning (*see also* Disturbance, sensation) 782.0
    tongue 529.6
  choking 784.99
  loss of (*see also* Disturbance, sensation) 782.0
  prickling (*see also* Disturbance, sensation) 782.0
  tingling (*see also* Disturbance, sensation) 782.0
Sense loss (touch) (*see also* Disturbance,
    sensation) 782.0
  smell 781.1
  taste 781.1
Sensibility disturbance NEC (cortical) (deep)
    (vibratory) (*see also* Disturbance, sensation)
    782.0
Sensitive dentine 521.89
Sensitiver Beziehungswahn 297.8
Sensitivity, sensitization —*see also* Allergy
  autoerythrocyte 287.2
  carotid sinus 337.01
  child (excessive) 313.21
  cold, autoimmune 283.0
  methemoglobin 289.7
  suxamethonium 289.89
  tuberculin, without clinical or radiological
    symptoms 795.51
Sensory
  extinction 781.8
  neglect 781.8
Separation
  acromioclavicular—see Dislocation, shoulder
  anxiety, abnormal 309.21
  apophysis, traumatic—see Fracture, by site
  choroid 363.70
    hemorrhagic 363.72
    serous 363.71
  costochondral (simple) (traumatic)—*see*
    Dislocation, costochondral
  delayed
    umbilical cord 779.83
  epiphysis, epiphyseal
    nontraumatic 732.9
      upper femoral 732.2
    traumatic—*see* Fracture, by site
  fracture—*see* Fracture, by site
  infundibulum cardiac from right ventricle by a
    partition 746.83
  joint (current) (traumatic)—*see* Dislocation, by
    site
  placenta (normally implanted)—*see* Placenta,
    separation
  pubic bone, obstetrical trauma 665.6
  retina, retinal (*see also* Detachment, retina) 361.9
    layers 362.40
      sensory (*see also* Retinoschisis) 361.10
    pigment epithelium (exudative) 362.42
      hemorrhagic 362.43
  sternoclavicular (traumatic)—*see* Dislocation,
    sternoclavicular
  symphysis pubis, obstetrical trauma 665.6
  tracheal ring, incomplete (congenital) 748.3

Sepsis (generalized) 995.91
  with
    abortion—*see* Abortion, by type, with sepsis
    acute organ dysfunction 995.92
    ectopic pregnancy (*see also* categories
      633.0-633.9) 639.0
    molar pregnancy (*see also* categories 630-632)
      639.0
    multiple organ dysfunction (MOD) 995.92
  buccal 528.3
  complicating labor 659.3
  dental (pulpal origin) 522.4
  female genital organ NEC 614.9
  fetus (intrauterine) 771.81
  following
    abortion 639.0
    ectopic or molar pregnancy 639.0
    infusion, perfusion, or transfusion 999.39
  Friedländer's 038.49
  intra-abdominal 567.22
  intraocular 360.00
  localized—code to specific localized infection
    in operation wound 998.59
    skin (*see also* Abscess) 682.9
  malleus 024
  newborn (organism unspecified) NEC 771.81
  oral 528.3
  puerperal, postpartum, childbirth (pelvic) 670.2
  resulting from infusion, injection, transfusion, or
    vaccination 999.39
  severe 995.92
  skin, localized (*see also* Abscess) 682.9
  umbilical (newborn) (organism unspecified)
    771.89
    tetanus 771.3
  urinary 599.0
    meaning sepsis 995.91
    meaning urinary tract infection 599.0
Septate —*see also* Septum
Septic —*see also* condition
  adenoids 474.01
    and tonsils 474.02
  arm (with lymphangitis) 682.3
  embolus—*see* Embolism
  finger (with lymphangitis) 681.00
  foot (with lymphangitis) 682.7
  gallbladder (*see also* Cholecystitis) 575.8
  hand (with lymphangitis) 682.4
  joint (*see also* Arthritis, septic) 711.0
  kidney (*see also* Infection, kidney) 590.9
  leg (with lymphangitis) 682.6
  mouth 528.3
  nail 681.9
    finger 681.02
    toe 681.11
  shock (endotoxic) 785.52
    postoperative 998.02
  sore (*see also* Abscess) 682.9
    throat 034.0
      milk-borne 034.0
      streptococcal 034.0
  spleen (acute) 289.59
  teeth (pulpal origin) 522.4
  throat 034.0
  thrombus—*see* Thrombosis
  toe (with lymphangitis) 681.10
  tonsils 474.00
    and adenoids 474.02
  umbilical cord (newborn) (organism
    unspecified) 771.89
  uterus (*see also* Endometritis) 615.9

Septicemia, septicemic (generalized)
  (suppurative) 038.9
with
  abortion—*see* Abortion, by type, with sepsis
  ectopic pregnancy (*see also* categories
    633.0-633.9) 639.0
  molar pregnancy (*see also* categories 630-632)
    639.0
Aerobacter aerogenes 038.49
anaerobic 038.3
anthrax 022.3
Bacillus coli 038.42
Bacteroides 038.3
Clostridium 038.3
complicating labor 659.3
cryptogenic 038.9
enteric gram-negative bacilli 038.40
Enterobacter aerogenes 038.49
Erysipelothrix (insidiosa) (rhusiopathiae) 027.1
Escherichia coli 038.42
following
  abortion 639.0
  ectopic or molar pregnancy 639.0
  infusion, injection, transfusion, or vaccination
    999.39
Friedländer's (bacillus) 038.49
gangrenous 038.9
gonococcal 098.89
gram-negative (organism) 038.40
  anaerobic 038.3
Hemophilus influenzae 038.41
herpes (simplex) 054.5
herpetic 054.5
Listeria monocytogenes 027.0
meningeal—*see* Meningitis
meningococcal (chronic) (fulminating) 036.2
methicillin
  resistant Staphylococcus aureus (MRSA) 038.12
  susceptible Staphylococcus aureus (MSSA)
    038.11
MRSA (methicillin resistant Staphylococcus
  aureus) 038.12
MSSA (methicillin susceptible Staphylococcus
  aureus) 038.11
navel, newborn (organism unspecified) 771.89
newborn (organism unspecified) 771.81
plague 020.2
pneumococcal 038.2
postabortal 639.0
postoperative 998.59
Proteus vulgaris 038.49
Pseudomonas (aeruginosa) 038.43
puerperal, postpartum 670.2
Salmonella (aertrycke) (callinarum)
  (choleraesuis) (enteritidis) (suipestifer) 003.1
Serratia 038.44
Shigella (*see also* Dysentery, bacillary) 004.9
specified organism NEC 038.8
staphylococcal 038.10
  aureus 038.11
    methicillin
      resistant (MRSA) 038.12
      susceptible (MSSA) 038.11
  specified organism NEC 038.19
streptococcal (anaerobic) 038.0
suipestifer 003.1
umbilicus, newborn (organism unspecified) 771.89
viral 079.99
Yersinia enterocolitica 038.49

Septum, septate (congenital)—*see also*
  Anomaly, specified type NEC
anal 751.2
aqueduct of Sylvius 742.3
  with spina bifida (*see also* Spina bifida) 741.0
hymen 752.49
uterus (complete) (partial) 752.35
vagina
  in pregnancy or childbirth 654.7
    affecting fetus or newborn 763.89
    causing obstructed labor 660.2
      affecting fetus or newborn 763.1
  longitudinal (with or without obstruction) 752.47
  transverse 752.46
Sequestration
lung (congenital) (extralobar) (intralobar) 748.5
orbit 376.10
pulmonary artery (congenital) 747.39
splenic 289.52
Sequestrum
bone (*see also* Osteomyelitis) 730.1
  jaw 526.4
dental 525.8
jaw bone 526.4
sinus (accessory) (nasal) (*see also* Sinusitis) 473.9
  maxillary 473.0
Sequoiosis asthma 495.8
Serology for syphilis
doubtful
  with signs or symptoms—*see* Syphilis, by site
    and stage
  follow-up of latent syphilis—*see* Syphilis, latent
false positive 795.6
negative, with signs or symptoms—*see* Syphilis,
  by site and stage
positive 097.1
  with signs or symptoms—*see* Syphilis, by site
    and stage
  false 795.6
  follow-up of latent syphilis—*see* Syphilis, latent
  only finding—*see* Syphilis, latent
reactivated 097.1
Seroma (postoperative) (non-infected) 998.13
infected 998.51
post-traumatic 729.91
Seropurulent —*see* condition
Serositis, multiple 569.89
pericardial 423.2
peritoneal 568.82
pleural—*see* Pleurisy
Serotonin syndrome 333.99
Serous —*see* condition
Sertoli cell
adenoma (M8640/0)
  specified site—*see* Neoplasm, by site, benign
  unspecified site
    female 220
    male 222.0
carcinoma (M8640/3)
  specified site—*see* Neoplasm, by site,
    malignant
  unspecified site 186.9
syndrome (germinal aplasia) 606.0
tumor (M8640/0)
  with lipid storage (M8641/0)
    specified site—*see* Neoplasm, by site,
      benign
    unspecified site
      female 220
      male 222.0

Sertoli cell—*continued*
tumor—*continued*
specified site—*see* Neoplasm, by site, benign
unspecified site
female 220
male 222.0
Sertoli-Leydig cell tumor (M8631/0)
specified site—*see* Neoplasm, by site, benign
unspecified site
female 220
male 222.0
Serum
allergy, allergic reaction 999.59
shock 999.49
arthritis 999.59 *[713.6]*
complication or reaction NEC 999.59
disease NEC 999.59
hepatitis 070.3
intoxication 999.59
jaundice (homologous) *see* Hepatitis, viral
neuritis 999.59
poisoning NEC 999.59
rash NEC 999.59
reaction NEC 999.59
sickness NEC 999.59
Sesamoiditis 733.99
Seven-day fever 061
of
Japan 100.89
Queensland 100.89
Sever's disease or osteochondrosis (calcaneum) 732.5
Sex chromosome mosaics 758.81
Sex reassignment surgery status (*see also*
Trans-sexualism) 302.50
Sextuplet
affected by maternal complications of pregnancy
761.5
healthy liveborn—*see* Newborn, multiple
pregnancy (complicating delivery) NEC 651.8
with fetal loss and retention of one or more
fetus(es) 651.6
following (elective) fetal reduction 651.7
Sexual
anesthesia 302.72
deviation (*see also* Deviation, sexual) 302.9
disorder (*see also* Deviation, sexual) 302.9
frigidity (female) 302.72
function, disorder of (psychogenic) 302.70
specified type NEC 302.79
immaturity (female) (male) 259.0
impotence 607.84
organic origin NEC 607.84
psychogenic 302.72
precocity (constitutional) (cryptogenic) (female)
(idiopathic) (male) NEC 259.1
with adrenal hyperplasia 255.2
sadism 302.84
Sexuality, pathological (*see also* Deviation,
sexual) 302.9
Sézary's disease, reticulosis, or syndrome
(M9701/3) 202.2
Shadow, lung 793.19
Shaken infant syndrome 995.55
Shaking
head (tremor) 781.0
palsy or paralysis (*see also* Parkinsonism) 332.0
Shallowness, acetabulum 736.39
Shaver's disease or syndrome (bauxite
pneumoconiosis) 503
Shearing
artificial skin graft 996.55
decellularized allodermis graft 996.55

Sheath (tendon)—*see* condition
Shedding
nail 703.8
teeth, premature, primary (deciduous) 520.6
Sheehan's disease or syndrome (postpartum
pituitary necrosis) 253.2
Shelf, rectal 569.49
Shell
shock (current) (*see also* Reaction, stress, acute)
308.9
lasting state 300.16
teeth 520.5
Shield kidney 753.3
Shift, mediastinal 793.2
Shifting
pacemaker 427.89
sleep-work schedule (affecting sleep) 327.36
Shiga's
bacillus 004.0
dysentery 004.0
Shigella (dysentery) (*see also* Dysentery,
bacillary) 004.9
carrier (suspected) of V02.3
Shigellosis (*see also* Dysentery, bacillary) 004.9
Shingles (*see also* Herpes, zoster) 053.9
eye NEC 053.29
Shin splints 844.9
Shipyard eye or disease 077.1
Shirodkar suture, in pregnancy 654.5
Shock 785.50
with
abortion—*see* Abortion, by type, with shock
ectopic pregnancy (*see also* categories
633.0-633.9) 639.5
molar pregnancy (*see also* categories 630-632)
639.5
allergic—*see* Anaphylactic reaction or shock
anaclitic 309.21
anaphylactic—*see also* Anaphylactic reaction or
shock
due to administration of blood and blood
products 999.41
anaphylactoid—*see* Anaphylactic reaction or
shock
anesthetic
correct substance properly administered 995.4
overdose or wrong substance given 968.4
specified anesthetic—*see* Table of drugs and
chemicals
birth, fetus or newborn NEC 779.89
cardiogenic 785.51
chemical substance—*see* Table of drugs and
chemicals
circulatory 785.59
complicating
abortion—*see* Abortion, by type, with shock
ectopic pregnancy (*see also* categories
633.0-633.9) 639.5
labor and delivery 669.1
molar pregnancy (*see also* categories 630-632)
639.5
culture 309.29
due to
drug 995.0
correct substance properly administered 995.0
overdose or wrong substance given or taken
977.9
specified drug—*see* Table of drugs and
chemicals
food—*see* Anaphylactic shock, due to, food
during labor and delivery 669.1

Shock—*continued*
  electric 994.8
    from electroshock gun (taser) 994.8
  endotoxic 785.52
    due to surgical procedure 998.02
    postoperative 998.02
  following
    abortion 639.5
    ectopic or molar pregnancy 639.5
    injury (immediate) (delayed) 958.4
    labor and delivery 669.1
  gram-negative 785.52
    postoperative 998.02
  hematogenic 785.59
  hemorrhagic
    due to
      disease 785.59
      surgery (intraoperative) (postoperative) 998.09
      trauma 958.4
  hypovolemic NEC 785.59
    surgical 998.09
    traumatic 958.4
  insulin 251.0
    therapeutic misadventure 962.3
  kidney 584.5
    traumatic (following crushing) 958.5
  lightning 994.0
  lung 518.82
    related to trauma and surgery 518.52
  nervous (*see also* Reaction, stress, acute) 308.9
  obstetric 669.1
    with
      abortion—*see* Abortion, by type, with shock
      ectopic pregnancy (*see also* categories 633.0-633.9) 639.5
      molar pregnancy (*see also* categories 630-632) 639.5
    following
      abortion 639.5
      ectopic or molar pregnancy 639.5
  paralysis, paralytic (*see also* Disease, cerebrovascular, acute) 436
    late effect—*see* Late effect(s) (of) cerebrovascular disease
  pleural (surgical) 998.09
    due to trauma 958.4
  postoperative 998.00
    with
      abortion—*see* Abortion, by type, with shock
      ectopic pregnancy (*see also* categories 633.0-633.9) 639.5
      molar pregnancy (*see also* categories 630-632) 639.5
    cardiogenic 998.01
    following
      abortion 639.5
      ectopic or molar pregnancy 639.5
    hypovolemic 998.09
    specified NEC 998.09
    septic (endotoxic) (gram-negative) 998.02
  psychic (*see also* Reaction, stress, acute) 308.9
    past history (of) V15.49
  psychogenic (*see also* Reaction, stress, acute) 308.9
  septic 785.52
    with
      abortion—*see* Abortion, by type, with shock
      ectopic pregnancy (*see also* categories 633.0-633.9) 639.5
      molar pregnancy (*see also* categories 630-632) 639.5

Shock—*continued*
  septic—*continued*
    due to
      surgical procedure 998.02
      transfusion NEC 999.89
        bone marrow 996.85
    following
      abortion 639.5
      ectopic or molar pregnancy 639.5
      surgical procedure 998.02
      transfusion NEC 999.89
        bone marrow 996.85
    postoperative 998.02
  spinal—*see also* Injury, spinal, by site
    with spinal bone injury—*see* Fracture, vertebra, by site, with spinal cord injury
  surgical 998.00
  therapeutic misadventure NEC (*see also* Complications) 998.89
  thyroxin 962.7
  toxic 040.82
  transfusion—*see* Complications, transfusion
  traumatic (immediate) (delayed) 958.4
Shoemakers' chest 738.3
Short, shortening, shortness
  Achilles tendon (acquired) 727.81
  arm 736.89
    congenital 755.20
  back 737.9
  bowel syndrome 579.3
  breath 786.05
  cervical, cervix 649.7
    gravid uterus 649.7
    non-gravid uterus 622.5
      acquired 622.5
      congenital 752.49
  chain acyl CoA dehydrogenase deficiency (SCAD) 277.85
  common bile duct, congenital 751.69
  cord (umbilical) 663.4
    affecting fetus or newborn 762.6
  cystic duct, congenital 751.69
  esophagus (congenital) 750.4
  femur (acquired) 736.81
    congenital 755.34
  frenulum linguae 750.0
  frenum, lingual 750.0
  hamstrings 727.81
  hip (acquired) 736.39
    congenital 755.63
  leg (acquired) 736.81
    congenital 755.30
  metatarsus (congenital) 754.79
    acquired 736.79
  organ or site, congenital NEC—*see* Distortion
  palate (congenital) 750.26
  P-R interval syndrome 426.81
  radius (acquired) 736.09
    congenital 755.26
  round ligament 629.89
  sleeper 307.49
  stature, constitutional (hereditary) (idiopathic) 783.43
  tendon 727.81
    Achilles (acquired) 727.81
      congenital 754.79
    congenital 756.89
  thigh (acquired) 736.81
    congenital 755.34
  tibialis anticus 727.81
  umbilical cord 663.4
    affecting fetus or newborn 762.6

Short, shortening, shortness—*continued*
  urethra 599.84
  uvula (congenital) 750.26
  vagina 623.8
Shortsightedness 367.1
Shoshin (acute fulminating beriberi) 265.0
Shoulder —*see* condition
Shovel-shaped incisors 520.2
Shower, thromboembolic —*see* Embolism
Shunt (status)
  aortocoronary bypass V45.81
  arterial-venous (dialysis) V45.11
  arteriovenous, pulmonary (acquired) 417.0
    congenital 747.39
    traumatic (complication) 901.40
  cerebral ventricle (communicating) in situ V45.2
  coronary artery bypass V45.81
  surgical, prosthetic, with complications—*see*
    Complications, shunt
  vascular NEC V45.89
Shutdown, renal 586
  with
    abortion—*see* Abortion, by type, with renal
      failure
    ectopic pregnancy (*see also* categories
      633.0-633.9) 639.3
    molar pregnancy (*see also* categories 630-632)
      639.3
  complicating
    abortion 639.3
    ectopic or molar pregnancy 639.3
  following labor and delivery 669.3
Shwachman's syndrome 288.02
Shy-Drager syndrome (orthostatic hypotension
  with multisystem degeneration) 333.0
Sialadenitis (any gland) (chronic) (suppurative)
  527.2
  epidemic—*see* Mumps
Sialadenosis, periodic 527.2
Sialaporia 527.7
Sialectasia 527.8
Sialitis 527.2
Sialoadenitis (*see also* Sialadenitis) 527.2
Sialoangitis 527.2
Sialodochitis (fibrinosa) 527.2
Sialodocholithiasis 527.5
Sialolithiasis 527.5
Sialorrhea (*see also* Ptyalism) 527.7
  periodic 527.2
Sialosis 527.8
  rheumatic 710.2
Siamese twin 759.4
  complicating pregnancy 678.1
Sicard's syndrome 352.6
Sicca syndrome (keratoconjunctivitis) 710.2
Sick 799.9
  cilia syndrome 759.89
  or handicapped person in family V61.49
Sickle-cell
  anemia (*see also* Disease, sickle-cell) 282.60
  disease (*see also* Disease, sickle-cell) 282.60
  hemoglobin
    C disease (without crisis) 282.63
      with
        crisis 282.64
        vaso-occlusive pain 282.64
    D disease (without crisis) 282.68
      with crisis 282.69
    E disease (without crisis) 282.68
      with crisis 282.69

Sickle-cell—*continued*
  thalassemia (without crisis) 282.41
    with
      crisis 282.42
      vaso-occlusive pain 282.42
  trait 282.5
Sicklemia (*see also* Disease, sickle-cell) 282.60
  trait 282.5
Sickness
  air (travel) 994.6
  airplane 994.6
  alpine 993.2
  altitude 993.2
  Andes 993.2
  aviators' 993.2
  balloon 993.2
  car 994.6
  compressed air 993.3
  decompression 993.3
  green 280.9
  harvest 100.89
  milk 988.8
  morning 643.0
  motion 994.6
  mountain 993.2
    acute 289.0
  protein (*see also* Complications, vaccination)
    999.59
  radiation NEC 990
  roundabout (motion) 994.6
  sea 994.6
  serum NEC 999.59
  sleeping (African) 086.5
    by Trypanosoma 086.5
      gambiense 086.3
      rhodesiense 086.4
    Gambian 086.3
    late effect 139.8
    Rhodesian 086.4
  sweating 078.2
  swing (motion) 994.6
  train (railway) (travel) 994.6
  travel (any vehicle) 994.6
Sick sinus syndrome 427.81
Sideropenia (*see also* Anemia, iron deficiency)
  280.9
Siderosis (lung) (occupational) 503
  central nervous system (CNS) 437.8
  cornea 371.15
  eye (bulbi) (vitreous) 360.23
  lens 360.23
Siegal-Cattan-Mamou disease (periodic) 277.31
Siemens' syndrome
  ectodermal dysplasia 757.31
  keratosis follicularis spinulosa (decalvans)
    757.39
Sighing respiration 786.7
Sigmoid
  flexure—*see* condition
  kidney 753.3
Sigmoiditis —*see* Enteritis
Silfverskiöld's syndrome 756.50
Silicosis, sillicotic (complicated) (occupational)
  (simple) 502
  fibrosis, lung (confluent) (massive)
    (occupational) 502
  non-nodular 503
  pulmonum 502
Silicotuberculosis (*see also* Tuberculosis) 011.4
Silo fillers' disease 506.9
Silver's syndrome (congenital hemihypertrophy
  and short stature) 759.89

Silver wire arteries, retina 362.13
Silvestroni-Bianco syndrome (thalassemia
   minima) 282.49
Simian crease 757.2
Simmonds' cachexia or disease (pituitary
   cachexia) 253.2
Simons' disease or syndrome (progressive
   lipodystrophy) 272.6
Simple, simplex —*see* condition
Sinding-Larsen disease (juvenile osteopathia
   patellae) 732.4
Singapore hemorrhagic fever 065.4
Singers' node or nodule 478.5
Single
   atrium 745.69
   coronary artery 746.85
   umbilical artery 747.5
   ventricle 745.3
Singultus 786.8
   epidemicus 078.89
Sinus —*see also* Fistula
   abdominal 569.81
   arrest 426.6
   arrhythmia 427.89
   bradycardia 427.89
      chronic 427.81
   branchial cleft (external) (internal) 744.41
   coccygeal (infected) 685.1
      with abscess 685.0
   dental 522.7
   dermal (congenital) 685.1
      with abscess 685.0
   draining—*see* Fistula
   infected, skin NEC 686.9
   marginal, ruptured or bleeding 641.2
      affecting fetus or newborn 762.1
   pause 426.6
   pericranii 742.0
   pilonidal (infected) (rectum) 685.1
      with abscess 685.0
   preauricular 744.46
   rectovaginal 619.1
   sacrococcygeal (dermoid) (infected) 685.1
      with abscess 685.0
   skin
      infected NEC 686.9
      noninfected—*see* Ulcer, skin
   tachycardia 427.89
   tarsi syndrome 726.79
   testis 608.89
   tract (postinfectional)—*see* Fistula
   urachus 753.7
Sinuses, Rokitansky-Aschoff (*see also* Disease,
   gallbladder) 575.8
Sinusitis (accessory) (nasal) (hyperplastic)
   (nonpurulent) (purulent) (chronic) 473.9
   with influenza, flu, or grippe (*see also*
      Influenza) 487.1
   acute 461.9
      ethmoidal 461.2
      frontal 461.1
      maxillary 461.0
      specified type NEC 461.8
      sphenoidal 461.3
   allergic (*see also* Fever, hay) 477.9
   antrum—*see* Sinusitis, maxillary
   due to
      fungus, any sinus 117.9
      high altitude 993.1
   ethmoidal 473.2
      acute 461.2

Sinusitis—*continued*
   frontal 473.1
      acute 461.1
   influenzal (*see also* Influenza) 487.1
   maxillary 473.0
      acute 461.0
   specified site NEC 473.8
   sphenoidal 473.3
      acute 461.3
   syphilitic, any sinus 095.8
   tuberculous, any sinus (*see also* Tuberculosis) 012.8
Sinusitis-bronchiectasis-situs inversus
   (syndrome) (triad) 759.3
Sipple's syndrome (medullary thyroid
   carcinoma-pheochromocytoma) 258.02
SIRS (systemic inflammatory response
   syndrome) 995.90
   due to
      infectious process 995.91
         with acute organ dysfunction 995.92
      non-infectious process 995.93
         with acute organ dysfunction 995.94
Sirenomelia 759.89
Siriasis 992.0
Sirkari's disease 085.0
Siti 104.0
Sitophobia 300.29
Situation, psychiatric 300.9
Situational
   disturbance (transient) (*see also* Reaction,
      adjustment) 309.9
      acute 308.3
   maladjustment, acute (*see also* Reaction,
      adjustment) 309.9
   reaction (*see also* Reaction, adjustment) 309.9
      acute 308.3
Situs inversus or transversus 759.3
   abdominalis 759.3
   thoracis 759.3
Sixth disease
   due to
      human herpesvirus 6 058.11
      human herpesvirus 7 058.12
Sjögren (-Gougerot) syndrome or disease
   (keratoconjunctivitis sicca) 710.2
   with lung involvement 710.2 [517.8]
Sjögren-Larsson syndrome (ichthyosis
   congenita) 757.1
SJS-TEN (Stevens-Johnson syndrome-toxic
   epidermal necrolysis overlap syndrome) 695.14
Skeletal —*see* condition
Skene's gland —*see* condition
Skenitis (*see also* Urethritis) 597.89
   gonorrheal (acute) 098.0
      chronic or duration of 2 months or over 098.2
Skerljevo 104.0
Skevas-Zerfus disease 989.5
Skin —*see also* condition
   donor V59.1
   hidebound 710.9
SLAP lesion (superior glenoid labrum) 840.7
Slate-dressers' lung 502
Slate-miners' lung 502
Sleep
   deprivation V69.4
   disorder 780.50
      with apnea—*see* Apnea, sleep
      child 307.40
      movement, unspecified 780.58
      nonorganic origin 307.40
         specified type NEC 307.49

Sleep—*continued*
  disturbance 780.50
    with apnea—*see* Apnea, sleep
    nonorganic origin 307.40
      specified type NEC 307.49
  drunkenness 307.47
  movement disorder, unspecified 780.58
  paroxysmal (*see also* Narcolepsy) 347.00
  related movement disorder, unspecified 780.58
  rhythm inversion 327.39
    nonorganic origin 307.45
  walking 307.46
    hysterical 300.13
Sleeping sickness 086.5
  late effect 139.8
Sleeplessness (*see also* Insomnia) 780.52
  menopausal 627.2
  nonorganic origin 307.41
Slipped, slipping
  epiphysis (postinfectional) 732.9
    traumatic (old) 732.9
      current—*see* Fracture, by site
    upper femoral (nontraumatic) 732.2
  intervertebral disc—*see* Displacement,
    intervertebral disc
  ligature, umbilical 772.3
  patella 717.89
  rib 733.99
  sacroiliac joint 724.6
  tendon 727.9
  ulnar nerve, nontraumatic 354.2
  vertebra NEC (*see also* Spondylolisthesis) 756.12
Slocumb's syndrome 255.3
Sloughing (multiple) (skin) 686.9
  abscess—*see* Abscess, by site
  appendix 543.9
  bladder 596.89
  fascia 728.9
  graft—*see* Complications, graft
  phagedena (*see also* Gangrene) 785.4
  reattached extremity (*see also* Complications,
    reattached extremity) 996.90
  rectum 569.49
  scrotum 608.89
  tendon 727.9
  transplanted organ (*see also* Rejection,
    transplant, organ, by site) 996.80
  ulcer (*see also* Ulcer, skin) 707.9
Slow
  feeding newborn 779.31
  fetal, growth NEC 764.9
    affecting management of pregnancy 656.5
Slowing
  heart 427.89
  urinary stream 788.62
Sluder's neuralgia or syndrome 337.09
Slurred, slurring, speech 784.59
Small, smallness
  cardiac reserve—*see* Disease, heart
  for dates
    fetus or newborn 764.0
      with malnutrition 764.1
    affecting management of pregnancy 656.5
  infant, term 764.0
    with malnutrition 764.1
    affecting management of pregnancy 656.5
  introitus, vagina 623.3
  kidney, unknown cause 589.9
    bilateral 589.1
    unilateral 589.0
  ovary 620.8

Small, smallness—*continued*
  pelvis
    with disproportion (fetopelvic) 653.1
      affecting fetus or newborn 763.1
      causing obstructed labor 660.1
        affecting fetus or newborn 763.1
  placenta—*see* Placenta, insufficiency
  uterus 621.8
  white kidney 582.9
Small-for-dates (*see also* Light-for-dates) 764.0
  affecting management of pregnancy 656.5
Smallpox 050.9
  contact V01.3
  exposure to V01.3
  hemorrhagic (pustular) 050.0
  malignant 050.0
  modified 050.2
  vaccination
    complications—*see* Complications,
      vaccination
    prophylactic (against) V04.1
Smearing, fecal 787.62
Smith's fracture (separation) (closed) 813.41
  open 813.51
Smith-Lemli-Opitz syndrome
  (cerebrohepatorenal syndrome) 759.89
Smith-Magenis syndrome 758.33
Smith-Strang disease (oasthouse urine) 270.2
Smokers'
  bronchitis 491.0
  cough 491.0
  syndrome (*see also* Abuse, drugs,
    nondependent) 305.1
  throat 472.1
  tongue 528.6
Smoking complicating pregnancy, childbirth, or
    the puerperium 649.0
Smothering spells 786.09
Snaggle teeth, tooth 524.39
Snapping
  finger 727.05
  hip 719.65
  jaw 524.69
    temporomandibular joint sounds on opening or
      closing 524.64
  knee 717.9
  thumb 727.05
Sneddon-Wilkinson disease or syndrome
  (subcorneal pustular dermatosis) 694.1
Sneezing 784.99
  intractable 478.19
Sniffing
  cocaine (*see also* Dependence) 304.2
  ether (*see also* Dependence) 304.6
  glue (airplane) (*see also* Dependence) 304.6
Snoring 786.09
Snow blindness 370.24
Snuffles (nonsyphilitic) 460
  syphilitic (infant) 090.0
Social migrant V60.0
Sodoku 026.0
Soemmering's ring 366.51
Soft —*see also* condition
  enlarged prostate 600.00
    with
      other lower urinary tract symptoms (LUTS)
        600.01
      urinary
        obstruction 600.01
        retention 600.01
  nails 703.8

Softening
bone 268.2
brain (necrotic) (progressive) 348.89
  arteriosclerotic 437.0
  congenital 742.4
  due to cerebrovascular accident 438.89
  embolic (*see also* Embolism, brain) 434.1
  hemorrhagic (*see also* Hemorrhage, brain) 431
  occlusive 434.9
  thrombotic (*see also* Thrombosis, brain) 434.0
cartilage 733.92
cerebellar—*see* Softening, brain
cerebral—*see* Softening, brain
cerebrospinal—*see* Softening, brain
myocardial, heart (*see also* Degeneration,
  myocardial) 429.1
nails 703.8
spinal cord 336.8
stomach 537.89
Soiling, fecal 787.62
Solar fever 061
Soldier's
heart 306.2
patches 423.1
Solitary
cyst
  bone 733.21
  kidney 593.2
kidney (congenital) 753.0
tubercle, brain (*see also* Tuberculosis, brain) 013.2
ulcer, bladder 596.89
Somatization reaction, somatic reaction (*see
  also* Disorder, psychosomatic) 306.9
disorder 300.81
Somatoform disorder 300.82
atypical 300.82
severe 300.81
undifferentiated 300.82
Somnambulism 307.46
hysterical 300.13
Somnolence 780.09
nonorganic origin 307.43
periodic 349.89
Sonne dysentery 004.3
Soor 112.0
Sore
Delhi 085.1
desert (*see also* Ulcer, skin) 707.9
eye 379.99
Lahore 085.1
mouth 528.9
  canker 528.2
  due to dentures 528.9
muscle 729.1
Naga (*see also* Ulcer, skin) 707.9
oriental 085.1
pressure (*see also* Ulcer, pressure) 707.00
  with gangrene (*see also* Ulcer, pressure)
    707.00 [785.4]
skin NEC 709.9
soft 099.0
throat 462
  with influenza, flu, or grippe (*see also*
    Influenza) 487.1
  acute 462
  chronic 472.1
  clergyman's 784.49
  coxsackie (virus) 074.0
  diphtheritic 032.0
  epidemic 034.0
  gangrenous 462

Sore —*continued*
throat—*continued*
  herpetic 054.79
  influenzal (*see also* Influenza) 487.1
  malignant 462
  purulent 462
  putrid 462
  septic 034.0
  streptococcal (ulcerative) 034.0
  ulcerated 462
  viral NEC 462
    Coxsackie 074.0
tropical (*see also* Ulcer, skin) 707.9
veldt (*see also* Ulcer, skin) 707.9
Sotos' syndrome (cerebral gigantism) 253.0
Sounds
friction, pleural 786.7
succussion, chest 786.7
temporomandibular joint
  on opening or closing 524.64
South African cardiomyopathy syndrome
  425.2
South American
blastomycosis 116.1
trypanosomiasis—*see* Trypanosomiasis
Southeast Asian hemorrhagic fever 065.4
Spacing, teeth, abnormal 524.30
excessive 524.32
Spade-like hand (congenital) 754.89
Spading nail 703.8
congenital 757.5
Spanemia 285.9
Spanish collar 605
Sparganosis 123.5
Spasm, spastic, spasticity (*see also* condition)
  781.0
accommodation 367.53
ampulla of Vater (*see also* Disease, gallbladder)
  576.8
anus, ani (sphincter) (reflex) 564.6
  psychogenic 306.4
artery NEC 443.9
  basilar 435.0
  carotid 435.8
  cerebral 435.9
    specified artery NEC 435.8
  retinal (*see also* Occlusion, retinal, artery)
    362.30
  vertebral 435.1
  vertebrobasilar 435.3
Bell's 351.0
bladder (sphincter, external or internal) 596.89
bowel 564.9
  psychogenic 306.4
bronchus, bronchiole 519.11
cardia 530.0
cardiac—*see* Angina
carpopedal (*see also* Tetany) 781.7
cecum 564.9
  psychogenic 306.4
cerebral (arteries) (vascular) 435.9
  specified artery NEC 435.8
cerebrovascular 435.9
cervix, complicating delivery 661.4
  affecting fetus or newborn 763.7
ciliary body (of accommodation) 367.53
colon 564.1
  psychogenic 306.4
common duct (*see also* Disease, biliary) 576.8
compulsive 307.22
conjugate 378.82

Spasm, spastic, spasticity—*continued*
  convergence 378.84
  coronary (artery)—*see* Angina
  diaphragm (reflex) 786.8
    psychogenic 306.1
  duodenum, duodenal (bulb) 564.89
  esophagus (diffuse) 530.5
    psychogenic 306.4
  facial 351.8
  fallopian tube 620.8
  gait 781.2
  gastrointestinal (tract) 536.8
    psychogenic 306.4
  glottis 478.75
    hysterical 300.11
    psychogenic 306.1
      specified as conversion reaction 300.11
    reflex through recurrent laryngeal nerve
      478.75
  habit 307.20
    chronic 307.22
    transient (of childhood) 307.21
  heart—*see* Angina
  hourglass—*see* Contraction, hourglass
  hysterical 300.11
  infantile (*see also* Epilepsy) 345.6
  internal oblique, eye 378.51
  intestinal 564.9
    psychogenic 306.4
  larynx, laryngeal 478.75
    hysterical 300.11
    psychogenic 306.1
      specified as conversion reaction 300.11
  levator palpebrae superioris 333.81
  lightning (*see also* Epilepsy) 345.6
  mobile 781.0
  muscle 728.85
    back 724.8
    psychogenic 306.0
  nerve, trigeminal 350.1
  nervous 306.0
  nodding 307.3
    infantile (*see also* Epilepsy) 345.6
  occupational 300.89
  oculogyric 378.87
  ophthalmic artery 362.30
  orbicularis 781.0
  perineal 625.8
  peroneo-extensor (*see also* Flat, foot) 734
  pharynx (reflex) 478.29
    hysterical 300.11
    psychogenic 306.1
      specified as conversion reaction 300.11
  pregnant uterus, complicating delivery 661.4
  psychogenic 306.0
  pylorus 537.81
    adult hypertrophic 537.0
    congenital or infantile 750.5
    psychogenic 306.4
  rectum (sphincter) 564.6
    psychogenic 306.4
  retinal artery NEC (*see also* Occlusion, retina,
    artery) 362.30
  sacroiliac 724.6
  salaam (infantile) (*see also* Epilepsy) 345.6
  saltatory 781.0
  sigmoid 564.9
    psychogenic 306.4
  sphincter of Oddi (*see also* Disease, gallbladder)
    576.5

Spasm, spastic, spasticity—*continued*
  stomach 536.8
    neurotic 306.4
  throat 478.29
    hysterical 300.11
    psychogenic 306.1
      specified as conversion reaction 300.11
  tic 307.20
    chronic 307.22
    transient (of childhood) 307.21
  tongue 529.8
  torsion 333.6
  trigeminal nerve 350.1
    postherpetic 053.12
  ureter 593.89
  urethra (sphincter) 599.84
  uterus 625.8
    complicating labor 661.4
      affecting fetus or newborn 763.7
  vagina 625.1
    psychogenic 306.51
  vascular NEC 443.9
  vasomotor NEC 443.9
  vein NEC 459.89
  vesical (sphincter, external or internal) 596.89
  viscera 789.0
Spasmodic —*see* condition
Spasmophilia (*see also* Tetany) 781.7
Spasmus nutans 307.3
Spastic —*see also* Spasm
  child 343.9
Spasticity —*see also* Spasm
  cerebral, child 343.9
Speakers' throat 784.49
Specific, specified —*see* condition
Speech
  defect, disorder, disturbance, impediment NEC
    784.59
    psychogenic 307.9
  (language) therapy V57.3
Spells 780.39
  breath-holding 786.9
Spencer's disease (epidemic vomiting) 078.82
Spens' syndrome (syncope with heart block)
  426.9
Spermatic cord —*see* condition
Spermatocele 608.1
  congenital 752.89
Spermatocystitis 608.4
Spermatocytoma (M9063/3)
  specified site—*see* Neoplasm, by site, malignant
  unspecified site 186.9
Spermatorrhea 608.89
Sperm counts
  fertility testing V26.21
  following sterilization reversal V26.22
  postvasectomy V25.8
Sphacelus (*see also* Gangrene) 785.4
Sphenoidal —*see* condition
Sphenoiditis (chronic) (*see also* Sinusitis,
  sphenoidal) 473.3
Sphenopalatine ganglion neuralgia 337.09
Sphericity, increased, lens 743.36
Spherocytosis (congenital) (familial) (hereditary)
  282.0
  hemoglobin disease 287.7
  sickle-cell (disease) 282.60
Spherophakia 743.36
Sphincter —*see* condition
Sphincteritis, sphincter of Oddi (*see also*
  Cholecystitis) 576.8

Sphingolipidosis 272.7
Sphingolipodystrophy 272.7
Sphingomyelinosis 272.7
Spicule tooth 520.2
Spider
  finger 755.59
  nevus 448.1
  vascular 448.1
Spiegler-Fendt sarcoid 686.8
Spielmeyer-Stock disease 330.1
Spielmeyer-Vogt disease 330.1
Spina bifida (aperta) 741.9

> *Note—Use the following fifth-digit*
> *subclassification with category 741:*
> *0 unspecified region*
> *1 cervical region*
> *2 dorsal [thoracic] region*
> *3 lumbar region*

  with hydrocephalus 741.0
  fetal (suspected), affecting management of
      pregnancy 655.0
  occulta 756.17
Spindle, Krukenberg's 371.13
Spine, spinal *—see* condition
Spiradenoma (eccrine) (M8403/0)—*see*
      Neoplasm, skin, benign
Spirillosis NEC (*see also* Fever, relapsing) 087.9
Spirillum minus 026.0
Spirillum obermeieri infection 087.0
Spirochetal *—see* condition
Spirochetosis 104.9
  arthritic, arthritica 104.9 *[711.8]*
  bronchopulmonary 104.8
  icterohemorrhagica 100.0
  lung 104.8
Spitting blood (*see also* Hemoptysis) 786.30
Splanchnomegaly 569.89
Splanchnoptosis 569.89
Spleen, splenic *—see also* condition
  agenesis 759.0
  flexure syndrome 569.89
  neutropenia syndrome 289.53
  sequestration syndrome 289.52
Splenectasis (*see also* Splenomegaly) 789.2
Splenitis (interstitial) (malignant) (nonspecific)
      289.59
  malarial (*see also* Malaria) 084.6
  tuberculous (*see also* Tuberculosis) 017.7
Splenocele 289.59
Splenomegalia *—see* Splenomegaly
Splenomegalic *—see* condition
Splenomegaly 789.2
  Bengal 789.2
  cirrhotic 289.51
  congenital 759.0
  congestive, chronic 289.51
  cryptogenic 789.2
  Egyptian 120.1
  Gaucher's (cerebroside lipidosis) 272.7
  idiopathic 789.2
  malarial (*see also* Malaria) 084.6
  neutropenic 289.53
  Niemann-Pick (lipid histiocytosis) 272.7
  siderotic 289.51
  syphilitic 095.8
      congenital 090.0
  tropical (Bengal) (idiopathic) 789.2
Splenopathy 289.50
Splenopneumonia *—see* Pneumonia
Splenoptosis 289.59

Splinter *—see* Injury, superficial, by site
Split, splitting
  heart sounds 427.89
  lip, congenital (*see also* Cleft, lip) 749.10
  nails 703.8
  urinary stream 788.61
Spoiled child reaction (*see also* Disturbance,
      conduct) 312.1
Spondylarthritis (*see also* Spondylosis) 721.90
Spondylarthrosis (*see also* Spondylosis) 721.90
Spondylitis 720.9
  ankylopoietica 720.0
  ankylosing (chronic) 720.0
  atrophic 720.9
      ligamentous 720.9
  chronic (traumatic) (*see also* Spondylosis) 721.90
  deformans (chronic) (*see also* Spondylosis) 721.90
  gonococcal 098.53
  gouty 274.00
  hypertrophic (*see also* Spondylosis) 721.90
  infectious NEC 720.9
  juvenile (adolescent) 720.0
  Kümmell's 721.7
  Marie-Strümpell (ankylosing) 720.0
  muscularis 720.9
  ossificans ligamentosa 721.6
  osteoarthritica (*see also* Spondylosis) 721.90
  posttraumatic 721.7
  proliferative 720.0
  rheumatoid 720.0
  rhizomelica 720.0
  sacroiliac NEC 720.2
  senescent (*see also* Spondylosis) 721.90
  senile (*see also* Spondylosis) 721.90
  static (*see also* Spondylosis) 721.90
  traumatic (chronic) (*see also* Spondylosis) 721.90
  tuberculous (*see also* Tuberculosis) 015.0 *[720.81]*
  typhosa 002.0 *[720.81]*
Spondyloarthrosis (*see also* Spondylosis) 721.90
Spondylolisthesis (congenital) (lumbosacral)
      756.12
  with disproportion (fetopelvic) 653.3
      affecting fetus or newborn 763.1
      causing obstructed labor 660.1
          affecting fetus or newborn 763.1
  acquired 738.4
  degenerative 738.4
  traumatic 738.4
      acute (lumbar)—*see* Fracture, vertebra,
          lumbar
      site other than lumbosacral—*see* Fracture,
          vertebra, by site
Spondylolysis (congenital) 756.11
  acquired 738.4
  cervical 756.19
  lumbosacral region 756.11
      with disproportion (fetopelvic) 653.3
          affecting fetus or newborn 763.1
          causing obstructed labor 660.1
              affecting fetus or newborn 763.1
Spondylopathy
  inflammatory 720.9
      specified type NEC 720.89
  traumatic 721.7
Spondylose rhizomelique 720.0
Spondylosis 721.90
  with
      disproportion 653.3
          affecting fetus or newborn 763.1
          causing obstructed labor 660.1
              affecting fetus or newborn 763.1
      myelopathy NEC 721.91

Spondylosis—*continued*
cervical, cervicodorsal 721.0
  with myelopathy 721.1
  inflammatory 720.9
lumbar, lumbosacral 721.3
  with myelopathy 721.42
sacral 721.3
  with myelopathy 721.42
thoracic 721.2
  with myelopathy 721.41
traumatic 721.7
Sponge
divers' disease 989.5
inadvertently left in operation wound 998.4
kidney (medullary) 753.17
Spongioblastoma (M9422/3)
multiforme (M9440/3)
  specified site—*see* Neoplasm, by site, malignant
  unspecified site 191.9
polare (M9423/3)
  specified site—*see* Neoplasm, by site,
    malignant
  unspecified site 191.9
primitive polar (M9443/3)
  specified site—*see* Neoplasm, by site,
    malignant
  unspecified site 191.9
specified site—*see* Neoplasm, by site, malignant
unspecified site 191.9
Spongiocytoma (M9400/3)
specified site—*see* Neoplasm, by site, malignant
unspecified site 191.9
Spongioneuroblastoma (M9504/3)—*see*
Neoplasm, by site, malignant
Spontaneous —*see also* condition
fracture—*see* Fracture, pathologic
Spoon nail 703.8
congenital 757.5
Sporadic —*see* condition
Sporotrichosis (bones) (cutaneous)
  (disseminated) (epidermal) (lymphatic)
  (lymphocutaneous) (mucous membranes)
  (pulmonary) (skeletal) (visceral) 117.1
Sporotrichum schenckii infection 117.1
Spots, spotting
atrophic (skin) 701.3
Bitôt's (in the young child) 264.1
café au lait 709.09
cayenne pepper 448.1
complicating pregnancy 649.5
cotton wool (retina) 362.83
de Morgan's (senile angiomas) 448.1
Fúchs' black (myopic) 360.21
intermenstrual
  irregular 626.6
  regular 626.5
interpalpebral 372.53
Koplik's 055.9
liver 709.09
Mongolian (pigmented) 757.33
of pregnancy 649.5
purpuric 782.7
ruby 448.1
Spotted fever —*see* Fever, spotted
Sprain, strain (joint) (ligament) (muscle)
  (tendon) 848.9
abdominal wall (muscle) 848.8
Achilles tendon 845.09
acromioclavicular 840.0
ankle 845.00
  and foot 845.00

Sprain, strain—*continued*
anterior longitudinal, cervical 847.0
arm 840.9
  upper 840.9
  and shoulder 840.9
astragalus 845.00
atlanto-axial 847.0
atlanto-occipital 847.0
atlas 847.0
axis 847.0
back (*see also* Sprain, spine) 847.9
breast bone 848.40
broad ligament—*see* Injury, internal, broad
  ligament
calcaneofibular 845.02
carpal 842.01
carpometacarpal 842.11
cartilage
  costal, without mention of injury to sternum
    848.3
    involving sternum 848.42
  ear 848.8
  knee 844.9
    with current tear (*see also* Tear, meniscus)
      836.2
  semilunar (knee) 844.8
    with current tear (*see also* Tear, meniscus)
      836.2
  septal, nose 848.0
  thyroid region 848.2
  xiphoid 848.49
cervical, cervicodorsal, cervicothoracic 847.0
chondrocostal, without mention of injury to
  sternum 848.3
  involving sternum 848.42
chondrosternal 848.42
chronic (joint)—*see* Derangement, joint
clavicle 840.9
coccyx 847.4
collar bone 840.9
collateral, knee (medial) (tibial) 844.1
  lateral (fibular) 844.0
  recurrent or old 717.89
    lateral 717.81
    medial 717.82
coracoacromial 840.8
coracoclavicular 840.1
coracohumeral 840.2
coracoid (process) 840.9
coronary, knee 844.8
costal cartilage, without mention of injury to
  sternum 848.3
  involving sternum 848.42
cricoarytenoid articulation 848.2
cricothyroid articulation 848.2
cruciate
  knee 844.2
  old 717.89
    anterior 717.83
    posterior 717.84
deltoid
  ankle 845.01
  shoulder 840.8
dorsal (spine) 847.1
ear cartilage 848.8
elbow 841.9
  and forearm 841.9
  specified site NEC 841.8
femur (proximal end) 843.9
  distal end 844.9

Sprain, strain—*continued*
  fibula (proximal end) 844.9
    distal end 845.00
  fibulocalcaneal 845.02
  finger(s) 842.10
  foot 845.10
    and ankle 845.00
  forearm 841.9
    and elbow 841.9
    specified site NEC 841.8
  glenoid (shoulder) (*see also* SLAP lesion) 840.8
  hand 842.10
  hip 843.9
    and thigh 843.9
  humerus (proximal end) 840.9
    distal end 841.9
  iliofemoral 843.0
  infraspinatus 840.3
  innominate
    acetabulum 843.9
    pubic junction 848.5
    sacral junction 846.1
  internal
    collateral, ankle 845.01
    semilunar cartilage 844.8
      with current tear (*see also* Tear, meniscus)
        836.2
      old 717.5
  interphalangeal
    finger 842.13
    toe 845.13
  ischiocapsular 843.1
  jaw (cartilage) (meniscus) 848.1
    old 524.69
  knee 844.9
    and leg 844.9
    old 717.5
      collateral
        lateral 717.81
          medial 717.82
      cruciate
        anterior 717.83
          posterior 717.84
  late effect—*see* Late, effects (of), sprain
  lateral collateral, knee 844.0
    old 717.81
  leg 844.9
    and knee 844.9
  ligamentum teres femoris 843.8
  low back 846.9
  lumbar (spine) 847.2
  lumbosacral 846.0
    chronic or old 724.6
  mandible 848.1
    old 524.69
  maxilla 848.1
  medial collateral, knee 844.1
    old 717.82
  meniscus
    jaw 848.1
      old 524.69
    knee 844.8
      with current tear (*see also* Tear, meniscus)
        836.2
      old 717.5
    mandible 848.1
      old 524.69
    specified site NEC 848.8
  metacarpal 842.10
    distal 842.12
    proximal 842.11

Sprain, strain—*continued*
  metacarpophalangeal 842.12
  metatarsal 845.10
  metatarsophalangeal 845.12
  midcarpal 842.19
  midtarsal 845.19
  multiple sites, except fingers alone or toes alone
    848.8
  neck 847.0
  nose (septal cartilage) 848.0
  occiput from atlas 847.0
  old—*see* Derangement, joint
  orbicular, hip 843.8
  patella(r) 844.8
    old 717.89
  pelvis 848.5
  phalanx
    finger 842.10
    toe 845.10
  radiocarpal 842.02
  radiohumeral 841.2
  radioulnar 841.9
    distal 842.09
  radius, radial (proximal end) 841.9
    and ulna 841.9
      distal 842.09
    collateral 841.0
    distal end 842.00
  recurrent—*see* Sprain, by site
  rib (cage), without mention of injury to sternum
    848.3
    involving sternum 848.42
  rotator cuff (capsule) 840.4
  round ligament—*see also* Injury, internal, round
    ligament
    femur 843.8
  sacral (spine) 847.3
  sacrococcygeal 847.3
  sacroiliac (region) 846.9
    chronic or old 724.6
    ligament 846.1
    specified site NEC 846.8
  sacrospinatus 846.2
  sacrospinous 846.2
  sacrotuberous 846.3
  scaphoid bone, ankle 845.00
  scapula(r) 840.9
  semilunar cartilage (knee) 844.8
    with current tear (*see also* Tear, meniscus)
      836.2
    old 717.5
  septal cartilage (nose) 848.0
  shoulder 840.9
    and arm, upper 840.9
    blade 840.9
  specified site NEC 848.8
  spine 847.9
    cervical 847.0
    coccyx 847.4
    dorsal 847.1
    lumbar 847.2
    lumbosacral 846.0
      chronic or old 724.6
    sacral 847.3
    sacroiliac (*see also* Sprain, sacroiliac) 846.9
      chronic or old 724.6
    thoracic 847.1
  sternoclavicular 848.41
  sternum 848.40
  subglenoid (*see also* SLAP lesion) 840.8
  subscapularis 840.5

Sprain, strain—*continued*
  supraspinatus 840.6
  symphysis
    jaw 848.1
      old 524.69
    mandibular 848.1
      old 524.69
    pubis 848.5
  talofibular 845.09
  tarsal 845.10
  tarsometatarsal 845.11
  temporomandibular 848.1
    old 524.69
  teres
    ligamentum femoris 843.8
    major or minor 840.8
  thigh (proximal end) 843.9
    and hip 843.9
    distal end 844.9
  thoracic (spine) 847.1
  thorax 848.8
  thumb 842.10
  thyroid cartilage or region 848.2
  tibia (proximal end) 844.9
    distal end 845.00
  tibiofibular
    distal 845.03
    superior 844.3
  toe(s) 845.10
  trachea 848.8
  trapezoid 840.8
  ulna, ulnar (proximal end) 841.9
    collateral 841.1
    distal end 842.00
  ulnohumeral 841.3
  vertebrae (*see also* Sprain, spine) 847.9
    cervical, cervicodorsal, cervicothoracic 847.0
  wrist (cuneiform) (scaphoid) (semilunar) 842.00
  xiphoid cartilage 848.49
Sprengel's deformity (congenital) 755.52
Spring fever 309.23
Sprue 579.1
  celiac 579.0
  idiopathic 579.0
  meaning thrush 112.0
  nontropical 579.0
  tropical 579.1
Spur —*see also* Exostosis
  bone 726.91
    calcaneal 726.73
  calcaneal 726.73
  iliac crest 726.5
  nose (septum) 478.19
    bone 726.91
  septal 478.19
Spuria placenta —*see* Placenta, abnormal
Spurway's syndrome (brittle bones and blue
  sclera) 756.51
Sputum, abnormal (amount) (color) (excessive)
  (odor) (purulent) 786.4
  bloody 786.30
Squamous —*see also* condition
  cell metaplasia
    bladder 596.89
    cervix—*see* condition
  epithelium in
    cervical canal (congenital) 752.49
    uterine mucosa (congenital) 752.39
  metaplasia
    bladder 596.89
    cervix—*see* condition

Squashed nose 738.0
  congenital 754.0
Squeeze, divers' 993.3
Squint (*see also* Strabismus) 378.9
  accommodative (*see also* Esotropia) 378.00
  concomitant (*see also* Heterotropia) 378.30
Stab —*see also* Wound, open, by site
  internal organs—*see* Injury, internal, by site,
    with open wound
Staggering gait 781.2
  hysterical 300.11
Staghorn calculus 592.0
Stähl's
  ear 744.29
  pigment line (cornea) 371.11
Stähli's pigment lines (cornea) 371.11
Stain, staining
  meconium 779.84
  port wine 757.32
  tooth, teeth (hard tissues) 521.7
    due to
      accretions 523.6
      deposits (betel) (black) (green) (materia
        alba) (orange) (tobacco) 523.6
      metals (copper) (silver) 521.7
      nicotine 523.6
      pulpal bleeding 521.7
      tobacco 523.6
Stammering (see also Disorder, fluency) 315.35
Standstill
  atrial 426.6
  auricular 426.6
  cardiac (*see also* Arrest, cardiac) 427.5
  sinoatrial 426.6
  sinus 426.6
  ventricular (*see also* Arrest, cardiac) 427.5
Stannosis 503
Stanton's disease (melioidosis) 025
Staphylitis (acute) (catarrhal) (chronic)
  (gangrenous) (membranous) (suppurative)
  (ulcerative) 528.3
Staphylococcemia 038.10
  aureus 038.11
  specified organism NEC 038.19
Staphylococcus, staphylococcal —*see* condition
Staphyloderma (skin) 686.00
Staphyloma 379.11
  anterior, localized 379.14
  ciliary 379.11
  cornea 371.73
  equatorial 379.13
  posterior 379.12
  posticum 379.12
  ring 379.15
  sclera NEC 379.11
Starch eating 307.52
Stargardt's disease 362.75
Starvation (inanition) (due to lack of food) 994.2
  edema 262
  voluntary NEC 307.1
Stasis
  bile (duct) (*see also* Disease, biliary) 576.8
  bronchus (*see also* Bronchitis) 490
  cardiac (*see also* Failure, heart) 428.0
  cecum 564.89
  colon 564.89
  dermatitis (*see also* Varix, with stasis
    dermatitis) 454.1
  duodenal 536.8
  eczema (*see also* Varix, with stasis dermatitis)
    454.1

Stasis—*continued*
  edema (*see also* Hypertension, venous) 459.30
  foot 991.4
  gastric 536.3
  ileocecal coil 564.89
  ileum 564.89
  intestinal 564.89
  jejunum 564.89
  kidney 586
  liver 571.9
    cirrhotic—*see* Cirrhosis, liver
  lymphatic 457.8
  pneumonia 514
  portal 571.9
  pulmonary 514
  rectal 564.89
  renal 586
    tubular 584.5
  stomach 536.3
  ulcer
    with varicose veins 454.0
    without varicose veins 459.81
  urine NEC (*see also* Retention, urine) 788.20
  venous 459.81
State
  affective and paranoid, mixed, organic psychotic 294.8
  agitated 307.9
    acute reaction to stress 308.2
  anxiety (neurotic) (*see also* Anxiety) 300.00
    specified type NEC 300.09
  apprehension (*see also* Anxiety) 300.00
    specified type NEC 300.09
  climacteric, female 627.2
    following induced menopause 627.4
  clouded
    epileptic (*see also* Epilepsy) 345.9
    paroxysmal (idiopathic) (*see also* Epilepsy) 345.9
  compulsive (mixed) (with obsession) 300.3
  confusional 298.9
    acute 293.0
      with
        arteriosclerotic dementia 290.41
        presenile brain disease 290.11
        senility 290.3
      alcoholic 291.0
      drug-induced 292.81
    epileptic 293.0
    postoperative 293.9
    reactive (emotional stress) (psychological trauma) 298.2
    subacute 293.1
  constitutional psychopathic 301.9
  convulsive (*see also* Convulsions) 780.39
  depressive NEC 311
    induced by drug 292.84
    neurotic 300.4
  dissociative 300.15
  hallucinatory 780.1
    induced by drug 292.12
  hypercoagulable (primary) 289.81
    secondary 289.82
  hyperdynamic beta-adrenergic circulatory 429.82
  locked-in 344.81
  menopausal 627.2
    artificial 627.4
    following induced menopause 627.4
  neurotic NEC 300.9
    with depersonalization episode 300.6

State—*continued*
  obsessional 300.3
  oneiroid (*see also* Schizophrenia) 295.4
  panic 300.01
  paranoid 297.9
    alcohol-induced 291.5
    arteriosclerotic 290.42
    climacteric 297.2
    drug-induced 292.11
    in
      presenile brain disease 290.12
      senile brain disease 290.20
    involutional 297.2
    menopausal 297.2
    senile 290.20
    simple 297.0
  postleukotomy 310.0
  pregnant (*see also* Pregnancy) V22.2
  psychogenic, twilight 298.2
  psychotic, organic (*see also* Psychosis, organic) 294.9
    mixed paranoid and affective 294.8
    senile or presenile NEC 290.9
    transient NEC 293.9
      with
        anxiety 293.84
        delusions 293.81
        depression 293.83
        hallucinations 293.82
  residual schizophrenic (*see also* Schizophrenia) 295.6
  tension (*see also* Anxiety) 300.9
  transient organic psychotic 293.9
    anxiety type 293.84
    depressive type 293.83
    hallucinatory type 293.83
    paranoid type 293.81
    specified type NEC 293.89
  twilight
    epileptic 293.0
    psychogenic 298.2
  vegetative (persistent) 780.03
Status (post)
  absence
    epileptic (*see also* Epilepsy) 345.2
    of organ, acquired (postsurgical)—*see* Absence, by site, acquired
  administration of tPA (rtPA) in a different institution within the last 24 hours prior to admission to facility V45.88
  anastomosis of intestine (for bypass) V45.3
  angioplasty, percutaneous transluminal coronary V45.82
  anginosus 413.9
  ankle prosthesis V43.66
  aortocoronary bypass or shunt V45.81
  arthrodesis V45.4
  artificially induced condition NEC V45.89
  artificial opening (of) V44.9
    gastrointestinal tract NEC V44.4
    specified site NEC V44.8
    urinary tract NEC V44.6
    vagina V44.7
  aspirator V46.0
  asthmaticus (*see also* Asthma) 493.9
  awaiting organ transplant V49.83
  bariatric surgery V45.86
    complicating pregnancy, childbirth, or the puerperium 649.2
  bed confinement V49.84

Status—*continued*
  breast
    correction V43.82
    implant removal V45.83
    reconstruction V43.82
  cardiac
    device (in situ) V45.00
      defibrillator, automatic implantable (with
        synchronous cardiac pacemaker) V45.02
      pacemaker V45.01
        fitting or adjustment V53.3
      carotid sinus V45.09
        fitting or adjustment V53.3
    carotid sinus stimulator V45.09
    cataract extraction V45.61
  chemotherapy V66.2
    current V58.69
  circumcision, female 629.20
  clitorectomy (female genital mutilation type I) 629.21
    with excision of labia minora (female genital mutilation type II) 629.22
  colonization — *see* Carrier (suspected) of
  colostomy V44.3
  contraceptive device V45.59
    intrauterine V45.51
    subdermal V45.52
  convulsivus idiopathicus (*see also* Epilepsy) 345.3
  coronary artery bypass or shunt V45.81
  cutting
    female genital 629.20
      specified NEC 629.29
      type I 629.21
      type II 629.22
      type III 629.23
      type IV 629.29
  cystostomy V44.50
    appendico-vesicostomy V44.52
    cutaneous-vesicostomy V44.51
    specified type NEC V44.59
  defibrillator, automatic implantable cardiac (with synchronous cardiac pacemaker) V45.02
  delinquent immunization V15.83
  dental crowns V45.84
  dental fillings V45.84
  dental restoration V45.84
  dental sealant V49.82
  dialysis (hemo) (peritoneal) V45.11
  do not resuscitate V49.86
  donor V59.9
  drug therapy or regimen V67.59
    high-risk medication NEC V67.51
  elbow prosthesis V43.62
  embedded
    fragment — *see* Foreign body, retained
    splinter — *see* Foreign body, retained
  enterostomy V44.4
  epileptic, epilepticus (absence) (grand mal) (*see also* Epilepsy) 345.3
  focal motor 345.7
  partial 345.7
  petit mal 345.2
  psychomotor 345.7
  temporal lobe 345.7
  estrogen receptor
    negative [ER-] V86.1
    positive [ER+] V86.0
  explantation of joint prosthesis NEC V88.29
    hip V88.21
    knee V88.22

Status—*continued*
  eye (adnexa) surgery V45.69
  female genital
    cutting 629.20
      specified NEC 629.29
      type I 629.21
      type II 629.22
      type III 629.23
      type IV 629.29
    mutilation 629.20
      type IV 629.29
  filtering bleb (eye) (postglaucoma) V45.69
    with rupture or complication 997.99
    postcataract extraction (complication) 997.99
  finger joint prosthesis V43.69
  foster care V60.81
  gastric
    banding V45.86
      complicating pregnancy, childbirth, or the puerperium 649.2
    bypass for obesity V45.86
      complicating pregnancy, childbirth, or the puerperium 649.2
  gastrostomy V44.1
  grand mal 345.3
  heart valve prosthesis V43.3
  hemodialysis V45.11
  hip prosthesis (joint) (partial) (total) V43.64
    explantation V88.21
  hysterectomy V88.01
    partial with remaining cervical stump V88.02
    total V88.01
  ileostomy V44.2
  infibulation (female genital mutilation type III) 629.23
  insulin pump V45.85
  intestinal bypass V45.3
  intrauterine contraceptive device V45.51
  jejunostomy V44.4
  joint prosthesis NEC V43.69
    explantation V88.29
  knee joint prosthesis V43.65
    explantation V88.22
  lacunaris 437.8
  lacunosis 437.8
  lapsed immunization schedule V15.83
  low birth weight V21.30
    less than 500 grams V21.31
    500-999 grams V21.32
    1000-1499 grams V21.33
    1500-1999 grams V21.34
    2000-2500 grams V21.35
  lymphaticus 254.8
  malignant neoplasm, ablated or excised—*see* History, malignant neoplasm
  marmoratus 333.79
  military deployment V62.22
  mutilation, female 629.20
    type I 629.21
    type II 629.22
    type III 629.23
    type IV 629.29
  nephrostomy V44.6
  neuropacemaker NEC V45.89
    brain V45.89
    carotid sinus V45.09
    neurologic NEC V45.89
  obesity surgery V45.86
    complicating pregnancy, childbirth, or the puerperium 649.2

Status—*continued*
organ replacement
by artificial or mechanical device or prosthesis of
artery V43.4
artificial skin V43.83
bladder V43.5
blood vessel V43.4
breast V43.82
eye globe V43.0
heart
assist device V43.21
fully implantable artificial heart V43.22
valve V43.3
intestine V43.89
joint V43.60
ankle V43.66
elbow V43.62
finger V43.69
hip (partial) (total) V43.64
knee V43.65
shoulder V43.61
specified NEC 43.69
wrist V43.63
kidney V43.89
larynx V43.81
lens V43.1
limb(s) V43.7
liver V43.89
lung V43.89
organ NEC V43.89
pancreas V43.89
skin (artificial) V43.83
tissue NEC V43.89
vein V43.4
by organ transplant (heterologous)
(homologous)—*see* Status, transplant
pacemaker
brain V45.89
cardiac V45.01
carotid sinus V45.09
neurologic NEC V45.89
specified site NEC V45.89
percutaneous transluminal coronary angioplasty
V45.82
peritoneal dialysis V45.11
petit mal 345.2
physical restraints V49.87
postcommotio cerebri 310.2
postmenopausal (age related) (natural) V49.81
postoperative NEC V45.89
postpartum NEC V24.2
care immediately following delivery V24.0
routine follow-up V24.2
postsurgical NEC V45.89
renal dialysis V45.11
noncompliance V45.12
respirator (ventilator) V46.11
encounter
during
mechanical failure V46.14
power failure V46.12
for weaning V46.13
retained foreign body—*see* Foreign body, retained
reversed jejunal transposition (for bypass) V45.3
sex reassignment surgery status (*see also*
Trans-sexualism) 302.50
shoulder prosthesis V43.61

Status—*continued*
shunt
aortocoronary bypass V45.81
arteriovenous (for dialysis) V45.11
cerebrospinal fluid V45.2
vascular NEC V45.89
aortocoronary (bypass) V45.81
ventricular (communicating) (for drainage)
V45.2
sterilization
tubal ligation V26.51
vasectomy V26.52
subdermal contraceptive device V45.52
thymicolymphaticus 254.8
thymicus 254.8
thymolymphaticus 254.8
tooth extraction 525.10
tracheostomy V44.0
transplant
blood vessel V42.89
bone V42.4
marrow V42.81
cornea V42.5
heart V42.1
valve V42.2
intestine V42.84
kidney V42.0
liver V42.7
lung V42.6
organ V42.9
removal (due to complication, failure,
rejection or infection) V45.87
specified site NEC V42.89
pancreas V42.83
peripheral stem cells V42.82
skin V42.3
stem cells, peripheral V42.82
tissue V42.9
specified type NEC V42.89
vessel, blood V42.89
tubal ligation V26.51
underimmunization V15.83
ureterostomy V44.6
urethrostomy V44.6
vagina, artificial V44.7
vasectomy V26.52
vascular shunt NEC V45.89
aortocoronary (bypass) V45.81
ventilator (respirator) V46.11
encounter
during
mechanical failure V46.14
power failure V46.12
for weaning V46.13
wheelchair confinement V46.3
wrist prosthesis V43.63
Stave fracture —*see* Fracture, metacarpus,
metacarpal bone(s)
Steal
subclavian artery 435.2
vertebral artery 435.1
Stealing, solitary, child problem (*see also*
Disturbance, conduct) 312.1
Steam burn —*see* Burn, by site
Steatocystoma multiplex 706.2
Steatoma (infected) 706.2
eyelid (cystic) 374.84
infected 373.13

Steatorrhea (chronic) 579.8
  with lacteal obstruction 579.2
  idiopathic 579.0
    adult 579.0
    infantile 579.0
  pancreatic 579.4
  primary 579.0
  secondary 579.8
  specified cause NEC 579.8
  tropical 579.1
Steatosis 272.8
  heart (*see also* Degeneration, myocardial) 429.1
  kidney 593.89
  liver 571.8
Steele-Richardson (-Olszewski) Syndrome 333.0
Stein's syndrome (polycystic ovary) 256.4
Stein-Leventhal syndrome (polycystic ovary) 256.4
Steinbrocker's syndrome (*see also* Neuropathy, peripheral, autonomic) 337.9
Steinert's disease 359.21
STEMI (ST elevation myocardial infarction) (*see also* Infarct, myocardium, ST elevation) 410.9
Stenocardia (*see also* Angina) 413.9
Stenocephaly 756.0
Stenosis (cicatricial)—*see also* Stricture
  ampulla of Vater 576.2
    with calculus, cholelithiasis, or stones—*see* Choledocholithiasis
  anus, anal (canal) (sphincter) 569.2
    congenital 751.2
  aorta (ascending) 747.22
    arch 747.10
    arteriosclerotic 440.0
    calcified 440.0
  aortic (valve) 424.1
    with
      mitral (valve)
        insufficiency or incompetence 396.2
        stenosis or obstruction 396.0
      atypical 396.0
    congenital 746.3
    rheumatic 395.0
      with
        insufficiency, incompetency or regurgitation 395.2
          with mitral (valve) disease 396.8
        mitral (valve)
          disease (stenosis) 396.0
          insufficiency or incompetence 396.2
          stenosis or obstruction 396.0
    specified cause, except rheumatic 424.1
    syphilitic 093.22
  aqueduct of Sylvius (congenital) 742.3
    with spina bifida (*see also* Spina bifida) 741.0
    acquired 331.4
  artery NEC (*see also* Arteriosclerosis) 447.1
    basilar—*see* Narrowing, artery, basilar
    carotid (common) (internal)—*see* Narrowing, artery, carotid
    celiac 447.4
    cerebral 437.0
      due to
        embolism (*see also* Embolism, brain) 434.1
        thrombus (*see also* Thrombosis, brain) 434.0
    extremities 440.20
    precerebral—*see* Narrowing, artery, precerebral
    pulmonary (congenital) 747.31
      acquired 417.8
    renal 440.1
    vertebral—*see* Narrowing, artery, vertebral

Stenosis—*continued*
  bile duct or biliary passage (*see also* Obstruction, biliary) 576.2
    congenital 751.61
  bladder neck (acquired) 596.0
    congenital 753.6
  brain 348.89
  bronchus 519.19
    syphilitic 095.8
  cardia (stomach) 537.89
    congenital 750.7
  cardiovascular (*see also* Disease, cardiovascular) 429.2
  carotid artery—*see* Narrowing, artery, carotid
  cervix, cervical (canal) 622.4
    congenital 752.49
    in pregnancy or childbirth 654.6
      affecting fetus or newborn 763.89
      causing obstructed labor 660.2
        affecting fetus or newborn 763.1
  colon (*see also* Obstruction, intestine) 560.9
    congenital 751.2
  colostomy 569.62
  common bile duct (*see also* Obstruction, biliary) 576.2
    congenital 751.61
  coronary (artery) —*see* Arteriosclerosis, coronary
  cystic duct (*see also* Obstruction, gallbladder) 575.2
    congenital 751.61
  due to (presence of) any device, implant, or graft classifiable to 996.0-996.5—*see* Complications, due to (presence of) any device, implant, or graft classified to 996.0-996.5 NEC
  duodenum 537.3
    congenital 751.1
  ejaculatory duct NEC 608.89
  endocervical os—*see* Stenosis, cervix
  enterostomy 569.62
  esophagostomy 530.87
  esophagus 530.3
    congenital 750.3
    syphilitic 095.8
      congenital 090.5
  external ear canal 380.50
    secondary to
      inflammation 380.53
      surgery 380.52
      trauma 380.51
  gallbladder (*see also* Obstruction, gallbladder) 575.2
  glottis 478.74
  heart valve (acquired)—*see also* Endocarditis
    congenital NEC 746.89
      aortic 746.3
      mitral 746.5
      pulmonary 746.02
      tricuspid 746.1
  hepatic duct (*see also* Obstruction, biliary) 576.2
  hymen 623.3
  hypertrophic subaortic (idiopathic) 425.11
  infundibulum cardiac 746.83
  intestine (*see also* Obstruction, intestine) 560.9
    congenital (small) 751.1
      large 751.2
  lacrimal
    canaliculi 375.53
    duct 375.56
      congenital 743.65

Stenosis—*continued*
  lacrimal—*continued*
    punctum 375.52
      congenital 743.65
    sac 375.54
      congenital 743.65
  lacrimonasal duct 375.56
    congenital 743.65
    neonatal 375.55
  larynx 478.74
    congenital 748.3
    syphilitic 095.8
      congenital 090.5
  mitral (valve) (chronic) (inactive) 394.0
    with
      aortic (valve)
        disease (insufficiency) 396.1
        insufficiency or incompetence 396.1
        stenosis or obstruction 396.0
      incompetency, insufficiency or regurgitation
        394.2
        with aortic valve disease 396.8
    active or acute 391.1
      with chorea (acute) (rheumatic)
        (Sydenham's) 392.0
    congenital 746.5
    specified cause, except rheumatic 424.0
    syphilitic 093.21
  myocardium, myocardial (*see also*
      Degeneration, myocardial) 429.1
    hypertrophic subaortic (idiopathic) 425.11
  nares (anterior) (posterior) 478.19
    congenital 748.0
  nasal duct 375.56
    congenital 743.65
  nasolacrimal duct 375.56
    congenital 743.65
    neonatal 375.55
  organ or site, congenital NEC—*see* Atresia
  papilla of Vater 576.2
    with calculus, cholelithiasis, or stones—*see*
      Choledocholithiasis
  pulmonary (artery) (congenital) 747.31
    with ventricular septal defect, dextraposition
      of aorta and hypertrophy of right ventricle
      745.2
    acquired 417.8
    infundibular 746.83
    in tetralogy of Fallot 745.2
    subvalvular 746.83
    valve (*see also* Endocarditis, pulmonary) 424.3
      congenital 746.02
    vein 747.49
      acquired 417.8
    vessel NEC 417.8
  pulmonic (congenital) 746.02
    infundibular 746.83
    subvalvular 746.83
  pylorus (hypertrophic) 537.0
    adult 537.0
    congenital 750.5
    infantile 750.5
  rectum (sphincter) (*see also* Stricture, rectum) 569.2
  renal artery 440.1
  salivary duct (any) 527.8
  sphincter of Oddi (*see also* Obstruction, biliary) 576.2
  spinal 724.00
    cervical 723.0
    lumbar, lumbosacral (without neurogenic
      claudication) 724.02
      with neurogenic claudication 724.03

Stenosis—*continued*
  spinal—*continued*
    nerve (root) NEC 724.9
      specified region NEC 724.09
    thoracic, thoracolumbar 724.01
  stomach, hourglass 537.6
  subaortic 746.81
    hypertrophic (idiopathic) 425.11
  supra (valvular)-aortic 747.22
  trachea 519.19
    congenital 748.3
    syphilitic 095.8
    tuberculous (*see also* Tuberculosis) 012.8
  tracheostomy 519.02
  tricuspid (valve) (*see also* Endocarditis,
      tricuspid) 397.0
    congenital 746.1
    nonrheumatic 424.2
  tubal 628.2
  ureter (*see also* Stricture, ureter) 593.3
    congenital 753.29
  urethra (*see also* Stricture, urethra) 598.9
  vagina 623.2
    congenital 752.49
    in pregnancy or childbirth 654.7
      affecting fetus or newborn 763.89
      causing obstructed labor 660.2
        affecting fetus or newborn 763.1
  valve (cardiac) (heart) (*see also* Endocarditis) 424.90
    congenital NEC 746.89
      aortic 746.3
      mitral 746.5
      pulmonary 746.02
      tricuspid 746.1
      urethra 753.6
  valvular (*see also* Endocarditis) 424.90
    congenital NEC 746.89
      urethra 753.6
  vascular graft or shunt 996.1
    atherosclerosis —*see* Arteriosclerosis,
      extremities
    embolism 996.74
    occlusion NEC 996.74
    thrombus 996.74
  vena cava (inferior) (superior) 459.2
    congenital 747.49
  ventricular shunt 996.2
  vulva 624.8
Stent jail 996.72
Stercolith (*see also* Fecalith) 560.32
  appendix 543.9
Stercoraceous, stercoral ulcer 569.82
  anus or rectum 569.41
Stereopsis, defective
  with fusion 368.33
  without fusion 368.32
Stereotypies NEC 307.3
Sterility
  female—*see* Infertility, female
  male (*see also* Infertility, male) 606.9
Sterilization, admission for V25.2
  status
    tubal ligation V26.51
    vasectomy V26.52
Sternalgia (*see also* Angina) 413.9
Sternopagus 759.4
Sternum bifidum 756.3
Sternutation 784.99

Steroid
  effects (adverse) (iatrogenic)
    cushingoid
      correct substance properly administered 255.0
      overdose or wrong substance given or taken
        962.0
    diabetes—*see* Diabetes, secondary
      correct substance properly administered 251.8
      overdose or wrong substance given or taken
        962.0
    due to
      correct substance properly administered 255.8
      overdose or wrong substance given or taken
        962.0
    fever
      correct substance properly administered 780.60
      overdose or wrong substance given or taken
        962.0
    withdrawal
      correct substance properly administered 255.41
      overdose or wrong substance given or taken
        962.0
  responder 365.03
Stevens-Johnson disease or syndrome (erythema
    multiforme exudativum) 695.13
  toxic epidermal necrolysis overlap (SJS-TEN
    overlap syndrome) 695.14
Stewart-Morel syndrome (hyperostosis frontalis
    interna) 733.3
Sticker's disease (erythema infectiosum) 057.0
Stickler syndrome 759.89
Sticky eye 372.03
Stieda's disease (calcification, knee joint) 726.62
Stiff
  back 724.8
  neck (*see also* Torticollis) 723.5
Stiff-baby 759.89
Stiff-man syndrome 333.91
Stiffness, joint NEC 719.50
  ankle 719.57
  back 724.8
  elbow 719.52
  finger 719.54
  hip 719.55
  knee 719.56
  multiple sites 719.59
  sacroiliac 724.6
  shoulder 719.51
  specified site NEC 719.58
  spine 724.9
  surgical fusion V45.4
  wrist 719.53
Stigmata, congenital syphilis 090.5
Still's disease or syndrome 714.30
  adult onset 714.2
Still-Felty syndrome (rheumatoid arthritis with
    splenomegaly and leukopenia) 714.1
Stillbirth, stillborn NEC 779.9
Stiller's disease (asthenia) 780.79
Stilling-Türk-Duane syndrome (ocular
    retraction syndrome) 378.71
Stimulation, ovary 256.1
Sting (animal) (bee) (fish) (insect) (jellyfish)
    (Portuguese man-o-war) (wasp) (venomous)
    989.5
  anaphylactic shock or reaction 989.5
  plant 692.6
Stippled epiphyses 756.59

Stitch
  abscess 998.59
  burst (in external operation wound) (*see also*
    Dehiscence) 998.32
    internal 998.31
  in back 724.5
Stojano's (subcostal) syndrome 098.86
Stokes' disease (exophthalmic goiter) 242.0
Stokes-Adams syndrome (syncope with heart
    block) 426.9
Stokvis' (-Talma) disease (enterogenous
    cyanosis) 289.7
Stomach —*see* condition
Stoma malfunction
  colostomy 569.62
  cystostomy 596.82
    infection 596.81
    mechanical 596.82
    specified complication NEC 596.83
  enterostomy 569.62
  esophagostomy 530.87
  gastrostomy 536.42
  ileostomy 569.62
  nephrostomy 997.5
  tracheostomy 519.02
  ureterostomy 997.5
Stomatitis 528.00
  angular 528.5
    due to dietary or vitamin deficiency 266.0
  aphthous 528.2
  bovine 059.11
  candidal 112.0
  catarrhal 528.00
  denture 528.9
  diphtheritic (membranous) 032.0
  due to
    dietary deficiency 266.0
    thrush 112.0
    vitamin deficiency 266.0
  epidemic 078.4
  epizootic 078.4
  follicular 528.00
  gangrenous 528.1
  herpetic 054.2
  herpetiformis 528.2
  malignant 528.00
  membranous acute 528.00
  monilial 112.0
  mycotic 112.0
  necrotic 528.1
    ulcerative 101
  necrotizing ulcerative 101
  parasitic 112.0
  septic 528.00
  specified NEC 528.09
  spirochetal 101
  suppurative (acute) 528.00
  ulcerative 528.00
    necrotizing 101
  ulceromembranous 101
  vesicular 528.00
    with exanthem 074.3
  Vincent's 101
Stomatocytosis 282.8
Stomatomycosis 112.0
Stomatorrhagia 528.9
Stone(s) —*see also* Calculus
  bladder 594.1
    diverticulum 594.0
  cystine 270.0

Stone(s)—*continued*
  heart syndrome (*see also* Failure, ventricular, left) 428.1
  kidney 592.0
  prostate 602.0
  pulp (dental) 522.2
  renal 592.0
  salivary duct or gland (any) 527.5
  ureter 592.1
  urethra (impacted) 594.2
  urinary (duct) (impacted) (passage) 592.9
    bladder 594.1
      diverticulum 594.0
    lower tract NEC 594.9
    specified site 594.8
  xanthine 277.2
Stonecutters' lung 502
  tuberculous (*see also* Tuberculosis) 011.4
Stonemasons'
  asthma, disease, or lung 502
    tuberculous (*see also* Tuberculosis) 011.4
  phthisis (*see also* Tuberculosis) 011.4
Stoppage
  bowel (*see also* Obstruction, intestine) 560.9
  heart (*see also* Arrest, cardiac) 427.5
  intestine (*see also* Obstruction, intestine) 560.9
  urine NEC (*see also* Retention, urine) 788.20
Storm, thyroid (apathetic) (*see also* Thyrotoxicosis) 242.9
Strabismus (alternating) (congenital) (nonparalytic) 378.9
  concomitant (*see also* Heterotropia) 378.30
    convergent (*see also* Esotropia) 378.00
    divergent (*see also* Exotropia) 378.10
  convergent (*see also* Esotropia) 378.00
  divergent (*see also* Exotropia) 378.10
  due to adhesions, scars—*see* Strabismus, mechanical
  in neuromuscular disorder NEC 378.73
  intermittent 378.20
    vertical 378.31
  latent 378.40
    convergent (esophoria) 378.41
    divergent (exophoria) 378.42
    vertical 378.43
  mechanical 378.60
    due to
      Brown's tendon sheath syndrome 378.61
      specified musculofascial disorder NEC 378.62
  paralytic 378.50
    third or oculomotor nerve (partial) 378.51
      total 378.52
    fourth or trochlear nerve 378.53
    sixth or abducens nerve 378.54
  specified type NEC 378.73
  vertical (hypertropia) 378.31
Strain —*see also* Sprain, by site
  eye NEC 368.13
  heart—*see* Disease, heart
  meaning gonorrhea—*see* Gonorrhea
  on urination 788.65
  physical NEC V62.89
  postural 729.90
  psychological NEC V62.89
Strands
  conjunctiva 372.62
  vitreous humor 379.25
Strangulation, strangulated 994.7
  appendix 543.9
  asphyxiation or suffocation by 994.7

Strangulation, strangulated—*continued*
  bladder neck 596.0
  bowel—*see* Strangulation, intestine
  colon—*see* Strangulation, intestine
  cord (umbilical)—*see* Compression, umbilical cord
  due to birth injury 767.8
  food or foreign body (*see also* Asphyxia, food) 933.1
  hemorrhoids 455.8
    external 455.5
    internal 455.2
  hernia—*see also* Hernia, by site, with obstruction
    gangrenous—*see* Hernia, by site, with gangrene
  intestine (large) (small) 560.2
    with hernia—*see also* Hernia, by site, with obstruction
      gangrenous—*see* Hernia, by site, with gangrene
    congenital (small) 751.1
      large 751.2
  mesentery 560.2
  mucus (*see also* Asphyxia, mucus) 933.1
    newborn 770.18
  omentum 560.2
  organ or site, congenital NEC—*see* Atresia
  ovary 620.8
    due to hernia 620.4
  penis 607.89
    foreign body 939.3
  rupture (*see also* Hernia, by site, with obstruction) 552.9
    gangrenous (*see also* Hernia, by site, with gangrene) 551.9
  stomach, due to hernia (*see also* Hernia, by site, with obstruction) 552.9
    with gangrene (*see also* Hernia, by site, with gangrene) 551.9
  umbilical cord—*see* Compression, umbilical cord
  vesicourethral orifice 596.0
Strangury 788.1
Strawberry
  gallbladder (*see also* Disease, gallbladder) 575.6
  mark 757.32
  tongue (red) (white) 529.3
Straw itch 133.8
Streak, ovarian 752.0
Strephosymbolia 315.01
  secondary to organic lesion 784.69
Streptobacillary fever 026.1
Streptobacillus moniliformis 026.1
Streptococcemia 038.0
Streptococcicosis —*see* Infection, streptococcal
Streptococcus, streptococcal —*see* condition
Streptoderma 686.00
Streptomycosis —*see* Actinomycosis
Streptothricosis —*see* Actinomycosis
Streptothrix —*see* Actinomycosis
Streptotrichosis —*see* Actinomycosis
Stress 308.9
  fracture—*see* Fracture, stress
  polycythemia 289.0
  reaction (gross) (*see also* Reaction, stress, acute) 308.9
Stretching, nerve —*see* Injury, nerve, by site
Striae (albicantes) (atrophicae) (cutis distensae) (distensae) 701.3
Striations of nails 703.8

Stricture (*see also* Stenosis) 799.89
  ampulla of Vater 576.2
    with calculus, cholelithiasis, or stones—*see*
      Choledocholithiasis
  anus (sphincter) 569.2
    congenital 751.2
    infantile 751.2
  aorta (ascending) 747.22
    arch 747.10
    arteriosclerotic 440.0
    calcified 440.0
  aortic (valve) (*see also* Stenosis, aortic) 424.1
    congenital 746.3
  aqueduct of Sylvius (congenital) 742.3
    with spina bifida (*see also* Spina bifida) 741.0
    acquired 331.4
  artery 447.1
    basilar—*see* Narrowing, artery, basilar
    carotid (common) (internal)—*see* Narrowing,
      artery, carotid
    celiac 447.4
    cerebral 437.0
      congenital 747.81
      due to
        embolism (*see also* Embolism, brain) 434.1
        thrombus (*see also* Thrombosis, brain)
          434.0
    congenital (peripheral) 747.60
      cerebral 747.81
      coronary 746.85
      gastrointestinal 747.61
      lower limb 747.64
      renal 747.62
      retinal 743.58
      specified NEC 747.69
      spinal 747.82
      umbilical 747.5
      upper limb 747.63
    coronary —*see* Arteriosclerosis, coronary
      congenital 746.85
    precerebral—*see* Narrowing, artery,
      precerebral NEC
    pulmonary (congenital) 747.31
      acquired 417.8
    renal 440.1
    vertebral—*see* Narrowing, artery, vertebral
  auditory canal (congenital) (external) 744.02
    acquired (*see also* Stricture, ear canal,
      acquired) 380.50
  bile duct or passage (any) (postoperative) (*see
    also* Obstruction, biliary) 576.2
    congenital 751.61
  bladder 596.89
    congenital 753.6
    neck 596.0
      congenital 753.6
  bowel (*see also* Obstruction, intestine) 560.9
  brain 348.89
  bronchus 519.19
    syphilitic 095.8
  cardia (stomach) 537.89
    congenital 750.7
  cardiac—*see also* Disease, heart
    orifice (stomach) 537.89
  cardiovascular (*see also* Disease,
    cardiovascular) 429.2
  carotid artery—*see* Narrowing, artery, carotid
  cecum (*see also* Obstruction, intestine) 560.9
  cervix, cervical (canal) 622.4
    congenital 752.49

Stricture—*continued*
  cervix—*continued*
    in pregnancy or childbirth 654.6
      affecting fetus or newborn 763.89
      causing obstructed labor 660.2
        affecting fetus or newborn 763.1
  colon (*see also* Obstruction, intestine) 560.9
    congenital 751.2
  colostomy 569.62
  common bile duct (*see also* Obstruction, biliary)
    576.2
    congenital 751.61
  coronary (artery) —*see* Arteriosclerosis,
    coronary
    congenital 746.85
  cystic duct (*see also* Obstruction, gallbladder)
    575.2
    congenital 751.61
  cystostomy 596.83
  digestive organs NEC, congenital 751.8
  duodenum 537.3
    congenital 751.1
  ear canal (external) (congenital) 744.02
    acquired 380.50
      secondary to
        inflammation 380.53
        surgery 380.52
        trauma 380.51
  ejaculatory duct 608.85
  enterostomy 569.62
  esophagostomy 530.87
  esophagus (corrosive) (peptic) 530.3
    congenital 750.3
    syphilitic 095.8
      congenital 090.5
  Eustachian tube (*see also* Obstruction,
    Eustachian tube) 381.60
    congenital 744.24
  fallopian tube 628.2
    gonococcal (chronic) 098.37
      acute 098.17
    tuberculous (*see also* Tuberculosis) 016.6
  gallbladder (*see also* Obstruction, gallbladder)
    575.2
    congenital 751.69
  glottis 478.74
  heart—*see also* Disease, heart
    congenital NEC 746.89
    valve—*see also* Endocarditis
      congenital NEC 746.89
        aortic 746.3
        mitral 746.5
        pulmonary 746.02
        tricuspid 746.1
  hepatic duct (*see also* Obstruction, biliary) 576.2
  hourglass, of stomach 537.6
  hymen 623.3
  hypopharynx 478.29
  intestine (*see also* Obstruction, intestine) 560.9
    congenital (small) 751.1
      large 751.2
    ischemic 557.1
  lacrimal
    canaliculi 375.53
      congenital 743.65
    punctum 375.52
      congenital 743.65
    sac 375.54
      congenital 743.65
  lacrimonasal duct 375.56
    congenital 743.65
    neonatal 375.55

Stricture—*continued*
  larynx 478.79
    congenital 748.3
    syphilitic 095.8
      congenital 090.5
  lung 518.89
  meatus
    ear (congenital) 744.02
      acquired (*see also* Stricture, ear canal,
        acquired) 380.50
    osseous (congenital) (ear) 744.03
      acquired (*see also* Stricture, ear canal,
        acquired) 380.50
    urinarius (*see also* Stricture, urethra) 598.9
      congenital 753.6
  mitral (valve) (*see also* Stenosis, mitral) 394.0
    congenital 746.5
    specified cause, except rheumatic 424.0
  myocardium, myocardial (*see also*
      Degeneration, myocardial) 429.1
    hypertrophic subaortic (idiopathic) 425.11
  nares (anterior) (posterior) 478.19
    congenital 748.0
  nasal duct 375.56
    congenital 743.65
    neonatal 375.55
  nasolacrimal duct 375.56
    congenital 743.65
    neonatal 375.55
  nasopharynx 478.29
    syphilitic 095.8
  nephrostomy 997.5
  nose 478.19
    congenital 748.0
  nostril (anterior) (posterior) 478.19
    congenital 748.0
  organ or site, congenital NEC—*see* Atresia
  osseous meatus (congenital) (ear) 744.03
    acquired (*see also* Stricture, ear canal,
      acquired) 380.50
  os uteri (*see also* Stricture, cervix) 622.4
  oviduct—*see* Stricture, fallopian tube
  pelviureteric junction 593.3
  pharynx (dilation) 478.29
  prostate 602.8
  pulmonary, pulmonic
    artery (congenital) 747.31
      acquired 417.8
      noncongenital 417.8
    infundibulum (congenital) 746.83
    valve (*see also* Endocarditis, pulmonary)
      424.3
      congenital 746.02
    vein (congenital) 747.49
      acquired 417.8
    vessel NEC 417.8
  punctum lacrimale 375.52
    congenital 743.65
  pylorus (hypertrophic) 537.0
    adult 537.0
    congenital 750.5
    infantile 750.5
  rectosigmoid 569.89
  rectum (sphincter) 569.2
    congenital 751.2
    due to
      chemical burn 947.3
      irradiation 569.2
      lymphogranuloma venereum 099.1
      gonococcal 098.7
      inflammatory 099.1

Stricture—*continued*
  rectum—*continued*
    syphilitic 095.8
    tuberculous (*see also* Tuberculosis) 014.8
  renal artery 440.1
  salivary duct or gland (any) 527.8
  sigmoid (flexure) (*see also* Obstruction,
      intestine) 560.9
  spermatic cord 608.85
  stoma (following) (of)
    colostomy 569.62
    cystostomy 596.83
    enterostomy 569.62
    esophagostomy 530.87
    gastrostomy 536.42
    ileostomy 569.62
    nephrostomy 997.5
    tracheostomy 519.02
    ureterostomy 997.5
  stomach 537.89
    congenital 750.7
    hourglass 537.6
  subaortic 746.81
    hypertrophic (acquired) (idiopathic) 425.11
  subglottic 478.74
  syphilitic NEC 095.8
  tendon (sheath) 727.81
  trachea 519.19
    congenital 748.3
    syphilitic 095.8
    tuberculous (*see also* Tuberculosis) 012.8
  tracheostomy 519.02
  tricuspid (valve) (*see also* Endocarditis,
      tricuspid) 397.0
    congenital 746.1
    nonrheumatic 424.2
  tunica vaginalis 608.85
  ureter (postoperative) 593.3
    congenital 753.29
    tuberculous (*see also* Tuberculosis) 016.2
  ureteropelvic junction 593.3
    congenital 753.21
  ureterovesical orifice 593.3
    congenital 753.22
  urethra (anterior) (meatal) (organic) (posterior)
      (spasmodic) 598.9
    associated with schistosomiasis (*see also*
      Schistosomiasis) 120.9 [598.01]
    congenital (valvular) 753.6
    due to
      infection 598.00
        syphilis 095.8 [598.01]
      trauma 598.1
    gonococcal 098.2 [598.01]
    gonorrheal 098.2 [598.01]
    infective 598.00
    late effect of injury 598.1
    postcatheterization 598.2
    postobstetric 598.1
    postoperative 598.2
    specified cause NEC 598.8
    syphilitic 095.8 [598.01]
    traumatic 598.1
    valvular, congenital 753.6
  urinary meatus (*see also* Stricture, urethra)
      598.9
    congenital 753.6
  uterus, uterine 621.5
    os (external) (internal)—see Stricture, cervix
  vagina (outlet) 623.2
    congenital 752.49

Stricture—*continued*
  valve (cardiac) (heart) (*see also* Endocarditis) 424.90
    congenital (cardiac) (heart) NEC 746.89
      aortic 746.3
      mitral 746.5
      pulmonary 746.02
      tricuspid 746.1
      urethra 753.6
  valvular (*see also* Endocarditis) 424.90
  vascular graft or shunt 996.1
    atherosclerosis —*see* Arteriosclerosis, extremities
    embolism 996.74
    occlusion NEC 996.74
    thrombus 996.74
  vas deferens 608.85
    congenital 752.89
  vein 459.2
  vena cava (inferior) (superior) NEC 459.2
    congenital 747.49
  ventricular shunt 996.2
  vesicourethral orifice 596.0
    congenital 753.6
  vulva (acquired) 624.8
Stridor 786.1
  congenital (larynx) 748.3
Stridulous —*see* condition
Strippling of nails 703.8
Stroke 434.91
  apoplectic (*see also* Disease, cerebrovascular, acute) 436
  brain—*see* Infarct, brain
  embolic 434.11
  epileptic—*see* Epilepsy
  healed or old V12.54
  heart—*see* Disease, heart
  heat 992.0
  hemorrhagic—*see* Hemorrhage, brain
  iatrogenic 997.02
  in evolution 434.91
  ischemic 434.91
  late effect—*see* Late effect(s) (of) cerebrovascular disease
  lightning 994.0
  paralytic—*see* Infarct, brain
  postoperative 997.02
  progressive 435.9
  thrombotic 434.01
Stromatosis, endometrial (M8931/1) 236.0
Strong pulse 785.9
Strongyloides stercoralis infestation 127.2
Strongyloidiasis 127.2
Strongyloidosis 127.2
Strongylus (gibsoni) infestation 127.7
Strophulus (newborn) 779.89
  pruriginosus 698.2
Struck by lightning 994.0
Struma (*see also* Goiter) 240.9
  fibrosa 245.3
  Hashimoto (struma lymphomatosa) 245.2
  lymphomatosa 245.2
  nodosa (simplex) 241.9
    endemic 241.9
    multinodular 241.1
    sporadic 241.9
    toxic or with hyperthyroidism 242.3
      multinodular 242.2
      uninodular 242.1
    toxicosa 242.3
      multinodular 242.2
      uninodular 242.1

Struma—*continued*
  uninodular 241.0
  ovarii (M9090/0) 220
    and carcinoid (M9091/1) 236.2
    malignant (M9090/3) 183.0
  Riedel's (ligneous thyroiditis) 245.3
  scrofulous (*see also* Tuberculosis) 017.2
  tuberculous (*see also* Tuberculosis) 017.2
    abscess 017.2
    adenitis 017.2
    lymphangitis 017.2
    ulcer 017.2
Strumipriva cachexia (*see also* Hypothyroidism) 244.9
Strümpell-Marie disease or spine (ankylosing spondylitis) 720.0
Strümpell-Westphal pseudosclerosis (hepatolenticular degeneration) 275.1
Stuart's disease (congenital factor X deficiency) (*see also* Defect, coagulation) 286.3
Stuart-Prower factor deficiency (congenital factor X deficiency) (*see also* Defect, coagulation) 286.3
Students' elbow 727.2
Stuffy nose 478.19
Stump —*see also* Amputation
  cervix, cervical (healed) 622.8
Stupor 780.09
  catatonic (*see also* Schizophrenia) 295.2
  circular (*see also* Psychosis, manic-depressive, circular) 296.7
  manic 296.89
  manic-depressive (*see also* Psychosis, affective) 296.89
  mental (anergic) (delusional) 298.9
  psychogenic 298.8
  reaction to exceptional stress (transient) 308.2
  traumatic NEC—*see also* Injury, intracranial
    with spinal (cord)
      lesion—*see* Injury, spinal, by site
      shock—*see* Injury, spinal, by site
Sturge (-Weber) (-Dimitri) disease or syndrome (encephalocutaneous angiomatosis) 759.6
Sturge-Kalischer-Weber syndrome (encephalocutaneous angiomatosis) 759.6
Stuttering 315.35
  adult onset 307.0
  childhood onset 315.35
  due to late effect of cerebrovascular disease (see also Late effect(s) (of) cerebrovascular disease) 438.14
  in conditions classified elsewhere 784.52
Sty, stye 373.11
  external 373.11
  internal 373.12
  meibomian 373.12
Subacidity, gastric 536.8
  psychogenic 306.4
Subacute —*see* condition
Subarachnoid —*see* condition
Subclavian steal syndrome 435.2
Subcortical —*see* condition
Subcostal syndrome 098.86
  nerve compression 354.8
Subcutaneous, subcuticular —*see* condition
Subdelirium 293.1
Subdural —*see* condition
Subendocardium —*see* condition
Subependymoma (M9383/1) 237.5
Suberosis 495.3
Subglossitis —*see* Glossitis

Subhemophilia 286.0
Subinvolution (uterus) 621.1
  breast (postlactational) (postpartum) 611.89
  chronic 621.1
  puerperal, postpartum 674.8
Sublingual —*see* condition
Sublinguitis 527.2
Subluxation —*see also* Dislocation, by site
  congenital NEC—*see also* Malposition,
    congenital
  hip (unilateral) 754.32
    with dislocation of other hip 754.35
    bilateral 754.33
  joint
    lower limb 755.69
    shoulder 755.59
    upper limb 755.59
  lower limb (joint) 755.69
  shoulder (joint) 755.59
  upper limb (joint) 755.59
  lens 379.32
    anterior 379.33
    posterior 379.34
  radial head 832.2
  rotary, cervical region of spine—*see* Fracture,
    vertebra, cervical
Submaxillary —*see* condition
Submersion (fatal) (nonfatal) 994.1
Submissiveness (undue), in child 313.0
Submucous —*see* condition
Subnormal, subnormality
  accommodation (*see also* Disorder,
    accommodation) 367.9
  mental (*see also* Disability, intellectual) 319
    mild 317
    moderate 318.0
    profound 318.2
    severe 318.1
  temperature (accidental) 991.6
    not associated with low environmental
      temperature 780.99
Subphrenic —*see* condition
Subscapular nerve —*see* condition
Subseptus uterus 752.35
Subsiding appendicitis 542
Substance abuse in family V61.42
Substernal thyroid (*see also* Goiter) 240.9
  congenital 759.2
Substitution disorder 300.11
Subtentorial —*see* condition
Subtertian
  fever 084.0
  malaria (fever) 084.0
Subthyroidism (acquired) (*see also*
  Hypothyroidism) 244.9
  congenital 243
Succenturiata placenta —*see* Placenta,
  abnormal
Succussion sounds, chest 786.7
Sucking thumb, child 307.9
Sudamen 705.1
Sudamina 705.1
Sudanese kala-azar 085.0
Sudden
  death, cause unknown (less than 24 hours) 798.1
    cardiac (SCD)
      family history of V17.41
      personal history of, successfully resuscitated
        V12.53
    during childbirth 669.9
    infant 798.0

Sudden—*continued*
  death—*continued*
    puerperal, postpartum 674.9
  hearing loss NEC 388.2
  heart failure (*see also* Failure, heart) 428.9
  infant death syndrome 798.0
Sudeck's atrophy, disease, or syndrome 733.7
SUDS (Sudden unexplained death) 798.2
Suffocation (*see also* Asphyxia) 799.01
  by
    bed clothes 994.7
    bunny bag 994.7
    cave-in 994.7
    constriction 994.7
    drowning 994.1
    inhalation
      food or foreign body (*see also* Asphyxia,
        food or foreign body) 933.1
      oil or gasoline (*see also* Asphyxia, food or
        foreign body) 933.1
    overlying 994.7
    plastic bag 994.7
    pressure 994.7
    strangulation 994.7
  during birth 768.1
  mechanical 994.7
Sugar
  blood
    high 790.29
    low 251.2
  in urine 791.5
Suicide, suicidal (attempted)
  by poisoning—*see* Table of drugs and chemicals
  ideation V62.84
  risk 300.9
  tendencies 300.9
  trauma NEC (*see also* nature and site of injury)
    959.9
Suipestifer infection (*see also* Infection,
  Salmonella) 003.9
Sulfatidosis 330.0
Sulfhemoglobinemia, sulphemoglobinemia
  (acquired) (congenital) 289.7
Sumatran mite fever 081.2
Summer —*see* condition
Sunburn 692.71
  dermatitis 692.71
  due to
    other ultraviolet radiation 692.82
    tanning bed 692.82
  first degree 692.71
  second degree 692.76
  third degree 692.77
SUNCT (Short-lasting Unilateral Neuralgiform
  headache with Conjunctival injection and
  Tearing) 339.05
Sunken
  acetabulum 718.85
  fontanels 756.0
Sunstroke 992.0
Superfecundation 651.9
  with fetal loss and retention of one or more
    fetus(es) 651.6
  following (elective) fetal reduction 651.7
Superfetation 651.9
  with fetal loss and retention of one or more
    fetus(es) 651.6
  following (elective) fetal reduction 651.7
Supernumerary (congenital)
  aortic cusps 746.89
  auditory ossicles 744.04

Supernumerary—*continued*
  bone 756.9
  breast 757.6
  carpal bones 755.56
  cusps, heart valve NEC 746.89
    mitral 746.5
    pulmonary 746.09
  digit(s) 755.00
    finger 755.01
    toe 755.02
  ear (lobule) 744.1
  fallopian tube 752.19
  finger 755.01
  hymen 752.49
  kidney 753.3
  lacrimal glands 743.64
  lacrimonasal duct 743.65
  lobule (ear) 744.1
  mitral cusps 746.5
  muscle 756.82
  nipples 757.6
  organ or site NEC—*see* Accessory
  ossicles, auditory 744.04
  ovary 752.0
  oviduct 752.19
  pulmonic cusps 746.09
  rib 756.3
    cervical or first 756.2
      syndrome 756.2
  roots (of teeth) 520.2
  spinal vertebra 756.19
  spleen 759.0
  tarsal bones 755.67
  teeth 520.1
    causing crowding 524.31
  testis 752.89
  thumb 755.01
  toe 755.02
  uterus 752.2
  vagina 752.49
  vertebra 756.19
Supervision (of)
  contraceptive method previously prescribed V25.40
    intrauterine device V25.42
    oral contraceptive (pill) V25.41
    specified type NEC V25.49
    subdermal implantable contraceptive V25.43
  dietary (for) V65.3
    allergy (food) V65.3
    colitis V65.3
    diabetes mellitus V65.3
    food allergy intolerance V65.3
    gastritis V65.3
    hypercholesterolemia V65.3
    hypoglycemia V65.3
    intolerance (food) V65.3
    obesity V65.3
    specified NEC V65.3
  lactation V24.1
  newborn health
    8 to 28 days old V20.32
    under 8 days old V20.31
  pregnancy—*see* Pregnancy, supervision of
Supplemental teeth 520.1
  causing crowding 524.31
Suppression
  binocular vision 368.31
  lactation 676.5
  menstruation 626.8
  ovarian secretion 256.39
  renal 586

Suppression—*continued*
  urinary secretion 788.5
  urine 788.5
Suppuration, suppurative —*see also* condition
  accessory sinus (chronic) (*see also* Sinusitis)
    473.9
  adrenal gland 255.8
  antrum (chronic) (*see also* Sinusitis, maxillary)
    473.0
  bladder (*see also* Cystitis) 595.89
  bowel 569.89
  brain 324.0
    late effect 326
  breast 611.0
    puerperal, postpartum 675.1
  dental periosteum 526.5
  diffuse (skin) 686.00
  ear (middle) (*see also* Otitis media) 382.4
    external (*see also* Otitis, externa) 380.10
    internal 386.33
  ethmoidal (sinus) (chronic) (*see also* Sinusitis,
    ethmoidal) 473.2
  fallopian tube (*see also* Salpingo-oophoritis)
    614.2
  frontal (sinus) (chronic) (*see also* Sinusitis,
    frontal) 473.1
  gallbladder (*see also* Cholecystitis, acute) 575.0
  gum 523.30
  hernial sac—*see* Hernia, by site
  intestine 569.89
  joint (*see also* Arthritis, suppurative) 711.0
  labyrinthine 386.33
  lung 513.0
  mammary gland 611.0
    puerperal, postpartum 675.1
  maxilla, maxillary 526.4
    sinus (chronic) (*see also* Sinusitis, maxillary)
      473.0
  muscle 728.0
  nasal sinus (chronic) (*see also* Sinusitis) 473.9
  pancreas 577.0
  parotid gland 527.2
  pelvis, pelvic
    female (*see also* Disease, pelvis,
      inflammatory) 614.4
      acute 614.3
    male (*see also* Peritonitis) 567.21
  pericranial (*see also* Osteomyelitis) 730.2
  salivary duct or gland (any) 527.2
  sinus (nasal) (*see also* Sinusitis) 473.9
  sphenoidal (sinus) (chronic) (*see also* Sinusitis,
    sphenoidal) 473.3
  thymus (gland) 254.1
  thyroid (gland) 245.0
  tonsil 474.8
  uterus (*see also* Endometritis) 615.9
  vagina 616.10
  wound—*see also* Wound, open, by site,
    complicated
    dislocation—*see* Dislocation, by site,
      compound
    fracture—*see* Fracture, by site, open
    scratch or other superficial injury—*see* Injury,
      superficial, by site
Supraeruption, teeth 524.34
Supraglottitis 464.50
  with obstruction 464.51
Suprapubic drainage 596.89
Suprarenal (gland)—*see* condition

Suprascapular nerve —*see* condition
Suprasellar —*see* condition
Supraspinatus syndrome 726.10
Surfer knots 919.8
  infected 919.9
Surgery
  cosmetic NEC V50.1
    breast reconstruction following mastectomy
      V51.0
    following healed injury or operation V51.8
    hair transplant V50.0
  elective V50.9
    breast
      augmentation or reduction V50.1
      reconstruction following mastectomy V51.0
    circumcision, ritual or routine (in absence of
      medical indication) V50.2
    cosmetic NEC V50.1
    ear piercing V50.3
    face-lift V50.1
    following healed injury or operation V51.8
    hair transplant V50.0
  not done because of
    contraindication V64.1
    patient's decision V64.2
    specified reason NEC V64.3
  plastic
    breast
      augmentation or reduction V50.1
      reconstruction following mastectomy V51.0
    cosmetic V50.1
    face-lift V50.1
    following healed injury or operation V51.8
    repair of scarred tissue (following healed
      injury or operation) V51.8
    specified type NEC V50.8
  previous, in pregnancy or childbirth
    cervix 654.6
      affecting fetus or newborn (*see also*
        Newborn, affected by) 760.63
      causing obstructed labor 660.2
        affecting fetus or newborn 763.1
    pelvic soft tissues NEC 654.9
      affecting fetus or newborn (*see also*
        Newborn, affected by) 760.63
      causing obstructed labor 660.2
        affecting fetus or newborn 763.1
    perineum or vulva 654.8
    uterus NEC 654.9
      affecting fetus or newborn (*see also*
        Newborn, affected by) 760.63
      causing obstructed labor 660.2
        affecting fetus or newborn 763.1
      due to previous cesarean delivery 654.2
    vagina 654.7
Surgical
  abortion—*see* Abortion, legal
  emphysema 998.81
  kidney (*see also* Pyelitis) 590.80
  operation NEC 799.9
  procedures, complication or misadventure—*see*
    Complications, surgical procedure
  shock 998.00
Survey
  fetal anatomic V28.81

Susceptibility
  genetic
    to
      MEN (multiple endocrine neoplasia) V84.81
      neoplasia
        multiple endocrine (MEN) V84.81
      neoplasm
        malignant, of
          breast V84.01
          endometrium V84.04
          other V84.09
          ovary V84.02
          prostate V84.03
        specified disease NEC V84.89
Suspected condition, ruled out (*see also*
  Observation, suspected) V71.9
  specified condition NEC V71.89
Suspended uterus, in pregnancy or childbirth
  654.4
  affecting fetus or newborn 763.89
  causing obstructed labor 660.2
    affecting fetus or newborn 763.1
Sutton's disease 709.09
Sutton and Gull's disease (arteriolar
  nephrosclerosis) (*see also* Hypertension,
  kidney) 403.90
Suture
  burst (in external operation wound) (*see also*
    Dehiscence) 998.32
    internal 998.31
  inadvertently left in operation wound 998.4
  removal V58.32
  Shirodkar, in pregnancy (with or without
    cervical incompetence) 654.5
Swab inadvertently left in operation wound
  998.4
Swallowed, swallowing
  difficulty (*see also* Dysphagia) 787.20
  foreign body NEC (*see also* Foreign body) 938
Swamp fever 100.89
Swan neck hand (intrinsic) 736.09
Sweat (s), sweating
  disease or sickness 078.2
  excessive (*see also* Hyperhidrosis) 780.8
  fetid 705.89
  fever 078.2
  gland disease 705.9
    specified type NEC 705.89
  miliary 078.2
  night 780.8
Sweeley-Klionsky disease (angiokeratoma
  corporis diffusum) 272.7
Sweet's syndrome (acute febrile neutrophilic
  dermatosis) 695.89
Swelling 782.3
  abdominal (not referable to specific organ)
    789.3
  adrenal gland, cloudy 255.8
  ankle 719.07
  anus 787.99
  arm 729.81
  breast 611.72
  Calabar 125.2
  cervical gland 785.6
  cheek 784.2
  chest 786.6
  ear 388.8
  epigastric 789.3
  extremity (lower) (upper) 729.81

Swelling—*continued*
eye 379.92
female genital organ 625.8
finger 729.81
foot 729.81
glands 785.6
gum 784.2
hand 729.81
head 784.2
inflammatory—*see* Inflammation
joint (*see also* Effusion, joint) 719.0
   tuberculous—*see* Tuberculosis, joint
kidney, cloudy 593.89
leg 729.81
limb 729.81
liver 573.8
lung 786.6
lymph nodes 785.6
mediastinal 786.6
mouth 784.2
muscle (limb) 729.81
neck 784.2
nose or sinus 784.2
palate 784.2
pelvis 789.3
penis 607.83
perineum 625.8
rectum 787.99
scrotum 608.86
skin 782.2
splenic (*see also* Splenomegaly) 789.2
substernal 786.6
superficial, localized (skin) 782.2
testicle 608.86
throat 784.2
toe 729.81
tongue 784.2
tubular (*see also* Disease, renal) 593.9
umbilicus 789.3
uterus 625.8
vagina 625.8
vulva 625.8
wandering, due to Gnathostoma (spinigerum)
   128.1
white—*see* Tuberculosis, arthritis
Swift's disease 985.0
Swimmers'
ear (acute) 380.12
itch 120.3
Swimming in the head 780.4
Swollen —*see also* Swelling
glands 785.6
Swyer-James syndrome (unilateral hyperlucent
   lung) 492.8
Swyer's syndrome (XY pure gonadal
   dysgenesis) 752.7
Sycosis 704.8
barbae (not parasitic) 704.8
contagiosa 110.0
lupoid 704.8
mycotic 110.0
parasitic 110.0
vulgaris 704.8
Sydenham's chorea —*see* Chorea, Sydenham's
Sylvatic yellow fever 060.0
Sylvest's disease (epidemic pleurodynia) 074.1
Symblepharon 372.63
congenital 743.62
Symonds' syndrome 348.2
Sympathetic —*see* condition
Sympatheticotonia (*see also* Neuropathy,
   peripheral, autonomic) 337.9

Sympathicoblastoma (M9500/3)
specified site—*see* Neoplasm, by site, malignant
unspecified site 194.0
Sympathicogonioma (M9500/3)—*see*
   Sympathicoblastoma
Sympathoblastoma (M9500/3)—*see*
   Sympathicoblastoma
Sympathogonioma (M9500/3)—*see*
   Sympathicoblastoma
Symphalangy (*see also* Syndactylism) 755.10
Symptoms, specified (general) NEC 780.99
abdomen NEC 789.9
bone NEC 733.90
breast NEC 611.79
cardiac NEC 785.9
cardiovascular NEC 785.9
chest NEC 786.9
cognition 799.59
development NEC 783.9
digestive system NEC 787.99
emotional state NEC 799.29
eye NEC 379.99
gastrointestinal tract NEC 787.99
genital organs NEC
   female 625.9
   male 608.9
head and neck NEC 784.99
heart NEC 785.9
jaw 784.92
joint NEC 719.60
   ankle 719.67
   elbow 719.62
   foot 719.67
   hand 719.64
   hip 719.65
   knee 719.66
   multiple sites 719.69
   pelvic region 719.65
   shoulder (region) 719.61
   specified site NEC 719.68
   temporomandibular 524.69
   wrist 719.63
larynx NEC 784.99
limbs NEC 729.89
lymphatic system NEC 785.9
maxilla 784.92
menopausal 627.2
metabolism NEC 783.9
mouth NEC 528.9
muscle NEC 728.9
musculoskeletal NEC 781.99
   limbs NEC 729.89
nervous system NEC 781.99
neurotic NEC 300.9
nutrition, metabolism, and development NEC 783.9
pelvis NEC 789.9
   female 625.9
peritoneum NEC 789.9
respiratory system NEC 786.9
skin and integument NEC 782.9
subcutaneous tissue NEC 782.9
throat NEC 784.99
tonsil NEC 784.99
urinary system NEC 788.99
vascular NEC 785.9
Sympus 759.89
Synarthrosis 719.80
ankle 719.87
elbow 719.82
foot 719.87
hand 719.84

Synarthrosis—*continued*
  hip 719.85
  knee 719.86
  multiple sites 719.89
  pelvic region 719.85
  shoulder (region) 719.81
  specified site NEC 719.88
  wrist 719.83
Syncephalus 759.4
Synchondrosis 756.9
  abnormal (congenital) 756.9
  ischiopubic (van Neck's) 732.1
Synchysis (senile) (vitreous humor) 379.21
  scintillans 379.22
Syncope (near) (pre-) 780.2
  anginosa 413.9
  bradycardia 427.89
  cardiac 780.2
  carotid sinus 337.01
  complicating delivery 669.2
  due to lumbar puncture 349.0
  fatal 798.1
  heart 780.2
  heat 992.1
  laryngeal 786.2
  tussive 786.2
  vasoconstriction 780.2
  vasodepressor 780.2
  vasomotor 780.2
  vasovagal 780.2
Syncytial infarct —*see* Placenta, abnormal
Syndactylism, syndactyly (multiple sites) 755.10
  fingers (without fusion of bone) 755.11
    with fusion of bone 755.12
  toes (without fusion of bone) 755.13
    with fusion of bone 755.14
Syndrome —*see also* Disease
  5q minus 238.74
  abdominal
    acute 789.0
    migraine 346.2
    muscle deficiency 756.79
  Abercrombie's (amyloid degeneration) 277.39
  abnormal innervation 374.43
  abstinence
    alcohol 291.81
    drug 292.0
    neonatal 779.5
  Abt-Letterer-Siwe (acute histiocytosis X)
    (M9722/3) 202.5
  Achard-Thiers (adrenogenital) 255.2
  acid pulmonary aspiration 997.39
    obstetric (Mendelson's) 668.0
  acquired immune deficiency 042
  acquired immunodeficiency 042
  acrocephalosyndactylism 755.55
  acute abdominal 789.0
  acute chest 517.3
  acute coronary 411.1
  Adair-Dighton (brittle bones and blue sclera,
    deafness) 756.51
  Adams-Stokes (-Morgagni) (syncope with heart
    block) 426.9
  addisonian 255.41
  Adie (-Holmes) (pupil) 379.46
  adiposogenital 253.8
  adrenal
    hemorrhage 036.3
    meningococcic 036.3
  adrenocortical 255.3

Syndrome—*continued*
  adrenogenital (acquired) (congenital) 255.2
    feminizing 255.2
    iatrogenic 760.79
    virilism (acquired) (congenital) 255.2
  affective organic NEC 293.89
    drug-induced 292.84
  afferent loop NEC 537.89
  African macroglobulinemia 273.3
  Ahumada-Del Castillo (nonpuerperal
    galactorrhea and amenorrhea) 253.1
  air blast concussion—*see* Injury, internal, by site
  Alagille 759.89
  Albright (-Martin) (pseudohypoparathyroidism)
    275.49
  Albright-McCune-Sternberg (osteitis fibrosa
    disseminata) 756.59
  alcohol withdrawal 291.81
  Alder's (leukocyte granulation anomaly) 288.2
  Aldrich (-Wiskott) (eczema-thrombocytopenia)
    279.12
  Alibert-Bazin (mycosis, fungoides) (M9700/3)
    202.1
  Alice in Wonderland 293.89
  alien hand 781.8
  Allen-Masters 620.6
  Alligator baby (ichthyosis congenita) 757.1
  Alport's (hereditary hematuria-nephropathy-
    deafness) 759.89
  Alvarez (transient cerebral ischemia) 435.9
  alveolar capillary block 516.8
  Alzheimer's 331.0
    with dementia—*see* Alzheimer's, dementia
  amnestic (confabulatory) 294.0
    alcohol-induced persisting 291.1
    drug-induced 292.83
    posttraumatic 294.0
  amotivational 292.89
  amyostatic 275.1
  amyotrophic lateral sclerosis 335.20
  androgen insensitivity 259.51
    partial 259.52
  Angelman 759.89
  angina (*see also* Angina) 413.9
  ankyloglossia superior 750.0
  anterior
    chest wall 786.52
    compartment (tibial) 958.8
    spinal artery 433.8
      compression 721.1
    tibial (compartment) 958.8
  antibody deficiency 279.00
    agammaglobulinemic 279.00
    congenital 279.04
    hypogammaglobulinemic 279.00
  anticardiolipin antibody 289.81
  antimongolism 758.39
  antiphospholipid antibody 289.81
  Anton (-Babinski) (hemiasomatognosia) 307.9
  anxiety (*see also* Anxiety) 300.00
    organic 293.84
  aortic
    arch 446.7
    bifurcation (occlusion) 444.09
    ring 747.21
  Apert's (acrocephalosyndactyly) 755.55
  Apert-Gallais (adrenogenital) 255.2
  aphasia-apraxia-alexia 784.69
  apical ballooning 429.83
  "approximate answers" 300.16
  arcuate ligament (-celiac axis) 447.4

Syndrome—*continued*
arcus aortae 446.7
arc-welders' 370.24
argentaffin, argintaffinoma 259.2
Argonz-Del Castillo (nonpuerperal galactorrhea and amenorrhea) 253.1
Argyll Robertson's (syphilitic) 094.89
  nonsyphilitic 379.45
arm-shoulder (*see also* Neuropathy, peripheral, autonomic) 337.9
Armenian 277.31
Arnold-Chiari (*see also* Spina bifida) 741.0
  type I 348.4
  type II 741.0
  type III 742.0
  type IV 742.2
Arrillaga-Ayerza (pulmonary artery sclerosis with pulmonary hypertension) 416.0
arteriomesenteric duodenum occlusion 537.89
arteriovenous steal 996.73
arteritis, young female (obliterative brachiocephalic) 446.7
aseptic meningitis—*see* Meningitis, aseptic
Asherman's 621.5
Asperger's 299.8
asphyctic (*see also* Anxiety) 300.00
aspiration, of newborn (massive) 770.18
  meconium 770.12
ataxia-telangiectasia 334.8
Audry's (acropachyderma) 757.39
auriculotemporal 350.8
autoimmune lymphoproliferative (ALPS) 279.41
autosomal—*see also* Abnormal, autosomes NEC
  deletion 758.39
    5p 758.31
    22q11.2 758.32
Avellis' 344.89
Axenfeld's 743.44
Ayerza (-Arrillaga) (pulmonary artery sclerosis with pulmonary hypertension) 416.0
Baader's (erythema multiforme exudativum) 695.19
Baastrup's 721.5
Babinski (-Vaquez) (cardiovascular syphilis) 093.89
Babinski-Fröhlich (adiposogenital dystrophy) 253.8
Babinski-Nageotte 344.89
Bagratuni's (temporal arteritis) 446.5
Bakwin-Krida (craniometaphyseal dysplasia) 756.89
Balint's (psychic paralysis of visual disorientation) 368.16
Ballantyne (-Runge) (postmaturity) 766.22
ballooning posterior leaflet 424.0
Banti's—*see* Cirrhosis, liver
Bard-Pic's (carcinoma, head of pancreas) 157.0
Bardet-Biedl (obesity, polydactyly, and intellectual disabilities) 759.89
Barlow's (mitral valve prolapse) 424.0
Barlow (-Möller) (infantile scurvy) 267
Baron Munchausen's 301.51
Barré-Guillain 357.0
Barré-Liéou (posterior cervical sympathetic) 723.2
Barrett's (chronic peptic ulcer of esophagus) 530.85
Bársony-Polgár (corkscrew esophagus) 530.5
Bársony-Teschendorf (corkscrew esophagus) 530.5

Syndrome—*continued*
Barth 759.89
Bartter's (secondary hyperaldosteronism with juxtaglomerular hyperplasia) 255.13
basal cell nevus 759.89
Basedow's (exophthalmic goiter) 242.0
basilar artery 435.0
basofrontal 377.04
Bassen-Kornzweig (abetalipoproteinemia) 272.5
Batten-Steinert 359.21
battered
  adult 995.81
  baby or child 995.54
  spouse 995.81
Baumgarten-Cruveilhier (cirrhosis of liver) 571.5
Beals 759.82
Bearn-Kunkel (-Slater) (lupoid hepatitis) 571.49
Beau's (*see also* Degeneration, myocardial) 429.1
Bechterew-Strümpell-Marie (ankylosing spondylitis) 720.0
Beck's (anterior spinal artery occlusion) 433.8
Beckwith (-Wiedemann) 759.89
Behçet's 136.1
Bekhterev-Strümpell-Marie (ankylosing spondylitis) 720.0
Benedikt's 344.89
Béquez César (-Steinbrinck-Chédiak-Higashi) (congenital gigantism of peroxidase granules) 288.2
Bernard-Horner (*see also* Neuropathy, peripheral, autonomic) 337.9
Bernard-Sergent (acute adrenocortical insufficiency) 255.41
Bernhardt-Roth 355.1
Bernheim's (*see also* Failure, heart) 428.0
Bertolotti's (sacralization of fifth lumbar vertebra) 756.15
Besnier-Boeck-Schaumann (sarcoidosis) 135
Bianchi's (aphasia-apraxia-alexia syndrome) 784.69
Biedl-Bardet (obesity, polydactyly, and intellectual disabilities) 759.89
Biemond's (obesity, polydactyly, and intellectual disabilities) 759.89
big spleen 289.4
bilateral polycystic ovarian 256.4
Bing-Horton's 339.00
Biörck (-Thorson) (malignant carcinoid) 259.2
Birt-Hogg-Dube 759.89
Blackfan-Diamond (congenital hypoplastic anemia) 284.01
black lung 500
black widow spider bite 989.5
bladder neck (*see also* Incontinence, urine) 788.30
blast (concussion)—*see* Blast, injury
blind loop (postoperative) 579.2
Bloch-Siemens (incontinentia pigmenti) 757.33
Bloch-Sulzberger (incontinentia pigmenti) 757.33
Bloom (-Machacek) (-Torre) 757.39
Blount-Barber (tibia vara) 732.4
blue
  bloater 491.20
    with
      acute bronchitis 491.22
      exacerbation (acute) 491.21
  diaper 270.0
  drum 381.02
  sclera 756.51
  toe 445.02

Syndrome—*continued*
  Boder-Sedgwick (ataxia-telangiectasia) 334.8
  Boerhaave's (spontaneous esophageal rupture)
    530.4
  Bonnevie-Ullrich 758.6
  Bonnier's 386.19
  Borjeson-Forssman-Lehmann 759.89
  Bouillaud's (rheumatic heart disease) 391.9
  Bourneville (-Pringle) (tuberous sclerosis) 759.5
  Bouveret (-Hoffmann) (paroxysmal tachycardia)
    427.2
  brachial plexus 353.0
  Brachman-de Lange (Amsterdam dwarf,
    intellectual disabilities, and brachycephaly)
    759.89
  bradycardia-tachycardia 427.81
  Brailsford-Morquio (dystrophy)
    (mucopolysaccharidosis IV) 277.5
  brain (acute) (chronic) (nonpsychotic) (organic)
    (with behavioral reaction) (with neurotic
    reaction) 310.9
    with
      presenile brain disease (*see also* Dementia,
        presenile) 290.10
      psychosis, psychotic reaction (*see also*
        Psychosis, organic) 294.9
    chronic alcoholic 291.2
    congenital (*see also* Disability, intellectual)
      319
    postcontusional 310.2
    posttraumatic
      nonpsychotic 310.2
      psychotic 293.9
        acute 293.0
        chronic (*see also* Psychosis, organic) 294.8
        subacute 293.1
    psycho-organic (*see also* Syndrome,
      psycho-organic) 310.9
    psychotic (*see also* Psychosis, organic) 294.9
    senile (*see also* Dementia, senile) 290.0
  branchial arch 744.41
  Brandt's (acrodermatitis enteropathica) 686.8
  Brennemann's 289.2
  Briquet's 300.81
  Brissaud-Meige (infantile myxedema) 244.9
  broad ligament laceration 620.6
  Brock's (atelectasis due to enlarged lymph
    nodes) 518.0
  broken heart 429.83
  Brown's tendon sheath 378.61
  Brown-Séquard 344.89
  brown spot 756.59
  Brugada 746.89
  Brugsch's (acropachyderma) 757.39
  bubbly lung 770.7
  Buchem's (hyperostosis corticalis) 733.3
  Budd-Chiari (hepatic vein thrombosis) 453.0
  Büdinger-Ludloff-Läwen 717.89
  bulbar 335.22
    lateral (*see also* Disease, cerebrovascular,
      acute) 436
  Bullis fever 082.8
  bundle of Kent (anomalous atrioventricular
    excitation) 426.7
  Bürger-Grütz (essential familial hyperlipemia)
    272.3
  Burke's (pancreatic insufficiency and chronic
    neutropenia) 577.8
  Burnett's (milk-alkali) 275.42
  Burnier's (hypophyseal dwarfism) 253.3
  burning feet 266.2

Syndrome—*continued*
  Bywaters' 958.5
  Caffey's (infantile cortical hyperostosis) 756.59
  Calvé-Legg-Perthes (osteochondrosis, femoral
    capital) 732.1
  Caplan (-Colinet) syndrome 714.81
  capsular thrombosis (*see also* Thrombosis,
    brain) 434.0
  carbohydrate-deficient glycoprotein (CDGS) 271.8
  carcinogenic thrombophlebitis 453.1
  carcinoid 259.2
  cardiac asthma (*see also* Failure, ventricular,
    left) 428.1
  cardiacos negros 416.0
  cardiofaciocutaneous 759.89
  cardiopulmonary obesity 278.03
  cardiorenal (*see also* Hypertension, cardiorenal)
    404.90
  cardiorespiratory distress (idiopathic), newborn
    769
  cardiovascular renal (*see also* Hypertension,
    cardiorenal) 404.90
  cardiovasorenal 272.7
  Carini's (ichthyosis congenita) 757.1
  carotid
    artery (internal) 435.8
    body or sinus 337.01
  carpal tunnel 354.0
  Carpenter's 759.89
  Cassidy (-Scholte) (malignant carcinoid) 259.2
  cat-cry 758.31
  cauda equina 344.60
  causalgia 355.9
    lower limb 355.71
    upper limb 354.4
  cavernous sinus 437.6
  celiac 579.0
    artery compression 447.4
    axis 447.4
  central pain 338.0
  cerebellomedullary malformation (*see also*
    Spina bifida) 741.0
  cerebral gigantism 253.0
  cerebrohepatorenal 759.89
  cervical (root) (spine) NEC 723.8
    disc 722.71
    posterior, sympathetic 723.2
    rib 353.0
    sympathetic paralysis 337.09
    traumatic (acute) NEC 847.0
  cervicobrachial (diffuse) 723.3
  cervicocranial 723.2
  cervicodorsal outlet 353.2
  Céstan's 344.89
  Céstan (-Raymond) 433.8
  Céstan-Chenais 344.89
  chancriform 114.1
  Charcot's (intermittent claudication) 443.9
    angina cruris 443.9
    due to atherosclerosis 440.21
  Charcot-Marie-Tooth 356.1
  Charcot-Weiss-Baker 337.01
  CHARGE association 759.89
  Cheadle (-Möller) (-Barlow) (infantile scurvy)
    267
  Chédiak-Higashi (-Steinbrinck) (congenital
    gigantism of peroxidase granules) 288.2
  chest wall 786.52
  Chiari's (hepatic vein thrombosis) 453.0
  Chiari-Frommel 676.6
  chiasmatic 368.41

Syndrome—*continued*
  Chilaiditi's (subphrenic displacement, colon)
      751.4
  chondroectodermal dysplasia 756.55
  chorea-athetosis-agitans 275.1
  Christian's (chronic histiocytosis X) 277.89
  chromosome 4 short arm deletion 758.39
  chronic pain 338.4
  Churg-Strauss 446.4
  Clarke-Hadfield (pancreatic infantilism) 577.8
  Claude's 352.6
  Claude Bernard-Horner (*see also* Neuropathy,
      peripheral, autonomic) 337.9
  Clérambault's
    automatism 348.89
    erotomania 297.8
  Clifford's (postmaturity) 766.22
  climacteric 627.2
  Clouston's (hidrotic ectodermal dysplasia)
      757.31
  clumsiness 315.4
  Cockayne's (microencephaly and dwarfism)
      759.89
  Cockayne-Weber (epidermolysis bullosa)
      757.39
  Coffin-Lowry 759.89
  Cogan's (nonsyphilitic interstitial keratitis)
      370.52
  cold injury (newborn) 778.2
  Collet (-Sicard) 352.6
  combined immunity deficiency 279.2
  compartment(al) (anterior) (deep) (posterior) 958.8
    nontraumatic
      abdomen 729.73
      arm 729.71
      buttock 729.72
      fingers 729.71
      foot 729.72
      forearm 729.71
      hand 729.71
      hip 729.72
      leg 729.72
      lower extremity 729.72
      shoulder 729.71
      specified site NEC 729.79
      thigh 729.72
      toes 729.72
      upper extremity 729.71
      wrist 729.71
    post-surgical (see also Syndrome,
        compartment, non-traumatic) 998.89
    traumatic 958.90
      abdomen 958.93
      arm 958.91
      buttock 958.92
      fingers 958.91
      foot 958.92
      forearm 958.91
      hand 958.91
      hip 958.92
      leg 958.92
      lower extremity 958.92
      shoulder 958.91
      specified site NEC 958.99
      thigh 958.92
      tibial 958.92
      toes 958.92
      upper extremity 958.91
      wrist 958.91

Syndrome—*continued*
  complex regional pain — *see* also, Dystrophy,
      sympathetic
    type I — *see* Dystrophy, sympathetic
        (posttraumatic) (reflex)
    type II — *see* Causalgia
  compression 958.5
    cauda equina 344.60
      with neurogenic bladder 344.61
  concussion 310.2
  congenital
    affecting more than one system 759.7
      specified type NEC 759.89
    congenital central alveolar hypoventilation
        327.25
    facial diplegia 352.6
    muscular hypertrophy-cerebral 759.89
  congestion-fibrosis (pelvic) 625.5
  conjunctivourethrosynovial 099.3
  Conn (-Louis) (primary aldosteronism) 255.12
  Conradi (-Hünermann) (chondrodysplasia
      calcificans congenita) 756.59
  conus medullaris 336.8
  Cooke-Apert-Gallais (adrenogenital) 255.2
  Cornelia de Lange's (Amsterdam dwarf,
      intellectual disabilities, and brachycephaly)
      759.8
  coronary insufficiency or intermediate 411.1
  cor pulmonale 416.9
  corticosexual 255.2
  Costen's (complex) 524.60
  costochondral junction 733.6
  costoclavicular 353.0
  costovertebral 253.0
  Cotard's (paranoia) 297.1
  Cowden 759.6
  craniovertebral 723.2
  Creutzfeldt-Jakob 046.19
    with dementia
      with behavioral disturbance 046.19
          [294.11]
      without behavioral disturbance 046.19
          [294.10]
    variant 046.11
      with dementia
        with behavioral disturbance 046.11
            [294.11]
        without behavioral disturbance 046.11
            [294.10]
  crib death 798.0
  cricopharyngeal 787.20
  cri-du-chat 758.31
  Crigler-Najjar (congenital hyperbilirubinemia)
      277.4
  crocodile tears 351.8
  Cronkhite-Canada 211.3
  croup 464.4
  CRST (cutaneous systemic sclerosis) 710.1
  crush 958.5
  crushed lung (*see also* Injury, internal, lung) 861.20
  Cruveilhier-Baumgarten (cirrhosis of liver)
      571.5
  cubital tunnel 354.2
  Cuiffini-Pancoast (M8010/3) (carcinoma,
      pulmonary apex) 162.3
  Curschmann (-Batten) (-Steinert) 359.21
  Cushing's (iatrogenic) (idiopathic) (pituitary
      basophilism) (pituitary-dependent) 255.0
    overdose or wrong substance given or taken
        962.0
  Cyriax's (slipping rib) 733.99

Syndrome—*continued*
cystic duct stump 576.0
Da Costa's (neurocirculatory asthenia) 306.2
Dameshek's (erythroblastic anemia) 282.49
Dana-Putnam (subacute combined sclerosis with
    pernicious anemia) 281.0 *[336.2]*
Danbolt (-Closs) (acrodermatitis enteropathica)
    686.8
Dandy-Walker (atresia, foramen of Magendie)
    742.3
    with spina bifida (*see also* Spina bifida) 741.0
Danlos' 756.83
Davies-Colley (slipping rib) 733.99
dead fetus 641.3
defeminization 255.2
defibrination (*see also* Fibrinolysis) 286.6
Degos' 447.8
Deiters' nucleus 386.19
Déjérine-Roussy 338.0
Déjérine-Thomas 333.0
de Lange's (Amsterdam dwarf, intellectual
    disabilities, and brachycephaly) (Cornelia)
    759.89
Del Castillo's (germinal aplasia) 606.0
deletion chromosomes 758.39
delusional
    induced by drug 292.11
dementia-aphonia, of childhood (*see also*
    Psychosis, childhood) 299.1
demyelinating NEC 341.9
denial visual hallucination 307.9
depersonalization 300.6
de Quervain's 259.51
Dercum's (adiposis dolorosa) 272.8
de Toni-Fanconi (-Debré) (cystinosis) 270.0
diabetes-dwarfism-obesity (juvenile) 258.1
diabetes mellitus-hypertension-nephrosis 250.4
    [581.81]
    due to secondary diabetes 249.4 *[581.81]*
diabetes mellitus in newborn infant 775.1
diabetes-nephrosis 250.4 *[581.81]*
    due to secondary diabetes 249.4 *[581.81]*
diabetic amyotrophy 250.6 *[353.5]*
    due to secondary diabetes 249.6 [353.5]
Diamond-Blackfan (congenital hypoplastic
    anemia) 284.01
Diamond-Gardener (autoerythrocyte
    sensitization) 287.2
DIC (diffuse or disseminated intravascular
    coagulopathy) (*see also* Fibrinolysis) 286.6
diencephalohypophyseal NEC 253.8
diffuse cervicobrachial 723.3
diffuse obstructive pulmonary 496
DiGeorge's (thymic hypoplasia) 279.11
Dighton's 756.51
Di Guglielmo's (erythremic myelosis)
    (M9841/3) 207.0
disequilibrium 276.9
disseminated platelet thrombosis 446.6
Ditthomska 307.81
Doan-Wiseman (primary splenic neutropenia)
    289.53
Döhle body-panmyelopathic 288.2
Donohue's (leprechaunism) 259.8
dorsolateral medullary (*see also* Disease,
    cerebrovascular, acute) 436
double athetosis 333.71
double whammy 360.81
Down's (mongolism) 758.0
Dresbach's (elliptocytosis) 282.1

Syndrome—*continued*
Dressler's (postmyocardial infarction) 411.0
    hemoglobinuria 283.2
    postcardiotomy 429.4
drug withdrawal, infant, of dependent mother
    779.5
dry skin 701.1
eye 375.15
DSAP (disseminated superficial actinic
    porokeratosis) 692.75
Duane's (retraction) 378.71
Duane-Stilling-Türk (ocular retraction
    syndrome) 378.71
Dubin-Johnson (constitutional
    hyperbilirubinemia) 277.4
Dubin-Sprinz (constitutional
    hyperbilirubinemia) 277.4
Duchenne's 335.22
due to abnormality
    autosomal NEC (*see also* Abnormal,
        autosomes NEC) 758.5
    13 758.1
    18 758.2
    21 or 22 758.0
    D_1 758.1
    E_3 758.2
    G 758.0
    chromosomal 758.89
    sex 758.81
dumping 564.2
    nonsurgical 536.8
Duplay's 726.2
Dupré's (meningism) 781.6
Dyke-Young (acquired macrocytic hemolytic
    anemia) 283.9
dyspraxia 315.4
dystocia, dystrophia 654.9
Eagle-Barrett 756.71
Eales' 362.18
Eaton-Lambert (*see also* Syndrome,
    Lambert-Eaton) 358.30
Ebstein's (downward displacement, tricuspid
    valve into right ventricle) 746.2
ectopic ACTH secretion 255.0
eczema-thrombocytopenia 279.12
Eddowes' (brittle bones and blue sclera) 756.51
Edwards' 758.2
efferent loop 537.89
effort (aviators') (psychogenic) 306.2
Ehlers-Danlos 756.83
Eisenmenger's (ventricular septal defect) 745.4
Ekbom's (restless legs) 333.94
Ekman's (brittle bones and blue sclera) 756.51
electric feet 266.2
Elephant man 237.71
Ellison-Zollinger (gastric hypersecretion with
    pancreatic islet cell tumor) 251.5
Ellis-van Creveld (chondroectodermal
    dysplasia) 756.55
embryonic fixation 270.2
empty sella (turcica) 253.8
endocrine-hypertensive 255.3
Engel-von Recklinghausen (osteitis fibrosa
    cystica) 252.01
enteroarticular 099.3
entrapment—*see* Neuropathy, entrapment
eosinophilia myalgia 710.5
epidemic vomiting 078.82
Epstein's—*see* Nephrosis
Erb (-Oppenheim) -Goldflam 358.00
Erdheim-Chester 277.89

Syndrome—*continued*
Erdheim's (acromegalic macrospondylitis) 253.0
Erlacher-Blount (tibia vara) 732.4
erythrocyte fragmentation 283.19
euthyroid sick 790.94
Evans' (thrombocytopenic purpura) 287.32
excess cortisol, iatrogenic 255.0
exhaustion 300.5
extrapyramidal 333.90
eyelid-malar-mandible 756.0
eye retraction 378.71
Faber's (achlorhydric anemia) 280.9
Fabry (-Anderson) (angiokeratoma corporis
     diffusum) 272.7
facet 724.8
Fallot's 745.2
falx (*see also* Hemorrhage, brain) 431
familial eczema-thrombocytopenia 279.12
Fanconi's (anemia) (congenital pancytopenia)
     284.09
Fanconi (-de Toni) (-Debré) (cystinosis) 270.0
Farber (-Uzman) (disseminated
     lipogranulomatosis) 272.8
fatigue NEC 300.5
   chronic 780.71
faulty bowel habit (idiopathic megacolon) 564.7
FDH (focal dermal hypoplasia) 757.39
fecal reservoir 560.39
Feil-Klippel (brevicollis) 756.16
Felty's (rheumatoid arthritis with splenomegaly
     and leukopenia) 714.1
fertile eunuch 257.2
fetal alcohol 760.71
   late effect 760.71
fibrillation-flutter 427.32
fibrositis (periarticular) 729.0
Fiedler's (acute isolated myocarditis) 422.91
Fiessinger-Leroy (-Reiter) 099.3
Fiessinger-Rendu (erythema multiforme
     exudativum) 695.19
first arch 756.0
fish odor 270.8
Fisher's 357.0
Fitz's (acute hemorrhagic pancreatitis) 577.0
Fitz-Hugh and Curtis 098.86
   due to
       Chlamydia trachomatis 099.56
       Neisseria gonorrhoeae (gonococcal
            peritonitis) 098.86
Flajani (-Basedow) (exophthalmic goiter) 242.0
flat back
   acquired 737.29
   postprocedural 738.5
floppy
   infant 781.99
   iris 364.81
   valve (mitral) 424.0
flush 259.2
Foix-Alajouanine 336.1
Fong's (hereditary osteo-onychodysplasia)
     756.89
foramen magnum 348.4
Forbes-Albright (nonpuerperal amenorrhea and
     lactation associated with pituitary tumor)
     253.1
Foster-Kennedy 377.04
Foville's (peduncular) 344.89
Fragile X 759.83
Franceschetti's (mandibulofacial dysostosis)
     756.0
Fraser's 759.89

Syndrome—*continued*
Freeman-Sheldon 759.89
Frey's (auriculotemporal) 705.22
Friderichsen-Waterhouse 036.3
Friedrich-Erb-Arnold (acropachyderma) 757.39
Fröhlich's (adiposogenital dystrophy) 253.8
Froin's 336.8
Frommel-Chiari 676.6
frontal lobe 310.0
Fuller Albright's (osteitis fibrosa disseminata)
     756.59
Fukuhara 277.87
functional
   bowel 564.9
   prepubertal castrate 752.89
Gaisböck's (polycythemia hypertonica) 289.0
ganglion (basal, brain) 333.90
   geniculi 351.1
Ganser's, hysterical 300.16
Gardner-Diamond (autoerythrocyte
     sensitization) 287.2
gastroesophageal junction 530.0
gastroesophageal laceration-hemorrhage 530.7
gastrojejunal loop obstruction 537.89
Gayet-Wernicke's (superior hemorrhagic
     polioencephalitis) 265.1
Gee-Herter-Heubner (nontropical sprue) 579.0
Gélineau's (*see also* Narcolepsy) 347.00
genito-anorectal 099.1
Gerhardt's (vocal cord paralysis) 478.30
Gerstmann's (finger agnosia) 784.69
Gerstmann-Sträussler-Scheinker (GSS) 046.71
Giannotti Crosti 057.8
   due to known virus—*see* Infection, virus
   due to unknown virus 057.8
Gilbert's 277.4
Gilford (-Hutchinson) (progeria) 259.8
Gilles de la Tourette's 307.23
Gillespie's (dysplasia oculodentodigitalis)
     759.89
Glénard's (enteroptosis) 569.89
Glinski-Simmonds (pituitary cachexia) 253.2
glucuronyl transferase 277.4
glue ear 381.20
Goldberg (-Maxwell) (-Morris) (testicular
     feminization) 259.51
Goldenhar's (oculoauriculovertebral dysplasia)
     756.0
Goldflam-Erb 358.00
Goltz-Gorlin (dermal hypoplasia) 757.39
Good's 279.06
Goodpasture's (pneumorenal) 446.21
Gopalan's (burning feet) 266.2
Gorlin-Chaudhry-Moss 759.89
Gorlin's 759.89
Gougerot (-Houwer) -Sjögren
     (keratoconjunctivitis sicca) 710.2
Gougerot-Blum (pigmented purpuric lichenoid
     dermatitis) 709.1
Gougerot-Carteaud (confluent reticulate
     papillomatosis) 701.8
Gouley's (constrictive pericarditis) 423.2
Gowers' (vasovagal attack) 780.2
Gowers-Paton-Kennedy 377.04
Gradenigo's 383.02
Gray or grey (chloramphenicol) (newborn) 779.4
Greig's (hypertelorism) 756.0
GSS (Gerstmann-Sträussler-Scheinker) 046.71
Gubler-Millard 344.89
Guérin-Stern (arthrogryposis multiplex
     congenita) 754.89

Syndrome—*continued*
Guillain-Barré (-Strohl) 357.0
Gunn's (jaw-winking syndrome) 742.8
Günther's (congenital erythropoietic porphyria)
   277.1
gustatory sweating 350.8
H3O 759.81
Hadfield-Clarke (pancreatic infantilism) 577.8
Haglund-Läwen-Fründ 717.89
hairless women 257.8
hair tourniquet—*see also* Injury, superficial, by
   site
  finger 915.8
   infected 915.9
  penis 911.8
   infected 911.9
  toe 917.8
   infected 917.9
Hallermann-Streiff 756.0
Hallervorden-Spatz 333.0
Hamman's (spontaneous mediastinal
   emphysema) 518.1
Hamman-Rich (diffuse interstitial pulmonary
   fibrosis) 516.33
Hand-Schüller-Christian (chronic histiocytosis
   X) 277.89
hand-foot 693.0
Hanot-Chauffard (-Troisier) (bronze diabetes)
   275.01
Harada's 363.22
Hare's (M8010/3) (carcinoma, pulmonary apex)
   162.3
Harkavy's 446.0
harlequin color change 779.89
Harris' (organic hyperinsulinism) 251.1
Hart's (pellagra-cerebellar ataxia-renal
   aminoaciduria) 270.0
Hayem-Faber (achlorhydric anemia) 280.9
Hayem-Widal (acquired hemolytic jaundice) 283.9
headache — *see* Headache, syndrome
Heberden's (angina pectoris) 413.9
Hedinger's (malignant carcinoid) 259.2
Hegglin's 288.2
Heller's (infantile psychosis) (*see also*
   Psychosis, childhood) 299.1
H.E.L.L.P. 642.5
hemolytic-uremic (adult) (child) 283.11
hemophagocytic 288.4
  infection-associated 288.4
Hench-Rosenberg (palindromic arthritis) (*see
   also* Rheumatism, palindromic) 719.3
Henoch-Schönlein (allergic purpura) 287.0
hepatic flexure 569.89
hepatopulmonary 573.5
hepatorenal 572.4
  due to a procedure 997.49
  following delivery 674.8
hepatourologic 572.4
Herrick's (hemoglobin S disease) 282.61
Herter (-Gee) (nontropical sprue) 579.0
Heubner-Herter (nontropical sprue) 579.0
Heyd's (hepatorenal) 572.4
HHHO 759.81
high grade myelodysplastic 238.73
  with 5q deletion 238.73
Hilger's 337.09
histiocytic 288.4
Hoffa (-Kastert) (liposynovitis prepatellaris) 272.8
Hoffmann's 244.9 *[359.5]*
Hoffmann-Bouveret (paroxysmal tachycardia)
   427.2

Syndrome—*continued*
Hoffmann-Werdnig 335.0
Holländer-Simons (progressive lipodystrophy)
   272.6
Holmes' (visual disorientation) 368.16
Holmes-Adie 379.46
Hoppe-Goldflam 358.00
Yorner's (sde also Neuropathy, peripheral,
   autonomic) 337.9
  traumatic—*see* Injury, nerve, cervical
   sympathetic
hospital addiction 301.51
hungry bone 275.5
Hunt's (herpetic geniculate ganglionitis) 053.11
  dyssynergia cerebellaris myoclonica 334.2
Hunter (-Hurler) (mucopolysaccharidosis II)
   277.5
hunterian glossitis 529.4
Hurler (-Hunter) (mucopolysaccharidosis II)
   277.5
Hutchinson's incisors or teeth 090.5
Hutchinson-Boeck (sarcoidosis) 135
Hutchinson-Gilford (progeria) 259.8
hydralazine
  correct substance properly administered 695.4
  overdose or wrong substance given or taken
   972.6
hydraulic concussion (abdomen) (*see also*
   Injury, internal, abdomen) 868.00
hyperabduction 447.8
hyperactive bowel 564.9
hyperaldosteronism with hypokalemic alkalosis
   (Bartter's) 255.13
hypercalcemic 275.42
hypercoagulation NEC 289.89
hypereosinophilic (idiopathic) 288.3
hyperfusion 997.01
hyperkalemic 276.7
hyperkinetic—*see also* Hyperkinesia
  heart 429.82
hyperlipemia-hemolytic anemia-icterus 571.1
hypermobility 728.5
hypernatremia 276.0
hyperosmolarity 276.0
hypersomnia-bulimia 349.89
hypersplenic 289.4
hypersympathetic (*see also* Neuropathy,
   peripheral, autonomic) 337.9
hypertransfusion, newborn 776.4
hyperventilation, psychogenic 306.1
hyperviscosity (of serum) NEC 273.3
  polycythemic 289.0
  sclerothymic 282.8
hypoglycemic (familial) (neonatal) 251.2
  functional 251.1
hypokalemic 276.8
hypophyseal 253.8
hypophyseothalamic 253.8
hypopituitarism 253.2
hypoplastic left heart 746.7
hypopotassemia 276.8
hyposmolality 276.1
hypotension, maternal 669.2
hypothenar hammer 443.89
hypotonia-hypomentia-hypogonadism-obesity
   759.81
ICF (intravascular coagulation-fibrinolysis) (*see
   also* Fibrinolysis) 286.6
idiopathic cardiorespiratory distress, newborn 769
idiopathic nephrotic (infantile) 581.9

Syndrome—*continued*

Imerslund (-Gräsbeck) (anemia due to familial selective vitamin B₁₂ malabsorption) 281.1
immobility (paraplegic) 728.3
immune reconstitution inflammatory (IRIS) 995.90
immunity deficiency, combined 279.2
impending coronary 411.1
impingement
    shoulder 726.2
    vertebral bodies 724.4
inappropriate secretion of antidiuretic hormone (ADH) 253.6
incomplete
    mandibulofacial 756.0
infant
    death, sudden (SIDS) 798.0
    Hercules 255.2
    of diabetic mother 775.0
    shaken 995.55
infantilism 253.3
inferior vena cava 459.2
influenza-like (*see also* Influenza) 487.1
inspissated bile, newborn 774.4
insufficient sleep 307.44
intermediate coronary (artery) 411.1
internal carotid artery (*see also* Occlusion, artery, carotid) 433.1
interspinous ligament 724.8
intestinal
    carcinoid 259.2
    gas 787.3
    knot 560.2
intraoperative floppy iris (IFIS) 364.81
intravascular
    coagulation-fibrinolysis (ICF) (*see also* Fibrinolysis) 286.6
    coagulopathy (*see also* Fibrinolysis) 286.6
inverted Marfan's 759.89
IRDS (idiopathic respiratory distress, newborn) 769
irritable
    bowel 564.1
    heart 306.2
    weakness 300.5
ischemic bowel (transient) 557.9
    chronic 557.1
    due to mesenteric artery insufficiency 557.1
Itsenko-Cushing (pituitary basophilism) 255.0
IVC (intravascular coagulopathy) (*see also* Fibrinolysis) 286.6
Ivemark's (asplenia with congenital heart disease) 759.0
Jaccoud's 714.4
Jackson's 344.89
Jadassohn-Lewandowski (pachyonychia congenita) 757.5
Jaffe-Lichtenstein (-Uehlinger) 252.01
Jahnke's (encephalocutaneous angiomatosis) 759.6
Jakob-Creutzfeldt 046.19
    with dementia
        with behavioral disturbance 046.19 *[294.11]*
        without behavioral disturbance 046.19 *[294.10]*
    variant
        with dementia
            with behavioral disturbance 046.11 *[294.11]*
            without behavioral disturbance 046.11 *[294.10]*
Jaksch's (pseudoleukemia infantum) 285.8

Syndrome—*continued*

Jaksch-Hayem (-Luzet) (pseudoleukemia infantum) 285.8
jaw-winking 742.8
jejunal 564.2
Jervell-Lange-Nielsen 426.82
jet lag 327.35
Jeune's (asphyxiating thoracic dystrophy of newborn) 756.4
Job's (chronic granulomatous disease) 288.1
Jordan's 288.2
Joseph-Diamond-Blackfan (congenital hypoplastic anemia) 284.01
Joubert 759.89
jugular foramen 352.6
Kabuki 759.89
Kahler's (multiple myeloma) (M9730/3) 203.0
Kalischer's (encephalocutaneous angiomatosis) 759.6
Kallmann's (hypogonadotropic hypogonadism with anosmia) 253.4
Kanner's (autism) (*see also* Psychosis, childhood) 299.0
Kartagener's (sinusitis, bronchiectasis, situs inversus) 759.3
Kasabach-Merritt (capillary hemangioma associated with thrombocytopenic purpura) 287.39
Kast's (dyschondroplasia with hemangiomas) 756.4
Kaznelson's (congenital hypoplastic anemia) 284.01
Kearns-Sayre 277.87
Kelly's (sideropenic dysphagia) 280.8
Kimmelstiel-Wilson (intercapillary glomerulosclerosis) 250.4 *[581.81]*
    due to secondary diabetes 249.4 *[581.81]*
Klauder's (erythema multiforme exudativum) 695.19
Klein-Waardenburg (ptosis-epicanthus) 270.2
Kleine-Levin 327.13
Klinefelter's 758.7
Klippel-Feil (brevicollis) 756.16
Klippel-Trenaunay 759.89
Klumpke (-Déjérine) (injury to brachial plexus at birth) 767.6
Klüver-Bucy (-Terzian) 310.0
Köhler-Pellegrini-Stieda (calcification, knee joint) 726.62
König's 564.89
Korsakoff's (nonalcoholic) 294.0
    alcoholic 291.1
Korsakoff (-Wernicke) (nonalcoholic) 294.0
    alcoholic 291.1
Kostmann's (infantile genetic agranulocytosis) 288.01
Krabbe's
    congenital muscle hypoplasia 756.89
    cutaneocerebral angioma 759.6
Kunkel (lupoid hepatitis) 571.49
labyrinthine 386.50
laceration, broad ligament 620.6
Lambert-Eaton 358.30
    in
        diseases classified elsewhere 358.39
        neoplastic disease 358.31
Landau-Kleffner 345.8
Langdon Down (mongolism) 758.0
Larsen's (flattened facies and multiple congenital dislocations) 755.8

Syndrome—*continued*
  lateral
    cutaneous nerve of thigh 355.1
    medullary (*see also* Disease, cerebrovascular
      acute) 436
  Launois' (pituitary gigantism) 253.0
  Launois-Cléret (adiposogenital dystrophy) 253.8
  Laurence-Moon (-Bardet) -Biedl (obesity,
    polydactyly, and intellectual disabilities)
    759.8
  Lawford's (encephalocutaneous angiomatosis) 759.6
  lazy
    leukocyte 288.09
    posture 728.3
  Lederer-Brill (acquired infectious hemolytic
    anemia) 283.19
  Legg-Calvé-Perthes (osteochondrosis capital
    femoral) 732.1
  Lemiere 451.89
  Lennox's (*see also* Epilepsy) 345.0
  Lennox-Gastaut syndrome 345.0
    with tonic seizures 345.1
  lenticular 275.1
  Léopold-Lévi's (paroxysmal thyroid instability)
    242.9
  Lepore hemoglobin 282.45
  Léri-Weill 756.59
  Leriche's (aortic bifurcation occlusion) 444.09
  Lermoyez's (*see also* Disease, Ménière's)
    386.00
  Lesch-Nyhan (hypoxanthine-guanine-
    phosphoribosyltransferase deficiency) 277.2
  leukoencephalopathy, reversible, posterior 348.5
  Lev's (acquired complete heart block) 426.0
  Levi's (pituitary dwarfism) 253.3
  Lévy-Roussy 334.3
  Lichtheim's (subacute combined sclerosis with
    pernicious anemia) 281.0 *[336.2]*
  Li-Fraumeni V84.01
  Lightwood's (renal tubular acidosis) 588.89
  Lignac (-de Toni) (-Fanconi) (-Debré)
    (cystinosis) 270.0
  Likoff's (angina in menopausal women) 413.9
  liver-kidney 572.4
  Lloyd's 258.1
  lobotomy 310.0
  Löffler's (eosinophilic pneumonitis) 518.3
  Löfgren's (sarcoidosis) 135
  long arm 18 or 21 deletion 758.39
  Looser (-Debray) -Milkman (osteomalacia with
    pseudofractures) 268.2
  Lorain-Levi (pituitary dwarfism) 253.3
  Louis-Bar (ataxia-telangiectasia) 334.8
  low
    atmospheric pressure 993.2
    back 724.2
      psychogenic 306.0
    output (cardiac) (*see also* Failure, heart) 428.9
  Lowe's (oculocerebrorenal dystrophy) 270.8
  Lowe-Terrey-MacLachlan (oculocerebrorenal
    dystrophy) 270.8
  lower radicular, newborn 767.4
  Lown (-Ganong)-Levine (short P-R interval,
    normal QRS complex, and supraventricular
    tachycardia) 426.81
  Lucey-Driscoll (jaundice due to delayed
    conjugation) 774.30
  Luetscher's (dehydration) 276.51
  lumbar vertebral 724.4
  Lutembacher's (atrial septal defect with mitral
    stenosis) 745.5

Syndrome—*continued*
  Lyell's (toxic epidermal necrolysis) 695.15
    due to drug
      correct substance properly administered
        695.15
      overdose or wrong substance given or taken
        977.9
      specified drug—*see* Table of drugs and
        chemicals
  MacLeod's 492.8
  macrogenitosomia praecox 259.8
  macroglobulinemia 273.3
  macrophage activation 288.4
  Maffucci's (dyschondroplasia with
    hemangiomas) 756.4
  Magenblase 306.4
  magnesium-deficiency 781.7
  Mal de Debarquement 780.4
  malabsorption 579.9
    postsurgical 579.3
    spinal fluid 331.3
  malignant carcinoid 259.2
  Mallory-Weiss 530.7
  mandibulofacial dysostosis 756.0
  manic-depressive (*see also* Psychosis, affective)
    296.80
  Mankowsky's (familial dysplastic osteopathy)
    731.2
  maple syrup (urine) 270.3
  Marable's (celiac artery compression) 447.4
  Marchesani (-Weill) (brachymorphism and
    ectopia lentis) 759.89
  Marchiafava-Bignami 341.8
  Marchiafava-Micheli (paroxysmal nocturnal
    hemoglobinuria) 283.2
  Marcus Gunn's (jaw-winking syndrome) 742.8
  Marfan's (arachnodactyly) 759.82
    meaning congenital syphilis 090.49
      with luxation of lens 090.49 *[379.32]*
  Marie's (acromegaly) 253.0
    primary or idiopathic (acropachyderma)
      757.39
    secondary (hypertrophic pulmonary
      osteoarthropathy) 731.2
  Markus-Adie 379.46
  Maroteaux-Lamy (mucopolysaccharidosis VI)
    277.5
  Martin's 715.27
  Martin-Albright (pseudohypoparathyroidism)
    275.49
  Martorell-Fabré (pulseless disease) 446.7
  massive aspiration of newborn 770.18
  Masters-Allen 620.6
  mastocytosis 757.33
  maternal hypotension 669.2
  maternal obesity 646.1
  May (-Hegglin) 288.2
  McArdle (-Schmid) (-Pearson) (glycogenosis V)
    271.0
  McCune-Albright (osteitis fibrosa disseminata)
    756.59
  McQuarrie's (idiopathic familial hypoglycemia)
    251.2
  meconium
    aspiration 770.12
    plug (newborn) NEC 777.1
  median arcuate ligament 447.4
  mediastinal fibrosis 519.3
  Meekeren-Ehlers-Danlos 756.83

Syndrome—*continued*
  Meige (blepharospasm-oromandibular dystonia)
    333.82
  -Milroy (chronic hereditary edema) 757.0
  MELAS (mitochondrial encephalopathy, lactic
    acidosis and stroke-like episodes) 277.87
  Melkersson (-Rosenthal) 351.8
  MEN (multiple endocrine neoplasia)
    type I 258.01
    type IIA 258.02
    type IIB 258.03
  Mende's (ptosis-epicanthus) 270.2
  Mendelson's (resulting from a procedure)
    997.32
    during labor 668.0
    obstetric 668.0
  Ménétrier's (hypertrophic gastritis) 535.2
  Ménière's (*see also* Disease, Ménière's) 386.00
  meningo-eruptive 047.1
  Menkes' 759.89
    glutamic acid 759.89
    maple syrup (urine) disease 270.3
  menopause 627.2
    postartificial 627.4
  menstruation 625.4
  MERRF (myoclonus with epilepsy and with
    ragged red fibers) 277.87
  mesenteric
    artery, superior 557.1
    vascular insufficiency (with gangrene) 557.1
  metabolic 277.7
  metastatic carcinoid 259.2
  Meyenburg-Altherr-Uehlinger 733.99
  Meyer-Schwickerath and Weyers (dysplasia
    oculodentodigitalis) 759.89
  Micheli-Rietti (thalassemia minor) 282.46
  Michotte's 721.5
  micrognathia-glossoptosis 756.0
  microphthalmos (congenital) 759.89
  midbrain 348.89
  middle
    lobe (lung) (right) 518.0
    radicular 353.0
  Miescher's
    familial acanthosis nigricans 701.2
    granulomatosis disciformis 709.3
  Mieten's 759.89
  migraine 346.0
  Mikity-Wilson (pulmonary dysmaturity) 770.7
  Mikulicz's (dryness of mouth, absent or
    decreased lacrimation) 527.1
  milk alkali (milk drinkers') 275.42
  Milkman (-Looser) (osteomalacia with
    pseudofractures) 268.2
  Millard-Gubler 344.89
  Miller-Dieker 758.33
  Miller Fisher's 357.0
  Milles' (encephalocutaneous angiomatosis) 759.6
  Minkowski-Chauffard (*see also* Spherocytosis)
    282.0
  Mirizzi's (hepatic duct stenosis) 576.2
    with calculus, cholelithiasis, or stones—*see*
      Choledocholithiasis
  mitochondrial neurogastrointestinal
    encephalopathy (MNGIE) 277.87
  mitral
    click (-murmur) 785.2
    valve prolapse 424.0
  MNGIE (mitochondrial neurogastrointestinal
    encephalopathy) 277.87

Syndrome—*continued*
  Möbius'
    congenital oculofacial paralysis 352.6
    ophthalmoplegic migraine 346.2
  Mohr's (Types I and II) 759.89
  monofixation 378.34
  Moore's (*see also* Epilepsy) 345.5
  Morel-Moore (hyperostosis frontalis interna) 733.3
  Morel-Morgagni (hyperostosis frontalis interna)
    733.3
  Morgagni (-Stewart-Morel) (hyperostosis
    frontalis interna) 733.3
  Morgagni-Adams-Stokes (syncope with heart
    block) 426.9
  Morquio (-Brailsford) (-Ullrich)
    (mucopolysaccharidosis IV) 277.5
  Morris (testicular feminization) 259.51
  Morton's (foot) (metatarsalgia) (metatarsal
    neuralgia) (neuralgia) (neuroma) (toe) 355.6
  Moschcowitz (-Singer-Symmers) (thrombotic
    thrombocytopenic purpura) 446.6
  Mounier-Kuhn 748.3
    with
      acute exacerbation 494.1
      bronchiectasis 494.0
        with (acute) exacerbation 494.1
      acquired 519.19
        with bronchiectasis 494.0
          with (acute) exacerbation 494.1
  Mucha-Haberman (acute parapsoriasis
    varioliformis) 696.2
  mucocutaneous lymph node (acute) (febrile)
    (infantile) (MCLS) 446.1
  multiple
    deficiency 260
    endocrine neoplasia [MEN]
      type I 258.01
      type IIA 258.02
      type IIB 258.03
    operations 301.51
  Munchausen's 301.51
  Münchmeyer's (exostosis luxurians) 728.11
  Murchison-Sanderson—*see* Disease, Hodgkin's
  myasthenic—*see* Myasthenia, syndrome
  myelodysplastic 238.75
    with 5q deletion 238.74
    high grade with 5q deletion 238.73
    lesions, low grade 238.72
    therapy-related 289.83
  myeloproliferative (chronic) (M9960/1) 238.79
  myofascial pain NEC 729.1
  Naffziger's 353.0
  Nager-de Reynier (dysostosis mandibularis)
    756.0
  nail-patella (hereditary osteo-onychodysplasia)
    756.89
  NARP (neuropathy, ataxia and retinitis
    pigmentosa) 277.87
  Nebécourt's 253.3
  Neill-Dingwall (microencephaly and dwarfism)
    759.89
  nephrotic (*see also* Nephrosis) 581.9
    diabetic 250.4 *[581.81]*
      due to secondary diabetes 249.4 *[581.81]*
  Netherton's (ichthyosiform erythroderma) 757.1
  neurocutaneous 759.6
  neuroleptic malignant 333.92
  Nezelof's (pure alymphocytosis) 279.13
  Niemann-Pick (lipid histiocytosis) 272.7
  Nonne-Milroy-Meige (chronic hereditary
    edema) 757.0
  nonsense 300.16

Syndrome—*continued*
  Noonan's 759.89
  Nothnagel's
    ophthalmoplegia-cerebellar ataxia 378.52
    vasomotor acroparesthesia 443.89
  nucleus ambiguous-hypoglossal 352.6
  OAV (oculoauriculovertebral dysplasia) 756.0
  obesity hypoventilation 278.03
  obsessional 300.3
  oculocutaneous 364.24
  oculomotor 378.81
  oculourethroarticular 099.3
  Ogilvie's (sympathicotonic colon obstruction)
    560.89
  ophthalmoplegia-cerebellar ataxia 378.52
  Oppenheim-Urbach (necrobiosis lipoidica
    diabeticorum) 250.8 *[709.3]*
    due to secondary diabetes 249.8 *[709.3]*
  oral-facial-digital 759.89
  organic
    affective NEC 293.83
      drug-induced 292.84
    anxiety 293.84
    delusional 293.81
      alcohol-induced 291.5
      drug-induced 292.11
      due to or associated with
        arteriosclerosis 290.42
        presenile brain disease 290.12
        senility 290.20
    depressive 293.83
      drug-induced 292.84
      due to or associated with
        arteriosclerosis 290.43
        presenile brain disease 290.13
        senile brain disease 290.21
    hallucinosis 293.82
      drug-induced 292.84
  organic affective 293.83
    induced by drug 292.84
  organic personality 310.1
    induced by drug 292.89
  Ormond's 593.4
  orodigitofacial 759.89
  orthostatic hypotensive-dysautonomic-
    dyskinetic 333.0
  Osler-Weber-Rendu (familial hemorrhagic
    telangiectasia) 448.0
  osteodermopathic hyperostosis 757.39
  osteoporosis-osteomalacia 268.2
  Österreicher-Turner (hereditary
    osteo-onychodysplasia) 756.89
  os trigonum 755.69
  Ostrum-Furst 756.59
  otolith 386.19
  otopalatodigital 759.89
  outlet (thoracic) 353.0
  ovarian remnant 620.8
  Owren's (*see also* Defect, coagulation) 286.3
  OX 758.6
  pacemaker 429.4
  Paget-Schroetter (intermittent venous
    claudication) 453.89
  pain—*see also* Pain
    central 338.0
    chronic 338.4

Syndrome—*continued*
  pain—*continued*
    complex regional 355.9
      type I 337.20
        lower limb 337.22
        specified site NEC 337.29
        upper limb 337.21
      type II
        lower limb 355.71
        upper limb 354.4
    myelopathic 338.0
    thalamic (hypersthetic) 338.0
  painful
    apicocostal vertebral (M8010/3) 162.3
    arc 726.19
    bruising 287.2
    feet 266.2
  Pancoast's (carcinoma, pulmonary apex)
    (M8010/3) 162.3
  panhypopituitary (postpartum) 253.2
  papillary muscle 429.81
    with myocardial infarction 410.8
  Papillon-Léage and Psaume (orodigitofacial
    dysostosis) 759.89
  parabiotic (transfusion)
    donor (twin) 772.0
    recipient (twin) 776.4
  paralysis agitans 332.0
  paralytic 344.9
    specified type NEC 344.89
  Paraneoplastic —*see* condition
  Parinaud's (paralysis of conjugate upward gaze)
    378.81
    oculoglandular 372.02
  Parkes Weber and Dimitri (encephalocutaneous
    angiomatosis) 759.6
  Parkinson's (*see* also Parkinsonism) 332.0
  parkinsonian (*see* also Parkinsonism) 332.0
  Parry's (exophthalmic goiter) 242.0
  Parry-Romberg 349.89
  Parsonage-Aldren-Turner 353.5
  Parsonage-Turner 353.5
  Patau's (trisomy D₁) 758.1
  patella clunk 719.66
  patellofemoral 719.46
  Paterson (-Brown) (-Kelly) (sideropenic
    dysphagia) 280.8
  Payr's (splenic flexure syndrome) 569.89
  pectoral girdle 447.8
  pectoralis minor 447.8
  Pelger-Huët (hereditary hyposegmentation)
    288.2
  pellagra-cerebellar ataxia-renal aminoaciduria
    270.0
  Pellegrini-Stieda 726.62
  pellagroid 265.2
  Pellizzi's (pineal) 259.8
  pelvic congestion (-fibrosis) 625.5
  Pendred's (familial goiter with deaf-mutism)
    243
  Penfield's (*see also* Epilepsy) 345.5
  Penta X 758.81
  peptic ulcer—*see* Ulcer, peptic 533.9
  perabduction 447.8
  periodic 277.31
  periurethral fibrosis 593.4
  persistent fetal circulation 747.83
  Petges-Cléjat (poikilodermatomyositis) 710.3
  Peutz-Jeghers 759.6
  Pfeiffer (acrocephalosyndactyly) 755.55

Syndrome—*continued*
  phantom limb 353.6
  pharyngeal pouch 279.11
  Pick's (pericardial pseudocirrhosis of liver) 423.2
    heart 423.2
    liver 423.2
  Pick-Herxheimer (diffuse idiopathic cutaneous atrophy) 701.8
  Pickwickian (cardiopulmonary obesity) 278.03
  PIE (pulmonary infiltration with eosinophilia) 518.3
  Pierre Marie-Bamberger (hypertrophic pulmonary osteoarthropathy) 731.2
  Pierre Mauriac's (diabetes-dwarfism-obesity) 258.1
  Pierre Robin 756.0
  pigment dispersion, iris 364.53
  pineal 259.8
  pink puffer 492.8
  pituitary 253.0
  placental
    dysfunction 762.2
    insufficiency 762.2
    transfusion 762.3
  plantar fascia 728.71
  plateau iris (without glaucoma) 364.82
    with glaucoma 365.23
  plica knee 727.83
  Plummer-Vinson (sideropenic dysphagia) 280.8
  pluricarential of infancy 260
  plurideficiency of infancy 260
  pluriglandular (compensatory) 258.8
  Poland 756.81
  polycarential of infancy 260
  polyglandular 258.8
  polysplenia 759.0
  pontine 433.8
  popliteal
    artery entrapment 447.8
    web 756.89
  postartificial menopause 627.4
  postcardiac injury
    postcardiotomy 429.4
    postmyocardial infarction 411.0
  postcardiotomy 429.4
  post-chemoembolization—code to associated conditions
  postcholecystectomy 576.0
  postcommissurotomy 429.4
  postconcussional 310.2
  postcontusional 310.2
  postencephalitic 310.89
  posterior
    cervical sympathetic 723.2
    fossa compression 348.4
    inferior cerebellar artery (*see also* Disease, cerebrovascular, acute) 436
    reversible encephalopathy (PRES) 348.39
  postgastrectomy (dumping) 564.2
  post-gastric surgery 564.2
  posthepatitis 780.79
  postherpetic (neuralgia) (zoster) 053.19
    geniculate ganglion 053.11
    ophthalmica 053.19
  postimmunization—*see* Complications, vaccination
  postinfarction 411.0
  postinfluenza (asthenia) 780.79
  postirradiation 990

Syndrome—*continued*
  postlaminectomy 722.80
    cervical, cervicothoracic 722.81
    lumbar, lumbosacral 722.83
    thoracic, thoracolumbar 722.82
  postleukotomy 310.0
  postlobotomy 310.0
  postmastectomy lymphedema 457.0
  postmature (of newborn) 766.22
  postmyocardial infarction 411.0
  postoperative NEC 998.9
    blind loop 579.2
  postpartum panhypopituitary 253.2
  postperfusion NEC 999.89
    bone marrow 996.85
  postpericardiotomy 429.4
  postphlebitic (asymptomatic) 459.10
    with
      complications NEC 459.19
      inflammation 459.12
        and ulcer 459.13
      stasis dermatitis 459.12
        with ulcer 459.13
      ulcer 459.11
        with inflammation 459.13
  postpolio (myelitis) 138
  postvagotomy 564.2
  postvalvulotomy 429.4
  postviral (asthenia) NEC 780.79
  Potain's (gastrectasis with dyspepsia) 536.1
  potassium intoxication 276.7
  Potter's 753.0
  Prader (-Labhart) -Willi (-Fanconi) 759.81
  preinfarction 411.1
  preleukemic 238.75
  premature senility 259.8
  premenstrual 625.4
  premenstrual tension 625.4
  pre ulcer 536.9
  Prinzmetal-Massumi (anterior chest wall syndrome) 786.52
  Profichet's 729.90
  progeria 259.8
  progressive pallidal degeneration 333.0
  prolonged gestation 766.22
  Proteus (dermal hypoplasia) 757.39
  prune belly 756.71
  prurigo-asthma 691.8
  pseudocarpal tunnel (sublimis) 354.0
  pseudohermaphroditism-virilism-hirsutism 255.2
  pseudoparalytica 358.00
  pseudo-Turner's 759.89
  psycho-organic 293.9
    acute 293.0
    anxiety type 293.84
    depressive type 293.83
    hallucinatory type 293.82
    nonpsychotic severity 310.1
      specified focal (partial) NEC 310.89
    paranoid type 293.81
    specified type NEC 293.89
    subacute 293.1
  pterygolymphangiectasia 758.6
  ptosis-epicanthus 270.2
  pulmonary
    arteriosclerosis 416.0
    hypoperfusion (idiopathic) 769
    renal (hemorrhagic) 446.21
  pulseless 446.7
  Putnam-Dana (subacute combined sclerosis with pernicious anemia) 281.0 *[336.2]*

Syndrome—*continued*
  pyloroduodenal 537.89
  pyramidopallidonigral 332.0
  pyriformis 355.0
  QT interval prolongation 426.82
  radicular NEC 729.2
    lower limbs 724.4
    upper limbs 723.4
      newborn 767.4
  Raeder-Harbitz (pulseless disease) 446.7
  Ramsay Hunt's
    dyssynergia cerebellaris myoclonica 334.2
    herpetic geniculate ganglionitis 053.11
  rapid time-zone change 327.35
  Raymond (-Céstan) 433.8
  Raynaud's (paroxysmal digital cyanosis) 443.0
  RDS (respiratory distress syndrome, newborn)
    769
  Refsum's (heredopathia atactica
    polyneuritiformis) 356.3
  Reichmann's (gastrosuccorrhea) 536.8
  Reifenstein's (hereditary familial
    hypogonadism, male) 259.51
  Reilly's (*see also* Neuropathy, peripheral,
    autonomic) 337.9
  Reiter's 099.3
  renal glomerulohyalinosis-diabetic 250.4
    [581.81]
    due to secondary diabetes 249.4 [581.81]
  Rendu-Osler-Weber (familial hemorrhagic
    telangiectasia) 448.0
  renofacial (congenital biliary fibroangiomatosis)
    753.0
  Rénon-Delille 253.8
  respiratory distress (idiopathic) (newborn) 769
    adult (following trauma and surgery) 518.52
      specified NEC 518.82
    type II 770.6
  restless legs (RLS) 333.94
  retinoblastoma (familial) 190.5
  retraction (Duane's) 378.71
  retroperitoneal fibrosis 593.4
  retroviral seroconversion (acute) V08
  Rett's 330.8
  Reye's 331.81
  Reye-Sheehan (postpartum pituitary necrosis)
    253.2
  Riddoch's (visual disorientation) 368.16
  Ridley's (*see also* Failure, ventricular, left)
    428.1
  Rieger's (mesodermal dysgenesis, anterior
    ocular segment) 743.44
  Rietti-Greppi-Micheli (thalassemia minor)
    282.46
  right ventricular obstruction—*see* Failure heart
  Riley-Day (familial dysautonomia) 742.8
  Robin's 756.0
  Rokitansky-Kuster-Hauser (congenital absence,
    vagina) 752.45
  Romano-Ward (prolonged QT interval
    syndrome) 426.82
  Romberg's 349.89
  Rosen-Castleman-Liebow (pulmonary
    proteinosis) 516.0
  rotator cuff, shoulder 726.10
  Roth's 355.1
  Rothmund's (congenital poikiloderma) 757.33
  Rotor's (idiopathic hyperbilirubinemia) 277.4
  Roussy-Lévy 334.3
  Roy (-Jutras) (acropachyderma) 757.39

Syndrome—*continued*
  rubella (congenital) 771.0
  Rubinstein-Taybi's (brachydactylia, short
    stature, and intellectual disabilities) 759.89
  Rud's (mental deficiency, epilepsy, and
    infantilism) 759.89
  Ruiter-Pompen (-Wyers) (angiokeratoma
    corporis diffusum) 272.7
  Runge's (postmaturity) 766.22
  Russell (-Silver) (congenital hemihypertrophy
    and short stature) 759.89
  Rytand-Lipsitch (complete atrioventricular
    block) 426.0
  sacralization-scoliosis-sciatica 756.15
  sacroiliac 724.6
  Saenger's 379.46
  salt
    depletion (*see also* Disease, renal) 593.9
      due to heat NEC 992.8
        causing heat exhaustion or prostration
          992.4
    low (*see also* Disease, renal) 593.9
    salt-losing (*see also* Disease, renal) 593.9
  Sanfilippo's (mucopolysaccharidosis III) 277.5
  Scaglietti-Dagnini (acromegalic
    macrospondylitis) 253.0
  scalded skin 695.81
  scalenus anticus (anterior) 353.0
  scapulocostal 354.8
  scapuloperoneal 359.1
  scapulovertebral 723.4
  Schaumann's (sarcoidosis) 135
  Scheie's (mucopolysaccharidosis IS) 277.5
  Scheuthauer-Marie-Sainton (cleidocranialis
    dysostosis) 755.59
  Schirmer's (encephalocutaneous angiomatosis)
    759.6
  schizophrenic, of childhood NEC (*see also*
    Psychosis, childhood) 299.9
  Schmidt's
    sphallo-pharyngo-laryngeal hemiplegia 352.6
    thyroid-adrenocortical insufficiency 258.1
    vagoaccessory 352.6
  Schneider's 047.9
  Schnitzler 273.1
  Scholte's (malignant carcinoid) 259.2
  Scholz (-Bielschowsky-Henneberg) 330.0
  Schroeder's (endocrine-hypertensive) 255.3
  Schüller-Christian (chronic histiocytosis X)
    277.89
  Schultz's (agranulocytosis) 288.09
  Schwachman's—*see* Syndrome, Shwachman's
  Schwartz (-Jampel) 359.23
  Schwartz-Bartter (inappropriate secretion of
    antidiuretic hormone) 253.6
  Scimitar (anomalous venous drainage, right lung
    to inferior vena cave) 747.49
  sclerocystic ovary 256.4
  sea-blue histiocyte 272.7
  Seabright-Bantam (pseudohypoparathyroidism)
    275.49
  Seckel's 759.89
  Secretan's (posttraumatic edema) 782.3
  secretoinhibitor (keratoconjunctivitis sicca)
    710.2
  Seeligmann's (ichthyosis congenita) 757.1
  Senear-Usher (pemphigus erythematosus) 694.4
  senilism 259.8
  seroconversion, retroviral (acute) V08
  serotonin 333.99

Syndrome—*continued*

serous meningitis 348.2
Sertoli cell (germinal aplasia) 606.0
sex chromosome mosaic 758.81
Sézary's (reticulosis) (M9701/3) 202.2
shaken infant 995.55
Shaver's (bauxite pneumoconiosis) 503
Sheehan's (postpartum pituitary necrosis) 253.2
shock (traumatic) 958.4
    kidney 584.5
        following crush injury 958.5
    lung 518.82
        related to trauma and surgery 518.52
    neurogenic 308.9
    psychic 308.9
Shone's 746.84
short
    bowel 579.3
    P-R interval 426.81
shoulder-arm (*see also* Neuropathy, peripheral, autonomic) 337.9
shoulder-girdle 723.4
shoulder-hand (*see also* Neuropathy, peripheral, autonomic) 337.9
Shwachman's 288.02
Shy-Drager (orthostatic hypotension with multisystem degeneration) 333.0
Sicard's 352.6
sicca (keratoconjunctivitis) 710.2
sick
    cell 276.1
    cilia 759.89
    sinus 427.81
sideropenic 280.8
Siemens'
    ectodermal dysplasia 757.31
    keratosis follicularis spinulosa (decalvans) 757.39
Silfverskiöld's (osteochondrodystrophy, extremities) 756.50
Silver's (congenital hemihypertrophy and short stature) 759.89
Silvestroni-Bianco (thalassemia minima) 282.46
Simons' (progressive lipodystrophy) 272.6
sinus tarsi 726.79
sinusitis-bronchiectasis-situs inversus 759.3
Sipple's (medullary thyroid carcinoma-pheochromocytoma) 258.02
Sjögren (-Gougerot) (keratoconjunctivitis sicca) 710.2
    with lung involvement 710.2 [517.8]
Sjögren-Larsson (ichthyosis congenita) 757.1
SJS-TEN (Stevens-Johnson syndrome-toxic epidermal necrolysis overlap) 695.14
Slocumb's 255.3
Sluder's 337.09
Smith-Lemli-Opitz (cerebrohepatorenal syndrome) 759.89
Smith-Magenis 758.33
smokers' 305.1
Sneddon-Wilkinson (subcorneal pustular dermatosis) 694.1
Sotos' (cerebral gigantism) 253.0
South African cardiomyopathy 425.2
spasmodic
    upward movement, eyes(s) 378.82
    winking 307.20
Spens' (syncope with heart block) 426.9
spherophakia-brachymorphia 759.89

Syndrome—*continued*

spinal cord injury—*see also* Injury, spinal, by site
    with fracture, vertebra—*see* Fracture, vertebra, by site, with spinal cord injury
    cervical—*see* Injury, spinal, cervical
    fluid malabsorption (acquired) 331.3
splenic
    agenesis 759.0
    flexure 569.89
    neutropenia 289.53
    sequestration 289.52
Spurway's (brittle bones and blue sclera) 756.51
staphylococcal scalded skin 695.81
Stein's (polycystic ovary) 256.4
Stein-Leventhal (polycystic ovary) 256.4
Steinbrocker's (*see also* Neuropathy, peripheral, autonomic) 337.9
Stevens-Johnson (erythema multiforme exudativum) 695.13
    toxic epidermal necrolysis overlap (SJS-TEN overlap syndrome) 695.14
Stewart-Morel (hyperostosis frontalis interna) 733.3
Stickler 759.89
stiff-baby 759.89
stiff-man 333.91
Still's (juvenile rheumatoid arthritis) 714.30
Still-Felty (rheumatoid arthritis with splenomegaly and leukopenia) 714.1
Stilling-Türk-Duane (ocular retraction syndrome) 378.71
Stojano's (subcostal) 098.86
Stokes (-Adams) (syncope with heart block) 426.9
Stokvis-Talma (enterogenous cyanosis) 289.7
stone heart (*see also* Failure, ventricular, left) 428.1
straight-back 756.19
stroke (*see also* Disease, cerebrovascular, acute) 436
    little 435.9
Sturge-Kalischer-Weber (encephalotrigeminal angiomatosis) 759.6
Sturge-Weber (-Dimitri) (encephalocutaneous angiomatosis) 759.6
subclavian-carotid obstruction (chronic) 446.7
subclavian steal 435.2
subcoracoid-pectoralis minor 447.8
subcostal 098.86
    nerve compression 354.8
subperiosteal hematoma 267
subphrenic interposition 751.4
sudden infant death (SIDS) 798.0
Sudeck's 733.7
Sudeck-Leriche 733.7
superior
    cerebellar artery (*see also* Disease, cerebrovascular, acute) 436
    mesenteric artery 557.1
    pulmonary sulcus (tumor) (M8010/3) 162.3
    semi-circular canal dehiscence 386.8
    vena cava 459.2
suprarenal cortical 255.3
supraspinatus 726.10
Susac 348.39
swallowed blood 777.3
sweat retention 705.1
Sweet's (acute febrile neutrophilic dermatosis) 695.89
Swyer-James (unilateral hyperlucent lung) 492.8

Syndrome—*continued*
Swyer's (XY pure gonadal dysgenesis) 752.7
Symonds' 348.2
sympathetic
  cervical paralysis 337.09
  pelvic 625.5
syndactylic oxycephaly 755.55
syphilitic-cardiovascular 093.89
systemic
  fibrosclerosing 710.8
  inflammatory response (SIRS) 995.90
    due to
      infectious process 995.91
        with acute organ dysfunction 995.92
      non-infectious process 995.93
        with acute organ dysfunction 995.94
systolic click (-murmur) 785.2
Tabagism 305.1
tachycardia-bradycardia 427.81
Takayasu (-Onishi) (pulseless disease) 446.7
Takotsubo 429.83
Tapia's 352.6
tarsal tunnel 355.5
Taussig-Bing (transposition, aorta and
  overriding pulmonary artery) 745.11
Taybi's (otopalatodigital) 759.89
Taylor's 625.5
teething 520.7
tegmental 344.89
telangiectasis-pigmentation-cataract 757.33
temporal 383.02
  lobectomy behavior 310.0
temporomandibular joint-pain-dysfunction
  [TMJ] NEC 524.60
  specified NEC 524.69
Terry's (*see also* Retinopathy of prematurity)
  362.21
testicular feminization 259.51
testis, nonvirilizing 257.8
tethered (spinal) cord 742.59
thalamic 338.0
Thibierge-Weissenbach (cutaneous systemic
  sclerosis) 710.1
Thiele 724.6
thoracic outlet (compression) 353.0
thoracogenous rheumatic (hypertrophic
  pulmonary osteoarthropathy) 731.2
Thorn's (*see also* Disease, renal) 593.9
Thorson-Biörck (malignant carcinoid) 259.2
thrombopenia-hemangioma 287.39
thyroid-adrenocortical insufficiency 258.1
Tietze's 733.6
time-zone (rapid) 327.35
Tobias' (carcinoma, pulmonary apex)
  (M8010/3) 162.3
toilet seat 926.0
Tolosa-Hunt 378.55
Toni-Fanconi (cystinosis) 270.0
Touraine's (hereditary osteo-onychodysplasia)
  756.89
Touraine-Solente-Golé (acropachyderma)
  757.39
toxic
  oil 710.5
  shock 040.82
transfusion
  fetal-maternal 772.0
  twin
    donor (infant) 772.0
    recipient (infant) 776.4
transient left ventricular apical ballooning 429.83

Syndrome—*continued*
Treacher Collins' (incomplete mandibulofacial
  dysostosis) 756.0
trigeminal plate 259.8
triple X female 758.81
trisomy NEC 758.5
  13 or D_1 758.1
  16-18 or E 758.2
  18 or E_3 758.2
  20 758.5
  21 or G (mongolism) 758.0
  22 or G (mongolism) 758.0
  G 758.0
Troisier-Hanot-Chauffard (bronze diabetes) 275.01
tropical wet feet 991.4
Trousseau's (thrombophlebitis migrans visceral
  cancer) 453.1
tumor lysis (following antineoplastic drug
  therapy) (spontaneous) 277.88
Türk's (ocular retraction syndrome) 378.71
Turner's 758.6
Turner-Varny 758.6
Twiddler's (due to)
  automatic implantable defibrillator 996.04
  pacemaker 996.01
twin-to-twin transfusion 762.3
  recipient twin 776.4
Uehlinger's (acropachyderma) 757.39
Ullrich (-Bonnevie) (-Turner) 758.6
Ullrich-Feichtiger 759.89
underwater blast injury (abdominal) (*see also*
  Injury, internal, abdomen) 868.00
universal joint, cervix 620.6
Unverricht (-Lundborg) 345.1
Unverricht-Wagner (dermatomyositis) 710.3
upward gaze 378.81
Urbach-Oppenheim (necrobiosis lipoidica
  diabeticorum) 250.8 *[709.3]*
  due to secondary diabetes 249.8 *[709.3]*
Urbach-Wiethe (lipoid proteinosis) 272.8
uremia, chronic 585.9
urethral 597.81
urethro-oculoarticular 099.3
urethro-oculosynovial 099.3
urohepatic 572.4
uveocutaneous 364.24
uveomeningeal, uveomeningitis 363.22
vagohypoglossal 352.6
vagovagal 780.2
van Buchem's (hyperostosis corticalis) 733.3
van der Hoeve's (brittle bones and blue sclera,
  deafness) 756.51
van der Hoeve-Halbertsma-Waardenburg
  (ptosis-epicanthus) 270.2
van der Hoeve-Waardenburg-Gualdi
  (ptosis-epicanthus) 270.2
van Neck-Odelberg (juvenile osteochondrosis)
  732.1
vanishing twin 651.33
vascular splanchnic 557.0
vasomotor 443.9
vasovagal 780.2
VATER 759.89
Velo-cardio-facial 758.32
vena cava (inferior) (superior) (obstruction)
  459.2
Verbiest's (claudicatio intermittens spinalis)
  435.1
Vernet's 352.6

Syndrome—*continued*
vertebral
  artery 435.1
    compression 721.1
  lumbar 724.4
  steal 435.1
vertebrogenic (pain) 724.5
vertiginous NEC 386.9
video display tube 723.8
Villaret's 352.6
Vinson-Plummer (sideropenic dysphagia) 280.8
virilizing adrenocortical hyperplasia, congenital 255.2
virus, viral 079.99
visceral larval migrans 128.0
visual disorientation 368.16
vitamin B$_6$ deficiency 266.1
vitreous touch 997.99
Vogt's (corpus striatum) 333.71
Vogt-Koyanagi 364.24
Volkmann's 958.6
von Bechterew-Strümpell (ankylosing spondylitis) 720.0
von Graefe's 378.72
von Hippel-Lindau (angiomatosis retinocerebellosa) 759.6
von Schroetter's (intermittent venous claudication) 453.89
von Willebrand (-Jürgens) (angiohemophilia) 286.4
Waardenburg-Klein (ptosis epicanthus) 270.2
Wagner (-Unverricht) (dermatomyositis) 710.3
Waldenström's (macroglobulinemia) 273.3
Waldenström-Kjellberg (sideropenic dysphagia) 280.8
Wallenberg's (posterior inferior cerebellar artery) (*see also* Disease, cerebrovascular, acute) 436
Waterhouse (-Friderichsen) 036.3
water retention 276.69
Weber's 344.89
Weber-Christian (nodular nonsuppurative panniculitis) 729.30
Weber-Cockayne (epidermolysis bullosa) 757.39
Weber-Dimitri (encephalocutaneous angiomatosis) 759.6
Weber-Gubler 344.89
Weber-Leyden 344.89
Weber-Osler (familial hemorrhagic telangiectasia) 448.0
Wegener's (necrotizing respiratory granulomatosis) 446.4
Weill-Marchesani (brachymorphism and ectopia lentis) 759.89
Weingarten's (tropical eosinophilia) 518.3
Weiss-Baker (carotid sinus syncope) 337.01
Weissenbach-Thibierge (cutaneous systemic sclerosis) 710.1
Werdnig-Hoffmann 335.0
Werlhof-Wichmann (*see also* Purpura, thrombocytopenic) 287.39
Wermer's (polyendocrine adenomatosis) 258.01
Werner's (progeria adultorum) 259.8
Wernicke's (nonalcoholic) (superior hemorrhagic polioencephalitis) 265.1

Syndrome—*continued*
Wernicke-Korsakoff (nonalcoholic) 294.0
  alcoholic 291.1
Westphal-Strümpell (hepatolenticular degeneration) 275.1
wet
  brain (alcoholic) 303.9
  feet (maceration) (tropical) 991.4
  lung
    adult 518.52
    newborn 770.6
whiplash 847.0
Whipple's (intestinal lipodystrophy) 040.2
"whistling face" (craniocarpotarsal dystrophy) 759.89
Widal (-Abrami) (acquired hemolytic jaundice) 283.9
Wilkie's 557.1
Wilkinson-Sneddon (subcorneal pustular dermatosis) 694.1
Willan-Plumbe (psoriasis) 696.1
Willebrand (-Jürgens) (angiohemophilia) 286.4
Willi-Prader (hypogenital dystrophy with diabetic tendency) 759.81
Wilson's (hepatolenticular degeneration) 275.1
Wilson-Mikity 770.7
Wiskott-Aldrich (eczema-thrombocytopenia) 279.12
withdrawal
  alcohol 291.81
  drug 292.0
  infant of dependent mother 779.5
Woakes' (ethmoiditis) 471.1
Wolff-Parkinson-White (anomalous atrioventricular excitation) 426.7
Wright's (hyperabduction) 447.8
X
  cardiac 413.9
  dysmetabolic 277.7
xiphoidalgia 733.99
XO 758.6
XXX 758.81
XXXXY 758.81
XXY 758.7
yellow vernix (placental dysfunction) 762.2
Zahorsky's 074.0
Zellweger 277.86
Zieve's (jaundice, hyperlipemia and hemolytic anemia) 571.1
Zollinger-Ellison (gastric hypersecretion with pancreatic islet cell tumor) 251.5
Zuelzer-Ogden (nutritional megaloblastic anemia) 281.2
Synechia (iris) (pupil) 364.70
  anterior 364.72
    peripheral 364.73
  intrauterine (traumatic) 621.5
  posterior 364.71
  vulvae, congenital 752.49
Synesthesia (*see also* Disturbance, sensation) 782.0
Synodontia 520.2
Synophthalmus 759.89
Synorchidism 752.89
Synorchism 752.89
Synostosis (congenital) 756.59
  astragaloscaphoid 755.67
  radioulnar 755.53
  talonavicular (bar) 755.67
  tarsal 755.67
Synovial —*see* condition

Synovioma (M9040/3)—*see also* Neoplasm, connective tissue, malignant
  benign (M9040/3)—*see* Neoplasm, connective tissue, benign
Synoviosarcoma (M9040/3)—*see* Neoplasm, connective tissue, malignant
Synovitis (*see also* Tenosynovitis) 727.00
  chronic crepitant, wrist 727.2
  due to crystals—*see* Arthritis, due to crystals
  gonococcal 098.51
  gouty 274.00
  specified NEC 727.09
  syphilitic 095.7
    congenital 090.0
  traumatic, current—*see* Sprain, by site
  tuberculous—*see* Tuberculosis, synovitis
  villonodular 719.20
    ankle 719.27
    elbow 719.22
    foot 719.27
    hand 719.24
    hip 719.25
    knee 719.26
    multiple sites 719.29
    pelvic region 719.25
    shoulder (region) 719.21
    specified site NEC 719.28
    wrist 719.23
Syphilide 091.3
  congenital 090.0
  newborn 090.0
  tubercular 095.8
    congenital 090.0
Syphilis, syphilitic (acquired) 097.9
  with lung involvement 095.1
  abdomen (late) 095.2
  acoustic nerve 094.86
  adenopathy (secondary) 091.4
  adrenal (gland) 095.8
    with cortical hypofunction 095.8
  age under 2 years NEC (*see also* Syphilis, congenital) 090.9
    acquired 097.9
  alopecia (secondary) 091.82
  anemia 095.8
  aneurysm (artery) (ruptured) 093.89
    aorta 093.0
    central nervous system 094.89
    congenital 090.5
  anus 095.8
    primary 091.1
    secondary 091.3
  aorta, aortic (arch) (abdominal) (insufficiency) (pulmonary) (regurgitation) (stenosis) (thoracic) 093.89
    aneurysm 093.0
  arachnoid (adhesive) 094.2
  artery 093.89
    cerebral 094.89
    spinal 094.89
  arthropathy (neurogenic) (tabetic) 094.0 *[713.5]*
  asymptomatic—*see* Syphilis, latent
  ataxia, locomotor (progressive) 094.0
  atrophoderma maculatum 091.3
  auricular fibrillation 093.89
  Bell's palsy 094.89
  bladder 095.8
  bone 095.5
    secondary 091.61
  brain 094.89
  breast 095.8

Syphilis, syphilitic—*continued*
  bronchus 095.8
  bubo 091.0
  bulbar palsy 094.89
  bursa (late) 095.7
  cardiac decompensation 093.89
  cardiovascular (early) (late) (primary) (secondary) (tertiary) 093.9
    specified type and site NEC 093.89
  causing death under 2 years of age (*see also* Syphilis, congenital) 090.9
    stated to be acquired NEC 097.9
  central nervous system (any site) (early) (late) (latent) (primary) (recurrent) (relapse) (secondary) (tertiary) 094.9
    with
      ataxia 094.0
      paralysis, general 094.1
        juvenile 090.40
      paresis (general) 094.1
        juvenile 090.40
      tabes (dorsalis) 094.0
        juvenile 090.40
      taboparesis 094.1
        juvenile 090.40
    aneurysm (ruptured) 094.87
    congenital 090.40
    juvenile 090.40
    remission in (sustained) 094.9
    serology doubtful, negative, or positive 094.9
    specified nature or site NEC 094.89
    vascular 094.89
  cerebral 094.89
    meningovascular 094.2
    nerves 094.89
    sclerosis 094.89
    thrombosis 094.89
  cerebrospinal 094.89
    tabetic 094.0
  cerebrovascular 094.89
  cervix 095.8
  chancre (multiple) 091.0
    extragenital 091.2
    Rollet's 091.0
  Charcot's joint 094.0 *[713.5]*
  choked disc 094.89 *[377.00]*
  chorioretinitis 091.51
    congenital 090.0 *[363.13]*
    late 094.83
  choroiditis 091.51
    congenital 090.0 *[363.13]*
    late 094.83
    prenatal 090.0 *[363.13]*
  choroidoretinitis (secondary) 091.51
    congenital 090.0 *[363.13]*
    late 094.83
  ciliary body (secondary) 091.52
    late 095.8 *[364.11]*
  colon (late) 095.8
  combined sclerosis 094.89
  complicating pregnancy, childbirth or puerperium 647.0
    affecting fetus or newborn 760.2
  condyloma (latum) 091.3

Syphilis, syphilitic—*continued*
congenital 090.9
  with
    encephalitis 090.41
    paresis (general) 090.40
    tabes (dorsalis) 090.40
    taboparesis 090.40
  chorioretinitis, choroiditis 090.0 *[363.13]*
  early or less than 2 years after birth NEC 090.2
    with manifestations 090.0
    latent (without manifestations) 090.1
      negative spinal fluid test 090.1
      serology, positive 090.1
    symptomatic 090.0
  interstitial keratitis 090.3
  juvenile neurosyphilis 090.40
  late or 2 years or more after birth NEC 090.7
    chorioretinitis, choroiditis 090.5 *[363.13]*
    interstitial keratitis 090.3
    juvenile neurosyphilis NEC 090.40
    latent (without manifestations) 090.6
      negative spinal fluid test 090.6
      serology, positive 090.6
    symptomatic or with manifestations NEC
      090.5
      interstitial keratitis 090.3
conjugal 097.9
  tabes 094.0
conjunctiva 095.8 *[372.10]*
contact V01.6
cord, bladder 094.0
cornea, late 095.8 *[370.59]*
coronary (artery) 093.89
  sclerosis 093.89
coryza 095.8
  congenital 090.0
cranial nerve 094.89
cutaneous—*see* Syphilis, skin
dacryocystitis 095.8
degeneration, spinal cord 094.89
d'emblée 095.8
dementia 094.1
  paralytica 094.1
  juvenilis 090.40
destruction of bone 095.5
dilatation, aorta 093.0
due to blood transfusion 097.9
dura mater 094.89
ear 095.8
  inner 095.8
    nerve (eighth) 094.86
    neurorecurrence 094.86
early NEC 091.0
  cardiovascular 093.9
  central nervous system 094.9
    paresis 094.1
    tabes 094.0
  latent (without manifestations) (less than 2
    years after infection) 092.9
    negative spinal fluid test 092.9
    serological relapse following treatment 092.0
    serology positive 092.9
  paresis 094.1
  relapse (treated, untreated) 091.7
  skin 091.3
  symptomatic NEC 091.89
    extragenital chancre 091.2
    primary, except extragenital chancre 091.0
    secondary (*see also* Syphilis, secondary) 091.3
      relapse (treated, untreated) 091.7
  tabes 094.0
  ulcer 091.3

Syphilis, syphilitic—*continued*
eighth nerve 094.86
endemic, nonvenereal 104.0
endocarditis 093.20
  aortic 093.22
  mitral 093.21
  pulmonary 093.24
  tricuspid 093.23
epididymis (late) 095.8
epiglottis 095.8
epiphysitis (congenital) 090.0
esophagus 095.8
Eustachian tube 095.8
exposure to V01.6
eye 095.8 *[363.13]*
  neuromuscular mechanism 094.85
eyelid 095.8 *[373.5]*
  with gumma 095.8 *[373.5]*
  ptosis 094.89
fallopian tube 095.8
fracture 095.5
gallbladder (late) 095.8
gastric 095.8
  crisis 094.0
  polyposis 095.8
general 097.9
  paralysis 094.1
    juvenile 090.40
genital (primary) 091.0
glaucoma 095.8
gumma (late) NEC 095.9
  cardiovascular system 093.9
  central nervous system 094.9
  congenital 090.5
  heart or artery 093.89
heart 093.89
  block 093.89
  decompensation 093.89
  disease 093.89
  failure 093.89
  valve (*see also* Syphilis, endocarditis) 093.20
hemianesthesia 094.89
hemianopsia 095.8
hemiparesis 094.89
hemiplegia 094.89
hepatic artery 093.89
hepatitis 095.3
hepatomegaly 095.3
  congenital 090.0
hereditaria tarda (*see also* Syphilis, congenital,
  late) 090.7
hereditary (*see also* Syphilis, congenital) 090.9
  interstitial keratitis 090.3
Hutchinson's teeth 090.5
hyalitis 095.8
inactive—*see* Syphilis, latent
infantum NEC (*see also* Syphilis, congenital)
  090.9
inherited—*see* Syphilis, congenital
internal ear 095.8
intestine (late) 095.8
iris, iritis (secondary) 091.52
  late 095.8 *[364.11]*
joint (late) 095.8
keratitis (congenital) (early) (interstitial) (late)
  (parenchymatous) (punctata profunda) 090.3
kidney 095.4
lacrimal apparatus 095.8
laryngeal paralysis 095.8
larynx 095.8

Syphilis, syphilitic—*continued*
late 097.0
  cardiovascular 093.9
  central nervous system 094.9
  latent or 2 years or more after infection
    (without manifestations) 096
    negative spinal fluid test 096
    serology positive 096
  paresis 094.1
  specified site NEC 095.8
  symptomatic or with symptoms 095.9
  tabes 094.0
latent 097.1
  central nervous system 094.9
  date of infection unspecified 097.1
  early or less than 2 years after infection 092.9
  late or 2 years or more after infection 096
  serology
    doubtful
      follow-up of latent syphilis 097.1
        central nervous system 094.9
        date of infection unspecified 097.1
        early or less than 2 years after infection
          092.9
        late or 2 years or more after infection
          096
      positive, only finding 097.1
        date of infection unspecified 097.1
        early or less than 2 years after infection
          097.1
        late or 2 years or more after infection 097.1
lens 095.8
leukoderma 091.3
  late 095.8
lienis 095.8
lip 091.3
  chancre 091.2
  late 095.8
  primary 091.2
Lissauer's paralysis 094.1
liver 095.3
  secondary 091.62
locomotor ataxia 094.0
lung 095.1
lymphadenitis (secondary) 091.4
lymph gland (early) (secondary) 091.4
  late 095.8
macular atrophy of skin 091.3
  striated 095.8
maternal, affecting fetus or newborn 760.2
  manifest syphilis in newborn—*see* Syphilis,
    congenital
mediastinum (late) 095.8
meninges (adhesive) (basilar) (brain) (spinal
  cord) 094.2
meningitis 094.2
  acute 091.81
  congenital 090.42
meningoencephalitis 094.2
meningovascular 094.2
  congenital 090.49
mesarteritis 093.89
  brain 094.89
  spine 094.89
middle ear 095.8
mitral stenosis 093.21
monoplegia 094.89
mouth (secondary) 091.3
  late 095.8
mucocutaneous 091.3
  late 095.8

Syphilis, syphilitic—*continued*
mucous
  membrane 091.3
    late 095.8
  patches 091.3
    congenital 090.0
mulberry molars 090.5
muscle 095.6
myocardium 093.82
myositis 095.6
nasal sinus 095.8
neonatorum NEC (*see also* Syphilis, congenital)
  090.9
nerve palsy (any cranial nerve) 094.89
nervous system, central 094.9
neuritis 095.8
  acoustic nerve 094.86
neurorecidive of retina 094.83
neuroretinitis 094.85
newborn (*see also* Syphilis, congenital) 090.9
nodular superficial 095.8
nonvenereal, endemic 104.0
nose 095.8
  saddle back deformity 090.5
  septum 095.8
    perforated 095.8
occlusive arterial disease 093.89
ophthalmic 095.8 *[363.13]*
ophthalmoplegia 094.89
optic nerve (atrophy) (neuritis) (papilla) 094.84
orbit (late) 095.8
orchitis 095.8
organic 097.9
osseous (late) 095.5
osteochondritis (congenital) 090.0
osteoporosis 095.5
ovary 095.8
oviduct 095.8
palate 095.8
  gumma 095.8
  perforated 090.5
pancreas (late) 095.8
pancreatitis 095.8
paralysis 094.89
  general 094.1
  juvenile 090.40
paraplegia 094.89
paresis (general) 094.1
  juvenile 090.40
paresthesia 094.89
Parkinson's disease or syndrome 094.82
paroxysmal tachycardia 093.89
pemphigus (congenital) 090.0
penis 091.0
  chancre 091.0
  late 095.8
pericardium 093.81
perichondritis, larynx 095.8
periosteum 095.5
  congenital 090.0
  early 091.61
  secondary 091.61
peripheral nerve 095.8
petrous bone (late) 095.5
pharynx 095.8
  secondary 091.3
pituitary (gland) 095.8
placenta 095.8
pleura (late) 095.8
pneumonia, white 090.0
pontine (lesion) 094.89

Syphilis, syphilitic—*continued*
portal vein 093.89
primary NEC 091.2
  anal 091.1
  and secondary (*see also* Syphilis, secondary)
    091.9
  cardiovascular 093.9
  central nervous system 094.9
  extragenital chancre NEC 091.2
  fingers 091.2
  genital 091.0
  lip 091.2
  specified site NEC 091.2
  tonsils 091.2
prostate 095.8
psychosis (intracranial gumma) 094.89
ptosis (eyelid) 094.89
pulmonary (late) 095.1
  artery 093.89
pulmonum 095.1
pyelonephritis 095.4
recently acquired, symptomatic NEC 091.89
rectum 095.8
respiratory tract 095.8
retina
  late 094.83
  neurorecidive 094.83
retrobulbar neuritis 094.85
salpingitis 095.8
sclera (late) 095.0
sclerosis
  cerebral 094.89
  coronary 093.89
  multiple 094.89
  subacute 094.89
scotoma (central) 095.8
scrotum 095.8
secondary (and primary) 091.9
  adenopathy 091.4
  anus 091.3
  bone 091.61
  cardiovascular 093.9
  central nervous system 094.9
  chorioretinitis, choroiditis 091.51
  hepatitis 091.62
  liver 091.62
  lymphadenitis 091.4
  meningitis, acute 091.81
  mouth 091.3
  mucous membranes 091.3
  periosteum 091.61
  periostitis 091.61
  pharynx 091.3
  relapse (treated) (untreated) 091.7
  skin 091.3
  specified form NEC 091.89
  tonsil 091.3
  ulcer 091.3
  viscera 091.69
  vulva 091.3
seminal vesicle (late) 095.8
seronegative
  with signs or symptoms—*see* Syphilis, by site
    and stage
seropositive
  with signs or symptoms—*see* Syphilis, by site
    and stage
  follow-up of latent syphilis—*see* Syphilis,
    latent
  only finding—*see* Syphilis, latent
seventh nerve (paralysis) 094.89

Syphilis, syphilitic—*continued*
sinus 095.8
sinusitis 095.8
skeletal system 095.5
skin (early) (secondary) (with ulceration) 091.3
  late or tertiary 095.8
small intestine 095.8
spastic spinal paralysis 094.0
spermatic cord (late) 095.8
spinal (cord) 094.89
  with
    paresis 094.1
    tabes 094.0
spleen 095.8
splenomegaly 095.8
spondylitis 095.5
staphyloma 095.8
stigmata (congenital) 090.5
stomach 095.8
synovium (late) 095.7
tabes dorsalis (early) (late) 094.0
  juvenile 090.40
tabetic type 094.0
  juvenile 090.40
taboparesis 094.1
  juvenile 090.40
tachycardia 093.89
tendon (late) 095.7
tertiary 097.0
  with symptoms 095.8
  cardiovascular 093.9
  central nervous system 094.9
  multiple NEC 095.8
  specified site NEC 095.8
testis 095.8
thorax 095.8
throat 095.8
thymus (gland) 095.8
thyroid (late) 095.8
tongue 095.8
tonsil (lingual) 095.8
  primary 091.2
  secondary 091.3
trachea 095.8
tricuspid valve 093.23
tumor, brain 094.89
tunica vaginalis (late) 095.8
ulcer (any site) (early) (secondary) 091.3
  late 095.9
  perforating 095.9
    foot 094.0
urethra (stricture) 095.8
urogenital 095.8
uterus 095.8
uveal tract (secondary) 091.50
  late 095.8 *[363.13]*
uveitis (secondary) 091.50
  late 095.8 *[363.13]*
uvula (late) 095.8
  perforated 095.8
vagina 091.0
  late 095.8
valvulitis NEC 093.20
vascular 093.89
  brain or cerebral 094.89
vein 093.89
  cerebral 094.89
ventriculi 095.8
vesicae urinariae 095.8
viscera (abdominal) 095.2
  secondary 091.69

Syphilis, syphilitic—*continued*
  vitreous (hemorrhage) (opacities) 095.8
  vulva 091.0
    late 095.8
    secondary 091.3
Syphiloma 095.9
  cardiovascular system 093.9
  central nervous system 094.9
  circulatory system 093.9
  congenital 090.5
Syphilophobia 300.29
Syringadenoma (M8400/0)—*see also* Neoplasm,
    skin, benign
  papillary (M8406/0)—*see* Neoplasm, skin,
    benign
Syringobulbia 336.0
Syringocarcinoma (M8400/3)—*see* Neoplasm,
    skin, malignant
Syringocystadenoma (M8400/0)—*see also*
    Neoplasm, skin, benign
  papillary (M8406/0)—*see* Neoplasm, skin,
    benign
Syringocystoma (M8407/0)—*see* Neoplasm,
    skin, benign
Syringoma (M8407/0)—*see also* Neoplasm, skin,
    benign
  chondroid (M8940/0)—*see* Neoplasm, by site,
    benign
Syringomyelia 336.0
Syringomyelitis 323.9
  late effect—*see* category 326
Syringomyelocele (*see also* Spina bifida) 741.9
Syringopontia 336.0
System, systemic —*see also* condition
  disease, combined—*see* Degeneration,
    combined
  fibrosclerosing syndrome 710.8
  inflammatory response syndrome (SIRS) 995.90
    due to
      infectious process 995.91
        with acute organ dysfunction 995.92
      non-infectious process 995.93
        with acute organ dysfunction 995.94
  lupus erythematosus 710.0
    inhibitor 795.79

T

Tab —*see* Tag
Tabacism 989.8
Tabacosis 989.8
Tabardillo 080
  flea-borne 081.0
  louse-borne 080
Tabes, tabetic
  with
    central nervous system syphilis 094.0
    Charcot's joint 094.0 *[713.5]*
    cord bladder 094.0
    crisis, viscera (any) 094.0
    paralysis, general 094.1
    paresis (general) 094.1
    perforating ulcer 094.0
  arthropathy 094.0 *[713.5]*
  bladder 094.0
  bone 094.0
  cerebrospinal 094.0
  congenital 090.40
  conjugal 094.0
  dorsalis 094.0
    neurosyphilis 094.0
  early 094.0
  juvenile 090.40
  latent 094.0
  mesenterica (*see also* Tuberculosis) 014.8
  paralysis insane, general 094.1
  peripheral (nonsyphilitic) 799.89
  spasmodic 094.0
    not dorsal or dorsalis 343.9
  syphilis (cerebrospinal) 094.0
Taboparalysis 094.1
Taboparesis (remission) 094.1
  with
    Charcot's joint 094.1 *[713.5]*
    cord bladder 094.1
    perforating ulcer 094.1
  juvenile 090.40
Tache noir 923.20
Tachyalimentation 579.3
Tachyarrhythmia, tachyrhythmia —*see also*
    Tachycardia
  paroxysmal with sinus bradycardia 427.81
Tachycardia 785.0
  atrial 427.89
  auricular 427.89
  AV nodal re-entry (re-entrant) 427.89
  newborn 779.82
  nodal 427.89
    nonparoxysmal atrioventricular 426.89
  nonparoxysmal atrioventricular (nodal) 426.89
  nonsustained 427.2
  paroxysmal 427.2
    with sinus bradycardia 427.81
    atrial (PAT) 427.0
      psychogenic 316 *[427.0]*
    atrioventricular (AV) 427.0
      psychogenic 316 *[427.0]*
    essential 427.2
    junctional ectopic 427.0
    nodal 427.0
    psychogenic 316 *[427.2]*
      atrial 316 *[427.0]*
      supraventricular 316 *[427.0]*
      ventricular 316 *[427.1]*

Tachycardia—*continued*
    supraventricular 427.0
      psychogenic 316 *[427.0]*
    ventricular 427.1
      psychogenic 316 *[427.1]*
  postoperative 997.1
  psychogenic 306.2
  sick sinus 427.81
  sinoauricular 427.89
  sinus 427.89
  supraventricular 427.89
  sustained 427.2
    supraventricular 427.0
    ventricular 427.1
  ventricular (paroxysmal) 427.1
    psychogenic 316 *[427.1]*
Tachygastria 536.8
Tachypnea 786.06
  hysterical 300.11
  newborn (idiopathic) (transitory) 770.6
  psychogenic 306.1
  transitory, of newborn 770.6
TACO (transfusion associated circulatory
    overload) 276.61
Taenia (infection) (infestation) (*see also*
    Infestation, taenia) 123.3
  diminuta 123.6
  echinococcal infestation (*see also*
    Echinococcus) 122.9
  nana 123.6
  saginata infestation 123.2
  solium (intestinal form) 123.0
    larval form 123.1
Taeniasis (intestine) (*see also* Infestation, Taenia)
    123.3
  saginata 123.2
  solium 123.0
Taenzer's disease 757.4
Tag (hypertrophied skin) (infected) 701.9
  adenoid 474.8
  anus 455.9
  endocardial (*see also* Endocarditis) 424.90
  hemorrhoidal 455.9
  hymen 623.8
  perineal 624.8
  preauricular 744.1
  rectum 455.9
  sentinel 455.9
  skin 701.9
    accessory 757.39
    anus 455.9
    congenital 757.39
    preauricular 744.1
    rectum 455.9
  tonsil 474.8
  urethra, urethral 599.84
  vulva 624.8
Tahyna fever 062.5
Takayasu (-Onishi) disease or syndrome
    (pulseless disease) 446.7
Takotsubo syndrome 429.83
Talc granuloma 728.82
  in operation wound 998.7
Talcosis 502
Talipes (congenital) 754.70
  acquired NEC 736.79
    planus 734

Talipes—*continued*
  asymmetric 754.79
    acquired 736.79
  calcaneovalgus 754.62
    acquired 736.76
  calcaneovarus 754.59
    acquired 736.76
  calcaneus 754.79
    acquired 736.76
  cavovarus 754.59
    acquired 736.75
  cavus 754.71
    acquired 736.73
  equinovalgus 754.69
    acquired 736.72
  equinovarus 754.51
    acquired 736.71
  equinus 754.79
    acquired, NEC 736.72
  percavus 754.71
    acquired 736.73
  planovalgus 754.69
    acquired 736.79
  planus (acquired) (any degree) 734
    congenital 754.61
    due to rickets 268.1
  valgus 754.60
    acquired 736.79
  varus 754.50
    acquired 736.79
Talma's disease 728.85
Talon noir 924.20
  hand 923.20
  heel 924.20
  toe 924.3
Tamponade heart (Rose's) (*see also*
    Pericarditis) 423.3
Tanapox 059.21
Tangier disease (familial high-density
    lipoprotein deficiency) 272.5
Tank ear 380.12
Tantrum (childhood) (*see also* Disturbance,
    conduct) 312.1
Tapeworm (infection) (infestation) (*see also*
    Infestation, tapeworm) 123.9
Tapia's syndrome 352.6
Tarantism 297.8
Target-oval cell anemia 285.8
  with thalassemia—*see* Thalassemia
Tarlov's cyst 355.9
Tarral-Besnier disease (pityriasis rubra pilaris)
    696.4
Tarsalgia 729.2
Tarsal tunnel syndrome 355.5
Tarsitis (eyelid) 373.00
  syphilitic 095.8 *[373.00]*
  tuberculous (*see also* Tuberculosis) 017.0 *[373.4]*
Tartar (teeth) 523.6
Tattoo (mark) 709.09
Taurodontism 520.2
Taussig-Bing defect, heart, or syndrome
    (transposition, aorta and overriding pulmonary
    artery) 745.11
Tay's choroiditis 363.41
Tay-Sachs
  amaurotic familial idiocy 330.1
  disease 330.1
Taybi's syndrome (otopalatodigital) 759.89
Taylor's
  disease (diffuse idiopathic cutaneous atrophy) 701.8
  syndrome 625.5

TBI (traumatic brain injury) (see also Injury,
    intracranial) 854.0
  with skull fracture —see Fracture, skull, by site
Tear, torn (traumatic)—*see also* Wound, open,
    by site
  annular fibrosis 722.51
  anus, anal (sphincter) 863.89
    with open wound in cavity 863.99
    complicating delivery (healed) (old) 654.8
      with mucosa 664.3
        not associated with third-degree perineal
          laceration 664.6
    nontraumatic, nonpuerperal (healed) (old)
      569.43
  articular cartilage, old (*see also* Disorder,
    cartilage, articular) 718.0
  bladder
    with
      abortion—*see* Abortion, by type, with
        damage to pelvic organs
      ectopic pregnancy (*see also* categories
        633.0-633.9) 639.2
      molar pregnancy (*see also* categories
        630-632) 639.2
    following
      abortion 639.2
      ectopic or molar pregnancy 639.2
    obstetrical trauma 665.5
  bowel
    with
      abortion—*see* Abortion, by type, with
        damage to pelvic organs
      ectopic pregnancy (*see also* categories
        633.0-633.9) 639.2
      molar pregnancy (*see also* categories
        630-632) 639.2
    following
      abortion 639.2
      ectopic or molar pregnancy 639.2
    obstetrical trauma 665.5
  broad ligament
    with
      abortion—*see* Abortion, by type, with
        damage to pelvic organs
      ectopic pregnancy (*see also* categories
        633.0-633.9) 639.2
      molar pregnancy (*see also* categories
        630-632) 639.2
    following
      abortion 639.2
      ectopic or molar pregnancy 639.2
    obstetrical trauma 665.6
  bucket handle (knee) (meniscus)—*see* Tear,
    meniscus
  capsule
    joint—*see* Sprain, by site
    spleen—*see* Laceration, spleen, capsule
  cartilage—*see also* Sprain, by site
    articular, old (*see also* Disorder, cartilage,
      articular) 718.0
    knee—*see* Tear, meniscus
    semilunar (knee) (current injury)—*see* Tear,
      meniscus
  cervix
    with
      abortion—*see* Abortion, by type, with
        damage to pelvic organs
      ectopic pregnancy (*see also* categories
        633.0-633.9) 639.2
      molar pregnancy (*see also* categories
        630-632) 639.2

Tear, torn—*continued*
  cervix—*continued*
    following
      abortion 639.2
      ectopic or molar pregnancy 639.2
      obstetrical trauma (current) 665.3
    old 622.3
  dural 349.31
    accidental puncture or laceration during a
      procedure 349.31
    incidental (inadvertent) 349.31
    nontraumatic NEC 349.39
  internal organ (abdomen, chest, or pelvis)—*see*
    Injury, internal, by site
  ligament—*see also* Sprain, by site
    with open wound—*see* Wound, open by site
  meniscus (knee) (current injury) 836.2
    bucket handle 836.0
      old 717.0
    lateral 836.1
      anterior horn 836.1
        old 717.42
      bucket handle 836.1
        old 717.41
      old 717.40
      posterior horn 836.1
        old 717.43
      specified site NEC 836.1
        old 717.49
    medial 836.0
      anterior horn 836.0
        old 717.1
      bucket handle 836.0
        old 717.0
      old 717.3
      posterior horn 836.0
        old 717.2
    old NEC 717.5
    site other than knee—*see* Sprain, by site
  muscle—*see also* Sprain, by site
    with open wound—*see* Wound, open by site
  pelvic
    floor, complicating delivery 664.1
    organ NEC
      with
        abortion—*see* Abortion, by type, with
          damage to pelvic organs
        ectopic pregnancy (*see also* categories
          633.0-633.9) 639.2
        molar pregnancy (*see also* categories
          630-632) 639.2
      following
        abortion 639.2
        ectopic or molar pregnancy 639.2
        obstetrical trauma 665.5
  perineum—*see also* Laceration, perineum
    obstetrical trauma 665.5
  periurethral tissue
    with
      abortion—*see* Abortion, by type, with
        damage to pelvic organs
      ectopic pregnancy (*see also* categories
        633.0-633.9) 639.2
      molar pregnancy (*see also* categories
        630-632) 639.2
    following
      abortion 639.2
      ectopic or molar pregnancy 639.2
      obstetrical trauma 664.8
  rectovaginal septum—*see* Laceration,
    rectovaginal septum

Tear, torn—*continued*
  retina, retinal (recent) (with detachment) 361.00
    without detachment 361.30
    dialysis (juvenile) (with detachment) 361.04
    giant (with detachment) 361.03
    horseshoe (without detachment) 361.32
    multiple (with detachment) 361.02
      without detachment 361.33
    old
      delimited (partial) 361.06
      partial 361.06
      total or subtotal 361.07
    partial (without detachment)
      giant 361.03
      multiple defects 361.02
      old (delimited) 361.06
      single defect 361.01
    round hole (without detachment) 361.31
    single defect (with detachment) 361.01
    total or subtotal (recent) 361.05
      old 361.07
  rotator cuff (traumatic) 840.4
    current injury 840.4
    degenerative 726.10
    nontraumatic (complete) 727.61
      partial 726.13
  semilunar cartilage, knee (*see also* Tear,
    meniscus) 836.2
    old 717.5
  tendon—*see also* Sprain, by site
    with open wound—*see* Wound, open by site
  tentorial, at birth 767.0
  umbilical cord
    affecting fetus or newborn 772.0
    complicating delivery 663.8
  urethra
    with
      abortion—*see* Abortion, by type, with
        damage to pelvic organs
      ectopic pregnancy (*see also* categories
        633.0-633.9) 639.2
      molar pregnancy (*see also* categories
        630-632) 639.2
    following
      abortion 639.2
      ectopic or molar pregnancy 639.2
      obstetrical trauma 665.5
  uterus—*see* Injury, internal, uterus
  vagina—*see* Laceration, vagina
  vessel, from catheter 998.2
  vulva, complicating delivery 664.0
Tear stone 375.57
Teeth, tooth —*see also* condition
  grinding 306.8
  prenatal 520.6
Teething 520.7
  syndrome 520.7
Tegmental syndrome 344.89
Telangiectasia, telangiectasis (verrucous) 448.9
  ataxic (cerebellar) 334.8
  familial 448.0
  hemorrhagic, hereditary (congenital) (senile) 448.0
  hereditary hemorrhagic 448.0
  retina 362.15
  spider 448.1
Telecanthus (congenital) 743.63
Telescoped bowel or intestine (*see also*
  Intussusception) 560.0
Teletherapy, adverse effect NEC 990
Telogen effluvium 704.02

Temperature
body, high (of unknown origin) (*see also*
    Pyrexia) 780.60
cold, trauma from 991.9
  newborn 778.2
  specified effect NEC 991.8
high
  body (of unknown origin) (*see also* Pyrexia)
    780.60
  trauma from—*see* Heat
Temper tantrum (childhood) (*see also*
  Disturbance, conduct) 312.1
Temple —*see* condition
Temporal —*see also* condition
lobe syndrome 310.0
Temporomandibular joint-pain-dysfunction
syndrome 524.60
Temporosphenoidal —*see* condition
Tendency
bleeding (*see also* Defect, coagulation) 286.9
homosexual, ego-dystonic 302.0
paranoid 301.0
suicide 300.9
Tenderness
abdominal (generalized) (localized) 789.6
rebound 789.6
skin 782.0
Tendinitis, tendonitis (*see also* Tenosynovitis)
  726.90
Achilles 726.71
adhesive 726.90
  shoulder 726.0
calcific 727.82
  shoulder 726.11
gluteal 726.5
patellar 726.64
peroneal 726.79
pes anserinus 726.61
psoas 726.5
tibialis (anterior) (posterior) 726.72
trochanteric 726.5
Tendon —*see* condition
Tendosynovitis —*see* Tenosynovitis
Tendovaginitis —*see* Tenosynovitis
Tenesmus 787.99
rectal 787.99
vesical 788.99
Tenia —*see* Taenia
Teniasis —*see* Taeniasis
Tennis elbow 726.32
Tenonitis —*see also* Tenosynovitis
eye (capsule) 376.04
Tenontosynovitis —*see* Tenosynovitis
Tenontothecitis —*see* Tenosynovitis
Tenophyte 727.9
Tenosynovitis (*see also* Synovitis) 727.00
adhesive 726.90
  shoulder 726.0
ankle 727.06
bicipital (calcifying) 726.12
buttock 727.09
due to crystals—*see* Arthritis, due to crystals
elbow 727.09
finger 727.05
foot 727.06
gonococcal 098.51
hand 727.05
hip 727.09
knee 727.09
radial styloid 727.04

Tenosynovitis—*continued*
shoulder 726.10
  adhesive 726.0
specified NEC 727.09
spine 720.1
supraspinatus 726.10
toe 727.06
tuberculous—*see* Tuberculosis, tenosynovitis
wrist 727.05
Tenovaginitis —*see* Tenosynovitis
Tension
arterial, high (*see also* Hypertension) 401.9
  without diagnosis of hypertension 796.2
headache 307.81
intraocular (elevated) 365.00
nervous 799.21
ocular (elevated) 365.00
pneumothorax 512.0
  iatrogenic 512.1
  postoperative 512.1
  spontaneous 512.0
premenstrual 625.4
state 300.9
Tentorium —*see* condition
Teratencephalus 759.89
Teratism 759.7
Teratoblastoma (malignant) (M9080/3)—*see*
  Neoplasm, by site, malignant
Teratocarcinoma (M9081/3)—*see also*
  Neoplasm, by site, malignant
liver 155.0
Teratoma (solid) (M9080/1)—*see also*
  Neoplasm, by site, uncertain behavior
adult (cystic) (M9080/0)—*see* Neoplasm, by
  site, benign
and embryonal carcinoma, mixed
  (M9081/3)—*see* Neoplasm, by site,
  malignant
benign (M9080/0)—*see* Neoplasm, by site,
  benign
combined with choriocarcinoma
  (M9101/3)—*see* Neoplasm, by site,
  malignant
cystic (adult) (M9080/0)—*see* Neoplasm, by
  site, benign
differentiated type (M9080/0)—*see* Neoplasm,
  by site, benign
embryonal (M9080/3)—*see also* Neoplasm, by
  site, malignant
  liver 155.0
fetal
  sacral, causing fetopelvic disproportion 653.7
immature (M9080/3)—*see* Neoplasm, by site,
  malignant
liver (M9080/3) 155.0
  adult, benign, cystic, differentiated type or
    mature (M9080/0) 211.5
malignant (M9080/3)—*see also* Neoplasm, by
  site, malignant
  anaplastic type (M9082/3)—*see* Neoplasm, by
    site, malignant
  intermediate type (M9083/3)—*see* Neoplasm,
    by site, malignant
  liver (M9080/3) 155.0
  trophoblastic (M9102/3)
    specified site—*see* Neoplasm, by site,
     malignant
    unspecified site 186.9
  undifferentiated type (M9082/3)—*see*
    Neoplasm, by site, malignant

Teratoma—*continued*
  mature (M9080/0)—*see* Neoplasm, by site, benign
    malignant (M9080/3) —see Neoplasm, by site,
      malignant
  ovary (M9080/0) 220
    embryonal, immature, or malignant (M9080/3)
      183.0
  suprasellar (M9080/3)—*see* Neoplasm, by site,
    malignant
  testis (M9080/3) 186.9
    adult, benign, cystic, differentiated type or
      mature (M9080/0) 222.0
    undescended 186.0
Terminal care V66.7
Termination
  anomalous—*see also* Malposition, congenital
    portal vein 747.49
    right pulmonary vein 747.42
  pregnancy (legal) (therapeutic) (*see* Abortion,
    legal) 635.9
    fetus NEC 779.6
    illegal (*see also* Abortion, illegal) 636.9
Ternidens diminutus infestation 127.7
Terrors, night (child) 307.46
Terry's syndrome (*see also* Retinopathy of
  prematurity) 362.21
Tertiary —*see* condition
Tessellated fundus, retina (tigroid) 362.89
Test(s)
  adequacy
    hemodialysis V56.31
    peritoneal dialysis V56.32
  AIDS virus V72.69
  allergen V72.7
  bacterial disease NEC (*see also* Screening, by
    name of disease) V74.9
  basal metabolic rate V72.69
  blood
    alcohol V70.4
    drug V70.4
      for therapeutic drug monitoring V58.83
      for routine general physical examination
        V72.62
      prior to treatment or procedure V72.63
    typing V72.86
      Rh typing V72.86
  developmental, infant or child V20.2
  Dick V74.8
  fertility V26.21
  genetic
    female V26.32
    for genetic disease carrier status
      female V26.31
      male V26.34
    male V26.39
  hearing V72.19
    following failed hearing screening V72.11
    routine, for infant and child V20.2
  HIV V72.69
  human immunodeficiency virus V72.69
  immunity status V72.61
  Kveim V82.89
  laboratory V72.60
    for medicolegal reason V70.4
    ordered as part of a routine general medical
      examination V72.62
    pre-operative V72.63
    pre-procedural V72.63
    specified NEC V72.69
  male partner of female with recurrent pregnancy
    loss V26.35

Test(s)—*continued*
  Mantoux (for tuberculosis) V74.1
  mycotic organism V75.4
  nuchal translucency V28.89
  parasitic agent NEC V75.8
  paternity V70.4
  peritoneal equilibration V56.32
  pregnancy
    negative result V72.41
    positive result V72.42
      first pregnancy V72.42
    unconfirmed V72.40
  preoperative V72.84
    cardiovascular V72.81
    respiratory V72.82
    specified NEC V72.83
  procreative management NEC V26.29
    genetic disease carrier status
      female V26.31
      male V26.34
  Rh typing V72.86
  sarcoidosis V82.89
  Schick V74.3
  Schultz-Charlton V74.8
  skin, diagnostic
    allergy V72.7
    bacterial agent NEC (*see also* Screening, by
      name of disease) V74.9
    Dick V74.8
    hypersensitivity V72.7
    Kveim V82.89
    Mantoux V74.1
    mycotic organism V75.4
    parasitic agent NEC V75.8
    sarcoidosis V82.89
    Schick V74.3
    Schultz-Charlton V74.8
    tuberculin V74.1
  specified type NEC V72.85
  tuberculin V74.1
  vision V72.0
    routine, for infant and child V20.2
  Wassermann
    positive (*see also* Serology for syphilis,
      positive) 097.1
    false 795.6
Testicle, testicular, testis —*see also* condition
  feminization (syndrome) 259.51
Tetanus, tetanic (cephalic) (convulsions) 037
  with
    abortion—*see* Abortion, by type, with sepsis
    ectopic pregnancy (*see also* categories
      633.0-633.9) 639.0
    molar pregnancy (*see* categories 630-632) 639.0
  following
    abortion 639.0
    ectopic or molar pregnancy 639.0
  inoculation V03.7
    reaction (due to serum)—*see* Complications,
      vaccination
  neonatorum 771.3
  puerperal, postpartum, childbirth 670.8
Tetany, tetanic 781.7
  alkalosis 276.3
  associated with rickets 268.0
  convulsions 781.7
    hysterical 300.11
  functional (hysterical) 300.11
  hyperkinetic 781.7
    hysterical 300.11

Tetany, tetanic—*continued*
  hyperpnea 786.01
    hysterical 300.11
    psychogenic 306.1
  hyperventilation 786.01
    hysterical 300.11
    psychogenic 306.1
  hypocalcemic, neonatal 775.4
  hysterical 300.11
  neonatal 775.4
  parathyroid (gland) 252.1
  parathyroprival 252.1
  postoperative 252.1
  postthyroidectomy 252.1
  pseudotetany 781.7
    hysterical 300.11
  psychogenic 306.1
    specified as conversion reaction 300.11
Tetralogy of Fallot 745.2
Tetraplegia —*see* Quadriplegia
Thailand hemorrhagic fever 065.4
Thalassanemia 282.40
Thalassemia (disease) 282.40
  with other hemoglobinopathy 282.49
  alpha (major) (severe) (triple gene defect)
    282.43
    silent carrier 282.46
  beta (homozygous) (major) (severe) 282.44
  delta-beta (homozygous) 282.45
  dominant 282.49
  Hb-S (without crisis) 282.41
    with
      crisis 282.42
      vaso-occlusive pain 282.42
  hemoglobin
    C (Hb-C) 282.49
    D (Hb-D) 282.49
    E (Hb-E) 282.49
    E-beta 282.47
    H (Hb-H) 282.49
    I (Hb-I) 282.49
  high fetal gene (see also Thalassemia) 282.40
  high fetal hemoglobin (see also Thalassemia)
    282.40
  intermedia 282.44
  major 282.44
  minor (alpha) (beta) 282.46
  mixed 282.49
  sickle-cell (without crisis) 282.41
    with
      crisis 282.42
      vaso-occlusive pain 282.42
  specified NEC 282.49
  trait (alpha) (beta) (delta-beta) 282.46
Thalassemic variants 282.49
Thaysen-Gee disease (nontropical sprue) 579.0
Thecoma (M8600/0) 220
  malignant (M8600/3) 183.0
Thelarche, precocious 259.1
Thelitis 611.0
  puerperal, postpartum 675.0
Therapeutic —*see* condition
Therapy V57.9
  blood transfusion, without reported diagnosis
    V58.2
  breathing V57.0
  chemotherapy, antineoplastic V58.11
    fluoride V07.31
    prophylactic NEC V07.39

Therapy—*continued*
  dialysis (intermittent) (treatment)
    extracorporeal V56.0
    peritoneal V56.8
    renal V56.0
    specified type NEC V56.8
  exercise NEC V57.1
    breathing V57.0
  extracorporeal dialysis (renal) V56.0
  fluoride prophylaxis V07.31
  hemodialysis V56.0
  hormone replacement (postmenopausal) V07.4
  immunotherapy, antineoplastic V58.12
  long term oxygen therapy V46.2
  occupational V57.21
  orthoptic V57.4
  orthotic V57.81
  peritoneal dialysis V56.8
  physical NEC V57.1
  postmenopausal hormone replacement V07.4
  radiation V58.0
  speech (-language) V57.3
  vocational V57.22
Thermalgesia 782.0
Thermalgia 782.0
Thermanalgesia 782.0
Thermanesthesia 782.0
Thermic —*see* condition
Thermography (abnormal) 793.99
  breast 793.89
Thermoplegia 992.0
Thesaurismosis
  amyloid 277.39
  bilirubin 277.4
  calcium 275.40
  cystine 270.0
  glycogen (*see also* Disease, glycogen storage)
    271.0
  kerasin 272.7
  lipoid 272.7
  melanin 255.41
  phosphatide 272.7
  urate 274.9
Thiaminic deficiency 265.1
  with beriberi 265.0
Thibierge-Weissenbach syndrome (cutaneous
  systemic sclerosis) 710.1
Thickened endometrium 793.5
Thickening
  bone 733.99
    extremity 733.99
  breast 611.79
  hymen 623.3
  larynx 478.79
  nail 703.8
    congenital 757.5
  periosteal 733.99
  pleura (*see also* Pleurisy) 511.0
  skin 782.8
  subepiglottic 478.79
  tongue 529.8
  valve, heart—*see* Endocarditis
Thiele syndrome 724.6
Thigh —*see* condition
Thinning vertebra (*see also* Osteoporosis) 733.00
Thirst, excessive 783.5
  due to deprivation of water 994.3
Thomsen's disease 359.22
Thomson's disease (congenital poikiloderma) 757.33

Thoracic —*see also* condition
kidney 753.3
outlet syndrome 353.0
stomach—*see* Hernia, diaphragm
Thoracogastroschisis (congenital) 759.89
Thoracopagus 759.4
Thoracoschisis 756.3
Thorax —*see* condition
Thorn's syndrome (*see also* Disease, renal) 593.9
Thornwaldt's, Tornwaldt's
bursitis (pharyngeal) 478.29
cyst 478.26
disease (pharyngeal bursitis) 478.29
Thoracoscopic surgical procedure converted to
open procedure V64.42
Thorson-Biörck syndrome (malignant
carcinoid) 259.2
Threadworm (infection) (infestation) 127.4
Threatened
abortion or miscarriage 640.0
with subsequent abortion (*see also* Abortion,
spontaneous) 634.9
affecting fetus 762.1
labor 644.1
affecting fetus or newborn 761.8
premature 644.0
miscarriage 640.0
affecting fetus 762.1
premature
delivery 644.2
affecting fetus or newborn 761.8
labor 644.0
before 22 completed weeks gestation 640.0
Three-day fever 066.0
Threshers' lung 495.0
Thrix annulata (congenital) 757.4
Throat —*see* condition
Thrombasthenia (Glanzmann's) (hemorrhagic)
(hereditary) 287.1
Thromboangiitis 443.1
obliterans (general) 443.1
cerebral 437.1
vessels
brain 437.1
spinal cord 437.1
Thromboarteritis —*see* Arteritis
Thromboasthenia (Glanzmann's) (hemorrhagic)
(hereditary) 287.1
Thrombocytasthenia (Glanzmann's) 287.1
Thrombocythemia (primary) (M9962/1) 238.71
essential 238.71
hemorrhagic 238.71
idiopathic (hemorrhagic) (M9962/1) 238.71
Thrombocytopathy (dystrophic) (granulopenic)
287.1
Thrombocytopenia, thrombocytopenic 287.5
with
absent radii (TAR) syndrome 287.33
giant hemangioma 287.39
amegakaryocytic, congenital 287.33
congenital 287.33
cyclic 287.39
dilutional 287.49
due to
drugs 287.49
extracorporeal circulation of blood 287.49
massive blood transfusion 287.49
platelet alloimmunization 287.49
essential 287.30
fetal 678.0

Thrombocytopenia— *continued*
heparin-induced (HIT) 289.84
hereditary 287.33
Kasabach-Merritt 287.39
neonatal, transitory 776.1
due to
exchange transfusion 776.1
idiopathic maternal thrombocytopenia 776.1
isoimmunization 776.1
primary 287.30
puerperal, postpartum 666.3
purpura (*see also* Purpura, thrombocytopenic)
287.30
thrombotic 446.6
secondary NEC 287.49
sex-linked 287.39
Thrombocytosis 238.71
essential 238.71
primary 238.71
Thromboembolism —*see* Embolism
Thrombopathy (Bernard-Soulier) 287.1
constitutional 286.4
Willebrand-Jürgens (angiohemophilia) 286.4
Thrombopenia (*see also* Thrombocytopenia) 287.5
Thrombophlebitis 451.9
antecubital vein 451.82
antepartum (superficial) 671.2
affecting fetus or newborn 760.3
deep 671.3
arm 451.89
deep 451.83
superficial 451.82
breast, superficial 451.89
cavernous (venous) sinus—*see*
Thrombophlebitis, intracranial venous sinus
cephalic vein 451.82
cerebral (sinus) (vein) 325
late effect—*see* category 326
nonpyogenic 437.6
in pregnancy or puerperium 671.5
late effect—*see* Late effect(s) (of)
cerebrovascular disease
due to implanted device—*see* Complications,
due to (presence of) any device, implant, or
graft classified to 996.0-996.5 NEC
during or resulting from a procedure NEC 997.2
femoral 451.11
femoropopliteal 451.19
following infusion, perfusion, or transfusion
999.2
hepatic (vein) 451.89
idiopathic, recurrent 453.1
iliac vein 451.81
iliofemoral 451.11
intracranial venous sinus (any) 325
late effect—*see* category 326
nonpyogenic 437.6
in pregnancy or puerperium 671.5
late effect—*see* Late effect(s) (of)
cerebrovascular disease
jugular vein 451.89
lateral (venous) sinus—*see* Thrombophlebitis,
intracranial venous sinus
leg 451.2
deep (vessels) 451.19
femoral vein 451.11
specified vessel NEC 451.19
superficial (vessels) 451.0
femoral vein 451.11
longitudinal (venous) sinus—*see*
Thrombophlebitis, intracranial venous sinus

Thrombophlebitis—*continued*
  lower extremity 451.2
    deep (vessels) 451.19
      femoral vein 451.11
      specified vessel NEC 451.19
    superficial (vessels) 451.0
  migrans, migrating 453.1
  pelvic
    with
      abortion—*see* Abortion, by type, with sepsis
      ectopic pregnancy (*see also* categories
        633.0-633.9) 639.0
      molar pregnancy (*see also* categories
        630-632) 639.0
    following
      abortion 639.0
      ectopic or molar pregnancy 639.0
    puerperal 671.4
  popliteal vein 451.19
  portal (vein) 572.1
  postoperative 997.2
  pregnancy (superficial) 671.2
    affecting fetus or newborn 760.3
    deep 671.3
  puerperal, postpartum, childbirth (extremities)
    (superficial) 671.2
    deep 671.4
    pelvic 671.4
    septic 670.3
    specified site NEC 671.5
  radial vein 451.83
  saphenous (greater) (lesser) 451.0
  sinus (intracranial)—*see* Thrombophlebitis,
    intracranial venous sinus
  specified site NEC 451.89
  tibial vein 451.19
Thrombosis, thrombotic (marantic) (multiple)
    (progressive) (vein) (vessel) 453.9
  with childbirth or during the puerperium—*see*
    Thrombosis, puerperal, postpartum
  antepartum—*see* Thrombosis, pregnancy
  aorta, aortic 444.1
    abdominal 444.09
      saddle 444.01
    bifurcation 444.09
    saddle 444.01
    terminal 444.09
    thoracic 444.1
    valve—*see* Endocarditis, aortic
  apoplexy (*see also* Thrombosis, brain) 434.0
    late effect—*see* Late effect(s) (of)
      cerebrovascular disease
  appendix, septic—*see* Appendicitis, acute
  arteriolar-capillary platelet, disseminated 446.6
  artery, arteries (postinfectional) 444.9
    auditory, internal 433.8
    basilar (*see also* Occlusion, artery, basilar) 433.0
    carotid (common) (internal) (*see also*
      Occlusion, artery, carotid) 433.1
      with other precerebral artery 433.3
    cerebellar (anterior inferior) (posterior
      inferior) (superior) 433.8
    cerebral (*see also* Thrombosis, brain) 434.0
    choroidal (anterior) 433.8
    communicating posterior 433.8
    coronary (*see also* Infarct, myocardium) 410.9
      due to syphilis 093.89
      healed or specified as old 412
      without myocardial infarction 411.81
    extremities 444.22
      lower 444.22
      upper 444.21

Thrombosis, thrombotic—*continued*
  artery, arteries—*continued*
    femoral 444.22
    hepatic 444.89
    hypophyseal 433.8
    meningeal, anterior or posterior 433.8
    mesenteric (with gangrene) 557.0
    ophthalmic (*see also* Occlusion, retina) 362.30
    pontine 433.8
    popliteal 444.22
    precerebral—*see* Occlusion, artery,
      precerebral NEC
    pulmonary 415.19
      iatrogenic 415.11
      personal history of V12.55
      postoperative 415.11
      septic 415.12
    renal 593.81
    retinal (*see also* Occlusion, retina) 362.30
    specified site NEC 444.89
    spinal, anterior or posterior 433.8
    traumatic (complication) (early) (*see also*
      Injury, blood vessel, by site) 904.9
    vertebral (*see also* Occlusion, artery,
      vertebral) 433.2
      with other precerebral artery 433.3
  atrial (endocardial) 424.90
    due to syphilis 093.89
    without endocarditis 429.89
  auricular (*see also* Infarct, myocardium) 410.9
  axillary (acute) (vein) 453.84
    chronic 453.74
    personal history of V12.51
  basilar (artery) (*see also* Occlusion, artery,
    basilar) 433.0
  bland NEC 453.9
  brain (artery) (stem) 434.0
    due to syphilis 094.89
    iatrogenic 997.02
    late effect—*see* Late effect(s) (of)
      cerebrovascular disease
    postoperative 997.02
    puerperal, postpartum, childbirth 674.0
    sinus (*see also* Thrombosis, intracranial
      venous sinus) 325
  capillary 448.9
    arteriolar, generalized 446.6
  cardiac (*see also* Infarct, myocardium) 410.9
    due to syphilis 093.89
    healed or specified as old 412
    valve—*see* Endocarditis
  carotid (artery) (common) (internal) (*see also*
    Occlusion, artery, carotid) 433.1
    with other precerebral artery 433.3
  cavernous sinus (venous)—*see* Thrombosis,
    intracranial venous sinus
  cerebellar artery (anterior inferior) (posterior
    inferior) (superior) 433.8
    late effect—*see* Late effect(s) (of)
      cerebrovascular disease
  cerebral (arteries) (*see also* Thrombosis, brain)
    434.0
    late effect—*see* Late effect(s) (of)
      cerebrovascular disease
  coronary (artery) (*see also* Infarct, myocardium)
    410.9
    due to syphilis 093.89
    healed or specified as old 412
    without myocardial infarction 411.81
  corpus cavernosum 607.82
  cortical (*see also* Thrombosis, brain) 434.0

Thrombosis, thrombotic—*continued*
  due to (presence of) any device, implant, or graft
    classifiable to 996.0-996.5—*see*
    Complications, due to (presence of) any
    device, implant, or graft classified to
    996.0-996.5 NEC
  effort 453.89
  endocardial—*see* Infarct, myocardium
  eye (*see also* Occlusion, retina) 362.30
  femoral (vein) 453.6
    with inflammation or phlebitis 451.11
    artery 444.22
    deep 453.41
    personal history of V12.51
  genital organ, male 608.83
  heart (chamber) (*see also* Infarct, myocardium)
    410.9
  hepatic (vein) 453.0
    artery 444.89
    infectional or septic 572.1
  iliac (acute) (vein) 453.41
    with inflammation or phlebitis 451.81
    artery (common) (external) (internal) 444.81
    chronic 453.51
    personal history of V12.51
  inflammation, vein—*see* Thrombophlebitis
  internal carotid artery (*see also* Occlusion,
    artery, carotid) 433.1
    with other precerebral artery 433.3
  intestine (with gangrene) 557.0
  intracranial (*see also* Thrombosis, brain) 434.0
    venous sinus (any) 325
      nonpyogenic origin 437.6
        in pregnancy or puerperium 671.5
  intramural (*see also* Infarct, myocardium) 410.9
    without
      cardiac condition 429.89
      coronary artery disease 429.89
      myocardial infarction 429.89
    healed or specified as old 412
  jugular (bulb)
    external (acute) 453.89
      chronic 453.79
    internal (acute) 453.86
      chronic 453.76
  kidney 593.81
    artery 593.81
  lateral sinus (venous)—*see* Thrombosis,
    intracranial venous sinus
  leg (see also Thrombosis, lower extremity)
    453.6
    with inflammation or phlebitis—*see*
      Thrombophlebitis
    deep (vessels) 453.40
      acute 453.40
        lower (distal) 453.42
        upper (proximal) 453.41
      chronic 453.50
        lower (distal) 453.52
        upper (proximal) 453.51
    personal history of V12.51
    superficial (vessels) 453.6
  liver (venous) 453.0
    artery 444.89
    infectional or septic 572.1
    portal vein 452
  longitudinal sinus (venous)—*see* Thrombosis,
    intracranial venous sinus

Thrombosis, thrombotic—*continued*
  lower extremity (superficial) 453.6
    deep vessels 453.40
      acute 453.40
        calf 453.42
        distal (lower leg) 453.42
        femoral 453.41
        iliac 453.41
        lower leg 453.42
        peroneal 453.42
        popliteal 453.41
        proximal (upper leg) 453.41
        thigh 453.41
        tibial 453.42
      chronic 453.50
        calf 453.52
        distal (lower leg) 453.52
        femoral 453.51
        iliac 453.51
        lower leg 453.52
        peroneal 453.52
        popliteal 453.51
        proximal (upper leg) 453.51
        thigh 453.51
        tibial 453.52
      personal history of V12.51
      saphenous (greater) (lesser) 453.6
      superficial 453.6
  lung 415.19
    iatrogenic 415.11
    personal history of V12.55
    postoperative 415.11
    septic 415.12
  marantic, dural sinus 437.6
  meninges (brain) (*see also* Thrombosis, brain)
    434.0
  mesenteric (artery) (with gangrene) 557.0
    vein (inferior) (superior) 557.0
  mitral—*see* Insufficiency, mitral
  mural (heart chamber) (*see also* Infarct,
    myocardium) 410.9
    without
      cardiac condition 429.89
      coronary artery disease 429.89
      myocardial infarction 429.89
    due to syphilis 093.89
    following myocardial infarction 429.79
    healed or specified as old 412
  omentum (with gangrene) 557.0
  ophthalmic (artery) (*see also* Occlusion, retina)
    362.30
  pampiniform plexus (male) 608.83
    female 620.8
  parietal (*see also* Infarct, myocardium) 410.9
  penis, penile 607.82
  peripheral arteries 444.22
    lower 444.22
    upper 444.21
  platelet 446.6
  portal 452
    due to syphilis 093.89
    infectional or septic 572.1
  precerebral artery—*see also* Occlusion, artery,
    precerebral NEC
  pregnancy 671.2
    deep (vein) 671.3
    superficial (vein) 671.2

Thrombosis, thrombotic—*continued*
puerperal, postpartum, childbirth 671.2
  brain (artery) 674.0
    venous 671.5
  cardiac 674.8
  cerebral (artery) 674.0
    venous 671.5
  deep (vein) 671.4
  intracranial sinus (nonpyogenic) (venous) 671.5
  pelvic 671.4
  pulmonary (artery) 673.2
  specified site NEC 671.5
  superficial 671.2
pulmonary (artery) (vein) 415.19
  iatrogenic 415.11
  personal history of V12.55
  postoperative 415.11
  septic 415.12
radial vein 451.83
renal (artery) 593.81
  vein 453.3
resulting from presence of shunt or other internal prosthetic device—*see* Complications, due to (presence of) any device, implant, or graft classified to 996.0-996.5 NEC
retina, retinal (artery) 362.30
  arterial branch 362.32
  central 362.31
  partial 362.33
  vein
    central 362.35
    tributary (branch) 362.36
saphenous vein (greater) (lesser) 453.6
scrotum 608.83
seminal vesicle 608.83
sigmoid (venous) sinus (*see* Thrombosis, intracranial venous sinus) 325
silent NEC 453.9
sinus, intracranial (venous) (any) (*see also* Thrombosis, intracranial venous sinus) 325
softening, brain (*see also* Thrombosis, brain) 434.0
specified site NEC (acute) 453.89
  chronic 453.79
spermatic cord 608.83
spinal cord 336.1
  due to syphilis 094.89
  in pregnancy or puerperium 671.5
  pyogenic origin 324.1
    late effect—*see* category 326
spleen, splenic 289.59
  artery 444.89
testis 608.83
traumatic (complication) (early) (*see also* Injury, blood vessel, by site) 904.9
tricuspid—*see* Endocarditis, tricuspid
tumor—*see* Neoplasm, by site
tunica vaginalis 608.83
umbilical cord (vessels) 663.6
  affecting fetus or newborn 762.6
upper extremity (acute) 453.83
  chronic 453.73
    deep 453.72
    superficial 453.71
  deep 453.82
  superficial 453.81
vas deferens 608.83

Thrombosis, thrombotic—*continued*
vein
  antecubital (acute) 453.81
    chronic 453.71
  axillary (acute) 453.84
    chronic 453.74
  basilic (acute) 453.81
    chronic 453.71
  brachial (acute) 453.82
    chronic 453.72
  brachiocephalic (innominate) (acute) 453.87
    chronic 453.77
  cephalic (acute) 453.81
    chronic 453.71
  deep 453.40
    personal history of V12.51
  internal jugular (acute) 453.86
    chronic 453.76
  lower extremity—*see* Thrombosis, lower extremity
  personal history of V12.51
  radial (acute) 453.82
    chronic 453.72
  saphenous (greater) (lesser) 453.6
  specified site NEC (acute) 453.89
    chronic 453.79
  subclavian (acute) 453.85
    chronic 453.75
  superior vena cava (acute) 453.87
    chronic 453.77
  thoracic (acute) 453.87
    chronic 453.77
  ulnar (acute) 453.82
    chronic 453.72
  upper extremity - see Thrombosis, upper extremity
vena cava
  inferior 453.2
  personal history of V12.51
  superior (acute) 453.87
    chronic 453.77
Thrombus —*see* Thrombosis
Thrush 112.0
newborn 771.7
Thumb —*see also* condition
gamekeeper's 842.12
sucking (child problem) 307.9
Thygeson's superficial punctate keratitis 370.21
Thymergasia (*see also* Psychosis, affective) 296.80
Thymitis 254.8
Thymoma (benign) (M8580/0) 212.6
malignant (M8580/3) 164.0
Thymus, thymic (gland)—*see* condition
Thyrocele (*see also* Goiter) 240.9
Thyroglossal —*see also* condition
cyst 759.2
duct, persistent 759.2
Thyroid (body) (gland)—*see also* condition
hormone resistance 246.8
lingual 759.2
Thyroiditis 245.9
acute (pyogenic) (suppurative) 245.0
  nonsuppurative 245.0
autoimmune 245.2
chronic (nonspecific) (sclerosing) 245.8
  fibrous 245.3
  lymphadenoid 245.2
  lymphocytic 245.2
  lymphoid 245.2

Thyroiditis—*continued*
  complicating pregnancy, childbirth, or
    puerperium 648.1
  de Quervain's (subacute granulomatous) 245.1
  fibrous (chronic) 245.3
  giant (cell) (follicular) 245.1
  granulomatous (de Quervain's) (subacute) 245.1
  Hashimoto's (struma lymphomatosa) 245.2
  iatrogenic 245.4
  invasive (fibrous) 245.3
  ligneous 245.3
  lymphocytic (chronic) 245.2
  lymphoid 245.2
  lymphomatous 245.2
  pseudotuberculous 245.1
  pyogenic 245.0
  radiation 245.4
  Riedel's (ligneous) 245.3
  subacute 245.1
  suppurative 245.0
  tuberculous (*see also* Tuberculosis) 017.5
  viral 245.1
  woody 245.3
Thyrolingual duct, persistent 759.2
Thyromegaly 240.9
Thyrotoxic
  crisis or storm (*see also* Thyrotoxicosis) 242.9
  heart failure (*see also* Thyrotoxicosis) 242.9 *[425.7]*
Thyrotoxicosis 242.9

Note—Use the following fifth-digit
subclassification with category 242:

0 without mention of thyrotoxic crisis or storm
1 with mention of thyrotoxic crisis or storm

---

  with
    goiter (diffuse) 242.0
      adenomatous 242.3
        multinodular 242.2
        uninodular 242.1
      nodular 242.3
        multinodular 242.2
        uninodular 242.1
    infiltrative
      dermopathy 242.0
      ophthalmopathy 242.0
    thyroid acropachy 242.0
  complicating pregnancy, childbirth, or
    puerperium 648.1
  due to
    ectopic thyroid nodule 242.4
    ingestion of (excessive) thyroid material 242.8
    specified cause NEC 242.8
  factitia 242.8
  heart 242.9 *[425.7]*
  neonatal (transient) 775.3
TIA (transient ischemic attack) 435.9
  with transient neurologic deficit 435.9
  late effect—*see* Late effect(s) (of)
    cerebrovascular disease
Tibia vara 732.4
Tic 307.20
  breathing 307.20
  child problem 307.21
  compulsive 307.22
  convulsive 307.20
  degenerative (generalized) (localized) 333.3
    facial 351.8
  douloureux (*see also* Neuralgia, trigeminal)
    350.1
    atypical 350.2

Tic —*continued*
  habit 307.20
    chronic (motor or vocal) 307.22
    transient (of childhood) 307.21
  lid 307.20
    transient (of childhood) 307.21
  motor-verbal 307.23
  occupational 300.89
  orbicularis 307.20
    transient (of childhood) 307.21
  organic origin 333.3
  postchoreic—*see* Chorea
  psychogenic 307.20
    compulsive 307.22
  salaam 781.0
  spasm 307.20
    chronic (motor or vocal) 307.22
    transient (of childhood) 307.21
Tick (-borne) fever NEC 066.1
  American mountain 066.1
  Colorado 066.1
  hemorrhagic NEC 065.3
    Crimean 065.0
    Kyasanur Forest 065.2
    Omsk 065.1
  mountain 066.1
  nonexanthematous 066.1
Tick-bite fever NEC 066.1
  African 087.1
  Colorado (virus) 066.1
  Rocky Mountain 082.0
Tick paralysis 989.5
Tics and spasms, compulsive 307.22
Tietze's disease or syndrome 733.6
Tight, tightness
  anus 564.89
  chest 786.59
  fascia (lata) 728.9
  foreskin (congenital) 605
  hymen 623.3
  introitus (acquired) (congenital) 623.3
  rectal sphincter 564.89
  tendon 727.81
    Achilles (heel) 727.81
  urethral sphincter 598.9
Tilting vertebra 737.9
Timidity, child 313.21
Tinea (intersecta) (tarsi) 110.9
  amiantacea 110.0
  asbestina 110.0
  barbae 110.0
  beard 110.0
  black dot 110.0
  blanca 111.2
  capitis 110.0
  corporis 110.5
  cruris 110.3
  decalvans 704.09
  flava 111.0
  foot 110.4
  furfuracea 111.0
  imbricata (Tokelau) 110.5
  lepothrix 039.0
  manuum 110.2
  microsporic (*see also* Dermatophytosis) 110.9
  nigra 111.1
  nodosa 111.2
  pedis 110.4
  scalp 110.0
  specified site NEC 110.8
  sycosis 110.0

Tinea—*continued*
tonsurans 110.0
trichophytic (*see also* Dermatophytosis) 110.9
unguium 110.1
versicolor 111.0
Tingling sensation (*see also* Disturbance, sensation) 782.0
Tin-miners' lung 503
Tinnitus (aurium) 388.30
audible 388.32
objective 388.32
subjective 388.31
Tipped, teeth 524.33
Tipping
pelvis 738.6
with disproportion (fetopelvic) 653.0
affecting fetus or newborn 763.1
causing obstructed labor 660.1
affecting fetus or newborn 763.1
teeth 524.33
Tiredness 780.79
Tissue —*see* condition
Tobacco
abuse (affecting health) NEC (*see also* Abuse, drugs, nondependent) 305.1
heart 989.8
use disorder complicating pregnancy, childbirth, or the puerperium 649.0
Tobias' syndrome (carcinoma, pulmonary apex) (M8010/3) 162.3
Tocopherol deficiency 269.1
Todd's
cirrhosis—*see* Cirrhosis, biliary
paralysis (postepileptic transitory paralysis) 344.89
Toe —*see* condition
Toilet, artificial opening (*see also* Attention to, artificial, opening) V55.9
Tokelau ringworm 110.5
Tollwut 071
Tolosa-Hunt syndrome 378.55
Tommaselli's disease
correct substance properly administered 599.70
overdose or wrong substance given or taken 961.4
Tongue —*see also* condition
worms 134.1
Tongue tie 750.0
Toni-Fanconi syndrome (cystinosis) 270.0
Tonic pupil 379.46
Tonsil —*see* condition
Tonsillitis (acute) (catarrhal) (croupous) (follicular) (gangrenous) (infective) (lacunar) (lingual) (malignant) (membranous) (phlegmonous) (pneumococcal) (pseudomembranous) (purulent) (septic) (staphylococcal) (subacute) (suppurative) (toxic) (ulcerative) (vesicular) (viral) 463
with influenza, flu, or grippe (*see also* Influenza) 487.1
chronic 474.00
diphtheritic (membranous) 032.0
hypertrophic 474.00
influenzal (*see also* Influenza) 487.1
parenchymatous 475
streptococcal 034.0
tuberculous (*see also* Tuberculosis) 012.8
Vincent's 101
Tonsillopharyngitis 465.8
Tooth, teeth —*see* condition
Toothache 525.9
Topagnosis 782.0

Tophi (gouty) 274.03
ear 274.81
heart 274.82
specified site NEC 274.82
TORCH infection (—see also Infection, congenital) 760.2
Torn —*see* Tear, torn
Tornwaldt's bursitis (disease) (pharyngeal bursitis) 478.29
cyst 478.26
Torpid liver 573.9
Torsion
accessory tube 620.5
adnexa (female) 620.5
aorta (congenital) 747.29
acquired 447.1
appendix
epididymis 608.24
testis 608.23
bile duct 576.8
with calculus, choledocholithiasis or stones—*see* Choledocholithiasis
congenital 751.69
bowel, colon, or intestine 560.2
cervix (*see* Malposition, uterus)
duodenum 537.3
dystonia—*see* Dystonia, torsion
epididymis 608.24
appendix 608.24
fallopian tube 620.5
gallbladder (*see also* Disease, gallbladder) 575.8
congenital 751.69
gastric 537.89
hydatid of Morgagni (female) 620.5
kidney (pedicle) 593.89
Meckel's diverticulum (congenital) 751.0
mesentery 560.2
omentum 560.2
organ or site, congenital NEC—*see* Anomaly, specified type NEC
ovary (pedicle) 620.5
congenital 752.0
oviduct 620.5
penis 607.89
congenital 752.69
renal 593.89
spasm—*see* Dystonia, torsion
spermatic cord 608.22
extravaginal 608.21
intravaginal 608.22
spleen 289.59
testicle, testis 608.20
appendix 608.23
tibia 736.89
umbilical cord—*see* Compression, umbilical cord
uterus (*see also* Malposition, uterus) 621.6
Torticollis (intermittent) (spastic) 723.5
congenital 754.1
sternomastoid 754.1
due to birth injury 767.8
hysterical 300.11
ocular 781.93
psychogenic 306.0
specified as conversion reaction 300.11
rheumatic 723.5
rheumatoid 714.0
spasmodic 333.83
traumatic, current NEC 847.0

Tortuous
artery 447.1
fallopian tube 752.19
organ or site, congenital NEC—*see* Distortion
renal vessel, congenital 747.62
retina vessel (congenital) 743.58
acquired 362.17
ureter 593.4
urethra 599.84
vein—*see* Varicose, vein
Torula, torular (infection) 117.5
histolytica 117.5
lung 117.5
Torulosis 117.5
Torus
fracture
fibula 823.41
with tibia 823.42
humerus 812.49
radius (alone) 813.45
with ulna 813.47
tibia 823.40
with fibula 823.42
ulna (alone) 813.46
with radius 813.47
mandibularis 526.81
palatinus 526.81
Touch, vitreous 997.99
Touraine's syndrome (hereditary
osteo-onychodysplasia) 756.89
Touraine-Solente-Golé syndrome
(acropachyderma) 757.39
Tourette's disease (motor-verbal tic) 307.23
Tower skull 756.0
with exophthalmos 756.0
Toxemia 799.89
with abortion—*see* Abortion, by type, with toxemia
bacterial—*see* Septicemia
biliary (*see also* Disease, biliary) 576.8
burn—*see* Burn, by site
congenital NEC 779.89
eclamptic 642.6
with pre-existing hypertension 642.7
erysipelatous (*see also* Erysipelas) 035
fatigue 799.89
fetus or newborn NEC 779.89
food (*see also* Poisoning, food) 005.9
gastric 537.89
gastrointestinal 558.2
intestinal 558.2
kidney (*see also* Disease, renal) 593.9
lung 518.89
malarial NEC (*see also* Malaria) 084.6
maternal (of pregnancy), affecting fetus or
newborn 760.0
myocardial—*see* Myocarditis, toxic
of pregnancy (mild) (pre-eclamptic) 642.4
with
convulsions 642.6
pre-existing hypertension 642.7
affecting fetus or newborn 760.0
severe 642.5
pre-eclamptic—*see* Toxemia, of pregnancy
puerperal, postpartum—*see* Toxemia, of
pregnancy
pulmonary 518.89
renal (*see also* Disease, renal) 593.9
septic (*see also* Septicemia) 038.9
small intestine 558.2

Toxemia—*continued*
staphylococcal 038.10
aureus 038.11
due to food 005.0
specified organism NEC 038.19
stasis 799.89
stomach 537.89
uremic (*see also* Uremia) 586
urinary 586
Toxemica cerebropathia psychica
(nonalcoholic) 294.0
alcoholic 291.1
Toxic (poisoning)—*see also* condition
from drug or poison—*see* Table of drugs and
chemicals
oil syndrome 710.5
shock syndrome 040.82
thyroid (gland) (*see also* Thyrotoxicosis) 242.9
Toxicemia —*see* Toxemia
Toxicity
dilantin
asymptomatic 796.0
symptomatic—*see* Table of Drugs and Chemicals
drug
asymptomatic 796.0
symptomatic—*see* Table of Drugs and Chemicals
fava bean 282.2
from drug or poison
asymptomatic 796.0
symptomatic—*see* Table of Drugs and
Chemicals
Toxicosis (*see also* Toxemia) 799.89
capillary, hemorrhagic 287.0
Toxinfection 799.89
gastrointestinal 558.2
Toxocariasis 128.0
Toxoplasma infection, generalized 130.9
Toxoplasmosis (acquired) 130.9
with pneumonia 130.4
congenital, active 771.2
disseminated (multisystemic) 130.8
maternal
with suspected damage to fetus affecting
management of pregnancy 655.4
affecting fetus or newborn 760.2
manifest toxoplasmosis in fetus or newborn
771.2
multiple sites 130.8
multisystemic disseminated 130.8
specified site NEC 130.7
Trabeculation, bladder 596.89
Trachea —*see* condition
Tracheitis (acute)(catarrhal)(infantile)
(membranous) (plastic) (pneumococcal)
(septic) (suppurative) (viral) 464.10
with
bronchitis 490
acute or subacute 466.0
chronic 491.8
tuberculosis—*see* Tuberculosis, pulmonary
laryngitis (acute) 464.20
with obstruction 464.21
chronic 476.1
tuberculous (*see also* Tuberculosis, larynx) 012.3
obstruction 464.11
chronic 491.8
with
bronchitis (chronic) 491.8
laryngitis (chronic) 476.1
due to external agent—*see* Condition,
respiratory, chronic, due to

Tracheitis—*continued*
 diphtheritic (membranous) 032.3
  due to external agent—*see* Inflammation,
   respiratory, upper, due to
 edematous 464.11
 influenzal (*see also* Influenza) 487.1
 streptococcal 034.0
 syphilitic 095.8
 tuberculous (*see also* Tuberculosis) 012.8
Trachelitis (nonvenereal) (*see also* Cervicitis) 616.0
 trichomonal 131.09
Tracheobronchial —*see* condition
Tracheobronchitis (*see also* Bronchitis) 490
 acute or subacute 466.0
  with bronchospasm or obstruction 466.0
 chronic 491.8
 influenzal (*see also* Influenza) 487.1
 senile 491.8
Tracheobronchomegaly (congenital) 748.3
 with bronchiectasis 494.0
  with (acute) exacerbation 494.1
 acquired 519.19
  with bronchiectasis 494.0
   with (acute) exacerbation 494.1
Tracheobronchopneumonitis —*see* Pneumonia,
 broncho
Tracheocele (external) (internal) 519.19
 congenital 748.3
Tracheomalacia 519.19
 congenital 748.3
Tracheopharyngitis (acute) 465.8
 chronic 478.9
  due to external agent—*see* Condition,
   respiratory, chronic, due to
  due to external agent—*see* Inflammation,
   respiratory, upper, due to
Tracheostenosis 519.19
 congenital 748.3
Tracheostomy
 attention to V55.0
 complication 519.00
 granuloma 519.09
 hemorrhage 519.09
 infection 519.01
 malfunctioning 519.02
 obstruction 519.09
 sepsis 519.01
 status V44.0
 stenosis 519.02
Trachoma, trachomatous 076.9
 active (stage) 076.1
 contraction of conjunctiva 076.1
 dubium 076.0
 healed or late effect 139.1
 initial (stage) 076.0
 Türck's (chronic catarrhal laryngitis) 476.0
Trachyphonia 784.49
Traction, vitreomacular 379.27
Training
 insulin pump V65.46
 orthoptic V57.4
 orthotic V57.81
Train sickness 994.6
Trait
 hemoglobin
  abnormal NEC 282.7
   with thalassemia 282.46
  C (*see also* Disease, hemoglobin, C) 282.7
   with elliptocytosis 282.7
  S (Hb-S) 282.5

Trait—*continued*
 Lepore 282.49
  with other abnormal hemoglobin NEC 282.49
 paranoid 301.0
 sickle-cell 282.5
  with
   elliptocytosis 282.5
   spherocytosis 282.5
  thalassemia (alpha) (beta) (delta-beta) 282.46
Traits, paranoid 301.0
Tramp V60.0
Trance 780.09
 hysterical 300.13
Transaminasemia 790.4
Transfusion, blood
 donor V59.01
  stem cells V59.02
 fetal twin to twin 678.0
 incompatible (*see also* Complications,
  transfusion) 999.80
  ABO (*see also* Complications, transfusion)
   999.60
  minor blood group 999.89
  non-ABO (*see also* Complications,
   transfusion) 999.75
  Rh (antigen) (C) (c) (D) (E) (e) (*see also*
   Complications, transfusion) 999.70
 reaction or complication—*see* Complications,
  transfusion
 related acute lung injury (TRALI) 518.7
 syndrome
  fetomaternal 772.0
  twin-to-twin
   blood loss (donor twin) 772.0
   recipient twin 776.4
 twin to twin fetal 678.0
 without reported diagnosis V58.2
Transient —*see also* condition
 alteration of awareness 780.02
 blindness 368.12
 deafness (ischemic) 388.02
 global amnesia 437.7
 hyperglycemia (post-procedural) 790.29
 hypoglycemia (post-procedural) 251.2
 person (homeless) NEC V60.0
Transitional, lumbosacral joint of vertebra
 756.19
Translocation
 autosomes NEC 758.5
  13-15 758.1
  16-18 758.2
  21 or 22 758.0
  balanced in normal individual 758.4
  D₁ 758.1
  E₃ 758.2
  G 758.0
 balanced autosomal in normal individual 758.4
 chromosomes NEC 758.89
 Down's syndrome 758.0
Translucency, iris 364.53
Transmission of chemical substances through
  the placenta (affecting fetus or newborn)
  760.70
 alcohol 760.71
 anticonvulsants 760.77
 antifungals 760.74
 anti-infective agents 760.74
 antimetabolics 760.78
 cocaine 760.75
 "crack" 760.75
 diethylstilbestrol [DES] 760.76
 hallucinogenic agents 760.73

Transmission —*continued*
  medicinal agents NEC 760.79
  narcotics 760.72
  obstetric anesthetic or analgesic drug 763.5
  specified agent NEC 760.79
  suspected, affecting management of pregnancy 655.5
Transplant(ed)
  bone V42.4
    marrow V42.81
  complication—*see also* Complications, due to (presence of) any device, implant, or graft classified to 996.0-996.5 NEC
    bone marrow 996.85
    corneal graft NEC 996.79
      infection or inflammation 996.69
      reaction 996.51
      rejection 996.51
    organ (failure) (immune or nonimmune cause) (infection) (rejection) 996.80
      bone marrow 996.85
      heart 996.83
      intestines 996.87
      kidney 996.81
      liver 996.82
      lung 996.84
      pancreas 996.86
      specified NEC 996.89
    previously removed due to complication, failure, rejection or infection V45.87
    removal status V45.87
    skin NEC 996.79
      infection or inflammation 996.69
      rejection 996.52
        artificial 996.55
        decellularized allodermis 996.55
    stem cell(s) 996.88
      from
        peripheral blood 996.88
        umbilical blood 996.88
  cornea V42.5
  hair V50.0
  heart V42.1
    valve V42.2
  intestine V42.84
  kidney V42.0
  liver V42.7
  lung V42.6
  organ V42.9
    specified NEC V42.89
  pancreas V42.83
  peripheral stem cells V42.82
  skin V42.3
  stem cells, peripheral V42.82
  tissue V42.9
    specified NEC V42.89
Transplants, ovarian, endometrial 617.1
Transposed —*see* Transposition
Transposition (congenital)—*see also* Malposition, congenital
  abdominal viscera 759.3
  aorta (dextra) 745.11
  appendix 751.5
  arterial trunk 745.10
  colon 751.5
  great vessels (complete) 745.10
    both originating from right ventricle 745.11
    corrected 745.12
    double outlet right ventricle 745.11
    incomplete 745.11
    partial 745.11
    specified type NEC 745.19

Transposition—*continued*
  heart 746.87
    with complete transposition of viscera 759.3
  intestine (large) (small) 751.5
  pulmonary veins 747.49
  reversed jejunal (for bypass) (status) V45.3
  scrotal 752.81
  stomach 750.7
    with general transposition of viscera 759.3
  teeth, tooth 524.30
  vessels (complete) 745.10
    partial 745.11
  viscera (abdominal) (thoracic) 759.3
Trans-sexualism 302.50
  with
    asexual history 302.51
    heterosexual history 302.53
    homosexual history 302.52
Transverse —*see also* condition
  arrest (deep), in labor 660.3
    affecting fetus or newborn 763.1
  lie 652.3
    before labor, affecting fetus or newborn 761.7
    causing obstructed labor 660.0
      affecting fetus or newborn 763.1
    during labor, affecting fetus or newborn 763.1
Transvestism, transvestitism (transvestic fetishism) 302.3
Trapped placenta (with hemorrhage) 666.0
  without hemorrhage 667.0
Trauma, traumatism (*see also* Injury, by site) 959.9
  birth—*see* Birth, injury NEC
  causing hemorrhage of pregnancy or delivery 641.8
  complicating
    abortion—*see* Abortion, by type, with damage to pelvic organs
    ectopic pregnancy (*see also* categories 633.0-633.9) 639.2
    molar pregnancy (*see also* categories 630-632) 639.2
  during delivery NEC 665.9
  following
    abortion 639.2
    ectopic or molar pregnancy 639.2
  maternal, during pregnancy, affecting fetus or newborn 760.5
  neuroma—*see* Injury, nerve, by site
  previous major, affecting management of pregnancy, childbirth, or puerperium V23.8
  psychic (current)—*see also* Reaction, adjustment
    previous (history) V15.49
  psychologic, previous (affecting health) V15.49
  transient paralysis—*see* Injury, nerve, by site
Traumatic —*see also* condition
  brain injury (TBI) (see also Injury, intracranial) 854.0
    with skull fracture - see Fracture, skull, by site
Treacher Collins' syndrome (incomplete facial dysostosis) 756.0
Treitz's hernia —*see* Hernia, Treitz's
Trematode infestation NEC 121.9
Trematodiasis NEC 121.9
Trembles 988.8
Trembling paralysis (*see also* Parkinsonism) 332.0
Tremor 781.0
  essential (benign) 333.1
  familial 333.1

Tremor—*continued*
  flapping (liver) 572.8
  hereditary 333.1
  hysterical 300.11
  intention 333.1
  medication-induced postural 333.1
  mercurial 985.0
  muscle 728.85
  Parkinson's (*see also* Parkinsonism) 332.0
  psychogenic 306.0
    specified as conversion reaction 300.11
  senilis 797
  specified type NEC 333.1
Trench
  fever 083.1
  foot 991.4
  mouth 101
  nephritis—*see* Nephritis, acute
Treponema pallidum infection (*see also*
  Syphilis) 097.9
Treponematosis 102.9
  due to
    T. pallidum—*see* Syphilis
    T. pertenue (yaws) (*see also* Yaws) 102.9
Triad
  Kartagener's 759.3
  Reiter's (complete) (incomplete) 099.3
  Saint's (*see also* Hernia, diaphragm) 553.3
Trichiasis 704.2
  cicatricial 704.2
  eyelid 374.05
    with entropion (*see also* Entropion) 374.00
Trichinella spiralis (infection) (infestation) 124
Trichinelliasis 124
Trichinellosis 124
Trichiniasis 124
Trichinosis 124
Trichobezoar 938
  intestine 936
  stomach 935.2
Trichocephaliasis 127.3
Trichocephalosis 127.3
Trichocephalus infestation 127.3
Trichoclasis 704.2
Trichoepithelioma (M8100/0)—*see also*
  Neoplasm, skin, benign
  breast 217
  genital organ NEC—*see* Neoplasm, by site,
    benign
  malignant (M8100/3)—*see* Neoplasm, skin,
    malignant
Trichofolliculoma (M8101/0)—*see* Neoplasm,
  skin, benign
Tricholemmoma (M8102/0)—*see* Neoplasm,
  skin, benign
Trichomatosis 704.2
Trichomoniasis 131.9
  bladder 131.09
  cervix 131.09
  intestinal 007.3
  prostate 131.03
  seminal vesicle 131.09
  specified site NEC 131.8
  urethra 131.02
  urogenitalis 131.00
  vagina 131.01
  vulva 131.01
  vulvovaginal 131.01

Trichomycosis 039.0
  axillaris 039.0
  nodosa 111.2
  nodularis 111.2
  rubra 039.0
Trichonocardiosis (axillaris) (palmellina) 039.0
Trichonodosis 704.2
Trichophytid, trichophyton infection (*see also*
  Dermatophytosis) 110.9
Trichophytide —*see* Dermatophytosis
Trichophytobezoar 938
  intestine 936
  stomach 935.2
Trichophytosis —*see* Dermatophytosis
Trichoptilosis 704.2
Trichorrhexis (nodosa) 704.2
Trichosporosis nodosa 111.2
Trichostasis spinulosa (congenital) 757.4
Trichostrongyliasis (small intestine) 127.6
Trichostrongylosis 127.6
Trichostrongylus (instabilis) infection 127.6
Trichotillomania 312.39
Trichromat, anomalous (congenital) 368.59
Trichromatopsia, anomalous (congenital)
  368.59
Trichuriasis 127.3
Trichuris trichiura (any site) (infection)
  (infestation) 127.3
Tricuspid (valve)—*see* condition
Trifid —*see also* Accessory
  kidney (pelvis) 753.3
  tongue 750.13
Trigeminal neuralgia (*see also* Neuralgia,
  trigeminal) 350.1
Trigeminoencephaloangiomatosis 759.6
Trigeminy 427.89
  postoperative 997.1
Trigger finger (acquired) 727.03
  congenital 756.89
Trigonitis (bladder) (chronic)
  (pseudomembranous) 595.3
  tuberculous (*see also* Tuberculosis) 016.1
Trigonocephaly 756.0
Trihexosidosis 272.7
Trilobate placenta —*see* Placenta, abnormal
Trilocular heart 745.8
Trimethylaminuria 270.8
Tripartita placenta —*see* Placenta, abnormal
Triple —*see also* Accessory
  kidneys 753.3
  uteri 752.2
  X female 758.81
Triplegia 344.89
  congenital or infantile 343.8
Triplet
  affected by maternal complications of pregnancy
    761.5
  healthy liveborn—*see* Newborn, multiple
  pregnancy (complicating delivery) NEC 651.1
    with fetal loss and retention of one or more
      fetus(es) 651.4
    following (elective) fetal reduction 651.7
Triplex placenta —*see* Placenta, abnormal
Triplication —*see* Accessory
Trismus 781.0
  neonatorum 771.3
  newborn 771.3
Trisomy (syndrome) NEC 758.5
  13 (partial) 758.1
  16-18 758.2

Trisomy—*continued*
  18 (partial) 758.2
  21 (partial) 758.0
  22 758.0
  autosomes NEC 758.5
  D$_1$ 758.1
  E$_3$ 758.2
  G (group) 758.0
  group D$_1$ 758.1
  group E 758.2
  group G 758.0
Tritanomaly 368.53
Tritanopia 368.53
Troisier-Hanot-Chauffard syndrome (bronze diabetes) 275.01
Trombidiosis 133.8
Trophedema (hereditary) 757.0
  congenital 757.0
Trophoblastic disease (*see also* Hydatidiform mole) 630
  previous, affecting management of pregnancy V23.1
Tropholymphedema 757.0
Trophoneurosis NEC 356.9
  arm NEC 354.9
  disseminated 710.1
  facial 349.89
  leg NEC 355.8
  lower extremity NEC 355.8
  upper extremity NEC 354.9
Tropical —*see also* condition
  maceration feet (syndrome) 991.4
  wet foot (syndrome) 991.4
Trouble —*see also* Disease
  bowel 569.9
  heart—*see* Disease, heart
  intestine 569.9
  kidney (*see also* Disease, renal) 593.9
  nervous 799.21
  sinus (*see also* Sinusitis) 473.9
Trousseau's syndrome (thrombophlebitis migrans) 453.1
Truancy, childhood —*see also* Disturbance, conduct
  socialized 312.2
  undersocialized, unsocialized 312.1
Truncus
  arteriosus (persistent) 745.0
  common 745.0
  communis 745.0
Trunk —*see* condition
Trychophytide —*see* Dermatophytosis
Trypanosoma infestation —*see* Trypanosomiasis
Trypanosomiasis 086.9
  with meningoencephalitis 086.9 *[323.2]*
  African 086.5
    due to Trypanosoma 086.5
      gambiense 086.3
      rhodesiense 086.4
  American 086.2
    with
      heart involvement 086.0
      other organ involvement 086.1
    without mention of organ involvement 086.2
  Brazilian—*see* Trypanosomiasis, American
  Chagas'—*see* Trypanosomiasis, American
  due to Trypanosoma
    cruzi—*see* Trypanosomiasis, American
    gambiense 086.3
    rhodesiense 086.4

Trypanosomiasis—*continued*
  gambiensis, Gambian 086.3
  North American—*see* Trypanosomiasis, American
  rhodesiensis, Rhodesian 086.4
  South American—*see* Trypanosomiasis, American
T-shaped incisors 520.2
Tsutsugamushi fever 081.2
Tube, tubal, tubular —*see also* condition
  ligation, admission for V25.2
Tubercle —*see also* Tuberculosis
  brain, solitary 013.2
  Darwin's 744.29
  epithelioid noncaseating 135
  Ghon, primary infection 010.0
Tuberculid, tuberculide (indurating) (lichenoid) (miliary) (papulonecrotic) (primary) (skin) (subcutaneous) (*see also* Tuberculosis) 017.0
Tuberculoma —*see also* Tuberculosis
  brain (any part) 013.2
  meninges (cerebral) (spinal) 013.1
  spinal cord 013.4
Tuberculosis, tubercular, tuberculous
  (calcification) (calcified) (caseous) (chromogenic acid-fast bacilli) (congenital) (degeneration) (disease) (fibrocaseous) (fistula) (gangrene) (interstitial) (isolated circumscribed lesions) (necrosis) (parenchymatous) (ulcerative) 011.9

Note—Use the following fifth-digit subclassification with categories 010-018:

0 unspecified
1 bacteriological or histological examination not done
2 bacteriological or histological examination unknown (at present)
3 tubercle bacilli found (in sputum) by microscopy
4 tubercle bacilli not found (in sputum) by microscopy, but found by bacterial culture
5 tubercle bacilli not found by bacteriological examination, but tuberculosis confirmed histologically
6 tubercle bacilli not found by bacteriological or histological examination, but tuberculosis confirmed by other methods [inoculation of animals]

For tuberculous conditions specified as late effects or sequelae, see category 137.

---

  abdomen 014.8
    lymph gland 014.8
  abscess 011.9
    arm 017.9
    bone (*see also* Osteomyelitis, due to, tuberculosis) 015.9 *[730.8]*
      hip 015.1 *[730.85]*
      knee 015.2 *[730.86]*
      sacrum 015.0 *[730.88]*
      specified site NEC 015.7 *[730.88]*
      spinal 015.0 *[730.88]*
      vertebra 015.0 *[730.88]*
    brain 013.3
    breast 017.9
    Cowper's gland 016.5
    dura (mater) 013.8
      brain 013.3
      spinal cord 013.5

Tuberculosis, tubercular—*continued*
  abscess—*continued*
    epidural 013.8
      brain 013.3
      spinal cord 013.5
    frontal sinus—*see* Tuberculosis, sinus
    genital organs NEC 016.9
      female 016.7
      male 016.5
    genitourinary NEC 016.9
    gland (lymphatic)—*see* Tuberculosis, lymph
      gland
    hip 015.1
    iliopsoas 015.0 *[730.88]*
    intestine 014.8
    ischiorectal 014.8
    joint 015.9
      hip 015.1
      knee 015.2
      specified joint NEC 015.8
      vertebral 015.0 *[730.88]*
    kidney 016.0 *[590.81]*
    knee 015.2
    lumbar 015.0 *[730.88]*
    lung 011.2
      primary, progressive 010.8
    meninges (cerebral) (spinal) 013.0
    pelvic 016.9
      female 016.7
      male 016.5
    perianal 014.8
      fistula 014.8
    perinephritic 016.0 *[590.81]*
    perineum 017.9
    perirectal 014.8
    psoas 015.0 *[730.88]*
    rectum 014.8
    retropharyngeal 012.8
    sacrum 015.0 *[730.88]*
    scrofulous 017.2
    scrotum 016.5
    skin 017.0
      primary 017.0
    spinal cord 013.5
    spine or vertebra (column) 015.0 *[730.88]*
    strumous 017.2
    subdiaphragmatic 014.8
    testis 016.5
    thigh 017.9
    urinary 016.3
      kidney 016.0 *[590.81]*
    uterus 016.7
  accessory sinus—*see* Tuberculosis, sinus
  Addison's disease 017.6
  adenitis (*see also* Tuberculosis, lymph gland)
    017.2
  adenoids 012.8
  adenopathy (*see also* Tuberculosis, lymph
    gland) 017.2
    tracheobronchial 012.1
      primary progressive 010.8
  adherent pericardium 017.9 *[420.0]*
  adnexa (uteri) 016.7
  adrenal (capsule) (gland) 017.6
  air passage NEC 012.8
  alimentary canal 014.8
  anemia 017.9
  ankle (joint) 015.8
    bone 015.5 *[730.87]*
  anus 014.8
  apex (*see also* Tuberculosis, pulmonary) 011.9

Tuberculosis, tubercular—*continued*
  apical (*see also* Tuberculosis, pulmonary) 011.9
  appendicitis 014.8
  appendix 014.8
  arachnoid 013.0
  artery 017.9
  arthritis (chronic) (synovial) 015.9 *[711.40]*
    ankle 015.8 *[730.87]*
    hip 015.1 *[711.45]*
    knee 015.2 *[711.46]*
    specified site NEC 015.8 *[711.48]*
    spine or vertebra (column) 015.0 *[720.81]*
    wrist 015.8 *[730.83]*
  articular—*see* Tuberculosis, joint
  ascites 014.0
  asthma (*see also* Tuberculosis, pulmonary)
    011.9
  axilla, axillary 017.2
    gland 017.2
  bilateral (*see also* Tuberculosis, pulmonary)
    011.9
  bladder 016.1
  bone (*see also* Osteomyelitis, due to,
    tuberculosis) 015.9 *[730.8]*
    hip 015.1 *[730.85]*
    knee 015.2 *[730.86]*
    limb NEC 015.5 *[730.88]*
    sacrum 015.0 *[730.88]*
    specified site NEC 015.7 *[730.88]*
    spinal or vertebral column 015.0 *[730.88]*
  bowel 014.8
    miliary 018.9
  brain 013.2
  breast 017.9
  broad ligament 016.7
  bronchi, bronchial, bronchus 011.3
    ectasia, ectasis 011.5
    fistula 011.3
      primary, progressive 010.8
    gland 012.1
      primary, progressive 010.8
    isolated 012.2
    lymph gland or node 012.1
      primary, progressive 010.8
  bronchiectasis 011.5
  bronchitis 011.3
  bronchopleural 012.0
  bronchopneumonia, bronchopneumonic 011.6
  bronchorrhagia 011.3
  bronchotracheal 011.3
    isolated 012.2
  bronchus—*see* Tuberculosis, bronchi
  bronze disease (Addison's) 017.6
  buccal cavity 017.9
  bulbourethral gland 016.5
  bursa (*see also* Tuberculosis, joint) 015.9
  cachexia NEC (*see also* Tuberculosis,
    pulmonary) 011.9
  cardiomyopathy 017.9 *[425.8]*
  caries (*see also* Tuberculosis, bone) 015.9
    [730.8]
  cartilage (*see also* Tuberculosis, bone) 015.9
    [730.8]
    intervertebral 015.0 *[730.88]*
  catarrhal (*see also* Tuberculosis, pulmonary)
    011.9
  cecum 014.8
  cellular tissue (primary) 017.0
  cellulitis (primary) 017.0
  central nervous system 013.9
    specified site NEC 013.8

Tuberculosis, tubercular—*continued*
  cerebellum (current) 013.2
  cerebral (current) 013.2
    meninges 013.0
  cerebrospinal 013.6
    meninges 013.0
  cerebrum (current) 013.2
  cervical 017.2
    gland 017.2
    lymph nodes 017.2
  cervicitis (uteri) 016.7
  cervix 016.7
  chest (*see also* Tuberculosis, pulmonary) 011.9
  childhood type or first infection 010.0
  choroid 017.3 *[363.13]*
  choroiditis 017.3 *[363.13]*
  ciliary body 017.3 *[364.11]*
  colitis 014.8
  colliers' 011.4
  colliquativa (primary) 017.0
  colon 014.8
    ulceration 014.8
  complex, primary 010.0
  complicating pregnancy, childbirth, or
      puerperium 647.3
    affecting fetus or newborn 760.2
  congenital 771.2
  conjunctiva 017.3 *[370.31]*
  connective tissue 017.9
    bone—*see* Tuberculosis, bone
  contact V01.1
  converter (tuberculin skin test) (without disease)
      795.51
  cornea (ulcer) 017.3 *[370.31]*
  Cowper's gland 016.5
  coxae 015.1 *[730.85]*
  coxalgia 015.1 *[730.85]*
  cul-de-sac of Douglas 014.8
  curvature, spine 015.0 *[737.40]*
  cutis (colliquativa) (primary) 017.0
  cyst, ovary 016.6
  cystitis 016.1
  dacryocystitis 017.3 *[375.32]*
  dactylitis 015.5
  diarrhea 014.8
  diffuse (*see also* Tuberculosis, miliary) 018.9
    lung—*see* Tuberculosis, pulmonary
    meninges 013.0
  digestive tract 014.8
  disseminated (*see also* Tuberculosis, miliary)
      018.9
    meninges 013.0
  duodenum 014.8
  dura (mater) 013.9
    abscess 013.8
      cerebral 013.3
      spinal 013.5
  dysentery 014.8
  ear (inner) (middle) 017.4
    bone 015.6
    external (primary) 017.0
    skin (primary) 017.0
  elbow 015.8
  emphysema—*see* Tuberculosis, pulmonary
  empyema 012.0
  encephalitis 013.6
  endarteritis 017.9
  endocarditis (any valve) 017.9 *[424.91]*
  endocardium (any valve) 017.9 *[424.91]*
  endocrine glands NEC 017.9
  endometrium 016.7

Tuberculosis, tubercular—*continued*
  enteric, enterica 014.8
  enteritis 014.8
  enterocolitis 014.8
  epididymis 016.4
  epididymitis 016.4
  epidural abscess 013.8
    brain 013.3
    spinal cord 013.5
  epiglottis 012.3
  episcleritis 017.3 *[379.00]*
  erythema (induratum) (nodosum) (primary) 017.1
  esophagus 017.8
  Eustachian tube 017.4
  exposure to V01.1
  exudative 012.0
    primary, progressive 010.1
  eye 017.3
  eyelid (primary) 017.0
    lupus 017.0 *[373.4]*
  fallopian tube 016.6
  fascia 017.9
  fauces 012.8
  finger 017.9
  first infection 010.0
  fistula, perirectal 014.8
  Florida 011.6
  foot 017.9
  funnel pelvis 137.3
  gallbladder 017.9
  galloping (*see also* Tuberculosis, pulmonary)
      011.9
  ganglionic 015.9
  gastritis 017.9
  gastrocolic fistula 014.8
  gastroenteritis 014.8
  gastrointestinal tract 014.8
  general, generalized 018.9
    acute 018.0
    chronic 018.8
  genital organs NEC 016.9
    female 016.7
    male 016.5
  genitourinary NEC 016.9
  genu 015.2
  glandulae suprarenalis 017.6
  glandular, general 017.2
  glottis 012.3
  grinders' 011.4
  groin 017.2
  gum 017.9
  hand 017.9
  heart 017.9 *[425.8]*
  hematogenous—*see* Tuberculosis, miliary
  hemoptysis (*see also* Tuberculosis, pulmonary)
      011.9
  hemorrhage NEC (*see also* Tuberculosis,
      pulmonary) 011.9
  hemothorax 012.0
  hepatitis 017.9
  hilar lymph nodes 012.1
    primary, progressive 010.8
  hip (disease) (joint) 015.1
    bone 015.1 *[730.85]*
  hydrocephalus 013.8
  hydropneumothorax 012.0
  hydrothorax 012.0
  hypoadrenalism 017.6
  hypopharynx 012.8
  ileocecal (hyperplastic) 014.8
  ileocolitis 014.8

Tuberculosis, tubercular—*continued*
ileum 014.8
iliac spine (superior) 015.0 *[730.88]*
incipient NEC (*see also* Tuberculosis,
pulmonary) 011.9
indurativa (primary) 017.1
infantile 010.0
infection NEC 011.9
without clinical manifestation 010.0
infraclavicular gland 017.2
inguinal gland 017.2
inguinalis 017.2
intestine (any part) 014.8
iris 017.3 *[364.11]*
iritis 017.3 *[364.11]*
ischiorectal 014.8
jaw 015.7 *[730.88]*
jejunum 014.8
joint 015.9
hip 015.1
knee 015.2
specified site NEC 015.8
vertebral 015.0 *[730.88]*
keratitis 017.3 *[370.31]*
interstitial 017.3 *[370.59]*
keratoconjunctivitis 017.3 *[370.31]*
kidney 016.0
knee (joint) 015.2
kyphoscoliosis 015.0 *[737.43]*
kyphosis 015.0 *[737.41]*
lacrimal apparatus, gland 017.3
laryngitis 012.3
larynx 012.3
latent 795.51
leptomeninges, leptomeningitis (cerebral)
(spinal) 013.0
lichenoides (primary) 017.0
linguae 017.9
lip 017.9
liver 017.9
lordosis 015.0 *[737.42]*
lung—*see* Tuberculosis, pulmonary
luposa 017.0
eyelid 017.0 *[373.4]*
lymphadenitis—*see* Tuberculosis, lymph gland
lymphangitis—*see* Tuberculosis, lymph gland
lymphatic (gland) (vessel)—*see* Tuberculosis,
lymph gland
lymph gland or node (peripheral) 017.2
abdomen 014.8
bronchial 012.1
primary, progressive 010.8
cervical 017.2
hilar 012.1
primary, progressive 010.8
intrathoracic 012.1
primary, progressive 010.8
mediastinal 012.1
primary, progressive 010.8
mesenteric 014.8
peripheral 017.2
retroperitoneal 014.8
tracheobronchial 012.1
primary, progressive 010.8
malignant NEC (*see also* Tuberculosis,
pulmonary) 011.9
mammary gland 017.9
marasmus NEC (*see also* Tuberculosis,
pulmonary) 011.9
mastoiditis 015.6
maternal, affecting fetus or newborn 760.2

Tuberculosis, tubercular—*continued*
mediastinal (lymph) gland or node 012.1
primary, progressive 010.8
mediastinitis 012.8
primary, progressive 010.8
mediastinopericarditis 017.9 *[420.0]*
mediastinum 012.8
primary, progressive 010.8
medulla 013.9
brain 013.2
spinal cord 013.4
melanosis, Addisonian 017.6
membrane, brain 013.0
meninges (cerebral) (spinal) 013.0
meningitis (basilar) (brain) (cerebral)
(cerebrospinal) (spinal) 013.0
meningoencephalitis 013.0
mesentery, mesenteric 014.8
lymph gland or node 014.8
miliary (any site) 018.9
acute 018.0
chronic 018.8
specified type NEC 018.8
millstone makers' 011.4
miners' 011.4
moulders' 011.4
mouth 017.9
multiple 018.9
acute 018.0
chronic 018.8
muscle 017.9
myelitis 013.6
myocarditis 017.9 *[422.0]*
myocardium 017.9 *[422.0]*
nasal (passage) (sinus) 012.8
nasopharynx 012.8
neck gland 017.2
nephritis 016.0 *[583.81]*
nerve 017.9
nose (septum) 012.8
ocular 017.3
old NEC 137.0
without residuals V12.01
omentum 014.8
oophoritis (acute) (chronic) 016.6
optic 017.3 *[377.39]*
nerve trunk 017.3 *[377.39]*
papilla, papillae 017.3 *[377.39]*
orbit 017.3
orchitis 016.5 *[608.81]*
organ, specified NEC 017.9
orificialis (primary) 017.0
osseous (*see also* Tuberculosis, bone) 015.9
[730.8]
osteitis (*see also* Tuberculosis, bone) 015.9
[730.8]
osteomyelitis (*see also* Tuberculosis, bone)
015.9 *[730.8]*
otitis (media) 017.4
ovaritis (acute) (chronic) 016.6
ovary (acute) (chronic) 016.6
oviducts (acute) (chronic) 016.6
pachymeningitis 013.0
palate (soft) 017.9
pancreas 017.9
papulonecrotic (primary) 017.0
parathyroid glands 017.9
paronychia (primary) 017.0
parotid gland or region 017.9
pelvic organ NEC 016.9
female 016.7
male 016.5

Tuberculosis, tubercular—*continued*
  pelvis (bony) 015.7 *[730.85]*
  penis 016.5
  peribronchitis 011.3
  pericarditis 017.9 *[420.0]*
  pericardium 017.9 *[420.0]*
  perichondritis, larynx 012.3
  perineum 017.9
  periostitis (*see also* Tuberculosis, bone) 015.9
    [730.8]
  periphlebitis 017.9
    eye vessel 017.3 *[362.18]*
    retina 017.3 *[362.18]*
  perirectal fistula 014.8
  peritoneal gland 014.8
  peritoneum 014.0
  peritonitis 014.0
  pernicious NEC (*see also* Tuberculosis,
    pulmonary) 011.9
  pharyngitis 012.8
  pharynx 012.8
  phlyctenulosis (conjunctiva) 017.3 *[370.31]*
  phthisis NEC (*see also* Tuberculosis,
    pulmonary) 011.9
  pituitary gland 017.9
  placenta 016.7
  pleura, pleural, pleurisy, pleuritis (fibrinous)
    (obliterative) (purulent) (simple plastic)
    (with effusion) 012.0
    primary, progressive 010.1
  pneumonia, pneumonic 011.6
  pneumothorax 011.7
  polyserositis 018.9
    acute 018.0
    chronic 018.8
  potters' 011.4
  prepuce 016.5
  primary 010.9
    complex 010.0
    complicated 010.8
      with pleurisy or effusion 010.1
    progressive 010.8
      with pleurisy or effusion 010.1
    skin 017.0
  proctitis 014.8
  prostate 016.5 *[601.4]*
  prostatitis 016.5 *[601.4]*
  pulmonaris (*see also* Tuberculosis, pulmonary)
    011.9
  pulmonary (artery) (incipient) (malignant)
    (multiple round foci) (pernicious)
    (reinfection stage) 011.9
    cavitated or with cavitation 011.2
      primary, progressive 010.8
    childhood type or first infection 010.0
    chromogenic acid-fast bacilli 795.39
    fibrosis or fibrotic 011.4
    infiltrative 011.0
      primary, progressive 010.9
    nodular 011.1
    specified NEC 011.8
    sputum positive only 795.39
    status following surgical collapse of lung NEC
      011.9
  pyelitis 016.0 *[590.81]*
  pyelonephritis 016.0 *[590.81]*
  pyemia—*see* Tuberculosis, miliary
  pyonephrosis 016.0
  pyopneumothorax 012.0
  pyothorax 012.0

Tuberculosis, tubercular—*continued*
  rectum (with abscess) 014.8
    fistula 014.8
  reinfection stage (*see also* Tuberculosis,
    pulmonary) 011.9
  renal 016.0
  renis 016.0
  reproductive organ 016.7
  respiratory NEC (*see also* Tuberculosis,
    pulmonary) 011.9
    specified site NEC 012.8
  retina 017.3 *[363.13]*
  retroperitoneal (lymph gland or node) 014.8
    gland 014.8
  retropharyngeal abscess 012.8
  rheumatism 015.9
  rhinitis 012.8
  sacroiliac (joint) 015.8
  sacrum 015.0 *[730.88]*
  salivary gland 017.9
  salpingitis (acute) (chronic) 016.6
  sandblasters' 011.4
  sclera 017.3 *[379.09]*
  scoliosis 015.0 *[737.43]*
  scrofulous 017.2
  scrotum 016.5
  seminal tract or vesicle 016.5 *[608.81]*
  senile NEC (*see also* Tuberculosis, pulmonary)
    011.9
  septic NEC (*see also* Tuberculosis, miliary)
    018.9
  shoulder 015.8
    blade 015.7 *[730.8]*
  sigmoid 014.8
  sinus (accessory) (nasal) 012.8
    bone 015.7 *[730.88]*
    epididymis 016.4
  skeletal NEC (*see also* Osteomyelitis, due to
    tuberculosis) 015.9 *[730.8]*
  skin (any site) (primary) 017.0
  small intestine 014.8
  soft palate 017.9
  spermatic cord 016.5
  spinal
    column 015.0 *[730.88]*
    cord 013.4
    disease 015.0 *[730.88]*
    medulla 013.4
    membrane 013.0
    meninges 013.0
  spine 015.0 *[730.88]*
  spleen 017.7
  splenitis 017.7
  spondylitis 015.0 *[720.81]*
  spontaneous pneumothorax—*see* Tuberculosis,
    pulmonary
  sternoclavicular joint 015.8
  stomach 017.9
  stonemasons' 011.4
  struma 017.2
  subcutaneous tissue (cellular) (primary) 017.0
  subcutis (primary) 017.0
  subdeltoid bursa 017.9
  submaxillary 017.9
    region 017.9
  supraclavicular gland 017.2
  suprarenal (capsule) (gland) 017.6
  swelling, joint (*see also* Tuberculosis, joint)
    015.9
  symphysis pubis 015.7 *[730.88]*

Tuberculosis, tubercular—*continued*
  synovitis 015.9 *[727.01]*
    hip 015.1 *[727.01]*
    knee 015.2 *[727.01]*
    specified site NEC 015.8 *[727.01]*
    spine or vertebra 015.0 *[727.01]*
  systemic—*see* Tuberculosis, miliary
  tarsitis (eyelid) 017.0 *[373.4]*
    ankle (bone) 015.5 *[730.87]*
  tendon (sheath)—*see* Tuberculosis,
    tenosynovitis
  tenosynovitis 015.9 *[727.01]*
    hip 015.1 *[727.01]*
    knee 015.2 *[727.01]*
    specified site NEC 015.8 *[727.01]*
    spine or vertebra 015.0 *[727.01]*
  testis 016.5 *[608.81]*
  throat 012.8
  thymus gland 017.9
  thyroid gland 017.5
  toe 017.9
  tongue 017.9
  tonsil (lingual) 012.8
  tonsillitis 012.8
  trachea, tracheal 012.8
    gland 012.1
      primary, progressive 010.8
    isolated 012.2
  tracheobronchial 011.3
    glandular 012.1
      primary, progressive 010.8
    isolated 012.2
    lymph gland or node 012.1
      primary, progressive 010.8
  tubal 016.6
  tunica vaginalis 016.5
  typhlitis 014.8
  ulcer (primary) (skin) 017.0
    bowel or intestine 014.8
    specified site NEC—*see* Tuberculosis, by site
  unspecified site—*see* Tuberculosis, pulmonary
  ureter 016.2
  urethra, urethral 016.3
  urinary organ or tract 016.3
    kidney 016.0
  uterus 016.7
  uveal tract 017.3 *[363.13]*
  uvula 017.9
  vaccination, prophylactic (against) V03.2
  vagina 016.7
  vas deferens 016.5
  vein 017.9
  verruca (primary) 017.0
  verrucosa (cutis) (primary) 017.0
  vertebra (column) 015.0 *[730.88]*
  vesiculitis 016.5 *[608.81]*
  viscera NEC 014.8
  vulva 016.7 *[616.51]*
  wrist (joint) 015.8
    bone 015.5 *[730.83]*
Tuberculum
  auriculae 744.29
  occlusal 520.2
  paramolare 520.2
Tuberosity
  jaw, excessive 524.07
  maxillary, entire 524.07
Tuberous sclerosis (brain) 759.5
Tubo-ovarian —*see* condition
Tuboplasty, after previous sterilization V26.0
Tubotympanitis 381.10

Tularemia 021.9
  with
    conjunctivitis 021.3
    pneumonia 021.2
  bronchopneumonic 021.2
  conjunctivitis 021.3
  cryptogenic 021.1
  disseminated 021.8
  enteric 021.1
  generalized 021.8
  glandular 021.8
  intestinal 021.1
  oculoglandular 021.3
  ophthalmic 021.3
  pneumonia 021.2
  pulmonary 021.2
  specified NEC 021.8
  typhoidal 021.1
  ulceroglandular 021.0
  vaccination, prophylactic (against) V03.4
Tularensis conjunctivitis 021.3
Tumefaction —*see also* Swelling
  liver (*see also* Hypertrophy, liver) 789.1
Tumor (M8000/1)—*see also* Neoplasm, by site,
    unspecified nature
  Abrikossov's (M9580/0)—*see also* Neoplasm,
    connective tissue, benign
    malignant (M9580/3)—*see* Neoplasm,
      connective tissue, malignant
  acinar cell (M8550/1)—*see* Neoplasm, by site,
    uncertain behavior
  acinic cell (M8550/1)—*see* Neoplasm, by site,
    uncertain behavior
  adenomatoid (M9054/0)—*see also* Neoplasm,
    by site, benign
    odontogenic (M9300/0) 213.1
      upper jaw (bone) 213.0
  adnexal (skin) (M8390/0)—*see* Neoplasm, skin,
    benign
  adrenal
    cortical (benign) (M8370/0) 227.0
      malignant (M8370/3) 194.0
    rest (M8671/0)—*see* Neoplasm, by site, benign
  alpha cell (M8152/0)
    malignant (M8152/3)
      pancreas 157.4
      specified site NEC—*see* Neoplasm, by site,
        malignant
      unspecified site 157.4
    pancreas 211.7
    specified site NEC—*see* Neoplasm, by site,
      benign
    unspecified site 211.7
  aneurysmal (*see also* Aneurysm) 442.9
  aortic body (M8691/1) 237.3
    malignant (M8691/3) 194.6
  argentaffin (M8241/1)—*see* Neoplasm, by site,
    uncertain behavior
  basal cell (M8090/1)—*see also* Neoplasm, skin,
    uncertain behavior
  benign (M8000/0)—*see* Neoplasm, by site, benign
  beta cell (M8151/0)
    malignant (M8151/3)
      pancreas 157.4
      specified site—*see* Neoplasm, by site,
        malignant
      unspecified site 157.4
    pancreas 211.7
    specified site NEC—*see* Neoplasm, by site,
      benign
    unspecified site 211.7
  blood—*see* Hematoma

Tumor—*continued*
brenner (M9000/0) 220
  borderline malignancy (M9000/1) 236.2
  malignant (M9000/3) 183.0
  proliferating (M9000/1) 236.2
Brooke's (M8100/0)—*see* Neoplasm, skin, benign
brown fat (M8880/0)—*see* Lipoma, by site
Burkitt's (M9750/3) 200.2
calcifying epithelial odontogenic (M9340/0) 213.1
  upper jaw (bone) 213.0
carcinoid (M8240/1) 209.60
  benign 209.60
    appendix 209.51
    ascending colon 209.53
    bronchus 209.61
    cecum 209.52
    colon 209.50
    descending colon 209.55
    duodenum 209.41
    foregut 209.65
    hindgut 209.67
    ileum 209.43
    jejunum 209.42
    kidney 209.64
    large intestine 209.50
    lung 209.61
    midgut 209.66
    rectum 209.57
    sigmoid colon 209.56
    small intestine 209.40
    specified NEC 209.69
    stomach 209.63
    thymus 209.62
    transverse colon 209.54
  malignant (of) 209.20
    appendix 209.11
    ascending colon 209.13
    bronchus 209.21
    cecum 209.12
    colon 209.10
    descending colon 209.15
    duodenum 209.01
    foregut 209.25
    hindgut 209.27
    ileum 209.03
    jejunum 209.02
    kidney 209.24
    large intestine 209.10
    lung 209.21
    midgut 209.26
    rectum 209.17
    sigmoid colon 209.16
    small intestine 209.00
    specified NEC 209.29
    stomach 209.23
    thymus 209.22
    transverse colon 209.14
  secondary—*see* Tumor, neuroendocrine,
    secondary
carotid body (M8692/1) 237.3
  malignant (M8692/3) 194.5
Castleman's (mediastinal lymph node
  hyperplasia) 785.6
cells (M8001/1)—*see also* Neoplasm, by site,
  unspecified nature
  benign (M8001/0)—*see* Neoplasm, by site,
    benign
  malignant (M8001/3)—*see* Neoplasm, by site,
    malignant
  uncertain whether benign or malignant
    (M8001/1)—*see* Neoplasm, by site,
    uncertain nature

Tumor—*continued*
cervix
  in pregnancy or childbirth 654.6
    affecting fetus or newborn 763.89
    causing obstructed labor 660.2
      affecting fetus or newborn 763.1
chondromatous giant cell (M9230/0)—*see*
  Neoplasm, bone, benign
chromaffin (M8700/0)—*see also* Neoplasm, by
  site, benign
  malignant (M8700/3)—*see* Neoplasm, by site,
    malignant
Cock's peculiar 706.2
Codman's (benign chondroblastoma)
  (M9230/0)—*see* Neoplasm, bone, benign
dentigerous, mixed (M9282/0) 213.1
  upper jaw (bone) 213.0
dermoid (M9084/0)—*see* Neoplasm, by site,
  benign
  with malignant transformation (M9084/3)
    183.0
desmoid (extra-abdominal) (M8821/1)—*see
  also* Neoplasm, connective tissue, uncertain
  behavior
  abdominal (M8822/1)—*see* Neoplasm,
    connective tissue, uncertain behavior
embryonal (mixed) (M9080/1)—*see also*
  Neoplasm, by site, uncertain behavior
  liver (M9080/3) 155.0
endodermal sinus (M9071/3)
  specified site—*see* Neoplasm, by site,
    malignant
  unspecified site
    female 183.0
    male 186.9
epithelial
  benign (M8010/0)—*see* Neoplasm, by site,
    benign
  malignant (M8010/3)—*see* Neoplasm, by site,
    malignant
Ewing's (M9260/3)—*see* Neoplasm, bone,
  malignant
fatty—*see* Lipoma
fetal, causing disproportion 653.7
  causing obstructed labor 660.1
fibroid (M8890/0)—*see* Leiomyoma
G cell (M8153/1)
  malignant (M8153/3)
    pancreas 157.4
    specified site NEC—*see* Neoplasm, by site,
      malignant
    unspecified site 157.4
  specified site—*see* Neoplasm, by site,
    uncertain behavior
  unspecified site 235.5
giant cell (type) (M8003/1)—*see also*
  Neoplasm, by site, unspecified nature
  bone (M9250/1) 238.0
    malignant (M9250/3)—*see* Neoplasm, bone,
      malignant
  chondromatous (M9230/0)—*see* Neoplasm,
    bone, benign
  malignant (M8003/3)—*see* Neoplasm, by site,
    malignant
  peripheral (gingiva) 523.8
  soft parts (M9251/1)—*see also* Neoplasm,
    connective tissue, uncertain behavior
    malignant (M9251/3)—*see* Neoplasm,
      connective tissue, malignant
  tendon sheath 727.02

Tumor—*continued*

glomus (M8711/0)—*see also* Hemangioma, by
site
jugulare (M8690/1) 237.3
malignant (M8690/3) 194.6
gonadal stromal (M8590/1)—*see* Neoplasm, by
site, uncertain behavior
granular cell (M9580/0)—*see also* Neoplasm,
connective tissue, benign
malignant (M9580/3)—*see* Neoplasm,
connective tissue, malignant
granulosa cell (M8620/1) 236.2
malignant (M8620/3) 183.0
granulosa cell-theca cell (M8621/1) 236.2
malignant (M8621/3) 183.0
Grawitz's (hypernephroma) (M8312/3) 189.0
hazard-crile (M8350/3) 193
hemorrhoidal—*see* Hemorrhoids
hilar cell (M8660/0) 220
hurthle cell (benign) (M8290/0) 226
malignant (M8290/3) 193
hydatid (*see also* Echinococcus) 122.9
hypernephroid (M8311/1)—*see also* Neoplasm,
by site, uncertain behavior
interstitial cell (M8650/1)—*see also* Neoplasm,
by site, uncertain behavior
benign (M8650/0)—*see* Neoplasm, by site,
benign
malignant (M8650/3)—*see* Neoplasm, by site,
malignant
islet cell (M8150/0)
malignant (M8150/3)
pancreas 157.4
specified site—*see* Neoplasm, by site,
malignant
unspecified site 157.4
pancreas 211.7
specified site NEC—*see* Neoplasm, by site,
benign
unspecified site 211.7
juxtaglomerular (M8361/1) 236.91
Krukenberg's (M8490/6) 198.6
Leydig cell (M8650/1)
benign (M8650/0)
specified site—*see* Neoplasm, by site,
benign
unspecified site
female 220
male 220.0
malignant (M8650/3)
specified site—*see* Neoplasm, by site,
malignant
unspecified site
female 183.0
male 186.9
specified site—*see* Neoplasm, by site,
uncertain behavior
unspecified site
female 236.2
male 236.4
lipid cell, ovary (M8670/0) 220
lipoid cell, ovary (M8670/0) 220
lymphomatous, benign (M9590/0)—*see also*
Neoplasm, by site, benign
lysis syndrome (following antineoplastic drug
therapy) (spontaneous) 277.88
Malherbe's (M8110/0)—*see* Neoplasm, skin,
benign

Tumor—*continued*

malignant (M8000/3)—*see also* Neoplasm, by
site, malignant
fusiform cell (type) (M8004/3)—*see*
Neoplasm, by site, malignant
giant cell (type) (M8003/3)—*see* Neoplasm,
by site, malignant
mixed NEC (M8940/3)—*see* Neoplasm, by
site, malignant
small cell (type) (M8002/3)—*see* Neoplasm,
by site, malignant
spindle cell (type) (M8004/3)—*see* Neoplasm,
by site, malignant
mast cell (M9740/1) 238.5
malignant (M9740/3) 202.6
melanotic, neuroectodermal (M9363/0)—*see*
Neoplasm, by site, benign
Merkel cell—*see* Carcinoma, Merkel cell
mesenchymal
malignant (M8800/3)—*see* Neoplasm,
connective tissue, malignant
mixed (M8990/1)—*see* Neoplasm, connective
tissue, uncertain behavior
mesodermal, mixed (M8951/3)—*see also*
Neoplasm, by site, malignant
liver 155.0
mesonephric (M9110/1)—*see also* Neoplasm,
by site, uncertain behavior
malignant (M9110/3)—*see* Neoplasm, by site,
malignant
metastatic
from specified site (M8000/3)—*see*
Neoplasm, by site, malignant
to specified site (M8000/6)—*see* Neoplasm,
by site, malignant, secondary
mixed NEC (M8940/0)—*see also* Neoplasm, by
site, benign
malignant (M8940/3)—*see* Neoplasm, by site,
malignant
mucocarcinoid, malignant (M8243/3)—*see*
Neoplasm, by site, malignant
mucoepidermoid (M8430/1)—*see* Neoplasm, by
site, uncertain behavior
Müllerian, mixed (M8950/3)—*see* Neoplasm,
by site, malignant
myoepithelial (M8982/0)—*see* Neoplasm, by
site, benign
neuroendocrine 209.60
malignant poorly differentiated 209.30
secondary 209.70
bone 209.73
distant lymph nodes 209.71
liver 209.72
peritoneum 209.74
site specified NEC 209.79
neurogenic olfactory (M9520/3) 160.0
nonencapsulated sclerosing (M8350/3) 193
odontogenic (M9270/1) 238.0
adenomatoid (M9300/0) 213.1
upper jaw (bone) 213.0
benign (M9270/0) 213.1
upper jaw (bone) 213.0
calcifying epithelial (M9340/0) 213.1
upper jaw (bone) 213.0
malignant (M9270/3) 170.1
upper jaw (bone) 170.0
squamous (M9312/0) 213.1
upper jaw (bone) 213.0
ovarian stromal (M8590/1) 236.2

Tumor—*continued*
  ovary
    in pregnancy or childbirth 654.4
      affecting fetus or newborn 763.89
      causing obstructed labor 660.2
        affecting fetus or newborn 763.1
  pacinian (M9507/0)—*see* Neoplasm, skin,
    benign
  Pancoast's (M8010/3) 162.3
  papillary—*see* Papilloma
  pelvic, in pregnancy or childbirth 654.9
    affecting fetus or newborn 763.89
    causing obstructed labor 660.2
      affecting fetus or newborn 763.1
  phantom 300.11
  plasma cell (M9731/1) 238.6
    benign (M9731/0)—*see* Neoplasm, by site,
      benign
    malignant (M9731/3) 203.8
  polyvesicular vitelline (M9071/3)
    specified site—*see* Neoplasm, by site,
      malignant
    unspecified site
      female 183.0
      male 186.9
  Pott's puffy (*see also* Osteomyelitis) 730.2
  Rathke's pouch (M9350/1) 237.0
  regaud's (M8082/3)—*see* Neoplasm,
    nasopharynx, malignant
  rete cell (M8140/0) 222.0
  retinal anlage (M9363/0)—*see* Neoplasm, by
    site, benign
  Rokitansky's 620.2
  salivary gland type, mixed (M8940/0)—*see also*
    Neoplasm, by site, benign
    malignant (M8940/3)—*see* Neoplasm, by site,
      malignant
  Sampson's 617.1
  Schloffer's (*see also* Peritonitis) 567.29
  Schmincke (M8082/3)—*see* Neoplasm,
    nasopharynx, malignant
  sebaceous (*see also* Cyst, sebaceous) 706.2
  secondary (M8000/6)—*see* Neoplasm, by site,
    secondary
    carcinoid — *see* Tumor, neuroendocrine,
      secondary
    neuroendocrine — *see* Tumor,
      neuroendocrine, secondary
  Sertoli cell (M8640/0)
    with lipid storage (M8641/0)
      specified site—*see* Neoplasm, by site,
        benign
      unspecified site
        female 220
        male 222.0
    specified site—*see* Neoplasm, by site, benign
    unspecified site
      female 220
      male 222.0
  Sertoli-Leydig cell (M8631/0)
    specified site—*see* Neoplasm, by site, benign
    unspecified site
      female 220
      male 222.0
  sex cord (-stromal) (M8590/1)—*see* Neoplasm,
    by site, uncertain behavior
  skin appendage (M8390/0)—*see* Neoplasm,
    skin, benign

Tumor—*continued*
  soft tissue
    benign (M8800/0)—*see* Neoplasm, connective
      tissue, benign
    malignant (M8800/3)—*see* Neoplasm,
      connective tissue, malignant
  sternomastoid 754.1
  stromal
    abdomen
      benign 215.5
      malignant NEC 171.5
      uncertain behavior 238.1
    digestive system 238.1
      benign 215.5
      malignant NEC 171.5
      uncertain behavior 238.1
    endometrium (endometrial) 236.0
    gastric 238.1
      benign 215.5
      malignant NEC 171.5
      uncertain behavior 238.1
    gastrointestinal 238.1
      benign 215.5
      malignant NEC 171.5
      uncertain behavior 238.1
    intestine (small) 238.1
      benign 215.5
      malignant 152.9
      uncertain behavior 238.1
    stomach 238.1
      benign 215.5
      malignant 151.9
      uncertain behavior 238.1
  superior sulcus (lung) (pulmonary) (syndrome)
    (M8010/3) 162.3
  suprasulcus (M8010/3) 162.3
  sweat gland (M8400/1)—*see also* Neoplasm,
    skin, uncertain behavior
    benign (M8400/0)—*see* Neoplasm, skin,
      benign
    malignant (M8400/3)—*see* Neoplasm, skin,
      malignant
  syphilitic brain 094.89
    congenital 090.49
  testicular stromal (M8590/1) 236.4
  theca cell (M8600/0) 220
  theca cell-granulosa cell (M8621/1) 236.2
  theca-lutein (M8610/0) 220
  turban (M8200/0) 216.4
  uterus
    in pregnancy or childbirth 654.1
      affecting fetus or newborn 763.89
      causing obstructed labor 660.2
        affecting fetus or newborn 763.1
  vagina
    in pregnancy or childbirth 654.7
      affecting fetus or newborn 763.89
      causing obstructed labor 660.2
        affecting fetus or newborn 763.1
  varicose (*see also* Varicose, vein) 454.9
  von Recklinghausen's (M9540/1) 237.71
  vulva
    in pregnancy or childbirth 654.8
      affecting fetus or newborn 763.89
      causing obstructed labor 660.2
        affecting fetus or newborn 763.1
  Warthin's (salivary gland) (M8561/0) 210.2
  white—*see also* Tuberculosis, arthritis
  White-Darier 757.39
  Wilms' (nephroblastoma) (M8960/3) 189.0

Tumor—*continued*
  yolk sac (M9071/3)
    specified site—*see* Neoplasm, by site, malignant
    unspecified site
      female 183.0
      male 186.9
Tumorlet (M8040/1)—*see* Neoplasm, by site,
  uncertain behavior
Tungiasis 134.1
Tunica vasculosa lentis 743.39
Tunnel vision 368.45
Turban tumor (M8200/0) 216.4
Türck's trachoma (chronic catarrhal laryngitis)
  476.0
Türk's syndrome (ocular retraction syndrome)
  378.71
Turner's
  hypoplasia (tooth) 520.4
  syndrome 758.6
  tooth 520.4
Turner-Kieser syndrome (hereditary
  osteo-onychodysplasia) 756.89
Turner-Varny syndrome 758.6
Turricephaly 756.0
Tussis convulsiva (*see also* Whooping cough) 033.9
Twiddler's syndrome (due to)
  automatic implantable defibrillator 996.04
  pacemaker 996.01
Twin
  affected by maternal complications of pregnancy
    761.5
  conjoined 759.4
    fetal 678.1
  healthy liveborn—*see* Newborn, twin
  pregnancy (complicating delivery) NEC 651.0
    with fetal loss and retention of one fetus 651.3
    conjoined 678.1
    following (elective) fetal reduction 651.7
Twinning, teeth 520.2
Twist, twisted
  bowel, colon, or intestine 560.2
  hair (congenital) 757.4
  mesentery 560.2
  omentum 560.2
  organ or site, congenital NEC—*see* Anomaly,
    specified type NEC
  ovarian pedicle 620.5
    congenital 752.0
  umbilical cord—*see* Compression, umbilical
    cord
Twitch 781.0
Tylosis 700
  buccalis 528.6
  gingiva 523.8
  linguae 528.6
  palmaris et plantaris 757.39
Tympanism 787.3
Tympanites (abdominal) (intestine) 787.3
Tympanitis —*see* Myringitis
Tympanosclerosis 385.00
  involving
    combined sites NEC 385.09
      with tympanic membrane 385.03
    tympanic membrane 385.01
      with ossicles 385.02
      and middle ear 385.03
Tympanum —*see* condition
Tympany
  abdomen 787.3
  chest 786.7
Typhlitis (*see also* Appendicitis) 541

Typhoenteritis 002.0
Typhogastric fever 002.0
Typhoid (abortive) (ambulant) (any site) (fever)
  (hemorrhagic) (infection) (intermittent)
  (malignant) (rheumatic) 002.0
  with pneumonia 002.0 *[484.8]*
  abdominal 002.0
  carrier (suspected) of V02.1
  cholecystitis (current) 002.0
  clinical (Widal and blood test negative) 002.0
  endocarditis 002.0 *[421.1]*
  inoculation reaction—*see* Complications,
    vaccination
  meningitis 002.0 *[320.7]*
  mesenteric lymph nodes 002.0
  myocarditis 002.0 *[422.0]*
  osteomyelitis (*see also* Osteomyelitis, due to,
    typhoid) 002.0 *[730.8]*
  perichondritis, larynx 002.0 *[478.71]*
  pneumonia 002.0 *[484.8]*
  spine 002.0 *[720.81]*
  ulcer (perforating) 002.0
  vaccination, prophylactic (against) V03.1
  Widal negative 002.0
Typhomalaria (fever) (*see also* Malaria) 084.6
Typhomania 002.0
Typhoperitonitis 002.0
Typhus (fever) 081.9
  abdominal, abdominalis 002.0
  African tick 082.1
  amarillic (*see also* Fever, Yellow) 060.9
  brain 081.9
  cerebral 081.9
  classical 080
  endemic (flea-borne) 081.0
  epidemic (louse-borne) 080
  exanthematic NEC 080
  exanthematicus SAI 080
    brillii SAI 081.1
    Mexicanus SAI 081.0
    pediculo vestimenti causa 080
    typhus murinus 081.0
  flea-borne 081.0
  Indian tick 082.1
  Kenya tick 082.1
  louse-borne 080
  Mexican 081.0
    flea-borne 081.0
    louse-borne 080
    tabardillo 080
  mite-borne 081.2
  murine 081.0
  North Asian tick-borne 082.2
  petechial 081.9
  Queensland tick 082.3
  rat 081.0
  recrudescent 081.1
  recurrent (*see also* Fever, relapsing) 087.9
  São Paulo 082.0
  scrub (China) (India) (Malaya) (New Guinea)
    081.2
  shop (of Malaya) 081.0
  Siberian tick 082.2
  tick-borne NEC 082.9
  tropical 081.2
  vaccination, prophylactic (against) V05.8
Tyrosinemia 270.2
  neonatal 775.89
Tyrosinosis (Medes) (Sakai) 270.2
Tyrosinuria 270.2
Tyrosyluria 270.2

U

Uehlinger's syndrome (acropachyderma) 757.39
Uhl's anomaly or disease (hypoplasia of
  myocardium, right ventricle) 746.84
Ulcer, ulcerated, ulcerating, ulceration,
  ulcerative 707.9
  with gangrene 707.9 *[785.4]*
  abdomen (wall) (*see also* Ulcer, skin) 707.8
  ala, nose 478.19
  alveolar process 526.5
  amebic (intestine) 006.9
    skin 006.6
  anastomotic—*see* Ulcer, gastrojejunal
  anorectal 569.41
  antral—*see* Ulcer, stomach
  anus (sphincter) (solitary) 569.41
    varicose—*see* Varicose, ulcer, anus
  aorta —*see* Aneurysm
  aphthous (oral) (recurrent) 528.2
    genital organ(s)
      female 616.50
      male 608.89
    mouth 528.2
  arm (*see also* Ulcer, skin) 707.8
  arteriosclerotic plaque—*see* Arteriosclerosis, by
    site
  artery NEC 447.2
    without rupture 447.8
  atrophic NEC—*see* Ulcer, skin
  Barrett's (chronic peptic ulcer of esophagus)
    530.85
  bile duct 576.8
  bladder (solitary) (sphincter) 596.89
    bilharzial (*see also* Schistosomiasis) 120.9
      [595.4]
    submucosal (*see also* Cystitis) 595.1
    tuberculous (*see also* Tuberculosis) 016.1
  bleeding NEC—*see* Ulcer, peptic, with
    hemorrhage
  bone 730.9
  bowel (*see also* Ulcer, intestine) 569.82
  breast 611.0
  bronchitis 491.8
  bronchus 519.19
  buccal (cavity) (traumatic) 528.9
  burn (acute)—*see* Ulcer, duodenum
  Buruli 031.1
  buttock (*see also* Ulcer, skin) 707.8
    decubitus (*see also* Ulcer, pressure) 707.00
  cancerous (M8000/3)—*see* Neoplasm, by site,
    malignant
  cardia—*see* Ulcer, stomach
  cardio-esophageal (peptic) 530.20
    with bleeding 530.21
  cecum (*see also* Ulcer, intestine) 569.82
  cervix (uteri) (trophic) 622.0
    with mention of cervicitis 616.0
  chancroidal 099.0
  chest (wall) (*see also* Ulcer, skin) 707.8
  Chiclero 085.4
  chin (pyogenic) (*see also* Ulcer, skin) 707.8
  chronic (cause unknown)—*see also* Ulcer, skin
    penis 607.89
  Cochin-China 085.1
  colitis—*see* Colitis, ulcerative
  colon (*see also* Ulcer, intestine) 569.82
  conjunctiva (acute) (postinfectional) 372.00

Ulcer, ulcerated, ulcerating—*continued*
  cornea (infectional) 370.00
    with perforation 370.06
    annular 370.02
    catarrhal 370.01
    central 370.03
    dendritic 054.42
    marginal 370.01
    mycotic 370.05
    phlyctenular, tuberculous (*see also*
      Tuberculosis) 017.3 *[370.31]*
    ring 370.02
    rodent 370.07
    serpent, serpiginous 370.04
    superficial marginal 370.01
    tuberculous (*see also* Tuberculosis) 017.3
      [370.31]
  corpus cavernosum (chronic) 607.89
  crural—*see* Ulcer, lower extremity
  Curling's—*see* Ulcer, duodenum
  Cushing's—*see* Ulcer, peptic
  cystitis (interstitial) 595.1
  decubitus (unspecified site) (*see also* Ulcer,
    pressure) 707.00
    with gangrene 707.00 *[785.4]*
    ankle 707.06
    back
      lower 707.03
      upper 707.02
    buttock 707.05
    coccyx 707.03
    elbow 707.01
    head 707.09
    heel 707.07
    hip 707.04
    other site 707.09
    sacrum 707.03
    shoulder blades 707.02
  dendritic 054.42
  diabetes, diabetic (mellitus) 250.8 *[707.9]*
    due to secondary diabetes 249.8 *[707.9]*
    lower limb 250.8 *[707.10]*
      due to secondary diabetes 249.8 *[707.10]*
      ankle 250.8 *[707.13]*
        due to secondary diabetes 249.8 *[707.13]*
      calf 250.8 *[707.12]*
        due to secondary diabetes 249.8 *[707.12]*
      foot 250.8 *[707.15]*
        due to secondary diabetes 249.8 *[707.15]*
      heel 250.8 *[707.14]*
        due to secondary diabetes 249.8 *[707.14]*
      knee 250.8 *[707.19]*
        due to secondary diabetes 249.8 *[707.19]*
      specified site NEC 250.8 *[707.19]*
        due to secondary diabetes 249.8 *[707.19]*
      thigh 250.8 *[707.11]*
        due to secondary diabetes 249.8 *[707.11]*
      toes 250.8 *[707.15]*
        due to secondary diabetes 249.8 *[707.15]*
    specified site NEC 250.8 *[707.8]*
      due to secondary diabetes 249.8 *[707.8]*
  Dieulafoy—*see* Lesion, Dieulafoy
  due to
    infection NEC—*see* Ulcer, skin
    radiation, radium—*see* Ulcer, by site
    trophic disturbance (any region)—*see* Ulcer,
      skin
    x-ray—*see* Ulcer, by site

Ulcer, ulcerated, ulcerating—*continued*
  duodenum, duodenal (eroded) (peptic) 532.9

> *Note*—*Use the following fifth-digit subclassification with categories 531-534:*
>
> 0 *without mention of obstruction*
> 1 *with obstruction*

    with
      hemorrhage (chronic) 532.4
        and perforation 532.6
      perforation (chronic) 532.5
        and hemorrhage 532.6
    acute 532.3
      with
        hemorrhage 532.0
          and perforation 532.2
        perforation 532.1
          and hemorrhage 532.2
    bleeding (recurrent)—*see* Ulcer, duodenum, with hemorrhage
    chronic 532.7
      with
        hemorrhage 532.4
          and perforation 532.6
        perforation 532.5
          and hemorrhage 532.6
    penetrating—*see* Ulcer, duodenum, with perforation
    perforating—*see* Ulcer, duodenum, with perforation
  dysenteric NEC 009.0
  elusive 595.1
  endocarditis (any valve) (acute) (chronic) (subacute) 421.0
  enteritis —*see* Colitis, ulcerative
  enterocolitis 556.0
  epiglottis 478.79
  esophagus (peptic) 530.20
    with bleeding 530.21
    due to ingestion
      aspirin 530.20
      chemicals 530.20
      medicinal agents 530.20
    fungal 530.20
    infectional 530.20
    varicose (*see also* Varix, esophagus) 456.1
      bleeding (*see also* Varix, esophagus, bleeding) 456.0
  eye NEC 360.00
    dendritic 054.42
  eyelid (region) 373.01
  face (*see also* Ulcer, skin) 707.8
  fauces 478.29
  Fenwick (-Hunner) (solitary) (*see also* Cystitis) 595.1
  fistulous NEC—*see* Ulcer, skin
  foot (indolent) (*see also* Ulcer, lower extremity) 707.15
    perforating 707.15
      leprous 030.1
      syphilitic 094.0
    trophic 707.15
    varicose 454.0
      inflamed or infected 454.2
  frambesial, initial or primary 102.0
  gallbladder or duct 575.8
  gall duct 576.8
  gangrenous (*see also* Gangrene) 785.4
  gastric—*see* Ulcer, stomach
  gastrocolic—*see* Ulcer, gastrojejunal

Ulcer, ulcerated, ulcerating—*continued*
  gastroduodenal—*see* Ulcer, peptic
  gastroesophageal—*see* Ulcer, stomach
  gastrohepatic—*see* Ulcer, stomach
  gastrointestinal—*see* Ulcer, gastrojejunal
  gastrojejunal (eroded) (peptic) 534.9

> *Note*—*Use the following fifth-digit subclassification with categories 531-534:*
>
> 0 *without mention of obstruction*
> 1 *with obstruction*

    with
      hemorrhage (chronic) 534.4
        and perforation 534.6
      perforation 534.5
        and hemorrhage 534.6
    acute 534.3
      with
        hemorrhage 534.0
          and perforation 534.2
        perforation 534.1
          and hemorrhage 534.2
    bleeding (recurrent)—*see* Ulcer, gastrojejunal, with hemorrhage
    chronic 534.7
      with
        hemorrhage 534.4
          and perforation 534.6
        perforation 534.5
          and hemorrhage 534.6
    penetrating—*see* Ulcer, gastrojejunal, with perforation
    perforating—*see* Ulcer, gastrojejunal, with perforation
  gastrojejunocolic—*see* Ulcer, gastrojejunal
  genital organ
    female 629.89
    male 608.89
  gingiva 523.8
  gingivitis 523.10
  glottis 478.79
  granuloma of pudenda 099.2
  groin (*see also* Ulcer, skin) 707.8
  gum 523.8
  gumma, due to yaws 102.4
  hand (*see also* Ulcer, skin) 707.8
  hard palate 528.9
  heel (*see also* Ulcer, lower extremity) 707.14
    decubitus (*see also* Ulcer, pressure) 707.07
  hemorrhoids 455.8
    external 455.5
    internal 455.2
  hip (*see also* Ulcer, skin) 707.8
    decubitus (*see also* Ulcer, pressure) 707.04
  Hunner's 595.1
  hypopharynx 478.29
  hypopyon (chronic) (subacute) 370.04
  hypostaticum—*see* Ulcer, varicose
  ileocolitis 556.1
  ileum (*see also* Ulcer, intestine) 569.82
  intestine, intestinal 569.82
    with perforation 569.83
    amebic 006.9
    duodenal—*see* Ulcer, duodenum
    granulocytopenic (with hemorrhage) 288.09
    marginal 569.82
    perforating 569.83
    small, primary 569.82
    stercoraceous 569.82
    stercoral 569.82

Ulcer, ulcerated, ulcerating—*continued*
  tuberculous (*see also* Tuberculosis) 014.8
  typhoid (fever) 002.0
  varicose 456.8
  ischemic 707.9
    lower extremity (*see also* Ulcer, lower
      extremity) 707.10
      ankle 707.13
      calf 707.12
      foot 707.15
      heel 707.14
      knee 707.19
      specified site NEC 707.19
      thigh 707.11
      toes 707.15
  jejunum, jejunal—*see* Ulcer, gastrojejunal
  keratitis (*see also* Ulcer, cornea) 370.00
  knee—*see* Ulcer, lower extremity
  labium (majus) (minus) 616.50
  laryngitis (*see also* Laryngitis) 464.00
    with obstruction 464.01
  larynx (aphthous) (contact) 478.79
    diphtheritic 032.3
  leg—*see* Ulcer, lower extremity
  lip 528.5
  Lipschütz's 616.50
  lower extremity (atrophic) (chronic)
    (neurogenic) (perforating) (pyogenic)
    (trophic) (tropical) 707.10
    with gangrene (*see also* Ulcer, lower
      extremity) 707.10 *[785.4]*
      arteriosclerotic 440.24
    ankle 707.13
    arteriosclerotic 440.23
      with gangrene 440.24
    calf 707.12
    decubitus (*see also* Ulcer, pressure) 707.00
      with gangrene 707.00 *[785.4]*
      ankle 707.06
      buttock 707.05
      heel 707.07
      hip 707.04
    foot 707.15
    heel 707.14
    knee 707.19
    specified site NEC 707.19
    thigh 707.11
    toes 707.15
    varicose 454.0
      inflamed or infected 454.2
  luetic—*see* Ulcer, syphilitic
  lung 518.89
    tuberculous (*see also* Tuberculosis) 011.2
  malignant (M8000/3)—*see* Neoplasm, by site,
    malignant
  marginal NEC—*see* Ulcer, gastrojejunal
  meatus (urinarius) 597.89
  Meckel's diverticulum 751.0
  Meleney's (chronic undermining) 686.09
  Mooren's (cornea) 370.07
  mouth (traumatic) 528.9
  mycobacterial (skin) 031.1
  nasopharynx 478.29
  navel cord (newborn) 771.4
  neck (*see also* Ulcer, skin) 707.8
    uterus 622.0
  neurogenic NEC—*see* Ulcer, skin

Ulcer, ulcerated, ulcerating—*continued*
  nose, nasal (infectional) (passage) 478.19
    septum 478.19
      varicose 456.8
    skin—*see* Ulcer, skin
    spirochetal NEC 104.8
  oral mucosa (traumatic) 528.9
  palate (soft) 528.9
  penetrating NEC—*see* Ulcer, peptic, with
    perforation
  penis (chronic) 607.89
  peptic (site unspecified) 533.9

> *Note—Use the following fifth-digit*
> *subclassification with categories 531-534:*
>
> 0 *without mention of obstruction*
> 1 *with obstruction*

    with
      hemorrhage 533.4
        and perforation 533.6
      perforation (chronic) 533.5
        and hemorrhage 533.6
    acute 533.3
      with
        hemorrhage 533.0
          and perforation 533.2
        perforation 533.1
          and hemorrhage 533.2
    bleeding (recurrent)—*see* Ulcer, peptic, with
      hemorrhage
    chronic 533.7
      with
        hemorrhage 533.4
          and perforation 533.6
        perforation 533.5
          and hemorrhage 533.6
    penetrating—*see* Ulcer, peptic, with
      perforation
  perforating NEC (*see also* Ulcer, peptic, with
    perforation) 533.5
    skin 707.9
  perineum (*see also* Ulcer, skin) 707.8
  peritonsillar 474.8
  phagedenic (tropical) NEC—*see* Ulcer, skin
  pharynx 478.29
  phlebitis—*see* Phlebitis
  plaster (*see also* Ulcer, pressure) 707.00
  popliteal space—*see* Ulcer, lower extremity
  postpyloric—*see* Ulcer, duodenum
  prepuce 607.89
  prepyloric—*see* Ulcer, stomach
  pressure 707.00
    with
      abrasion, blister, partial thickness skin loss
        involving epidermis and/or dermis
        707.22
      full thickness skin loss involving damage or
        necrosis of subcutaneous tissue 707.23
      gangrene 707.00 [785.4]
      necrosis of soft tissues through to underlying
        muscle, tendon, or bone 707.24
    ankle 707.06
    back
      lower 707.03
      upper 707.02
    buttock 707.05
    coccyx 707.03
    elbow 707.01
    head 707.09
    healed — omit code
    healing — code to Ulcer, pressure, by stage

Ulcer, ulcerated, ulcerating—*continued*
  heel 707.07
  hip 707.04
  other site 707.09
  sacrum 707.03
  shoulder blades 707.02
  stage
    I (healing) 707.21
    II (healing) 707.22
    III (healing) 707.23
    IV (healing) 707.24
    unspecified (healing) 707.20
  unstageable 707.25
 primary of intestine 569.82
  with perforation 569.83
 proctitis 556.2
  with ulcerative sigmoiditis 556.3
 prostate 601.8
 pseudopeptic—*see* Ulcer, peptic
 pyloric—*see* Ulcer, stomach
 rectosigmoid 569.82
  with perforation 569.83
 rectum (sphincter) (solitary) 569.41
  stercoraceous, stercoral 569.41
  varicose—*see* Varicose, ulcer, anus
 retina (*see also* Chorioretinitis) 363.20
 rodent (M8090/3)—*see also* Neoplasm, skin,
   malignant
  cornea 370.07
 round—*see* Ulcer, stomach
 sacrum (region) (*see also* Ulcer, skin) 707.8
 Saemisch's 370.04
 scalp (*see also* Ulcer, skin) 707.8
 sclera 379.09
 scrofulous (*see also* Tuberculosis) 017.2
 scrotum 608.89
  tuberculous (*see also* Tuberculosis) 016.5
  varicose 456.4
 seminal vesicle 608.89
 sigmoid 569.82
  with perforation 569.83
 skin (atrophic) (chronic) (neurogenic)
   (non-healing) (perforating) (pyogenic)
   (trophic) 707.9
  with gangrene 707.9 *[785.4]*
  amebic 006.6
  decubitus (*see also* Ulcer, pressure) 707.00
   with gangrene 707.00 *[785.4]*
  in granulocytopenia 288.09
  lower extremity (*see also* Ulcer, lower
    extremity) 707.10
   with gangrene 707.10 *[785.4]*
    arteriosclerotic 440.24
   ankle 707.13
   arteriosclerotic 440.23
    with gangrene 440.24
   calf 707.12
   foot 707.15
   heel 707.14
   knee 707.19
   specified site NEC 707.19
   thigh 707.11
   toes 707.15
  mycobacterial 031.1
  syphilitic (early) (secondary) 091.3
  tuberculous (primary) (*see also* Tuberculosis)
   017.0
  varicose—*see* Ulcer, varicose
 sloughing NEC—*see* Ulcer, skin
 soft palate 528.9
 solitary, anus or rectum (sphincter) 569.41

Ulcer, ulcerated, ulcerating—*continued*
 sore throat 462
  streptococcal 034.0
 spermatic cord 608.89
 spine (tuberculous) 015.0 *[730.88]*
 stasis (leg) (venous) 454.0
  with varicose veins 454.0
  inflamed or infected 454.2
  without varicose veins 459.81
 stercoral, stercoraceous 569.82
  with perforation 569.83
  anus or rectum 569.41
 stoma, stomal—*see* Ulcer, gastrojejunal
 stomach (eroded) (peptic) (round) 531.9

> Note—*Use the following fifth-digit*
> *subclassification with categories 531-534:*
>
> 0 *without mention of obstruction*
> 1 *with obstruction*

  with
   hemorrhage 531.4
    and perforation 531.6
   perforation (chronic) 531.5
    and hemorrhage 531.6
  acute 531.3
   with
    hemorrhage 531.0
     and perforation 531.2
    perforation 531.1
     and hemorrhage 531.2
  bleeding (recurrent)—*see* Ulcer, stomach,
   with hemorrhage
  chronic 531.7
   with
    hemorrhage 531.4
     and perforation 531.6
    perforation 531.5
     and hemorrhage 531.6
  penetrating—*see* Ulcer, stomach, with
   perforation
  perforating—*see* Ulcer, stomach, with
   perforation
 stomatitis 528.00
 stress—*see* Ulcer, peptic
 strumous (tuberculous) (*see also* Tuberculosis)
  017.2
 submental (*see also* Ulcer, skin) 707.8
 submucosal, bladder 595.1
 syphilitic (any site) (early) (secondary) 091.3
  late 095.9
  perforating 095.9
   foot 094.0
 testis 608.89
 thigh—*see* Ulcer, lower extremity
 throat 478.29
  diphtheritic 032.0
 toe—*see* Ulcer, lower extremity
 tongue (traumatic) 529.0
 tonsil 474.8
  diphtheritic 032.0
 trachea 519.19
 trophic—*see* Ulcer, skin
 tropical NEC (*see also* Ulcer, skin) 707.9
 tuberculous—*see* Tuberculosis, ulcer
 tunica vaginalis 608.89
 turbinate 730.9
 typhoid (fever) 002.0
  perforating 002.0
 umbilicus (newborn) 771.4
 unspecified site NEC—*see* Ulcer, skin

Ulcer, ulcerated, ulcerating—*continued*
  urethra (meatus) (*see also* Urethritis) 597.89
  uterus 621.8
    cervix 622.0
      with mention of cervicitis 616.0
    neck 622.0
      with mention of cervicitis 616.0
  vagina 616.89
  valve, heart 421.0
  varicose (lower extremity, any part) 454.0
    anus—*see* Varicose, ulcer, anus
    broad ligament 456.5
    esophagus (*see also* Varix, esophagus) 456.1
      bleeding (*see also* Varix, esophagus,
        bleeding) 456.0
    inflamed or infected 454.2
    nasal septum 456.8
    perineum 456.6
    rectum—*see* Varicose, ulcer, anus
    scrotum 456.4
    specified site NEC 456.8
    sublingual 456.3
    vulva 456.6
  vas deferens 608.89
  vesical (*see also* Ulcer, bladder) 596.89
  vulva (acute) (infectional) 616.50
    Behçet's syndrome 136.1 *[616.51]*
    herpetic 054.12
    tuberculous 016.7 *[616.51]*
  vulvobuccal, recurring 616.50
  x-ray—*see* Ulcer, by site
  yaws 102.4
Ulcerosa scarlatina 034.1
Ulcus —*see also* Ulcer
  cutis tuberculosum (*see also* Tuberculosis)
    017.0
  duodeni—*see* Ulcer, duodenum
  durum 091.0
    extragenital 091.2
  gastrojejunale—*see* Ulcer, gastrojejunal
  hypostaticum—*see* Ulcer, varicose
  molle (cutis) (skin) 099.0
  serpens cornea (pneumococcal) 370.04
  ventriculi—*see* Ulcer, stomach
Ulegyria 742.4
Ulerythema
  acneiforma 701.8
  centrifugum 695.4
  ophryogenes 757.4
Ullrich (-Bonnevie) (-Turner) syndrome 758.6
Ullrich-Feichtiger syndrome 759.89
Ulnar —*see* condition
Ulorrhagia 523.8
Ulorrhea 523.8
Umbilicus, umbilical —*see also* condition
  cord necrosis, affecting fetus or newborn 762.6
Unacceptable
  existing dental restoration
    contours 525.65
    morphology 525.65
Unavailability of medical facilities (at) V63.9
  due to
    investigation by social service agency V63.8
    lack of services at home V63.1
    remoteness from facility V63.0
    waiting list V63.2
  home V63.1
  outpatient clinic V63.0
  specified reason NEC V63.8
Uncinaria americana infestation 126.1
Uncinariasis (*see also* Ancylostomiasis) 126.9
Unconscious, unconsciousness 780.09

Underdevelopment —*see also* Undeveloped
  sexual 259.0
Underfill, endodontic 526.63
Undernourishment 269.9
Undernutrition 269.9
Under observation —*see* Observation
Underweight 783.22
  for gestational age—*see* Light-for-dates
Underwood's disease (sclerema neonatorum)
  778.1
Undescended —*see also* Malposition, congenital
  cecum 751.4
  colon 751.4
  testis 752.51
Undetermined diagnosis or cause 799.9
Undeveloped, undevelopment —*see also*
  Hypoplasia
  brain (congenital) 742.1
  cerebral (congenital) 742.1
  fetus or newborn 764.9
  heart 746.89
  lung 748.5
  testis 257.2
  uterus 259.0
Undiagnosed (disease) 799.9
Undulant fever (*see also* Brucellosis) 023.9
Unemployment, anxiety concerning V62.0
Unequal leg (acquired) (length) 736.81
  congenital 755.30
Unerupted teeth, tooth 520.6
Unextracted dental root 525.3
Unguis incarnatus 703.0
Unicornis uterus 752.33
Unicornuate uterus (with or without a separate
  uterine horn) 752.33
Unicorporeus uterus 752.39
Uniformis uterus 752.39
Unilateral —*see also* condition
  development, breast 611.89
  organ or site, congenital NEC—*see* Agenesis
  vagina 752.49
Unilateralis uterus 752.39
Unilocular heart 745.8
Uninhibited (neurogenic) bladder 596.54
  with cauda equina syndrome 344.61
  neurogenic—*see* Neurogenic, bladder 596.54
Union, abnormal —*see also* Fusion
  divided tendon 727.89
  larynx and trachea 748.3
Universal
  joint, cervix 620.6
  mesentery 751.4
Unknown
  cause of death 799.9
  diagnosis 799.9
Unna's disease (seborrheic dermatitis) 690.10
Unresponsiveness, adrenocorticotropin
  (ACTH) 255.41
Unsoundness of mind (*see also* Psychosis) 298.9
Unspecified cause of death 799.9
Unsatisfactory
  cytology smear
    anal 796.78
    cervical 795.08
    vaginal 795.18
  restoration, tooth (existing) 525.60
    specified NEC 525.69
Unstable
  back NEC 724.9
  colon 569.89
  joint—*see* Instability, joint

Unstable—*continued*
lie 652.0
  affecting fetus or newborn (before labor) 761.7
  causing obstructed labor 660.0
    affecting fetus or newborn 763.1
  lumbosacral joint (congenital) 756.19
    acquired 724.6
  sacroiliac 724.6
  spine NEC 724.9
Untruthfulness, child problem (*see also*
  Disturbance, conduct) 312.0
Unverricht (-Lundborg) disease, syndrome, or
  epilepsy 345.1
Unverricht-Wagner syndrome
  (dermatomyositis) 710.3
Upper respiratory —*see* condition
Upset
  gastric 536.8
    psychogenic 306.4
  gastrointestinal 536.8
    psychogenic 306.4
    virus (*see also* Enteritis, viral) 008.8
  intestinal (large) (small) 564.9
    psychogenic 306.4
  menstruation 626.9
  mental 300.9
  stomach 536.8
    psychogenic 306.4
Urachus —*see also* condition
  patent 753.7
  persistent 753.7
Uratic arthritis 274.00
Urbach's lipoid proteinosis 272.8
Urbach-Oppenheim disease or syndrome
  (necrobiosis lipoidica diabeticorum) 250.8
  [709.3]
  due to secondary diabetes 249.8 *[709.3]*
Urbach-Wiethe disease or syndrome (lipoid
  proteinosis) 272.8
Urban yellow fever 060.1
Urea, blood, high —*see* Uremia
Uremia, uremic (absorption) (amaurosis)
  (amblyopia) (aphasia) (apoplexy) (coma)
  (delirium) (dementia) (dropsy) (dyspnea)
  (fever) (intoxication) (mania) (paralysis)
  (poisoning) (toxemia) (vomiting) 586
  with
    abortion—*see* Abortion, by type, with renal
      failure
    ectopic pregnancy (*see also* categories
      633.0-633.9) 639.3
    hypertension (*see also* Hypertension, kidney)
      403.91
    molar pregnancy (*see also* categories 630-632)
      639.3
  chronic 585.9
  complicating
    abortion 639.3
    ectopic or molar pregnancy 639.3
    hypertension (*see also* Hypertension, kidney)
      403.91
    labor and delivery 669.3
  congenital 779.89
  extrarenal 788.99
  hypertensive (chronic) (*see also* Hypertension,
    kidney) 403.91
  maternal NEC, affecting fetus or newborn 760.1
  neuropathy 585.9 *[357.4]*
  pericarditis 585.9 *[420.0]*
  prerenal 788.99
  pyelitic (*see also* Pyelitis) 590.80

Ureter, ureteral —*see* condition
Ureteralgia 788.0
Ureterectasis 593.89
Ureteritis 593.89
  cystica 590.3
  due to calculus 592.1
  gonococcal (acute) 098.19
    chronic or duration of 2 months or over 098.39
  nonspecific 593.89
Ureterocele (acquired) 593.89
  congenital 753.23
Ureterolith 592.1
Ureterolithiasis 592.1
Ureterostomy status V44.6
  with complication 997.5
Urethra, urethral —*see* condition
Urethralgia 788.99
Urethritis (abacterial) (acute) (allergic) (anterior)
  (chronic) (nonvenereal) (posterior) (recurrent)
  (simple) (subacute) (ulcerative)
  (undifferentiated) 597.80
  diplococcal (acute) 098.0
    chronic or duration of 2 months or over 098.2
  due to Trichomonas (vaginalis) 131.02
  gonococcal (acute) 098.0
    chronic or duration of 2 months or over 098.2
  nongonococcal (sexually transmitted) 099.40
    Chlamydia trachomatis 099.41
    Reiter's 099.3
    specified organism NEC 099.49
  nonspecific (sexually transmitted) (*see also*
    Urethritis, nongonococcal) 099.40
  not sexually transmitted 597.80
  Reiter's 099.3
  trichomonal or due to Trichomonas (vaginalis)
    131.02
  tuberculous (*see also* Tuberculosis) 016.3
  venereal NEC (*see also* Urethritis,
    nongonococcal) 099.40
Urethrocele
  female 618.03
    with uterine prolapse 618.4
      complete 618.3
      incomplete 618.2
  male 599.5
Urethrolithiasis 594.2
Urethro-oculoarticular syndrome 099.3
Urethro-oculosynovial syndrome 099.3
Urethrorectal —*see* condition
Urethrorrhagia 599.84
Urethrorrhea 788.7
Urethrostomy status V44.6
  with complication 997.5
Urethrotrigonitis 595.3
Urethrovaginal —*see* condition
Urgency
  fecal 787.63
  hypertensive—*see* Hypertension
Urhidrosis, uridrosis 705.89
Uric acid
  diathesis 274.9
  in blood 790.6
Uricacidemia 790.6
Uricemia 790.6
Uricosuria 791.9
Urination
  frequent 788.41
  painful 788.1
  urgency 788.63

Urine, urinary —*see also* condition
  abnormality NEC 788.69
  blood in (*see also* Hematuria) 599.70
  discharge, excessive 788.42
  enuresis 788.30
    nonorganic origin 307.6
  extravasation 788.8
  frequency 788.41
  hesitancy 788.64
  incontinence 788.30
    active 788.30
    female 788.30
      stress 625.6
        and urge 788.33
    male 788.30
      stress 788.32
        and urge 788.33
    mixed (stress and urge) 788.33
    neurogenic 788.39
    nonorganic origin 307.6
    overflow 788.38
    stress (female) 625.6
      male NEC 788.32
  intermittent stream 788.61
  pus in 791.9
  retention or stasis NEC 788.20
    bladder, incomplete emptying 788.21
    psychogenic 306.53
    specified NEC 788.29
  secretion
    deficient 788.5
    excessive 788.42
    frequency 788.41
  strain 788.65
  stream
    intermittent 788.61
    slowing 788.62
    splitting 788.61
    weak 788.62
  urgency 788.63
Urinemia —*see* Uremia
Urinoma NEC 599.9
  bladder 596.89
  kidney 593.89
  renal 593.89
  ureter 593.89
  urethra 599.84
Uroarthritis, infectious 099.3
Urodialysis 788.5
Urolithiasis 592.9
Uronephrosis 593.89
Uropathy 599.9
  obstructive 599.60
Urosepsis 599.0
  meaning sepsis 995.91
  meaning urinary tract infection 599.0
Urticaria 708.9
  with angioneurotic edema 995.1
    hereditary 277.6
  allergic 708.0
  cholinergic 708.5
  chronic 708.8
  cold, familial 708.2
  dermatographic 708.3
  due to
    cold or heat 708.2
    drugs 708.0
    food 708.0
    inhalants 708.0
    plants 708.8
    serum 999.59

Uritcaria—*continued*
  factitial 708.3
  giant 995.1
    hereditary 277.6
  gigantea 995.1
    hereditary 277.6
  idiopathic 708.1
  larynx 995.1
    hereditary 277.6
  neonatorum 778.8
  nonallergic 708.1
  papulosa (Hebra) 698.2
  perstans hemorrhagica 757.39
  pigmentosa 757.33
  recurrent periodic 708.8
  serum 999.59
  solare 692.72
  specified type NEC 708.8
  thermal (cold) (heat) 708.2
  vibratory 708.4
Urticarioides acarodermatitis 133.9
Use of
  agents affecting estrogen receptors and estrogen
      levels NEC V07.59
  anastrozole (Arimidex) V07.52
  aromatase inhibitors V07.52
  estrogen receptor downregulators V07.59
  exemestane (Aromasin) V07.52
  fulvestrant (Faslodex) V07.59
  gonadotropin-releasing hormone (GnRH)
      agonist V07.59
  goserelin acetate (Zoladex) V07.59
  letrozole (Femara) V07.52
  leuprolide acetate (leuprorelin) (Lupron) V07.59
  megestrol acetate (Megace) V07.59
  methadone 304.00
  nonprescribed drugs (*see also* Abuse, drugs,
      nondependent) 305.9
  patent medicines (*see also* Abuse, drugs,
      nondependent) 305.9
  raloxifene (Evista) V07.51
  selective estrogen receptor modulators (SERMs)
      V07.51
  tamoxifen (Nolvadex) V07.51
  toremifene (Fareston) V07.51
Usher-Senear disease (pemphigus
    erythematosus) 694.4
Uta 085.5
Uterine size-date discrepancy 649.6
Uteromegaly 621.2
Uterovaginal —*see* condition
Uterovesical —*see* condition
Uterus —*see also* condition
  with only one functioning horn 752.33
Utriculitis (utriculus prostaticus) 597.89
Uveal —*see* condition
Uveitis (anterior) (*see also* Iridocyclitis) 364.3
  acute or subacute 364.00
    due to or associated with
      gonococcal infection 098.41
      herpes (simplex) 054.44
        zoster 053.22
    primary 364.01
    recurrent 364.02
    secondary (noninfectious) 364.04
      infectious 364.03
  allergic 360.11

Uveitis—*continued*
  chronic 364.10
    due to or associated with
      sarcoidosis 135 *[364.11]*
      tuberculosis (*see also* Tuberculosis) 017.3
        [364.11]
  due to
    operation 360.11
    toxoplasmosis (acquired) 130.2
      congenital (active) 771.2
  granulomatous 364.10
  heterochromic 364.21
  lens-induced 364.23
  nongranulomatous 364.00
  posterior 363.20
    disseminated—*see* Chorioretinitis,
      disseminated
    focal—*see* Chorioretinitis, focal
  recurrent 364.02
  sympathetic 360.11
  syphilitic (secondary) 091.50
    congenital 090.0 *[363.13]*
    late 095.8 *[363.13]*
  tuberculous (*see also* Tuberculosis) 017.3
    [364.11]
Uveoencephalitis 363.22
Uveokeratitis (*see also* Iridocyclitis) 364.3
Uveoparotid fever 135
Uveoparotitis 135
Uvula —*see* condition
Uvulitis (acute) (catarrhal) (chronic)
  (gangrenous) (membranous) (suppurative)
  (ulcerative) 528.3

V

Vaccination
complication or reaction—*see* Complications, vaccination
delayed V64.00
not carried out V64.00
  because of
    acute illness V64.01
    allergy to vaccine or component V64.04
    caregiver refusal V64.05
    chronic illness V64.02
    guardian refusal V64.05
    immune compromised state V64.03
    parent refusal V64.05
    patient had disease being vaccinated against V64.08
    patient refusal V64.06
    reason NEC V64.09
    religious reasons V64.07
prophylactic (against) V05.9
  arthropod-borne viral
    disease NEC V05.1
    encephalitis V05.0
  chickenpox V05.4
  cholera (alone) V03.0
    with typhoid-paratyphoid (cholera + TAB) V06.0
  common cold V04.7
  diphtheria (alone) V03.5
    with
      poliomyelitis (DTP + polio) V06.3
      tetanus V06.5
        pertussis combined [DTP] [DTaP] V06.1
      typhoid-paratyphoid (DTP + TAB) V06.2
  disease (single) NEC V05.9
    bacterial NEC V03.9
      specified type NEC V03.89
    combinations NEC V06.9
      specified type NEC V06.8
    specified type NEC V05.8
  encephalitis, viral, arthropod-borne V05.0
  Hemophilus influenzae, type B [Hib] V03.81
  hepatitis, viral V05.3
  influenza V04.81
    with
      Streptococcus pneumoniae [pneumococcus] V06.6
  leishmaniasis V05.2
  measles (alone) V04.2
    with mumps-rubella (MMR) V06.4
  mumps (alone) V04.6
    with measles and rubella (MMR) V06.4
  pertussis alone V03.6
  plague V03.3
  poliomyelitis V04.0
    with diphtheria-tetanus-pertussis (DTP + polio) V06.3
  rabies V04.5
  respiratory syncytial virus (RSV) V04.82
  rubella (alone) V04.3
    with measles and mumps (MMR) V06.4
  smallpox V04.1
  Streptococcus pneumoniae [pneumococcus] V03.82
    with
      influenza V06.6
  tetanus toxoid (alone) V03.7
    with diphtheria [Td] [DT] V06.5
      with
        pertussis [DTP] [DTaP] V06.1

Vaccination—*continued*
      with poliomyelitis (DTP + polio) V06.3
  tuberculosis (BCG) V03.2
  tularemia V03.4
  typhoid-paratyphoid (TAB) (alone) V03.1
    with diphtheria-tetanus-pertussis (TAB + DTP) V06.2
  varicella V05.4
  viral
    disease NEC V04.89
    encephalitis, arthropod-borne V05.0
    hepatitis V05.3
  yellow fever V04.4
Vaccinia (generalized) 999.0
  congenital 771.2
  conjunctiva 999.39
  eyelids 999.0 *[373.5]*
  localized 999.39
  nose 999.39
  not from vaccination 051.02
    eyelid 051.02 *[373.5]*
  sine vaccinatione 051.02
  without vaccination 051.02
Vacuum
  extraction of fetus or newborn 763.3
  in sinus (accessory) (nasal) (*see also* Sinusitis) 473.9
Vagabond V60.0
Vagabondage V60.0
Vagabonds' disease 132.1
Vagina, vaginal —*see also* condition
  high risk human papillomavirus (HPV) DNA test positive 795.15
  low risk human papillomavirus (HPV) DNA test positive 795.19
Vaginalitis (tunica) 608.4
Vaginismus (reflex) 625.1
  functional 306.51
  hysterical 300.11
  psychogenic 306.51
Vaginitis (acute) (chronic) (circumscribed) (diffuse) (emphysematous) (Hemophilus vaginalis) (nonspecific) (nonvenereal) (ulcerative) 616.10
  with
    abortion—*see* Abortion, by type, with sepsis
    ectopic pregnancy (*see also* categories 633.0-633.9) 639.0
    molar pregnancy (*see also* categories 630-632) 639.0
  adhesive, congenital 752.49
  atrophic, postmenopausal 627.3
  bacterial 616.10
  blennorrhagic (acute) 098.0
    chronic or duration of 2 months or over 098.2
  candidal 112.1
  chlamydial 099.53
  complicating pregnancy or puerperium 646.6
    affecting fetus or newborn 760.8
  congenital (adhesive) 752.49
  due to
    C. albicans 112.1
    Trichomonas (vaginalis) 131.01
  following
    abortion 639.0
    ectopic or molar pregnancy 639.0

Vaginitis—*continued*
  gonococcal (acute) 098.0
    chronic or duration of 2 months or over 098.2
  granuloma 099.2
  Monilia 112.1
  mycotic 112.1
  pinworm 127.4 *[616.11]*
  postirradiation 616.10
  postmenopausal atrophic 627.3
  senile (atrophic) 627.3
  syphilitic (early) 091.0
    late 095.8
  trichomonal 131.01
  tuberculous (*see also* Tuberculosis) 016.7
  venereal NEC 099.8
Vaginosis —*see* Vaginitis
Vagotonia 352.3
Vagrancy V60.0
VAIN I (vaginal intraepithelial neoplasia I) 623.0
VAIN II (vaginal intraepithelial neoplasia II) 623.0
VAIN III (vaginal intraepithelial neoplasia III) 233.31
Vallecula —*see* condition
Valley fever 114.0
Valsuani's disease (progressive pernicious anemia, puerperal) 648.2
Valve, valvular (formation)—*see also* condition
  cerebral ventricle (communicating) in situ V45.2
  cervix, internal os 752.49
  colon 751.5
  congenital NEC—*see* Atresia
  formation, congenital NEC—*see* Atresia
  heart defect—*see* Anomaly, heart, valve
  ureter 753.29
    pelvic junction 753.21
    vesical orifice 753.22
  urethra 753.6
Valvulitis (chronic) (*see also* Endocarditis) 424.90
  rheumatic (chronic) (inactive) (with chorea) 397.9
    active or acute (aortic) (mitral) (pulmonary) (tricuspid) 391.1
  syphilitic NEC 093.20
    aortic 093.22
    mitral 093.21
    pulmonary 093.24
    tricuspid 093.23
Valvulopathy —*see* Endocarditis
van Bogaert's leukoencephalitis (sclerosing) (subacute) 046.2
van Bogaert-Nijssen (-Peiffer) disease 330.0
van Buchem's syndrome (hyperostosis corticalis) 733.3
Vancomycin (glycopeptide)
  intermediate staphylococcus aureus (VISA/GISA) V09.8
  resistant
    enterococcus (VRE) V09.8
    staphylococcus aureus (VRSA/GRSA) V09.8
van Creveld-von Gierke disease (glycogenosis I) 271.0
van den Bergh's disease (enterogenous cyanosis) 289.7
van der Hoeve's syndrome (brittle bones and blue sclera, deafness) 756.51
van der Hoeve-Halbertsma-Waardenburg syndrome (ptosis-epicanthus) 270.2

van der Hoeve-Waardenburg-Gualdi syndrome (ptosis epicanthus) 270.2
Vanillism 692.89
Vanishing lung 492.0
Vanishing twin 651.33
van Neck (-Odelberg) disease or syndrome (juvenile osteochondrosis) 732.1
Vapor asphyxia or suffocation NEC 987.9
  specified agent—*see* Table of drugs and chemicals
Vaquez's disease (M9950/1) 238.4
Vaquez-Osler disease (polycythemia vera) (M9950/1) 238.4
Variance, lethal ball, prosthetic heart valve 996.02
Variants, thalassemic 282.49
Variations in hair color 704.3
Varicella 052.9
  with
    complication 052.8
      specified NEC 052.7
    pneumonia 052.1
  exposure to V01.71
  vaccination and inoculation (prophylactic) V05.4
Varices —*see* Varix
Varicocele (scrotum) (thrombosed) 456.4
  ovary 456.5
  perineum 456.6
  spermatic cord (ulcerated) 456.4
Varicose
  aneurysm (ruptured) (*see also* Aneurysm) 442.9
  dermatitis (lower extremity)—*see* Varicose, vein, inflamed or infected
  eczema—*see* Varicose, vein
  phlebitis—*see* Varicose, vein, inflamed or infected
  placental vessel—*see* Placenta, abnormal
  tumor—*see* Varicose, vein
  ulcer (lower extremity, any part) 454.0
    anus 455.8
      external 455.5
      internal 455.2
    esophagus (*see also* Varix, esophagus) 456.1
      bleeding (*see also* Varix, esophagus, bleeding) 456.0
    inflamed or infected 454.2
    nasal septum 456.8
    perineum 456.6
    rectum—*see* Varicose, ulcer, anus
    scrotum 456.4
    specified site NEC 456.8
  vein (lower extremity) (ruptured) (*see also* Varix) 454.9
    with
      complications NEC 454.8
      edema 454.8
      inflammation or infection 454.1
        ulcerated 454.2
      pain 454.8
      stasis dermatitis 454.1
        with ulcer 454.2
      swelling 454.8
      ulcer 454.0
        inflamed or infected 454.2
    anus—*see* Hemorrhoids
    broad ligament 456.5
    congenital (peripheral) NEC 747.60
      gastrointestinal 747.61
      lower limb 747.64
      renal 747.62

Varicose—*continued*
   specified NEC 747.69
   upper limb 747.63
  esophagus (ulcerated) (*see also* Varix,
    esophagus) 456.1
   bleeding (*see also* Varix, esophagus,
    bleeding) 456.0
  inflamed or infected 454.1
   with ulcer 454.2
  in pregnancy or puerperium 671.0
   vulva or perineum 671.1
  nasal septum (with ulcer) 456.8
  pelvis 456.5
  perineum 456.6
   in pregnancy, childbirth, or puerperium
    671.1
  rectum—*see* Hemorrhoids
  scrotum (ulcerated) 456.4
  specified site NEC 456.8
  sublingual 456.3
  ulcerated 454.0
   inflamed or infected 454.2
  umbilical cord, affecting fetus or newborn
   762.6
  urethra 456.8
  vulva 456.6
   in pregnancy, childbirth, or puerperium
    671.1
  vessel—*see also* Varix
  placenta—*see* Placenta, abnormal
Varicosis, varicosities, varicosity (*see also*
  Varix) 454.9
Variola 050.9
  hemorrhagic (pustular) 050.0
  major 050.0
  minor 050.1
  modified 050.2
Varioloid 050.2
Variolosa, purpura 050.0
Varix (lower extremity) (ruptured) 454.9
  with
   complications NEC 454.8
   edema 454.8
   inflammation or infection 454.1
    with ulcer 454.2
   pain 454.8
   stasis dermatitis 454.1
    with ulcer 454.2
   swelling 454.8
   ulcer 454.0
    with inflammation or infection 454.2
  aneurysmal (*see also* Aneurysm) 442.9
  anus—*see* Hemorrhoids
  arteriovenous (congenital) (peripheral) NEC
   747.60
   gastrointestinal 747.61
   lower limb 747.64
   renal 747.62
   specified NEC 747.69
   spinal 747.82
   upper limb 747.63
  bladder 456.5
  broad ligament 456.5
  congenital (peripheral) NEC 747.60
  esophagus (ulcerated) 456.1
   bleeding 456.0
    in
     cirrhosis of liver 571.5 *[456.20]*
     portal hypertension 572.3 *[456.20]*
   congenital 747.69

Varix—*continued*
  in
   cirrhosis of liver 571.5 *[456.21]*
    with bleeding 571.5 *[456.20]*
   portal hypertension 572.3 *[456.21]*
    with bleeding 572.3 *[456.20]*
  gastric 456.8
  inflamed or infected 454.1
   ulcerated 454.2
  in pregnancy or puerperium 671.0
   perineum 671.1
   vulva 671.1
  labia (majora) 456.6
  orbit 456.8
   congenital 747.69
  ovary 456.5
  papillary 448.1
  pelvis 456.5
  perineum 456.6
   in pregnancy or puerperium 671.1
  pharynx 456.8
  placenta—*see* Placenta, abnormal
  prostate 456.8
  rectum—*see* Hemorrhoids
  renal papilla 456.8
  retina 362.17
  scrotum (ulcerated) 456.4
  sigmoid colon 456.8
  specified site NEC 456.8
  spinal (cord) (vessels) 456.8
  spleen, splenic (vein) (with phlebolith) 456.8
  sublingual 456.3
  ulcerated 454.0
   inflamed or infected 454.2
  umbilical cord, affecting fetus or newborn 762.6
  uterine ligament 456.5
  vocal cord 456.8
  vulva 456.6
   in pregnancy, childbirth, or puerperium 671.1
Vasa previa 663.5
  affecting fetus or newborn 762.6
  hemorrhage from, affecting fetus or newborn 772.0
Vascular —*see also* condition
  loop on papilla (optic) 743.57
  sheathing, retina 362.13
  spasm 443.9
  spider 448.1
Vascularity, pulmonary, congenital 747.39
Vascularization
  choroid 362.16
  cornea 370.60
   deep 370.63
   localized 370.61
  retina 362.16
  subretinal 362.16
Vasculitis 447.6
  allergic 287.0
  cryoglobulinemic 273.2
  disseminated 447.6
  kidney 447.8
  leukocytoclastic 446.29
  nodular 695.2
  retinal 362.18
  rheumatic—*see* Fever, rheumatic
Vasculopathy
  cardiac allograft 996.83
Vas deferens —*see* condition
Vas deferentitis 608.4
Vasectomy, admission for V25.2

Vasitis 608.4
  nodosa 608.4
  scrotum 608.4
  spermatic cord 608.4
  testis 608.4
  tuberculous (*see also* Tuberculosis) 016.5
  tunica vaginalis 608.4
  vas deferens 608.4
Vasodilation 443.9
Vasomotor —*see* condition
Vasoplasty, after previous sterilization V26.0
Vasoplegia, splanchnic (*see also* Neuropathy, peripheral, autonomic) 337.9
Vasospasm 443.9
  cerebral (artery) 435.9
    with transient neurologic deficit 435.9
  coronary 413.1
  nerve
    arm NEC 354.9
    autonomic 337.9
    brachial plexus 353.0
    cervical plexus 353.2
    leg NEC 355.8
    lower extremity NEC 355.8
    peripheral NEC 355.9
    spinal NEC 355.9
    sympathetic 337.9
    upper extremity NEC 354.9
  peripheral NEC 443.9
  retina (artery) (*see also* Occlusion, retinal, artery) 362.30
Vasospastic —*see* condition
Vasovagal attack (paroxysmal) 780.2
  psychogenic 306.2
Vater's ampulla —*see* condition
VATER syndrome 759.89
vCJD (variant Creutzfeldt-Jakob disease) 046.11
Vegetation, vegetative
  adenoid (nasal fossa) 474.2
  consciousness (persistent) 780.03
  endocarditis (acute) (any valve) (chronic) (subacute) 421.0
  heart (mycotic) (valve) 421.0
  state (persistent) 780.03
Veil
  Jackson's 751.4
  over face (causing asphyxia) 768.9
Vein, venous —*see* condition
Veldt sore (*see also* Ulcer, skin) 707.9
Velo-cardio-facial syndrome 758.32
Velpeau's hernia —*see* Hernia, femoral
Venereal
  balanitis NEC 099.8
  bubo 099.1
  disease 099.9
    specified nature or type NEC 099.8
  granuloma inguinale 099.2
  lymphogranuloma (Durand-Nicolas-Favre), any site 099.1
  salpingitis 098.37
  urethritis (*see also* Urethritis, nongonococcal) 099.40
  vaginitis NEC 099.8
  warts 078.11
Vengefulness, in child (*see also* Disturbance, conduct) 312.0
Venofibrosis 459.89
Venom, venomous
  bite or sting (animal or insect) 989.5
  poisoning 989.5
Venous —*see* condition

Ventouse delivery NEC 669.5
  affecting fetus or newborn 763.3
Ventral —*see* condition
Ventricle, ventricular —*see also* condition
  escape 427.69
  standstill (*see also* Arrest, cardiac) 427.5
Ventriculitis, cerebral (*see also* Meningitis) 322.9
Ventriculostomy status V45.2
Verbiest's syndrome (claudicatio intermittens spinalis) 435.1
Vernet's syndrome 352.6
Verneuil's disease (syphilitic bursitis) 095.7
Verruca (filiformis) 078.10
  acuminata (any site) 078.11
  necrogenica (primary) (*see also* Tuberculosis) 017.0
  peruana 088.0
  peruviana 088.0
  plana (juvenilis) 078.19
  plantaris 078.12
  seborrheica 702.19
    inflamed 702.11
  senilis 702.0
  tuberculosa (primary) (*see also* Tuberculosis) 017.0
  venereal 078.11
  viral 078.10
    specified NEC 078.19
  vulgaris 078.10
Verrucosities (*see also* Verruca) 078.10
Verrucous endocarditis (acute) (any valve) (chronic) (subacute) 710.0 *[424.91]*
  nonbacterial 710.0 *[424.91]*
Verruga
  peruana 088.0
  peruviana 088.0
Verse's disease (calcinosis intervertebralis) 275.49 *[722.90]*
Version
  before labor, affecting fetus or newborn 761.7
  cephalic (correcting previous malposition) 652.1
    affecting fetus or newborn 763.1
  cervix (*see* Version, uterus)
  uterus (postinfectional) (postpartal, old) (*see also* Malposition, uterus) 621.6
    forward—*see* Anteversion, uterus
    lateral—*see* Lateroversion, uterus
Vertebra, vertebral —*see* condition
Vertigo 780.4
  auditory 386.19
  aural 386.19
  benign paroxysmal positional 386.11
  central origin 386.2
  cerebral 386.2
  Dix and Hallpike (epidemic) 386.12
  endemic paralytic 078.81
  epidemic 078.81
    Dix and Hallpike 386.12
    Gerlier's 078.81
    Pedersen's 386.12
    vestibular neuronitis 386.12
  epileptic—*see* Epilepsy
  Gerlier's (epidemic) 078.81
  hysterical 300.11
  labyrinthine 386.10
  laryngeal 786.2
  malignant positional 386.2
  Ménière's (*see also* Disease, Ménière's) 386.00
  menopausal 627.2
  otogenic 386.19

Vertigo—*continued*
paralytic 078.81
paroxysmal positional, benign 386.11
Pedersen's (epidemic) 386.12
peripheral 386.10
specified type NEC 386.19
positional
benign paroxysmal 386.11
malignant 386.2
Verumontanitis (chronic) (*see also* Urethritis) 597.89
Vesania (*see also* Psychosis) 298.9
Vesical —*see* condition
Vesicle
cutaneous 709.8
seminal—*see* condition
skin 709.8
Vesicocolic —*see* condition
Vesicoperineal —*see* condition
Vesicorectal —*see* condition
Vesicourethrorectal —*see* condition
Vesicovaginal —*see* condition
Vesicular —*see* condition
Vesiculitis (seminal) 608.0
amebic 006.8
gonorrheal (acute) 098.14
chronic or duration of 2 months or over 098.34
trichomonal 131.09
tuberculous (*see also* Tuberculosis) 016.5 [608.81]
Vestibulitis (ear) (*see also* Labyrinthitis) 386.30
nose (external) 478.19
vulvar 625.71
Vestibulopathy, acute peripheral (recurrent) 386.12
Vestige, vestigial —*see also* Persistence
branchial 744.41
structures in vitreous 743.51
Vibriosis NEC 027.9
Vidal's disease (lichen simplex chronicus) 698.3
Video display tube syndrome 723.8
Vienna type encephalitis 049.8
Villaret's syndrome 352.6
Villous —*see* condition
VIN I (vulvar intraepithelial neoplasia I) 624.01
VIN II (vulvar intraepithelial neoplasia II) 624.02
VIN III (vulvar intraepithelial neoplasia III) 233.32
Vincent's
angina 101
bronchitis 101
disease 101
gingivitis 101
infection (any site) 101
laryngitis 101
stomatitis 101
tonsillitis 101
Vinson-Plummer syndrome (sideropenic dysphagia) 280.8
Viosterol deficiency (*see also* Deficiency, calciferol) 268.9
Virchow's disease 733.99
Viremia 790.8
Virilism (adrenal) (female) NEC 255.2
with
3-beta-hydroxysteroid dehydrogenase defect 255.2
11-hydroxylase defect 255.2
21-hydroxylase defect 255.2

Virilism—*continued*
adrenal
hyperplasia 255.2
insufficiency (congenital) 255.2
cortical hyperfunction 255.2
Virilization (female) (suprarenal) (*see also* Virilism) 255.2
isosexual 256.4
Virulent bubo 099.0
Virus, viral —*see also* condition
infection NEC (*see also* Infection, viral) 079.99
septicemia 079.99
yaba monkey tumor 059.22
VISA (vancomycin intermediate staphylococcus aureus) V09.8
Viscera, visceral —*see* condition
Visceroptosis 569.89
Visible peristalsis 787.4
Vision, visual
binocular, suppression 368.31
blurred, blurring 368.8
hysterical 300.11
defect, defective (*see also* Impaired, vision) 369.9
disorientation (syndrome) 368.16
disturbance NEC (*see also* Disturbance, vision) 368.9
hysterical 300.11
examination V72.0
field, limitation 368.40
fusion, with defective steropsis 368.33
hallucinations 368.16
halos 368.16
loss 369.9
both eyes (*see also* Blindness, both eyes) 369.3
complete (*see also* Blindness, both eyes) 369.00
one eye 369.8
sudden 368.16
low (both eyes) 369.20
one eye (other eye normal) (*see also* Impaired, vision) 369.70
blindness, other eye 369.10
perception, simultaneous without fusion 368.32
tunnel 368.45
Vitality, lack or want of 780.79
newborn 779.89
Vitamin deficiency NEC (*see also* Deficiency, vitamin) 269.2
Vitelline duct, persistent 751.0
Vitiligo 709.01
due to pinta (carate) 103.2
eyelid 374.53
vulva 624.8
Vitium cordis —*see* Disease, heart
Vitreous —*see also* condition
touch syndrome 997.99
VLCAD (long chain/very long chain acyl CoA dehydrogenase deficiency, LCAD) 277.85
Vocal cord —*see* condition
Vocational rehabilitation V57.22
Vogt's (Cecile) disease or syndrome 333.7
Vogt-Koyanagi syndrome 364.24
Vogt-Spielmeyer disease (amaurotic familial idiocy) 330.1
Voice
change (*see also* Dysphonia) 784.49
loss (*see also* Aphonia) 784.41
Volhard-Fahr disease (malignant nephrosclerosis) 403.00

Volhynian fever 083.1
Volkmann's ischemic contracture or paralysis
(complicating trauma) 958.6
Voluntary starvation 307.1
Volvulus (bowel) (colon) (intestine) 560.2
with
hernia—*see also* Hernia, by site, with
obstruction
gangrenous—*see* Hernia, by site, with
gangrene
perforation 560.2
congenital 751.5
duodenum 537.3
fallopian tube 620.5
oviduct 620.5
stomach (due to absence of gastrocolic
ligament) 537.89
Vomiting 787.03
with nausea 787.01
allergic 535.4
asphyxia 933.1
bilious (cause unknown) 787.04
following gastrointestinal surgery 564.3
newborn 779.32
blood (*see also* Hematemesis) 578.0
causing asphyxia, choking, or suffocation (*see
also* Asphyxia, food) 933.1
cyclical 536.2
associated with migraine 346.2
psychogenic 306.4
epidemic 078.82
fecal matter 569.87
following gastrointestinal surgery 564.3
functional 536.8
psychogenic 306.4
habit 536.2
hysterical 300.11
nervous 306.4
neurotic 306.4
newborn 779.33
bilious 779.32
of or complicating pregnancy 643.9
due to
organic disease 643.8
specific cause NEC 643.8
early—*see* Hyperemesis, gravidarum
late (after 22 completed weeks of gestation)
643.2
pernicious or persistent 536.2
complicating pregnancy—*see* Hyperemesis,
gravidarum
psychogenic 306.4
physiological 787.03
bilious 787.04
psychic 306.4
psychogenic 307.54
stercoral 569.89
uncontrollable 536.2
psychogenic 306.4
uremic—*see* Uremia
winter 078.82
von Bechterew (-Strumpell) disease or syndrome
(ankylosing spondylitis) 720.0
von Bezold's abscess 383.01
von Economo's disease (encephalitis lethargica)
049.8
von Eulenburg's disease (congenital
paramyotonia) 359.29
von Gierke's disease (glycogenosis I) 271.0
von Gies' joint 095.8
von Graefe's disease or syndrome 378.72

von Hippel (-Lindau) disease or syndrome
(retinocerebral angiomatosis) 759.6
von Jaksch's anemia or disease
(pseudoleukemia infantum) 285.8
von Recklinghausen's
disease or syndrome (nerves) (skin) (M9540/1)
237.71
bones (osteitis fibrosa cystica) 252.01
tumor (M9540/1) 237.71
von Recklinghausen-Applebaum disease
(hemochromatosis) (*see also*
Hemochromatosis) 275.03
von Schroetter's syndrome (intermittent venous
claudication) 453.89
von Willebrand (-Jürgens) (-Minot) disease or
syndrome (angiohemophilia) 286.4
von Zambusch's disease (lichen sclerosus et
atrophicus) 701.0
Voorhoeve's disease or dyschondroplasia 756.4
Vossius' ring 921.3
late effect 366.21
Voyeurism 302.82
VRE (vancomycin resistant enterococcus) V09.8
Vrolik's disease (osteogenesis imperfecta) 756.51
VRSA (vancomycin resistant staphylococcus
aureus) V09.8
Vulva —*see* condition
Vulvismus 625.1
Vulvitis (acute) (allergic) (chronic) (gangrenous)
(hypertrophic) (intertriginous) 616.10
with
abortion—*see* Abortion, by type, with sepsis
ectopic pregnancy (*see also* categories
633.0-633.9) 639.0
molar pregnancy (*see also* categories 630-632)
639.0
adhesive, congenital 752.49
blennorrhagic (acute) 098.0
chronic or duration of 2 months or over 098.2
chlamydial 099.53
complicating pregnancy or puerperium 646.6
due to Ducrey's bacillus 099.0
following
abortion 639.0
ectopic or molar pregnancy 639.0
gonococcal (acute) 098.0
chronic or duration of 2 months or over 098.2
herpetic 054.11
leukoplakic 624.09
monilial 112.1
puerperal, postpartum, childbirth 646.6
syphilitic (early) 091.0
late 095.8
trichomonal 131.01
Vulvodynia 625.70
specified NEC 625.79
Vulvorectal —*see* condition
Vulvovaginitis (*see also* Vulvitis) 616.10
amebic 006.8
chlamydial 099.53
gonococcal (acute) 098.0
chronic or duration of 2 months or over 098.2
herpetic 054.11
monilial 112.1
trichomonal (Trichomonas vaginalis) 131.01

W

Waardenburg's syndrome 756.89
  meaning ptosis-epicanthus 270.2
Waardenburg-Klein syndrome
  (ptosis-epicanthus) 270.2
Wagner's disease (colloid milium) 709.3
Wagner (-Unverricht) syndrome
  (dermatomyositis) 710.3
Waiting list, person on V63.2
  undergoing social agency investigation V63.8
Wakefulness disorder (*see also* Hypersomnia)
  780.54
  nonorganic origin 307.43
Waldenström's
  disease (osteochondrosis, capital femoral) 732.1
  hepatitis (lupoid hepatitis) 571.49
  hypergammaglobulinemia 273.0
  macroglobulinemia 273.3
  purpura, hypergammaglobulinemic 273.0
  syndrome (macroglobulinemia) 273.3
Waldenström-Kjellberg syndrome (sideropenic
  dysphagia) 280.8
Walking
  difficulty 719.7
    psychogenic 307.9
  sleep 307.46
    hysterical 300.13
Wall, abdominal —*see* condition
Wallenberg's syndrome (posterior inferior
  cerebellar artery) (*see also* Disease,
  cerebrovascular, acute) 436
Wallgren's
  disease (obstruction of splenic vein with
    collateral circulation) 459.89
  meningitis (*see also* Meningitis, aseptic) 047.9
Wandering
  acetabulum 736.39
  gallbladder 751.69
  in diseases classified elsewhere V40.31
  kidney, congenital 753.3
  organ or site, congenital NEC—*see* Malposition,
    congenital
  pacemaker (atrial) (heart) 427.89
  spleen 289.59
Wardrop's disease (with lymphangitis) 681.9
  finger 681.02
  toe 681.11
War neurosis 300.16
Wart (digitate) (filiform) (infectious) (juvenile)
  (plantar) (viral) 078.10
  common 078.19
  external genital organs (venereal) 078.11
  fig 078.19
  flat 078.19
  genital 078.11
  Hassall-Henle's (of cornea) 371.41
  Henle's (of cornea) 371.41
  juvenile 078.19
  moist 078.10
  Peruvian 088.0
  plantar 078.12
  prosector (*see also* Tuberculosis) 017.0
  seborrheic 702.19
    inflamed 702.11
  senile 702.0
  specified NEC 078.19
  syphilitic 091.3
  tuberculous (*see also* Tuberculosis) 017.0
  venereal (female) (male) 078.11

Warthin's tumor (salivary gland) (M8561/0) 210.2
Washerwoman's itch 692.4
Wassilieff's disease (leptospiral jaundice) 100.0
Wasting
  disease 799.4
    due to malnutrition 261
  extreme (due to malnutrition) 261
  muscular NEC 728.2
  palsy, paralysis 335.21
  pelvic muscle 618.83
Water
  clefts 366.12
  deprivation of 994.3
  in joint (*see also* Effusion, joint) 719.0
  intoxication 276.69
  itch 120.3
  lack of 994.3
  loading 276.69
  on
    brain—*see* Hydrocephalus
    chest 511.89
  poisoning 276.69
Waterbrash 787.1
Water-hammer pulse (*see also* Insufficiency,
  aortic) 424.1
Waterhouse (-Friderichsen) disease or syndrome
  036.3
Water-losing nephritis 588.89
Watermelon stomach 537.82
  with hemorrhage 537.83
  without hemorrhage 537.82
Wax in ear 380.4
Waxy
  degeneration, any site 277.39
  disease 277.39
  kidney 277.39 *[583.81]*
  liver (large) 277.39
  spleen 277.39
Weak, weakness (generalized) 780.79
  arches (acquired) 734
    congenital 754.61
  bladder sphincter 596.59
  congenital 779.89
  eye muscle—*see* Strabismus
  facial 781.94
  foot (double)—*see* Weak, arches
  heart, cardiac (*see also* Failure, heart) 428.9
    congenital 746.9
  mind 317
  muscle (generalized) 728.87
  myocardium (*see also* Failure, heart) 428.9
  newborn 779.89
  pelvic fundus
    pubocervical tissue 618.81
    rectovaginal tissue 618.82
  pulse 785.9
  senile 797
  valvular—*see* Endocarditis
Wear, worn, tooth, teeth (approximal) (hard
  tissues) (interproximal) (occlusal)—*see also*
  Attrition, teeth 521.10
Weather, weathered
  effects of
    cold NEC 991.9
      specified effect NEC 991.8
    hot (*see also* Heat) 992.9
  skin 692.74

WXYZ

Web, webbed (congenital)—*see also* Anomaly,
    specified type NEC
  canthus 743.63
  digits (*see also* Syndactylism) 755.10
  duodenal 751.5
  esophagus 750.3
  fingers (*see also* Syndactylism, fingers) 755.11
  larynx (glottic) (subglottic) 748.2
  neck (pterygium colli) 744.5
  Paterson-Kelly (sideropenic dysphagia) 280.8
  popliteal syndrome 756.89
  toes (*see also* Syndactylism, toes) 755.13
Weber's paralysis or syndrome 344.89
Weber-Christian disease or syndrome (nodular
    nonsuppurative panniculitis) 729.30
Weber-Cockayne syndrome (epidermolysis
    bullosa) 757.39
Weber-Dimitri syndrome 759.6
Weber-Gubler syndrome 344.89
Weber-Leyden syndrome 344.89
Weber-Osler syndrome (familial hemorrhagic
    telangiectasia) 448.0
Wedge-shaped or wedging vertebra (*see also*
    Osteoporosis) 733.00
Wegener's granulomatosis or syndrome 446.4
Wegner's disease (syphilitic osteochondritis)
    090.0
Weight
  gain (abnormal) (excessive) 783.1
    during pregnancy 646.1
      insufficient 646.8
  less than 1000 grams at birth 765.0
  loss (cause unknown) 783.21
Weightlessness 994.9
Weil's disease (leptospiral jaundice) 100.00
Weill-Marchesani syndrome (brachymorphism
    and ectopia lentis) 759.89
Weingarten's syndrome (tropical eosinophilia)
    518.3
Weir Mitchell's disease (erythromelalgia)
    443.82
Weiss-Baker syndrome (carotid sinus syncope)
    337.01
Weissenbach-Thibierge syndrome (cutaneous
    systemic sclerosis) 710.1
Wen (*see also* Cyst, sebaceous) 706.2
Wenckebach's phenomenon, heart block
    (second degree) 426.13
Werdnig-Hoffmann syndrome (muscular
    atrophy) 335.0
Werlhof's disease (*see also* Purpura,
    thrombocytopenic) 287.39
Werlhof-Wichmann syndrome (*see also*
    Purpura, thrombocytopenic) 287.39
Wermer's syndrome or disease (polyendocrine
    adenomatosis) 258.01
Werner's disease or syndrome (progeria
    adultorum) 259.8
Werner-His disease (trench fever) 083.1
Werner-Schultz disease (agranulocytosis)
    288.09
**Wernicke's encephalopathy, disease or
    syndrome** (superior hemorrhagic
    polioencephalitis) 265.1
Wernicke-Korsakoff syndrome or psychosis
    (nonalcoholic) 294.0
  alcoholic 291.1
Wernicke-Posadas disease (*see also*
    Coccidioidomycosis) 114.9
Wesselsbron fever 066.3
West African fever 084.8

West Nile
  encephalitis 066.41
  encephalomyelitis 066.41
  fever 066.40
    with
      cranial nerve disorders 066.42
      encephalitis 066.41
      optic neuritis 066.42
      other complications 066.49
      other neurologic manifestations 066.42
      polyradiculitis 066.42
  virus 066.40
Westphal-Strümpell syndrome
    (hepatolenticular degeneration) 275.1
Wet
  brain (alcoholic) (*see also* Alcoholism) 303.9
  feet, tropical (syndrome) (maceration) 991.4
  lung (syndrome)
    adult 518.52
    newborn 770.6
Wharton's duct —*see* condition
Wheal 709.8
Wheelchair confinement status V46.3
Wheezing 786.07
Whiplash injury or syndrome 847.0
Whipple's disease or syndrome (intestinal
    lipodystrophy) 040.2
Whipworm 127.3
"Whistling face" syndrome (craniocarpotarsal
    dystrophy) 759.89
White —*see also* condition
  kidney
    large—*see* Nephrosis
    small 582.9
  leg, puerperal, postpartum, childbirth 671.4
    nonpuerperal 451.19
  mouth 112.0
  patches of mouth 528.6
  sponge nevus of oral mucosa 750.26
  spot lesions, teeth 521.01
White's disease (congenital) (keratosis
    follicularis) 757.39
Whitehead 706.2
Whitlow (with lymphangitis) 681.01
  herpetic 054.6
Whitmore's disease or fever (melioidosis) 025
Whooping cough 033.9
  with pneumonia 033.9 *[484.3]*
  due to
    Bordetella
      bronchoseptica 033.8
        with pneumonia 033.8 *[484.3]*
      parapertussis 033.1
        with pneumonia 033.1 *[484.3]*
      pertussis 033.0
        with pneumonia 033.0 *[484.3]*
    specified organism NEC 033.8
      with pneumonia 033.8 *[484.3]*
  vaccination, prophylactic (against) V03.6
Wichmann's asthma (laryngismus stridulus)
    478.75
Widal (-Abrami) syndrome (acquired hemolytic
    jaundice) 283.9
Widening aorta (*see also* Ectasia, aortic) 447.70
  with aneurysm 441.9
  ruptured 441.5
Wilkie's disease or syndrome 557.1
Wilkinson-Sneddon disease or syndrome
    (subcorneal pustular dermatosis) 694.1
Willan's lepra 696.1
Willan-Plumbe syndrome (psoriasis) 696.1

Willebrand (-Jürgens) syndrome or
thrombopathy (angiohemophilia) 286.4
Willi-Prader syndrome (hypogenital dystrophy
with diabetic tendency) 759.81
Willis' disease (diabetes mellitus) (*see also*
Diabetes) 250.0
due to secondary diabetes 249.0
Wilms' tumor or neoplasm (nephroblastoma)
(M8960/3) 189.0
Wilson's
disease or syndrome (hepatolenticular
degeneration) 275.1
hepatolenticular degeneration 275.1
lichen ruber 697.0
Wilson-Brocq disease (dermatitis exfoliativa)
695.89
Wilson-Mikity syndrome 770.7
Window —*see also* Imperfect, closure
aorticopulmonary 745.0
Winged scapula 736.89
Winter —*see also* condition
vomiting disease 078.82
Wise's disease 696.2
Wiskott-Aldrich syndrome
(eczema-thrombocytopenia) 279.12
Withdrawal symptoms, syndrome
alcohol 291.81
delirium (acute) 291.0
chronic 291.1
newborn 760.71
drug or narcotic 292.0
newborn, infant of dependent mother 779.5
steroid NEC
correct substance properly administered 255.41
overdose or wrong substance given or taken
962.0
Withdrawing reaction, child or adolescent
313.22
Witts' anemia (achlorhydric anemia) 280.9
Witzelsucht 301.9
Woakes' syndrome (ethmoiditis) 471.1
Wohlfart-Kugelberg-Welander disease 335.11
Woillez's disease (acute idiopathic pulmonary
congestion) 518.52
Wolff-Parkinson-White syndrome (anomalous
atrioventricular excitation) 426.7
Wolhynian fever 083.1
Wolman's disease (primary familial
xanthomatosis) 272.7
Wood asthma 495.8
Woolly, wooly hair (congenital) (nevus) 757.4
Wool-sorters' disease 022.1
Word
blindness (congenital) (developmental) 315.01
secondary to organic lesion 784.61
deafness (secondary to organic lesion) 784.69
developmental 315.31
Worm (s) (colic) (fever) (infection) (infestation)
(*see also* Infestation) 128.9
guinea 125.7
in intestine NEC 127.9
Worm-eaten soles 102.3
Worn out (*see also* Exhaustion) 780.79
artificial heart valve 996.02
cardiac defibrillator (with synchronous cardiac
pacemaker) V53.32
cardiac pacemaker lead or battery V53.31
joint prosthesis (see also Complications,
mechanical, device NEC, prosthetic NEC,
joint) 996.46
"Worried well" V65.5

Wound, open (by cutting or piercing instrument)
(by firearms) (cut) (dissection) (incised)
(laceration) (penetration) (perforating)
(puncture) (with initial hemorrhage, not
internal) 879.8

---

*Note—For fracture with open wound, see
Fracture. For laceration, traumatic rupture,
tear or penetrating wound of internal organs,
such as heart, lung, liver, kidney, pelvic organs,
etc., whether or not accompanied by open
wound or fracture in the same region, see
Injury, internal. For contused wound, see
Contusion. For crush injury, see Crush. For
abrasion, insect bite (nonvenomous), blister, or
scratch, see Injury, superficial.*

Complicated includes wounds with:
  delayed healing
  delayed treatment
  foreign body
  primary infection

*For late effect of open wound, see Late, effect,
wound, open, by site.*

---

abdomen, abdominal (external) (muscle) 879.2
complicated 879.3
wall (anterior) 879.2
complicated 879.3
lateral 879.4
complicated 879.5
alveolar (process) 873.62
complicated 873.72
ankle 891.0
with tendon involvement 891.2
complicated 891.1
anterior chamber, eye (*see also* Wound, open,
intraocular) 871.9
anus 863.89
arm 884.0
with tendon involvement 884.2
complicated 884.1
forearm 881.00
with tendon involvement 881.20
complicated 881.10
multiple sites—*see* Wound, open, multiple,
upper limb
upper 880.03
with tendon involvement 880.23
complicated 880.13
multiple sites (with axillary or shoulder
regions) 880.09
with tendon involvement 880.29
complicated 880.19
artery—*see* Injury, blood vessel, by site
auditory
canal (external) (meatus) 872.02
complicated 872.12
ossicles (incus) (malleus) (stapes) 872.62
complicated 872.72
auricle, ear 872.01
complicated 872.11
axilla 880.02
with tendon involvement 880.22
complicated 880.12
with tendon involvement 880.29
involving other sites of upper arm 880.09
complicated 880.19
back 876.0
complicated 876.1

Wound, open—*continued*
  bladder—*see* Injury, internal, bladder
  blood vessel—*see* Injury, blood vessel, by site
  brain—*see* Injury, intracranial, with open
      intracranial wound
  breast 879.0
    complicated 879.1
  brow 873.42
    complicated 873.52
  buccal mucosa 873.61
    complicated 873.71
  buttock 877.0
    complicated 877.1
  calf 891.0
    with tendon involvement 891.2
    complicated 891.1
  canaliculus lacrimalis 870.8
    with laceration of eyelid 870.2
  canthus, eye 870.8
    laceration—*see* Laceration, eyelid
  cavernous sinus—*see* Injury, intracranial
  cerebellum—*see* Injury, intracranial
  cervical esophagus 874.4
    complicated 874.5
  cervix—*see* Injury, internal, cervix
  cheek(s) (external) 873.41
    complicated 873.51
    internal 873.61
      complicated 873.71
  chest (wall) (external) 875.0
    complicated 875.1
  chin 873.44
    complicated 873.54
  choroid 363.63
  ciliary body (eye) (*see also* Wound, open,
      intraocular) 871.9
  clitoris 878.8
    complicated 878.9
  cochlea 872.64
    complicated 872.74
  complicated 879.9
  conjunctiva—*see* Wound, open, intraocular
  cornea (nonpenetrating) (*see also* Wound, open,
      intraocular) 871.9
  costal region 875.0
    complicated 875.1
  Descemet's membrane (*see also* Wound, open,
      intraocular) 871.9
  digit(s)
    foot 893.0
      with tendon involvement 893.2
      complicated 893.1
    hand 883.0
      with tendon involvement 883.2
      complicated 883.1
  drumhead, ear 872.61
    complicated 872.71
  ear 872.8
    canal 872.02
      complicated 872.12
    complicated 872.9
    drum 872.61
      complicated 872.71
    external 872.00
      complicated 872.10
    multiple sites 872.69
      complicated 872.79
    ossicles (incus) (malleus) (stapes) 872.62
      complicated 872.72
    specified part NEC 872.69
      complicated 872.79

Wound, open—*continued*
  elbow 881.01
    with tendon involvement 881.21
    complicated 881.11
  epididymis 878.2
    complicated 878.3
  epigastric region 879.2
    complicated 879.3
  epiglottis 874.01
    complicated 874.11
  esophagus (cervical) 874.4
    complicated 874.5
    thoracic—*see* Injury, internal, esophagus
  Eustachian tube 872.63
    complicated 872.73
  extremity
    lower (multiple) NEC 894.0
      with tendon involvement 894.2
      complicated 894.1
    upper (multiple) NEC 884.0
      with tendon involvement 884.2
      complicated 884.1
  eye(s) (globe)—*see* Wound, open, intraocular
  eyeball NEC 871.9
    laceration (*see also* Laceration, eyeball) 871.4
    penetrating (*see also* Penetrating wound,
        eyeball) 871.7
  eyebrow 873.42
    complicated 873.52
  eyelid NEC 870.8
    laceration—*see* Laceration, eyelid
  face 873.40
    complicated 873.50
    multiple sites 873.49
      complicated 873.59
    specified part NEC 873.49
      complicated 873.59
  fallopian tube—*see* Injury, internal, fallopian
      tube
  finger(s) (nail) (subungual) 883.0
    with tendon involvement 883.2
    complicated 883.1
  flank 879.4
    complicated 879.5
  foot (any part except toe(s) alone) 892.0
    with tendon involvement 892.2
    complicated 892.1
  forearm 881.00
    with tendon involvement 881.20
    complicated 881.10
  forehead 873.42
    complicated 873.52
  genital organs (external) NEC 878.8
    complicated 878.9
    internal—*see* Injury, internal, by site
  globe (eye) (*see also* Wound, open, eyeball)
      871.9
  groin 879.4
    complicated 879.5
  gum(s) 873.62
    complicated 873.72
  hand (except finger(s) alone) 882.0
    with tendon involvement 882.2
    complicated 882.1
  head NEC 873.8
    with intracranial injury—*see* Injury,
        intracranial
    due to or associated with skull fracture—*see*
        Fracture, skull
    complicated 873.9
  scalp—*see* Wound, open, scalp

Wound, open—*continued*
  heel 892.0
    with tendon involvement 892.2
    complicated 892.1
  high-velocity (grease gun)—*see* Wound, open,
    complicated, by site
  hip 890.0
    with tendon involvement 890.2
    complicated 890.1
  hymen 878.6
    complicated 878.7
  hypochondrium 879.4
    complicated 879.5
  hypogastric region 879.2
    complicated 879.3
  iliac (region) 879.4
    complicated 879.5
  incidental to
    dislocation—*see* Dislocation, open, by site
    fracture—*see* Fracture, open, by site
    intracranial injury—*see* Injury, intracranial,
      with open intracranial wound
    nerve injury—*see* Injury, nerve, by site
  inguinal region 879.4
    complicated 879.5
  instep 892.0
    with tendon involvement 892.2
    complicated 892.1
  interscapular region 876.0
    complicated 876.1
  intracranial—*see* Injury, intracranial, with open
    intracranial wound
  intraocular 871.9
    with
      partial loss (of intraocular tissue) 871.2
      prolapse or exposure (of intraocular tissue)
        871.1
    laceration (*see also* Laceration, eyeball) 871.4
    penetrating 871.7
      with foreign body (nonmagnetic) 871.6
        magnetic 871.5
    without prolapse (of intraocular tissue) 871.0
  iris (*see also* Wound, open, eyeball) 871.9
  jaw (fracture not involved) 873.44
    with fracture—*see* Fracture, jaw
    complicated 873.54
  knee 891.0
    with tendon involvement 891.2
    complicated 891.1
  labium (majus) (minus) 878.4
    complicated 878.5
  lacrimal apparatus, gland, or sac 870.8
    with laceration of eyelid 870.2
  larynx 874.01
    with trachea 874.00
      complicated 874.10
    complicated 874.11
  leg (multiple) 891.0
    with tendon involvement 891.2
    complicated 891.1
    lower 891.0
      with tendon involvement 891.2
      complicated 891.1
    thigh 890.0
      with tendon involvement 890.2
      complicated 890.1
    upper 890.0
      with tendon involvement 890.2
      complicated 890.1
  lens (eye) (alone) (*see also* Cataract, traumatic)
    366.20

Wound, open—*continued*
    with involvement of other eye structures—*see*
      Wound, open, eyeball
  limb
    lower (multiple) NEC 894.0
      with tendon involvement 894.2
      complicated 894.1
    upper (multiple) NEC 884.0
      with tendon involvement 884.2
      complicated 884.1
  lip 873.43
    complicated 873.53
  loin 876.0
    complicated 876.1
  lumbar region 876.0
    complicated 876.1
  malar region 873.41
    complicated 873.51
  mastoid region 873.49
    complicated 873.59
  mediastinum—*see* Injury, internal, mediastinum
  midthoracic region 875.0
    complicated 875.1
  mouth 873.60
    complicated 873.70
    floor 873.64
      complicated 873.74
    multiple sites 873.69
      complicated 873.79
    specified site NEC 873.69
      complicated 873.79
  multiple, unspecified site(s) 879.8

> *Note—Multiple open wounds of sites classifiable to the same four-digit category should be classified to that category unless they are in different limbs.*
>
> *Multiple open wounds of sites classifiable to different four-digit categories, or to different limbs, should be coded separately.*

    complicated 879.9
    lower limb(s) (one or both) (sites classifiable
      to more than one three-digit category in
      890 to 893) 894.0
      with tendon involvement 894.2
      complicated 894.1
    upper limb(s) (one or both) (sites classifiable
      to more than one three-digit category in
      880 to 883) 884.0
      with tendon involvement 884.2
      complicated 884.1
  muscle—*see* Sprain, by site
  nail
    finger(s) 883.0
      complicated 883.1
    thumb 883.0
      complicated 883.1
    toe(s) 893.0
      complicated 893.1
  nape (neck) 874.8
    complicated 874.9
    specified part NEC 874.8
      complicated 874.9
  nasal—*see also* Wound, open, nose
    cavity 873.22
      complicated 873.32
    septum 873.21
      complicated 873.31
    sinuses 873.23
      complicated 873.33

Wound, open—*continued*
- nasopharynx 873.22
  - complicated 873.32
- neck 874.8
  - complicated 874.9
  - nape 874.8
    - complicated 874.9
  - specified part NEC 874.8
    - complicated 874.9
- nerve—*see* Injury, nerve, by site
- non-healing surgical 998.83
- nose 873.20
  - complicated 873.30
  - multiple sites 873.29
    - complicated 873.39
  - septum 873.21
    - complicated 873.31
  - sinuses 873.23
    - complicated 873.33
- occipital region—*see* Wound, open, scalp
- ocular NEC 871.9
  - adnexa 870.9
    - specified region NEC 870.8
  - laceration (*see also* Laceration, ocular) 871.4
  - muscle (extraocular) 870.3
    - with foreign body 870.4
    - eyelid 870.1
    - intraocular—*see* Wound, open, eyeball
  - penetrating (*see also* Penetrating wound, ocular) 871.7
- orbit 870.8
  - penetrating 870.3
    - with foreign body 870.4
- orbital region 870.9
- ovary—*see* Injury, internal, pelvic organs
- palate 873.65
  - complicated 873.75
- palm 882.0
  - with tendon involvement 882.2
  - complicated 882.1
- parathyroid (gland) 874.2
  - complicated 874.3
- parietal region—*see* Wound, open, scalp
- pelvic floor or region 879.6
  - complicated 879.7
- penis 878.0
  - complicated 878.1
- perineum 879.6
  - complicated 879.7
- periocular area 870.8
  - laceration of skin 870.0
- pharynx 874.4
  - complicated 874.5
- pinna 872.01
  - complicated 872.11
- popliteal space 891.0
  - with tendon involvement 891.2
  - complicated 891.1
- prepuce 878.0
  - complicated 878.1
- pubic region 879.2
  - complicated 879.3
- pudenda 878.8
  - complicated 878.9
- rectovaginal septum 878.8
  - complicated 878.9
- sacral region 877.0
  - complicated 877.1
- sacroiliac region 877.0
  - complicated 877.1
- salivary (ducts) (glands) 873.69
  - complicated 873.79

Wound, open—*continued*
- scalp 873.0
  - complicated 873.1
- scalpel, fetus or newborn 767.8
- scapular region 880.01
  - with tendon involvement 880.21
  - complicated 880.11
  - involving other sites of upper arm 880.09
    - with tendon involvement 880.29
    - complicated 880.19
- sclera (*see also* Wound, open, intraocular) 871.9
- scrotum 878.2
  - complicated 878.3
- seminal vesicle—*see* Injury, internal, pelvic organs
- shin 891.0
  - with tendon involvement 891.2
  - complicated 891.1
- shoulder 880.00
  - with tendon involvement 880.20
  - complicated 880.10
  - involving other sites of upper arm 880.09
    - with tendon involvement 880.29
    - complicated 880.19
- skin NEC 879.8
  - complicated 879.9
- skull—*see also* Injury, intracranial, with open intracranial wound
  - with skull fracture—*see* Fracture, skull
- spermatic cord (scrotal) 878.2
  - complicated 878.3
  - pelvic region—*see* Injury, internal, spermatic cord
- spinal cord—*see* Injury, spinal
- sternal region 875.0
  - complicated 875.1
- subconjunctival—*see* Wound, open, intraocular
- subcutaneous NEC 879.8
  - complicated 879.9
- submaxillary region 873.44
  - complicated 873.54
- submental region 873.44
  - complicated 873.54
- subungual
  - finger(s) (thumb)—*see* Wound, open, finger
  - toe(s)—*see* Wound, open, toe
- supraclavicular region 874.8
  - complicated 874.9
- supraorbital 873.42
  - complicated 873.52
- surgical, non-healing 998.83
- temple 873.49
  - complicated 873.59
- temporal region 873.49
  - complicated 873.59
- testis 878.2
  - complicated 878.3
- thigh 890.0
  - with tendon involvement 890.2
  - complicated 890.1
- thorax, thoracic (external) 875.0
  - complicated 875.1
- throat 874.8
  - complicated 874.9
- thumb (nail) (subungual) 883.0
  - with tendon involvement 883.2
  - complicated 883.1
- thyroid (gland) 874.2
  - complicated 874.3
- toe(s) (nail) (subungual) 893.0
  - with tendon involvement 893.2

Wound, open—*continued*
  complicated 893.1
 tongue 873.64
  complicated 873.74
 tonsil—*see* Wound, open, neck
 trachea (cervical region) 874.02
  with larynx 874.00
   complicated 874.10
  complicated 874.12
  intrathoracic—*see* Injury, internal, trachea
 trunk (multiple) NEC 879.6
  complicated 879.7
  specified site NEC 879.6
   complicated 879.7
 tunica vaginalis 878.2
  complicated 878.3
 tympanic membrane 872.61
  complicated 872.71
 tympanum 872.61
  complicated 872.71
 umbilical region 879.2
  complicated 879.3
 ureter—*see* Injury, internal, ureter
 urethra—*see* Injury, internal, urethra
 uterus—*see* Injury, internal, uterus
 uvula 873.69
  complicated 873.79
 vagina 878.6
  complicated 878.7
 vas deferens—*see* Injury, internal, vas deferens
 vitreous (humor) 871.2
 vulva 878.4
  complicated 878.5
 wrist 881.02
  with tendon involvement 881.22
  complicated 881.12
Wright's syndrome (hyperabduction) 447.8
 pneumonia 390 *[517.1]*
Wringer injury —*see* Crush injury, by site
Wrinkling of skin 701.8
Wrist —*see also* condition
 drop (acquired) 736.05
Wrong drug (given in error) NEC 977.9
 specified drug or substance—*see* Table of drugs
  and chemicals
Wry neck —*see also* Torticollis
 congenital 754.1
Wuchereria infestation 125.0
 bancrofti 125.0
 Brugia malayi 125.1
 malayi 125.1
Wuchereriasis 125.0
Wuchereriosis 125.0
Wuchernde struma langhans (M8332/3) 193

X

Xanthelasma 272.2
  eyelid 272.2 *[374.51]*
  palpebrarum 272.2 *[374.51]*
Xanthelasmatosis (essential) 272.2
Xanthelasmoidea 757.33
Xanthine stones 277.2
Xanthinuria 277.2
Xanthofibroma (M8831/0)—*see* Neoplasm,
  connective tissue, benign
Xanthoma(s), xanthomatosis 272.2
  with
    hyperlipoproteinemia
      type I 272.3
      type III 272.2
      type IV 272.1
      type V 272.3
  bone 272.7
  craniohypophyseal 277.89
  cutaneotendinous 272.7
  diabeticorum 250.8 *[272.2]*
    due to secondary diabetes 249.8 *[272.2]*
  disseminatum 272.7
  eruptive 272.2
  eyelid 272.2 *[374.51]*
  familial 272.7
  hereditary 272.7
  hypercholesterinemic 272.0
  hypercholesterolemic 272.0
  hyperlipemic 272.4
  hyperlipidemic 272.4
  infantile 272.7
  joint 272.7
  juvenile 272.7
  multiple 272.7
  multiplex 272.7
  primary familial 272.7
  tendon (sheath) 272.7
  tuberosum 272.2
  tuberous 272.2
  tubo-eruptive 272.2
Xanthosis 709.09
  surgical 998.81
Xenophobia 300.29
Xeroderma (congenital) 757.39
  acquired 701.1
    eyelid 373.33
  eyelid 373.33
  pigmentosum 757.33
  vitamin A deficiency 264.8
Xerophthalmia 372.53
  vitamin A deficiency 264.7
Xerosis
  conjunctiva 372.53
    with Bitôt's spot 372.53
      vitamin A deficiency 264.1
    vitamin A deficiency 264.0
  cornea 371.40
    with corneal ulceration 370.00
      vitamin A deficiency 264.3
    vitamin A deficiency 264.2
  cutis 706.8
  skin 706.8
Xerostomia 527.7
Xiphodynia 733.90
Xiphoidalgia 733.90
Xiphoiditis 733.99
Xiphopagus 759.4

XO syndrome 758.6
X-ray
  effects, adverse, NEC 990
  of chest
    for suspected tuberculosis V71.2
    routine V72.5
XXX syndrome 758.81
XXXXY syndrome 758.81
XXY syndrome 758.7
Xyloketosuria 271.8
Xylosuria 271.8
Xylulosuria 271.8
XYY syndrome 758.81

Y

Yaba monkey tumor virus 059.22
Yawning 786.09
   psychogenic 306.1
Yaws 102.9
   bone or joint lesions 102.6
   butter 102.1
   chancre 102.0
   cutaneous, less than five years after infection
      102.2
   early (cutaneous) (macular) (maculopapular)
      (micropapular) (papular) 102.2
      frambeside 102.2
      skin lesions NEC 102.2
   eyelid 102.9 *[373.4]*
   ganglion 102.6
   gangosis, gangosa 102.5
   gumma, gummata 102.4
      bone 102.6
   gummatous
      frambeside 102.4
      osteitis 102.6
      periostitis 102.6
   hydrarthrosis 102.6
   hyperkeratosis (early) (late) (palmar) (plantar)
      102.3
   initial lesions 102.0
   joint lesions 102.6
   juxta-articular nodules 102.7
   late nodular (ulcerated) 102.4
   latent (without clinical manifestations) (with
      positive serology) 102.8
   mother 102.0
   mucosal 102.7
   multiple papillomata 102.1
   nodular, late (ulcerated) 102.4
   osteitis 102.6
   papilloma, papillomata (palmar) (plantar) 102.1
   periostitis (hypertrophic) 102.6
   ulcers 102.4
   wet crab 102.1
Yeast infection (*see also* Candidiasis) 112.9
Yellow
   atrophy (liver) 570
      chronic 571.8
      resulting from administration of blood,
         plasma, serum, or other biological
         substance (within 8 months of
         administration)—*see* Hepatitis, viral
   fever—*see* Fever, yellow
   jack (*see also* Fever, yellow) 060.9
   jaundice (*see also* Jaundice) 782.4
Yersinia septica 027.8

Z

Zagari's disease (xerostomia) 527.7
Zahorsky's disease (exanthema subitum) (*see
   also* Exanthem subitum) 058.10
   syndrome (herpangina) 074.0
Zellweger syndrome 277.86
Zenker's diverticulum (esophagus) 530.6
Ziehen-Oppenheim disease 333.6
Zieve's syndrome (jaundice, hyperlipemia, and
   hemolytic anemia) 571.1
Zika fever 066.3
Zollinger-Ellison syndrome (gastric
   hypersecretion with pancreatic islet cell
   tumor) 251.5
Zona (*see also* Herpes, zoster) 053.9
Zoophilia (erotica) 302.1
Zoophobia 300.29
Zoster (herpes) (*see also* Herpes, zoster) 053.9
Zuelzer (-Ogden) anemia or syndrome
   (nutritional megaloblastic anemia) 281.2
Zygodactyly (*see also* Syndactylism) 755.10
Zygomycosis 117.7
Zymotic —*see* condition

SECTION 2

ALPHABETIC INDEX TO POISONING AND EXTERNAL CAUSES OF ADVERSE EFFECTS OF DRUGS AND OTHER CHEMICAL SUBSTANCES

TABLE OF DRUGS AND CHEMICALS

This table contains a classification of drugs and other chemical substances to identify poisoning states and external causes of adverse effects.

Each of the listed substances in the table is assigned a code according to the poisoning classification (960–989). These codes are used when there is a statement of poisoning, overdose, wrong substance given or taken, or intoxication.

The table also contains a listing of external causes of adverse effects. An adverse effect is a pathologic manifestation due to ingestion or exposure to drugs or other chemical substances (e.g., dermatitis, hypersensitivity reaction, aspirin gastritis). The adverse effect is to be identified by the appropriate code found in Section 1, Index to Diseases and Injuries. An external cause code can then be used to identify the circumstances involved. The table headings pertaining to external causes are defined below:

> **Accidental poisoning (E850–E869)**—accidental overdose of drug, wrong substance given or taken, drug taken inadvertently, accidents in the usage of drugs and biologicals in medical and surgical procedures, and to show external causes of poisonings classifiable to 980–989.

> **Therapeutic use (E930–E949)**—a correct substance properly administered in therapeutic or prophylactic dosage as the external cause of adverse effects.

> **Suicide attempt (E950–E952)**—instances in which self–inflicted injuries or poisonings are involved.

> **Assault (E961–E962)**—injury or poisoning inflicted by another person with the intent to injure or kill.

> **Undetermined (E980–E982)**—to be used when the intent of the poisoning or injury cannot be determined whether it was intentional or accidental.

The American Hospital Formulary Service list numbers are included in the table to help classify new drugs not identified in the table by name. The AHFS list numbers are keyed to the continually revised American Hospital Formulary Service (AHFS).* These listings are found in the table under the main term **Drug**.

Excluded from the table are radium and other radioactive substances. The classification of adverse effects and complications pertaining to these substances will be found in Section 1, Index to Diseases and Injuries, and Section 3, Index to External Causes of Injuries.

Although certain substances are indexed with one or more subentries, the majority are listed according to one use or state. It is recognized that many substances may be used in various ways, in medicine and in industry, and may cause adverse effects whatever the state of the agent (solid, liquid, or fumes arising from a liquid). In cases in which the reported data indicates a use or state not in the table, or which is clearly different from the one listed, an attempt should be made to classify the substance in the form which most nearly expresses the reported facts.

DRUGS & CHEMICALS

*American Hospital Formulary Service, 2 vol. (Washington, DC: American Society of Hospital Pharmacists, 1959)

Substance	Poisoning	Accident	Therapeutic Use	Suicide Attempt	Assault	Undetermined
				External Cause (E-Code)		
1–propanol	980.3	E860.4	—	E950.9	E962.1	E980.9
2–propanol	980.2	E860.3	—	E950.9	E962.1	E980.9
2, 4–D (dichlorophenoxyacetic acid)	989.4	E863.5	—	E950.6	E962.1	E980.7
2, 4–toluene diisocyanate	983.0	E864.0	—	E950.7	E962.1	E980.6
2, 4, 5–T (trichlorophenoxyacetic acid)	989.2	E863.5	—	E950.6	E962.1	E980.7
14–hydroxydihydromorphinone	965.09	E850.2	E935.2	E950.0	E962.0	E980.0
ABOB	961.7	E857	E931.7	E950.4	E962.0	E980.4
Abrus (seed)	988.2	E865.3	—	E950.9	E962.1	E980.9
Absinthe	980.0	E860.1	—	E950.9	E962.1	E980.9
beverage	980.0	E860.0	—	E950.9	E962.1	E980.9
Acenocoumarin, acenocoumarol	964.2	E858.2	E934.2	E950.4	E962.0	E980.4
Acepromazine	969.1	E853.0	E939.1	E950.3	E962.0	E980.3
Acetal	982.8	E862.4	—	E950.9	E962.1	E980.9
Acetaldehyde (vapor)	987.8	E869.8	—	E952.8	E962.2	E982.8
liquid	989.89	E866.8	—	E950.9	E962.1	E980.9
Acetaminophen	965.4	E850.4	E935.4	E950.0	E962.0	E980.0
Acetaminosalol	965.1	E850.3	E935.3	E950.0	E962.0	E980.0
Acetanilid(e)	965.4	E850.4	E935.4	E950.0	E962.0	E980.0
Acetarsol, acetarsone	961.1	E857	E931.1	E950.4	E962.0	E980.4
Acetazolamide	974.2	E858.5	E944.2	E950.4	E962.0	E980.4
Acetic						
acid	983.1	E864.1	—	E950.7	E962.1	E980.6
with sodium acetate (ointment)	976.3	E858.7	E946.3	E950.4	E962.0	E980.4
irrigating solution	974.5	E858.5	E944.5	E950.4	E962.0	E980.4
lotion	976.2	E858.7	E946.2	E950.4	E962.0	E980.4
anhydride	983.1	E864.1	—	E950.7	E962.1	E980.6
ether (vapor)	982.8	E862.4	—	E950.9	E962.1	E980.9
Acetohexamide	962.3	E858.0	E932.3	E950.4	E962.0	E980.4
Acetomenaphthone	964.3	E858.2	E934.3	E950.4	E962.0	E980.4
Acetomorphine	965.01	E850.0	E935.0	E950.0	E962.0	E980.0
Acetone (oils) (vapor)	982.8	E862.4	—	E950.9	E962.1	E980.9
Acetophenazine (maleate)	969.1	E853.0	E939.1	E950.3	E962.0	E980.3
Acetophenetidin	965.4	E850.4	E935.4	E950.0	E962.0	E980.0
Acetophenone	982.0	E862.4	—	E950.9	E962.1	E980.9
Acetorphine	965.09	E850.2	E935.2	E950.0	E962.0	E980.0
Acetosulfone (sodium)	961.8	E857	E931.8	E950.4	E962.0	E980.4
Acetrizoate (sodium)	977.8	E858.8	E947.8	E950.4	E962.0	E980.4
Acetylcarbromal	967.3	E852.2	E937.3	E950.2	E962.0	E980.2
Acetylcholine (chloride)	971.0	E855.3	E941.0	E950.4	E962.0	E980.4
Acetylcysteine	975.5	E858.6	E945.5	E950.4	E962.0	E980.4
Acetyldigitoxin	972.1	E858.3	E942.1	E950.4	E962.0	E980.4
Acetyldihydrocodeine	965.09	E850.2	E935.2	E950.0	E962.0	E980.0
Acetyldihydrocodeinone	965.09	E850.2	E935.2	E950.0	E962.0	E980.0
Acetylene (gas) (industrial)	987.1	E868.1	—	E951.8	E962.2	E981.8
incomplete combustion of — see Carbon monoxide, fuel, utility						
tetrachloride (vapor)	982.3	E862.4	—	E950.9	E962.1	E980.9
Acetyliodosalicylic acid	965.1	E850.3	E935.3	E950.0	E962.0	E980.0
Acetylphenylhydrazine	965.8	E850.8	E935.8	E950.0	E962.0	E980.0
Acetylsalicylic acid	965.1	E850.3	E935.3	E950.0	E962.0	E980.0
Achromycin	960.4	E856	E930.4	E950.4	E962.0	E980.4
ophthalmic preparation	976.5	E858.7	E946.5	E950.4	E962.0	E980.4
topical NEC	976.0	E858.7	E946.0	E950.4	E962.0	E980.4
Acidifying agents	963.2	E858.1	E933.2	E950.4	E962.0	E980.4
Acids (corrosive) NEC	983.1	E864.1	—	E950.7	E962.1	E980.6
Aconite (wild)	988.2	E865.4	—	E950.9	E962.1	E980.9
Aconitine (liniment)	976.8	E858.7	E946.8	E950.4	E962.0	E980.4
Aconitum ferox	988.2	E865.4	—	E950.9	E962.1	E980.9
Acridine	983.0	E864.0	—	E950.7	E962.1	E980.6
vapor	987.8	E869.8	—	E952.8	E962.2	E982.8

Substance	Poisoning	Accident	Therapeutic Use	Suicide Attempt	Assault	Undetermined
			External Cause (E-Code)			
Acriflavine	961.9	E857	E931.9	E950.4	E962.0	E980.4
Acrisorcin	976.0	E858.7	E946.0	E950.4	E962.0	E980.4
Acrolein (gas)	987.8	E869.8	—	E952.8	E962.2	E982.8
liquid	989.89	E866.8	—	E950.9	E962.1	E980.9
Actaea spicata	988.2	E865.4	—	E950.9	E962.1	E980.9
Acterol	961.5	E857	E931.5	E950.4	E962.0	E980.4
ACTH	962.4	E858.0	E932.4	E950.4	E962.0	E980.4
Acthar	962.4	E858.0	E932.4	E950.4	E962.0	E980.4
Actinomycin (C) (D)	960.7	E856	E930.7	E950.4	E962.0	E980.4
Adalin (acetyl)	967.3	E852.2	E937.3	E950.2	E962.0	E980.2
Adenosine (phosphate)	977.8	E858.8	E947.8	E950.4	E962.0	E980.4
Adhesives	989.89	E866.6	—	E950.9	E962.1	E980.9
ADH	962.5	E858.0	E932.5	E950.4	E962.0	E980.4
Adicillin	960.0	E856	E930.0	E950.4	E962.0	E980.4
Adiphenine	975.1	E855.6	E945.1	E950.4	E962.0	E980.4
Adjunct, pharmaceutical	977.4	E858.8	E947.4	E950.4	E962.0	E980.4
Adrenal (extract, cortex or medulla) (glucocorticoids) (hormones) (mineralocorticoids)	962.0	E858.0	E932.0	E950.4	E962.0	E980.4
ENT agent	976.6	E858.7	E946.6	E950.4	E962.0	E980.4
ophthalmic preparation	976.5	E858.7	E946.5	E950.4	E962.0	E980.4
topical NEC	976.0	E858.7	E946.0	E950.4	E962.0	E980.4
Adrenalin	971.2	E855.5	E941.2	E950.4	E962.0	E980.4
Adrenergic blocking agents	971.3	E855.6	E941.3	E950.4	E962.0	E980.4
Adrenergics	971.2	E855.5	E941.2	E950.4	E962.0	E980.4
Adrenochrome (derivatives)	972.8	E858.3	E942.8	E950.4	E962.0	E980.4
Adrenocorticotropic hormone	962.4	E858.0	E932.4	E950.4	E962.0	E980.4
Adrenocorticotropin	962.4	E858.0	E932.4	E950.4	E962.0	E980.4
Adriamycin	960.7	E856	E930.7	E950.4	E962.0	E980.4
Aerosol spray — *see* Sprays						
Aerosporin	960.8	E856	E930.8	E950.4	E962.0	E980.4
ENT agent	976.6	E858.7	E946.6	E950.4	E962.0	E980.4
ophthalmic preparation	976.5	E858.7	E946.5	E950.4	E962.0	E980.4
topical NEC	976.0	E858.7	E946.0	E950.4	E962.0	E980.4
Aethusa cynapium	988.2	E865.4	—	E950.9	E962.1	E980.9
Afghanistan black	969.6	E854.1	E939.6	E950.3	E962.0	E980.3
Aflatoxin	989.7	E865.9	—	E950.9	E962.1	E980.9
African boxwood	988.2	E865.4	—	E950.9	E962.1	E980.9
Agar (–agar)	973.3	E858.4	E943.3	E950.4	E962.0	E980.4
Agricultural agent NEC	989.89	E863.9	—	E950.6	E962.1	E980.7
Agrypnal	967.0	E851	E937.0	E950.1	E962.0	E980.1
Air contaminant(s), source or type not specified	987.9	E869.9	—	E952.9	E962.2	E982.9
specified type — *see* specific substance						
Akee	988.2	E865.4	—	E950.9	E962.1	E980.9
Akrinol	976.0	E858.7	E946.0	E950.4	E962.0	E980.4
Alantolactone	961.6	E857	E931.6	E950.4	E962.0	E980.4
Albamycin	960.8	E856	E930.8	E950.4	E962.0	E980.4
Albumin (normal human serum)	964.7	E858.2	E934.7	E950.4	E962.0	E980.4
Albuterol	975.7	E858.6	E945.7	E950.4	E962.0	E980.4
Alcohol	980.9	E860.9	—	E950.9	E962.1	E980.9
absolute	980.0	E860.1	—	E950.9	E962.1	E980.9
beverage	980.0	E860.0	E947.8	E950.9	E962.1	E980.9
amyl	980.3	E860.4	—	E950.9	E962.1	E980.9
antifreeze	980.1	E860.2	—	E950.9	E962.1	E980.9
butyl	980.3	E860.4	—	E950.9	E962.1	E980.9
dehydrated	980.0	E860.1	—	E950.9	E862.1	E980.9
beverage	980.0	E860.0	E947.8	E950.9	E962.1	E980.9
denatured	980.0	E860.1	—	E950.9	E962.1	E980.9
deterrents	977.3	E858.8	E947.3	E950.4	E962.0	E980.4
diagnostic (gastric function)	977.8	E858.8	E947.8	E950.4	E962.0	E980.4

Substance	Poisoning	Accident	Therapeutic Use	Suicide Attempt	Assault	Undetermined
			External Cause (E-Code)			
ethyl 980.0	E860.1	—	E950.9	E962.1	E980.9
beverage 980.0	E860.0	E947.8	E950.9	E962.1	E980.9
grain 980.0	E860.1	—	E950.9	E962.1	E980.9
beverage 980.0	E860.0	E947.8	E950.9	E962.1	E980.9
industrial 980.9	E860.9	—	E950.9	E962.1	E980.9
isopropyl 980.2	E860.3	—	E950.9	E962.1	E980.9
methyl 980.1	E860.2	—	E950.9	E962.1	E980.9
preparation for consumption 980.0	E860.0	E947.8	E950.9	E962.1	E980.9
propyl 980.3	E860.4	—	E950.9	E962.1	E980.9
secondary 980.2	E860.3	—	E950.9	E962.1	E980.9
radiator 980.1	E860.2	—	E950.9	E962.1	E980.9
rubbing 980.2	E860.3	—	E950.9	E962.1	E980.9
specified type NEC 980.8	E860.8	—	E950.9	E962.1	E980.9
surgical 980.9	E860.9	—	E950.9	E962.1	E980.9
vapor (from any type of alcohol) 987.8	E869.8	—	E952.8	E962.2	E982.8
wood 980.1	E860.2	—	E950.9	E962.1	E980.9
Alcuronium chloride 975.2	E858.6	E945.2	E950.4	E962.0	E980.4
Aldactone 974.4	E858.5	E944.4	E950.4	E962.0	E980.4
Aldicarb 989.3	E863.2	—	E950.6	E962.1	E980.7
Aldomet 972.6	E858.3	E942.6	E950.4	E962.0	E980.4
Aldosterone 962.0	E858.0	E932.0	E950.4	E962.0	E980.4
Aldrin (dust) 989.2	E863.0	—	E950.6	E962.1	E980.7
Algeldrate 973.0	E858.4	E943.0	E950.4	E962.0	E980.4
Alidase 963.4	E858.1	E933.4	E950.4	E962.0	E980.4
Aliphatic thiocyanates 989.0	E866.8	—	E950.9	E962.1	E980.9
Alkaline antiseptic solution (aromatic) 976.6	E858.7	E946.6	E950.4	E962.0	E980.4
Alkalinizing agents (medicinal) 963.3	E858.1	E933.3	E950.4	E962.0	E980.4
Alkalis, caustic 983.2	E864.2	—	E950.7	E962.1	E980.6
Alkalizing agents (medicinal) 963.3	E858.1	E933.3	E950.4	E962.0	E980.4
Alka–seltzer 965.1	E850.3	E935.3	E950.0	E962.0	E980.0
Alkavervir 972.6	E858.3	E942.6	E950.4	E962.0	E980.4
Allegron 969.05	E854.0	E939.0	E950.3	E962.0	E980.3
Alleve see Naproxen					
Allobarbital, allobarbitone 967.0	E851	E937.0	E950.1	E962.0	E980.1
Allopurinol 974.7	E858.5	E944.7	E950.4	E962.0	E980.4
Allylestrenol 962.2	E858.0	E932.2	E950.4	E962.0	E980.4
Allylisopropylacetylurea 967.8	E852.8	E937.8	E950.2	E962.0	E980.2
Allylisopropylmalonylurea 967.0	E851	E937.0	E950.1	E962.0	E980.1
Allyltribromide 967.3	E852.2	E937.3	E950.2	E962.0	E980.2
Aloe, aloes, aloin 973.1	E858.4	E943.1	E950.4	E962.0	E980.4
Alosetron 973.8	E858.4	E943.8	E950.4	E962.0	E980.4
Aloxidone 966.0	E855.0	E936.0	E950.4	E962.0	E980.4
Aloxiprin 965.1	E850.3	E935.3	E950.0	E962.0	E980.0
Alpha amylase 963.4	E858.1	E933.4	E950.4	E962.0	E980.4
Alpha-1 blockers 971.3	E855.6	E941.3	E950.4	E962.0	E980.4
Alpha tocopherol 963.5	E858.1	E933.5	E950.4	E962.0	E980.4
Alphaprodine (hydrochloride) 965.09	E850.2	E935.2	E950.0	E962.0	E980.0
Alseroxylon 972.6	E858.3	E942.6	E950.4	E962.0	E980.4
Alum (ammonium) (potassium) 983.2	E864.2	—	E950.7	E962.1	E980.6
medicinal (astringent) NEC 976.2	E858.7	E946.2	E950.4	E962.0	E980.4
Aluminium, aluminum (gel) (hydroxide) . . . 973.0	E858.4	E943.0	E950.4	E962.0	E980.4
acetate solution 976.2	E858.7	E946.2	E950.4	E962.0	E980.4
aspirin 965.1	E850.3	E935.3	E950.0	E962.0	E980.0
carbonate 973.0	E858.4	E943.0	E950.4	E962.0	E980.4
glycinate 973.0	E858.4	E943.0	E950.4	E962.0	E980.4
nicotinate 972.2	E858.3	E942.2	E950.4	E962.0	E980.4
ointment (surgical) (topical) 976.3	E858.7	E946.3	E950.4	E962.0	E980.4
phosphate 973.0	E858.4	E943.0	E950.4	E962.0	E980.4
subacetate 976.2	E858.7	E946.2	E950.4	E962.0	E980.4
topical NEC 976.3	E858.7	E946.3	E950.4	E962.0	E980.4

TABLE OF DRUGS AND CHEMICALS

Substance	Poisoning	Accident	Therapeutic Use	Suicide Attempt	Assault	Undetermined
				External Cause (E-Code)		
Alurate	967.0	E851	E937.0	E950.1	E962.0	E980.1
Alverine (citrate)	975.1	E858.6	E945.1	E950.4	E962.0	E980.4
Alvodine	965.09	E850.2	E935.2	E950.0	E962.0	E980.0
Amanita phalloides	988.1	E865.5	—	E950.9	E962.1	E980.9
Amantadine (hydrochloride)	966.4	E855.0	E936.4	E950.4	E962.0	E980.4
Ambazone	961.9	E857	E931.9	E950.4	E962.0	E980.4
Ambenonium	971.0	E855.3	E941.0	E950.4	E962.0	E980.4
Ambutonium bromide	971.1	E855.4	E941.1	E950.4	E962.0	E980.4
Ametazole	977.8	E858.8	E947.8	E950.4	E962.0	E980.4
Amethocaine (infiltration) (topical)	968.5	E855.2	E938.5	E950.4	E962.0	E980.4
nerve block (peripheral) (plexus)	968.6	E855.2	E938.6	E950.4	E962.0	E980.4
spinal	968.7	E855.2	E938.7	E950.4	E962.0	E980.4
Amethopterin	963.1	E858.1	E933.1	E950.4	E962.0	E980.4
Amfepramone	977.0	E858.8	E947.0	E950.4	E962.0	E980.4
Amidon	965.02	E850.1	E935.1	E950.0	E962.0	E980.0
Amidopyrine	965.5	E850.5	E935.5	E950.0	E962.0	E980.0
Aminacrine	976.0	E858.7	E946.0	E950.4	E962.0	E980.4
Aminitrozole	961.5	E857	E931.5	E950.4	E962.0	E980.4
Aminoacetic acid	974.5	E858.5	E944.5	E950.4	E962.0	E980.4
Amino acids	974.5	E858.5	E944.5	E950.4	E962.0	E980.4
Aminocaproic acid	964.4	E858.2	E934.4	E950.4	E962.0	E980.4
Aminoethylisothiourium	963.8	E858.1	E933.8	E950.4	E962.0	E980.4
Aminoglutethimide	966.3	E855.0	E936.3	E950.4	E962.0	E980.4
Aminometradine	974.3	E858.5	E944.3	E950.4	E962.0	E980.4
Aminopentamide	971.1	E855.4	E941.1	E950.4	E962.0	E980.4
Aminophenazone	965.5	E850.5	E935.5	E950.0	E962.0	E980.0
Aminophenol	983.0	E864.0	—	E950.7	E962.1	E980.6
Aminophenylpyridone	969.5	E853.8	E939.5	E950.3	E962.0	E980.3
Aminophyllin	975.7	E858.6	E945.7	E950.4	E962.0	E980.4
Aminopterin	963.1	E858.1	E933.1	E950.4	E962.0	E980.4
Aminopyrine	965.5	E850.5	E935.5	E950.0	E962.0	E980.0
Aminosalicylic acid	961.8	E857	E931.8	E950.4	E962.0	E980.4
Amiphenazole	970.1	E854.3	E940.1	E950.4	E962.0	E980.4
Amiquinsin	972.6	E858.3	E942.6	E950.4	E962.0	E980.4
Amisometradine	974.3	E858.5	E944.3	E950.4	E962.0	E980.4
Amitriptyline	969.05	E854.0	E939.0	E950.3	E962.0	E980.3
Ammonia (fumes) (gas) (vapor)	987.8	E869.8	—	E952.8	E962.2	E982.8
liquid (household) NEC	983.2	E861.4	—	E950.7	E962.1	E980.6
spirit, aromatic	970.89	E854.3	E940.8	E950.4	E962.0	E980.4
Ammoniated mercury	976.0	E858.7	E946.0	E950.4	E962.0	E980.4
Ammonium						
carbonate	983.2	E864.2	—	E950.7	E962.1	E980.6
chloride (acidifying agent)	963.2	E858.1	E933.2	E950.4	E962.0	E980.4
expectorant	975.5	E858.6	E945.5	E950.4	E962.0	E980.4
compounds (household) NEC	983.2	E861.4	—	E950.7	E962.1	E980.6
fumes (any usage)	987.8	E869.8	—	E952.8	E962.2	E982.8
industrial	983.2	E864.2	—	E950.7	E962.1	E980.6
ichthyosulfonate	976.4	E858.7	E946.4	E950.4	E962.0	E980.4
mandelate	961.9	E857	E931.9	E950.4	E962.0	E980.4
Amobarbital	967.0	E851	E937.0	E950.1	E962.0	E980.1
Amodiaquin(e)	961.4	E857	E931.4	E950.4	E962.0	E980.4
Amopyroquin(e)	961.4	E857	E931.4	E950.4	E962.0	E980.4
Amphenidone	969.5	E853.8	E939.5	E950.3	E962.0	E980.3
Amphetamine	969.72	E854.2	E939.7	E950.3	E962.0	E980.3
Amphomycin	960.8	E856	E930.8	E950.4	E962.0	E980.4
Amphotericin B	960.1	E856	E930.1	E950.4	E962.0	E980.4
topical	976.0	E858.7	E946.0	E950.4	E962.0	E980.4
Ampicillin	960.0	E856	E930.0	E950.4	E962.0	E980.4
Amprotropine	971.1	E855.4	E941.1	E950.4	E962.0	E980.4
Amygdalin	977.8	E858.8	E947.8	E950.4	E962.0	E980.4
Amyl						

Substance	Poisoning	Accident	Therapeutic Use	Suicide Attempt	Assault	Undetermined
			External Cause (E-Code)			
acetate (vapor)	982.8	E862.4	—	E950.9	E962.1	E980.9
alcohol	980.3	E860.4	—	E950.9	E962.1	E980.9
nitrite (medicinal)	972.4	E858.3	E942.4	E950.4	E962.0	E980.4
Amylase (alpha)	963.4	E858.1	E933.4	E950.4	E962.0	E980.4
Amylene hydrate	980.8	E860.8	—	E950.9	E962.1	E980.9
Amylobarbitone	967.0	E851	E937.0	E950.1	E962.0	E980.1
Amylocaine	968.9	E855.2	E938.9	E950.4	E962.0	E980.4
infiltration (subcutaneous)	968.5	E855.2	E938.5	E950.4	E962.0	E980.4
nerve block (peripheral) (plexus)	968.6	E855.2	E938.6	E950.4	E962.0	E980.4
spinal	968.7	E855.2	E938.7	E950.4	E962.0	E980.4
topical (surface)	968.5	E855.2	E938.5	E950.4	E962.0	E980.4
Amytal (sodium)	967.0	E851	E937.0	E950.1	E962.0	E980.1
Analeptics	970.0	E854.3	E940.0	E950.4	E962.0	E980.4
Analgesics	965.9	E850.9	E935.9	E950.0	E962.0	E980.0
aromatic NEC	965.4	E850.4	E935.4	E950.0	E962.0	E980.0
non–narcotic NEC	965.7	E850.7	E935.7	E950.0	E962.0	E980.0
specified NEC	965.8	E850.8	E935.8	E950.0	E962.0	E980.0
Anamirta cocculus	988.2	E865.3	—	E950.9	E962.1	E980.9
Ancillin	960.0	E856	E930.0	E950.4	E962.0	E980.4
Androgens (anabolic congeners)	962.1	E858.0	E932.1	E950.4	E962.0	E980.4
Androstalone	962.1	E858.0	E932.1	E950.4	E962.0	E980.4
Androsterone	962.1	E858.0	E932.1	E950.4	E962.0	E980.4
Anemone pulsatilla	988.2	E865.4	—	E950.9	E962.1	E980.9
Anesthesia, anesthetic (general) NEC	968.4	E855.1	E938.4	E950.4	E962.0	E980.4
block (nerve) (plexus)	968.6	E855.2	E938.6	E950.4	E962.0	E980.4
gaseous NEC	968.2	E855.1	E938.2	E950.4	E962.0	E980.4
halogenated hydrocarbon derivatives NEC	968.2	E855.1	E938.2	E950.4	E962.0	E980.4
infiltration (intradermal) (subcutaneous) (submucosal)	968.5	E855.2	E938.5	E950.4	E962.0	E980.4
intravenous	968.3	E855.1	E938.3	E950.4	E962.0	E980.4
local NEC	968.9	E855.2	E938.9	E950.4	E962.0	E980.4
nerve blocking (peripheral) (plexus)	968.6	E855.2	E938.6	E950.4	E962.0	E980.4
rectal NEC	968.3	E855.1	E938.3	E950.4	E962.0	E980.4
spinal	968.7	E855.2	E938.7	E950.4	E962.0	E980.4
surface	968.5	E855.2	E938.5	E950.4	E962.0	E980.4
topical	968.5	E855.2	E938.5	E950.4	E962.0	E980.4
Aneurine	963.5	E858.1	E933.5	E950.4	E962.0	E980.4
Angio–Conray	977.8	E858.8	E947.8	E950.4	E962.0	E980.4
Anginine *see* Glyceryl trinitrate						
Angiotensin	971.2	E855.5	E941.2	E950.4	E962.0	E980.4
Anhydrohydroxyprogesterone	962.2	E858.0	E932.2	E950.4	E962.0	E980.4
Anhydron	974.3	E858.5	E944.3	E950.4	E962.0	E980.4
Anileridine	965.09	E850.2	E935.2	E950.0	E962.0	E980.0
Aniline (dye) (liquid)	983.0	E864.0	—	E950.7	E962.1	E980.6
analgesic	965.4	E850.4	E935.4	E950.0	E962.0	E980.0
derivatives, therapeutic NEC	965.4	E850.4	E935.4	E950.0	E962.0	E980.0
vapor	987.8	E869.8	—	E952.8	E962.2	E982.8
Anisindione	964.2	E858.2	E934.2	E950.4	E962.0	E980.4
Anisotropine	971.1	E855.4	E941.1	E950.4	E962.0	E980.4
Anorexic agents	977.0	E858.8	E947.0	E950.4	E962.0	E980.4
Ant (bite) (sting)	989.5	E905.5	—	E950.9	E962.1	E980.9
Antabuse	977.3	E858.8	E947.3	E950.4	E962.0	E980.4
Antacids	973.0	E858.4	E943.0	E950.4	E962.0	E980.4
Antazoline	963.0	E858.1	E933.0	E950.4	E962.0	E980.4
Anthelmintics	961.6	E857	E931.6	E950.4	E962.0	E980.4
Anthralin	976.4	E858.7	E946.4	E950.4	E962.0	E980.4
Anthramycin	960.7	E856	E930.7	E950.4	E962.0	E980.4
Antiadrenergics	971.3	E855.6	E941.3	E950.4	E962.0	E980.4
Antiallergic agents	963.0	E858.1	E933.0	E950.4	E962.0	E980.4

Substance	Poisoning	Accident	Therapeutic Use	Suicide Attempt	Assault	Undetermined
				External Cause (E-Code)		
Antianemic agents NEC	964.1	E858.2	E934.1	E950.4	E962.0	E980.4
Antiaris toxicaria	988.2	E865.4	—	E950.9	E962.1	E980.9
Antiarteriosclerotic agents	972.2	E858.3	E942.2	E950.4	E962.0	E980.4
Antiasthmatics	975.7	E858.6	E945.7	E950.4	E962.0	E980.4
Antibiotics	960.9	E856	E930.9	E950.4	E962.0	E980.4
antifungal	960.1	E856	E930.1	E950.4	E962.0	E980.4
antimycobacterial	960.6	E856	E930.6	E950.4	E962.0	E980.4
antineoplastic	960.7	E856	E930.7	E950.4	E962.0	E980.4
cephalosporin (group)	960.5	E856	E930.5	E950.4	E962.0	E980.4
chloramphenicol (group)	960.2	E856	E930.2	E950.4	E962.0	E980.4
macrolides	960.3	E856	E930.3	E950.4	E962.0	E980.4
specified NEC	960.8	E856	E930.8	E950.4	E962.0	E980.4
tetracycline (group)	960.4	E856	E930.4	E950.4	E962.0	E980.4
Anticancer agents NEC	963.1	E858.1	E933.1	E950.4	E962.0	E980.4
antibiotics	960.7	E856	E930.7	E950.4	E962.0	E980.4
Anticholinergics	971.1	E855.4	E941.1	E950.4	E962.0	E980.4
Anticholinesterase (organophosphorus) (reversible)	971.0	E855.3	E941.0	E950.4	E962.0	E980.4
Anticoagulants	964.2	E858.2	E934.2	E950.4	E962.0	E980.4
antagonists	964.5	E858.2	E934.5	E950.4	E962.0	E980.4
Anti–common cold agents NEC	975.6	E858.6	E945.6	E950.4	E962.0	E980.4
Anticonvulsants NEC	966.3	E855.0	E936.3	E950.4	E962.0	E980.4
Antidepressants	969.00	E854.0	E939.0	E950.3	E962.0	E980.3
monoamine oxidase inhibitors (MAOI)	969.01	E854.0	E939.0	E950.3	E962.0	E980.3
specified type NEC	969.09	E854.0	E939.0	E950.3	E962.0	E980.3
SSNRI (selective serotonin and norepinephrine reuptake inhibitors)	969.02	E854.0	E939.0	E950.3	E962.0	E980.3
SSRI (selective serotonin reuptake inhibitors)	969.03	E854.0	E939.0	E950.3	E962.0	E980.3
tetracyclic	969.04	E854.0	E939.0	E950.3	E962.0	E980.3
tricyclic	969.05	E854.0	E939.0	E950.3	E962.0	E980.3
Antidiabetic agents	962.3	E858.0	E932.3	E950.4	E962.0	E980.4
Antidiarrheal agents	973.5	E858.4	E943.5	E950.4	E962.0	E980.4
Antidiuretic hormone	962.5	E858.0	E932.5	E950.4	E962.0	E980.4
Antidotes NEC	977.2	E858.8	E947.2	E950.4	E962.0	E980.4
Antiemetic agents	963.0	E858.1	E933.0	E950.4	E962.0	E980.4
Antiepilepsy agent NEC	966.3	E855.0	E936.3	E950.4	E962.0	E980.4
Antifertility pills	962.2	E858.0	E932.2	E950.4	E962.0	E980.4
Antiflatulents	973.8	E858.4	E943.8	E950.4	E962.0	E980.4
Antifreeze	989.89	E866.8	—	E950.9	E962.1	E980.9
alcohol	980.1	E860.2	—	E950.9	E962.1	E980.9
ethylene glycol	982.8	E862.4	—	E950.9	E962.1	E980.9
Antifungals (nonmedicinal) (sprays)	989.4	E863.6	—	E950.6	E962.1	E980.7
medicinal NEC	961.9	E857	E931.9	E950.4	E962.0	E980.4
antibiotic	960.1	E856	E930.1	E950.4	E962.0	E980.4
topical	976.0	E858.7	E946.0	E950.4	E962.0	E980.4
Antigastric secretion agents	973.0	E858.4	E943.0	E950.4	E962.0	E980.4
Antihelmintics	961.6	E857	E931.6	E950.4	E962.0	E980.4
Antihemophilic factor (human)	964.7	E858.2	E934.7	E950.4	E962.0	E980.4
Antihistamine	963.0	E858.1	E933.0	E950.4	E962.0	E980.4
Antihypertensive agents NEC	972.6	E858.3	E942.6	E950.4	E962.0	E980.4
Anti–infectives NEC	961.9	E857	E931.9	E950.4	E962.0	E980.4
antibiotics	960.9	E856	E930.9	E950.4	E962.0	E980.4
specified NEC	960.8	E856	E930.8	E950.4	E962.0	E980.4
antihelmintic	961.6	E857	E931.6	E950.4	E962.0	E980.4
antimalarial	961.4	E857	E931.4	E950.4	E962.0	E980.4
antimycobacterial NEC	961.8	E857	E931.8	E950.4	E962.0	E980.4
antibiotics	960.6	E856	E930.6	E950.4	E962.0	E980.4
antiprotozoal NEC	961.5	E857	E931.5	E950.4	E962.0	E980.4
blood	961.4	E857	E931.4	E950.4	E962.0	E980.4
antiviral	961.7	E857	E931.7	E950.4	E962.0	E980.4
arsenical	961.1	E857	E931.1	E950.4	E962.0	E980.4

Substance	Poisoning	Accident	Therapeutic Use	Suicide Attempt	Assault	Undetermined
			External Cause (E-Code)			
ENT agents	976.6	E858.7	E946.6	E950.4	E962.0	E980.4
heavy metals NEC	961.2	E857	E931.2	E950.4	E962.0	E980.4
local	976.0	E858.7	E946.0	E950.4	E962.0	E980.4
ophthalmic preparation	976.5	E858.7	E946.5	E950.4	E962.0	E980.4
topical NEC	976.0	E858.7	E946.0	E950.4	E962.0	E980.4
Anti–inflammatory agents (topical)	976.0	E858.7	E946.0	E950.4	E962.0	E980.4
Antiknock (tetraethyl lead)	984.1	E862.1	—	E950.9	E962.1	E980.9
Antilipemics	972.2	E858.3	E942.2	E950.4	E962.0	E980.4
Antimalarials	961.4	E857	E931.4	E950.4	E962.0	E980.4
Antimony (compounds) (vapor) NEC	985.4	E866.2	—	E950.9	E962.1	E980.9
anti–infectives	961.2	E857	E931.2	E950.4	E962.0	E980.4
pesticides (vapor)	985.4	E863.4	—	E950.6	E962.2	E980.7
potassium tartrate	961.2	E857	E931.2	E950.4	E962.0	E980.4
tartrated	961.2	E857	E931.2	E950.4	E962.0	E980.4
Antimuscarinic agents	971.1	E855.4	E941.1	E950.4	E962.0	E980.4
Antimycobacterials NEC	961.8	E857	E931.8	E950.4	E962.0	E980.4
antibiotics	960.6	E856	E930.6	E950.4	E962.0	E980.4
Antineoplastic agents	963.1	E858.1	E933.1	E950.4	E962.0	E980.4
antibiotics	960.7	E856	E930.7	E950.4	E962.0	E980.4
Anti–Parkinsonism agents	966.4	E855.0	E936.4	E950.4	E962.0	E980.4
Antiphlogistics	965.69	E850.6	E935.6	E950.0	E962.0	E980.0
Antiprotozoals NEC	961.5	E857	E931.5	E950.4	E962.0	E980.4
blood	961.4	E857	E931.4	E950.4	E962.0	E980.4
Antipruritics (local)	976.1	E858.7	E946.1	E950.4	E962.0	E980.4
Antipsychotic agents NEC	969.3	E853.8	E939.3	E950.3	E962.0	E980.3
Antipyretics	965.9	E850.9	E935.9	E950.0	E962.0	E980.0
specified NEC	965.8	E850.8	E935.8	E950.0	E962.0	E980.0
Antipyrine	965.5	E850.5	E935.5	E950.0	E962.0	E980.0
Antirabies serum (equine)	979.9	E858.8	E949.9	E950.4	E962.0	E980.4
Antirheumatics	965.69	E850.6	E935.6	E950.0	E962.0	E980.0
Antiseborrheics	976.4	E858.7	E946.4	E950.4	E962.0	E980.4
Antiseptics (external) (medicinal)	976.0	E858.7	E946.0	E950.4	E962.0	E980.4
Antistine	963.0	E858.1	E933.0	E950.4	E962.0	E980.4
Antithyroid agents	962.8	E858.0	E932.8	E950.4	E962.0	E980.4
Antitoxin, any	979.9	E858.8	E949.9	E950.4	E962.0	E980.4
Antituberculars	961.8	E857	E931.8	E950.4	E962.0	E980.4
antibiotics	960.6	E856	E930.6	E950.4	E962.0	E980.4
Antitussives	975.4	E858.6	E945.5	E950.4	E962.0	E980.4
Antivaricose agents (sclerosing)	972.7	E858.3	E942.7	E950.4	E962.0	E980.4
Antivenin (crotaline) (spider–bite)	979.9	E858.8	E949.9	E950.4	E962.0	E980.4
Antivert	963.0	E858.1	E933.0	E950.4	E962.0	E980.4
Antivirals NEC	961.7	E857	E931.7	E950.4	E962.0	E980.4
Ant poisons — *see* Pesticides						
Antrol	989.4	E863.4	—	E950.6	E962.1	E980.7
fungicide	989.4	E863.6	—	E950.6	E962.1	E980.7
Apomorphine hydrochloride (emetic)	973.6	E858.4	E943.6	E950.4	E962.0	E980.4
Appetite depressants, central	977.0	E858.8	E947.0	E950.4	E962.0	E980.4
Apresoline	972.6	E858.3	E942.6	E950.4	E962.0	E980.4
Aprobarbital, aprobarbitone	967.0	E851	E937.0	E950.1	E962.0	E980.1
Apronalide	967.8	E852.8	E937.8	E950.2	E962.0	E980.2
Aqua fortis	983.1	E864.1	—	E950.7	E962.1	E980.6
Arachis oil (topical)	976.3	E858.7	E946.3	E950.4	E962.0	E980.4
cathartic	973.2	E858.4	E943.2	E950.4	E962.0	E980.4
Aralen	961.4	E857	E931.4	E950.4	E962.0	E980.4
Arginine salts	974.5	E858.5	E944.5	E950.4	E962.0	E980.4
Argyrol	976.0	E858.7	E946.0	E950.4	E962.0	E980.4
ENT agent	976.6	E858.7	E946.6	E950.4	E962.0	E980.4
ophthalmic preparation	976.5	E858.7	E946.5	E950.4	E962.0	E980.4
Aristocort	962.0	E858.0	E932.0	E950.4	E962.0	E980.4
ENT agent	976.6	E858.7	E946.6	E950.4	E962.0	E980.4

Substance	Poisoning	Accident	Therapeutic Use	Suicide Attempt	Assault	Undetermined
			External Cause (E-Code)			
ophthalmic preparation	976.5	E858.7	E946.5	E950.4	E962.0	E980.4
topical NEC	976.0	E858.7	E946.0	E950.4	E962.0	E980.4
Aromatics, corrosive	983.0	E864.0	—	E950.7	E962.1	E980.6
disinfectants	983.0	E861.4	—	E950.7	E962.1	E980.6
Arsenate of lead (insecticide)	985.1	E863.4	—	E950.8	E962.1	E980.8
herbicide	985.1	E863.5	—	E950.8	E962.1	E980.8
Arsenic, arsenicals (compounds) (dust) (fumes) (vapor) NEC	985.1	E866.3	—	E950.8	E962.1	E980.8
anti–infectives	961.1	E857	E931.1	E950.4	E962.0	E980.4
pesticide (dust) (fumes)	985.1	E863.4	—	E950.8	E962.1	E980.8
Arsine (gas)	985.1	E866.3	—	E950.8	E962.1	E980.8
Arsphenamine (silver)	961.1	E857	E931.1	E950.4	E962.0	E980.4
Arsthinol	961.1	E857	E931.1	E950.4	E962.0	E980.4
Artane	971.1	E855.4	E941.1	E950.4	E962.0	E980.4
Arthropod (venomous) NEC	989.5	E905.5	—	E950.9	E962.1	E980.9
Asbestos	989.81	E866.8	—	E950.9	E962.1	E980.9
Ascaridole	961.6	E857	E931.6	E950.4	E962.0	E980.4
Ascorbic acid	963.5	E858.1	E933.5	E950.4	E962.0	E980.4
Asiaticoside	976.0	E858.7	E946.0	E950.4	E962.0	E980.4
Aspidium (oleoresin)	961.6	E857	E931.6	E950.4	E962.0	E980.4
Aspirin	965.1	E850.3	E935.3	E950.0	E962.0	E980.0
Astringents (local)	976.2	E858.7	E946.2	E950.4	E962.0	E980.4
Atabrine	961.3	E857	E931.3	E950.4	E962.0	E980.4
Ataractics	969.5	E853.8	E939.5	E950.3	E962.0	E980.3
Atonia drug, intestinal	973.3	E858.4	E943.3	E950.4	E962.0	E980.4
Atophan	974.7	E858.5	E944.7	E950.4	E962.0	E980.4
Atropine	971.1	E855.4	E941.1	E950.4	E962.0	E980.4
Attapulgite	973.5	E858.4	E943.5	E950.4	E962.0	E980.4
Attenuvax	979.4	E858.8	E949.4	E950.4	E962.0	E980.4
Aureomycin	960.4	E856	E930.4	E950.4	E962.0	E980.4
ophthalmic preparation	976.5	E858.7	E946.5	E950.4	E962.0	E980.4
topical NEC	976.0	E858.7	E946.0	E950.4	E962.0	E980.4
Aurothioglucose	965.69	E850.6	E935.6	E950.0	E962.0	E980.0
Aurothioglycanide	965.69	E850.6	E935.6	E950.0	E962.0	E980.0
Aurothiomalate	965.69	E850.6	E935.6	E950.0	E962.0	E980.0
Automobile fuel	981	E862.1	—	E950.9	E962.1	E980.9
Autonomic nervous system agents NEC . . .	971.9	E855.9	E941.9	E950.4	E962.0	E980.4
Avlosulfon	961.8	E857	E931.8	E950.4	E962.0	E980.4
Avomine	967.8	E852.8	E937.8	E950.2	E962.0	E980.2
Azacyclonol	969.5	E853.8	E939.5	E950.3	E962.0	E980.3
Azapetine	971.3	E855.6	E941.3	E950.4	E962.0	E980.4
Azaribine	963.1	E858.1	E933.1	E950.4	E962.0	E980.4
Azaserine	960.7	E856	E930.7	E950.4	E962.0	E980.4
Azathioprine	963.1	E858.1	E933.1	E950.4	E962.0	E980.4
Azosulfamide	961.0	E857	E931.0	E950.4	E962.0	E980.4
Azulfidine	961.0	E857	E931.0	E950.4	E962.0	E980.4
Azuresin	977.8	E858.8	E947.8	E950.4	E962.0	E980.4
Bacimycin	976.0	E858.7	E946.0	E950.4	E962.0	E980.4
ophthalmic preparation	976.5	E858.7	E946.5	E950.4	E962.0	E980.4
Bacitracin	960.8	E856	E930.8	E950.4	E962.0	E980.4
ENT agent	976.6	E858.7	E946.6	E950.4	E962.0	E980.4
ophthalmic preparation	976.5	E858.7	E946.5	E950.4	E962.0	E980.4
topical NEC	976.0	E858.7	E946.0	E950.4	E962.0	E980.4
Baking soda	963.3	E858.1	E933.3	E950.4	E962.0	E980.4
BAL	963.8	E858.1	E933.8	E950.4	E962.0	E980.4
Bamethan (sulfate)	972.5	E858.3	E942.5	E950.4	E962.0	E980.4
Bamipine	963.0	E858.1	E933.0	E950.4	E962.0	E980.4
Baneberry	988.2	E865.4	—	E950.9	E962.1	E980.9
Banewort	988.2	E865.4	—	E950.9	E962.1	E980.9
Barbenyl	967.0	E851	E937.0	E950.1	E962.0	E980.1
Barbital, barbitone	967.0	E851	E937.0	E950.1	E962.0	E980.1

Substance	Poisoning	Accident	Therapeutic Use	Suicide Attempt	Assault	Undetermined
			External Cause (E-Code)			

Barbiturates, barbituric acid 967.0	E851	E937.0	E950.1	E962.0	E980.1
anesthetic (intravenous) 968.3	E855.1	E938.3	E950.4	E962.0	E980.4
Barium (carbonate) (chloride) (sulfate) 985.8	E866.4	—	E950.9	E962.1	E980.9
diagnostic agent 977.8	E858.8	E947.8	E950.4	E962.0	E980.4
pesticide. 985.8	E863.4	—	E950.6	E962.1	E980.7
rodenticide. 985.8	E863.7	—	E950.6	E962.1	E980.7
Barrier cream 976.3	E858.7	E946.3	E950.4	E962.0	E980.4
Battery acid or fluid 983.1	E864.1	—	E950.7	E962.1	E980.6
Bay rum 980.8	E860.8	—	E950.9	E962.1	E980.9
BCG vaccine 978.0	E858.8	E948.0	E950.4	E962.0	E980.4
Bearsfoot 988.2	E865.4	—	E950.9	E962.1	E980.9
Beclamide. 966.3	E855.0	E936.3	E950.4	E962.0	E980.4
Bee (sting) (venom). 989.5	E905.3	—	E950.9	E962.1	E980.9
Belladonna (alkaloids). 971.1	E855.4	E941.1	E950.4	E962.0	E980.4
Bemegride. 970.0	E854.3	E940.0	E950.4	E962.0	E980.4
Benactyzine 969.8	E855.8	E939.8	E950.3	E962.0	E980.3
Benadryl 963.0	E858.1	E933.0	E950.4	E962.0	E980.4
Bendrofluazide. 974.3	E858.5	E944.3	E950.4	E962.0	E980.4
Bendroflumethiazide 974.3	E858.5	E944.3	E950.4	E962.0	E980.4
Benemid 974.7	E858.5	E944.7	E950.4	E962.0	E980.4
Benethamine penicillin G 960.0	E856	E930.0	E950.4	E962.0	E980.4
Benisone 976.0	E858.7	E946.0	E950.4	E962.0	E980.4
Benoquin 976.8	E858.7	E946.8	E950.4	E962.0	E980.4
Benoxinate 968.5	E855.2	E938.5	E950.4	E962.0	E980.4
Bentonite 976.3	E858.7	E946.3	E950.4	E962.0	E980.4
Benzalkonium (chloride). 976.0	E858.7	E946.0	E950.4	E962.0	E980.4
ophthalmic preparation. 976.5	E858.7	E946.5	E950.4	E962.0	E980.4
Benzamidosalicylate (calcium) 961.8	E857	E931.8	E950.4	E962.0	E980.4
Benzathine penicillin 960.0	E856	E930.0	E950.4	E962.0	E980.4
Benzcarbimine 963.1	E858.1	E933.1	E950.4	E962.0	E980.4
Benzedrex. 971.2	E855.5	E941.2	E950.4	E962.0	E980.4
Benzedrine (amphetamine) 969.72	E854.2	E939.7	E950.3	E962.0	E980.3
Benzene (acetyl) (dimethyl) (methyl) (solvent) (vapor). 982.0	E862.4	—	E950.9	E962.1	E980.9
hexachloride (gamma) (insecticide) (vapor). 989.2	E863.0	—	E950.6	E962.1	E980.7
Benzethonium 976.0	E858.7	E946.0	E950.4	E962.0	E980.4
Benzhexol (chloride) 966.4	E855.0	E936.4	E950.4	E962.0	E980.4
Benzilonium 971.1	E855.4	E941.1	E950.4	E962.0	E980.4
Benzin(e) — *see* Ligroin					
Benziodarone 972.4	E858.3	E942.4	E950.4	E962.0	E980.4
Benzocaine 968.5	E855.2	E938.5	E950.4	E962.0	E980.4
Benzodiapin 969.4	E853.2	E939.4	E950.3	E962.0	E980.3
Benzodiazepines (tranquilizers) NEC. 969.4	E853.2	E939.4	E950.3	E962.0	E980.3
Benzoic acid (with salicylic acid) (anti–infective) 976.0	E858.7	E946.0	E950.4	E962.0	E980.4
Benzoin. 976.3	E858.7	E946.3	E950.4	E962.0	E980.4
Benzol (vapor) 982.0	E862.4	—	E950.9	E962.1	E980.9
Benzomorphan 965.09	E850.2	E935.2	E950.0	E962.0	E980.0
Benzonatate 975.4	E858.6	E945.4	E950.4	E962.0	E980.4
Benzothiadiazides. 974.3	E858.5	E944.3	E950.4	E962.0	E980.4
Benzoylpas 961.8	E857	E931.8	E950.4	E962.0	E980.4
Benzperidol 969.5	E853.8	E939.5	E950.3	E962.0	E980.3
Benzphetamine. 977.0	E858.8	E947.0	E950.4	E962.0	E980.4
Benzpyrinium 971.0	E855.3	E941.0	E950.4	E962.0	E980.4
Benzquinamide. 963.0	E858.1	E933.0	E950.4	E962.0	E980.4
Benzthiazide. 974.3	E858.5	E944.3	E950.4	E962.0	E980.4
Benztropine 971.1	E855.4	E941.1	E950.4	E962.0	E980.4
Benzyl acetate 982.8	E862.4	—	E950.9	E962.1	E980.9

TABLE OF DRUGS AND CHEMICALS

Substance	Poisoning	Accident	Therapeutic Use	Suicide Attempt	Assault	Undetermined
			External Cause (E-Code)			
benzoate (anti–infective)	976.0	E858.7	E946.0	E950.4	E962.0	E980.4
morphine	965.09	E850.2	E935.2	E950.0	E962.0	E980.0
penicillin	960.0	E856	E930.0	E950.4	E962.0	E980.4
Bephenium hydroxynapthoate	961.6	E857	E931.6	E950.4	E962.0	E980.4
Bergamot oil	989.89	E866.8	—	E950.9	E962.1	E980.9
Berries, poisonous	988.2	E865.3	—	E950.9	E962.1	E980.9
Beryllium (compounds) (fumes)	985.3	E866.4	—	E950.9	E962.1	E980.9
Beta–carotene	976.3	E858.7	E946.3	E950.4	E962.0	E980.4
Beta–Chlor	967.1	E852.0	E937.1	E950.2	E962.0	E980.2
Betamethasone	962.0	E858.0	E932.0	E950.4	E962.0	E980.4
topical	976.0	E858.7	E946.0	E950.4	E962.0	E980.4
Betazole	977.8	E858.8	E947.8	E950.4	E962.0	E980.4
Bethanechol	971.0	E855.3	E941.0	E950.4	E962.0	E980.4
Bethanidine	972.6	E858.3	E942.6	E950.4	E962.0	E980.4
Betula oil	976.3	E858.7	E946.3	E950.4	E962.0	E980.4
Bhang	969.6	E854.1	E939.6	E950.3	E962.0	E980.3
Bialamicol	961.5	E857	E931.5	E950.4	E962.0	E980.4
Bichloride of mercury — *see* Mercury, chloride						
Bichromates (calcium) (crystals) (potassium) (sodium)	983.9	E864.3	—	E950.7	E962.1	E980.6
fumes	987.8	E869.8	—	E952.8	E962.2	E982.8
Biguanide derivatives, oral	962.3	E858.0	E932.3	E950.4	E962.0	E980.4
Biligrafin	977.8	E858.8	E947.8	E950.4	E962.0	E980.4
Bilopaque	977.8	E858.8	E947.8	E950.4	E962.0	E980.4
Bioflavonoids	972.8	E858.3	E942.8	E950.4	E962.0	E980.4
Biological substance NEC	979.9	E858.8	E949.9	E950.4	E962.0	E980.4
Biperiden	966.4	E855.0	E936.4	E950.4	E962.0	E980.4
Bisacodyl	973.1	E858.4	E943.1	E950.4	E962.0	E980.4
Bishydroxycoumarin	964.2	E858.2	E934.2	E950.4	E962.0	E980.4
Bismarsen	961.1	E857	E931.1	E950.4	E962.0	E980.4
Bismuth (compounds) NEC	985.8	E866.4	—	E950.9	E962.1	E980.9
anti–infectives	961.2	E857	E931.2	E950.4	E962.0	E980.4
subcarbonate	973.5	E858.4	E943.5	E950.4	E962.0	E980.4
sulfarsphenamine	961.1	E857	E931.1	E950.4	E962.0	E980.4
Bisphosphonates						
intravenous	963.1	E858.1	E933.7	E950.4	E962.0	E980.4
oral	963.1	E858.1	E933.6	E950.4	E962.0	E980.4
Bithionol	961.6	E857	E931.6	E950.4	E962.0	E980.4
Bitter almond oil	989.0	E866.8	—	E950.9	E962.1	E980.9
Bittersweet	988.2	E865.4	—	E950.9	E962.1	E980.9
Black						
flag	989.4	E863.4	—	E950.6	E962.1	E980.7
henbane	988.2	E865.4	—	E950.9	E962.1	E980.9
leaf (40)	989.4	E863.4	—	E950.6	E962.1	E980.7
widow spider (bite)	989.5	E905.1	—	E950.9	E962.1	E980.9
antivenin	979.9	E858.8	E949.9	E950.4	E962.0	E980.4
Blast furnace gas (carbon monoxide from)	986	E868.8	—	E952.1	E962.2	E982.1
Bleach NEC	983.9	E864.3	—	E950.7	E962.1	E980.6
Bleaching solutions	983.9	E864.3	—	E950.7	E962.1	E980.6
Bleomycin (sulfate)	960.7	E856	E930.7	E950.4	E962.0	E980.4
Blockain	968.9	E855.2	E938.9	E950.4	E962.0	E980.4
infiltration (subcutaneous)	968.5	E855.2	E938.5	E950.4	E962.0	E980.4
nerve block (peripheral) (plexus)	968.6	E855.2	E938.6	E950.4	E962.0	E980.4
topical (surface)	968.5	E855.2	E938.5	E950.4	E962.0	E980.4
Blood (derivatives) (natural) (plasma) (whole)	964.7	E858.2	E934.7	E950.4	E962.0	E980.4
affecting agent	964.9	E858.2	E934.9	E950.4	E962.0	E980.4
specified NEC	964.8	E858.2	E934.8	E950.4	E962.0	E980.4
substitute (macromolecular)	964.8	E858.2	E934.8	E950.4	E962.0	E980.4
Blue velvet	965.09	E850.2	E935.2	E950.0	E962.0	E980.0

Substance	Poisoning	Accident	Therapeutic Use	Suicide Attempt	Assault	Undetermined
			External Cause (E-Code)			

Substance	Poisoning	Accident	Therapeutic Use	Suicide Attempt	Assault	Undetermined
Bone meal	989.89	E866.5	—	E950.9	E962.1	E980.9
Bonine	963.0	E858.1	E933.0	E950.4	E962.0	E980.4
Boracic acid	976.0	E858.7	E946.0	E950.4	E962.0	E980.4
ENT agent	976.6	E858.7	E946.6	E950.4	E962.0	E980.4
ophthalmic preparation	976.5	E858.7	E946.5	E950.4	E962.0	E980.4
Borate (cleanser) (sodium)	989.6	E861.3	—	E950.9	E962.1	E980.9
Borax (cleanser)	989.6	E861.3	—	E950.9	E962.1	E980.9
Boric acid	976.0	E858.7	E946.0	E950.4	E962.0	E980.4
ENT agent	976.6	E858.7	E946.6	E950.4	E962.0	E980.4
ophthalmic preparation	976.5	E858.7	E946.5	E950.4	E962.0	E980.4
Boron hydride NEC	989.89	E866.8	—	E950.9	E962.1	E980.9
fumes or gas	987.8	E869.8	—	E952.8	E962.2	E982.8
Botox	975.3	E858.6	E945.3	E950.4	E962.0	E980.4
Brake fluid vapor	987.8	E869.8	—	E952.8	E962.2	E982.8
Brass (compounds) (fumes)	985.8	E866.4	—	E950.9	E962.1	E980.9
Brasso	981	E861.3	—	E950.9	E962.1	E980.9
Bretylium (tosylate)	972.6	E858.3	E942.6	E950.4	E962.0	E980.4
Brevital (sodium)	968.3	E855.1	E938.3	E950.4	E962.0	E980.4
British antilewisite	963.8	E858.1	E933.8	E950.4	E962.0	E980.4
Bromal (hydrate)	967.3	E852.2	E937.3	E950.2	E962.0	E980.2
Bromelains	963.4	E858.1	E933.4	E950.4	E962.0	E980.4
Bromides NEC	967.3	E852.2	E937.3	E950.2	E962.0	E980.2
Bromine (vapor)	987.8	E869.8	—	E952.8	E962.2	E982.8
compounds (medicinal)	967.3	E852.2	E937.3	E950.2	E962.0	E980.2
Bromisovalum	967.3	E852.2	E937.3	E950.2	E962.0	E980.2
Bromobenzyl cyanide	987.5	E869.3	—	E952.8	E962.2	E982.8
Bromodiphenhydramine	963.0	E858.1	E933.0	E950.4	E962.0	E980.4
Bromoform	967.3	E852.2	E937.3	E950.2	E962.0	E980.2
Bromophenol blue reagent	977.8	E858.8	E947.8	E950.4	E962.0	E980.4
Bromosalicylhydroxamic acid	961.8	E857	E931.8	E950.4	E962.0	E980.4
Bromo–seltzer	965.4	E850.4	E935.4	E950.0	E962.0	E980.0
Brompheniramine	963.0	E858.1	E933.0	E950.4	E962.0	E980.4
Bromural	967.3	E852.2	E937.3	E950.2	E962.0	E980.2
Brown spider (bite) (venom)	989.5	E905.1	—	E950.9	E962.1	E980.9
Brucia	988.2	E865.3	—	E950.9	E962.1	E980.9
Brucine	989.1	E863.7	—	E950.6	E962.1	E980.7
Brunswick green — *see* Copper						
Bruten — *see* Ibuprofen						
Bryonia (alba) (dioica)	988.2	E865.4	—	E950.9	E962.1	E980.9
Buclizine	969.5	E853.8	E939.5	E950.3	E962.0	E980.3
Bufferin	965.1	E850.3	E935.3	E950.0	E962.0	E980.0
Bufotenine	969.6	E854.1	E939.6	E950.3	E962.0	E980.3
Buphenine	971.2	E855.5	E941.2	E950.4	E962.0	E980.4
Bupivacaine	968.9	E855.2	E938.9	E950.4	E962.0	E980.4
infiltration (subcutaneous)	968.5	E855.2	E938.5	E950.4	E962.0	E980.4
nerve block (peripheral) (plexus)	968.6	E855.2	E938.6	E950.4	E962.0	E980.4
Busulfan	963.1	E858.1	E933.1	E950.4	E962.0	E980.4
Butabarbital (sodium)	967.0	E851	E937.0	E950.1	E962.0	E980.1
Butabarbitone	967.0	E851	E937.0	E950.1	E962.0	E980.1
Butabarpal	967.0	E851	E937.0	E950.1	E962.0	E980.1
Butacaine	968.5	E855.2	E938.5	E950.4	E962.0	E980.4
Butallylonal	967.0	E851	E937.0	E950.1	E962.0	E980.1
Butane (distributed in mobile container)	987.0	E868.0	—	E951.1	E962.2	E981.1
distributed through pipes	987.0	E867	—	E951.0	E962.2	E981.0
incomplete combustion of — *see* Carbon monoxide, butane						
Butanol	980.3	E860.4	—	E950.9	E962.1	E980.9
Butanone	982.8	E862.4	—	E950.9	E962.1	E980.9
Butaperazine	969.1	E853.0	E939.1	E950.3	E962.0	E980.3
Butazolidin	965.5	E850.5	E935.5	E950.0	E962.0	E980.0

Substance	Poisoning	Accident	Therapeutic Use	Suicide Attempt	Assault	Undetermined
			External Cause (E-Code)			
Butethal	967.0	E851	E937.0	E950.1	E962.0	E980.1
Butethamate	971.1	E855.4	E941.1	E950.4	E962.0	E980.4
Buthalitone (sodium)	968.3	E855.1	E938.3	E950.4	E962.0	E980.4
Butisol (sodium)	967.0	E851	E937.0	E950.1	E962.0	E980.1
Butobarbital, butobarbitone.	967.0	E851	E937.0	E950.1	E962.0	E980.1
Butriptyline	969.05	E854.0	E939.0	E950.3	E962.0	E980.3
Buttercups.	988.2	E865.4	—	E950.9	E962.1	E980.9
Butter of antimony — *see* Antimony						
Butyl						
acetate (secondary)	982.8	E862.4	—	E950.9	E962.1	E980.9
alcohol	980.3	E860.4	—	E950.9	E962.1	E980.9
carbinol	980.8	E860.8	—	E950.9	E962.1	E980.9
carbitol	982.8	E862.4	—	E950.9	E962.1	E980.9
cellosolve	982.8	E862.4	—	E950.9	E962.1	E980.9
chloral (hydrate)	967.1	E852.0	E937.1	E950.2	E962.0	E980.2
formate	982.8	E862.4	—	E950.9	E962.1	E980.9
scopolammonium bromide	971.1	E855.4	E941.1	E950.4	E962.0	E980.4
Butyn	968.5	E855.2	E938.5	E950.4	E962.0	E980.4
Butyrophenone (–based tranquilizers) . . .	969.2	E853.1	E939.2	E950.3	E962.0	E980.3
Cacodyl, cacodylic acid — *see* Arsenic						
Cactinomycin	960.7	E856	E930.7	E950.4	E962.0	E980.4
Cade oil	976.4	E858.7	E946.4	E950.4	E962.0	E980.4
Cadmium (chloride) (compounds) (dust)						
(fumes) (oxide)	985.5	E866.4	—	E950.9	E962.1	E980.9
sulfide (medicinal) NEC	976.4	E858.7	E946.4	E950.4	E962.0	E980.4
Caffeine	969.71	E854.2	E939.7	E950.3	E962.0	E980.3
Calabar bean.	988.2	E865.4	—	E950.9	E962.1	E980.9
Caladium seguinium	988.2	E865.4	—	E950.9	E962.1	E980.9
Calamine (liniment) (lotion)	976.3	E858.7	E946.3	E950.4	E962.0	E980.4
Calciferol	963.5	E858.1	E933.5	E950.4	E962.0	E980.4
Calcium (salts) NEC	974.5	E858.5	E944.5	E950.4	E962.0	E980.4
acetylsalicylate	965.1	E850.3	E935.3	E950.0	E962.0	E980.0
benzamidosalicylate	961.8	E857	E931.8	E950.4	E962.0	E980.4
carbaspirin	965.1	E850.3	E935.3	E950.0	E962.0	E980.0
carbamide (citrated)	977.3	E858.8	E947.3	E950.4	E962.0	E980.4
carbonate (antacid)	973.0	E858.4	E943.0	E950.4	E962.0	E980.4
cyanide (citrated)	977.3	E858.8	E947.3	E950.4	E962.0	E980.4
dioctyl sulfosuccinate	973.2	E858.4	E943.2	E950.4	E962.0	E980.4
disodium edathamil	963.8	E858.1	E933.8	E950.4	E962.0	E980.4
disodium edetate	963.8	E858.1	E933.8	E950.4	E962.0	E980.4
EDTA.	963.8	E858.1	E933.8	E950.4	E962.0	E980.4
hydrate, hydroxide	983.2	E864.2	—	E950.7	E962.1	E980.6
mandelate	961.9	E857	E931.9	E950.4	E962.0	E980.4
oxide	983.2	E864.2	—	E950.7	E962.1	E980.6
Calomel — *see* Mercury, chloride						
Caloric agents NEC.	974.5	E858.5	E944.5	E950.4	E962.0	E980.4
Calusterone	963.1	E858.1	E933.1	E950.4	E962.0	E980.4
Camoquin	961.4	E857	E931.4	E950.4	E962.0	E980.4
Camphor (oil)	976.1	E858.7	E946.1	E950.4	E962.0	E980.4
Candeptin	976.0	E858.7	E946.0	E950.4	E962.0	E980.4
Candicidin	976.0	E858.7	E946.0	E950.4	E962.0	E980.4
Cannabinols	969.6	E854.1	E939.6	E950.3	E962.0	E980.3
Cannabis (derivatives) (indica) (sativa)	969.6	E854.1	E939.6	E950.3	E962.0	E980.3
Canned heat	980.1	E860.2	—	E950.9	E962.1	E980.9
Cantharides, cantharidin, cantharis.	976.8	E858.7	E946.8	E950.4	E962.0	E980.4
Capillary agents	972.8	E858.3	E942.8	E950.4	E962.0	E980.4
Capreomycin	960.6	E856	E930.6	E950.4	E962.0	E980.4
Captodiame, captodiamine	969.5	E853.8	E939.5	E950.3	E962.0	E980.3
Caramiphen (hydrochloride)	971.1	E855.4	E941.1	E950.4	E962.0	E980.4
Carbachol.	971.0	E855.3	E941.0	E950.4	E962.0	E980.4
Carbacrylamine resins	974.5	E858.5	E944.5	E950.4	E962.0	E980.4

Substance	Poisoning	Accident	Therapeutic Use	Suicide Attempt	Assault	Undetermined
			External Cause (E-Code)			
Carbamate (sedative)	967.8	E852.8	E937.8	E950.2	E962.0	E980.2
herbicide	989.3	E863.5	—	E950.6	E962.1	E980.7
insecticide	989.3	E863.2	—	E950.6	E962.1	E980.7
Carbamazepine	966.3	E855.0	E936.3	E950.4	E962.0	E980.4
Carbamic esters	967.8	E852.8	E937.8	E950.2	E962.0	E980.2
Carbamide	974.4	E858.5	E944.4	E950.4	E962.0	E980.4
topical	976.8	E858.7	E946.8	E950.4	E962.0	E980.4
Carbamylcholine chloride	971.0	E855.3	E941.0	E950.4	E962.0	E980.4
Carbarsone	961.1	E857	E931.1	E950.4	E962.0	E980.4
Carbaryl	989.3	E863.2	—	E950.6	E962.1	E980.7
Carbaspirin	965.1	E850.3	E935.3	E950.0	E962.0	E980.0
Carbazochrome	972.8	E858.3	E942.8	E950.4	E962.0	E980.4
Carbenicillin	960.0	E856	E930.0	E950.4	E962.0	E980.4
Carbenoxolone	973.8	E858.4	E943.8	E950.4	E962.0	E980.4
Carbetapentane	975.4	E858.6	E945.4	E950.4	E962.0	E980.4
Carbimazole	962.8	E858.0	E932.8	E950.4	E962.0	E980.4
Carbinol	980.1	E860.2	—	E950.9	E962.1	E980.9
Carbinoxamine	963.0	E858.1	E933.0	E950.4	E962.0	E980.4
Carbitol	982.8	E862.4	—	E950.9	E962.1	E980.9
Carbocaine	968.9	E855.2	E938.9	E950.4	E962.0	E980.4
infiltration (subcutaneous)	968.5	E855.2	E938.5	E950.4	E962.0	E980.4
nerve block (peripheral) (plexus)	968.6	E855.2	E938.6	E950.4	E962.0	E980.4
topical (surface)	968.5	E855.2	E938.5	E950.4	E962.0	E980.4
Carbol–fuchsin solution	976.0	E858.7	E946.0	E950.4	E962.0	E980.4
Carbolic acid (*see also* Phenol)	983.0	E864.0	—	E950.7	E962.1	E980.6
Carbomycin	960.8	E856	E930.8	E950.4	E962.0	E980.4
Carbon						
bisulfide (liquid) (vapor)	982.2	E862.4	—	E950.9	E962.1	E980.9
dioxide (gas)	987.8	E869.8	—	E952.8	E962.2	E982.8
disulfide (liquid) (vapor)	982.2	E862.4	—	E950.9	E962.1	E980.9
monoxide (from incomplete combustion of) (in) NEC	986	E868.9	—	E952.1	E962.2	E982.1
blast furnace gas	986	E868.8	—	E952.1	E962.2	E982.1
butane (distributed in mobile container)	986	E868.0	—	E951.1	E962.2	E981.1
distributed through pipes	986	E867	—	E951.0	E962.2	E981.0
charcoal fumes	986	E868.3	—	E952.1	E962.2	E982.1
coal						
gas (piped)	986	E867	—	E951.0	E962.2	E981.0
solid (in domestic stoves, fireplaces)	986	E868.3	—	E952.1	E962.2	E982.1
coke (in domestic stoves, fireplaces)	986	E868.3	—	E952.1	E962.2	E982.1
exhaust gas (motor) not in transit	986	E868.2	—	E952.0	E962.2	E982.0
combustion engine, any not in watercraft	986	E868.2	—	E952.0	E962.2	E982.0
farm tractor, not in transit	986	E868.2	—	E952.0	E962.2	E982.0
gas engine	986	E868.2	—	E952.0	E962.2	E982.0
motor pump	986	E868.2	—	E952.0	E962.2	E982.0
motor vehicle, not in transit	986	E868.2	—	E952.0	E962.2	E982.0
fuel (in domestic use)	986	E868.3	—	E952.1	E962.2	E982.1
gas (piped)	986	E867	—	E951.0	E962.2	E981.0
in mobile container	986	E868.0	—	E951.1	E962.2	E981.1
utility	986	E868.1	—	E951.8	E962.2	E981.1
in mobile container	986	E868.0	—	E951.1	E962.2	E981.1
piped (natural)	986	E867	—	E951.0	E962.2	E981.0
illuminating gas	986	E868.1	—	E951.8	E962.2	E981.8
industrial fuels or gases, any	986	E868.8	—	E952.1	E962.2	E982.1
kerosene (in domestic stoves, fireplaces)	986	E868.3	—	E952.1	E962.2	E982.1
kiln gas or vapor	986	E868.8	—	E952.1	E962.2	E982.1

Substance	Poisoning	Accident	Therapeutic Use	Suicide Attempt	Assault	Undetermined
			External Cause (E-Code)			
motor exhaust gas, not in transit	986	E868.2	—	E952.0	E962.2	E982.0
piped gas (manufactured) (natural)	986	E867	—	E951.0	E962.2	E981.0
producer gas	986	E868.8	—	E952.1	E962.2	E982.1
propane (distributed in mobile container)	986	E868.0	—	E951.1	E962.2	E981.1
distributed through pipes	986	E867	—	E951.0	E962.2	E981.0
specified source NEC	986	E868.8	—	E952.1	E962.2	E982.1
stove gas	986	E868.1	—	E951.8	E962.2	E981.8
piped	986	E867	—	E951.0	E962.2	E981.0
utility gas	986	E868.1	—	E951.8	E962.2	E981.8
piped	986	E867	—	E951.0	E962.2	E981.0
water gas	986	E868.1	—	E951.8	E962.2	E981.8
wood (in domestic stoves, fireplaces)	986	E868.3	—	E952.1	E962.2	E982.1
tetrachloride (vapor) NEC	987.8	E869.8	—	E952.8	E962.2	E982.8
liquid (cleansing agent) NEC	982.1	E861.3	—	E950.9	E962.1	E980.9
solvent	982.1	E862.4	—	E950.9	E962.1	E980.9
Carbonic acid (gas)	987.8	E869.8	—	E952.8	E962.2	E982.8
anhydrase inhibitors	974.2	E858.5	E944.2	E950.4	E962.0	E980.4
Carbowax	976.3	E858.7	E946.3	E950.4	E962.0	E980.4
Carbrital	967.0	E851	E937.0	E950.1	E962.0	E980.1
Carbromal (derivatives)	967.3	E852.2	E937.3	E950.2	E962.0	E980.2
Cardiac						
depressants	972.0	E858.3	E942.0	E950.4	E962.0	E980.4
rhythm regulators	972.0	E858.3	E942.0	E950.4	E962.0	E980.4
Cardiografin	977.8	E858.8	E947.8	E950.4	E962.0	E980.4
Cardio–green	977.8	E858.8	E947.8	E950.4	E962.0	E980.4
Cardiotonic glycosides	972.1	E858.3	E942.1	E950.4	E962.0	E980.4
Cardiovascular agents NEC	972.9	E858.3	E942.9	E950.4	E962.0	E980.4
Cardrase	974.2	E858.5	E944.2	E950.4	E962.0	E980.4
Carfusin	976.0	E858.7	E946.0	E950.4	E962.0	E980.4
Carisoprodol	968.0	E855.1	E938.0	E950.4	E962.0	E980.4
Carmustine	963.1	E858.1	E933.1	E950.4	E962.0	E980.4
Carotene	963.5	E858.1	E933.5	E950.4	E962.0	E980.4
Carphenazine (maleate)	969.1	E853.0	E939.1	E950.3	E962.0	E980.3
Carter's Little Pills	973.1	E858.4	E943.1	E950.4	E962.0	E980.4
Cascara (sagrada)	973.1	E858.4	E943.1	E950.4	E962.0	E980.4
Cassava	988.2	E865.4	—	E950.9	E962.1	E980.9
Castellani's paint	976.0	E858.7	E946.0	E950.4	E962.0	E980.4
Castor						
bean	988.2	E865.3	—	E950.9	E962.1	E980.9
oil	973.1	E858.4	E943.1	E950.4	E962.0	E980.4
Caterpillar (sting)	989.5	E905.5	—	E950.9	E962.1	E980.9
Catha (edulis)	970.89	E854.3	E940.8	E950.4	E962.0	E980.4
Cathartics NEC	973.3	E858.4	E943.3	E950.4	E962.0	E980.4
contact	973.1	E858.4	E943.1	E950.4	E962.0	E980.4
emollient	973.2	E858.4	E943.2	E950.4	E962.0	E980.4
intestinal irritants	973.1	E858.4	E943.1	E950.4	E962.0	E980.4
saline	973.3	E858.4	E943.3	E950.4	E962.0	E980.4
Cathomycin	960.8	E856	E930.8	E950.4	E962.0	E980.4
Caustic(s)	983.9	E864.4	—	E950.7	E962.1	E980.6
alkali	983.2	E864.2	—	E950.7	E962.1	E980.6
hydroxide	983.2	E864.2	—	E950.7	E962.1	E980.6
potash	983.2	E864.2	—	E950.7	E962.1	E980.6
soda	983.2	E864.2	—	E950.7	E962.1	E980.6
specified NEC	983.9	E864.3	—	E950.7	E962.1	E980.6
Ceepryn	976.0	E858.7	E946.0	E950.4	E962.0	E980.4
ENT agent	976.6	E858.7	E946.6	E950.4	E962.0	E980.4
lozenges	976.6	E858.7	E946.6	E950.4	E962.0	E980.4
Celestone	962.0	E858.0	E932.0	E950.4	E962.0	E980.4
topical	976.0	E858.7	E946.0	E950.4	E962.0	E980.4
Cellosolve	982.8	E862.4	—	E950.9	E962.1	E980.9

Substance	Poisoning	Accident	Therapeutic Use	Suicide Attempt	Assault	Undetermined
			External Cause (E-Code)			
Cell stimulants and proliferants	976.8	E858.7	E946.8	E950.4	E962.0	E980.4
Cellulose derivatives, cathartic	973.3	E858.4	E943.3	E950.4	E962.0	E980.4
nitrates (topical)	976.3	E858.7	E946.3	E950.4	E962.0	E980.4
Centipede (bite)	989.5	E905.4	—	E950.9	E962.1	E980.9
Central nervous system						
depressants	968.4	E855.1	E938.4	E950.4	E962.0	E980.4
anesthetic (general) NEC	968.4	E855.1	E938.4	E950.4	E962.0	E980.4
gases NEC	968.2	E855.1	E938.2	E950.4	E962.0	E980.4
intravenous	968.3	E855.1	E938.3	E950.4	E962.0	E980.4
barbiturates	967.0	E851	E937.0	E950.1	E962.0	E980.1
bromides	967.3	E852.2	E937.3	E950.2	E962.0	E980.2
cannabis sativa	969.6	E854.1	E939.6	E950.3	E962.0	E980.3
chloral hydrate	967.1	E852.0	E937.1	E950.2	E962.0	E980.2
hallucinogenics	969.6	E854.1	E939.6	E950.3	E962.0	E980.3
hypnotics	967.9	E852.9	E937.9	E950.2	E962.0	E980.2
specified NEC	967.8	E852.8	E937.8	E950.2	E962.0	E980.2
muscle relaxants	968.0	E855.1	E938.0	E950.4	E962.0	E980.4
paraldehyde	967.2	E852.1	E937.2	E950.2	E962.0	E980.2
sedatives	967.9	E852.9	E937.9	E950.2	E962.0	E980.2
mixed NEC	967.6	E852.5	E937.6	E950.2	E962.0	E980.2
specified NEC	967.8	E852.8	E937.8	E950.2	E962.0	E980.2
muscle–tone depressants	968.0	E855.1	E938.0	E950.4	E962.0	E980.4
stimulants	970.9	E854.3	E940.9	E950.4	E962.0	E980.4
amphetamines	969.72	E854.2	E939.7	E950.3	E962.0	E980.3
analeptics	970.0	E854.3	E940.0	E950.4	E962.0	E980.4
antidepressants	969.00	E854.0	E939.0	E950.3	E962.0	E980.3
opiate antagonists	970.1	E854.3	E940.0	E950.4	E962.0	E980.4
specified NEC	970.89	E854.3	E940.8	E950.4	E962.0	E980.4
Cephalexin	960.5	E856	E930.5	E950.4	E962.0	E980.4
Cephaloglycin	960.5	E856	E930.5	E950.4	E962.0	E980.4
Cephaloridine	960.5	E856	E930.5	E950.4	E962.0	E980.4
Cephalosporins NEC	960.5	E856	E930.5	E950.4	E962.0	E980.4
N (adicillin)	960.0	E856	E930.0	E950.4	E962.0	E980.4
Cephalothin (sodium)	960.5	E856	E930.5	E950.4	E962.0	E980.4
Cerbera (odallam)	988.2	E865.4	—	E950.9	E962.1	E980.9
Cerberin	972.1	E858.3	E942.1	E950.4	E962.0	E980.4
Cerebral stimulants	970.9	E854.3	E940.9	E950.4	E962.0	E980.4
psychotherapeutic	969.79	E854.2	E939.7	E950.3	E962.0	E980.3
specified NEC	970.89	E854.3	E940.8	E950.4	E962.0	E980.4
Cetalkonium (chloride)	976.0	E858.7	E946.0	E950.4	E962.0	E980.4
Cetoxime	963.0	E858.1	E933.0	E950.4	E962.0	E980.4
Cetrimide	976.2	E858.7	E946.2	E950.4	E962.0	E980.4
Cetylpyridinium	976.0	E858.7	E946.0	E950.4	E962.0	E980.4
ENT agent	976.6	E858.7	E946.6	E950.4	E962.0	E980.4
lozenges	976.6	E858.7	E946.6	E950.4	E962.0	E980.4
Cevadilla — see Sabadilla						
Cevitamic acid	963.5	E858.1	E933.5	E950.4	E962.0	E980.4
Chalk, precipitated	973.0	E858.4	E943.0	E950.4	E962.0	E980.4
Charcoal						
fumes (carbon monoxide)	986	E868.3	—	E952.1	E962.2	E982.1
industrial	986	E868.8	—	E952.1	E962.2	E982.1
medicinal (activated)	973.0	E858.4	E943.0	E950.4	E962.0	E980.4
Chelating agents NEC	977.2	E858.8	E947.2	E950.4	E962.0	E980.4
Chelidonium majus	988.2	E865.4	—	E950.9	E962.1	E980.9
Chemical substance	989.9	E866.9	—	E950.9	E962.1	E980.9
specified NEC	989.89	E866.8	—	E950.9	E962.1	E980.9
Chemotherapy, antineoplastic	963.1	E858.1	E933.1	E950.4	E962.0	E980.4
Chenopodium (oil)	961.6	E857	E931.6	E950.4	E962.0	E980.4
Cherry laurel	988.2	E865.4	—	E950.9	E962.1	E980.9
Chiniofon	961.3	E857	E931.3	E950.4	E962.0	E980.4

Substance	Poisoning	Accident	Therapeutic Use	Suicide Attempt	Assault	Undetermined
			External Cause (E-Code)			
Chlophedianol 975.4	E858.6	E945.4	E950.4	E962.0	E980.4
Chloral (betaine) (formamide) (hydrate) . . . 967.1	E852.0	E937.1	E950.2	E962.0	E980.2
Chloralamide 967.1	E852.0	E937.1	E950.2	E962.0	E980.2
Chlorambucil 963.1	E858.1	E933.1	E950.4	E962.0	E980.4
Chloramphenicol 960.2	E856	E930.2	E950.4	E962.0	E980.4
ENT agent. 976.6	E858.7	E946.6	E950.4	E962.0	E980.4
ophthalmic preparation 976.5	E858.7	E946.5	E950.4	E962.0	E980.4
topical NEC 976.0	E858.7	E946.0	E950.4	E962.0	E980.4
Chlorate(s) (potassium) (sodium) NEC 983.9	E864.3	—	E950.7	E962.1	E980.6
herbicides 989.4	E863.5	—	E950.6	E962.1	E980.7
Chlorcyclizine 963.0	E858.1	E933.0	E950.4	E962.0	E980.4
Chlordan(e) (dust) 989.2	E863.0	—	E950.6	E962.1	E980.7
Chlordantoin. 976.0	E858.7	E946.0	E950.4	E962.0	E980.4
Chlordiazepoxide. 969.4	E853.2	E939.4	E950.3	E962.0	E980.3
Chloresium 976.8	E858.7	E946.8	E950.4	E962.0	E980.4
Chlorethiazol 967.1	E852.0	E937.1	E950.2	E962.0	E980.2
Chlorethyl — *see* Ethyl, chloride					
Chloretone 967.1	E852.0	E937.1	E950.2	E962.0	E980.2
Chlorex 982.3	E862.4	—	E950.9	E962.1	E980.9
Chlorhexadol 967.1	E852.0	E937.1	E950.2	E962.0	E980.2
Chlorhexidine (hydrochloride). 976.0	E858.7	E946.0	E950.4	E962.0	E980.4
Chlorhydroxyquinolin 976.0	E858.7	E946.0	E950.4	E962.0	E980.4
Chloride of lime (bleach) 983.9	E864.3	—	E950.7	E962.1	E980.6
Chlorinated					
camphene 989.2	E863.0	—	E950.6	E962.1	E980.7
diphenyl. 989.89	E866.8	—	E950.9	E962.1	E980.9
hydrocarbons NEC 989.2	E863.0	—	E950.6	E962.1	E980.7
solvent. 982.3	E862.4	—	E950.9	E962.1	E980.9
lime (bleach). 983.9	E864.3	—	E950.7	E962.1	E980.6
naphthalene — *see* Naphthalene					
pesticides NEC 989.2	E863.0	—	E950.6	E962.1	E980.7
soda — *see* Sodium, hypochlorite					
Chlorine (fumes) (gas). 987.6	E869.8	—	E952.8	E962.2	E982.8
bleach. 983.9	E864.3	—	E950.7	E962.1	E980.6
compounds NEC 983.9	E864.3	—	E950.7	E962.1	E980.6
disinfectant 983.9	E861.4	—	E950.7	E962.1	E980.6
releasing agents NEC 983.9	E864.3	—	E950.7	E962.1	E980.6
Chlorisondamine 972.3	E858.3	E942.3	E950.4	E962.0	E980.4
Chlormadinone. 962.2	E858.0	E932.2	E950.4	E962.0	E980.4
Chlormerodrin 974.0	E858.5	E944.0	E950.4	E962.0	E980.4
Chlormethiazole 967.1	E852.0	E937.1	E950.2	E962.0	E980.2
Chlormethylenecycline. 960.4	E856	E930.4	E950.4	E962.0	E980.4
Chlormezanone. 969.5	E853.8	E939.5	E950.3	E962.0	E980.3
Chloroacetophenone. 987.5	E869.3	—	E952.8	E962.2	E982.8
Chloroaniline 983.0	E864.0	—	E950.7	E962.1	E980.6
Chlorobenzene, chlorobenzol 982.0	E862.4	—	E950.9	E962.1	E980.9
Chlorobutanol 967.1	E852.0	E937.1	E950.2	E962.0	E980.2
Chlorodinitrobenzene 983.0	E864.0	—	E950.7	E962.1	E980.6
dust or vapor. 987.8	E869.8	—	E952.8	E962.2	E982.8
Chloroethane — *see* Ethyl, chloride					
Chloroform (fumes) (vapor) 987.8	E869.8	—	E952.8	E962.2	E982.8
anesthetic (gas) 968.2	E855.1	E938.2	E950.4	E962.0	E980.4
liquid NEC 968.4	E855.1	E938.4	E950.4	E962.0	E980.4
solvent 982.3	E862.4	—	E950.9	E962.1	E980.9
Chloroguanide 961.4	E857	E931.4	E950.4	E962.0	E980.4
Chloromycetin 960.2	E856	E930.2	E950.4	E962.0	E980.4
ENT agent. 976.6	E858.7	E946.6	E950.4	E962.0	E980.4
ophthalmic preparation 976.5	E858.7	E946.5	E950.4	E962.0	E980.4
otic solution 976.6	E858.7	E946.6	E950.4	E962.0	E980.4
topical NEC 976.0	E858.7	E946.0	E950.4	E962.0	E980.4
Chloronitrobenzene 983.0	E864.0	—	E950.7	E962.1	E980.6

Substance	Poisoning	Accident	Therapeutic Use	Suicide Attempt	Assault	Undetermined
			External Cause (E-Code)			
dust or vapor.	987.8	E869.8	—	E952.8	E962.2	E982.8
Chlorophenol	983.0	E864.0	—	E950.7	E962.1	E980.6
Chlorophenothane	989.2	E863.0	—	E950.6	E962.1	E980.7
Chlorophyll (derivatives).	976.8	E858.7	E946.8	E950.4	E962.0	E980.4
Chloropicrin (fumes)	987.8	E869.8	—	E952.8	E962.2	E982.8
fumigant.	989.4	E863.8	—	E950.6	E962.1	E980.7
fungicide	989.4	E863.6	—	E950.6	E962.1	E980.7
pesticide (fumes)	989.4	E863.4	—	E950.6	E962.1	E980.7
Chloroprocaine	968.9	E855.2	E938.9	E950.4	E962.0	E980.4
infiltration (subcutaneous)	968.5	E855.2	E938.5	E950.4	E962.0	E980.4
nerve block (peripheral) (plexus). . . .	968.6	E855.2	E938.6	E950.4	E962.0	E980.4
Chloroptic.	976.5	E858.7	E946.5	E950.4	E962.0	E980.4
Chloropurine.	963.1	E858.1	E933.1	E950.4	E962.0	E980.4
Chloroquine (hydrochloride) (phosphate) . . .	961.4	E857	E931.4	E950.4	E962.0	E980.4
Chlorothen	963.0	E858.1	E933.0	E950.4	E962.0	E980.4
Chlorothiazide	974.3	E858.5	E944.3	E950.4	E962.0	E980.4
Chlorotrianisene	962.2	E858.0	E932.2	E950.4	E962.0	E980.4
Chlorovinyldichloroarsine	985.1	E866.3	—	E950.8	E962.1	E980.8
Chloroxylenol	976.0	E858.7	E946.0	E950.4	E962.0	E980.4
Chlorphenesin (carbamate)	968.0	E855.1	E938.0	E950.4	E962.0	E980.4
topical (antifungal)	976.0	E858.7	E946.0	E950.4	E962.0	E980.4
Chlorpheniramine	963.0	E858.1	E933.0	E950.4	E962.0	E980.4
Chlorphenoxamine.	966.4	E855.0	E936.4	E950.4	E962.0	E980.4
Chlorphentermine	977.0	E858.8	E947.0	E950.4	E962.0	E980.4
Chlorproguanil	961.4	E857	E931.4	E950.4	E962.0	E980.4
Chlorpromazine	969.1	E853.0	E939.1	E950.3	E962.0	E980.3
Chlorpropamide	962.3	E858.0	E932.3	E950.4	E962.0	E980.4
Chlorprothixene	969.3	E853.8	E939.3	E950.3	E962.0	E980.3
Chlorquinaldol	976.0	E858.7	E946.0	E950.4	E962.0	E980.4
Chlortetracycline	960.4	E856	E930.4	E950.4	E962.0	E980.4
Chlorthalidone	974.4	E858.5	E944.4	E950.4	E962.0	E980.4
Chlortrianisene.	962.2	E858.0	E932.2	E950.4	E962.0	E980.4
Chlor–Trimeton	963.0	E858.1	E933.0	E950.4	E962.0	E980.4
Chlorzoxazone	968.0	E855.1	E938.0	E950.4	E962.0	E980.4
Choke damp	987.8	E869.8	—	E952.8	E962.2	E982.8
Cholebrine	977.8	E858.8	E947.8	E950.4	E962.0	E980.4
Cholera vaccine	978.2	E858.8	E948.2	E950.4	E962.0	E980.4
Cholesterol–lowering agents	972.2	E858.3	E942.2	E950.4	E962.0	E980.4
Cholestyramine (resin).	972.2	E858.3	E942.2	E950.4	E962.0	E980.4
Cholic acid	973.4	E858.4	E943.4	E950.4	E962.0	E980.4
Choline						
dihydrogen citrate	977.1	E858.8	E947.1	E950.4	E962.0	E980.4
salicylate	965.1	E850.3	E935.3	E950.0	E962.0	E980.0
theophyllinate	974.1	E858.5	E944.1	E950.4	E962.0	E980.4
Cholinergics	971.0	E855.3	E941.0	E950.4	E962.0	E980.4
Cholografin	977.8	E858.8	E947.8	E950.4	E962.0	E980.4
Chorionic gonadotropin	962.4	E858.0	E932.4	E950.4	E962.0	E980.4
Chromates.	983.9	E864.3	—	E950.7	E962.1	E980.6
dust or mist	987.8	E869.8	—	E952.8	E962.2	E982.8
lead	984.0	E866.0	—	E950.9	E962.1	E980.9
paint	984.0	E861.5	—	E950.9	E962.1	E980.9
Chromic acid	983.9	E864.3	—	E950.7	E962.1	E980.6
dust or mist	987.8	E869.8	—	E952.8	E962.2	E982.8
Chromium.	985.6	E866.4	—	E950.9	E962.1	E980.9
compounds — *see* Chromates						
Chromonar	972.4	E858.3	E942.4	E950.4	E962.0	E980.4
Chromyl chloride.	983.9	E864.3	—	E950.7	E962.1	E980.6
Chrysarobin (ointment)	976.4	E858.7	E946.4	E950.4	E962.0	E980.4
Chrysazin	973.1	E858.4	E943.1	E950.4	E962.0	E980.4
Chymar	963.4	E858.1	E933.4	E950.4	E962.0	E980.4

Substance	Poisoning	Accident	Therapeutic Use	Suicide Attempt	Assault	Undetermined
			External Cause (E-Code)			
ophthalmic preparation	976.5	E858.7	E946.5	E950.4	E962.0	E980.4
Chymotrypsin	963.4	E858.1	E933.4	E950.4	E962.0	E980.4
ophthalmic preparation	976.5	E858.7	E946.5	E950.4	E962.0	E980.4
Cicuta maculata or virosa	988.2	E865.4	—	E950.9	E962.1	E980.9
Cigarette lighter fluid	981	E862.1	—	E950.9	E962.1	E980.9
Cinchocaine (spinal)	968.7	E855.2	E938.7	E950.4	E962.0	E980.4
topical (surface)	968.5	E855.2	E938.5	E950.4	E962.0	E980.4
Cinchona	961.4	E857	E931.4	E950.4	E962.0	E980.4
Cinchonine alkaloids	961.4	E857	E931.4	E950.4	E962.0	E980.4
Cinchophen	974.7	E858.5	E944.7	E950.4	E962.0	E980.4
Cinnarizine	963.0	E858.1	E933.0	E950.4	E962.0	E980.4
Citanest	968.9	E855.2	E938.9	E950.4	E962.0	E980.4
infiltration (subcutaneous)	968.5	E855.2	E938.5	E950.4	E962.0	E980.4
nerve block (peripheral) (plexus)	968.6	E855.2	E938.6	E950.4	E962.0	E980.4
Citric acid	989.89	E866.8	—	E950.9	E962.1	E980.9
Citrovorum factor	964.1	E858.2	E934.1	E950.4	E962.0	E980.4
Claviceps purpurea	988.2	E865.4	—	E950.9	E962.1	E980.9
Cleaner, cleansing agent type not specified	989.89	E861.9	—	E950.9	E962.1	E980.9
of paint or varnish	982.8	E862.9	—	E950.9	E962.1	E980.9
specified type NEC	989.89	E861.3	—	E950.9	E962.1	E980.9
Clematis vitalba	988.2	E865.4	—	E950.9	E962.1	E980.9
Clemizole	963.0	E858.1	E933.0	E950.4	E962.0	E980.4
penicillin	960.0	E856	E930.0	E950.4	E962.0	E980.4
Clidinium	971.1	E855.4	E941.1	E950.4	E962.0	E980.4
Clindamycin	960.8	E856	E930.8	E950.4	E962.0	E980.4
Cliradon	965.09	E850.2	E935.2	E950.0	E962.0	E980.0
Clocortolone	962.0	E858.0	E932.0	E950.4	E962.0	E980.4
Clofedanol	975.4	E858.6	E945.4	E950.4	E962.0	E980.4
Clofibrate	972.2	E858.3	E942.2	E950.4	E962.0	E980.4
Clomethiazole	967.1	E852.0	E937.1	E950.2	E962.0	E980.2
Clomiphene	977.8	E858.8	E947.8	E950.4	E962.0	E980.4
Clonazepam	969.4	E853.2	E939.4	E950.3	E962.0	E980.3
Clonidine	972.6	E858.3	E942.6	E950.4	E962.0	E980.4
Clopamide	974.3	E858.5	E944.3	E950.4	E962.0	E980.4
Clorazepate	969.4	E853.2	E939.4	E950.3	E962.0	E980.3
Clorexolone	974.4	E858.5	E944.4	E950.4	E962.0	E980.4
Clorox (bleach)	983.9	E864.3	—	E950.7	E962.1	E980.6
Clortermine	977.0	E858.8	E947.0	E950.4	E962.0	E980.4
Clotrimazole	976.0	E858.7	E946.0	E950.4	E962.0	E980.4
Cloxacillin	960.0	E856	E930.0	E950.4	E962.0	E980.4
Coagulants NEC	964.5	E858.2	E934.5	E950.4	E962.0	E980.4
Coal (carbon monoxide from) — *see also* Carbon, monoxide, coal						
oil — *see* Kerosene						
tar NEC	983.0	E864.0	—	E950.7	E962.1	E980.6
fumes	987.8	E869.8	—	E952.8	E962.2	E982.8
medicinal (ointment)	976.4	E858.7	E946.4	E950.4	E962.0	E980.4
analgesics NEC	965.5	E850.5	E935.5	E950.0	E962.0	E980.0
naphtha (solvent)	981	E862.0	—	E950.9	E962.1	E980.9
Cobalt (fumes) (industrial)	985.8	E866.4	—	E950.9	E962.1	E980.9
Cobra (venom)	989.5	E905.0	—	E950.9	E962.1	E980.9
Coca (leaf)	970.81	E854.3	E940.8	E950.4	E962.0	E980.4
Cocaine (hydrochloride) (salt)	970.81	E854.3	E940.8	E950.4	E962.0	E980.4
topical anesthetic	968.5	E855.2	E938.5	E950.4	E962.0	E980.4
Coccidioidin	977.8	E858.8	E947.8	E950.4	E962.0	E980.4
Cocculus indicus	988.2	E865.3	—	E950.9	E962.1	E980.9
Cochineal	989.89	E866.8	—	E950.9	E962.1	E980.9
medicinal products	977.4	E858.8	E947.4	E950.4	E962.0	E980.4
Codeine	965.09	E850.2	E935.2	E950.0	E962.0	E980.0
Coffee	989.89	E866.8	—	E950.9	E962.1	E980.9
Cogentin	971.1	E855.4	E941.1	E950.4	E962.0	E980.4

Substance		Poisoning	Accident	Therapeutic Use	Suicide Attempt	Assault	Undetermined
					External Cause (E-Code)		
Coke fumes or gas (carbon monoxide)	986	E868.3	—		E952.1	E962.2	E982.1
industrial use	986	E868.8	—		E952.1	E962.2	E982.1
Colace	973.2	E858.4	E943.2	E950.4	E962.0	E980.4	
Colchicine	974.7	E858.5	E944.7	E950.4	E962.0	E980.4	
Colchicum	988.2	E865.3	—	E950.9	E962.1	E980.9	
Cold cream	976.3	E858.7	E946.3	E950.4	E962.0	E980.4	
Colestipol	972.2	E858.3	E942.2	E950.4	E962.0	E980.4	
Colistimethate	960.8	E856	E930.8	E950.4	E962.0	E980.4	
Colistin	960.8	E856	E930.8	E950.4	E962.0	E980.4	
Collagen	977.8	E866.8	E947.8	E950.9	E962.1	E980.9	
Collagenase	976.8	E858.7	E946.8	E950.4	E962.0	E980.4	
Collodion (flexible)	976.3	E858.7	E946.3	E950.4	E962.0	E980.4	
Colocynth	973.1	E858.4	E943.1	E950.4	E962.0	E980.4	
Coloring matter — *see* Dye(s)							
Combustion gas — *see* Carbon, monoxide							
Compazine	969.1	E853.0	E939.1	E950.3	E962.0	E980.3	
Compound							
42 (warfarin)	989.4	E863.7	—	E950.6	E962.1	E980.7	
269 (endrin)	989.2	E863.0	—	E950.6	E962.1	E980.7	
497 (dieldrin)	989.2	E863.0	—	E950.6	E962.1	E980.7	
1080 (sodium fluoroacetate)	989.4	E863.7	—	E950.6	E962.1	E980.7	
3422 (parathion)	989.3	E863.1	—	E950.6	E962.1	E980.7	
3911 (phorate)	989.3	E863.1	—	E950.6	E962.1	E980.7	
3956 (toxaphene)	989.2	E863.0	—	E950.6	E962.1	E980.7	
4049 (malathion)	989.3	E863.1	—	E950.6	E962.1	E980.7	
4124 (dicapthon)	989.4	E863.4	—	E950.6	E962.1	E980.7	
E (cortisone)	962.0	E858.0	E932.0	E950.4	E962.0	E980.4	
F (hydrocortisone)	962.0	E858.0	E932.0	E950.4	E962.0	E980.4	
Congo red	977.8	E858.8	E947.8	E950.4	E962.0	E980.4	
Coniine, conine	965.7	E850.7	E935.7	E950.0	E962.0	E980.0	
Conium (maculatum)	988.2	E865.4	—	E950.9	E962.1	E980.9	
Conjugated estrogens (equine)	962.2	E858.0	E932.2	E950.4	E962.0	E980.4	
Contac	975.6	E858.6	E945.6	E950.4	E962.0	E980.4	
Contact lens solution	976.5	E858.7	E946.5	E950.4	E962.0	E980.4	
Contraceptives (oral)	962.2	E858.0	E932.2	E950.4	E962.0	E980.4	
vaginal	976.8	E858.7	E946.8	E950.4	E962.0	E980.4	
Contrast media (roentgenographic)	977.8	E858.8	E947.8	E950.4	E962.0	E980.4	
Convallaria majalis	988.2	E865.4	—	E950.9	E962.1	E980.9	
Copper (dust) (fumes) (salts) NEC	985.8	E866.4	—	E950.9	E962.1	E980.9	
arsenate, arsenite	985.1	E866.3	—	E950.8	E962.1	E980.8	
insecticide	985.1	E863.4	—	E950.8	E962.1	E980.8	
emetic	973.6	E858.4	E943.6	E950.4	E962.0	E980.4	
fungicide	985.8	E863.6	—	E950.6	E962.1	E980.7	
insecticide	985.8	E863.4	—	E950.6	E962.1	E980.7	
oleate	976.0	E858.7	E946.0	E950.4	E962.0	E980.4	
sulfate	983.9	E864.3	—	E950.7	E962.1	E980.6	
fungicide	983.9	E863.6	—	E950.7	E962.1	E980.6	
cupric	973.6	E858.4	E943.6	E950.4	E962.0	E980.4	
cuprous	983.9	E864.3	—	E950.7	E962.1	E980.6	
Copperhead snake (bite) (venom)	989.5	E905.0	—	E950.9	E962.1	E980.9	
Coral (sting)	989.5	E905.6	—	E950.9	E962.1	E980.9	
snake (bite) (venom)	989.5	E905.0	—	E950.9	E962.1	E980.9	
Cordran	976.0	E858.7	E946.0	E950.4	E962.0	E980.4	
Corn cures	976.4	E858.7	E946.4	E950.4	E962.0	E980.4	
Cornhusker's lotion	976.3	E858.7	E946.3	E950.4	E962.0	E980.4	
Corn starch	976.3	E858.7	E946.3	E950.4	E962.0	E980.4	
Corrosive	983.9	E864.4	—	E950.7	E962.1	E980.6	
acids NEC	983.1	E864.1	—	E950.7	E962.1	E980.6	
aromatics	983.0	E864.0	—	E950.7	E962.1	E980.6	
disinfectant	983.0	E861.4	—	E950.7	E962.1	E980.6	

Substance	Poisoning	Accident	Therapeutic Use	Suicide Attempt	Assault	Undetermined
			External Cause (E-Code)			
fumes NEC	987.9	E869.9	—	E952.9	E962.2	E982.9
specified NEC	983.9	E864.3	—	E950.7	E962.1	E980.6
sublimate — *see* Mercury, chloride						
Cortate	962.0	E858.0	E932.0	E950.4	E962.0	E980.4
Cort–Dome	962.0	E858.0	E932.0	E950.4	E962.0	E980.4
ENT agent	976.6	E858.7	E946.6	E950.4	E962.0	E980.4
ophthalmic preparation	976.5	E858.7	E946.5	E950.4	E962.0	E980.4
topical NEC	976.0	E858.7	E946.0	E950.4	E962.0	E980.4
Cortef	962.0	E858.0	E932.0	E950.4	E962.0	E980.4
ENT agent	976.6	E858.7	E946.6	E950.4	E962.0	E980.4
ophthalmic preparation	976.5	E858.7	E946.5	E950.4	E962.0	E980.4
topical NEC	976.0	E858.7	E946.0	E950.4	E962.0	E980.4
Corticosteroids (fluorinated)	962.0	E858.0	E932.0	E950.4	E962.0	E980.4
ENT agent	976.6	E858.7	E946.6	E950.4	E962.0	E980.4
ophthalmic preparation	976.5	E858.7	E946.5	E950.4	E962.0	E980.4
topical NEC	976.0	E858.7	E946.0	E950.4	E962.0	E980.4
Corticotropin	962.4	E858.0	E932.4	E950.4	E962.0	E980.4
Cortisol	962.0	E858.0	E932.0	E950.4	E962.0	E980.4
ENT agent	976.6	E858.7	E946.6	E950.4	E962.0	E980.4
ophthalmic preparation	976.5	E858.7	E946.5	E950.4	E962.0	E980.4
topical NEC	976.0	E858.7	E946.0	E950.4	E962.0	E980.4
Cortisone derivatives (acetate)	962.0	E858.0	E932.0	E950.4	E962.0	E980.4
ENT agent	976.6	E858.7	E946.6	E950.4	E962.0	E980.4
ophthalmic preparation	976.5	E858.7	E946.5	E950.4	E962.0	E980.4
topical NEC	976.0	E858.7	E946.0	E950.4	E962.0	E980.4
Cortogen	962.0	E858.0	E932.0	E950.4	E962.0	E980.4
ENT agent	976.6	E858.7	E946.6	E950.4	E962.0	E980.4
ophthalmic preparation	976.5	E858.7	E946.5	E950.4	E962.0	E980.4
Cortone	962.0	E858.0	E932.0	E950.4	E962.0	E980.4
ENT agent	976.6	E858.7	E946.6	E950.4	E962.0	E980.4
ophthalmic preparation	976.5	E858.7	E946.5	E950.4	E962.0	E980.4
Cortril	962.0	E858.0	E932.0	E950.4	E962.0	E980.4
ENT agent	976.6	E858.7	E946.6	E950.4	E962.0	E980.4
ophthalmic preparation	976.5	E858.7	E946.5	E950.4	E962.0	E980.4
topical NEC	976.0	E858.7	E946.0	E950.4	E962.0	E980.4
Cosmetics	989.89	E866.7	—	E950.9	E962.1	E980.9
Cosyntropin	977.8	E858.8	E947.8	E950.4	E962.0	E980.4
Cotarnine	964.5	E858.2	E934.5	E950.4	E962.0	E980.4
Cottonseed oil	976.3	E858.7	E946.3	E950.4	E962.0	E980.4
Cough mixtures (antitussives)	975.4	E858.6	E945.4	E950.4	E962.0	E980.4
containing opiates	965.09	E850.2	E935.2	E950.0	E962.0	E980.0
expectorants	975.5	E858.6	E945.5	E950.4	E962.0	E980.4
Coumadin	964.2	E858.2	E934.2	E950.4	E962.0	E980.4
rodenticide	989.4	E863.7	—	E950.6	E962.1	E980.7
Coumarin	964.2	E858.2	E934.2	E950.4	E962.0	E980.4
Coumetarol	964.2	E858.2	E934.2	E950.4	E962.0	E980.4
Cowbane	988.2	E865.4	—	E950.9	E962.1	E980.9
Cozyme	963.5	E858.1	E933.5	E950.4	E962.0	E980.4
Crack	970.81	E854.3	E940.8	E950.4	E962.0	E980.4
Creolin	983.0	E864.0	—	E950.7	E962.1	E980.6
disinfectant	983.0	E861.4	—	E950.7	E962.1	E980.6
Creosol (compound)	983.0	E864.0	—	E950.7	E962.1	E980.6
Creosote (beechwood) (coal tar)	983.0	E864.0	—	E950.7	E962.1	E980.6
medicinal (expectorant)	975.5	E858.6	E945.5	E950.4	E962.0	E980.4
syrup	975.5	E858.6	E945.5	E950.4	E962.0	E980.4
Cresol	983.0	E864.0	—	E950.7	E962.1	E980.6
disinfectant	983.0	E861.4	—	E950.7	E962.1	E980.6
Cresylic acid	983.0	E864.0	—	E950.7	E962.1	E980.6
Cropropamide	965.7	E850.7	E935.7	E950.0	E962.0	E980.0
with crotethamide	970.0	E854.3	E940.0	E950.4	E962.0	E980.4
Crotamiton	976.0	E858.7	E946.0	E950.4	E962.0	E980.4

Substance	Poisoning	Accident	Therapeutic Use	Suicide Attempt	Assault	Undetermined
		External Cause (E-Code)				
Crotethamide 965.7	E850.7	E935.7	E950.0	E962.0	E980.0
with cropropamide 970.0	E854.3	E940.0	E950.4	E962.0	E980.4
Croton (oil) 973.1	E858.4	E943.1	E950.4	E962.0	E980.4
chloral 967.1	E852.0	E937.1	E950.2	E962.0	E980.2
Crude oil 981	E862.1	—	E950.9	E962.1	E980.9
Cryogenine 965.8	E850.8	E935.8	E950.0	E962.0	E980.0
Cryolite (pesticide) 989.4	E863.4	—	E950.6	E962.1	E980.7
Cryptenamine 972.6	E858.3	E942.6	E950.4	E962.0	E980.4
Crystal violet 976.0	E858.7	E946.0	E950.4	E962.0	E980.4
Cuckoopint 988.2	E865.4	—	E950.9	E962.1	E980.9
Cumetharol 964.2	E858.2	E934.2	E950.4	E962.0	E980.4
Cupric sulfate 973.6	E858.4	E943.6	E950.4	E962.0	E980.4
Cuprous sulfate 983.9	E864.3	—	E950.7	E962.1	E980.6
Curare, curarine 975.2	E858.6	E945.2	E950.4	E962.0	E980.4
Cyanic acid — see Cyanide(s)					
Cyanide(s) (compounds) (hydrogen)					
(potassium) (sodium) NEC 989.0	E866.8	—	E950.9	E962.1	E980.9
dust or gas (inhalation) NEC 987.7	E869.8	—	E952.8	E962.2	E982.8
fumigant. 989.0	E863.8	—	E950.6	E962.1	E980.7
mercuric — see Mercury					
pesticide (dust) (fumes) 989.0	E863.4	—	E950.6	E962.1	E980.7
Cyanocobalamin 964.1	E858.2	E934.1	E950.4	E962.0	E980.4
Cyanogen (chloride) (gas) NEC . . . 987.8	E869.8	—	E952.8	E962.2	E982.8
Cyclaine 968.5	E855.2	E938.5	E950.4	E962.0	E980.4
Cyclamen europaeum 988.2	E865.4	—	E950.9	E962.1	E980.9
Cyclandelate. 972.5	E858.3	E942.5	E950.4	E962.0	E980.4
Cyclazocine 965.09	E850.2	E935.2	E950.0	E962.0	E980.0
Cyclizine 963.0	E858.1	E933.0	E950.4	E962.0	E980.4
Cyclobarbital, cyclobarbitone 967.0	E851	E937.0	E950.1	E962.0	E980.1
Cycloguanil 961.4	E857	E931.4	E950.4	E962.0	E980.4
Cyclohexane. 982.0	E862.4	—	E950.9	E962.1	E980.9
Cyclohexanol 980.8	E860.8	—	E950.9	E962.1	E980.9
Cyclohexanone. 982.8	E862.4	—	E950.9	E962.1	E980.9
Cyclomethycaine 968.5	E855.2	E938.5	E950.4	E962.0	E980.4
Cyclopentamine 971.2	E855.5	E941.2	E950.4	E962.0	E980.4
Cyclopenthiazide 974.3	E858.5	E944.3	E950.4	E962.0	E980.4
Cyclopentolate 971.1	E855.4	E941.1	E950.4	E962.0	E980.4
Cyclophosphamide 963.1	E858.1	E933.1	E950.4	E962.0	E980.4
Cyclopropane 968.2	E855.1	E938.2	E950.4	E962.0	E980.4
Cycloserine 960.6	E856	E930.6	E950.4	E962.0	E980.4
Cyclothiazide 974.3	E858.5	E944.3	E950.4	E962.0	E980.4
Cycrimine. 966.4	E855.0	E936.4	E950.4	E962.0	E980.4
Cymarin 972.1	E858.3	E942.1	E950.4	E962.0	E980.4
Cyproheptadine 963.0	E858.1	E933.0	E950.4	E962.0	E980.4
Cyprolidol. 969.09	E854.0	E939.0	E950.3	E962.0	E980.3
Cytarabine 963.1	E858.1	E933.1	E950.4	E962.0	E980.4
Cytisus					
laburnum 988.2	E865.4	—	E950.9	E962.1	E980.9
scoparius 988.2	E865.4	—	E950.9	E962.1	E980.9
Cytomel 962.7	E858.0	E932.7	E950.4	E962.0	E980.4
Cytosine (antineoplastic) 963.1	E858.1	E933.1	E950.4	E962.0	E980.4
Cytoxan. 963.1	E858.1	E933.1	E950.4	E962.0	E980.4
Dacarbazine 963.1	E858.1	E933.1	E950.4	E962.0	E980.4
Dactinomycin 960.7	E856	E930.7	E950.4	E962.0	E980.4
DADPS 961.8	E857	E931.8	E950.4	E962.0	E980.4
Dakin's solution (external) 976.0	E858.7	E946.0	E950.4	E962.0	E980.4
Dalmane 969.4	E853.2	E939.4	E950.3	E962.0	E980.3
DAM. 977.2	E858.8	E947.2	E950.4	E962.0	E980.4
Danilone 964.2	E858.2	E934.2	E950.4	E962.0	E980.4
Danthron 973.1	E858.4	E943.1	E950.4	E962.0	E980.4

Substance	Poisoning	Accident	Therapeutic Use	Suicide Attempt	Assault	Undetermined
			External Cause (E-Code)			
Dantrolene	975.2	E858.6	E945.2	E950.4	E962.0	E980.4
Daphne (gnidium) (mezereum)	988.2	E865.4	—	E950.9	E962.1	E980.9
berry	988.2	E865.3	—	E950.9	E962.1	E980.9
Dapsone	961.8	E857	E931.8	E950.4	E962.0	E980.4
Daraprim	961.4	E857	E931.4	E950.4	E962.0	E980.4
Darnel	988.2	E865.3	—	E950.9	E962.1	E980.9
Darvon	965.8	E850.8	E935.8	E950.0	E962.0	E980.0
Daunorubicin	960.7	E856	E930.7	E950.4	E962.0	E980.4
DBI	962.3	E858.0	E932.3	E950.4	E962.0	E980.4
D–Con (rodenticide)	989.4	E863.7	—	E950.6	E962.1	E980.7
DDS	961.8	E857	E931.8	E950.4	E962.0	E980.4
DDT	989.2	E863.0	—	E950.6	E962.1	E980.7
Deadly nightshade	988.2	E865.4	—	E950.9	E962.1	E980.9
berry	988.2	E865.3	—	E950.9	E962.1	E980.9
Deanol	969.79	E854.2	E939.7	E950.3	E962.0	E980.3
Debrisoquine	972.6	E858.3	E942.6	E950.4	E962.0	E980.4
Decaborane	989.89	E866.8	—	E950.9	E962.1	E980.9
fumes	987.8	E869.8	—	E952.8	E962.2	E982.8
Decadron	962.0	E858.0	E932.0	E950.4	E962.0	E980.4
ENT agent	976.6	E858.7	E946.6	E950.4	E962.0	E980.4
ophthalmic preparation	976.5	E858.7	E946.5	E950.4	E962.0	E980.4
topical NEC	976.0	E858.7	E946.0	E950.4	E962.0	E980.4
Decahydronaphthalene	982.0	E862.4	—	E950.9	E962.1	E980.9
Decalin	982.0	E862.4	—	E950.9	E962.1	E980.9
Decamethonium	975.2	E858.6	E945.2	E950.4	E962.0	E980.4
Decholin	973.4	E858.4	E943.4	E950.4	E962.0	E980.4
sodium (diagnostic)	977.8	E858.8	E947.8	E950.4	E962.0	E980.4
Declomycin	960.4	E856	E930.4	E950.4	E962.0	E980.4
Deferoxamine	963.8	E858.1	E933.8	E950.4	E962.0	E980.4
Dehydrocholic acid	973.4	E858.4	E943.4	E950.4	E962.0	E980.4
Dekalin	982.0	E862.4	—	E950.9	E962.1	E980.9
Delalutin	962.2	E858.0	E932.2	E950.4	E962.0	E980.4
Delphinium	988.2	E865.3	—	E950.9	E962.1	E980.9
Deltasone	962.0	E858.0	E932.0	E950.4	E962.0	E980.4
Deltra	962.0	E858.0	E932.0	E950.4	E962.0	E980.4
Delvinal	967.0	E851	E937.0	E950.1	E962.0	E980.1
Demecarium (bromide)	971.0	E855.3	E941.0	E950.4	E962.0	E980.4
Demeclocycline	960.4	E856	E930.4	E950.4	E962.0	E980.4
Demecolcine	963.1	E858.1	E933.1	E950.4	E962.0	E980.4
Demelanizing agents	976.8	E858.7	E946.8	E950.4	E962.0	E980.4
Demerol	965.09	E850.2	E935.2	E950.0	E962.0	E980.0
Demethylchlortetracycline	960.4	E856	E930.4	E950.4	E962.0	E980.4
Demethyltetracycline	960.4	E856	E930.4	E950.4	E962.0	E980.4
Demeton	989.3	E863.1	—	E950.6	E962.1	E980.7
Demulcents	976.3	E858.7	E946.3	E950.4	E962.0	E980.4
Demulen	962.2	E858.0	E932.2	E950.4	E962.0	E980.4
Denatured alcohol	980.0	E860.1	—	E950.9	E962.1	E980.9
Dendrid	976.5	E858.7	E946.5	E950.4	E962.0	E980.4
Dental agents, topical	976.7	E858.7	E946.7	E950.4	E962.0	E980.4
Deodorant spray (feminine hygiene)	976.8	E858.7	E946.8	E950.4	E962.0	E980.4
Deoxyribonuclease	963.4	E858.1	E933.4	E950.4	E962.0	E980.4
Depressants						
appetite, central	977.0	E858.8	E947.0	E950.4	E962.0	E980.4
cardiac	972.0	E858.3	E942.0	E950.4	E962.0	E980.4
central nervous system (anesthetic)	968.4	E855.1	E938.4	E950.4	E962.0	E980.4
psychotherapeutic	969.5	E853.9	E939.5	E950.3	E962.0	E980.3
Dequalinium	976.0	E858.7	E946.0	E950.4	E962.0	E980.4
Dermolate	976.2	E858.7	E946.2	E950.4	E962.0	E980.4
DES	962.2	E858.0	E932.2	E950.4	E962.0	E980.4
Desenex	976.0	E858.7	E946.0	E950.4	E962.0	E980.4
Deserpidine	972.6	E858.3	E942.6	E950.4	E962.0	E980.4

Substance	Poisoning	Accident	Therapeutic Use	Suicide Attempt	Assault	Undetermined
			External Cause (E-Code)			
Desipramine	969.05	E854.0	E939.0	E950.3	E962.0	E980.3
Deslanoside	972.1	E858.3	E942.1	E950.4	E962.0	E980.4
Desocodeine	965.09	E850.2	E935.2	E950.0	E962.0	E980.0
Desomorphine	965.09	E850.2	E935.2	E950.0	E962.0	E980.0
Desonide	976.0	E858.7	E946.0	E950.4	E962.0	E980.4
Desoxycorticosterone derivatives	962.0	E858.0	E932.0	E950.4	E962.0	E980.4
Desoxyephedrine	969.72	E854.2	E939.7	E950.3	E962.0	E980.3
DET	969.6	E854.1	E939.6	E950.3	E962.0	E980.3
Detergents (ingested) (synthetic)	989.6	E861.0	—	E950.9	E962.1	E980.9
external medication	976.2	E858.7	E946.2	E950.4	E962.0	E980.4
Deterrent, alcohol	977.3	E858.8	E947.3	E950.4	E962.0	E980.4
Detrothyronine	962.7	E858.0	E932.7	E950.4	E962.0	E980.4
Dettol (external medication)	976.0	E858.7	E946.0	E950.4	E962.0	E980.4
Dexamethasone	962.0	E858.0	E932.0	E950.4	E962.0	E980.4
ENT agent	976.6	E858.7	E946.6	E950.4	E962.0	E980.4
ophthalmic preparation	976.5	E858.7	E946.5	E950.4	E962.0	E980.4
topical NEC	976.0	E858.7	E946.0	E950.4	E962.0	E980.4
Dexamphetamine	969.72	E854.2	E939.7	E950.3	E962.0	E980.3
Dexedrine	969.72	E854.2	E939.7	E950.3	E962.0	E980.3
Dexpanthenol	963.5	E858.1	E933.5	E950.4	E962.0	E980.4
Dextran	964.8	E858.2	E934.8	E950.4	E962.0	E980.4
Dextriferron	964.0	E858.2	E934.0	E950.4	E962.0	E980.4
Dextroamphetamine	969.72	E854.2	E939.7	E950.3	E962.0	E980.3
Dextro calcium pantothenate	963.5	E858.1	E933.5	E950.4	E962.0	E980.4
Dextromethorphan	975.4	E858.6	E945.4	E950.4	E962.0	E980.4
Dextromoramide	965.09	E850.2	E935.2	E950.0	E962.0	E980.0
Dextro pantothenyl alcohol	963.5	E858.1	E933.5	E950.4	E962.0	E980.4
topical	976.8	E858.7	E946.8	E950.4	E962.0	E980.4
Dextropropoxyphene (hydrochloride)	965.8	E850.8	E935.8	E950.0	E962.0	E980.0
Dextrorphan	965.09	E850.2	E935.2	E950.0	E962.0	E980.0
Dextrose NEC	974.5	E858.5	E944.5	E950.4	E962.0	E980.4
Dextrothyroxin	962.7	E858.0	E932.7	E950.4	E962.0	E980.4
DFP	971.0	E855.3	E941.0	E950.4	E962.0	E980.4
DHE–45	972.9	E858.3	E942.9	E950.4	E962.0	E980.4
Diabinese	962.3	E858.0	E932.3	E950.4	E962.0	E980.4
Diacetyl monoxime	977.2	E858.8	E947.2	E950.4	E962.0	E980.4
Diacetylmorphine	965.01	E850.0	E935.0	E950.0	E962.0	E980.0
Diagnostic agents	977.8	E858.8	E947.8	E950.4	E962.0	E980.4
Dial (soap)	976.2	E858.7	E946.2	E950.4	E962.0	E980.4
sedative	967.0	E851	E937.0	E950.1	E962.0	E980.1
Diallylbarbituric acid	967.0	E851	E937.0	E950.1	E962.0	E980.1
Diaminodiphenylsulfone	961.8	E857	E931.8	E950.4	E962.0	E980.4
Diamorphine	965.01	E850.0	E935.0	E950.0	E962.0	E980.0
Diamox	974.2	E858.5	E944.2	E950.4	E962.0	E980.4
Diamthazole	976.0	E858.7	E946.0	E950.4	E962.0	E980.4
Diaphenylsulfone	961.8	E857	E931.8	E950.4	E962.0	E980.4
Diasone (sodium)	961.8	E857	E931.8	E950.4	E962.0	E980.4
Diazepam	969.4	E853.2	E939.4	E950.3	E962.0	E980.3
Diazinon	989.3	E863.1	—	E950.6	E962.1	E980.7
Diazomethane (gas)	987.8	E869.8	—	E952.8	E962.2	E982.8
Diazoxide	972.5	E858.3	E942.5	E950.4	E962.0	E980.4
Dibenamine	971.3	E855.6	E941.3	E950.4	E962.0	E980.4
Dibenzheptropine	963.0	E858.1	E933.0	E950.4	E962.0	E980.4
Dibenzyline	971.3	E855.6	E941.3	E950.4	E962.0	E980.4
Diborane (gas)	987.8	E869.8	—	E952.8	E962.2	E982.8
Dibromomannitol	963.1	E858.1	E933.1	E950.4	E962.0	E980.4
Dibucaine (spinal)	968.7	E855.2	E938.7	E950.4	E962.0	E980.4
topical (surface)	968.5	E855.2	E938.5	E950.4	E962.0	E980.4
Dibunate sodium	975.4	E858.6	E945.4	E950.4	E962.0	E980.4
Dibutoline	971.1	E855.4	E941.1	E950.4	E962.0	E980.4

Substance	Poisoning	Accident	Therapeutic Use	Suicide Attempt	Assault	Undetermined
			External Cause (E-Code)			
Dicapthon 989.4	E863.4	—	E950.6	E962.1	E980.7
Dichloralphenazone 967.1	E852.0	E937.1	E950.2	E962.0	E980.2
Dichlorodifluoromethane 987.4	E869.2	—	E952.8	E962.2	E982.8
Dichloroethane 982.3	E862.4	—	E950.9	E962.1	E980.9
Dichloroethylene 982.3	E862.4	—	E950.9	E962.1	E980.9
Dichloroethyl sulfide 987.8	E869.8	—	E952.8	E962.2	E982.8
Dichlorohydrin 982.3	E862.4	—	E950.9	E962.1	E980.9
Dichloromethane (solvent) (vapor) 982.3	E862.4	—	E950.9	E962.1	E980.9
Dichlorophen(e) 961.6	E857	E931.6	E950.4	E962.0	E980.4
Dichlorphenamide 974.2	E858.5	E944.2	E950.4	E962.0	E980.4
Dichlorvos 989.3	E863.1	—	E950.6	E962.1	E980.7
Diclofenac sodium 965.69	E850.6	E935.6	E950.0	E962.0	E980.0
Dicoumarin, dicumarol 964.2	E858.2	E934.2	E950.4	E962.0	E980.4
Dicyanogen (gas) 987.8	E869.8	—	E952.8	E962.2	E982.8
Dicyclomine 971.1	E855.4	E941.1	E950.4	E962.0	E980.4
Dieldrin (vapor) 989.2	E863.0	—	E950.6	E962.1	E980.7
Dienestrol 962.2	E858.0	E932.2	E950.4	E962.0	E980.4
Dietetics 977.0	E858.8	E947.0	E950.4	E962.0	E980.4
Diethazine 966.4	E855.0	E936.4	E950.4	E962.0	E980.4
Diethyl					
barbituric acid 967.0	E851	E937.0	E950.1	E962.0	E980.1
carbamazine 961.6	E857	E931.6	E950.4	E962.0	E980.4
carbinol 980.8	E860.8	—	E950.9	E962.1	E980.9
carbonate 982.8	E862.4	—	E950.9	E962.1	E980.9
ether (vapor) — *see* Ether(s)					
propion 977.0	E858.8	E947.0	E950.4	E962.0	E980.4
stilbestrol 962.2	E858.0	E932.2	E950.4	E962.0	E980.4
Diethylene					
dioxide 982.8	E862.4	—	E950.9	E962.1	E980.9
glycol (monoacetate) (monoethyl ether) . . . 982.8	E862.4	—	E950.9	E962.1	E980.9
Diethylsulfone–diethylmethane 967.8	E852.8	E937.8	E950.2	E962.0	E980.2
Difencloxazine 965.09	E850.2	E935.2	E950.0	E962.0	E980.0
Diffusin 963.4	E858.1	E933.4	E950.4	E962.0	E980.4
Diflos 971.0	E855.3	E941.0	E950.4	E962.0	E980.4
Digestants 973.4	E858.4	E943.4	E950.4	E962.0	E980.4
Digitalin(e) 972.1	E858.3	E942.1	E950.4	E962.0	E980.4
Digitalis glycosides 972.1	E858.3	E942.1	E950.4	E962.0	E980.4
Digitoxin 972.1	E858.3	E942.1	E950.4	E962.0	E980.4
Digoxin 972.1	E858.3	E942.1	E950.4	E962.0	E980.4
Dihydrocodeine 965.09	E850.2	E935.2	E950.0	E962.0	E980.0
Dihydrocodeinone 965.09	E850.2	E935.2	E950.0	E962.0	E980.0
Dihydroergocristine 972.9	E858.3	E942.9	E950.4	E962.0	E980.4
Dihydroergotamine 972.9	E858.3	E942.9	E950.4	E962.0	E980.4
Dihydroergotoxine 972.9	E858.3	E942.9	E950.4	E962.0	E980.4
Dihydrohydroxycodeinone 965.09	E850.2	E935.2	E950.0	E962.0	E980.0
Dihydrohydroxymorphinone 965.09	E850.2	E935.2	E950.0	E962.0	E980.0
Dihydroisocodeine 965.09	E850.2	E935.2	E950.0	E962.0	E980.0
Dihydromorphine 965.09	E850.2	E935.2	E950.0	E962.0	E980.0
Dihydromorphinone 965.09	E850.2	E935.2	E950.0	E962.0	E980.0
Dihydrostreptomycin 960.6	E856	E930.6	E950.4	E962.0	E980.4
Dihydrotachysterol 962.6	E858.0	E932.6	E950.4	E962.0	E980.4
Dihydroxyanthraquinone 973.1	E858.4	E943.1	E950.4	E962.0	E980.4
Dihydroxycodeinone 965.09	E850.2	E935.2	E950.0	E962.0	E980.0
Diiodohydroxyquin 961.3	E857	E931.3	E950.4	E962.0	E980.4
topical 976.0	E858.7	E946.0	E950.4	E962.0	E980.4
Diiodohydroxyquinoline 961.3	E857	E931.3	E950.4	E962.0	E980.4
Dilantin 966.1	E855.0	E936.1	E950.4	E962.0	E980.4
Dilaudid 965.09	E850.2	E935.2	E950.0	E962.0	E980.0
Diloxanide 961.5	E857	E931.5	E950.4	E962.0	E980.4
Dimefline 970.0	E854.3	E940.0	E950.4	E962.0	E980.4
Dimenhydrinate 963.0	E858.1	E933.0	E950.4	E962.0	E980.4

Substance	Poisoning	Accident	Therapeutic Use	Suicide Attempt	Assault	Undetermined
			External Cause (E-Code)			
Dimercaprol 963.8	E858.1	E933.8	E950.4	E962.0	E980.4
Dimercaptopropanol. 963.8	E858.1	E933.8	E950.4	E962.0	E980.4
Dimetane 963.0	E858.1	E933.0	E950.4	E962.0	E980.4
Dimethicone 976.3	E858.7	E946.3	E950.4	E962.0	E980.4
Dimethindene 963.0	E858.1	E933.0	E950.4	E962.0	E980.4
Dimethisoquin 968.5	E855.2	E938.5	E950.4	E962.0	E980.4
Dimethisterone 962.2	E858.0	E932.2	E950.4	E962.0	E980.4
Dimethoxanate 975.4	E858.6	E945.4	E950.4	E962.0	E980.4
Dimethyl					
arsine, arsinic acid — see Arsenic					
carbinol 980.2	E860.3	—	E950.9	E962.1	E980.9
diguanide 962.3	E858.0	E932.3	E950.4	E962.0	E980.4
ketone 982.8	E862.4	—	E950.9	E962.1	E980.9
vapor 987.8	E869.8	—	E952.8	E962.2	E982.8
meperidine. 965.09	E850.2	E935.2	E950.0	E962.0	E980.0
parathion 989.3	E863.1	—	E950.6	E962.1	E980.7
polysiloxane 973.8	E858.4	E943.8	E950.4	E962.0	E980.4
sulfate (fumes) 987.8	E869.8	—	E952.8	E962.2	E982.8
liquid 983.9	E864.3	—	E950.7	E962.1	E980.6
sulfoxide NEC 982.8	E862.4	—	E950.9	E962.1	E980.9
medicinal 976.4	E858.7	E946.4	E950.4	E962.0	E980.4
triptamine 969.6	E854.1	E939.6	E950.3	E962.0	E980.3
tubocurarine 975.2	E858.6	E945.2	E950.4	E962.0	E980.4
Dindevan 964.2	E858.2	E934.2	E950.4	E962.0	E980.4
Dinitro (–ortho–) cresol (herbicide) (spray) . . 989.4	E863.5	—	E950.6	E962.1	E980.7
insecticide 989.4	E863.4	—	E950.6	E962.1	E980.7
Dinitrobenzene. 983.0	E864.0	—	E950.7	E962.1	E980.6
vapor 987.8	E869.8	—	E952.8	E962.2	E982.8
Dinitro–orthocresol (herbicide) 989.4	E863.5	—	E950.6	E962.1	E980.7
insecticide 989.4	E863.4	—	E950.6	E962.1	E980.7
Dinitrophenol (herbicide) (spray) 989.4	E863.5	—	E950.6	E962.1	E980.7
insecticide 989.4	E863.4	—	E950.6	E962.1	E980.7
Dinoprost 975.0	E858.6	E945.0	E950.4	E962.0	E980.4
Dioctyl sulfosuccinate (calcium) (sodium). . 973.2	E858.4	E943.2	E950.4	E962.0	E980.4
Diodoquin. 961.3	E857	E931.3	E950.4	E962.0	E980.4
Dione derivatives NEC 966.3	E855.0	E936.3	E950.4	E962.0	E980.4
Dionin 965.09	E850.2	E935.2	E950.0	E962.0	E980.0
Dioxane. 982.8	E862.4	—	E950.9	E962.1	E980.9
Dioxin — see herbicide					
Dioxyline 972.5	E858.3	E942.5	E950.4	E962.0	E980.4
Dipentene 982.8	E862.4	—	E950.9	E962.1	E980.9
Diphemanil 971.1	E855.4	E941.1	E950.4	E962.0	E980.4
Diphenadione 964.2	E858.2	E934.2	E950.4	E962.0	E980.4
Diphenhydramine. 963.0	E858.1	E933.0	E950.4	E962.0	E980.4
Diphenidol 963.0	E858.1	E933.0	E950.4	E962.0	E980.4
Diphenoxylate 973.5	E858.4	E943.5	E950.4	E962.0	E980.4
Diphenylchloroarsine 985.1	E866.3	—	E950.8	E962.1	E980.8
Diphenylhydantoin (sodium) 966.1	E855.0	E936.1	E950.4	E962.0	E980.4
Diphenylpyraline 963.0	E858.1	E933.0	E950.4	E962.0	E980.4
Diphtheria					
antitoxin. 979.9	E858.8	E949.9	E950.4	E962.0	E980.4
toxoid. 978.5	E858.8	E948.5	E950.4	E962.0	E980.4
with tetanus toxoid 978.9	E858.8	E948.9	E950.4	E962.0	E980.4
with pertussis component 978.6	E858.8	E948.6	E950.4	E962.0	E980.4
vaccine 978.5	E858.8	E948.5	E950.4	E962.0	E980.4
Dipipanone 965.09	E850.2	E935.2	E950.0	E962.0	E980.0
Diplovax 979.5	E858.8	E949.5	E950.4	E962.0	E980.4
Diprophylline 975.1	E858.6	E945.1	E950.4	E962.0	E980.4
Dipyridamole 972.4	E858.3	E942.4	E950.4	E962.0	E980.4
Dipyrone 965.5	E850.5	E935.5	E950.0	E962.0	E980.0

Substance	Poisoning	Accident	Therapeutic Use	Suicide Attempt	Assault	Undetermined
			External Cause (E-Code)			
Diquat	989.4	E863.5	—	E950.6	E962.1	E980.7
Disinfectant NEC.	983.9	E861.4	—	E950.7	E962.1	E980.6
alkaline	983.2	E861.4	—	E950.7	E962.1	E980.6
aromatic.	983.0	E861.4	—	E950.7	E962.1	E980.6
Disipal	966.4	E855.0	E936.4	E950.4	E962.0	E980.4
Disodium edetate.	963.8	E858.1	E933.8	E950.4	E962.0	E980.4
Disulfamide	974.4	E858.5	E944.4	E950.4	E962.0	E980.4
Disulfanilamide	961.0	E857	E931.0	E950.4	E962.0	E980.4
Disulfiram.	977.3	E858.8	E947.3	E950.4	E962.0	E980.4
Dithiazanine	961.6	E857	E931.6	E950.4	E962.0	E980.4
Dithioglycerol	963.8	E858.1	E933.8	E950.4	E962.0	E980.4
Dithranol	976.4	E858.7	E946.4	E950.4	E962.0	E980.4
Diucardin	974.3	E858.5	E944.3	E950.4	E962.0	E980.4
Diupres.	974.3	E858.5	E944.3	E950.4	E962.0	E980.4
Diuretics NEC	974.4	E858.5	E944.4	E950.4	E962.0	E980.4
carbonic acid anhydrase inhibitors	974.2	E858.5	E944.2	E950.4	E962.0	E980.4
mercurial	974.0	E858.5	E944.0	E950.4	E962.0	E980.4
osmotic.	974.4	E858.5	E944.4	E950.4	E962.0	E980.4
purine derivatives	974.1	E858.5	E944.1	E950.4	E962.0	E980.4
saluretic.	974.3	E858.5	E944.3	E950.4	E962.0	E980.4
Diuril.	974.3	E858.5	E944.3	E950.4	E962.0	E980.4
Divinyl ether	968.2	E855.1	E938.2	E950.4	E962.0	E980.4
D–lysergic acid diethylamide	969.6	E854.1	E939.6	E950.3	E962.0	E980.3
DMCT	960.4	E856	E930.4	E950.4	E962.0	E980.4
DMSO	982.8	E862.4	—	E950.9	E962.1	E980.9
DMT.	969.6	E854.1	E939.6	E950.3	E962.0	E980.3
DNOC	989.4	E863.5	—	E950.6	E962.1	E980.7
DOCA	962.0	E858.0	E932.0	E950.4	E962.0	E980.4
Dolophine.	965.02	E850.1	E935.1	E950.0	E962.0	E980.0
Doloxene	965.8	E850.8	E935.8	E950.0	E962.0	E980.0
DOM.	969.6	E854.1	E939.6	E950.3	E962.0	E980.3
Domestic gas — *see* Gas, utility						
Domiphen (bromide) (lozenges)	976.6	E858.7	E946.6	E950.4	E962.0	E980.4
Dopa (levo)	966.4	E855.0	E936.4	E950.4	E962.0	E980.4
Dopamine	971.2	E855.5	E941.2	E950.4	E962.0	E980.4
Doriden.	967.5	E852.4	E937.5	E950.2	E962.0	E980.2
Dormiral	967.0	E851	E937.0	E950.1	E962.0	E980.1
Dormison	967.8	E852.8	E937.8	E950.2	E962.0	E980.2
Dornase.	963.4	E858.1	E933.4	E950.4	E962.0	E980.4
Dorsacaine	968.5	E855.2	E938.5	E950.4	E962.0	E980.4
Dothiepin hydrochloride	969.05	E854.0	E939.0	E950.3	E962.0	E980.3
Doxapram	970.0	E854.3	E940.0	E950.4	E962.0	E980.4
Doxepin	969.05	E854.0	E939.0	E950.3	E962.0	E980.3
Doxorubicin	960.7	E856	E930.7	E950.4	E962.0	E980.4
Doxycycline	960.4	E856	E930.4	E950.4	E962.0	E980.4
Doxylamine	963.0	E858.1	E933.0	E950.4	E962.0	E980.4
Dramamine	963.0	E858.1	E933.0	E950.4	E962.0	E980.4
Drano (drain cleaner)	983.2	E864.2	—	E950.7	E962.1	E980.6
Dromoran	965.09	E850.2	E935.2	E950.0	E962.0	E980.0
Dromostanolone	962.1	E858.0	E932.1	E950.4	E962.0	E980.4
Droperidol.	969.2	E853.1	E939.2	E950.3	E962.0	E980.3
Drotrecogin alfa	964.2	E858.2	E934.2	E950.4	E962.0	E980.4
Drug	977.9	E858.9	E947.9	E950.5	E962.0	E980.5
specified NEC	977.8	E858.8	E947.8	E950.4	E962.0	E980.4
AHFS List						
4:00 antihistamine drugs	963.0	E858.1	E933.0	E950.4	E962.0	E980.4
8:04 amebacides	961.5	E857	E931.5	E950.4	E962.0	E980.4
arsenical anti–infectives.	961.1	E857	E931.1	E950.4	E962.0	E980.4
quinoline derivatives	961.3	E857	E931.3	E950.4	E962.0	E980.4
8:08 anthelmintics.	961.6	E857	E931.6	E950.4	E962.0	E980.4
quinoline derivatives	961.3	E857	E931.3	E950.4	E962.0	E980.4

Substance	Poisoning	Accident	Therapeutic Use	Suicide Attempt	Assault	Undetermined
			External Cause (E-Code)			
8:12.04 antifungal antibiotics	960.1	E856	E930.1	E950.4	E962.0	E980.4
8:12.06 cephalosporins	960.5	E856	E930.5	E950.4	E962.0	E980.4
8:12.08 chloramphenicol	960.2	E856	E930.2	E950.4	E962.0	E980.4
8:12.12 erythromycins	960.3	E856	E930.3	E950.4	E962.0	E980.4
8:12.16 penicillins	960.0	E856	E930.0	E950.4	E962.0	E980.4
8:12.20 streptomycins	960.6	E856	E930.6	E950.4	E962.0	E980.4
8:12.24 tetracyclines	960.4	E856	E930.4	E950.4	E962.0	E980.4
8:12.28 other antibiotics	960.8	E856	E930.8	E950.4	E962.0	E980.4
antimycobacterial	960.6	E856	E930.6	E950.4	E962.0	E980.4
macrolides	960.3	E856	E930.3	E950.4	E962.0	E980.4
8:16 antituberculars	961.8	E857	E931.8	E950.4	E962.0	E980.4
antibiotics	960.6	E856	E930.6	E950.4	E962.0	E980.4
8:18 antivirals	961.7	E857	E931.7	E950.4	E962.0	E980.4
8:20 plasmodicides (antimalarials)	961.4	E857	E931.4	E950.4	E962.0	E980.4
8:24 sulfonamides	961.0	E857	E931.0	E950.4	E962.0	E980.4
8:26 sulfones	961.8	E857	E931.8	E950.4	E962.0	E980.4
8:28 treponemicides	961.2	E857	E931.2	E950.4	E962.0	E980.4
8:32 trichomonacides	961.5	E857	E931.5	E950.4	E962.0	E980.4
quinoline derivatives	961.3	E857	E931.3	E950.4	E962.0	E980.4
nitrofuran derivatives	961.9	E857	E931.9	E950.4	E962.0	E980.4
8:36 urinary germicides	961.9	E857	E931.9	E950.4	E962.0	E980.4
quinoline derivatives	961.3	E857	E931.3	E950.4	E962.0	E980.4
8:40 other anti–infectives	961.9	E857	E931.9	E950.4	E962.0	E980.4
10:00 antineoplastic agents	963.1	E858.1	E933.1	E950.4	E962.0	E980.4
antibiotics	960.7	E856	E930.7	E950.4	E962.0	E980.4
progestogens	962.2	E858.0	E932.2	E950.4	E962.0	E980.4
12:04 parasympathomimetic (cholinergic) agents	971.0	E855.3	E941.0	E950.4	E962.0	E980.4
12:08 parasympatholytic (cholinergic –blocking) agents	971.1	E855.4	E941.1	E950.4	E962.0	E980.4
12:12 Sympathomimetic (adrenergic) agents	971.2	E855.5	E941.2	E950.4	E962.0	E980.4
12:16 sympatholytic (adrenergic– blocking) agents	971.3	E855.6	E941.3	E950.4	E962.0	E980.4
12:20 skeletal muscle relaxants central nervous system muscle-tone depressants	968.0	E855.1	E938.0	E950.4	E962.0	E980.4
myoneural blocking agents	975.2	E858.6	E945.2	E950.4	E962.0	E980.4
16:00 blood derivatives	964.7	E858.2	E934.7	E950.4	E962.0	E980.4
20:04 antianemia drugs	964.1	E858.2	E934.1	E950.4	E962.0	E980.4
20:04.04 iron preparations	964.0	E858.2	E934.0	E950.4	E962.0	E980.4
20:04.08 liver and stomach preparations	964.1	E858.2	E934.1	E950.4	E962.0	E980.4
20:12.04 anticoagulants	964.2	E858.2	E934.2	E950.4	E962.0	E980.4
20:12.08 antiheparin agents	964.5	E858.2	E934.5	E950.4	E962.0	E980.4
20:12.12 coagulants	964.5	E858.2	E934.5	E950.4	E962.0	E980.4
20:12.16 hemostatics NEC	964.5	E858.2	E934.5	E950.4	E962.0	E980.4
capillary active drugs	972.8	E858.3	E942.8	E950.4	E962.0	E980.4
24:04 cardiac drugs	972.9	E858.3	E942.9	E950.4	E962.0	E980.4
cardiotonic agents	972.1	E858.3	E942.1	E950.4	E962.0	E980.4
rhythm regulators	972.0	E858.3	E942.0	E950.4	E962.0	E980.4
24:06 antilipemic agents	972.2	E858.3	E942.2	E950.4	E962.0	E980.4
thyroid derivatives	962.7	E858.0	E932.7	E950.4	E962.0	E980.4
24:08 hypotensive agents	972.6	E858.3	E942.6	E950.4	E962.0	E980.4
adrenergic blocking agents	971.3	E855.6	E941.3	E950.4	E962.0	E980.4
ganglion blocking agents	972.3	E858.3	E942.3	E950.4	E962.0	E980.4
vasodilators	972.5	E858.3	E942.5	E950.4	E962.0	E980.4
24:12 vasodilating agents NEC	972.5	E858.3	E942.5	E950.4	E962.0	E980.4
coronary	972.4	E858.3	E942.4	E950.4	E962.0	E980.4
nicotinic acid derivatives	972.2	E858.3	E942.2	E950.4	E962.0	E980.4
24:16 sclerosing agents	972.7	E858.3	E942.7	E950.4	E962.0	E980.4

Substance	Poisoning	Accident	Therapeutic Use	Suicide Attempt	Assault	Undetermined
		External Cause (E-Code)				
28:04 general anesthetics	968.4	E855.1	E938.4	E950.4	E962.0	E980.4
gaseous anesthetics	968.2	E855.1	E938.2	E950.4	E962.0	E980.4
halothane	968.1	E855.1	E938.1	E950.4	E962.0	E980.4
intravenous anesthetics	968.3	E855.1	E938.3	E950.4	E962.0	E980.4
28:08 analgesics and antipyretics	965.9	E850.9	E935.9	E950.0	E962.0	E980.0
antirheumatics	965.69	E850.6	E935.6	E950.0	E962.0	E980.0
aromatic analgesics	965.4	E850.4	E935.4	E950.0	E962.0	E980.0
non–narcotic NEC	965.7	E850.7	E935.7	E950.0	E962.0	E980.0
opium alkaloids	965.00	E850.2	E935.2	E950.0	E962.0	E980.0
heroin	965.01	E850.0	E935.0	E950.0	E962.0	E980.0
methadone	965.02	E850.1	E935.1	E950.0	E962.0	E980.0
specified type NEC	965.09	E850.2	E935.2	E950.0	E962.0	E980.0
pyrazole derivatives	965.5	E850.5	E935.5	E950.0	E962.0	E980.0
salicylates	965.1	E850.3	E935.3	E950.0	E962.0	E980.0
specified NEC	965.8	E850.8	E935.8	E950.0	E962.0	E980.0
28:10 narcotic antagonists	970.1	E854.3	E940.1	E950.4	E962.0	E980.4
28:12 anticonvulsants	966.3	E855.0	E936.3	E950.4	E962.0	E980.4
barbiturates	967.0	E851	E937.0	E950.1	E962.0	E980.1
benzodiazepine–based tranquilizers	969.4	E853.2	E939.4	E950.3	E962.0	E980.3
bromides	967.3	E852.2	E937.3	E950.2	E962.0	E980.2
hydantoin derivatives	966.1	E855.0	E936.1	E950.4	E962.0	E980.4
oxazolidine (derivatives)	966.0	E855.0	E936.0	E950.4	E962.0	E980.4
succinimides	966.2	E855.0	E936.2	E950.4	E962.0	E980.4
28:16.04 anti-depressants	969.00	E854.0	E939.0	E950.3	E962.0	E980.3
28:16.08 tranquilizers	969.5	E853.9	E939.5	E950.3	E962.0	E980.3
benzodiazepine–based	969.4	E853.2	E939.4	E950.3	E962.0	E980.3
butyrophenone–based	969.2	E853.1	E939.2	E950.3	E962.0	E980.3
major NEC	969.3	E853.8	E939.3	E950.3	E962.0	E980.3
phenothiazine–based	969.1	E853.0	E939.1	E950.3	E962.0	E980.3
28:16.12 other psychotherapeutic agents	969.8	E855.8	E939.8	E950.3	E962.0	E980.3
28:20 respiratory and cerebral stimulants	970.9	E854.3	E940.9	E950.4	E962.0	E980.4
analeptics	970.0	E854.3	E940.0	E950.4	E962.0	E980.4
anorexigenic agents	977.0	E858.8	E947.0	E950.4	E962.0	E980.4
psychostimulants	969.70	E854.2	E939.7	E950.3	E962.0	E980.3
specified NEC	970.89	E854.3	E940.8	E950.4	E962.0	E980.4
28:24 sedatives and hypnotics	967.9	E852.9	E937.9	E950.2	E962.0	E980.2
barbiturates	967.0	E851	E937.0	E950.1	E962.0	E980.1
benzodiazepine–based tranquilizers	969.4	E853.2	E939.4	E950.3	E962.0	E980.3
chloral hydrate (group)	967.1	E852.0	E937.1	E950.2	E962.0	E980.2
glutethamide group	967.5	E852.4	E937.5	E950.2	E962.0	E980.2
intravenous anesthetics	968.3	E855.1	E938.3	E950.4	E962.0	E980.4
methaqualone (compounds)	967.4	E852.3	E937.4	E950.2	E962.0	E980.2
paraldehyde	967.2	E852.1	E937.2	E950.2	E962.0	E980.2
phenothiazine–based tranquilizers	969.1	E853.0	E939.1	E950.3	E962.0	E980.3
specified NEC	967.8	E852.8	E937.8	E950.2	E962.0	E980.2
thiobarbiturates	968.3	E855.1	E938.3	E950.4	E962.0	E980.4
tranquilizer NEC	969.5	E853.9	E939.5	E950.3	E962.0	E980.3
36:04 to 36:88 diagnostic agents	977.8	E858.8	E947.8	E950.4	E962.0	E980.4
40:00 electrolyte, caloric, and water balance agents NEC	974.5	E858.5	E944.5	E950.4	E962.0	E980.4
40:04 acidifying agents	963.2	E858.1	E933.2	E950.4	E962.0	E980.4
40:08 alkalinizing agents	963.3	E858.1	E933.3	E950.4	E962.0	E980:4
40:10 ammonia detoxicants	974.5	E858.5	E944.5	E950.4	E962.0	E980.4
40:12 replacement solutions	974.5	E858.5	E944.5	E950.4	E962.0	E980.4
plasma expanders	964.8	E852.8	E934.8	E950.4	E962.0	E980.4
40:16 sodium–removing resins	974.5	E858.5	E944.5	E950.4	E962.0	E980.4
40:18 potassium–removing resins	974.5	E858.5	E944.5	E950.4	E962.0	E980.4
40:20 caloric agents	974.5	E858.5	E944.5	E950.4	E962.0	E980.4
40:24 salt and sugar substitutes	974.5	E858.5	E944.5	E950.4	E962.0	E980.4
40:28 diuretics NEC	974.4	E858.5	E944.4	E950.4	E962.0	E980.4

Substance	Poisoning	Accident	Therapeutic Use	Suicide Attempt	Assault	Undetermined
			External Cause (E-Code)			
carbonic acid anhydrase inhibitors 974.2		E858.5	E944.2	E950.4	E962.0	E980.4
mercurials 974.0		E858.5	E944.0	E950.4	E962.0	E980.4
purine derivatives 974.1		E858.5	E944.1	E950.4	E962.0	E980.4
saluretics. 974.3		E858.5	E944.3	E950.4	E962.0	E980.4
thiazides 974.3		E858.5	E944.3	E950.4	E962.1	E980.4
40:36 irrigating solutions 974.5		E858.5	E944.5	E950.4	E962.0	E980.4
40:40 uricosuric agents. 974.7		E858.5	E944.7	E950.4	E962.0	E980.4
44:00 enzymes 963.4		E858.1	E933.4	E950.4	E962.0	E980.4
fibrinolysis–affecting agents 964.4		E858.2	E934.4	E950.4	E962.0	E980.4
gastric agents. 973.4		E858.4	E943.4	E950.4	E962.0	E980.4
48:00 expectorants and cough preparations						
antihistamine agents 963.0		E858.1	E933.0	E950.4	E962.0	E980.4
antitussives. 975.4		E858.6	E945.4	E950.4	E962.0	E980.4
codeine derivatives. 965.09		E850.2	E935.2	E950.0	E962.0	E980.0
expectorants 975.5		E858.6	E945.5	E950.4	E962.0	E980.4
narcotic agents NEC 965.09		E850.2	E935.2	E950.0	E962.0	E980.0
52:04 anti–infectives (EENT)						
ENT agent 976.6		E858.7	E946.6	E950.4	E962.0	E980.4
ophthalmic preparation 976.5		E858.7	E946.5	E950.4	E962.0	E980.4
52:04.04 antibiotics (EENT)						
ENT agent 976.6		E858.7	E946.6	E950.4	E962.0	E980.4
ophthalmic preparation 976.5		E858.7	E946.5	E950.4	E962.0	E980.4
52:04.06 antivirals (EENT)						
ENT agent 976.6		E858.7	E946.6	E950.4	E962.0	E980.4
ophthalmic preparation 976.5		E858.7	E946.5	E950.4	E962.0	E980.4
52:04.08 sulfonamides (EENT)						
ENT agent 976.6		E858.7	E946.6	E950.4	E962.0	E980.4
ophthalmic preparation 976.5		E858.7	E946.5	E950.4	E962.0	E980.4
52:04.12 miscellaneous anti–infectives (EENT)						
ENT agent 976.6		E858.7	E946.6	E950.4	E962.0	E980.4
ophthalmic preparation 976.5		E858.7	E946.5	E950.4	E962.0	E980.4
52:08 anti–inflammatory agents (EENT)						
ENT agent 976.6		E858.7	E946.6	E950.4	E962.0	E980.4
ophthalmic preparation 976.5		E858.7	E946.5	E950.4	E962.0	E980.4
52:10 carbonic anhydrase inhibitors . . . 974.2		E858.5	E944.2	E950.4	E962.0	E980.4
52:12 contact lens solutions. 976.5		E858.7	E946.5	E950.4	E962.0	E980.4
52:16 local anesthetics (EENT) 968.5		E855.2	E938.5	E950.4	E962.0	E980.4
52:20 miotics. 971.0		E855.3	E941.0	E950.4	E962.0	E980.4
52:24 mydriatics						
adrenergics. 971.2		E855.5	E941.2	E950.4	E962.0	E980.4
anticholinergics 971.1		E855.4	E941.1	E950.4	E962.0	E980.4
antimuscarinics 971.1		E855.4	E941.1	E950.4	E962.0	E980.4
parasympatholytics. 971.1		E855.4	E941.1	E950.4	E962.0	E980.4
spasmolytics 971.1		E855.4	E941.1	E950.4	E962.0	E980.4
sympathomimetics 971.2		E855.5	E941.2	E950.4	E962.0	E980.4
52:28 mouth washes and gargles. 976.6		E858.7	E946.6	E950.4	E962.0	E980.4
52:32 vasoconstrictors (EENT) 971.2		E855.5	E941.2	E950.4	E962.0	E980.4
52:36 unclassified agents (EENT)						
ENT agent 976.6		E858.7	E946.6	E950.4	E962.0	E980.4
ophthalmic preparation 976.5		E858.7	E946.5	E950.4	E962.0	E980.4
56:04 antacids and adsorbents 973.0		E858.4	E943.0	E950.4	E962.0	E980.4
56:08 antidiarrhea agents 973.5		E858.4	E943.5	E950.4	E962.0	E980.4
56:10 antiflatulents 973.8		E858.4	E943.8	E950.4	E962.0	E980.4
56:12 cathartics NEC 973.3		E858.4	E943.3	E950.4	E962.0	E980.4
emollients 973.2		E858.4	E943.2	E950.4	E962.0	E980.4
irritants 973.1		E858.4	E943.1	E950.4	E962.0	E980.4
56:16 digestants 973.4		E858.4	E943.4	E950.4	E962.0	E980.4
56:20 emetics and antiemetics						
antiemetics 963.0		E858.1	E933.0	E950.4	E962.0	E980.4
emetics 973.6		E858.4	E943.6	E950.4	E962.0	E980.4

Substance	Poisoning	Accident	Therapeutic Use	Suicide Attempt	Assault	Undetermined
			External Cause (E-Code)			
56:24 lipotropic agents	977.1	E858.8	E947.1	E950.4	E962.0	E980.4
56:40 miscellaneous G.I. drugs	973.8	E858.4	E943.8	E950.4	E962.0	E980.4
60:00 gold compounds	965.69	E850.6	E935.6	E950.0	E962.0	E980.0
64:00 heavy metal antagonists	963.8	E858.1	E933.8	E950.4	E962.0	E980.4
68:04 adrenals	962.0	E858.0	E932.0	E950.4	E962.0	E980.4
68:08 androgens	962.1	E858.0	E932.1	E950.4	E962.0	E980.4
68:12 contraceptives, oral	962.2	E858.0	E932.2	E950.4	E962.0	E980.4
68:16 estrogens	962.2	E858.0	E932.2	E950.4	E962.0	E980.4
68:18 gonadotropins	962.4	E858.0	E932.4	E950.4	E962.0	E980.4
68:20 insulins and antidiabetic agents	962.3	E858.0	E932.3	E950.4	E962.0	E980.4
68:20.08 insulins	962.3	E858.0	E932.3	E950.4	E962.0	E980.4
68:24 parathyroid	962.6	E858.0	E932.6	E950.4	E962.0	E980.4
68:28 pituitary (posterior)	962.5	E858.0	E932.5	E950.4	E962.0	E980.4
anterior	962.4	E858.0	E932.4	E950.4	E962.0	E980.4
68:32 progestogens	962.2	E858.0	E932.2	E950.4	E962.0	E980.4
68:34 other corpus luteum hormones NEC	962.2	E858.0	E932.2	E950.4	E962.0	E980.4
68:36 thyroid and antithyroid antithyroid	962.8	E858.0	E932.8	E950.4	E962.0	E980.4
thyroid (derivatives)	962.7	E858.0	E932.7	E950.4	E962.0	E980.4
72:00 local anesthetics NEC	968.9	E855.2	E938.9	E950.4	E962.0	E980.4
topical (surface)	968.5	E855.2	E938.5	E950.4	E962.0	E980.4
infiltration (intradermal) (subcutaneous) (submucosal)	968.5	E855.2	E938.5	E950.4	E962.0	E980.4
nerve blocking (peripheral) (plexus) (regional)	968.6	E855.2	E938.6	E950.4	E962.0	E980.4
spinal	968.7	E855.2	E938.7	E950.4	E962.0	E980.4
76:00 oxytocics	975.0	E858.6	E945.0	E950.4	E962.0	E980.4
78:00 radioactive agents	990	—	—	—	—	—
80:04 serums NEC	979.9	E858.8	E949.9	E950.4	E962.0	E980.4
immune gamma globulin (human)	964.6	E858.2	E934.6	E950.4	E962.0	E980.4
80:08 toxoids NEC	978.8	E858.8	E948.8	E950.4	E962.0	E980.4
diphtheria	978.5	E858.8	E948.5	E950.4	E962.0	E980.4
and tetanus	978.9	E858.8	E948.9	E950.4	E962.0	E980.4
with pertussis component	978.6	E858.8	E948.6	E950.4	E962.0	E980.4
tetanus	978.4	E858.8	E948.4	E950.4	E962.0	E980.4
and diphtheria	978.9	E858.8	E948.9	E950.4	E962.0	E980.4
with pertussis component	978.6	E858.8	E948.6	E950.4	E962.0	E980.4
80:12 vaccines	979.9	E858.8	E949.9	E950.4	E962.0	E980.4
bacterial NEC	978.8	E858.8	E948.8	E950.4	E962.0	E980.4
with other bacterial components	978.9	E858.8	E948.9	E950.4	E962.0	E980.4
pertussis component	978.6	E858.8	E948.6	E950.4	E962.0	E980.4
viral and rickettsial components	979.7	E858.8	E949.7	E950.4	E962.0	E980.4
rickettsial NEC	979.6	E858.8	E949.6	E950.4	E962.0	E980.4
with bacterial component	979.7	E858.8	E949.7	E950.4	E962.0	E980.4
pertussis component	978.6	E858.8	E948.6	E950.4	E962.0	E980.4
viral component	979.7	E858.8	E949.7	E950.4	E962.0	E980.4
viral NEC	979.6	E858.8	E949.6	E950.4	E962.0	E980.4
with bacterial component	979.7	E858.8	E949.7	E950.4	E962.0	E980.4
pertussis component	978.6	E858.8	E948.6	E950.4	E962.0	E980.4
rickettsial component	979.7	E858.8	E949.7	E950.4	E962.0	E980.4
84:04.04 antibiotics (skin and mucous membrane)	976.0	E858.7	E946.0	E950.4	E962.0	E980.4
84:04.08 fungicides (skin and mucous membrane)	976.0	E858.7	E946.0	E950.4	E962.0	E980.4
84:04.12 scabicides and pediculicides (skin and mucous membrane)	976.0	E858.7	E946.0	E950.4	E962.0	E980.4

Substance	Poisoning	Accident	Therapeutic Use	Suicide Attempt	Assault	Undetermined
			External Cause (E-Code)			
84:04.16 miscellaneous local anti–infectives (skin and mucous membrane) 976.0	E858.7	E946.0	E950.4	E962.0	E980.4
84:06 anti–inflammatory agents (skin and mucous membrane). 976.0	E858.7	E946.0	E950.4	E962.0	E980.4
84:08 antipruritics and local anesthetics antipruritics. 976.1	E858.7	E946.1	E950.4	E962.0	E980.4
local anesthetics. 968.5	E855.2	E938.5	E950.4	E962.0	E980.4
84:12 astringents 976.2	E858.7	E946.2	E950.4	E962.0	E980.4
84:16 cell stimulants and proliferants. . . . 976.8	E858.7	E946.8	E950.4	E962.0	E980.4
84:20 detergents 976.2	E858.7	E946.2	E950.4	E962.0	E980.4
84:24 emollients, demulcents, and protectants 976.3	E858.7	E946.3	E950.4	E962.0	E980.4
84:28 keratolytic agents 976.4	E858.7	E946.4	E950.4	E962.0	E980.4
84:32 keratoplastic agents 976.4	E858.7	E946.4	E950.4	E962.0	E980.4
84:36 miscellaneous agents (skin and mucous membrane). 976.8	E858.7	E946.8	E950.4	E962.0	E980.4
86:00 spasmolytic agents 975.1	E858.6	E945.1	E950.4	E962.0	E980.4
antiasthmatics. 975.7	E858.6	E945.7	E950.4	E962.0	E980.4
papaverine 972.5	E858.3	E942.5	E950.4	E962.0	E980.4
theophylline 974.1	E858.5	E944.1	E950.4	E962.0	E980.4
88:04 vitamin A 963.5	E858.1	E933.5	E950.4	E962.0	E980.4
88:08 vitamin B complex. 963.5	E858.1	E933.5	E950.4	E962.0	E980.4
hematopoietic vitamin 964.1	E858.2	E934.1	E950.4	E962.0	E980.4
nicotinic acid derivatives 972.2	E858.3	E942.2	E950.4	E962.0	E980.4
88:12 vitamin C 963.5	E858.1	E933.5	E950.4	E962.0	E980.4
88:16 vitamin D 963.5	E858.1	E933.5	E950.4	E962.0	E980.4
88:20 vitamin E 963.5	E858.1	E933.5	E950.4	E962.0	E980.4
88:24 vitamin K activity 964.3	E858.2	E934.3	E950.4	E962.0	E980.4
88:28 multivitamin preparations 963.5	E858.1	E933.5	E950.4	E962.0	E980.4
92:00 unclassified therapeutic agents . . . 977.8	E858.8	E947.8	E950.4	E962.0	E980.4
Duboisine. 971.1	E855.4	E941.1	E950.4	E962.0	E980.4
Dulcolax 973.1	E858.4	E943.1	E950.4	E962.0	E980.4
Duponol (C) (EP) 976.2	E858.7	E946.2	E950.4	E962.0	E980.4
Durabolin 962.1	E858.0	E932.1	E950.4	E962.0	E980.4
Dyclone. 968.5	E855.2	E938.5	E950.4	E962.0	E980.4
Dyclonine 968.5	E855.2	E938.5	E950.4	E962.0	E980.4
Dydrogesterone 962.2	E858.0	E932.2	E950.4	E962.0	E980.4
Dyes NEC 989.89	E866.8	—	E950.9	E962.1	E980.9
diagnostic agents 977.8	E858.8	E947.8	E950.4	E962.0	E980.4
pharmaceutical NEC. 977.4	E858.8	E947.4	E950.4	E962.0	E980.4
Dyfols 971.0	E855.3	E941.0	E950.4	E962.0	E980.4
Dymelor 962.3	E858.0	E932.3	E950.4	E962.0	E980.4
Dynamite 989.89	E866.8	—	E950.9	E962.1	E980.9
fumes 987.8	E869.8	—	E952.8	E962.2	E982.8
Dyphylline 975.1	E858.6	E945.1	E950.4	E962.0	E980.4
Ear preparations 976.6	E858.7	E946.6	E950.4	E962.0	E980.4
Echothiopate, ecothiopate 971.0	E855.3	E941.0	E950.4	E962.0	E980.4
Ecstasy 969.72	E854.2	E939.7	E950.3	E962.0	E980.3
Ectylurea 967.8	E852.8	E937.8	E950.2	E962.0	E980.2
Edathamil disodium. 963.8	E858.1	E933.8	E950.4	E962.0	E980.4
Edecrin 974.4	E858.5	E944.4	E950.4	E962.0	E980.4
Edetate, disodium (calcium) 963.8	E858.1	E933.8	E950.4	E962.0	E980.4
Edrophonium 971.0	E855.3	E941.0	E950.4	E962.0	E980.4
Elase 976.8	E858.7	E946.8	E950.4	E962.0	E980.4
Elaterium 973.1	E858.4	E943.1	E950.4	E962.0	E980.4
Elder 988.2	E865.4	—	E950.9	E962.1	E980.9
berry (unripe) 988.2	E865.3	—	E950.9	E962.1	E980.9
Electrolytes NEC. 974.5	E858.5	E944.5	E950.4	E962.0	E980.4
Electrolytic agent NEC 974.5	E858.5	E944.5	E950.4	E962.0	E980.4

Substance	Poisoning	Accident	Therapeutic Use	Suicide Attempt	Assault	Undetermined
			External Cause (E-Code)			
Embramine	963.0	E858.1	E933.0	E950.4	E962.0	E980.4
Emetics	973.6	E858.4	E943.6	E950.4	E962.0	E980.4
Emetine (hydrochloride)	961.5	E857	E931.5	E950.4	E962.0	E980.4
Emollients	976.3	E858.7	E946.3	E950.4	E962.0	E980.4
Emylcamate	969.5	E853.8	E939.5	E950.3	E962.0	E980.3
Encyprate	969.09	E854.0	E939.0	E950.3	E962.0	E980.3
Endocaine	968.5	E855.2	E938.5	E950.4	E962.0	E980.4
Endrin	989.2	E863.0	—	E950.6	E962.1	E980.7
Enflurane	968.2	E855.1	E938.2	E950.4	E962.0	E980.4
Enovid	962.2	E858.0	E932.2	E950.4	E962.0	E980.4
ENT preparations (anti–infectives)	976.6	E858.7	E946.6	E950.4	E962.0	E980.4
Enzodase	963.4	E858.1	E933.4	E950.4	E962.0	E980.4
Enzymes NEC	963.4	E858.1	E933.4	E950.4	E962.0	E980.4
Epanutin	966.1	E855.0	E936.1	E950.4	E962.0	E980.4
Ephedra (tincture)	971.2	E855.5	E941.2	E950.4	E962.0	E980.4
Ephedrine	971.2	E855.5	E941.2	E950.4	E962.0	E980.4
Epiestriol	962.2	E858.0	E932.2	E950.4	E962.0	E980.4
Epilim — *see* Sodium valproate						
Epinephrine	971.2	E855.5	E941.2	E950.4	E962.0	E980.4
Epsom salt	973.3	E858.4	E943.3	E950.4	E962.0	E980.4
Equanil	969.5	E853.8	E939.5	E950.3	E962.0	E980.3
Equisetum (diuretic)	974.4	E858.5	E944.4	E950.4	E962.0	E980.4
Ergometrine	975.0	E858.6	E945.0	E950.4	E962.0	E980.4
Ergonovine	975.0	E858.6	E945.0	E950.4	E962.0	E980.4
Ergot NEC	988.2	E865.4	—	E950.9	E962.1	E980.9
medicinal (alkaloids)	975.0	E858.6	E945.0	E950.4	E962.0	E980.4
Ergotamine (tartrate) (for migraine) NEC	972.9	E858.3	E942.9	E950.4	E962.0	E980.4
Ergotrate	975.0	E858.6	E945.0	E950.4	E962.0	E980.4
Erythrityl tetranitrate	972.4	E858.3	E942.4	E950.4	E962.0	E980.4
Erythrol tetranitrate	972.4	E858.3	E942.4	E950.4	E962.0	E980.4
Erythromycin	960.3	E856	E930.3	E950.4	E962.0	E980.4
ophthalmic preparation	976.5	E858.7	E946.5	E950.4	E962.0	E980.4
topical NEC	976.0	E858.7	E946.0	E950.4	E962.0	E980.4
Eserine	971.0	E855.3	E941.0	E950.4	E962.0	E980.4
Eskabarb	967.0	E851	E937.0	E950.1	E962.0	E980.1
Eskalith	969.8	E855.8	E939.8	E950.3	E962.0	E980.3
Estradiol (cypionate) (dipropionate) (valerate)	962.2	E858.0	E932.2	E950.4	E962.0	E980.4
Estriol	962.2	E858.0	E932.2	E950.4	E962.0	E980.4
Estrogens (with progestogens)	962.2	E858.0	E932.2	E950.4	E962.0	E980.4
Estrone	962.2	E858.0	E932.2	E950.4	E962.0	E980.4
Etafedrine	971.2	E855.5	E941.2	E950.4	E962.0	E980.4
Ethacrynate sodium	974.4	E858.5	E944.4	E950.4	E962.0	E980.4
Ethacrynic acid	974.4	E858.5	E944.4	E950.4	E962.0	E980.4
Ethambutol	961.8	E857	E931.8	E950.4	E962.0	E980.4
Ethamide	974.2	E858.5	E944.2	E950.4	E962.0	E980.4
Ethamivan	970.0	E854.3	E940.0	E950.4	E962.0	E980.4
Ethamsylate	964.5	E858.2	E934.5	E950.4	E962.0	E980.4
Ethanol	980.0	E860.1	—	E950.9	E962.1	E980.9
beverage	980.0	E860.0	—	E950.9	E962.1	E980.9
Ethchlorvynol	967.8	E852.8	E937.8	E950.2	E962.0	E980.2
Ethebenecid	974.7	E858.5	E944.7	E950.4	E962.0	E980.4
Ether(s) (diethyl) (ethyl) (vapor)	987.8	E869.8	—	E952.8	E962.2	E982.8
anesthetic	968.2	E855.1	E938.2	E950.4	E962.0	E980.4
petroleum — *see* Ligroin						
solvent	982.8	E862.4	—	E950.9	E962.1	E980.9
Ethidine chloride (vapor)	987.8	E869.8	—	E952.8	E962.2	E982.8
liquid (solvent)	982.3	E862.4	—	E950.9	E962.1	E980.9
Ethinamate	967.8	E852.8	E937.8	E950.2	E962.0	E980.2
Ethinylestradiol	962.2	E858.0	E932.2	E950.4	E962.0	E980.4
Ethionamide	961.8	E857	E931.8	E950.4	E962.0	E980.4

Substance	Poisoning	Accident	Therapeutic Use	Suicide Attempt	Assault	Undetermined
			External Cause (E-Code)			
Ethisterone	962.2	E858.0	E932.2	E950.4	E962.0	E980.4
Ethobral	967.0	E851	E937.0	E950.1	E962.0	E980.1
Ethocaine (infiltration) (topical)	968.5	E855.2	E938.5	E950.4	E962.0	E980.4
nerve block (peripheral) (plexus)	968.6	E855.2	E938.6	E950.4	E962.0	E980.4
spinal	968.7	E855.2	E938.7	E950.4	E962.0	E980.4
Ethoheptazine (citrate)	965.7	E850.7	E935.7	E950.0	E962.0	E980.0
Ethopropazine	966.4	E855.0	E936.4	E950.4	E962.0	E980.4
Ethosuximide	966.2	E855.0	E936.2	E950.4	E962.0	E980.4
Ethotoin	966.1	E855.0	E936.1	E950.4	E962.0	E980.4
Ethoxazene	961.9	E857	E931.9	E950.4	E962.0	E980.4
Ethoxzolamide	974.2	E858.5	E944.2	E950.4	E962.0	E980.4
Ethyl						
acetate (vapor)	982.8	E862.4	—	E950.9	E962.1	E980.9
alcohol	980.0	E860.1	—	E950.9	E962.1	E980.9
beverage	980.0	E860.0	—	E950.9	E962.1	E980.9
aldehyde (vapor)	987.8	E869.8	—	E952.8	E962.2	E982.8
liquid	989.89	E866.8	—	E950.9	E962.1	E980.9
aminobenzoate	968.5	E855.2	E938.5	E950.4	E962.0	E980.4
biscoumacetate	964.2	E858.2	E934.2	E950.4	E962.0	E980.4
bromide (anesthetic)	968.2	E855.1	E938.2	E950.4	E962.0	E980.4
carbamate (antineoplastic)	963.1	E858.1	E933.1	E950.4	E962.0	E980.4
carbinol	980.3	E860.4	—	E950.9	E962.1	E980.9
chaulmoograte	961.8	E857	E931.8	E950.4	E962.0	E980.4
chloride (vapor)	987.8	E869.8	—	E952.8	E962.2	E982.8
anesthetic (local)	968.5	E855.2	E938.5	E950.4	E962.0	E980.4
inhaled	968.2	E855.1	E938.2	E950.4	E962.0	E980.4
solvent	982.3	E862.4	—	E950.9	E962.1	E980.9
estranol	962.1	E858.0	E932.1	E950.4	E962.0	E980.4
ether — *see* Ether(s)						
formate (solvent) NEC	982.8	E862.4	—	E950.9	E962.1	E980.9
iodoacetate	987.5	E869.3	—	E952.8	E962.2	E982.8
lactate (solvent) NEC	982.8	E862.4	—	E950.9	E962.1	E980.9
methylcarbinol	980.8	E860.8	—	E950.9	E962.1	E980.9
morphine	965.09	E850.2	E935.2	E950.0	E962.0	E980.0
Ethylene (gas)	987.1	E869.8	—	E952.8	E962.2	E982.8
anesthetic (general)	968.2	E855.1	E938.2	E950.4	E962.0	E980.4
chlorohydrin (vapor)	982.3	E862.4	—	E950.9	E962.1	E980.9
dichloride (vapor)	982.3	E862.4	—	E950.9	E962.1	E980.9
glycol(s) (any) (vapor)	982.8	E862.4	—	E950.9	E962.1	E980.9
Ethylidene						
chloride NEC	982.3	E862.4	—	E950.9	E962.1	E980.9
diethyl ether	982.8	E862.4	—	E950.9	E962.1	E980.9
Ethynodiol	962.2	E858.0	E932.2	E950.4	E962.0	E980.4
Etidocaine	968.9	E855.2	E938.9	E950.4	E962.0	E980.4
infiltration (subcutaneous)	968.5	E855.2	E938.5	E950.4	E962.0	E980.4
nerve (peripheral) (plexus)	968.6	E855.2	E938.6	E950.4	E962.0	E980.4
Etilfen	967.0	E851	E937.0	E950.1	E962.0	E980.1
Etomide	965.7	E850.7	E935.7	E950.0	E962.0	E980.0
Etorphine	965.09	E850.2	E935.2	E950.0	E962.0	E980.0
Etoval	967.0	E851	E937.0	E950.1	E962.0	E980.1
Etryptamine	969.01	E854.0	E939.0	E950.3	E962.0	E980.3
Eucaine	968.5	E855.2	E938.5	E950.4	E962.0	E980.4
Eucalyptus (oil) NEC	975.5	E858.6	E945.5	E950.4	E962.0	E980.4
Eucatropine	971.1	E855.4	E941.1	E950.4	E962.0	E980.4
Eucodal	965.09	E850.2	E935.2	E950.0	E962.0	E980.0
Euneryl	967.0	E851	E937.0	E950.1	E962.0	E980.1
Euphthalmine	971.1	E855.4	E941.1	E950.4	E962.0	E980.4
Eurax	976.0	E858.7	E946.0	E950.4	E962.0	E980.4
Euresol	976.4	E858.7	E946.4	E950.4	E962.0	E980.4
Euthroid	962.7	E858.0	E932.7	E950.4	E962.0	E980.4

Substance	Poisoning	Accident	Therapeutic Use	Suicide Attempt	Assault	Undetermined
		External Cause (E-Code)				
Evans blue	977.8	E858.8	E947.8	E950.4	E962.0	E980.4
Evipal	967.0	E851	E937.0	E950.1	E962.0	E980.1
sodium	968.3	E855.1	E938.3	E950.4	E962.0	E980.4
Evipan	967.0	E851	E937.0	E950.1	E962.0	E980.1
sodium	968.3	E855.1	E938.3	E950.4	E962.0	E980.4
Exalgin	965.4	E850.4	E935.4	E950.0	E962.0	E980.0
Excipients, pharmaceutical	977.4	E858.8	E947.4	E950.4	E962.0	E980.4
Exhaust gas — *see* Carbon, monoxide						
Ex–Lax (phenolphthalein)	973.1	E858.4	E943.1	E950.4	E962.0	E980.4
Expectorants	975.5	E858.6	E945.5	E950.4	E962.0	E980.4
External medications (skin) (mucous membrane)	976.9	E858.7	E946.9	E950.4	E962.0	E980.4
dental agent	976.7	E858.7	E946.7	E950.4	E962.0	E980.4
ENT agent	976.6	E858.7	E946.6	E950.4	E962.0	E980.4
ophthalmic preparation	976.5	E858.7	E946.5	E950.4	E962.0	E980.4
specified NEC	976.8	E858.7	E946.8	E950.4	E962.0	E980.4
Eye agents (anti–infective)	976.5	E858.7	E946.5	E950.4	E962.0	E980.4
Factor IX complex (human)	964.5	E858.2	E934.5	E950.4	E962.0	E980.4
Fecal softeners	973.2	E858.4	E943.2	E950.4	E962.0	E980.4
Fenbutrazate	977.0	E858.8	E947.0	E950.4	E962.0	E980.4
Fencamfamin	970.89	E854.3	E940.8	E950.4	E962.0	E980.4
Fenfluramine	977.0	E858.8	E947.0	E950.4	E962.0	E980.4
Fenoprofen	965.61	E850.6	E935.6	E950.0	E962.0	E980.0
Fentanyl	965.09	E850.2	E935.2	E950.0	E962.0	E980.0
Fentazin	969.1	E853.0	E939.1	E950.3	E962.0	E980.3
Fenticlor, fentichlor	976.0	E858.7	E946.0	E950.4	E962.0	E980.4
Fer de lance (bite) (venom)	989.5	E905.0	—	E950.9	E962.1	E980.9
Ferric — *see* Iron						
Ferrocholinate	964.0	E858.2	E934.0	E950.4	E962.0	E980.4
Ferrous fumerate, gluconate, lactate, salt NEC, sulfate (medicinal)	964.0	E858.2	E934.0	E950.4	E962.0	E980.4
Ferrum — *see* Iron						
Fertilizers NEC	989.89	E866.5	—	E950.9	E962.1	E980.4
with herbicide mixture	989.4	E863.5	—	E950.6	E962.1	E980.7
Fibrinogen (human)	964.7	E858.2	E934.7	E950.4	E962.0	E980.4
Fibrinolysin	964.4	E858.2	E934.4	E950.4	E962.0	E980.4
Fibrinolysis–affecting agents	964.4	E858.2	E934.4	E950.4	E962.0	E980.4
Filix mas	961.6	E857	E931.6	E950.4	E962.0	E980.4
Fiorinal	965.1	E850.3	E935.3	E950.0	E962.0	E980.0
Fire damp	987.1	E869.8	—	E952.8	E962.2	E982.8
Fish, nonbacterial or noxious	988.0	E865.2	—	E950.9	E962.1	E980.9
shell	988.0	E865.1	—	E950.9	E962.1	E980.9
Flagyl	961.5	E857	E931.5	E950.4	E962.0	E980.4
Flavoxate	975.1	E858.6	E945.1	E950.4	E962.0	E980.4
Flaxedil	975.2	E858.6	E945.2	E950.4	E962.0	E980.4
Flaxseed (medicinal)	976.3	E858.7	E946.3	E950.4	E962.0	E980.4
Flomax	971.3	E855.6	E941.3	E950.4	E962.0	E980.4
Florantyrone	973.4	E858.4	E943.4	E950.4	E962.0	E980.4
Floraquin	961.3	E857	E931.3	E950.4	E962.0	E980.4
Florinef	962.0	E858.0	E932.0	E950.4	E962.0	E980.4
ENT agent	976.6	E858.7	E946.6	E950.4	E962.0	E980.4
ophthalmic preparation	976.5	E858.7	E946.5	E950.4	E962.0	E980.4
topical NEC	976.0	E858.7	E946.0	E950.4	E962.0	E980.4
Flowers of sulfur	976.4	E858.7	E946.4	E950.4	E962.0	E980.4
Floxuridine	963.1	E858.1	E933.1	E950.4	E962.0	E980.4
Flucytosine	961.9	E857	E931.9	E950.4	E962.0	E980.4
Fludrocortisone	962.0	E858.0	E932.0	E950.4	E962.0	E980.4
ENT agent	976.6	E858.7	E946.6	E950.4	E962.0	E980.4
ophthalmic preparation	976.5	E858.7	E946.5	E950.4	E962.0	E980.4
topical NEC	976.0	E858.7	E946.0	E950.4	E962.0	E980.4
Flumethasone	976.0	E858.7	E946.0	E950.4	E962.0	E980.4

Substance	Poisoning	Accident	Therapeutic Use	Suicide Attempt	Assault	Undetermined
			External Cause (E-Code)			
Flumethiazide	974.3	E858.5	E944.3	E950.4	E962.0	E980.4
Flumidin	961.7	E857	E931.7	E950.4	E962.0	E980.4
Flunitrazepam	969.4	E853.2	E939.4	E950.3	E962.0	E980.3
Fluocinolone	976.0	E858.7	E946.0	E950.4	E962.0	E980.4
Fluocortolone	962.0	E858.0	E932.0	E950.4	E962.0	E980.4
Fluohydrocortisone	962.0	E858.0	E932.0	E950.4	E962.0	E980.4
ENT agent	976.6	E858.7	E946.6	E950.4	E962.0	E980.4
ophthalmic preparation	976.5	E858.7	E946.5	E950.4	E962.0	E980.4
topical NEC	976.0	E858.7	E946.0	E950.4	E962.0	E980.4
Fluonid	976.0	E858.7	E946.0	E950.4	E962.0	E980.4
Fluopromazine	969.1	E853.0	E939.1	E950.3	E962.0	E980.3
Fluoracetate	989.4	E863.7	—	E950.6	E962.1	E980.7
Fluorescein (sodium)	977.8	E858.8	E947.8	E950.4	E962.0	E980.4
Fluoride(s) (pesticides) (sodium) NEC	989.4	E863.4	—	E950.6	E962.1	E980.7
hydrogen — see Hydrofluoric acid						
medicinal	976.7	E858.7	E946.7	E950.4	E962.0	E980.4
not pesticide NEC	983.9	E864.4	—	E950.7	E962.1	E980.6
stannous	976.7	E858.7	E946.7	E950.4	E962.0	E980.4
Fluorinated corticosteroids	962.0	E858.0	E932.0	E950.4	E962.0	E980.4
Fluorine (compounds) (gas)	987.8	E869.8	—	E952.8	E962.2	E982.8
salt — see Fluoride(s)						
Fluoristan	976.7	E858.7	E946.7	E950.4	E962.0	E980.4
Fluoroacetate	989.4	E863.7	—	E950.6	E962.1	E980.7
Fluorodeoxyuridine	963.1	E858.1	E933.1	E950.4	E962.0	E980.4
Fluorometholone (topical) NEC	976.0	E858.7	E946.0	E950.4	E962.0	E980.4
ophthalmic preparation	976.5	E858.7	E946.5	E950.4	E962.0	E980.4
Fluorouracil	963.1	E858.1	E933.1	E950.4	E962.0	E980.4
Fluothane	968.1	E855.1	E938.1	E950.4	E962.0	E980.4
Fluoxetine hydrochloride	969.03	E854.0	E939.0	E950.3	E962.0	E980.3
Fluoxymesterone	962.1	E858.0	E932.1	E950.4	E962.0	E980.4
Fluphenazine	969.1	E853.0	E939.1	E950.3	E962.0	E980.3
Fluprednisolone	962.0	E858.0	E932.0	E950.4	E962.0	E980.4
Flurandrenolide	976.0	E858.7	E946.0	E950.4	E962.0	E980.4
Flurazepam (hydrochloride)	969.4	E853.2	E939.4	E950.3	E962.0	E980.3
Flurbiprofen	965.61	E850.6	E935.6	E950.0	E962.0	E980.0
Flurobate	976.0	E858.7	E946.0	E950.4	E962.0	E980.4
Flurothyl	969.8	E855.8	E939.8	E950.3	E962.0	E980.3
Fluroxene	968.2	E855.1	E938.2	E950.4	E962.0	E980.4
Folacin	964.1	E858.2	E934.1	E950.4	E962.0	E980.4
Folic acid	964.1	E858.2	E934.1	E950.4	E962.0	E980.4
Follicle stimulating hormone	962.4	E858.0	E932.4	E950.4	E962.0	E980.4
Food, foodstuffs, nonbacterial or noxious	988.9	E865.9	—	E950.9	E962.1	E980.9
berries, seeds	988.2	E865.3	—	E950.9	E962.1	E980.9
fish	988.0	E865.2	—	E950.9	E962.1	E980.9
mushrooms	988.1	E865.5	—	E950.9	E962.1	E980.9
plants	988.2	E865.9	—	E950.9	E962.1	E980.9
specified type NEC	988.2	E865.4	—	E950.9	E962.1	E980.9
shellfish	988.0	E865.1	—	E950.9	E962.1	E980.9
specified NEC	988.8	E865.8	—	E950.9	E962.1	E980.9
Fool's parsley	988.2	E865.4	—	E950.9	E962.1	E980.9
Formaldehyde (solution)	989.89	E861.4	—	E950.9	E962.1	E980.9
fungicide	989.4	E863.6	—	E950.6	E962.1	E980.7
gas or vapor	987.8	E869.8	—	E952.8	E962.2	E982.8
Formalin	989.89	E861.4	—	E950.9	E962.1	E980.9
fungicide	989.4	E863.6	—	E950.6	E962.1	E980.7
vapor	987.8	E869.8	—	E952.8	E962.2	E982.8
Formic acid	983.1	E864.1	—	E950.7	E962.1	E980.6
vapor	987.8	E869.8	—	E952.8	E962.2	E982.8
Fowler's solution	985.1	E866.3	—	E950.8	E962.1	E980.8
Foxglove	988.2	E865.4	—	E950.9	E962.1	E980.9

Substance	Poisoning	Accident	Therapeutic Use	Suicide Attempt	Assault	Undetermined
			External Cause (E-Code)			
Fox green 977.8	E858.8	E947.8	E950.4	E962.0	E980.4
Framycetin 960.8	E856	E930.8	E950.4	E962.0	E980.4
Frangula (extract). 973.1	E858.4	E943.1	E950.4	E962.0	E980.4
Frei antigen 977.8	E858.8	E947.8	E950.4	E962.0	E980.4
Freons 987.4	E869.2	—	E952.8	E962.2	E982.8
Fructose 974.5	E858.5	E944.5	E950.4	E962.0	E980.4
Frusemide 974.4	E858.5	E944.4	E950.4	E962.0	E980.4
FSH 962.4	E858.0	E932.4	E950.4	E962.0	E980.4
Fuel					
automobile. 981	E862.1	—	E950.9	E962.1	E980.9
exhaust gas, not in transit. 986	E868.2	—	E952.0	E962.2	E982.0
vapor NEC 987.1	E869.8	—	E952.8	E962.2	E982.8
gas (domestic use) — see also Carbon, monoxide, fuel					
utility 987.1	E868.1	—	E951.8	E962.2	E981.8
incomplete combustion of — see Carbon, monoxide, fuel, utility					
in mobile container. 987.0	E868.0	—	E951.1	E962.2	E981.1
piped (natural). 987.1	E867	—	E951.0	E962.2	E981.0
industrial, incomplete combustion 986	E868.3	—	E952.1	E962.2	E982.1
Fugillin 960.8	E856	E930.8	E950.4	E962.0	E980.4
Fulminate of mercury 985.0	E866.1	—	E950.9	E962.1	E980.9
Fulvicin. 960.1	E856	E930.1	E950.4	E962.0	E980.4
Fumadil. 960.8	E856	E930.8	E950.4	E962.0	E980.4
Fumagillin 960.8	E856	E930.8	E950.4	E962.0	E980.4
Fumes (from) 987.9	E869.9	—	E952.9	E962.2	E982.9
carbon monoxide — see Carbon, monoxide					
charcoal (domestic use) 986	E868.3	—	E952.1	E962.2	E982.1
chloroform — see Chloroform					
coke (in domestic stoves, fireplaces) 986	E868.3	—	E952.1	E962.2	E982.1
corrosive NEC 987.8	E869.8	—	E952.8	E962.2	E982.8
ether — see Ether(s)					
freons 987.4	E869.2	—	E952.8	E962.2	E982.8
hydrocarbons 987.1	E869.8	—	E952.8	E962.2	E982.8
petroleum (liquefied) 987.0	E868.0	—	E951.1	E962.2	E981.1
distributed through pipes (pure or mixed with air) 987.0	E867	—	E951.0	E962.2	E981.0
lead — see Lead					
metals — see specified metal					
nitrogen dioxide 987.2	E869.0	—	E952.8	E962.2	E982.8
pesticides — see Pesticides					
petroleum (liquefied) 987.0	E868.0	—	E951.1	E962.2	E981.1
distributed through pipes (pure or mixed with air) 987.0	E867	—	E951.0	E962.2	E981.0
polyester 987.8	E869.8	—	E952.8	E962.2	E982.8
specified source, other (see also substance specified) 987.8	E869.8	—	E952.8	E962.2	E982.8
sulfur dioxide 987.3	E869.1	—	E952.8	E962.2	E982.8
Fumigants 989.4	E863.8	—	E950.6	E962.1	E980.7
Fungi, noxious, used as food 988.1	E865.5	—	E950.9	E962.1	E980.9
Fungicides (see also Antifungals) 989.4	E863.6	—	E950.6	E962.1	E980.7
Fungizone. 960.1	E856	E930.1	E950.4	E962.0	E980.4
topical 976.0	E858.7	E946.0	E950.4	E962.0	E980.4
Furacin 976.0	E858.7	E946.0	E950.4	E962.0	E980.4
Furadantin. 961.9	E857	E931.9	E950.4	E962.0	E980.4
Furazolidone 961.9	E857	E931.9	E950.4	E962.0	E980.4
Furnace (coal burning) (domestic), gas from 986	E868.3	—	E952.1	E962.2	E982.1
industrial 986	E868.8	—	E952.1	E962.2	E982.1
Furniture polish 989.89	E861.2	—	E950.9	E962.1	E980.9
Furosemide 974.4	E858.5	E944.4	E950.4	E962.0	E980.4

TABLE OF DRUGS AND CHEMICALS

Substance	Poisoning	Accident	Therapeutic Use	Suicide Attempt	Assault	Undetermined
			External Cause (E-Code)			
Furoxone 961.9	E857	E931.9	E950.4	E962.0	E980.4	
Fusel oil (amyl) (butyl) (propyl). 980.3	E860.4	—	E950.9	E962.1	E980.9	
Fusidic acid 960.8	E856	E930.8	E950.4	E962.0	E980.4	
Gallamine 975.2	E858.6	E945.2	E950.4	E962.0	E980.4	
Gallotannic acid 976.2	E858.7	E946.2	E950.4	E962.0	E980.4	
Gamboge 973.1	E858.4	E943.1	E950.4	E962.0	E980.4	
Gamimune 964.6	E858.2	E934.6	E950.4	E962.0	E980.4	
Gamma–benzene hexachloride (vapor) 989.2	E863.0	—	E950.6	E962.1	E980.7	
Gamma globulin 964.6	E858.2	E934.6	E950.4	E962.0	E980.4	
Gamma Hydroxy Butyrate (GHB) 968.4	E855.1	E938.4	E950.4	E962.0	E980.4	
Gamulin 964.6	E858.2	E934.6	E950.4	E962.0	E980.4	
Ganglionic blocking agents. 972.3	E858.3	E942.3	E950.4	E962.0	E980.4	
Ganja. 969.6	E854.1	E939.6	E950.3	E962.0	E980.3	
Garamycin 960.8	E856	E930.8	E950.4	E962.0	E980.4	
ophthalmic preparation. 976.5	E858.7	E946.5	E950.4	E962.0	E980.4	
topical NEC 976.0	E858.7	E946.0	E950.4	E962.0	E980.4	
Gardenal 967.0	E851	E937.0	E950.1	E962.0	E980.1	
Gardepanyl 967.0	E851	E937.0	E950.1	E962.0	E980.1	
Gas 987.9	E869.9	—	E952.9	E962.2	E982.9	
acetylene 987.1	E868.1	—	E951.8	E962.2	E981.8	
incomplete combustion of — see Carbon, monoxide, fuel, utility						
air contaminants, source or type not specified 987.9	E869.9	—	E952.9	E962.2	E982.9	
anesthetic (general) NEC. 968.2	E855.1	E938.2	E950.4	E962.0	E980.4	
blast furnace 986	E868.8	—	E952.1	E962.2	E982.1	
butane — see Butane						
carbon monoxide — see Carbon, monoxide						
chlorine 987.6	E869.8	—	E952.8	E962.2	E982.8	
coal — see Carbon, monoxide, coal						
cyanide 987.7	E869.8	—	E952.8	E962.2	E982.8	
dicyanogen. 987.8	E869.8	—	E952.8	E962.2	E982.8	
domestic — see Gas, utility						
exhaust — see Carbon, monoxide, exhaust gas						
from wood– or coal–burning stove or fireplace 986	E868.3	—	E952.1	E962.2	E982.1	
fuel (domestic use) — see also Carbon, monoxide, fuel						
industrial use 986	E868.8	—	E952.1	E962.2	E982.1	
utility 987.1	E868.1	—	E951.8	E962.2	E981.8	
incomplete combustion of — see Carbon, monoxide, fuel, utility						
in mobile container. 987.0	E868.0	—	E951.1	E962.2	E981.1	
piped (natural). 987.1	E867	—	E951.0	E962.2	E981.0	
garage 986	E868.2	—	E952.0	E962.2	E982.0	
hydrocarbon NEC. 987.1	E869.8	—	E952.8	E962.2	E982.8	
incomplete combustion of — see Carbon, monoxide, fuel, utility						
liquefied (mobile container) 987.0	E868.0	—	E951.1	E962.2	E981.1	
piped 987.0	E867	—	E951.0	E962.2	E981.0	
hydrocyanic acid 987.7	E869.8	—	E952.8	E962.2	E982.8	
illuminating — see Gas, utility						
incomplete combustion, any — see Carbon, monoxide						
kiln. 986	E868.8	—	E952.1	E962.2	E982.1	
lacrimogenic 987.5	E869.3	—	E952.8	E962.2	E982.8	
marsh. 987.1	E869.8	—	E952.8	E962.2	E982.8	
motor exhaust, not in transit 986	E868.8	—	E952.1	E962.2	E982.1	
mustard — see Mustard, gas						
natural 987.1	E867	—	E951.0	E962.2	E981.0	

Substance	Poisoning	Accident	Therapeutic Use	Suicide Attempt	Assault	Undetermined
			External Cause (E-Code)			
nerve (war) 987.9	E869.9	—	E952.9	E962.2	E982.9
oils. 981	E862.1	—	E950.9	E962.1	E980.9
petroleum (liquefied) (distributed in					
mobile containers) 987.0	E868.0	—	E951.1	E962.2	E981.1
piped (pure or mixed with air). 987.0	E867	—	E951.1	E962.2	E981.1
piped (manufactured) (natural) NEC 987.1	E867	—	E951.0	E962.2	E981.0
producer. 986	E868.8	—	E952.1	E962.2	E982.1
propane — see Propane					
refrigerant (freon). 987.4	E869.2	—	E952.8	E962.2	E982.8
not freon. 987.9	E869.9	—	E952.9	E962.2	E982.9
sewer 987.8	E869.8	—	E952.8	E962.2	E982.8
specified source NEC (see also substance					
specified). 987.8	E869.8	—	E952.8	E962.2	E982.8
stove — see Gas, utility					
tear. 987.5	E869.3	—	E952.8	E962.2	E982.8
utility (for cooking, heating, or lighting)					
(piped) NEC 987.1	E868.1	—	E951.8	E962.2	E981.8
incomplete combustion of — see Carbon,					
monoxide, fuel, utility					
in mobile container 987.0	E868.0	—	E951.1	E962.2	E981.1
piped (natural) 987.1	E867	—	E951.0	E962.2	E981.0
water 987.1	E868.1	—	E951.8	E962.2	E981.8
incomplete combustion of — see Carbon,					
monoxide, fuel, utility					
Gaseous substance — see Gas					
Gasoline, gasolene 981	E862.1	—	E950.9	E962.1	E980.9
vapor 987.1	E869.8	—	E952.8	E962.2	E982.8
Gastric enzymes 973.4	E858.4	E943.4	E950.4	E962.0	E980.4
Gastrografin 977.8	E858.8	E947.8	E950.4	E962.0	E980.4
Gastrointestinal agents. 973.9	E858.4	E943.9	E950.4	E962.0	E980.4
specified NEC 973.8	E858.4	E943.8	E950.4	E962.0	E980.4
Gaultheria procumbens 988.2	E865.4	—	E950.9	E962.1	E980.9
Gelatin (intravenous) 964.8	E858.2	E934.8	E950.4	E962.0	E980.4
absorbable (sponge). 964.5	E858.2	E934.5	E950.4	E962.0	E980.4
Gelfilm 976.8	E858.7	E946.8	E950.4	E962.0	E980.4
Gelfoam 964.5	E858.2	E934.5	E950.4	E962.0	E980.4
Gelsemine. 970.89	E854.3	E940.8	E950.4	E962.0	E980.4
Gelsemium (sempervirens) 988.2	E865.4	—	E950.9	E962.1	E980.9
Gemonil 967.0	E851	E937.0	E950.1	E962.0	E980.1
Gentamicin 960.8	E856	E930.8	E950.4	E962.0	E980.4
ophthalmic preparation. 976.5	E858.7	E946.5	E950.4	E962.0	E980.4
topical NEC 976.0	E858.7	E946.0	E950.4	E962.0	E980.4
Gentian violet 976.0	E858.7	E946.0	E950.4	E962.0	E980.4
Gexane 976.0	E858.7	E946.0	E950.4	E962.0	E980.4
Gila monster (venom) 989.5	E905.0	—	E950.9	E962.1	E980.9
Ginger, Jamaica 989.89	E866.8	—	E950.9	E962.1	E980.9
Gitalin 972.1	E858.3	E942.1	E950.4	E962.0	E980.4
Gitoxin 972.1	E858.3	E942.1	E950.4	E962.0	E980.4
Glandular extract (medicinal) NEC 977.9	E858.9	E947.9	E950.5	E962.0	E980.5
Glaucarubin 961.5	E857	E931.5	E950.4	E962.0	E980.4
Globin zinc insulin 962.3	E858.0	E932.3	E950.4	E962.0	E980.4
Glucagon 962.3	E858.0	E932.3	E950.4	E962.0	E980.4
Glucochloral. 967.1	E852.0	E937.1	E950.2	E962.0	E980.2
Glucocorticoids 962.0	E858.0	E932.0	E950.4	E962.0	E980.4
Glucose. 974.5	E858.5	E944.5	E950.4	E962.0	E980.4
oxidase reagent 977.8	E858.8	E947.8	E950.4	E962.0	E980.4
Glucosulfone sodium 961.8	E857	E931.8	E950.4	E962.0	E980.4
Glue(s) 989.89	E866.6	—	E950.9	E962.1	E980.9
Glutamic acid (hydrochloride) 973.4	E858.4	E943.4	E950.4	E962.0	E980.4
Glutaraldehyde 989.89	E861.4	—	E950.9	E962.1	E980.9
Glutathione 963.8	E858.1	E933.8	E950.4	E962.0	E980.4

Substance	Poisoning	Accident	Therapeutic Use	Suicide Attempt	Assault	Undetermined
			External Cause (E-Code)			
Glutethimide (group)	967.5	E852.4	E937.5	E950.2	E962.0	E980.2
Glycerin (lotion)	976.3	E858.7	E946.3	E950.4	E962.0	E980.4
Glycerol (topical)	976.3	E858.7	E946.3	E950.4	E962.0	E980.4
Glyceryl						
guaiacolate	975.5	E858.6	E945.5	E950.4	E962.0	E980.4
triacetate (topical)	976.0	E858.7	E946.0	E950.4	E962.0	E980.4
trinitrate	972.4	E858.3	E942.4	E950.4	E962.0	E980.4
Glycine	974.5	E858.5	E944.5	E950.4	E962.0	E980.4
Glycobiarsol	961.1	E857	E931.1	E950.4	E962.0	E980.4
Glycols (ether)	982.8	E862.4	—	E950.9	E962.1	E980.9
Glycopyrrolate	971.1	E855.4	E941.1	E950.4	E962.0	E980.4
Glymidine	962.3	E858.0	E932.3	E950.4	E962.0	E980.4
Gold (compounds) (salts)	965.69	E850.6	E935.6	E950.0	E962.0	E980.0
Golden sulfide of antimony	985.4	E866.2	—	E950.9	E962.1	E980.9
Goldylocks	988.2	E865.4	—	E950.9	E962.1	E980.9
Gonadal tissue extract	962.9	E858.0	E932.9	E950.4	E962.0	E980.4
female	962.2	E858.0	E932.2	E950.4	E962.0	E980.4
male	961.1	E858.0	E932.1	E950.4	E962.0	E980.4
Gonadotropin	962.4	E858.0	E932.4	E950.4	E962.0	E980.4
Grain alcohol	980.0	E860.1	—	E950.9	E962.1	E980.9
beverage	980.0	E860.0	—	E950.9	E962.1	E980.9
Gramicidin	960.8	E856	E930.8	E950.4	E962.0	E980.4
Gratiola officinalis	988.2	E865.4	—	E950.9	E962.1	E980.9
Grease	989.89	E866.8	—	E950.9	E962.1	E980.9
Green hellebore	988.2	E865.4	—	E950.9	E962.1	E980.9
Green soap	976.2	E858.7	E946.2	E950.4	E962.0	E980.4
Grifulvin	960.1	E856	E930.1	E950.4	E962.0	E980.4
Griseofulvin	960.1	E856	E930.1	E950.4	E962.0	E980.4
Growth hormone	962.4	E858.0	E932.4	E950.4	E962.0	E980.4
Guaiacol	975.5	E858.6	E945.5	E950.4	E962.0	E980.4
Guaiac reagent	977.8	E858.8	E947.8	E950.4	E962.0	E980.4
Guaifenesin	975.5	E858.6	E945.5	E950.4	E962.0	E980.4
Guaiphenesin	975.5	E858.6	E945.5	E950.4	E962.0	E980.4
Guanatol	961.4	E857	E931.4	E950.4	E962.0	E980.4
Guanethidine	972.6	E858.3	E942.6	E950.4	E962.0	E980.4
Guano	989.89	E866.5	—	E950.9	E962.1	E980.9
Guanochlor	972.6	E858.3	E942.6	E950.4	E962.0	E980.4
Guanoctine	972.6	E858.3	E942.6	E950.4	E962.0	E980.4
Guanoxan	972.6	E858.3	E942.6	E950.4	E962.0	E980.4
Hair treatment agent NEC	976.4	E858.7	E946.4	E950.4	E962.0	E980.4
Halcinonide	976.0	E858.7	E946.0	E950.4	E962.0	E980.4
Halethazole	976.0	E858.7	E946.0	E950.4	E962.0	E980.4
Hallucinogens	969.6	E854.1	E939.6	E950.3	E962.0	E980.3
Haloperidol	969.2	E853.1	E939.2	E950.3	E962.0	E980.3
Haloprogin	976.0	E858.7	E946.0	E950.4	E962.0	E980.4
Halotex	976.0	E858.7	E946.0	E950.4	E962.0	E980.4
Halothane	968.1	E855.1	E938.1	E950.4	E962.0	E980.4
Halquinols	976.0	E858.7	E946.0	E950.4	E962.0	E980.4
Hand sanitizer	976.0	E858.7	E946.0	E950.4	E962.0	E980.4
Harmonyl	972.6	E858.3	E942.6	E950.4	E962.0	E980.4
Hartmann's solution	974.5	E858.5	E944.5	E950.4	E962.0	E980.4
Hashish	969.6	E854.1	E939.6	E950.3	E962.0	E980.3
Hawaiian wood rose seeds	969.6	E854.1	E939.6	E950.3	E962.0	E980.3
Headache cures, drugs, powders NEC	977.9	E858.9	E947.9	E950.5	E962.0	E980.9
Heavenly Blue (morning glory)	969.6	E854.1	E939.6	E950.3	E962.0	E980.3
Heavy metal						
antagonists	963.8	E858.1	E933.8	E950.4	E962.0	E980.4
anti–infectives	961.2	E857	E931.2	E950.4	E962.0	E980.4
Hedaquinium	976.0	E858.7	E946.0	E950.4	E962.0	E980.4
Hedge hyssop	988.2	E865.4	—	E950.9	E962.1	E980.9

TABLE OF DRUGS AND CHEMICALS

Substance	Poisoning	Accident	Therapeutic Use	Suicide Attempt	Assault	Undetermined
			External Cause (E-Code)			
Heet 976.8	E858.7	E946.8	E950.4	E962.0	E980.4
Helenin 961.6	E857	E931.6	E950.4	E962.0	E980.4
Hellebore (black) (green) (white) 988.2	E865.4	—	E950.9	E962.1	E980.9
Hemlock 988.2	E865.4	—	E950.9	E962.1	E980.9
Hemostatics 964.5	E858.2	E934.5	E950.4	E962.0	E980.4
capillary active drugs 972.8	E858.3	E942.8	E950.4	E962.0	E980.4
Henbane 988.2	E865.4	—	E950.9	E962.1	E980.9
Heparin (sodium) 964.2	E858.2	E934.2	E950.4	E962.0	E980.4
Heptabarbital, heptabarbitone 967.0	E851	E937.0	E950.1	E962.0	E980.1
Heptachlor 989.2	E863.0	—	E950.6	E962.1	E980.7
Heptalgin 965.09	E850.2	E935.2	E950.0	E962.0	E980.0
Herbicides 989.4	E863.5	—	E950.6	E962.1	E980.7
Heroin 965.01	E850.0	E935.0	E950.0	E962.0	E980.0
Herplex 976.5	E858.7	E946.5	E950.4	E962.0	E980.4
HES 964.8	E858.2	E934.8	E950.4	E962.0	E980.4
Hetastarch 964.8	E858.2	E934.8	E950.4	E962.0	E980.4
Hexachlorocyclohexane 989.2	E863.0	—	E950.6	E962.1	E980.7
Hexachlorophene 976.2	E858.7	E946.2	E950.4	E962.0	E980.4
Hexadimethrine (bromide) 964.5	E858.2	E934.5	E950.4	E962.0	E980.4
Hexafluorenium 975.2	E858.6	E945.2	E950.4	E962.0	E980.4
Hexa–germ 976.2	E858.7	E946.2	E950.4	E962.0	E980.4
Hexahydrophenol 980.8	E860.8	—	E950.9	E962.1	E980.9
Hexalin 980.8	E860.8	—	E950.9	E962.1	E980.9
Hexamethonium 972.3	E858.3	E942.3	E950.4	E962.0	E980.4
Hexamethyleneamine 961.9	E857	E931.9	E950.4	E962.0	E980.4
Hexamine 961.9	E857	E931.9	E950.4	E962.0	E980.4
Hexanone 982.8	E862.4	—	E950.9	E962.1	E980.9
Hexapropymate 967.8	E852.8	E937.8	E950.2	E962.0	E980.2
Hexestrol 962.2	E858.0	E932.2	E950.4	E962.0	E980.4
Hexethal (sodium) 967.0	E851	E937.0	E950.1	E962.0	E980.1
Hexetidine 976.0	E858.7	E946.0	E950.4	E962.0	E980.4
Hexobarbital, hexobarbitone 967.0	E851	E937.0	E950.1	E962.0	E980.1
sodium (anesthetic) 968.3	E855.1	E938.3	E950.4	E962.0	E980.4
soluble 968.3	E855.1	E938.3	E950.4	E962.0	E980.4
Hexocyclium 971.1	E855.4	E941.1	E950.4	E962.0	E980.4
Hexoestrol 962.2	E858.0	E932.2	E950.4	E962.0	E980.4
Hexone 982.8	E862.4	—	E950.9	E962.1	E980.9
Hexylcaine 968.5	E855.2	E938.5	E950.4	E962.0	E980.4
Hexylresorcinol 961.6	E857	E931.6	E950.4	E962.0	E980.4
Hinkle's pills 973.1	E858.4	E943.1	E950.4	E962.0	E980.4
Histalog 977.8	E858.8	E947.8	E950.4	E962.0	E980.4
Histamine (phosphate) 972.5	E858.3	E942.5	E950.4	E962.0	E980.4
Histoplasmin 977.8	E858.8	E947.8	E950.4	E962.0	E980.4
Holly berries 988.2	E865.3	—	E950.9	E962.1	E980.9
Homatropine 971.1	E855.4	E941.1	E950.4	E962.0	E980.4
Homo–tet 964.6	E858.2	E934.6	E950.4	E962.0	E980.4
Hormones (synthetic substitute) NEC 962.9	E858.0	E932.9	E950.4	E962.0	E980.4
adrenal cortical steroids 962.0	E858.0	E932.0	E950.4	E962.0	E980.4
antidiabetic agents 962.3	E858.0	E932.3	E950.4	E962.0	E980.4
follicle stimulating 962.4	E858.0	E932.4	E950.4	E962.0	E980.4
gonadotropic 962.4	E858.0	E932.4	E950.4	E962.0	E980.4
growth 962.4	E858.0	E932.4	E950.4	E962.0	E980.4
ovarian (substitutes) 962.2	E858.0	E932.2	E950.4	E962.0	E980.4
parathyroid (derivatives) 962.6	E858.0	E932.6	E950.4	E962.0	E980.4
pituitary (posterior) 962.5	E858.0	E932.5	E950.4	E962.0	E980.4
anterior 962.4	E858.0	E932.4	E950.4	E962.0	E980.4
thyroid (derivative) 962.7	E858.0	E932.7	E950.4	E962.0	E980.4
Hornet (sting) 989.5	E905.3	—	E950.9	E962.1	E980.9
Horticulture agent NEC 989.4	E863.9	—	E950.6	E962.1	E980.7
Hyaluronidase 963.4	E858.1	E933.4	E950.4	E962.0	E980.4
Hyazyme 963.4	E858.1	E933.4	E950.4	E962.0	E980.4

Substance	Poisoning	Accident	Therapeutic Use	Suicide Attempt	Assault	Undetermined
			External Cause (E-Code)			
Hycodan	965.09	E850.2	E935.2	E950.0	E962.0	E980.0
Hydantoin derivatives	966.1	E855.0	E936.1	E950.4	E962.0	E980.4
Hydeltra	962.0	E858.0	E932.0	E950.4	E962.0	E980.4
Hydergine	971.3	E855.6	E941.3	E950.4	E962.0	E980.4
Hydrabamine penicillin	960.0	E856	E930.0	E950.4	E962.0	E980.4
Hydralazine, hydrallazine	972.6	E858.3	E942.6	E950.4	E962.0	E980.4
Hydrargaphen	976.0	E858.7	E946.0	E950.4	E962.0	E980.4
Hydrazine	983.9	E864.3	—	E950.7	E962.1	E980.6
Hydriodic acid	975.5	E858.6	E945.5	E950.4	E962.0	E980.4
Hydrocarbon gas	987.1	E869.8	—	E952.8	E962.2	E982.8
incomplete combustion of — see						
Carbon, monoxide, fuel, utility						
liquefied (mobile container)	987.0	E868.0	—	E951.1	E962.2	E981.1
piped (natural)	987.0	E867	—	E951.0	E962.2	E981.0
Hydrochloric acid (liquid)	983.1	E864.1	—	E950.7	E962.1	E980.6
medicinal	973.4	E858.4	E943.4	E950.4	E962.0	E980.4
vapor	987.8	E869.8	—	E952.8	E962.2	E982.8
Hydrochlorothiazide	974.3	E858.5	E944.3	E950.4	E962.0	E980.4
Hydrocodone	965.09	E850.2	E935.2	E950.0	E962.0	E980.0
Hydrocortisone	962.0	E858.0	E932.0	E950.4	E962.0	E980.4
ENT agent	976.6	E858.7	E946.6	E950.4	E962.0	E980.4
ophthalmic preparation	976.5	E858.7	E946.5	E950.4	E962.0	E980.4
topical NEC	976.0	E858.7	E946.0	E950.4	E962.0	E980.4
Hydrocortone	962.0	E858.0	E932.0	E950.4	E962.0	E980.4
ENT agent	976.6	E858.7	E946.6	E950.4	E962.0	E980.4
ophthalmic preparation	976.5	E858.7	E946.5	E950.4	E962.0	E980.4
topical NEC	976.0	E858.7	E946.0	E950.4	E962.0	E980.4
Hydrocyanic acid — see Cyanide(s)						
Hydroflumethiazide	974.3	E858.5	E944.3	E950.4	E962.0	E980.4
Hydrofluoric acid (liquid)	983.1	E864.1	—	E950.7	E962.1	E980.6
vapor	987.8	E869.8	—	E952.8	E962.2	E982.8
Hydrogen	987.8	E869.8	—	E952.8	E962.2	E982.8
arsenide	985.1	E866.3	—	E950.8	E962.1	E980.8
arseniureted	985.1	E866.3	—	E950.8	E962.1	E980.8
cyanide (salts)	989.0	E866.8	—	E950.9	E962.1	E980.9
gas	987.7	E869.8	—	E952.8	E962.2	E982.8
fluoride (liquid)	983.1	E864.1	—	E950.7	E962.1	E980.6
vapor	987.8	E869.8	—	E952.8	E962.2	E982.8
peroxide (solution)	976.6	E858.7	E946.6	E950.4	E962.0	E980.4
phosphureted	987.8	E869.8	—	E952.8	E962.2	E982.8
sulfide (gas)	987.8	E869.8	—	E952.8	E962.2	E982.8
arseniureted	985.1	E866.3	—	E950.8	E962.1	E980.8
sulfureted	987.8	E869.8	—	E952.8	E962.2	E982.8
Hydromorphinol	965.09	E850.2	E935.2	E950.0	E962.0	E980.0
Hydromorphinone	965.09	E850.2	E935.2	E950.0	E962.0	E980.0
Hydromorphone	965.09	E850.2	E935.2	E950.0	E962.0	E980.0
Hydromox	974.3	E858.5	E944.3	E950.4	E962.0	E980.4
Hydrophilic lotion	976.3	E858.7	E946.3	E950.4	E962.0	E980.4
Hydroquinone	983.0	E864.0	—	E950.7	E962.1	E980.6
vapor	987.8	E869.8	—	E952.8	E962.2	E982.8
Hydrosulfuric acid (gas)	987.8	E869.8	—	E952.8	E962.2	E982.8
Hydrous wool fat (lotion)	976.3	E858.7	E946.3	E950.4	E962.0	E980.4
Hydroxide, caustic	983.2	E864.2	—	E950.7	E962.1	E980.6
Hydroxocobalamin	964.1	E858.2	E934.1	E950.4	E962.0	E980.4
Hydroxyamphetamine	971.2	E855.5	E941.2	E950.4	E962.0	E980.4
Hydroxychloroquine	961.4	E857	E931.4	E950.4	E962.0	E980.4
Hydroxydihydrocodeinone	965.09	E850.2	E935.2	E950.0	E962.0	E980.0
Hydroxyethyl starch	964.8	E858.2	E934.8	E950.4	E962.0	E980.4
Hydroxyphenamate	969.5	E853.8	E939.5	E950.3	E962.0	E980.3
Hydroxyphenylbutazone	965.5	E850.5	E935.5	E950.0	E962.0	E980.0

Substance	Poisoning	Accident	Therapeutic Use	Suicide Attempt	Assault	Undetermined
			External Cause (E-Code)			
Hydroxyprogesterone 962.2	E858.0	E932.2	E950.4	E962.0	E980.4
Hydroxyquinoline derivatives 961.3	E857	E931.3	E950.4	E962.0	E980.4
Hydroxystilbamidine 961.5	E857	E931.5	E950.4	E962.0	E980.4
Hydroxyurea. 963.1	E858.1	E933.1	E950.4	E962.0	E980.4
Hydroxyzine. 969.5	E853.8	E939.5	E950.3	E962.0	E980.3
Hyoscine (hydrobromide) 971.1	E855.4	E941.1	E950.4	E962.0	E980.4
Hyoscyamine 971.1	E855.4	E941.1	E950.4	E962.0	E980.4
Hyoscyamus (albus) (niger) 988.2	E865.4	—	E950.9	E962.1	E980.9
Hypaque 977.8	E858.8	E947.8	E950.4	E962.0	E980.4
Hypertussis 964.6	E858.2	E934.6	E950.4	E962.0	E980.4
Hypnotics NEC 967.9	E852.9	E937.9	E950.2	E962.0	E980.2
Hypochlorites — see Sodium, hypochlorite					
Hypotensive agents NEC. 972.6	E858.3	E942.6	E950.4	E962.0	E980.4
Ibufenac 965.69	E850.6	E935.6	E950.0	E962.0	E980.0
ibuprofen 965.61	E850.6	E935.6	E950.0	E962.0	E980.0
ICG 977.8	E858.8	E947.8	E950.4	E962.0	E980.4
Ichthammol 976.4	E858.7	E946.4	E950.4	E962.0	E980.4
Ichthyol. 976.4	E858.7	E946.4	E950.4	E962.0	E980.4
Idoxuridine 976.5	E858.7	E946.5	E950.4	E962.0	E980.4
IDU 976.5	E858.7	E946.5	E950.4	E962.0	E980.4
Iletin 962.3	E858.0	E932.3	E950.4	E962.0	E980.4
Ilex 988.2	E865.4	—	E950.9	E962.1	E980.9
Illuminating gas — see Gas, utility					
Ilopan 963.5	E858.1	E933.5	E950.4	E962.0	E980.4
Ilotycin 960.3	E856	E930.3	E950.4	E962.0	E980.4
ophthalmic preparation. 976.5	E858.7	E946.5	E950.4	E962.0	E980.4
topical NEC 976.0	E858.7	E946.0	E950.4	E962.0	E980.4
Imipramine 969.05	E854.0	E939.0	E950.3	E962.0	E980.3
Immu–G 964.6	E858.2	E934.6	E950.4	E962.0	E980.4
Immuglobin 964.6	E858.2	E934.6	E950.4	E962.0	E980.4
Immune serum globulin 964.6	E858.2	E934.6	E950.4	E962.0	E980.4
Immunosuppressive agents 963.1	E858.1	E933.1	E950.4	E962.0	E980.4
Immu–tetanus 964.6	E858.2	E934.6	E950.4	E962.0	E980.4
Indandione (derivatives) 964.2	E858.2	E934.2	E950.4	E962.0	E980.4
Inderal 972.0	E858.3	E942.0	E950.4	E962.0	E980.4
Indian					
hemp 969.6	E854.1	E939.6	E950.3	E962.0	E980.3
tobacco 988.2	E865.4	—	E950.9	E962.1	E980.9
Indigo carmine 977.8	E858.8	E947.8	E950.4	E962.0	E980.4
Indocin 965.69	E850.6	E935.6	E950.0	E962.0	E980.0
Indocyanine green 977.8	E858.8	E947.8	E950.4	E962.0	E980.4
Indomethacin 965.69	E850.6	E935.6	E950.0	E962.0	E980.0
Industrial					
alcohol 980.9	E860.9	—	E950.9	E962.1	E980.9
fumes. 987.8	E869.8	—	E952.8	E962.2	E982.8
solvents (fumes) (vapors). 982.8	E862.9	—	E950.9	E962.1	E980.9
Influenza vaccine. 979.6	E858.8	E949.6	E950.4	E962.0	E982.8
Ingested substances NEC 989.9	E866.9	—	E950.9	E962.1	E980.9
INH (isoniazid) 961.8	E857	E931.8	E950.4	E962.0	E980.4
Inhalation, gas (noxious) — see Gas					
Ink. 989.89	E866.8	—	E950.9	E962.1	E980.9
Innovar 967.6	E852.5	E937.6	E950.2	E962.0	E980.2
Inositol niacinate 972.2	E858.3	E942.2	E950.4	E962.0	E980.4
Inproquone 963.1	E858.1	E933.1	E950.4	E962.0	E980.4
Insect (sting), venomous 989.5	E905.5	—	E950.9	E962.1	E980.9
Insecticides (see also Pesticides) 989.4	E863.4	—	E950.6	E962.1	E980.7
chlorinated. 989.2	E863.0	—	E950.6	E962.1	E980.7
mixtures. 989.4	E863.3	—	E950.6	E962.1	E980.7
organochlorine (compounds) 989.2	E863.0	—	E950.6	E962.1	E980.7
organophosphorus (compounds) 989.3	E863.1	—	E950.6	E962.1	E980.7
Insular tissue extract 962.3	E858.0	E932.3	E950.4	E962.0	E980.4

Substance	Poisoning	Accident	Therapeutic Use	Suicide Attempt	Assault	Undetermined
			External Cause (E-Code)			
Insulin (amorphous) (globin) (isophane) (Lente) (NPH) (protamine) (Semilente) (Ultralente) (zinc) 962.3		E858.0	E932.3	E950.4	E962.0	E980.4
Intranarcon 968.3		E855.1	E938.3	E950.4	E962.0	E980.4
Inulin. 977.8		E858.8	E947.8	E950.4	E962.0	E980.4
Invert sugar 974.5		E858.5	E944.5	E950.4	E962.0	E980.4
Inza—*see* Naproxen						
Iodide NEC (*see also* Iodine). 976.0		E858.7	E946.0	E950.4	E962.0	E980.4
mercury (ointment) 976.0		E858.7	E946.0	E950.4	E962.0	E980.4
methylate 976.0		E858.7	E946.0	E950.4	E962.0	E980.4
potassium (expectorant) NEC 975.5		E858.6	E945.5	E950.4	E962.0	E980.4
Iodinated glycerol 975.5		E858.6	E945.5	E950.4	E962.0	E980.4
Iodine (antiseptic, external) (tincture)						
NEC 976.0		E858.7	E946.0	E950.4	E962.0	E980.4
diagnostic 977.8		E858.8	E947.8	E950.4	E962.0	E980.4
for thyroid conditions (antithyroid) 962.8		E858.0	E932.8	E950.4	E962.0	E980.4
vapor 987.8		E869.8	—	E952.8	E962.2	E982.8
Iodized oil 977.8		E858.8	E947.8	E950.4	E962.0	E980.4
Iodobismitol 961.2		E857	E931.2	E950.4	E962.0	E980.4
Iodochlorhydroxyquin 961.3		E857	E931.3	E950.4	E962.0	E980.4
topical 976.0		E858.7	E946.0	E950.4	E962.0	E980.4
Iodoform 976.0		E858.7	E946.0	E950.4	E962.0	E980.4
Iodopanoic acid 977.8		E858.8	E947.8	E950.4	E962.0	E980.4
Iodophthalein 977.8		E858.8	E947.8	E950.4	E962.0	E980.4
Ion exchange resins 974.5		E858.5	E944.5	E950.4	E962.0	E980.4
Iopanoic acid 977.8		E858.8	E947.8	E950.4	E962.0	E980.4
Iophendylate 977.8		E858.8	E947.8	E950.4	E962.0	E980.4
Iothiouracil 962.8		E858.0	E932.8	E950.4	E962.0	E980.4
Ipecac 973.6		E858.4	E943.6	E950.4	E962.0	E980.4
Ipecacuanha 973.6		E858.4	E943.6	E950.4	E962.0	E980.4
Ipodate 977.8		E858.8	E947.8	E950.4	E962.0	E980.4
Ipral 967.0		E851	E937.0	E950.1	E962.0	E980.1
Ipratropium 975.1		E858.6	E945.1	E950.4	E962.0	E980.4
Iproniazid 969.01		E854.0	E939.0	E950.3	E962.0	E980.3
Iron (compounds) (medicinal)						
(preparations) 964.0		E858.2	E934.0	E950.4	E962.0	E980.4
dextran 964.0		E858.2	E934.0	E950.4	E962.0	E980.4
nonmedicinal (dust) (fumes) NEC 985.8		E866.4	—	E950.9	E962.1	E980.9
Irritant drug 977.9		E858.9	E947.9	E950.5	E962.0	E980.5
Ismelin 972.6		E858.3	E942.6	E950.4	E962.0	E980.4
Isoamyl nitrite 972.4		E858.3	E942.4	E950.4	E962.0	E980.4
Isobutyl acetate 982.8		E862.4	—	E950.9	E962.1	E980.9
Isocarboxazid 969.01		E854.0	E939.0	E950.3	E962.0	E980.3
Isoephedrine 971.2		E855.5	E941.2	E950.4	E962.0	E980.4
Isoetharine 971.2		E855.5	E941.2	E950.4	E962.0	E980.4
Isofluorophate 971.0		E855.3	E941.0	E950.4	E962.0	E980.4
Isoniazid (INH) 961.8		E857	E931.8	E950.4	E962.0	E980.4
Isopentaquine 961.4		E857	E931.4	E950.4	E962.0	E980.4
Isophane insulin 962.3		E858.0	E932.3	E950.4	E962.0	E980.4
Isopregnenone 962.2		E858.0	E932.2	E950.4	E962.0	E980.4
Isoprenaline 971.2		E855.5	E941.2	E950.4	E962.0	E980.4
Isopropamide 971.1		E855.4	E941.1	E950.4	E962.0	E980.4
Isopropanol 980.2		E860.3	—	E950.9	E962.1	E980.9
topical (germicide) 976.0		E858.7	E946.0	E950.4	E962.0	E980.4
Isopropyl						
acetate 982.8		E862.4	—	E950.9	E962.1	E980.9
alcohol 980.2		E860.3	—	E950.9	E962.1	E980.9
topical (germicide). 976.0		E858.7	E946.0	E950.4	E962.0	E980.4
ether 982.8		E862.4	—	E950.9	E962.1	E980.9
Isoproterenol. 971.2		E855.5	E941.2	E950.4	E962.0	E980.4

Substance	Poisoning	Accident	Therapeutic Use	Suicide Attempt	Assault	Undetermined
			External Cause (E-Code)			
Isosorbide dinitrate 972.4	E858.3	E942.4	E950.4	E962.0	E980.4
Isothipendyl 963.0	E858.1	E933.0	E950.4	E962.0	E980.4
Isoxazolyl penicillin. 960.0	E856	E930.0	E950.4	E962.0	E980.4
Isoxsuprine hydrochloride 972.5	E858.3	E942.5	E950.4	E962.0	E980.4
I–thyroxine sodium 962.7	E858.0	E932.7	E950.4	E962.0	E980.4
Jaborandi (pilocarpus) (extract) 971.0	E855.3	E941.0	E950.4	E962.0	E980.4
Jalap 973.1	E858.4	E943.1	E950.4	E962.0	E980.4
Jamaica					
dogwood (bark). 965.7	E850.7	E935.7	E950.0	E962.0	E980.0
ginger. 989.89	E866.8	—	E950.9	E962.1	E980.9
Jatropha. 988.2	E865.4	—	E950.9	E962.1	E980.9
curcas. 988.2	E865.3	—	E950.9	E962.1	E980.9
Jectofer 964.0	E858.2	E934.0	E950.4	E962.0	E980.4
Jellyfish (sting). 989.5	E905.6	—	E950.9	E962.1	E980.9
Jequirity (bean) 988.2	E865.3	—	E950.9	E962.1	E980.9
Jimson weed. 988.2	E865.4	—	E950.9	E962.1	E980.9
seeds 988.2	E865.3	—	E950.9	E962.1	E980.9
Juniper tar (oil) (ointment) 976.4	E858.7	E946.4	E950.4	E962.0	E980.4
Kallikrein 972.5	E858.3	E942.5	E950.4	E962.0	E980.4
Kanamycin 960.6	E856	E930.6	E950.4	E962.0	E980.4
Kantrex 960.6	E856	E930.6	E950.4	E962.0	E980.4
Kaolin 973.5	E858.4	E943.5	E950.4	E962.0	E980.4
Karaya (gum) 973.3	E858.4	E943.3	E950.4	E962.0	E980.4
Kemithal 968.3	E855.1	E938.3	E950.4	E962.0	E980.4
Kenacort 962.0	E858.0	E932.0	E950.4	E962.0	E980.4
Keratolytics 976.4	E858.7	E946.4	E950.4	E962.0	E980.4
Keratoplastics 976.4	E858.7	E946.4	E950.4	E962.0	E980.4
Kerosene, kerosine (fuel) (solvent) NEC . . . 981	E862.1	—	E950.9	E962.1	E980.9
insecticide 981	E863.4	—	E950.6	E962.1	E980.7
vapor 987.1	E869.8	—	E952.8	E962.2	E982.8
Ketamine 968.3	E855.1	E938.3	E950.4	E962.0	E980.4
Ketobemidone 965.09	E850.2	E935.2	E950.0	E962.0	E980.0
Ketols 982.8	E862.4	—	E950.9	E962.1	E980.9
Ketone oils 982.8	E862.4	—	E950.9	E962.1	E980.9
Ketoprofen 965.61	E850.6	E935.6	E950.0	E962.0	E980.0
Kiln gas or vapor (carbon monoxide) 986	E868.8	—	E952.1	E962.2	E982.1
Konsyl 973.3	E858.4	E943.3	E950.4	E962.0	E980.4
Kosam seed 988.2	E865.3	—	E950.9	E962.1	E980.9
Krait (venom) 989.5	E905.0	—	E950.9	E962.1	E980.9
Kwell (insecticide) 989.2	E863.0	—	E950.6	E962.1	E980.7
anti–infective (topical) 976.0	E858.7	E946.0	E950.4	E962.0	E980.4
Laburnum (flowers) (seeds) 988.2	E865.3	—	E950.9	E962.1	E980.9
leaves 988.2	E865.4	—	E950.9	E962.1	E980.9
Lacquers 989.89	E861.6	—	E950.9	E962.1	E980.9
Lacrimogenic gas. 987.5	E869.3	—	E952.8	E962.2	E982.8
Lactic acid 983.1	E864.1	—	E950.7	E962.1	E980.6
Lactobacillus acidophilus 973.5	E858.4	E943.5	E950.4	E962.0	E980.4
Lactoflavin 963.5	E858.1	E933.5	E950.4	E962.0	E980.4
Lactuca (virosa) (extract) 967.8	E852.8	E937.8	E950.2	E962.0	E980.2
Lactucarium 967.8	E852.8	E937.8	E950.2	E962.0	E980.2
Laevulose 974.5	E858.5	E944.5	E950.4	E962.0	E980.4
Lanatoside(C) 972.1	E858.3	E942.1	E950.4	E962.0	E980.4
Lanolin (lotion) 976.3	E858.7	E946.3	E950.4	E962.0	E980.4
Largactil 969.1	E853.0	E939.1	E950.3	E962.0	E980.3
Larkspur 988.2	E865.3	—	E950.9	E962.1	E980.9
Laroxyl 969.05	E854.0	E939.0	E950.3	E962.0	E980.3
Lasix 974.4	E858.5	E944.4	E950.4	E962.0	E980.4
Latex 989.82	E866.8	—	E950.9	E962.1	E980.9
Lathyrus (seed). 988.2	E865.3	—	E950.9	E962.1	E980.9
Laudanum. 965.09	E850.2	E935.2	E950.0	E962.0	E980.0
Laudexium 975.2	E858.6	E945.2	E950.4	E962.0	E980.4

Substance	Poisoning	Accident	Therapeutic Use	Suicide Attempt	Assault	Undetermined
			External Cause (E-Code)			
Laurel, black or cherry	988.2	E865.4	—	E950.9	E962.1	E980.9
Laurolinium	976.0	E858.7	E946.0	E950.4	E962.0	E980.4
Lauryl sulfoacetate	976.2	E858.7	E946.2	E950.4	E962.0	E980.4
Laxatives NEC	973.3	E858.4	E943.3	E950.4	E962.0	E980.4
emollient	973.2	E858.4	E943.2	E950.4	E962.0	E980.4
L–dopa	966.4	E855.0	E936.4	E950.4	E962.0	E980.4
L Tryptophan—*see* amino acid						
Lead (dust) (fumes) (vapor) NEC	984.9	E866.0	—	E950.9	E962.1	E980.9
acetate (dust)	984.1	E866.0	—	E950.9	E962.1	E980.9
anti–infectives	961.2	E857	E931.2	E950.4	E962.0	E980.4
antiknock compound (tetraethyl)	984.1	E862.1	—	E950.9	E962.1	E980.9
arsenate, arsenite (dust) (insecticide)						
(vapor)	985.1	E863.4	—	E950.8	E962.1	E980.8
herbicide	985.1	E863.5	—	E950.8	E962.1	E980.8
carbonate	984.0	E866.0	—	E950.9	E962.1	E980.9
paint	984.0	E861.5	—	E950.9	E962.1	E980.9
chromate	984.0	E866.0	—	E950.9	E962.1	E980.9
paint	984.0	E861.5	—	E950.9	E962.1	E980.9
dioxide	984.0	E866.0	—	E950.9	E962.1	E980.9
inorganic (compound)	984.0	E866.0	—	E950.9	E962.1	E980.9
paint	984.0	E861.5	—	E950.9	E962.1	E980.9
iodine	984.0	E866.0	—	E950.9	E962.1	E980.9
pigment (paint)	984.0	E861.5	—	E950.9	E962.1	E980.9
monoxide (dust)	984.0	E866.0	—	E950.9	E962.1	E980.9
paint	984.0	E861.5	—	E950.9	E962.1	E980.9
organic	984.1	E866.0	—	E950.9	E962.1	E980.9
oxide	984.0	E866.0	—	E950.9	E962.1	E980.9
paint	984.0	E861.5	—	E950.9	E962.1	E980.9
paint	984.0	E861.5	—	E950.9	E962.1	E980.9
salts	984.0	E866.0	—	E950.9	E962.1	E980.9
specified compound NEC	984.8	E866.0	—	E950.9	E962.1	E980.9
tetra–ethyl	984.1	E862.1	—	E950.9	E962.1	E980.9
Lebanese red	969.6	E854.1	E939.6	E950.3	E962.0	E980.3
Lente Iletin (insulin)	962.3	E858.0	E932.3	E950.4	E962.0	E980.4
Leptazol	970.0	E854.3	E940.0	E950.4	E962.0	E980.4
Leritine	965.09	E850.2	E935.2	E950.0	E962.0	E980.0
Letter	962.7	E858.0	E932.7	E950.4	E962.0	E980.4
Lettuce opium	967.8	E852.8	E937.8	E950.2	E962.0	E980.2
Leucovorin (factor)	964.1	E858.2	E934.1	E950.4	E962.0	E980.4
Leukeran	963.1	E858.1	E933.1	E950.4	E962.0	E980.4
Levalbuterol	975.7	E858.6	E945.7	E950.4	E962.0	E980.4
Levallorphan	970.1	E854.3	E940.1	E950.4	E962.0	E980.4
Levanil	967.8	E852.8	E937.8	E950.2	E962.0	E980.2
Levarterenol	971.2	E855.5	E941.2	E950.4	E962.0	E980.4
Levodopa	966.4	E855.0	E936.4	E950.4	E962.0	E980.4
Levo–dromoran	965.09	E850.2	E935.2	E950.0	E962.0	E980.0
Levoid	962.7	E858.0	E932.7	E950.4	E962.0	E980.4
Levo–iso–methadone	965.02	E850.1	E935.1	E950.0	E962.0	E980.0
Levomepromazine	967.8	E852.8	E937.8	E950.2	E962.0	E980.2
Levoprome	967.8	E852.8	E937.8	E950.2	E962.0	E980.2
Levopropoxyphene	975.4	E858.6	E945.4	E950.4	E962.0	E980.4
Levorphan, levophanol	965.09	E850.2	E935.2	E950.0	E962.0	E980.0
Levothyroxine (sodium)	962.7	E858.0	E932.7	E950.4	E962.0	E980.4
Levsin	971.1	E855.4	E941.1	E950.4	E962.0	E980.4
Levulose	974.5	E858.5	E944.5	E950.4	E962.0	E980.4
Lewisite (gas)	985.1	E866.3	—	E950.8	E962.1	E980.8
Librium	969.4	E853.2	E939.4	E950.3	E962.0	E980.3
Lidex	976.0	E858.7	E946.0	E950.4	E962.0	E980.4
Lidocaine (infiltration) (topical)	968.5	E855.2	E938.5	E950.4	E962.0	E980.4
nerve block (peripheral) (plexus)	968.6	E855.2	E938.6	E950.4	E962.0	E980.4

Substance	Poisoning	Accident	Therapeutic Use	Suicide Attempt	Assault	Undetermined
			External Cause (E-Code)			
spinal 968.7	E855.2	E938.7	E950.4	E962.0	E980.4
Lighter fluid 981	E862.1	—	E950.9	E962.1	E980.9
Lignocaine (infiltration) (topical) 968.5	E855.2	E938.5	E950.4	E962.0	E980.4
nerve block (peripheral) (plexus) 968.6	E855.2	E938.6	E950.4	E962.0	E980.4
spinal 968.7	E855.2	E938.7	E950.4	E962.0	E980.4
Ligroin(e) (solvent) 981	E862.0	—	E950.9	E962.1	E980.9
vapor 987.1	E869.8	—	E952.8	E962.2	E982.8
Ligustrum vulgare 988.2	E865.3	—	E950.9	E962.1	E980.9
Lily of the valley 988.2	E865.4	—	E950.9	E962.1	E980.9
Lime (chloride) 983.2	E864.2	—	E950.7	E962.1	E980.6
solution, sulferated 976.4	E858.7	E946.4	E950.4	E962.0	E980.4
Limonene 982.8	E862.4	—	E950.9	E962.1	E980.9
Lincomycin 960.8	E856	E930.8	E950.4	E962.0	E980.4
Lindane (insecticide) (vapor) 989.2	E863.0	—	E950.6	E962.1	E980.7
anti–infective (topical) 976.0	E858.7	E946.0	E950.4	E962.0	E980.4
Liniments NEC 976.9	E858.7	E946.9	E950.4	E962.0	E980.4
Linoleic acid 972.2	E858.3	E942.2	E950.4	E962.0	E980.4
Liothyronine 962.7	E858.0	E932.7	E950.4	E962.0	E980.4
Liotrix 962.7	E858.0	E932.7	E950.4	E962.0	E980.4
Lipancreatin 973.4	E858.4	E943.4	E950.4	E962.0	E980.4
Lipo–Lutin 962.2	E858.0	E932.2	E950.4	E962.0	E980.4
Lipotropic agents 977.1	E858.8	E947.1	E950.4	E962.0	E980.4
Liquefied petroleum gases 987.0	E868.0	—	E951.1	E962.2	E981.1
piped (pure or mixed with air) 987.0	E867	—	E951.0	E962.2	E981.0
Liquid petrolatum 973.2	E858.4	E943.2	E950.4	E962.0	E980.4
substance 989.9	E866.9	—	E950.9	E962.1	E980.9
specified NEC 989.89	E866.8	—	E950.9	E962.1	E980.9
Lirugen 979.4	E858.8	E949.4	E950.4	E962.0	E980.4
Lithane 969.8	E855.8	E939.8	E950.3	E962.0	E980.3
Lithium 985.8	E866.4	—	E950.9	E962.1	E980.9
carbonate 969.8	E855.8	E939.8	E950.3	E962.0	E980.3
Lithonate 969.8	E855.8	E939.8	E950.3	E962.0	E980.3
Liver (extract) (injection) (preparations) . . . 964.1	E858.2	E934.1	E950.4	E962.0	E980.4
Lizard (bite) (venom) 989.5	E905.0	—	E950.9	E962.1	E980.9
LMD 964.8	E858.2	E934.8	E950.4	E962.0	E980.4
Lobelia 988.2	E865.4	—	E950.9	E962.1	E980.9
Lobeline 970.0	E854.3	E940.0	E950.4	E962.0	E980.4
Locorten 976.0	E858.7	E946.0	E950.4	E962.0	E980.4
Lolium temulentum 988.2	E865.3	—	E950.9	E962.1	E980.9
Lomotil 973.5	E858.4	E943.5	E950.4	E962.0	E980.4
Lomustine 963.1	E858.1	E933.1	E950.4	E962.0	E980.4
Lophophora williamsii 969.6	E854.1	E939.6	E950.3	E962.0	E980.3
Lorazepam 969.4	E853.2	E939.4	E950.3	E962.0	E980.3
Lotions NEC 976.9	E858.7	E946.9	E950.4	E962.0	E980.4
Lotronex 973.8	E858.4	E943.8	E950.4	E962.0	E980.4
Lotusate 967.0	E851	E937.0	E950.1	E962.0	E980.1
Lowila 976.2	E858.7	E946.2	E950.4	E962.0	E980.4
Loxapine 969.3	E853.8	E939.3	E950.3	E962.0	E980.3
Lozenges (throat) 976.6	E858.7	E946.6	E950.4	E962.0	E980.4
LSD (25) 969.6	E854.1	E939.6	E950.3	E962.0	E980.3
Lubricating oil NEC 981	E862.2	—	E950.9	E962.1	E980.9
Lucanthone 961.6	E857	E931.6	E950.4	E962.0	E980.4
Luminal 967.0	E851	E937.0	E950.1	E962.0	E980.1
Lung irritant (gas) NEC 987.9	E869.9	—	E952.9	E962.2	E982.9
Lutocylol 962.2	E858.0	E932.2	E950.4	E962.0	E980.4
Lutromone 962.2	E858.0	E932.2	E950.4	E962.0	E980.4
Lututrin 975.0	E858.6	E945.0	E950.4	E962.0	E980.4
Lye (concentrated) 983.2	E864.2	—	E950.7	E962.1	E980.6
Lygranum (skin test) 977.8	E858.8	E947.8	E950.4	E962.0	E980.4
Lymecycline 960.4	E856	E930.4	E950.4	E962.0	E980.4
Lymphogranuloma venereum antigen 977.8	E858.8	E947.8	E950.4	E962.0	E980.4

Substance	Poisoning	Accident	Therapeutic Use	Suicide Attempt	Assault	Undetermined
			External Cause (E-Code)			
Lynestrenol	962.2	E858.0	E932.2	E950.4	E962.0	E980.4
Lyovac Sodium Edecrin	974.4	E858.5	E944.4	E950.4	E962.0	E980.4
Lypressin	962.5	E858.0	E932.5	E950.4	E962.0	E980.4
Lysergic acid (amide) (diethylamide)	969.6	E854.1	E939.6	E950.3	E962.0	E980.3
Lysergide	969.6	E854.1	E939.6	E950.3	E962.0	E980.3
Lysine vasopressin	962.5	E858.0	E932.5	E950.4	E962.0	E980.4
Lysol	983.0	E864.0	—	E950.7	E962.1	E980.6
Lytta (vitatta)	976.8	E858.7	E946.8	E950.4	E962.0	E980.4
Mace	987.5	E869.3	—	E952.8	E962.2	E982.8
Macrolides (antibiotics)	960.3	E856	E930.3	E950.4	E962.0	E980.4
Mafenide	976.0	E858.7	E946.0	E950.4	E962.0	E980.4
Magaldrate	973.0	E858.4	E943.0	E950.4	E962.0	E980.4
Magic mushroom	969.6	E854.1	E939.6	E950.3	E962.0	E980.3
Magnamycin	960.8	E856	E930.8	E950.4	E962.0	E980.4
Magnesia magma	973.0	E858.4	E943.0	E950.4	E962.0	E980.4
Magnesium (compounds) (fumes) NEC	985.8	E866.4	—	E950.9	E962.1	E980.9
antacid	973.0	E858.4	E943.0	E950.4	E962.0	E980.4
carbonate	973.0	E858.4	E943.0	E950.4	E962.0	E980.4
cathartic	973.3	E858.4	E943.3	E950.4	E962.0	E980.4
citrate	973.3	E858.4	E943.3	E950.4	E962.0	E980.4
hydroxide	973.0	E858.4	E943.0	E950.4	E962.0	E980.4
oxide	973.0	E858.4	E943.0	E950.4	E962.0	E980.4
sulfate (oral)	973.3	E858.4	E943.3	E950.4	E962.0	E980.4
intravenous	966.3	E855.0	E936.3	E950.4	E962.0	E980.4
trisilicate	973.0	E858.4	E943.0	E950.4	E962.0	E980.4
Malathion (insecticide)	989.3	E863.1	—	E950.6	E962.1	E980.7
Male fern (oleoresin)	961.6	E857	E931.6	E950.4	E962.0	E980.4
Mandelic acid	961.9	E857	E931.9	E950.4	E962.0	E980.4
Manganese compounds (fumes) NEC	985.2	E866.4	—	E950.9	E962.1	E980.9
Mannitol (diuretic) (medicinal) NEC	974.4	E858.5	E944.4	E950.4	E962.0	E980.4
hexanitrate	972.4	E858.3	E942.4	E950.4	E962.0	E980.4
mustard	963.1	E858.1	E933.1	E950.4	E962.0	E980.4
Mannomustine	963.1	E858.1	E933.1	E950.4	E962.0	E980.4
MAO inhibitors	969.01	E854.0	E939.0	E950.3	E962.0	E980.3
Mapharsen	961.1	E857	E931.1	E950.4	E962.0	E980.4
Marcaine	968.9	E855.2	E938.9	E950.4	E962.0	E980.4
infiltration (subcutaneous)	968.5	E855.2	E938.5	E950.4	E962.0	E980.4
nerve block (peripheral) (plexus)	968.6	E855.2	E938.6	E950.4	E962.0	E980.4
Marezine	963.0	E858.1	E933.0	E950.4	E962.0	E980.4
Marihuana, marijuana (derivatives)	969.6	E854.1	E939.6	E950.3	E962.0	E980.3
Marine animals or plants (sting)	989.5	E905.6	—	E950.9	E962.1	E980.9
Marplan	969.01	E854.0	E939.0	E950.3	E962.0	E980.3
Marsh gas	987.1	E869.8	—	E952.8	E962.2	E982.8
Marsilid	969.01	E854.0	E939.0	E950.3	E962.0	E980.3
Matulane	963.1	E858.1	E933.1	E950.4	E962.0	E980.4
Mazindol	977.0	E858.8	E947.0	E950.4	E962.0	E980.4
MDMA	969.72	E854.2	E939.7	E950.3	E962.0	E980.3
Meadow saffron	988.2	E865.3	—	E950.9	E962.1	E980.9
Measles vaccine	979.4	E858.8	E949.4	E950.4	E962.0	E980.4
Meat, noxious or nonbacterial	988.8	E865.0	—	E950.9	E962.1	E980.9
Mebanazine	969.01	E854.0	E939.0	E950.3	E962.0	E980.3
Mebaral	967.0	E851	E937.0	E950.1	E962.0	E980.1
Mebendazole	961.6	E857	E931.6	E950.4	E962.0	E980.4
Mebeverine	975.1	E858.6	E945.1	E950.4	E962.0	E980.4
Mebhydroline	963.0	E858.1	E933.0	E950.4	E962.0	E980.4
Mebrophenhydramine	963.0	E858.1	E933.0	E950.4	E962.0	E980.4
Mebutamate	969.5	E853.8	E939.5	E950.3	E962.0	E980.3
Mecamylamine (chloride)	972.3	E858.3	E942.3	E950.4	E962.0	E980.4
Mechlorethamine hydrochloride	963.1	E858.1	E933.1	E950.4	E962.0	E980.4
Meclizene (hydrochloride)	963.0	E858.1	E933.0	E950.4	E962.0	E980.4

Substance	Poisoning	Accident	Therapeutic Use	Suicide Attempt	Assault	Undetermined
			External Cause (E-Code)			
Meclofenoxate	970.0	E854.3	E940.0	E950.4	E962.0	E980.4
Meclozine (hydrochloride)	963.0	E858.1	E933.0	E950.4	E962.0	E980.4
Medazepam	969.4	E853.2	E939.4	E950.3	E962.0	E980.3
Medicine, medicinal substance	977.9	E858.9	E947.9	E950.5	E962.0	E980.5
specified NEC	977.8	E858.8	E947.8	E950.4	E962.0	E980.4
Medinal	967.0	E851	E937.0	E950.1	E962.0	E980.1
Medomin	967.0	E851	E937.0	E950.1	E962.0	E980.1
Medroxyprogesterone	962.2	E858.0	E932.2	E950.4	E962.0	E980.4
Medrysone	976.5	E858.7	E946.5	E950.4	E962.0	E980.4
Mefenamic acid	965.7	E850.7	E935.7	E950.0	E962.0	E980.0
Megahallucinogen	969.6	E854.1	E939.6	E950.3	E962.0	E980.3
Megestrol	962.2	E858.0	E932.2	E950.4	E962.0	E980.4
Meglumine	977.8	E858.8	E947.8	E950.4	E962.0	E980.4
Meladinin	976.3	E858.7	E946.3	E950.4	E962.0	E980.4
Melanizing agents	976.3	E858.7	E946.3	E950.4	E962.0	E980.4
Melarsoprol	961.1	E857	E931.1	E950.4	E962.0	E980.4
Melia azedarach	988.2	E865.3	—	E950.9	E962.1	E980.9
Mellaril	969.1	E853.0	E939.1	E950.3	E962.0	E980.3
Meloxine	976.3	E858.7	E946.3	E950.4	E962.0	E980.4
Melphalan	963.1	E858.1	E933.1	E950.4	E962.0	E980.4
Menadiol sodium diphosphate	964.3	E858.2	E934.3	E950.4	E962.0	E980.4
Menadione (sodium bisulfate)	964.3	E858.2	E934.3	E950.4	E962.0	E980.4
Menaphthone	964.3	E858.2	E934.3	E950.4	E962.0	E980.4
Meningococcal vaccine	978.8	E858.8	E948.8	E950.4	E962.0	E980.4
Menningovax–C	978.8	E858.8	E948.8	E950.4	E962.0	E980.4
Menotropins	962.4	E858.0	E932.4	E950.4	E962.0	E980.4
Menthol NEC	976.1	E858.7	E946.1	E950.4	E962.0	E980.4
Mepacrine	961.3	E857	E931.3	E950.4	E962.0	E980.4
Meparfynol	967.8	E852.8	E937.8	E950.2	E962.0	E980.2
Mepazine	969.1	E853.0	E939.1	E950.3	E962.0	E980.3
Mepenzolate	971.1	E855.4	E941.1	E950.4	E962.0	E980.4
Meperidine	965.09	E850.2	E935.2	E950.0	E962.0	E980.0
Mephenamin(e)	966.4	E855.0	E936.4	E950.4	E962.0	E980.4
Mephenesin (carbamate)	968.0	E855.1	E938.0	E950.4	E962.0	E980.4
Mephenoxalone	969.5	E853.8	E939.5	E950.3	E962.0	E980.3
Mephentermine	971.2	E855.5	E941.2	E950.4	E962.0	E980.4
Mephenytoin	966.1	E855.0	E936.1	E950.4	E962.0	E980.4
Mephobarbital	967.0	E851	E937.0	E950.1	E962.0	E980.1
Mepiperphenidol	971.1	E855.4	E941.1	E950.4	E962.0	E980.4
Mepivacaine	968.9	E855.2	E938.9	E950.4	E962.0	E980.4
infiltration (subcutaneous)	968.5	E855.2	E938.5	E950.4	E962.0	E980.4
nerve block (peripheral) (plexus)	968.6	E855.2	E938.6	E950.4	E962.0	E980.4
topical (surface)	968.5	E855.2	E938.5	E950.4	E962.0	E980.4
Meprednisone	962.0	E858.0	E932.0	E950.4	E962.0	E980.4
Meprobam	969.5	E853.8	E939.5	E950.3	E962.0	E980.3
Meprobamate	969.5	E853.8	E939.5	E950.3	E962.0	E980.3
Mepyramine (maleate)	963.0	E858.1	E933.0	E950.4	E962.0	E980.4
Meralluride	974.0	E858.5	E944.0	E950.4	E962.0	E980.4
Merbaphen	974.0	E858.5	E944.0	E950.4	E962.0	E980.4
Merbromin	976.0	E858.7	E946.0	E950.4	E962.0	E980.4
Mercaptomerin	974.0	E858.5	E944.0	E950.4	E962.0	E980.4
Mercaptopurine	963.1	E858.1	E933.1	E950.4	E962.0	E980.4
Mercumatilin	974.0	E858.5	E944.0	E950.4	E962.0	E980.4
Mercuramide	974.0	E858.5	E944.0	E950.4	E962.0	E980.4
Mercuranin	976.0	E858.7	E946.0	E950.4	E962.0	E980.4
Mercurochrome	976.0	E858.7	E946.0	E950.4	E962.0	E980.4
Mercury, mercuric, mercurous (compounds) (cyanide) (fumes) (nonmedicinal) (vapor) NEC	985.0	E866.1	—	E950.9	E962.1	E980.9
ammoniated	976.0	E858.7	E946.0	E950.4	E962.0	E980.4
anti–infective	961.2	E857	E931.2	E950.4	E962.0	E980.4

Substance	Poisoning	Accident	Therapeutic Use	Suicide Attempt	Assault	Undetermined
			External Cause (E-Code)			
topical	976.0	E858.7	E946.0	E950.4	E962.0	E980.4
chloride (antiseptic) NEC	976.0	E858.7	E946.0	E950.4	E962.0	E980.4
fungicide	985.0	E863.6	—	E950.6	E962.1	E980.7
diuretic compounds	974.0	E858.5	E944.0	E950.4	E962.0	E980.4
fungicide	985.0	E863.6	—	E950.6	E962.1	E980.7
organic (fungicide)	985.0	E863.6	—	E950.6	E962.1	E980.7
Merethoxylline	974.0	E858.5	E944.0	E950.4	E962.0	E980.4
Mersalyl	974.0	E858.5	E944.0	E950.4	E962.0	E980.4
Merthiolate (topical)	976.0	E858.7	E946.0	E950.4	E962.0	E980.4
ophthalmic preparation	976.5	E858.7	E946.5	E950.4	E962.0	E980.4
Meruvax	979.4	E858.8	E949.4	E950.4	E962.0	E980.4
Mescal buttons	969.6	E854.1	E939.6	E950.3	E962.0	E980.3
Mescaline (salts)	969.6	E854.1	E939.6	E950.3	E962.0	E980.3
Mesoridazine besylate	969.1	E853.0	E939.1	E950.3	E962.0	E980.3
Mestanolone	962.1	E858.0	E932.1	E950.4	E962.0	E980.4
Mestranol	962.2	E858.0	E932.2	E950.4	E962.0	E980.4
Metacresylacetate	976.0	E858.7	E946.0	E950.4	E962.0	E980.4
Metaldehyde (snail killer) NEC	989.4	E863.4	—	E950.6	E962.1	E980.7
Metals (heavy) (nonmedicinal) NEC	985.9	E866.4	—	E950.9	E962.1	E980.9
dust, fumes, or vapor NEC	985.9	E866.4	—	E950.9	E962.1	E980.9
light NEC	985.9	E866.4	—	E950.9	E962.1	E980.9
dust, fumes, or vapor NEC	985.9	E866.4	—	E950.9	E962.1	E980.9
pesticides (dust) (vapor)	985.9	E863.4	—	E950.6	E962.1	E980.7
Metamucil	973.3	E858.4	E943.3	E950.4	E962.0	E980.4
Metaphen	976.0	E858.7	E946.0	E950.4	E962.0	E980.4
Metaproterenol	975.1	E858.6	E945.1	E950.4	E962.0	E980.4
Metaraminol	972.8	E858.3	E942.8	E950.4	E962.0	E980.4
Metaxalone	968.0	E855.1	E938.0	E950.4	E962.0	E980.4
Metformin	962.3	E858.0	E932.3	E950.4	E962.0	E980.4
Methacycline	960.4	E856	E930.4	E950.4	E962.0	E980.4
Methadone	965.02	E850.1	E935.1	E950.0	E962.0	E980.0
Methallenestril	962.2	E858.0	E932.2	E950.4	E962.0	E980.4
Methamphetamine	969.72	E854.2	E939.7	E950.3	E962.0	E980.3
Methandienone	962.1	E858.0	E932.1	E950.4	E962.0	E980.4
Methandriol	962.1	E858.0	E932.1	E950.4	E962.0	E980.4
Methandrostenolone	962.1	E858.0	E932.1	E950.4	E962.0	E980.4
Methane gas	987.1	E869.8	—	E952.8	E962.2	E982.8
Methanol	980.1	E860.2	—	E950.9	E962.1	E980.9
vapor	987.8	E869.8	—	E952.8	E962.2	E982.8
Methantheline	971.1	E855.4	E941.1	E950.4	E962.0	E980.4
Methaphenilene	963.0	E858.1	E933.0	E950.4	E962.0	E980.4
Methapyrilene	963.0	E858.1	E933.0	E950.4	E962.0	E980.4
Methaqualone (compounds)	967.4	E852.3	E937.4	E950.2	E962.0	E980.2
Metharbital, metharbitone	967.0	E851	E937.0	E950.1	E962.0	E980.1
Methazolamide	974.2	E858.5	E944.2	E950.4	E962.0	E980.4
Methdilazine	963.0	E858.1	E933.0	E950.4	E962.0	E980.4
Methedrine	969.72	E854.2	E939.7	E950.3	E962.0	E980.3
Methenamine (mandelate)	961.9	E857	E931.9	E950.4	E962.0	E980.4
Methenolone	962.1	E858.0	E932.1	E950.4	E962.0	E980.4
Methergine	975.0	E858.6	E945.0	E950.4	E962.0	E980.4
Methiacil	962.8	E858.0	E932.8	E950.4	E962.0	E980.4
Methicillin (sodium)	960.0	E856	E930.0	E950.4	E962.0	E980.4
Methimazole	962.8	E858.0	E932.8	E950.4	E962.0	E980.4
Methionine	977.1	E858.8	E947.1	E950.4	E962.0	E980.4
Methisazone	961.7	E857	E931.7	E950.4	E962.0	E980.4
Methitural	967.0	E851	E937.0	E950.1	E962.0	E980.1
Methixene	971.1	E855.4	E941.1	E950.4	E962.0	E980.4
Methobarbital, methobarbitone	967.0	E851	E937.0	E950.1	E962.0	E980.1
Methocarbamol	968.0	E855.1	E938.0	E950.4	E962.0	E980.4
Methohexital, methohexitone (sodium)	968.3	E855.1	E938.3	E950.4	E962.0	E980.4

Substance	Poisoning	Accident	Therapeutic Use	Suicide Attempt	Assault	Undetermined
			External Cause (E-Code)			
Methoin.	966.1	E855.0	E936.1	E950.4	E962.0	E980.4
Methopholine	965.7	E850.7	E935.7	E950.0	E962.0	E980.0
Methorate	975.4	E858.6	E945.4	E950.4	E962.0	E980.4
Methoserpidine.	972.6	E858.3	E942.6	E950.4	E962.0	E980.4
Methotrexate.	963.1	E858.1	E933.1	E950.4	E962.0	E980.4
Methotrimeprazine	967.8	E852.8	E937.8	E950.2	E962.0	E980.2
Methoxa–Dome	976.3	E858.7	E946.3	E950.4	E962.0	E980.4
Methoxamine	971.2	E855.5	E941.2	E950.4	E962.0	E980.4
Methoxsalen.	976.3	E858.7	E946.3	E950.4	E962.0	E980.4
Methoxybenzyl penicillin	960.0	E856	E930.0	E950.4	E962.0	E980.4
Methoxychlor	989.2	E863.0	—	E950.6	E962.1	E980.7
Methoxyflurane	968.2	E855.1	E938.2	E950.4	E962.0	E980.4
Methoxyphenamine	971.2	E855.5	E941.2	E950.4	E962.0	E980.4
Methoxypromazine	969.1	E853.0	E939.1	E950.3	E962.0	E980.3
Methoxypsoralen	976.3	E858.7	E946.3	E950.4	E962.0	E980.4
Methscopolamine (bromide)	971.1	E855.4	E941.1	E950.4	E962.0	E980.4
Methsuximide	966.2	E855.0	E936.2	E950.4	E962.0	E980.4
Methyclothiazide.	974.3	E858.5	E944.3	E950.4	E962.0	E980.4
Methyl						
acetate	982.8	E862.4	—	E950.9	E962.1	E980.9
acetone	982.8	E862.4	—	E950.9	E962.1	E980.9
alcohol	980.1	E860.2	—	E950.9	E962.1	E980.9
amphetamine	969.72	E854.2	E939.7	E950.3	E962.0	E980.3
androstanolone	962.1	E858.0	E932.1	E950.4	E962.0	E980.4
atropine	971.1	E855.4	E941.1	E950.4	E962.0	E980.4
benzene	982.0	E862.4	—	E950.9	E962.1	E980.9
bromide (gas)	987.8	E869.8	—	E952.8	E962.2	E982.8
fumigant	987.8	E863.8	—	E950.6	E962.2	E980.7
butanol	980.8	E860.8	—	E950.9	E962.1	E980.9
carbinol	980.1	E860.2	—	E950.9	E962.1	E980.9
cellosolve	982.8	E862.4	—	E950.9	E962.1	E980.9
cellulose.	973.3	E858.4	E943.3	E950.4	E962.0	E980.4
chloride (gas)	987.8	E869.8	—	E952.8	E962.2	E982.8
cyclohexane	982.8	E862.4	—	E950.9	E962.1	E980.9
cyclohexanone	982.8	E862.4	—	E950.9	E962.1	E980.9
dihydromorphinone	965.09	E850.2	E935.2	E950.0	E962.0	E980.0
ergometrine	975.0	E858.6	E945.0	E950.4	E962.0	E980.4
ergonovine	975.0	E858.6	E945.0	E950.4	E962.0	E980.4
ethyl ketone	982.8	E862.4	—	E950.9	E962.1	E980.9
hydrazine	983.9	E864.3	—	E950.7	E962.1	E980.6
isobutyl ketone	982.8	E862.4	—	E950.9	E962.1	E980.9
morphine NEC	965.09	E850.2	E935.2	E950.0	E962.0	E980.0
parafynol	967.8	E852.8	E937.8	E950.2	E962.0	E980.2
parathion	989.3	E863.1	—	E950.6	E962.1	E980.7
pentynol NEC	967.8	E852.8	E937.8	E950.2	E962.0	E980.2
peridol	969.2	E853.1	E939.2	E950.3	E962.0	E980.3
phenidate	969.73	E854.2	E939.7	E950.3	E962.0	E980.3
prednisolone	962.0	E858.0	E932.0	E950.4	E962.0	E980.4
ENT agent	976.6	E858.7	E946.6	E950.4	E962.0	E980.4
ophthalmic preparation	976.5	E858.7	E946.5	E950.4	E962.0	E980.4
topical NEC	976.0	E858.7	E946.0	E950.4	E962.0	E980.4
propylcarbinol	980.8	E860.8	—	E950.9	E962.1	E980.9
rosaniline NEC	976.0	E858.7	E946.0	E950.4	E962.0	E980.4
salicylate NEC	976.3	E858.7	E946.3	E950.4	E962.0	E980.4
sulfate (fumes)	987.8	E869.8	—	E952.8	E962.2	E982.8
liquid	983.9	E864.3	—	E950.7	E962.1	E980.6
sulfonal	967.8	E852.8	E937.8	E950.2	E962.0	E980.2
testosterone	962.1	E858.0	E932.1	E950.4	E962.0	E980.4
thiouracil	962.8	E858.0	E932.8	E950.4	E962.0	E980.4
Methylated spirit	980.0	E860.1	—	E950.9	E962.1	E980.9
Methyldopa	972.6	E858.3	E942.6	E950.4	E962.0	E980.4

Substance	Poisoning	Accident	Therapeutic Use	Suicide Attempt	Assault	Undetermined
			External Cause (E-Code)			

Substance						
Methylene						
blue	961.9	E857	E931.9	E950.4	E962.0	E980.4
chloride or dichloride (solvent) NEC	982.3	E862.4	—	E950.9	E962.1	E980.9
Methylhexabital	967.0	E851	E937.0	E950.1	E962.0	E980.1
Methylparaben (ophthalmic)	976.5	E858.7	E946.5	E950.4	E962.0	E980.4
Methyprylon	967.5	E852.4	E937.5	E950.2	E962.0	E980.2
Methysergide	971.3	E855.6	E941.3	E950.4	E962.0	E980.4
Metoclopramide	963.0	E858.1	E933.0	E950.4	E962.0	E980.4
Metofoline	965.7	E850.7	E935.7	E950.0	E962.0	E980.0
Metopon	965.09	E850.2	E935.2	E950.0	E962.0	E980.0
Metronidazole	961.5	E857	E931.5	E950.4	E962.0	E980.4
Metycaine	968.9	E855.2	E938.9	E950.4	E962.0	E980.4
infiltration (subcutaneous)	968.5	E855.2	E938.5	E950.4	E962.0	E980.4
nerve block (peripheral) (plexus)	968.6	E855.2	E938.6	E950.4	E962.0	E980.4
topical (surface)	968.5	E855.2	E938.5	E950.4	E962.0	E980.4
Metyrapone	977.8	E858.8	E947.8	E950.4	E962.0	E980.4
Mevinphos	989.3	E863.1	—	E950.6	E962.1	E980.7
Mezereon (berries)	988.2	E865.3	—	E950.9	E962.1	E980.9
Micatin	976.0	E858.7	E946.0	E950.4	E962.0	E980.4
Miconazole	976.0	E858.7	E946.0	E950.4	E962.0	E980.4
Midol	965.1	E850.3	E935.3	E950.0	E962.0	E980.0
Mifepristone	962.9	E858.0	E932.9	E950.4	E962.0	E980.4
Milk of magnesia	973.0	E858.4	E943.0	E950.4	E962.0	E980.4
Millipede (tropical) (venomous)	989.5	E905.4	—	E950.9	E962.1	E980.9
Miltown	969.5	E853.8	E939.5	E950.3	E962.0	E980.3
Mineral						
oil (medicinal)	973.2	E858.4	E943.2	E950.4	E962.0	E980.4
nonmedicinal	981	E862.1	—	E950.9	E962.1	E980.9
topical	976.3	E858.7	E946.3	E950.4	E962.0	E980.4
salts NEC	974.6	E858.5	E944.6	E950.4	E962.0	E980.4
spirits	981	E862.0	—	E950.9	E962.1	E980.9
Minocycline	960.4	E856	E930.4	E950.4	E962.0	E980.4
Mithramycin (antineoplastic)	960.7	E856	E930.7	E950.4	E962.0	E980.4
Mitobronitol	963.1	E858.1	E933.1	E950.4	E962.0	E980.4
Mitomycin (antineoplastic)	960.7	E856	E930.7	E950.4	E962.0	E980.4
Mitotane	963.1	E858.1	E933.1	E950.4	E962.0	E980.4
Moderil	972.6	E858.3	E942.6	E950.4	E962.0	E980.4
Mogadon—see Nitrazepam						
Molindone	969.3	E853.8	E939.3	E950.3	E962.0	E980.3
Monistat	976.0	E858.7	E946.0	E950.4	E962.0	E980.4
Monkshood	988.2	E865.4	—	E950.9	E962.1	E980.9
Monoamine oxidase inhibitors	969.01	E854.0	E939.0	E950.3	E962.0	E980.3
Monochlorobenzene	982.0	E862.4	—	E950.9	E962.1	E980.9
Monosodium glutamate	989.89	E866.8	—	E950.9	E962.1	E980.9
Monoxide, carbon — see Carbon, monoxide						
Moperone	969.2	E853.1	E939.2	E950.3	E962.0	E980.3
Morning glory seeds	969.6	E854.1	E939.6	E950.3	E962.0	E980.3
Moroxydine (hydrochloride)	961.7	E857	E931.7	E950.4	E962.0	E980.4
Morphazinamide	961.8	E857	E931.8	E950.4	E962.0	E980.4
Morphinans	965.09	E850.2	E935.2	E950.0	E962.0	E980.0
Morphine NEC	965.09	E850.2	E935.2	E950.0	E962.0	E980.0
antagonists	970.1	E854.3	E940.1	E950.4	E962.0	E980.4
Morpholinylethylmorphine	965.09	E850.2	E935.2	E950.0	E962.0	E980.0
Morrhuate sodium	972.7	E858.3	E942.7	E950.4	E962.0	E980.4
Moth balls (see also Pesticides)	989.4	E863.4	—	E950.6	E962.1	E980.7
naphthalene	983.0	E863.4	—	E950.7	E962.1	E980.6
Motor exhaust gas — see Carbon, monoxide, exhaust gas						
Mouth wash	976.6	E858.7	E946.6	E950.4	E962.0	E980.4
Mucolytic agent	975.5	E858.6	E945.5	E950.4	E962.0	E980.4

Substance	Poisoning	Accident	Therapeutic Use	Suicide Attempt	Assault	Undetermined
			External Cause (E-Code)			
Mucomyst. 975.5	E858.6	E945.5	E950.4	E962.0	E980.4
Mucous membrane agents (external) 976.9	E858.7	E946.9	E950.4	E962.0	E980.4
specified NEC 976.8	E858.7	E946.8	E950.4	E962.0	E980.4
Mumps					
immune globulin (human) 964.6	E858.2	E934.6	E950.4	E962.0	E980.4
skin test antigen 977.8	E858.8	E947.8	E950.4	E962.0	E980.4
vaccine 979.6	E858.8	E949.6	E950.4	E962.0	E980.4
Mumpsvax 979.6	E858.8	E949.6	E950.4	E962.0	E980.4
Muriatic acid — *see* Hydrochloric acid					
Muscarine 971.0	E855.3	E941.0	E950.4	E962.0	E980.4
Muscle affecting agents NEC 975.3	E858.6	E945.3	E950.4	E962.0	E980.4
oxytocic 975.0	E858.6	E945.0	E950.4	E962.0	E980.4
relaxants 975.3	E858.6	E945.3	E950.4	E962.0	E980.4
central nervous system 968.0	E855.1	E938.0	E950.4	E962.0	E980.4
skeletal 975.2	E858.6	E945.2	E950.4	E962.0	E980.4
smooth 975.1	E858.6	E945.1	E950.4	E962.0	E980.4
Mushrooms, noxious 988.1	E865.5	—	E950.9	E962.1	E980.9
Mussel, noxious 988.0	E865.1	—	E950.9	E962.1	E980.9
Mustard (emetic) 973.6	E858.4	E943.6	E950.4	E962.0	E980.4
gas 987.8	E869.8	—	E952.8	E962.2	E982.8
nitrogen 963.1	E858.1	E933.1	E950.4	E962.0	E980.4
Mustine 963.1	E858.1	E933.1	E950.4	E962.0	E980.4
M–vac 979.4	E858.8	E949.4	E950.4	E962.0	E980.4
Mycifradin 960.8	E856	E930.8	E950.4	E962.0	E980.4
topical 976.0	E858.7	E946.0	E950.4	E962.0	E980.4
Mycitracin 960.8	E856	E930.8	E950.4	E962.0	E980.4
ophthalmic preparation 976.5	E858.7	E946.5	E950.4	E962.0	E980.4
Mycostatin 960.1	E856	E930.1	E950.4	E962.0	E980.4
topical 976.0	E858.7	E946.0	E950.4	E962.0	E980.4
Mydriacyl 971.1	E855.4	E941.1	E950.4	E962.0	E980.4
Myelobromal 963.1	E858.1	E933.1	E950.4	E962.0	E980.4
Myleran 963.1	E858.1	E933.1	E950.4	E962.0	E980.4
Myochrysin(e) 965.69	E850.6	E935.6	E950.0	E962.0	E980.0
Myoneural blocking agents 975.2	E858.6	E945.2	E950.4	E962.0	E980.4
Myristica fragrans 988.2	E865.3	—	E950.9	E962.1	E980.9
Myristicin 988.2	E865.3	—	E950.9	E962.1	E980.9
Mysoline 966.3	E855.0	E936.3	E950.4	E962.0	E980.4
Nafcillin (sodium) 960.0	E856	E930.0	E950.4	E962.0	E980.4
Nail polish remover 982.8	E862.4	—	E950.9	E962.1	E980.9
Nalidixic acid 961.9	E857	E931.9	E950.4	E962.0	E980.4
Nalorphine 970.1	E854.3	E940.1	E950.4	E962.0	E980.4
Naloxone 970.1	E854.3	E940.1	E950.4	E962.0	E980.4
Nandrolone (decanoate) (phenproprioate) . . . 962.1	E858.0	E932.1	E950.4	E962.0	E980.4
Naphazoline 971.2	E855.5	E941.2	E950.4	E962.0	E980.4
Naphtha (painter's) (petroleum) 981	E862.0	—	E950.9	E962.1	E980.9
solvent 981	E862.0	—	E950.9	E962.1	E980.9
vapor 987.1	E869.8	—	E952.8	E962.2	E982.8
Naphthalene (chlorinated) 983.0	E864.0	—	E950.7	E962.1	E980.6
insecticide or moth repellent 983.0	E863.4	—	E950.7	E962.1	E980.6
vapor 987.8	E869.8	—	E952.8	E962.2	E982.8
Naphthol 983.0	E864.0	—	E950.7	E962.1	E980.6
Naphthylamine 983.0	E864.0	—	E950.7	E962.1	E980.6
Naprosyn—*see* Naproxen					
Naproxen 965.61	E850.6	E935.6	E950.0	E962.0	E980.0
Narcotic (drug) 967.9	E852.9	E937.9	E950.2	E962.0	E980.2
analgesic NEC 965.8	E850.8	E935.8	E950.0	E962.0	E980.0
antagonist 970.1	E854.3	E940.1	E950.4	E962.0	E980.4
specified NEC 967.8	E852.8	E937.8	E950.2	E962.0	E980.2
Narcotine 975.4	E858.6	E945.4	E950.4	E962.0	E980.4
Nardil 969.01	E854.0	E939.0	E950.3	E962.0	E980.3
Natrium cyanide — *see* Cyanide(s)					

Substance	Poisoning	Accident	Therapeutic Use	Suicide Attempt	Assault	Undetermined
			External Cause (E-Code)			
Natural						
blood (product)	964.7	E858.2	E934.7	E950.4	E962.0	E980.4
gas (piped)	987.1	E867	—	E951.0	E962.2	E981.0
incomplete combustion	986	E867	—	E951.0	E962.2	E981.0
Nealbarbital, nealbarbitone	967.0	E851	E937.0	E950.1	E962.0	E980.1
Nectadon	975.4	E858.6	E945.4	E950.4	E962.0	E980.4
Nematocyst (sting)	989.5	E905.6	—	E950.9	E962.1	E980.9
Nembutal	967.0	E851	E937.0	E950.1	E962.0	E980.1
Neoarsphenamine	961.1	E857	E931.1	E950.4	E962.0	E980.4
Neocinchophen	974.7	E858.5	E944.7	E950.4	E962.0	E980.4
Neomycin	960.8	E856	E930.8	E950.4	E962.0	E980.4
ENT agent	976.6	E858.7	E946.6	E950.4	E962.0	E980.4
ophthalmic preparation	976.5	E858.7	E946.5	E950.4	E962.0	E980.4
topical NEC	976.0	E858.7	E946.0	E950.4	E962.0	E980.4
Neonal	967.0	E851	E937.0	E950.1	E962.0	E980.1
Neoprontosil	961.0	E857	E931.0	E950.4	E962.0	E980.4
Neosalvarsan	961.1	E857	E931.1	E950.4	E962.0	E980.4
Neosilversalvarsan	961.1	E857	E931.1	E950.4	E962.0	E980.4
Neosporin	960.8	E856	E930.8	E950.4	E962.0	E980.4
ENT agent	976.6	E858.7	E946.6	E950.4	E962.0	E980.4
ophthalmic preparation	976.5	E858.7	E946.5	E950.4	E962.0	E980.4
topical NEC	976.0	E858.7	E946.0	E950.4	E962.0	E980.4
Neostigmine	971.0	E855.3	E941.0	E950.4	E962.0	E980.4
Neraval	967.0	E851	E937.0	E950.1	E962.0	E980.1
Neravan	967.0	E851	E937.0	E950.1	E962.0	E980.1
Nerium oleander	988.2	E865.4	—	E950.9	E962.1	E980.9
Nerve gases (war)	987.9	E869.9	—	E952.9	E962.2	E982.9
Nesacaine	968.9	E855.2	E938.9	E950.4	E962.0	E980.4
infiltration (subcutaneous)	968.5	E855.2	E938.5	E950.4	E962.0	E980.4
nerve block (peripheral) (plexus)	968.6	E855.2	E938.6	E950.4	E962.0	E980.4
Neurobarb	967.0	E851	E937.0	E950.1	E962.0	E980.1
Neuroleptics NEC	969.3	E853.8	E939.3	E950.3	E962.0	E980.3
Neuroprotective agent	977.8	E858.8	E947.8	E950.4	E962.0	E980.4
Neutral spirits	980.0	E860.1	—	E950.9	E962.1	E980.9
beverage	980.0	E860.0	—	E950.9	E962.1	E980.9
Niacin, niacinamide	972.2	E858.3	E942.2	E950.4	E962.0	E980.4
Nialamide	969.01	E854.0	E939.0	E950.3	E962.0	E980.3
Nickle (carbonyl) (compounds) (fumes) (tetracarbonyl) (vapor)	985.8	E866.4	—	E950.9	E962.1	E980.9
Niclosamide	961.6	E857	E931.6	E950.4	E962.0	E980.4
Nicomorphine	965.09	E850.2	E935.2	E950.0	E962.0	E980.0
Nicotinamide	972.2	E858.3	E942.2	E950.4	E962.0	E980.4
Nicotine (insecticide) (spray) (sulfate) NEC	989.4	E863.4	—	E950.6	E962.1	E980.7
not insecticide	989.89	E866.8	—	E950.9	E962.1	E980.9
Nicotinic acid (derivatives)	972.2	E858.3	E942.2	E950.4	E962.0	E980.4
Nicotinyl alcohol	972.2	E858.3	E942.2	E950.4	E962.0	E980.4
Nicoumalone	964.2	E858.2	E934.2	E950.4	E962.0	E980.4
Nifenazone	965.5	E850.5	E935.5	E950.0	E962.0	E980.0
Nifuraldezone	961.9	E857	E931.9	E950.4	E962.0	E980.4
Nightshade (deadly)	988.2	E865.4	—	E950.9	E962.1	E980.9
Nikethamide	970.0	E854.3	E940.0	E950.4	E962.0	E980.4
Nilstat	960.1	E856	E930.1	E950.4	E962.0	E980.4
topical	976.0	E858.7	E946.0	E950.4	E962.0	E980.4
Nimodipine	977.8	E858.8	E947.8	E950.4	E962.0	E980.4
Niridazole	961.6	E857	E931.6	E950.4	E962.0	E980.4
Nisentil	965.09	E850.2	E935.2	E950.0	E962.0	E980.0
Nitrates	972.4	E858.3	E942.4	E950.4	E962.0	E980.4
Nitrazepam	969.4	E853.2	E939.4	E950.3	E962.0	E980.3
Nitric						
acid (liquid)	983.1	E864.1	—	E950.7	E962.1	E980.6

Substance	Poisoning	Accident	Therapeutic Use	Suicide Attempt	Assault	Undetermined
			External Cause (E-Code)			
vapor	987.8	E869.8	—	E952.8	E962.2	E982.8
oxide (gas)	987.2	E869.0	—	E952.8	E962.2	E982.8
Nitrite, amyl (medicinal) (vapor)	972.4	E858.3	E942.4	E950.4	E962.0	E980.4
Nitroaniline	983.0	E864.0	—	E950.7	E962.1	E980.6
vapor	987.8	E869.8	—	E952.8	E962.2	E982.8
Nitrobenzene, nitrobenzol	983.0	E864.0	—	E950.7	E962.1	E980.6
vapor	987.8	E869.8	—	E952.8	E962.2	E982.8
Nitrocellulose	976.3	E858.7	E946.3	E950.4	E962.0	E980.4
Nitrofuran derivatives	961.9	E857	E931.9	E950.4	E962.0	E980.4
Nitrofurantoin	961.9	E857	E931.9	E950.4	E962.0	E980.4
Nitrofurazone	976.0	E858.7	E946.0	E950.4	E962.0	E980.4
Nitrogen (dioxide) (gas) (oxide)	987.2	E869.0	—	E952.8	E962.2	E982.8
mustard (antineoplastic)	963.1	E858.1	E933.1	E950.4	E962.0	E980.4
Nitroglycerin, nitroglycerol (medicinal)	972.4	E858.3	E942.4	E950.4	E962.0	E980.4
nonmedicinal	989.89	E866.8	—	E950.9	E962.1	E980.9
fumes	987.8	E869.8	—	E952.8	E962.2	E982.8
Nitrohydrochloric acid	983.1	E864.1	—	E950.7	E962.1	E980.6
Nitromersol	976.0	E858.7	E946.0	E950.4	E962.0	E980.4
Nitronaphthalene	983.0	E864.0	—	E950.7	E962.2	E980.6
Nitrophenol	983.0	E864.0	—	E950.7	E962.2	E980.6
Nitrothiazol	961.6	E857	E931.6	E950.4	E962.0	E980.4
Nitrotoluene, nitrotoluol	983.0	E864.0	—	E950.7	E962.1	E980.6
vapor	987.8	E869.8	—	E952.8	E962.2	E982.8
Nitrous	968.2	E855.1	E938.2	E950.4	E962.0	E980.4
acid (liquid)	983.1	E864.1	—	E950.7	E962.1	E980.6
fumes	987.2	E869.0	—	E952.8	E962.2	E982.8
oxide (anesthetic) NEC	968.2	E855.1	E938.2	E950.4	E962.0	E980.4
Nitrozone	976.0	E858.7	E946.0	E950.4	E962.0	E980.4
Noctec	967.1	E852.0	E937.1	E950.2	E962.0	E980.2
Noludar	967.5	E852.4	E937.5	E950.2	E962.0	E980.2
Noptil	967.0	E851	E937.0	E950.1	E962.0	E980.1
Noradrenalin	971.2	E855.5	E941.2	E950.4	E962.0	E980.4
Noramidopyrine	965.5	E850.5	E935.5	E950.0	E962.0	E980.0
Norepinephrine	971.2	E855.5	E941.2	E950.4	E962.0	E980.4
Norethandrolone	962.1	E858.0	E932.1	E950.4	E962.0	E980.4
Norethindrone	962.2	E858.0	E932.2	E950.4	E962.0	E980.4
Norethisterone	962.2	E858.0	E932.2	E950.4	E962.0	E980.4
Norethynodrel	962.2	E858.0	E932.2	E950.4	E962.0	E980.4
Norlestrin	962.2	E858.0	E932.2	E950.4	E962.0	E980.4
Norlutin	962.2	E858.0	E932.2	E950.4	E962.0	E980.4
Normison—see Benzodiazepines						
Normorphine	965.09	E850.2	E935.2	E950.0	E962.0	E980.0
Nortriptyline	969.05	E854.0	E939.0	E950.3	E962.0	E980.3
Noscapine	975.4	E858.6	E945.4	E950.4	E962.0	E980.4
Nose preparations	976.6	E858.7	E946.6	E950.4	E962.0	E980.4
Novobiocin	960.8	E856	E930.8	E950.4	E962.0	E980.4
Novocain (infiltration) (topical)	968.5	E855.2	E938.5	E950.4	E962.0	E980.4
nerve block (peripheral) (plexus)	968.6	E855.2	E938.6	E950.4	E962.0	E980.4
spinal	968.7	E855.2	E938.7	E950.4	E962.0	E980.4
Noxythiolin	961.9	E857	E931.9	E950.4	E962.0	E980.4
NPH Iletin (insulin)	962.3	E858.0	E932.3	E950.4	E962.0	E980.4
Numorphan	965.09	E850.2	E935.2	E950.0	E962.0	E980.0
Nunol	967.0	E851	E937.0	E950.1	E962.0	E980.1
Nupercaine (spinal anesthetic)	968.7	E855.2	E938.7	E950.4	E962.0	E980.4
topical (surface)	968.5	E855.2	E938.5	E950.4	E962.0	E980.4
Nutmeg oil (liniment)	976.3	E858.7	E946.3	E950.4	E962.0	E980.4
Nux vomica	989.1	E863.7	—	E950.6	E962.1	E980.7
Nydrazid	961.8	E857	E931.8	E950.4	E962.0	E980.4
Nylidrin	971.2	E855.5	E941.2	E950.4	E962.0	E980.4
Nystatin	960.1	E856	E930.1	E950.4	E962.0	E980.4
topical	976.0	E858.7	E946.0	E950.4	E962.0	E980.4

Substance	Poisoning	Accident	Therapeutic Use	Suicide Attempt	Assault	Undetermined
			External Cause (E-Code)			
Nytol	963.0	E858.1	E933.0	E950.4	E962.0	E980.4
Oblivion	967.8	E852.8	E937.8	E950.2	E962.0	E980.2
Octyl nitrite	972.4	E858.3	E942.4	E950.4	E962.0	E980.4
Oestradiol (cypionate) (dipropionate) (valerate)	962.2	E858.0	E932.2	E950.4	E962.0	E980.4
Oestriol	962.2	E858.0	E932.2	E950.4	E962.0	E980.4
Oestrone	962.2	E858.0	E932.2	E950.4	E962.0	E980.4
Oil (of) NEC	989.89	E866.8	—	E950.9	E962.1	E980.9
bitter almond	989.0	E866.8	—	E950.9	E962.1	E980.9
camphor	976.1	E858.7	E946.1	E950.4	E962.0	E980.4
colors	989.89	E861.6	—	E950.9	E962.1	E980.9
fumes	987.8	E869.8	—	E952.8	E962.2	E982.8
lubricating	981	E862.2	—	E950.9	E962.1	E980.9
specified source, other — *see* substance specified						
vitriol (liquid)	983.1	E864.1	—	E950.7	E962.1	E980.6
fumes	987.8	E869.8	—	E952.8	E962.2	E982.8
wintergreen (bitter) NEC	976.3	E858.7	E946.3	E950.4	E962.0	E980.4
Ointments NEC	976.9	E858.7	E946.9	E950.4	E962.0	E980.4
Oleander	988.2	E865.4	—	E950.9	E962.1	E980.9
Oleandomycin	960.3	E856	E930.3	E950.4	E962.0	E980.4
Oleovitamin A	963.5	E858.1	E933.5	E950.4	E962.0	E980.4
Oleum ricini	973.1	E858.4	E943.1	E950.4	E962.0	E980.4
Olive oil (medicinal) NEC	973.2	E858.4	E943.2	E950.4	E962.0	E980.4
OMPA	989.3	E863.1	—	E950.6	E962.1	E980.7
Oncovin	963.1	E858.1	E933.1	E950.4	E962.0	E980.4
Ophthaine	968.5	E855.2	E938.5	E950.4	E962.0	E980.4
Ophthetic	968.5	E855.2	E938.5	E950.4	E962.0	E980.4
Opiates, opioids, opium NEC	965.00	E850.2	E935.2	E950.0	E962.0	E980.0
antagonists	970.1	E854.3	E940.1	E950.4	E962.0	E980.4
Oracon	962.2	E858.0	E932.2	E950.4	E962.0	E980.4
Oragrafin	977.8	E858.8	E947.8	E950.4	E962.0	E980.4
Oral contraceptives	962.2	E858.0	E932.2	E950.4	E962.0	E980.4
Orciprenaline	975.1	E858.6	E945.1	E950.4	E962.0	E980.4
Organidin	975.5	E858.6	E945.5	E950.4	E962.0	E980.4
Organophosphates	989.3	E863.1	—	E950.6	E962.1	E980.7
Orimune	979.5	E858.8	E949.5	E950.4	E962.0	E980.4
Orinase	962.3	E858.0	E932.3	E950.4	E962.0	E980.4
Orphenadrine	966.4	E855.0	E936.4	E950.4	E962.0	E980.4
Ortal (sodium)	967.0	E851	E937.0	E950.1	E962.0	E980.1
Orthoboric acid	976.0	E858.7	E946.0	E950.4	E962.0	E980.4
ENT agent	976.6	E858.7	E946.6	E950.4	E962.0	E980.4
ophthalmic preparation	976.5	E858.7	E946.5	E950.4	E962.0	E980.4
Orthocaine	968.5	E855.2	E938.5	E950.4	E962.0	E980.4
Ortho–Novum	962.2	E858.0	E932.2	E950.4	E962.0	E980.4
Orthotolidine (reagent)	977.8	E858.8	E947.8	E950.4	E962.0	E980.4
Osmic acid (liquid)	983.1	E864.1	—	E950.7	E962.1	E980.6
fumes	987.8	E869.8	—	E952.8	E962.2	E982.8
Osmotic diuretics	974.4	E858.5	E944.4	E950.4	E962.0	E980.4
Ouabain	972.1	E858.3	E942.1	E950.4	E962.0	E980.4
Ovarian hormones (synthetic substitutes)	962.2	E858.0	E932.2	E950.4	E962.0	E980.4
Ovral	962.2	E858.0	E932.2	E950.4	E962.0	E980.4
Ovulation suppressants	962.2	E858.0	E932.2	E950.4	E962.0	E980.4
Ovulen	962.2	E858.0	E932.2	E950.4	E962.0	E980.4
Oxacillin (sodium)	960.0	E856	E930.0	E950.4	E962.0	E980.4
Oxalic acid	983.1	E864.1	—	E950.7	E962.1	E980.6
Oxanamide	969.5	E853.8	E939.5	E950.3	E962.0	E980.3
Oxandrolone	962.1	E858.0	E932.1	E950.4	E962.0	E980.4
Oxaprozin	965.61	E850.6	E935.6	E950.0	E962.0	E980.0
Oxazepam	969.4	E853.2	E939.4	E950.3	E962.0	E980.3

Substance	Poisoning	Accident	Therapeutic Use	Suicide Attempt	Assault	Undetermined
			External Cause (E-Code)			
Oxazolidine derivatives	966.0	E855.0	E936.0	E950.4	E962.0	E980.4
Ox bile extract	973.4	E858.4	E943.4	E950.4	E962.0	E980.4
Oxedrine	971.2	E855.5	E941.2	E950.4	E962.0	E980.4
Oxeladin	975.4	E858.6	E945.4	E950.4	E962.0	E980.4
Oxethazaine NEC	968.5	E855.2	E938.5	E950.4	E962.0	E980.4
Oxidizing agents NEC	983.9	E864.3	—	E950.7	E962.1	E980.6
Oxolinic acid	961.3	E857	E931.3	E950.4	E962.0	E980.4
Oxophenarsine	961.1	E857	E931.1	E950.4	E962.0	E980.4
Oxsoralen	976.3	E858.7	E946.3	E950.4	E962.0	E980.4
Oxtriphylline	975.7	E858.6	E945.7	E950.4	E962.0	E980.4
Oxybuprocaine	968.5	E855.2	E938.5	E950.4	E962.0	E980.4
Oxybutynin	975.1	E858.6	E945.1	E950.4	E962.0	E980.4
Oxycodone	965.09	E850.2	E935.2	E950.0	E962.0	E980.0
Oxygen	987.8	E869.8	—	E952.8	E962.2	E982.8
Oxylone	976.0	E858.7	E946.0	E950.4	E962.0	E980.4
ophthalmic preparation	976.5	E858.7	E946.5	E950.4	E962.0	E980.4
Oxymesterone	962.1	E858.0	E932.1	E950.4	E962.0	E980.4
Oxymetazoline	971.2	E855.5	E941.2	E950.4	E962.0	E980.4
Oxymetholone	962.1	E858.0	E932.1	E950.4	E962.0	E980.4
Oxymorphone	965.09	E850.2	E935.2	E950.0	E962.0	E980.0
Oxypertine	969.09	E854.0	E939.0	E950.3	E962.0	E980.3
Oxyphenbutazone	965.5	E850.5	E935.5	E950.0	E962.0	E980.0
Oxyphencyclimine	971.1	E855.4	E941.1	E950.4	E962.0	E980.4
Oxyphenisatin	973.1	E858.4	E943.1	E950.4	E962.0	E980.4
Oxyphenonium	971.1	E855.4	E941.1	E950.4	E962.0	E980.4
Oxyquinoline	961.3	E857	E931.3	E950.4	E962.0	E980.4
Oxytetracycline	960.4	E856	E930.4	E950.4	E962.0	E980.4
Oxytocics	975.0	E858.6	E945.0	E950.4	E962.0	E980.4
Oxytocin	975.0	E858.6	E945.0	E950.4	E962.0	E980.4
Ozone	987.8	E869.8	—	E952.8	E962.2	E982.8
PABA	976.3	E858.7	E946.3	E950.4	E962.0	E980.4
Packed red cells	964.7	E858.2	E934.7	E950.4	E962.0	E980.4
Paint NEC	989.89	E861.6	—	E950.9	E962.1	E980.9
cleaner	982.8	E862.9	—	E950.9	E962.1	E980.9
fumes NEC	987.8	E869.8	—	E952.8	E962.1	E982.8
lead (fumes)	984.0	E861.5	—	E950.9	E962.1	E980.9
solvent NEC	982.8	E862.9	—	E950.9	E962.1	E980.9
stripper	982.8	E862.9	—	E950.9	E962.1	E980.9
Palfium	965.09	E850.2	E935.2	E950.0	E962.0	E980.0
Palivizumab	979.9	E858.8	E949.6	E950.4	E962.0	E980.4
Paludrine	961.4	E857	E931.4	E950.4	E962.0	E980.4
PAM	977.2	E855.8	E947.2	E950.4	E962.0	E980.4
Pamaquine (naphthoate)	961.4	E857	E931.4	E950.4	E962.0	E980.4
Pamprin	965.1	E850.3	E935.3	E950.0	E962.0	E980.0
Panadol	965.4	E850.4	E935.4	E950.0	E962.0	E980.0
Pancreatic dornase (mucolytic)	963.4	E858.1	E933.4	E950.4	E962.0	E980.4
Pancreatin	973.4	E858.4	E943.4	E950.4	E962.0	E980.4
Pancrelipase	973.4	E858.4	E943.4	E950.4	E962.0	E980.4
Pangamic acid	963.5	E858.1	E933.5	E950.4	E962.0	E980.4
Panthenol	963.5	E858.1	E933.5	E950.4	E962.0	E980.4
topical	976.8	E858.7	E946.8	E950.4	E962.0	E980.4
Pantopaque	977.8	E858.8	E947.8	E950.4	E962.0	E980.4
Pantopon	965.00	E850.2	E935.2	E950.0	E962.0	E980.0
Pantothenic acid	963.5	E858.1	E933.5	E950.4	E962.0	E980.4
Panwarfin	964.2	E858.2	E934.2	E950.4	E962.0	E980.4
Papain	973.4	E858.4	E943.4	E950.4	E962.0	E980.4
Papaverine	972.5	E858.3	E942.5	E950.4	E962.0	E980.4
Para–aminobenzoic acid	976.3	E858.7	E946.3	E950.4	E962.0	E980.4
Para–aminophenol derivatives	965.4	E850.4	E935.4	E950.0	E962.0	E980.0
Para–aminosalicylic acid (derivatives)	961.8	E857	E931.8	E950.4	E962.0	E980.4
Paracetaldehyde (medicinal)	967.2	E852.1	E937.2	E950.2	E962.0	E980.2

Substance	Poisoning	Accident	Therapeutic Use	Suicide Attempt	Assault	Undetermined
			External Cause (E-Code)			
Paracetamol	965.4	E850.4	E935.4	E950.0	E962.0	E980.0
Paracodin	965.09	E850.2	E935.2	E950.0	E962.0	E980.0
Paradione	966.0	E855.0	E936.0	E950.4	E962.0	E980.4
Paraffin(s) (wax)	981	E862.3	—	E950.9	E962.1	E980.9
liquid (medicinal)	973.2	E858.4	E943.2	E950.4	E962.0	E980.4
nonmedicinal (oil)	981	E962.1	—	E950.9	E962.1	E980.9
Paraldehyde (medicinal)	967.2	E852.1	E937.2	E950.2	E962.0	E980.2
Paramethadione	966.0	E855.0	E936.0	E950.4	E962.0	E980.4
Paramethasone	962.0	E858.0	E932.0	E950.4	E962.0	E980.4
Paraquat	989.4	E863.5	—	E950.6	E962.1	E980.7
Parasympatholytics	971.1	E855.4	E941.1	E950.4	E962.0	E980.4
Parasympathomimetics	971.0	E855.3	E941.0	E950.4	E962.0	E980.4
Parathion	989.3	E863.1	—	E950.6	E962.1	E980.7
Parathormone	962.6	E858.0	E932.6	E950.4	E962.0	E980.4
Parathyroid (derivatives)	962.6	E858.0	E932.6	E950.4	E962.0	E980.4
Paratyphoid vaccine	978.1	E858.8	E948.1	E950.4	E962.0	E980.4
Paredrine	971.2	E855.5	E941.2	E950.4	E962.0	E980.4
Paregoric	965.00	E850.2	E935.2	E950.0	E962.0	E980.0
Pargyline	972.3	E858.3	E942.3	E950.4	E962.0	E980.4
Paris green	985.1	E866.3	—	E950.8	E962.1	E980.8
insecticide	985.1	E863.4	—	E950.8	E962.1	E980.8
Parnate	969.01	E854.0	E939.0	E950.3	E962.0	E980.3
Paromomycin	960.8	E856	E930.8	E950.4	E962.0	E980.4
Paroxypropione	963.1	E858.1	E933.1	E950.4	E962.0	E980.4
Parzone	965.09	E850.2	E935.2	E950.0	E962.0	E980.0
PAS	961.8	E857	E931.8	E950.4	E962.0	E980.4
PCBs	981	E862.3	—	E950.9	E962.1	E980.9
PCP (pentachlorophenol)	989.4	E863.6	—	E950.6	E962.1	E980.7
herbicide	989.4	E863.5	—	E950.6	E962.1	E980.7
insecticide	989.4	E863.4	—	E950.6	E962.1	E980.7
phencyclidine	968.3	E855.1	E938.3	E950.4	E962.0	E980.4
Peach kernel oil (emulsion)	973.2	E858.4	E943.2	E950.4	E962.0	E980.4
Peanut oil (emulsion) NEC	973.2	E858.4	E943.2	E950.4	E962.0	E980.4
topical	976.3	E858.7	E946.3	E950.4	E962.0	E980.4
Pearly Gates (morning glory seeds)	969.6	E854.1	E939.6	E950.3	E962.0	E980.3
Pecazine	969.1	E853.0	E939.1	E950.3	E962.0	E980.3
Pecilocin	960.1	E856	E930.1	E950.4	E962.0	E980.4
Pectin (with kaolin) NEC	973.5	E858.4	E943.5	E950.4	E962.0	E980.4
Pelletierine tannate	961.6	E857	E931.6	E950.4	E962.0	E980.4
Pemoline	969.79	E854.2	E939.7	E950.3	E962.0	E980.3
Pempidine	972.3	E858.3	E942.3	E950.4	E962.0	E980.4
Penamecillin	960.0	E856	E930.0	E950.4	E962.0	E980.4
Penethamate hydriodide	960.0	E856	E930.0	E950.4	E962.0	E980.4
Penicillamine	963.8	E858.1	E933.8	E950.4	E962.0	E980.4
Penicillin (any type)	960.0	E856	E930.0	E950.4	E962.0	E980.4
Penicillinase	963.4	E858.1	E933.4	E950.4	E962.0	E980.4
Pentachlorophenol (fungicide)	989.4	E863.6	—	E950.6	E962.1	E980.7
herbicide	989.4	E863.5	—	E950.6	E962.1	E980.7
insecticide	989.4	E863.4	—	E950.6	E962.1	E980.7
Pentaerythritol	972.4	E858.3	E942.4	E950.4	E962.0	E980.4
chloral	967.1	E852.0	E937.1	E950.2	E962.0	E980.2
tetranitrate NEC	972.4	E858.3	E942.4	E950.4	E962.0	E980.4
Pentagastrin	977.8	E858.8	E947.8	E950.4	E962.0	E980.4
Pentalin	982.3	E862.4	—	E950.9	E962.1	E980.9
Pentamethonium (bromide)	972.3	E858.3	E942.3	E950.4	E962.0	E980.4
Pentamidine	961.5	E857	E931.5	E950.4	E962.0	E980.4
Pentanol	980.8	E860.8	—	E950.9	E962.1	E980.9
Pentaquine	961.4	E857	E931.4	E950.4	E962.0	E980.4
Pentazocine	965.8	E850.8	E935.8	E950.0	E962.0	E980.0
Penthienate	971.1	E855.4	E941.1	E950.4	E962.0	E980.4

Substance	Poisoning	Accident	Therapeutic Use	Suicide Attempt	Assault	Undetermined
			External Cause (E-Code)			
Pentobarbital, pentobarbitone (sodium) 967.0	E851	E937.0	E950.1	E962.0	E980.1
Pentolinium (tartrate) 972.3	E858.3	E942.3	E950.4	E962.0	E980.4
Pentothal 968.3	E855.1	E938.3	E950.4	E962.0	E980.4
Pentylenetetrazol 970.0	E854.3	E940.0	E950.4	E962.0	E980.4
Pentylsalicylamide 961.8	E857	E931.8	E950.4	E962.0	E980.4
Pepsin 973.4	E858.4	E943.4	E950.4	E962.0	E980.4
Peptavlon 977.8	E858.8	E947.8	E950.4	E962.0	E980.4
Percaine (spinal) 968.7	E855.2	E938.7	E950.4	E962.0	E980.4
topical (surface) 968.5	E855.2	E938.5	E950.4	E962.0	E980.4
Perchloroethylene (vapor) 982.3	E862.4	—	E950.9	E962.1	E980.9
medicinal 961.6	E857	E931.6	E950.4	E962.0	E980.4
Percodan 965.09	E850.2	E935.2	E950.0	E962.0	E980.0
Percogesic 965.09	E850.2	E935.2	E950.0	E962.0	E980.0
Percorten 962.0	E858.0	E932.0	E950.4	E962.0	E980.4
Pergonal 962.4	E858.0	E932.4	E950.4	E962.0	E980.4
Perhexiline 972.4	E858.3	E942.4	E950.4	E962.0	E980.4
Periactin 963.0	E858.1	E933.0	E950.4	E962.0	E980.4
Periclor 967.1	E852.0	E937.1	E950.2	E962.0	E980.2
Pericyazine 969.1	E853.0	E939.1	E950.3	E962.0	E980.3
Peritrate 972.4	E858.3	E942.4	E950.4	E962.0	E980.4
Permanganates NEC 983.9	E864.3	—	E950.7	E962.1	E980.6
potassium (topical) 976.0	E858.7	E946.0	E950.4	E962.0	E980.4
Pernocton 967.0	E851	E937.0	E950.1	E962.0	E980.1
Pernoston 967.0	E851	E937.0	E950.1	E962.0	E980.1
Peronin(e) 965.09	E850.2	E935.2	E950.0	E962.0	E980.0
Perphenazine 969.1	E853.0	E939.1	E950.3	E962.0	E980.3
Pertofrane 969.05	E854	E939.0	E950.3	E962.0	E980.3
Pertussis					
immune serum (human) 964.6	E858.2	E934.6	E950.4	E962.0	E980.4
vaccine (with diphtheria toxoid) (with tetanus toxoid) 978.6	E858.8	E948.6	E950.4	E962.0	E980.4
Peruvian balsam 976.8	E858.7	E946.8	E950.4	E962.0	E980.4
Pesticides (dust) (fumes) (vapor) 989.4	E863.4	—	E950.6	E962.1	E980.7
arsenic 985.1	E863.4	—	E950.8	E962.1	E980.8
chlorinated 989.2	E863.0	—	E950.6	E962.1	E980.7
cyanide 989.0	E863.4	—	E950.6	E962.1	E980.7
kerosene 981	E863.4	—	E950.6	E962.1	E980.7
mixture (of compounds) 989.4	E863.3	—	E950.6	E962.1	E980.7
naphthalene 983.0	E863.4	—	E950.7	E962.1	E980.6
organochlorine (compounds) 989.2	E863.0	—	E950.6	E962.1	E980.7
petroleum (distillate) (products)					
NEC 981	E863.4	—	E950.6	E962.1	E980.7
specified ingredient NEC 989.4	E863.4	—	E950.6	E962.1	E980.7
strychnine 989.1	E863.4	—	E950.6	E962.1	E980.7
thallium 985.8	E863.7	—	E950.6	E962.1	E980.7
Pethidine (hydrochloride) 965.09	E850.2	E935.2	E950.0	E962.0	E980.0
Petrichloral 967.1	E852.0	E937.1	E950.2	E962.0	E980.2
Petrol 981	E862.1	—	E950.9	E962.1	E980.9
vapor 987.1	E869.8	—	E952.8	E962.2	E982.8
Petrolatum (jelly) (ointment) 976.3	E858.7	E946.3	E950.4	E962.0	E980.4
hydrophilic 976.3	E858.7	E946.3	E950.4	E962.0	E980.4
liquid 973.2	E858.4	E943.2	E950.4	E962.0	E980.4
topical 976.3	E858.7	E946.3	E950.4	E962.0	E980.4
nonmedicinal 981	E862.1	—	E950.9	E962.1	E980.9
Petroleum (cleaners) (fuels) (products)					
NEC 981	E862.1	—	E950.9	E962.1	E980.9
benzin(e) — see Ligroin					
ether — see Ligroin					
jelly — see Petrolatum					
naphtha — see Ligroin					
pesticide 981	E863.4	—	E950.6	E962.1	E980.7

Substance	Poisoning	Accident	Therapeutic Use	Suicide Attempt	Assault	Undetermined
			External Cause (E-Code)			
solids	981	E862.3	—	E950.9	E962.1	E980.9
solvents	981	E862.0	—	E950.9	E962.1	E980.9
vapor	987.1	E869.8	—	E952.8	E962.2	E982.8
Peyote	969.6	E854.1	E939.6	E950.3	E962.0	E980.3
Phanodorm, phanodorn	967.0	E851	E937.0	E950.1	E962.0	E980.1
Phanquinone, phanquone	961.5	E857	E931.5	E950.4	E962.0	E980.4
Pharmaceutical excipient or adjunct	977.4	E858.8	E947.4	E950.4	E962.0	E980.4
Phenacemide	966.3	E855.0	E936.3	E950.4	E962.0	E980.4
Phenacetin	965.4	E850.4	E935.4	E950.0	E962.0	E980.0
Phenadoxone	965.09	E850.2	E935.2	E950.0	E962.0	E980.0
Phenaglycodol	969.5	E853.8	E939.5	E950.3	E962.0	E980.3
Phenantoin	966.1	E855.0	E936.1	E950.4	E962.0	E980.4
Phenaphthazine reagent	977.8	E858.8	E947.8	E950.4	E962.0	E980.4
Phenazocine	965.09	E850.2	E935.2	E950.0	E962.0	E980.0
Phenazone	965.5	E850.5	E935.5	E950.0	E962.0	E980.0
Phenazopyridine	976.1	E858.7	E946.1	E950.4	E962.0	E980.4
Phenbenicillin	960.0	E856	E930.0	E950.4	E962.0	E980.4
Phenbutrazate	977.0	E858.8	E947.0	E950.4	E962.0	E980.4
Phencyclidine	968.3	E855.1	E938.3	E950.4	E962.0	E980.4
Phendimetrazine	977.0	E858.8	E947.0	E950.4	E962.0	E980.4
Phenelzine	969.01	E854.0	E939.0	E950.3	E962.0	E980.3
Phenergan	967.8	E852.8	E937.8	E950.2	E962.0	E980.2
Phenethicillin (potassium)	960.0	E856	E930.0	E950.4	E962.0	E980.4
Phenetsal	965.1	E850.3	E935.3	E950.0	E962.0	E980.0
Pheneturide	966.3	E855.0	E936.3	E950.4	E962.0	E980.4
Phenformin	962.3	E858.0	E932.3	E950.4	E962.0	E980.4
Phenglutarimide	971.1	E855.4	E941.1	E950.4	E962.0	E980.4
Phenicarbazide	965.8	E850.8	E935.8	E950.0	E962.0	E980.0
Phenindamine (tartrate)	963.0	E858.1	E933.0	E950.4	E962.0	E980.4
Phenindione	964.2	E858.2	E934.2	E950.4	E962.0	E980.4
Pheniprazine	969.01	E854.0	E939.0	E950.3	E962.0	E980.3
Pheniramine (maleate)	963.0	E858.1	E933.0	E950.4	E962.0	E980.4
Phenmetrazine	977.0	E858.8	E947.0	E950.4	E962.0	E980.4
Phenobal	967.0	E851	E937.0	E950.1	E962.0	E980.1
Phenobarbital	967.0	E851	E937.0	E950.1	E962.0	E980.1
Phenobarbitone	967.0	E851	E937.0	E950.1	E962.0	E980.1
Phenoctide	976.0	E858.7	E946.0	E950.4	E962.0	E980.4
Phenol (derivatives) NEC	983.0	E864.0	—	E950.7	E962.1	E980.6
disinfectant	983.0	E864.0	—	E950.7	E962.1	E980.6
pesticide	989.4	E863.4	—	E950.6	E962.1	E980.7
red	977.8	E858.8	E947.8	E950.4	E962.0	E980.4
Phenolphthalein	973.1	E858.4	E943.1	E950.4	E962.0	E980.4
Phenolsulfonphthalein	977.8	E858.8	E947.8	E950.4	E962.0	E980.4
Phenomorphan	965.09	E850.2	E935.2	E950.0	E962.0	E980.0
Phenonyl	967.0	E851	E937.0	E950.1	E962.0	E980.1
Phenoperidine	965.09	E850.2	E935.2	E950.0	E962.0	E980.0
Phenoquin	974.7	E858.5	E944.7	E950.4	E962.0	E980.4
Phenothiazines (tranquilizers) NEC	969.1	E853.0	E939.1	E950.3	E962.0	E980.3
insecticide	989.3	E863.4	—	E950.6	E962.1	E980.7
Phenoxybenzamine	971.3	E855.6	E941.3	E950.4	E962.0	E980.4
Phenoxymethyl penicillin	960.0	E856	E930.0	E950.4	E962.0	E980.4
Phenprocoumon	964.2	E858.2	E934.2	E950.4	E962.0	E980.4
Phensuximide	966.2	E855.0	E936.2	E950.4	E962.0	E980.4
Phentermine	977.0	E858.8	E947.0	E950.4	E962.0	E980.4
Phentolamine	971.3	E855.6	E941.3	E950.4	E962.0	E980.4
Phenyl						
butazone	965.5	E850.5	E935.5	E950.0	E962.0	E980.0
enediamine	983.0	E864.0	—	E950.7	E962.1	E980.6
hydrazine	983.0	E864.0	—	E950.7	E962.1	E980.6
antineoplastic	963.1	E858.1	E933.1	E950.4	E962.0	E980.4

Substance	Poisoning	Accident	Therapeutic Use	Suicide Attempt	Assault	Undetermined
			External Cause (E-Code)			
mercuric compounds — *see* Mercury						
salicylate	976.3	E858.7	E946.3	E950.4	E962.0	E980.4
Phenylephrin.	971.2	E855.5	E941.2	E950.4	E962.0	E980.4
Phenylethybiguanide	962.3	E858.0	E932.3	E950.4	E962.0	E980.4
Phenylpropanolamine	971.2	E855.5	E941.2	E950.4	E962.0	E980.4
Phenylsulfthion.	989.3	E863.1	—	E950.6	E962.1	E980.7
Phenyramidol, phenyramidon	965.7	E850.7	E935.7	E950.0	E962.0	E980.0
Phenytoin	966.1	E855.0	E936.1	E950.4	E962.0	E980.4
pHisoHex	976.2	E858.7	E946.2	E950.4	E962.0	E980.4
Pholcodine	965.09	E850.2	E935.2	E950.0	E962.0	E980.0
Phorate	989.3	E863.1	—	E950.6	E962.1	E980.7
Phosdrin	989.3	E863.1	—	E950.6	E962.1	E980.7
Phosgene (gas).	987.8	E869.8	—	E952.8	E962.2	E982.8
Phosphate (tricresyl)	989.89	E866.8	—	E950.9	E962.1	E980.9
organic	989.3	E863.1	—	E950.6	E962.1	E980.7
solvent	982.8	E862.4	—	E950.9	E926.1	E980.9
Phosphine	987.8	E869.8	—	E952.8	E962.2	E982.8
fumigant.	987.8	E863.8	—	E950.6	E962.2	E980.7
Phospholine	971.0	E855.3	E941.0	E950.4	E962.0	E980.4
Phosphoric acid	983.1	E864.1	—	E950.7	E962.1	E980.6
Phosphorus (compounds) NEC	983.9	E864.3	—	E950.7	E962.1	E980.6
rodenticide.	983.9	E863.7	—	E950.7	E962.1	E980.6
Phthalimidogluarimide.	967.8	E852.8	E937.8	E950.2	E962.0	E980.2
Phthalylsulfathiazole	961.0	E857	E931.0	E950.4	E962.0	E980.4
Phylloquinone	964.3	E858.2	E934.3	E950.4	E962.0	E980.4
Physeptone	965.02	E850.1	E935.1	E950.0	E962.0	E980.0
Physostigma venenosum	988.2	E865.4	—	E950.9	E962.1	E980.9
Physostigmine	971.0	E855.3	E941.0	E950.4	E962.0	E980.4
Phytolacca decandra.	988.2	E865.4	—	E950.9	E962.1	E980.9
Phytomenadione	964.3	E858.2	E934.3	E950.4	E962.0	E980.4
Phytonadione	964.3	E858.2	E934.3	E950.4	E962.0	E980.4
Picric (acid)	983.0	E864.0	—	E950.7	E962.1	E980.6
Picrotoxin	970.0	E854.3	E940.0	E950.4	E962.0	E980.4
Pilocarpine	971.0	E855.3	E941.0	E950.4	E962.0	E980.4
Pilocarpus (jaborandi) extract	971.0	E855.3	E941.0	E950.4	E962.0	E980.4
Pimaricin	960.1	E856	E930.1	E950.4	E962.0	E980.4
Piminodine	965.09	E850.2	E935.2	E950.0	E962.0	E980.0
Pine oil, pinesol (disinfectant)	983.9	E861.4	—	E950.7	E962.1	E980.6
Pinkroot	961.6	E857	E931.6	E950.4	E962.0	E980.4
Pipadone	965.09	E850.2	E935.2	E950.0	E962.0	E980.0
Pipamazine	963.0	E858.1	E933.0	E950.4	E962.0	E980.4
Pipazethate	975.4	E858.6	E945.4	E950.4	E962.0	E980.4
Pipenzolate	971.1	E855.4	E941.1	E950.4	E962.0	E980.4
Piperacetazine	969.1	E853.0	E939.1	E950.3	E962.0	E980.3
Piperazine NEC	961.6	E857	E931.6	E950.4	E962.0	E980.4
estrone sulfate	962.2	E858.0	E932.2	E950.4	E962.0	E980.4
Piper cubeba.	988.2	E865.4	—	E950.9	E962.1	E980.9
Piperidione	975.4	E858.6	E945.4	E950.4	E962.0	E980.4
Piperidolate	971.1	E855.4	E941.1	E950.4	E962.0	E980.4
Piperocaine	968.9	E855.2	E938.9	E950.4	E962.0	E980.4
infiltration (subcutaneous)	968.5	E855.2	E938.5	E950.4	E962.0	E980.4
nerve block (peripheral) (plexus). . . .	968.6	E855.2	E938.6	E950.4	E962.0	E980.4
topical (surface)	968.5	E855.2	E938.5	E950.4	E962.0	E980.4
Pipobroman	963.1	E858.1	E933.1	E950.4	E962.0	E980.4
Pipradrol	970.89	E854.3	E940.8	E950.4	E962.0	E980.0
Piscidia (bark) (erythrina)	965.7	E850.7	E935.7	E950.0	E962.0	E980.0
Pitch	983.0	E864.0	—	E950.7	E962.1	E980.6
Pitkin's solution	968.7	E855.2	E938.7	E950.4	E962.0	E980.4
Pitocin	975.0	E858.6	E945.0	E950.4	E962.0	E980.4
Pitressin (tannate)	962.5	E858.0	E932.5	E950.4	E962.0	E980.4
Pituitary extracts (posterior)	962.5	E858.0	E932.5	E950.4	E962.0	E980.4

Substance	Poisoning	Accident	Therapeutic Use	Suicide Attempt	Assault	Undetermined
			External Cause (E-Code)			
anterior 962.4	E858.0	E932.4	E950.4	E962.0	E980.4
Pituitrin. 962.5	E858.0	E932.5	E950.4	E962.0	E980.4
Placental extract 962.9	E858.0	E932.9	E950.4	E962.0	E980.4
Placidyl. 967.8	E852.8	E937.8	E950.2	E962.0	E980.2
Plague vaccine. 978.3	E858.8	E948.3	E950.4	E962.0	E980.4
Plant foods or fertilizers NEC 989.89	E866.5	—	E950.9	E962.1	E980.9
mixed with herbicides 989.4	E863.5	—	E950.6	E962.1	E980.7
Plants, noxious, used as food 988.2	E865.9	—	E950.9	E962.1	E980.9
berries and seeds 988.2	E865.3	—	E950.9	E962.1	E980.9
specified type NEC 988.2	E865.4	—	E950.9	E962.1	E980.9
Plasma (blood). 964.7	E858.2	E934.7	E950.4	E962.0	E980.4
expanders 964.8	E858.2	E934.8	E950.4	E962.0	E980.4
Plasmanate 964.7	E858.2	E934.7	E950.4	E962.0	E980.4
Plegicil 969.1	E853.0	E939.1	E950.3	E962.0	E980.3
Podophyllin 976.4	E858.7	E946.4	E950.4	E962.0	E980.4
Podophyllum resin 976.4	E858.7	E946.4	E950.4	E962.0	E980.4
Poison NEC 989.9	E866.9	—	E950.9	E962.1	E980.9
Poisonous berries 988.2	E865.3	—	E950.9	E962.1	E980.9
Pokeweed (any part) 988.2	E865.4	—	E950.9	E962.1	E980.9
Poldine 971.1	E855.4	E941.1	E950.4	E962.0	E980.4
Poliomyelitis vaccine 979.5	E858.8	E949.5	E950.4	E962.0	E980.4
Poliovirus vaccine 979.5	E858.8	E949.5	E950.4	E962.0	E980.4
Polish (car) (floor) (furniture) (metal) (silver) 989.89	E861.2	—	E950.9	E962.1	E980.9
abrasive 989.89	E861.3	—	E950.9	E962.1	E980.9
porcelain 989.89	E861.3	—	E950.9	E962.1	E980.9
Poloxalkol. 973.2	E858.4	E943.2	E950.4	E962.0	E980.4
Polyaminostyrene resins 974.5	E858.5	E944.5	E950.4	E962.0	E980.4
Polychlorinated biphenyl—see PCBs					
Polycycline 960.4	E856	E930.4	E950.4	E962.0	E980.4
Polyester resin hardener 982.8	E862.4	—	E950.9	E962.1	E980.9
fumes. 987.8	E869.8	—	E952.8	E962.2	E982.8
Polyestradiol (phosphate) 962.2	E858.0	E932.2	E950.4	E962.0	E980.4
Polyethanolamine alkyl sulfate 976.2	E858.7	E946.2	E950.4	E962.0	E980.4
Polyethylene glycol 976.3	E858.7	E946.3	E950.4	E962.0	E980.4
Polyferose. 964.0	E858.2	E934.0	E950.4	E962.0	E980.4
Polymyxin B 960.8	E856	E930.8	E950.4	E962.0	E980.4
ENT agent. 976.6	E858.7	E946.6	E950.4	E962.0	E980.4
ophthalmic preparation. 976.5	E858.7	E946.5	E950.4	E962.0	E980.4
topical NEC 976.0	E858.7	E946.0	E950.4	E962.0	E980.4
Polynoxylin(e) 976.0	E858.7	E946.0	E950.4	E962.0	E980.4
Polyoxymethyleneurea. 976.0	E858.7	E946.0	E950.4	E962.0	E980.4
Polytetrafluoroethylene (inhaled) 987.8	E869.8	—	E952.8	E962.2	E982.8
Polythiazide 974.3	E858.5	E944.3	E950.4	E962.0	E980.4
Polyvinylpyrrolidone 964.8	E858.2	E934.8	E950.4	E962.0	E980.4
Pontocaine (hydrochloride) (infiltration) (topical) 968.5	E855.2	E938.5	E950.4	E962.0	E980.4
nerve block (peripheral) (plexus). 968.6	E855.2	E938.6	E950.4	E962.0	E980.4
spinal 968.7	E855.2	E938.7	E950.4	E962.0	E980.4
Pot. 969.6	E854.1	E939.6	E950.3	E962.0	E980.3
Potash (caustic) 983.2	E864.2	—	E950.7	E962.1	E980.6
Potassic saline injection (lactated) 974.5	E858.5	E944.5	E950.4	E962.0	E980.4
Potassium (salts) NEC. 974.5	E858.5	E944.5	E950.4	E962.0	E980.4
aminosalicylate 961.8	E857	E931.8	E950.4	E962.0	E980.4
arsenite (solution). 985.1	E866.3	—	E950.8	E962.1	E980.8
bichromate. 983.9	E864.3	—	E950.7	E962.1	E980.6
bisulfate 983.9	E864.3	—	E950.7	E962.1	E980.6
bromide (medicinal) NEC 967.3	E852.2	E937.3	E950.2	E962.0	E980.2
carbonate 983.2	E864.2	—	E950.7	E962.1	E980.6
chlorate NEC. 983.9	E864.3	—	E950.7	E962.1	E980.6

Substance	Poisoning	Accident	Therapeutic Use	Suicide Attempt	Assault	Undetermined
			External Cause (E-Code)			
cyanide — *see* Cyanide						
hydroxide	983.2	E864.2	—	E950.7	E962.1	E980.6
iodide (expectorant) NEC	975.5	E858.6	E945.5	E950.4	E962.0	E980.4
nitrate	989.89	E866.8	—	E950.9	E962.1	E980.9
oxalate	983.9	E864.3	—	E950.7	E962.1	E980.6
perchlorate NEC	977.8	E858.8	E947.8	E950.4	E962.0	E980.4
antithyroid	962.8	E858.0	E932.8	E950.4	E962.0	E980.4
permanganate	976.0	E858.7	E946.0	E950.4	E962.0	E980.4
nonmedicinal	983.9	E864.3	—	E950.7	E962.1	E980.6
Povidone–iodine (anti–infective) NEC	976.0	E858.7	E946.0	E950.4	E962.0	E980.4
Practolol	972.0	E858.3	E942.0	E950.4	E962.0	E980.4
Pralidoxime (chloride)	977.2	E858.8	E947.2	E950.4	E962.0	E980.4
Pramoxine	968.5	E855.2	E938.5	E950.4	E962.0	E980.4
Prazosin	972.6	E858.3	E942.6	E950.4	E962.0	E980.4
Prednisolone	962.0	E858.0	E932.0	E950.4	E962.0	E980.4
ENT agent	976.6	E858.7	E946.6	E950.4	E962.0	E980.4
ophthalmic preparation	976.5	E858.7	E946.5	E950.4	E962.0	E980.4
topical NEC	976.0	E858.7	E946.0	E950.4	E962.0	E980.4
Prednisone	962.0	E858.0	E932.0	E950.4	E962.0	E980.4
Pregnanediol	962.2	E858.0	E932.2	E950.4	E962.0	E980.4
Pregneninolone	962.2	E858.0	E932.2	E950.4	E962.0	E980.4
Preludin	977.0	E858.8	E947.0	E950.4	E962.0	E980.4
Premarin	962.2	E858.0	E932.2	E950.4	E962.0	E980.4
Prenylamine	972.4	E858.3	E942.4	E950.4	E962.0	E980.4
Preparation H	976.8	E858.7	E946.8	E950.4	E962.0	E980.4
Preservatives	989.89	E866.8	—	E950.9	E962.1	E980.9
Pride of China	988.2	E865.3	—	E950.9	E962.1	E980.9
Prilocaine	968.9	E855.2	E938.9	E950.4	E962.0	E980.4
infiltration (subcutaneous)	968.5	E855.2	E938.5	E950.4	E962.0	E980.4
nerve block (peripheral) (plexus)	968.6	E855.2	E938.6	E950.4	E962.0	E980.4
Primaquine	961.4	E857	E931.4	E950.4	E962.0	E980.4
Primidone	966.3	E855.0	E936.3	E950.4	E962.0	E980.4
Primula (veris)	988.2	E865.4	—	E950.9	E962.1	E980.9
Prinadol	965.09	E850.2	E935.2	E950.0	E962.0	E980.0
Priscol, Priscoline	971.3	E855.6	E941.3	E950.4	E962.0	E980.4
Privet	988.2	E865.4	—	E950.9	E962.1	E980.9
Privine	971.2	E855.5	E941.2	E950.4	E962.0	E980.4
Pro–Banthine	971.1	E855.4	E941.1	E950.4	E962.0	E980.4
Probarbital	967.0	E851	E937.0	E950.1	E962.0	E980.1
Probenecid	974.7	E858.5	E944.7	E950.4	E962.0	E980.4
Procainamide (hydrochloride)	972.0	E858.3	E942.0	E950.4	E962.0	E980.4
Procaine (hydrochloride) (infiltration) (topical)	968.5	E855.2	E938.5	E950.4	E962.0	E980.4
nerve block (peripheral) (plexus)	968.6	E855.2	E938.6	E950.4	E962.0	E980.4
penicillin G	960.0	E856	E930.0	E950.4	E962.0	E980.4
spinal	968.7	E855.2	E938.7	E950.4	E962.0	E980.4
Procalmidol	969.5	E853.8	E939.5	E950.3	E962.0	E980.3
Procarbazine	963.1	E858.1	E933.1	E950.4	E962.0	E980.4
Prochlorperazine	969.1	E853.0	E939.1	E950.3	E962.0	E980.3
Procyclidine	966.4	E855.0	E936.4	E950.4	E962.0	E980.4
Producer gas	986	E868.8	—	E952.1	E962.2	E982.1
Profenamine	966.4	E855.0	E936.4	E950.4	E962.0	E980.4
Profenil	975.1	E858.6	E945.1	E950.4	E962.0	E980.4
Progesterones	962.2	E858.0	E932.2	E950.4	E962.0	E980.4
Progestin	962.2	E858.0	E932.2	E950.4	E962.0	E980.4
Progestogens (with estrogens)	962.2	E858.0	E932.2	E950.4	E962.0	E980.4
Progestone	962.2	E858.0	E932.2	E950.4	E962.0	E980.4
Proguanil	961.4	E857	E931.4	E950.4	E962.0	E980.4
Prolactin	962.4	E858.0	E932.4	E950.4	E962.0	E980.4
Proloid	962.7	E858.0	E932.7	E950.4	E962.0	E980.4
Proluton	962.2	E858.0	E932.2	E950.4	E962.0	E980.4

Substance	Poisoning	Accident	Therapeutic Use	Suicide Attempt	Assault	Undetermined
			External Cause (E-Code)			
Promacetin	961.8	E857	E931.8	E950.4	E962.0	E980.4
Promazine	969.1	E853.0	E939.1	E950.3	E962.0	E980.3
Promedol	965.09	E850.2	E935.2	E950.0	E962.0	E980.0
Promethazine	967.8	E852.8	E937.8	E950.2	E962.0	E980.2
Promin	961.8	E857	E931.8	E950.4	E962.0	E980.4
Pronestyl (hydrochloride)	972.0	E858.3	E942.0	E950.4	E962.0	E980.4
Pronetalol, pronethalol	972.0	E858.3	E942.0	E950.4	E962.0	E980.4
Prontosil	961.0	E857	E931.0	E950.4	E962.0	E980.4
Propamidine isethionate	961.5	E857	E931.5	E950.4	E962.0	E980.4
Propanal (medicinal)	967.8	E852.8	E937.8	E950.2	E962.0	E980.2
Propane (gas) (distributed in mobile container)	987.0	E868.0	—	E951.1	E962.2	E981.1
distributed through pipes	987.0	E867	—	E951.0	E962.2	E981.0
incomplete combustion of – *see* Carbon monoxide, Propane						
Propanidid	968.3	E855.1	E938.3	E950.4	E962.0	E980.4
Propanol	980.3	E860.4	—	E950.9	E962.1	E980.9
Propantheline	971.1	E855.4	E941.1	E950.4	E962.0	E980.4
Proparacaine	968.5	E855.2	E938.5	E950.4	E962.0	E980.4
Propatyl nitrate	972.4	E858.3	E942.4	E950.4	E962.0	E980.4
Propicillin	960.0	E856	E930.0	E950.4	E962.0	E980.4
Propiolactone (vapor)	987.8	E869.8	—	E952.8	E962.2	E982.8
Propiomazine	967.8	E852.8	E937.8	E950.2	E962.0	E980.2
Propionaldehyde (medicinal)	967.8	E852.8	E937.8	E950.2	E962.0	E980.2
Propionate compound	976.0	E858.7	E946.0	E950.4	E962.0	E980.4
Propion gel	976.0	E858.7	E946.0	E950.4	E962.0	E980.4
Propitocaine	968.9	E855.2	E938.9	E950.4	E962.0	E980.4
infiltration (subcutaneous)	968.5	E855.2	E938.5	E950.4	E962.0	E980.4
nerve block (peripheral) (plexus)	968.6	E855.2	E938.6	E950.4	E962.0	E980.4
Propoxur	989.3	E863.2	—	E950.6	E962.1	E980.7
Propoxycaine	968.9	E855.2	E938.9	E950.4	E962.0	E980.4
infiltration (subcutaneous)	968.5	E855.2	E938.5	E950.4	E962.0	E980.4
nerve block (peripheral) (plexus)	968.6	E855.2	E938.6	E950.4	E962.0	E980.4
topical (surface)	968.5	E855.2	E938.5	E950.4	E962.0	E980.4
Propoxyphene (hydrochloride)	965.8	E850.8	E935.8	E950.0	E962.0	E980.0
Propranolol	972.0	E858.3	E942.0	E950.4	E962.0	E980.4
Propyl						
alcohol	980.3	E860.4	—	E950.9	E962.1	E980.9
carbinol	980.3	E860.4	—	E950.9	E962.1	E980.9
hexadrine	971.2	E855.5	E941.2	E950.4	E962.0	E980.4
iodone	977.8	E858.8	E947.8	E950.4	E962.0	E980.4
thiouracil	962.8	E858.0	E932.8	E950.4	E962.0	E980.4
Propylene	987.1	E869.8	—	E952.8	E962.2	E982.8
Propylparaben (ophthalmic)	976.5	E858.7	E946.5	E950.4	E962.0	E980.4
Proscillaridin	972.1	E858.3	E942.1	E950.4	E962.0	E980.4
Prostaglandins	975.0	E858.6	E945.0	E950.4	E962.0	E980.4
Prostigmin	971.0	E855.3	E941.0	E950.4	E962.0	E980.4
Protamine (sulfate)	964.5	E858.2	E934.5	E950.4	E962.0	E980.4
zinc insulin	962.3	E858.0	E932.3	E950.4	E962.0	E980.4
Protectants (topical)	976.3	E858.7	E946.3	E950.4	E962.0	E980.4
Protein hydrolysate	974.5	E858.5	E944.5	E950.4	E962.0	E980.4
Prothiaden—*see* Dothiepin hydrochloride						
Prothionamide	961.8	E857	E931.8	E950.4	E962.0	E980.4
Prothipendyl	969.5	E853.8	E939.5	E950.3	E962.0	E980.3
Protokylol	971.2	E855.5	E941.2	E950.4	E962.0	E980.4
Protopam	977.2	E858.8	E947.2	E950.4	E962.0	E980.4
Protoveratrine(s) (A) (B)	972.6	E858.3	E942.6	E950.4	E962.0	E980.4
Protriptyline	969.05	E854.0	E939.0	E950.3	E962.0	E980.3
Provera	962.2	E858.0	E932.2	E950.4	E962.0	E980.4
Provitamin A	963.5	E858.1	E933.5	E950.4	E962.0	E980.4

Substance	Poisoning	Accident	Therapeutic Use	Suicide Attempt	Assault	Undetermined
			External Cause (E-Code)			
Proxymetacaine	968.5	E855.2	E938.5	E950.4	E962.0	E980.4
Proxyphylline	975.1	E858.6	E945.1	E950.4	E962.0	E980.4
Prozac—*see* Fluoxetine hydrochloride						
Prunus						
laurocerasus	988.2	E865.4	—	E950.9	E962.1	E980.9
virginiana	988.2	E865.4	—	E950.9	E962.1	E980.9
Prussic acid	989.0	E866.8	—	E950.9	E962.1	E980.9
vapor	987.7	E869.8	—	E952.8	E962.2	E982.8
Pseudoephedrine	971.2	E855.5	E941.2	E950.4	E962.0	E980.4
Psilocin	969.6	E854.1	E939.6	E950.3	E962.0	E980.3
Psilocybin	969.6	E854.1	E939.6	E950.3	E962.0	E980.3
PSP	977.8	E858.8	E947.8	E950.4	E962.0	E980.4
Psychedelic agents	969.6	E854.1	E939.6	E950.3	E962.0	E980.3
Psychodysleptics	969.6	E854.1	E939.6	E950.3	E962.0	E980.3
Psychostimulants	969.70	E854.2	E939.7	E950.3	E962.0	E980.3
Psychotherapeutic agents	969.9	E855.9	E939.9	E950.3	E962.0	E980.3
antidepressants	969.00	E854.0	E939.0	E950.3	E962.0	E980.3
specified NEC	969.8	E855.8	E939.8	E950.3	E962.0	E980.3
tranquilizers NEC	969.5	E853.9	E939.5	E950.3	E962.0	E980.3
Psychotomimetic agents	969.6	E854.1	E939.6	E950.3	E962.0	E980.3
Psychotropic agents	969.9	E854.8	E939.9	E950.3	E962.0	E980.3
specified NEC	969.8	E854.8	E939.8	E950.3	E962.0	E980.3
Psyllium	973.3	E858.4	E943.3	E950.4	E962.0	E980.4
Pteroylglutamic acid	964.1	E858.2	E934.1	E950.4	E962.0	E980.4
Pteroyltriglutamate	963.1	E858.1	E933.1	E950.4	E962.0	E980.4
PTFE	987.8	E869.8	—	E952.8	E962.2	E982.8
Pulsatilla	988.2	E865.4	—	E950.9	E962.1	E980.9
Purex (bleach)	983.9	E864.3	—	E950.7	E962.1	E980.6
Purine diuretics	974.1	E858.5	E944.1	E950.4	E962.0	E980.4
Purinethol	963.1	E858.1	E933.1	E950.4	E962.0	E980.4
PVP	964.8	E858.2	E934.8	E950.4	E962.0	E980.4
Pyrabital	965.7	E850.7	E935.7	E950.0	E962.0	E980.0
Pyramidon	965.5	E850.5	E935.5	E950.0	E962.0	E980.0
Pyrantel (pamoate)	961.6	E857	E931.6	E950.4	E962.0	E980.4
Pyrathiazine	963.0	E858.1	E933.0	E950.4	E962.0	E980.4
Pyrazinamide	961.8	E857	E931.8	E950.4	E962.0	E980.4
Pyrazinoic acid (amide)	961.8	E857	E931.8	E950.4	E962.0	E980.4
Pyrazole (derivatives)	965.5	E850.5	E935.5	E950.0	E962.0	E980.0
Pyrazolone (analgesics)	965.5	E850.5	E935.5	E950.0	E962.0	E980.0
Pyrethrins, pyrethrum	989.4	E863.4	—	E950.6	E962.1	E980.7
Pyribenzamine	963.0	E858.1	E933.0	E950.4	E962.0	E980.4
Pyridine (liquid) (vapor)	982.0	E862.4	—	E950.9	E962.1	E980.9
aldoxime chloride	977.2	E858.8	E947.2	E950.4	E962.0	E980.4
Pyridium	976.1	E858.7	E946.1	E950.4	E962.0	E980.4
Pyridostigmine	971.0	E855.3	E941.0	E950.4	E962.0	E980.4
Pyridoxine	963.5	E858.1	E933.5	E950.4	E962.0	E980.4
Pyrilamine	963.0	E858.1	E933.0	E950.4	E962.0	E980.4
Pyrimethamine	961.4	E857	E931.4	E950.4	E962.0	E980.4
Pyrogallic acid	983.0	E864.0	—	E950.7	E962.1	E980.6
Pyroxylin	976.3	E858.7	E946.3	E950.4	E962.0	E980.4
Pyrrobutamine	963.0	E858.1	E933.0	E950.4	E962.0	E980.4
Pyrrocaine	968.5	E855.2	E938.5	E950.4	E962.0	E980.4
Pyrvinium (pamoate)	961.6	E857	E931.6	E950.4	E962.0	E980.4
PZI	962.3	E858.0	E932.3	E950.4	E962.0	E980.4
Quaalude	967.4	E852.3	E937.4	E950.2	E962.0	E980.2
Quaternary ammonium derivatives	971.1	E855.4	E941.1	E950.4	E962.0	E980.4
Quicklime	983.2	E864.2	—	E950.7	E962.1	E980.6
Quinacrine	961.3	E857	E931.3	E950.4	E962.0	E980.4
Quinaglute	972.0	E858.3	E942.0	E950.4	E962.0	E980.4
Quinalbarbitone	967.0	E851	E937.0	E950.1	E962.0	E980.1
Quinestradiol	962.2	E858.0	E932.2	E950.4	E962.0	E980.4

Substance	Poisoning	Accident	Therapeutic Use	Suicide Attempt	Assault	Undetermined
		External Cause (E-Code)				
Quinethazone 974.3		E858.5	E944.3	E950.4	E962.0	E980.4
Quinidine (gluconate) (polygalacturonate)						
(salts) (sulfate) 972.0		E858.3	E942.0	E950.4	E962.0	E980.4
Quinine. 961.4		E857	E931.4	E950.4	E962.0	E980.4
Quiniobine 961.3		E857	E931.3	E950.4	E962.0	E980.4
Quinolines 961.3		E857	E931.3	E950.4	E962.0	E980.4
Quotane. 968.5		E855.2	E938.5	E950.4	E962.0	E980.4
Rabies						
immune globulin (human) 964.6		E858.2	E934.6	E950.4	E962.0	E980.4
vaccine 979.1		E858.8	E949.1	E950.4	E962.0	E980.4
Racemoramide 965.09		E850.2	E935.2	E950.0	E962.0	E980.0
Racemorphan 965.09		E850.2	E935.2	E950.0	E962.0	E980.0
Radiator alcohol 980.1		E860.2	—	E950.9	E962.1	E980.9
Radio–opaque (drugs) (materials) . . . 977.8		E858.8	E947.8	E950.4	E962.0	E980.4
Ranunculus 988.2		E865.4	—	E950.9	E962.1	E980.9
Rat poison 989.4		E863.7	—	E950.6	E962.1	E980.7
Rattlesnake (venom) 989.5		E905.0	—	E950.9	E962.1	E980.9
Raudixin 972.6		E858.3	E942.6	E950.4	E962.0	E980.4
Rautensin 972.6		E858.3	E942.6	E950.4	E962.0	E980.4
Rautina 972.6		E858.3	E942.6	E950.4	E962.0	E980.4
Rautotal 972.6		E858.3	E942.6	E950.4	E962.0	E980.4
Rauwiloid 972.6		E858.3	E942.6	E950.4	E962.0	E980.4
Rauwoldin. 972.6		E858.3	E942.6	E950.4	E962.0	E980.4
Rauwolfia (alkaloids) 972.6		E858.3	E942.6	E950.4	E962.0	E980.4
Realgar. 985.1		E866.3	—	E950.8	E962.1	E980.8
Red cells, packed 964.7		E858.2	E934.7	E950.4	E962.0	E980.4
Reducing agents, industrial NEC 983.9		E864.3	—	E950.7	E962.1	E980.6
Refrigerant gas (freon) 987.4		E869.2	—	E952.8	E962.2	E982.8
not freon 987.9		E869.9	—	E952.9	E962.2	E982.9
Regroton 974.4		E858.5	E944.4	E950.4	E962.0	E980.4
Rela 968.0		E855.1	E938.0	E950.4	E962.0	E980.4
Relaxants, skeletal muscle (autonomic). . . 975.2		E858.6	E945.2	E950.4	E962.0	E980.4
central nervous system. 968.0		E855.1	E938.0	E950.4	E962.0	E980.4
Renese 974.3		E858.5	E944.3	E950.4	E962.0	E980.4
Renografin 977.8		E858.8	E947.8	E950.4	E962.0	E980.4
Replacement solutions. 974.5		E858.5	E944.5	E950.4	E962.0	E980.4
Rescinnamine 972.6		E858.3	E942.6	E950.4	E962.0	E980.4
Reserpine 972.6		E858.3	E942.6	E950.4	E962.0	E980.4
Resorcin, resorcinol. 976.4		E858.7	E946.4	E950.4	E962.0	E980.4
Respaire 975.5		E858.6	E945.5	E950.4	E962.0	E980.4
Respiratory agents NEC 975.8		E858.6	E945.8	E950.4	E962.0	E980.4
Retinoic acid 976.8		E858.7	E946.8	E950.4	E962.0	E980.4
Retinol 963.5		E858.1	E933.5	E950.4	E962.0	E980.4
Rh₀ (D) immune globulin (human). 964.6		E858.2	E934.6	E950.4	E962.0	E980.4
Rhodine. 965.1		E850.3	E935.3	E950.0	E962.0	E980.0
RhoGAM 964.6		E858.2	E934.6	E950.4	E962.0	E980.4
Riboflavin. 963.5		E858.1	E933.5	E950.4	E962.0	E980.4
Ricin. 989.89		E866.8	—	E950.9	E962.1	E980.9
Ricinus communis 988.2		E865.3	—	E950.9	E962.1	E980.9
Rickettsial vaccine NEC 979.6		E858.8	E949.6	E950.4	E962.0	E980.4
with viral and bacterial vaccine 979.7		E858.8	E949.7	E950.4	E962.0	E980.4
Rifampin 960.6		E856	E930.6	E950.4	E962.0	E980.4
Rimifon. 961.8		E857	E931.8	E950.4	E962.0	E980.4
Ringer's injection (lactated) 974.5		E858.5	E944.5	E950.4	E962.0	E980.4
Ristocetin 960.8		E856	E930.8	E950.4	E962.0	E980.4
Ritalin 969.73		E854.2	E939.7	E950.3	E962.0	E980.3
Roach killers — *see* Pesticides						
Rocky Mountain spotted fever vaccine 979.6		E858.8	E949.6	E950.4	E962.0	E980.4
Rodenticides. 989.4		E863.7	—	E950.6	E962.1	E980.7
Rohypnol 969.4		E853.2	E939.4	E950.3	E962.0	E980.3

Substance	Poisoning	Accident	Therapeutic Use	Suicide Attempt	Assault	Undetermined
			External Cause (E-Code)			
Rolaids	973.0	E858.4	E943.0	E950.4	E962.0	E980.4
Rolitetracycline	960.4	E856	E930.4	E950.4	E962.0	E980.4
Romilar	975.4	E858.6	E945.4	E950.4	E962.0	E980.4
Rose water ointment	976.3	E858.7	E946.3	E950.4	E962.0	E980.4
Rotenone	989.4	E863.7	—	E950.6	E962.1	E980.7
Rotoxamine	963.0	E858.1	E933.0	E950.4	E962.0	E980.4
Rough–on–rats	989.4	E863.7	—	E950.6	E962.1	E980.7
Rubbing alcohol	980.2	E860.3	—	E950.9	E962.1	E980.9
Rubella virus vaccine	979.4	E858.8	E949.4	E950.4	E962.0	E980.4
Rubelogen	979.4	E858.8	E949.4	E950.4	E962.0	E980.4
Rubeovax	979.4	E858.8	E949.4	E950.4	E962.0	E980.4
Rubidomycin	960.7	E856	E930.7	E950.4	E962.0	E980.4
Rue	988.2	E865.4	—	E950.9	E962.1	E980.9
RU486	962.9	E858.0	E932.9	E950.4	E962.0	E980.4
Ruta	988.2	E865.4	—	E950.9	E962.1	E980.9
Sabadilla (medicinal)	976.0	E858.7	E946.0	E950.4	E962.0	E980.4
pesticide	989.4	E863.4	—	E950.6	E962.1	E980.7
Sabin oral vaccine	979.5	E858.8	E949.5	E950.4	E962.0	E980.4
Saccharated iron oxide	964.0	E858.2	E934.0	E950.4	E962.0	E980.4
Saccharin	974.5	E858.5	E944.5	E950.4	E962.0	E980.4
Safflower oil	972.2	E858.3	E942.2	E950.4	E962.0	E980.4
Salbutamol sulfate	975.7	E858.6	E945.7	E950.4	E962.0	E980.4
Salicylamide	965.1	E850.3	E935.3	E950.0	E962.0	E980.0
Salicylate(s)	965.1	E850.3	E935.3	E950.0	E962.0	E980.0
methyl	976.3	E858.7	E946.3	E950.4	E962.0	E980.4
theobromine calcium	974.1	E858.5	E944.1	E950.4	E962.0	E980.4
Salicylazosulfapyridine	961.0	E857	E931.0	E950.4	E962.0	E980.4
Salicylhydroxamic acid	976.0	E858.7	E946.0	E950.4	E962.0	E980.4
Salicylic acid (keratolytic) NEC	976.4	E858.7	E946.4	E950.4	E962.0	E980.4
congeners	965.1	E850.3	E935.3	E950.0	E962.0	E980.0
salts	965.1	E850.3	E935.3	E950.0	E962.0	E980.0
Saliniazid	961.8	E857	E931.8	E950.4	E962.0	E980.4
Salol	976.3	E858.7	E946.3	E950.4	E962.0	E980.4
Salt (substitute) NEC	974.5	E858.5	E944.5	E950.4	E962.0	E980.4
Saluretics	974.3	E858.5	E944.3	E950.4	E962.0	E980.4
Saluron	974.3	E858.5	E944.3	E950.4	E962.0	E980.4
Salvarsan 606 (neosilver) (silver)	961.1	E857	E931.1	E950.4	E962.0	E980.4
Sambucus canadensis	988.2	E865.4	—	E950.9	E962.1	E980.9
berry	988.2	E865.3	—	E950.9	E962.1	E980.9
Sandril	972.6	E858.3	E942.6	E950.4	E962.0	E980.4
Sanguinaria canadensis	988.2	E865.4	—	E950.9	E962.1	E980.9
Saniflush (cleaner)	983.9	E861.3	—	E950.7	E962.1	E980.6
Santonin	961.6	E857	E931.6	E950.4	E962.0	E980.4
Santyl	976.8	E858.7	E946.8	E950.4	E962.0	E980.4
Sarkomycin	960.7	E856	E930.7	E950.4	E962.0	E980.4
Saroten	969.05	E854.0	E939.0	E950.3	E962.0	E980.3
Saturnine – *see* Lead						
Savin (oil)	976.4	E858.7	E946.4	E950.4	E962.0	E980.4
Scammony	973.1	E858.4	E943.1	E950.4	E962.0	E980.4
Scarlet red	976.8	E858.7	E946.8	E950.4	E962.0	E980.4
Scheele's green	985.1	E866.3	—	E950.8	E962.1	E980.8
insecticide	985.1	E863.4	—	E950.8	E962.1	E980.8
Schradan	989.3	E863.1	—	E950.6	E962.1	E980.7
Schweinfurt (h) green	985.1	E866.3	—	E950.8	E962.1	E980.8
insecticide	985.1	E863.4	—	E950.8	E962.1	E980.8
Scilla — *see* Squill						
Sclerosing agents	972.7	E858.3	E942.7	E950.4	E962.0	E980.4
Scopolamine	971.1	E855.4	E941.1	E950.4	E962.0	E980.4
Scouring powder	989.89	E861.3	—	E950.9	E962.1	E980.9
Sea						
anemone (sting)	989.5	E905.6	—	E950.9	E962.1	E980.9

Substance	Poisoning	Accident	Therapeutic Use	Suicide Attempt	Assault	Undetermined
			External Cause (E-Code)			
cucumber (sting)	989.5	E905.6	—	E950.9	E962.1	E980.9
snake (bite) (venom)	989.5	E905.0	—	E950.9	E962.1	E980.9
urchin spine (puncture)	989.5	E905.6	—	E950.9	E962.1	E980.9
Secbutabarbital	967.0	E851	E937.0	E950.1	E962.0	E980.1
Secbutabaritone	967.0	E851	E937.0	E950.1	E962.0	E980.1
Secobarbital	967.0	E851	E937.0	E950.1	E962.0	E980.1
Seconal	967.0	E851	E937.0	E950.1	E962.0	E980.1
Secretin	977.8	E858.8	E947.8	E950.4	E962.0	E980.4
Sedatives, nonbarbiturate	967.9	E852.9	E937.9	E950.2	E962.0	E980.2
specified NEC	967.8	E852.8	E937.8	E950.2	E962.0	E980.2
Sedormid	967.8	E852.8	E937.8	E950.2	E962.0	E980.2
Seed (plant)	988.2	E865.3	—	E950.9	E962.1	E980.9
disinfectant or dressing	989.89	E866.5	—	E950.9	E962.1	E980.9
Selective serotonin and norepinephrine reuptake inhibitors (SSNRI)	969.02	E854.0	E939.0	E950.3	E962.0	E980.3
Selective serotonin reuptake inhibitors (SSRI)	969.03	E854.0	E939.0	E950.3	E962.0	E980.3
Selenium (fumes) NEC	985.8	E866.4	—	E950.9	E962.1	E980.9
disulfide or sulfide	976.4	E858.7	E946.4	E950.4	E962.0	E980.4
Selsun	976.4	E858.7	E946.4	E950.4	E962.0	E980.4
Senna	973.1	E858.4	E943.1	E950.4	E962.0	E980.4
Septisol	976.2	E858.7	E946.2	E950.4	E962.0	E980.4
Serax	969.4	E853.2	E939.4	E950.3	E962.0	E980.3
Serenesil	967.8	E852.8	E937.8	E950.2	E962.0	E980.2
Serenium (hydrochloride)	961.9	E857	E931.9	E950.4	E962.0	E980.4
Serepax—see Oxazepam						
Sernyl	968.3	E855.1	E938.3	E950.4	E962.0	E980.4
Serotonin	977.8	E858.8	E947.8	E950.4	E962.0	E980.4
Serpasil	972.6	E858.3	E942.6	E950.4	E962.0	E980.4
Sewer gas	987.8	E869.8	—	E952.8	E962.2	E982.8
Shampoo	989.6	E861.0	—	E950.9	E962.1	E980.9
Shellfish, nonbacterial or noxious	988.0	E865.1	—	E950.9	E962.1	E980.9
Silicones NEC	989.83	E866.8	E947.8	E950.9	E962.1	E980.9
Silvadene	976.0	E858.7	E946.0	E950.4	E962.0	E980.4
Silver (compound) (medicinal) NEC	976.0	E858.7	E946.0	E950.4	E962.0	E980.4
anti–infectives	976.0	E858.7	E946.0	E950.4	E962.0	E980.4
arsphenamine	961.1	E857	E931.1	E950.4	E962.0	E980.4
nitrate	976.0	E858.7	E946.0	E950.4	E962.0	E980.4
ophthalmic preparation	976.5	E858.7	E946.5	E950.4	E962.0	E980.4
toughened (keratolytic)	976.4	E858.7	E946.4	E950.4	E962.0	E980.4
nonmedicinal (dust)	985.8	E866.4	—	E950.9	E962.1	E980.9
protein (mild) (strong)	976.0	E858.7	E946.0	E950.4	E962.0	E980.4
salvarsan	961.1	E857	E931.1	E950.4	E962.0	E980.4
Simethicone	973.8	E858.4	E943.8	E950.4	E962.0	E980.4
Sinequan	969.05	E854.0	E939.0	E950.3	E962.0	E980.3
Singoserp	972.6	E858.3	E942.6	E950.4	E962.0	E980.4
Sintrom	964.2	E858.2	E934.2	E950.4	E962.0	E980.4
Sitosterols	972.2	E858.3	E942.2	E950.4	E962.0	E980.4
Skeletal muscle relaxants	975.2	E858.6	E945.2	E950.4	E962.0	E980.4
Skin						
agents (external)	976.9	E858.7	E946.9	E950.4	E962.0	E980.4
specified NEC	976.8	E858.7	E946.8	E950.4	E962.0	E980.4
test antigen	977.8	E858.8	E947.8	E950.4	E962.0	E980.4
Sleep–eze	963.0	E858.1	E933.0	E950.4	E962.0	E980.4
Sleeping draught (drug) (pill) (tablet)	967.9	E852.9	E937.9	E950.2	E962.0	E980.2
Smallpox vaccine	979.0	E858.8	E949.0	E950.4	E962.0	E980.4
Smelter fumes NEC	985.9	E866.4	—	E950.9	E962.1	E980.9
Smog	987.3	E869.1	—	E952.8	E962.2	E982.8
Smoke NEC	987.9	E869.9	—	E952.9	E962.2	E982.9
Smooth muscle relaxant	975.1	E858.6	E945.1	E950.4	E962.0	E980.4
Snail killer	989.4	E863.4	—	E950.6	E962.1	E980.7

Substance	Poisoning	Accident	Therapeutic Use	Suicide Attempt	Assault	Undetermined
		External Cause (E-Code)				
Snake (bite) (venom)	989.5	E905.0	—	E950.9	E962.1	E980.9
Snuff	989.89	E866.8	—	E950.9	E962.1	E980.9
Soap (powder) (product)	989.6	E861.1	—	E950.9	E962.1	E980.9
medicinal, soft	976.2	E858.7	E946.2	E950.4	E962.0	E980.4
Soda (caustic)	983.2	E864.2	—	E950.7	E962.1	E980.6
bicarb.	963.3	E858.1	E933.3	E950.4	E962.0	E980.4
chlorinated — Sodium, hypochlorite						
Sodium						
acetosulfone	961.8	E857	E931.8	E950.4	E962.0	E980.4
acetrizoate	977.8	E858.8	E947.8	E950.4	E962.0	E980.4
amytal	967.0	E851	E937.0	E950.1	E962.0	E980.1
arsenate — see Arsenic						
bicarbonate	963.3	E858.1	E933.3	E950.4	E962.0	E980.4
bichromate	983.9	E864.3	—	E950.7	E962.1	E980.6
biphosphate	963.2	E858.1	E933.2	E950.4	E962.0	E980.4
bisulfate	983.9	E864.3	—	E950.7	E962.1	E980.6
borate (cleanser)	989.6	E861.3	—	E950.9	E962.1	E980.9
bromide NEC	967.3	E852.2	E937.3	E950.2	E962.0	E980.2
cacodylate (nonmedicinal) NEC	978.8	E858.8	E948.8	E950.4	E962.0	E980.4
anti–infective	961.1	E857	E931.1	E950.4	E962.0	E980.4
herbicide	989.4	E863.5	—	E950.6	E962.1	E980.7
calcium edetate	963.8	E858.1	E933.8	E950.4	E962.0	E980.4
carbonate NEC	983.2	E864.2	—	E950.7	E962.1	E980.6
chlorate NEC	983.9	E864.3	—	E950.7	E962.1	E980.6
herbicide	983.9	E863.5	—	E950.7	E962.1	E980.6
chloride NEC	974.5	E858.5	E944.5	E950.4	E962.0	E980.4
chromate	983.9	E864.3	—	E950.7	E962.1	E980.6
citrate	963.3	E858.1	E933.3	E950.4	E962.0	E980.4
cyanide — see Cyanide(s)						
cyclamate	974.5	E858.5	E944.5	E950.4	E962.0	E980.4
diatrizoate	977.8	E858.8	E947.8	E950.4	E962.0	E980.4
dibunate	975.4	E858.6	E945.4	E950.4	E962.0	E980.4
dioctyl sulfosuccinate	973.2	E858.4	E943.2	E950.4	E962.0	E980.4
edetate	963.8	E858.1	E933.8	E950.4	E962.0	E980.4
ethacrynate	974.4	E858.5	E944.4	E950.4	E962.0	E980.4
fluoracetate (dust) (rodenticide)	989.4	E863.7	—	E950.6	E962.1	E980.7
fluoride — see Fluoride(s)						
free salt	974.5	E858.5	E944.5	E950.4	E962.0	E980.4
glucosulfone	961.8	E857	E931.8	E950.4	E962.0	E980.4
hydroxide	983.2	E864.2	—	E950.7	E962.1	E980.6
hypochlorite (bleach) NEC	983.9	E864.3	—	E950.7	E962.1	E980.6
disinfectant	983.9	E861.4	—	E950.7	E962.1	E980.6
medicinal (anti–infective) (external)	976.0	E858.7	E946.0	E950.4	E962.0	E980.4
vapor	987.8	E869.8	—	E952.8	E962.2	E982.8
hyposulfite	976.0	E858.7	E946.0	E950.4	E962.0	E980.4
indigotindisulfonate	977.8	E858.8	E947.8	E950.4	E962.0	E980.4
iodide	977.8	E858.8	E947.8	E950.4	E962.0	E980.4
iothalamate	977.8	E858.8	E947.8	E950.4	E962.0	E980.4
iron edetate	964.0	E858.2	E934.0	E950.4	E962.0	E980.4
lactate	963.3	E858.1	E933.3	E950.4	E962.0	E980.4
lauryl sulfate	976.2	E858.7	E946.2	E950.4	E962.0	E980.4
L–triiodothyronine	962.7	E858.0	E932.7	E950.4	E962.0	E980.4
metrizoate	977.8	E858.8	E947.8	E950.4	E962.0	E980.4
monofluoroacetate (dust) (rodenticide)	989.4	E863.7	—	E950.6	E962.1	E980.7
morrhuate	972.7	E858.3	E942.7	E950.4	E962.0	E980.4
nafcillin	960.0	E856	E930.0	E950.4	E962.0	E980.4
nitrate (oxidizing agent)	983.9	E864.3	—	E950.7	E962.1	E980.6
nitrite (medicinal)	972.4	E858.3	E942.4	E950.4	E962.0	E980.4
nitroferricyanide	972.6	E858.3	E942.6	E950.4	E962.0	E980.4
nitroprusside	972.6	E858.3	E942.6	E950.4	E962.0	E980.4
para–aminohippurate	977.8	E858.8	E947.8	E950.4	E962.0	E980.4

Substance	Poisoning	Accident	Therapeutic Use	Suicide Attempt	Assault	Undetermined
				External Cause (E-Code)		
perborate (non-medicinal) NEC	989.89	E866.8	—	E950.9	E962.1	E980.9
medicinal	976.6	E858.7	E946.6	E950.4	E962.0	E980.4
soap	989.6	E861.1	—	E950.9	E962.1	E980.9
percarbonate — *see* Sodium, perborate						
phosphate	973.3	E858.4	E943.3	E950.4	E962.0	E980.4
polystyrene sulfonate	974.5	E858.5	E944.5	E950.4	E962.0	E980.4
propionate	976.0	E858.7	E946.0	E950.4	E962.0	E980.4
psylliate	972.7	E858.3	E942.7	E950.4	E962.0	E980.4
removing resins	974.5	E858.5	E944.5	E950.4	E962.0	E980.4
salicylate	965.1	E850.3	E935.3	E950.0	E962.0	E980.0
sulfate	973.3	E858.4	E943.3	E950.4	E962.0	E980.4
sulfoxone	961.8	E857	E931.8	E950.4	E962.0	E980.4
tetradecyl sulfate	972.7	E858.3	E942.7	E950.4	E962.0	E980.4
thiopental	968.3	E855.1	E938.3	E950.4	E962.0	E980.4
thiosalicylate	965.1	E850.3	E935.3	E950.0	E962.0	E980.0
thiosulfate	976.0	E858.7	E946.0	E950.4	E962.0	E980.4
tolbutamide	977.8	E858.8	E947.8	E950.4	E962.0	E980.4
tyropanoate	977.8	E858.8	E947.8	E950.4	E962.0	E980.4
valproate	966.3	E855.0	E936.3	E950.4	E962.0	E980.4
Solanine	977.8	E858.8	E947.8	E950.4	E962.0	E980.4
Solanum dulcamara	988.2	E865.4	—	E950.9	E962.1	E980.9
Solapsone	961.8	E857	E931.8	E950.4	E962.0	E980.4
Solasulfone	961.8	E857	E931.8	E950.4	E962.0	E980.4
Soldering fluid	983.1	E864.1	—	E950.7	E962.1	E980.6
Solid substance	989.9	E866.9	—	E950.9	E962.1	E980.9
specified NEC	989.9	E866.8	—	E950.9	E962.1	E980.9
Solvents, industrial	982.8	E862.9	—	E950.9	E962.1	E980.9
naphtha	981	E862.0	—	E950.9	E962.1	E980.9
petroleum	981	E862.0	—	E950.9	E962.1	E980.9
specified NEC	982.8	E862.4	—	E950.9	E962.1	E980.9
Soma	968.0	E855.1	E938.0	E950.4	E962.0	E980.4
Somatotropin	962.4	E858.0	E932.4	E950.4	E962.0	E980.4
Sominex	963.0	E858.1	E933.0	E950.4	E962.0	E980.4
Somnos	967.1	E852.0	E937.1	E950.2	E962.0	E980.2
Somonal	967.0	E851	E937.0	E950.1	E962.0	E980.1
Soneryl	967.0	E851	E937.0	E950.1	E962.0	E980.1
Soothing syrup	977.9	E858.9	E947.9	E950.5	E962.0	E980.5
Sopor	967.4	E852.3	E937.4	E950.2	E962.0	E980.2
Soporific drug	967.9	E852.9	E937.9	E950.2	E962.0	E980.2
specified type NEC	967.8	E852.8	E937.8	E950.2	E962.0	E980.2
Sorbitol NEC	977.4	E858.8	E947.4	E950.4	E962.0	E980.4
Sotradecol	972.7	E858.3	E942.7	E950.4	E962.0	E980.4
Spacoline	975.1	E858.6	E945.1	E950.4	E962.0	E980.4
Spanish fly	976.8	E858.7	E946.8	E950.4	E962.0	E980.4
Sparine	969.1	E853.0	E939.1	E950.3	E962.0	E980.3
Sparteine	975.0	E858.6	E945.0	E950.4	E962.0	E980.4
Spasmolytics	975.1	E858.6	E945.1	E950.4	E962.0	E980.4
anticholinergics	971.1	E855.4	E941.1	E950.4	E962.0	E980.4
Spectinomycin	960.8	E856	E930.8	E950.4	E962.0	E980.4
Speed	969.72	E854.2	E939.7	E950.3	E962.0	E980.3
Spermicides	976.8	E858.7	E946.8	E950.4	E962.0	E980.4
Spider (bite) (venom)	989.5	E905.1	—	E950.9	E962.1	E980.9
antivenin	979.9	E858.8	E949.9	E950.4	E962.0	E980.4
Spigelia (root)	961.6	E857	E931.6	E950.4	E962.0	E980.4
Spiperone	969.2	E853.1	E939.2	E950.3	E962.0	E980.3
Spiramycin	960.3	E856	E930.3	E950.4	E962.0	E980.4
Spirilene	969.5	E853.8	E939.5	E950.3	E962.0	E980.3
Spirit(s) (neutral) NEC	980.0	E860.1	—	E950.9	E962.1	E980.9
beverage	980.0	E860.0	—	E950.9	E962.1	E980.9
industrial	980.9	E860.9	—	E950.9	E962.1	E980.9

Substance	Poisoning	Accident	Therapeutic Use	Suicide Attempt	Assault	Undetermined
			External Cause (E-Code)			
mineral 981	E862.0	—	E950.9	E962.1	E980.9
of salt — *see* Hydrochloric acid					
surgical 980.9	E860.9	—	E950.9	E962.1	E980.9
Spironolactone 974.4	E858.5	E944.4	E950.4	E962.0	E980.4
Sponge, absorbable (gelatin) 964.5	E858.2	E934.5	E950.4	E962.0	E980.4
Sporostacin 976.0	E858.7	E946.0	E950.4	E962.0	E980.4
Sprays (aerosol) 989.89	E866.8	—	E950.9	E962.1	E980.9
cosmetic. 989.89	E866.7	—	E950.9	E962.1	E980.9
medicinal NEC 977.9	E858.9	E947.9	E950.5	E962.0	E980.5
pesticides — *see* Pesticides					
specified content — *see* substance					
specified					
Spurge flax 988.2	E865.4	—	E950.9	E962.1	E980.9
Spurges. 988.2	E865.4	—	E950.9	E962.1	E980.9
Squill (expectorant) NEC 975.5	E858.6	E945.5	E950.4	E962.0	E980.4
rat poison 989.4	E863.7	—	E950.6	E962.1	E980.7
Squirting cucumber (cathartic) 973.1	E858.4	E943.1	E950.4	E962.0	E980.4
SSNRI (selective serotonin and					
norepinephrine reuptake inhibitors) . . . 969.02	E854.0	E939.0	E950.3	E962.0	E980.3
SSRI (selective serotonin reuptake inhibitors) . 969.03	E854.0	E939.0	E950.3	E962.0	E980.3
Stains 989.89	E866.8	—	E950.9	E962.1	E980.9
Stannous — *see also* Tin					
fluoride. 976.7	E858.7	E946.7	E950.4	E962.0	E980.4
Stanolone 962.1	E858.0	E932.1	E950.4	E962.0	E980.4
Stanozolol. 962.1	E853.0	E932.1	E950.4	E962.0	E980.4
Staphisagria or stavesacre (pediculicide) . . . 976.0	E858.7	E946.0	E950.4	E962.0	E980.4
Stelazine 969.1	E853.0	E939.1	E950.3	E962.0	E980.3
Stemetil. 969.1	E853.0	E939.1	E950.3	E962.0	E980.3
Sterculia (cathartic) (gum) 973.3	E858.4	E943.3	E950.4	E962.0	E980.4
Sternutator gas 987.8	E869.8	—	E952.8	E962.2	E982.8
Steroids NEC 962.0	E858.0	E932.0	E950.4	E962.0	E980.4
ENT agent. 976.6	E858.7	E946.6	E950.4	E962.0	E980.4
ophthalmic preparation. 976.5	E858.7	E946.5	E950.4	E962.0	E980.4
topical NEC 976.0	E858.7	E946.0	E950.4	E962.0	E980.4
Stibine 985.8	E866.4	—	E950.9	E962.1	E980.9
Stibophen 961.2	E857	E931.2	E950.4	E962.0	E980.4
Stilbamide, stilbamidine 961.5	E857	E931.5	E950.4	E962.0	E980.4
Stilbestrol 962.2	E858.0	E932.2	E950.4	E962.0	E980.4
Stimulants (central nervous system) 970.9	E854.3	E940.9	E950.4	E962.0	E980.4
analeptics 970.0	E854.3	E940.0	E950.4	E962.0	E980.4
opiate antagonist 970.1	E854.3	E940.1	E950.4	E962.0	E980.4
psychotherapeutic NEC 969.09	E854.0	E939.0	E950.3	E962.0	E980.3
specified NEC 970.89	E854.3	E940.8	E950.4	E962.0	E980.4
Storage batteries (acid) (cells) 983.1	E864.1	—	E950.7	E962.1	E980.6
Stovaine 968.9	E855.2	E938.9	E950.4	E962.0	E980.4
infiltration (subcutaneous) 968.5	E855.2	E938.5	E950.4	E962.0	E980.4
nerve block (peripheral) (plexus). 968.6	E855.2	E938.6	E950.5	E962.0	E980.4
spinal. 968.7	E855.2	E938.7	E950.4	E962.0	E980.4
topical (surface) 968.5	E855.2	E938.5	E950.4	E962.0	E980.4
Stovarsal 961.1	E857	E931.1	E950.4	E962.0	E980.4
Stove gas — *see* Gas, utility					
Stoxil. 976.5	E858.7	E946.5	E950.4	E962.0	E980.4
STP 969.6	E854.1	E939.6	E950.3	E962.0	E980.3
Stramonium (medicinal) NEC. 971.1	E855.4	E941.1	E950.4	E962.0	E980.4
natural state 988.2	E865.4	—	E950.9	E962.1	E980.9
Streptodornase 964.4	E858.2	E934.4	E950.4	E962.0	E980.4
Streptoduocin 960.6	E856	E930.6	E950.4	E962.0	E980.4
Streptokinase 964.4	E858.2	E934.4	E950.4	E962.0	E980.4
Streptomycin 960.6	E856	E930.6	E950.4	E962.0	E980.4
Streptozocin 960.7	E856	E930.7	E950.4	E962.0	E980.4
Stripper (paint) (solvent) 982.8	E862.9	—	E950.9	E962.1	E980.9

Substance	Poisoning	Accident	Therapeutic Use	Suicide Attempt	Assault	Undetermined
			External Cause (E-Code)			
Strobane	989.2	E863.0	—	E950.6	E962.1	E980.7
Strophanthin	972.1	E858.3	E942.1	E950.4	E962.0	E980.4
Strophanthus hispidus or kombe	988.2	E865.4	—	E950.9	E962.1	E980.9
Strychnine (rodenticide) (salts)	989.1	E863.7	—	E950.6	E962.1	E980.7
medicinal NEC	970.89	E854.3	E940.8	E950.4	E962.0	E980.4
Strychnos (ignatii) — *see* Strychnine						
Styramate	968.0	E855.1	E938.0	E950.4	E962.0	E980.4
Styrene	983.0	E864.0	—	E950.7	E962.1	E980.6
Succinimide (anticonvulsant)	966.2	E855.0	E936.2	E950.4	E962.0	E980.4
mercuric — *see* Mercury						
Succinylcholine	975.2	E858.6	E945.2	E950.4	E962.0	E980.4
Succinylsulfathiazole	961.0	E857	E931.0	E950.4	E962.0	E980.4
Sucrose	974.5	E858.5	E944.5	E950.4	E962.0	E980.4
Sulfacetamide	961.0	E857	E931.0	E950.4	E962.0	E980.4
ophthalmic preparation	976.5	E858.7	E946.5	E950.4	E962.0	E980.4
Sulfachlorpyridazine	961.0	E857	E931.0	E950.4	E962.0	E980.4
Sulfacytine	961.0	E857	E931.0	E950.4	E962.0	E980.4
Sulfadiazine	961.0	E857	E931.0	E950.4	E962.0	E980.4
silver (topical)	976.0	E858.7	E946.0	E950.4	E962.0	E980.4
Sulfadimethoxine	961.0	E857	E931.0	E950.4	E962.0	E980.4
Sulfadimidine	961.0	E857	E931.0	E950.4	E962.0	E980.4
Sulfaethidole	961.0	E857	E931.0	E950.4	E962.0	E980.4
Sulfafurazole	961.0	E857	E931.0	E950.4	E962.0	E980.4
Sulfaguanidine	961.0	E857	E931.0	E950.4	E962.0	E980.4
Sulfamerazine	961.0	E857	E931.0	E950.4	E962.0	E980.4
Sulfameter	961.0	E857	E931.0	E950.4	E962.0	E980.4
Sulfamethizole	961.0	E857	E931.0	E950.4	E962.0	E980.4
Sulfamethoxazole	961.0	E857	E931.0	E950.4	E962.0	E980.4
Sulfamethoxydiazine	961.0	E857	E931.0	E950.4	E962.0	E980.4
Sulfamethoxypyridazine	961.0	E857	E931.0	E950.4	E962.0	E980.4
Sulfamethylthiazole	961.0	E857	E931.0	E950.4	E962.0	E980.4
Sulfamylon	976.0	E858.7	E946.0	E950.4	E962.0	E980.4
Sulfan blue (diagnostic dye)	977.8	E858.8	E947.8	E950.4	E962.0	E980.4
Sulfanilamide	961.0	E857	E931.0	E950.4	E962.0	E980.4
Sulfanilylguanidine	961.0	E857	E931.0	E950.4	E962.0	E980.4
Sulfaphenazole	961.0	E857	E931.0	E950.4	E962.0	E980.4
Sulfaphenylthiazole	961.0	E857	E931.0	E950.4	E962.0	E980.4
Sulfaproxyline	961.0	E857	E931.0	E950.4	E962.0	E980.4
Sulfapyridine	961.0	E857	E931.0	E950.4	E962.0	E980.4
Sulfapyrimidine	961.0	E857	E931.0	E950.4	E962.0	E980.4
Sulfarsphenamine	961.1	E857	E931.1	E950.4	E962.0	E980.4
Sulfasalazine	961.0	E857	E931.0	E950.4	E962.0	E980.4
Sulfasomizole	961.0	E857	E931.0	E950.4	E962.0	E980.4
Sulfasuxidine	961.0	E857	E931.0	E950.4	E962.0	E980.4
Sulfinpyrazone	974.7	E858.5	E944.7	E950.4	E962.0	E980.4
Sulfisoxazole	961.0	E857	E931.0	E950.4	E962.0	E980.4
ophthalmic preparation	976.5	E858.7	E946.5	E950.4	E962.0	E980.4
Sulfomyxin	960.8	E856	E930.8	E950.4	E962.0	E980.4
Sulfonal	967.8	E852.8	E937.8	E950.2	E962.0	E980.2
Sulfonamides (mixtures)	961.0	E857	E931.0	E950.4	E962.0	E980.4
Sulfones	961.8	E857	E931.8	E950.4	E962.0	E980.4
Sulfonethylmethane	967.8	E852.8	E937.8	E950.2	E962.0	E980.2
Sulfonmethane	967.8	E852.8	E937.8	E950.2	E962.0	E980.2
Sulfonphthal, sulfonphthol	977.8	E858.8	E947.8	E950.4	E962.0	E980.4
Sulfonylurea derivatives, oral	962.3	E858.0	E932.3	E950.4	E962.0	E980.4
Sulfoxone	961.8	E857	E931.8	E950.4	E962.0	E980.4
Sulfur, sulfureted, sulfuric, sulfurous, sulfuryl (compounds) NEC	989.89	E866.8	—	E950.9	E962.1	E980.9
acid	983.1	E864.1	—	E950.7	E962.1	E980.6
dioxide	987.3	E869.1	—	E952.8	E962.2	E982.8

Substance	Poisoning	Accident	Therapeutic Use	Suicide Attempt	Assault	Undetermined
			External Cause (E-Code)			
ether — *see* Ether(s)						
hydrogen	987.8	E869.8	—	E952.8	E962.2	E982.8
medicinal (keratolytic) (ointment) NEC . . .	976.4	E858.7	E946.4	E950.4	E962.0	E980.4
pesticide (vapor)	989.4	E863.4	—	E950.6	E962.1	E980.7
vapor NEC.	987.8	E869.8	—	E952.8	E962.2	E982.8
Sulkowitch's reagent	977.8	E858.8	E947.8	E950.4	E962.0	E980.4
Sulph — *see also* Sulf–						
Sulphadione	961.8	E857	E931.8	E950.4	E962.0	E980.4
Sulthiame, sultiame	966.3	E855.0	E936.3	E950.4	E962.0	E980.4
Superinone	975.5	E858.6	E945.5	E950.4	E962.0	E980.4
Suramin.	961.5	E857	E931.5	E950.4	E962.0	E980.4
Surfacaine.	968.5	E855.2	E938.5	E950.4	E962.0	E980.4
Surital	968.3	E855.1	E938.3	E950.4	E962.0	E980.4
Sutilains	976.8	E858.7	E946.8	E950.4	E962.0	E980.4
Suxamethoniam (bromide) (chloride)						
(iodide)	975.2	E858.6	E945.2	E950.4	E962.0	E980.4
Suxethonium (bromide)	975.2	E858.6	E945.2	E950.4	E962.0	E980.4
Sweet oil (birch)	976.3	E858.7	E946.3	E950.4	E962.0	E980.4
Sym–dichloroethyl ether	982.3	E862.4	—	E950.9	E962.1	E980.9
Sympatholytics.	971.3	E855.6	E941.3	E950.4	E962.0	E980.4
Sympathomimetics	971.2	E855.5	E941.2	E950.4	E962.0	E980.4
Synagis	979.6	E858.8	E949.6	E950.4	E962.0	E980.4
Synalar	976.0	E858.7	E946.0	E950.4	E962.0	E980.4
Synthroid	962.7	E858.0	E932.7	E950.4	E962.0	E980.4
Syntocinon	975.0	E858.6	E945.0	E950.4	E962.0	E950.4
Syrosingopine	972.6	E858.3	E942.6	E950.4	E962.0	E980.4
Systemic agents (primarily)	963.9	E858.1	E933.9	E950.4	E962.0	E980.4
specified NEC	963.8	E858.1	E933.8	E950.4	E962.0	E980.4
Tablets (*see also* specified substance)	977.9	E858.9	E947.9	E950.5	E962.0	E980.5
Tace	962.2	E858.0	E932.2	E950.4	E962.0	E980.4
Tacrine	971.0	E855.3	E941.0	E950.4	E962.0	E980.4
Talbutal	967.0	E851	E937.0	E950.1	E962.0	E980.1
Talc	976.3	E858.7	E946.3	E950.4	E962.0	E980.4
Talcum	976.3	E858.7	E946.3	E950.4	E962.0	E980.4
Tamsulosin	971.3	E855.6	E941.3	E950.4	E962.0	E980.4
Tandearil, tanderil	965.5	E850.5	E935.5	E950.0	E962.0	E980.0
Tannic acid	983.1	E864.1	—	E950.7	E962.1	E980.6
medicinal (astringent)	976.2	E858.7	E946.2	E950.4	E962.0	E980.4
Tannin — *see* Tannic acid						
Tansy.	988.2	E865.4	—	E950.9	E962.1	E980.9
TAO	960.3	E856	E930.3	E950.4	E962.0	E980.4
Tapazole	962.8	E858.0	E932.8	E950.4	E962.0	E980.4
Tar NEC	983.0	E864.0	—	E950.7	E962.1	E980.6
camphor — *see* Naphthalene						
fumes	987.8	E869.8	—	E952.8	E962.2	E982.8
Taractan	969.3	E853.8	E939.3	E950.3	E962.0	E980.3
Tarantula (venomous)	989.5	E905.1	—	E950.9	E962.1	E980.9
Tartar emetic (anti–infective)	961.2	E857	E931.2	E950.4	E962.0	E980.4
Tartaric acid	983.1	E864.1	—	E950.7	E962.1	E980.6
Tartrated antimony (anti–infective).	961.2	E857	E931.2	E950.4	E962.0	E980.4
TCA — *see* Trichloroacetic acid						
TDI	983.0	E864.0	—	E950.7	E962.1	E980.6
vapor	987.8	E869.8	—	E952.8	E962.2	E982.8
Tear gas	987.5	E869.3	—	E952.8	E962.2	E982.8
Teclothiazide.	974.3	E858.5	E944.3	E950.4	E962.0	E980.4
Tegretol.	966.3	E855.0	E936.3	E950.4	E962.0	E980.4
Telepaque	977.8	E858.8	E947.8	E950.4	E962.0	E980.4
Tellurium	985.8	E866.4	—	E950.9	E962.1	E980.9
fumes	985.8	E866.4	—	E950.9	E962.1	E980.9
TEM	963.1	E858.1	E933.1	E950.4	E962.0	E980.4
Temazepan—*see* Benzodiazepines						

Substance	Poisoning	Accident	Therapeutic Use	Suicide Attempt	Assault	Undetermined
		External Cause (E-Code)				
TEPA	963.1	E858.1	E933.1	E950.4	E962.0	E980.4
TEPP	989.3	E863.1	—	E950.6	E962.1	E980.7
Terbutaline	971.2	E855.5	E941.2	E950.4	E962.0	E980.4
Teroxalene	961.6	E857	E931.6	E950.4	E962.0	E980.4
Terpin hydrate	975.5	E858.6	E945.5	E950.4	E962.0	E980.4
Terramycin	960.4	E856	E930.4	E950.4	E962.0	E980.4
Tessalon	975.4	E858.6	E945.4	E950.4	E962.0	E980.4
Testosterone	962.1	E858.0	E932.1	E950.4	E962.0	E980.4
Tetanus (vaccine)	978.4	E858.8	E948.4	E950.4	E962.0	E980.4
antitoxin	979.9	E858.8	E949.9	E950.4	E962.0	E980.4
immune globulin (human)	964.6	E858.2	E934.6	E950.4	E962.0	E980.4
toxoid	978.4	E858.8	E948.4	E950.4	E962.0	E980.4
with diphtheria toxoid	978.9	E858.8	E948.9	E950.4	E962.0	E980.4
with pertussis	978.6	E858.8	E948.6	E950.4	E962.0	E980.4
Tetrabenazine	969.5	E853.8	E939.5	E950.3	E962.0	E980.3
Tetracaine (infiltration) (topical)	968.5	E855.2	E938.5	E950.4	E962.0	E980.4
nerve block (peripheral) (plexus)	968.6	E855.2	E938.6	E950.4	E962.0	E980.4
spinal	968.7	E855.2	E938.7	E950.4	E962.0	E980.4
Tetrachlorethylene—see Tetrachloroethylene						
Tetrachlormethiazide	974.3	E858.5	E944.3	E950.4	E962.0	E980.4
Tetrachloroethane (liquid) (vapor)	982.3	E862.4	—	E950.9	E962.1	E980.9
paint or varnish	982.3	E861.6	—	E950.9	E962.1	E980.9
Tetrachloroethylene (liquid) (vapor)	982.3	E862.4	—	E950.9	E962.1	E980.9
medicinal	961.6	E857	E931.6	E950.4	E962.0	E980.4
Tetrachloromethane — see Carbon, tetrachloride						
Tetracycline	960.4	E856	E930.4	E950.4	E962.0	E980.4
ophthalmic preparation	976.5	E858.7	E946.5	E950.4	E962.0	E980.4
topical NEC	976.0	E858.7	E946.0	E950.4	E962.0	E980.4
Tetraethylammonium chloride	972.3	E858.3	E942.3	E950.4	E962.0	E980.4
Tetraethyl lead (antiknock compound)	984.1	E862.1	—	E950.9	E962.1	E980.9
Tetraethyl pyrophosphate	989.3	E863.1	—	E950.6	E962.1	E980.7
Tetraethylthiuram disulfide	977.3	E858.8	E947.3	E950.4	E962.0	E980.4
Tetrahydroaminoacridine	971.0	E855.3	E941.0	E950.4	E962.0	E980.4
Tetrahydrocannabinol	969.6	E854.1	E939.6	E950.3	E962.0	E980.3
Tetrahydronaphthalene	982.0	E862.4	—	E950.9	E962.1	E980.9
Tetrahydrozoline	971.2	E855.5	E941.2	E950.4	E962.0	E980.4
Tetralin	982.0	E862.4	—	E950.9	E962.1	E980.9
Tetramethylthiuram (disulfide) NEC	989.4	E863.6	—	E950.6	E962.1	E980.7
medicinal	976.2	E858.7	E946.2	E950.4	E962.0	E980.4
Tetronal	967.8	E852.8	E937.8	E950.2	E962.0	E980.2
Tetryl	983.0	E864.0	—	E950.7	E962.1	E980.6
Thalidomide	967.8	E852.8	E937.8	E950.2	E962.0	E980.2
Thallium (compounds) (dust) NEC	985.8	E866.4	—	E950.9	E962.1	E980.9
pesticide (rodenticide)	985.8	E863.7	—	E950.6	E962.1	E980.7
THC	969.6	E854.1	E939.6	E950.3	E962.0	E980.3
Thebacon	965.09	E850.2	E935.2	E950.0	E962.0	E980.0
Thebaine	965.09	E850.2	E935.2	E950.0	E962.0	E980.0
Theobromine (calcium salicylate)	974.1	E858.5	E944.1	E950.4	E962.0	E980.4
Theophylline (diuretic)	974.1	E858.5	E944.1	E950.4	E962.0	E980.4
ethylenediamine	975.7	E858.6	E945.7	E950.4	E962.0	E980.4
Thiabendazole	961.6	E857	E931.6	E950.4	E962.0	E980.4
Thialbarbital, thialbarbitone	968.3	E855.1	E938.3	E950.4	E962.0	E980.4
Thiamine	963.5	E858.1	E933.5	E950.4	E962.0	E980.4
Thiamylal (sodium)	968.3	E855.1	E938.3	E950.4	E962.0	E980.4
Thiazesim	969.09	E854.0	E939.0	E950.3	E962.0	E980.3
Thiazides (diuretics)	974.3	E858.5	E944.3	E950.4	E962.0	E980.4
Thiethylperazine	963.0	E858.1	E933.0	E950.4	E962.0	E980.4
Thimerosal (topical)	976.0	E858.7	E946.0	E950.4	E962.0	E980.4
ophthalmic preparation	976.5	E858.7	E946.5	E950.4	E962.0	E980.4

1672

Substance	Poisoning	Accident	Therapeutic Use	Suicide Attempt	Assault	Undetermined
		External Cause (E-Code)				
Thioacetazone 961.8	E857	E931.8	E950.4	E962.0	E980.4
Thiobarbiturates 968.3	E855.1	E938.3	E950.4	E962.0	E980.4
Thiobismol 961.2	E857	E931.2	E950.4	E962.0	E980.4
Thiocarbamide 962.8	E858.0	E932.8	E950.4	E962.0	E980.4
Thiocarbarsone 961.1	E857	E931.1	E950.4	E962.0	E980.4
Thiocarlide 961.8	E857	E931.8	E950.4	E962.0	E980.4
Thioguanine 963.1	E858.1	E933.1	E950.4	E962.0	E980.4
Thiomercaptomerin 974.0	E858.5	E944.0	E950.4	E962.0	E980.4
Thiomerin 974.0	E858.5	E944.0	E950.4	E962.0	E980.4
Thiopental, thiopentone (sodium) . . . 968.3	E855.1	E938.3	E950.4	E962.0	E980.4
Thiopropazate 969.1	E853.0	E939.1	E950.3	E962.0	E980.3
Thioproperazine 969.1	E853.0	E939.1	E950.3	E962.0	E980.3
Thioridazine 969.1	E853.0	E939.1	E950.3	E962.0	E980.3
Thio–TEPA, thiotepa 963.1	E858.1	E933.1	E950.4	E962.0	E980.4
Thiothixene 969.3	E853.8	E939.3	E950.3	E962.0	E980.3
Thiouracil 962.8	E858.0	E932.8	E950.4	E962.0	E980.4
Thiourea 962.8	E858.0	E932.8	E950.4	E962.0	E980.4
Thiphenamil 971.1	E855.4	E941.1	E950.4	E962.0	E980.4
Thiram NEC 989.4	E863.6	—	E950.6	E962.1	E980.7
medicinal 976.2	E858.7	E946.2	E950.4	E962.0	E980.4
Thonzylamine 963.0	E858.1	E933.0	E950.4	E962.0	E980.4
Thorazine 969.1	E853.0	E939.1	E950.3	E962.0	E980.3
Thornapple 988.2	E865.4	—	E950.9	E962.1	E980.9
Throat preparation (lozenges) NEC 976.6	E858.7	E946.6	E950.4	E962.0	E980.4
Thrombin 964.5	E858.2	E934.5	E950.4	E962.0	E980.4
Thrombolysin 964.4	E858.2	E934.4	E950.4	E962.0	E980.4
Thymol 983.0	E864.0	—	E950.7	E962.1	E980.6
Thymus extract 962.9	E858.0	E932.9	E950.4	E962.0	E980.4
Thyroglobulin 962.7	E858.0	E932.7	E950.4	E962.0	E980.4
Thyroid (derivatives) (extract) 962.7	E858.0	E932.7	E950.4	E962.0	E980.4
Thyrolar 962.7	E858.0	E932.7	E950.4	E962.0	E980.4
Thyrothrophin, thyrotropin 977.8	E858.8	E947.8	E950.4	E962.0	E980.4
Thyroxin(e) 962.7	E858.0	E932.7	E950.4	E962.0	E980.4
Tigan 963.0	E858.1	E933.0	E950.4	E962.0	E980.4
Tigloidine 968.0	E855.1	E938.0	E950.4	E962.0	E980.4
Tin (chloride) (dust) (oxide) NEC 985.8	E866.4	—	E950.9	E962.1	E980.9
anti–infectives 961.2	E857	E931.2	E950.4	E962.0	E980.4
Tinactin 976.0	E858.7	E946.0	E950.4	E962.0	E980.4
Tincture, iodine — *see* Iodine					
Tindal 969.1	E853.0	E939.1	E950.3	E962.0	E980.3
Titanium (compounds) (vapor) 985.8	E866.4	—	E950.9	E962.1	E980.9
ointment 976.3	E858.7	E946.3	E950.4	E962.0	E980.4
Titroid 962.7	E858.0	E932.7	E950.4	E962.0	E980.4
TMTD — *see* Tetramethylthiuram disulfide					
TNT 989.89	E866.8	—	E950.9	E962.1	E980.9
fumes 987.8	E869.8	—	E952.8	E962.2	E982.8
Toadstool 988.1	E865.5	—	E950.9	E962.1	E980.9
Tobacco NEC 989.84	E866.8	—	E950.9	E962.1	E980.9
Indian 988.2	E865.4	—	E950.9	E962.1	E980.9
smoke, second-hand 987.8	E869.4	—	—	—	—
Tocopherol 963.5	E858.1	E933.5	E950.4	E962.0	E980.4
Tocosamine 975.0	E858.6	E945.0	E950.4	E962.0	E980.4
Tofranil 969.05	E854.0	E939.0	E950.3	E962.0	E980.3
Toilet deodorizer 989.8	E866.8	—	E950.9	E962.1	E980.9
Tolazamide 962.3	E858.0	E932.3	E950.4	E962.0	E980.4
Tolazoline 971.3	E855.6	E941.3	E950.4	E962.0	E980.4
Tolbutamide 962.3	E858.0	E932.3	E950.4	E962.0	E980.4
sodium 977.8	E858.8	E947.8	E950.4	E962.0	E980.4
Tolmetin 965.69	E850.6	E935.6	E950.0	E962.0	E980.0
Tolnaftate 976.0	E858.7	E946.0	E950.4	E962.0	E980.4
Tolpropamine 976.1	E858.7	E946.1	E950.4	E962.0	E980.4

Substance	Poisoning	Accident	Therapeutic Use	Suicide Attempt	Assault	Undetermined
		External Cause (E-Code)				
Tolserol	968.0	E855.1	E938.0	E950.4	E962.0	E980.4
Toluene (liquid) (vapor)	982.0	E862.4	—	E950.9	E962.1	E980.9
diisocyanate	983.0	E864.0	—	E950.7	E962.1	E980.6
Toluidine	983.0	E864.0	—	E950.7	E962.1	E980.6
vapor	987.8	E869.8	—	E952.8	E962.2	E982.8
Toluol (liquid) (vapor)	982.0	E862.4	—	E950.9	E962.1	E980.9
Tolylene–2,4–diisocyanate	983.0	E864.0	—	E950.7	E962.1	E980.6
Tonics, cardiac	972.1	E858.3	E942.1	E950.4	E962.0	E980.4
Toxaphene (dust) (spray)	989.2	E863.0	—	E950.6	E962.1	E980.7
Toxoids NEC	978.8	E858.8	E948.8	E950.4	E962.0	E980.4
Tractor fuel NEC	981	E862.1	—	E950.9	E962.1	E980.9
Tragacanth	973.3	E858.4	E943.3	E950.4	E962.0	E980.4
Tramazoline	971.2	E855.5	E941.2	E950.4	E962.0	E980.4
Tranquilizers	969.5	E853.9	E939.5	E950.3	E962.0	E980.3
benzodiazepine–based	969.4	E853.2	E939.4	E950.3	E962.0	E980.3
butyrophenone–based	969.2	E853.1	E939.2	E950.3	E962.0	E980.3
major NEC	969.3	E853.8	E939.3	E950.3	E962.0	E980.3
phenothiazine–based	969.1	E853.0	E939.1	E950.3	E962.0	E980.3
specified NEC	969.5	E853.8	E939.5	E950.3	E962.0	E980.3
Trantoin	961.9	E857	E931.9	E950.4	E962.0	E980.4
Tranxene	969.4	E853.2	E939.4	E950.3	E962.0	E980.3
Tranylcypromine (sulfate)	969.01	E854.0	E939.0	E950.3	E962.0	E980.3
Trasentine	975.1	E858.6	E945.1	E950.4	E962.0	E980.4
Travert	974.5	E858.5	E944.5	E950.4	E962.0	E980.4
Trecator	961.8	E857	E931.8	E950.4	E962.0	E980.4
Tretinoin	976.8	E858.7	E946.8	E950.4	E962.0	E980.4
Triacetin	976.0	E858.7	E946.0	E950.4	E962.0	E980.4
Triacetyloleandomycin	960.3	E856	E930.3	E950.4	E962.0	E980.4
Triamcinolone	962.0	E858.0	E932.0	E950.4	E962.0	E980.4
ENT agent	976.6	E858.7	E946.6	E950.4	E962.0	E980.4
ophthalmic preparation	976.5	E858.7	E946.5	E950.4	E962.0	E980.4
topical NEC	976.0	E858.7	E946.0	E950.4	E962.0	E980.4
Triamterene	974.4	E858.5	E944.4	E950.4	E962.0	E980.4
Triaziquone	963.1	E858.1	E933.1	E950.4	E962.0	E980.4
Tribromacetaldehyde	967.3	E852.2	E937.3	E950.2	E962.0	E980.2
Tribromoethanol	968.2	E855.1	E938.2	E950.4	E962.0	E980.4
Tribromomethane	967.3	E852.2	E937.3	E950.2	E962.0	E980.2
Trichlorethane	982.3	E862.4	—	E950.9	E962.1	E980.9
Trichlormethiazide	974.3	E858.5	E944.3	E950.4	E962.0	E980.4
Trichloroacetic acid	983.1	E864.1	—	E950.7	E962.1	E980.6
medicinal (keratolytic)	976.4	E858.7	E946.4	E950.4	E962.0	E980.4
Trichloroethanol	967.1	E852.0	E937.1	E950.2	E962.0	E980.2
Trichloroethylene (liquid) (vapor)	982.3	E862.4	—	E950.9	E962.1	E980.9
anesthetic (gas)	968.2	E855.1	E938.2	E950.4	E962.0	E980.4
Trichloroethyl phosphate	967.1	E852.0	E937.1	E950.2	E962.0	E980.2
Trichlorofluoromethane NEC	987.4	E869.2	—	E952.8	E962.2	E982.8
Trichlorotriethylamine	963.1	E858.1	E933.1	E950.4	E962.0	E980.4
Trichomonacides NEC	961.5	E857	E931.5	E950.4	E962.0	E980.4
Trichomycin	960.1	E856	E930.1	E950.4	E962.0	E980.4
Triclofos	967.1	E852.0	E937.1	E950.2	E962.0	E980.2
Tricresyl phosphate	989.89	E866.8	—	E950.9	E962.1	E980.9
solvent	982.8	E862.4	—	E950.9	E962.1	E980.9
Tricyclamol	966.4	E855.0	E936.4	E950.4	E962.0	E980.4
Tridesilon	976.0	E858.7	E946.0	E950.4	E962.0	E980.4
Tridihexethyl	971.1	E855.4	E941.1	E950.4	E962.0	E980.4
Tridione	966.0	E855.0	E936.0	E950.4	E962.0	E980.4
Triethanolamine NEC	983.2	E864.2	—	E950.7	E962.1	E980.6
detergent	983.2	E861.0	—	E950.7	E962.1	E980.6
trinitrate	972.4	E858.3	E942.4	E950.4	E962.0	E980.4
Triethanomelamine	963.1	E858.1	E933.1	E950.4	E962.0	E980.4

Substance	Poisoning	Accident	Therapeutic Use	Suicide Attempt	Assault	Undetermined
			External Cause (E-Code)			
Triethylene melamine	963.1	E858.1	E933.1	E950.4	E962.0	E980.4
Triethylenephosphoramide	963.1	E858.1	E933.1	E950.4	E962.0	E980.4
Triethylenethiophosphoramide	963.1	E858.1	E933.1	E950.4	E962.0	E980.4
Trifluoperazine	969.1	E853.0	E939.1	E950.3	E962.0	E980.3
Trifluperidol	969.2	E853.1	E939.2	E950.3	E962.0	E980.3
Triflupromazine	969.1	E853.0	E939.1	E950.3	E962.0	E980.3
Trihexyphenidyl	971.1	E855.4	E941.1	E950.4	E962.0	E980.4
Triiodothyronine	962.7	E858.0	E932.7	E950.4	E962.0	E980.4
Trilene	968.2	E855.1	E938.2	E950.4	E962.0	E980.4
Trimeprazine	963.0	E858.1	E933.0	E950.4	E962.0	E980.4
Trimetazidine	972.4	E858.3	E942.4	E950.4	E962.0	E980.4
Trimethadione	966.0	E855.0	E936.0	E950.4	E962.0	E980.4
Trimethaphan	972.3	E858.3	E942.3	E950.4	E962.0	E980.4
Trimethidinium	972.3	E858.3	E942.3	E950.4	E962.0	E980.4
Trimethobenzamide	963.0	E858.1	E933.0	E950.4	E962.0	E980.4
Trimethylcarbinol	980.8	E860.8	—	E950.9	E962.1	E980.9
Trimethylpsoralen	976.3	E858.7	E946.3	E950.4	E962.0	E980.4
Trimeton	963.0	E858.1	E933.0	E950.4	E962.0	E980.4
Trimipramine	969.05	E854.0	E939.0	E950.3	E962.0	E980.3
Trimustine	963.1	E858.1	E933.1	E950.4	E962.0	E980.4
Trinitrin	972.4	E858.3	E942.4	E950.4	E962.0	E980.4
Trinitrophenol	983.0	E864.0	—	E950.7	E962.1	E980.6
Trinitrotoluene	989.89	E866.8	—	E950.9	E962.1	E980.9
fumes	987.8	E869.8	—	E952.8	E962.2	E982.8
Trional	967.8	E852.8	E937.8	E950.2	E962.0	E980.2
Trioxide of arsenic — *see* Arsenic						
Trioxsalen	976.3	E858.7	E946.3	E950.4	E962.0	E980.4
Tripelennamine	963.0	E858.1	E933.0	E950.4	E962.0	E980.4
Triperidol	969.2	E853.1	E939.2	E950.3	E962.0	E980.3
Triprolidine	963.0	E858.1	E933.0	E950.4	E962.0	E980.4
Trisoralen	976.3	E858.7	E946.3	E950.4	E962.0	E980.4
Troleandomycin	960.3	E856	E930.3	E950.4	E962.0	E980.4
Trolnitrate (phosphate)	972.4	E858.3	E942.4	E950.4	E962.0	E980.4
Trometamol	963.3	E858.1	E933.3	E950.4	E962.0	E980.4
Tromethamine	963.3	E858.1	E933.3	E950.4	E962.0	E980.4
Tronothane	968.5	E855.2	E938.5	E950.4	E962.0	E980.4
Tropicamide	971.1	E855.4	E941.1	E950.4	E962.0	E980.4
Troxidone	966.0	E855.0	E936.0	E950.4	E962.0	E980.4
Tryparsamide	961.1	E857	E931.1	E950.4	E962.0	E980.4
Trypsin	963.4	E858.1	E933.4	E950.4	E962.0	E980.4
Tryptizol	969.05	E854.0	E939.0	E950.3	E962.0	E980.3
Tuaminoheptane	971.2	E855.5	E941.2	E950.4	E962.0	E980.4
Tuberculin (old)	977.8	E858.8	E947.8	E950.4	E962.0	E980.4
Tubocurare	975.2	E858.6	E945.2	E950.4	E962.0	E980.4
Tubocurarine	975.2	E858.6	E945.2	E950.4	E962.0	E980.4
Turkish green	969.6	E854.1	E939.6	E950.3	E962.0	E980.3
Turpentine (spirits of) (liquid) (vapor)	982.8	E862.4	—	E950.9	E962.1	E980.9
Tybamate	969.5	E853.8	E939.5	E950.3	E962.0	E980.3
Tyloxapol	975.5	E858.6	E945.5	E950.4	E962.0	E980.4
Tymazoline	971.2	E855.5	E941.2	E950.4	E962.0	E980.4
Typhoid vaccine	978.1	E858.8	E948.1	E950.4	E962.0	E980.4
Typhus vaccine	979.2	E858.8	E949.2	E950.4	E962.0	E980.4
Tyrothricin	976.0	E858.7	E946.0	E950.4	E962.0	E980.4
ENT agent	976.6	E858.7	E946.6	E950.4	E962.0	E980.4
ophthalmic preparation	976.5	E858.7	E946.5	E950.4	E962.0	E980.4
Undecenoic acid	976.0	E858.7	E946.0	E950.4	E962.0	E980.4
Undecylenic acid	976.0	E858.7	E946.0	E950.4	E962.0	E980.4
Unna's boot	976.3	E858.7	E946.3	E950.4	E962.0	E980.4
Uracil mustard	963.1	E858.1	E933.1	E950.4	E962.0	E980.4
Uramustine	963.1	E858.1	E933.1	E950.4	E962.0	E980.4
Urari	975.2	E858.6	E945.2	E950.4	E962.0	E980.4

Substance	Poisoning	Accident	Therapeutic Use	Suicide Attempt	Assault	Undetermined
			External Cause (E-Code)			
Urea	974.4	E858.5	E944.4	E950.4	E962.0	E980.4
topical	976.8	E858.7	E946.8	E950.4	E962.0	E980.4
Urethan(e) (antineoplastic)	963.1	E858.1	E933.1	E950.4	E962.0	E980.4
Urginea (maritima) (scilla) — *see* Squill						
Uric acid metabolism agents NEC	974.7	E858.5	E944.7	E950.4	E962.0	E980.4
Urokinase	964.4	E858.2	E934.4	E950.4	E962.0	E980.4
Urokon	977.8	E858.8	E947.8	E950.4	E962.0	E980.4
Urotropin	961.9	E857	E931.9	E950.4	E962.0	E980.4
Urtica	988.2	E865.4	—	E950.9	E962.1	E980.9
Utility gas — *see* Gas, utility						
Vaccine NEC	979.9	E858.8	E949.9	E950.4	E962.0	E980.4
bacterial NEC	978.8	E858.8	E948.8	E950.4	E962.0	E980.4
with						
other bacterial component	978.9	E858.8	E948.9	E950.4	E962.0	E980.4
pertussis component	978.6	E858.8	E948.6	E950.4	E962.0	E980.4
viral–rickettsial component	979.7	E858.8	E949.7	E950.4	E962.0	E980.4
mixed NEC	978.9	E858.8	E948.9	E950.4	E962.0	E980.4
BCG	978.0	E858.8	E948.0	E950.4	E962.0	E980.4
cholera	978.2	E858.8	E948.2	E950.4	E962.0	E980.4
diphtheria	978.5	E858.8	E948.5	E950.4	E962.0	E980.4
influenza	979.6	E858.8	E949.6	E950.4	E962.0	E980.4
measles	979.4	E858.8	E949.4	E950.4	E962.0	E980.4
meningococcal	978.8	E858.8	E948.8	E950.4	E962.0	E980.4
mumps	979.6	E858.8	E949.6	E950.4	E962.0	E980.4
paratyphoid	978.1	E858.8	E948.1	E950.4	E962.0	E980.4
pertussis (with diphtheria toxoid) (with tetanus toxoid)	978.6	E858.8	E948.6	E950.4	E962.0	E980.4
plague	978.3	E858.8	E948.3	E950.4	E962.0	E980.4
poliomyelitis	979.5	E858.8	E949.5	E950.4	E962.0	E980.4
poliovirus	979.5	E858.8	E949.5	E950.4	E962.0	E980.4
rabies	979.1	E858.8	E949.1	E950.4	E962.0	E980.4
respiratory syncytial virus	979.6	E858.8	E949.6	E950.4	E962.0	E980.4
rickettsial NEC	979.6	E858.8	E949.6	E950.4	E962.0	E980.4
with						
bacterial component	979.7	E858.8	E949.7	E950.4	E962.0	E980.4
pertussis component	978.6	E858.8	E948.6	E950.4	E962.0	E980.4
viral component	979.7	E858.8	E949.7	E950.4	E962.0	E980.4
Rocky Mountain spotted fever	979.6	E858.8	E949.6	E950.4	E962.0	E980.4
rotavirus	979.6	E858.8	E949.6	E950.4	E962.0	E980.4
rubella virus	979.4	E858.8	E949.4	E950.4	E962.0	E980.4
sabin oral	979.5	E858.8	E949.5	E950.4	E962.0	E980.4
smallpox	979.0	E858.8	E949.0	E950.4	E962.0	E980.4
tetanus	978.4	E858.8	E948.4	E950.4	E962.0	E980.4
typhoid	978.1	E858.8	E948.1	E950.4	E962.0	E980.4
typhus	979.2	E858.8	E949.2	E950.4	E962.0	E980.4
viral NEC	979.6	E858.8	E949.6	E950.4	E962.0	E980.4
with						
bacterial component	979.7	E858.8	E949.7	E950.4	E962.0	E980.4
pertussis component	978.6	E858.8	E948.6	E950.4	E962.0	E980.4
rickettsial component	979.7	E858.8	E949.7	E950.4	E962.0	E980.4
yellow fever	979.3	E858.8	E949.3	E950.4	E962.0	E980.4
Vaccinia immune globulin (human)	964.6	E858.2	E934.6	E950.4	E962.0	E980.4
Vaginal contraceptives	976.8	E858.7	E946.8	E950.4	E962.0	E980.4
Valethamate	971.1	E855.4	E941.1	E950.4	E962.0	E980.4
Valisone	976.0	E858.7	E946.0	E950.4	E962.0	E980.4
Valium	969.4	E853.2	E939.4	E950.3	E962.0	E980.3
Valmid	967.8	E852.8	E937.8	E950.2	E962.0	E980.2
Vanadium	985.8	E866.4	—	E950.9	E962.1	E980.9
Vancomycin	960.8	E856	E930.8	E950.4	E962.0	E980.4
Vapor (*see also* Gas)	987.9	E869.9	—	E952.9	E962.2	E982.9

Substance	Poisoning	Accident	Therapeutic Use	Suicide Attempt	Assault	Undetermined
				External Cause (E-Code)		
kiln (carbon monoxide)	986	E868.8	—	E952.1	E962.2	E982.1
lead — *see* Lead						
specified source NEC (*see also*						
specific substance)	987.8	E869.8	—	E952.8	E962.2	E982.8
Varidase	964.4	E858.2	E934.4	E950.4	E962.0	E980.4
Varnish	989.89	E861.6	—	E950.9	E962.1	E980.9
cleaner	982.8	E862.9	—	E950.9	E962.1	E980.9
Vaseline	976.3	E858.7	E946.3	E950.4	E962.0	E980.4
Vasodilan	972.5	E858.3	E942.5	E950.4	E962.0	E980.4
Vasodilators NEC.	972.5	E858.3	E942.5	E950.4	E962.0	E980.0
coronary.	972.4	E858.3	E942.4	E950.4	E962.0	E980.4
Vasopressin	962.5	E858.0	E932.5	E950.4	E962.0	E980.4
Vasopressor drugs	962.5	E858.0	E932.5	E950.4	E962.0	E980.4
Venom, venomous (bite) (sting)	989.5	E905.9	—	E950.9	E962.1	E980.9
arthropod NEC	989.5	E905.5	—	E950.9	E962.1	E980.9
bee	989.5	E905.3	—	E950.9	E962.1	E980.9
centipede	989.5	E905.4	—	E950.9	E962.1	E980.9
hornet	989.5	E905.3	—	E950.9	E962.1	E980.9
lizard	989.5	E905.0	—	E950.9	E962.1	E980.9
marine animals or plants	989.5	E905.6	—	E950.9	E962.1	E980.9
millipede (topical)	989.5	E905.4	—	E950.9	E962.1	E980.9
plant NEC	989.5	E905.7	—	E950.9	E962.1	E980.9
marine	989.5	E905.6	—	E950.9	E962.1	E980.9
scorpion	989.5	E905.2	—	E950.9	E962.1	E980.9
snake	989.5	E905.0	—	E950.9	E962.1	E980.9
specified NEC	989.5	E905.8	—	E950.9	E962.1	E980.9
spider	989.5	E905.1	—	E950.9	E962.1	E980.9
wasp	989.5	E905.3	—	E950.9	E962.1	E980.9
Ventolin—*see* Salbutamol sulfate						
Veramon	967.0	E851	E937.0	E950.1	E962.0	E980.1
Veratrum						
album	988.2	E865.4	—	E950.9	E962.1	E980.9
alkaloids	972.6	E858.3	E942.6	E950.4	E962.0	E980.4
viride	988.2	E865.4	—	E950.9	E962.1	E980.9
Verdigris (*see also* Copper)	985.8	E866.4	—	E950.9	E962.1	E980.9
Veronal	967.0	E851	E937.0	E950.1	E962.0	E980.1
Veroxil	961.6	E857	E931.6	E950.4	E962.0	E980.4
Versidyne	965.7	E850.7	E935.7	E950.0	E962.0	E980.0
Viagra	972.5	E858.3	E942.5	E950.4	E962.0	E980.4
Vienna						
green	985.1	E866.3	—	E950.8	E962.1	E980.8
insecticide	985.1	E863.4	—	E950.6	E962.1	E980.7
red	989.89	E866.8	—	E950.9	E962.1	E980.9
pharmaceutical dye	977.4	E858.8	E947.4	E950.4	E962.0	E980.4
Vinbarbital, vinbarbitone	967.0	E851	E937.0	E950.1	E962.0	E980.1
Vinblastine	963.1	E858.1	E933.1	E950.4	E962.0	E980.4
Vincristine	963.1	E858.1	E933.1	E950.4	E962.0	E980.4
Vinesthene, vinethene	968.2	E855.1	E938.2	E950.4	E962.0	E980.4
Vinyl						
bital	967.0	E851	E937.0	E950.1	E962.0	E980.1
ether	968.2	E855.1	E938.2	E950.4	E962.0	E980.4
Vioform	961.3	E857	E931.3	E950.4	E962.0	E980.4
topical	976.0	E858.7	E946.0	E950.4	E962.0	E980.4
Viomycin	960.6	E856	E930.6	E950.4	E962.0	E980.4
Viosterol	963.5	E858.1	E933.5	E950.4	E962.0	E980.4
Viper (venom)	989.5	E905.0	—	E950.9	E962.1	E980.9
Viprynium (embonate)	961.6	E857	E931.6	E950.4	E962.0	E980.4
Virugon	961.7	E857	E931.7	E950.4	E962.0	E980.4
Visine	976.5	E858.7	E946.5	E950.4	E962.0	E980.4
Vitamins NEC	963.5	E858.1	E933.5	E950.4	E962.0	E980.4
B$_{12}$	964.1	E858.2	E934.1	E950.4	E962.0	E980.4

Substance	Poisoning	Accident	Therapeutic Use	Suicide Attempt	Assault	Undetermined
			External Cause (E-Code)			
hematopoietic 964.1	E858.2	E934.1	E950.4	E962.0	E980.4
K 964.3	E858.2	E934.3	E950.4	E962.0	E980.4
Vleminckx's solution 976.4	E858.7	E946.4	E950.4	E962.0	E980.4
Voltaren—*see* Diclofenac sodium					
Warfarin (potassium) (sodium) 964.2	E858.2	E934.2	E950.4	E962.0	E980.4
rodenticide. 989.4	E863.7	—	E950.6	E962.1	E980.7
Wasp (sting). 989.5	E905.3	—	E950.9	E962.1	E980.9
Water					
balance agents NEC 974.5	E858.5	E944.5	E950.4	E962.0	E980.4
gas 987.1	E868.1	—	E951.8	E962.2	E981.8
incomplete combustion of — *see*					
Carbon, monoxide, fuel, utility					
hemlock 988.2	E865.4	—	E950.9	E962.1	E980.9
moccasin (venom). 989.5	E905.0	—	E950.9	E962.1	E980.9
Wax (paraffin) (petroleum) 981	E862.3	—	E950.9	E962.1	E980.9
automobile. 989.89	E861.2	—	E950.9	E962.1	E980.9
floor 981	E862.0	—	E950.9	E962.1	E980.9
Weed killers NEC 989.4	E863.5	—	E950.6	E962.1	E980.7
Welldorm 967.1	E852.0	E937.1	E950.2	E962.0	E980.2
White					
arsenic — *see* Arsenic					
hellebore 988.2	E865.4	—	E950.9	E962.1	E980.9
lotion (keratolytic) 976.4	E858.7	E946.4	E950.4	E962.0	E980.4
spirit 981	E862.0	—	E950.9	E962.1	E980.9
Whitewashes. 989.89	E861.6	—	E950.9	E962.1	E980.9
Whole blood. 964.7	E858.2	E934.7	E950.4	E962.0	E980.4
Wild					
black cherry 988.2	E865.4	—	E950.9	E962.1	E980.9
poisonous plants NEC 988.2	E865.4	—	E950.9	E962.1	E980.9
Window cleaning fluid 989.89	E861.3	—	E950.9	E962.1	E980.9
Wintergreen (oil) 976.3	E858.7	E946.3	E950.4	E962.0	E980.4
Witch hazel 976.2	E858.7	E946.2	E950.4	E962.0	E980.4
Wood					
alcohol 980.1	E860.2	—	E950.9	E962.1	E980.9
spirit 980.1	E860.2	—	E950.9	E962.1	E980.9
Woorali 975.2	E858.6	E945.2	E950.4	E962.0	E980.4
Wormseed, American 961.6	E857	E931.6	E950.4	E962.0	E980.4
Xanthine diuretics 974.1	E858.5	E944.1	E950.4	E962.0	E980.4
Xanthocillin 960.0	E856	E930.0	E950.4	E962.0	E980.4
Xanthotoxin 976.3	E858.7	E946.3	E950.4	E962.0	E980.4
Xigris 964.2	E858.2	E934.2	E950.4	E962.0	E980.4
Xylene (liquid) (vapor) 982.0	E862.4	—	E950.9	E962.1	E980.9
Xylocaine (infiltration) (topical) 968.5	E855.2	E938.5	E950.4	E962.0	E980.4
nerve block (peripheral) (plexus) . . . 968.6	E855.2	E938.6	E950.4	E962.0	E980.4
spinal 968.7	E855.2	E938.7	E950.4	E962.0	E980.4
Xylol (liquid) (vapor) 982.0	E862.4	—	E950.9	E962.1	E980.9
Xylometazoline 971.2	E855.5	E941.2	E950.4	E962.0	E980.4
Yellow					
fever vaccine 979.3	E858.8	E949.3	E950.4	E962.0	E980.4
jasmine 988.2	E865.4	—	E950.9	E962.1	E980.9
Yew 988.2	E865.4	—	E950.9	E962.1	E980.9
Zactane 965.7	E850.7	E935.7	E950.0	E962.0	E980.0
Zaroxolyn 974.3	E858.5	E944.3	E950.4	E962.0	E980.4
Zephiran (topical) 976.0	E858.7	E946.0	E950.4	E962.0	E980.4
ophthalmic preparation 976.5	E858.7	E946.5	E950.4	E962.0	E980.4
Zerone 980.1	E860.2	—	E950.9	E962.1	E980.9
Zinc (compounds) (fumes) (salts)					
(vapor) NEC 985.8	E866.4	—	E950.9	E962.1	E980.9
anti–infectives 976.0	E858.7	E946.0	E950.4	E962.0	E980.4
antivaricose 972.7	E858.3	E942.7	E950.4	E962.0	E980.4

Substance	Poisoning	Accident	Therapeutic Use	Suicide Attempt	Assault	Undetermined
			External Cause (E-Code)			
bacitracin	976.0	E858.7	E946.0	E950.4	E962.0	E980.4
chloride	976.2	E858.7	E946.2	E950.4	E962.0	E980.4
gelatin	976.3	E858.7	E946.3	E950.4	E962.0	E980.4
oxide	976.3	E858.7	E946.3	E950.4	E962.0	E980.4
peroxide	976.0	E858.7	E946.0	E950.4	E962.0	E980.4
pesticides	985.8	E863.4	—	E950.6	E962.1	E980.7
phosphide (rodenticide)	985.8	E863.7	—	E950.6	E962.1	E980.7
stearate	976.3	E858.7	E946.3	E950.4	E962.0	E980.4
sulfate (antivaricose)	972.7	E858.3	E942.7	E950.4	E962.0	E980.4
ENT agent	976.6	E858.7	E946.6	E950.4	E962.0	E980.4
ophthalmic solution	976.5	E858.7	E946.5	E950.4	E962.0	E980.4
topical NEC	976.0	E858.7	E946.0	E950.4	E962.0	E980.4
undecylenate	976.0	E858.7	E946.0	E950.4	E962.0	E980.4
Zovant	964.2	E858.2	E934.2	E950.4	E962.0	E980.4
Zoxazolamine	968.0	E855.1	E938.0	E950.4	E962.0	E980.4
Zygadenus (venenosus)	988.2	E865.4	—	E950.9	E962.1	E980.9
Zyprexa	969.3	E853.8	E939.3	E950.3	E962.0	E980.3

TABLE OF DRUGS AND CHEMICALS

Substance	Poisoning	Accident	Therapeutic Use	Suicide Attempt	Assault	Undetermined
		External Cause (E-Code)				

SECTION 3

ALPHABETIC INDEX TO EXTERNAL CAUSES
OF INJURY AND POISONING (E CODE)

This section contains the index to the codes which classify environmental events, circumstances, and other conditions as the cause of injury and other adverse effects. Where a code from the section Supplementary Classification of External Causes of Injury and Poisoning (E800-E998) is applicable, it is intended that the E code shall be used in addition to a code from the main body of the classification, Chapters 1-17.

The alphabetic index to the E codes is organized by main terms which describe the *accident, circumstance, event,* or specific *agent* which caused the injury or other adverse effect.

> *Note—Transport accidents (E800-E848) include accidents involving:*
> *aircraft and space craft (E840-E845)*
> *watercraft (E830-E838)*
> *motor vehicle (E810-E825)*
> *railway (E800-E807)*
> *other road vehicles (E826-E829)*
>
> *For definitions and examples related to transport accidents—see Volume 1, pages 571-585.*
>
> *The fourth-digit subdivisions for use with categories E800-E848 to identify the injured person are found on pages 1447-1451.*
>
> *For identifying the place in which an accident or poisoning occurred (circumstances classifiable to categories E850-E869 and E880-E928)— see the listing in this section under "Accident, occurring"*

See the Table of Drugs and Chemicals (Section 2 of this volume) for identifying the specific agent involved in drug overdose or a wrong substance given or taken in error, and for intoxication or poisoning by a drug or other chemical substance.

The specific adverse effect, reaction, or localized toxic effect to a correct drug or substance properly administered in therapeutic or prophylactic dosage should be classified according to the nature of the adverse effect (e.g.: allergy, dermatitis, tachycardia) listed in Section 1 of this volume.

External
Causes
Injury

A

Abandonment
causing exposure to weather conditions—*see* Exposure
child, with intent to injure or kill E968.4
helpless person, infant, newborn E904.0
 with intent to injure or kill E968.4
Abortion, criminal, injury to child E968.8
Abuse, (alleged) (suspected)
adult
 by
  child E967.4
  ex-partner E967.3
  ex-spouse E967.3
  father E967.0
  grandchild E967.7
  grandparent E967.6
  mother E967.2
  non-related caregiver E967.8
  other relative E967.7
  other specified person(s) E967.1
  partner E967.3
  sibling E967.5
  spouse E967.3
  stepfather E967.0
  stepmother E967.2
  unspecified person E967.9
child
 by
  boyfriend of parent or guardian E967.0
  child E967.4
  father E967.0
  female partner of parent or guardian E967.2
  girlfriend of parent or guardian E967.2
  grandchild E967.7
  grandparent E967.6
  male partner of parent or guardian E967.0
  mother E967.2
  non-related caregiver E967.8
  other relative E967.7
  other specified person(s) E967.1
  sibling E967.5
  stepfather E967.0
  stepmother E967.2
   ⁻ified person E967.9
) E928.9
   transit) (powered) E841
  g, take-off E840
  aused by cataclysm—*see* categories
  , E909
  ⁻t of E929.1
  ⁻ed (*see also* Collision, aircraft,
   ⁻wered) E842
 while alighting, boarding E843
amphibious vehicle
 on
  land—*see* Accident, motor vehicle
  water—*see* Accident, watercraft
animal, ridden NEC E828
animal-drawn vehicle NEC E827
balloon (*see also* Collision, aircraft, unpowered) E842
caused by, due to
 abrasive wheel (metalworking) E919.3
 animal NEC E906.9
  being ridden (in sport or transport) E828
 avalanche NEC E909.2
 band saw E919.4
 bench saw E919.4

Accident—*continued*
bore, earth-drilling or mining (land) (seabed) E919.1
bulldozer E919.7
cataclysmic
 earth surface movement or eruption E909.9
 storm E908.9
chain
 hoist E919.2
  agricultural operations E919.0
  mining operations E919.1
 saw E920.1
circular saw E919.4
cold (excessive) (*see also* Cold, exposure to) E901.9
combine E919.0
conflagration—*see* Conflagration
corrosive liquid, substance NEC E924.1
cotton gin E919.8
crane E919.2
 agricultural operations E919.0
 mining operations E919.1
cutting or piercing instrument (*see also* Cut) E920.9
dairy equipment E919.8
derrick E919.2
 agricultural operations E919.0
 mining operations E919.1
drill E920.1
 earth (land) (seabed) E919.1
 hand (powered) E920.1
  not powered E920.4
 metalworking E919.3
 woodworking E919.4
earth(-)
 drilling machine E919.1
 moving machine E919.7
 scraping machine E919.7
electric
 current (*see also* Electric shock) E925.9
 motor—*see also* Accident, machine, by type of machine
  current (of)—*see* Electric shock
elevator (building) (grain) E919.2
 agricultural operations E919.0
 mining operations E919.1
environmental factors NEC E928.9
excavating machine E919.7
explosive material (*see also* Explosion) E923.9
farm machine E919.0
fire, flames—*see also* Fire
 conflagration—*see* Conflagration
firearm missile—*see* Shooting
forging (metalworking) machine E919.3
forklift (truck) E919.2
 agricultural operations E919.0
 mining operations E919.1
gas turbine E919.5
harvester E919.0
hay derrick, mower, or rake E919.0
heat (excessive) (*see also* Heat) E900.9
hoist (*see also* Accident, caused by, due to, lift) E919.2
 chain—*see* Accident, caused by, due to, chain
 shaft E919.1

Accident—*continued*
  hot
    liquid E924.0
      caustic or corrosive E924.1
      object (not producing fire or flames)
        E924.8
    substance E924.9
      caustic or corrosive E924.1
      liquid (metal) NEC E924.0
      specified type NEC E924.8
  human bite E928.3
  ignition—*see* Ignition
  internal combustion engine E919.5
  landslide NEC E909.2
  lathe (metalworking) E919.3
    turnings E920.8
    woodworking E919.4
  lift, lifting (appliances) E919.2
    agricultural operations E919.0
    mining operations E919.1
    shaft E919.1
  lightning NEC E907
  machine, machinery—*see also* Accident,
    machine
    drilling, metal E919.3
    manufacturing, for manufacture of
      beverages E919.8
      clothing E919.8
      foodstuffs E919.8
      paper E919.8
      textiles E919.8
    milling, metal E919.3
    moulding E919.4
    power press, metal E919.3
    printing E919.8
    rolling mill, metal E919.3
    sawing, metal E919.3
    specified type NEC E919.8
    spinning E919.8
    weaving E919.8
  natural factor NEC E928.9
  overhead plane E919.4
  plane E920.4
    overhead E919.4
  powered
    hand tool NEC E920.1
    saw E919.4
      hand E920.1
  printing machine E919.8
  pulley (block) E919.2
    agricultural operations E919.0
    mining operations E919.1
    transmission E919.6
  radial saw E919.4
  radiation—*see* Radiation
  reaper E919.0
  road scraper E919.7
    when in transport under its own
      power—*see* categories E810—E825
  roller coaster E919.8
  sander E919.4
  saw E920.4
    band E919.4
    bench E919.4
    chain E920.1
    circular E919.4
    hand E920.4
      powered E920.1
    powered, except hand E919.4
    radial E919.4
  sawing machine, metal E919.3

Accident—*continued*
  shaft
    hoist E919.1
    lift E919.1
    transmission E919.6
  shears E920.4
    hand E920.4
      powered E920.1
    mechanical E919.3
  shovel E920.4
    steam E919.7
  spinning machine E919.8
  steam—*see also* Burning, steam
    engine E919.5
    shovel E919.7
  thresher E919.0
  thunderbolt NEC E907
  tractor E919.0
    when in transport under its own
      power—*see* categories E810-E825
  transmission belt, cable, chain, gear, pinion,
    pulley, shaft E919.6
  turbine (gas) (water driven) E919.5
  under-cutter E919.1
  weaving machine E919.8
  winch E919.2
    agricultural operations E919.0
    mining operations E919.1
  diving E883.0
    with insufficient air supply E913.2
  glider (hang) (*see also* Collision, aircraft,
    unpowered) E842
  hovercraft
    on
      land—*see* Accident, motor vehicle
      water—*see* Accident, watercraft
  ice yacht (*see also* Accident, vehicle NEC)
    E848
  in
    medical, surgical procedure
      as, or due to misadventure—*see*
        Misadventure
      causing an abnormal reaction or later
        complication without mention of
        misadventure—*see* Reaction, abnormal
  kite carrying a person (*see also* Collision,
    aircraft, unpowered) E842
  land yacht (*see also* Accident, vehicle NEC)
    E848
  late effect of—*see* Late effect
  launching pad E845
  machine, machinery (*see also* Accident,
    caused by, due to, by specific type of
    machine) E919.9
    agricultural including animal-powered
      E919.0
    earth-drilling E919.1
    earth moving or scraping E919.7
    excavating E919.7
    involving transport under own power on
      highway or transport vehicle—*see*
      categories E810-E825, E840-E845
    lifting (appliances) E919.2
    metalworking E919.3
    mining E919.1
    prime movers, except electric motors E919.5
      electric motors—*see* Accident, machine, by
        specific type of machine
    recreational E919.8
    specified type NEC E919.8

Accident—*continued*
transmission E919.6
watercraft (deck) (engine room) (galley)
(laundry) (loading) E836
woodworking or forming E919.4
motor vehicle (on public highway) (traffic)
E819
due to cataclysm—*see* categories E908,
E909
involving
collision (*see also* Collision, motor
vehicle) E812
nontraffic, not on public highway—*see*
categories E820-E825
not involving collision—*see* categories
E816-E819
nonmotor vehicle NEC E829
nonroad—*see* Accident, vehicle NEC
road, except pedal cycle, animal-drawn
vehicle, or animal being ridden E829
nonroad vehicle NEC—*see* Accident, vehicle
NEC
not elsewhere classifiable involving
cable car (not on rails) E847
on rails E829
coal car in mine E846
hand truck—*see* Accident, vehicle NEC
logging car E846
sled(ge), meaning snow or ice vehicle E848
tram, mine or quarry E846
truck
mine or quarry E846
self-propelled, industrial E846
station baggage E846
tub, mine or quarry E846
vehicle NEC E848
snow and ice E848
used only on industrial premises E846
wheelbarrow E848
occurring (at) (in)
apartment E849.0
baseball field, diamond E849.4
construction site, any E849.3
dock E849.8
yard E849.3
dormitory E849.7
factory (building) (premises) E849.3
farm E849.1
buildings E849.1
house E849.0
football field E849.4
forest E849.8
garage (place of work) E849.3
private (home) E849.0
gravel pit E849.2
gymnasium E849.4
highway E849.5
home (private) (residential) E849.0
institutional E849.7
hospital E849.7
hotel E849.6
house (private) (residential) E849.0
movie E849.6
public E849.6
institution, residential E849.7
jail E849.7
mine E849.2
motel E849.6
movie house E849.6
office (building) E849.6

Accident—*continued*
orphanage E849.7
park (public) E849.4
mobile home E849.8
trailer E849.8
parking lot or place E849.8
place
industrial NEC E849.3
parking E849.8
public E849.8
specified place NEC E849.5
recreational NEC E849.4
sport NEC E849.4
playground (park) (school) E849.4
prison E849.6
public building NEC E849.6
quarry E849.2
railway
line NEC E849.8
yard E849.3
residence
home (private) E849.0
resort (beach) (lake) (mountain) (seashore)
(vacation) E849.4
restaurant E849.6
sand pit E849.2
school (building) (private) (public) (state)
E849.6
reform E849.7
riding E849.4
seashore E849.8
resort E849.4
shop (place of work) E849.3
commercial E849.6
skating rink E849.4
sports palace E849.4
stadium E849.4
store E849.6
street E849.5
swimming pool (public) E849.4
private home or garden E849.0
tennis court E849.4
theatre, theater E849.6
trailer court E849.8
tunnel E849.8
under construction E849.2
warehouse E849.3
yard
dock E849.3
industrial E849.3
private (home) E849.0
railway E849.3
off-road type motor vehicle (not on public
highway) NEC E821
on public highway—*see* categories
E810-E819
pedal cycle E826
railway E807
due to cataclysm—*see* categories E908,
E909
involving
avalanche E909.2
burning by engine, locomotive, train (*see
also* Explosion, railway engine) E803
collision (*see also* Collision, railway) E800
derailment (*see also* Derailment, railway)
E802
explosion (*see also* Explosion, railway
engine) E803
fall (*see also* Fall, from, railway rolling
stock) E804

Accident—*continued*

    fire (*see also* Explosion, railway engine)
        E803
    hitting by, being struck by
        object falling in, on, from, rolling stock,
            train, vehicle E806
        rolling stock, train, vehicle E805
    overturning, railway rolling stock, train,
        vehicle (*see also* Derailment, railway)
        E802
    running off rails, railway (*see also*
        Derailment, railway) E802
    specified circumstances NEC E806
    train or vehicle hit by
        avalanche E909
        falling object (earth, rock, tree) E806
        due to cataclysm—*see* categories E908,
            E909
        landslide E909
  roller skate E885.1
  scooter (nonmotorized) E885.0
  skateboard E885.2
  ski(ing) E885.3
    jump E884.9
    lift or tow (with chair or gondola) E847
  snowboard E885.4
  snow vehicle, motor driven (not on public
    highway) E820
  on public highway—*see* categories
    E810-E819
  spacecraft E845
  specified cause NEC E928.8
  street car E829
  traffic NEC E819
  vehicle NEC (with pedestrian) E848
    battery powered
        airport passenger vehicle E846
        truck (baggage) (mail) E846
    powered commercial or industrial (with other
        vehicle or object within commercial or
        industrial premises) E846
  watercraft E838
    with
        drowning or submersion resulting from
            accident other than to watercraft E832
            accident to watercraft E830
        injury, except drowning or submersion,
            resulting from
            accident other than to watercraft—*see*
                categories E833-E838
            accident to watercraft E831
    due to, caused by cataclysm—*see* categories
        E908, E909
    machinery E836
Acid throwing E961
Acosta syndrome E902.0
Activity (involving) E030
  aerobic and step exercise (class) E009.2
  alpine skiing E003.2
  animal care NEC E019.9
  arts and handcrafts NEC E012.9
  athletics NEC E008.9
    played
        as a team or group NEC E007.9
        individually NEC E006.9
  baking E015.2
  ballet E005.0
  barbells E010.2
  BASE (Building, Antenna, Span, Earth)
    jumping E004.2
  baseball E007.3

Activity—*continued*

  basketball E007.6
  bathing (personal) E013.0
  beach volleyball E007.7
  bike riding E006.4
  boogie boarding E002.7
  bowling E006.3
  boxing E008.0
  brass instrument playing E018.3
  building and construction E016.2
  bungee jumping E004.3
  calisthenics E009.1
  canoeing (in calm and turbulent water) E002.5
  capture the flag E007.8
  cardiorespiratory exercise NEC E009.9
  caregiving (providing) NEC E014.9
    bathing E014.0
    lifting E014.1
  cellular
    communication device E011.1
    telephone E011.1
  challenge course E009.4
  cheerleading E005.4
  circuit training E009.3
  cleaning
    floor E013.4
  climbing NEC E004.9
    mountain E004.0
    rock E004.0
    wall climbing E004.0
  combatives E008.4
  computer
    keyboarding E011.0
    technology NEC E011.9
  confidence course E009.4
  construction (building) E016.2
  cooking and baking E015.2
  cooking and grilling NEC E015.9
  cool down exercises E009.1
  cricket E007.9
  crocheting E012.0
  cross country skiing E003.3
  dancing (all types) E005.0
  digging
    dirt E016.0
  dirt digging E016.0
  dishwashing E015.0
  diving (platform) (springboard) E002.1
    underwater E002.4
  dodge ball E007.8
  downhill skiing E003.2
  drum playing E018.1
  dumbbells E010.2
  electronic
    devices NEC E011.9
        hand held interactive E011.1
    game playing (using) (with)
        interactive device E011.1
        keyboard or other stationary device E011.0
  elliptical machine E009.0
  exercise(s)
    machines ((primarily) for)
        cardiorespiratory conditioning E009.0
        muscle strengthening E010.0
    muscle strengthening (non-machine) NEC
        E010.9
  external motion NEC E017.9
    roller coaster E017.0
  field hockey E007.4
  figure skating (pairs) (singles) E003.0
  flag football E007.1

Activity—*continued*
　floor mopping and cleaning E013.4
　food preparation and clean up E015.0
　football (American) NOS E007.0
　　flag E007.1
　　tackle E007.0
　　touch E007.1
　four square E007.8
　free weights E010.2
　frisbee (ultimate) E008.3
　furniture
　　building E012.2
　　finishing E012.2
　　repair E012.2
　game playing (electronic)
　　using
　　　interactive device E011.1
　　　keyboard or other stationary device E011.0
　gardening E016.1
　golf E006.2
　grass drills E009.5
　grilling and smoking food E015.1
　grooming and shearing an animal E019.2
　guerilla drills E009.5
　gymnastics (rhythmic) E005.2
　handball E008.2
　handcrafts NEC E012.9
　hand held interactive electronic device E011.1
　hang gliding E004.4
　hiking (on level or elevated terrain) E001.0
　hockey (ice) E003.1
　　field E007.4
　horseback riding E006.1
　household maintenance NEC E013.9
　ice NEC E003.9
　　dancing E003.0
　　hockey E003.1
　　skating E003.0
　inline roller skating E006.0
　ironing E013.3
　judo E008.4
　jumping (off) NEC E004.9
　　BASE (Building, Antenna, Span, Earth) E004.2
　　bungee E004.3
　　jacks E009.1
　　rope E006.5
　jumping jacks E009.1
　jumping rope E006.5
　karate E008.4
　kayaking (in calm and turbulent water) E002.5
　keyboarding (computer) E011.0
　kickball E007.8
　knitting E012.0
　lacrosse E007.4
　land maintenance NEC E016.9
　landscaping E016.1
　laundry E013.1
　machines (exercise) primarily for cardiorespiratory conditioning E009.0
　maintenance
　　building E016.9
　　household NEC E013.9
　　land E016.9
　　property E016.9
　marching (on level or elevated terrain) E001.0
　martial arts E008.4
　microwave oven E015.2
　mopping (floor) E013.4
　mountain climbing E004.0
　milking an animal E019.1

Activity—*continued*
　muscle strengthening
　　exercises (non-machine) NEC E010.9
　　machines E010.0
　musical keyboard (electronic) playing E018.0
　nordic skiing E003.3
　obstacle course E009.4
　oven (microwave) E015.2
　packing up and unpacking in moving to a new residence E013.5
　parasailing E002.9
　percussion instrument playing NEC E018.1
　personal
　　bathing and showering E013.0
　　hygiene NEC E013.8
　　showering E013.0
　physical
　　games generally associated with school recess, summer camp and children 007.8
　　training NEC E009.9
　piano playing E018.0
　pilates E010.3
　platform diving E002.1
　playing musical instrument
　　brass instrument E018.3
　　drum E018.1
　　musical keyboard (electronic) E018.0
　　percussion instrument NEC E018.1
　　piano E018.0
　　string instrument E018.2
　　wind instrument E018.3
　property maintenance NEC E016.9
　pruning (garden and lawn) E016.1
　pull-ups E010.1
　push-ups E010.1
　racquetball E008.2
　rafting (in calm and turbulent water) E002.5
　raking (leaves) E016.0
　rappelling E004.1
　refereeing a sports activity E029.0
　residential relocation E013.5
　rhythmic
　　gymnastics E005.2
　　movement NEC E005.9
　riding
　　horseback E006.1
　　roller coaster E017.0
　rock climbing E004.0
　roller coaster riding E017.0
　roller skating (inline) E006.0
　rough housing and horseplay E029.2
　rowing (in calm and turbulent water) E002.5
　rugby E007.2
　running E001.1
　SCUBA diving E002.4
　sewing E012.1
　shoveling E016.0
　　dirt E016.0
　　snow E016.0
　showering (personal) E013.0
　sit-ups E010.1
　skateboarding E006.0
　skating (ice) E003.0
　　roller E006.0
　skiing (alpine) (downhill) E003.2
　　cross country E003.3
　　nordic E003.3
　sledding (snow) E003.2
　smoking and grilling food E015.1
　snorkeling E002.4

Activity—*continued*
snow NEC E003.9
  boarding E003.2
  shoveling E016.0
  sledding E003.2
  tubing E003.2
soccer E007.5
softball E007.3
specified NEC E029.9
spectator at an event E029.1
sports NEC E008.9
sports played as a team or group NEC E007.9
sports played individually NEC E006.9
springboard diving E002.1
squash E008.2
stationary bike E009.0
step (stepping) exercise (class) E009.2
stepper machine E009.0
stove E015.2
string instrument playing E018.2
surfing E002.7
swimming E002.0
tackle football E007.0
tap dancing E005.0
tennis E008.2
tobogganing E003.2
touch football E007.1
track and field events (non-running) E006.6
  running E001.1
trampoline E005.3
treadmill E009.0
trimming shrubs E016.1
tubing (in calm and turbulent water) E002.5
  snow E003.2
ultimate frisbee E008.3
underwater diving E002.4
unpacking in moving to a new residence E013.5
use of stove, oven and microwave oven E015.2
vacuuming E013.2
volleyball (beach) (court) E007.7
wake boarding E002.6
walking an animal E019.0
walking (on level or elevated terrain) E001.0
  an animal E019.0
wall climbing E004.0
warm up and cool down exercises E009.1
water NEC E002.9
  aerobics E002.3
  craft NEC E002.9
  exercise E002.3
  polo E002.2
  skiing E002.6
  sliding E002.8
  survival training and testing E002.9
weeding (garden and lawn) E016.1
wind instrument playing E018.3
windsurfing E002.7
wrestling E008.1
yoga E005.1
Activity status E000.9
child assisting in compensated work of other family member E000.8
civilian
  done for
    financial or other compensation E000.0
    pay or income E000.0
family member assisting in compensated work of other family member E000.8
for income E000.0

Activity status—*continued*
hobby or leisure E000.8
off duty military E000.8
military E000.1
  off duty E000.8
recreation E000.8
specified NEC E000.8
sport not for income E000.8
student E000.8
volunteer E000.2
Aeroneurosis E902.1
Aero-otitis media —*see* Effects of, air pressure
Aerosinusitis —*see* Effects of, air pressure
After-effect, late —*see* Late effect
Air
blast
  in
    terrorism E979.2
    war operations E993.9
embolism (traumatic) NEC E928.9
  in
    infusion or transfusion E874.1
    perfusion E874.2
sickness E903
Alpine sickness E902.0
Altitude sickness —*see* Effects of, air pressure
Anaphylactic shock, anaphylaxis (*see also* Table of drugs and chemicals) E947.9
due to bite or sting (venomous)—*see* Bite, venomous
Andes disease E902.0
Apoplexy heat—*see* Heat
Arachnidism E905.1
Arson E968.0
Asphyxia, asphyxiation
by
  chemical
    in
      terrorism E979.7
      war operations E997.2
  explosion—*see* Explosion
  food (bone) (regurgitated food) (seed) E911
  foreign object, except food E912
  fumes
    in
      terrorism (chemical weapons) E979.7
      war operations E997.2
  gas—*see also* Table of drugs and chemicals
    in
      terrorism E979.7
      war operations E997.2
  legal
    execution E978
    intervention (tear) E972
    tear E972
  mechanical means (*see also* Suffocation) E913.9
from
  conflagration—*see* Conflagration
  fire—*see also* Fire E899
    in
      terrorism E979.3
      war operations E990.9
  ignition—*see* Ignition
Aspiration
foreign body—*see* Foreign body, aspiration
mucus, not of newborn (with asphyxia, obstruction respiratory passage, suffocation) E912
phlegm (with asphyxia, obstruction respiratory passage, suffocation) E912

Aspiration—*continued*
  vomitus (with asphyxia, obstruction respiratory
      passage, suffocation) (*see also* Foreign
      body, aspiration, food) E911
Assassination (attempt) (*see also* Assault)
    E968.9
Assault (homicidal) (by) (in) E968.9
  acid E961
    swallowed E962.1
  air gun E968.6
  BB gun E968.6
  bite NEC E968.8
    of human being E968.7
  bomb ((placed in) car or house) E965.8
    antipersonnel E965.5
    letter E965.7
    petrol E965.7
  brawl (hand) (fists) (foot) E960.0
  burning, burns (by fire) E968.0
    acid E961
      swallowed E962.1
    caustic, corrosive substance E961
      swallowed E962.1
    chemical from swallowing caustic, corrosive
        substance NEC E962.1
    hot liquid E968.3
    scalding E968.3
    vitriol E961
      swallowed E962.1
  caustic, corrosive substance E961
    swallowed E962.1
  cut, any part of body E966
  dagger E966
  drowning E964
  explosive(s) E965.9
    bomb (*see also* Assault, bomb) E965.8
    dynamite E965.8
  fight (hand) (fists) (foot) E960.0
    with weapon E968.9
      blunt or thrown E968.2
      cutting or piercing E966
      firearm—*see* Shooting, homicide
  fire E968.0
  firearm(s)—*see* Shooting, homicide
  garrotting E963
  gunshot (wound)—*see* Shooting, homicide
  hanging E963
  injury NEC E968.9
  knife E966
  late effect of E969
  ligature E963
  poisoning E962.9
    drugs or medicinals E962.0
    gas(es) or vapors, except drugs and
        medicinals E962.2
    solid or liquid substances, except drugs and
        medicinals E962.1
  puncture, any part of body E966
  pushing
    before moving object, train, vehicle E968.5
    from high place E968.1
  rape E960.1
  scalding E968.3
  shooting—*see* Shooting, homicide
  sodomy E960.1
  stab, any part of body E966
  strangulation E963
  submersion E964
  suffocation E963
  transport vehicle E968.5
  violence NEC E968.9

Assault—*continued*
  vitriol E961
    swallowed E962.1
  weapon E968.9
    blunt or thrown E968.2
    cutting or piercing E966
    firearm—*see* Shooting, homicide
  wound E968.9
    cutting E966
    gunshot—*see* Shooting, homicide
    knife E966
    piercing E966
    puncture E966
    stab E966
Attack by animal NEC E906.9
Avalanche E909.2
  falling on or hitting
    motor vehicle (in motion) (on public
        highway) E909.2
    railway train E909.2
Aviators' disease E902.1

B

**Barotitis, barodontalgia, barosinusitis,
    barotrauma** (otitic) (sinus)—*see* Effects of,
    air pressure
Battered
  baby or child (syndrome)—*see* Abuse, child;
      category E967
  person other than baby or child—*see* Assault
Bayonet wound (*see also* Cut, by bayonet)
    E920.3
  in
    legal intervention E974
    terrorism E979.8
    war operations E995.2
Bean in nose E912
Bed set on fire NEC E898.0
Beheading (by guillotine)
  homicide E966
  legal execution E978
Bending, injury
  due to
    repetitive movement E927.3
    sudden strenuous movement E927.0
Bends E902.0
Bite
  animal (nonvenomous) NEC E906.5
    venomous NEC E905.9
  arthropod (nonvenomous) NEC E906.4
    venomous—*see* Sting
  black widow spider E905.1
  cat E906.3
  centipede E905.4
  cobra E905.0
  copperhead snake E905.0
  coral snake E905.0
  dog E906.0
  fer de lance E905.0
  gila monster E905.0
  human being
    accidental E928.3
    assault E968.7
  insect (nonvenomous) E906.4
    venomous—*see* Sting
  krait E905.0
  late effect of—*see* Late effect
  lizard E906.2
    venomous E905.0

Bite *—continued*
  mamba E905.0
  marine animal
    nonvenomous E906.3
      snake E906.2
    venomous E905.6
      snake E905.0
  millipede E906.4
    venomous E905.4
  moray eel E906.3
  rat E906.1
  rattlesnake E905.0
  rodent, except rat E906.3
  serpent—*see* Bite, snake
  shark E906.3
  snake (venomous) E905.0
    nonvenomous E906.2
    sea E905.0
  spider E905.1
    nonvenomous E906.4
  tarantula (venomous) E905.1
  venomous NEC E905.9
  by specific animal—*see* category E905
  viper E905.0
  water moccasin E905.0
Blast (air)
  from nuclear explosion E996
  in
    terrorism E979.2
      from nuclear explosion E979.5
      underwater E979.0
    war operations E993.9
      from nuclear explosion—*see* War
        operations, injury due to, nuclear
        weapons
      underwater E992.9
  underwater E992
Blizzard E908.3
Blow E928.9
  by law-enforcing agent, police (on duty) E975
    with blunt object (baton) (nightstick) (stave)
      (truncheon) E973
Blowing up (*see also* Explosion) E923.9
Brawl (hand) (fists) (foot) E960.0
Breakage (accidental)
  cable of cable car not on rails E847
  ladder (causing fall) E881.0
  part (any) of
    animal-drawn vehicle E827
    ladder (causing fall) E881.0
    motor vehicle
      in motion (on public highway) E818
        not on public highway E825
    nonmotor road vehicle, except animal-drawn
      vehicle or pedal cycle E829
    off-road type motor vehicle (not on public
      highway) NEC E821
      on public highway E818
    pedal cycle E826
    scaffolding (causing fall) E881.1
    snow vehicle, motor-driven (not on public
      highway) E820
      on public highway E818
    vehicle NEC—*see* Accident, vehicle
Broken
  glass
    fall on E888.0
    injury by E920.8
  power line (causing electric shock) E925.1

Bumping against, into (accidentally)
  object (moving) E917.9
    caused by crowd E917.1
      with subsequent fall E917.6
    furniture E917.3
      with subsequent fall E917.7
    in
      running water E917.2
      sports E917.0
        with subsequent fall E917.5
    stationary E917.4
      with subsequent fall E917.8
  person(s) E917.9
    with fall E886.9
      in sports E886.0
    as, or caused by, a crowd E917.1
      with subsequent fall E917.6
    in sports E917.0
      with fall E886.0
Burning, burns (accidental) (by) (from) (on)
  E899
  acid (any kind) E924.1
    swallowed—*see* Table of drugs and
      chemicals
  airgun E928.7
  bedclothes (*see also* Fire, specified NEC)
    E898.0
  blowlamp (*see also* Fire, specified NEC)
    E898.1
  blowtorch (*see also* Fire, specified NEC)
    E898.1
  boat, ship, watercraft—*see* categories E830,
    E831, E837
  bonfire (controlled) E897
    uncontrolled E892
  candle (*see also* Fire, specified NEC) E898.1
  caustic liquid, substance E924.1
    swallowed—*see* Table of drugs and
      chemicals
  chemical E924.1
    from swallowing caustic, corrosive
      substance—*see* Table of drugs and
      chemicals
    in
      terrorism E979.7
      war operations E997.2
  cigar(s) or cigarette(s) (*see also* Fire, specified
    NEC) E898.1
  clothes, clothing, nightdress—*see* Ignition,
    clothes
    with conflagration—*see* Conflagration
  conflagration—*see* Conflagration
  corrosive liquid, substance E924.1
    swallowed—*see* Table of drugs and
      chemicals
  electric current (*see also* Electric shock)
    E925.9
  fire, flames (*see also* Fire) E899
  firearm E928.7
  flare, Verey pistol E922.8
  heat
    from appliance (electrical) E924.8
    in local application or packing during
      medical or surgical procedure E873.5
  homicide (attempt) (*see also* Assault, burning)
    E968.0
  hot
    liquid E924.0
      caustic or corrosive E924.1
    object (not producing fire or flames) E924.8
    substance E924.9
      caustic or corrosive E924.1

Burning, burns—*continued*
    liquid (metal) NEC E924.0
        specified type NEC E924.8
        tap water E924.2
    ignition—*see also* Ignition
    clothes, clothing, nightdress—*see also*
        Ignition, clothes
        with conflagration—*see* Conflagration
    highly inflammable material (benzine) (fat)
        (gasoline) (kerosene) (paraffin) (petrol)
        E894
    inflicted by other person
        stated as
            homicidal, intentional (*see also* Assault,
                burning) E968.0
            undetermined whether accidental or
                intentional (*see also* Burn, stated as
                undetermined whether accidental or
                intentional) E988.1
    internal, from swallowed caustic, corrosive
        liquid, substance—*see* Table of drugs and
        chemicals
    in
        from nuclear explosion E996
        petrol bomb E990.0
        terrorism E979.3
            from nuclear explosion E979.5
            petrol bomb E979.3
        war operations (from fire-producing device
            or conventional weapon) E990.9
            from nuclear explosion (see also War
                operations, injury due to, nuclear
                weapons) E996.2
            incendiary bomb E990.0
            petrol bomb E990.0
    lamp (*see also* Fire, specified NEC) E898.1
    late effect of NEC E929.4
    lighter (cigar) (cigarette) (*see also* Fire,
        specified NEC) E898.1
    lightning E907
    liquid (boiling) (hot) (molten) E924.0
        caustic, corrosive (external) E924.1
        swallowed—*see* Table of drugs and
            chemicals
    local application of externally applied
        substance in medical or surgical care
        E873.5
    machinery—*see* Accident, machine
    matches (*see also* Fire, specified NEC) E898.1
    medicament, externally applied E873.5
    metal, molten E924.0
    object (hot) E924.8
        producing fire or flames—*see* Fire
    oven (electric) (gas) E924.8
    pipe (smoking) (*see also* Fire, specified NEC)
        E898.1
    radiation—*see* Radiation
    railway engine, locomotive, train (*see also*
        Explosion, railway engine) E803
    self-inflicted (unspecified whether accidental
        or intentional) E988.1
        caustic or corrosive substance NEC E988.7
        stated as intentional, purposeful E958.1
            caustic or corrosive substance NEC E958.7
        stated as undetermined whether accidental or
        intentional E988.1
        caustic or corrosive substance NEC E988.7
    steam E924.0
        pipe E924.8

Burning, burns—*continued*
    substance (hot) E924.9
        boiling or molten E924.0
        caustic, corrosive (external) E924.1
        swallowed—*see* Table of drugs and
            chemicals
    suicidal (attempt) NEC E958.1
        caustic substance E958.7
        late effect of E959
    tanning bed E926.2
    therapeutic misadventure
        overdose of radiation E873.2
    torch, welding (*see also* Fire, specified NEC)
        E898.1
    trash fire (*see also* Burning, bonfire) E897
    vapor E924.0
    vitriol E924.1
    x-rays E926.3
        in medical, surgical procedure—*see*
            Misadventure, failure, in dosage,
            radiation
Butted by animal E906.8

C

Cachexia, lead or saturnine E866.0
    from pesticide NEC (*see also* Table of drugs
        and chemicals) E863.4
Caisson disease E902.2
Capital punishment (any means) E978
Car sickness E903
Casualty (not due to war) NEC E928.9
    terrorism E979.8
    war (*see also* War operations) E995.9
Cat
    bite E906.3
    scratch E906.8
Cataclysmic (any injury)
    earth surface movement or eruption E909.9
        specified type NEC E909.8
    storm or flood resulting from storm E908.9
        specified type NEC E909.8
Catching fire —*see* Ignition
Caught
    between
        objects (moving) (stationary and moving)
        E918
        and machinery—*see* Accident, machine
    by cable car, not on rails E847
    in
        machinery (moving parts of)—*see* Accident,
        machine
        object E918
Cave-in (causing asphyxia, suffocation (by
    pressure)) (*see also* Suffocation, due to,
    cave-in) E913.3
Cave-in—*continued*
    with injury other than asphyxia or suffocation
        E916
        with asphyxia or suffocation (*see also*
            Suffocation, due to, cave-in) E913.3
    struck or crushed by E916
        with asphyxia or suffocation (*see also*
            Suffocation, due to, cave-in) E913.3
Change(s) in air pressure—*see also* Effects of,
    air pressure
    sudden, in aircraft (ascent) (descent) (causing
        aeroneurosis or aviators' disease) E902.1
Chilblains E901.0
    due to manmade conditions E901.1

Choking (on) (any object except food or
   vomitus) E912
   apple E911
   bone E911
   food, any type (regurgitated) E911
   mucus or phlegm E912
   seed E911
Civil insurrection —*see* War operations
Cloudburst E908.8
Cold, exposure to (accidental) (excessive)
   (extreme) (place) E901.9
   causing chilblains or immersion foot E901.0
   due to
      manmade conditions E901.1
      specified cause NEC E901.8
      weather (conditions) E901.0
   late effect of NEC E929.5
   self-inflicted (undetermined whether accidental
      or intentional) E988.3
   suicidal E958.3
   suicide E958.3
Colic, lead, painters', or saturnine —*see*
   category E866
Collapse
   building E916
      burning (uncontrolled fire) E891.8
         in terrorism E979.3
         private E890.8
   dam E909.3
   due to heat—*see* Heat
   machinery—*see* Accident, machine
   man-made structure E909.3
   postoperative NEC E878.9
   structure, burning NEC E891.8
      burning (uncontrolled fire)
         in terrorism E979.3
Collision (accidental)

> Note—In the case of collisions between different
> types of vehicles, persons and objects, priority in
> classification is in the following order:
>
>   Aircraft
>   Watercraft
>   Motor vehicle
>   Railway vehicle
>   Pedal Cycle
>   Animal-drawn vehicle
>   Animal being ridden
>   Streetcar or other nonmotor road vehicle
>   Other vehicle
>   Pedestrian or person using pedestrian
>   conveyance
>   Object (except where falling from or set in
>   motion by vehicle etc. listed above)
>
> In the listing below, the combinations are listed
> only under the vehicle etc. having priority. For
> definitions, *see* E code introduction.

   aircraft (with object or vehicle) (fixed)
      (movable) (moving) E841
      with
         person (while landing, taking off) (without
            accident to aircraft) E844
         powered (in transit) (with unpowered
            aircraft) E841
            while landing, taking off E840
         unpowered E842
            while landing, taking off E840

Collision—*continued*
   animal being ridden (in sport or transport)
      E828
      and
         animal (being ridden) (herded)
            (unattended) E828
         nonmotor road vehicle, except pedal cycle
            or animal-drawn vehicle E828
         object (fallen) (fixed) (movable) (moving)
            not falling from or set in motion by
            vehicle of higher priority E828
         pedestrian (conveyance or vehicle) E828
   animal-drawn vehicle E827
      and
         animal (being ridden) (herded)
            (unattended) E827
         nonmotor road vehicle, except pedal cycle
            E827
         object (fallen) (fixed) (movable) (moving)
            not falling from or set in motion by
            vehicle of higher priority E827
         pedestrian (conveyance or vehicle) E827
         streetcar E827
   motor vehicle (on public highway) (traffic
      accident) E812
      after leaving, running off, public highway
         (without antecedent collision) (without
         re-entry) E816
      with antecedent collision on public
         highway—*see* categories E810-E815
      with re-entrance collision with another
         motor vehicle E811
      and
         abutment (bridge) (overpass) E815
         animal (herded) (unattended) E815
            carrying person, property E813
         animal-drawn vehicle E813
         another motor vehicle (abandoned)
            (disabled) (parked) (stalled) (stopped)
            E812
            with, involving re-entrance (on same
               roadway) (across median strip) E811
         any object, person, or vehicle off the
            public highway resulting from a
            noncollision motor vehicle nontraffic
            accident E816
         avalanche, fallen or not moving E815
            falling E909
         boundary fence E815
         culvert E815
         fallen
            stone E815
            tree E815
         falling E909.2
         guard post or guard rail E815
         inter-highway divider E815
         landslide, fallen or not moving E815
            moving E909
         machinery (road) E815
         moving E909.2
         nonmotor road vehicle NEC E813
         object (any object, person, or vehicle off
            the public highway resulting from a
            noncollision motor vehicle nontraffic
            accident) E815
            off, normally not on, public highway
               resulting from a noncollision motor
               vehicle traffic accident E816
         pedal cycle E813
         pedestrian (conveyance) E814
         person (using pedestrian conveyance) E814

Collision—*continued*

post or pole (lamp) (light) (signal) (telephone) (utility) E815
railway rolling stock, train, vehicle E810
safety island E815
street car E813
traffic signal, sign, or marker (temporary) E815
tree E815
tricycle E813
wall of cut made for road E815
due to cataclysm—*see* categories E908, E909
not on public highway, nontraffic accident E822
and
    animal (carrying person, property) (herded) (unattended) E822
    animal-drawn vehicle E822
    another motor vehicle (moving), except off-road motor vehicle E822
      stationary E823
    avalanche, fallen, not moving E823
      moving E909
    landslide, fallen, not moving E823
      moving E909
    nonmotor vehicle (moving) E822
      stationary E823
    object (fallen) (normally) (fixed) (movable but not in motion) (stationary) E823
    moving, except when falling from, set in motion by, aircraft or cataclysm E822
    pedal cycle (moving) E822
      stationary E823
    pedestrian (conveyance) E822
    person (using pedestrian conveyance) E822
    railway rolling stock, train, vehicle (moving) E822
      stationary E823
    road vehicle (any) (moving) E822
      stationary E823
    tricycle (moving) E822
      stationary E823
    moving E909.2
off-road type motor vehicle (not on public highway) E821
and
    animal (being ridden) (-drawn vehicle) E821
    another off-road motor vehicle, except snow vehicle E821
    other motor vehicle, not on public highway E821
    other object or vehicle NEC, fixed or movable, not set in motion by aircraft, motor vehicle on highway, or snow vehicle, motor-driven E821
    pedal cycle E821
    pedestrian (conveyance) E821
    railway train E821
on public highway—*see* Collision, motor vehicle
pedal cycle E826
and
    animal (carrying person, property) (herded) (unherded) E826
    animal-drawn vehicle E826

Collision—*continued*

    another pedal cycle E826
    nonmotor road vehicle E826
    object (fallen) (fixed) (movable) (moving) not falling from or set in motion by aircraft, motor vehicle, or railway train NEC E826
    pedestrian (conveyance) E826
    person (using pedestrian conveyance) E826
    street car E826
pedestrian(s) (conveyance) E917.9
with fall E886.9
    in sports E886.0
and
    crowd, human stampede E917.1
      with subsequent fall E917.6
    furniture E917.3
      with subsequent fall E917.7
    machinery—*see* Accident, machine
    object (fallen) (moving) not falling from or set in motion by any vehicle classifiable to E800-E848, E917.9
    caused by a crowd E917.1
      with subsequent fall E917.6
    furniture E917.3
      with subsequent fall E917.7
    in
      running water E917.2
        with drowning or submersion—*see* Submersion
      sports E917.0
        with subsequent fall E917.5
      stationary E917.4
        with subsequent fall E917.8
    vehicle, nonmotor, nonroad E848
in
    running water E917.2
      with drowning or submersion—*see* Submersion
    sports E917.0
      with fall E886.0
person(s) (using pedestrian conveyance) (*see also* Collision, pedestrian) E917.9
railway (rolling stock) (train) (vehicle) (with (subsequent) derailment, explosion, fall or fire) E800
with antecedent derailment E802
and
    animal (carrying person) (herded) (unattended) E801
    another railway train or vehicle E800
    buffers E801
    fallen tree on railway E801
    farm machinery, nonmotor (in transport) (stationary) E801
    gates E801
    nonmotor vehicle E801
    object (fallen) (fixed) (movable) (moving) not falling from, set in motion by, aircraft or motor vehicle NEC E801
    pedal cycle E801
    pedestrian (conveyance) E805
    person (using pedestrian conveyance) E805
    platform E801
    rock on railway E801
    street car E801

Collision—*continued*
snow vehicle, motor-driven (not on public
highway) E820
and
animal (being ridden) (-drawn vehicle)
E820
another off-road motor vehicle E820
other motor vehicle, not on public highway
E820
other object or vehicle NEC, fixed or
movable, not set in motion by aircraft
or motor vehicle on highway E820
pedal cycle E820
pedestrian (conveyance) E820
railway train E820
on public highway—*see* Collision, motor
vehicle
street car(s) E829
and
animal, herded, not being ridden,
unattended E829
nonmotor road vehicle NEC E829
object (fallen) (fixed) (movable) (moving)
not falling from or set in motion by
aircraft, animal-drawn vehicle, animal
being ridden, motor vehicle, pedal
cycle, or railway train E829
pedestrian (conveyance) E829
person (using pedestrian conveyance) E829
vehicle
animal-drawn—*see* Collision, animal-drawn
vehicle
motor—*see* Collision, motor vehicle
nonmotor
nonroad E848
and
another nonmotor, nonroad vehicle
E848
object (fallen) (fixed) (movable)
(moving) not falling from or set in
motion by aircraft, animal-drawn
vehicle, animal being ridden, motor
vehicle, nonmotor road vehicle,
pedal cycle, railway train, or
streetcar E848
road, except animal being ridden,
animal-drawn vehicle, or pedal cycle
E829
and
animal, herded, not being ridden,
unattended E829
another nonmotor road vehicle, except
animal being ridden, animal-drawn
vehicle, or pedal cycle E829
object (fallen) (fixed) (movable)
(moving) not falling from or set in
motion by, aircraft, animal-drawn
vehicle, animal being ridden, motor
vehicle, pedal cycle, or railway
train E829
pedestrian (conveyance) E829
person (using pedestrian conveyance)
E829
vehicle, nonmotor, nonroad E829
watercraft E838
and
person swimming or water skiing E838
causing
drowning, submersion E830
injury except drowning, submersion E831
Combustion, spontaneous —*see* Ignition

**Complication of medical or surgical
procedure or treatment**
as an abnormal reaction—*see* Reaction,
abnormal
delayed, without mention of
misadventure—*see* Reaction, abnormal
due to misadventure—*see* Misadventure
Compression
divers' squeeze E902.2
trachea by
food E911
foreign body, except food E912
Conflagration
building or structure, except private dwelling
(barn) (church) (convalescent or residential
home) (factory) (farm outbuilding)
(hospital) (hotel) (institution) (educational)
(dormitory) (residential) (school) (shop)
(store) (theatre) E891.9
with or causing (injury due to)
accident or injury NEC E891.9
specified circumstance NEC E891.8
burns, burning E891.3
carbon monoxide E891.2
fumes E891.2
polyvinylchloride (PVC) or similar
material E891.1
smoke E891.2
causing explosion E891.0
in terrorism E979.3
not in building or structure E892
private dwelling (apartment) (boarding house)
(camping place) (caravan) (farmhouse)
(home (private)) (house) (lodging house)
(private garage) (rooming house)
(tenement) E890.9
with or causing (injury due to)
accident or injury NEC E890.9
specified circumstance NEC E890.8
burns, burning E890.3
carbon monoxide E890.2
fumes E890.2
polyvinylchloride (PVC) or similar
material E890.1
smoke E890.2
causing explosion E890.0
Constriction, external
caused by
hair E928.4
other object E928.5
Contact with
dry ice E901.1
liquid air, hydrogen, nitrogen E901.1
Cramp(s)
Heat—*see* Heat
swimmers (*see also* category E910) E910.2
not in recreation or sport E910.3
Cranking (car) (truck) (bus) (engine), injury
by E917.9
Crash
aircraft (in transit) (powered) E841
at landing, take-off E840
in
terrorism E979.1
war operations E994.9
on runway NEC E840
stated as
homicidal E968.8
suicidal E958.6
undetermined whether accidental or
intentional E988.6
unpowered E842

Crash—*continued*
  glider E842
  motor vehicle—*see also* Accident, motor
    vehicle
    homicidal E968.5
    suicidal E958.5
    undetermined whether accidental or
      intentional E988.5
Crushed (accidentally) E928.9
  between
    boat(s), ship(s), watercraft (and dock or pier)
      (without accident to watercraft) E838
      after accident to, or collision, watercraft
        E831
    objects (moving) (stationary and moving)
      E918
  by
    avalanche NEC E909.2
    boat, ship, watercraft after accident to,
      collision, watercraft E831
    cave-in E916
      with asphyxiation or suffocation (*see also*
        Suffocation, due to, cave-in) E913.3
    crowd, human stampede E917.1
    falling
      aircraft (*see also* Accident, aircraft) E841
      in
        terrorism E979.1
        war operations E994.8
      earth, material E916
        with asphyxiation or suffocation (*see
          also* Suffocation, due to, cave-in)
          E913.3
      object E916
        on ship, watercraft E838
        while loading, unloading watercraft E838
    firearm E928.7
    landslide NEC E909.2
    lifeboat after abandoning ship E831
    machinery—*see* Accident, machine
    railway rolling stock, train, vehicle (part of)
      E805
    slide trigger mechanism, scope or other part
      of gun E928.7
    street car E829
    vehicle NEC—*see* Accident, vehicle NEC
  in
    machinery—*see* Accident, machine
    object E918
    transport accident—*see* categories
      E800-E848
  late effect of NEC E929.9
Cut, cutting (any part of body) (accidental)
  E920.9
  by
    arrow E920.8
    axe E920.4
    bayonet (*see also* Bayonet wound) E920.3
      in war operations E995.2
    blender E920.2
    broken glass E920.8
      following fall E888.0
    can opener E920.4
      powered E920.2
    chisel E920.4
    circular saw E919.4
    cutting or piercing instrument—*see also*
      category E920
      following fall E888.0
      late effect of E929.8
    dagger E920.3

Cut, cutting—*continued*
  dart E920.8
  drill—*see* Accident, caused by drill
  edge of stiff paper E920.8
  electric
    beater E920.2
    fan E920.2
    knife E920.2
    mixer E920.2
  firearm component E928.7
  fork E920.4
  garden fork E920.4
  hand saw or tool (not powered) E920.4
    powered E920.1
  hedge clipper E920.4
    powered E920.1
  hoe E920.4
  ice pick E920.4
  knife E920.3
    electric E920.2
    in war operations E995.2
  lathe turnings E920.8
  lawn mower E920.4
    powered E920.0
    riding E919.8
  machine—*see* Accident, machine
  meat
    grinder E919.8
    slicer E919.8
  nails E920.8
  needle E920.4
    hypodermic E920.5
  object, edged, pointed, sharp—*see* category
    E920
    following fall E888.0
  paper cutter E920.4
  piercing instrument—*see also* category E920
    late effect of E929.8
  pitchfork E920.4
  powered
    can opener E920.2
    garden cultivator E920.1
      riding E919.8
    hand saw E920.1
    hand tool NEC E920.1
    hedge clipper E920.1
    household appliance or implement E920.2
    lawn mower (hand) E920.0
      riding E919.8
    rivet gun E920.1
    staple gun E920.1
  rake E920.4
  saw
    circular E919.4
    hand E920.4
  scissors E920.4
  screwdriver E920.4
  sewing machine (electric) (powered) E920.2
    not powered E920.4
  shears E920.4
  shovel E920.4
  slide trigger mechanism, scope or other part
    of gun E928.7
  spade E920.4
  splinters E920.8
  sword E920.3
    in war operations E995.2
  tin can lid E920.8
  wood slivers E920.8
  homicide (attempt) E966

Cut, cutting—*continued*
inflicted by other person
stated as
intentional, homicidal E966
undetermined whether accidental or
intentional E986
late effect of NEC E929.8
legal
execution E978
intervention E974
self-inflicted (unspecified whether accidental
or intentional) E986
stated as intentional, purposeful E956
stated as undetermined whether accidental or
intentional E986
suicidal (attempt) E956
terrorism E979.8
war operations E995.2
Cyclone E908.1

D

**Death due to injury occurring one year or
more previous** —*see* Late effect
Decapitation (accidental circumstances) NEC
E928.9
homicidal E966
legal execution (by guillotine) E978
Deprivation —*see also* Privation
homicidal intent E968.4
Derailment (accidental)
railway (rolling stock) (train) (vehicle) (with
subsequent collision) E802
with
collision (antecedent) (*see also* Collision,
railway) E800
Derailment (accidental)—*continued*
explosion (subsequent) (without antecedent
collision) E802
antecedent collision E803
fall (without collision (antecedent)) E802
fire (without collision (antecedent)) E802
street car E829
Descent
parachute (voluntary) (without accident to
aircraft) E844
due to accident to aircraft—*see* categories
E840-E842
Desertion
child, with intent to injure or kill E968.4
helpless person, infant, newborn E904.0
with intent to injure or kill E968.4
Destitution —*see* Privation
Dirty bomb (*see also* War operations, injury
due to, nuclear weapons) E996.9
Disability, late effect or sequela of injury
—*see* Late effect
Disease
Andes E902.0
aviators' E902.1
caisson E902.2
range E902.0
Divers' disease, palsy, paralysis, squeeze
E902.0
Dog bite E906.0
Dragged by
cable car (not on rails) E847
on rails E829
motor vehicle (on highway) E814
not on highway, nontraffic accident E825
street car E829

Drinking poison (accidental) —*see* Table of
drugs and chemicals
Drowning —*see* Submersion
Dust in eye E914\

E

Earth falling (on) (with asphyxia or suffocation
(by pressure)) (*see also* Suffocation, due to,
cave-in) E913.3
as, or due to, a cataclysm (involving any
transport vehicle)—*see* categories E908,
E909
not due to cataclysmic action E913.3
motor vehicle (in motion) (on public
highway) E818
not on public highway E825
nonmotor road vehicle NEC E829
pedal cycle E826
railway rolling stock, train, vehicle E806
street car E829
struck or crushed by E916
with asphyxiation or suffocation E913.3
with injury other than asphyxia,
suffocation E916
Earthquake (any injury) E909.0
Effect(s) (adverse) of
air pressure E902.9
at high altitude E902.9
in aircraft E902.1
residence or prolonged visit (causing
conditions classifiable to E902.0)
E902.0
due to
diving E902.2
specified cause NEC E902.8
in aircraft E902.1
cold, excessive (exposure to) (*see also* Cold,
exposure to) E901.9
heat (excessive) (*see also* Heat) E900.9
hot
place—*see* Heat
weather E900.0
insulation—*see* Heat
late—*see* Late effect of
motion E903
nuclear explosion or weapon
in
terrorism E979.5
war operations (*see also* War operations,
injury due to, nuclear weapons) E996.9
radiation—*see* Radiation
terrorism, secondary E979.9
travel E903
Electric shock, electrocution (accidental) (from
exposed wire, faulty appliance, high voltage
cable, live rail, open socket) (by) (in) E925.9
appliance or wiring
domestic E925.0
factory E925.2
farm (building) E925.8
house E925.0
home E925.0
industrial (conductor) (control apparatus)
(transformer) E925.2
outdoors E925.8
public building E925.8
residential institution E925.8
school E925.8
specified place NEC E925.8

Electric shock, electrocution—*continued*
  caused by other person
    stated as
      intentional, homicidal E968.8
      undetermined whether accidental or
        intentional E988.4
  electric power generating plant, distribution
    station E925.1
  electroshock gun (taser) (stun gun) E925.8
    caused by other person E968.8
      legal intervention E975
      stated as accidental E925.8
      stated as intentional E968.8
    due to legal intervention E975
    stated as intentional self-harm (suicidal
      (attempt)) E958.4
    stated as undetermined whether accidental or
      intentional E988.4
    suicide (attempt) E958.4
  homicidal (attempt) E968.8
  legal execution E978
  lightning E907
  machinery E925.9
    domestic E925.0
    factory E925.2
    farm E925.8
    home E925.0
  misadventure in medical or surgical procedure
    in electroshock therapy E873.4
  self-inflicted (undetermined whether accidental
    or intentional) E988.4
    stated as intentional E958.4
  stated as undetermined whether accidental or
    intentional E988.4
  suicidal (attempt) E958.4
  transmission line E925.1
Electrocution —*see* Electric shock
Embolism
  air (traumatic) NEC—*see* Air, embolism
Encephalitis
  lead or saturnine E866.0
  from pesticide NEC E863.4
Entanglement
  in
    bedclothes, causing suffocation E913.0
    wheel of pedal cycle E826
Entry of foreign body, material, any —*see*
  Foreign body
Execution, legal (any method) E978
Exertion, excessive physical, from prolonged
  activity E927.2
Exhaustion
  cold—*see* Cold, exposure to
  due to excessive exertion E927.2
  heat—*see* Heat
Explosion (accidental) (in) (of) (on) E923.9
  acetylene E923.2
  aerosol can E921.8
  aircraft (in transit) (powered) E841
    at landing, take-off E840
    in
      terrorism E979.1
      war operations
        from
          enemy fire or explosive(s) (device
            placed on aircraft) E994.0
          own onboard explosives E994.1
    unpowered E842
  air tank (compressed) (in machinery) E921.1
  anesthetic gas in operating theatre E923.2

Explosion—*continued*
  automobile tire NEC E921.8
    causing transport accident—*see* categories
      E810-E825
  blasting (cap) (materials) E923.1
  boiler (machinery), not on transport vehicle
    E921.0
    steamship—*see* Explosion, watercraft
  bomb E923.8
    in
      terrorism E979.2
      war operations E993.8
        after cessation of hostilities E998.1
        atom, hydrogen or nuclear (*see also* War
          operations, injury due to, nuclear
          weapons) E996.9
        injury by fragments from E991.9
          antipersonnel bomb E991.3
  butane E923.2
  caused by
    other person
      stated as
        intentional, homicidal—*see* Assault,
          explosive
        undetermined whether accidental or
          homicidal E985.5
  coal gas E923.2
  detonator E923.1
  dynamite E923.1
  explosive (material) NEC E923.9
    gas(es) E923.2
    missile E923.8
      in
        terrorism E979.2
        war operations E993.1
          injury by fragments from E991.9
            antipersonnel bomb E991.3
    used in blasting operations E923.1
  fire-damp E923.2
  fireworks E923.0
  gas E923.2
    cylinder (in machinery) E921.1
    pressure tank (in machinery) E921.1
  gasoline (fumes) (tank) not in moving motor
    vehicle E923.2
  grain store (military) (munitions) E923.8
  grenade E923.8
    in
      terrorism E979.2
      war operations E993.8
        injury by fragments from E991.4
  homicide (attempt)—*see* Assault, explosive
  hot water heater, tank (in machinery) E921.0
  in mine (of explosive gases) NEC E923.2
  late effect of NEC E929.8
  machinery—*see also* Accident, machine
    pressure vessel—*see* Explosion, pressure
      vessel
  methane E923.2
  missile E923.8
    in
      terrorism E979.2
      war operations E993.1
        injury by fragments from E991.4
  motor vehicle (part of)
    in motion (on public highway) E818
      not on public highway E825
  munitions (dump) (factory) E923.8
    in
      terrorism E979.2
      war operations E993.9

Explosion—*continued*
of mine E923.8
  in
    terrorism
      at sea or in harbor E979.0
      land E979.2
      marine E979.0
    war operations
      after cessation of hostilities E998.0
      at sea or in harbor E992.2
      land E993.8
        after cessation of hostilities E998.0
        injury by fragments from E991.4
      marine E992.2
own weapons
  in
    terrorism (*see also* Suicide) E979.2
    war operations E993.7
      injury by fragments from E991.9
        antipersonnel bomb E991.3
pressure
  cooker E921.8
  gas tank (in machinery) E921.1
  vessel (in machinery) E921.9
    on transport vehicle—*see* categories
      E800-E848
    specified type NEC E921.8
propane E923.2
railway engine, locomotive, train (boiler) (with
  subsequent collision, derailment, fall) E803
  with
    collision (antecedent) (*see also* Collision,
      railway) E800
    derailment (antecedent) E802
    fire (without antecedent collision or
      derailment) E803
secondary fire resulting from—*see* Fire
self-inflicted (unspecified whether accidental
  or intentional) E985.5
  stated as intentional, purposeful E955.5
shell (artillery) E923.8
  in
    terrorism E979.2
    war operations E993.2
      injury by fragments from E991.4
stated as undetermined whether caused
  accidentally or purposely inflicted E985.5
steam or water lines (in machinery) E921.0
suicide (attempted) E955.5
terrorism—*see* Terrorism, explosion
torpedo E923.8
  in
    terrorism E979.0
    war operations E992.0
transport accident—*see* categories E800-E848
war operations—*see* War operations, explosion
watercraft (boiler) E837
  causing drowning, submersion (after jumping
    from watercraft) E830
Exposure (weather) (conditions) (rain) (wind)
  E904.3
  with homicidal intent E968.4

Exposure—*continued*
environmental
  to
    algae bloom E928.6
    blue-green algae bloom E928.6
    brown tide E928.6
    cyanobacteria bloom E928.6
    Florida red tide E928.6
    harmful algae
      and toxins E928.6
      bloom E928.6
    pfiesteria piscicida E928.6
    red tide E928.6
excessive E904.3
  cold (*see also* Cold, exposure to) E901.9
    self-inflicted—*see* Cold, exposure to,
      self-inflicted
  heat (*see also* Heat) E900.9
fire—*see* Fire
helpless person, infant, newborn due to
  abandonment or neglect E904.0
noise E928.1
prolonged in deep-freeze unit or refrigerator
  E901.1
radiation—*see* Radiation
resulting from transport accident—*see*
  categories E800-E848
smoke from, due to
  fire—*see* Fire
  tobacco, second-hand E869.4
vibration E928.2
External cause status E000.9
child assisting in compensated work of other
  family member E000.8
civilian
  done for
    financial or other compensation E000.0
    pay or income E000.0
family member assisting in compensated work
  of other family member E000.8
for income E000.0
hobby or leisure E000.8
off duty military E000.8
military E000.1
  off duty E000.8
recreation E000.8
specified NEC E000.8
sport not for income E000.8
student E000.8
volunteer E000.2

F

Fall, falling (accidental) E888.9
building E916
  burning E891.8
    private E890.8
down
  escalator E880.0
  ladder E881.0
    in boat, ship, watercraft E833
  staircase E880.9
  stairs, steps—*see* Fall, from, stairs
earth (with asphyxia or suffocation (by
  pressure)) (*see also* Earth, falling) E913.3
from, off
  aircraft (at landing, take-off) (in-transit)
    (while alighting, boarding) E843
    resulting from accident to aircraft—*see*
      categories E840-E842

Fall, falling—*continued*
  animal (in sport or transport) E828
  animal-drawn vehicle E827
  balcony E882
  bed E884.4
  bicycle E826
  boat, ship, watercraft (into water) E832
    after accident to, collision, fire on E830
      and subsequently struck by (part of) boat
        E831
    and subsequently struck by (part of) boat
      E838
    burning, crushed, sinking E830
      and subsequently struck by (part of) boat
        E831
  bridge E882
  building E882
    burning (uncontrolled fire) E891.8
      in terrorism E979.3
      private E890.8
  bunk in boat, ship, watercraft E834
    due to accident to watercraft E831
  cable car (not on rails) E847
    on rails E829
  car—*see* Fall from motor vehicle
  chair E884.2
  cliff E884.1
  commode E884.6
  curb (sidewalk) E880.1
  elevation aboard ship E834
    due to accident to ship E831
  embankment E884.9
  escalator E880.0
  fire escape E882
  flagpole E882
  furniture NEC E884.5
  gangplank (into water) (*see also* Fall, from,
    boat) E832
    to deck, dock E834
  hammock on ship E834
    due to accident to watercraft E831
  haystack E884.9
  heelies E885.1
  high place NEC E884.9
    stated as undetermined whether accidental
      or intentional—*see* Jumping, from, high
      place
  horse (in sport or transport) E828
  in-line skates E885.1
  ladder E881.0
    in boat, ship, watercraft E833
      due to accident to watercraft E831
  machinery—*see also* accident, machine
    not in operation E884.9
  motor vehicle (in motion) (on public
    highway) E818
    not on public highway E825
      stationary, except while alighting,
        boarding, entering, leaving E884.9
      while alighting, boarding, entering,
        leaving E824
    stationary, except while alighting, boarding,
      entering, leaving E884.9
    while alighting, boarding, entering, leaving,
      except off-road type motor vehicle
      E817
    off-road type—*see* Fall, from, off-road
      type motor vehicle
  motorized
    mobility scooter E884.3
    wheelchair E884.3

Fall, falling—*continued*
  nonmotor road vehicle (while alighting,
    boarding) NEC E829
    stationary, except while alighting, boarding,
      entering, leaving E884.9
  off road type motor vehicle (not on public
    highway) NEC E821
    on public highway E818
      while alighting, boarding, entering,
        leaving E817
  snow vehicle—*see* Fall from snow vehicle,
    motor-driven
  one
    deck to another on ship E834
      due to accident to ship E831
    level to another NEC E884.9
      boat, ship, or watercraft E834
        due to accident to watercraft E831
  pedal cycle E826
  playground equipment E884.0
  railway rolling stock, train, vehicle (while
    alighting, boarding) E804
    with
      collision (*see also* Collision, railway)
        E800
      derailment (*see also* Derailment, railway)
        E802
      explosion (*see also* Explosion, railway
        engine) E803
  rigging (aboard ship) E834
    due to accident to watercraft E831
  roller skates E885.1
  scaffolding E881.1
  scooter (nonmotorized) E885.0
    motorized mobility E884.3
  sidewalk (curb) E880.1
    moving E885.9
  skateboard E885.2
  skis E885.3
  snowboard E885.4
  snow vehicle, motor-driven (not on public
    highway) E820
    on public highway E818
      while alighting, boarding, entering,
        leaving E817
  stairs, steps E880.9
    boat, ship, watercraft E833
      due to accident to watercraft E831
    motor bus, motor vehicle—*see* Fall, from,
      motor vehicle, while alighting,
      boarding
    street car E829
  stationary vehicle NEC E884.9
  stepladder E881.0
  street car (while boarding, alighting) E829
    stationary, except while boarding or
      alighting E884.9
  structure NEC E882
    burning (uncontrolled fire) E891.8
      in terrorism E979.3
  table E884.9
  toilet E884.6
  tower E882
  tree E884.9
  turret E882
  vehicle NEC—*see also* Accident, vehicle
    NEC
    stationary E884.9
  viaduct E882
  wall E882
  wheelchair (electric) (motorized) E884.3

Fall, falling—*continued*
  wheelies E885.1
  window E882
  in, on
    aircraft (at landing, take-off) (in-transit)
      E843
      resulting from accident to aircraft—*see*
        categories E840-E842
    boat, ship, watercraft E835
      due to accident to watercraft E831
      one level to another NEC E834
      on ladder, stairs E833
    cutting or piercing instrument or machine
      E888.0
    deck (of boat, ship, watercraft) E835
      due to accident to watercraft E831
    escalator E880.0
    gangplank E835
    glass, broken E888.0
    knife E888.0
    ladder E881.0
      in boat, ship, watercraft E833
        due to accident to watercraft E831
    object
      edged, pointed or sharp E888.0
      other E888.1
    pitchfork E888.0
    railway rolling stock, train, vehicle (while
      alighting, boarding) E804
      with
        collision (*see also* Collision, railway) E800
        derailment (*see also* Derailment, railway)
          E802
        explosion (*see also* Explosion, railway
          engine) E803
    scaffolding E881.1
    scissors E888.0
    staircase, stairs, steps (*see also* Fall, from,
      stairs) E880.9
    street car E829
    water transport (*see also* Fall, in, boat) E835
  into
    cavity E883.9
    dock E883.9
      from boat, ship, watercraft (*see also* Fall,
        from, boat) E832
    hold (of ship) E834
      due to accident to watercraft E831
    hole E883.9
    manhole E883.2
    moving part of machinery—*see* Accident,
      machine
    opening in surface NEC E883.9
    pit E883.9
    quarry E883.9
    shaft E883.9
    storm drain E883.2
    tank E883.9
    water (with drowning or submersion) E910.9
    well E883.1
  late effect of NEC E929.3
  object (*see also* Hit by, object, falling) E916
  other E888.8
  over
    animal E885.9
    cliff E884.1
    embankment E884.9
    small object E885.9
  overboard (*see also* Fall, from, boat) E832
  resulting in striking against object E888.1
    sharp E888.0
  rock E916

Fall, falling—*continued*
  same level NEC E888.9
    aircraft (any kind) E843
      resulting from accident to aircraft—*see*
        categories E840-E842
    boat, ship, watercraft E835
    due to accident to, collision, watercraft E831
  from
    collision, pushing, shoving, by or with
      other person(s) E886.9
    as, or caused by, a crowd E917.6
    in sports E886.0
    in-line skates E885.1
    roller skates E885.1
    scooter (nonmotorized) E885.0
    skateboard E885.2
    skis E885.3
    slipping, stumbling, tripping E885.9
    snowboard E885.4
  snowslide E916
    as avalanche E909.2
  stone E916
  through
    hatch (on ship) E834
      due to accident to watercraft E831
    roof E882
    window E882
  timber E916
  while alighting from, boarding, entering,
    leaving
    aircraft (any kind) E843
    motor bus, motor vehicle—*see* Fall, from,
      motor vehicle, while alighting, boarding
    nonmotor road vehicle NEC E829
    railway train E804
    street car E829
Fallen on by
  animal (horse) (not being ridden) E906.8
  being ridden (in sport or transport) E828
Fell or jumped from high place, so stated
  —*see* Jumping, from, high place
Felo-de-se (*see also* Suicide) E958.9
Fever
  heat—*see* Heat
  thermic—*see* Heat
Fight (hand) (fist) (foot) (*see also* Assault,
  fight) E960.0
Fire (accidental) (caused by great heat from
  appliance (electrical), hot object or hot
  substance) (secondary, resulting from
  explosion) E899
  conflagration—*see* Conflagration
  controlled, normal (in brazier, fireplace,
    furnace, or stove) (charcoal) (coal) (coke)
    (electric) (gas) (wood)
  bonfire E897
  brazier, not in building or structure E897
  in building or structure, except private
    dwelling (barn) (church) (convalescent or
    residential home) (factory) (farm
    outbuilding) (hospital) (hotel) (institution
    (educational) (dormitory) (residential))
    (private garage) (school) (shop) (store)
    (theatre) E896
  in private dwelling (apartment) (boarding
    house) (camping place) (caravan)
    (farmhouse) (home (private)) (house)
    (lodging house) (rooming house)
    (tenement) E895
  not in building or structure E897
  trash E897

Fire —*continued*
forest (uncontrolled) E892
grass (uncontrolled) E892
hay (uncontrolled) E892
homicide (attempt) E968.0
late effect of E969
in, of, on, starting in E892
aircraft (in transit) (powered) E841
at landing, take-off E840
stationary E892
unpowered (balloon) (glider) E842
balloon E842
boat, ship, watercraft—*see* categories E830,
E831, E837
building or structure, except private dwelling
(barn) (church) (convalescent or
residential home) (factory) (farm
outbuilding) (hospital) (hotel) (institution
(educational) (dormitory) (residential))
(school) (shop) (store) (theatre) (*see also*
Conflagration, building or structure,
except private dwelling) E891.9
forest (uncontrolled) E892
glider E842
grass (uncontrolled) E892
hay (uncontrolled) E892
lumber (uncontrolled) E892
machinery—*see* Accident, machine
mine (uncontrolled) E892
motor vehicle (in motion) (on public
highway) E818
not on public highway E825
stationary E892
prairie (uncontrolled) E892
private dwelling (apartment) (boarding
house) (camping place) (caravan)
(farmhouse) (home (private)) (house)
(lodging house) (private garage) (rooming
house) (tenement) (*see also*
Conflagration, private dwelling) E890.9
railway rolling stock, train, vehicle (*see also*
Explosion, railway engine) E803
stationary E892
room NEC E898.1
street car (in motion) E829
stationary E892
terrorism (by fire-producing device) E979.3
fittings or furniture (burning building)
(uncontrolled fire) E979.3
from nuclear explosion E979.5
transport vehicle, stationary NEC E892
tunnel (uncontrolled) E892
war operations (by fire-producing device or
conventional weapon) E990.9
from nuclear explosion (*see also* War
operations, injury due to, nuclear
weapons) E996.2
incendiary bomb E990.0
petrol bomb E990.0
late effect of NEC E929.4
lumber (uncontrolled) E892
mine (uncontrolled) E892
prairie (uncontrolled) E892
self-inflicted (unspecified whether accidental
or intentional) E988.1
stated as intentional, purposeful E958.1

Fire —*continued*
specified NEC E898.1
with
conflagration—*see* Conflagration
ignition (of)
clothing—*see* Ignition, clothes
highly inflammable material (benzine)
(fat) (gasoline) (kerosene) (paraffin)
(petrol) E894
started by other person
stated as
with intent to injure or kill E968.0
undetermined whether or not with intent to
injure or kill E988.1
suicide (attempted) E958.1
late effect of E959
tunnel (uncontrolled) E892
Fireball effects from nuclear explosion
in
terrorism E979.5
war operations (see also War operations,
injury due to, nuclear weapons) E996.2
Fireworks (explosion) E923.0
Flash burns from explosion (*see also*
Explosion) E923.9
Flood (any injury) (resulting from storm)
E908.2
caused by collapse of dam or manmade
structure E909.3
Forced landing (aircraft) E840
Foreign body, object or material (entrance into
(accidental)
air passage (causing injury) E915
with asphyxia, obstruction, suffocation E912
food or vomitus E911
nose (with asphyxia, obstruction, suffocation)
E912
causing injury without asphyxia,
obstruction, suffocation E915
alimentary canal (causing injury) (with
obstruction) E915
with asphyxia, obstruction respiratory
passage, suffocation E912
food E911
mouth E915
with asphyxia, obstruction, suffocation
E912
food E911
pharynx E915
with asphyxia, obstruction, suffocation
E912
food E911
aspiration (with asphyxia, obstruction
respiratory passage, suffocation) E912
causing injury without asphyxia, obstruction
respiratory passage, suffocation E915
food (regurgitated) (vomited) E911
causing injury without asphyxia,
obstruction respiratory passage,
suffocation E915
mucus (not of newborn) E912
phlegm E912
bladder (causing injury or obstruction) E915
bronchus, bronchi—*see* Foreign body, air
passages
conjunctival sac E914
digestive system—*see* Foreign body,
alimentary canal
ear (causing injury or obstruction) E915
esophagus (causing injury or obstruction) (*see
also* Foreign body, alimentary canal) E915

Foreign body—*continued*
  eye (any part) E914
  eyelid E914
  hairball (stomach) (with obstruction) E915
  ingestion—*see* Foreign body, alimentary canal
  inhalation—*see* Foreign body, aspiration
  intestine (causing injury or obstruction) E915
  iris E914
  lacrimal apparatus E914
  larynx—*see* Foreign body, air passage
  late effect of NEC E929.8
  lung—*see* Foreign body, air passage
  mouth—*see* Foreign body, alimentary canal,
    mouth
  nasal passage—*see* Foreign body, air passage,
    nose
  nose—*see* Foreign body, air passage, nose
  ocular muscle E914
  operation wound (left in)—*see* Misadventure,
    foreign object
  orbit E914
  pharynx—*see* Foreign body, alimentary canal,
    pharynx
  rectum (causing injury or obstruction) E915
  stomach (hairball) (causing injury or
    obstruction) E915
  tear ducts or glands E914
  trachea—*see* Foreign body, air passage
  urethra (causing injury or obstruction) E915
  vagina (causing injury or obstruction) E915
Found dead, injured
  from exposure (to)—*see* Exposure
  on
    public highway E819
    railway right of way E807
Fracture (circumstances unknown or
    unspecified) E887
  due to specified external means—*see* manner
    of accident
  late effect of NEC E929.3
  occurring in water transport NEC E835
Freezing —*see* Cold, exposure to
Frostbite E901.0
  due to manmade conditions E901.1
Frozen —*see* Cold, exposure to

G

Garrotting, homicidal (attempted) E963
Gored E906.8
Gunshot wound (*see also* Shooting) E922.9

H

Hailstones, injury by E904.3
Hairball (stomach) (with obstruction) E915
Hanged himself (*see also* Hanging,
  self-inflicted) E983.0
Hang gliding E842
Hanging (accidental) E913.8
  caused by other person
    in accidental circumstances E913.8
    stated as
      intentional, homicidal E963
      undetermined whether accidental or
        intentional E983.0
  homicide (attempt) E963
  in bed or cradle E913.0
  legal execution E978

Hanging—*continued*
  self-inflicted (unspecified whether accidental
    or intentional) E983.0
    in accidental circumstances E913.8
    stated as intentional, purposeful E953.0
  stated as undetermined whether accidental or
    intentional E983.0
  suicidal (attempt) E953.0
Heat (apoplexy) (collapse) (cramps) (effects of)
    (excessive) (exhaustion) (fever) (prostration)
    (stroke) E900.9
  due to
    manmade conditions (listed in E900.1,
      except boat, ship, watercraft) E900.1
    weather (conditions) E900.0
  from
    electric heating apparatus causing burning E924.8
    nuclear explosion
      in
        terrorism E979.5
        war operations (see also War operations,
          injury due to, nuclear weapons)
          E996.2
  generated in, boiler, engine, evaporator, fire
    room of boat, ship, watercraft E838
  inappropriate in local application or packing in
    medical or surgical procedure E873.5
  late effect of NEC E989
Hemorrhage
  delayed following medical or surgical
    treatment without mention of
    misadventure—*see* Reaction, abnormal
  during medical or surgical treatment as
    misadventure—*see* Misadventure, cut
High
  altitude, effects E902.9
  level of radioactivity, effects—*see* Radiation
  pressure effects—*see also* Effects of, air
    pressure
    from rapid descent in water (causing caisson
      or divers' disease, palsy, or paralysis)
      E902.2
  temperature, effects—*see* Heat
Hit, hitting (accidental) by
  aircraft (propeller) (without accident to
    aircraft) E844
    unpowered E842
  avalanche E909.2
  being thrown against object in or part of
    motor vehicle (in motion) (on public
      highway) E818
    not on public highway E825
    nonmotor road vehicle NEC E829
    street car E829
  boat, ship, watercraft
    after fall from watercraft E838
    damaged, involved in accident E831
    while swimming, water skiing E838
  bullet (*see also* Shooting) E922.9
    from air gun E922.4
    in
      terrorism E979.4
      war operations E991.2
        rubber E991.0
  flare, Very pistol (*see also* Shooting) E922.8
  hailstones E904.3
  landslide E909.2
  law-enforcing agent (on duty) E975
    with blunt object (baton) (night stick) (stave)
      (truncheon) E973
  machine—*see* Accident, machine

Hit, hitting—*continued*
  missile
    firearm (*see also* Shooting) E922.9
    in
      terrorism—*see* Terrorism, missle
      war operations—*see* War operations,
        missile
  motor vehicle (on public highway) (traffic
      accident) E814
    not on public highway, nontraffic accident
      E822
  nonmotor road vehicle NEC E829
  object
    falling E916
      from, in, on
        aircraft E844
          due to accident to aircraft—*see*
            categories E840-E842
          unpowered E842
        boat, ship, watercraft E838
          due to accident to watercraft E831
        building E916
          burning E891.8
            in terrorism E979.3
            private E890.8
        cataclysmic
          earth surface movement or eruption
            E909.9
          storm E908.9
        cave-in E916
          with asphyxiation or suffocation (*see
            also* Suffocation, due to, cave-in)
            E913.3
        earthquake E909.0
        motor vehicle (in motion) (on public
          highway) E818
          not on public highway E825
          stationary E916
        nonmotor road vehicle NEC E829
        pedal cycle E826
        railway rolling stock, train, vehicle E806
        street car E829
        structure, burning NEC E891.8
        vehicle, stationary E916
      moving NEC—*see* Striking against, object
      projected NEC—*see* Striking against, object
      set in motion by
        compressed air or gas, spring, striking,
          throwing—*see* Striking against, object
        explosion—*see* Explosion
      thrown into, on, or towards
        motor vehicle (in motion) (on public
          highway) E818
          not on public highway E825
        nonmotor road vehicle NEC E829
        pedal cycle E826
        street car E829
  off-road type motor vehicle (not on public
      highway) E821
    on public highway E814
  other person(s) E917.9
    with blunt or thrown object E917.9
      in sports E917.0
        with subsequent fall E917.5
      intentionally, homicidal E968.2
    as, or caused by, a crowd E917.1
      with subsequent fall E917.6
    in sports E917.0
  pedal cycle E826

Hit, hitting—*continued*
  police (on duty) E975
    with blunt object (baton) (nightstick) (stave)
      (truncheon) E973
  railway, rolling stock, train, vehicle (part of)
    E805
  shot—*see* Shooting
  snow vehicle, motor-driven (not on public
    highway) E820
    on public highway E814
  street car E829
  vehicle NEC—*see* Accident, vehicle NEC
Homicide, homicidal (attempt) (justifiable) (*see
  also* Assault) E968.9
Hot
  liquid, object, substance, accident caused
    by—*see also* Accident, caused by, hot, by
    type of substance
  late effect of E929.8
  place, effects—*see* Heat
  weather, effects E900.0
Humidity, causing problem E904.3
Hunger E904.1
  resulting from
    abandonment or neglect E904.0
    transport accident—*see* categories
      E800-E848
Hurricane (any injury) E908.0
Hypobarism, hypobaropathy —*see* Effects of,
  air pressure
Hypothermia —*see* Cold, exposure to

I

Ictus
  caloris—*see* Heat
  solaris E900.0
Ignition (accidental)
  anesthetic gas in operating theatre E923.2
  bedclothes
    with
      conflagration—*see* Conflagration
      ignition (of)
        clothing—*see* Ignition, clothes
        highly inflammable material (benzine)
          (fat) (gasoline) (kerosene) (paraffin)
          (petrol) E894
  benzine E894
  clothes, clothing (from controlled fire) (in
      building) E893.9
    with conflagration—*see* Conflagration
    from
      bonfire E893.2
      highly inflammable material E894
      sources or material as listed in E893.8
      trash fire E893.2
      uncontrolled fire—*see* Conflagration
    in
      private dwelling E893.0
      specified building or structure, except
        private dwelling E893.1
      not in building or structure E893.2
  explosive material—*see* Explosion
  fat E894
  gasoline E894
  kerosene E894
  material
    explosive—*see* Explosion
    highly inflammable E894
      with conflagration—*see* Conflagration
      with explosion E923.2

Ignition—*continued*
nightdress—*see* Ignition, clothes
paraffin E894
petrol E894
Immersion —*see* Submersion
Implantation of quills of porcupine E906.8
Inanition (from) E904.9
hunger—*see* Lack of, food
resulting from homicidal intent E968.4
thirst—*see* Lack of, water
Inattention after, at birth E904.0
homicidal, infanticidal intent E968.4
Infanticide (*see also* Assault)
Ingestion
foreign body (causing injury) (with
obstruction)—*see* Foreign body, alimentary
canal
poisonous substance NEC—*see* Table of drugs
and chemicals
Inhalation
excessively cold substance, manmade E901.1
foreign body—*see* Foreign body, aspiration
liquid air, hydrogen, nitrogen E901.1
mucus, not of newborn (with asphyxia,
obstruction respiratory passage,
suffocation) E912
phlegm (with asphyxia, obstruction respiratory
passage, suffocation) E912
poisonous gas—*see* Table of drugs and chemicals
smoke from, due to
fire —*see* Fire
tobacco, second-hand E869.4
vomitus (with asphyxia, obstruction respiratory
passage, suffocation) E911
Injury, injured (accidental(ly)) NEC E928.9
by, caused by, from
air rifle (B-B gun) E922.4
animal (not being ridden) NEC E906.9
being ridden (in sport or transport) E828
assault (*see also* Assault) E968.9
avalanche E909.2
bayonet (*see also* Bayonet wound) E920.3
being thrown against some part of, or object in
motor vehicle (in motion) (on public
highway) E818
not on public highway E825
nonmotor road vehicle NEC E829
off-road motor vehicle NEC E821
railway train E806
snow vehicle, motor-driven E820
street car E829
bending
due to
repetitive movement E927.3
sudden strenuous movement E927.0
bite, human E928.3
broken glass E920.8
bullet—*see* Shooting
cave-in (*see also* Suffocation, due to,
cave-in) E913.3
without asphyxiation or suffocation E916
cloudburst E908.8
component of firearm or air gun E928.7
cutting or piercing instrument (*see also* Cut)
E920.9
cyclone E908.1
earth surface movement or eruption E909.9
earthquake E909.0
electric current (*see also* Electric shock) E925.9
explosion (*see also* Explosion) E923.9
of gun part E928.7
fire—*see* Fire

Injury, injured—*continued*
by —*continued*
flare, Very pistol E922.8
flood E908.2
foreign body—*see* Foreign body
gun recoil E928.7
hailstones E904.3
hurricane E908.0
landslide E909.2
law-enforcing agent, police, in course of
legal intervention—*see* Legal intervention
lightning E907
live rail or live wire—*see* Electric shock
machinery—*see also* Accident, machine
aircraft, without accident to aircraft E844
boat, ship, watercraft (deck) (engine room)
(galley) (laundry) (loading) E836
mechanism of firearm or air gun E928.7
missile
explosive E923.8
firearm—*see* Shooting
in
terrorism—*see* Terrorism, missile
war operations—*see* War operations,
missile
moving part of motor vehicle (in motion)
(on public highway) E818
not on public highway, nontraffic accident
E825
while alighting, boarding, entering,
leaving—*see* Fall, from, motor vehicle,
while alighting, boarding
nail E920.8
needle (sewing) E920.4
hypodermic E920.5
noise E928.1
object
fallen on
motor vehicle (in motion) (on public
highway) E818
not on public highway E825
falling—*see* Hit by, object, falling
paintball gun E922.5
radiation—*see* Radiation
railway rolling stock, train, vehicle (part of)
E805
door or window E806
recoil of firearm E928.7
rotating propeller, aircraft E844
rough landing of off-road type motor vehicle
(after leaving ground or rough terrain)
E821
snow vehicle E820
saber (*see also* Wound, saber) E920.3
shot—*see* Shooting
sound waves E928.1
splinter or sliver, wood E920.8
storm E908.9
straining
due to
repetitive movement E927.3
sudden strenuous movement E927.0
street car (door) E829
suicide (attempt) E958.9
sword E920.3
terrorism—*see* Terrorism
third rail—*see* Electric shock
thunderbolt E907
tidal wave E909.4
caused by storm E908.0

Injury, injured—*continued*
 by —*continued*
  tornado E908.1
  torrential rain E908.2
  twisting
   due to
    repetitive movement E927.3
    sudden strenuous movement E927.0
  vehicle NEC—*see* Accident, vehicle NEC
  vibration E928.2
  volcanic eruption E909.1
  weapon burst, in war operations E993.9
  weightlessness (in spacecraft, real or
    simulated) E928.0
  wood splinter or sliver E920.8
 due to
  civil insurrection—*see* War operations
   occurring after cessation of hostilities
    E998.9
  terrorism—*see* Terrorism
  war operations—*see* War operations
   occurring after cessation of hostilities
    E998.9
  weapon of mass destruction [WMD] E997.3
 homicidal (*see also* Assault) E968.9
 in, on
  civil insurrection—*see* War operations
  fight E960.0
  parachute descent (voluntary) (without
    accident to aircraft) E844
   with accident to aircraft—*see* categories
    E840-E842
  public highway E819
  railway right of way E807
  terrorism—*see* Terrorism
  war operations—*see* War operations
 inflicted (by)
  in course of arrest (attempted), suppression
    of disturbance, maintenance of order, by
    law-enforcing agents—*see* Legal
    intervention
  law-enforcing agent (on duty)—*see* Legal
    intervention
  other person
   stated as
    accidental E928.9
    homicidal, intentional—*see* Assault
    undetermined whether accidental or
      intentional—*see* Injury, stated as
      undetermined
  police (on duty)—*see* Legal intervention
 late effect of E929.9
 purposely (inflicted) by other person(s)—*see*
   Assault
 self-inflicted (unspecified whether accidental
   or intentional) E988.9
  stated as
   accidental E928.9
   intentionally, purposely E958.9
 specified cause NEC E928.8

Injury, injured—*continued*
 stated as
  undetermined whether accidentally or
    purposely inflicted (by) E988.9
  cut (any part of body) E986
  cutting or piercing instrument (classifiable
    to E920) E986
  drowning E984
  explosive(s) (missile) E985.5
  falling from high place E987.9
   manmade structure, except residential E987.1
   natural site E987.2
   residential premises E987.0
  hanging E983.0
  knife E986
  late effect of E989
  puncture (any part of body) E986
  shooting—*see* Shooting, stated as undetermined
    whether accidental or intentional
  specified means NEC E988.8
  stab (any part of body) E986
  strangulation—*see* Suffocation, stated as
    undetermined whether accidental or
    intentional
  submersion E984
  suffocation—*see* Suffocation, stated as
    undetermined whether accidental or
    intentional
 to child due to criminal abortion E968.8
Insufficient nourishment —*see also* Lack of,
  food
 homicidal intent E968.4
Insulation, effects —*see* Heat
Interruption of respiration by
 food lodged in esophagus E911
 foreign body, except food, in esophagus E912
Intervention, legal —*see* Legal intervention
Intoxication, drug or poison —*see* Table of
  drugs and chemicals
Irradiation —*see* Radiation

J

Jammed (accidentally)
 between objects (moving) (stationary and
   moving) E918
 in object E918
Jumped or fell from high place, so stated
 —*see* Jumping, from, high place, stated as
 in undetermined circumstances
Jumping
 before train, vehicle or other moving object
   (unspecified whether accidental or
   intentional) E988.0
 stated as
  intentional, purposeful E958.0
  suicidal (attempt) E958.0
 from
  aircraft
   by parachute (voluntarily) (without
     accident to aircraft) E844
   due to accident to aircraft—*see* categories
     E840-E842
  boat, ship, watercraft (into water)
   after accident to, fire on, watercraft E830
    and subsequently struck by (part of) boat
      E831
   burning, crushed, sinking E830
    and subsequently struck by (part of) boat
      E831

Jumping—*continued*
  voluntarily, without accident (to boat) with
    injury other than drowning or
    submersion E883.0
  building—*see also* Jumping, from, high
    place
    burning (uncontrolled fire) E891.8
     in terrorism E979.3
     private E890.8
  cable car (not on rails) E847
    on rails E829
  high place
    in accidental circumstances or in
     sport—*see* categories E880-E884
    stated as
     with intent to injure self E957.9
      man-made structures NEC E957.1
      natural sites E957.2
      residential premises E957.0
     in undetermined circumstances E987.9
      man-made structures NEC E987.1
      natural sites E987.2
      residential premises E987.0
     suicidal (attempt) E957.9
      man-made structures NEC E957.1
      natural sites E957.1
      residential premises E957.0
  motor vehicle (in motion) (on public
    highway)—*see* Fall, from, motor vehicle
  nonmotor road vehicle NEC E829
  street car E829
  structure—*see also* Jumping, from, high
    place
    burning NEC (uncontrolled fire) E891.8
     in terrorism E979.3
  into water
    with injury other than drowning or
     submersion E883.0
    drowning or submersion—*see* Submersion
  from, off, watercraft—*see* Jumping, from,
    boat
Justifiable homicide —*see* Assault

K

Kicked by
  animal E906.8
  person(s) (accidentally) E917.9
    with intent to injure or kill E960.0
    as, or caused by a crowd E917.1
     with subsequent fall E917.6
    in fight E960.0
    in sports E917.0
     with subsequent fall E917.5
Kicking against
  object (moving) E917.9
    in sports E917.0
     with subsequent fall E917.5
    stationary E917.4
     with subsequent fall E917.8
  person—*see* Striking against, person
Killed, killing (accidentally) NEC (*see also*
  Injury) E928.9
  in
    action—*see* War operations
    brawl, fight (hand) (fists) (foot) E960.0
     by weapon—*see also* Assault
      cutting, piercing E966
      firearm—*see* Shooting, homicide

Killed, killing—*continued*
  self
    stated as
     accident E928.9
     suicide—*see* Suicide
    unspecified whether accidental or suicidal
     E988.9
Knocked down (accidentally) (by) NEC E928.9
  animal (not being ridden) E906.8
    being ridden (in sport or transport) E828
  blast from explosion (*see also* Explosion)
    E923.9
  crowd, human stampede E917.6
  late effect of—*see* Late effect
  person (accidentally) E917.9
    in brawl, fight E960.0
    in sports E917.5
  transport vehicle—*see* vehicle involved under
    Hit by
  while boxing E917.5

L

Laceration NEC E928.9
Lack of
  air (refrigerator or closed place), suffocation
    by E913.2
  care (helpless person) (infant) (newborn)
    E904.0
    homicidal intent E968.4
  food except as result of transport accident
    E904.1
    helpless person, infant, newborn due to
     abandonment or neglect E904.0
  water except as result of transport accident
    E904.2
    helpless person, infant, newborn due to
     abandonment or neglect E904.0
Landslide E909.2
  falling on, hitting
    motor vehicle (any) (in motion) (on or off
     public highway) E909.2
    railway rolling stock, train, vehicle E909.2
Late effect of
  accident NEC (accident classifiable to E928.9)
    E929.9
    specified NEC (accident classifiable to
     E910-E928.8) E929.8
  assault E969
  fall, accidental (accident classifiable to
    E880-E888) E929.3
  fire, accident caused by (accident classifiable
    to E890-E899) E929.4
  homicide, attempt (any means) E969
  injury due to terrorism E999.1
  injury undetermined whether accidentally or
    purposely inflicted (injury classifiable to
    E980-E988) E989
  legal intervention (injury classifiable to
    E970-E976) E977
  medical or surgical procedure, test or therapy
    as, or resulting in, or from
     abnormal or delayed reaction or
      complication—*see* Reaction, abnormal
     misadventure—*see* Misadventure
  motor vehicle accident (accident classifiable to
    E810-E825) E929.0
  natural or environmental factor, accident due
    to (accident classifiable to E900-E909)
    E929.5

Late effect of—*continued*

poisoning, accidental (accident classifiable to E850-E858, E860-E869) E929.2

suicide, attempt (any means) E959

transport accident NEC (accident classifiable to E800-E807, E826-E838, E840-E848) E929.1

war operations, injury due to (injury classifiable to E990-E998) E999.0

Launching pad accident E845

Legal

execution, any method E978

intervention (by) (injury from) E976

baton E973

bayonet E974

blow E975

blunt object (baton) (nightstick) (stave) (truncheon) E973

cutting or piercing instrument E974

dynamite E971

execution, any method E973

explosive(s) (shell) E971

firearms(s) E970

gas (asphyxiation) (poisoning) (tear) E972

grenade E971

late effect of E977

machine gun E970

manhandling E975

mortar bomb E971

nightstick E973

revolver E970

rifle E970

specified means NEC E975

stabbing E974

stave E973

truncheon E973

Lifting, injury

due to

repetitive movement E927.3

sudden strenuous movement E927.0

Lightning (shock) (stroke) (struck by) E907

Liquid (noncorrosive) in eye E914

corrosive E924.1

Loss of control

motor vehicle (on public highway) (without antecedent collision) E816

with

antecedent collision on public highway —*see* Collision, motor vehicle

involving any object, person or vehicle not on public highway E816

on public highway—*see* Collision, motor vehicle

not on public highway, nontraffic accident E825

with antecedent collision—*see* Collision, motor vehicle, not on public highway

off-road type motor vehicle (not on public highway) E821

on public highway—*see* Loss of control, motor vehicle

snow vehicle, motor-driven (not on public highway) E820

on public highway—*see* Loss of control, motor vehicle

Lost at sea E832

with accident to watercraft E830

in war operations E995.8

Low

pressure, effects—*see* Effects of, air pressure

temperature, effects—*see* Cold, exposure to

Lying before train, vehicle or other moving object (unspecified whether accidental or intentional) E988.0

stated as intentional, purposeful, suicidal (attempt) E958.0

Lynching (*see also* Assault) E968.9

M

Malfunction, atomic power plant in water transport E838

Mangled (accidentally) NEC E928.9

Manhandling (in brawl, fight) E960.0

legal intervention E975

Manslaughter (nonaccidental)—*see* Assault

Marble in nose E912

Mauled by animal E906.8

Medical procedure, complication of

delayed or as an abnormal reaction without mention of misadventure—*see* Reaction, abnormal

due to or as a result of misadventure—*see* Misadventure

Melting of fittings and furniture in burning in terrorism E979.3

Minamata disease E865.2

Misadventure(s) to patient(s) during surgical or medical care E876.9

contaminated blood, fluid, drug or biological substance (presence of agents and toxins as listed in E875) E875.9

administered (by) NEC E875.9

infusion E875.0

injection E875.1

specified means NEC E875.2

transfusion E875.0

vaccination E875.1

cut, cutting, puncture, perforation or hemorrhage (accidental) (inadvertent) (inappropriate) (during) E870.9

aspiration of fluid or tissue (by puncture or catheterization, except heart) E870.5

biopsy E870.8

needle (aspirating) E870.5

blood sampling E870.5

catheterization E870.5

heart E870.6

dialysis (kidney) E870.2

endoscopic examination E870.4

enema E870.7

infusion E870.1

injection E870.3

lumbar puncture E870.5

needle biopsy E870.5

paracentesis, abdominal E870.5

perfusion E870.2

specified procedure NEC E870.8

surgical operation E870.0

thoracentesis E870.5

transfusion E870.1

vaccination E870.3

excessive amount of blood or other fluid during transfusion or infusion E873.0

failure

in dosage E873.9

electroshock therapy E873.4

inappropriate temperature (too hot or too cold) in local application and packing E873.5

Misadventure(s)—*continued*

infusion
excessive amount of fluid E873.0
incorrect dilution of fluid E873.1
insulin-shock therapy E873.4
nonadministration of necessary drug or
medicinal E873.6
overdose—*see also* Overdose
radiation, in therapy E873.2
radiation
inadvertent exposure of patient (receiving
radiation for test or therapy) E873.3
not receiving radiation for test or
therapy—*see* Radiation
overdose E873.2
specified procedure NEC 873.8
transfusion
excessive amount of blood E873.0
mechanical, of instrument or apparatus
(during procedure) E874.9
aspiration of fluid or tissue (by puncture or
catheterization, except of heart) E874.4
biopsy E874.8
needle (aspirating) E874.4
blood sampling E874.4
catheterization E874.4
heart E874.5
dialysis (kidney) E874.2
endoscopic examination E874.3
enema E874.8
infusion E874.1
injection E874.8
lumbar puncture E874.4
needle biopsy E874.4
paracentesis, abdominal E874.4
perfusion E874.2
specified procedure NEC E874.8
surgical operation E874.0
thoracentesis E874.4
transfusion E874.1
vaccination E874.8
sterile precautions (during procedure) E872.9
aspiration of fluid or tissue (by puncture or
catheterization, except heart) E872.5
biopsy E872.8
needle (aspirating) E872.5
blood sampling E872.5
catheterization E872.5
heart E872.6
dialysis (kidney) E872.2
endoscopic examination E872.4
enema E872.8
infusion E872.1
injection E872.3
lumbar puncture E872.5
needle biopsy E872.5
paracentesis, abdominal E872.5
perfusion E872.2
removal of catheter or packing E872.8
specified procedure NEC E872.8
surgical operation E872.0
thoracentesis E872.5
transfusion E872.1
vaccination E872.3
suture or ligature during surgical procedure
E876.2
to introduce or to remove tube or instrument
E876.4
foreign object left in body—*see*
Misadventure, foreign object

Misadventure(s)—*continued*

foreign object left in body (during procedure)
E871.9
aspiration of fluid or tissue (by puncture or
catheterization, except heart) E871.5
biopsy E871.8
needle (aspirating) E871.5
blood sampling E871.5
catheterization E871.5
heart E871.6
dialysis (kidney) E871.2
endoscopic examination E871.4
enema E871.8
infusion E871.1
injection E871.3
lumbar puncture E871.5
needle biopsy E871.5
paracentesis, abdominal E871.5
perfusion E871.2
removal of catheter or packing E871.7
specified procedure NEC E871.8
surgical operation E871.0
thoracentesis E871.5
transfusion E871.1
vaccination E871.3
hemorrhage—*see* Misadventure, cut
inadvertent exposure of patient to radiation
(being received for test or therapy) E873.3
inappropriate
temperature (too hot or too cold) in local
application or packing E873.5
infusion—*see also* Misadventure, by specific
type, infusion
excessive amount of fluid E873.0
incorrect dilution of fluid E873.1
wrong fluid E876.1
mismatched blood in transfusion E876.0
nonadministration of necessary drug or
medicinal E873.6
overdose—*see also* Overdose
radiation, in therapy E873.2
perforation—*see* Misadventure, cut
performance of correct operation (procedure)
on wrong
body part E876.7
side E876.7
site E876.7
performance of operation (procedure)
intended for another patient E876.6
on patient not scheduled for surgery E876.6
on wrong patient E876.6
performance of wrong operation on correct
patient E876.5
puncture—*see* Misadventure, cut
specified type NEC E876.8
failure
suture or ligature during surgical operation
E876.2
to introduce or to remove tube or
instrument E876.4
foreign object left in body E871.9
infusion of wrong fluid E876.1
transfusion of mismatched blood E876.0
wrong
fluid in infusion E876.1
placement of endotracheal tube during
anesthetic procedure E876.3
transfusion—*see also* Misadventure, by
specific type, transfusion
excessive amount of blood E873.0
mismatched blood E876.0

Misadventure(s)—*continued*
wrong
  device implanted into correct surgical site
    E876.5
  procedure (operation) performed on the
    correct patient E876.5
  drug given in error—*see* Table of drugs and
    chemicals
  fluid in infusion E876.1
  placement of endotracheal tube during
    anesthetic procedure E876.3
Motion (effects) E903
  sickness E903
Mountain sickness E902.0
**Mucus aspiration or inhalation, not of
  newborn** (with asphyxia, obstruction
  respiratory passage, suffocation) E912
Mudslide of cataclysmic nature E909.2
Murder (attempt) (*see also* Assault) E968.9

N

Nail, injury by E920.8
Needlestick (sewing needle) E920.4
  hypodermic E920.5
Neglect —*see also* Privation
  criminal E968.4
  homicidal intent E968.4
Noise (causing injury) (pollution) E928.1
Nuclear weapon (see also War operations,
  injury due to, nuclear weapons) E996.9

O

Object
falling
  from, in, on, hitting
    aircraft E844
      due to accident to aircraft—*see*
        categories E840-E842
    machinery—*see also* Accident, machine
      not in operation E916
    motor vehicle (in motion) (on public
      highway) E818
      not on public highway E825
      stationary E916
    nonmotor road vehicle NEC E829
    pedal cycle E826
    person E916
    railway rolling stock, train, vehicle E806
    street car E829
    watercraft E838
      due to accident to watercraft E831
set in motion by
  accidental explosion of pressure vessel—*see*
    category E921
  firearm—*see* category E922
  machine(ry)—*see* Accident, machine
  transport vehicle—*see* categories E800-E848
thrown from, in, on, towards
  aircraft E844
  cable car (not on rails) E847
    on rails E829
  motor vehicle (in motion) (on public
    highway) E818
    not on public highway E825
  nonmotor road vehicle NEC E829
  pedal cycle E826
  street car E829
  vehicle NEC—*see* Accident, vehicle NEC

Obstruction
air passages, larynx, respiratory passages
  by
    external means NEC—*see* Suffocation
    food, any type (regurgitated) (vomited)
      E911
    material or object, except food E912
    mucus E912
    phlegm E912
    vomitus E911
digestive tract, except mouth or pharynx
  by
    food, any type E915
    foreign body (any) E915
esophagus
  food E911
  foreign body, except food E912
  without asphyxia or obstruction of
    respiratory passage E915
mouth or pharynx
  by
    food, any type E911
    material or object, except food E912
respiration—*see* Obstruction, air passages
Oil in eye E914
Overdose
anesthetic (drug)—*see* Table of drugs and
  chemicals
drug—*see* Table of drugs and chemicals
Overexertion E927.9
from
  lifting
    repetitive movement E927.3
    sudden strenuous movement E927.0
  maintaining prolonged positions E927.1
    holding E927.1
    sitting E927.1
    standing E927.1
  prolonged static position E927.1
  pulling
    repetitive movement E927.3
    sudden strenuous movement E927.0
  pushing
    repetitive movement E927.3
    sudden strenuous movement E927.0
  specified NEC E927.8
  sudden strenuous movement E927.0
Overexposure (accidental) (to)
cold (*see also* Cold, exposure to) E901.9
  due to manmade conditions E901.1
heat (*see also* Heat) E900.9
radiation—*see* Radiation
radioactivity—*see* Radiation
sun, except sunburn E900.0
weather—*see* Exposure
wind—*see* Exposure
Overheated (*see also* Heat) E900.9
Overlaid E913.0
Overturning (accidental)
animal-drawn vehicle E827
boat, ship, watercraft
  causing
    drowning, submersion E830
    injury except drowning, submersion E831
machinery—*see* Accident, machine
motor vehicle (*see also* Loss of control, motor
  vehicle) E816
  with antecedent collision on public
    highway—*see* Collision, motor vehicle
  not on public highway, nontraffic accident
    E825

Overturning—*continued*
  with antecedent collision—*see* Collision,
    motor vehicle, not on public highway
  nonmotor road vehicle NEC E829
  off-road type motor vehicle—*see* Loss of
    control, off-road type motor vehicle
  pedal cycle E826
  railway rolling stock, train, vehicle (*see also*
    Derailment, railway) E802
  street car E829
  vehicle NEC—*see* Accident, vehicle NEC

P

Palsy, divers' E902.2
Parachuting (voluntary) (without accident to
  aircraft) E844
  due to accident to aircraft—*see* categories
    E840-E842
Paralysis
  divers' E902.2
  lead or saturnine E866.0
  from pesticide NEC E863.4
Pecked by bird E906.8
Performance of correct operation (procedure)
  on wrong
  body part E876.7
  side E876.7
  site E876.7
Performance of operation (procedure)
  intended for another patient E876.6
  on patient not scheduled for surgery E876.6
  on wrong patient E876.6
Performance of wrong operation on correct
  patient E876.5
Phlegm aspiration or inhalation (with
  asphyxia, obstruction respiratory passage,
  suffocation) E912
Piercing (*see also* Cut) E920.9
  by slide trigger mechanism, scope or other
    part of gun E928.7
Pinched
  between objects (moving) (stationary and
    moving) E918
  by slide trigger mechanism, scope or other
    part of gun E928.7
  in object E918
Pinned under
  machine(ry)—*see* Accident, machine
Place of occurrence of accident —*see*
  Accident (to), occurring (at) (in)
Plumbism E866.0
  from insecticide NEC E863.4
Poisoning (accidental) (by)—*see also* Table of
  drugs and chemicals
  carbon monoxide
    generated by
      aircraft in transit E844
      motor vehicle
        in motion (on public highway) E818
        not on public highway E825
      watercraft (in transit) (not in transit) E838
  caused by injection of poisons or toxins into
    or through skin by plant thorns, spines, or
    other mechanism E905.7
    marine or sea plants E905.6
  fumes or smoke due to
    conflagration—*see* Conflagration
    explosion or fire—*see* Fire
    ignition—*see* Ignition

Poisoning—*continued*
  gas
    in legal intervention E972
    legal execution, by E978
    on watercraft E838
    used as anesthetic—*see* Table of drugs and
      chemicals
  in
    terrorism (chemical weapons) E979.7
    war operations E997.2
  late effect of—*see* Late effect
  legal
    execution E978
    intervention
      by gas E972
Pressure, external, causing asphyxia,
  suffocation (*see also* Suffocation) E913.9
Privation E904.9
  food (*see also* Lack of, food) E904.1
  helpless person, infant, newborn due to
    abandonment or neglect E904.0
  late effect of NEC E929.5
  resulting from transport accident—*see*
    categories E800-E848
  water (*see also* Lack of, water) E904.2
Projected objects, striking against or struck
  by —*see* Striking against, object
Prolonged stay in
  high altitude (causing conditions as listed in
    E902.0) E902.0
  weightless environment E928.0
Prostration
  heat—*see* Heat
Pulling, injury
  due to
    repetitive movement E927.3
    sudden strenuous movement E927.0
Puncture, puncturing (*see also* Cut) E920.9
  by
    plant thorns or spines E920.8
      toxic reaction E905.7
        marine or sea plants E905.6
    sea-urchin spine E905.6
Pushing (injury in) (overexertion) E927.8
  by other person(s) (accidental) E917.9
    as, or caused by, a crowd, human stampede
      E917.1
      with subsequent fall E917.6
    before moving vehicle or object
      stated as
        intentional, homicidal E968.5
        undetermined whether accidental or
          intentional E988.8
    from
      high place
        in accidental circumstances—*see*
          categories E880-E884
        stated as
          intentional, homicidal E968.1
          undetermined whether accidental or
            intentional E987.9
          man-made structure, except
            residential E987.1
          natural site E987.2
          residential E987.0
      motor vehicle (*see also* Fall, from, motor
        vehicle) E818
        stated as
          intentional, homicidal E968.5
          undetermined whether accidental or
            intentional E988.8

Pushing—*continued*
  by other person—*continued*
    in sports E917.0
      with fall E886.0
    with fall E886.9
      in sports E886.0
  due to
    repetitive movement E927.3
    sudden strenuous movement E927.0

R

Radiation (exposure to) E926.9
  abnormal reaction to medical test or therapy
    E879.2
  arc lamps E926.2
  atomic power plant (malfunction) NEC E926.9
    in water transport E838
  electromagnetic, ionizing E926.3
  gamma rays E926.3
  in
    terrorism (from or following nuclear
      explosion) (direct) (secondary) E979.5
      laser E979.8
    war operations (see also War operations,
      injury due to, nuclear weapons) E996.3
      laser(s) E997.0
    water transport E838
  inadvertent exposure of patient (receiving test
    or therapy) E873.3
  infrared (heaters and lamps) E926.1
    excessive heat E900.1
  ionized, ionizing (particles, artificially
    accelerated) E926.8
    electromagnetic E926.3
  isotopes, radioactive—*see* Radiation,
    radioactive isotopes
  laser(s) E926.4
    in
      terrorism E979.8
      war operations E997.0
  misadventure in medical care—*see*
    Misadventure, failure, in dosage,
    radiation
  late effect of NEC E929.8
    excessive heat from—*see* Heat
  light sources (visible) (ultraviolet) E926.2
  misadventure in medical or surgical
    procedure—*see* Misadventure, failure, in
    dosage, radiation
  overdose (in medical or surgical procedure)
    E873.2
  radar E926.0
  radioactive isotopes E926.5
    atomic power plant malfunction E926.5
      in water transport E838
    misadventure in medical or surgical
      treatment—*see* Misadventure, failure, in
      dosage, radiation
  radiobiologicals—*see* Radiation, radioactive
    isotopes
  radiofrequency E926.0
  radiopharmaceuticals—*see* Radiation,
    radioactive isotopes
  radium NEC E926.9
  sun E926.2
    excessive heat from E900.0
  tanning bed E926.2
  welding arc or torch E926.2
    excessive heat from E900.1

Radiation—*continued*
  x-rays (hard) (soft) E926.3
    misadventure in medical or surgical
      treatment—*see* Misadventure, failure, in
      dosage, radiation
Rape E960.1
Reaction —abnormal to or following(medical or
    surgical procedure) E879.9
  amputation (of limbs) E878.5
  anastomosis (arteriovenous) (blood vessel)
    (gastrojejunal) (skin) (tendon) (natural,
    artificial material, tissue) E878.2
    external stoma, creation of E878.3
  aspiration (of fluid) E879.4
    tissue E879.8
  biopsy E879.8
  blood
    sampling E879.7
    transfusion
      procedure E879.8
  bypass—*see* Reaction, abnormal, anastomosis
  catheterization
    cardiac E879.0
    urinary E879.6
  colostomy E878.3
  cystostomy E878.3
  dialysis (kidney) E879.1
  drugs or biologicals—*see* Table of drugs and
    chemicals
  duodenostomy E878.3
  electroshock therapy E879.3
  formation of external stoma E878.3
  gastrostomy E878.3
  graft—*see* Reaction, abnormal, anastomosis
  hypothermia E879.8
  implant, implantation (of)
    artificial
      internal device (cardiac pacemaker)
        (electrodes in brain) (heart valve
        prosthesis) (orthopedic) E878.1
      material or tissue (for anastomosis or
        bypass) E878.2
        with creation of external stoma E878.3
      natural tissues (for anastomosis or bypass)
        E878.2
        as transplantion—*see* Reaction, abnormal,
          transplant
        with creation of external stoma E878.3
  infusion
    procedure E879.8
  injection
    procedure E879.8
  insertion of gastric or duodenal sound E879.5
  insulin-shock therapy E879.3
  lumbar puncture E879.4
  perfusion E879.1
  procedures other than surgical operation (*see
    also* Reaction, abnormal, by specific type
    of procedure) E879.9
  specified procedure NEC E879.8
  radiological procedure or therapy E879.2
  removal of organ (partial) (total) NEC E878.6
    with
      anastomosis, bypass or graft E878.2
      formation of external stoma E878.3
      implant of artificial internal device E878.1
  transplant(ation)
    partial organ E878.4
    whole organ E878.0

Reaction—*continued*
sampling
  blood E879.7
  fluid NEC E879.4
  tissue E879.8
shock therapy E879.3
surgical operation (*see also* Reaction,
  abnormal, by specified type of operation)
  E878.9
  restorative NEC E878.4
  with
    anastomosis, bypass or graft E878.2
    formation of external stoma E878.3
    implant(ation)—*see* Reaction, abnormal,
     implant
    transplant(ation)—*see* Reaction,
     abnormal, transplant
  specified operation NEC E878.8
thoracentesis E879.4
transfusion
  procedure E879.8
transplant, transplantation (heart) (kidney)
  (liver) E878.0
  partial organ E878.4
ureterostomy E878.3
vaccination E879.8
Reduction in
atmospheric pressure—*see also* Effects of, air
  pressure
while surfacing from
  deep water diving causing caisson or
   divers' disease, palsy or paralysis
   E902.2
  underground E902.8
Repetitive movements NEC E927.8
Residual (effect)—*see* Late effect
Rock falling on or hitting (accidentally)
motor vehicle (in motion) (on public highway)
  E818
  not on public highway E825
nonmotor road vehicle NEC E829
pedal cycle E826
person E916
railway rolling stock, train, vehicle E806
Running off, away
animal (being ridden) (in sport or transport)
  E828
  not being ridden E906.8
animal-drawn vehicle E827
rails, railway (*see also* Derailment) E802
roadway
  motor vehicle (without antecedent collision)
   E816
   nontraffic accident E825
    with antecedent collision—*see* Collision,
     motor vehicle, not on public highway
   with
    antecedent collision—*see* Collision motor
     vehicle
    subsequent collision
     involving any object, person or vehicle
      not on public highway E816
      on public highway E811
  nonmotor road vehicle NEC E829
  pedal cycle E826
Run over (accidentally) (by)
animal (not being ridden) E906.8
  being ridden (in sport or transport) E828
animal-drawn vehicle E827
machinery—*see* Accident, machine

Run over—*continued*
motor vehicle (on public highway)—*see* Hit
  by, motor vehicle
nonmotor road vehicle NEC E829
railway train E805
street car E829
vehicle NEC E848

S

Saturnism E866.0
from insecticide NEC E863.4
Scald, scalding (accidental) (by) (from) (in)
  E924.0
acid—*see* Scald, caustic
boiling tap water E924.2
caustic or corrosive liquid, substance E924.1
  swallowed—*see* Table of drugs and
   chemicals
homicide (attempt)—*see* Assault, burning
inflicted by other person
  stated as
   intentional or homicidal E968.3
   undetermined whether accidental or
    intentional E988.2
late effect of NEC E929.8
liquid (boiling) (hot) E924.0
local application of externally applied
  substance in medical or surgical care
  E873.5
molten metal E924.0
self-inflicted (unspecified whether accidental
  or intentional) E988.2
  stated as intentional, purposeful E958.2
stated as undetermined whether accidental or
  intentional E988.2
steam E924.0
tap water (boiling) E924.2
transport accident—*see* categories E800-E848
vapor E924.0
Scratch, cat E906.8
Sea
sickness E903
Self-mutilation —*see* Suicide
Sequelai (of)
in
  terrorism E999.1
  war operations E999.0
Shock
anaphylactic (*see also* Table of drugs and
  chemicals) E947.9
  due to
   bite (venomous)—*see* Bite, venomous NEC
   sting—*see* Sting
electric (*see also* Electric shock) E925.9
from electric appliance or current (*see also*
  Electric shock) E925.9
Shooting, shot (accidental(ly)) E922.9
air gun E922.4
BB gun E922.4
hand gun (pistol) (revolver) E922.0
himself (*see also* Shooting, self-inflicted)
  E985.4
  hand gun (pistol) (revolver) E985.0
  military firearm, except hand gun E985.3
   hand gun (pistol) (revolver) E985.0
  rifle (hunting) E985.2
   military E985.3
  shotgun (automatic) E985.1
  specified firearm NEC E985.4
  Verey pistol E985.4

Shooting, shot—*continued*
 homicide (attempt) E965.4
  air gun E968.6
  BB gun E968.6
  hand gun (pistol) (revolver) E965.0
  military firearm, except hand gun E965.3
   hand gun (pistol) (revolver) E965.0
  paintball gun E965.4
  rifle (hunting) E965.2
   military E965.3
  shotgun (automatic) E965.1
  specified firearm NEC E965.4
  Verey pistol E965.4
 inflicted by other person
  in accidental circumstances E922.9
   hand gun (pistol) (revolver) E922.0
   military firearm, except hand gun E922.3
    hand gun (pistol) (revolver) E922.0
   rifle (hunting) E922.2
    military E922.3
   shotgun (automatic) E922.1
   specified firearm NEC E922.8
   Verey pistol E922.8
  stated as
   intentional, homicidal E965.4
    hand gun (pistol) (revolver) E965.0
    military firearm, except hand gun E965.3
     hand gun (pistol) (revolver) E965.0
    paintball gun E965.4
    rifle (hunting) E965.2
     military E965.3
    shotgun (automatic) E965.1
    specified firearm E965.4
    Verey pistol E965.4
   undetermined whether accidental or
     intentional E985.4
    air gun E985.6
    BB gun E985.6
    hand gun (pistol) (revolver) E985.0
    military firearm, except hand gun E985.3
     hand gun (pistol) (revolver) E985.0
    paintball gun E985.7
    rifle (hunting) E985.2
    shotgun (automatic) E985.1
    specified firearm NEC E985.4
    Verey pistol E985.4
 in
  terrorism—*see* Terrorism, shooting
  war operations—*see* War operations,
    shooting
 legal
  execution E978
  intervention E970
 military firearm, except hand gun E922.3
  hand gun (pistol) (revolver) E922.0
 paintball gun E922.5
 rifle (hunting) 922.2
  military E922.3
 self-inflicted (unspecified whether accidental
   or intentional) E985.4
  air gun E985.6
  BB gun E985.6
  hand gun (pistol) (revolver) E985.0
  military firearm, except hand gun E985.3
   hand gun (pistol) (revolver) E985.0
  paintball gun E985.7
  rifle (hunting) E985.2
   military E985.3
  shotgun (automatic) E985.1
  specified firearm NEC E985.4

Shooting, shot—*continued*
 stated as
  accidental E922.9
   hand gun (pistol) (revolver) E922.0
   military firearm, except hand gun E922.3
    hand gun (pistol) (revolver) E922.0
   paintball gun E922.5
   rifle (hunting) E922.2
    military E922.3
   shotgun (automatic) E922.1
   specified firearm NEC E922.8
   Verey pistol E922.8
  intentional, purposeful E955.4
   hand gun (pistol) (revolver) E955.0
   military firearm, except hand gun E955.3
    hand gun (pistol) (revolver) E955.0
   paintball gun E955.7
   rifle (hunting) E955.2
    military E955.3
   shotgun (automatic) E955.1
   specified firearm NEC E955.4
   Verey pistol E955.4
 shotgun (automatic) E922.1
 specified firearm NEC E922.8
 stated as undetermined whether accidental or
   intentional E985.4
  hand gun (pistol) (revolver) E985.0
  military firearm, except hand gun E985.3
   hand gun (pistol) (revolver) E985.0
  paintball gun E985.7
  rifle (hunting) E985.2
   military E985.3
  shotgun (automatic) E985.1
  specified firearm NEC E985.4
  Verey pistol E985.4
 suicidal (attempt) E955.4
  air gun E955.6
  BB gun E955.6
  hand gun (pistol) (revolver) E955.0
  military firearm, except hand gun E955.3
   hand gun (pistol) (revolver) E955.0
  paintball gun E955.7
  rifle (hunting) E955.2
   military E955.3
  shotgun (automatic) E955.1
  specified firearm NEC E955.4
  Verey pistol E955.4
 Verey pistol E922.8
Shoving (accidentally) by other person (*see also*
  Pushing by other person) E917.9
Sickness
 air E903
 alpine E902.0
 car E903
 motion E903
 mountain E902.0
 sea E903
 travel E903
Sinking (accidental)
 boat, ship, watercraft (causing drowning,
   submersion) E830
 causing injury except drowning, submersion
   E831
Siriasis E900.0
Skydiving E844
Slashed wrists (*see also* Cut, self-inflicted) E986
Slipping (accidental)
 on
  deck (of boat, ship, watercraft) (icy) (oily)
    (wet) E835
  ice E885.9

Slipping (on)—*continued*
  ladder of ship E833
    due to accident to watercraft E831
  mud E885.9
  oil E885.9
  snow E885.9
  stairs of ship E833
    due to accident to watercraft E831
  surface
    slippery E885.9
    wet E885.9
Sliver, wood, injury by E920.8
Smothering, smothered (*see also* Suffocation)
  E913.9
Smouldering building or structure in
  terrorism E979.3
Sodomy (assault) E960.1
Solid substance in eye (any part) or adnexa E914
Sound waves (causing injury) E928.1
Splinter, injury by E920.8
Stab, stabbing E966
  accidental—*see* Cut
Starvation E904.1
  helpless person, infant, newborn—*see* Lack of
    food
  homicidal intent E968.4
  late effect of NEC E929.5
  resulting from accident connected with
    transport—*see* categories E800-E848
Stepped on
  by
    animal (not being ridden) E906.8
      being ridden (in sport or transport) E828
    crowd E917.1
    person E917.9
      in sports E917.0
  in sports E917.0
Stepping on
  object (moving) E917.9
    in sports E917.0
      with subsequent fall E917.5
    stationary E917.4
      with subsequent fall E917.8
  person E917.9
    as, or caused by a crowd E917.1
      with subsequent fall E917.6
    in sports E917.0
Sting E905.9
  ant E905.5
  bee E905.3
  caterpillar E905.5
  coral E905.6
  hornet E905.3
  insect NEC E905.5
  jelly fish E905.6
  marine animal or plant E905.6
  nematocysts E905.6
  scorpion E905.2
  sea anemone E905.6
  sea cucumber E905.6
  wasp E905.3
  yellow jacket E905.3
Storm E908.9
  specified type NEC E908.8
Straining, injury
  due to
    repetitive movement E927.3
    sudden strenuous movement E927.0
Strangling —*see* Suffocation
Strangulation —*see* Suffocation
Strenuous movements (in recreational or other
  activities) NEC E927.8

Striking against
  bottom (when jumping or diving into water)
    E883.0
  object (moving) E917.9
    caused by crowd E917.1
      with subsequent fall E917.6
    furniture E917.3
      with subsequent fall E917.7
    in
      running water E917.2
        with drowning or submersion—*see*
          Submersion
      sports E917.0
        with subsequent fall E917.5
    stationary E917.4
      with subsequent fall E917.8
  person(s) E917.9
    with fall E886.9
      in sports E886.0
    as, or caused by, a crowd E917.1
      with subsequent fall E917.6
    in sports E917.0
      with fall E886.0
Stroke
  heat—*see* Heat
  lightning E907
Struck by —*see also* Hit by
  bullet
    in
      terrorism E979.4
      war operation E991.2
        rubber E991.0
  lightning E907
  missile
    in terrorism—*see* Terrorism, missile
  object
    falling
      from, in, on
        building
          burning (uncontrolled fire)
            in terrorism E979.3
  thunderbolt E907
Stumbling over animal, carpet, curb, rug or
  (small) object (with fall) E885.9
  without fall—*see* Striking against, object
Submersion (accidental) E910.8
  boat, ship, watercraft (causing drowning,
    submersion) E830
    causing injury except drowning, submersion
      E831
  by other person
    in accidental circumstances—*see* category
      E910
    intentional, homicidal E964
    stated as undetermined whether accidental or
      intentional E984
  due to
    accident
      machinery—*see* Accident, machine
      to boat, ship, watercraft E830
      transport—*see* categories E800-E848
    avalanche E909.2
    cataclysmic
      earth surface movement or eruption E909.9
      storm E908.9
    cloudburst E908.8
    cyclone E908.1

Submersion—*continued*
  fall
    from
      boat, ship, watercraft (not involved in
          accident) E832
        burning, crushed E830
        involved in accident, collision E830
      gangplank (into water) E832
      overboard NEC E832
    flood E908.2
    hurricane E908.0
    jumping into water E910.8
      from boat, ship, watercraft
        burning, crushed, sinking E830
        involved in accident, collision E830
        not involved in accident, for swim
            E910.2
      in recreational activity (without diving
          equipment) E910.2
        with or using diving equipment E910.1
      to rescue another person E910.3
  homicide (attempt) E964
  in
    bathtub E910.4
    specified activity, not sport, transport or
        recreational E910.3
    sport or recreational activity (without diving
        equipment) E910.2
      with or using diving equipment E910.1
      water skiing E910.0
    swimming pool NEC E910.8
    terrorism E979.8
    war operations E995.4
      intentional E995.3
    water transport E832
      due to accident to boat, ship, watercraft
          E830
  landslide E909.2
    overturning boat, ship, watercraft E909.2
    sinking boat, ship, watercraft E909.2
    submersion boat, ship, watercraft E909.2
    tidal wave E909.4
      caused by storm E908.0
    torrential rain E908.2
  late effect of NEC E929.8
  quenching tank E910.8
  self-inflicted (unspecified whether accidental
      or intentional) E984
    in accidental circumstances—*see* category
        E910
    stated as intentional, purposeful E954
  stated as undetermined whether accidental or
      intentional E984
  suicidal (attempted) E954
  while
    attempting rescue of another person E910.3
    engaged in
      marine salvage E910.3
      underwater construction or repairs E910.3
    fishing, not from boat E910.2
    hunting, not from boat E910.2
    ice skating E910.2
    pearl diving E910.3
    placing fishing nets E910.3
    playing in water E910.2
    scuba diving E910.1
      nonrecreational E910.3
    skin diving E910.1
    snorkel diving E910.2
    spear fishing underwater E910.1
    surfboarding E910.2

Submersion—*continued*
  swimming (swimming pool) E910.2
  wading (in water) E910.2
  water skiing E910.0
Sucked
  into
    jet (aircraft) E844
Suffocation (accidental) (by external means) (by
    pressure) (mechanical) E913.9
  caused by other person
    in accidental circumstances—*see* category
        E913
    stated as
      intentional, homicidal E963
      undetermined whether accidental or
          intentional E983.9
        by, in
          hanging E983.0
          plastic bag E983.1
          specified means NEC E983.3
  due to, by
    avalanche E909.2
    bedclothes E913.0
    bib E913.0
    blanket E913.0
    cave-in E913.3
      caused by cataclysmic earth surface
          movement or eruption E909.9
    conflagration—*see* Conflagration
    explosion—*see* Explosion
    falling earth, other substance E913.3
    fire—*see* Fire
    food, any type (ingestion) (inhalation)
        (regurgitated) (vomited) E911
    foreign body, except food (ingestion)
        (inhalation) E912
    ignition—*see* Ignition
    landslide E909.2
    machine(ry)—*see* Accident, machine
    material, object except food entering by nose
        or mouth, ingested, inhaled E912
    mucus (aspiration) (inhalation), not of
        newborn E912
    phlegm (aspiration) (inhalation) E912
    pillow E913.0
    plastic bag—*see* Suffocation, in, plastic bag
    sheet (plastic) E913.0
    specified means NEC E913.8
    vomitus (aspiration) (inhalation) E911
  homicidal (attempt) E963
    in war operations E995.3
  in
    airtight enclosed place E913.2
    baby carriage E913.0
    bed E913.0
    closed place E913.2
    cot, cradle E913.0
    perambulator E913.0
    plastic bag (in accidental circumstances)
        E913.1
      homicidal, purposely inflicted by other
          person E963
      self-inflicted (unspecified whether
          accidental or intentional) E983.1
        in accidental circumstances E913.1
        intentional, suicidal E953.1
      stated as undetermined whether
          accidentally or purposely inflicted
          E983.1
      suicidal, purposely self-inflicted E953.1
    refrigerator E913.2
    war operations E995.3

Suffocation—*continued*
self-inflicted—*see also* Suffocation, stated as
undetermined whether accidental or
intentional E953.9
in accidental circumstances—*see* category E913
stated as intentional, purposeful—*see*
Suicide, suffocation
stated as undetermined whether accidental or
intentional E983.9
by, in
hanging E983.0
plastic bag E983.1
specified means NEC E983.8
suicidal—*see* Suicide, suffocation
Suicide, suicidal (attempted) (by) E958.9
burning, burns E958.1
caustic substance E958.7
poisoning E950.7
swallowed E950.7
cold, extreme E958.3
cut (any part of body) E956
cutting or piercing instrument (classifiable to
E920) E956
drowning E954
electrocution E958.4
explosive(s) (classifiable to E923) E955.5
fire E958.1
firearm (classifiable to E922)—*see* Shooting,
suicidal
hanging E953.0
jumping
before moving object, train, vehicle E958.0
from high place—*see* Jumping, from, high
place, stated as, suicidal
knife E956
late effect of E959
motor vehicle, crashing of E958.5
poisoning—*see* Table of drugs and chemicals
puncture (any part of body) E956
scald E958.2
shooting—*see* Shooting, suicidal
specified means NEC E958.8
stab (any part of body) E956
strangulation—*see* Suicide, suffocation
submersion E954
suffocation E953.9
by, in
hanging E953.0
plastic bag E953.1
specified means NEC E953.8
wound NEC E958.9
Sunburn E926.2
Sunstroke E900.0
Supersonic waves (causing injury) E928.1
Surgical procedure, complication of
delayed or as an abnormal reaction without
mention of misadventure—*see* Reaction,
abnormal
due to or as a result of misadventure—*see*
Misadventure
Swallowed, swallowing
foreign body—*see* Foreign body, alimentary
canal
poison—*see* Table of drugs and chemicals
substance
caustic—*see* Table of drugs and chemicals
corrosive—*see* Table of drugs and chemicals
poisonous—*see* Table of drugs and
chemicals
Swimmers cramp (*see also* category E910)
E910.2
not in recreation or sport E910.3

Syndrome, battered
baby or child—*see* Abuse, child
wife—*see* Assault

T

Tackle in sport E886.0
Terrorism (injury) (by) (in) E979.8
air blast E979.2
aircraft burned, destroyed, exploded, shot
down E979.1
used as a weapon E979.1
anthrax E979.6
asphyxia from
chemical (weapons) E979.7
fire, conflagration (caused by fire-producing
device) E979.3
from nuclear explosion E979.5
gas or fumes E979.7
bayonet E979.8
biological agents E979.6
blast (air) (effects) E979.2
from nuclear explosion E979.5
underwater E979.0
Terrorism—*continued*
bomb (antipersonnel) (mortor) (explosion)
(fragments) E979.2
bullet(s) (from carbine, machine gun, pistol,
rifle, shotgun) E979.4
burn from
chemical E979.7
fire, conflagration (caused by fire-producing
device) E979.3
from nuclear explosion E979.5
gas E979.7
burning aircraft E979.1
chemical E979.7
cholera E979.6
conflagration E979.3
crushed by falling aircraft E979.1
depth charge E979.0
destruction of aircraft E979.1
disability, as seqelae one year or more after
injury E999.1
drowning E979.8
effect
of nuclear weapon (direct) (secondary)
E979.5
secondary NEC E979.9
sequelae E999.1
explosion (artillery shell) (breech-block)
(cannon block) E979.2
aircraft E979.1
bomb (antipersonnel) (mortor) E979.2
nuclear (atom) (hydrogen) E979.5
depth-charge E979.0
grenade E979.2
injury by fragments from E979.2
land-mine E979.2
marine weapon E979.0
mine (land) E979.2
at sea or in harbor E979.0
marine E979.0
missile (explosive) NEC E979.2
munitions (dump) (factory) E979.2
nuclear (weapon) E979.5
other direct and secondary effects of
E979.5
sea-based artillery shell E979.0
torpedo E979.0

Terrorism—*continued*
exposure to ionizing radiation from nuclear
explosion E979.5
falling aircraft E979.1
fire or fire-producing device E979.3
firearms E979.4
fireball effects from nuclear explosion E979.5
fragments from artillery shell, bomb NEC,
grenade, guided missile, land-mine, rocket,
shell, shrapnel E979.2
gas or fumes E979.7
grenade (explosion) (fragments) E979.2
guided missile (explosion) (fragments) E979.2
nuclear E979.5
heat from nuclear explosion E979.5
hot substances E979.3
hydrogen cyanide E979.7
land-mine (explosion) (fragments) E979.2
laser(s) E979.8
late effect of E999.1
lewisite E979.7
lung irritant (chemical) (fumes) (gas) E979.7
marine mine E979.0
mine E979.2
at sea E979.0
in harbor E979.0
land (explosion) (fragments) E979.2
marine E979.0
missile (explosion) (fragments) (guided)
E979.2
marine E979.0
nuclear E979.5
mortar bomb (explosion) (fragments) E979.2
mustard gas E979.7
nerve gas E979.7
nuclear weapons E979.5
pellets (shotgun) E979.4
petrol bomb E979.3
piercing object E979.8
phosgene E979.7
poisoning (chemical) (fumes) (gas) E979.7
radiation, ionizing from nuclear explosion
E979.5
rocket (explosion) (fragments) E979.2
saber, sabre E979.8
sarin E979.7
screening smoke E979.7
sequelae effect (of) E999.1
shell (aircraft) (artillery) (cannon) (land-based)
(explosion) (fragments) E979.2
sea-based E979.0
shooting E979.4
bullet(s) E979.4
pellet(s) (rifle) (shotgun) E979.4
shrapnel E979.2
smallpox E979.7
stabbing object(s) E979.8
submersion E979.8
torpedo E979.0
underwater blast E979.0
vesicant (chemical) (fumes) (gas) E979.7
weapon burst E979.2
Thermic fever E900.9
Thermoplegia E900.9
Thirst —*see also* Lack of water
resulting from accident connected with
transport—*see* categories E800-E848

Thrown (accidently)
against object in or part of vehicle
by motion of vehicle
aircraft E844
boat, ship, watercraft E838
motor vehicle (on public highway) E818
not on public highway E825
off-road type (not on public highway)
E821
on public highway E818
snow vehicle E820
on public highway E818
nonmotor road vehicle NEC E829
railway rolling stock, train, vehicle E806
street car E829
from
animal (being ridden) (in sport or transport)
E828
high place, homicide (attempt) E968.1
machinery—*see* Accident, machine
vehicle NEC—*see* Accident, vehicle NEC
off—*see* Thrown, from
overboard (by motion of boat, ship, watercraft)
E832
by accident to boat, ship, watercraft E830
Thunderbolt NEC E907
Tidal wave (any injury) E909.4
caused by storm E908.0
Took
overdose of drug—*see* Table of drugs and
chemicals
poison—*see* Table of drugs and chemicals
Tornado (any injury) E908.1
Torrential rain (any injury) E908.2
Traffic accident NEC E819
Trampled by animal E906.8
being ridden (in sport or transport) E828
Trapped (accidentally)
between
objects (moving) (stationary and moving)
E918
by
door of
elevator E918
motor vehicle (on public highway) (while
alighting, boarding)—*see* Fall, from,
motor vehicle, while alighting
railway train (underground) E806
street car E829
subway train E806
in object E918
Trauma
cumulative
from
repetitive
impact E927.4
motion or movements E927.3
sudden from strenuous movements E927.0
Travel (effects) E903
sickness E903
Tree
falling on or hitting E916
motor vehicle (in motion) (on public
highway) E818
not on public highway E825
nonmotor road vehicle NEC E829
pedal cycle E826
person E916
railway rolling stock, train, vehicle E806
street car E829
Trench foot E901.0

Tripping over animal, carpet, curb, rug, or
small object (with fall) E885.9
without fall—*see* Striking against, object
Tsunami E909.4
Twisting, injury
due to
repetitive movement E927.3
sudden strenuous movement E927.0

V

Violence, nonaccidental (*see also* Assault)
E968.9
Volcanic eruption (any injury) E909.1
Vomitus in air passages (with asphyxia,
obstruction or suffocation) E911

W

War operations (during hostilities) (injury) (by)
(in) E995.9
after cessation of hostilities, injury due to
E998.9
air blast E993.9
aircraft burned, destroyed, exploded, shot
down E994
asphyxia from
chemical E997.2
fire, conflagration (caused by fire-producing
device or conventional weapon) E990.9
from nuclear explosion (see also War
operations, injury due to, nuclear
weapons) E996.8
incendiary bomb E990.0
petrol bomb E990.0
fumes E997.2
gas E997.2
baton (nightstick) E995.1
battle wound NEC E995.8
bayonet E995.2
biological warfare agents E997.1
blast (air) (effects) E993.9
from nuclear explosion—*see* War operations,
injury due to, nuclear weapons
underwater E992.9
bomb (mortar) (explosion) E993.2
after cessation of hostilities E998.1
fragments, injury by E991.4
antipersonnel E991.3
bullet(s) (from carbine, machine gun, pistol,
rifle, shotgun) E991.2
rubber E991.0
burn from
chemical E997.2
fire, conflagration (caused by fire-producing
device or conventional weapon) E990.9
from
conventional weapon E990.3
flamethrower E990.1
incendiary bomb E990.0
incendiary bullet E990.2
nuclear explosion E996.2
petrol bomb E990.0
gas E997.2
burning aircraft E994.3
chemical E997.2
chlorine E997.2
conventional warfare, specified form NEC E995.8
crushing by falling aircraft E994.8

War operations—*continued*
depth charge E992.1
destruction of aircraft E994.9
detonation of own munitions (ammunition)
(artillery) (mortars), unintentional E993.6
disability as sequela one year or more after
injury E999.0
discharge of own munitions launch device
(autocannons) (automatic grenade
launchers) (missile launchers) (small arms),
unintentional E993.7
drowning E995.4
effect, nuclear weapon (see also War
operations, injury due to, nuclear weapons)
E996.9
explosion (breech block) (cannon shell)
E993.9
after cessation of hostilities
bomb placed in war E998.1
mine placed in war E998.0
aircraft E994.1
due to
enemy fire or explosives E994.0
own onboard explosives E994.1
artillery shell E993.2
bomb (mortar) E993.2
aerial E993.0
atom (*see also* War operations, injury due
to, nuclear weapons) E996.9
hydrogen (*see also* War operations, injury
due to, nuclear weapons) E996.9
injury by fragments from E991.4
antipersonnel E991.3
nuclear (*see also* War operations, injury
due to, nuclear weapons) E996.9
depth charge E992.1
injury by fragments from E991.4
antipersonnel E991.3
marine weapon NEC E992.8
mine
at sea or in harbor E992.2
land E993.8
injury by fragments from E991.4
marine E992.2
missle, guided E993.1
mortar E993.2
munitions (accidental) (being used in war)
(dump) (factory) E993.9
own E993.7
launch device (autocannons) (automatic
grenade launchers) (missile launchers)
(small arms) E993.7
nuclear (weapon) (*see also* War operations,
injury due to, nuclear weapons) E996.9
own weapons (accidental) E993.7
injury by fragments from E991.9
antipersonnel E991.3
sea-based artillery shell E992.3
specified NEC E993.8
torpedo E992.0
exposure to ionizing radiation from nuclear
explosion (*see also* War operations, injury
due to, nuclear weapons) E996.3
falling aircraft E994.8
fire or fire-producing device E990.9
flamethrower E990.1
incendiary bomb E990.0
incendiary bullet E990.2
indirectly caused from conventional weapon
E990.3
petrol bomb E990.0

War operations—*continued*
fireball effects from nuclear explosion E996.2
fragments from
  antipersonnel bomb E991.3
  artillery shell E991.4
  bomb NEC E991.4
  grenade E991.4
  guided missile E991.4
  land mine E991.4
  rocket E991.4
  shell E991.4
  shrapnel E991.9
fumes E997.2
gas E997.2
grenade (explosion) E993.8
  fragments, injury by E991.4
guided missile (explosion) E993.1
  fragments, injury by E991.4
nuclear (*see also* War operations, injury due
  to, nuclear weapons) E996.9
heat from nuclear explosion E996.2
injury due to
  aerial bomb E993.0
  air blast E993.9
  aircraft shot down E994.0
injury due to—*continued*
  artillery shell E993.2
  blast E993.9
    wave E993.9
    wind E993.9
  bomb E993.8
  but occurring after cessation of hostilities
    explosion of bombs E998.1
    explosion of mines E998.0
    specified NEC E998.8
  conventional warfare E995.9
    specified form NEC E995.8
  depth charge E992.1
  destruction of aircraft E994.9
    due to
      air to air missile E994.0
      collision with other aircraft E994.2
      enemy fire or explosives E994.0
      on board explosion (explosives) E994.1
      on board fire E994.3
      rocket propelled grenade [RPG] E994.0
      small arms fire E994.0
      surface to air missile E994.0
    specified NEC E994.8
  dirty bomb (see also War operations, injury
    due to, nuclear weapons) E996.9
  drowning E995.4
  explosion (direct pressure) (indirect pressure)
    (due to) E993.9
    depth charge E992.1
    improvised explosive device [IED]
      person borne E993.3
      roadside E993.5
      specified NEC E993.5
      transport vehicle (air) (land) (water)
        borne E993.4
      vehicle (air) (land) (water) borne E993.4
    marine mines (in harbor) (at sea) E992.2
    marine weapons E992.9
      specified NEC E992.8
    sea based artillery shell E992.3
    specified NEC E993.8
    torpedo E992.0

War operations—*continued*
unintentional (of own)
  autocannons E993.7
  automatic grenade launchers E993.7
  launch device discharge E993.7
  munitions detonation (ammunition)
    (artillery) (mortars) E993.6
  missile launchers E993.7
  small arms E993.7
fragments (from) E991.9
  artillery E991.8
  artillery shells E991.4
  autocannons E991.8
  automatic grenade launchers [AGL] E991.8
  bombs E991.4
    antipersonnel E991.3
  detonation of unexploded ordnance [UXO]
    E991.4
  grenade E991.4
  guided missile E991.4
  improvised explosive device [IED]
    person borne E991.5
    roadside E991.7
    specified NEC E991.7
    transport vehicle (air) (land) (water)
      borne E991.6
    vehicle (air) (land) (water) borne E991.6
  land mine E991.4
  missile launchers E991.8
  mortars E991.8
  munitions (artillery shells) (bombs)
    (grenades) (rockets) (shells) E991.4
  rockets E991.4
  shells E991.4
  small arms E991.8
  specified NEC E991.9
  weapons (artillery) (autocannons) (mortars)
    (small arms) E991.8
grenade E993.8
guided missile E993.1
hand to hand combat, unarmed E995.0
improvised explosive device [IED]
  person borne E993.3
  roadside E993.5
  specified NEC E993.5
  transport vehicle (air) (land) (water) borne
    E993.4
  vehicle (air) (land) (water) borne E993.4
inability to surface or obtain air E995.4
land mine E993.8
marine mines (in harbor) (at sea) E992.2
marine weapons E992.9
  specified NEC E992.8
mortar E993.2
nuclear weapons E996.9
  beta burns E996.3
  blast debris E996.1
  blast pressure E996.0
  burns due to thermal radiation E996.2
  direct blast effect E996.0
  fallout exposure E996.3
  fireball effect E996.2
  flash burns E996.2
  heat effect E996.2
  indirect blast effect E996.1
  nuclear radiation effects E996.3
  radiation exposure (acute) E996.3
  radiation sickness E996.3
  secondary effects E996.3
  specified effects NEC E996.8
  thermal radiation effect E996.2

War operations—*continued*
  piercing object E995.2
  restriction of airway, intentional E995.3
  sea based artillery shell E992.3
  shrapnel E991.9
  stave E995.1
  strangulation E995.3
  strike by blunt object (baton) (nightstick)
    (stave) E995.1
  submersion (accidental) (unintentional)
    E995.4
    intentional E995.3
  suffocation E995.3
    accidental E995.4
  torpedo E992.0
  underwater blast E992.9
  weapon of mass destruction [WMD] E997.3
  knife E995.2
  lacrimator (gas) (chemical) E997.2
  land mine (explosion) E993.8
    after cessation of hostilities E998.0
    fragments, injury by E991.4
  laser(s) E997.0
  late effect of E999.0
  lewisite E997.2
  lung irritant (chemical) (fumes) (gas) E997.2
  marine mine E992.2
  mine
    after cessation of hostilities E998.0
    at sea E992.2
    in harbor E992.2
    land (explosion) E993.8
      fragments, injury by E991.4
    marine E992.2
  missile (guided) (explosion) E993.1
    fragments, injury by E991.4
    marine E992.8
    nuclear (*see also* War operations, injury due
      to, nuclear weapons) E996.9
  mortar bomb (explosion) E993.2
    fragments, injury by E991.4
  mustard gas E997.2
  nerve gas E997.2
  phosgene E997.2
  piercing object E995.2
  poisoning (chemical) (fumes) (gas) E997.2
  radiation, ionizing from nuclear explosion (*see*
    also War operations, injury due to, nuclear
    weapons) E996.3
  rocket (explosion) E993.8
    fragments, injury by E991.4
  saber, sabre E995.2
  screening smoke E997.8
  shell (aircraft) (artillery) (cannon) (land based)
    (explosion) E993.2
    fragments, injury by E991.4
    sea-based E992.3
  shooting E991.2
    after cessation of hostilities E998.8
    bullet(s) E991.2
      rubber E991.0
    pellet(s) (rifle) E991.1
  shrapnel E991.9
  stave E995.2
  strike by blunt object (baton) (nightstick)
    (stave) E995.1
  submersion E995.4
    intentional E995.3
  sword E995.2
  torpedo E992.0

War operations—*continued*
  unconventional warfare, except by nuclear
    weapon E997.9
    biological (warfare) E997.1
    gas, fumes, chemicals E997.2
    laser(s) E997.0
    specified type NEC E997.8
  underwater blast E992.9
  vesicant (chemical) (fumes) (gas) E997.2
  weapon burst E993.9
Washed
  away by flood—*see* Flood
  away by tidal wave—*see* Tidal wave
  off road by storm (transport vehicle) E908.9
  overboard E832
Weapon of mass destruction [WMD] E997.3
Weather exposure —*see also* Exposure
  cold E901.0
  hot E900.0
Weightlessness (causing injury) (effects of) (in
  spacecraft, real or simulated) E928.0
Wound (accidental) NEC (*see also* Injury)
  E928.9
  battle (*see also* War operation) E995.9
  bayonet E920.3
  in
    legal intervention E974
    war operations E995.2
  gunshot—*see* Shooting
  incised—*see* Cut
  saber, sabre E920.3
    in war operations E995.2
Wrong
  body part, performance of correct operation
    (procedure) on E876.7
  device implanted into correct surgical site
    E876.5
  patient, performance of operation (procedure)
    on E876.6
  procedure (operation) performed on correct
    patient E876.5
  side, performance of correct operation
    (procedure) on E876.7
  site, performance of correct operation
    (procedure) on E876.7

RAILWAY ACCIDENTS (E800–E807)

The following fourth-digit subdivisions are for use with categories E800-E807 to identify the injured person.

.0 Railway employee

Any person who by virtue of his employment in connection with a railway, whether by the railway company or not, is at increased risk of involvement in a railway accident, such as:

catering staff on train	postal staff on train
driver	railway fireman
guard	shunter
porter	sleeping car attendant

.1 Passenger on railway

Any authorized person traveling on a train, except a railway employee

Excludes: intending passenger waiting at station (.8)
unauthorized rider on railway vehicle (.8)

.2 Pedestrian

See definition (r), Vol. 1, E code introduction

.3 Pedal cyclist

See definition (p), Vol. 1, E code introduction

.8 Other specified person

Intending passenger waiting at station

Unauthorized rider on railway vehicle

.9 Unspecified person

MOTOR VEHICLE TRAFFIC AND NONTRAFFIC ACCIDENTS
(E810–825)

The following fourth–digit subdivisions are for use with categories E810–E819 and E820–E825 to identify the injured person:

.0 Driver of motor vehicle other than motorcycle

See definition (l), Vol. 1, E code introduction

.1 Passenger in motor vehicle other than motorcycle

See definition (l), Vol. 1, E code introduction

.2 Motorcyclist

See definition (l), Vol. 1, E code introduction

.3 Passenger on motorcycle

See definition (l), Vol. 1, E code introduction

.4 Occupant of streetcar

.5 Rider of animal; occupant of animal–drawn vehicle

.6 Pedal cyclist

See definition (p), Vol. 1, E code introduction

.7 Pedestrian

See definition (r), Vol. 1, E code introduction

.8 Other specified person

Occupant of vehicle other than above

Person in railway train involved in accident

Unauthorized rider of motor vehicle

.9 Unspecified person

OTHER ROAD VEHICLE ACCIDENTS (E826–E829)

(animal–drawn vehicle, streetcar, pedal cycle, and other nonmotor road vehicle accidents)

The following fourth–digit subdivisions are for use with categories E826–E829 to identify the injured person:

.0 Pedestrian

See definition (r), Vol. 1, E code introduction

.1 Pedal cyclist (does not apply to codes E827, E828, E829)

See definition (p), Vol. 1, E code introduction

.2 Rider of animal (does not apply to code E829)

.3 Occupant of animal–drawn vehicle (does not apply to codes E828, E829)

.4 Occupant of streetcar

.8 Other specified person

.9 Unspecified person

WATER TRANSPORT ACCIDENTS (E830–E838)

The following fourth–digit subdivisions are for use with categories E830–E838 to identify the injured person:

.0 Occupant of small boat, unpowered

.1 Occupant of small boat, powered

See definition (t), Vol. 1, E code introduction

Excludes: water skier (.4)

.2 Occupant of other watercraft — crew

Persons:

engaged in operation of watercraft

providing passenger services [cabin attendants, ship's physician, catering personnel]

working on ship during voyage in other capacity [musician in band, operators of shops and beauty parlors]

.3 Occupant of other watercraft — other than crew

Passenger

Occupant of lifeboat, other than crew, after abandoning ship

.4 Water skier

.5 Swimmer

.6 Dockers, stevedores

Longshoreman employed on the dock in loading and unloading ships

.8 Other specified person

Immigration and custom officials on board ship

Person:
accompanying passenger or member of crew
visiting boat

Pilot (guiding ship into port)

.9 Unspecified person

AIR AND SPACE TRANSPORT ACCIDENTS (E840–E845)

The following fourth–digit subdivisions are for use with categories E840–E845 to identify the injured person:

.0 Occupant of spacecraft

.1 Occupant of military aircraft, any

Crew in military aircraft [air force] [army] [national guard] [navy]

Passenger (civilian) (military) in military aircraft [air force] [army] [national guard] [navy]

Troops in military aircraft [air force] [army] [national guard] [navy]

Excludes: occupants of aircraft operated under jurisdiction of police departments (.5) parachutist (.7).

.2 Crew of commercial aircraft (powered) in surface to surface transport

.3 Other occupant of commercial aircraft (powered) in surface to surface transport

Flight personnel:
   not part of crew
   on familiarization flight

Passenger on aircraft (powered) NOS

.4 Occupant of commercial aircraft (powered) in surface to air transport

Occupant [crew] [passenger] of aircraft (powered) engaged in activities, such as:
      aerial spraying (crops) (fire retardants)
      air drops of emergency supplies
      air drops of parachutists, except from military craft
      crop dusting
      lowering of construction material [bridge or telephone pole]
      sky writing

.5 Occupant of other powered aircraft

Occupant [crew] [passenger] of aircraft (powered) engaged in activities, such as:
      aerobatic flying
      aircraft racing
      rescue operation
      storm surveillance
      traffic surveillance

Occupant of private plane NOS

.6 Occupant of unpowered aircraft, except parachutist

Occupant of aircraft classifiable to E842

.7 Parachutist (military) (other)

Person making voluntary descent

Excludes: person making descent after accident to aircraft (.1–.6)

.8 Ground crew, airline employee

Persons employed at airfields (civil) (military) or launching pads, not occupants of aircraft

.9 Other person

010.0 Primary tuberculous infection
Revise exclusion terms

017.0 Skin and subcutaneous cellular tissue
Revise exclusion terms

041.41 Shiga toxin-producing Escherichia coli [E. coli] (STEC) O157
New code

041.42 Other specified Shiga toxin-producing Escherichia coli [E. coli] (STEC)
New code

041.43 Shiga toxin-producing Escherichia coli [E. coli] (STEC), unspecified
New code

041.49 Other and unspecified Escherichia coli [E. coli]
New code

099.3 Reiter's disease
Add inclusion term

140 Malignant neoplasm of lip
Revise exclusion terms

154.2 Anal canal
Revise exclusion terms

154.3 Anus, unspecified
Revise exclusion terms

160.0 Nasal cavities
Revise exclusion terms

160.1 Auditory tube, middle ear, and mastoid air cells
Revise exclusion terms

173 Other and unspecified malignant neoplasm of skin
Revise code, add exclusion term

173.0 Other and unspecified malignant neoplasm of skin of lip
Revise subcategory

173.00 Unspecified malignant neoplasm of skin of lip
New code

173.01 Basal cell carcinoma of skin of lip
New code

173.02 Squamous cell carcinoma of skin of lip
New code

173.09 Other specified malignant neoplasm of skin of lip
New code

173.1 Other and unspecified malignant neoplasm of eyelid, including canthus
Revise subcategory

173.10 Unspecified malignant neoplasm of eyelid, including canthus
New code

173.11 Basal cell carcinoma of eyelid, including canthus
New code

173.12 Squamous cell carcinoma of eyelid, including canthus
New code

173.19 Other specified malignant neoplasm of eyelid, including canthus
New code

173.2 Other and unspecified malignant neoplasm of skin of ear and external auditory canal
Revise subcategory

173.20 Unspecified malignant neoplasm of skin of ear and external auditory canal
New code

173.21 Basal cell carcinoma of skin of ear and external auditory canal
New code

173.22 Squamous cell carcinoma of skin of ear and external auditory canal
New code

173.29 Other specified malignant neoplasm of skin of ear and external auditory canal
New code

173.3 Other and unspecified malignant neoplasm of skin of other and unspecified parts of face
Revise subcategory

173.30 Unspecified malignant neoplasm of skin of other and unspecified parts of face
New code

173.31 Basal cell carcinoma of skin of other and unspecified parts of face
New code

173.32 Squamous cell carcinoma of skin of other and unspecified parts of face
New code

173.39 Other specified malignant neoplasm of skin of other and unspecified parts of face
New code

173.4 Other and unspecified malignant neoplasm of scalp and skin of neck
Revise subcategory

173.40 Unspecified malignant neoplasm of scalp and skin of neck
New code

173.41 Basal cell carcinoma of scalp and skin of neck
New code

173.42 Squamous cell carcinoma of scalp and skin of neck
New code

173.49 Other specified malignant neoplasm of scalp and skin of neck
New code

173.5 Other and unspecified malignant neoplasm of skin of trunk, except scrotum
Revise subcategory

173.50 Unspecified malignant neoplasm of skin of trunk, except scrotum
New code

173.51 Basal cell carcinoma of skin of trunk, except scrotum
New code

173.52 Squamous cell carcinoma of skin of trunk, except scrotum
New code

173.59 Other specified malignant neoplasm of skin of trunk, except scrotum
New code

173.6 Other and unspecified malignant neoplasm of skin of upper limb, including shoulder
Revise subcategory

173.60 Unspecified malignant neoplasm of skin of upper limb, including shoulder
New code

173.61 Basal cell carcinoma of skin of upper limb, including shoulder
New code

173.62 Squamous cell carcinoma of skin of upper limb, including shoulder
New code

173.69 Other specified malignant neoplasm of skin of upper limb, including shoulder
New code

173.7 Other and unspecified malignant neoplasm of skin of lower limb, including hip
Revise subcategory

173.70 Unspecified malignant neoplasm of skin of lower limb, including hip
New code

173.71 Basal cell carcinoma of skin of lower limb, including hip
New code

173.72 Squamous cell carcinoma of skin of lower limb, including hip
New code

173.79 Other specified malignant neoplasm of skin of lower limb, including hip
New code

173.8 Other and unspecified malignant neoplasm of other specified sites of skin
Revise subcategory

173.80 Unspecified malignant neoplasm of other specified sites of skin
New code

173.81 Basal cell carcinoma of other specified sites of skin
New code

173.82 Squamous cell carcinoma of other specified sites of skin
New code

173.89 Other specified malignant neoplasm of other specified sites of skin
New code

173.9 Other and unspecified malignant neoplasm of skin, site unspecified
Revise subcategory

173.90 Unspecified malignant neoplasm of skin, site unspecified
New code

173.91 Basal cell carcinoma of skin, site unspecified
New code

173.92 Squamous cell carcinoma of skin, site unspecified
New code

173.99 Other specified malignant neoplasm of skin, site unspecified
New code

174 Malignant neoplasm of female breast
Revise exclusion terms

175 Malignant neoplasm of male breast
Revise exclusion terms

190 Malignant neoplasm of eye
Revise exclusion terms

202.5 Letterer-Siwe disease
Add exclusion term

209.71 Secondary neuroendocrine tumor of distant lymph nodes
Delete inclusion term

209.74 Secondary neuroendocrine tumor of peritoneum
Add inclusion term

236.1 Placenta
Add, revise inclusion terms

243 Congenital hypothyroidism
Revise "Use additional" note

249.8 Secondary diabetes mellitus with other specified manifestations
Revise "Use additional" note

250.8 Diabetes mellitus with other specified manifestations
Revise "Use additional" note

276.5 Volume depletion
Revise exclusion term

277.89 Other specified disorders of metabolism
Add exclusion term

282.40 Thalassemia, unspecified
New code

282.41 Sickle-cell thalassemia without crisis
Add inclusion term

282.43 Alpha thalassemia
New code

282.44 Beta thalassemia
New code

282.45 Delta-beta thalassemia
New code

282.46 Thalassemia minor
New code

282.47 Hemoglobin E-beta thalassemia
New code

282.49 Other thalassemia
New code

282.5 Sickle-cell trait
Revise exclusion term

282.7 Other hemoglobinopathies
Add exclusion terms

283.11 Hemolytic-uremic syndrome
Add "Use additional code" notes

284.1 Pancytopenia
Delete exclusion term

284.11 Antineoplastic chemotherapy induced pancytopenia
New code

284.12 Other drug induced pancytopenia
New code

284.19 Other pancytopenia
New code

286.5 Hemorrhagic disorder due to intrinsic circulating anticoagulants, antibodies, or inhibitors
Revise subcategory

286.52 **Acquired hemophilia**
New code

286.53 **Antiphospholipid antibody with hemorrhagic disorder**
New code

286.59 **Other hemorrhagic disorder due to intrinsic circulating anticoagulants, antibodies, or inhibitors**
New code

289.81 **Primary hypercoagulable state**
Add/revise inclusion terms; add exclusion terms

Ch. 5 **MENTAL, BEHAVIORAL AND NEURODEVELOPMENTAL DISORDERS (290-319)**
Revise Chapter Title

290.0 **Senile dementia, uncomplicated**
Revise exclusion term

294.1 **Dementia in conditions classified elsewhere**
Revise "Code first" note

294.11 **Dementia in conditions classified elsewhere with behavioral disturbance**
Delete inclusion term, add "Use additional" note

294.2 **Dementia, unspecified**
New subcategory

294.20 **Dementia, unspecified, without behavioral disturbance**
New code

294.21 **Dementia, unspecified, with behavioral disturbance**
New code

294.8 **Other persistent mental disorders due to conditions classified elsewhere**
Delete inclusion term, revise exclusion term

310.2 **Postconcussion syndrome**
Revise exclusion term

310.8 **Other specified nonpsychotic mental disorders following organic brain damage**
Delete inclusion terms

310.81 **Pseudobulbar affect**
New code

310.89 **Other specified nonpsychotic mental disorders following organic brain damage**
New code

317 **Mild intellectual disabilities**
Revise title

318 **Other specified intellectual disabilities**
Revise title

318.0 **Moderate intellectual disabilities**
Revise title

318.1 **Severe intellectual disabilities**
Revise title

318.2 **Profound intellectual disabilities**
Revise title

319 **Unspecified intellectual disabilities**
Revise title

323.0 **Encephalitis, myelitis, and encephalomyelitis in viral diseases classified elsewhere**
Add "Code first" note

323.4 **Other encephalitis, myelitis, and encephalomyelitis due to other infections classified elsewhere**
Revise title

323.41 **Other encephalitis and encephalomyelitis due to other infections classified elsewhere**
Revise title

323.42 **Other myelitis due to other infections classified elsewhere**
Revise title

330 **Cerebral degenerations usually manifest in childhood**
Revise "Use additional code" note

331.6 **Corticobasal degeneration**
New code

331.83 **Mild cognitive impairment, so stated**
Revise exclusion terms

345.8 **Other forms of epilepsy and recurrent seizures**
Delete inclusion term

345.9 **Epilepsy, unspecified**
Delete inclusion term

346 **Migraine**
Revise 5th digit classification

348.82 **Brain death**
New code

348.89 **Other conditions of brain**
Add exclusion term

358.1 **Myasthenic syndromes in diseases classified elsewhere**
Delete inclusion term

358.3 **Lambert-Eaton syndrome**
New subcategory

358.30 **Lambert-Eaton syndrome, unspecified**
New code

358.31 **Lambert-Eaton syndrome in neoplastic disease**
New code

358.39 **Lambert-Eaton syndrome in other diseases classified elsewhere**
New code

365.01 **Open angle with borderline findings, low risk**
Revise code title, revise inclusion terms

365.02 **Anatomical narrow angle**
Add inclusion term

365.05 **Open angle with borderline findings, high risk**
New code

365.06 **Primary angle closure without glaucoma damage**
New code

365.10 **Open-angle glaucoma, unspecified**
Add "Use additional code" note

365.11 **Primary open angle glaucoma**
Add "Use additional code" note

365.12 **Low tension glaucoma**
Add "Use additional code" note

365.13 **Pigmentary glaucoma**
Add "Use additional code" note

365.20 **Primary angle-closure glaucoma, unspecified**
Add "Use additional code" note

365.22 **Acute angle-closure glaucoma**
Add inclusion terms

365.23 **Chronic angle-closure glaucoma**
Add inclusion terms, add "Use additional code" note

365.31 **Glaucomatous stage**
Add "Use additional code" note

365.52 **Pseudoexfoliation glaucoma**
Add "Use additional code" note

365.62 **Glaucoma associated with ocular inflammations**
Add "Use additional code" note

365.63 **Glaucoma associated with vascular disorders**
Add "Use additional code" note

365.65 **Glaucoma associated with ocular trauma**
Add "Use additional code" note

365.7 **Glaucoma stage**
New subcategory

365.70 **Glaucoma stage, unspecified**
New code

365.71 **Mild stage glaucoma**
New code

365.72 **Moderate stage glaucoma**
New code

365.73 **Severe stage glaucoma**
New code

365.74 **Indeterminate stage glaucoma**
New code

379.27 **Vitreomacular adhesion**
New code

414.4 **Coronary atherosclerosis due to calcified coronary lesion**
New code

415.1 **Pulmonary embolism and infarction**
Revise exclusion term

415.13 **Saddle embolus of pulmonary artery**
New code

416.2 **Chronic pulmonary embolism**
Revise exclusion term

417.0 **Arteriovenous fistula of pulmonary vessels**
Revise exclusion term

417.1 **Aneurysm of pulmonary artery**
Revise exclusion terms

424.1 **Aortic valve disorders**
Revise exclusion term

425.1 **Hypertrophic cardiomyopathy**
Revise title, delete inclusion term, add exclusion term

425.11 **Hypertrophic obstructive cardiomyopathy**
New code

425.18 **Other hypertrophic cardiomyopathy**
New code

425.4 **Other primary cardiomyopathies**
Delete inclusion terms

430 **Subarachnoid hemorrhage**
Add exclusion term

440.23 **Atherosclerosis of the extremities with ulceration**
Revise "Use additional code" note

440.24 **Atherosclerosis of the extremities with gangrene**
Revise "Use additional code" note

444.0 **Of abdominal aorta**
Delete inclusion terms

444.01 **Saddle embolus of abdominal aorta**
New code

444.09 **Other arterial embolism and thrombosis of abdominal aorta**
New code

444.89 **Other**
Revise exclusion term

449 **Septic arterial embolism**
Revise "Use additional code" note

459.81 **Venous (peripheral) insufficiency, unspecified**
Revise "Use additional code" note

466.1 **Acute bronchiolitis**
Add exclusion term

487 **Influenza**
Revise exclusion terms

488 **Influenza due to certain identified influenza viruses**
Revise exclusion term

488.1 **Influenza due to identified 2009 H1N1 influenza virus**
Revise title, revise inclusion terms, add exclusion terms

488.11 **Influenza due to identified 2009 H1N1 influenza virus with pneumonia**
Revise title, revise inclusion terms

488.12 **Influenza due to identified 2009 H1N1 influenza virus with other respiratory manifestations**
Revise title, revise inclusion terms

488.19 **Influenza due to identified 2009 H1N1 influenza virus with other manifestations**
Revise title, revise inclusion terms

488.8 **Influenza due to novel influenza A**
New subcategory

488.81 **Influenza due to identified novel influenza A virus with pneumonia**
New code

488.82 **Influenza due to identified novel influenza A virus with other respiratory manifestations**
New code

488.89 **Influenza due to identified novel influenza A virus with other manifestations**
New code

506 **Respiratory conditions due to chemical fumes and vapors**
Add "Use additional code" note

507 **Pneumonitis due to solids and liquids**
Add exclusion term

508 **Respiratory conditions due to other and unspecified external agents**
Add "Use additional code" note

508.2 **Respiratory conditions due to smoke inhalation**
New code

512 **Pneumothorax and air leak**
Revise title

512.2 **Postoperative air leak**
New code

512.8 **Other pneumothorax and air leak**
Revise title, delete inclusion terms

512.81	**Primary spontaneous pneumothorax** New code		**518.51**	**Acute respiratory failure following trauma and surgery** New code
512.82	**Secondary spontaneous pneumothorax** New code		**518.52**	**Other pulmonary insufficiency, not elsewhere classified, following trauma and surgery** New code
512.83	**Chronic pneumothorax** New code		**518.53**	**Acute and chronic respiratory failure following trauma and surgery** New code
512.84	**Other air leak** New code			
512.89	**Other pneumothor** New code		**518.81**	**Acute respiratory failure** Add exclusion term
514	**Pulmonary congestion and hypostasis** Revise exclusion term		**518.82**	**Other pulmonary insufficiency, not elsewhere classified** Revise exclusion terms
516.3	**Idiopathic interstitial pneumonia** Revise title, delete inclusion terms		**518.84**	**Acute and chronic respiratory failure** Add exclusion term
516.30	**Idiopathic interstitial pneumonia, not otherwise specified** New code		**536.3**	**Gastroparesis** Revise "Code first" note
516.31	**Idiopathic pulmonary fibrosis** New code		**539**	**Complications of bariatric procedures** New category
516.32	**Idiopathic non-specific interstitial pneumonitis** New code		**539.0**	**Complications of gastric band procedure** New subcategory
516.33	**Acute interstitial pneumonitis** New code		**539.01**	**Infection due to gastric band procedure** New code
516.34	**Respiratory bronchiolitis interstitial lung disease** New code		**539.09**	**Other complications of gastric band procedure** New code
516.35	**Idiopathic lymphoid interstitial pneumonia** New code		**539.8**	**Complications of other bariatric procedure** New subcategory
516.36	**Cryptogenic organizing pneumonia** New code		**539.81**	**Infection due to other bariatric procedure** New code
516.37	**Desquamative interstitial pneumonia** New code		**539.89**	**Other complications of other bariatric procedure** New code
516.4	**Lymphangioleiomyomatosis** New code		**569.49**	**Other** Revise "Use additional code" note
516.5	**Adult pulmonary Langerhans cell histiocytosis** New code		**572.8**	**Other sequelae of chronic liver disease** Add exclusion term
516.6	**Interstitial lung diseases of childhood** New subcategory		**573.5**	**Hepatopulmonary syndrome** New code
516.61	**Neuroendocrine cell hyperplasia of infancy** New code		**574**	**Cholelithiasis** Add exclusion term
516.62	**Pulmonary interstitial glycogenosis** New code		**590**	**Infections of kidney** Revise "Use additional code" note
516.63	**Surfactant mutations of the lung** New code		**595**	**Cystitis** Revise "Use additional code" note
516.64	**Alveolar capillary dysplasia with vein misalignment** New code		**596.8**	**Other specified disorders of bladder** Delete inclusion terms
516.69	**Other interstitial lung diseases of childhood** New code		**596.81**	**Infection of cystostomy** New code
516.8	**Other specified alveolar and parietoalveolar pneumonopathies** Revise inclusion terms, add "Code first" note, add "Use additional" note, add exclusion terms		**596.82**	**Mechanical complication of cystostomy** New code
			596.83	**Other complication of cystostomy** New code
518.3	**Pulmonary eosinophilia** Add exclusion term		**596.89**	**Other specified disorders of bladder** New code
518.5	**Pulmonary insufficiency following trauma and surgery** Delete inclusion terms		**599.0**	**Urinary tract infection, site not specified** Revise "Use additional code" note

604	**Orchitis and epididymitis** Revise "Use additional code" note
616.10	**Vaginitis and vulvovaginitis, unspecified** Revise "Use additional code" note
618.04	**Rectocele** Revise "Use additional code" note
629.3	**Complication of implanted vaginal mesh and other prosthetic materials** New subcategory
629.31	**Erosion of implanted vaginal mesh and other prosthetic materials to surrounding organ or tissue** New code
629.32	**Exposure of implanted vaginal mesh and other prosthetic materials into vagina** New code
631	**Other abnormal product of conception** Delete inclusion terms
631.0	**Inappropriate change in quantitative human chorionic gonadotropin (hCG) in early pregnancy** New code
631.8	**Other abnormal products of conception** New code
632	**Missed abortion** Revise exclusion terms
646.7	**Liver and biliary tract disorders in pregnancy** Revise title
649.8	**Onset (spontaneous) of labor after 37 completed weeks of gestation but before 39 completed weeks gestation, with delivery by (planned) cesarean section** New subcategory
704.4	**Pilar and trichilemmal cysts** New subcategory
704.41	**Pilar cyst** New code
704.42	**Trichilemmal cyst** New code
706.2	**Sebaceous cyst** Add exclusion terms
713.6	**Arthropathy associated with hypersensitivity reaction** Revise "Code first" note
718.6	**Unspecified intrapelvic protrusion of acetabulum** Revise valid fifth digits
726.13	**Partial tear of rotator cuff** New code
727.61	**Complete rupture of rotator cuff** Add exclusion term
747.3	**Anomalies of pulmonary artery** Delete inclusion terms
747.31	**Pulmonary artery coarctation and atresia** New code
747.32	**Pulmonary arteriovenous malformation** New code

747.39	**Other anomalies of pulmonary artery and pulmonary circulation** New code
747.6	**Other anomalies of peripheral vascular system** Revise exclusion term
747.89	**Other** Revise exclusion terms
780.93	**Memory loss** Revise exclusion term
785.52	**Septic shock** Revise "Code first" notes
785.59	**Other** Revise exclusion terms
786.09	**Other** Revise exclusion terms
793.1	**Lung field** Delete inclusion terms
793.11	**Solitary pulmonary nodule** New code
793.19	**Other nonspecific abnormal finding of lung field** New code
795.5	**Nonspecific reaction to test for tuberculosis** Revise title, delete inclusion terms
795.51	**Nonspecific reaction to tuberculin skin test without active tuberculosis** New code
795.52	**Nonspecific reaction to cell mediated immunity measurement of gamma interferon antigen response without active tuberculosis** New code
799.1	**Respiratory arrest** Revise exclusion terms
808.43	**Multiple closed pelvic fractures with disruption of pelvic circle** Revise title, add inclusion term
808.44	**Multiple closed pelvic fractures without disruption of pelvic circle** New code
808.53	**Multiple open pelvic fractures with disruption of pelvic circle** Revise title, add inclusion term
808.54	**Multiple open pelvic fractures without disruption of pelvic circle** New code
958	**Certain early complications of trauma** Revise exclusion terms
958.4	**Traumatic shock** Revise exclustion terms
964.7	**Natural blood and blood products** Revise exclusion terms
968.5	**Surface (topical) and infiltration anesthetics** Revise titlte, revise inclusion term
995.0	**Other anaphylactic reaction** Revise title, add inclusion terms, revise exclusion terms
995.1	**Angioneurotic edema** Add inclusion term, revise exclusion term
995.4	**Shock due to anesthesia** Revise exclusion term

995.6 Anaphylactic reaction due to food
Revise title, revise inclusion terms

995.60 Anaphylactic reaction due to unspecified food
Revise title

995.61 Anaphylactic reaction due to peanuts
Revise title

995.62 Anaphylactic reaction due to crustaceans
Revise title

995.63 Anaphylactic reaction due to fruits and vegetables
Revise title

995.64 Anaphylactic reaction due to tree nuts and see
Revise title

995.65 Anaphylactic reaction due to fish
Revise title

995.66 Anaphylactic reaction due to food additives
Revise title

995.67 Anaphylactic reaction due to milk products
Revise title

995.68 Anaphylactic reaction due to eggs
Revise title

995.69 Anaphylactic reaction due to other specified food
Revise title

995.7 Other adverse food reactions, not elsewhere classified
Revise exclusion term

996 Complications peculiar to certain specified procedures
Revise exclusion term

996.39 Other
Delete inclusion term, revise exclusion term

996.62 Due to vascular device, implant and graft
Revise exclusion terms

996.64 Due to indwelling urinary catheter
Add exclusion terms

996.7 Other complications of internal (biological) (synthetic) prosthetic device, implant, and graft
Revise exclusion term

996.76 Due to genitourinary device, implant, and graft
Add exclusion term

996.88 Stem cell
New code

997 Complications affecting specified body systems, not elsewhere classified
Revise exclusion term

997.3 Respiratory complications
Revise exclusion terms

997.32 Postprocedural aspiration pneumonia
New code

997.39 Other respiratory complications
New code

997.4 Digestive system complications
Add exclusion terms

997.41 Retained cholelithiasis following cholecystectomy
New code

997.49 Other digestive system complications
New code

997.5 Urinary complications
Delete inclusion term, add exclusion terms

998.0 Postoperative shock
Revise inclusion and exclusion terms

998.00 Postoperative shock, unspecified
New code

998.01 Postoperative shock, cardiogenic
New code

998.02 Postoperative shock, septic
New code

998.09 Postoperative shock, other
New code

998.31 Disruption of internal operation (surgical) wound
Revise exclusion term

999.31 Other and unspecified infection due to central venous catheter
Revise code title and inclusion terms

999.32 Bloodstream infection due to central venous catheter
New code

999.33 Local infection due to central venous catheter
New code

999.34 Acute infection following transfusion, infusion, or injection of blood and blood products
New code

999.4 Anaphylactic reaction due to serum
Revise code title, revise inclusion and exclusion terms

999.41 Anaphylactic reaction due to administration of blood and blood products
New code

999.42 Anaphylactic reaction due to vaccination
New code

999.49 Anaphylactic reaction due to other serum
New code

999.51 Other serum reaction due to administration of blood and blood products
New code

999.52 Other serum reaction due to vaccination
New code

999.59 Other serum reaction
New code

999.6 ABO incompatibility reaction due to transfusion of blood or blood products
Revise exclusion term

999.8 Other and unspecified infusion and transfusion reaction
Revise exclusion term

V12.21 Gestational diabetes
New code

V12.29 Other endocrine, metabolic, and immunity disorders
New code

V12.5 Diseases of circulatory system
Add exclusion term

V12.51 Venous thrombosis and embolism
Delete inclusion term, add exclusion term

V12.55 Pulmonary embolism
New code

V13.81 Anaphylaxis
New code

V13.89 Other specified diseases
New code

V17.0 Psychiatric condition
Revise exclusion term

V18.4 Intellectual disabilities
Revise code title

V19.11 Glaucoma
New code

V19.19 Other specified eye disorder
New code

V23.42 Pregnancy with history of ectopic pregnancy
New code

V23.87 Pregnancy with inconclusive fetal viability
New code

V40.31 Wandering in diseases classified elsewhere
New code

V40.39 Other specified behavioral problem
New code

V54.82 Aftercare following explantation of joint prosthesis
New code

V55 Attention to artificial openings
Revise exclusion term

V58.68 Long term (current) use of bisphosphonates
New code

V58.69 Long-term (current) use of other medications
Revise inclusion term, add exclusion terms

V79.2 Intellectual disabilities
Revise code title

V84 Genetic susceptibility to disease
Add exclusion term

V84.81 Genetic susceptibility to multiple endocrine neoplasia [MEN]
Add exclusion term

V87.02 Contact with and (suspected) exposure to uranium
New code

V88.2 Acquired absence of joint
New subcategory

V88.21 Acquired absence of hip joint
New code

V88.22 Acquired absence of knee joint
New code

V88.29 Acquired absence of other joint
New code

PROCEDURES: TABULAR LIST AND ALPHABETIC INDEX

VOLUME 3

1.   **OPERATIONS ON THE NERVOUS SYSTEM (01-05)**

00   **Procedures and interventions, Not Elsewhere Classified**

      00.0   **Therapeutic ultrasound**

> | Excludes: | *diagnostic ultrasound (non-invasive) (88.71-88.79)* |
> |---|---|
> | | *intracardiac echocardiography [ICE] (heart chamber(s)) (37.28)* |
> | | *intravascular imaging (adjunctive) (00.21-00.29)* |

           00.01   **Therapeutic ultrasound of vessels of head and neck**
Anti-restenotic ultrasound
Intravscular non-ablative ultrasound

> | Excludes: | *diagnostic ultrasound of:* |
> |---|---|
> | | *eye (95.13)* |
> | | *head and neck (88.71)* |
> | | *that of inner ear (20.79)* |
> | | *ultrasonic:* |
> | | *angioplasty of non-coronary vessel (39.50)* |
> | | *embolectomy (38.01, 38.02)* |
> | | *endarterectomy (38.11, 38.12)* |
> | | *thrombectomy (38.01, 38.02)* |

           00.02   **Therapeutic ultrasound of heart**
Note: real-time imaging of lumen of blood vessel(s) using sound waves
Anti-restenotic ultrasound
Intravascular non-ablative ultrasound

> | Excludes: | *diagnostic ultrasound of heart (88.72)* |
> |---|---|
> | | *ultrasonic angioplasty of coronary vessels (00.66, 36.09)* |
> | | *ultrasound ablation of heart lesion (37.34)* |

           00.03   **Therapeutic ultrasound of peripheral vascular vessels**
Anti-restenotic ultrasound
Intravascular non-ablative ultrasound

> | Excludes: | *diagnostic ultrasound of peripheral vascular system (88.77)* |
> |---|---|
> | | *ultrasonic angioplasty of:* |
> | | *non-coronary vessel (39.50)* |

           00.09   **Other therapeutic ultrasound**

> | Excludes: | *ultrasonic:* |
> |---|---|
> | | *fragmentation of urinary stones (59.95)* |
> | | *percutaneous nephrostomy with fragmentation (55.04)* |
> | | *physical therapy (93.35)* |
> | | *transurethral guided laser induced prostatectomy (TULIP) (60.21)* |

      00.1   **Pharmaceuticals**

           00.10   **Implantation of chemotherapeutic agent**
Brain wafer chemotherapy
Interstitial / intracavitary

> | Excludes: | *injection of infusion of cancer chemotherapeutic substance (99.25)* |
> |---|---|

           00.11   **Infusion of drotrecogin alfa (activated)**
Infusion of recombinant protein

           00.12   **Administration of inhaled nitric oxide**
Nitric oxide therapy

           00.13   **Injection or infusion of nesiritide**
Human B-type natriuretic peptide (hBNP)

           00.14   **Injection or infusion of oxazolidinone class of antibiotics**
Linezolid injection

           00.15   **High-dose infusion interleukin-2 [IL-2]**
Infusion (IV bolus, CIV) interleukin
Injection of aldesleukin

> | Excludes: | *low-dose infusion interleukin-2 (99.28)* |
> |---|---|

           00.16   **Pressurized treatment of venous bypass graft [conduit] with pharmaceutical substance**
Ex-vivo treatment vessel
Hyperbaric pressurized graft [conduit]

           00.17   **Infusion of vasopressor agent**

VOL 3
PROCEDURES

	Valid O.R. procedure		Non-O.R. procedure		Nonspecific O.R. procedure		Noncovered O.R. procedure

00.18 Infusion of immunosuppressive antibody therapy
Monoclonal antibody therapy
Polyclonal antibody therapy
Includes: during induction phase of solid organ transplantation

00.19 Disruption of blood brain barrier via infusion [BBBD]
Infusion of substance to disrupt blood brain barrier
Code also chemotherapy (99.25)

Excludes: *other perfusion (39.97)*

00.2 Intravascular imaging of blood vessels
Endovascular ultrasonography
Intravascular [ultrasound] imaging of blood vessels
Intravascular ultrasound (IVUS)
Virtual histology intravascular ultrasound [VH-IVUS]
Note: real-time imaging of lumen of blood vessel(s) using sound waves
Code also any synchronous diagnostic or therapeutic procedures

Excludes: *adjunct vascular system procedures, number of vessels (00.40-00.43)*
diagnostic procedures on blood vessels treated (38.21-38.29)
diagnostic ultrasound of peripheral vascular system (88.77)
intravascular imaging of vessel(s) by OCT (38.24-38.25)
magnetic resonance imaging (MRI) (88.91-88.97)
therapeutic ultrasound (00.01-00.09)

00.21 Intravascular imaging of extracranial cerebral vessels
Common carotid vessels and branches
Intravascular ultrasound (IVUS), extracranial cerebral vessels

Excludes: *diagnostic ultrasound (non-invasive) of head and neck (88.71)*

00.22 Intravascular imaging of intrathoracic vessels
Aorta and aortic arch
Intravascular ultrasound (IVUS), intrathoracic vessels
Vena cava (superior) (inferior)

Excludes: *diagnostic ultrasound (non-invasive) of other sites of thorax (88.73)*

00.23 Intravascular imaging of peripheral vessels
Imaging of:
  vessels of arm(s)
  vessels of leg(s)
Intravascular ultrasound (IVUS), peripheral vessels

Excludes: *diagnostic ultrasound (non-invasive) of peripheral vascular system (88.77)*

00.24 Intravascular imaging of coronary vessels
Intravascular ultrasound (IVUS), coronary vessels

Excludes: *diagnostic ultrasound, (non-invasive) of heart (88.72)*
intracardiac echocardiography [ICE] (ultrasound of heart chamber(s)) (37.28)

00.25 Intravascular imaging of renal vessels
Intravascular ultrasound (IVUS), renal vessels
Renal artery

Excludes: *diagnostic ultrasound (non-invasive) of urinary system (88.75)*

00.28 Intravascular imaging, other specified vessel(s)

00.29 Intravascular imaging, unspecified vessel(s)

00.3 Computer assisted surgery [CAS]
CT-free navigation
Image guided navigation (IGN)
Image guided surgery (IGS)
Imageless navigation
That without the use of robotic(s) technology
Code also diagnostic or therapeutic procedure

Excludes: *robotic assisted procedures (17.41-17.49)*
stereotactic frame application only (93.59)

00.31 Computer assisted surgery with CT/CTA

00.32 Computer assisted surgery with MR/MRA

00.33 Computer assisted surgery with fluoroscopy

00.34 Imageless computer assisted surgery

● Code new
to this edition

▲ Revision of
existing code

④ ⑤ Fourth or fifth
digit required

00.35 Computer assisted surgery with multiple datasets

00.39 Other computer assisted surgery
Computer assisted surgery NOS

00.4 Adjunct vascular system procedures
Note: These codes can apply to both coronary and peripheral vessels. These codes are to be used in conjunction with other therapeutic procedure codes to provide additional information on the number of vessels upon which a procedure was performed and/or the number of stents inserted. As appropriate, code both the number of vessels operated on (00.40-00.43), and the number of stents inserted (00.45-00.48).

Code also any:
angioplasty (00.61-00.62, 00.66, 39.50)
atherectomy (17.53-17.56)
endarterectomy (38.10-38.18)
insertion of vascular stent(s) (00.55, 00.63-00.65, 36.06-36.07, 39.90)
other removal of coronary artery obstruction (36.09)

00.40 Procedure on single vessel
Number of vessels, unspecified

Excludes:	(aorto)coronary bypass (36.10-36.19)
	intravascular imaging of blood vessels (00.21-00.29)

00.41 Procedure on two vessels

Excludes:	(aorto)coronary bypass (36.10-36.19)
	intravascular imaging of blood vessels (00.21-00.29)

00.42 Procedure on three vessels

Excludes:	(aorto)coronary bypass (36.10-36.19)
	intravascular imaging of blood vessels (00.21-00.29)

00.43 Procedure on four or more vessels

Excludes:	(aorto)coronary bypass (36.10-36.19)
	intravascular imaging of blood vessels (00.21-00.29)

00.44 Procedure on vessel bifurcation
Note: This code is to be used to identify the presence of a vessel bifurcation; it does not describe a specific bifurcation stent. Use this code only once per operative episode, irrespective of the number of bifurcations in vessels.

00.45 Insertion of one vascular stent
Number of stents, unspecified

00.46 Insertion of two vascular stents

00.47 Insertion of three vascular stents

00.48 Insertion of four or more vascular stents

00.49 SuperSaturated oxygen therapy
Aqueous oxygen (AO) therapy
SSO_2
SuperOxygenation infusion therapy

Code also any:
injection or infusion of thrombolytic agent (99.10)
insertion of coronary artery stent(s) (36.06-36.07)
intracoronary artery thrombolytic infusion (36.04)
number of vascular stents inserted (00.45-00.48)
number of vessels treated (00.40-00.43)
open chest coronary artery angioplasty (36.03)
other removal of coronary obstruction (37.09)
percutaneous transluminal coronary angioplasty [PCTA] (00.66)
procedure on vessel bifurcation (00.44)
transluminal coronary atherectomy (17.55)

Excludes:	other oxygen enrichment (93.96)
	other perfusion (39.97)

00.5 Other cardiovascular procedures

	Valid O.R. procedure		Non-O.R. procedure		Nonspecific O.R. procedure		Noncovered O.R. procedure

00.50 **Implantation of cardiac resynchronization pacemaker without mention of defibrillation, total system [CRT-P]**

Note: Device testing during procedure—*omit code*

Biventricular pacemaker
BiV pacemaker
Biventricular pacing without internal cardiac defibrillator
Implantation of cardiac resynchronization (biventricular) pulse generator pacing device, formation of pocket, transvenous leads including placement of lead into left ventricular coronary venous system, and intraoperative procedures for evaluation of lead signals
That with CRT-P generator and one or more leads

Excludes: *implantation of cardiac resynchronization defibrillator, total system [CRT-D] (00.51)*
insertion or replacement of any type pacemaker device (37.80-37.87)
replacement of cardiac resynchronization defibrillator pulse generator only [CRT-D] (00.54)
replacement of cardiac resynchronization pacemaker pulse generator only [CRT-P] (00.53)

00.51 **Implantation of cardiac resynchronization defibrillator, total system [CRT-D]**

Note: Device testing during procedure—*omit code*

BiV defibrillator
Biventricular defibrillator
BiV ICD
BiV pacemaker with defibrillator
BiV pacing with defibrillator
Biventricular pacing with internal cardiac defibrillator
Implantation of a cardiac resynchronization (biventricular) pulse generator with defibrillator [AICD], formation of pocket, transvenous leads, including placement of lead into left ventricular coronary venous system, intraoperative procedures for evaluation of lead signals, and obtaining defibrillator threshold measurements
That with CRT-D generator and one or more leads

Excludes: *implantation of cardiac resynchronization pacemaker, total system [CRT-P] (00.50)*
implantation or replacement of automatic cardioverter/defibrillator, total system [AICD] (37.94)
replacement of cardiac resynchronization defibrillator pulse generator only, [CRT-D] (00.54)

00.52 **Implantation or replacement of transvenous lead [electrode] into left ventricular coronary venous sytem**

Excludes: *implantation of cardiac resynchronization defibrillator, total system [CRT-D] (00.51)*
implantation of cardiac resynchronization pacemeker, total system [CRT-P] (00.50)
initial insertion of transvenous lead [electrode] (37.70-37.72)
replacement of transvenous atrial and/or ventricular lead(s) [electrodes] (37.76)

00.53 **Implantation or replacement of cardiac resynchronization pacemaker pulse generator only [CRT-P]**

Note: Device testing during procedure—*omit code*

Implantation of CRT-P device with removal of any existing CRT-P or other pacemaker device

Excludes: *implantation of cardiac resynchronization pacemaker, total system [CRT-P] (00.50)*
implantation or replacement of cardiac resynchronization defibrillator pulse generator only [CRT-D] (00.54)
insertion or replacement of any type pacemaker device (37.80-37.87)

● Code new
to this edition

▲ Revision of
existing code

④ ⑤ Fourth or fifth
digit required

00.54 Implantation or replacement of cardiac resynchronization defibrillator pulse generator device only [CRT-D]

Note: Device testing during procedure—*omit code*

Implantation of CRT-D device with removal of any existing CRT-D, CRT-P, pacemaker, or defibrillator device

> *Excludes:* *implantation of automatic cardioverter/defibrillator pulse generator only (37.96)*
> *implantation of cardiac resynchronization defibrillator, total system [CRT-D] (00.51)*
> *implantation or replacement of cardiac resynchronization pacemaker pulse generator only [CRT-P] (00.53)*

00.55 Insertion of drug-eluting stent(s) of other peripheral vessel(s)

Endograft(s)
Endovascular graft(s)
Stent graft(s)

Code also any:
angioplasty of other non-coronary vessel(s) (39.50)
atherectomy of other non-coronary vessel(s) (17.56)
number of vascular stents inserted (00.45-00.48)
number of vessels treated (00.40-00.43)
procedure on vessel bifurcation (00.44)

> *Excludes:* *drug-coated peripheral stents, e.g., heparin coated (39.90)*
> *insertion of cerebrovascular stent(s) (00.63-00.65)*
> *insertion of drug-eluting coronary artery stent (36.07)*
> *insertion of drug-eluting stent(s) of superficial femoral artery (00.60)*
> *insertion of non-drug-eluting stent(s):*
> *coronary artery (36.06)*
> *peripheral vessel (39.90)*
> *that for other endovascular procedure (39.71-39.79)*

▲ **00.56 Insertion or replacement of implantable pressure sensor with lead for intracardiac or great vessel hemodynamic monitoring**

Note: The sensor is physically connected by a lead to a separately implanted monitor

Code also any associated implantation or replacement of subcutaneous monitor (00.57)

> *Excludes:* *circulatory monitoring (blood gas, arterial or venous pressure, cardiac output and coronary blood flow) (89.60-89.69)*
> *insertion of implantable pressure sensor without lead for intracardiac or great vessel hemodynamic monitoring (38.26)*

00.57 Implantation or replacement of subcutaneous device for intracardiac or great vessel hemodynamic monitoring

Implantation of monitoring device with formation of subcutaneous pocket and connection to intracardiac pressure sensor via lead

Code also any associated insertion or replacement of implanted pressure sensor with lead (00.56)

00.58 Insertion of intra-aneurysm sac pressure monitoring device (intraoperative)

Insertion of pressure sensor during endovascular repair of abdominal or thoracic aortic aneurysm(s)

00.59 Intravascular pressure measurement of coronary arteries

Includes: fractional flow reserve (FFR)

Code also any synchronous diagnostic or therapeutic procedures

> *Excludes:* *intravascular pressure measurement of intrathoracic arteries (00.67)*

00.6 Procedures on blood vessels

00.60 Insertion of drug-eluting stent(s) of superficial femoral artery

Code also any:
angioplasty of other non-coronary vessel(s) (39.50)
atherectomy of other non-coronary vessel(s) (17.56)
non-drug-eluting peripheral stents (39.90)
number of vascular stents inserted (00.45-00.48)
number of vessels treated (00.40-00.43)
procedure on vessel bifurcation (00.44)

> *Excludes:* *insertion of drug-eluting stent(s) of other peripheral vessel (00.55)*
> *that for other endovascular procedure (39.71-39.79)*

| | Valid O.R. procedure | | Non-O.R. procedure | | Nonspecific O.R. procedure | | Noncovered O.R. procedure |

▲ **00.61** **Percutaneous angioplasty of extracranial vessel(s)**
    Carotid
    Vertebral

    Code also any:
      injection or infusion of thrombolytic agent (99.10)
      number of vascular stents inserted (00.45-00.48)
      number of vessels treated (00.40-00.43)
      percutaneous atherectomy of extracranial vessel(s) (17.53)
      percutaneous insertion of carotid artery stent(s) (00.63)
      percutaneous insertion of other extracranial artery stent(s) (00.64)
      procedure on vessel bifurcation (00.44)

    | Excludes: | *angioplasty of other non-coronary vessel(s) (39.50)* |

            atherectomy of other non-coronary vessel(s) (17.56)
            removal of cerebrovascular obstruction of vessel(s) by open approach
                (38.01-38.02, 38.11-38.12, 38.31-38.32, 38.41-38.42)

▲ **00.62** **Percutaneous angioplasty of intracranial vessel(s)**
    Basilar artery
    Intracranial portion of vertebral artery

    Code also any:
      injection or infusion of thrombolytic agent (99.10)
      number of vascular stents inserted (00.45-00.48)
      number of vessels treated (00.40-00.43)
      percutaneous atherectomy of intracranial vessel(s) (17.54)
      percutaneous insertion of intracranial stent(s) (00.65)
      procedure on vessel bifurcation (00.44)

    | Excludes: | *angioplasty of other non-coronary vessel(s) (39.50)* |

            atherectomy of other non-coronary vessel(s) (17.56)
            removal of cerebrovascular obstruction of vessel(s) by open approach
                (38.01-38.02, 38.11-38.12, 38.31-38.32, 38.41-38.42)

00.63 **Percutaneous insertion of carotid artery stent(s)**
    Includes the use of any embolic protection device, distal protection device, filter
      device, or stent delivery system
    Non-drug-eluting stent

    Code also any:
      number of vascular stents inserted (00.45-00.48)
      number of vessels treated (00.40-00.43)
      percutaneous angioplasty of extracranial vessel(s) (00.61)
      percutaneous atherectomy of extracranial vessel(s) (17.53)
      procedure on vessel bifurcation (00.44)

    | Excludes: | *angioplasty of other non-coronary vessel(s) (39.50)* |

            atherectomy of other non-coronary vessel(s) (17.56)
            insertion of coil-retention or embolization stent (39.72)
            insertion of drug-eluting peripheral vessel stent(s) (00.55)

▲ **00.64** **Percutaneous insertion of other extracranial artery stent(s)**
    Includes the use of any embolic protection device, distal protection device, filter
      device, or stent delivery system
    Vertebral stent

    Code also any:
      number of vascular stents inserted (00.45-00.48)
      number of vessels treated (00.40-00.43)
      percutaneous angioplasty of extracranial vessel(s) (00.61)
      percutaneous atherectomy of extracranial vessel(s) (17.53)
      procedure on vessel bifurcation (00.44)

    | Excludes: | *angioplasty of other non-coronary vessel(s) (39.50)* |

            atherectomy of other non-coronary vessel(s) (17.56)
            insertion of coil-retention or embolization stent (39.72)
             insertion of drug-eluting peripheral vessel stent(s) (00.55)

● Code new
  to this edition
    ▲ Revision of
      existing code
    ④ ⑤ Fourth or fifth
        digit required

00.65 Percutaneous insertion of intracranial vascular stent(s)

Basilar stent

Includes the use of any embolic protection device, distal protection device, filter device, or stent delivery system

Code also any:
number of vascular stents inserted (00.45-00.48)
number of vessels treated (00.40-00.43)
percutaneous angioplasty of intracranial vessel(s) (00.62)
percutaneous atherectomy of intracranial vessel(s) (17.54)
procedure on vessel bifurcation (00.44)

Excludes: *angioplasty of other non-coronary vessel(s) (39.50)*
atherectomy of other non-coronary vessel(s) (17.56)
insertion of coil-retention or embolization stent (39.72)
insertion of drug-eluting peripheral vessel stent(s) (00.55)

▲ **00.66 Percutaneous transluminal coronary angioplasty [PTCA]**

Balloon angioplasty of coronary artery
Percutaneous coronary angioplasty NOS
PTCA NOS

Code also any:
injection or infusion of thrombolytic agent (99.10)
insertion of coronary artery stent(s) (36.06-36.07)
intracoronary artery thrombolytic infusion (36.04)
number of vascular stents inserted (00.45-00.48)
number of vessels treated (00.40-00.43)
procedure on vessel bifurcation (00.44)
SuperSaturated oxygen therapy (00.49)
transluminal coronary atherectomy (17.55)

00.67 Intravascular pressure measurement of intrathoracic arteries

Assessment of:
aorta and aortic arch
carotid

Code also any synchronous diagnostic or therapeutic procedures

00.68 Intravascular pressure measurement of peripheral arteries

Assessment of:
other peripheral vessels
vessels of arm(s)
vessels of leg(s)

Code also any synchronous diagnostic or therapeutic procedures

00.69 Intravascular pressure measurement, other specified and unspecified vessels

Iliac vessels
Intra-abdominal vessels
Mesenteric vessels
Renal vessels

Code also any synchronous diagnostic or therapeutic procedures

Excludes: *intravascular pressure measurement of:*
coronary arteries (00.59)
intrathoracic arteries (00.67)
peripheral arteries (00.68)

00.7 Other hip procedures

00.70 Revision of hip replacement, both acetabular and femoral components

Total hip revision

Code also any:
removal of (cement) (joint) spacer (84.57)
type of bearing surface, if known (00.74-00.77)

Excludes: *revision of hip replacement, acetabular component only (00.71)*
revision of hip replacement, femoral component only (00.72)
revision of hip replacement, Not Otherwise Specified (81.53)
revision with replacement of acetabular liner and/or femoral head only (00.73)

| Valid O.R. procedure | Non-O.R. procedure | Nonspecific O.R. procedure | Noncovered O.R. procedure |

00.71 Revision of hip replacement, acetabular component
Partial, acetabular component only
That with:
exchange of acetabular cup and liner
exchange of femoral head
Code also any type of bearing surface, if known (00.74-00.77)

> Excludes: *revision of hip replacement, both acetabular and femoral components (00.70)*
> *revision of hip replacement, femoral component (00.72)*
> *revision of hip replacement, Not Otherwise Specified (81.53)*
> *revision with replacement of acetabular liner and/or femoral head only (00.73)*

00.72 Revision of hip replacement, femoral component
Partial, femoral component only
That with:
exchange of acetabular liner
exchange of femoral stem and head
Code also any type of bearing surface, if known (00.74-00.77)

> Excludes: *revision of hip replacement, acetabular component (00.71)*
> *revision of hip replacement, both acetabular and femoral components (00.70)*
> *revision of hip replacement, not otherwise specified (81.53)*
> *revision with replacement of acetabular liner and/or femoral head only (00.73)*

00.73 Revision of hip replacement, acetabular liner and/or femoral head only
Code also any type of bearing surface, if known (00.74-00.77)

00.74 Hip bearing surface, metal-on-polyethylene

00.75 Hip bearing surface, metal-on-metal

00.76 Hip bearing surface, ceramic-on-ceramic

00.77 Hip bearing surface, ceramic-on-polyethylene
Hip bearing surface, oxidized zirconium-on-polyethylene

00.8 Other knee and hip procedures
Note: Report up to two components using 00.81-00.83 to describe revision of knee replacements. If all three components are revised, report 00.80.

00.80 Revision of knee replacement, total (all components)
Replacement of femoral, tibial, and patellar components (all components)
Code also any removal of (cement) (joint) spacer (84.57)

> Excludes: *revision of only one or two components (tibial, femoral or patellar component) (00.81-00.84)*

00.81 Revision of knee replacement, tibial component
Replacement of tibial baseplate and tibial insert (liner)

> Excludes: *revision of knee replacement, total (all components) (00.80)*

00.82 Revision of knee replacement, femoral component
That with replacement of tibial insert (liner)

> Excludes: *revision of knee replacement, total (all components) (00.80)*

00.83 Revision of knee replacement, patellar component

> Excludes: *revision of knee replacement, total (all components) (00.80)*

00.84 Revision of total knee replacement, tibial insert (liner)
Replacement of tibial insert (liner)

> Excludes: *that with replacement of tibial component (tibial baseplate and liner) (00.81)*

00.85 Resurfacing hip, total, acetabulum and femoral head
Hip resurfacing arthroplasty, total

00.86 Resurfacing hip, partial, femoral head
Hip resurfacing arthroplasty, NOS
Hip resurfacing arthroplasty, partial, femoral head

> Excludes: *that with resurfacing of acetabulum (00.85)*

00.87 Resurfacing hip, partial, acetabulum
Hip resurfacing arthroplasty, partial, acetabulum

> Excludes: *that with resurfacing of femoral head (00.85)*

● Code new to this edition   ▲ Revision of existing code   ④ ⑤ Fourth or fifth digit required

00.9   **Other procedures and interventions**

    00.91   **Transplant from live related donor**
        Code also organ transplant procedure

    00.92   **Transplant from live non-related donor**
        Code also organ transplant procedure

    00.93   **Transplant from cadaver**
        Code also organ transplant procedure

    00.94   **Intra-operative neurophysiologic monitoring**
        Includes: Cranial nerve, peripheral nerve and spinal cord testing performed intra-operatively

        Intra-operative neurophysiologic testing
        IOM
        Nerve monitoring
        Neuromonitoring
        That by:
          brainstem auditory evoked potentials [BAEP]
          electroencephalogram [EEG]
          electromyogram [EMG]
          motor evoked potentials [MEP]
          nerve conduction study
          somatosensory evoked potentials [SSEP]
          transcranial Doppler

        | Excludes: | *brain temperature monitoring (01.17)* |
        intracranial oxygen monitoring (01.16)
        intracranial pressure monitoring (01.10)
        plethysmogram (89.58)

01   **Incision and excision of skull, brain, and cerebral meninges**

  01.0   **Cranial puncture**

    01.01   **Cisternal puncture**
        Cisternal tap

        | Excludes: | *pneumocisternogram (87.02)* |

    01.02   **Ventriculopuncture through previously implanted catheter**
        Puncture of ventricular shunt tubing

    01.09   **Other cranial puncture**
        Aspiration of
          subarachnoid space
          subdural space
        Cranial aspiration NOS
        Puncture of anterior fontanel
        Subdural tap (through fontanel)

  01.1   **Diagnostic procedures on skull, brain, and cerebral meninges**

    01.10   **Intracranial pressure monitoring**
        Includes: insertion of catheter or probe for monitoring

    01.11   **Closed [percutaneous] [needle] biopsy of cerebral meninges**
        Burr hole approach

    01.12   **Open biopsy of cerebral meninges**

    01.13   **Closed [percutaneous] [needle] biopsy of brain**
        Burr hole approach
        Stereotactic method

    01.14   **Open biopsy of brain**

    01.15   **Biopsy of skull**

    01.16   **Intracranial oxygen monitoring**
        Includes: insertion of catheter or probe for monitoring
        Partial pressure of brain oxygen ($PbtO_2$)

    01.17   **Brain temperature monitoring**
        Includes: insertion of catheter or probe for monitoring

| | Valid O.R. procedure | | Non-O.R. procedure | | Nonspecific O.R. procedure | | Noncovered O.R. procedure |

01.18 Other diagnostic procedures on brain and cerebral meninges

> Excludes: *brain temperature monitoring (01.17)*
> *cerebral:*
>   *arteriography (88.41)*
>   *thermography (88.81)*
> *contrast radiogram of brain (87.01-87.02)*
> *echoencephalogram (88.71)*
> *electroencephalogram (89.14)*
> *intracranial oxygen monitoring (01.16)*
> *intracranial pressure monitoring (01.10)*
> *microscopic examination of specimen from nervous system and of*
>   *spinal fluid (90.01-90.09)*
> *neurologic examination (89.13)*
> *phlebography of head and neck (88.61)*
> *pneumoencephalogram (87.01)*
> *radioisotope scan:*
>   *cerebral (92.11)*
>   *head NEC (92.12)*
> *tomography of head:*
>   *C.A.T. scan (87.03)*
>   *other (87.04)*

01.19 Other diagnostic procedures on skull

> Excludes: *transillumination of skull (89.16)*
> *x-ray of skull (87.17)*

01.2 Craniotomy and craniectomy

> Excludes: *decompression of skull fracture (02.02)*
> *exploration of orbit (16.01-16.09)*
> *that as operative approach—omit code*

01.20 Cranial implantation or replacement of neurostimulator pulse generator
Code also any associated lead implantation (02.93)

> Excludes: *implantation or replacement of subcutaneous neurostimulator pulse*
> *generator (86.94 -86.98)*

01.21 Incision and drainage of cranial sinus

01.22 Removal of intracranial neurostimulator lead(s)
Code also any removal of neurostimulator pulse generator (86.05)

> Excludes: *removal with synchronous replacement (02.93)*

01.23 Reopening of craniotomy site

01.24 Other craniotomy
Cranial decompression
Cranial exploration
Cranial trephination
Craniotomy NOS
Craniotomy with removal of epidural abscess
Craniotomy with removal of extradural hematoma
Craniotomy with removal of foreign body of skull

> Excludes: *removal of foreign body with incision into brain (01.39)*

01.25 Other craniectomy
Debridement of skull NOS
Sequestrectomy of skull

> Excludes: *debridement of compound fracture of skull (02.02)*
> *strip craniectomy (02.01)*

01.26 Insertion of catheter(s) into cranial cavity or tissue
Code also any concomitant procedure (e.g. resection (01.59))

> Excludes: *placement of intracerebral catheter(s) via burr hole(s) (01.28)*

01.27 Removal of catheter(s) from cranial cavity or tissue

01.28 Placement of intracerebral catheter(s) via burr hole(s)
Convection enhanced delivery
Stereotactic placement of intracerebral catheter(s)
Code also infusion of medication

> Excludes: *insertion of catheter(s) into cranial cavity or tissue(s) (01.26)*

● Code new
to this edition ▲ Revision of
existing code ④ ⑤ Fourth or fifth
digit required

01.29 Removal of cranial neurostimulator pulse generator

01.3 Incision of brain and cerebral meninges

01.31 Incision of cerebral meninges
Drainage of:
intracranial hygroma
subarachnoid abscess (cerebral)
subdural empyema

01.32 Lobotomy and tractotomy
Division of:
brain tissue
cerebral tracts
Percutaneous (radio frequency) cingulotomy

01.39 Other incision of brain
Amygdalohippocampotomy
Drainage of intracerebral hematoma
Incision of brain NOS

Excludes: *division of cortical adhesions (02.91)*

01.4 Operations on thalamus and globus pallidus

01.41 Operations on thalamus
Chemothalamectomy
Thalamotomy

Excludes: *that by stereotactic radiosurgery (92.30-92.39)*

01.42 Operations on globus pallidus
Pallidoansectomy
Pallidotomy

Excludes: *that by stereotactic radiosurgery (92.30-92.39)*

01.5 Other excision or destruction of brain and meninges

01.51 Excision of lesion or tissue of cerebral meninges
Decortication of (cerebral) meninges
Resection of (cerebral) meninges
Stripping of subdural membrane of (cerebral) meninges

Excludes: *biopsy of cerebral meninges (01.11-01.12)*

01.52 Hemispherectomy

01.53 Lobectomy of brain

01.59 Other excision or destruction of lesion or tissue of brain
Amygdalohippocampectomy
Curettage of brain
Debridement of brain
Marsupialization of brain cyst
Transtemporal (mastoid) excision of brain tumor

Excludes: *biopsy of brain (01.13-01.14)*
laser interstitial thermal therapy [LITT] of lesion or tissue of brain under guidance (17.61)
that by stereotactic radiosurgery (92.30-92.39)

01.6 Excision of lesion of skull
Removal of granulation tissue of cranium

Excludes: *biopsy of skull (01.15)*
sequestrectomy (01.25)

02 Other operations on skull, brain, and cerebral meninges

02.0 Cranioplasty

Excludes: *that with synchronous repair of encephalocele (02.12)*

02.01 Opening of cranial suture
Linear craniectomy
Strip craniectomy

02.02 Elevation of skull fracture fragments
Debridement of compound fracture of skull
Decompression of skull fracture
Reduction of skull fracture

Code also any synchronous debridement of brain (01.59)

Excludes: *debridement of skull NOS (01.25)*
removal of granulation tissue of cranium (01.6)

Valid O.R. procedure | Non-O.R. procedure | Nonspecific O.R. procedure | Noncovered O.R. procedure

02.03 Formation of cranial bone flap
Repair of skull with flap

02.04 Bone graft to skull
Pericranial graft (autogenous) (heterogenous)

02.05 Insertion of skull plate
Replacement of skull plate

02.06 Other cranial osteoplasty
Repair of skull NOS
Revision of bone flap of skull

02.07 Removal of skull plate
Excludes: removal with synchronous replacement (02.05)

02.1 Repair of cerebral meninges
Excludes: marsupialization of cerebral lesion (01.59)

02.11 Simple suture of dura mater of brain

02.12 Other repair of cerebral meninges
Closure of fistula of cerebrospinal fluid
Dural graft
Repair of encephalocele including synchronous cranioplasty
Repair of meninges NOS
Subdural patch

02.13 Ligation of meningeal vessel
Ligation of:
longitudinal sinus
middle meningeal artery

02.14 Choroid plexectomy
Cauterization of choroid plexus

● **02.2 Ventriculostomy**

● **02.21 Insertion or replacement of external ventricular drain [EVD]**
External ventricular drainage [EVD] setup
Replacement of external ventricular drain
Ventricular catheter placement for:
drainage of cerebrospinal fluid [CSF]
injection of medication or other substance
sampling of cerebrospinal fluid [CSF]
Excludes: extracranial ventricular shunt (02.31-02.35, 02.39)
intracranial ventricular shunt (02.22)
other cranial puncture (01.09)
ventricular shunt replacement (02.41-02.43)

● **02.22 Intracranial ventricular shunt or anastomosis**
Anastomosis of ventricle to:
cervical subarachnoid space
cistern magna
Insertion of Holter valve into intracranial system
Shunt between two intracranial ventricles
That by endoscopy
Third ventriculostomy
Ventriculocisternostomy

02.3 Extracranial ventricular shunt
Includes: that with insertion of valve

02.31 Ventricular shunt to structure in head and neck
Ventricle to nasopharynx shunt
Ventriculomastoid anastomosis

02.32 Ventricular shunt to circulatory system
Ventriculoatrial anastomosis
Ventriculocaval shunt

02.33 Ventricular shunt to thoracic cavity
Ventriculopleural anastomosis

02.34 Ventricular shunt to abdominal cavity and organs
Ventriculocholecystostomy
Ventriculoperitoneostomy

02.35 Ventricular shunt to urinary system
Ventricle to ureter shunt

● Code new to this edition   ▲ Revision of existing code   ④ ⑤ Fourth or fifth digit required

▲ **02.39** **Ventricular shunt to extracranial site NEC**
Ventricle to bone marrow shunt

02.4 **Revision, removal, and irrigation of ventricular shunt**

Excludes: *revision of distal catheter of ventricular shunt (54.95)*

02.41 **Irrigation and exploration of ventricular shunt**
Exploration of ventriculoperitoneal shunt at ventricular site
Re-programming of ventriculoperitoneal shunt

02.42 **Replacement of ventricular shunt**
Reinsertion of Holter valve
Revision of ventriculoperitoneal shunt at ventricular site

02.43 **Removal of ventricular shunt**

02.9 **Other operations on skull, brain, and cerebral meninges**

Excludes: *operations on:*
pineal gland (07.17, 07.51-07.59)
pituitary gland [hypophysis] (07.13-07.15, 07.61-07.79)

02.91 **Lysis of cortical adhesions**

02.92 **Repair of brain**

02.93 **Implantation or replacement of intracranial neurostimulator lead(s)**
Implantation, insertion, placement, or replacement of intracranial:
brain pacemaker [neuropacemaker]
depth electrodes
electroencephalographic receiver
epidural pegs
foramen ovale electrodes
intracranial electrostimulator
subdural grids
subdural strips

Code also any:
insertion of cranial implantation or replacement of neurostimulator pulse generator
(01.20)
insertion of subcutaneous neurostimulator pulse generator (86.94-86.98)

02.94 **Insertion or replacement of skull tongs or halo traction device**

02.95 **Removal of skull tongs or halo traction device**

02.96 **Insertion of sphenoidal electrodes**

02.99 **Other**

Excludes: *chemical shock therapy (94.24)*
electroshock therapy:
subconvulsive (94.26)
other (94.27)

03 **Operations on spinal cord and spinal canal structures**
Code also any application or administration of an adhesion barrier substance (99.77)

03.0 **Exploration and decompression of spinal canal structures**

03.01 **Removal of foreign body from spinal canal**

03.02 **Reopening of laminectomy site**

03.09 **Other exploration and decompression of spinal canal**
Decompression:
laminectomy
laminotomy
Expansile laminoplasty
Exploration of spinal nerve root
Foraminotomy

*Code also any synchronous insertion, replacement and revision of posterior spinal
motion preservation device(s), if performed (84.80 - 84.85)*

Excludes: *drainage of spinal fluid by anastomosis (03.71-03.79)*
laminectomy with excision of intervertebral disc (80.51)
spinal tap (03.31)
that as operative approach—omit code

03.1 **Division of intraspinal nerve root**
Rhizotomy

	Valid O.R. procedure		Non-O.R. procedure		Nonspecific O.R. procedure		Noncovered O.R. procedure

03.2   Chordotomy

03.21   Percutaneous chordotomy
Stereotactic chordotomy

03.29   Other chordotomy
Chordotomy NOS
Tractotomy (one-stage) (two-stage) of spinal cord
Transection of spinal cord tracts

03.3   Diagnostic procedures on spinal cord and spinal canal structures

03.31   Spinal tap
Lumbar puncture for removal of dye

> *Excludes:*   *lumbar puncture for injection of dye [myelogram] (87.21)*

03.32   Biopsy of spinal cord or spinal meninges

03.39   Other diagnostic procedures on spinal cord and spinal canal structures

> *Excludes:*   *microscopic examination of specimen from nervous system or of spinal*
> *fluid (90.01-90.09)*
> *x-ray of spine (87.21-87.29)*

03.4   Excision or destruction of lesion of spinal cord or spinal meninges
Curettage of spinal cord or spinal meninges
Debridement of spinal cord or spinal meninges
Marsupialization of cyst of spinal cord or spinal meninges
Resection of spinal cord or spinal meninges

> *Excludes:*   *biopsy of spinal cord or meninges (03.32)*

03.5   Plastic operations on spinal cord structures

03.51   Repair of spinal meningocele
Repair of meningocele NOS

03.52   Repair of spinal myelomeningocele

03.53   Repair of vertebral fracture
Elevation of spinal bone fragments
Reduction of fracture of vertebrae
Removal of bony spicules from spinal canal

> *Excludes:*   *percutaneous vertebral augmentation (81.66)*
> *percutaneous vertebroplasty (81.65)*

03.59   Other repair and plastic operations on spinal cord structures
Repair of:
diastematomyelia
spina bifida NOS
spinal cord NOS
spinal meninges NOS
vertebral arch defect

03.6   Lysis of adhesions of spinal cord and nerve roots

03.7   Shunt of spinal theca
Includes: that with valve

03.71   Spinal subarachnoid-peritoneal shunt

03.72   Spinal subarachnoid-ureteral shunt

03.79   Other shunt of spinal theca
Lumbar-subarachnoid shunt NOS
Pleurothecal anastomosis
Salpingothecal anastomosis

03.8   Injection of destructive agent into spinal canal

03.9   Other operations on spinal cord and spinal canal structures

03.90   Insertion of catheter into spinal canal for infusion of therapeutic or palliative
substances
Insertion of catheter into epidural, subarachnoid, or subdural space of spine with
intermittent or continuous infusion of drug (with creation of any reservoir)
Code also any implantation of infusion pump (86.06)

03.91   Injection of anesthetic into spinal canal for analgesia

> *Excludes:*   *that for operative anesthesia—omit code*

● Code new
to this edition
▲ Revision of
existing code
④ ⑤ Fourth or fifth
digit required

03.92 **Injection of other agent into spinal canal**
Intrathecal injection of steroid
Subarachnoid perfusion of refrigerated saline

Excludes: *injection of:*
contrast material for myelogram (87.21)
destructive agent into spinal canal (03.8)

03.93 **Implantation or replacement of spinal neurostimulator lead(s)**
Code also any insertion of neurostimulator pulse generator (86.94-86.98)

03.94 **Removal of spinal neurostimulator lead(s)**
Code also any removal of neurostimulator pulse generator (86.05)

03.95 **Spinal blood patch**

03.96 **Percutaneous denervation of facet**

03.97 **Revision of spinal thecal shunt**

03.98 **Removal of spinal thecal shunt**

03.99 **Other**

04 **Operations on cranial and peripheral nerves**

04.0 **Incision, division, and excision of cranial and peripheral nerves**

Excludes: *opticociliary neurectomy (12.79)*
sympathetic ganglionectomy (05.21-05.29)

04.01 **Excision of acoustic neuroma**
That by craniotomy

Excludes: *that by stereotactic radiosurgery (92.3)*

04.02 **Division of trigeminal nerve**
Retrogasserian neurotomy

04.03 **Division or crushing of other cranial and peripheral nerves**

Excludes: *that of:*
glossopharyngeal nerve (29.92)
laryngeal nerve (31.91)
nerves to adrenal glands (07.42)
phrenic nerve for collapse of lung (33.31)
vagus nerve (44.00-44.03)

04.04 **Other incision of cranial and peripheral nerves**

04.05 **Gasserian ganglionectomy**

04.06 **Other cranial or peripheral ganglionectomy**

Excludes: *sympathetic ganglionectomy (05.21-05.29)*

04.07 **Other excision or avulsion of cranial and peripheral nerves**
Curettage of peripheral nerve
Debridement of peripheral nerve
Resection of peripheral nerve
Excision of peripheral neuroma [Morton's]

Excludes: *biopsy of cranial or peripheral nerve (04.11-04.12)*

04.1 **Diagnostic procedures on peripheral nervous system**

04.11 **Closed [percutaneous] [needle] biopsy of cranial or peripheral nerve or ganglion**

04.12 **Open biopsy of cranial or peripheral nerve or ganglion**

04.19 **Other diagnostic procedures on cranial and peripheral nerves and ganglia**

Excludes: *microscopic examination of specimen from nervous system*
(90.01-90.09)
neurologic examination (89.13)

04.2 **Destruction of cranial and peripheral nerves**
Destruction of cranial or peripheral nerves by:
cryoanalgesia
injection of neurolytic agent
radiofrequency
Radiofrequency ablation

04.3 **Suture of cranial and peripheral nerves**

04.4 **Lysis of adhesions and decompression of cranial and peripheral nerves**

04.41 **Decompression of trigeminal nerve root**

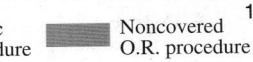

Valid O.R.
procedure

Non-O.R.
procedure

Nonspecific
O.R. procedure

Noncovered
O.R. procedure

04.42 Other cranial nerve decompression

04.43 Release of carpal tunnel

04.44 Release of tarsal tunnel

04.49 Other peripheral nerve or ganglion decompression or lysis of adhesions
Peripheral nerve neurolysis NOS

04.5 Cranial or peripheral nerve graft

04.6 Transposition of cranial and peripheral nerves
Nerve transplantation

04.7 Other cranial or peripheral neuroplasty

04.71 Hypoglossal-facial anastomosis

04.72 Accessory-facial anastomosis

04.73 Accessory-hypoglossal anastomosis

04.74 Other anastomosis of cranial or peripheral nerve

04.75 Revision of previous repair of cranial and peripheral nerves

04.76 Repair of old traumatic injury of cranial and peripheral nerves

04.79 Other neuroplasty

04.8 Injection into peripheral nerve

Excludes: *destruction of nerve (by injection of neurolytic agent) (04.2)*

04.80 Peripheral nerve injection, not otherwise specified

04.81 Injection of anesthetic into peripheral nerve for analgesia

Excludes: *that for operative anesthesia—omit code*

04.89 Injection of other agent, except neurolytic

Excludes: *injection of neurolytic agent (04.2)*

04.9 Other operations on cranial and peripheral nerves

04.91 Neurectasis

04.92 Implantation or replacement of peripheral neurostimulator lead(s)

Code also any insertion of neurostimulator pulse generator (86.94-86.98)

Excludes: *implantation or replacement of carotid sinus stimulation lead(s) (39.82)*

04.93 Removal of peripheral neurostimulator lead(s)

Code also any removal of neurostimulator pulse generator (86.05)

04.99 Other

05 Operations on sympathetic nerves or ganglia

Excludes: *paracervical uterine denervation (69.3)*

05.0 Division of sympathetic nerve or ganglion

Excludes: *that of nerves to adrenal glands (07.42)*

05.1 Diagnostic procedures on sympathetic nerves or ganglia

05.11 Biopsy of sympathetic nerve or ganglion

05.19 Other diagnostic procedures on sympathetic nerves or ganglia

05.2 Sympathectomy

05.21 Sphenopalatine ganglionectomy

05.22 Cervical sympathectomy

05.23 Lumber sympathectomy

05.24 Presacral sympathectomy

05.25 Periarterial sympathectomy

05.29 Other sympathectomy and ganglionectomy
Excision or avulsion of sympathetic nerve NOS
Sympathetic ganglionectomy NOS

Excludes: *biopsy of sympathetic nerve or ganglion (05.11)*
opticociliary neurectomy (12.79)
periarterial sympathectomy (05.25)
tympanosympathectomy (20.91)

● Code new to this edition   ▲ Revision of existing code   ④ ⑤ Fourth or fifth digit required

05.3   Injection into sympathetic nerve or ganglion

     Excludes: *injection of ciliary sympathetic ganglion (12.79)*

     05.31   Injection of anesthetic into sympathetic nerve for analgesia

     05.32   Injection of neurolytic agent into sympathetic nerve

     05.39   Other injection into sympathetic nerve or ganglion

05.8   Other operations on sympathetic nerves or ganglion

     05.81   Repair of sympathetic nerve or ganglion

     05.89   Other

05.9   Other operations on nervous system

| Valid O.R. procedure | Non-O.R. procedure | Nonspecific O.R. procedure | Noncovered O.R. procedure |

This page intentionally left blank.

● Code new
to this edition

▲ Revision of
existing code

④ ⑤ Fourth or fifth
digit required

2. OPERATIONS ON THE ENDOCRINE SYSTEM (06-07)

06 Operations on thyroid and parathyroid glands
Includes: incidental resection of hyoid bone

06.0 Incision of thyroid field

> *Excludes:* *division of isthmus (06.91)*

06.01 Aspiration of thyroid field
Percutaneous or needle drainage of thyroid field

> *Excludes:* *aspiration biopsy of thyroid (06.11)*
> *drainage by incision (06.09)*
> *postoperative aspiration of field (06.02)*

06.02 Reopening of wound of thyroid field
Reopening of wound of thyroid field for:
control of (postoperative) hemorrhage
examination
exploration
removal of hematoma

06.09 Other incision of thyroid field
Drainage of hematoma by incision
Drainage of thyroglossal tract by incision
Exploration by incision:
    neck
    thyroid (field)
Removal of foreign body by incision
Thyroidotomy NOS by incision

> *Excludes:* *postoperative exploration (06.02)*
> *removal of hematoma by aspiration (06.01)*

06.1 Diagnostic procedures on thyroid and parathyroid glands

06.11 Closed [percutaneous] [needle] biopsy of thyroid gland
Aspiration biopsy of thyroid

06.12 Open biopsy of thyroid gland

06.13 Biopsy of parathyroid gland

06.19 Other diagnostic procedures on thyroid and parathyroid glands

> *Excludes:* *radioisotope scan of:*
> *parathyroid (92.13)*
> *thyroid (92.01)*
> *soft tissue x-ray of thyroid field (87.09)*

06.2 Unilateral thyroid lobectomy
Complete removal of one lobe of thyroid (with removal of isthmus or portion of other lobe)
Hemithyroidectomy

> *Excludes:* *partial substernal thyroidectomy (06.51)*

06.3 Other partial thyroidectomy

06.31 Excision of lesion of thyroid

> *Excludes:* *biopsy of thyroid (06.11-06.12)*
> *laser interstitial thermal therapy [LITT] of lesion or tissue of neck*
> *under guidance (17.62)*

06.39 Other
Isthmectomy
Partial thyroidectomy NOS

> *Excludes:* *partial substernal thyroidectomy (06.51)*

06.4 Complete thyroidectomy

> *Excludes:* *complete substernal thyroidectomy (06.52)*
> *that with laryngectomy (30.3-30.4)*

06.5 Substernal thyroidectomy

06.50 Substernal thyroidectomy, not otherwise specified

06.51 Partial substernal thyroidectomy

06.52 Complete substernal thyroidectomy

Valid O.R. procedure   Non-O.R. procedure   Nonspecific O.R. procedure   Noncovered O.R. procedure

06.6 **Excision of lingual thyroid**
Excision of thyroid by:
submental route
transoral route

06.7 **Excision of thyroglossal duct or tract**

06.8 **Parathyroidectomy**

> **06.81** **Complete parathyroidectomy**

> **06.89** **Other parathyroidectomy**
> Parathyroidectomy NOS
> Partial parathyroidectomy
>
> > *Excludes:* *biopsy of parathyroid (06.13)*

06.9 **Other operations on thyroid (region) and parathyroid**

> **06.91** **Division of thyroid isthmus**
> Transection of thyroid isthmus

> **06.92** **Ligation of thyroid vessels**

> **06.93** **Suture of thyroid gland**

> **06.94** **Thyroid tissue reimplantation**
> Autotransplantation of thyroid tissue

> **06.95** **Parathyroid tissue reimplantation**
> Autotransplantation of parathyroid tissue

> **06.98** **Other operations on thyroid glands**

> **06.99** **Other operations on parathyroid glands**

07 **Operations on other endocrine glands**
Includes: operations on:
adrenal glands
pineal gland
pituitary gland
thymus

> *Excludes:* *operations on:*
> *aortic and carotid bodies (39.81-39.89)*
> *ovaries (65.0-65.99)*
> *pancreas (52.01-52.99)*
> *testes (62.0-62.99)*

07.0 **Exploration of adrenal field**

> *Excludes:* *incision of adrenal gland (07.41)*

> **07.00** **Exploration of adrenal field, not otherwise specified**

> **07.01** **Unilateral exploration of adrenal field**

> **07.02** **Bilateral exploration of adrenal field**

07.1 **Diagnostic procedures on adrenal glands, pituitary gland, pineal gland, and thymus**

> **07.11** **Closed [percutaneous] [needle] biopsy of adrenal gland**

> **07.12** **Open biopsy of adrenal gland**

> **07.13** **Biopsy of pituitary gland, transfrontal approach**

> **07.14** **Biopsy of pituitary gland, transsphenoidal approach**

> **07.15** **Biopsy of pituitary gland, unspecified approach**

> **07.16** **Biopsy of thymus**

> **07.17** **Biopsy of pineal gland**

> **07.19** **Other diagnostic procedures on adrenal glands, pituitary gland, pineal gland, and thymus**
>
> > *Excludes:* *microscopic examination of specimen from endocrine gland (90.11-90.19)*
> > *radioisotope scan of pituitary gland (92.11)*

07.2 **Partial adrenalectomy**

> **07.21** **Excision of lesion of adrenal gland**
>
> > *Excludes:* *biopsy of adrenal gland (07.11-07.12)*

> **07.22** **Unilateral adrenalectomy**
> Adrenalectomy NOS
>
> > *Excludes:* *excision of remaining adrenal gland (07.3)*

● Code new
to this edition ▲ Revision of
existing code ④ ⑤ Fourth or fifth
digit required

07.29 Other partial adrenalectomy
Partial adrenalectomy NOS

07.3 Bilateral adrenalectomy
Excision of remaining adrenal gland

> Excludes: bilateral partial adrenalectomy (07.29)

07.4 Other operations on adrenal glands, nerves, and vessels

07.41 Incision of adrenal gland
Adrenalotomy (with drainage)

07.42 Division of nerves to adrenal glands

07.43 Ligation of adrenal vessels

07.44 Repair of adrenal gland

07.45 Reimplantation of adrenal tissue
Autotransplantation of adrenal tissue

07.49 Other

07.5 Operations on pineal gland

07.51 Exploration of pineal field

> Excludes: that with incision of pineal gland (07.52)

07.52 Incision of pineal gland

07.53 Partial excision of pineal gland

> Excludes: biopsy of pineal gland (07.17)

07.54 Total excision of pineal gland
Pinealectomy (complete) (total)

07.59 Other operations on pineal gland

07.6 Hypophysectomy

07.61 Partial excision of pituitary gland, transfrontal approach
Cryohypophysectomy, partial, transfrontal approach
Division of hypophyseal stalk, transfrontal approach
Excision of lesion of pituitary [hypophysis], transfrontal approach
Hypophysectomy, subtotal, transfrontal approach
Infundibulectomy, hypophyseal, transfrontal approach

> Excludes: biopsy of pituitary gland, transfrontal approach (07.13)

07.62 Partial excision of pituitary gland, transsphenoidal approach

> Excludes: biopsy of pituitary gland, transsphenoidal approach (07.14)

07.63 Partial excision of pituitary gland, unspecified approach

> Excludes: biopsy of pituitary gland NOS (07.15)

07.64 Total excision of pituitary gland, transfrontal approach
Ablation of pituitary by implantation (strontium-yttrium) (Y), transfrontal approach
Cryohypophysectomy, complete, transfrontal approach

07.65 Total excision of pituitary gland, transsphenoidal approach

07.68 Total excision of pituitary gland, other specified approach

07.69 Total excision of pituitary gland, unspecified approach
Hypophysectomy NOS
Pituitectomy NOS

07.7 Other operations on hypophysis

07.71 Exploration of pituitary fossa

> Excludes: exploration with incision of pituitary gland (07.72)

07.72 Incision of pituitary gland
Aspiration of:
craniobuccal pouch
craniopharyngioma
hypophysis
pituitary gland
Rathke's pouch

07.79 Other
Insertion of pack into sella turcica

07.8 Thymectomy

07.80 **Thymectomy, not otherwise specified**

07.81 **Other partial excision of thymus**
Open partial excision of thymus

> Excludes: *biopsy of thymus (07.16)*
> *thoracoscopic partial excision of thymus (07.83)*

07.82 **Other total excision of thymus**
Open total excision of thymus

> Excludes: *thoracoscopic total excision of thymus (07.84)*

07.83 **Thoracoscopic partial excision of thymus**

> Excludes: *other partial excision of thymus (07.81)*

07.84 **Thoracoscopic total excision of thymus**

> Excludes: *other total excision of thymus (07.82)*

07.9 **Other operations on thymus**

07.91 **Exploration of thymus field**

> Excludes: *exploration with incision of thymus (07.92)*

07.92 **Other incision of thymus**
Open incision of thymus

> Excludes: *thoracoscopic incision of thymus (07.95)*

07.93 **Repair of thymus**

07.94 **Transplantation of thymus**

07.95 **Thoracoscopic incision of thymus**

> Excludes: *other incision of thymus (07.92)*

07.98 **Other and unspecified thoracoscopic operations on thymus**

07.99 **Other and unspecified operations on thymus**
Transcervical thymectomy

> Excludes: *other thoracoscopic operations on thymus (07.98)*

3. **OPERATIONS ON THE EYE (08-16)**

08 **Operations on eyelids**
    Includes: operations on the eyebrow

    08.0 **Incision of eyelid**

        08.01 **Incision of lid margin**

        08.02 **Severing of blepharorrhaphy**

        08.09 **Other incision of eyelid**

    08.1 **Diagnostic procedures on eyelid**

        08.11 **Biopsy of eyelid**

        08.19 **Other diagnostic procedures on eyelid**

    08.2 **Excision or destruction of lesion or tissue of eyelid**
    Code also any synchronous reconstruction (08.61-08.74)
    Excludes: *biopsy of eyelid (08.11)*

        08.20 **Removal of lesion of eyelid, not otherwise specified**
    Removal of meibomian gland NOS

        08.21 **Excision of chalazion**

        08.22 **Excision of other minor lesion of eyelid**
    Excision of:
    verruca
    wart

        08.23 **Excision of major lesion of eyelid, partial-thickness**
    Excision involving one-fourth or more of lid margin, partial-thickness

        08.24 **Excision of major lesion of eyelid, full-thickness**
    Excision involving one-fourth or more of lid margin, full-thickness
    Wedge resection of eyelid

        08.25 **Destruction of lesion of eyelid**

    08.3 **Repair of blepharoptosis and lid retraction**

        08.31 **Repair of blepharoptosis by frontalis muscle technique with suture**

        08.32 **Repair of blepharoptosis by frontalis muscle technique with fascial sling**

        08.33 **Repair of blepharoptosis by resection or advancement of levator muscle or aponeurosis**

        08.34 **Repair of blepharoptosis by other levator muscle techniques**

        08.35 **Repair of blepharoptosis by tarsal technique**

        08.36 **Repair of blepharoptosis by other techniques**
    Correction of eyelid ptosis NOS
    Orbicularis oculi muscle sling for correction of blepharoptosis

        08.37 **Reduction of overcorrection of ptosis**

        08.38 **Correction of lid retraction**

    08.4 **Repair of entropion or ectropion**

        08.41 **Repair of entropion or ectropion by thermocauterization**

        08.42 **Repair of entropion or ectropion by suture technique**

        08.43 **Repair of entropion or ectropion with wedge resection**

        08.44 **Repair of entropion or ectropion with lid reconstruction**

        08.49 **Other repair of entropion or ectropion**

    08.5 **Other adjustment of lid position**

        08.51 **Canthotomy**
    Enlargement of palpebral fissure

        08.52 **Blepharorrhaphy**
    Canthorrhaphy
    Tarsorrhaphy

        08.59 **Other**
    Canthoplasty NOS
    Repair of epicanthal fold

    08.6 **Reconstruction of eyelid with flaps or grafts**
    Excludes: *that associated with repair of entropion and ectropion (08.44)*

| Valid O.R. procedure | Non-O.R. procedure | Nonspecific O.R. procedure | Noncovered O.R. procedure |

08.61 Reconstruction of eyelid with skin flap or graft

08.62 Reconstruction of eyelid with mucous membrane flap or graft

08.63 Reconstruction of eyelid with hair follicle graft

08.64 Reconstruction of eyelid with tarsoconjunctival flap
Transfer of tarsoconjunctival flap from opposing lid

08.69 Other reconstruction of eyelid with flap or graft

08.7 Other reconstruction of eyelid

Excludes: *that associated with repair of entropion and ectropion (08.44)*

08.70 Reconstruction of eyelid, not otherwise specified

08.71 Reconstruction of eyelid involving lid margin, partial-thickness

08.72 Other reconstruction of eyelid, partial-thickness

08.73 Reconstruction of eyelid involving lid margin, full-thickness

08.74 Other reconstruction of eyelid, full-thickness

08.8 Other repair of eyelid

08.81 Linear repair of laceration of eyelid or eyebrow

08.82 Repair of laceration involving lid margin, partial-thickness

08.83 Other repair of laceration of eyelid, partial-thickness

08.84 Repair of laceration involving lid margin, full-thickness

08.85 Other repair of laceration of eyelid, full-thickness

08.86 Lower eyelid rhytidectomy

08.87 Upper eyelid rhytidectomy

08.89 Other eyelid repair

08.9 Other operations on eyelids

08.91 Electrosurgical epilation of eyelid

08.92 Cryosurgical epilation of eyelid

08.93 Other epilation of eyelid

08.99 Other

09 Operations on lacrimal system

09.0 Incision of lacrimal gland
Incision of lacrimal cyst (with drainage)

09.1 Diagnostic procedures on lacrimal system

09.11 Biopsy of lacrimal gland

09.12 Biopsy of lacrimal sac

09.19 Other diagnostic procedures on lacrimal system

Excludes: *contrast dacryocystogram (87.05)*
soft tissue x-ray of nasolacrimal duct (87.09)

09.2 Excision of lesion or tissue of lacrimal gland

09.20 Excision of lacrimal gland, not otherwise specified

09.21 Excision of lesion of lacrimal gland

Excludes: *biopsy of lacrimal gland (09.11)*

09.22 Other partial dacryoadenectomy

Excludes: *biopsy of lacrimal gland (09.11)*

09.23 Total dacryoadenectomy

09.3 Other operations on lacrimal gland

09.4 Manipulation of lacrimal passage
Includes: removal of calculus
that with dilation

Excludes: *contrast dacryocystogram (87.05)*

09.41 Probing of lacrimal punctum

09.42 Probing of lacrimal canaliculi

09.43 Probing of nasolacrimal duct

Excludes: *that with insertion of tube or stent (09.44)*

● Code new
to this edition

▲ Revision of
existing code

④ ⑤ Fourth or fifth
digit required

09.44 Intubation of nasolacrimal duct
Insertion of stent into nasolacrimal duct

09.49 Other manipulation of lacrimal passage

09.5 **Incision of lacrimal sac and passages**

09.51 Incision of lacrimal punctum

09.52 Incision of lacrimal canaliculi

09.53 Incision of lacrimal sac

09.59 Other incision of lacrimal passages
Incision (and drainage) of nasolacrimal duct NOS

09.6 Excision of lacrimal sac and passage
Excludes: *biopsy of lacrimal sac (09.12)*

09.7 **Repair of canaliculus and punctum**
Excludes: *repair of eyelid (08.81-08.89)*

09.71 Correction of everted punctum

09.72 Other repair of punctum

09.73 Repair of canaliculus

09.8 **Fistulization of lacrimal tract to nasal cavity**

09.81 Dacryocystorhinostomy [DCR]

09.82 Conjunctivocystorhinostomy
Conjunctivodacryocystorhinostomy [CDCR]
Excludes: *that with insertion of tube or stent (09.83)*

09.83 Conjunctivorhinostomy with insertion of tube or stent

09.9 **Other operations on lacrimal system**

09.91 Obliteration of lacrimal punctum

09.99 Other

10 **Operations on conjunctiva**

10.0 Removal of embedded foreign body from conjunctiva by incision
Excludes: removal of:
embedded foreign body without incision (98.22)
superficial foreign body (98.21)

10.1 Other incision of conjunctiva

10.2 Diagnostic procedures on conjunctiva

10.21 Biopsy of conjunctiva

10.29 Other diagnostic procedures on conjunctiva

10.3 Excision or destruction of lesion or tissue of conjunctiva

10.31 Excision of lesion or tissue of conjunctiva
Excision of ring of conjunctiva around cornea
Excludes: *biopsy of conjunctiva (10.21)*

10.32 Destruction of lesion of conjunctiva
Excludes: *excision of lesion (10.31)*
thermocauterization for entropion (08.41)

10.33 Other destructive procedures on conjunctiva
Removal of trachoma follicles

10.4 Conjunctivoplasty

10.41 Repair of symblepharon with free graft

10.42 Reconstruction of conjunctival cul-de-sac with free graft
Excludes: *revision of enucleation socket with graft (16.63)*

10.43 Other reconstruction of conjunctival cul-de-sac
Excludes: *revision of enucleation socket (16.64)*

10.44 Other free graft to conjunctiva

10.49 Other conjunctivoplasty
Excludes: *repair of cornea with conjunctival flap (11.53)*

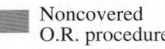

Valid O.R. procedure   Non-O.R. procedure   Nonspecific O.R. procedure   Noncovered O.R. procedure

10.5 **Lysis of adhesions of conjunctiva and eyelid**
Division of symblepharon (with insertion of conformer)

10.6 **Repair of laceration of conjunctiva**
| Excludes: | *that with repair of sclera (12.81)* |

10.9 **Other operations on conjunctiva**

10.91 **Subconjunctival injection**

10.99 **Other**

11 **Operations on cornea**

11.0 **Magnetic removal of embedded foreign body from cornea**
| Excludes: | *that with incision (11.1)* |

11.1 **Incision of cornea**
Incision of cornea for removal of foreign body

11.2 **Diagnostic procedures on cornea**

11.21 **Scraping of cornea for smear or culture**

11.22 **Biopsy of cornea**

11.29 **Other diagnostic procedures on cornea**

11.3 **Excision of pterygium**

11.31 **Transposition of pterygium**

11.32 **Excision of pterygium with corneal graft**

11.39 **Other excision of pterygium**

11.4 **Excision or destruction of tissue or other lesion of cornea**

11.41 **Mechanical removal of corneal epithelium**
That by chemocauterization
| Excludes: | *that for smear or culture (11.21)* |

11.42 **Thermocauterization of corneal lesion**

11.43 **Cryotherapy of corneal lesion**

11.49 **Other removal or destruction of corneal lesion**
Excision of cornea NOS
| Excludes: | *biopsy of cornea (11.22)* |

11.5 **Repair of cornea**

11.51 **Suture of corneal laceration**

11.52 **Repair of postoperative wound dehiscence of cornea**

11.53 **Repair of corneal laceration or wound with conjunctival flop**

11.59 **Other repair of cornea**

11.6 **Corneal transplant**
| Excludes: | *excision of pterygium with corneal graft (11.32)* |

11.60 **Corneal transplant, not otherwise specified**
Keratoplasty NOS
Note: To report donor source —*see* codes 00.91-00.93

11.61 **Lamellar keratoplasty with autograft**

11.62 **Other lamellar keratoplasty**

11.63 **Penetrating keratoplasty with autograft**
Perforating keratoplasty with autograft

11.64 **Other penetrating keratoplasty**
Perforating keratoplasty (with homograft)

11.69 **Other corneal transplant**

11.7 **Other reconstructive and refractive surgery on cornea**

11.71 **Keratomileusis**

11.72 **Keratophakia**

11.73 **Keratoprosthesis**

11.74 **Thermokeratoplasty**

11.75 **Radial keratotomy**

11.76 **Epikeratophakia**

● Code new to this edition   ▲ Revision of existing code   ④ ⑤ Fourth or fifth digit required

11.79 Other

11.9 **Other operations on cornea**

    11.91 **Tattooing of cornea**

    11.92 **Removal of artificial implant from cornea**

    11.99 **Other**

12 **Operation on iris, ciliary body, sclera, and anterior chamber**

> *Excludes:* *operations on cornea (11.0-11.99)*

12.0 **Removal of intraocular foreign body from anterior segment of eye**

    12.00 **Removal of intraocular foreign body from anterior segment of eye, not otherwise specified**

    12.01 **Removal of intraocular foreign body from anterior segment of eye with use of magnet**

    12.02 **Removal of intraocular foreign body from anterior segment of eye without use of magnet**

12.1 **Iridotomy and simple iridectomy**

> *Excludes:* *iridectomy associated with:*
> *cataract extraction (13.11-13.69)*
> *removal of lesion (12.41-12.42)*
> *scleral fistulization (12.61-12.69)*

    12.11 **Iridotomy with transfixion**

    12.12 **Other iridotomy**
        Corectomy
        Discission of iris
        Iridotomy NOS

    12.13 **Excision of prolapsed iris**

    12.14 **Other iridectomy**
        iridectomy (basal) (peripheral) (total)

12.2 **Diagnostic procedures on iris, ciliary body, sclera, and anterior chamber**

    12.21 **Diagnostic aspiration of anterior chamber of eye**

    12.22 **Biopsy of iris**

    12.29 **Other diagnostic procedures on iris, ciliary body, sclera, and anterior chamber**

12.3 **Iridoplasty and coreoplasty**

    12.31 **Lysis of goniosynechiae**
        Lysis of goniosynechiae by injection of air or liquid

    12.32 **Lysis of other anterior synechiae**
        Lysis of anterior synechiae:
          NOS
          by injection of air or liquid

    12.33 **Lysis of posterior synechiae**
        Lysis of iris adhesions NOS

    12.34 **Lysis of corneovitreal adhesions**

    12.35 **Coreoplasty**
        Needling of pupillary membrane

    12.39 **Other iridoplasty**

12.4 **Excision or destruction of lesion of iris and ciliary body**

    12.40 **Removal of lesion of anterior segment of eye, not otherwise specified**

    12.41 **Destruction of lesion of iris, nonexcisional**
        Destruction of lesion of iris by:
          cauterization
          cryotherapy
          photocoagulation

    12.42 **Excision of lesion of iris**

> *Excludes:* *biopsy of iris (12.22)*

    12.43 **Destruction of lesion of ciliary body, nonexcisional**

    12.44 **Excision of lesion of ciliary body**

12.5 **Facilitation of intraocular circulation**

    12.51 **Goniopuncture without goniotomy**

	Valid O.R. procedure		Non-O.R. procedure		Nonspecific O.R. procedure		Noncovered O.R. procedure

12.52 Goniotomy without goniopuncture

12.53 Goniotomy with goniopuncture

12.54 Trabeculotomy ab externo

12.55 Cyclodialysis

12.59 Other facilitation of intraocular circulation

12.6 Scleral fistulization

> Excludes: *exploratory sclerotomy (12.89)*

12.61 Trephination of sclera with iridectomy

12.62 Thermocauterization of sclera with iridectomy

12.63 Iridencleisis and iridotasis

12.64 Trabeculectomy ab externo

12.65 Other scleral fistulization with iridectomy

12.66 Postoperative revision of scleral fistulization procedure
Revision of filtering bleb

> Excludes: *repair of fistula (12.82)*

● **12.67** Insertion of aqueous drainage device
Anterior chamber drainage device
Aqueous drainage shunt or stent
Eye valve implant
Filtration canal shunt or device

12.69 Other fistulizing procedure

12.7 Other procedures for relief of elevated intraocular pressure

12.71 Cyclodiathermy

12.72 Cyclocryotherapy

12.73 Cyclophotocoagulation

12.74 Diminution of ciliary body, not otherwise specified

12.79 Other glaucoma procedures

12.8 Operations on sclera

> Excludes: *those associated with:*
> *retinal reattachment (14.41-14.59)*
> *scleral fistulization (12.61-12.69)*

12.81 Suture of laceration of sclera
Suture of sclera with synchronous repair of conjunctiva

12.82 Repair of scleral fistula

> Excludes: *postoperative revision of scleral fistulization procedure (12.66)*

12.83 Revision of operative wound of anterior segment, not elsewhere classified

> Excludes: *postoperative revision of scleral fistulization procedure (12.66)*

12.84 Excision or destruction of lesion of sclera

12.85 Repair of scleral staphyloma with graft

12.86 Other repair of scleral staphyloma

12.87 Scleral reinforcement with graft

12.88 Other scleral reinforcement

12.89 Other operations on sclera
Exploratory sclerotomy

12.9 Other operations on iris, ciliary body, and anterior chamber

12.91 Therapeutic evacuation of anterior chamber
Paracentesis of anterior chamber

> Excludes: *diagnostic aspiration (12.21)*

12.92 Injection into anterior chamber
Injection of:
air into anterior chamber
liquid into anterior chamber
medication into anterior chamber

12.93 **Removal or destruction of epithelial downgrowth from anterior chamber**

Excludes: *that with iridectomy (12.41-12.42)*

12.97 **Other operations on iris**

12.98 **Other operations on ciliary body**

12.99 **Other operations on anterior chamber**

13 Operations on lens

13.0 **Removal of foreign body from lens**

Excludes: *removal of pseudophakos (13.8)*

13.00 **Removal of foreign body from lens, not otherwise specified**

13.01 **Removal of foreign body from lens with use of magnet**

13.02 **Removal of foreign body from lens without use of magnet**

13.1 **Intracapsular extraction of lens**

Code also any synchronous insertion of pseudophakos (13.71)

13.11 **Intracapsular extraction of lens by temporal inferior route**

13.19 **Other intracapsular extraction of lens**
Cataract extraction NOS
Cryoextraction of lens
Erysiphake extraction of cataract
Extraction of lens NOS

13.2 **Extracapsular extraction of lens by linear extraction technique**

Code also any synchronous insertion of pseudophakos (13.71)

13.3 **Extracapsular extraction of lens by simple aspiration (and irrigation) technique**
Irrigation of traumatic cataract
Code also any synchronous insertion of pseudophakos (13.71)

13.4 **Extracapsular extraction of lens by fragmentation and aspiration technique**

Code also any synchronous insertion of pseudophakos (13.71)

13.41 **Phacoemulsification and aspiration of cataract**

13.42 **Mechanical phacofragmentation and aspiration of cataract by posterior route**

Code also any synchronous vitrectomy (14.74)

13.43 **Mechanical phacofragmentation and other aspiration of cataract**

13.5 **Other extracapsular extraction of lens**

Code also any synchronous insertion of pseudophakos (13.71)

13.51 **Extracapsular extraction of lens by temporal inferior route**

13.59 **Other extracapsular extraction of lens**

13.6 **Other cataract extraction**

Code also any synchronous insertion of pseudophakos (13.71)

13.64 **Discission of secondary membrane [after cataract]**

13.65 **Excision of secondary membrane [after cataract]**
Capsulectomy

13.66 **Mechanical fragmentation of secondary membrane [after cataract]**

13.69 **Other cataract extraction**

13.7 **Insertion of prosthetic lens [pseudophakos]**

Excludes: *implantation of intraocular telescope prosthesis (13.91)*

13.70 **Insertion of pseudophakos, not otherwise specified**

13.71 **Insertion of intraocular lens prosthesis at time of cataract extraction, one-stage**

Code also synchronous extraction of cataract (13.11-13.69)

13.72 **Secondary insertion of intraocular lens prosthesis**

13.8 **Removal of implanted lens**
Removal of pseudophakos

13.9 **Other operations on lens**

13.90 **Operation on lens, not elsewhere classified (NEC)**

13.91 **Implantation of intraocular telescope prosthesis**
Includes: removal of lens, any method
Implantable miniature telescope

Excludes: *secondary insertion of ocular implant (16.61)*

Valid O.R. procedure | Non-O.R. procedure | Nonspecific O.R. procedure | Noncovered O.R. procedure

14   **Operations on retina, choroid, vitreous, and posterior chamber**

     14.0   **Removal of foreign body from posterior segment of eye**

         Excludes: *removal of surgically implanted material (14.6)*

         14.00   **Removal of foreign body from posterior segment of eye, not otherwise specified**

         14.01   **Removal of foreign body from posterior segment of eye with use of magnet**

         14.02   **Removal of foreign body from posterior segment of eye without use of magnet**

     14.1   **Diagnostic procedures on retina, choroid, vitreous, and posterior chamber**

         14.11   **Diagnostic aspiration of vitreous**

         14.19   **Other diagnostic procedures on retina, choroid, vitreous, and posterior chamber**

     14.2   **Destruction of lesion of retina and choroid**
         Includes: destruction of chorioretinopathy or isolated chorioretinal lesion

         Excludes: *that for repair of retina (14.31-14.59)*

         14.21   **Destruction of chorioretinal lesion by diathermy**

         14.22   **Destruction of chorioretinal lesion by cryotherapy**

         14.23   **Destruction of chorioretinal lesion by xenon arc photocoagulation**

         14.24   **Destruction of chorioretinal lesion by laser photocoagulation**

         14.25   **Destruction of chorioretinal lesion by photocoagulation of unspecified type**

         14.26   **Destruction of chorioretinal lesion by radiation therapy**

         14.27   **Destruction of chorioretinal lesion by implantation of radiation source**

         14.29   **Other destruction of chorioretinal lesion**
           Destruction of lesion of retina and choroid NOS

     14.3   **Repair of retinal tear**
         Includes: repair of retinal defect

         Excludes: *repair of retinal detachment (14.41-14.59)*

         14.31   **Repair of retinal tear by diathermy**

         14.32   **Repair of retinal tear by cryotherapy**

         14.33   **Repair of retinal tear by xenon arc photocoagulation**

         14.34   **Repair of retinal tear by laser photocoagulation**

         14.35   **Repair of retinal tear by photocoagulation of unspecified type**

         14.39   **Other repair of retinal tear**

     14.4   **Repair of retinal detachment with scleral buckling and implant**

         14.41   **Scleral buckling with implant**

         14.49   **Other scleral buckling**
           Scleral buckling with:
             air tamponade
             resection of sclera
             vitrectomy

     14.5   **Other repair of retinal detachment**
         Includes: that with drainage

         14.51   **Repair of retinal detachment with diathermy**

         14.52   **Repair of retinal detachment with cryotherapy**

         14.53   **Repair of retinal detachment with xenon arc photocoagulation**

         14.54   **Repair of retinal detachment with laser photocoagulation**

         14.55   **Repair of retinal detachment with photocoagulation of unspecified type**

         14.59   **Other**

     14.6   **Removal of surgically implanted material from posterior segment of eye**

     14.7   **Operations on vitreous**

         14.71   **Removal of vitreous, anterior approach**
           Open sky technique
           Removal of vitreous, anterior approach (with replacement)

         14.72   **Other removal of vitreous**
           Aspiration of vitreous by posterior sclerotomy

         14.73   **Mechanical vitrectomy by anterior approach**

         14.74   **Other mechanical vitrectomy**
           Posterior approach

● Code new to this edition   ▲ Revision of existing code   ④ ⑤ Fourth or fifth digit required

14.75 Injection of vitreous substitute

Excludes: *that associated with removal (14.71-14.72)*

14.79 Other operations on vitreous

14.9 Other operations on retina, choroid, and posterior chamber

15 Operations on extraocular muscles

15.0 Diagnostic procedures on extraocular muscles or tendons

15.01 Biopsy of extraocular muscle or tendon

15.09 Other diagnostic procedures on extraocular muscles and tendons

15.1 Operations on one extraocular muscle involving temporary detachment from globe

15.11 Recession of one extraocular muscle

15.12 Advancement of one extraocular muscle

15.13 Resection of one extraocular muscle

15.19 Other operations on one extraocular muscle involving temporary detachment from globe

Excludes: *transposition of muscle (15.5)*

15.2 Other operations on one extraocular muscle

15.21 Lengthening procedure on one extraocular muscle

15.22 Shortening procedure on one extraocular muscle

15.29 Other

15.3 Operations on two or more extraocular muscles involving temporary detachment from globe, one or both eyes

15.4 Other operations on two or more extraocular muscles, one or both eyes

15.5 Transposition of extraocular muscles

Excludes: *that for correction of ptosis (08.31-08.36)*

15.6 Revision of extraocular muscle surgery

15.7 Repair of injury of extraocular muscle
Freeing of entrapped extraocular muscle
Lysis of adhesions of extraocular muscle
Repair of laceration of extraocular muscle, tendon, or Tenon's capsule

15.9 Other operations on extraocular muscles and tendon

16 Operations on orbit and eyeball

Excludes: *reduction of fracture of orbit (76.78-76.79)*

16.0 Orbitotomy

16.01 Orbitotomy with bone flap
Orbitotomy with lateral approach

16.02 Orbitotomy with insertion of orbital implant

Excludes: *that with bone flap (16.01)*

16.09 Other orbitotomy

16.1 Removal of penetrating foreign body from eye, not otherwise specified

Excludes: *removal of nonpenetrating foreign body (98.21)*

16.2 Diagnostic procedures on orbit and eyeball

16.21 Ophthalmoscopy

16.22 Diagnostic aspiration of orbit

16.23 Biopsy of eyeball and orbit

16.29 Other diagnostic procedures on orbit and eyeball

Excludes: *examination of form and structure of eye (95.11-95.16)*
general and subjective eye examination (95.01-95.09)
microscopic examination of specimen from eye (90.21-90.29)
objective functional tests of eye (95.21-95.26)
ocular thermography (88.82)
tonometry (89.11)
X-ray of orbit (87.14, 87.16)

16.3 Evisceration of eyeball

16.31 Removal of ocular contents with synchronous implant into scleral shell

	Valid O.R. procedure		Non-O.R. procedure		Nonspecific O.R. procedure		Noncovered O.R. procedure

16.39 Other evisceration of eyeball

16.4 **Enucleation of eyeball**

16.41 Enucleation of eyeball with synchronous implant into Tenon's capsule with attachment of muscles
Integrated implant of eyeball

16.42 Enucleation of eyeball with other synchronous implant

16.49 Other enucleation of eyeball
Removal of eyeball NOS

16.5 **Exenteration of orbital contents**

16.51 Exenteration of orbit with removal of adjacent structures
Radical orbitomaxillectomy

16.52 Exenteration of orbit with therapeutic removal of orbital bone

16.59 Other exenteration of orbit
Evisceration of orbit NOS
Exenteration of orbit with temporalis muscle transplant

16.6 **Secondary procedures after removal of eyeball**

> Excludes: *that with synchronous:*
> *enucleation of eyeball (16.41-16.42)*
> *evisceration of eyeball (16.31)*

16.61 Secondary insertion of ocular implant

16.62 Revision and reinsertion of ocular implant

16.63 Revision of enucleation socket with graft

16.64 Other revision of enucleation socket

16.65 Secondary graft to exenteration cavity

16.66 Other revision of exenteration cavity

16.69 Other secondary procedures after removal of eyeball

16.7 **Removal of ocular or orbital implant**

16.71 Removal of ocular implant

16.72 Removal of orbital implant

16.8 **Repair of injury of eyeball and orbit**

16.81 Repair of wound of orbit

> Excludes: *reduction of orbital fracture (76.78-76.79)*
> *repair of extraocular muscles (15.7)*

16.82 Repair of rupture of eyeball
Repair of multiple structures of eye

> Excludes: *repair of laceration of:*
> *cornea (11.51-11.59)*
> *sclera (12.81)*

16.89 Other repair of injury of eyeball or orbit

16.9 **Other operations on orbit and eyeball**

> Excludes: *irrigation of eye (96.51)*
> *prescription and fitting of low vision aids (95.31-95.33)*
> *removal of:*
> *eye prosthesis NEC (97.31)*
> *nonpenetrating foreign body from eye without incision (98.21)*

16.91 Retrobulbar injection of therapeutic agent

> Excludes: *injection of radiographic contrast material (87.14)*
> *opticociliary injection (12.79)*

16.92 Excision of lesion of orbit

> Excludes: *biopsy of orbit (16.23)*

16.93 Excision of lesion of eye, unspecified structure

> Excludes: *biopsy of eye NOS (16.23)*

16.98 Other operations on orbit

16.99 Other operations on eyeball

● Code new
to this edition ▲ Revision of
existing code ④ ⑤ Fourth or fifth
digit required

3A   OTHER MISCELLANEOUS DIAGNOSTIC AND THERAPEUTIC PROCEDURES (17)

17   Other miscellaneous procedures

17.1   Laparoscopic unilateral repair of inguinal hernia

Excludes: *other and open unilateral repair of hernia (53.00-53.05)*

17.11   Laparoscopic repair of direct inguinal hernia with graft or prosthesis
Laparoscopic repair of direct and indirect inguinal hernia with graft or prosthesis

17.12   Laparoscopic repair of indirect inguinal hernia with graft or prosthesis

17.13   Laparoscopic repair of inguinal hernia with graft or prosthesis, not otherwise specified

17.2   Laparoscopic bilateral repair of inguinal hernia

Excludes: *other and open bilateral repair of hernia (53.10-53.17)*

17.21   Laparoscopic bilateral repair of direct inguinal hernia with graft or prosthesis

17.22   Laparoscopic bilateral repair of indirect inguinal hernia with graft or prosthesis

17.23   Laparoscopic bilateral repair of inguinal hernia, one direct and one indirect, with graft or prosthesis

17.24   Laparoscopic bilateral repair of inguinal hernia with graft or prosthesis, not otherwise specified

17.3   Laparoscopic partial excision of large intestine

Excludes: *other and open partial excision of large intestine (45.71-45.79)*

17.31   Laparoscopic multiple segmental resection of large intestine

17.32   Laparoscopic cecectomy

17.33   Laparoscopic right hemicolectomy

17.34   Laparoscopic resection of transverse colon

17.35   Laparoscopic left hemicolectomy

17.36   Laparoscopic sigmoidectomy

17.39   Other laparoscopic partial excision of large intestine

17.4   Robotic assisted procedures
Computer assisted robotic surgery
Computer-enhanced robotic surgery
Robotic procedure with computer assistance
Surgeon-controlled robotic surgery

Code first primary procedure

Excludes: *computer assisted surgery (00.31-00.35, 00.39)*

Note: This category includes use of a computer console with (3-D) imaging, software, camera(s), visualization and instrumentation *combined* with use of robotic arms, device(s), or system(s) at the time of the procedure

17.41   Open robotic assisted procedure
Robotic assistance in open procedure

17.42   Laparoscopic robotic assisted procedure
Robotic assistance in laparoscopic procedure

17.43   Percutaneous robotic assisted procedure
Robotic assistance in percutaneous procedure

17.44   Endoscopic robotic assisted procedure
Robotic assistance in endoscopic procedure

17.45   Thoracoscopic robotic assisted procedure
Robotic assistance in thoracoscopic procedure

17.49   Other and unspecified robotic assisted procedure
Robotic assistance in other and unspecified procedure

Excludes: *endoscopic robotic assisted procedure (17.44)*
laparoscopic robotic assisted procedure (17.42)
open robotic assisted procedure (17.41)
percutaneous robotic assisted procedure (17.43)
thoracoscopic robotic assisted procedure (17.45)

Valid O.R. procedure   Non-O.R. procedure   Nonspecific O.R. procedure   Noncovered O.R. procedure

17.5 Additional cardiovascular procedures

17.51 **Implantation of rechargeable cardiac contractility modulation [CCM], total system**

Note: Device testing during procedure – omit code

Implantation of CCM system includes formation of pocket, transvenous leads, including placement of leads, placement of catheter into left ventricle, intraoperative procedures for evaluation of lead signals, obtaining sensing threshold measurements, obtaining defibrillator threshold measurements.

Includes implantation of device with removal of existing device

Code also any concomitant:
coronary bypass (36.10 – 36.19)
extracorporeal circulation (39.61)
insertion or replacement of automatic cardioverter/defibrillator, total system [AICD] (37.94)

> Excludes: *implantation of CCM pulse generator only (17.52)*

17.52 **Implantation or replacement of cardiac contractility modulation [CCM] rechargeable pulse generator only**

Note: Device testing during procedure – omit code

Implantation of CCM device with removal of any existing CCM device

Code also any concomitant:
revision of device pocket (37.79)
revision of lead [electrode] (37.75)

● **17.53** **Percutaneous arherectomy of extracranial vessel(s)**
Directional atherectomy
Excimer laser atherectomy
Rotational atherectomy
That by laser
That by transluminal extraction

Code also any:
injection or infusion of thrombolytic agent (99.10)
number of vascular stents inserted (00.45-00.48)
number of vessels treated (00.40-00.43)
percutaneous insertion of carotid artery stent(s) (00.63)
percutaneous insertion of other extracranial artery stent(s) (00.64)
procedure on vessel bifurcation (00.44)

> Excludes: *angioplasty of other non-coronary vessel(s) (39.50)*
> *atherectomy of intracranial vessel(s) (17.54)*
> *atherectomy of other non-coronary vessel(s) (17.56)*
> *removal of cerebrovascular obstruction of vessel(s) by open approach (38.01-38.02, 38.11-38.12, 38.31-38.32, 38.41-38.42)*

● **17.54** **Percutaneous atherectomy of intracranial vessel(s)**
Directional atherectomy
Excimer laser atherectomy
Rotational atherectomy
That by laser
That by transluminal extraction

Code also any:
injection or infusion of thrombolytic agent (99.10)
number of vascular stents inserted (00.45-00.48)
number of vessels treated (00.40-00.43)
percutaneous insertion of intracranial vascular stent(s) (00.65)
procedure on vessel bifurcation (00.44)

> Excludes: *angioplasty of other non-coronary vessel(s) (39.50)*
> *atherectomy of extracranial vessel(s) (17.53)*
> *atherectomy of other non-coronary vessel(s) (17.56)*
> *removal of cerebrovascular obstruction of vessel(s) by open approach (38.01-38.02, 38.11-38.12, 38.31-38.32, 38.41-38.42)*

● Code new to this edition	▲ Revision of existing code	④ ⑤ Fourth or fifth digit required

- **17.55 Transluminal coronary atherectomy**
  Directional atherectomy
  Excimer laser atherectomy
  Rotational atherectomy
  That by laser
  That by percutaneous approach
  That by transluminal extraction

  Code also any:
  injection or infusion of thrombolytic agent (99.10)
  insertion of coronary artery stent (36.06-36.07)
  intracoronary artery thrombolytic infusion (36.04)
  number of vascular stents inserted (00.45-00.48)
  number of vessels treated (00.40-00.43)
  procedure on vessel bifurcation (00.44)
  SuperSaturated oxygen therapy (00.49)
  transluminal coronary angioplasty (00.66)

- **17.56 Atherectomy of other non-coronary vessel(s)**
  Percutaneous transluminal atherectomy of:
      lower extremity vessels
      mesenteric artery
      renal artery
      upper extremity vessels
  Includes:
      Directional atherectomy
      Excimer laser atherectomy
      Rotational atherectomy
      That by laser
      That by transluminal extraction

  Code also any:
  injection or infusion of thrombolytic agent (99.10)
  insertion of drug-eluting peripheral vessel stent (00.55)
  insertion of non-drug-eluting peripheral vessel stent(s) or stent graft(s) (39.90)
  number of vascular stents inserted (00.45-00.48)
  number of vessels treated (00.40-00.43)
  procedure on vessel bifurcation (00.44)

Excludes:	*percutaneous angioplasty of extracranial or intracranial vessel(s) (00.61-00.62)*
	percutaneous angioplasty of other non-coronary vessel(s) (39.50)
	percutaneous atherectomy of extracranial vessel(s) (17.53)
	percutaneous atherectomy of intracranial vessel(s) (17.54)

17.6 Laser interstitial thermal therapy [LITT] under guidance
Focused laser interstitial thermal therapy [f-LITT] under MRI guidance
MRI-guided LITT

17.61 Laser interstitial thermal therapy [LITT] of lesion or tissue of brain under guidance
Focused laser interstitial thermal therapy [f-LITT] under MRI guidance
MRI-guided LITT of lesion or tissue of brain

Excludes:	*laser interstitial thermal therapy [LITT] of lesion or tissue of head under guidance (17.62)*

17.62 Laser interstitial thermal therapy [LITT] of lesion or tissue of head and neck under guidance
Focused laser interstitial thermal therapy [f-LITT] under MRI guidance
MRI-guided LITT of lesion or tissue of head and neck

Excludes:	*laser interstitial thermal therapy [LITT] of lesion or tissue of brain under guidance (17.61)*

17.63 Laser interstitial thermal therapy [LITT] of lesion or tissue of liver under guidance
Focused laser interstitial thermal therapy [f-LITT] under MRI guidance
MRI-guided LITT of lesion or tissue of liver

17.69 **Laser interstitial thermal therapy [LITT] of lesion or tissue of other and unspecified site under guidance**
Focused laser interstitial thermal therapy [f-LITT] under MRI guidance
MRI-guided LITT of lesion or tissue of breast
MRI-guided LITT of lesion or tissue of lung
MRI-guided LITT of lesion or tissue of prostate

Excludes:	*laser interstitial thermal therapy [LITT] of lesion or tissue of brain under guidance (17.61)*
	laser interstitial thermal therapy [LITT] of lesion or tissue of head and neck under guidance (17.62)
	laser interstitial thermal therapy [LITT] of lesion or tissue of liver under guidance (17.63)

17.7 **Other diagnostic and therapeutic procedures**

17.70 **Intravenous infusion of clofarabine**

| Excludes: | *injection or infusion of cancer chemotherapeutic substance (99.25)* |

17.71 **Non-coronary intra-operative fluorescence vascular angiography [IFVA]**
Intraoperative laser arteriogram
SPY arteriogram
SPY arteriography

| Excludes: | *intra-operative coronary fluorescence vascular angiography (88.59)* |

● **17.8** **Other adjunct procedures**
Note: These codes are to be used in conjunction with other therapeutic procedure codes to provide additional information on devices used as part of a procedure.

● **17.81** **Insertion of antimicrobial envelope**
Use of anti-microbial (mesh) (prophylactic antibiotics embedded) envelope with the insertion of cardiovascular implantable electronic devices (CIED)

Code first primary procedure:
Insertion of cardiovascular implantable electronic device(s) [CIED] (00.51, 00.53, 00.54, 37.94, 37.96, 37.98)

● Code new to this edition   ▲ Revision of existing code   ④ ⑤ Fourth or fifth digit required

4.   OPERATIONS ON THE EAR (18-20)

18   Operations on external ear
Includes: operations on:
external auditory canal
skin and cartilage of:
auricle
meatus

18.0   Incision of external ear

Excludes: *removal of intraluminal foreign body (98.11)*

18.01   Piercing of ear lobe
Piercing of pinna

18.02   Incision of external auditory canal

18.09   Other incision of external ear

18.1   Diagnostic procedures on external ear

18.11   Otoscopy

18.12   Biopsy of external ear

18.19   Other diagnostic procedures on external ear

Excludes: *microscopic examination of specimen from ear (90.31-90.39)*

18.2   Excision or destruction of lesion of external ear

18.21   Excision of preauricular sinus
Radical excision of preauricular sinus or cyst

Excludes: *excision of preauricular remnant [appendage] (18.29)*

18.29   Excision or destruction of other lesion of external ear
Cauterization of external car
Coagulation of external car
Cryosurgery of external car
Curettage of external car
Electrocoagulation of external car
Enucleation of external car
Excision of:
exostosis of external auditory canal
preauricular remnant [appendage]
Partial excision of ear

Excludes: *biopsy of external ear (18.12)*
radical excision of lesion (18.31)
removal of cerumen (96.52)

18.3   Other excision of external ear

Excludes: *biopsy of external ear (18.12)*

18.31   Radical excision of lesion of external ear

Excludes: *radical excision of preauricular sinus (18.21)*

18.39   Other
Amputation of external ear

Excludes: *excision of lesion (18.21-18.29, 18.31)*

18.4   Suture of laceration of external ear

18.5   Surgical correction of prominent ear
Ear:
pinning
setback

18.6   Reconstruction of external auditory canal
Canaloplasty of external auditory meatus
Construction [reconstruction] of external meatus of ear:
osseous portion
skin-lined portion (with skin graft)

18.7   Other plastic repair of external ear

18.71   Construction of auricle of ear
Prosthetic appliance for absent ear
Reconstruction:
auricle
ear

| | Valid O.R. procedure | | Non-O.R. procedure | | Nonspecific O.R. procedure | | Noncovered O.R. procedure |

18.72 Reattachment of amputated ear

18.79 Other plastic repair of external ear
Otoplasty NOS
Postauricular skin graft
Repair of lop ear

18.9 Other operations on external ear

> *Excludes:* irrigation of ear (96.52)
> packing of external auditory canal (96.11)
> removal of:
>   cerumen (96.52)
>   foreign body (without incision) (98.11)

19 Reconstructive operations on middle ear

19.0 Stapes mobilization

Division, otosclerotic:	Remobilization of stapes
material	Stapediolysis
process	Transcrural stapes mobilization

> *Excludes:* that with synchronous stapedectomy (19.11-19.19)

19.1 Stapedectomy

> *Excludes:* revision of previous stapedectomy (19.21-19.29)
> stapes mobilization only (19.0)

19.11 Stapedectomy with incus replacement
Stapedectomy with incus:
  homograft
  prosthesis

19.19 Other stapedectomy

19.2 Revision of stapedectomy

19.21 Revision of stapedectomy with incus replacement

19.29 Other revision of stapedectomy

19.3 Other operations on ossicular chain
Incudectomy NOS
Ossiculectomy NOS
Reconstruction of ossicles, second stage

19.4 Myringoplasty
Epitympanic, type I
Myringoplasty by:
  cauterization
  graft
Tympanoplasty (type I)

19.5 Other tympanoplasty

19.52 Type II tympanoplasty
Closure of perforation with graft against incus or malleus

19.53 Type III tympanoplasty
Graft placed in contact with mobile and intact stapes

19.54 Type IV tympanoplasty
Mobile footplate left exposed with air pocket between round window and graft

19.55 Type V tympanoplasty
Fenestra in horizontal semicircular canal covered by graft

19.6 Revision of tympanoplasty

19.9 Other repair of middle ear
Closure of mastoid fistula
Mastoid myoplasty
Obliteration of tympanomastoid cavity

20 Other operations on middle and inner ear

20.0 Myringotomy

20.01 Myringotomy with insertion of tube
Myringostomy

20.09 Other myringotomy
Aspiration of middle ear NOS

20.1 Removal of tympanostomy tube

20.2 Incision of mastoid and middle ear

● Code new
to this edition   ▲ Revision of
existing code   ④ ⑤ Fourth or fifth
digit required

20.21 Incision of mastoid

20.22 Incision of petrous pyramid air cells

20.23 Incision of middle ear
Atticotomy
Division of tympanum
Lysis of adhesions of middle ear

> *Excludes:* *divisions of otosclerotic process (19.0)*
> *stapediolysis (19.0)*
> *that with stapedectomy (19.11-19.19)*

20.3 Diagnostic procedures on middle and inner ear

20.31 Electrocochleography

20.32 Biopsy of middle and inner ear

20.39 Other diagnostic procedures on middle and inner ear

> *Excludes:* *auditory and vestibular function tests (89.13, 95.41-95.49)*
> *microscopic examination of specimen from ear (90.31-90.39)*

20.4 Mastoidectomy
Code also any:
skin graft (18.79)
tympanoplasty (19.4-19.55)

> *Excludes:* *that with implantation of cochlear prosthetic device (20.96-20.98)*

20.41 Simple mastoidectomy

20.42 Radical mastoidectomy

20.49 Other mastoidectomy
Atticoantrotomy
Mastoidectomy:
  NOS
  modified radical

20.5 Other excision of middle ear

> *Excludes:* *that with synchronous mastoidectomy (20.41-20.49)*

20.51 Excision of lesion of middle ear

> *Excludes:* *biopsy of middle ear (20.32)*

20.59 Other
Apicectomy of petrous pyramid
Tympanectomy

20.6 Fenestration of inner ear

20.61 Fenestration of inner ear (initial)
Fenestration of labyrinth with graft (skin) (vein)
Fenestration of semicircular canals with graft (skin) (vein)
Fenenstration of vestibule with graft (skin) (vein)

> *Excludes:* *that with tympanoplasty type V (19.55)*

20.62 Revision of fenestration of inner ear

20.7 Incision, excision, and destruction of inner ear

20.71 Endolymphatic shunt

20.72 Injection into inner ear
Destruction by injection (alcohol):
  inner ear
  semicircular canals
  vestibule

20.79 Other incision, excision and destruction of inner ear
Decompression of labyrinth
Drainage of inner ear
Fistulization:
  endolymphatic sac
  labyrinth
Incision of endolymphatic sac
Labyrinthectomy (transtympanic)
Opening of bony labyrinth
Perilymphatic tap

> *Excludes:* *biopsy of inner ear (20.32)*

| ▧ | Valid O.R. procedure | ▧ | Non-O.R. procedure | ▧ | Nonspecific O.R. procedure | ▧ | Noncovered O.R. procedure |

20.8 **Operations on Eustachian tube**
Catheterization of Eustachian tube
Inflation of Eustachian tube
Injection (Teflon paste) of Eustachian tube
Insufflation (boric acid-salicylic acid) of Eustachian tube
Intubation of Eustachian tube
Politzerization of Eustachian tube

20.9 **Other operations on inner and middle ear**

20.91 **Tympanosympathectomy**

20.92 **Revision of mastoidectomy**

20.93 **Repair of oval and round windows**
Closure of fistula:
oval window
perilymph
round window

20.94 **Injection of tympanum**

20.95 **Implantation of electromagnetic bearing device**
Bone conduction hearing device

> | Excludes: | *cochlear prosthetic device (20.96-20.98)*

20.96 **Implantation or replacement of cochlear prosthetic device, not otherwise specified**
Implantation of receiver (within skull) and insertion of electrode(s) in the cochlea
Includes: mastoidectomy

> | Excludes: | *electromagnetic hearing device (20.95)*

20.97 **Implantation or replacement of cochlear prosthetic device, single channel**
Implantation of receiver (within skull) and insertion of electrode in the cochlea
Includes: mastoidectomy

> | Excludes: | *electromagnetic hearing device (20.95)*

20.98 **Implantation or replacement of cochlear prosthetic device, multiple channel**
Implantation of receiver (within skull) and insertion of electrodes in the cochlea
Includes: mastoidectomy

> | Excludes: | *electromagnetic hearing device (20.95)*

20.99 **Other operations on middle and inner ear**
Attachment of percutaneous abutment (screw) for prosthetic device
Repair or removal of cochlear prosthetic device (receiver) (electrode)

> | Excludes: | *adjustment (external components) of cochlear prosthetic device (95.49)*
> *fitting of hearing aid (95.48)*

● Code new
to this edition
▲ Revision of
existing code
④ ⑤ Fourth or fifth
digit required

5. OPERATIONS ON THE NOSE, MOUTH, AND PHARYNX (21-29)

21 Operation on nose
Includes: operations on:
bone of nose
skin of nose

21.0 Control of epistaxis

21.00 Control of epistaxis, not otherwise specified

21.01 Control of epistaxis by anterior nasal packing

21.02 Control of epistaxis by posterior (and anterior) packing

21.03 Control of epistaxis by cauterization (and packing)

21.04 Control of epistaxis by ligation of ethmoidal arteries

21.05 Control of epistaxis by (transantral) ligation of the maxillary artery

21.06 Control of epistaxis by ligation of the external carotid artery

21.07 Control of epistaxis by excision of nasal mucosa and skin grafting on septum and lateral nasal wall

21.09 Control of epistaxis by other means

21.1 Incision of nose
Chondrotomy
Incision of skin of nose
Nasal septotomy

21.2 Diagnostic procedures on nose

21.21 Rhinoscopy

21.22 Biopsy of nose

21.29 Other diagnostic procedures on nose
Excludes: *microscopic examination of specimen from nose (90.31-90.39)*
nasal:
function study (89.12)
x-ray (87.16)
rhinomanometry (89.12)

21.3 Local excision or destruction of lesion of nose
Excludes: *biopsy of nose (21.22)*
nasal fistulectomy (21.82)

21.30 Excision or destruction of nose, not otherwise specified

21.31 Local excision or destruction of intranasal lesion
Nasal polypectomy

21.32 Local excision or destruction of other lesion of nose

21.4 Resection of nose
Amputation of nose

21.5 Submucous resection of nasal septum

21.6 Turbinectomy

21.61 Turbinectomy by diathermy or cryosurgery

21.62 Fracture of the turbinates

21.69 Other turbinectomy
Excludes: *turbinectomy associated with sinusectomy (22.31-22.39, 22.42, 22.60-22.64)*

21.7 Reduction of nasal fracture

21.71 Closed reduction of nasal fracture

21.72 Open reduction of nasal fracture

21.8 Repair and plastic operations on the nose

21.81 Suture of laceration of nose

21.82 Closure of nasal fistula
Nasolabial fistulectomy
Nasopharyngeal fistulectomy
Oronasal fistulectomy

	Valid O.R. procedure		Non-O.R. procedure		Nonspecific O.R. procedure		Noncovered O.R. procedure

21.83 Total nasal reconstruction
Reconstruction of nose with:
   arm flap
   forehead flap

21.84 Revision rhinoplasty
Rhinoseptoplasty
Twisted nose rhinoplasty

21.85 Augmentation rhinoplasty
Augmentation rhinoplasty with:
   graft
   synthetic implant

21.86 Limited rhinoplasty
Plastic repair of nasolabial flaps
Tip rhinoplasty

21.87 Other rhinoplasty
Rhinoplasty NOS

21.88 Other septoplasty
Crushing of nasal septum
Repair of septal perforation

> | Excludes: | *septoplasty associated with submucous resection of septum (21.5)*

21.89 Other repair and plastic operations on nose
Reattachment of amputated nose

21.9 Other operations on nose

21.91 Lysis of adhesions of nose
Posterior nasal scrub

21.99 Other

> | Excludes: | *dilation of frontonasal duct (96.21)*
> *irrigation of nasal passages (96.53)*
> *removal of:*
>   *intraluminal foreign body without incision (98.12)*
>   *nasal packing (97.32)*
> *replacement of nasal packing (97.21)*

22 Operations on nasal sinuses

22.0 Aspiration and lavage of nasal sinus

22.00 Aspiration and lavage of nasal sinus, not otherwise specified

22.01 Puncture of nasal sinus for aspiration or lavage

22.02 Aspiration or lavage of nasal sinus through natural ostium

22.1 Diagnostic procedures on nasal sinus

22.11 Closed [endoscopic] [needle] biopsy of nasal sinus

22.12 Open biopsy of nasal sinus

22.19 Other diagnostic procedures on nasal sinuses
Endoscopy without biopsy

> | Excludes: | *transillumination of sinus (89.35)*
> *x-ray of sinus (87.15-87.16)*

22.2 Intranasal antrotomy

> | Excludes: | *antrotomy with external approach (22.31-22.39)*

22.3 External maxillary antrotomy

22.31 Radical maxillary antrotomy
Removal of lining membrane of maxillary sinus using Caldwell-Luc approach

22.39 Other external maxillary antrotomy
Exploration of maxillary antrum with Caldwell-Luc approach

22.4 Frontal sinusotomy and sinusectomy

22.41 Frontal sinusotomy

22.42 Frontal sinusectomy
Excision of lesion of frontal sinus
Obliteration of frontal sinus (with fat)

> | Excludes: | *biopsy of nasal sinus (22.11-22.12)*

● Code new
  to this edition
▲ Revision of
  existing code
④ ⑤ Fourth or fifth
  digit required

22.5 Other nasal sinusotomy

22.50 Sinusotomy, not otherwise specified

22.51 Ethmoidotomy

22.52 Sphenoidotomy

22.53 Incision of multiple nasal sinuses

22.6 Other nasal sinusectomy
Includes: that with incidental turbinectomy

Excludes: *biopsy of nasal sinus (22.11-22.12)*

22.60 Sinusectomy, not otherwise specified

22.61 Excision of lesion of maxillary sinus with Caldwell-Luc approach

22.62 Excision of lesion of maxillary sinus with other approach

22.63 Ethmoidectomy

22.64 Sphenoidectomy

22.7 Repair of nasal sinus

22.71 Closure of nasal sinus fist
Repair of oro-antral fistula

22.79 Other repair of nasal sinus
Reconstruction of frontonasal duct
Repair of bone of accessory sinus

22.9 Other operations on nasal sinuses
Exteriorization of maxillary sinus
Fistulization of sinus

Excludes: *dilation of frontonasal duct (96.21)*

23 Removal and restoration of teeth

23.0 Forceps extraction of tooth

23.01 Extraction of deciduous tooth

23.09 Extraction of other tooth
Extraction of tooth NOS

23.1 Surgical removal of tooth

23.11 Removal of residual root

23.19 Other surgical extraction of tooth
Odontectomy NOS
Removal of impacted tooth
Tooth extraction with elevation of mucoperiosteal flap

23.2 Restoration of tooth by filling

23.3 Restoration of tooth by inlay

23.4 Other dental restoration

23.41 Application of crown

23.42 Insertion of fixed bridge

23.43 Insertion of removable bridge

23.49 Other

23.5 Implantation of tooth

23.6 Prosthetic dental implant
Endosseous dental implant

23.7 Apicoectomy and root canal therapy

23.70 Root canal not otherwise specified

23.71 Root canal therapy with irrigation

23.72 Root canal therapy with apicoectomy

23.73 Apicoectomy

24 Other operations on teeth, gums, and alveoli

24.0 Incision of gum or alveolar bone
Apical alveolotomy

24.1 Diagnostic procedures on teeth, gums, and alveoli

24.11 Biopsy of gum

24.12 Biopsy of alveoli

| Valid O.R. procedure | Non-O.R. procedure | Nonspecific O.R. procedure | Noncovered O.R. procedure |

24.19 Other diagnostic procedures on teeth, gums, and alveoli

Excludes: *dental:*
examination (89.31)
x-ray:
full-mouth (87.11)
other (87.12)
microscopic examination of dental specimen (90.81-90.89)

24.2 Gingivoplasty
Gingivoplasty with bone or soft tissue graft

24.3 Other operations on gum

24.31 Excision of lesion or tissue of gum

Excludes: *biopsy of gum (24.11)*
excision of odontogenic lesion (24.4)

24.32 Suture of laceration of gum

24.39 Other

24.4 Excision of dental lesion of jaw
Excision of odontogenic lesion

24.5 Alveoloplasty
Alveolectomy (interradicular) (intraseptal) (radical) (simple) (with graft or implant)

Excludes: *biopsy of alveolus (24.12)*
en bloc resection of alveolar process and palate (27.32)

24.6 Exposure of tooth

24.7 Application of orthodontic appliance
Application, insertion, or fitting of:
arch bars
orthodontic obturator
orthodontic wiring
periodontal splint

Excludes: *nonorthodontic dental wiring (93.55)*

24.8 Other orthodontic operation
Closure of diastema (alveolar) (dental)
Occlusal adjustment
Removal of arch bars
Repair of dental arch

Excludes: *removal of nonorthodontic wiring (97.33)*

24.9 Other dental operations

24.91 Extension or deepening of buccolabial or lingual sulcus

24.99 Other

Excludes: *dental:*
debridement (96.54)
examination (89.31)
prophylaxis (96.54)
scaling and polishing (96.54)
wiring (93.55)
fitting of dental appliance [denture] (99.97)
microscopic examination of dental specimen (90.81-90.89)
removal of dental:
packing (97.34)
prosthesis (97.35)
wiring (97.33)
replacement of dental packing (97.22)

25 Operations on tongue

25.0 Diagnostic procedures on tongue

25.01 Closed [needle] biopsy of tongue

25.02 Open biopsy of tongue
Wedge biopsy

25.09 Other diagnostic procedures on tongue

● Code new
to this edition

▲ Revision of
existing code

④ ⑤ Fourth or fifth
digit required

25.1   **Excision or destruction of lesion or tissue of tongue**

> Excludes: *biopsy of tongue (25.01-25.02)*
> *frenumectomy:*
> *labial (27.41)*
> *lingual (25.92)*

25.2   **Partial glossectomy**

25.3   **Complete glossectomy**
     Glossectomy NOS
     Code also any neck dissection (40.40-40.42)

25.4   **Radical glossectomy**
     Code also any:
       neck dissection (40.40-40.42)
       tracheostomy (31.1-31.29)

25.5   **Repair of tongue and glossoplasty**

     25.51   **Suture of laceration of tongue**

     25.59   **Other repair and plastic operations on tongue**
         Fascial sling of tongue
         Fusion of tongue (to lip)
         Graft of mucosa or skin to tongue

> Excludes: *lysis of adhesions of tongue (25.93)*

25.9   **Other operations on tongue**

     25.91   **Lingual frenotomy**

> Excludes: *labial frenotomy (27.91)*

     25.92   **Lingual frenectomy**

> Excludes: *labial frenectomy (27.41)*

     25.93   **Lysis of adhesions of tongue**

     25.94   **Other glossotomy**

     25.99   **Other**

26   **Operations on salivary glands and ducts**
     Includes: operations on:
         lesser salivary gland and duct
         parotid gland and duct
         sublingual gland and duct
         submaxillary gland and duct

   Code also any neck dissection (40.40-40.42)

26.0   **Incision of salivary gland or duct**

26.1   **Diagnostic procedures on salivary glands and ducts**

     26.11   **Closed [needle] biopsy of salivary gland or duct**

     26.12   **Open biopsy of salivary gland or duct**

     26.19   **Other diagnostic procedures on salivary glands and ducts**

> Excludes: *x-ray of salivary gland (87.09)*

26.2   **Excision of lesion of salivary gland**

     26.21   **Marsupialization of salivary gland cyst**

     26.29   **Other excision of salivary gland lesion**

> Excludes: *biopsy of salivary gland (26.11-26.12)*
> *salivary fistulectomy (26.42)*

26.3   **Sialoadenectomy**

     26.30   **Sialoadenectomy, not otherwise specified**

     26.31   **Partial sialoadenectomy**

     26.32   **Complete sialoadenectomy**
         En bloc excision of salivary gland lesion
         Radical sialoadenectomy

26.4   **Repair of salivary gland or duct**

     26.41   **Suture of laceration of salivary gland**

     26.42   **Closure of salivary fistula**

	Valid O.R. procedure		Non-O.R. procedure		Nonspecific O.R. procedure		Noncovered O.R. procedure

26.49 **Other repair and plastic operations on salivary gland or duct**
Fistulization of salivary gland
Plastic repair of salivary gland or duct NOS
Transplantation of salivary duct opening

26.9 **Other operations on salivary gland or duct**

26.91 **Probing of salivary duct**

26.99 **Other**

27 **Other operations on mouth and face**
Includes: operations on:
lips
palate
soft tissue of face and mouth, except tongue and gingiva

Excludes   *operations on:*
gingiva (24.0-24.99)
tongue (25.01-25.99)

27.0 **Drainage of face and floor of mouth**
Drainage of:
facial region (abscess)
fascial compartment of face
Ludwig's angina
Excludes: *drainage of thyroglossal tract (06.09)*

27.1 **Incision of palate**

27.2 **Diagnostic procedures on oral cavity**

27.21 **Biopsy of bony palate**

27.22 **Biopsy of uvula and soft palate**

27.23 **Biopsy of lip**

27.24 **Biopsy of mouth, unspecified structure**

27.29 **Other diagnostic procedures on oral cavity**
Excludes: *soft tissue x-ray (87.09)*

27.3 **Excision of lesion or tissue of bony palate**

27.31 **Local excision or destruction of lesion or tissue of bony palate**
Local excision or destruction of palate by:
cautery
chemotherapy
cryotherapy
Excludes: *biopsy of bony palate (27.21)*

27.32 **Wide excision or destruction of lesion or tissue of bony palate**
En bloc resection of alveolar process and palate

27.4 **Excision of other parts of mouth**

27.41 **Labial frenectomy**
Excludes: *division of labial frenum (27.91)*

27.42 **Wide excision of lesion of lip**

27.43 **Other excision of lesion or tissue of lip**

27.49 **Other excision of mouth**
Excludes: *biopsy of mouth NOS (27.24)*
excision of lesion of:
palate (27.31-27.32)
tongue (25.1)
uvula (27.72)
fistulectomy of mouth (27.53)
frenectomy of:
lip (27.41)
tongue (25.92)

27.5 **Plastic repair of lip and mouth**
Excludes: *palatoplasty (27.61-27.69)*

27.51 **Suture of laceration of lip**

27.52 **Suture of laceration of other part of mouth**

● Code new
to this edition   ▲ Revision of
existing code   ④ ⑤ Fourth or fifth
digit required

27.53 Closure of fistula of mouth

> *Excludes:* fistulectomy:
>> nasolabial (21.82)
>> oro-antral (22.71)
>> oronasal (21.82)

27.54 Repair of cleft lip

27.55 Full-thickness skin graft to lip and mouth

27.56 Other skin graft to lip and mouth

27.57 Attachment of pedicle or flap graft to lip and mouth

27.59 Other plastic repair of mouth

27.6 Palatoplasty

27.61 Suture of laceration of palate

27.62 Correction of cleft palate
Correction of cleft palate by push-back operation

> *Excludes:* revision of cleft palate repair (27.63)

27.63 Revision of cleft palate repair
Secondary:
  attachment of pharyngeal flap
  lengthening of palate

27.64 Insertion of palatal implant

27.69 Other plastic repair of palate
Code also any insertion of palatal implant (27.64)

> *Excludes:* fistulectomy of mouth (27.53)

27.7 Operations on uvula

27.71 Incision of uvula

27.72 Excision of uvula

> *Excludes:* biopsy of uvula (27.22)

27.73 Repair of uvula

> *Excludes:* that with synchronous cleft palate repair (27.62)
> uranostaphylorrhaphy (27.62)

27.79 Other operations on uvula

27.9 Other operations on mouth and face

27.91 Labial frenotomy
Division of labial frenum

> *Excludes:* lingual frenotomy (25.91)

27.92 Incision of mouth, unspecified structure

> *Excludes:* incision of:
>> gum (24.0)
>> palate (27.1)
>> salivary gland or duct (26.0)
>> tongue (25.94)
>> uvula (27.71)

27.99 Other operations on oral cavity
Graft of buccal sulcus

> *Excludes:* removal of:
>> intraluminal foreign body (98.01)
>> penetrating foreign body from mouth without incision (98.22)

28 Operations on tonsils and adenoids

28.0 Incision and drainage of tonsil and peritonsillar structures
Drainage (oral) (transcervical) of:
  parapharyngeal abscess
  peritonsillar abscess
  retropharyngeal abscess
  tonsillar abscess

28.1 Diagnostic procedures on tonsils and adenoids

28.11 Biopsy of tonsils and adenoids

 Valid O.R. procedure

 Non-O.R. procedure

 Nonspecific O.R. procedure

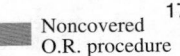 Noncovered O.R. procedure

28.19 Other diagnostic procedures on tonsils and adenoids
> *Excludes:* soft tissue x-ray (87.09)

28.2 Tonsillectomy without adenoidectomy

28.3 Tonsillectomy with adenoidectomy

28.4 Excision of tonsil tag

28.5 Excision of lingual tonsil

28.6 Adenoidectomy without tonsillectomy
Excision of adenoid tag

28.7 Control of hemorrhage after tonsillectomy and adenoidectomy

28.9 Other operations on tonsils and adenoids

28.91 Removal of foreign body from tonsil and adenoid by incision
> *Excludes:* that without incision (98.13)

28.92 Excision of lesion of tonsil and adenoid
> *Excludes:* biopsy of tonsil and adenoid (28.11)

28.99 Other

29 Operation on pharynx
Includes: operations on:
hypopharynx
nasopharynx
oropharynx
pharyngeal pouch
pyriform sinus

29.0 Pharyngotomy
Drainage of pharyngeal bursa
> *Excludes:* incision and drainage of retropharyngeal abscess (28.0)
> removal of foreign body (without incision) (98.13)

29.1 Diagnostic procedures on pharynx

29.11 Pharyngoscopy

29.12 Pharyngeal biopsy
Biopsy of supraglottic mass

29.19 Other diagnostic procedures on pharynx
> *Excludes:* x-ray of nasopharynx:
> contrast (87.06)
> other (87.09)

29.2 Excision of branchial cleft cyst or vestige
> *Excludes:* branchial cleft fistulectomy (29.52)

29.3 Excision or destruction of lesion or tissue of pharynx

29.31 Cricopharyngeal myotomy
> *Excludes* that with pharyngeal diverticulectomy (29.32)

29.32 Pharyngeal diverticulectomy

29.33 Pharyngectomy (partial)
> *Excludes* laryngopharyngectomy (30.3)

29.39 Other excision or destruction of lesion or tissue of pharynx

29.4 Plastic operation on pharynx
Correction of nasopharyngeal atresia
> *Excludes:* pharyngoplasty associated with cleft palate repair (27.62-27.63)

29.5 Other repair of pharynx

29.51 Suture of laceration of pharynx

29.52 Closure of branchial cleft fistula

29.53 Closure of other fistula of pharynx
Pharyngoesophageal fistulectomy

29.54 Lysis of pharyngeal adhesions

29.59 Other

● Code new to this edition   ▲ Revision of existing code   ④ ⑤ Fourth or fifth digit required

29.9 **Other operations on pharynx**

    29.91 **Dilation of pharynx**
         Dilation of nasopharynx

    29.92 Division of glossopharyngeal nerve

    29.99 Other

         | Excludes: | *insertion of radium into pharynx and nasopharynx (92.27)*
                        removal of intraluminal foreign body (98.13)

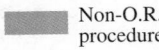
Valid O.R. procedure

Non-O.R. procedure

Nonspecific O.R. procedure

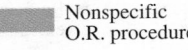
Noncovered O.R. procedure

This page intentionally left blank.

● Code new
 to this edition

▲ Revision of
 existing code

④ ⑤ Fourth or fifth
 digit required

6. OPERATIONS ON THE RESPIRATORY SYSTEM (30-34)

30 Excision of larynx

30.0 Excision or destruction of lesion or tissue of larynx

30.01 Marsupialization of laryngeal cyst

30.09 Other excision or destruction of lesion or tissue of larynx
Stripping of vocal cords

Excludes: biopsy of larynx (31.43)
laryngeal fistulectomy (31.62)
laryngotracheal fistulectomy (31.62)

30.1 Hemilaryngectomy

30.2 Other partial laryngectomy

30.21 Epiglottidectomy

30.22 Vocal cordectomy
Excision of vocal cords

30.29 Other partial laryngectomy
Excision of laryngeal cartilage

30.3 Complete laryngectomy
Block dissection of larynx (with thyroidectomy) (with synchronous tracheostomy)
Laryngopharyngectomy

Excludes: that with radical neck dissection (30.4)

30.4 Radical laryngectomy
Complete [total] laryngectomy with radical neck dissection (with thyroidectomy) (with
synchronous tracheostomy)

31 Other operations on larynx and trachea

31.0 Injection of larynx
Injection of inert material into larynx or vocal cords

31.1 Temporary tracheostomy
Temporary percutaneous dilatational tracheostomy [PDT]
Tracheotomy for assistance in breathing
Code also any synchronous bronchoscopy, if performed (33.21-33.24, 33.27)

31.2 Permanent tracheostomy

31.21 Mediastinal tracheostomy

31.29 Other permanent tracheostomy
Permanent percutaneous dilatational tracheostomy [PDT]
Code also any synchronous bronchoscopy, if performed (33.21-33.24, 33.27)

Excludes: that with laryngectomy (30.3-30.4)

31.3 Other incision of larynx or trachea

Excludes: that for assistance in breathing (31.1-31.29)

31.4 Diagnostic procedures on larynx and trachea

31.41 Tracheoscopy through artificial stoma

Excludes: that with biopsy (31.43-31.44)

31.42 Laryngoscopy and other tracheoscopy

Excludes: that with biopsy (31.43-31.44)

31.43 Closed [endoscopic] biopsy of larynx

31.44 Closed [endoscopic] biopsy of trachea

31.45 Open biopsy of larynx or trachea

31.48 Other diagnostic procedures on larynx

Excludes: contrast laryngogram (87.07)
microscopic examination of specimen from larynx (90.31-90.39)
soft tissue x-ray of larynx NEC (87.09)

31.49 Other diagnostic procedures on trachea

Excludes: microscopic examination of specimen from trachea (90.41-90.49)
x-ray of trachea (87.49)

Valid O.R. procedure	Non-O.R. procedure	Nonspecific O.R. procedure	Noncovered O.R. procedure

31.5 **Local excision or destruction of lesion or tissue of trachea**
> *Excludes:* *biopsy of trachea (31.44-31.45)*
> *laryngotracheal fistulectomy (31.62)*
> *tracheoesophageal fistulectomy (31.73)*

31.6 **Repair of larynx**

31.61 **Suture of laceration of larynx**

31.62 **Closure of fistula of larynx**
Laryngotracheal fistulectomy
Take-down of laryngostomy

31.63 **Revision of laryngostomy**

31.64 **Repair of laryngeal fracture**

31.69 **Other repair of larynx**
Arytenoidopexy
Graft of larynx
Transposition of vocal cords
> *Excludes:* *construction of artificial larynx (31.75)*

31.7 **Repair and plastic operations on trachea**

31.71 **Suture of laceration of trachea**

31.72 **Closure of external fistula of trachea**
Closure of tracheotomy

31.73 **Closure of other fistula of trachea**
Tracheoesophageal fistulectomy
> *Excludes:* *laryngotracheal fistulectomy (31.62)*

31.74 **Revision of tracheostomy**

31.75 **Reconstruction of trachea and construction of artificial larynx**
Tracheoplasty with artificial larynx

31.79 **Other repair and plastic operations on trachea**

31.9 **Other operations on larynx and trachea**

31.91 **Division of laryngeal nerve**

31.92 **Lysis of adhesions of trachea or larynx**

31.93 **Replacement of laryngeal or tracheal stent**

31.94 **Injection of locally-acting therapeutic substance into trachea**

31.95 **Tracheoesophageal fistulization**

31.98 **Other operations on larynx**
Dilation of larynx
Division of congenital web of larynx
Removal of keel or stent of larynx
> *Excludes:* *removal of intraluminal foreign body from larynx without incision (98.14)*

31.99 **Other operations on trachea**
> *Excludes:* *removal of:*
> *intraluminal foreign body from trachea without incision (98.15)*
> *tracheostomy tube (97.37)*
> *replacement of tracheostomy tube (97.23)*
> *tracheostomy toilette (96.35)*

32 **Excision of lung and bronchus**
Includes: rib resection as operative approach
sternotomy as operative approach
sternum-splitting incision as operative approach
thoracotomy as operative approach
Code also any synchronous bronchoplasty (33.48)

32.0 **Local excision or destruction of lesion or tissue of bronchus**
> *Excludes:* *biopsy of bronchus (33.24-33.25)*
> *bronchial fistulectomy (33.42)*

32.01 **Endoscopic excision or destruction of lesion or tissue of bronchus**

32.09 **Other local excision or destruction of lesion or tissue of bronchus**
> *Excludes:* *that by endoscopic approach (32.01)*

● Code new to this edition ▲ Revision of existing code ④ ⑤ Fourth or fifth digit required

32.1 **Other excision of bronchus**
Resection (wide sleeve) of bronchus

> Excludes: radical dissection [excision] of bronchus (32.6)

32.2 **Local excision or destruction of lesion or tissue of lung**

32.20 **Thoracoscopic excision of lesion or tissue of lung**
Thoracoscopic wedge resection

32.21 **Plication of emphysematous bleb**

32.22 **Lung volume reduction surgery**

32.23 **Open ablation of lung lesion or tissue**

32.24 **Percutaneous ablation of lung lesion or tissue**

32.25 **Thoracoscopic ablation of lung lesion or tissue**

> Excludes: thoracoscopic excision of lesion or tissue of lung (32.20)

32.26 **Other and unspecified ablatin of lung lesion or tissue**

> Excludes: bronchoscopic bronchial thermoplasty, ablation of smooth airway muscle (32.27)

32.27 **Bronchoscopic bronchial thermoplasty, ablation of smooth airway muscle**

32.28 **Endoscopic excision or destruction of lesion or tissue of lung**

> Excludes: ablation of lung lesion or tissue:
> open (32.23)
> other (32.26)
> percutaneous (32.24)
> thoracoscopic (32.25)
> biopsy of lung (33.26-33.27)

32.29 **Other local excision or destruction of lesion or tissue of lung**
Resection of lung:
NOS
wedge

> Excludes: ablation of lung lesion or tissue:
> open (32.23)
> other (32.26)
> percutaneous (32.24)
> thoracoscopic (32.25)
> biopsy of lung (33.26-33.27)
> laser interstitial thermal therapy [LITT] of lesion or tissue of lung under guidance (17.69)
> that by endoscopic approach (32.28)
> thoracoscopic excision of lesion or tissue of lung (32.20)
> wide excision of lesion of lung (32.3)

32.3 **Segmental resection of lung**
Partial lobectomy

32.30 **Thoracoscopic segmental resection of lung**

32.39 **Other and unspecified segmental resection of lung**

> Excludes: thoracoscopic segmental resection of lung (32.30)

32.4 **Lobectomy of lung**
Lobectomy with segmental resection of adjacent lobes of lung

> Excludes: that with radical dissection [excision] of thoracic structures (32.6)

32.41 **Thoracoscopic lobectomy of lung**

32.49 **Other lobectomy of lung**

> Excludes: thoracoscopic lobectomy of lung (32.41)

32.5 **Pneumonectomy**
Excision of lung NOS
Pneumonectomy (with mediastinal dissection)

32.50 **Thoracoscopic pneumonectomy**

32.59 **Other and unspecified pneumonectomy**

> Excludes: thoracoscopic pneumonectomy (32.50)

32.6 **Radical dissection of thoracic structures**
Block [en bloc] dissection of bronchus, lobe of lung, brachial plexus, intercostal structure, ribs (transverse process), and sympathetic nerves

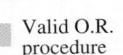

| | Valid O.R. procedure | | Non-O.R. procedure | | Nonspecific O.R. procedure | | Noncovered O.R. procedure |

32.9   Other excision of lung

> | Excludes: | biopsy of lung and bronchus *(33.24-33.27)*
> pulmonary decortication *(34.51)*

33   **Other operations on lung and bronchus**
Includes: rib resection as operative approach
sternotomy as operative approach
sternum-splitting incision as operative approach
thoracotomy as operative approach

33.0   **Incision of bronchus**

33.1   **Incision of lung**

> | Excludes: | puncture of lung *(33.93)*

33.2   **Diagnostic procedures on lung and bronchus**

33.20   **Thoracoscopic lung biopsy**

> | Excludes: | closed endoscopic biopsy of lung *(33.27)*
> closed [percutaneous] [needle] biopsy of lung *(33.26)*
> open biopsy of lung *(33.28)*

33.21   **Bronchoscopy through artificial stoma**

> | Excludes: | that with biopsy *(33.24, 33.27)*

33.22   **Fiber-optic bronchoscopy**

> | Excludes: | that with biopsy *(33.24. 33.27)*

33.23   **Other bronchoscopy**

> | Excludes: | that for:
> aspiration *(96.05)*
> biopsy *(33.24, 33.27)*

33.24   **Closed [endoscopic] biopsy of bronchus**
Bronchoscopy (fiberoptic) (rigid) with:
brush biopsy of "lung"
brushing or washing for specimen collection
excision (bite) biopsy
Diagnostic bronchoalveolar lavage (BAL)
Mini-bronchoalveolar lavage [mini-BAL]
Transbronchoscopic needle aspiration [TBNA] of bronchus

> | Excludes: | closed biopsy of lung, other than brush biopsy of "lung" *(33.26, 33.27)*
> whole lung lavage *(33.99)*

33.25   **Open biopsy of bronchus**

> | Excludes: | open biopsy of lung *(33.28)*

33.26   **Closed [percutaneous] [needle] biopsy of lung**
Fine needle aspiration (FNA) of lung
Transthoracic needle biopsy of lung (TTNB)

> | Excludes: | endoscopic biopsy of lung *(33.27)*
> thoracoscopic lung biopsy *(33.20)*

33.27   **Closed endoscopic biopsy of lung**
Fiberoptic (flexible) bronchoscopy with fluoroscopic guidance with biopsy
Transbronchial lung biopsy
Transbronchoscopic needle aspiration [TBNA] of lung

> | Excludes: | brush biopsy of lung *(33.24)*
> percutaneous biopsy of lung *(33.26)*
> thoracoscopic lung biopsy *(33.20)*

33.28   **Open biopsy of lung**

● Code new
to this edition   ▲ Revision of
existing code   ④ ⑤ Fourth or fifth
digit required

33.29 Other diagnostic procedures on lung and bronchus

Excludes: *bronchoalveolar lavage [BAL] (33.24)*
contrast bronchogram:
endotracheal (87.31)
other (87.32)
endoscopic pulmonary airway flow measurement (33.72)
lung scan (92.15)
magnetic resonance imaging (88.92)
microscopic examination of specimen from bronchus or lung
(90.41-90.49)
routine chest x-ray (87.44)
ultrasonography of lung (88.73)
vital capacity determination (89.37)
x-ray of bronchus or lung NOS (87.49)

33.3 Surgical collapse of lung

33.31 Destruction of phrenic nerve for collapse of lung

33.32 Artificial pneumothorax for collapse of lung
Thoracotomy for collapse of lung

33.33 Pneumoperitoneum for collapse of lung

33.34 Thoracoplasty

33.39 Other surgical collapse of lung
Collapse of lung NOS

33.4 Repair and plastic operation on lung and bronchus

33.41 Suture of laceration of bronchus

33.42 Closure of bronchial fistula
Closure of bronchostomy
Fistulectomy:
bronchocutaneous
bronchoesophageal
bronchovisceral

Excludes: *closure of fistula:*
bronchomediastinal (34.73)
bronchopleural (34.73)
bronchopleuromediastinal (34.73)

33.43 Closure of laceration of lung

33.48 Other repair and plastic operation on bronchus

33.49 Other repair ad plastic operations on lung

Excludes: *closure of pleural fistula (34.73)*

33.5 Lung transplant
Code also cardiopulmonary bypass [extracorporeal circulation] [heart-lung machine]
39.61
Note: To report donor source—*see* codes 00.91-00.93

Excludes: *Combined heart-lung transplantation (33.6)*

33.50 Lung transplantation, not otherwise specified

33.51 Unilateral lung transplantation

33.52 Bilateral lung transplantation
Double-lung transplantation
En bloc transplantation

33.6 Combined heart-lung transplantation
Code also cardiopulmonary bypass [extracorporeal circulation] [heart-lung machine]
(39.61)
Note: To report donor source—*see* codes 00.91-00.93

33.7 Other endoscopic procedures in bronchus or lung

Excludes: *insertion of tracheobronchial stent (96.05)*

33.71 Endoscopic insertion or replacement of bronchial valve(s), single lobe
Endobronchial airflow redirection valve
Intrabronchial airflow redirection valve

Excludes: *endoscopic insertion or replacement of bronchial valve(s), multiple*
lobes (33.73)

	Valid O.R. procedure		Non-O.R. procedure		Nonspecific O.R. procedure		Noncovered O.R. procedure

33.72 Endoscopic pulmonary airway flow measurement
Assessment of pulmonary airway flow

Code also any diagnostic or therapeutic procedure if performed

33.73 Endoscopic insertion or replacement of bronchial valve(s), multiple lobes
Endobronchial airflow redirection valve
Intrabronchial airflow redirection valve

Excludes: *endoscopic insertion or replacement of bronchial valve(s), single lobe (33.71)*

33.78 Endoscopic removal of bronchial device(s) or substances

33.79 Endoscopic insertion of other bronchial device or substances
Biologic Lung Volume Reduction NOS (BLVR)

33.9 Other operations on lung and bronchus

33.91 Bronchial dilation

33.92 Ligation of bronchus

33.93 Puncture of lung

Excludes: *needle biopsy (33.26)*

33.98 Other operations on bronchus

Excludes: *bronchial lavage (96.56)*
removal of intraluminal foreign body from bronchus without incision (98.15)

33.99 Other operations on lung
Whole lung lavage

Excludes: *other continuous mechanical ventilation (96.70-96.72)*
respiratory therapy (93.90-93.99)

34 Operations on chest wall, pleura, mediastinum, and diaphragm

Excludes: *operations on breast (85.0-85.99)*

34.0 Incision of chest wall and pleura

Excludes: *that as operative approach—omit code*

34.01 Incision of chest wall
Extrapleural drainage

Excludes: *incision of pleura (34.09)*

34.02 Exploratory thoracotomy

34.03 Reopening of recent thoracotomy site

34.04 Insertion of intercostal catheter for drainage
Chest tube
Closed chest drainage
Revision of intercostal catheter (chest tube) (with lysis of adhesions)

Excludes: *thoracoscopic drainage of pleural cavity (34.06)*

34.05 Creation of pleuroperitoneal shunt

34.06 Thoracoscopic drainage of pleural cavity
Evacuation of empyema

34.09 Other incision of pleura
Creation of pleural window for drainage
Intercostal stab
Open chest drainage

Excludes: *thoracoscopy (34.21)*
thoracotomy for collapse of lung (33.32)

34.1 Incision of mediastinum

Code also any biopsy, if performed

Excludes: *mediastinoscopy (34.22)*
mediastinotomy associated with pneumonectomy (32.5)

34.2 Diagnostic procedures on chest wall, pleura, mediastinum, and diaphragm

34.20 Thoracoscopic pleural biopsy

34.21 Transpleural thoracoscopy

34.22 Mediastinoscopy

Code also any biopsy, if performed

● Code new to this edition   ▲ Revision of existing code   ④ ⑤ Fourth or fifth digit required

34.23 Biopsy of chest wall

34.24 Other pleural biopsy

> Excludes: *thoracoscopic pleural biopsy (34.20)*

34.25 Closed [percutaneous] [needle] biopsy of mediastinum

34.26 Open biopsy of mediastinum

34.27 Biopsy of diaphragm

34.28 Other diagnostic procedures on chest wall, pleura, and diaphragm

> Excludes: *angiocardiography (88.50-88.58)*
> *aortography (88.42)*
> *arteriography of:*
>   *intrathoracic vessels NEC (88.44)*
>   *pulmonary arteries (88.43)*
> *microscopic examination of specimen from chest wall. pleura, and*
>   *diaphragm (90.41-90.49)*
> *phlebography of:*
>   *intrathoracic vessels NEC (88.63)*
>   *pulmonary veins (88.62)*
> *radiological examinations of thorax:*
>   *C.A.T. scan (87.41)*
>   *diaphragmatic x-ray (87.49)*
>   *intrathoracic lymphangiogram (87.34)*
>   *routine chest x-ray (87.44)*
>   *sinogram of chest wall (87.38)*
>   *soft tissue x-ray of chest wall NEC (87.39)*
>   *tomogram of thorax NEC (87. 42)*
>   *ultrasonography of thorax (88.73)*

34.29 Other diagnostic procedures on mediastinum

> Excludes: *mediastinal:*
> *pneumogram (87.33)*
> *x-ray NEC (87.49)*

34.3 Excision or destruction of lesion or tissue of mediastinum

> Excludes: *biopsy or mediastinum (34.25-34.26)*
> *mediastinal fistulectomy (34.73)*

34.4 Excision or destruction of lesion of chest wall
Excision of lesion of chest wall NOS (with excision of ribs)

> Excludes: *biopsy of chest wall (34.23)*
> *costectomy not incidental to thoracic procedure (77. 91)*
> *excision of lesion of:*
>   *breast (85.20-85.25)*
>   *cartilage (80.89)*
>   *skin (86.2-86.3)*
> *fistulectomy (34. 73)*

34.5 Pleurectomy

34.51 Decortication of lung

> Excludes: *thoracoscopic decortication of lung (34.52)*

34.52 Thoracoscopic decortication of lung

34.59 Other excision of pleura
Excision of pleural lesion

> Excludes: *biopsy of pleura (34.24)*
> *pleural fistulectomy (34.73)*

34.6 Scarification of pleura
Pleurosclerosis

> Excludes: *injection of sclerosing agent (34.92)*

34.7 Repair of chest wall

34.71 Suture of laceration of chest wall

> Excludes: *suture of skin and subcutaneous tissue alone (86.59)*

34.72 Closure of thoracostomy

Valid O.R. procedure	Non-O.R. procedure	Nonspecific O.R. procedure	Noncovered O.R. procedure

34.73 **Closure of other fistula of thorax**
Closure of:
 bronchopleural fistula
 bronchopleurocutaneous fistula
 bronchopleuromediastinal fistula

34.74 **Repair of pectus deformity**
Repair of:
 pectus carinatum (with implant)
 pectus excavatum (with implant)

34.79 **Other repair of chest wall**
Repair of chest wall NOS

34.8 **Operations on diaphragm**

34.81 **Excision of lesion or tissue of diaphragm**
Excludes: biopsy of diaphragm (34.27)

34.82 **Suture of laceration of diaphragm**

34.83 **Closure of fistula of diaphragm**
Thoracicoabdominal fistulectomy
Thoracicogastric fistulectomy
Thoracicointestinal fistulectomy

34.84 **Other repair of diaphragm**
Excludes: repair of diaphragmatic hernia (53.7-53.82)

34.85 **Implantation of diaphragmatic pacemaker**

34.89 **Other operations on diaphragm**

34.9 **Other operations on thorax**

34.91 **Thoracentesis**

34.92 **Injection into thoracic cavity**
Chemical pleurodesis
Injection of cytotoxic agent or tetracycline
Instillation into thoracic cavity
Requires additional code for any cancer chemotherapeutic substance (99.25)
Excludes: that for collapse of lung (33.32)

34.93 **Repair of pleura**

34.99 **Other**
Excludes: removal of:
 mediastinal drain (97.42)
 sutures (97.43)
 thoracotomy tube (97.41)

● Code new
 to this edition
▲ Revision of
 existing code
④ ⑤ Fourth or fifth
 digit required

7. **OPERATIONS ON THE CARDIOVASCULAR SYSTEM (35-39)**

35 **Operations on valves and septa of heart**
   Includes: sternotomy (median) (transverse) as operative approach
            thoracotomy as operative approach
   Code also any cardiopulmonary bypass [extracorporeal circulation] [heart-lung machine] (39.61)

▲ **35.0   Closed heart valvotomy or transcatheter replacement of heart valve**

  Excludes: *percutaneous (balloon) valvuloplasty (35.96)*

   35.00 Closed heart valvotomy, unspecified valve
   35.01 Closed heart valvotomy, aortic valve
   35.02 Closed heart valvotomy, mitral valve
   35.03 Closed heart valvotomy, pulmonary valve
   35.04 Closed heart valvotomy, tricuspid valve

● **35.05 Endovascular replacement of aortic valve**
   Note: Includes that with any balloon valvuloplasty; do not code separately
      Implantation of transcatheter aortic valve
      Replacement of aortic valve with tissue graft (autograft) (bioprosthetic)
         (heterograft) (homograft):
         transarterial approach
         transfemoral approach
      TAVI (transcatheter aortic valve implantation)
      TAVR (transcatheter aortic valve replacement)
      Excludes: *open and other replacement of heart valve (35.20-35.28)*

● **35.06 Transapical replacement of aortic valve**
   Note: Includes that with any balloon valvuloplasty; do not code separately
      Implantation of transcatheter aortic valve
      Replacement of aortic valve with tissue graft (autograft) (bioprosthetic)
         (heterograft) (homograft):
         intercostal approach
         transventricular approach
      That via transthoracic exposure, i.e. thoracotomy, sternotomy, or subxiphoid
         approach
      Excludes: *open and other replacement of heart valve (35.20-35.28)*

● **35.07 Endovascular replacement of pulmonary valve**
   Note: Includes that with any balloon valvuloplasty; do not code separately
      Implantation of transcatheter pulmonary valve
      PPVI (percutaneous pulmonary valve implantation)
      Replacement of pulmonary valve:
         transfemoral approach
         transvenous approach
      That within previously created right ventricle-to pulmonary artery conduit
      TPVI (transcatheter pulmonary valve implantation)
      Excludes: *open and other replacement of heart valve (35.20-35.28)*

● **35.08 Transapical replacement of pulmonary valve**
   Note: Includes that with any balloon valvuloplasty; do not code separately
      Implantation of transcatheter pulmonary valve
      Replacement of pulmonary valve:
         intercostal approach
         transventricular approach
      That via transthoracic exposure, i.e. thoracotomy, sternotomy, or subxiphoid
         approach
      Excludes: *open and other replacement of heart valve (35.20-35.28)*

● **35.09 Endovascular replacement of unspecified heart valve**
   Note: Includes that with any balloon valvuloplasty; do not code separately
      Replacement of valve via:
         intercostal approach
         transventricular approach
      Excludes: *open and other replacement of heart valve (35.20-35.28)*

	Valid O.R. procedure		Non-O.R. procedure		Nonspecific O.R. procedure		Noncovered O.R. procedure

35.1 Open heart valvuloplasty without replacement
Includes: open heart valvotomy

> Excludes: *that associated with repair of:*
> > *endocardial cushion defect (35.54, 35.63, 35.73)*
> > *percutaneous (balloon) valvuloplasty (35.96)*
> > *valvular defect associated with atrial and ventricular septal defects (35.54, 35.63, 35.73)*

> *Code also cardiopulmonary bypass, if performed [extracorporeal circulation] [heart-lung machine] (39.61)*

35.10 Open heart valvuloplasty without replacement, unspecified valve
35.11 Open heart valvuloplasty of aortic valve without replacement
35.12 Open heart valvuloplasty of mitral valve without replacement
35.13 Open heart valvuloplasty of pulmonary valve without replacement
35.14 Open heart valvuloplasty of tricuspid valve without replacement

▲ **35.2 Open and other replacement of heart valve**
Includes: excision of heart valve with replacement

> *Code also cardiopulmonary bypass [extracorporeal circulation] [heart-lung machine] (39.61)*

> Excludes: *that associated with repair of:*
> > *endocardial cushion defect (35.54, 35.63, 35.73)*
> > *valvular defect associated with atrial and ventricular septal defects (35.54, 35.63, 35.73)*
> > *transapical replacement of heart valve (35.06, 35.08)*
> > *transcatheter replacement of heart valve (35.05, 35.07)*

▲ **35.20 Open and other replacement of unspecified heart valve**
That with tissue graft or prosthetic implant

> Excludes: *endovascular replacement of unspecified heart valve (35.09)*

▲ **35.21 Open and other replacement of aortic valve with tissue graft**
Includes that by:
  autograft
  heterograft
  homograft

> Excludes: *endovascular replacement of aortic valve (35.05)*
> *transapical replacement of aortic valve (35.06)*

▲ **35.22 Open and other replacement of aortic valve**
Replacement of aortic valve NOS
That with prosthetic (partial) (synthetic) (total)

> Excludes: *endovascular replacement of aortic valve (35.05)*
> *transapical replacement of aortic valve (35.06)*

▲ **35.23 Open and other replacement of mitral valve with tissue graft**
Includes that by:
  autograft
  heterograft
  homograft

▲ **35.24 Open and other replacement of mitral valve**
Replacement of mitral valve NOS
That with prosthetic (partial) (synthetic) (total)

> Excludes: *percutaneous repair with implant or leaflet clip (35.97)*

▲ **35.25 Open and other replacement of pulmonary valve with tissue graft**
Includes that by:
  autograft
  heterograft
  homograft

> Excludes: *endovascular replacement of pulmonary valve (35.07)*
> *transapical replacement of pulmonary valve (35.08)*

▲ **35.26 Open and other replacement of pulmonary valve**
Replacement of pulmonary valve, NOS
That with prosthetic (partial) (synthetic) (total)

> Excludes: *endovascular replacement of pulmonary valve (35.07)*
> *transapical replacement of pulmonary valve (35.08)*

● Code new
to this edition
▲ Revision of
existing code
④ ⑤ Fourth or fifth
digit required

▲ 35.27 **Open and other replacement of tricuspid valve with tissue graft**
Includes that by:
autograft
heterograft
homograft

▲ 35.28 **Open and other replacement of tricuspid valve**
Replacement of tricuspid valve, NOS
That with prosthetic (partial) (synthetic) (total)

35.3 **Operations on structures adjacent to heart valves**
Code also cardiopulmonary bypass [extracorporeal circulation] [heart-lung machine] (39.61)

35.31 **Operations on papillary muscle**
Division of papillary muscle
Reattachment of papillary muscle
Repair of papillary muscle

35.32 **Operations on chordae tendineae**
Division of chordae tendineae
Repair of chordae tendineae

35.33 **Annuloplasty**
Plication of annulus

35.34 **Infundibulectomy**
Right ventricular infundibulectomy

35.35 **Operations on trabeculae carneae cordis**
Division of trabeculae carneae cordis
Excision of trabeculae carneae cordis
Excision of aortic subvalvular ring

35.39 **Operations on other structures adjacent to valves of heart**
Repair of sinus of Valsalva (aneurysm)

35.4 **Production of septal defect in heart**

35.41 **Enlargement of existing atrial septal defect**
Rashkind procedure
Septostomy (atrial) (balloon)

35.42 **Creation of septal defect in heart**
Blalock-Hanlon operation

35.5 **Repair of atrial and ventricular septa with prosthesis**
Includes: repair of septa with synthetic implant of patch
Code also cardiopulmonary bypass [extracorporeal circulation] [heart-lung machine] (39.61)

35.50 **Repair of unspecified septal defect of heart with prosthesis**

Excludes: *that associated with repair of:*
endocardial cushion defect (35.54)
septal defect associated with valvular defect (35.54)

35.51 **Repair of atrial septal defect with prosthesis, open technique**
Atrioseptoplasty with prosthesis
Correction of atrial septal defect with prosthesis
Repair:
foramen ovale (patent) with prosthesis
ostium secundum defect with prosthesis

Excludes: *that associated with repair of:*
atrial septal defect associated with valvular and ventricular septal defects (35.54)
endocardial cushion defect (35.54)

35.52 **Repair of atrial septal defect with prosthesis, closed technique**
Insertion of atrial septal umbrella [King-Mills]

35.53 **Repair of ventricular septal defect with prosthesis, open technique**
Correction of ventricular septal defect with prosthesis
Repair of supracristal defect with prosthesis

Excludes: *that associated with repair of:*
endocardial cushion defect (35.54)
ventricular defect associated with valvular and atrial septal defects (35.54)

 Valid O.R. procedure
 Non-O.R. procedure
 Nonspecific O.R. procedure
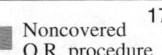 Noncovered O.R. procedure

35.54 Repair of endocardial cushion defect with prosthesis
Repair:
atrioventricular canal with prosthesis (grafted to septa)
ostium primum defect with prosthesis (grafted to septa)
valvular defect associated with atrial and ventricular septal defects with prosthesis
(grafted to septa)

Excludes:	*repair of isolated:*
	atrial septal defect (35.51-35.52)
	valvular defect (35.20, 35.22, 35.24, 35.26. 35.28)
	ventricular septal defect (35.53)

35.55 Repair of ventricular septal defect with prosthesis, closed technique

35.6 Repair of atrial and ventricular septa with tissue graft
Code also cardiopulmonary bypass [extracorporeal circulation] [heart-lung machine]
(39.61)

35.60 Repair of unspecified septal defect of heart with tissue graft

Excludes:	*that associated with repair of:*
	endocardial cushion defect (35.63)
	septal defect associated with valvular, defect (33.63)

35.61 Repair of atrial septal defect with tissue graft
Atrioseptoplasty with tissue graft
Correction of atrial septal defect with tissue graft
Repair:
foramen ovale (patent) with tissue graft
ostium secundum defect with tissue graft

Excludes:	*that associated with repair of:*
	atrial septal defect associated with valvular and ventricular septal
	defects (35.63)
	endocardial cushion defect (35.63)

35.62 Repair of ventricular septal defect with tissue graft
Correction of ventricular septal defect with tissue graft
Repair of supracristal defect with tissue graft

Excludes:	*that associated with repair of:*
	endocardial cushion defect (35.63)
	ventricular defect associated with valvular and atrial septal defects
	(35.63)

35.63 Repair of endocardial cushion defect with tissue graft
Repair of:
atrioventricular canal with tissue graft
ostium primum defect with tissue graft
valvular defect associated with atrial and ventricular septal defects, with tissue
graft

Excludes:	*repair of isolated*
	atrial septal defect (35.61)
	valvular defect (35.20-35.21. 35.23, 35.25. 35.27)
	ventricular septal defect (35.62)

35.7 Other and unspecified repair of atrial and ventricular septa
Code also cardiopulmonary bypass [extracorporeal circulation] [heart-lung machine]
(39.61)

35.70 Other and unspecified repair of unspecified septal defect of heart
Repair of septal defect NOS

Excludes:	*that associated with repair of:*
	endocardial cushion defect (35.73)
	septal defect associated with valvular defect (35.73)

● Code new
to this edition

▲ Revision of
existing code

④ ⑤ Fourth or fifth
digit required

35.71 Other and unspecified repair of atrial septal defect

Repair NOS:
atrial septum
foramen ovale (patent)
ostium secundum defect

Excludes: *that associated with repair of:*
atrial septal defect associated with valvular and ventricular septal defects (35.73)
endocardial cushion defect (35.73)

35.72 Other and unspecified repair of ventricular septal defect

Repair NOS:
supracristal defect
ventricular septum

Excludes: *that associated with repair of:*
endocardial cushion defect (35.73)
ventricular septal defect associated with valvular and atrial septal defects (35.73)

35.73 Other and unspecified repair of endocardial cushion defect

Repair NOS:
atrioventricular canal
ostium primum defect
valvular defect associated with atrial and ventricular septal defects

Excludes: *repair of isolated:*
atrial septal defect (35.71)
valvular defect (35.20, 35.22, 35.24, 35.26, 35.28)
ventricular septal defect (35.72)

35.8   Total repair of certain congenital cardiac anomalies

Note: For partial repair of defect [e.g. repair of atrial septal defect in tetralogy of Fallot]— code to specific procedure

35.81 Total repair of tetralogy of Fallot

One-stage total correction of tetralogy of Fallot with or without:
commissurotomy of pulmonary valve
infundibulectomy
outflow tract prosthesis
patch graft of outflow tract
prosthetic tube for pulmonary artery
repair of ventricular septal defect (with prosthesis)
take-down of previous systemic-pulmonary artery anastomosis

35.82 Total repair of total anomalous pulmonary venous connection

One-stage total correction of total anomalous pulmonary venous connection with or without:
anastomosis between (horizontal) common pulmonary trunk and posterior wall of left atrium (side-to-side)
enlargement of foramen ovale
incision [excision] of common wall between posterior left atrium and coronary sinus and roofing of resultant defect with patch graft (synthetic)
ligation of venous connection (descending anomalous vein) (to left innominate vein) (to superior vena cava)
repair of atrial septal defect (with prosthesis)

35.83 Total repair of truncus arteriosus

One-stage total correction of truncus arteriosus with or without:
construction (with aortic homograft) (with prosthesis) of a pulmonary artery placed from right ventricle to arteries supplying the lung
ligation of connections between aorta and pulmonary artery
repair of ventricular septal defect (with prosthesis)

35.84 Total correction of transposition of great vessels, not elsewhere classified

Arterial switch operation [Jatene]
Total correction of transposition of great arteries at the arterial level by switching the great arteries, including the left or both coronary arteries, implanted in the wall of the pulmonary artery

Excludes: *baffle operation [Mustard] [Senning] (35.91)*
creation of shunt between right ventricle and pulmonary artery [Rastelli] (35.92)

Valid O.R. procedure   Non-O.R. procedure   Nonspecific O.R. procedure   Noncovered O.R. procedure

35.9 **Other operations on valves and septa of heart**

Code also cardiopulmonary bypass, if performed [extracorporeal circulation] [heart-lung machine] (39.61)

35.91 **Interatrial transposition of venous return**

Baffle:
 atrial
 interatrial
Mustard's operation
Resection of atrial septum and insertion of patch to direct systemic venous return to tricuspid valve and pulmonary venous return to mitral valve

35.92 **Creation of conduit between right ventricle and pulmonary artery**

Creation of shunt between right ventricle and (distal) pulmonary artery

 Excludes: *that associated with total repair of truncus arteriosus (35.83)*

35.93 **Creation of conduit between left ventricle and aorta**

Creation of apicoaortic shunt
Shunt between apex of left ventricle and aorta

35.94 **Creation of conduit between atrium and pulmonary artery**

Fontan procedure

35.95 **Revision of corrective procedure on heart**

Replacement of prosthetic heart valve poppet
Resuture or prosthesis of:
 septum
 valve

 Excludes: *complete revision—code to specific procedure*
  replacement of prosthesis or graft of:
   septum (35.50-35.63)
   valve (35.20-35.28)

35.96 **Percutaneous balloon valvuloplasty**

Balloon dilation of valve

 Excludes: *endovascular replacement of heart valve (35.05, 35.07)*
  mitral valve repair with implant (35.97)
  transapical replacement of heart valve (35.06, 35.08)

35.97 **Percutaneous mitral valve repair with implant**

Endovascular mitral valve repair
Implantation of mitral valve leaflet clip
Transcatheter mitral valve repair

Code also any transesophageal echocardiography [TEE] (88.72)

 Excludes: *percutaneous balloon valvuloplasty (35.96)*

35.98 **Other operations on septa of heart**

35.99 **Other operations on valves of heart**

36 **Operations on vessels of heart**

Includes: sternotomy (median) (transverse) as operative approach
 thoracotomy as operative approach

Code also any:
 injection or infusion of platelet inhibitor (99.20)
 injection or infusion of thrombolytic agent (99.10)
Code also cardiopulmonary bypass, if performed [extracorporeal circulation] [heart-lung machine] (39.61)

36.0 **Removal of coronary artery obstruction and insertion of stent(s)**

36.03 **Open chest coronary artery angioplasty**

Coronary (artery):
 endarterectomy (with patch graft)
 thromboendarterectomy (with patch graft)
Open surgery for direct relief of coronary artery obstruction

Code also any:
 insertion of drug-eluting coronary stent(s) (36.07)
 insertion of non-drug-eluting coronary stent(s) (36.06)
 number of vascular stents inserted (00.45-00.48)
 number of vessels treated (00.40-00.43)
 procedure on vessel bifurcation (00.44)

 Excludes: *that with coronary artery bypass graft (36.10-36.19)*

● Code new
   to this edition

▲ Revision of
   existing code

④ ⑤ Fourth or fifth
   digit required

36.04   Intracoronary artery thrombolytic infusion
That by direct coronary artery injection, infusion, or catheterization
enzyme infusion
platelet inhibitor

Excludes: *infusion of platelet inhibitor (99.20)*
infusion of thrombolytic agent (99.10)
that associated with any procedure in 36.03

36.06   Insertion of non-drug-eluting coronary artery stent(s)
Bare stent(s)
Bonded stent(s)
Drug-coated stent(s), i.e. heparin coated
Endograft(s)
Endovascular graft(s)
Stent graft(s)

Code also any:
number of vascular stents inserted (00.45-00.48)
number of vessels treated (00.40-00.43)
open chest coronary artery angioplasty (36.03)
percutaneous transluminal coronary angioplasty [PTCA] (00.66)
procedure on vessel bifurcation (00.44)
transluminal coronary atherectomy (17.55)

Excludes: *insertion of drug-eluting coronary artery stent(s) (36.07)*

36.07   Insertion of drug-eluting coronary artery stent(s)
Endograft(s)
Endovascular graft(s)
Stent graft(s)

Code also any:
number of vascular stents inserted (00.45-00.48)
number of vessels treated (00.40-00.43)
open chest coronary artery angioplasty (36.03)
percutaneous transluminal coronary angioplasty [PTCA] (00.66)
procedure on vessel bifurcation (00.44)
transluminal coronary atherectomy (17.55)

Excludes: *drug-coated stent(s), e.g., heparin coated (36.06)*
insertion of non-drug-eluting coronary artery stent(s) (36.06)

36.09   Other removal of coronary artery obstruction
Coronary angioplasty NOS

Code also any:
number of vascular stents inserted (00.45-00.48)
number of vessels treated (00.40-00.43)
procedure on vessel bifurcation (00.44)

Excludes: *that by open angioplasty (36.03)*
that by percutaneous transluminal coronary angioplasty [PTCA]
(00.66)
transluminal coronary atherectomy (17.55)

36.1   Bypass anastomosis for heart revascularization
Note: Do not assign codes from series 00.40-00.43 with codes from series 36.10-36.19

Code also:
cardiopulmonary bypass [extracorporeal circulation] [heart-lung machine] (39.61)
pressurized treatment of venous bypass graft [conduit] with pharmaceutical substance, if
performed (00.16)

36.10   Aortocoronary bypass for heart revascularization, not otherwise specified
Direct revascularization:
cardiac with catheter stent, prosthesis, or vein graft
coronary with catheter stent, prosthesis, or vein graft
heart muscle with catheter stent, prosthesis, or vein graft
myocardial with catheter stent, prosthesis, or vein graft
Heart revascularization NOS

36.11   (Aorto)coronary bypass of one coronary artery

36.12   (Aorto)coronary bypass of two coronary arteries

36.13   (Aorto)coronary bypass of three coronary arteries

36.14   (Aorto)coronary bypass of four or more coronary arteries

Valid O.R.
procedure

Non-O.R.
procedure

Nonspecific
O.R. procedure

Noncovered
O.R. procedure

36.15 Single internal mammary-coronary artery bypass
Anastomosis (single):
mammary artery to coronary artery
thoracic artery to coronary artery

36.16 Double internal mammary-coronary artery bypass
Anastomosis (double):
mammary artery to coronary artery
thoracic artery to coronary artery

36.17 Abdominal-coronary artery bypass
Anastomosis:
gastroepiploic artery to coronary artery

36.19 Other bypass anastomosis for heart revascularization

36.2 Heart revascularization by arterial implant
Implantation of:
aortic branches [ascending aortic branches] into heart muscle
blood vessels into myocardium
internal mammary artery [internal thoracic artery] into:
heart muscle
myocardium
ventricle
ventricular wall
Indirect heart revascularization NOS

36.3 Other heart revascularization

36.31 Open chest transmyocardial revascularization

36.32 Other transmyocardial revascularization

36.33 Endoscopic transmyocardial revascularization
Thorascopic transmyocardial revascularization

36.34 Percutaneous transmyocardial revascularization
Endovascular transmyocardial revascularization

36.39 Other heart revascularization
Abrasion of epicardium
Cardio-omentopexy
Intrapericardial poudrage
Myocardial graft:
mediastinal fat
omentum
pectoral muscles

36.9 Other operations on vessels of heart
Code also cardiopulmonary bypass [extracorporeal circulation] [heart-lung machine] (39.61)

36.91 Repair of aneurysm of coronary vessel

36.99 Other operations on vessel of heart
Exploration of coronary artery
Incision of coronary artery
Ligation of coronary artery
Repair of arteriovenous fistula

37 Other operations on heart and pericardium
Code also any injection or infusion of platelet inhibitor (99.20)

37.0 Pericardiocentesis

37.1 Cardiotomy and pericardiotomy
Code also cardiopulmonary bypass [extracorporeal circulation] [heart-lung machine] (39.61)

37.10 Incision of heart, not otherwise specified
Cardiolysis NOS

37.11 Cardiotomy
Incision of:
atrium
endocardium
myocardium
ventricle

37.12 Pericardiotomy
Pericardial window operation
Pericardiolysis
Pericardiotomy

● Code new
to this edition

▲ Revision of
existing code

④ ⑤ Fourth or fifth
digit required

37.2   Diagnostic procedures on heart and pericardium

37.20   Noninvasive programmed electrical stimulation [NIPS]

> Excludes: that as part of intraoperative testing—omit code
> catheter based invasive electrophysiologic testing (37.26)
> device interrogation only without arrhythmia induction (bedside check) (89.45-89.49)

37.21   Right heart cardiac catheterization
Cardiac catheterization NOS

> Excludes: that with catheterization of left heart (37.23)

37.22   Left heart cardiac catheterization

> Excludes: that with catheterization of right heart (37.23)

37.23   Combined right and left heart cardiac catheterization

37.24   Biopsy of pericardium

37.25   Biopsy of heart

37.26   Catheter based invasive electrophysiologic testing
Electrophysiologic studies (EPS)

Code also any concomitant procedure

> Excludes: that as part of intraoperative testing—omit code
> device interrogation only without arrhythmia induction (bedside check) (89.45-89.49)
> His bundle recording (37.29)
> noninvasive programmed electrical stimulation (NIPS) (37.20)

37.27   Cardiac mapping

Code also any concomitant procedure

> Excludes: electrocardiogram (89.52)
> His bundle recording (37.29)

37.28   Intracardiac echocardiography [ICE]
Echocardiography of heart chambers

Code also any synchronous Doppler flow mapping (88.72)

> Excludes: intravascular imaging of coronary vessels (intravascular ultrasound) (IVUS) (00.24)

37.29   Other diagnostic procedures on heart and pericardium

> Excludes: angiocardiography (88.50-88.58)
> cardiac function tests (89.41-89.69)
> cardiovascular radioisotopic scan and function study (92.05)
> coronary arteriography (88.55-88.57)
> diagnostic pericardiocentesis (37.0)
> diagnostic ultrasound of heart (88.72)
> x-ray of heart (87.49)

37.3   Pericardiectomy and excision of lesion of heart

Code also cardiopulmonary bypass [extracorporeal circulation] [heart-lung machine], if performed (39.61)

37.31   Pericardiectomy
Excision of:
    adhesions of pericardium
    constricting scar of: epicardium
                              pericardium

37.32   Excision of aneurysm of heart
Repair of aneurysm of heart

37.33   Excision or destruction of other lesion or tissue of heart, open approach
Ablation or incision of heart tissue (cryoablation) (electrocurrent) (laser) (microwave) (radiofrequency) (resection) (ultrasound), open chest approach
Cox-maze procedure
Maze procedure
That by median sternotomy
That by thoracotomy without use of thoracoscope

> Excludes: ablation, excision or destruction of lesion or tissue of heart:
> endovascular approach (37.34)
> thoracoscopic approach (37.37)
> excision or destuction of left atrial appendage (LAA) (37.36)

Valid O.R. procedure	Non-O.R. procedure	Nonspecific O.R. procedure	Noncovered O.R. procedure

37.34 Excision or destruction of other lesion or tissue of heart, endovascular approach
Ablation of heart tissue (cryoablation) (electrocurrent) (laser) (microwave)
(radiofrequency) (ultrasound), via peripherally inserted catheter
Modified maze procedure, percutaneous approach

> *Excludes:* *ablation, excision or destruction of lesion of tissue of heart:*
> *open approach (37.33)*
> *thoracoscopic approach (37.37)*

37.35 Partial ventriculectomy
Ventricular reduction surgery
Ventricular remodeling

> *Code also any synchronous:*
> *mitral valve repair (35.02, 35.12)*
> *mitral valve replacement (35.23-35.24)*

▲ **37.36 Excision, destruction, or exclusion of left atrial appendage (LAA)**
Includes: thoracoscopic approach, minithoracotomy approach, percutaneous
approach, endovascular approach, or subxiphoid approach
Clipping of left atrial appendage
Oversewing of left atrial appendage
Stapling of left atrial appendage
That by fastener or suture

> *Code also any:*
> *concomitant procedure performed*
> *fluoroscopy (87.49)*
> *transesophageal echocardiography (TEE) (88.72)*

> *Excludes:* *ablation, excision or destruction of lesion or tissue of heart,*
> *endovascular approach (37.34)*
> *excision or destruction of other lesion or tissue of heart, thoracoscopic*
> *approach (37.37)*
> *insertion of left atrial appendage device (37.90)*

37.37 Excision or destruction of other lesion or tissue of heart, thoracoscopic approach
Ablation or incision of heart tissue (cryoablation) (electrocautery) (laser)
(microwave) (radiofrequency) (resection) (ultrasound) , via thoracoscope
Modified maze procedure, thoracoscopic approach
That via thoracoscopically-assisted approach (without thoracotomy) (with port
access) (with sub-xiphoid incision)

> *Excludes:* *ablation, excision or destruction of lesion or tissue of heart:*
> *open approach (37.33)*
> *endovascular approach (37.34)*
> *thoracoscopic excision or destruction of left atrial appendage [LAA]*
> *(37.36)*

37.4 Repair of heart and pericardium

37.41 Implantation of prosthetic cardiac support device around the heart
Cardiac support device (CSD)
Epicardial support device
Fabric (textile) (mesh) device
Ventricular support device on surface of heart

> *Code also any:*
> *cardiopulmonary bypass [extracorporeal circulation] [heart-lung machine] if*
> *performed (39.61)*
> *mitral valve repair (35.02, 35.12)*
> *mitral valve replacement (35.23-35.24)*
> *transesophageal echocardiography (88.72)*

> *Excludes:* *circulatory assist systems (37.61-37.68)*

37.49 Other repair of heart and pericardium

37.5 Heart replacement procedures

37.51 Heart transplantation

> *Excludes:* *combined heart-lung transplantation (33.6)*

37.52 Implantation of total internal biventricular heart replacement system
Artificial heart

> *Excludes:* *implantation of heart assist system [VAD] (37.62, 37.65, 37.66, 37.68)*

Note: This procedure includes substantial removal of part or all of the biological heart.
Both ventricles are resected, and the native heart is no longer intact. Ventriculectomy
is included in this procedure; do not code separately.

● Code new
to this edition   ▲ Revision of
existing code   ④ ⑤ Fourth or fifth
digit required

37.53 **Replacement or repair of thoracic unit of (total) replacement heart system**

> Excludes: *replacement and repair of heart assist system [VAD] (37.63)*

37.54 **Replacement or repair of other implantable component of (total) replacement heart system**
Implantable battery
Implantable controller
Transcutaneous energy transfer [TET] device

> Excludes: *replacement or repair of heart assist system [VAD] (37.63)*
> *replacement or repair of thoracic unit of (total) replacement heart system (37.53)*

37.55 **Removal of internal biventricular heart replacement system**
Explantation of artificial heart

Code also any concomitant procedure, such as:
combined heart-lung transplantation (33.6)
heart transplantation (37.51)
implantation of internal biventricular heart replacement system (37.52)

> Excludes: *explantation [removal] of external heart assist system (37.64)*
> *explantation [removal] of percutaneous external heart assist device (97.44)*
> *nonoperative removal of heart assist system (97.44)*
> *that with replacement or repair of heart replacement system (37.53, 37.54)*

37.6 **Implantation of heart and circulatory assist system(s)**

> Excludes: *implantation of prosthetic cardiac support system (37.41)*

37.60 **Implantation or insertion of biventricular external heart assist system**
Temporary cardiac support for both left and right ventricles, inserted in the same operative episode
Includes: open chest (sternotomy) procedure for cannulae attachments
Note: Device (outside the body but connected to heart) with external circulation pump. Ventriculotomy is included; do not code separately

> Excludes: *implantation of internal biventricular heart replacement system (artificial heart) (37.52)*
> *implant of pulsation balloon (37.61)*
> *insertion of percutaneous external heart assist device (37.68)*
> *insertion of temporary non-implantable extracorporeal circulatory assist device (37.62)*

37.61 **Implant of pulsation balloon**

37.62 **Insertion of temporary non-implantable extracorporeal circulatory assist device**
Insertion of:
heart assist system, NOS
heart pump

> Excludes: *implantation of total internal biventricular heart replacement system [artificial heart] (37.52)*
> *implant of external heart assist system (37.65)*
> *insertion of implantable extracorporeal heart assist system (37.66)*
> *insertion of percutaneous external heart assist device (37.68)*
> *removal of heart assist system (37.64)*

Note: Includes explantation of this device; do not code separately

37.63 **Repair of heart assist system**
Replacement of parts of an existing ventricular assist device (VAD)

> Excludes: *replacement or repair of other implantable component of (total) replacement heart system [artificial heart] (37.54)*
> *replacement or repair of thoracic unit of (total) replacement heart system [artificial heart] (37.53)*

37.64 **Removal of external heart assist system(s) or device(s)**
Explantation of external device(s) providing left and right ventricular support
Explantation of single external device and cannulae

> Excludes: *explantation [removal] of percutaneous external heart assist device (97.44)*
> *nonoperative removal of heart assist system (97.44)*
> *temporary non-implantable extracorporeal circulatory assist device (37.62)*
> *that with replacement of implant (37.63)*

Valid O.R. procedure   Non-O.R. procedure   Nonspecific O.R. procedure   Noncovered O.R. procedure

37.65 **Implant of single ventricular (extracorporeal) external heart assist system**
Insertion of one device into one ventricle
Note: Device (outside the body but connected to heart) with external circulation and pump.
Note: Insertion or implantation of one external VAD for left or right heart support.
Includes open chest (sternotomy) procedure for cannulae attachments

Excludes: *implant of pulsation balloon (37.61)*
implantation of total internal biventricular heart replacement system (37.52)
insertion of implantable heart assist system (37.66)
insertion or implantation of two external VADs for simultaneous right and left heart support (37.60)
insertion of percutaneous external heart assist device (37.68)
that without sternotomy (37.62)

37.66 **Insertion of implantable heart assist system**
Note: Device directly connected to the heart and implanted in the upper left quadrant of peritoneal cavity
Note: This device can be used for either destination therapy (DT) or bridge-to-transplant (BTT)
Axial flow heart assist system
Diagonal pump heart assist system
Left ventricular assist device (LVAD)
Pulsatile heart assist system
Right ventricular assist device (RVAD)
Rotary pump heart assist system
Transportable, implantable heart assist system
Ventricular assist device (VAD) not otherwise specified

Excludes: *implant of pulsation balloon (37.61)*
implantation of total internal biventricular heart replacement system [artificial heart] (37.52)
insertion of percutaneous external heart assist device (37.68)

37.67 **Implantation of cardiomyostimulation system**
Note: Two-step open procedure consisting of transfer of one end of the latissimus dorsi muscle; wrapping it around the heart; rib resection; implantation of epicardial cardiac pacing leads into the right ventricle; tunneling and pocket creation for the cardiomyostimulator.

37.68 **Insertion of percutaneous external heart assist device**
Includes percutaneous [femoral] insertion of cannulae attachments
Circulatory assist device
Extrinsic heart assist device
pVAD
Percutaneous heart assist device

37.7 **Insertion, revision, replacement and removal of leads; insertion of temporary pacemaker system; or revision of cardiac device pocket**
Code also any insertion and replacement of pacemaker device (37.80-37.87)

Excludes: *implantation or replacement of transvenous lead [electrode] into left ventricular cardiac venous system (00.52)*

37.70 **Initial insertion of lead [electrode], not otherwise specified**

Excludes: *insertion of temporary transvenous pacemaker system (37.78)*
replacement of atrial and/or ventricular lead(s) (37.76)

37.71 **Initial insertion of transvenous lead [electrode] into ventricle**

Excludes: *insertion of temporary transvenous pacemaker system (37.78)*
replacement of atrial and/or ventricular lead(s) (37.76)

37.72 **Initial insertion of transvenous leads [electrodes] into atrium and ventricle**

Excludes: *insertion of temporary transvenous pacemaker system (37.78)*
replacement of atrial and/or ventricular lead(s) (37.76)

37.73 **Initial insertion of transvenous lead [electrode] into atrium**

Excludes: *insertion of temporary transvenous pacemaker system (37.78)*
replacement of atrial and/or ventricular lead(s) (37.76)

● Code new to this edition   ▲ Revision of existing code   ④ ⑤ Fourth or fifth digit required

37.74 Insertion or replacement of epicardial lead [electrode] into epicardium

Insertion or replacement of epicardial lead by:
sternotomy
thoracotomy

> Excludes: *replacement of atrial and/or ventricular lead(s) (37.76)*

37.75 Revision of lead [electrode]

Repair of electrode [removal with re-insertion]
Repositioning of lead(s) (AICD) (cardiac device) (CRT-D) (CRT-P) (defibrillator) (pacemaker) (pacing) (sensing) [electrode]
Revision of lead NOS

> Excludes: *repositioning of temporary transvenous pacemaker system—omit code*

37.76 Replacement of transvenous atrial and/or ventricular lead(s) [electrode]

Removal or abandonment of existing transvenous or epicardial lead(s) with transvenous lead(s) replacement

> Excludes: *replacement of epicardial lead [electrode] (37.74)*

37.77 Removal of lead(s) [electrode] without replacement

Removal:
epicardial lead (transthoracic approach)
transvenous lead(s)

> Excludes: *removal of temporary transvenous pacemaker system—omit code*
> *that with replacement of:*
> *atrial and/or ventricular lead(s) [electrode] (37.76)*
> *epicardial lead [electrode] (37.74)*

37.78 Insertion of temporary transvenous pacemaker system

> Excludes: *intraoperative cardiac pacemaker (39.64)*

37.79 Revision or relocation of cardiac device pocket

Debridement and reforming pocket (skin and subcutaneous tissue)
Insertion of loop recorder
Relocation of pocket [creation of new pocket] pacemaker or CRT-P
Removal of cardiac device/pulse generator without replacement
Removal of the implantable hemodynamic pressure sensor (lead) and monitor device
Removal without replacement of cardiac resynchronization defibrillator device
Repositioning of implantable hemodynamic pressure sensor (lead) and monitor device
Repositioning of pulse generator
Revision of cardioverter/defibrillator (automatic) pocket
Revision of pocket for intracardiac hemodynamic monitoring
Revision or relocation of CRT-D pocket
Revision or relocation of pacemaker, defibrillator, or other implanted cardiac device pocket

> Excludes: *removal of loop recorder (86.05)*

37.8 Insertion, replacement, removal, and revision of pacemaker device

Note: Device testing during procedure—omit code

> *Code also any lead insertion, lead replacement, lead removal and/or lead revision (37.70-37.77)*

> Excludes: *implantation of cardiac resynchronication pacemaker [CRT-P] (00.50)*
> *implantation or replacement of cardiac resynchronization pacemaker pulse generator only [CRT-P] (00.53)*

37.80 Insertion of permanent pacemaker, initial or replacement, type of device not specified

37.81 Initial insertion of single-chamber device, not specified as rate responsive

> Excludes: *replacement of existing pacemaker device (37.85-37.87)*

37.82 Initial insertion of a single-chamber device, rate responsive

Rate responsive to physiologic stimuli other than atrial rate

> Excludes: *replacement of existing pacemaker device (37.85-37.87)*

37.83 Initial insertion of dual-chamber device

Atrial ventricular sequential device

> Excludes: *replacement of existing pacemaker device (37.85-37.87)*

	Valid O.R. procedure		Non-O.R. procedure		Nonspecific O.R. procedure		Noncovered O.R. procedure

37.85 **Replacement of any type pacemaker device with single-chamber device, not specified as rate responsive**

37.86 **Replacement of any type pacemaker device with single-chamber device, rate responsive**
Rate responsive to physiologic stimuli other than atrial rate

37.87 **Replacement of any type pacemaker device with dual-chamber device**
Atrial ventricular sequential device

37.89 **Revision or removal of pacemaker device**
Removal without replacement of cardiac resynchronization pacemaker device [CRT-P]
Repair of pacemaker device

> Excludes: *removal of temporary transvenous pacemaker system—omit code*
> *replacement of existing pacemaker device (37.85-37.87)*
> *replacement of existing pacemaker device with CRT-P pacemaker device (00.53)*

37.9 **Other operations on heart and pericardium**

37.90 **Insertion of left atrial appendage device**
Left atrial filter
Left atrial occluder
Transseptal catheter technique

37.91 **Open chest cardiac massage**

> Excludes: *closed chest cardiac massage (99.63)*

37.92 **Injection of therapeutic substance into heart**

37.93 **Injection of therapeutic substance into pericardium**

37.94 **Implantation or replacement of automatic cardioverter/defibrillator, total system [AICD]**
Implantation of defibrillator with leads (epicardial patches), formation of pocket (abdominal fascia) (subcutaneous), any transvenous leads, intraoperative procedures for evaluation of lead signals, and obtaining defibrillator threshold measurements
Techniques:
lateral thoracotomy
medial sternotomy
subxiphoid procedure
Note: Device testing during procedure—*omit code*
Code also extracorporeal circulation, if performed (39.61)
Code also any concomitant procedure [e.g., coronary bypass (36.10-36.19) or CCM, total system (17.51)]

> Excludes: *implantation of cardiac resynchronization defibrillator, total system [CRT-D] (00.51)*

37.95 **Implantation of automatic cardioverter/defibrillator lead(s) only**

37.96 **Implantation of automatic cardioverter/defibrillator pulse generator only**
Note: Device testing during procedure—*omit code*

> Excludes: *implantation or replacement of cardiac resynchronization defibrillator, pulse generator device only [CRT-D] (00.54)*

37.97 **Replacement of automatic cardioverter/defibrillator lead(s) only**

> Excludes: *replacement of epicardial lead [electrode] into epicardium (37.74)*
> *replacement of transvenous lead [electrode] into left ventricular coronary venous system (00.52)*

37.98 **Replacement of automatic cardioverter/defibrillator pulse generator only**
Note: Device testing during procedure—*omit code*

> Excludes: *replacement of cardiac resynchronization defibrillator, pulse generator device only [CRT-D] (00.54)*

● Code new to this edition   ▲ Revision of existing code   ④ ⑤ Fourth or fifth digit required

37.99 Other

Excludes: *cardiac retraining (93.36)*
conversion of cardiac rhythm (99.60-99.69)
implantation of prosthetic cardiac support device (37.41)
insertion of left atrial appendage device (37.90)
maze procedure (Cox-maze), open (37.33)
maze procedure, endovascular approach (37.34)
repositioning of pulse generator (37.79)
revision of lead(s) (37.75)
*revision or relocation of pacemaker, defibrillator or other implanted
cardiac device pocket (37.79)*

38 Incision, excision, and occlusion of vessels

Code also any application or administration of an adhesion barrier substance (99.77)
Code also cardiopulmonary bypass [extracorporeal circulation] [heart-lung machine] (39.61)

Excludes: *that of coronary vessels (00.66, 36.03, 36.04, 36.09, 36.10-36.99)*

The following fourth-digit subclassification is for use with appropriate categories in sections 38.0,
38.1, 38.3, 38.5, 38.6, 38.8 and 38.9, which are marked with a symbol④ to identify the site.
Valid fourth digits are in [brackets] under each code.

0 unspecified site
1 intracranial vessels
Cerebral (anterior) (middle)
Circle of Willis
Posterior communicating artery
2 other vessels of head and neck
Carotid artery (common) (external) (internal)
Jugular vein (external) (internal)
3 upper limb vessels
Axillary	Radial
Brachial	Ulnar

4 aorta
5 other thoracic vessels
Innominate	Subclavian
Pulmonary (artery) (vein)	Vena cava, superior

6 abdominal arteries
Celiac	Mesenteric
Gastric	Renal
Hepatic	Splenic
Iliac	Umbilical

Excludes: *abdominal aorta (4)*
7 abdominal veins
Iliac	Splenic
Portal	Vena cava(inferior)
Renal	

8 lower limb arteries
Femoral (common) (superficial)
Popliteal
Tibial
9 lower limb veins
Femoral	Saphenous
Popliteal	Tibial

④ **38.0 Incision of vessel**
[0-9] Embolectomy
Thrombectomy

Excludes: *endovascular removal of obstruction from head and neck vessel(s) (39.74)*
puncture or catheterization of any:
artery (38.91, 38.98)
vein (38.92-38.95, 38.99)

④ **38.1** **Endarterectomy**
[0-6,8] Endarterectomy with:
  embolectomy
  patch graft
  temporary bypass during procedure
  thrombectomy

Code also any:
  number of vascular stents inserted (00.45-00.48)
  number of vessels treated (00.40-00.43)
  procedure on vessel bifurcation (00.44)

38.2 **Diagnostic procedures on blood vessels**

Excludes: *adjunct vascular system procedures (00.40-00.43)*

38.21 **Biopsy of blood vessel**

38.22 **Percutaneous angioscopy**

Excludes: *angioscopy of eye (95.12)*

38.23 **Intravascular spectroscopy**
  Includes: spectroscopy of both coronary and peripheral vessels
  Intravascular chemography
  Near infrared (NIR) spectroscopy

Excludes: *intravascular imaging of:*
  coronary vessels (00.24, 38.24)
  peripheral vessels (00.23, 38.25)

38.24 **Intravascular imaging of coronary vessel(s) by optical coherence tomography [OCT]**

38.25 **Intravascular imaging of non-coronary vessel(s) by optical coherence tomography [OCT]**

Excludes: *intravascular imaging of coronary vessel(s) by OCT (38.24)*

● **38.26** **Insertion of implantable pressure sensor without lead for intracardiac or great vessel hemodynamic monitoring**
  Note: The sensor is a standalone device and is not physically connected to a separately implanted monitor.

  Leadless pressure sensor not physically connected to a separately implanted monitor
  Single device combination leadless pressure sensor with integral monitor for intracardiac or great vessel (or branch thereof) hemodynamic monitoring
  With or without internal batteries
  Without leads

Excludes: *circulatory monitoring (blood gas, arterial or venous pressure, cardiac output and coronary blood flow) (89.60-89.69)*
  hemodynamic monitoring system with sensor and separately implanted monitor (00.56 – 00.57)
  insertion or replacement of implantable pressure sensor with lead for intracardiac or great vessel hemodynamic monitoring (00.56)

38.29 **Other diagnostic procedures on blood vessels**

Excludes: *blood vessel thermography (88.86)*
  circulatory monitoring (89.61-89.69)
  contrast:
  angiocardiography (88.50-88.58)
  arteriography (88.40-88.49)
  phlebography (88.60-88.67)
  impedance phlebography (88.68)
  peripheral vascular ultrasonography (88.77)
  plethysmogram (89.58)

④ **38.3** **Resection of vessel with anastomosis**
[0-9] Angiectomy with anastomosis
  Excision of:
  aneurysm (arteriovenous) with anastomosis
  blood vessel (lesion) with anastomosis

● Code new
to this edition

▲ Revision of
existing code

④ ⑤ Fourth or fifth
digit required

④ **38.4** **Resection of vessel with replacement**
[0-9]   Angiectomy with replacement
         Excision of
           aneurysm (arteriovenous) with replacement
           blood vessel (lesion) with replacement
         Partial resection with replacement

| Excludes: | *endovascular repair of aneurysm (39.71-39.79)* |

Requires the use of one of the following fourth-digit subclassifications to identify site:

0 unspecified site
1 intracranial vessels
  Cerebral (anterior) (middle)
  Circle of Willis
  Posterior communicating artery
2 other vessels of head and neck
  Carotid artery (common) (external) (internal)
  Jugular vein (external) (internal)
3 upper limb vessels
  Axillary   Radial
  Brachial   Ulnar
4 aorta, abdominal
  Code also any thoracic vessel involvement (thoracoabdominal procedure) (38.45)
5 thoracic vessel
  Aorta (thoracic)   Subclavian
  Innominate   Vena cava (superior)
  Pulmonary (artery) (vein)
  Code also any abdominal aorta involvement (thoracoabdominal procedure) (38.44)
6 abdominal arteries
  Celiac   Mesenteric
  Gastric   Renal
  Hepatic   Splenic
  Iliac   Umbilical

| Excludes: | *abdominal aorta (4)* |

7 abdominal veins
  Iliac   Splenic
  Portal   Vena cava (inferior)
  Renal
8 lower limb arteries
  Femoral (common) (superficial)
  Tibial

9 lower limb veins
  Femoral   Saphenous
  Popliteal   Tibial

④ **38.5** **Ligation and stripping of varicose veins**
[0-3,5,7,9]

Excludes:	*ligation of varices:*
	esophageal (42.91)
	gastric (44.91)

④ **38.6** **Other excision of vessels**
[0-9]   Excision of blood vessel (lesion) NOS

Excludes:	*excision of vessel for aortocoronary bypass (36.10-36.14)*
	excision with:
	anastomosis (38.30-38.39)
	graft replacement (38.40-38.49)
	implant (38.40-38.49)

38.7 **Interruption of vena cava**
         Insertion of implant or sieve in vena cava
         Ligation of vena cava (inferior) (superior)
         Plication of vena cava

| Valid O.R. procedure | Non-O.R. procedure | Nonspecific O.R. procedure | Noncovered O.R. procedure |

④ **38.8** **Other surgical occlusion of vessels**
[0-9] Clamping of blood vessel
Division of blood vessel
Ligation of blood vessel
Occlusion of blood vessel

> *Excludes:* *adrenal vessels (07.43)*
> *esophageal varices (42.91)*
> *gastric or duodenal vessel for ulcer (44.40-44.49)*
> *gastric varices (44.91)*
> *meningeal vessel (02.13)*
> *percutaneous transcatheter infusion embolization (99.29)*
> *spermatic vein for varicocele (63.1)*
> *surgical occlusion of vena cava (38.7)*
> *that for chemoembolization (99.25)*
> *that for control of (postoperative) hemorrhage:*
> *anus (49.95)*
> *bladder (57.93)*
> *following vascular procedure (39.41)*
> *nose (21.00-21.09)*
> *prostate (60.94)*
> *tonsil (28.7)*
> *thyroid vessel (06.92)*

38.9 **Puncture of vessel**

> *Excludes:* *that for circulatory monitoring (89.60-89.69)*

38.91 **Arterial catheterization**

38.92 **Umbilical vein catheterization**

38.93 **Venous catheterization, not elsewhere classified**

> *Excludes:* *that for cardiac catheterization (37.21-37.23)*
> *that for renal dialysis (38.95)*
> *that with guidance (electrocardiogram) (fluoroscopy) (ultrasound) (38.97)*

38.94 **Venous cutdown**

38.95 **Venous catheterization for renal dialysis**

> *Excludes:* *insertion of totally implantable vascular access device [VAD] 86.07*

38.97 **Central venous catheter placement with guidance**
Includes guidance by:
electrocardiogram
fluoroscopy
ultrasound

38.98 **Other puncture of artery**

> *Excludes:* *that for:*
> *arteriography (88.40-88.49)*
> *coronary arteriography (88.55-88.57)*

38.99 **Other puncture of vein**
Phlebotomy

> *Excludes:* *that for:*
> *angiography of veins (88.60-88.68)*
> *extracorporeal circulation (39.61, 50.92)*
> *injection or infusion of:*
> *sclerosing solution (39.92)*
> *therapeutic or prophylactic substance (99.11-99.29)*
> *perfusion (39.96-39.97)*
> *phlebography (88.60-88.68)*
> *transfusion (99.01-99.09)*

39 **Other operations on vessels**

> *Excludes:* *those on coronary vessels (36.03-36.99)*

39.0 **Systemic to pulmonary artery shunt**
Descending aorta-pulmonary artery anastomosis (graft)
Left to right anastomosis (graft)
Subclavian-pulmonary anastomosis (graft)

> *Code also cardiopulmonary bypass [extracorporeal circulation] [heart-lung machine] (39.61)*

● Code new to this edition   ▲ Revision of existing code   ④ ⑤ Fourth or fifth digit required

39.1   Intra-abdominal venous shunt
Anastomosis:
  mesocaval
  portacaval
  portal vein to inferior vena cava
  splenic and renal veins
  transjugular intrahepatic portosystemic shunt (TIPS)

Excludes: *peritoneovenous shunt (54.94)*

39.2   Other shunt or vascular bypass
Code also pressurized treatment of venous bypass graft [conduit] with pharmaceutical substance, if performed (00.16)

39.21   Caval-pulmonary artery anastomosis
Code also cardiopulmonary bypass (39.61)

39.22   Aorta-subclavian-carotid bypass
Bypass (arterial):
  aorta to carotid and brachial
  aorta to subclavian and carotid
  carotid to subclavian

39.23   Other intrathoracic vascular shunt or bypass
Intrathoracic (arterial) bypass graft NOS

Excludes: *coronary artery bypass (36.10-36.19)*

39.24   Aorta-renal bypass

39.25   Aorta-iliac-femoral bypass
Bypass:
  aortofemoral
  aortoiliac
  aortoiliac to popliteal
  aortopopliteal
  iliofemoral [iliac-femoral]

39.26   Other intra-abdominal vascular shunt or bypass
Bypass:
  aortoceliac
  aortic-superior mesenteric
  common hepatic-common iliac-renal
Intra-abdominal arterial bypass graft NOS

Excludes: *peritoneovenous shunt (54.94)*

39.27   Arteriovenostomy for renal dialysis
Anastomosis for renal dialysis
Formation of (peripheral) arteriovenous fistula for renal (kidney] dialysis
Code also any renal dialysis (39.95)

39.28   Extracranial-intracranial (EC-IC) vascular bypass

39.29   Other (peripheral) vascular shunt or bypass
Bypass (graft):
  axillary-brachial
  axillary-femoral [axillofemoral] (superficial)
  brachial
  femoral-femoral
  femoroperoneal
  femoropopliteal (arteries)
  femorotibial (anterior) (posterior)
  popliteal
  vascular NOS

Excludes: *peritoneovenous shunt (54.94)*

39.3   Suture of vessel
Repair of laceration of blood vessel

Excludes: *any other vascular puncture closure device—omit code*
  suture of aneurysm (39.52)
  that for control of hemorrhage (postoperative):
    anus (49.95)
    bladder (57.93)
    following vascular procedure (39.41)
    nose (21.00-21.09)
    prostate (60.94)
    tonsil (28.7)

Valid O.R. procedure   Non-O.R. procedure   Nonspecific O.R. procedure   Noncovered O.R. procedure

39.30 Suture of unspecified blood vessel

39.31 Suture of artery

39.32 Suture of vein

39.4 Revision of vascular procedure

39.41 Control of hemorrhage following vascular surgery

> *Excludes:* *that for control of hemorrhage (postoperative):*
> *anus (49.95)*
> *bladder (57.93)*
> *nose (21.00-21.09)*
> *prostate (60.94)*
> *tonsil (28.7)*

39.42 Revision of arteriovenous shunt for renal dialysis
Conversion of renal dialysis:
end-to-end anastomosis to end-to-side
end-to-side anastomosis to end-to-end
vessel-to-vessel cannula to arteriovenous shunt
Removal of old arteriovenous shunt and creation of new shunt

> *Excludes:* *replacement of vessel-to-vessel cannula (39.94)*

39.43 Removal of arteriovenous shunt for renal dialysis

> *Excludes:* *that with replacement [revision] of shunt (39.42)*

39.49 Other revision of vascular procedure
Declotting (graft)
Revision of:
anastomosis of blood vessel
vascular procedure (previous)

39.5 Other repair of vessels

▲ **39.50** Angioplasty of other non-coronary vessel(s)
Percutaneous transluminal angioplasty (PTA) of non-coronary vessel:
lower extremity vessels
mesenteric artery
renal artery
upper extremity vessels

> *Code also any:*
> *atherectomy of other non-coronary vessel(s) (17.56)*
> *injection or infusion of thrombolytic agent (99.10)*
> *insertion of drug-eluting peripheral vessel stent (00.55)*
> *insertion of non-drug-eluting peripheral vessel stent(s) or stent graft(s) (39.90)*
> *number of vascular stents inserted (00.45-00.48)*
> *number of vessels treated (00.40-00.43)*
> *procedure on vessel bifurcation (00.44)*

> *Excludes:* *percutaneous angioplasty of extracranial or intracranial vessel(s)*
> *(00.61-00.62)*
> *percutaneous atherectomy of extracranial or intracranial vessel(s)*
> *(17.53-17.54)*

39.51 Clipping of aneurysm

> *Excludes:* *clipping of arteriovenous fistula (39.53)*

39.52 Other repair of aneurysm
Repair of aneurysm by:
coagulation
electrocoagulation
filipuncture
methyl methacrylate
suture
wiring
wrapping

> *Excludes:* *endovascular repair of aneurysm (39.71-39.79)*
> *re-entry operation (aorta) (39.54)*
> *that with:*
> *graft replacement (38.40-38.49)*
> *resection (38.30-38.49, 38.60-38.69)*

● Code new
to this edition
▲ Revision of
existing code
④ ⑤ Fourth or fifth
digit required

39.53 Repair of arteriovenous fistula
Embolization of carotid cavernous fistula
Repair of arteriovenous fistula by:
  clipping
  coagulation
  ligation and division

> Excludes: repair of:
> arteriovenous shunt for renal dialysis (39.42)
> head and neck vessels, endovascular approach (39.72)
> that with:
> graft replacement (38.40-38.49)
> resection (38.30-38.49, 38.60-38.69)

39.54 Re-entry operation (aorta)
Fenestration of dissecting aneurysm of thoracic aorta

> Code also cardiopulmonary bypass [extracorporeal circulation] [heart-lung machine] (39.61)

39.55 Reimplantation of aberrant renal vessel

39.56 Repair of blood vessel with tissue patch graft

> Excludes: that with resection (38.40-38.49)

39.57 Repair of blood vessel with synthetic patch graft

> Excludes: that with resection (38.40-38.49)

39.58 Repair of blood vessel with unspecified type of patch graft

> Excludes: that with resection (38.40-38.49)

39.59 Other repair of vessel
Aorticopulmonary window operation
Arterioplasty NOS
Construction of venous valves (peripheral)
Plication of vein (peripheral)
Reimplantation of artery

> Code also cardiopulmonary bypass [extracorporeal circulation] [heart-lung machine] (39.61)

> Excludes: interruption of the vena cava (38.7)
> reimplantation of renal artery (39.55)
> that with:
> graft (39.56-39.58)
> resection (38.30-38.49, 38.60-38.69)

39.6 Extracorporeal circulation and procedures auxiliary to heart surgery

39.61 Extracorporeal circulation auxiliary to open heart surgery
Artificial heart and lung
Cardiopulmonary bypass
Pump oxygenator

> Excludes: extracorporeal hepatic assistance (50.92)
> extracorporeal membrane oxygenation [ECMO] (39.65)
> hemodialysis (39.95)
> percutaneous cardiopulmonary bypass (39.66)

39.62 Hypothermia (systemic) incidental to open heart surgery

39.63 Cardioplegia
Arrest:
  anoxic
  circulatory

39.64 Intraoperative cardiac pacemaker
Temporary pacemaker used during and immediately following cardiac surgery

39.65 Extracorporeal membrane oxygenation (ECMO)

> Excludes: extracorporeal circulation auxiliary to open heart surgery (39.61)
> percutaneous cardiopulmonary bypass (39.66)

39.66 Percutaneous cardiopulmonary bypass
Closed chest

> Excludes: extracorporeal circulation auxiliary to open heart surgery (39.61)
> extracorporeal hepatic assistance (50.92)
> extracorporeal membrane oxygenation [ECMO] (39.65)
> hemodialysis (39.95)

Valid O.R. procedure   Non-O.R. procedure   Nonspecific O.R. procedure   Noncovered O.R. procedure

39.7 Endovascular procedures on vessel(s)
Embolization
Endoluminal repair
Implantation
Occlusion
Removal
Repair

> Excludes: angioplasty of other non-coronary vessel(s) (39.50)
> atherectomy of other non-coronary vessel(s) (17.56)
> insertion of non-drug-eluting peripheral vessel stent(s) (39.90)
> other repair of aneurysm (39.52)
> percutaneous insertion of carotid artery stent(s) (00.63)
> percutaneous insertion of intracranial stent(s) (00.65)
> percutaneous insertion of other precerebral artery stent(s) (00.64)
> resection of abdominal aorta with replacement (38.44)
> resection of lower limb arteries with replacement (38.48)
> resection of thoracic aorta with replacement (38.45)
> resection of upper limb vessels with replacement (38.43)
> temporary therapeutic partial occlusion of vessel (39.77)

▲ **39.71 Endovascular implantation of other graft in abdominal aorta**
Endovascular repair of abdominal aortic aneurysm with graft
Stent graft(s)

> *Code also intra-aneurysm sac pressure monitoring (intraoperative) (00.58)*

> Excludes: endovascular implantation of branching or fenestrated graft in aorta
> (39.78)

▲ **39.72 Endovascular (total) embolization or occlusion of head and neck vessels**
Coil-retention stent
Embolization stent
Endograft(s)
Endovascular grafts(s)
Liquid tissue adhesive (glue) embolization or occlusion
Other implant or substance for repair, embolization or occlusion
That for repair of aneurysm, arteriovenous malformation [AVM] or fistula

> Excludes: embolization of head or neck vessels using bare coils (39.75)
> embolization of head or neck vessels using bioactive coils (39.76)
> mechanical thrombectomy of pre-cerebral and cerebral vessels (39.74)

39.73 Endovascular implantation of graft in thoracic aorta
Endograft(s)
Endovascular graft(s)
Endovascular repair of defect of thoracic aorta with graft(s) or device(s)
Stent graft(s) or device(s)
That for repair of aneurysm, dissection, or injury

> *Code also intra-aneurysm sac pressure monitoring (intraoperative) (00.58)*

> Excludes: fenestration of dissecting aneurysm of thoracic aorta (39.54)

39.74 Endovascular removal of obstruction from head and neck vessel(s)
Endovascular embolectomy
Endovascular thrombectomy of pre-cerebral and cerebral vessels
Mechanical embolectomy or thrombectomy

> *Code also:*
> any injection or infusion of thrombolytic agent (99.10)
> number of vessels treated (00.40-00.43)
> procedure on vessel bifurcation (00.44)

> Excludes: endarterectomy of intracranial vessels and other vessels of head and
> neck (38.11-38.12)
> occlusive endovascular embolization of head or neck vessel(s) using
> bare coils (39.75)
> occlusive endovascular embolization of head or neck vessel(s) using
> bioactive coils (39.76)
> open embolectomy or thrombectomy (38.01- 38.02)

**39.75 Endovascular embolization or occlusion of vessel(s) of head or neck using bare
coils**
Bare metal coils
Bare platinum coils [BPC]
That for treatment of aneurysm, arteriovenous malformation [AVM] or fistula

● Code new
to this edition   ▲ Revision of
existing code   ④ ⑤ Fourth or fifth
digit required

39.76 Endovascular embolization or occlusion of vessel(s) of head or neck using bioactive coils
Biodegradable inner luminal polymer coils
Coil embolization or occlusion utilizing bioactive coils
Coils containing polyglycolic acid [PGA]
That for treatment of aneurysm, arteriovenous malformation [AVM] or fistula

● **39.77 Temporary (partial) therapeutic endovascular occlusion of vessel**
Includes that of aorta
That by balloon catheter

Code also any: diagnostic arteriogram (88.40-88.49)

Excludes: *any endovascular head or neck vessel procedure (39.72, 39.74-39.76)*
diagnostic procedures on blood vessels (38.21-38.29)
permanent endovascular procedure (39.79)

● **39.78 Endovascular implantation of branching or fenestrated graft(s) in aorta**

39.79 Other endovascular procedures on other vessels
Endograft(s)
Endovascular graft(s)
Liquid tissue adhesive (glue) embolization or occlusion
Other coil embolization or occlusion
Other implant or substance for repair, embolization or occlusion
Repair of aneurysm

Excludes: *abdominal aortic aneurysm resection [AAA] (38.44)*
endovascular implantation of graft in abdominal aorta (39.71)
endovascular implantation of graft in thoracic aorta (39.73)
endovascular embolization or occlusion of head and neck vessels, bare metal coils (39.75)
endovascular embolization or occlusion of head and neck vessels, bioactive coils (39.76)
insertion of drug-eluting peripheral vessel stent(s) (00.55)
insertion of non-drug-eluting peripheral vessel stent(s) (for other than aneurysm repair) (39.90)
non-endovascular repair of arteriovenous fistula (39.53)
other surgical occlusion of vessels—see category 38.8
percutaneous transcatheter infusion (99.29)
thoracic aortic aneurysm resection (38.45)
transcatheter embolization for gastric or duodenal bleeding (44.44)
uterine artery embolization with coils (68.24)

39.8 Operations on carotid body, carotid sinus and other vascular bodies

Excludes: *excision of glomus jugulare (20.51)*

39.81 Implantation or replacement of carotid sinus stimulation device, total system
Carotid sinus baroreflex activation device
Implantation of carotid sinus stimulator and lead(s)
Includes: carotid explorations

Excludes: *implantation or replacement of carotid sinus stimulation lead(s) only (39.82)*
implantation or replacement of carotid sinus stimulation pulse generator only (39.83)

39.82 Implantation or replacement of carotid sinus stimulation lead(s) only

Excludes: *implantation or replacement of carotid sinus stimulation device, total system (39.81)*

39.83 Implantation or replacement of carotid sinus stimulation pulse generator only

Excludes: *implantation or replacement of carotid sinus stimulation device, total system (39.81)*

39.84 Revision of carotid sinus stimulation lead(s) only
Repair of electrode [removal with re-insertion]
Repositioning of lead(s) [electrode]

39.85 Revision of carotid sinus stimulation pulse generator
Debridement and reforming pocket (skin and subcutaneous tissue)
Relocation of pocket [creation of new pocket]
Repositioning of pulse generator
Revision of carotid sinus stimulation pulse generator pocket

39.86 Removal of carotid sinus stimulation device, total system

39.87 Removal of carotid sinus stimulation lead(s) only

39.88 Removal of carotid sinus stimulation pulse generator only

Valid O.R. procedure   Non-O.R. procedure   Nonspecific O.R. procedure   Noncovered O.R. procedure

39.89 **Other operations on carotid body, carotid sinus and other vascular bodies**
Chemodectomy
Denervation of:
  aortic body
  carotid body
Glomectomy, carotid

> Excludes: excision of glomus jugulare (20.51)

39.9 **Other operations on vessels**

39.90 **Insertion of non-drug-eluting peripheral (non-coronary) vessel stent(s)**
Bare stent(s)
Bonded stent(s)
Drug-coated stent(s), i.e., heparing coated
Endograft(s)
Endovascular graft(s)
Endovascular recanalization techniques
Stent graft(s)
Code also any:
  non-coronary angioplasty or atherectomy (39.50)
  number of vascular stents inserted (00.45-00.48)
  number of vessels treated (00.40-00.43)
  procedure on vessel bifurcation (00.44)

> Excludes: *that for aneurysm repair (39.71-39.79)*
> *insertion of drug-eluting peripheral vessel stent(s) (00.55)*
> *percutaneous insertion of carotid artery stent(s) (00.63)*
> *percutaneous insertion of intracranial stent(s) (00.65)*
> *percutaneous insertion of other precerebral artery stent(s) (00.64)*

39.91 **Freeing of vessel**
Dissection and freeing of adherent tissue:
  artery-vein-nerve bundle
  vascular bundle

39.92 **Injection of sclerosing agent into vein**

> Excludes: *injection:*
> *esophageal varices (42.33)*
> *hemorrhoids (49.42)*

39.93 **Insertion of vessel-to-vessel cannula**
Formation of arteriovenous:
  fistula by external cannula
  shunt by external cannula
Code also any renal dialysis (39.95)

39.9 4 **Replacement of vessel-to-vessel cannula**
Revision of vessel-to-vessel cannula

39.95 **Hemodialysis**
Artificial kidney   Hemofiltration
Hemodiafiltration   Renal dialysis

> Excludes: *peritoneal dialysis (54.98)*

39.96 **Total body perfusion**
Code also substance perfused (99.21-99.29)

39.97 **Other perfusion**
Perfusion NOS
Perfusion, local [regional] of:
  carotid artery
  coronary artery
  head
  lower limb
  neck
  upper limb
Code also substance perfused (99.21-99.29)

> Excludes: *perfusion of:*
> *kidney (55.95)*
> *large intestine (46.96)*
> *liver (50.93)*
> *small intestine (46.95)*
> *SuperSaturated oxygen therapy (00.49)*

● Code new   ▲ Revision of   ④ ⑤ Fourth or fifth
to this edition   existing code   digit required

39.98 **Control of hemorrhage, not otherwise specified**
Angiotripsy
Control of postoperative hemorrhage NOS
Venotripsy

Excludes: *control of hemorrhage (postoperative):*
anus (49.95)
bladder (57.93)
following vascular procedure (39.41)
nose (21.00-21.09)
prostate (60.94)
tonsil (28.7)
that by:
ligation (38.80-38.89)
suture (39.30-39.32)

39.99 **Other operations on vessels**

Excludes: *injection or infusion of therapeutic or prophylactic substance*
(99.11-99.29)
transfusion of blood and blood components (99.01-99.09)

This page intentionally left blank.

● Code new
to this edition

▲ Revision of
existing code

④ ⑤ Fourth or fifth
digit required

8. OPERATIONS ON THE HEMIC AND LYMPHATIC SYSTEM (40-41)

40   Operations on lymphatic system

40.0   Incision of lymphatic structures

40.1   Diagnostic procedures on lymphatic structures

40.11   Biopsy of lymphatic structure
Transbronchoscopic needle aspiration [TBNA] of lymph node

40.19   Other diagnostic procedures on lymphatic structures

Excludes: lymphangiogram
    abdominal (88.04)
    cervical (87.08)
    intrathoracic (87.34)
    lower limb (88.36)
    upper limb (88.34)
  microscopic examination of specimen (90.71-90.79)
  radioisotope scan (92.16)
  thermography (88.89)

40.2   Simple excision of lymphatic structure

Excludes: biopsy of lymphatic structure (40.11)

40.21   Excision of deep cervical lymph node

40.22   Excision of internal mammary lymph node

40.23   Excision of axillary lymph node

40.24   Excision of inguinal lymph mode

40.29   Simple excision of other lymphatic structure
Excision of:
  cystic hygroma
  lymphangioma
Simple lymphadenectomy

40.3   Regional lymph node excision
Extended regional lymph node excision
Regional lymph node excision with excision of lymphatic drainage area including skin, subcutaneous tissue, and fat

40.4   Radical excision of cervical lymph nodes
Resection of cervical lymph nodes down to muscle and deep fascia

Excludes: that associated with radical laryngectomy (30.4)

40.40   Radical neck dissection, not otherwise specified

40.41   Radical neck dissection, unilateral

40.42   Radical neck dissection, bilateral

40.5   Radical excision of other lymph nodes

Excludes: that associated with radical mastectomy (85.45-85.48)

40.50   Radical excision of lymph nodes, not otherwise specified
Radical (lymph) node dissection NOS

40.51   Radical excision of axillary lymph nodes

40.52   Radical excision of periaortic lymph nodes

40.53   Radical excision of iliac lymph nodes

40.54   Radical groin dissection

40.59   Radical excision of other lymph nodes

Excludes: radical neck dissection (40.40-40.42)

40.6   Operations on thoracic duct

40.61   Cannulation of thoracic duct

40.62   Fistulization of thoracic duct

40.63   Closure of fistula of thoracic duct

40.64   Ligation of thoracic duct

40.69   Other operations on thoracic duct

 Valid O.R. procedure

 Non-O.R. procedure

 Nonspecific O.R. procedure

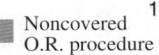 Noncovered O.R. procedure

40.9 **Other operations on lymphatic structures**
Anastomosis of peripheral lymphatics
Dilation of peripheral lymphatics
Ligation of peripheral lymphatics
Obliteration of peripheral lymphatics
Reconstruction of peripheral lymphatics
Repair of peripheral lymphatics
Transplantation of peripheral lymphatics
Correction of lymphedema of limb, NOS

Excludes: *reduction of elephantiasis of scrotum (61.3)*

41 **Operations on bone marrow and spleen**

41.0 **Bone marrow or hematopoietic stem cell transplant**
Note: To report donor source—*see* codes 00.91-00.93

Excludes: *aspiration of bone marrow from donor (41.91)*

41.00 **Bone marrow transplant, not otherwise specified**

41.01 **Autologous bone marrow transplant without purging**

Excludes: *that with purging (41.09)*

41.02 **Allogeneic bone marrow transplant with purging**
Allograft of bone marrow with in vitro removal (purging) of T-cells

41.03 **Allogeneic bone marrow transplant without purging**
Allograft of bone marrow NOS

41.04 **Autologous hematopoietic stem cell transplant without purging**

Excludes: *that with purging (41.07)*

41.05 **Allogeneic hematopoietic stem cell transplant without purging**

Excludes: *that with purging (41.08)*

41.06 **Cord blood stem cell transplant**

41.07 **Autologous hematopoietic stem cell transplant with purging**
Cell depletion

41.08 **Allogeneic hematopoietic stem cell transplant with purging**
Cell depletion

41.09 **Autologous bone marrow transplant with purging**
With extracorporeal purging of malignant cells from marrow
Cell depletion

41.1 **Puncture of spleen**

Excludes: *aspiration biopsy of spleen (41.32)*

41.2 **Splenotomy**

41.3 **Diagnostic procedures on bone marrow and spleen**

41.31 **Biopsy of bone marrow**

41.32 **Closed [aspiration] [percutaneous] biopsy of spleen**
Needle biopsy of spleen

41.33 **Open biopsy of spleen**

41.38 **Other diagnostic procedures on bone marrow**

Excludes: *microscopic examination of specimen from bone marrow (90.61-90.69)*
radioisotope scan (92.05)

41.39 **Other diagnostic procedures on spleen**

Excludes: *microscopic examination of specimen from spleen (90.61-90.69)*
radioisotope scan (92.05)

41.4 **Excision or destruction of lesion or tissue of spleen**
Code also any application or administration of an adhesion barrier substance (99.77)

Excludes: *excision of accessory spleen (41.93)*

41.41 **Marsupialization of splenic cyst**

41.42 **Excision of lesion or tissue of spleen**

Excludes: *biopsy of spleen (41.32-41.33)*

41.43 **Partial splenectomy**

● Code new
to this edition
▲ Revision of
existing code
④ ⑤ Fourth or fifth
digit required

41.5 **Total splenectomy**

Code also any application or administration of an adhesion barrier substance (99.77)

Splenectomy NOS

41.9 **Other operations on spleen and bone marrow**

Code also any application or administration of an adhesion barrier substance (99.77)

41.91 **Aspiration of bone marrow from donor for transplant**

Excludes: *biopsy of bone marrow (41.31)*

41.92 **Injection into bone marrow**

Excludes: *bone marrow transplant (41.00-41.03)*

41.93 **Excision of accessory spleen**

41.94 **Transplantation of spleen**

41.95 **Repair and plastic operations on spleen**

41.98 **Other operations on bone marrow**

41.99 **Other operations on spleen**

Valid O.R. procedure   Non-O.R. procedure   Nonspecific O.R. procedure   Noncovered O.R. procedure

This page intentionally left blank.

● Code new
to this edition
▲ Revision of
existing code
④ ⑤ Fourth or fifth
digit required

9. OPERATIONS ON THE DIGESTIVE SYSTEM (42-54)

42 Operations on esophagus

42.0 Esophagotomy

    42.01 Incision of esophageal web

    42.09 Other incision of esophagus
        Esophagotomy NOS

        | Excludes: | *esophagomyotomy (42.7)* |
        esophagostomy (42.10-42.19)

42.1 Esophagostomy

    42.10 Esophagostomy, not otherwise specified

    42.11 Cervical esophagostomy

    42.12 Exteriorization of esophageal pouch

    42.19 Other external fistulization of esophagus
        Thoracic esophagostomy
        Code also any resection (42.40-42.42)

42.2 Diagnostic procedures on esophagus

    42.21 Operative esophagoscopy by incision

    42.22 Esophagoscopy through artificial stoma

        | Excludes: | *that with biopsy (42.24)* |

    42.23 Other esophagoscopy

        | Excludes: | *that with biopsy (42.24)* |

    42.24 Closed [endoscopic] biopsy of esophagus
        Brushing or washing for specimen collection
        Esophagoscopy with biopsy
        Suction biopsy of the esophagus

        | Excludes: | *esophagogastroduodenoscopy [EGD] with closed biopsy (45.16)* |

    42.25 Open biopsy of esophagus

    42.29 Other diagnostic procedures on esophagus

        | Excludes: | *barium swallow (87.61)* |
        esophageal manometry (89.32)
        microscopic examination of specimen from esophagus (90.81-90.89)

42.3 Local excision or destruction of lesion or tissue of esophagus

    42.31 Local excision of esophageal diverticulum

    42.32 Local excision of other lesion or tissue of esophagus

        | Excludes: | *biopsy of esophagus (42.24-42.25)* |
        esophageal fistulectomy (42.84)

    42.33 Endoscopic excision or destruction of lesion or tissue of esophagus
        Ablation of esophageal neoplasm by endoscopic approach
        Control of esophageal bleeding by endoscopic approach
        Esophageal polypectomy by endoscopic approach
        Esophageal varices by endoscopic approach
        Injection of esophageal varices by endoscopic approach

        | Excludes: | *biopsy of esophagus (42.24-42.25)* |
        fistulectomy (42.84)
        open ligation of esophageal varices (42.91)

    42.39 Other destruction of lesion or tissue of esophagus

        | Excludes: | *that by endoscopic approach (42.33)* |

42.4 Excision of esophagus

    | Excludes: | *esophagogastrectomy NOS (43.99)* |

    42.40 Esophagectomy, not otherwise specified

Valid O.R. procedure   Non-O.R. procedure   Nonspecific O.R. procedure   Noncovered O.R. procedure

42.41 Partial esophagectomy

Code also any synchronous:
anastomosis other than end-to-end (42.51-42.69)
esophagostomy (42.10-42.19)
gastrostomy (43.11-43.19)

42.42 Total esophagectomy

Code also any synchronous:
gastrostomy (43.11-43.19)
interposition or anastomosis other than end-to-end (42.51-42.69)

Excludes: *esophagogastrectomy (43.99)*

42.5 Intrathoracic anastomosis of esophagus

Code also any synchronous:
esophagectomy (42.40-42.42)
gastrostomy (43.1)

42.51 Intrathoracic esophagoesophagostomy

42.52 Intrathoracic esophagogastrostomy

42.53 Intrathoracic esophageal anastomosis with interposition of small bowel

42.54 Other intrathoracic esophagoenterostomy
Anastomosis of esophagus to intestinal segment NOS

42.55 Intrathoracic esophageal anastomosis with interposition of colon

42.56 Other intrathoracic esophagocolostomy
Esophagocolostomy NOS

42.58 Intrathoracic esophageal anastomosis with other interposition
Construction of artificial esophagus
Retrosternal formation of reversed gastric tube

42.59 Other intrathoracic anastomosis of esophagus

42.6 Antesternal anastomosis of esophagus

Code also any synchronous:
esophagectomy (42.40-42.42)
gastrostomy (43.1)

42.61 Antesternal esophagoesophagostomy

42.62 Antesternal esophagogastrostomy

42.63 Antesternal esophageal anastomosis with interposition of small bowel

42.64 Other antesternal esophagoenterostomy
Antethoracic:
esophagoenterostomy
esophagoileostomy
esophagojejunostomy

42.65 Antesternal esophageal anastomosis with interposition of colon

42.66 Other antesternal esophagocolostomy
Antethoracic esophagocolostomy

42.68 Other antesternal esophageal anastomosis with interposition

42.69 Other antesternal anastomosis of esophagus

42.7 Esophagomyotomy

42.8 Other repair of esophagus

42.81 Insertion of permanent tube into esophagus

42.82 Suture of laceration of esophagus

42.83 Closure of esophagostomy

42.84 Repair of esophageal fistula, not elsewhere classified

Excludes: *repair of fistula:*
bronchoesophageal (33.42)
esophagopleurocutaneous (34.73)
pharyngoesophageal (29.53)
tracheoesophageal (31.73)

42.85 Repair of esophageal stricture

42.86 Production of subcutaneous tunnel without esophageal anastomosis

42.87 Other graft of esophagus

> | Excludes: | antesternal esophageal anastomosis with interposition of:
> colon (42.65)
> small bowel (42.63)
> antesternal esophageal anastomosis with other interposition (42.68)
> intrathoracic esophageal anastomosis with interposition of:
> colon (42.55)
> small bowel (42.53)
> intrathoracic esophageal anastomosis with other interposition (42.58)

42.89 Other repair of esophagus

42.9 Other operations on esophagus

42.91 Ligation of esophageal varices

> | Excludes: | that by endoscopic approach (42.33)

42.92 Dilation of esophagus
Dilation of cardiac sphincter

> | Excludes: | intubation of esophagus (96.03, 96.06-96.08)

42.99 Other

> | Excludes: | insertion of Sengstaken tube (96.06)
> intubation of esophagus (96.03, 96.06-96.08)
> removal of intraluminal foreign body from esophagus without incision (98.02)
> tamponade of esophagus (96.06)

43 Incision and excision of stomach
Code also any application or administration of an adhesion barrier substance (99.77)

43.0 Gastrotomy

> | Excludes: | gastrostomy (43.11-43.19)
> that for control of hemorrhage (44.49)

43.1 Gastrostomy

43.11 Percutaneous [endoscopic] gastrostomy [PEG]
Percutaneous transabdominal gastrostomy

43.19 Other gastrostomy

> | Excludes: | percutaneous [endoscopic] gastrostomy [PEG] (43.11)

43.3 Pyloromyotomy

43.4 Local excision or destruction of lesion or tissue of stomach

43.41 Endoscopic excision or destruction of lesion or tissue of stomach
Gastric polypectomy by endoscopic approach
Gastric varices by endoscopic approach

> | Excludes: | biopsy of stomach (44.14-44.15)
> control of hemorrhage (44.43)
> open ligation of gastric varices (44.91)

43.42 Local excision of other lesion or tissue of stomach

> | Excludes: | biopsy of stomach (44.14-44.15)
> gastric fistulectomy (44.62-44.63)
> partial gastrectomy (43.5-43.89)

43.49 Other destruction of lesion or tissue of stomach

> | Excludes: | that by endoscopic approach (43.41)

43.5 Partial gastrectomy with anastomosis to esophagus
Proximal gastrectomy

43.6 Partial gastrectomy with anastomosis to duodenum
Billroth I operation
Distal gastrectomy
Gastropylorectomy

43.7 Partial gastrectomy with anastomosis to jejunum
Billroth II operation

43.8 Other partial gastrectomy

43.81 Partial gastrectomy with jejunal transposition
Henley jejunal transposition operation
Code also any synchronous intestinal resection (45.51)

Valid O.R. procedure   Non-O.R. procedure   Nonspecific O.R. procedure   Noncovered O.R. procedure

● **43.82 Laparoscopic vertical (sleeve) gastrectomy**
> *Excludes:* *laparoscopic banding (44.95)*
> *laparoscopic gastric restrictive procedure (44.95)*

▲ **43.89 Open and other partial gastrectomy**
Partial gastrectomy with bypass gastrogastrostomy
Sleeve resection of stomach
> *Excludes:* *laparoscopic sleeve gastrectomy (43.82)*

43.9 Total gastrectomy

43.91 Total gastrectomy with intestinal interposition

43.99 Other total gastrectomy
Complete gastroduodenectomy
Esophagoduodenostomy with complete gastrectomy
Esophagogastrectomy NOS
Esophagojejunostomy with complete gastrectomy
Radical gastrectomy

44 Other operations on stomach
Code also any application or administration of an adhesion barrier substance (99.77)

44.0 Vagotomy

44.00 Vagotomy, not otherwise specified
Division of vagus nerve NOS

44.01 Truncal vagotomy

44.02 Highly selective vagotomy
Parietal cell vagotomy
Selective proximal vagotomy

44.03 Other selective vagotomy

44.1 Diagnostic procedures on stomach

44.11 Transabdominal gastroscopy
Intraoperative gastroscopy
> *Excludes:* *that with biopsy (44.14)*

44.12 Gastroscopy through artificial stoma
> *Excludes:* *that with biopsy (44.14)*

44.13 Other gastroscopy
> *Excludes:* *that with biopsy (44.14)*

44.14 Closed [endoscopic] biopsy of stomach
Brushing or washing for specimen collection
> *Excludes:* *esophagogastroduodenoscopy [EGD] with closed biopsy (45.16)*

44.15 Open biopsy of stomach

44.19 Other diagnostic procedures on stomach
> *Excludes:* *gastric lavage (96.33)*
> *microscopic examination of specimen from stomach (90.81-90.89)*
> *upper GI series (87.62)*

44.2 Pyloroplasty

44.21 Dilation of pylorus by incision

44.22 Endoscopic dilation of pylorus
Dilation with balloon endoscope
Endoscopic dilation of gastrojejunostomy site

44.29 Other pyloroplasty
Pyloroplasty NOS
Revision of pylorus

44.3 Gastroenterostomy without gastrectomy

44.31 High gastric bypass
Printen and Mason gastric bypass

44.32 Percutaneous [endoscopic] gastrojejunostomy
Bypass:
gastroduodenostomy
PEGJJ
> *Excludes:* *percutaneous (endoscopic) feeding jejunostomy (46.32)*

● Code new to this edition   ▲ Revision of existing code   ④ ⑤ Fourth or fifth digit required

44.38 Laparoscopic gastroenterostomy
Bypass:
    gastroduodenostomy
    gastroenterostomy
    gastrogastrostomy
Laparoscopic gastrojejunostomy without gastrectomy NEC

> Excludes: gastroenterostomy, open approach (44.39)

44.39 Other gastroenterostomy
Bypass:
    gastroduodenostomy
    gastroenterostomy
    gastrogastrostomy
Gastrojejunostomy without gastrectomy NOS

44.4 Control of hemorrhage and suture of ulcer of stomach or duodenum

44.40 Suture of peptic ulcer, not otherwise specified

44.41 Suture of gastric ulcer site

> Excludes: ligation of gastric varices (44.91)

44.42 Suture of duodenal ulcer site

44.43 Endoscopic control of gastric or duodenal bleeding

44.44 Transcatheter embolization for gastric or duodenal bleeding

> Excludes: surgical occlusion of abdominal vessels (38.86-38.87)

44.49 Other control of hemorrhage of stomach or duodenum
That with gastrotomy

44.5 Revision of gastric anastomosis
Closure of:
    gastric anastomosis
    gastroduodenostomy
    gastrojejunostomy
Pantaloon operation

44.6 Other repair of stomach

44.61 Suture of laceration of stomach

> Excludes: that of ulcer site(44.41)

44.62 Closure of gastrostomy

44.63 Closure of other gastric fistula
Closure of:
    gastrocolic fistula
    gastrojejunocolic fistula

44.64 Gastropexy

44.65 Esophagogastroplasty
Belsey operation
Esophagus and stomach cardioplasty

44.66 Other procedures for creation of esophagogastric sphincteric competence
Fundoplication
Gastric cardioplasty
Nissen's fundoplication
Restoration of cardio-esophageal angle

> Excludes: that by laparoscopy (44.67)

44.67 Laparoscopic procedures for creation of esophagogastric sphincteric competence
Fundoplication
Gastric cardioplasty
Nissen's fundoplication
Restoration of cardio-esophageal angle

44.68 Laparoscopic gastroplasty
Banding
Silastic vertical banding
Vertical banded gastroplasty (VBG)

Code also any synchronous laparoscopic gastroenterostomy (44.38)

> Excludes: insertion, laparoscopic adjustable gastric band (restrictive procedure)
>   (44.95)
>   other repair of stomach, open approach (44.61-44.65, 44.69)

Valid O.R.
procedure

Non-O.R.
procedure

Nonspecific
O.R. procedure

Noncovered
O.R. procedure

44.69 Other
Inversion of gastric diverticulum
Repair of stomach NOS

44.9 **Other operations on stomach**

44.91 **Ligation of gastric varices**

Excludes: that by endoscopic approach (43.41)

44.92 **Intraoperative manipulation of stomach**
Reduction of gastric volvulus

44.93 **Insertion of gastric bubble [balloon]**

44.94 **Removal of gastric bubble [balloon]**

44.95 **Laparoscopic gastric restrictive procedure**
Adjustable gastric band and port insertion

Excludes: laparoscoipc gastroplasty (44.68)
other repair of stomach (44.69)

44.96 **Laparoscopic revision of gastric restrictive procedure**
Revision or replacement of:
adjustable gastric band
subcutaneous gastric port device

44.97 **Laparoscopic removal of gastric restrictive device(s)**
Removal of either or both:
adjustable gastric band
subcutaneous port device

Excludes: nonoperative removal of gastric restrictive device(s) (97.86)
open removal of gastric restrictive device(s) (44.99)

44.98 **(Laparoscopic) adjustment of size of adjustable gastric restrictive device**
Infusion of saline for device tightening
Withdrawal of saline for device loosening

Code also any:
abdominal ultrasound (88.76)
abdominal wall fluoroscopy (88.09)
barium swallaw (87.61)

44.99 **Other**

Excludes: change of gastrostomy tube (97.02)
dilation of cardiac sphincter (42.92)
gastric:
cooling (96.31)
freezing (96.32)
gavage (96.35)
hypothermia (96.31)
lavage (96.33)
insertion of nasogastric tube (96.07)
irrigation of gastrostomy (96.36)
irrigation of nasogastric tube (96.34)
removal of:
gastrostomy tube (97.51)
intraluminal foreign body from stomach without incision (98.03)
replacement of:
gastrostomy tube (97.02)
(naso-)gastric tube (97.01)

45 **Incision, excision, and anastomosis of intestine**
Code also any application or administration of an adhesion barrier substance (99.77)

45.0 **Enterotomy**

Excludes: duodenocholedochotomy (51.41-51.42, 51.51)
that for destruction of lesion (45.30-45.34)
that of exteriorized intestine (46.14, 46.24, 46.31)

45.00 **Incision of intestine, not otherwise specified**

45.01 **Incision of duodenum**

45.02 **Other incision of small intestine**

45.03 **Incision of large intestine**

Excludes: proctotomy (48.0)

● Code new
to this edition
▲ Revision of
existing code
④ ⑤ Fourth or fifth
digit required

45.1   Diagnostic procedures on small intestine
Code also any laparotomy (54.11-54.19)

> **45.11   Transabdominal endoscopy of small intestine**
> Intraoperative endoscopy of small intestine
>
> > | Excludes: | that with biopsy (45.14) |

> **45.12   Endoscopy of small intestine through artificial stoma**
>
> > | Excludes: | that with biopsy (45.14) |

> **45.13   Other endoscopy of small intestine**
> Esophagogastroduodenoscopy [EGD]
>
> > | Excludes: | that with biopsy (45.14, 45.16) |

> **45.14   Closed [endoscopic] biopsy of small intestine**
> Brushing or washing for specimen collection
>
> > | Excludes: | esophagogastroduodenoscopy [EGD] with closed biopsy (45.16) |

> **45.15   Open biopsy of small intestine**

> **45.16   Esophagogastroduodenoscopy [EGD] with closed biopsy**
> Biopsy of one or more sites involving esophagus, stomach, and/or duodenum

> **45.19   Other diagnostic procedures on small intestine**
>
> > | Excludes: | microscopic examination of specimen from small intestine (90.91-90.99) |
> > | | radioisotope scan (92.04) |
> > | | ultrasonography (88.74) |
> > | | x-ray (87.61-87.69) |

45.2   Diagnostic procedures on large intestine
Code also any laparotomy (54.11-54.19)

> **45.21   Transabdominal endoscopy of large intestine**
> Intraoperative endoscopy of large intestine
>
> > | Excludes: | that with biopsy (45.25) |

> **45.22   Endoscopy of large intestine through artificial stoma**
>
> > | Excludes: | that with biopsy (45.25) |

> **45.23   Colonoscopy**
> Flexible fiberoptic colonoscopy
>
> > | Excludes: | endoscopy of large intestine through artificial stoma (45.22) |
> > | | flexible sigmoidoscopy (45.24) |
> > | | rigid proctosigmoidoscopy (48.23) |
> > | | transabdominal endoscopy of large intestine (45.21) |

> **45.24   Flexible sigmoidoscopy**
> Endoscopy of descending colon
>
> > | Excludes: | rigid proctosigmoidoscopy (48.23) |

> **45.25   Closed [endoscopic] biopsy of large intestine**
> Biopsy, closed, of unspecified intestinal site
> Brushing or washing for specimen collection
> Colonoscopy with biopsy
>
> > | Excludes: | proctosigmoidoscopy with biopsy (48.24) |

> **45.26   Open biopsy of large intestine**

> **45.27   Intestinal biopsy, site unspecified**

> **45.28   Other diagnostic procedures on large intestine**

> **45.29   Other diagnostic procedures on intestine, site unspecified**
>
> > | Excludes: | microscopic examination of specimen (90.91-90.99) |
> > | | scan and radioisotope function study (92.04) |
> > | | ultrasonography (88.74) |
> > | | x-ray (87.61-87.69) |

45.3   Local excision or destruction of lesion or tissue of small intestine

> **45.30   Endoscopic excision or destruction of lesion of duodenum**
>
> > | Excludes: | biopsy of duodenum (45.14-45.15) |
> > | | control of hemorrhage (44.43) |
> > | | fistulectomy (46.72) |

| Valid O.R. procedure | Non-O.R. procedure | Nonspecific O.R. procedure | Noncovered O.R. procedure |

45.31 **Other local excision of lesion of duodenum**

> Excludes: | *biopsy of duodenum (45.14-45.15)*
> *fistulectomy (46.72)*
> *multiple segmental resection (45.61)*
> *that by endoscopic approach (45.30)*

45.32 **Other destruction of lesion of duodenum**

> Excludes: | *that by endoscopic approach (45.30)*

45.33 **Local excision of lesion or tissue of small intestine, except duodenum**
Excision of redundant mucosa of ileostomy

> Excludes: | *biopsy of small intestine (45.14-45.15)*
> *fistulectomy (46.74)*
> *multiple segmental resection (45.61)*

45.34 **Other destruction of lesion of small intestine, except duodenum**

45.4 **Local excision or destruction of lesion or tissue of large intestine**

45.41 **Excision of lesion or tissue of large intestine**
Excision of redundant mucosa of colostomy

> Excludes: | *biopsy of large intestine (45.25-45.27)*
> *endoscopic polypectomy of large intestine (45.42)*
> *fistulectomy (46.76)*
> *multiple segmental resection (17.31, 45.71)*
> *that by endoscopic approach (45.42-45.43)*

45.42 **Endoscopic polypectomy of large intestine**

> Excludes: | *that by open approach (45.41)*

45.43 **Endoscopic destruction of other lesion or tissue of large intestine**
Endoscopic ablation of tumor of large intestine
Endoscopic control of colonic bleeding

> Excludes: | *endoscopic polypectomy of large intestine (45.42)*

45.49 **Other destruction of lesion of large intestine**

> Excludes: | *that by endoscopic approach (45.43)*

45.5 **Isolation of intestinal segment**
Code also any synchronous:
anastomosis other than end-to-end (45.90-45.94)
enterostomy (46.10-46.39)

45.50 **Isolation of intestinal segment not otherwise specified**
Isolation of intestinal pedicle flap
Reversal of intestinal segment

45.51 **Isolation of segment of small intestine**
Isolation of ileal loop
Resection of small intestine for interposition

45.52 **Isolation of segment of large intestine**
Resection of colon for interposition

45.6 **Other excision of small intestine**
Code also any synchronous:
anastomosis other than end-to-end (45.90-45.93, 45.95)
colostomy (46.10-46.13)
enterostomy (46.10-46.39)

> Excludes: | *cecectomy (17.32, 45.72)*
> *enterocolectomy (17.39, 45.79)*
> *gastroduodenectomy (43.6-43.99)*
> *ileocolectomy (17.33, 45.73)*
> *pancreatoduodenectomy (52.51-52.7)*

45.61 **Multiple segmental resection of small intestine**
Segmental resection for multiple traumatic lesions of small intestine

45.62 **Other partial resection of small intestine**
Duodenectomy   Jejunectomy
Ileectomy

> Excludes: | *duodenectomy with synchronous pancreatectomy (52.51-52.7)*
> *resection of cecum and terminal ileum (17.32, 45.72)*

45.63 **Total removal of small intestine**

● Code new
to this edition   ▲ Revision of
existing code   ④ ⑤ Fourth or fifth
digit required

45.7 **Open and other partial excision of large intestine**
Code also any synchronous:
anastomosis other than end-to-end (45.92-45.94)
enterostomy (46.10-46.39)

Excludes: *laparoscopic partial excision of large intestine (17.31-17.39)*

45.71 **Open and other multiple segmental resection of large intestine**
Segmental resection for multiple traumatic lesions of large intestine

45.72 **Open and other cecectomy**
Resection of cecum and terminal ileum

45.73 **Open and other right hemicolectomy**
Ileocolectomy
Right radical colectomy

45.74 **Open and other resection of transverse colon**

45.75 **Open and other left hemicolectomy**

Excludes: *proctosigmoidectomy (48.41-48.69)*
second stage Mikulicz operation (46.04)

45.76 **Open and other sigmoidectomy**

45.79 **Other and unspecified partial excision of large intestine**
Enterocolectomy NEC

45.8 **Total intra-abdominal colectomy**
Excision of cecum, colon, and sigmoid

Excludes: *coloproctectomy (48.41-48.69)*

45.81 **Laparoscopic total intra-abdominal colectomy**

45.82 **Open total intra-abdominal colectomy**

45.83 **Other and unspecified total intra-abdominal colectomy**

45.9 **Intestinal anastomosis**
Code also any synchronous resection (45.31-45.8, 48.41-48.69)

Excludes: *end-to-end anastomosis – omit code*

45.90 **Intestinal anastomosis, not otherwise specified**

45.91 **Small-to-small intestinal anastomosis**

45.92 **Anastomosis of small intestine to rectal stump**
Hampton procedure

45.93 **Other small-to-large intestinal anastomosis**

45.94 **Large-to-large intestinal anastomosis**

Excludes: *rectorectostomy (48.74)*

45.95 **Anastomosis to anus**
Formation of endorectal ileal pouch (J-pouch) (H-pouch) (S-pouch) with
anastomosis of small intestine to anus

46 **Other operations on intestine**
Code also any application or administration of an adhesion barrier substance (99.77)

46.0 **Exteriorization of intestine**
Includes: loop enterostomy
multiple stage resection of intestine

46.01 **Exteriorization of small intestine**
Loop ileostomy

46.02 **Resection of exteriorized segment of small intestine**

46.03 **Exteriorization of large intestine**
Exteriorization of intestine NOS
First stage Mikulicz exteriorization of intestine
Loop colostomy

46.04 **Resection of exteriorized segment of large intestine**
Resection of exteriorized segment of intestine NOS
Second stage Mikulicz operation

| | Valid O.R.
procedure | | Non-O.R.
procedure | | Nonspecific
O.R. procedure | | Noncovered
O.R. procedure |

46.1 Colostomy

Code also any synchronous resection (45.49, 45.71-45.79, 45.8)

> *Excludes:* loop colostomy (46.03)
> that with abdominoperineal resection of rectum (48.5)
> that with synchronous anterior rectal resection (48.62)

46.10 Colostomy, not otherwise specified

46.11 Temporary colostomy

46.13 Other permanent colostomy

46.14 Delayed opening of colostomy

46.2 Ileostomy

Code also any synchronous resection (45.34, 45.61-45.63)

> *Excludes:* loop ileostomy (46.01)

46.20 Ileostomy, not otherwise specified

46.21 Temporary ileostomy

46.22 Continent ileostomy

46.23 Other permanent ileostomy

46.24 Delayed opening of ileostomy

46.3 Other enterostomy

Code also any synchronous resection (45.61-45.8)

46.31 Delayed opening of other enterostomy

46.32 Percutaneous [endoscopic] jejunostomy [PEJ]
Endoscopic conversion of gastrostomy to jejunostomy
Percutaneous (endoscopic) feeding enterostomy

> *Excludes:* percutaneous [endoscopic] gastrojejunostomy (bypass) (44.32)

46.39 Other
Duodenostomy
Feeding enterostomy

46.4 Revision of intestinal stoma

46.40 Revision of intestinal stoma, not otherwise specified
Plastic enlargement of intestinal stoma
Reconstruction of stoma of intestine
Release of scar tissue of intestinal stoma

> *Excludes:* excision of redundant mucosa (45.41)

46.41 Revision of stoma of small intestine

> *Excludes:* excision of redundant mucosa (45.33)

46.42 Repair of pericolostomy hernia

46.43 Other revision of stoma of large intestine

> *Excludes:* excision of redundant mucosa (45.41)

46.5 Closure of intestinal stoma

Code also any synchronous resection (45.34, 45.49, 45.61-45.8)

46.50 Closure of intestinal stoma, not otherwise specified

46.51 Closure of stoma of small intestine

46.52 Closure of stoma of large intestine
Closure or take-down of:
   cecostomy
   colostomy
   sigmoidostomy

46.6 Fixation of intestine

46.60 Fixation of intestine, not otherwise specified
Fixation of intestine to abdominal wall

46.61 Fixation of small intestine to abdominal wall
Ileopexy

46.62 Other fixation of small intestine
Noble plication of small intestine
Plication of jejunum

● Code new to this edition   ▲ Revision of existing code   ④ ⑤ Fourth or fifth digit required

46.63 Fixation of large intestine to abdominal wall
Cecocoloplicopexy
Sigmoidopexy (Moschowitz)

46.64 Other fixation of large intestine
Cecofixation
Colofixation

46.7 Other repair of intestine

Excludes: closure of:
ulcer of duodenum (44.42)
vesicoenteric fistula (57.83)

46.71 Suture of laceration of duodenum

46.72 Closure of fistula of duodenum

46.73 Suture of laceration of small intestine, except duodenum

46.74 Closure of fistula of small intestine, except duodenum

Excludes: closure of:
artificial stoma (46.51)
vaginal fistula (70.74)
repair of gastrojejunocolic fistula (44.63)

46.75 Suture of laceration of large intestine

46.76 Closure of fistula of large intestine

Excludes: closure of:
gastrocolic fistula (44.63)
rectal fistula (48.73)
sigmoidovesical fistula (57.83)
stoma (46.52)
vaginal fistula (70.72-70.73)
vesicocolic fistula (57.83)
vesicosigmoidovaginal fistula (57.83)

46.79 Other repair of intestine
Duodenoplasty

46.8 Dilation and manipulation of intestine

46.80 Intra-abdominal manipulation of intestine, not otherwise specified
Correction of intestinal malrotation
Reduction of:
intestinal torsion
intestinal volvulus
intussusception

Excludes: reduction of intussusception with:
fluoroscopy (96.29)
ionizing radiation enema (96.29)
ultrasonography guidance (96.29)

46.81 Intra-abdominal manipulation of small intestine

46.82 Intra-abdominal manipulation of large intestine

46.85 Dilation of intestine
Dilation (balloon) of duodenum
Dilation (balloon) of jejunum
Endoscopic dilation (balloon) of large intestine
That through rectum or colostomy

Excludes: with insertion of colonic stent (46.86-46.87)

46.86 Endoscopic insertion of colonic stent(s)
Colonoscopy (flexible) (through stoma) with transendoscopic stent placement
Combined with fluoroscopic-guided insertion
Stent endoprosthesis of colon
Through the scope [TTS] technique

Excludes: other non-endoscopic insertion of colonic stent (46.87)

	Valid O.R. procedure		Non-O.R. procedure		Nonspecific O.R. procedure		Noncovered O.R. procedure

46.87   Other insertion of colonic stent(s)
Includes: that by:
fluoroscopic guidance only
rectal guiding tube
Non-endoscopic insertion

Code also any synchronous diagnostic procedure(s)

Excludes: *endoscopic insertion of colonic stent (46.86)*

46.9   Other operations on intestines

46.91   Myotomy of sigmoid colon

46.92   Myotomy of other parts of colon

46.93   Revision of anastomosis of small intestine

46.94   Revision of anastomosis of large intestine

46.95   Local perfusion of small intestine
Code also substance perfused (99.21-99.29)

46.96   Local perfusion of large intestine
Code also substance perfused (99.21-99.29)

46.97   Transplant of intestine
Note: To report donor source—*see* codes 00.91-00.93

46.99   Other
Ileoentectropy

Excludes: *diagnostic procedures on intestine (45.11-45.29)*
dilation of enterostomy stoma (96.24)
intestinal intubation (96.08)
removal of:
intraluminal foreign body from intestine without incision (98.04)
intraluminal foreign body from small intestine without incision
(98.03)
tube from large intestine (97.53)
tube from small intestine (97.52)
replacement of:
large intestine tube or enterostomy device (97.04)
small intestine tube or enterostomy device (97.03)

47   Operations on appendix
Includes: appendiceal stump

Code also any application or administration of an adhesion barrier substance (99.77)

47.0   Appendectomy

Excludes: *incidental appendectomy, so described (47.11, 47.19)*

47.01   Laparoscopic appendectomy

47.09   Other appendectomy

47.1   Incidental appendectomy

47.11   Laparoscopic incidental appendectomy

47.19   Other incidental appendectomy

47.2   Drainage of appendiceal abscess

Excludes: *that with appendectomy (47.0)*

47.9   Other operations on appendix

47.91   Appendicostomy

47.92   Closure of appendiceal fistula

47.99   Other
Anastomosis of appendix

Excludes: *diagnostic procedures on appendix (45.21-45.29)*

48   Operations on rectum, rectosigmoid, and perirectal tissue
Code also any application or administration of an adhesion barrier substance (99.77)

48.0   Proctotomy
Decompression of imperforate anus
Panas' operation [linear proctotomy]

Excludes: *incision of perirectal tissue (48.81)*

● Code new   ▲ Revision of   ④ ⑤ Fourth or fifth
to this edition   existing code   digit required

48.1   **Proctostomy**

48.2   **Diagnostic procedures on rectum, rectosigmoid, and perirectal tissue**

    48.21   **Transabdominal proctosigmoidoscopy**
Intraoperative proctosigmoidoscopy

        | Excludes: | *that with biopsy (48.24)*

    48.22   **Proctosigmoidoscopy through artificial stoma**

        | Excludes: | *that with biopsy (48.24)*

    48.23   **Rigid proctosigmoidoscopy**

        | Excludes: | *flexible sigmoidoscopy (45.24)*

    48.24   **Closed [endoscopic] biopsy of rectum**
Brushing or washing for specimen collection
Proctosigmoidoscopy with biopsy

    48.25   **Open biopsy of rectum**

    48.26   **Biopsy of perirectal tissue**

    48.29   **Other diagnostic procedures on rectum, rectosigmoid and perirectal tissue**

        | Excludes: | *digital examination of rectum (89.34)*
lower GI series (87.64)
microscopic examination of specimen from rectum (90.91-90.99)

48.3   **Local excision or destruction of lesion or tissue of rectum**

    48.31   **Radical electrocoagulation of rectal lesion or tissue**

    48.32   **Other electrocoagulation of rectal lesion or tissue**

    48.33   **Destruction of rectal lesion or tissue by laser**

    48.34   **Destruction of rectal lesion or tissue by cryosurgery**

    48.35   **Local excision of rectal lesion or tissue**

        | Excludes: | *biopsy of rectum (48.24-48.25)*
[endoscopic] polypectomy of rectum (48.36)
excision of perirectal tissue (48.82)
hemorrhoidectomy (49.46)
rectal fistulectomy (48.73)

    48.36   **[Endoscopic] polypectomy of rectum**

48.4   **Pull-through resection of rectum**
Code also any synchronous anastomosis other than end-to-end (45.90, 45.92-45.95)

    48.40   **Pull-through resection of rectum, not otherwise specified**
Pull-through resection NOS

        | Excludes: | *Abdominoperineal pull-through NOS (48.50)*

    48.41   **Soave submucosal resection of rectum**
Endorectal pull-through operation

    48.42   **Laparoscopic pull-through resection of rectum**

    48.43   **Open pull-through resection of rectum**

    48.49   **Other pull-through resection of rectum**
Abdominoperineal pull-through
Altemeier operation   Swenson proctectomy

        | Excludes: | *Duhamel abdominoperineal pull-through (48.65)*
laparoscopic pull-through resection of rectum (48.42)
open pull-through resection of rectum (48.43)
pull-through resection of rectum, not otherwise specified (48.40)

48.5   **Abdominoperineal resection of rectum**
Includes: with synchronous colostomy
Combined abdominoendorectal resection
Complete proctectomy
Code also any synchronous anastomosis other than end-to-end (45.90, 45.92-45.95)

    | Excludes: | *Duhamel abdominoperineal pull-through (48.65)*
that as part of pelvic exenteration (68.8)

    48.50   **Abdominoperineal resection of the rectum, not otherwise specified**

    48.51   **Laparoscopic abdominoperineal resection of the rectum**

    48.52   **Open abdominoperineal resection of the rectum**

1837

| Valid O.R. procedure | Non-O.R. procedure | Nonspecific O.R. procedure | Noncovered O.R. procedure |

48.59 Other abdominoperineal resection of the rectum

> Excludes: *abdominoperineal resection of the rectum, NOS (48.50)*
> *laparoscopic abdominoperineal resection of the rectum (48.51)*
> *open abdominoperineal resection of the rectum (48.52)*

48.6 Other resection of rectum

> *Code also any synchronous anastomosis other than end-to-end (45.90, 45.92-45.95)*

48.61 Transsacral rectosigmoidectomy

48.62 Anterior resection of rectum with synchronous colostomy

48.63 Other anterior resection of rectum

> Excludes: *that with synchronous colostomy (48.62)*

48.64 Posterior resection of rectum

48.65 Duhamel resection of rectum
Duhamel abdominoperineal pull-through

48.69 Other
Partial proctectomy
Rectal resection NOS

48.7 Repair of rectum

> Excludes: *repair of:*
> *current obstetric laceration (75.62)*
> *vaginal rectocele (70.50, 70.52, 70.53, 70.55)*

48.71 Suture of laceration of rectum

48.72 Closure of proctostomy

48.73 Closure of other rectal fistula

> Excludes: *fistulectomy:*
> *perirectal (48.93)*
> *rectourethral (58.43)*
> *rectovaginal (70.73)*
> *rectovesical (57.83)*
> *rectovesicovaginal (57.83)*

48.74 Rectorectostomy
Rectal anastomosis NOS
Stapled transanal rectal resection (STARR)

48.75 Abdominal proctopexy
Frickman procedure
Ripstein repair of rectal prolapse

48.76 Other proctopexy
Delorme repair of prolapsed rectum
Proctosigmoidopexy
Puborectalis sling operation

> Excludes: *manual reduction of rectal prolapse (96.26)*

48.79 Other repair of rectum
Repair of old obstetric laceration of rectum

> Excludes: *anastomosis to:*
> *large intestine (45.94)*
> *small intestine (45.92-45.93)*
> *repair of:*
> *current obstetrical laceration (75.62)*
> *vaginal rectocele (70.50, 70.52)*

48.8 Incision or excision of perirectal tissue or lesion
Includes: pelvirectal tissue
rectovaginal septum

48.81 Incision of perirectal tissue
Incision of rectovaginal septum

48.82 Excision of perirectal tissue

> Excludes: *perirectal biopsy (48.26)*
> *perirectofistulectomy (48.93)*
> *rectal fistulectomy (48.73)*

48.9 Other operations on rectum and perirectal tissue

48.91 Incision of rectal stricture

● Code new
to this edition

▲ Revision of
existing code

④ ⑤ Fourth or fifth
digit required

48.92 Anorectal myectomy

48.93 Repair of perirectal fistula

> Excludes: *that opening into rectum (48.73)*

48.99 Other

> Excludes: *digital examination of rectum (89.34)*
> *dilation of rectum (96.22)*
> *insertion of rectal tube (96.09)*
> *irrigation of rectum (96.38-96.39)*
> *manual reduction of rectal prolapse (96.26)*
> *proctoclysis (96.37)*
> *rectal massage (99.93)*
> *rectal packing (96.19)*
> *removal of:*
>   *impacted feces (96.38)*
>   *intraluminal foreign body from rectum without incision (98.05)*
>   *rectal packing (97.59)*
> *transanal enema (96.39)*

49 Operations on anus

Code also any application or administration of an adhesion barrier substance (99.77)

49.0 Incision or excision of perianal tissue

49.01 Incision of perianal abscess

49.02 Other incision of perianal tissue
Undercutting of perianal tissue

> Excludes: *anal fistulotomy (49.11)*

49.03 Excision of perianal skin tags

49.04 Other excision of perianal tissue

> Excludes: *anal fistulectomy (49.12)*
> *biopsy of perianal tissue (49.22)*

49.1 Incision or excision of anal fistula

> Excludes: *closure of anal fistula (49.73)*

49.11 Anal fistulotomy

49.12 Anal fistulectomy

49.2 Diagnostic procedures on anus and perianal tissue

49.21 Anoscopy

49.22 Biopsy of perianal tissue

49.23 Biopsy of anus

49.29 Other diagnostic procedures on anus and perianal tissue

> Excludes: *microscopic examination of specimen from anus (90.91-90.99)*

49.3 Local excision or destruction of other lesion or tissue of anus
Anal cryptotomy
Cauterization of lesion of anus

> Excludes: *biopsy of anus (49.23)*
> *control of (postoperative) hemorrhage of anus (49.95)*
> *hemorrhoidectomy (49.46)*

49.31 Endoscopic excision or destruction of lesion or tissue of anus

49.39 Other local excision or destruction of lesion or tissue of anus

> Excludes: *that by endoscopic approach (49.31)*

49.4 Procedures on hemorrhoids

49.41 Reduction of hemorrhoids

49.42 Injection of hemorrhoids

49.43 Cauterization of hemorrhoids
Clamp and cautery of hemorrhoids

49.44 Destruction of hemorrhoids by cryotherapy

49.45 Ligation of hemorrhoids

49.46 Excision of hemorrhoids
Hemorrhoidectomy NOS

49.47 Evacuation of thrombosed hemorrhoids

1839

▨ Valid O.R. procedure	▨ Non-O.R. procedure	▨ Nonspecific O.R. procedure	▨ Noncovered O.R. procedure

49.49 **Other procedures on hemorrhoids**
Lord procedure

49.5 **Division of anal sphincter**

49.51 **Left lateral anal sphincterotomy**

49.52 **Posterior anal sphincterotomy**

49.59 **Other anal sphincterotomy**
Division of sphincter NOS

49.6 **Excision of anus**

49.7 **Repair of anus**

Excludes: *repair of current obstetric laceration (75.62)*

49.71 **Suture of laceration of anus**

49.72 **Anal cerclage**

49.73 **Closure of anal fistula**

Excludes: *excision of anal fistula (49.12)*

49.74 **Gracilis muscle transplant for anal incontinence**

49.75 **Implantation or revision of artificial anal sphincter**
Removal with subsequent replacement
Replacement during same or subsequent operative episode

49.76 **Removal of artificial anal sphincter**
Explanation or removal without replacement

Excludes: *revision with implantation during same operative episode (49.75)*

49.79 **Other repair of anal sphincter**
Repair of old obstetric laceration of anus

Excludes: *anoplasty with synchronous*
hemorrhoidectomy (49.46)
repair of current obstetric laceration (75.62)

49.9 **Other operations on anus**

Excludes: *dilation of anus (sphincter) (96.23)*

49.91 **Incision of anal septum**

49.92 **Insertion of subcutaneous electrical anal stimulator**

49.93 **Other incision of anus**
Removal of:
foreign body from anus with incision
seton from anus

Excludes: *anal fistulotomy (49.11)*
removal of intraluminal foreign body without incision (98.05)

49.94 **Reduction of anal prolapse**

Excludes: *manual reduction of rectal prolapse (96.26)*

49.95 **Control of (postoperative) hemorrhage of anus**

49.99 **Other**

50 **Operations on liver**
Code also any application or administration of an adhesion barrier substance (99.77)

50.0 **Hepatotomy**
Incision of abscess of liver
Removal of gallstones from liver
Stromeyer-Little operation

50.1 **Diagnostic procedures on liver**

50.11 **Closed (percutaneous) [needle] biopsy of liver**
Diagnostic aspiration of liver

50.12 **Open biopsy of liver**
Wedge biopsy

50.13 **Transjugular liver biopsy**
Transvenous liver biopsy

Excludes: *closed (percutaneous) [needle] biopsy of liver (50.11)*
laparoscopic liver biopsy (50.14)

50.14 Laparoscopic liver biopsy

> Excludes: *closed (percutaneous) [needle] biopsy of liver (50.11)*
> *open biopsy of liver (50.12)*
> *transjugular liver biopsy (50.13)*

50.19 Other diagnostic procedures on liver

> Excludes: *laparoscopic liver biopsy (50.14)*
> *liver scan and radioisotope function study (92.02)*
> *microscopic examination of specimen from liver (91.01-91.09)*
> *transjugular liver biopsy (50.13)*

50.2 Local excision or destruction of liver tissue or lesion

50.21 Marsupialization of lesion of liver

50.22 Partial hepatectomy
Wedge resection of liver

> Excludes: *biopsy of liver, (50.11-50.12)*
> *hepatic lobectomy (50.3)*

50.23 Open ablation of liver lesion or tissue

50.24 Percutaneous ablation of liver lesion or tissue

50.25 Laparoscopic ablation of liver lesion or tissue

50.26 Other and unspecified ablation of liver lesion or tissue

50.29 Other destruction of lesion of liver
Cauterization of hepatic lesion
Enucleation of hepatic lesion
Evacuation of hepatic lesion

> Excludes: *ablation of liver lesion or tissue:*
> *laparoscopic (50.25)*
> *open (50.23)*
> *other (50.26)*
> *percutaneous (50.24)*
> *laser interstitial thermal therapy [LITT] of lesion or tissue of liver*
> *under guidance (17.63)*
> *percutaneous aspiration of lesion (50.91)*

50.3 Lobectomy of liver
Total hepatic lobectomy with partial excision of other lobe

50.4 Total hepatectomy

50.5 Liver transplant
Note: To report donor source—*see* codes 00.91-00.93

50.51 Auxiliary liver transplant
Auxiliary hepatic transplantation leaving patient's own liver in situ

50.59 Other transplant of liver

50.6 Repair of liver

50.61 Closure of laceration of liver

50.69 Other repair of liver
Hepatopexy

50.9 Other operations on liver

> Excludes: *lysis of adhesions (54.5)*

50.91 Percutaneous aspiration of liver

> Excludes: *percutaneous biopsy (50.11)*

50.92 Extracorporeal hepatic assistance
Liver dialysis

50.93 Localized perfusion of liver

50.94 Other injection of therapeutic substance into liver

50.99 Other

| Valid O.R. procedure | Non-O.R. procedure | Nonspecific O.R. procedure | Noncovered O.R. procedure |

51   Operations on gallbladder and biliary tract

Code also any application or administration of an adhesion barrier substance (99.77)

Includes: operations on:
ampulla of Vater
common bile duct
cystic duct
hepatic duct
intrahepatic bile duct
sphincter of Oddi

51.0   Cholecystotomy and cholecystostomy

51.01   Percutaneous aspiration of gallbladder
Percutaneous cholecystotomy for drainage
That by: needle or catheter

> Excludes: *needle biopsy (51.12)*

51.02   Trocar cholecystostomy

51.03   Other cholecystostomy

51.04   Other cholecystotomy
Cholelithotomy NOS

51.1   Diagnostic procedures on biliary tract

> Excludes: *that for endoscopic procedures classifiable to 51.64, 51.84-51.88, 52.14,*
> *52.21, 52.93-52.94, 52.97-52.98*

51.10   Endoscopic retrograde cholangiopancreatography [ERCP]

> Excludes: *endoscopic retrograde:*
> *cholangiography [ERC] (51.11)*
> *pancreatography [ERP] (52.13)*

51.11   Endoscopic retrograde cholangiography [ERC]
Laparoscopic exploration of common bile duct

> Excludes: *endoscopic retrograde:*
> *cholangiopancreatography [ERCP] (51.10)*
> *pancreatography [ERP] (52.13)*

51.12   Percutaneous biopsy of gallbladder or bile ducts
Needle biopsy of gallbladder

51.13   Open biopsy of gallbladder or bile ducts

51.14   Other closed [endoscopic] biopsy of biliary duct or sphincter of Oddi
Brushing or washing for specimen collection
Closed biopsy of biliary duct or sphincter of Oddi by procedures classifiable to
51.10-51.11, 52.13

51.15   Pressure measurement of sphincter of Oddi
Pressure measurement of sphincter by procedures classifiable to 51.10-51.11, 52.13

51.19   Other diagnostic procedures on biliary tract

> Excludes: *biliary tract x-ray (87.51-87.59)*
> *microscopic examination of specimen from biliary tract (91.01-91.09)*

51.2   Cholecystectomy

51.21   Other partial cholecystectomy
Revision of prior cholecystectomy

> Excludes: *that by laparoscope (51.24)*

51.22   Cholecystectomy

> Excludes: *laparoscopic cholecystectomy (51.23)*

51.23   Laparoscopic cholecystectomy
That by laser

51.24   Laparoscopic partial cholecystectomy

51.3   Anastomosis of gallbladder or bile duct

> Excludes: *resection with end-to-end anastomosis (51.61-51.69)*

51.31   Anastomosis of gallbladder to hepatic ducts

51.32   Anastomosis of gallbladder to intestine

51.33   Anastomosis of gallbladder to pancreas

51.34   Anastomosis of gallbladder to stomach

● Code new
to this edition

▲ Revision of
existing code

④ ⑤ Fourth or fifth
digit required

51.35 Other gallbladder anastomosis
Gallbladder anastomosis NOS

51.36 Choledochoenterostomy

51.37 Anastomosis of hepatic duct to gastrointestinal tract
Kasai portoenterostomy

51.39 Other bile duct anastomosis
Anastomosis of bile duct NOS
Anastomosis of unspecified bile duct to:
  intestine
  liver
  pancreas
  stomach

51.4 Incision of bile duct for relief of obstruction

51.41 Common duct exploration for removal of calculus
  Excludes: percutaneous extraction (51.96)

51.42 Common duct exploration for relief of other obstruction

51.43 Insertion of choledochohepatic tube for decompression
Hepatocholedochostomy

51.49 Incision of other bile ducts for relief of obstruction

51.5 Other incision of bile duct
  Excludes: that for relief of obstruction (51.41-51.49)

51.51 Exploration of common duct
Incision of common bile duct

51.59 Incision of other bile duct

51.6 Local excision or destruction of lesion or tissue of biliary ducts and sphincter of Oddi
Code also anastomosis other than end-to-end (51.31, 51.36-51.39)
  Excludes: biopsy of bile duct (51.12-51.13)

51.61 Excision of cystic duct remnant

51.62 Excision of ampulla of Vater (with reimplantation of common duct)

51.63 Other excision of common duct
Choledochectomy
  Excludes: fistulectomy (51.72)

51.64 Endoscopic excision or destruction of lesion of biliary ducts or sphincter of Oddi
Excision or destruction of lesion of biliary duct by procedures classifiable to
  51.10-51.11, 52.13

51.69 Excision of other bile duct
Excision of lesion of bile duct NOS
  Excludes: fistulectomy (51.79)

51.7 Repair of bile ducts

51.71 Simple suture of common bile duct

51.72 Choledochoplasty
Repair of fistula of common bile duct

51.79 Repair of other bile ducts
Closure of artificial opening of bile duct NOS
Suture of bile duct NOS
  Excludes: operative removal of prosthetic device (51.95)

51.8 Other operations on biliary ducts and sphincter of Oddi

51.81 Dilation of sphincter of Oddi
Dilation of ampulla of Vater
  Excludes: that by endoscopic approach (51.84)

51.82 Pancreatic sphincterotomy
Incision of pancreatic sphincter
Transduodenal ampullary sphincterotomy
  Excludes: that by endoscopic approach (51.85)

51.83 Pancreatic sphincteroplasty

51.84 Endoscopic dilation of ampulla and biliary duct
Dilation of ampulla and biliary duct by procedures classifiable to 51.10-51.11, 52.13

Valid O.R. procedure   Non-O.R. procedure   Nonspecific O.R. procedure   Noncovered O.R. procedure

51.85 **Endoscopic sphincterotomy and papillotomy**
Sphincterotomy and papillotomy by procedures classifiable to 51.10-51.11, 52.13

51.86 **Endoscopic insertion of nasobiliary drainage tube**
Insertion of nasobiliary tube by procedures classifiable to 51.10-51.11, 52.13

51.87 **Endoscopic insertion of stent (tube) into bile duct**
Endoprosthesis of bile duct
Insertion of stent into bile duct by procedures classifiable to 51.10-51.11, 52.13

> *Excludes:* *nasobiliary drainage tube (51.86)*
> *replacement of stent (tube) (97.05)*

51.88 **Endoscopic removal of stone(s) from biliary tract**
Laparoscopic removal of stone(s) from biliary tract
Removal of biliary tract stone(s) by procedures classifiable to 51.10-51.11, 52.13

> *Excludes:* *percutaneous extraction of common duct stones (51.96)*

51.89 **Other operations on sphincter of Oddi**

51.9 **Other operations on biliary tract**

51.91 **Repair of laceration of gallbladder**

51.92 **Closure of cholecystostomy**

51.93 **Closure of other biliary fistula**
Cholecystogastroenteric fistulectomy

51.94 **Revision of anastomosis of biliary tract**

51.95 **Removal of prosthetic device from bile duct**

> *Excludes:* *nonoperative removal (97.55)*

51.96 **Percutaneous extraction of common duct stones**

51.98 **Other percutaneous procedures on biliary tract**
Percutaneous biliary endoscopy via existing T-tube or other tract for:
dilation of biliary duct stricture
exploration (postoperative)
removal of stone(s) except common duct stone
Percutaneous transhepatic biliary drainage

> *Excludes:* *percutaneous aspiration of gallbladder (51.01)*
> *percutaneous biopsy and/or collection of specimen by brushing or*
>   *washing (51.12)*
> *percutaneous removal of common duct stone(s) (51.96)*

51.99 **Other**
Insertion or replacement of biliary tract prosthesis

> *Excludes:* *biopsy of gallbladder (51.12-51.13)*
> *irrigation of cholecystostomy and other biliary tube (96.41)*
> *lysis of peritoneal adhesions (54.5)*
> *nonoperative removal of:*
>   *cholecystostomy tube (97.54)*
>   *tube from biliary tract or liver (97.55)*

52 **Operations on pancreas**
Includes: operations on pancreatic duct
Code also any application or administration of an adhesion barrier substance (99.77)

52.0 **Pancreatotomy**

52.01 **Drainage of pancreatic cyst by catheter**

52.09 **Other pancreatotomy**
Pancreatolithotomy

> *Excludes:* *drainage by anastomosis (52.4, 52.96)*
> *incision of pancreatic sphincter (51.82)*
> *marsupialization of cyst (52.3)*

52.1 **Diagnostic procedures on pancreas**

52.11 **Closed [aspiration] [needle] [percutaneous] biopsy of pancreas**

52.12 **Open biopsy of pancreas**

52.13 **Endoscopic retrograde pancreatography [EPR]**

> *Excludes:* *endoscopic retrograde:*
> *cholangiography [ERC] (51.11)*
> *cholangiopancreatography [ERCP] (51.10)*
> *that for procedures classifiable to 51.14-51.15, 51.64, 51.84-51.88,*
>   *52.14, 52.21, 52.92-52.94, 52.97-52.98*

● Code new
to this edition
▲ Revision of
existing code
④ ⑤ Fourth or fifth
digit required

52.14 Closed [endoscopic] biopsy of pancreatic duct
Closed biopsy of pancreatic duct by procedures classifiable to 51.10-51.11, 52.13

52.19 Other diagnostic procedure on pancreas

> *Excludes:* *contrast pancreatogram (87.66)*
> *endoscopic retrograde pancreatography [ERP] (52.13))*
> *microscopic examination of specimen from pancreas (91.01-91.09)*

52.2 Local excision or destruction of pancreas and pancreatic duct

> *Excludes:* *biopsy of pancreas (52.11-52.12, 52.14)*
> *pancreatic fistulectomy (52.95)*

52.21 Endoscopic excision or destruction of lesion or tissue of pancreatic duct
Excision or destruction of lesion or tissue of pancreatic duct by procedures classifiable to 51.10-51.11, 52.13

52.22 Other excision or destruction of lesion or tissue of pancreas or pancreatic duct

52.3 Marsupialization of pancreatic cyst

> *Excludes:* *drainage of cyst by catheter (52.01)*

52.4 Internal drainage of pancreatic cyst
Pancreaticocystoduodenostomy
Pancreaticocystogastrostomy
Pancreaticocystojejunostomy

52.5 Partial pancreatectomy

> *Excludes:* *pancreatic fistulectomy (52.95)*

52.51 Proximal pancreatectomy
Excision of head of pancreas (with part of body)
Proximal pancreatectomy with synchronous duodenectomy

52.52 Distal pancreatectomy
Excision of tail of pancreas (with part of body)

52.53 Radical subtotal pancreatectomy

52.59 Other partial pancreatectomy

52.6 Total pancreatectomy
Pancreatectomy with synchronous duodenectomy

52.7 Radical pancreaticoduodenectomy
One-stage pancreaticoduodenal resection with choledochojejunal anastomosis, pancreaticojejunal anastomosis, and gastrojejunostomy
Two-stage pancreaticoduodenal resection (first stage) (second stage)
Radical resection of the pancreas
Whipple procedure

> *Excludes:* *radical subtotal pancreatectomy (52.53)*

52.8 Transplant of pancreas
Note: To report donor source—*see* codes 00.91-00.93

52.80 Pancreatic transplant, not otherwise specified

52.81 Reimplantation of pancreatic tissue

52.82 Homotransplant of pancreas

52.83 Heterotransplant of pancreas

52.84 Autotransplantation of cells of Islets of Langerhans
Homotransplantation of islet cells of pancreas

52.85 Allotransplantation of cells of Islets of Langerhans
Heterotransplantation of islet cells of pancreas

52.86 Transplantation of cells of Islets of Langerhans, not otherwise specified

52.9 Other operations on pancreas

52.92 Cannulation of pancreatic duct

> *Excludes:* *that by endoscopic approach (52.93)*

52.93 Endoscopic insertion of stent (tube) into pancreatic duct
Insertion of cannula or stent into pancreatic duct by procedures classifiable to 51.10-51.11, 52.13

> *Excludes:* *endoscopic insertion of nasopancreatic drainage tube (52.97)*
> *replacement of stent (tube) (97.05)*

52.94 Endoscopic removal of stone(s) from pancreatic duct
Removal of stone(s) from pancreatic duct by procedures classifiable to 51.10-51.11, 52.13

52.95 Other repair of pancreas
Fistulectomy of pancreas
Simple suture of pancreas

52.96 Anastomosis of pancreas
Anastomosis of pancreas (duct) to:
intestine
jejunum
stomach

Excludes: *anastomosis to:*
bile duct (51.39)
gallbladder (51.33)

52.97 Endoscopic insertion of nasopancreatic drainage tube
Insertion of nasopancreatic drainage tube by procedures classifiable to 51.10-51.11, 52.13

Excludes: *drainage of pancreatic cyst by catheter (52.01)*
replacement of stent (tube) (97.05)

52.98 Endoscopic dilation of pancreatic duct
Dilation of Wirsung's duct by procedures classifiable to 51.10-51.11,52.13

52.99 Other
Dilation of pancreatic [Wirsung's] duct by open approach
Repair of pancreatic [Wirsung's] duct by open approach

Excludes: *irrigation of pancreatic tube (96.42)*
removal of pancreatic tube (97.56)

53   Repair of hernia

Code also any application or administration of an adhesion barrier substance (99.77)
Includes: hernioplasty
herniorrhaphy
herniotomy

Excludes: *manual reduction of hernia (96.27)*

53.0   Other unilateral repair of inguinal hernia

Excludes: *laparoscopic unilateral repair of inguinal hernia (17.11-17.13)*

53.00 Unilateral repair of inguinal hernia, not otherwise specified
Inguinal herniorrhaphy NOS

53.01 Other and open repair of direct inguinal hernia
Direct and indirect inguinal hernia

53.02 Other and open repair of indirect inguinal hernia

53.03 Other and open repair of direct inguinal hernia with graft or prosthesis

53.04 Other and open repair of indirect inguinal hernia with graft or prosthesis

53.05 Repair of inguinal hernia with graft or prosthesis, not otherwise specified

53.1   Other bilateral repair of inguinal hernia

Excludes: *laparoscopic bilateral repair of inguinal hernia (17.21-17.24)*

53.10 Bilateral repair of inguinal hernia, not otherwise specified

53.11 Other and open bilateral repair of direct inguinal hernia

53.12 Other and open bilateral repair of indirect inguinal hernia

53.13 Other and open bilateral repair of inguinal hernia, one direct and one indirect

53.14 Other and open bilateral repair of direct inguinal hernia with graft or prosthesis

53.15 Other and open bilateral repair of indirect inguinal hernia with graft or prosthesis

53.16 Other and open bilateral repair of inguinal hernia, one direct and one indirect, with graft or prosthesis

53.17 Bilateral inguinal hernia repair with graft or prosthesis, not otherwise specified

53.2   Unilateral repair of femoral hernia

53.21 Unilateral repair of femoral hernia with graft or prosthesis

53.29 Other unilateral femoral herniorrhaphy

● Code new
to this edition
▲ Revision of
existing code
④ ⑤ Fourth or fifth
digit required

53.3   **Bilateral repair of femoral hernia**

   53.31   Bilateral repair of femoral hernia with graft or prosthesis

   53.39   Other bilateral femoral herniorrhaphy

53.4   **Repair of umbilical hernia**

   Excludes: repair of gastroschisis (54.71)

   53.41   Other and open repair of umbilical hernia with graft or prosthesis

   53.42   Laparoscopic repair of umbilical hernia with graft or prosthesis

   53.43   Other laparoscopic umbilical herniorrhaphy

   53.49   Other open umbilical herniorrhaphy

     Excludes: other laparoscopic umbilical herniorrhaphy (53.43)
                   repair of umbilical hernia with graft or prosthesis (53.41, 53.42)

53.5   **Repair of other hernia of anterior abdominal wall (without graft or prosthesis)**

   53.51   Incisional hernia repair

   53.59   Repair of other hernia of anterior abdominal wall
     Repair of hernia:
      epigastric
      hypogastric
      spigelian
      ventral
     That by laparoscopic approach

53.6   **Repair of other hernia of anterior abdominal wall with graft or prosthesis**

   53.61   Other open incisional hernia repair with graft or prosthesis

     Excludes: laparoscopic incisional hernia repair with graft or prosthesis (53.62)

   53.62   Laparoscopic incisional hernia repair with graft or prosthesis

   53.63   Other laparoscopic repair of other hernia of anterior abdominal wall with graft or prosthesis

   53.69   Other and open repair of other hernia of anterior abdominal wall with graft or prosthesis

     Excludes: other laparoscopic repair of other hernia of anterior abdominal wall with graft or prosthesis (53.63)

53.7   **Repair of diaphragmatic hernia, abdominal approach**

   53.71   Laparoscopic repair of diaphragmatic hernia, abdominal approach

   53.72   Other and open repair of diaphragmatic hernia, abdominal approach

   53.75   Repair of diaphragmatic hernia, abdominal approach, not otherwise specified

     Excludes: laparoscopic repair of diaphragmatic hernia (53.71)
                   other and open repair of diaphragmatic hernia (53.72)

53.8   **Repair of diaphragmatic hernia, thoracic approach**

   53.80   Repair of diaphragmatic hernia with thoracic approach, not otherwise specified
     Thoracoabdominal repair of diaphragmatic hernia

   53.81   Plication of the diaphragm

   53.82   Repair of parasternal hernia

   53.83   Laparoscopic repair of diaphragmatic hernia, with thoracic approach

   53.84   Other and open repair of diaphragmatic hernia, with thoracic approach

     Excludes: repair of diaphragmatic hernia with thoracic approach NOS (53.80)

53.9   **Other hernia repair**
   Repair of hernia:
     ischiatic   omental
     ischiorectal   retroperitoneal
     lumbar   sciatic
     obturator

     Excludes: relief of strangulated hernia with exteriorization of intestine (46.01, 46.03)
                   repair of pericolostomy hernia (46.42)
                   repair of vaginal enterocele (70.92)

Valid O.R. procedure   Non-O.R. procedure   Nonspecific O.R. procedure   Noncovered O.R. procedure

54   Other operations on abdominal region

Code also any application or administration of an adhesion barrier substance (99.77)

Includes: operations on:

epigastric region	mesentery
flank	omentum
groin region	pelvic cavity
hypochondrium	peritoneum
inguinal region	retroperitoneal tissue space
loin region	

Excludes: *hernia repair (53.00-53.9)*
obliteration of cul-de-sac (70.92)
retroperitoneal tissue dissection (59.00-59.09)
skin and subcutaneous tissue of abdominal wall (86.01-86.99)

54.0   Incision of abdominal wall

Drainage of:
abdominal wall
extraperitoneal abscess
retroperitoneal abscess

Excludes: *incision of peritoneum (54.95)*
laparotomy (54.11-54.19)

54.1   Laparotomy

54.11   Exploratory laparotomy

Excludes: *exploration incidental to intra-abdominal surgery—omit code*

54.12   Reopening of recent laparotomy site

Reopening of recent laparotomy site for:
control of hemorrhage
exploration
incision of hematoma

54.19   Other laparotomy

Drainage of intraperitoneal abscess or hematoma

Excludes: *culdocentesis (70.0)*
drainage of appendiceal abscess (47.2)
exploration incidental to intra-abdominal surgery—omit code
Ladd operation (54.95)
percutaneous drainage of abdomen (54.91)
removal of foreign body (54.92)

54.2   Diagnostic procedures of abdominal region

54.21   Laparoscopy

Peritoneoscopy

Excludes: *laparoscopic cholecystectomy (51.23)*
that incidental to destruction of fallopian tubes (66.21-66.29)

54.22   Biopsy or abdominal wall or umbilicus

54.23   Biopsy of peritoneum

Biopsy of:
mesentery
omentum
peritoneal implant

Excludes: *closed biopsy of:*
omentum (54.24)
peritoneum (54.24)

54.24   Closed [percutaneous] [needle] biopsy of intra-abdominal mass

Closed biopsy of:
omentum
peritoneal implant
peritoneum

Excludes: *that of:*
fallopian tube (66.11)
ovary (65.11)
uterine ligaments (68.15)
uterus (68.16)

54.25   Peritoneal lavage

Diagnostic peritoneal lavage

Excludes: *peritoneal dialysis (54.98)*

● Code new
to this edition

▲ Revision of
existing code

④ ⑤ Fourth or fifth
digit required

54.29 **Other diagnostic procedures on abdominal region**

> Excludes: *abdominal lymphangiogram (88.04)*
> *abdominal x-ray NEC (88.19)*
> *angiocardiography of venae cavae (88.51)*
> *C.A.T. scan of abdomen (88.01)*
> *contrast x-ray of abdominal cavity (88.11-88.15)*
> *intra-abdominal arteriography NEC (88.47)*
> *microscopic examination of peritoneal and retroperitoneal specimen*
> *   (91.11-91.19)*
> *phlebography of:*
> *   intra-abdominal vessels NEC (88.65)*
> *   portal venous system (88.64)*
> *sinogram of abdominal wall (88.03)*
> *soft tissue x-ray of abdominal wall NEC (88.09)*
> *tomography of abdomen NEC(88.02)*
> *ultrasonography of abdomen and retroperitoneum (88.76)*

54.3 **Excision or destruction of lesion or tissue of abdominal wall or umbilicus**
Debridement of abdominal wall
Omphalectomy

> Excludes: *biopsy of abdominal wall or umbilicus (54.22)*
> *size reduction operation (86.83)*
> *that of skin of abdominal wall (86.22, 86.26, 86.3)*

54.4 **Excision or destruction of peritoneal tissue**
Excision of:
    appendices epiploicae
    falciform ligament
    gastrocolic ligament
    lesion of:
        mesentery
        omentum
        peritoneum
    presacral lesion NOS
    retroperitoneal lesion NOS

> Excludes: *biopsy of peritoneum (54.23)*
> *endometrectomy of cul-de-sac (70.32)*

54.5 **Lysis of peritoneal adhesions**
Freeing of adhesions of:
    biliary tract
    intestines
    liver
    pelvic peritoneum
    peritoneum
    spleen
    uterus

> Excludes: *lysis of adhesions of:*
> *   bladder (59.11)*
> *   fallopian tube and ovary (65.81, 65.89)*
> *   kidney (59.02)*
> *   ureter (59.01-59.02)*

54.51 **Laparoscopic lysis of peritoneal adhesions**

54.59 **Other lysis of peritoneal adhesions**

54.6 **Suture of abdominal wall and peritoneum**

54.61 **Reclosure of postoperative disruption of abdominal wall**

54.62 **Delayed closure of granulating abdomen wound**
Tertiary subcutaneous wound closure

54.63 **Other suture of abdominal wall**
Suture of laceration of abdominal wall

> Excludes: *closure of operative wound—omit code*

54.64 **Suture of peritoneum**
Secondary suture of peritoneum

> Excludes: *closure of operative wound—omit code*

54.7 **Other repair of abdominal wall and peritoneum**

54.71 **Repair of gastroschisis**

| Valid O.R. procedure | Non-O.R. procedure | Nonspecific O.R. procedure | Noncovered O.R. procedure |

54.72 Other repair of abdominal wall

54.73 Other repair of peritoneum
Suture of gastrocolic ligament

54.74 Other repair of omentum
Epiplorrhaphy
Graft of omentum
Omentopexy
Reduction of torsion of omentum
> Excludes: cardio-omentopexy (36.39)

54.75 Other repair of mesentery
Mesenteric plication
Mesenteropexy

54.9 Other operations of abdominal region
> Excludes: removal of ectopic pregnancy (69.11, 74.3)

54.91 Percutaneous abdominal drainage
Paracentesis
> Excludes: creation of cutaneoperitoneal fistula (54.93)

54.92 Removal of foreign body from peritoneal cavity

54.93 Creation of cutaneoperitoneal fistula

54.94 Creation of peritoneovascular shunt
Peritoneovenous shunt

54.95 Incision of peritoneum
Exploration of ventriculoperitoneal shunt at peritoneal site
Ladd operation
Revision of distal catheter of ventricular shunt
Revision of ventriculoperitoneal shunt at peritoneal site
> Excludes: that incidental to laparotomy (54.11-54.19)

54.96 Injection of air into peritoneal cavity
Pneumoperitoneum
> Excludes: that for:
> collapse of lung (33.33)
> radiography (88.12-88.13, 88.15)

54.97 Injection of locally-acting therapeutic substance into peritoneal cavity
> Excludes: peritoneal dialysis (54.98)

54.98 Peritoneal dialysis
> Excludes: peritoneal lavage (diagnostic) (54.25)

54.99 Other
> Excludes: removal of:
> abdominal wall sutures (97.83)
> peritoneal drainage device (97.82)
> retroperitoneal drainage device (97.81)

10. OPERATIONS ON THE URINARY SYSTEM (55-59)

55 Operations on kidney

Code also any application or administration of an adhesion barrier substance (99.77)
Includes: operations on renal pelvis

> Excludes: *perirenal tissue (59.00-59.09, 59.21-59.29, 59.91-59.92)*

55.0 Nephrotomy and nephrostomy

> Excludes: *drainage by:*
> *anastomosis (55.86)*
> *aspiration (55.92)*
> *incision of kidney pelvis (55.11-55.12)*

55.01 Nephrotomy
Evacuation of renal cyst
Exploration of kidney
Nephrolithotomy

55.02 Nephrostomy

55.03 Percutaneous nephrostomy without fragmentation
Nephrostolithotomy, percutaneous (nephroscopic)
Percutaneous removal of kidney stone(s) by:
  basket extraction
  forceps extraction (nephroscopic)
Pyelostolithotomy, percutaneous (nephroscopic)
With placement of catheter down ureter

> Excludes: *percutaneous removal by fragmentation (55.04)*
> *repeat nephroscopic removal during current episode (55.92)*

55.04 Percutaneous nephrostomy with fragmentation
Percutaneous nephrostomy with disruption of kidney stone by ultrasonic energy and
  extraction (suction) through endoscope
With placement of catheter down ureter
With fluoroscopic guidance

> Excludes: *repeat fragmentation during current episode (59.95)*

55.1 Pyelotomy and pyelostomy

> Excludes: *drainage by anastomosis (55.86)*
> *percutaneous pyelostolithotomy (55.03)*
> *removal of calculus without incision (56.0)*

55.11 Pyelotomy
Exploration of renal pelvis
Pyelolithotomy

55.12 Pyelostomy
Insertion of drainage tube into renal pelvis

55.2 Diagnostic procedures on kidney

55.21 Nephroscopy

55.22 Pyeloscopy

55.23 Closed [percutaneous] [needle] biopsy of kidney
Endoscopic biopsy via existing nephrostomy, nephrotomy, pyelostomy, or
  pyelotomy

55.24 Open biopsy of kidney

55.29 Other diagnostic procedures on kidney

> Excludes: *microscopic examination of specimen from kidney (91.21-91.29)*
> *pyelogram:*
> *intravenous (87.73)*
> *percutaneous (87.75)*
> *retrograde (87.74)*
> *radioisotope scan (92.03)*
> *renal arteriography (88.45)*
> *tomography:*
> *C.A.T. scan (87.71)*
> *other (87.72)*

55.3 Local excision or destruction of lesion or tissue of kidney

55.31 Marsupialization of kidney lesion

55.32 Open ablation of renal lesion or tissue

55.33 Percutaneous ablation of renal lesion or tissue

| | Valid O.R. procedure | | Non-O.R. procedure | | Nonspecific O.R. procedure | | Noncovered O.R. procedure |

55.34 **Laparoscopic ablation of renal lesion or tissue**

55.35 **Other and unspecified ablation of renal lesion or tissue**

55.39 **Other local destruction or excision of renal lesion or tissue**
Obliteration of calyceal diverticulum

> Excludes: *ablation of renal lesion or tissue:*
> *laparoscopic (55.34)*
> *open (55.32)*
> *other (55.35)*
> *percutaneous (55.33)*
> *biopsy of kidney (55.23-55.24)*
> *partial nephrectomy (55.4)*
> *percutaneous aspiration of kidney (55.92)*
> *wedge resection of kidney (55.4)*

55.4 Partial nephrectomy
Calycectomy
Wedge resection of kidney

Code also any synchronous resection of ureter (56.40-56.42)

55.5 Complete nephrectomy
Code also any synchronous excision of:
adrenal gland (07.21-07.3)
bladder segment (57.6)
lymph nodes (40.3, 40.52-40.59)

55.51 **Nephroureterectomy**
Nephroureterectomy with bladder cuff
Total nephrectomy (unilateral)

> Excludes: *removal of transplanted kidney (55.53)*

55.52 **Nephrectomy of remaining kidney**
Removal of solitary kidney

> Excludes: *removal of transplanted kidney (55.53)*

55.53 **Removal of transplanted or rejected kidney**

55.54 **Bilateral nephrectomy**

> Excludes: *complete nephrectomy NOS (55.51)*

55.6 Transplant of kidney
Note: To report donor source—*see* codes 00.91-00.93

55.61 **Renal autotransplantation**

55.69 **Other kidney transplantation**

55.7 Nephropexy
Fixation or suspension of movable [floating] kidney

55.8 Other repair of kidney

55.81 **Suture of laceration of kidney**

55.82 **Closure of nephrostomy and pyelostomy**

55.83 **Closure of other fistula of kidney**

55.84 **Reduction of torsion of renal pedicle**

55.85 **Symphysiotomy for horseshoe kidney**

55.86 **Anastomosis of kidney**
Nephropyeloureterostomy
Pyeloureterovesical anastomosis
Ureterocalyceal anastomosis

> Excludes: *nephrocystanastomosis NOS (56.73)*

55.87 **Correction of ureteropelvic junction**

55.89 **Other**

55.9 Other operations on kidney

> Excludes: *lysis of perirenal adhesions (59.02)*

55.91 **Decapsulation of kidney**
Capsulectomy of kidney
Decortication of kidney

● Code new
to this edition

▲ Revision of
existing code

④ ⑤ Fourth or fifth
digit required

55.92 **Percutaneous aspiration of kidney (pelvis)**
Aspiration of renal cyst
Renipuncture
> Excludes: *percutaneous biopsy of kidney (55.23)*

55.93 **Replacement of nephrostomy tube**

55.94 **Replacement of pyelostomy tube**

55.95 **Local perfusion of kidney**

55.96 **Other Injection of therapeutic substance into kidney**
Injection into renal cyst

55.97 **Implantation or replacement of mechanical kidney**

55.98 **Removal of mechanical kidney**

55.99 **Other**
> Excludes: *removal of pyelostomy or nephrostomy tube (97.61)*

56 Operations on ureter
Code also any application or administration of an adhesion barrier substance (99.77)

56.0 **Transurethral removal of obstruction from ureter and renal pelvis**
Removal of:
    blood clot from ureter or renal pelvis without incision
    calculus from ureter or renal pelvis without incision
    foreign body from ureter or renal pelvis without incision
> Excludes: *manipulation without removal of obstruction (59.8)*
> *that by incision (55.11, 56.2)*
> *transurethral insertion of ureteral stent for passage of calculus (59.8)*

56.1 **Ureteral meatotomy**

56.2 **Ureterotomy**
Incision of ureter for:
    drainage
    exploration
    removal of calculus
> Excludes: *cutting of ureterovesical orifice (56.1)*
> *removal of calculus without incision (56.0)*
> *transurethral insertion of ureteral stent for passage of calculus (59.8)*
> *urinary diversion (56.51-56.79)*

56.3 **Diagnostic procedures on ureter**

56.31 **Ureteroscopy**

56.32 **Closed percutaneous biopsy of ureter**
> Excludes: *endoscopic biopsy of ureter (56.33)*

56.33 **Closed endoscopic biopsy of ureter**
Cystourethroscopy with ureteral biopsy
Transurethral biopsy of ureter
Ureteral endoscopy with biopsy through ureterotomy
Ureteroscopy with biopsy
> Excludes: *percutaneous biopsy of ureter (56.32)*

56.34 **Open biopsy of ureter**

56.35 **Endoscopy (cystoscopy) (looposcopy) of ileal conduit**

56.39 **Other diagnostic procedures on ureter**
> Excludes: *microscopic examination of specimen from ureter (91.21-91.29)*

56.4 **Ureterectomy**
Code also anastomosis other than end-to-end (56.51-56.79)
> Excludes: *fistulectomy (56.84)*
> *nephroureterectomy (55.51-55.54)*

56.40 **Ureterectomy, not otherwise specified**

56.41 **Partial ureterectomy**
Excision of lesion of ureter
Shortening of ureter with reimplantation
> Excludes: *biopsy of ureter (56.32-56.34)*

56.42 **Total ureterectomy**

	Valid O.R. procedure		Non-O.R. procedure		Nonspecific O.R. procedure		Noncovered O.R. procedure

56.5   **Cutaneous uretero-ileostomy**

     56.51   **Formation of cutaneous uretero-ileostomy**
          Construction of ileal conduit
          External ureteral ileostomy
          Formation of open ileal bladder
          Ileal loop operation
          Ileoureterostomy (Bricker's) (ileal bladder)
          Transplantation of ureter into ileum with external diversion

          | Excludes: | *closed ileal bladder (57.87)*
                         replacement of ureteral defect by ileal segment (56.89)

     56.52   **Revision of cutaneous uretero-ileostomy**

56.6   **Other external urinary diversion**

     56.61   **Formation of other cutaneous ureterostomy**
          Anastomosis of ureter to skin
          Ureterostomy NOS

     56.62   **Revision of other cutaneous ureterostomy**
          Revision of ureterostomy stoma

          | Excludes: | *nonoperative removal of ureterostomy tube (97.62)*

56.7   **Other anastomosis or bypass of ureter**

     | Excludes: | *ureteropyelostomy (55.86)*

     56.71   **Urinary diversion to intestine**
          Anastomosis of ureter to intestine
          Internal urinary diversion NOS
          Code also any synchronous colostomy (46.10-46.13)

          | Excludes: | *external ureteral ileostomy (56.51)*

     56.72   **Revision of ureterointestinal anastomosis**

          | Excludes: | *revision of external ureteral ileostomy (56.52)*

     56.73   **Nephrocystanastomosis, not otherwise specified**

     56.74   **Ureteroneocystostomy**
          Replacement of ureter with bladder flap
          Ureterovesical anastomosis

     56.75   **Transureteroureterostomy**

          | Excludes: | *ureteroureterostomy associated with partial resection (56.41)*

     56.79   **Other**

56.8   **Repair of ureter**

     56.81   **Lysis of intraluminal adhesions of ureter**

          | Excludes: | *lysis of periureteral adhesions (59.02-59.03)*
                         ureterolysis (59.02-59.03)

     56.82   **Suture of laceration of ureter**

     56.83   **Closure of ureterostomy**

     56.84   **Closure of other fistula of ureter**

     56.85   **Ureteropexy**

     56.86   **Removal of ligature from ureter**

     56.89   **Other repair of ureter**
          Graft of ureter
          Replacement of ureter with ileal segment implanted into bladder
          Ureteroplication

56.9   **Other operations on ureter**

     56.91   **Dilation of ureteral meatus**

     56.92   **Implantation of electronic ureteral stimulator**

     56.93   **Replacement of electronic ureteral stimulator**

     56.94   **Removal of electronic ureteral stimulator**

          | Excludes: | *that with synchronous replacement (56.93)*

     56.95   **Ligation of ureter**

   ● Code new
        to this edition
              ▲ Revision of
                 existing code
                    ④ ⑤ Fourth or fifth
                       digit required

56.99 Other

> *Excludes:* *removal of ureterostomy tube and ureteral catheter (97.62)*
> *ureteral catheterization (59.8)*

57 Operations on urinary bladder

Code also any application or administration of an adhesion barrier substance (99.77)

> *Excludes:* *perivesical tissue (59.11-59.29, 59.91-59.92)*
> *ureterovesical orifice (56.0-56.99)*

57.0 Transurethral clearance of bladder

Drainage of bladder without incision
Removal of:
    blood clots from bladder without incision
    calculus from bladder without incision
    foreign body from bladder without incision

> *Excludes:* *that by incision (57.19)*

57.1 Cystotomy and cystostomy

> *Excludes:* *cystotomy and cystostomy as operative approach—omit code*

57.11 Percutaneous aspiration of bladder

57.12 Lysis of intraluminal adhesion with incision into bladder

> *Excludes:* *transurethral lysis of intraluminal adhesions (57.41)*

57.17 Percutaneous cystostomy

Closed cystostomy
Percutaneous suprapubic cystostomy

> *Excludes:* *removal of cystostomy tube (97.63)*
> *replacement of cystostomy tube (59.94)*

57.18 Other suprapubic cystostomy

> *Excludes* *percutaneous cystostomy (57.17)*
> *removal of cystostomy tube (97.63)*
> *replacement of cystostomy tube (59.94)*

57.19 Other cystotomy

Cystolithotomy

> *Excludes:* *percutaneous cystostomy (57.17)*
> *suprapubic cystostomy (57.18)*

57.2 Vesicostomy

> *Excludes:* *percutaneous cystostomy (57.17)*
> *suprapubic cystostomy (57.18)*

57.21 Vesicostomy

Creation of permanent opening from bladder to skin using a bladder flap

57.22 Revision or closure of vesicostomy

> *Excludes:* *closure of cystostomy (57.82)*

57.3 Diagnostic procedures on bladder

57.31 Cystoscopy through artificial stoma

57.32 Other cystoscopy

Transurethral cystoscopy

> *Excludes:* *cystourethroscopy with ureteral biopsy (56.33)*
> *retrograde pyelogram (87.74)*
> *that for control of hemorrhage (postoperative):*
>   *bladder (57.93)*
>   *prostate (60.94)*

57.33 Closed [transurethral] biopsy of bladder

57.34 Open biopsy of bladder

57.39 Other diagnostic procedures on bladder

> *Excludes:* *cystogram NEC (87.77)*
> *microscopic examination of specimen from bladder (91.31-91.39)*
> *retrograde cystourethrogram (87.76)*
> *therapeutic distention of bladder (96.25)*

57.4 Transurethral excision or destruction of bladder tissue

57.41 Transurethral lysis of intraluminal adhesions

Valid O.R. procedure	Non-O.R. procedure	Nonspecific O.R. procedure	Noncovered O.R. procedure

57.49 **Other transurethral excision or destruction of lesion or tissue of bladder**
Endoscopic resection of bladder lesion

Excludes: *transurethral biopsy of bladder (57.33)*
transurethral fistulectomy (57.83-57.84)

57.5 **Other excision or destruction of bladder tissue**

Excludes: *that with transurethral approach (57.41-57.49)*

57.51 **Excision of urachus**
Excision of urachal sinus of bladder

Excludes: *excision of urachal cyst of abdominal wall (54.3)*

57.59 **Open excision or destruction of other lesion or tissue of bladder**
Endometrectomy of bladder
Suprapubic excision of bladder lesion

Excludes: *biopsy of bladder (57.33-57.34)*
fistulectomy of bladder (57.83-57.84)

57.6 **Partial cystectomy**
Excision of bladder dome
Trigonectomy
Wedge resection of bladder

57.7 **Total cystectomy**
Includes: total cystectomy with urethrectomy

57.71 **Radical cystectomy**
Pelvic exenteration in male
Removal of bladder, prostate, seminal vesicles, and fat
Removal of bladder, urethra, and fat in a female

Code also any:
lymph node dissection (40.3, 40.5)
urinary diversion (56.51-56.79)

Excludes: *that as part of pelvic exenteration in female (68.8)*

57.79 **Other total cystectomy**

57.8 **Other repair of urinary bladder**

Excludes: *repair of:*
current obstetric laceration (75.61)
cystocele (70.50-70.51)
that for stress incontinence (59.3-59.79)

57.81 **Suture of laceration of bladder**

57.82 **Closure of cystostomy**

57.83 **Repair of fistula involving bladder and intestine**
Rectovesicovaginal fistulectomy
Vesicosigmoidovaginal fistulectomy

57.84 **Repair of other fistula of bladder**
Cervicovesical fistulectomy
Urethroperineovesical fistulectomy
Uterovesical fistulectomy
Vaginovesical fistulectomy

Excludes: *vesicoureterovaginal fistulectomy (56.84)*

57.85 **Cystourethroplasty and plastic repair of bladder neck**
Plication of sphincter of urinary bladder
V-Y plasty of bladder neck

57.86 **Repair of bladder exstrophy**

57.87 **Reconstruction of urinary bladder**
Anastomosis of bladder with isolated segment of ileum
Augmentation of bladder
Replacement of bladder with ileum or sigmoid [closed ileal bladder]

Code also resection of intestine (45.50-45.52)

57.88 **Other anastomosis of bladder**
Anastomosis of bladder to intestine NOS
Cystocolic anastomosis

Excludes: *formation of closed ileal bladder (5787)*

● Code new
to this edition

▲ Revision of
existing code

④ ⑤ Fourth or fifth
digit required

57.89 Other repair of bladder
Bladder suspension, not elsewhere classified
Cystopexy NOS
Repair of old obstetric laceration of bladder

> Excludes: *repair of current obstetric laceration (75.61)*

57.9 Other operations on bladder

57.91 Sphincterotomy of bladder
Division of bladder neck

57.92 Dilation of bladder neck

57.93 Control of (postoperative) hemorrhage of bladder

57.94 Insertion of indwelling urinary catheter

57.95 Replacement of indwelling urinary catheter

57.96 Implantation of electronic bladder stimulator

57.97 Replacement of electronic bladder stimulator

57.98 Removal of electronic bladder stimulator

> Excludes: *that with synchronous replacement (57.97)*

57.99 Other

> Excludes: *irrigation of:*
> *cystostomy (96.47)*
> *other indwelling urinary catheter (96.48)*
> *lysis of external adhesions (59.11)*
> *removal of:*
> *cystostomy tube (97.63)*
> *other urinary drainage device (97.64)*
> *therapeutic distention of bladder (96.25)*

58 Operations on urethra
Code also any application or administration of an adhesion barrier substance (99.77)
Includes: operations on:
bulbourethral gland [Cowper's gland]
periurethral tissue

58.0 Urethrotomy
Excision of urethral septum
Formation of urethrovaginal fistula
Perineal urethrostomy
Removal of calculus from urethra by incision

> Excludes: *drainage of bulbourethral gland or periurethral tissue (58.91)*
> *internal urethral meatotomy (58.5)*
> *removal of urethral calculus without incision (58.6)*

58.1 Urethral meatotomy

> Excludes: *internal urethral meatotomy (58.5)*

58.2 Diagnostic procedures on urethra

58.21 Perineal urethroscopy

58.22 Other urethroscopy

58.23 Biopsy of urethra

58.24 Biopsy of periurethral tissue

58.29 Other diagnostic procedures on urethra and periurethral tissue

> Excludes: *microscopic examination of specimen from urethra (91.31-91.39)*
> *retrograde cystourethrogram (87.76)*
> *urethral pressure profile (89.25)*
> *urethral sphincter electromyogram (89.23)*

58.3 Excision or destruction of lesion or tissue of urethra

> Excludes: *biopsy of urethra (58.23)*
> *excision of bulbourethral gland (58.92)*
> *fistulectomy (58.43)*
> *urethrectomy as part of:*
> *complete cystectomy (57.79)*
> *pelvic evisceration (68.8)*
> *radical cystectomy (57.71)*

58.31 Endoscopic excision or destruction of lesion or tissue of urethra
Fulguration of urethral lesion

| | Valid O.R. procedure | | Non-O.R. procedure | | Nonspecific O.R. procedure | | Noncovered O.R. procedure |

58.39 **Other local excision or destruction of lesion or tissue of urethra**
Excision of:
congenital valve of urethra
lesion of urethra
stricture of urethra
Urethrectomy

Excludes: *that by endoscopic approach (58.31)*

58.4 **Repair of urethra**

Excludes: *repair of current obstetric laceration (75.61)*

58.41 **Suture of laceration of urethra**

58.42 **Closure of urethrostomy**

58.43 **Closure of other fistula of urethra**

Excludes: *repair of urethroperineovesical fistula (57.84)*

58.44 **Reanastomosis of urethra**
Anastomosis of urethra

58.45 **Repair of hypospadias or epispadias**

58.46 **Other reconstruction of urethra**
Urethral construction

58.47 **Urethral meatoplasty**

58.49 **Other repair of urethra**
Benenenti rotation of bulbous urethra
Repair of old obstetric laceration of urethra
Urethral plication

Excludes: *repair of:*
current obstetric laceration (75.61)
urethrocele (70.50-70.51)

58.5 **Release of urethral stricture**
Cutting of urethra] sphincter
Internal urethral meatotomy
Urethrolysis

58.6 **Dilation of urethra**
Dilation of urethrovesical junction
Passage of sounds through urethra
Removal of calculus from urethra without incision

Excludes: *urethral calibration (89.29)*

58.9 **Other operations on urethra and periurethral tissue**

58.91 **Incision of periurethral tissue**
Drainage of bulbourethral gland

58.92 **Excision of periurethral tissue**

Excludes: *biopsy of periurethral tissue (58.24)*
lysis of periurethral adhesions (59.11-59.12)

58.93 **Implantation of artificial urinary sphincter [AUS]**
Placement of inflatable:
bladder sphincter
urethral sphincter
Removal with replacement of sphincter device [AUS]
With pump and/or reservoir

58.99 **Other**
Removal of inflatable urinary sphincter without replacement
Repair of inflatable sphincter pump and/or reservoir
Surgical correction of hydraulic pressure of inflatable sphincter device

Excludes: *removal of:*
intraluminal foreign body from urethra without incision (98.19)
urethral stent (97.65)

59 **Other operations on urinary tract**
Code also any application or administration of an adhesion barrier substance (99.77)

59.0 **Dissection of retroperitoneal tissue**

59.00 **Retroperitoneal dissection, not otherwise specified**

● Code new
to this edition
▲ Revision of
existing code
④ ⑤ Fourth or fifth
digit required

59.02 **Other lysis of perirenal or periureteral adhesions**

> Excludes: *that by laparoscope (59.03)*

59.03 **Laparoscopic lysis of perirenal or periureteral adhesions**

59.09 **Other incision of perirenal or periureteral tissue**
Exploration of perinephric area
Incision of perirenal abscess

59.1 **Incision of perivesical tissue**

59.11 **Other lysis of perivesical adhesions**

59.12 **Laparoscopic lysis of perivesical adhesions**

59.19 **Other incision of perivesical tissue**
Exploration of perivesical tissue
Incision of hematoma of space of Retzius
Retropubic exploration

59.2 **Diagnostic procedures on perirenal and perivesical tissue**

59.21 **Biopsy of perirenal or perivesical tissue**

59.29 **Other diagnostic procedures on perirenal tissue, perivesical tissue, and
retroperitoneum**

> Excludes: *microscopic examination of specimen from:*
> *perirenal tissue (91.21-91.29)*
> *perivesical tissue (91.31-91.39)*
> *retroperitoneum NEC (91.11-91.19)*
> *retroperitoneal x-ray (88.14-88.16)*

59.3 **Plication of urethrovesical junction**
Kelly-Kennedy operation on urethra
Kelly-Stoeckel urethral plication

59.4 **Suprapubic sling operation**
Goebel-Frangenheim-Stoeckel urethrovesical suspension
Millin-Read urethrovesical suspension
Oxford operation for urinary incontinence
Urethrocystopexy by suprapubic suspension

59.5 **Retropubic urethral suspension**
Burch procedure
Marshall-Marchetti-Krantz operation
Suture of periurethral tissue to symphysis pubis
Urethral suspension NOS

59.6 **Paraurethral suspension**
Pereyra paraurethral suspension
Periurethral suspension

59.7 **Other repair of urinary stress incontinence**

59.71 **Levator muscle operation for urethrovesical suspension**
Cystourethropexy with levator muscle sling
Gracilis muscle transplant for urethrovesical suspension
Pubococcygeal sling

59.72 **Injection of implant into urethra and/or bladder neck**
Collagen implant
Endoscopic injection of implant
Fat implant
Polytef implant

59.79 **Other**
Anterior urethropexy
Augmentation urethroplasty
Repair of stress incontinence NOS
Tudor "rabbit ear" urethropexy

59.8 **Ureteral catheterization**
Drainage of kidney by catheter
Insertion of ureteral stent
Ureterovesical orifice dilation

> *Code also any synchronous ureterotomy (56.2)*

> Excludes: *that for:*
> *retrograde pyelogram (87.74)*
> *transurethral removal of calculus or clot from ureter and renal pelvis (56.0)*

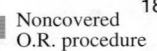

| | Valid O.R. procedure | | Non-O.R. procedure | | Nonspecific O.R. procedure | | Noncovered O.R. procedure |

59.9 **Other operations on urinary system**

> Excludes: *nonoperative removal of therapeutic device (97.61-97.69)*

59.91 **Excision of perirenal or perivesical tissue**

> Excludes: *biopsy of perirenal or perivesical tissue (59.21)*

59.92 **Other operations on perirenal or perivesical tissue**

59.93 **Replacement of ureterostomy tube**
Change of ureterostomy tube
Reinsertion of ureterostomy tube

> Excludes: *nonoperative removal of ureterostomy tube (97.62)*

59.94 **Replacement of cystostomy tube**

> Excludes: *nonoperative removal of cystostomy tube (97.63)*

59.95 **Ultrasonic fragmentation of urinary stones**
Shattered urinary stones

> Excludes: *percutaneous nephrostomy with fragmentation (55.04)*
> *shockwave disintegration (98.51)*

59.99 **Other**

> Excludes: *instillation of medication into urinary tract (96.49)*
> *irrigation of urinary tract (96.45-96.48)*

● Code new
to this edition

▲ Revision of
existing code

④ ⑤ Fourth or fifth
digit required

11. OPERATIONS ON THE MALE GENITAL ORGANS (60-64)

60 Operations on prostate and seminal vesicles
Code also any application or administration of an adhesion barrier substance (99.77)
Includes: operations on periprostatic tissue

> *Excludes:* *that associated with radical cystectomy (57.71)*

60.0 Incision of prostate
Drainage of prostatic abscess
Prostatolithotomy

> *Excludes:* *drainage of periprostatic tissue only (60.81)*

60.1 Diagnostic procedures on prostate and seminal vesicles

60.11 Closed [percutaneous] [needle] biopsy of prostate
Approach:
 transrectal
 transurethral
Punch biopsy

60.12 Open biopsy of prostate

60.13 Closed [percutaneous] biopsy of seminal vesicles
Needle biopsy of seminal vesicles

60.14 Open biopsy of seminal vesicles

60.15 Biopsy of periprostatic tissue

60.18 Other diagnostic procedures on prostate and periprostatic tissue

> *Excludes:* *microscopic examination of specimen from prostate (91.31-91.39)*
> *x-ray of prostate (87.92)*

60.19 Other diagnostic procedures on seminal vesicles

> *Excludes:* *microscopic examination of specimen from seminal vesicles (91.31-91.39)*
> *x-ray:*
> *contrast seminal vesiculogram (87.91)*
> *other (87.92)*

60.2 Transurethral prostatectomy

> *Excludes:* *local excision of lesion of prostate (60.61)*

60.21 Transurethral (ultrasound) guided laser induced prostatectomy (TULIP)
Ablation (contact) (noncontact) by laser

60.29 Other transurethral prostatectomy
Excision of median bar by transurethral approach
Transurethral electrovaporization of prostate (TEVAP)
Transurethral enucleative procedure
Transurethral prostatectomy NOS
Transurethral resection of prostate (TURP)

60.3 Suprapubic prostatectomy
Transvesical prostatectomy

> *Excludes:* *local excision of lesion of prostate (60.61)*
> *radical prostatectomy (60.5)*

60.4 Retropubic prostatectomy

> *Excludes:* *local excision of lesion of prostate (60.61)*
> *radical prostatectomy (60.5)*

60.5 Radical prostatectomy
Prostatovesiculectomy
Radical prostatectomy by any approach

> *Excludes:* *cystoprostatectomy (57.71)*

60.6 Other prostatectomy

60.61 Local excision of lesion of prostate

> *Excludes:* *biopsy of prostate (60.11-60 12)*
> *laser interstitial thermal therapy [LITT] of lesion or tissue of prostate under guidance (17.69)*

| Valid O.R. procedure | Non-O.R. procedure | Nonspecific O.R. procedure | Noncovered O.R. procedure |

60.62 **Perineal prostatectomy**
Cryoablation of prostate
Cryoprostatectomy
Cryosurgery of prostate
Radical cryosurgical ablation of prostate (RCSA)

> *Excludes:* *local excision of lesion of prostate (60.61)*

60.69 **Other**

60.7 **Operations on seminal vesicles**

60.71 **Percutaneous aspiration of seminal vesicle**

> *Excludes:* *needle biopsy of seminal vesicle (60.13)*

60.72 **Incision of seminal vesicle**

60.73 **Excision of seminal vesicle**
Excision of Mullerian duct cyst
Spermatocystectomy

> *Excludes:* *biopsy of seminal vesicle (60.13-60.14)*
> *prostatovesiculectomy (60.5)*

60.79 **Other operations on seminal vesicles**

60.8 **Incision or excision of periprostatic tissue**

60.81 **Incision of periprostatic tissue**
Drainage of periprostatic abscess

60.82 **Excision of periprostatic tissue**
Excision of lesion of periprostatic tissue

> *Excludes:* *biopsy of periprostatic tissue (60.15)*

60.9 **Other operations on prostate**

60.91 **Percutaneous aspiration of prostate**

> *Excludes:* *needle biopsy of prostate (60.11)*

60.92 **Injection into prostate**

60.93 **Repair of prostate**

60.94 **Control of (postoperative) hemorrhage of prostate**
Coagulation of prostatic bed
Cystoscopy for control of prostate hemorrhage

60.95 **Transurethral balloon dilation of the prostatic urethra**

60.96 **Transurethral destruction of prostate tissue by microwave thermotherapy**
Transurethral microwave thermotherapy (TUMT) of prostate

> *Excludes:* *Prostatectomy:*
> *other (60.61-60.69)*
> *radical (60.5)*
> *retropubic (60.4)*
> *suprapubic (60.3)*
> *transurethral (60.21-60.29)*

60.97 **Other transurethral destruction of prostate tissue by other thermotherapy**
Radiofrequency thermotherapy
Transurethral needle ablation (TUNA) of prostate

> *Excludes:* *Prostatectomy:*
> *other (60.61-60.69)*
> *radical (60.5)*
> *retropubic (60.4)*
> *suprapubic (60.3)*
> *transurethral (60.21-60.29)*

60.99 **Other**

> *Excludes:* *prostatic massage (99.94)*

61 **Operations on scrotum and tunica vaginalis**

61.0 **Incision and drainage of scrotum and tunica vaginalis**

> *Excludes:* *percutaneous aspiration of hydrocele (61.91)*

61.1 **Diagnostic procedures on scrotum and tunica vaginalis**

61.11 **Biopsy of scrotum or tunica vaginalis**

61.19 **Other diagnostic procedures on scrotum and tunica vaginalis**

● Code new to this edition   ▲ Revision of existing code   ④ ⑤ Fourth or fifth digit required

61.2 **Excision of hydrocele (of tunica vaginalis)**
Bottle repair of hydrocele of tunica vaginalis

Excludes: *percutaneous aspiration of hydrocele (61.91)*

61.3 **Excision or destruction of lesion or tissue of scrotum**
Fulguration of lesion of scrotum
Reduction of elephantiasis of scrotum
Partial scrotectomy of scrotum

Excludes: *biopsy of scrotum (61.11)*
scrotal fistulectomy (61.42)

61.4 **Repair of scrotum and tunica vaginalis**

61.41 **Suture of laceration of scrotum and tunica vaginalis**

61.42 **Repair of scrotal fistula**

61.49 **Other repair of scrotum and tunica vaginalis**
Reconstruction with rotational or pedicle flaps

61.9 **Other operations on scrotum and tunica vaginalis**

61.91 **Percutaneous aspiration of tunics vaginalis**
Aspiration of hydrocele of tunica vaginalis

61.92 **Excision of lesion of tunica vaginalis other than hydrocele**
Excision of hematocele of tunica vaginalis

61.99 **Other**

Excludes: *removal of foreign body from scrotum without incision (98.24)*

62 **Operations on testes**

62.0 **Incision of testis**

62.1 **Diagnostic procedures on testes**

62.11 **Closed [percutaneous] [needle] biopsy of testis**

62.12 **Open biopsy or testis**

62.19 **Other diagnostic procedures on testes**

62.2 **Excision or destruction of testicular lesion**
Excision of appendix testis
Excision of cyst of Morgagni in the male

Excludes: *biopsy of testis (62.11-62.12)*

62.3 **Unilateral orchiectomy**
Orchidectomy (with epididymectomy) NOS

62.4 **Bilateral orchiectomy**
Male castration
Radical bilateral orchiectomy (with epididymectomy)
Code also any synchronous lymph node dissection (40.3, 40.5)

62.41 **Removal of both testes at same operative episode**
Bilateral orchidectomy NOS

62.42 **Removal of remaining testis**
Removal of solitary testis

62.5 **Orchiopexy**
Mobilization and replacement of testis in scrotum
Orchiopexy with detorsion of testis
Torek (-Bevan) operation (orchidopexy) (first stage) (second stage)
Transplantation to and fixation of testis in scrotum

62.6 **Repair of testes**

Excludes: *reduction of torsion (63.52)*

62.61 **Suture of laceration of testis**

62.69 **Other repair of testis**
Testicular graft

62.7 **Insertion of testicular prosthesis**

62.9 **Other operations on testis**

62.91 **Aspiration of testis**

Excludes: *percutaneous biopsy of testis (62.11)*

62.92 **Injection of therapeutic substance into testis**

62.99 **Other**

| Valid O.R. procedure | Non-O.R. procedure | Nonspecific O.R. procedure | Noncovered O.R. procedure |

63   Operations on spermatic cord, epididymis, and vas deferens

    63.0   Diagnostic procedures on spermatic cord, epididymis and vas deferens

        63.01   Biopsy of spermatic cord, epididymis, or vas deferens

        63.09   Other diagnostic procedures on spermatic cord, epididymis, and vas deferens

            | Excludes: | *contrast epididymogram (87.93)* |
            contrast vasogram (87.94)
            other x-ray of epididymis and vas deferens (87.95)

    63.1   Excision of varicocele and hydrocele of spermatic cord
        High ligation of spermatic vein
        Hydrocelectomy of canal of Nuck

    63.2   Excision of cyst of epididymis
        Spermatocelectomy

    63.3   Excision of other lesion or tissue of spermatic cord and epididymis
        Excision of appendix epididymis

        | Excludes: | *biopsy of spermatic cord or epididymis (63.01)* |

    63.4   Epididymectomy

        | Excludes: | *that synchronous with orchiectomy (62.3-62.42)* |

    63.5   Repair of spermatic cord and epididymis

        63.51   Suture of laceration of spermatic cord and epididymis

        63.52   Reduction of torsion of testis or spermatic cord

            | Excludes: | *that associated with orchiopexy (62.5)* |

        63.53   Transplantation of spermatic cord

        63.59   Other repair of spermatic cord and epididymis

    63.6   Vasotomy
        Vasostomy

    63.7   Vasectomy and ligation of vas deferens

        63.70   Male sterilization procedure not otherwise specified

        63.71   Ligation of vas deferens
            Crushing of vas deferens
            Division of vas deferens

        63.72   Ligation of spermatic cord

        63.73   Vasectomy

    63.8   Repair of vas deferens and epididymis

        63.81   Suture of laceration of vas deferens and epididymis

        63.82   Reconstruction of surgically divided vas deferens

        63.83   Epididymovasostomy

        63.84   Removal of ligature from vas deferens

        63.85   Removal of valve from vas deferens

        63.89   Other repair of vas deferens and epididymis

    63.9   Other operations on spermatic cord, epididymis and vas deferens

        63.91   Aspiration of spermatocele

        63.92   Epididymotomy

        63.93   Incision of spermatic cord

        63.94   Lysis of adhesions of spermatic cord

        63.95   Insertion of valve in vas deferens

        63.99   Other

64   Operations on penis
    Includes: operations on:
            corpora cavernosa
            glans penis
            prepuce

    64.0   Circumcision

    64.1   Diagnostic procedures on the penis

        64.11   Biopsy of penis

        64.19   Other diagnostic procedures on penis

    ● Code new
      to this edition   ▲ Revision of
         existing code   ④ ⑤ Fourth or fifth
         digit required

64.2   **Local excision or destruction of lesion of penis**

     Excludes: *biopsy of penis (64.11)*

64.3   **Amputation of penis**

64.4   **Repair and plastic operation on penis**

     64.41   **Suture of laceration of penis**

     64.42   **Release of chordee**

     64.43   **Construction of penis**

     64.44   **Reconstruction of penis**

     64.45   **Replantation of penis**
          Reattachment of amputated penis

     64.49   **Other repair of penis**

          Excludes: *repair of epispadias and hypospadias (58.45)*

64.5   **Operations for sex transformation, not otherwise classified.**

64.9   **Other operations on male genital organs**

     64.91   **Dorsal or lateral slit of prepuce**

     64.92   **Incision of penis**

     64.93   **Division of penile adhesions**

     64.94   **Fitting of external prosthesis of penis**
          Penile prosthesis NOS

     64.95   **insertion or replacement of non-inflatable penile prosthesis**
          Insertion of semi-rigid rod prosthesis into shaft of penis

          Excludes: *external penile prosthesis (64.94)*
                 inflatable penile prosthesis (64.97)
                 plastic repair, penis (64.43-64.49)
                 that associated with:
                     construction (64.43)
                     reconstruction (64.44)

     64.96   **Removal of internal prosthesis of penis**
          Removal without replacement of non-inflatable or inflatable penile prosthesis

     64.97   **Insertion or replacement or inflatable penile prosthesis**
          Insertion of cylinders into shaft of penis and placement of pump and reservoir

          Excludes: *external penile prosthesis (64.94)*
                 non-inflatable penile prosthesis (64.95)
                 plastic repair, penis (64.43-64.49)

     64.98   **Other operations on penis**
          Corpora cavernosa-corpus spongiosum shunt
          Corpora-saphenous shunt
          Irrigation of corpus cavernosum

          Excludes: *removal of foreign body:*
                 intraluminal (98.19)
                 without incision (98.24)
                 stretching of foreskin (99.95)

     64.99   **Other**

          Excludes: *collection of sperm for artificial insemination (99.96)*

| Valid O.R. procedure | Non-O.R. procedure | Nonspecific O.R. procedure | Noncovered O.R. procedure |

This page intentionally left blank.

12. OPERATIONS ON THE FEMALE GENITAL ORGANS (65-71)

65 Operations on ovary

Code also any application or administration of an adhesion barrier substance (99.77)

65.0 Oophorotomy
Salpingo-oophorotomy

65.01 Laparoscopic oophorotomy

65.09 Other oophorotomy

65.1 Diagnostic procedures on ovaries

65.11 Aspiration biopsy of ovary

65.12 Other biopsy of ovary

65.13 Laparoscopic biopsy of ovary

65.14 Other laparoscopic diagnostic procedures on ovaries

65.19 Other diagnostic procedure on ovaries

> Excludes: *microscopic examination of specimen from ovary (91.41-91-49)*

65.2 Local excision or destruction of ovarian lesion or tissue

65.21 Marsupialization of ovarian cyst

> Excludes: *that by laparoscope (65.23)*

65.22 Wedge resection of ovary

> Excludes: *that by laparoscope (65.24)*

65.23 Laparoscopic marsupialization of ovarian cyst

65.24 Laparoscopic wedge resection of ovary

65.25 Other laparoscopic local excision or destruction of ovary

65.29 Other local excision or destruction of ovary
Bisection of ovary
Cauterization of ovary
Partial excision of ovary

> Excludes: *biopsy of ovary (65.11-65.13)*
> *that by laparoscope (65.25)*

65.3 Unilateral oophorectomy

65.31 Laparoscopic unilateral oophorectomy

65.39 Other unilateral oophorectomy

> Excludes: *that by laparoscope (65.31)*

65.4 Unilateral salpingo-oophorectomy

65.41 Laparoscopic unilateral salpingo-oophorectomy

65.49 Other unilateral salpingo-oophorectomy

65.5 Bilateral oophorectomy

65.51 Other removal of both ovaries at same operative episode
Female castration

> Excludes: *that by laparoscope (65.53)*

65.52 Other removal of remaining ovary
Removal of solitary ovary

> Excludes: *that by laparoscope (65.54)*

65.53 Laparoscopic removal of both ovaries at same operative episode

65.54 Laparoscopic removal of remaining ovary

65.6 Bilateral salpingo-oophorectomy

65.61 Other removal of both ovaries and tubes at same operative episode

> Excludes: *that by laparoscope (65.63)*

65.62 Other removal of remaining ovary and tube
Removal of solitary ovary and tube

> Excludes: *that by laparoscope (65.64)*

65.63 Laparoscopic removal of both ovaries and tubes at same operative episode

65.64 Laparoscopic removal of remaining ovary and tube

| | Valid O.R. procedure | | Non-O.R. procedure | | Nonspecific O.R. procedure | | Noncovered O.R. procedure |

65.7 **Repair of ovary**

    Excludes: *salpingo-oophorostomy (66.72)*

    65.71 **Other simple suture of ovary**

        Excludes: *that by laparoscope (65.74)*

    65.72 **Other reimplantation of ovary**

        Excludes: *that by laparoscope (65.75)*

    65.73 **Other salpingo-oophoroplasty**

        Excludes: *that by laparoscope (65.76)*

    65.74 **Laparoscopic simple suture of ovary**

    65.75 **Laparoscopic reimplantation of ovary**

    65.76 **Laparoscopic salpingo-oophoroplasty**

    65.79 **Other repair of ovary**
        Oophoropexy

65.8 **Lysis of adhesions of ovary and fallopian tube**

    65.81 **Laparoscopic lysis of adhesions of ovary and fallopian tube**

    65.89 **Other lysis of adhesions of ovary and fallopian tube**

        Excludes: *that by laparoscope (65.81)*

65.9 **Other operations on ovary**

    65.91 **Aspiration of ovary**

        Excludes: *aspiration biopsy of ovary (65.11)*

    65.92 **Transplantation of ovary**

        Excludes: *reimplantation of ovary (65.72, 65.75)*

    65.93 **Manual rupture of ovarian cyst**

    65.94 **Ovarian denervation**

    65.95 **Release of torsion of ovary**

    65.99 **Other**
        Ovarian drilling

66 **Operations on fallopian tubes**

    Code also any application or administration of an adhesion barrier substance (99.77)

66.0 **Salpingotomy and salpingostomy**

    66.01 **Salpingotomy**

    66.02 **Salpingostomy**

66.1 **Diagnostic procedures on fallopian tubes**

    66.11 **Biopsy of fallopian tube**

    66.19 **Other diagnostic procedures on fallopian tubes**

        Excludes: *microscopic examination of specimen from fallopian tubes*
            (91.41-91.49)
            radiography of fallopian tubes (87.82-87.83, 87.85)
            Rubin's test (66.8)

66.2 **Bilateral endoscopic destruction or occlusion of fallopian tubes**
    Includes: bilateral endoscopic destruction or occlusion of fallopian tubes by:
            culdoscopy
            endoscopy
            hysteroscopy
            laparoscopy
            peritoneoscopy
        endoscopic destruction of solitary fallopian tube

    66.21 **Bilateral endoscopic ligation and crushing of fallopian tubes**

    66.22 **Bilateral endoscopic ligation and division of fallopian tubes**

    66.29 **Other bilateral endoscopic destruction or occlusion of fallopian tubes**

66.3 **Other bilateral destruction or occlusion of fallopian tubes**
    Includes: destruction of solitary fallopian tube

    Excludes: *endoscopic destruction or occlusion of fallopian tubes (66.21-66.29)*

    66.31 **Other bilateral ligation and crushing of fallopian tubes**

● Code new
to this edition

▲ Revision of
existing code

④ ⑤ Fourth or fifth
digit required

66.32 Other bilateral ligation and division of fallopian tubes
Pomeroy operation

66.39 Other bilateral destruction or occlusion of fallopian tubes
Female sterilization operation NOS

66.4 Total unilateral salpingectomy

66.5 Total bilateral salpingectomy

Excludes: *bilateral partial salpingectomy for sterilization (66.39)*
that with oophorectomy (65.61-65.64)

66.51 Removal of both fallopian tubes at same operative episode

66.52 Removal of remaining fallopian tube
Removal of solitary fallopian tube

66.6 Other salpingectomy
Includes: salpingectomy by:
cauterization
coagulation
electrocoagulation
excision

Excludes: *fistulectomy (66.73)*

66.61 Excision or destruction of lesion of fallopian tube

Excludes: *biopsy of fallopian tube (66.11)*

66.62 Salpingectomy with removal of tubal pregnancy
Code also any synchronous oophorectomy (65.31, 65.39)

66.63 Bilateral partial salpingectomy, not otherwise specified

66.69 Other partial salpingectomy

66.7 Repair of fallopian tube

66.71 Simple suture of fallopian tube

66.72 Salpingo-oophorostomy

66.73 Salpingo-salpingostomy

66.74 Salpingo-uterostomy

66.79 Other repair of fallopian tube
Graft of fallopian tube
Reopening of divided fallopian tube
Salpingoplasty

66.8 Insufflation of fallopian tube
Insufflation of fallopian tube with:
air
dye
gas
saline
Rubin's test

Excludes: *insufflation of therapeutic agent (66.95)*
that for hysterosalpingography (87.82-87.83)

66.9 Other operations on fallopian tubes

66.91 Aspiration of fallopian tube

66.92 Unilateral destruction or occlusion of fallopian tube

Excludes: *that of solitary tube (66.21-66.39)*

66.93 Implantation or replacement of prosthesis of fallopian tube

66.94 Removal of prosthesis of fallopian tube

66.95 Insufflation of therapeutic agent into fallopian tubes

66.96 Dilation of fallopian tube

66.97 Burying of fimbriae in uterine wall

66.99 Other

Excludes: *lysis of adhesions of ovary and tube (65.81, 65.89)*

67 Operations on cervix
Code also any application or administration of an adhesion barrier substance (99.77)

Valid O.R.
procedure

Non-O.R.
procedure

Nonspecific
O.R. procedure

Noncovered
O.R. procedure

67.0 **Dilation of cervical canal**

> Excludes: *dilation and curettage (69.01-69.09)*
> *that for induction of labor (73.1)*

67.1 **Diagnostic procedures on cervix**

67.11 **Endocervical biopsy**

> Excludes: *conization of cervix (67.2)*

67.12 **Other cervical biopsy**
Punch biopsy of cervix NOS

> Excludes: *conization of cervix (67.2)*

67.19 **Other diagnostic procedures on cervix**

> Excludes: *microscopic examination of specimen from cervix (91.41-91.49)*

67.2 **Conization of cervix**

> Excludes: *that by:*
> *cryosurgery (67.33)*
> *electrosurgery (67.32)*

67.3 **Other excision or destruction of lesion or tissue of cervix**

67.31 **Marsupialization of cervical cyst**

67.32 **Destruction of lesion of cervix by cauterization**
Electroconization of cervix
LEEP (loop electrosurgical excision procedure)
LLETZ (large loop excision of the transformation zone)

67.33 **Destruction of lesion of cervix by cryosurgery**
Cryoconization of cervix

67.39 **Other excision or destruction of lesion or tissue of cervix**

> Excludes: *biopsy of cervix (67.11-67.12)*
> *cervical fistulectomy (67.62)*
> *conization of cervix (67.2)*

67.4 **Amputation of cervix**
Cervicectomy with synchronous colporrhaphy

67.5 **Repair of internal cervical os**

67.51 **Transabdominal cerclage of cervix**

67.59 **Other repair of internal cervical os**
Cerclage of isthmus uteri
McDonald operation
Shirodkar operation
Transvaginal cerclage

> Excludes: *laparoscopically assisted supracervical hysterectomy [LASH] (68.31)*
> *transabdominal cerclage of cervix (67.51)*

67.6 **Other repair of cervix**

> Excludes: *repair of current obstetric laceration (75.51)*

67.61 **Suture of laceration of cervix**

67.62 **Repair of fistula of cervix**
Cervicosigmoidal fistulectomy

> Excludes: *fistulectomy:*
> *cervicovesical (57.84)*
> *ureterocervical (56.84)*
> *vesicocervicovaginal (57.84)*

67.69 **Other repair of cervix**
Repair of old obstetric laceration of cervix

68 **Other incision and excision of uterus**

Code also any application or administration of an adhesion barrier substance (99.77)

68.0 **Hysterotomy**
Hysterotomy with removal of hydatidiform mole

> Excludes: *hysterotomy for termination of pregnancy (74.91)*

68.1 **Diagnostic procedures on uterus and supporting structures**

● Code new
to this edition   ▲ Revision of
existing code   ④ ⑤ Fourth or fifth
digit required

68.11 Digital examination of uterus

> Excludes: *pelvic examination, so described (89.26)*
> *postpartal manual exploration of uterine cavity (75.7)*

68.12 Hysteroscopy

> Excludes: *that with biopsy (68.16)*

68.13 Open biopsy of uterus

> Excludes: *closed biopsy of uterus (68.16)*

68.14 Open biopsy of uterine ligaments

> Excludes: *closed biopsy of uterine ligaments (68.15)*

68.15 Closed biopsy of uterine ligaments

Endoscopic (laparoscopy) biopsy of uterine adnexa, except ovary and fallopian tube

68.16 Closed biopsy of uterus

Endoscopic (laparoscopy) (hysteroscopy) biopsy of uterus

> Excludes: *open biopsy of uterus (68.13)*

68.19 Other diagnostic procedures on uterus and supporting structures

> Excludes: *diagnostic:*
> *aspiration curettage (69.59)*
> *dilation and curettage (69.09)*
> *microscopic examination of specimen from uterus (91.41-91.49)*
> *pelvic examination (89.26)*
> *radioisotope scan of:*
> *placenta (92.17)*
> *uterus (92.19)*
> *ultrasonography of uterus (88.78-88.79)*
> *x-ray of uterus (87.81-87.89)*

68.2 Excision or destruction of lesion or tissue of uterus

68.21 Division of endometrial synechiae

Lysis of intraluminal uterine adhesions

68.22 Incision or excision of congenital septum of uterus

68.23 Endometrial ablation

Dilation and curettage
Hysteroscopic endometrial ablation

● **68.24 Uterine artery embolization [UAE] with coils**

> Excludes: *that without coils (68.25)*

● **68.25 Uterine artery embolization [UAE] without coils**

Includes that by:
gelatin sponge
gelfoam
microspheres
particulate agent NOS
polyvinyl alcohol [PVA]
spherical embolics

> Excludes: *that with coils (68.24)*

68.29 Other excision or destruction of lesion of uterus

Uterine myomectomy

> Excludes: *biopsy of uterus (68.13)*
> *uterine fistulectomy (69.42)*

68.3 Subtotal abdominal hysterectomy

68.31 Laparoscopic supracervical hysterectomy [LSH]

Classic infrafascial SEMM hysterectomy [CISH]
Laparoscopically assisted supracervical hysterectomy [LASH]

68.39 Other and unspecified subtotal abdominal hysterectomy

Supracervical hysterectomy

> Excludes: *classic infrafascial SEMM hysterectomy [CISH] (68.31)*
> *laparoscopic supracervical hysterectomy [LSH] (68.31)*

	Valid O.R. procedure		Non-O.R. procedure		Nonspecific O.R. procedure		Noncovered O.R. procedure

68.4   Total abdominal hysterectomy
Hysterectomy:
extended

Code also any synchronous removal of tubes and ovaries (65.31-65.64)

Excludes: *radical abdominal hysterectomy, any approach (68.61-68.69)*

68.41   Laparoscopic total abdominal hysterectomy
Total laparoscopic hysterectomy [TLH]

68.49   Other and unspecified total abdominal hysterectomy
Hysterectomy:
Extended

Excludes: *laparoscopic total abdominal hysterectomy (68.41)*

68.5   Vaginal hysterectomy
Code also any synchronous:
removal of tubes and ovaries (65.31-65.64)
repair of cystocele or rectocele (70.50-70.52)
repair of pelvic floor (70.79)

68.51   Laparoscopically assisted vaginal hysterectomy (LAVH)

68.59   Other and unspecified vaginal hysterectomy

Excludes: *laparoscopically assisted vaginal hysterectomy (LAVH) (68.51)*
radical vaginal hysterectomy (68.7)

68.6   Radical abdominal hysterectomy
Code also any synchronous:
lymph gland dissection (40.3, 40.5)
removal of tubes and ovaries (65.61-65.64)

Excludes: *pelvic evisceration (68.8)*

68.61   Laparoscopic radical abdominal hysterectomy
Laparoscopic modified radical hysterectomy
Total laparoscopic radical hysterectomy [TLRH]

68.69   Other and unspecified radical abdominal hysterectomy
Modified radical hysterectomy
Wertheim's operation

Excludes: *laparoscopic total abdominal hysterectomy (68.41)*
laparoscopic radical abdominal hysterectomy (68.61)

68.7   Radical vaginal hysterectomy
Code also any synchronous:
lymph gland dissection (40.3, 40.5)
removal of tubes and ovaries (65.61-65.64)

Excludes: *abdominal hysterectomy, any approach (68.31-68.39, 68.41-68.49,*
68.61-68.69, 68.9)

68.71   Laparoscopic radical vaginal hysterectomy [LRVH]

68.79   Other and unspecified radical vaginal hysterectomy
Hysterocolpectomy
Schauta operation

68.8   Pelvic evisceration
Removal of ovaries, tubes, uterus, vagina, bladder and urethra (with removal of sigmoid
colon and rectum)

Code also any synchronous:
colostomy (46.12-46.13)
lymph gland dissection (40.3, 40.5)
urinary diversion (56.51-56.79)

68.9   Other and unspecified hysterectomy
Hysterectomy, NOS

Excludes: *abdominal hysterectomy, any approach (68.31-68.39, 68.41-68.49,*
68.61-68.69)
vaginal hysterectomy, any approach (68.51-68.59, 68.71-68.79)

69   Other operations on uterus and supporting structures
Code also any application or administration of an adhesion barrier substance (99.77)

69.0   Dilation and curettage of uterus

Excludes: *aspiration curettage of uterus (69.51-69.59)*

69.01 Dilation and curettage for termination of pregnancy

69.02 Dilation and curettage following delivery or abortion

69.09 Other dilation and curettage
Diagnostic D and C

69.1 Excision or destruction of lesion or tissue of uterus and supporting structures

69.19 Other excision or destruction of uterus and supporting structures

Excludes: *biopsy of uterine ligament (68.14)*

69.2 Repair of uterine supporting structures

69.21 Interposition operation
Watkins procedure

69.22 Other uterine suspension
Hysteropexy
Manchester operation
Plication of uterine ligament

69.23 Vaginal repair of chronic inversion of uterus

69.29 Other repair of uterus and supporting structures

69.3 Paracervical uterine denervation

69.4 Uterine repair

Excludes: *repair of current obstetric laceration (75.50-75.52)*

69.41 Suture of laceration of uterus

69.42 Closure of fistula of uterus

Excludes: *uterovesical fistulectomy (57.84)*

69.49 Other repair of uterus
Repair of old obstetric laceration of uterus

69.5 Aspiration curettage of uterus

Excludes: *menstrual extraction (69.6)*

69.51 Aspiration curettage of uterus for termination of pregnancy
Therapeutic abortion NOS

69.52 Aspiration curettage following delivery or abortion

69.59 Other aspiration curettage of uterus

69.6 Menstrual extraction or regulation

69.7 Insertion of intrauterine contraceptive device

69.9 Other operations on uterus, cervix, and supporting structures

Excludes: *obstetric dilation or incision of cervix (73.1, 73.93)*

69.91 Insertion of therapeutic device into uterus

Excludes: *insertion of:*
intrauterine contraceptive device (69.7)
laminaria (69.93)
obstetric insertion of bag, bougie, or pack (73.1)

69.92 Artificial insemination

69.93 Insertion of laminaria

69.94 Manual replacement of inverted uterus

Excludes: *that in immediate postpartal period (75.94)*

69.95 Incision of cervix

Excludes: *that to assist delivery (73.93)*

69.96 Removal of cerclage material from cervix

69.97 Removal of other penetrating foreign body from cervix

Excludes: *removal of intraluminal foreign body from cervix (98.16)*

69.98 Other operations on supporting structures of uterus

Excludes: *biopsy of uterine ligament (68.14)*

| Valid O.R. procedure | Non-O.R. procedure | Nonspecific O.R. procedure | Noncovered O.R. procedure |

69.99 **Other operations on cervix and uterus**

> Excludes: removal of:
> foreign body (98.16)
> intrauterine contraceptive device (97.71)
> obstetric bag, bougie, or pack (97.72)
> packing (97.72)

70 **Operations on vagina and cul-de-sac**

Code also any application or administration of an adhesion barrier substance (99.77)

70.0 **Culdocentesis**

70.1 **Incision of vagina and cul-de-sac**

70.11 **Hymenotomy**

70.12 **Culdotomy**

70.13 **Lysis of intraluminal adhesion of vagina**

70.14 **Other vaginotomy**
Division of vaginal septum
Drainage of hematoma of vaginal cuff

70.2 **Diagnostic procedures on vagina and cul-de-sac**

70.21 **Vaginoscopy**

70.22 **Culdoscopy**

70.23 **Biopsy of cul-de-sac**

70.24 **Vaginal biopsy**

70.29 **Other diagnostic procedures on vagina and cul-de-sac**

70.3 **Local excision or destruction of vagina and cul-de-sac**

70.31 **Hymenectomy**

70.32 **Excision or destruction of lesion of cul-de-sac**
Endometrectomy of cul-de-sac

> Excludes: biopsy of cul-de-sac (70.23)

70.33 **Excision or destruction of lesion of vagina**

> Excludes: biopsy of vagina (70.24)
> vaginal fistulectomy (70.72-70.75)

70.4 **Obliteration and total excision of vagina**
Vaginectomy

> Excludes: obliteration of vaginal vault (70.8)

70.5 **Repair of cystocele and rectocele**

70.50 **Repair of cystocele and rectocele**

> Excludes: repair of cystocele and rectocele with graft or prosthesis (70.53)

70.51 **Repair of cystocele**
Anterior colporrhaphy (with urethrocele repair)

> Excludes: repair of cystocele and rectocele with graft or prosthesis (70.53)
> repair of cystocele with graft or prosthesis (70.54)

70.52 **Repair of rectocele**
Posterior colporrhaphy

> Excludes: repair of cystocele and rectocele with graft or prosthesis (70.53)
> repair of rectocele with graft or prosthesis (70.55)
> STARR procedure (48.74)

70.53 **Repair of cystocele and rectocele with graft or prosthesis**
Use additional code for biological substance (70.94) or synthetic substance (70.95), if known

70.54 **Repair of cystocele with graft or prosthesis**
Anterior colporrhaphy (with urethrocele repair)
Use additional code for biological substance (70.94) or synthetic substance (70.95), if known

70.55 **Repair of rectocele with graft or prosthesis**
Posterior colporrhaphy
Use additional code for biological substance (70.94) or synthetic substance (70.95), if known

● Code new to this edition   ▲ Revision of existing code   ④ ⑤ Fourth or fifth digit required

70.6   **Vaginal construction and reconstruction**

    70.61   **Vaginal construction**

    70.62   **Vaginal reconstruction**

    70.63   **Vaginal construction with graft or prosthesis**

        Use additional code for biological substance (70.94) or synthetic substance (70.95), if known

        | *Excludes:* | *vaginal construction (70.61)* |

    70.64   **Vaginal reconstruction with graft or prosthesis**

        Use additional code for biological substance (70.94) or synthetic substance (70.95), if known

        | *Excludes:* | *vaginal reconstruction (70.62)* |

70.7   **Other repair of vagina**

    | *Excludes:* | *lysis of intraluminal adhesions (70.13)* |
        repair of current obstetric laceration (75.69)
        that associated with cervical amputation (67.4)

    70.71   **Suture of laceration of vagina**

    70.72   **Repair of colovaginal fistula**

    70.73   **Repair of rectovaginal fistula**

    70.74   **Repair of other vaginoenteric fistula**

    70.75   **Repair of other fistula of vagina**

        | *Excludes:* | *repair of fistula:* |
            rectovesicovaginal (57.83)
            ureterovaginal (56.84)
            urethrovaginal (58.43)
            uterovaginal (69.42)
            vesicocervicovaginal (57.84)
            vesicosigmoidovaginal (57.83)
            vesicoureterovaginal (56.84)
            vesicovaginal (57.84)

    70.76   **Hymenorrhaphy**

    70.77   **Vaginal suspension and fixation**

    70.78   **Vaginal suspension and fixation with graft or prosthesis**

        Use additional code for biological substance (70.94) or synthetic substance (70.95), if known

    70.79   **Other repair of vagina**
        Colpoperineoplasty
        Repair of old obstetric laceration of vagina

70.8   **Obliteration of vaginal vault**
    LeFort operation

70.9   **Other operations on vagina and cul-de-sac**

    70.91   **Other operations on vagina**

        | *Excludes:* | *insertion of:* |
            diaphragm (96.17)
            mold (96.15)
            pack (96.14)
            pessary (96.18)
            suppository (96.49)
           removal of:
            diaphragm (97.73)
            foreign body (98.17)
            pack (97.75)
            pessary (97.74)
           replacement of:
            diaphragm (97.24)
            pack (97.26)
            pessary (97.25)
           vaginal dilation (96.16)
           vaginal douche (96.44)

| Valid O.R. procedure | Non-O.R. procedure | Nonspecific O.R. procedure | Noncovered O.R. procedure |

70.92 Other operations on cul-de-sac
Obliteration of cul-de-sac
Repair of vaginal enterocele

70.93 Other operations on cul-de-sac with graft or prosthesis
Repair of vaginal enterocele with graft or prosthesis

*Use additional code for biological substance (70.94) or synthetic substance (70.95),
if known*

70.94 Insertion of biological graft
Allogenic material or substance
Allograft
Autograft
Autologous material or substance
Heterograft
Xenogenic material or substance

Code first these procedures when done with graft or prosthesis:
Other operations on cul-de-sac (70.93)
Repair of cystocele (70.54)
Repair of cystocele and rectocele (70.53)
Repair of rectocele (70.55)
Vaginal construction (70.63)
Vaginal reconstruction (70.64)
Vaginal suspension and fixation (70.78)

70.95 Insertion of synthetic graft or prosthesis
Artificial tissue

Code first these procedures when done with graft or prosthesis:
Other operations on cul-de-sac (70.93)
Repair of cystocele (70.54)
Repair of cystocele and rectocele (70.53)
Repair of rectocele (70.55)
Vaginal construction (70.63)
Vaginal reconstruction (70.64)
Vaginal suspension and fixation (70.78)

71 Operations on vulva and perineum
Code also any application or administration of an adhesion barrier substance (99.77)

71.0 Incision of vulva and perineum

71.01 Lysis of vulvar adhesions

71.09 Other incision of vulva and perineum
Enlargement of introitus NOS

Excludes: *removal of foreign body without incision (98.23)*

71.1 Diagnostic procedures on vulva

71.11 Biopsy of vulva

71.19 Other diagnostic procedures on vulva

71.2 Operations on Bartholin's gland

71.21 Percutaneous aspiration of Bartholin's gland (cyst)

71.22 Incision of Bartholin's gland (cyst)

71.23 Marsupialization of Bartholin's gland (cyst)

71.24 Excision or other destruction of Bartholin's gland (cyst)

71.29 Other operations on Bartholin's gland

71.3 Other local excision or destruction of vulva and perineum
Division of Skene's gland

Excludes: *biopsy of vulva (71.11)*
vulvar fistulectomy (71.72)

71.4 Operations on clitoris
Amputation of clitoris
Clitoridotomy
Female circumcision

71.5 Radical vulvectomy
Code also any synchronous lymph gland dissection (40.3, 40.5)

71.6 Other vulvectomy

71.61 Unilateral vulvectomy

● Code new
to this edition
▲ Revision of
existing code
④ ⑤ Fourth or fifth
digit required

71.62 **Bilateral vulvectomy**
Vulvectomy NOS

71.7 **Repair of vulva and perineum**

> Excludes: repair of current obstetric laceration (75.69)

71.71 **Suture of laceration of vulva or perineum**

71.72 **Repair of fistula of vulva or perineum**

> Excludes: repair of fistula:
> urethroperineal (58.43)
> urethroperineovesical (57.84)
> vaginoperineal (70.75)

71.79 **Other repair of vulva and perineum**
Repair of old obstetric laceration of vulva or perineum

71.8 **Other operations on vulva**

> Excludes: removal of:
> foreign body without incision (98.23)
> packing (97.75)
> replacement of packing (97.26)

71.9 **Other operations on female genital organs**

Valid O.R.
procedure

Non-O.R.
procedure

Nonspecific
O.R. procedure

Noncovered
O.R. procedure

This page intentionally left blank.

● Code new
to this edition

▲ Revision of
existing code

④ ⑤ Fourth or fifth
digit required

13. OBSTETRICAL PROCEDURES (72-75)

72 **Forceps, vacuum, and breech delivery**

72.0 **Low forceps operation**
Outlet forceps operation

72.1 **Low forceps operation with episiotomy**
Outlet forceps operation with episiotomy

72.2 **Mid forceps operation**

72.21 **Mid forceps operation with episiotomy**

72.29 **Other mid forceps operation**

72.3 **High forceps operation**

72.31 **High forceps operation with episiotomy**

72.39 **Other high forceps operation**

72.4 **Forceps rotation of fetal head**
DeLee maneuver
Key-in-lock rotation
Kielland rotation
Scanzoni's maneuver
Code also any associated forceps extraction (72.0-72.39)

72.5 **Breech extraction**

72.51 **Partial breech extraction with forceps to aftercoming head**

72.52 **Other partial breech extraction**

72.53 **Total breech extraction with forceps to aftercoming head**

72.54 **Other total breech extraction**

72.6 **Forceps application to aftercoming head**
Piper forceps operation

> *Excludes:* partial breech extraction with forceps to aftercoming head (72.51)
> total breech extraction with forceps to aftercoming head (72.53)

72.7 **Vacuum extraction**
Includes: Malström's extraction

72.71 **Vacuum extraction with episiotomy**

72.79 **Other vacuum extraction**

72.8 **Other specified instrumental delivery**

72.9 **Unspecified instrumental delivery**

73 **Other procedures inducing or assisting delivery**

73.0 **Artificial rupture of membranes**

73.01 **Induction of labor by artificial rupture of membranes**
Surgical induction NOS

> *Excludes:* artificial rupture of membranes after onset of labor (73.09)

73.09 **Other artificial rupture of membranes**
Artificial rupture of membranes at time of delivery

73.1 **Other surgical induction of labor**
Induction by cervical dilation

> *Excludes:* injection for abortion (75.0)
> insertion of suppository for abortion (96.49)

73.2 **Internal and combined version and extraction**

73.21 **Internal and combined version without extraction**
Version NOS

73.22 **Internal and combined version with extraction**

73.3 **Failed forceps**
Application of forceps without delivery
Trial forceps

73.4 **Medical induction of labor**

> *Excludes:* medication to augment active labor—omit code

73.5 **Manually assisted delivery**

73.51 **Manual rotation of fetal head**

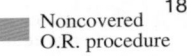

| Valid O.R. procedure | Non-O.R. procedure | Nonspecific O.R. procedure | Noncovered O.R. procedure |

73.59 Other manually assisted delivery
Assisted spontaneous delivery
Crede maneuver

73.6 Episiotomy
Episioproctotomy
Episiotomy with subsequent episiorrhaphy

Excludes: *that with:*
high forceps (72.31)
low forceps (72.1)
mid forceps (72.21)
outlet forceps (72.1)
vacuum extraction (72.71)

73.8 Operations on fetus to facilitate delivery
Clavicotomy on fetus
Destruction of fetus
Needling of hydrocephalic head

73.9 Other operations assisting delivery

73.91 External version

73.92 Replacement of prolapsed umbilical cord

73.93 Incision of cervix to assist delivery
Dührssen's incisions

73.94 Pubiotomy to assist delivery
Obstetrical symphysiotomy

73.99 Other

Excludes: *dilation of cervix obstetrical, to induce labor (73.1)*
insertion of bag or bougie to induce labor (73.1)
removal of cerclage material (69.96)

74   Cesarean section and removal of fetus
Code also any synchronous:
hysterectomy (68.3-68.4, 68.6, 68.8)
myomectomy (68.29)
sterilization (66.31-66.39, 66.63)

74.0 Classical cesarean section
Transperitoneal classical cesarean section

74.1 Low cervical cesarean section
Lower uterine segment cesarean section

74.2 Extraperitoneal cesarean section
Supravesical cesarean section

74.3 Removal of extratubal ectopic pregnancy
Removal of:
ectopic abdominal pregnancy
fetus from peritoneal or extraperitoneal cavity following uterine or tubal rupture

Excludes: *that by salpingostomy (66.02)*
that by salpingotomy (66.01)
that with synchronous salpingectomy (66.62)

74.4 Cesarean section of other specified type
Peritoneal exclusion cesarean section
Transperitoneal cesarean section NOS
Vaginal cesarean section

74.9 Cesarian section of unspecified type

74.91 Hysterotomy to terminate pregnancy
Therapeutic abortion by hysterotomy

74.99 Other cesarean section of unspecified type
Cesarean section NOS
Obstetrical abdominouterotomy
Obstetrical hysterotomy

● Code new
to this edition
▲ Revision of
existing code
④ ⑤ Fourth or fifth
digit required

75   Other obstetric operations

    75.0   Intra-amniotic injection for abortion
       Injection of:
          prostaglandin for induction of abortion
          saline for induction of abortion
       Termination of pregnancy by intrauterine injection

         | Excludes: | *insertion of prostaglandin suppository for abortion (96.49)*

    75.1   Diagnostic amniocentesis

    75.2   Intrauterine transfusion
       Exchange transfusion in utero
       Insertion of catheter into abdomen of fetus for transfusion
       Code also any hysterotomy approach (68.0)

    75.3   Other intrauterine operations on fetus and amnion
       Code also any hysterotomy approach (68.0)

        75.31   Amnioscopy
           Fetoscopy
           Laparoamnioscopy

        75.32   Fetal EKG (scalp)

        75.33   Fetal blood sampling and biopsy

        75.34   Other fetal monitoring
           Antepartum fetal nonstress test
           Fetal monitoring, not otherwise specified

           | Excludes: | *fetal pulse oximetry (75.38)*

        75.35   Other diagnostic procedures on fetus and amnion
           Intrauterine pressure determination

           | Excludes: | *amniocentesis (75.1)*
                diagnostic procedures on gravid uterus
                  and placenta (87.81, 88.46, 88.78, 92.17)

        75.36   Correction of fetal defect

        75.37   Amnioinfusion
           Code also injection of antibiotic (99.21)

        75.38   Fetal pulse oximetry
           Transcervical fetal oxygen saturation monitoring
           Transcervical fetal SpO$_2$ monitoring

    75.4   Manual removal of retained placenta

       | Excludes: | *aspiration curettage (69.52)*
               dilation and curettage (69.02)

    75.5   Repair of current obstetric laceration of uterus

        75.50   Repair of current obstetric laceration of uterus not otherwise specified

        75.51   Repair of current obstetric laceration of cervix

        75.52   Repair of current obstetric laceration of corpus uteri

    75.6   Repair of other current obstetric laceration
       Code also episiotomy, if performed (73.6)

        75.61   Repair of current obstetric laceration of bladder and urethra

        75.62   Repair of current obstetric laceration of rectum and sphincter ani

        75.69   Repair of other current obstetric laceration
           Episioperineorrhaphy
           Repair of:
             pelvic floor
             perineum
             vagina
             vulva
           Secondary repair of episiotomy

    75.7   Manual exploration of uterine cavity, postpartum

    75.8   Obstetric tamponade of uterus or vagina

       | Excludes: | *antepartum tamponade (73.1)*

    75.9   Other obstetric operations

Valid O.R. procedure   Non-O.R. procedure   Nonspecific O.R. procedure   Noncovered O.R. procedure

75.91 **Evacuation of obstetrical incision hematoma of perineum**
Evacuation of hematoma of:
episiotomy
perineorrhaphy

75.92 **Evacuation of other hematoma of vulva or vagina**

75.93 **Surgical correction of inverted uterus**
Spintelli operation

Excludes: *vaginal repair of chronic inversion of uterus (69.23)*

75.94 **Manual replacement of inverted uterus**

75.99 **Other**

● Code new
to this edition

▲ Revision of
existing code

④ ⑤ Fourth or fifth
digit required

14. OPERATIONS ON THE MUSCULOSKELETAL SYSTEM (76-84)

76 Operations on facial bones and joints

> Excludes: *accessory sinuses (22.00-22.9)*
> *nasal bones (21.00-21.99)*
> *skull (01.01-02.99)*

76.0 Incision of facial bone without division

76.01 Sequestrectomy of facial bone
Removal of necrotic bone chip from facial bone

76.09 Other incision of facial bone
Reopening of osteotomy site of facial bone

> Excludes: *osteotomy associated with orthognathic surgery (76.61-76.69)*
> *removal of internal fixation device (76.97)*

76.1 Diagnostic procedures on facial bones and joints

76.11 Biopsy of facial bone

76.19 Other diagnostic procedures on facial bones and joints

> Excludes: *contrast arthrogram of temporomandibular joint (87.13)*
> *other x-ray (87.11-87.12 87.14-87.16)*

76.2 Local excision or destruction of lesion of facial bone

> Excludes: *biopsy of facial bone (76.11)*
> *excision of odontogenic lesion (24.4)*

76.3 Partial ostectomy of facial bone

76.31 Partial mandibulectomy
Hemimandibulectomy

> Excludes: *that associated with temporomandibular arthroplasty (76.5)*

76.39 Partial ostectomy of other facial bone
Hemimaxillectomy (with bone graft or prosthesis)

76.4 Excision and reconstruction of facial bones

76.41 Total mandibulectomy with synchronous reconstruction

76.42 Other total mandibulectomy

76.43 Other reconstruction of mandible

> Excludes: *genioplasty (76.67-76.68)*
> *that with synchronous total mandibulectomy (76.41)*

76.44 Total ostectomy of other facial bone with synchronous reconstruction

76.45 Other total ostectomy of other facial bone

76.46 Other reconstruction of other facial bone

> Excludes: *that with synchronous total ostectomy (76.44)*

76.5 Temporomandibular arthroplasty

76.6 Other facial bone repair and orthognathic surgery

> *Code also any synchronous:*
> bone graft (76.91)
> synthetic implant (76.92)

> Excludes: *reconstruction of facial bones (76.41-76.46)*

76.61 Closed osteoplasty [osteotomy] of mandibular ramus
Gigli saw osteotomy

76.62 Open osteoplasty [osteotomy] of mandibular ramus

76.63 Osteoplasty [osteotomy] of body of mandible

76.64 Other orthognathic surgery on mandible
Mandibular osteoplasty NOS
Segmental or subapical osteotomy

76.65 Segmental osteoplasty [osteotomy] of maxilla
Maxillary osteoplasty NOS

76.66 Total osteoplasty [osteotomy] of maxilla

76.67 Reduction genioplasty
Reduction mentoplasty

	Valid O.R. procedure		Non-O.R. procedure	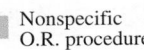	Nonspecific O.R. procedure	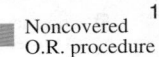	Noncovered O.R. procedure

76.68 Augmentation genioplasty
Mentoplasty:
NOS
with graft or implant

76.69 Other facial bone repair
Osteoplasty of facial bone NOS

76.7 Reduction of facial fracture
Includes: internal fixation

Code also any synchronous:
bone graft (76.91)
synthetic implant (76.92)

Excludes: *that of nasal bones (21.71-21.72)*

76.70 Reduction of facial fracture, not otherwise specified

76.71 Closed reduction of malar and zygomatic fracture

76.72 Open reduction of malar and zygomatic fracture

76.73 Closed reduction of maxillary fracture

76.74 Open reduction of maxillary fracture

76.75 Closed reduction of mandibular fracture

76.76 Open reduction of mandibular fracture

76.77 Open reduction of alveolar fracture
Reduction of alveolar fracture with stabilization of teeth

76.78 Other closed reduction of facial fracture
Closed reduction of orbital fracture

Excludes: *nasal bone (21.71)*

76.79 Other open reduction of facial fracture
Open reduction of orbit rim or wall

Excludes: *nasal bone (21.72)*

76.9 Other operations on facial bones and joints

76.91 Bone graft to facial bone
Autogenous graft to facial bone
Bone bank graft to facial bone
Heterogenous graft to facial bone

76.92 Insertion of synthetic implant in facial bone
Alloplastic implant to facial bone

76.93 Closed reduction of temporomandibular dislocation

76.94 Open reduction of temporomandibular dislocation

76.95 Other manipulation of temporomandibular joint

76.96 Injection of therapeutic substance into temporomandibular joint

76.97 Removal of internal fixation device from facial bone

Excludes: *removal of:*
dental wiring (97.33)
external mandibular fixation device NEC (97.36)

76.99 Other

● Code new
to this edition

▲ Revision of
existing code

④ ⑤ Fourth or fifth
digit required

77 Incision, excision, and division of other bones

> Excludes: *laminectomy for decompression (03.09)*
> *operations on:*
> *accessory sinuses (22.00-22.9)*
> *ear ossicles (19.0-19.55)*
> *facial bones (76.01-76.99)*
> *joint structures (80.00-81.99)*
> *mastoid (19.9-20.99)*
> *nasal bones (21.00-21.99)*
> *skull (01.01-02.99)*

The following fourth-digit subclassification is for use with appropriate categories in section 77, marked with a symbol to identify the site. Valid fourth-digit categories are in [brackets] under each code.

  0 **unspecified site**
  1 **scapula, clavicle, and thorax [ribs and sternum]**
  2 **humerus**
  3 **radius and ulna**
  4 **carpals and metacarpals**
  5 **femur**
  6 **patella**
  7 **tibia and fibula**
  8 **tarsals and metatarsals**
  9 **other**
     Pelvic bones
     Phalanges (of foot) (of hand)
     Vertebrae

④ **77.0 Sequestrectomy**
[0-9]

④ **77.1 Other incision of bone without division**
[0-9] Reopening of osteotomy site

> Excludes: *aspiration of bone marrow (41.31,41.91)*
> *removal of internal fixation device (78.60-78.69)*

④ **77.2 Wedge osteotomy**
[0-9] > Excludes: *that for hallux valgus (77.51)*

④ **77.3 Other division of bone**
[0-9] Osteoarthrotomy

> Excludes: *clavicotomy of fetus (73.8)*
> *laminotomy or incision of vertebra (03.01-03.09)*
> *pubiotomy to assist delivery (73.94)*
> *sternotomy incidental to thoracic operation—omit code*

④ **77.4 Biopsy of bone**
[0-9]

77.5 Excision and repair of bunion and other toe deformities

77.51 Bunionectomy with soft tissue correction and osteotomy of the first metatarsal

77.52 Bunionectomy with soft tissue correction and arthrodesis

77.53 Other bunionectomy with soft tissue correction

77.54 Excision or correction of bunionette
That with osteotomy

77.56 Repair of hammer toe
Fusion of hammer toe
Phalangectomy (partial) of hammer toe
Filleting of hammer toe

77.57 Repair of claw toe
Fusion of claw toe
Phalangectomy (partial) of claw toe
Capsulotomy of claw toe
Tendon lengthening of claw toe

77.58 Other excision, fusion, and repair of toes
Cockup toe repair
Overlapping toe repair
That with use of prosthetic materials

77.59 Other bunionectomy
Resection of hallux valgus joint with insertion of prosthesis

	Valid O.R. procedure		Non-O.R. procedure		Nonspecific O.R. procedure		Noncovered O.R. procedure

④ **77.6** **Local excision of lesion or tissue of bone**
[0-9] | *Excludes:* | *biopsy of bone (77.40-77.49)*

debridement of compound fracture (79.60-79.69)

④ **77.7** **Excision of bone for graft**
[0-9]

④ **77.8** **Other partial ostectomy**
[0-9]   Condylectomy
| *Excludes:* | *amputation (84.00-84.19,84.91)*
arthrectomy (80.90-80.99)
excision of bone ends associated with:
  arthrodesis (81.00-81.39, 81.62-81.66)
  arthroplasty (81.40-81.59, 81.71-81.85)
excision of cartilage (80.5-80.6, 80.80-80.99)
excision of head of femur with synchronous replacement (00.70-00.73,
  81.51-81.53)
hemilaminectomy (03.01-03.09)
laminectomy (03.01-03.09)
ostectomy for hallux valgus (77.51-77.59)
partial amputation:
  finger (84.01)
  thumb (84.02)
  toe (84.11)
resection of ribs incidental to thoracic operation—omit code
that incidental to other operation—omit code

④ **77.9** **Total ostectomy**
[0-9] | *Excludes:* | *amputation of limb (84.00-84.19, 84.91)*

that incidental to other operation—omit code

78 **Other operations on bones, except facial bones**
| *Excludes:* | *operations on:*
  accessory sinuses (22.00-22.9)
  facial bones (76.01-76.99)
  joint structures (80.00-81.99)
  nasal bones (21.00-21.99)
  skull (01.01-02.99)

The following fourth-digit subclassification is for use with categories in section 78 to identify the
site. Valid fourth-digit categories are in [brackets] under each code.

0 unspecified site
1 scapula, clavicle, and thorax (ribs and sternum]
2 humerus
3 radius and ulna
4 carpals and metacarpals
5 femur
6 patella
7 tibia and fibulas
8 tarsals and metatarsals
9 other
     Pelvic bones
     Phalanges (of foot) (of hand)
     Vertebrae

④ **78.0** **Bone graft**
[0-9]   Bone:
     bank graft
     graft (autogenous) (heterogenous)
     That with debridement of bone graft site (removal of sclerosed, fibrous, or necrotic bone or
       tissue)
     Transplantation of bone
     Code also any excision of bone for graft (77.70-77.79)
     | *Excludes:* | *that for bone lengthening (78.30-78.39)*

④ **78.1** **Application of external fixator device**
[0-9]   Fixator with insertion of pins/wires/screws into bone
     Code also any type of fixator device, if known (84.71-84.73)
     | *Excludes:* | *other immobilization, pressure, and attention to wound (93.51-93.59)*

● Code new   ▲ Revision of   ④ ⑤ Fourth or fifth
      to this edition   existing code   digit required

④ **78.2** **Limb shortening procedures**
[0,2-5,7-9] Epiphyseal stapling
Open epiphysiodesis
Percutaneous epiphysiodesis
Resection/osteotomy

④ **78.3** **Limb lengthening procedures**
[0,2-5,7-9] Bone graft with or without internal fixation devices or osteotomy
Distraction technique with or without corticotomy/osteotomy
Code also any application of an external fixation device (78.10-78.19)

④ **78.4** **Other repair or plastic operations on bone**
[0-9] Other operation on bone NEC
Repair of malunion or nonunion fracture NEC

Excludes:	*application of external fixation device (78.10-78.19)*
	limb lengthening procedures (78.30-78.39)
	limb shortening procedures (78.20-78.29)
	osteotomy (77.3)
	reconstruction of thumb (82.61-82.69)
	repair of pectus deformity (34.74)
	repair with bone graft (78.00-78.09)

④ **78.5** **Internal fixation of bone without fracture reduction**
[0-9] Internal fixation of bone (prophylactic)
Reinsertion of internal fixation device
Revision of displaced or broken fixation device

Excludes:	*arthroplasty and arthrodesis (81.00-81.85)*
	bone graft (78.00-78.09)
	insertion of sternal fixation device with rigid plates (84.94)
	limb shortening procedures (78.20-78.29)
	that for fracture reduction (79.10-79.19, 79.30-79.59)

④ **78.6** **Removal of implanted devices from bone**
[0-9] External fixator device (invasive)
Internal fixation device
Removal of bone growth stimulator (invasive)
Removal of internal limb lengthening device
Removal of pedicle screw(s) used in spinal fusion

Excludes:	*removal of cast, splint, and traction device (Kirschner wire) (Steinmann pin)*
	(97.88)
	removal of posterior spinal motion preservation (facet replacement,
	pedicle-based dynamic stabilization, interspinous process) device(s)
	(80.09)
	removal of skull tongs or halo traction device (02.95)

④ **78.7** **Osteoclasis**
[0-9]

④ **78.8** **Diagnostic procedures on bone, not elsewhere classified**
[0-9]

Excludes:	*biopsy of bone (77.40-77.49)*
	magnetic resonance imaging (88.94)
	microscopic examination of specimen from
	bone (91.51-91.59)
	radioisotope scan (92.14)
	skeletal x-ray (87.21-87.29, 87.43, 88.21-88.33)
	thermography (88.83)

④ **78.9** **Insertion of bone growth stimulator**
(0-9) Insertion of:
bone stimulator (electrical) to aid bone healing
osteogenic electrodes for bone growth stimulation
totally implanted device (invasive)

Excludes:	*non-invasive (transcutaneous) (surface) stimulator (99.86)*

79   Reduction of fracture and dislocation

  Includes: application of cast or splint
                      reduction with insertion of traction device (Kirschner wire) (Steinmann pin)

  Code also any:
    application of external fixator device (78.10-78.19)
    type of fixator device, if known (84.71-84.73)

Excludes:	*external fixation alone for immobilization of fracture (93.51-93.56,93.59)*

          internal fixation without reduction of fracture (78.50-78.59)
          operations on:
            facial bones (76.70-76.79)
            nasal bones (21.71-21.72)
            orbit (76.78-76.79)
            skull (02.02)
            vertebrae (03.53)
          removal of cast or splint (97.88)
          replacement of cast or splint (97.11-97.14)
          traction alone for reduction of fracture (93.41-93.46)

  The following fourth-digit subclassification is for use with appropriate categories in section 79, marked with a symbol to identify the site. Valid fourth-digit codes are in [brackets] under each code.

    0 unspecified site
    1 humerus
    2 radius and ulna
      Arm NOS
    3 carpals and metacarpals
      Hand NOS
    4 phalanges of hand
    5 femur
    6 tibia and fibula
      Leg NOS
    7 tarsals and metatarsals
      Foot NOS
    8 phalanges of foot
    9 other specified bone

④ **79.0   Closed reduction of fracture without internal fixation**
[0-9] | Excludes: | *that for separation of epiphysis (79.40-79.49)* |

④ **79.1   Closed reduction of fracture with internal fixation**
[0-9] | Excludes: | *that for separation of epiphysis (79.40-79.49)* |

④ **79.2   Open reduction of fracture without internal fixation**
[0-9] | Excludes: | *that for separation of epiphysis (79.50-79.59)* |

④ **79.3   Open reduction of fracture with internal fixation**
[0-9] | Excludes: | *that for separation of epiphysis (79.50-79.59)* |

④ **79.4   Closed reduction of separated epiphysis**
[0-2,5,6,9]   Reduction with or without internal fixation

④ **79.5   Open reduction of separated epiphysis**
[0-2,5,6,9]   Reduction with or without internal fixation

④ **79.6   Debridement of open fracture site**
[0-9]   Debridement of compound fracture

79.7   Closed reduction of dislocation
  Includes: closed reduction (with external traction device)

  | Excludes: | *closed reduction of dislocation of temporomandibular joint (76.93)* |

  79.70   Closed reduction of dislocation of unspecified site
  79.71   Closed reduction of dislocation of shoulder
  79.72   Closed reduction of dislocation of elbow
  79.73   Closed reduction of dislocation of wrist
  79.74   Closed reduction of dislocation of hand and finger
  79.75   Closed reduction of dislocation of hip
  79.76   Closed reduction of dislocation of knee
  79.77   Closed reduction of dislocation of ankle
  79.78   Closed reduction of dislocation of foot and toe

● Code new to this edition   ▲ Revision of existing code   ④ ⑤ Fourth or fifth digit required

79.79   Closed reduction of dislocation of other specified sites

79.8   Open reduction of dislocation
Includes: open reduction (with internal and external fixation devices)

> Excludes: *open reduction of dislocation of temporomandibular joint (76.94)*

79.80   Open reduction of dislocation of unspecified site

79.81   Open reduction of dislocation of shoulder

79.82   Open reduction of dislocation of elbow

79.83   Open reduction of dislocation of wrist

79.84   Open reduction of dislocation of hand and finger

79.85   Open reduction of dislocation of hip

79.86   Open reduction of dislocation of knee

79.87   Open reduction of dislocation of ankle

79.88   Open reduction of dislocation of foot and toe

79.89   Open reduction or dislocation of other specified sites

④ **79.9   Unspecified operation on bone injury**
[0-9]

80   Incision and excision of joint structures
Includes: operations on:
        capsule of joint
        cartilage
        condyle
        ligament
        meniscus
        synovial membrane

> Excludes: *cartilage of:*
>   *ear (18.01-18.9)*
>   *nose (21.00-21.99)*
>   *temporomandibular joint (76.01-76.99)*

The following fifth-digit subclassification is for use with appropriate categories in section 80, that are marked with a symbol to identify the site:

  0   unspecified site
  1   shoulder
  2   elbow
  3   wrist
  4   hand and finger
  5   hip
  6   knee
  7   ankle
  8   foot and toe
  9   other specified sites
     Spine

④ **80.0   Arthrotomy for removal of prosthesis, without replacement**
Includes: removal of posterior spinal motion preservation (dynamic stabilization, facet replacement, interspinous process) device(s)

Code also any:
insertion of (cement) (joint) (methylmethacrylate) spacer (84.56)
removal of (cement) (joint) (methylmethacrylate) spacer (84.57)

> Excludes: *removal of pedicle screws used in spinal fusion (78.69)*

80.00   Arthrotomy for removal of prosthesis without replacement, unspecified site

80.01   Arthrotomy for removal of prosthesis without replacement, shoulder

80.02   Arthrotomy for removal of prosthesis without replacement, elbow

80.03   Arthrotomy for removal of prosthesis without replacement, wrist

80.04   Arthrotomy for removal of prosthesis without replacement, hand and finger

80.05   Arthrotomy for removal of prosthesis without replacement, hip

80.06   Arthrotomy for removal of prosthesis without replacement, knee

80.07   Arthrotomy for removal of prosthesis without replacement, ankle

80.08   Arthrotomy for removal of prosthesis without replacement, foot and toe

80.09   Arthrotomy for removal of prosthesis without replacement, other specified sites

④ **80.1** **Other arthrotomy**
Arthrostomy

> Excludes: *that for:*
> *arthrography (88.32)*
> *arthroscopy (80.20-80.29)*
> *injection of drug (81.92)*
> *operative approach—omit code*

④ **80.2** **Arthroscopy**

④ **80.3** **Biopsy of joint structure**
Aspiration biopsy

④ **80.4** **Division of joint capsule, ligament, or cartilage**
Goldner clubfoot release
Heyman-Herndon(-Strong) correction of metatarsus varus
Release of:
  adherent or constrictive joint capsule
  joint
  ligament

> Excludes: *symphysiotomy to assist delivery (73.94)*
> *that for:*
> *carpal tunnel syndrome (04.43)*
> *tarsal tunnel syndrome (04.44)*

80.5 **Excision, destruction and other repair of intervertebral disc**

80.50 **Excision or destruction of intervertebral disc, unspecified**
Unspecified as to excision or destruction

80.51 **Excision of intervertebral disc**
Diskectomy
Levels:
  cervical
  lumbar (lumbosacral)
  thoracic
Removal of herniated nucleus pulposus
That by laminotomy or hemilaminectomy
That with decompression of spinal nerve root at same level
Requires additional code for any concomitant decompression of spinal nerve root at
  different level from excision site

Code also any concurrent spinal fusion (81.00-81.09)

Code also any repair of the anulus fibrosus (80.53-80.54)

> Excludes: *intervertebral chemonucleolysis (80.52)*
> *laminectomy for exploration of intraspinal canal (03.09)*
> *laminotomy for decompression of spinal nerve root only (03.09)*
> *that for insertion of (non-fusion) spinal disc replacement device*
>   *(84.60-84.69)*
> *that with corpectomy, (vertebral) (80.99)*

80.52 **Intervertebral chemonucleolysis**
Injection of proteolytic enzyme into intervertebral space (chymopapain)
With aspiration of disc fragments
With diskography

> Excludes: *injection of anesthetic substance (03.91)*
> *injection of other substances (03.92)*

80.53 **Repair of the anulus fibrosus with graft or prosthesis**
Anular disc repair
Closure (sealing) of the anulus fibrosus defect
Includes:
  microsurgical suture repair with fascial autograft
  soft tissue re-approximation repair with tension bands
  surgical mesh repair

Code also any"
  application or administration of adhesion barrier substance, if performed (99.77)
  intervertebral discectomy, if performed (80.51)
  locally harvested fascia for graft (83.43)

● Code new
  to this edition

▲ Revision of
  existing code

④ ⑤ Fourth or fifth
  digit required

80.54 Other and unspecified repair of the anulus fibrosus
Anular disc repair
Closure (sealing) of the anulus fibrosus defect
Microsurgical suture repair without fascial autograft
Percutaneous repair of the anulus fibrosus

Code also any:
  application or administration of adhesion barrier substance, if performed (99.77)
  intervertebral discectomy, if performed (80.51)

80.59 Other destruction of intervertebral disc
Destruction NEC
That by laser

80.6 Excision of semilunar cartilage of knee
Excision of meniscus of knee

④ **80.7 Synovectomy**
Complete or partial resection of synovial membrane

| Excludes: | excision of Baker's cyst (83.39) |

④ **80.8 Other local excision or destruction of lesion of joint**

④ **80.9 Other excision of joint**

| Excludes: | cheilectomy of joint (77.80-77.89) |
| | excision of bone ends (77.80-77.89) |

81 Repair and plastic operations on joint structures

81.0 Spinal fusion
Note: Spinal fusion is classified by the anatomic portion (column) fused and the technique
(approach) used to perform the fusion.

For the anterior column, the body (corpus) of adjacent vertebrae are fused (interbody
fusion). The anterior column can be fused using an anterior, lateral, or posterior technique.

For the posterior column, posterior structures of adjacent vertebrae are fused (pedicle,
lamina, facet, transverse process, or "gutter" fusion). A posterior column fusion can be
performed using a posterior, posterolateral, or lateral transverse technique.

Code also any insertion of interbody spinal fusion device (84.51)
Code also any insertion of recombinant bone morphogenetic protein (84.52)
Code also any synchronous excision of (locally) harvested bone for graft (77.70-77.79)
Code also the total number of vertebrae fused (81.62-81.64)
Includes: arthrodesis of spine with:
                bone graft
                internal fixation

| Excludes: | correction of pseudarthrosis of spine (81.30-81.39) |
| | refusion of spine (81.30-81.39) |

81.00 Spinal fusion, not otherwise specified

81.01 Atlas-axis spinal fusion
Craniocervical fusion by anterior transoral or posterior technique
C1-C2 fusion by anterior transoral or posterior technique
Occiput-C2 fusion by anterior transoral or posterior technique

81.02 Other cervical fusion of the anterior column, anterior technique
Arthrodesis of C2 level or below:
  anterior interbody fusion
  anterolateral technique

81.03 Other cervical fusion of the posterior column, posterior technique
Arthrodesis of C2 level or below, posterolateral technique

81.04 Dorsal and dorsolumbar fusion of the anterior column, anterior technique
Arthrodesis of thoracic or thoracolumbar region:
  anterior interbody fusion
  anterolateral technique
Extracavitary technique

81.05 Dorsal and dorsolumbar fusion of the posterior column, posterior technique
Arthrodesis of thoracic or thoracolumbar region, posterolateral technique

| | Valid O.R. procedure | | Non-O.R. procedure | | Nonspecific O.R. procedure | | Bilateral procedure |

81.06 Lumbar and lumbosacral fusion of the anterior column, anterior technique
> Anterior lumbar interbody fusion (ALIF)
> Arthrodesis of lumbar or lumbosacral region:
>> anterior interbody fusion
>> anterolateral technique
>> retroperitoneal
>> transperitoneal
> Direct lateral interbody fusion [DLIF]
> Extreme lateral interbody fusion [XLIF]

81.07 Lumbar and lumbosacral fusion of the posterior column, posterior technique
> Facet fusion
> Posterolateral technique
> Transverse process technique

81.08 Lumbar and lumbosacral fusion of the anterior column, posterior technique
> Arthrodesis of lumbar or lumbosacral region, posterior interbody fusion
> Axial lumbar interbody fusion [AxiaLIF]
> Posterior lumbar interbody fusion (PLIF)
> Transforaminal lumbar interbody fusion (TLIF)

81.1 Arthrodesis and arthroereisis of foot and ankle
> Includes: arthrodesis of foot and ankle with:
>> bone graft
>> external fixation device

81.11 Ankle fusion
> Tibiotalar fusion

81.12 Triple arthrodesis
> Talus to calcaneus and calcaneus to cuboid and navicular

81.13 Subtalar fusion
> Excludes: *arthroereisis (81.18)*

81.14 Midtarsal fusion

81.15 Tarsometatarsal fusion

81.16 Metatarsophalangeal fusion

81.17 Other fusion of foot

81.18 Subtalar joint arthroereisis

81.2 Arthrodesis of other joint
> Includes: arthrodesis with:
>> bone graft
>> external fixation device
>> excision of bone ends and compression

81.20 Arthrodesis of unspecified joint

81.21 Arthrodesis of hip

81.22 Arthrodesis of knee

81.23 Arthrodesis of shoulder

81.24 Arthrodesis of elbow

81.25 Carporadial fusion

81.26 Metacarpocarpal fusion

81.27 Metacarpophalangeal fusion

81.28 Interphalangeal fusion

81.29 Arthrodesis of other specified joints

● Code new
  to this edition
▲ Revision of
  existing code
④ ⑤ Fourth or fifth
  digit required

81.3   Refusion of spine

Note: Spine fusion is classified by the anatomic portion (column) fused and the technique (approach) used to perform the fusion.

For the anterior column, the body (corpus) of adjacent vertebrae are fused (interbody fusion). The anterior column can be fused using an anterior, lateral, or posterior technique.

For the posterior column, posterior structures of adjacent vertebrae are fused (pedicle, lamina, facet, transverse process, or "gutter" fusion). A posterior column fusion can be performed using a posterior, posterolateral, or lateral transverse technique.

Includes: arthrodesis of spine with:
　　　　　　　bone graft
　　　　　　　internal fixation
　　　　　　correction of pseudarthrosis of spine

Code also any insertion of interbody spinal fusion device (84.51)
Code also any insertion of recombinant bone morphogenetic protein (84.52)
Code also any synchronous excision of (locally) harvested bone for graft (77.70-77.79)
Code also the total number of vertebrae fused (81.62-81.64)

81.30   Refusion of spine, not otherwise specified

81.31   Refusion of atlas-axis spine
Craniocervical fusion by anterior, transoral or posterior technique
C1-C2 fusion by anterior, transoral or posterior technique
Occiput C2 fusion by anterior, transoral or posterior technique

81.32   Refusion of other cervical spine, anterior column, anterior technique
Arthrodesis of C2 level or below:
　anterior interbody fusion
　anterolateral technique

81.33   Refusion of other cervical spine, posterior column, posterior technique
Arthrodesis of C2 level or below, posterolateral technique

81.34   Refusion of dorsal and dorsolumbar spine, anterior column, anterior technique
Arthrodesis of thoracic or thoracolumbar region, anterior interbody fusion
Extracavitary technique

81.35   Refusion of dorsal and dorsolumbar spine, posterior column, posterior technique
Arthrodesis of thoracic and thoracolumbar region, posterolateral technique

81.36   Refusion of lumbar and lumbosacral spine, anterior column, anterior technique
Anterior lumbar interbody fusion (ALIF)
Arthrodesis of lumbar or lumbosacral region:
　anterior interbody fusion
　anterolateral technique
　retroperitoneal
　transperitoneal
Direct lateral interbody fusion [DLIF]
Extreme lateral interbody fusion [XLIF]

81.37   Refusion of lumbar and lumbosacral spine, posterior column, posterior technique
Facet fusion
Posterolateral technique
Transverse process technique

81.38   Refusion of lumbar and lumbosacral spine, anterior column, posterior technique
Arthrodesis of lumbar or lumbosacral region, posterior interbody fusion
Axial lumbar interbody fusion [AxiaLIF]
Posterior lumbar interbody fusion (PLIF)
Transforaminal lumbar interbody fusion (TLIF)

81.39   Refusion of spine, not elsewhere classified

81.4   Other repair of joint of lower extremity
Includes: arthroplasty of lower extremity with:
　　　　　　　external traction or fixation
　　　　　　　graft of bone chips or cartilage
　　　　　　　internal fixation device

81.40   Repair of hip, not elsewhere classified

81.42   Five-in-one repair of knee
Medial meniscectomy, medial collateral ligament repair, vastus medialis advancement, semitendinosus advancement, and pes anserinus transfer

---

Valid O.R. procedure　　Non-O.R. procedure　　Nonspecific O.R. procedure　　Noncovered O.R. procedure

81.43 Triad knee repair
Medial meniscectomy with repair of the anterior cruciate ligament and the medial
collateral ligament
O'Donoghue procedure

81.44 Patellar stabilization
Roux-Goldthwait operation for recurrent dislocation of patella

81.45 Other repair of the cruciate ligaments

81.46 Other repair of the collateral ligaments

81.47 Other repair of knee

81.49 Other repair of ankle

81.5   Joint replacement of lower extremity
Note: Removal of prior prosthesis — *omit code*
Includes: arthroplasty of lower extremity with:
external traction or fixation
graft of bone (chips) or cartilage
internal fixation device or prosthesis

81.51 Total hip replacement
Replacement of both femoral head and acetabulum by prosthesis
Total reconstruction of hip
Code also any type of bearing surface, if known (00.74-00.77)

81.52 Partial hip replacement
Bipolar endoprosthesis
Code also any type of bearing surface, if known (00.74-00.77)

81.53 Revision of hip replacement, not otherwise specified
Revision of hip replacement, not specified as to component(s) replaced, (acetabular,
femoral or both)
Code also any:
removal of (cement) (joint) spacer (84.57)
type of bearing surface, if known (00.74-00.77)

| Excludes: | *revision of hip replacement, components specified (00.70-00.73)* |

81.54 Total knee replacement
Bicompartmental
Partial knee replacement
Tricompartmental
Unicompartmental (hemijoint)

81.55 Revision of knee replacement, not otherwise specified
Code also any removal of (cement) spacer (84.57)

| Excludes: | *arthrodesis of knee (81.22)* |
| | *revision of knee replacement, components specified (00.80-00.84)* |

81.56 Total ankle replacement

81.57 Replacement of joint of foot and toe

81.59 Revision of joint replacement of lower extremity, not elsewhere classified

81.6   Other procedures on spine
Note: Number of vertebrae
The vertebral spine consists of 25 vertebrae in the following order and number:
Cervical: C1 (atlas), C2 (axis), C3, C4, C5, C6, C7
Thoracic or Dorsal: T1, T2, T3, T4, T5, T6, T7, T8, T9, T10, T11, T12
Lumbar or Sacral: L1, L2, L3, L4, L5, S1

Coders should report only one code from the series 81.62 or 81.63 or 81.64 to show the
total number of vertebrae fused on the patient.
Code also the level and approach of the fusion or refusion (81.00-81.08, 81.30-81.39)

81.62 Fusion or refusion of 2-3 vertebrae

81.63 Fusion or refusion of 4-8 vertebrae

81.64 Fusion or refusion of 9 or more vertebrae

81.65 Percutaneous vertebroplasty
Injection of bone void filler (cement) (polymethylmethacrylate) (PMMA) into the
diseased or fractured vertebral body

| Excludes: | *kyphoplasty (81.66)* |
| | *percutaneous vertebral augmentation (81.66)* |

● Code new
to this edition   ▲ Revision of
existing code   ④ ⑤ Fourth or fifth
digit required

81.66 **Percutaneous vertebral augmentation**

Insertion of inflatable balloon, bone tamp, or other device displacing (removing) (compacting) bone to create a space (cavity) (void) prior to the injection of bone void filler (cement) (polymethylmethacrylate) (PMMA) or other substance

Arcuplasty
Kyphoplasty
SKyphoplasty
Spineoplasty

Excludes: percutaneous vertebroplasty (81.65)

81.7 **Arthroplasty and repair of hand, fingers, and wrist**

Includes: arthroplasty of hand and finger with:
external traction or fixation
graft of bone (chips) or cartilage
internal fixation device or prosthesis

Excludes: operations on muscle, tendon, and fascia of hand (82.01-82.99)

81.71 **Arthroplasty of metacarpophalangeal and interphalangeal joint with implant**

81.72 **Arthroplasty of metacarpophalangeal and interphalangeal joint without implant**

81.73 **Total wrist replacement**

81.74 **Arthroplasty of carpocarpal or carpometacarpal joint with implant**

81.75 **Arthroplasty of carpocarpal or carpometacarpal joint without implant**

81.79 **Other repair of hand, fingers, and wrist**

81.8 **Arthroplasty and repair of shoulder and elbow**

Includes: arthroplasty of upper limb NEC with:
external traction or fixation
graft of bone (chips) or cartilage
internal fixation device or prosthesis

81.80 **Other total shoulder replacement**

Excludes: reverse total shoulder replacement (81.88)

81.81 **Partial shoulder replacement**

81.82 **Repair of recurrent dislocation of shoulder**

81.83 **Other repair of shoulder**

81.84 **Total elbow replacement**
Partial elbow replacement

81.85 **Other repair of elbow**

81.88 **Reverse total shoulder replacement**
Reverse ball-and-socket of the shoulder

Excludes: conversion of prior (failed) total shoulder replacement (arthroplasty) to reverse total shoulder replacement (81.97)

81.9 **Other operations on joint structures**

81.91 **Arthrocentesis**
Joint aspiration

Excludes: that for:
arthrography (88.32)
biopsy of joint structure (80.30-80.39)
injection of drug (81.92)

81.92 **Injection of therapeutic substance into joint or ligament**

81.93 **Suture of capsule or ligament of upper extremity**

Excludes: that associated with arthroplasty (81.71-81.75, 81.80-81.81, 81.84)

81.94 **Suture of capsule or ligament of ankle and foot**

Excludes: that associated with arthroplasty (81.56-81.59)

81.95 **Suture of capsule or ligament of other lower extremity**

Excludes: that associated with arthroplasty (81.51-81.55, 81.59)

81.96 **Other repair of joint**

81.97 **Revision of joint replacement of upper extremity**
Partial   Total
Revision of arthroplasty of shoulder
Includes: removal of cement spacer

Valid O.R. procedure   Non-O.R. procedure   Nonspecific O.R. procedure   Noncovered O.R. procedure

81.98 Other diagnostic procedures on joint structures

> *Excludes:* *arthroscopy (80.20-80.29)*
> *biopsy of joint structure (80.30-80.39)*
> *microscopic examination of specimen from joint (91.51-91.59)*
> *thermography (88.83)*
> *x-ray (87.21-87.29, 88.21-88.33)*

81.99 Other

82 Operations on muscle, tendon, and fascia of hand
Includes: operations on:
aponeurosis
synovial membrane (tendon sheath)
tendon sheath

82.0   Incision of muscle, tendon, fascia, and bursa of hand

82.01 Exploration of tendon sheath of hand
Incision of tendon sheath of hand
Removal of rice bodies in tendon sheath of hand

> *Excludes:* *division of tendon (82.11)*

82.02 Myotomy of hand

> *Excludes:* *myotomy for division (82.19)*

82.03 Bursotomy of hand

82.04 Incision and drainage of palmar or thenar space

82.09 Other incision of soft tissue of hand

> *Excludes:* *incision of skin and subcutaneous tissue alone (86.01-86.09)*

82.1   Division of muscle, tendon, and fascia of hand

82.11 Tenotomy of hand
Division of tendon of hand

82.12 Fasciotomy of hand
Division of fascia of hand

82.19 Other division of soft tissue of hand
Division of muscle of hand

82.2   Excision of lesion of muscle, tendon, and fascia of hand

82.21 Excision of lesion of tendon sheath of hand
Ganglionectomy of tendon sheath (wrist)

82.22 Excision of lesion of muscle of hand

82.29 Excision of other lesion of soft tissue of hand

> *Excludes:* *excision of lesion of skin and subcutaneous tissue (86.21-86.3)*

82.3   Other excision of soft tissue of hand
Code also any skin graft (86.61-86.62, 86.73)

> *Excludes:* *excision of skin and subcutaneous tissue (86.21-86.3)*

82.31 Bursectomy of hand

82.32 Excision of tendon of hand for graft

82.33 Other tenonectomy of hand
Tenosynovectomy of hand

> *Excludes:* *excision of lesion of:*
> *tendon (82.29)*
> *sheath (82.21)*

82.34 Excision of muscle or fascia of hand for graft

82.35 Other fasciectomy of hand
Release of Dupuytren's contracture

> *Excludes:* *excision of lesion of fascia (82.29)*

82.36 Other myectomy of hand

> *Excludes:* *excision of lesion of muscle (82.22)*

82.39 Other excision of soft tissue of hand

> *Excludes:* *excision of skin (86.21-86.3)*
> *excision of soft tissue lesion (82.29)*

82.4   Suture of muscle, tendon, and fascia of hand

● Code new   ▲ Revision of   ④ ⑤ Fourth or fifth
     to this edition   existing code   digit required

82.41 **Suture of tendon sheath of hand**

82.42 **Delayed suture of flexor tendon of hand**

82.43 **Delayed suture of other tendon of hand**

82.44 **Other suture of flexor tendon of hand**

Excludes: *delayed suture of flexor tendon of hand (82.42)*

82.45 **Other suture of other tendon of hand**

Excludes: *delayed suture of other tendon of hand (82.43)*

82.46 **Suture of muscle or fascia of hand**

82.5 **Transplantation of muscle and tendon of hand**

82.51 **Advancement of tendon of hand**

82.52 **Recession of tendon of hand**

82.53 **Reattachment of tendon of hand**

82.54 **Reattachment of muscle of hand**

82.55 **Other change in hand muscle or tendon length**

82.56 **Other hand tendon transfer or transplantation**

Excludes: *pollicization of thumb (82.61)*
transfer of finger, except thumb (82.81)

82.57 **Other hand tendon transposition**

82.58 **Other hand muscle transfer or transplantation**

82.59 **Other hand muscle transposition**

82.6 **Reconstruction of thumb**
Includes: digital transfer to act as thumb
Code also any amputation for digital transfer (84.01, 84.11)

82.61 **Pollicization operation carrying over nerves and blood supply**

82.69 **Other reconstruction of thumb**
"Cocked-hat" procedure [skin flap and bone]
Grafts:
bone to thumb
skin (pedicle) to thumb

82.7 **Plastic operation on hand with graft or implant**

82.71 **Tendon pulley reconstruction**
Reconstruction for opponensplasty

82.72 **Plastic operation on hand with graft of muscle or fascia**

82.79 **Plastic operation on hand with other graft or implant**
Tendon graft to hand

82.8 **Other plastic operations on hand**

82.81 **Transfer of finger, except thumb**

Excludes: *pollicization of thumb (82.61)*

82.82 **Repair of cleft hand**

82.83 **Repair of macrodactyly**

82.84 **Repair of mallet finger**

82.85 **Other tenodesis of hand**
Tendon fixation of hand NOS

82.86 **Other tenoplasty of hand**
Myotenoplasty of hand

82.89 **Other plastic operations on hand**
Plication of fascia
Repair of fascial hernia

Excludes: *that with graft or implant (82.71-82.79)*

82.9 **Other operations on muscle, tendon, and fascia of hand**

Excludes: *diagnostic procedures on soft tissue of hand (83.21-83.29)*

82.91 **Lysis of adhesions of hand**
Freeing of adhesions of fascia, muscle, and tendon of hand

Excludes: *decompression of carpal tunnel (04.43)*
that by stretching or manipulation only (93.26)

Valid O.R. procedure   Non-O.R. procedure   Nonspecific O.R. procedure   Noncovered O.R. procedure

82.92 **Aspiration of bursa of hand**

82.93 **Aspiration of other soft tissue of hand**

> Excludes: *skin and subcutaneous tissue (86.01)*

82.94 **Injection of therapeutic substance into bursa of hand**

82.95 **Injection of therapeutic substance into tendon of hand**

82.96 **Other injection of locally-acting therapeutic substance into soft tissue of hand**

> Excludes: *subcutaneous or intramuscular injection (99.11-99.29)*

82.99 **Other operations on muscle, tendon, and fascia of hand**

83 **Operations on muscle, tendon, fascia, and bursa, except hand**

Includes: operations on:
aponeurosis
synovial membrane of bursa and tendon sheaths
tendon sheaths

> Excludes: *diaphragm (34.81-34.89)*
> *hand (82.01-82.99)*
> *muscles of eye (15.01-15.9).*

83.0 **Incision of muscle, tendon, fascia, and bursa**

83.01 **Exploration of tendon sheath**
Incision of tendon sheath
Removal of rice bodies from tendon sheath

83.02 **Myotomy**

> Excludes: *cricopharyngeal myotomy (29.31)*

83.03 **Bursotomy**
Removal of calcareous deposit of bursa

> Excludes: *aspiration of bursa (percutaneous) (83.94)*

83.09 **Other incision of soft tissue**
Incision of fascia

> Excludes: *incision of skin and subcutaneous tissue alone (86.01-86.09)*

83.1 **Division of muscle, tendon, and fascia**

83.11 **Achillotenotomy**

83.12 **Adductor tenotomy of hip**

83.13 **Other tenotomy**
Aponeurotomy
Division of tendon
Tendon release
Tendon transection
Tenotomy for thoracic outlet decompression

83.14 **Fasciotomy**
Division of fascia
Division of iliotibial band
Fascia stripping
Release of Volkmann's contracture by fasciotomy

83.19 **Other division of soft tissue**
Division of muscle
Muscle release
Myotomy for thoracic outlet decompression
Myotomy with division
Scalenotomy
Transection of muscle

83.2 **Diagnostic procedures on muscle, tendon, fascia, and bursa, including that of hand**

83.21 **Open biopsy of soft tissue**

> Excludes: *biopsy of chest wall (34.23)*
> *closed biopsy of skin and subcutaneous tissue (86.11)*

83.29 **Other diagnostic procedures on muscle, tendon, fascia, and bursa, including that of hand**

> Excludes: *microscopic examination of specimen (91.51-91.59)*
> *soft tissue x-ray (87.09, 87.38-87.39, 88.09, 88.35, 88.37)*
> *thermography of muscle (88.84)*

● Code new
to this edition
▲ Revision of
existing code
④ ⑤ Fourth or fifth
digit required

83.3 **Excision of lesion of muscle, tendon, fascia, and bursa**

> Excludes: biopsy of soft tissue (83.21)

83.31 **Excision of lesion of tendon sheath**
Excision of ganglion of tendon sheath, except of hand

83.32 **Excision of lesion of muscle**
Excision of:
    heterotopic bone
    muscle scar for release of Volkmann's contracture
    myositis ossificans

83.39 **Excision of lesion of other soft tissue**
Excision of Baker's cyst

> Excludes: bursectomy (83.5)
> excision of lesion of skin and subcutaneous tissue (86.3)
> synovectomy (80.70-80.79)

83.4 **Other excision of muscle, tendon, and fascia**

83.41 **Excision of tendon for graft**

83.42 **Other tenonectomy**
Excision of:
    aponeurosis
    tendon sheath
Tenosynovectomy

83.43 **Excision of muscle or fascia for graft**

83.44 **Other fasciectomy**

83.45 **Other myectomy**
Debridement of muscle NOS
Scalenectomy

83.49 **Other excision of soft tissue**

83.5 **Bursectomy**

83.6 **Suture of muscle, tendon, and fascia**

83.61 **Suture of tendon sheath**

83.62 **Delayed suture of tendon**

83.63 **Rotator cuff repair**

83.64 **Other suture of tendon**
Achillorrhaphy
Aponeurorrhaphy

> Excludes: delayed suture of tendon (83.62)

83.65 **Other suture of muscle or fascia**
Repair of diastasis recti

83.7 **Reconstruction of muscle and tendon**

> Excludes: reconstruction of muscle and tendon associated with arthroplasty

83.71 **Advancement of tendon**

83.72 **Recession of tendon**

83.73 **Reattachment of tendon**

83.74 **Reattachment of muscle**

83.75 **Tendon transfer or transplantation**

83.76 **Other tendon transposition**

83.77 **Muscle transfer or transplantation**
Release of Volkmann's contracture by muscle transplantation

83.79 **Other muscle transposition**

83.8 **Other plastic operations on muscle, tendon, and fascia**

> Excludes: plastic operations on muscle, tendon, and fascia associated with arthroplasty

83.81 **Tendon graft**

83.82 **Graft of muscle or fascia**

83.83 **Tendon pulley reconstruction**

83.84 **Release of clubfoot, not elsewhere classified**
Evans operation on clubfoot

	Valid O.R. procedure		Non-O.R. procedure		Nonspecific O.R. procedure		Noncovered O.R. procedure

83.85 **Other change in muscle or tendon length**
Hamstring lengthening
Heel cord shortening
Plastic achillotenotomy
Tendon plication

83.86 **Quadricepsplasty**

83.87 **Other plastic operations on muscle**
Musculoplasty
Myoplasty

83.88 **Other plastic operations on tendon**
Myotenoplasty
Tendon fixation
Tenodesis
Tenoplasty

83.89 **Other plastic operations on fascia**
Fascia lengthening
Fascioplasty
Plication of fascia

83.9 **Other operations on muscle, tendon, fascia, and bursa**

Excludes: *nonoperative:*
manipulation (93.25-93.29)
stretching (93.27-93.29)

83.91 **Lysis of adhesions of muscle, tendon, fascia,and bursa**

Excludes: *that for tarsal tunnel syndrome (04.44)*

83.92 **Insertion or replacement of skeletal muscle stimulator**
Implantation, insertion, placement, or replacement of skeletal muscle:
electrodes
stimulator

83.93 **Removal of skeletal muscle stimulator**

83.94 **Aspiration of bursa**

83.95 **Aspiration of other soft tissue**

Excludes: *that of skin and subcutaneous tissue (86.01)*

83.96 **Injection of therapeutic substance into bursa**

83.97 **Injection of therapeutic substance into tendon**

83.98 **Injection of locally-acting therapeutic substance into other soft tissue**

Excludes: *subcutaneous or intramuscular injection (99.11-99.29)*

83.99 **Other operations on muscle, tendon, fascia and bursa**
Suture of bursa

84 **Other procedures on musculoskeletal system**

84.0 **Amputation of upper limb**

Excludes: *revision of amputation stump (84.3)*

84.00 **Upper limb amputation, not otherwise specified**
Closed flap amputation of upper limb NOS
Kineplastic amputation of upper limb NOS
Open or guillotine amputation of upper limb NOS
Revision of current traumatic amputation of upper limb NOS

84.01 **Amputation and disarticulation of finger**

Excludes: *ligation of supernumerary finger (86.26)*

84.02 **Amputation and disarticulation of thumb**

84.03 **Amputation through hand**
Amputation through carpals

84.04 **Disarticulation of wrist**

84.05 **Amputation through forearm**
Forearm amputation

84.06 **Disarticulation of elbow**

84.07 **Amputation through humerus**
Upper arm amputation

84.08 **Disarticulation of shoulder**

● Code new
to this edition
▲ Revision of
existing code
④ ⑤ Fourth or fifth
digit required

84.09 Interthoracoscapular amputation
Forequarter amputation

84.1 Amputation of lower limb

> Excludes: *revision of amputation stump (84.3)*

84.10 Lower limb amputation, not otherwise specified
Closed flap amputation of lower limb NOS
Kineplastic amputation of lower limb NOS
Open or guillotine amputation of lower limb NOS
Revision of current traumatic amputation of lower limb NOS

84.11 Amputation of toe
Amputation through metatarsophalangeal joint
Disarticulation of toe
Metatarsal head amputation
Ray amputation of foot (disarticulation of the metatarsal head of the toe extending across the forefoot just proximal to the metatarsophalangeal crease)

> Excludes: *ligation of supernumerary toe (86.26)*

84.12 Amputation through foot
Amputation of forefoot
Amputation through middle of foot
Chopart's amputation
Midtarsal amputation
Transmetatarsal amputation (amputation of the forefoot, including all the toes)

> Excludes: *ray amputation of foot (84.11)*

84.13 Disarticulation of ankle

84.14 Amputation of ankle through malleoli of tibia and fibula

84.15 Other amputation below knee
Amputation of leg through tibia and fibula NOS

84.16 Disarticulation of knee
Batch, Spitler, and McFaddin amputation
Mazet amputation
S.P. Roger's amputation

84.17 Amputation above knee
Amputation of leg through femur
Amputation of thigh
Conversion of below-knee amputation into above-knee amputation
Supracondylar above-knee amputation

84.18 Disarticulation of hip

84.19 Abdominopelvic amputation
Hemipelvectomy
Hindquarter amputation

84.2 Reattachment of extremity

84.21 Thumb reattachment

84.22 Finger reattachment

84.23 Forearm, wrist, or hand reattachment

84.24 Upper arm reattachment
Reattachment of arm NOS

84.25 Toe reattachment

84.26 Foot reattachment

84.27 Lower leg or ankle reattachment
Reattachment of leg NOS

84.28 Thigh reattachment

84.29 Other reattachment

84.3 Revision of amputation stump
Reamputation of stump
Secondary closure of stump
Trimming of stump

> Excludes: *revision of current traumatic amputation [revision by further amputation of current injury] (84.00-84.19, 84.91)*

84.4 Implantation or fitting of prosthetic limb device

84.40 Implantation or fitting of prosthetic limb device not otherwise specified

Valid O.R. procedure	Non-O.R. procedure	Nonspecific O.R. procedure	Noncovered O.R. procedure

84.41   Fitting of prosthesis of upper arm and shoulder

84.42   Fitting of prosthesis of lower arm and hand

84.43   Fitting of prosthesis of arm, not otherwise specified

84.44   Implantation of prosthetic device of arm

84.45   Fitting of prosthesis above knee

84.46   Fitting of prosthesis below knee

84.47   Fitting of prosthesis of leg, not otherwise specified

84.48   Implantation of prosthetic device of leg

84.5   **Implantation of other musculoskeletal devices and substances**

84.51   **Insertion of interbody spinal fusion device**
Insertion of:
  cages (carbon, ceramic, metal, plastic, or titanium)
  interbody fusion cage
  synthetic cages or spacers
  threaded bone dowels
Code also refusion of spine (81.30-81.39)
Code also spinal fusion (81.00-81.08)
Excludes: *insertion of (non-fusion) spinal disc replacement device (84.60-84.69)*

84.52   **Insertion of recombinant bone morphogenetic protein rhBMP**
That via collagen sponge, coral, ceramic and other carriers
Code also primary procedure performed:
  fracture repair (79.00-79.99)
  spinal fusion (81.00-81.08)
  spinal refusion (81.30-81.39)

84.53   **Implantation of internal limb lengthening device with kinetic distraction**
Code also limb lengthening procedure (78.30-78.39)

84.54   **Implantation of other internal limb lengthening device**
Implantation of internal limb lengthening device, not otherwise specified (NOS)
Code also limb lengthening procedure (78.30-78.39)

84.55   **Insertion of bone void filler**
Insertion of:
  acrylic cement (PMMA)
  bone void cement
  calcium based bone void filler
  polymethylmethacrylate (PMMA)
Excludes: *that with percutaneous vertebral augmentation (81.66)*
          that with percutaneous vertebroplasty (81.65)

84.56   **Insertion or replacement of (cement) spacer**
Insertion or replacement of joint (methylmethacrylate) spacer

84.57   **Removal of (cement) spacer**
Removal of joint (methylmethacrylate) spacer

84.59   **Insertion of other spinal devices**
Excludes: *initial insertion of pedicle screws with spinal fusion-omit code*
          insertion of facet replacement device(s) (84.84)
          insertion of interspinous process device(s) (84.80)
          insertion of pedicle-based dynamic stabilization device(s) (84.82)

84.6   **Replacement of spinal disc**
Includes: non-fusion arthroplasty of the spine with insertion of artificial disc prosthesis

84.60   **Insertion of spinal disc prosthesis, not otherwise specified**
Replacement of spinal disc, NOS
Includes: diskectomy (discectomy)

84.61   **Insertion of partial spinal disc prosthesis, cervical**
Nuclear replacement device, cervical
Partial artificial disc prosthesis (flexible), cervical
Replacement of nuclear disc (nucleus pulposus), cervical
Includes: diskectomy (discectomy)

84.62   **Insertion of total spinal disc prosthesis, cervical**
Replacement of cervial spinal disc, NOS
Replacement of total spinal disc, cervical
Total artificial disc prosthesis (flexible), cervical
Includes: diskectomy (discectomy)

● Code new to this edition   ▲ Revision of existing code   ④ ⑤ Fourth or fifth digit required

84.63 Insertion of spinal disc prosthesis, thoracic
Artificial disc prosthesis (flexible), thoracic
Replacement of thoracic spinal disc, partial or total
Includes: diskectomy (discectomy)

84.64 Insertion of partial spinal disc prosthesis, lumbosacral
Nuclear replacement device, lumbar
Partial artificial disc prosthesis (flexible), lumbar
Replacement of nuclear disc (nucleus pulposus), lumbar
Includes: diskectomy (discectomy)

84.65 Insertion of total spinal disc prosthesis, lumbosacral
Replacement of lumbar spinal disc, NOS
Replacement of total spinal disc, lumbar
Total artificial disc prosthesis (flexible), lumbar
Includes: diskectomy (discectomy)

84.66 Revision or replacement of artificial spinal disc prosthesis, cervical
Removal of (partial) (total) spinal disc prosthesis with synchronous insertion of new (partial) (total) spinal disc prosthesis, cervical
Repair of previously inserted spinal disc prosthesis, cervical

84.67 Revision or replacement of artificial spinal disc prosthesis, thoracic
Removal of (partial) (total) spinal disc prosthesis with synchronous insertion of new (partial) (total) spinal disc prosthesis, thoracic
Repair of previously inserted spinal disc prosthesis, thoracic

84.68 Revision or replacement of artificial spinal disc prosthesis, lumbosacral
Removal of (partial) (total) spinal disc prosthesis with synchronous insertion of new (partial) (total) spinal disc prosthesis, lumbosacral
Repair of previously inserted spinal disc prosthesis, lumbosacral

84.69 Revision or replacement of artificial spinal disc prosthesis, not otherwise specified
Removal of (partial) (total) spinal disc prosthesis with synchronous insertion of new (partial) (total) spinal disc prosthesis
Repair of previously inserted spinal disc prosthesis

84.7 Adjunct codes for external fixator devices
Code also any primary procedure performed:
application of external fixator device (78.10, 78.12-78.13, 78.15, 78.17-78.19)
reduction of fracture and dislocation (79.00-79.89)

84.71 Application of external fixator device, monoplanar system
Excludes: *other hybrid device or system (84.73)*
ring device or system (84.72)

84.72 Application of external fixator device, ring system
Ilizarov type
Sheffield type
Excludes: *monoplanar device or system (84.71)*
other hybrid device or system (84.73)

84.73 Application of hybrid external fixator device
Computer (assisted) (dependent) external fixator device
Hybrid system using both ring and monoplanar devices
Excludes: *monoplanar device or system, when used alone (84.71)*
ring device or system, when used alone (84.72)

84.8 Insertion, replacement and revision of posterior spinal motion preservation device(s)
Dynamic spinal stabilization device(s)
Includes: any synchronous facetectomy (partial, total) performed at the same level
Code also any synchronous surgical decompression (foraminotomy, laminectomy, laminotomy), if performed (03.09)
Excludes: *fusion of spine (81.00 – 81.08, 81.30-81.39)*
insertion of artificial disc prosthesis (84.60-84.69)
insertion of interbody spinal fusion device (84.51)

84.80 Insertion or replacement of interspinous process device(s)
Interspinous process decompression device(s)
Interspinous process distraction device(s)
Excludes: *insertion or replacement of facet replacement device (84.84)*
insertion or replacement of pedicle-based dynamic stabilization device (84.82)

	Valid O.R. procedure		Non-O.R. procedure		Nonspecific O.R. procedure		Noncovered O.R. procedure

84.81 Revision of interspinous process device(s)
Repair of previously inserted interspinous process device(s)

> Excludes: revision of facet replacement device(s) (84.85)
> revision of pedicle-based dynamic stabilization device (84.83)

84.82 Insertion or replacement of pedicle-based dynamic stabilization device(s)

> Excludes: initial insertion of pedicle screws with spinal fusion – omit code
> insertion or replacement of facet replacement device(s) (84.84)
> insertion or replacement of interspinous process device(s) (84.80)
> replacement of pedicle screws used in spinal fusion (78.59)

84.83 Revision of pedicle-based dynamic stabilization device(s)
Repair of previously inserted pedicle-based dynamic stabilization device(s)

> Excludes: removal of pedicle screws used in spinal fusion (78.69)
> replacement of pedicle screws used in spinal fusion (78.59)
> revision of facet replacement device(s) (84.85)
> revision of interspinous process device(s) (84.81)

84.84 Insertion or replacement of facet replacement device(s)
Facet arthroplasty

> Excludes: initial insertion of pedicle screws with spinal fusion-omit code
> insertion or replacement of interspinous process device(s) (84.80)
> insertion or replacement of pedicle-based dynamic stabilization device(s) (84.82)
> replacement of pedicle screws used in spinal fusion (78.59)

84.85 Revision of facet replacement device(s)
Repair of previously inserted facet replacement device(s)

> Excludes: removal of pedicle screws used in spinal fusion (78.69)
> replacement of pedicle screws used in spinal fusion (78.59)
> revision of interspinous process device(s) (84.81)
> revision of pedicle-based dynamic stabilization device(s) (84.83)

84.9 Other operations on musculoskeletal system

> Excludes: nonoperative manipulation (93.25-93.29)

84.91 Amputation, not otherwise specified

84.92 Separation of equal conjoined twins

84.93 Separation of unequal conjoined twins
Separation of conjoined twins NOS

84.94 Insertion of sternal fixation device with rigid plates

> Excludes: insertion of sternal fixation device for internal fixation of fracture (79.39)
> internal fixation of bone without fracture reduction (78.59)

84.99 Other

● Code new to this edition ▲ Revision of existing code ④ ⑤ Fourth or fifth digit required

15. OPERATIONS ON THE INTEGUMENTARY SYSTEM (85-86)

85   Operations on the breast
Includes: operations on the skin and subcutaneous tissue of:
breast, female or male
previous mastectomy site, female or male
revision of previous mastectomy site

85.0   Mastotomy
Incision of breast (skin)
Mammotomy

Excludes: *aspiration of breast (85.91)*
removal of implant (85.94)

85.1   Diagnostic procedures on breast

85.11   Closed [percutaneous] [needle] biopsy of breast

85.12   Open biopsy of breast

85.19   Other diagnostic procedures on breast

Excludes: *mammary ductogram (87.35)*
mammography NEC (87.37)
manual examination (89.36)
microscopic examination of specimen (91.61-91.69)
thermography (88.85)
ultrasonography (88.73)
xerography (87.36)

85.2   Excision or destruction of breast tissue

Excludes: *mastectomy (85.41-85.48)*
reduction mammoplasty (85.31-85.32)

85.20   Excision or destruction of breast tissue, not otherwise specified

Excludes: *laser interstitial thermal therapy [LITT] of lesion or tissue of breast*
under guidance (17.69)

85.21   Local excision of lesion of breast
Lumpectomy
Removal of area of fibrosis from breast

Excludes: *biopsy of breast (85.11-8.5.12)*

85.22   Resection of quadrant of breast

85.23   Subtotal mastectomy

Excludes: *quadrant resection (85.22)*

85.24   Excision of ectopic breast tissue
Excision of accessory nipple

85.25   Excision of nipple

Excludes: *excision of accessory nipple (85.24)*

85.3   Reduction mammoplasty and subcutaneous mammectomy

85.31   Unilateral reduction mammoplasty
Unilateral:
amputative mammoplasty
size reduction mammoplasty

85.32   Bilateral reduction mammoplasty
Amputative mammoplasty
Reduction mammoplasty (for gynecomastia)

85.33   Unilateral subcutaneous mammectomy with synchronous implant

Excludes: *that without synchronous implant (85.34)*

85.34   Other unilateral subcutaneous mammectomy
Removal of breast tissue with preservation of skin and nipple
Subcutaneous mammectomy NOS

85.35   Bilateral subcutaneous mammectomy with synchronous implant

Excludes: *that without synchronous implant (85.36)*

85.36   Other bilateral subcutaneous mammectomy

Valid O.R.
procedure

Non-O.R.
procedure

Nonspecific
O.R. procedure

Noncovered
O.R. procedure

85.4   Mastectomy

  85.41 Unilateral simple mastectomy
  Mastectomy:
    NOS
    complete

  85.42 Bilateral simple mastectomy
  Bilateral complete mastectomy

  85.43 Unilateral extended simple mastectomy
  Extended simple mastectomy NOS
  Modified radical mastectomy
  Simple mastectomy with excision of regional lymph nodes

  85.44 Bilateral extended simple mastectomy

  85.45 Unilateral radical mastectomy
  Excision of breast, pectoral muscles, and regional lymph nodes [axillary, clavicular, supraclavicular]
  Radical mastectomy NOS

  85.46 Bilateral radical mastectomy

  85.47 Unilateral extended radical mastectomy
  Excision of breast, muscles, and lymph nodes [axillary, clavicular, supraclavicular, internal mammary, and mediastinal]
  Extended radical mastectomy NOS

  85.48 Bilateral extended radical mastectomy

85.5   Augmentation mammoplasty
  Excludes: that associated with subcutaneous mammectomy (85.33, 85.35)

  85.50 Augmentation mammoplasty, not otherwise specified

  85.51 Unilateral injection into breast for augmentation
    Excludes: injection of fat graft of breast (85.55)

  85.52 Bilateral injection into breast for augmentation
  Injection into breast for augmentation NOS
    Excludes: injection of fat graft of breast (85.55)

  85.53 Unilateral breast implant

  85.54 Bilateral breast implant
  Breast implant NOS

  85.55 Fat graft to breast
  Includes: extraction of fat for autologous graft
  Autologous fat transplantation or transfer
  Fat graft to breast NOS
  Fat graft to breast with or without use of enriched graft
  Micro-fat grafting
    Excludes: that with reconstruction of breast (85.70 –85.79)

85.6   Mastopexy

85.7   Total reconstruction of breast

  85.70 Total reconstruction of breast, not otherwise specified
  Perforator flap, free

  85.71 Latissimus dorsi myocutaneous flap

  85.72 Transverse rectus abdominus myocutaneous (TRAM) flap, pedicled
    Excludes: transverse rectus abdominis myocutaneous (TRAM) flap, free (85.73)

  85.73 Transverse rectus abdominis myocutaneous (TRAM) flap, free
    Excludes: transverse rectus abdominis myocutaneous (TRAM) flap, pedicled (85.72)

  85.74 Deep inferior epigastric artery perforator (DIEP) flap, free

  85.75 Superficial inferior epigastric artery (SIEA) flap, free

  85.76 Gluteal artery perforator (GAP) flap, free

● Code new to this edition   ▲ Revision of existing code   ④ ⑤ Fourth or fifth digit required

85.79 Other total reconstruction of breast

> *Excludes:* *deep inferior epigastric artery perforator (DIEP) flap, free (85.74)*
> *gluteal artery perforator (GAP) flap, free (85.76)*
> *latissimus dorsi myocutaneous flap (85.71)*
> *perforator flap, free (85.70)*
> *superficial inferior epigastric artery (SIEA) flap, free (85.75)*
> *total reconstruction of breast, NOS (85.70)*
> *transverse rectus abdominus myocutaneous (TRAM) flap, free (85.73)*
> *transverse rectus abdominis myocutaneous (TRAM) flap, pedicled (85.72)*

85.8 Other repair and plastic operations on breast

> *Excludes:* *that for:*
> *augmentation (85.50-85.54)*
> *reconstruction (85.70-85.76, 85.79)*
> *reduction (85.31-85.32)*

85.81 Suture of laceration of breast

85.82 Split-thickness graft to breast

85.83 Full-thickness graft to breast

85.84 Pedicle graft to breast

85.85 Muscle flap graft to breast

85.86 Transposition of nipple

85.87 Other repair or reconstruction of nipple

85.89 Other mammoplasty

85.9 Other operations on the breast

85.91 Aspiration of breast

> *Excludes:* *percutaneous biopsy of breast (85.11)*

85.92 Injection of therapeutic agent into breast

> *Excludes:* *that for augmentation of breast (85.51-85.52, 85.55)*

85.93 Revision of implant of breast

85.94 Removal of implant of breast

85.95 Insertion of breast tissue expander

Insertion (soft tissue) of tissue expander (one or more) under muscle or platysma to develop skin flaps for donor use

85.96 Removal of breast tissue expander(s)

85.99 Other

86 Operations on skin and subcutaneous tissue

Includes: operations on:
hair follicles
male perineum
nails
sebaceous glands
subcutaneous fat pads
sudoriferous glands
superficial fossae

> *Excludes:* *those on skin of:*
> *anus (49.01-49.99)*
> *breast (mastectomy site) (85.0-85.99)*
> *ear (18.01-18.9)*
> *eyebrow (08.01-08.99)*
> *eyelid (08.01-08.99)*
> *female perineum (71.01-71.9)*
> *lips (27.0-27.99)*
> *nose (21.00-21.99)*
> *penis (64.0-64.99)*
> *scrotum (61.0-61.99)*
> *vulva (71.01-71.9)*

Valid O.R. procedure	Non-O.R. procedure	Nonspecific O.R. procedure	Noncovered O.R. procedure

86.0 Incision of skin and subcutaneous tissue

86.01 Aspiration of skin and subcutaneous tissue
Aspiration of:
  abscess of nail, skin, or subcutaneous tissue
  hematoma of nail, skin, or subcutaneous tissue
  seroma of nail, skin, or subcutaneous tissue

86.02 Injection or tattooing of skin lesion or defect
Injection of filling material
Insertion of filling material
Pigmenting of skin

86.03 Incision of pilonidal sinus or cyst
Excludes: *marsupialization (86.21)*

86.04 Other incision with drainage of skin and subcutaneous tissue
Excludes: *drainage of:*
    fascial compartments of face and mouth (27.0)
    palmar or thenar space (82.04)
    pilonidal sinus or cyst (86.03)

86.05 Incision with removal of foreign body or device from skin and subcutaneous tissue
Removal of carotid sinus baroreflex activation device
Removal of loop recorder
Removal of neurostimulator pulse generator (single array, dual array)
Removal of tissue expander(s) from skin or soft tissue other than breast tissue
Excludes: *removal of foreign body without incision (98.20-98.29)*

86.06 Insertion of totally implantable infusion pump
Code also any associated catheterization
Excludes: *insertion of totally implantable vascular access device (86.07)*

86.07 Insertion of totally implantable vascular access device [VAD]
Totally implanted port
Excludes: *insertion of totally implantable infusion pump (86.06)*

86.09 Other incision of skin and subcutaneous tissue
Creation of thalamic stimulator pulse generator pocket, new site
Escharotomy
Exploration:
  sinus tract, skin
  superficial fossa
Relocation of subcutaneous device pocket NEC
Reopening subcutaneous pocket for device revision without replacement
Undercutting of hair follicle
Excludes: *creation of loop recorder pocket, new site and insertion/relocation of*
      device (37.79)
    creation of pocket for implantable, patient-activated cardiac event
      recorder and insertion/relocation of device (37.79)
    removal of catheter from cranial cavity (01.27)
    that for drainage (86.04)
    that of cardiac pacemaker pocket, new site (37.79)
    that of fascial compartments of face and mouth (27.0)

86.1 Diagnostic procedures on skin and subcutaneous tissue

86.11 Closed biopsy of skin and subcutaneous tissue

86.19 Other diagnostic procedures on skin and subcutaneous tissue
Excludes: *microscopic examination of specimen from skin and subcutaneous*
      tissue (91.61-91.79)

86.2 Excision or destruction of lesion or tissue of skin and subcutaneous tissue

86.21 Excision of pilonidal cyst or sinus
Marsupialization of cyst
Excludes: *incision of pilonidal cyst or sinus (86.03)*

● Code new
  to this edition
▲ Revision of
  existing code
④ ⑤ Fourth or fifth
  digit required

86.22 Excisional debridement of wound, infection, or burn
Removal by excision of:
    devitalized tissue
    necrosis
    slough

> *Excludes:*   *debridement of:*
>   *abdominal all (wound) (54.3)*
>   *bone (77.60-77.69)*
>   *muscle (83.45) of hand (82.36)*
>   *nail (bed) (fold) (86.27)*
>   *nonexcisional debridement of wound, infection, or burn (86.28)*
>   *open fracture site (79.60-79.69)*
>   *pedicle or flap graft (86.75)*

86.23 Removal of nail, nailbed, or nail fold

86.24 Chemosurgery of skin
Chemical peel of skin

86.25 Dermabrasion
That with laser

> *Excludes:*   *dermabrasion of wound to remove embedded debris (86.28)*

86.26 Ligation of dermal appendage

> *Excludes:*   *excision of preauricular appendage (18.29)*

86.27 Debridement of nail, nail bed, or nail fold
Removal of:
    necrosis
    slough

> *Excludes:*   *removal of nail, nail bed, or nail fold (86.23)*

86.28 Nonexcisional debridement of wound, infection, or burn
Debridement NOS
Maggot therapy
Removal of devitalized tissue, necrosis, and slough by such methods as:
    brushing
    irrigation (under pressure)
    scrubbing
    washing
Ultrasonic debridement
Water scalpel (jet)

86.3 Other local excision or destruction of lesion or tissue of skin and subcutaneous tissue
Destruction of skin by:
    cauterization
    cryosurgery
    fulguration
    laser beam
That with Z-plasty

> *Excludes:*   *adipectomy (86.83)*
>   *biopsy of skin (86.11)*
>   *wide or radical excision of skin (86.4)*
>   *Z-plasty without excision (86.84)*

86.4 Radical excision of skin lesion
Wide excision of skin lesion involving underlying or adjacent structure
Code also any lymph node dissection (40.3-40.5)

86.5 Suture or other closure of skin and subcutaneous tissue

86.51 Replantation of scalp

86.59 Closure of skin and subcutaneous tissue of other sites
Adhesives (surgical) (tissue)
Staples
Sutures

> *Excludes:*   *application of adhesive strips (butterfly)—omit code*

86.6 Free skin graft
Includes: excision of skin for autogenous graft

> *Excludes:*   *construction or reconstruction of:*
>   *penis (64.43-64.44)*
>   *trachea (31.75)*
>   *vagina (70.61-70.64)*

| Valid O.R. procedure | Non-O.R. procedure | Nonspecific O.R. procedure | Noncovered O.R. procedure |

86.60 Free skin graft, not otherwise specified

86.61 Full-thickness skin graft to hand

> *Excludes:* heterograft (86.65)
> homograft (86.66)

86.62 Other skin graft to hand

> *Excludes:* heterograft (86.65)
> homograft (86.66)

86.63 Full-thickness skin graft to other sites

> *Excludes:* heterograft (86.65)
> homograft (86.66)

86.64 Hair transplant

> *Excludes:* hair follicle transplant to eyebrow or eyelash (08.63)

86.65 Heterograft to skin
Pigskin graft
Porcine graft

> *Excludes:* application of dressing only (93.57)

86.66 Homograft to skin
Graft to skin of amnionic membrane from donor
Graft to skin of skin from donor

86.67 Dermal regenerative graft
Artificial skin, NOS
Creation of "neodermis"
Decellularized allodermis
Integumentary matrix implants
Prosthetic implant of dermal layer of skin
Regenerate dermal layer of skin

> *Excludes:* heterograft to skin (86.65)
> homograft to skin (86.66)

86.69 Other skin graft to other sites

> *Excludes:* heterograft (86.65)
> homograft (86.66)

86.7 Pedicle grafts or flaps

> *Excludes:* construction or reconstruction of:
> penis (64.43-64.44)
> trachea (31.75)
> vagina (70.61-70.64)

86.70 Pedicle or flap graft, not otherwise specified

86.71 Cutting and preparation of pedicle grafts or flaps
Elevation of pedicle from its bed
Flap design and raising
Partial cutting of pedicle or tube
Pedicle delay

> *Excludes:* pollicization or digital transfer (82.61, 82.81)
> revision of pedicle (86.75)

86.72 Advancement of pedicle graft

86.73 Attachment of pedicle or flap graft to hand

> *Excludes:* pollicization or digital transfer (82.61, 82.81)

86.74 Attachment of pedicle or flap graft to other sites
Attachment by: Attachment by:
  advanced flap   rotating flap
  double pedicled flap   sliding flop
  pedicle graft   tube graft

86.75 Revision of pedicle or flap graft
Debridement of pedicle or flap graft
Defatting of pedicle or flap graft

86.8 Other repair and reconstruction of skin and subcutaneous tissue

86.81 Repair for facial weakness

● Code new to this edition   ▲ Revision of existing code   ④ ⑤ Fourth or fifth digit required

86.82 **Facial rhytidectomy**
Face lift

> Excludes: *rhytidectomy of eyelid (08.86-08.87)*

86.83 **Size reduction plastic operation**
Liposuction
Reduction of adipose tissue of:
abdominal wall (pendulous)
arms (batwing)
buttock
thighs (trochanteric lipomatosis)

> Excludes: *breast (85.31-85.32)*
> *liposuction to harvest fat graft (86.90)*

86.84 **Relaxation of scar or web contracture of skin**
Z-plasty of skin

> Excludes: *Z-plasty with excision of lesion (86.3)*

86.85 **Correction of syndactyly**

86.86 **Onychoplasty**

86.87 **Fat graft of skin and subcutaneous tissue**
Includes: extraction of fat for autologous graft
Autologous fat transplantation or transfer
Fat graft NOS
Fat graft of skin and subcutaneous tissue with or without use of enriched graft
Micro-fat grafting

> Excludes: *fat graft to breast (85.55)*

86.89 **Other repair and reconstruction of skin and subcutaneous tissue**

> Excludes: *mentoplasty (76.67-76.68)*

86.9 **Other operations on skin and subcutaneous tissue**

86.90 **Extraction of fat for graft or banking**
Harvest of fat for extraction of cells for future use
Liposuction to harvest fat graft

> Excludes: *that with graft at same operative episode (85.55, 86.87)*

86.91 **Excision of skin for graft**
Excision of skin with closure of donor site

> Excludes: *that with graft at same operative episode (86.60-86.69)*

86.92 **Electrolysis and other epilation of skin**

> Excludes: *epilation of eyelid (08.91-08.93)*

86.93 **Insertion of tissue expander**
Insertion (subcutaneous) (soft tissue) of expander (one or more) in scalp (subgaleal
space), face, neck, trunk except breast, and upper and lower extremities for
development of skin flaps for donor use

> Excludes: *flap graft preparation (86.71)*
> *tissue expander, breast (85.95)*

86.94 **Insertion or replacement of single array neurostimulator pulse generator, not
specified as rechargeable**
Pulse generator (single array, single channel, single port) for intracranial, spinal, and
peripheral neurostimulator
Code also any associated lead implantation (02.93, 03.93, 04.92)

> Excludes: *cranial implantation or replacement of neurostimulator pulse*
> *generator (01.20)*
> *insertion or replacement of single array rechargeable neurostimulator*
> *pulse generator (86.97)*

▲ **86.95** **Insertion or replacement of multiple array neurostimulator pulse generator, not
specified as rechargeable**
Pulse generator (multiple array, multiple channel, multiple port) for intracranial,
spinal, and peripheral neurostimulator
Code also any associated lead implantation (02.93, 03.93, 04.92)

> Excludes: *cranial implantation or replacement of neurostimulator pulse*
> *generator (01.20)*
> *insertion or replacement of multiple array rechargeable*
> *neurostimulator pulse generator (86.98)*

| | Valid O.R. procedure | | Non-O.R. procedure | | Nonspecific O.R. procedure | | Noncovered O.R. procedure |

86.96 **Insertion or replacement of other neurostimulator pulse generator**

Code also any associated lead implantation (02.93, 03.93, 04.92)

Excludes: *cranial implantation or replacement of neurostimulator pulse generator (01.20)*

insertion of multiple array neurostimulator pulse generator (86.95, 86.98)

insertion of single array neurostimulator pulse generator (86.94, 86.97)

86.97 **Insertion or replacement of single array rechargeable neurostimulator pulse generator**

Rechargeable pulse generator (single array, single channel, single port) for intracranial, spinal, and peripheral neurostimulator

Code also any associated lead implantation (02.93, 03.93, 04.92)

Excludes: *cranial implantation or replacement of neurostimulator pulse generator (01.20)*

▲ **86.98** **Insertion or replacement of multiple array (two or more) rechargeable neurostimulator pulse generator**

Rechargeable pulse generator (multiple array, multiple channel, multiple port) for intracranial, spinal, and peripheral neurostimulator

Code also any associated lead implantation (02.93, 03.93, 04.92)

Excludes: *cranial implantation or replacement of neurostimulator pulse generator (01.20)*

86.99 **Other**

Excludes: *removal of sutures from:*
  abdomen (97.83)
  head and neck (97.38)
  thorax (97.43)
  trunk NEC (97.84)
wound catheter:
  irrigation (96.58)
  replacement (97.15)

● Code new
to this edition

▲ Revision of
existing code

④ ⑤ Fourth or fifth
digit required

16. MISCELLANEOUS DIAGNOSTIC AND THERAPEUTIC PROCEDURES (87-99)

87 Diagnostic Radiology

87.0 Soft tissue x-ray of face, head, and neck

> Excludes: *angiography (88.40-88.68)*

87.01 Pneumoencephalogram

87.02 Other contrast radiogram of brain and skull
Pneumocisternogram
Pneumoventriculogram
Posterior fossa myelogram

87.03 Computerized axial tomography of head
C.A.T. scan of head

87.04 Other tomography of head

87.05 Contrast dacryocystogram

87.06 Contrast radiogram of nasopharynx

87.07 Contrast laryngogram

87.08 Cervical lymphangiogram

87.09 Other soft tissue x-ray of face, head, and neck
Noncontrast x-ray of:
adenoid
larynx
nasolacrimal duct
nasopharynx
salivary gland
thyroid region
uvula

> Excludes: *x-ray study of eye (95.14)*

87.1 Other x-ray of face, head, and neck

> Excludes: *angiography (88.40-88.68)*

87.11 Full-mouth x-ray of teeth

87.12 Other dental x-ray
Orthodontic cephalogram or cephalometrics
Panorex examination of mandible
Root canal x-ray

87.13 Temporomandibular contrast arthrogram

87.14 Contrast radiogram of orbit

87.15 Contrast radiogram of sinus

87.16 Other x-ray of facial bones
X-ray of:
frontal area
mandible
maxilla
nasal sinuses
nose
orbit
supraorbital area
symphysis menti
zygomaticomaxillary complex

87.17 Other x-ray of skull
Lateral projection of skull
Sagittal projection of skull
Tangential projection of skull

87.2 X-ray of spine

87.21 Contrast myelogram

87.22 Other x-ray of cervical spine

87.23 Other x-ray of thoracic spine

87.24 Other x-ray of lumbosacral spine
Sacrococcygeal x-ray

87.29 Other x-ray of spine
Spinal x-ray NOS

| | Valid O.R. procedure | | Non-O.R. procedure | | Nonspecific O.R. procedure | | Noncovered O.R. procedure |

87.3   Soft tissue x-ray of thorax
> *Excludes:* angiocardiography (88.50-88.58)
>   angiography (88.40-88.68)

87.31   Endotracheal bronchogram

87.32   Other contrast bronchogram
Transcricoid bronchogram

87.33   Mediastinal pneumogram

87.34   Intrathoracic lymphangiogram

87.35   Contrast radiogram of mammary ducts

87.36   Xerography of breast

87.37   Other mammography

87.38   Sinogram of chest wall
Fistulogram of chest wall

87.39   Other soft tissue x-ray of chest wall

87.4   Other x-ray of thorax
> *Excludes:* angiocardiography (88.50-88.58)
>   angiography (88.40-88.68)

87.41   Computerized axial tomography of thorax
C.A.T. scan of heart
C.A.T. scan of thorax
Crystal linea scan of x-ray beam of thorax
Electronic substraction of thorax
Photoelectric response of thorax
Tomography with use of computer, x-rays, and camera of thorax

87.42   Other tomography of thorax
Cardiac tomogram
> *Excludes:* C.A.T. scan of heart (87.41)

87.43   X-ray of ribs, sternum, and clavicle
Examination for:
  cervical rib
  fracture

87.44   Routine chest x-ray, so described
X-ray of chest NOS

87.49   Other chest x-ray
X-ray of:
  bronchus NOS
  diaphragm NOS
  heart NOS
  lung NOS
  mediastinum NOS
  trachea NOS

87.5   Biliary tract x-ray

87.51   Percutaneous hepatic cholangiogram

87.52   Intravenous cholangiogram

87.53   Intraoperative cholangiogram

87.54   Other cholangiogram

87.59   Other biliary tract x-ray
Cholecystogram

87.6   Other x-ray of digestive system

87.61   Barium swallow

87.62   Upper GI series

87.63   Small bowel series

87.64   Lower GI series

87.65   Other x-ray of intestine

87.66   Contrast pancreatogram

87.69   Other digestive tract x-ray

87.7   X-ray of urinary system
> *Excludes:* angiography of renal vessels (88.45, 88.65)

● Code new to this edition   ▲ Revision of existing code   ④ ⑤ Fourth or fifth digit required

87.71 Computerized axial tomography of kidney
C.A.T. scan of kidney

87.72 Other nephrotomogram

87.73 Intravenous pyelogram
Diuretic infusion pyelogram

87.74 Retrograde pyelogram

87.75 Percutaneous pyelogram

87.76 Retrograde cystourethrogram

87.77 Other cystogram

87.78 Ileal conduitogram

87.79 Other x-ray of the urinary system
KUB x-ray

87.8 X-ray of female genital organs

87.81 X-ray of gravid uterus
Intrauterine cephalometry by x-ray

87.82 Gas contrast hysterosalpingogram

87.83 Opaque dye contrast hysterosalpingogram

87.84 Percutaneous hysterogram

87.85 Other x-ray of fallopian tubes and uterus

87.89 Other x-ray of female genital organs

87.9 X-ray of male genital organs

87.91 Contrast seminal vesiculogram

87.92 Other x-ray of prostate and seminal vesicles

87.93 Contrast epididymogram

87.94 Contrast vasogram

87.95 Other x-ray of epididymis and vas deferens

87.99 Other x-ray of male genital organs

88 Other diagnostic radiology and related techniques

88.0 Soft tissue x-ray of abdomen

> Excludes: *angiography (88.40-88.68)*

88.01 Computerized axial tomography of abdomen
C.A.T. scan of abdomen

> Excludes: *C.A.T. scan of kidney (87.71)*

88.02 Other abdomen tomography

> Excludes: *nephrotomogram (87.72)*

88.03 Sinogram of abdominal wall
Fistulogram of abdominal wall

88.04 Abdominal lymphangiogram

88.09 Other soft tissue x-ray of abdominal wall

88.1 Other x-ray of abdomen

88.11 Pelvic opaque dye contrast radiography

88.12 Pelvic gas contrast radiography
Pelvic pneumoperitoneum

88.13 Other peritoneal pneumogram

88.14 Retroperitoneal fistulogram

88.15 Retroperitoneal pneumogram

88.16 Other retroperitoneal x-ray

88.19 Other x-ray of abdomen
Flat plate of abdomen

88.2 Skeletal x-ray of extremities and pelvis

> Excludes: *contrast radiogram of joint (88.32)*

88.21 Skeletal x-ray of shoulder and upper arm

88.22 Skeletal x-ray of elbow and forearm

88.23 Skeletal x-ray of wrist and hand

| | Valid O.R. procedure | | Non-O.R. procedure | | Nonspecific O.R. procedure | | Noncovered O.R. procedure |

88.24 Skeletal x-ray of upper limb, not otherwise specified

88.25 Pelvimetry

88.26 Other skeletal x-ray of pelvis and hip

88.27 Skeletal x-ray of thigh, knee, and lower leg

88.28 Skeletal x-ray of ankle and foot

88.29 Skeletal x-ray of lower limb, not otherwise specified

88.3 Other x-ray

88.31 Skeletal series
X-ray of whole skeleton

88.32 Contrast arthrogram

> Excludes: that of temporomandibular joint (87.13)

88.33 Other skeletal x-ray

> Excludes: skeletal x-ray of:
> extremities and pelvis (88.21-88.29)
> face, head, and neck (87.11-87.17)
> spine (87.21-87.29)
> thorax (87.43)

88.34 Lymphangiogram of upper limb

88.35 Other soft tissue x-ray of upper limb

88.36 Lymphangiogram of lower limb

88.37 Other soft tissue x-ray of lower limb

> Excludes: femoral angiography (88.48, 88.66)

88.38 Other computerized axial tomography
C.A.T. scan NOS

> Excludes: C.A.T. scan of:
> abdomen (88.01)
> head (87.03)
> heart (87.41)
> kidney (87.71)
> thorax (87.41)

88.39 X-ray, other and unspecified

88.4 Arteriography using contrast material
Includes: angiography of arteries
arterial puncture for injection of contrast material
radiography of arteries (by fluoroscopy)
retrograde arteriography
Note: The fourth-digit subclassification identifies the site to be viewed, not the site of injection.

> Excludes: arteriography using:
> radioisotopes or radionuclides (92.01-92.19)
> ultrasound (88.71-88.79)
> fluorescein angiography of eye (95.12)

88.40 Arteriography using contrast material, unspecified site

88.41 Arteriography of cerebral arteries
Angiography of:
basilar artery
carotid (internal)
posterior cerebral circulation
vertebral artery

88.42 Aortography
Arteriography of aorta and aortic arch

88.43 Arteriography of pulmonary arteries

88.44 Arteriography of other intrathoracic vessels

> Excludes: angiocardiography (88.50-88.58)
> arteriography of coronary arteries (88.55-88.57)

88.45 Arteriography of renal arteries

88.46 Arteriography of placenta
Placentogram using contrast material

88.47 Arteriography of other intra-abdominal arteries

● Code new to this edition ▲ Revision of existing code ④ ⑤ Fourth or fifth digit required

88.48 Arteriography of femoral and other lower extremity arteries

88.49 Arteriography of other specified sites

88.5 **Angiocardiography using contrast material**

Includes: arterial puncture and insertion of arterial catheter for injection of contrast
material
cineangiocardiography
selective angiocardiography

Code also synchronous cardiac catheterization (37.21-37.23)

Excludes: *angiography of pulmonary vessels (88.43, 88.62)*

88.50 **Angiocardiography, not otherwise specified**

88.51 **Angiocardiography of venae cavae**
Interior vena cavography
Phlebography of vena cava (inferior) (superior)

88.52 **Angiocardiography of right heart structures**
Angiocardiography of:
pulmonary valve
right atrium
right ventricle (outflow tract)

Excludes: *intra-operative fluorescence vascular angiography (88.59)*
that combined with left heart angiocardiography (88.54)

88.53 **Angiocardiography of left heart structures**
Angiocardiography of:
aortic valve
left atrium
left ventricle (outflow tract)

Excludes: *intra-operative fluorescence vascular angiography (88.59)*
that combined with right heart angiocardiography (88.54)

88.54 **Combined right and left heart angiocardiography**

Excludes: *intra-operative fluorescence vascular angiography (88.59)*

88.55 **Coronary arteriography using a single catheter**
Coronary arteriography by Sones technique
Direct selective coronary arteriography using a single catheter

Excludes: *intra-operative fluorescence vascular angiography (88.59)*

88.56 **Coronary arteriography using two catheters**
Coronary arteriography by:
Judkins technique
Ricketts and Abrams technique
Direct selective coronary arteriography using two catheters

Excludes: *intra-operative fluorescence vascular angiography (88.59)*

88.57 **Other and unspecified coronary arteriography**
Coronary arteriography NOS

Excludes: *intra-operative fluorescence vascular angiography (88.59)*

88.58 **Negative-contrast cardiac roentgenography**
Cardiac roentgenography with injection of carbon dioxide

88.59 **Intra-operative coronary fluorescence vascular angiography**
Intraoperative laser arteriogram (SPY)
SPY arteriogram
SPY arteriography

88.6 **Phlebography**
Includes: angiography of veins
radiography of veins (by fluoroscopy)
retrograde phlebography
venipuncture for injection of contrast material
venography using contrast material

Note: The fourth-digit subclassification (88.60-88.67) identifies the site to be viewed, not
the site of injection.

Excludes: *angiography using:*
radioisotopes or radionuclides (92.01-92.19)
ultrasound (88.71-88.79)
fluorescein angiography of eye (95.12)

88.60 **Phlebography using contrast material, unspecified site**

	Valid O.R. procedure		Non-O.R. procedure		Nonspecific O.R. procedure		Noncovered O.R. procedure

88.61 Phlebography of veins of head and neck using contrast material

88.62 Phlebography of pulmonary veins using contrast material

88.63 Phlebography of other intrathoracic veins using contrast material

88.64 Phlebography of the portal venous system using contrast material
Splenoportogram (by splenic arteriography)

88.65 Phlebography of other intra-abdominal veins using contrast material

88.66 Phlebography of femoral and other lower extremity veins using contrast material

88.67 Phlebography of other specified sites using contrast material

88.68 Impedance phlebography

88.7 **Diagnostic ultrasound**
Includes: echography
non-invasive ultrasound
ultrasonic angiography
ultrasonography

Excludes: *intravascular imaging (adjunctive) (IVUS) (00.21-00.29)*
that for intraoperative monitoring (00.94)
therapeutic ultrasound (00.01-00.09)

88.71 **Diagnostic ultrasound of head and neck**
Determination of midline shift of brain
Echoencephalography

Excludes: *eye (95.13)*

88.72 **Diagnostic ultrasound of heart**
Echocardiography
Transesophageal echocardiography

Excludes: *echocardiography of heart chambers (37.28)*
intracardiac echocardiography (ICE) (37.28)
intravascular (IVUS) imaging of coronary vessels (00.24)

88.73 **Diagnostic ultrasound of other sites of thorax**
Aortic arch ultrasonography
Breast ultrasonography
Lung ultrasonography

88.74 **Diagnostic ultrasound of digestive system**

88.75 **Diagnostic ultrasound of urinary system**

88.76 **Diagnostic ultrasound of abdomen and retroperitoneum**

88.77 **Diagnostic ultrasound of peripheral vascular system**
Deep vein thrombosis ultrasonic scanning

Excludes: *adjunct vascular system procedures (00.40-00.43)*

88.78 **Diagnostic ultrasound of gravid uterus**
Intrauterine cephalometry:
echo
ultrasonic
Placental localization by ultrasound

88.79 **Other diagnostic ultrasound**
Ultrasonography of:
multiple sites
nongravid uterus
total body

88.8 **Thermography**

88.81 **Cerebral thermography**

88.82 **Ocular thermography**

88.83 **Bone thermography**
Osteoarticular thermography

88.84 **Muscle thermography**

88.85 **Breast thermography**

88.86 **Blood vessel thermography**
Deep vein thermography

88.89 **Thermography of other sites**
Lymph gland thermography
Thermography NOS

● Code new to this edition   ▲ Revision of existing code   ④ ⑤ Fourth or fifth digit required

88.9 **Other diagnostic imaging**

    88.90 **Diagnostic imaging, not elsewhere classified**

    88.91 **Magnetic resonance imaging of brain and brain stem**

> Excludes: *intraoperative magnetic resonance imaging (88.96)*
> *laser interstitial thermal therapy [LITT] of lesion or tissue of brain under guidance (17.61)*
> *real-time magnetic resonance imaging (88.96)*

    88.92 **Magnetic resonance imaging of chest and myocardium**
        For evaluation of hilar and mediastinal lymphadenopathy

> Excludes: *laser interstitial thermal therapy [LITT] of lesion or tissue of breast under guidance (17.69)*
> *laser interstitial thermal therapy [LITT] of lesion or tissue of lung under guidance (17.69)*

    88.93 **Magnetic resonance imaging of spinal canal**
        Levels:
          cervical
          lumbar (lumbosacral)
          thoracic
        Spinal cord
        Spine

    88.94 **Magnetic resonance imaging of musculoskeletal**
        Bone marrow blood supply
        Extremities (upper) (lower)

    88.95 **Magnetic resonance imaging of pelvis, prostate, and bladder**

> Excludes: *laser interstitial thermal therapy [LITT] of lesion or tissue of prostate under guidance (17.69)*

    88.96 **Other intraoperative magnetic resonance imaging**
        iMRI
        Real-time magnetic resonance imaging

    88.97 **Magnetic resonance imaging of other and unspecified sites**
        abdomen   neck
        face   eye orbit

> Excludes: *laser interstitial thermal therapy [LITT] of lesion or tissue of other and unspecified site under guidance (17.69)*

    88.98 **Bone mineral density studies**
        Dual photon absorptiometry
        Quantitative computed tomography (CT) studies
        Radiographic densitometry
        Single photon absorptiometry

89 **Interview, evaluation, consultation, and examination**

    89.0 **Diagnostic interview, consultation, and evaluation**

> Excludes: *psychiatric diagnostic interview (94.11-94.19)*

    89.01 **Interview and evaluation, described as brief**
        Abbreviated history and evaluation

    89.02 **Interview and evaluation, described as limited**
        Interval history and evaluation

    89.03 **Interview and evaluation, described as comprehensive**
        History and evaluation of new problem

    89.04 **Other interview and evaluation**

    89.05 **Diagnostic interview and evaluation, not otherwise specified**

    89.06 **Consultation, described as limited**
        Consultation on a single organ system

    89.07 **Consultation, described as comprehensive**

    89.08 **Other consultation**

    89.09 **Consultation, not otherwise specified**

    89.1 **Anatomic and physiologic measurements and manual examinations—nervous system and sense organs**

> Excludes: *ear examination (95.41-95.49)*
> *eye examination (95.01-95.26)*
> *the listed procedures when done as part of a general physical examination (89.7)*

89.10 Intracarotid amobarbital test
Wada test

89.11 Tonometry

89.12 Nasal function study
Rhinomanometry

89.13 Neurologic examination

89.14 Electroencephalogram

Excludes: *that with polysomnogram (89.17)*

89.15 Other nonoperative neurologic function tests

89.16 Transillumination of newborn skull

89.17 Polysomnogram
Sleep recording

89.18 Other sleep disorder function tests
Multiple sloop latency test [MSLT]

89.19 Video and radio-telemetered electroencephalographic monitoring
Radiographic EEG monitoring
Video EEG monitoring

Excludes: *intraoperative monitoring (00.94)*

89.2 Anatomic and physiologic measurements and manual examinations—genitourinary system

Excludes: *the listed procedures when done as part of a general physical examination (89.7)*

89.21 Urinary manometry
Manometry through:
indwelling urethral catheter
nephrostomy
pyelostomy
ureterostomy

89.22 Cystometrogram

89.23 Urethral sphincter electromyogram

89.24 Uroflowmetry [UFR]

89.25 Urethral pressure profile [UPP]

89.26 Gynecological examination
Pelvic examination

89.29 Other nonoperative genitourinary system measurements
Bioassay of urine
Renal clearance
Urine chemistry

89.3 Other anatomic and physiologic measurements and manual examinations

Excludes: *the listed procedures when done as part of a general physical examination (89.7)*

89.31 Dental examination
Oral mucosal survey
Periodontal survey

89.32 Esophageal manometry

89.33 Digital examination of enterostomy stoma
Digital examination of colostomy stoma

89.34 Digital examination of rectum

89.35 Transillumination of nasal sinuses

89.36 Manual examination of breast

89.37 Vital capacity determination

Excludes: *endoscopic pulmonary airway flow measurement (33.72)*

89.38 Other nonoperative respiratory measurements
Plethysmography for measurement of respiratory function
Thoracic impedance plethysmography

Excludes: *endoscopic pulmonary airway flow measurement (33.72)*

● Code new
to this edition
▲ Revision of
existing code
④ ⑤ Fourth or fifth
digit required

89.39 Other nonoperative measurements and examinations
Basal metabolic rate [BMR]
14 C-Urea breath test
Gastric:
  analysis
  function NEC

> Excludes: *body measurements (93.07)*
> *cardiac tests (89.41-89.69)*
> *fundus photography (95.11)*
> *limb length measurement (93.06)*

89.4   Cardiac stress tests, pacemaker and defibrillator checks

89.41 Cardiovascular stress test using treadmill

89.42 Masters' two-step stress test

89.43 Cardiovascular stress test using bicycle ergometer

89.44 Other cardiovascular stress test
Thallium stress test with or without transesophageal pacing

89.45 Artificial pacemaker rate check
Artificial pacemaker function check NOS
Bedside device check of pacemaker or cardiac resynchronization pacemaker
  [CRT-P]
Interrogation only without arrhythmia induction

> Excludes: *catheter based invasive electrophysiologic testing (37.26)*
> *noninvasive programmed electrical stimulation [NIPS] (arrhythmia induction) (37.20)*

89.46 Artificial pacemaker artifact wave form check

89.47 Artificial pacemaker electrode impedance check

89.48 Artificial pacemaker voltage or amperage threshold check

89.49 Automatic implantable cardioverter/defibrillator (AICD) check
Bedside check of an AICD or cardiac resynchronization defibrillator [CRT-D]
Checking pacing thresholds of device
Interrogation only without arrhythmia induction

> Excludes: *catheter based invasive electrophysiologic testing (37.26)*
> *noninvasive programmed electrical stimulation [NIPS] (arrhythmia induction) (37.20)*

89.5   Other nonoperative cardiac and vascular diagnostic procedures

> Excludes: *fetal EKG (75.32)*

89.50 Ambulatory cardiac monitoring
Analog devices [Holter-type]

89.51 Rhythm electrocardiogram
Rhythm EKG (with one to three leads)

89.52 Electrocardiogram
ECG NOS
EKG (with 12 or more leads)

89.53 Vectorcardiogram (with ECG)

89.54 Electrographic monitoring
Telemetry

> Excludes: *ambulatory cardiac monitoring (89.50)*
> *electrographic monitoring during surgery—omit code*

89.55 Phonocardiogram with ECG lead

89.56 Carotid pulse tracing with ECG lead

> Excludes: *oculoplethysmography (89.58)*

89.57 Apexcardiogram (with ECG lead)

89.58 Plethysmogram
Penile plethysmography with nerve stimulation

> Excludes: *plethysmography (for):*
> *measurement of respiratory function (89.38)*
> *thoracic impedance (89.38)*

89.59 Other nonoperative cardiac and vascular measurements

Valid O.R.   Non-O.R.   Nonspecific   Noncovered
procedure   procedure   O.R. procedure   O.R. procedure

89.6 Circulatory monitoring

> *Excludes:* *electrocardiographic monitoring during surgery—omit code*
> *implantation or replacement of subcutaneous device for intracardiac*
> *hemodynamic monitoring (00.57)*
> *insertion or replacement of implantable pressure sensor (lead) for*
> *intracardiac hemodynamic monitoring (00.56)*

89.60 Continuous intra-arterial blood gas monitoring
Insertion of blood gas monitoring system and continuous monitoring of blood gases through an intra-arterial sensor

89.61 Systemic arterial pressure monitoring

> *Excludes:* *intra-aneurysm sac pressure monitoring (intraoperative) (00.58)*
> *intravascular pressure measurement of intrathoracic arteries (00.67)*
> *intravascular pressure measurement of peripheral arteries (00.68)*

89.62 Central venous pressure monitoring

> *Excludes:* *intravascular pressure measurement, other specified and unspecified*
> *vessels (00.69)*

89.63 Pulmonary artery pressure monitoring

> *Excludes:* *pulmonary artery wedge monitoring (89.64)*

89.64 Pulmonary artery wedge monitoring
Pulmonary capillary wedge [PCW] monitoring
Swan-Ganz catheterization

89.65 Measurement of systemic arterial blood gases

> *Excludes:* *continuous intra-arterial blood gas monitoring (89.60)*

89.66 Measurement of mixed venous blood gases

89.67 Monitoring of cardiac output by oxygen consumption technique
Fick method

89.68 Monitoring of cardiac output by other technique
Cardiac output monitor by thermodilution indicator

89.69 Monitoring of coronary blood flow
Coronary blood flow monitoring by coincidence counting technique

> *Excludes:* *intravascular pressure measurement of coronary arteries (00.59)*

89.7 General physical examination

89.8 Autopsy

90 Microscopic examination—I
The following fourth-digit subclassification is for use with categories in section 90 to identify type of examination:

    1 bacterial smear
    2 culture
    3 culture and sensitivity
    4 parasitology
    5 toxicology
    6 cell block and Papanicolaou smear
    9 other microscopic examination

④ **90.0 Microscopic examination of specimen from nervous system and of spinal fluid**

④ **90.1 Microscopic examination of specimen from endocrine gland, not elsewhere classified**

④ **90.2 Microscopic examination of specimen from eye**

④ **90.3 Microscopic examination of specimen from ear, nose, throat, and larynx**

④ **90.4 Microscopic examination of specimen from trachea, bronchus, pleura, lung, and other thoracic specimen, and of sputum**

④ **90.5 Microscopic examination of blood**

④ **90.6 Microscopic examination of specimen from spleen and of bone marrow**

④ **90.7 Microscopic examination of specimen from lymph node and of lymph**

④ **90.8 Microscopic examination of specimen from upper gastrointestinal tract and of vomitus**

④ **90.9 Microscopic examination of specimen from lower gastrointestinal tract and of stool**

91 Microscopic examination—II

The following fourth-digit subclassification is for use with categories in section 91 to identify type of examination:

1 bacterial smear
2 culture
3 culture and sensitivity
4 parasitology
5 toxicology
6 cell block and Papanicolaou smear
9 other microscopic examination

④ **91.0 Microscopic examination of specimen from liver, biliary trace and pancreas**

④ **91.1 Microscopic examination of peritoneal and retroperitoneal specimen**

④ **91.2 Microscopic examination of specimen from kidney, ureter, perirenal and periureteral tissue**

④ **91.3 Microscopic examination of specimen from bladder, urethra, prostate, seminal vesicle, perivesical tissue, and of urine and semen**

④ **91.4 Microscopic examination of specimen from female genital tract**
Amnionic sac
Fetus

④ **91.5 Microscopic examination of specimen from musculoskeletal system and of joint fluid**
Microscopic examination of:

bone	ligament
bursa	muscle
cartilage	synovial membrane
fascia	tendon

④ **91.6 Microscopic examination of specimen from skin and other integument**
Microscopic examination of:
hair
nails
skin

> Excludes: *mucous membrane—code to organ site*
> *that of operative wound (91.71-91.79)*

④ **91.7 Microscopic examination of specimen from operative wound**

④ **91.8 Microscopic examination of specimen from other site**

④ **91.9 Microscopic examination of specimen from unspecified site**

92 Nuclear Medicine

92.0 Radioisotope scan and function study

92.01 Thyroid scan and radioisotope function studies
Iodine-131 uptake
Protein-bound iodine
Radio-iodine uptake

92.02 Liver scan and radioisotope function study

92.03 Renal scan and radioisotope function study
Renal clearance study

92.04 Gastrointestinal scan and radioisotope function study
Radio-cobalt B_{12} Schilling test
Radio-iodinated triolein study

92.05 Cardiovascular and hematopoietic scan and radioisotope function study
Bone marrow scan or function study
Cardiac output scan or function study
Circulation time scan or function study
Radionuclide cardiac
ventriculogram scan or function study
Spleen scan or function study

92.09 Other radioisotope function studies

92.1 Other radioisotope scan

92.11 Cerebral scan
Pituitary

92.12 Scan of other sites of head
> Excludes: *eye (95.16)*

92.13 Parathyroid scan

92.14 Bone scan

	Valid O.R. procedure		Non-O.R. procedure		Nonspecific O.R. procedure		Noncovered O.R. procedure

92.15 Pulmonary scan

92.16 Scan of lymphatic system

92.17 Placental scan

92.18 Total body scan

92.19 Scan of other sites

92.2 Therapeutic radiology and nuclear medicine

> Excludes: that for:
>> ablation of pituitary gland (07.64-07.69)
>> destruction of chorioretinal lesion (14.26-14.27)

92.20 Infusion of liquid brachytherapy radioisotope
I-125 radioisotope
Intracavitary brachytherapy
Includes: removal of radioisotope

92.21 Superficial radiation
Contact radiation [up to 150 KVP]

92.22 Orthovoltage radiation
Deep radiation [200-300 KVP]

92.23 Radioisotopic teleradiotherapy
Teleradiotherapy using:
  cobalt-60
  iodine-125
  radioactive cesium

92.24 Teleradiotherapy using photons
Megavoltage NOS
Supervoltage NOS
Use of:
  Betatron
  linear accelerator

92.25 Teleradiotherapy using electrons
Beta particles

> Excludes: intra-operative electron radiation therapy (92.41)

92.26 Teleradiotherapy of other particulate radiation
Neutrons   Protons NOS

92.27 Implantation or insertion of radioactive elements
Intravascular brachytherapy

Code also incision of site

> Excludes: infusion of liquid brachytherapy radioisotope (92.20)

92.28 Injection or instillation of radioisotopes
Injection or infusion of radioimmunoconjugate
Intracavitary injection or instillation
Intravenous injection or instillation
Iodine-131 [I-131] tositumomab
Radioimmunotherapy
Ytrium-90 [Y-90] ibritumomab tiuxetan

> Excludes: infusion of liquid brachytherapy radioisotope (92.20)

92.29 Other radiotherapeutic procedure

92.3 Stereotactic radiosurgery

> Excludes: stereotactic biopsy

Code also stereotactic head frame application (93.59)

92.30 Stereotactic radiosurgery, not otherwise specified

92.31 Single source photon radiosurgery
High energy x-rays
Linear accelerator (LINAC)

92.32 Multi-source photon radiosurgery
Cobalt 60 radiation
Gamma irradiation

92.33 Particulate radiosurgery
Particle beam radiation (cyclotron)
Proton accelerator

● Code new
   to this edition

▲ Revision of
   existing code

④ ⑤ Fourth or fifth
       digit required

92.39 Stereotactic radiosurgery, not elsewhere classified

92.4 **Intra-operative radiation procedures**

92.41 **Intra-operative electron radiation therapy**
IOERT
That using a mobile linear accelerator

93 **Physical therapy, respiratory therapy, rehabilitation, and related procedures**

93.0 **Diagnostic physical therapy**

93.01 **Functional evaluation**

93.02 **Orthotic evaluation**

93.03 **Prosthetic evaluation**

93.04 **Manual testing of muscle function**

93.05 **Range of motion testing**

93.06 **Measurement of limb length**

93.07 **Body measurement**
Girth measurement
Measurement of skull circumference

93.08 **Electromyography**

Excludes:	eye EMG (95.25)
	that for intraoperative monitoring (00.94)
	that with polysomnogram (89.17)
	urethral sphincter EMG (89.23)

93.09 **Other diagnostic physical therapy procedure**

93.1 **Physical therapy exercises**

93.11 **Assisting exercise**

Excludes:	assisted exercise in pool (93.31)

93.12 **Other active musculoskeletal exercise**

93.13 **Resistive exercise**

93.14 **Training in joint movements**

93.15 **Mobilization of spine**

93.16 **Mobilization of other joints**

Excludes:	manipulation of temporomandibular joint (76.95)

93.17 **Other passive musculoskeletal exercise**

93.18 **Breathing exercise**

93.19 **Exercise, not elsewhere classified**

93.2 **Other physical therapy musculoskeletal manipulation**

93.21 **Manual and mechanical traction**

Excludes:	skeletal traction (93.43-93.44)
	skin traction (93.45-93.46)
	spinal traction (93.41-93.42)

93.22 **Ambulation and gait training**

93.23 **Fitting of orthotic device**

93.24 **Training in use of prosthetic or orthotic device**
Training in crutch walking

93.25 **Forced extension of limb**

93.26 **Manual rupture of joint adhesions**

93.27 **Stretching of muscle or tendon**

93.28 **Stretching of fascia**

93.29 **Other forcible correction of deformity**

93.3 **Other physical therapy therapeutic procedures**

93.31 **Assisted exercise in pool**

93.32 **Whirlpool treatment**

93.33 **Other hydrotherapy**

93.34 **Diathermy**

Valid O.R. procedure	Non-O.R. procedure	Nonspecific O.R. procedure	Noncovered O.R. procedure

93.35 Other heat therapy
Acupuncture with smouldering moxa
Hot packs
Hyperthermia NEC
Infrared irradiation
Moxibustion
Paraffin bath

Excludes: *hyperthermia for treatment of cancer (99.85)*

93.36 Cardiac retraining

93.37 Prenatal training
Training for natural childbirth

93.38 Combined physical therapy without mention of the components

93.39 Other physical therapy

93.4 Skeletal traction and other traction

93.41 Spinal traction using skull device
Traction using:
caliper tongs
Crutchfield tongs
halo device
Vinke tongs

Excludes: *insertion of tongs or halo traction device (02.94)*

93.42 Other spinal traction
Cotrel's traction

Excludes: *cervical collar (93.52)*

93.43 Intermittent skeletal traction

93.44 Other skeletal traction
Bryant's traction
Dunlop's traction
Lyman Smith traction
Russell's traction

93.45 Thomas' splint traction

93.46 Other skin traction of limbs
Adhesive tape traction
Boot traction
Buck's traction
Gallows traction

93.5 Other immobilization, pressure, and attention to wound

Excludes: *external fixator device (84.71-84.73)*
wound cleansing (96.58-96.59)

93.51 Application of plaster jacket

Excludes: *Minerva jacket (93.52)*

93.52 Application of neck support
Application of:
cervical collar
Minerva jacket
molded neck support

93.53 Application of other cast

93.54 Application of splint
Plaster splint   Tray splint

Excludes: *periodontal splint (24.7)*

93.55 Dental wiring

Excludes: *that for orthodontia (24.7)*

93.56 Application of pressure dressing
Application of:
Gibney bandage
Robert Jones' bandage
Shanz dressing

93.57 Application of other wound dressing
Porcine wound dressing

● Code new   ▲ Revision of   ④ ⑤ Fourth or fifth
to this edition   existing code   digit required

93.58 Application of pressure trousers
Application of:
anti-shock trousers
MAST trousers
vasopneumatic device

93.59 Other immobilization, pressure and attention to wound
Elastic stockings
Electronic gaiter
Intermittent pressure device
Oxygenation of wound (hyperbaric)
Stereotactic head frame application
Strapping (non-traction)
Velpeau dressing

93.6 Osteopathic manipulative treatment

93.61 Osteopathic manipulative treatment for general mobilization
General articulatory treatment

93.62 Osteopathic manipulative treatment using high-velocity low-amplitude forces
Thrusting forces

93.63 Osteopathic manipulative treatment using low-velocity high-amplitude forces
Springing forces

93.64 Osteopathic manipulative treatment using isotonic, isometric forces

93.65 Osteopathic manipulative treatment using indirect forces

93.66 Osteopathic manipulative treatment to move tissue fluids
Lymphatic pump

93.67 Other specified osteopathic manipulative treatment

93.7 Speech and reading rehabilitation and rehabilitation of the blind

93.71 Dyslexia training

93.72 Dysphasia training

93.73 Esophageal speech training

93.74 Speech defect training

93.75 Other speech training and therapy

93.76 Training in use of lead dog for the blind

93.77 Training in braille or Moon

93.78 Other rehabilitation for the blind

93.8 Other rehabilitation therapy

93.81 Recreation therapy
Diversional therapy
Play therapy

> Excludes: play psychotherapy (94.36)

93.82 Educational therapy
Education of bed-bound children
Special schooling for the handicapped

93.83 Occupational therapy
Daily living activities therapy

> Excludes: training in activities of daily living for the blind (93.78)

93.84 Music therapy

93.85 Vocational rehabilitation
Sheltered employment
Vocational:
assessment
retraining
training

93.89 Rehabilitation, not elsewhere classified

93.9 Respiratory therapy

> Excludes: insertion of airway (96.01-96.05)
> other continuous invasive (through endotracheal tube or tracheostomy)
> mechanical ventilation (96.70-96.72)

Valid O.R. procedure   Non-O.R. procedure   Nonspecific O.R. procedure   Noncovered O.R. procedure

93.90 **Non-invasive mechanical ventilation**
Bi-level airway pressure
BiPAP without (delivery through) endotracheal tube or tracheostomy
CPAP without (delivery through) endotracheal tube or tracheostomy
Mechanical ventilation NOS
Non-invasive positive pressure (NIPPV)
Non-invasive PPV
NPPV
That delivered by non-invasive interface:
  face mask
  nasal mask
  nasal pillow
  oral mouthpiece
  oronasal mask

> Excludes: invasive (through endotracheal tube or tracheostomy) continuous mechanical ventilation (96.70-96.72)

Note: Patients admitted on *non-invasive* mechanical ventilation that subsequently require *invasive* mechanical ventilation; code both types of mechanical ventilation

93.91 **Intermittent positive pressure breathing [IPPB]**

93.93 **Nonmechanical methods of resuscitation**
Artificial respiration
Manual resuscitation
Mouth-to-mouth resuscitation

93.94 **Respiratory medication administered by nebulizer**
Mist therapy

93.95 **Hyperbaric oxygenation**

> Excludes: oxygenation of wound (93.59)

93.96 **Other oxygen enrichment**
Catalytic oxygen therapy
Cytoreductive effect
Oxygenators
Oxygen therapy

> Excludes: oxygenation of wound (93.59)
> SuperSaturated oxygen therapy (00.49)

93.97 **Decompression chamber**

93.98 **Other control of atmospheric pressure and composition**
Antigen-free air conditioning
Helium therapy

> Excludes: inhaled nitric oxide therapy (INO) (00.12)

93.99 **Other respiratory procedures**
Continuous negative pressure ventilation [CNP]
Postural drainage

94 **Procedures related to the psyche**

94.0 **Psychologic evaluation and testing**

94.01 **Administration of intelligence test**
Administration of:
  Stanford-Binet
  Wechsler Adult Intelligence Scale
  Wechsler Intelligence Scale for Children

94.02 **Administration of psychologic test**
Administration of:
  Bender Visual - Motor Gestalt Test
  Benton Visual Retention Test
  Minnesota Multiphasic Personality Inventory
  Wechsler Memory Scale

94.03 **Character analysis**

94.08 **Other psychologic evaluation and testing**

94.09 **Psychologic mental status determination, not otherwise specified**

94.1 **Psychiatric interviews, consultations, and evaluations**

● Code new
to this edition

▲ Revision of
existing code

④ ⑤ Fourth or fifth
digit required

94.11 Psychiatric mental status determination
Clinical psychiatric mental status determination
Evaluation for criminal responsibility
Evaluation for testimentary capacity
Medicolegal mental status determination
Mental status determination NOS

94.12 Routine psychiatric visit, not otherwise specified

94.13 Psychiatric commitment evaluation
Pre-commitment interview

94.19 Other psychiatric interview and evaluation
Follow-up psychiatric interview NOS

94.2 Psychiatric somatotherapy

94.21 Narcoanalysis
Narcosynthesis

94.22 Lithium therapy

94.23 Neuroleptic therapy

94.24 Chemical shock therapy

94.25 Other psychiatric drug therapy

94.26 Subconvulsive electroshock therapy

94.27 Other electroshock therapy
Electroconvulsive therapy (ECT)
EST

94.29 Other psychiatric somatotherapy

94.3 Individual psychotherapy

94.31 Psychoanalysis

94.32 Hypnotherapy
Hypnodrome
Hypnosis

94.33 Behavior therapy
Aversion therapy
Behavior modification
Desensitization therapy
Extinction therapy
Relaxation training
Token economy

94.34 Individual therapy for psychosexual dysfunction

> Excludes: that performed in group setting (94.41)

94.35 Crisis intervention

94.36 Play psychotherapy

94.37 Exploratory verbal psychotherapy

94.38 Supportive verbal psychotherapy

94.39 Other individual psychotherapy
Biofeedback

94.4 Psychotherapy and counselling

94.41 Group therapy for psychosexual dysfunction

94.42 Family therapy

94.43 Psychodrama

94.44 Other group therapy

94.45 Drug addiction counselling

94.46 Alcoholism counselling

94.49 Other counselling

94.5 Referral for psychologic rehabilitation

94.51 Referral for psychotherapy

94.52 Referral for psychiatric aftercare
That in:
  halfway house
  outpatient (clinic) facility

 Valid O.R. procedure   Non-O.R. procedure 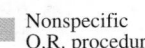 Nonspecific O.R. procedure Noncovered O.R. procedure

94.53 Referral for alcoholism rehabilitation

94.54 Referral for drug addiction rehabilitation

94.55 Referral for vocational rehabilitation

94.59 Referral for other psychologic rehabilitation

94.6 Alcohol and drug rehabilitation and detoxification

94.61 Alcohol rehabilitation

94.62 Alcohol detoxification

94.63 Alcohol rehabilitation and detoxification

94.64 Drug rehabilitation

94.65 Drug detoxification

94.66 Drug rehabilitation and detoxification

94.67 Combined alcohol and drug rehabilitation

94.68 Combined alcohol and drug detoxification

94.69 Combined alcohol and drug rehabilitation and detoxification

95 Ophthalmologic and otologic diagnosis and treatment

95.0 General and subjective eye examination

95.01 Limited eye examination
Eye examination with prescription of spectacles

95.02 Comprehensive eye examination
Eye examination covering all aspects of the visual system

95.03 Extended ophthalmologic work-up
Examination (for):
glaucoma
neuro-ophthalmology
retinal disease

95.04 Eye examination under anesthesia
Code also type of examination

95.05 Visual field study

95.06 Color vision study

95.07 Dark adaptation study

95.09 Eye examination, not otherwise specified
Vision check NOS

95.1 Examinations of form and structure of eye

95.11 Fundus photography

95.12 Fluorescein angiography or angioscopy of eye

95.13 Ultrasound study of eye

95.14 X-ray study of eye

95.15 Ocular motility study

95.16 P^{32} and other tracer studies of eye

95.2 Objective functional tests of eye

Excludes: *that with polysomnogram (89.17)*

95.21 Electroretinogram [ERG]

95.22 Electro-oculogram [EOG]

95.23 Visual evoked potential [VEP]

95.24 Electronystagmogram [ENG]

95.25 Electromyogram of eye [EMG]

95.26 Tonography, provocative tests, and other glaucoma testing

95.3 Special vision services

95.31 Fitting and dispensing of spectacles

95.32 Prescription, fitting, and dispensing of contact lens

95.33 Dispensing of other low vision aids

95.34 Ocular prosthetics

95.35 Orthoptic training

● Code new
to this edition

▲ Revision of
existing code

④ ⑤ Fourth or fifth
digit required

95.36 Ophthalmologic counselling and instruction
Counselling in:
  adaptation to visual loss
  use of low vision aids

95.4 Nonoperative procedures related to hearing

95.41 Audiometry
Békésy 5-tone audiometry
Impedance audiometry
Stapedial reflex response
Subjective audiometry
Tympanogram

95.42 Clinical test of hearing
Tuning fork test
Whispered speech test

95.43 Audiological evaluation
Audiological evaluation by:
  Barany noise machine
  blindfold test
  delayed feedback
  masking
  Weber lateralization

95.44 Clinical vestibular function tests
Thermal test of vestibular function

95.45 Rotation tests
Barany chair

95.46 Other auditory and vestibular function tests

95.47 Hearing examination, not otherwise specified

95.48 Fitting of hearing aid
> *Excludes:* *implantation of electromagnetic hearing device (20.95)*

95.49 Other nonoperative procedures related to hearing
Adjustment (external components) of cochlear prosthetic device

96 Nonoperative intubation and irrigation

96.0 Nonoperative intubation of gastrointestinal and respiratory tracts

96.01 Insertion of nasopharyngeal airway

96.02 Insertion of oropharyngeal airway

96.03 Insertion of esophageal obturator airway

96.04 Insertion of endotracheal tube

96.05 Other intubation of respiratory tract
> *Excludes:* *endoscopic insertion or replacement of bronchial device or substance (33.71, 33.79)*

96.06 Insertion of Sengstaken tube
Esophageal tamponade

96.07 Insertion of other (naso-)gastric tube
Intubation for decompression
> *Excludes:* *that for enteral infusion of nutritional substances (96.6)*

96.08 Insertion of (naso-)intestinal tube
Miller-Abbott tube (for decompression)

96.09 Insertion of rectal tube
Replacement of rectal tube

96.1 Other nonoperative insertion
> *Excludes:* *nasolacrimal intubation (09.44)*

96.11 Packing of external auditory canal

96.14 Vaginal packing

96.15 Insertion of vaginal mold

96.16 Other vaginal dilation

96.17 Insertion of vaginal diaphragm

96.18 Insertion of other vaginal pessary

96.19 Rectal packing

Valid O.R. procedure   Non-O.R. procedure   Nonspecific O.R. procedure   Noncovered O.R. procedure

96.2 **Nonoperative dilation and manipulation**

96.21 **Dilation of frontonasal duct**

96.22 **Dilation of rectum**

96.23 **Dilation of anal sphincter**

96.24 **Dilation and manipulation of enterostomy stoma**

96.25 **Therapeutic distention of bladder**
Intermittent distention of bladder

96.26 **Manual reduction of rectal prolapse**

96.27 **Manual reduction of hernia**

96.28 **Manual reduction of enterostomy prolapse**

96.29 **Reduction with intussusception of alimentary tract**
With:
Fluoroscopy
Ionizing radiation enema
Ultrasonography guidance
Hydrostatic reduction
Pneumantic reduction

> *Excludes:* *intra-abdominal manipulation of intestine, not otherwise specified (46.80)*

96.3 **Nonoperative alimentary tract irrigation, cleaning, and local instillation**

96.31 **Gastric cooling**
Gastric hypothermia

96.32 **Gastric freezing**

96.33 **Gastric lavage**

96.34 **Other irrigation of (naso-)gastric tube**

96.35 **Gastric gavage**

96.36 **Irrigation of gastrostomy or enterostomy**

96.37 **Proctoclysis**

96.38 **Removal of impacted feces**
Removal of impaction:
by flushing
manually

96.39 **Other transanal enema**
Rectal irrigation

> *Excludes:* *reduction of intussusception of alimentary tract by ionizing radiation enema (96.29)*

96.4 **Nonoperative irrigation, cleaning, and local instillation of other digestive and genitourinary organs**

96.41 **Irrigation of cholecystostomy and other biliary tube**

96.42 **Irrigation of pancreatic tube**

96.43 **Digestive tract instillation, except gastric gavage**

96.44 **Vaginal douche**

96.45 **Irrigation of nephrostomy and pyelostomy**

96.46 **Irrigation of ureterostomy and ureteral catheter**

96.47 **Irrigation of cystostomy**

96.48 **Irrigation of other indwelling urinary catheter**

96.49 **Other genitourinary instillation**
Insertion of prostaglandin suppository

96.5 **Other nonoperative irrigation and cleaning**

96.51 **Irrigation of eye**
Irrigation of cornea

> *Excludes:* *irrigation with removal of foreign body (98.21)*

96.52 **Irrigation of ear**
Irrigation with removal of cerumen

96.53 **Irrigation of nasal passages**

96.54 **Dental scaling, polishing, and debridement**
Dental prophylaxis
Plaque removal

● Code new
to this edition

▲ Revision of
existing code

④ ⑤ Fourth or fifth
digit required

96.55 **Tracheostomy toilette**

96.56 **Other lavage of bronchus and trachea**

> Excludes: *diagnostic bronchoalveolar lavage (BAL) (33.24)*
> *whole lung lavage (33.99)*

96.57 **Irrigation of vascular catheter**

96.58 **Irrigation of wound catheter**

96.59 **Other irrigation of wound**
Wound cleaning NOS

> Excludes: *debridement (86.22, 86.27-86.28)*

96.6 **Enteral infusion of concentrated nutritional substances**

96.7 **Other continuous invasive mechanical ventilation**
Includes: BiPAP delivered through endotracheal tube or tracheostomy (invasive interface)
CPAP delivered through endotracheal tube or tracheostomy (invasive interface)
Endotracheal respiratory assistance
Invasive positive pressure ventilation [IPPV]
Mechanical ventilation through invasive interface
That by tracheostomy
Weaning of an intubated (endotracheal tube) patient

> Excludes: *continuous negative pressure ventilation [CNP] (iron lung) (cuirass) (93.99)*
> *intermittent positive pressure breathing [IPPB] (93.91)*
> *non-invasive bi-level positive airway pressure (BiPAP) (93.90)*
> *non-invasive continuous positive airway pressure [CPAP] (93.90)*
> *non-invasive positive pressure (NIPPV) (93.90)*
> *that by face mask (93.90-93.99)*
> *that by nasal cannula (93.90-93.99)*
> *that by nasal catheter (93.90-93.99)*

Code also any associated:
endotracheal tube insertion (96.04)
tracheostomy (31.1-31.29)

Note: Endotracheal Intubation
To calculate the number of hours (duration) of continuous mechanical ventilation during a hospitalization, begin the count from the start of the (endotracheal) intubation. The duration ends with (endotracheal) extubation.

If the patient is intubated prior to admission, begin counting the duration from the time of admission. If a patient is transferred (discharged) while intubated, the duration would end at the time of transfer (discharge).

For patients who begin on (endotracheal) intubation and subsequently have a tracheostomy performed for mechanical ventilation, the duration begins with the (endotracheal) intubation and ends when the mechanical ventilation is turned off (after the weaning period).

Tracheostomy
To calculate the number of hours of continuous mechanical ventilation during a hospitalization, begin counting the duration when mechanical ventilation is started. The duration ends when the mechanical ventilator is turned off (after the weaning period).

If a patient has received a tracheostomy prior to admission and is on mechanical ventilation at the time of admission, begin counting the duration from the time of admission. If a patient is transferred (discharged) while still on mechanical ventilation via tracheostomy, the duration would end at the time of the transfer (discharge).

96.70 **Continuous invasive mechanical ventilation of unspecified duration**
Invasive mechanical ventilation NOS

96.71 **Continuous invasive mechanical ventilation for less than 96 consecutive hours**

96.72 **Continuous invasive mechanical ventilation for 96 consecutive hours or more**

97 **Replacement and removal of therapeutic appliances**

97.0 **Nonoperative replacement of gastrointestinal appliance**

97.01 **Replacement of (naso-)gastric or esophagostomy tube**

97.02 **Replacement of gastrostomy tube**

97.03 **Replacement of tube or enterostomy device of small intestine**

97.04 **Replacement of tube or enterostomy device of large intestine**

97.05 **Replacement of stent (tube) in biliary or pancreatic duct**

Valid O.R. procedure	Non-O.R. procedure	Nonspecific O.R. procedure	Noncovered O.R. procedure

97.1 Nonoperative replacement of musculoskeletal and integumentary system appliance

97.11 Replacement of cast on upper limb

97.12 Replacement of cast on lower limb

97.13 Replacement of other cast

97.14 Replacement of other device for musculoskeletal immobilization
Splinting
Strapping

97.15 Replacement of wound catheter

97.16 Replacement of wound packing or drain

Excludes: repacking of:
dental wound (97.22)
vulvar wound (97.26)

97.2 Other nonoperative replacement

97.21 Replacement of nasal packing

97.22 Replacement of dental packing

97.23 Replacement of tracheostomy tube

97.24 Replacement and refitting of vaginal diaphragm

97.25 Replacement of other vaginal pessary

97.26 Replacement of vaginal or vulvar packing or drain

97.29 Other nonoperative replacements

97.3 Nonoperative removal of therapeutic device from head and neck

97.31 Removal of eye prosthesis

Excludes: removal of ocular implant (16.71)
removal of orbital implant (16.72)

97.32 Removal of nasal packing

97.33 Removal of dental wiring

97.34 Removal of dental packing

97.35 Removal of dental prosthesis

97.36 Removal of other external mandibular fixation device

97.37 Removal of tracheostomy tube

97.38 Removal of sutures from head and neck

97.39 Removal of other therapeutic device from head and neck

Excludes: removal of skull tongs (02.94)

97.4 Nonoperative removal of therapeutic device from thorax

97.41 Removal of thoracotomy tube or pleural cavity drain

97.42 Removal of mediastinal drain

97.43 Removal of sutures from thorax

97.44 Nonoperative removal of heart assist system
Explantation [removal] of circulatory assist device
Explantation [removal] of percutaneous external heart assist device
Intra-aortic balloon pump [IABP]
Removal of extrinsic heart assist device
Removal of pVAD
Removal of percutaneous heart assist device

97.49 Removal of other device from thorax

Excludes: endoscopic removal of bronchial device(s) or substances (33.78)

97.5 Nonoperative removal of therapeutic device from digestive system

97.51 Removal of gastrostomy tube

97.52 Removal of tube from small intestine

97.53 Removal of tube from large intestine or appendix

97.54 Removal of cholecystostomy tube

97.55 Removal of T-tube, other bile duct tube, or liver tube
Removal of bile duct stent

97.56 Removal of pancreatic tube or drain

● Code new to this edition   ▲ Revision of existing code   ④ ⑤ Fourth or fifth digit required

97.59 **Removal of other device from digestive system**
Removal of rectal packing

97.6 **Nonoperative removal of therapeutic device from urinary system**

97.61 **Removal of pyelostomy and nephrostomy tube**

97.62 **Removal of ureterostomy tube and ureteral catheter**

97.63 **Removal of cystostomy tube**

97.64 **Removal of other urinary drainage device**
Removal of indwelling urinary catheter

97.65 **Removal of urethral stent**

97.69 **Removal of other device from urinary system**

97.7 **Nonoperative removal of therapeutic device from genital system**

97.71 **Removal of intrauterine contraceptive device**

97.72 **Removal of intrauterine pack**

97.73 **Removal of vaginal diaphragm**

97.74 **Removal of other vaginal pessary**

97.75 **Removal of vaginal or vulva packing**

97.79 **Removal of other device from genital tract**
Removal of sutures

97.8 **Other nonoperative removal of therapeutic device**

97.81 **Removal of retroperitoneal drainage device**

97.82 **Removal of peritoneal drainage device**

97.83 **Removal of abdominal wall sutures**

97.84 **Removal of sutures from trunk, not elsewhere classified**

97.85 **Removal of packing from trunk, not elsewhere classified**

97.86 **Removal of other device from abdomen**

97.87 **Removal of other device from trunk**

97.88 **Removal of external immobilization device**
Removal of:
  brace
  cast
  splint

97.89 **Removal of other therapeutic device**

98 **Nonoperative removal of foreign body or calculus**

98.0 **Removal of intraluminal foreign body from digestive system without incision**
> Excludes: *removal of therapeutic device (97.51-97.59)*

98.01 **Removal of intraluminal foreign body from mouth without incision**

98.02 **Removal of intraluminal foreign body from esophagus without incision**

98.03 **Removal of intraluminal foreign body from stomach and small intestine without incision**

98.04 **Removal of intraluminal foreign body from large intestine without incision**

98.05 **Removal of intraluminal foreign body from rectum and anus without incision**

98.1 **Removal of intraluminal foreign body from other sites without incision**
> Excludes: *removal of therapeutic device (97.31-97.49, 97.61-97.89)*

98.11 **Removal of intraluminal foreign body from ear without incision**

98.12 **Removal of intraluminal foreign body from nose without incision**

98.13 **Removal of intraluminal foreign body from pharynx without incision**

98.14 **Removal of intraluminal foreign body from larynx without incision**

98.15 **Removal of intraluminal foreign body from trachea and bronchus without incision**
> Excludes: *endoscopic removal of bronchial device(s) or substances (33.78)*

98.16 **Removal of intraluminal foreign body from uterus without incision**
> Excludes: *removal of intrauterine contraceptive device (97.71)*

98.17 **Removal of intraluminal foreign body from vagina without incision**

98.18 **Removal of intraluminal foreign body from artificial stoma without incision**

	Valid O.R. procedure		Non-O.R. procedure		Nonspecific O.R. procedure		Noncovered O.R. procedure

98.19 Removal of intraluminal foreign body from urethra without incision

98.2 **Removal of other foreign body without incision**

> Excludes: *removal of intraluminal foreign body (98.01-98.19)*

98.20 Removal of foreign body, not otherwise specified

98.21 Removal of superficial foreign body from eye without incision

98.22 Removal of other foreign body without incision from head and neck
Removal of embedded foreign body from eyelid or conjunctiva without incision

98.23 Removal of foreign body from vulva without incision

98.24 Removal of foreign body from scrotum or penis without incision

98.25 Removal of other foreign body without incision from trunk except scrotum, penis, or vulva

98.26 Removal of foreign body from hand without incision

98.27 Removal of foreign body without incision from upper limb, except hand

98.28 Removal of foreign body from foot without incision

98.29 Removal of foreign body without incision from lower limb, except foot

98.5 **Extracorporeal shockwave lithotripsy [ESWL]**
Lithotriptor tank procedure
Disintegration of stones by extracorporeal induced shockwaves
That with insertion of stent

98.51 Extracorporeal shockwave lithotripsy [ESWL] of the kidney, ureter and/or bladder

98.52 Extracorporeal shockwave lithotripsy [ESWL] of the gallbladder and/or bile duct

98.59 Extracorporeal shockwave lithotripsy of other sites

99 **Other nonoperative procedures**

99.0 **Transfusion of blood and blood components**
Use additional code for that done via catheter or cutdown (38.92-38.94)

99.00 Perioperative autologous transfusion of whole blood or blood components
Intraoperative blood collection
Postoperative blood collection
Salvage

99.01 Exchange transfusion
Transfusion:
exsanguination
replacement

99.02 Transfusion of previously collected autologous blood
Blood component

99.03 Other transfusion of whole blood
Transfusion:
NOS
blood NOS
hemodilution

99.04 Transfusion of packed cells

99.05 Transfusion of platelets
Transfusion of thrombocytes

99.06 Transfusion of coagulation factors
Transfusion of antihemophilic factor

99.07 Transfusion of other serum
Transfusion of plasma

> Excludes: *injection [transfusion] of:*
> *antivenin (99.16)*
> *gamma globulin (99.14)*

99.08 Transfusion of blood expander
Transfusion of Dextran

99.09 Transfusion of other substance
Transfusion of:
blood surrogate
granulocytes

> Excludes: *transplantation [transfusion] of bone marrow (41.00-41.09)*

● Code new to this edition   ▲ Revision of existing code   ④ ⑤ Fourth or fifth digit required

99.1   Injection or Infusion of therapeutic or prophylactic substance

Includes: injection or infusion given:
hypodermically acting locally or systemically
intramuscularly acting locally or systemically
intravenously acting locally or systemically

99.10   Injection or infusion of thrombolytic agent

Alteplase
Anistreplase
Reteplase
Streptokinase
Tenecteplase
Tissue plasminogen activator (TPA)
Urokinase

Excludes: *aspirin—omit code*
GP IIB/IIIa platelet inhibitors (99.20)
heparin (99.19)
SuperSaturated oxygen therapy (00.49)
warfarin—omit code

99.11   Injection of Rh immune globulin

Injection of:
Anti-D (Rhesus) globulin
RhoGAM

99.12   Immunization for allergy

Desensitization

99.13   Immunization for autoimmune disease

99.14   Injection or infusion of immunoglobulin

Injection of immune sera
Injection or infusion of gamma globulin

99.15   Parenteral infusion of concentrated nutritional substances

Hyperalimentation
Peripheral parenteral nutrition [PPN]
Total parenteral nutrition [TPN]

99.16   Injection of antidote

Injection of:
antivenin
heavy metal antagonist

99.17   Injection of insulin

99.18   Injection or infusion of electrolytes

99.19   Injection of anticoagulant

Excludes: *infusion of drotrecogin alfa (activated) (00.11)*

99.2   Injection or infusion of other therapeutic or prophylactic substance

Includes: injection or infusion given:
hypodermically acting locally or systemically
intramuscularly acting locally or systemically
intravenously acting locally or systemically

Use additional code for:
injection (into):
breast (85.92)
bursa (82.94, 83.96)
intraperitoneal (cavity) (54.97)
intrathecal (03.92)
joint (76.96, 81.92)
kidney (55.96)
liver (50.94)
orbit (16.91)
other sites—see Alphabetic Index
perfusion:
NOS (39.97)
intestine (46.95, 46.96)
kidney (55.95)
liver (50.93)
total body (39.96)

Excludes: *SuperSaturated oxygen therapy (00.49)*

Valid O.R.   Non-O.R.   Nonspecific   Noncovered
procedure   procedure   O.R. procedure   O.R. procedure

99.20 Injection or infusion of platelet inhibitor
Glycoprotein IIB/IIIa inhibitor
GP IIB/IIIa inhibitor
GP IIB-IIIa inhibitor

> Excludes: *infusion of heparin (99.19)*
> *injection or infusion of thrombolytic agent (99.10)*

99.21 Injection of antibiotic

> Excludes: *injection or infusion of oxazolidinone class of antibiotics (00.14)*

99.22 Injection of other anti-infective

> Excludes: *injection or infusion of oxazolidinone class of antibiotics (00.14)*

99.23 Injection of steroid
Injection of cortisone
Subdermal implantation of progesterone

99.24 Injection of other hormone

99.25 Injection or infusion of cancer chemotherapeutic substance
Chemoembolization
Injection or infusion of antineoplastic agent

Use additional code for disruption of blood brain barrier, if performed [BBBD] (00.19)

> Excludes: *immunotherapy, antineoplastic (00.15, 99.28)*
> *implantation of chemotherapeutic agent (00.10)*
> *injection or infusion of biological response modifier [BRM] as an antineoplastic agent (99.28)*
> *injection of radioisotopes (92.28)*
> *intravenous infusion of clofarabine (17.70)*

99.26 Injection of tranquilizer

99.27 Iontophoresis

99.28 Injection or infusion of biological response modifier [BRM] as an antineoplastic agent
Low-dose interleukin-2 (IL-2) therapy
Immunotherapy, antineoplastic
Infusion of cintredekin besudotox
Interleukin therapy
Tumor vaccine

> Excludes: *high-dose infusion interleukin-2 [IL-2] (00.15)*

99.29 Injection or infusion of other therapeutic or prophylactic substance

> Excludes: *administration of neuroprotective agent (99.75)*
> *immunization (99.31-99.59)*
> *infusion of blood brain barrier disruption substance (00.19)*
> *injection of sclerosing agent into:*
>   *esophageal varices (42.33)*
>   *hemorrhoids (49.42)*
>   *veins (39.92)*
> *injection or infusion of human B-type natriuretic peptide (hBNP) (00.13)*
> *injection or infusion of nesiritide (00.13)*
> *injection or infusion of platelet inhibitor (99.20)*
> *injection or infusion of thrombolytic agent (99.10)*
> *uterine artery embolization without coils (68.25)*

99.3 Prophylactic vaccination and inoculation against certain bacterial diseases

99.31 Vaccination against cholera

99.32 Vaccination against typhoid and paratyphoid fever
Administration of TAB vaccine

99.33 Vaccination against tuberculosis
Administration of BCG vaccine

99.34 Vaccination against plague

99.35 Vaccination against tularemia

99.36 Administration of diphtheria toxoid

> Excludes: *administration of:*
>   *diphtheria antitoxin (99.58)*
>   *diphtheria-tetanus-pertussis combined (99.39)*

99.37 **Vaccination against pertussis**

> Excludes: *administration of diphtheria-tetanus-pertussis, combined (99.39)*

99.38 **Administration of tetanus toxoid**

> Excludes: *administration of:*
> *diphtheria-tetanus-pertussis combined (99.39)*
> *tetanus antitoxin (99.56)*

99.39 **Administration of diphtheria-tetanus-pertussis, combined**

99.4 **Prophylactic vaccination and inoculation against certain viral diseases**

99.41 **Administration of poliomyelitis vaccine**

99.42 **Vaccination against smallpox**

99.43 **Vaccination against yellow fever**

99.44 **Vaccination against rabies**

99.45 **Vaccination against measles**

> Excludes: *administration of measles-mumps-rubella vaccine (99.48)*

99.46 **Vaccination against mumps**

> Excludes: *administration of measles-mumps-rubella vaccine (99.48)*

99.47 **Vaccination against rubella**

> Excludes: *administration of measles-mumps-rubella vaccine (99.48)*

99.48 **Administration of measles-mumps-rubella vaccine**

99.5 **Other vaccination and inoculation**

99.51 **Prophylactic vaccination against the common cold**

99.52 **Prophylactic vaccination against influenza**

99.53 **Prophylactic vaccination against arthropod-borne viral encephalitis**

99.54 **Prophylactic vaccination against other arthropod-borne viral diseases**

99.55 **Prophylactic administration of vaccine against other disease**
Vaccination against:
anthrax
brucellosis
Rocky Mountain spotted fever
Staphylococcus
Streptococcus
typhus

99.56 **Administration of tetanus antitoxin**

99.57 **Administration of botulism antitoxin**

99.58 **Administration of other antitoxins**
Administration of:
diphtheria antitoxin
gas gangrene antitoxin
scarlet fever antitoxin

99.59 **Other vaccination and inoculation**
Vaccination NOS

> Excludes: *injection of:*
> *gamma globulin (99.14)*
> *Rh immune globulin (99.11)*
> *immunization for:*
> *allergy (99.12)*
> *autoimmune disease (99.13)*

99.6 **Conversion of cardiac rhythm**

> Excludes: *open chest cardiac:*
> *electric stimulation (37.91)*
> *massage (37.91)*

99.60 **Cardiopulmonary resuscitation, not otherwise specified**

99.61 **Atrial cardioversion**

Valid O.R. procedure

Non-O.R. procedure

Nonspecific O.R. procedure

Noncovered O.R. procedure

99.62 Other electric countershock of heart
   Cardioversion:
     NOS
     external
   Conversion to sinus rhythm
   Defibrillation
   External electrode stimulation

99.63 Closed chest cardiac massage
   Cardiac massage NOS
   Manual external cardiac massage

99.64 Carotid sinus stimulation

99.69 Other conversion of cardiac rhythm

99.7 Therapeutic apheresis or other injection, administration, or infusion of other therapeutic or prophylactic substance

99.71 Therapeutic plasmapheresis

   | Excludes: | *extracorporeal immunoadsorption [ECI] (99.76)* |

99.72 Therapeutic leukopheresis
   Therapeutic leukocytapheresis

99.73 Therapeutic erythrocytapheresis
   Therapeutic erythropheresis

99.74 Therapeutic plateletpheresis

99.75 Administration of neuroprotective agent

99.76 Extracorporeal immunoadsorption
   Removal of antibodies from plasma with protein A columns

99.77 Application or administraion of adhesion barrier substance

99.78 Aquapheresis
   Plasma water removal
   Ultrafiltration [for water removal]

Excludes:	*hemodiafiltration (39.95)*
	hemodialysis (39.95)
	therapeutic plasmapheresis (99.71)

99.79 Other
   Apheresis (harvest) of stem cells
   Leech therapy

99.8 Miscellaneous physical procedures

99.81 Hypothermia (central) (local)

Excludes:	*gastric cooling (96.31)*
	gastric freezing (96.32)
	that incidental to open heart surgery (39.62)

99.82 Ultraviolet light therapy
   Actinotherapy

99.83 Other phototherapy
   Phototherapy of the newborn

   | Excludes: | *extracorporeal photochemotherapy (99.88)* |
   | | *photocoagulation of retinal lesion (14.23-14.25, 14.33-14.35, 14.53-14.55)* |

99.84 Isolation
   Isolation after contact with infectious disease
   Protection of individual from his surroundings
   Protection of surroundings from individual

99.85 Hyperthermia for treatment of cancer
   Hyperthermia (adjunct therapy) induced by microwave, ultrasound, low energy radiofrequency, probes (interstitial), or other means in the treatment of cancer
   Code also any concurrent chemotherapy or radiation therapy

99.86 Non-invasive placement of bone growth stimulator
   Transcutaneous (surface) placement of pads or patches for stimulation to aid bone healing

   | Excludes: | *insertion of invasive or semi-invasive bone growth stimulators (device) (percutaneous electrodes) (78.90-78.99)* |

● Code new to this edition   ▲ Revision of existing code   ④ ⑤ Fourth or fifth digit required

99.88 Therapeutic photopheresis

Extracorporeal photochemotherapy

Extracorporeal photopheresis

> Excludes: other phototherapy (99.83)
> ultraviolet light therapy (99.82)

99.9 Other miscellaneous procedures

99.91 Acupuncture for anesthesia

99.92 Other acupuncture

> Excludes: that with smouldering moxa (93.35)

99.93 Rectal massage (for levator spasm)

99.94 Prostatic massage

99.95 Stretching of foreskin

99.96 Collection of sperm for artificial insemination

99.97 Fitting of denture

99.98 Extraction of milk from lactating breast

99.99 Other

Leech therapy

Valid O.R. procedure	Non-O.R. procedure	Nonspecific O.R. procedure	Noncovered O.R. procedure

This page intentionally left blank.

● Code new
   to this edition

▲ Revision of
   existing code

④ ⑤ Fourth or fifth
   digit required

A

Abbe operation
construction of vagina 70.61
  with graft or prosthesis 70.63
intestinal anastomosis—*see* Anastomosis
  intestine
Abciximab, infusion 99.20
Abdominocentesis 54.91
Abdominohysterectomy 68.49
laparoscopic 68.41
Abdominoplasty 86.83
Abdominoscopy 54.21
Abdominouterotomy 68.0
obstetrical 74.99
Abduction, arytenoid 31.69
AbioCor® total replacement heart 37.52
Ablation
biliary ducts (lesion) by ERCP 51.64
endometrial (hysteroscopic) 68.23
inner ear (cryosurgery) (ultrasound) 20.79
  by injection 20.72
lesion
  esophagus 42.39
    endoscopic 42.33
  heart
    by peripherally inserted catheter 37.34
    endovascular approach 37.34
    Maze procedure (Cox-maze)
      endovascular approach 37.34
      open approach 37.33
      thoracoscopic approach 37.37
    thoracoscopic approach 37.37
  liver 50.26
    laparoscopic 50.25
    open 50.23
    percutaneous 50.24
  lung 32.26
    bronchoscopic thermoplasty 32.27
    open 32.23
    percutaneous 32.24
    thoracoscopic 32.25
  renal 55.35
    laparoscopic 55.34
    open 55.32
    percutaneous 55.33
intestine
  large 45.49
    endoscopic 45.43
large intestine 45.49
  endoscopic 45.43
pituitary 07.69
  by
    Cobalt-60 92.32
    implantation (strontium-yttrium) (Y) NEC
      07.68
      transfrontal approach 07.64
      transphenoidal approach 07.65
    proton beam (Bragg peak) 92.33
prostate, by
    cryoablation 60.62
    laser, transurethral 60.21
    radical cryosurgical ablation (RCSA) 60.62
    radiofrequency thermotherapy 60.97
    transurethral needle ablation (TUNA) 60.97
tissue
    heart—*see* Ablation, lesion, heart
    liver—*see* Ablation, lesion, liver
    lung—*see* Ablation, lesion, lung
    renal—*see* Ablation, lesion, renal

Abortion, therapeutic 69.51
by
  aspiration curettage 69.51
  dilation and curettage 69.01
  hysterectomy—*see* Hysterectomy
  hysterotomy 74.91
  insertion
    laminaria 69.93
    prostaglandin suppository 96.49
  intra-amniotic injection (saline) 75.0
Abrasion
corneal epithelium 11.41
  for smear or culture 11.21
epicardial surface 36.39
pleural 34.6
skin 86.25
Abscission, cornea 11.49
Absorptiometry
photon (dual) (single) 88.98
Aburel operation (intra-amniotic injection for
  abortion) 75.0
Accouchement forcé 73.99
Acetabulectomy 77.85
Acetabuloplasty NEC 81.40
with prosthetic implant 81.52
Achillorrhaphy 83.64
delayed 83.62
Achillotenotomy 83.11
plastic 83.85
Achillotomy 83.11
plastic 83.85
Acid peel, skin 86.24
Acromionectomy 77.81
Acromioplasty 81.83
for recurrent dislocation of shoulder 81.82
partial replacement 81.81
total replacement, NEC 81.80
  other 81.80
  reverse 81.88
Actinotherapy 99.82
Activities of daily living (ADL)
therapy 93.83
training for the blind 93.78
Acupuncture 99.92
with smouldering moxa 93.35
for anesthesia 99.91
Adams operation
advancement of round ligament 69.22
crushing of nasal septum 21.88
excision of palmar fascia 82.35
Adenectomy —*see also* Excision, by site
prostate NEC 60.69
retropubic 60.4
Adenoidectomy (without tonsillectomy) 28.6
with tonsillectomy 28.3
Adhesiolysis —*see also* Lysis, adhesions
for collapse of lung 33.39
middle ear 20.23
Adipectomy 86.83
Adjustment
cardiac pacemaker program
  (reprogramming)—*omit code*
cochlear prosthetic device (external components)
  95.49
dental 99.97
gastric restrictive device (laparoscopic) 44.98
occlusal 24.8

Adjustment—*continued*
  orthopedic device (noninvasive)
    external fixator – omit code
  spectacles 95.31
Administration (of)—*see also* Injection
  Activase® 99.10
  adhesion barrier substance 99.77
  Alteplase (tPA, generic) 99.10
  Anistreplase (tPA, generic) 99.10
  antitoxins NEC 99.58
    botulism 99.57
    diphtheria 99.58
    gas gangrene 99.58
    scarlet fever 99.58
    tetanus 99.56
  Bender Visual-Motor Gestalt test 94.02
  Benton Visual Retention test 94.02
  DrotAA 00.11
  Eminase® 99.10
  inhaled nitric oxide 00.12
  intelligence test or scale (Stanford-Binet)
      (Wechsler) (adult) (children) 94.01
  Minnesota Multiphasic Personality Inventory
      (MMPI) 94.02
  MMPI (Minnesota Multiphasic Personality
      Inventory) 94.02
  neuroprotective agent 99.75
  Proleukin® (low-dose) 99.28
    high-dose 00.15
  psychologic test 94.02
  Retavase® 99.10
  Reteplase (tPA, generic) 99.10
  Stanford-Binet test 94.01
  Streptase® 99.10
  Streptokinase (tPA, generic) 99.10
  Tenecteplase (tPA, generic) 99.10
  TNKase™ 99.10
  toxoid
    diphtheria 99.36
      with tetanus and pertussis, combined (DTP)
        99.39
    tetanus 99.38
      with diphtheria and pertussis, combined
        (DTP) 99.39
  vaccine—*see also* Vaccination
    BCG 99.33
    measles-mumps-rubella (MMR) 99.48
    poliomyelitis 99.41
    TAB 99.32
  Wechsler
    Intelligence Scale (adult) (children) 94.01
    Memory Scale 94.02
  Xigris® 00.11
Adrenalectomy (unilateral) 07.22
  with partial removal of remaining gland 07.29
  bilateral 07.3
    partial 07.29
    subtotal 07.29
  complete 07.3
  partial NEC 07.29
  remaining gland 07.3
  subtotal NEC 07.29
  total 07.3
Adrenalorrhaphy 07.44
Adrenalotomy (with drainage) 07.41
Advancement
  extraocular muscle 15.12
    multiple (with resection or recession) 15.3
  eyelid muscle 08.59
  eye muscle 15.12
    multiple (with resection or recession) 15.3

Advancement—*continued*
  graft—*see* Graft
  leaflet (heart) 35.10
  pedicle (flap) 86.72
  profundus tendon (Wagner) 82.51
  round ligament 69.22
  tendon 83.71
    hand 82.51
    profundus (Wagner) 82.51
    Wagner (profundus tendon) 82.51
AESOP® (Automated Endoscopic System for
    Optimal Positioning) –*see* category 17.4
Albee operation
  bone peg, femoral neck 78.05
  graft for slipping patella 78.06
  sliding inlay graft, tibia 78.07
Albert operation (arthrodesis of knee) 81.22
Aldridge (Studdiford) operation (urethral sling)
    59.5
Alexander operation
  prostatectomy
    perineal 60.62
    suprapubic 60.3
  shortening of round ligaments 69.22
Alexander-Adams operation (shortening of
    round ligaments) 69.22
Alimentation, parenteral 99.29
Allograft —*see* Graft
Almoor operation (extrapetrosal drainage)
    20.22
Altemeier operation (perineal rectal
    pull-through) 48.49
Alveolectomy (interradicular) (intraseptal)
    (radical) (simple) (with graft) (with implant)
    24.5
Alveoloplasty (with graft or implant) 24.5
Alveolotomy (apical) 24.0
Ambulatory cardiac monitoring (ACM) 89.50
Ammon operation (dacryocystotomy) 09.53
Amniocentesis (transuterine) (diagnostic) 75.1
  with intra-amniotic injection of saline 75.0
Amniography 87.81
Amnioinfusion 75.37
Amnioscopy, internal 75.31
Amniotomy 73.09
  to induce labor 73.01
Amputation (cineplastic) (closed flap)
    (guillotine) (kineplastic) (open) 84.91
  abdominopelvic 84.19
  above-elbow 84.07
  above-knee (AK) 84.17
  ankle (disarticulation) 84.13
    through malleoli of tibia and fibula 84.14
  arm NEC 84.00
    through
      carpals 84.03
      elbow (disarticulation) 84.06
      forearm 84.05
      humerus 84.07
      shoulder (disarticulation) 84.08
      wrist (disarticulation) 84.04
    upper 84.07
  Batch-Spittler-McFaddin (knee disarticulation)
    84.16
  below-knee (BK) NEC 84.15
    conversion into above-knee amputation 84.17
  Boyd (hip disarticulation) 84.18
  Callander's (knee disarticulation) 84.16
  carpals 84.03
  cervix 67.4
  Chopart's (midtarsal) 84.12

Amputation—*continued*
clitoris 71.4
Dieffenbach (hip disarticulation) 84.18
Dupuytren's (shoulder disarticulation) 84.08
ear, external 18.39
elbow (disarticulation) 84.06
finger, except thumb 84.01
  thumb 84.02
foot (middle) 84.12
forearm 84.05
forefoot 84.12
forequarter 84.09
Gordon-Taylor (hindquarter) 84.19
Gritti-Stokes (knee disarticulation) 84.16
Guyon (ankle) 84.13
hallux 84.11
hand 84.03
Hey's (foot) 84.12
hindquarter 84.19
hip (disarticulation) 84.18
humerus 84.07
interscapulothoracic 84.09
interthoracoscapular 84.09
King-Steelquist (hindquarter) 84.19
Kirk (thigh) 84.17
knee (disarticulation) 84.16
Kutler (revision of current traumatic amputation
  of finger) 84.01
Larry (shoulder disarticulation) 84.08
leg NEC 84.10
  above knee (AK) 84.17
  below knee (BK) 84.15
  through
    ankle (disarticulation) 84.13
    femur (AK) 84.17
    foot 84.12
    hip (disarticulation) 84.18
    tibia and fibula (BK) 84.15
Lisfranc
  foot 84.12
  shoulder (disarticulation) 84.08
Littlewood (forequarter) 84.09
lower limb NEC (*see also* Amputation, leg) 84.10
Mazet (knee disarticulation) 84.16
metacarpal 84.03
metatarsal 84.11
  head (bunionectomy) 77.59
metatarsophalangeal (joint) 84.11
midtarsal 84.12
nose 21.4
penis (circle) (complete) (flap) (partial) (radical)
  64.3
Pirogoff's (ankle amputation through malleoli of
  tibia and fibula) 84.14
ray
  finger 84.01
  foot 84.11
  toe (metatarsal head) 84.11
root (tooth) (apex) 23.73
  with root canal therapy 23.72
shoulder (disarticulation) 84.08
Sorondo-Ferré (hindquarter) 84.19
S.P. Rogers (knee disarticulation) 84.16
supracondylar, above-knee 84.17
supramalleolar, foot 84.14
Syme's (ankle amputation through malleoli of
  tibia and fibula) 84.14
thigh 84.17
thumb 84.02
toe (through metatarsophalangeal joint) 84.11
transcarpal 84.03
transmetatarsal 84.12

Amputation—*continued*
upper limb NEC (*see also* Amputation, arm)
  84.00
wrist (disarticulation) 84.04
Amygdalohippocampectomy 01.59
Amygdalohippocampotomy 01.39
Amygdalotomy 01.39
Analysis
cardiac rhythm device (CRT-D) (CRT-P) (AICD)
  (pacemaker)—*see* Interrogation
character 94.03
gastric 89.39
psychologic 94.31
transactional
  group 94.44
  individual 94.39
Anastomosis
abdominal artery to coronary artery 36.17
accessory-facial nerve 04.72
accessory-hypoglossal nerve 04.73
anus (with formation of endorectal deal pouch)
  45.95
aorta (descending)—pulmonary (artery) 39.0
aorta-renal artery 39.24
aorta-subclavian artery 39.22
aortoceliac 39.26
aorto(ilio)femoral 39.25
aortomesenteric 39.26
appendix 47.99
arteriovenous NEC 39.29
  for renal dialysis 39.27
artery (suture of distal to proximal end) 39.31
  with
    bypass graft 39.29
      extracranial-intracranial [EC-IC] 39.28
    excision or resection of vessel—*see*
      Arteriectomy, with anastomosis, by site
    revision 39.49
bile ducts 51.39
bladder NEC 57.88
  with
    isolated segment of intestine 57.87 *[45.50]*
    colon (sigmoid) 57.87 *[45.52]*
    ileum 57.87 *[45.51]*
    open loop of ileum 57.87 *[45.51]*
  to intestine 57.88
    ileum 57.87 *[45.51]*
bowel—(*see also* Anastomosis, intestine) 45.90
bronchotracheal 33.48
bronchus 33.48
carotid-subclavian artery 39.22
caval-mesenteric vein 39.1
caval-pulmonary artery 39.21
cervicoesophageal 42.59
colohypopharyngeal (intrathoracic) 42.55
  antesternal or antethoracic 42.65
common bile duct 51.39
common pulmonary trunk and left atrium
  (posterior wall) 35.82
cystic bile duct 51.39
cystocolic 57.88
epididymis to vas deferens 63.83
esophagocolic (intrathoracic) NEC 42.56
  with interposition 42.55
  antesternal or antethoracic NEC 42.66
    with interposition 42.65
esophagocologastric (intrathoracic) 42.55
  antesternal or antethoracic 42.65
esophagoduodenal (intrathoracic) NEC 42.54
  with interposition 42.53

Anastomosis—*continued*
  esophagoenteric (intrathoracic) NEC *see also*
    Anastomosis, esophagus to intestinal
    segment) 42.54
    antesternal or antethoracic NEC (*see also*
      Anastomosis, esophagus, antesternal, to
      intestinal segment) 42.64
  esophagoesophageal (intrathoracic) 42.51
    antesternal or antethoracic 42.61
  esophagogastric (intrathoracic) 42.52
    antesternal or antethoracic 42.62
  esophagus (intrapleural) (intrathoracic)
    (retrosternal) NEC 42.59
    with
      gastrectomy (partial) 43.5
        complete or total 43.99
      interposition (of) NEC 42.58
        colon 42.55
        jejunum 42.53
        small bowel 42.53
    antesternal or antethoracic NEC 42.69
    with
      interposition (of) NEC 42.68
        colon 42.65
        jejunal loop 42.63
        small bowel 42.63
        rubber tube 42.68
    to intestinal segment NEC 42.64
      with interposition 42.68
      colon NEC 42.66
        with interposition 42.65
      small bowel NEC 42.64
        with interposition 42.63
    to intestinal segment (intrathoracic) NEC 42.54
      with interposition 42.58
      antesternal or antethoracic NEC 42.64
        with interposition 42.68
      colon (intrathoracic) NEC 42.56
        with interposition 42.55
        antesternal or antethoracic 42.66
          with interposition 42.65
      small bowel NEC 42.54
        with interposition 42.53
        antesternal or antethoracic 42.64
          with interposition 42.63
  facial-accessory nerve 04.72
  facial-hypoglossal nerve 04.71
  fallopian tube 66.73
    by reanastomosis 66.79
  gallbladder 51.35
    to
      hepatic ducts 51.31
      intestine 51.32
      pancreas 51.33
      stomach 51.34
  gastroepiploic artery (to)
    coronary artery 36.17
  hepatic duct 51.39
  hypoglossal-accessory nerve 04.73
  hypoglossal-facial nerve 04.71
  ileal loop to bladder 57.87 *[45.51]*
  ileoanal 45.95
  ileorectal 45.93
  inferior vena cava and portal vein 39.1
  internal mammary artery (to)
    coronary artery (single vessel) 36.15
      double vessel 36.16
    myocardium 36.2

Anastomosis—*continued*
  intestine 45.90
    large-to-anus 45.95
    large-to-large 45.94
    large-to-rectum 45.94
    large-to-small 45.93
    small-to-anus 45.95
    small-to-large 45.93
    small-to-rectal stump 45.92
    small-to-small 45.91
  intrahepatic 51.79
  intrathoracic vessel NEC 39.23
  kidney (pelvis) 55.86
  lacrimal sac to conjunctiva 09.82
  left-to-right (systemic-pulmonary artery) 39.0
  lymphatic (channel) (peripheral) 40.9
  mesenteric-caval 39.1
  mesocaval 39.1
  nasolacrimal 09.81
  nerve (cranial) (peripheral) NEC 04.74
    accessory-facial 04.72
    accessory-hypoglossal 04.73
    hypoglossal-facial 04.71
  pancreas (duct) (to) 52.96
    bile duct 51.39
    gall bladder 51.33
    intestine 52.96
    jejunum 52.96
    stomach 52.96
  pleurothecal (with valve) 03.79
  portacaval 39.1
  portal vein to inferior vena cava 39.1
  pulmonary-aortic (Pott's) 39.0
  pulmonary artery and superior vena cava 39.21
  pulmonary-innominate artery (Blalock) 39.0
  pulmonary-subclavian artery (Blalock-Taussig)
    39.0
  pulmonary vein and azygos vein 39.23
  pyeloileocutaneous 56.51
  pyeloureterovesical 55.86
  radial artery 36.19
  rectum, rectal NEC 48.74
    stump to small intestine 45.92
  renal (pelvis) 55.86
    vein and splenic vein 39.1
  renoportal 39.1
  salpingothecal (with valve) 03.79
  splenic to renal veins 39.1
  splenorenal (venous) 39.1
    arterial 39.26
  subarachnoid-peritoneal (with valve) 03.71
  subarachnoid-ureteral (with valve) 03.72
  subclavian-aortic 39.22
  superior vena cava to pulmonary artery 39.21
  systemic-pulmonary artery 39.0
  thoracic artery (to)
    coronary artery (single) 36.15
      double 36.16
    myocardium 36.2
  ureter (to) NEC 56.79
    bladder 56.74
    colon 56.71
    ileal pouch (bladder) 56.51
    ileum 56.71
    intestine 56.71
    skin 56.61
  ureterocalyceal 55.86
  ureterocolic 56.71
  ureterovesical 56.74
  urethra (end-to-end) 58.44
  vas deferens 63.82

Anastomosis—*continued*
  veins (suture of proximal to distal end) (with
      bypass graft) 39.29
    with excision or resection of vessel—*see*
        Phlebectomy, with anastomosis, by site
    mesenteric to vena cava 39.1
    portal to inferior vena cava 39.1
    revision 39.49
    splenic and renal 39.1
  ventricle, ventricular (intracerebral) (with valve)
      (*see also* Shunt, ventricular) 02.22
  ventriculoatrial (with valve) 02.32
  ventriculocaval (with valve) 02.32
  ventriculomastoid (with valve) 02.31
  ventriculopleural (with valve) 02.33
  vesicle—*see* Anastomosis, bladder
Anderson operation (tibial lengthening) 78.37
Anel operation (dilation of lacrimal duct) 09.42
Anesthesia
  acupuncture for 99.91
  cryoanalgesia
    nerve (cranial) (peripheral) 04.2
  spinal—*omit code*
Aneurysmectomy 38.60
  with
    anastomosis 38.30
      abdominal
        artery 38.36
        vein 38.37
      aorta (arch) (ascending) (descending) 38.34
      head and neck NEC 38.32
      intracranial NEC 38.31
      lower limb
        artery 38.38
        vein 38.39
      thoracic NEC 38.35
      upper limb (artery) (vein) 38.33
    graft replacement (interposition) 38.40
      abdominal
        aorta
          endovascular approach 39.71
            fenestrated (branching) graft 39.78
          open approach 38.44
          Zenith® Renu™ AAA graft 39.71
        artery 38.46
        vein 38.47
      aorta (arch) (ascending) (descending thoracic)
        abdominal 38.44
        thoracic 38.45
        thoracoabdominal 38.45 *[38.44]*
      head and neck NEC 38.42
      intracranial NEC 38.41
      lower limb
        artery 38.48
        vein 38.49
      thoracic NEC 38.45
      upper limb (artery) (vein) 38.43
  abdominal
    artery 38.66
    vein 38.67
  aorta (arch) (ascending) (descending) 38.64
  atrial, auricular 37.32
  head and neck NEC 38.62
  heart 37.32
  intracranial NEC 38.61
  lower limb
    artery 38.68
    vein 38.69
  sinus of Valsalva 35.39
  thoracic NEC 38.65
  upper limb (artery) (vein) 38.63
  ventricle (myocardium) 37.32

Aneurysmoplasty —*see* Aneurysmorrhaphy
Aneurysmorrhaphy NEC 39.52
  by or with
    Anastomosis—*see* Aneurysmectomy, with
        anastomosis, by site
    clipping 39.51
    coagulation 39.52
    electrocoagulation 39.52
    endovascular graft
      abdominal aorta 39.71
        fenestrated (branching) graft 39.78
      lower extremity artery(s) 39.79
      thoracic aorta 39.73
      upper extremity artery(s) 39.79
    excision or resection—*see also*
        Aneurysmectomy, by site
      with
        anastomosis—*see* Aneurysmectomy, with
            anastomosis, by site
        graft replacement—*see* Aneurysmectomy,
            with graft replacement, by site
    filipuncture 39.52
    graft replacement—*see* Aneurysmectomy, with
        graft replacement, by site
    methyl methacrylate 39.52
    suture 39.52
    wiring 39.52
    wrapping 39.52
  Matas' 39.52
Aneurysmotomy —*see* Aneurysmectomy
Angiectomy
  with
    anastomosis 38.30
      abdominal
        artery 38.36
        vein 38.37
      aorta (arch) (ascending) (descending) 38.34
      head and neck NEC 38.32
      intracranial NEC 38.31
      lower limb
        artery 38.38
        vein 38.39
      thoracic vessel NEC 38.35
      upper limb (artery) (vein) 38.33
    graft replacement (interposition) 38.40
      abdominal
        aorta 38.44
        artery 38.46
        vein 38.47
      aorta (arch) (ascending) (descending thoracic)
        abdominal 38.44
        thoracic 38.45
        thoracoabdominal 38.45 *[38.44]*
      head and neck NEC 38.42
      intracranial NEC 38.41
      lower limb
        artery 38.48
        vein 38.49
      thoracic vessel NEC 38.45
      upper limb (artery) (vein) 38.43
Angiocardiography (selective) 88.50
  carbon dioxide (negative contrast) 88.58
  combined right and left heart 88.54
  intra-operative coronary fluorescence vascular
      88.59
  left heart (aortic valve) (atrium) (ventricle)
      (ventricular outflow tract) 88.53
    combined with right heart 88.54
  right heart (atrium) (pulmonary valve) (ventricle)
      (ventricular outflow tract) 88.52
    combined with left heart 88.54

Angiocardiography—*continued*
SPY, coronary 88.59
vena cava (inferior) (superior) 88.51
Angiography (arterial) (*see also* Arteriography)
88.40
basilar 88.41
brachial 88.49
by C.A.T. —*see* Scan, C.A.T., by site
by computed tomography —*see* Scan, C.A.T., by site
by magnetic resonance – *see* Imaging, magnetic resonance, by site
by radioisotope—*see* Scan, radioisotope, by site
by ultrasound—*see* Ultrasonography, by site
carotid (internal) 88.41
celiac 88.47
cerebral (posterior circulation) 88.41
coronary NEC 88.57
intra-operative fluorescence vascular 88.59
eye (fluorescein) 95.12
femoral 88.48
heart 88.50
intra-abdominal NEC 88.47
intracranial 88.41
intrathoracic vessels NEC 88.44
lower extremity NEC 88.48
neck 88.41
non-coronary, intra-operative fluorescence 17.71
placenta 88.46
pulmonary 88.43
renal 88.45
specified artery NEC 88.49
transfemoral 88.48
upper extremity NEC 88.49
veins—*see* Phlebography
vertebral 88.41
Angioplasty (laser) —*see also* Repair, blood vessel

Note: Also use 00.40, 00.41, 00.42, or 00.43 to show the total number of vessels treated. Use code 00.44 once to show procedure on a bifurcated vessel. In addition, use 00.45, 00.46, 00.47, or 00.48 to show the number of vascular stents inserted.

balloon (percutaneous transluminal) NEC 39.50
coronary artery 00.66
coronary 36.09
open chest approach 36.03
percutaneous transluminal (balloon) 00.66
percutaneous transluminal (balloon)
basilar 00.62
carotid 00.61
cerebrovascular
extracranial 00.62
intracranial 00.61
carotid 00.61
coronary (balloon) 00.66
extracranial 00.61
femoropopliteal 39.50
iliac 39.50
intracranial 00.62
lower extremity NOS 39.50
mesenteric 39.50
peripheral NEC 39.50
renal 39.50
subclavian 39.50
upper extremity NOS 39.50
vertebral 00.61
intracranial portion 00.62

Angioplasty (laser)—*continued*
specified site NEC 39.50
cerebrovascular
extracranial 00.62
intracranial 00.61
peripheral 39.50
Angiorrhaphy 39.30
artery 39.31
vein 39.32
Angioscopy, percutaneous 38.22
eye (fluorescein) 95.12
Angiotomy 38.00
abdominal
artery 38.06
vein 38.07
aorta (arch) (ascending) (descending) 38.04
head and neck NEC 38.02
intracranial NEC 38.01
lower limb
artery 38.08
vein 38.09
thoracic NEC 38.05
upper limb (artery) (vein) 38.03
Angiotripsy 39.98
Ankylosis, production of —*see* Arthrodesis
Annuloplasty (heart) (posteromedial) 35.33
Anoplasty 49.79
with hemorrhoidectomy 49.46
Anoscopy 49.21
Antibiogram —*see* Examination, microscopic
Antiembolic filter, vena cava 38.7
Antiphobic treatment 94.39
Antrectomy
mastoid 20.49
maxillary 22.39
radical 22.31
pyloric 43.6
Antrostomy —*see* Antrotomy
Antrotomy (exploratory) (nasal sinus) 22.2
Caldwell-Luc (maxillary sinus) 22.39
with removal of membrane lining 22.31
intranasal 22.2
with external approach (Caldwell-Luc) 22.39
radical 22.31
maxillary (simple) 22.2
with Caldwell-Luc approach 22.39
with removal of membrane lining 22.31
external (Caldwell-Luc approach) 22.39
with removal of membrane lining 22.31
radical (with removal of membrane lining) 22.31
Antrum window operation —*see* Antrotomy, maxillary
Aorticopulmonary window operation 39.59
Aortogram, aortography (abdominal) (retrograde) (selective) (translumbar) 88.42
Aortoplasty (aortic valve) (gusset type) 35.11
Aortotomy 38.04
Apexcardiogram (with ECG lead) 89.57
Apheresis, therapeutic —*see category* 99.7
Apicectomy
lung 32.39
thoracoscopic 32.30
petrous pyramid 20.59
tooth (root) 23.73
with root canal therapy 23.72
Apicoectomy 23.73
with root canal therapy 23.72
Apicolysis (lung) 33.39
Apicostomy, alveolar 24.0
Aponeurectomy 83.42
hand 82.33

Aponeurorrhaphy (*see also* Suture, tendon)
   83.64
   hand (*see also* Suture, tendon, hand) 82.45
Aponeurotomy 83.13
   hand 82.11
Appendectomy (with drainage) 47.09
   incidental 47.19
      laparoscopic 47.11
   laparoscopic 47.01
Appendicocecostomy 47.91
Appendicoenterostomy 47.91
Appendicolysis 54.59
   with appendectomy 47.01, 47.09
   laparoscopic 54.51
Appendicostomy 47.91
   closure 47.92
Appendicotomy 47.2
Application
   adhesion barrier substance 99.77
   anti-shock trousers 93.58
   arch bars (orthodontic) 24.7
      for immobilization (fracture) 93.55
   barrier substance, adhesion 99.77
   Barton's tongs (skull) (with synchronous skeletal
      traction) 02.94
   bone growth stimulator (surface) (transcutaneous)
      99.86
   bone morphogenetic protein (Infuse™) (OP-1™)
      (recombinant) (rhBMP) 84.52
   Bryant's traction 93.44
      with reduction of fracture or dislocation—*see*
         Reduction, fracture and Reduction,
         dislocation
   Buck's traction 93.46
   caliper tongs (skull) (with synchronous skeletal
      traction) 02.94
   cast (fiberglass) (plaster) (plastic) NEC 93.53
      with reduction of fracture or dislocation—*see*
         Reduction, fracture and Reduction,
         dislocation
      spica 93.51
   cervical collar 93.52
      with reduction of fracture or dislocation—*see*
         Reduction, fracture and Reduction,
         dislocation
   clamp, cerebral aneurysm (Crutchfield)
      (Silverstone) 39.51
   croupette, croup tent 93.94
   crown (artificial) 23.41
   Crutchfield tongs (skull) (with synchronous
      skeletal traction) 02.94
   Dunlop's traction 93.44
      with reduction of fracture or dislocation—*see*
         Reduction, fracture and Reduction,
         dislocation
   elastic stockings 93.59
   electronic gaiter 93.59
   external fixator device (bone) 78.10
      carpal, metacarpal 78.14
      clavicle 78.11
      computer assisted (dependent) 84.73
      femur 78.15
      fibula 78.17
      humerus 78.12
      hybrid device or system 84.73
      Ilizarov 84.72
      monoplanar system or device 84.71
      patella 78.16
      pelvic 78.19
      phalanges (foot) (hand) 78.19
      radius 78.13

Application—*continued*
      ring device or system 84.72
      scapula 78.11
      Sheffield type 84.72
      specified site NEC 78.19
      tarsal, metatarsal 78.18
      thorax (ribs) (sternum) 78.11
      tibia 78.17
      ulna 78.13
      vertebrae 78.19
   forceps, with delivery—*see* Delivery, forceps
   graft—*see* Graft
   gravity (G.) suit 93.59
   intermittent pressure device 93.59
   Jewett extension brace 93.59
   Jobst pumping unit (reduction of edema) 93.59
   Lyman Smith traction 93.44
      with reduction of fracture or dislocation—*see*
         Reduction, fracture and Reduction,
         dislocation
   MAST (military anti-shock trousers) 93.58
   Minerva jacket 93.52
   minifixator device (bone)—*see category* 78.1
   neck support (molded) 93.52
   obturator (orthodontic) 24.7
   orthodontic appliance (obturator) (wiring) 24.7
   pelvic sling 93.44
      with reduction of fracture or dislocation—*see*
         Reduction, fracture and Reduction,
         dislocation
   peridontal splint (orthodontic) 24.7
   plaster jacket 93.51
      Minerva 93.52
   pressure
      dressing (bandage) (Gibney) (Robert Jones')
         (Shanz) 93.56
      trousers (anti-shock) (MAST) 93.58
   prosthesis for missing ear 18.71
   Russell's traction 93.44
      with reduction of fracture or dislocation—*see*
         Reduction, fracture and Reduction,
         dislocation
   splint, for immobilization (plaster) (pneumatic)
      (tray) 93.54
      with fracture reduction—*see* Reduction, fracture
   stereotactic head frame 93.59
   strapping (non-traction) 93.59
   substance, adhesion barrier 99.77
   Thomas collar 93.52
      with reduction of fracture or dislocation—*see*
         Reduction, fracture and Reduction,
         dislocation
   traction
      with reduction of fracture or dislocation—*see*
         Reduction, fracture and Reduction,
         dislocation
      adhesive tape (skin) 93.46
      boot 93.46
      Bryant's 93.44
      Buck's 93.46
      Cotrel's 93.42
      Dunlop's 93.44
      gallows 93.46
      Lyman Smith 93.44
      Russell's 93.44
      skeletal NEC 93.44
         intermittent 93.43
      skin, limbs NEC 93.46

Application—*continued*
  spinal NEC 93.42
    with skull device (halo) (caliper)
      (Crutchfield) (Gardner-Wells) (Vinke)
      (tongs) 93.41
      with synchronous insertion 02.94
    Thomas' splint 93.45
  Unna's paste boot 93.53
  vasopneumatic device 93.58
  Velpeau dressing 93.59
  Vinke tongs (skull) (with synchronous skeletal
    traction) 02.94
  wound dressing 93.57
Aquapheresis 99.78
Arc lamp —*see* Photocoagulation
Arcuplasty 81.66
Arrest
  bone growth (epiphyseal) 78.20
    by stapling—see Stapling, epiphyseal plate
    femur 78.25
    fibula 78.27
    humerus 78.22
    radius 78.23
    tibia 78.27
    ulna 78.23
  cardiac, induced (anoxic) (circulatory) 39.63
  circulatory, induced (anoxic) 39.63
  hemorrhage—*see* Control, hemorrhage
Arslan operation (fenestration of inner ear) 20.61
Arteriectomy 38.60
  with
    anastomosis 38.30
      abdominal 38.36
      aorta (arch) (ascending) (descending) 38.34
      head and neck NEC 38.32
      intracranial NEC 38.31
      lower limb 38.38
      thoracic NEC 38.35
      upper limb 38.33
    graft replacement (interposition) 38.40
      abdominal
        aorta 38.44
        aorta (arch) (ascending) (descending thoracic)

        abdominal 38.44
        thoracic 38.45
        thoracoabdominal 38.45 *[38.44]*
      head and neck NEC 38.42
      intracranial NEC 38.41
      lower limb 38.48
      thoracic NEC 38.45
      upper limb 38.43
    abdominal 38.66
    aorta (arch) (ascending) (descending) 38.64
    head and neck NEC 38.62
    intracranial NEC 38.61
    lower limb 38.68
    thoracic NEC 38.65
    upper limb 38.63
Arteriography (contrast) (fluoroscopic)
    (retrograde) 88.40
  by
    radioisotope—*see* Scan, radioisotope
    ultrasound (Doppler)—*see* Ultrasonography, by
      site
  aorta (arch) (ascending) (descending) 88.42
  basilar 88.41
  brachial 88.49
  carotid (internal) 88.41
  cerebral (posterior circulation) 88.41

Arteriography—*continued*
  coronary (direct) (selective) NEC 88.57
    double catheter technique (Judkins) (Ricketts
      and Abrams) 88.56
    intra-operative fluorescence vascular 88.59
    single catheter technique (Sones) 88.55
  Doppler (ultrasonic)—*see* Ultrasonography, by
    site
  femoral 88.48
  head and neck 88.41
  intra-abdominal NEC 88.47
  intrathoracic NEC 88.44
  lower extremity 88.48
  placenta 88.46
  pulmonary 88.43
  radioisotope—*see* Scan, radioisotope
  renal 88.45
  specified site NEC 88.49
  SPY, coronary 88.59
  superior mesenteric artery 88.47
  transfemoral 88.48
  ultrasound—*see* Ultrasonography, by site
  upper extremity 88.49
Arterioplasty —*see* Repair, artery
Arteriorrhaphy 39.31
Arteriotomy 38.00
  abdominal 38.06
  aorta (arch) (ascending) (descending) 38.04
  head and neck NEC 38.02
  intracranial NEC 38.01
  lower limb 38.08
  thoracic NEC 38.05
  upper limb 38.03
Arteriovenostomy 39.29
  for renal dialysis 39.27
Arthrectomy 80.90
  ankle 80.97
  elbow 80.92
  foot and toe 80.98
  hand and finger 80.94
  hip 80.95
  intervertebral disc—see category 80.5
  knee 80.96
    semilunar cartilage 80.6
  shoulder 80.91
  specified site NEC 80.99
  spine NEC 80.99
  wrist 80.93
Arthrocentesis 81.91
  for arthrography—*see* Arthrogram
Arthrodesis (compression) (extra-articular)
    (intra-articular) (with bone graft) (with
    fixation device) 81.20
  ALIF (anterior lumbar interbody fusion) 81.06
  ankle 81.11
  carporadial 81.25
  cricoarytenoid 31.69
  elbow 81.24
  finger 81.28
  foot NEC 81.17
  hip 81.21
  interphalangeal
    finger 81.28
    toe NEC 77.58
      claw toe repair 77.57
      hammer toe repair 77.56
  ischiofemoral 81.21
  knee 81.22

Arthrodesis—*continued*
  lumbosacral, lumbar NEC 81.08
    anterior column (interbody)
      anterolateral (anterior) technique 81.06
      posterior technique 81.08
    axial lumbar interbody fusion [AxiaLIF] 81.08
    direct lateral interbody fusion [DLIF} 81.06
    extreme lateral interbody fusion [XLIF] 81.06
    facet 81.07
    lateral transverse process technique 81.07
  McKeever (metatarsophalangeal) 81.16
  metacarpocarpal 81.26
  metacarpophalangeal 81.27
  metatarsophalangeal 81.16
  midtarsal 81.14
  pantalar 81.11
  PLIF (posterior lumbar interbody fusion) 81.08
  sacroiliac 81.08
  shoulder 81.23
  specified joint NEC 81.29
  spinal (*see also* Fusion, spinal) 81.00
  subtalar 81.13
  tarsometatarsal 81.15
  tibiotalar 81.11
  TLIF (transforaminal lumbar interbody fusion) 81.08
  toe NEC 77.58
    claw toe repair 77.57
    hammer toe repair 77.56
  triple 81.12
  wrist 81.26
Arthroendoscopy —*see* Arthroscopy
Arthroereisis, subtalar joint 81.18
Arthrogram, arthrography 88.32
  temporomandibular 87.13
Arthrolysis 93.26
Arthroplasty (with fixation device) (with prosthesis) (with traction) 81.96
  ankle 81.49
  carpals 81.75
    with prosthetic implant 81.74
  carpocarpal, carpometacarpal 81.75
    with prosthetic implant 81.74
  Carroll and Taber (proximal interphalangeal joint) 81.72
  cup (partial hip) 81.52
  Curtis (interphalangeal joint) 81.72
  elbow 81.85
    with prosthetic replacement (partial) (total) 81.84
  femoral head NEC 81.40
    with prosthetic implant 81.52
  finger(s) 81.72
    with prosthetic implant 81.71
  foot (metatarsal) with joint replacement 81.57
  Fowler (metacarpophalangeal joint) 81.72
  hand (metacarpophalangeal) (interphalangeal) 81.72
    with prosthetic implant 81.71
  hip (with bone graft) 81.40
    cup (partial hip) 81.52
    femoral head NEC 81.40
      with prosthetic implant 81.52
        with total replacement 81.51
    partial replacement 81.52
    total replacement 81.51
  interphalangeal joint 81.72
    with prosthetic implant 81.71
  Kessler (carpometacarpal joint) 81.74

Arthroplasty—*continued*
  knee (*see also* Repair, knee) 81.47
    prosthetic replacement (bicompartmental) (hemijoint) (partial) (total) (tricompartmental) (unicompartmental) 81.54
    revision 81.55
  metacarpophalangeal joint 81.72
    with prosthetic implant 81.71
  shoulder 81.83
    prosthetic replacement (partial) 81.81
      total, NEC 81.80
        other 81.80
        reverse 81.88
    for recurrent dislocation 81.82
  temporomandibular 76.5
  toe NEC 77.58
    with prosthetic replacement 81.57
    for hallux valgus repair 77.59
  wrist 81.75
    with prosthetic implant 81.74
    total replacement 81.73
Arthroscopy 80.20
  ankle 80.27
  elbow 80.22
  finger 80.24
  foot 80.28
  hand 80.24
  hip 80.25
  knee 80.26
  shoulder 80.21
  specified site NEC 80.29
  toe 80.28
  wrist 80.23
Arthrostomy (*see also* Arthrotomy) 80.10
Arthrotomy 80.10
  as operative approach—*omit code*
  with
    arthrography—*see* Arthrogram
    arthroscopy—*see* Arthroscopy
    injection of drug 81.92
    removal of prosthesis without replacement —*see* Removal, prosthesis, joint structures
  ankle 80.17
  elbow 80.12
  foot and toe 80.18
  hand and finger 80.14
  hip 80.15
  knee 80.16
  shoulder 80.11
  specified site NEC 80.19
  spine 80.19
  wrist 80.13
Artificial
  heart 37.52
    AbioCor® 37.52
    CardioWest™ (TAH-t) 37.52
  insemination 69.92
  kidney 39.95
  rupture of membranes 73.09
Arytenoidectomy 30.29
Arytenoidopexy 31.69
Asai operation (larynx) 31.75
Aspiration
  abscess—*see* Aspiration, by site
  anterior chamber, eye (therapeutic) 12.91
    diagnostic 12.21
  aqueous (eye) (humor) (therapeutic) 12.91
    diagnostic 12.21
  ascites 54.91
  Bartholin's gland (cyst) (percutaneous) 71.21

Aspiration—*continued*
  biopsy—*see* Biopsy, by site
  bladder (catheter) 57.0
    percutaneous (needle) 57.11
  bone marrow (for biopsy) 41.31
    from donor for transplant 41.91
    stem cell 99.79
  branchial cleft cyst 29.0
  breast 85.91
  bronchus 96.05
    with lavage 96.56
  bursa (percutaneous) 83.94
    hand 82.92
  calculus, bladder 57.0
  cataract 13.3
    with
      phacoemulsification 13.41
      phacofragmentation 13.43
        posterior route 13.42
  chest 34.91
  cisternal 01.01
  cranial (puncture) 01.09
  craniobuccal pouch 07.72
  craniopharyngioma 07.72
  cul-de-sac (abscess) 70.0
  curettage, uterus 69.59
    after abortion or delivery 69.52
    diagnostic 69.59
    to terminate pregnancy 69.51
  cyst—*see* Aspiration, by site
  diverticulum, pharynx 29.0
  endotracheal 96.04
    with lavage 96.56
  extradural 01.09
  eye (anterior chamber) (therapeutic) 12.91
    diagnostic 12.21
  fallopian tube 66.91
  fascia 83.95
    hand 82.93
  gallbladder (percutaneous) 51.01
  hematoma—*see also* Aspiration, by site
    obstetrical 75.92
      incisional 75.91
  hydrocele, tunica vaginalis 61.91
  hygroma—*see* Aspiration, by site
  hyphema 12.91
  hypophysis 07.72
  intracranial space (epidural) (extradural)
      (subarachnoid) (subdural) (ventricular) 01.09
    through previously implanted catheter or
      reservoir (Ommaya) (Rickham) 01.02
  joint 81.91
    for arthrography—*see* Arthrogram
  kidney (cyst) (pelvis) (percutaneous)
      (therapeutic) 55.92
    diagnostic 55.23
  liver (percutaneous) 50.91
  lung (percutaneous) (puncture) (needle) (trocar)
      33.93
  middle ear 20.09
    with intubation 20.01
  muscle 83.95
    hand 82.93
  nail 86.01
  nasal sinus 22.00
    by puncture 22.01
    through natural ostium 22.02
  nasotracheal 96.04
    with lavage 96.56
  orbit, diagnostic 16.22
  ovary 65.91

Aspiration—*continued*
  percutaneous—*see* Aspiration, by site
  pericardium (wound) 37.0
  pituitary gland 07.72
  pleural cavity 34.91
  prostate (percutaneous) 60.91
  Rathke's pouch 07.72
  seminal vesicles 60.71
  seroma—*see* Aspiration, by site
  skin 86.01
  soft tissue NEC 83.95
    hand 82.93
  spermatocele 63.91
  spinal (puncture) 03.31
  spleen (cyst) 41.1
  stem cell 99.79
  subarachnoid space (cerebral) 01.09
  subcutaneous tissue 86.01
  subdural space (cerebral) 01.09
  tendon 83.95
    hand 82.93
  testis 62.91
  thymus 07.92
    thoracoscopic 07.95
  thyroid (field) (gland) 06.01
    postoperative 06.02
  trachea 96.04
    with lavage 96.56
    percutaneous 31.99
  tunica vaginalis (hydrocele) (percutaneous) 61.91
  vitreous (and replacement) 14.72
    diagnostic 14.11
Assessment
  fitness to testify 94.11
  mental status 94.11
  nutritional status 89.39
  personality 94.03
  temperament 94.02
  vocational 93.85
Assistance
  cardiac—(*see also* Resuscitation, cardiac
    extracorporeal circulation) 39.61
  endotracheal respiratory—*see category* 96.7
  hepatic, extracorporeal 50.92
  respiratory (endotracheal) (mechanical)—*see*
    Ventilation, mechanical
  respiratory (mechanical) NEC —*see category*
    93.9
Astragalectomy 77.98
Asymmetrogammagram —*see* Scan,
    radioisotope
Atherectomy
  cerebrovascular
    percutaneous
      extracranial vessel(s) 17.53
      intracranial vessel(s) 17.54
  coronary
    percutaneous transluminal 17.55
  peripheral (noncoronary) 17.56
Atriocommissuropexy (mitral valve) 35.12
Atrioplasty NEC 37.99
  combined with repair of valvular and ventricular
    septal defects—*see* Repair, endocardial
    cushion defect
  septum (heart) NEC 35.71
Atrioseptopexy (*see also* Repair, atrial septal
    defect) 35.71
Atrioseptoplasty (*see also* Repair, atrial septal
    defect) 35.71
Atrioseptostomy (balloon) 35.41
Atriotomy 37.11
Atrioventriculostomy (cerebral-heart) 02.32

Attachment
  abutment (screw) for prosthetic ear device
      percutaneous 20.99
  eye muscle
      orbicularis oculi to eyebrow 08.36
      rectus to frontalis 15.9
  pedicle (flap) graft 86.74
      hand 86.73
      lip 27.57
      mouth 27.57
  pharyngeal flap (for cleft palate repair) 27.62
      secondary or subsequent 27.63
  prosthetic ear device, abutment 20.99
  retina—*see* Reattachment, retina
Atticoantrostomy (ear) 20.49
Atticoantrotomy (ear) 20.49
Atticotomy (ear) 20.23
Audiometry (Békésy 5-tone) (impedance)
      (stapedial reflex response) (subjective) 95.41
Augmentation
  bladder 57.87
  breast—*see* Mammoplasty, augmentation
  buttock ("fanny-lift") 86.89
  chin 76.68
  genioplasty 76.68
Augmentation—*continued*
  mammoplasty—*see* Mammoplasty, augmentation
  outflow tract (pulmonary valve) (gusset type)
      35.26
      in total repair of tetralogy or Fallot 35.81
  vocal cord(s) 31.0
Auriculectomy 18.39
Autograft —*see* Graft
Autologous —*see* Blood, transfusion
Autopsy 89.8
Autotransfusion (whole blood)—*see* Blood,
      transfusion
Autotransplant, autotransplantation —*see also*
      Reimplantation
  adrenal tissue (heterotopic) (orthotopic) 07.45
  kidney 55.61
  lung—*see* Transplant, transplantation, lung
  ovary 65.72
      laparoscopic 65.75
  pancreatic tissue 52.81
  parathyroid tissue (heterotopic) (orthotopic) 06.95
  thyroid tissue (heterotopic) (orthotopic) 06.94
  tooth 23.5
Avulsion, nerve (cranial) (peripheral) NEC 04.07
  acoustic 04.01
  phrenic 33.31
  sympathetic 05.29
Azygography 88.63

B

Bacterial smear —*see* Examination, microscopic
Baffes operation (interatrial transposition of venous return) 35.91
Baffle, atrial or interatrial 35.91
Balanoplasty 64.49
Baldy-Webster operation (uterine suspension) 69.22
Ballistocardiography 89.59
Balloon
  angioplasty—*see* Angioplasty, balloon
  dilation of pylorus 44.22
  pump, intra-aortic 37.61
  systostomy (atrial) 35.41
  valvuloplasty, percutaneous 35.96
Ball operation
  herniorrhaphy—*see* Repair, hernia, inguinal
  undercutting 49.02
Bandage 93.57
  elastic 93.56
Banding
  gastric 44.68
    vertical 44.68
  pulmonary artery 38.85
Bankhart operation (capsular repair into glenoid, for shoulder dislocation) 81.82
Bardenheurer operation (ligation of innominate artery) 38.85
Barium swallow 87.61
Barkan operation (goniotomy) 12.52
  with goniopuncture 12.53
Barr operation (transfer of tibialis posterior tendon) 83.75
Barsky operation (closure of cleft hand) 82.82
Basal metabolic rate 89.39
Basiotripsy 73.8
Bassett operation (vulvectomy with inguinal lymph node dissection) 71.5 *[40.3]*
Bassini operation —*see* Repair, hernia, inguinal
Batch-Spittler-McFaddin operation (knee disarticulation) 84.16
Batista operation (partial ventriculectomy) (ventricular reduction) (ventricular remodeling) 37.35
Bearing surface, hip
  ceramic-on-ceramic 00.76
  ceramic-on-polyethylene 00.77
  metal-on-metal 00.75
  metal on polyethylene 00.74
  oxidized zirconium -on-polyethylene 00.77
Beck operation
  aorta-coronary sinus shunt 36.39
  epicardial poudrage 36.39
Beck-Jianu operation (permanent gastrostomy) 43.19
Behavior modification 94.33
Bell-Beuttner operation (subtotal abdominal hysterectomy) 68.39
  laparoscopic 68.31
Belsey operation (esophagogastric sphincter) 44.65
Benenenti operation (rotation of bulbous urethra) 58.49
Berke operation (levator resection of eyelid) 08.33
Bicuspidization of heart valve 35.10
  aortic 35.11
  mitral 35.12

Bicycle dynamometer 93.01
Biesenberger operation (size reduction of breast, bilateral) 85.32
  unilateral 85.31
Bifurcation, bone (*see also* Osteotomy) 77.30
Bigelow operation (litholapaxy) 57.0
Bililite therapy (ultraviolet) 99.82
Billroth I operation (partial gastrectomy with gastroduodenostomy) 43.6
Billroth II operation (partial gastrectomy with gastrojejunostomy) 43.7
Binnie operation (hepatopexy) 50.69
Biofeedback, psychotherapy 94.39
Biopsy
  abdominal wall 54.22
  adenoid 28.11
  adrenal gland NEC 07.11
    closed 07.11
    open 07.12
    percutaneous (aspiration) (needle) 07.11
  alveolus 24.12
  anus 49.23
  appendix 45.26
  artery (any site) 38.21
  aspiration—*see* Biopsy, by site
  bile ducts 51.14
    closed (endoscopic) 51.14
    open 51.13
    percutaneous (needle) 51.12
  bladder 57.33
    closed 57.33
    open 57.34
    transurethral 57.33
  blood vessel (any site) 38.21
  bone 77.40
    carpal, metacarpal 77.44
    clavicle 77.41
    facial 76.11
    femur 77.45
    fibula 77.47
    humerus 77.42
    marrow 41.31
    patella 77.46
    pelvic 77.49
    phalanges (foot) (hand) 77.49
    radius 77.43
    scapula 77.41
    specified site NEC 77.49
    tarsal, metatarsal 77.48
    thorax (ribs) (sternum) 77.41
    tibia 77.47
    ulna 77.43
    vertebrae 77.49
  bowel—*see* Biopsy, intestine
  brain NEC 01.13
    closed 01.13
    open 01.14
    percutaneous (needle) 01.13
  breast 85.11
    blind 85.11
    closed 85.11
    open 85.12
    percutaneous (needle) (Vimm-Silverman) 85.11
  bronchus NEC 33.24
    brush 33.24
    closed (endoscopic) 33.24
    open 33.25

Biopsy—*continued*
  transbronchoscopic needle aspiration (TBNA)
    33.24
  Wang needle (transbronchoscopic) 33.24
  washings 33.24
 bursa 83.21
 cardioesophageal (junction) 44.14
  closed (endoscopic) 44.14
  open 44.15
 cecum 45.25
  brush 45.25
  closed (endoscopic) 45.25
  open 45.26
 cerebral meninges NEC 01.11
  closed 01.11
  open 01.12
  percutaneous (needle) 01.11
 cervix (punch) 67.12
  conization (sharp) 67.2
 chest wall 34.23
 clitoris 71.11
 colon 45.25
  brush 45.25
  closed (endoscopic) 45.25
  open 45.26
 conjunctiva 10.21
 cornea 11.22
 cul-de-sac 70.23
 diaphragm 34.27
 duodenum 45.14
  brush 45.14
  closed (endoscopic) 45.14
  open 45.15
 ear (external) 18.12
  middle or inner 20.32
 endocervix 67.11
 endometrium NEC 68.16
  by
    aspiration curettage 69.59
    dilation and curettage 69.09
  closed (endoscopic) 68.16
  open 68.13
 epididymis 63.01
 esophagus 42.24
  closed (endoscopic) 42.24
  open 42.25
 extraocular muscle or tendon 15.01
 eye 16.23
  muscle (oblique) (rectus) 15.01
 eyelid 08.11
 fallopian tube 66.11
 fascia 83.21
 fetus 75.33
 gallbladder 51.12
  closed (endoscopic) 51.14
  open 51.13
  percutaneous (needle) 51.12
 ganglion (cranial) (peripheral) NEC 04.11
  closed 04.11
  open 04.12
  percutaneous (needle) 04.11
  sympathetic nerve 05.11
 gum 24.11
 heart 37.25
 hypophysis (*see also* Biopsy, pituitary gland)
  07.15
 ileum 45.14
  brush 45.14
  closed (endoscopic) 45.14
  open 45.15

Biopsy—*continued*
 intestine NEC 45.27
  large 45.25
   brush 45.25
   closed (endoscopic) 45.25
   open 45.26
  small 45.14
   brush 45.14
   closed (endoscopic) 45.14
   open 45.15
 intra-abdominal mass 54.24
  closed 54.24
  percutaneous (needle) 54.24
 iris 12.22
 jejunum 45.14
  brush 45.14
  closed (endoscopic) 45.14
  open 45.15
 joint structure (aspiration) 80.30
  ankle 80.37
  elbow 80.32
  foot and toe 80.38
  hand and finger 80.34
  hip 80.35
  knee 80.36
  shoulder 80.31
  specified site NEC 80.39
  spine 80.39
  wrist 80.33
 kidney 55.23
  closed 55.23
  open 55.24
  percutaneous (aspiration) (needle) 55.23
 labia 71.11
 lacrimal
  gland 09.11
  sac 09.12
 larynx 31.43
  brush 31.43
  closed (endoscopic) 31.43
  open 31.45
 lip 27.23
 liver 50.11
  closed 50.11
  laparoscopic 50.14
  open 50.12
  percutaneous (aspiration) (needle) 50.11
  transjugular 50.13
  transvenous 50.13
 lung NEC 33.27
  brush 33.24
  closed (percutaneous) (needle) 33.26
   brush 33.24
   endoscopic 33.27
    brush 33.24
   endoscopic 33.27
    brush 33.24
   open 33.28
   thoracoscopic 33.20
   transbronchial 33.27
   transthoracic 33.26
 lymphatic structure (channel) (node) (vessel)
  40.11
 mediastinum NEC 34.25
  closed 34.25
  open 34.26
  percutaneous (needle) 34.25
 meninges (cerebral) NEC 01.11
  closed 01.11
  open 01.12
  percutaneous (needle) 01.11
  spinal 03.32

Biopsy—*continued*
  mesentery 54.23
  mouth NEC 27.24
  muscle 83.21
    extraocular 15.01
    ocular 15.01
  nasopharynx 29.12
  nerve (cranial) (peripheral) NEC 04.11
    closed 04.11
    open 04.12
    percutaneous (needle) 04.11
    sympathetic 05.11
  nose, nasal 21.22
    sinus 22.11
      closed (endoscopic) (needle) 22.11
      open 22.12
  ocular muscle or tendon 15.01
  omentum
    closed 54.24
    open 54.23
    percutaneous (needle) 54.24
  orbit 16.23
    by aspiration 16.22
  ovary 65.12
    by aspiration 65.11
    laparoscopic 65.13
  palate (bony) 27.21
    soft 27.22
  pancreas 52.11
    closed (endoscopic) 52.11
    open 52.12
    percutaneous (aspiration) (needle) 52.11
  pancreatic duct 52.14
    closed (endoscopic) 52.14
    percutaneous (aspiration) (needle) 52.11
  parathyroid gland 06.13
  penis 64.11
  perianal tissue 49.22
  pericardium 37.24
  periprostatic 60.15
  perirectal tissue 48.26
  perirenal tissue 59.21
  peritoneal implant
    closed 54.24
    open 54.23
    percutaneous (needle) 54.24
  peritoneum
    closed 54.24
    open 54.23
    percutaneous (needle) 54.24
  periurethral tissue 58.24
  perivesical tissue 59.21
  pharynx, pharyngeal 29.12
  pineal gland 07.17
  pituitary gland 07.15
    transfrontal approach 07.13
    transsphenoidal approach 07.14
  pleura, pleural 34.24
    thoracoscopic 34.20
  prostate NEC 60.11
    closed (transurethral) 60.11
    open 60.12
    percutaneous (needle) 60.11
    transrectal 60.11
  rectum 48.24
    brush 48.24
    closed (endoscopic) 48.24
    open 48.25
  retroperitoneal tissue 54.24
  salivary gland or duct 26.11
    closed (needle) 26.11
    open 26.12

Biopsy—*continued*
  scrotum 61.11
  seminal vesicle NEC 60.13
    closed 60.13
    open 60.14
    percutaneous (needle) 60.13
  sigmoid colon 45.25
    brush 45.25
    closed (endoscopic) 45.25
    open 45.26
  sinus, nasal 22.11
    closed (endoscopic) (needle) 22.11
    open 22.12
  skin (punch) 86.11
  skull 01.15
  soft palate 27.22
  soft tissue NEC 86.11
    closed (needle) (punch) 86.11
    open 83.21
  spermatic cord 63.01
  sphincter of Oddi 51.14
    closed (endoscopic) 51.14
    open 51.13
  spinal cord (meninges) 03.32
  spleen 41.32
    closed 41.32
    open 41.33
    percutaneous (aspiration) (needle) 41.32
  stomach 44.14
    brush 44.14
    closed (endoscopic) 44.14
    open 44.15
  subcutaneous tissue (punch) 86.11
  supraglottic mass 29.12
  sympathetic nerve 05.11
  tendon 83.21
    extraocular 15.01
    ocular 15.01
  testis NEC 62.11
    closed 62.11
    open 62.12
    percutaneous (needle) 62.11
  thymus 07.16
  thyroid gland NEC 06.11
    closed 06.11
    open 06.12
    percutaneous (aspiration) (needle) 06.11
  tongue 25.01
    closed (needle) 25.01
    open 25.02
  tonsil 28.11
  trachea 31.44
    brush 31.44
    closed (endoscopic) 31.44
    open 31.45
  tunica vaginalis 61.11
  umbilicus 54.22
  ureter 56.33
    closed (percutaneous) 56.32
      endoscopic 56.33
    open 56.34
    transurethral 56.33
  urethra 58.23
  uterus, uterine (endometrial) 68.16
    by
      aspiration curettage 69.59
      dilation and curettage 69.09
    closed (endoscopic) 68.16
    ligaments 68.15
      closed (endoscopic) 68.15
      open 68.14
    open 68.13

Biopsy—*continued*
 uvula 27.22
 vagina 70.24
 vas deferens 63.01
 vein (any site) 38.21
 vulva 71.11
BiPAP 93.90
 delivered by
 endotracheal tube —*see* category 96.7
 tracheostomy —*see* category 96.7
BIS (bispectral index) monitoring 00.94
 [89.14]
Bischoff operation (ureteroneocystostomy) 56.74
Bisection —*see also* Excision
 hysterectomy 68.39
 laparoscopic 68.31
 ovary 65.29
 laparoscopic 65.25
 stapes foot plate 19.19
 with incus replacement 19.11
Bischoff operation (spinal myelotomy) 03.29
Blalock operation (systemic-pulmonary
 anastomosis) 39.0
Blalock-Hanlon operation (creation of atrial
 septal defect) 35.42
Blalock-Taussig operation
 (subclavian-pulmonary anastomosis) 39.0
Blascovic operation (resection and advancement
 of levator palpebrae superioris) 08.33
Blepharectomy 08.20
Blepharoplasty (*see also* Reconstruction, eyelid)
 08.70
 extensive 08.44
Blepharorrhaphy 08.52
 division or severing 08.02
Blepharotomy 08.09
Blind rehabilitation therapy NEC 93.78
Block
 caudal—*see* Injection, spinal
 celiac ganglion or plexus 05.31
 dissection
 breast
 bilateral 85.46
 unilateral 85.45
 bronchus 32.6
 larynx 30.3
 lymph nodes 40.50
 neck 40.40
 vulva 71.5
 epidural, spinal—*see* Injection, spinal
 gasserian ganglion 04.81
 intercostal nerves 04.81
 intrathecal—*see* Injection, spinal
 nerve (cranial) (peripheral) NEC 04.81
 paravertebral stellate ganglion 05.31
 peripheral nerve 04.81
 spinal nerve root (intrathecal)—*see* Injection,
 spinal
 stellate (ganglion) 05.31
 subarachnoid, spinal—*see* Injection, spinal
 sympathetic nerve 05.31
 trigeminal nerve 04.81
Blood
 flow study, Doppler-type (ultrasound)—*see*
 Ultrasonography
 patch, spine (epidural) 03.95

Blood—*continued*
 transfusion
 antihemophilic factor 99.06
 autologous
 collected prior to surgery 99.02
 intraoperative 99.00
 perioperative 99.00
 postoperative 99.00
 previously collected 99.02
 salvage 99.00
 blood expander 99.08
 blood surrogate 99.09
 coagulation factors 99.06
 exchange 99.01
 granulocytes 99.09
 hemodilution 99.03
 other substance 99.09
 packed cells 99.04
 plasma 99.07
 platelets 99.05
 serum, other 99.07
 thrombocytes 99.05
Blount operation
 femoral shortening (with blade plate) 78.25
 by epiphyseal stapling 78.25
Boari operation (bladder flap) 56.74
Bobb operation (cholelithotomy) 51.04
Bone
 age studies 88.33
 mineral density study 88.98
Bonney operation (abdominal hysterectomy)
 68.49
 laparoscopic 68.41
Borthen operation (iridotasis) 12.63
Boot operation
 plantar dissection 80.48
 radiocarpal fusion 81.26
Bosworth operation
 arthroplasty for acromioclavicular separation 81.83
 fusion of posterior lumbar and lumbosacral spine
 81.08
 for pseudarthrosis 81.38
 resection of radial head ligaments (for tennis
 elbow) 80.92
 shelf procedure, hip 81.40
Bottle repair of hydrocele, tunics vaginalis 61.2
Boyd operation (hip disarticulation) 84.18
Brachytherapy intravascular 92.27
Brauer operation (cardiolysis) 37.10
Breech extraction —*see* Extraction, breech
Bricker operation (ileoureterostomy) 56.51
Brisement (force) 93.26
Bristow operation (repair of shoulder
 dislocation) 81.82
Brock operation (pulmonary valvotomy) 35.03
Brockman operation (soft tissue release for
 clubfoot) 83.84
Bronchogram, bronchography 87.32
 endotracheal 87.31
 transcricoid 87.32
Bronchoplasty 33.48
Bronchorrhaphy 33.41
Bronchoscopy NEC 33.23
 with biopsy 33.24
 lung 33.27
 brush 33.24
 fiberoptic 33.22
 with biopsy 33.24
 lung 33.27
 brush 33.24

Bronchoscopy—*continued*
through tracheostomy 33.21
with biopsy 33.24
lung 33.27
brush 33.24
Bronchospirometry 89.38
Bronchostomy 33.0
closure 33.42
Bronchotomy 33.0
Browne (Denis) operation (hypospadias repair)
58.45
Brunschwig operation (temporary gastrostomy)
43.19
Buckling, scleral 14.49
with
air tamponade 14.49
implant (silicone) (vitreous) 14.41
resection of sclera 14.49
vitrectomy 14.49
vitreous implant (silicone) 14.41
Bunionectomy (radical) 77.59
with
arthrodesis 77.52
osteotomy of first metatarsal 77.51
resection of joint with prosthetic implant 77.59
soft tissue correction NEC 77.53
Bunnell operation (tendon transfer) 82.56
Burch procedure (retropubic urethral suspension
for urinary stress incontinence) 59.5
Burgess operation (amputation of ankle) 84.14
Burn dressing 93.57
Burr holes 01.24
Bursectomy 83.5
hand 82.31
Bursocentesis 83.94
hand 82.92
Bursotomy 83.03
hand 82.03
Burying of fimbriae in uterine wall 66.97
Bypass
abdominal-coronary artery 36.17
aortocoronary (catheter stent) (with prosthesis)
(with saphenous graft) (with vein graft) 36.10
one coronary vessel 36.11
two coronary vessels 36.12
three coronary vessels 36.13
four coronary vessels 36.14
arterial (graft) (mandril grown graft) (vein graft)
NEC 39.29
carotid-cerebral 39.28
carotid-vertebral 39.28
extracranial-intracranial [EC-IC] 39.28
intra-abdominal NEC 39.26
intrathoracic NEC 39.23
peripheral NEC 39.29
cardiopulmonary 39.61
open 39.61
percutaneous (closed) 39.66
carotid-cerebral 39.28
carotid-vertebral 39.28
coronary (*see also* Bypass, aortocoronary) 36.10
extracranial-intracranial [EC-IC] 39.28
gastric 44.39
high 44.31
laparoscopic 44.38
Printen and Mason 44.31
gastroduodenostomy (Jaboulay's) 44.39
laparoscopic 44.38
percutaneous [endoscopic] 44.32

Bypass—*continued*
gastroenterostomy 44.39
laparoscopic 44.38
gastroepiploic-coronary artery 36.17
gastrogastrostomy 44.39
laparoscopic 44.38
graft, pressurized treatment 00.16
heart-lung (complete) (partial) 39.61
open 39.61
percutaneous (closed) 39.66
high gastric 44.31
ileo-jejunal 45.91
internal mammary-coronary artery (single) 36.15
double vessel 36.16
jejunal-ileum 45.91
pulmonary 39.61
open 39.61
percutaneous (closed) 39.66
shunt
intestine
large-to-large 45.94
small-to-large 45.93
small-to-small 45.91
stomach 44.39
high gastric 44.31
laparoscopic 44.38
terminal ileum 45.93
vascular (arterial) (graft) (mandril grown graft)
(vein graft) NEC 39.29
aorta-carotid-brachial 39.22
aorta-iliac-femoral 39.25
aorta-renal 39.24
aorta-subclavian-carotid 39.22
aortic-superior mesenteric 39.26
aortocarotid 39.22
aortoceliac 39.26
aortocoronary (*see also* Bypass, aortocoronary)
36.10
aortofemoral 39.25
aortofemoral-popliteal 39.25
aortoiliac 39.25
to popliteal 39.25
aortoiliofemoral 39.25
aortomesenteric 39.26
aortopopliteal 39.25
aortorenal 39.24
aortosubclavian 39.22
axillary-brachial 39.29
axillary-femoral (superficial) 39.29
axillofemoral (superficial) 39.29
carotid to subclavian artery 39.22
carotid-cerebral 39.28
carotid-vertebral 39.28
common hepatic-common iliac-renal 39.26
coronary (*see also* Bypass, aortocoronary)
36.10
extracranial-intracranial [EC-IC] 39.28
femoral-femoral 39.29
femoroperoneal 39.29
femoropopliteal (reversed saphenous vein)
(saphenous) 39.29
femorotibial (anterior) (posterior) 39.29
iliofemoral 39.25
ilioiliac 39.26
internal mammary-coronary artery (single)
36.15
double vessel 36.16
intra-abdominal (arterial) NEC 39.26
venous NEC 39.1
intrathoracic NEC 39.23
peripheral artery NEC 39.29

Bypass—*continued*
  popliteal-tibial 39.29
  renal artery 39.24
  splenorenal (venous) 39.1
    arterial 39.26
  subclavian-axillary 39.29
  subclavian-carotid 39.22
  subclavian-subclavian 39.22
  Y graft to renal arteries 39.24

Caldwell operation (sulcus extension) 24.91
Caldwell-Luc operation (maxillary sinusotomy) 22.39
  with removal of membrane lining 22.31
Calibration, urethra 89.29
Calicectomy (renal) 55.4
Callander operation (knee disarticulation) 84.16
Caloric test, vestibular function 95.44
Calycectomy (renal) 55.4
Calyco-ileoneocystostomy 55.86
Calycotomy (renal) 55.11
Campbell operation
  bone block, ankle 81.11
  fasciotomy (iliac crest) 83.14
  reconstruction of anterior cruciate ligament 81.45
Campimetry 95.05
Canaliculodacryocystorhinostomy 09.81
Canaliculoplasty 09.73
Canaliculorhinostomy 09.81
Canaloplasty, external auditory meatus 18.6
Cannulation —*see also* Insertion, catheter
  ampulla of Vater 51.99
  antrum 22.01
  arteriovenous 39.93
  artery 38.91
  caval-mesenteric vein 39.1
  cisterna chyli 40.61
  Eustachian tube 20.8
  lacrimal apparatus 09.42
  lymphatic duct, left (thoracic) 40.61
  nasal sinus (by puncture) 22.01
    through natural ostium 22.02
  pancreatic duct 52.92
    by retrograde endoscopy (ERP) 52.93
  renoportal 39.1
  sinus (nasal) (by puncture) 22.01
    through natural ostium 22.02
  splenorenal (venous) 39.1
    arterial 39.26
  thoracic duct (cervical approach) (thoracic approach) 40.61
Cannulization —*see* Cannulation
Canthocystostomy 09.82
Canthoplasty 08.59
Canthorrhaphy 08.52
  division or severing 08.02
Canthotomy 08.51
Capsulectomy
  joint (*see also* Arthrectomy) 80.90
  kidney 55.91
  lens 13.65
    with extraction of lens 13.51
  ovary 65.29
    laparoscopic 65.25
Capsulo-iridectomy 13.65
Capsuloplasty —*see* Arthroplasty
Capsulorrhaphy 81.96
  with arthroplasty—*see* Arthroplasty
  ankle 81.94
  foot 81.94
  lower extremity NEC 81.95
  upper extremity 81.93
Capsulotomy
  joint (*see also* Division, joint capsule) 80.40
    for claw toe repair 77.57

Capsulotomy—*continued*
  lens 13.64
    with
      discission of lens 13.2
      removal of foreign body 13.02
        by magnet extraction 13.01
Cardiac
  mapping 37.27
  massage (external) (closed chest) 99.63
    open chest 37.91
  retraining 93.36
Cardiac support device (CSD) 37.41
Cardiectomy (stomach) 43.5
Cardiocentesis 37.0
Cardiography (*see also* Angiocardiography) 88.50
Cardiolysis 37.10
Cardiomyopexy 36.39
Cardiomyotomy 42.7
Cardio-omentopexy 36.39
Cardiopericardiopexy 36.39
Cardioplasty (stomach and esophagus) 44.65
  stomach alone 44.66
    laparoscopic 44.67
Cardioplegia 39.63
Cardiopneumopexy 36.39
Cardiorrhaphy 37.49
Cardioschisis 37.12
Cardiosplenopexy 36.39
Cardiotomy (exploratory) 37.11
Cardiovalvulotomy —*see* Valvulotomy, heart
Cardioversion (external) 99.62
  atrial 99.61
CardioWest™ Total Temporary Artificial Heart (TAH-t) 37.52
Carotid pulse tracing with ECG lead 89.56
Carpectomy (partial) 77.84
  total 77.94
Carroll and Taber arthroplasty (proximal interphalangeal joint) 81.72
Casting (for immobilization) NEC 93.53
  with fracture-reduction—*see* Reduction, fracture
Castration
  female (oophorectomy, bilateral) 65.51
    laparoscopic 65.53
  male 62.41
C.A.T. (computerized axial tomography) (*see also* Scan, C.A.T.) 88.38
Catheterization —*see also* Insertion, catheter
  arteriovenous 39.93
  artery 38.91
  bladder, indwelling 57.94
    percutaneous (cystostomy) 57.17
    suprapubic NEC 57.18
  bronchus 96.05
    with lavage 96.56
  cardiac (right) 37.21
    combined left and right 37.23
    left 37.22
      combined with right heart 37.23
    right 37.21
      combined with left heart 37.23
  central venous NEC 38.93
    peripherally inserted central catheter (PICC) 38.93

Catheterization—*continued*
chest 34.04
revision (with lysis of adhesions) 34.04
thoracoscopic 34.06
thoracoscopic 34.06
Eustachian tube 20.8
heart (right) 37.21
combined left and right 37.23
left 37.22
combined with right heart 37.23
right 37.21
combined with left heart 37.23
hepatic vein 38.93
inferior vena cava 38.93
intercostal space (with water seal), for drainage 34.04
revision (with lysis of adhesions) 34.04
thoracoscopic 34.06
thoracoscopic 34.06
lacrimonasal duct 09.44
laryngeal 96.05
nasolacrimal duct 09.44
pancreatic cyst 52.01
renal vein 38.93
Swan-Ganz (pulmonary) 89.64
transtracheal for oxygenation 31.99
umbilical vein 38.92
ureter (to kidney) 59.8
for retrograde pyelogram 87.74
urethra, indwelling 57.94
vein NEC 38.93
for renal dialysis 38.95
Cattell operation (herniorrhaphy) 53.51
Cauterization —*see also* Destruction, lesion, by site
anus NEC 49.39
endoscopic 49.31
Bartholin's gland 71.24
broad ligament 69.19
bronchus 32.09
endoscopic 32.01
canaliculi 09.73
cervix 67.32
chalazion 08.25
choroid plexus 02.14
conjunctiva 10.33
lesion 10.32
cornea (fistula) (ulcer) 11.42
ear, external 18.29
endometrial implant—*see* Excision, lesion, by site
entropion 08.41
esophagus 42.39
endoscopic 42.33
eyelid 08.25
for entropion or ectropion 08.41
fallopian tube 66.61
by endoscopy (hysteroscopy) (laparoscopy) 66.29
hemorrhoids 49.43
iris 12.41
lacrimal
gland 09.21
punctum 09.72
for eversion 09.71
sac 09.6
larynx 30.09
liver 50.29
lung 32.29
endoscopic 32.28
meibomian gland 08.25

Cauterization—*continued*
nose, for epistaxis (with packing) 21.03
ovary 65.29
laparoscopic 65.25
palate (bony) 27.31
pannus (superficial) 11.42
pharynx 29.39
punctum, lacrimal 09.72
for eversion 09.71
rectum 48.32
radical 48.31
round ligament 69.19
sclera 12.84
with iridectomy 12.62
skin 86.3
subcutaneous tissue 86.3
tonsillar fossa 28.7
urethra 58.39
endoscopic 58.31
uterosacral ligament 69.19
uterotubal ostia 66.61
uterus 68.29
vagina 70.33
vocal cords 30.09
vulva 71.3
Cavernoscopy 34.21
Cavernostomy 33.1
Cavernotomy, kidney 55.39
Cavography (inferior vena cava) 88.51
CCM (implantation of cardiac contractility modulation)
rechargeable pulse generator only 17.52
total system 17.51
Cecectomy (with resection of terminal ileum)
laparoscopic 17.32
open and other 45.72
Cecil operation (urethral reconstruction) 58.46
Cecocoloplicopexy 46.63
Cecocolostomy 45.94
Cecofixation 46.64
Ceco-ileostomy 45.93
Cecopexy 46.64
Cecoplication 46.62
Cecorrhaphy 46.75
Cecosigmoidostomy 45.94
Cecostomy (tube) (*see also* Colostomy) 46.10
Cecotomy 45.03
Celiocentesis 54.91
Celioscopy 54.21
Celiotomy, exploratory 54.11
Cell block and Papanicolaou smear —*see* Examination, microscopic
CentriMag® acute circulatory support device 37.62
Cephalogram 87.17
dental 87.12
orthodontic 87.12
Cephalometry, cephalometrics 87.17
echo 88.78
orthodontic 87.12
ultrasound (sonar) 88.78
x-ray 87.81
Cephalotomy, fetus 73.8
Cerclage
anus 49.72
cervix 67.59
transabdominal 67.51
transvaginal 67.59
isthmus uteri (cervix) 67.59
retinal reattachment (*see also* Buckling, scleral) 14.49
sclera (*see also* Buckling, scleral) 14.49

Cervicectomy (with synchronous colporrhaphy) 67.4
Cervicoplasty 67.69
Cesarean section 74.99
 classical 74.0
 corporeal 74.0
 extraperitoneal 74.2
 fundal 74.0
 laparotrachelotomy 74.1
 Latzko 74.2
 low cervical 74.1
 lower uterine segment 74.1
 peritoneal exclusion 74.4
 specified type NEC 74.4
 supravesical 74.2
 transperitoneal 74.4
  classical 74.0
  low cervical 74.1
 upper uterine segment 74.0
 vaginal 74.4
 Waters 74.2
Chamberlain procedure —*see* Mediastinotomy
Chandler operation (hip fusion) 81.21
Change —*see also* Replacement
 cast NEC 97.13
  lower limb 97.12
  upper limb 97.11
 cystostomy catheter or tube 59.94
 gastrostomy tube 97.02
 length
  bone—*see either category* 78.2 Shortening, bone *or category* 78.3 Lengthening, bone
  muscle 83.85
   hand 82.55
  tendon 83.85
   hand 82.55
 nephrostomy catheter or tube 55.93
 pyelostomy catheter or tube 55.94
 splint 97.14
 tracheostomy tube 97.23
 ureterostomy catheter or tube 59.93
 urethra] catheter, indwelling 57.95
Character analysis, psychologic 94.03
Charles operation (correction of lymphedema) 40.9
Charnley operation (compression arthrodesis)
 ankle 81.11
 hip 81.21
 knee 81.22
Cheatle-Henry operation —*see* Repair, hernia, femoral
Check
 automatic implantable cardioverter/defibrillator (AICD) (interrogation only) 89.49
 CRT-D (cardiac resynchronization defibrillator) (interrogation only) 89.49
 CRT-P (cardiac resynchronization pacemaker) (interrogation only) 89.45
 pacemaker, artificial (cardiac) (function) (interrogation only) (rate) 89.45
  amperage threshold 89.48
  artifact wave form 89.46
  electrode impedance 89.47
  voltage threshold 89.48
 vision NEC 95.09
Cheiloplasty 27.59
Cheilorrhaphy 27.51
Cheilostomatoplasty 27.59
Cheilotomy 27.0
Chemical peel, skin 86.24

Chemocauterization —*see also* Destruction, lesion, by site
 corneal epithelium 11.41
 palate 27.31
Chemodectomy 39.89
Chemoembolization 99.25
Chemolysis
 nerve (peripheral) 04.2
 spinal canal structure 03.8
Chemoneurolysis 04.2
Chemonucleolysis (nucleus pulposus) 80.52
Chemopallidectomy 01.42
Chemopeel (skin) 86.24
Chemosurgery
 esophagus 42.39
  endoscopic 42.33
 Mohs' 86.24
 skin (superficial) 86.24
 stomach 43.49
  endoscopic 43.41
Chemothalamectomy 01.41
Chemotherapy —*see also* Immunotherapy
 Antabuse 94.25
 for cancer NEC 99.25
  brain wafer implantation 00.10
  CLO 17.70
  clofarabine 17.70
  CLOLAR® 17.70
  implantation of chemotherapeutic agent 00.10
  interstitial implantation 00.10
  intracavitary implantation 00.10
  wafer chemotherapy 00.10
 lithium 94.22
 methadone 94.25
 palate (bony) 27.31
Chevalier-Jackson operation (partial laryngectomy) 30.29
Child operation (radical subtotal pancreatectomy) 52.53
Cholangiocholangiostomy 51.39
Cholangiocholecystocholedochectomy 51.22
Cholangio-enterostomy 51.39
Cholangiogastrostomy 51.39
Cholangiogram 87.54
 endoscopic retrograde (ERC) 51.11
 intraoperative 87.53
 intravenous 87.52
 percutaneous hepatic 87.51
 transhepatic 87.53
Cholangiography (*see also* Cholangiogram) 87.54
Cholangiojejunostomy (intrahepatic) 51.39
Cholangiopancreatography
 endoscopic retrograde 51.10
Cholangiostomy 51.59
Cholangiotomy 51.59
Cholecystectomy (total) 51.22
 laparoscopic 51.23
 partial 51.21
  laparoscopic 51.24
Cholecystenterorrhaphy 51.91
Cholecystocecostomy 51.32
Cholecystocholangiogram 87.59
Cholecystocolostomy 51.32
Cholecystoduodenostomy 51.32
Cholecystoenterostomy (Winiwater) 51.32
Cholecystogastrostomy 51.34
Cholecystogram 87.59
Cholecystoileostomy 51.32
Cholecystojejunostomy (Roux-en-Y) (with jejunojejunostomy) 51.32
Cholecystopancreatostomy 51.33
Cholecystopexy 51.99

Cholecystorrhaphy 51.91
Cholecystostomy NEC 51.03
  by trocar 51.02
Cholecystotomy 51.04
  percutaneous 51.01
Choledochectomy 51.63
Choledochoduodenostomy 51.36
Choledochoenterostomy 51.36
Choledochojejunostomy 51.36
Choledocholithotomy 51.41
  endoscopic 51.88
Choledocholithotripsy 51.41
  endoscopic 51.88
Choledochopancreatostomy 51.39
Choledochoplasty 51.72
Choledochorrhaphy 51.71
Choledochoscopy 51.11
Choledochostomy 51.51
Choledochotomy 51.51
Cholelithotomy 51.04
Chondrectomy 80.90
  ankle 80.97
  elbow 80.92
  foot and toe 80.98
  hand and finger 80.94
  hip 80.95
  intervertebral cartilage see category 80.5
  knee (semilunar cartilage) 80.6
  nasal (submucous) 21.5
  semilunar cartilage (knee) 80.6
  shoulder 80.91
  specified site NEC 80.99
  spine see category 80.5
  wrist 80.93
Chondroplasty —see Arthroplasty
Chondrosternoplasty (for pectus excavatum
    repair) 34.74
Chondrotomy (see also Division, cartilage) 80.40
  nasal 21.1
Chopart operation (midtarsal amputation) 84.12
Chordectomy, vocal 30.22
Chordotomy (spinothalmic) (anterior) (posterior)
    NEC 03.29
  percutaneous 03.21
  stereotactic 03.21
Ciliarotomy 12.55
Ciliectomy (ciliary body) 12.44
  eyelid margin 08.20
Cinch, cinching
  for scleral buckling (see also Buckling, scleral)
    14.49
  ocular muscle (oblique) (rectus) 15.22
    multiple (two or more muscles) 15.4
Cineangiocardiography (see also
    Angiocardiography) 88.50
Cineplasty, cineplastic prosthesis
  amputation—see Amputation
  arm 84.44
  biceps 84.44
  extremity 84.40
    lower 84.48
    upper 84.44
  leg 84.48
Cineradiography —see Radiography
Cingulumotomy (brain) (percutaneous radio
    frequency) 01.32
Circumcision (male) 64.0
  female 71.4
CISH [classic infrafascial SEMM hysterectomy]
    68.31

Clagett operation (closure of chest wall
    following open flap drainage) 34.72
Clamp and cautery, hemorrhoids 49.43
Clamping
  aneurysm (cerebral) 39.51
  blood vessel—see Ligation, blood vessel
  ventricular shunt 02.43
Clavicotomy 77.31
  fetal 73.8
Claviculectomy (partial) 77.81
  total 77.91
Clayton operation (resection of metatarsal heads
    and bases of phalanges) 77.88
Cleaning, wound 96.59
Clearance
  bladder (transurethral) 57.0
  pelvic
    female 68.8
    male 57.71
  prescalene fat pad 40.21
  renal pelvis (transurethral) 56.0
  ureter (transurethral) 56.0
Cleft lip 86.21
Cleidotomy 77.31
  fetal 73.8
Clipping
  aneurysm (basilar) (carotid) (cerebellar)
      (cerebellopontine) (communicating artery)
      (vertebral) 39.51
  arteriovenous fistula 39.53
  frenulum, frenum
    labia (lips) 27.91
    lingual (tongue) 25.91
  left atrial appendage 37.36
  tip of uvula 27.72
Clitoridectomy 71.4
Clitoridotomy 71.4
Clivogram 87.02
Closure —see also Repair
  abdominal wall 54.63
    delayed (granulating wound) 54.62
    secondary 54.61
    tertiary 54.62
  amputation stump, secondary 84.3
  anular disc 80.54
    with graft or prosthesis 80.53
  anulus fibrosus 80.54
    with graft or prosthesis 80.53
  aorticopulmonary fenestration (fistula) 39.59
  appendicostomy 47.92
  artificial opening
    bile duct 51.79
    bladder 57.82
    bronchus 33.42
    common duct 51.72
    esophagus 42.83
    gallbladder 51.92
    hepatic duct 51.79
    intestine 46.50
      large 46.52
      small 46.51
    kidney 55.82
    larynx 31.62
    rectum 48.72
    stomach 44.62
    thorax 34.72
    trachea 31.72
    ureter 56.83
    urethra 58.42

Closure—*continued*
  atrial septal defect (*see also* Repair, atrial septal
    defect) 35.71
    with umbrella device (King-Mills type) 35.52
    combined with repair of valvular and
      ventricular septal defects—*see* Repair,
      endocardial cushion defect
  bronchostomy 33.42
  cecostomy 46.52
  cholecystostomy 51.92
  cleft hand 82.82
  colostomy 46.52
  cystostomy 57.82
  diastema (alveolar) (dental) 24.8
  disrupted abdominal wall (postoperative) 54.61
  duodenostomy 46.51
  encephalocele 02.12
  endocardial cushion defect (*see also* Repair,
    endocardial cushion defect) 35.73
  enterostomy 46.50
  esophagostomy 42.83
  fenestration
    aorticopulmonary 39.59
    septal, heart (*see also* Repair, heart, septum)
      35.70
  filtering bleb, corneoscleral (postglaucoma) 12.66
  fistula
    abdominothoracic 34.83
    anorectal 48.73
    anovaginal 70.73
    antrobuccal 22.71
    anus 49.73
    aorticopulmonary (fenestration) 39.59
    aortoduodenal 39.59
    appendix 47.92
    biliary tract 51.79
    bladder NEC 57.84
    branchial cleft 29.52
    bronchocutaneous 33.42
    bronchoesophageal 33.42
    bronchomediastinal 34.73
    bronchopleural 34.73
    bronchopleurocutaneous 34.73
    bronchopleuromediastinal 34.73
    bronchovisceral 33.42
    bronchus 33.42
    cecosigmoidal 46.76
    cerebrospinal fluid 02.12
    cervicoaural 18.79
    cervicosigmoidal 67.62
    cervicovesical 57.84
    cervix 67.62
    cholecystocolic 51.93
    cholecystoduodenal 51.93
    cholecystoenteric 51.93
    cholecystogastric 51.93
    cholecystojejunal 51.93
    cisterna chyli 40.63
    colon 46.76
    colovaginal 70.72
    common duct 51.72
    cornea 11.49
      with lamellar graft (homograft) 11.62
        autograft 11.61
    diaphragm 34.83
    duodenum 46.72
    ear, middle 19.9
    ear drum 19.4
    enterocolic 46.74
    enterocutaneous 46.74
    enterouterine 69.42

Closure—*continued*
    enterovaginal 70.74
    enterovesical 57.83
    esophagobronchial 33.42
    esophagocutaneous 42.84
    esophagopleurocutaneous 34.73
    esophagotracheal 31.73
    esophagus NEC 42.84
    fecal 46.79
    gallbladder 51.93
    gastric NEC 44.63
    gastrocolic 44.63
    gastroenterocolic 44.63
    gastroesophageal 42.84
    gastrojejunal 44.63
    gastrojejunocolic 44.63
    heart valve—*see* Repair, heart, valve
    hepatic duct 51.79
    hepatopleural 34.73
    hepatopulmonary 34.73
    ileorectal 46.74
    ileosigmoidal 46.74
    ileovesical 57.83
    ileum 46.74
    in ano 49.73
    intestine 46.79
      large 46.76
      small NEC 46.74
    intestinocolonic 46.74
    intestinoureteral 56.84
    intestinouterine 69.42
    intestinovaginal 70.74
    intestinovesical 57.83
    jejunum 46.74
    kidney 55.83
    lacrimal 09.99
    laryngotracheal 31.62
    larynx 31.62
    lymphatic duct, left (thoracic) 40.63
    mastoid (antrum) 19.9
    mediastinobronchial 34.73
    mediastinocutaneous 34.73
    mouth (external) 27.53
    nasal 21.82
      sinus 22.71
    nasolabial 21.82
    nasopharyngeal 21.82
    oroantral 22.71
    oronasal 21.82
    oval window (ear) 20.93
    pancreaticoduodenal 52.95
    perilymph 20.93
    perineorectal 48.73
    perineosigmoidal 46.76
    perineourethroscrotal 58.43
    perineum 71.72
    perirectal 48.93
    pharyngoesophageal 29.53
    pharynx NEC 29.53
    pleura, pleural NEC 34.93
    pleurocutaneous 34.73
    pleuropericardial 37.49
    pleuroperitoneal 34.83
    pulmonoperitoneal 34.83
    rectolabial 48.73
    rectoureteral 56.84
    rectourethral 58.43
    rectovaginal 70.73
    rectovesical 57.83
    rectovesicovaginal 57.83
    rectovulvar 48.73

Closure—*continued*
  rectum NEC 48.73
  renal 55.83
  reno-intestinal 55.83
  round window 20.93
  salivary (gland) (duct) 26.42
  scrotum 61.42
  sigmoidovaginal 70.74
  sigmoidovesical 57.83
  splenocolic 41.95
  stomach NEC 44.63
  thoracic duct 40.63
  thoracoabdominal 34.83
  thoracogastric 34.83
  thoracointestinal 34.83
  thorax NEC 34.71
  trachea NEC 31.73
  tracheoesophageal 31.73
  tympanic membrane (*see also* Tympanoplasty)
    19.4
  umbilicourinary 57.51
  ureter 56.84
  ureterocervical 56.84
  ureterorectal 56.84
  ureterosigmoidal 56.84
  ureterovaginal 56.84
  ureterovesical 56.84
  urethra 58.43
  urethroperineal 58.43
  urethroperineovesical 57.84
  urethrorectal 58.43
  urethroscrotal 58.43
  urethrovaginal 58.43
  uteroenteric 69.42
  uterointestinal 69.42
  uterorectal 69.42
  uteroureteric 56.84
  uterovaginal 69.42
  uterovesical 57.84
  vagina 70.75
  vaginocutaneous 70.75
  vaginoenteric 70.74
  vaginoperineal 70.75
  vaginovesical 57.84
  vesicocervicovaginal 57.84
  vesicocolic 57.83
  vesicocutaneous 57.84
  vesicoenteric 57.83
  vesicometrorectal 57.83
  vesicoperineal 57.84
  vesicorectal 57.83
  vesicosigmoidal 57.83
  vesicosigmoidovaginal 57.83
  vesicoureteral 56.84
  vesicoureterovaginal 56.84
  vesicourethral 57.84
  vesicourethrorectal 57.83
  vesicouterine 57.84
  vesicovaginal 57.84
  vulva 71.72
  vulvorectal 48.73
foramen ovale (patent) 35.71
  with
    prosthesis (open heart technique) 35.51
      closed heart technique 35.52
    tissue graft 35.61
gastroduodenostomy 44.5
gastrojejunostomy 44.5
gastrostomy 44.62
ileostomy 46.51
jejunostomy 46.51

Closure—*continued*
  laceration—*see also* Suture, by site
    liver 50.61
  laparotomy, delayed 54.62
  meningocele (spinal) 03.51
    cerebral 02.12
  myelomeningocele 03.52
  nephrostomy 55.82
  palmar cleft 82.82
  patent ductus arteriosus 38.85
  pelviostomy 55.82
  peptic ulcer (bleeding) (perforated) 44.40
  perforation
    ear drum (*see also* Tympanoplasty) 19.4
    esophagus 42.82
    nasal septum 21.88
    tympanic membrane (*see also* Tympanoplasty) 19.4
  proctostomy 48.72
  punctum, lacrimal (papilla) 09.91
  pyelostomy 55.82
  rectostomy 48.72
  septum defect (heart) (*see also* Repair, heart,
      septum) 35.70
  sigmoidostomy 46.52
  skin (V-Y type) 86.59
  stoma
    bile duct 51.79
    bladder 57.82
    bronchus 33.42
    common duct 51.72
    esophagus 42.83
    gallbladder 51.92
    hepatic duct 51.79
    intestine 46.50
      large 46.52
      small 46.51
    kidney 55.82
    larynx 31.62
    rectum 48.72
    stomach 44.62
    thorax 34.72
    trachea 31.72
    ureter 56.83
    urethra 58.42
  thoracostomy 34.72
  tracheostomy 31.72
  ulcer (bleeding) (peptic) (perforated) 44.40
    duodenum 44.42
    gastric 44.41
    intestine (perforated) 46.79
    skin 86.59
    stomach 44.41
  ureterostomy 56.83
  urethrostomy 58.42
  vagina 70.8
  vascular
    percutaneous puncture—*omit code*
  vesicostomy 57.22
  wound—*see also* Suture, by site
    with graft—*see* Graft
    with tissue adhesive 86.59
Coagulation, electrocoagulation —*see also*
  Destruction, lesion, by site
  aneurysm (cerebral) (peripheral vessel) 39.52
  arteriovenous fistula 39.53
  brain tissue (incremental) (radio frequency) 01.59
  broad ligament 69.19
  cervix 67.32
  ear
    external 18.29
    inner 20.79
    middle 20.51

Coagulation, electrocoagulation—*continued*
  fallopian tube 66.61
  gasserian ganglion 04.05
  nose, for epistaxis (with packing) 21.03
  ovary 65.29
    laparoscopic 65.25
  pharynx (by diathermy) 29.39
  prostatic bed 60.94
  rectum (polyp) 48.32
    radical 48.31
  retina (for)
    destruction of lesion 14.21
    reattachment 14.51
    repair of tear 14.31
  round ligament 69.19
  semicircular canals 20.79
  spinal cord (lesion) 03.4
  urethrovesical junction, transurethral 57.49
  uterosacral ligament 69.19
  uterus 68.29
  vagina 70.33
  vulva 71.3
Coating, aneurysm of brain 39.52
Cobalt-60 therapy (treatment) 92.23
Coccygectomy (partial) 77.89
  total 77.99
Coccygotomy 77.39
"Cocked hat" procedure (metacarpal lengthening and transfer of local flap) 82.69
Cockett operation (varicose vein)
  lower limb 38.59
  upper limb 38.53
Cody tack (perforation of footplate) 19.0
Coffey operation (uterine suspension) (Meig's modification) 69.22
Cole operation (anterior tarsal wedge osteotomy) 77.28
Colectomy (partial) (segmental) (subtotal)
  cecum (with terminal ileum)
    laparoscopic 17.32
    open and other 45.72
  laparoscopic 17.39
  left (Hartmann) (lower) (radical)
    laparoscopic 17.35
    open and other 45.75
  multiple segmental
    laparoscopic 17.31
    open and other 45.71
  open and other 45.79
  right (radical)
    laparoscopic 17.33
    open and other 45.73
  sigmoid
    laparoscopic 17.36
    open and other 45.76
  terminal ileum with cecum
    laparoscopic 17.32
    open and other 45.72
  total
    laparoscopic 45.81
    open 45.82
    other 45.83
    unspecified 45.83
  transverse
    laparoscopic 17.34
    open and other 45.74
Collapse, lung, surgical 33.39
  by
    destruction of phrenic nerve 33.31
    pneumoperitoneum 33.33
    pneumothorax, artificially-induced 33.32
  thoracoplasty 33.34

Collection, sperm for artificial insemination 99.96
Collis-Nissen operation (hiatal hernia repair with esophagogastroplasty) 53.80
Colocentesis 45.03
Colocolostomy 45.94
  proximal to distal segment 45.79
Colocystoplasty 57.87 *[45.52]*
Colofixation 46.64
Coloileotomy 45.00
Colonna operation
  adductor tenotomy (first stage) 83.12
  hip arthroplasty (second stage) 81.40
  reconstruction of hip (second stage) 81.40
Colonoscopy 45.23
  with
    biopsy 45.25
      rectum 48.24
    stent —*see* Insertion, stent, colon
  fiberoptic (flexible) 45.23
  intraoperative 45.21
  through stoma (artificial) 45.22
  transabdominal 45.21
Colopexy 46.63
Coloplication 46.64
Coloproctostomy 45.94
Colorectosigmoidostomy 45.94
Colorectostomy 45.94
Colorrhaphy 46.75
Coloscopy —*see* Colonoscopy
Colosigmoidostomy 45.94
Colostomy (ileo-ascending) (ileotransverse) (perineal) (transverse) 46.10
  with anterior rectal resection 48.62
  delayed opening 46.14
  loop 46.03
  permanent (magnetic) 46.13
  temporary 46.11
Colotomy 45.03
Colpectomy 70.4
Colpoceliocentesis 70.0
Colpocentesis 70.0
Colpocleisis (complete) (partial) 70.8
Colpohysterectomy 68.59
  laparoscopically assisted (LAVH) 68.51
Colpoperineoplasty 70.79
  with repair of urethrocele 70.51
    with graft or prosthesis 70.53
Colpoperineorrhaphy 70.71
  following delivery 75.69
Colpopexy 70.77
  with graft or prosthesis 70.78
Colpoplasty 70.79
Colpopoiesis 70.61
  vaginal construction 70.61
    with graft or prosthesis 70.63
Colporrhaphy 70.71
  anterior (cystocele repair) 70.51
    with graft or prosthesis 70.54
  for repair of
    cystocele 70.51
      with rectocele 70.50
        with graft or prosthesis 70.53
    enterocele 70.92
      with graft or prosthesis 70.93
    rectocele 70.52
      with cystocele 70.50
        with graft or prosthesis 70.53
    urethrocele 70.51
      with graft or prosthesis 70.54

Colporrhaphy—*continued*
posterior (rectocele repair) 70.52
with graft or prosthesis 70.55
Colposcopy 70.21
Colpotomy 70.14
for pelvic peritoneal drainage 70.12
Commando operation (radical glossectomy)
25.4
Commissurotomy
closed heart technique—*see* Valvulotomy, heart
open heart technique—*see* Valvuloplasty, heart
Compression, trigeminal nerve 04.02
Conchectomy 21.69
Conchotomy 21.1
Conduction study, nerve 89.15
Conduitogram, ileum 87.78
Condylectomy —*see* category 77.8
mandible 76.5
Condylotomy NEC (*see also* Division, joint
capsule) 80.40
mandible (open) 76.62
closed 76.61
Conization
cervix (knife) (sharp) (biopsy) 67.2
by
cryosurgery 67.33
electroconization 67.32
Conjunctivocystorhinostomy 09.82
with insertion of tube or stent 09.83
Conjunctivodacryocystorhinostomy (CDCR)
09.82
with insertion of tube or stent 09.83
Conjunctivodacryocystostomy 09.82
with insertion of tube or stent 09.83
Conjunctivoplasty 10.49
Conjunctivorhinostomy 09.82
with insertion of tube or stent 09.83
Constriction of globe, for scleral buckling (*see
also* Buckling, scleral) 14.49
Construction
auricle, ear (with graft) (with implant) 18.71
ear
auricle (with graft) (with implant) 18.71
meatus (osseous) (skin-lined) 18.6
endorectal ileal pouch (J-pouch) (H-pouch)
(S-pouch) (with anastomosis to anus) 45.95
esophagus, artificial—*see* Anastomosis,
esophagus
ileal bladder (open) 56.51
closed 57.87 *[45.51]*
ileal conduit 56.51
larynx, artificial 31.75
patent meatus (ear) 18.6
penis (rib graft) (skin graft) (myocutaneous flap)
64.43
pharyngeal valve, artificial 31.75
urethra 58.46
vagina, artificial 70.61
with graft or prosthesis 70.63
venous valves (peripheral) 39.59
Consultation 89.09
comprehensive 89.07
limited (single organ system) 89.06
specified type NEC 89.08
Continuous positive airway pressure [CPAP]
(noninvasive) 93.90
delivered by
endotracheal tube —*see* category 96.7
tracheostomy —*see* category 96.7

Control
atmospheric pressure and composition NEC
93.98
antigen-free air conditioning 93.98
decompression chamber 93.97
mountain sanatorium 93.98
epistaxis 21.00
by
cauterization (and packing) 21.03
coagulation (with packing) 21.03
electrocoagulation (with packing) 21.03
excision of nasal mucosa with grafting 21.07
ligation of artery 21.09
ethmoidal 21.04
external carotid 21.06
maxillary (transantral) 21.05
packing (nasal) (anterior) 21.01
posterior (and anterior) 21.02
specified means NEC 21.09
hemorrhage 39.98
abdominal cavity 54.19
adenoids (postoperative) 28.7
anus (postoperative) 49.95
bladder (postoperative) 57.93
chest 34.09
colon 45.49
endoscopic 45.43
duodenum (ulcer) 44.49
by
embolization (transcatheter) 44.44
suture (ligation) 44.42
endoscopic 44.43
esophagus 42.39
endoscopic 42.33
gastric (ulcer) 44.49
by
embolization (transcatheter) 44.44
suture (ligation) 44.41
endoscopic 44.43
intrapleural 34.09
postoperative (recurrent) 34.03
laparotomy site 54.12
nose (*see also* Control, epistaxis) 21.00
peptic (ulcer) 44.49
by
embolization (transcatheter) 44.44
suture (ligation) 44.40
endoscopic 44.43
pleura, pleural cavity 34.09
postoperative (recurrent) 34.03
postoperative NEC 39.98
postvascular surgery 39.41
prostate 60.94
specified site NEC 39.98
stomach (*see* Control, hemorrhage, gastric)
thorax NEC 34.09
postoperative (recurrent) 34.03
thyroid (postoperative) 06.02
tonsils (postoperative) 28.7
Conversion
anastomosis—*see* Revision, anastomosis
atrial rhythm (to sinus rhythm) 99.61
cardiac rhythm NEC 99.69
to sinus rhythm 99.62
gastrostomy to jejunostomy (endoscopic)
for feeding tube placement 46.32
obstetrical position—*see* Version
Cooling, gastric 96.31
CorCap™ 37.41
Cordectomy, vocal 30.22
Cordopexy, vocal 31.69

Cordotomy
spinal (bilateral) NEC 03.29
  percutaneous 03.21
vocal 31.3
Corectomy 12.12
Corelysis 12.35
Coreoplasty 12.35
Corneoconjunctivoplasty 11.53
Corpectomy (vertebral) 80.99
with diskectomy 80.99
Correction —*see also* Repair
atresia
  esophageal 42.85
    by magnetic forces 42.99
  external meatus (ear) 18.6
  nasopharynx, nasopharyngeal 29.4
  rectum 48.0
  tricuspid 35.94
atrial septal defect (*see also* Repair, atrial septal
    defect) 35.71
  combined with repair of valvular and
      ventricular septal defects—*see* Repair,
      endocardial cushion defect
blepharoptosis (*see also* Repair, blepharoptosis)
    08.36
bunionette (with osteotomy) 77.54
chordee 64.42
claw toe 77.57
cleft
  lip 27.54
  palate 27.62
clubfoot NEC 83.84
coarctation of aorta
  with
    anastomosis 38.34
    graft replacement 38.44
cornea NEC 11.59
  refractive NEC 11.79
    epikeratophakia 11.76
    keratomileusis 11.71
    keratophakia 11.72
    radial keratotomy 11.75
esophageal atresia 42.85
  by magnetic forces 42.99
everted lacrimal punctum 09.71
eyelid
  ptosis (*see also* Repair, blepharoptosis) 08.36
  retraction 08.38
fetal defect 75.36
forcible, of musculoskeletal deformity
    NEC 93.29
hammer toe 77.56
hydraulic pressure, open surgery (for) penile
    prosthesis, inflatable 64.99
  urinary sphincter, artificial 58.99
intestinal malrotation 46.80
  large 46.82
  small 46.81
inverted uterus—*see* Repair, inverted uterus
lymphedema (of limb) 40.9
  excision with graft 40.9
  obliteration of lymphatics 40.9
  transplantation of autogenous lymphatics 40.9
nasopharyngeal atresia 29.4
overlapping toes 77.58
palate (cleft) 27.62
prognathism NEC 76.64
prominent ear 18.5
punctum (everted) 09.71
spinal pseudarthrosis —*see* Refusion, spinal
syndactyly 86.85

Correction—*continued*
tetralogy of Fallot
  one-stage 35.81
  partial—*see specific procedure*
  total 35.81
total anomalous pulmonary venous connection
  one-stage 35.82
  partial—*see specific procedure*
  total 35.82
transposition, great arteries, total 35.84
tricuspid atresia 35.94
truncus arteriosus
  one-stage 35.83
  partial—*see specific procedure*
  total 35.83
ureteropelvic junction 55.87
ventricular septal defect (*see also* Repair,
    ventricular septal defect) 35.72
  combined with repair of valvular and atrial
      septal defects—*see* Repair, endocardial
      cushion defect
Costectomy 77.91
with lung excision—*see* Excision, lung
associated with thoracic operation—*omit code*
Costochondrectomy 77.91
associated with thoracic operation—*omit code*
Costosternoplasty (pectus excavatum repair)
    34.74
Costotomy 77.31
Costotransversectomy 77.91
associated with thoracic operation—*omit code*
Counseling (for) NEC 94.49
  alcoholism 94.46
  drug addiction 94.45
  employers 94.49
  family (medical) (social) 94.49
  marriage 94.49
  ophthalmologic (with instruction) 95.36
  pastoral 94.49
Countershock, cardiac NEC 99.62
Coventry Operation (tibial wedge osteotomy)
    77.27
CPAP (continuous positive airway pressure)
    93.90
delivered by
  endotracheal tube —*see category* 96.7
  tracheostomy —*see category* 96.7
Craniectomy 01.25
linear (opening of cranial suture) 02.01
reopening of site 01.23
strip (opening of cranial suture) 02.01
Cranioclasis, fetal 73.8
Cranioplasty 02.06
with synchronous repair of encephalocele 02.12
Craniotomy 01.24
as operative approach—*omit code*
fetal 73.8
for decompression of fracture 02.02
reopening of site 01.23
Craterization, bone (*see also* Excision, lesion,
    bone) 77.60
Crawford operation (tarso-frontalis sling of
    eyelid) 08.32
Creation —*see also* Formation
cardiac device (defibrillator) (pacemaker) pocket
  with initial insertion of cardiac device—*omit
    code*
  new site (skin) (subcutaneous) 37.79

Creation—*continued*
  conduit
    apical-aortic (AAC) 35.93
    ileal (urinary) 56.51
    left ventricle and aorta 35.93
    right atrium and pulmonary artery 35.94
    right ventricle and pulmonary (distal) artery
        35.92
    in repair of
      pulmonary artery atresia 35.92
      transposition of great vessels 35.92
      truncus arteriosus 35.83
  endorectal ileal pouch (J-pouch) (H-pouch)
      (S-pouch) (with anastomosis to anus) 45.95
  esophagogastric sphincteric competence NEC
      44.66
    laparoscopic 44.67
  Hartmann pouch—*see* Colectomy, by site
  interatrial fistula 35.42
  pericardial window 37.12
  pleural window, for drainage 34.09
  pocket
    cardiac device (defibrillator) (pacemaker)
      with initial insertion of cardiac device—*omit
          code*
      new site (skin) (subcutaneous) 37.79
    loop recorder 37.79
    thalamic stimulator pulse generator
      with initial insertion of battery package
          —*omit code*
      new site (skin) (subcutaneous) 86.09
  shunt—*see also* Shunt
    arteriovenous fistula, for dialysis 39.93
    left-to-right (systemic to pulmonary circulation)
        39.0
  subcutaneous tunnel for esophageal anastomosis
      42.86
    with anastomosis—*see* Anastomosis,
        esophagus, antesternal
  syndactyly (ringer) (toe) 86.89
  thalamic stimulator pulse generator pocket
    with initial insertion of battery package—*omit
        code*
    new site (skin) (subcutaneous) 86.09
  tracheoesophageal fistula 31.95
  window
    pericardial 37.12
    pleura, for drainage 34.09
Credé maneuver 73.59
Cricoidectomy 30.29
Cricothyreotomy (for assistance in breathing)
    31.1
Cricothyroidectomy 30.29
Cricothyrostomy 31.1
Cricothyrotomy (for assistance in breathing)
    31.1
Cricotomy (for assistance in breathing) 31.1
Cricotracheotomy (for assistance in breathing)
    31.1
Crisis Intervention 94.35
Croupette, croup tent 93.94
Crown, dental (ceramic) (gold) 23.41
Crushing
  bone—*see category* 78.4
  calculus
    bile (hepatic) passage 51.49
      endoscopic 51.88
    bladder (urinary) 57.0
    pancreatic duct 52.09
      endoscopic 52.94
  fallopian tube (*see also* Ligation, fallopian tube)
      66.39

Crushing—*continued*
  ganglion—*see* Crushing, nerve
  hemorrhoids 49.45
  nasal septum 21.88
  nerve (cranial) (peripheral) NEC 04.03
    acoustic 04.01
    auditory 04.01
    phrenic 04.03
      for collapse of lung 33.31
    sympathetic 05.0
    trigeminal 04.02
    vestibular 04.01
  vas deferens 63.71
Cryoablation —*see* Ablation
Cryoanalgesia
  nerve (cranial) (peripheral) 04.2
Cryoconization, cervix 67.33
Cryodestruction —*see* Destruction, lesion, by site
Cryoextraction, lens (*see also* Extraction,
    cataract, intracapsular) 13.19
Cryohypophysectomy (complete) (total) (*see
    also* Hypophysectomy) 07.69
Cryoleucotomy 01.32
Cryopexy, retinal —*see* Cryotherapy, retina
Cryoprostatectomy 60.62
Cryoretinopexy (for)
  reattachment 14.52
  repair of tear or defect 14.32
Cryosurgery —*see* Cryotherapy
Cryothalamectomy 01.41
Cryotherapy —*see also* Destruction, lesion, by
    site
  bladder 57.59
  brain 01.59
  cataract 13.19
  cervix 67.33
  choroid—*see* Cryotherapy, retina
  ciliary body 12.72
  corneal lesion (ulcer) 11.43
    to reshape cornea 11.79
  ear
    external 18.29
    inner 20.79
  esophagus 42.39
    endoscopic 42.33
  eyelid 08.25
  hemorrhoids 49.44
  iris 12.41
  nasal turbinates 21.61
  palate (bony) 27.31
  prostate 60.62
  retina (for)
    destruction of lesion 14.22
    reattachment 14.52
    repair of tear 14.32
  skin 86.3
  stomach 43.49
    endoscopic 43.41
  subcutaneous tissue 86.3
  turbinates (nasal) 21.61
  warts 86.3
    genital 71.3
Cryptectomy (anus) 49.39
  endoscopic 49.31
Cryptorchidectomy (unilateral) 62.3
  bilateral 62.41
Cryptotomy (anus) 49.39
  endoscopic 49.31
Cuirass 93.99
Culdocentesis 70.0

Culdoplasty 70.92
  with graft or prosthesis 70.93
Culdoscopy (exploration) (removal of foreign
  body or lesion) 70.22
Culdotomy 70.12
Culp-Deweerd operation (spiral flap
  pyeloplasty) 55.87
Culp-Scardino operation (ureteral flap
  pyeloplasty) 55.87
Culture (and sensitivity)—*see* Examination,
  microscopic
Curettage (with packing) (with secondary
  closure)—*see also* Dilation and curettage
  adenoids 28.6
  anus 49.39
    endoscopic 49.31
  bladder 57.59
    transurethral 57.49
  bone (*see also* Excision, lesion, bone) 77.60
  brain 01.59
  bursa 83.39
    hand 82.29
  cartilage (*see also* Excision, lesion, joint) 80.80
  cerebral meninges 01.51
  chalazion 08.25
  conjunctiva (trachoma follicles) 10.33
  corneal epithelium 11.41
    for smear or culture 11.21
  ear, external 18.29
  eyelid 08.25
  joint (*see also* Excision, lesion, joint) 80.80
  meninges (cerebral) 01.51
    spinal 03.4
  muscle 83.32
    hand 82.22
  nerve (peripheral) 04.07
    sympathetic 05.29
  sclera 12.84
  skin 86.3
  spinal cord (meninges) 03.4
  subgingival 24.31
  tendon 83.39
    hand 82.29
    sheath 83.31
      hand 82.21
  uterus (with dilation) 69.09
    aspiration (diagnostic) NEC 69.59
      after abortion or delivery 69.52
      to terminate pregnancy 69.51
    following delivery or abortion 69.02
Curette evacuation, lens 13.2
Curtis operation (interphalangeal joint
  arthroplasty) 81.72
Cutaneolipectomy 86.83
Cutdown, venous 38.94
Cutting
  nerve (crania]) (peripheral) NEC 04.03
    acoustic 04.01
    auditory 04.01
    root, spinal 03.1
    sympathetic 05.0
    trigeminal 04.02
    vestibular 04.01
  pedicle (flap) graft 86.71
  pylorus (with wedge resection) 43.3
  spinal nerve root 03.1
  ureterovesical orifice 56.1
  urethral sphincter 58.5

CVP (central venous pressure monitoring) 89.62
Cyclectomy (ciliary body) 12.44
  eyelid margin 08.20
Cyclicotomy 12.55
Cycloanemization 12.74
Cyclocryotherapy 12.72
Cyclodialysis (initial) (subsequent) 12.55
Cyclodiathermy (penetrating) (surface) 12.71
Cycloelectrolysis 12.71
Cyclophotocoagulation 12.73
Cyclotomy 12.55
Cystectomy —*see also* Excision, lesion, by site
  gallbladder—*see* Cholecystectomy
  urinary (partial) (subtotal) 57.6
    complete (with urethrectomy) 57.79
    radical 57.71
      with pelvic exenteration (female) 68.8
    total (with urethrectomy) 57.79
Cystocolostomy 57.88
Cystogram, cystography NEC 87.77
Cystolitholapaxy 57.0
Cystolithotomy 57.19
Cystometrogram 89.22
Cystopexy NEC 57.89
Cystoplasty NEC 57.89
Cystoproctostomy 57.88
Cystoprostatectomy, radical 57.71
Cystopyelography 87.74
Cystorrhaphy 57.81
Cystoscopy (transurethral) 57.32
  with biopsy 57.33
  for
    control of hemorrhage
      bladder 57.93
      prostate 60.94
    retrograde pyelography 87.74
  ileal conduit 56.35
  through stoma (artificial) 57.31
Cystostomy
  closed (suprapubic) (percutaneous) 57.17
  open (suprapubic) 57.18
  percutaneous (closed) (suprapubic) 57.17
  suprapubic
    closed 57.17
    open 57.18
Cystotomy (open) (for removal of calculi) 57.19
Cystourethrogram (retrograde) (voiding) 87.76
Cystourethropexy (by) 59.79
  levator muscle sling 59.71
  retropubic suspension 59.5
  suprapubic suspension 59.4
Cystourethroplasty 57.85
Cystourethroscopy 57.32
  with biopsy
    bladder 57.33
    ureter 56.33
Cytology —*see* Examination, microscopic

D

Dacryoadenectomy 09.20
  partial 09.22
  total 09.23
Dacryoadenotomy 09.0
Dacryocystectomy (complete) (partial) 09.6
Dacryocystogram 87.05
Dacryocystorhinostomy (DCR) (by intubation)
  (external) (intranasal) 09.81
Dacryocystostomy 09.53
Dacryocystosyringotomy 09.53
Dacryocystotomy 09.53
Dahlman operation (excision of esophageal
  diverticulum) 42.31
Dana operation (posterior rhizotomy) 03.1
Danforth operation (fetal) 73.8
Darrach operation (ulnar resection) 77.83
da Vinci® (S HD) Surgical System —see
  category 17.4
Davis operation (intubated ureterotomy) 56.2
Deaf training 95.49
Debridement NOS 86.28
  excisional, NOS 86.22
    abdominal wall 54.3
    bone (*see also* Excision, lesion, bone) 77.60
      fracture—*see* Debridement, open fracture
    brain 01.59
    burn (skin) 86.22
    bursa 83.5
    cerebral meninges 01.51
    fascia 83.44
    flap graft 86.75
    graft (flap) (pedicle) 86.75
    heart valve (calcified)—*see* Valvuloplasty,
      heart
    infection (skin) 86.22
      nail bed or nail fold 86.27
    joint—*see* Excision, lesion, joint
    meninges (cerebral) 01.51
      spinal 03.4
    muscle 83.45
      hand 82.36
    nail 86.27
    nerve (peripheral) 04.07
    open fracture (compound) 79.60
      arm NEC 79.62
      carpal, metacarpal 79.63
      facial bone 76.2
      femur 79.65
      fibula 79.66
      foot NEC 79.67
      hand NEC 79.63
      humerus 79.61
      leg NEC 79.66
      phalanges
        foot 79.68
        hand 79.64
      radius 79.62
      specified site NEC 79.69
      tarsal, metatarsal 79.67
      tibia 79.66
      ulna 79.62
    patella 77.66
    pedicle graft 86.75
    skin or subcutaneous tissue (burn) (infection)
      (wound) 86.22
    cardioverter/defibrillator (automatic) pocket
      37.79

Debridement—*continued*
  graft 86.75
  nail, nail bed, or nail fold 86.27
  pacemaker pocket 37.79
  pocket
    cardiac device NEC 37.79
    cardiac pacemaker 37.79
    cardioverter/defibrillator (automatic) 37.79
  skull 01.25
    compound fracture 02.02
  spinal cord (meninges) 03.4
  tendon 83.39
  wound (skin) 86.22
  nonexcisional, NOS 86.28
    burn (skin) 86.28
    dental 96.54
    infection (skin) 86.28
    skin or subcutaneous tissue (burn) (infection)
      (wound) 86.28
    ultrasonic, ultrasound 86.28
    VersaJet™ 86.28
    wound (skin) 86.28
Decapitation, fetal 73.8
Decapsulation, kidney 55.91
Declotting —*see also* Removal, thrombus
  arteriovenous cannula or shunt 39.49
Decompression
  anus (imperforate) 48.0
  biliary tract 51.49
    by intubation 51.43
      endoscopic 51.87
      percutaneous 51.98
  brain 01.24
  carpal tunnel 04.43
  cauda equina 03.09
  chamber 93.97
  colon 96.08
    by incision 45.03
    endoscopic (balloon) 46.85
  common bile duct 51.42
    by intubation 51.43
      endoscopic 51.87
      percutaneous 51.98
  cranial 01.24
    for skull fracture 02.02
  endolymphatic sac 20.79
  ganglion (peripheral) NEC 04.49
    cranial NEC 04.42
  gastric 96.07
  heart 37.0
  intestine 96.08
    by incision 45.00
      endoscopic (balloon) 46.85
  intracranial 01.24
  labyrinth 20.79
  laminectomy 03.09
  laminotomy 03.09
  median nerve 04.43
  muscle 83.02
    hand 82.02
  nerve (peripheral) NEC 04.49
    auditory 04.42
    cranial NEC 04.42
    median 04.43
    trigeminal (root) 04.41
  orbit (*see also* Orbitotomy) 16.09
  pancreatic duct 52.92
    endoscopic 52.93

Decompression—*continued*
pericardium 37.0
rectum 48.0
skull fracture 02.02
spinal cord (canal) 03.09
tarsal tunnel 04.44
tendon (sheath) 83.01
hand 82.01
thoracic outlet
by
myotomy (division of scalenus anticus
muscle) 83.19
tenotomy 83.13
trigeminal (nerve root) 04.41
Decortication
arterial 05.25
brain 01.51
cerebral meninges 01.51
heart 37.31
kidney 55.91
lung (partial) (total) 34.51
thoracoscopic 34.52
nasal turbinates—*see* Turbinectomy
nose 21.89
ovary 65.29
laparoscopic 65.25
periarterial 05.25
pericardium 37.31
ventricle, heart (complete) 37.31
Decoy, E2F 00.16
Deepening
alveolar ridge 24.5
buccolabial sulcus 24.91
lingual sulcus 24.91
Defatting, flap or pedicle graft 86.75
Defibrillation, electric (external) (internal) 99.62
automatic cardioverter/defibrillator —*see*
category 37.9
de Grandmont operation (tarsectomy) 08.35
Delaying of pedicle graft 86.71
Delivery (with)
assisted spontaneous 73.59
breech extraction (assisted) 72.52
partial 72.52
with forceps to aftercoming head 72.51
total 72.54
with forceps to aftercoming head 72.53
unassisted (spontaneous delivery)—*omit code*
cesarean section—*see* Cesarean section
Credé maneuver 73.59
De Lee maneuver 72.4
forceps 72.9
application to aftercoming head (Piper) 72.6
with breech extraction
partial 72.51
total 72.53
Barton's 72.4
failed 73.3
high 72.39
with episiotomy 72.31
low (outlet) 72.0
with episiotomy 72.1
mid 72.29
with episiotomy 72.21
outlet (low) 72.0
with episiotomy 72.1
rotation of fetal head 72.4
trial 73.3
instrumental NEC 72.9
specified NEC 72.8
key-in-lock rotation 72.4

Delivery—*continued*
Kielland rotation 72.4
Malström's extraction 72.79
with episiotomy 72.71
manually assisted (spontaneous) 73.59
spontaneous (unassisted) 73.59
assisted 73.59
vacuum extraction 72.79
with episiotomy 72.71
Delorme operation
pericardiectomy 37.31
proctopexy 48.76
repair of prolapsed rectum 48.76
thoracoplasty 33.34
Denervation
aortic body 39.89
carotid body 39.89
facet, percutaneous (radio frequency) 03.96
ovarian 65.94
paracervical uterine 69.3
uterosacral 69.3
Denker operation (radical maxillary antrotomy)
22.31
Dennis-Barco operation —*see* Repair, hernia,
femoral
Denonvillier operation (limited rhinoplasty)
21.86
Densitometry, bone (serial)
(radiographic) 88.98
Depilation, skin 86.92
Derlacki operation (tympanoplasty) 19.4
Dermabond 86.59
Dermabrasion (laser) 86.25
for wound debridement 86.28
Derotation —*see* Reduction, torsion
Desensitization
allergy 99.12
psychologic 94.33
Desmotomy (*see also* Division, ligament) 80.40
Destruction
breast 85.20
chorioretinopathy (*see also* Destruction, lesion,
choroid) 14.29
ciliary body 12.74
epithelial downgrowth, anterior chamber 12.93
fallopian tube 66.39
with
crushing (and ligation) 66.31
by endoscopy laparoscopy) 66.21
division (and ligation) 66.32
by endoscopy (culdoscopy) (hysteroscopy)
(laparoscopy) (peritoneoscopy) 66.22
ligation 66.39
with
crushing 66.31
by endoscopy (laparoscopy) 66.21
division 66.32
by endoscopy (culdoscopy)
(hysteroscopy) (laparoscopy)
(peritoneoscopy) 66.22
unilateral 66.92
fetus 73.8
hemorrhoids 49.49
by
cryotherapy 49.44
sclerotherapy 49.42
inner ear NEC 20.79
by injection 20.72
intervertebral disc NOS 80.50
by injection 80.52
by other specified method 80.59

Destruction—*continued*
  herniated (nucleus pulposus) 80.51
  LAA 37.36
  lacrimal sac 09.6
  left atrial appendage 37.36
  lesion (local)
    anus 49.39
      endoscopic 49.31
    Bartholin's gland 71.24
      by
        aspiration 71.21
        excision 71.24
        incision 71.22
        marsupialization 71.23
    biliary ducts 51.69
      endoscopic 51.64
    bladder 57.59
      transurethral 57.49
    bone—*see* Excision, lesion, bone
    bowel—*see* Destruction, lesion, intestine
    brain (transtemporal approach) NEC 01.59
      by stereotactic radiosurgery 92.30
        cobalt 60 92.32
        linear accelerator (LINAC) 92.31
        multi-source 92.32
        particle beam (92.33)
        particulate (92.33)
        radiosurgery NEC (92.39)
        single source photon (92.31)
    breast NEC 85.20
    bronchus NEC 32.09
      endoscopic 32.01
    cerebral NEC 01.59
      meninges 01.51
    cervix 67.39
      by
        cauterization 67.32
        cryosurgery, cryoconization 67.33
        electroconization 67.32
    choroid 14.29
      by
        cryotherapy 14.22
        diathermy 14.21
        implantation of radiation source 14.27
        photocoagulation 14.25
          laser 14.24
          xenon arc 14.23
        radiation therapy 14.26
    ciliary body (nonexcisional) 12.43
      by excision 12.44
    conjunctiva 10.32
      by excision 10.31
    cornea NEC 11.49
      by
        cryotherapy 11.43
        electrocauterization 11.42
        thermocauterization 11.42
    cul-de-sac 70.32
    duodenum NEC 45.32
      by excision 45.31
        endoscopic 45.30
      endoscopic 45.30
    esophagus (chemosurgery) (cryosurgery)
        (electroresection) (fulguration) NEC 42.39
      by excision 42.32
        endoscopic 42.33
      endoscopic 42.33
    eye NEC 16.93
    eyebrow 08.25
    eyelid 08.25
      excisional—*see* Excision, lesion, eyelid

Destruction—*continued*
  heart
    by catheter ablation 37.34
    by endovascular approach 37.34
    by open approach 37.33
    by thoracoscopic approach 37.37
    left atrial appendage 37.36
  intestine (large) 45.49
    by excision 45.41
      endoscopic 45.43
        polypectomy 45.42
    endoscopic 45.43
      polypectomy 45.42
    small 45.34
      by excision 45.33
  intranasal 21.31
  iris (nonexcisional) NEC 12.41
    by excision 12.42
  kidney 55.39
    by marsupialization 55.31
  lacrimal sac 09.6
  larynx 30.09
  liver 50.29
  lung 32.29
    endoscopic 32.28
  meninges (cerebral) 01.51
    spinal 03.4
  nerve (peripheral) 04.07
    sympathetic 05.29
  nose 21.30
    intranasal 21.31
    specified NEC 21.32
  ovary
    by aspiration 65.91
    by excision 65.29
      laparoscopic 65.25
    cyst by rupture (manual) 65.93
  palate (bony) (local) 27.31
    wide 27.32
  pancreas 52.22
    by marsupialization 52.3
    endoscopic 52.21
  pancreatic duct 52.22
    endoscopic 52.21
  penis 64.2
  pharynx (excisional) 29.39
  pituitary gland
    by stereotactic radiosurgery 92.30
      cobalt 60 92.32
      linear accelerator (LINAC) 92.31
      multi-source 92.32
      particle beam 92.33
      particulate 92.33
      radiosurgery NEC 92.39
      single source photon 92.31
  rectum (local) 48.32
    by
      cryosurgery 48.34
      electrocoagulation 48.32
      excision 48.35
      fulguration 48.32
      laser (Argon) 48.33
    polyp 48.36
    radical 48.31
  retina 14.29
    by
      cryotherapy 14.22
      diathermy 14.21
      implantation of radiation source 14.27
      photocoagulation 14.25
        laser 14.24
        xenon arc 14.23

Destruction—*continued*
  radiation therapy 14.26
  salivary gland NEC 26.29
    by marsupialization 26.21
  sclera 12.84
  scrotum 61.3
  skin NEC 86.3
  sphincter of Oddi 51.69
    endoscopic 51.64
  spinal cord (meninges) 03.4
  spleen 41.42
    by marsupialization 41.41
  stomach NEC 43.49
    by excision 43.42
      endoscopic 43.41
    endoscopic 43.41
  subcutaneous tissue NEC 86.3
  testis 62.2
  tongue 25.1
  urethra (excisional) 58.39
    endoscopic 58.31
  uterus 68.29
  nerve (cranial) (peripheral) (by cryoanalgesia) (by radio frequency) 04.2
  sympathetic, by injection of neurolytic agent 05.32
  neuroma 04.07
    acoustic
      by craniotomy 04.01
      by radiosurgery 04.07
    cranial 04.07
    Morton's 04.07
    peripheral
      Morton's 04.07
  neuroma
    acoustic 04.01
      by craniotomy 04.01
      by stereotactic radiosurgery 92.30
        cobalt 60 92.32
        linear accelerator (LINAC) 92.31
        multi-source 92.32
        particle beam 92.33
        particulate 92.33
        radiosurgery NEC 92.39
        single source photon 92.31
  prostate (prostatic tissue)
    by
      cryotherapy 60.62
      microwave 60.96
      radiofrequency 60.97
    transurethral microwave thermotherapy (TUMT) 60.96
    transurethral needle ablation (TUNA) 60.97
    TULIP (transurethral (ultrasound) guided laser induced prostatectomy) 60.21
    TUMT (transurethral microwave thermotherapy) 60.96
    TUNA (transurethral needle ablation) 60.97
  semicircular canals, by injection 20.72
  tissue of heart —*see* Excision, lesion, heart
  vestibule, by injection 20.72
Detachment, uterosacral ligaments 69.3
Determination
  mental status (clinical) (medicolegal) (psychiatric) NEC 94.11
  psychologic NEC 94.09
  vital capacity (pulmonary) 89.37
Detorsion
  intestine (twisted) (volvulus) 46.80
    large 46.82
      endoscopic (balloon) 46.85
    small 46.81

Detorsion—*continued*
  kidney 55.84
  ovary 65.95
  spermatic cord 63.52
    with orchiopexy 62.5
  testis 63.52
    with orchiopexy 62.5
  volvulus 46.80
    endoscopic (balloon) 46.85
Detoxification therapy 94.25
  alcohol 94.62
    with rehabilitation 94.63
    combined alcohol and drug 94.68
      with rehabilitation 94.69
  drug 94.65
    with rehabilitation 94.66
    combined alcohol and drug 94.68
      with rehabilitation 94.69
Devascularization, stomach 44.99
Device
  CorCap™ 37.41
  external fixator—*see* Fixator, external
Dewebbing
  esophagus 42.01
  syndactyly (fingers) (toes) 86.85
Dextrorotation —*see* Reduction, torsion
Dialysis
  hemodiafiltration, hemofiltration (extracorporeal) 39.95
  kidney (extracorporeal) 39.95
  liver 50.92
  peritoneal 54.98
  renal (extracorporeal) 39.95
Diaphanoscopy
  nasal sinuses 89.35
  skull (newborn) 89.16
Diaphysectomy —*see* category 77.8
Diathermy 93.34
  choroid—*see* Diathermy, retina
  nasal turbinates 21.61
  retina
    for
      destruction of lesion 14.21
      reattachment 14.51
      repair of tear 14.31
  surgical—*see* Destruction, lesion, by site
  turbinates (nasal) 21.61
Dickson operation (fascial transplant) 83.82
Dickson-Diveley operation (tendon transfer and arthrodesis to correct claw toe) 77.57
Dieffenbach operation (hip disarticulation) 84.18
Dilation
  achalasia 42.92
  ampulla of Vater 51.81
    endoscopic 51.84
  anus, anal (sphincter) 96.23
  biliary duct
    endoscopic 51.84
    pancreatic duct 52.99
      endoscopic 52.98
    percutaneous (endoscopy) 51.98
    sphincter
      of Oddi 51.81
        endoscopic 51.84
      pancreatic 51.82
        endoscopic 51.85
  bladder 96.25
    neck 57.92
  bronchus 33.91
  cervix (canal) 67.0
    obstetrical 73.1

Dilation—*continued*
  to assist delivery 73.1
  choanae (nasopharynx) 29.91
  colon, (endoscopic) (balloon) 46.85
    with insertion of colonic stent
      endoscopic 46.86
      other 46.87
  colostomy stoma 96.24
  duodenum, (endoscopic) (balloon) 46.85
    with insertion of colonic stent
      endoscopic 46.86
      other 46.87
  endoscopic—*see* Dilation, by site
  enterostomy stoma 96.24
  esophagus (by bougie) (by sound) 42.92
  fallopian tube 66.96
  foreskin (newborn) 99.95
  frontonasal duct 96.21
  gastrojejunostomy site, endoscopic 44.22
  heart valve—*see* Valvulotomy, heart
  ileostomy stoma 96.24
  ileum (endoscopic) (balloon) 46.85
    with insertion of colonic stent
      endoscopic 46.86
      other 46.87
  intestinal stoma (artificial) 96.24
  intestine (endoscopic) (balloon) 46.85
    with insertion of colonic stent
      endoscopic 46.86
      other 46.87
  jejunum (endoscopic) (balloon) 46.85
    with insertion of colonic stent
      endoscopic 46.86
      other 46.87
  lacrimal
    duct 09.42
    punctum 09.41
  larynx 31.98
  lymphatic structure(s) (peripheral) 40.9
  nares 21.99
  nasolacrimal duct (retrograde) 09.43
    with insertion of tube or stent 09.44
  nasopharynx 29.91
  pancreatic duct 52.99
    endoscopic 52.98
  pharynx 29.91
  prostatic urethra (transurethral) (balloon) 60.95
  punctum, lacrimal papilla 09.41
  pylorus
    by incision 44.21
    endoscopic 44.22
  rectum 96.22
  salivary duct 26.91
  sphenoid ostia 22.52
  sphincter
    anal 96.23
    cardiac 42.92
    of Oddi 51.81
      endoscopic 51.84
    pancreatic 51.82
      endoscopic 51.85
    pylorus (endoscopic) 44.22
      by incision 44.21
  Stenson's duct 26.91
  trachea 31.99
  ureter 59.8
    meatus 56.91
  ureterovesical orifice 59.8
  urethra 58.6
    prostatic (transurethral))balloon) 60.95

Dilation—*continued*
  urethrovesical junction 58.6
  vagina (instrumental) (manual) NEC 96.16
  vesical neck 57.92
  Wharton's duct 26.91
  Wirsung's duct 52.99
    endoscopic 52.98
Dilation and curettage, uterus (diagnostic) 69.09
  after
    abortion 69.02
    delivery 69.02
  to terminate pregnancy 69.01
Diminution, ciliary body 12.74
Disarticulation 84.91
  ankle 84.13
  elbow 84.06
  finger, except thumb 84.01
    thumb 84.02
  hip 84.18
  knee 84.16
  shoulder 84.08
  thumb 84.02
  toe 84.11
  wrist 84.04
Discectomy —*see* Diskectomy
Discission
  capsular membrane 13.64
  cataract (Wheeler knife) (Ziegler knife) 13.2
    congenital 13.69
    secondary membrane 13.64
  iris 12.12
  lens (capsule) (Wheeler knife) (Ziegler knife)
    (with capsulotomy) 13.2
  orbitomaxillary, radical 16.51
  pupillary 13.2
  secondary membrane (after cataract) 13.64
  vitreous strands (posterior approach) 14.74
    anterior approach 14.73
Discogram, diskogram 87.21
Discolysis (by injection) 80.52
Diskectomy (discectomy), intervertebral 80.51
  herniated (nucleus pulposus) 80.51
    percutaneous 80.59
  with corpectomy 80.99
Dispensing (with fitting)
  contact lens 95.32
  low vision aids NEC 95.33
  spectacles 95.31
Disruption
  blood brain barrier via infusion [BBBD] 00.19
Dissection —*see also* Excision
  aneurysm 38.60
  artery-vein-nerve bundle 39.91
  branchial cleft fistula or sinus 29.52
  bronchus 32.1
  femoral hernia 53.29
  groin, radical 40.54
  larynx block (en bloc) 30.3
  mediastinum with pneumonectomy 32.59
    thoracoscopic 32.50
  neck, radical 40.40
    with laryngectomy 30.4
    bilateral 40.42
    unilateral 40.41
  orbital fibrous bands 16.92
  pterygium (with reposition) 11.31
  radical neck—*see* Dissection, neck, radical
  retroperitoneal NEC 59.00
  thoracic structures (block) (en bloc) (radical)
    (brachial plexus, bronchus, lobe of lung, ribs,
    and sympathetic nerves) 32.6
  vascular bundle 39.91

Distention, bladder (therapeutic) (intermittent)
    96.25
Diversion
    biliopancreatic (BPD) 43.7 *[45.51] [45.91]*
        with duodenal switch 43.89 *[45.51] [45.91]*
    cutaneous 56.61
    ileal conduit 56.51
    internal NEC 56.71
    ureter to
        intestine 56.71
        skin 56.61
    uretero-ileostomy 56.51
    urinary
        cutaneous 56.61
        ileal conduit 56.51
        internal NEC 56.71
        ureter to
            intestine 56.71
            skin 56.61
        uretero-ileostomy 56.51
Diversional therapy 93.81
Diverticulectomy
    bladder (suprapubic) 57.59
        transurethral approach 57.49
    duodenum 45.31
        endoscopic 45.30
    esophagus 42.31
        endoscopic 42.33
    esophagomyotomy 42.7
    hypopharyngeal (by cricopharyngeal myotomy)
        29.32
    intestine
        large 45.41
            endoscopic 45.43
        small 45.33
    kidney 55.39
    Meckel's 45.33
    pharyngeal (by cricopharyngeal myotomy) 29.32
    pharyngoesophageal (by cricopharyngeal
        myotomy) 29.32
    stomach 43.42
        endoscopic 43.41
    urethra 58.39
        endoscopic 58.31
Division
    Achilles tendon 83.11
    adductor tendon (hip) 83.12
    adhesions—*see* Lysis, adhesions
    angle of mandible (open) 76.62
        closed 76.61
    anterior synechiae 12.32
    aponeurosis 83.13
    arcuate ligament (spine)—omit
    arteriovenous fistula (with ligation) 39.53
    artery (with ligation) 38.80
        abdominal 38.86
        aorta (arch) (ascending) (descending) 38.84
        head and neck NEC 38.82
        intracranial NEC 38.81
        lower limb 38.88
        thoracic NEC 38.85
        upper limb 38.83
    bladder neck 57.91
    blepharorrhaphy 08.02
    blood vessels, cornea 10.1
    bone (*see also* Osteotomy) 77.30
    brain tissue 01.32
        cortical adhesions 02.91
    canaliculus 09.52
    canthorrhaphy 08.02

Division—*continued*
    cartilage 80.40
        ankle 80.47
        elbow 80.42
        foot and toe 80.48
        hand and finger 80.44
        hip 80.45
        knee 80.46
        shoulder 80.41
        specified site NEC 80.49
        spine 80.49
        wrist 80.43
    cerebral tracts 01.32
    chordae tendineae 35.32
    common wall between posterior left atrium and
        coronary sinus (with roofing of resultant
        defect with patch graft) 35.82
    congenital web
        larynx 31.98
        pharynx 29.54
    endometrial synechiae 68.21
    fallopian tube—*see* Ligation, fallopian tube
    fascia 83.14
        hand 82.12
    frenulum, frenum
        labial 27.91
        lingual 25.91
        tongue 25.91
    ganglion, sympathetic 05.0
    glossopharyngeal nerve 29.92
    goniosynechiae 12.31
    hypophyseal stalk (*see also* Hypophysectomy,
        partial) 07.63
    iliotibial band 83.14
    isthmus
        horseshoe kidney 55.85
        thyroid 06.91
    joint capsule 80.40
        ankle 80.47
        elbow 80.42
        foot and toe 80.48
        hand and finger 80.44
        hip 80.45
        knee 80.46
        shoulder 80.41
        specified site NEC 80.49
        wrist 80.43
    labial frenum 27.91
    lacrimal ductules 09.0
    laryngeal nerve (external) (recurrent) (superior)
        31.91
    ligament 80.40
        ankle 80.47
        arcuate (spine)—*omit code*
        canthal 08.36
        elbow 80.42
        foot and toe 80.48
        hand and finger 80.44
        hip 80.45
        knee 80.46
        palpebrae 08.36
        shoulder 80.41
        specified site NEC 80.49
        spine 80.49
            arcuate—*omit code*
            flavum—*omit code*
        uterosacral 69.3
        wrist 80.43
    ligamentum flavum (spine)—*omit code*
    meninges (cerebral) 01.31

Division—*continued*
muscle 83.19
  hand 82.19
nasolacrimal duct stricture (with drainage) 09.59
nerve (cranial) (peripheral) NEC 04.03
  acoustic 04.01
  adrenal gland 07.42
  auditory 04.01
  glossopharyngeal 29.92
  lacrimal branch 05.0
  laryngeal (external) (recurrent) (superior) 31.91
  vestibular 04.01
phrenic 04.03
  for collapse of lung 33.31
root, spinal or intraspinal 03.1
sympathetic 05.0
tracts
  cerebral 01.32
  spinal cord 03.29
    percutaneous 03.21
  trigeminal 04.02
  vagus (*see also* Vagotomy) 44.00
  vestibular 04.01
otosclerotic process or material, middle ear 19.0
papillary muscle (heart) 35.31
patent ductus arteriosus 38.85
penile adhesions 64.93
posterior synechiae 12.33
pylorus (with wedge resection) 43.3
rectum (stricture) 48.91
scalenus anticus muscle 83.19
Skene's gland 71.3
soft tissue NEC 83.19
  hand 82.19
sphincter
  anal (external) (internal) 49.59
    left lateral 49.51
    posterior 49.52
  cardiac 42.7
  of Oddi 51.82
    endoscopic 51.85
  pancreatic 51.82
    endoscopic 51.85
spinal
  cord tracts 03.29
    percutaneous 03.21
  nerve root 03.1
symblepharon (with insertion of conformer) 10.5
synechiae
  endometrial 68.21
  iris (posterior) 12.33
    anterior 12.32
tarsorrhaphy 08.02
tendon 83.13
  Achilles 83.11
  adductor (hip) 83.12
  hand 82.11
trabeculae carneae cordis (heart) 35.35
tympanum 20.23
uterosacral ligaments 69.3
vaginal septum 70.14
vas deferens 63.71
vein (with ligation) 38.80
  abdominal 38.87
  head and neck NEC 38.82
  intracranial NEC 38.81
  lower limb 38.89
    varicose 38.59
  thoracic NEC 38.85
  upper limb 38.83

Division—*continued*
varicose 38.50
  abdominal 38.57
  head and neck NEC 38.52
  intracranial NEC 38.51
  lower limb 38.59
  thoracic NEC 38.55
  upper limb 39.53
vitreous, cicatricial bands (posterior approach) 14.74
  anterior approach 14.73
Doleris operation (shortening of round ligaments) 69.22
D'Ombrain operation (excision of pterygium with corneal graft) 11.32
Domestic tasks therapy 93.83
Dopplergram, Doppler flow mapping —*see also* Ultrasonography
aortic arch 88.73
head and neck 88.71
heart 88.72
intraoperative transcranial 00.94
thorax NEC 88.73
Dorrance operation (push-back operation for cleft palate) 27.62
Dotter operation (transluminal angioplasty) 39.59
Douche, vagina 96.44
Douglas operation (suture of tongue to lip for micrognathia) 25.59
Downstream® System (AO therapy) (aqueous oxygen) 00.49
Doyle operation (paracervical uterine denervation) 69.3
Drainage
by
  anastomosis—*see* Anastomosis
  aspiration—*see* Aspiration
  incision—*see* Incision
abdomen 54.19
  percutaneous 54.91
abscess—*see also* Drainage, by site and Incision, by site
  appendix 47.2
    with appendectomy 47.09
      laparoscopic 47.01
  parapharyngeal (oral) (transcervical) 28.0
  peritonsillar (oral) (transcervical) 28.0
  retropharyngeal (oral) (transcervical) 28.0
  thyroid (field) (gland) 06.09
    percutaneous (needle) 06.01
    postoperative 06.02
  tonsil, tonsillar (oral) (transcervical) 28.0
antecubital fossa 86.04
appendix 47.91
  with appendectomy 47.09
    laparoscopic 47.01
  abscess 47.2
    with appendectomy 47.09
      laparoscopic 47.01
axilla 86.04
bladder (without incision) 57.0
  by indwelling catheter 57.94
    percutaneous suprapubic (closed) 57.17
    suprapubic NEC 57.18
buccal space 27.0

Drainage—*continued*
bursa 83.03
  by aspiration 83.94
    hand 82.92
  hand 82.03
    by aspiration 82.92
  radial 82.03
  ulnar 82.03
cerebrum, cerebral (meninges) (ventricle)
  (incision) (trephination) 01.39
  by
    anastomosis—*see* Shunt, ventricular
    aspiration 01.09
    through previously implanted catheter 01.02
chest (closed) 34.04
  open (by incision) 34.09
  thoracoscopic 34.06
crania] sinus (incision) (trephination) 01.21
  by aspiration 01.09
cul-de-sac 70.12
  by aspiration 70.0
cyst—*see also* Drainage, by site and incision, by
  site
  pancreas (by catheter) 52.01
    by marsupialization 52.3
    internal (anastomosis) 52.4
  pilonidal 86.03
  spleen, splenic (by marsupialization) 41.41
duodenum (tube) 46.39
  by incision 45.01
ear
  external 18.09
  inner 20.79
  middle (by myringotomy) 20.09
    with intubation 20.01
epidural space, cerebral (incision) (trephination)
  01.24
  by aspiration 01.09
extradural space, cerebral (incision) (trephination)
  01.24
  by aspiration 01.09
extraperitoneal 54.0
facial region 27.0
fascial compartments, head and neck 27.0
fetal hydrocephalic head (needling) (trocar) 73.8
fluid (blood) (cerebrospinal) (CSF)
  by
    external ventricular drain (EVD) placement
      02.21
gallbladder 51.04
  by
    anastomosis 51.35
    aspiration 51.01
    incision 51.04
groin region (abdominal wall) (inguinal) 54.0
  skin 86.04
  subcutaneous tissue 86.04
hematoma—*see* Drainage, by site and Incision,
  by site
hydrocephalic head (needling) (trocar) 73.8
hypochondrium 54.0
  intra-abdominal 54.19
iliac fossa 54.0
infratemporal fossa 27.0
intracranial space (epidural) (extradural)
  (incision) (trephination) 01.24
  by aspiration 01.09
  subarachnoid or subdural (incision)
    (trephination) 01.31
    by aspiration 01.09
intraperitoneal 54.19
  percutaneous 54.91

Drainage—*continued*
kidney (by incision) 55.01
  by
    anastomosis 55.86
    catheter 59.8
  pelvis (by incision) 55.11
liver 50.0
  by aspiration 50.91
Ludwig's angina 27.0
lung (by incision) 33.1
  by punch (needle) (trocar) 33.93
midpalmar space 82.04
mouth floor 27.0
mucocele, nasal sinus 22.00
  by puncture 22.01
  through natural ostium 22.02
omentum 54.19
  percutaneous 54.91
ovary (aspiration) 65.91
  by incision 65.09
    laparoscopic 65.01
palmar space (middle) 82.04
pancreas (by catheter) 52.01
  by anastomosis 52.96
parapharyngeal 28.0
paronychia 86.04
parotid space 27.0
pelvic peritoneum (female) 70.12
  male 54.19
pericardium 37.0
perigastric 54.19
  percutaneous 54.91
perineum
  female 71.09
  male 86.04
perisplenic tissue 54.19
  percutaneous 54.91
peritoneum 54.19
  pelvic (female) 70.12
  percutaneous 54.91
peritonsillar 28.0
pharyngeal space, lateral 27.0
pilonidal cyst or sinus 86.03
pleura (closed) 34.04
  open (by incision) 34.09
  thoracoscopic 34.06
popliteal space 86.04
postural 93.99
postzygomatic space 27.0
pseudocyst, pancreas 52.3
  by anastomosis 52.4
pterygopalatine fossa 27.0
retropharyngeal 28.0
scrotum 61.0
skin 86.04
spinal (canal) (cord) 03.09
  by anastomosis—*see* Shunt, spinal
  diagnostic 03.31
spleen 41.2
  cyst (by marsupialization) 41.41
subarachnoid space, cerebral (incision)
  (trephination) 01.31
  by aspiration 01.09
subcutaneous tissue 86.04
subdiaphragmatic 54.91
  percutaneous 54.91
subdural space, cerebral (incision) (trephination)
  01.31
  by aspiration 01.09
subhepatic space 54.19
  percutaneous 54.91

Drainage—*continued*
sublingual space 27.0
submental space 27.0
subphrenic space 54.19
  percutaneous 54.91
supraclavicular fossa 86.04
temporal pouches 27.0
tendon (sheath) 83.01
  hand 82.01
thenar space 82.04
thorax (closed) 34.04
  open (by incision) 34.09
  thoracoscopic 34.06
thyroglossal tract (by incision) 06.09
  by aspiration 06.01
thyroid (field) (gland) (by incision) 06.09
  by aspiration 06.01
  postoperative 06.02
tonsil 28.0
tunica vaginalis 61.0
ureter (by catheter) 59.8
  by
    anastomosis NEC (*see also* Anastomosis,
      ureter) 56.79
    incision 56.2
ventricle (cerebral) (incision)
  by
    anastomosis—*see* Shunt, ventricular
    aspiration 01.09
      through previously implanted catheter 01.02
    extracranial ventricular shunt —*see* category
      02.3
vertebral column 03.09
Drawing test 94.08
Dressing
burn 93.57
ulcer 93.56
wound 93.57
Drilling
bone—*see also* Incision, bone 77.10
ovary 65.99
Drotrecogin alfa (activated), infusion 00.11
Ductogram, mammary 87.35
Duhamel operation (abdominoperineal
  pull-through) 48.65
Dührssen's
incisions (cervix, to assist delivery) 73.93
operation (vaginofixation of uterus) 69.22
Dunn operation (triple arthrodesis) 81.12
Duodenectomy 45.62
with
  gastrectomy—*see* Gastrectomy
  pancreatectomy—*see* Pancreatectomy
Duodenocholedochotomy 51.51
Duodenoduodenostomy 45.91
proximal to distal segment 45.62
Duodenoileostomy 45.91
Duodenojejunostomy 45.91
Duodenoplasty 46.79
Duodenorrhaphy 46.71
Duodenoscopy 45.13
through stoma (artificial) 45.12
transabdominal (operative) 45.11
Duodenostomy 46.39
Duodenotomy 45.01
Dupuytren operation
fasciectomy 82.35
fasciotomy 82.12
  with excision 82.35
shoulder disarticulation 84.08
Durabond 86.59

Duraplasty 02.12
Durham (Caldwell) operation (transfer of biceps
  femoris tendon) 83.75
DuToit and Roux operation (staple
  capsulorrhaphy of shoulder) 81.82
DuVries operation (tenoplasty) 83.88
Dwyer operation
fasciotomy 83.14
soft tissue release NEC 83.84
wedge osteotomy, calcaneus 77.28

E2F decoy 00.16
Eagleton operation (extrapetrosal drainage)
  20.22
ECG —*see* Electrocardiogram
Echocardiography 88.72
  intracardiac (heart chambers) (ICE) 37.28
  intravascular (coronary vessels) 00.24
  transesophageal 88.72
    monitoring (Doppler) (ultrasound) 89.68
Echoencephalography 88.71
Echography —*see* Ultrasonography
Echogynography 88.79
Echoplacentogram 88.78
ECMO (extracorporeal membrane oxygenation)
  39.65
Eden-Hybinette operation (glenoid bone block)
  78.01
Educational therapy (bed-bound children)
  (handicapped) 93.82
EEG (electroencephalogram) 89.14
  monitoring (radiographic) (video) 89.19
Effler operation (heart) 36.2
Effleurage 93.39
EGD (esophagogastroduodenoscopy) 45.13
  with closed biopsy 45.16
Eggers operation
  tendon release (patellar retinacula) 83.13
  tendon transfer (biceps femoris tendon)
    (hamstring tendon) 83.75
EKG (*see also* Electrocardiogram) 89.52
Elastic hosiery 93.59
Electrocardiogram (with 12 or more leads)
  89.52
  with vectorcardiogram 89.53
  fetal (scalp), intrauterine 75.32
  rhythm (with one to three leads) 89.51
Electrocautery —*see also* Cauterization
  cervix 67.32
  corneal lesion (ulcer) 11.42
  esophagus 42.39
    endoscopic 42.33
Electrocoagulation —*see also* Destruction,
  lesion, by site
  aneurysm (cerebral) (peripheral vessels) 39.52
  cervix 67.32
  cystoscopic 57.49
  ear
    external 18.29
    inner 20.79
    middle 20.51
  fallopian tube (lesion) 66.61
    for tubal ligation—*see* Ligation, fallopian tube
  gasserian ganglion 04.02
  nasal turbinates 21.61
  nose, for epistaxis (with packing) 21.03
  ovary 65.29
    laparoscopic 65.25
  prostatic bed 60.94
  rectum (polyp) 48.32
    radical 48.31
  retina (for)
    destruction of lesion 14.21
    reattachment 14.51
    repair of tear 14.31
  round ligament 69.19
  semicircular canals 20.79
  urethrovesical junction, transurethral 57.49

Electrocoagulation—*continued*
  uterine ligament 69.19
  uterosacral ligament 69.19
  uterus 68.29
  vagina 70.33
  vulva 71.3
Electrocochleography 20.31
Electroconization, cervix 67.32
Electroconvulsive therapy (ECT) 94.27
Electroencephalogram (EEG) 89.14
  monitoring (radiographic) (video) 89.19
    intraoperative 00.94
Electrogastrogram 44.19
Electrokeratotomy 11.49
Electrolysis
  ciliary body 12.71
  hair follicle 86.92
  retina (for)
    destruction of lesion 14.21
    reattachment 14.51
    repair of tear 14.31
  skin 86.92
  subcutaneous tissue 86.92
Electromyogram, electromyography (EMG)
  muscle) 93.08
  eye 95.25
  urethral sphincter 89.23
Electronarcosis 94.29
Electronic gaiter 93.59
Electronystagmogram (ENG) 95.24
Electrooculogram (EOG) 95.22
Electroresection —*see also* Destruction, lesion,
  by site
  bladder neck (transurethral) 57.49
  esophagus 42.39
    endoscopic 42.33
  prostate (transurethral) 60.29
  stomach 43.49
    endoscopic 43.41
Electroretinogram (ERG) 95.21
Electroshock therapy (EST) 94.27
  subconvulsive 94.26
Elevation
  bone fragments (fractured)
    orbit 76.79
    sinus (nasal)
      frontal 22.79
      maxillary 22.79
    skull (with debridement) 02.02
    spinal 03.53
  pedicle graft 86.71
Elliot operation (scleral trephination with
  iridectomy) 12.61
Ellis Jones operation (repair of peroneal tendon)
  83.88
Ellison operation (reinforcement of collateral
  ligament) 81.44
Elmslie-Cholmeley operation (tarsal wedge
  osteotomy) 77.28
Eloesser operation
  thoracoplasty 33.34
  thoracostomy 34.09
Elongation —*see* Lengthening
Embolectomy 38.00
  with endarterectomy—*see* Endarterectomy
  abdominal
    artery 38.06
    vein 38.07

Embolectomy—*continued*
  aorta (arch) (ascending) (descending) 38.04
  arteriovenous shunt or cannula 39.49
  bovine graft 39.49
  head and neck NEC 38.02
  intracranial NEC 38.01
  lower limb
    artery 38.08
    vein 38.09
  mechanical
    endovascular
      head and neck 39.74
  pulmonary (artery) (vein) 38.05
  thoracic NEC 38.05
  upper limb (artery) (vein) 38.03
Embolization (transcatheter)
  adhesive (glue) 39.79
    head and neck 39.72
  arteriovenous fistula 39.53
    endovascular 39.72
  artery (selective) 38.80
    by
      endovascular approach 39.79
        head and neck vessels 39.72
          bare coils 39.75
          bioactive coils 39.76
          partial occlusion (balloon) (temporary)
            39.77
      percutaneous transcatheter infusion 99.29
    abdominal NEC 38.86
      duodenal (transcatheter) 44.44
      gastric (transcatheter) 44.44
      renal (transcatheter) 38.86
    aorta (arch) (ascending) (descending) 38.84
      temporary therapeutic endovascular (balloon)
        (partial occlusion) 39.77
    duodenal (transcatheter) 44.44
    gastric (transcatheter) 44.44
    head and neck NEC 38.82
    intracranial NEC 38.81
    lower limb 38.88
    renal (transcatheter) 38.86
    thoracic NEC 38.85
    upper limb 38.83
    uterine (gelatin sponge) (gelfoam)
      (microspheres) (PVA) (spherical embolics)
      (without coil(s)) 68.25
  AVM, intracranial, endovascular approach 39.72
  carotid cavernous fistula 39.53
  chemoembolization 99.25
  coil, endovascular 39.79
    head and neck 39.75
      bare coils 39.75
      bioactive coils 39.76
    uterine artery 68.24
  vein (selective) 38.80
    abdominal NEC 38.87
      duodenal (transcatheter) 44.44
      gastric (transcatheter) 44.44
    by
      endovascular approach 39.79
        head and neck 39.72
        partial occlusion (balloon) (temporary)
          39.77
    duodenal (transcatheter) 44.44
    gastric (transcatheter) 44.44
Embryotomy 73.8
EMG —*see* Electromyogram
Emmet operation (cervix) 67.61
Encephalocentesis (*see also* Puncture) 01.09
  fetal head, transabdominal 73.8

Encephalography (cisternal puncture)
  (fractional) (lumbar) (pneumoencephalogram)
  87.01
Encephalopuncture 01.09
Encircling procedure —*see also* Cerclage
  sclera, for buckling 14.49
    with implant 14.41
Endarterectomy (gas) (with patch graft) 38.10
  abdominal 38.16
  aorta (arch) (ascending) (descending) 38.14
  coronary artery—*see* category 36.0
    open chest approach 36.03
  head and neck (open) 38.12

> *Note: Also use 00.40, 00.41, 00.42, or 00.43 to show the total number of vessels treated. Use code 00.44 once to show procedure on a bifurcated vessel. In addition, use 00.45, 00.46, 00.47, or 00.48 to show the number of vascular stents inserted.*

    percutaneous approach, extracranial vessel(s)
      00.61
    percutaneous approach, intracranial vessel(s)
      00.62
  intracranial (open) NEC 38.11
    percutaneous approach, intracranial vessel(s)
      00.62

> *Note: Also use 00.40, 00.41, 00.42, or 00.43 to show the total number of vessels treated. Use code 00.44 once to show procedure on a bifurcated vessel. In addition, use 00.45, 00.46, 00.47, or 00.48 to show the number of vascular stents inserted.*

  lower limb 38.18
  thoracic NEC 38.15
  upper limb 38.13
Endoaneurysmorrhaphy (*see also*
  Aneurysmorrhaphy) 39.52
  by or with
    endovascular graft
      abdominal aorta 39.71
        fenestrated (branching) graft 39.78
      lower extremity artery(s) 39.79
      thoracic aorta 39.73
      upper extremity artery(s) 39.79
Endolymphatic (subarachnoid) shunt 20.71
Endometrectomy (uterine) (internal) 68.29
  bladder 57.59
  cul-de-sac 70.32
Endoprosthesis
  bile duct 51.87
  femoral head (bipolar) 81.52
Endoscopy
  with biopsy—*see* Biopsy, by site, closed
  anus 49.21
  biliary tract (operative) 51.11
    by retrograde cholangiography (ERC) 51.11
    by retrograde cholangiopancreatography
      (ERCP) 51.10
    intraoperative 51.11
    percutaneous (via T-tube or other tract) 51.98
      with removal of common duct stones 51.96
  bladder 57.32
    through stoma (artificial) 57.31
  bronchus NEC 33.23
    with biopsy 33.24
    fiberoptic 33.22
    through stoma (artificial) 33.21

Endoscopy—*continued*
  colon 45.23
    through stoma (artificial) 45.22
    transabdominal (operative) 45.21
  cul-de-sac 70.22
  ear 18.11
  esophagus NEC 42.23
    through stoma (artificial) 42.22
    transabdominal (operative) 42.21
  ileum 45.13
    through stoma (artificial) 45.12
    transabdominal (operative) 45.11
  intestine NEC 45.24
    large 45.24
      fiberoptic (flexible) 45.23
      through stoma (artificial) 45.22
      transabdominal (intraoperative) 45.21
    small 45.13
      esophagogastroduodenoscopy (EGD) 45.13
        with closed biopsy 45.16
      through stoma (artificial) 45.12
      transabdominal (operative) 45.11
  jejunum 45.13
    through stoma (artificial) 45.12
    transabdominal (operative) 45.11
  kidney 55.21
  larynx 31.42
    through stoma (artificial) 31.41
  lung—*see* Bronchoscopy
  mediastinum (transpleural) 34.22
  nasal sinus 22.19
  nose 21.21
  pancreatic duct 52.13
  pelvis 55.22
  peritoneum 54.21
  pharynx 29.11
  rectum 48.23
    through stoma (artificial) 48.22
    transabdominal (operative) 48.21
  sinus, nasal 22.19
  stomach NEC 44.13
    through stoma (artificial) 44.12
    transabdominal (operative) 44.11
  thorax (transpleural) 34.21
  trachea NEC 31.42
    through stoma (artificial) 31.41
  transpleural
    mediastinum 34.22
    thorax 34.21
  ureter 56.31
  urethra 58.22
  uterus 68.12
  vagina 70.21
Enema (transanal) NEC 96.39
  for removal of impacted feces 96.38
ENG (electronystagmogram) 95.24
Enlargement
  aortic lumen, thoracic 38.14
  atrial septal defect (pre-existing) 35.41
    in repair of total anomalous pulmonary venous
      connection 35.82
  eye socket 16.64
  foramen ovale (pre-existing) 35.41
    in repair of total anomalous pulmonary venous
      connection 35.82
  intestinal stoma 46.40
    large intestine 46.43
    small intestine 46.41
  introitus 96.16
  orbit (eye) 16.64
  palpebral fissure 08.51

Enlargement—*continued*
  punctum 09.41
  sinus tract (skin) 86.89
Enterectomy NEC 45.63
Enteroanastomosis
  large-to-large intestine 45.94
  small-to-large intestine 45.93
  small-to-small intestine 45.91
Enterocelectomy 53.9
  female 70.92
    with graft or prosthesis 70.93
  vaginal 70.92
    with graft or prosthesis 70.93
Enterocentesis 45.00
  duodenum 45.01
  large intestine 45.03
  small intestine NEC 45.02
Enterocholecystostomy 51.32
Enteroclysis (small bowel) 96.43
Enterocolectomy NEC 45.79
Enterocolostomy 45.93
Enteroentectropy 46.99
Enteroenterostomy 45.90
  small-to-large intestine 45.93
  small-to-small intestine 45.91
Enterogastrostomy 44.39
  laparoscopic 44.38
Enterolithotomy 45.00
Enterolysis 54.59
  laparoscopic 54.51
Enteropancreatostomy 52.96
Enterorrhaphy 46.79
  large intestine 46.75
  small intestine 46.73
Enterostomy NEC 46.39
  cecum (*see also* Colostomy) 46.10
  colon (transverse) (*see also* Colostomy) 46.10
    loop 46.03
  delayed opening 46.31
  duodenum 46.39
    loop 46.01
  feeding NEC 46.39
    percutaneous (endoscopic) 46.32
  ileum (Brooke) (Dragstedt) 46.20
    loop 46.01
  jejunum (feeding) 46.39
    loop 46.01
    percutaneous (endoscopic) 46.32
  sigmoid colon (*see also* Colostomy) 46.10
    loop 46.03
  transverse colon (*see also* Colostomy) 46.10
    loop 46.03
Enterotomy 45.00
  large intestine 45.03
  small intestine 45.02
Enucleation —*see also* Excision, lesion, by site
  cyst
    broad ligament 69.19
    dental 24.4
    liver 50.29
    ovarian 65.29
      laparoscopic 65.25
    parotid gland 26.29
    salivary gland 26.29
    skin 86.3
    subcutaneous tissue 86.3
  eyeball 16.49
    with implant (into Tenon's capsule) 16.42
      with attachment of muscles 16.41
EOG (electro-oculogram) 95.22
Epicardiectomy 36.39

Epididymectomy 63.4
  with orchidectomy (unilateral) 62.3
    bilateral 62.41
Epididymogram 87.93
Epididymoplasty 63.59
Epididymorrhaphy 63.81
Epididymotomy 63.92
Epididymovasostomy 63.83
Epiglottidectomy 30.21
Epikeratophakia 11.76
Epilation
  eyebrow (forceps) 08.93
    cryosurgical 08.92
    electrosurgical 08.91
  eyelid (forceps) NEC 08.93
    cryosurgical 08.92
    electrosurgical 08.91
  skin 86.92
Epiphysiodesis (*see also* Arrest, bone
    growth)—*see* category 78.2
Epiphysiolysis (*see also* Arrest, bone
    growth)—*see* 78.2
Epiploectomy 54.4
Epiplopexy 54.74
Epiplorrhaphy 54.74
Episioperineoplasty 71.79
Episioperineorrhaphy 71.71
  obstetrical 75.69
Episioplasty 71.79
Episioproctotomy 73.6
Episiorrhaphy 71.71
  following episiotomy—*see* Episiotomy
  for obstetrical laceration 75.69
Episiotomy (with subsequent episiorrhaphy) 73.6
  high forceps 72.31
  low forceps 72.1
  mid forceps 72.21
  nonobstetrical 71.09
  outlet forceps 72.1
EPS (electrophysiologic stimulation)
  as part of intraoperative testing —*omit code*
  catheter based invasive electrophysiologic testing
    37.26
  device interrogation only without arrhythmia
    induction (bedside check) 89.45-89.49
  noninvasive programmed electrical stimulation
    (NIPS) 37.20
Eptifibatide, infusion 99.20
Equalization, leg
  lengthening—*see* category 78.3
  shortening—*see* category 78.2
Equilibration (occlusal) 24.8
Equiloudness balance 95.43
ERC (endoscopic) retrograde cholangiography
    51.11
ERCP (endoscopic retrograde
    cholangiopancreatography) 51.10
  cannulation of pancreatic duct 52.93
ERG (electroretinogram) 95.21
ERP (endoscopic retrograde pancreatography)
    52.13
Eruption, tooth, surgical 24.6
Erythrocytapheresis, therapeutic 99.73
Escharectomy 86.22
Escharotomy 86.09
Esophageal voice training (postlaryngectomy)
    93.73
Esophagectomy 42.40
  abdominothoracocervical (combined)
    (synchronous) 42.42

Esophagectomy—*continued*
  partial or subtotal 42.41
  total 42.42
Esophagocologastrostomy (intrathoracic) 42.55
  antesternal or antethoracic 42.65
Esophagocolostomy (intrathoracic) NEC 42.56
  with interposition of Colon 42.55
  antesternal or antethoracic NEC 42.66
    with interposition of colon 42.65
Esophagoduodenostomy (intrathoracic) NEC
    42.54
  with
    complete gastrectomy 43.99
    interposition of small bowel 42.53
Esophagoenterostomy (intrathoracic) NEC (*see
    also* Anastomosis, esophagus, to intestinal
    segment) 42.54
  antesternal or antethoracic (*see also* Anastomosis,
    esophagus, antesternal, to intestinal segment)
    42.64
Esophagoesophagostomy (intrathoracic) 42.51
  antesternal or antethoracic 42.61
Esophagogastrectomy 43.99
Esophagogastroduodenoscopy (EGD) 45.13
  with closed biopsy 45.16
  through stoma (artificial) 45.12
  transabdominal (operative) 45.11
Esophagogastromyotomy 42.7
Esophagogastropexy 44.65
Esophagogastroplasty 44.65
Esophagogastroscopy NEC 44.13
  through stoma (artificial) 44.12
  transabdominal (operative) 44.11
Esophagogastrostomy (intrathoracic) 42.52
  with partial gastrectomy 43.5
  antesternal or antethoracic 42.62
Esophagoileostomy (intrathoracic) NEC 42.54
  with interposition of small bowel 42.53
  antesternal or antethoracic NEC 42.64
    with interposition of small bowel 42.63
Esophagojejunostomy (intrathoracic) NEC 42.54
  with
    complete gastrectomy 43.99
    interposition of small bowel 42.53
  antesternal or antethoracic NEC 42.64
    with interposition of small bowel 42.63
Esophagomyotomy 42.7
Esophagoplasty NEC 42.89
Esophagorrhaphy 42.82
Esophagoscopy NEC 42.23
  with closed biopsy 42.24
  by incision (operative) 42.21
  through stoma (artificial) 42.22
  transabdominal (operative) 42.21
Esophagostomy 42.10
  cervical 42.11
  thoracic 42.19
Esophagotomy NEC 42.09
Estes operation (ovary) 65.72
  laparoscopic 65.75
Estlander operation (thoracoplasty) 33.34
ESWL (extracorporeal shock wave lithotripsy)
    NEC 98.59
  bile duct 98.52
  bladder 98.51
  gallbladder 98.52
  kidney 98.51
  Kock pouch (urinary diversion) 98.51
  renal pelvis 98.51
  specified site NEC 98.59
  ureter 98.51

Ethmoidectomy 22.63
Ethmoidotomy 22.51
Evacuation
  abscess—*see* Drainage, by site
  anterior chamber (eye) (aqueous) (hyphema)
    12.91
Evacuation—*continued*
  cyst—*see also* Excision, lesion, by site
    breast 85.91
    kidney 55.01
    liver 50.29
  hematoma—*see also* Incision, hematoma
    obstetrical 75.92
      incisional 75.91
  hemorrhoids (thrombosed) 49.47
  pelvic blood clot (by incision) 54.19
    by
      culdocentesis 70.0
      culdoscopy 70.22
  retained placenta
    with curettage 69.02
    manual 75.4
  streptothrix from lacrimal duct 09.42
Evaluation (of)
  audiological 95.43
  cardiac rhythm device (CRT-D) (CRT-P) (AICD)
    (pacemaker)—*see* Interrogation
  criminal responsibility, psychiatric 94.11
  functional (physical therapy) 93.01
  hearing NEC 95.49
  orthotic (for brace fitting) 93.02
  prosthetic (for artificial limb fitting) 93.03
  psychiatric NEC 94.19
    commitment 94.13
  psychologic NEC 94.08
  testimentary capacity, psychiatric 94.11
Evans operation (release of clubfoot) 83.84
Evisceration
  eyeball 16.39
    with implant (into scleral shell) 16.31
  ocular contents 16.39
    with implant (into scleral shell) 16.31
  orbit (*see also* Exenteration, orbit) 16.59
  pelvic (anterior) (posterior) (partial) (total)
    (female) 68.8
    male 57.71
Evulsion
  nail (bed) (fold) 86.23
  skin 86.3
  subcutaneous tissue 86.3
Examination (for)
  breast
    manual 89.36
    radiographic NEC 87.37
    thermographic 88.85
    ultrasonic 88.73
  cervical rib (by x-ray) 87.43
  colostomy stoma (digital) 89.33
  dental (oral mucosa) (peridontal) 89.31
    radiographic NEC 87.12
  enterostomy stoma (digital) 89.33
  eye 95.09
    color vision 95.06
    comprehensive 95.02
    dark adaptation 95.07
    limited (with prescription of spectacles) 95.01
    under anesthesia 95.04
  fetus, intrauterine 75.35
  general physical 89.7
  glaucoma 95.03
  gynecological 89.26
  hearing 95.47

Examination—*continued*
  microscopic (specimen) (of) 91.9

> *Note—Use the following fourth-digit*
> *subclassification with categories 90-91 to*
> *identify type of examination:*
>
> *1 bacterial smear*
> *2 culture*
> *3 culture and sensitivity*
> *4 parasitology*
> *5 toxicology*
> *6 cell block and Papanicolaou smear*
> *9 other microscopic examination*

  adenoid 90.3
  adrenal gland 90.1
  amnion 91.4
  anus 90.9
  appendix 90.9
  bile ducts 91.0
  bladder 91.3
  blood 90.5
  bone 91.5
    marrow 90.6
  brain 90.0
  breast 91.6
  bronchus 90.4
  bursa 91.5
  cartilage 91.5
  cervix 91.4
  chest wall 90.4
  chorion 91.4
  colon 90.9
  cul-de-sac 91.1
  dental 90.8
  diaphragm 90.4
  duodenum 90.8
  ear 90.3
  endocrine gland NEC 90.1
  esophagus 90.8
  eye 90.2
  fallopian tube 91.4
  fascia 91.5
  female genital tract 91.4
  fetus 91.4
  gallbladder 91.0
  hair 91.6
  ileum 90.9
  jejunum 90.9
  joint fluid 91.5
  kidney 91.2
  large intestine 90.9
  larynx 90.3
  ligament 91.5
  liver 91.0
  lung 90.4
  lymph (node) 90.7
  meninges 90.0
  mesentery 91.1
  mouth 90.8
  muscle 91.5
  musculoskeletal system 91.5
  nails 91.6
  nerve 90.0
  nervous system 90.0
  nose 90.3
  omentum 91.1
  operative wound 91.7
  ovary 91.4
  pancreas 91.0

Examination—*continued*
  parathyroid gland 90.1
  penis 91.3
  perirenal tissue 91.2
  peritoneum (fluid) 91.1
  periureteral tissue 91.2
  perivesical (tissue) 91.3
  pharynx 90.3
  pineal gland 90.1
  pituitary gland 90.1
  placenta 91.4
  pleura (fluid) 90.4
  prostate 91.3
  rectum 90.9
  retroperitoneum 91.1
  semen 91.3
  seminal vesicle 91.3
  sigmoid 90.9
  skin 91.6
  small intestine 90.9
  specified site NEC 91.8
  spinal fluid 90.0
  spleen 90.6
  sputum 90.4
  stomach 90.8
  stool 90.9
  synovial membrane 91.5
  tendon 91.5
  thorax NEC 90.4
  throat 90.3
  thymus 90.1
  thyroid gland 90.1
  tonsil 90.3
  trachea 90.4
  ureter 91.2
  urethra 91.3
  urine 91.3
  uterus 91.4
  vagina 91.4
  vas deferens 91.3
  vomitus 90.8
  vulva 91.4
 neurologic 89.13
 neuro-ophthalmology 95.03
 ophthalmoscopic 16.21
 panorex, mandible 87.12
 pelvic (manual) 89.26
   instrumental (by pelvimeter) 88.25
   pelvimetric 88.25
 physical, general 89.7
 postmortem 89.8
 rectum (digital) 89.34
   endoscopic 48.23
     through stoma (artificial) 48.22
     transabdominal 48.21
 retinal disease 95.03
 specified type (manual) NEC 89.39
 thyroid field, postoperative 06.02
 uterus (digital) 68.11
   endoscopic 68.12
 vagina 89.26
   endoscopic 70.21
 visual field 95.05
Exchange transfusion 99.01
 intrauterine 75.2
Excision
 aberrant tissue—*see* Excision, lesion, by site of
   tissue origin
 abscess—*see* Excision, lesion, by site

Excision—*continued*
 accessory tissue—*see also* Excision, lesion, by
   site of tissue origin
   lung 32.29
     endoscopic 32.28
     thoracoscopic 32.20
   spleen 41.93
 adenoids (tag) 28.6
   with tonsillectomy 28.3
 adenoma—*see* Excision, lesion, by site
 adrenal gland (*see also* Adrenalectomy) 07.22
 ampulla of Vater (with reimplantation of
   common duct) 51.62
 anal papilla 49.39
   endoscopic 49.31
 aneurysm (arteriovenous) (*see also*
   Aneurysmectomy) 38.60
   coronary artery 36.91
   heart 37.32
   myocardium 37.32
   sinus of Valsalva 35.39
   ventricle (heart) 37.32
 anus (complete) (partial) 49.6
 aortic subvalvular ring 35.35
 apocrine gland 86.3
 aponeurosis 83.42
   hand 82.33
 appendage, left atrial 37.36
 appendiceal stump 47.01-47.09
 appendices epiploicae 54.4
 appendix (*see also* Appendectomy) 47.01, 47.09
   epididymis 63.3
   testis 62.2
 arcuate ligament (spine)—*omit code*
 arteriovenous fistula (*see also* Aneurysmectomy)
   38.60
 artery (*see also* Arteriectomy) 38.60
 Baker's cyst, knee 83.39
 Bartholin's gland 71.24
 basal ganglion 01.59
 bile duct 51.69
   endoscopic 51.64
 bladder—*see also* Cystectomy
 bleb (emphysematous), lung 32.29
   endoscopic 32.28
   thoracoscopic 32.20
 blood vessel (*see also* Angiectomy) 38.60
 bone (ends) (partial), except facial—*see* category
   77.8
   facial NEC 76.39
     total 76.45
       with reconstruction 76.44
   for graft (autograft) (homograft)—*see* category
     77.7
   fragments (chips) (*see also* Incision, bone)
     77.10
   joint (*see also* Arthrotomy) 80.10
   necrotic (*see also* Sequestrectomy, bone)
     77.00
 heterotopic, from
   muscle 83.32
     hand 82.22
   skin 86.3
   tendon 83.31
     hand 82.21
 mandible 76.31
   with arthrodesis—*see* Arthrodesis
   total 76.42
     with reconstruction 76.41
 spur—*see* Excision, lesion, bone

Excision—*continued*
    total, except facial—*see* category 77.9
      facial NEC 76.45
        with reconstruction 76.44
        mandible 76.42
        with reconstruction 76.41
    brain 01.59
      hemisphere 01.52
      lobe 01.53
    branchial cleft cyst or vestige 29.2
    breast (*see also* Mastectomy) 85.41
      aberrant tissue 85.24
      accessory 85.24
      ectopic 85.24
      nipple 85.25
        accessory 85.24
      segmental 85.23
      supernumerary 85.24
      wedge 85.21
    broad ligament 69.19
    bronchogenic cyst 32.09
      endoscopic 32.01
    bronchus (wide sleeve) NEC 32.1
    buccal mucosa 27.49
    bulbourethral gland 58.92
    bulbous tuberosities (mandible) (maxilla)
      (fibrous) (osseous) 24.31
    bunion (*see also* Bunionectomy) 77.59
    bunionette (with osteotomy) 77.54
    bursa 83.5
      hand 82.31
    canal of Nuck 69.19
    cardioma 37.33
    carotid body (lesion) (partial) (total) 39.89
    cartilage (*see also* Chondrectomy) 80.90
      intervertebral—*see* category 80.5
      knee (semilunar) 80.6
      larynx 30.29
      nasal (submucous) 21.5
    caruncle, urethra 58.39
      endoscopic 58.31
    cataract (*see also* Extraction, cataract) 13.19
      secondary membrane (after cataract) 13.65
    cervical
      rib 77.91
      stump 67.4
    cervix (stump) NEC 67.4
      cold (knife) 67.2
      conization 67.2
      cryoconization 67.33
      electroconization 67.32
    chalazion (multiple) (single) 08.21
    cholesteatoma—*see* Excision, lesion, by site
    choroid plexus 02.14
    cicatrix (skin) 86.3
    cilia base 08.20
    ciliary body, prolapsed 12.98
    clavicle (head) (partial) 77.81
      total (complete) 77.91
    clitoris 71.4
    coarctation of aorta (end-to-end anastomosis)
      38.64
      with
        graft replacement (interposition)
          abdominal 38.44
          thoracic 38.45
          thoracoabdominal 38.45 *[38.44]*

Excision—*continued*
  common
    duct 51.63
    wall between posterior and coronary sinus (with
      roofing of resultant defect with patch graft)
      35.82
  condyle—*see* 77.8
    mandible 76.5
  conjunctival ring 10.31
  cornea 11.49
    epithelium (with chemocauterization) 11.41
      for smear or culture 11.21
  costal cartilage 80.99
  cul-de-sac (Douglas') 70.92
    with graft or prosthesis 70.93
  cusp, heart valve 35.10
    aortic 35.11
    mitral 35.12
    tricuspid 35.14
  cyst—*see also* Excision, lesion, by site
    apical (tooth) 23.73
      with root canal therapy 23.72
    Baker's (popliteal) 83.39
    breast 85.21
    broad ligament 69.19
    bronchogenic 32.09
      endoscopic 32.01
    cervix 67.39
    dental 24.4
    dentigerous 24.4
    epididymis 63.2
    fallopian tube 66.61
    Gartner's duct 70.33
    hand 82.29
    labia 71.3
    lung 32.29
      endoscopic 32.28
      thoracoscopic 32.20
    mesonephric duct 69.19
    Morgagni
      female 66.61
      male 62.2
    mullerian duct 60.73
    nasolabial 27.49
    nasopalatine 27.31
      by wide excision 27.32
    ovary 65.29
      laparoscopic 65.25
    parovarian 69.19
    pericardium 37.31
    periodontal (apical) (lateral) 24.4
    popliteal (Baker's), knee 83.39
    radicular 24.4
    spleen 41.42
    synovial (membrane) 83.39
    thyroglossal (with resection of hyoid bone) 06.7
    urachal (bladder) 57.51
      abdominal wall 54.3
    vagina (Gartner's duct) 70.33
  cystic
    duct remnant 51.61
    hygroma 40.29
  dentinoma 24.4
  diaphragm 34.81
  disc, intervertebral NOS 80.50
    herniated (nucleus pulposus) 80.51
    other specified (diskectomy) 80.51

Excision—*continued*
diverticulum
  ampulla of Vater 51.62
  anus 49.39
    endoscopic 49.31
  bladder 57.59
    transurethral 57.49
  duodenum 45.31
    endoscopic 45.30
  esophagus (local) 42.31
    endoscopic 42.33
  hypopharyngeal (by cricopharyngeal myotomy)
    29.32
  intestine
    large 45.41
      endoscopic 45.43
    small NEC 45.33
  Meckel's 45.33
  pharyngeal (by cricopharyngeal myotomy)
    29.32
  pharyngoesophageal (by cricopharyngeal
    myotomy) 29.32
  stomach 43.42
    endoscopic 43.41
  urethra 58.39
    endoscopic 58.31
  ventricle, heart 37.33
duct
  mullerian 69.19
  paramesonephric 69.19
  thyroglossal (with resection of hyoid bone) 06.7
ear, external (complete) NEC 18.39
  partial 18.29
    radical 18.31
ectopic
  abdominal fetus 74.3
  tissue—*see also* Excision, lesion, by site of
    tissue origin
    bone, from muscle 83.32
    breast 85.24
    lung 32.29
      endoscopic 32.28
      thoracoscopic 32.20
    spleen 41.93
empyema pocket, lung 34.09
epididymis 63.4
epiglottis 30.21
epithelial downgrowth, anterior chamber (eye)
  12.93
epulis (gingiva) 24.31
esophagus (*see also* Esophagectomy) 42.40
exostosis (*see also* Excision, lesion, bone) 77.60
  auditory canal, external 18.29
  facial bone 76.2
  first metatarsal (hallux valgus repair)—*see*
    Bunionectomy
eye 16.49
  with implant (into Tenon's capsule) 16.42
  with attachment of muscles 16.41
eyelid 08.20
  redundant skin 08.86
falciform ligament 54.4
fallopian tube—*see* Salpingectomy
fascia 83.44
  for graft 83.43
  hand 82.34
  hand 82.35
  for graft 82.34
fat pad NEC 86.3
  knee (infrapatellar) (prepatellar) 86.3
  scalene 40.21

Excision—*continued*
fibroadenoma, breast 85.21
fissure, anus 49.39
  endoscopic 49.31
fistula—*see also* Fistulectomy
  anal 49.12
  arteriovenous (*see also* Aneurysmectomy)
    38.60
  ileorectal 46.74
  lacrimal
    gland 09.21
    sac 09.6
  rectal 48.73
  vesicovaginal 57.84
frenulum, frenum
  labial (lip) 27.41
  lingual (tongue) 25.92
ganglion (hand) (tendon sheath) (wrist) 82.21
  gasserian 04.05
  site other than hand or nerve 83.31
  sympathetic nerve 05.29
  trigeminal nerve 04.05
gastrocolic ligament 54.4
gingiva 24.31
glomus jugulare tumor 20.51
goiter—*see* Thyroidectomy
gum 24.31
hamartoma, mammary 85.21
hallux valgus—*see also* Bunionectomy with
  prosthetic implant 77.59
heart assist system—*see* Removal
hematocele, tunica vaginalis 61.92
hematoma—*see* Drainage, by site
hemorrhoids (external) (internal) (tag) 49.46
heterotopic bone, from
  muscle 83.32
    hand 82.22
  skin 86.3
  tendon 83.31
    hand 82.21
hydatid of Morgagni
  female 66.61
  male 62.2
hydatid cyst, liver 50.29
hydrocele
  canal of Nuck (female) 69.19
  male 63.1
  round ligament 69.19
  spermatic cord 63.1
  tunica vaginalis 61.2
hygroma, cystic 40.29
hymen (tag) 70.31
hymeno-urethral fusion 70.31
intervertebral disc—*see* Excision, disc,
  intervertebral (NOS) 80.50
intestine (*see also* Resection, intestine)
  for interposition 45.50
    large 45.52
    small 45.51
  large (total)
    for interposition 45.52
    laparoscopic 45.81
    local 45.41
      endoscopic 45.43
    open 45.82
    other 45.83
    segmental
      laparoscopic 17.39
      multiple
        laparoscopic 17.31
        open and other 45.71

Excision—*continued*
    open and other 45.79
    unspecified 45.83
  small (total) 45.63
    for interposition 45.51
    local 45.33
    partial 45.62
    segmental 45.62
      multiple 45.61
intraductal papilloma 85.21
iris prolapse 12.13
joint (*see also* Arthrectomy) 80.90
keloid (scar), skin 86.3
LAA 37.36
labia—*see* Vulvectomy
lacrimal
  gland 09.20
    partial 09.22
    total 09.23
  passage 09.6
  sac 09.6
left atrial appendage 37.36
lesion (local)
  abdominal wall 54.3
  accessory sinus—*see* Excision, lesion, nasal
    sinus
  adenoids 28.92
  adrenal gland(s) 07.21
  alveolus 24.4
  ampulla of Vater 51.62
  anterior chamber (eye) NEC 12.40
  anus 49.39
    endoscopic 49.31
  apocrine gland 86.3
  artery 38.60
    abdominal 38.66
    aorta (arch) (ascending) (descending thoracic)
      38.64
    with end-to-end anastomosis 38.45
      abdominal 38.44
      thoracic 38.45
      thoracoabdominal 38.45 *[38.44]*
    with interposition graft replacement 38.45
      abdominal 38.44
      thoracic 38.45
      thoracoabdominal 38.45 *[38.44]*
    head and neck NEC 38.62
    intracranial NEC 38.61
    lower limb 38.68
    thoracic NEC 38.65
    upper limb 38.63
  atrium 37.33
  auditory canal or meatus, external 18.29
    radical 18.31
  auricle, ear 18.29
    radical 18.31
  biliary ducts 51.69
    endoscopic 51.64
  bladder (transurethral) 57.49
    open 57.59
    suprapubic 57.59
  blood vessel 38.60
    abdominal
      artery 38.66
      vein 38.67
    aorta (arch) (ascending) (descending) 38.64
    head and neck NEC 38.62
    intracranial NEC 38.61
    lower limb
      artery 38.68
      vein 38.69

Excision—*continued*
    thoracic NEC 38.65
    upper limb (artery) (vein) 38.63
  bone 77.60
    carpal, metacarpal 77.64
    clavicle 77.61
    facial 76.2
    femur 77.65
    fibula 77.67
    humerus 77.62
    jaw 76.2
      dental 24.4
    patella 77.66
    pelvic 77.69
    phalanges (foot) (hand) 77.69
    radius 77.63
    scapula 77.61
    skull 01.6
    specified site NEC 77.69
    tarsal, metatarsal 77.68
    thorax (ribs) (sternum) 77.61
    tibia 77.67
    ulna 77.63
    vertebrae 77.69
  brain (transtemporal approach) NEC 01.59
    by stereotactic radiosurgery 92.30
      cobalt 60 92.32
      linear accelerator (LINAC) 92.31
      multi-source 92.32
      particle beam 92.33
      particulate 92.33
      radiosurgery NEC 92.39
      single source photon 92.31
  breast (segmental) (wedge) 85.21
  broad ligament 69.19
  bronchus NEC 32.09
    endoscopic 32.01
  cerebral (cortex) NEC 01.59
    meninges 01.51
  cervix (myoma) 67.39
  chest wall 34.4
  choroid plexus 02.14
  ciliary body 12.44
  colon 45.41
    endoscopic NEC 45.43
    polypectomy 45.42
  conjunctive 10.31
  cornea 11.49
  cranium 01.6
  cul-de-sac (Douglas) 70.32
  dental (jaw) 24.4
  diaphragm 34.81
  duodenum (local) 45.31
    endoscopic 45.30
  ear, external 18.29
    radical 18.31
  endometrium 68.29
  epicardium 37.31
  epididymis 63.3
  epiglottis 30.09
  esophagus NEC 42.32
    endoscopic 42.33
  eye, eyeball 16.93
    anterior segment NEC 12.40
  eyebrow (skin) 08.20
  eyelid 08.20
    by
      halving procedure 08.24
      wedge resection 08.24

Excision—*continued*
- major
  - full-thickness 08.24
  - partial-thickness 08.23
  - minor 08.22
- fallopian tube 66.61
- fascia 83.39
  - hand 82.29
- groin region (abdominal wall) (inguinal) 54.3
  - skin 86.3
  - subcutaneous tissue 86.3
- gum 24.31
- heart 37.34
  - Cox-maze, open 37.33
  - maze, modified, endovascular 37.34
  - maze, modified, open 37.33
  - open 37.33
  - other approach, closed 37.34
- hepatic duct 51.69
- inguinal canal 54.3
- intestine
  - large 45.41
    - endoscopic NEC 45.43
    - polypectomy 45.42
  - small NEC 45.33
- intracranial NEC 01.59
- intranasal 21.31
- intraspinal 03.4
- iris 12.42
- jaw 76.2
  - dental 24.4
- joint 80.80
  - ankle 80.87
  - elbow 80.82
  - foot and toe 80.88
  - hand and finger 80.84
  - hip 80.85
  - knee 80.86
  - shoulder 80.81
  - specified site NEC 80.89
  - spine 80.89
  - wrist 80.83
- kidney 55.39
  - with partial nephrectomy 55.4
- labia 71.3
- lacrimal
  - gland (frontal approach) 09.21
  - passage 09.6
  - sac 09.6
- larynx 30.09
- ligament (joint) (*see also* Excision, lesion, joint) 80.80
  - broad 69.19
  - round 69.19
  - uterosacral 69.19
- lip 27.43
  - by wide excision 27.42
- liver 50.29
- lung NEC 32.29
  - by wide excision 32.39
    - thoracoscopic 32.30
  - endoscopic 32.28
  - thoracoscopic 32.20
- lymph structure(s) (channel) (vessel) NEC 40.29
  - node—*see* Excision, lymph, node
- mammary duct 85.21
- mastoid (bone) 20.49
- mediastinum 34.3
- meninges (cerebral) 01.51
  - spinal 03.4
- mesentery 54.4

Excision—*continued*
- middle ear 20.51
- mouth NEC 27.49
- muscle 83.32
  - hand 82.22
  - ocular 15.13
- myocardium 37.33
- nail 86.23
- nasal sinus 22.60
  - antrum 22.62
    - with Caldwell-Luc approach 22.61
    - specified approach NEC 22.62
  - ethmoid 22.63
  - frontal 22.42
  - maxillary 22.62
    - with Caldwell-Luc approach 22.61
    - specified approach NEC 22.62
  - sphenoid 22.64
- nasopharynx 29.3
- nerve (cranial) (peripheral) 04.07
  - sympathetic 05.29
- nonodontogenic 24.31
- nose 21.30
  - intranasal 21.31
  - polyp 21.31
  - skin 21.32
  - specified site NEC 21.32
- odontogenic 24.4
- omentum 54.4
- orbit 16.92
- ovary 65.29
  - by wedge resection 65.22
    - laparoscopic 65.24
  - that by laparoscope 65.25
- palate (bony) 27.31
  - by wide excision 27.32
  - soft 27.49
- pancreas (local) 52.22
  - endoscopic 52.21
- parathyroid 06.89
- parotid gland or duct NEC 26.29
- pelvic wall 54.3
- pelvirectal tissue 48.82
- penis 64.2
- pericardium 37.31
- perineum (female) 71.3
  - male 86.3
- periprostatic tissue 60.82
- perirectal tissue 48.82
- perirenal tissue 59.91
- peritoneum 54.4
- perivesical tissue 59.91
- pharynx 29.39
  - diverticulum 29.32
- pineal gland 07.53
- pinna 18.29
  - radical 18.31
- pituitary (gland) (*see also* Hypophysectomy, partial) 07.63
  - by stereotactic radiosurgery 92.30
    - cobalt 60 92.32
    - linear accelerator (LINAC) 92.31
    - multi-source 92.32
    - particle beam 92.33
    - particulate 92.33
    - radiosurgery NEC 92.39
    - single source photon 92.31
- pleura 34.59
- pouch of Douglas 70.32
- preauricular (ear) 18.21
- presacral 54.4
- prostate (transurethral) 60.61

Excision—*continued*
  pulmonary (fibrosis) 32.29
    endoscopic 32.28
    thoracoscopic 32.20
  rectovaginal septum 48.82
  rectum 48.35
    polyp (endoscopic) 48.36
  retroperitoneum 54.4
  salivary gland or duct NEC 26.29
    en bloc 26.32
  sclera 12.84
  scrotum 61.3
  sinus (nasal)—*see* Excision, lesion, nasal sinus
  Skene's gland 71.3
  skin 86.3
    breast 85.21
    nose 21.32
    radical (wide) (involving underlying or
        adjacent structure) (with flap closure)
        86.4
    scrotum 61.3
  skull 01.6
  soft tissue NEC 83.39
    hand 82.29
  spermatic cord 63.3
  sphincter of Oddi 51.62
    endoscopic 51.64
  spinal cord (meninges) 03.4
  spleen (cyst) 41.42
  stomach NEC 43.42
    endoscopic 43.41
      polyp 43.41
    polyp (endoscopic) 43.41
  subcutaneous tissue 86.3
    breast 85.21
  subgingival 24.31
  sweat gland 86.3
  tendon 83.39
    hand 82.29
    ocular 15.13
    sheath 83.31
      hand 82.21
  testis 62.2
  thorax 34.4
  thymus
    partial (open) (other) 07.81
      thoracoscopic 07.83
    total (open) (other) 07.82
      thoracoscopic 07.84
  thyroid 06.31
    substernal or transsternal route 06.51
  tongue 25.1
  tonsil 28.92
  trachea 31.5
  tunica vaginalis 61.92
  ureter 56.41
  urethra 58.39
    endoscopic 58.31
  uterine ligament 69.19
  uterosacral ligament 69.19
  uterus 68.29
  vagina 70.33
  vein 38.60
    abdominal 38.67
    head and neck NEC 38.62
    intracranial NEC 38.61
    lower limb 38.69
    thoracic NEC 38.65
    upper limb 38.63
  ventricle (heart) 37.33
  vocal cords 30.09

Excision—*continued*
  vulva 71.3
  ligament (*see also* Arthrectomy) 80.90
    broad 69.19
    round 69.19
    uterine 69.19
    uterosacral 69.19
  ligamentum flavum (spine)—*omit code*
  lingual tonsil 28.5
  lip 27.43
  liver (partial) 50.22
  loose body
    bone—*see* Sequestrectomy, bone
    joint 80.10
  lung (with mediastinal dissection) 32.59
    accessory or ectopic tissue 32.29
      endoscopic 32.28
      thoracoscopic 32.20
    segmental 32.39
      thoracoscopic 32.30
    specified type NEC 32.29
      endoscopic 32.28
      thoracoscopic 32.20
    thoracoscopic 32.50
    volume reduction surgery 32.22
      biologic lung volume reduction (BLVR)
        —*see* category 33.7
    wedge 32.29
      thoracoscopic 32.20
  lymph, lymphatic
    drainage area 40.29
      radical—*see* Excision, lymph, node, radical
      regional (with lymph node, skin,
          subcutaneous tissue, and fat) 40.3
    node (simple) NEC 40.29
      with
        lymphatic drainage area (including skin,
            subcutaneous tissue, and fat) 40.3
        mastectomy—*see* Mastectomy, radical
        muscle and deep fascia—*see* Excision,
            lymph, node, radical
      axillary 40.23
        radical 40.51
        regional (extended) 40.3
      cervical (deep) (with excision of scalene fat
          pad) 40.21
        with laryngectomy 30.4
        radical (including muscle and deep fascia)
            40.40
          bilateral 40.42
          unilateral 40.41
        regional (extended) 40.3
        superficial 40.29
      groin 40.24
        radical 40.54
        regional (extended) 40.3
      iliac 40.29
        radical 40.53
        regional (extended) 40.3
      inguinal (deep) (superficial) 40.24
        radical 40.54
        regional (extended) 40.3
      jugular—*see* Excision, lymph, node, cervical
      mammary (internal) 40.22
        external 40.29
          radical 40.59
          regional (extended) 40.3
        radical 40.59
        regional (extended) 40.3
      paratracheal—*see* Excision, lymph, node,
          cervical

Excision—*continued*

  periaortic 40.29
    radical 40.52
    regional (extended) 40.3
  radical 40.50
    with mastectomy—*see* Mastectomy, radical
    specified site NEC 40.59
    regional (extended) 40.3
    sternal—*see* Excision, lymph, node,
      mammary
  structure(s) (simple) NEC 40.29
    radical 40.59
    regional (extended) 40.3
  lymphangioma (simple)—*see also* Excision,
    lymph, lymphatic, node 40.29
  lymphocele 40.29
  mastoid (*see also* Mastoidectomy) 20.49
  median bar, transurethral approach 60.29
  meibomian gland 08.20
  meniscus (knee) 80.6
    acromioclavicular 80.91
    jaw 76.5
    sternoclavicular 80.91
    temporomandibular (joint) 76.5
    wrist 80.93
  müllerian duct cyst 60.73
  muscle 83.45
    for graft 83.43
      hand 82.34
    hand 82.36
      for graft 82.34
  myositis ossificans 83.32
    hand 82.22
  nail (bed) (fold) 86.23
  nasolabial cyst 27.49
  nasopalatine cyst 27.31
    by wide excision 27.32
  neoplasm—*see* Excision, lesion, by site
  nerve (cranial) (peripheral) NEC 04.07
    sympathetic 05.29
  neuroma (Morton's) (peripheral nerve) 04.07
    acoustic
      by craniotomy 04.01
      by stereotactic radiosurgery 92.30
        cobalt 60 92.32
        linear accelerator (LINAC) 92.31
        multi-source 92.32
        particle beam 92.33
        particulate 92.33
        radiosurgery NEC 92.39
        single source photon 92.31
    sympathetic nerve 05.29
  nipple 85.25
    accessory 85.24
  odontoma 24.4
  orbital contents (*see also* Exenteration, orbit)
    16.59
  osteochondritis dissecans (*see also* Excision,
    lesion, joint) 80.80
  ovary—*see also* Oophorectomy
    partial 65.29
      by wedge resection 65.22
        laparoscopic 65.24
      that by laparoscope 65.25
  Pancoast tumor (lung) 32.6

Excision—*continued*

  pancreas (total) (with synchronous
    duodenectomy) 52.6
    partial NEC 52.59
      distal (tail) (with part of body) 52.52
      proximal (head) (with pan of body) (with
        synchronous duodenectomy) 52.51
      radical subtotal 52.53
    radical (one-stage) (two-stage) 52.7
    subtotal 52.53
  paramesonephric duct 69.19
  parathyroid gland (partial) (subtotal) NEC (*see*
    also Parathyroidectomy) 06.89
  parotid gland (*see also* Excision, salivary
    gland) 26.30
  parovarian cyst 69.19
  patella (complete) 77.96
    partial 77.86
  pelvirectal tissue 48.82
  perianal tissue 49.04
    skin tags 49.03
  pericardial adhesions 37.31
  periprostatic tissue 60.82
  perirectal tissue 48.82
  perirenal tissue 59.91
  periurethral tissue 58.92
  perivesical tissue 59.91
  petrous apex cells 20.59
  pharyngeal bands 29.54
  pharynx (partial) 29.33
  pilonidal cyst or sinus (open) (with partial
    closure) 86.21
  pineal gland (complete) (total) 07.54
    partial 07.53
  pituitary gland (complete) (total) (*see also*
    Hypophysectomy) 07.69
  pleura NEC 34.59
  polyp—*see also* Excision, lesion, by site
    esophagus 42.32
      endoscopic 42.33
    large intestine 45.41
      endoscopic 45.42
    nose 21.31
    rectum (endoscopic) 48.36
    stomach (endoscopic) 43.41
  preauricular
    appendage (remnant) 18.29
    cyst, fistula, or sinus (congenital) 18.21
    remnant 18.29
  prolapsed iris (in wound) 12.13
  prostate—*see* Prostatectomy
  pterygium (simple) 11.39
    with corneal graft 11.32
  radius (head) (partial) 77.83
    total 77.93
  ranula, salivary gland NEC 26.29
  rectal mucosa 48.35
  rectum—*see* Resection, rectum
  redundant mucosa
    colostomy 45.41
      endoscopic 45.43
    duodenostomy 45.31
      endoscopic 45.30
    ileostomy 45.33
    jejunostomy 45.33
    perineum 71.3
    rectum 48.35
    vulva 71.3

Excision—*continued*
renal vessel, aberrant 38.66
rib (cervical) 77.91
ring of conjunctiva around cornea 10.31
round ligament 69.19
salivary gland 26.30
  complete 26.32
  partial 26.31
  radical 26.32
scalene fat pad 40.21
scar—*see also* Excision, lesion, by site
  epicardium 37.31
  mastoid 20.92
  pericardium 37.31
  pleura 34.59
  skin 86.3
  thorax 34.4
secondary membrane, lens 13.65
seminal vesicle 60.73
  with radical prostatectomy 60.5
septum—*see also* Excision, by site
  uterus (congenital) 68.22
  vagina 70.33
sinus—*see also* Excision, lesion, by site
  nasal—*see* Sinusectomy
  pilonidal 86.21
  preauricular (ear) (radical) 18.21
  tarsi 80.88
  thyroglossal (with resection of hyoid bone) 06.7
  urachal (bladder) 57.51
    abdominal wall 54.3
Skene's gland 71.3
skin (local) 86.3
  for graft (with closure of donor site) 86.91
  radical (wide) (involving underlying or adjacent structure) (with flap closure) 86.4
  tags
    perianal 49.03
    periauricular 18.29
soft tissue NEC 83.49
  hand 82.39
spermatocele 63.2
spinous process 77.89
spleen (total) 41.5
  accessory 41.93
  partial 41.43
stomach—*see* Gastrectomy
sublingual gland (salivary) (*see also* Excision, salivary gland) 26.30
submaxillary Stand (*see also* Excision, salivary gland) 26.30
supernumerary
  breast 85.24
  digits 86.26
sweat gland 86.3
synechiae—*see also* Lysis, synechiae endometrial 68.21
tarsal plate (eyelid) 08.20
  by wedge resection 08.24
tattoo 86.3
  by dermabrasion 86.25
tendon (sheath) 83.42
  for graft 83.41
    hand 82.32
  hand 82.33
    for graft 82.32
thymus (*see also* Thymectomy) 07.80
thyroglossal duct or tract (with resection of hyoid bone) 06.7
thyroid NEC (*see also* Thyroidectomy) 06.39

Excision—*continued*
tongue (complete) (total) 25.3
  partial or subtotal 25.2
  radical 25.4
tonsil 28.2
  with adenoidectomy 28.3
  lingual 28.5
  tag 28.4
tooth NEC (*see also* Removal, tooth, surgical) 23.19
  from nasal sinus 22.60
torus
  lingual 76.2
  mandible, mandibularis 76.2
  palate, palatinus 27.31
    by wide excision 27.32
trabeculae carneae cordis (heart) 35.35
trochanteric lipomatosis 86.83
tumor—*see* Excision, lesion, by site
ulcer—*see also* Excision, lesion, by site
  duodenum 45.31
    endoscopic 45.30
  stomach 43.42
    endoscopic 43.41
umbilicus 54.3
urachus, urachal (cyst) (bladder) 57.51
  abdominal wall 54.3
ureter, ureteral 56.40
  with nephrectomy—*see* Nephrectomy
  partial 56.41
  stricture 56.41
  total 56.42
ureterocele 56.41
urethra, urethral 58.39
  endoscopic 58.31
  with complete cystectomy 57.79
  septum 58.0
  stricture 58.39
    endoscopic 58.31
  valve (congenital) 58.39
    endoscopic (transurethral) (transvesical) 58.31
urethrovaginal septum 70.33
uterus (corpus) (*see also* Hysterectomy) 68.9
  cervix 67.4
    lesion 67.39
  lesion 68.29
  septum 68.22
uvula 27.72
vagina (total) 70.4
varicocele, spermatic cord 63.1
vein (*see also* Phlebectomy) 38.60
  varicose 38.50
    abdominal 38.57
    head and neck NEC 38.52
    intracranial NEC 38.51
    lower limb 38.59
    ovarian 38.67
    thoracic NEC 38.55
    upper limb 38.53
verruca—*see also* Excision, lesion, by site
  eyelid 08.22
vesicovaginal septum 70.33
vitreous opacity 14.74
  anterior approach 14.73
vocal cord(s) (submucous) 30.22
vulva (bilateral) (simple) (*see also* Vulvectomy) 71.62
wart—*see also* Excision, lesion, by site
  eyelid 08.22
wolffian duct 69.19

Excision—*continued*
  xanthoma (tendon sheath, hand) 82.21
    site other than hand 83.31
Excisional biopsy —*see* Biopsy
Exclusion
  LAA 37.36
  laparoscopic 44.38
  left atrial appendage 37.36
    percutaneous 37.36
    TigerPaw™ System 37.36
  pyloric
    laparoscopic 44.38
    open 44.39
Exenteration
  ethmoid air cells 22.63
  orbit 16.59
    with
      removal of adjacent structures 16.51
      temporalis muscle transplant 16.59
      therapeutic removal of bone 16.52
  pelvic (organs) (female) 68.8
    male 57.71
  petrous pyramid air cells 20.59
Exercise (physical therapy) NEC 93.19
  active musculoskeletal NEC 93.12
  assisting 93.11
    in pool 93.31
  breathing 93.18
  musculoskeletal
    active NEC 93.12
    passive NEC 93.17
  neurologic 89.13
  passive musculoskeletal NEC 93.17
  resistive 93.13
Exfoliation, skin, by chemical 86.24
Exostectomy (*see also* Excision, lesion, bone) 77.60
  first metatarsal (hallux valgus repair)—*see*
    Bunionectomy
  hallux valgus repair (with wedge
    osteotomy)—*see* Bunionectomy
Expiratory flow rate 89.38
Explant, explantation —*see* Removal
Exploration —*see* also Incision
  abdomen 54.11
  abdominal wall 54.0
  adrenal (gland) 07.41
    field 07.00
      bilateral 07.02
      unilateral 07.01
  artery 38.00
    abdominal 38.06
    aorta (arch) (ascending) (descending) 38.04
    head and neck NEC 38.02
    intracranial NEC 38.01
    lower limb 38.08
    thoracic NEC 38.05
    upper limb 38.03
  auditory canal, external 18.02
  axilla 86.09
  bile duct(s) 51.59
    common duct 51.51
      endoscopic 51.11
      for relief of obstruction 51.42
        endoscopic 51.84
      for removal of calculus 51.41
        endoscopic 51.88
      laparoscopic 51.11
    for relief of obstruction 51.49
      endoscopic 51.84

Exploration—*continued*
  bladder (by incision) 57.19
    endoscopic 57.32
      through stoma (artificial) 57.31
  bone (*see also* Incision, bone) 77.10
  brain (tissue) 01.39
  breast 85.0
  bronchus 33.0
    endoscopic—*see* Bronchoscopy
  bursa 83.03
    hand 82.03
  carotid body 39.89
  carpal tunnel 04.43
  choroid 14.9
  ciliary body 12.44
  colon 45.03
  common bile duct 51.51
    endoscopic 51.11
    for
      relief of obstruction 51.42
        endoscopic 51.84
      removal of calculus 51.41
        endoscopic 51.88
  coronary artery 36.99
  cranium 01.24
  cul-de-sac 70.12
    endoscopic 70.22
  disc space 03.09
  duodenum 45.01
  endoscopic—*see* Endoscopy, by site
  epididymis 63.92
  esophagus (by incision) NEC 42.09
    endoscopic—*see* Esophagoscopy
  ethmoid sinus 22.51
  eyelid 08.09
  fallopian tube 66.01
  fascia 83.09
    hand 82.09
  flank 54.0
  fossa (superficial) NEC 86.09
    pituitary 07.71
  frontal sinus 22.41
  frontonasal duct 96.21
  gallbladder 51.04
  groin (region) (abdominal wall) (inguinal) 54.0
    skin and subcutaneous tissue 86.09
  heart 37.11
  hepatic duct 51.59
  hypophysis 07.72
  ileum 45.02
  inguinal canal (groin) 54.0
  intestine (by incision) NEC 45.00
    large 45.03
    small 45.02
  intrathoracic 34.02
  jejunum 45.02
  joint structures (*see also* Arthrotomy) 80.10
  kidney 55.01
    pelvis 55.11
  labia 71.09
  lacrimal
    gland 09.0
    sac 09.53
  laparotomy site 54.12
  larynx (by incision) 31.3
    endoscopic 31.42
  liver 50.0
  lung (by incision) 33.1
  lymphatic structure(s) (channel) (node) (vessel)
    40.0
  mastoid 20.21

Exploration—*continued*
  maxillary antrum or sinus (Caldwell-Luc
    approach) 22.39
  mediastinum 34.1
    endoscopic 34.22
  middle ear (transtympanic) 20.23
  muscle 83.02
    hand 82.02
  neck (*see also* Exploration, thyroid) 06.09
  nerve (cranial) (peripheral) NEC 04.04
    auditory 04.01
    root (spinal) 03.09
  nose 21.1
  orbit (*see also* Orbitotomy) 16.09
  pancreas 52.09
    endoscopic 52.13
  pancreatic duct 52.09
    endoscopic 52.13
  pelvis (by laparotomy) 54.11
    by colpotomy 70.12
  penis 64.92
  perinephric area 59.09
  perineum (female) 71.09
    male 86.09
  peripheral vessels
    lower limb
      artery 38.08
      vein 38.09
    upper limb (artery) (vein) 38.03
  periprostatic tissue 60.81
  perirenal tissue 59.09
  perivesical tissue 59.19
  petrous pyramid air cells 20.22
  pilonidal sinus 86.03
  pineal (gland) 07.52
    field 07.51
  pituitary (gland) 07.72
    fossa 07.71
  pleura 34.09
  popliteal space 86.09
  prostate 60.0
  rectum (*see also* Proctoscopy) 48.23
    by incision 48.0
  retroperitoneum 54.0
  retropubic 59.19
  salivary gland 26.0
  sclera (by incision) 12.89
  scrotum 61.0
  shunt
    ventriculoperitoneal at
      peritoneal site 54.95
      ventricular site 02.41
  sinus
    ethmoid 22.51
    frontal 22.41
    maxillary (Caldwell-Luc approach) 22.39
    sphenoid 22.52
    tract, skin and subcutaneous tissue 86.09
  skin 86.09
  soft tissue NEC 83.09
    hand 82.09
  spermatic cord 63.93
  sphenoidal sinus 22.52
  spinal (canal) (nerve rook) 03.09
  spleen 41.2
  stomach (by incision) 43.0
    endoscopic—*see* Gastroscopy
  subcutaneous tissue 86.09
  subdiaphragmatic space 54.11
  superficial fossa 86.09
  tarsal tunnel 04.44

Exploration—*continued*
  tendon (sheath) 83.01
    hand 82.01
  testes 62.0
  thymus (gland) 07.92
    field 07.91
    thoracoscopic 07.95
  thyroid (field) (gland) (by incision) 06.09
    postoperative 06.02
  trachea (by incision) 31.3
    endoscopic—*see* Tracheoscopy
  tunica vaginalis 61.0
  tympanum 20.09
    transtympanic route 20.23
  ureter (by incision) 56.2
    endoscopic 56.31
  urethra (by incision) 58.0
    endoscopic 58.22
  uterus (corpus) 68.0
    cervix 69.95
    digital 68.11
    postpartal, manual 75.7
  vagina (by incision) 70.14
    endoscopic 70.21
  vas deferens 63.6
  vein 38.00
    abdominal 38.07
    head and neck NEC 38.02
    intracranial NEC 38.01
    lower limb 38.09
    thoracic NEC 38.05
    upper limb 38.03
  vulva (by incision) 71.09
Exposure —*see also* Incision, by site
  tooth (for orthodontic treatment) 24.6
Expression, trachoma follicles 10.33
Exsanguination transfusion 99.01
Extension
  buccolabial sulcus 24.91
  limb, forced 93.25
  lingual sulcus 24.91
  mandibular ridge 76.43
Exteriorization
  esophageal pouch 42.12
  intestine 46.03
    large 46.03
    small 46.01
  maxillary sinus 22.9
  pilonidal cyst or sinus (open excision) (with
    partial closure) 86.21
Extirpation —*see also* Excision, by site
  aneurysm—*see* Aneurysmectomy
  arteriovenous fistula—*see* Aneurysmectomy
  lacrimal sac 09.6
  larynx 30.3
    with radical neck dissection (with synchronous
      thyroidectomy) (with synchronous
      tracheostomy) 30.4
  nerve, tooth (*see also* Therapy, root canal) 23.70
  varicose vein (peripheral) (lower limb) 38.59
    upper limb 38.53
Extracorporeal
  circulation (regional), except hepatic 39.61
    hepatic 50.92
    percutaneous 39.66
  hemodialysis 39.95
  membrane oxygenation (ECMO) 39.65
  photopheresis, therapeutic 99.88

Extracorporeal—*continued*
  shock wave lithotripsy (ESWL) NEC 98.59
    bile duct 98.52
    bladder 98.51
    gallbladder 98.52
    kidney 98.51
    renal pelvis 98.51
    specified site NEC 98.59
    ureter 98.51
Extracranial-intracranial bypass [EC-IC]
  39.28
Extraction
  breech (partial) 72.52
    with forceps to aftercoming head 72.51
      total 72.54
        with forceps to aftercoming head 72.53
  cataract 13.19
    after cataract (by)
      capsulectomy 13.65
      capsulotomy 13.64
      discission 13.64
      excision 13.65
      iridocapsulectomy 13.65
      mechanical fragmentation 13.66
      needling 13.64
      phacofragmentation (mechanical) 13.66
    aspiration (simple) (with irrigation) 13.3
    cryoextraction (intracapsular approach) 13.19
      temporal inferior route (in presence of
        fistulization bleb) 13.11
    curette evacuation (extracapsular approach)
      13.2
    emulsification (and aspiration) 13.41
    erysiphake (intracapsular approach) 13.19
      temporal inferior route (in presence of
        fistulization bleb) 13.11
    extracapsular approach (with iridectomy) NEC
      13.59
    by temporal inferior route (in presence of
      fistulization bleb) 13.51
    aspiration (simple) (with irrigation) 13.3
    curette evacuation 13.2
    emulsification (and aspiration) 13.41
    linear extraction 13.2
    mechanical fragmentation with aspiration by
      posterior route 13.42
      specified route NEC 13.43
    phacoemulsification (ultrasonic) (with
      aspiration) 13.41
    phacofragmentation (mechanical)
      with aspiration by
        posterior route 13.42
        specified route NEC 13.43
      ultrasonic (with aspiration) 13.41
    rotoextraction (mechanical) with aspiration
      by
      posterior route 13.42
      specified route NEC 13.43
    intracapsular (combined) (simple) (with
      iridectomy) (with suction) (with
      zonulolysis) 13.19
    by temporal inferior route (in presence of
      fistulization bleb) 13.11
    linear extraction (extracapsular approach) 13.2
    phacoemulsification (and aspiration) 13.41
    phacofragmentation (mechanical)
      with aspiration by
        posterior route 13.42
        specified route NEC 13.43
      ultrasonic 13.41

Extraction—*continued*
  rotoextraction (mechanical)
    with aspiration by
      posterior route 13.42
      specified route NEC 13.43
  secondary membranous (after cataract) (by)
    capsulectomy 13.65
    capsulotomy 13.64
    discission 13.64
    excision 13.65
    iridocapsulectomy 13.65
    mechanical fragmentation 13.66
    needling 13.64
    phacofragmentation (mechanical) 13.66
  common duct stones (percutaneous) (through
    sinus tract) (with basket) 51.96
  fat for grafting or banking 86.90
  foreign body—*see* Removal, foreign body
  kidney stone(s), percutaneous 55.03
    with fragmentation procedure 55.04
  lens (eye) (*see also* Extraction, cataract) 13.19
  Malström's 72.79
    with episiotomy 72.71
  menstrual, menses 69.6
  milk from lactating breast (manual) (pump) 99.98
  tooth (by forceps) (multiple) (single) NEC 23.09
    with mucoperiosteal flap elevation 23.19
    deciduous 23.01
    surgical NEC (*see also* Removal, tooth,
      surgical) 23.19
  vacuum, fetus 72.79
    with episiotomy 72.71
  vitreous (*see also* Removal, vitreous) 14.72

F

Face lift 86.82
Facetectomy 77.89
Facilitation, Intraocular circulation NEC 12.59
Failed (trial) forceps 73.3
Family
    counselling (medical) (social) 94.49
    therapy 94.42
Farabeuf operation (ischiopubiotomy) 77.39
Fasanella-Servatt operation
    (blepharoptosis repair) 08.35
Fasciaplasty —*see* Fascioplasty
Fascia sling operation —*see* Operation, sling
Fasciectomy 83.44
    for graft 83.43
        hand 82.34
    hand 82.35
        for graft 82.34
    palmar (release of Dupuytren's contracture) 82.35
Fasciodesis 83.89
    hand 82.89
Fascioplasty (*see also* Repair, fascia) 83.89
    hand (*see also* Repair, fascia, hand) 82.89
Fasciorrhaphy —*see* Suture, fascia
Fasciotomy 83.14
    Dupuytren's 82.12
        with excision 82.35
    Dwyer 83.14
    hand 82.12
    Ober-Yount 83.14
    orbital (*see also* Orbitotomy) 16.09
    palmar (release of Dupuytren's
        contracture) 82.12
        with excision 82.35
Fenestration
    aneurysm (dissecting), thoracic aorta 39.54
    aortic aneurysm 39.54
    cardiac valve 35.10
    chest wall 34.01
    ear
        inner (with graft) 20.61
            revision 20.62
        tympanic 19.55
    labyrinth (with graft) 20.61
    Lempert's (endaural) 19.9
    operation (aorta) 39.54
    oval window, ear canal 19.55
    palate 27.1
    pericardium 37.12
    semicircular canals (with graft) 20.61
    stapes foot plate (with vein graft) 19.19
        with incus replacement 19.11
    tympanic membrane 19.55
    vestibule (with graft) 20.61
Ferguson operation (hernia repair) 53.00
Fetography 87.81
Fetoscopy 75.31
Fiberoscopy —*see* Endoscopy, by site
Fibroidectomy, uterine 68.29
Fick operation (perforation of foot plate) 19.0
Filipuncture (aneurysm) (cerebral) 39.52
Filleting
    hammer toe 77.56
    pancreas 52.3
Filling, tooth (amalgam) (plastic) (silicate) 23.2
    root canal (*see also* Therapy, root canal) 23.70

Fimbriectomy (*see also* Salpingectomy, partial)
    66.69
    Uchida (with tubal ligation) 66.32
Finney operation (pyloroplasty) 44.29
Fissurectomy, anal 49.39
    endoscopic 49.31
    skin (subcutaneous tissue) 49.04
Fistulectomy —*see also* Closure, fistula, by site
    abdominothoracic 34.83
    abdominouterine 69.42
    anus 49.12
    appendix 47.92
    bile duct 51.79
    biliary tract NEC 51.79
    bladder (transurethral approach) 57.84
    bone (*see also* Excision, lesion, bone) 77.60
    branchial cleft 29.52
    bronchocutaneous 33.42
    bronchoesophageal 33.42
    bronchomediastinal 34.73
    bronchopleural 34.73
    bronchopleurocutaneous 34.73
    bronchopleuromediastinal 34.73
    bronchovisceral 33.42
    cervicosigmoidal 67.62
    cholecystogastroenteric 51.93
    cornea 11.49
    diaphragm 34.83
    enterouterine 69.42
    esophagopleurocutaneous 34.73
    esophagus NEC 42.84
    fallopian tube 66.73
    gallbladder 51.93
    gastric NEC 44.63
    hepatic duct 51.79
    hepatopleural 34.73
    hepatopulmonary 34.73
    intestine
        large 46.76
        small 46.74
    intestinouterine 69.42
    joint (*see also* Excision, lesion, joint) 80.80
    lacrimal
        gland 09.21
        sac 09.6
    laryngotracheal 31.62
    larynx 31.62
    mediastinocutaneous 34.73
    mouth NEC 27.53
    nasal 21.82
        sinus 22.71
    nasolabial 21.82
    nasopharyngeal 21.82
    oroantral 22.71
    oronasal 21.82
    pancreas 52.95
    perineorectal 71.72
    perineosigmoidal 71.72
    perirectal, not opening into rectum 48.93
    pharyngoesophageal 29.53
    pharynx NEC 29.53
    pleura 34.73
    rectolabial 71.72
    rectourethral 58.43
    rectouterine 69.42
    rectovaginal 70.73
    rectovesical 57.83
    rectovulvar 71.72

Fistulectomy—*continued*
rectum 48.73
salivary (duct) (gland) 26.42
scrotum 61.42
skin 86.3
stomach NEC 44.63
subcutaneous tissue 86.3
thoracoabdominal 34.83
thoracogastric 34.83
thoracointestinal 34.83
thorax NEC 34.73
trachea NEC 31.73
tracheoesophageal 31.73
ureter 56.84
urethra 58.43
uteroenteric 69.42
uterointestinal 69.42
uterorectal 69.42
uterovaginal 69.42
vagina 70.75
vesicosigmoidovaginal 57.83
vocal cords 31.62
vulvorectal 71.72
Fistulization
appendix 47.91
arteriovenous 39.27
cisterna chyli 40.62
endolymphatic sac (for decompression) 20.79
esophagus, external 42.10
cervical 42.11
specified technique NEC 42.19
interatrial 35.41
labyrinth (for decompression) 20.79
lacrimal sac into nasal cavity 09.81
larynx 31.29
lymphatic duct, left (thoracic) 40.62
orbit 16.09
peritoneal 54.93
salivary gland 26.49
sclera 12.69
by trephination 12.61
with iridectomy 12.65
sinus, nasal NEC 22.9
subarachnoid space 02.22
thoracic duct 40.62
trachea 31.29
tracheoesophageal 31.95
urethrovaginal 58.0
ventricle, cerebral—*see also* Shunt, ventricular 02.22
Fistulogram
abdominal wall 88.03
chest wall 87.38
retroperitoneum 88.14
specified site NEC 88.49
Fistulotomy, anal 49.11
Fitting
arch bars (orthodontic) 24.7
for immobilization (fracture) 93.55
artificial limb 84.40
contact lens 95.32
denture (total) 99.97
bridge (fixed) 23.42
removable 23.43
partial (fixed) 23.42
removable 23.43
hearing aid 95.48
obturator (orthodontic) 24.7
ocular prosthetics 95.34
orthodontic
appliance 24.7

Fitting—*continued*
obturator 24.7
wiring 24.7
orthotic device 93.23
periodontal splint (orthodontic) 24.7
prosthesis, prosthetic device
above knee 84.45
arm 84.43
lower (and hand) 84.42
upper (and shoulder) 84.41
below knee 84.46
hand (and lower arm) 84.42
leg 84.47
above knee 84.45
below knee 84.46
limb NEC 84.40
ocular 95.34
penis (external) 64.94
shoulder (and upper arm) 84.41
spectacles 95.31
Five-in-one repair, knee 81.42
Fixation
bone
external, without reduction 93.59
with fracture reduction—*see* Reduction, fracture
cast immobilization NEC 93.53
external fixator—*see* Fixator, external
splint 93.54
traction (skeletal) NEC 93.44
intermittent 93.43
internal (without fracture-reduction) 78.50
with fracture-reduction—*see* Reduction, fracture
carpal, metacarpal 78.54
clavicle 78.51
femur 78.55
fibula 78.57
humerus 78.52
patella 78.56
pelvic 78.59
phalanges (foot) (hand) 78.59
radius 78.53
scapula 78.51
specified site NEC 78.59
tarsal, metatarsal 78.58
thorax (ribs) (sternum) 78.51
sternal fixation device with rigid plates 84.94
tibia 78.57
ulna 78.53
vertebrae 78.59
breast (pendulous) 85.6
cardinal ligaments 69.22
cervical collar 93.52
duodenum 46.62
to abdominal wall 46.61
external (without manipulation for reduction) 93.59
with fracture-reduction—*see* Reduction, fracture
cast immobilization NEC 93.53
pressure dressing 93.56
splint 93.54
traction (skeletal) NEC 93.44
intermittent 93.43
strapping (non-traction) 93.59
hip 81.40
ileum 46.62
to abdominal wall 46.61

Fixation—*continued*
internal
  with fracture-reduction—*see* Reduction,
    fracture
  without fracture-reduction—*see* Fixation, bone,
    internal
intestine 46.60
  large 46.64
    to abdominal wall 46.63
  small 46.62
    to abdominal wall 46.61
    to abdominal wall 46.60
iris (bombé) 12.11
jejunum 46.62
  to abdominal wall 46.61
joint—*see* Arthroplasty
kidney 55.7
ligament
  cardinal 69.22
  palpebrae 08.36
omentum 54.74
parametrial 69.22
plaster jacket 93.51
  other cast 93.53
rectum (sling) 48.76
spine, with fusion (*see also* Fusion, spinal) 81.00
spleen 41.95
splint 93.54
tendon 83.88
  hand 82.85
testis in scrotum 62.5
tongue 25.59
urethrovaginal (to Cooper's ligament) 70.77
  with graft or prosthesis 70.78
uterus (abdominal) (vaginal) (ventrofixation)
  69.22
vagina 70.77
  with graft or prosthesis 70.78

Fixator, external
computer assisted (dependent) 84.73
hybrid device or system 84.73
Ilizarov type 84.72
monoplanar system 84.71
ring device or system 84.72
Sheffield type 84.72

Flooding (psychologic desensitization) 94.33
Flowmetry, Doppler (ultrasonic)—*see also*
  Ultrasonography
aortic arch 88.73
head and neck 88.71
heart 88.72
thorax NEC 88.73

Fluoroscopy —*see* Radiography
Fog therapy (respiratory) 93.94
Folding, eye muscle 15.22
multiple (two or more muscles) 15.4
Foley operation (pyeloplasty) 55.87
Fontan operation (creation of conduit between
  right atrium and pulmonary artery) 35.94
Foraminotomy 03.09
Forced extension, limb 93.25
Forceps delivery —*see* Delivery, forceps
Formation
adhesions
  pericardium 36.39
  pleura 34.6
anus, artificial —*see* Colostomy
  duodenostomy 46.39
  ileostomy —*see* Ileostomy
  jejunostomy 46.39
    percutaneous (endoscopic) (PEJ) 46.32

Formation—*continued*
arteriovenous fistula (for kidney dialysis)
  (peripheral) (shunt) 39.27
  external cannula 39.93
bone flap, cranial 02.03
cardiac device (defibrillator) (pacemaker) pocket
  with initial insertion of cardiac device—*omit*
    code
  new site (skin) (subcutaneous) 37.79
colostomy —*see* Colostomy
conduit
  apical-aortic (AAC) 35.93
  ileal (urinary) 56.51
  left ventricle and aorta 35.93
  right atrium and pulmonary artery 35.94
  right ventricle and pulmonary (distal) artery
    35.92
  in repair of
    pulmonary artery atresia 35.92
    transposition of great vessels 35.92
    truncus arteriosus 35.83
endorectal ileal pouch (J-pouch) (H-pouch)
  (S-pouch) (with anastomosis to anus) 45.95
fistula
  arteriovenous (for kidney dialysis) (peripheral)
    shunt) 39.27
    external cannula 39.93
  bladder to skin NEC 57.18
    with bladder flap 57.21
    percutaneous 57.17
  cutaneoperitoneal 54.93
  gastric 43.19
    percutaneous (endoscopic)
      (transabdominal) 43.11
  mucous —*see* Colostomy
  rectovaginal 48.99
  tracheoesophageal 31.95
  tubulovalvular (Beck-Jianu) (Frank's)
    (Janeway) (Spivack's) (Ssabanejew-Frank)
    43.19
  urethrovaginal 58.0
ileal
  bladder
    closed 57.87 *[45.51]*
    open 56.51
  conduit 56.51
interatrial fistula 35.42
mucous fistula —*see* Colostomy
pericardial
  baffle, interatrial 35.91
  window 37.12
pleural window (for drainage) 34.09
pocket
  cardiac device (defibrillator) (pacemaker)
    with initial insertion of cardiac device—*omit*
      code
    new site (skin) (subcutaneous) 37.79
  loop recorder 37.79
  thalamic stimulator pulse generator
    with initial insertion of battery package—*omit*
      code
    new site (skin) (subcutaneous) 86.09
pupil 12.39
  by iridectomy 12.14
rectovaginal fistula 48.99
reversed gastric tube (intrathoracic) (retrosternal)
  42.58
  antesternal or antethoracic 42.68
septal defect, interatrial 35.42
shunt
  abdominovenous 54.94
  arteriovenous 39.93

Formation—*continued*
  peritoneojugular 54.94
  peritoneo-vascular 54.94
  pleuroperitoneal 34.05
  transjugular intrahepatic portosystemic (TIPS) 39.1
  subcutaneous tunnel
    esophageal 42.86
      with anastomosis—*see* Anastomosis, esophagus, antesternal
    pulse generator lead wire 86.99
      with initial procedure—*omit code*
    thalamic stimulator pulse generator pocket
      with insertion of battery package—*omit code*
    new site (skin) (subcutaneous) 86.09
  syndactyly (finger) (toe) 86.89
  tracheoesophageal 31.95
  tubulovalvular fistula (Beck-Jianu) (Frank's) (Janeway) (Spivack's) (Ssabanejew-Frank) 43.19
  uretero-ileostomy, cutaneous 56.51
  ureterostomy, cutaneous 56.61
    ileal 56.51
  urethrovaginal fistula 58.0
  window
    pericardial 37.12
    pleural (for drainage) 34.09
      thoracoscopic 34.06
Fothergill (Donald) operation (uterine suspension) 69.22
Fowler operation
  arthroplasty of metacarpophalangeal joint 81.72
  release (mallet ringer repair) 82.84
  tenodesis (hand) 82.85
  thoracoplasty 33.34
Fox operation (entropion repair with wedge resection) 08.43
Fracture, surgical (*see also* Osteoclasis) 78.70
  turbinates (nasal) 21.62
Fragmentation
  lithotriptor—*see* Lithotripsy
  mechanical
    cataract (with aspiration) 13.43
      posterior route 13.42
      secondary membrane 13.66
    secondary membrane (after cataract) 13.66
  ultrasonic
    cataract (with aspiration) 13.41
    stones, urinary (Kock pouch) 59.95
    percutaneous nephrostomy 55.04
Franco operation (suprapubic cystotomy) 57.18
Frank operation 43.19
Frazier (Spiller) operation (subtemporal trigeminal rhizotomy) 04.02
Fredet-Ramstedt operation (pyloromyotomy) (with wedge resection) 43.3
Freeing
  adhesions—*see* Lysis, adhesions
  anterior synechiae (with injection of air or liquid) 12.32
  artery-vein-nerve bundle 39.91
  extraocular muscle, entrapped 15.7
  goniosynechiae (with injection of air or liquid) 12.31
  intestinal segment for interposition 45.50
    large 45.52
    small 45.51
  posterior synechiae 12.33
  synechiae (posterior) 12.33
    anterior (with injection of air or liquid) 12.32
  vascular bundle 39.91
  vessel 39.91

Freezing
  gastric 96.32
  prostate 60.62
Frenckner operation (intrapetrosal drainage) 20.22
Frenectomy
  labial 27.41
  lingual 25.92
  lip 27.41
  maxillary 27.41
  tongue 25.92
Frenotomy
  labial 27.91
  lingual 25.91
Frenulumectomy —*see* Frenectomy
Frickman operation (abdominal proctopexy) 48.75
Frommel operation (shortening of uterosacral ligaments) 69.22
Fulguration —*see also* Electrocoagulation *and* Destruction, lesion, by site
  adenoid fossa 28.7
  anus 49.39
    endoscopic 49.31
  bladder (transurethral) 57.49
    suprapubic 57.59
  choroid 14.21
  duodenum 45.32
    endoscopic 45.30
  esophagus 42.39
    endoscopic 42.33
  large intestine 45.49
    endoscopic 45.43
      polypectomy 45.42
  penis 64.2
  perineum, female 71.3
  prostate, transurethral 60.29
  rectum 48.32
    radical 48.31
  retina 14.21
  scrotum 61.3
  Skene's gland 71.3
  skin 86.3
  small intestine NEC 45.34
    duodenum 45.32
      endoscopic 45.30
  stomach 43.49
    endoscopic 43.41
  subcutaneous tissue 86.3
  tonsillar fossa 28.7
  urethra 58.39
    endoscopic 58.31
  vulva 71.3
Function
  study—*see also* Scan, radioisotope
    gastric 89.39
    muscle 93.08
      ocular 95.25
    nasal 89.12
    pulmonary—*see* categories 89.37-89.38
    renal 92.03
    thyroid 92.01
    urethral sphincter 89.23
Fundectomy, uterine 68.39
Fundoplication (esophageal) (Nissen's) 44.66
  laparoscopic 44.67
Fundusectomy, gastric 43.89

Fusion
  atlas-axis (spine) —*see* Fusion, spinal, atlas-axis
  bone (*see also* Osteoplasty) 78.40
  cervical (spine) (C2 level or below) —*see* Fusion,
    spinal, cervical
  claw toe 77.57
  craniocervical —*see* Fusion, spinal,
    craniocervical
  dorsal, dorsolumbar —*see* Fusion, spinal, dorsal,
    dorsolumbar
  epiphyseal-diaphyseal (*see also* Arrest, bone
    growth) 78.20
  epiphysiodesis (*see also* Arrest, bone growth)
    78.20
  hammer toe 77.56
  joint (with bone graft) (*see also* Arthrodesis)
    81.20
    ankle 81.11
    claw toe 77.57
    foot NEC 81.17
    hammer toe 77.56
    hip 81.21
    interphalangeal, finger 81.28
    ischiofemoral 81.21
    metatarsophalangeal 81.16
    midtarsal 81.14
    overlapping toe(s) 77.58
    pantalar 81.11
    spinal (*see also* Fusion, spinal) 81.00
    subtalar 81.13
    tarsal joints NEC 81.17
    tarsometatarsal 81.15
    tibiotalar 81.11
    toe NEC 77.58
      claw toe 77.57
      hammer toe 77.56
      overlapping toe(s) 77.58
  lip to tongue 25.59
  lumbar, lumbosacral —*see* Fusion, spinal,
    lumbar, lumbosacral
  occiput-C2 (spinal)—*see* Fusion, spinal, occiput
  spinal, NOS (with graft) (with internal fixation)
    (with instrumentation) 81.00
    anterior lumbar interbody fusion (ALIF) 81.06
    atlas-axis (anterior) (transoral) (posterior) 81.01
      for pseudarthrosis 81.31
    axial lumbar interbody fusion [AxiaLIF] 81.08
    cervical (C2 level or below) NEC 81.02
      anterior column (interbody) anterolateral
        (anterior) technique 81.02
        for pseudarthrosis 81.32
      C1-C2 level (anterior) (posterior) 81.01
        for pseudarthrosis 81.31
      for pseudarthrosis 81.32
      posterior column, posterolateral (posterior)
        technique 81.03
        for pseudarthrosis 81.33
    craniocervical (anterior transoral) (posterior)
      81.01
      for pseudarthrosis NEC 81.31
    direct lateral interbody fusion [DLIF] 81.06
    dorsal, dorsolumbar NEC 81.05
      anterior column (interbody) anterolateral
        (anterior) (extracavitary) technique 81.04
        for pseudarthrosis 81.34
        for pseudarthrosis 81.35
      posterior column, posterolateral (posterior)
        technique 81.05
        for pseudarthrosis 81.35
    extreme lateral interbody fusion [XLIF] 81.06
    facet 81.07

Fusion—*continued*
  lumbar, lumbosacral NEC 81.08
    anterior column (interbody)
      anterolateral (anterior) technique 81.06
      for pseudarthrosis 81.36
      posterior technique 81.08
        for pseudarthrosis 81.38
    lateral transverse process technique 81.07
      for pseudarthrosis 81.37
    posterior column, posterior (posterolateral)
      (transverse process) technique 81.07
    number of vertebrae —*see* codes 81.62-81.64
    occiput-C2 (anterior) (transoral) (posterior)
      81.01
      for pseudarthrosis 81.31

> *Note: Also use either 81.62, 81.63 or 81.64 as*
> *an additional code to show the total number of*
> *vertebrae fused*

    posterior lumbar interbody fusion (PLIF) 81.08
    transforaminal lumbar interbody fusion (TLIF)
      81.08
  tongue (to lip) 25.59

G

Gait training 93.22
Galeaplasty 86.89
Galvanoionization 99.27
Games
  competitive 94.39
  organized 93.89
Gamma irradiation, stereotactic 92.32
Ganglionectomy
  gasserian 04.05
  lumbar sympathetic 05.23
  nerve (cranial) (peripheral) NEC 04.06
    sympathetic 05.29
  sphenopalatine (Meckel's) 05.21
  tendon sheath (wrist) 82.21
    site other than hand 83.31
  trigeminal 04.05
Ganglionotomy, trigeminal (radio frequency)
  04.02
Gant operation (wedge osteotomy of trochanter)
  77.25
Garceau operation (tibial tendon transfer) 83.75
Gardner operation (spinal meningocele repair)
  03.51
Gas endarterectomy 38.10
  abdominal 38.16
  aorta (arch) (ascending) (descending) 38.14
  coronary artery 36.09
  head and neck NEC 38.12
  intracranial NEC 38.11
  lower limb 38.18
  thoracic NEC 38.15
  upper limb 38.13
Gastrectomy (partial) (sleeve) (subtotal) NEC
  43.89
  with
    anastomosis (to) NEC 43.89
      duodenum 43.6
      esophagus 43.5
      gastrogastric 43.89
      jejunum 43.7
    esophagogastrostomy 43.5
    gastroduodenostomy (bypass) 43.6
    gastroenterostomy (bypass) 43.7
    gastrogastrostomy (bypass) 43.89
    gastrojejunostomy (bypass) 43.7
    jejunal transposition 43.81
  complete NEC 43.99
    with intestinal interposition 43.91
  distal 43.6
  Hofmeister 43.7
  laparoscopic, vertical (sleeve) 43.82
  Polya 43.7
  proximal 43.5
  radical NEC 43.99
    with intestinal interposition 43.91
  sleeve
    laparoscopic 43.82
  total NEC 43.99
    with intestinal interposition 43.91
Gastrocamera 44.19
Gastroduodenectomy —*see* Gastrectomy
Gastroduodenoscopy 45.13
  through stoma (artificial) 45.12
  transabdominal (operative) 45.11
Gastroduodenostomy (bypass) (Jaboulay's)
  44.39
  laparoscopic 44.38
  with partial gastrectomy 43.6

Gastroenterostomy (bypass) NEC 44.39
  laparoscopic 44.38
  with partial gastrectomy 43.7
Gastrogastrostomy (bypass) 44.39
  laparoscopic 44.38
  with partial gastrectomy 43.89
Gastrojejunostomy (bypass) 44.39
  with partial gastrectomy 43.7
  laparoscopic 44.38
  percutaneous (endoscopic)
    for bypass 44.32
    for feeding tube placement 46.32
Gastrolysis 54.59
  laparoscopic 54.51
Gastropexy 44.64
Gastroplasty NEC 44.69
  laparoscopic 44.68
  vertical banded gastroplasty (VGB) 44.68
Gastroplication 44.69
  laparoscopic 44.68
Gastropylorectomy 43.6
Gastrorrhaphy 44.61
Gastroscopy NEC 44.13
  through stoma (artificial) 44.12
  transabdominal (operative) 44.11
Gastrostomy (Brunschwig's) (decompression)
  (fine caliber tube) (Kader) (permanent)
  (Stamm) (Stamm-Kader) (temporary) (tube)
  (Witzel) 43.19
  Beck-Jianu 43.19
  Frank's 43.19
  Janeway 43.19
  percutaneous (endoscopic) (PEG) 43.11
  Spivack's 43.19
  Ssabanejew-Frank 43.19
Gastrotomy 43.0
  for control of hemorrhage 44.49
Gavage, gastric 96.35
Gelman operation (release of clubfoot) 83.84
Genioplasty (augmentation) (with graft) (with
  implant) 76.68
  reduction 76.67
Ghormley operation (hip fusion) 81.21
Gifford operation
  destruction of lacrimal sac 09.6
  keratotomy (delimiting) 11.1
    radial (refractive) 11.75
Gill operation
  arthrodesis of shoulder 81.23
  laminectomy 03.09
Gill-Stein operation (carporadial arthrodesis)
  81.25
Gilliam operation (uterine suspension) 69.22
Gingivectomy 24.31
Gingivoplasty (with bone graft) (with soft tissue
  graft) 24.2
Girdlestone operation
  laminectomy with spinal fusion 81.00
  muscle transfer for claw toe repair 77.57
  resection of femoral head and neck (without
    insertion of joint prosthesis) 77.85
    with replacement prosthesis—*see* Implant,
      joint, hip
  resection of hip prosthesis 80.05
    with replacement prosthesis—*see* Implant,
      joint, hip
Girdlestone-Taylor operation (muscle transfer
  for claw toe repair) 77.57

Glenn operation (anastomosis of superior vena
   cava to right pulmonary artery) 39.21
Glenoplasty, shoulder 81.83
  with
    partial replacement 81.81
    total replacement, NEC 81.80
     other 81.80
     reverse 81.88
    for recurrent dislocation 81.82
Glomectomy
  carotid 39.89
  jugulare 20.51
Glossectomy (complete) (total) 25.3
  partial or subtotal 25.2
  radical 25.4
Glossopexy 25.59
Glossoplasty NEC 25.59
Glossorrhaphy 25.51
Glossotomy NEC 25.94
  for tongue tic 25.91
Glycoprotein IIB/IIIa inhibitor 99.20
Goebel-Frangenheim-Stoeckel operation
  (urethrovesical suspension) 59.4
Goldner operation (clubfoot release) 80.48
Goldthwaite operation
  ankle stabilization 81.11
  patellar stabilization 81.44
  tendon transfer for stabilization of patella 81.44
Gonadectomy
  ovary
    bilateral 65.51
     laparoscopic 65.53
    unilateral 65.39
     laparoscopic 65.31
  testis 62.3
Goniopuncture 12.51
  with goniotomy 12.53
Gonioscopy 12.29
Goniopasis 12.59
Goniotomy (Barkan's) 12.52
  with goniopuncture 12.53
Goodal-Power operation (vagina) 70.8
Gordon-Taylor operation (hindquarter
  amputation) 84.19
GP IIB/IIIa inhibitor, infusion 99.20
Graber-Duvernay operation (drilling of femoral
  head) 77.15
Graft, grafting
  aneurysm 39.52
    endovascular
     abdominal aorta 39.71
      fenestrated (branching) graft 39.78
     lower extremity artery(s) 39.79
     thoracic aorta 39.73
     upper extremity artery(s) 39.79
  artery, arterial (patch) 39.58
    with
     excision or resection of vessel—*see*
      Arteriectomy, with graft replacement
     synthetic patch (Dacron) (Teflon) 39.57
     tissue patch (vein) (autogenous) (homograft)
      39.56
  blood vessel (patch) 39.58
    with
     excision or resection of vessel—*see*
      Angiectomy, with graft replacement
     synthetic patch (Dacron) (Teflon) 39.57
     tissue patch (vein) (autogenous) (homograft)
      39.56

Graft, grafting—*continued*
  bone (autogenous) (bone bank) (dual onlay)
    (heterogenous) (inlay) (massive onlay)
    (multiple) (osteoperiosteal) (peg)
    (subperiosteal) (with metallic fixation) 78.00
    with
     arthrodesis—*see* Arthrodesis
     arthroplasty—*see* Arthroplasty
     gingivoplasty 24.2
     lengthening—*see* Lengthening, bone
    carpals, metacarpals 78.04
    clavicle 78.01
    facial NEC 76.91
     with total ostectomy 76.44
    femur 78.05
    fibula 78.07
    humerus 78.02
    joint—*see* Arthroplasty
     mandible 76.91
    with total mandibulectomy 76.41
    marrow—*see* Transplant, bone, marrow
    nose—*see* Graft, nose
    patella 78.06
    pelvic 78.09
    pericranial 02.04
    phalanges (foot) (hand) 78.09
    radius 78.03
    scapula 78.01
    skull 02.04
    specified site NEC 78.09
    spine 78.09
     with fusion—*see* Fusion, spinal
    tarsal, metatarsal 78.08
    thorax (ribs) (sternum) 78.01
    thumb (with transfer of skin nap) 82.69
    tibia 78.07
    ulna 78.03
    vertebrae 78.09
     with fusion—*see* Fusion, spinal
  breast (*see also* Mammoplasty) 85.89
    fat graft 85.55
  buccal sulcus 27.99
  cartilage (joint)—*see also* Arthroplasty
    nose—*see* Graft, nose
  chest wall (mesh) (silastic) 34.79
  conjunctiva (free) (mucosa) 10.44
    for symblepharon repair 10.41
  cornea (*see also* Keratoplasty) 11.60
  dermal-fat 86.69
  dermal regenerative 86.67
  dura 02.12
  ear
    auricle 18.79
    external auditory meatus 18.6
    inner 20.61
    pedicle preparation 86.71
  esophagus NEC 42.87
    with interposition (intrathoracic) NEC 42.58
     antesternal or antethoracic NEC 42.68
     colon (intrathoracic) 42.55
      antesternal or antethoracic 42.65
     small bowel (intrathoracic) 42.53
      antesternal or antethoracic 42.63
  eyebrow (*see also* Reconstruction, eyelid, with
    graft) 08.69
  eyelid (*see also* Reconstruction, eyelid, with
    graft) 08.69
    free mucous membrane 08.62
  eye socket (skin) (cartilage) (bone) 16.63
  fallopian tube 66.79

Graft, grafting—*continued*
  fascia 83.82
    with hernia repair—*see* Repair, hernia
    eyelid 08.32
    hand 82.72
    tarsal cartilage 08.69
  fat pad NEC 86.89
    with skin graft—*see* Graft, skin, full-thickness
  flap (advanced) (rotating) (sliding)—*see also*
    Graft, skin, pedicle
    tarsoconjunctival 08.64
  hair-bearing skin 86.64
  hand
    fascia 82.72
    free skin 86.62
    muscle 82.72
    pedicle (flap) 86.73
    tendon 82.79
  heart, for revascularization—*see* category 36.3
  joint—*see* Arthroplasty
  larynx 31.69
  lip 27.56
    full-thickness 27.55
  lymphatic structure(s) (channel) (node) (vessel)
    40.9
  mediastinal fat to myocardium 36.39
  meninges (cerebral) 02.12
  mouth, except palate 27.56
    full-thickness 27.55
  muscle 83.82
    hand 82.72
  myocardium, for revascularization 36.39
  nasolabial flaps 21.86
  nerve (cranial) (peripheral) 04.5
  nipple 85.86
  nose 21.89
    with
      augmentation 21.85
      rhinoplasty—*see* Rhinoplasty
      total reconstruction 21.83
    septum 21.88
    tip 21.86
  omentum 54.74
    to myocardium 36.39
  orbit (bone) (cartilage) (skin) 16.63
  outflow tract (patch) (pulmonary valve) 35.26
    in total repair of tetralogy of Fallot 35.81
  ovary 65.92
  palate 27.69
    for cleft palate repair 27.62
  pedicle—*see* Graft, skin, pedicle
  penis (rib) (skin) 64.49
  pigskin 86.65
  pinch—*see* Graft, skin, free
  pocket—*see* Graft, skin, pedicle
  porcine 86.65
  postauricular (Wolff) 18.79
  razor—*see* Graft, skin, free
  rope—*see* Graft, skin, pedicle
  saphenous vein in aortocoronary bypass—*see*
    Bypass, aortocoronary
  scrotum 61.49
  skin (partial-thickness) (split-thickness) 86.69
    amniotic membrane 86.66
    auditory meatus (ear) 18.6
    dermal-fat 86.69
      for breast augmentation 85.50
    dermal regenerative 86.67
    ear
      auditory meatus 18.6
      postauricular 18.79
    eyelid 08.61

Graft, grafting—*continued*
  fat 86.87
  flap—*see* Graft, skin, pedicle
  free (autogenous) NEC 86.60
    breast
      deep inferior epigastric artery perforator
        (DIEP) flap, free 85.74
      gluteal artery perforator [GAP] flap, free
        85.76
      superficial inferior epigastric artery (SIEA)
        flap, free 85.75
      transverse rectus abdominis
        musculocutaneous (TRAM) flap, free
        85.73
    lip 27.56
    thumb 86.62
      for
        pollicization 82.61
        reconstruction 82.69
  full-thickness 86.63
    breast 85.83
    hand 86.61
  hair-bearing 86.64
    eyelid or eyebrow 08.63
  hand 86.62
    full-thickness 86.61
  heterograft 86.65
  homograft 86.66
  island flap 86.70
  mucous membrane 86.69
    eyelid 08.62
  nose—*see* Graft, nose
  pedicle (flap) (tube) 86.70
    advancement 86.72
    attachment to site (advanced) (double)
      (rotating) (sliding) 86.74
      hand (cross finger) (pocket) 86.73
      lip 27.57
      mouth 27.57
      thumb 86.73
        for
          pollicization 82.61
          reconstruction NEC 82.69
    breast 85.84
      deep inferior epigastric artery perforator
        (DIEP) flap, free 85.74
      gluteal artery perforator (GAP) flap, free
        85.76
      latissimus dorsi myocutaneous flap 85.71
      superficial inferior epigastric artery (SIEA)
        flap, free 85.75
      transverse rectus abdominis musculo-
        cutaneous (TRAM) flap, free 85.73
      transverse rectus abdominis myocutaneous
        (TRAM) flap, pedicled 85.72
    defatting 86.75
    delayed 86.71
    design and raising 86.71
    elevation 86.71
    preparation of (cutting) 86.71
    revision 86.75
    sculpturing 86.71
    transection 86.71
    transfer 86.74
    trimming 86.71
  postauricular 18.79
  rotation flap 86.70
  specified site NEC 86.69
    full-thickness 86.63

Graft, grafting—*continued*
  tarsal cartilage 08.69
  temporalis muscle to orbit 16.63
    with exenteration of orbit 16.59
  tendon 83.81
    for joint repair—*see* Arthroplasty
    hand 82.79
  testicle 62.69
  thumb (for reconstruction) NEC 82.69
  tongue (mucosal) (skin) 25.59
  trachea 31.79
  tubular (tube)—*see* Graft, skin, pedicle
  tunnel—*see* Graft, skin, pedicle
  tympanum (*see also* Tympanoplasty) 19.4
  ureter 56.89
  vagina
    biological 70.94
    synthetic 70.95
  vein (patch) 39.58
    with
      excision or resection of vessel—*see*
        Phlebectomy, with graft replacement
      synthetic patch (Dacron) (Teflon) 39.57
      tissue patch (vein) (autogenous) (homograft)
        39.56
  vermilion border (lip) 27.56
Grattage, conjunctive 10.31
Green operation (scapulopexy) 78.41
Grice operation (subtalar arthrodesis) 81.13
Grip, strength 93.04
Gritti-Stokes operation (knee disarticulation)
  84.16
Gross operation (herniorrhaphy)
  laparoscopic 53.43
    with graft or prosthesis 53.42
  other and open with graft or prosthesis 53.41
  other open 53.49
Group therapy 94.44
Guttering, bone (*see also* Excision, lesion, bone)
  77.60
Guyon operation (amputation of ankle) 84.13

H

Hagner operation (epididymotomy) 63.92
Halsted operation —*see* Repair, hernia, inguinal
Hampton operation (anastomosis small intestine
  to rectal stump) 45.92
Hanging hip operation (muscle release) 83.19
Harelip operation 27.54
Harrison-Richardson operation (vaginal
  suspension) 70.77
  with graft or prosthesis 70.78
Hartmann resection (of intestine) (with
  pouch)—*see* Colectomy, by site
Harvesting
  bone marrow 41.91
  fat for grafting or banking 86.90
  stem cells 99.79
Hauser operation
  achillotenotomy 83.11
  bunionectomy with adductor tendon transfer
    77.53
  stabilization of patella 81.44
Heaney operation (vaginal hysterectomy) 68.59
  laparoscopically assisted (LAVH) 68.51
Hearing aid (with battery replacement) 95.49
Hearing test 95.47
HeartMate® implantable heart assist system
  37.66
HeartMate® II left ventricular assist system
  [LVAS] 37.66
Hegar operation (perineorrhaphy) 71.79
Heine operation (cyclodialysis) 12.55
Heineke-Mikulicz operation (pyloroplasty)
  44.29
Heller operation (esophagomyotomy) 42.7
Hellstöm operation (transplantation of aberrant
  renal vessel) 39.55
Hemicolectomy
  left
    laparoscopic 17.35
    open and other 45.75
  right (extended)
    laparoscopic 17.33
    open and other 45.73
Hemicystectomy 57.6
Hemigastrectomy —*see* Gastrectomy
Hemiglossectomy 25.2
Hemilaminectomy (decompression)
  (exploration) 03.09
Hemilaryngectomy (anterior) (lateral) (vertical)
  30.1
Hemimandibulectomy 76.31
Hemimastectomy (radical) 85.23
Hemimaxillectomy (with bone graft) (with
  prosthesis) 76.39
Heminephrectomy 55.4
Hemipelvectomy 84.19
Hemispherectomy (cerebral) 01.52
Hemithyroidectomy (with removal of isthmus)
  (with removal of portion of remaining lobe)
  06.2
Hemodiafiltration (extracorporeal) 39.95
Hemodialysis (extracorporeal) 39.95
Hemodilution 99.03
Hemofiltration (extracorporeal) 39.95
Hemorrhage control —*see* Control, hemorrhage

Hemorrhoidectomy 49.46
  by
    cautery, cauterization 49.43
    crushing 49.45
    cryotherapy, cryosurgery 49.44
    excision 49.46
    injection 49.42
    ligation 49.45
Hemostasis —*see* Control, hemorrhage
Henley operation (jejunal transposition) 43.81
Hepatectomy (complete) (total) 50.4
  partial or subtotal 50.22
Hepatic assistance, extracorporeal 50.92
Hepaticocholangiojejunostomy 51.37
Hepaticocystoduodenostomy 51.37
Hepaticodochotomy 51.59
Hepaticoduodenostomy 51.37
Hepaticojejunostomy 51.37
Hepaticolithectomy 51.49
  endoscopic 51.88
Hepaticolithotomy 51.49
  endoscopic 51.88
Hepaticostomy 51.59
Hepaticotomy 51.59
Hepatocholangiocystoduodenostomy 51.37
Hepatocholedochostomy 51.43
  endoscopic 51.87
Hepatoduodenostomy 50.69
Hepatogastrostomy 50.69
Hepatojejunostomy 50.69
Hepatolithotomy
  hepatic duct 51.49
  liver 50.0
Hepatopexy 50.69
Hepatorrhaphy 50.61
Hepatostomy (external) (internal) 50.69
Hepatotomy (with packing) 50.0
Hernioplasty —*see* Repair, hernia
Herniorrhaphy —*see* Repair, hernia
Herniotomy —*see* Repair, hernia
Heterograft —*see* Graft
Heterotransplant, heterotransplantation
  —*see* Transplant
Hey operation (amputation of foot) 84.12
Hey-Groves operation (reconstruction of
  anterior cruciate ligament) 81.45
Heyman operation (soft tissue release for
  clubfoot) 83.84
Heyman-Herndon (Strong) operation (correction
  of metatarsus varus) 80.48
Hibbs operation (lumbar spinal fusion)—*see*
  Fusion, lumbar
Higgins operation —*see* Repair, hernia, femoral
High forceps delivery 72.39
  with episiotomy 72.31
Hill-Allison operation (hiatal hernia repair,
  transpleural approach) 53.80
Hinging, mitral valve 35.12
His bundle recording 37.29
Hitchcock operation (anchoring tendon of
  biceps) 83.88
Hofmeister operation (gastrectomy) 43.7
Hoke operation
  midtarsal fusion 81.14
  triple arthrodesis 81.12

Holth operation
  iridencleisis 12.63
  sclerectomy 12.65
Homan operation (correction of lymphedema)
  40.9
Homograft —*see* Graft
Homotransplant, homotransplantation —*see*
  Transplant
Hosiery, elastic 93.59
Hutch operation (ureteroneocystostomy) 56.74
Hybinette-Eden operation (glenoid bone block)
  78.01
Hydrocelectomy
  canal of Nuck (female) 69.19
    male 63.1
  round ligament 69.19
  spermatic cord 63.1
  tunica vaginalis 61.2
Hydrotherapy 93.33
  assisted exercise in pool 93.31
  whirlpool 93.32
Hymenectomy 70.31
Hymenoplasty 70.76
Hymenorrhaphy 70.76
Hymenotomy 70.11
Hyperalimentation 99.15
Hyperbaric oxygenation 93.95
  wound 93.59
Hyperextension, joint 93.25
Hyperthermia NEC 93.35
  for cancer treatment (interstitial) (local)
    (radiofrequency) (regional) (ultrasound)
    (whole-body) 99.85
Hypnodrama, psychiatric 94.32
Hypnosis (psychotherapeutic) 94.32
  for anesthesia—*omit code*
Hypnotherapy 94.32
Hypophysectomy (complete) (total) 07.69
  partial or subtotal 07.63
    transfrontal approach 07.61
    transsphenoidal approach 07.62
  specified approach NEC 07.68
  transfrontal approach (complete) (total) 07.64
    partial 07.61
  transsphenoidal approach (complete) (total) 07.65
    partial 07.62
Hypothermia (central) (local) 99.81
  gastric (cooling) 96.31
    freezing 96.32
  systemic (in open heart surgery) 39.62
Hypotympanotomy 20.23
Hysterectomy NOS 68.9
  abdominal
    laparoscopic (total) (TLH) 68.41
    other (total) 68.49
    partial or subtotal (supracervical)
      (supravaginal) 68.39
    radical (modified) (Wertheim's) 68.69
      laparoscopic (total) [TLRH] 68.61
  laparoscopic
    abdominal
      radical (total) (TLRH) 68.61
      total (TLH) 68.41
    supracervical (LASH) (LSH) 68.31
    total (TLH) 68.41
    vaginal, assisted (LAVH) 68.51
      radical (LRVH) 68.71

Hysterectomy—*continued*
  radical
    abdominal
      laparoscopic 68.61
      other (modified) (Wertheim's) 68.69
    vaginal
      laparoscopic (LRVH) 68.71
      other 68.79
        subterm other 68.79
  supracervical 68.39
    classic infrafascial SEMM hysterectomy
      [CISH] 68.31
    laparoscopically assisted [LASH] 68.31
  vaginal (complete) (partial) (subtotal) (total)
    68.59
    laparoscopically assisted (LAVH) 68.51
    radical (Schauta) 68.79
      laparoscopic [LRVH] 68.71
Hysterocolpectomy (radical) (vaginal) 68.79
  abdominal 68.69
    laparoscopic 68.61
  laparoscopic 68.71
Hysterogram NEC 87.85
  percutaneous 87.84
Hysterolysis 54.59
  laparoscopic 54.51
Hysteromyomectomy 68.29
Hysteropexy 69.22
Hysteroplasty 69.49
Hysterorrhaphy 69.41
Hysterosalpingography
  gas (contrast) 87.82
  opaque dye (contrast) 87.83
Hysterosalpingostomy 66.74
Hysteroscopy 68.12
  ablation
    endometrial 68.23
  with biopsy 68.16
Hysterotomy (with removal of foreign body)
    (with removal of hydatidiform mole) 68.0
  for intrauterine transfusion 75.2
  obstetrical 74.99
    for termination of pregnancy 74.91
Hysterotrachelectomy 67.4
Hysterotracheloplasty 69.49
Hysterotrachelorrhaphy 69.41
Hysterotrachelotomy 69.95

I

IAEMT (intraoperative anesthetic effect monitoring and titration) 00.94 *[89.14]*
ICCE (intracapsular cataract extraction) 13.19
Ileal
  bladder
    closed 57.87 *[45.51]*
    open (ileoureterostomy) 56.51
    conduit (ileoureterostomy) 56.51
Ileocecostomy 45.93
Ileocolectomy
  laparoscopic 17.33
  open and other 45.73
Ileocolostomy 45.93
Ileocolotomy 45.00
Ileocystoplasty (isolated segment anastomosis) (open loop) 57.87 *[45.51]*
Ileoduodenotomy 45.01
Ileoectomy (partial) 45.62
  with cecectomy
    laparoscopic 17.32
    open and other 45.72
Ileoentectropy 46.99
Ileoesophagostomy 42.54
Ileoileostomy 45.91
  proximal to distal segment 45.62
Ileoloopogram 87.78
Ileopancreatostomy 52.96
Ileopexy 46.61
Ileoproctostomy 45.93
Ileorectostomy 45.93
Ileorrhaphy 46.73
Ileoscopy 45.13
  through stoma (artificial) 45.12
  transabdominal (operative) 45.11
Ileosigmoidostomy 45.93
Ileostomy 46.20
  continent (permanent) 46.22
  delayed opening 46.24
  Hendon (temporary) 46.21
  loop 46.01
  Paul (temporary) 46.21
  permanent 46.23
    continent 46.22
  repair 46.41
  revision 46.41
  tangential (temporary) 46.21
  temporary 46.21
  transplantation to new site 46.23
  tube (temporary) 46.21
  ureteral
    external 56.51
    internal 56.71
Ileotomy 45.02
Ileotransversostomy 45.93
Ileoureterostomy (Bricker's) (ileal bladder) 56.51
Imaging (diagnostic)
  by
    optical coherence tomography (OCT) —*see* OCT and Tomography, optical coherence
  diagnostic, not elsewhere classified 88.90
  endovascular ultrasound—*see* Imaging, intravascular ultrasound
  intraoperative
    iMRI—*see* Imaging, magnetic resonance
    intravascular—*see* Imaging, intravascular ultrasound

Imaging—*continued*
  intravascular ultrasound (IVUS) 00.29
    aorta 00.22
    aortic arch 00.22
    carotid vessel 00.21
    cerebral vessel, extracranial 00.21
    coronary vessel 00.24
    intrathoracic vessel 00.22
    other specified vessel 00.28
    peripheral vessel 00.23
    renal vessel 00.25
    vena cava (inferior) (superior) 00.22
  magnetic resonance (nuclear), (proton) NEC 88.97
    abdomen 88.97
    bladder (urinary) 88.95
    bone marrow blood supply 88.94
    brain (brain stem) 88.91
      intraoperative (iMRI) 88.96
      real-time 88.96
    chest (hilar) (mediastinal) 88.92
    computer assisted surgery (CAS) with MR/MRA 00.32
    extremity (upper) (lower) 88.94
    eye orbit 88.97
    face 88.97
    head NEC 88.97
    musculoskeletal 88.94
    myocardium 88.92
    neck 88.97
    orbit of eye 88.97
    prostate 88.95
    specified site NEC 88.97
    spinal canal (cord) (spine) 88.93
  VH™-IVUS — *see* Imaging (diagnostic), intravascular ultrasound (IVUS), by site
  virtual histology intravascular ultrasound — *see* Imaging (diagnostic), intravascular ultrasound (IVUS), by site
Immobilization (by)
  with fracture-reduction—*see* Reduction, fracture
  bandage 93.59
  bone 93.53
  cast NEC 93.53
    with reduction of fracture or dislocation—*see* Reduction, fracture, *and* Reduction, dislocation
  device NEC 93.59
  pressure dressing 93.56
  splint (plaster) (tray) 93.54
    with reduction of fracture or dislocation—*see* Reduction, fracture, *and* Reduction, dislocation
  stereotactic head frame 93.59
  strapping (non-traction) 93.59
Immunization —*see also* Vaccination
  allergy 99.12
  autoimmune disease 99.13
  BCG 99.33
  brucellosis 99.55
  cholera 99.31
  diphtheria 99.36
  DPT 99.39
  epidemic parotitis 99.46
  German measles 99.47
  Hemophilus influenzae 99.52
  influenza 99.52
  measles 99.45
  meningococcus 99.55

Immunization—*continued*
  mumps 99.46
  pertussis 99.37
  plague 99.34
  poliomyelitis 99.41
  rabies 99.44
  rubella 99.47
  salmonella 99.55
  smallpox 99.42
  staphylococcus 99.55
  TAB 99.32
  tetanus 99.38
  triple vaccine 99.48
  tuberculosis 99.33
  tularemia 99.35
  typhoid-paratyphoid 99.32
  typhus 99.55
  viral NEC 99.55
  whooping cough 99.37
  yellow fever 99.43
Immunoadsorption
  extracorporeal (ECI) 99.76
Immunotherapy, antineoplastic 99.28
  C-Parvum 99.28
  Interferon 99.28
  Interleukin-2 (low-dose) 99.28
    high-dose 00.15
  Levamisole 99.28
  Proleukin (low-dose) 99.28
    high-dose 00.15
  Thymosin 99.28
Impella® percutaneous external heart assist
  device 37.68
Implant, implantation
  abdominal artery to coronary artery 36.17
  artery
    aortic branches to heart muscle 36.2
    mammary to ventricular wall (Vineberg) 36.2
  baffle, atrial or interatrial 35.91
  biliary fistulous tract into stomach or intestine
    51.39
  bipolar endoprosthesis (femoral head) 81.52
  bladder sphincter, artificial (inflatable) 58.93
  blood vessels to myocardium 36.2
  bone growth stimulator (invasive) (percutaneous)
    (semi-invasive)—*see* category 78.9
  bone morphogenetic protein (Infuse™) (OP-1™)
    (recombinant) (rhBMP) 84.52
  bone void filler 84.55
    that with percutaneous vertebral augmentation
      81.66
    that with percutaneous vertebroplasty 81.65
  breast (for augmentation) (bilateral) 85.54
    unilateral 85.53
  cardiac contractility modulation (CCM)
    rechargeable pulse generator only 17.52
    total system 17.51
  cardiac resynchronization device
    defibrillator (biventricular) (BiV ICD) (BiV
      pacemaker with defibrillator) (BiV pacing
      with defibrillator) (CRT-D) (device and one
      or more leads) (total system) 00.51
      left ventricular coronary venous lead only 00.52
      pulse generator only 00.54
    pacemaker (BiV) (biventricular) (CRT-P)
      (device and one or more leads) (total
      system) 00.50
      left ventricular coronary venous lead only 00.52
      pulse generator only 00.54
  cardiac support device (CSD) 37.41

Implant, implantation—*continued*
  CCM (cardiac contractility modulation)
    rechargeable pulse generator only 17.52
    total system 17.51
  chemotherapeutic agent 00.10
  coil(s), endovascular 39.79
    head or neck vessels
      bare metal 39.75
      bioactive 39.76
  CorCap™ 37.41
  CRT-D (biventricular defibrillator) (BiV ICD)
    (BiV pacemaker with defibrillator) (BiV
    pacing with defibrillator) (cardiac
    resynchronization defibrillator) (device and
    one or more leads) 00.51
    left ventricular coronary venous lead only 00.52
    pulse generator only 00.53
  CRT-P (biventricular pacemaker) (BiV
    pacemaker) (cardiac resynchronization
    pacemaker) (device and one or more leads)
    00.50
    left ventricular coronary venous lead only 00.52
    pulse generator only 00.53
  cardiomyostimulation system 37.67
  cardioverter/defibrillator, automatic 37.94
    leads only (patch electrodes) (sensing) (pacing)
      37.95
    pulse generator only 37.96
    total system 37.94
  chest wall (mesh) (silastic) 34.79
  chin (polyethylene) (silastic) 76.68
  cochlea (electrode) 20.96
    prosthetic device (electrode and receiver) 20.96
      channel (single) 20.97
        multiple 20.98
      electrode only 20.99
      internal coil only 20.99
  cornea 11.73
  custodis eye 14.41
  dental (endosseous) (prosthetic) 23.6
  device
    adjustable gastric band and port 44.95
    bronchial device NOS 33.79
    bronchial substance NOS 33.79
    bronchial valve(s)
      multiple lobes 33.73
      single lobe 33.71
    cardiac support device (CSD) 37.41
    CorCap™ 37.41
    epicardial support device 37.41
    Lap-Band™ 44.95
    left atrial appendage 37.90
    left atrial filter 37.90
    left atrial occluder 37.90
    MitraClip® percutaneous mitral valve leaflet
      clip 35.97
    prosthetic cardiac support device 37.41
    sternal fixation device with rigid plates 84.94
    subcutaneous for intracardiac or great vessel
      hemodynamic monitoring 00.57
    vascular access 86.07
    ventricular support device 37.41
  diaphragmatic pacemaker 34.85
  Dynesys® 84.82
  electrode(s)
    brain 02.93
      depth 02.93
      foramen ovale 02.93
      sphenoidal 02.96

Implant, implantation—*continued*
  cardiac (initial) (transvenous) 37.70
    atrium (initial) 37.73
      replacement 37.76
    atrium and ventricle (initial) 37.72
      replacement 37.76
    epicardium (sternotomy or thoracotomy
      approach) 37.74
    left ventricular coronary venous system 00.52
    temporary transvenous pacemaker system
      37.78
      during and immediately following cardiac
        surgery 39.64
    ventricle (initial) 37.71
      replacement 37.76
  carotid sinus 39.82
    with synchronous pulse generator
      implantation (total system) 39.81
  depth 02.93
  foramen ovale 02.93
  gastric 04.92
  heart (*see also* Implant, electrode(s), cardiac)
    37.70
  intracranial 02.93
  osteogenic (invasive) for bone growth
    stimulation—*see* category 78.9
  peripheral nerve 04.92
  sacral nerve 04.92
  sphenoidal 02.96
  spine 03.93
  electroencephalographic receiver
    brain 02.93
    intracranial 02.93
  electronic stimulator
    anus (subcutaneous) 49.92
    bladder 57.96
    bone growth stimulator (invasive)
      (percutaneous) (semi-invasive) 78.9
    brain—*see* Implant, neurostimulator, brain
    carotid sinus 39.83
    with synchronous lead(s) implantation (total
      system) 39.81
    cochlear 20.96
      channel (single) 20.97
        multiple 20.98
    gastric 04.92
    intracranial—*see* Implant, neurostimulator,
      intracranial
    peripheral nerve—*see* Implant, neurostimulator,
      peripheral nerve
    phrenic nerve 34.85
    skeletal muscle 83.92
    spine—*see* Implant, neurostimulator, spine
    ureter 56.92
  electrostimulator—*see* Implant, electronic
    stimulator, by site
  endoprosthesis
    bile duct 51.87
    femoral head (bipolar) 81.52
    pancreatic duct 52.93
  endosseous (dental) 23.6
  epidural pegs 02.93
  epikeratoprosthesis 11.73
  estradiol (pellet) 99.23
  eye (Iowa type) 16.61
    integrated 16.41
  facial bone, synthetic (alloplastic) 76.92
  fallopian tube (Mulligan hood) (silastic tube)
    (stent) 66.93
    into uterus 66.74
  gastroepiploic artery to coronary artery 36.17
  hearing device, electromagnetic 20.95

Implant, implantation—*continued*
  heart
    artificial 37.52
      total internal biventricular replacement
        system 37.52
      AbioCor® 37.52
      CardioWest™ (TAH-t) 37.52
    assist system
      CentriMag® —*see* Insertion, circulatory
        support device
      external heart assist device, percutaneous
        —*see* Insertion, circulatory support
        device
      external heart assist system, open approach
        37.65
      extrinsic 37.68
      HeartMate® implantable heart assist system
        37.66
      HeartMate® II left ventricular assist system
        [LVAS] 37.66
      Impella® percutaneous external circulatory
        assist device —*see* Insertion, circulatory
        support device
      implantable 37.66
      non-implantable—*see* Insertion, circulatory
        support device
      percutaneous external circulatory assist
        device—*see* Insertion, circulatory support
        device
      pulsation balloon 37.61
      pVAD (percutaneous VAD) —*see* Insertion,
        circulatory support device
      TandemHeart® —*see* Insertion, circulatory
        support device
      temporary non-implantable circulatory assist
        device—*see* Insertion, circulatory support
        device
      that for destination therapy (DT) 37.66
    auxiliary ventricle 37.62
    cardiac support device (CSD) 37.41
    circulatory assist system—*see* Implant, heart,
      assist system
    CorCap™ 37.41
    epicardial support device 37.41
    pacemaker (*see also* Implant, pacemaker,
      cardiac) 37.80
    prosthetic cardiac support device 37.41
    total internal biventricular replacement system
      37.52
    valve(s)
      prosthesis or synthetic device (partial)
        (synthetic) (total) 35.20
        aortic 35.22
        mitral 35.24
        pulmonary 35.26
        tricuspid 35.28
      tissue graft 35.20
        aortic 35.21
        mitral 35.23
        pulmonary 35.25
        tricuspid 35.27
    ventricular support device 37.41
  inert material
    breast (for augmentation) (bilateral) 85.54
      unilateral 85.53
    larynx 31.0
    nose 21.85
    orbit (eye socket) 16.69
      reinsertion 16.62
    scleral shell (cup) (with evisceration of eyeball)
      16.31
      reinsertion 16.62

Implant, implantation—*continued*
  Tenon's capsule (with enucleation of eyeball) 16.42
    with attachment of muscles 16.41
    reinsertion 16.62
  urethra 59.79
  vocal cord(s) 31.0
  infusion pump 86.06
  interbody spinal fusion device 84.51
  intracardiac or great vessel hemodynamic
    monitor, subcutaneous 00.57
  joint (prosthesis) (silastic) (Swanson type) NEC
    81.96
    ankle (total) 81.56
      revision 81.59
    carpocarpal, carpometacarpal 81.74
    elbow (total) 81.84
      revision 81.97
    extremity (bioelectric) (cineplastic)
      (kineplastic) 84.40
      lower 84.48
        revision 81.59
      upper 84.44
        revision 81.97
    femoral (bipolar endoprosthesis) 81.52
      revision NOS 81.53
        acetabular and femoral components (total)
          00.70
        acetabular component only 00.71
        acetabular liner and/or femoral head only
          00.73
        femoral component only 00.72
        femoral head only and/or acetabular liner
          00.73
        total (acetabular and femoral components)
          00.70
    finger 81.71
    hand (metacarpophalangeal) (interphalangeal)
      81.71
      revision 81.97
    hip (partial) 81.52
      revision NOS 81.53
        acetabular and femoral components (total)
          00.70
        acetabular component only 00.71
        acetabular liner and/or femoral head only
          00.73
        femoral component only 00.72
        femoral head only and/or acetabular liner
          00.73
        partial
          acetabular component only 00.71
          acetabular liner and/or femoral head only
            00.73
          femoral component only 00.72
          femoral head only and/or acetabular liner
            00.73
          total (acetabular and femoral components)
            00.70
        total 81.51
          revision (acetabular and femoral
            components) 00.70
    interphalangeal 81.71
      revision 81.97

Implant, implantation—*continued*
    knee (partial) (total) 81.54
      revision NOS 81.55
        femoral component 00.82
        partial
          femoral component 00.82
          patellar component 00.83
          tibial component 00.81
          tibial insert 00.84
        patellar component 00.83
        tibial component 00.81
        tibial insert 00.84
        total (all components) 00.80
    metacarpophalangeal 81.71
      revision 81.97
    shoulder (partial) 81.81
      revision 81.97
      total replacement, NEC 81.80
        other 81.80
        reverse 81.88
    toe 81.57
      for hallux valgus repair 77.59
      revision 81.59
    wrist (partial) 81.74
      revision 81.97
      total replacement 81.73
  kidney, mechanical 55.97
  Lap-Band™ 44.95
  larynx 31.0
  leads (cardiac)—*see* Implant, electrode(s) cardiac
  limb lengthening device, internal (NOS) 84.54
    with kinetic distraction 84.53
  mammary artery
    in ventricle (Vineberg) 36.2
    to coronary artery (single vessel) 36.15
      double vessel 36.16
  M-Brace™ 84.82
  Mulligan hood, fallopian tube 66.93
  nerve (peripheral) 04.79
  neuropacemaker—*see* Implant, neurostimulator,
    by site
  neurostimulator
    brain 02.93
    electrodes
      brain 02.93
      gastric 04.92
      intracranial 02.93
      peripheral nerve 04.92
      sacral nerve 04.92
      spine 03.93
    intracranial 02.93
    peripheral nerve 04.92
    pulse generator (subcutaneous) 86.96
      cranial 01.20
      multiple array 86.95
        rechargeable 86.98
      single array 86.94
        rechargeable 86.97
    spine 03.93
  nose 21.85
  Ommaya reservoir 02.22
  orbit 16.69
    reinsertion 16.62
  outflow tract prosthesis (heart) (gusset type)
    in
      pulmonary valvuloplasty 35.26
      total repair of tetralogy of Fallot 35.81
  ovary into uterine cavity 65.72
    laparoscoic 65.75

Implant, implantation—*continued*
pacemaker
  brain—*see* Implant, neurostimulator, brain
  cardiac (device) (initial) (permanent)
    (replacement) 37.80
    dual-chamber device (initial) 37.83
      replacement 37.87
    resynchronization device (biventricular
      pacemaker) (BiV pacemaker) (CRT-P)
      device only (initial) (replacement) 00.53
      total system (device and one or more leads)
        00.50
      transvenous lead into left ventricular
        coronary venous system 00.52
    single-chamber device (initial) 37.81
      rate responsive 37.82
      replacement 37.85
        rate responsive 37.86
    temporary transvenous pacemaker system
      37.78
      during and immediately following cardiac
        surgery 39.64
  carotid sinus 39.89
  diaphragm 34.85
  gastric 04.92
  intracranial—*see* Implant, neurostimulator,
    intracranial
  neural—*see* Implant, neurostimulator, by site
  peripheral nerve—*see* Implant, neurostimulator,
    peripheral nerve
  spine—*see* Implant, neurostimulator, spine
pancreas (duct) 52.96
penis, prosthetic (internal)
  inflatable 64.97
  non-inflatable 64.95
port, vascular access device 86.07
premaxilla 76.68
progesterone (subdermal) 99.23
prosthesis, prosthetic device
  acetabulum (Aufranc-Turner) 81.52
  ankle (total) 81.56
  arm (bioelectric) (cineplastic) (kineplastic)
    84.44
  breast (Cronin) (Dow-Coming)
    (Perras-Pappillon) (bilateral) 85.54
    unilateral 85.53
  cardiac support device (CSD) (CorCap™)
    37.41
  cochlear 20.96
    channel (single) 20.97
      multiple 20.98
  extremity (bioelectric) (cineplastic)
    (kineplastic) 84.40
    lower 84.48
    upper 84.44
  fallopian tube (Mulligan hood) (stent) 66.93
  femoral head (Austin-Moore) (bipolar) (Eicher)
    (Thompson) 81.52
    revision NOS 81.53
      acetabular and femoral components (total)
        00.70
      acetabular component only 00.71
      acetabular liner and/or femoral head only
        00.73
      femoral component only 00.72
      femoral head only and/or acetabular liner
        00.73
      partial
        acetabular component only 00.71
        acetabular liner and/or femoral head only
          00.73

Implant, implantation—*continued*
      femoral component only 00.72
      femoral head only and/or acetabular liner
        00.73
      total (acetabular and femoral components)
        00.70
  joint (Swanson type) NEC 81.96
    ankle (total) 81.56
    carpocarpal, carpometacarpal 81.74
    elbow (total) 81.84
    finger 81.71
    hand (metacarpophalangeal) (interphalangeal)
      81.71
    hip (partial) 81.52
      revision NOS 81.53
        acetabular and femoral components (total)
          00.70
        acetabular component only 00.71
        acetabular liner and/or femoral head only
          00.73
        femoral component only 00.72
        femoral head only and/or acetabular liner
          00.73
        partial
          acetabular component only 00.71
          acetabular liner and/or femoral head
            only 00.73
          femoral component only 00.72
          femoral head only and/or acetabular
            liner 00.73
        total (acetabular and femoral components)
          00.70
    total 81.51
      revision (acetabular and femoral
        components) 00.70
    interphalangeal 81.71
    knee (partial) (total) 81.54
      revision NOS 81.55
        femoral component 00.82
        partial
          femoral component 00.82
          patellar component 00.83
          tibial component 00.81
          tibial insert 00.84
        patellar component 00.83
        tibial component 00.81
        tibial insert 00.84
        total (all components) 00.80
    metacarpophalangeal 81.71
    shoulder (partial) 81.81
      total, NEC 81.80
        other 81.80
        reverse 81.88
    toe 81.57
      for hallux valgus repair 77.59
    wrist (partial) 81.74
      total 81.73
  leg (bioelectric) (cineplastic) (kineplastic) 84.48
  lens 13.91
  outflow tract (heart) (gusset type)
    in
      pulmonary valvuloplasty 35.26
      total repair of tetralogy of Fallot 35.81
  penile (non-inflatable) (internal) 64.95
    inflatable (internal) 64.97
  skin (dermal regenerative) (matrix) 86.67
  testicular (bilateral) (unilateral) 62.7
pulsation balloon (phase-shift) 37.61
pump, infusion 86.06
radial artery 36.19
radioactive isotope 92.27

Implant, implantation—*continued*
  radium (radon) 92.27
  retinal attachment 14.41
    with buckling 14.41
  Rheos™ carotid sinus baroreflex activation
      device 39.81
  Rickham reservoir 02.22
  silicone
    breast (bilateral) 85.54
      unilateral 85.53
    skin (for filling of defect) 86.02
      for augmentation NEC 86.89
  spine NEC 84.59
    facet replacement device(s) 84.84
    interspinous process decompression device
        84.80
    pedicle-based dynamic stabilization device(s)
        84.82
    posterior motion preservation device(s) —*see*
        category 84.8
  stimoceiver—*see* Implant, neurostimulator, by
      site
  stimulator
    electrodes
      carotid sinus (baroreflex activation device)
          39.82
        with synchronous pulse generator
            implantation (total system) 39.81
      pulse generator
        carotid sinus (baroreflex activation device)
            39.83
          with synchronous electrode(s) implantation
              (total system) 39.81
  subdural
    grids 02.93
    strips 02.93
  Swanson prosthesis (joint) (silastic) NEC 81.96
    carpocarpal, carpometacarpal 81.74
    finger 81.71
    hand (metacarpophalangeal) (interphalangeal)
        81.71
    interphalangeal 81.71
    knee (partial) (total) 81.54
      revision 81.55
    metacarpophalangeal 81.71
    toe 81.57
      for hallux valgus repair 77.59
    wrist (partial) 81.74
      total 81.73
  systemic arteries into myocardium (Vineberg
      type operation) 36.2
  Tandem™ heart 37.68
  telescope (IMT) (miniature) 13.91
  testicular prosthesis (bilateral) (unilateral) 62.7
  tissue expander (skin) NEC 86.93
    breast 85.95
  tissue mandril (for vascular graft) 39.99
    with
      blood vessel repair 39.56
      vascular bypass or shunt—*see* Bypass,
          vascular
  tooth (bud) (germ) 23.5
    prosthetic 23.6
  umbrella, vena cava 38.7
  ureters into
    bladder 56.74
    intestine 56.71
      external diversion 56.51
    skin 56.61
  urethan sphincter, artificial (inflatable) 58.93

Implant, implantation—*continued*
  urethra
    for repair of urinary stress incontinence
      collagen 59.72
      fat 59.72
      polytef 59.72
  urinary sphincter, artificial (inflatable) 58.93
  valve(s)
    endovascular—*see* Replacement, heart valve,
        by site
  vascular access device 86.07
  vitreous (silicone) 14.75
    for retinal reattachment 14.41
      with buckling 14.41
  vocal cord(s) (paraglottic) 31.98
  X Stop™ 84.80
Implosion (psychologic desensitization) 94.33
Incision (and drainage)
  with
    exploration—*see* Exploration
    removal of foreign body—*see* Removal, foreign
        body
  abdominal wall 54.0
    as operative approach—*omit code*
  abscess—*see also* Incision, by site
    antecubital fossa 86.04
    appendix 47.2
      with appendectomy 47.09
        laparoscopic 47.01
    axilla 86.04
    cheek 86.04
    extraperitoneal 54.0
    face 86.04
    gluteal 86.04
    groin region (abdominal wall) (inguinal) 54.0
      skin 86.04
      subcutaneous tissue 86.04
    hair follicle 86.04
    ischiorectal 49.01
    lip 27.0
    nailbed or nailfold 86.04
    neck 86.04
    omental 54.19
    paronychia 86.04
    perianal 49.01
    perigastric 54.19
    perineum (female) 71.09
      male 86.04
    perisplenic 54.19
    peritoneal NEC 54.19
      pelvic (female) 70.12
    popliteal space 86.04
    retroperitoneal 54.0
    sclera 12.89
    skin 86.04
    subcutaneous tissue 86.04
    subdiaphragmatic 54.19
    subhepatic 54.19
    submaxillary 86.04
    subphrenic 54.19
    supraclavicular fossa 86.04
    vas deferens 63.6
  adrenal gland 07.41
  alveolus, alveolar bone 24.0
  antecubital fossa 86.09
  anus NEC 49.93
    fistula 49.11
    septum 49.91
  appendix 47.2

Incision—*continued*

artery 38.00
  abdominal 38.06
  aorta (arch) (ascending) (descending) 38.04
  head and neck NEC 38.02
  intracranial NEC 38.01
  lower limb 38.08
  thoracic NEC 38.05
  upper limb 38.03
atrium (heart) 37.11
auditory canal or meatus, external 18.02
auricle 18.09
axilla 86.09
Bartholin's gland or cyst 71.22
bile duct (with T or Y tube insertion)
  NEC 51.59
  common (exploratory) 51.51
    for
      relief of obstruction NEC 51.42
      removal of calculus 51.41
  for
    exploration 51.59
    relief of obstruction 51.49
bladder 57.19
  neck (transurethral) 57.91
  percutaneous suprapubic (closed) 57.17
  suprapubic NEC 57.18
blood vessel (*see also* Angiotomy) 38.00
bone 77.10
  alveolus, alveolar 24.0
  carpals, metacarpals 77.14
  clavicle 77.11
  facial 76.09
  femur 77.15
  fibula 77.17
  humerus 77.12
  patella 77.16
  pelvic 77.19
  phalanges (foot) (hand) 77.19
  radius 77.13
  scapula 77.11
  skull 01.24
  specified site NEC 77.19
  tarsals, metatarsals 77.18
  thorax (ribs) (sternum) 77.11
  tibia 77.17
  ulna 77.13
  vertebrae 77.19
brain 01.39
  cortical adhesions 02.91
breast (skin) 85.0
  with removal of tissue expander 85.96
bronchus 33.0
buccal space 27.0
bulbourethral gland 58.91
bursa 83.03
  hand 82.03
  pharynx 29.0
carotid body 39.89
cerebral (meninges) 01.39
  epidural or extradural space 01.24
  subarachnoid or subdural space 01.31
cerebrum 01.39
cervix 69.95
  to
    assist delivery 73.93
    replace inverted uterus 75.93
chalazion 08.09
  with removal of capsule 08.21
cheek 86.09

Incision—*continued*

chest wall (for extrapleural drainage) (for
  removal of foreign body) 34.01
  as operative approach—*omit code*
common bile duct (for exploration) 51.51
  for
    relief of obstruction 51.42
    removal of calculus 51.41
common wall between posterior left atrium and
  coronary sinus (with roofing of resultant
  defect with patch graft) 35.82
conjunctiva 10.1
cornea 11.1
  radial (refractive) 11.75
cranial sinus 01.21
craniobuccal pouch 07.72
cul-de-sac 70.12
cyst
  dentigerous 24.0
  radicular (apical) (periapical) 24.0
Dührssen's (cervix, to assist delivery) 73.93
duodenum 45.01
ear
  external 18.09
  inner 20.79
  middle 20.23
endocardium 37.11
endolymphatic sac 20.79
epididymis 63.92
epidural space, cerebral 01.24
epigastric region 54.0
  intra-abdominal 54.19
esophagus, esophageal NEC 42.09
  web 42.01
exploratory—*see* Exploration
extradural space (cerebral) 01.24
extrapleural 34.01
eyebrow 08.09
eyelid 08.09
  margin (trichiasis) 08.01
face 86.09
fallopian tube 66.01
fascia 83.09
  with division 83.14
    hand 82.12
  hand 82.09
    with division 82.12
fascial compartments, head and neck 27.0
fistula, anal 49.11
flank 54.0
furuncle—*see* Incision, by site
gallbladder 51.04
gingiva 24.0
gluteal 86.09
groin region (abdominal wall) (inguinal) 54.0
  skin 86.09
  subcutaneous tissue 86.09
gum 24.0
hair follicles 86.09
heart 37.10
  valve—*see* Valvulotomy
hematoma—*see also* Incision, by site
  axilla 86.04
  broad ligament 69.98
  ear 18.09
  episiotomy site 75.91
  fossa (superficial) NEC 86.04
  groin region (abdominal wall) (inguinal) 54.0
    skin 86.04
    subcutaneous tissue 86.04
  laparotomy site 54.12

Incision—*continued*
   mediastinum 34.1
   perineum (female) 71.09
      male 86.04
   popliteal space 86.04
   scrotum 61.0
   skin 86.04
   space of Retzius 59.19
   subcutaneous tissue 86.04
   vagina (cuff) 70.14
      episiotomy site 75.91
      obstetrical NEC 75.92
  hepatic ducts 51.59
  hordeolum 08.09
  hygroma—*see also* Incision, by site
   cystic 40.0
  hymen 70.11
  hypochondrium 54.0
   intra-abdominal 54.19
  hypophysis 07.72
  iliac fossa 54.0
  infratemporal fossa 27.0
  ingrown nail 86.09
  intestine 45.00
   large 45.03
   small 45.02
  intracerebral 01.39
  intracranial (epidural space) (extradural space)
     01.24
   subarachnoid or subdural space 01.31
  intraperitoneal 54.19
  ischiorectal tissue 49.02
   abscess 49.01
  joint structures (*see also* Arthrotomy) 80.10
  kidney 55.01
   pelvis 55.11
  labia 71.09
  lacrimal
   canaliculus 09.52
   gland 09.0
   passage NEC 09.59
   punctum 09.51
   sac 09.53
  larynx NEC 31.3
  ligamentum flavum (spine)—*omit code*
  liver 50.0
  lung 33.1
  lymphangioma 40.0
  lymphatic structure (channel) (node) (vessel) 40.0
  mastoid 20.21
  mediastinum 34.1
  meibomian gland 08.09
  meninges (cerebral) 01.31
   spinal 03.09
  midpalmar space 82.04
  mouth NEC 27.92
   floor 27.0
  muscle 83.02
   with division 83.19
     hand 82.19
   hand 82.02
     with division 82.19
  myocardium 37.11
  nailbed or nailfold 86.09
  nasolacrimal duct (stricture) 09.59
  neck 86.09
  nerve (cranial) (peripheral) NEC 04.04
   root (spinal) 03.1
  nose 21.1
  omentum 54.19
  orbit (*see also* Orbitotomy) 16.09

Incision—*continued*
  ovary 65.09
   laparoscopic 65.01
  palate 27.1
  palmar space (middle) 82.04
  pancreas 52.09
  pancreatic sphincter 51.82
   endoscopic 51.85
  parapharyngeal (oral) (transcervical) 28.0
  paronychia 86.09
  parotid
   gland or duct 26.0
   space 27.0
  pelvirectal tissue 48.81
  penis 64.92
  perianal (skin) (tissue) 49.02
   abscess 49.01
  perigastric 54.19
  perineum (female) 71.09
   male 86.09
  peripheral vessels
   lower limb
     artery 38.08
     vein 38.09
   upper limb (artery) (vein) 38.03
  periprostatic tissue 60.81
  perirectal tissue 48.81
  perirenal tissue 59.09
  perisplenic 54.19
  peritoneum 54.95
   by laparotomy 54.19
   pelvic (female) 70.12
     male 54.19
  periureteral tissue 59.09
  periurethral tissue 58.91
  perivesical tissue 59.19
  petrous pyramid (air cells) (apex)
     (mastoid) 20.22
  pharynx, pharyngeal (bursa) 29.0
   space, lateral 27.0
  pilonidal sinus (cyst) 86.03
  pineal gland 07.52
  pituitary (gland) 07.72
  pleura NEC 34.09
  popliteal space 86.09
  postzygomatic space 27.0
  pouch of Douglas 70.12
  prostate (perineal approach) (transurethral
     approach) 60.0
  pterygopalatine fossa 27.0
  pulp canal (tooth) 24.0
  Rathke's pouch 07.72
  rectovaginal septum 48.81
  rectum 48.0
   stricture 48.91
  renal pelvis 55.11
  retroperitoneum 54.0
  retropharyngeal (oral) (transcervical) 28.0
  salivary gland or duct 26.0
  sclera 12.89
  scrotum 61.0
  sebaceous cyst 86.04
  seminal vesicle 60.72
  sinus—*see* Sinusotomy
  Skene's duct or gland 71.09
  skin 86.09
   with drainage 86.04
   breast 85.0
   cardiac pacemaker pocket, new site 37.79
   ear 18.09
   nose 21.1

Incision—*continued*

subcutaneous tunnel for pulse generator lead wire 86.99
  with initial procedure—*omit code*
thalamic stimulator pulse generator pocket, new site 86.09
  with initial insertion of battery package—*omit code*
tunnel, subcutanous for pulse generator lead wire 86.99
  with initial procedure —*omit code*
skull (bone) 01.24
soft tissue NEC 83.09
  with division 83.19
    hand 82.19
  hand 82.09
    with division 82.19
space of Retzius 59.19
spermatic cord 63.93
sphincter of Oddi 51.82
  endoscopic 51.85
spinal
  cord 03.09
  nerve root 03.1
spleen 41.2
stomach 43.0
stye 08.09
subarachnoid space, cerebral 01.31
subcutaneous tissue 86.09
  with drainage 86.04
  tunnel
    esophageal 42.86
      with anastomosis—*see* Anastomosis, esophagus, antesternal
    pulse generator lead wire 86.99
      with initial procedure—*omit code*
subdiaphragmatic space 54.19
subdural space, cerebral 01.31
sublingual space 27.0
submandibular space 27.0
submaxillary 86.09
  with drainage 86.04
submental space 27.0
subphrenic space 54.19
supraclavicular fossa 86.09
  with drainage 86.04
sweat glands, skin 86.04
temporal pouches 27.0
tendon (sheath) 83.01
  with division 83.13
    hand 82.11
  hand 82.01
    with division 82.11
testis 62.0
thenar space 82.04
thymus (open) (other) 07.92
  thoracoscopic 07.95
thyroid (field) (gland) NEC 06.09
  postoperative 06.02
tongue NEC 25.94
  for tongue tic 25.91
tonsil 28.0
trachea NEC 31.3
tunica vaginalis 61.0
umbilicus 54.0
urachal cyst 54.0
ureter 56.2
urethra 58.0
uterus (corpus) 68.0
  cervix 69.95
  for termination of pregnancy 74.91
  septum (congenital) 68.22

Incision—*continued*

uvula 27.71
vagina (cull) (septum) (stenosis) 70.14
  for
    incisional hematoma (episiotomy) 75.91
    obstetrical hematoma NEC 75.92
    pelvic abscess 70.12
vas deferens 63.6
vein 38.00
  abdominal 38.07
  head and neck NEC 38.02
  intracranial NEC 38.01
  lower limb 38.09
  thoracic NEC 38.05
  upper limb 38.03
  vertebral column 03.09
vulva 71.09
  obstetrical 75.92
web, esophageal 42.01
Incudectomy NEC 19.3
  with
    stapedectomy (*see also* Stapedectomy) 19.19
    Tympanoplasty—*see* Tympanoplasty
Incudopexy 19.19
Incudostapediopexy 19.19
  with incus replacement 19.11
Indentation, sclera, for buckling (*see also* Buckling, scleral) 14.49
Indicator dilution flow measurement 89.68
Induction
  abortion
    by
      D and C 69.01
      insertion of prostaglandin suppository 96.49
      intra-amniotic injection (prostaglandin) (saline) 75.0
  labor
    medical 73.4
    surgical 73.01
      intra- and extra-amniotic injection 73.1
      stripping of membranes 73.1
Inflation
  belt wrap 93.99
  Eustachian tube 20.8
  fallopian tube 66.8
    with injection of therapeutic agent 66.95
Infolding sclera, for buckling (*see also* Buckling, scleral) 14.49
Infraction, turbinates (nasal) 21.62
Infundibulectomy
  hypophyseal (*see also* Hypophysectomy, partial) 07.63
  ventricle (heart) (right) 35.34
    in total repair of tetralogy of Fallot 35.81
Infusion (intra-arterial) (intravenous)
  with
    disruption of blood brain barrier [BBBD] 00.19
  Abciximab 99.20
  antibiotic
    oxazolidinone class 00.14
  antineoplastic agent (chemotherapeutic) 99.25
    biological response modifier [BRM] 99.28
    cintredekin besudotox 99.28
    CLO 17.70
    clofarabine 17.70
    CLOLAR® 17.70
    high-dose interleukin-2 00.15
    low-dose interleukin-2 99.28

Infusion—*continued*
  biological response modifier [BRM],
      antineoplastic agent 99.28
    cintredekin besudotox 99.28
    high-dose interleukin-2 00.15
    low-dose interleukin-2 99.28
  cancer chemotherapy agent NEC 99.25
  cintredekin besudotox 99.28
  CLO 17.70
  clofarabine 17.70
  CLOLAR® 17.70
  drotrecogin alfa (activated) 00.11
  electrolytes 99.18
  enzymes, thrombolytic (streptokinase) (tissue
      plasminogen activator) (TPA) (urokinase)
    direct coronary artery 36.04
    intravenous 99.10
  Eptifibatide 99.20
  gamma globulin 99.14
  GP IIB/IIIa inhibitor 99.20
  hormone substance NEC 99.24
  human B-type natriuretic peptide (hBNP) 00.13
  IgG (immunoglobulin) 99.14
  immunoglobulin (IgG) (IVIG) (IVIg) 99.14
  immunosuppressive antibody therapy 00.18
  interleukin-2
    high-dose 00.15
    low-dose 99.28
  IVIG (immunoglobulin) (IVIg) 99.14
  lymphocyte 99.09
  nesiritide 00.13
  neuroprotective agent 99.75
  nimodipine 99.75
  nutritional substance (*see* Nutrition)
  platelet inhibitor
    direct coronary artery 36.04
    intravenous 99.20
  Proleukin (low-dose) 99.28
    high-dose 00.15
  prophylactic substance NEC 99.29
  radioimmunoconjugate 92.28
  radioimmunotherapy 92.28
  radioisotope (liquid brachytherapy) (liquid I-125)
      92.20
  recombinant protein 00.11
  reteplase 99.10
  therapeutic substance NEC 99.29
  thrombolytic agent (enzyme) (streptokinase)
      99.10
    with percutaneous transluminal angioplasty

  Note: Also use 00.40, 00.41, 00.42, or 00.43 to
  show the total number of vessels treated.

      coronary 00.66
      non-coronary vessel(s) 39.50
      specified site NEC 39.50
    direct intracoronary artery 36.04
  tirofiban (HCl) 99.20
  vaccine
    tumor 99.28
  vasopressor 00.17
Injection (into) (hypodermically)
    (intramuscularly) (intravenously) (acting
    locally or systemically)
  Actinomycin D, for cancer chemotherapy 99.25
  adhesion barrier substance 99.77
  alcohol
    nerve—*see* Injection, nerve
    spinal 03.8
  anterior chamber, eye (air) (liquid) (medication)
      12.92

Injection—*continued*
  antibiotic 99.21
    oxazolidinone class 00.14
  anticoagulant 99.19
  anti-D (Rhesus) globulin 99.11
  antidote NEC 99.16
  anti-infective NEC 99.22
  antineoplastic agent (chemotherapeutic) 99.25
    biological response modifier [BRM] 99.28
    cintredekin besudotox 99.28
    high-dose interleukin-2 00.15
    low-dose interleukin-2 99.28
  antivenin 99.16
  barrier substance, adhesion 99.77
  BCG
    for chemotherapy 99.25
    vaccine 99.33
  biological response modifier [BRM],
      antineoplastic agent 99.28
    cintredekin besudotox 99.28
    high-dose interleukin-2 00.15
    low-dose interleukin-2 99.28
  bone marrow 41.92
    transplant—*see* Transplant, bone, marrow
  breast (therapeutic agent) 85.92
    inert material (silicone) (bilateral) 85.52
      unilateral 85.51
  bursa (therapeutic agent) 83.96
    hand 82.94
  cancer chemotherapeutic agent 99.25
  caudal—*see* Injection, spinal
  cintredekin besudotox 99.28
  cortisone 99.23
  costochondral junction 81.92
  dinoprost-tromethine, intra-amniotic 75.0
  ear, with alcohol 20.72
  electrolytes 99.18
  enzymes, thrombolytic (streptokinase) (tissue
      plasminogen activator) (TPA) (urokinase)
    direct coronary artery 36.04
    intravenous 99.10
  epidural, spinal—*see* Injection, spinal
  esophageal varices or blood vessel
      (endoscopic)(sclerosing agent) 42.33
  Eustachian tube (inert material) 20.8
  eye (orbit) (retrobulbar) 16.91
    anterior chamber 12.92
    subconjunctival 10.91
  fascia 83.98
    hand 82.96
  gamma globulin 99.14
  ganglion, sympathetic 05.39
    ciliary 12.79
    paravertebral stellate 05.39
  gel, adhesion barrier—*see* Injection, adhesion
      barrier substance
  globulin
    anti-D (Rhesus) 99.11
    gamma 99.14
    Rh immune 99.11
  heart 37.92
  heavy metal antagonist 99.16
  hemorrhoids (sclerosing agent) 49.42
  hormone NEC 99.24
  human B-type natriuretic peptide (hBNP) 00.13
  IgG (immunoglobulin) 99.14
  immune sera 99.14
  immunoglobulin (IgG) (IVIG) (IVIg) 99.14
  inert material—*see* Implant, inert material
  inner ear, for destruction 20.72
  insulin 99.17

Injection—*continued*
intervertebral space for herniated disc 80.52
intra-amniotic
  for induction of
    abortion 75.0
    labor 73.1
intrathecal—*see* Injection, spinal
IVIG (immunoglobulin) (IVIg) 99.14
joint (therapeutic agent) 81.92
  temporomandibular 76.96
kidney (cyst) (therapeutic substance) NEC 55.96
larynx 31.0
ligament (joint) (therapeutic substance) 81.92
liver 50.94
lung, for surgical collapse 33.32
Methotrexate, for cancer chemotherapy 99.25
nerve (cranial) (peripheral) 04.80
  agent NEC 04.89
    alcohol 04.2
    anesthetic for analgesia 04.81
      for operative anesthesia—*omit code*
    neurolytic 04.2
    phenol 04.2
  laryngeal (external) (recurrent) (superior) 31.91
  optic 16.91
  sympathetic 05.39
    alcohol 05.32
    anesthetic for analgesia 05.31
    neurolytic agent 05.32
    phenol 05.32
nesiritide 00.13
neuroprotective agent 99.75
nimodipine 99.75
orbit 16.91
pericardium 37.93
peritoneal cavity
  air 54.96
  locally-acting therapeutic substance 54.97
platelet inhibitor
  direct coronary artery 36.04
  intravenous 99.20
prophylactic substance NEC 99.29
prostate 60.92
radioimmunoconjugate 92.28
radioimmunotherapy 92.28
radioisotopes (intracavitary) (intravenous) 92.28
renal pelvis (cyst) 55.96
retrobulbar (therapeutic substance) 16.91
  for anesthesia—*omit code*
Rh immune globulin 99.11
RhoGAM 99.11
sclerosing agent NEC 99.29
  esophageal varices 42.33
  hemorrhoids 49.42
  pleura 34.92
    treatment of malignancy (cytotoxic agent)
      34.92 *[99.25]*
      with tetracycline 34.92 *[99.21]*
  varicose vein 39.92
  vein NEC 39.92
semicircular canals, for destruction 20.72
silicone—*see* Implant, inert material
skin (sclerosing agent) (filling material) 86.02
soft tissue 83.98
  hand 82.96
spinal (canal) NEC 03.92
  alcohol 03.8
  anesthetic agent for analgesia 03.91
    for operative anesthesia—*omit code*
  contrast material (for myelogram) 87.21
  destructive agent NEC 03.8
  neurolytic agent NEC 03.8

Injection—*continued*
  phenol 03.8
  proteolytic enzyme (chemopapain)
    (chemodiactin) 80.52
  saline (hypothermic) 03.92
  steroid 03.92
spinal nerve root (intrathecal)—*see* Injection,
  spinal
steroid NEC 99.23
subarachnoid, spinal—*see* Injection, spinal
subconjunctival 10.91
tendon 83.97
  hand 82.95
testis 62.92
therapeutic agent NEC 99.29
thoracic cavity 34.92
thrombolytic agent (enzyme) (streptokinase)
  99.10
  with percutaneous transluminal angioplasty

> *Note: Also use 00.40, 00.41, 00.42, or 00.43 to show the total number of vessels treated.*

    coronary 00.66
    direct intracoronary artery 36.04
    non-coronary vessel(s) 39.50
    specified site NEC 39.50
trachea 31.94
tranquilizer 99.26
tunica vaginalis (with aspiration) 61.91
tympanum 20.94
urethra (inert material)
  for repair of urinary stress incontinence
    collagen implant 59.72
    endoscopic injection of implant 59.72
    fat implant 59.72
    polytef implant 59.72
vaccine
  tumor 99.28
varices, esophagus (endoscopic) (sclerosing
  agent) 42.33
varicose vein (sclerosing agent) 39.92
  esophagus 42.33
vestibule, for destruction 20.72
vitreous substitute (silicone) 14.75
  for reattachment of retina 14.59
vocal cords 31.0
Inlay, tooth 23.3
Inoculation
  antitoxins—*see* Administration, antitoxins
  toxoids—*see* Administration, toxoids
  vaccine—*see* Administration, vaccine
Insemination, artificial 69.92
Insertion
  airway
    esophageal obturator 96.03
    nasopharynx 96.01
    oropharynx 96.02
  Allen-Brown cannula 39.93
  antimicrobial envelope 17.81
  aqueous drainage device (shunt) (stent) 12.67
  arch bars (orthodontic) 24.7
    for immobilization (fracture) 93.55
  atrial septal umbrella 35.52
  Austin-Moore prosthesis 81.52
  baffle, heart (atrial) (interatrial) (intra-atrial)
    35.91
  bag, cervix (nonobstetrical) 67.0
    after delivery or abortion 75.8
    to assist delivery or induce labor 73.1
  Baker's (tube) (for stenting) 46.85

Insertion—*continued*

balloon
  gastric 44.93
  heart (pulsation-type) (Kantrowitz) 37.61
  intestine (for decompression) (for dilation) 46.85
    with insertion of colonic stent
      endoscopic 46.86
      other 46.87
band (adjustable)
  gastric, laparoscopic 44.95
  Lap-Band™ 44.95
Barton's tongs (skull) (with synchronous skeletal traction) 02.94
bipolar endoprosthesis (femoral head) 81.52
bladder sphincter, artificial (inflatable) 58.93
Blakemore-Sengstaken tube 96.06
bone growth stimulator (invasive) (percutaneous) (semi-invasive)—*see* category 78.9
bone morphogenetic protein (Infuse™) (OP-1™) (recombinant) (rhBMP) 84.52
bone void filler 84.55
  that with percutaneous vertebral augmentation 81.66
  that with percutaneous vertebroplasty 81.65
bougie, cervix, nonobstetrical 67.0
  to assist delivery or induce labor 73.1
breast implant (for augmentation) (bilateral) 85.54
  unilateral 85.53
bridge (dental) (fixed) 23.42
  removable 23.43
bubble (balloon), stomach 44.93
caliper tongs (skull) (with synchronous skeletal traction) 02.94
cannula
  Allen-Brown 39.93
  for extracorporeal membrane oxygenation (ECMO)—*omit code*
  nasal sinus (by puncture) 22.01
    through natural ostium 22.02
  pancreatic duct 52.92
    endoscopic 52.93
  vessel to vessel 39.93
cardiac resynchronization device
  defibrillator (biventricular defibrillator) (BiV ICD) (BiV pacemaker with defibrillator) (BiV pacing with defibrillator) (CRT-D) (device and one or more leads) (total system) 00.51
    left ventricular coronary venous lead only 00.52
    pulse generator only 00.53
  pacemaker (biventricular pacemaker) (BiV pacemaker) (CRT-P) (device and one or more leads) (total system) 00.50
    left ventricular coronary venous lead only 00.52
    pulse generator only 00.53
cardiac support device (CSD) (CorCap™) 37.41
carotid artery stent(s) (stent graft) 00.63

Note: Also use 00.40, 00.41, 00.42, or 00.43 to show the total number of vessels treated. Use code 00.44 once to show procedure on a bifurcated vessel. In addition, use 00.45, 00.46, 00.47, or 00.48 to show the number of vascular stents inserted.

Insertion—*continued*

catheter
  abdomen of fetus, for intrauterine transfusion 75.2
  anterior chamber (eye), for permanent drainage (glaucoma) 12.79
  artery 38.91
  bile duct(s) 51.59
    common 51.51
      endoscopic 51.87
    endoscopic 51.87
  bladder, indwelling 57.94
    suprapubic 57.18
      percutaneous (closed) 57.17
  bronchus 96.05
    with lavage 96.56
  central venous NEC 38.93
    for
      hemodialysis 38.95
      pressure monitoring 89.62
    peripherally inserted central catheter (PICC) 38.93
    with guidance 38.97
  chest 34.04
    revision (with lysis of adhesions) 34.04
      thoracoscopic 34.06
    thoracoscopic 34.06
  cranial cavity 01.26
    placement via burr hole(s) 01.28
  esophagus (nonoperative) 96.06
    permanent tube 42.81
  intercostal (with water seal), for drainage 34.04
    revision (with lysis of adhesions) 34.04
      thoracoscopic 34.06
    thoracoscopic 34.06
  intracerebral 01.26
    placement via burr hole(s) 01.28
  NeuroFlo™ (partial abdominal aorta occlusion) 39.77
  spinal canal space (epidural) (subarachnoid) (subdural) for infusion of therapeutic or palliative substances 03.90
  Swan-Ganz (pulmonary) 89.64
  temporary occlusion, abdominal aorta 39.77
  transtracheal for oxygenation 31.99
  vein NEC 38.93
    for renal dialysis 38.95
chest tube 34.04
  thoracoscopic 34.06
choledochohepatic tube (for decompression) 51.43
  endoscopic 51.87
circulatory support device
  CentriMag® 37.62
  external heart assist device
    biventricular 37.60
    Impella® 37.68
    percutaneous 37.68
    temporary 37.62
  non-implantable 37.62
  pVAD (percutaneous VAD) 37.68
  TandemHeart® 37.68
  temporary non-implantable circulatory assist device 37.62
cochlear prosthetic device—*see* Implant, cochlea, prosthetic device
contraceptive device (intrauterine) 69.7
CorCap™ 37.41
cordis cannula 54.98

Insertion—*continued*
coronary (artery)

> *Note: Also use 00.40, 00.41, 00.42, or 00.43 to show the total number of vessels treated. Use code 00.44 once to show procedure on a bifurcated vessel. In addition, use 00.45, 00.46, 00.47, or 00.48 to show the number of vascular stents inserted.*

stent, drug-eluting 36.07
stent, non-drug-eluting 36.06
Crosby-Cooney button 54.98
CRT-D (biventricular defibrillator) (BiV ICD) (BiV pacemaker with defibrillator) (BiV pacing with defibrillator) (cardiac resynchronization defibrillator) (device and one or more leads) 00.51
left ventricular coronary venous lead only 00.52
pulse generator only 00.54
CRT-P (biventricular pacemaker) (BiV pacemaker) (cardiac resynchronization pacemaker) (device and one or more leads) 00.50
left ventricular coronary venous lead only 00.52
pulse generator only 00.53
Crutchfield tongs (skull) (with synchronous skeletal traction) 02.94
Davidson button 54.98
denture (total) 99.97
device
adjustable gastric band and port 44.95
bronchial device NOS 33.79
bronchial substance NOS 33.79
bronchial valve(s)
multiple lobes 33.73
single lobe 33.71
cardiac resynchronization —*see* Insertion, cardiac resynchronization device
cardiac support device (CSD) 37.41
CorCap™ 37.41
epicardial support device 37.41
Lap-Band™ 44.95
left atrial appendage 37.90
left atrial filter 37.90
left atrial occluder 37.90
MitraClip® mitral leaflet clip 35.97
prosthetic cardiac support device 37.41
sternal fixation device with rigid plates 84.94
vascular access 86.07
ventricular support device 37.41
diaphragm, vagina 96.17
drainage tube
kidney 55.02
pelvis 55.12
renal pelvis 55.12
Dynesys® 84.82
elbow prosthesis (total) 81.84
revision 81.97
electrode(s)
bone growth stimulator (invasive) (percutaneous) (semi-invasive)—*see* category 78.9
brain 02.93
depth 02.93
foramen ovale 02.93
sphenoidal 02.96
depth 02.93
foramen ovale 02.93
gastric 04.92

Insertion—*continued*
heart (initial) (transvenous) 37.70
atrium (initial) 37.73
replacement 37.76
atrium and ventricle (initial) 37.72
replacement 37.76
epicardium (sternotomy or thoracotomy approach) 37.74
left ventricular coronary venous system 00.52
temporary transvenous pacemaker system 37.78
during and immediately following cardiac surgery 39.64
ventricle (initial) 37.71
replacement 37.76
intracranial 02.93
osteogenic (for bone growth stimulation)—*see* category 78.9
peripheral nerve 04.92
sacral nerve 04.92
sphenoidal 02.96
spine 03.93
electroencephalographic receiver—*see* Implant, electroencephalographic receiver, by site
electronic stimulator—*see* Implant, electronic stimulator, by site
electrostimulator—*see* Implant, electronic stimulator, by site
endograft(s), endovascular graft(s)
endovascular, abdominal aorta 39.71
fenestrated (branching) 39.78
endovascular, head and neck vessels 39.72
endovascular, other vessels (for aneurysm) 39.79
endovascular, thoracic aorta 39.73
endoprosthesis
bile duct 51.87
femoral head (bipolar) 81.52
pancreatic duct 52.93
envelope, antimicrobial 17.81
epidural pegs 02.93
external fixation device (bone)—*see* category 78.1
eye valve implant 12.67
facial bone implant (alloplastic) (synthetic) 76.92
filling material, skin (filling of defect) 86.02
filter
vena cava (inferior) (superior) (transvenous) 38.7
fixator, mini device (bone)—*see* category 78.1
frame (stereotactic)
for radiosurgery 93.59
Gardner Wells tongs (skull) (with synchronous skeletal traction) 02.94
gastric bubble (balloon) 44.93
globe, into eye socket 16.69
Greenfield filter 38.7
halo device (skull) (with synchronous skeletal traction) 02.94
Harrington rod—*see also* Fusion, spinal, by level
with dorsal, dorsolumbar fusion 81.05
Harris pin 79.15
heart
assist system—*see* Implant, heart assist system
cardiac support device (CSD) 37.41
circulatory assist system—*see* Implant, heart assist system
CorCap™ 37.41
epicardial support device 37.41
Impella® 37.68

Insertion—*continued*

pacemaker—*see* Insertion, pacemaker, cardiac
prosthetic cardiac support device 37.41
pump (Kantrowitz) 37.62
valve—*see* Replacement, heart valve
ventricular support device 37.41
hip prosthesis (partial) 81.52
    revision NOS 81.53
        acetabular and femoral components (total)
            00.70
        acetabular component only 00.71
        acetabular liner and/or femoral head only
            00.73
        femoral component only 00.72
        femoral head only and/or acetabular liner
            00.73
        partial
            acetabular component only 00.71
            acetabular liner and/or femoral head only
                00.73
            femoral component only 00.72
            femoral head only and/or acetabular liner
                00.73
        total (acetabular and femoral components)
            00.70
    total 81.51
        revision
            acetabular and femoral components (total)
                00.70
            total (acetabular and femoral components)
                00.70
Holter valve 02.22
Hufnagel valve—*see* Replacement, heart valve
implant—*see* Insertion, prosthesis
infusion pump 86.06
interbody spinal fusion device 84.51
intercostal catheter (with water seal) for drainage
    34.04
    revision (with lysis of adhesions) 34.04
    thoracoscopic 34.06
intra-arterial blood gas monitoring system 89.60
intrauterine
    contraceptive device 69.7
    radium (intracavitary) 69.91
    tamponade (nonobstetric) 69.91
Kantrowitz
    heart pump 37.62
    pulsation balloon (phase-shift) 37.61
keratoprosthesis 11.73
King-Mills umbrella device (heart) 35.52
Kirschner wire 93.44
    with reduction of fracture or dislocation—*see*
        Reduction, fracture *and* Reduction,
        dislocation
knee prosthesis (partial) (total) 81.54
    revision NOS 81.55
        femoral component 00.82
        partial
            femoral component 00.82
            patellar component 00.83
            tibial component 00.81
            tibial insert 00.84
        patellar component 00.83
        tibial component 00.81
        tibial insert 00.84
        total (all components) 00.80
laminaria, cervix 69.93
Lap-Band™ 44.95
larynx, valved tube 31.75
leads—*see* Insertion, electrode(s)

Insertion—*continued*

lens, prosthetic (intraocular) 13.70
    with cataract extraction, one-stage 13.71
    secondary (subsequent to cataract extraction)
        13.72
limb lengthening device, internal, NOS 84.54
    with kinetic distraction 84.53
loop recorder 37.79
M-Brace™ 84.82
metal staples into epiphyseal plate (*see also*
    Stapling, epiphyseal plate) 78.20
minifixator device (bone)—*see* category 78.1
Mobitz-Uddin umbrella, vena cava 38.7
mold, vagina 96.15
Moore (cup) 81.52
myringotomy device (button) (tube) 20.01
    with intubation 20.01
nasobiliary drainage tube (endoscopic) 51.86
nasogastric tube
    for
        decompression, intestinal 96.07
        feeding 96.6
naso-intestinal tube 96.08
nasolacrimal tube or stent 09.44
nasopancreatic drainage tube (endoscopic) 52.97
neuropacemaker—*see* Implant, neurostimulator,
    by site
neurostimulator—*see* Implant, neurostimulator,
    by site
non-coronary vessel
    stent(s) (stent graft)

> *Note: Also use 00.40, 00.41, 00.42, or 00.43 to show the total number of vessels treated. Use code 00.44 once to show procedure on a bifurcated vessel. In addition, use 00.45, 00.46, 00.47, or 00.48 to show the number of vascular stents inserted.*

        basilar 00.64
        carotid 00.63
        extracranial 00.64
        intracranial 00.65
        peripheral 39.90
            bare, drug-coated 39.90
            drug-eluting 00.55
        vertebral 00.64
        with
            angioplasty 39.50
            atherectomy 17.56
            bypass—*omit code*
non-invasive (transcutaneous) (surface)
    stimulator 99.86
obturator (orthodontic) 24.7
ocular implant
    with synchronous
        enucleation 16.42
            with muscle attachment to implant 16.41
        evisceration 16.31
    following or secondary to
        enucleation 16.61
        evisceration 16.61
Ommaya reservoir 02.22
orbital implant (stent) (outside muscle cone)
    16.69
    with orbitotomy 16.02
orthodontic appliance (obturator) (wiring) 24.7
outflow tract prosthesis (gusset type) (heart)
    in
        pulmonary valvuloplasty 35.26
        total repair of tetralogy of Fallot 35.81

Insertion—*continued*
pacemaker
brain—*see* Implant, neurostimulator, brain
cardiac (device) (initial) (permanent)
(replacement) 37.80
dual-chamber device (initial) 37.83
replacement 37.87
during and immediately following cardiac
surgery 39.64
resynchronization (biventricular pacemaker)
(BiV pacemaker) (CRT-P) (device)
device only (initial) (replacement) 00.53
total system (device and one or more leads)
00.50
transvenous lead into left ventricular
coronary venous system 00.52
single-chamber device (initial) 37.81
rate responsive 37.82
replacement 37.85
rate responsive 37.86
temporary transvenous pacemaker system
37.78
during and immediately following cardiac
surgery 39.64
carotid 39.89
gastric 04.92
heart—*see* Insertion, pacemaker, cardiac
intracranial—*see* Implant, neurostimulator,
intracranial
neural—*see* Implant, neurostimulator, by site
peripheral nerve—*see* Implant, neurostimulator,
peripheral nerve
spine—*see* Implant, neurostimulator, spine
pacing catheter—*see* Insertion, pacemaker,
cardiac
pack
auditory canal, external 96.11
cervix (nonobstetrical) 67.0
after delivery or abortion 75.8
to assist delivery or induce labor 73.1
rectum 96.19
sella turcica 07.79
vagina (nonobstetrical) 96.14
after delivery or abortion 75.8
palatal implant 27.64
penis, prosthetic (non-inflatable) (internal) 64.95
inflatable (internal) 64.97
peridontal splint (orthodontic) 24.7
peripheral blood vessel—*see* non-coronary
pessary
cervix 96.18
to assist delivery or induce labor 73.1
vagina 96.18
pharyngeal valve, artificial 31.75
port, vascular access 86.07
prostaglandin suppository (for abortion) 96.49

Insertion—*continued*
prosthesis, prosthetic device
acetabulum (partial) 81.52
hip 81.52
revision NOS 81.53
acetabular and femoral components (total)
00.70
acetabular component only 00.71
acetabular liner and/or femoral head only
00.73
femoral component only 00.72
femoral head only and/or acetabular liner
00.73
partial
acetabular component only 00.71
acetabular liner and/or femoral head
only 00.73
femoral component only 00.72
femoral head only and/or acetabular
liner 00.73
total (acetabular and femoral components)
00.70
ankle (total) 81.56
arm (bioelectric) (cineplastic) (kineplastic)
84.44
biliary tract 51.99
breast (bilateral) 85.54
unilateral 85.53
cardiac support device (CSD) (CorCap™)
37.41
chin (polyethylene) (silastic) 76.68
elbow (total) 81.84
revision 81.97
extremity (bioelectric) (cineplastic)
(kineplastic) 84.40
lower 84.48
upper 84.44
fallopian tube 66.93
femoral head (Austin-Moore) (bipolar) (Eicher)
(Thompson) 81.52
hip (partial) 81.52
revision NOS 81.53
acetabular and femoral components (total)
00.70
acetabular component only 00.71
acetabular liner and/or femoral head only
00.73
femoral component only 00.72
femoral head only and/or acetabular liner
00.73
partial
acetabular component only 00.71
acetabular liner and/or femoral head
only 00.73
femoral component only 00.72
femoral head only and/or acetabular
liner 00.73
total (acetabular and femoral components)
00.70
total 81.51
revision
acetabular and femoral components (total)
00.70
total (acetabular and femoral components)
00.70
joint—*see* Arthroplasty

Insertion—*continued*

knee (partial) (total) 81.54
  revision NOS 81.55
    femoral component 00.82
    partial
      femoral component 00.82
      patellar component 00.83
      tibial component 00.81
      tibial insert 00.84
    patellar component 00.83
    tibial component 00.81
    tibial insert 00.84
    total (all components) 00.80
leg (bioelectric) (cineplastic) (kineplastic) 84.48
lens 13.91
ocular (secondary) 16.61
  with orbital exenteration 16.42
outflow tract (gusset type) (heart)
  in
    pulmonary valvuloplasty 35.26
    total repair of tetralogy of Fallot 35.81
penile (non-inflatable) (internal) 64.95
  inflatable (internal) 64.97
  with
    construction 64.43
    reconstruction 64.44
Rosen (for urinary incontinence) 59.79
shoulder
  partial 81.81
  revision 81.97
  total, NEC 81.80
    other 81.80
    reverse 81.88
spine
  artificial disc, NOS 84.60
    cervical 84.62
      nucleus 84.61
      partial 84.61
      total 84.62
    lumbar, lumbosacral 84.65
      nucleus 84.64
      partial 84.64
      total 84.65
    thoracic (partial) (total) 84.63
    other device 84.59
testicular (bilateral) (unilateral) 62.7
toe 81.57
  for hallux valgus repair 77.59
vagina
  synthetic 70.95
pseudophakos (*see also* Insertion, lens) 13.70
pump, infusion 86.06
radioactive isotope 92.27
radium 92.27
radon seeds 92.27
Reuter bobbin (with intubation) 20.01
Rickham, reservoir 02.22
Rosen prosthesis (for urinary incontinence) 59.79
Scribner shunt 39.93
Sengstaken-Blakemore tube 96.06
sensor (lead)
  intra-aneurysm sac pressure monitoring device
    00.58
  intra-arterial, for continuous blood gas
    monitoring 89.60
  intracardiac or great vessel hemodynamic
    monitoring
    with lead 00.56
    without lead 38.26
shunt—*see* Shunt
sieve, vena cava 38.7
skeletal muscle stimulator 83.92

Insertion—*continued*

skull
  plate 02.05
  stereotactic frame 93.59
  tongs (Barton) (caliper) (Garder Wells) (Vinke)
    (with synchronous skeletal traction) 02.94
spacer (cement) (joint) (methylmethacrylate)
  84.56
spine 84.51
sphenoidal electrodes 02.96
spine
  bone void filler
    that with percutaneous vertebral
      augmentation 81.66
    that with percutaneous vertebroplasty 81.65
  cage (BAK) 84.51
  facet replacement device(s) 84.84
  interbody spinal fusion device 84.51
  interspinous process decompression device
    84.80
  non-fusion stabilization device —*see* category
    84.8
  pedicle-based dynamic stabilization device(s)
    84.82
  posterior motion preservation device(s) —*see*
    category 84.8
  spacer 84.51
Spitz-Holter valve 02.2
Steinmann pin 93.44
  with reduction of fracture or dislocation—*see*
    Reduction, fracture *and* Reduction,
    dislocation
stent(s) (stent graft)
  aqueous drainage 12.67
  artery (bare) (bonded) (drug-coated)
    (non-drug-eluting)

> *Note: Also use 00.40, 00.41, 00.42, or 00.43 to show the total number of vessels treated. Use code 00.44 once to show procedure on a bifurcated vessel. In addition, use 00.45, 00.46, 00.47, or 00.48 to show the number of vascular stents inserted.*

    basilar 00.64
    carotid 00.63
    cerebrovascular
      cerebral (intracranial) 00.65
      precerebral (extracranial) 00.64
        carotid 00.63
    coronary (bare) (bonded) (drug-coated)
      (non-drug-eluting) 36.06
      drug-eluting 36.07
    extracranial 00.64
      carotid 00.63
    femoral artery, superficial 39.90
      drug-eluting 00.60
      non-drug eluting 39.90
    intracranial 00.65
    non-coronary vessel
      basilar 0.64
      carotid 00.63
      extracranial 00.64
      femoral artery, superficial 39.90
        drug eluting 00.60
        non-drug eluting 39.90
      intracranial 00.65
    peripheral 39.90
      bare, drug-coated 39.90
      drug-eluting 00.55
      femoral artery, superficial, drug eluting
        00.60
    vertebral 00.64

Insertion—*continued*
  bile duct 51.43
    endoscopic 51.87
    percutaneous transhepatic 51.98
  colon
    endoscopic (fluoroscopic guidance) 46.86
    other 46.87
  coronary (artery) (bare) (bonded) (drug-coated)
    (non-drug-eluting) 36.06

Note: Also use 00.40, 00.41, 00.42, or 00.43 to show the total number of vessels treated. Use code 00.44 once to show procedure on a bifurcated vessel. In addition, use 00.45, 00.46, 00.47, or 00.48 to show the number of vascular stents inserted.

    drug-eluting 36.07
  esophagus (endoscopic) (fluoroscopic) 42.81
  mesenteric 39.90
    bare, drug-coated 39.90
    drug-eluting 00.55
  non-coronary vessel

Note: Also use 00.40, 00.41, 00.42, or 00.43 to show the total number of vessels treated. Use code 00.44 once to show procedure on a bifurcated vessel. In addition, use 00.45, 00.46, 00.47, or 00.48 to show the number of vascular stents inserted.

    basilar 00.64
    carotid 00.63
    extracranial 00.64
    intracranial 00.65
    mesenteric 39.90
      bare, drug-coated 39.90
      drug-eluting 00.55
    peripheral 39.90
      bare, drug-coated 39.90
      drug-eluting 00.55
    renal 39.90
      bare, drug-coated 39.90
      drug-eluting 00.55
    vertebral 00.64
      with angioplasty or atherectomy 39.50
  pancreatic duct 52.92
    endoscopic 52.93
  peripheral 39.90

Note: Also use 00.40, 00.41, 00.42, or 00.43 to show the total number of vessels treated. Use code 00.44 once to show procedure on a bifurcated vessel. In addition, use 00.45, 00.46, 00.47, or 00.48 to show the number of vascular stents inserted.

    bare, drug-coated 39.90
    drug-eluting 00.55
  precerebral 00.64

Note: Also use 00.40, 00.41, 00.42, or 00.43 to show the total number of vessels treated. Use code 00.44 once to show procedure on a bifurcated vessel. In addition, use 00.45, 00.46, 00.47, or 00.48 to show the number of vascular stents inserted.

  renal 39.90
    bare, drug-coated 39.90
    drug-eluting 00.55

Insertion—*continued*
  subclavian 39.90

Note: Also use 00.40, 00.41, 00.42, or 00.43 to show the total number of vessels treated. Use code 00.44 once to show procedure on a bifurcated vessel. In addition, use 00.45, 00.46, 00.47, or 00.48 to show the number of vascular stents inserted.

    bare, drug-coated 39.90
    drug-eluting 00.55
  tracheobronchial 96.05
  vertebral 00.64

Note: Also use 00.40, 00.41, 00.42, or 00.43 to show the total number of vessels treated. Use code 00.44 once to show procedure on a bifurcated vessel. In addition, use 00.45, 00.46, 00.47, or 00.48 to show the number of vascular stents inserted.

  sternal fixation device with rigid plates 84.94
  stimoceiver—*see* Implant, neurostimulator, by
    site
  stimulator for bone growth—*see* category 78.9
  subdural
    grids 02.93
    strips 02.93
  suppository
    prostaglandin (for abortion) 96.49
    vagina 96.49
  Swan-Ganz catheter (pulmonary) 89.64
  tampon
    esophagus 96.06
    uterus 69.91
    vagina 96.14
      after delivery or abortion 75.8
  Tandem™ heart 37.68
  telescope (IMT) (miniature) 13.91
  testicular prosthesis (bilateral) (unilateral) 62.7
  tissue expander (skin) NEC 86.93
    breast 85.95
  tissue mandril (peripheral vessel) (Dacron)
    (Spark's type) 39.99
    with
      blood vessel repair 39.56
      vascular bypass or shunt—*see* Bypass,
        vascular
  tongs, skull (with synchronous skeletal traction)
    02.94
  totally implanted device for bone growth
    (invasive)—*see* category 78.9
  tube—*see also* Catheterization *and* Intubation
    bile duct 51.43
      endoscopic 51.87
    chest 34.04
      revision (with lysis of adhesions) 34.04
        thoracoscopic 34.06
      thoracoscopic 34.06
    endotracheal 96.04
    esophagus (nonoperative) (Sengstaken) 96.06
      permanent (silicone) (Souttar) 42.81
    feeding
      esophageal 42.81
      gastric 96.6
      nasogastric 96.6
    gastric
      by gastrostomy—*see* category 43.1
      for
        decompression, intestinal 96.07
        feeding 96.6

Insertion—*continued*
   intercostal catheter (with water seal), for
      drainage 34.04
      revision (with lysis of adhesions) 34.04
      thoracoscopic 34.06
   Miller-Abbott (for intestinal decompression)
      96.08
   nasobiliary (drainage) 51.86
   nasogastric (for intestinal decompression) NEC
      96.07
   naso-intestinal 96.08
   nasopancreatic drainage (endoscopic) 52.97
   pancreatic duct 52.92
      endoscopic 52.93
   rectum 96.09
   stomach (nasogastric) (for intestinal
      decompression) NEC 96.07
      for feeding 96.6
   tracheobronchial 96.05
  umbrella device
   atrial septum (King-Nos) 35.52
   vena cava (Mobitz-Uddin) 38.7
  ureteral stent (transurethral) 59.8
   with ureterotomy 59.8 *[56.2]*
  urinary sphincter, artificial (AUS) (inflatable)
     58.93
  vaginal mold 96.15
  valve(s)
   bronchus
    multiple lobes 33.73
    single lobe 33.71
   Holter 02.22
   Hufnagel—*see* Replacement, heart valve
   pharyngeal (artificial) 31.75
   Spitz-Holter 02.22
   vas deferens 63.95
  vascular access device, totally implantable 86.07
  vena cava sieve or umbrella 38.7
  Vinke tongs (skull) (with synchronous skeletal
     traction) 02.94
  X Stop™ 84.80
Instillation
  bladder 96.49
  digestive tract, except gastric gavage 96.43
  genitourinary NEC 96.49
  radioisotope (intracavitary) (intravenous) 92.28
  thoracic cavity 34.92
Insufflation
  Eustachian tube 20.8
  fallopian tube (air) (dye) (gas) (saline) 66.8
   for radiography—*see* Hysterosalpingography
   therapeutic substance 66.95
  lumbar retroperitoneal, bilateral 88.15
Intercricothyroidotomy (for assistance in
    breathing) 31.1
Interleukin-2, infusion
  high-dose 00.15
  low-dose 99.28
Intermittent positive pressure breathing
   (IPPB) 93.91
Interposition operation
  esophageal reconstruction (intrathoracic)
    (retrosternal) NEC (*see also* Anastomosis,
    esophagus, with, interposition) 42.58
   antesternal or antethoracic NEC (*see also*
    Anastomosis, esophagus, antesternal, with,
    interposition) 42.68
  uterine suspension 69.21

Interrogation
  cardioverter-defibrillator, automatic (AICD)
   with catheter based invasive electrophysiologic
    testing 37.26
   with NIPS (arrhythmia induction) 37.20
   interrogation only (bedside device check) 89.49
  CRT-D (cardiac resynchronization defibrillator)
   with catheter based invasive electrophysiologic
    testing 37.26
   with NIPS (arrhythmia induction) 37.20
   interrogation only (bedside device check) 89.49
  CRT-P (cardiac resynchronization pacemaker)
   with catheter based invasive electrophysiologic
    testing 37.26
   with NIPS (arrhythmia induction) 37.20
   interrogation only (bedside device check) 89.45
  pacemaker
   with catheter based invasive electrophysiologic
    testing 37.26
   with NIPS (arrhythmia induction) 37.20
   interrogation only (bedside device check) 89.45
Interruption
  vena cava (inferior) (superior) 38.7
Interview (evaluation) (diagnostic)
  medical, except psychiatric 89.05
   brief (abbreviated history) 89.01
   comprehensive (history and evaluation of new
    problem) 89.03
   limited (interval history) 89.02
   specified type NEC 89.04
  psychiatric NEC 94.19
   follow-up 94.19
   initial 94.19
   pre-commitment 94.13
Intimectomy 38.10
  abdominal 38.16
  aorta (arch) (ascending) (descending) 38.14
  head and neck NEC 38.12
  intracranial NEC 38.11
  lower limb 38.18
  thoracic NEC 38.15
  upper limb 38.13
Intraoperative anesthetic effect monitoring and
   titration (IAEMT) 00.94 *[89.14]*
Introduction
  orthodontic appliance 24.7
  therapeutic substance (acting locally or
    systemically) NEC 99.29
   bursa 83.96
    hand 82.94
   fascia 83.98
    hand 82.96
   heart 37.92
   joint 81.92
    temporomandibular 76.96
   ligament (joint) 81.92
   pericardium 37.93
   soft tissue NEC 83.98
    hand 82.96
   tendon 83.97
    hand 82.95
   vein 39.92
Intubation —*see also* Catheterization *and*
   Insertion
  bile duct(s) 51.59
   common 51.51
    endoscopic 51.87
   endoscopic 51.87
  esophagus (nonoperative) (Sengstaken) 96.06
   permanent tube (silicone) (Souttar) 42.81
  Eustachian tube 20.8

Intubation—*continued*
intestine (for decompression) 96.08
lacrimal for
  dilation 09.42
    tear drainage, intranasal 09.81
larynx 96.05
nasobiliary (drainage) 51.86
nasogastric
  for
    decompression, intestinal 96.07
    feeding 96.6
naso-intestinal 96.08
nasolacrimal (duct) (with irrigation) 09.44
nasopancreatic drainage (endoscopic) 52.97
respiratory tract NEC 96.05
small intestine (Miller-Abbott) 96.08
stomach (nasogastric) (for intestinal
  decompression) NEC 96.07
  for feeding 96.6
trachea 96.04
ventriculocisternal 02.22
Invagination, diverticulum
gastric 44.69
  laparoscopic 44.68
pharynx 29.59
stomach 44.69
  laparoscopic 44.68
Inversion
appendix 47.99
diverticulum
  gastric 44.69
    laparoscopic 44.68
  intestine
    large 45.49
      endoscopic 45.43
    small 45.34
  stomach 44.69
    laparoscopic 44.68
tunica vaginalis 61.49
IOERT (intra-operative electron radiation
  therapy) 92.41
IOM (intra-operative neurophysiologic
  monitoring) 00.94
Ionization, medical 99.27
Iontherapy 99.27
Iontophoresis 99.27
Iridectomy (basal) (buttonhole) (optical)
  (peripheral) (total) 12.14
  with
    capsulectomy 13.65
    cataract extraction—*see* Extraction, cataract
    filtering operation (for glaucoma) NEC 12.65
    scleral
      fistulization 12.65
      thermocauterization 12.62
      trephination 12.61
Iridencleisis 12.63
Iridesis 12.63
Irido-capsulectomy 13.65
Iridocyclectomy 12.44
Iridocystectomy 12.42
Iridodesis 12.63
Iridoplasty NEC 12.39
Iridosclerectomy 12.65
Iridosclerotomy 12.69
Iridotasis 12.63
Iridotomy 12.12
  by photocoagulation 12.12
  with transfixion 12.11
  for iris bombé 12.11
  specified type NEC 12.12

Iron lung 93.99
Irradiation
gamma, stereotactic 92.32
Irrigation
anterior chamber (eye) 12.91
bronchus NEC 96.56
canaliculus 09.42
catheter
  ureter 96.46
  urinary, indwelling NEC 96.48
  vascular 96.57
  ventricular 02.41
  wound 96.58
cholecystostomy 96.41
cornea 96.51
  with removal of foreign body 98.21
corpus cavernosum 64.98
cystostomy 96.47
ear (removal of cerumen) 96.52
enterostomy 96.36
eye 96.51
  with removal of foreign body 98.21
gastrostomy 96.36
lacrimal
  canaliculi 09.42
  punctum 09.41
muscle 83.02
  hand 82.02
nasal
  passages 96.53
  sinus 22.00
nasolacrimal duct 09.43
  with insertion of tube or stent 09.44
nephrostomy 96.45
peritoneal 54.25
pyelostomy 96.45
rectal 96.39
stomach 96.33
tendon (sheath) 83.01
  hand 82.01
trachea NEC 96.56
traumatic cataract 13.3
tube
  biliary NEC 96.41
  nasogastric NEC 96.34
  pancreatic 96.42
ureterostomy 96.46
ventricular shunt 02.41
wound (cleaning) NEC 96.59
Irving operation (tubal ligation) 66.32
Irwin operation (*see also* Osteotomy) 77.30
Ischiectomy (partial) 77.89
total 77.99
Ischiopubiotomy 77.39
Isolation
after contact with infectious disease 99.84
ileal loop 45.51
intestinal segment or pedicle nap
  large 45.52
  small 45.51
Isthmectomy, thyroid (*see also* Thyroidectomy,
  partial) 06.39
IVUS —see Ultrasound, intravascular, by site

J-K

Joulay operation (gastroduodenostomy) 44.39
  laparoscopic 44.38
Janeway operation (permanent gastrostomy)
  43.19
Jatene operation (arterial switch) 35.84
Jejunectomy 45.62
Jejunocecostomy 45.93
Jejunocholecystostomy 51.32
Jejunocolostomy 45.93
Jejunoileostomy 45.91
Jejunojejunostomy 45.91
Jejunopexy 46.61
Jejunorrhaphy 46.73
Jejunostomy (feeding) 46.39
  delayed opening 46.31
  loop 46.01
  percutaneous (endoscopic) (PEJ) 46.32
  revision 46.41
Jejunotomy 45.02
Johanson operation (urethral reconstruction)
  58.46
Jones operation
  claw toe (transfer of extensor hallucis longus
    tendon) 77.57
    modified (with arthrodesis) 77.57
  dacryocystorhinostomy 09.81
  hammer toe (interphalangeal fusion) 77.56
    modified (tendon transfer with arthrodesis) 77.57
  repair of peroneal tendon 83.88
Joplin operation (exostectomy with tendon
  transfer) 77.53

Kader operation (temporary gastrostomy) 43.19
Kasai portoenterostomy 51.37
Kaufman operation (for urinary stress
  incontinence) 59.79
Kazanjiian operation (buccal vestibular sulcus
  extension) 24.91
Kehr operation (hepatopexy) 50.69
Keller operation (bunionectomy) 77.59
Kelly (Kennedy) operation (urethrovesical
  plication) 59.3
Kelly-Stoeckel operation (urethrovesical
  plication) 59.3
Kelotomy 53.9
Keratectomy (complete) (partial) (superficial)
  11.49
  for pterygium 11.39
    with corneal graft 11.32
Keratocentesis (for hyphema) 12.91
Keratomileusis 11.71
Keratophakia 11.72
Keratoplasty (tectonic) (with autograft) (with
  homograft) 11.60
  lamellar (nonpenetrating) (with homograft) 11.62
    with autograft 11.61
  penetrating (full-thickness) (with homograft)
    11.64
    with autograft 11.63
  perforating—*see* Keratoplasty, penetrating
  refractive 11.71
  specified type NEC 11.69
Keratoprosthesis 11.73
Keratotomy (delimiting) (posterior) 11.1
  radial (refractive) 11.75
Kerr operation (low cervical cesarean section)
  74.1
Kessler operation (arthroplasty, carpometacarpal
  joint) 81.74
Kidner operation (excision of accessory
  navicular bone) (with tendon transfer) 77.98
Killian operation (frontal sinusotomy) 22.41
Kineplasty —*see* Cineplasty
King-Steelquist operation (hindquarter
  amputation) 84.19
Kirk operation (amputation through thigh) 84.17
Kock pouch operation
  bowel anastomosis—*omit code*
  continent ileostomy 46.22
  cutaneous uretero-ileostomy 56.51
  ESWL (extracorporeal shockwave lithotripsy)
    98.51
  removal, calculus 57.19
  revision, cutaneous uretero-ileostomy 56.52
  urinary diversion procedure 56.51
Kondoleon operation (correction of
  lymphedema) 40.9
Krause operation (sympathetic denervation)
  05.29
Kroener operation (partial salpingectomy) 66.69
Kroenlein operation (lateral orbitotomy) 16.01
Krönig operation (low cervical cesarean section)
  74.1
Krukenberg operation (reconstruction of
  below-elbow amputation) 82.89
Kuhnt-Szymanowski operation (ectropion
  repair with lid reconstruction) 08.44
Kyphoplasty 81.66

L

Labbe operation (gastrotomy) 43.0
Labiectomy (bilateral) 71.62
  unilateral 71.61
Labyrinthectomy (transtympanic) 20.79
Labyrinthotomy (transtympanic) 20.79
Ladd operation (mobilization of intestine) 54.95
Lagrange operation (iridosclerectomy) 12.65
Lambrinudi operation (triple arthrodesis) 81.12
Laminectomy (decompression) (for exploration)
  03.09
  as operative approach—*omit code*
  with
    excision of herniated intervertebral disc
      (nucleus pulposus) 80.51
    excision of other intraspinal lesion (tumor) 03.4
  reopening of site 03.02
Laminography —*see* Radiography
Laminoplasty, expansile 03.09
Laminotomy (decompression) (for exploration)
  03.09
  as operative approach—*omit code*
  reopening of site 03.02
Langenbeck operation (cleft palate repair) 27.62
Laparoamnioscopy 75.31
Laparorrhaphy 54.63
Laparoscopy 54.21
  with
    biopsy (intra-abdominal) 54.24
      uterine ligaments 68.15
      uterus 68.16
    destruction of fallopian tubes—*see* Destruction,
      fallopian tube
Laparotomy NEC 54.19
  as operative approach—*omit code*
  exploratory (pelvic) 54.11
  reopening of recent operative site (for control of
    hemorrhage) (for exploration) (for incision of
    hematoma) 54.12
Laparotrachelotomy 74.1
Lapidus operation (bunionectomy with
  metatarsal osteotomy) 77.51
Larry operation (shoulder disarticulation) 84.08
Laryngectomy
  with radical neck dissection (with synchronous
    thyroidectomy) (with synchronous
    tracheostomy) 30.4
  complete (with partial laryngectomy) (with
    synchronous tracheostomy) 30.3
    with radical neck dissection (with synchronous
      thyroidectomy) (with synchronous
      tracheostomy) 30.4
  frontolateral partial (extended) 30.29
  glottosupraglottic partial 30.29
  lateral partial 30.29
  partial (frontolateral) (glottosupraglottic) (lateral)
    (submucous) (supraglottic) (vertical) 30.29
  radical (with synchronous thyroidectomy) (with
    synchronous tracheostomy) 30.4
  submucous (partial) 30.29
  supraglottic partial 30.29
  total (with partial pharyngectomy) (with
    synchronous tracheostomy) 30.3
    with radical neck dissection (with synchronous
      thyroidectomy) (with synchronous
      tracheostomy) 30.4
  vertical partial 30.29
  wide field 30.3

Laryngocentesis 31.3
Laryngoesophagectomy 30.4
Laryngofissure 30.29
Laryngogram 87.09
  contrast 87.07
Laryngopharyngectomy (with synchronous
  tracheostomy) 30.3
  radical (with synchronous thyroidectomy) 30.4
Laryngopharyngoesophagectomy (with
  synchronous tracheostomy) 30.3
  with radical neck dissection (with synchronous
    thyroidectomy) 30.4
Laryngoplasty 31.69
Laryngorrhaphy 31.61
Laryngoscopy (suspension) (through artificial
  stoma) 31.42
Laryngostomy (permanent) 31.29
  revision 31.63
  temporary (emergency) 31.1
Laryngotomy 31.3
Laryngotracheobronchoscopy 33.23
  with biopsy 33.24
Laryngotracheoscopy 31.42
Laryngotracheostomy (permanent) 31.29
  temporary (emergency) 31.1
Laryngotracheotomy (temporary) 31.1
  permanent 31.29
Laser —*see also* Coagulation, Destruction, *and*
  Photocoagulation by site
  angioplasty, percutaneous transluminal 39.59
  coronary—*see* angioplasty, coronary
Laser interstitial thermal therapy (LITT)
  under guidance
  lesion
    brain 17.61
    breast 17.69
    head and neck 17.62
    liver 17.63
    lung 17.69
    prostate 17.69
    thyroid 17.62
Lash operation
  internal cervical os repair 67.59
  laparoscopic supracervical hysterectomy 68.31
LASIK (Laser-assisted in situ keratomileusis)
  11.71
Latzko operation
  cesarean section 74.2
  colpocleisis 70.8
Lavage
  antral 22.00
  bronchus NEC 96.56
    diagnostic (endoscopic) bronchoalveolar lavage
      (BAL) (Mini-BAL) 33.24
  endotracheal 96.56
  gastric 96.33
  lung (total) (whole) 33.99
    diagnostic (endoscopic) bronchoalveolar lavage
      (BAL) 33.24
  nasal sinus(es) 22.00
    by puncture 22.01
    through natural ostium 22.02
  peritoneal (diagnostic) 54.25
  trachea NEC 96.56
Leadbetter operation (urethral reconstruction)
  58.46
Leadbetter-Politano operation
  (ureteroneocystostomy) 56.74

LEEP (loop elecrosurgical excision procedure) of cervix 67.32
Le Fort operation (colpocleisis) 70.8
LeMesurier operation (cleft lip repair) 27.54
Lengthening
  bone (with bone graft) 78.30
    femur 78.35
    for reconstruction of thumb 82.69
    specified site NEC (*see also* category 78.3) 78.39
    tibia 78.37
    ulna 78.33
  extraocular muscle NEC 15.21
    multiple (two or more muscles) 15.4
  fascia 83.89
    hand 82.89
  hamstring NEC 83.85
  heel cord 83.85
  leg
    femur 78.35
    tibia 78.37
  levator palpebrae muscle 08.38
  muscle 83.85
    extraocular 15.21
      multiple (two or more muscles) 15.4
    hand 82.55
  palate 27.62
    secondary or subsequent 27.63
  tendon 83.85
    for claw toe repair 77.57
    hand 82.55
Leriche operation (periarterial sympathectomy) 05.25
Leucotomy, leukotomy 01.32
Leukopheresis, therapeutic 99.72
Lid suture operation (blepharoptosis) 08.31
Ligation
  adrenal vessel (artery) (vein) 07.43
  aneurysm 39.52
  appendages, dermal 86.26
  arteriovenous fistula 39.53
    coronary artery 36.99
  artery 38.80
    abdominal 38.86
    adrenal 07.43
    aorta (arch) (ascending) (descending) 38.84
    coronary (anomalous) 36.99
    ethmoidal 21.04
    external carotid 21.06
    for control of epistaxis—*see* Control, epistaxis
    head and neck NEC 38.82
    intracranial NEC 38.81
    lower limb 38.88
    maxillary (transantral) 21.05
    middle meningeal 02.13
    thoracic NEC 38.85
    thyroid 06.92
    upper limb 38.83
  atrium, heart 37.99
  auricle, heart 37.99
  bleeding vessel—*see* Control, hemorrhage
  blood vessel 38.80
    abdominal
      artery 38.86
      vein 38.87
    adrenal 07.43
    aorta (arch) (ascending) (descending) 38.84
    esophagus 42.91
      endoscopic 42.33
    head and neck NEC 38.82
    intracranial NEC 38.81

Ligation—*continued*
  lower limb
    artery 38.88
    vein 38.89
  meningeal (artery) (longitudinal sinus) 02.13
  thoracic NEC 38.85
  thyroid 06.92
  upper limb (artery) (vein) 38.83
  bronchus 33.92
  cisterna chyli 40.64
  coronary
    artery (anomalous) 36.99
    sinus 36.39
  dermal appendage 86.26
  ductus arteriosus, patent 38.85
  esophageal vessel 42.91
    endoscopic 42.33
  ethmoidal artery 21.04
  external carotid artery 21.06
  fallopian tube (bilateral) (remaining) (solitary) 66.39
    by endoscopy (culdoscopy) (hysteroscopy) (laparoscopy) (peritoneoscopy) 66.29
    with
      crushing 66.31
        by endoscopy (laparoscopy) 66.21
      division 66.32
        by endoscopy (culdoscopy) (laparoscopy) (peritoneoscopy) 66.22
      Falope ring 66.39
        by endoscopy (laparoscopy) 66.29
    unilateral 66.92
  fistula, arteriovenous 39.53
    coronary artery 36.99
  gastric
    artery 38.86
    varices 44.91
      endoscopic 43.41
  hemorrhoids 49.45
  longitudinal sinus (superior) 02.13
  lymphatic (channel) (peripheral) 40.9
    thoracic duct 40.64
  maxillary artery 21.05
  meningeal vessel 02.13
  spermatic
    cord 63.72
      varicocele 63.1
    vein (high) 63.1
  splenic vessels 38.86
  subclavian artery 38.85
  superior longitudinal sinus 02.13
  supernumerary digit 86.26
  thoracic duct 40.64
  thyroid vessel (artery) (vein) 06.92
  toes (supernumerary) 86.26
  tooth 93.55
    impacted 24.6
  ulcer (peptic) (base) (bed) (bleeding vessel) 44.40
    duodenal 44.42
    gastric 44.41
  ureter 56.95
  varices
    esophageal 42.91
      endoscopic 42.33
    gastric 44.91
      endoscopic 43.41
    peripheral vein (lower limb) 38.59
      upper limb 38.53
  varicocele 63.1
  vas deferens 63.71

Ligation—*continued*
vein 38.80
  abdominal 38.87
  adrenal 07.43
  head and neck NEC 38.82
  intracranial NEC 38.81
  lower limb 38.89
  spermatic, high 63.1
  thoracic NEC 38.85
  thyroid 06.92
  upper limb 38.83
  varicose 38.50
    abdominal 38.57
    esophagus 42.91
      endoscopic 42.33
    gastric 44.91
      endoscopic 43.41
    head and neck NEC 38.52
    intracranial NEC 38.51
    lower limb 38.59
    stomach 44.91
    thoracic NEC 38.55
    upper limb 38.53
  vena cava, inferior 38.7
  venous connection between anomalous
    vein to
    left innominate vein 35.82
    superior vena cava 35.82
  wart 86.26
Light coagulation —*see* Photocoagulation
Lindholm operation (repair of ruptured tendon)
  83.88
Lingulectomy, lung 32.39
Linton operation (varicose vein) 38.59
Lipectomy (subcutaneous tissue) (abdominal)
  (submental) 86.83
Liposuction 86.83
Lip reading training 95.49
Lip shave 27.43
Lisfranc operation
  foot amputation 84.12
  shoulder disarticulation 84.08
Litholapaxy, bladder 57.0
  by incision 57.19
Lithotomy
  bile passage 51.49
  bladder (urinary) 57.19
  common duct 51.41
    percutaneous 51.96
  gallbladder 51.04
  hepatic duct 51.49
  kidney 55.01
    percutaneous 55.03
  ureter 56.2
Lithotripsy
  bile duct NEC 51.49
    extracorporeal shockwave (ESWL) 98.52
  bladder 57.0
    extracorporeal shockwave (ESWL) 98.51
    with ultrasonic fragmentation 57.0 *[59.95]*
  extracorporeal shockwave (ESWL) NEC 98.59
    bile duct 98.52
    bladder (urinary) 98.51
    gallbladder 98.52
    kidney 98.51
    Kock pouch 98.51
    renal pelvis 98.51
    specified site NEC 98.59
    ureter 98.51
  gallbladder NEC 51.04
    endoscopic 51.88

Lithotripsy—*continued*
  extracorporeal shockwave (ESWL) 98.52
  kidney 56.0
    extracorporeal shock wave (EWSL) 98.51
    percutaneous nephrostomy with fragmentation
      (laser) (ultrasound) 55.04
  renal pelvis 56.0
    extracorporeal shock wave (EWSL) 98.51
    percutaneous nephrostomy with fragmentation
      (laser) (ultrasound) 55.04
  ureter 56.0
    extracorporeal shockwave (ESWL) 98.51
LITT (laser interstitial thermal therapy)
  under guidance
  lesion
    brain 17.61
    breast 17.69
    head and neck 17.62
    liver 17.63
    lung 17.69
    prostate 17.69
    thyroid 17.62
Littlewood operation (forequarter amputation)
  84.09
LLETZ (large loop excision of the
  transformation zone) of cervix 67.32
Lloyd-Davies operation (abdominoperineal
  resection), NOS 48.50
  laparoscopic 48.51
  open 48.52
  other 48.59
Lobectomy
  brain 01.53
    partial 01.59
  liver (with partial excision of adjacent lobes) 50.3
  lung (complete) 32.49
    partial 32.39
      thoracoscopic 32.30
    segmental (with resection of adjacent lobes)
      32.49
      thoracoscopic 32.41
    thoracoscopic 32.41
  thyroid (total) (unilateral) (with removal of
    isthmus) (with removal of portion of
    remaining lobe) 06.2
    partial (*see also* Thyroidectomy, partial) 06.39
    substernal 06.51
    subtotal (*see also* Thyroidectomy, partial) 06.39
Lobotomy, brain 01.32
Localization, placenta 88.78
  by RISA injection 92.17
Longmire operation (bile duct anastomosis)
  51.39
Loop ileal stoma (*see also* Ileostomy) 46.01
Loopogram 87.78
Looposcopy (ileal conduit) 56.35
Lord operation
  dilation of anal canal for hemorrhoids 49.49
  hemorrhoidectomy 49.49
  orchidopexy 62.5
Lower GI series (x-ray) 87.64
Lucas and Murray operation (knee arthrodesis
  with place) 81.22
Lumpectomy
  breast 85.21
  specified site—*see* Excision, lesion, by site
Lymphadenectomy (simple) (*see also* Excision,
  lymph, node) 40.29
Lymphadenotomy 40.0
Lymphangiectomy (radical) (*see also* Excision,
  lymph, node, by site, radical) 40.50

Lymphangiogram
abdominal 88.04
cervical 87.08
intrathoracic 87.34
lower limb 88.36
pelvic 88.04
upper limb 88.34
Lymphangioplasty 40.9
Lymphangiorrhaphy 40.9
Lymphangiotomy 40.0
Lymphaticostomy 40.9
thoracic duct 40.62
Lysis
adhesions

> *Note:*
> *blunt — omit code*
> *digital — omit code*
> *manual — omit code*
> *mechanical — omit code*
> *without instrumentation — omit code*

abdominal 54.59
laparoscopic 54.51
appendiceal 54.59
laparoscopic 54.51
artery-vein-nerve bundle 39.91
biliary tract 54.59
laparoscopic 54.51
bladder (neck) (intraluminal) 57.12
external 59.11
laparoscopic 59.12
transurethral 57.41
blood vessels 39.91
bone—*see* category 78.4
bursa 83.91
by stretching or manipulation 93.28
hand 82.91
cartilage of joint 93.26
chest wall 33.99
choanae (nasopharynx) 29.54
conjunctiva 10.5
corneovitreal 12.34
cortical (brain) 02.91
ear, middle 20.23
Eustachian tube 20.8
extraocular muscle 15.7
extrauterine 54.59
laparoscopic 54.51
eyelid 08.09
and conjunctiva 10.5
eye muscle 15.7
fallopian tube 65.89
laparoscopic 65.81
fascia 83.91
hand 82.91
by stretching or manipulation 93.26
gallbladder 54.59
laparoscopic 54.51
ganglion (peripheral) NEC 04.49
cranial NEC 04.42
hand 82.91
by stretching or manipulation 93.26
heart 37.10
intestines 54.59
laparoscopic 54.51
iris (posterior) 12.33
anterior 12.32
joint (capsule) (structure) (*see also* Division, joint capsule) 80.40
kidney 59.02
laparoscopic 59.03

Lysis—*continued*
labia (vulva) 71.01
larynx 31.92
liver 54.59
laparoscopic 54.51
lung (for collapse of lung) 33.39
mediastinum 34.99
meninges (spinal) 03.6
cortical 02.91
middle ear 20.23
muscle 83.91
by stretching or manipulation 93.27
extraocular 15.7
hand 82.91
by stretching or manipulation 93.26
nasopharynx 29.54
nerve (peripheral) NEC 04.49
cranial NEC 04.42
roots, spinal 03.6
trigeminal 04.41
nose, nasal 21.91
ocular muscle 15.7
ovary 65.89
laparoscopic 65.81
pelvic 54.59
laparoscopic 54.51
penile 64.93
pericardium 37.12
perineal (female) 71.01
peripheral vessels 39.91
perirectal 48.81
perirenal 59.02
laparoscopic 59.03
peritoneum (pelvic) 54.59
laparoscopic 54.51
periureteral 59.02
laparoscopic 59.03
perivesical 59.11
laparoscopic 59.12
pharynx 29.54
pleura (for collapse of lung) 33.39
spermatic cord 63.94
spinal (cord) (meninges) (nerve roots) 03.6
spleen 54.59
laparoscopic 54.51
tendon 83.91
by stretching or manipulation 93.27
hand 82.91
by stretching or manipulation 93.26
thorax 34.99
tongue 25.93
trachea 31.92
tubo-ovarian 65.89
laparoscopic 65.81
ureter 59.02
with freeing or repositioning of ureter 59.02
intraluminal 56.81
laparoscopic 59.03
urethra (intraluminal) 58.5
uterus 54.59
intraluminal 68.21
laparoscopic 54.51
peritoneal 54.59
laparoscopic 54.51
vagina (intraluminal) 70.13
vitreous (posterior approach) 14.74
anterior approach 14.73
vulva 71.01
goniosynechiae (with injection of air or liquid) 12.31
synechiae (posterior) 12.33
anterior (with injection of air or liquid) 12.32

M

Madlener operation (tubal ligation) 66.31
Magnet extraction
foreign body
  anterior chamber, eye 12.01
  choroid 14.01
  ciliary body 12.01
  conjunctiva 98.22
  cornea 11.0
  eye, eyeball NEC 98.21
    anterior segment 12.01
    posterior segment 14.01
  intraocular (anterior segment) 12.01
  iris 12.01
  lens 13.01
  orbit 98.21
  retina 14.01
  sclera 12.01
  vitreous 14.01
Magnetic resonance imaging (nuclear) *see*
  Imaging, magnetic resonance
Magnuson (Stack) operation (arthroplasty for
  recurrent shoulder dislocation) 81.82
Mako Tactile Guidance System™ [TSG]—*see*
  category 17.4
Malleostapediopexy 19.19
  with incus replacement 19.11
Malström's vacuum extraction 72.79
  with episiotomy 72.71
Mammaplasty —*see* Mammoplasty
Mammectomy —*see also* Mastectomy
  subcutaneous (unilateral) 85.34
    with synchronous implant 85.33
    bilateral 85.36
      with synchronous implant 85.35
Mammilliplasty 85.87
Mammography NEC 87.37
Mammoplasty 85.89
  with
    full-thickness graft 85.83
    muscle flap 85.85
    pedicle graft 85.84
    split-thickness graft 85.82
  amputative (reduction) (bilateral) 85.32
    unilateral 85.31
  augmentation 85.50
    with
      breast implant (bilateral) 85.54
        unilateral 85.53
      injection into breast (bilateral) 85.52
        unilateral 85.51
  reduction (bilateral) 85.32
    unilateral 85.31
  revision 85.89
  size reduction (gynecomastia) (bilateral) 85.32
    unilateral 85.31
Mammotomy 85.0
Manchester (Donald) (Fothergill) operation
  (uterine suspension) 69.22
Mandibulectomy (partial) 76.31
  total 76.42
    with reconstruction 76.41
Maneuver (method)
  Bracht 72.52
  Credé 73.59
  De Lee (key-in-lock) 72.4
  Kristeller 72.54

Maneuver—*continued*
  Lovset's (extraction of arms
    in breech birth) 72.52
  Mauriceau (Smellie-Veit) 72.52
  Pinard (total breech extraction) 72.54
  Prague 72.52
  Ritgen 73.59
  Scanzoni (rotation) 72.4
  Van Hoorn 72.52
  Wigand-Martin 72.52
Manipulation
  with reduction of fracture or dislocation—*see*
    Reduction, fracture *and* Reduction,
    dislocation
  enterostomy stoma (with dilation) 96.24
  intestine (intra-abdominal) 46.80
    large 46.82
    small 46.81
  joint
    adhesions 93.26
      temporomandibular 76.95
    dislocation—*see* Reduction, dislocation
  lacrimal passage (tract) NEC 09.49
  muscle structures 93.27
  musculoskeletal (physical therapy) NEC 93.29
  nasal septum, displaced 21.88
  osteopathic NEC 93.67
    for general mobilization (general articulation)
      93.61
    high-velocity, low-amplitude forces (thrusting)
      93.62
    indirect forces 93.65
    isotonic, isometric forces 93.64
    low-velocity, high-amplitude forces (springing)
      93.63
    to move tissue fluids 93.66
  rectum 96.22
  salivary duct 26.91
  stomach, intraoperative 44.92
  temporomandibular joint NEC 76.95
  ureteral calculus by catheter
    with removal 56.0
    without removal 59.8
  uterus NEC 69.98
    gravid 75.99
    inverted
      manual replacement (following delivery)
        75.94
      surgical—*see* Repair, inverted uterus
Manometry
  esophageal 89.32
  spinal fluid 89.15
  urinary 89.21
Manual arts therapy 93.81
Mapping
  cardiac (electrophysiologic) 37.27
    doppler (flow) 88.72
  electrocardiogram only 89.52
Marckwald operation (cervical os repair) 67.59
Marshall-Marchetti (Krantz) operation
  (retropubic urethral suspension) 59.5
Marsupialization —*see also* Destruction, lesion,
  by site
  cyst
    Bartholin's 71.23
    brain 01.59
    cervical (nabothian) 67.31

Marsupialization—*continued*
  dental 24.4
  dentigerous 24.4
  kidney 55.31
  larynx 30.01
  liver 50.21
  ovary 65.21
    laparoscopic 65.23
  pancreas 52.3
  pilonidal (open excision) (with partial closure)
      86.21
  salivary gland 26.21
  spinal (intraspinal) (meninges) 03.4
  spleen, splenic 41.41
  lesion
    brain 01.59
    cerebral 01.59
    liver 50.21
  pilonidal cyst or sinus (open excision) (with
      partial closure) 86.21
  pseudocyst, pancreas 52.3
  ranula, salivary gland 26.21
Massage
  cardiac (external) (manual) (closed) 99.63
    open 37.91
  prostatic 99.94
  rectal (for levator spasm) 99.93
MAST (military anti-shock trousers) 93.58
Mastectomy (complete) (prophylactic) (simple)
    (unilateral) 85.41
  with
    excision of regional lymph nodes 85.43
      bilateral 85.44
    preservation of skin and nipple 85.34
      with synchronous implant 85.33
      bilateral 85.36
        with synchronous implant 85.35
    bilateral 85.42
    extended
      radical (Urban) (unilateral) 85.47
        bilateral 85.48
      simple (with regional lymphadenectomy)
          (unilateral) 85.43
        bilateral 85.44
  modified radical (unilateral) 85.43
    bilateral 85.44
  partial 85.23
  radical (Halsted) (Meyer) (unilateral) 85.45
    bilateral 85.46
    extended (Urban) (unilateral) 85.47
      bilateral 85.48
    modified (unilateral) 85.43
      bilateral 85.44
  subcutaneous 85.34
    with synchronous implant 85.33
    bilateral 85.36
      with synchronous implant 85.35
  subtotal 85.23
Masters' stress test (two-step) 89.42
Mastoidectomy (cortical) (conservative) 20.49
  complete (simple) 20.41
  modified radical 20.49
  radical 20.42
    modified 20.49
  simple (complete) 20.41
Mastoidotomy 20.21
Mastoidotympanectomy 20.42
Mastopexy 85.6
Mastoplasty —*see* Mammoplasty
Mastorrhaphy 85.81
Mastotomy 85.0
Matas operation (aneurysmorrhaphy) 39.52

Mayo operation
  bunionectomy 77.59
  herniorrhaphy
    laparoscopic 53.43
      with graft or prosthesis 53.42
    other and open with graft or prosthesis 53.41
    other open 53.49
  vaginal hysterectomy 68.59
    laparoscopically assisted (LAVH) 68.51
Maze procedure
  Cox-maze, open 37.33
  maze, modified, endovascular 37.34
  maze, modified, open 37.33
Mazet operation (knee disarticulation) 84.16
McBride operation (bunionectomy with soft
    tissue correction) 77.53
McBurney operation —*see* Repair, hernia,
    inguinal
McCall operation (enterocele repair) 70.92
McCauley operation (release of clubfoot) 83.84
McDonald operation (encirclement suture,
    cervix) 67.59
McIndoe operation (vaginal construction) 70.61
  with graft or prosthesis 70.63
McKeever operation (fusion of first
    metatarsophalangeal joint for hallux valgus
    repair) 77.52
McKissock operation (breast reduction) 85.33
McReynolds operation (transposition of
    pterygium) 11.31
McVay operation
  femoral hernia—*see* Repair, hernia, femoral
  inguinal hernia—*see* Repair, hernia, inguinal
Measurement
  airway resistance 89.38
  anatomic NEC 89.39
  arterial blood gases 89.65
    blood gases
      arterial 89.65
        continuous intra-arterial 89.60
      venous 89.66
  basal metabolic rate (BMR) 89.39
  blood gases
    arterial 89.65
    venous 89.66
  body 93.07
  cardiac output (by)
    Fick method 89.67
    indicator dilution technique 89.68
    oxygen consumption technique 89.67
    thermodilution indicator 89.68
  cardiovascular NEC 89.59
  central venous pressure 89.62
  coronary blood flow 89.69
    fractional flow reserve (FFR) 00.59
    intravascular pressure measurement 00.59
  gastric function NEC 89.39
  girth 93.07
  intelligence 94.01
  intracranial pressure 01.10
  intraocular tension or pressure 89.11
    as part of extended ophthalmologic work-up
        95.03
  intrauterine pressure 75.35
  intravascular pressure 00.69
    coronary 00.59
    iliac 00.69
    intra-abdominal 00.69
    intrathoracic 00.67
      aorta 00.67
      aortic arch 00.67
      carotid 00.67

Measurement—*continued*
  mesenteric 00.69
  peripheral 00.68
  renal 00.69
limb length 93.06
lung volume 89.37
mixed venous blood gases 89.66
physiologic NEC 89.39
portovenous pressure 89.62
pulmonary airway flow, endoscopic 33.72
range of motion 93.05
renal clearance 89.29
respiratory NEC 89.38
skin fold thickness 93.07
skull circumference 93.07
sphincter of Oddi pressure 51.15
systemic arterial
  blood gases 89.65
    continuous intra-arterial 89.60
  pressure 89.61
urine (bioassay) (chemistry) 89.29
vascular 89.59
venous blood gases 89.66
vital capacity (pulmonary) 89.37
Meatoplasty
  ear 18.6
  urethra 58.47
Meatotomy
  ureter 56.1
  urethra 58.1
    internal 58.5
Mechanical ventilation —*see* Ventilation
Mediastinectomy 34.3
Mediastinoscopy 34.22
Mediastinotomy (Chamberlain procedure) 34.1
  with pneumonectomy 32.59
    thoracoscopic 32.50
Meloplasty, facial 86.82
Meningeorrhaphy (cerebral) 02.12
  spinal NEC 03.59
    for
      meningocele 03.51
      myelomeningocele 03.52
Meniscectomy (knee) NEC 80.6
  acromioclavicular 80.91
  sternoclavicular 80.91
  temporomandibular (joint) 76.5
  wrist 80.93
Menstrual extraction or regulation 69.6
Mentoplasty (augmentation) (with graft) (with implant) 76.68
  reduction 76.67
Mesenterectomy 54.4
Mesenteriopexy 54.75
Mesenteriplication 54.75
Mesocoloplication 54.75
Mesopexy 54.75
Metatarsectomy 77.98
Metroplasty 69.49
Mid forceps delivery 72.29
Mikulicz operation (exteriorization of intestine) (first stage) 46.03
  second stage 46.04
Miles operation (proctectomy), NOS 48.50
  laparoscopic 48.51
  open 48.52
  other 48.59
Military anti-shock trousers (MAST) 93.58
Millard operation (cheiloplasty) 27.54
Miller operation
  midtarsal arthrodesis 81.14
  urethrovesical suspension 59.4

Millin-Read operation (urethrovesical suspension) 59.4
Mist therapy 93.94
Mitchell operation (hallux valgus repair) 77.51
MitraClip® mitral valve leaflet clip 35.97
Mobilization
  joint NEC 93.16
  mandible 76.95
  neostrophingic (mitral valve) 35.12
  spine 93.15
  stapes (transcrural) 19.0
  testis in scrotum 62.5
Mohs operation (chemosurgical excision of skin) 86.24
Molegraphy 87.81
Monitoring
  BIS (bispectral index) monitoring 00.94 *[89.14]*
  brain temperature 01.17
  cardiac output (by)
    ambulatory (ACM) 89.50
    electrographic 89.54
      during surgery—*omit code*
    Fick method 89.67
    Holter-type device 89.50
    indicator dilution technique 89.68
    intracardiac or great vessel hemodynamic
      sensor with lead 00.56
      sensor without lead 38.26
      subcutaneous device 00.57
    oxygen consumption technique 89.67
    specified technique NEC 89.68
    telemetry (cardiac) 89.54
    thermodilution indicator 89.68
    transesophageal (Doppler) (ultrasound) 89.68
  central venous pressure 89.62
  circulatory NEC 89.69
  continuous intra-arterial blood gas 89.60
  coronary blood flow (coincidence counting technique) 89.69
    fractional flow reserve (FFR) 00.59
    intravascular pressure measurement 00.59
  electroencephalographic 89.19
    intraoperative 00.94
    radio-telemetered 89.19
    video 89.19
  fetus (fetal heart)
    antepartum
      nonstress (fetal activity acceleration determinations) 75.34
      oxytocin challenge (contraction stress test) 75.35
      ultrasonography (early pregnancy) (Doppler) 88.78
    intrapartum (during labor) (extrauterine) (external) 75.34
      auscultatory (stethoscopy)—*omit code*
      internal (with contraction measurements) (ECG) 75.32
      intrauterine (direct) (ECG) 75.32
      phonocardiographic (extrauterine) 75.34
      pulsed ultrasound (Doppler) 88.78
      transcervical fetal oxygen saturation monitoring 75.38
      transcervical fetal SpO$_2$ monitoring 75.38
  Holter-type device (cardiac) 89.50
  IAEMT (intraoperative anesthetic effect monitoring and titration) 00.94 *[89.14]*
  intra-aneurysm sac pressure 00.58
  intracranial oxygen 01.16
  intracranial pressure 01.10

Monitoring—*continued*
  intraoperative
    anesthetic effect monitoring and titration
      (IAEMT) 00.94 *[89.14]*
    neurophysiologic (BAEP) (brainstem auditory
      evoked potentials) (EEG)
      (electroencephalogram) (electromyogram)
      (EMG) (MEP) (motor evoked potentials)
      (nerve conduction study) (somatosensory
      evoked potentials) (SSEP) (transcranial
      Doppler) 00.94
  intravascular pressure 00.69
    coronary 00.59
    iliac 00.69
    intra-abdominal 00.69
    intrathoracic 00.67
      aorta 00.67
      aortic arch 00.67
      carotid 00.67
    mesenteric 00.69
    peripheral 00.68
    renal 00.69
  neurophysiologic
    intra-operative 00.94
  partial pressure of brain oxygen (PbtO₂) 01.16
  pulmonary artery
    pressure 89.63
    wedge 89.64
  sleep (recording)—*see* categories 89.17-89.18
  systemic arterial pressure 89.61
    intra-aneurysm sac pressure 00.58
  telemetry (cardiac) 89.54
  transesophageal cardiac output (Doppler) 89.68
  ventricular pressure (cardiac) 89.62
Moore operation (arthroplasty) 81.52
Moschowitz
  enterocele repair 70.92
    with graft or prosthesis 70.93
  herniorrhaphy—*see* Repair, hernia, femoral
  sigmoidopexy 46.63
Mountain resort sanitarium 93.98
Mouth-to-mouth resuscitation 93.93
Moxibustion 93.35
MRI —*see* Imaging, magnetic resonance
Muller operation (banding of pulmonary artery)
  38.85
Multiple sleep latency test (MSLT) 89.18
Mumford operation (partial claviculectomy)
  77.81
Musculoplasty (*see also* Repair, muscle) 83.87
  hand (*see also* Repair, muscle, hand) 82.89
Music therapy 93.84
Mustard operation (interatrial transposition of
  venous return) 35.91
Myectomy 83.45
  anorectal 48.92
  eye muscle 15.13
    multiple 15.3
  for graft 83.43
    hand 82.34
  hand 82.36
    for graft 82.34
  levator palpebrae 08.33
  rectal 48.92
Myelogram, myelography (air) (gas) 87.21
  posterior fossa 87.02
Myelotomy
  spine, spinal (cord) (tract) (one-stage) (two-stage)
    03.29
    percutaneous 03.21
Myocardiectomy (infarcted area) 37.33
Myocardiotomy 37.11

Myoclasis 83.99
  hand 82.99
Myomectomy (uterine) 68.29
  broad ligament 69.19
Myoplasty (*see also* Repair, muscle) 83.87
  hand (*see also* Repair, muscle, hand) 82.89
  mastoid 19.9
Myorrhaphy 83.65
  hand 82.46
Myosuture 83.65
  hand 82.46
Myotasis 93.27
Myotenontoplasty (*see also* Repair, tendon)
  83.88
  hand 82.86
Myotenoplasty (*see also* Repair, tendon) 83.88
  hand 82.86
Myotenotomy 83.13
  hand 82.11
Myotomy 83.02
  with division 83.19
    hand 82.19
  colon NEC 46.92
    sigmoid 46.91
  cricopharyngeal 29.31
    that for pharyngeal (pharyngoesophageal)
      diverticulectomy 29.32
  esophagus 42.7
  eye (oblique) (rectus) 15.21
    multiple (two or more muscles) 15.4
  hand 82.02
    with division 82.19
  levator palpebrae 08.38
  sigmoid (colon) 46.91
Myringectomy 20.59
Myringodectomy 20.59
Myringomalleolabyrinthopexy 19.52
Myringoplasty (epitympanic, type I) (by
  cauterization) (by graft) 19.4
  revision 19.6
Myringostapediopexy 19.53
Myringostomy 20.01
Myringotomy (with aspiration) (with drainage)
  20.09
  with insertion of tube or drainage device (button)
    (grommet) 20.01

N

Nailing, intramedullary
  with fracture reduction—*see* Reduction, fracture
    with internal fixation
  internal (without fracture reduction) 78.50
Narcoanalysis 94.21
Narcosynthesis 94.21
Narrowing, palpebral fissure 08.51
Nasopharyngogram 87.09
  contrast 87.06
Necropsy 89.8
Needleoscopy (fetus) 75.31
Needling
  Bartholin's gland (cyst) 71.21
  cataract (secondary) 13.64
  fallopian tube 66.91
  hydrocephalic head 73.8
  lens (capsule) 13.2
  pupillary membrane (iris) 12.35
Nephrectomy (complete) (total) (unilateral)
    55.51
  bilateral 55.54
  partial (wedge) 55.4
  remaining or solitary kidney 55.52
  removal transplanted kidney 55.53
Nephrocolopexy 55.7
Nephrocystanastomosis NEC 56.73
Nephrolithotomy 55.01
Nephrolysis 59.02
  laparoscopic 59.03
Nephropexy 55.7
Nephroplasty 55.89
Nephropyeloplasty 55.87
Nephropyeloureterostomy 55.86
Nephrorrhaphy 55.81
Nephroscopy 55.21
Nephrostolithotomy, percutaneous 55.03
Nephrostomy (with drainage tube) 55.02
  closure 55.82
  percutaneous 55.03
    with fragmentation (ultrasound) 55.04
Nephrotomogram, nephrotomography NEC
    87.72
Nephrotomy 55.01
Nephroureterectomy (with bladder cuff) 55.51
Nephroureterocystectomy 55.51 *[57.79]*
Nerve block (cranial) (peripheral) NEC (*see also*
    Block, by site) 04.81
Neurectasis (cranial) (peripheral) 04.91
Neurectomy (cranial) (infraorbital) (occipital)
    (peripheral) (spinal) NEC 04.07
  gastric (vagus) (*see also* Vagotomy) 44.00
  opticociliary 12.79
  paracervical 05.22
  presacral 05.24
  retrogasserian 04.07
  sympathetic—*see* Sympathectomy
  trigeminal 04.07
  tympanic 20.91
Neurexeresis NEC 04.07
Neuroablation
  radiofrequency 04.2
Neuroanastomosis (cranial) (peripheral) NEC
    04.74
  accessory-facial 04.72
  accessory-hypoglossal 04.73
  hypoglossal-facial 04.71

NeuroFlo™ catheter for partial (temporary)
    abdominal aorta occlusion 39.77
Neurolysis (peripheral nerve) NEC 04.49
  carpal tunnel 04.43
  cranial nerve NEC 04.42
  spinal (cord) (nerve roots) 03.6
  tarsal tunnel 04.44
  trigeminal nerve 04.41
Neuromonitoring
  intra-operative 00.94
Neuroplasty (cranial) (peripheral) NEC 04.79
  of old injury (delayed repair) 04.76
  revision 04.75
Neurorrhaphy (cranial) (peripheral) 04.3
Neurotomy (cranial) (peripheral) (spinal) NEC
    04.04
  acoustic 04.01
  glossopharyngeal 29.92
  lacrimal branch 05.0
  retrogasserian 04.02
  sympathetic 05.0
  vestibular 04.01
Neurotripsy (peripheral) NEC 04.03
  trigeminal 04.02
Nicola operation (tenodesis for recurrent
    dislocation of shoulder) 81.82
Nimodipine, infusion 99.75
NIPS (noninvasive programmed electrical
    stimulation) 37.20
Nissen operation (fundoplication of stomach)
    44.66
  laparoscopic 44.67
Noble operation (plication of small intestine)
    46.62
Norman Miller operation (vaginopexy) 70.77
  with graft or prosthesis 70.78
Norton operation (extraperitoneal cesarean
    section) 74.2
Nuclear magnetic resonance imaging
    —*see* Imaging, magnetic resonance
Nutrition , concentration substances
  enteral infusion (of) 96.6
  parenteral, total 99.15
    peripheral 99.15

O

Ober (Yount) operation (gluteal-iliotibial fasciotomy) 83.14

Obliteration
bone cavity (*see also* Osteoplasty) 78.40
calyceal diverticulum 55.39
canaliculi 09.6
cerebrospinal fistula 02.12
cul-de-sac 70.92
  with graft or prosthesis 70.93
frontal sinus (with fat) 22.42
lacrimal punctum 09.91
lumbar pseudomeningocele 03.51
lymphatic structure(s) (peripheral) 40.9
maxillary sinus 22.31
meningocele (sacral) 03.51
pelvic 68.8
pleural cavity 34.6
sacral meningocele 03.51
Skene's gland 71.3
tympanomastoid cavity 19.9
vagina, vaginal (partial) (total) 70.4
  vault 70.8

Occlusal molds (dental) 89.31

Occlusion
artery
  by embolization—*see* Embolization, artery
  by endovascular approach—*see* Embolization, artery
  by ligation—*see* Ligation, artery
fallopian tube—*see* Ligation, fallopian tube
patent ductus arteriosus (PDA) 38.85
vein
  by embolization—*see* Embolization, vein
  by endovascular approach—*see* Embolization, vein
  by ligation—*see* Ligation, vein
vena cava (surgical) 38.7

Occupational therapy 93.83

OCT (optical coherence tomography) (intravascular imaging)
coronary vessel(s) 38.24
non-coronary vessel(s) 38.25

O'Donoghue operation (triad knee repair) 81.43

Odontectomy NEC (*see also* Removal, tooth, surgical) 23.19

Oleothorax 33.39

Olshausen operation (uterine suspension) 69.22

Omentectomy 54.4

Omentofixation 54.74

Omentopexy 54.74

Omentoplasty 54.74

Omentorrhaphy 54.74

Omentotomy 54.19

Omphalectomy 54.3

Onychectomy 86.23

Onychoplasty 86.86

Onychotomy 86.09
with drainage 86.04

Oophorectomy (unilateral) 65.39
with salpingectomy 65.49
  laparoscopic 65.41
bilateral (same operative episode) 65.51
  laparoscopic 65.53
  with salpingectomy 65.61
    laparoscopic 65.63
laparoscopic 65.31

Oophorectomy—*continued*
partial 65.29
  laparoscopic 65.25
  wedge 65.22
    that by laparoscope 65.24
remaining ovary 65.52
  laparoscopic 65.54
  with tube 65.62
    laparoscopic 65.64

Oophorocystectomy 65.29
laparoscopic 65.25

Oophoropexy 65.79

Oophoroplasty 65.79

Oophororrhaphy 65.71
laparoscopic 65.74

Oophorostomy 65.09
laparoscopic 65.01

Oophorotomy 65.09
laparoscopic 65.01

Opening
bony labyrinth (ear) 20.79
cranial suture 02.01
heart valve
  closed heart technique—*see* Valvulotomy, by site
  open heart technique—*see* Valvuloplasty, by site
spinal dura 03.09

Operation
Abbe
  construction of vagina 70.61
    with graft or prosthesis 70.63
  intestinal anastomosis—*see* Anastomosis, intestine
abdominal (region) NEC 54.99
abdominoperineal, NOS 48.50
  laparoscopic 48.51
  open 48.52
  other 48.59
Aburel (intra-amniotic injection for abortion) 75.0
Adams
  advancement of round ligament 69.22
  crushing of nasal septum 21.88
  excision of palmar fascia 82.35
adenoids NEC 28.99
adrenal (gland) (nerve) (vessel) NEC 07.49
Albee
  bone peg, femoral neck 78.05
  graft for slipping patella 78.06
  sliding inlay graft, tibia 78.07
Albert (arthrodesis, knee) 81.22
Aldridge (Studdiford) (urethral sling) 59.5
Alexander
  prostatectomy
    perineal 60.62
    suprapubic 60.3
  shortening of round ligaments of uterus 69.22
Alexander-Adams (shortening of round ligaments of uterus) 69.22
Almoor (extrapetrosal drainage) 20.22
Altemeier (perineal rectal pull-through) 48.49
Ammon (dacryocystotomy) 09.53
Anderson (tibial lengthening) 78.37
Anel (dilation of lacrimal duct) 09.42
anterior chamber (eye) NEC 12.99
anti-incontinence NEC 59.79
antrum window (nasal sinus) 22.2
  with Caldwell-Luc approach 22.39

Operation—*continued*
anus NEC 49.99
aortic body NEC 39.89
aorticopulmonary window 39.59
appendix NEC 47.99
Arslan (fenestration of inner ear) 20.61
artery NEC 39.99
Asai (larynx) 31.75
Baffes (interatrial transposition of venous return) 35.91
Baldy-Webster (uterine suspension) 69.22
Ball
  herniorrhaphy—*see* Repair, hernia, inguinal
  undercutting 49.02
Bankhart (capsular repair into glenoid, for shoulder dislocation) 81.82
Bardenheurer (ligation of innominate artery) 38.85
Barkan (goniotomy) 12.52
  with goniopuncture 12.53
Barr (transfer of tibialis posterior tendon) 83.75
Barsky (closure of cleft hand) 82.82
Bassett (vulvectomy with inguinal lymph node dissection) 71.5 *[40.3]*
Bassini (herniorrhaphy)—*see* Repair, hernia, inguinal
Batch-Spittler-McFaddin (knee disarticulation) 84.16
Batista (partial ventriculectomy) (ventricular reduction) (ventricular remodeling) 37.35
Beck I (epicardial poudrage) 36.39
Beck II (aorta-coronary sinus shunt) 36.39
Beck-Jianu (permanent gastrostomy) 43.19
Bell-Beuttner (subtotal abdominal hysterectomy) 68.39
Belsey (esophagogastric sphincter) 44.65
Benenenti (rotation of bulbous urethra) 58.49
Berke (levator resection eyelid) 08.33
Biesenberger (size reduction of breast, bilateral) 85.32
  unilateral 85.31
Bigelow (litholapaxy) 57.0
biliary (duct) (tract) NEC 51.99
Billroth I (partial gastrectomy with gastroduodenostomy) 43.6
Billroth II (partial gastrectomy with gastrojejunostomy) 43.7
Binnie (hepatopexy) 50.69
Bischoff (ureteroneocystostomy) 56.74
bisection hysterectomy 68.39
  laparoscopic 68.31
Bishoff (spinal myelotomy) 03.29
bladder NEC 57.99
  flap 56.74
Blalock (systemic-pulmonary anastomosis) 39.0
Blalock-Hanlon (creation of atrial septal defect) 35.42
Blalock-Taussig (subclavian-pulmonary anastomosis) 39.0
Blascovic (resection and advancement of levator palpebrae superioris) 08.33
blood vessel NEC 39.99
Blount
  femoral shortening (with blade plate) 78.25
    by epiphyseal stapling 78.25
Boari (bladder flap) 56.74
Bobb (cholelithotomy) 51.04
bone NEC—*see* category 78.4
  facial 76.99
  injury NEC—*see* category 79.9
  marrow NEC 41.98
  skull NEC 02.99

Operation—*continued*
Bonney (abdominal hysterectomy) 68.49
  laparoscopic 68.41
Borthen (iridotasis) 12.63
Bost
  plantar dissection 80.48
  radiocarpal fusion 81.26
Bosworth
  arthroplasty for acromioclavicular separation 81.83
  fusion of posterior lumbar spine 81.08
    for pseudarthrosis 81.38
  resection of radial head ligaments (for tennis elbow) 80.92
  shelf procedure, hip 81.40
bottle (repair of hydrocele of tunica vaginalis) 61.2
Boyd (hip disarticulation) 84.18
brain NEC 02.99
Brauer (cardiolysis) 37.10
breast NEC 85.99
Bricker (ileoureterostomy) 56.51
Bristow (repair of shoulder dislocation) 81.82
Brock (pulmonary valvulotomy) 35.03
Brockman (soft tissue release for clubfoot) 83.84
bronchus NEC 33.98
Browne (Denis) (hypospadias repair) 58.45
Brunschwig (temporary gastrostomy) 43.19
buccal cavity NEC 27.99
Bunnell (tendon transfer) 82.56
Burch procedure (retropubic urethral suspension for urinary stress incontinence) 59.5
Burgess (amputation of ankle) 84.14
bursa NEC 83.99
  hand 82.99
bypass—*see* Bypass
Caldwell (sulcus extension) 24.91
Caldwell-Luc (maxillary sinusotomy) 22.39
  with removal of membrane lining 22.31
Callander (knee disarticulation) 84.16
Campbell
  bone block, ankle 81.11
  fasciotomy (iliac crest) 83.14
  reconstruction of anterior cruciate ligaments 81.45
canthus NEC 08.99
cardiac NEC 37.99
  septum NEC 35.98
  valve NEC 35.99
carotid body or gland NEC 39.89
Carroll and Taber (arthroplasty proximal interphalangeal joint) 81.72
Cattell (herniorrhaphy) 53.51
Cecil (urethral reconstruction) 58.46
cecum NEC 46.99
cerebral (meninges) NEC 02.99
cervix NEC 69.99
Chandler (hip fusion) 81.21
Charles (correction of lymphedema) 40.9
Charnley (compression arthrodesis)
  ankle 81.11
  hip 81.21
  knee 81.22
Cheatle-Henry—*see* Repair, hernia, femoral
chest cavity NEC 34.99
Chevalier-Jackson (partial laryngectomy) 30.29
Child (radical subtotal pancreatectomy) 52.53
Chopart (midtarsal amputation) 84.12
chordae tendineae NEC 35.32
choroid NEC 14.9
ciliary body NEC 12.98
cisterna chyli NEC 40.69

Operation—*continued*

Clagett (closure of chest wall following open flap drainage) 34.72
Clayton (resection of metatarsal heads and bases of phalanges) 77.88
clitoris NEC 71.4
cocked hat (metacarpal lengthening and transfer of local flap) 82.69
Cockett (varicose vein)
  lower limb 38.59
  upper limb 38.53
Cody tack (perforation of footplate) 19.0
Coffey (uterine suspension) (Meigs' modification) 69.22
Cole (anterior tarsal wedge osteotomy) 77.28
Collis-Nissen (hiatal hernia repair) 53.80
colon NEC 46.99
Colonna
  adductor tenotomy (first stage) 83.12
  hip arthroplasty (second stage) 81.40
  reconstruction of hip (second stage) 81.40
commando (radical glossectomy) 25.4
conjunctive NEC 10.99
  destructive NEC 10.33
cornea NEC 11.99
Coventry (tibial wedge osteotomy) 77.27
Cox-maze procedure (ablation or destruction of heart tissue) —*see* maze procedure
Crawford (tarso-frontalis sling of eyelid) 08.32
cul-de-sac NEC 70.92
Culp-Deweerd (spiral flap pyeloplasty) 55.87
Culp-Scardino (ureteral flap pyeloplasty) 55.87
Curtis (interphalangeal joint arthroplasty) 81.72
cystocele NEC 70.51
Dahlman (excision of esophageal diverticulum) 42.31
Dana (posterior rhizotomy) 03.1
Danforth (fetal) 73.8
Darrach (ulnar resection) 77.83
Davis (intubated ureterotomy) 56.2
de Grandmont (tarsectomy) 08.35
Delorme
  pericardiectomy 37.31
  proctopexy 48.76
  repair of prolapsed rectum 48.76
  thoracoplasty 33.34
Denker (radical maxillary antrotomy) 22.31
Dennis-Varco (herniorrhaphy)—*see* Repair, hernia, femoral
Denonvillier (limited rhinoplasty) 21.86
dental NEC 24.99
  orthodontic NEC 24.8
Derlacki (tympanoplasty) 19.4
diaphragm NEC 34.89
Dickson (fascial transplant) 83.82
Dickson-Diveley (tendon transfer and arthrodesis to correct claw toe) 77.57
Dieffenbach (hip disarticulation) 84.18
digestive tract NEC 46.99
Doleris (shortening of round ligaments) 69.22
D'Ombrain (excision of pterygium with corneal graft) 11.32
Dorrance (push-back operation for cleft palate) 27.62
Dotter (transluminal angioplasty) 39.59
Douglas (suture of tongue to lip for micrognathia) 25.59
Doyle (paracervical uterine denervation) 69.3
Duhamel (abdominoperineal pull-through) 48.65
Duhrssen (vaginofixation of uterus) 69.22
Dunn (triple arthrodesis) 81.12
duodenum NEC 46.99

Operation—*continued*

Dupuytren
  fasciectomy 82.35
  fasciotomy 82.12
    with excision 82.35
  shoulder disarticulation 84.08
Durham (Caldwell) (transfer of biceps femoris tendon) 83.75
DuToit and Roux (staple capsulorrhaphy of shoulder) 81.82
DuVries (tenoplasty) 83.88
Dwyer
  fasciotomy 83.14
  soft tissue release NEC 83.84
  wedge osteotomy, calcaneus 77.28
Eagleton (extrapetrosal drainage) 20.22
ear (external) NEC 18.9
  middle or inner NEC 20.99
Eden-Hybinette (glenoid bone block) 78.01
Effler (heart) 36.2
Eggers
  tendon release (patellar retinacula) 83.13
  tendon transfer (biceps femoris tendon) (hamstring tendon) 83.75
Elliot (scleral trephination with iridectomy) 12.61
Ellis Jones (repair of peroneal tendon) 83.88
Ellison (reinforcement of collateral ligament) 81.44
Elmslie-Cholmeley (tarsal wedge osteotomy) 77.28
Eloesser
  thoracoplasty 33.34
  thoracostomy 34.09
Emmet (cervix) 67.61
endorectal pull-through 48.41
epididymis NEC 63.99
esophagus NEC 42.99
Estes (ovary) 65.72
  laparoscopic 65.75
Estlander (thoracoplasty) 33.34
Evans (release of clubfoot) 83.84
extraocular muscle NEC 15.9
  multiple (two or more muscles) 15.4
    with temporary detachment from globe 15.3
  revision 15.6
  single 15.29
    with temporary detachment from globe 15.19
eyeball NEC 16.99
eyelid(s) NEC 08.99
face NEC 27.99
facial bone or joint NEC 76.99
fallopian tube NEC 66.99
Farabeuf (ischiopubiotomy) 77.39
Fasanella-Servatt (blepharoptosis repair) 08.35
fascia NEC 83.99
  hand 82.99
female (genital organs) NEC 71.9
  hysterectomy NEC 68.9
fenestration (aorta) 39.54
Ferguson (hernia repair) 53.00
Fick (perforation of footplate) 19.0
filtering (for glaucoma) 12.79
  with iridectomy 12.65
Finney (pyloroplasty) 44.2
fistulizing, sclera NEC 12.69
Foley (pyeloplasty) 55.87
Fontan (creation of conduit between right atrium and pulmonary artery) 35.94
Fothergill (Donald) (uterine suspension) 69.22

Operation—*continued*
Fowler
  arthroplasty of metacarpophalangeal joint 81.72
  release (mallet finger repair) 82.84
  tenodesis (hand) 82.85
  thoracoplasty 33.34
Fox (entropion repair with wedge resection)
  08.43
Franco (suprapubic cystotomy) 57.19
Frank (permanent gastrostomy) 43.19
Frazier (Spiller) (subtemporal trigeminal
  rhizotomy) 04.02
Fredet-Ramstedt (pyloromyotomy) (with wedge
  resection) 43.3
Frenckner (intrapetrosal drainage) 20.22
Frickman (abdominal proctopexy) 48.75
Frommel (shortening of uterosacral ligaments)
  69.22
Gabriel (abdominoperineal resection of rectum),
  NOS 48.50
  laparoscopic 48.51
  open 48.52
  other 48.59
gallbladder NEC 51.99
ganglia NEC 04.99
  sympathetic 05.89
Gant (wedge osteotomy of trochanter) 77.25
Garceau (tibial tendon transfer) 83.75
Gardner (spinal meningocele repair) 03.51
gastric NEC 44.99
Gelman (release of clubfoot) 83.84
genital organ NEC
  female 71.9
  male 64.99
Ghormley (hip fusion) 81.21
Gifford
  destruction of lacrimal sac 09.6
  keratotomy (delimiting) 11.1
Gill
  arthrodesis of shoulder 81.23
  laminectomy 03.09
Gill-Stein (carporadial arthrodesis) 81.25
Gilliam (uterine suspension) 69.22
Girdlestone
  laminectomy with spinal fusion 81.00
  muscle transfer for claw toe 77.57
  resection of femoral head and neck (without
    insertion of joint prosthesis) 77.85
    with replacement prosthesis—*see* Implant,
      joint, hip
  resection of hip prosthesis 80.05
    with replacement prosthesis—*see* Implant,
      joint, hip
Girdlestone-Taylor (muscle transfer for claw toe
  repair) 77.57
glaucoma NEC 12.79
Glenn (anastomosis of superior vena cava to right
  pulmonary artery) 39.21
globus pallidus NEC 01.42
Goebel-Frangenheim-Stoeckel (urethrovesical
  suspension) 59.4
Goldner (clubfoot release) 80.48
Goldthwait
  ankle stabilization 81.11
  patella stabilization 81.44
  tendon transfer for patella dislocation 81.44
Goodall-Power (vagina) 70.4
Gordon-Taylor (hindquarter amputation) 84.19
Graber-Duvernay (drilling femoral head) 77.15
Green (scapulopexy) 78.41
Grice (subtalar arthrodesis) 81.13
Gritti-Stokes (knee disarticulation) 84.16

Operation—*continued*
Gross (herniorrhaphy)
  laparoscopic 53.43
    with graft or prosthesis 53.42
  other and open with graft or prosthesis 53.41
  other open 53.49
gum NEC 24.39
Guyon (amputation of ankle) 84.13
Hagner (epididymotomy) 63.92
Halsted—*see* Repair, hernia, inguinal
Halsted mastectomy 85.45
Hampton (anastomosis small intestine to rectal
  stump) 45.92
hanging hip (muscle release) 83.19
harelip 27.54
Harrison-Richardson (vaginal suspension) 70.77
  with graft or prosthesis 70.78
Hartmann—*see* Colectomy, by site
Hauser
  achillotenotomy 83.11
  bunionectomy with adductor tendon transfer
    77.53
  stabilization of patella 81.44
Heaney (vaginal hysterectomy) 68.59
  laparoscopically assisted (LAVH) 68.51
heart NEC 37.99
  valve NEC 35.99
    adjacent structure NEC 35.39
Hegar (perineorrhaphy) 71.79
Heine (cyclodialysis) 12.55
Heineke-Mikulicz (pyloroplasty) 44.2
Heller (esophagomyotomy) 42.7
Hellstrom (transplantation of aberrant renal
  vessel) 39.55
hemorrhoids NEC 49.49
Henley jejunal transposition) 43.81
hepatic NEC 50.99
hernia—*see* Repair, hernia
Hey (amputation of foot) 84.12
Hey-Groves (reconstruction of anterior
  cruciate ligament) 81.45
Heyman (soft tissue release for clubfoot) 83.84
Heyman-Herndon (Strong) (correction of
  metatarsus varus) 80.48
Hibbs (lumbar spinal fusion)—*see* Fusion, lumbar
Higgins—*see* Repair, hernia, femoral
Hill-Allison (hiatal hernia repair, transpleural
  approach) 53.80
Hitchcock (anchoring tendon of biceps) 83.88
Hofmeister (gastrectomy) 43.7
Hoke
  midtarsal fusion 81.14
  triple arthrodesis 81.12
Holth
  iridencleisis 12.63
  sclerectomy 12.65
Homan (correction of lymphedema) 40.9
Hutch (ureteroneocystostomy) 56.74
Hybinette-eden (glenoid bone block) 78.01
hymen NEC 70.91
hypopharynx NEC 29.99
hypophysis NEC 07.79
ileal loop 56.51
ileum NEC 46.99
intestine NEC 46.99
iris NEC 12.97
  inclusion 12.63
Irving (tubal ligation) 66.32
Irwin (*see also* Osteotomy) 77.30
Jaboulay (gastroduodenostomy) 44.39
  laparoscopic 44.38

Operation—*continued*

Janeway (permanent gastrostomy) 43.19
Jatene (arterial switch) 35.84
jejunum NEC 46.99
Johanson (urethral reconstruction) 58.46
joint (capsule) (ligament) (structure) NEC 81.99
   facial NEC 76.99
Jones
   claw toe (transfer of extensor hallucis longus
      tendon) 77.57
     modified (with arthrodesis) 77.57
   dacryocystorhinostomy 09.81
   hammer toe (interphalangeal fusion) 77.56
     modified (tendon transfer with arthrodesis)
      77.57
   repair of peroneal tendon 83.88
Joplin (exostectomy with tendon transfer) 77.53
Kader (temporary gastrostomy) 43.19
Kaufman (for urinary stress incontinence) 59.79
Kazanjiian (buccal vestibular sulcus extension)
   24.91
Kehr (hepatopexy) 50.69
Keller (bunionectomy) 77.59
Kelly (Kennedy) (urethrovesical plication) 59.3
Kelly-Stoeckel (urethrovesical plication) 59.3
Kerr (cesarean section) 74.1
Kessler (arthroplasty, carpometacarpal joint)
   81.74
Kidner (excision of accessory navicular bone)
   (with tendon transfer) 77.98
kidney NEC 55.99
Killian (frontal sinusotomy) 22.41
King-Steelquist (hindquarter amputation) 84.19
Kirk (amputation through thigh) 84.17
Kock pouch
   bowel anastomosis—*omit code*
   continent ileostomy 46.22
   cutaneous uretero-ileostomy 56.51
   ESWL (extracorporeal shockwave lithotripsy)
     98.51
   removal, calculus 57.19
   revision, cutaneous uretero-ileostomy 56.52
   urinary diversion procedure 56.51
Kondoleon (correction of lymphedema) 40.9
Krause (sympathetic denervation) 05.29
Kroener (partial salpingectomy) 66.69
Kroenlein (lateral orbitotomy) 16.01
Kronig (low cervical cesarean section) 74.1
Krukenberg (reconstruction of below-elbow
   amputation) 82.89
Kuhnt-Szymanowski (ectropion repair with lid
   reconstruction) 08.44
Labbe (gastrotomy) 43.0
labia NEC 71.8
lacrimal
   gland 09.3
   system NEC 09.99
Ladd (mobilization of intestine) 54.95
Lagrange (iridosclerectomy) 12.65
Lambrinudi (triple arthrodesis) 81.12
Langenbeck (cleft palate repair) 27.62
Lapidus (bunionectomy with metatarsal
   osteotomy) 77.51
Larry (shoulder disarticulation) 84.08
larynx NEC 31.98
Lash
   internal cervical os repair 67.59
   laparoscopic supracervical hysterectomy 68.31
Latzko
   cesarean section, extraperitoneal 74.2
   colpocleisis 70.8

Operation—*continued*

Leadbetter (urethral reconstruction) 58.46
Leadbetter-Politano (ureteroneocystostomy)
   56.74
Le Fort (colpocleisis) 70.8
LeMesurier (cleft lip repair) 27.54
lens NEC 13.90
Leriche (periarterial sympathectomy) 05.25
levator muscle sling
   eyelid ptosis repair 08.33
   urethrovesical suspension 59.71
   urinary stress incontinence 59.71
lid suture (blepharoptosis) 08.31
ligament NEC 81.99
   broad NEC 69.98
   round NEC 69.98
   uterine NEC 69.98
Lindholm (repair of ruptured tendon) 83.88
Linton (varicose vein) 38.59
lip NEC 27.99
Lisfranc
   foot amputation 84.12
   shoulder disarticulation 84.08
Littlewood (forequarter amputation) 84.09
liver NEC 50.99
Lloyd-Davies (abdominoperineal resection), NOS
   48.50
   laparoscopic 48.51
   open 48.52
   other 48.59
Longmire (bile duct anastomosis) 51.39
Lord
   dilation of anal canal for hemorrhoids 49.49
   hemorrhoidectomy 49.49
   orchidopexy 62.5
Lucas and Murray (knee arthrodesis with plate)
   81.22
lung NEC 33.99
lung volume reduction 32.22
   biologic lung volume reduction (BLVR)—*see
     category* 33.7
lymphatic structure(s) NEC 40.9
   duct, left (thoracic) NEC 40.69
Madlener (tubal ligation) 66.31
Magnuson (Stack) (arthroplasty for recurrent
   shoulder dislocation) 81.82
male genital organs NEC 64.99
Manchester (Donald) (Fothergill), (uterine
   suspension) 69.22
mandible NEC 76.99
   orthognathic 76.64
Marckwald (cervical os repair) 67.59
Marshall-Marchetti (Krantz) (retropubic urethral
   suspension) 59.5
Matas (aneurysmorrhaphy) 39.52
Mayo
   bunionectomy 77.59
   herniorrhaphy
     laparoscopic 53.43
       with graft or prosthesis 53.42
     other and open with graft or prosthesis 53.41
     other open 53.49
   vaginal hysterectomy 68.59
     laparoscopically assisted (LAVH) 68.51
Maze procedure (ablation or destruction of heart
   tissue)
   by incision (open) 37.33
   by median sternotomy 37.33
   by peripherally inserted catheter 37.34
   by thoracotomy without thoracoscope 37.33
   endovascular approach 37.34
Mazet (knee disarticulation) 84.16

Operation—*continued*

McBride (bunionectomy with soft tissue correction) 77.53

McBurney—*see* Repair, hernia, inguinal

McCall (enterocele repair) 70.92
  with graft or prosthesis 70.93

McCauley (release of clubfoot) 83.84

McDonald (encirclement suture, cervix) 67.59

McIndoe (vaginal construction) 70.61
  with graft or prosthesis 70.63

McKeever (fusion of first metatarsophalangeal joint for hallux valgus repair) 77.52

McKissock (breast reduction) 85.33

McReynolds (transposition of pterygium) 11.31

McVay
  femoral hernia—*see* Repair, hernia, femoral
  inguinal hernia—*see* Repair, hernia, inguinal

meninges (spinal) NEC 03.99
  cerebral NEC 02.99

mesentery NEC 54.99

Mikulicz (exteriorization of intestine) (first stage) 46.03
  second stage 46.04

Miles (complete proctectomy), NOS 48.50
  laparoscopic 48.51
  open 48.52
  other 48.59

Millard (cheiloplasty) 27.54

Miller
  midtarsal arthrodesis 81.14
  urethrovesical suspension 59.4

Millin-Read (urethrovesical suspension) 59.4

Mitchell (hallux valgus repair) 77.51

Mohs (chemosurgical excision of skin) 86.24

Moore (arthroplasty) 81.52

Moschowitz
  enterocele repair 70.92
    with graft or prosthesis 70.93
  herniorrhaphy—*see* Repair, hernia, femoral
  sigmoidopexy 46.63

mouth NEC 27.99

Muller (banding of pulmonary artery) 38.85

Mumford (partial claviculectomy) 77.81

muscle NEC 83.99
  extraocular—*see* Operation, extraocular
  hand NEC 82.99
  papillary heart NEC 35.31

musculoskeletal system NEC 84.99

Mustard (interatrial transposition of venous return) 35.91

nail (finger) (toe) NEC 86.99

nasal sinus NEC 22.9

nasopharynx NEC 29.99

nerve (cranial) (peripheral) NEC 04.99
  adrenal NEC 07.49
  sympathetic NEC 05.89

nervous system NEC 05.9

Nicola (tenodesis for recurrent dislocation of shoulder) 81.82

nipple NEC 85.99

Nissen (fundoplication of stomach) 44.66
  laparoscopic 44.67

Noble (plication of small intestine) 46.62

node (lymph) NEC 40.9

Norman Miller (vaginopexy) 70.77
  with graft or prosthesis 70.78

Norton (extraperitoneal cesarean operation) 74.2

nose, nasal NEC 21.99
  sinus NEC 22.9

Ober (Yount) (gluteal-iliotibial fasciotomy) 83.14

obstetric NEC 75.99

Operation—*continued*

ocular NEC 16.99
  muscle—*see* Operation, extraocular muscle

O'Donoghue (triad knee repair) 81.43

Olshausen (uterine suspension) 69.22

omentum NEC 54.99

ophthalmologic NEC 16.99

oral cavity NEC 27.99

orbicularis muscle sling 08.36

orbit NEC 16.98

oropharynx NEC 29.99

orthodontic NEC 24.8

orthognathic NEC 76.69

Oscar Miller (midtarsal arthrodesis) 81.14

Osmond-Clark (soft tissue release with peroneus brevis tendon transfer) 83.75

ovary NEC 65.99

Oxford (for urinary incontinence) 59.4

palate NEC 27.99

palpebral ligament sling 08.36

Panas (linear proctotomy) 48.0

Pancoast (division of trigeminal nerve at foramen ovale) 04.02

pancreas NEC 52.99

pantaloon (revision of gastric anastomosis) 44.5

papillary muscle (heart) NEC 35.31

Paquin (ureteroneocystostomy) 56.74

parathyroid gland(s) NEC 06.99

parotid gland or duct NEC 26.99

Partsch (marsupialization of dental cyst) 24.4

Pattee (auditory canal) 18.6

Peet (splanchnic resection) 05.29

Pemberton
  osteotomy of ilium 77.39
  rectum (mobilization and fixation for prolapse repair) 48.76

penis NEC 64.98

Pereyra (paraurethral suspension) 59.6

pericardium NEC 37.99

perineum (female) NEC 71.8
  male NEC 86.99

perirectal tissue NEC 48.99

perirenal tissue NEC 59.92

peritoneum NEC 54.99

periurethral tissue NEC 58.99

perivesical tissue NEC 59.92

pharyngeal flap (cleft palate repair) 27.62
  secondary or subsequent 27.63

pharynx, pharyngeal (pouch) NEC 29.99

pineal gland NEC 07.59

Pinsker (obliteration of nasoseptal telangiectasia) 21.07

Piper (forceps) 72.6

Pirogoff (ankle amputation through malleoli of tibia and fibula) 84.14

pituitary gland NEC 07.79

plastic—*see* Repair, by site

pleural cavity NEC 34.99

Politano-Leadbetter (ureteroneocystostomy) 56.74

pollicization (with nerves and blood supply) 82.61

Polya (gastrectomy) 43.7

Pomeroy (ligation and division of fallopian tubes) 66.32

Poncet
  lengthening of Achilles tendon 83.85
  urethrostomy, perineal 58.0

Porro (cesarean section) 74.99

posterior chamber (eye) NEC 14.9

Operation—*continued*
Potts-Smith (descending aorta-left pulmonary
    artery anastomosis) 39.0
Printen and Mason (high gastric bypass) 44.31
prostate NEC (*see also* Prostatectomy) 60.69
    specified type 60.99
pterygium 11.39
    with corneal graft 11.32
Puestow (pancreaticojejunostomy) 52.96
pull-through NEC 48.49
pulmonary NEC 33.99
push-back (cleft palate repair) 27.62
Putti-Platt (capsulorrhaphy of shoulder for
    recurrent dislocation) 81.82
pyloric exclusion 44.39
    laparoscopic 44.38
pyriform sinus NEC 29.99
"rabbit ear" (anterior urethropexy) (Tudor) 59.79
Ramadier (intrapetrosal drainage) 20.22
Ramstedt (pyloromyotomy) (with wedge
    resection) 43.3
Rankin
    exteriorization of intestine 46.03
    proctectomy (complete), NOS 48.50
        laparoscopic 48.51
        open 48.52
        other 48.59
Rashkind (balloon septostomy) 35.41
Rastelli (creation of conduit between right
    ventricle and pulmonary artery) 35.92
    in repair of
        pulmonary artery atresia 35.92
        transposition of great vessels 35.92
        truncus arteriosus 35.83
Raz-Pereyra procedure (bladder neck suspension)
    59.79
rectal NEC 48.99
rectocele NEC 70.52
re-entry (aorta) 39.54
renal NEC 55.99
respiratory (tract) NEC 33.99
retina NEC 14.9
Ripstein (repair of rectal prolapse) 48.75
Rodney Smith (radical subtotal pancreatectomy)
    52.53
Roux-en-Y
    bile duct 51.36
    cholecystojejunostomy 51.32
    esophagus (intrathoracic) 42.54
    gastroenterostomy 44.39
        laparoscopic 44.38
    gastrojejunostomy 44.39
        laparoscopic 44.38
    pancreaticojejunostomy 52.96
Roux-Goldthwait (repair of patellar dislocation)
    81.44
Roux-Herzen-Judine (jejunal loop interposition)
    42.63
Ruiz-Mora (proximal phalangectomy for hammer
    toe) 77.99
Russe (bone graft of scaphoid) 78.04
Saemisch (corneal section) 11.1
salivary gland or duct NEC 26.99
Salter (innominate osteotomy) 77.39
Sauer-Bacon (abdominoperineal resection), NOS
    48.50
    laparoscopic 48.51
    open 48.52
    other 48.59
Schanz (femoral osteotomy) 77.35

Operation—*continued*
Schauta (-Amreich) (radical vaginal
    hysterectomy) 68.79
    laparoscopic 68.71
Schede (thoracoplasty) 33.34
Scheie
    cautery of sclera 12.62
    sclerostomy 12.62
Schlatter (total gastrectomy) 43.99
Schroeder (endocervical excision) 67.39
Schuchardt (nonobstetrical episiotomy) 71.09
Schwartze (simple mastoidectomy) 20.41
sclera NEC 12.89
Scott
    intestinal bypass for obesity 45.93
    jejunocolostomy (bypass) 45.93
scrotum NEC 61.99
Seddon-Brooks (transfer of pectoralis major
    tendon) 83.75
Semb (apicolysis of lung) 33.39
seminal vesicle NEC 60.79
Senning (correction of transposition of great
    vessels) 35.91
Sever (division of soft tissue of arm) 83.19
Sewell (heart) 36.2
sex transformation NEC 64.5
Sharrard (iliopsoas muscle transfer) 83.77
shelf (hip arthroplasty) 81.40
Shirodkar (encirclement suture, cervix) 67.59
sigmoid NEC 46.99
Silver (bunionectomy) 77.59
Sistrunk (excision of thyroglossal cyst) 06.7
Skene's gland NEC 71.8
skin NEC 86.99
skull NEC 02.99
sling
    eyelid
        fascia lata, palpebral 08.36
        frontalis fascial 08.32
        levator muscle 08.33
        orbicularis muscle 08.36
        palpebrae ligament, fascia lata 08.36
        tarsus muscle 08.35
    fascial (fascia lata)
        eye 08.32
        for facial weakness (trigeminal nerve
            paralysis) 86.81
        palpebral ligament 08.36
        tongue 25.59
    tongue (fascial) 25.59
    urethra (suprapubic) 59.4
        retropubic 59.5
    urethrovesical 59.5
Slocum (pes anserinus transfer) 81.47
Sluder (tonsillectomy) 28.2
Smith (open osteotomy of mandible) 76.62
Smith-Peterson (radiocarpal arthrodesis) 81.25
Smithwick (sympathectomy) 05.29
Soave (endorectal pull-through) 48.41
soft tissue NEC 83.99
    hand 82.99
Sonneberg (inferior maxillary neurectomy) 04.07
Sorondo-Ferré (hindquarter amputation) 84.19
Soutter (iliac crest fasciotomy) 83.14
Spalding-Richardson (uterine suspension) 69.22
spermatic cord NEC 63.99
sphincter of Oddi NEC 51.89
spinal (canal) (cord) (structures) NEC 03.99
Spinelli (correction of inverted uterus) 75.93
Spivack (permanent gastrostomy) 43.19
spleen NEC 41.99

Operation—*continued*
S.P. Rogers (knee disarticulation) 84.16
Ssabanejew-Frank (permanent gastrostomy) 43.19
Stacke (simple mastoidectomy) 20.41
Stallard (conjunctivocystorhinostomy) 09.82
  with insertion of tube or stent 09.83
Stamm (Kader) (temporary gastrostomy) 43.19
Steinberg 44.5
Steindler
  fascia stripping (for cavus deformity) 83.14
  flexorplasty (elbow) 83.77
  muscle transfer 83.77
sterilization NEC
  female (*see also* specific operation) 66.39
  mate (*see also* Ligation, vas deferens) 63.70
Stewart (renal plication with pyeloplasty) 55.87
stomach NEC 44.99
Stone (anoplasty) 49.79
Strassman (metroplasty) 69.49
  metroplasty (Jones modification) 69.49
  uterus 68.22
Strayer (gastrocnemius recession) 83.72
stress incontinence—*see* Repair, stress incontinence
Stromeyer-Little (hepatotomy) 50.0
Strong (unbridling of celiac artery axis) 39.91
Sturmdorf (conization of cervix) 67.2
subcutaneous tissue NEC 86.99
sublingual gland or duct NEC 26.99
submaxillary gland or duct NEC 26.99
Summerskill (dacryocystorhinostomy by intubation) 09.81
Surmay (jejunostomy) 46.39
Swenson
  bladder reconstruction 57.87
  proctectomy 48.49
Swinney (urethral reconstruction) 58.46
Syme
  ankle amputation through malleoli of tibia and fibula 84.14
  urethrotomy, external 58.0
sympathetic nerve NEC 05.89
Taarnhoj (trigeminal nerve root decompression) 04.41
Tack (sacculotomy) 20.79
Talma-Morison (omentopexy) 54.74
Tanner (devascularization of stomach) 44.99
TAPVC NEC 35.82
tarsus NEC 08.99
  muscle sling 08.35
tendon NEC 83.99
  extraocular NEC 15.9
  hand NEC 82.99
testis NEC 62.99
tetralogy of Fallot
  partial repair—*see* specific procedure
  total (one-stage) 35.81
Thal (repair of esophageal stricture) 42.85
thalamus (stereotactic) 01.41
  by stereotactic radiosurgery 92.32
    cobalt 60 92.32
    linear accelerator (LINAC) 92.31
    multi-source 92.32
    particle beam 92.33
    particulate 92.33
    radiosurgery NEC 92.39
    single source proton 92.31

Operation—*continued*
Thiersch
  anus 49.79
  skin graft 86.69
    hand 86.62
Thompson
  cleft lip repair 27.54
  correction of lymphedema 40.9
  quadricepsplasty 83.86
  thumb apposition with bone graft 82.69
thoracic duct NEC 40.69
thorax NEC 34.99
Thorek (partial cholecystectomy) 51.21
three-snip, punctum 09.51
thymus NEC 07.99
  thoracoscopic, NEC 07.98
thyroid gland NEC 06.98
TKP (thermokeratoplasty) 11.74
Tomkins (metroplasty) 69.49
tongue NEC 25.99
  flap, palate 27.62
  tie 25.91
tonsil NEC 28.99
Torek (Bevan) (orchidopexy) (first stage) (second stage) 62.5
Torkildsen (ventriculocisternal shunt) 02.22
Torpin (cul-de-sac resection) 70.92
Toti (dacryocystorhinostomy) 09.81
Touchas 86.83
Touroff (ligation of subclavian artery) 38.85
trabeculae corneae cordis (heart) NEC 35.35
trachea NEC 31.99
Trauner (lingual sulcus extension) 24.91
truncus arteriosus NEC 35.83
Tsuge (macrodactyly repair) 82.83
Tudor "rabbit ear" (anterior urethropexy) 59.79
Tuffier
  apicolysis of lung 33.39
  vaginal hysterectomy 68.59
    laparoscopically assisted (LAVH) 68.51
  tunica vaginalis NEC 61.99
Turco (release of joint capsules in clubfoot) 80.48
Uchida (tubal ligation with or without fimbriectomy) 66.32
umbilicus NEC 54.99
urachus NEC 57.51
Urban (mastectomy) (unilateral) 85.47
  bilateral 85.48
ureter NEC 56.99
urethra NEC 58.99
urinary system NEC 59.99
uterus NEC 69.99
  supporting structures NEC 69.98
uvula NEC 27.79
vagina NEC 70.91
vascular NEC 39.99
vas deferens NEC 63.99
  ligation NEC 63.71
vein NEC 39.99
vena cava sieve 38.7
vertebra NEC 78.49
vesical (bladder) NEC 57.99
vessel NEC 39.99
  cardiac NEC 36.99
Vicq d'Azyr (larynx) 31.1
Vidal (varicocele ligation) 63.1
Vineberg (implantation of mammary artery into ventricle) 36.2
vitreous NEC 14.79
vocal cord NEC 31.98

Operation—*continued*
von Kraske (proctectomy) 48.64
Voss (hanging hip operation) 83.19
Vulpius (Compere) (lengthening of
   gastrocnemius muscle) 83.85
vulva NEC 71.8
Ward-Mayo (vaginal hysterectomy) 68.59
   laparoscopically assisted (LAVH) 68.51
Wardill (cleft palate) 27.62
Waters (extraperitoneal cesarean section) 74.2
Waterston (aorta-right pulmonary artery
   anastomosis) 39.0
Watkins (Wertheim) (uterus interposition) 69.21
Watson-Jones
   hip arthrodesis 81.21
   reconstruction of lateral ligaments, ankle 81.49
   shoulder arthrodesis (extra-articular) 81.23
   tenoplasty 83.88
Weir
   appendicostomy 47.91
   correction of nostrils 21.86
Wertheim (radical hysterectomy) 68.69
   laparoscopic 68.61
West (dacryocystorhinostomy) 09.81
Wheeler
   entropion repair 08.44
   halving procedure (eyelid) 08.24
Whipple (radical pancreaticoduodenectomy) 52.7
   Child modification (radical subtotal
     pancreatectomy) 52.53
   Rodney Smith modification (radical subtotal
     pancreatectomy) 52.53
While (lengthening of tendo calcaneus by
   incomplete tenotomy) 83.11
Whitehead
   glossectomy, radical 25.4
   hemorrhoidectomy 49.46
Whitman
   foot stabilization (talectomy) 77.98
   hip reconstruction 81.40
   repair of serratus anterior muscle 83.87
   talectomy 77.98
   trochanter wedge osteotomy 77.25
Wier (entropion repair) 08.44
Williams-Richardson (vaginal construction)
   70.61
   with graft or prosthesis 70.63
Wilms (thoracoplasty) 33.34
Wilson (angulation osteotomy for hallux valgus)
   77.51
window
   antrum (nasal sinus)—*see* Antrotomy, maxillary
   aorticopulmonary 39.59
   bone cortex (*see also* Incision, bone) 77.10
     facial 76.09
   nasoantral—*see* Antrotomy, maxillary
   pericardium 37.12
   pleural 34.09
Winiwarter (cholecystoenterostomy) 51.32
Witzel (temporary gastrostomy) 43.19
Woodward (release of high riding scapula) 81.83
Young
   epispadias repair 58.45
   tendon transfer (anterior tibialis) (repair of flat
     foot) 83.75
Yount (division of iliotibial band) 83.14
Zancolli
   capsuloplasty 81.72
   tendon transfer (biceps) 82.56
Ziegler (iridectomy) 12.14

Operculectomy 24.6
Ophthalmectomy 16.49
   with implant (into Tenon's capsule) 16.42
   with attachment of muscles 16.41
Ophthalmoscopy 16.21
Opponensplasty (hand) 82.56
Optical coherence tomography (OCT)
   (intravascular imaging)
   coronary vessel(s) 38.24
   non-coronary vessel(s) 38.25
Orbitomaxillectomy, radical 16.51
Orbitotomy (anterior) (frontal) (temporofrontal)
   (transfrontal) NEC 16.09
   with
     bone flap 16.01
     insertion of implant 16.02
   Kroenlein (lateral) 16.01
   lateral 16.01
Orchidectomy (with epididymectomy)
   (unilateral) 62.3
   bilateral (radical) 62.41
   remaining or solitary testis 62.42
Orchidopexy 62.5
Orchidoplasty 62.69
Orchidorrhaphy 62.61
Orchidotomy 62.0
Orchiectomy (with epididymectomy) (unilateral)
   62.3
   bilateral (radical) 62.41
   remaining or solitary testis 62.42
Orchiopexy 62.5
Orchioplasty 62.69
Orthoroentgenography —*see* Radiography
Oscar Miller operation (midtarsal arthrodesis)
   81.14
Osmond-Clark operation (soft tissue release
   with peroneus brevis tendon transfer) 83.75
Ossiculectomy NEC 19.3
   with
     stapedectomy (*see also* Stapedectomy) 19.19
     stapes mobilization 19.0
     tympanoplasty 19.53
       revision 19.6
Ossiculotomy NEC 19.3
Ostectomy (partial), except facial—*see also*
   category 77.8
   facial NEC 76.39
     total 76.45
       with reconstruction 76.44
   first metatarsal head—*see* Bunionectomy
   for graft (autograft) (homograft)—*see also*
     category 77.7
   mandible 76.31
     total 76.42
       with reconstruction 76.41
   total, except facial—*see also* category 77.9
     facial NEC 76.45
       with reconstruction 76.44
     mandible 76.42
       with reconstruction 76.41
Osteoarthrotomy (*see also* Osteotomy) 77.30
Osteoclasis 78.70
   carpal, metacarpal 78.74
   clavicle 78.71
   ear 20.79
   femur 78.75
   fibula 78.77
   humerus 78.72
   patella 78.76
   pelvic 78.79
   phalanges (foot) (hand) 78.79

Osteoclasis—*continued*
radius 78.73
scapula 78.71
specified site NEC 78.79
tarsal, metatarsal 78.78
thorax (ribs) (sternum) 78.71
tibia 78.77
ulna 78.73
vertebrae 78.79
Osteolysis —*see* category 78.4
Osteopathic manipulation (*see also*
Manipulation, osteopathic) 93.67
Osteoplasty NEC—*see* category 78.4
with bone graft—*see* Graft, bone
for
bone lengthening—*see* Lengthening, bone
bone shortening—*see* Shortening, bone
repair of malunion or nonunion of fracture—*see*
Repair, fracture, malunion or nonunion
carpal, metacarpal 78.44
clavicle 78.41
cranium NEC 02.06
with
flap (bone) 02.03
graft (bone) 02.04
facial bone NEC 76.69
femur 78.45
fibula 78.47
humerus 78.42
mandible, mandibular NEC 76.64
body 76.63
ramus (open) 76.62
closed 76.61
maxilla (segmental) 76.65
total 76.66
nasal bones 21.89
patella 78.46
pelvic 78.49
phalanges (foot) (hand) 78.49
radius 78.43
scapula 78.41
skull NEC 02.06
with
flap (bone) 02.03
graft (bone) 02.04
specified site NEC 78.49
tarsal, metatarsal 78.48
thorax (ribs) (sternum) 78.41
tibia 78.47
ulna 78.43
vertebrae 78.49
Osteorrhaphy (*see also* Osteoplasty) 78.40
Osteosynthesis (fracture) —*see* Reduction,
fracture
Osteotomy (adduction) (angulation) (block)
(derotational) (displacement) (partial)
(rotational) 77.30
carpals, metacarpals 77.34
wedge 77.24
clavicle 77.31
wedge 77.21
facial bone NEC 76.69
femur 77.35
wedge 77.25
fibula 77.37
wedge 77.27
humerus 77.32
wedge 77.22
mandible (segmental) (subapical) 76.64
angle (open) 76.62
closed 76.61
body 76.63

Osteotomy—*continued*
Gigli saw 76.61
ramus (open) 76.62
closed 76.61
maxilla (segmental) 76.65
total 76.66
metatarsal 77.38
wedge 77.28
for hallux valgus repair 77.51
patella 77.36
wedge 77.26
pelvic 77.39
wedge 77.29
phalanges (foot) (hand) 77.39
for repair of
bunion—*see* Bunionectomy
bunionette 77.54
hallux valgus—*see* Bunionectomy
wedge 77.29
for repair of
bunion—*see* Bunionectomy
bunionette 77.54
hallux valgus—*see* Bunionectomy
radius 77.33
wedge 77.23
scapula 77.31
wedge 77.21
specified site NEC 77.39
wedge 77.29
tarsal 77.38
wedge 77.28
thorax (ribs) (sternum) 77.31
wedge 77.21
tibia 77.37
wedge 77.27
toe 77.39
for repair of
bunion—*see* Bunionectomy
bunionette 77.54
hallux valgus—*see* Bunionectomy
wedge 77.29
for repair of
bunion—*see* bunionectomy
bunionette 77.54
hallux valgus—*see* Bunionectomy
ulna 77.33
wedge 77.23
vertebrae 77.39
wedge 77.29
Otonecrectomy (inner ear) 20.79
Otoplasty (external) 18.79
auditory canal or meatus 18.6
auricle 18.79
cartilage 18.79
reconstruction 18.71
prominent or protruding 18.5
Otoscopy 18.11
Outfolding, sclera, for buckling (*see also*
Buckling, scleral) 14.49
Outfracture, turbinates (nasal) 21.62
Output and clearance, circulatory 92.05
Overdistension, bladder (therapeutic) 96.25
Overlapping, sclera, for buckling (*see also*
Buckling, scleral) 14.49
Oversewing
left atrial appendage (LAA) 37.36
pleural bleb 32.21
ulcer crater (peptic) 44.40
duodenum 44.42
stomach 44.41
Oxford operation (for urinary incontinence) 59.4
Oximetry fetal pulse 75.38

Oxygenation 93.96
   extracorporeal membrane (ECMO) 39.65
   hyperbaric 93.95
     wound 93.59
   infusion therapy, Super 00.49
Oxygen therapy (catalytic) (pump) 93.96
   hyperbaric 93.95
   SuperSaturated 00.49

P

Pacemaker
  cardiac—*see also* Insertion, pacemaker, cardiac
    intraoperative (temporary) 39.64
    temporary (during and immediately following
      cardiac surgery) 39.64
Packing —*see also* Insertion, pack
  auditory canal 96.11
  nose, for epistaxis (anterior) 21.01
    posterior (and anterior) 21.02
  rectal 96.19
  sella turcica 07.79
  vaginal 96.14
Palatoplasty 27.69
  for cleft palate 27.62
    secondary or subsequent 27.63
Palatorrhaphy 27.61
  for cleft palate 27.62
Pallidectomy 01.42
Pallidoansotomy 01.42
Pallidotomy 01.42
  by stereotactic radiosurgery 92.32
    cobalt 60 92.32
    linear accelerator (LINAC) 92.31
    multi-source 92.32
    particle beam 92.33
    particulate 92.33
    radiosurgery NEC 92.39
    single source proton 92.31
Panas operation (linear proctotomy) 48.0
Pancoast operation (division of trigeminal nerve
    at foramen ovale) 04.02
Pancreatectomy (total) (with synchronous
    duodenectomy) 52.6
  partial NEC 52.59
    distal (tail) (with part of body) 52.52
    proximal (head) (with part of body) (with
      synchronous duodenectomy) 52.51
    radical 52.53
      subtotal 52.53
    radical 52.7
      subtotal 52.53
Pancreaticocystoduodenostomy 52.4
Pancreaticocystoenterostomy 52.4
Pancreaticocystogastrostomy 52.4
Pancreaticocystojejunostomy 52.4
Pancreaticoduodenectomy (total) 52.6
  partial NEC 52.59
    proximal 52.51
    radical subtotal 52.53
  radical (one-stage) (two-stage) 52.7
    subtotal 52.53
Pancreaticoduodenostomy 52.96
Pancreaticoenterostomy 52.96
Pancreaticogastrostomy 52.96
Pancreaticoileostomy 52.96
Pancreaticojejunostomy 52.96
Pancreatoduodenectomy (total) 52.6
  partial NEC 52.59
  radical (one-stage) (two-stage) 52.7
    subtotal 52.53
Pancreatogram 87.66
  endoscopic retrograde (ERP) 52.13
Pancreatolithotomy 52.09
  endoscopic 52.94
Pancreatotomy 52.09
Pancreatolithotomy 52.09
  endoscopic 52.94

Panendoscopy 57.32
  specified site, other than bladder—*see*
    Endoscopy, by site
  through artificial stoma 57.31
Panhysterectomy (abdominal) 68.49
  laparoscopic 68.41
  vaginal 68.59
    laparoscopically assisted (LAVH) 68.51
Panniculectomy 86.83
Panniculotomy 86.83
Pantaloon operation (revision of gastric
    anastomosis) 44.5
Papillectomy, anal 49.39
  endoscopic 49.31
Papillotomy (pancreas) 51.82
  endoscopic 51.85
Paquin operation (ureteroneocystostomy) 56.74
Paracentesis
  abdominal (percutaneous) 54.91
  anterior chamber, eye 12.91
  bladder 57.11
  cornea 12.91
  eye (anterior chamber) 12.91
  thoracic, thoracis 34.91
  tympanum 20.09
    with intubation 20.01
Parasitology —*see* Examination, microscopic
Parathyroidectomy (partial) (subtotal) NEC
    06.89
  complete 06.81
  ectopic 06.89
  global removal 06.81
  mediastinal 06.89
  total 06.81
Parenteral nutrition, total 99.15
  peripheral 99.15
Parotidectomy 26.30
  complete 26.32
  partial 26.31
  radical 26.32
Partsch operation (marsupialization of dental
    cyst) 24.4
Passage —*see* Insertion and Intubation
Passage of sounds, urethra 58.6
Patch
  blood, spinal (epidural) 03.95
  graft—*see* Graft
  spinal, blood (epidural) 03.95
  subdural, brain 02.12
Patellapexy 78.46
Patellaplasty NEC 78.46
Patellectomy 77.96
  partial 77.86
Pattee operation (auditory canal) 18.6
PDT (percutaneous dilatational tracheostomy)
    —*see* Tracheostomy
Pectenotomy (*see also* Sphincterotomy, anal)
    49.59
Pedicle flap —*see* Graft, skin, pedicle
Peet operation (splanchnic resection) 05.29
PEG (percutaneous endoscopic gastrostomy)
    43.11
PEGJJ (percutaneous [endoscopic]
    gastrojejunostomy) 44.32
PEJ (percutaneous endoscopic jejunostomy)
    46.32
Pelvectomy, kidney (partial) 55.4

Pelvimetry 88.25
  gynecological 89.26
Pelviolithotomy 55.11
Pelvioplasty, kidney 55.87
Pelviostomy 55.12
  closure 55.82
Pelviotomy 77.39
  to assist delivery 73.94
Pelvi-ureteroplasty 55.87
Pemberton operation
  osteotomy of ilium 77.39
  rectum (mobilization and fixation for prolapse
    repair) 48.76
Penectomy 64.3
Pereyra operation (paraurethral suspension) 59.6
Perforation
  stapes footplate 19.0
Perfusion NEC 39.97
  carotid artery 39.97
  coronary artery 39.97
  for
    chemotherapy NEC 99.25
    hormone therapy NEC 99.24
  head 39.97
  hyperthermic (lymphatic), localized region
    or site 93.35
  intestine (large) (local) 46.96
    small 46.95
  kidney, local 55.95
  limb (lower) (upper) 39.97
  liver, localized 50.93
  neck 39.97
  subarachnoid (spinal cord) (refrigerated saline)
    03.92
  total body 39.96
Pericardiectomy 37.31
Pericardiocentesis 37.0
Pericardiolysis 37.12
Pericardioplasty 37.49
Pericardiorrhaphy 37.49
Pericardiostomy (tube) 37.12
pericardiotomy 37.12
Peridectomy 10.31
Perilimbal suction 89.11
Perimetry 95.05
Perineoplasty 71.79
Perineorrhaphy 71.71
  obstetrical laceration (current) 75.69
Perineotomy (nonobstetrical) 71.09
  to assist delivery—*see* Episiotomy
Periosteotomy (*see also* Incision, bone) 77.10
  facial bone 76.09
Perirectofistulectomy 48.93
Peritectomy 10.31
Peritomy 10.1
Peritoneocentesis 54.91
Peritoneoscopy 54.21
Peritoneotomy 54.19
Peritoneumectomy 54.4
Phacoemulsification (ultrasonic) (with
  aspiration) 13.41
Phacofragmentation (mechanical) (with
  aspiration) 13.43
  posterior route 13.42
  ultrasonic 13.41
Phalangectomy (partial) 77.89
  claw toe 77.57
  cockup toe 77.58
  hammer toe 77.56
  overlapping toe 77.58
  total 77.99

Phalangization (fifth metacarpal) 82.81
Pharyngeal flop operation (cleft palate repair)
  27.62
  secondary or subsequent 27.63
Pharyngectomy (partial) 29.33
  with laryngectomy 30.3
Pharyngogram 87.09
  contrast 87.06
Pharyngolaryngectomy 30.3
Pharyngoplasty (with silastic implant) 29.4
  for cleft palate 27.62
    secondary or subsequent 27.63
Pharyngorrhaphy 29.51
  for cleft palate 27.62
Pharyngoscopy 29.11
Pharyngotomy 29.0
Phenopeel (skin) 86.24
Phlebectomy 38.60
  with
    anastomosis 38.30
      abdominal 38.37
      head and neck NEC 38.32
      intracranial NEC 38.31
      lower limb 38.39
      thoracic NEC 38.35
      upper limb 38.33
    graft replacement 38.40
      abdominal 38.47
      head and neck NEC 38.42
      intracranial NEC 38.41
      lower limb 38.49
      thoracic NEC 38.45
      upper limb 38.43
  abdominal 38.67
  head and neck NEC 38.62
  intracranial NEC 38.61
  lower limb 38.69
  thoracic NEC 38.65
  upper limb 38.63
  varicose 38.50
    abdominal 38.57
    head and neck NEC 38.52
    intracranial NEC 38.51
    lower limb 38.59
    thoracic NEC 38.55
    upper limb 38.53
Phlebogoniostomy 12.52
Phlebography (contrast) (retrograde) 88.60
  by radioisotope—*see* Scan, radioisotope, by site
  adrenal 88.65
  femoral 88.66
  head 88.61
  hepatic 88.64
  impedance 88.68
  intra-abdominal NEC 88.65
  intrathoracic NEC 88.63
  lower extremity NEC 88.66
  neck 88.61
  portal system 88.64
  pulmonary 88.62
  specified site NEC 88.67
  vena cava (inferior) (superior) 88.51
Phleborrhaphy 39.32
Phlebotomy 38.99
Phonocardiogram, with ECG lead 89.55
Photochemotherapy NEC 99.83
  extracorporeal 99.88
Photocoagulation
  ciliary body 12.73
  eye, eyeball 16.99

Photocoagulation—*continued*
iris 12.41
macular hole—*see* Photocoagulation, retina
orbital lesion 16.92
retina
  for
    destruction of lesion 14.25
    reattachment 14.55
    repair of tear or defect 14.35
  laser (beam)
    for
      destruction of lesion 14.24
      reattachment 14.54
      repair of tear or defect 14.34
  xenon arc
    for
      destruction of lesion 14.23
      reattachment 14.53
      repair of tear or defect 14.33
Photography 89.39
  fundus 95.11
Photopheresis, therapeutic 99.88
Phototherapy NEC 99.83
  newborn 99.83
  ultraviolet 99.82
Phrenemphraxis 04.03
  for collapse of lung 33.31
Phrenicectomy 04.03
  for collapse of lung 33.31
Phrenicoexeresis 04.03
  for collapse of lung 33.31
Phrenicotomy 04.03
  for collapse of lung 33.31
Phrenicotripsy 04.03
  for collapse of lung 33.31
Phrenoplasty 34.84
Physical medicine —*see* Therapy, physical
Physical therapy —*see* Therapy, physical
Physiotherapy, chest 93.99
PICC (peripherally inserted central catheter)
  38.93
Piercing ear, external (pinna) 18.01
Pigmenting, skin 86.02
Pilojection (aneurysm) (Gallagher) 39.52
Pinealectomy (complete) (total) 07.54
  partial 07.53
Pinealotomy (with drainage) 07.52
Pinning
  bone—*see* Fixation, bone, internal
  ear 18.5
Pinsker operation (obliteration of nasoseptal
  telangiectasia) 21.07
Piper operation (forceps) 72.6
Pirogoff operation (ankle amputation through
  malleoli of tibia and fibula) 84.14
Pituitectomy (complete) (total) (*see also*
  Hypophysectomy) 07.69
Placentogram, placentography 88.46
  with radioisotope (RISA) 92.17
Planing, skin 86.25
Plantation, tooth (bud) (germ) 23.5
  prosthetic 23.6
Plasma exchange 99.07
Plasmapheresis, therapeutic 99.71
Plastic repair —*see* Repair, by site
Plasty —*see also* Repair, by site
  bladder neck (V-Y) 57.85
  skin (without graft) 86.89
  subcutaneous tissue 86.89
Platelet inhibitor (GP IIB/IIIa inhibitor only),
  infusion 99.20

Plateletpheresis, therapeutic 99.74
Play
  psychotherapy 94.36
  therapy 93.81
Pleating
  eye muscle 15.22
    multiple (two or more muscles) 15.4
  sclera, for buckling (*see also* Buckling, scleral)
    14.49
Plethysmogram (carotid) 89.58
  air-filled (pneumatic) 89.58
  capacitance 89.58
  cerebral 89.58
  differential 89.58
  oculoplethysmogram 89.58
  penile 89.58
  photoelectric 89.58
  regional 89.58
  respiratory function measurement (body) 89.38
  segmental 89.58
  strain-gauge 89.58
  thoracic impedance 89.38
  venous occlusion 89.58
  water-filled 89.58
Plethysmography penile 89.58
  CaverMap™ 89.58
Pleurectomy NEC 34.59
Pleurocentesis 34.91
Pleurodesis 34.6
  chemical 34.92
    with cancer chemotherapy substance 34.92
      [99.25]
    tetracycline 34.92 *[99.21]*
Pleurolysis (for collapse of lung) 33.39
Pleuropexy 34.99
Pleurosclerosis 34.6
  chemical 34.92
    with cancer chemotherapy substance 34.92
      [99.25]
    tetracycline 34.92 *[99.21]*
Pleurotomy 34.09
Plexectomy
  choroid 02.14
  hypogastric 05.24
Plication
  aneurysm, heart 37.32
  annulus, heart valve 35.33
  bleb (emphysematous), lung 32.21
  broad ligament 69.22
  diaphragm (for hernia repair) (thoracic approach)
    (thoracoabdominal approach) 53.81
  eye muscle (oblique) (rectus) 15.22
    multiple (two or more muscles) 15.4
  fascia 83.89
    hand 82.89
  inferior vena cava 38.7
  intestine (jejunum) (Noble) 46.62
  Kelly (Stoeckel) (urethrovesical junction) 59.3
  levator, for blepharoptosis 08.34
  ligament (*see also* Arthroplasty) 81.96
    broad 69.22
    round 69.22
    uterosacral 69.22
  mesentery 54.75
  round ligament 69.22
  sphincter, urinary bladder 57.85
  stomach 44.69
    laparoscopic 44.68
  superior vena cava 38.7
  tendon 83.85
    hand 82.55

Plication—*continued*
  tricuspid valve (with repositioning) 35.14
  ureter 56.89
  urethra 58.49
  urethrovesical junction 59.3
  vein (peripheral) 39.59
  vena cava (inferior) (superior) 38.7
  ventricle (heart)
    aneurysm 37.32
Plicotomy, tympanum 20.23
Plombage, lung 33.39
Pneumocentesis 33.93
Pneumocisternogram 87.02
Pneumoencephalogram 87.01
Pneumogram, pneumography
  extraperitoneal 88.15
  mediastinal 87.33
  orbit 87.14
  pelvic 88.13
  peritoneum NEC 88.13
  presacral 88.15
  retroperitoneum 88.15
Pneumogynecography 87.82
Pneumomediastinography 87.33
Pneumonectomy (extended) (radical) (standard)
  (total) (with mediastinal dissection) 32.59
  partial
    complete excision, one lobe 32.49
    resection (wedge), one lobe 32.39
  thoracoscopic 32.50
Pneumonolysis (for collapse of lung) 33.39
Pneumonotomy (with exploration) 33.1
Pneumoperitoneum (surgically-induced) 54.96
  for collapse of lung 33.33
  pelvic 88.12
Pneumothorax (artificial) (surgical) 33.32
  intrapleural 33.32
Pneumoventriculogram 87.02
Politano-Leadbetter operation
  (ureteroneocystostomy) 56.74
Politzerization, Eustachian tube 20.8
Pollicization (with carry over of nerves and blood
  supply) 82.61
Polya operation (gastrectomy) 43.7
Polypectomy —*see also* Excision, lesion, by site
  esophageal 42.32
    endoscopic 42.33
  gastric (endoscopic) 43.41
  large intestine (colon) 45.42
  nasal 21.31
  rectum (endoscopic) 48.36
Polysomnogram 89.17
Pomeroy operation (ligation and division of
  fallopian tubes) 66.32
Poncet operation
  lengthening of Achilles tendon 83.85
  urethrostomy, perineal 58.0
Porro operation (cesarean section) 74.99
Portoenterostomy (Kasai) 51.37
Positrocephalogram 92.11
Positron emission tomography (PET) —*see*
  Scan, radioisotope
Postmortem examination 89.8
Potts-Smith operation (descending aorta-left
  pulmonary artery anastomosis) 39.0
Poudrage
  intrapericardial 36.39
  pleural 34.6
PPN (peripheral parenteral nutrition) 99.15
PPVI (percutaneous pulmonary valve
  implantation) 35.07

Preparation (cutting), pedicle (flap) graft 86.71
Preputiotomy 64.91
Prescription for glasses 95.31
Pressurized
  graft treatment 00.16
Printen and Mason operation (high gastric
  bypass) 44.31
Probing
  canaliculus, lacrimal (with irrigation) 09.42
  lacrimal
    canaliculi 09.42
    punctum (with irrigation) 09.41
  nasolacrimal duct (with irrigation) 09.43
    with insertion of tube or stent 09.44
  salivary duct (for dilation of duct) (for removal of
    calculus) 26.91
    with incision 26.0
Procedure —*see also* specific procedure
  diagnostic NEC
    abdomen (region) 54.29
    adenoid 28.19
    adrenal gland 07.19
    alveolus 24.19
    amnion 75.35
    anterior chamber, eye 12.29
    anus 49.29
    appendix 45.28
    biliary tract 51.19
    bladder 57.39
    blood vessel (any site) 38.29
    bone 78.80
      carpal, metacarpal 78.84
      clavicle 78.81
      facial 76.19
      femur 78.85
      fibula 78.87
      humerus 78.82
      marrow 41.38
      patella 78.86
      pelvic 78.89
      phalanges (foot) (hand) 78.89
      radius 78.83
      scapula 78.81
      specified site NEC 78.89
      tarsal, metatarsal 78.88
      thorax (ribs) (sternum) 78.81
      tibia 78.87
      ulna 78.83
      vertebrae 78.89
    brain 01.18
    breast 85.19
    bronchus 33.29
    buccal 27.24
    bursa 83.29
    canthus 08.19
    cecum 45.28
    cerebral meninges 01.18
    cervix 67.19
    chest wall 34.28
    choroid 14.19
    ciliary body 12.29
    clitoris 71.19
    colon 45.28
    conjunctiva 10.29
    cornea 11.29
    cul-de-sac 70.29
    dental 24.19
    diaphragm 34.28
    duodenum 45.19

Procedure—*continued*

ear
  external 18.19
  inner and middle 20.39
epididymis 63.09
esophagus 42.29
Eustachian tube 20.39
extraocular muscle or tendon 15.09
eye 16.29
  anterior chamber 12.29
  posterior chamber 14.19
eyeball 16.29
eyelid 08.19
fallopian tube 66.19
fascia (any site) 83.29
fetus 75.35
gallbladder 51.19
ganglion (cranial) (peripheral) 04.19
  sympathetic 05.19
gastric 44.19
globus pallidus 01.18
gum 24.19
heart 37.29
hepatic 50.19
hypophysis 07.19
ileum 45.19
intestine 45.29
  large 45.28
  small 45.19
iris 12.29
jejunum 45.19
joint (capsule) (ligament) (structure) NEC
    81.98
  facial 76.19
kidney 55.29
labia 71.19
lacrimal (system) 09.19
large intestine 45.28
larynx 31.48
ligament 81.98
  uterine 68.19
liver 50.19
lung 33.29
lymphatic structure (channel) (gland) (node)
    (vessel) 40.19
mediastinum 34.29
meninges (cerebral) 01.18
  spinal 03.39
mouth 27.29
muscle 83.29
  extraocular (oblique) (rectus) 15.09
  papillary (heart) 37.29
nail 86.19
nasopharynx 29.19
nerve (cranial) (peripheral) NEC 04.19
  sympathetic 05.19
nipple 85.19
nose, nasal 21.29
  sinus 22.19
ocular 16.29
  muscle 15.09
omentum 54.29
ophthalmologic 16.29
oral (cavity) 27.29
orbit 16.29
orthodontic 24.19
ovary 65.19
  laparoscopic 65.14
palate 27.29
pancreas 52.19
papillary muscle (heart) 37.29

Procedure—*continued*

parathyroid gland 06.19
penis 64.19
perianal tissue 49.29
pericardium 37.29
periprostatic tissue 60.18
perirectal tissue 48.29
perirenal tissue 59.29
peritoneum 54.29
periurethral tissue 58.29
perivesical tissue 59.29
pharynx 29.19
pineal gland 07.19
pituitary gland 07.19
pleura 34.28
posterior chamber, eye 14.19
prostate 60.18
pulmonary 33.29
rectosigmoid 48.29
rectum 48.29
renal 55.29
respiratory 33.29
retina 14.19
retroperitoneum 59.29
salivary gland or duct 26.19
sclera 12.29
scrotum 61.19
seminal vesicle 60.19
sigmoid 45.28
sinus, nasal 22.19
skin 86.19
skull 01.19
soft tissue 83.29
spermatic cord 63.09
sphincter of Oddi 51.19
spine, spinal (canal) (Cord) (meninges)
    (structure) 03.39
spleen 41.39
stomach 44.19
subcutaneous tissue 86.19
sympathetic nerve 05.19
tarsus 09.19
tendon NEC 83.29
  extraocular 15.09
testicle 62.19
thalamus 01.18
thoracic duct 40.19
thorax 34.28
thymus 07.19
thyroid gland 06.19
tongue 25.09
tonsils 28.19
tooth 24.19
trachea 31.49
tunica vaginalis 61.19
ureter 56.39
urethra 58.29
uterus and supporting structures 68.19
uvula 27.29
vagina 70.29
vas deferens 63.09
vesical 57.39
vessel (blood) (any site) 38.2
vitreous 14.19
vulva 71.19
fistulizing, sclera NEC 12.69
miscellaneous (nonoperative) NEC 99.99
respiratory (nonoperative) NEC 93.99
surgical—*see* Operation
Proctectasis 96.22

Proctectomy (partial) (*see also* Resection, rectum) 48.69
  abdominoperineal, NOS 48.50
    laparoscopic 48.51
    open 48.52
    other 48.59
  complete (Miles) (Rankin), NOS 48.50
    laparoscopic 48.51
    open 48.52
    other 48.59
  pull-through
    laparoscopic 48.42
    not otherwise specified 48.40
    open 48.43
    other 48.49
Proctoclysis 96.37
Proctoclysis 48.99
Proctopexy (Delorme) 48.76
  abdominal (Ripstein) 48.75
Proctoplasty 48.79
Proctorrhaphy 48.71
Proctoscopy 48.23
  with biopsy 48.24
  through stoma (artificial) 48.22
  transabdominal approach 48.21
Proctosigmoidectomy (*see also* Resection, rectum) 48.69
Proctosigmoidopexy 48.76
Proctosigmoidoscopy (rigid) 48.23
  with biopsy 48.24
  flexible 45.24
  through stoma (artificial) 48.22
  transabdominal approach 48.21
Proctostomy 48.1
Proctotomy (decompression) (linear) 48.0
Production —*see also* Formation *and* Creation
  atrial septal defect 35.42
  subcutaneous tunnel for esophageal anastomosis 42.86
    with anastomosis—*see* Anastomosis, esophagus, antesternal
Prognathic recession 76.64
Prophylaxis, dental (scaling) (polishing) 96.54
Prostatectomy (complete) (partial) NEC 60.69
  loop 60.29
  perineal 60.62
  radical (any approach) 60.5
  retropubic (punch) (transcapsular) 60.4
  suprapubic (punch) (transvesical) 60.3
  transcapsular NEC 60.69
    retropubic 60.4
  transperineal 60.62
  transurethral 60.29
    ablation (contact) (noncontact) by laser 60.21
    electrovaporization 60.29
    enucleative 60.29
    resection of prostate (TURP) 60.29
    ultrasound guided laser induced (TULIP) 60.21
  transvesical punch (suprapubic) 60.3
Prostatocystotomy 60.0
Prostatolithotomy 60.0
Prostatotomy (perineal) 60.0
Prostatovesiculectomy 60.5
Protection (of)
  individual from his surroundings 99.84
  surroundings from individual 99.84
Psychoanalysis 94.31
Psychodrama 94.43

Psychotherapy NEC 94.39
  biofeedback 94.39
  exploratory verbal 94.37
  group 94.44
    for psychosexual dysfunctions 94.41
  play 94.36
  psychosexual dysfunctions 94.34
  supportive verbal 94.38
PTCA (percutaneous transluminal coronary angioplasty)—*see* Angioplasty, balloon, coronary
Ptyalectasis 26.91
Ptyalithotomy 26.0
Ptyalolithotomy 26.0
Pubiotomy 77.39
  assisting delivery 73.94
Pubococcygeoplasty 59.71
Puestow operation (pancreaticojejunostomy) 52.96
Pull-through
  abdomino-anal 48.49
  abdominoperineal 48.49
    Duhamel type 48.65
  endorectal 48.41
Pulmowrap 93.99
Pulpectomy (*see also* Therapy, root canal) 23.70
Pulpotomy (*see also* Therapy, root canal) 23.70
Pump-oxygenator for extracorporeal circulation 39.61
  percutaneous 39.66
Punch
  operation
    bladder neck, transurethral 57.49
    prostate—*see* Prostatectomy
  resection, vocal cords 30.22
Puncture
  antrum (nasal) (bilateral) (unilateral) 22.01
  artery NEC 38.98
    for
      arteriography (*see also* Arteriography) 88.40
      coronary arteriography (*see also* Arteriography, coronary) 88.57
    percutaneous vascular closure—*omit code*
  bladder, suprapubic (for drainage) NEC 57.18
    needle 57.11
    percutaneous (suprapubic) 57.17
  bursa 83.94
    hand 82.92
  cisternal 01.01
    with contrast media 87.02
  cranial 01.09
    with contrast media 87.02
  craniobuccal pouch 07.72
  craniopharyngioma 07.72
  fallopian tube 66.91
  fontanel, anterior 01.09
  heart 37.0
    for intracardiac injection 37.92
  hypophysis 07.72
  iris 12.12
  joint 81.91
  kidney (percutaneous) 55.92
  larynx 31.98
  lumbar (diagnostic) (removal of dye) 03.31
  lung (for aspiration) 33.93
  nasal sinus 22.01
  pericardium 37.0
  pituitary gland 07.72
  pleural cavity 34.91
  Rathke's pouch 07.72
  spinal 03.31

Puncture—*continued*
   spleen 41.1
      for biopsy 41.32
      sternal (for bone marrow biopsy) 41.31
         donor for bone marrow transplant 41.91
      vein NEC 38.99
         for
            phlebography (*see also* Phlebography) 88.60
            transfusion—*see* Transfusion
      ventricular shunt tubing 01.02
Pupillotomy 12.35
Push-back operation (cleft palate repair) 27.62
Putti-Platt operation (capsulorrhaphy of
      shoulder for recurrent dislocation) 81.82
pVAD (percutaneous ventricular assist device)
      37.68
Pyelogram (intravenous) 87.73
   infusion (continuous) (diuretic) 87.73
   percutaneous 87.75
   retrograde 87.74
Pyeloileostomy 56.71
Pyelolithotomy 55.11
Pyeloplasty 55.87
Pyelorrhaphy 55.81
Pyeloscopy 55.22
Pyelostolithotomy, percutaneous 55.03
Pyelostomy 55.12
   closure 55.82
Pyelotomy 55.11
Pyeloureteroplasty 55.87
Pylorectomy 43.6
Pyloroduodenotomy —*see* category 44.2
Pyloromyotomy (Ramstedt) (with wedge
      resection) 43.3
Pyloroplasty (Finney) (Heineke-Mikulicz) 44.29
   dilation, endoscopic 44.22
      by incision 44.21
   not elsewhere classified 44.29
   revision 44.29
Pylorostomy —*see* Gastrostomy

Q-R

Quadrant resection of breast 85.22
Quadricepsplasty (Thompson) 83.86
Quarantine 99.84
Quenuthoracoplasty 77.31
Quotient, respiratory 89.38

Rachicentesis 03.31
Rachitomy 03.09
Radiation therapy —*see also* Therapy, radiation
  teleradiotheraphy—*see* Teleradiotherapy
Radical neck dissection —*see* Dissection, neck
Radicotomy 03.1
Radiculectomy 03.1
Radiculotomy 03.1
Radiography (diagnostic) NEC 88.39
  abdomen, abdominal (flat plate) NEC 88.19
    wall (soft tissue) NEC 88.09
  adenoid 87.09
  ankle (skeletal) 88.28
    soft tissue 88.37
  bone survey 88.31
  bronchus 87.49
  chest (routine) 87.44
    wall NEC 87.39
  clavicle 87.43
  computer assisted surgery (CAS) with
      fluoroscopy 00.33
  contrast (air) (gas) (radio-opaque substance) NEC
    abdominal wall 88.03
    arteries (by fluoroscopy)—*see* Arteriography
    bile ducts NEC 87.54
    bladder NEC 87.77
    brain 87.02
    breast 87.35
    bronchus NEC (transcricoid) 87.32
      endotracheal 87.31
    epididymis 87.93
    esophagus 87.61
    fallopian tubes
      gas 87.82
      opaque dye 87.83
    fistula (sinus tract)—*see also* Radiography,
        contrast, by site
      abdominal wall 88.03
      chest wall 87.38
    gallbladder NEC 87.59
    intervertebral disc(s) 87.21
    joints 88.32
    larynx 87.07
    lymph—*see* Lymphangiogram
    mammary ducts 87.35
    mediastinum 87.33
    nasal sinuses 87.15
    nasolacrimal ducts 87.05
    nasopharynx 87.06
    orbit 87.14
    pancreas 87.66
    pelvis
      gas 88.12
      opaque dye 88.11
    peritoneum NEC 88.13
    retroperitoneum NEC 88.15
    seminal vesicles 87.91
    sinus tract—*see also* Radiography, contrast, by
        site
      abdominal wall 88.03
      chest wall 87.38
      nose 87.15
    skull 87.02
    spinal disc(s) 87.21
    trachea 87.32
    uterus
      gas 87.82
      opaque dye 87.83

Radiography—*continued*
  vas deferens 87.94
  veins (by fluoroscopy)—*see* Phlebography
  vena cava (inferior) (superior) 88.51
  dental NEC 87.12
  diaphragm 87.49
  digestive tract NEC 87.69
    barium swallow 87.61
    lower GI series 87.64
    small bowel series 87.63
    upper GI series 87.62
  elbow (skeletal) 88.22
    soft tissue 88.35
  epididymis NEC 87.95
  esophagus 87.69
    barium-swallow 87.61
  eye 95.14
  face, head, and neck 87.09
  facial bones 87.16
  fallopian tubes 87.85
  foot 88.28
  forearm (skeletal) 88.22
    soft tissue 88.35
  frontal area, facial 87.16
  genital organs
    female NEC 87.89
    male NEC 87.99
  hand (skeletal) 88.23
    soft tissue 88.35
  head NEC 87.09
  heart 87.49
  hip (skeletal) 88.26
    soft tissue 88.37
  intestine NEC 87.65
  kidney-ureter-bladder (KUB) 87.79
  knee (skeletal) 88.27
    soft tissue 88.37
  KUB (kidney-ureter-bladder) 87.79
  larynx 87.09
  lower leg (skeletal) 88.27
    soft tissue 88.37
  lower limb (skeletal) NEC 88.29
    soft tissue NEC 88.37
  lung 87.49
  mandible 87.16
  maxilla 87.16
  mediastinum 87.49
  nasal sinuses 87.16
  nasolacrimal duct 87.09
  nasopharynx 87.09
  neck NEC 87.09
  nose 87.16
  orbit 87.16
  pelvis (skeletal) 88.26
    pelvimetry 88.25
    soft tissue 88.19
  prostate NEC 87.92
  retroperitoneum NEC 88.16
  ribs 87.43
  root canal 87.12
  salivary gland 87.09
  seminal vesicles NEC 87.92
  shoulder (skeletal) 88.21
    soft tissue 88.35
  skeletal NEC 88.33
    series (whole or complete) 88.31
  skull (lateral, sagittal or tangential projection)
    NEC 87.17
  spine NEC 87.29
    cervical 87.22
    lumbosacral 87.24

Radiography—*continued*
  sacrococcygeal 87.24
  thoracic 87.23
  sternum 87.43
  supraorbital area 87.16
  symphysis menti 87.16
  teeth NEC 87.12
    full-mouth 87.11
  thigh (skeletal) 88.27
    soft tissue 88.37
  thyroid region 87.09
  tonsils and adenoids 87.09
  trachea 87.49
  ultrasonic—*see* Ultrasonography
  upper arm (skeletal) 88.21
    soft tissue 88.35
  upper limb (skeletal) NEC 88.24
    soft tissue NEC 88.35
  urinary system NEC 87.79
  uterus NEC 87.85
    gravid 87.81
  uvula 87.09
  vas deferens NEC 87.95
  wrist 88.23
  zygomaticomaxillary complex 87.16
Radioimmunotherapy 92.28
Radioisotope
  scanning—*see* Scan, radioisotope
  therapy—*see* Therapy, radioisotope
Radiology
  diagnostic—*see* Radiography
  therapeutic—*see* Therapy, radiation
Radiosurgery, stereotactic 92.30
  cobalt 60 92.32
  linear accelerator (LINAC) 92.31
  multi-source 92.32
  particle beam 92.33
  particulate 92.33
  radiosurgry NEC 92.39
  single source photon 92.31
Raising, pedicle graft 86.71
Ramadier operation (intrapetrosal drainage)
  20.22
Ramisection (sympathetic) 05.0
Ramstedt operation (pyeloromyotomy) (with
  wedge resection) 43.3
Range of motion testing 93.05
Rankin operation
  exteriorization of intestine 46.03
  proctectomy (complete), NOS 48.50
    laparoscopic 48.51
    open 48.52
    other 48.59
Rashkind operation (balloon septostomy) 35.41
Rastelli operation (creation of conduit between
  right ventricle and pulmonary artery) 35.92
  in repair of
    pulmonary artery atresia 35.92
    transposition of great vessels 35.92
    truncus arteriosus 35.83
Raz-Pereyra procedure (Bladder neck
  suspension) 59.79
RCSA (radical cryosurgical ablation) of
  prostate 60.62
Readjustment —*see* Adjustment
Reamputation, stump 84.3
Reanastomosis —*see* Anastomosis
Reattachment
  amputated ear 18.72
  ankle 84.27
  arm (upper) NEC 84.24

Reattachment—*continued*
choroid and retina NEC 14.59
  by
    cryotherapy 14.52
    diathermy 14.51
    electrocoagulation 14.51
    photocoagulation 14.55
      laser 14.54
      xenon arc 14.53
ear (amputated) 18.72
extremity 84.29
  ankle 84.27
  arm (upper) NEC 84.24
  fingers, except thumb 84.22
    thumb 84.21
  foot 84.26
  forearm 84.23
  hand 84.23
  leg (lower) NEC 84.27
  thigh 84.28
  thumb 84.21
  toe 84.25
  wrist 84.23
finger 84.22
  thumb 84.21
foot 84.26
forearm 84.23
hand 84.23
joint capsule (*see also* Arthroplasty) 81.96
leg (lower) NEC 84.27
ligament—*see also* Arthroplasty
  uterosacral 69.22
muscle 83.74
  hand 82.54
  papillary (heart) 35.31
nerve (peripheral) 04.79
nose (amputated) 21.89
papillary muscle (heart) 35.31
penis (amputated) 64.45
retina (and choroid) NEC 14.59
  by
    cryotherapy 14.52
    diathermy 14.51
    electrocoagulation 14.51
    photocoagulation 14.55
      laser 14.54
      xenon arc 14.53
tendon (to tendon) 83.73
  hand 82.53
  to skeletal attachment 83.88
    hand 82.85
thigh 84.28
thumb 84.21
toe 84.25
tooth 23.5
uterosacral ligament(s) 69.22
vessels (peripheral) 39.59
  renal, aberrant 39.55
wrist 84.23
Recession
extraocular muscle 15.11
  multiple (two or more muscles) (with
    advancement or resection) 15.3
gastrocnemius tendon (Strayer operation) 83.72
levator palpebrae (superioris) muscle 08.38
prognathic jaw 76.64
tendon 83.72
  hand 82.52
Reclosure —*see also* Closure
disrupted abdominal wall (postoperative) 54.61

Reconstruction (plastic)—*see also* Construction
  and Repair, by site
alveolus, alveolar (process) (ridge) (with graft or
  implant) 24.5
artery (graft)—*see* Graft, artery
artificial stoma, intestine 46.40
auditory canal (external) 18.6
auricle (ear) 18.71
bladder 57.87
  with
    ileum 57.87 *[45.51]*
    sigmoid 57.87 *[45.52]*
bone, except facial (*see also* Osteoplasty) 78.40
  facial NEC 76.46
    with total ostectomy 76.44
  mandible 76.43
    with total mandibulectomy 76.41
breast, total, NOS 85.70
  deep inferior epigastric artrey perforator (DIEP)
    flap, free 85.74
  gluteal artery perforator (GAP) flap, free 85.76
  latissimus dorsi myocutaneous flap 85.71
  other 85.79
  superficial inferior epigastric artery (SIEA)
    flap, free 85.75
  transverse rectus abdominis musculocutaneous
    (TRAM) flap, free 85.73
  transverse rectus abdominis myocutaneous
    (TRAM) flap, pedicled 85.72
bronchus 33.48
canthus (lateral) 08.59
cardiac annulus 35.33
chest wall (mesh) (silastic) 34.79
cleft lip 27.54
conjunctival cul-de-sac 10.43
  with graft (buccal mucous membrane) (free)
    10.42
cornea NEC 11.79
diaphragm 34.84
ear (external) (auricle) 18.71
  external auditory canal 18.6
  meatus (new) (osseous skin-lined) 18.6
  ossicles 19.3
  prominent or protruding 18.5
eyebrow 08.70
eyelid 08.70
  with graft or flap 08.69
    hair follicle 08.63
    mucous membrane 08.62
    skin 08.61
    tarsoconjunctival (one-stage) (two-stage)
      08.64
  full-thickness 08.74
    involving lid margin 08.73
  partial-thickness 08.72
    involving lid margin 08.71
eye socket 16.64
  with graft 16.63
fallopian tube 66.79
foot and toes (with fixation device) 81.57
  with prosthetic implant 81.57
frontonasal duct 22.79
hip (total) (with prosthesis) 81.51
intraoral 27.59
joint—*see* Arthroplasty
lymphatic (by transplantation) 40.9
mandible 76.43
  with total mandibulectomy 76.41
mastoid cavity 19.9
mouth 27.59
nipple NEC 85.87

Reconstruction—*continued*
  nose (total) (with arm flap) (with forehead flap)
    21.83
  ossicles (graft) (prosthesis) NEC 19.3
    with
      stapedectomy 19.19
      tympanoplasty 19.53
  pelvic floor 71.79
  penis (rib graft) (skin graft)
    (myocutaneous flap) 64.44
  pharynx 29.4
  scrotum (with pedicle flap) (with rotational flap)
    61.49
  skin (plastic) (without graft) NEC 86.89
    with graft—*see* Graft, skin
  subcutaneous tissue (plastic) (without skin graft)
    NEC 86.89
    with graft—*see* Graft, skin
  tendon pulley (with graft) (with local tissue)
    83.83
    for opponensplasty 82.71
    hand 82.71
  thumb (osteoplastic) (with bone graft)
    (with skin graft) 82.69
  trachea (with graft) 31.75
  umbilicus
    laparoscopic 53.43
      with graft or prosthesis 53.42
    other and open with graft or prosthesis 53.41
    other open 53.49
  ureteropelvic junction 55.87
  urethra 58.46
  vagina 70.62
    with graft or prosthesis 70.64
  vas deferens, surgically divided 63.82
Recontour, gingiva 24.2
Recreational therapy 93.81
Rectectomy (*see also* Resection, rectum) 48.69
Rectopexy (Delorme) 48.76
  abdominal (Ripstein) 48.75
Rectoplasty 48.79
Rectorectostomy 48.74
Rectorrhaphy 48.71
Rectosigmoidectomy (*see also* Resection,
  rectum) 48.69
  transsacral 48.61
Rectosigmoidostomy 45.94
Rectostomy 48.1
  closure 48.72
Red cell survival studies 92.05
Reduction —*see also* Excision, by site
  adipose tissue 86.83
  batwing arms 86.83
  breast (bilateral) 85.32
    unilateral 85.31
  bulbous tuberosities (mandible) (maxilla)
    (fibrous) (osseous) 24.31
  buttocks 86.83
  diastasis, ankle mortise (closed) 79.77
    open 79.87
  dislocation (of joint) (manipulation) (with cast)
    (with splint) (with traction device) (closed)
    79.70
    with fracture—*see* Reduction, fracture, by site
    ankle (closed) 79.77
      open 79.87
    elbow (closed) 79.72
      open 79.82
    finger (closed) 79.74
      open 79.84

Reduction—*continued*
    foot (closed) 79.78
      open 79.88
    hand (closed) 79.74
      open 79.84
    hip (closed) 79.75
      open 79.85
    knee (closed) 79.76
      open 79.86
    open (with external fixation) (with internal
      fixation) 79.80
      specified site NEC 79.89
    shoulder (closed) 79.71
      open 79.81
    specified site (closed) NEC 79.79
      open 79.89
    temporomandibular (closed) 76.93
      open 76.94
    toe (closed) 79.78
      open 79.88
    wrist (closed) 79.73
      open 79.83
  elephantiasis, scrotum 61.3
  epistaxis (*see also* Control, epistaxis) 21.00
  fracture (bone) (with cast) (with splint) (with
    traction device) (closed) 79.00
    with internal fixation 79.10
    alveolar process (with stabilization of teeth)
      mandible (closed) 76.75
        open 76.77
      maxilla (closed) 76.73
        open 76.77
      open 76.77
    ankle—*see* Reduction, fracture, leg
    arm (closed) NEC 79.02
      with internal fixation 79.12
      open 79.22
        with internal fixation 79.32
    blow-out—*see* Reduction, fracture, orbit
    carpal, metacarpal (closed) 79.03
      with internal fixation 79.13
      open 79.23
        with internal fixation 79.33
    epiphysis—*see* Reduction, separation
    facial (bone) NEC 76.70
      closed 76.78
      open 76.79
    femur (closed) 79.05
      with internal fixation 79.15
      open 79.25
        with internal fixation 79.35
    fibula (closed) 79.06
      with internal fixation 79.16
      open 79.26
        with internal fixation 79.36
    foot (closed) NEC 79.07
      with internal fixation 79.17
      open 79.27
        with internal fixation 79.37
    hand (closed) NEC 79.03
      with internal fixation 79.13
      open 79.23
        with internal fixation 79.33
    humerus (closed) 79.01
      with internal fixation 79.11
      open 79.21
        with internal fixation 79.31
    jaw (lower)—*see also* Reduction, fracture,
      mandible
    upper—*see* Reduction, fracture, maxilla

Reduction—*continued*
  larynx 31.64
  leg (closed) NEC 79.06
    with internal fixation 79.16
    open 79.26
      with internal fixation 79.36
  malar (closed) 76.71
    open 76.72
  mandible (with dental wiring) (closed) 76.75
    open 76.76
  maxilla (with dental wiring) (closed) 76.73
    open 76.74
  nasal (closed) 21.71
    open 21.72
  open 79.20
    with internal fixation 79.30
    specified site NEC 79.29
      with internal fixation 79.39
  orbit (rim) (wall) (closed) 76.78
    open 76.79
  patella (open) (with internal fixation) 79.36
  phalanges
    foot (closed) 79.08
      with internal fixation 79.18
      open 79.28
        with internal fixation 79.38
    hand (closed) 79.04
      with internal fixation 79.14
      open 79.24
        with internal fixation 79.34
  radius (closed) 79.02
    with internal fixation 79.12
    open 79.22
      with internal fixation 79.32
  skull 02.02
  specified site (closed) NEC 79.09
    with internal fixation 79.19
    open 79.29
      with internal fixation 79.39
  spine 03.53
  tarsal, metatarsal (closed) 79.07
    with internal fixation 79.17
    open 79.27
      with internal fixation 79.37
  tibia (closed) 79.06
    with internal fixation 79.16
    open 79.26
      with internal fixation 79.36
  ulna (closed) 79.02
    with internal fixation 79.12
    open 79.22
      with internal fixation 79.32
  vertebra 03.53
  zygoma, zygomatic arch (closed) 76.71
    open 76.72
fracture-dislocation—*see* Reduction, fracture
heart volume 37.35
hemorrhoids (manual) 49.41
hernia—*see also* Repair, hernia
  manual 96.27
intussusception (open) 46.80
  with
    fluoroscopy 96.29
    ionizing radiation enema 96.29
    ultrasonography guidance 96.29
  hydrostatic 96.29
  large intestine 46.82
    endoscopic (balloon) 46.85
  pneumatic 96.29
  small intestine 46.81
lung volume 32.22

Reduction—*continued*
  biologic lung volume reduction (BLVR) —*see*
    category 33.7
  malrotation, intestine (manual) (surgical) 46.80
    large 46.82
      endoscopic (balloon) 46.85
    small 46.81
  mammoplasty (bilateral) 85.32
    unilateral 85.31
  prolapse
    anus (operative) 49.94
    colostomy (manual) 96.28
    enterostomy (manual) 96.28
    ileostomy (manual) 96.28
    rectum (manual) 96.26
    uterus
      by pessary 96.18
      surgical 69.22
  ptosis overcorrection 08.37
  retroversion, uterus by pessary 96.18
  separation, epiphysis (with internal fixation)
    (closed) 79.40
    femur (closed) 79.45
      open 79.55
    fibula (closed) 79.46
      open 79.56
    humerus (closed) 79.41
      open 79.51
    open 79.50
    specified site (closed) NEC—*see also* category
      79.4
      open—*see* category 79.5
    tibia (closed) 79.46
      open 79.56
  size
    abdominal wall (adipose) (pendulous) 86.83
    arms (adipose) (batwing) 86.83
    breast (bilateral) 85.32
      unilateral 85.31
    buttocks (adipose) 86.83
    finger (macrodactyly repair) 82.83
    skin 86.83
    subcutaneous tissue 86.83
    thighs (adipose) 86.83
  torsion
    intestine (manual) (surgical) 46.80
      large 46.82
        endoscopic (balloon) 46.85
      small 46.81
    kidney pedicle 55.84
    omentum 54.74
    spermatic cord 63.52
      with orchiopexy 62.5
    testis 63.52
      with orchiopexy 62.5
    uterus NEC 69.98
      gravid 75.99
  ventricular 37.35
  volvulus
    intestine 46.80
      large 46.82
        endoscopic (balloon) 46.85
      small 46.81
    stomach 44.92
Reefing, joint capsule (*see also* Arthroplasty)
  81.96
Re-entry operation (aorta) 39.54
Re-establishment, continuity —*see also*
  Anastomosis
  bowel 46.50
  fallopian tube 66.79
  vas deferens 63.82

Referral (for)
  psychiatric aftercare (halfway house) (outpatient clinic) 94.52
  psychotherapy 94.51
  rehabilitation
    alcoholism 94.53
    drug addiction 94.54
    psychologic NEC 94.59
    vocational 94.55
Reformation
  cardiac pacemaker pocket, new site (skin) (subcutaneous) 37.79
  cardioverter/defibrillator (automatic) pocket, new site (skin) (subcutaneous) 37.79
  chamber of eye 12.99
Refracture
  bone (for faulty union) (*see also* Osteoclasis) 78.70
  nasal bones 21.88
Refusion
  spinal NOS 81.30
    atlas-axis (anterior) (transoral) (posterior) 81.31
    axial lumbar interbody fusion [AxiaLIF] 81.38
    cervical (C2 level or below) NEC 81.32
      anterior column (interbody), anterolateral (anterior) technique 81.32
      C1-C2 level (anterior) (posterior) 81.31
      posterior column, posterolateral (posterior) technique 81.33
    craniocervical (anterior) (transoral) (posterior) 81.31
    direct lateral interbody fusion [DLIF] 81.36
    dorsal, dorsolumbar NEC 81.35
      anterior column (interbody), anterolateral (anterior) (extracavitary) technique 81.34
      posterior column, posterolateral (posterior) technique 81.35
    extreme lateral interbody fusion [XLIF] 81.36
    facet 81.37
    lumbar, lumbosacral NEC 81.38
      anterior column (interbody)
        anterolateral (anterior) technique 81.36
        posterior technique 81.38
      anterior lumbar interbody fusion (ALIF) 81.36
      lateral transverse process technique 81.37
      posterior column, posterior (posterolateral) (transverse process) technique 81.37
      transforaminal lumbar interbody fusion (TLIF) 81.38
    number of vertebrae —*see* codes 81.62-81.64
    occiput — C2 (anterior) (transoral) (posterior) 81.31
    refusion NEC 81.39

Note: Also use either 81.62, 81.63 or 81.64 as an additional code to show the total number of vertebrae fused

---

Regional blood flow study 92.05
Regulation, menstrual 69.6
Rehabilitation programs NEC 93.89
  alcohol 94.61
    with detoxification 94.63
    combined alcohol and drug 94.67
      with detoxification 94.69
  drug 94.64
    with detoxification 94.66
    combined drug and alcohol 94.67
      with detoxification 94.69
  sheltered employment 93.85
  vocational 93.85

Reimplantation
  adrenal tissue (heterotopic) (orthotopic) 07.45
  artery 39.59
    renal, aberrant 39.55
  bile ducts following excision of ampulla of Vater 51.62
  extremity—*see* Reattachment, extremity
  fallopian tube into uterus 66.74
  kidney 55.61
  lung 33.5
  ovary 65.72
    laparoscopic 65.75
  pancreatic tissue 52.81
  parathyroid tissue (heterotopic) (orthotopic) 06.95
  pulmonary artery for hemitruncus repair 35.83
  renal vessel, aberrant 39.55
  testis in scrotum 62.5
  thyroid tissue (heterotopic) (orthotopic) 06.94
  tooth 23.5
  ureter into bladder 56.74
Reinforcement —*see also* Repair, by site
  sclera NEC 12.88
    with graft 12.87
Reinsertion —*see also* Insertion *or* Revision
  cystostomy tube 59.94
  fixation device (internal) (*see also* Fixation, bone, internal) 78.50
  heart valve (prosthetic) 35.95
  Holter (Spitz) valve 02.42
  implant (expelled) (extruded)
    eyeball (with conjunctival graft) 16.62
    orbital 16.62
  nephrostomy tube 55.93
  pyelostomy tube 55.94
  ureteral stent (transurethral) 59.8
    with ureterotomy 59.8 *[56.2]*
  ureterostomy tube 59.93
  valve
    heart (prosthetic) 35.95
    ventricular (cerebral) 02.42
Relaxation —(*see also* Release)
  training 94.33
Release
  carpal tunnel (for nerve decompression) 04.43
  celiac artery axis 39.91
  central slip, extensor tendon hand (mallet finger repair) 82.84
  chordee 64.42
  clubfoot NEC 83.84
  de Quervain's tenosynovitis 82.01
  Dupuytren's contracture (by palmar fasciectomy) 82.35
    by fasciotomy (subcutaneous) 82.12
    with excision 82.35
  Fowler (mallet finger repair) 82.84
  joint (capsule) (adherent) (constrictive) (*see also* Division, joint capsule) 80.40
  laryngeal 31.92
  ligament (*see also* Division, ligament) 80.40
    median arcuate 39.91
  median arcuate ligament 39.91
  muscle (division) 83.19
    hand 82.19
  nerve (peripheral) NEC 04.49
    cranial NEC 04.42
    trigeminal 04.41
  pressure, intraocular 12.79
  scar tissue
    skin 86.84
  stoma—*see* Revision, stoma
  tarsal tunnel 04.44

Release—*continued*
  tendon 83.13
    hand 82.11
      extensor, central slip (repair mallet finger)
        82.84
      sheath 83.01
        hand 82.01
  tenosynovitis 83.01
    abductor pollicis longus 82.01
    de Quervain's 82.01
    external pollicis brevis 82.01
    hand 82.01
  torsion
    intestine 46.80
      large 46.82
        endoscopic (balloon) 46.85
      small 46.81
    kidney pedicle 55.84
    ovary 65.95
    testes 63.52
  transverse carpal ligament (for nerve
      decompression) 04.43
  trigger finger or thumb 82.01
  urethral stricture 58.5
  Volkmann's contracture
    excision of scar, muscle 83.32
    fasciotomy 83.14
    muscle transplantation 83.77
  web contracture (skin) 86.84
Relief —*see* Release
Relocation —*see also* Revision
  cardiac device (CRT-D) (CRT-P) (defibrillator)
      (pacemaker) pocket, new site (skin)
      (subcutaneous) 37.79
  CRT-D pocket 37.79
  CRT-P pocket 37.79
  subcutaneous device pocket NEC 86.09
Remobilization
  joint 93.16
  stapes 19.0
Remodel ventricle 37.35
Removal —*see also* Excision
  Abrams bar (chest wall) 34.01
  abscess—*see* Incision, by site
  adenoid tag(s) 28.6
  anal sphincter
    with revision 49.75
    without revision 49.76
  arch bars (orthodontic) 24.8
    immobilization device 97.33
  arterial graft or prosthesis 39.49
  arteriovenous shunt (device) 39.43
    with creation of new shunt 39.42
  artificial heart
    internal biventricular replacement system 37.55
  Barton's tongs (skull) 02.95
    with synchronous replacement 02.94
  bladder sphincter, artificial 58.99
    with replacement 58.93
  blood clot—*see also* Incision, by site
    bladder (by incision) 57.19
      without incision 57.0
    kidney (without incision) 56.0
      by incision 55.01
    ureter (by catheter) (without incision) 56.0
      by incision 56.2
  bone fragment (chip) (*see also* Incision, bone)
      77.10
    joint (*see also* Arthrotomy) 80.10
    necrotic (*see also* Sequestrectomy, bone) 77.00
      joint (*see also* Arthrotomy) 80.10
    skull 01.25

Removal—*continued*
    with debridement compound fracture 02.02
  bone growth stimulator—*see* category 78.6
  bony spicules, spinal canal 03.53
  brace 97.88
  breast implant 85.94
    tissue expander 85.96
  bronchial device or substance
    endoscopic 33.78
  calcareous deposit
    bursa 83.03
      hand 82.03
    tendon, intratendinous 83.39
      hand 82.29
  calcification, heart valve leaflets—*see*
    Valvuloplasty, heart
  calculus
    bile duct (by incision) 51.49
      endoscopic 51.88
      laparoscopic 51.88
      percutaneous 51.98
    bladder (by incision) 57.19
      without incision 57.0
    common duct (by incision) 51.41
      endoscopic 51.88
      laparoscopic 51.88
      percutaneous 51.96
    gallbladder 51.04
      endoscopic 51.88
      laparoscopic 51.88
    kidney (by incision) 55.01
      without incision 56.0
      percutaneous 55.03
        with fragmentation (ultrasound) 55.04
      renal pelvis (by incision) 55.11
        percutaneous nephrostomy 55.03
          with fragmentation (ultrasound) 55.04
        transurethral 56.0
    lacrimal
      canaliculi 09.42
        by incision 09.52
      gland 09.3
        by incision 09.0
      passage(s) 09.49
        by incision 09.59
      punctum 09.41
        by incision 09.51
      sac 09.49
        by incision 09.53
    pancreatic duct (by incision) 52.09
      endoscopic 52.94
    perirenal tissue 59.09
    pharynx 29.39
    prostate 60.0
    salivary gland (by incision) 26.0
      by probe 26.91
    ureter (by incision) 56.2
      without incision 56.0
    urethra (by incision) 58.0
      without incision 58.6
  caliper tongs (skull) 02.95
  cannula
    for extracorporeal membrane oxygenation
      (ECMO)—*omit code*
  cardiac pacemaker (device) (initial) (permanent)   .
      (cardiac resynchronization device, CRT-P)
      37.89
    with replacement
      cardiac resynchronization pacemaker
        (CRT-P)
        device only 00.53
        total system 00.50

Removal—*continued*
    dual-chamber device 37.87
    single-chamber device 37.85
        rate responsive 37.86
    cardioverter/defibrillator pulse generator
        without replacement (cardiac resynchronization
            defibrillator device (CRT-D)) 37.79
    cast 97.88
        with reapplication 97.13
            lower limb 97.12
            upper limb 97.11
    catheter (indwelling)—*see also* Removal, tube
        bladder 97.64
        cranial cavity 01.27
        middle ear (tympanum) 20.1
        ureter 97.62
        urinary 97.64
    CCM (cardiac contractility modulation) without
        replacement (rechargeable pulse generator)
        (total system) 37.79
    cerclage material, cervix 69.96
    cerumen, ear 96.52
    corneal epithelium 11.41
        for smear or culture 11.21
    coronary artery obstruction (thrombus) 36.09
        direct intracoronary artery infusion 36.04
        open chest approach 36.03
        percutaneous transluminal (balloon) 00.66

---

*Note: Also use 00.40, 00.41, 00.42, or 00.43 to
show the total number of vessels treated. Use
code 00.44 once to show procedure on a
bifurcated vessel. In addition, use 00.45, 00.46,
00.47, or 00.48 to show the number of vascular
stents inserted.*

    Crutchfield tongs (skull) 02.95
        with synchronous replacement 02.94
    cyst—*see also* Excision, lesion, by site
        dental 24.4
        lung 32.29
            endoscopic 32.28
            thoracoscopic 32.20
    cystic duct remnant 51.61
    decidua (by)
        aspiration curettage 69.52
        curettage (D and C) 69.02
        manual 75.4
    dental wiring (immobilization device) 97.33
        orthodontic 24.8
    device (therapeutic) NEC 97.89
        abdomen NEC 97.86
        bronchus 33.78
            valve 33.78
        digestive system NEC 97.59
        drainage—*see* Removal, tube
        for musculoskeletal immobilization NEC 97.88
        fixation device external 97.88
            mandibular NEC 97.36
            minifixator (bone) —*see* category 78.6
        genital tract NEC 97.79
        head and neck NEC 97.39
        intrauterine contraceptive 97.71
        minifixator—*see* category 78.6
        spine 80.09
        thorax NEC 97.49
        trunk NEC 97.87
        urinary system NEC 97.69
    diaphragm, vagina 97.73
    drainage device—*see* Removal, tube
    dye, spinal canal 03.31

Removal—*continued*
    ectopic fetus (from) 66.02
        abdominal cavity 74.3
        extraperitoneal (intraligamentous) 74.3
        fallopian tube (by salpingostomy) 66.02
            by salpingotomy 66.01
            with salpingectomy 66.62
        intraligamentous 74.3
        ovarian 74.3
        peritoneal (following uterine or tubal rupture)
            74.3
        site NEC 74.3
        tubal (by salpingostomy) 66.02
            by salpingotomy 66.01
            with salpingectomy 66.62
    electrodes
        bone growth stimulator—*see* category 78.6
        brain 01.22
            depth 01.22
                with synchronous replacement 02.93
            foramen ovale 01.22
                with synchronous replacement 02.93
            sphenoidal—*omit code*
                with synchronous replacement 02.96
        cardiac pacemaker (atrial) (transvenous)
            (ventricular) 37.77
            with replacement 37.76
        carotid sinus 39.87
            with synchronous pulse generator removal
                (total system) 39.86
            with synchronous replacement 39.82
        depth 01.22
            with synchronous replacement 02.93
        epicardial (myocardial) 37.77
            with replacement (by)
                atrial and/or ventricular lead(s)
                    (electrode) 37.76
                epicardial lead 37.74
        epidural pegs 01.22
            with synchronous replacement 02.93
        foramen ovale 01.22
            with synchronous replacement 02.93
        gastric 04.93
            with synchronous replacement 04.92
        intracranial 01.22
            with synchronous replacement 02.93
        peripheral nerve 04.93
            with synchronous replacement 04.92
        sacral nerve 04.93
        sphenoidal—*omit code*
            with synchronous replacement 02.96
        spinal 03.94
            with synchronous replacement 03.93
        temporary transvenous pacemaker
            system—*omit code*
    electroencephalographic receiver (brain)
        (intracranial) 01.22
        with synchronous replacement 02.93
    electronic
        stimulator—*see* Removal, neurostimulator, by
            site
            bladder 57.98
            bone 78.6
    electrostimulator—*see* Removal, electronic,
        stimulator, by site
    embolus 38.00
        with endarterectomy—*see* Endarterectomy
        abdominal
            artery 38.06
            vein 38.07
        aorta (arch) (ascending) (descending) 38.04
        arteriovenous shunt or cannula 39.49

Removal—*continued*
  bovine graft 39.49
  head and neck vessel
    endovascular approach 39.74
    open approach, intracranial vessels 38.01
    open approach, other vessels of head and
      neck 38.02
  intracranial vessel
    endovascular approach 39.74
    open approach, intracranial vessels 38.01
    open approach, other vessels of head and
      neck 38.02
  lower limb
    artery 38.08
    vein 38.09
  pulmonary (artery) (vein) 38.05
  thoracic vessel NEC 38.05
  upper limb (artery) (vein) 38.03
  embryo—*see* Removal, ectopic fetus
  encircling tube, eye (episcleral) 14.6
  epithelial downgrowth, anterior chamber 12.93
  external fixation device 97.88
    mandibular NEC 97.36
    minifixator (bone)—*see* category 78.6
  extrauterine embryo—*see* Removal, ectopic fetus
  eyeball 16.49
    with implant 16.42
    with attachment of muscles 16.41
  fallopian tube—*see* Salpingectomy
  feces (impacted) (by flushing) (manual) 96.38
  fetus, ectopic—*see* Removal, ectopic fetus
  fingers, supernumerary 86.26
  fixation device
    external 97.88
      mandibular NEC 97.36
      minifixator (bone)—*see* category 78.6
    internal 78.60
      carpal, metacarpal 78.64
      clavicle 78.61
      facial (bone) 76.97
      femur 78.65
      fibula 78.67
      humerus 78.62
      patella 78.66
      pelvic 78.69
      phalanges—(foot) (hand) 78.69
      radius 78.63
      scapula 78.61
      specified site NEC 78.69
      tarsal metatarsal 78.68
      thorax (ribs) (sternum) 78.61
      tibia 78.67
      ulna 78.63
      vertebrae 78.69
  foreign body NEC (*see also* Incision, by site)
    98.20
    abdominal (cavity) 54.92
      wall 54.0
    adenoid 98.13
      by incision 28.91
    alveolus, alveolar bone 98.22
      by incision 24.0
    antecubital fossa 98.27
      by incision 86.05
    anterior chamber 12.00
      by incision 12.02
        with use of magnet 12.01
    anus (intraluminal) 98.05
      by incision 49.93
    artificial stoma (intraluminal) 98.18
    auditory canal, external 18.02

Removal—*continued*
  axilla 98.27
    by incision 86.05
  bladder (without incision) 57.0
    by incision 57.19
  bone, except fixation device (*see also* Incision,
    bone) 77.10
    alveolus, alveolar 98.22
      by incision 24.0
  brain 01.39
    without incision into brain 01.24
  breast 85.0
  bronchus (intraluminal) 98.15
    by incision 33.0
  bursa 83.03
    hand 82.03
  canthus 98.22
    by incision 08.51
  cerebral meninges 01.31
  cervix (intraluminal) NEC 98.16
    penetrating 69.97
  choroid (by incision) 14.00
    with use of magnet 14.01
    without use of magnet 14.02
  ciliary body (by incision) 12.00
    with use of magnet 12.01
    without use of magnet 12.02
  conjunctiva (by magnet) 98.22
    by incision 10.0
  cornea 98.21
    by incision 11.1
    by magnet 11.0
  duodenum 98.03
    by incision 45.01
  ear (intraluminal) 98.11
    with incision 18.09
  epididymis 63.92
  esophagus (intraluminal) 98.02
    by incision 42.09
  extrapleural (by incision) 34.01
  eye, eyeball (by magnet) 98.21
    anterior segment (by incision) 12.00
      with use of magnet 12.01
      without use of magnet 12.02
    posterior segment (by incision) 14.00
      with use of magnet 14.01
      without use of magnet 14.02
    superficial 98.21
  eyelid 98.22
    by incision 08.09
  fallopian tube
    by salpingostomy 66.02
    by salpingotomy 66.01
  fascia 83.09
    hand 82.09
  foot 98.28
  gall bladder 51.04
  groin region (abdominal wall) (inguinal) 54.0
  gum 98.22
    by incision 24.0
  hand 98.26
  head and neck NEC 98.22
  heart 37.11
  internal fixation, device—*see* Removal, fixation
    device, internal
  intestine
    by incision 45.00
    large (intraluminal) 98.04
      by incision 45.03
    small (intraluminal) 98.03
      by incision 45.02

Removal—*continued*
 intraocular (by incision) 12.00
  with use of magnet 12.01
  without use of magnet 12.02
 iris (by incision) 12.00
  with use of magnet 12.01
  without use of magnet 12.02
 joint structure (*see also* Arthrotomy) 80.10
 kidney (transurethral) (by endoscopy) 56.0
  by incision 55.01
  pelvis (transurethral) 56.0
   by incision 55.11
 labia 98.23
  by incision 71.09
 lacrimal
  canaliculi 09.42
   by incision 09.52
  gland 09.3
   by incision 09.0
  passage(s) 09.49
   by incision 09.59
  punctum 09.41
   by incision 09.51
  sac 09.49
   by incision 09.53
 large intestine (intraluminal) 98.04
  by incision 45.03
 larynx (intraluminal) 98.14
  by incision 31.3
 lens 13.00
  by incision 13.02
  with use of magnet 13.01
 liver 50.0
 lower limb, except foot 98.29
  foot 98.28
 lung 33.1
 mediastinum 34.1
 meninges (cerebral) 01.31
  spinal 03.01
 mouth (intraluminal) 98.01
  by incision 27.92
 muscle 83.02
  hand 82.02
 nasal sinus 22.50
  antrum 22.2
   with Caldwell-Luc approach 22.39
  ethmoid 22.51
  frontal 22.41
  maxillary 22.2
   with Caldwell-Luc approach 22.39
  sphenoid 22.52
 nerve (cranial) (peripheral) NEC 04.04
  root 03.01
 nose (intraluminal) 98.12
  by incision 21.1
 oral cavity (intraluminal) 98.01
  by incision 27.92
 orbit (by magnet) 98.21
  by incision 16.1
 palate (penetrating) 98.22
  by incision 27.1
 pancreas 52.09
 penis 98.24
  by incision 64.92
 pericardium 37.12
 perineum (female) 98.23
  by incision 71.09
  male 98.25
   by incision 86.05
 perirenal tissue 59.09
 peritoneal cavity 54.92

Removal—*continued*
 perivesical tissue 59.19
 pharynx (intraluminal) 98.13
  by pharyngotomy 29.0
 pleura (by incision) 34.09
 popliteal space 98.29
  by incision 86.05
 rectum (intraluminal) 98.05
  by incision 48.0
 renal pelvis (transurethral) 56.0
  by incision 56.1
 retina (by incision) 14.00
  with use of magnet 14.01
  without use of magnet 14.02
 retroperitoneum 54.92
 sclera (by incision) 12.00
  with use of magnet 12.01
  without use of magnet 12.02
 scrotum 98.24
  by incision 61.0
 sinus (nasal) 22.50
  antrum 22.2
   with Caldwell-Luc approach 22.39
  ethmoid 22.51
  frontal 22.41
  maxillary 22.2
   with Caldwell-Luc approach 22.39
  sphenoid 22.52
 skin NEC 98.20
  by incision 86.05
 skull 01.24
  with incision into brain 01.39
 small intestine (intraluminal) 98.03
  by incision 45.02
 soft tissue NEC 83.09
  hand 82.09
 spermatic cord 63.93
 spinal (canal) (cord) (meninges) 03.01
 stomach (intraluminal) 98.03
  bubble (balloon) 44.94
  by incision 43.0
 subconjunctival (by magnet) 98.22
  by incision 10.0
 subcutaneous tissue NEC 98.20
  by incision 86.05
 supraclavicular fossa 98.27
  by incision 86.05
 tendon (sheath) 83.01
  hand 82.01
 testis 62.0
 thorax (by incision) 34.09
 thyroid (field) (gland) (by incision) 06.09
 tonsil 98.13
  by incision 28.91
 trachea (intraluminal) 98.15
  by incision 31.3
 trunk NEC 98.25
 tunica vaginalis 98.24
 upper limb, except hand 98.27
  hand 98.26
 ureter (transurethral) 56.0
  by incision 56.2
 urethra (intraluminal) 98.19
  by incision 58.0
 uterus (intraluminal) 98.16
 vagina (intraluminal) 98.17
  by incision 70.14
 vas deferens 63.6
 vitreous (by incision) 14.00
  with use of magnet 14.01
  without use of magnet 14.02

Removal—*continued*
  vulva 98.23
    by incision 71.09
  gallstones
    bile duct (by incision) NEC 51.49
      endoscopic 51.88
    common duct (by incision) 51.41
      endoscopic 51.88
      percutaneous 51.96
    duodenum 45.01
    gallbladder 51.04
      endoscopic 51.88
      laparoscopic 51.88
    hepatic ducts 51.49
      endoscopic 51.88
    intestine 45.00
      large 45.03
      small NEC 45.02
    liver 50.0
  Gardner Wells tongs (skull) 02.95
    with synchronous replacement 02.94
  gastric band (adjustable), laparoscopic 44.97
  gastric bubble (balloon) 44.94
  granulation tissue—*see also* Excision, lesion, by
      site
    with repair—*see* Repair, by site
    cranial 01.6
    skull 01.6
  halo traction device (skull) 02.95
    with synchronous replacement 02.94
  heart assist system
    with replacement 37.63
    intra-aortic balloon pump (IABP) 97.44
    nonoperative 97.44
    open removal 37.64
    percutaneous external device 97.44
  heart replacement system
    internal biventricular 37.55
  hematoma—*see* Drainage, by site
  Hoffman minifixator device (bone)—*see* category
      78.6
  hydatidiform mole 68.0
  impacted
    feces (rectum) (by flushing) (manual) 96.38
    tooth 23.19
      from nasal sinus (maxillary) 22.61
  implant
    breast 85.94
    cochlear prosthetic device 20.99
    cornea 11.92
    lens (prosthetic) 13.8
    middle ear NEC 20.99
    ocular 16.71
      posterior segment 14.6
    orbit 16.72
    retina 14.6
    tympanum 20.1
  implantable hemodynamic sensor (lead) and
      monitor device 37.79
  internal biventricular heart replacement system
      37.55
  internal fixation device—*see* Removal, fixation
      device, internal
  intra-aortic balloon pump (IABP) 97.44
  intrauterine contraceptive device (IUD) 97.71
  joint (structure) NOS 80.90
    ankle 80.97
    elbow 80.92
    foot and toe 80.98
    hand and finger 80.94
    hip 80.95

Removal—*continued*
    knee 80.96
    other specified sites 80.99
    shoulder 80.91
    spine 80.99
    toe 80.98
    wrist 80.93
  Kantrowitz heart pump 37.64
    nonoperative 97.44
  keel (tantalum plate), larynx 31.98
  kidney—*see also* Nephrectomy
    mechanical 55.98
    transplanted or rejected 55.53
  laminaria (tent), uterus 97.79
  leads (cardiac)—*see* Removal, electrodes, cardiac
      pacemaker
  lesion—*see* Excision, lesion, by site
  ligamentum flavum (spine)—*omit code*
  ligature
    fallopian tube 66.79
    ureter 56.86
    vas deferens 63.84
  limb lengthening device, internal—*see* category
      78.6
  loop recorder 86.05
  loose body
    bone—*see* Sequestrectomy, bone
    joint 80.10
    mesh (surgical)—*see* Removal, foreign body,
        by site
  lymph node—*see* Excision, lymph, node
  minifixator device (bone)—*see* category 78.6
    external fixation device 97.88
  Mulligan hood, fallopian tube 66.94
    with synchronous replacement 66.93
  muscle stimulator (skeletal) 83.93
    with replacement 83.92
  myringotomy device or tube 20.1
  nail (bed) (fold) 86.23
    internal fixation device—*see* Removal, fixation
        device, internal
  necrosis
    skin 86.28
      excisional 86.22
  neuropacemaker—*see* Removal, neurostimulator,
      by site
  neurostimulator
    brain 01.22
      with synchronous replacement 02.93
    electrodes
      brain 01.22
        with synchronous replacement 02.93
      gastric 04.93
        with synchronous replacement 04.92
      intracranial 01.22
        with synchronous replacement 02.93
      peripheral nerve 04.93
        with synchronous replacement 04.92
      sacral nerve 04.93
        with synchronous replacement 04.92
      spinal 03.94
        with synchronous replacement 03.93
    intracranial 01.22
      with synchronous replacement 02.93
    peripheral nerve 04.93
      with synchronous replacement 04.92

Removal—*continued*
  pulse generator (subcutaneous single array, multiple array) 86.05
    with synchronous replacement 86.96
      multiple array 86.95
        rechargeable 86.98
      single array 86.94
        rechargeable 86.97
    cranial 01.29
      with synthronous replacement 01.20
    spinal 03.94
      with synchronous replacement 03.93
  nonabsorbable surgical material NEC—*see* Removal, foreign body, by site
  odontoma (tooth) 24.4
  orbital implant 16.72
  osteocartilaginous loose body, joint structures (*see also* Arthrotomy) 80.10
  outer attic wall (middle ear) 20.59
  ovo-testis (unilateral) 62.3
    bilateral 62.41
  pacemaker
    brain (intracranial)—*see* Removal, neurostimulator
    cardiac (device) (initial) (permanent) 37.89
      with replacement
        dual-chamber device 37.87
        single-chamber device 37.85
          rate responsive 37.86
      electrodes (atrial) (transvenous) (ventricular) 37.77
        with replacement 37.76
      epicardium (myocardium) 37.77
        with replacement (by)
          atrial and/or ventricular lead(s) (electrode) 37.76
          epicardial lead 37.74
      temporary transvenous pacemaker system—*omit code*
    intracranial—*see* Removal, neurostimulator
    neural—*see* Removal, neurostimulator
    peripheral nerve—*see* Removal, neurostimulator
    spine—*see* Removal, neurostimulator
  pack, packing
    dental 97.34
    intrauterine 97.72
    nasal 97.32
    rectum 97.59
    trunk NEC 97.85
    vagina 97.75
    vulva 97.75
  pantopaque dye, spinal canal 03.31
  patella (complete) 77.96
    partial 77.86
  pectus deformity implant device 34.01
  pelvic viscera, en masse (female) 68.8
    male 57.71
  pessary, vagina NEC 97.74
  pharynx (partial) 29.33
  phlebolith—*see* Removal, embolus
  placenta (by)
    aspiration curettage 69.52
    D and C 69.02
    manual 75.4
  plaque, dental 96.54
  plate, skull 02.07
    with synchronous replacement 02.05

Removal—*continued*
  polyp—*see also* Excision, lesion, by site
    esophageal 42.32
      endoscopic 42.33
    gastric (endoscopic) 43.41
    intestine 45.41
      endoscopic 45.42
    nasal 21.31
  prosthesis
    bile duct 51.95
      nonoperative 97.55
    cochlear prosthetic device 20.99
    dental 97.35
    eye 97.31
    facial bone 76.99
    fallopian tue 66.94
      with synchronous replacement 66.93
    joint structures
      with replacement —*see* Revision, joint replacement, by site
      without replacement
        ankle 80.07
        elbow 80.02
        foot and toe 80.08
        hand and finger 80.04
        hip 80.05
        knee 80.06
        shoulder 80.01
        specified site NEC 80.09
        spine 80.09
        unspecified site 80.00
        wrist 80.03
    lens 13.8
    penis (internal) without replacement 64.96
    Rosen (urethra) 59.99
    testicular, by incision 62.0
    urinary sphincter, artificial 58.99
      with replacement 58.93
  pseudophakos 13.8
  pterygium 11.39
    with corneal graft 11.32
  pulse generator
    cardiac pacemaker 37.86
    cardioverter/defibrillator 37.79
    carotid sinus 39.88
      with synchronous electrode removal (total system) 39.86
      with synchronous replacement 39.83
    neurostimulator—*see* Removal, neurostimulator, pulse generator
  pump assist device, heart 37.64
    with replacement 37.63
    nonoperative 97.44
  radioactive material—*see* Removal, foreign body, by site
  redundant skin, eyelid 08.86
  rejected organ
    kidney 55.53
    testis 62.42
  reservoir, ventricular (Ommaya) (Rickham) 02.43
    with synchronous replacement 02.42
  retained placenta (by)
    aspiration curettage 69.52
    D and C 69.02
    manual 75.4
  retinal implant 14.6
  Rheos™ carotid sinus baroreflex activation device 86.05
  rhinolith 21.31
  rice bodies, tendon sheaths 83.01
    hand 82.01

Removal—*continued*

Roger-Anderson minifixator device (bone)—*see* category 78.6

root, residual (tooth) (buried) (retained) 23.11

Rosen prosthesis (urethra) 59.99

Scribner shunt 39.43

scleral buckle or implant 14.6

secondary membranous cataract (with iridectomy) 13.65

secundines (by)
  aspiration curettage 69.52
  D and C 69.02
  manual 75.4

sequestrum—*see* Sequestrectomy

seton, anus 49.93

Shepard's tube (ear) 20.1

Shirodkar suture, cervix 69.96

shunt
  arteriovenous 39.43
    with creation of new shunt 39.42
  lumbar-subarachnoid NEC 03.98
  pleurothecal 03.98
  salpingothecal 03.98
  spinal (thecal) NEC 03.98
  subarachnoid-peritoneal 03.98
  subarachnoid-ureteral 03.98

silastic tubes
  ear 20.1
  fallopian tubes 66.94
    with synchronous replacement 66.93

skin
  necrosis or slough 86.28
    excisional 86.22
  superficial layer (by dermabrasion) 86.25

skull tongs 02.95
  with synchronous replacement 02.94

spacer (cement) (joint) (methylmethacrylate) 84.57

splint 97.88

stent
  bile duct 97.55
  larynx 31.98
  ureteral 97.62
  urethral 97.65

stimoceiver—*see* Removal, neurostimulator

subdural
  grids 01.22
  strips 01.22

supernumerary digit(s) 86.26

suture(s) NEC 97.89
  abdominal wall 97.83
  by incision—*see* Incision, by site
  genital tract 97.79
  head and neck 97.38
  thorax 97.43
  trunk NEC 97.84

symblepharon—*see* Repair, symblepharon

temporary transvenous pacemaker system—*omit code*

testis (unilateral) 62.3
  bilateral 62.41
  remaining or solitary 62.42

Removal—*continued*

thrombus 38.00
  with endarterectomy—*see* Endarterectomy
  abdominal
    artery 38.06
    vein 38.07
  aorta (arch) (ascending) (descending) 38.04
  arteriovenous shunt or cannula 39.49
  bovine graft 39.49
  coronary artery 36.09
  head and neck vessel NEC 38.02
  intracranial vessel NEC 38.01
  lower limb
    artery 38.08
    vein 38.09
  pulmonary (artery) (vein) 38.05
  thoracic vessel NEC 38.05
  upper limb (artery) (vein) 38.0

tissue expander (skin) NEC 86.05
  breast 85.96

toes, supernumerary 86.26

tongs, skull 02.95
  with synchronous replacement 02.94

tonsil tag 28.4

tooth (by forceps) (multiple) (single NEC 23.09
  deciduous 23.01
  surgical NEC 23.19
    impacted 23.19
    residual root 23.11
    root apex 23.73
      with root canal therapy 23.72

trachoma follicles 10.33

T-tube (bile duct) 97.55

tube
  appendix 97.53
  bile duct (T-tube) NEC 97.55
  cholecystostomy 97.54
  cranial cavity 01.27
  cystostomy 97.63
  ear (button) 20.1
  gastrostomy 97.51
  large intestine 97.53
  liver 97.55
  mediastinum 97.42
  nephrostomy 97.61
  pancreas 97.56
  peritoneum 97.82
  pleural cavity 97.41
  pyelostomy 97.61
  retroperitoneum 97.81
  small intestine 97.52
  thoracotomy 97.41
  tracheostomy 97.37
  tympanostomy 20.1
  tympanum 20.1
  ureterostomy 97.62

ureteral splint (stent) 97.62

urethral sphincter, artificial 58.99
  with replacement 58.93

urinary sphincter, artificial 58.99
  with replacement 58.93

utricle 20.79

valve
  vas deferens 63.85
  ventricular (cerebral) 02.43

vascular graft or prosthesis 39.49

ventricular shunt or reservoir 02.43
  with synchronous replacement 02.42

Vinke tongs (skull) 02.95
  with synchronous replacement 02.94

Removal—*continued*
  vitreous (with replacement) 14.72
    anterior approach (partial) 14.71
    open sky technique 14.71
  Wagner-Brooker minifixator device (bone)—*see*
    category 78.6
  wiring, dental (immobilization device) 97.33
    orthodontic 24.8
Renipuncture (percutaneous) 55.92
Renogram 92.03
Renotransplantation NEC 55.69
  Note: To report donor source:
    cadaver 00.93
    live non-related donor 00.92
    live related donor 00.91
    live unrelated donor 00.92
Reopening —*see also* Incision, by site
  blepharorrhaphy 08.02
  canthorrhaphy 08.02
  cilia base 08.71
  craniotomy or craniectomy site 01.23
  fallopian tube (divided) 66.79
  iris in anterior chambers 12.97
  laminectomy or laminotomy site 03.02
  laparotomy site 54.12
  osteotomy site (*see also* Incision, bone) 77.10
    facial bone 76.09
  tarsorrhaphy 08.02
  thoracotomy site (for control of hemorrhage) (for
    examination) (for exploration) 34.03
  thyroid field wound (for control of hemorrhage)
    (for examination) (for exploration) (for
    removal of hematoma) 06.02
Repacking —*see* Replacement, pack, by site
Repair
  abdominal wall 54.72
  adrenal gland 07.44
  alveolus, alveolar (process) (ridge) (with graft)
    (with implant) 24.5
  anal sphincter 49.79
    artificial sphincter
      implantation 49.75
      revision 49.75
    laceration (by suture) 49.71
      obstetric (current) 75.62
      old 49.79
  aneurysm (false) (true) 39.52
    by or with
      clipping 39.51
      coagulation 39.52
      coil, NEC (endovascular approach) 39.79
        head and neck
          bare coils 39.75
          bioactive coils 39.76
      electrocoagulation 39.52
      endovascular graft 39.79
        abdominal aorta 39.71
          fenestrated (branching) graft 39.78
        head and neck 39.72
        lower extremity artery(s) 39.79
        thoracic aorta 39.73
        upper extremity artery(s) 39.79
      excision or resection of vessel—*see also*
        Aneurysmectomy, by site
        with
          anastomosis—*see* Aneurysmectomy, with
            anastomosis, by site
          graft replacement—*see* Aneurysmectomy,
            with graft replacement, by site
    filipuncture 39.52

Repair—*continued*
    graft replacement—*see* Aneurysmectomy,
      with graft replacement, by site
  ligation 39.52
  liquid tissue adhesive (glue) 39.79
    endovascular approach 39.79
      head and neck 39.72
  methyl methacrylate 39.52
    endovascular approach 39.79
      head and neck 39.72
  occlusion 39.52
    endovascular approach 39.79
      head and neck 39.72
  suture 39.52
  trapping 39.52
  wiring 39.52
  wrapping (gauze) (methyl methacrylate)
    (plastic) 39.52
coronary artery 36.91
sinus of Valsalva 35.39
thoracic aorta (dissecting), by fenestration
  39.54
anomalous pulmonary venous connection (total)
  one-stage 35.82
  partial—*see* specific procedure
  total 35.82
anular disc 80.54
  with graft or prosthesis 80.53
anulus fibrosus 80.54
  with graft or prosthesis 80.53
anus 49.79
  laceration (by suture) 49.71
    obstetric (current) 75.62
    old 49.79
aorta 39.31
aorticopulmonary window 39.59
arteriovenous fistula 39.53
  by or with
    clipping 39.53
    coagulation 39.53
    coil, NEC (endovascular approach) 39.79
      head and neck vessels
        bare coils 39.75
        bioactive coils 39.76
    division 39.53
    excision or resection—*see also*
      Aneurysmectomy, by site
      with
        anastomosis—*see* Aneurysmectomy,
          with anastomosis, by site
        graft replacement—*see*
          Aneurysmectomy, with graft
          replacement, by site
    ligation 39.53
      coronary artery 36.99
    occlusion 39.53
      endovascular approach 39.79
        head and neck 39.72
    suture 39.53
artery NEC 39.59
  by
    endovascular approach
      abdominal aorta 39.71
        fenestrated (branching) graft 39.78
      head and neck (total embolization or
        occlusion) 39.72
      other repair (of aneurysm) 39.79

Repair—*continued*
  percutaneous repair of intracranial vessel(s)
    (for stent insertion) 00.62

Note: Also use 00.40, 00.41, 00.42, or 00.43 to show the total number of vessels treated. Use code 00.44 once to show procedure on a bifurcated vessel. In addition, use 00.45, 00.46, 00.47, or 00.48 to show the number of vascular stents inserted.

  percutaneous repair of extracranial vessel(s)
    (for stent insertion) 00.61

Note: Also use 00.40, 00.41, 00.42, or 00.43 to show the total number of vessels treated. Use code 00.44 once to show procedure on a bifurcated vessel. In addition, use 00.45, 00.46, 00.47, or 00.48 to show the number of vascular stents inserted.

  non-coronary percutaneous transluminal
    approach

Note: Also use 00.40, 00.41, 00.42, or 00.43 to show the total number of vessels treated. Use code 00.44 once to show procedure on a bifurcated vessel. In addition, use 00.45, 00.46, 00.47, or 00.48 to show the number of vascular stents inserted.

  angioplasty
    basilar 00.62
    carotid 00.61
    femoropopliteal 39.50
    iliac 39.50
    lower extremity NOS 39.50
    mesenteric 39.50
    renal 39.50
    upper extremity NOS 39.50
    vertebral 00.61
      intracranial portion 00.62
    atherectomy 17.56
  coronary NEC 36.99
    by angioplasty—*see* Angioplasty, coronary
    by atherectomy
      percutaneous transluminal 17.55
  with
    patch graft 39.58
      with excision or resection of vessel—*see*
        Arteriectomy, with graft replacement,
        by site
      synthetic (Dacron) (Teflon) 39.57
      tissue (vein) (autogenous) (homograft)
        39.56
    suture 39.31
  artificial opening—*see* Repair, stoma
  atrial septal defect 35.71
    with
      prosthesis (open heart technique) 35.51
        closed heart technique 35.52
      tissue graft 35.61
    combined with repair of valvular and
      ventricular septal defects—*see* Repair,
      endocardial cushion defect
    in total repair of total anomalous pulmonary
      venous connection 35.82
  atrioventricular canal defect (any type) 35.73
    with
      prosthesis 35.54
      tissue graft 35.63
  bifid digit (finger) 82.89

Repair—*continued*
  bile duct NEC 51.79
    laceration (by suture) NEC 51.79
      common bile duct 51.71
  bladder NEC 57.89
    exstrophy 57.86
    for stress incontinence—*see* Repair, stress
      incontinence
    laceration (by suture) 57.81
      obstetric (current) 75.61
        old 57.89
    neck 57.85
  blepharophimosis 08.59
  blepharoptosis 08.36
    by
      frontalis muscle technique (with)
        fascial sling 08.32
        suture 08.31
      levator muscle technique 08.34
        with resection or advancement 08.33
      orbicularis oculi muscle sling 08.36
      tarsal technique 08.35
  blood vessel NEC 39.59
    with
      patch graft 39.58
        with excision or resection—*see*
          Angiectomy, with graft replacement
        synthetic (Dacron) (Teflon) 39.57
        tissue (vein) (autogenous) (homograft)
          39.56
      resection—*see* Angiectomy
      suture 39.30
    coronary artery NEC 36.99
      by angioplasty—*see* Angioplasty, coronary
      by atherectomy
        percutaneous transluminal 17.55
    peripheral vessel NEC 39.59
      by angioplasty 39.50

Note: Also use 00.40, 00.41, 00.42, or 00.43 to show the total number of vessels treated. Use code 00.44 once to show procedure on a bifurcated vessel. In addition, use 00.45, 00.46, 00.47, or 00.48 to show the number of vascular stents inserted.

      by atherectomy 17.56

Note: Also use 00.40, 00.41, 00.42, or 00.43 to show the total number of vessels treated. Use code 00.44 once to show procedure on a bifurcated vessel. In addition, use 00.45, 00.46, 00.47, or 00.48 to show the number of vascular stents inserted.

      by endovascular approach 39.79
  bone NEC (*see also* Osteoplasty) —*see* category
    78.4
    accessory sinus 22.79
    by synostosis technique—*see* Arthrodesis
    cranium NEC 02.06
      with
        flap (bone) 02.03
        graft (bone) 02.04
    for malunion, nonunion, or delayed union of
      fracture—*see* Repair, fracture, malunion or
      nonunion
    nasal 21.89
    skull NEC 02.06
      with
        flap (bone) 02.03
        graft (bone) 02.04

Repair—*continued*

bottle, hydrocele of tunica vaginalis 61.2
brain (trauma) NEC 02.92
breast (plastic) (*see also* Mammoplasty) 85.89
broad ligament 69.29
bronchus NEC 33.48
  laceration (by suture) 33.41
bunionette (with osteotomy) 77.54
canaliculus, lacrimal 09.73
canthus (lateral) 08.59
cardiac pacemaker NEC 37.89
  electrode (s) (lead) NEC 37.75
cardioverter/defibrillator (automatic) pocket
  (skin) (subcutaneous) 37.99
cerebral meninges 02.12
cervix 67.69
  internal os 67.59
    transabdominal 67.51
    transvaginal 67.59
  laceration (by suture) 67.61
    obstetric (current) 75.51
    old 67.69
chest wall (mesh) (silastic) NEC 34.79
chordae tendineae 35.32
choroid NEC 14.9
  with retinal repair—*see* Repair, retina
cisterna chyli 40.69
claw toe 77.57
cleft
  hand 82.82
  laryngotracheal 31.69
  lip 27.54
  palate 27.62
    secondary or subsequent 27.63
coarctation of aorta—*see* Excision, coarctation of
  aorta
cochlear prosthetic device 20.99
  external components only 95.49
cockup toe 77.58
colostomy 46.43
conjunctiva NEC 10.49
  with scleral repair 12.81
  laceration 10.6
    with repair of sclera 12.81
  late effect of trachoma 10.49
cornea NEC 11.59
  with
    conjunctiva flap 11.53
    transplant—*see* Keratoplasty
  postoperative dehiscence 11.52
coronary artery NEC 36.99
  by angioplasty—*see* Angioplasty, coronary
  by atherectomy
    percutaneous transluminal 17.55
cranium NEC 02.06
  with
    flap (bone) 02.03
    graft (bone) 02.04
cusp, valve—*see* Repair, heart, valve
cystocele 70.51
  with graft or prosthesis 70.54
  and rectocele 70.50
    with graft or prosthesis 70.53
dental arch 24.8
diaphragm NEC 34.84
diastasis recti 83.65
diastematomyelia 03.59

Repair—*continued*

ear (external) 18.79
  auditory canal or meatus 18.6
  auricle NEC 18.79
  cartilage NEC 18.79
  laceration (by suture) 18.4
  lop ear 18.79
  middle NEC 19.9
  prominent or protruding 18.5
ectropion 08.49
  by or with
    lid reconstruction 08.44
    suture (technique) 08.42
    thermocauterization 08.41
    wedge resection 08.43
encephalocele (cerebral) 02.12
endocardial cushion defect 35.73
  with
    prosthesis (grafted to septa) 35.54
    tissue graft 35.63
enterocele (female) 70.92
  with graft or prosthesis 70.93
  male 53.9
enterostomy 46.40
entropion 08.49
  by or with
    lid reconstruction 08.44
    suture (technique) 08.42
    thermocauterization 08.41
    wedge resection 08.43
epicanthus (fold) 08.59
epididymis (and spermatic cord) NEC 63.59
  with vas deferens 63.89
epiglottis 31.69
episiotomy
  routine following delivery—*see* Episiotomy
  secondary 75.69
epispadias 58.45
esophagus, esophageal NEC 42.89
  fistula NEC 42.84
  stricture 42.85
exstrophy of bladder 57.86
eye, eyeball 16.89
  multiple structures 16.82
  rupture 16.82
  socket 16.64
    with graft 16.63
eyebrow 08.89
  linear 08.81
eyelid 08.89
  full-thickness 08.85
    involving lid margin 08.84
  laceration 08.81
    full-thickness 08.85
      involving lid margin 08.84
    partial-thickness 08.83
      involving lid margin 08.82
    linear 08.81
    partial-thickness 08.83
      involving lid margin 08.82
  retraction 08.38
fallopian tube (with prosthesis) 66.79
  by
    anastomosis 66.73
    reanastomosis 66.79
    reimplantation into
      ovary 66.72
      uterus 66.74
    suture 66.71
false aneurysm—*see* Repair, aneurysm

Repair—*continued*
  fascia 83.89
    by or with
      arthroplasty—*see* Arthroplasty
      graft (fascial) (muscle) 83.82
        hand 82.72
        tendon 83.81
          hand 82.79
      suture (direct) 83.65
        hand 82.46
    hand 82.89
      by
        graft NEC 82.79
          fascial 82.72
          muscle 82.72
        suture (direct) 82.46
    joint—*see* Arthroplasty
  filtering bleb (corneal) (scleral) (by excision) 12.82
    by
      corneal graft (*see also* Keratoplasty) 11.60
      scleroplasty 12.82
      suture 11.51
    with conjunctival flap 11.53
  fistula—*see also* Closure, fistula
    anovaginal 70.73
    arteriovenous 39.53
      clipping 39.53
      coagulation 39.53
        endovascular approach 39.79
          head and neck 39.72
      division 39.53
      excision or resection—*see also*
        Aneurysmectomy, by site
        with
          anastomosis—*see* Aneurysmectomy, with
            anastomosis, by site
          graft replacement—*see* Aneurysmectomy,
            with graft replacement, by site
      ligation 39.53
        coronary artery 36.99
      occlusion 39.53
        endovascular approach 39.79
          head and neck 39.72
      suture 39.53
    cervicovesical 57.84
    cervix 67.62
    choledochoduodenal 51.72
    colovaginal 70.72
    enterovaginal 70.74
    enterovesical 57.83
    esophagocutaneous 42.84
    ileovesical 57.83
    intestinovaginal 70.74
    intestinovesical 57.83
    oroantral 22.71
    perirectal 48.93
    pleuropericardial 37.49
    rectovaginal 70.73
    rectovesical 57.83
    rectovesicovaginal 57.83
    scrotum 61.42
    sigmoidovaginal 70.74
    sinus
      nasal 22.71
      of Valsalva 35.39
    splenocolic 41.95
    urethroperineovesical 57.84
    urethrovesical 57.84
    urethrovesicovaginal 57.84
    uterovesical 57.84

Repair—*continued*
    vagina NEC 70.75
    vaginocutaneous 70.75
    vaginoenteric NEC 70.74
    vaginoileal 70.74
    vaginoperineal 70.75
    vaginovesical 57.84
    vesicocervicovaginal 57.84
    vesicocolic 57.83
    vesicocutaneous 57.84
    vesicoenteric 57.83
    vesicointestinal 57.83
    vesicometrorectal 57.83
    vesicoperineal 57.84
    vesicorectal 57.83
    vesicosigmoidal 57.83
    vesicosigmoidovaginal 57.83
    vesicourethral 57.84
    vesicourethrorectal 57.83
    vesicouterine 57.84
    vesicovaginal 57.84
    vulva 71.72
    vulvorectal 48.73
  foramen ovale (patent) 35.71
    with
      prosthesis (open heart technique) 35.51
        closed heart technique 35.52
      tissue graft 35.61
  fracture—*see also* Reduction, fracture
    larynx 31.64
    malunion or nonunion (delayed) NEC—*see*
      category 78.4
    with
      graft—*see* Graft, bone
      insertion (of)
        bone growth stimulator (invasive)—*see*
          category 78.9
        internal fixation device 78.5
      manipulation for realignment—*see*
        Reduction, fracture, by site, closed
    osteotomy
      with
        correction of alignment—*see* category
          77.3
          with internal fixation device—*see*
            categories 77.3 *[78.5]*
          with intramedullary rod—*see*
            categories 77.3 *[78.5]*
        replacement arthroplasty—*see* Arthroplasty
        sequestrectomy—*see* category 77.0
        Sofield type procedure—*see* categories 77.3
          [78.5]
        synostosis technique—*see* Arthrodesis
    vertebra 03.53
  funnel chest (with implant) 34.74
  gallbladder 51.91
  gastroschisis 54.71
  great vessels NEC 39.59
    laceration (by suture) 39.30
      artery 39.31
      vein 39.32
  hallux valgus NEC 77.59
    resection of joint with prosthetic implant 77.59
  hammer toe 77.56
  hand 82.89
    with graft or implant 82.79
      fascia 82.72
      muscle 82.72
      tendon 82.79

Repair—*continued*
  heart 37.49
    assist system 37.63
    septum 35.70
      with
        prosthesis 35.50
        tissue graft 35.60
      atrial 35.71
        with
          prosthesis (open heart technique) 35.51
            closed heart technique 35.52
          tissue graft 35.61
          combined with repair of valvular and
            ventricular septal defects—*see* Repair,
            endocardial cushion defect
          in total repair of
            tetralogy of Fallot 35.81
            total anomalous pulmonary venous
              connection 35.82
            truncus arteriosus 35.83
        combined with repair of valvular defect—*see*
          Repair, endocardial cushion defect
      ventricular 35.72
        with
          prosthesis (open heart technique) 35.53
            closed heart technique 35.55
          tissue graft 35.62
          combined with repair of valvular and atrial
            septal defects—*see* Repair, endocardial
            cushion defect
          in total repair of
            tetralogy of Fallot 35.81
            total anomalous pulmonary venous
              connection 35.82
            truncus arteriosus 35.83
    valve (cusps) (open heart technique) 35.10
      aortic (without replacement) 35.11
        combined with repair of atrial and ventricular
          septal defects—*see* Repair, endocardial
          cushion defect
      mitral (without replacement) 35.12
        with
          leaflet clip implant 35.97
          MitrClip® 35.97
        balloon, percutaneous 35.96
        endovascular repair with implant 35.97
        percutaneous with leaflet clip implant 35.97
      pulmonary (without replacement) 35.13
        in total repair of tetralogy of Fallot 35.81
      tricuspid (without replacement) 35.14
    total internal biventricular replacement system
      37.52
      implantable battery 37.54
      implantable controller 37.54
      thoracic unit 37.53
      transcutaneous energy transfer [TET] device
        37.54
  hepatic duct 51.79

Repair—*continued*
  hernia NEC 53.9
    anterior abdominal wall NEC (laparoscopic
      without graft or prosthesis) 53.59
      with prosthesis or graft
        laparoscopic 53.63
        other and open 53.69
    colostomy 46.42
    crural 53.29
    cul-de-sac (Douglas') 70.92
    diaphragmatic
      abdominal approach
        laparoscopic 53.71
        other and open 53.72
        unspecified 53.75
      thoracic, thoracoabdominal approach 53.80
        laparoscopic 53.83
        other and open 53.84
    epigastric 53.59
      with prosthesis or graft 53.69
    esophageal hiatus
      abdominal approach
        laparoscopic 53.71
        other and open 53.72
        unspecified 53.75
      thoracic, thoracoabdominal approach 53.80
    fascia 83.89
      hand 82.89
    femoral (unilateral) 53.29
      with prosthesis or graft 53.21
      bilateral 53.39
        with prosthesis or graft 53.31
    Ferguson 53.00
    Halsted 53.00
    Hill-Allison (hiatal hernia repair, transpleural
      approach) 53.80
    hypogastric 53.59
      with prosthesis or graft 53.69
    incisional 53.51
      laparoscopic with prosthesis or graft 53.62
      other open with prosthesis or graft 53.61
    inguinal (unilateral) 53.00
      with prosthesis or graft 53.05
      bilateral 53.10
        with prosthesis or graft 53.17
          laparoscopic 17.24
        direct
          laparoscopic with graft or prosthesis
            17.21
          other and open (laparoscopic without
            graft or prosthesis) 53.11
            with prosthesis or graft 53.14
        direct and indirect
          laparoscopic with graft or prosthesis
            17.23
          other and open (laparoscopic without
            graft or prosthesis) 53.13
            with prosthesis or graft 53.16
        indirect
          laparoscopic with graft or prosthesis
            17.22
          other and open (laparoscopic without
            graft or prosthesis) 53.12
            with prosthesis or graft 53.15

Repair—*continued*

  direct (unilateral)

    with prosthesis or graft 53.03

    and indirect (unilateral)

      laparoscopic with graft or prosthesis 17.11

      other and open (laparoscopic without graft or prosthesis) 53.01

        with prosthesis or graft 53.03

    laparoscopic with graft or prosthesis 17.11

    other and open (laparoscopic without graft or prosthesis) 53.01

      with prosthesis or graft 53.03

  indirect (unilateral)

    laparoscopic with graft or prosthesis 17.12

    other and open (laparoscopic without graft or prosthesis) 53.02

      with prosthesis or graft 53.04

  laparoscopic with graft or prosthesis, NOS 17.13

  internal 53.9

  ischiatic 53.9

  ischiorectal 53.9

  lumbar 53.9

  manual 96.27

  obturator 53.9

  omental 53.9

  paraesophageal

    laparoscopic 53.71

    other and open 53.72

    unspecified 53.75

  parahiatal

    laparoscopic 53.71

    other and open 53.72

    unspecified 53.75

  paraileostomy 46.41

  parasternal 53.82

  paraumbilical

    laparoscopic 53.43

      with graft or prosthesis 53.42

    other and open with graft or prosthesis 53.41

    other open 53.49

  pericolostomy 46.42

  perineal (enterocele) 53.9

  preperitoneal 53.29

  pudendal 53.9

  retroperitoneal 53.9

  sciatic 53.9

  scrotal—*see* Repair, hernia, inguinal

  spigelian 53.59

    with prosthesis or graft 53.69

  umbilical

    laparoscopic 53.43

      with graft or prosthesis 53.42

    other and open with graft or prosthesis 53.41

    other open 53.49

  uveal 12.39

  ventral (laparoscopic without graft or prosthesis) 53.59

    with prosthesis or graft

      laparoscopic 53.63

      other and open 53.69

    incisional 53.51

      laparoscopic without graft or prosthesis 53.59

      other open with prosthesis or graft 53.61

hydrocele

  round ligament 69.19

  spermatic cord 63.1

  tunica vaginalis 61.2

hymen 70.76

Repair—*continued*

  hypospadias 58.45

  ileostomy 46.41

  ingrown toenail 86.23

  intestine, intestinal NEC 46.79

    fistula—*see* Closure, fistula, intestine

    laceration

      large intestine 46.75

      small intestine NEC 46.73

    stoma—*see* Repair, stoma

  inverted uterus NEC 69.29

    manual

      nonobstetric 69.94

      obstetric 75.94

    obstetrical

      manual 75.94

      surgical 75.93

    vaginal approach 69.23

  iris (rupture) NEC 12.39

  jejunostomy 46.41

  joint (capsule) (cartilage) NEC (*see also* Arthroplasty) 81.96

  kidney NEC 55.89

  knee (joint) NEC 81.47

    collateral ligaments 81.46

    cruciate ligaments 81.45

    five-in-one 81.42

    triad 81.43

  labia—*see* Repair, vulva

  laceration—*see* Suture, by site

  lacrimal system NEC 09.99

    canaliculus 09.73

    punctum 09.72

      for eversion 09.71

  laryngostomy 31.62

  laryngotracheal cleft 31.69

  larynx 31.69

    fracture 31.64

    laceration 31.61

  leads (cardiac) NEC 37.75

  ligament (*see also* Arthroplasty) 81.96

    broad 69.29

    collateral, knee NEC 81.46

    cruciate, knee NEC 81.45

    round 69.29

    uterine 69.29

  lip NEC 27.59

    cleft 27.54

    laceration (by suture) 27.51

  liver NEC 50.69

    laceration 50.61

  lop ear 18.79

  lung NEC 33.49

  lymphatic (channel) (peripheral) NEC 40.9

    duct, left (thoracic) NEC 40.69

  macrodactyly 82.83

  mallet finger 82.84

  mandibular ridge 76.64

  mastoid (antrum) (cavity) 19.9

  meninges (cerebral) NEC 02.12

    spinal NEC 03.59

      meningocele 03.51

      myelomeningocele 03.52

  meningocele (spinal) 03.51

    cranial 02.12

  mesentery 54.75

  mouth NEC 27.59

    laceration NEC 27.52

Repair—*continued*
 muscle NEC 83.87
  by
   graft or implant (fascia) (muscle) 83.82
    hand 82.72
    tendon 83.81
     hand 82.79
   suture (direct) 83.65
    hand 82.46
   transfer or transplantation (muscle) 83.77
    hand 82.58
  hand 82.89
   by
    graft or implant NEC 82.79
     fascia 82.72
    suture (direct) 82.46
    transfer or transplantation (muscle) 82.58
 musculotendinous cuff, shoulder 83.63
 myelomeningocele 03.52
 nasal
  septum (perforation) NEC 21.88
  sinus NEC 22.79
   fistula 22.71
 nasolabial flaps (plastic) 21.86
 nasopharyngeal atresia 29.4
 nerve (cranial) (peripheral) NEC 04.79
  old injury 04.76
  revision 04.75
  sympathetic 05.81
 nipple NEC 85.87
 nose (external) (internal) (plastic) NEC (*see also*
   Rhinoplasty) 21.89
  laceration (by suture) 21.81
 notched lip 27.59
 omentum 54.74
 omphalocele
  laparoscopic 53.43
   with graft or prosthesis 53.42
  other and open with graft or prosthesis 53.41
  other open 53.49
 orbit 16.89
  wound 16.81
 ostium
  primum defect 35.73
   with prosthesis 35.54
   with tissue graft 35.63
  secundum defect 35.71
   with
    prosthesis (open heart technique) 35.51
     closed heart technique 35.52
    tissue graft 35.61
 ovary 65.79
  with tube 65.73
   laparoscopic 65.76
 overlapping toe 77.58
 pacemaker
  cardiac
   device (permanent) 37.89
   electrode(s) (lead) NEC 37.75
   pocket (skin) (subcutaneous) 37.79
 palate NEC 27.69
  cleft 27.62
   secondary or subsequent 27.63
  laceration (by suture) 27.61

Repair—*continued*
 pancreas NEC 52.95
  Wirsung's duct 52.99
 papillary muscle (heart) 35.31
 patent ductus arteriosus 38.85
 pectus deformity (chest) (carinatum) (excavatum)
   34.74
 pelvic floor NEC 70.79
  obstetric laceration (current) 75.69
   old 70.79
 penis NEC 64.49
  for epispadias or hypospadias 58.45
  inflatable prosthesis 64.99
  laceration 64.41
 pericardium 37.49
 perineum (female) 71.79
  laceration (by suture) 71.71
   obstetric (current) 75.69
    old 71.79
  male NEC 86.89
   laceration (by suture) 86.59
 peritoneum NEC 54.73
  by suture 54.64
 pharynx NEC 29.59
  laceration (by suture) 29.51
  plastic 29.4
 pleura NEC 34.93
 postcataract wound dehiscence 11.52
  with conjunctival flap 11.53
 pouch of Douglas 70.52
 primum ostium defect 35.73
  with
   prosthesis 35.54
   tissue graft 35.63
 prostate 60.93
 ptosis, eyelid—*see* Repair, blepharoptosis
 punctum, lacrimal NEC 09.72
  for correction of eversion 09.71
 quadriceps (mechanism) 83.86
 rectocele (posterior colporrhaphy) 70.52
  with graft or prosthesis 70.55
  and cystocele 70.50
   with graft or prosthesis 70.53
 rectum NEC 48.79
  laceration (by suture) 48.71
  prolapse NEC 48.76
   abdominal approach 48.75
   STARR procedure 48.74
 retina, retinal
  detachment 14.59
   by
    cryotherapy 14.52
    diathermy 14.51
    photocoagulation 14.55
     laser 14.54
     xenon arc 14.53
    scleral buckling (*see also* Buckling, scleral)
      14.49
  tear or defect 14.39
   by
    cryotherapy 14.32
    diathermy 14.31
    photocoagulation 14.35
     laser 14.34
     xenon arc 14.33
 retroperitoneal tissue 54.73
 rotator cuff (graft) (suture) 83.63

Repair—*continued*
  round ligament 69.29
  ruptured tendon NEC 83.88
    hand 82.86
  salivary gland or duct NEC 26.49
  sclera, scleral 12.89
    fistula 12.82
    staphyloma NEC 12.86
      with graft 12.85
  scrotum 61.49
  sinus
    nasal NEC 22.79
    of Valsalva (aneurysm) 35.39
  skin (plastic) (without graft) 86.89
    laceration (by suture) 86.59
  skull NEC 02.06
    with
      flap (bone) 02.03
      graft (bone) 02.04
  spermatic cord NEC 63.59
    laceration (by suture) 63.51
  sphincter ani 49.79
    laceration (by suture) 49.71
      obstetric (current) 75.62
      old 49.79
  spina bifida NEC 03.59
    meningocele 03.51
    myelomeningocele 03.52
  spinal (cord) (meninges) (structures) NEC 03.59
    meningocele 03.51
    myelomeningocele 03.52
  spleen 41.95
  sternal defect 78.41
  stoma
    bile duct 51.79
    bladder 57.22
    bronchus 33.42
    common duct 51.72
    esophagus 42.89
    gallbladder 51.99
    hepatic duct 51.79
    intestine 46.40
      large 46.43
      small 46.41
    kidney 55.89
    larynx 31.63
    rectum 48.79
    stomach 44.69
      laparoscopic 44.68
    thorax 34.79
    trachea 31.74
    ureter 56.62
    urethra 58.49
  stomach NEC 44.69
    laceration (by suture) 44.61
    laparoscopic 44.68
  stress incontinence (urinary) NEC 59.79
    by
      anterior urethropexy 59.79
      Burch 59.5
      cystourethropexy (with levator muscle sling) 59.71
      gracilis muscle transplant 59.71
      injection of implant (collagen) (fat) (polytef) 59.72
      levator muscle sling 59.71
      paraurethral suspension (Pereyra) 59.6
      periurethral suspension 59.6
      plication of urethrovesical junction 59.3
      pubococcygeal sling 59.71
      retropubic urethral suspension 59.5

Repair—*continued*
    suprapubic sling 59.4
    tension free vaginal tape 59.79
    urethrovesical suspension 59.4
  subcutaneous tissue (plastic) (without skin graft) 86.89
    laceration (by suture) 86.59
  supracristal defect (heart) 35.72
    with
      prosthesis (open heart technique) 35.53
        closed heart technique 35.55
      tissue graft 35.62
  symblepharon NEC 10.49
    by division (with insertion of conformer) 10.5
    with free graft 10.41
  syndactyly 86.85
  synovial membrane, joint—*see* Arthroplasty
  telecanthus 08.59
  tendon 83.88
    by or with
      arthroplasty—*see* Arthroplasty
      graft or implant (tendon) 83.81
        fascia 83.82
          hand 82.72
        hand 82.79
        muscle 83.82
          hand 82.72
      suture (direct) (immediate) (primary) (*see also* Suture, tendon) 83.64
        hand 82.45
      transfer or transplantation (tendon) 83.75
        hand 82.56
    hand 82.86
      by
        graft or implant (tendon) 82.79
        suture (direct) (immediate) (primary) (*see also* Suture, tendon, hand) 82.45
        transfer or transplantation (tendon) 82.56
    rotator cuff (direct suture) 83.63
    ruptured NEC 83.88
      hand 82.86
    sheath (direct suture) 83.61
      hand 82.41
  testis NEC 62.69
  tetralogy of Fallot
    partial—*see* specific procedure
    total (one-stage) 35.81
  thoracic duct NEC 40.69
  thoracostomy 34.72
  thymus (gland) 07.93
  tongue NEC 25.59
  tooth NEC 23.2
    by
      crown (artificial) 23.41
      filling (amalgam) (plastic) (silicate) 23.2
      inlay 23.3
  total anomalous pulmonary venous connection
    partial—*see* specific procedure
    total (one-stage) 35.82
  trachea NEC 31.79
    laceration (by suture) 31.71
  tricuspid atresia 35.94
  truncus arteriosus
    partial—*see* specific procedure
    total (one-stage) 35.83
  tunica vaginalis 61.49
    laceration (by suture) 61.41
  tympanum—*see* Tympanoplasty
  ureter NEC 56.89
    laceration (by suture) 56.82

Repair—*continued*
  ureterocele 56.89
  urethra NEC 58.49
    laceration (by suture) 58.41
      obstetric (current) 75.61
      old 58.49
    meatus 58.47
  urethrocele (anterior colporrhaphy) (female)
      70.51
    with graft or prosthesis 70.54
    and rectocele 70.50
      with graft or prosthesis 70.53
  urinary sphincter, artificial (component) 58.99
  urinary stress incontinence—*see* Repair, stress
      incontinence
  uterus, uterine 69.49
    inversion—*see* Repair, inverted uterus
    laceration (by suture) 69.41
      obstetric (current) 75.50
      old 69.49
    ligaments 69.29
      by
        interposition 69.21
        plication 69.22
  uvula 27.73
    with synchronous cleft palate repair 27.62
  vagina, vaginal (cuff) (wall) NEC 70.79
    anterior 70.51
      with graft or prosthesis 70.54
      with posterior repair 70.50
        with graft or prosthesis 70.53
    cystocele 70.51
      with graft or prosthesis 70.54
      and rectocele 70.50
        with graft or prosthesis 70.53
    enterocele 70.92
      with graft or prosthesis 70.93
    laceration (by suture) 70.71
      obstetric (current) 75.69
      old 70.79
    posterior 70.52
      with anterior repair 70.50
        with graft or prosthesis 70.53
    rectocele 70.52
      with graft or prosthesis 70.55
      and cystocele 70.50
        with graft or prosthesis 70.53
    urethrocele 70.51
      with graft or prosthesis 70.54
      and rectocele 70.50
        with graft or prosthesis 70.53
  varicocele 63.1
  vas deferens 63.89
    by
      anastomosis 63.82
        to epididymis 63.83
      reconstruction 63.82
    laceration (by suture) 63.81
  vein NEC 39.59
    by
      endovascular approach
        head and neck (embolization or occlusion)
          39.72
    with
      patch graft 39.58
        with excision or resection of vessel—*see*
          Phlebectomy, with graft replacement,
          by site
        synthetic (Dacron) (Teflon) 39.57
        tissue (vein) (autogenous) (homograft) 39.56
    suture 39.32

Repair—*continued*
  ventricular septal defect 35.72
    with
      prosthesis (open heart technique) 35.53
        closed heart technique 35.55
        in total repair of tetralogy of Fallot 35.81
      tissue graft 35.62
    combined with repair of valvular and atrial
        septal defects—*see* Repair, endocardial
        cushion defect
    in total repair of
      tetralogy of Fallot 35.81
      truncus arteriosus 35.83
  vertebral arch defect (spina bifida) 03.59
  vulva NEC 71.79
    laceration (by suture) 71.71
      obstetric (current) 75.69
      old 71.79
  Wirsung's duct 52.99
  wound (skin) (without graft) 86.59
    abdominal wall 54.63
      dehiscence 54.61
    postcataract dehiscence (corneal) 11.52
Replacement
  acetabulum (with prosthesis) 81.52
  ankle, total 81.56
    revision 81.59
  aortic valve, NOS 35.22
    with
      prosthesis 35.22
      tissue graft 35.21
        endovascular 35.05
      endovascular (TAVI) (TAVR) (transarterial)
        (transcatheter) (transfemoral) (with tissue
        graft) 35.05
      transapical (intercostal) (transcatheter)
        (transthoracic) (transventricular) (with
        tissue graft) 35.06
  artery—*see* Graft, artery
  bag—*see* Replacement, pack or bag
  Barton's tongs (skull) 02.94
  bladder
    with
      ileal loop 57.87 *[45.51]*
      sigmoid 57.87 *[45.52]*
    sphincter, artificial 58.93
  bronchial device NOS 33.79
  bronchial substance NOS 33.79
  bronchial valve(s)
    multiple lobes 33.73
    single lobe 33.71
  caliper tongs (skull) 02.94
  cannula
    arteriovenous shunt 39.94
    pancreatic duct 97.05
    vessel-to-vessel (arteriovenous) 39.94
  cardiac contractility modulation (CCM)
    rechargeable pulse generator only 17.52
    total system 17.51
  cardiac resynchronization device
    defibrillator (biventricular defibrillator) (BiV
      ICD) (BiV pacemaker with defibrillator)
      (BiV pacing with defibrillator) (CRT-D)
      (device and one or more leads) (total
      system) 00.51
      left ventricular coronary venous lead only 00.52
      pulse generator only 00.54
    pacemaker (biventricular pacemaker) (BiV
      pacemaker) (CRT-P) (device and one or
      more leads) (total system) 00.50
      left ventricular coronary venous lead only 00.52
      pulse generator only 00.53

Replacement—*continued*
  cardioverter/defibrillator (total system) 37.94
    leads only (electrodes) (sensing) (pacing) 37.97
    pulse generator only 37.98
  cast NEC 97.13
    lower limb 97.12
    upper limb 97.11
  catheter
    bladder (indwelling) 57.95
    cystostomy 59.94
    external ventricular drain 02.21
    ventricular shunt (cerebral) 02.42
    wound 97.15
  CCM (cardiac contractility modulation)
    rechargeable pulse generator only 17.52
    total system 17.51
  CRT-D (biventricular defibrillator) (BiV ICD)
    (BiV pacemaker with defibrillator) (BiV
    pacing with defibrillator) (cardiac
    resynchronization defibrillator) (device and
    one or more leads) 00.51
    left ventricular coronary venous lead only 00.52
    pulse generator only 00.54
  CRT-P (biventricular pacemaker) (BiV
    pacemaker) (cardiac resynchronization
    pacemaker) (device and one or more leads)
    00.50
    left ventricular coronary venous lead only 00.52
    pulse generator only 00.53
  Crutchfield tongs (skull) 02.94
  cystostomy tube (catheter) 59.94
  device
    subcutaneous for intracardiac or great vessel
      hemodynamic monitoring 00.57
  diaphragm, vagina 97.24
  disc—*see* Replacement, intervertebral disc
  drain—*see also* Replacement, tube
    vagina 97.26
    vulva 97.26
    wound, musculoskeletal or skin 97.16
  ear (prosthetic) 18.71
  elbow (joint), total 81.84
  electrode(s)—*see* Implant, electrode or lead, by
      site or name of device
    brain
      depth 02.93
      foramen ovale 02.93
      sphenoidal 02.96
    carotid sinus 39.82
      with synchronous pulse generator
        replacement (total system) 39.81
    depth 02.93
    foramen ovale 02.93
    gastric 04.92
    intracranial 02.93
    pacemaker—*see* Replacement, pacemaker,
      electrode(s)
    peripheral nerve 04.92
    sacral nerve 04.92
    sphenoidal 02.96
    spine 03.93
  electroencephalographic receiver (brain)
      (intracranial) 02.93
  electronic
    cardioverter/defibrillator—*see* Replacement,
      cardioverter/defibrillator
    leads (electrodes)—*see* Replacement,
      electrode(s)

Replacement—*continued*
  stimulator—*see also* Implant, electronic
      stimulator, by site
    bladder 57.97
    muscle (skeletal) 83.92
    ureter 56.93
  electrostimulator—*see* Implant, electronic
      stimulator, by site
  enterostomy device (tube)
    large intestine 97.04
    small intestine 97.03
  epidural pegs 02.93
  femoral head, by prosthesis 81.52
    revision 81.53
  Gardner Wells tongs (skull) 02.94
  gastric band, laparoscopic 44.96
  gastric port device (subcutaneous) 44.96
  graft—*see* Graft
  halo traction device (skull) 02.94
  Harrington rod (with refusion of spine)—*see*
      Refusion, spinal
  heart
    artificial
      total internal biventricular replacement
        system 37.52
      implantable battery 37.54
      implantable controller 37.54
      thoracic unit 37.53
      transcutaneous energy transfer [TET]
        device 37.54
    total internal biventricular replacement system
      37.52
      implantable battery 37.54
      implantable controller 37.54
      thoracic unit 37.53
      transcutaneous energy transfer [TET] device
        37.54
    valve, NOS (with prosthesis) (with tissue graft)
      35.20
      aortic, NOS 35.22
        with
          prosthesis 35.22
          tissue graft 35.21
            endovascular 35.05
          endovascular (TAVI) (TAVR)
            (transarterial) (transcatheter)
            (transfemoral) (with tissue graft) 35.05
          transapical (intercostal) (transcatheter)
            (transthoracic) (transventricular) (with
            tissue graft) 35.06
      endovascular, NOS 35.09
      mitral, NOS 35.24
        with
          prosthesis 35.24
          tissue graft 35.23
      poppet (prosthetic) 35.95
      pulmonary, NOS 35.26
        with
          prosthesis 35.26
          tissue graft 35.25
          endovascular (percutaneous) (PPVI)
            (TPVR) (transcatheter) (transfemoral)
            (transvenous) 35.07
          in total repair of tetralogy of Fallot 35.81
          transapical (intercostal) (transcatheter)
            (transthoracic) (transventricular) 35.08
      tricuspid, NOS 35.28
        with
          prosthesis 35.28
          tissue graft 35.27

Replacement—*continued*
hip (partial) (with fixation device) (with
    prosthesis) (with traction) 81.52
  acetabulum 81.52
    revision 81.53
  femoral head 81.52
    revision 81.53
  total 81.51
    revision 81.53
intervertebral disc
  artificial, NOS 84.60
    cervical 84.62
      nucleus 84.61
      partial 84.61
      total 84.62
    lumbar, lumbosacral 84.65
      nucleus 84.64
      partial 84.64
      total 84.65
    thoracic (partial) (total) 84.63
inverted uterus—*see* Repair, inverted uterus
iris NEC 12.39
kidney, mechanical 55.97
knee, (bicompartmental) (hemijoint) (partial)
    (total) (tricompartmental) (unicompartmental)
    81.54
  revision 81.55
laryngeal stent 31.93
leads (electrode) (s)—*see* Replacement,
    electrode(s)
mechanical kidney 55.97
mitral valve, NOS 35.24
  with
    prosthesis 35.24
    tissue graft 35.23
Mulligan hood, fallopian tube 66.93
muscle stimulator (skeletal) 83.92
nephrostomy tube 55.93
neuropacemaker—*see* Implant, neurostimulator,
    by site
neurostimulator—*see* Implant, neurostimulator,
    by site
  skeletal muscle 83.92
pacemaker
  brain—*see* Implant, neurostimulator, brain
  cardiac device (initial) (permanent)
    dual-chamber device 37.87
    single-chamber device 37.85
    rate responsive 37.86
    resynchronization—*see* Replacement, CRT-P
  electrode(s), cardiac (atrial) (transvenous)
    (ventricular) 37.76
    epicardium (myocardium) 37.74
    left ventricular coronary venous system 00.52
  gastric —*see* Implant, neurostimulator, gastric
  intracranial—*see* Implant, neurostimulator,
    intracranial
  neural—*see* Implant, neurostimulator, by site
  peripheral nerve—*see* Implant, neurostimulator,
    peripheral nerve
  sacral nerve—*see* Implant, neurostimulator,
    sacral nerve
  spine—*see* Implant, neurostimulator, spine
  temporary transvenous pacemaker system 37.78
pack or bag
  nose 97.21
  teeth, tooth 97.22
  vagina 97.26
  vulva 97.26
  wound 97.16

Replacement—*continued*
pessary, vagina NEC 97.25
prosthesis
  acetabulum 81.53
  arm (bioelectric) (cineplastic) (kineplastic)
    84.44
  biliary tract 51.99
  cochlear 20.96
  channel (single) 20.97
    multiple 20.98
  elbow 81.97
  extremity (bioelectric) (cineplastic)
    (kineplastic) 84.40
    lower 84.48
    upper 84.44
  fallopian tube (Mulligan hood) (stent) 66.93
  femur 81.53
  knee 81.55
  leg (bioelectric) (cineplastic) (kineplastic) 84.48
  penis (non-inflatable) (internal) 64.95
    inflatable (internal) 64.97
  shoulder NEC 81.83
    partial 81.81
    total 81.80
  urinary sphincter, artificial 58.93
pulmonary valve, NOS 35.26
  with
    prosthesis 35.26
    tissue graft 35.25
  endovascular (percutaneous) (PPVI) (TPVR)
    (transcatheter) (transfemoral) (transvenous)
    35.07
  transapical (intercostal) (transcatheter)
    (transthoracic) (transventricular) 35.08
  in total repair tetrology of Fallot 35.81
pyelostomy tube 55.94
rectal tube 96.09
Rheos™ carotid sinus baroreflex activation
    device 39.81
sensor (lead)
  intracardiac or great vessel hemodynamic
    monitoring 00.56
shoulder NEC 81.83
  partial 81.81
  total, NEC 81.80
    other 81.80
    reverse 81.88
skull
  plate 02.05
  tongs 02.94
spacer (cement) (joint) (methylmethacrylate)
    84.56
specified appliance or device NEC 97.29
spinal motion preservation device
  facet replacement device(s) 84.84
  interspinous process device(s) 84.80
  pedicle-based dynamic stabilization device(s)
    84.82
splint 97.14
stent
  bile duct 97.05
  fallopian tube 66.93
  larynx 31.93
  pancreatic duct 97.05
  trachea 31.93
stimoceiver—*see* Implant, stimoceiver, by site

Replacement—*continued*
stimulator
  electrode(s)
    carotid sinus 39.82
      with synchronous pulse generator
        replacement (total system) 39.81
    pulse generator
      carotid sinus 39.83
        with synchronous electrode(s) replacement
          (total system) 39.81
subdural
  grids 02.93
  strips 02.93
testis in scrotum 62.5
tongs, skull 02.94
tracheal stent 31.93
tricuspid valve (with prosthesis) 35.28
  with tissue graft 35.27
tube
  bile duct 97.05
  bladder 57.95
  cystostomy 59.94
  esophagostomy 97.01
  gastrostomy 97.02
  large intestine 97.04
  nasogastric 97.01
  nephrostomy 55.93
  pancreatic duct 97.05
  pyelostomy 55.94
  rectal 96.09
  small intestine 97.03
  tracheostomy 97.23
  ureterostomy 59.93
  ventricular (cerebral) 02.42
umbilical cord, prolapsed 73.92
ureter (with)
  bladder flap 56.74
  ileal segment implanted into bladder 56.89
    [45.51]
ureterostomy tube 59.93
urethral sphincter, artificial 58.93
urinary sphincter, artificial 58.93
valve
  heart—*see also* Replacement, heart valve
    poppet (prosthetic) 35.95
  ventricular (cerebral) 02.42
  ventricular shunt (valve) 02.42
Vinke tongs (skull) 02.94
vitreous (silicone) 14.75
  for retinal reattachment 14.59
Replant, replantation —*see also* Reattachment
extremity—*see* Reattachment, extremity
penis 64.45
scalp, 86.51
tooth 23.5
Reposition
cardiac pacemaker
  electrode(s) (atrial) (transvenous) (ventricular)
    37.75
  pocket 37.79
cardiac resynchronization defibrillator (CRT-D)
  —*see* Revision, cardiac resynchronization
  defibrillator
cardiac resynchronization pacemaker (CRT-P)
  —*see* Revision, cardiac resynchronization
  pacemaker
cardioverter/defibrillator
  lead(s) (epicardial patch) (pacing) (sensing) 37.75
  pocket 37.79
  pulse generator 37.79
cilia base 08.71

Reposition—*continued*
implantable hemodynamic sensor (lead) and
    monitor device 37.7
iris 12.39
neurostimulator
  leads
    subcutaneous, without device replacement
      86.09
    within brain 02.93
    within or over gastric nerve 04.92
    within or over peripheral nerve 04.92
    within or over sacral nerve 04.92
    within spine 03.93
  pulse generator
    subcutaneous, without device replacement
      86.09
subcutaneous device pocket NEC 86.09
renal vessel, aberrant 39.55
thyroid tissue 06.94
tricuspid valve (with plication) 35.14
Resection —*see also* Excision, by site
abdominoendorectal (combined), NOS 48.50
  laparoscopic 48.51
  open 48.52
  other 48.59
abdominoperineal (rectum), NOS 48.50
  pull-through (Altmeier) (Swenson) NEC 48.49
    Duhamel type 48.65
    laparoscopic 48.42
    not otherwise specified 48.40
    open 48.43
alveolar process and palate (en bloc) 27.32
aneurysm—*see* Aneurysmectomy
aortic valve (for subvalvular stenosis) 35.11
artery—*see* Arteriectomy
bile duct NEC 51.69
  common duct NEC 51.63
bladder (partial) (segmental) (transvesical)
    (wedge) 57.6
  complete or total 57.79
  lesion NEC 57.59
    transurethral approach 57.49
  neck 57.59
    transurethral approach 57.49
blood vessel—*see* Angiectomy
brain 01.59
  by
    stereotactic radiosurgery 92.30
      cobalt 60 92.32
      linear accelerator (LINAC) 92.31
      multi-source 92.32
      particle beam 92.33
      particulate 92.33
      radiosurgery NEC 92.39
      single source photon 92.31
  hemisphere 01.52
  lobe 01.53
breast—*see also* Mastectomy
  quadrant 85.22
  segmental 85.23
broad ligament 69.19
bronchus (sleeve) (wide sleeve) 32.1
block (en bloc) (with radical dissection of
    brachial plexus, bronchus, lobe of lung, ribs,
    and sympathetic nerves) 32.6
bursa 83.5
  hand 82.31
cecum (and terminal ileum)
  laparoscopic 17.32
  open and other 45.72
cerebral meninges 01.51

Resection—*continued*
  chest wall 34.4
  clavicle 77.81
  clitoris 71.4
  colon (partial) (segmental)
    ascending (cecum and terminal ileum)
      laparoscopic 17.32
      open and other 45.72
    cecum (and terminal ileum)
      laparoscopic 17.32
      open and other 45.72
    complete
      laparoscopic 45.81
      open 45.82
      other 45.83
      unspecified 45.83
    descending (sigmoid)
      laparoscopic 17.36
      open and other 45.76
    for interposition 45.52
    Hartmann
      laparoscopic 17.35
      open and other 45.75
    hepatic flexure
      laparoscopic 17.33
      open and other 45.73
    laparoscopic 17.39
    left radical (hemicolon)
      laparoscopic 17.35
      open and other 45.75
    multiple segmental
      laparoscopic 17.31
      open and other 45.71
    open and other 45.79
    right radical (hemicolon) (ileocolectomy)
      laparoscopic 17.33
      open and other 45.73
    segmental NEC
      laparoscopic 17.39
      multiple
        laparoscopic 17.31
        open and other 45.71
    open and other 45.79
    sigmoid
      laparoscopic 17.36
      open and other 45.76
    splenic flexure
      laparoscopic 17.35
      open and other 45.75
    total
      laparoscopic 45.81
      open 45.82
      other 45.83
      unspecified 45.83
    transverse
      laparoscopic 17.34
      open and other 45.74
  conjunctiva, for pterygium 11.39
    corneal graft 11.32
  cornual (fallopian tube) (unilateral) 66.69
    bilateral 66.63
  diaphragm 34.81
  endaural 20.79
  endorectal (pull-through) (Soave) 48.41
    combined abdominal, NOS 48.50
      laparoscopic 48.51
      open 48.52
      other 48.59
  esophagus (partial) (subtotal) (*see also*
      Esophagectomy) 42.41
    total 42.42

Resection—*continued*
  exteriorized intestine—*see* Resection, intestine,
      exteriorized
  fascia 83.44
    for graft 83.43
      hand 82.34
    hand 82.35
      for graft 82.34
  gallbladder (total) 51.22
  gastric (partial) (sleeve) (subtotal) NEC (*see also*
      Gastrectomy) 43.89
    with anastomosis NEC 43.89
      esophagogastric 43.5
      gastroduodenal 43.6
      gastrogastric 43.89
      gastrojejunal 43.7
    complete or total NEC 43.99
      with intestinal interposition 43.91
    laparoscopic 43.82
    radical NEC 43.99
      with intestinal interposition 43.91
    wedge 43.42
      endoscopic 43.41
  hallux valgus (joint)—*see also* Bunionectomy
    with prosthetic implant 77.59
  hepatic
    duct 51.69
    flexure (colon)
      laparoscopic 17.33
      open and other 45.73
  infundibula, heart (right) 35.34
  intestine (partial) NEC
    cecum (with terminal ileum)
      laparoscopic 17.32
      open and other 45.72
    exteriorized (large intestine) 46.04
      small intestine 46.02
    for interposition 45.50
      large intestine 45.52
      small intestine 45.51
    hepatic flexure
      laparoscopic 17.33
      open and other 45.73
    ileum 45.62
      with cecum
        laparoscopic 17.32
        open and other 45.72
    laparoscopic 17.39
    large (partial) (segmental) NEC
      for interposition 45.52
      laparoscopic 17.39
      multiple segmental
        laparoscopic 17.31
        open and other 45.71
      other 45.79
      total
        laparoscopic 45.81
        open 45.82
        other 45.83
        unspecified 45.83
      unspecified 45.79
    left hemicolon
      laparoscopic 17.35
      open and other 45.75
    multiple segmental (large intestine)
      laparoscopic 17.31
      open and other 45.71
      small intestine 45.61
    open and other 45.79

Resection—*continued*
 right hemicolon
  laparoscopic 17.33
  open and other 45.73
 segmental (large intestine)
  laparoscopic 17.39
  multiple
   laparoscopic 17.31
   open and other 45.71
  open and other 45.79
  small intestine 45.62
   multiple 45.61
 sigmoid
  laparoscopic 17.36
  open and other 45.76
 small (partial) (segmental) NEC 45.62
  for interposition 45.51
  multiple segmental 45.61
  total 45.63
 total
  large intestine
   laparoscopic 45.81
   open 45.82
   other 45.83
   unspecified 45.83
  small intestine 45.63
 joint structure NEC (*see also* Arthrectomy) 80.90
 kidney (segmental) (wedge) 55.4
 larynx—*see also* Laryngectomy
  submucous 30.29
 lesion—*see* Excision, lesion, by site
 levator palpebrae muscle 08.33
 ligament (*see also* Arthrectomy) 80.90
  broad 69.19
  round 69.19
  uterine 69.19
 lip (wedge) 27.43
 liver (partial) (wedge) 50.22
  lobe (total) 50.3
  total 50.4
 lung (wedge) NEC 32.29
  endoscopic 32.28
  segmental (any part) 32.39
   thoracoscopic 32.30
  thoracoscopic 32.20
  volume reduction 32.22
   biologic lung volume reduction (BLVR)
    —*see* category 33.7
 meninges (cerebral) 01.51
  spinal 03.4
 mesentery 54.4
 muscle 83.45
  extraocular 15.13
   with
    advancement or recession of other eye
     muscle 15.3
    suture of original insertion 15.13
   levator palpebrae 08.33
   Müller's for blepharoptosis 08.35
   orbicularis oculi 08.20
   tarsal, for blepharoptosis 08.35
  for graft 83.43
   hand 82.34
  hand 82.36
   for graft 82.34
  ocular—*see* Resection, muscle, extraocular
 myocardium 37.33
 nasal septum (submucous) 21.5

Resection—*continued*
 nerve (cranial) (peripheral) NEC 04.07
  phrenic 04.03
   for collapse of lung 33.31
  sympathetic 05.29
  vagus—*see* Vagotomy
 nose (complete) (extended) (partial)
   (radical) 21.4
 omentum 54.4
 orbitomaxillary, radical 16.51
 ovary—(*see also* Oophorectomy)
  wedge 65.22
   laparoscopic 65.24
 palate (bony) (local) 27.31
  by wide excision 27.32
  soft 27.49
 pancreas (total) (with synchronous
   duodenectomy) 52.6
  partial NEC 52.59
   distal (tail) (with part of body) 52.52
   proximal (head) (with part or body) (with
    synchronous duodenectomy) 52.51
   radical subtotal 52.53
  radical (one-stage) (two-stage) 52.7
  subtotal 52.53
 pancreaticoduodenal (*see also* Pancreatectomy)
   52.6
 pelvic viscera (en masse) (female) 68.8
  male 57.71
 penis 64.3
 pericardium (partial) (for)
  chronic constrictive pericarditis 37.31
  drainage 37.12
  removal of adhesions 37.31
 peritoneum 54.4
 pharynx (partial) 29.33
 phrenic nerve 04.03
  for collapse of lung 33.31
 prostate—*see also* Prostatectomy
  transurethral (punch) 60.29
 pterygium 11.39
 radial head 77.83
 rectosigmoid (*see also* Resection, rectum) 48.69
 rectum (partial) NEC 48.69
  with
   pelvic exenteration 68.8
   transsacral sigmoidectomy 48.61
  abdominoendorectal (combined), NOS 48.50
   laparoscopic 48.51
   open 48.52
   other 48.59
  abdominoperineal, NOS 48.50
   laparoscopic 48.51
   open 48.52
   other 48.59
   pull-through NEC 48.49
    laparoscopic 48.42
    not otherwise specified 48.40
    open 48.43
    Duhamel type 48.65
  anterior 48.63
   with colostomy (synchronous) 48.62
  Duhamel 48.65
  endorectal 48.41
   combined abdominal, NOS 48.50
    laparoscopic 48.51
    open 48.52
    other 48.59
  posterior 48.64

Resection—*continued*
  pull-through NEC 48.49
    endorectal 48.41
    laparosopic 48.42
    not otherwise specified 48.40
    open 48.43
    STARR procedure 48.74
    submucosal (Soave) 48.41
      combined abdominal, NOS 48.50
        laparoscopic 48.51
        open 48.52
        other 48.59
  rib (transaxillary) 77.91
    as operative approach—*omit code*
    incidental to thoracic operation—*omit code*
  right ventricle (heart), for infundibular
    stenosis 35.34
  root (tooth) (apex) 23.73
    with root canal therapy 23.72
    residual or retained 23.11
  round ligament 69.19
  sclera 12.65
    with scleral buckling (*see also* Buckling,
      scleral) 14.49
    lamellar (for retinal reattachment) 14.49
      with implant 14.41
  scrotum 61.3
  soft tissue NEC 83.49
    hand 82.39
  sphincter of Oddi 51.89
  spinal cord (meninges) 03.4
  splanchnic 05.29
  splenic flexure (colon) 45.75
  sternum 77.81
  stomach (partial) (sleeve) (subtotal) NEC (*see
    also* Gastrectomy) 43.89
    with anastomosis NEC 43.89
      esophagogastric 43.5
      gastroduodenal 43.6
      gastrogastric 43.89
      gastrojejunal 43.7
    complete or total NEC 43.99
      with intestinal interposition 43.91
    fundus 43.89
    laparoscopic 43.82
    radical NEC 43.99
      with intestinal interposition 43.91
    wedge 43.42
      endoscopic 43.41
  submucous
    larynx 30.29
    nasal septum 21.5
    vocal cords 30.22
  synovial membrane (complete) (partial) (*see also*
    Synovectomy) 80.70
  tarsolevator 08.33
  tendon 83.42
    hand 82.33
  thoracic structures (block) (en bloc) (radical)
    (brachial plexus, bronchus, lobes of lung, ribs,
    and sympathetic nerves) 32.6
  thorax 34.4
  tongue 25.2
    wedge 25.1
  tooth root 23.73
    with root canal therapy 23.72
    apex (abscess) 23.73
      with root canal therapy 23.72
    residual or retained 23.11
  trachea 31.5

Resection—*continued*
  transurethral
    bladder NEC 57.49
    prostate 60.29
  transverse colon
    laparoscopic 17.34
    open and other 45.74
  turbinates—*see* Turbinectomy
  ureter (partial) 56.41
    total 56.42
  uterus—*see* Hysterectomy
  vein—*see* Phlebectomy
  ventricle (heart) 37.35
    infundibula 35.34
  vesical neck 57.59
    transurethral 57.49
  vocal cords (punch) 30.22
Respirator, volume-controlled (Bennett)
  (Byrd)—*see* Ventilation
Restoration
  cardioesophageal angle 44.66
    laparoscopic 44.67
  dental NEC 23.49
    by
      application of crown (artificial) 23.41
      insertion of bridge (fixed) 23.42
        removable 23.43
    extremity—*see* Reattachment, extremity
  eyebrow 08.70
    with graft 08.63
  eye socket 16.64
    with graft 16.63
  tooth NEC 23.2
    by
      crown (artificial) 23.41
      filling (amalgam) (plastic) (silicate) 23.2
      inlay 23.3
Restrictive
  gastric band, laparoscopic 44.95
Resurfacing hip 00.86
  acetabulum 00.87
    with femoral head 00.85
  femoral head 00.86
    with acetabulum 00.85
  partial NOS 00.85
    acetabulum 00.87
    femoral head 00.86
  total (acetabulum and femoral head) 00.85
Resuscitation
  artificial respiration 93.93
  cardiac 99.60
    cardioversion 99.62
      atrial 99.61
    defibrillation 99.62
    external massage 99.63
      open chest 37.91
    intracardiac injection 37.92
  cardiopulmonary 99.60
  endotracheal intubation 96.04
  manual 93.93
  mouth-to-mouth 93.93
  pulmonary 93.93
Resuture
  abdominal wall 54.61
  cardiac septum prosthesis 35.95
  chest wall 34.71
  heart valve prosthesis (poppet) 35.95
  wound (skin and subcutaneous tissue) (without
    graft) NEC 86.59
Retavase, infusion 99.10
Reteplase, infusion 99.10

Retightening (noninvasive)
  external fixator device — *omit code*
Retinaculotomy NEC (*see also* Division,
    ligament) 80.40
  carpal tunnel (flexor) 04.43
Retraining
  cardiac 93.36
    vocational 93.85
Retrogasserian neurotomy 04.02
Revascularization
  cardiac (heart muscle) (myocardium) (direct)
    36.10
    with
      bypass anastomosis
        abdominal artery to coronary artery 36.17
        aortocoronary (catheter stent) (homograft)
          (prosthesis) (saphenous vein graft)
          36.10
          one coronary vessel 36.11
          two coronary vessels 36.12
          three coronary vessels 36.13
          four coronary vessels 36.14
        gastroepiploic artery to coronary artery
          36.17
        internal mammary-coronary artery (single
          vessel) 36.15
          double vessel 36.16
        specified type NEC 36.19
        thoracic artery-coronary artery (single
          vessel) 36.15
          double vessel 36.16
      implantation of artery into heart (muscle)
        (myocardium) (ventricle) 36.2
    indirect 36.2
    specified type NEC 36.39
    transmyocardial
      endoscopic 36.33
      endovascular 36.34
      open chest 36.31
      percutaneous 36.34
      specified type NEC 36.32
      thoracoscopic 36.33
Reversal, intestinal segment 45.50
  large 45.52
  small 45.51
Revision
  amputation stump 84.3
    current traumatic—*see* Amputation
  anastomosis
    biliary tract 51.94
    blood vessel 39.49
    gastric, gastrointestinal (with jejunal
      interposition) 44.5
    intestine (large) 46.94
      small 46.93
    pleurothecal 03.97
    pyelointestinal 56.72
    salpingothecal 03.97
    subarachnoid-peritoneal 03.97
    subarachnoid-ureteral 03.97
    ureterointestinal 56.72
  ankle replacement (prosthesis) 81.59
  anterior segment (eye) wound (operative) NEC
    12.83
  arteriovenous shunt (cannula) (for dialysis) 39.42
  arthroplasty—*see* Arthroplasty
  bone flap, skull 02.06
  breast implant 85.93
  bronchostomy 33.42

Revision—*continued*
  bypass graft (vascular) 39.49
    abdominal-coronary artery 36.17
    aortocoronary (catheter stent) (with prosthesis)
      (with saphenous vein graft) (with vein graft)
      36.10
      one coronary vessel 36.11
      two coronary vessels 36.12
      three coronary vessels 36.13
      four coronary vessels 36.14
    CABG—*see* Revision, aortocoronary bypass
      graft
    chest tube—*see* intercostal catheter
    coronary artery bypass graft (CABG)—*see*
      Revision, aortocoronary bypass graft,
      abdominal-coronary artery bypass, and
      internal mammary-coronary artery bypass
    intercostal catheter (with lysis of adhesions)
      34.04
      thoracoscopic 34.06
    internal mammary-coronary artery (single)
      36.15
      double vessel 36.16
  cannula, vessel-to-vessel (arteriovenous) 39.94
  canthus, lateral 08.59
  cardiac pacemaker
    device (permanent) 37.89
    electrode(s) (atrial) (transvenous) (ventricular)
      37.75
    pocket 37.79
  cardiac resynchronization defibrillator (CRT-D)
    device 37.79
    electrode(s) 37.75
    pocket 37.79
  cardiac resynchronization pacemaker (CRT-P)
    device (permanent) 37.89
    electrode(s) (atrial) (transvenous) (ventricular)
      37.75
    pocket 37.79
  cardioverter/defibrillator (automatic)
    pocket 37.79
  cholecystostomy 51.99
  cleft palate repair 27.63
  colostomy 46.43
  conduit, urinary 56.52
  cystostomy (stoma) 57.22
  disc—*see* Revision, intervertebral disc
  elbow replacement (prosthesis) 81.97
  enterostomy (stoma) 46.40
    large intestine 46.43
    small intestine 46.41
  enucleation socket 16.64
    with graft 16.63
  esophagostomy 42.83
  exenteration cavity 16.66
    with secondary graft 16.65
  extraocular muscle surgery 15.6
  fenestration, inner ear 20.62
  filtering bleb 12.66
  fixation device (broken) (displaced) (*see also*
    Fixation, bone, internal) 78.50
  flap or pedicle graft (skin) 86.75
  foot replacement (prosthesis) 81.59
  gastric anastomosis (with jejunal interposition) 44.5
  gastric band, laparoscopic 44.96
  gastric port device
    laparoscopic 44.96
  gastroduodenostomy (with jejunal interposition) 44.5
  gastrointestinal anastomosis (with jejunal
    interposition) 44.5
  gastrojejunostomy 44.5

Revision—*continued*
  gastrostomy 44.69
    laparoscopic 44.68
  hand replacement (prosthesis) 81.97
  heart procedure NEC 35.95
  hip replacement NOS 81.53
    acetabular and femoral components (total) 00.70
    acetabular component only 00.71
    acetabular liner and/or femoral head only 00.73
    femoral component only 00.72
    femoral head only and/or acetabular liner 00.73
    partial
      acetabular component only 00.71
      acetabular liner and/or femoral head only 00.73
      femoral component only 00.72
      femoral head only and/or acetabular liner 00.73
    total (acetabular and femoral components) 00.70
  Holter (Spitz) valve 02.42
  ileal conduit 56.52
  ileostomy 46.41
  intervertebral disc, artificial (partial) (total) NOS
      84.69
    cervical 84.66
    lumbar, lumbosacral 84.68
    thoracic 84.67
  jejunoileal bypass 46.93
  jejunostomy 46.41
  joint replacement 81.59
    acetabular and femoral components (total) 00.70
    acetabular component only 00.71
    acetabular liner and/or femoral head only 00.73
    ankle 81.59
    elbow 81.97
    femoral component only 00.72
    femoral head only and/or acetabular liner 00.73
    foot 81.59
    hand 81.97
    hip 81.53
      acetabular and femoral components (total) 00.70
      acetabular component only 00.71
      acetabular liner and/or femoral head only 00.73
      femoral component only 00.72
      femoral head only and/or acetabular liner 00.73
      partial
        acetabular component only 00.71
        acetabular liner and/or femoral head only 00.73
        femoral component only 00.72
        femoral head only and/or acetabular liner 00.73
      total (acetabular and femoral components) 00.70
    knee replacement NOS 81.55
      femoral component 00.82
      partial
        femoral component 00.82
        patellar component 00.83
        tibial component 00.81
        tibial insert 00.84
      patellar component 00.83
      tibial component 00.81
      tibial insert 00.84
      total (all components) 00.80
    lower extremity NEC 81.59
    toe 81.59
    upper extremity 81.97
    wrist 81.97

Revision—*continued*
  knee replacement (prosthesis) NOS 81.55
    femoral component 00.82
    partial
      femoral component 00.82
      patellar component 00.83
      tibial component 00.81
      tibial insert 00.84
    patellar component 00.83
    tibial component 00.81
    tibial insert 00.84
    total (all components) 00.80
  laryngostomy 31.63
  lateral canthus 08.59
  mallet finger 82.84
  mastoid antrum 19.9
  mastoidectomy 20.92
  nephrostomy 55.89
  neuroplasty 04.75
  ocular implant 16.62
  orbital implant 16.62
  pocket
    cardiac device (defibrillator) (pacemaker)
      with initial insertion of cardiac device—*omit
        code*
      new site (cardiac device pocket) (skin)
        (subcutaneous) 37.79
    carotid sinus stimulation pulse generator 39.85
      with initial insertion of pulse generator—*omit
        code*
    intracardiac hemodynamic monitoring 37.79
    subcutaneous device pocket NEC
      with initial insertion of generator or
        device—*omit code*
      new site 86.09
    thalamic stimulator pulse generator
      with initial insertion of battery
        package—*omit code*
      new site (skin) (subcutaneous) 86.09
  previous mastectomy site—*see* categories
      85.0-85.99
  proctostomy 48.79
  prosthesis
    acetabular and femoral components (total)
        00.70
    acetabular component only 00.71
    acetabular liner and/or femoral head only 00.73
    ankle 81.59
    breast 85.93
    elbow 81.97
    femoral component only 00.72
    femoral head only and/or acetabular liner 00.73
    foot 81.59
    hand 81.97
    heart valve (poppet) 35.95
    hip 81.53
      acetabular and femoral components (total)
          00.70
      acetabular component only 00.71
      acetabular liner and/or femoral head only
          00.73
      femoral component only 00.72
      femoral head only and/or acetabular liner
          00.73
      partial
        acetabular component only 00.71
        acetabular liner and/or femoral head only
            00.73
        femoral component only 00.72
        femoral head only and/or acetabular liner
            00.73

Revision—*continued*
    total (acetabular and femoral components)
        00.70
    knee NOS 81.55
      femoral component 00.82
      partial
        femoral component 00.82
        patellar component 00.83
        tibial component 00.81
        tibial insert 00.84
      patellar component 00.83
      tibial component 00.81
      tibial insert 00.84
      total (all components) 00.80
    lower extremity NEC 81.59
    shoulder 81.97
    spine
      facet replacement device 84.85
      interspinous process device(s) 84.81
      pedicle-based dynamic stabilization device(s)
        84.83
    toe 81.59
    upper extremity 81.97
    wrist 81.97
ptosis overcorrection 08.37
pyelostomy 55.12
pyloroplasty 44.29
rhinoplasty 21.84
scar
    skin 86.84
      with excision 86.3
scleral fistulization 12.66
shoulder replacement (prosthesis) 81.97
shunt
    arteriovenous (cannula) (for dialysis) 39.42
    lumbar-subarachnoid NEC 03.97
    peritoneojugular 54.99
    peritoneovascular 54.99
    pleurothecal 03.97
    salpingothecal 03.97
    spinal (thecal) NEC 03.97
    subarachnoid-peritoneal 03.97
    subarachnoid-ureteral 03.97
    ventricular (cerebral) 02.42
    ventriculoperitoneal
      at peritoneal site 54.95
      at ventricular site 02.42
stapedectomy NEC 19.29
    with incus replacement (homograft) (prosthesis)
      19.21
stimulator
    electrode(s)
      carotid sinus 39.84
    pulse generator
      carotid sinus 39.85
stoma
    bile duct 51.79
    bladder (vesicostomy) 57.22
    bronchus 33.42
    common duct 51.72
    esophagus 42.89
    gallbladder 51.99
    hepatic duct 51.79
    intestine 46.40
      large 46.43
      small 46.41
    kidney 55.89
    larynx 31.63
    rectum 48.79
    stomach 44.69
      laparoscopic 44.68

Revision—*continued*
    thorax 34.79
    trachea 31.74
    ureter 56.62
    urethra 58.4
  tack operation 20.79
  toe replacement (prosthesis) 81.59
  tracheostomy 31.74
  tunnel
    pulse generator lead wire 86.99
      with initial procedure—*omit code*
  tympanoplasty 19.6
  uretero-ileostomy, cutaneous 56.52
  ureterostomy (cutaneous) (stoma) NEC 56.62
    ileal 56.52
  urethrostomy 58.49
  urinary conduit 56.52
  vascular procedure (previous) NEC 39.49
  ventricular shunt (cerebral) 02.42
  vesicostomy stoma 57.22
  wrist replacement (prosthesis) 81.97
Rhinectomy 21.4
Rhinocheiloplasty 27.59
  cleft lip 27.54
Rhinomanometry 89.12
Rhinoplasty (external) (internal) NEC 21.87
  augmentation (with graft) (with synthetic
    implant) 21.85
  limited 21.86
  revision 21.84
  tip 21.86
  twisted nose 21.84
Rhinorrhaphy (external) (internal) 21.81
  for epistaxis 21.09
Rhinoscopy 21.21
Rhinoseptoplasty 21.84
Rhinotomy 21.1
Rhizotomy (radio frequency) (spinal) 03.1
  acoustic 04.01
  trigeminal 04.02
Rhytidectomy (facial) 86.82
  eyelid
    lower 08.86
    upper 08.87
Rhytidoplasty (facial) 86.82
Ripstein operation (repair of prolapsed rectum)
  48.75
Robotic assisted surgery
  endoscopic 17.44
  laparosopic 17.42
  open 17.41
  other and unspecified 17.49
  percutaneous 17.43
  thoracoscopic 17.45
Rodney Smith operation (radical subtotal
  pancreatectomy) 52.53
Roentgenography —*see also* Radiography
  cardiac, negative contrast 88.58
Rolling of conjunctiva 10.33
Root
  canal (tooth) (therapy) 23.70
    with
      apicoectomy 23.72
      irrigation 23.71
  resection (tooth) (apex) 23.73
    with root canal therapy 23.72
    residual or retained 23.11
Rotation of fetal head
  forceps (instrumental) (Kielland) (Scanzoni)
    (key-in-lock) 72.4
  manual 73.51

Routine
 chest x-ray 87.44
 psychiatric visit 94.12
Roux-en-Y operation
 bile duct 51.36
 cholecystojejunostomy 51.32
 esophagus (intrathoracic) 42.54
 gastroenterostomy 44.39
  laparoscopic 44.38
 gastrojejunostomy 44.39
  laparoscopic 44.38
 pancreaticojejunostomy 52.96
Roux-Goldthwait operation (repair of recurrent
  patellar dislocation) 81.44
Roux-Herzen-Judine operation (jejunal loop
  interposition) 42.63
Rubin test (insufflation of fallopian tube) 66.8
Ruiz-Mora operation (proximal phalangectomy
  for hammer toe) 77.99
Rupture
 esophageal web 42.01
 joint adhesions, manual 93.26
 membranes, artificial 73.09
  for surgical induction of labor 73.01
 ovarian cyst, manual 65.93
Russe operation (bone graft of scaphoid) 78.04

S

Sacculotomy (lack) 20.79
Sacrectomy (partial) 77.89
　　total 77.99
Saemisch operation (corneal section) 11.1
Salpingectomy (bilateral) (total) (transvaginal)
　　66.51
　　with oophorectomy 65.61
　　　laparoscopic 65.63
　　partial (unilateral) 66.69
　　　with removal of tubal pregnancy 66.62
　　　bilateral 66.63
　　　　for sterilization 66.39
　　　　by endoscopy 66.29
　　　remaining or solitary tube 66.52
　　　　with ovary 65.62
　　　　　laparoscopic 65.64
　　　unilateral (total) 66.4
　　　　with
　　　　　oophorectomy 65.49
　　　　　　laparoscopic 65.41
　　　　　removal of tubal pregnancy 66.62
　　　　　partial 66.69
Salpingography 87.85
Salpingohysterostomy 66.74
Salpingo-oophorectomy (unilateral) 65.49
　　that by laparoscope 65.41
　　bilateral (same operative episode) 65.61
　　　laparoscopic 65.63
　　remaining or solitary tube and ovary 65.62
　　　laparoscopic 65.64
Salpingo-oophoroplasty 65.73
　　laparoscopic 65.76
Salpingo-oophororrhaphy 65.79
Salpingo-oophorostomy 66.72
Salpingo-oophorotomy 65.09
　　laparoscopic 65.01
Salpingoplasty 66.79
Salpingorrhaphy 66.71
Salpingosalpingostomy 66.73
Salpingostomy (for removal of non-ruptured
　　ectopic pregnancy) 66.02
Salpingotomy 66.01
Salpingo-uterostomy 66.74
Salter operation (innominate osteotomy) 77.39
Salvage (autologous blood) (intraoperative)
　　(perioperative) (postoperative) 99.00
Sampling, blood for genetic determination of
　　fetus 75.33
Sandpapering (skin) 86.25
Saucerization
　　bone (see also Excision, lesion, bone) 77.60
　　rectum 48.99
Sauer-Bacon operation (abdominoperineal
　　resection), NOS 48.50
　　laparoscopic 48.51
　　open 48.52
　　other 48.59
Scalenectomy 83.45
Scalenotomy 83.19
Scaling and polishing, dental 96.54
Scan, scanning
　　C.A.T. (computerized axial tomography) 88.38
　　　abdomen 88.01
　　　bone 88.38
　　　　mineral density 88.98
　　　brain 87.03
　　　cardiac 87.41

Scan, scanning—continued
　　coronary 87.41
　　head 87.03
　　kidney 87.71
　　skeletal 88.38
　　　mineral density 88.98
　　thorax 87.41
　　with computer assisted surgery (CAS) 00.31
　　computerized axial tomography (C.A.T.) (see
　　　also Scan, C.A.T.) 88.38
　　C.T.—see Scan, C.A.T.
　　gallium—see Scan, radioisotope
　　liver 92.02
　　MUGA (multiple gated acquisition) —see Scan,
　　　radioisotope
　　positron emission tomography (PET)—see Scan,
　　　radioisotope
　　radioisotope
　　　adrenal 92.09
　　　bone 92.14
　　　　marrow 92.05
　　　bowel 92.04
　　　cardiac output 92.05
　　　cardiovascular 92.05
　　　cerebral 92.11
　　　circulation time 92.05
　　　eye 95.16
　　　gastrointestinal 92.04
　　　head NEC 92.12
　　　hematopoietic 92.05
　　　intestine 92.04
　　　iodine-131 92.01
　　　kidney 92.03
　　　liver 92.02
　　　lung 92.15
　　　lymphatic system 92.16
　　　myocardial infarction 92.05
　　　pancreatic 92.04
　　　parathyroid 92.13
　　　pituitary 92.11
　　　placenta 92.17
　　　protein-bound iodine 92.01
　　　pulmonary 92.15
　　　radio-iodine uptake 92.01
　　　renal 92.03
　　　specified site NEC 92.19
　　　spleen 92.05
　　　thyroid 92.01
　　　total body 92.18
　　　uterus 92.19
　　renal 92.03
　　thermal—see Thermography
Scapulectomy (partial) 77.81
　　total 77.91
Scapulopexy 78.41
Scarification
　　conjunctiva 10.33
　　nasal veins (with packing) 21.03
　　pericardium 36.39
　　pleura 34.6
　　　chemical 34.92
　　　　with cancer chemotherapy substance 34.92
　　　　　[99.25]
　　　　tetracycline 34.92 [99.21]
Schanz operation (femoral osteotomy) 77.35
Schauta (-Amreich) operation (radical vaginal
　　hysterectomy) 68.79
　　laparoscopic 68.71

Schede operation (thoracoplasty) 33.34
Scheie operation
  cautery of sclera 12.62
  sclerostomy 12.62
Schlatter operation (total gastrectomy) 43.99
Schroeder operation (endocervical excision)
  67.39
Schuchardt operation (nonobstetrical
  episiotomy) 71.09
Schwartze operation (simple mastoidectomy)
  20.41
Scintiphotography —*see* Scan, radioisotope
Scintiscan —*see* Scan, radioisotope
Sclerectomy (punch) (scissors) 12.65
  for retinal reattachment 14.49
  Holth's 12.65
  trephine 12.61
    with implant 14.41
Scleroplasty 12.89
Sclerostomy (Scheie's) 12.62
Sclerotherapy
  esophageal varices (endoscopic) 42.33
  hemorrhoids 49.42
  pleura 34.92
    treatment of malignancy (cytotoxic agent)
      34.92 *[99.25]*
    with tetracycline 34.92 *[99.21]*
  varicose vein 39.92
  vein NEC 39.92
Sclerotomy (exploratory) 12.89
  anterior 12.89
    with
      iridectomy 12.65
      removal of vitreous 14.71
  posterior 12.89
    with
      iridectomy 12.65
      removal of vitreous 14.72
Scott operation
  intestinal bypass for obesity 45.93
  jejunocolostomy (bypass) 45.93
Scraping
  corneal epithelium 11.41
    for smear or culture 11.21
  trachoma follicles 10.33
Scrotectomy (partial) 61.3
Scrotoplasty 61.49
Scrotorrhaphy 61.41
Scrototomy 61.0
Scrub, posterior nasal (adhesions) 21.91
Sculpturing, heart valve —*see* Valvuloplasty,
  heart
Section —*see also* Division *and* Incision
  cesarean—*see* Cesarean section
  ganglion, sympathetic 05.0
  hypophyseal stalk (*see also* Hypophysectomy,
    partial) 07.63
  ligamentum flavum (spine)—*omit code*
  nerve (cranial) (peripheral) NEC 04.03
    acoustic 04.01
    spinal root (posterior) 03.1
    sympathetic 05.0
    trigeminal tract 04.02
  Saemisch (corneal) 11.1
  spinal ligament 80.49
    arcuate—*omit code*
    flavum—*omit code*
  tooth (impacted) 23.19
Seddon-Brooks operation (transfer of pectoralis
  major tendon) 83.75
Semb operation (apicolysis of lung) 33.39

Senning operation (correction of transposition of
  great vessels) 35.91
Separation
  twins (attached) (conjoined) (Siamese) 84.93
    asymmetrical (unequal) 84.93
    symmetrical (equal) 84.92
Septectomy
  atrial (closed) 35.41
    open 35.42
    transvenous method (balloon) 35.41
  submucous (nasal) 21.5
Septoplasty NEC 21.88
  with submucous resection of septum 21.5
Septorhinoplasty 21.84
Septostomy (atrial) (balloon) 35.41
Septotomy, nasal 21.1
Sequestrectomy
  bone 77.00
    carpals, metacarpals 77.04
    clavicle 77.01
    facial 76.01
    femur 77.05
    fibula 77.07
    humerus 77.02
    nose 21.32
    patella 77.06
    pelvic 77.09
    phalanges (foot) (hand) 77.09
    radius 77.03
    scapula 77.01
    skull 01.25
    specified site NEC 77.09
    tarsals, metatarsals 77.08
    thorax (ribs) (sternum) 77.01
    tibia 77.07
    ulna 77.03
    vertebrae 77.09
  nose 21.32
  skull 01.25
Sesamoidectomy 77.98
Setback, ear 18.5
Sever operation (division of soft tissue of arm)
  83.19
Severing of blepharorrhaphy 08.02
Sewell operation (heart) 36.2
Sharrard operation (iliopsoas muscle transfer)
  83.77
Shaving
  bone (*see also* Excision, lesion, bone) 77.60
  cornea (epithelium) 11.41
    for smear or culture 11.21
  patella 77.66
Shelf operation (hip arthroplasty) 81.40
Shirodkar operation (encirclement suture,
  cervix) 67.59
Shock therapy
  chemical 94.24
  electroconvulsive 94.27
  electrotonic 94.27
  insulin 94.24
  subconvulsive 94.26
Shortening
  bone (fusion) 78.20
    femur 78.25
    specified site NEC (*see* category 78.2)
    tibia 78.27
    ulna 78.23
  endopelvic fascia 69.22
  extraocular muscle NEC 15.22
    multiple (two or more muscles) 15.4
  eyelid margin 08.71
  eye muscle NEC 15.22

Shortening—*continued*
  multiple (two or more muscles) (with
    lengthening) 15.4
  finger (macrodactyly repair) 82.83
  heel cord 83.85
  levator palpebrae muscle 08.33
  ligament—*see also* Arthroplasty
    round 69.22
    uterosacral 69.22
  muscle 83.85
    extraocular 15.22
      multiple (two or more muscles) 15.4
    hand 82.55
  sclera (for repair of retinal detachment) 14.59
    by scleral buckling (*see also* Buckling, scleral)
      14.49
  tendon 83.85
    hand 82.55
  ureter (with reimplantation) 56.41
Shunt —*see also* Anastomosis *and* Bypass,
  vascular
  abdominovenous 54.94
  aorta-coronary sinus 36.39
  aorta (descending) pulmonary (artery) 39.0
  aortocarotid 39.22
  aortoceliac 39.26
  aortofemoral 39.25
  aortoiliac 39.25
  aortoiliofemoral 39.25
  aortomesenteric 39.26
  aorto-myocardial (graft) 36.2
  aortorenal 39.24
  aortosubclavian 39.22
  apicoaortic 35.93
  aqueous drainage 12.67
  arteriovenous NEC 39.29
    for renal dialysis (by)
      anastomosis 39.27
      external cannula 39.93
  ascending aorta to pulmonary artery (Waterston)
    39.0
  axillary-femoral 39.29
  carotid-carotid 39.22
  carotid-subclavian 39.22
  caval-mesenteric 39.1
  corpora cavernosa-corpus spongiosum 64.98
  corpora-saphenous 64.98
  descending aorta to pulmonary artery
    (Potts-Smith) 39.0
  endolymphatic (subarachnoid) 20.71
  endolymph-perilymph 20.71
  extracranial-intracranial (EC-IC) 39.28
  femoroperoneal 39.29
  femoropopliteal 39.29
  iliofemoral 39.25
  ilioiliac 39.25
  intestinal
    large-to-large 45.94
    small-to-large 45.93
    small-to-small 45.91
  left subclavian to descending aorta
    (Blalock-Park) 39.0
  left-to-right (systemic-pulmonary artery) 39.0
  left ventricle (heart) (apex) and aorta 35.93
  lienorenal 39.1
  lumbar-subarachnoid (with valve) NEC 03.79
  mesocaval 39.1
  peritoneal-jugular 54.94
  peritoneo-vascular 54.94
  peritoneovenous 54.94
  pleuroperitoneal 34.05
  pleurothecal (with valve) 03.79

Shunt—*continued*
  portacaval (double) 39.1
  portal-systemic 39.1
  portal vein to vena cava 39.1
  pulmonary-innominate 39.0
  pulmonary vein to atrium 35.82
  renoportal 39.1
  right atrium and pulmonary artery 35.94
  right ventricle and pulmonary artery (distal) 35.92
    in repair of
      pulmonary artery atresia 35.92
      transposition of great vessels 35.92
      truncus arteriosus 35.83
  salpingothecal (with valve) 03.79
  semicircular-subarachnoid 20.71
  spinal (thecal) (with valve) NEC 03.79
  subarachnoid-peritoneal 03.71
  subarachnoid-ureteral 03.72
  splenorenal (venous) 39.1
    arterial 39.26
  subarachnoid-peritoneal (with valve) 03.71
  subarachnoid-ureteral (with valve) 03.72
  subclavian-pulmonary 39.0
  subdural-peritoneal (with valve) 02.34
  superior mesenteric-caval 39.1
  systemic-pulmonary artery 39.0
  transjugular intrahepatic portosystemic (TIPS) 39.1
  vena cava to pulmonary artery (Green) 39.21
  ventricular (cerebral) (with valve) 02.22
    to
      abdominal cavity or organ 02.34
      bone marrow 02.39
      cervical subarachnoid space 02.22
      circulatory system 02.32
      cisterna magna 02.22
      extracranial site NEC 02.39
      gallbladder 02.34
      head or neck structure 02.31
      intracerebral site NEC 02.22
      lumbar site 02.39
      mastoid 02.31
      nasopharynx 02.31
      peritoneal 02.34
      thoracic cavity 02.33
      ureter 02.35
      urinary system 02.35
      venous system 02.35
  ventriculoatrial (with valve) 02.32
  ventriculocaval (with valve) 02.32
  ventriculocisternal (with valve) 02.22
  ventriculolumbar (with valve) 02.39
  ventriculomastoid (with valve) 02.31
  ventriculonasopharyngeal 02.31
  ventriculopleural (with valve) 02.33
Sialoadenectomy (parotid) (sublingual)
  (submaxillary) 26.30
  complete 26.32
  partial 26.31
  radical 26.32
Sialoadenolithotomy 26.0
Sialoadenotomy 26.0
Sialodochoplasty NEC 26.49
Sialogram 87.09
Sialolithotomy 26.0
Sieve, vena cava 38.7
Sigmoid bladder 57.87 *[45.52]*
Sigmoidectomy
  laparoscopic 17.36
  open and other 45.76
Sigmoidomyotomy 46.91
Sigmoidopexy (Moschowitz) 46.63

Sigmoidoproctectomy (*see also* Resection, rectum) 48.69
Sigmoidoproctostomy 45.94
Sigmoidorectostomy 45.94
Sigmoidorrhaphy 46.75
Sigmoidoscopy (rigid) 48.23
  with biopsy 45.25
  flexible 45.24
  through stoma (artificial) 45.22
  transabdominal 45.21
Sigmoidosigmoidostomy 45.94
  proximal to distal segment
    laparoscopic 17.36
    open and other 45.76
Sigmoidostomy (*see also* Colostomy) 46.10
Sigmoidotomy 45.03
Sign language 93.75
Silver operation (bunionectomy) 77.59
Sinogram
  abdominal wall 88.03
  chest wall 87.38
  retroperitoneum 88.14
Sinusectomy (nasal) (complete) (partial) (with turbinectomy) 22.60
  antrum 22.62
    with Caldwell-Luc approach 22.61
  ethmoid 22.63
  frontal 22.42
  maxillary 22.62
    with Caldwell-Luc approach 22.61
  sphenoid 22.64
Sinusotomy (nasal) 22.50
  antrum (intranasal) 22.2
    with external approach (Caldwell-Luc) 22.39
      radical (with removal of membrane lining) 22.31
  ethmoid 22.51
  frontal 22.41
  maxillary (intranasal) 22.2
    external approach (Caldwell-Luc) 22.39
      radical (with removal of membrane lining) 22.31
  multiple 22.53
  perinasal 22.50
  sphenoid 22.52
Sistrunk operation (excision of thyroglossal cyst) 06.7
Size reduction
  abdominal wall (adipose) (pendulous) 86.83
  arms (adipose) (batwing) 86.83
  breast (bilateral) 85.32
    unilateral 85.31
  buttocks (adipose) 86.83
  skin 86.83
  subcutaneous tissue 86.83
  thighs (adipose) 86.83
Skeletal series (x-ray) 88.31
SKyphoplasty 81.66
Sling —*see also* Operation, sling
  fascial (fascia lata)
    for facial weakness (trigeminal nerve paralysis) 86.81
    mouth 86.81
    orbicularis (mouth) 86.81
    tongue 25.59
  levator muscle (urethrocystopexy) 59.71
  pubococcygeal 59.71
  rectum (puborectalis) 48.76
  tongue (fascial) 25.59

Slitting
  canaliculus for
    passage of tube 09.42
    removal of streptothrix 09.42
  lens 13.2
  prepuce (dorsal) (lateral) 64.91
Slocum operation (pes anserinus transfer) 81.47
Sluder operation (tonsillectomy) 28.2
Small bowel series (x-ray) 87.63
Smith operation (open osteotomy of mandible) 76.62
Smith-Peterson operation (radiocarpal arthrodesis) 81.25
Smithwick operation (sympathectomy) 05.29
Snaring, polyp, colon (endoscopic) 45.42
Snip, punctum (with dilation) 09.51
Soave operation (endorectal pull-through) 48.41
Somatotherapy, psychiatric NEC 94.29
Sonneberg operation (inferior maxillary neurectomy) 04.07
Sorondo-Ferré operation (hindquarter amputation) 84.19
Soutter operation (iliac crest fasciotomy) 83.14
Spaulding-Richardson operation (uterine suspension) 69.22
Spectrophotometry NEC 89.39
  blood 89.39
  placenta 89.29
  urine 89.29
Spectroscopy
  intravascular 38.23
  near infrared (NIR) 38.23
Speech therapy NEC 93.75
Spermatocelectomy 63.2
Spermatocystectomy 60.73
Spermatocystotomy 60.72
Sphenoidectomy 22.64
Sphenoidotomy 22.52
Sphincterectomy, anal 49.6
Sphincteroplasty
  anal 49.79
    obstetrical laceration (current) 75.62
      old 49.79
  bladder neck 57.85
  pancreas 51.83
  sphincter of Oddi 51.83
Sphincterorrhaphy, anal 49.71
  obstetrical laceration (current) 75.62
    old 49.79
Sphincterotomy
  anal (external) (internal) 49.59
    left lateral 49.51
    posterior 49.52
  bladder (neck) (transurethral) 57.91
  choledochal 51.82
    endoscopic 51.85
  iris 12.12
  pancreatic 51.82
    endoscopic 51.85
  sphincter of Oddi 51.82
    endoscopic 51.85
  transduodenal ampullary 51.82
    endoscopic 51.85
Spinal anesthesia —*omit code*
Spinelli operation (correction of inverted uterus) 75.93
Spineoplasty 81.66
Spirometry (incentive) (respiratory) 89.37
Spivack operation (permanent gastrostomy) 43.19
Splanchnicectomy 05.29
Splanchnicotomy 05.0

Splenectomy (complete) (total) 41.5
  partial 41.43
Splenogram 88.64
  radioisotope 92.05
Splenolysis 54.59
  laparoscopic 54.51
Splenopexy 41.95
Splenoplasty 41.95
Splenoportogram (by splenic arteriography)
  88.64
Splenorrhaphy 41.95
Splenotomy 41.2
Splinting
  dental (for immobilization) 93.55
    orthodontic 24.7
  musculoskeletal 93.54
  ureteral 56.2
Splitting —*see also* Division
  canaliculus 09.52
  lacrimal papilla 09.51
  spinal cord tracts 03.29
    percutaneous 03.21
  tendon sheath 83.01
    hand 82.01
Spondylosyndesis (*see also* Fusion, spinal) 81.00
S.P. Rogers operation (knee disarticulation)
  84.16
Ssabanejew-Frank operation (permanent
  gastrostomy) 43.19
Stab, intercostal 34.09
Stabilization, joint —*see also* Arthrodesis
  patella (for recurrent dislocation) 81.44
Stacke operation (simple mastoidectomy) 20.41
Stallard operation (conjunctivocystorhinostomy)
  09.82
  with insertion of tube or stent 09.83
Stamm (Kader) operation (temporary
  gastrostomy) 43.19
Stapedectomy 19.19
  with incus replacement (homograft) (prosthesis)
    19.11
  revision 19.29
    with incus replacement 19.21
Stapediolysis 19.0
Stapling
  artery 39.31
  blebs, lung (emphysematous) 32.21
  diaphysis (*see also* Stapling, epiphyseal plate)
    78.20
  epiphyseal plate 78.20
    femur 78.25
    fibula 78.27
    humerus 78.22
    radius 78.23
    specified site NEC 78.29
    tibia 78.27
    ulna 78.23
  gastric varices 44.91
  graft—*see* Graft
  left atrial appendage 37.36
  vein 39.32
STARR (stapled transanal rectal resection) 48.74
StaXx® FX Structural Kyphoplasty System
  81.66
Steinberg operation 44.5
Steindler operation
  fascia stripping (for cavus deformity) 83.14
  flexorplasty (elbow) 83.77
  muscle transfer 83.77
Stereotactic head frame application 93.59

Stereotactic radiosurgery 92.30
  cobalt 60 92.32
  linear accelerator (LINAC) 92.31
  multi-source 92.32
  particle beam 92.33
  particulate 92.33
  radiosurgery NEC 92.39
  single source photon 92.31
Sterilization
  female (*see also* specific operation) 66.39
  male NEC (*see also* Ligation, vas deferens) 63.70
Sternotomy 77.31
  as operative approach—*omit code*
  for bone marrow biopsy 41.31
Stewart operation (renal plication with
  pyeloplasty) 55.87
Stimulation (electronic) —*see also* Implant,
  electronic stimulator
  bone growth (percutaneous)—*see* category 78.9
    transcutaneous (surface) 99.86
  cardiac (external) 99.62
    internal 37.91
  carotid sinus 99.64
  CaverMap™ 89.58
  defibrillator
    as part of intraoperative testing —*omit code*
    catheter based invasive electrophysiologic
      testing 37.26
    device interrogation only without arrhythmia
      induction (bedside check) 89.45-89.49
    noninvasive programmed electrical stimulation
      (NIPS) 37.20
  electrophysiologic, cardiac
    as part of intraoperative testing —*omit code*
    catheter based invasive electrophysiologic
      testing 37.26
    device interrogation only without arrhythmia
      induction (bedside check) 89.45-89.49
    noninvasive programmed electrical stimulation
      (NIPS) 37.20
  nerve
    CaverMap™ 89.58
    penile 89.58
    peripheral or spinal cord, transcutaneous 93.39
Stitch, Kelly-Stoeckel (urethra) 59.3
Stomatoplasty 27.59
Stomatorrhaphy 27.52
Stone operation (anoplasty) 49.79
Strapping (non-traction) 93.59
Strassman operation (metroplasty) 69.49
Strayer operation (gastrocnemius recession)
  83.72
Stretching
  eyelid (with elongation) 08.71
  fascia 93.28
  foreskin 99.95
  iris 12.63
  muscle 93.27
  nerve (cranial) (peripheral) 04.91
  tendon 93.27
Stripping
  bone (*see also* Incision, bone) 77.10
  carotid sinus 39.89
  cranial suture 02.01
  fascia 83.14
    hand 82.12
  membranes for surgical induction of labor 73.1
  meninges (cerebral) 01.51
    spinal 03.4
  saphenous vein, varicose 38.59

Stripping—*continued*
  subdural membrane (cerebral) 01.51
    spinal 03.4
  varicose veins (lower limb) 38.59
    upper limb 38.53
  vocal cords 30.09
Stromeyer-Little operation (hepatotomy) 50.0
Strong operation (unbridling of celiac artery
  axis) 39.91
Stryker frame 93.59
Study
  bone mineral density 88.98
  bundle of His 37.29
  color vision 95.06
  conduction, nerve (median) 89.15
  dark adaptation, eye 95.07
  electrophysiologic stimulation and recording,
    cardiac
    as part of intraoperative testing —*omit code*
    catheter based invasive electrophysiologic
      testing 37.26
    device interrogation only without arrhythmia
      induction (bedside check) 89.45-89.49
    noninvasive programmed electrical stimulation
      (NIPS) 37.20
  function—*see also* Function, study
  radioisotope—*see* Scan, radioisotope
  lacrimal flow (radiographic) 87.05
  ocular motility 95.15
  pulmonary
    airway flow measurement, endoscopic 33.72
    function —*see* categories 89.37-89.38
  radiographic—*see* Radiography
  radio-iodinated triolein 92.04
  renal clearance 92.03
  spirometer 89.37
  tracer—*see also* Scan, radioisotope
    eye (P^{32}) 95.16
  ultrasonic—*see* Ultrasonography
  visual field 95.05
  xenon flow NEC 92.19
    cardiovascular 92.05
    pulmonary 92.15
Sturmdorf operation (conization of cervix) 67.2
Submucous resection
  larynx 30.29
  nasal septum 21.5
Summerskill operation
  (dacryocystorhinostomy by intubation) 09.81
Surgery
  computer assisted (CAS) 00.39
    with robotics —*see* category 17.4
    CAS with CT/CTA 00.31
    CAS with fluoroscopy 00.33
    CAS with MR/MRA 00.32
    CAS with multiple datasets 00.35
      imageless 00.34
      other CAS 00.39
  IGS—*see* Surgery, computer assisted
  image guided—*see* Surgery, computer assisted
  navigation (CT-free, IGN image guided,
    imageless)—*see* Surgery, computer assisted
  robotic assisted —*see* category 17.4
Surmay operation (jejunostomy) 46.39
Suspension
  balanced, for traction 93.45
  bladder NEC 57.89
  diverticulum, pharynx 29.59
  kidney 55.7
  Olshausen (uterus) 69.22
  ovary 65.79

Suspension—*continued*
  paraurethral (Pereyra) 59.6
  periurethral 59.6
  urethra (retropubic) (sling) 59.5
  urethrovesical
    Goebel-Frangenheim-Stoeckel 59.4
    gracilis muscle transplant 59.71
    levator muscle sling 59.71
    Marshall-Marchetti (Krantz) 59.5
    Millin-Read 59.4
    suprapubic 59.4
  uterus (abdominal or vaginal approach) 69.22
  vagina 70.77
    with graft or prosthesis 70.78
Suture (laceration)
  abdominal wall 54.63
    secondary 54.61
  adenoid fossa 28.7
  adrenal (gland) 07.44
  aneurysm (cerebral) (peripheral) 39.52
  anus 49.71
    obstetric laceration (current) 75.62
      old 49.79
  aorta 39.31
  aponeurosis (*see also* Suture, tendon) 83.64
  arteriovenous fistula 39.53
  artery 39.31
    percutaneous puncture closure—*omit code*
  bile duct 51.79
  bladder 57.81
    obstetric laceration (current) 75.61
  blood vessel NEC 39.30
    artery 39.31
    percutaneous puncture closure—*omit code*
    vein 39.32
  breast (skin) 85.81
  bronchus 33.41
  bursa 83.99
    hand 82.99
  canaliculus 09.73
  cecum 46.75
  cerebral meninges 02.11
  cervix (traumatic laceration) 67.61
    internal os, encirclement 67.59
    obstetric laceration (current) 75.51
      old 67.69
  chest wall 34.71
  cleft palate 27.62
  clitoris 71.4
  colon 46.75
  common duct 51.71
  conjunctiva 10.6
  cornea 11.51
    with conjunctival flap 11.53
  corneoscleral 11.51
    with conjunctival flap 11.53
  diaphragm 34.82
  duodenum 46.71
    ulcer (bleeding) (perforated) 44.42
      endoscopic 44.43
  dura mater (cerebral) 02.11
    spinal 03.59
  ear, external 18.4
  enterocele 70.92
    with graft or prosthesis 70.93
  entropion 08.42
  epididymis (and)
    spermatic cord 63.51
    vas deferens 63.81
  episiotomy—*see* Episiotomy
  esophagus 42.82

Suture—*continued*
  eyeball 16.89
  eyebrow 08.81
  eyelid 08.81
    with entropion or ectropion repair 08.42
  fallopian tube 66.71
  fascia 83.65
    hand 82.46
    to skeletal attachment 83.89
      hand 82.89
  gallbladder 51.91
  ganglion, sympathetic 05.81
  gingiva 24.32
  great vessel 39.30
    artery 39.31
    vein 39.32
  gum 24.32
  heart 37.49
  hepatic duct 51.79
  hymen 70.76
  ileum 46.73
  intestine 46.79
    large 46.75
    small 46.73
  jejunum 46.73
  joint capsule 81.96
    with arthroplasty—*see* Arthroplasty
    ankle 81.94
    foot 81.94
    lower extremity NEC 81.95
    upper extremity 81.93
  kidney 55.81
  labia 71.71
  laceration—*see* Suture, by site
  larynx 31.61
  ligament 81.96
    with arthroplasty—*see* Arthroplasty
    ankle 81.94
    broad 69.29
    Cooper's 54.64
    foot and toes 81.94
    gastrocolic 54.73
    knee 81.95
    lower extremity NEC 81.95
    sacrouterine 69.29
    upper extremity 81.93
    uterine 69.29
  ligation—*see* Ligation
  lip 27.51
  liver 50.61
  lung 33.43
  meninges (cerebral) 02.11
    spinal 03.59
  mesentery 54.75
  mouth 27.52
  muscle 83.65
    hand 82.46
    ocular (oblique) (rectus) 15.7
  nerve (cranial) (peripheral) 04.3
    sympathetic 05.81
  nose (external) (internal) 21.81
    for epistaxis 21.09
  obstetric laceration NEC 75.69
    bladder 75.61
    cervix 75.51
    corpus uteri 75.52
    pelvic floor 75.69
    perineum 75.69
    periurethral 75.69
    rectum 75.62
    sphincter ani 75.62
    urethra 75.61

Suture—*continued*
  uterus 75.50
  vagina 75.69
  vulva 75.69
  omentum 54.64
  ovary 65.71
    laparoscopic 65.74
  palate 27.61
    cleft 27.62
  palpebral fissure 08.59
  pancreas 52.95
  pelvic floor 71.71
    obstetric laceration (current) 75.69
  penis 64.41
  peptic ulcer (bleeding) (perforated) 44.40
  pericardium 37.49
  perineum (female) 71.71
    after delivery 75.69
      episiotomy repair—*see* Episiotomy
    male 86.59
  periosteum 78.20
    carpal, metacarpal 78.24
    femur 78.25
    fibula 78.27
    humerus 78.22
    pelvic 78.29
    phalanxes (foot) (hand) 78.29
    radius 78.23
    specified site NEC 78.29
    tarsal metatarsal 78.28
    tibia 78.27
    ulna 78.23
    vertebrae 78.29
  peritoneum 54.64
  periurethral tissue to symphysis pubis 59.5
  pharynx 29.51
  pleura 34.93
  rectum 48.71
    obstetric laceration (current) 75.62
  retina (for reattachment) 14.59
  sacrouterine ligament 69.29
  salivary gland 26.41
  scalp 86.59
    replantation 86.51
  sclera (with repair of conjunctive) 12.81
  scrotum (skin) 61.41
  secondary
    abdominal wall 54.61
    episiotomy 75.69
    peritoneum 54.64
  sigmoid 46.75
  skin (mucous membrane) (without graft) 86.59
    with graft—*see* Graft, skin
    breast 85.81
    ear 18.4
    eyebrow 08.81
    eyelid 08.81
    nose 21.81
    penis 64.41
    scalp 86.59
      replantation 86.51
    scrotum 61.41
    vulva 71.71
  specified site NEC—*see* Repair, by site
  spermatic cord 63.51
  sphincter ani 49.71
    obstetric laceration (current) 75.62
      old 49.79
  spinal meninges 03.59
  spleen 41.95

Suture—*continued*
  stomach 44.61
    ulcer (bleeding) (perforated) 44.41
      endoscopic 44.43
  subcutaneous tissue (without skin graft) 86.59
    with graft—*see* Graft, skin
  tendon (direct) (immediate) (primary) 83.64
    delayed (secondary) 83.62
      hand NEC 82.43
        flexors 82.42
    hand NEC 82.45
      delayed (secondary) 82.43
      flexors 82.44
        delayed (secondary) 82.42
    ocular 15.7
    rotator cuff 83.63
    sheath 83.61
      hand 82.41
    supraspinatus (rotator cuff repair) 83.63
    to skeletal attachment 83.88
      hand 82.85
  Tenon's capsule 15.7
  testis 62.61
  thymus 07.93
  thyroid gland 06.93
  tongue 25.51
  tonsillar fossa 28.7
  trachea 31.71
  tunics vaginalis 61.41
  ulcer (bleeding) (perforated) (peptic) 44.40
    duodenum 44.42
      endoscopic 44.43
    gastric 44.41
      endoscopic 44.43
    intestine 46.79
    skin 86.59
    stomach 44.41
      endoscopic 44.43
  ureter 56.82
  urethra 58.41
    obstetric laceration (current) 75.61
  uterosacral ligament 69.29
  uterus 69.41
    obstetric laceration (current) 75.50
      old 69.49
  uvula 27.73
  vagina 70.71
    obstetric laceration (current) 75.69
      old 70.79
  vas deferens 63.81
  vein 39.32
  vulva 71.71
    obstetric laceration (current) 75.69
      old 71.79
Suture-ligation —*see also* Ligation
  blood vessel—*see* Ligation, blood vessel
Sweep, anterior iris 12.97
Swenson operation
  bladder reconstruction 57.87
  proctectomy 48.49
Swinney operation (urethral reconstruction)
  58.46
Switch, switching
  coronary arteries 35.84
  great arteries, total 35.84
Syme operation
  ankle amputation through malleoli of tibia and
    fibula 84.14
  urethrotomy, external 58.0

Sympathectomy NEC 05.29
  cervical 05.22
  cervicothoracic 05.22
  lumbar 05.23
  periarterial 05.25
  presacral 05.24
  renal 05.29
  thoracolumbar 05.23
  tympanum 20.91
Sympatheticotripsy 05.0
Symphysiotomy 77.39
  assisting delivery (obstetrical) 73.94
  kidney (horseshoe) 55.85
Symphysis, pleural 34.6
Synchondrotomy (*see also* Division, cartilage)
  80.40
Syndactylization 86.89
Syndesmotomy (*see also* Division, ligament)
  80.40
Synechiotomy
  endometrium 68.21
  iris (posterior) 12.33
    anterior 12.32
Synovectomy (joint) (complete) (partial) 80.70
  ankle 80.77
  elbow 80.72
  foot and toe 80.78
  hand and finger 80.74
  hip 80.75
  knee 80.76
  shoulder 80.71
  specified site NEC 80.79
  spine 80.79
  tendon sheath 83.42
    hand 82.33
  wrist 80.73
Syringing
  lacrimal duct or sac 09.43
  nasolacrimal duct 09.43
    with
      dilation 09.43
      insertion of tube or stent 09.44

T

Taarnhoj operation (trigeminal nerve root decompression) 04.41
Tack operation (sacculotomy) 20.79
Tactile Guidance System ™ [TGS]—*see* category 17.4
Take-down
 anastomosis
  arterial 39.49
  blood vessel 39.49
  gastric, gastrointestinal 44.5
  intestine 46.93
  stomach 44.5
  vascular 39.49
  ventricular 02.43
 arterial bypass 39.49
 arteriovenous shunt 39.43
  with creation of new shunt 39.42
 cecostomy 46.52
 colostomy 46.52
 duodenostomy 46.51
 enterostomy 46.50
 esophagostomy 42.83
 gastroduodenostomy 44.5
 gastrojejunostomy 44.5
 ileostomy 46.51
 intestinal stoma 46.50
  large 46.52
  small 46.51
 jejunoileal bypass 46.93
 jejunostomy 46.51
 laryngostomy 31.62
 sigmoidostomy 46.52
 stoma
  bile duct 51.79
  bladder 57.82
  bronchus 33.42
  common duct 51.72
  esophagus 42.83
  gall bladder 51.92
  hepatic duct 51.79
  intestine 46.50
   large 46.52
   small 46.51
  kidney 55.82
  larynx 31.62
  rectum 48.72
  stomach 44.62
  thorax 34.72
  trachea 31.72
  ureter 56.83
  urethra 58.42
 systemic-pulmonary artery anastomosis 39.49
  in total repair of tetralogy of Fallot 35.81
 tracheostomy 31.72
 vascular anastomosis or bypass 39.49
 ventricular shunt (cerebral) 02.43
Talectomy 77.98
Talma-Morison operation (omentopexy) 54.74
Tamponade
 esophageal 96.06
 intrauterine (nonobstetric) 69.91
  after delivery or abortion 75.8
  antepartum 73.1
 vagina 96.14
  after delivery or abortion 75.8
  antepartum 73.1
Tanner operation (devascularization of stomach) 44.99

Tap
 abdomen 54.91
 chest 34.91
 cisternal 01.01
 crania] 01.09
 joint 81.91
 lumbar (diagnostic) (removal of dye) 03.31
 perilymphatic 20.79
 spinal (diagnostic) 03.31
 subdural (through fontanel) 01.09
 thorax 34.91
Tarsectomy 08.20
 de Grandmont 08.35
Tarsoplasty (*see also* Reconstruction, eyelid) 08.70
Tarsorrhaphy (lateral) 08.52
 division or severing 08.02
Tattooing
 cornea 11.91
 skin 86.02
Tautening, eyelid for entropion 08.42
TAVI (transcatheter aortic valve implantation) 35.05
TAVR (transcatheter aortic valve replacement) 35.05
Telemetry (cardiac) 89.54
Teleradiotherapy
 beta particles 92.25
  intra-operative 92.41
 Betatron 92.24
 cobalt-60 92.23
 electrons 92.25
  intra-operative 92.41
 iodine-125 92.23
 linear accelerator 92.24
 neutrons 92.26
 particulate radiation NEC 92.26
 photons 92.24
 protons 92.26
 radioactive cesium 92.23
 radioisotopes NEC 92.23
Temperature gradient study (*see also* Thermography) 88.89
Temperament assessment 94.02
Tendinoplasty —*see* Repair, tendon
Tendinosuture (immediate) (primary) (*see also* Suture, tendon) 83.64
 hand (*see also* Suture, tendon, hand) 82.45
Tendolysis 83.91
 hand 82.91
Tendoplasty —*see* Repair, tendon
Tenectomy 83.39
 eye 15.13
  levator palpebrae 08.33
  multiple (two or more tendons) 15.3
 hand 82.29
 levator palpebrae 08.33
 tendon sheath 83.31
  hand 82.21
Tenodesis (tendon fixation to skeletal attachment) 83.88
 Fowler 82.85
 hand 82.85
Tenolysis 83.91
 hand 82.91
Tenomyoplasty (*see also* Repair, tendon) 83.88
 hand (*see also* Repair, tendon, hand) 82.86
Tenomyotomy —*see* Tenonectomy

Tenonectomy 83.42
  for graft 83.41
    hand 82.32
  hand 82.33
    for graft 82.32
Tenontomyoplasty —*see* Repair, tendon
Tenontoplasty —*see* Repair, tendon
Tenoplasty (*see also* Repair, tendon) 83.88
  hand (*see also* Repair, tendon, hand) 82.86
Tenorrhaphy (*see also* Suture, tendon) 83.64
  hand (*see also* Suture, tendon, hand) 82.45
  to skeletal attachment 83.88
    hand 82.85
Tenosuspension 83.88
  hand 82.86
Tenosuture (*see also* Suture, tendon) 83.64
  hand (*see also* Suture, tendon, hand) 82.45
  to skeletal attachment 83.88
    hand 82.85
Tenosynovectomy 83.42
  hand 82.33
Tenotomy 83.13
  Achilles tendon 83.11
  adductor (hip) (subcutaneous) 83.12
  eye 15.12
    levator palpebrae 08.38
    multiple (two or more tendons) 15.4
  hand 82.11
  levator palpebrae 08.38
  pectoralis minor tendon (decompression thoracic
    outlet) 83.13
  stapedius 19.0
  tensor tympani 19.0
Tenovaginotomy —*see* Tenotomy
Tensing, orbicularis oculi 08.59
Termination of pregnancy
  by
    aspiration curettage 69.51
    dilation and curettage 69.01
    hysterectomy—*see* Hysterectomy
    hysterotomy 74.91
    intra-amniotic injection (saline) 75.0
Test, testing (for)
  auditory function NEC 95.46
  Bender Visual-Motor Gestalt 94.02
  Benton Visual Retention 94.02
  14 C-Urea breath 89.39
  cardiac (vascular)
    function NEC 89.59
    stress 89.44
      bicycle ergometer 89.43
      Masters' two-step 89.42
      treadmill 89.41
  Denver developmental (screening) 94.02
  fetus, fetal
    nonstress (fetal activity acceleration
      determinations) 75.34
    oxytocin challenge (contraction stress) 75.35
    sensitivity (to oxytocin)—*omit code*
  function
    cardiac NEC 89.59
    hearing NEC 95.46
    muscle (by)
      electromyography 93.08
      manual 93.04
    neurologic NEC 89.15
    vestibular 95.46
      clinical 95.44
  glaucoma NEC 95.26
  hearing 95.47
    clinical NEC 95.42

Test, testing—*continued*
  intelligence 94.01
  internal jugular-subclavian venous reflux 89.6
  intracarotid amobarbital (Wada) 89.10
  Masters' two-step stress (cardiac) 89.42
  muscle function (by)
    electromyography 93.08
    manual 93.04
  neurologic function NEC 89.15
  neurophysiologic monitoring
    intra-operative 00.94
  nocturnal penile tumescence 89.29
  provocative, for glaucoma 95.26
  psychologic NEC 94.08
  psychometric 94.01
  radio-cobalt B_{12} Schilling 92.04
  range of motion 93.05
  rotation (Barany chair) (hearing) 95.45
  sleep disorder function—*see* categories
    89.17-89.18
  Stanford-Binet 94.01
  Thallium stress (transesophageal pacing) 89.44
  tuning fork (hearing) 95.42
  Urea breath, (14 C) 89.39
  vestibular function NEC 95.46
    thermal 95.44
  Wada (hemispheric function) 89.10
  whispered speech (hearing) 95.42
TEVAP (transurethral electrovaporization of
  prostate) 60.29
Thalamectomy 01.41
Thalamotomy 01.41
  by stereotactic radiosurgery 92.32
    cobalt 60 92.32
    linear accelerator (LINAC) 92.31
    multi-source 92.32
    particle beam 92.33
    particulate 92.33
    radiosurgery NEC 92.39
    single source proton 92.31
Thal operation (repair of esophageal stricture)
  42.85
Theleplasty 85.87
Therapy
  Antabuse 94.25
  aqueous oxygen (AO) 00.49
  art 93.89
  aversion 94.33
  behavior 94.33
  Bennett respirator—*see* category 96.7
  blind rehabilitation NEC 93.78
  Byrd respirator—*see* category 96.7
  carbon dioxide 94.25
  cobalt-60 92.23
  conditioning, psychiatric 94.33
  continuous positive airway pressure (CPAP)
    93.90
    delivered by
      endotracheal tube —*see* category 96.7
      tracheostomy —*see* category 96.7
  croupette, croup tent 93.94
  daily living activities 93.83
    for the blind 93.78
  dance 93.89
  desensitization 94.33
  detoxification 94.25
  diversional 93.81
  domestic tasks 93.83
    for the blind 93.78
  Downstream® system 00.49

Therapy—*continued*
  educational (bed-bound children) (handicapped)
    93.82
  electroconvulsive (ECT) 94.27
  electroshock (EST) 94.27
    subconvulsive 94.26
  electrotonic (ETT) 94.27
  encounter group 94.44
  extinction 94.33
  family 94.42
  fog (inhalation) 93.94
  gamma ray 92.23
  group NEC 94.44
    for psychosexual dysfunction 94.41
  hearing NEC 95.49
  heat NEC 93.35
    for cancer treatment 99.85
  helium 93.98
  hot pack(s) 93.35
  hyperbaric oxygen 93.95
    wound 93.59
  hyperthermia NEC 93.35
    for cancer treatment 99.85
  individual, psychiatric NEC 94.39
    for psychosexual dysfunction 94.34
  industrial 93.89
  infrared irradiation 93.35
  inhalation NEC 93.96
    nitric oxide 00.12
  insulin shock 94.24
  intermittent positive pressure breathing (IPPB)
    93.91
  IPPB (intermittent positive pressure breathing)
    93.91
  leech 99.99
  lithium 94.22
  LITT (laser interstitial thermal therapy) under
    guidance
    lesion
      brain 17.61
      breast 17.69
      head and neck 17.62
      liver 17.63
      lung 17.69
      prostate 17.69
      thyroid 17.62
  maggot 86.28
  manipulative, osteopathic (*see also* Manipulation,
    osteopathic) 93.67
  manual arts 93.81
  methadone 94.25
  mist (inhalation) 93.94
  music 93.84
  nebulizer 93.94
  neuroleptic 94.23
  nitric oxide 00.12
  occupational 93.83
  oxygen 93.96
    aqueous 00.49
    catalytic 93.96
    hyperbaric 93.95
      wound 93.59
    SuperSaturated 00.49
    wound (hyperbaric) 93.59
  paraffin bath 93.35
  physical NEC 93.39
    combined (without mention of components)
      93.38
    diagnostic NEC 93.09
  play 93.81
    psychotherapeutic 94.36

Therapy—*continued*
  positive and expiratory pressure—*see* category 96.7
  psychiatric NEC 94.39
    drug NEC 94.25
    lithium 94.22
  radiation 92.29
    contact (150 KVP or less) 92.21
    deep (200-300 KVP) 92.22
    electron, intra-operative 92.41
    high voltage (200-300 KVP) 92.22
    low voltage (150 KVP or less) 92.21
    megavoltage 92.24
    orthovoltage 92.22
    particle source NEC 92.26
    photon 92.24
    radioisotope (teleradiotherapy) 92.23
    retinal lesion 14.26
    superficial (150 KVP or less) 92.21
    supervoltage 92.24
  radioisotope, radioisotopic NEC 92.29
    implantation or insertion 92.27
    injection or instillation 92.28
    teleradiotherapy 92.23
  radium (radon) 92.23
  recreational 93.81
  rehabilitation NEC 93.89
  respiratory NEC 93.99
    bi-level positive airway pressure [BiPAP] 93.90
      delivered by
        endotracheal tube—*see* category 96.7
        tracheostomy—*see* category 96.7
    continuous positive airway pressure [CPAP]
      93.90
      delivered by
        endotracheal tube—*see* category 96.7
        tracheostomy—*see* category 96.7
    endotracheal respiratory assistance—*see*
      category 96.7
    intermittent positive pressure breathing [IPPB]
      93.91
    negative pressure (continuous) [CNP] 93.99
    nitric oxide 00.12
    non-invasive positive pressure (NIPPV) 93.90
    other continuous invasive (unspecified
      duration) 96.70
      for less than 96 consecutive hours 96.71
      for 96 consecutive hours or more 96.72
    positive and expiratory pressure [PEEP]
      invasive—*see* category 96.7
      noninvasive 93.90
  root canal 23.70
    with
      apicoectomy 23.72
      irrigation 23.71
  shock
    chemical 94.24
    electric 94.27
      subconvulsive 94.26
    insulin 94.24
  speech 93.75
    for correction of defect 93.74
  SuperOxygenation (SSO2) 00.49
  SuperSaturated oxygen 00.49
  ultrasound
    heat therapy 93.35
    hyperthermia for cancer treatment 99.85
    physical therapy 93.35
    therapeutic—*see* Ultrasound
  ultraviolet light 99.82
Thermocautery —*see* Cauterization

Thermography 88.89
  blood vessel 88.86
  bone 88.83
  breast 88.85
  cerebral 88.81
  eye 88.82
  lymph gland 88.89
  muscle 88.84
  ocular 88.82
  osteoarticular 88.83
  specified site NEC 88.89
  vein, deep 88.86
Thermokeratoplasty 11.74
Thermoplasty
  bronchoscopic, bronchial (lung) 32.27
Thermosclerectomy 12.62
Thermotherapy (hot packs) (paraffin bath) NEC
  93.35
  prostate
    by
      microwave 60.96
      radiofrequency 60.97
    transurethral microwave thermotherapy
      (TUMT) 60.96
    transurethral needle ablation (TUNA) 60.97
    TUMT (transurethral microwave
      thermotherapy) 60.96
    TUNA (transurethral needle ablation) 60.97
Thiersch operation
  anus 49.79
  skin graft 86.69
    hand 86.62
Thompson operation
  cleft lip repair 27.54
  correction of lymphedema 40.9
  quadricepsplasty 83.86
  thumb apposition with bone graft 82.69
Thoracectomy 34.09
  for lung collapse 33.34
Thoracentesis 34.91
Thoracocentesis 34.91
Thoracolysis (for collapse of lung) 33.39
Thoracoplasty (anterior) (extrapleural)
  (paravertebral) (posterolateral) (complete)
  (partial) 33.34
Thoracoscopy, transpleural (for exploration)
  34.21
Thoracostomy 34.09
  for lung collapse 33.32
Thoracotomy (with drainage) 34.09
  exploratory 34.02
Thoratec® implantable ventricular assist device
  (IVAD™) 37.66
Thoratec® ventricular assist device (VAD)
  system 37.66
Three-snip operation, punctum 09.51
Thrombectomy 38.00
  with endarterectomy—*see* Endarterectomy
  abdominal
    artery 38.06
    vein 38.07
  aorta (arch) (ascending) (descending) 38.04
  arteriovenous shunt or cannula 39.49
  bovine graft 39.49
  coronary artery 36.09
  head and neck vessel NEC 38.02
  intracranial vessel NEC 38.01
  lower limb
    artery 38.08
    vein 38.09

Thrombectomy—*continued*
  mechanical
    endovascular
      head and neck 39.74
    pulmonary vessel 38.05
    thoracic vessel NEC 38.05
    upper limb (artery) (vein) 38.03
Thromboendarterectomy 38.10
  abdominal 38.16
  aorta (arch) (ascending) (descending) 38.14
  coronary artery 36.09
    open chest approach 36.03
  head and neck NEC 38.12
  intracranial NEC 38.11
  lower limb 38.18
  thoracic NEC 38.15
  upper limb 38.13
Thymectomy 07.80
  partial (open) (other) 07.81
    thoracoscopic 07.83
  total (open) (other) 07.82
    thoracoscopic 07.84
  transcervical 07.99
Thyrochondrotomy 31.3
Thyrocricoidectomy 30.29
Thyrocricotomy (for assistance in breathing) 31.1
Thyroidectomy NEC 06.39
  by mediastinotomy (*see also* Thyroidectomy,
    substernal) 06.50
  with laryngectomy—*see* Laryngectomy
  complete or total 06.4
    substernal (by mediastinotomy) (transsternal
      route) 06.52
    transoral route (lingual) 06.6
  lingual (complete) (partial) (subtotal) (total) 06.6
  partial or subtotal NEC 06.39
    with complete removal of remaining lobe 06.2
    submental route (lingual) 06.6
    substernal (by mediastinotomy) (transsternal
      route) 06.51
  remaining tissue 06.4
  submental route (lingual) 06.6
  substernal (by mediastinotomy)
    (transsternal route) 06.50
    complete or total 06.52
    partial or subtotal 06.51
  transoral route (lingual) 06.6
  transsternal route (*see also* Thyroidectomy,
    substernal) 06.50
  unilateral (with removal of isthmus) (with
    removal of portion of other lobe) 06.2
Thyroidorrhaphy 06.93
Thyroidotomy (field) (gland) NEC 06.09
  postoperative 06.02
Thyrotomy 31.3
  with tantalum plate 31.69
Tirofiban (HCl), infusion 99.20
Toilette
  skin—*see* Debridement, skin or subcutaneous
    tissue
  tracheostomy 96.55
Token economy (behavior therapy) 94.33
Tomkins operation (metroplasty) 69.49
Tomography —*see also* Radiography
  abdomen NEC 88.02
  cardiac 87.42

Tomography—*continued*
computerized axial NEC 88.38
  abdomen 88.01
  bone 88.38
    quantitative 88.98
  brain 87.03
  cardiac 87.41
  coronary 87.41
  head 87.03
  kidney 87.71
  skeletal 88.38
    quantitative 88.98
  thorax 87.41
 head NEC 87.04
 kidney NEC 87.72
 lung 87.42
 optical coherence (intravascular imaging)
  coronary vessel(s) 38.24
  non-coronary vessel(s) 38.25
 thorax NEC 87.42
Tongue tie operation 25.91
Tonography 95.26
Tonometry 89.11
Tonsillectomy 28.2
 with adenoidectomy 28.3
Tonsillotomy 28.0
Topectomy 01.32
Torek (Bevan) operation (orchidopexy) (first stage) (second stage) 62.5
Torkildsen operation (ventriculocisternal shunt) 02.2
Torpin operation (cul-de-sac resection) 70.92
Toti operation (dacryocystorhinostomy) 09.81
Touchas operation 86.83
Touroff operation (ligation of subclavian artery) 38.85
Toxicology —*see* Examination, microscopic
TPN (total parenteral nutrition) 99.15
Trabeculectomy ab externo 12.64
Trabeculodialysis 12.59
Trabeculotomy ab externo 12.54
Trachelectomy 67.4
Trachelopexy 69.22
Tracheloplasty 67.69
Trachelorrhaphy (Emmet) (suture) 67.61
 obstetrical 75.51
Trachelotomy 69.95
 obstetrical 73.93
Tracheocricotomy (for assistance breathing) 31.1
Tracheofissure 31.1
Tracheography 87.32
Tracheolaryngotomy (emergency) 31.1
 permanent opening 31.29
Tracheoplasty 31.79
 with artificial larynx 31.75
Tracheorrhaphy 31.71
Tracheoscopy NEC 31.42
 through tracheotomy (stoma) 31.41
Tracheostomy (emergency) (temporary) (for assistance in breathing) 31.1
 mediastinal 31.21
 percutaneous dilatational
  other permanent 31.29
  temporary 31.1
 permanent NEC 31.29
 revision 31.74

Tracheotomy (emergency) (temporary) (for assistance in breathing) 31.1
 percutaneous dilatational
  other permanent 31.29
  temporary 31.1
 permanent 31.29
Tracing, carotid pulse with ECG lead 89.56
Traction
 with reduction of fracture or dislocation—*see* Reduction, fracture *and* Reduction, dislocation
 adhesive tape (skin) 93.46
 boot 93.46
 Bryant's (skeletal) 93.44
 Buck's 93.46
 caliper tongs 93.41
  with synchronous insertion of device 02.94
 Cortel's (spinal) 93.42
 Crutchfield tongs 93.41
  with synchronous insertion of device 02.94
 Dunlop's (skeletal) 93.44
 gallows 93.46
 Gardner Wells 93.41
  with synchronous insertion of device 02.94
 halo device, skull 93.41
  with synchronous insertion of device 02.94
 Lyman Smith (skeletal) 93.44
 manual, intermittent 93.21
 mechanical, intermittent 93.21
 Russell's (skeletal) 93.44
 skeletal NEC 93.44
  intermittent 93.43
 skin, limbs NEC 93.46
 spinal NEC 93.42
  with skull device (halo) (caliper) (Crutchfield) (Gardner Wells) (Vinke) (tongs) 93.41
   with synchronous insertion of device 02.94
 Thomas' splint 93.45
 Vinke tongs 93.41
  with synchronous insertion of device 02.94
Tractotomy
 brain 01.32
 medulla oblongata 01.32
 mesencephalon 01.32
 percutaneous 03.21
 spinal cord (one-stage) (two-stage) 03.29
 trigeminal (percutaneous) (radio frequency) 04.02
Training (for) (in)
 ADL (activities of daily living) 93.83
  for the blind 93.78
 ambulation 93.22
 braille 93.77
 crutch walking 93.24
 dyslexia 93.71
 dysphasia 93.72
 esophageal speech (postlaryngectomy) 93.73
 gait 93.22
 joint movements 93.14
 lip reading 93.75
 Moon (blind reading) 93.77
 orthoptic 95.35
 prenatal (natural childbirth) 93.37
 prosthetic or orthotic device usage 93.24
 relaxation 94.33
 speech NEC 93.75
  esophageal 93.73
  for correction of defect 93.74
 use of lead dog for the blind 93.76
 vocational 93.85

TRAM (transverse rectus abdominis
musculocutaneous) flap of breast
free 85.73
pedicled 85.72
Transactional analysis
group 94.44
individual 94.39
Transection —*see also* Division
artery (with ligation) (*see also* Division, artery)
38.80
renal, aberrant (with reimplantation) 39.55
bone (*see also* Osteotomy) 77.30
fallopian tube (bilateral) (remaining)
(solitary) 66.39
by endoscopy 66.22
unilateral 66.92
isthmus, thyroid 06.91
muscle 83.19
eye 15.13
multiple (two or more muscles) 15.3
hand 82.19
nerve (cranial) (peripheral) NEC 04.03
acoustic 04.01
root (spinal) 03.1
sympathetic 05.0
tracts in spinal cord 03.29
trigeminal 04.02
vagus (transabdominal) (*see also* Vagotomy)
44.00
pylorus (with wedge resection) 43.3
renal vessel, aberrant (with reimplantation) 39.55
spinal
cord tracts 03.29
nerve root 03.1
tendon 83.13
hand 82.11
uvula 27.71
vas deferens 63.71
vein (with ligation) (*see also* Division, vein)
38.80
renal, aberrant (with reimplantation) 39.55
varicose (lower limb) 38.59
Transfer, transference
bone shaft, fibula into tibia 78.47
digital (to replace absent thumb) 82.69
finger (to thumb) (same hand) 82.61
to
finger, except thumb 82.81
opposite hand (with amputation) 82.69
[84.01]
toe (to thumb) (with amputation) 82.69 *[84.11]*
to finger, except thumb 82.81 *[84.11]*
fat pad NEC 86.89
with skin graft—*see* Graft, skin, full-thickness
finger (to replace absent thumb) (same hand)
82.61
to
finger, except thumb 82.81
opposite hand (with amputation) 82.69
[84.01]
muscle origin 83.77
hand 82.58
nerve (cranial) (peripheral) (radial anterior)
(ulnar) 04.6
pedicle graft 86.74
pes anserinus (tendon) (repair of knee) 81.47
tarsoconjunctival flap, from opposing lid 08.64
tendon 83.75
hand 82.56
pes anserinus (repair of knee) 81.47
toe-to-thumb (free) (pedicle) (with amputation)
82.69 *[84.11]*

Transfixion —*see also* Fixation
iris (bombe) 12.11
Transfusion (of) 99.03
antihemophilic factor 99.06
antivenin 99.16
autologous blood
collected prior to surgery 99.02
intraoperative 99.00
perioperative 99.00
postoperative 99.00
previously collected 99.02
salvage 99.00
blood (whole) NOS 99.03
expander 99.08
surrogate 99.09
bone marrow 41.00
allogeneic 41.03
with purging 41.02
allograft 41.03
with purging 41.02
autograft 41.01
with purging 41.09
autologous 41.01
with purging 41.09
coagulation factors 99.06
Dextran 99.08
exchange 99.01
intraperitoneal 75.2
in utero (with hysterotomy) 75.2
exsanguination 99.01
gamma globulin 99.14
granulocytes 99.09
hemodilution 99.03
intrauterine 75.2
packed cells 99.04
plasma 99.07
platelets 99.05
replacement, total 99.01
serum NEC 99.07
substitution 99.01
thrombocytes 99.05
Transillumination
nasal sinuses 89.35
skull (newborn) 89.16
Translumbar aortogram 88.42
Transplant, transplantation
Note: To report donor source:
cadaver 00.93
live non-related donor 00.92
live related donor 00.91
live unrelated donor 00.92
artery 39.59
renal, aberrant 39.55
autotransplant—*see* Reimplantation
blood vessel 39.59
renal, aberrant 39.55
bone (*see also* Graft, bone) 78.00
marrow 41.00
allogeneic 41.03
with purging 41.02
allograft 41.03
with purging 41.02
autograft 41.01
with purging 41.09
autologous 41.01
with purging 41.09
stem cell
allogeneic (hematopoietic) 41.05
with purging 41.08
autologous (hematopoietic) 41.04
with purging 41.07

Transplant, transplantation—*continued*
    cord blood 41.06
    stem cell
        allogeneic (hematopoietic) 41.05
           with purging 41.08
        autologous (hematopoietic) 41.04
           with purging 41.07
        cord blood 41.06
    combined heart-lung 33.6
    conjunctiva, for pterygium 11.39
    corneal (*see also* Keratoplasty) 11.60
    dura 02.12
    fascia 83.82
        hand 82.72
    finger (replacing absent thumb) (same hand)
        82.61
    to
        finger, except thumb 82.81
        opposite hand (with amputation) 82.69
           [84.01]
    gracilis muscle (for) 83.77
        anal incontinence 49.74
        urethrovesical suspension 59.71
    hair follicles
        eyebrow 08.63
        eyelid 08.63
        scalp 86.64
    heart (orthotopic) 37.51
        combined with lung 33.6
    ileal stoma to new site 46.23
    intestine 46.97
    Islets of Langerhans (cells) 52.86
        allotransplantation of cells 52.85
        autotransplantation of cells 52.84
        heterotransplantation 52.85
        homotransplantation 52.84
    kidney NEC 55.69
    liver 50.59
        auxiliary (permanent) (temporary) (recipient's
           liver in situ) 50.51
        cells into spleen via percutaneous
           catheterization 38.91
    lung 33.50
        bilateral 33.52
        combined with heart 33.6
        double 33.52
        single 33.51
        unilateral 33.51
    lymphatic structure(s) (peripheral) 40.9
    mammary artery to myocardium or ventricular
        wall 36.2
    muscle 83.77
        gracilis (for) 83.77
           anal incontinence 49.74
           urethrovesical suspension 59.71
        hand 82.58
        temporalis 83.77
           with orbital exenteration 16.59
    nerve (cranial) (peripheral) 04.6
    ovary 65.92
    pancreas 52.80
        heterotransplant 52.83
        homotransplant 52.82
        Islets of Langerhans (cells) 52.86
           allotransplantation of cells 52.85
           autotransplantation of cells 52.84
           heterotransplantation of cells 52.85
           homotransplantation of cells 52.84
        reimplantation 52.81
    pes anserinus (tendon) (repair of knee) 81.47

Transplant, transplantation—*continued*
    renal NEC 55.69
        vessel, aberrant 39.55
    salivary duct opening 26.49
    skin—*see* Graft, skin
    spermatic cord 63.53
    spleen 41.94
    stem cell
        allogeneic (hematopoietic) 41.05
           with purging 41.08
        autologous (hematopoietic) 41.04
           with purging 41.07
        cord blood 41.06
    tendon 83.75
        hand 82.56
        pes anserinus (repair of knee) 81.47
        superior rectus (blepharoptosis) 08.36
    testis to scrotum 62.5
    thymus 07.94
    thyroid tissue 06.94
    toe (replacing absent thumb) (with amputation)
        82.69 *[84.11]*
        to finger, except thumb 82.81 *[84.11]*
    tooth 23.5
    ureter to
        bladder 56.74
        ileum (external diversion) 56.51
           internal diversion only 56.71
        intestine 56.71
        skin 56.61
    vein (peripheral) 39.59
        renal, aberrant 39.55
    vitreous 14.72
        anterior approach 14.71
Transposition
    extraocular muscles 15.5
    eyelash naps 08.63
    eye muscle (oblique) (rectus) 15.5
    finger (replacing absent thumb) (same hand)
        82.61
    to
        finger, except thumb 82.81
        opposite hand (with amputation) 82.69
           [84.01]
    interatrial venous return 35.91
    jejunal (Henley) 43.81
    joint capsule (*see also* Arthroplasty) 81.96
    muscle NEC 83.79
        extraocular 15.5
        hand 82.59
    nerve (cranial) (peripheral) (radial anterior)
        (ulnar) 04.6
    nipple 85.86
    pterygium 11.31
    tendon NEC 83.76
        hand 82.57
    vocal cords 31.69
Transureteroureterostomy 56.75
Transversostomy (*see also* Colostomy) 46.10
Trapping, aneurysm (cerebral) 39.52
Trauner operation (lingual sulcus extension)
    24.91
Trephination, trephining
    accessory sinus—*see* Sinusotomy
    corneoscleral 12.89
    cranium 01.24
    nasal sinus—*see* Sinusotomy
    sclera (with iridectomy) 12.61
Trial (failed) forceps 73.3
Trigonectomy 57.6
Trimming, amputation stump 84.3
Triple arthrodesis 81.12

Trochanterplasty 81.40
Tsuge operation (macrodactyly repair) 82.83
Tuck, tucking —*see also* Plication
  eye muscle 15.22
    multiple (two or more muscles) 15.4
  levator palpebrae, for blepharoptosis 08.34
Tudor "rabbit ear" operation (anterior
    urethropexy) 59.79
Tuffier operation
  apicolysis of lung 33.39
  vaginal hysterectomy 68.59
    laparoscopically assisted (LAVH) 68.51
TULIP (transurethral ultrasound guided laser
    induced prostatectomy) 60.21
TUMT (transurethral microwave thermotherapy)
    of prostate 60.96
TUNA (transurethral needle ablation) of prostate
    60.97
TURP (transurethral resection of prostate) 60.29
Tunnel, subcutaneous (antethoracic) 42.86
  esophageal 42.86
    with anastomosis—*see* Anastomosis,
        esophagus, antesternal
  pulse generator lead wire 86.99
    with initial procedure—*omit code*
Turbinectomy (complete) (partial) NEC 21.69
  by
    cryosurgery 21.61
    diathermy 21.61
  with sinusectomy—*see* Sinusectomy
Turco operation (release of joint capsules in
    clubfoot) 80.48
Tylectomy (breast) (partial) 85.21
Tympanectomy 20.59
  with tympanoplasty—*see* Tympanoplasty
Tympanogram 95.41
Tympanomastoidectomy 20.42
Tympanoplasty (type I) (with graft) 19.4
  with
    air pocket over round window 19.54
    fenestra in semicircular canal 19.55
    graft against
      incus or malleus 19.52
      mobile and intact stapes 19.53
    incudostapediopexy 19.52
  epitympanic, type I 19.4
  revision 19.6
  type
    II (graft against incus or malleus) 19.52
    III (graft against mobile and intact stapes) 19.53
    IV (air pocket over round window) 19.54
    V (fenestra in semicircular canal) 19.55
Tympanosympathectomy 20.91
Tympanotomy 20.09
  with intubation 20.01

U

UAE (uterine artery embolization), NOS 68.25
with
  coils 68.24
  particulate agent (gelatin sponge) (gelfoam)
    (microspheres) (polyvinyl alcohol) (PVA)
    (spherical embolics) 68.25
Uchida operation (tubal ligation with or without
  fimbriectomy) 66.32
UFR (uroflowmetry) 89.24
Ultrafiltration 99.78
  hemodiafiltration 39.95
  hemodialysis (kidney) 39.95
  removal, plasma water 99.78
  therapeutic plasmapheresis 99.71
Ultrasonography
  abdomen 88.76
  aortic arch 88.73
  biliary tract 88.74
  breast 88.73
  deep vein thrombosis 88.77
  digestive system 88.74
  eye 95.13
  head and neck 88.71
  heart
  intestine 88.74
  intravascular—*see* Ultrasound, intravascular
    (IVUS)
  lung 88.73
  midline shift, brain 88.71
  multiple sites 88.79
  peripheral vascular system 88.77
  retroperitoneum 88.76
  therapeutic—*see* Ultrasound
  thorax NEC 88.73
  total body 88.79
  urinary system 88.75
  uterus 88.79
    gravid 88.78
Ultrasound
  diagnostic—*see* Ultrasonography
  fragmentation (of)
    cataract (with aspiration) 13.41
    urinary calculus, stones (Kock pouch) 59.95
  heart
    intracardiac (heart chambers) (ICE) 37.28
    intravascular (coronary vessels) (IVUS) 00.24
    non-invasive 88.72
  inner ear 20.79
  intravascular (IVUS) (VH™-IVUS) 00.29
    aorta 00.22
    aortic arch 00.22
    cerebral vessel, extracranial 00.21
    coronary vessel 00.24
    intrathoracic vessel 00.22
    other specified vessel 00.28
    peripheral vessel 00.23
    renal vessel 00.23
    vena cava (inferior) (superior) 00.22
  therapeutic
    head 00.01
    heart 00.02
    neck 00.01
    other therapeutic ultrasuond 00.09
    peripheral vascular vessels 00.03
    vessels of head and neck 00.01
  therapy 93.35

Ultrasound—*continued*
  VH™-IVUS– *see* Ultrasound, intravascular, by
    site
  virtual histology intravascular ultrasound – *see*
    Ultrasound, intravascular, by site
Umbilectomy 54.3
Unbridling
  blood vessel, peripheral 39.91
  celiac artery axis 39.91
Uncovering —*see* Incision, by site
Undercutting
  hair follicle 86.09
  perianal tissue 49.02
Unroofing —*see also* Incision, by site
  external
    auditory canal 18.02
    ear NEC 18.09
  kidney cyst 55.39
UPP (urethral pressure profile) 89.25
UPPP (uvulopalatopharyngoplasty) 27.69 *[29.4]*
Upper GI series (x-ray) 87.62
Uranoplasty (for cleft palate repair) 27.62
Uranorrhaphy (for cleft palate repair) 27.62
Uranostaphylorrhaphy 27.62
Urban operation (mastectomy) (unilateral) 85.47
  bilateral 85.48
Ureterectomy 56.40
  with nephrectomy 55.51
  partial 56.41
  total 56.42
Ureterocecostomy 56.71
Ureterocelectomy 56.41
Ureterocolostomy 56.71
Ureterocystostomy 56.74
Ureteroenterostomy 56.71
Ureteroileostomy (internal diversion) 56.71
  external diversion 56.51
Ureterolithotomy 56.2
Ureterolysis 59.02
  with freeing or repositioning of ureter 59.02
  laparoscopic 59.03
Ureteroneocystostomy 56.74
Ureteropexy 56.85
Ureteroplasty 56.89
Ureteroplication 56.89
Ureteroproctostomy 56.71
Ureteropyelography (intravenous) (diuretic
  infusion) 87.73
  percutaneous 87.75
  retrograde 87.74
Ureteropyeloplasty 55.87
Ureteropyelostomy 55.86
Ureterorrhaphy 56.82
Ureteroscopy 56.31
  with biopsy 56.33
Ureterosigmoidostomy 56.71
Ureterostomy (cutaneous) (external) (tube) 56.61
  closure 56.83
  ileal 56.51
Ureterotomy 56.2
Ureteroureterostomy (crossed) 56.75
  lumbar 56.41
  resection with end-to-end anastomosis 56.41
  spatulated 56.41
Urethral catheterization, indwelling 57.94
Urethral pressure profile (UPP) 89.25

Urethrectomy (complete) (partial) (radical) 58.39
  with
    complete cystectomy 57.79
    pelvic exenteration 68.8
    radical cystectomy 57.71
Urethrocystography (retrograde) (voiding) 87.76
Urethrocystopexy (by) 59.79
  levator muscle sling 59.71
  retropubic suspension 59.5
  suprapubic suspension 59.4
Urethrolithotomy 58.0
Urethrolysis 58.5
Urethropexy 58.49
  anterior 59.79
Urethroplasty 58.49
  augmentation 59.79
    collagen implant 59.72
    fat implant 59.72
    injection (endoscopic) of implant into urethra
        59.72
    polytef implant 59.72
Urethrorrhaphy 58.41
Urethroscopy 58.22
  for control of hemorrhage of prostate 60.94
  perineal 58.21
Urethrostomy (perineal) 58.0
Urethrotomy (external) 58.0
  internal (endoscopic) 58.5
Uroflowmetry (UFR) 89.24
Urography (antegrade) (excretory) (intravenous)
        87.73
  retrograde 87.74
Uteropexy (abdominal approach) (vaginal
        approach) 69.22
UVP (uvulopalatopharyngoplasty) 27.69 *[29.4]*
Uvulectomy 27.72
Uvulopalatopharyngoplasty (UPPP) 27.69
  [29.4]
Uvulotomy 27.71

V

Vaccination (prophylactic) (against) 99.59
  anthrax 99.55
  brucellosis 99.55
  cholera 99.31
  common cold 99.51
  disease NEC 99.55
    arthropod-borne viral NEC 99.54
  encephalitis, arthropod-borne viral 99.53
  German measles 99.47
  hydrophobia 99.44
  infectious parotitis 99.46
  influenza 99.52
  measles 99.45
  mumps 99.46
  paratyphoid fever 99.32
  pertussis 99.37
  plague 99.34
  poliomyelitis 99.41
  rabies 99.44
  Rocky Mountain spotted fever 99.55
  rubella 99.47
  rubeola 99.45
  smallpox 99.42
  Staphylococcus 99.55
  Streptococcus 99.55
  tuberculosis 99.33
  tularemia 99.35
  typhoid 99.32
  typhus 99.55
  tumor 99.28
  undulant fever 99.55
  yellow fever 99.43
Vacuum extraction, fetal head 72.79
  with episiotomy 72.71
VAD
  vascular access device —*see* Vascular access
    device, totally implantable
  ventricular assist device —*see* Implant, heart
    assist system
Vagectomy (subdiaphragmatic) (*see also*
  Vagotomy) 44.00
Vaginal douche 96.44
Vaginectomy 70.4
Vaginofixation 70.77
  with graft or prosthesis 70.78
Vaginoperineotomy 70.14
Vaginoplasty 70.79
Vaginorrhaphy 70.71
  obstetrical 75.69
Vaginoscopy 70.21
Vaginotomy 70.14
  for
    culdocentesis 70.0
    pelvic abscess 70.12
Vagotomy (gastric) 44.00
  parietal cell 44.02
  selective NEC 44.03
    highly 44.02
    Holle's 44.02
    proximal 44.02
  truncal 44.01
Valvotomy —*see* Valvulotomy
Valvulectomy, heart —*see* Valvuloplasty, heart

Valvuloplasty
  heart, unspecified (without valve replacement)
    35.10
    with prosthesis or tissue graft—*see*
      Replacement, heart, valve, by site
  aortic valve 35.11
    percutaneous (balloon) 35.96
  balloon, percutaneous 35.96
  combined with repair of atrial and ventricular
    septal defects—*see* Repair, endocardial
    cushion defect
  mitral valve
    balloon, percutaneous repair 35.96
    endovascular repair with implant 35.97
    open, without replacement 35.12
    percutaneous repair
      with implant (leaflet clip) 35.97
    transcatheter repair with implant 35.97
  open heart technique 35.10
  percutaneous (balloon) 35.96
  pulmonary valve 35.13
    in total repair of tetralogy of Fallot 35.81
    percutaneous (balloon) 35.96
  tricuspid valve 35.14
Valvulotomy
  heart (closed heart technique) (transatrial)
    (transventricular) 35.00
  aortic valve 35.01
  mitral valve 35.02
  open heart technique—*see* Valvuloplasty, heart
  pulmonary valve 35.03
    in total repair of tetralogy of Fallot 35.81
  tricuspid valve 35.04
Varicocelectomy, spermatic cord 63.1
Varicotomy, peripheral vessels (lower limb)
  38.59
  upper limb 38.53
Vascular access device (VAD), totally
  implantable 86.07
Vascular closure, percutaneous puncture—*omit
  code*
Vascularization —*see* Revascularization
Vasectomy (complete) (partial) 63.73
Vasogram 87.94
Vasoligation 63.71
  gastric 38.86
Vasorrhaphy 63.81
Vasostomy 63.6
Vasotomy 63.6
Vasotripsy 63.71
Vasovasostomy 63.82
Vectorcardiogram (VCG) (with ECG) 89.53
Vectra® vascular access graft 86.07
Venectomy —*see* Phlebectomy
Venipuncture NEC 38.99
  for injection of contrast material—*see*
    Phlebography
Venography —*see* Phlebography
Venorrhaphy 39.32
Venotomy 38.00
  abdominal 38.07
  head and neck NEC 38.02
  intracranial NEC 38.01
  lower limb 38.09
  thoracic NEC 38.05
  upper limb 38.03
Venotripsy 39.98

Venovenostomy 39.29
Ventilation
bi-level positive airway pressure [BiPAP] 93.90
  delivered by
    endotracheal tube —*see* category 96.7
    tracheostomy —*see* category 96.7
continuous positive airway pressure [CPAP]
  93.90
  delivered by
    endotracheal tube —*see* category 96.7
    tracheostomy —*see* category 96.7
endotracheal respiratory assistance—*see* category
  96.7
mechanical, NOS 93.90
  by endotracheal tube —*see* category 96.7
  by tracheostomy —*see* category 96.7
  endotracheal respiratory assistance—*see*
    category 96.7
  invasive —see category 96.7
  non-invasive [NIPPV] 93.90
  other continuous invasive (unspecified
    duration) 96.70
    for less than 96 consecutive hours 96.71
    for 96 consecutive hours or more 96.72
  non-invasive positive pressure (NIPPV) 93.90
  positive and expiratory pressure [PEEP]
    invasive —see category 96.7
    non-invasive [NIPPV] 93.90
  negative pressure (continuous) [CNP] 93.99
Ventriculectomy, heart partial 37.35
Ventriculocholecystostomy 02.34
Ventriculocisternostomy 02.22
Ventriculocordectomy 30.29
Ventriculogram, Ventriculography (cerebral)
  87.02
cardiac
  left ventricle (outflow tract) 88.53
    combined with right heart 88.54
  right ventricle (outflow tract) 88.52
    combined with left heart 88.54
radionuclide cardiac 92.05
Ventriculomyocardiotomy 37.11
Ventriculoperitoneostomy 02.34
Ventriculopuncture 01.09
through previously implanted catheter or
  reservoir (Ommaya) (Rickham) 01.02
Ventriculoseptopexy (*see also* Repair,
  ventricular septal defect) 35.72
Ventriculoseptoplasty (*see also* Repair,
  ventricular septal defect) 35.72
Ventriculostomy
for
  external ventricular drainage (EVD) 02.21
  placement of ventricular catheter 02.21
  third (endoscopic) 02.22
Ventriculotomy
cerebral 02.22
heart 37.11
Ventriculoureterostomy 02.35
Ventriculovenostomy 02.32
Ventrofixation, uterus 69.22
Ventrohysteropexy 69.22
Ventrosuspension, uterus 69.22
VEP (visual evoked potential) 95.23

Version, obstetrical (bimanual) (cephalic)
  (combined) (internal) (podalic) 73.21
with extraction 73.22
Braxton Hicks 73.21
  with extraction 73.22
external (bipolar) 73.91
Potter's (podalic) 73.21
  with extraction 73.22
Wigand's (external) 73.91
Wright's (cephalic) 73.21
  with extraction 73.22
Vertebroplasty, percutaneous 81.65
Vesicolithotomy (suprapubic) 57.19
Vesicostomy 57.21
Vesicourethroplasty 57.85
Vesiculectomy 60.73
with radical prostatectomy 60.5
Vesiculogram, seminal 87.92
contrast 87.91
Vesiculotomy 60.72
Vestibuloplasty (buccolabial) (lingual) 24.91
Vestibulotomy 20.79
VH™-IVUS —*see* Ultrasound, intravascular, by site
Vicq D'azyr operation (larynx) 31.1
Vidal operation (varicocele ligation) 63.1
Vidianectomy 05.21
Villusectomy (*see also* Synovectomy) 80.70
Vision check 95.09
Visual evoked potential (VEP) 95.23
Vitrectomy (mechanical) (posterior approach)
  14.74
with scleral buckling 14.49
anterior approach 14.73
Vocational
assessment 93.85
retraining 93.85
schooling 93.82
Voice training (postlaryngectomy) 93.73
von Kraske operation (proctectomy) 48.64
Voss operation (hanging hip operation) 83.19
Vulpius (-Compere) operation (lengthening of
  gastrocnemius muscle) 83.85
Vulvectomy (bilateral) (simple) 71.62
partial (unilateral) 71.61
radical (complete) 71.5
unilateral 71.61
V-Y operation (repair)
bladder 57.89
  neck 57.85
ectropion 08.44
lip 27.59
skin (without graft) 86.89
subcutaneous tissue (without skin graft) 86.89
tongue 25.59

W

Wada test (hemispheric function) 89.10
Wang needle aspiration biopsy
   bronchus 33.24
   lung 33.27
Ward-Mayo operation (vaginal hysterectomy)
      68.59
   laparoscopically assisted (LAVH) 68.51
Washing —*see* Lavage *and* Irrigation
Waterston operation (aorta-right pulmonary
      artery anastomosis) 39.0
Watkins (Wertheim) **operation** (uterus
      interposition) 69.21
Watson-Jones operation
   hip arthrodesis 81.21
   reconstruction of lateral ligaments, ankle 81.49
   shoulder arthrodesis (extra-articular) 81.23
   tenoplasty 83.88
Webbing (syndactylization) 86.89
Weir operation
   appendicostomy 47.91
   correction of nostrils 21.86
Wertheim operation (radical hysterectomy) 68.69
   laparoscopic 68.61
West operation (dacryocystorhinostomy) 09.81
Wheeler operation
   entropion repair 08.44
   halving procedure (eyelid) 08.24
Whipple operation (radical
      pancreaticoduodenectomy) 52.7
   Child modification (radical subtotal
      pancreatectomy) 52.53
   Rodney Smith modification (radical subtotal
      pancreatectomy) 52.53
White operation (lengthening of tendon
      calcaneus by incomplete tenotomy) 83.11
Whitehead operation
   glossectomy, radical 25.4
   hemorrhoidectomy 49.46
Whitman operation
   foot stabilization (talectomy) 77.98
   hip reconstruction 81.40
   repair of serratus anterior muscle 83.87
   talectomy 77.98
   trochanter wedge osteotomy 77.25
Wier operation (entropion repair) 08.44
Williams-Richardson operation (vaginal
      construction) 70.61
   with graft or prosthesis 70.63
Wilms operation (thoracoplasty) 33.34
Wilson operation (angulation osteotomy for
      hallux valgus) 77.51
Window operation
   antrum (nasal sinus)—*see* Antrotomy, maxillary
   aorticopulmonary 39.59
   bone cortex (*see also* Incision, bone) 77.10
      facial 76.09
   nasoantral—*see* Antrotomy, maxillary
   pericardium 37.12
   pleura 34.09
Winiwarter operation (cholecystoenterostomy)
      51.32
Wiring
   aneurysm 39.52
   dental (for immobilization) 93.55
      with fracture-reduction—*see* Reduction, fracture
   orthodontic 24.7
Wirsungojejunostomy 52.96
Witzel operation (temporary gastrostomy) 43.19

Woodward operation (release of high riding
      scapula) 81.83
Wrapping, aneurysm (gauze) (methyl
      methacrylate) (plastic) 39.52

X

Xenograft 86.65
Xerography, breast 87.36
Xeromammogmphy 87.36
Xiphoidectomy 77.81
X-ray
   chest (routine) 87.44
      wail NEC 87.39
   contrast—*see* Radiography, contrast
   diagnostic—*see* Radiography
   injection of radio-opaque substance—*see*
      Radiography, contrast
   skeletal series, whole or complete 88.31
   therapeutic—*see* Therapy, radiation

Y

Young operation
   epispadias repair 58.45
   tendon transfer (anterior tibialis) (repair of flat
      foot) 83.75
Yount operation (division of iliotibial band)
      83.14

Z

Zancolli operation
   capsuloplasty 81.72
   tendon transfer (biceps) 82.56
Zeus® Robotic Surgical System —*see* category
      17.4
Ziegler operation (iridectomy) 12.14
Zonulolysis (with lens extraction) (*see also*
      Extraction, cataract, intracapsular) 13.19
Z-plasty
   epicanthus 08.59
   eyelid (*see also* Reconstruction, eyelid) 08.70
   hypopharynx 29.4
   skin (scar) (web contracture) 86.84
      with excision of lesion 86.3

SUMMARY OF ADDITIONS, DELETIONS AND REVISIONS TO VOLUME 3 IN FY2012

00.4   **Adjunct vascular system procedures**
Revise code also note; add code also note

00.49   **SuperSaturated oxygen therapy**
Add code also note

00.55   **Insertion of drug-eluting stent(s) of other peripheral vessel(s)**
Revise code also note, add code also note

00.56   **Insertion or replacement of implantable pressure sensor with lead for intracardiac or great vessel hemodynamic monitoring**
Revise code title, add note, revise code also note, add exclusion term

00.57   **Implantation or replacement of subcutaneous device for intracardiac or great vessel hemodynamic monitoring**
Revise inclusion term, revise code also note

00.60   **Insertion of drug-eluting stent(s) of superficial femoral artery**
Revise code also note, add code also note

00.61   **Percutaneous angioplasty of extracranial vessel(s)**
Revise code title, delete inclusion term, add/revise code also note, add/revise exclusion terms

00.62   **Percutaneous angioplasty of intracranial vessel(s)**
Revise code title, add inclusion terms, add code also note, revise/add exclusion terms

00.63   **Percutaneous insertion of carotid artery stent(s)**
Revise/add code also notes, revise/add exclusion terms

00.64   **Percutaneous insertion of other extracranial artery stent(s)**
Revise code title, delete inclusion term, revise/add code also notes, revise/add exclusion terms

00.65   **Percutaneous insertion of intracranial vascular stent(s)**
Add inclusion term, revise/add code also notes, revise/add exclusion terms

00.66   **Percutaneous transluminal coronary angioplasty [PTCA]**
Revise code title, delete inclusion term, add code also note

00.77   **Hip bearing surface, ceramic-on-polyethylene**
Add inclusion term

00.94   **Intra-operative neurophysiologic monitoring**
Add inclusion terms

02.2   **Ventriculostomy**
New subcategory, delete inclusion terms

02.21   **Insertion or replacement of external ventricular drain [EVD]**
New code

02.22   **Intracranial ventricular shunt or anastomosis**
New code

02.39   **Ventricular shunt to extracranial site NEC**
Revise code title, delete inclusion term

02.42   **Replacement of ventricular shunt**
Delete inclusion term

12.67   **Insertion of aqueous drainage device**
New code

13.65   **Excision of secondary membrane [after cataract]**
Revise code title, add inclusion term

17.53   **Percutaneous atherectomy of extracranial vessel(s)**
New code

17.54   **Percutaneous atherectomy of intracranial vessel(s)**
New code

17.55   **Transluminal coronary atherectomy**
New code

17.56   **Atherectomy of other non-coronary vessel(s)**
New code

17.8   **Other adjunct procedures**
New subcategory

17.81   **Insertion of antimicrobial envelope**
New code

33.24   **Closed [endoscopic] biopsy of bronchus**
Add inclusion term, delete exclusion term

35   **Operations on valves and septa of heart**
Revise code also note

35.0   **Closed heart valvotomy or transcatheter replacement of heart valve**
Revise subcategory title

35.05   **Endovascular replacement of aortic valve**
New code

35.06   **Transapical replacement of aortic valve**
New code

35.07   **Endovascular replacement of pulmonary valve**
New code

35.08   **Transapical replacement of pulmonary valve**
New code

35.09   **Endovascular replacement of unspecified heart valve**
New code

35.2 **Open and other replacement of heart valve**
Revise subcategory title, , add exclusion terms

35.20 **Open and other replacement of unspecified heart valve**
Revise code title, delete/add inclusion terms, add exclusion term

35.21 **Open and other replacement of aortic valve with tissue graft**
Revise code title, delete/add inclusion terms, add exclusion terms

35.22 **Open and other replacement of aortic valve**
Revise code title, delete/add inclusion terms, add exclusion terms

35.23 **Open and other replacement of mitral valve with tissue graft**
Revise code title, delete/add inclusion terms

35.24 **Open and other replacement of mitral valve**
Revise code title, delete/add inclusion terms

35.25 **Open and other replacement of pulmonary valve with tissue graft**
Revise code title, delete/add inclusion terms, add exclusion terms

35.26 **Open and other replacement of pulmonary valve**
Revise code title, delete/add inclusion terms, add exclusion terms

35.27 **Open and other replacement of tricuspid valve with tissue graft**
Revise code title, delete/add inclusion terms

35.28 **Open and other replacement of tricuspid valve**
Revise code title, delete/add inclusion terms

35.96 **Percutaneous balloon valvuloplasty**
Add exclusion terms

36.06 **Insertion of non-drug eluting coronary artery stent(s)**
Revise/add code also notes

36.07 **Insertion of drug-eluting coronary artery stent(s)**
Revise/add code also notes

36.09 **Other removal of coronary artery obstruction**
Revise/add exclusion terms

37.36 **Excision, destruction, or exclusion of left atrial appendage (LAA)**
Revise code title, revise/add/delete inclusion terms, revise/add code also notes, add exclusion term

38.26 **Insertion of implantable pressure sensor without lead for intracardiac or great vessel hemodynamic monitoring**
New code

39.50 **Angioplasty of other non-coronary vessel(s)**
Revise code title, add code also note, revise/add exclusion terms

39.7 **Endovascular procedures on vessel(s)**
Revise/add exclusion terms

39.71 **Endovascular implantation of other graft in abdominal aorta**
Revise code title, add exclusion term

39.72 **Endovascular (total) embolization or occlusion of head and neck vessels**
Revise code title, add inclusion terms

39.77 **Temporary (partial) therapeutic endovascular occlusion of vessel**
New code

39.78 **Endovascular implantation of branching or fenestrated graft(s) in aorta**
New code

39.79 **Other endovascular procedures on other vessels**
Add exclusion term

43.82 **Laparoscopic vertical (sleeve) gastrectomy**
New code

43.89 **Open and other partial gastrectomy**
Revise code title, add exclusion term

68.24 **Uterine artery embolization [UAE] with coils**
New code

68.25 **Uterine artery embolization [UAE] without coils**
New code

68.4 **Total abdominal hysterectomy**
Delete exclusion term

68.49 **Other and unspecified total abdominal hysterectomy**
Add exclusion term

86.28 **Nonexcisional debridement of wound, infection, or burn**
Add inclusion term

86.94 **Insertion or replacement of single array neurostimulator pulse generator, not specified as rechargeable**
Revise inclusion term

86.95 **Insertion or replacement of multiple array neurostimulator pulse generator, not specified as rechargeable**
Revise code title, revise inclusion term, revise exclusion term

86.96 **Insertion or replacement of other neurostimulator pulse generator**
Revise exclusion term

86.97 **Insertion or replacement of single array rechargeable neurostimulator pulse generator**
Revise inclusion term

86.98 **Insertion or replacement of multiple array (two or more) rechargeable neurostimulator pulse generator**
Revise code title, revise inclusion term

88.7   **Diagnostic ultrasound**
Add exclusion term

89.19   **Video and radio-telemetered
electroencephalographic monitoring**
Add exclusion term

93.08   **Electromyography**
Add exclusion term

99.09   **Transfusion of other substance**
Revise exclusion term

99.29   **Injection or infusion of other
therapeutic or prophylactic substance**
Add exclusion term